Mark frequently used sections in your code book with these color-coded flags.

ICD-10-CM Code Book

2022

Anne B. Casto, RHIA, CCS
Consulting Editor

AHIMA
American Health Information
Management Association®

Softbound
ISBN: 978-1-58426-843-7
AHIMA Product No.: AC221021

Spiralbound
ISBN: 978-1-58426-843-7
AHIMA Product No.: AC221121

AHIMA Staff:
Rachel Schratz, MA, Assistant Editor
Christine Scheid, Content Development Manager
Megan Grennan, Director, Content Production and AHIMA Press
James Pinnick, Vice President, Content and Product Development

Cover image: © knikola, Shutterstock

The Centers for Medicare and Medicaid Services (CMS) and the National Center for Health Statistics (NCHS), two departments within the US Federal Government's Department of Health and Human Services (HHS) provide the *International Classification of Diseases, Tenth Revision, Clinical Modification* (ICD-10-CM) for coding and reporting. ICD-10-CM is the US modification to the World Health Organization's (WHO) International Classification of Diseases, Tenth Revision (ICD-10).

Coding Clinic for ICD-10-CM and ICD-10-PCS is a publication of the American Hospital Association (AHA).

Unless otherwise noted, art pieces were created by Jason Isley and Cognition Studio, Inc, and are all copyright of the American Health Information Management Association.

The websites listed in this book were current and valid as of the date of publication. However, webpage addresses and the information on them may change at any time. The user is encouraged to perform his or her own general web searches to locate any site addresses listed here that are no longer valid.

For more information about AHIMA Press publications, including updates, visit https://www.ahima.org/education-events/education-by-product/books/.

American Health Information Management Association
233 North Michigan Avenue, 21st Floor
Chicago, Illinois 60601-5809
ahima.org

Contents

About the Consulting Editor

Anne B. Casto, RHIA, CCS, is the president of Casto Consulting, LLC. Casto Consulting, LLC is a consulting firm that provides services to hospitals and other healthcare stakeholders primarily in the areas of reimbursement and coding. Casto Consulting, LLC specializes in linking coding and billing practices to positive revenue cycle outcomes. Additionally, the firm provides guidance to consulting firms, healthcare organizations and healthcare insurers regarding reimbursement methodologies and Medicare regulations.

Additionally, Ms. Casto is a lecturer in the HIMS department at The Ohio State University, School of Health and Rehabilitation Sciences. Over the past 20 years, Ms. Casto has taught numerous courses in the areas of healthcare reimbursement, coding, healthcare data trending, and coding analytics.

Prior to her current roles, Ms. Casto was the vice president of clinical information for Cleverley & Associates where she worked very closely with APC regulations and guidelines, preparing hospitals for the implementation of the Medicare OPPS. Ms. Casto was also the clinical information product manager for CHIPS/Ingenix. She joined CHIPS/Ingenix in 1998 and spent the majority of her time developing coding compliance products for the inpatient and outpatient settings.

Ms. Casto has been responsible for inpatient and outpatient coding activities in several large hospitals including Mt. Sinai Medical Center (NYC), Beth Israel Medical Center (NYC), and The Ohio State University. She has worked extensively with CMI, quality measures, physician documentation, and coding accuracy efforts at these facilities.

Ms. Casto received her degree in Health Information Management at The Ohio State University in 1995. She received her Certified Coding Specialist credential in 1998 from the American Health Information Management Association. In 2009 Ms. Casto received her ICD-10-CM/PCS Trainer certificate from AHIMA. Ms. Casto is the co-author of an AHIMA published text book entitled *Principles of Healthcare Reimbursement*. Additionally, Ms. Casto was a contributing author to the published AHIMA books: *Severity DRGs and Reimbursement; A MS-DRG Primer* and *Effective Management of Coding Services.*

Ms. Casto received the AHIMA Legacy Award, part of the FORE Triumph Awards, in 2007 which honors a significant contribution to the knowledge base of the HIM field through an insightful publication. Additionally, Ms. Casto was honored with the Ohio Health Information Management Association's Distinguished Member Award in 2008 and the Ohio Health Information Management Association's Professional Achievement Award in 2011.

Acknowledgments

Many thanks to my family for their support during this project. Thanks to Dr. Susan White, The Ohio State University; your data manipulation skills are second to none. Thanks to Drew Beverick for providing valuable insight from the student perspective. Many thanks to Linda Hyde, RHIA, and Rachael D'Andrea, MS, RHIA, CDIP, CHTS-TR, CPHQ, for their very thorough technical review of the book.

Introduction

ICD-10-CM History and Background

The International Classification of Diseases, Tenth Revision, Clinical Modification (ICD-10-CM) is the United Stated modification to the World Health Organization's (WHO) International Classification of Diseases, Tenth Revision (ICD-10). The WHO adopted the tenth revision in 1990. Since that time, several countries, including Australia and Canada, have developed their own modification to ICD-10 and have implemented it for use.

In 1994, the National Center for Health Statistics (NCHS) began the process of determining the viability of ICD-10 and the applicability of a clinical modification of the code set for the United States. The NCHS has made draft versions of ICD-10-CM available since 2002. NCHS continued to refine and update the code set for use in the United States while the healthcare community waited for adoption of the code set by Congress. On August 22, 2008, the long-awaited official Notice of Proposed Rule Making (NPRM) regarding the adopting of the ICD-10-CM and ICD-10-PCS classifications was published in the *Federal Register*. On January 16, 2009, the Centers for Medicare and Medicaid Services (CMS) published the Final Rule for adoption of the ICD-10-CM and ICD-10-PCS code sets udders rules, 45 CFR Parts 160 and 162 of the Health Insurance Portability and Accountability Act of 1996 (HIPAA). Within this rule, a compliance (implementation) date of October 1, 2013 was released. The compliance date was revised and ICD-10-CM was successfully implemented on October 1, 2015.

Characteristics of ICD-10-CM

ICD-10-CM far exceeds its predecessors in the number of codes provided. The disease classification has been expanded to include health-related conditions and to provide greater specificity at the seventh-character level of detail. When available, these seventh characters are not optional; they are intended for use in recording the information substantiated in the clinical record.

The ICD-10-CM/PCS Coordination and Maintenance Committee

Annual modifications are made to ICD-10-CM through the ICD-10-CM Coordination and Maintenance Committee (C&M). The Committee is made up of representatives from two US federal government agencies, the National Center for Health Statistics, and the Centers for Medicare and Medicaid Services (CMS). C&M holds meetings twice a year, which are open to the public. Modification proposals submitted to C&M for consideration are presented at the meetings for public discussion. An open comment period follows each of these meetings. Those modification proposals which are approved are incorporated into the official government version of ICD-10-CM and become effective for use on October 1 of each year.

Guidance in the Use of ICD10-CM

To code accurately, it is necessary to have a working knowledge of medical terminology and to understand the characteristics, code book terminology, and conventions of ICD-10-CM. Transforming verbal descriptions of diseases, injuries, and conditions into numerical designations (coding) is a complex activity and should not be undertaken without proper training.

Originally, coding was accomplished to provide access to health records by diagnoses and operations through retrieval for medical research education and administration. Today, medical codes are utilized to facilitate payment of health services, evaluate utilization patterns, and study the appropriateness of healthcare costs. Coding also provides the basis for epidemiological studies and research into the quality of healthcare.

Coding must be performed correctly and consistently to produce meaningful statics to aid in planning for the health needs of the nation.

Official Conventions

ICD-10-CM Official Guidelines for Coding and Reporting 2022

(October 1, 2021 - September 30, 2022)

Narrative changes appear in bold text

Items <u>underlined</u> have been moved within the guidelines since the 2021 version

***Italics* are used to indicate revisions to heading changes**

The Centers for Medicare and Medicaid Services (CMS) and the National Center for Health Statistics (NCHS), two departments within the US Federal Government's Department of Health and Human Services (HHS) provide the following guidelines for coding and reporting using the International Classification of Diseases, Tenth Revision, Clinical

Modification (ICD-10-CM). These guidelines should be used as a companion document to the official version of the ICD-10-CM as published on the NCHS website. The ICD-10-CM is a morbidity classification published by the United States for classifying diagnoses and reason for visits in all healthcare settings. The ICD-10-CM is based on the ICD-10, the statistical classification of disease published by the World Health Organization (WHO).

These guidelines have been approved by the four organizations that make up the Cooperating Parties for the ICD-10-CM: the American Hospital Association (AHA), the American Health Information Management Association (AHIMA), CMS, and NCHS.

These guidelines are a set of rules that have been developed to accompany and complement the official conventions and instructions provided within the ICD-10-CM itself. The instructions and conventions of the classification take precedence over guidelines. These guidelines are based on the coding and sequencing instructions in the Tabular List and Alphabetic Index of ICD-10-CM, but provide additional instruction. Adherence to these guidelines when assigning ICD-10-CM diagnosis codes is required under the Health Insurance Portability and Accountability Act (HIPAA). The diagnosis codes (Tabular List and Alphabetic Index) have been adopted under HIPAA for all healthcare settings. A joint effort between the healthcare provider and the coder is essential to achieve complete and accurate documentation, code assignment, and reporting of diagnoses and procedures. These guidelines have been developed to assist both the healthcare provider and the coder in identifying those diagnoses that are to be reported. The importance of consistent, complete documentation in the medical record cannot be overemphasized. Without such documentation accurate coding cannot be achieved. The entire record should be reviewed to determine the specific reason for the encounter and the conditions treated.

The term encounter is used for all settings, including hospital admissions. In the context of these guidelines, the term provider is used throughout the guidelines to mean physician or any qualified healthcare practitioner who is legally accountable for establishing the patient's diagnosis. Only this set of guidelines, approved by the Cooperating Parties, is official.

The guidelines are organized into sections. Section I includes the structure and conventions of the classification and general guidelines that apply to the entire classification, and chapter-specific guidelines that correspond to the chapters as they are arranged in the classification. Section II includes guidelines for selection of principal diagnosis for non-outpatient settings. Section III includes guidelines for reporting additional diagnoses in non-outpatient settings. Section IV is for outpatient coding and reporting. It is necessary to review all sections of the guidelines to fully understand all of the rules and instructions needed to code properly.

Section I. Conventions, General Coding Guidelines and Chapter Specific Guidelines

The conventions, general guidelines and chapter-specific guidelines are applicable to all healthcare settings unless otherwise indicated. The conventions and instructions of the classification take precedence over guidelines.

A. Conventions for the ICD-10-CM

The conventions for the ICD-10-CM are the general rules for use of the classification independent of the guidelines. These conventions are incorporated within the Alphabetic Index and Tabular List of the ICD-10-CM as instructional notes.

1. The Alphabetic Index and Tabular List

The ICD-10-CM is divided into the Alphabetic Index, an alphabetical list of terms and their corresponding code, and the Tabular List, a structured list of codes divided into chapters based on body system or condition. The Alphabetic Index consists of the following parts: the Index of Diseases and Injury, the Index of External Causes of Injury, the Table of Neoplasms, and the Table of Drugs and Chemicals.

See Section I.C2. General guidelines

See Section I.C.19. Adverse effects, poisoning, underdosing and toxic effects

2. Format and Structure

The ICD-10-CM Tabular List contains categories, subcategories and codes. Characters for categories, subcategories and codes may be either a letter or a number. All categories are 3 characters. A three-character category that has no further subdivision is equivalent to a code. Subcategories are either 4 or 5 characters. Codes may be 3, 4, 5, 6, or 7 characters. That is, each level of subdivision after a category is a subcategory. The final level of subdivision is a code. Codes that have applicable 7th characters are still referred to as codes, not subcategories. A code that has an applicable 7th character is considered invalid without the 7th character.

The ICD-10-CM uses an indented format for ease in reference.

3. Use of Codes for Reporting Purposes

For reporting purposes only codes are permissible, not categories or subcategories, and any applicable 7th character is required.

Official Coding Guidelines

4. Placeholder Character

The ICD-10-CM utilizes a placeholder character X. The X is used as a placeholder at certain codes to allow for future expansion. An example of this is at the poisoning, adverse effect and underdosing codes, categories T36–T50. Where a placeholder exists, the X must be used in order for the code to be considered a valid code.

5. 7th Characters

Certain ICD-10-CM categories have applicable 7th characters. The applicable 7th character is required for all codes within the category, or as the notes in the Tabular List instruct. The 7th character must always be the 7th character in the data field. If a code that requires a 7th character is not 6 characters, a placeholder X must be used to fill in the empty characters.

6. Abbreviations

a. Alphabetic Index Abbreviations

NEC "Not elsewhere classifiable"
This abbreviation in the Alphabetic Index represents "other specified". When a specific code is not available for a condition, the Alphabetic Index directs the coder to the "other specified" code in the Tabular List.

NOS "Not otherwise specified"
This abbreviation is the equivalent of unspecified.

b. Tabular List Abbreviations

NEC "Not elsewhere classifiable"
This abbreviation in the Tabular List represents "other specified". When a specific code is not available for a condition the Tabular List includes an NEC entry under a code to identify the code as the "other specified" code.

NOS "Not otherwise specified"
This abbreviation is the equivalent of unspecified.

7. Punctuation

[ ] Brackets are used in the Tabular List to enclose synonyms, alternative wording or explanatory phrases. Brackets are used in the Alphabetic Index to identify manifestation codes.

( ) Parentheses are used in both the Alphabetic Index and Tabular List to enclose supplementary words that may be present or absent in the statement of a disease or procedure without affecting the code number to which it is assigned. The terms within the parentheses are referred to as nonessential modifiers. The nonessential modifiers in the Alphabetic Index to Diseases apply to subterms following a main term except when a nonessential modifier and a subentry are mutually exclusive, the subentry takes precedence. For example, in the ICD-10-CM Alphabetic Index under the main term Enteritis, "acute" is a nonessential modifier and "chronic" is a subentry. In this case, the nonessential modifier "acute" does not apply to the subentry "chronic".

: Colons are used in the Tabular List after an incomplete term which needs one or more of the modifiers following the colon to make it assignable to a given category.

8. Use of "and"

See Section I.A.14. Use of the term "And"

9. Other and Unspecified Codes

a. "Other" Codes

Codes titled "other" or "other specified" are for use when the information in the medical record provides detail for which a specific code does not exist. Alphabetic Index entries with NEC in the line designate "other" codes in the Tabular List. These Alphabetic Index entries represent specific disease entities for which no specific code exists so the term is included within an "other" code.

b. "Unspecified" Codes

Codes titled "unspecified" are for use when the information in the medical record is insufficient to assign a more specific code. For those categories for which an unspecified code is not provided, the "other specified" code may represent both other and unspecified.

See Section I.B.18 Use of Signs/Symptom/Unspecified Codes

10. Includes Notes

This note appears immediately under a three character code title to further define, or give examples of, the content of the category.

11. Inclusion Terms

List of terms is included under some codes. These terms are the conditions for which that code is to be used. The terms may be synonyms of the code title, or, in the case of "other specified" codes, the terms are a list of the various conditions assigned to that code. The inclusion terms are not necessarily exhaustive. Additional terms found only in the Alphabetic Index may also be assigned to a code.

12. Excludes Notes

The ICD-10-CM has two types of excludes notes. Each type of note has a different definition for use but they are all similar in that they indicate that codes excluded from each other are independent of each other.

a. Excludes1

A type 1 Excludes note is a pure excludes note. It means "NOT CODED HERE!" An Excludes1 note indicates that the code excluded should never be used at the same time as the code above the Excludes1 note. An Excludes1 is used when two conditions cannot occur together, such as a congenital form versus an acquired form of the same condition.

An exception to the Excludes1 definition is the circumstance when the two conditions are unrelated to each other. If it is not clear whether the two conditions involving an Excludes1 note are related or not, query the provider. For example, code F45.8, Other somatoform disorders, has an Exlcudes1 note for "sleep related teeth grinding (G47.63)," because "teeth grinding" is an inclusion term under F45.8. Only one of these two codes should be assigned for teeth grinding. However, psychogenic dysmenorrhea is also an inclusion term under F45.8, and a patient could have both this conditions and sleep related teeth grinding. In this case, the two conditions are clearly unrelated to each other, and do it would be appropriate to report F45.8 and G47.63 together.

b. Excludes2

A type 2 Excludes note represents "Not included here". An Excludes2 note indicates that the condition excluded is not part of the condition represented by the code, but a patient may have both conditions at the same time. When an Excludes2 note appears under a code, it is acceptable to use both the code and the excluded code together, when appropriate.

13. Etiology/Manifestation Convention ("Code first", "Use additional code" and "In Diseases Classified Elsewhere" Notes)

Certain conditions have both an underlying etiology and multiple body system manifestations due to the underlying etiology. For such conditions, the ICD-10-CM has a coding convention that requires the underlying condition be sequenced first, if applicable, followed by the manifestation. Wherever such a combination exists, there is a "use additional code" note at the etiology code, and a "code first" note at the manifestation code. These instructional notes indicate the proper sequencing order of the codes, etiology followed by manifestation.

In most cases the manifestation codes will have in the code title, "in diseases classified elsewhere." Codes with this title are a component of the etiology/manifestation convention. The code title indicates that it is a manifestation code. "In diseases classified elsewhere" codes are never permitted to be used as first-listed or principal diagnosis codes. They must be used in conjunction with an underlying condition code and they must be listed following the underlying condition. See category F02, Dementia in other diseases classified elsewhere, for an example of this convention.

There are manifestation codes that do not have "in diseases classified elsewhere" in the title. For such codes, there is a "use additional code" note at the etiology code and a "code first" note at the manifestation code and the rules for sequencing apply.

In addition to the notes in the Tabular List, these conditions also have a specific Alphabetic Index entry structure. In the Alphabetic Index both conditions are listed together with the etiology code first followed by the manifestation codes in brackets. The code in brackets is always to be sequenced second.

An example of the etiology/manifestation convention is dementia in Parkinson's disease. In the Alphabetic Index, code G20 is listed first, followed by code F02.80 or F02.81 in brackets. Code G20 represents the underlying etiology, Parkinson's disease, and must be sequenced first, whereas codes F02.80 and F02.81 represent the manifestation of dementia in diseases classified elsewhere, with or without behavioral disturbance.

"Code first" and "Use additional code" notes are also used as sequencing rules in the classification for certain codes that are not part of an etiology/ manifestation combination.

See Section I.B. 7. Multiple coding for a single condition.

14. "And"

The word "and" should be interpreted to mean either "and" or "or" when it appears in a title.

For example, cases of "tuberculosis of bones", "tuberculosis of joints" and "tuberculosis of bones and joints" are classified to subcategory A18.0, Tuberculosis of bones and joints.

15. "With"

The word "with" or "in" should be interpreted to mean "associated with" or "due to" when it appears in a code title, the Alphabetic Index (either under a main term or subterm), or an instructional note in the Tabular List. The classification presumes a causal relationship between the two conditions linked by these terms in the Alphabetic Index or Tabular List. These conditions should be coded as related even in the absence of provider documentation explicitly linking them, unless the documentation clearly states the conditions are unrelated or when another guideline exists that specifically requires a documented linkage between two conditions (e.g., sepsis guideline for "acute organ dysfunction that is not clearly associated with the sepsis"). For conditions not specifically linked by these relational terms in the classification or when a guideline requires that a linkage between two conditions be explicitly documented, provider documentation must link the conditions in order to code them as related.

The word "with" in the Alphabetic Index is sequenced immediately following the main term or subterm, not in alphabetical order.

16. "See" and "See Also"

The "see" instruction following a main term in the Alphabetic Index indicates that another term should be referenced. It is necessary to go to the main term referenced with the "see" note to locate the correct code.

A "see also" instruction following a main term in the Alphabetic Index instructs that there is another main term that may also be referenced that may provide additional Alphabetic Index entries that may be useful. It is not necessary to follow the "see also" note when the original main term provides the necessary code.

17. "Code Also Note"

A "code also" note instructs that two codes may be required to fully describe a condition, but this note does not provide sequencing direction. The sequencing depends on the circumstances of the encounter.

18. Default Codes

A code listed next to a main term in the ICD-10-CM Alphabetic Index is referred to as a default code. The default code represents that condition that is most commonly associated with the main term, or is the unspecified code for the condition. If a condition is documented in a medical record (for example, appendicitis) without any additional information, such as acute or chronic, the default code should be assigned.

19. Code Assignment and Clinical Criteria

The assignment of a diagnosis code is based on the provider's diagnostic statement that the condition exists. The provider's statement that the patient has a particular condition is sufficient. Code assignment is not based on clinical criteria used by the provider to establish the diagnosis.

B. General Coding Guidelines

1. Locating a Code in the ICD-10-CM

To select a code in the classification that corresponds to a diagnosis or reason for visit documented in a medical record, first locate the term in the Alphabetic Index, and then verify the code in the Tabular List. Read and be guided by instructional notations that appear in both the Alphabetic Index and the Tabular List.

It is essential to use both the Alphabetic Index and Tabular List when locating and assigning a code. The Alphabetic Index does not always provide the full code. Selection of the full code, including laterality and any applicable 7th character can only be done in the Tabular List. A dash (-) at the end of an Alphabetic Index entry indicates that additional characters are required. Even if a dash is not included at the Alphabetic Index entry, it is necessary to refer to the Tabular List to verify that no 7th character is required.

2. Level of Detail in Coding

Diagnosis codes are to be used and reported at their highest number of characters available **and to the highest level of specificity documented in the medical record.**

ICD-10-CM diagnosis codes are composed of codes with 3, 4, 5, 6, or 7 characters. Codes with three characters are included in ICD-10-CM as the heading of a category of codes that may be further subdivided by the use of fourth and/or fifth characters and/or sixth characters, which provide greater detail.

A three-character code is to be used only if it is not further subdivided. A code is invalid if it has not been coded to the full number of characters required for that code, including the 7th character, if applicable.

3. Code or Codes from A00.0–T88.9, Z00–Z99.8, *U00–U85*

The appropriate code or codes from A00.0–T88.9, Z00–Z99.8, **and U00–U85** must be used to identify diagnoses, symptoms, conditions, problems, complaints or other reason(s) for the encounter/visit.

4. Signs and Symptoms

Codes that describe symptoms and signs, as opposed to diagnoses, are acceptable for reporting purposes when a related definitive diagnosis has not been established (confirmed) by the provider. Chapter 18 of ICD-10-CM, Symptoms, Signs, and Abnormal Clinical and Laboratory Findings, Not Elsewhere Classified (codes R00.0–R99) contains many, but not all codes for symptoms.

See Section I.B.18 Use of Signs/Symptom/Unspecified Codes

5. Conditions that are an Integral Part of a Disease Process

Signs and symptoms that are associated routinely with a disease process should not be assigned as additional codes, unless otherwise instructed by the classification.

6. Conditions that are not an Integral Part of a Disease Process

Additional signs and symptoms that may not be associated routinely with a disease process should be coded when present.

7. Multiple Coding for a Single Condition

In addition to the etiology/manifestation convention that requires two codes to fully describe a single condition that affects multiple body systems, there are other single conditions that also require more than one code. "Use additional code" notes are found in the Tabular List at codes that are not part of an etiology/manifestation pair where a secondary code is useful to fully describe a condition. The sequencing rule is the same as the etiology/manifestation pair, "use additional code" indicates that a secondary code should be added, if known.

For example, for bacterial infections that are not included in chapter 1, a secondary code from category B95, Streptococcus, Staphylococcus, and Enterococcus, as the cause of diseases classified elsewhere, or B96, Other bacterial agents as the cause of diseases classified elsewhere, may be required to identify the bacterial organism causing the infection. A "use additional code" note will normally be found at the infectious disease code, indicating a need for the organism code to be added as a secondary code.

"Code first" notes are also under certain codes that are not specifically manifestation codes but may be due to an underlying cause. When there is a "code first" note and an underlying condition is present, the underlying condition should be sequenced first, if known.

"Code, if applicable, any causal condition first", notes indicate that this code may be assigned as a principal diagnosis when the causal condition is unknown or not applicable. If a causal condition is known, the code for that condition should be sequenced as the principal or first-listed diagnosis.

Multiple codes may be needed for sequela, complication codes and obstetric codes to more fully describe a condition. See the specific guidelines for these conditions for further instruction.

8. Acute and Chronic Conditions

If the same condition is described as both acute (subacute) and chronic, and separate subentries exist in the Alphabetic Index at the same indentation level, code both and sequence the acute (subacute) code first.

9. Combination Code

A combination code is a single code used to classify:

- Two diagnoses, or
- A diagnosis with an associated secondary process (manifestation)
- A diagnosis with an associated complication

Combination codes are identified by referring to subterm entries in the Alphabetic Index and by reading the inclusion and exclusion notes in the Tabular List.

Assign only the combination code when that code fully identifies the diagnostic conditions involved or when the Alphabetic Index so directs. Multiple coding should not be used when the classification provides a combination code that clearly identifies all of the elements documented in the diagnosis. When the combination code lacks necessary specificity in describing the manifestation or complication, an additional code should be used as a secondary code.

10. Sequela (Late Effects)

A sequela is the residual effect (condition produced) after the acute phase of an illness or injury has terminated. There is no time limit on when a sequela code can be used. The residual may be apparent early, such as in cerebral infarction, or it may occur months or years later, such as that due to a previous injury. Examples of sequela include: scar formation resulting from a burn, deviated septum due to a nasal fracture, and infertility due to tubal occlusion from old tuberculosis.

Coding of sequela generally requires two codes sequenced in the following order: The condition or nature of the sequela is sequenced first. The sequela code is sequenced second.

An exception to the above guidelines are those instances where the code for the sequela is followed by a manifestation code identified in the Tabular List and title, or the sequela code has been expanded (at the fourth, fifth or sixth, character levels) to include the manifestation(s). The code for the acute phase of an illness or injury that led to the sequela is never used with a code for the late effect.

- *See Section I.C.9. Sequelae of cerebrovascular disease*
- *See Section I.C.15. Sequelae of complication of pregnancy, childbirth and the puerperium*
- *See Section I.C.19. Application of 7th characters for Chapter 19*

11. Impending or Threatened Condition

Code any condition described at the time of discharge as "impending" or "threatened" as follows:

- If it did occur, code as confirmed diagnosis.
- If it did not occur, reference the Alphabetic Index to determine if the condition has a subentry term for "impending" or "threatened" and also reference main term entries for "Impending" and for "Threatened."
- If the subterms are listed, assign the given code.
- If the subterms are not listed, code the existing underlying condition(s) and not the condition described as impending or threatened.

12. Reporting Same Diagnosis Code More than Once

Each unique ICD-10-CM diagnosis code may be reported only once for an encounter. This applies to bilateral conditions when there are no distinct codes identifying laterality or two different conditions classified to the same ICD-10-CM diagnosis code.

13. Laterality

Some ICD-10-CM codes indicate laterality, specifying whether the condition occurs on the left, right or is bilateral. If no bilateral code is provided and the condition is bilateral, assign separate codes for both the left and right side. If the side is not identified in the medical record, assign the code for the unspecified side.

When a patient has a bilateral condition and each side is treated during separate encounters, assign the "bilateral" code (as the conditions still exists on both sides), including for the encounter to treat the first side. For the second encounter for treatment after one side has previously been treated and the condition no longer exists on that side, assign the appropriate unilateral code for the side where the conditions still exists (e.g., cataract surgery performed on each eye in separate encounters). The bilateral code would not be assigned for the subsequent encounter, as the patient no longer has the condition in the previously-treated site. If the treatment on the first side did not completely resolve the condition, then the bilateral code would still be appropriate.

When laterality is not documented by the patient's provider, code assignment for the affected side may be based on medical record documentation from other clinicians. If there is conflicting medical record documentation regarding the affected side, the patient's attending provider should be queried for clarification. Codes for "unspecified" side should rarely be used, such as when the documentation in the record is insufficient to determine the affected side and it is not possible to obtain clarification.

14. Documentation by Clinicians Other than the Patient's Provider

Code assignment is based on the documentation by **the** patient's provider (i.e., physician or other qualified healthcare practitioner legally accountable for establishing the patient's diagnosis). There are a few exceptions **when** code assignment may be based on medical record documentation from clinicians who are not the patient's provider (i.e., physician, or other qualified healthcare practitioner legally accountable for establishing the patient's diagnosis). **In this context, "clinicians" other than the patient's provider refer to healthcare professionals permitted, based on regulatory or accreditation requirements or internal hospital policies, to document in a patient's official medical record.**

These exceptions include codes for:

- **Body Mass Index (BMI)**
- **Depth of non-pressure chronic ulcers**
- **Pressure ulcer stage**
- **Coma scale**
- **NIH stroke scale (NIHSS)**

- **Social determinants of health (SDOH)**
- **Laterality**
- **Blood alcohol level**

This information is typically**, or may be,** documented by other clinicians involved in the care of the patient (e.g., a dietitian often documents the BMI, a nurse often documents the pressure ulcer stages, and an emergency medical technician often documents the coma scale). However, the associated diagnosis (such as overweight, obesity, acute stroke pressure ulcer, **or a condition classifiable to category F10, Alcohol related disorders**) must be documented by the patient's provider. If there is conflicting medical record documentation, either from the same clinician or different clinicians, the patient's attending provider should be queried for clarification.

The BMI, coma scale, and NIHSS codes **blood alcohol level codes,** and **codes for social determinants of health** should only be reported as secondary diagnoses.

See Section I.C.21.c.17 for additional information regarding coding social determinants of health

15. Syndromes

Follow the Alphabetic Index guidance when coding syndromes. In the absence of Alphabetic Index guidance, assign codes for the documented manifestations of the syndrome. Additional codes for manifestations that are not an integral part of the disease process may also be assigned when the condition does not have a unique code.

16. Documentation of Complications of Care

Code assignment is based on the provider's documentation of the relationship between the condition and the care or procedure, unless otherwise instructed by the classification. The guideline extends to any complications of care, regardless of the chapter the code is located in. It is important to note that not all conditions that occur during or following medical care or surgery are classified as complications. There must be a cause-and-effect relationship between the care provided and the condition, and an indication in the documentation that it is a complication. Query the provider for clarification, if the complication is not clearly documented.

17. Borderline Diagnosis

If the provider documents a "borderline" diagnosis at the time of discharge, the diagnosis is coded as confirmed, unless the classification provides a specific entry (e.g., borderline diabetes). If a borderline condition has a specific index entry in ICD-10-CM, it should be coded as such. Since borderline conditions are not uncertain diagnoses, no distinction is made between the care setting (inpatient versus outpatient). Whenever the documentation is unclear regarding a borderline condition, coders are encouraged to query for clarification.

18. Use of Sign/Symptom/Unspecified Codes

Sign/symptom and "unspecified" codes have acceptable, even necessary, uses. While specific diagnosis codes should be reported when they are supported by the available medical record documentation and clinical knowledge of the patient's health condition, there are instances when signs/symptoms or unspecified codes are the best choices for accurately reflecting the healthcare encounter. Each healthcare encounter should be coded to the level of certainty known for that encounter.

As stated in the introductory section of these official coding guidelines, a joint effort between the healthcare provider and the coder is essential to achieve complete and accurate documentation, code assignment, and reporting of diagnoses and procedures. The importance of consistent, complete documentation in the medical record cannot be overemphasized. Without such documentation accurate coding cannot be achieved. The entire record should be reviewed to determine the specific reason for the encounter and the conditions treated.

If a definitive diagnosis has not been established by the end of the encounter, it is appropriate to report codes for sign(s) and/or symptom(s) in lieu of a definitive diagnosis. When sufficient clinical information isn't known or available about a particular health condition to assign a more specific code, it is acceptable to report the appropriate "unspecified" code (e.g., a diagnosis of pneumonia has been determined, but not the specific type). Unspecified codes should be reported when they are the codes that most accurately reflects what is known about the patient's condition at the time of that particular encounter. It would be inappropriate to select a specific code that is not supported by the medical record documentation or conduct medically unnecessary diagnostic testing in order to determine a more specific code.

19. Coding for Healthcare Encounters in Hurricane Aftermath

a. Use of External Cause of Morbidity Codes

An external cause of morbidity code should be assigned to identify the cause of the injury(ies) incurred as a result of the hurricane. The use of external cause of morbidity codes is supplemental to the application of ICD-10-CM codes. External cause of morbidity codes are never to be recorded as a principal diagnosis (first-listed in non-inpatient settings). The appropriate injury code should be sequenced before any external cause codes. The external cause of morbidity codes capture how the injury or health condition happened (cause), the intent (unintentional or accidental; or intentional, such as suicide or assault), the place where the event occurred, the activity of the patient at the time of the event, and the person's status (e.g., civilian, military). They should not be assigned for encounters to treat hurricane victims' medical conditions when no injury, adverse effect or poisoning is involved. External cause of morbidity codes should be assigned for each encounter for care and treatment of the injury. External cause of morbidity codes may be assigned in all health care settings. For the purpose of capturing complete and accurate ICD-10-CM data in the aftermath of the hurricane, a healthcare setting should be considered as any location where medical care is provided by licensed healthcare professionals.

b. Sequencing of External Causes of Morbidity Codes

Codes for cataclysmic events, such as hurricane, take priority over all other external cause codes except child and adult abuse and terrorism and should be sequenced before other external cause of injury codes. Assign as many external cause of morbidity codes as necessary to fully explain each cause. For example, if an injury occurs as a result of a building collapse during the hurricane, external cause codes for both the hurricane and the building collapse should be assigned with the external causes code for hurricane being sequenced as the first external cause code. For injuries incurred as a direct result of the hurricane, assign the appropriate code(s) for the injuries, followed by the code X37.0-, Hurricane (with the appropriate 7th character), and any other applicable external cause of injury codes. Code X37.0- also should be assigned when an injury is incurred as a result of flooding caused by a levee breaking related to the hurricane. Code X38.-, Flood (with appropriate 7th character), should be assigned when an injury is from flooding resulting directly from the storm. Code X36.0-, Collapse of dam or man-made structure, should not be assigned when the cause of the collapse is due to the hurricane. Use of code X36.0- is limited to collapses of man-made structures due to earth surface movements, not due to storm surges directly from a hurricane.

c. Other External Causes of Morbidity Code Issues

For injuries that are not a direct result of the hurricane, such as an evacuee that has incurred an injury as a result of a motor vehicle accident, assign the appropriate external cause of morbidity code(s) to describe the cause of the injury, but do not assign code X37.0-, Hurricane. If it is not clear whether the injury was a direct result of the hurricane, assume the injury is due to the hurricane and assign code X37.0-, Hurricane, as well as any other applicable external cause of morbidity codes. In addition to code X37.0-, Hurricane, other possible applicable external cause of morbidity codes include:

- W54.0-, Bitten by dog
- X30-, Exposure to excessive natural heat
- X31-, Exposure to excessive natural cold
- X38-, Flood

d. Use of Z codes

Z codes (other reasons for healthcare encounters) may be assigned as appropriate to further explain the reasons for presenting for healthcare services, including transfers between healthcare facilities, **or provide additional information relevant to a patient encounter**. The ICD-10-CM Official Guidelines for Coding and Reporting identify which codes may be assigned as principal or first-listed diagnosis only, secondary diagnosis only, or principal/first-listed or secondary (depending on the circumstances). Possible applicable Z codes include:

- Z59.0. Homelessness
- Z59.1-, Inadequate housing
- Z59.5-, Extreme poverty
- Z75.1-, Person awaiting admission to adequate facility elsewhere
- Z75.3-, Unavailability and inaccessibility of health-care facilities
- Z74.4-, Unavailability and inaccessibility of other helping agencies
- Z76.2-, Encounter for health supervision and care of other healthy infant and child
- Z99.12-, Encounter for respirator [ventilator] dependence during power failure

The external cause of morbidity codes and the Z codes listed above are not an all-inclusive list. Other codes may be applicable to the encounter based upon the documentation. Assign as many codes as necessary to fully explain each healthcare encounter. Since patient history information may be very limited, use any available documentation to assign the appropriate external cause of morbidity and Z codes.

C. Chapter-Specific Coding Guidelines

Consulting Editor Note

In this book the Chapter-Specific Coding Guidelines are included here and in the Tabular List of Diseases and Injuries at the beginning of the chapter for which they are applicable.

Additionally, notes have been added throughout the Diagnosis and Procedure Tabular to alert the coder when the code under review is included in a chapter specific coding guideline. The user can then reference the coding guideline prior to making their final code selection. For example:

A41 Other sepsis

Review coding guideline C.1.d

This note alerts the coder to reference the chapter specific coding guidelines (C), chapter 1, guideline d, before making the final code selection. The guidelines for chapter 1, Certain Infectious and Parasitic Diseases, is located at the beginning of Chapter 1 in the Diagnosis Tabular. Please note that the coding guideline notes may be provided at the category, sub-category, or sub-classification level, whichever is applicable to the coding guidance.

In addition to general coding guidelines, there are guidelines for specific diagnoses and/or conditions in the classification. Unless otherwise indicated, these guidelines apply to all health care settings. Please refer to Section II for guidelines on the selection of principal diagnosis.

1. Chapter 1: Certain Infectious and Parasitic Diseases (A00-B99), U07.1 U09.9

a. Human Immunodeficiency Virus (HIV) Infections

1) Code only confirmed cases

Code only confirmed cases of HIV infection/illness. This is an exception to the hospital inpatient guideline Section II, H.

In this context, "confirmation" does not require documentation of positive serology or culture for HIV; the provider's diagnostic statement that the patient is HIV positive, or has an HIV-related illness is sufficient.

2) Selection and sequencing of HIV codes

(a) Patient admitted for HIV-related condition

If a patient is admitted for an HIV-related condition, the principal diagnosis should be B20, Human immunodeficiency virus [HIV] disease followed by additional diagnosis codes for all reported HIV-related conditions.

(b) Patient with HIV disease admitted for unrelated condition

If a patient with HIV disease is admitted for an unrelated condition (such as a traumatic injury), the code for the unrelated condition (e.g., the nature of injury code) should be the principal diagnosis. Other diagnoses would be B20 followed by additional diagnosis codes for all reported HIV-related conditions.

(c) Whether the patient is newly diagnosed

Whether the patient is newly diagnosed or has had previous admissions/encounters for HIV conditions is irrelevant to the sequencing decision.

(d) Asymptomatic human immunodeficiency virus

Z21, Asymptomatic human immunodeficiency virus [HIV] infection status, is to be applied when the patient without any documentation of symptoms is listed as being "HIV positive," "known HIV," "HIV test positive," or similar terminology. Do not use this code if the term "AIDS" is used or if the patient is treated for any HIV-related illness or is described as having any condition(s) resulting from his/her HIV positive status; use B20 in these cases.

(e) Patients with inconclusive HIV serology

Patients with inconclusive HIV serology, but no definitive diagnosis or manifestations of the illness, may be assigned code R75, Inconclusive laboratory evidence of human immunodeficiency virus [HIV].

(f) Previously diagnosed HIV-related illness

Patients with any known prior diagnosis of an HIV-related illness should be coded to B20. Once a patient has developed an HIV-related illness, the patient should always be assigned code B20 on every subsequent admission/encounter. Patients previously diagnosed with any HIV illness (B20) should never be assigned to R75 or Z21, Asymptomatic human immunodeficiency virus [HIV] infection status.

(g) HIV Infection in Pregnancy, Childbirth and the Puerperium

During pregnancy, childbirth or the puerperium, a patient admitted (or presenting for a health care encounter) because of an HIV-related illness should receive a principal diagnosis code of O98.7-, Human immunodeficiency [HIV] disease complicating pregnancy, childbirth and the puerperium, followed by B20 and the code(s) for the HIV-related illness(es). Codes from Chapter 15 always take sequencing priority. Patients with asymptomatic HIV infection status admitted (or presenting for a health care encounter) during pregnancy, childbirth, or the puerperium should receive codes of O98.7- and Z21.

(h) Encounters for testing for HIV

If a patient is being seen to determine his/her HIV status, use code Z11.4, Encounter for screening for human immunodeficiency virus [HIV]. Use additional codes for any associated high risk behavior.

If a patient with signs or symptoms is being seen for HIV testing, code the signs and symptoms. An additional counseling code Z71.7, Human immunodeficiency virus [HIV] counseling, may be used if counseling is provided during the encounter for the test.

When a patient returns to be informed of his/her HIV test results and the test result is negative, use code Z71.7, Human immunodeficiency virus [HIV] counseling.

If the results are positive, see previous guidelines and assign codes as appropriate.

(i) History of HIV managed by medication

If a patient with documented history of HIV disease is currently managed on antiretroviral medications, assign code B20, Human immunodeficiency virus [HIV] disease. Code Z79.899, Other long term (current) drug therapy, may be assigned as an additional code to identify the long-term (current) use of antiretroviral medications.

b. Infectious agents as the cause of diseases classified to other chapters

Certain infections are classified in chapters other than Chapter 1 and no organism is identified as part of the infection code. In these instances, it is necessary to use an additional code from Chapter 1 to identify the organism. A code from category B95, Streptococcus, Staphylococcus, and Enterococcus as the cause of diseases classified to other chapters, B96, Other bacterial agents as the cause of diseases classified to other chapters, or B97, Viral agents as the cause of diseases classified to other chapters, is to be used as an additional code to identify the organism. An instructional note will be found at the infection code advising that an additional organism code is required.

c. Infections resistant to antibiotics

Many bacterial infections are resistant to current antibiotics. It is necessary to identify all infections documented as antibiotic resistant. Assign a code from category Z16, Resistance to antimicrobial drugs, following the infection code only if the infection code does not identify drug resistance.

d. Sepsis, Severe Sepsis, and Septic Shock

1) Coding of Sepsis and Severe Sepsis

(a) Sepsis

For a diagnosis of sepsis, assign the appropriate code for the underlying systemic infection. If the type of infection or causal organism is not further specified, assign code A41.9, Sepsis, unspecified organism.

A code from subcategory R65.2, Severe sepsis, should not be assigned unless severe sepsis or an associated acute organ dysfunction is documented.

(i) Negative or inconclusive blood cultures and sepsis

Negative or inconclusive blood cultures do not preclude a diagnosis of sepsis in patients with clinical evidence of the condition, however, the provider should be queried.

(ii) Urosepsis

The term urosepsis is a nonspecific term. It is not to be considered synonymous with sepsis. It has no default code in the Alphabetic Index. Should a provider use this term, he/she must be queried for clarification.

(iii) Sepsis with organ dysfunction

If a patient has sepsis and associated acute organ dysfunction or multiple organ dysfunction (MOD), follow the instructions for coding severe sepsis.

(iv) Acute organ dysfunction that is not clearly associated with the sepsis

If a patient has sepsis and an acute organ dysfunction, but the medical record documentation indicates that the acute organ dysfunction is related to a medical condition other than the sepsis, do not assign a code from subcategory R65.2, Severe sepsis. An acute organ dysfunction must be associated with the sepsis in order to assign the severe sepsis code. If the documentation is not clear as to whether an acute organ dysfunction is related to the sepsis or another medical condition, query the provider.

(b) Severe sepsis

The coding of severe sepsis requires a minimum of 2 codes: first a code for the underlying systemic infection, followed by a code from subcategory R65.2, Severe sepsis. If the causal organism is not documented, assign code A41.9, Sepsis, unspecified organism, for the infection. Additional code(s) for the associated acute organ dysfunction are also required.

Due to the complex nature of severe sepsis, some cases may require querying the provider prior to assignment of the codes.

2) Septic shock

(a) Septic shock generally refers to circulatory failure associated with severe sepsis, and therefore, it represents a type of acute organ dysfunction.

For cases of septic shock, the code for the systemic infection should be sequenced first, followed by code R65.21, Severe sepsis with septic shock or code T81.12, Postprocedural septic shock. Any additional codes for the other acute organ dysfunctions should also be assigned. As noted in the sequencing instructions in the Tabular List, the code for septic shock cannot be assigned as a principal diagnosis.

3) Sequencing of severe sepsis

If severe sepsis is present on admission, and meets the definition of principal diagnosis, the underlying systemic infection should be assigned as principal diagnosis followed by the appropriate code from subcategory R65.2 as required by the sequencing rules in the Tabular List. A code from subcategory R65.2 can never be assigned as a principal diagnosis.

When severe sepsis develops during an encounter (it was not present on admission) the underlying systemic infection and the appropriate code from subcategory R65.2 should be assigned as secondary diagnoses.

Severe sepsis may be present on admission but the diagnosis may not be confirmed until sometime after admission. If the documentation is not clear whether severe sepsis was present on admission, the provider should be queried.

4) Sepsis or severe sepsis with a localized infection

If the reason for admission is both sepsis or severe sepsis and a localized infection, such as pneumonia or cellulitis, a code(s) for the underlying systemic infection should be assigned first and the code for the localized infection should be assigned as a secondary diagnosis. If the patient has severe sepsis, a code from subcategory R65.2 should also be assigned as a secondary diagnosis. If the patient is admitted with a localized infection, such as pneumonia, and sepsis/severe sepsis doesn't develop until after admission, the localized infection should be assigned first, followed by the appropriate sepsis/severe sepsis codes.

5) Sepsis due to a postprocedural infection

(a) Documentation of causal relationship

As with all postprocedural complications, code assignment is based on the provider's documentation of the relationship between the infection and the procedure.

(b) Sepsis due to a postprocedural infection

For infections following a procedure, a code from T81.40, to T81.43, Infection following a procedure, or a code from O86.00 to O86.03, Infection of obstetric surgical wound, that identifies the site of the infection should be coded first, if known. Assign an additional code for sepsis following a procedure (T81.44) or sepsis following an obstetrical procedure (O86.04). Use an additional code to identify the infectious agent. If the patient has severe sepsis the appropriate code from subcategory R65.2 should also be assigned with the additional code(s) for any acute organ dysfunction.

For infections following infusion, transfusion, therapeutic injection, or immunization, a code from subcategory T80.2, Infections following infusion, transfusion, and therapeutic injection, or code T88.0-, Infection following immunization, should be coded first, followed by the code for the specific infection. If the patient has severe sepsis, the appropriate code from subcategory R65.2 should also be assigned, with the additional code(s) for any acute organ dysfunction.

(c) Postprocedural infection and postprocedural septic shock

If a postprocedural infection has resulted in postprocedural septic shock, assign the codes indicated above for sepsis due to a postprocedural infection, followed by code T81.12-, Postprocedural septic shock. Do not assign code R65.21, Severe sepsis with septic shock. Additional code(s) should be assigned for any acute organ dysfunction.

6) Sepsis and severe sepsis associated with a noninfectious process (condition)

In some cases a noninfectious process (condition), such as trauma, may lead to an infection which can result in sepsis or severe sepsis. If sepsis or severe sepsis is documented as associated with a noninfectious condition, such as a burn or serious injury, and this condition meets the definition for principal diagnosis, the code for the noninfectious condition should be sequenced first, followed by the code for the resulting infection. If severe sepsis, is present a code from subcategory R65.2 should also be assigned with any associated organ dysfunction(s) codes. It is not necessary to assign a code from subcategory R65.1, Systemic inflammatory response syndrome (SIRS) of non-infectious origin, for these cases.

If the infection meets the definition of principal diagnosis it should be sequenced before the non-infectious condition. When both the associated non-infectious condition and the infection meet the definition of principal diagnosis either may be assigned as principal diagnosis.

Only one code from category R65, Symptoms and signs specifically associated with systemic inflammation and infection, should be assigned. Therefore, when a non-infectious condition leads to an infection resulting in severe sepsis, assign the appropriate code from subcategory R65.2, Severe sepsis. Do not additionally assign a code from subcategory R65.1, Systemic inflammatory response syndrome (SIRS) of non-infectious origin.

See Section I.C.18. SIRS due to non-infectious process

7) Sepsis and septic shock complicating abortion, pregnancy, childbirth, and the puerperium

See Section I.C.15. Sepsis and septic shock complicating abortion, pregnancy, childbirth and the puerperium

8) Newborn sepsis

See Section I.C.16. f. Bacterial sepsis of Newborn

e. Methicillin Resistant Staphylococcus aureus (MRSA) Conditions

1) Selection and sequencing of MRSA codes

(a) Combination codes for MRSA infection

When a patient is diagnosed with an infection that is due to methicillin resistant Staphylococcus aureus (MRSA), and that infection has a combination code that includes the causal organism (e.g., sepsis, pneumonia) assign the appropriate combination code for the condition (e.g., code A41.02, Sepsis due to Methicillin resistant Staphylococcus aureus or code J15.212, Pneumonia due to Methicillin resistant Staphylococcus aureus). Do not assign code B95.62, Methicillin resistant Staphylococcus aureus infection as the cause of diseases classified elsewhere, as an additional code because the combination code includes the type of infection and the MRSA organism. Do not assign a code from subcategory Z16.11, Resistance to penicillins, as an additional diagnosis.

See Section C.1. for instructions on coding and sequencing of sepsis and severe sepsis.

(b) Other codes for MRSA infection

When there is documentation of a current infection (e.g., wound infection, stitch abscess, urinary tract infection) due to MRSA, and that infection does not have a combination code that includes the causal organism, assign the appropriate code to identify the condition along with code B95.62, Methicillin resistant Staphylococcus aureus infection as the cause of diseases classified elsewhere for the MRSA infection. Do not assign a code from subcategory Z16.11, Resistance to penicillins.

(c) Methicillin susceptible Staphylococcus aureus (MSSA) and MRSA colonization

The condition or state of being colonized or carrying MSSA or MRSA is called colonization or carriage, while an individual person is described as being colonized or being a carrier. Colonization means that MSSA or MSRA is present on or in the body without necessarily causing illness. A positive MRSA colonization test might be documented by the provider as "MRSA screen positive" or "MRSA nasal swab positive".

Assign code Z22.322, Carrier or suspected carrier of Methicillin resistant Staphylococcus aureus, for patients documented as having MRSA colonization. Assign code Z22.321, Carrier or suspected carrier of Methicillin susceptible Staphylococcus aureus, for patient documented as having MSSA colonization. Colonization is not necessarily indicative of a disease process or as the cause of a specific condition the patient may have unless documented as such by the provider.

(d) MRSA colonization and infection

If a patient is documented as having both MRSA colonization and infection during a hospital admission, code Z22.322, Carrier or suspected carrier of Methicillin resistant Staphylococcus aureus, and a code for the MRSA infection may both be assigned.

f. Zika virus infections

1) Code only confirmed cases

Code only a confirmed diagnosis of Zika virus (A92.5, Zika virus disease) as documented by the provider. This is an exception to the hospital inpatient guideline Section II, H. In this context, "confirmation" does not require documentation of the type of test performed; the provider's diagnostic statement that the condition is confirmed is sufficient. This code should be assigned regardless of the stated mode of transmission.

If the provider documents "suspected", "possible" or "provable" Zika, do not assign code A92.5. Assign a code(s) explaining the reason for encounter (such as fever, rash, or joint pain) or Z20.821, Contact with and (suspected) exposure to Zika virus.

g. Coronavirus infections

1) COVID-19 infection (infection due to SARS-CoV-2)

(a) Code only confirmed cases

Code only a confirmed diagnosis of the 2019 novel coronavirus disease (COVID-19) as documented by the provider or documentation of a positive COVID-19 test result. For a confirmed diagnosis, assign code U07.1, COVID-19. This is an exception to the hospital inpatient guideline Section II, H. In this context, "confirmation" does not require documentation of a positive test result for COVID-19; the provider's documentation that the individual has COVID-19 is sufficient.

If the provider documents "suspected," "possible," "probable," or "inconclusive" COVID-19, do not assign code U07.1. Instead, code the signs and symptoms reported.

See guideline I.C.1.g.1.g.

(b) Sequencing of codes

When COVID-19 meets the definition of principle diagnosis, code U07.1, COVID-19, should be sequenced first, followed by the appropriate codes for associated manifestations, except when another guideline requires that certain codes be sequenced first, such as obstetrics, sepsis, or transplant complications.

For a COVID-19 infection that progresses to sepsis, see Section I.C.1.d Sepsis, Severe Sepsis, and Septic Shock

See Section I.C.15.s. for COVID-19 infection in pregnancy, childbirth, and the puerperium

See Section I.C.16.h. for COVID-19 infection in newborn

For a COVID-19 infection in a lung transplant patient, see Section I.C.19.g.3.a. Transplant complications other than kidney

(c) Acute respiratory manifestations of COVID-19

When the reason for the encounter/admission is a respiratory manifestation of COVID-19, assign code U07.1, COVID-19, as the principal/first-listed diagnosis and assign code(s) for the respiratory manifestation(s) as additional diagnoses.

The following conditions are examples of common respiratory manifestations of COVID-19.

(i) Pneumonia

For a patient with pneumonia confirmed as due to COVID-19, assign codes U07.1, COVID-19, and J12.82, Pneumonia due to coronavirus disease 2019.

(ii) Acute bronchitis

For a patient with acute bronchitis confirmed as due to COVID-19, assign codes U07.1, and J20.8, Acute bronchitis due to other specified organisms.

Bronchitis not otherwise specified (NOS) due to COVID-19 should be coded using code U07.1 and J40, Bronchitis, not specified as acute or chronic.

(iii) Lower respiratory infection

If the COVID-19 is documented as being associated with lower respiratory infection, not otherwise specified (NOS), or an acute respiratory infection, NOS, codes U07.1 and J22, Unspecified acute lower respiratory infection, should be assigned.

If the COVID-19 is documented as being associated with a respiratory infection, NOS, codes U07.1 and J98.8, Other specified respiratory disorders, should be assigned.

(iv) Acute respiratory distress syndrome

For acute respiratory distress syndrome (ARDS) due to COVID-19, assign codes U07.1 and J80, Acute respiratory distress syndrome

(v) Acute respiratory failure

For acute respiratory failure due to COVID-19, assign code U07.1 and code J96.0-, Acute respiratory failure.

(d) Non-respiratory manifestations of COVID-19

When the reason for the encounter/admission is a non-respiratory manifestation (e.g., viral enteritis) of COVID-19, assign code U07.1, COVID-19, as the principal/first-listed diagnosis and assign code(s) for the manifestation(s) as additional diagnoses.

(e) Exposure to COVID-19

For asymptomatic individuals with actual or suspected exposure to COVID-19, assign code Z20.822, Contact with and (suspected) exposure to COVID-19.

For symptomatic individuals with actual or suspected exposure to COVID-19 and the infection has been ruled out, or test results are inconclusive or unknown, assign code Z20.822, Contact with and (suspected) exposure to COVID-19.

See guidelines I.C.21.c.1, Contact/Exposure, for additional guidance regarding the use of category Z20 codes.

If COVID-19 is confirmed, see guidelines I.C.1.g.1.a.

(f) Screening for COVID-19

During the COVID-19 pandemic, a screening code is generally not appropriate. Do not assign code Z11.52, Encounter for screening for COVID-19. For encounters for COVID-19 testing, including preoperative testing, code as exposure to COVID-19 (guideline I.C.1.g.1.e).

Coding guidance will be updated as new information concerning any changes in the pandemic status becomes available.

(g) Signs and symptoms without definitive diagnosis of COVID-19

For patient presenting with any signs/symptoms associated with COVID-19 (such as fever, etc.) but a definitive diagnosis has not been established, assign the appropriate code(s) for each of the presenting signs and symptoms such as:

- R05.**1, Acute** cough, **or R05.9, Cough, unspecified**
- R06.02 Shortness of breath
- R50.9 Fever, unspecified

If a patient with signs/symptoms associated with COVID-19 also has an actual or suspected contact with or exposure to COVID-19, assign Z20.828, Contact with and (suspected) exposure to other viral communicable diseases, as an additional code.

(h) Asymptomatic individuals who test positive for COVID-19

For asymptomatic individuals who test positive for COVID-19, *see guideline I.C.1.g.1.a.* Although the individual is asymptomatic, the individual has tested positive and is considered to have a COVID-19 infection.

(i) Personal history of COVID-19

For patients with a history of COVID-19, assign code Z86.16, Personal history of COVID-19.

(j) Follow-up visits after COVID-19 infection has resolved

For individuals who previously had COVID-19, **without residual symptom(s) or condition(s)** and are being seen for follow-up evaluation, and COVID-19 test results are negative, assign codes Z09, Encounter for follow-up examination after completed treatment for conditions other than malignant neoplasm, and Z86.16, Personal history of COVID-19. **For follow-up visits for individuals with symptom(s) or condition(s) related to a previous COVID-19 infection, see guideline I.C.1.g.l.m.**

See Section I.C.21.c.8, Factors influencing health states and contact with health services, Follow-up

(k) Encounter for antibody testing

For an encounter for antibody testing that is not being performed to confirm a current COVID-19 infection, nor is a follow-up test after resolution of COVID-19, assign Z01.84, Encounter for antibody response examination.

Follow the applicable guidelines above if the individual is being tested to confirm a current COVID-19 infection.

For follow-up testing after a COVID-19 infection, see guideline I.C.1.g.1.j.

(l) Multisystem Inflammatory Syndrome

For individuals with multisystem inflammatory syndrome (MIS) and COVID-19, assign code U07.1, COVID-19, as the principal/first-listed diagnosis and assign code M35.81, Multisystem inflammatory syndrome, as an additional diagnosis.

If an individual with a history of COVID-19 develops MIS, assign codes M35.81, Multisystem inflammatory syndrome, and **U09.9, Post COVID-19 condition, unspecified**.

If an individual with a known or suspected exposure to COVID-19, and no current COVID-19 infection or history of COVID-19, develops MIS, assign codes M5.81, Muyltisystem Inflammatory Syndrome, and Z20.822, Contact with and (suspected) exposure to COVID-19.

Additional codes should be assigned for any associated complications of MIS.

(m) Post COVID-19 Condition

For sequela of COVID-19, or associated symptoms or conditions that develop following a previous COVID-19 infection, assign a code(s) for the specific symptom(s) or condition(s) related to the previous COVID-19 infection, if known, and code U09.9, Post COVID-19 condition, unspecified.

Code U09.9 should not be assigned for manifestations of an active (current) COVID-19 infection.

If a patient has a condition(s) associated with a previous COVID-19 infection and develops a new active (current) COVID-19 infection, code U09.9 may be assigned in conjunction with code U07.1, COVID-19, to identify that the patient also has a condition(s) associated with a previous COVID-19 infection. Code(s) for the specific condition(s) associated with the previous COVID-19 infection and code(s) for manifestation(s) of the new active (current) COVID-19 infection should also be assigned.

2. Chapter 2: Neoplasms (C00-D49)

General guidelines

Chapter 2 of the ICD-10-CM contains the codes for most benign and all malignant neoplasms. Certain benign neoplasms, such as prostatic adenomas, may be found in the specific body system chapters. To properly code a neoplasm it is necessary to determine from the record if the neoplasm is benign, in-situ, malignant, or of uncertain histologic behavior. If malignant, any secondary (metastatic) sites should also be determined.

Primary malignant neoplasms overlapping site boundaries

A primary malignant neoplasm that overlaps two or more contiguous (next to each other) sites should be classified to the subcategory/code .8 ('overlapping lesion'), unless the combination is specifically indexed elsewhere. For multiple neoplasms of the same site that are not contiguous such as tumors in different quadrants of the same breast, codes for each site should be assigned.

Malignant neoplasm of ectopic tissue

Malignant neoplasms of ectopic tissue are to be coded to the site of origin mentioned, e.g., ectopic pancreatic malignant neoplasms involving the stomach are coded to malignant neoplasm of pancreas, unspecified (C25.9).

The neoplasm table in the Alphabetic Index should be referenced first. However, if the histological term is documented, that term should be referenced first, rather than going immediately to the Neoplasm Table, in order to determine which column in the Neoplasm Table is appropriate. For example, if the documentation indicates "adenoma," refer to the term in the Alphabetic Index to review the entries under this term and the instructional note to "see also neoplasm, by site, benign." The table provides the proper code based on the type of neoplasm and the site. It is important to select the proper column in the table that corresponds to the type of neoplasm. The Tabular List should then be referenced to verify that the correct code has been selected from the table and that a more specific site code does not exist.

See Section I.C.21. Factors influencing health status and contact with health services, Status, for information regarding Z15.0, codes for genetic susceptibility to cancer.

a. Treatment directed at the malignancy

If the treatment is directed at the malignancy, designate the malignancy as the principal diagnosis.

The only exception to this guideline is if a patient admission/encounter is solely for the administration of chemotherapy, immunotherapy or external beam radiation therapy, assign the appropriate Z51.-- code as the first-listed or principal diagnosis, and the diagnosis or problem for which the service is being performed as a secondary diagnosis.

b. Treatment of secondary site

When a patient is admitted because of a primary neoplasm with metastasis and treatment is directed toward the secondary site only, the secondary neoplasm is designated as the principal diagnosis even though the primary malignancy is still present.

c. Coding and sequencing of complications

Coding and sequencing of complications associated with the malignancies or with the therapy thereof are subject to the following guidelines:

1) Anemia associated with malignancy

When admission/encounter is for management of an anemia associated with the malignancy, and the treatment is only for anemia, the appropriate code for the malignancy is sequenced as the principal or first-listed diagnosis followed by the appropriate code for the anemia (such as code D63.0, Anemia in neoplastic disease).

2) Anemia associated with chemotherapy, immunotherapy and radiation therapy

When the admission/encounter is for management of an anemia associated with an adverse effect of the administration of chemotherapy or immunotherapy and the only treatment is for the anemia, the anemia code is sequenced first followed by the appropriate codes for the neoplasm and the adverse effect (T45.1X5, Adverse effect of antineoplastic and immunosuppressive drugs).

When the admission/encounter is for management of an anemia associated with an adverse effect of radiotherapy, the anemia code should be sequenced first, followed by the appropriate neoplasm code and code Y84.2, Radiological procedure and radiotherapy as the cause of abnormal reaction of the patient, or of later complication, without mention of misadventure at the time of the procedure.

3) Management of dehydration due to the malignancy

When the admission/encounter is for management of dehydration due to the malignancy and only the dehydration is being treated (intravenous rehydration), the dehydration is sequenced first, followed by the code(s) for the malignancy.

4) Treatment of a complication resulting from a surgical procedure

When the admission/encounter is for treatment of a complication resulting from a surgical procedure, designate the complication as the principal or first-listed diagnosis if treatment is directed at resolving the complication.

d. Primary malignancy previously excised

When a primary malignancy has been previously excised or eradicated from its site and there is no further treatment directed to that site and there is no evidence of any existing primary malignancy at that site, a code from category Z85, Personal history of malignant neoplasm, should be used to indicate the former site of the malignancy. Any mention of extension, invasion, or metastasis to another site is coded as a secondary malignant neoplasm to that site. The secondary site may be the principal or first-listed diagnosis with the Z85 code used as a secondary code.

e. Admissions/Encounters involving chemotherapy, immunotherapy and radiation therapy

1) Episode of care involves surgical removal of neoplasm

When an episode of care involves the surgical removal of a neoplasm, primary or secondary site, followed by adjunct chemotherapy or radiation treatment during the same episode of care, the code for the neoplasm should be assigned as principal or first-listed diagnosis.

2) Patient admission/encounter solely for administration of chemotherapy, immunotherapy and radiation therapy

If a patient admission/encounter is solely for the administration of chemotherapy, immunotherapy or external beam radiation therapy assign code Z51.0, Encounter for antineoplastic radiation therapy, or Z51.11, Encounter for antineoplastic chemotherapy, or Z51.12, Encounter for antineoplastic immunotherapy as the first-listed or principal diagnosis. If a patient receives more than one of these therapies during the same admission more than one of these codes may be assigned, in any sequence.

The malignancy for which the therapy is being administered should be assigned as a secondary diagnosis.

If a patient admission/encounter is for the insertion or implantation of radioactive elements (e.g., brachytherapy) the appropriate code for the malignancy is sequenced as the principal or first-listed diagnosis. Code Z51.0 should not be assigned.

3) Patient admitted for radiation therapy, chemotherapy or immunotherapy and develops complications

When a patient is admitted for the purpose of external beam radiotherapy, immunotherapy or chemotherapy and develops complications such as uncontrolled nausea and vomiting or dehydration, the principal or first-listed diagnosis is Z51.0, Encounter for antineoplastic radiation therapy, or Z51.11, Encounter for antineoplastic chemotherapy, or Z51.12, Encounter for antineoplastic immunotherapy followed by any codes for the complications.

When a patient is admitted for the purpose of insertion or implantation of radioactive elements (e.g., brachytherapy) and develops complications such as uncontrolled nausea and vomiting or dehydration, the principal or first-listed diagnosis is the appropriate code for the malignancy followed by any codes for the complications.

f. Admission/encounter to determine extent of malignancy

When the reason for admission/encounter is to determine the extent of the malignancy, or for a procedure such as paracentesis or thoracentesis, the primary malignancy or appropriate metastatic site is designated as the principal or first-listed diagnosis, even though chemotherapy or radiotherapy is administered.

g. Symptoms, signs, and abnormal findings listed in Chapter 18 associated with neoplasms

Symptoms, signs, and ill-defined conditions listed in Chapter 18 characteristic of, or associated with, an existing primary or secondary site malignancy cannot be used to replace the malignancy as principal or first-listed diagnosis, regardless of the number of admissions or encounters for treatment and care of the neoplasm.

See section I.C.21. Factors influencing health status and contact with health services, Encounter for prophylactic organ removal.

h. Admission/encounter for pain control/management

See Section I.C.6. for information on coding admission/encounter for pain control/management.

i. Malignancy in two or more noncontiguous sites

A patient may have more than one malignant tumor in the same organ. These tumors may represent different primaries or metastatic disease, depending on the site. Should the documentation be unclear, the provider should be queried as to the status of each tumor so that the correct codes can be assigned.

j. Disseminated malignant neoplasm, unspecified

Code C80.0, Disseminated malignant neoplasm, unspecified, is for use only in those cases where the patient has advanced metastatic disease and no known primary or secondary sites are specified. It should not be used in place of assigning codes for the primary site and all known secondary sites.

k. Malignant neoplasm without specification of site

Code C80.1, Malignant (primary) neoplasm, unspecified, equates to Cancer, unspecified. This code should only be used when no determination can be made as to the primary site of a malignancy. This code should rarely be used in the inpatient setting.

l. Sequencing of neoplasm codes

1) Encounter for treatment of primary malignancy

If the reason for the encounter is for treatment of a primary malignancy, assign the malignancy as the principal/first-listed diagnosis. The primary site is to be sequenced first, followed by any metastatic sites.

2) Encounter for treatment of secondary malignancy

When an encounter is for a primary malignancy with metastasis and treatment is directed toward the metastatic (secondary) site(s) only, the metastatic site(s) is designated as the principal/first-listed diagnosis. The primary malignancy is coded as an additional code.

3) Malignant neoplasm in a pregnant patient

When a pregnant woman has a malignant neoplasm, a code from subcategory O9A.1-, Malignant neoplasm complicating pregnancy, childbirth, and the puerperium, should be sequenced first, followed by the appropriate code from Chapter 2 to indicate the type of neoplasm.

4) Encounter for complication associated with a neoplasm

When an encounter is for management of a complication associated with a neoplasm, such as dehydration, and the treatment is only for the complication, the complication is coded first, followed by the appropriate code(s) for the neoplasm.

The exception to this guideline is anemia. When the admission/encounter is for management of an anemia associated with the malignancy, and the treatment is only for anemia, the appropriate code for the malignancy is sequenced as the principal or first-listed diagnosis followed by code D63.0, Anemia in neoplastic disease.

5) Complication from surgical procedure for treatment of a neoplasm

When an encounter is for treatment of a complication resulting from a surgical procedure performed for the treatment of the neoplasm, designate the complication as the principal/first-listed diagnosis. See the guideline regarding the coding of a current malignancy versus personal history to determine if the code for the neoplasm should also be assigned.

6) Pathologic fracture due to a neoplasm

When an encounter is for a pathological fracture due to a neoplasm, and the focus of treatment is the fracture, a code from subcategory M84.5, Pathological fracture in neoplastic disease, should be sequenced first, followed by the code for the neoplasm.

If the focus of treatment is the neoplasm with an associated pathological fracture, the neoplasm code should be sequenced first, followed by a code from M84.5 for the pathological fracture.

m. Current malignancy versus personal history of malignancy

When a primary malignancy has been excised but further treatment, such as an additional surgery for the malignancy, radiation therapy or chemotherapy is directed to that site, the primary malignancy code should be used until treatment is completed.

When a primary malignancy has been previously excised or eradicated from its site, there is no further treatment (of the malignancy) directed to that site, and there is no evidence of any existing primary malignancy at that site, a code from category Z85, Personal history of malignant neoplasm, should be used to indicate the former site of the malignancy.

Subcategories Z85.0-Z85.7 should only be assigned for the former site of a primary malignancy, not the site of a secondary malignancy. Codes from subcategory Z85.8-, may be assigned for the former site(s) of either a primary or secondary malignancy included in this subcategory.

See Section I.C.21. Factors influencing health status and contact with health services, History (of)

n. Leukemia, Multiple Myeloma, and Malignant Plasma Cell Neoplasms in remission versus personal history

The categories for leukemia, and category C90, Multiple myeloma and malignant plasma cell neoplasms, have codes indicating whether or not the leukemia has achieved remission. There are also codes Z85.6, Personal history of leukemia, and Z85.79, Personal history of other malignant neoplasms of lymphoid, hematopoietic and related tissues. If the documentation is unclear, as to whether the leukemia has achieved remission, the provider should be queried.

See Section I.C.21. Factors influencing health status and contact with health services, History (of)

o. Aftercare following surgery for neoplasm

See Section I.C.21. Factors influencing health status and contact with health services, Aftercare

p. Follow-up care for completed treatment of a malignancy

See Section I.C.21. Factors influencing health status and contact with health services, Follow-up

q. Prophylactic organ removal for prevention of malignancy

See Section I.C. 21, Factors influencing health status and contact with health services, Prophylactic organ removal

r. Malignant neoplasm associated with transplanted organ

A malignant neoplasm of a transplanted organ should be coded as a transplant complication. Assign first the appropriate code from category T86.-, Complications of transplanted organs and tissue, followed by code C80.2, Malignant neoplasm associated with transplanted organ. Use an additional code for the specific malignancy.

s. Breast Implant Associated Anaplastic Large Cell Lymphoma

Breast implant associated anaplastic large cell lymphoma (BIA-ALCL) is a type of lymphoma that can develop around breast implants. Assign code C84.7A, Anaplastic large cell lymphoma, ALK-negative, breast, for BIA-ALCL. Do not assign a complication code from chapter 19.

3. Chapter 3: Diseases of the Blood and Blood-Forming Organs and Certain Disorders Involving the Immune Mechanism (D50-D89)

Reserved for future guideline expansion

4. Chapter 4: Endocrine, Nutritional and Metabolic Diseases (E00-E89)

a. Diabetes mellitus

The diabetes mellitus codes are combination codes that include the type of diabetes mellitus, the body system affected, and the complications affecting that body system. As many codes within a particular category as are necessary to describe all of the complications of the disease may be used. They should be sequenced based on the reason for a particular encounter. Assign as many codes from categories E08 – E13 as needed to identify all of the associated conditions that the patient has.

1) Type of diabetes

The age of a patient is not the sole determining factor, though most type 1 diabetics develop the condition before reaching puberty. For this reason type 1 diabetes mellitus is also referred to as juvenile diabetes.

2) Type of diabetes mellitus not documented

If the type of diabetes mellitus is not documented in the medical record the default is E11.-, Type 2 diabetes mellitus.

3) Diabetes mellitus and the use of insulin and oral hypoglycemics

If the documentation in a medical record does not indicate the type of diabetes but does indicate that the patient uses insulin, code E11-, Type 2 diabetes mellitus, should be assigned. **Additional** code(s) should be assigned from category Z79 to identify the long-term (current) use of insulin, oral hypoglycemic drugs, **or injectable non-insulin antidiabetic, as follows:**

If the patient is treated with both oral medications and insulin, **both code Z79.4, Long term (current) use of insulin, and code Z79.84, Long term (current) use of oral hypoglycemic drugs,** should be assigned. If the patient is treated with both insulin and an injectable non-insulin antidiabetic drug, assign codes Z79.4, Long-term (current) use of insulin, and Z79.899, Other long term (current) drug therapy. If the patient is treated with both oral hypoglycemic drugs and an injectable non-insulin antidiabetic drug, assign codes Z79.84, Long-term (current) use of oral hypoglycemic drugs, and Z79.899, Other long-term (current) drug therapy. Code Z79.4 should not be assigned if insulin is given temporarily to bring a type 2 patient's blood sugar under control during an encounter.

4) Diabetes mellitus in pregnancy and gestational diabetes

See Section I.C.15. Diabetes mellitus in pregnancy.

See Section I.C.15. Gestational (pregnancy induced) diabetes

5) Complications due to insulin pump malfunction

(a) Underdose of insulin due to insulin pump failure

An underdose of insulin due to an insulin pump failure should be assigned to a code from subcategory T85.6, Mechanical complication of other specified internal and external prosthetic devices, implants and grafts, that specifies the type of pump malfunction, as the principal or first-listed code, followed by code T38.3x6-, Underdosing of insulin and oral hypoglycemic [antidiabetic] drugs. Additional codes for the type of diabetes mellitus and any associated complications due to the underdosing should also be assigned.

(b) Overdose of insulin due to insulin pump failure

The principal or first-listed code for an encounter due to an insulin pump malfunction resulting in an overdose of insulin, should also be T85.6-, Mechanical complication of other specified internal and external prosthetic devices, implants and grafts, followed by code T38.3x1-, Poisoning by insulin and oral hypoglycemic [antidiabetic] drugs, accidental (unintentional).

6) Secondary diabetes mellitus

Codes under categories E08, Diabetes mellitus due to underlying condition, E09, Drug or chemical induced diabetes mellitus, and E13, Other specified diabetes mellitus, identify complications/manifestations associated with secondary diabetes mellitus. Secondary diabetes is always caused by another condition or event (e.g., cystic fibrosis, malignant neoplasm of pancreas, pancreatectomy, adverse effect of drug, or poisoning).

(a) Secondary diabetes mellitus and the use of insulin or *oral* hypoglycemic drugs

For patients with secondary diabetes mellitus who routinely use insulin or oral hypoglycemic drugs, **or injectable non-insulin drugs,** an additional code from category Z79 should be assigned to identify the long-term (current) use of insulin, oral hypoglycemic drugs, **or non-injectable non-insulin drugs as follows:**

If the patient is treated with both oral medications and insulin, **both code Z79.4, Long term (current) use of insulin, and code Z79.84, Long term (current) use of oral hypoglycemic drugs,** should be assigned. If the patient is treated with both insulin and an injectable non-insulin antidiabetic drug, assign codes Z79.4, Long-term (current) use of insulin, and Z79.899, Other long term (current) drug therapy. If the patient is treated with both oral hypoglycemic drugs and an injectable non-insulin antidiabetic drug, assign codes Z79.84, Long-term (current) use of oral hypoglycemic drugs, and Z79.899, Other long-term (current) drug therapy. Code Z79.4 should not be assigned if insulin is given temporarily to bring a secondary diabetic patient's blood sugar under control during an encounter.

(b) Assigning and sequencing secondary diabetes codes and its causes

The sequencing of the secondary diabetes codes in relationship to codes for the cause of the diabetes is based on the Tabular List instructions for categories E08, E09 and E13.

(i) Secondary diabetes mellitus due to pancreatectomy

For postpancreatectomy diabetes mellitus (lack of insulin due to the surgical removal of all or part of the pancreas), assign code E89.1, Postprocedural hypoinsulinemia. Assign a code from category E13 and a code from subcategory Z90.41-, Acquired absence of pancreas, as additional codes.

(ii) Secondary diabetes due to drugs

Secondary diabetes may be caused by an adverse effect of correctly administered medications, poisoning or sequela of poisoning.

See section I.C.19.e for coding of adverse effects and poisoning, and section I.C.20 for external cause code reporting.

5. Chapter 5: Mental, Behavioral and Neurodevelopmental Disorders (F01-F99)

a. Pain disorders related to psychological factors

Assign code F45.41, for pain that is exclusively related to psychological disorders. As indicated by the Excludes 1 note under category G89, a code from category G89 should not be assigned with code F45.41

Code F45.42, Pain disorders with related psychological factors, should be used with a code from category G89, Pain, not elsewhere classified, if there is documentation of a psychological component for a patient with acute or chronic pain.

See Section I.C.6. Pain

b. Mental and behavioral disorders due to psychoactive substance use

1) In Remission

Selection of codes for "in remission" for categories F10-F19, Mental and behavioral disorders due to psychoactive substance use (categories F10-F19 with -.11, -.21) requires the provider's clinical judgment. The appropriate codes for "in remission" are assigned only on the basis of provider documentation (as defined in the Official

Guidelines for Coding and Reporting), unless otherwise instructed by the classification.

Mild substance use disorders in early or sustained remission are classified to the appropriate codes for substance abuse in remission, and moderate or severe substance use disorders in early or sustained remission are classified to the appropriate codes for substance dependence in remission.

2) Psychoactive Substance Use, Abuse And Dependence

When the provider documentation refers to use, abuse and dependence of the same substance (e.g. alcohol, opioid, cannabis, etc.), only one code should be assigned to identify the pattern of use based on the following hierarchy:

- If both use and abuse are documented, assign only the code for abuse
- If both abuse and dependence are documented, assign only the code for dependence
- If use, abuse and dependence are all documented, assign only the code for dependence
- If both use and dependence are documented, assign only the code for dependence.

3) Psychoactive Substance Use Unspecified

As with all other unspecified diagnoses, the codes for unspecified psychoactive substance use disorders (F10.9-, F11.9-, F12.9-, F13.9-, F14.9-, F15.9-, F16.9-, F18.9-, F19.9-) should only be assigned based on provider documentation and when they meet the definition of a reportable diagnosis (see Section III, Reporting Additional Diagnoses). These codes are to be used only when the psychoactive substance use is associated with a **substance related** disorder (chapter 5 **disorders** such as sexual dysfunction, sleep disorder, or a mental or behavioral disorder) **or medical condition**, mental or behavioral disorder, and such a relationship is documented by the provider.

4) Medical Conditions Due to Psychoactive Substance Use, Abuse and Dependence

Medical conditions due to substance use, abuse, and dependence are not classified as substance-induced disorders. Assign the diagnosis code for the medical condition as directed by the Alphabetical Index along with the appropriate psychoactive substance use, abuse or dependence code. For example, for alcoholic pancreatitis due to alcohol dependence, assign the appropriate code from subcategory K85.2, Alcohol induced acute pancreatitis, and the appropriate code from subcategory F10.2, such as code F10.20, Alcohol dependence, uncomplicated. It would not be appropriate to assign code F10.288, Alcohol dependence with other alcohol-induced disorder.

5) Blood Alcohol Level

A code from category Y90, Evidence of alcohol involvement determined by blood alcohol level, may be assigned when this information is documented and the patient's provider has documented a condition classifiable to category F10, Alcohol related disorders. The blood alcohol level does not need to be documented by the patient's provider in order for it to be coded.

c. Factitious Disorder

Factitious disorder imposed on self or Munchausen's syndrome is a disorder in which a person falsely reports or causes his or her own physical or psychological signs or symptoms. For patients with documented factitious disorder on self or Munchausen's syndrome, assign the appropriate code from subcategory F68.1-, Factitious disorder imposed on self.

Munchausen's syndrome by proxy (MSBP) is a disorder in which a caregiver (perpetrator) falsely reports or causes an illness or injury in another person (victim) under his or her care, such as a child, an elderly adult, or a person who has a disability. The conditions is also referred to as "factitious disorder imposed on another" or "factitious disorder by proxy." The perpetrator, not the victim, receives this diagnosis. Assign code F68.A, Factitious disorder imposed on another, to the perpetrator's record. For the victim of a patient suffering from MSBP, assign the appropriate code from categories T74, Adult and child abuse, neglect and other maltreatment, confirmed, or T76, Adult and child abuse, neglect and other maltreatment, suspected.

See Section I.C.19.f. Adult and child abuse, neglect and other maltreatment

6. Chapter 6: Diseases of the Nervous System (G00-G99)

a. Dominant/nondominant side

Codes from category G81, Hemiplegia and hemiparesis, and subcategories, G83.1, Monoplegia of lower limb, G83.2, Monoplegia of upper limb, and G83.3, Monoplegia, unspecified, identify whether the dominant or nondominant side is affected. Should the affected side be documented, but not specified as dominant or nondominant, and the classification system does not indicate a default, code selection is as follows:

- For ambidextrous patients, the default should be dominant.
- If the left side is affected, the default is non-dominant.
- If the right side is affected, the default is dominant.

b. Pain-Category G89

1) General coding information

Codes in category G89, Pain, not elsewhere classified, may be used in conjunction with codes from other categories and chapters to provide more detail about acute or chronic pain and neoplasm-related pain, unless otherwise indicated below.

If the pain is not specified as acute or chronic, post- thoracotomy, post procedural, or neoplasm-related, do not assign codes from category G89.

A code from category G89 should not be assigned if the underlying (definitive) diagnosis is known, unless the reason for the encounter is pain control/management and not management of the underlying condition.

When an admission or encounter is for a procedure aimed at treating the underlying condition (e.g., spinal fusion, kyphoplasty), a code for the underlying condition (e.g., vertebral fracture, spinal stenosis) should be assigned as the principal diagnosis. No code from category G89 should be assigned.

(a) Category G89 Codes as Principal or First-Listed Diagnosis

Category G89 codes are acceptable as principal diagnosis or the first-listed code:

- When pain control or pain management is the reason for the admission/encounter (e.g., a patient with displaced intervertebral disc, nerve impingement and severe back pain presents for injection of steroid into the spinal canal). The underlying cause of the pain should be reported as an additional diagnosis, if known.
- When a patient is admitted for the insertion of a neurostimulator for pain control, assign the appropriate pain code as the principal or first-listed diagnosis. When an admission or encounter is for a procedure aimed at treating the underlying condition and a neurostimulator is inserted for pain control during the same admission/encounter, a code for the underlying condition should be assigned as the principal diagnosis and the appropriate pain code should be assigned as a secondary diagnosis.

(b) Use of Category G89 Codes in Conjunction with Site Specific Pain Codes

(i) Assigning Category G89 and Site-Specific Pain Codes

Codes from category G89 may be used in conjunction with codes that identify the site of pain (including codes from chapter 18) if the category G89 code provides additional information. For example, if the code describes the site of the pain, but does not fully describe whether the pain is acute or chronic, then both codes should be assigned.

(ii) Sequencing of Category G89 Codes with Site- Specific Pain Codes

The sequencing of category G89 codes with site-specific pain codes (including chapter 18 codes), is dependent on the circumstances of the encounter/admission as follows:

- If the encounter is for pain control or pain management, assign the code from category G89 followed by the code identifying the specific site of pain (e.g., encounter for pain management for acute neck pain from trauma is assigned code G89.11, Acute pain due to trauma, followed by code M54.2, Cervicalgia, to identify the site of pain).
- If the encounter is for any other reason except pain control or pain management, and a related definitive diagnosis has not been established (confirmed) by the provider, assign the code for the specific site of pain first, followed by the appropriate code from category G89.

2) Pain due to devices, implants and grafts

See Section I.C.19. Pain due to medical devices

3) Postoperative Pain

The provider's documentation should be used to guide the coding of postoperative pain, as well as *Section III. Reporting Additional Diagnoses and Section IV. Diagnostic Coding* and *Reporting in the Outpatient Setting.*

The default for post-thoracotomy and other postoperative pain not specified as acute or chronic is the code for the acute form.

Routine or expected postoperative pain immediately after surgery should not be coded.

(a) Postoperative pain not associated with specific postoperative complication

Postoperative pain not associated with a specific postoperative complication is assigned to the appropriate postoperative pain code in category G89.

(b) Postoperative pain associated with specific postoperative complication

Postoperative pain associated with a specific postoperative complication (such as painful wire sutures) is assigned to the appropriate code(s) found in Chapter 19, Injury, poisoning, and certain other consequences of external causes. If appropriate, use additional code(s) from category G89 to identify acute or chronic pain (G89.18 or G89.28).

4) **Chronic pain**

Chronic pain is classified to subcategory G89.2. There is no time frame defining when pain becomes chronic pain. The provider's documentation should be used to guide use of these codes.

5) **Neoplasm Related Pain**

Code G89.3 is assigned to pain documented as being related, associated or due to cancer, primary or secondary malignancy, or tumor. This code is assigned regardless of whether the pain is acute or chronic.

This code may be assigned as the principal or first- listed code when the stated reason for the admission/encounter is documented as pain control/pain management. The underlying neoplasm should be reported as an additional diagnosis.

When the reason for the admission/encounter is management of the neoplasm and the pain associated with the neoplasm is also documented, code G89.3 may be assigned as an additional diagnosis. It is not necessary to assign an additional code for the site of the pain.

See Section I.C.2 for instructions on the sequencing of neoplasms for all other stated reasons for the admission/encounter (except for pain control/pain management).

6) **Chronic pain syndrome**

Central pain syndrome (G89.0) and chronic pain syndrome (G89.4) are different than the term "chronic pain," and therefore codes should only be used when the provider has specifically documented this condition.

See Section I.C.5. Pain disorders related to psychological factors

7. Chapter 7: Diseases of the Eye and Adnexa (H00-H59)

a. Glaucoma

1) **Assigning Glaucoma Codes**

Assign as many codes from category H40, Glaucoma, as needed to identify the type of glaucoma, the affected eye, and the glaucoma stage.

2) **Bilateral glaucoma with same type and stage**

When a patient has bilateral glaucoma and both eyes are documented as being the same type and stage, and there is a code for bilateral glaucoma, report only the code for the type of glaucoma, bilateral, with the seventh character for the stage.

When a patient has bilateral glaucoma and both eyes are documented as being the same type and stage, and the classification does not provide a code for bilateral glaucoma (i.e. subcategories H40.10, H40.11 and H40.20) report only one code for the type of glaucoma with the appropriate seventh character for the stage.

3) **Bilateral glaucoma stage with different types or stages**

When a patient has bilateral glaucoma and each eye is documented as having a different type or stage, and the classification distinguishes laterality, assign the appropriatecode for each eye rather than the code for bilateral glaucoma.

When a patient has bilateral glaucoma and each eye is documented as having a different type, and the classification does not distinguish laterality (i.e. subcategories H40.10, H40.11 and H40.20), assign one code for each type of glaucoma with the appropriate seventh character for the stage.

When a patient has bilateral glaucoma and each eye is documented as having the same type, but different stage, and the classification does not distinguish laterality (i.e. subcategories H40.10, H40.11 and H40.20), assign a code for the type of glaucoma for each eye with the seventh character for the specific glaucoma stage documented for each eye.

4) **Patient admitted with glaucoma and stage evolves during the admission**

If a patient is admitted with glaucoma and the stage progresses during the admission, assign the code for highest stage documented.

5) **Indeterminate stage glaucoma**

Assignment of the seventh character "4" for "indeterminate stage" should be based on the clinical documentation. The seventh character "4" is used for glaucomas whose stage cannot be clinically determined. This seventh character should not be confused with the seventh character "0", unspecified, which should be assigned when there is no documentation regarding the stage of the glaucoma.

b. Blindness

If "blindness" or "low vision" of both eyes is documented but the visual impairment category is not documented, assign code H54.3, Unqualified visual loss, both eyes. If "blindness" or "low vision" in one eye is documented but the visual impairment category is not documented, assign a code from H54.6-, Unqualified visual loss, one eye. If "blindness" or "visual loss" is documented without any information about whether one or both eyes are affected, assign code H54.7, Unspecified visual loss.

8. Chapter 8: Diseases of the Ear and Mastoid Process (H60-H95)

Reserved for future guideline expansion

9. Chapter 9: Diseases of the Circulatory System (I00-I99)

a. Hypertension

The classification presumes a causal relationship between hypertension and heart involvement and between hypertension and kidney involvement, as the two conditions are linked by the term "with" in the Alphabetic Index. These conditions should be coded as related even in the absence of provider documentation explicitly linking them, unless the documentation clearly states the conditions are unrelated.

For hypertension and conditions not specifically linked by relational terms such as "with," "associated with" or "due to" in the classification, provider documentation must link the conditions in order to code them as related.

1) Hypertension with Heart Disease

Hypertension with heart conditions classified to I50.- or I51.4-I51.7, I51.89, I51.9, are assigned to, a code from category I11, Hypertensive heart disease. Use an additional code(s) from category I50, Heart failure, to identify the type(s) of heart failure in those patients with heart failure.

The same heart conditions (I50.-, I51.4-I51.7, I51.89, I51.9) with hypertension are coded separately if the provider has documented they are unrelated to the hypertension. Sequence according to the circumstances of the admission/ encounter.

2) Hypertensive Chronic Kidney Disease

Assign codes from category I12, Hypertensive chronic kidney disease, when both hypertension and a condition classifiable to category N18, Chronic kidney disease (CKD), are present. CKD should not be coded as hypertensive if the provider indicates the CKD is not related to the hypertension.

The appropriate code from category N18 should be used as a secondary code with a code from category I12 to identify the stage of chronic kidney disease.

See Section I.C.14. Chronic kidney disease.

If a patient has hypertensive chronic kidney disease and acute renal failure, the acute renal failure should also be coded. Sequence according to the circumstances of the admission/encounter.

3) Hypertensive Heart and Chronic Kidney Disease

Assign codes from combination category I13, Hypertensive heart and chronic kidney disease, when there is hypertension with both heart and kidney involvement. If heart failure is present, assign an additional code from category I50 to identify the type of heart failure.

The appropriate code from category N18, Chronic kidney disease, should be used as a secondary code with a code from category I13 to identify the stage of chronic kidney disease.

See Section I.C.14. Chronic kidney disease.

The codes in category I13, Hypertensive heart and chronic kidney disease, are combination codes that include hypertension, heart disease and chronic kidney disease. The Includes note at I13 specifies that the conditions included at I11 and I12 are included together in I13. If a patient has hypertension, heart disease and chronic kidney disease then a code from I13 should be used, not individual codes for hypertension, heart disease and chronic kidney disease, or codes from I11 or I12.

For patients with both acute renal failure and chronic kidney disease the acute renal failure should also be coded. Sequence according to the circumstances of the admission/encounter.

4) Hypertensive Cerebrovascular Disease

For hypertensive cerebrovascular disease, first assign the appropriate code from categories I60-I69, followed by the appropriate hypertension code.

5) Hypertensive Retinopathy

Subcategory H35.0, Background retinopathy and retinal vascular changes, should be used with a code from category I10 – I15, Hypertensive disease to include the systemic hypertension. The sequencing is based on the reason for the encounter.

6) Hypertension, Secondary

Secondary hypertension is due to an underlying condition. Two codes are required: one to identify the underlying etiology and one from category I15 to identify the hypertension. Sequencing of codes is determined by the reason for admission/encounter.

7) **Hypertension, Transient**

Assign code R03.0, Elevated blood pressure reading without diagnosis of hypertension, unless patient has an established diagnosis of hypertension. Assign code O13.-, Gestational [pregnancy-induced] hypertension without significant proteinuria, or O14.-, Pre-eclampsia, for transient hypertension of pregnancy.

8) **Hypertension, Controlled**

This diagnostic statement usually refers to an existing state of hypertension under control by therapy. Assign the appropriate code from categories I10-I15, Hypertensive diseases.

9) **Hypertension, Uncontrolled**

Uncontrolled hypertension may refer to untreated hypertension or hypertension not responding to current therapeutic regimen. In either case, assign the appropriate code from categories I10-I15, Hypertensive diseases.

10) **Hypertensive Crisis**

Assign a code from category I16, Hypertensive crisis, for documented hypertensive urgency, hypertensive emergency or unspecified hypertensive crisis. Code also any identified hypertensive disease (I10-I15). The sequencing is based on the reason for the encounter.

11) **Pulmonary Hypertension**

Pulmonary hypertension is classified to category I27, Other pulmonary heart diseases. For secondary pulmonary hypertension (I27.1, I27.2-), code also any associated conditions or adverse effects of drugs or toxins. The sequencing is based on the reason for the encounter, except for adverse effects of drugs (See Section I.C.19.e).

b. Atherosclerotic Coronary Artery Disease and Angina

ICD-10-CM has combination codes for atherosclerotic heart disease with angina pectoris. The subcategories for these codes are I25.11, Atherosclerotic heart disease of native coronary artery with angina pectoris and I25.7, Atherosclerosis of coronary artery bypass graft(s) and coronary artery of transplanted heart with angina pectoris.

When using one of these combination codes it is not necessary to use an additional code for angina pectoris. A causal relationship can be assumed in a patient with both atherosclerosis and angina pectoris, unless the documentation indicates the angina is due to something other than the atherosclerosis.

If a patient with coronary artery disease is admitted due to an acute myocardial infarction (AMI), the AMI should be sequenced before the coronary artery disease.

See Section I.C.9. Acute myocardial infarction (AMI)

c. Intraoperative and Postprocedural Cerebrovascular Accident

Medical record documentation should clearly specify the cause- and-effect relationship between the medical intervention and the cerebrovascular accident in order to assign a code for intraoperative or postprocedural cerebrovascular accident.

Proper code assignment depends on whether it was an infarction or hemorrhage and whether it occurred intraoperatively or postoperatively. If it was a cerebral hemorrhage, code assignment depends on the type of procedure performed.

d. Sequelae of Cerebrovascular Disease

1) **Category I69, Sequelae of Cerebrovascular disease**

Category I69 is used to indicate conditions classifiable to categories I60-I67 as the causes of sequela (neurologic deficits), themselves classified elsewhere. These "late effects" include neurologic deficits that persist after initial onset of conditions classifiable to categories I60-I67. The neurologic deficits caused by cerebrovascular disease may be present from the onset or may arise at any time after the onset of the condition classifiable to categories I60-I67.

Codes from category I69, Sequelae of cerebrovascular disease, that specify hemiplegia, hemiparesis and monoplegia identify whether the dominant or nondominant side is affected. Should the affected side be documented, but not specified as dominant or nondominant, and the classification system does not indicate a default, code selection is as follows:

- For ambidextrous patients, the default should be dominant.
- If the left side is affected, the default is non-dominant.
- If the right side is affected, the default is dominant.

2) **Codes from category I69 with codes from I60-I67**

Codes from category I69 may be assigned on a health care record with codes from I60-I67, if the patient has a current cerebrovascular disease and deficits from an old cerebrovascular disease.

3) Codes from category I69 and Personal history of transient ischemic attack (TIA) and cerebral infarction (Z86.73)

Codes from category I69 should not be assigned if the patient does not have neurologic deficits.

See Section I.C.21. 4. History (of) for use of personal history codes

e. Acute myocardial infarction (AMI)

1) ST elevation myocardial infarction (STEMI) and non ST elevation myocardial infarction (NSTEMI)

The ICD-10-CM codes for type 1 acute myocardial infarction (AMI) identify the site, such as anterolateral wall or true posterior wall. Subcategories I21.0-I21.2 and code I21.3 are used for type 1 ST elevation myocardial infarction (STEMI). Code I21.4, Non-ST elevation (NSTEMI) myocardial infarction, is used for type 1 non ST elevation myocardial infarction (NSTEMI) and nontransmural MIs.

If a type 1 NSTEMI evolves to STEMI, assign the STEMI code. If a type 1 STEMI converts to NSTEMI due to thrombolytic therapy, it is still coded as STEMI.

For encounters occurring while the myocardial infarction is equal to, or less than, four weeks old, including transfers to another acute setting or a postacute setting, and the myocardial infarction meets the definition for "other diagnoses" (see Section III, Reporting Additional Diagnoses), codes from category I21 may continue to be reported. For encounters after the 4 week time frame and the patient is still receiving care related to the myocardial infarction, the appropriate aftercare code should be assigned, rather than a code from category I21. For old or healed myocardial infarctions not requiring further care, code I25.2, Old myocardial infarction, may be assigned.

2) Acute myocardial infarction, unspecified

Code I21.9, Acute myocardial infarction, unspecified, is the default for unspecified acute myocardial infarction or unspecified type. If only type 1 STEMI or transmural MI without the site is documented, assign code I21.3, ST elevation (STEMI) myocardial infarction of unspecified site.

3) AMI documented as nontransmural or subendocardial but site provided

If an AMI is documented as nontransmural or subendocardial, but the site is provided, it is still coded as a subendocardial AMI.

See Section I.C.21.3 for information on coding status post administration of tPA in a different facility within the last 24 hours.

4) Subsequent acute myocardial infarction

A code from category I22, Subsequent ST elevation (STEMI) and non-ST elevation (NSTEMI) myocardial infarction, is to be used when a patient who has suffered a type 1 or unspecified AMI has a new AMI within the 4 week time frame of the initial AMI. A code from category I22 must be used in conjunction with a code from category I21. The sequencing of the I22 and I21 codes depends on the circumstances of the encounter.

Do not assign code I22 for subsequent myocardial infarctions other than type 1 or unspecified. For subsequent type 2 AMI assign only code I21.A1. For subsequent type 4 or type 5 AMI, assign only code I21.A9.

If a subsequent myocardial infarction of one type occurs within 4 weeks of a myocardial infarction of a different type, assign the appropriate codes from category I21 to identify each type. Do not assign a code from I22. Codes from category I22 should only be assigned if both the initial and subsequent myocardial infarctions are type 1 or unspecified.

5) Other Types of Myocardial Infarction

The ICD-10-CM provides codes for different types of myocardial infarction. Type 1 myocardial infarctions are assigned to codes I21.0-I21.4.

Type 2 myocardial infarction (myocardial infarction due to demand ischemia or secondary to ischemic imbalance) is assigned to code I21.A1, Myocardial infarction type 2 with the underlying cause coded first. Do not assign code I24.8, Other forms of acute ischemic heart disease, for the demand ischemia. If a type 2 AMI is described as NSTEMI or STEMI, only assign code I21.A1. Codes I21.0-I21.4 should only be assigned for type 1 AMIs.

Acute myocardial infarctions type 3, 4a, 4b, 4c and 5 are assigned to code I21.A9, Other myocardial infarction type.

The "Code also" and "Code first" notes should be followed related to complications, and for coding of postprocedural myocardial infarctions during or following cardiac surgery.

10. Chapter 10: Diseases of the Respiratory System (J00-J99), U07.0

a. Chronic Obstructive Pulmonary Disease [COPD] and Asthma

1) Acute exacerbation of chronic obstructive bronchitis and asthma

The codes in categories J44 and J45 distinguish between uncomplicated cases and those in acute exacerbation. An acute exacerbation is a worsening or a decompensation of a chronic condition. An acute exacerbation is not equivalent to an infection superimposed on a chronic condition, though an exacerbation may be triggered by an infection.

b. Acute Respiratory Failure

1) Acute respiratory failure as principal diagnosis

A code from subcategory J96.0, Acute respiratory failure, or subcategory J96.2, Acute and chronic respiratory failure, may be assigned as a principal diagnosis when it is the condition established after study to be chiefly responsible for occasioning the admission to the hospital, and the selection is supported by the Alphabetic Index and Tabular List. However, chapter- specific coding guidelines (such as obstetrics, poisoning, HIV, newborn) that provide sequencing direction take precedence.

2) Acute respiratory failure as secondary diagnosis

Respiratory failure may be listed as a secondary diagnosis if it occurs after admission, or if it is present on admission, but does not meet the definition of principal diagnosis.

3) Sequencing of acute respiratory failure and another acute condition

When a patient is admitted with respiratory failure and another acute condition, (e.g., myocardial infarction, cerebrovascular accident, aspiration pneumonia), the principal diagnosis will not be the same in every situation. This applies whether the other acute condition is a respiratory or nonrespiratory condition. Selection of the principal diagnosis will be dependent on the circumstances of admission. If both the respiratory failure and the other acute condition are equally responsible for occasioning the admission to the hospital, and there are no chapter-specific sequencing rules, the guideline regarding two or more diagnoses that equally meet the definition for principal diagnosis *(Section II, C.)* may be applied in these situations.

If the documentation is not clear as to whether acute respiratory failure and another condition are equally responsible for occasioning the admission, query the provider for clarification.

c. Influenza due to certain identified influenza viruses

Code only confirmed cases of influenza due to certain identified influenza viruses (category J09), and due to other identified influenza virus (category J10). This is an exception to the hospital inpatient guideline Section II, H. (Uncertain Diagnosis).

In this context, "confirmation" does not require documentation of positive laboratory testing specific for avian or other novel influenza A or other identified influenza virus. However, coding should be based on the provider's diagnostic statement that the patient has avian influenza, or other novel influenza A, for category J09, or has another particular identified strain of influenza, such as H1N1 or H3N2, but not identified as novel or variant, for category J10.

If the provider records "suspected" or "possible" or "probable" avian influenza, or novel influenza, or other identified influenza, then the appropriate influenza code from category J11, Influenza due to unidentified influenza virus, should be assigned. A code from category J09, Influenza due to certain identified influenza viruses, should not be assigned nor should a code from category J10, Influenza due to other identified influenza virus.

d. Ventilator associated Pneumonia

1) Documentation of Ventilator associated Pneumonia

As with all procedural or postprocedural complications, code assignment is based on the provider's documentation of the relationship between the condition and the procedure.

Code J95.851, Ventilator associated pneumonia, should be assigned only when the provider has documented ventilator associated pneumonia (VAP). An additional code to identify the organism (e.g., Pseudomonas aeruginosa, code B96.5) should also be assigned. Do not assign an additional code from categories J12-J18 to identify the type of pneumonia.

Code J95.851 should not be assigned for cases where the patient has pneumonia and is on a mechanical ventilator and the provider has not specifically stated that the pneumonia is ventilator-associated pneumonia. If the documentation is unclear as to whether the patient has a pneumonia that is a complication attributable to the mechanical ventilator, query the provider.

2) Ventilator associated Pneumonia Develops after Admission

A patient may be admitted with one type of pneumonia (e.g., code J13, Pneumonia due to Streptococcus pneumonia) and subsequently develop VAP. In this instance, the principal diagnosis would be the appropriate code from categories J12- J18 for the pneumonia diagnosed at the time of admission. Code J95.851, Ventilator associated pneumonia, would be assigned as an additional diagnosis when the provider has also documented the presence of ventilator associated pneumonia.

e. Vaping-related disorders

For patients presenting with condition(s) related to vaping, assign code U07.0, Vaping-related disorder, as the principal diagnosis. For lung injury due to vaping, assign only code U07.0. Assign additional codes for other manifestations, such as acute respiratory failure (subcategory J96.0-) or pneumonitis (code J68.0).

Associated respiratory signs and symptoms due to vaping, such as cough, shortness of breath, etc., are not coded separately, when a definitive diagnosis has been established. However, it would be appropriate to code separately any gastrointestinal symptoms, such as diarrhea and abdominal pain.

See Section I.C.1.g.1.c.i. for Pneumonia confirmed as due to COVID-19

11. Chapter 11: Diseases of the Digestive System (K00-K95)

Reserved for future guideline expansion

12. Chapter 12: Diseases of the Skin and Subcutaneous Tissue (L00-L99)

a. Pressure ulcer stage codes

1) Pressure ulcer stages

Codes in category L89, Pressure ulcer, identify the site and stage of the pressure ulcer.

The ICD-10-CM classifies pressure ulcer stages based on severity, which is designated by stages 1-4, deep tissue pressure injury, unspecified stage and unstageable.

Assign as many codes from category L89 as needed to identify all the pressure ulcers the patient has, if applicable.

See Section I.B.14 for pressure ulcer stage documentation by clinicians other than patient's provider.

2) Unstageable pressure ulcers

Assignment of the code for unstageable pressure ulcer (L89.--0) should be based on the clinical documentation. These codes are used for pressure ulcers whose stage cannot be clinically determined (e.g., the ulcer is covered by eschar or has been treated with a skin or muscle graft) and pressure ulcers that are documented as deep tissue injury but not documented as due to trauma. This code should not be confused with the codes for unspecified stage (L89.--9). When there is no documentation regarding the stage of the pressure ulcer, assign the appropriate code for unspecified stage (L89.--9).

If during an encounter, the stage of an unstageable pressure ulcer is revealed after debridement, assign only the code for the stage revealed following debridement.

3) Documented pressure ulcer stage

Assignment of the pressure ulcer stage code should be guided by clinical documentation of the stage or documentation of the terms found in the Alphabetic Index. For clinical terms describing the stage that are not found in the Alphabetic Index, and there is no documentation of the stage, the provider should be queried.

4) Patients admitted with pressure ulcers documented as healed

No code is assigned if the documentation states that the pressure ulcer is completely healed at the time of admission.

5) Patients admitted with pressure ulcers documented as healing

Pressure ulcers described as healing should be assigned the appropriate pressure ulcer stage code based on the documentation in the medical record. If the documentation does not provide information about the stage of the healing pressure ulcer, assign the appropriate code for unspecified stage.

If the documentation is unclear as to whether the patient has a current (new) pressure ulcer or if the patient is being treated for a healing pressure ulcer, query the provider.

For ulcers that were present on admission but healed at the time of discharge, assign the code for the site and stage of the pressure ulcer at the time of admission.

6) Patient admitted with pressure ulcer evolving into another stage during the admission

If a patient is admitted to an inpatient hospital with a pressure ulcer at one stage and it progresses to a higher stage, two separate codes should be assigned: one code for the site and stage of the ulcer on admission and a second code for the same ulcer site and the highest stage reported during the stay.

7) Pressure-induced deep tissue damage

For pressure-induced deep tissue damage or deep tissue pressure injury, assign only the appropriate code for pressure-induced deep tissue damage (L89.--6).

b. Non-Pressure Chronic Ulcers

1) Patients admitted with non-pressure ulcers documented as healed

No code is assigned if the documentation states that the non-pressure ulcer is completely healed at the time of admission.

2) Patients admitted with non-pressure ulcers documented as healing

Non-pressure ulcers described as healing should be assigned the appropriate non-pressure ulcer code based on the documentation in the medical record. If the documentation does not provide information about the severity of the healing non-pressure ulcer, assign the appropriate code unspecified severity.

If the documentation is unclear as to whether the patient has a current (new) non-pressure ulcer or if the patient is being treated for a healing non-pressure ulcer, query the provider.

For ulcers that were present on admission but healed at the time of discharge, assign the code for the site and severity of the non-pressure ulcer at the time of admission.

3) Patient admitted with non-pressure ulcer that progresses to another severity level during the admission

If a patient is admitted to an inpatient hospital with a non-pressure ulcer at one severity level and it progresses to a higher severity level, two separate codes should be assigned; one code for the site and severity level of the ulcer on admission and a second code for the same ulcer site and the highest severity level reported during the stay.

See Section I.B.14 for pressure ulcer stage documentation by clinicians other than patient's provider.

13. Chapter 13: Diseases of the Musculoskeletal System and Connective Tissue (M00-M99)

a. Site and laterality

Most of the codes within Chapter 13 have site and laterality designations. The site represents the bone, joint or the muscle involved. For some conditions where more than one bone, joint or muscle is usually involved, such as osteoarthritis, there is a "multiple sites" code available. For categories where no multiple site code is provided and more than one bone, joint or muscle is involved, multiple codes should be used to indicate the different sites involved.

1) Bone versus joint

For certain conditions, the bone may be affected at the upper or lower end, (e.g., avascular necrosis of bone, M87, Osteoporosis, M80, M81). Though the portion of the bone affected may be at the joint, the site designation will be the bone, not the joint.

b. Acute traumatic versus chronic or recurrent musculoskeletal conditions

Many musculoskeletal conditions are a result of previous injury or trauma to a site, or are recurrent conditions. Bone, joint or muscle conditions that are the result of a healed injury are usually found in chapter 13. Recurrent bone, joint or muscle conditions are also usually found in chapter 13. Any current, acute injury should be coded to the appropriate injury code from chapter 19. Chronic or recurrent conditions should generally be coded with a code from chapter 13. If it is difficult to determine from the documentation in the record which code is best to describe a condition, query the provider.

c. Coding of Pathologic Fractures

7th character A is for use as long as the patient is receiving active treatment for the fracture. While the patient may be seen by a new or different provider over the course of treatment for a pathological fracture, assignment of the 7th character is based on whether the patient is undergoing active treatment and not whether the provider is seeing the patient for the first time.

7th character, D is to be used for encounters after the patient has completed active treatment for the fracture and is receiving routine care for the fracture during the healing or recovery phase. The other 7th characters, listed under each subcategory in the Tabular List, are to be used for subsequent encounters for routine care of fractures during the healing and recovery phase as well as treatment of problems associated with the healing, such as malunions, nonunions, and sequelae.

Care for complications of surgical treatment for fracture repairs during the healing or recovery phase should be coded with the appropriate complication codes.

See Section I.C.19. Coding of traumatic fractures.

d. Osteoporosis

Osteoporosis is a systemic condition, meaning that all bones of the musculoskeletal system are affected. Therefore, site is not a component of the codes under category M81, Osteoporosis without current pathological fracture. The site codes under category M80, Osteoporosis with current pathological fracture, identify the site of the fracture, not the osteoporosis.

1) Osteoporosis without pathological fracture

Category M81, Osteoporosis without current pathological fracture, is for use for patients with osteoporosis who do not currently have a pathologic fracture due to the osteoporosis, even if they have had a fracture in the past. For patients with a history of osteoporosis fractures, status code Z87.310, Personal history of (healed) osteoporosis fracture, should follow the code from M81.

2) Osteoporosis with current pathological fracture

Category M80, Osteoporosis with current pathological fracture, is for patients who have a current pathologic fracture at the time of an encounter. The codes under M80 identify the site of the fracture. A code from category

M80, not a traumatic fracture code, should be used for any patient with known osteoporosis who suffers a fracture, even if the patient had a minor fall or trauma, if that fall or trauma would not usually break a normal, healthy bone.

e. Multisystem Inflammatory Syndrome

See Section I.C.1.g.1.l for Multisystem Inflammatory Syndrome

14. Chapter 14: Diseases of the Genitourinary System (N00-N99)

a. Chronic kidney disease

1) Stages of chronic kidney disease (CKD)

The ICD-10-CM classifies CKD based on severity. The severity of CKD is designated by stages 1-5. Stage 2, code N18.2, equates to mild CKD; stage 3, code N18.3, equates to moderate CKD; and stage 4, code N18.4, equates to severe CKD. Code N18.6, End stage renal disease (ESRD), is assigned when the provider has documented end-stage-renal disease (ESRD).

If both a stage of CKD and ESRD are documented, assign code N18.6 only.

2) Chronic kidney disease and kidney transplant status

Patients who have undergone kidney transplant may still have some form of chronic kidney disease (CKD) because the kidney transplant may not fully restore kidney function. Therefore, the presence of CKD alone does not constitute a transplant complication. Assign the appropriate N18 code for the patient's stage of CKD and code Z94.0, Kidney transplant status. If a transplant complication such as failure or rejection or other transplant complication is documented, see section I.C.19.g for information on coding complications of a kidney transplant. If the documentation is unclear as to whether the patient has a complication of the transplant, query the provider.

3) Chronic kidney disease with other conditions

Patients with CKD may also suffer from other serious conditions, most commonly diabetes mellitus and hypertension. The sequencing of the CKD code in relationship to codes for other contributing conditions is based on the conventions in the Tabular List.

See I.C.9. Hypertensive chronic kidney disease.

See I.C.19. Chronic kidney disease and kidney transplant complications.

15. Chapter 15: Pregnancy, Childbirth and the Puerperium (O00-O9A)

a. General Rules for Obstetric Cases

1) Codes from chapter 15 and sequencing priority

Obstetric cases require codes from chapter 15, codes in the range O00-O9A, Pregnancy, Childbirth, and the Puerperium. Chapter 15 codes have sequencing priority over codes from other chapters. Additional codes from other chapters may be used in conjunction with chapter 15 codes to further specify conditions. Should the provider document that the pregnancy is incidental to the encounter, then code Z33.1, Pregnant state, incidental, should be used in place of any chapter 15 codes. It is the provider's responsibility to state that the condition being treated is not affecting the pregnancy.

2) Chapter 15 codes used only on the maternal record

Chapter 15 codes are to be used only on the maternal record, never on the record of the newborn.

3) Final character for trimester

The majority of codes in Chapter 15 have a final character indicating the trimester of pregnancy. The timeframes for the trimesters are indicated at the beginning of the chapter. If trimester is not a component of a code it is because the condition always occurs in a specific trimester, or the concept of trimester of pregnancy is not applicable. Certain codes have characters for only certain trimesters because the condition does not occur in all trimesters, but it may occur in more than just one.

Assignment of the final character for trimester should be based on the provider's documentation of the trimester (or number of weeks) for the current admission/encounter. This applies to the assignment of trimester for pre-existing conditions as well as those that develop during or are due to the pregnancy. The provider's documentation of the number of weeks may be used to assign the appropriate code identifying the trimester.

Whenever delivery occurs during the current admission, and there is an "in childbirth" option for the obstetric complication being coded, the "in childbirth" code should be assigned. **When the classification does not provide an obstetric code with an "in childbirth" option, it is appropriate to assign a code describing the current trimester.**

4) Selection of trimester for inpatient admissions that encompass more than one trimester

In instances when a patient is admitted to a hospital for complications of pregnancy during one trimester and remains in the hospital into a subsequent trimester, the trimester character for the antepartum complication code should be assigned on the basis of the trimester when the complication developed, not the trimester of the discharge. If the condition developed prior to the current admission/encounter or represents a pre-existing condition, the trimester character for the trimester at the time of the admission/encounter should be assigned.

5) Unspecified trimester

Each category that includes codes for trimester has a code for "unspecified trimester." The "unspecified trimester" code should rarely be used, such as when the documentation in the record is insufficient to determine the trimester and it is not possible to obtain clarification.

6) 7th character for Fetus Identification

Where applicable, a 7th character is to be assigned for certain categories (O31, O32, O33.3 - O33.6, O35, O36, O40, O41, O60.1, O60.2, O64, and O69) to identify the fetus for which the complication code applies.

Assign 7th character "0":

- For single gestations
- When the documentation in the record is insufficient to determine the fetus affected and it is not possible to obtain clarification.
- When it is not possible to clinically determine which fetus is affected.

b. Selection of OB Principal or First-listed Diagnosis

1) Routine outpatient prenatal visits

For routine outpatient prenatal visits when no complications are present, a code from category Z34, Encounter for supervision of normal pregnancy, should be used as the first-listed diagnosis. These codes should not be used in conjunction with chapter 15 codes.

2) Supervision of High-Risk Pregnancy

Codes from category O09, Supervision of high-risk pregnancy, are intended for use only during the prenatal period. For complications during the labor or delivery episode as a result of a high-risk pregnancy, assign the applicable complication codes from Chapter 15. If there are no complications during the labor or delivery episode, assign code O80, Encounter for full-term uncomplicated delivery.

For routine prenatal outpatient visits for patients with high-risk pregnancies, a code from category O09, Supervision of high-risk pregnancy, should be used as the first-listed diagnosis. Secondary chapter 15 codes may be used in conjunction with these codes if appropriate.

3) Episodes when no delivery occurs

In episodes when no delivery occurs, the principal diagnosis should correspond to the principal complication of the pregnancy which necessitated the encounter. Should more than one complication exist, all of which are treated or monitored, any of the complications codes may be sequenced first.

4) When a delivery occurs

When an obstetric patient is admitted and delivers during that admission, the condition that prompted the admission should be sequenced as the principal diagnosis. If multiple conditions prompted the admission, sequence the one most related to the delivery as the principal diagnosis. A code for any complication of the delivery should be assigned as an additional diagnosis. In cases of cesarean delivery, if the patient was admitted with a condition that resulted in the performance of a cesarean procedure, that condition should be selected as the principal diagnosis. If the reason for the admission was unrelated to the condition resulting in the cesarean delivery, the condition related to the reason for the admission should be selected as the principal diagnosis.

5) Outcome of delivery

A code from category Z37, Outcome of delivery, should be included on every maternal record when a delivery has occurred. These codes are not to be used on subsequent records or on the newborn record.

c. Pre-existing conditions versus conditions due to the pregnancy

Certain categories in Chapter 15 distinguish between conditions of the mother that existed prior to pregnancy (pre-existing) and those that are a direct result of pregnancy. When assigning codes from Chapter 15, it is important to assess if a condition was pre-existing prior to pregnancy or developed during or due to the pregnancy in order to assign the correct code.

Categories that do not distinguish between pre-existing and pregnancy- related conditions may be used for either. It is acceptable to use codes specifically for the puerperium with codes complicating pregnancy and childbirth if a condition arises postpartum during the delivery encounter.

d. Pre-existing hypertension in pregnancy

Category O10, Pre-existing hypertension complicating pregnancy, childbirth and the puerperium, includes codes for hypertensive heart and hypertensive chronic kidney disease. When assigning one of the O10 codes that includes hypertensive heart disease or hypertensive chronic kidney disease, it is necessary to add a secondary code from the appropriate hypertension category to specify the type of heart failure or chronic kidney disease.

See Section I.C.9. Hypertension.

e. Fetal Conditions Affecting the Management of the Mother

1) Codes from categories O35 and O36

Codes from categories O35, Maternal care for known or suspected fetal abnormality and damage, and O36, Maternal care for other fetal problems, are assigned only when the fetal condition is actually responsible for modifying the management of the mother, i.e., by requiring diagnostic studies, additional observation, special care, or termination of pregnancy. The fact that the fetal condition exists does not justify assigning a code from this series to the mother's record.

2) In utero surgery

In cases when surgery is performed on the fetus, a diagnosis code from category O35, Maternal care for known or suspected fetal abnormality and damage, should be assigned identifying the fetal condition. Assign the appropriate procedure code for the procedure performed.

No code from Chapter 16, the perinatal codes, should be used on the mother's record to identify fetal conditions. Surgery performed in utero on a fetus is still to be coded as an obstetric encounter.

f. HIV Infection in Pregnancy, Childbirth and the Puerperium

During pregnancy, childbirth or the puerperium, a patient admitted because of an HIV-related illness should receive a principal diagnosis from subcategory O98.7-, Human immunodeficiency [HIV] disease complicating pregnancy, childbirth and the puerperium, followed by the code(s) for the HIV-related illness(es).

Patients with asymptomatic HIV infection status admitted during pregnancy, childbirth, or the puerperium should receive codes of O98.7- and Z21, Asymptomatic human immunodeficiency virus [HIV] infection status.

g. Diabetes mellitus in pregnancy

Diabetes mellitus is a significant complicating factor in pregnancy. Pregnant women who are diabetic should be assigned a code from category O24, Diabetes mellitus in pregnancy, childbirth, and the puerperium, first, followed by the appropriate diabetes code(s) (E08- E13) from Chapter 4.

h. Long term use of insulin and oral hypoglycemics

See section I.C.4.a.3 for information on the long term use of insulin and oral hypoglycemic.

i. Gestational (pregnancy induced) diabetes

Gestational (pregnancy induced) diabetes can occur during the second and third trimester of pregnancy in **patients** who were not diabetic prior to pregnancy. Gestational diabetes can cause complications in the pregnancy similar to those of pre-existing diabetes mellitus. It also puts the **patient** at greater risk of developing diabetes after the pregnancy. Codes for gestational diabetes are in subcategory O24.4, Gestational diabetes mellitus. No other code from category O24, Diabetes mellitus in pregnancy, childbirth, and the puerperium, should be used with a code from O24.4

The codes under subcategory O24.4 include diet controlled, insulin controlled, and controlled by oral hypoglycemic drugs. If a patient with gestational diabetes is treated with both diet and insulin, only the code for insulin-controlled is required. If a patient with gestational diabetes is treated with both diet and oral hypoglycemic medications, only the code for "controlled by oral hypoglycemic drugs" is required. Code Z79.4, Long-term (current) use of insulin or code Z79.84, Long-term (current) use of oral hypoglycemic drugs, should not be assigned with codes from subcategory O24.4.

An abnormal glucose tolerance in pregnancy is assigned a code from subcategory O99.81, Abnormal glucose complicating pregnancy, childbirth, and the puerperium.

j. Sepsis and septic shock complicating abortion, pregnancy, childbirth and the puerperium

When assigning a chapter 15 code for sepsis complicating abortion, pregnancy, childbirth, and the puerperium, a code for the specific type of infection should be assigned as an additional diagnosis. If severe sepsis is present, a code from subcategory R65.2, Severe sepsis, and code(s) for associated organ dysfunction(s) should also be assigned as additional diagnoses.

k. Puerperal sepsis

Code O85, Puerperal sepsis, should be assigned with a secondary code to identify the causal organism (e.g., for a bacterial infection, assign a code from category B95-B96, Bacterial infections in conditions classified elsewhere). A code from category A40, Streptococcal sepsis, or A41, Other sepsis, should not be used for puerperal sepsis. If applicable, use additional codes to identify severe sepsis (R65.2-) and any associated acute organ dysfunction.

Code O85 should not be assigned for sepsis following an obstetrical procedure (*See Section I.C.1.d.5b., Sepsis due to a postprocedural infection*).

l. Alcohol, tobacco and drug use during pregnancy, childbirth and the puerperium

1) Alcohol use during pregnancy, childbirth and the puerperium

Codes under subcategory O99.31, Alcohol use complicating pregnancy, childbirth, and the puerperium, should be assigned for any pregnancy case when a **patient** uses alcohol during the pregnancy or postpartum. A secondary code from category F10, Alcohol related disorders, should also be assigned to identify manifestations of the alcohol use.

2) Tobacco use during pregnancy, childbirth and the puerperium

Codes under subcategory O99.33, Smoking (tobacco) complicating pregnancy, childbirth, and the puerperium, should be assigned for any pregnancy case when a mother uses any type of tobacco product during the pregnancy or postpartum. A secondary code from category F17, Nicotine dependence, should also be assigned to identify the type of nicotine dependence.

3) Drug use during pregnancy, childbirth and the puerperium

Codes under subcategory O99.32, Drug use complicating pregnancy, childbirth, and the puerperium, should be assigned for any pregnancy case when a **patient** uses drugs during the pregnancy or postpartum. This can involve illegal drugs, or inappropriate use or abuse of prescription drugs. Secondary code(s) from categories F11-F16 and F18-F19 should also be assigned to identify manifestations of the drug use.

m. Poisoning, toxic effects, adverse effects and underdosing in a pregnant patient

A code from subcategory O9A.2, Injury, poisoning and certain other consequences of external causes complicating pregnancy, childbirth, and the puerperium, should be sequenced first, followed by the appropriate injury, poisoning, toxic effect, adverse effect or underdosing code, and then the additional code(s) that specifies the condition caused by the poisoning, toxic effect, adverse effect or underdosing.

See Section I.C.19. Adverse effects, poisoning, underdosing and toxic effects.

n. Normal Delivery, Code O80

1) Encounter for full term uncomplicated delivery

Code O80 should be assigned when a **patient** is admitted for a full-term normal delivery and delivers a single, healthy infant without any complications antepartum, during the delivery, or postpartum during the delivery episode. Code O80 is always a principal diagnosis. It is not to be used if any other code from chapter 15 is needed to describe a current complication of the antenatal, delivery, or postnatal period. Additional codes from other chapters may be used with code O80 if they are not related to or are in any way complicating the pregnancy.

2) Uncomplicated delivery with resolved antepartum complication

Code O80 may be used if the patient had a complication at some point during the pregnancy, but the complication is not present at the time of the admission for delivery.

3) Outcome of delivery for O80

Z37.0, Single live birth, is the only outcome of delivery code appropriate for use with O80.

o. The Peripartum and Postpartum Periods

1) Peripartum and Postpartum periods

The postpartum period begins immediately after delivery and continues for six weeks following delivery. The peripartum period is defined as the last month of pregnancy to five months postpartum.

2) Peripartum and postpartum complication

A postpartum complication is any complication occurring within the six-week period.

3) Pregnancy-related complications after 6 week period

Chapter 15 codes may also be used to describe pregnancy-related complications after the peripartum or postpartum period if the provider documents that a condition is pregnancy related.

4) Admission for routine postpartum care following delivery outside hospital

When the mother delivers outside the hospital prior to admission and is admitted for routine postpartum care and no complications are noted, code Z39.0, Encounter for care and examination of mother immediately after delivery, should be assigned as the principal diagnosis.

5) Pregnancy associated cardiomyopathy

Pregnancy associated cardiomyopathy, code O90.3, is unique in that it may be diagnosed in the third trimester of pregnancy but may continue to progress months after delivery. For this reason, it is referred to as peripartum cardiomyopathy. Code O90.3 is only for use when the cardiomyopathy develops as a result of pregnancy in a woman who did not have pre-existing heart disease.

p. Code O94, Sequelae of complication of pregnancy, childbirth, and the puerperium

1) Code O94

Code O94, Sequelae of complication of pregnancy, childbirth, and the puerperium, is for use in those cases when an initial complication of a pregnancy develops a sequelae requiring care or treatment at a future date.

2) After the initial postpartum period

This code may be used at any time after the initial postpartum period.

3) Sequencing of Code O94

This code, like all sequela codes, is to be sequenced following the code describing the sequelae of the complication.

q. Termination of Pregnancy and Spontaneous abortions

1) Abortion with Liveborn Fetus

When an attempted termination of pregnancy results in a liveborn fetus, assign code Z33.2, Encounter for elective termination of pregnancy and a code from category Z37, Outcome of Delivery.

2) Retained Products of Conception following an abortion

Subsequent encounters for retained products of conception following a spontaneous abortion or elective termination of pregnancy, without complications are assigned O03.4, Incomplete spontaneous, abortion without complication, or codes O07.4, Failed attempted termination of pregnancy without complication. This advice is appropriate even when the patient was discharged previously with a discharge diagnosis of complete abortion. If the patient has a specific complication associated with the spontaneous abortion or elective termination of pregnancy in addition to retained products of conception, assign the appropriate complication code (e.g., O03.-, O04.-, O07.-) instead of code O03.4 or O07.4.

3) Complications leading to abortion

Codes from Chapter 15 may be used as additional codes to identify any documented complications of the pregnancy in conjunction with codes in categories in O04, O07 and O08.

r. Abuse in a pregnant patient

For suspected or confirmed cases of abuse of a pregnant patient, a code(s) from subcategories O9A.3, Physical abuse complicating pregnancy, childbirth, and the puerperium, O9A.4, Sexual abuse complicating pregnancy, childbirth, and the puerperium, and O9A.5, Psychological abuse complicating pregnancy, childbirth, and the puerperium, should be sequenced first, followed by the appropriate codes (if applicable) to identify any associated current injury due to physical abuse, sexual abuse, and the perpetrator of abuse.

See Section I.C.19. Adult and child abuse, neglect and other maltreatment.

s. COVID-19 infection in pregnancy, childbirth, and the puerperium

During pregnancy, childbirth or the puerperium, when COVID-19 is the reason for admission/encounter, code O98.5-, Other viral diseases complicating pregnancy, childbirth and the puerperium, should be sequenced as the principal/first-listed diagnosis, and code U07.1, COVID-19, and the appropriate codes for associated manifestation(s) should be assigned as additional diagnoses. Codes from Chapter 15 always take sequencing priority.

If the reason for admission/encounter is unrelated to COVID-19 but the patient tests positive for COVID-19 during the admission/encounter, the appropriate code for the reason for admission/encounter should be sequenced as the principal/first-listed diagnosis, and code O98.5- and U07.1, as well as the appropriate codes for associated COVID-19 manifestations, should be assigned as additional diagnoses.

16. Chapter 16: Certain Conditions Originating in the Perinatal Period (P00-P96)

For coding and reporting purposes the perinatal period is defined as before birth through the 28th day following birth. The following guidelines are provided for reporting purposes

a. General Perinatal Rules

1) Use of Chapter 16 Codes

Codes in this chapter are <u>never</u> for use on the maternal record. Codes from Chapter 15, the obstetric chapter, are never permitted on the newborn record. Chapter 16 codes may be used throughout the life of the patient if the condition is still present.

2) Principal Diagnosis for Birth Record

When coding the birth episode in a newborn record, assign a code from category Z38, Liveborn infants according to place of birth and type of delivery, as the principal diagnosis. A code from category Z38 is assigned only once, to a newborn at the time of birth. If a newborn is transferred to another institution, a code from category Z38 should not be used at the receiving hospital.

A code from category Z38 is used only on the newborn record, not on the mother's record.

3) **Use of Codes from other Chapters with Codes from Chapter 16**

Codes from other chapters may be used with codes from chapter 16 if the codes from the other chapters provide more specific detail. Codes for signs and symptoms may be assigned when a definitive diagnosis has not been established. If the reason for the encounter is a perinatal condition, the code from chapter 16 should be sequenced first.

4) **Use of Chapter 16 Codes after the Perinatal Period**

Should a condition originate in the perinatal period, and continue throughout the life of the patient, the perinatal code should continue to be used regardless of the patient's age.

5) **Birth process or community acquired conditions**

If a newborn has a condition that may be either due to the birth process or community acquired and the documentation does not indicate which it is, the default is due to the birth process and the code from Chapter 16 should be used. If the condition is community-acquired, a code from Chapter 16 should not be assigned.

For COVID-19 infection in a newborn, see guideline I.C.16.h

6) **Code all clinically significant conditions**

All clinically significant conditions noted on routine newborn examination should be coded. A condition is clinically significant if it requires:

- clinical evaluation; or
- therapeutic treatment; or
- diagnostic procedures; or
- extended length of hospital stay; or
- increased nursing care and/or monitoring; or
- has implications for future health care needs

Note: The perinatal guidelines listed above are the same as the general coding guidelines for "additional diagnoses", except for the final point regarding implications for future health care needs. Codes should be assigned for conditions that have been specified by the provider as having implications for future health care needs.

b. Observation and Evaluation of Newborns for Suspected Conditions not Found

1) **Use of Z05 codes**

Assign a code from category Z05, Observation and evaluation of newborns and infants for suspected conditions ruled out, to identify those instances when a healthy newborn is evaluated for a suspected condition that is determined after study not to be present. Do not use a code from category Z05 when the patient has identified signs or symptoms of a suspected problem; in such cases code the sign or symptom.

2) **Z05 on Other than the Birth Record**

A code from category Z05 may also be assigned as a principal or first-listed code for readmissions or encounters when the code from category Z38 code no longer applies. Codes from category Z05 are fur use only for healthy newborns and infants for which no condition after study is found to be present.

3) **Z05 on a birth record**

A code from category Z05 is to be used as a secondary code after the code from category Z38, Liveborn infants according to place of birth and type of delivery.

c. Coding Additional Perinatal Diagnoses

1) **Assigning codes for conditions that require treatment**

Assign codes for conditions that require treatment or further investigation, prolong the length of stay, or require resource utilization.

2) **Codes for conditions specified as having implications for future health care needs**

Assign codes for conditions that have been specified by the provider as having implications for future health care needs.

Note: This guideline should not be used for adult patients.

d. Prematurity and Fetal Growth Retardation

Providers utilize different criteria in determining prematurity. A code for prematurity should not be assigned unless it is documented. Assignment of codes in categories P05, Disorders of newborn related to slow fetal growth and fetal malnutrition, and P07, Disorders of newborn related to short gestation and low birth weight, not elsewhere classified, should be based on the recorded birth weight and estimated gestational age.

When both birth weight and gestational age are available, two codes from category P07 should be assigned, with the code for birth weight sequenced before the code for gestational age.

e. Low birth weight and immaturity status

Codes from category P07, Disorders of newborn related to short gestation and low birth weight, not elsewhere classified, are for use for a child or adult who was premature or had a low birth weight as a newborn and this is affecting the patient's current health status.

See Section I.C.21. Factors influencing health status and contact with health services, Status.

f. Bacterial Sepsis of Newborn

Category P36, Bacterial sepsis of newborn, includes congenital sepsis. If a perinate is documented as having sepsis without documentation of congenital or community acquired, the default is congenital and a code from category P36 should be assigned. If the P36 code includes the causal organism, an additional code from category B95, Streptococcus, Staphylococcus, and Enterococcus as the cause of diseases classified elsewhere, or B96, Other bacterial agents as the cause of diseases classified elsewhere, should not be assigned. If the P36 code does not include the causal organism, assign an additional code from category B96. If applicable, use additional codes to identify severe sepsis (R65.2-) and any associated acute organ dysfunction.

g. Stillbirth

Code P95, Stillbirth, is only for use in institutions that maintain separate records for stillbirths. No other code should be used with P95. Code P95 should not be used on the mother's record.

h. COVID-19 Infection in Newborn

For a newborn that tests positive for COVID-19, assign code U07.1, COVID-19, and the appropriate codes for associated manifestation(s) in neonates/newborns in the absence of documentation indicating a specific type of transmission. For a newborn that tests positive for COVID-19 and the provider documents the condition was contracted in utero or during the birth process, assign codes P35.8, Other congenital viral diseases, and U07.1, COVID-19. When coding the birth episode in a newborn record, the appropriate code from category Z38, Liveborn infants according to place of birth and type of delivery, should be assigned as the principal diagnosis.

17. Chapter 17: Congenital Malformations, Deformations and Chromosomal Abnormalities (Q00-Q99)

Assign an appropriate code(s) from categories Q00-Q99, Congenital malformations, deformations, and chromosomal abnormalities when a malformation/deformation or chromosomal abnormality is documented. A malformation/deformation or chromosomal abnormality may be the principal/first-listed diagnosis on a record or a secondary diagnosis.

When a malformation/deformation or chromosomal abnormality does not have a unique code assignment, assign additional code(s) for any manifestations that may be present.

When the code assignment specifically identifies the malformation/deformation or chromosomal abnormality, manifestations that are an inherent component of the anomaly should not be coded separately. Additional codes should be assigned for manifestations that are not an inherent component.

Codes from Chapter 17 may be used throughout the life of the patient. If a congenital malformation or deformity has been corrected, a personal history code should be used to identify the history of the malformation or deformity. Although present at birth, a malformation/deformation or chromosomal abnormality may not be identified until later in life. Whenever the condition is diagnosed by the provider, it is appropriate to assign a code from codes Q00-Q99. For the birth admission, the appropriate code from category Z38, Liveborn infants, according to place of birth and type of delivery, should be sequenced as the principal diagnosis, followed by any congenital anomaly codes, Q00-Q99.

18. Chapter 18: Symptoms, Signs, and Abnormal Clinical and Laboratory Findings, Not Elsewhere Classified (R00-R99)

Chapter 18 includes symptoms, signs, abnormal results of clinical or other investigative procedures, and ill-defined conditions regarding which no diagnosis classifiable elsewhere is recorded. Signs and symptoms that point to a specific diagnosis have been assigned to a category in other chapters of the classification.

a. Use of symptom codes

Codes that describe symptoms and signs are acceptable for reporting purposes when a related definitive diagnosis has not been established (confirmed) by the provider.

b. Use of a symptom code with a definitive diagnosis code

Codes for signs and symptoms may be reported in addition to a related definitive diagnosis when the sign or symptom is not routinely associated with that diagnosis, such as the various signs and symptoms associated with complex syndromes. The definitive diagnosis code should be sequenced before the symptom code.

Signs or symptoms that are associated routinely with a disease process should not be assigned as additional codes, unless otherwise instructed by the classification.

c. Combination codes that include symptoms

ICD-10-CM contains a number of combination codes that identify both the definitive diagnosis and common symptoms of that diagnosis. When using one of these combination codes, an additional code should not be assigned for the symptom.

d. Repeated falls

Code R29.6, Repeated falls, is for use for encounters when a patient has recently fallen and the reason for the fall is being investigated.

Code Z91.81, History of falling, is for use when a patient has fallen in the past and is at risk for future falls. When appropriate, both codes R29.6 and Z91.81 may be assigned together.

Code R40.20, Unspecified coma, may be assigned in conjunction with codes for any medical condition.

e. Coma

Code R40.20, Unspecified coma, may be assigned in conjunction with codes for any medical condition.

Do not report codes for unspecified coma, individual or total Glasgow coma scale scores for a patient with a medically induced coma or a sedated patient.

1) Coma Scale

The coma scale codes (R40.2**1- to R40.24-**) can be used in conjunction with traumatic brain injury codes, acute cerebrovascular disease or sequelae of cerebrovascular disease codes. These codes are primarily for use by trauma registries, but they may be used in any setting where this information is collected. The coma scale codes should be sequenced after the diagnosis code(s).

These codes, one from each subcategory, are needed to complete the scale. The 7th character indicates when the scale was recorded. The 7th character should match for all three codes.

At a minimum, report the initial score documented on presentation at your facility. This may be a score from the emergency medicine technician (EMT) or in the emergency department. If desired, a facility may choose to capture multiple coma scale scores.

Assign code R40.24, Glasgow coma scale, total score, when only the total score is documented in the medical record and not the individual score(s).

If multiple coma scores are captured within the first 24 hours after hospital admission, assign only the code for the score at the time of admission. ICD-10-CM does not classify coma scores that are reported after admission but less than 24 hours later.

See Section I.B.14 for coma scale documentation by clinicians other than the patient's provider.

f. Functional quadriplegia

GUIDELINE HAS BEEN DELETED EFFECTIVE OCTOBER 1, 2017

g. SIRS due to Non-Infectious Process

The systemic inflammatory response syndrome (SIRS) can develop as a result of certain non-infectious disease processes, such as trauma, malignant neoplasm, or pancreatitis. When SIRS is documented with a noninfectious condition, and no subsequent infection is documented, the code for the underlying condition, such as an injury, should be assigned, followed by code R65.10, Systemic inflammatory response syndrome (SIRS) of non-infectious origin without acute organ dysfunction, or code R65.11, Systemic inflammatory response syndrome (SIRS) of non-infectious origin with acute organ dysfunction. If an associated acute organ dysfunction is documented, the appropriate code(s) for the specific type of organ dysfunction(s) should be assigned in addition to code R65.11. If acute organ dysfunction is documented, but it cannot be determined if the acute organ dysfunction is associated with SIRS or due to another condition (e.g., directly due to the trauma), the provider should be queried.

h. Death NOS

Code R99, Ill-defined and unknown cause of mortality, is only for use in the very limited circumstance when a patient who has already died is brought into an emergency department or other healthcare facility and is pronounced dead upon arrival. It does not represent the discharge disposition of death.

i. NIHSS Stroke Scale

The NIH stroke scale (NIHSS) codes (R29.7--) can be used in conjunction with acute stroke codes (I63) to identify the patient's neurological status and the severity of the stroke. The stroke scale codes should be sequenced after the acute stroke diagnosis code(s).

At a minimum, report the initial score documented. If desired, a facility may choose to capture multiple stroke scale scores.

See Section I.B.14 for NIHSS stroke scale documentation by clinicians other than patient's provider.

19. Chapter 19: Injury, Poisoning and Certain Other Consequences of External Causes (S00-T88)

a. Application of 7th Characters in Chapter 19

Most categories in chapter 19 have a 7th character requirement for each applicable code. Most categories in this chapter have three 7th character values (with the exception of fractures): A, initial encounter, D, subsequent encounter and S, sequela. Categories for traumatic fractures have additional 7th character values. While the patient may be seen by a new or different provider over the course of treatment for an injury, assignment of the 7th character is based on whether the patient is undergoing active treatment and not whether the provider is seeing the patient for the first time.

For complication codes, active treatment refers to treatment for the condition described by the code, even though it may be related to an earlier precipitating problem. For example, code T84.50XA, Infection and inflammatory reaction due to unspecified internal joint prosthesis, initial encounter, is used when active treatment is provided for the infection, even though the condition relates to the prosthetic device, implant or graft that was placed at a previous encounter.

7th character "A", initial encounter is used for each encounter where the patient is receiving active treatment for the condition.

7th character "D" subsequent encounter is used for encounters after the patient has completed active treatment of the condition and is receiving routine care for the condition during the healing or recovery phase.

The aftercare Z codes should not be used for aftercare for conditions such as injuries or poisonings, where 7th characters are provided to identify subsequent care. For example, for aftercare of an injury, assign the acute injury code with the 7th character "D" (subsequent encounter).

7th character "S", sequela, is for use for complications or conditions that arise as a direct result of a condition, such as scar formation after a burn. The scars are sequelae of the burn. When using 7th character "S", it is necessary to use both the injury code that precipitated the sequela and the code for the sequela itself. The "S" is added only to the injury code, not the sequela code. The 7th character "S" identifies the injury responsible for the sequela. The specific type of sequela (e.g. scar) is sequenced first, followed by the injury code.

See Section I.B.10 Sequela (Late Effects)

b. Coding of Injuries

When coding injuries, assign separate codes for each injury unless a combination code is provided, in which case the combination code is assigned. Codes from category T07, Unspecified multiple injuries should not be assigned in the inpatient setting unless information for a more specific code is not available. Traumatic injury codes (S00-T14.9) are not to be used for normal, healing surgical wounds or to identify complications of surgical wounds.

The code for the most serious injury, as determined by the provider and the focus of treatment, is sequenced first.

1) Superficial injuries

Superficial injuries such as abrasions or contusions are not coded when associated with more severe injuries of the same site.

2) Primary injury with damage to nerves/blood vessels

When a primary injury results in minor damage to peripheral nerves or blood vessels, the primary injury is sequenced first with additional code(s) for injuries to nerves and spinal cord (such as category S04), and/or injury to blood vessels (such as category S15). When the primary injury is to the blood vessels or nerves, that injury should be sequenced first.

3) Iatrogenic injuries

Injury codes from Chapter 19 should not be assigned for injuries that occur during, or as a result of, a medical intervention. Assign the appropriate complication code(s).

c. Coding of Traumatic Fractures

The principles of multiple coding of injuries should be followed in coding fractures. Fractures of specified sites are coded individually by site in accordance with both the provisions within categories S02, S12, S22, S32, S42, S49, S52, S59, S62, S72, S79, S82, S89, S92 and the level of detail furnished by medical record content.

A fracture not indicated as open or closed should be coded to closed. A fracture not indicated whether displaced or not displaced should be coded to displaced.

More specific guidelines are as follows:

1) Initial vs. Subsequent Encounter for Fractures

Traumatic fractures are coded using the appropriate 7th character for initial encounter (A, B, C) for each encounter where the patient is receiving active treatment for the fracture. The appropriate 7th character for initial encounter should also be assigned for a patient who delayed seeking treatment for the fracture or nonunion.

Fractures are coded using the appropriate 7th character for subsequent care for encounters after the patient has completed active treatment of the fracture and is receiving routine care for the fracture during the healing or recovery phase.

Care for complications of surgical treatment for fracture repairs during the healing or recovery phase should be coded with the appropriate complication codes.

Care of complications of fractures, such as malunion and nonunion, should be reported with the appropriate 7th character for subsequent care with nonunion (K, M, N,) or subsequent care with malunion (P, Q, R).

Malunion/nonunion: The appropriate 7th character for initial encounter should also be assigned for a patient who delayed seeking treatment for the fracture or nonunion.

The open fracture designations in the assignment of the 7th character for fractures of the forearm, femur and lower leg, including ankle are based on the Gustilo open fracture classification. When the Gustilo classification type is not specified for an open fracture, the 7th character for open fracture type I or II should be assigned (B, E, H, M, Q).

A code from category M80, not a traumatic fracture code, should be used for any patient with known osteoporosis who suffers a fracture, even if the patient had a minor fall or trauma, if that fall or trauma would not usually break a normal, healthy bone.

See Section I.C.13. Osteoporosis.

The aftercare Z codes should not be used for aftercare for traumatic fractures. For aftercare of a traumatic fracture, assign the acute fracture code with the appropriate 7th character.

2) Multiple fractures sequencing

Multiple fractures are sequenced in accordance with the severity of the fracture.

3) Physeal fractures

For physeal fractures, assign only the code identifying the type of physeal fracture. Do not assign a separate code to identify the specific bone that is fractured.

d. Coding of Burns and Corrosions

The ICD-10-CM makes a distinction between burns and corrosions. The burn codes are for thermal burns, except sunburns, that come from a heat source, such as a fire or hot appliance. The burn codes are also for burns resulting from electricity and radiation. Corrosions are burns due to chemicals. The guidelines are the same for burns and corrosions.

Current burns (T20-T25) are classified by depth, extent and by agent (X code). Burns are classified by depth as first degree (erythema), second degree (blistering), and third degree (full-thickness involvement). Burns of the eye and internal organs (T26-T28) are classified by site, but not by degree.

1) Sequencing of burn and related condition codes

Sequence first the code that reflects the highest degree of burn when more than one burn is present.

a. When the reason for the admission or encounter is for treatment of external multiple burns, sequence first the code that reflects the burn of the highest degree.

b. When a patient has both internal and external burns, the circumstances of admission govern the selection of the principal diagnosis or first-listed diagnosis.

c. When a patient is admitted for burn injuries and other related conditions such as smoke inhalation and/or respiratory failure, the circumstances of admission govern the selection of the principal or first-listed diagnosis.

2) Burns of the same anatomic site

Classify burns of the same anatomic site and on the same side but of different degrees to the subcategory identifying the highest degree recorded in the diagnosis (e.g., for second and third degree burns of right thigh, assign only code T24.311-).

3) Non-healing burns

Non-healing burns are coded as acute burns.

Necrosis of burned skin should be coded as a non-healed burn.

4) Infected Burn

For any documented infected burn site, use an additional code for the infection.

5) Assign separate codes for each burn site

When coding burns, assign separate codes for each burn site. Category T30, Burn and corrosion, body region unspecified is extremely vague and should rarely be used.

Codes for burns of "multiple sites" should only be assigned when the medical record documentation does not specify the individual sites.

6) Burns and Corrosions Classified According to Extent of Body Surface Involved

Assign codes from category T31, Burns classified according to extent of body surface involved, or T32, Corrosions classified according to extent of body surface involved, for **acute burns or corrosions** when the site of the burn **or corrosion** is not specified or when there is a need for additional data. It is advisable to use category T31 as additional coding when needed to provide data for evaluating burn mortality, such as that needed by burn units. It is also advisable to use category T31 as an additional code for reporting purposes when there is mention of a third-degree burn involving 20 percent or more of the body surface. **Codes from categories T31 and T32 should not be used for sequelae of burns or corrosions.**

Categories T31 and T32 are based on the classic "rule of nines" in estimating body surface involved: head and neck are assigned nine percent, each arm nine percent, each leg 18 percent, the anterior trunk 18 percent, posterior trunk 18 percent, and genitalia one percent. Providers may change these percentage assignments where necessary to accommodate infants and children who have proportionately larger heads than adults, and patients who have large buttocks, thighs, or abdomen that involve burns.

7) Encounters for treatment of sequela of burns

Encounters for the treatment of the late effects of burns or corrosions (i.e., scars or joint contractures) should be coded with a burn or corrosion code with the 7th character "S" for sequela.

8) Sequelae with a late effect code and current burn

When appropriate, both a code for a current burn or corrosion with 7th character "A" or "D" and a burn or corrosion code with 7th character "S" may be assigned on the same record (when both a current burn and sequelae of an old burn exist). Burns and corrosions do not heal at the same rate and a current healing wound may still exist with sequela of a healed burn or corrosion.

See Section I.B.10 Sequela (Late Effects)

9) Use of an external cause code with burns and corrosions

An external cause code should be used with burns and corrosions to identify the source and intent of the burn, as well as the place where it occurred.

e. Adverse Effects, Poisoning, Underdosing and Toxic Effects

Codes in categories T36-T65 are combination codes that include the substance that was taken as well as the intent. No additional external cause code is required for poisonings, toxic effects, adverse effects and underdosing codes.

1) Do not code directly from the Table of Drugs

Do not code directly from the Table of Drugs and Chemicals. Always refer back to the Tabular List.

2) Use as many codes as necessary to describe

Use as many codes as necessary to describe completely all drugs, medicinal or biological substances.

3) If the same code would describe the causative agent

If the same code would describe the causative agent for more than one adverse reaction, poisoning, toxic effect or underdosing, assign the code only once.

4) If two or more drugs, medicinal or biological substances

If two or more drugs, medicinal or biological substances are taken, code each individually unless a combination code is listed in the Table of Drugs and Chemicals.

If multiple unspecified drugs, medicinal or biological substances were taken, assign the appropriate code from subcategory T50.91, Poisoning by, adverse effect of and underdosing of multiple unspecified drugs, medicaments and biological substances.

5) The occurrence of drug toxicity is classified in ICD-10-CM as follows:

(a) Adverse Effect

When coding an adverse effect of a drug that has been correctly prescribed and properly administered, assign the appropriate code for the nature of the adverse effect followed by the appropriate code for the adverse effect of the drug (T36-T50). The code for the drug should have a 5th or 6th character "5" (for example T36.0X5-) Examples of the nature of an adverse effect are tachycardia, delirium, gastrointestinal hemorrhaging, vomiting, hypokalemia, hepatitis, renal failure, or respiratory failure.

(b) Poisoning

When coding a poisoning or reaction to the improper use of a medication (e.g., overdose, wrong substance given or taken in error, wrong route of administration), first assign the appropriate code from categories T36-T50. The poisoning codes have an associated intent as their 5th or 6th character (accidental, intentional self-harm, assault and undetermined.) If the intent of the poisoning is unknown or unspecified, code the intent as accidental intent. The undetermined intent is only for use if the documentation in the record specifies that the intent cannot be determined. Use additional code(s) for all manifestations of poisonings.

If there is also a diagnosis of abuse or dependence of the substance, the abuse or dependence is assigned as an additional code.

Examples of poisoning include:

(i) Error was made in drug prescription

Errors made in drug prescription or in the administration of the drug by provider, nurse, patient, or other person.

(ii) Overdose of a drug intentionally taken

If an overdose of a drug was intentionally taken or administered and resulted in drug toxicity, it would be coded as a poisoning.

(iii) Nonprescribed drug taken with correctly prescribed and properly administered drug

If a nonprescribed drug or medicinal agent was taken in combination with a correctly prescribed and properly administered drug, any drug toxicity or other reaction resulting from the interaction of the two drugs would be classified as a poisoning.

(iv) Interaction of drug(s) and alcohol

When a reaction results from the interaction of a drug(s) and alcohol, this would be classified as poisoning.

See Section I.C.4. if poisoning is the result of insulin pump malfunctions.

(c) Underdosing

Underdosing refers to taking less of a medication than is prescribed by a provider or a manufacturer's instruction. Discontinuing the use of a prescribed medication on the patient's own initiative (not directed by the patient's provider) is also classified as an underdosing. For underdosing, assign the code from categories T36-T50 (fifth or sixth character "6").

Codes for underdosing should never be assigned as principal or first-listed codes. If a patient has a relapse or exacerbation of the medical condition for which the drug is prescribed because of the reduction in dose, then the medical condition itself should be coded.

Noncompliance (Z91.12-, Z91.13- and Z91.14-) or complication of care (Y63.6-Y63.9) codes are to be used with an underdosing code to indicate intent, if known.

(d) Toxic Effects

When a harmful substance is ingested or comes in contact with a person, this is classified as a toxic effect. The toxic effect codes are in categories T51-T65.

Toxic effect codes have an associated intent: accidental, intentional self-harm, assault and undetermined.

f. Adult and child abuse, neglect and other maltreatment

Sequence first the appropriate code from categories T74.- (Adult and child abuse, neglect and other maltreatment, confirmed) or T76.- (Adult and child abuse, neglect and other maltreatment, suspected) for abuse, neglect and other maltreatment, followed by any accompanying mental health or injury code(s).

If the documentation in the medical record states abuse or neglect it is coded as confirmed (T74.-). It is coded as suspected if it is documented as suspected (T76.-).

For cases of confirmed abuse or neglect an external cause code from the assault section (X92-Y09) should be added to identify the cause of any physical injuries. A perpetrator code (Y07) should be added when the perpetrator of the abuse is known. For suspected cases of abuse or neglect, do not report external cause or perpetrator code.

If a suspected case of abuse, neglect or mistreatment is ruled out during an encounter code Z04.71, Encounter for examination and observation following alleged physical adult abuse, ruled out, or code Z04.72, Encounter for examination and observation following alleged child physical abuse, ruled out, should be used, not a code from T76.

If a suspected case of alleged rape or sexual abuse is ruled out during an encounter code Z04.41, Encounter for examination and observation following alleged adult rape or code Z04.42, Encounter for examination and observation following alleged child rape, should be used, not a code from T76.

If a suspected case of forced sexual exploitation or forced labor exploitation is ruled out during an encounter, code Z04.81, Encounter for examination and observation of victim following forced sexual exploitation, or code Z04.82, Encounter for examination and observation of victim following forced labor exploitation, should be used, not a code from T76.

See Section I.C.15. Abuse in a pregnant patient.

g. **Complications of care**

1) **General guidelines for complications of care**

(a) **Documentation of complications of care**

See Section I.B.16. for information on documentation of complications of care.

2) **Pain due to medical devices**

Pain associated with devices, implants or grafts left in a surgical site (for example painful hip prosthesis) is assigned to the appropriate code(s) found in Chapter 19, Injury, poisoning, and certain other consequences of external causes. Specific codes for pain due to medical devices are found in the T code section of the ICD-10-CM. Use additional code(s) from category G89 to identify acute or chronic pain due to presence of the device, implant or graft (G89.18 or G89.28).

3) **Transplant complications**

(a) **Transplant complications other than kidney**

Codes under category T86, Complications of transplanted organs and tissues, are for use for both complications and rejection of transplanted organs. A transplant complication code is only assigned if the complication affects the function of the transplanted organ. Two codes are required to fully describe a transplant complication: the appropriate code from category T86 and a secondary code that identifies the complication.

Pre-existing conditions or conditions that develop after the transplant are not coded as complications unless they affect the function of the transplanted organs.

See I.C.21. for transplant organ removal status.

See I.C.2. for malignant neoplasm associated with transplanted organ.

(b) **Kidney transplant complications**

Patients who have undergone kidney transplant may still have some form of chronic kidney disease (CKD) because the kidney transplant may not fully restore kidney function. Code T86.1- should be assigned for documented complications of a kidney transplant, such as transplant failure or rejection or other transplant complication. Code T86.1- should not be assigned for post kidney transplant patients who have chronic kidney (CKD) unless a transplant complication such as transplant failure or rejection is documented. If the documentation is unclear as to whether the patient has a complication of the transplant, query the provider.

Conditions that affect the function of the transplanted kidney, other than CKD, should be assigned a code from subcategory T86.1, Complications of transplanted organ, Kidney, and a secondary code that identifies the complication.

For patients with CKD following a kidney transplant, but who do not have a complication such as failure or rejection, *see section I.C.14. Chronic kidney disease and kidney transplant status.*

4) **Complication codes that include the external cause**

As with certain other T codes, some of the complications of care codes have the external cause included in the code. The code includes the nature of the complication as well as the type of procedure that caused the complication. No external cause code indicating the type of procedure is necessary for these codes.

5) **Complications of care codes within the body system chapters**

Intraoperative and postprocedural complication codes are found within the body system chapters with codes specific to the organs and structures of that body system. These codes should be sequenced first, followed by a code(s) for the specific complication, if applicable.

Complication codes from the body system chapters should be assigned for intraoperative and postprocedural complications (e.g., the appropriate complication code from chapter 9 would be assigned for a vascular intraoperative or postprocedural complication) unless the complication is specifically indexed to a T code in chapter 19.

20. Chapter 20: External Causes of Morbidity (V00-Y99)

The external causes of morbidity codes should never be sequenced as the first-listed or principal diagnosis.

External cause codes are intended to provide data for injury research and evaluation of injury prevention strategies. These codes capture how the injury or health condition happened (cause), the intent (unintentional or accidental; or intentional, such as suicide or assault), the place where the event occurred the activity of the patient at the time of the event, and the person's status (e.g., civilian, military).

There is no national requirement for mandatory ICD-10-CM external cause code reporting. Unless a provider is subject to a state-based external cause code reporting mandate or these codes are required by a particular payer, reporting of ICD-10-CM codes in Chapter 20, External Causes of Morbidity, is not required. In the absence of a mandatory reporting requirement, providers are encouraged to voluntarily report external cause codes, as they provide valuable data for injury research and evaluation of injury prevention strategies.

a. General External Cause Coding Guidelines

1) Used with any code in the range of A00.0-T88.9, Z00-Z99

An external cause code may be used with any code in the range of A00.0-T88.9, Z00-Z99, classification that represents a health condition due to an external cause. Though they are most applicable to injuries, they are also valid for use with such things as infections or diseases due to an external source, and other health conditions, such as a heart attack that occurs during strenuous physical activity.

2) External cause code used for length of treatment

Assign the external cause code, with the appropriate 7th character (initial encounter, subsequent encounter or sequela) for each encounter for which the injury or condition is being treated.

Most categories in chapter 20 have a 7th character requirement for each applicable code. Most categories in this chapter have three 7th character values: A, initial encounter, D, subsequent encounter and S, sequela. While the patient may be seen by a new or different provider over the course of treatment for an injury or condition, assignment of the 7th character for external cause should match the 7th character of the code assigned for the associated injury or condition for the encounter.

3) Use the full range of external cause codes

Use the full range of external cause codes to completely describe the cause, the intent, the place of occurrence, and if applicable, the activity of the patient at the time of the event, and the patient's status, for all injuries, and other health conditions due to an external cause.

4) Assign as many external cause codes as necessary

Assign as many external cause codes as necessary to fully explain each cause. If only one external code can be recorded, assign the code most related to the principal diagnosis.

5) The selection of the appropriate external cause code

The selection of the appropriate external cause code is guided by the Alphabetic Index of External Causes and by Inclusion and Exclusion notes in the Tabular List.

6) External cause code can never be a principal diagnosis

An external cause code can never be a principal (first-listed) diagnosis.

7) Combination external cause codes

Certain of the external cause codes are combination codes that identify sequential events that result in an injury, such as a fall which results in striking against an object. The injury may be due to either event or both. The combination external cause code used should correspond to the sequence of events regardless of which caused the most serious injury.

8) No external cause code needed in certain circumstances

No external cause code from Chapter 20 is needed if the external cause and intent are included in a code from another chapter (e.g. T36.0X1- Poisoning by penicillins, accidental (unintentional)).

b. Place of Occurrence Guideline

Codes from category Y92, Place of occurrence of the external cause, are secondary codes for use after other external cause codes to identify the location of the patient at the time of injury or other condition.

Generally, a place of occurrent code is assigned only once, at the initial encounter for treatment. However, in the rare instance that a new injury occurs during hospitalization, an additional place of occurrence code may be assigned. No 7th characters are used for Y92.

Do not use place of occurrence code Y92.9 if the place is not stated or is not applicable.

c. Activity Code

Assign a code from category Y93, Activity code, to describe the activity of the patient at the time the injury or other health condition occurred.

An activity code is used only once, at the initial encounter for treatment. Only one code from Y93 should be recorded on a medical record.

The activity codes are not applicable to poisonings, adverse effects, misadventures or sequela.

Do not assign Y93.9, Unspecified activity, if the activity is not stated.

A code from category Y93 is appropriate for use with external cause and intent codes if identifying the activity provides additional information about the event.

d. Place of Occurrence, Activity, and Status Codes Used with other External Cause Code

When applicable, place of occurrence, activity, and external cause status codes are sequenced after the main external cause code(s). Regardless of the number of external cause codes assigned, generally there should be only one place of occurrence code, one activity code, and one external cause status code assigned to an encounter. However, in the rare instance that a new injury occurs during hospitalization, an additional place of occurrence code may be assigned.

e. If the Reporting Format Limits the Number of External Cause Codes

If the reporting format limits the number of external cause codes that can be used in reporting clinical data, report the code for the cause/intent most related to the principal diagnosis. If the format permits capture of additional external cause codes, the cause/intent, including medical misadventures, of the additional events should be reported rather than the codes for place, activity, or external status.

f. Multiple External Cause Coding Guidelines

More than one external cause code is required to fully describe the external cause of an illness or injury. The assignment of external cause codes should be sequenced in the following priority:

If two or more events cause separate injuries, an external cause code should be assigned for each cause. The first-listed external cause code will be selected in the following order:

External codes for child and adult abuse take priority over all other external cause codes.

See Section I.C.19., Child and Adult abuse guidelines.

External cause codes for terrorism events take priority over all other external cause codes except child and adult abuse.

External cause codes for cataclysmic events take priority over all other external cause codes except child and adult abuse and terrorism.

External cause codes for transport accidents take priority over all other external cause codes except cataclysmic events, child and adult abuse and terrorism.

Activity and external cause status codes are assigned following all causal (intent) external cause codes.

The first-listed external cause code should correspond to the cause of the most serious diagnosis due to an assault, accident, or self-harm, following the order of hierarchy listed above.

g. Child and Adult Abuse Guideline

Adult and child abuse, neglect and maltreatment are classified as assault. Any of the assault codes may be used to indicate the external cause of any injury resulting from the confirmed abuse.

For confirmed cases of abuse, neglect and maltreatment, when the perpetrator is known, a code from Y07, Perpetrator of maltreatment and neglect, should accompany any other assault codes.

See Section I.C.19. Adult and child abuse, neglect and other maltreatment

h. Unknown or Undetermined Intent Guideline

If the intent (accident, self-harm, assault) of the cause of an injury or other condition is unknown or unspecified, code the intent as accidental intent. All transport accident categories assume accidental intent.

1) Use of undetermined intent

External cause codes for events of undetermined intent are only for use if the documentation in the record specifies that the intent cannot be determined.

i. Sequelae (Late Effects) of External Cause Guidelines

1) Sequelae external cause codes

Sequela are reported using the external cause code with the 7th character "S" for sequela. These codes should be used with any report of a late effect or sequela resulting from a previous injury.

See Section I.B.10 Sequela (Late Effects)

2) Sequela external cause code with a related current injury

A sequela external cause code should never be used with a related current nature of injury code.

3) Use of sequela external cause codes for subsequent visits

Use a late effect external cause code for subsequent visits when a late effect of the initial injury is being treated. Do not use a late effect external cause code for subsequent visits for follow- up care (e.g., to assess healing, to receive rehabilitative therapy) of the injury when no late effect of the injury has been documented.

j. Terrorism Guidelines

1) Cause of injury identified by the Federal Government (FBI) as terrorism

When the cause of an injury is identified by the Federal Government (FBI) as terrorism, the first-listed external cause code should be a code from category Y38, Terrorism. The definition of terrorism employed by the FBI is found at the inclusion note at the beginning of category Y38. Use additional code for place of occurrence (Y92.-). More than one Y38 code may be assigned if the injury is the result of more than one mechanism of terrorism.

2) Cause of an injury is suspected to be the result of terrorism

When the cause of an injury is suspected to be the result of terrorism a code from category Y38 should not be assigned. Suspected cases should be classified as assault.

3) Code Y38.9, Terrorism, secondary effects

Assign code Y38.9, Terrorism, secondary effects, for conditions occurring subsequent to the terrorist event. This code should not be assigned for conditions that are due to the initial terrorist act.

It is acceptable to assign code Y38.9 with another code from Y38 if there is an injury due to the initial terrorist event and an injury that is a subsequent result of the terrorist event.

k. External cause status

A code from category Y99, External cause status, should be assigned whenever any other external cause code is assigned for an encounter, including an Activity code, except for the events noted below. Assign a code from category Y99, External cause status, to indicate the work status of the person at the time the event occurred. The status code indicates whether the event occurred during military activity, whether a non-military person was at work, whether an individual including a student or volunteer was involved in a non-work activity at the time of the causal event.

A code from Y99, External cause status, should be assigned, when applicable, with other external cause codes, such as transport accidents and falls. The external cause status codes are not applicable to poisonings, adverse effects, misadventures or late effects. Do not assign a code from category Y99 if no other external cause codes (cause, activity) are applicable for the encounter.

An external cause status code is used only once, at the initial encounter for treatment. Only one code from Y99 should be recorded on a medical record.

Do not assign code Y99.9, Unspecified external cause status, if the status is not stated.

21. Chapter 21: Factors Influencing Health Status and Contact with Health Services (Z00-Z99)

NOTE The chapter specific guidelines provide additional information about the use of Z codes for specified encounters.

a. Use of Z codes in any healthcare setting

Z codes are for use in any healthcare setting. Z codes may be used as either a first-listed (principal diagnosis code in the inpatient setting) or secondary code, depending on the circumstances of the encounter. Certain Z codes may only be used as first-listed or principal diagnosis.

b. Z Codes indicate a reason for an encounter *or Provide Additional Information about a Patient Encounter*

Z codes are not procedure codes. A corresponding procedure code must accompany a Z code to describe any procedure performed.

c. Categories of Z Codes

1) Contact/Exposure

Category Z20 indicates contact with, and suspected exposure to, communicable diseases. These codes are for patients who do not show any sign or symptom of a disease but are suspected to have been exposed to it by close personal contact with an infected individual or are in an area where a disease is epidemic.

Category Z77, Other contact with and (suspected) exposures hazardous to health, indicates contact with and suspected exposures hazardous to health.

Contact/exposure codes may be used as a first-listed code to explain an encounter for testing, or, more commonly, as a secondary code to identify a potential risk.

2) Inoculations and vaccinations

Code Z23 is for encounters for inoculations and vaccinations. It indicates that a patient is being seen to receive a prophylactic inoculation against a disease. Procedure codes are required to identify the actual administration of the injection and the type(s) of immunizations given. Code Z23 may be used as a secondary code if the inoculation is given as a routine part of preventive health care, such as a well-baby visit.

3) Status

Status codes indicate that a patient is either a carrier of a disease or has the sequelae or residual of a past disease or condition. This includes such things as the presence of prosthetic or mechanical devices resulting from past treatment. A status code is informative, because the status may affect the course of treatment and its outcome. A status code is distinct from a history code. The history code indicates that the patient no longer has the condition.

A status code should not be used with a diagnosis code from one of the body system chapters, if the diagnosis code includes the information provided by the status code. For example, code Z94.1, Heart transplant status, should not be used with a code from subcategory T86.2, Complications of heart transplant. The status code does not provide additional information. The complication code indicates that the patient is a heart transplant patient.

For encounters for weaning from a mechanical ventilator, assign a code from subcategory J96.1, Chronic respiratory failure, followed by code Z99.11, Dependence on respirator [ventilator] status.

The status Z codes/categories are:

Z14 Genetic carrier

Genetic carrier status indicates that a person carries a gene, associated with a particular disease, which may be passed to offspring who may develop that disease. The person does not have the disease and is not at risk of developing the disease.

Z15 Genetic susceptibility to disease

Genetic susceptibility indicates that a person has a gene that increases the risk of that person developing the disease.

Codes from category Z15 should not be used as principal or first-listed codes. If the patient has the condition to which he/she is susceptible, and that condition is the reason for the encounter, the code for the current condition should be sequenced first. If the patient is being seen for follow-up after completed treatment for this condition, and the condition no longer exists, a follow-up code should be sequenced first, followed by the appropriate personal history and genetic susceptibility codes. If the purpose of the encounter is genetic counseling associated with procreative management, code Z31.5, Encounter for genetic counseling, should be assigned as the first-listed code, followed by a code from category Z15. Additional codes should be assigned for any applicable family or personal history.

Z16 Resistance to antimicrobial drugs

This code indicates that a patient has a condition that is resistant to antimicrobial drug treatment. Sequence the infection code first.

Z17 Estrogen receptor status

Z18 Retained foreign body fragments

Z19 Hormone sensitivity malignancy status

Z21 Asymptomatic HIV infection status

This code indicates that a patient has tested positive for HIV but has manifested no signs or symptoms of the disease.

Z22 Carrier of infectious disease

Carrier status indicates that a person harbors the specific organisms of a disease without manifest symptoms and is capable of transmitting the infection.

Z28.3 Underimmunization status

Z33.1 Pregnant state, incidental

This code is a secondary code only for use when the pregnancy is in no way complicating the reason for visit. Otherwise, a code from the obstetric chapter is required.

Z66 Do not resuscitate

This code may be used when it is documented by the provider that a patient is on do not resuscitate status at any time during the stay.

Z67 Blood type

Z68 Body mass index (BMI)

BMI codes should only be assigned when there is an associated, reportable diagnosis (such as obesity). Do not assign BMI codes during pregnancy.

See Section I.B.14 for BMI documentation by clinicians other than the patient's provider.

Z74.01 Bed confinement status

Z76.82 Awaiting organ transplant status

Z78 Other specified health status

Code Z78.1, Physical restraint status, may be used when it is documented by the provider that a patient has been put in restraints during the current encounter. Please note that this code should not be reported when it is documented by the provider that a patient is temporarily restrained during a procedure.

Z79 Long-term (current) drug therapy

Codes from this category indicate a patient's continuous use of a prescribed drug (including such things as aspirin therapy) for the long-term treatment of a condition or for prophylactic use. It is not for use for patients who have addictions to drugs. This subcategory is not for use of medications for detoxification or maintenance programs to prevent withdrawal symptoms in patients with drug dependence (e.g., methadone maintenance for opiate dependence). Assign the appropriate code for the drug dependence instead.

Assign a code from Z79 if the patient is receiving a medication for an extended period as a prophylactic measure (such as for the prevention of deep vein thrombosis) or as treatment of a chronic condition (such as arthritis) or a disease requiring a lengthy course of treatment (such as cancer). Do not assign a code from category Z79 for medication being administered for a brief period of time to treat an acute illness or injury (such as a course of antibiotics to treat acute bronchitis).

Z88 Allergy status to drugs, medicaments and biological substances

Except: Z88.9, Allergy status to unspecified drugs, medicaments and biological substances status

Z89 Acquired absence of limb

Z90 Acquired absence of organs, not elsewhere classified

Z91.0- Allergy status, other than to drugs and biological substances

Z92.82 Status post administration of tPA (rtPA) in a different facility within the last 24 hours prior to admission to a current facility

Assign code Z92.82, Status post administration of tPA (rtPA) in a different facility within the last 24 hours prior to admission to current facility, as a secondary diagnosis when a patient is received by transfer into a facility and documentation indicates they were administered tissue plasminogen activator (tPA) within the last 24 hours prior to admission to the current facility.

This guideline applies even if the patient is still receiving the tPA at the time they are received into the current facility.

The appropriate code for the condition for which the tPA was administered (such as cerebrovascular disease or myocardial infarction) should be assigned first.

Code Z92.82 is only applicable to the receiving facility record and not to the transferring facility record.

Z93 Artificial opening status

Z94 Transplanted organ and tissue status

Z95 Presence of cardiac and vascular implants and grafts

Z96 Presence of other functional implants

Z97 Presence of other devices

Z98 Other postprocedural states

Assign code Z98.85, Transplanted organ removal status, to indicate that a transplanted organ has been previously removed. This code should not be assigned for the encounter in which the transplanted organ is removed. The complication necessitating removal of the transplant organ should be assigned for that encounter.

See section I.C19. for information on the coding of organ transplant complications.

Z99 Dependence on enabling machines and devices, not elsewhere classified

NOTE Categories Z89-Z90 and Z93-Z99 are for use only if there are no complications or malfunctions of the organ or tissue replaced, the amputation site or the equipment on which the patient is dependent.

4) History (of)

There are two types of history Z codes, personal and family. Personal history codes explain a patient's past medical condition that no longer exists and is not receiving any treatment, but that has the potential for recurrence, and therefore may require continued monitoring.

Family history codes are for use when a patient has a family member(s) who has had a particular disease that causes the patient to be at higher risk of also contracting the disease.

Personal history codes may be used in conjunction with follow- up codes and family history codes may be used in conjunction with screening codes to explain the need for a test or procedure. History codes are also acceptable on any medical record regardless of the reason for visit. A history of an illness, even if no longer present, is important information that may alter the type of treatment ordered.

The reason for the encounter (for example, screening or counseling) should be sequenced first and the appropriate personal and/or family history code(s) should be assigned as additional diagnos(es).

The history Z code categories are:

Z80 Family history of primary malignant neoplasm

Z81 Family history of mental and behavioral disorders

Z82	Family history of certain disabilities and chronic diseases (leading to disablement)
Z83	Family history of other specific disorders
Z84	Family history of other conditions
Z85	Personal history of malignant neoplasm
Z86	Personal history of certain other diseases
Z87	Personal history of other diseases and conditions
Z91.4-	Personal history of psychological trauma, not elsewhere classified
Z91.5	Personal history of self-harm
Z91.81	History of falling
Z91.82	Personal history of military deployment
Z92	Personal history of medical treatment
	Except: Z92.0, Personal history of contraception Except: Z92.82, Status post administration of tPA (rtPA) in a different facility within the last 24 hours prior to admission to a current facility

5) Screening

Screening is the testing for disease or disease precursors in seemingly well individuals so that early detection and treatment can be provided for those who test positive for the disease (e.g., screening mammogram).

The testing of a person to rule out or confirm a suspected diagnosis because the patient has some sign or symptom is a diagnostic examination, not a screening. In these cases, the sign or symptom is used to explain the reason for the test.

A screening code may be a first-listed code if the reason for the visit is specifically the screening exam. It may also be used as an additional code if the screening is done during an office visit for other health problems. A screening code is not necessary if the screening is inherent to a routine examination, such as a pap smear done during a routine pelvic examination.

Should a condition be discovered during the screening then the code for the condition may be assigned as an additional diagnosis.

The Z code indicates that a screening exam is planned. A procedure code is required to confirm that the screening was performed.

The screening Z codes/categories:

Z11	Encounter for screening for infectious and parasitic diseases
Z12	Encounter for screening for malignant neoplasms
Z13	Encounter for screening for other diseases and disorders
	Except: Z13.9, Encounter for screening, unspecified
Z36	Encounter for antenatal screening for mother

6) Observation

There are three observation Z code categories. They are for use in very limited circumstances when a person is being observed for a suspected condition that is ruled out. The observation codes are not for use if an injury or illness or any signs or symptoms related to the suspected condition are present. In such cases the diagnosis/symptom code is used with the corresponding external cause code.

The observation codes are primarily to be used as principal/first-listed diagnosis. An observation code may be assigned as a secondary diagnosis code when the patient is being observed for a condition that is ruled out and is unrelated to the principal/first-listed diagnosis (e.g., patient presents for treatment following injuries sustained in a motor vehicle accident and is also observed for suspected COVID-19 infection that is subsequently ruled out). Also, when the principal diagnosis is required to be a code from category Z38, Liveborn infants according to place of birth and type of delivery, then a code form category Z05, Encounter for observation and evaluation of newborn for suspected diseases and conditions ruled out, is sequenced after the Z38 code. Additional codes may be used in addition to the observation code but only if they are unrelated to the suspected condition being observed.

Codes from subcategory Z03.7, Encounter for suspected maternal and fetal conditions ruled out, may either be used as a first-listed or as an additional code assignment depending on the case. They are for use in very limited circumstances on a maternal record when an encounter is for a suspected maternal or fetal condition that is ruled out during that encounter (for example, a maternal or fetal condition may be suspected due to an abnormal test result). These codes should not be used when the condition is confirmed. In those cases, the confirmed condition should be coded. In addition, these codes are not for use if an illness or any signs or symptoms related to the suspected condition or problem are present. In such cases the diagnosis/symptom code is used.

Additional codes may be used in addition to the code from subcategory Z03.7, but only if they are unrelated to the suspected condition being evaluated.

Codes from subcategory Z03.7 may not be used for encounters for antenatal screening of mother. *See Section I.C.21. Screening.*

For encounters for suspected fetal condition that are inconclusive following testing and evaluation, assign the appropriate code from category O35, O36, O40 or O41.

The observation Z code categories:

Z03	Encounter for medical observation for suspected diseases and conditions ruled out
Z04	Encounter for examination and observation for other reasons
	Except: Z04.9, Encounter for examination and observation for unspecified reason
Z05	Encounter for observation and evaluation of newborn for suspected diseases and conditions ruled out

7) Aftercare

Aftercare visit codes cover situations when the initial treatment of a disease has been performed and the patient requires continued care during the healing or recovery phase, or for the long-term consequences of the disease. The aftercare Z code should not be used if treatment is directed at a current, acute disease. The diagnosis code is to be used in these cases. Exceptions to this rule are codes Z51.0, Encounter for antineoplastic radiation therapy, and codes from subcategory Z51.1, Encounter for antineoplastic chemotherapy and immunotherapy. These codes are to be first-listed, followed by the diagnosis code when a patient's encounter is solely to receive radiation therapy, chemotherapy, or immunotherapy for the treatment of a neoplasm. If the reason for the encounter is more than one type of antineoplastic therapy, code Z51.0 and a code from subcategory Z51.1 may be assigned together, in which case one of these codes would be reported as a secondary diagnosis.

The aftercare Z codes should also not be used for aftercare for injuries. For aftercare of an injury, assign the acute injury code with the appropriate 7th character (for subsequent encounter).

The aftercare codes are generally first-listed to explain the specific reason for the encounter. An aftercare code may be used as an additional code when some type of aftercare is provided in addition to the reason for admission and no diagnosis code is applicable. An example of this would be the closure of a colostomy during an encounter for treatment of another condition.

Aftercare codes should be used in conjunction with other aftercare codes or diagnosis codes to provide better detail on the specifics of an aftercare encounter visit, unless otherwise directed by the classification. Should a patient receive multiple types of antineoplastic therapy during the same encounter, code Z51.0, Encounter for antineoplastic radiation therapy, and codes from subcategory Z51.1, Encounter for antineoplastic chemotherapy and immunotherapy, may be used together on a record. The sequencing of multiple aftercare codes depends on the circumstances of the encounter.

Certain aftercare Z code categories need a secondary diagnosis code to describe the resolving condition or sequelae. For others, the condition is included in the code title.

Additional Z code aftercare category terms include fitting and adjustment, and attention to artificial openings.

Status Z codes may be used with aftercare Z codes to indicate the nature of the aftercare. For example code Z95.1, Presence of aortocoronary bypass graft, may be used with code Z48.812, Encounter for surgical aftercare following surgery on the circulatory system, to indicate the surgery for which the aftercare is being performed. A status code should not be used when the aftercare code indicates the type of status, such as using Z43.0, Encounter for attention to tracheostomy, with Z93.0, Tracheostomy status.

The aftercare Z category/codes:

Z42	Encounter for plastic and reconstructive surgery following medical procedure or healed injury
Z43	Encounter for attention to artificial openings
Z44	Encounter for fitting and adjustment of external prosthetic device
Z45	Encounter for adjustment and management of implanted device
Z46	Encounter for fitting and adjustment of other devices
Z47	Orthopedic aftercare
Z48	Encounter for other postprocedural aftercare
Z49	Encounter for care involving renal dialysis
Z51	Encounter for other aftercare and medical care

8) Follow-up

The follow-up codes are used to explain continuing surveillance following completed treatment of a disease, condition, or injury. They imply that the condition has been fully treated and no longer exists. They should not be confused with aftercare codes, or injury codes with a 7th character for subsequent encounter, that explain ongoing care of a healing condition or its sequelae. Follow-up codes may be used in conjunction with history codes to provide the full picture of the healed condition and its treatment. The follow-up code is sequenced first, followed by the history code.

A follow-up code may be used to explain multiple visits. Should a condition be found to have recurred on the follow-up visit, then the diagnosis code for the condition should be assigned in place of the follow-up code.

The follow-up Z code categories:

Z08	Encounter for follow-up examination after completed treatment for malignant neoplasm
Z09	Encounter for follow-up examination after completed treatment for conditions other than malignant neoplasm
Z39	Encounter for maternal postpartum care and examination

9) Donor

Codes in category Z52, Donors of organs and tissues, are used for living individuals who are donating blood or other body tissue. These codes are only for individuals donating for others, not for self-donations. They are not used to identify cadaveric donations.

10) Counseling

Counseling Z codes are used when a patient or family member receives assistance in the aftermath of an illness or injury, or when support is required in coping with family or social problems.

The counseling Z codes/categories:

Z30.0-	Encounter for general counseling and advice on contraception
Z31.5	Encounter for procreative genetic counseling
Z31.6-	Encounter for general counseling and advice on procreation
Z32.2	Encounter for childbirth instruction
Z32.3	Encounter for childcare instruction
Z69	Encounter for mental health services for victim and perpetrator of abuse
Z70	Counseling related to sexual attitude, behavior and orientation
Z71	Persons encountering health services for other counseling and medical advice, not elsewhere classified

NOTE Code Z71.84, Encounter for health counseling related to travel, is to be used for health risk and safety counseling for future travel purposes.

Code Z71.85, Encounter for immunization safety counseling, is to be used for counseling of the patient or caregiver regarding the safety of a vaccine. This code should not be used for the provision of general information regarding risks and potential side effects during routine encounters for the administration of vaccines.

Z76.81	Expectant mother prebirth pediatrician visit

11) Encounters for Obstetrical and Reproductive Services

See Section I.C.15. Pregnancy, Childbirth, and the Puerperium, for further instruction on the use of these codes.

Z codes for pregnancy are for use in those circumstances when none of the problems or complications included in the codes from the Obstetrics chapter exist (a routine prenatal visit or postpartum care). Codes in category Z34, Encounter for supervision of normal pregnancy, are always first-listed and are not to be used with any other code from the OB chapter.

Codes in category Z3A, Weeks of gestation, may be assigned to provide additional information about the pregnancy. Category Z3A codes should not be assigned for pregnancies with abortive outcomes (categories O00-O08), elective termination of pregnancy (code Z33.2), nor for postpartum conditions, as category Z3A is not applicable to these conditions. The date of the admission should be used to determine weeks of gestation for inpatient admissions that encompass more than one gestational week.

The outcome of delivery, category Z37, should be included on all maternal delivery records. It is always a secondary code. Codes in category Z37 should not be used on the newborn record.

Z codes for family planning (contraceptive) or procreative management and counseling should be included on an obstetric record either during the pregnancy or the postpartum stage, if applicable.

Z codes/categories for obstetrical and reproductive services:

Z30	Encounter for contraceptive management
Z31	Encounter for procreative management
Z32.2	Encounter for childbirth instruction
Z32.3	Encounter for childcare instruction
Z33	Pregnant state
Z34	Encounter for supervision of normal pregnancy
Z36	Encounter for antenatal screening of mother
Z3A	Weeks of gestation
Z37	Outcome of delivery
Z39	Encounter for maternal postpartum care and examination
Z76.81	Expectant mother prebirth pediatrician visit

12) Newborns and Infants

See Section I.C.16. Newborn (Perinatal) Guidelines, for further instruction on the use of these codes.

Newborn Z codes/categories:

Z76.1	Encounter for health supervision and care of foundling
Z00.1-	Encounter for routine child health examination
Z38	Liveborn infants according to place of birth and type of delivery

13) Routine and administrative examinations

The Z codes allow for the description of encounters for routine examinations, such as, a general check-up, or, examinations for administrative purposes, such as, a pre-employment physical. The codes are not to be used if the examination is for diagnosis of a suspected condition or for treatment purposes. In such cases the diagnosis code is used. During a routine exam, should a diagnosis or condition be discovered, it should be coded as an additional code. Pre-existing and chronic conditions and history codes may also be included as additional codes as long as the examination is for administrative purposes and not focused on any particular condition.

Some of the codes for routine health examinations distinguish between "with" and "without" abnormal findings. Code assignment depends on the information that is known at the time the encounter is being coded. For example, if no abnormal findings were found during the examination, but the encounter is being coded before test results are back, it is acceptable to assign the code for "without abnormal findings." When assigning a code for "with abnormal findings," additional code(s) should be assigned to identify the specific abnormal finding(s).

Pre-operative examination and pre-procedural laboratory examination Z codes are for use only in those situations when a patient is being cleared for a procedure or surgery and no treatment is given.

The Z codes/categories for routine and administrative examinations:

Z00	Encounter for general examination without complaint, suspected or reported diagnosis
Z01	Encounter for other special examination without complaint, suspected or reported diagnosis
Z02	Encounter for administrative examination
	Except: Z02.9, Encounter for administrative examinations, unspecified
Z32.0-	Encounter for pregnancy test

14) Miscellaneous Z codes

The miscellaneous Z codes capture a number of other health care encounters that do not fall into one of the other categories. Certain of these codes identify the reason for the encounter; others are for use as additional codes that provide useful information on circumstances that may affect a patient's care and treatment.

Prophylactic Organ Removal

For encounters specifically for prophylactic removal of an organ (such as prophylactic removal of breasts due to a genetic susceptibility to cancer or a family history of cancer), the principal or first-listed code should be a code from category Z40, Encounter for prophylactic surgery, followed by the appropriate codes to identify the associated risk factor (such as genetic susceptibility or family history).

If the patient has a malignancy of one site and is having prophylactic removal at another site to prevent either a new primary malignancy or metastatic disease, a code for the malignancy should also be assigned in addition to a code from subcategory Z40.0, Encounter for prophylactic surgery for risk factors related to malignant neoplasms. A Z40.0 code should not be assigned if the patient is having organ removal for treatment of a malignancy, such as the removal of the testes for the treatment of prostate cancer.

Miscellaneous Z codes/categories:

Z28	Immunization not carried out
	Except: Z28.3, Underimmunization status
Z29	Encounter for other prophylactic measures
Z40	Encounter for prophylactic surgery
Z41	Encounter for procedures for purposes other than remedying health state
	Except: Z41.9, Encounter for procedure for purposes other than remedying health state, unspecified
Z53	Persons encountering health services for specific procedures and treatment, not carried out
Z55	Problems related to education and literacy
Z56	Problems related to employment and unemployment
Z57	Occupational exposure to risk factors
Z58	Problems related to physical environment
Z59	Problems related to housing and economic circumstances
Z60	Problems related to social environment
Z62	Problems related to upbringing
Z63	Other problems related to primary support group, including family circumstances
Z64	Problems related to certain psychosocial circumstances
Z65	Problems related to other psychosocial circumstances
Z72	Problems related to lifestyle
	Note: These codes should be assigned only when the documentation specifies that the patient has an associated problem.
Z73	Problems related to life management difficulty
Z74	Problems related to care provider dependency
	Except: Z74.01, Bed confinement status
Z75	Problems related to medical facilities and other health care
Z76.0	Encounter for issue of repeat prescription
Z76.3	Healthy person accompanying sick person
Z76.4	Other boarder to healthcare facility
Z76.5	Malingerer [conscious simulation]
Z91.1-	Patient's noncompliance with medical treatment and regimen
Z91.83	Wandering in diseases classified elsewhere
Z91.84-	Oral health risk factors
Z91.89	Other specified personal risk factors, not elsewhere classified

See Section I.B.14 for Z55-Z65 Persons with potential health hazards related to socioeconomic and psychosocial circumstances, documentation by clinicians other than the patient's provider.

15) Nonspecific Z codes

Certain Z codes are so non-specific, or potentially redundant with other codes in the classification, that there can be little justification for their use in the inpatient setting. Their use in the outpatient setting should be limited to those instances when there is no further documentation to permit more precise coding. Otherwise, any sign or symptom or any other reason for visit that is captured in another code should be used.

Nonspecific Z codes/categories:

Z02.9	Encounter for administrative examinations, unspecified
Z04.9	Encounter for examination and observation for unspecified reason
Z13.9	Encounter for screening, unspecified
Z41.9	Encounter for procedure for purposes other than remedying health state, unspecified
Z52.9	Donor of unspecified organ or tissue
Z86.59	Personal history of other mental and behavioral disorders
Z88.9	Allergy status to unspecified drugs, medicaments and biological substances status
Z92.0	Personal history of contraception

16) Z Codes That May Only be Principal/First-Listed Diagnosis

The following Z codes/categories may only be reported as the principal/first-listed diagnosis, except when there are multiple encounters on the same day and the medical records for the encounters are combined:

Z00	Encounter for general examination without complaint, suspected or reported diagnosis Except: Z00.6
Z01	Encounter for other special examination without complaint, suspected or reported diagnosis
Z02	Encounter for administrative examination
Z03	Encounter for medical observation for suspected diseases and conditions ruled out
Z04	Encounter for examination and observation for other reasons
Z33.2	Encounter for elective termination of pregnancy
Z31.81	Encounter for male factor infertility in female patient
Z31.83	Encounter for assisted reproductive fertility procedure cycle
Z31.84	Encounter for fertility preservation procedure
Z34	Encounter for supervision of normal pregnancy
Z39	Encounter for maternal postpartum care and examination
Z38	Liveborn infants according to place of birth and type of delivery
Z40	Encounter for prophylactic surgery
Z42	Encounter for plastic and reconstructive surgery following medical procedure or healed injury
Z51.0	Encounter for antineoplastic radiation therapy
Z51.1-	Encounter for antineoplastic chemotherapy and immunotherapy
Z52	Donors of organs and tissues Except: Z52.9, Donor of unspecified organ or tissue
Z76.1	Encounter for health supervision and care of foundling
Z76.2	Encounter for health supervision and care of other healthy infant and child
Z99.12	Encounter for respirator [ventilator] dependence during power failure

17) Social Determinants of Health

Codes describing social determinants of health (SDOH) should be assigned when this information is documented.

For social determinants of health, such as information found in categories Z55-Z65, Persons with potential health hazards related to socioeconomic and psychosocial circumstances, code assignment may be based on medical record documentation from clinicians involved in the care of the patient who are not the patient's provider since this information represents social information, rather than medical diagnoses. **For example, coding professionals may utilize documentation of social information from social workers, community health workers, case managers, or nurses, if their documentation is included in the official medical record.**

Patient self-reported documentation may be used to assign codes for social determinants of health, as long as the patient self-reported information is signed-off by and incorporated into the medical record by either a clinician or provider.

Social determinants of health codes are located primarily in these Z code categories:

Z55	**Problems related to education and literacy**
Z56	**Problems related to employment and unemployment**
Z57	**Occupational exposure to risk factors**
Z58	**Problems related to physical environment**
Z59	**Problems related to housing and economic circumstances**
Z60	**Problems related to social environment**
Z62	**Problems related to upbringing**
Z63	**Other problems related to primary support group, including family circumstances**
Z64	**Problems related to certain psychosocial circumstances**
Z65	**Problems related to other psychosocial circumstances**

See Section I.B.14. Documentation by Clinicians Other than the Patient's Provider.

22. **Chapter 22: Codes for Special Purposes (U00-U85)**

U07.0 Vaping-related disorder (*see Section I.C.10.e, Vaping-related disorders*)

U07.1 COVID-19 (*see Section I.C.1.g.1., COVID-19 infection*)

U09.9 Post COVID-19 condition, unspecified (*see Section I.C.1.g.1.m*)

Section II. Selection of Principal Diagnosis

The circumstances of inpatient admission always govern the selection of principal diagnosis. The principal diagnosis is defined in the Uniform Hospital Discharge Data Set (UHDDS) as "that condition established after study to be chiefly responsible for occasioning the admission of the patient to the hospital for care."

The UHDDS definitions are used by hospitals to report inpatient data elements in a standardized manner. These data elements and their definitions can be found in the July 31, 1985, Federal Register (Vol. 50, No, 147), pp. 31038–40.

Since that time the application of the UHDDS definitions has been expanded to include all non-outpatient settings (acute care, short term, long term care and psychiatric hospitals; home health agencies; rehab facilities; nursing homes, etc). The UHDDS definitions also apply to hospice services (all levels of care).

In determining principal diagnosis, coding conventions in the ICD-10-CM, the Tabular List and Alphabetic Index take precedence over these official coding guidelines.
(See Section I.A., Conventions for the ICD-10-CM)

The importance of consistent, complete documentation in the medical record cannot be overemphasized. Without such documentation the application of all coding guidelines is a difficult, if not impossible, task.

A. Codes for Symptoms, Signs, and Ill-Defined Conditions

Codes for symptoms, signs, and ill-defined conditions from Chapter 18 are not to be used as principal diagnosis when a related definitive diagnosis has been established.

B. Two or More Interrelated Conditions, Each Potentially Meeting the Definition for Principal Diagnosis

When there are two or more interrelated conditions (such as diseases in the same ICD-10-CM chapter or manifestations characteristically associated with a certain disease) potentially meeting the definition of principal diagnosis, either condition may be sequenced first, unless the circumstances of the admission, the therapy provided, the Tabular List, or the Alphabetic Index indicate otherwise.

C. Two or More Diagnoses that Equally Meet the Definition for Principal Diagnosis

In the unusual instance when two or more diagnoses equally meet the criteria for principal diagnosis as determined by the circumstances of admission, diagnostic workup and/or therapy provided, and the Alphabetic Index, Tabular List, or another coding guidelines does not provide sequencing direction, any one of the diagnoses may be sequenced first.

D. Two or More Comparative or Contrasting Conditions

In those rare instances when two or more contrasting or comparative diagnoses are documented as "either/or" (or similar terminology), they are coded as if the diagnoses were confirmed and the diagnoses are sequenced according to the circumstances of the admission. If no further determination can be made as to which diagnosis should be principal, either diagnosis may be sequenced first.

E. A Symptom(s) Followed by Contrasting/Comparative Diagnoses

GUIDELINE HAS BEEN DELETED EFFECTIVE OCTOBER 1, 2014.

F. Original Treatment Plan not Carried out

Sequence as the principal diagnosis the condition, which after study occasioned the admission to the hospital, even though treatment may not have been carried out due to unforeseen circumstances.

G. Complications of Surgery and Other Medical Care

When the admission is for treatment of a complication resulting from surgery or other medical care, the complication code is sequenced as the principal diagnosis. If the complication is classified to the T80–T88 series and the code lacks the necessary specificity in describing the complication, an additional code for the specific complication should be assigned.

H. Uncertain Diagnosis

If the diagnosis documented at the time of discharge is qualified as "probable", "suspected", "likely", "questionable", "possible", or "still to be ruled out," "compatible with," "consistent with," or other similar terms indicating uncertainty, code the condition as if it existed or was established. The bases for these guidelines are the diagnostic workup, arrangements for further workup or observation, and initial therapeutic approach that correspond most closely with the established diagnosis.

Note: This guideline is applicable only to inpatient admissions to short-term, acute, long-term care and psychiatric hospitals.

I. Admission from Observation Unit

1. Admission Following Medical Observation

When a patient is admitted to an observation unit for a medical condition, which either worsens or does not improve, and is subsequently admitted as an inpatient of the same hospital for this same medical condition, the principal diagnosis would be the medical condition which led to the hospital admission.

2. Admission Following Post-Operative Observation

When a patient is admitted to an observation unit to monitor a condition (or complication) that develops following outpatient surgery, and then is subsequently admitted as an inpatient of the same hospital, hospitals should apply the Uniform Hospital Discharge Data Set (UHDDS) definition of principal diagnosis as "that condition established after study to be chiefly responsible for occasioning the admission of the patient to the hospital for care."

J. Admission from Outpatient Surgery

When a patient receives surgery in the hospital's outpatient surgery department and is subsequently admitted for continuing inpatient care at the same hospital, the following guidelines should be followed in selecting the principal diagnosis for the inpatient admission:

- If the reason for the inpatient admission is a complication, assign the complication as the principal diagnosis.
- If no complication, or other condition, is documented as the reason for the inpatient admission, assign the reason for the outpatient surgery as the principal diagnosis.
- If the reason for the inpatient admission is another condition unrelated to the surgery, assign the unrelated condition as the principal diagnosis.

K. Admissions/Encounters for Rehabilitation

When the purpose for the admission/encounter is rehabilitation, sequence first the code for the condition for which the service is being performed. For example, for an admission/encounter for rehabilitation for rightsided dominant hemiplegia following a cerebrovascular infarction, report code I69.351, Hemiplegia and hemiparesis following cerebral infarction affecting right dominant side, as the first-listed or principal diagnosis.

If the condition for which the rehabilitation service is being provided is no longer present, report the appropriate aftercare code as the first-listed or principal diagnosis, unless the rehabilitation service is being provided following an injury. For rehabilitation services following active treatment of an injury, assign the injury code with the appropriate seventh character for subsequent encounter as the first-listed or principal diagnosis. For example, if a patient with severe degenerative osteoarthritis of the hip, underwent hip replacement and the current encounter/admission is for rehabilitation, report code Z47.1, Aftercare following joint replacement surgery, as the first-listed or principal diagnosis. If the patient requires rehabilitation post hip replacement for right intertrochanteric femur fracture, report code S72.141D, Displaced intertrochanteric fracture of right femur, subsequent encounter for closed fracture with routine healing, as the first-listed or principal diagnosis.

See Section I.C.21.c.7, Factors influencing health states and contact with health services, Aftercare.
See Section I.C.19.a for additional information about the use of 7th characters for injury codes.

Section III. Reporting Additional Diagnoses

GENERAL RULES FOR OTHER (ADDITIONAL) DIAGNOSES

For reporting purposes the definition for "other diagnoses" is interpreted as additional conditions that affect patient care in terms of requiring:

- clinical evaluation; or
- therapeutic treatment; or
- diagnostic procedures; or
- extended length of hospital stay; or
- increased nursing care and/or
- monitoring

The UHDDS item #11-b defines Other Diagnoses as "all conditions that coexist at the time of admission, that develop subsequently, or that affect the treatment received and/or the length of stay. Diagnoses that relate to an earlier episode

Official Coding Guidelines

which have no bearing on the current hospital stay are to be excluded." UHDDS definitions apply to inpatients in acute-care, short-term, long term care and psychiatric hospital setting. The UHDDS definitions are used by acute-care shortterm hospitals to report inpatient data elements in a standardized manner. These data elements and their definitions can be found in the July 31, 1985, *Federal Register* (Vol. 50, No, 147), pp. 31038–40.

Since that time the application of the UHDDS definitions has been expanded to include all nonoutpatient settings (acute-care, short-term, long-term care and psychiatric hospitals; home health agencies; rehab facilities; nursing homes, etc). The UHDDS definitions also apply to hospice services (all levels of care).

The following guidelines are to be applied in designating "other diagnoses" when neither the Alphabetic Index nor the Tabular List in ICD-10-CM provide direction. The listing of the diagnoses in the patient record is the responsibility of the attending provider.

A. Previous Conditions

If the provider has included a diagnosis in the final diagnostic statement, such as the discharge summary or the face sheet, it should ordinarily be coded. Some providers include in the diagnostic statement resolved conditions or diagnoses and status-post procedures from previous admission that have no bearing on the current stay. Such conditions are not to be reported and are coded only if required by hospital policy.

However, history codes (categories Z80–Z87) may be used as secondary codes if the historical condition or family history has an impact on current care or influences treatment.

B. Abnormal Findings

Abnormal findings (laboratory, x-ray, pathologic, and other diagnostic results) are not coded and reported unless the provider indicates their clinical significance. If the findings are outside the normal range and the attending provider has ordered other tests to evaluate the condition or prescribed treatment, it is appropriate to ask the provider whether the abnormal finding should be added.

Please note: This differs from the coding practices in the outpatient setting for coding encounters for diagnostic tests that have been interpreted by a provider.

C. Uncertain Diagnosis

If the diagnosis documented at the time of discharge is qualified as "probable", "suspected", "likely", "questionable", "possible", or "still to be ruled out," "compatible with," "consistent with," or other similar terms indicating uncertainty, code the condition as if it existed or was established. The bases for these guidelines are the diagnostic workup, arrangements for further workup or observation, and initial therapeutic approach that correspond most closely with the established diagnosis.

Note: This guideline is applicable only to inpatient admissions to short-term, acute-care, long-term care and psychiatric hospitals.

Section IV. Diagnostic Coding and Reporting Guidelines for Outpatient Services

These coding guidelines for outpatient diagnoses have been approved for use by hospitals/ providers in coding and reporting hospital-based outpatient services and provider-based office visits. Guidelines in Section I, Conventions, general coding guidelines and chapter-specific guidelines, should also be applied for outpatient services and office visits.

Information about the use of certain abbreviations, punctuation, symbols, and other conventions used in the ICD-10-CM Tabular List (code numbers and titles), can be found in Section IA of these guidelines, under "Conventions Used in the Tabular List." Section I.B. contains general guidelines that apply to the entire classification. Section I.C. contains chapter-specific guidelines that correspond to the chapters as they are arranged in the classification. Information about the correct sequence to use in finding a code is also described in Section I.

The terms encounter and visit are often used interchangeably in describing outpatient service contacts and, therefore, appear together in these guidelines without distinguishing one from the other.

Though the conventions and general guidelines apply to all settings, coding guidelines for outpatient and provider reporting of diagnoses will vary in a number of instances from those for inpatient diagnoses, recognizing that:

The Uniform Hospital Discharge Data Set (UHDDS) definition of principal diagnosis does not apply to hospital-based outpatient services and provider-based office visits.

Coding guidelines for inconclusive diagnoses (probable, suspected, rule out, etc.) were developed for inpatient reporting and do not apply to outpatients.

A. Selection of First-Listed Condition

In the outpatient setting, the term first-listed diagnosis is used in lieu of principal diagnosis.

In determining the first-listed diagnosis the coding conventions of ICD-10-CM, as well as the general and disease specific guidelines take precedence over the outpatient guidelines.

Diagnoses often are not established at the time of the initial encounter/visit. It may take two or more visits before the diagnosis is confirmed.

The most critical rule involves beginning the search for the correct code assignment through the Alphabetic Index. Never begin searching initially in the Tabular List as this will lead to coding errors.

1. Outpatient Surgery

When a patient presents for outpatient surgery (same day surgery), code the reason for the surgery as the first-listed diagnosis (reason for the encounter), even if the surgery is not performed due to a contraindication.

2. Observation Stay

When a patient is admitted for observation for a medical condition, assign a code for the medical condition as the first-listed diagnosis.

When a patient presents for outpatient surgery and develops complications requiring admission to observation, code the reason for the surgery as the first reported diagnosis (reason for the encounter), followed by codes for the complications as secondary diagnoses.

B. Codes from A00.0–T88.9, Z00–Z99, *U00–U85*

The appropriate code(s) from A00.0–T88.9, Z00–Z99 **and U00–U85** must be used to identify diagnoses, symptoms, conditions, problems, complaints, or other reason(s) for the encounter/visit.

C. Accurate Reporting of ICD-10-CM Diagnosis Codes

For accurate reporting of ICD-10-CM diagnosis codes, the documentation should describe the patient's condition, using terminology which includes specific diagnoses as well as symptoms, problems, or reasons for the encounter. There are ICD-10-CM codes to describe all of these.

D. Codes that Describe Symptoms and Signs

Codes that describe symptoms and signs, as opposed to diagnoses, are acceptable for reporting purposes when a diagnosis has not been established (confirmed) by the provider. Chapter 18 of ICD-10-CM, Symptoms, Signs, and Abnormal Clinical, and Laboratory Findings Not Elsewhere Classified (codes R00–R99) contain many, but not all codes for symptoms.

E. Encounters for Circumstances Other than a Disease or Injury

ICD-10-CM provides codes to deal with encounters for circumstances other than a disease or injury. The Factors Influencing Health Status and Contact with Health Services codes (Z00–Z99) are provided to deal with occasions when circumstances other than a disease or injury are recorded as diagnosis or problems.

See Section I.C.21. Factors influencing health status and contact with health services.

F. Level of Detail in Coding

1. ICD-10-CM Codes with 3, 4, 5, 6, Or 7 Characters

ICD-10-CM is composed of codes with 3, 4, 5, 6, or 7 characters. Codes with three characters are included in ICD-10-CM as the heading of a category of codes that may be further subdivided by the use of fourth, fifth, sixth, or seventh characters to provide greater specificity.

2. Use of Full Number of Characters Required for a Code

A three-character code is to be used only if it is not further subdivided. A code is invalid if it has not been coded to the full number of characters required for that code, including the 7th character, if applicable.

3. Highest level of specificity

Code to the highest level of specificity when supported by the medical record documentation.

G. ICD-10-CM Code for the Diagnosis, Condition, Problem, or Other Reason for Encounter/Visit

List first the ICD-10-CM code for the diagnosis, condition, problem, or other reason for encounter/visit shown in the medical record to be chiefly responsible for the services provided. List additional codes that describe any coexisting conditions. In some cases the first-listed diagnosis may be a symptom when a diagnosis has not been established (confirmed) by the provider.

H. Uncertain Diagnosis

Do not code diagnoses documented as "probable", "suspected," "questionable," "rule out," "compatible with," "consistent with," or "working diagnosis" or other similar terms indicating uncertainty. Rather, code the condition(s) to the highest degree of certainty for that encounter/visit, such as symptoms, signs, abnormal test results, or other reason for the visit.

Please note: This differs from the coding practices used by short-term, acute-care, long-term care and psychiatric hospitals.

I. Chronic Diseases

Chronic diseases treated on an ongoing basis may be coded and reported as many times as the patient receives treatment and care for the condition(s).

J. Code All Documented Conditions that Coexist

Code all documented conditions that coexist at the time of the encounter/visit, and require or affect patient care treatment or management. Do not code conditions that were previously treated and no longer exist. However, history codes (categories Z80–Z87) may be used as secondary codes if the historical condition or family history has an impact on current care or influences treatment.

K. Patients Receiving Diagnostic Services Only

For patients receiving diagnostic services only during an encounter/visit, sequence first the diagnosis, condition, problem, or other reason for encounter/visit shown in the medical record to be chiefly responsible for the outpatient services provided during the encounter/visit. Codes for other diagnoses (e.g., chronic conditions) may be sequenced as additional diagnoses.

For encounters for routine laboratory/radiology testing in the absence of any signs, symptoms, or associated diagnosis, assign Z01.89, Encounter for other specified special examinations. If routine testing is performed during the same encounter as a test to evaluate a sign, symptom, or diagnosis, it is appropriate to assign both the Z code and the code describing the reason for the non-routine test.

For outpatient encounters for diagnostic tests that have been interpreted by a physician, and the final report is available at the time of coding, code any confirmed or definitive diagnosis(es) documented in the interpretation. Do not code related signs and symptoms as additional diagnoses.

Please note: This differs from the coding practice in the hospital inpatient setting regarding abnormal findings on test results.

L. Patients Receiving Therapeutic Services Only

For patients receiving therapeutic services only during an encounter/visit, sequence first the diagnosis, condition, problem, or other reason for encounter/visit shown in the medical record to be chiefly responsible for the outpatient services provided during the encounter/visit. Codes for other diagnoses (e.g., chronic conditions) may be sequenced as additional diagnoses.

The only exception to this rule is that when the primary reason for the admission/encounter is chemotherapy or radiation therapy, the appropriate Z code for the service is listed first, and the diagnosis or problem for which the service is being performed listed second.

M. Patients Receiving Preoperative Evaluations Only

For patients receiving preoperative evaluations only, sequence first a code from subcategory Z01.81, Encounter for pre-procedural examinations, to describe the pre-op consultations. Assign a code for the condition to describe the reason for the surgery as an additional diagnosis. Code also any findings related to the pre-op evaluation.

N. Ambulatory Surgery

For ambulatory surgery, code the diagnosis for which the surgery was performed. If the postoperative diagnosis is known to be different from the preoperative diagnosis at the time the diagnosis is confirmed, select the postoperative diagnosis for coding, since it is the most definitive.

O. Routine Outpatient Prenatal Visits

See Section I.C.15. Routine outpatient prenatal visits.

P. Encounters for General Medical Examinations with Abnormal Findings

The subcategories for encounters for general medical examinations, Z00.0- and encounter for routine child health examination, Z00.12-, provide codes for with and without abnormal findings. Should a general medical examination result in an abnormal finding, the code for general medical examination with abnormal finding should be assigned as the first-listed diagnosis. An examination with abnormal findings refers to a condition/diagnosis that is newly identified or a change in severity of a chronic condition (such as uncontrolled hypertension, or an acute exacerbation of chronic obstructive pulmonary disease) during a routine physical examination. A secondary code for the abnormal finding should also be coded.

Q. Encounters for Routine Health Screenings

See Section I.C.21. Factors influencing health status and contact with health services, Screening

Appendix I. Present on Admission Reporting Guidelines

Introduction

These guidelines are to be used as a supplement to the *ICD-10-CM Official Guidelines for Coding and Reporting* to facilitate the assignment of the Present on Admission (POA) indicator for each diagnosis and external cause of injury code reported on claim forms (UB-04 and 837 Institutional).

These guidelines are not intended to replace any guidelines in the main body of the *ICD-10-CM Official Guidelines for Coding and Reporting*. The POA guidelines are not intended to provide guidance on when a condition should be coded, but rather, how to apply the POA indicator to the final set of diagnosis codes that have been assigned in accordance with Sections I, II, and III of the official coding guidelines. Subsequent to the assignment of the ICD-10-CM codes, the POA indicator should then be assigned to those conditions that have been coded.

As stated in the Introduction to the ICD-10-CM Official Guidelines for Coding and Reporting, a joint effort between the healthcare provider and the coder is essential to achieve complete and accurate documentation, code assignment, and reporting of diagnoses and procedures. The importance of consistent, complete documentation in the medical record cannot be overemphasized. Medical record documentation from any provider involved in the care and treatment of the patient may be used to support the determination of whether a condition was present on admission or not. In the context of the official coding guidelines, the term "provider" means a physician or any qualified healthcare practitioner who is legally accountable for establishing the patient's diagnosis.

These guidelines are not a substitute for the provider's clinical judgment as to the determination of whether a condition was or was not present on admission. The provider should be queried regarding issues related to the linking of signs/symptoms, timing of test results, and the timing of findings.

Please see the CDC website for the detailed list of ICD-10-CM codes that do not require the use of a POA indicator (https://www.cdc.gov/nchs/icd/icd10cm.htm). The codes and categories on this exempt list are for circumstances regarding the healthcare encounter or factors influencing health status that do not represent a current disease or injury or that describe conditions that are always present on admission.

General Reporting Requirements

All claims involving inpatient admissions to general acute-care hospitals or other facilities that are subject to a law or regulation mandating collection of present on admission information.

Present on admission is defined as present at the time the order for inpatient admission occurs—conditions that develop during an outpatient encounter, including emergency department, observation, or outpatient surgery, are considered as present on admission.

POA indicator is assigned to principal and secondary diagnoses (as defined in Section II of the Official Guidelines for Coding and Reporting) and the external cause of injury codes.

Issues related to inconsistent, missing, conflicting or unclear documentation must still be resolved by the provider.

If a condition would not be coded and reported based on UHDDS definitions and current official coding guidelines, then the POA indicator would not be reported.

Reporting Options

Y—Yes
N—No
U—Unknown
W—Clinically undetermined
Unreported/Not used—(Exempt from POA reporting)

Reporting Definitions

Y = present at the time of inpatient admission
N = not present at the time of inpatient admission
U = documentation is insufficient to determine if condition is present on admission
W = provider is unable to clinically determine whether condition was present on admission or not

Timeframe for POA Identification and Documentation

There is no required timeframe as to when a provider (per the definition of "provider" used in these guidelines) must identify or document a condition to be present on admission. In some clinical situations, it may not be possible for a provider to make a definitive diagnosis (or a condition may not be recognized or reported by the patient) for a period of time after admission. In some cases it may be several days before the provider arrives at a definitive diagnosis. This does not mean that the condition was not present on admission. Determination of whether the condition was present on admission or not will be based on the applicable POA guideline as identified in this document, or on the provider's best clinical judgment.

If at the time of code assignment the documentation is unclear as to whether a condition was present on admission or not, it is appropriate to query the provider for clarification.

Assigning the POA Indicator

Condition is on the "Exempt from Reporting" list

Leave the "present on admission" field blank if the condition is on the list of ICD-10-CM codes for which this field is not applicable. This is the only circumstance in which the field may be left blank.

POA Explicitly Documented

Assign "Y" for any condition the provider explicitly documents as being present on admission.

Assign "N" for any condition the provider explicitly documents as not present at the time of admission.

Conditions diagnosed prior to inpatient admission

Assign "Y" for conditions that were diagnosed prior to admission (example: hypertension, diabetes mellitus, asthma)

Conditions diagnosed during the admission but clearly present before admission

Assign "Y" for conditions diagnosed during the admission that were clearly present but not diagnosed until after admission occurred.

Diagnoses subsequently confirmed after admission are considered present on admission if at the time of admission they are documented as suspected, possible, rule out, differential diagnosis, or constitute an underlying cause of a symptom that is present at the time of admission.

Condition develops during outpatient encounter prior to inpatient admission

Assign "Y" for any condition that develops during an outpatient encounter prior to a written order for inpatient admission.

Documentation does not indicate whether condition was present on admission

Assign "U" when the medical record documentation is unclear as to whether the condition was present on admission. "U" should not be routinely assigned and used only in very limited circumstances. Coders are encouraged to query the providers when the documentation is unclear.

Documentation states that it cannot be determined whether the condition was or was not present on admission

Assign "W" when the medical record documentation indicates that it cannot be clinically determined whether or not the condition was present on admission.

Chronic condition with acute exacerbation during the admission

If a single code identifies both the chronic condition and the acute exacerbation, see POA guidelines pertaining to codes that contain multiple clinical concepts.

If a single code only identifies the chronic condition and not the acute exacerbation (e.g., acute exacerbation of chronic leukemia), assign "Y."

Conditions documented as possible, probable, suspected, or rule out at the time of discharge

If the final diagnosis contains a possible, probable, suspected, or rule out diagnosis, and this diagnosis was based on signs, symptoms or clinical findings suspected at the time of inpatient admission, assign "Y."

If the final diagnosis contains a possible, probable, suspected, or rule out diagnosis, and this diagnosis was based on signs, symptoms or clinical findings that were not present on admission, assign "N".

Conditions documented as impending or threatened at the time of discharge

If the final diagnosis contains an impending or threatened diagnosis, and this diagnosis is based on symptoms or clinical findings that were present on admission, assign "Y".

If the final diagnosis contains an impending or threatened diagnosis, and this diagnosis is based on symptoms or clinical findings that were not present on admission, assign "N".

Acute and Chronic Conditions

Assign "Y" for acute conditions that are present at time of admission and N for acute conditions that are not present at time of admission.

Assign "Y" for chronic conditions, even though the condition may not be diagnosed until after admission.

If a single code identifies both an acute and chronic condition, see the POA guidelines for codes that contain multiple clinical concepts.

Codes That Contain Multiple Clinical Concepts

Assign "N" if at least one of the clinical concepts included in the code was not present on admission (e.g., COPD with acute exacerbation and the exacerbation was not present on admission; gastric ulcer that does not start bleeding until after admission; asthma patient develops status asthmaticus after admission)

Assign "Y" if all parts of the clinical concepts included in the code were present on admission (e.g., duodenal ulcer that perforates prior to admission)

For infection codes that include the causal organism, assign "Y" if the infection (or signs of the infection) were present on admission, even though the culture results may not be known until after admission (e.g., patient is admitted with pneumonia and the provider documents pseudomonas as the causal organism a few days later).

Same Diagnosis Code for Two or More Conditions

When the same ICD-10-CM diagnosis code applies to two or more conditions during the same encounter (e.g. two separate conditions classified to the same ICD-10-CM diagnosis code):

Assign "Y" if all conditions represented by the single ICD-10-CM code were present on admission (e.g. bilateral unspecified age-related cataracts).

Assign "N" if any of the conditions represented by the single ICD-10-CM code was not present on admission (e.g. traumatic secondary and recurrent hemorrhage and seroma is assigned to a single code T79.2, but only one of the conditions was present on admission).

Obstetrical Conditions

Whether or not the patient delivers during the current hospitalization does not affect assignment of the POA indicator. The determining factor for POA assignment is whether the pregnancy complication or obstetrical condition described by the code was present at the time of admission or not.

If the pregnancy complication or obstetrical condition was present on admission (e.g., patient admitted in preterm labor), assign "Y".

If the pregnancy complication or obstetrical condition was not present on admission (e.g., 2nd degree laceration during delivery, postpartum hemorrhage that occurred during current hospitalization, fetal distress develops after admission), assign "N".

If the obstetrical code includes more than one diagnosis and any of the diagnoses identified by the code were not present on admission assign "N" (e.g., Category O11, Pre-existing hypertension with pre-eclampsia).

Perinatal Conditions

Newborns are not considered to be admitted until after birth. Therefore, any condition present at birth or that developed in utero is considered present at admission and should be assigned "Y". This includes conditions that occur during delivery (e.g., injury during delivery, meconium aspiration, exposure to streptococcus B in the vaginal canal).

Congenital Conditions and Anomalies

Assign "Y" for congenital conditions and anomalies except for categories Q00–Q99, Congenital anomalies, which are on the exempt list. Congenital conditions are always considered present on admission.

External Cause of Injury Codes

Assign "Y" for any external cause code representing an external cause of morbidity that occurred prior to inpatient admission (e.g., patient fell out of bed at home, patient fell out of bed in emergency room prior to admission).

Assign "N" for any external cause code representing an external cause of morbidity that occurred during inpatient hospitalization (e.g., patient fell out of hospital bed during hospital stay, patient experienced an adverse reaction to a medication administered after inpatient admission).

Consulting Editor's Note

The Official Coding Guidelines Appendix I, Present on Admission Reporting Guidelines, no longer provides a listing of Present on Admission (POA) exempt codes by category/sub-category. Instead interested parties can view a full list of the POA exempt code list via the National Center for Health Statistics webpage.

Here we are providing an updated 2022 POA exempt code list by category/sub-category to be used as a reference guide for the users of this code book. Users, including educators, can use this list to provide examples of the types of codes included on the POA exempt code list.

B90–B94	Sequelae of infectious and parasitic diseases
E64	Sequelae of malnutrition and other nutritional deficiencies
I25.2	Old myocardial infarction
I69	Sequelae of cerebrovascular disease

M84.7	Nontraumatic fracture, NEC (excluding codes ending in 7th character A)
M97	Periprosthetic fracture around internal prosthetic joint (excluding codes ending in 7th character A)
O09	Supervision of high risk pregnancy
O66.5	Attempted application of vacuum extractor and forceps
O80	Encounter for full-term uncomplicated delivery
O94	Sequelae of complication of pregnancy, childbirth, and the puerperium
P00	Newborn affected by maternal conditions that may be unrelated to present pregnancy
P29.3	Persistent fetal circulation
P78.84	Gestational alloimmune liver disease
P83.8	Other specified conditions of integument specific to newborn
P91.81	Neonatal encephalopathy
P91.82-	Neonatal cerebral infarction
P91.88	Other specified disturbances of cerebral status of newborn
Q00–Q99	Congenital malformations, deformations and chromosomal abnormalities
S00–T88.9	Injury, poisoning and certain other consequences of external causes with 7th character representing subsequent encounter or sequela
V00–V09	Pedestrian injured in transport accident Except V00.81-, Accident with wheelchair (powered) V00.83-, Accident with motorized mobility scooter
V10–V19	Pedal cycle rider injured in transport accident
V20–V29	Motorcycle rider injured in transport accident
V30–V39	Occupant of three-wheeled motor vehicle injured in transport accident
V40–V49	Car occupant injured in transport accident
V50–V59	Occupant of pick-up truck or van injured in transport accident
V60–V69	Occupant of heavy transport vehicle injured in transport accident
V70–V79	Bus occupant injured in transport accident
V80–V89	Other land transport accidents
V90–V94	Water transport accidents
V95–V97	Air and space transport accidents
V98–V99	Other and unspecified transport accidents
W09	Fall on and from playground equipment (except codes ending in 7th character A)
W14	Fall from tree
W15	Fall from cliff
W16	Fall, jump or diving into water (excluding codes that end in 7th character A)
W17.0	Fall into well
W17.1	Fall into storm drain or manhole
W17.3	Fall into empty swimming pool
W17.4	Fall from dock
W17.8	Other fall from one level to another
W18.00	Striking against unspecified object with subsequent fall (excluding codes ending in 7th character A)
W18.01	Striking against sports equipment with subsequent fall
W18.02	Striking against glass with subsequent fall (except codes ending in 7th character A)
W18.09	Striking against other object with subsequent fall (except codes ending in 7th character A)
W18.1	Fall from or off toilet (except codes ending in 7th character A)
W18.2	Fall in (into) shower or empty bathtub (except codes ending in 7th character A)
W18.3	Other and unspecified fall on same level (except codes ending in 7th character A)
W18.4	Slipping, tripping and stumbling without falling (except codes ending in 7th character A)

W21	Striking against or struck by sports equipment
W22.01	Walked into wall (except codes ending in 7th character A)
W22.02	Walked into lamppost
W22.03	Walked into furniture (except codes ending in 7th character A)
W22.04	Striking against wall of swimming pool (except codes ending in 7th character A)
W22.09	Striking against other stationary object (except codes ending in 7th character A)
W22.1	Striking against or struck by automobile airbag
W22.8	Striking against or struck by other objects
W24.0	Contact with lifting devices, not elsewhere classified (except codes ending in 7th character A)
W24.1	Contact with transmission devices, NEC
W26.1–W26.9	Contact with knife, sword or dagger
W27.0	Contact with workbench
W27.1	Contact with garden tool
W27.2	Contact with scissors (except codes ending in 7th character A)
W27.3	Contact with needle (except codes ending in 7th character A)
W27.4	Contact with kitchen utensil (except codes ending in 7th character A)
W27.5	Contact with paper-cutter (except codes ending in 7th character A)
W27.8	Contact with other nonpowered hand tool
W28	Contact with powered lawn mower
W29	Contact with other powered hand tools and household machinery
W30	Contact with agricultural machinery
W31	Contact with other and unspecified machinery
W32–W34	Accidental handgun discharge and malfunction
W35–W40	Exposure to inanimate mechanical forces
W42.0	Exposure to supersonic waves
W42.9	Exposure to other noise (except codes ending in 7th character A)
W45.0	Nail entering through skin
W49	Exposure to other inanimate mechanical forces (except codes ending in 7th character A)
W52	Crushed, pushed or stepped on by crowd or human stampede
W53	Contact with rodent
W54	Contact with dog
W55	Contact with other mammals
W56	Contact with nonvenomous marine animal
W57	Bitten or stung by nonvenomous insect and other nonvenomous arthropods (except codes ending in 7th character A)
W58	Contact with crocodile or alligator
W59.01	Bitten by nonvenomous lizards (except codes ending in 7th character A)
W59.02–W59.8	Contact with other nonvenomous reptiles
W60	Contact with nonvenomous plant thorns and spines and sharp leaves
W61	Contact with birds (domestic) (wild)
W62	Contact with nonvenomous amphibians
W64	Exposure to other animate mechanical forces
W65	Accidental drowning and submersion while in bath-tub (except codes ending in 7th character A)
W67	Accidental drowning and submersion while in swimming pool (except codes ending in 7th character A)
W69	Accidental drowning and submersion while in natural water
W73	Other specified cause of accidental non-transport drowning and submersion
W74	Unspecified cause of accidental drowning and submersion

W85	Exposure to electric transmission lines (except codes ending in 7th character A)
W86	Exposure to other specified electric current (except codes ending in 7th character A)
W88	Exposure to ionizing radiation (except codes ending in 7th character A)
W89	Exposure to man-made visible and ultraviolet light
W90	Exposure to other nonionizing radiation (except codes ending in 7th character A)
W92	Exposure to excessive heat of man-made origin
W93	Exposure to excessive cold of man-made origin
W94	Exposure to high and low air pressure and changes in air pressure
W99	Exposure to other man-made environmental factors
X02	Exposure to controlled fire in building or structure (except codes ending in 7th character A)
X03	Exposure to controlled fire, not in building or structure (except codes ending in 7th character A)
X04	Exposure to ignition of highly flammable material
X30	Exposure to excessive natural heat
X31	Exposure to excessive natural cold
X32	Exposure to sunlight
X34	Earthquake (except codes ending in 7th character A)
X35	Volcanic eruption
X36	Avalanche, landslide and other earth movements (except codes ending in 7th character A)
X37	Cataclysmic storm (except codes ending in 7th character A)
X38	Flood (except codes ending in 7th character A)
X39	Exposure to other forces of nature
X50	Overexertion and strenuous or repetitive movements
X52	Prolonged stay in weightless environment
X71	Intentional self-harm by drowning and submersion (except codes ending in 7th character A) Except X71.0-, Intentional self-harm by drowning and submersion while in bath tub
X72	Intentional self-harm by handgun discharge
X73	Intentional self-harm by rifle, shotgun and larger firearm discharge
X74	Intentional self-harm by other and unspecified firearm and gun discharge
X75	Intentional self-harm by explosive material
X76	Intentional self-harm by smoke, fire and flames
X77	Intentional self-harm by steam, hot vapors and hot objects
X81	Intentional self-harm by jumping or lying in front of moving object
X82	Intentional self-harm by crashing of motor vehicle
X83	Intentional self-harm by other specified means
X92	Assault by drowning and submersion (except codes ending in 7th character A)
X93	Assault by handgun discharge (except codes ending in 7th character A)
X94	Assault by rifle, shotgun and larger firearm discharge (except codes ending in 7th character A)
X95	Assault by other and unspecified firearm and gun discharge (except codes ending in 7th character A)
X96	Assault by explosive material (except codes ending in 7th character A)
X97	Assault by smoke, fire and flames (except codes ending in 7th character A)
X98	Assault by steam, hot vapors and hot objects (except codes ending in 7th character A)
X99	Assault by sharp object (except codes ending in 7th character A)
Y00	Assault by blunt object (except codes ending in 7th character A)
Y01	Assault by pushing from high place (except codes ending in 7th character A)
Y02	Assault by pushing or placing victim in front of moving object
Y03	Assault by crashing of motor vehicle

Y04	Assault by bodily force (except codes ending in 7th character A)
Y07	Perpetrator of assault, maltreatment and neglect
Y08	Assault by other specified means
Y21	Drowning and submersion, undetermined intent
Y22	Handgun discharge, undetermined intent (except codes ending in 7th character A)
Y23	Rifle, shotgun and larger firearm discharge, undetermined intent (except codes ending in 7th character A)
Y24	Other and unspecified firearm discharge, undetermined intent (except Y24.9, Unspecified firearm discharge, undetermined intent, initial encounter)
Y30	Falling, jumping or pushed from a high place, undetermined intent
Y32	Assault by crashing of motor vehicle, undetermined intent
Y35	Legal intervention (except codes ending in 7th character A)
Y36	Operations of war
Y37	Military operations
Y38	Terrorism (except codes ending in 7th character A)
Y92	Place of occurrence of the external cause (except Y92.23-, Y92.530 and Y92.538)
Y93.12–Y93.9	Activity code
Y99	External cause status
Z00	Encounter for general examination without complaint, suspected or reported diagnosis
Z01	Encounter for other special examination without complaint, suspected or reported diagnosis
Z02	Encounter for administrative examination
Z03	Encounter for medical observation for suspected diseases and conditions ruled out
Z04.8-	Encounter for examination and observation for other specified reasons
Z05	Encounter for observation and evaluation of newborn for suspected diseases and conditions ruled out
Z08	Encounter for follow-up examination following completed treatment for malignant neoplasm
Z09	Encounter for follow-up examination after completed treatment for conditions other than malignant neoplasm
Z11	Encounter for screening for infectious and parasitic diseases
Z11.8	Encounter for screening for other infectious and parasitic diseases
Z12	Encounter for screening for malignant neoplasms
Z13	Encounter for screening for other diseases and disorders
Z14	Genetic carrier
Z15	Genetic susceptibility to disease
Z17	Estrogen receptor status
Z18	Retained foreign body fragments
Z19	Hormone sensitivity malignancy status
Z20.821	Contact with and (suspected) exposure to Zika virus
Z22	Carrier of infectious disease
Z23	Encounter for immunization
Z28	Immunization not carried out and underimmunization status
Z29	Encounter for prophylactic measures
Z30	Encounter for contraceptive management
Z31	Encounter for procreative management
Z34	Encounter for supervision of normal pregnancy
Z3A	Weeks of gestation
Z36	Encounter for antenatal screening of mother
Z37	Outcome of delivery
Z38	Liveborn infants according to place of birth and type of delivery
Z39	Encounter for maternal postpartum care and examination

Z40.3	Encounter for prophylactic removal of fallopian tube(s)
Z41	Encounter for procedures for purposes other than remedying health state
Z42	Encounter for plastic and reconstructive surgery following medical procedure or healed injury
Z43	Encounter for attention to artificial openings
Z44	Encounter for fitting and adjustment of external prosthetic device
Z45	Encounter for adjustment and management of implanted device
Z46	Encounter for fitting and adjustment of other devices
Z47	Orthopedic aftercare
Z48	Encounter for other postprocedural aftercare
Z49	Encounter for care involving renal dialysis
Z51	Encounter for other aftercare (except Z51.5, Encounter for palliative care)
Z52	Donors of organs and tissues
Z53.3	Procedure converted to open procedure
Z55	Problems related to education and literacy
Z56	Problems related to employment and unemployment
Z57	Occupational exposure to risk factors
Z58.6	Inadequate drinking-water supply
Z59	Problems related to housing and economic circumstances
Z62.813	Personal history of forced labor or sexual exploitation in childhood
Z63	Other problems related to primary support group, including family circumstances
Z64	Problems related to certain psychosocial circumstances
Z65	Problems related to other psychosocial circumstances
Z65.8	Other specified problems related to psychosocial circumstances
Z67.1–Z67.9	Blood type
Z68	Body mass index (BMI)
Z69	Encounter for mental health services for victim and perpetrator of abuse
Z70	Counseling related to sexual attitude, behavior and orientation
Z71	Persons encountering health services for other counseling and medical advice, NEC
Z72	Problems related to lifestyle
Z73	Problems related to life management difficulty
Z74.01	Bed confinement status
Z75	Problems related to medical facilities and other health care
Z76	Persons encountering health services in other circumstances
Z77.110–Z77.128	Environmental pollution and hazards in the physical environment
Z78	Other specified health status
Z79	Long-term (current) drug therapy
Z80	Family history of primary malignant neoplasm
Z81	Family history of mental and behavioral disorders
Z82	Family history of certain disabilities and chronic diseases (leading to disablement)
Z83	Family history of other specific disorders
Z84	Family history of other conditions
Z85	Personal history of primary malignant neoplasm
Z86	Personal history of certain other diseases
Z87	Personal history of other diseases and conditions
Z87.828	Personal history of other (healed) physical injury and trauma
Z87.891	Personal history of nicotine dependence
Z88	Allergy status to drugs, medicaments and biological substances
Z89	Acquired absence of limb

Z90	Acquired absence of organs, NEC
Z91	Personal risk factors, NEC
Z92	Personal history of medical treatment
Z93	Artificial opening status
Z94	Transplanted organ and tissue status
Z95	Presence of cardiac and vascular implants and grafts
Z96.82	Presence of neurostimulator
Z97	Presence of other devices
Z98	Other postprocedural states
Z99	Dependence on enabling machines and devices, not elsewhere classified

Additional Conventions

The use of symbols and color-coding has been added to this code book to alert the user to Medicare reimbursement logic and edits that are impacted by diagnosis coding. Although some third-party payers have adopted Medicare's reimbursement methodology, others have not. Therefore, it is important to review your facilities payer reporting requirements for non-Medicare payers prior to diagnosis coding.

Some codes may be included in multiple reimbursement issues and, therefore, may have more than one symbol or color-coding feature. For a quick reference review, the legend at the bottom of each page of the Tabular as well as the inside cover of the code book. The symbols and color-coding features are described in detail here.

Tabular Enhancements

In an effort to make the Tabular more user-friendly, the following symbols and color-coding features have been added. These features are indented to help the user in selecting a complete and accurate diagnosis code.

Final Character Indicator

ICD-10-CM codes range in length from 3 to 7 characters. In order for a code to be "valid" it must be listed to the fullest character length available. For example, if a fourth character is available, a three-character code is considered invalid.

To help users comply with this convention, a red plus sign (+) is listed to the left of any subcategory or subclassification code that requires an additional character. For example:

+ **J45.2 Mild intermittent asthma**

The assignment of the seventh character can, at times, be tricky. There are designated categories of codes that require a seventh character even though the code may not already have six characters present. For these codes, the user must insert the placeholder character of X after the code to fill any open characters prior to the seventh character.

To help users comply with this convention, in this book, the phrase **X+7th** is in red and is located to the left of the code that requires the placeholder of X and/or the seventh character. For example:

X+7th M80.00 Age-related osteoporosis with current pathological fracture

Additionally, there are six character codes that require the application of a seventh character. For these codes a placeholder X is not required. To help users differentiate these codes, in this book, the phrase **+7th** is in red and is located to the left of the code that requires the seventh character. For example:

+7th S72.021 Displaced fracture of epiphysis (separation) (upper) of right femur

Lastly, there are some codes that have only three characters. They require no further specification with additional characters and are therefore valid codes. The following note: Valid 3-character code, no further characters required is located below the code description in this book. This note alerts the coder that the three-character code is valid and can be used for reporting.

Color Identification

The Tabular section of this code book contains many instructional notes for the user. In order to help navigate the various types of instructional notes, a color-coding system has been applied:

- Category block headers are presented in dark green font.
- Category codes (three characters) are presented in blue font.
- Includes notes have a gray color bar over the **Includes**
- Excludes1 notes have a yellow color bar over the ***Excludes1***
- Excludes2 notes have a bright green color bar over the ***Excludes2***

- Notes have a maroon color bar over the **NOTE**
- *Use additional code* notes are presented in orange font
- *Code also* notes are presented in orange font
- *Code first* notes are presented in orange font
- Seventh character options are presented in a box and are highlighted in gray

The following excerpt from the Tabular illustrates the color-coding applied in this code book.

Disorders of bone density and structure (M80–M85)

M80 Osteoporosis with current pathological fracture

Includes: osteoporosis with current fragility fracture

Use additional code to identify major osseous defect, if applicable (M89.7-)

Excludes1: *collapsed vertebra NOS (M48.5)*
pathological fracture NOS (M84.4)
wedging of vertebra NOS (M48.5)

Excludes2: *personal history of (healed) osteoporosis fracture (Z87.310)*

The appropriate 7th character is to be added to each code from category M80:
A initial encounter for fracture
D subsequent encounter for fracture with routine healing
G subsequent encounter for fracture with delayed healing
K subsequent encounter for fracture with nonunion
P subsequent encounter for fracture with malunion
S sequela

Medicare Code Edits

Hospital inpatient Medicare claims paid under the Inpatient Prospective payment System (IPPS) are processed through the Medicare Code Editor (MCE) prior to payment by the Medicare administrative contractor (MAC). The code edits are intended to ensure that all claims processed by the MAC are accurate and complete. The information in this manual is based on the MCE v39.

Several of the MCE edits pertain to diagnoses. We have identified the codes included in these edits throughout the Tabular section this manual to assist users with preparing accurate and complete claims. The MCE edits included in this manual:

- Age conflict
- Sex Conflict Edit
- Manifestation codes not allowed as principal diagnosis
- Unacceptable principal diagnoses

Note: It is important to remember these edits are Medicare edits and may not apply to other third-party payers claim processing.

Age Conflict

The age conflict edit is activated when the age of the patient and the type diagnosis code reported does not match. The following symbols are used to identify the four age conflict categories.

- Newborn diagnosis age 0: This symbol appears to the left of the applicable code in the Tabular.
- Pediatric diagnosis age 0–17: This symbol appears to the left of the applicable code in the Tabular.
- Maternity diagnosis age 12–55: This symbol appears to the left of the applicable code in the Tabular.
- Adult diagnosis age 15–124: This symbol appears to the left of the applicable code in the Tabular.

Sex Conflict Edit

The sex conflict edit is activated when the sex of the patient and the diagnosis reported does not match. The following symbols are used to identify female-only and male-only diagnoses.

♀ Female-only diagnosis: This symbol appears to the left of the applicable code in the Tabular.

♂ Male-only diagnosis: This symbol appears to the left of the applicable code in the Tabular.

Manifestation Code Not Allowed as Principal Diagnosis

Manifestation codes are used to report the manifestation of an underlying disease, not to report the disease itself. Therefore, within ICD-10-CM the manifestation should not be reported as the principal diagnosis; rather it should always be reported as a secondary diagnosis.

Manifestation codes are identified with a light green color bar over the code in the Tabular. For example:

D63.0 Anemia in neoplastic disease

Unacceptable Principal Diagnosis

There are specified codes that describe a circumstance which influences an individual's health status but not a current illness or injury, or codes that are not specific manifestations but may be due to an underlying cause. These codes are considered unacceptable as a principal diagnosis.

Unacceptable principal diagnosis codes are identified with a light blue color bar over the code in the Tabular:

B60.13 Keratoconjunctivitis due to Acanthamoeba

MS-DRG Diagnosis Designations

The MS-DRG system is utilized within the IPPS to determine the unadjusted reimbursement amount for Medicare hospital inpatient claims. The MS-DRG Definitions Manual includes the logic for MS-DRG refinement and selection as well as logic based on the IPPS final rules released each August. The information in this book is based on the MS-DRG v39. *Note:* It is important to remember that these edits are Medicare edits and may not apply to other third-party payers claim processing.

CC and MCC Codes

Within the MS-DRG system, one of the refinement pathways is whether there is a complication/comorbidity (CC) or major complication/comorbidity (MCC) code reported as a secondary diagnosis. For some of the MS-DRG families, the presence of a CC or MCC allows for an MS-DRG assignment that has a higher relative weight and, therefore, a higher reimbursement amount. There are exceptions to the application of the CC or MCC codes and the exceptions are referred to as *CC Exclusions* or *MCC Exclusions*. If exclusions apply, the CC/MCC code is assigned a principal diagnosis collection. Within this collection are the codes that, when reported as principal diagnosis, excludes the CC/MCC status from the secondary diagnosis code under review. Essentially, it takes away the CC/MCC code's ability to influence the MS-DRG assignment.

Codes that are considered CC codes have a purple **CC** to the left of the code in the Tabular. The principal diagnosis collection for each CC code is provided in Appendix A. Coding professionals may review the principal diagnosis collection identified if required for the task at hand. If the code requires a seventh character, the characters that are eligible for CC status are included within Appendix A.

Codes that are considered MCC codes have a purple **MCC** to the left of the code in the Tabular. The principal diagnosis collection for each MCC code is provided in Appendix A. Coding professionals may review the principal diagnosis collection identified if required for the task at hand. If the code requires a seventh character, the characters that are eligible for MCC status are included within Appendix A.

Hospital-Acquired Conditions Related Diagnoses

As part of the Medicare Value-Based Purchasing program, CMS has implemented a Paying for Value program entitled Hospital-Acquired Conditions (HACs) Present on Admission Indicator Program. This program is designed to reduce reimbursements to facilities where the value of the medical or surgical services have been comprised due to preventable conditions. Reimbursement for admissions that meet the HAC Present on Admission Indicator Program criteria will be reduced. In this manual, the HAC-associated procedures are identified with an orange rectangle **HAC** with HAC. The orange rectangle is located below the code description in the code listing. If there is conditional logic for the diagnosis code, it is included in Appendix B.

AHA *Coding Clinic for ICD-10-CM and ICD-10-PCS*

The American Hospital Association began publishing coding guidance for ICD-10-CM and ICD-10-PCS in the fourth quarter of 2012. In this code book we identify diagnosis codes that are discussed in the *Coding Clinic* guidance fourth quarter 2012 through second quarter 2021. Within the Tabular the following sky-blue note alerts the coder to review the AHA *Coding Clinic* prior to assignment of the code to ensure appropriate and accurate reporting. The quarter of publication, year, and page number(s) are provided in the note.

AHA CC: 4Q; 2012; pg#-pg#

CMS Hierarchical Condition Categories Risk Adjustment System

Since 2004, Medicare has utilized the CMS Hierarchical Condition Categories (CMS-HCC) model to risk adjust within the Medicare Advantage capitation payment system. Using the CMS-HCC model Medicare uses large pools of data to predict average costs for a predetermined set of factors; one of the factors is individual disease groups. The HCC diagnosis code listing is utilized to determine the individual disease groups from Medicare claims data. Additionally, CMS-HCC model is utilized in accountable care organizations payment methodologies (inpatient and outpatient settings) and in Medicare's inpatient acute care (IPPS) value-based purchasing program. The use of the CMS-HCC model for risk adjustment within payment systems continues to grow. Therefore, it is imperative that coding professionals in all settings are familiar with the reporting of HCC diagnosis codes. The most current list of CMS-HCC model diagnosis codes are identified in this code book. The CMS-HCC model is updated each year with an effective date of January 1.

CMS-HCC diagnosis codes are identified with a lavender color bar over the code in the Tabular:

E11.21 Type 2 diabetes mellitus with diabetic nephropathy

Basic Steps in ICD-10-CM Coding

To code each disease or condition completely and accurately, the coder should:

1. Identify all main terms included in the diagnostic statement.
2. Locate each main term in the Alphabetic Index.
3. Refer to any subterms indented under the main term. The subterms form individual line entries and describe essential differences by site, etiology, or clinical type.
4. Follow the instructions (see, see also) provided in the Alphabetic Index if the needed code is not located under the first main entry consulted.
5. Verify the code selected in the Tabular List.
6. Read and be guided by any instructional terms in the Tabular List.
7. Assign codes to their highest level of specificity, up to a total of seven characters if applicable.
8. Continue coding the diagnostic statement until all the component elements are fully identified.

(*Source:* Schraffenberger, L.A. *Basic ICD-10-CM/PCS Coding*, 2020 Edition, pp. 43–44. AHIMA.)

Index to Diseases and Injuries

A

- **Aarskog's syndrome** Q87.19
- **Abandonment** *—see* Maltreatment
- **Abasia** (-astasia) (hysterical) F44.4
- **Abderhalden-Kaufmann-Lignac syndrome** (cystinosis) E72.04
- **Abdomen, abdominal** *—see also* condition
  - acute R10.0
  - angina K55.1
  - muscle deficiency syndrome Q79.4
- **Abdominalgia** *—see* Pain, abdominal
- **Abduction contracture, hip or other joint** *—see* Contraction, joint
- **Aberrant** (congenital) *—see also* Malposition, congenital
  - adrenal gland Q89.1
  - artery (peripheral) Q27.8
    - basilar NEC Q28.1
    - cerebral Q28.3
    - coronary Q24.5
    - digestive system Q27.8
    - eye Q15.8
    - lower limb Q27.8
    - precerebral Q28.1
    - pulmonary Q25.79
    - renal Q27.2
    - retina Q14.1
    - specified site NEC Q27.8
    - subclavian Q27.8
    - upper limb Q27.8
    - vertebral Q28.1
  - breast Q83.8
  - endocrine gland NEC Q89.2
  - hepatic duct Q44.5
  - pancreas Q45.3
  - parathyroid gland Q89.2
  - pituitary gland Q89.2
  - sebaceous glands, mucous membrane, mouth, congenital Q38.6
  - spleen Q89.09
  - subclavian artery Q27.8
  - thymus (gland) Q89.2
  - thyroid gland Q89.2
  - vein (peripheral) NEC Q27.8
    - cerebral Q28.3
    - digestive system Q27.8
    - lower limb Q27.8
    - precerebral Q28.1
    - specified site NEC Q27.8
    - upper limb Q27.8
- **Aberration**
  - distantial *—see* Disturbance, visual
  - mental F99
- **Abetalipoproteinemia** E78.6
- **Abiotrophy** R68.89
- **Ablatio, ablation**
  - retinae *—see* Detachment, retina
- **Ablepharia, ablepharon** Q10.3
- **Abnormal, abnormality, abnormalities** *—see also* Anomaly
  - acid-base balance (mixed) E87.4
  - albumin R77.0
  - alphafetoprotein R77.2
  - alveolar ridge K08.9
  - anatomical relationship Q89.9
  - apertures, congenital, diaphragm Q79.1
  - auditory perception H93.29-

Abnormal, abnormality, abnormalities *(continued)*

  - auditory perception *(continued)*
    - diplacusis *—see* Diplacusis
    - hyperacusis *—see* Hyperacusis
    - recruitment *—see* Recruitment, auditory
    - threshold shift *—see* Shift, auditory threshold
  - autosomes Q99.9
    - fragile site Q95.5
  - basal metabolic rate R94.8
  - biosynthesis, testicular androgen E29.1
  - bleeding time R79.1
  - blood amino-acid level R79.83
  - blood-gas level R79.81
  - blood level (of)
    - cobalt R79.0
    - copper R79.0
    - iron R79.0
    - lithium R78.89
    - magnesium R79.0
    - mineral NEC R79.0
    - zinc R79.0
  - blood pressure
    - elevated R03.0
    - low reading (nonspecific) R03.1
  - blood sugar R73.09
  - bowel sounds R19.15
    - absent R19.11
    - hyperactive R19.12
  - brain scan R94.02
  - breathing R06.9
  - caloric test R94.138
  - cerebrospinal fluid R83.9
    - cytology R83.6
    - drug level R83.2
    - enzyme level R83.0
    - hormones R83.1
    - immunology R83.4
    - microbiology R83.5
    - nonmedicinal level R83.3
    - specified type NEC R83.8
  - chemistry, blood R79.9
    - C-reactive protein R79.82
    - drugs *—see* Findings, abnormal, in blood
    - gas level R79.81
    - minerals R79.0
    - pancytopenia D61.818
    - PTT R79.1
    - specified NEC R79.89
    - toxins *—see* Findings, abnormal, in blood
  - chest sounds (friction) (rales) R09.89
  - chromosome, chromosomal Q99.9
    - with more than three X chromosomes, female Q97.1
    - analysis result R89.8
      - bronchial washings R84.8
      - cerebrospinal fluid R83.8
      - cervix uteri NEC R87.89
      - nasal secretions R84.8
      - nipple discharge R89.8
      - peritoneal fluid R85.89
      - pleural fluid R84.8
      - prostatic secretions R86.8
      - saliva R85.89
      - seminal fluid R86.8
      - sputum R84.8
      - synovial fluid R89.8
      - throat scrapings R84.8
      - vagina R87.89
      - vulva R87.89
      - wound secretions R89.8

Abnormal, abnormality, abnormalities *(continued)*

  - chromosome *(continued)*
    - dicentric replacement Q93.2
    - ring replacement Q93.2
    - sex Q99.8
      - female phenotype Q97.9
        - specified NEC Q97.8
      - male phenotype Q98.9
        - specified NEC Q98.8
      - structural male Q98.6
    - specified NEC Q99.8
  - clinical findings NEC R68.89
  - coagulation D68.9
    - newborn, transient P61.6
    - profile R79.1
    - time R79.1
  - communication *—see* Fistula
  - conjunctiva, vascular H11.41-
  - coronary artery Q24.5
  - cortisol-binding globulin E27.8
  - course, eustachian tube Q17.8
  - creatinine clearance R94.4
  - cytology
    - anus R85.619
      - atypical squamous cells
        - cannot exclude high grade squamous intraepithelial lesion (ASC-H) R85.611
      - atypical squamous cells of undetermined significance (ASC-US) R85.610
      - cytologic evidence of malignancy R85.614
      - high grade squamous intraepithelial lesion (HGSIL) R85.613
      - human papillomavirus (HPV) DNA test
        - high risk positive R85.81
        - low risk postive R85.82
      - inadequate smear R85.615
      - low grade squamous intraepithelial lesion (LGSIL) R85.612
      - satisfactory anal smear but lacking transformation zone R85.616
      - specified NEC R85.618
      - unsatisfactory smear R85.615
    - female genital organs *—see* Abnormal, Papanicolaou (smear)
  - dark adaptation curve H53.61
  - dentofacial NEC *—see* Anomaly, dentofacial
  - development, developmental Q89.9
    - central nervous system Q07.9
  - diagnostic imaging
    - abdomen, abdominal region NEC R93.5
    - biliary tract R93.2
    - bladder R93.41
    - breast R92.8
    - central nervous system NEC R90.89
    - cerebrovascular NEC R90.89
    - coronary circulation R93.1
    - digestive tract NEC R93.3
    - gastrointestinal (tract) R93.3
    - genitourinary organs R93.89
    - head R93.0
    - heart R93.1
    - intrathoracic organ NEC R93.89
    - kidney R93.42-

Abnormal, abnormality, abnormalities *(continued)*

  - diagnostic imaging *(continued)*
    - limbs R93.6
    - liver R93.2
    - lung (field) R91.8
    - musculoskeletal system NEC R93.7
    - renal pelvis R93.41
    - retroperitoneum R93.5
    - site specified NEC R93.89
    - skin and subcutaneous tissue R93.89
    - skull R93.0
    - testis R93.81-
    - urinary organs specified NEC R93.49
    - ureter R93.41
  - direction, teeth, fully erupted M26.30
  - ear ossicles, acquired NEC H74.39-
    - ankylosis *—see* Ankylosis, ear ossicles
    - discontinuity *—see* Discontinuity, ossicles, ear
    - partial loss *—see* Loss, ossicles, ear (partial)
  - Ebstein Q22.5
  - echocardiogram R93.1
  - echoencephalogram R90.81
  - echogram *—see* Abnormal, diagnostic imaging
  - electrocardiogram [ECG] [EKG] R94.31
  - electroencephalogram [EEG] R94.01
  - electrolyte *—see* Imbalance, electrolyte
  - electromyogram [EMG] R94.131
  - electro-oculogram [EOG] R94.110
  - electrophysiological intracardiac studies R94.39
  - electroretinogram [ERG] R94.111
  - erythrocytes
    - congenital, with perinatal jaundice D58.9
  - feces (color) (contents) (mucus) R19.5
  - finding *—see* Findings, abnormal, without diagnosis
  - fluid
    - amniotic *—see* Abnormal, specimen, specified
    - cerebrospinal *—see* Abnormal, cerebrospinal fluid
    - peritoneal *—see* Abnormal, specimen, digestive organs
    - pleural *—see* Abnormal, specimen, respiratory organs
    - synovial *—see* Abnormal, specimen, specified
    - thorax (bronchial washings) (pleural fluid) *—see* Abnormal, specimen, respiratory organs
    - vaginal *—see* Abnormal, specimen, female genital organs
  - form
    - teeth K00.2
    - uterus *—see* Anomaly, uterus
  - function studies
    - auditory R94.120
    - bladder R94.8
    - brain R94.09

Abnormal, abnormality, abnormalities *(continued)*
- function studies *(continued)*
  - cardiovascular R94.30
  - ear R94.128
  - endocrine NEC R94.7
  - eye NEC R94.118
  - kidney R94.4
  - liver R94.5
  - nervous system
    - central NEC R94.09
    - peripheral NEC R94.138
  - pancreas R94.8
  - placenta R94.8
  - pulmonary R94.2
  - special senses NEC R94.128
  - spleen R94.8
  - thyroid R94.6
  - vestibular R94.121
- gait *—see* Gait
  - hysterical F44.4
- gastrin secretion E16.4
- globulin R77.1
  - cortisol-binding E27.8
  - thyroid-binding E07.89
- glomerular, minor (*see also* N00-N07 with fourth character .0) N05.0
- glucagon secretion E16.3
- glucose tolerance (test) (non-fasting) R73.09
- gravitational (G) forces or states (effect of) T75.81
- hair (color) (shaft) L67.9
  - specified NEC L67.8
- hard tissue formation in pulp (dental) K04.3
- head movement R25.0
- heart
  - rate R00.9
    - specified NEC R00.8
  - shadow R93.1
  - sounds NEC R01.2
- hemoglobin (disease) *—see also* Disease, hemoglobin D58.2
  - trait *—see* Trait, hemoglobin, abnormal
- histology NEC R89.7
- immunological findings R89.4
  - in serum R76.9
    - specified NEC R76.8
- increase in appetite R63.2
- involuntary movement *—see* Abnormal, movement, involuntary
- jaw closure M26.51
- karyotype R89.8
- kidney function test R94.4
- knee jerk R29.2
- leukocyte (cell) (differential) NEC D72.9
- liver function test (*see also* Elevated, liver function, test) R79.89
- loss of
  - height R29.890
  - weight R63.4
- mammogram NEC R92.8
  - calcification (calculus) R92.1
  - microcalcification R92.0
- Mantoux test R76.11
- movement (disorder) *—see also* Disorder, movement
  - head R25.0
  - involuntary R25.9
    - fasciculation R25.3
    - of head R25.0
    - spasm R25.2
    - specified type NEC R25.8
    - tremor R25.1

Abnormal, abnormality, abnormalities *(continued)*
- myoglobin (Aberdeen) (Annapolis) R89.7
- neonatal screening P09.9
  - for
    - congenital adrenal hyperplasia P09.2
    - congenital endocrine disease P09.2
    - congenital hematologic disorders P09.3
    - critical congenital heart disease P09.5
    - cystic fibrosis P09.4
    - hemoglobinothies P09.3
    - hypothyroidism P09.2
    - inborn errors of metabolism P09.1
    - neonatal hearing loss P09.6
    - red cell membrane defects P09.3
    - sickle cell P09.3
    - specified NEC P09.8
- oculomotor study R94.113
- palmar creases Q82.8
- Papanicolaou (smear)
  - anus R85.619
    - atypical squamous cells cannot exclude high grade squamous intraepithelial lesion (ASC-H) R85.611
    - atypical squamous cells of undetermined significance (ASC-US) R85.610
    - cytologic evidence of malignancy R85.614
    - high grade squamous intraepithelial lesion (HGSIL) R85.613
    - human papillomavirus (HPV) DNA test
      - high risk positive R85.81
      - low risk postive R85.82
    - inadequate smear R85.615
    - low grade squamous intraepithelial lesion (LGSIL) R85.612
    - satisfactory anal smear but lacking transformation zone R85.616
    - specified NEC R85.618
    - unsatisfactory smear R85.615
  - bronchial washings R84.6
  - cerebrospinal fluid R83.6
  - cervix R87.619
    - atypical squamous cells cannot exclude high grade squamous intraepithelial lesion (ASC-H) R87.611
    - atypical squamous cells of undetermined significance (ASC-US) R87.610
    - cytologic evidence of malignancy R87.614
    - high grade squamous intraepithelial lesion (HGSIL) R87.613
    - inadequate smear R87.615
    - low grade squamous intraepithelial lesion (LGSIL) R87.612
    - non-atypical endometrial cells R87.618
    - satisfactory cervical smear but lacking transformation zone R87.616
    - specified NEC R87.618
    - thin preparaton R87.619

Abnormal, abnormality, abnormalities *(continued)*
- Papanicolaou *(continued)*
  - cervix *(continued)*
    - unsatisfactory smear R87.615
  - nasal secretions R84.6
  - nipple discharge R89.6
  - peritoneal fluid R85.69
  - pleural fluid R84.6
  - prostatic secretions R86.6
  - saliva R85.69
  - seminal fluid R86.6
  - sites NEC R89.6
  - sputum R84.6
  - synovial fluid R89.6
  - throat scrapings R84.6
  - vagina R87.629
    - atypical squamous cells cannot exclude high grade squamous intraepithelial lesion (ASC-H) R87.621
    - atypical squamous cells of undetermined significance (ASC-US) R87.620
    - cytologic evidence of malignancy R87.624
    - high grade squamous intraepithelial lesion (HGSIL) R87.623
    - inadequate smear R87.625
    - low grade squamous intraepithelial lesion (LGSIL) R87.622
    - specified NEC R87.628
    - thin preparation R87.629
    - unsatisfactory smear R87.625
  - vulva R87.69
  - wound secretions R89.6
- partial thromboplastin time (PTT) R79.1
- pelvis (bony) *—see* Deformity, pelvis
- percussion, chest (tympany) R09.89
- periods (grossly) *—see* Menstruation
- phonocardiogram R94.39
- plantar reflex R29.2
- plasma
  - protein R77.9
    - specified NEC R77.8
  - viscosity R70.1
- pleural (folds) Q34.0
- posture R29.3
- product of conception O02.9
  - specified type NEC O02.89
- prothrombin time (PT) R79.1
- pulmonary
  - artery, congenital Q25.79
  - function, newborn P28.89
  - test results R94.2
- pulsations in neck R00.2
- pupillary H21.56-
  - function (reaction) (reflex) *—see* Anomaly, pupil, function
- radiological examination *—see* Abnormal, diagnostic imaging
- red blood cell(s) (morphology) (volume) R71.8
- reflex *—see* Reflex
- renal function test R94.4
- response to nerve stimulation R94.130
- retinal correspondence H53.31
- retinal function study R94.111
- rhythm, heart *—see also* Arrhythmia
- saliva *—see* Abnormal, specimen, digestive organs
- scan
  - kidney R94.4
  - liver R93.2

Abnormal, abnormality, abnormalities *(continued)*
- scan *(continued)*
  - thyroid R94.6
- secretion
  - gastrin E16.4
  - glucagon E16.3
- semen, seminal fluid *—see* Abnormal, specimen, male genital organs
- serum level (of)
  - acid phosphatase R74.8
  - alkaline phosphatase R74.8
  - amylase R74.8
  - enzymes R74.9
    - specified NEC R74.8
  - lipase R74.8
  - triacylglycerol lipase R74.8
- shape
  - gravid uterus *—see* Anomaly, uterus
- sinus venosus Q21.1
- size, tooth, teeth K00.2
- spacing, tooth, teeth, fully erupted M26.30
- specimen
  - digestive organs (peritoneal fluid) (saliva) R85.9
    - cytology R85.69
    - drug level R85.2
    - enzyme level R85.0
    - histology R85.7
    - hormones R85.1
    - immunology R85.4
    - microbiology R85.5
    - nonmedicinal level R85.3
    - specified type NEC R85.89
  - female genital organs (secretions) (smears) R87.9
    - cytology R87.69
      - cervix R87.619
        - human papillomavirus (HPV) DNA test
          - high risk positive R87.810
          - low risk positive R87.820
        - inadequate (unsatisfactory) smear R87.615
        - non-atypical endometrial cells R87.618
        - specified NEC R87.618
      - vagina R87.629
        - human papillomavirus (HPV) DNA test
          - high risk positive R87.811
          - low risk positive R87.821
        - inadequate (unsatisfactory) smear R87.625
      - vulva R87.69
    - drug level R87.2
    - enzyme level R87.0
    - histological R87.7
    - hormones R87.1
    - immunology R87.4
    - microbiology R87.5
    - nonmedicinal level R87.3
    - specified type NEC R87.89
  - male genital organs (prostatic secretions) (semen) R86.9
    - cytology R86.6
    - drug level R86.2
    - enzyme level R86.0
    - histological R86.7
    - hormones R86.1
    - immunology R86.4
    - microbiology R86.5

Abnormal, abnormality, abnormalities *(continued)*
- specimen *(continued)*
  - male genital organs *(continued)*
    - nonmedicinal level R86.3
    - specified type NEC R86.8
  - nipple discharge *—see* Abnormal, specimen, specified
  - respiratory organs (bronchial washings) (nasal secretions) (pleural fluid) (sputum) R84.9
    - cytology R84.6
    - drug level R84.2
    - enzyme level R84.0
    - histology R84.7
    - hormones R84.1
    - immunology R84.4
    - microbiology R84.5
    - nonmedicinal level R84.3
    - specified type NEC R84.8
  - specified organ, system and tissue NOS R89.9
    - cytology R89.6
    - drug level R89.2
    - enzyme level R89.0
    - histology R89.7
    - hormones R89.1
    - immunology R89.4
    - microbiology R89.5
    - nonmedicinal level R89.3
    - specified type NEC R89.8
  - synovial fluid *—see* Abnormal, specimen, specified
  - thorax (bronchial washings) (pleural fluids) *—see* Abnormal, specimen, respiratory organs
  - vagina (secretion) (smear) R87.629
  - vulva (secretion) (smear) R87.69
  - wound secretion *—see* Abnormal, specimen, specified
- spermatozoa *—see* Abnormal, specimen, male genital organs
- sputum (amount) (color) (odor) R09.3
- stool (color) (contents) (mucus) R19.5
  - bloody K92.1
  - guaiac positive R19.5
- synchondrosis Q78.8
- thermography *—see also* Abnormal, diagnostic imaging R93.89
- thyroid-binding globulin E07.89
- tooth, teeth (form) (size) K00.2
- toxicology (findings) R78.9
- transport protein E88.09
- tumor marker NEC R97.8
- ultrasound results *—see* Abnormal, diagnostic imaging
- umbilical cord complicating delivery O69.9
- urination NEC R39.198
- urine (constituents) R82.90
  - bile R82.2
  - cytological examination R82.89
  - drugs R82.5
  - fat R82.0
  - glucose R81
  - heavy metals R82.6
  - hemoglobin R82.3
  - histological examination R82.89
  - ketones R82.4
  - microbiological examination (culture) R82.79
  - myoglobin R82.1
  - positive culture R82.79
  - protein *—see* Proteinuria

Abnormal, abnormality, abnormalities *(continued)*
- urine *(continued)*
  - specified substance NEC R82.998
    - chromoabnormality NEC R82.91
  - substances nonmedical R82.6
- uterine hemorrhage *—see* Hemorrhage, uterus
- vectorcardiogram R94.39
- visually evoked potential (VEP) R94.112
- white blood cells D72.9
  - specified NEC D72.89
- X-ray examination *—see* Abnormal, diagnostic imaging

Abnormity (any organ or part) *—see* Anomaly

Abocclusion M26.29
- hemolytic disease (newborn) P55.1
- incompatibility reaction ABO *—see* Complication(s), transfusion, incompatibility reaction, ABO

Abolition, language R48.8

Aborter, habitual or recurrent *—see* Loss (of), pregnancy, recurrent

Abortion (complete) (spontaneous) O03.9
- with
  - retained products of conception *—see* Abortion, incomplete
- attempted (elective) (failed) O07.4
  - complicated by O07.30
    - afibrinogenemia O07.1
    - cardiac arrest O07.36
    - chemical damage of pelvic organ(s) O07.34
    - circulatory collapse O07.31
    - cystitis O07.38
    - defibrination syndrome O07.1
    - electrolyte imbalance O07.33
    - embolism (air) (amniotic fluid) (blood clot) (fat) (pulmonary) (septic) (soap) O07.2
    - endometritis O07.0
    - genital tract and pelvic infection O07.0
    - hemolysis O07.1
    - hemorrhage (delayed) (excessive) O07.1
    - infection
      - genital tract or pelvic O07.0
      - urinary tract tract O07.38
    - intravascular coagulation O07.1
    - laceration of pelvic organ(s) O07.34
    - metabolic disorder O07.33
    - oliguria O07.32
    - oophoritis O07.0
    - parametritis O07.0
    - pelvic peritonitis O07.0
    - perforation of pelvic organ(s) O07.34
    - renal failure or shutdown O07.32
    - salpingitis or salpingo-oophoritis O07.0
    - sepsis O07.37
    - shock O07.31
    - specified condition NEC O07.39
    - tubular necrosis (renal) O07.32

Abortion *(continued)*
- attempted *(continued)*
  - complicated *(continued)*
    - uremia O07.32
    - urinary tract infection O07.38
    - venous complication NEC O07.35
      - embolism (air) (amniotic fluid) (blood clot) (fat) (pulmonary) (septic) (soap) O07.2
- complicated (by) (following) O03.80
  - afibrinogenemia O03.6
  - cardiac arrest O03.86
  - chemical damage of pelvic organ(s) O03.84
  - circulatory collapse O03.81
  - cystitis O03.88
  - defibrination syndrome O03.6
  - electrolyte imbalance O03.83
  - embolism (air) (amniotic fluid) (blood clot) (fat) (pulmonary) (septic) (soap) O03.7
  - endometritis O03.5
  - genital tract and pelvic infection O03.5
  - hemolysis O03.6
  - hemorrhage (delayed) (excessive) O03.6
  - infection
    - genital tract or pelvic O03.5
    - urinary tract O03.88
  - intravascular coagulation O03.6
  - laceration of pelvic organ(s) O03.84
  - metabolic disorder O03.83
  - oliguria O03.82
  - oophoritis O03.5
  - parametritis O03.5
  - pelvic peritonitis O03.5
  - perforation of pelvic organ(s) O03.84
  - renal failure or shutdown O03.82
  - salpingitis or salpingo-oophoritis O03.5
  - sepsis O03.87
  - shock O03.81
  - specified condition NEC O03.89
  - tubular necrosis (renal) O03.82
  - uremia O03.82
  - urinary tract infection O03.88
  - venous complication NEC O03.85
    - embolism (air) (amniotic fluid) (blood clot) (fat) (pulmonary) (septic) (soap) O03.7
- failed *—see* Abortion, attempted
- habitual or recurrent N96
  - with current abortion *—see* categories O03-O04
  - without current pregnancy N96
  - care in current pregnancy O26.2-
- incomplete (spontaneous) O03.4
  - complicated (by) (following) O03.30
    - afibrinogenemia O03.1
    - cardiac arrest O03.36
    - chemical damage of pelvic organ(s) O03.34
    - circulatory collapse O03.31
    - cystitis O03.38
    - defibrination syndrome O03.1
    - electrolyte imbalance O03.33
    - embolism (air) (amniotic fluid) (blood clot) (fat) (pulmonary) (septic) (soap) O03.2
    - endometritis O03.0

Abortion *(continued)*
- incomplete *(continued)*
  - complicated *(continued)*
    - genital tract and pelvic infection O03.0
    - hemolysis O03.1
    - hemorrhage (delayed) (excessive) O03.1
    - infection
      - genital tract or pelvic O03.0
      - urinary tract O03.38
    - intravascular coagulation O03.1
    - laceration of pelvic organ(s) O03.34
    - metabolic disorder O03.33
    - oliguria O03.32
    - oophoritis O03.0
    - parametritis O03.0
    - pelvic peritonitis O03.0
    - perforation of pelvic organ(s) O03.34
    - renal failure or shutdown O03.32
    - salpingitis or salpingo-oophoritis O03.0
    - sepsis O03.37
    - shock O03.31
    - specified condition NEC O03.39
    - tubular necrosis (renal) O03.32
    - uremia O03.32
    - urinary infection O03.38
    - venous complication NEC O03.35
      - embolism (air) (amniotic fluid) (blood clot) (fat) (pulmonary) (septic) (soap) O03.2
- induced (encounter for) Z33.2
  - complicated by O04.80
    - afibrinogenemia O04.6
    - cardiac arrest O04.86
    - chemical damage of pelvic organ(s) O04.84
    - circulatory collapse O04.81
    - cystitis O04.88
    - defibrination syndrome O04.6
    - electrolyte imbalance O04.83
    - embolism (air) (amniotic fluid) (blood clot) (fat) (pulmonary) (septic) (soap) O04.7
    - endometritis O04.5
    - genital tract and pelvic infection O04.5
    - hemolysis O04.6
    - hemorrhage (delayed) (excessive) O04.6
    - infection
      - genital tract or pelvic O04.5
      - urinary tract O04.88
    - intravascular coagulation O04.6
    - laceration of pelvic organ(s) O04.84
    - metabolic disorder O04.83
    - oliguria O04.82
    - oophoritis O04.5
    - parametritis O04.5
    - pelvic peritonitis O04.5
    - perforation of pelvic organ(s) O04.84
    - renal failure or shutdown O04.82
    - salpingitis or salpingo-oophoritis O04.5
    - sepsis O04.87
    - shock O04.81
    - specified condition NEC O04.89
    - tubular necrosis (renal) O04.82

Abortion *(continued)*
  induced *(continued)*
    complicated *(continued)*
      uremia O04.82
      urinary tract infection O04.88
      venous complication NEC O04.85
        embolism (air) (amniotic fluid) (blood clot) (fat) (pulmonary) (septic) (soap) O04.7
  inevitable O03.4
  missed O02.1
  spontaneous —*see* Abortion (complete) (spontaneous)
    threatened O20.0
  threatened (spontaneous) O20.0
  tubal O00.10-
    with intrauterine pregnancy O00.11-

Abortus fever A23.1

Aboulomania F60.7

Abrami's disease D59.8

Abramov-Fiedler myocarditis(acute isolated myocarditis) I40.1

Abrasion T14.8
  abdomen, abdominal (wall) S30.811
  alveolar process S00.512
  ankle S90.51-
  antecubital space —*see* Abrasion, elbow
  anus S30.817
  arm (upper) S40.81-
  auditory canal —*see* Abrasion, ear
  auricle —*see* Abrasion, ear
  axilla —*see* Abrasion, arm
  back, lower S30.810
  breast S20.11-
  brow S00.81
  buttock S30.810
  calf —*see* Abrasion, leg
  canthus —*see* Abrasion, eyelid
  cheek S00.81
    internal S00.512
  chest wall —*see* Abrasion, thorax
  chin S00.81
  clitoris S30.814
  cornea S05.0-
  costal region —*see* Abrasion, thorax
  dental K03.1
  digit(s)
    foot —*see* Abrasion, toe
    hand —*see* Abrasion, finger
  ear S00.41-
  elbow S50.31-
  epididymis S30.813
  epigastric region S30.811
  epiglottis S10.11
  esophagus (thoracic) S27.818
    cervical S10.11
  eyebrow —*see* Abrasion, eyelid
  eyelid S00.21-
  face S00.81
  finger(s) S60.41-
    index S60.41-
    little S60.41-
    middle S60.41-
    ring S60.41-
  flank S30.811
  foot (except toe(s) alone) S90.81-
    toe —*see* Abrasion, toe
  forearm S50.81-
    elbow only —*see* Abrasion, elbow
  forehead S00.81
  genital organs, external
    female S30.816
    male S30.815

Abrasion *(continued)*
  groin S30.811
  gum S00.512
  hand S60.51-
  head S00.91
    ear —*see* Abrasion, ear
    eyelid —*see* Abrasion, eyelid
    lip S00.511
    nose S00.31
    oral cavity S00.512
    scalp S00.01
    specified site NEC S00.81
  heel —*see* Abrasion, foot
  hip S70.21-
  inguinal region S30.811
  interscapular region S20.419
  jaw S00.81
  knee S80.21-
  labium (majus) (minus) S30.814
  larynx S10.11
  leg (lower) S80.81-
    knee —*see* Abrasion, knee
    upper —*see* Abrasion, thigh
  lip S00.511
  lower back S30.810
  lumbar region S30.810
  malar region S00.81
  mammary —*see* Abrasion, breast
  mastoid region S00.81
  mouth S00.512
  nail
    finger —*see* Abrasion, finger
    toe —*see* Abrasion, toe
  nape S10.81
  nasal S00.31
  neck S10.91
    specified site NEC S10.81
    throat S10.11
  nose S00.31
  occipital region S00.01
  oral cavity S00.512
  orbital region —*see* Abrasion, eyelid
  palate S00.512
  palm —*see* Abrasion, hand
  parietal region S00.01
  pelvis S30.810
  penis S30.812
  perineum
    female S30.814
    male S30.810
  periocular area —*see* Abrasion, eyelid
  phalanges
    finger —*see* Abrasion, finger
    toe —*see* Abrasion, toe
  pharynx S10.11
  pinna —*see* Abrasion, ear
  popliteal space —*see* Abrasion, knee
  prepuce S30.812
  pubic region S30.810
  pudendum
    female S30.816
    male S30.815
  sacral region S30.810
  scalp S00.01
  scapular region —*see* Abrasion, shoulder
  scrotum S30.813
  shin —*see* Abrasion, leg
  shoulder S40.21-
  skin NEC T14.8
  sternal region S20.319
  submaxillary region S00.81
  submental region S00.81
  subungual
    finger(s) —*see* Abrasion, finger
    toe(s) —*see* Abrasion, toe
  supraclavicular fossa S10.81
  supraorbital S00.81

Abrasion *(continued)*
  temple S00.81
  temporal region S00.81
  testis S30.813
  thigh S70.31-
  thorax, thoracic (wall) S20.91
    back S20.41-
    front S20.31-
  throat S10.11
  thumb S60.31-
  toe(s) (lesser) S90.416
    great S90.41-
  tongue S00.512
  tooth, teeth (dentifrice) (habitual) (hard tissues) (occupational) (ritual) (traditional) K03.1
  trachea S10.11
  tunica vaginalis S30.813
  tympanum, tympanic membrane —*see* Abrasion, ear
  uvula S00.512
  vagina S30.814
  vocal cords S10.11
  vulva S30.814
  wrist S60.81-

Abrism —*see* Poisoning, food, noxious, plant

Abruptio placentae O45.9-
  with
    afibrinogenemia O45.01-
    coagulation defect O45.00-
      specified NEC O45.09-
    disseminated intravascular coagulation O45.02-
    hypofibrinogenemia O45.01-
  specified NEC O45.8-

Abruption, placenta —*see* Abruptio placentae

Abscess (connective tissue) (embolic) (fistulous) (infective) (metastatic) (multiple) (pernicious) (pyogenic) (septic) L02.91
  with
    diverticular disease (intestine) K57.80
      with bleeding K57.81
      large intestine K57.20
        with
          bleeding K57.21
          small intestine K57.40
            with bleeding K57.41
      small intestine K57.00
        with
          bleeding K57.01
          large intestine K57.40
            with bleeding K57.41
    lymphangitis - code by site under Abscess
  abdomen, abdominal
    cavity K65.1
    wall L02.211
  abdominopelvic K65.1
  accessory sinus —*see* Sinusitis
  adrenal (capsule) (gland) E27.8
  alveolar K04.7
    with sinus K04.6
  amebic A06.4
    brain (and liver or lung abscess) A06.6
    genitourinary tract A06.82
    liver (without mention of brain or lung abscess) A06.4
    lung (and liver) (without mention of brain abscess) A06.5
    specified site NEC A06.89
    spleen A06.89
  anerobic A48.0
  ankle —*see* Abscess, lower limb

Abscess *(continued)*
  anorectal K61.2
  antecubital space —*see* Abscess, upper limb
  antrum (chronic) (Highmore) —*see* Sinusitis, maxillary
  anus K61.0
  apical (tooth) K04.7
    with sinus (alveolar) K04.6
  appendix K35.33
  areola (acute) (chronic) (nonpuerperal) N61.1
    puerperal, postpartum or gestational —*see* Infection, nipple
  arm (any part) —*see* Abscess, upper limb
  artery (wall) I77.89
  atheromatous I77.2
  auricle, ear —*see* Abscess, ear, external
  axilla (region) L02.41-
    lymph gland or node L04.2
  back (any part, except buttock) L02.212
  Bartholin's gland N75.1
    with
      abortion —*see* Abortion, by type complicated by, sepsis
      ectopic or molar pregnancy O08.0
    following ectopic or molar pregnancy O08.0
  Bezold's —*see* Mastoiditis, acute
  bilharziasis B65.1
  bladder (wall) —*see* Cystitis, specified type NEC
  bone (subperiosteal) —*see also* Osteomyelitis, specified type NEC
    accessory sinus (chronic) —*see* Sinusitis
    chronic or old —*see* Osteomyelitis, chronic
    jaw (lower) (upper) M27.2
    mastoid —*see* Mastoiditis, acute, subperiosteal
    petrous —*see* Petrositis
    spinal (tuberculous) A18.01
      nontuberculous —*see* Osteomyelitis, vertebra
  bowel K63.0
  brain (any part) (cystic) (otogenic) G06.0
    amebic (with abscess of any other site) A06.6
    gonococcal A54.82
    pheomycotic (chromomycotic) B43.1
    tuberculous A17.81
  breast (acute) (chronic) (nonpuerperal) N61.1
    newborn P39.0
    puerperal, postpartum, gestational —*see* Mastitis, obstetric, purulent
  broad ligament N73.2
    acute N73.0
    chronic N73.1
  Brodie's (localized) (chronic) M86.8X-
  bronchi J98.09
  buccal cavity K12.2
  bulbourethral gland N34.0
  bursa M71.00
    ankle M71.07-
    elbow M71.02-
    foot M71.07-
    hand M71.04-
    hip M71.05-
    knee M71.06-

Abscess *(continued)*
- bursa *(continued)*
  - multiple sites M71.09
  - pharyngeal J39.1
  - shoulder M71.01-
  - specified site NEC M71.08
  - wrist M71.03-
- buttock L02.31
- canthus *—see* Blepharoconjunctivitis
- cartilage *—see* Disorder, cartilage, specified type NEC
- cecum K35.33
- cerebellum, cerebellar G06.0
  - sequelae G09
- cerebral (embolic) G06.0
  - sequelae G09
- cervical (meaning neck) L02.11
  - lymph gland or node L04.0
- cervix (stump) (uteri) *—see* Cervicitis
- cheek (external) L02.01
  - inner K12.2
- chest J86.9
  - with fistula J86.0
  - wall L02.213
- chin L02.01
- choroid *—see* Inflammation, chorioretinal
- circumtonsillar J36
- cold (lung) (tuberculous) *—see also* Tuberculosis, abscess, lung
  - articular *—see* Tuberculosis, joint
- colon (wall) K63.0
- colostomy K94.02
- conjunctiva *—see* Conjunctivitis, acute
- cornea H16.31-
- corpus
  - cavernosum N48.21
  - luteum *—see* Oophoritis
- Cowper's gland N34.0
- cranium G06.0
- cul-de-sac (Douglas') (posterior) *—see* Peritonitis, pelvic, female
- cutaneous *—see* Abscess, by site
- dental K04.7
  - with sinus (alveolar) K04.6
- dentoalveolar K04.7
  - with sinus K04.6
- diaphragm, diaphragmatic K65.1
- Douglas' cul-de-sac or pouch *—see* Peritonitis, pelvic, female
- Dubois A50.59
- ear (middle) *—see also* Otitis, media, suppurative
  - acute *—see* Otitis, media, suppurative, acute
  - external H60.0-
- entamebic *—see* Abscess, amebic
- enterostomy K94.12
- epididymis N45.4
- epidural G06.2
  - brain G06.0
  - spinal cord G06.1
- epiglottis J38.7
- epiploon, epiploic K65.1
- erysipelatous *—see* Erysipelas
- esophagus K20.80
- ethmoid (bone) (chronic) (sinus) J32.2
- external auditory canal *—see* Abscess, ear, external
- extradural G06.2
  - brain G06.0
    - sequelae G09
  - spinal cord G06.1
- extraperitoneal K68.19
- eye *—see* Endophthalmitis, purulent

Abscess *(continued)*
- eyelid H00.03-
- face (any part, except ear, eye and nose) L02.01
- fallopian tube *—see* Salpingitis
- fascia M72.8
- fauces J39.1
- fecal K63.0
- femoral (region) *—see* Abscess, lower limb
- filaria, filarial *—see* Infestation, filarial
- finger (any) *—see also* Abscess, hand
  - nail *—see* Cellulitis, finger
- foot L02.61-
- forehead L02.01
- frontal sinus (chronic) J32.1
- gallbladder K81.0
- genital organ or tract
  - female (external) N76.4
  - male N49.9
    - multiple sites N49.8
    - specified NEC N49.8
- gestational mammary O91.11-
- gestational subareolar O91.11-
- gingival *— see* Periodontitis, localized
- gland, glandular (lymph) (acute) *—see* Lymphadenitis, acute
- gluteal (region) L02.31
- gonorrheal *—see* Gonococcus
- groin L02.214
- gum *— see* Periodontitis, localized
- hand L02.51-
- head NEC L02.811
  - face (any part, except ear, eye and nose) L02.01
- heart *—see* Carditis
- heel *—see* Abscess, foot
- helminthic *—see* Infestation, helminth
- hepatic (cholangitic) (hematogenic) (lymphogenic) (pylephlebitic) K75.0
  - amebic A06.4
- horseshoe K61.31
- hip (region) *—see* Abscess, lower limb
- ileocecal K35.33
- ileostomy (bud) K94.12
- iliac (region) L02.214
  - fossa K35.33
- infraclavicular (fossa) *—see* Abscess, upper limb
- inguinal (region) L02.214
  - lymph gland or node L04.1
- intersphincteric K61.4
- intestine, intestinal NEC K63.0
  - rectal K61.1
- intra-abdominal (*see also* Abscess, peritoneum) K65.1
  - following procedure T81.43
    - obstetrical O86.03
  - postprocedural T81.43
    - retroperitoneal K68.11
- intracranial G06.0
- intramammary *—see* Abscess, breast
- intramuscular, following procedure T81.42
  - obstetrical O86.02
- intraorbital *—see* Abscess, orbit
- intraperitoneal K65.1
- intrasphincteric (anus) K61.4
- intraspinal G06.1
- intratonsillar J36
- ischiorectal (fossa) (specified NEC) K61.39
- jaw (bone) (lower) (upper) M27.2

Abscess *(continued)*
- joint *—see* Arthritis, pyogenic or pyemic
  - spine (tuberculous) A18.01
    - nontuberculous *—see* Spondylopathy, infective
- kidney N15.1
  - with calculus N20.0
    - with hydronephrosis N13.6
  - puerperal (postpartum) O86.21
- knee *—see also* Abscess, lower limb
  - joint M00.9
- labium (majus) (minus) N76.4
- lacrimal
  - caruncle *—see* Inflammation, lacrimal, passages, acute
  - gland *—see* Dacryoadenitis
  - passages (duct) (sac) *—see* Inflammation, lacrimal, passages, acute
- lacunar N34.0
- larynx J38.7
- lateral (alveolar) K04.7
  - with sinus K04.6
- leg (any part) *—see* Abscess, lower limb
- lens H27.8
- lingual K14.0
  - tonsil J36
- lip K13.0
- Littre's gland N34.0
- liver (cholangitic) (hematogenic) (lymphogenic) (pylephlebitic) (pyogenic) K75.0
  - amebic (due to Entamoeba histolytica) (dysenteric) (tropical) A06.4
    - with
      - brain abscess (and liver or lung abscess) A06.6
      - lung abscess A06.5
- loin (region) L02.211
- lower limb L02.41-
- lumbar (tuberculous) A18.01
  - nontuberculous L02.212
- lung (miliary) (putrid) J85.2
  - with pneumonia J85.1
    - due to specified organism (*see* Pneumonia, in (due to))
  - amebic (with liver abscess) A06.5
    - with
      - brain abscess A06.6
      - pneumonia A06.5
- lymph, lymphatic, gland or node (acute) *—see also* Lymphadenitis, acute
  - mesentery I88.0
- malar M27.2
- mammary gland *—see* Abscess, breast
- marginal, anus K61.0
- mastoid *—see* Mastoiditis, acute
- maxilla, maxillary M27.2
  - molar (tooth) K04.7
    - with sinus K04.6
  - premolar K04.7
  - sinus (chronic) J32.0
- mediastinum J85.3
- meibomian gland *—see* Hordeolum
- meninges G06.2
- mesentery, mesenteric K65.1
- mesosalpinx *—see* Salpingitis
- mons pubis L02.215
- mouth (floor) K12.2
- muscle *—see* Myositis, infective
- myocardium I40.0
- nabothian (follicle) *—see* Cervicitis
- nasal J32.9
- nasopharyngeal J39.1

Abscess *(continued)*
- navel L02.216
  - newborn P38.9
    - with mild hemorrhage P38.1
    - without hemorrhage P38.9
- neck (region) L02.11
  - lymph gland or node L04.0
- nephritic *—see* Abscess, kidney
- nipple N61.1
  - associated with
    - lactation *—see* Pregnancy, complicated by
    - pregnancy *—see* Pregnancy, complicated by
- nose (external) (fossa) (septum) J34.0
  - sinus (chronic) *—see* Sinusitis
- omentum K65.1
- operative wound T81.49
- orbit, orbital *—see* Cellulitis, orbit
- otogenic G06.0
- ovary, ovarian (corpus luteum) *—see* Oophoritis
- oviduct *—see* Oophoritis
- palate (soft) K12.2
  - hard M27.2
- palmar (space) *—see* Abscess, hand
- pancreas (duct) *—see* Pancreatitis, acute
- parafrenal N48.21
- parametric, parametrium N73.2
  - acute N73.0
  - chronic N73.1
- paranephric N15.1
- parapancreatic *—see* Pancreatitis, acute
- parapharyngeal J39.0
- pararectal K61.1
- parasinus *—see* Sinusitis
- parauterine *—see also* Disease, pelvis, inflammatory N73.2
- paravaginal *—see* Vaginitis
- parietal region (scalp) L02.811
- parodontal *—see* Periodontitis, aggressive, localized
- parotid (duct) (gland) K11.3
  - region K12.2
- pectoral (region) L02.213
- pelvis, pelvic
  - female *—see* Disease, pelvis, inflammatory
  - male, peritoneal K65.1
- penis N48.21
  - gonococcal (accessory gland) (periurethral) A54.1
- perianal K61.0
- periapical K04.7
  - with sinus (alveolar) K04.6
- periappendicular K35.33
- pericardial I30.1
- pericecal K35.33
- pericemental *—see* Periodontitis, aggressive, localized
- pericholecystic *—see* Cholecystitis, acute
- pericoronal *—see* Periodontitis, aggressive, localized
- peridental *—see* Periodontitis, aggressive, localized
- perimetric *—see also* Disease, pelvis, inflammatory N73.2
- perinephric, perinephritic *—see* Abscess, kidney
- perineum, perineal (superficial) L02.215
  - urethra N34.0
- periodontal (parietal) *—see* Periodontitis, aggressive, localized
  - apical K04.7

Abscess *(continued)*
- periosteum, periosteal *—see also* Osteomyelitis, specified type NEC
    - with osteomyelitis *—see also* Osteomyelitis, specified type NEC
        - acute *—see* Osteomyelitis, acute
        - chronic *—see* Osteomyelitis, chronic
- peripharyngeal J39.0
- peripleuritic J86.9
    - with fistula J86.0
- periprostatic N41.2
- perirectal K61.1
- perirenal (tissue) *—see* Abscess, kidney
- perisinuous (nose) *—see* Sinusitis
- peritoneum, peritoneal (perforated) K66.0 (ruptured) K65.1
    - with appendicitis (*see also* Appendicitis) K35.33
    - pelvic
        - female *—see* Peritonitis, pelvic, female
        - male K65.1
    - postoperative T81.49
    - puerperal, postpartum, childbirth O85
    - tuberculous A18.31
- peritonsillar J36
- perityphlic K35.33
- periureteral N28.89
- periurethral N34.0
    - gonococcal (accessory gland) (periurethral) A54.1
- periuterine *—see also* Disease, pelvis, inflammatory N73.2
- perivesical *—see* Cystitis, specified type NEC
- petrous bone *—see* Petrositis
- phagedenic NOS L02.91
    - chancroid A57
- pharynx, pharyngeal (lateral) J39.1
- pilonidal L05.01
- pituitary (gland) E23.6
- pleura J86.9
    - with fistula J86.0
- popliteal *—see* Abscess, lower limb
- postcecal K35.33
- postlaryngeal J38.7
- postnasal J34.0
- postoperative (any site) (*see also* Infection, postoperative wound) T81.49
    - retroperitoneal K68.11
- postpharyngeal J39.0
- posttonsillar J36
- post-typhoid A01.09
- pouch of Douglas *—see* Peritonitis, pelvic, female
- premammary *—see* Abscess, breast
- prepatellar *—see* Abscess, lower limb
- presacral K68.19
- prostate N41.2
    - gonococcal (acute) (chronic) A54.22
- psoas muscle K68.12
- puerperal - code by site under Puerperal, abscess
- pulmonary *—see* Abscess, lung
- pulp, pulpal (dental) K04.01
    - irreversible K04.02
    - reversible K04.01
- rectovaginal septum K63.0
- rectovesical *—see* Cystitis, specified type NEC
- rectum K61.1

Abscess *(continued)*
- renal *—see* Abscess, kidney
- retina *—see* Inflammation, chorioretinal
- retrobulbar *—see* Abscess, orbit
- retrocecal K65.1
- retrolaryngeal J38.7
- retromammary *—see* Abscess, breast
- retroperitoneal NEC K68.19
    - postprocedural K68.11
- retropharyngeal J39.0
- retrouterine *—see* Peritonitis, pelvic, female
- retrovesical *—see* Cystitis, specified type NEC
- root, tooth K04.7
    - with sinus (alveolar) K04.6
- round ligament *—see also* Disease, pelvis, inflammatory N73.2
- rupture (spontaneous) NOS L02.91
- sacrum (tuberculous) A18.01
    - nontuberculous M46.28
- salivary (duct) (gland) K11.3
- scalp (any part) L02.811
- scapular *—see* Osteomyelitis, specified type NEC
- sclera *—see* Scleritis
- scrofulous (tuberculous) A18.2
- scrotum N49.2
- seminal vesicle N49.0
- septal, dental K04.7
    - with sinus (alveolar) K04.6
- serous *—see* Periostitis
- shoulder (region) *—see* Abscess, upper limb
- sigmoid K63.0
- sinus (accessory) (chronic) (nasal) *—see also* Sinusitis
    - intracranial venous (any) G06.0
- Skene's duct or gland N34.0
- skin *—see* Abscess, by site
- specified site NEC L02.818
- spermatic cord N49.1
- sphenoidal (sinus) (chronic) J32.3
- spinal cord (any part) (staphylococcal) G06.1
    - tuberculous A17.81
- spine (column) (tuberculous) A18.01
    - epidural G06.1
    - nontuberculous *—see* Osteomyelitis, vertebra
- spleen D73.3
    - amebic A06.89
- stitch T81.41
    - following an obstetrical procedure O86.01
- subarachnoid G06.2
    - brain G06.0
    - spinal cord G06.1
- subareolar *—see* Abscess, breast
- subcecal K35.33
- subcutaneous *—see also* Abscess, by site
    - following procedure T81.41
        - obstetrical O86.01
    - pheomycotic (chromomycotic) B43.2
- subdiaphragmatic K65.1
- subdural G06.2
    - brain G06.0
        - sequelae G09
    - spinal cord G06.1
- sub-fascial, following an obstetrical procedure O86.02
- subgaleal L02.811
- subhepatic K65.1
- sublingual K12.2
    - gland K11.3
- submammary *—see* Abscess, breast

Abscess *(continued)*
- submandibular (region) (space) (triangle) K12.2
    - gland K11.3
- submaxillary (region) L02.01
    - gland K11.3
- submental L02.01
    - gland K11.3
- subperiosteal *—see* Osteomyelitis, specified type NEC
- subphrenic K65.1
    - following an obstetrical procedure O86.03
    - postoperative T81.43
- suburethral N34.0
- sudoriparous L75.8
- supraclavicular (fossa) *—see* Abscess, upper limb
- supralevator K61.5
- suprapelvic, acute N73.0
- suprarenal (capsule) (gland) E27.8
- sweat gland L74.8
- tear duct *—see* Inflammation, lacrimal, passages, acute
- temple L02.01
- temporal region L02.01
- temporosphenoidal G06.0
- tendon (sheath) M65.00
    - ankle M65.07-
    - foot M65.07-
    - forearm M65.03-
    - hand M65.04-
    - lower leg M65.06-
    - pelvic region M65.05-
    - shoulder region M65.01-
    - specified site NEC M65.08
    - thigh M65.05-
    - upper arm M65.02-
- testis N45.4
- thigh *—see* Abscess, lower limb
- thorax J86.9
    - with fistula J86.0
- throat J39.1
- thumb *—see also* Abscess, hand
    - nail *—see* Cellulitis, finger
- thymus (gland) E32.1
- thyroid (gland) E06.0
- toe (any) *—see also* Abscess, foot
    - nail *—see* Cellulitis, toe
- tongue (staphylococcal) K14.0
- tonsil(s) (lingual) J36
- tonsillopharyngeal J36
- tooth, teeth (root) K04.7
    - with sinus (alveolar) K04.6
    - supporting structures NEC *— see* Periodontitis, aggressive, localized
- trachea J39.8
- trunk L02.219
    - abdominal wall L02.211
    - back L02.212
    - chest wall L02.213
    - groin L02.214
    - perineum L02.215
    - umbilicus L02.216
- tubal *—see* Salpingitis
- tuberculous *—see* Tuberculosis, abscess
- tubo-ovarian *—see* Salpingo-oophoritis
- tunica vaginalis N49.1
- umbilicus L02.216
- upper
    - limb L02.41-
    - respiratory J39.8
- urethral (gland) N34.0
- urinary N34.0
- uterus, uterine (wall) *—see also* Endometritis
    - ligament *—see also* Disease, pelvis, inflammatory N73.2

Absence *(continued)*
- uterus, uterine *(continued)*
    - neck *—see* Cervicitis
- uvula K12.2
- vagina (wall) *—see* Vaginitis
- vaginorectal *—see* Vaginitis
- vas deferens N49.1
- vermiform appendix K35.33
- vertebra (column) (tuberculous) A18.01
    - nontuberculous *—see* Osteomyelitis, vertebra
- vesical *—see* Cystitis, specified type NEC
- vesico-uterine pouch *—see* Peritonitis, pelvic, female
- vitreous (humor) *—see* Endophthalmitis, purulent
- vocal cord J38.3
- von Bezold's *—see* Mastoiditis, acute
- vulva N76.4
- vulvovaginal gland N75.1
- web space *—see* Abscess, hand
- wound T81.49
- wrist *—see* Abscess, upper limb

Absence (of) (organ or part) (complete or partial)
- adrenal (gland) (congenital) Q89.1
    - acquired E89.6
- albumin in blood E88.09
- alimentary tract (congenital) Q45.8
    - upper Q40.8
- alveolar process (acquired) *—see* Anomaly, alveolar
- ankle (acquired) Z89.44-
- anus (congenital) Q42.3
    - with fistula Q42.2
- aorta (congenital) Q25.41
- appendix, congenital Q42.8
- arm (acquired) Z89.20-
    - above elbow Z89.22-
        - congenital (with hand present) *—see* Agenesis, arm, with hand present
            - and hand *—see* Agenesis, forearm, and hand
    - below elbow Z89.21-
        - congenital (with hand present) *—see* Agenesis, arm, with hand present
            - and hand *—see* Agenesis, forearm, and hand
    - congenital *—see* Defect, reduction, upper limb
    - shoulder (following explantation of shoulder joint prosthesis) (joint) (with or without presence of antibiotic-impregnated cement spacer) Z89.23-
        - congenital (with hand present) *—see* Agenesis, arm, with hand present
- artery (congenital) (peripheral) Q27.8
    - brain Q28.3
    - coronary Q24.5
    - pulmonary Q25.79
    - specified NEC Q27.8
    - umbilical Q27.0
- atrial septum (congenital) Q21.1
- auditory canal (congenital) (external) Q16.1
- auricle (ear), congenital Q16.0
- bile, biliary duct, congenital Q44.5
- bladder (acquired) Z90.6
    - congenital Q64.5
- bowel sounds R19.11
- brain Q00.0
    - part of Q04.3

Absence *(continued)*
- breast(s) (and nipple(s)) (acquired) Z90.1-
  - congenital Q83.8
- broad ligament Q50.6
- bronchus (congenital) Q32.4
- canaliculus lacrimalis, congenital Q10.4
- cerebellum (vermis) Q04.3
- cervix (acquired) (with uterus) Z90.710
  - with remaining uterus Z90.712
  - congenital Q51.5
- chin, congenital Q18.8
- cilia (congenital) Q10.3
  - acquired —*see* Madarosis
- clitoris (congenital) Q52.6
- coccyx, congenital Q76.49
- cold sense R20.8
- congenital
  - lumen —*see* Atresia
  - organ or site NEC —*see* Agenesis
  - septum —*see* Imperfect, closure
- corpus callosum Q04.0
- cricoid cartilage, congenital Q31.8
- diaphragm (with hernia), congenital Q79.1
- digestive organ(s) or tract, congenital Q45.8
  - acquired NEC Z90.49
  - upper Q40.8
- ductus arteriosus Q28.8
- duodenum (acquired) Z90.49
  - congenital Q41.0
- ear, congenital Q16.9
  - acquired H93.8-
  - auricle Q16.0
  - external Q16.0
  - inner Q16.5
  - lobe, lobule Q17.8
  - middle, except ossicles Q16.4
    - ossicles Q16.3
  - ossicles Q16.3
- ejaculatory duct (congenital) Q55.4
- endocrine gland (congenital) NEC Q89.2
  - acquired E89.89
- epididymis (congenital) Q55.4
  - acquired Z90.79
- epiglottis, congenital Q31.8
- esophagus (congenital) Q39.8
  - acquired (partial) Z90.49
- eustachian tube (congenital) Q16.2
- extremity (acquired) Z89.9
  - congenital Q73.0
  - knee (following explantation of knee joint prosthesis) (joint) (with or without presence of antibiotic-impregnated cement spacer) Z89.52-
  - lower (above knee) Z89.619
    - below knee Z89.51-
  - upper —*see* Absence, arm
- eye (acquired) Z90.01
  - congenital Q11.1
  - muscle (congenital) Q10.3
- eyeball (acquired) Z90.01
- eyelid (fold) (congenital) Q10.3
  - acquired Z90.01
- face, specified part NEC Q18.8
- fallopian tube(s) (acquired) Z90.79
  - congenital Q50.6
- family member (causing problem in home) NEC —*see also* Disruption, family Z63.32
- femur, congenital —*see* Defect, reduction, lower limb, longitudinal, femur
- fibrinogen (congenital) D68.2
  - acquired D65

Absence *(continued)*
- finger(s) (acquired) Z89.02-
  - congenital —*see* Agenesis, hand
- foot (acquired) Z89.43-
  - congenital —*see* Agenesis, foot
- forearm (acquired) —*see* Absence, arm, below elbow
- gallbladder (acquired) Z90.49
  - congenital Q44.0
- gamma globulin in blood D80.1
  - hereditary D80.0
- genital organs
  - acquired (female) (male) Z90.79
  - female, congenital Q52.8
    - external Q52.71
    - internal NEC Q52.8
  - male, congenital Q55.8
- genitourinary organs, congenital NEC
  - female Q52.8
  - male Q55.8
- globe (acquired) Z90.01
  - congenital Q11.1
- glottis, congenital Q31.8
- hand and wrist (acquired) Z89.11-
  - congenital —*see* Agenesis, hand
- head, part (acquired) NEC Z90.09
- heat sense R20.8
- hip (following explantation of hip joint prosthesis) (joint) (with or without presence of antibiotic-impregnated cement spacer) Z89.62-
- hymen (congenital) Q52.4
- ileum (acquired) Z90.49
  - congenital Q41.2
- immunoglobulin, isolated NEC D80.3
  - IgA D80.2
  - IgG D80.3
  - IgM D80.4
- incus (acquired) —*see* Loss, ossicles, ear
  - congenital Q16.3
- inner ear, congenital Q16.5
- intestine (acquired) (small) Z90.49
  - congenital Q41.9
    - specified NEC Q41.8
  - large Z90.49
    - congenital Q42.9
      - specified NEC Q42.8
- iris, congenital Q13.1
- jejunum (acquired) Z90.49
  - congenital Q41.1
- joint
  - acquired
    - hip (following explantation of hip joint prosthesis) (with or without presence of antibiotic-impregnated cement spacer) Z89.62-
    - knee (following explantation of knee joint prosthesis) (with or without presence of antibiotic-impregnated cement spacer) Z89.52-
    - shoulder (following explantation of shoulder joint prosthesis) (with or without presence of antibiotic-impregnated cement spacer) Z89.23-
  - congenital NEC Q74.8
- kidney(s) (acquired) Z90.5
  - congenital Q60.2
    - bilateral Q60.1
    - unilateral Q60.0

Absence *(continued)*
- knee (following explantation of knee joint prosthesis) (joint) (with or without presence of antibiotic-impregnated cement spacer) Z89.52-
- labyrinth, membranous Q16.5
- larynx (congenital) Q31.8
  - acquired Z90.02
- leg (acquired) (above knee) Z89.61-
  - below knee (acquired) Z89.51-
  - congenital —*see* Defect, reduction, lower limb
- lens (acquired) —*see also* Aphakia
  - congenital Q12.3
  - post cataract extraction Z98.4-
- limb (acquired) —*see* Absence, extremity
- lip Q38.6
- liver (congenital) Q44.7
- lung (fissure) (lobe) (bilateral) (unilateral) (congenital) Q33.3
  - acquired (any part) Z90.2
- menstruation —*see* Amenorrhea
- muscle (congenital) (pectoral) Q79.8
  - ocular Q10.3
- neck, part Q18.8
- neutrophil —*see* Agranulocytosis
- nipple(s) (with breast(s)) (acquired) Z90.1-
  - congenital Q83.2
- nose (congenital) Q30.1
  - acquired Z90.09
- organ
  - of Corti, congenital Q16.5
  - or site, congenital NEC Q89.8
    - acquired NEC Z90.89
- osseous meatus (ear) Q16.4
- ovary (acquired)
  - bilateral Z90.722
  - congenital
    - bilateral Q50.02
    - unilateral Q50.01
  - unilateral Z90.721
- oviduct (acquired)
  - bilateral Z90.722
  - congenital Q50.6
  - unilateral Z90.721
- pancreas (congenital) Q45.0
  - acquired Z90.410
    - complete Z90.410
    - partial Z90.411
    - total Z90.410
- parathyroid gland (acquired) E89.2
  - congenital Q89.2
- patella, congenital Q74.1
- penis (congenital) Q55.5
  - acquired Z90.79
- pericardium (congenital) Q24.8
- pituitary gland (congenital) Q89.2
  - acquired E89.3
- prostate (acquired) Z90.79
  - congenital Q55.4
- pulmonary valve Q22.0
- punctum lacrimale (congenital) Q10.4
- radius, congenital —*see* Defect, reduction, upper limb, longitudinal, radius
- rectum (congenital) Q42.1
  - with fistula Q42.0
  - acquired Z90.49
- respiratory organ NOS Q34.9
- rib (acquired) Z90.89
  - congenital Q76.6
- sacrum, congenital Q76.49
- salivary gland(s), congenital Q38.4
- scrotum, congenital Q55.29
- seminal vesicles (congenital) Q55.4
  - acquired Z90.79

Absence *(continued)*
- septum
  - atrial (congenital) Q21.1
  - between aorta and pulmonary artery Q21.4
  - ventricular (congenital) Q20.4
- sex chromosome
  - female phenotype Q97.8
  - male phenotype Q98.8
- skull bone (congenital) Q75.8
  - with
    - anencephaly Q00.0
    - encephalocele —*see* Encephalocele
    - hydrocephalus Q03.9
      - with spina bifida —*see* Spina bifida, by site, with hydrocephalus
    - microcephaly Q02
- spermatic cord, congenital Q55.4
- spine, congenital Q76.49
- spleen (congenital) Q89.01
  - acquired Z90.81
- sternum, congenital Q76.7
- stomach (acquired) (partial) Z90.3
  - congenital Q40.2
- superior vena cava, congenital Q26.8
- teeth, tooth (congenital) K00.0
  - acquired (complete) K08.109
    - class I K08.101
    - class II K08.102
    - class III K08.103
    - class IV K08.104
    - due to
      - caries K08.139
        - class I K08.131
        - class II K08.132
        - class III K08.133
        - class IV K08.134
      - periodontal disease K08.129
        - class I K08.121
        - class II K08.122
        - class III K08.123
        - class IV K08.124
      - specified NEC K08.199
        - class I K08.191
        - class II K08.192
        - class III K08.193
        - class IV K08.194
      - trauma K08.119
        - class I K08.111
        - class II K08.112
        - class III K08.113
        - class IV K08.114
  - partial K08.409
    - class I K08.401
    - class II K08.402
    - class III K08.403
    - class IV K08.404
    - due to
      - caries K08.439
        - class I K08.431
        - class II K08.432
        - class III K08.433
        - class IV K08.434
      - periodontal disease K08.429
        - class I K08.421
        - class II K08.422
        - class III K08.423
        - class IV K08.424
      - specified NEC K08.499
        - class I K08.491
        - class II K08.492
        - class III K08.493
        - class IV K08.494
      - trauma K08.419
        - class I K08.411
        - class II K08.412
        - class III K08.413
        - class IV K08.414

Absence *(continued)*
tendon (congenital) Q79.8
testis (congenital) Q55.0
acquired Z90.79
thumb (acquired) Z89.01-
congenital —*see* Agenesis, hand
thymus gland Q89.2
thyroid (gland) (acquired) E89.0
cartilage, congenital Q31.8
congenital E03.1
toe(s) (acquired) Z89.42-
with foot —*see* Absence, foot and ankle
congenital —*see* Agenesis, foot
great Z89.41-
tongue, congenital Q38.3
trachea (cartilage), congenital Q32.1
transverse aortic arch, congenital Q25.49
tricuspid valve Q22.4
umbilical artery, congenital Q27.0
upper arm and forearm with hand present, congenital —*see* Agenesis, arm, with hand present
ureter (congenital) Q62.4
acquired Z90.6
urethra, congenital Q64.5
uterus (acquired) Z90.710
with cervix Z90.710
with remaining cervical stump Z90.711
congenital Q51.0
uvula, congenital Q38.5
vagina, congenital Q52.0
vas deferens (congenital) Q55.4
acquired Z90.79
vein (peripheral) congenital NEC Q27.8
cerebral Q28.3
digestive system Q27.8
great Q26.8
lower limb Q27.8
portal Q26.5
precerebral Q28.1
specified site NEC Q27.8
upper limb Q27.8
vena cava (inferior) (superior), congenital Q26.8
ventricular septum Q20.4
vertebra, congenital Q76.49
vulva, congenital Q52.71
wrist (acquired) Z89.12-

Absorbent system disease I87.8

Absorption
carbohydrate, disturbance K90.49
chemical —*see* Table of Drugs and Chemicals
through placenta (newborn) P04.9
environmental substance P04.6
nutritional substance P04.5
obstetric anesthetic or analgesic drug P04.0
drug NEC —*see* Table of Drugs and Chemicals
addictive
through placenta (newborn) (*see also* Newborn, affected by, maternal, use of) P04.40
cocaine P04.41
hallucinogens P04.42
specified drug NEC P04.49
medicinal
through placenta (newborn) P04.19

Absorption *(continued)*
drug NEC *(continued)*
through placenta (newborn) P04.19
obstetric anesthetic or analgesic drug P04.0
fat, disturbance K90.49
pancreatic K90.3
noxious substance —*see* Table of Drugs and Chemicals
protein, disturbance K90.49
starch, disturbance K90.49
toxic substance —*see* Table of Drugs and Chemicals
uremic —*see* Uremia

Abstinence symptoms, syndrome
alcohol F10.239
with delirium F10.231
cocaine F14.23
neonatal P96.1
nicotine —*see* Dependence, drug, nicotine, with, withdrawal
opioid F11.93
with dependence F11.23
psychoactive NEC F19.939
with
delirium F19.931
dependence F19.239
with
delirium F19.231
perceptual disturbance F19.232
uncomplicated F19.230
perceptual disturbance F19.932
uncomplicated F19.930
sedative F13.939
with
delirium F13.931
dependence F13.239
with
delirium F13.231
perceptual disturbance F13.232
uncomplicated F13.230
perceptual disturbance F13.932
uncomplicated F13.930
stimulant NEC F15.93
with dependence F15.23

Abulia R68.89

Abulomania F60.7

Abuse
adult —*see* Maltreatment, adult
as reason for
couple see king advice (including offender) Z63.0
alcohol (non-dependent) F10.10
with
anxiety disorder F10.180
intoxication F10.129
with delirium F10.121
uncomplicated F10.120
mood disorder F10.14
other specified disorder F10.188
psychosis F10.159
delusions F10.150
hallucinations F10.151
sexual dysfunction F10.181
sleep disorder F10.182
unspecified disorder F10.19
withdrawal F10.139
with
perceptual disturbance F10.132
delirium F10.131
uncomplicated F10.130
counseling and surveillance Z71.41

Abuse *(continued)*
alcohol *(continued)*
in remission (early) (sustained) F10.11
amphetamine (or related substance) —*see also* Abuse, drug, stimulant NEC
stimulant NEC F15.10
with
anxiety disorder F15.180
intoxication F15.129
with
delirium F15.121
perceptual disturbance F15.122
withdrawal F15.13
analgesics (non-prescribed) (over the counter) F55.8
antacids F55.0
antidepressants —*see* Abuse, drug, psychoactive NEC
anxiolytic —*see* Abuse, drug, sedative
barbiturates —*see* Abuse, drug, sedative
caffeine —*see* Abuse, drug, stimulant NEC
cannabis, cannabinoids —*see* Abuse, drug, cannabis
child —*see* Maltreatment, child
cocaine —*see* Abuse, drug, cocaine
drug NEC (non-dependent) F19.10
with sleep disorder F19.182
amphetamine type —*see* Abuse, drug, stimulant NEC
analgesics (non-prescribed) (over the counter) F55.8
antacids F55.0
antidepressants —*see* Abuse, drug, psychoactive NEC
anxiolytics —*see* Abuse, drug, sedative
barbiturates —*see* Abuse, drug, sedative
caffeine —*see* Abuse, drug, stimulant NEC
cannabis F12.10
with
anxiety disorder F12.180
intoxication F12.129
with
delirium F12.121
perceptual disturbance F12.122
uncomplicated F12.120
other specified disorder F12.188
psychosis F12.159
delusions F12.150
hallucinations F12.151
unspecified disorder F12.19
withdrawal F12.13
in remission (early) (sustained) F12.11
cocaine F14.10
with
anxiety disorder F14.180
intoxication F14.129
with
delirium F14.121
perceptual disturbance F14.122
uncomplicated F14.120
mood disorder F14.14
other specified disorder F14.188
psychosis F14.159
delusions F14.150
hallucinations F14.151
sexual dysfunction F14.181
sleep disorder F14.182

Abuse *(continued)*
drug NEC *(continued)*
cocaine *(continued)*
with *(continued)*
unspecified disorder F14.19
withdrawal F14.13
in remission (early) (sustained) F14.11
counseling and surveillance Z71.51
hallucinogen F16.10
with
anxiety disorder F16.180
flashbacks F16.183
intoxication F16.129
with
delirium F16.121
perceptual disturbance F16.122
uncomplicated F16.120
mood disorder F16.14
other specified disorder F16.188
perception disorder, persisting F16.183
psychosis F16.159
delusions F16.150
hallucinations F16.151
unspecified disorder F16.19
in remission (early) (sustained) F16.11
hashish —*see* Abuse, drug, cannabis
herbal or folk remedies F55.1
hormones F55.3
hypnotics —*see* Abuse, drug, sedative
inhalant F18.10
with
anxiety disorder F18.180
dementia, persisting F18.17
intoxication F18.129
with delirium F18.121
uncomplicated F18.120
mood disorder F18.14
other specified disorder F18.188
psychosis F18.159
delusions F18.150
hallucinations F18.151
unspecified disorder F18.19
in remission (early) (sustained) F18.11
laxatives F55.2
in remission (early) (sustained) F19.11
LSD —*see* Abuse, drug, hallucinogen
marihuana —*see* Abuse, drug, cannabis
morphine type (opioids) —*see* Abuse, drug, opioid
opioid F11.10
with
intoxication F11.129
with
delirium F11.121
perceptual disturbance F11.122
uncomplicated F11.120
mood disorder F11.14
other specified disorder F11.188
psychosis F11.159
delusions F11.150
hallucinations F11.151
sexual dysfunction F11.181
sleep disorder F11.182
unspecified disorder F11.19

Abuse *(continued)*
- drug NEC *(continued)*
  - opioid *(continued)*
    - with *(continued)*
      - withdrawal F11.13
    - in remission (early) (sustained) F11.11
  - PCP (phencyclidine) (or related substance) —*see* Abuse, drug, hallucinogen
  - psychoactive NEC F19.10
    - with
      - amnestic disorder F19.16
      - anxiety disorder F19.180
      - dementia F19.17
      - intoxication F19.129
        - with
          - delirium F19.121
          - perceptual disturbance F19.122
        - uncomplicated F19.120
      - mood disorder F19.14
      - other specified disorder F19.188
      - psychosis F19.159
        - delusions F19.150
        - hallucinations F19.151
      - sexual dysfunction F19.181
      - sleep disorder F19.182
      - unspecified disorder F19.19
      - withdrawal F19.139
        - with
          - perceptual disturbance F19.132
        - delirium F19.131
        - uncomplicated F19.130
  - sedative, hypnotic or anxiolytic F13.10
    - with
      - anxiety disorder F13.180
      - intoxication F13.129
        - with delirium F13.121
        - uncomplicated F13.120
      - mood disorder F13.14
      - other specified disorder F13.188
      - psychosis F13.159
        - delusions F13.150
        - hallucinations F13.151
      - sexual dysfunction F13.181
      - sleep disorder F13.182
      - unspecified disorder F13.19
      - withdrawal F13.139
        - with
          - perceptual disturbance F13.132
        - delirium F13.131
        - uncomplicated F13.130
    - in remission (early) (sustained) F13.11
  - solvent —*see* Abuse, drug, inhalant
  - steroids F55.3
  - stimulant NEC F15.10
    - with
      - anxiety disorder F15.180
      - intoxication F15.129
        - with
          - delirium F15.121
          - perceptual disturbance F15.122
        - uncomplicated F15.120
      - mood disorder F15.14
      - other specified disorder F15.188
      - psychosis F15.159
        - delusions F15.150
        - hallucinations F15.151
      - sexual dysfunction F15.181
      - sleep disorder F15.182
      - unspecified disorder F15.19

Abuse *(continued)*
- drug NEC *(continued)*
  - stimulant *(continued)*
    - with *(continued)*
      - withdrawal F15.13
    - in remission (early) (sustained) F15.11
  - tranquilizers —*see* Abuse, drug, sedative
  - vitamins F55.4
- hallucinogens —*see* Abuse, drug, hallucinogen
- hashish —*see* Abuse, drug, cannabis
- herbal or folk remedies F55.1
- hormones F55.3
- hypnotic —*see* Abuse, drug, sedative
- inhalant —*see* Abuse, drug, inhalant
- laxatives F55.2
- LSD —*see* Abuse, drug, hallucinogen
- marihuana —*see* Abuse, drug, cannabis
- morphine type (opioids) —*see* Abuse, drug, opioid
- non-psychoactive substance NEC F55.8
  - antacids F55.0
  - folk remedies F55.1
  - herbal remedies F55.1
  - hormones F55.3
  - laxatives F55.2
  - steroids F55.3
  - vitamins F55.4
- opioids —*see* Abuse, drug, opioid
- PCP (phencyclidine) (or related substance) —*see* Abuse, drug, hallucinogen
- physical (adult) (child) —*see* Maltreatment
- psychoactive substance —*see* Abuse, drug, psychoactive NEC
- psychological (adult) (child) —*see* Maltreatment
- sedative —*see* Abuse, drug, sedative
- sexual —*see* Maltreatment
- solvent —*see* Abuse, drug, inhalant
- steroids F55.3
- vitamins F55.4

Acalculia R48.8
- developmental F81.2

Acanthamebiasis (with) B60.10
- conjunctiva B60.12
- keratoconjunctivitis B60.13
- meningoencephalitis B60.11
- other specified B60.19

Acanthocephaliasis B83.8

Acanthocheilonemiasis B74.4

Acanthocytosis E78.6

Acantholysis L11.9

Acanthosis (acquired) (nigricans) L83
- benign Q82.8
- congenital Q82.8
- seborrheic L82.1
  - inflamed L82.0
- tongue K14.3

Acapnia E87.3

Acarbia E87.2

Acardia, acardius Q89.8

Acardiacus amorphus Q89.8

Acardiotrophia I51.4

Acariasis B88.0
- scabies B86

Acarodermatitis (urticarioides) B88.0

Acarophobia F40.218

Acatalasemia, acatalasia E80.3

Acathisia (drug induced) G25.71

Accelerated atrioventricular conduction I45.6

Accentuation of personality traits (type A) Z73.1

Accessory (congenital)
- adrenal gland Q89.1
- anus Q43.4
- appendix Q43.4
- atrioventricular conduction I45.6
- auditory ossicles Q16.3
- auricle (ear) Q17.0
- biliary duct or passage Q44.5
- bladder Q64.79
- blood vessels NEC Q27.9
  - coronary Q24.5
- bone NEC Q79.8
- breast tissue, axilla Q83.1
- carpal bones Q74.0
- cecum Q43.4
- chromosome(s) NEC (nonsex) Q92.9
  - with complex rearrangements NEC Q92.5
    - seen only at prometaphase Q92.8
  - partial Q92.9
  - sex
    - female phenotype Q97.8
  - 13 —*see* Trisomy, 13
  - 18 —*see* Trisomy, 18
  - 21 —*see* Trisomy, 21
- coronary artery Q24.5
- cusp(s), heart valve NEC Q24.8
  - pulmonary Q22.3
- cystic duct Q44.5
- digit(s) Q69.9
- ear (auricle) (lobe) Q17.0
- endocrine gland NEC Q89.2
- eye muscle Q10.3
- eyelid Q10.3
- face bone(s) Q75.8
- fallopian tube (fimbria) (ostium) Q50.6
- finger(s) Q69.0
- foreskin N47.8
- frontonasal process Q75.8
- gallbladder Q44.1
- genital organ(s)
  - female Q52.8
    - external Q52.79
    - internal NEC Q52.8
  - male Q55.8
- genitourinary organs NEC Q89.8
  - female Q52.8
  - male Q55.8
- hallux Q69.2
- heart Q24.8
  - valve NEC Q24.8
    - pulmonary Q22.3
- hepatic ducts Q44.5
- hymen Q52.4
- intestine (large) (small) Q43.4
- kidney Q63.0
- lacrimal canal Q10.6
- leaflet, heart valve NEC Q24.8
- ligament, broad Q50.6
- liver Q44.7
  - duct Q44.5
- lobule (ear) Q17.0
- lung (lobe) Q33.1
- muscle Q79.8
- navicular of carpus Q74.0
- nervous system, part NEC Q07.8
- nipple Q83.3
- nose Q30.8
- organ or site not listed —*see* Anomaly, by site
- ovary Q50.31

Accessory *(continued)*
- oviduct Q50.6
- pancreas Q45.3
- parathyroid gland Q89.2
- parotid gland (and duct) Q38.4
- pituitary gland Q89.2
- preauricular appendage Q17.0
- prepuce N47.8
- renal arteries (multiple) Q27.2
- rib Q76.6
  - cervical Q76.5
- roots (teeth) K00.2
- salivary gland Q38.4
- sesamoid bones Q74.8
  - foot Q74.2
  - hand Q74.0
- skin tags Q82.8
- spleen Q89.09
- sternum Q76.7
- submaxillary gland Q38.4
- tarsal bones Q74.2
- teeth, tooth K00.1
- tendon Q79.8
- thumb Q69.1
- thymus gland Q89.2
- thyroid gland Q89.2
- toes Q69.2
- tongue Q38.3
- tooth, teeth K00.1
- tragus Q17.0
- ureter Q62.5
- urethra Q64.79
- urinary organ or tract NEC Q64.8
- uterus Q51.28
- vagina Q52.10
- valve, heart NEC Q24.8
  - pulmonary Q22.3
- vertebra Q76.49
- vocal cords Q31.8
- vulva Q52.79

Accident
- birth —*see* Birth, injury
- cardiac —*see* Infarct, myocardium
- cerebral I63.9
- cerebrovascular (embolic) (ischemic) (thrombotic) I63.9
  - aborted I63.9
  - hemorrhagic —*see* Hemorrhage, intracranial, intracerebral
  - old (without sequelae) Z86.73
    - with sequelae (of) —*see* Sequelae, infarction, cerebral
- coronary —*see* Infarct, myocardium
- craniovascular I63.9
- vascular, brain I63.9

Accidental —*see* condition

Accommodation (disorder) —*see also* condition
- hysterical paralysis of F44.89
- insufficiency of H52.4
- paresis —*see* Paresis, of accommodation
- spasm —*see* Spasm, of accommodation

Accouchement —*see* Delivery

Accreta placenta O43.21-

Accretio cordis (nonrheumatic) I31.0

Accretions, tooth, teeth K03.6

Acculturation difficulty Z60.3

Accumulation secretion, prostate N42.89

Acephalia, acephalism, acephalus, acephaly Q00.0

Acephalobrachia monster Q89.8

Acephalochirus monster Q89.8

Acephalogaster Q89.8

Acephalostomus monster Q89.8

Acephalothorax Q89.8
Acerophobia F40.298
Acetonemia R79.89
  in Type 1 diabetes E10.10
    with coma E10.11
Acetonuria R82.4
Achalasia (cardia) (esophagus) K22.0
  congenital Q39.5
  pylorus Q40.0
  sphincteral NEC K59.89
Ache(s) —*see* Pain
Acheilia Q38.6
Achillobursitis —*see* Tendinitis, Achilles
Achillodynia —*see* Tendinitis, Achilles
Achlorhydria, achlorhydric (neurogenic) K31.83
  anemia D50.8
  diarrhea K31.83
  psychogenic F45.8
  secondary to vagotomy K91.1
Achluophobia F40.228
Acholia K82.8
Acholuric jaundice (familial) (splenomegalic) —*see also* Spherocytosis
  acquired D59.8
Achondrogenesis Q77.0
Achondroplasia (osteosclerosis congenita) Q77.4
Achroma, cutis L80
Achromat (ism), achromatopsia (acquired) (congenital) H53.51
Achromia, congenital —*see* Albinism
Achromia parasitica B36.0
Achylia gastrica K31.89
  psychogenic F45.8
Acid
  burn —*see* Corrosion
  deficiency
    amide nicotinic E52
    ascorbic E54
    folic E53.8
    nicotinic E52
    pantothenic E53.8
  intoxication E87.2
  peptic disease K30
  phosphatase deficiency E83.39
  stomach K30
    psychogenic F45.8
Acidemia E87.2
  argininosuccinic E72.22
  isovaleric E71.110
  metabolic (newborn) P19.9
    first noted before onset of labor P19.0
    first noted during labor P19.1
    noted at birth P19.2
  methylmalonic E71.120
  pipecolic E72.3
  propionic E71.121
Acidity, gastric (high) K30
  psychogenic F45.8
Acidocytopenia —*see* Agranulocytosis
Acidocytosis D72.10
Acidopenia —*see* Agranulocytosis
Acidosis (lactic) (respiratory) E87.2
  in Type 1 diabetes E10.10
    with coma E10.11
  kidney, tubular N25.89
  lactic E87.2
  metabolic NEC E87.2
    with respiratory acidosis E87.4
    hyperchloremic, of newborn P74.421

Acidosis *(continued)*
  metabolic *(continued)*
    late, of newborn P74.0
  mixed metabolic and respiratory, newborn P84
  newborn P84
  renal (hyperchloremic) (tubular) N25.89
  respiratory E87.2
    complicated by
      metabolic
        acidosis E87.4
        alkalosis E87.4
Aciduria
  4-hydroxybutyric E72.81
  argininosuccinic E72.22
  gamma-hydroxybutyric E72.81
  glutaric (type I) E72.3
    type II E71.313
    type III E71.5-
  orotic (congenital) (hereditary) (pyrimidine deficiency) E79.8
    anemia D53.0
Acladiosis (skin) B36.0
Aclasis, diaphyseal Q78.6
Acleistocardia Q21.1
Aclusion —*see* Anomaly, dentofacial, malocclusion
Acne L70.9
  artificialis L70.8
  atrophica L70.2
  cachecticorum (Hebra) L70.8
  conglobata L70.1
  cystic L70.0
  decalvans L66.2
  excoriée (des jeunes filles) L70.5
  frontalis L70.2
  indurata L70.0
  infantile L70.4
  keloid L73.0
  lupoid L70.2
  necrotic, necrotica (miliaris) L70.2
  neonatal L70.4
  nodular L70.0
  occupational L70.8
  picker's L70.5
  pustular L70.0
  rodens L70.2
  rosacea L71.9
  specified NEC L70.8
  tropica L70.3
  varioliformis L70.2
  vulgaris L70.0
Acnitis (primary) A18.4
Acosta's disease T70.29
Acoustic —*see* condition
Acousticophobia F40.298
ACPO (acute colonic pseudo-obstruction) K59.81
Acquired —*see also* condition
  immunodeficiency syndrome (AIDS) B20
Acrania Q00.0
Acroangiodermatitis I78.9
Acroasphyxia, chronic I73.89
Acrobystitis N47.7
Acrocephalopolysyndactyly Q87.0
Acrocephalosyndactyly Q87.0
Acrocephaly Q75.0
Acrochondrohyperplasia —*see* Syndrome, Marfan's
Acrocyanosis I73.89
  newborn P28.2
    meaning transient blue hands and feet - omit code

Acrodermatitis L30.8
  atrophicans (chronica) L90.4
  continua (Hallopeau) L40.2
  enteropathica (hereditary) E83.2
  Hallopeau's L40.2
  infantile papular L44.4
  perstans L40.2
  pustulosa continua L40.2
  recalcitrant pustular L40.2
Acrodynia —*see* Poisoning, mercury
Acromegaly, acromegalia E22.0
Acromelalgia I73.81
Acromicria, acromikria Q79.8
Acronyx L60.0
Acropachy, thyroid —*see* Thyrotoxicosis
Acroparesthesia (simple) (vasomotor) I73.89
Acropathy, thyroid —*see* Thyrotoxicosis
Acrophobia F40.241
Acroposthitis N47.7
Acroscleriasis, acroscleroderma, acrosclerosis —*see* Sclerosis, systemic
Acrosphacelus I96
Acrospiroma, eccrine —*see* Neoplasm, skin, benign
Acrostealgia —*see* Osteochondropathy
Acrotrophodynia —*see* Immersion
ACTH ectopic syndrome E24.3
Actinic —*see* condition
Actinobacillosis, actinobacillus A28.8
  mallei A24.0
  muris A25.1
Actinomyces israelii (infection) —*see* Actinomycosis
Actinomycetoma (foot) B47.1
Actinomycosis, actinomycotic A42.9
  with pneumonia A42.0
  abdominal A42.1
  cervicofacial A42.2
  cutaneous A42.89
  gastrointestinal A42.1
  pulmonary A42.0
  sepsis A42.7
  specified site NEC A42.89
Actinoneuritis G62.82
Action, heart
  disorder I49.9
  irregular I49.9
    psychogenic F45.8
Activated protein C resistance D68.51
Activation
  mast cell (disorder) (syndrom) D89.40
    idiopathic D89.42
    monoclonal D89.41
    secondary D89.43
    specified type NEC D89.49
Active —*see* condition
Acute —*see also* condition
  abdomen R10.0
  gallbladder —*see* Cholecystitis, acute
Acyanotic heart disease (congenital) Q24.9
Acystia Q64.5

Adair-Dighton syndrome (brittle bones and blue sclera, deafness) Q78.0
Adamantinoblastoma —*see* Ameloblastoma
Adamantinoma —*see also* Cyst, calcifying odontogenic
  long bones C40.90
    lower limb C40.2-
    upper limb C40.0-
  malignant C41.1
    jaw (bone) (lower) C41.1
      upper C41.0
  tibial C40.2-
Adamantoblastoma —*see* Ameloblastoma
Adams-Stokes (-Morgagni) **disease or syndrome** I45.9
Adaption reaction —*see* Disorder, adjustment
Addiction —*see also* Dependence F19.20
  alcohol, alcoholic (ethyl) (methyl) (wood) (without remission) F10.20
    with remission F10.21
  drug —*see* Dependence, drug
  ethyl alcohol (without remission) F10.20
    with remission F10.21
  heroin —*see* Dependence, drug, opioid
  methyl alcohol (without remission) F10.20
    with remission F10.21
  methylated spirit (without remission) F10.20
    with remission F10.21
  morphine(-like substances) —*see* Dependence, drug, opioid
  nicotine —*see* Dependence, drug, nicotine
  opium and opioids —*see* Dependence, drug, opioid
  tobacco —*see* Dependence, drug, nicotine
Addisonian crisis E27.2
Addison's
  anemia (pernicious) D51.0
  disease (bronze) or syndrome E27.1
    tuberculous A18.7
  keloid L94.0
Addison-Biermer anemia (pernicious) D51.0
Addison-Schilder complex E71.528
Additional —*see also* Accessory
  chromosome(s) Q99.8
    sex —*see* Abnormal, chromosome, sex
    21 —*see* Trisomy, 21
Adduction contracture, hip or other joint —*see* Contraction, joint
Adenitis —*see also* Lymphadenitis
  acute, unspecified site L04.9
  axillary I88.9
    acute L04.2
    chronic or subacute I88.1
  Bartholin's gland N75.8
  bulbourethral gland —*see* Urethritis
  cervical I88.9
    acute L04.0
    chronic or subacute I88.1
  chancroid (Hemophilus ducreyi) A57
  chronic, unspecified site I88.1
  Cowper's gland —*see* Urethritis

Adenitis *(continued)*
due to Pasteurella multocida (P. septica) A28.0
epidemic, acute B27.09
gangrenous L04.9
gonorrheal NEC A54.89
groin I88.9
acute L04.1
chronic or subacute I88.1
infectious (acute) (epidemic) B27.09
inguinal I88.9
acute L04.1
chronic or subacute I88.1
lymph gland or node, except mesenteric I88.9
acute —*see* Lymphadenitis, acute
chronic or subacute I88.1
mesenteric (acute) (chronic) (nonspecific) (subacute) I88.0
parotid gland (suppurative) —*see* Sialoadenitis
salivary gland (any) (suppurative) —*see* Sialoadenitis
scrofulous (tuberculous) A18.2
Skene's duct or gland —*see* Urethritis
strumous, tuberculous A18.2
subacute, unspecified site I88.1
sublingual gland (suppurative) —*see* Sialoadenitis
submandibular gland (suppurative) —*see* Sialoadenitis
submaxillary gland (suppurative) —*see* Sialoadenitis
tuberculous —*see* Tuberculosis, lymph gland
urethral gland —*see* Urethritis
Wharton's duct (suppurative) —*see* Sialoadenitis

Adenoacanthoma —*see* Neoplasm, malignant, by site

Adenoameloblastoma —*see* Cyst, calcifying odontogenic

Adenocarcinoid (tumor) —*see* Neoplasm, malignant, by site

Adenocarcinoma —*see also* Neoplasm, malignant, by site
acidophil
specified site —*see* Neoplasm, malignant, by site
unspecified site C75.1
adrenal cortical C74.0-
alveolar —*see* Neoplasm, lung, malignant
apocrine
breast —*see* Neoplasm, breast, malignant
in situ
breast D05.8-
specified site NEC —*see* Neoplasm, skin, in situ
unspecified site D04.9
specified site NEC —*see* Neoplasm, skin, malignant
unspecified site C44.99
basal cell
specified site —*see* Neoplasm, skin, malignant
unspecified site C08.9
basophil
specified site —*see* Neoplasm, malignant, by site
unspecified site C75.1
bile duct type C22.1
liver C22.1
specified site NEC —*see* Neoplasm, malignant, by site
unspecified site C22.1

Adenocarcinoma *(continued)*
bronchiolar —*see* Neoplasm, lung, malignant
bronchioloalveolar —*see* Neoplasm, lung, malignant
ceruminous C44.29-
cervix, in situ —*see also* Carcinoma, cervix uteri, in situ D06.9
chromophobe
specified site —*see* Neoplasm, malignant, by site
unspecified site C75.1
diffuse type
specified site —*see* Neoplasm, malignant, by site
unspecified site C16.9
duct
infiltrating
with Paget's disease —*see* Neoplasm, breast, malignant
specified site —*see* Neoplasm, malignant, by site
unspecified site (female) 50.91-
male C50.92-
specified site —*see* Neoplasm, malignant, by site
unspecified site
female C56.9
male C61
eosinophil
specified site —*see* Neoplasm, malignant, by site
unspecified site C75.1
follicular
with papillary C73
moderately differentiated C73
specified site —*see* Neoplasm, malignant, by site
trabecular C73
unspecified site C73
well differentiated C73
Hurthle cell C73
in
adenomatous
polyposis coli C18.9
infiltrating duct
with Paget's disease —*see* Neoplasm, breast, malignant
specified site —*see* Neoplasm, by site, malignant
unspecified site (female) C50.91-
male C50.92-
inflammatory
specified site —*see* Neoplasm, by site, malignant
unspecified site (female) C50.91-
male C50.92-
intestinal type
specified site —*see* Neoplasm, by site, malignant
unspecified site C16.9
intracystic papillary
intraductal
breast D05.1-
noninfiltrating
breast D05.1-
papillary
with invasion
specified site —*see* Neoplasm, by site, malignant
unspecified site (female) C50.91-
male C50.92-
breast D05.1-
specified site NEC —*see* Neoplasm, in situ, by site
unspecified site D05.1-

Adenocarcinoma *(continued)*
intraductal *(continued)*
noninfiltrating *(continued)*
specified site NEC —*see* Neoplasm, in situ, by site
unspecified site D05.1-
papillary
with invasion
specified site —*see* Neoplasm, malignant, by site
unspecified site (female) C50.91-
male C50.92-
breast D05.1-
specified site —*see* Neoplasm, in situ, by site
unspecified site D05.1-
specified site NEC —*see* Neoplasm, in situ, by site
unspecified site D05.1-
islet cell
with exocrine, mixed
specified site —*see* Neoplasm, malignant, by site
unspecified site C25.9
pancreas C25.4
specified site NEC —*see* Neoplasm, malignant, by site
unspecified site C25.4
lobular
in situ
breast D05.0-
specified site NEC —*see* Neoplasm, in situ, by site
unspecified site D05.0-
specified site —*see* Neoplasm, malignant, by site
unspecified site (female) C50.91-
male C50.92-
mucoid —*see also* Neoplasm, malignant, by site
cell
specified site —*see* Neoplasm, malignant, by site
unspecified site C75.1
nonencapsulated sclerosing C73
papillary
with follicular C73
follicular variant C73
intraductal (noninfiltrating)
with invasion
specified site —*see* Neoplasm, malignant, by site
unspecified site (female) C50.91-
male C50.92-
breast D05.1-
specified site NEC —*see* Neoplasm, in situ, by site
unspecified site D05.1-
serous
specified site —*see* Neoplasm, malignant, by site
unspecified site C56.9
papillocystic
specified site —*see* Neoplasm, malignant, by site
unspecified site C56.9
pseudomucinous
specified site —*see* Neoplasm, malignant, by site
unspecified site C56.9
renal cell C64-
sebaceous —*see* Neoplasm, skin, malignant

Adenocarcinoma *(continued)*
serous —*see also* Neoplasm, malignant, by site
papillary
specified site —*see* Neoplasm, malignant, by site
unspecified site C56.9
sweat gland —*see* Neoplasm, skin, malignant
water-clear cell C75.0

Adenocarcinoma-in-situ —*see also* Neoplasm, in situ, by site
breast D05.9-

Adenofibroma
clear cell —*see* Neoplasm, benign, by site
endometrioid D27.9
borderline malignancy D39.10
malignant C56-
mucinous
specified site —*see* Neoplasm, benign, by site
unspecified site D27.9
papillary
specified site —*see* Neoplasm, benign, by site
unspecified site D27.9
prostate —*see* Enlargement, enlarged, prostate
serous
specified site —*see* Neoplasm, benign, by site
unspecified site D27.9
specified site —*see* Neoplasm, benign, by site
unspecified site D27.9

Adenofibrosis
breast —*see* Fibroadenosis, breast
endometrioid N80.0

Adenoiditis (chronic) J35.02
with tonsillitis J35.03
acute J03.90
recurrent J03.91
specified organism NEC J03.80
recurrent J03.81
staphylococcal J03.80
recurrent J03.81
streptococcal J03.00
recurrent J03.01

Adenoids —*see* condition

Adenolipoma —*see* Neoplasm, benign, by site

Adenolipomatosis, Launois-Bensaude E88.89

Adenolymphoma
specified site —*see* Neoplasm, benign, by site
unspecified site D11.9

Adenoma —*see also* Neoplasm, benign, by site
acidophil
specified site —*see* Neoplasm, benign, by site
unspecified site D35.2
acidophil-basophil, mixed
specified site —*see* Neoplasm, benign, by site
unspecified site D35.2
adrenal (cortical) D35.00
clear cell D35.00
compact cell D35.00
glomerulosa cell D35.00
heavily pigmented variant D35.00
mixed cell D35.00
alpha-cell
pancreas D13.7
specified site NEC —*see* Neoplasm, benign, by site

Adenoma *(continued)*
- alpha-cell *(continued)*
  - unspecified site D13.7
- alveolar D14.30
- apocrine
  - breast D24-
  - specified site NEC *—see* Neoplasm, skin, benign, by site
  - unspecified site D23.9
- basal cell D11.9
- basophil
  - specified site *—see* Neoplasm, benign, by site
  - unspecified site D35.2
- basophil-acidophil, mixed
  - specified site *—see* Neoplasm, benign, by site
  - unspecified site D35.2
- beta-cell
  - pancreas D13.7
  - specified site NEC *—see* Neoplasm, benign, by site
  - unspecified site D13.7
- bile duct D13.4
  - common D13.5
  - extrahepatic D13.5
  - intrahepatic D13.4
  - specified site NEC *—see* Neoplasm, benign, by site
  - unspecified site D13.4
- black D35.00
- bronchial D38.1
  - cylindroid type *—see* Neoplasm, lung, malignant
- ceruminous D23.2-
- chief cell D35.1
- chromophobe
  - specified site *—see* Neoplasm, benign, by site
  - unspecified site D35.2
- colloid
  - specified site *—see* Neoplasm, benign, by site
  - unspecified site D34
- eccrine, papillary *—see* Neoplasm, skin, benign
- endocrine, multiple
  - single specified site *—see* Neoplasm, uncertain behavior, by site
  - two or more specified sites D44-
  - unspecified site D44.9
- endometrioid *—see also* Neoplasm, benign
  - borderline malignancy *—see* Neoplasm, uncertain behavior, by site
- eosinophil
  - specified site *—see* Neoplasm, benign, by site
  - unspecified site D35.2
- fetal
  - specified site *—see* Neoplasm, benign, by site
  - unspecified site D34
- follicular
  - specified site *—see* Neoplasm, benign, by site
  - unspecified site D34
- hepatocellular D13.4
- Hurthle cell D34
- islet cell
  - pancreas D13.7
  - specified site NEC *—see* Neoplasm, benign, by site
  - unspecified site D13.7
- liver cell D13.4
- macrofollicular
  - specified site *—see* Neoplasm, benign, by site
  - unspecified site D34

Adenoma *(continued)*
- malignant, malignum *—see* Neoplasm, malignant, by site
- microcystic
  - pancreas D13.6
  - specified site NEC *—see* Neoplasm, benign, by site
  - unspecified site D13.6
- microfollicular
  - specified site *—see* Neoplasm, benign, by site
  - unspecified site D34
- mucoid cell
  - specified site *—see* Neoplasm, benign, by site
  - unspecified site D35.2
- multiple endocrine
  - single specified site *—see* Neoplasm, uncertain behavior, by site
  - two or more specified sites D44-
  - unspecified site D44.9
- nipple D24-
- papillary *—see also* Neoplasm, benign, by site
  - eccrine *—see* Neoplasm, skin, benign, by site
- Pick's tubular
  - specified site *—see* Neoplasm, benign, by site
  - unspecified site
    - female D27.9
    - male D29.20
- pleomorphic
  - carcinoma in *—see* Neoplasm, salivary gland, malignant
    - specified site *—see* Neoplasm, malignant, by site
    - unspecified site C08.9
- polypoid *—see also* Neoplasm, benign
  - adenocarcinoma in *—see* Neoplasm, malignant, by site
  - adenocarcinoma in situ *—see* Neoplasm, in situ, by site
- prostate *—see* Neoplasm, benign, prostate
- rete cell D29.20
- sebaceous *—see* Neoplasm, skin, benign
- Sertoli cell
  - specified site *—see* Neoplasm, benign, by site
  - unspecified site
    - female D27.9
    - male D29.20
- skin appendage *—see* Neoplasm, skin, benign
- sudoriferous gland *—see* Neoplasm, skin, benign
- sweat gland *—see* Neoplasm, skin, benign
- testicular
  - specified site *—see* Neoplasm, benign, by site
  - unspecified site
    - female D27.9
    - male D29.20
- tubular *—see also* Neoplasm, benign, by site
  - adenocarcinoma in *—see* Neoplasm, malignant, by site
  - adenocarcinoma in situ *—see* Neoplasm, in situ, by site
  - Pick's
    - specified site *—see* Neoplasm, benign, by site
    - unspecified site
      - female D27.9
      - male D29.20

Adenoma *(continued)*
- tubulovillous *—see also* Neoplasm, benign, by site
  - adenocarcinoma in *—see* Neoplasm, malignant, by site
  - adenocarcinoma in situ *—see* Neoplasm, in situ, by site
- villous *—see* Neoplasm, uncertain behavior, by site
  - adenocarcinoma in *—see* Neoplasm, malignant, by site
  - adenocarcinoma in situ *—see* Neoplasm, in situ, by site
- water-clear cell D35.1

Adenomatosis
- endocrine (multiple) E31.20
  - single specified site *—see* Neoplasm, uncertain behavior, by site
- erosive of nipple D24-
- pluriendocrine *—see* Adenomatosis, endocrine
- pulmonary D38.1
  - malignant *—see* Neoplasm, lung, malignant
- specified site *—see* Neoplasm, benign, by site
- unspecified site D12.6

Adenomatous
- goiter (nontoxic) E04.9
  - with hyperthyroidism *—see* Hyperthyroidism, with, goiter, nodular
  - toxic *—see* Hyperthyroidism, with, goiter, nodular

Adenomyoma *—see also* Neoplasm, benign, by site
- prostate *—see* Enlarged, prostate

Adenomyometritis N80.0

Adenomyosis N80.0

Adenopathy (lymph gland) R59.9
- generalized R59.1
- inguinal R59.0
- localized R59.0
- mediastinal R59.0
- mesentery R59.0
- syphilitic (secondary) A51.49
- tracheobronchial R59.0
  - tuberculous A15.4
    - primary (progressive) A15.7
- tuberculous *—see also* Tuberculosis, lymph gland
  - tracheobronchial A15.4
    - primary (progressive) A15.7

Adenosalpingitis *—see* Salpingitis

Adenosarcoma *—see* Neoplasm, malignant, by site

Adenosclerosis I88.8

Adenosis (sclerosing) breast *—see* Fibroadenosis, breast

Adenovirus, as cause of disease classified elsewhere B97.0

Adentia (complete) (partial) *—see* Absence, teeth

Adherent *—see also* Adhesions
- labia (minora) N90.89
- pericardium (nonrheumatic) I31.0
  - rheumatic I09.2
- placenta (with hemorrhage) O72.0
  - without hemorrhage O73.0
- prepuce, newborn N47.0
- scar (skin) L90.5
- tendon in scar L90.5

Adhesions, adhesive (postinfective)
- with intestinal obstruction K56.50

Adhesions, adhesive *(continued)*
- with intestinal obstruction *(continued)*
  - complete K56.52
  - incomplete K56.51
  - partial K56.51
- abdominal (wall) *—see* Adhesions, peritoneum
- appendix K38.8
- bile duct (common) (hepatic) K83.8
- bladder (sphincter) N32.89
- bowel *—see* Adhesions, peritoneum
- cardiac I31.0
  - rheumatic I09.2
- cecum *—see* Adhesions, peritoneum
- cervicovaginal N88.1
  - congenital Q52.8
  - postpartal O90.89
    - old N88.1
- cervix N88.1
- ciliary body NEC *—see* Adhesions, iris
- clitoris N90.89
- colon *—see* Adhesions, peritoneum
- common duct K83.8
- congenital *—see also* Anomaly, by site
  - fingers *—see* Syndactylism, complex, fingers
  - omental, anomalous Q43.3
  - peritoneal Q43.3
  - tongue (to gum or roof of mouth) Q38.3
- conjunctiva (acquired) H11.21-
  - congenital Q15.8
- cystic duct K82.8
- diaphragm *—see* Adhesions, peritoneum
- due to foreign body *—see* Foreign body
- duodenum *—see* Adhesions, peritoneum
- ear
  - middle H74.1-
- epididymis N50.89
- epidural *—see* Adhesions, meninges
- epiglottis J38.7
- eyelid H02.59
- female pelvis N73.6
- gallbladder K82.8
- globe H44.89
- heart I31.0
  - rheumatic I09.2
- ileocecal (coil) *—see* Adhesions, peritoneum
- ileum *—see* Adhesions, peritoneum
- intestine *—see also* Adhesions, peritoneum
  - with obstruction K56.50
    - complete K56.52
    - incomplete K56.51
    - partial K56.51
- intra-abdominal *—see* Adhesions, peritoneum
- iris H21.50-
  - anterior H21.51-
  - goniosynechiae H21.52-
  - posterior H21.54-
  - to corneal graft T85.898
- joint *—see* Ankylosis
  - knee M23.8X
  - temporomandibular M26.61-
- labium (majus) (minus), congenital Q52.5
- liver *—see* Adhesions, peritoneum
- lung J98.4
- mediastinum J98.59
- meninges (cerebral) (spinal) G96.12

Adhesions, adhesive *(continued)*
meninges *(continued)*
congenital Q07.8
tuberculous (cerebral) (spinal) A17.0
mesenteric *—see* Adhesions, peritoneum
nasal (septum) (to turbinates) J34.89
ocular muscle *—see* Strabismus, mechanical
omentum *—see* Adhesions, peritoneum
ovary N73.6
congenital (to cecum, kidney or omentum) Q50.39
paraovarian N73.6
pelvic (peritoneal)
female N73.6
postprocedural N99.4
male *—see* Adhesions, peritoneum
postpartal (old) N73.6
tuberculous A18.17
penis to scrotum (congenital) Q55.8
periappendiceal *—see also* Adhesions, peritoneum
pericardium (nonrheumatic) I31.0
focal I31.8
rheumatic I09.2
tuberculous A18.84
pericholecystic K82.8
perigastric *—see* Adhesions, peritoneum
periovarian N73.6
periprostatic N42.89
perirectal *—see* Adhesions, peritoneum
perirenal N28.89
peritoneum, peritoneal (postinfective) K66.0
with obstruction (intestinal) K56.50
complete K56.52
incomplete K56.51
partial K56.51
congenital Q43.3
pelvic, female N73.6
postprocedural N99.4
postpartal, pelvic N73.6
postprocedural K66.0
to uterus N73.6
peritubal N73.6
periureteral N28.89
periuterine N73.6
perivesical N32.89
perivesicular (seminal vesicle) N50.89
pleura, pleuritic J94.8
tuberculous NEC A15.6
pleuropericardial J94.8
postoperative (gastrointestinal tract) K66.0
with obstruction (*see also* Obstruction, intestine, postoperative) K91.30
due to foreign body accidentally left in wound *—see* Foreign body, accidentally left during a procedure
pelvic peritoneal N99.4
urethra *—see* Stricture, urethra, postprocedural
vagina N99.2
postpartal, old (vulva or perineum) N90.89
preputial, prepuce N47.5
pulmonary J98.4
pylorus *—see* Adhesions, peritoneum

Adhesions, adhesive *(continued)*
sciatic nerve *—see* Lesion, nerve, sciatic
seminal vesicle N50.89
shoulder (joint) *—see* Capsulitis, adhesive
sigmoid flexure *—see* Adhesions, peritoneum
spermatic cord (acquired) N50.89
congenital Q55.4
spinal canal G96.12
stomach *—see* Adhesions, peritoneum
subscapular *—see* Capsulitis, adhesive
temporomandibular M26.61-
tendinitis *—see also* Tenosynovitis, specified type NEC
shoulder *—see* Capsulitis, adhesive
testis N44.8
tongue, congenital (to gum or roof of mouth) Q38.3
acquired K14.8
trachea J39.8
tubo-ovarian N73.6
tunica vaginalis N44.8
uterus N73.6
internal N85.6
to abdominal wall N73.6
vagina (chronic) N89.5
postoperative N99.2
vitreomacular H43.82-
vitreous H43.89
vulva N90.89

Adiaspiromycosis B48.88

Adie (-Holmes) **pupil or syndrome** *—see* Anomaly, pupil, function, tonic pupil

Adiponecrosis neonatorum P83.88

Adiposis *—see also* Obesity
cerebralis E23.6
dolorosa E88.2

Adiposity *—see also* Obesity
heart *—see* Degeneration, myocardial
localized E65

Adiposogenital dystrophy E23.6

Adjustment
disorder *—see* Disorder, adjustment
implanted device *—see* Encounter (for), adjustment (of)
prosthesis, external *—see* Fitting
reaction *—see* Disorder, adjustment

Administration of tPA (rtPA) **in a different facility within the last 24 hours prior to admission to current facility** Z92.82

Admission (for) *—see also* Encounter (for)
adjustment (of)
artificial
arm Z44.00-
complete Z44.01-
partial Z44.02-
eye Z44.2
leg Z44.10-
complete Z44.11-
partial Z44.12-
brain neuropacemaker Z46.2
implanted Z45.42
breast
implant Z45.81
prosthesis (external) Z44.3
colostomy belt Z46.89
contact lenses Z46.0
cystostomy device Z46.6
dental prosthesis Z46.3
device NEC
abdominal Z46.89

Admission *(continued)*
adjustment (of) *(continued)*
device NEC *(continued)*
implanted Z45.89
cardiac Z45.09
defibrillator (with synchronous cardiac pacemaker) Z45.02
pacemaker (cardiac resynchronization therapy (CRT-P)) Z45.018
pulse generator Z45.010
resynchronization therapy defibrillator (CRT-D) Z45.02
hearing device Z45.328
bone conduction Z45.320
cochlear Z45.321
infusion pump Z45.1
nervous system Z45.49
CSF drainage Z45.41
hearing device *—see* Admission, adjustment, device, implanted, hearing device
neuropacemaker Z45.42
visual substitution Z45.31
specified NEC Z45.89
vascular access Z45.2
visual substitution Z45.31
nervous system Z46.2
implanted *—see* Admission, adjustment, device, implanted, nervous system
orthodontic Z46.4
prosthetic Z44.9
arm *—see* Admission, adjustment, artificial, arm
breast Z44.3
dental Z46.3
eye Z44.2
leg *—see* Admission, adjustment, artificial, leg
specified type NEC Z44.8
substitution
auditory Z46.2
implanted *—see* Admission, adjustment, device, implanted, hearing device
nervous system Z46.2
implanted *—see* Admission, adjustment, device, implanted, nervous system
visual Z46.2
implanted Z45.31
urinary Z46.6
hearing aid Z46.1
implanted *—see* Admission, adjustment, device, implanted, hearing device
ileostomy device Z46.89
intestinal appliance or device NEC Z46.89
neuropacemaker (brain) (peripheral nerve) (spinal cord) Z46.2
implanted Z45.42
orthodontic device Z46.4
orthopedic (brace) (cast) (device) (shoes) Z46.89
pacemaker (cardiac resynchronization therapy (CRT-P))
cardiac Z45.018
pulse generator Z45.010
nervous system Z46.2
implanted Z45.42

Admission *(continued)*
pacemaker *(continued)*
portacath (port-a-cath) Z45.2
prosthesis Z44.9
arm *—see* Admission, adjustment, artificial, arm
breast Z44.3
dental Z46.3
eye Z44.2
leg *—see* Admission, adjustment, artificial, leg
specified NEC Z44.8
spectacles Z46.0
aftercare *—see also* Aftercare Z51.89
postpartum
immediately after delivery Z39.0
routine follow-up Z39.2
radiation therapy (antineoplastic) Z51.0
attention to artificial opening (of) Z43.9
artificial vagina Z43.7
colostomy Z43.3
cystostomy Z43.5
enterostomy Z43.4
gastrostomy Z43.1
ileostomy Z43.2
jejunostomy Z43.4
nephrostomy Z43.6
specified site NEC Z43.8
intestinal tract Z43.4
urinary tract Z43.6
tracheostomy Z43.0
ureterostomy Z43.6
urethrostomy Z43.6
breast augmentation or reduction Z41.1
breast reconstruction following mastectomy Z42.1
change of
dressing (nonsurgical) Z48.00
neuropacemaker device (brain) (peripheral nerve) (spinal cord) Z46.2
implanted Z45.42
surgical dressing Z48.01
circumcision, ritual or routine (in absence of diagnosis) Z41.2
clinical research investigation (control) (normal comparison) (participant) Z00.6
contraceptive management Z30.9
cosmetic surgery NEC Z41.1
counseling *—see also* Counseling
dietary Z71.3
gestational carrier Z31.7
HIV Z71.7
human immunodeficiency virus Z71.7
nonattending third party Z71.0
procreative management NEC Z31.69
delivery, full-term, uncomplicated O80
cesarean, without indication O82
desensitization to allergens Z51.6
dietary surveillance and counseling Z71.3
ear piercing Z41.3
examination at health care facility (adult) (*see also* Examination) Z00.00
with abnormal findings Z00.01
clinical research investigation (control) (normal comparison) (participant) Z00.6
dental Z01.20
with abnormal findings Z01.21
donor (potential) Z00.5

Admission *(continued)*
- examination at health care facility *(continued)*
  - ear Z01.10
    - with abnormal findings NEC Z01.118
  - eye Z01.00
    - with abnormal findings Z01.01
    - following failed vision screening Z01.020
      - with abnormal findings Z01.021
  - general, specified reason NEC Z00.8
  - hearing Z01.10
    - with abnormal findings NEC Z01.118
    - infant or child (over 28 days old) Z00.129
      - with abnormal findings Z00.121
  - postpartum checkup Z39.2
  - psychiatric (general) Z00.8
    - requested by authority Z04.6
  - vision Z01.00
    - with abnormal findings Z01.01
    - following failed vision screening Z01.020
      - with abnormal findings Z01.021
    - infant or child (over 28 days old) Z00.129
      - with abnormal findings Z00.121
- fitting (of)
  - artificial
    - arm *—see* Admission, adjustment, artificial, arm
    - eye Z44.2
    - leg *—see* Admission, adjustment, artificial, leg
  - brain neuropacemaker Z46.2
    - implanted Z45.42
  - breast prosthesis (external) Z44.3
  - colostomy belt Z46.89
  - contact lenses Z46.0
  - cystostomy device Z46.6
  - dental prosthesis Z46.3
  - dentures Z46.3
  - device NEC
    - abdominal Z46.89
    - nervous system Z46.2
      - implanted *—see* Admission, adjustment, device, implanted, nervous system
    - orthodontic Z46.4
    - prosthetic Z44.9
      - breast Z44.3
      - dental Z46.3
      - eye Z44.2
    - substitution
      - auditory Z46.2
        - implanted *—see* Admission, adjustment, device, implanted, hearing device
      - nervous system Z46.2
        - implanted *—see* Admission, adjustment, device, implanted, nervous system
      - visual Z46.2
        - implanted Z45.31
  - hearing aid Z46.1
  - ileostomy device Z46.89
  - intestinal appliance or device NEC Z46.89

Admission *(continued)*
- fitting (of) *(continued)*
  - neuropacemaker (brain) (peripheral nerve) (spinal cord) Z46.2
    - implanted Z45.42
  - orthodontic device Z46.4
  - orthopedic device (brace) (cast) (shoes) Z46.89
  - prosthesis Z44.9
    - arm *—see* Admission, adjustment, artificial, arm
    - breast Z44.3
    - dental Z46.3
    - eye Z44.2
    - leg *—see* Admission, adjustment, artificial, leg
    - specified type NEC Z44.8
  - spectacles Z46.0
- follow-up examination Z09
- intrauterine device management Z30.431
  - initial prescription Z30.014
- mental health evaluation Z00.8
  - requested by authority Z04.6
- observation *—see* Observation
- Papanicolaou smear, cervix Z12.4
  - for suspected malignant neoplasm Z12.4
- plastic and reconstructive surgery following medical procedure or healed injury NEC Z42.8
- plastic surgery, cosmetic NEC Z41.1
- postpartum observation
  - immediately after delivery Z39.0
  - routine follow-up Z39.2
- poststerilization (for restoration) Z31.0
  - aftercare Z31.42
- procreative management Z31.9
- prophylactic (measure) *—see also* Encounter, prophylactic measures
  - organ removal Z40.00
    - breast Z40.01
    - fallopian tube(s) Z40.03
      - with ovary(s) Z40.02
    - ovary(s) Z40.02
    - specified organ NEC Z40.09
    - testes Z40.09
  - vaccination Z23
- psychiatric examination (general) Z00.8
  - requested by authority Z04.6
- radiation therapy (antineoplastic) Z51.0
- reconstructive surgery following medical procedure or healed injury NEC Z42.8
- removal of
  - cystostomy catheter Z43.5
  - drains Z48.03
  - dressing (nonsurgical) Z48.00
  - implantable subdermal contraceptive Z30.46
  - intrauterine contraceptive device Z30.432
  - neuropacemaker (brain) (peripheral nerve) (spinal cord) Z46.2
    - implanted Z45.42
  - staples Z48.02
  - surgical dressing Z48.01
  - sutures Z48.02
  - ureteral stent Z46.6
- respirator [ventilator] use during power failure Z99.12
- restoration of organ continuity (poststerilization) Z31.0
  - aftercare Z31.42
- sensitivity test *—see also* Test, skin
  - allergy NEC Z01.82
  - Mantoux Z11.1

Admission *(continued)*
- tuboplasty following previous sterilization Z31.0
  - aftercare Z31.42
- vasoplasty following previous sterilization Z31.0
  - aftercare Z31.42
- vision examination Z01.00
  - with abnormal findings Z01.01
  - following failed vision screening Z01.020
    - with abnormal findings Z01.021
  - infant or child (over 28 days old) Z00.129
    - with abnormal findings Z00.121
- waiting period for admission to other facility Z75.1

Adnexitis (suppurative) *—see* Salpingo-oophoritis

Adolescent X-linked adrenoleukodystrophy E71.521

Adrenal (gland) *—see* condition

Adrenalism, tuberculous A18.7

Adrenalitis, adrenitis E27.8
- autoimmune E27.1
- meningococcal, hemorrhagic A39.1

Adrenarche, premature E27.0

Adrenocortical syndrome *—see* Cushing's, syndrome

Adrenogenital syndrome E25.9
- acquired E25.8
- congenital E25.0
- salt loss E25.0

Adrenogenitalism, congenital E25.0

Adrenoleukodystrophy E71.529
- neonatal E71.511
- X-linked E71.529
  - Addison only phenotype E71.528
  - Addison-Schilder E71.528
  - adolescent E71.521
  - adrenomyeloneuropathy E71.522
  - childhood cerebral E71.520
  - other specified E71.528

Adrenomyeloneuropathy E71.522

Adventitious bursa *—see* Bursopathy, specified type NEC

Adverse effect *—see* Table of Drugs and Chemicals, categories T36-T50, with 6th character 5

Advice *—see* Counseling

Adynamia (episodica) (hereditary) (periodic) G72.3

Aeration lung imperfect, newborn *—see* Atelectasis

Aerobullosis T70.3

Aerocele *—see* Embolism, air

Aerodermectasia
- subcutaneous (traumatic) T79.7

Aerodontalgia T70.29

Aeroembolism T70.3

Aerogenes capsulatus infection A48.0

Aero-otitis media T70.0

Aerophagy, aerophagia (psychogenic) F45.8

Aerophobia F40.228

Aerosinusitis T70.1

Aerotitis T70.0

Affection *—see* Disease

Afibrinogenemia (*see also* Defect, coagulation) D68.8
- acquired D65
- congenital D68.2

Afibrinogenemia *(continued)*
- following ectopic or molar pregnancy O08.1
- in abortion *—see* Abortion, by type, complicated by, afibrinogenemia
- puerperal O72.3

African
- sleeping sickness B56.9
- tick fever A68.1
- trypanosomiasis B56.9
  - gambian B56.0
  - rhodesian B56.1

Aftercare (*see also* Care) Z51.89
- following surgery (for) (on)
  - amputation Z47.81
  - attention to
    - drains Z48.03
    - dressings (nonsurgical) Z48.00
      - surgical Z48.01
    - sutures Z48.02
  - circulatory system Z48.812
  - delayed (planned) wound closure Z48.1
  - digestive system Z48.815
  - explantation of joint prosthesis (staged procedure)
    - hip Z47.32
    - knee Z47.33
    - shoulder Z47.31
  - genitourinary system Z48.816
  - joint replacement Z47.1
  - neoplasm Z48.3
  - nervous system Z48.811
  - oral cavity Z48.814
  - organ transplant
    - bone marrow Z48.290
    - heart Z48.21
    - heart-lung Z48.280
    - kidney Z48.22
    - liver Z48.23
    - lung Z48.24
    - multiple organs NEC Z48.288
    - specified NEC Z48.298
  - orthopedic NEC Z47.89
  - planned wound closure Z48.1
  - removal of internal fixation device Z47.2
  - respiratory system Z48.813
  - scoliosis Z47.82
  - sense organs Z48.810
  - skin and subcutaneous tissue Z48.817
  - specified body system
    - circulatory Z48.812
    - digestive Z48.815
    - genitourinary Z48.816
    - nervous Z48.811
    - oral cavity Z48.814
    - respiratory Z48.813
    - sense organs Z48.810
    - skin and subcutaneous tissue Z48.817
    - teeth Z48.814
  - specified NEC Z48.89
  - spinal Z47.89
  - teeth Z48.814
- fracture - code to fracture with seventh character D
- involving
  - removal of
    - drains Z48.03
    - dressings (nonsurgical) Z48.00
    - staples Z48.02
    - surgical dressings Z48.01
    - sutures Z48.02
- neuropacemaker (brain) (peripheral nerve) (spinal cord) Z46.2
  - implanted Z45.42

Aftercare *(continued)*
  orthopedic NEC Z47.89
  postprocedural *—see* Aftercare, following surgery

After-cataract *—see* Cataract, secondary

Agalactia (primary) O92.3
  elective, secondary or therapeutic O92.5

Agammaglobulinemia (acquired (secondary)) (nonfamilial) D80.1
  with
    immunoglobulin-bearing B-lymphocytes D80.1
    lymphopenia D81.9
  autosomal recessive (Swiss type) D80.0
  Bruton's X-linked D80.0
  common variable (CVAgamma) D80.1
  congenital sex-linked D80.0
  hereditary D80.0
  lymphopenic D81.9
  Swiss type (autosomal recessive) D80.0
  X-linked (with growth hormone deficiency) (Bruton) D80.0

Aganglionosis (bowel) (colon) Q43.1

Age (old) *—see* Senility

Agenesis
  adrenal (gland) Q89.1
  alimentary tract (complete) (partial) NEC Q45.8
    upper Q40.8
  anus, anal (canal) Q42.3
    with fistula Q42.2
  aorta Q25.41
  appendix Q42.8
  arm (complete) Q71.0-
    with hand present Q71.1-
  artery (peripheral) Q27.9
    brain Q28.3
    coronary Q24.5
    pulmonary Q25.79
    specified NEC Q27.8
    umbilical Q27.0
  auditory (canal) (external) Q16.1
  auricle (ear) Q16.0
  bile duct or passage Q44.5
  bladder Q64.5
  bone Q79.9
  brain Q00.0
    part of Q04.3
  breast (with nipple present) Q83.8
    with absent nipple Q83.0
  bronchus Q32.4
  canaliculus lacrimalis Q10.4
  carpus *—see* Agenesis, hand
  cartilage Q79.9
  cecum Q42.8
  cerebellum Q04.3
  cervix Q51.5
  chin Q18.8
  cilia Q10.3
  circulatory system, part NOS Q28.9
  clavicle Q74.0
  clitoris Q52.6
  coccyx Q76.49
  colon Q42.9
    specified NEC Q42.8
  corpus callosum Q04.0
  cricoid cartilage Q31.8
  diaphragm (with hernia) Q79.1
  digestive organ(s) or tract (complete) (partial) NEC Q45.8
    upper Q40.8
  ductus arteriosus Q28.8
  duodenum Q41.0

Agenesis *(continued)*
  ear Q16.9
    auricle Q16.0
    lobe Q17.8
  ejaculatory duct Q55.4
  endocrine (gland) NEC Q89.2
  epiglottis Q31.8
  esophagus Q39.8
  eustachian tube Q16.2
  eye Q11.1
    adnexa Q15.8
  eyelid (fold) Q10.3
  face
    bones NEC Q75.8
    specified part NEC Q18.8
  fallopian tube Q50.6
  femur *—see* Defect, reduction, lower limb, longitudinal, femur
  fibula *—see* Defect, reduction, lower limb, longitudinal, fibula
  finger (complete) (partial) *—see* Agenesis, hand
  foot (and toes) (complete) (partial) Q72.3-
  forearm (with hand present) *—see* Agenesis, arm, with hand present
    and hand Q71.2-
  gallbladder Q44.0
  gastric Q40.2
  genitalia, genital (organ(s))
    female Q52.8
      external Q52.71
      internal NEC Q52.8
    male Q55.8
  glottis Q31.8
  hair Q84.0
  hand(and fingers) (complete) (partial) Q71.3-
  heart Q24.8
    valve NEC Q24.8
      pulmonary Q22.0
  hepatic Q44.7
  humerus *—see* Defect, reduction, upper limb
  hymen Q52.4
  ileum Q41.2
  incus Q16.3
  intestine (small) Q41.9
    large Q42.9
      specified NEC Q42.8
  iris (dilator fibers) Q13.1
  jaw M26.09
  jejunum Q41.1
  kidney(s) (partial) Q60.2
    bilateral Q60.1
    unilateral Q60.0
  labium (majus) (minus) Q52.71
  labyrinth, membranous Q16.5
  lacrimal apparatus Q10.4
  larynx Q31.8
  leg (complete) Q72.0-
    with foot present Q72.1-
    lower leg (with foot present) *—see* Agenesis, leg, with foot present
      and foot Q72.2-
  lens Q12.3
  limb (complete) Q73.0
    lower *—see* Agenesis, leg
    upper *—see* Agenesis, arm
  lip Q38.0
  liver Q44.7
  lung (fissure) (lobe) (bilateral) (unilateral) Q33.3
  mandible, maxilla M26.09
  metacarpus *—see* Agenesis, hand
  metatarsus *—see* Agenesis, foot
  muscle Q79.8
    eyelid Q10.3
    ocular Q15.8
  musculoskeletal system NEC Q79.8

Agenesis *(continued)*
  nail(s) Q84.3
  neck, part Q18.8
  nerve Q07.8
  nervous system, part NEC Q07.8
  nipple Q83.2
  nose Q30.1
  nuclear Q07.8
  organ
    of Corti Q16.5
    or site not listed *—see* Anomaly, by site
  osseous meatus (ear) Q16.1
  ovary
    bilateral Q50.02
    unilateral Q50.01
  oviduct Q50.6
  pancreas Q45.0
  parathyroid (gland) Q89.2
  parotid gland(s) Q38.4
  patella Q74.1
  pelvic girdle (complete) (partial) Q74.2
  penis Q55.5
  pericardium Q24.8
  pituitary (gland) Q89.2
  prostate Q55.4
  punctum lacrimale Q10.4
  radioulnar *—see* Defect, reduction, upper limb
  radius *—see* Defect, reduction, upper limb, longitudinal, radius
  rectum Q42.1
    with fistula Q42.0
  renal Q60.2
    bilateral Q60.1
    unilateral Q60.0
  respiratory organ NEC Q34.8
  rib Q76.6
  roof of orbit Q75.8
  round ligament Q52.8
  sacrum Q76.49
  salivary gland Q38.4
  scapula Q74.0
  scrotum Q55.29
  seminal vesicles Q55.4
  septum
    atrial Q21.1
    between aorta and pulmonary artery Q21.4
    ventricular Q20.4
  shoulder girdle (complete) (partial) Q74.0
  skull (bone) Q75.8
    with
      anencephaly Q00.0
      encephalocele *—see* Encephalocele
      hydrocephalus Q03.9
        with spina bifida *—see* Spina bifida, by site, with hydrocephalus
      microcephaly Q02
  spermatic cord Q55.4
  spinal cord Q06.0
  spine Q76.49
  spleen Q89.01
  sternum Q76.7
  stomach Q40.2
  submaxillary gland(s) (congenital) Q38.4
  tarsus *—see* Agenesis, foot
  tendon Q79.8
  testicle Q55.0
  thymus (gland) Q89.2
  thyroid (gland) E03.1
    cartilage Q31.8
  tibia *—see* Defect, reduction, lower limb, longitudinal, tibia
  tibiofibular *—see* Defect, reduction, lower limb, specified type NEC

Agenesis *(continued)*
  toe (and foot) (complete) (partial) *—see* Agenesis, foot
  tongue Q38.3
  trachea (cartilage) Q32.1
  ulna *—see* Defect, reduction, upper limb, longitudinal, ulna
  upper limb *—see* Agenesis, arm
  ureter Q62.4
  urethra Q64.5
  urinary tract NEC Q64.8
  uterus Q51.0
  uvula Q38.5
  vagina Q52.0
  vas deferens Q55.4
  vein(s) (peripheral) Q27.9
    brain Q28.3
    great NEC Q26.8
    portal Q26.5
  vena cava (inferior) (superior) Q26.8
  vermis of cerebellum Q04.3
  vertebra Q76.49
  vulva Q52.71

Ageusia R43.2

Agitated *—see* condition

Agitation R45.1

Aglossia (congenital) Q38.3

Aglossia-adactylia syndrome Q87.0

Aglycogenosis E74.00

Agnosia (body image) (other senses) (tactile) R48.1
  developmental F88
  verbal R48.1
    auditory R48.1
      developmental F80.2
    developmental F80.2
  visual (object) R48.3

Agoraphobia F40.00
  with panic disorder F40.01
  without panic disorder F40.02

Agrammatism R48.8

Agranulocytopenia *—see* Agranulocytosis

Agranulocytosis (chronic) (cyclical) (genetic) (infantile) (periodic) (pernicious) *—see also* Neutropenia D70.9
  congenital D70.0
  cytoreductive cancer chemotherapy sequela D70.1
  drug-induced D70.2
    due to cytoreductive cancer chemotherapy D70.1
  due to infection D70.3
  secondary D70.4
    drug-induced D70.2
      due to cytoreductive cancer chemotherapy D70.1

Agraphia (absolute) R48.8
  with alexia R48.0
  developmental F81.81

Ague (dumb) *—see* Malaria

Agyria Q04.3

Ahumada-del Castillo syndrome E23.0

Aichomophobia F40.298

AIDS (related complex) B20

Ailment heart *—see* Disease, heart

Ailurophobia F40.218

AIN *—see* Neoplasia, intraepithelial, anal

Ainhum (disease) L94.6

AIPHI (acute idiopathic pulmonary hemorrhage in infants (over 28 days old)) R04.81

Air
- anterior mediastinum J98.2
- compressed, disease T70.3
- conditioner lung or pneumonitis J67.7
- embolism (artery) (cerebral) (any site) T79.0
  - with ectopic or molar pregnancy O08.2
  - due to implanted device NEC —*see* Complications, by site and type, specified NEC
  - following
    - abortion —*see* Abortion by type, complicated by, embolism
    - ectopic or molar pregnancy O08.2
    - infusion, therapeutic injection or transfusion T80.0
  - in pregnancy, childbirth or puerperium —*see* Embolism, obstetric
  - traumatic T79.0
- hunger, psychogenic F45.8
- rarefied, effects of —*see* Effect, adverse, high altitude
- sickness T75.3

Airplane sickness T75.3

Akathisia (drug-induced) (treatment-induced) G25.71
- neuroleptic induced (acute) G25.71
- tardive G25.71

Akinesia R29.898

Akinetic mutism R41.89

Akureyri's disease G93.3

Alactasia, congenital E73.0

Alagille's syndrome Q44.7

Alastrim B03

Albers-Schönberg syndrome Q78.2

Albert's syndrome —*see* Tendinitis, Achilles

Albinism, albino E70.30
- with hematologic abnormality E70.339
  - Chédiak-Higashi syndrome E70.330
  - Hermansky-Pudlak syndrome E70.331
  - other specified E70.338
- I E70.320
- II E70.321
- ocular E70.319
  - autosomal recessive E70.311
  - other specified E70.318
  - X-linked E70.310
- oculocutaneous E70.329
  - other specified E70.328
  - tyrosinase (ty) negative E70.320
  - tyrosinase (ty) positive E70.321
- other specified E70.39

Albinismus E70.30

Albright (-McCune) (-Sternberg) syndrome Q78.1

Albuminous —*see* condition

Albuminuria, albuminuric (acute) (chronic) (subacute) (*see also* Proteinuria) R80.9
- complicating pregnancy —*see* Proteinuria, gestational

Albuminuria, albuminuric *(continued)*
- complicating pregnancy *(continued)*
  - with
    - gestational hypertension —*see* Pre-eclampsia
    - pre-existing hypertension —*see* Hypertension, complicating pregnancy, pre-existing, with, pre-eclampsia
- gestational —*see* Proteinuria, gestational
  - with
    - gestational hypertension —*see* Pre-eclampsia
    - pre-existing hypertension —*see* Hypertension, complicating pregnancy, pre-existing, with, pre-eclampsia
- orthostatic R80.2
- postural R80.2
- pre-eclamptic —*see* Pre-eclampsia
- scarlatinal A38.8

Albuminurophobia F40.298

Alcaptonuria E70.29

Alcohol, alcoholic, alcohol-induced
- addiction (without remission) F10.20
  - with remission F10.21
- amnestic disorder, persisting F10.96
  - with dependence F10.26
- anxiety disorder F10.980
- bipolar and related disorder F10.94
- brain syndrome, chronic F10.97
  - with dependence F10.27
- cardiopathy I42.6
- counseling and surveillance Z71.41
  - family member Z71.42
- delirium (acute) (tremens) (withdrawal) F10.231
  - with intoxication F10.921
    - in
      - abuse F10.121
      - dependence F10.221
- dementia F10.97
  - with dependence F10.27
- depressive disorder F10.94
  - with dependence F10.27
- deterioration F10.97
- hallucinosis (acute) F10.951
  - in
    - abuse F10.151
    - dependence F10.251
- insanity F10.959
- intoxication (acute) (without dependence) F10.129
  - with
    - delirium F10.121
    - dependence F10.229
      - with delirium F10.221
      - uncomplicated F10.220
  - uncomplicated F10.120
- jealousy F10.988
- Korsakoff's, Korsakov's, Korsakow's F10.26
- liver K70.9
  - acute —*see* Disease, liver, alcoholic, hepatitis
- major neurocognitive disorder, amnestic-confabulatory type F10.96
- major neurocognitive disorder, nonamnestic-confabulatory type F10.97
- mania (acute) (chronic) F10.959
- mild neurocognitive disorder F10.988

Alcohol, alcoholic, alcohol-induced *(continued)*
- paranoia, paranoid (type) psychosis F10.950
- pellagra E52
- poisoning, accidental (acute) NEC —*see* Table of Drugs and Chemicals, alcohol, poisoning
- psychosis —*see* Psychosis, alcoholic
- psychotic disorder F10.959
- sexual dysfunction F10.981
- sleep disorder F10.982
- withdrawal (without convulsions) F10.239
  - with delirium F10.231

Alcoholism (chronic) (without remission) F10.20
- with
  - psychosis —*see* Psychosis, alcoholic
  - remission F10.21
- Korsakov's F10.96
  - with dependence F10.26

Alder (-Reilly) anomaly or syndrome (leukocyte granulation) D72.0

Aldosteronism E26.9
- familial (type I) E26.02
- glucocorticoid-remediable E26.02
- primary (due to (bilateral) adrenal hyperplasia) E26.09
- primary NEC E26.09
- secondary E26.1
- specified NEC E26.89

Aldosteronoma D44.10

Aldrich (-Wiskott) syndrome (eczema-thrombocytopenia) D82.0

Alektorophobia F40.218

Aleppo boil B55.1

Aleukemic —*see* condition

Aleukia
- congenital D70.0
- hemorrhagica D61.9
  - congenital D61.09
- splenica D73.1

Alexia R48.0
- developmental F81.0
- secondary to organic lesion R48.0

Algoneurodystrophy M89.00
- ankle M89.07-
- foot M89.07-
- forearm M89.03-
- hand M89.04-
- lower leg M89.06-
- multiple sites M89.0-
- shoulder M89.01-
- specified site NEC M89.08
- thigh M89.05-
- upper arm M89.02-

Algophobia F40.298

Alienation, mental —*see* Psychosis

Alkalemia E87.3

Alkalosis E87.3
- metabolic E87.3
  - with respiratory acidosis E87.4
  - of newborn P74.41
- respiratory E87.3

Alkaptonuria E70.29

Allen-Masters syndrome N83.8

Allergy, allergic (reaction) (to) T78.40
- air-borne substance NEC (rhinitis) J30.89

Allergy, allergic *(continued)*
- alveolitis (extrinsic) J67.9
  - due to
    - Aspergillus clavatus J67.4
    - Cryptostroma corticale J67.6
    - organisms (fungal, thermophilic actinomycete) growing in ventilation (air conditioning) systems J67.7
  - specified type NEC J67.8
- anaphylactic reaction or shock T78.2
- angioneurotic edema T78.3
- animal (dander) (epidermal) (hair) (rhinitis) J30.81
- bee sting (anaphylactic shock) —*see* Toxicity, venom, arthropod, bee
- biological —*see* Allergy, drug
- colitis (*see also* Colitis, allergic) K52.29
- dander (animal) (rhinitis) J30.81
- dandruff (rhinitis) J30.81
- dental restorative material (existing) K08.55
- dermatitis —*see* Dermatitis, contact, allergic
- diathesis —*see* History, allergy
- drug, medicament & biological (any) (external) (internal) T78.40
  - correct substance properly administered —*see* Table of Drugs and Chemicals, by drug, adverse effect
  - wrong substance given or taken NEC (by accident) —*see* Table of Drugs and Chemicals, by drug, poisoning
- due to pollen J30.1
- dust (house) (stock) (rhinitis) J30.89
  - with asthma —*see* Asthma, allergic extrinsic
- eczema —*see* Dermatitis, contact, allergic
- epidermal (animal) (rhinitis) J30.81
- feathers (rhinitis) J30.89
- food (any) (ingested) NEC T78.1
  - anaphylactic shock —*see* Shock, anaphylactic, due to food
  - dermatitis —*see* Dermatitis, due to, food
  - dietary counseling and surveillance Z71.3
  - in contact with skin L23.6
  - rhinitis J30.5
  - status (without reaction) Z91.018
    - beef Z91.014
    - lamb Z91.014
    - eggs Z91.012
    - mammalian meats Z91.04
    - milk products Z91.011
    - peanuts Z91.010
    - pork Z91.014
    - red meats Z91.04
    - seafood Z91.013
    - specified NEC Z91.018
- gastrointestinal —*see also* specific type of allergic reaction
  - meaning colitis (*see also* Colitis, allergic) K52.29
  - meaning gastroenteritis (*see also* Gastroenteritis, allergic) K52.29
  - meaning other adverse food reaction not elsewhere classified T78.1
- grain J30.1
- grass (hay fever) (pollen) J30.1
  - asthma —*see* Asthma, allergic extrinsic
- hair (animal) (rhinitis) J30.81
- history (of) —*see* History, allergy
- horse serum —*see* Allergy, serum

Allergy, allergic *(continued)*
inhalant (rhinitis) J30.89
pollen J30.1
kapok (rhinitis) J30.89
medicine —*see* Allergy, drug
milk protein (*see also* Allergy, food) Z91.011
anaphylactic reaction T78.07
dematitis L27.2
entercolitis syndrome K52.21
enteropathy K52.22
gastroenteritis K52.29
gastroesophageal reflux (*see also* Reaction, adverse, food) K21.9
with esophagitis (without bleeding) K21.00
with bleeding K21.01
proctocolitis K52.29
nasal, seasonal due to pollen J30.1
pneumonia J82.89
pollen (any) (hay fever) J30.1
asthma —*see* Asthma, allergic extrinsic
primrose J30.1
primula J30.1
proctocolitis K52.29
purpura D69.0
ragweed (hay fever) (pollen) J30.1
asthma —*see* Asthma, allergic extrinsic
rose (pollen) J30.1
seasonal NEC J30.2
Senecio jacobae (pollen) J30.1
serum (*see also* Reaction, serum) T80.69
anaphylactic shock T80.59
shock (anaphylactic) T78.2
due to
administration of blood and blood products T80.51
adverse effect of correct medicinal substance properly administered T88.6
immunization T80.52
serum NEC T80.59
vaccination T80.52
specific NEC T78.49
tree (any) (hay fever) (pollen) J30.1
asthma —*see* Asthma, allergic extrinsic
upper respiratory J30.9
urticaria L50.0
vaccine —*see* Allergy, serum
wheat —*see* Allergy, food

Allescheriasis B48.2

Alligator skin disease Q80.9

Allocheiria, allochiria R20.8

Almeida's disease —*see* Paracoccidioidomycosis

Alopecia (hereditaria) (seborrheica) L65.9
androgenic L64.9
drug-induced L64.0
specified NEC L64.8
areata L63.9
ophiasis L63.2
specified NEC L63.8
totalis L63.0
universalis L63.1
cicatricial L66.9
specified NEC L66.8
circumscripta L63.9
congenital, congenitalis Q84.0
due to cytotoxic drugs NEC L65.8
mucinosa L65.2
postinfective NEC L65.8
postpartum L65.0
premature L64.8

Alopecia *(continued)*
specific (syphilitic) A51.32
specified NEC L65.8
syphilitic (secondary) A51.32
totalis (capitis) L63.0
universalis (entire body) L63.1
X-ray L58.1

Alpers' disease G31.81

Alpine sickness T70.29

Alport syndrome Q87.81

ALTE (apparent life threatening event) in newborn and infant R68.13

Alteration (of), **Altered**
awareness
transient R40.4
unintended under general anesthesia, during procedure T88.53
mental status R41.82
pattern of family relationships affecting child Z62.898
sensation
following
cerebrovascular disease I69.998
cerebral infarction I69.398
intracerebral hemorrhage I69.198
nontraumatic intracranial hemorrhage NEC I69.298
specified disease NEC I69.898
subarachnoid hemorrhage I69.098

Alternating —*see* condition

Altitude, high (effects) —*see* Effect, adverse, high altitude

Aluminosis (of lung) J63.0

Alveolitis
allergic (extrinsic) —*see* Pneumonitis, hypersensitivity
due to
Aspergillus clavatus J67.4
Cryptostroma corticale J67.6
fibrosing (cryptogenic) (idiopathic) J84.112
jaw M27.3
sicca dolorosa M27.3

Alveolus, alveolar —*see* condition

Alymphocytosis D72.810
thymic (with immunodeficiency) D82.1

Alymphoplasia, thymic D82.1

Alzheimer's disease or sclerosis —*see* Disease, Alzheimer's

Amastia (with nipple present) Q83.8
with absent nipple Q83.0

Amathophobia F40.228

Amaurosis (acquired) (congenital) —*see also* Blindness
fugax G45.3
hysterical F44.6
Leber's congenital H35.50
uremic —*see* Uremia

Amaurotic idiocy (infantile) (juvenile) (late) E75.4

Amaxophobia F40.248

Ambiguous genitalia Q56.4

Amblyopia (congenital) (ex anopsia) (partial) (suppression) H53.00-
anisometropic —*see* Amblyopia, refractive
deprivation H53.01-
hysterical F44.6

Amblyopia *(continued)*
nocturnal —*see also* Blindness, night
vitamin A deficiency E50.5
refractive H53.02-
strabismic H53.03-
suspect H53.04-
tobacco H53.8
toxic NEC H53.8
uremic —*see* Uremia

Ameba, amebic (histolytica) —*see also* Amebiasis
abscess (liver) A06.4

Amebiasis A06.9
with abscess —*see* Abscess, amebic
acute A06.0
chronic (intestine) A06.1
with abscess —*see* Abscess, amebic
cutaneous A06.7
cutis A06.7
cystitis A06.81
genitourinary tract NEC A06.82
hepatic —*see* Abscess, liver, amebic
intestine A06.0
nondysenteric colitis A06.2
skin A06.7
specified site NEC A06.89

Ameboma (of intestine) A06.3

Amelia Q73.0
lower limb —*see* Agenesis, leg
upper limb —*see* Agenesis, arm

Ameloblastoma —*see also* Cyst, calcifying odontogenic
long bones C40.9-
lower limb C40.2-
upper limb C40.0-
malignant C41.1
jaw (bone) (lower) C41.1
upper C41.0
tibial C40.2-

Amelogenesis imperfecta K00.5
nonhereditaria (segmentalis) K00.4

Amenorrhea N91.2
hyperhormonal E28.8
primary N91.0
secondary N91.1

Amentia —*see* Disability,intellectual
Meynert's (nonalcoholic) F04

American
leishmaniasis B55.2
mountain tick fever A93.2

Ametropia —*see* Disorder, refraction

AMH (asymptomatic microscopic hematuria) R31.21

Amianthosis J61

Amimia R48.8

Amino-acid disorder E72.9
anemia D53.0

Aminoacidopathy E72.9

Aminoaciduria E72.9

Amnes(t)ic syndrome (post-traumatic) F04
induced by
alcohol F10.96
with dependence F10.26
psychoactive NEC F19.96
with
abuse F19.16
dependence F19.26
sedative F13.96
with dependence F13.26

Amnesia R41.3
anterograde R41.1
auditory R48.8

Amnesia *(continued)*
dissociative F44.0
with dissociative fugue F44.1
hysterical F44.0
postictal in epilepsy —*see* Epilepsy
psychogenic F44.0
retrograde R41.2
transient global G45.4

Amnion, amniotic —*see* condition

Amnionitis —*see* Pregnancy, complicated by

Amok F68.8

Amoral traits F60.89

Amphetamine (or other stimulant) -induced
anxiety disorder F15.980
bipolar and related disorder F15.94
delirium F15.921
depressive disorder F15.94
obsessive-compulsive and related disorder F15.988
psychotic disorder F15.959
sexual dysfunction F15.981
sleep disorder F15.982
stimulant withdrawal F15.23

Ampulla
lower esophagus K22.89
phrenic K22.89

Amputation —*see also* Absence, by site, acquired
neuroma (postoperative) (traumatic) —*see* Complications, amputation stump, neuroma
stump (surgical)
abnormal, painful, or with complication (late) —*see* Complications, amputation stump
healed or old NOS Z89.9
traumatic (complete) (partial)
arm (upper) (complete) S48.91-
at
elbow S58.01-
partial S58.02-
shoulder joint (complete) S48.01-
partial S48.02-
between
elbow and wrist (complete) S58.11-
partial S58.12-
shoulder and elbow (complete) S48.11-
partial S48.12-
partial S48.92-
breast (complete) S28.21-
partial S28.22-
clitoris (complete) S38.211
partial S38.212
ear (complete) S08.11-
partial S08.12-
finger (complete) (metacarpophalangeal) S68.11-
index S68.11-
little S68.11-
middle S68.11-
partial S68.12-
index S68.12-
little S68.12-
middle S68.12-
ring S68.12-
ring S68.11-
thumb —*see* Amputation, traumatic, thumb

Amputation *(continued)*
  traumatic *(continued)*
    finger *(continued)*
      transphalangeal (complete) S68.61-
        index S68.61-
        little S68.61-
        middle S68.61-
        partial S68.62-
          index S68.62-
          little S68.62-
          middle S68.62-
          ring S68.62-
        ring S68.61-
    foot (complete) S98.91-
      at ankle level S98.01-
        partial S98.02-
      midfoot S98.31-
        partial S98.32-
      partial S98.92-
    forearm (complete) S58.91-
      at elbow level (complete) S58.01-
        partial S58.02-
      between elbow and wrist (complete) S58.11-
        partial S58.12-
      partial S58.92-
    genital organ(s) (external)
      female (complete) S38.211
        partial S38.212
      male
        penis (complete) S38.221
          partial S38.222
        scrotum (complete) S38.231
          partial S38.232
        testes (complete) S38.231
          partial S38.232
    hand (complete) (wrist level) S68.41-
      finger(s) alone —*see* Amputation, traumatic, finger
      partial S68.42-
      thumb alone —*see* Amputation, traumatic, thumb
      transmetacarpal (complete) S68.71-
        partial S68.72-
    head
      ear —*see* Amputation, traumatic, ear
      nose (partial) S08.812
        complete S08.811
      part S08.89
        scalp S08.0
    hip (and thigh) (complete) S78.91-
      at hip joint (complete) S78.01-
        partial S78.02-
      between hip and knee (complete) S78.11-
        partial S78.12-
      partial S78.92-
    labium (majus) (minus) (complete) S38.21-
      partial S38.21-
    leg (lower) S88.91-
      at knee level S88.01-
        partial S88.02-
      between knee and ankle S88.11-
        partial S88.12-
      partial S88.92-
    nose (partial) S08.812
      complete S08.811
    penis (complete) S38.221
      partial S38.222
    scrotum (complete) S38.231
      partial S38.232

Amputation *(continued)*
  traumatic *(continued)*
    shoulder —*see* Amputation, traumatic, arm
      at shoulder joint —*see* Amputation, traumatic, arm, at shoulder joint
    testes (complete) S38.231
      partial S38.232
    thigh —*see* Amputation, traumatic, hip
    thorax, part of S28.1
      breast —*see* Amputation, traumatic, breast
    thumb (complete) (metacarpophalangeal) S68.01-
      partial S68.02-
      transphalangeal (complete) S68.51-
        partial S68.52-
    toe (lesser) S98.13-
      great S98.11-
        partial S98.12-
      more than one S98.21-
        partial S98.22-
      partial S98.14-
    vulva (complete) S38.211
      partial S38.212

Amputee (bilateral) (old) Z89.9

Amsterdam dwarfism Q87.19

Amusia R48.8
  developmental F80.89

Amyelencephalus, amyelencephaly Q00.0

Amyelia Q06.0

Amygdalitis —*see* Tonsillitis

Amygdalolith J35.8

Amyloid heart (disease) E85.4 *[I43]*

Amyloidosis (generalized) (primary) E85.9
  with lung involvement E85.4 *[J99]*
  familial E85.2
  genetic E85.2
  heart E85.4 *[I43]*
  hemodialysis-associated E85.3
  liver E85.4 *[K77]*
  light chain (AL) E85.81
  localized E85.4
  neuropathic heredofamilial E85.1
  non-neuropathic heredofamilial E85.0
  organ limited E85.4
  Portuguese E85.1
  pulmonary E85.4 *[J99]*
  secondary systemic E85.3
  senile systemic (SSA) E85.82
  skin (lichen) (macular) E85.4 *[L99]*
  specified NEC E85.89
  subglottic E85.4 *[J99]*
  wild-type transthyretin-related (ATTR) E85.82

Amylopectinosis (brancher enzyme deficiency) E74.03

Amylophagia —*see* Pica

Amyoplasia congenita Q79.8

Amyotonia M62.89
  congenita G70.2

Amyotrophia, amyotrophy, amyotrophic G71.8
  congenita Q79.8

Amyotrophia, amyotrophy, amyotrophic *(continued)*
  diabetic —*see* Diabetes, amyotrophy
  lateral sclerosis G12.21
  neuralgic G54.5
  spinal progressive G12.25

Anacidity, gastric K31.83
  psychogenic F45.8

Anaerosis of newborn P28.89

Analbuminemia E88.09

Analgesia —*see* Anesthesia

Analphalipoproteinemia E78.6

Anaphylactic
  purpura D69.0
  shock or reaction —*see* Shock, anaphylactic

Anaphylactoid shock or reaction —*see* Shock, anaphylactic

Anaphylactoid syndrome of pregnancy O88.01-

Anaphylaxis —*see* Shock, anaphylactic

Anaplasia cervix —*see also* Dysplasia, cervix N87.9

Anaplasmosis [A. phagocytophilum] (transfusion transmitted) A79.82
  human A77.49

Anarthria R47.1

Anasarca R60.1
  cardiac —*see* Failure, heart, congestive
  lung J18.2
  newborn P83.2
  nutritional E43
  pulmonary J18.2
  renal N04.9

Anastomosis
  aneurysmal —*see* Aneurysm
  arteriovenous ruptured brain I60.8
    intracerebral I61.8
    intraparenchymal I61.8
    intraventricular I61.5
    subarachnoid I60.8
  intestinal K63.89
    complicated NEC K91.89
      involving urinary tract N99.89
  retinal and choroidal vessels (congenital) Q14.8

Anatomical narrow angle H40.03-

Ancylostoma, ancylostomiasis (braziliense) (caninum) (ceylanicum) (duodenale) B76.0
  Necator americanus B76.1

Andersen's disease (glycogen storage) E74.09

Anderson-Fabry disease E75.21

Andes disease T70.29

Andrews' disease (bacterid) L08.89

Androblastoma
  benign
    specified site —*see* Neoplasm, benign, by site
    unspecified site
      female D27.9
      male D29.20
  malignant
    specified site —*see* Neoplasm, malignant, by site

Androblastoma *(continued)*
  malignant *(continued)*
    unspecified site
      female C56.9
      male C62.90
  specified site —*see* Neoplasm, uncertain behavior, by site
  tubular
    with lipid storage
      specified site —*see* Neoplasm, benign, by site
      unspecified site
        female D27.9
        male D29.20
    specified site —*see* Neoplasm, benign, by site
    unspecified site
      female D27.9
      male D29.20
  unspecified site
    female D39.10
    male D40.10

Androgen insensitivity syndrome —*see also* Syndrome, androgen insensitivity E34.50

Androgen resistance syndrome —*see also* Syndrome, androgen insensitivity E34.50

Android pelvis Q74.2
  with disproportion (fetopelvic) O33.3
    causing obstructed labor O65.3

Androphobia F40.290

Anectasis, pulmonary (newborn) —*see* Atelectasis

Anemia (essential) (general) (hemoglobin deficiency) (infantile) (primary) (profound) D64.9
  with (due to) (in)
    disorder of
      anaerobic glycolysis D55.29
      pentose phosphate pathway D55.1
    koilonychia D50.9
  achlorhydric D50.8
  achrestic D53.1
  Addison (-Biermer) (pernicious) D51.0
  agranulocytic —*see* Agranulocytosis
  amino-acid-deficiency D53.0
  aplastic D61.9
    congenital D61.09
    drug-induced D61.1
    due to
      drugs D61.1
      external agents NEC D61.2
      infection D61.2
      radiation D61.2
    idiopathic D61.3
    red cell (pure) D60.9
      chronic D60.0
      congenital D61.01
      specified type NEC D60.8
      transient D60.1
    specified type NEC D61.89
    toxic D61.2
  aregenerative
    congenital D61.09
  asiderotic D50.9
  atypical (primary) D64.9
  Baghdad spring D55.0
  Balantidium coli A07.0
  Biermer's (pernicious) D51.0
  blood loss (chronic) D50.0
    acute D62
  bothriocephalus B70.0 *[D63.8]*
  brickmaker's B76.9 *[D63.8]*

Anemia *(continued)*
- cerebral I67.89
- childhood D58.9
- chlorotic D50.8
- chronic
  - blood loss D50.0
  - hemolytic D58.9
    - idiopathic D59.9
  - simple D53.9
- chronica congenita aregenerativa D61.09
- combined system disease NEC D51.0 *[G32.0]*
  - due to dietary vitamin B12 deficiency D51.3 *[G32.0]*
- complicating pregnancy, childbirth or puerperium *—see* Pregnancy, complicated by (management affected by), anemia
- congenital P61.4
  - aplastic D61.09
  - due to isoimmunization NOS P55.9
  - dyserythropoietic, dyshematopoietic D64.4
  - following fetal blood loss P61.3
  - Heinz body D58.2
  - hereditary hemolytic NOS D58.9
  - pernicious D51.0
  - spherocytic D58.0
- Cooley's (erythroblastic) D56.1
- cytogenic D51.0
- deficiency D53.9
  - 2, 3 diphosphoglycurate mutase D55.29
  - 2, 3 PG D55.29
  - 6 phosphogluconate dehydrogenase D55.1
  - 6-PGD D55.1
  - amino-acid D53.0
  - combined B12 and folate D53.1
  - enzyme D55.9
    - drug-induced (hemolytic) D59.2
    - glucose-6-phosphate dehydrogenase (G6PD) D55.0
    - glycolytic D55.29
    - nucleotide metabolism D55.3
    - related to hexose monophosphate (HMP) shunt pathway NEC D55.1
    - specified type NEC D55.8
  - erythrocytic glutathione D55.1
  - folate D52.9
    - dietary D52.0
    - drug-induced D52.1
  - folic acid D52.9
    - dietary D52.0
    - drug-induced D52.1
  - G SH D55.1
  - GGS-R D55.1
  - glucose-6-phosphate dehydrogenase D55.0
  - glutathione reductase D55.1
  - glyceraldehyde phosphate dehydrogenase D55.29
  - G6PD D55.0
  - hexokinase D55.29
  - iron D50.9
    - secondary to blood loss (chronic) D50.0
  - nutritional D53.9
    - with
      - poor iron absorption D50.8
      - specified deficiency NEC D53.8
  - phosphofructo-aldolase D55.29
  - phosphoglycerate kinase D55.29
  - PK D55.21
  - protein D53.0

Anemia *(continued)*
- deficiency *(continued)*
  - pyruvate kinase D55.21
  - transcobalamin II D51.2
  - triose-phosphate isomerase D55.29
  - vitamin B12 NOS D51.9
    - dietary D51.3
    - due to
      - intrinsic factor deficiency D51.0
      - selective vitamin B12 malabsorption with proteinuria D51.1
    - pernicious D51.0
    - specified type NEC D51.8
- Diamond-Blackfan (congenital hypoplastic) D61.01
- dibothriocephalus B70.0 *[D63.8]*
- dimorphic D53.1
- diphasic D53.1
- Diphyllobothrium (Dibothriocephalus) B70.0 *[D63.8]*
- due to (in) (with)
  - antineoplastic chemotherapy D64.81
  - blood loss (chronic) D50.0
    - acute D62
  - chemotherapy, antineoplastic D64.81
  - chronic disease classified elsewhere NEC D63.8
  - chronic kidney disease D63.1
  - deficiency
    - amino-acid D53.0
    - copper D53.8
    - folate (folic acid) D52.9
      - dietary D52.0
      - drug-induced D52.1
    - molybdenum D53.8
    - protein D53.0
    - zinc D53.8
  - dietary vitamin B12 deficiency D51.3
  - disorder of
    - glutathione metabolism D55.1
    - nucleotide metabolism D55.3
  - drug *—see* Anemia, by type *—see also* Table of Drugs and Chemicals
  - end stage renal disease D63.1
  - enzyme disorder D55.9
  - fetal blood loss P61.3
  - fish tapeworm (D.latum) infestation B70.0 *[D63.8]*
  - hemorrhage (chronic) D50.0
    - acute D62
  - impaired absorption D50.9
  - loss of blood (chronic) D50.0
    - acute D62
  - myxedema E03.9 *[D63.8]*
  - Necator americanus B76.1 *[D63.8]*
  - prematurity P61.2
  - selective vitamin B12 malabsorption with proteinuria D51.1
  - transcobalamin II deficiency D51.2
- Dyke-Young type (secondary) (symptomatic) D59.19
- dyserythropoietic (congenital) D64.4
- dyshematopoietic (congenital) D64.4
- Egyptian B76.9 *[D63.8]*
- elliptocytosis *—see* Elliptocytosis
- enzyme-deficiency, drug-induced D59.2
- epidemic *—see also* Ancylostomiasis B76.9 *[D63.8]*

Anemia *(continued)*
- erythroblastic
  - familial D56.1
  - newborn (*see also* Disease, hemolytic) P55.9
  - of childhood D56.1
- erythrocytic glutathione deficiency D55.1
- erythropoietin-resistant anemia (EPO resistant anemia) D63.1
- Faber's (achlorhydric anemia) D50.9
- factitious (self-induced blood letting) D50.0
- familial erythroblastic D56.1
- Fanconi's (congenital pancytopenia) D61.09
- favism D55.0
- fish tapeworm (D. latum) infestation B70.0 *[D63.8]*
- folate (folic acid) deficiency D52.9
- glucose-6-phosphate dehydrogenase (G6PD) deficiency D55.0
- glutathione-reductase deficiency D55.1
- goat's milk D52.0
- granulocytic *—see* Agranulocytosis
- Heinz body, congenital D58.2
- hemolytic D58.9
  - acquired D59.9
    - with hemoglobinuria NEC D59.6
    - autoimmune NEC D59.19
    - infectious D59.4
    - specified type NEC D59.8
    - toxic D59.4
  - acute D59.9
    - due to enzyme deficiency
      - specified type NEC D55.8
    - Lederer's D59.19
  - autoimmune D59.10
    - cold D59.12
    - drug-induced D59.0
    - mixed D59.13
    - warm D59.11
  - chronic D58.9
    - idiopathic D59.9
  - cold type (primary) (secondary) (symptomatic) D59.12
  - congenital (spherocytic) *—see* Spherocytosis
  - due to
    - cardiac conditions D59.4
    - drugs (nonautoimmune) D59.2
      - autoimmune D59.0
    - enzyme disorder D55.9
      - drug-induced D59.2
    - presence of shunt or other internal prosthetic device D59.4
  - familial D58.9
  - hereditary D58.9
    - due to enzyme disorder D55.9
      - specified type NEC D55.8
    - specified type NEC D58.8
  - idiopathic (chronic) D59.9
  - mechanical D59.4
  - microangiopathic D59.4
  - mixed type (primary) (secondary) (symptomatic) D59.13
  - nonautoimmune D59.4
    - drug-induced D59.2
  - nonspherocytic
    - congenital or hereditary NEC D55.8
      - glucose-6-phosphate dehydrogenase deficiency D55.0
      - pyruvate kinase deficiency D55.21

Anemia *(continued)*
- hemolytic *(continued)*
  - nonspherocytic *(continued)*
    - congenital or hereditary *(continued)*
      - type
        - I D55.1
        - II D55.29
    - type
      - I D55.1
      - II D55.29
  - primary
    - autoimmune
      - cold type D59.12
      - mixed type D59.13
      - warm type D59.11
  - secondary D59.4
    - autoimmune
      - cold type D59.12
      - mixed type D59.13
      - warm type D59.11
  - specified (hereditary) type NEC D58.8
  - Stransky-Regala type (*see also* Hemoglobinopathy) D58.8
  - symptomatic D59.4
    - autoimmune
      - cold type D59.12
      - mixed type D59.13
      - warm type D59.11
  - toxic D59.4
  - warm type (primary) (secondary) (symptomatic) D59.11
- hemorrhagic (chronic) D50.0
  - acute D62
- Herrick's D57.1
- hexokinase deficiency D55.29
- hookworm B76.9 *[D63.8]*
- hypochromic (idiopathic) (microcytic) (normoblastic) D50.9
  - due to blood loss (chronic) D50.0
    - acute D62
  - familial sex-linked D64.0
  - pyridoxine-responsive D64.3
  - sideroblastic, sex-linked D64.0
- hypoplasia, red blood cells D61.9
  - congenital or familial D61.01
- hypoplastic (idiopathic) D61.9
  - congenital or familial (of childhood) D61.01
- hypoproliferative (refractive) D61.9
- idiopathic D64.9
  - aplastic D61.3
  - hemolytic, chronic D59.9
- in (due to) (with)
  - chronic kidney disease D63.1
  - end stage renal disease D63.1
  - failure, kidney (renal) D63.1
  - neoplastic disease (*see also* Neoplasm) D63.0
- intertropical *—see also* Ancylostomiasis D63.8
- iron deficiency D50.9
  - secondary to blood loss (chronic) D50.0
    - acute D62
  - specified type NEC D50.8
- Joseph-Diamond-Blackfan (congenital hypoplastic) D61.01
- Lederer's (hemolytic) D59.19
- leukoerythroblastic D61.82
- macrocytic D53.9
  - nutritional D52.0
  - tropical D52.8
- malarial (*see also* Malaria) B54 *[D63.8]*
- malignant (progressive) D51.0
- malnutrition D53.9
- marsh (*see also* Malaria) B54 *[D63.8]*

Anemia *(continued)*
- Mediterranean (with other hemoglobinopathy) D56.9
- megaloblastic D53.1
  - combined B12 and folate deficiency D53.1
  - hereditary D51.1
  - nutritional D52.0
  - orotic aciduria D53.0
  - refractory D53.1
  - specified type NEC D53.1
- megalocytic D53.1
- microcytic (hypochromic) D50.9
  - due to blood loss (chronic) D50.0
    - acute D62
  - familial D56.8
- microdrepanocytosis D57.40
- microelliptopoikilocytic (Rietti-Greppi- Micheli) D56.9
- miner's B76.9 *[D63.8]*
- myelodysplastic D46.9
- myelofibrosis D75.81
- myelogenous D64.89
- myelopathic D64.89
- myelophthisic D61.82
- myeloproliferative D47.Z9
- newborn P61.4
  - due to
    - ABO (antibodies, isoimmunization, maternal/fetal incompatibility) P55.1
    - Rh (antibodies, isoimmunization, maternal/fetal incompatibility) P55.0
  - following fetal blood loss P61.3
  - posthemorrhagic (fetal) P61.3
- nonspherocytic hemolytic —*see* Anemia, hemolytic, nonspherocytic
- normocytic (infectional) D64.9
  - due to blood loss (chronic) D50.0
    - acute D62
  - myelophthisic D61.82
- nutritional (deficiency) D53.9
  - with
    - poor iron absorption D50.8
    - specified deficiency NEC D53.8
  - megaloblastic D52.0
- of prematurity P61.2
- orotaciduric (congenital) (hereditary) D53.0
- osteosclerotic D64.89
- ovalocytosis (hereditary) —*see* Elliptocytosis
- paludal (*see also* Malaria) B54 *[D63.8]*
- pernicious (congenital) (malignant) (progressive) D51.0
- pleochromic D64.89
  - of sprue D52.8
- posthemorrhagic (chronic) D50.0
  - acute D62
  - newborn P61.3
- postoperative (postprocedural)
  - due to (acute) blood loss D62
    - chronic blood loss D50.0
  - specified NEC D64.89
- postpartum O90.81
- pressure D64.89
- progressive D64.9
  - malignant D51.0
  - pernicious D51.0
- protein-deficiency D53.0
- pseudoleukemica infantum D64.89
- pure red cell D60.9
  - congenital D61.01
- pyridoxine-responsive D64.3
- pyruvate kinase deficiency D55.21

Anemia *(continued)*
- refractory D46.4
  - with
    - excess of blasts D46.20
      - 1(RAEB 1) D46.21
      - 2(RAEB 2) D46.22
      - in transformation (RAEB T) —*see* Leukemia, acute myeloblastic
    - hemochromatosis D46.1
    - sideroblasts (ring) (RARS) D46.1
  - megaloblastic D53.1
  - sideroblastic D46.1
  - sideropenic D50.9
  - without ring sideroblasts, so stated D46.0
  - without sideroblasts without excess of blasts D46.0
- Rietti-Greppi-Micheli D56.9
- scorbutic D53.2
- secondary to
  - blood loss (chronic) D50.0
    - acute D62
  - hemorrhage (chronic) D50.0
    - acute D62
- semiplastic D61.89
- sickle-cell —*see* Disease, sickle-cell
- sideroblastic D64.3
  - hereditary D64.0
  - hypochromic, sex-linked D64.0
  - pyridoxine-responsive NEC D64.3
  - refractory D46.1
  - secondary (due to)
    - disease D64.1
    - drugs and toxins D64.2
  - specified type NEC D64.3
- sideropenic (refractory) D50.9
  - due to blood loss (chronic) D50.0
    - acute D62
- simple chronic D53.9
- specified type NEC D64.89
- spherocytic (hereditary) —*see* Spherocytosis
- splenic D64.89
- splenomegalic D64.89
- stomatocytosis D58.8
- syphilitic (acquired) (late) A52.79 *[D63.8]*
- target cell D64.89
- thalassemia D56.9
- thrombocytopenic —*see* Thrombocytopenia
- toxic D61.2
- tropical B76.9 *[D63.8]*
  - macrocytic D52.8
- tuberculous A18.89 *[D63.8]*
- vegan D51.3
- vitamin
  - B6-responsive D64.3
  - B12 deficiency (dietary)
    - pernicious D51.0
- von Jaksch's D64.89
- Witts' (achlorhydric anemia) D50.8

Anemophobia F40.228

Anencephalus, anencephaly Q00.0

Anergasia —*see* Psychosis, organic

Anesthesia, anesthetic R20.0
- complication or reaction NEC (*see also* Complications, anesthesia) T88.59
  - due to
    - correct substance properly administered —*see* Table of Drugs and Chemicals, by drug, adverse effect

Anesthesia, anesthetic *(continued)*
- complication or reaction *(continued)*
  - due to *(continued)*
    - overdose or wrong substance given —*see* Table of Drugs and Chemicals, by drug, poisoning
  - unintended awareness under general anesthesia during procedure T88.53
    - personal history of Z92.84
- cornea H18.81-
- dissociative F44.6
- functional (hysterical) F44.6
- hyperesthetic, thalamic G89.0
- hysterical F44.6
- local skin lesion R20.0
- sexual (psychogenic) F52.1
- shock (due to) T88.2
- skin R20.0
- testicular N50.9

Anetoderma (maculosum) (of) L90.8
- Jadassohn-Pellizzari L90.2
- Schweniger-Buzzi L90.1

Aneurin deficiency E51.9

Aneurysm (anastomotic) (artery) (cirsoid) (diffuse) (false) (fusiform) (multiple) (saccular) I72.9
- abdominal (aorta) I71.4
  - ruptured I71.3
  - syphilitic A52.01
- aorta, aortic (nonsyphilitic) I71.9
  - abdominal I71.4
    - ruptured I71.3
  - arch I71.2
    - ruptured I71.1
  - arteriosclerotic I71.9
    - ruptured I71.8
  - ascending I71.2
    - ruptured I71.1
  - congenital Q25.43
  - descending I71.9
    - abdominal I71.4
      - ruptured I71.3
    - ruptured I71.8
    - thoracic I71.2
      - ruptured I71.1
  - root Q25.43
  - ruptured I71.8
  - sinus, congenital Q25.43
  - syphilitic A52.01
  - thoracic I71.2
    - ruptured I71.1
  - thoracoabdominal I71.6
    - ruptured I71.5
  - thorax, thoracic (arch) I71.2
    - ruptured I71.1
    - root Q25.43
  - transverse I71.2
    - ruptured I71.1
  - valve (heart) (*see also* Endocarditis, aortic) I35.8
- arteriosclerotic I72.9
  - cerebral I67.1
    - ruptured —*see* Hemorrhage, intracranial, subarachnoid
- arteriovenous (congenital) —*see also* Malformation, arteriovenous
  - acquired I77.0
    - brain I67.1
      - ruptured —*see* Aneurysm, arteriovenous, brain, ruptured
    - coronary I25.41
    - pulmonary I28.0

Aneurysm *(continued)*
- arteriovenous *(continued)*
  - brain Q28.2
    - ruptured I60.8
      - intracerebral I61.8
      - intraparenchymal I61.8
      - intraventricular I61.5
      - subarachnoid I60.8
  - peripheral —*see* Malformation, arteriovenous, peripheral
  - precerebral vessels Q28.0
  - specified site NEC —*see also* Malformation, arteriovenous
    - acquired I77.0
- basal —*see* Aneurysm, brain
- basilar (trunk) I72.5
- berry (congenital) (nonruptured) I67.1
  - ruptured I60.7
- brain I67.1
  - arteriosclerotic I67.1
    - ruptured —*see* Hemorrhage, intracranial, subarachnoid
  - arteriovenous (congenital) (nonruptured) Q28.2
    - acquired I67.1
      - ruptured —*see* Aneurysm, arteriovenous, brain, ruptured I60.8-
    - ruptured —*see* Aneurysm, arteriovenous, brain, ruptured I60.8-
  - berry (congenital) (nonruptured) I67.1
    - ruptured (*see also* Hemorrhage, intracranial, subarachnoid) I60.7
  - congenital Q28.3
    - ruptured I60.7
  - meninges I67.1
    - ruptured I60.8
  - miliary (congenital) (nonruptured) I67.1
    - ruptured (*see also* Hemorrhage, intracranial, subarachnoid) I60.7
  - mycotic I33.0
  - ruptured —*see* Hemorrhage, intracranial, subarachnoid
  - syphilitic (hemorrhage) A52.05
- cardiac (false) (*see also* Aneurysm, heart) I25.3
- carotid artery (common) (external) I72.0
  - internal (intracranial) I67.1
    - extracranial portion I72.0
  - ruptured into brain I60.0-
  - syphilitic A52.09
    - intracranial A52.05
- cavernous sinus I67.1
  - arteriovenous (congenital) (nonruptured) Q28.3
    - ruptured I60.8
- celiac I72.8
- central nervous system, syphilitic A52.05
- cerebral —*see* Aneurysm, brain
- chest —*see* Aneurysm, thorax
- circle of Willis I67.1
  - congenital Q28.3
    - ruptured I60.6
  - ruptured I60.6
- common iliac artery I72.3
- congenital (peripheral) Q27.8
  - aorta (root) (sinus) Q25.43
  - brain Q28.3
    - ruptured I60.7
  - coronary Q24.5
  - digestive system Q27.8
  - lower limb Q27.8
  - pulmonary Q25.79
  - retina Q14.1

Aneurysm *(continued)*
- congenital *(continued)*
  - specified site NEC Q27.8
  - upper limb Q27.8
- conjunctiva *—see* Abnormality, conjunctiva, vascular
- conus arteriosus *—see* Aneurysm, heart
- coronary (arteriosclerotic) (artery) I25.41
  - arteriovenous, congenital Q24.5
  - congenital Q24.5
  - ruptured *—see* Infarct, myocardium
  - syphilitic A52.06
  - vein I25.89
- cylindroid (aorta) I71.9
  - ruptured I71.8
  - syphilitic A52.01
- ductus arteriosus Q25.0
- endocardial, infective (any valve) I33.0
- femoral (artery) (ruptured) I72.4
- gastroduodenal I72.8
- gastroepiploic I72.8
- heart (wall) (chronic or with a stated duration of over 4 weeks) I25.3
  - valve *—see* Endocarditis
- hepatic I72.8
- iliac (common) (artery) (ruptured) I72.3
- infective I72.9
  - endocardial (any valve) I33.0
- innominate (nonsyphilitic) I72.8
  - syphilitic A52.09
- interauricular septum *—see* Aneurysm, heart
- interventricular septum *—see* Aneurysm, heart
- intrathoracic (nonsyphilitic) I71.2
  - ruptured I71.1
  - syphilitic A52.01
- lower limb I72.4
- lung (pulmonary artery) I28.1
- mediastinal (nonsyphilitic) I72.8
  - syphilitic A52.09
- miliary (congenital) I67.1
  - ruptured *—see* Hemorrhage, intracerebral, subarachnoid, intracranial
- mitral (heart) (valve) I34.8
- mural *—see* Aneurysm, heart
- mycotic I72.9
  - endocardial (any valve) I33.0
  - ruptured, brain *—see* Hemorrhage, intracerebral, subarachnoid
- myocardium *—see* Aneurysm, heart
- neck I72.0
- pancreaticoduodenal I72.8
- patent ductus arteriosus Q25.0
- peripheral NEC I72.8
  - congenital Q27.8
    - digestive system Q27.8
    - lower limb Q27.8
    - specified site NEC Q27.8
    - upper limb Q27.8
- popliteal (artery) (ruptured) I72.4
- precerebral
  - congenital (nonruptured) Q28.1
  - specified site, NEC I72.5
- pulmonary I28.1
  - arteriovenous Q25.72
    - acquired I28.0
  - syphilitic A52.09
  - valve (heart) *—see* Endocarditis, pulmonary
- racemose (peripheral) I72.9
  - congenital *—see* Aneurysm, congenital
- radial I72.1
- Rasmussen NEC A15.0

Aneurysm *(continued)*
- renal (artery) I72.2
- retina *—see also* Disorder, retina, microaneurysms
  - congenital Q14.1
  - diabetic *—see* E08-E13 with .3-
- sinus of Valsalva Q25.49
- specified NEC I72.8
- spinal (cord) I72.8
  - syphilitic (hemorrhage) A52.09
- splenic I72.8
- subclavian (artery) (ruptured) I72.8
  - syphilitic A52.09
- superior mesenteric I72.8
- syphilitic (aorta) A52.01
  - central nervous system A52.05
  - congenital (late) A50.54 *[I79.0]*
  - spine, spinal A52.09
- thoracoabdominal (aorta) I71.6
  - ruptured I71.5
  - syphilitic A52.01
- thorax, thoracic (aorta) (arch) (nonsyphilitic) I71.2
  - ruptured I71.1
  - syphilitic A52.01
- traumatic (complication) (early), specified site *—see* Injury, blood vessel
- tricuspid (heart) (valve) I07.8
- ulnar I72.1
- upper limb (ruptured) I72.1
- valve, valvular *—see* Endocarditis
- venous (*see also* Varix) I86.8
  - congenital Q27.8
    - digestive system Q27.8
    - lower limb Q27.8
    - specified site NEC Q27.8
    - upper limb Q27.8
- ventricle *—see* Aneurysm, heart
- vertebral artery I72.6
- visceral NEC I72.8

Angelman syndrome Q93.51

Anger R45.4

Angiectasis, angiectopia I99.8

Angiitis I77.6
- allergic granulomatous M30.1
- hypersensitivity M31.0
- necrotizing M31.9
  - specified NEC M31.8
- nervous system, granulomatous I67.7

Angina (attack) (cardiac) (chest) (heart) (pectoris) (syndrome) (vasomotor) I20.9
- with
  - atherosclerotic heart disease *—see* Arteriosclerosis, coronary (artery),
  - documented spasm I20.1
- abdominal K55.1
- accelerated *—see* Angina, unstable
- agranulocytic *—see* Agranulocytosis
- angiospastic *—see* Angina, with documented spasm
- aphthous B08.5
- crescendo *—see* Angina, unstable
- croupous J05.0
- cruris I73.9
- de novo effort *—see* Angina, unstable
- diphtheritic, membranous A36.0
- equivalent I20.8
- exudative, chronic J37.0
- following acute myocardial infarction I23.7
- gangrenous diphtheritic A36.0
- intestinal K55.1
- Ludovici K12.2
- Ludwig's K12.2

Angina *(continued)*
- malignant diphtheritic A36.0
- membranous J05.0
  - diphtheritic A36.0
  - Vincent's A69.1
- mesenteric K55.1
- monocytic *—see* Mononucleosis, infectious
- of effort *—see* Angina, specified NEC
- phlegmonous J36
  - diphtheritic A36.0
- post-infarctional I23.7
- pre-infarctional *—see* Angina, unstable
- Prinzmetal *—see* Angina, with documented spasm
- progressive *—see* Angina, unstable
- pseudomembranous A69.1
- pultaceous, diphtheritic A36.0
- spasm-induced *—see* Angina, with documented spasm
- specified NEC I20.8
- stable I20.8
- stenocardia *—see* Angina, specified NEC
- stridulous, diphtheritic A36.2
- tonsil J36
- trachealis J05.0
- unstable I20.0
- variant *—see* Angina, with documented spasm
- Vincent's A69.1
- worsening effort *—see* Angina, unstable

Angioblastoma *—see* Neoplasm, connective tissue, uncertain behavior

Angiocholecystitis *—see* Cholecystitis, acute

Angiocholitis *—see also* Cholecystitis, acute K83.09

Angiodysgenesis spinalis G95.19

Angiodysplasia (cecum) (colon) K55.20
- with bleeding K55.21
- duodenum (and stomach) K31.819
  - with bleeding K31.811
- stomach (and duodenum) K31.819
  - with bleeding K31.811

Angioedema (allergic) (any site) (with urticaria) T78.3
- episodic, with eosinophilia D72.118
- hereditary D84.1

Angioendothelioma *—see* Neoplasm, uncertain behavior, by site
- benign D18.00
  - intra-abdominal D18.03
  - intracranial D18.02
  - skin D18.01
  - specified site NEC D18.09
- bone *—see* Neoplasm, bone, malignant
- Ewing's *—see* Neoplasm, bone, malignant

Angioendotheliomatosis C85.8-

Angiofibroma *—see also* Neoplasm, benign, by site
- juvenile
  - specified site *—see* Neoplasm, benign, by site
  - unspecified site D10.6

Angiohemophilia (A) (B) D68.0

Angioid streaks (choroid) (macula) (retina) H35.33

Angiokeratoma *—see* Neoplasm, skin, benign
- corporis diffusum E75.21

Angioleiomyoma *—see* Neoplasm, connective tissue, benign

Angiolipoma *—see also* Lipoma
- infiltrating *—see* Lipoma

Angioma *—see also* Hemangioma, by site
- capillary I78.1
- hemorrhagicum hereditaria I78.0
- intra-abdominal D18.03
- intracranial D18.02
- malignant *—see* Neoplasm, connective tissue, malignant
- plexiform D18.00
  - intra-abdominal D18.03
  - intracranial D18.02
  - skin D18.01
  - specified site NEC D18.09
- senile I78.1
- serpiginosum L81.7
- skin D18.01
- specified site NEC D18.09
- spider I78.1
- stellate I78.1
- venous Q28.3

Angiomatosis Q82.8
- bacillary A79.89
- encephalotrigeminal Q85.8
- hemorrhagic familial I78.0
- hereditary familial I78.0
- liver K76.4

Angiomyolipoma *—see* Lipoma

Angiomyoliposarcoma *—see* Neoplasm, connective tissue, malignant

Angiomyoma *—see* Neoplasm, connective tissue, benign

Angiomyosarcoma *—see* Neoplasm, connective tissue, malignant

Angiomyxoma *—see* Neoplasm, connective tissue, uncertain behavior

Angioneurosis F45.8

Angioneurotic edema (allergic) (any site) (with urticaria) T78.3
- hereditary D84.1

Angiopathia, angiopathy I99.9
- cerebral I67.9
  - amyloid E85.4 *[I68.0]*
- diabetic (peripheral) *—see* Diabetes, angiopathy
- peripheral I73.9
  - diabetic *—see* Diabetes, angiopathy
  - specified type NEC I73.89
- retinae syphilitica A52.05
- retinalis (juvenilis)
  - diabetic *—see* Diabetes, retinopathy
  - proliferative *—see* Retinopathy, proliferative

Angiosarcoma *—see also* Neoplasm, connective tissue, malignant
- liver C22.3

Angiosclerosis *—see* Arteriosclerosis

Angiospasm (peripheral) (traumatic) (vessel) I73.9
- brachial plexus G54.0
- cerebral G45.9
- cervical plexus G54.2

Angiospasm *(continued)*
- nerve
  - arm *—see* Mononeuropathy, upper limb
    - axillary G54.0
    - median *—see* Lesion, nerve, median
    - ulnar *—see* Lesion, nerve, ulnar
  - axillary G54.0
  - leg *—see* Mononeuropathy, lower limb
  - median *—see* Lesion, nerve, median
  - plantar *—see* Lesion, nerve, plantar
  - ulnar *—see* Lesion, nerve, ulnar

Angiospastic disease or edema I73.9

Angiostrongyliasis
- due to
  - Parastrongylus
    - cantonensis B83.2
    - costaricensis B81.3
- intestinal B81.3

Anguillulosis *—see* Strongyloidiasis

Angulation
- cecum *—see* Obstruction, intestine
- coccyx (acquired) (*see also* subcategory) M43.8
  - congenital NEC Q76.49
- femur (acquired) *—see also* Deformity, limb, specified type NEC, thigh
  - congenital Q74.2
- intestine (large) (small) *—see* Obstruction, intestine
- sacrum (acquired) (*see also* subcategory) M43.8
  - congenital NEC Q76.49
- sigmoid (flexure) *—see* Obstruction, intestine
- spine *—see* Dorsopathy, deforming, specified NEC
- tibia (acquired) *—see also* Deformity, limb, specified type NEC, lower leg
  - congenital Q74.2
- ureter N13.5
  - with infection N13.6
- wrist (acquired) *—see also* Deformity, limb, specified type NEC, forearm
  - congenital Q74.0

Angulus infectiosus (lips) K13.0

Anhedonia R45.84
- sexual F52.0

Anhidrosis L74.4

Anhydration E86.0

Anhydremia E86.0

Anidrosis L74.4

Aniridia (congenital) Q13.1

Anisakiasis (infection) (infestation) B81.0

Anisakis larvae infestation B81.0

Aniseikonia H52.32

Anisocoria (pupil) H57.02
- congenital Q13.2

Anisocytosis R71.8

Anisometropia (congenital) H52.31

Ankle *—see* condition

Ankyloblepharon (eyelid) (acquired) *—see also* Blepharophimosis
- filiforme (adnatum) (congenital) Q10.3
- total Q10.3

Ankyloglossia Q38.1

Ankylosis (fibrous) (osseous) (joint) M24.60
- ankle M24.67-
- arthrodesis status Z98.1
- cricoarytenoid (cartilage) (joint) (larynx) J38.7
- dental K03.5
- ear ossicles H74.31-
- elbow M24.62-
- foot M24.67-
- hand M24.64-
- hip M24.65-
- incostapedial joint (infectional) *—see* Ankylosis, ear ossicles
- jaw (temporomandibular) M26.61-
- knee M24.66-
- lumbosacral (joint) M43.27
- postoperative (status) Z98.1
- produced by surgical fusion, status Z98.1
- sacro-iliac (joint) M43.28
- shoulder M24.61-
- specified site NEC M24.69
- spine (joint) *—see also* Fusion, spine
  - spondylitic *—see* Spondylitis, ankylosing
- surgical Z98.1
- temporomandibular M26.61-
- tooth, teeth (hard tissues) K03.5
- wrist M24.63-

Ankylostoma *—see* Ancylostoma

Ankylostomiasis *—see* Ancylostomiasis

Ankylurethria *—see* Stricture, urethra

Annular *—see also* condition
- detachment, cervix N88.8
- organ or site, congenital NEC *—see* Distortion
- pancreas (congenital) Q45.1

Anodontia (complete) (partial) (vera) K00.0
- acquired K08.10

Anomaly, anomalous (congenital) (unspecified type) Q89.9
- abdominal wall NEC Q79.59
- acoustic nerve Q07.8
- adrenal (gland) Q89.1
- Alder (-Reilly) (leukocyte granulation) D72.0
- alimentary tract Q45.9
  - upper Q40.9
- alveolar M26.70
  - hyperplasia M26.79
    - mandibular M26.72
    - maxillary M26.71
  - hypoplasia M26.79
    - mandibular M26.74
    - maxillary M26.73
  - ridge (process) M26.79
  - specified NEC M26.79
- ankle (joint) Q74.2
- anus Q43.9
- aorta (arch) NEC Q25.40
  - coarctation (preductal) (postductal) Q25.1
- aortic cusp or valve Q23.9
- appendix Q43.8
- apple peel syndrome Q41.1
- aqueduct of Sylvius Q03.0
  - with spina bifida *—see* Spina bifida, with hydrocephalus
- arm Q74.0
- arteriovenous NEC
  - coronary Q24.5
  - gastrointestinal Q27.33
    - acquired *—see* Angiodysplasia
- artery (peripheral) Q27.9
  - basilar NEC Q28.1
  - cerebral Q28.3
  - coronary Q24.5
  - digestive system Q27.8
  - eye Q15.8
  - great Q25.9
    - specified NEC Q25.8
  - lower limb Q27.8
  - peripheral Q27.9
    - specified NEC Q27.8
  - pulmonary NEC Q25.79
  - renal Q27.2
  - retina Q14.1
  - specified site NEC Q27.8
  - subclavian Q27.8
    - origin Q25.48
  - umbilical Q27.0
  - upper limb Q27.8
  - vertebral NEC Q28.1
- aryteno-epiglottic folds Q31.8
- atrial
  - bands or folds Q20.8
  - septa Q21.1
- atrioventricular
  - excitation I45.6
  - septum Q21.0
- auditory canal Q17.8
- auricle
  - ear Q17.8
    - causing impairment of hearing Q16.9
  - heart Q20.8
- Axenfeld's Q15.0
- back Q89.9
- band
  - atrial Q20.8
  - heart Q24.8
  - ventricular Q24.8
- Bartholin's duct Q38.4
- biliary duct or passage Q44.5
- bladder Q64.70
  - absence Q64.5
  - diverticulum Q64.6
  - exstrophy Q64.10
    - cloacal Q64.12
    - extroversion Q64.19
    - specified type NEC Q64.19
    - supravesical fissure Q64.11
  - neck obstruction Q64.31
  - specified type NEC Q64.79
- bone Q79.9
  - arm Q74.0
  - face Q75.9
  - leg Q74.2
  - pelvic girdle Q74.2
  - shoulder girdle Q74.0
  - skull Q75.9
    - with
      - anencephaly Q00.0
      - encephalocele *—see* Encephalocele
      - hydrocephalus Q03.9
        - with spina bifida *—see* Spina bifida, by site, with hydrocephalus
      - microcephaly Q02
- brain (multiple) Q04.9
  - vessel Q28.3
- breast Q83.9
- broad ligament Q50.6
- bronchus Q32.4
- bulbus cordis Q21.9
- bursa Q79.9
- canal of Nuck Q52.4
- canthus Q10.3
- capillary Q27.9
- cardiac Q24.9
  - chambers Q20.9
    - specified NEC Q20.8
  - septal closure Q21.9
    - specified NEC Q21.8
  - valve NEC Q24.8
    - pulmonary Q22.3
- cardiovascular system Q28.8
- carpus Q74.0
- caruncle, lacrimal Q10.6
- cascade stomach Q40.2
- cauda equina Q06.3
- cecum Q43.9
- cerebral Q04.9
  - vessels Q28.3
- cervix Q51.9
- Chédiak-Higashi (-Steinbrinck) (congenital gigantism of peroxidase granules) E70.330
- cheek Q18.9
- chest wall Q67.8
  - bones Q76.9
- chin Q18.9
- chordae tendineae Q24.8
- choroid Q14.3
  - plexus Q07.8
- chromosomes, chromosomal Q99.9
  - D (1) *—see* condition, chromosome 13
  - E (3) *—see* condition, chromosome 18
  - G *—see* condition, chromosome 21
  - sex
    - female phenotype Q97.8
    - gonadal dysgenesis (pure) Q99.1
    - Klinefelter's Q98.4
    - male phenotype Q98.9
    - Turner's Q96.9
  - specified NEC Q99.8
- cilia Q10.3
- circulatory system Q28.9
- clavicle Q74.0
- clitoris Q52.6
- coccyx Q76.49
- colon Q43.9
- common duct Q44.5
- communication
  - coronary artery Q24.5
  - left ventricle with right atrium Q21.0
- concha (ear) Q17.3
- connection
  - portal vein Q26.5
  - pulmonary venous Q26.4
    - partial Q26.3
    - total Q26.2
  - renal artery with kidney Q27.2
- cornea (shape) Q13.4
- coronary artery or vein Q24.5
- cranium *—see* Anomaly, skull
- cricoid cartilage Q31.8
- cystic duct Q44.5
- dental
  - alveolar *—see* Anomaly, alveolar
  - arch relationship M26.20
    - specified NEC M26.29
- dentofacial M26.9
  - alveolar *—see* Anomaly, alveolar
  - dental arch relationship M26.20
    - specified NEC M26.29
  - functional M26.50
    - specified NEC M26.59
  - jaw-cranial base relationship M26.10
    - asymmetry M26.12
      - maxillary M26.11
    - specified type NEC M26.19

Anomaly, anomalous *(continued)*
- dentofacial *(continued)*
  - jaw size M26.00
    - macrogenia M26.05
    - mandibular
      - hyperplasia M26.03
      - hypoplasia M26.04
    - maxillary
      - hyperplasia M26.01
      - hypoplasia M26.02
    - microgenia M26.06
    - specified type NEC M26.09
  - malocclusion M26.4
    - dental arch relationship NEC M26.29
    - jaw-cranial base relationship —*see* Anomaly, dentofacial, jaw-cranial base relationship
    - jaw size —*see* Anomaly, dentofacial, jaw size
  - specified type NEC M26.89
  - temporomandibular joint M26.60-
    - adhesions M26.61-
    - ankylosis M26.61-
    - arthralgia M26.62-
    - articular disc M26.63-
    - specified type NEC M26.69
  - tooth position, fully erupted M26.30
    - specified NEC M26.39
- dermatoglyphic Q82.8
- diaphragm (apertures) NEC Q79.1
- digestive organ(s) or tract Q45.9
  - lower Q43.9
  - upper Q40.9
- distance, interarch (excessive) (inadequate) M26.25
- distribution, coronary artery Q24.5
- ductus
  - arteriosus Q25.0
  - botalli Q25.0
- duodenum Q43.9
- dura (brain) Q04.9
  - spinal cord Q06.9
- ear (external) Q17.9
  - causing impairment of hearing Q16.9
  - inner Q16.5
  - middle (causing impairment of hearing) Q16.4
  - ossicles Q16.3
- Ebstein's (heart) (tricuspid valve) Q22.5
- ectodermal Q82.9
- Eisenmenger's (ventricular septal defect) Q21.8
- ejaculatory duct Q55.4
- elbow Q74.0
- endocrine gland NEC Q89.2
- epididymis Q55.4
- epiglottis Q31.8
- esophagus Q39.9
- eustachian tube Q17.8
- eye Q15.9
  - anterior segment Q13.9
    - specified NEC Q13.89
  - posterior segment Q14.9
    - specified NEC Q14.8
  - ptosis (eyelid) Q10.0
  - specified NEC Q15.8
- eyebrow Q18.8
- eyelid Q10.3
  - ptosis Q10.0
- face Q18.9
  - bone(s) Q75.9
- fallopian tube Q50.6
- fascia Q79.9
- femur NEC Q74.2

Anomaly, anomalous *(continued)*
- fibula NEC Q74.2
- finger Q74.0
- fixation, intestine Q43.3
- flexion (joint) NOS Q74.9
  - hip or thigh Q65.89
- foot NEC Q74.2
  - varus (congenital) Q66.3-
- foramen
  - Botalli Q21.1
  - ovale Q21.1
- forearm Q74.0
- forehead Q75.8
- form, teeth K00.2
- fovea centralis Q14.1
- frontal bone —*see* Anomaly, skull
- gallbladder (position) (shape) (size) Q44.1
- Gartner's duct Q52.4
- gastrointestinal tract Q45.9
- genitalia, genital organ(s) or system
  - female Q52.9
    - external Q52.70
    - internal NOS Q52.9
  - male Q55.9
    - hydrocele P83.5
    - specified NEC Q55.8
- genitourinary NEC
  - female Q52.9
  - male Q55.9
- Gerbode Q21.0
- glottis Q31.8
- granulation or granulocyte, genetic (constitutional) (leukocyte) D72.0
- gum Q38.6
- gyri Q07.9
- hair Q84.2
- hand Q74.0
- hard tissue formation in pulp K04.3
- head —*see* Anomaly, skull
- heart Q24.9
  - auricle Q20.8
  - bands or folds Q24.8
  - fibroelastosis cordis I42.4
  - obstructive NEC Q22.6
  - patent ductus arteriosus (Botalli) Q25.0
  - septum Q21.9
    - auricular Q21.1
    - interatrial Q21.1
    - interventricular Q21.0
      - with pulmonary stenosis or atresia, dextraposition of aorta and hypertrophy of right ventricle Q21.3
    - specified NEC Q21.8
    - ventricular Q21.0
      - with pulmonary stenosis or atresia, dextraposition of aorta and hypertrophy of right ventricle Q21.3
  - tetralogy of Fallot Q21.3
  - valve NEC Q24.8
    - aortic
      - bicuspid valve Q23.1
      - insufficiency Q23.1
      - stenosis Q23.0
        - subaortic Q24.4
    - mitral
      - insufficiency Q23.3
      - stenosis Q23.2
    - pulmonary Q22.3
      - atresia Q22.0
      - insufficiency Q22.2
      - stenosis Q22.1
        - infundibular Q24.3
        - subvalvular Q24.3

Anomaly, anomalous *(continued)*
- heart *(continued)*
  - valve *(continued)*
    - tricuspid
      - atresia Q22.4
      - stenosis Q22.4
  - ventricle Q20.8
- heel NEC Q74.2
- Hegglin's D72.0
- hemianencephaly Q00.0
- hemicephaly Q00.0
- hemicrania Q00.0
- hepatic duct Q44.5
- hip NEC Q74.2
- hourglass stomach Q40.2
- humerus Q74.0
- hydatid of Morgagni
  - female Q50.5
  - male (epididymal) Q55.4
    - testicular Q55.29
- hymen Q52.4
- hypersegmentation of neutrophils, hereditary D72.0
- hypophyseal Q89.2
- ileocecal (coil) (valve) Q43.9
- ileum Q43.9
- ilium NEC Q74.2
- integument Q84.9
  - specified NEC Q84.8
- interarch distance (excessive) (inadequate) M26.25
- intervertebral cartilage or disc Q76.49
- intestine (large) (small) Q43.9
  - with anomalous adhesions, fixation or malrotation Q43.3
- iris Q13.2
- ischium NEC Q74.2
- jaw —*see* Anomaly, dentofacial
  - alveolar —*see* Anomaly, alveolar
- jaw-cranial base relationship —*see* Anomaly, dentofacial, jaw-cranial base relationship
- jejunum Q43.8
- joint Q74.9
  - specified NEC Q74.8
- Jordan's D72.0
- kidney(s) (calyx) (pelvis) Q63.9
  - artery Q27.2
  - specified NEC Q63.8
- Klippel-Feil (brevicollis) Q76.1
- knee Q74.1
- labium (majus) (minus) Q52.70
- labyrinth, membranous Q16.5
- lacrimal apparatus or duct Q10.6
- larynx, laryngeal (muscle) Q31.9
  - web (bed) Q31.0
- lens Q12.9
- leukocytes, genetic D72.0
  - granulation (constitutional) D72.0
- lid (fold) Q10.3
- ligament Q79.9
  - broad Q50.6
  - round Q52.8
- limb Q74.9
  - lower NEC Q74.2
    - reduction deformity —*see* Defect, reduction, lower limb
  - upper Q74.0
- lip Q38.0
- liver Q44.7
  - duct Q44.5
- lower limb NEC Q74.2
- lumbosacral (joint) (region) Q76.49
  - kyphosis —*see* Kyphosis, congenital
  - lordosis —*see* Lordosis, congenital
- lung (fissure) (lobe) Q33.9
- mandible —*see* Anomaly, dentofacial

Anomaly, anomalous *(continued)*
- maxilla —*see* Anomaly, dentofacial
- May (-Hegglin) D72.0
- meatus urinarius NEC Q64.79
- meningeal bands or folds Q07.9
  - constriction of Q07.8
  - spinal Q06.9
- meninges Q07.9
  - cerebral Q04.8
  - spinal Q06.9
- meningocele Q05.9
- mesentery Q45.9
- metacarpus Q74.0
- metatarsus NEC Q74.2
- middle ear Q16.4
  - ossicles Q16.3
- mitral (leaflets) (valve) Q23.9
  - insufficiency Q23.3
  - specified NEC Q23.8
  - stenosis Q23.2
- mouth Q38.6
- Müllerian —*see also* Anomaly, by site
  - uterus NEC Q51.818
- multiple NEC Q89.7
- muscle Q79.9
  - eyelid Q10.3
- musculoskeletal system, except limbs Q79.9
- myocardium Q24.8
- nail Q84.6
- narrowness, eyelid Q10.3
- nasal sinus (wall) Q30.8
- neck (any part) Q18.9
- nerve Q07.9
  - acoustic Q07.8
  - optic Q07.8
- nervous system (central) Q07.9
- nipple Q83.9
- nose, nasal (bones) (cartilage) (septum) (sinus) Q30.9
  - specified NEC Q30.8
- ocular muscle Q15.8
- omphalomesenteric duct Q43.0
- opening, pulmonary veins Q26.4
- optic
  - disc Q14.2
  - nerve Q07.8
- opticociliary vessels Q13.2
- orbit (eye) Q10.7
- organ Q89.9
  - of Corti Q16.5
- origin
  - artery
    - innominate Q25.48
    - pulmonary Q25.79
    - renal Q27.2
    - subclavian Q25.48
- osseous meatus (ear) Q16.1
- ovary Q50.39
- oviduct Q50.6
- palate (hard) (soft) NEC Q38.5
- pancreas or pancreatic duct Q45.3
- papillary muscles Q24.8
- parathyroid gland Q89.2
- paraurethral ducts Q64.79
- parotid (gland) Q38.4
- patella Q74.1
- Pelger-Huët (hereditary hyposegmentation) D72.0
- pelvic girdle NEC Q74.2
- pelvis (bony) NEC Q74.2
  - rachitic E64.3
- penis (glans) Q55.69
- pericardium Q24.8
- peripheral vascular system Q27.9
- Peter's Q13.4
- pharynx Q38.8
- pigmentation L81.9
  - congenital Q82.8
- pituitary (gland) Q89.2

Anomaly, anomalous *(continued)*
pleural (folds) Q34.0
portal vein Q26.5
connection Q26.5
position, tooth, teeth, fully erupted M26.30
specified NEC M26.39
precerebral vessel Q28.1
prepuce Q55.69
prostate Q55.4
pulmonary Q33.9
artery NEC Q25.79
valve Q22.3
atresia Q22.0
insufficiency Q22.2
specified type NEC Q22.3
stenosis Q22.1
infundibular Q24.3
subvalvular Q24.3
venous connection Q26.4
partial Q26.3
total Q26.2
pupil Q13.2
function H57.00
anisocoria H57.02
Argyll Robertson pupil H57.01
miosis H57.03
mydriasis H57.04
specified type NEC H57.09
tonic pupil H57.05-
pylorus Q40.3
radius Q74.0
rectum Q43.9
reduction (extremity) (limb)
femur (longitudinal) —*see* Defect, reduction, lower limb, longitudinal, femur
fibula (longitudinal) —*see* Defect, reduction, lower limb, longitudinal, fibula
lower limb —*see* Defect, reduction, lower limb
radius (longitudinal) —*see* Defect, reduction, upper limb, longitudinal, radius
tibia (longitudinal) —*see* Defect, reduction, lower limb, longitudinal, tibia
ulna (longitudinal) —*see* Defect, reduction, upper limb, longitudinal, ulna
upper limb —*see* Defect, reduction, upper limb
refraction —*see* Disorder, refraction
renal Q63.9
artery Q27.2
pelvis Q63.9
specified NEC Q63.8
respiratory system Q34.9
specified NEC Q34.8
retina Q14.1
rib Q76.6
cervical Q76.5
Rieger's Q13.81
rotation —*see* Malrotation
hip or thigh Q65.89
round ligament Q52.8
sacroiliac (joint) NEC Q74.2
sacrum NEC Q76.49
kyphosis —*see* Kyphosis, congenital
lordosis —*see* Lordosis, congenital
saddle nose, syphilitic A50.57
salivary duct or gland Q38.4
scapula Q74.0
scrotum —*see* Malformation, testis and scrotum
sebaceous gland Q82.9
seminal vesicles Q55.4

Anomaly, anomalous *(continued)*
sense organs NEC Q07.8
sex chromosomes NEC —*see also* Anomaly, chromosomes
female phenotype Q97.8
male phenotype Q98.9
shoulder (girdle) (joint) Q74.0
sigmoid (flexure) Q43.9
simian crease Q82.8
sinus of Valsalva Q25.49
skeleton generalized Q78.9
skin (appendage) Q82.9
skull Q75.9
with
anencephaly Q00.0
encephalocele —*see* Encephalocele
hydrocephalus Q03.9
with spina bifida —*see* Spina bifida, by site, with hydrocephalus
microcephaly Q02
specified organ or site NEC Q89.8
spermatic cord Q55.4
spine, spinal NEC Q76.49
column NEC Q76.49
kyphosis —*see* Kyphosis, congenital
lordosis —*see* Lordosis, congenital
cord Q06.9
nerve root Q07.8
spleen Q89.09
agenesis Q89.01
stenonian duct Q38.4
sternum NEC Q76.7
stomach Q40.3
submaxillary gland Q38.4
tarsus NEC Q74.2
tendon Q79.9
testis —*see* Malformation, testis and scrotum
thigh NEC Q74.2
thorax (wall) Q67.8
bony Q76.9
throat Q38.8
thumb Q74.0
thymus gland Q89.2
thyroid (gland) Q89.2
cartilage Q31.8
tibia NEC Q74.2
saber A50.56
toe Q74.2
tongue Q38.3
tooth, teeth K00.9
eruption K00.6
position, fully erupted M26.30
spacing, fully erupted M26.30
trachea (cartilage) Q32.1
tragus Q17.9
tricuspid (leaflet) (valve) Q22.9
atresia or stenosis Q22.4
Ebstein's Q22.5
Uhl's (hypoplasia of myocardium, right ventricle) Q24.8
ulna Q74.0
umbilical artery Q27.0
union
cricoid cartilage and thyroid cartilage Q31.8
thyroid cartilage and hyoid bone Q31.8
trachea with larynx Q31.8
upper limb Q74.0
urachus Q64.4
ureter Q62.8
obstructive NEC Q62.39
cecoureterocele Q62.32
orthotopic ureterocele Q62.31

Anomaly, anomalous *(continued)*
urethra Q64.70
absence Q64.5
double Q64.74
fistula to rectum Q64.73
obstructive Q64.39
stricture Q64.32
prolapse Q64.71
specified type NEC Q64.79
urinary tract Q64.9
uterus Q51.9
with only one functioning horn Q51.4
uvula Q38.5
vagina Q52.4
valleculae Q31.8
valve (heart) NEC Q24.8
coronary sinus Q24.5
inferior vena cava Q24.8
pulmonary Q22.3
sinus coronario Q24.5
venae cavae inferioris Q24.8
vas deferens Q55.4
vascular Q27.9
brain Q28.3
ring Q25.45
vein(s) (peripheral) Q27.9
brain Q28.3
cerebral Q28.3
coronary Q24.5
developmental Q28.3
great Q26.9
specified NEC Q26.8
vena cava (inferior) (superior) Q26.9
venous —*see* Anomaly, vein(s)
venous return Q26.8
ventricular
bands or folds Q24.8
septa Q21.0
vertebra Q76.49
kyphosis —*see* Kyphosis, congenital
lordosis —*see* Lordosis, congenital
vesicourethral orifice Q64.79
vessel(s) Q27.9
optic papilla Q14.2
precerebral Q28.1
vitelline duct Q43.0
vitreous body or humor Q14.0
vulva Q52.70
wrist (joint) Q74.0

Anomia R48.8

Anonychia (congenital) Q84.3
acquired L60.8

Anophthalmos, anophthalmus (congenital) (globe) Q11.1
acquired Z90.01

Anopia, anopsia H53.46-
quadrant H53.46-

Anorchia, anorchism, anorchidism Q55.0

Anorexia R63.0
hysterical F44.89
nervosa F50.00
atypical F50.9
binge-eating type F50.2
with purging F50.02
restricting type F50.01

Anorgasmy, psychogenic (female) F52.31
male F52.32

Anosmia R43.0
hysterical F44.6
postinfectional J39.8

Anosognosia R41.89

Anosteoplasia Q78.9

Anovulatory cycle N97.0

Anoxemia R09.02
newborn P84

Anoxia (pathological) R09.02
altitude T70.29
cerebral G93.1
complicating
anesthesia (general) (local) or other sedation T88.59
in labor and delivery O74.3
in pregnancy O29.21-
postpartum, puerperal O89.2
delivery (cesarean) (instrumental) O75.4
during a procedure G97.81
newborn P84
resulting from a procedure G97.82
due to
drowning T75.1
high altitude T70.29
heart —*see* Insufficiency, coronary
intrauterine P84
myocardial —*see* Insufficiency, coronary
newborn P84
spinal cord G95.11
systemic (by suffocation) (low content in atmosphere) —*see* Asphyxia, traumatic

Anteflexion —*see* Anteversion

Antenatal
care (normal pregnancy) Z34.90
screening (encounter for) of mother (*see also* Encounter, antenatal screening) Z36.9

Antepartum —*see* condition

Anterior —*see* condition

Antero-occlusion M26.220

Anteversion
cervix —*see* Anteversion, uterus
femur (neck), congenital Q65.89
uterus, uterine (cervix) (postinfectional) (postpartal, old) N85.4
congenital Q51.818
in pregnancy or childbirth —*see* Pregnancy, complicated by

Anthophobia F40.228

Anthracosilicosis J60

Anthracosis (lung) (occupational) J60
lingua K14.3

Anthrax A22.9
with pneumonia A22.1
cerebral A22.8
colitis A22.2
cutaneous A22.0
gastrointestinal A22.2
inhalation A22.1
intestinal A22.2
meningitis A22.8
pulmonary A22.1
respiratory A22.1
sepsis A22.7
specified manifestation NEC A22.8

Anthropoid pelvis Q74.2
with disproportion (fetopelvic) O33.0

Anthropophobia F40.10
generalized F40.11

Antibodies, maternal (blood group) —*see* Isoimmunization, affecting management of pregnancy
anti-D —*see* Isoimmunization, affecting management of pregnancy, Rh
newborn P55.0

Antibody
- anticardiolipin R76.0
  - with
    - hemorrhagic disorder D68.312
    - hypercoagulable state D68.61
- antiphosphatidylglycerol R76.0
  - with
    - hemorrhagic disorder D68.312
    - hypercoagulable state D68.61
- antiphosphatidylinositol R76.0
  - with
    - hemorrhagic disorder D68.312
    - hypercoagulable state D68.61
- antiphosphatidylserine R76.0
  - with
    - hemorrhagic disorder D68.312
    - hypercoagulable state D68.61
- antiphospholipid R76.0
  - with
    - hemorrhagic disorder D68.312
    - hypercoagulable state D68.61

Anticardiolipin syndrome D68.61

Anticoagulant, circulating (intrinsic) (*see also* Disorder, hemorrhagic) D68.318
- drug-induced (extrinsic) (*see also* Disorder, hemorrhagic) D68.32
- iatrogenic D68.32

Antidiuretic hormone syndrome E22.2

Antimonial cholera —*see* Poisoning, antimony

Antiphospholipid
- antibody
  - with hemorrhagic disorder D68.312
  - syndrome D68.61

Antisocial personality F60.2

Antithrombinemia —*see* Circulating anticoagulants

Antithromboplastinemia D68.318

Antithromboplastinogenemia D68.318

Antitoxin complication or reaction —*see* Complications, vaccination

Antlophobia F40.228

Antritis J32.0
- maxilla J32.0
  - acute J01.00
    - recurrent J01.01
- stomach K29.60
  - with bleeding K29.61

Antrum, antral —*see* condition

Anuria R34
- calculous (impacted) (recurrent) (*see also* Calculus, urinary) N20.9
- following
  - abortion —*see* Abortion by type complicated by, renal failure
  - ectopic or molar pregnancy O08.4
- newborn P96.0
- postprocedural N99.0
- postrenal N13.8
- traumatic (following crushing) T79.5

Anus, anal —*see* condition

Anusitis K62.89

Anxiety F41.9
- depression F41.8
- episodic paroxysmal F41.0
- generalized F41.1
- hysteria F41.8
- neurosis F41.1
- panic type F41.0
- reaction F41.1

Anxiety *(continued)*
- separation, abnormal (of childhood) F93.0
- specified NEC F41.8
- state F41.1

Aorta, aortic —*see* condition

Aortectasia —*see* Ectasia, aorta
- with aneurysm —*see* Aneurysm, aorta

Aortitis (nonsyphilitic) (calcific) I77.6
- arteriosclerotic I70.0
- Doehle-Heller A52.02
- luetic A52.02
- rheumatic —*see* Endocarditis, acute, rheumatic
- specific (syphilitic) A52.02
- syphilitic A52.02
  - congenital A50.54 *[I79.1]*

Apathetic thyroid storm —*see* Thyrotoxicosis

Apathy R45.3

Apeirophobia F40.228

Apepsia K30
- psychogenic F45.8

Aperistalsis, esophagus K22.0

Apertognathia M26.29

Apert's syndrome Q87.0

Aphagia R13.0
- psychogenic F50.9

Aphakia (acquired) (postoperative) H27.0-
- congenital Q12.3

Aphasia (amnestic) (global) (nominal) (semantic) (syntactic) R47.01
- acquired, with epilepsy (Landau-Kleffner syndrome) —*see* Epilepsy, specified NEC
- auditory (developmental) F80.2
- developmental (receptive type) F80.2
  - expressive type F80.1
  - Wernicke's F80.2
- following
  - cerebrovascular disease I69.920
    - cerebral infarction I69.320
    - intracerebral hemorrhage I69.120
    - nontraumatic intracranial hemorrhage NEC I69.220
    - specified disease NEC I69.820
    - subarachnoid hemorrhage I69.020
- primary progressive G31.01 *[F02.80]*
  - with behavioral disturbance G31.01 *[F02.81]*
- progressive isolated G31.01 *[F02.80]*
  - with behavioral disturbance G31.01 *[F02.81]*
- sensory F80.2
- syphilis, tertiary A52.19
- Wernicke's (developmental) F80.2

Aphonia (organic) R49.1
- hysterical F44.4
- psychogenic F44.4

Aphthae, aphthous —*see also* condition
- Bednar's K12.0
- cachectic K14.0
- epizootic B08.8
- fever B08.8
- oral (recurrent) K12.0
- stomatitis (major) (minor) K12.0

Aphthae, aphthous *(continued)*
- thrush B37.0
- ulcer (oral) (recurrent) K12.0
  - genital organ(s) NEC
    - female N76.6
    - male N50.89
  - larynx J38.7

Apical —*see* condition

Apiphobia F40.218

Aplasia —*see also* Agenesis
- abdominal muscle syndrome Q79.4
- alveolar process (acquired) —*see* Anomaly, alveolar
  - congenital Q38.6
- aorta (congenital) Q25.41
- axialis extracorticalis (congenita) E75.29
- bone marrow (myeloid) D61.9
  - congenital D61.01
- brain Q00.0
  - part of Q04.3
- bronchus Q32.4
- cementum K00.4
- cerebellum Q04.3
- cervix (congenital) Q51.5
- congenital pure red cell D61.01
- corpus callosum Q04.0
- cutis congenita Q84.8
- erythrocyte congenital D61.01
- extracortical axial E75.29
- eye Q11.1
- fovea centralis (congenital) Q14.1
- gallbladder, congenital Q44.0
- iris Q13.1
- labyrinth, membranous Q16.5
- limb (congenital) Q73.8
  - lower —*see* Defect, reduction, lower limb
  - upper —*see* Agenesis, arm
- lung, congenital (bilateral) (unilateral) Q33.3
- pancreas Q45.0
- parathyroid-thymic D82.1
- Pelizaeus-Merzbacher E75.29
- penis Q55.5
- prostate Q55.4
- red cell (with thymoma) D60.9
  - acquired D60.9
    - due to drugs D60.9
  - adult D60.9
  - chronic D60.0
  - congenital D61.01
  - constitutional D61.01
  - due to drugs D60.9
  - hereditary D61.01
  - of infants D61.01
  - primary D61.01
  - pure D61.01
    - due to drugs D60.9
  - specified type NEC D60.8
  - transient D60.1
- round ligament Q52.8
- skin Q84.8
- spermatic cord Q55.4
- spleen Q89.01
- testicle Q55.0
- thymic, with immunodeficiency D82.1
- thyroid (congenital) (with myxedema) E03.1
- uterus Q51.0
- ventral horn cell Q06.1

Apnea, apneic (of) (spells) R06.81
- newborn NEC P28.4
  - obstructive P28.4
  - sleep (central) (obstructive) (primary) P28.3
- prematurity P28.4

Apnea, apneic *(continued)*
- sleep G47.30
  - central (primary) G47.31
    - idiopathic G47.31
    - in conditions classified elsewhere G47.37
  - obstructive (adult) (pediatric) G47.33
    - hypopnea G47.33
  - primary central G47.31
  - specified NEC G47.39

Apneumatosis, newborn P28.0

Apocrine metaplasia (breast) —*see* Dysplasia, mammary, specified type NEC

Apophysitis (bone) —*see also* Osteochondropathy
- calcaneus M92.8
- juvenile M92.9

Apoplectiform convulsions (cerebral ischemia) I67.82

Apoplexia, apoplexy, apoplectic
- adrenal A39.1
- heart (auricle) (ventricle) —*see* Infarct, myocardium
- heat T67.01
- hemorrhagic (stroke) —*see* Hemorrhage, intracranial
- meninges, hemorrhagic —*see* Hemorrhage, intracranial, subarachnoid
- uremic N18.9 *[I68.8]*

Appearance
- bizarre R46.1
- specified NEC R46.89
- very low level of personal hygiene R46.0

Appendage
- epididymal (organ of Morgagni) Q55.4
- intestine (epiploic) Q43.8
- preauricular Q17.0
- testicular (organ of Morgagni) Q55.29

Appendicitis (pneumococcal) (retrocecal) K37
- with
  - gangrene K35.891
  - perforation NOS K35.32
  - peritoneal abscess K35.33
  - peritonitis NEC K35.33
    - generalized (with perforation or rupture) K35.20
      - with abscess K35.21
    - localized K35.30
      - with
        - gangrene K35.31
        - perforation K35.32
          - and abscess K35.33
  - rupture (with localized peritonitis) K35.32
- acute (catarrhal) (fulminating) (gangrenous) (obstructive) (retrocecal) (suppurative) K35.80
  - with
    - gangrene K35.891
    - peritoneal abscess K35.33
    - peritonitis NEC K35.33
      - generalized (with perforation or rupture) K35.20
        - with abscess K35.21
      - localized K35.30
        - with
          - gangrene K35.31
          - perforation K35.32
            - and abscess K35.33
  - specified NEC K35.890
    - with gangrene K35.891

Appendicitis *(continued)*
- amebic A06.89
- chronic (recurrent) K36
- exacerbation *—see* Appendicitis, acute
- gangrenous *—see* Appendicitis, acute
- healed (obliterative) K36
- interval K36
- neurogenic K36
- obstructive K36
- recurrent K36
- relapsing K36
- ruptured NOS (with localized peritonitis) K35.32
- subacute (adhesive) K36
- subsiding K36
- suppurative *—see* Appendicitis, acute
- tuberculous A18.32

Appendicopathia oxyurica B80

Appendix, appendicular *—see also* condition
- epididymis Q55.4
- Morgagni
  - female Q50.5
  - male (epididymal) Q55.4
    - testicular Q55.29
- testis Q55.29

Appetite
- depraved *—see* Pica
- excessive R63.2
- lack or loss (*see also* Anorexia) R63.0
  - nonorganic origin F50.89
  - psychogenic F50.89
- perverted (hysterical) *—see* Pica

Apple peel syndrome Q41.1

Apprehension state F41.1

Apprehensiveness, abnormal F41.9

Approximal wear K03.0

Apraxia (classic) (ideational) (ideokinetic) (ideomotor) (motor) (verbal) R48.2
- following
  - cerebrovascular disease I69.990
    - cerebral infarction I69.390
    - intracerebral hemorrhage I69.190
    - nontraumatic intracranial hemorrhage NEC I69.290
    - specified disease NEC I69.890
    - subarachnoid hemorrhage I69.090
- oculomotor, congenital H51.8

Aptyalism K11.7

Apudoma *—see* Neoplasm, uncertain behavior, by site

Aqueous misdirection H40.83-

Arabicum elephantiasis *—see* Infestation, filarial

Arachnitis *—see* Meningitis

Arachnodactyly *—see* Syndrome, Marfan's

Arachnoiditis (acute) (adhesive) (basal) (brain) (cerebrospinal) *—see* Meningitis

Arachnophobia F40.210

Arboencephalitis, Australian A83.4

Arborization block (heart) I45.5

ARC (AIDS-related complex) B20

Arch
- aortic Q25.49
- bovine Q25.49

Arches *—see* condition

Arcuate uterus Q51.810

Arcuatus uterus Q51.810

Arcus (cornea) **senilis** *—see* Degeneration, cornea, senile

Arc-welder's lung J63.4

Areflexia R29.2

Areola *—see* condition

Argentaffinoma *—see also* Neoplasm, uncertain behavior, by site
- malignant *—see* Neoplasm, malignant, by site
- syndrome E34.0

Argininemia E72.21

Arginosuccinic aciduria E72.22

Argyll Robertson phenomenon, pupil or syndrome (syphilitic) A52.19
- atypical H57.09
- nonsyphilitic H57.09

Argyria, argyriasis
- conjunctival H11.13-
- from drug or medicament *—see* Table of Drugs and Chemicals, by substance

Argyrosis, conjunctival H11.13-

Arhinencephaly Q04.1

Ariboflavinosis E53.0

Arm *—see* condition

Arnold-Chiari disease, obstruction or syndrome (type II) Q07.00
- with
  - hydrocephalus Q07.02
    - with spina bifida Q07.03
  - spina bifida Q07.01
    - with hydrocephalus Q07.03
- type III *—see* Encephalocele
- type IV Q04.8

Aromatic amino-acid metabolism disorder E70.9
- specified NEC E70.89

Arousals, confusional G47.51

Arrest, arrested
- cardiac I46.9
  - complicating
    - abortion *—see* Abortion, by type, complicated by, cardiac arrest
    - anesthesia (general) (local) or other sedation *—see* Table of Drugs and Chemicals, by drug,
      - in labor and delivery O74.2
      - in pregnancy O29.11-
      - postpartum, puerperal O89.1
    - delivery (cesarean) (instrumental) O75.4
  - due to
    - cardiac condition I46.2
    - specified condition NEC I46.8
  - intraoperative I97.71-
  - newborn P29.81
  - personal history, successfully resuscitated Z86.74
  - postprocedural I97.12-
    - obstetric procedure O75.4
- cardiorespiratory *—see* Arrest, cardiac
- circulatory *—see* Arrest, cardiac
- deep transverse O64.0

Arrest, arrested *(continued)*
- development or growth
  - bone *—see* Disorder, bone, development or growth
  - child R62.50
  - tracheal rings Q32.1
- epiphyseal
  - complete
    - femur M89.15-
    - humerus M89.12-
    - tibia M89.16-
    - ulna M89.13-
  - forearm M89.13-
    - specified NEC M89.13-
    - ulna *—see* Arrest, epiphyseal, by type, ulna
  - lower leg M89.16-
    - specified NEC M89.168
    - tibia *—see* Arrest, epiphyseal, by type, tibia
  - partial
    - femur M89.15-
    - humerus M89.12-
    - tibia M89.16-
    - ulna M89.13-
  - specified NEC M89.18
- granulopoiesis *—see* Agranulocytosis
- growth plate *—see* Arrest, epiphyseal
- heart *—see* Arrest, cardiac
- legal, anxiety concerning Z65.3
- physeal *—see* Arrest, epiphyseal
- respiratory R09.2
  - newborn P28.81
- sinus I45.5
- spermatogenesis (complete) *—see* Azoospermia
  - incomplete *—see* Oligospermia
- transverse (deep) O64.0

Arrhenoblastoma
- benign
  - specified site *—see* Neoplasm, benign, by site
  - unspecified site
    - female D27.9
    - male D29.20
- malignant
  - specified site *—see* Neoplasm, malignant, by site
  - unspecified site
    - female C56.9
    - male C62.90
- specified site *—see* Neoplasm, uncertain behavior, by site
- unspecified site
  - female D39.10
  - male D40.10

Arrhythmia (auricle)(cardiac) (juvenile)(nodal) (reflex) (supraventricular)(transitory) (ventricle) I49.9
- block I45.9
- extrasystolic I49.49
- newborn
  - bradycardia P29.12
  - occurring before birth P03.819
    - before onset of labor P03.810
    - during labor P03.811
  - tachycardia P29.11
- psychogenic F45.8
- sinus I49.8
- specified NEC I49.8
- vagal R55
- ventricular re-entry I47.0

Arrillaga-Ayerza syndrome (pulmonary sclerosis with pulmonary hypertension) I27.0

Arsenical pigmentation L81.8
- from drug or medicament *—see* Table of Drugs and Chemicals

Arsenism *—see* Poisoning, arsenic

Arterial *—see* condition

Arteriofibrosis *— see* Arteriosclerosis

Arteriolar sclerosis *—see* Arteriosclerosis

Arteriolith *—see* Arteriosclerosis

Arteriolitis I77.6
- necrotizing, kidney I77.5
- renal *—see* Hypertension, kidney

Arteriolosclerosis *—see* Arteriosclerosis

Arterionephrosclerosis *—see* Hypertension, kidney

Arteriopathy I77.9
- cerebral autosomal dominant, with subcortical infarcts and leukoencephalopathy (CADASIL) I67.850

Arteriosclerosis, arteriosclerotic (diffuse) (obliterans) (of) (senile) (with calcification) I70.90
- with
  - chronic limb-threatening ischemia *—see* Arteriosclerosis, with critical limb ischemia
  - critical limb ischemia
    - bypass graft I70.329
      - autologous vein graft I70.429
        - leg I70.429
          - with
            - gangrene (and intermittent claudication, rest pain, and ulcer) I70.469
            - rest pain (and intermittent claudication) I70.429
          - bilateral I70.423
            - with
              - gangrene (and intermittent claudication, rest pain, and ulcer) I70.463
              - rest pain (and intermittent claudication) I70.423
          - left I70.422
            - with
              - gangrene (and intermittent claudication, rest pain, and ulcer) I70.462
              - rest pain (and intermittent claudication) I70.422
              - ulceration (and intermittent claudication and rest pain) I70.449
                - ankle I70.443
                - calf I70.442

- **Arteriosclerosis, arteriosclerotic** *(continued)*
  - with *(continued)*
    - critical limb ischemia *(continued)*
      - bypass graft *(continued)*
        - specified graft *(continued)*
          - leg *(continued)*
            - left *(continued)*
              - with *(continued)*
                - gangrene (and intermittent claudication, rest pain, and ulcer) I70.762
                - rest pain (and intermittent claudication) I70.722
                - ulceration (and intermittent claudication and rest pain) I70.749
                  - ankle I70.743
                  - calf I70.742
                  - foot site NEC I70.745
                  - heel I70.744
                  - lower leg NEC I70.748
                  - mid foot I70.744
                  - thigh I70.741
            - right I70.721
              - with
                - gangrene (and intermittent claudication, rest pain, and ulcer) I70.761
                - rest pain (and intermittent claudication) I70.721
                - ulceration (and intermittent claudication and rest pain) I70.739
                  - ankle I70.733
                  - calf I70.732
                  - foot site NEC I70.735
                  - heel I70.734
                  - lower leg NEC I70.738
                  - mid foot I70.734
                  - thigh I70.731
      - leg I70.229
        - with
          - gangrene (and intermittent claudication, rest pain, and ulcer) I70.269
          - rest pain (and intermittent claudication) I70.229
        - bilateral I70.223
          - with
            - gangrene (and intermittent claudication, rest pain, and ulcer) I70.263
            - rest pain (and intermittent claudication) I70.223

Arteriosclerosis, arteriosclerotic *(continued)*

- with *(continued)*
  - critical limb ischemia *(continued)*
    - bypass graft *(continued)*
      - leg *(continued)*
        - left I70.222
          - with
            - gangrene (and intermittent claudication, rest pain, and ulcer) I70.262
            - rest pain (and intermittent claudication) I70.222
            - ulceration (and intermittent claudication and rest pain) I70.249
              - ankle I70.243
              - calf I70.242
              - foot site NEC I70.245
              - heel I70.244
              - lower leg NEC I70.248
              - mid foot I70.244
              - thigh I70.241
        - right I70.221
          - with
            - gangrene (and intermittent claudication, rest pain, and ulcer) I70.261
            - rest pain (and intermittent claudication) I70.221
            - ulceration (and intermittent claudication and rest pain) I70.239
              - ankle I70.233
              - calf I70.232
              - foot site NEC I70.235
              - heel I70.234
              - lower leg NEC I70.238
              - mid foot I70.234
              - thigh I70.231
- aorta I70.0
- arteries of extremities *—see* Arteriosclerosis, extremities
  - with
    - chronic limb-threatening ischemia *—see* Arteriosclerosis, with critical limb ischemia
    - critical limb ischemia *—see* Arteriosclerosis, with clinical limb ischemia
- brain I67.2
- bypass graft
  - with
    - chronic limb-threatening ischemia *—see* Arteriosclerosis, with critical limb ischemia
    - critical limb ischemia *—see* Arteriosclerosis, with clinical limb ischemia
  - coronary *—see* Arteriosclerosis, coronary, bypass graft
  - extremities *—see* Arteriosclerosis, extremities, bypass graft
- cardiac *—see* Disease, heart, ischemic, atherosclerotic

Arteriosclerosis, arteriosclerotic *(continued)*

- cardiopathy *—see* Disease, heart, ischemic, atherosclerotic
- cardiorenal *—see* Hypertension, cardiorenal
- cardiovascular *—see* Disease, heart, ischemic, atherosclerotic
- carotid (*see also* Occlusion, artery, carotid) I65.2-
- central nervous system I67.2
- cerebral I67.2
- cerebrovascular I67.2
- coronary (artery) I25.10
  - due to
    - calcified coronary lesion (severely) I25.84
    - lipid rich plaque I25.83
  - bypass graft I25.810
    - with
      - angina pectoris I25.709
        - with documented spasm I25.701
        - specified type NEC I25.708
        - unstable I25.700
      - ischemic chest pain I25.709
    - autologous artery I25.810
      - with
        - angina pectoris I25.729
          - with documented spasm I25.721
          - specified type I25.728
          - unstable I25.720
        - ischemic chest pain I25.729
    - autologous vein I25.810
      - with
        - angina pectoris I25.719
          - with documented spasm I25.711
          - specified type I25.718
          - unstable I25.710
        - ischemic chest pain I25.719
    - nonautologous biological I25.810
      - with
        - angina pectoris I25.739
          - with documented spasm I25.731
          - specified type I25.738
          - unstable I25.730
        - ischemic chest pain I25.739
    - specified type NEC I25.810
      - with
        - angina pectoris I25.799
          - with documented spasm I25.791
          - specified type I25.798
          - unstable I25.790
        - ischemic chest pain I25.799
  - native vessel
    - with
      - angina pectoris I25.119
        - with documented spasm I25.111
        - specified type NEC I25.118
        - unstable I25.110
      - ischemic chest pain I25.119
  - transplanted heart I25.811
    - bypass graft I25.812
      - with
        - angina pectoris I25.769
          - with documented spasm I25.761
          - specified type I25.768
          - unstable I25.760

Arteriosclerosis, arteriosclerotic *(continued)*

- coronary *(continued)*
  - transplanted heart *(continued)*
    - bypass graft *(continued)*
      - with *(continued)*
        - ischemic chest pain I25.769
    - native coronary artery I25.811
      - with
        - angina pectoris I25.759
          - with documented spasm I25.751
          - specified type I25.758
          - unstable I25.750
        - ischemic chest pain I25.759
- extremities (native arteries) I70.209
  - with
    - chronic limb-threatening ischemia *—see* Arteriosclerosis, with critical limb ischemia
    - critical limb ischemia *—see* Arteriosclerosis, with clinical limb ischemia
  - bypass graft I70.309
    - with
      - chronic limb-threatening ischemia *—see* Arteriosclerosis, with critical limb ischemia
      - critical limb ischemia *—see* Arteriosclerosis, with clinical limb ischemia
    - autologous vein graft I70.409
      - leg I70.409
        - with
          - gangrene (and intermittent claudication, rest pain and ulcer) I70.469
          - intermittent claudication I70.419
          - rest pain (and intermittent claudication) I70.429
        - bilateral I70.403
          - with
            - gangrene (and intermittent claudication, rest pain and ulcer) I70.463
            - intermittent claudication I70.413
            - rest pain (and intermittent claudication) I70.423
          - specified type NEC I70.493
        - left I70.402
          - with
            - gangrene (and intermittent claudication, rest pain and ulcer) I70.462
            - intermittent claudication I70.412
            - rest pain (and intermittent claudication) I70.422
            - ulceration (and intermittent claudication and rest pain) I70.449
              - ankle I70.443
              - calf I70.442

Arteriosclerosis, arteriosclerotic *(continued)*
- extremities *(continued)*
  - bypass graft *(continued)*
    - autologous vein graft *(continued)*
      - leg *(continued)*
        - left *(continued)*
          - with *(continued)*
            - ulceration *(continued)*
              - foot site NEC I70.445
              - heel I70.444
              - lower leg NEC I70.448
              - midfoot I70.444
              - thigh I70.441
          - specified type NEC I70.492
        - right I70.401
          - with
            - gangrene (and intermittent claudication, rest pain and ulcer) I70.461
            - intermittent claudication I70.411
            - rest pain (and intermittent claudication) I70.421
            - ulceration (and intermittent claudication and rest pain) I70.439
              - ankle I70.433
              - calf I70.432
              - foot site NEC I70.435
              - heel I70.434
              - lower leg NEC I70.438
              - midfoot I70.434
              - thigh I70.431
          - specified type NEC I70.491
        - specified type NEC I70.499
      - specified NEC I70.408
        - with
          - gangrene (and intermittent claudication, rest pain and ulcer) I70.468
          - intermittent claudication I70.418
          - rest pain (and intermittent claudication) I70.428
          - ulceration (and intermittent claudication and rest pain) I70.45
        - specified type NEC I70.498
    - leg I70.309
      - with
        - gangrene (and intermittent claudication, rest pain and ulcer) I70.369
        - intermittent claudication I70.319
        - rest pain (and intermittent claudication) I70.329

Arteriosclerosis, arteriosclerotic *(continued)*
- extremities *(continued)*
  - bypass graft *(continued)*
    - leg *(continued)*
      - bilateral I70.303
        - with
          - gangrene (and intermittent claudication, rest pain and ulcer) I70.363
          - intermittent claudication I70.313
          - rest pain (and intermittent claudication) I70.323
        - specified type NEC I70.393
      - left I70.302
        - with
          - gangrene (and intermittent claudication, rest pain and ulcer) I70.362
          - intermittent claudication I70.312
          - rest pain (and intermittent claudication) I70.322
          - ulceration (and intermittent claudication and rest pain) I70.349
            - ankle I70.343
            - calf I70.342
            - foot site NEC I70.345
            - heel I70.344
            - lower leg NEC I70.348
            - midfoot I70.344
            - thigh I70.341
        - specified type NEC I70.392
      - right I70.301
        - with
          - gangrene (and intermittent claudication, rest pain and ulcer) I70.361
          - intermittent claudication I70.311
          - rest pain (and intermittent claudication) I70.321
          - ulceration (and intermittent claudication and rest pain) I70.339
            - ankle I70.333
            - calf I70.332
            - foot site NEC I70.335
            - heel I70.334
            - lower leg NEC I70.338
            - midfoot I70.334
            - thigh I70.331
        - specified type NEC I70.391
      - specified type NEC I70.399

Arteriosclerosis, arteriosclerotic *(continued)*
- extremities *(continued)*
  - bypass graft *(continued)*
    - nonautologous biological graft I70.509
      - leg I70.509
        - with
          - gangrene (and intermittent claudication, rest pain and ulcer) I70.569
          - intermittent claudication I70.519
          - rest pain (and intermittent claudication) I70.529
        - bilateral I70.503
          - with
            - gangrene (and intermittent claudication, rest pain and ulcer) I70.563
            - intermittent claudication I70.513
            - rest pain (and intermittent claudication) I70.523
          - specified type NEC I70.593
        - left I70.502
          - with
            - gangrene (and intermittent claudication, rest pain and ulcer) I70.562
            - intermittent claudication I70.512
            - rest pain (and intermittent claudication) I70.522
            - ulceration (and intermittent claudication and rest pain) I70.549
              - ankle I70.543
              - calf I70.542
              - foot site NEC I70.545
              - heel I70.544
              - lower leg NEC I70.548
              - midfoot I70.544
              - thigh I70.541
          - specified type NEC I70.592
        - right I70.501
          - with
            - gangrene (and intermittent claudication, rest pain and ulcer) I70.561
            - intermittent claudication I70.511
            - rest pain (and intermittent claudication) I70.521

Arteriosclerosis, arteriosclerotic *(continued)*
- extremities *(continued)*
  - bypass graft *(continued)*
    - nonbiological graft *(continued)*
      - leg *(continued)*
        - right *(continued)*
          - with *(continued)*
            - ulceration (and intermittent claudication and rest pain) I70.539
              - ankle I70.533
              - calf I70.532
              - foot site NEC I70.535
              - heel I70.534
              - lower leg NEC I70.538
              - midfoot I70.534
              - thigh I70.531
          - specified type NEC I70.591
        - specified type NEC I70.599
      - specified NEC I70.508
        - with
          - gangrene (and intermittent claudication, rest pain and ulcer) I70.568
          - intermittent claudication I70.518
          - rest pain (and intermittent claudication) I70.528
          - ulceration (and intermittent claudication and rest pain) I70.55
        - specified type NEC I70.598
    - nonbiological graft I70.609
      - leg I70.609
        - with
          - gangrene (and intermittent claudication, rest pain and ulcer) I70.669
          - intermittent claudication I70.619
          - rest pain (and intermittent claudication) I70.629
        - bilateral I70.603
          - with
            - gangrene (and intermittent claudication, rest pain and ulcer) I70.663
            - intermittent claudication I70.613
            - rest pain(and intermittent claudication) I70.623
          - specified type NEC I70.693
        - left I70.602
          - with
            - gangrene (and intermittent claudication, rest pain and ulcer) I70.662

Arteriosclerosis, arteriosclerotic *(continued)*
- renal (arterioles) *—see also* Hypertension, kidney
  - artery I70.1
- retina (vascular) I70.8 *[H35.0]-*
- specified artery NEC I70.8
- spinal (cord) G95.19
- vertebral (artery) I67.2

Arteriospasm I73.9

Arteriovenous *—see* condition

Arteritis I77.6
- allergic M31.0
- aorta (nonsyphilitic) I77.6
  - syphilitic A52.02
- aortic arch M31.4
- brachiocephalic M31.4
- brain I67.7
  - syphilitic A52.04
- cerebral I67.7
  - in
    - diseases classified elsewhere I68.2
    - systemic lupus erythematosus M32.19
  - listerial A32.89
  - syphilitic A52.04
  - tuberculous A18.89
- coronary (artery) I25.89
  - rheumatic I01.8
    - chronic I09.89
  - syphilitic A52.06
- cranial (left) (right), giant cell M31.6
- deformans *—see* Arteriosclerosis
- giant cell NEC M31.6
  - with polymyalgia rheumatica M31.5
- necrosing or necrotizing M31.9
  - specified NEC M31.8
- nodosa M30.0
- obliterans *—see* Arteriosclerosis
- pulmonary I28.8
- rheumatic *—see* Fever, rheumatic
- senile *—see* Arteriosclerosis
- suppurative I77.2
- syphilitic (general) A52.09
  - brain A52.04
  - coronary A52.06
  - spinal A52.09
- temporal, giant cell M31.6
- young female aortic arch syndrome M31.4

Artery, arterial *—see also* condition
- abscess I77.89
- single umbilical Q27.0

Arthralgia (allergic) *—see also* Pain, joint
- in caisson disease T70.3
- temporomandibular M26.62-

Arthritis, arthritic (acute) (chronic) (nonpyogenic) (subacute) M19.90
- allergic *—see* Arthritis, specified form NEC
- ankylosing (crippling) (spine) *—see also* Spondylitis, ankylosing
  - sites other than spine *—see* Arthritis, specified form NEC
- atrophic *—see* Osteoarthritis
  - spine *—see* Spondylitis, ankylosing
- back *—see* Spondylopathy, inflammatory
- blennorrhagic (gonococcal) A54.42
- Charcot's *—see* Arthropathy, neuropathic
  - diabetic *—see* Diabetes, arthropathy, neuropathic
  - syringomyelic G95.0

Arthritis, arthritic *(continued)*
- chylous (filarial) (*see also* category M01) B74.9
- climacteric (any site) NEC *—see* Arthritis, specified form NEC
- crystal (-induced) *—see* Arthritis, in, crystals
- deformans *—see* Osteoarthritis
- degenerative *—see* Osteoarthritis
- due to or associated with
  - acromegaly E22.0
  - brucellosis *—see* Brucellosis
  - caisson disease T70.3
  - diabetes *—see* Diabetes, arthropathy
  - dracontiasis (*see also* category M01) B72
  - enteritis NEC
    - regional *—see* Enteritis, regional
  - erysipelas (*see also* category M01) A46
  - erythema
    - epidemic A25.1
    - nodosum L52
  - filariasis NOS B74.9
  - glanders A24.0
  - helminthiasis (*see also* category M01) B83.9
  - hemophilia D66 *[M36.2]*
  - Henoch-(Schönlein) purpura D69.0 *[M36.4]*
  - human parvovirus (*see also* category M01) B97.6
  - infectious disease NEC M01
  - leprosy (*see also* category M01) *—see also* Leprosy A30.9
  - Lyme disease A69.23
  - mycobacteria (*see also* category M01) A31.8
  - parasitic disease NEC (*see also* category M01) B89
  - paratyphoid fever (*see also* category M01) (*see also* Fever, paratyphoid) A01.4
  - rat bite fever (*see also* category M01) A25.1
  - regional enteritis *—see* Enteritis, regional
  - respiratory disorder NOS J98.9
  - serum sickness (*see also* Reaction, serum) T80.69
  - syringomyelia G95.0
  - typhoid fever A01.04
- epidemic erythema A25.1
- febrile *—see* Fever, rheumatic
- gonococcal A54.42
- gouty (acute) *—see* Gout
- in (due to)
  - acromegaly (*see also* subcategory M14.8-) E22.0
  - amyloidosis (*see also* subcategory M14.8-) E85.4
  - bacterial disease (*see also* subcategory M01) A49.9
  - Behçet's syndrome M35.2
  - caisson disease (*see also* subcategory M14.8-) T70.3
  - coliform bacilli (Escherichia coli) *—see* Arthritis, in, pyogenic organism NEC
  - crystals M11.9
    - dicalcium phosphate *—see* Arthritis, in, crystals, specified type NEC
    - hydroxyapatite M11.0-
    - pyrophosphate *—see* Arthritis, in, crystals, specified type NEC
    - specified type NEC M11.80
      - ankle M11.87-

Arthritis, arthritic *(continued)*
- in *(continued)*
  - crystals *(continued)*
    - specified type *(continued)*
      - elbow M11.82-
      - foot joint M11.87-
      - hand joint M11.84-
      - hip M11.85-
      - knee M11.86-
      - multiple sites M11.8-
      - shoulder M11.81-
      - vertebrae M11.88
      - wrist M11.83-
  - dermatoarthritis, lipoid E78.81
  - dracontiasis (dracunculiasis) (*see also* category M01) B72
  - endocrine disorder NEC (*see also* subcategory M14.8-) E34.9
  - enteritis, infectious NEC (*see also* category M01) A09
    - specified organism NEC (*see also* category M01) A08.8
  - erythema
    - multiforme (*see also* subcategory M14.8-) L51.9
    - nodosum (*see also* subcategory M14.8-) L52
  - facet joint (*see also* Spondylosis) M47.819
  - gout *—see* Gout
  - helminthiasis NEC (*see also* category M01) B83.9
  - hemochromatosis (*see also* subcategory M14.8-) E83.118
  - hemoglobinopathy NEC D58.2 *[M36.3]*
  - hemophilia NEC D66 *[M36.2]*
  - Hemophilus influenzae M00.8- *[B96.2]*
  - Henoch (-Schönlein) purpura D69.0 *[M36.4]*
  - hyperparathyroidism NEC (*see also* subcategory M14.8-) E21.3
  - hypersensitivity reaction NEC T78.49 *[M36.4]*
  - hypogammaglobulinemia (*see also* subcategory M14.8-) D80.1
  - hypothyroidism NEC (*see also* subcategory M14.8-) E03.9
  - infection *—see* Arthritis, pyogenic or pyemic
    - spine *—see* Spondylopathy, infective
  - infectious disease NEC M01
  - leprosy (*see also* category M01) A30.9
  - leukemia NEC C95.9- *[M36.1]*
  - lipoid dermatoarthritis E78.81
  - Lyme disease A69.23
  - Mediterranean fever, familial (*see also* subcategory M14.8-) M04.1
  - Meningococcus A39.83
  - metabolic disorder NEC (*see also* subcategory M14.8-) E88.9
  - multiple myelomatosis C90.0- *[M36.1]*
  - mumps B26.85
  - mycosis NEC (*see also* category M01) B49
  - myelomatosis (multiple) C90.0- *[M36.1]*
  - neurological disorder NEC G98.0
  - ochronosis (*see also* subcategory M14.8-) E70.29
  - O'nyong-nyong (*see also* category M01) A92.1
  - parasitic disease NEC (*see also* category M01) B89

Arthritis, arthritic *(continued)*
- in *(continued)*
  - paratyphoid fever (*see also* category M01) A01.4
  - Pseudomonas *—see* Arthritis, pyogenic, bacterial NEC
  - psoriasis L40.50
  - pyogenic organism NEC *—see* Arthritis, pyogenic, bacterial NEC
  - Reiter's disease *—see* Reiter's disease
  - respiratory disorder NEC (*see also* subcategory M14.8-) J98.9
  - reticulosis, malignant (*see also* subcategory M14.8-) C86.0
  - rubella B06.82
  - Salmonella (arizonae) (cholerae-suis) (enteritidis) (typhimurium) A02.23
  - sarcoidosis D86.86
  - specified bacteria NEC *—see* Arthritis, pyogenic, bacterial NEC
  - sporotrichosis B42.82
  - syringomyelia G95.0
  - thalassemia NEC D56.9 *[M36.3]*
  - tuberculosis *—see* Tuberculosis, arthritis
  - typhoid fever A01.04
  - urethritis, Reiter's *—see* Reiter's disease
  - viral disease NEC (*see also* category M01) B34.9
- infectious or infective *—see also* Arthritis, pyogenic or pyemic
  - spine *—see* Spondylopathy, infective
- juvenile M08.90
  - with systemic onset *—see* Still's disease
  - ankle M08.97-
  - elbow M08.92-
  - foot joint M08.97-
  - hand joint M08.94-
  - hip M08.95-
  - knee M08.96-
  - multiple site M08.99
  - pauciarticular M08.40
    - ankle M08.47-
    - elbow M08.42-
    - foot joint M08.47-
    - hand joint M08.44-
    - hip M08.45-
    - knee M08.46-
    - shoulder M08.41-
    - specified site NEC M08.4A
    - vertebrae M08.48
    - wrist M08.43-
  - psoriatic L40.54
  - rheumatoid *—see* Arthritis, rheumatoid, juvenile
  - shoulder M08.91-
  - specified site NEC M08.9A
  - specified type NEC M08.80
    - ankle M08.87-
    - elbow M08.82-
    - foot joint M08.87-
    - hand joint M08.84-
    - hip M08.85-
    - knee M08.86-
    - multiple site M08.89
    - shoulder M08.81-
    - specified joint NEC M08.88
    - vertebrae M08.88
    - wrist M08.83-
  - vertebra M08.98
  - wrist M08.93-

Arthritis, arthritic *(continued)*
meaning osteoarthritis *—see* Osteoarthritis
meningococcal A39.83
menopausal (any site) NEC *—see* Arthritis, specified form NEC
mutilans (psoriatic) L40.52
mycotic NEC (*see also* category M01) B49
neuropathic (Charcot) *—see* Arthropathy, neuropathic
diabetic *—see* Diabetes, arthropathy, neuropathic
nonsyphilitic NEC G98.0
syringomyelic G95.0
ochronotic (*see also* subcategory M14.8-) E70.29
palindromic (any site) *—see* Rheumatism, palindromic
pneumococcal M00.10
ankle M00.17-
elbow M00.12-
foot joint *—see* Arthritis, pneumococcal, ankle
hand joint M00.14-
hip M00.15-
knee M00.16-
multiple site M00.19
shoulder M00.11-
vertebra M00.18
wrist M00.13-
postdysenteric *—see* Arthropathy, postdysenteric
postmeningococcal A39.84
postrheumatic, chronic *—see* Arthropathy, postrheumatic, chronic
primary progressive *—see also* Arthritis, specified form NEC
spine *—see* Spondylitis, ankylosing
psoriatic L40.50
purulent (any site except spine) *—see* Arthritis, pyogenic or pyemic
spine *—see* Spondylopathy, infective
pyogenic or pyemic (any site except spine) M00.9
bacterial NEC M00.80
ankle M00.87-
elbow M00.82-
foot joint *—see* Arthritis, pyogenic, bacterial NEC, ankle
hand joint M00.84-
hip M00.85-
knee M00.86-
multiple site M00.89
shoulder M00.81-
vertebra M00.88
wrist M00.83-
pneumococcal *—see* Arthritis, pneumococcal
spine *—see* Spondylopathy, infective
staphylococcal *—see* Arthritis, staphylococcal
streptococcal *—see* Arthritis, streptococcal NEC
pneumococcal *—see* Arthritis, pneumococcal
reactive *—see* Reiter's disease
rheumatic *—see also* Arthritis, rheumatoid
acute or subacute *—see* Fever, rheumatic
rheumatoid M06.9
with
carditis *—see* Rheumatoid, carditis

Arthritis, arthritic *(continued)*
rheumatoid M06.9 *(continued)*
with *(continued)*
endocarditis *—see* Rheumatoid, carditis
heart involvement NEC *—see* Rheumatoid, carditis
lung involvement *—see* Rheumatoid, lung
myocarditis *—see* Rheumatoid, carditis
myopathy *—see* Rheumatoid, myopathy
pericarditis *—see* Rheumatoid, carditis
polyneuropathy *—see* Rheumatoid, polyneuropathy
rheumatoid factor *—see* Arthritis, rheumatoid, seropositive
splenoadenomegaly and leukopenia *—see* Felty's syndrome
vasculitis *—see* Rheumatoid, vasculitis
visceral involvement NEC *—see* Rheumatoid, arthritis, with involvement of organs NEC
juvenile (with or without rheumatoid factor) M08.00
with systemic onset *—see* Still's disease
ankle M08.07-
elbow M08.02-
foot joint M08.07-
hand joint M08.04-
hip M08.05-
knee M08.06-
multiple site M08.09
shoulder M08.01-
specified site NEC M08.0A
vertebra M08.08
wrist M08.03-
seronegative M06.00
ankle M06.07-
elbow M06.02-
foot joint M06.07-
hand joint M06.04-
hip M06.05-
knee M06.06-
multiple site M06.09
shoulder M06.01-
specified site NEC M06.0A
vertebra M06.08
wrist M06.03-
seropositive M05.9
specified NEC M05.80
ankle M05.87-
elbow M05.82-
foot joint M05.87-
hand joint M05.84-
hip M05.85-
knee M05.86-
multiple sites M05.89
shoulder M05.81-
specified site NEC M05.8A
vertebra *—see* Spondylitis, ankylosing
wrist M05.83-
without organ involvement M05.70
ankle M05.77-
elbow M05.72-
foot joint M05.77-
hand joint M05.74-
hip M05.75-
knee M05.76-
multiple sites M05.79
shoulder M05.71-
specified site NEC M05.7A

Arthritis, arthritic *(continued)*
rheumatoid *(continued)*
seropositive *(continued)*
without organ involvement *(continued)*
vertebra *—see* Spondylitis, ankylosing
wrist M05.73-
specified type NEC M06.80
ankle M06.87-
elbow M06.82-
foot joint M06.87-
hand joint M06.84-
hip M06.85-
knee M06.86-
multiple site M06.89
shoulder M06.81-
specified site NEC M06.8A
vertebra M06.88
wrist M06.83-
spine *—see* Spondylitis, ankylosing
rubella B06.82
scorbutic (*see also* subcategory M14.8-) E54
senile or senescent *—see* Osteoarthritis
septic (any site except spine) *—see* Arthritis, pyogenic or pyemic
spine *—see* Spondylopathy, infective
serum (nontherapeutic) (therapeutic) *—see* Arthropathy, postimmunization
specified form NEC M13.80
ankle M13.87-
elbow M13.82-
foot joint M13.87-
hand joint M13.84-
hip M13.85-
knee M13.86-
multiple site M13.89
shoulder M13.81-
specified joint NEC M13.88
wrist M13.83-
spine *—see also* Spondylosis
infectious or infective NEC *—see* Spondylopathy, infective
Marie-Strümpell *—see* Spondylitis, ankylosing
pyogenic *—see* Spondylopathy, infective
rheumatoid *—see* Spondylitis, ankylosing
traumatic (old) *—see* Spondylopathy, traumatic
tuberculous A18.01
staphylococcal M00.00
ankle M00.07-
elbow M00.02-
foot joint *—see* Arthritis, staphylococcal, ankle
hand joint M00.04-
hip M00.05-
knee M00.06-
multiple site M00.09
shoulder M00.01-
vertebra M00.08
wrist M00.03-
streptococcal NEC M00.20
ankle M00.27-
elbow M00.22-
foot joint *—see* Arthritis, streptococcal, ankle
hand joint M00.24-
hip M00.25-
knee M00.26-
multiple site M00.29
shoulder M00.21-
vertebra M00.28
wrist M00.23-

Arthritis, arthritic *(continued)*
suppurative *—see* Arthritis, pyogenic or pyemic
syphilitic (late) A52.16
congenital A50.55 *[M12.80]*
syphilitica deformans (Charcot) A52.16
temporomandibular M26.64-
toxic of menopause (any site) *—see* Arthritis, specified form NEC
transient *—see* Arthropathy, specified form NEC
traumatic (chronic) *—see* Arthropathy, traumatic
tuberculous A18.02
spine A18.01
uratic *—see* Gout
urethritica (Reiter's) *—see* Reiter's disease
vertebral *—see* Spondylopathy, inflammatory
villous (any site) *—see* Arthropathy, specified form NEC

Arthrocele *—see* Effusion, joint

Arthrodesis status Z98.1

Arthrodynia *—see also* Pain, joint

Arthrodysplasia Q74.9

Arthrofibrosis, joint *—see* Ankylosis

Arthrogryposis (congenital) Q68.8
multiplex congenita Q74.3

Arthrokatadysis M24.7

Arthropathy *—see also* Arthritis M12.9
Charcot's *—see* Arthropathy, neuropathic
diabetic *—see* Diabetes, arthropathy, neuropathic
syringomyelic G95.0
cricoarytenoid J38.7
crystal (-induced) *—see* Arthritis, in, crystals
diabetic NEC *—see* Diabetes, arthropathy
distal interphalangeal, psoriatic L40.51
enteropathic M07.60
ankle M07.67-
elbow M07.62-
foot joint M07.67-
hand joint M07.64-
hip M07.65-
knee M07.66-
multiple site M07.69
shoulder M07.61-
vertebra M07.68
wrist M07.63-
facet joint (*see* Spondylosis) M47.819
following intestinal bypass M02.00
ankle M02.07-
elbow M02.02-
foot joint M02.07-
hand joint M02.04-
hip M02.05-
knee M02.06-
multiple site M02.09
shoulder M02.01-
vertebra M02.08
wrist M02.03-
gouty *—see also* Gout
in (due to)
Lesch-Nyhan syndrome E79.1 *[M14.8-]*
sickle-cell disorders D57- *[M14.8-]*

Arthropathy *(continued)*
hemophilic NEC D66 *[M36.2]*
in (due to)
hyperparathyroidism NEC E21.3 *[M14.8-]*
metabolic disease NOS E88.9 *[M14.8-]*
in (due to)
acromegaly E22.0 *[M14.8-]*
amyloidosis E85.4 *[M14.8-]*
blood disorder NOS D75.9 *[M36.3]*
diabetes —*see* Diabetes, arthropathy
endocrine disease NOS E34.9 *[M14.8-]*
erythema
multiforme L51.9 *[M14.8-]*
nodosum L52 *[M14.8-]*
hemochromatosis E83.118 *[M14.8-]*
hemoglobinopathy NEC D58.2 *[M36.3]*
hemophilia NEC D66 *[M36.2]*
Henoch-Schönlein purpura D69.0 *[M36.4]*
hyperthyroidism E05.90 *[M14.8-]*
hypothyroidism E03.9 *[M14.8-]*
infective endocarditis I33.0 *[M12.80]*
leukemia NEC C95.9- *[M36.1]*
malignant histiocytosis C96.A *[M36.1]*
metabolic disease NOS E88.9 *[M14.8-]*
multiple myeloma C90.0- *[M36.1]*
neoplastic disease NOS (*see also* Neoplasm) D49.9 *[M36.1]*
nutritional deficiency (*see also* subcategory M14.8-) E63.9
psoriasis NOS L40.50
sarcoidosis D86.86
syphilis (late) A52.77
congenital A50.55 *[M12.80]*
thyrotoxicosis (*see also* subcategory M14.8-) E05.90
ulcerative colitis K51.90 *[M07.60]*
viral hepatitis (postinfectious) NEC B19.9 *[M12.80]*
Whipple's disease (*see also* subcategory M14.8-) K90.81
Jaccoud —*see* Arthropathy, postrheumatic, chronic
juvenile —*see* Arthritis, juvenile
psoriatic L40.54
mutilans (psoriatic) L40.52
neuropathic (Charcot) M14.60
ankle M14.67-
diabetic —*see* Diabetes, arthropathy, neuropathic
elbow M14.62-
foot joint M14.67-
hand joint M14.64-
hip M14.65-
knee M14.66-
multiple site M14.69
nonsyphilitic NEC G98.0
shoulder M14.61-
syringomyelic G95.0
vertebra M14.68
wrist M14.63-
osteopulmonary —*see* Osteoarthropathy, hypertrophic, specified NEC
postdysenteric M02.10
ankle M02.17-
elbow M02.12-
foot joint M02.17-
hand joint M02.14-
hip M02.15-

Arthropathy *(continued)*
postdysenteric *(continued)*
knee M02.16-
multiple site M02.19
shoulder M02.11-
vertebra M02.18
wrist M02.13-
postimmunization M02.20
ankle M02.27-
elbow M02.22-
foot joint M02.27-
hand joint M02.24-
hip M02.25-
knee M02.26-
multiple site M02.29
shoulder M02.21-
vertebra M02.28
wrist M02.23-
postinfectious NEC B99 *[M12.80]*
in (due to)
enteritis due to Yersinia enterocolitica A04.6 *[M12.80]*
syphilis A52.77
viral hepatitis NEC B19.9 *[M12.80]*
postrheumatic, chronic (Jaccoud) M12.00
ankle M12.07-
elbow M12.02-
foot joint M12.07-
hand joint M12.04-
hip M12.05-
knee M12.06-
multiple site M12.09
shoulder M12.01-
specified joint NEC M12.08
vertebrae M12.08
wrist M12.03-
psoriatic NEC L40.59
interphalangeal, distal L40.51
reactive M02.9
in (due to)
infective endocarditis I33.0 *[M02.9]*
specified type NEC M02.80
ankle M02.87-
elbow M02.82-
foot joint M02.87-
hand joint M02.84-
hip M02.85-
knee M02.86-
multiple site M02.89
shoulder M02.81-
vertebra M02.88
wrist M02.83-
specified form NEC M12.80
ankle M12.87-
elbow M12.82-
foot joint M12.87-
hand joint M12.84-
hip M12.85-
knee M12.86-
multiple site M12.89
shoulder M12.81-
specified joint NEC M12.88
vertebrae M12.88
wrist M12.83-
syringomyelic G95.0
tabes dorsalis A52.16
tabetic A52.16
temporomandibular joint M26.65-
transient —*see* Arthropathy, specified form NEC
traumatic M12.50
ankle M12.57-
elbow M12.52-
foot joint M12.57-
hand joint M12.54-
hip M12.55-
knee M12.56-
multiple site M12.59

Arthropathy *(continued)*
traumatic *(continued)*
shoulder M12.51-
specified joint NEC M12.58
vertebrae M12.58
wrist M12.53-

Arthropyosis —*see* Arthritis, pyogenic or pyemic

Arthrosis (deformans) (degenerative) (localized) —*see also* Osteoarthritis M19.90
spine —*see* Spondylosis

Arthus' phenomenon or reaction T78.41
due to
drug —*see* Table of Drugs and Chemicals, by drug

Articular —*see* condition

Articulation, reverse (teeth) M26.24

Artificial
insemination complication —*see* Complications, artificial, fertilization
opening status (functioning) (without complication) Z93.9
anus (colostomy) Z93.3
colostomy Z93.3
cystostomy Z93.50
appendico-vesicostomy Z93.52
cutaneous Z93.51
specified NEC Z93.59
enterostomy Z93.4
gastrostomy Z93.1
ileostomy Z93.2
intestinal tract NEC Z93.4
jejunostomy Z93.4
nephrostomy Z93.6
specified site NEC Z93.8
tracheostomy Z93.0
ureterostomy Z93.6
urethrostomy Z93.6
urinary tract NEC Z93.6
vagina Z93.8
vagina status Z93.8

Arytenoid —*see* condition

Asbestosis (occupational) J61

ASC-H (atypical squamous cells cannot exclude high grade squamous intraepithelial lesion on cytologic smear)
anus R85.611
cervix R87.611
vagina R87.621

ASC-US (atypical squamous cells of undetermined significance on cytologic smear)
anus R85.610
cervix R87.610
vagina R87.620

Ascariasis B77.9
with
complications NEC B77.89
intestinal complications B77.0
pneumonia, pneumonitis B77.81

Ascaridosis, ascaridiasis —*see* Ascariasis

Ascaris (infection) (infestation) (lumbricoides) —*see* Ascariasis

Ascending —*see* condition

Aschoff's bodies —*see* Myocarditis, rheumatic

Ascites (abdominal) R18.8
cardiac (*see also* Failure, heart, right) I50.810

Ascites *(continued)*
chylous (nonfilarial) I89.8
filarial —*see* Infestation, filarial
due to
cirrhosis, alcoholic K70.31
hepatitis
alcoholic K70.11
chronic active K71.51
S. japonicum B65.2
heart (*see also* Failure, heart, right) I50.810
malignant R18.0
pseudochylous R18.8
syphilitic A52.74
tuberculous A18.31

Aseptic —*see* condition

Asherman's syndrome N85.6

Asialia K11.7

Asiatic cholera —*see* Cholera

Asimultagnosia (simultanagnosia) R48.3

Askin's tumor —*see* Neoplasm, connective tissue, malignant

Asocial personality F60.2

Asomatognosia R41.4

Aspartylglucosaminuria E77.1

Asperger's disease or syndrome F84.5

Aspergilloma —*see* Aspergillosis

Aspergillosis (with pneumonia) B44.9
bronchopulmonary, allergic B44.81
disseminated B44.7
generalized B44.7
pulmonary NEC B44.1
allergic B44.81
invasive B44.0
specified NEC B44.89
tonsillar B44.2

Aspergillus (flavus) (fumigatus) (infection) (terreus) —*see* Aspergillosis

Aspermatogenesis —*see* Azoospermia

Aspermia (testis) —*see* Azoospermia

Asphyxia, asphyxiation (by) R09.01
antenatal P84
birth P84
bunny bag —*see* Asphyxia, due to, mechanical threat to breathing, trapped in bed clothes
crushing S28.0
drowning T75.1
gas, fumes, or vapor —*see* Table of Drugs and Chemicals
inhalation —*see* Inhalation
intrauterine P84
local I73.00
with gangrene I73.01
mucus —*see also* Foreign body, respiratory tract, causing asphyxia
newborn P84
pathological R09.01
postnatal P84
mechanical —*see* Asphyxia, due to, mechanical threat to breathing
prenatal P84
reticularis R23.1
strangulation —*see* Asphyxia, due to, mechanical threat to breathing
submersion T75.1

Asthma, asthmatic *(continued)*
- Rostan's I50.1
- sandblaster's J62.8
- sequoiosis J67.8
- severe persistent J45.50
  - with
    - exacerbation (acute) J45.51
    - status asthmaticus J45.52
- specified NEC J45.998
- stonemason's J62.8
- thymic E32.8
- tuberculous *—see* Tuberculosis, pulmonary
- Wichmann's (laryngismus stridulus) J38.5
- wood J67.8

Astigmatism (compound) (congenital) H52.20-
- irregular H52.21-
- regular H52.22-

Astraphobia F40.220

Astroblastoma
- specified site *—see* Neoplasm, malignant, by site
- unspecified site C71.9

Astrocytoma (cystic)
- anaplastic
  - specified site *—see* Neoplasm, malignant, by site
  - unspecified site C71.9
- fibrillary
  - specified site *—see* Neoplasm, malignant, by site
  - unspecified site C71.9
- fibrous
  - specified site *—see* Neoplasm, malignant, by site
  - unspecified site C71.9
- gemistocytic
  - specified site *—see* Neoplasm, malignant, by site
  - unspecified site C71.9
- juvenile
  - specified site *—see* Neoplasm, malignant, by site
  - unspecified site C71.9
- pilocytic
  - specified site *—see* Neoplasm, malignant, by site
  - unspecified site C71.9
- piloid
  - specified site *—see* Neoplasm, malignant, by site
  - unspecified site C71.9
- protoplasmic
  - specified site *—see* Neoplasm, malignant, by site
  - unspecified site C71.9
- specified site NEC *—see* Neoplasm, malignant, by site
- subependymal D43.2
  - giant cell
    - specified site *—see* Neoplasm, uncertain behavior, by site
    - unspecified site D43.2
  - specified site *—see* Neoplasm, uncertain behavior, by site
  - unspecified site D43.2
- unspecified site C71.9

Astroglioma
- specified site *—see* Neoplasm, malignant, by site
- unspecified site C71.9

Asymbolia R48.8

Asymmetry *—see also* Distortion
- between native and reconstructed breast N65.1
- face Q67.0

Asymmetry *(continued)*
- jaw (lower) *—see* Anomaly, dentofacial, jaw-cranial base relationship, asymmetry

Asynergia, asynergy R27.8
- ventricular I51.89

Asystole (heart) *—see* Arrest, cardiac

At risk
- for
  - dental caries Z91.849
    - high Z91.843
    - low Z91.841
    - moderate Z91.842
- falling Z91.81

Ataxia, ataxy, ataxic R27.0
- acute R27.8
- autosomal recessive Friedreich G11.11
- brain (hereditary) G11.9
- cerebellar (hereditary) G11.9
  - with defective DNA repair G11.3
  - alcoholic G31.2
  - early-onset G11.10
    - with
      - essential tremor G11.19
      - myoclonus [Hunt's ataxia] G11.19
      - retained tendon reflexes G11.19
  - in
    - alcoholism G31.2
    - myxedema E03.9 *[G13.2]*
    - neoplastic disease (*see also* Neoplasm) D49.9 *[G32.81]*
    - specified disease NEC G32.81
  - late-onset (Marie's) G11.2
- cerebral (hereditary) G11.9
- congenital nonprogressive G11.0
- family, familial *—see* Ataxia, hereditary
- following
  - cerebrovascular disease I69.993
    - cerebral infarction I69.393
    - intracerebral hemorrhage I69.193
    - nontraumatic intracranial hemorrhage NEC I69.293
    - specified disease NEC I69.893
    - subarachnoid hemorrhage I69.093
- Friedreich's (heredofamilial) (cerebellar) (spinal) (with retained reflexes) G11.11
- gait R26.0
  - hysterical F44.4
- general R27.8
- gluten M35.9 *[G32.81]*
  - with celiac disease K90.0 *[G32.81]*
- hereditary G11.9
  - with neuropathy G60.2
  - cerebellar *—see* Ataxia, cerebellar
  - spastic G11.4
  - specified NEC G11.8
  - spinal (Friedreich's) G11.11
- heredofamilial *—see* Ataxia, hereditary
- Hunt's G11.19
- hysterical F44.4
- locomotor (progressive) (syphilitic) (partial) (spastic) A52.11
  - diabetic *—see* Diabetes, ataxia
- Marie's (cerebellar) (heredofamilial) (late- onset) G11.2
- nonorganic origin F44.4
- nonprogressive, congenital G11.0
- psychogenic F44.4
- Roussy-Lévy G60.0
- Sanger-Brown's (hereditary) G11.2

Ataxia, ataxy, ataxic *(continued)*
- spastic hereditary G11.4
- spinal
  - hereditary (Friedreich's) G11.11
  - progressive (syphilitic) A52.11
- spinocerebellar, X-linked recessive G11.19
- telangiectasia (Louis-Bar) G11.3

Ataxia-telangiectasia (Louis-Bar) G11.3

Atelectasis (massive) (partial) (pressure) (pulmonary) J98.11
- newborn P28.10
  - due to resorption P28.11
  - partial P28.19
  - primary P28.0
  - secondary P28.19
- primary (newborn) P28.0
- tuberculous *—see* Tuberculosis, pulmonary

Atelocardia Q24.9

Atelomyelia Q06.1

Atheroembolism
- of
  - extremities
    - lower I75.02-
    - upper I75.01-
  - kidney I75.81
  - specified NEC I75.89

Atheroma, atheromatous *—see also* Arteriosclerosis I70.90
- aorta, aortic I70.0
  - valve *—see also* Endocarditis, aortic I35.8
- aorto-iliac I70.0
- artery *—see* Arteriosclerosis
- basilar (artery) I67.2
- carotid (artery) (common) (internal) I67.2
- cerebral (arteries) I67.2
- coronary (artery) I25.10
  - with angina pectoris *—see* Arteriosclerosis, coronary (artery),
- degeneration *—see* Arteriosclerosis
- heart, cardiac *—see* Disease, heart, ischemic, atherosclerotic
- mitral (valve) I34.8
- myocardium, myocardial *—see* Disease, heart, ischemic, atherosclerotic
- pulmonary valve (heart) (*see also* Endocarditis, pulmonary) I37.8
- tricuspid (heart) (valve) I36.8
- valve, valvular *—see* Endocarditis
- vertebral (artery) I67.2

Atheromatosis *—see* Arteriosclerosis

Atherosclerosis *—see also* Arteriosclerosis
- coronary
  - artery I25.10
    - with angina pectoris *—see* Arteriosclerosis, coronary (artery),
    - due to
      - calcified coronary lesion (severely) I25.84
      - lipid rich plaque I25.83
  - transplanted heart I25.811
    - bypass graft I25.812
      - with angina pectoris *—see* Arteriosclerosis, coronary (artery),
    - native coronary artery I25.811
      - with angina pectoris *—see* Arteriosclerosis, coronary (artery),

Athetosis (acquired) R25.8
- bilateral (congenital) G80.3
- congenital (bilateral) (double) G80.3
- double (congenital) G80.3
- unilateral R25.8

Athlete's
- foot B35.3
- heart I51.7

Athrepsia E41

Athyrea (acquired) *—see also* Hypothyroidism
- congenital E03.1

Atonia, atony, atonic
- bladder (sphincter) (neurogenic) N31.2
- capillary I78.8
- cecum K59.89
  - psychogenic F45.8
- colon *—see* Atony, intestine
- congenital P94.2
- esophagus K22.89
- intestine K59.89
  - psychogenic F45.8
- stomach K31.89
  - neurotic or psychogenic F45.8
- uterus (during labor) O62.2
  - with hemorrhage (postpartum) O72.1
  - postpartum (with hemorrhage) O72.1
    - without hemorrhage O75.89

Atopy *—see* History, allergy

Atransferrinemia, congenital E88.09

Atresia, atretic
- alimentary organ or tract NEC Q45.8
  - upper Q40.8
- ani, anus, anal (canal) Q42.3
  - with fistula Q42.2
- aorta (ring) Q25.29
- aortic (orifice) (valve) Q23.0
  - arch Q25.21
  - congenital with hypoplasia of ascending aorta and defective development of left ventricle (with mitral stenosis) Q23.4
  - in hypoplastic left heart syndrome Q23.4
- aqueduct of Sylvius Q03.0
  - with spina bifida *—see* Spina bifida, with hydrocephalus
- artery NEC Q27.8
  - cerebral Q28.3
  - coronary Q24.5
  - digestive system Q27.8
  - eye Q15.8
  - lower limb Q27.8
  - pulmonary Q25.5
  - specified site NEC Q27.8
  - umbilical Q27.0
  - upper limb Q27.8
- auditory canal (external) Q16.1
- bile duct (common) (congenital) (hepatic) Q44.2
  - acquired *—see* Obstruction, bile duct
- bladder (neck) Q64.39
  - obstruction Q64.31
- bronchus Q32.4
- cecum Q42.8
- cervix (acquired) N88.2
  - congenital Q51.828
  - in pregnancy or childbirth *—see* Anomaly, cervix, in pregnancy or childbirth
    - causing obstructed labor O65.5

Atresia, atretic *(continued)*
- choana Q30.0
- colon Q42.9
  - specified NEC Q42.8
- common duct Q44.2
- cricoid cartilage Q31.8
- cystic duct Q44.2
  - acquired K82.8
    - with obstruction K82.0
- digestive organs NEC Q45.8
- duodenum Q41.0
- ear canal Q16.1
- ejaculatory duct Q55.4
- epiglottis Q31.8
- esophagus Q39.0
  - with tracheoesophageal fistula Q39.1
- eustachian tube Q17.8
- fallopian tube (congenital) Q50.6
  - acquired N97.1
- follicular cyst N83.0-
- foramen of
  - Luschka Q03.1
    - with spina bifida *—see* Spina bifida, with hydrocephalus
  - Magendie Q03.1
    - with spina bifida *—see* Spina bifida, with hydrocephalus
- gallbladder Q44.1
- genital organ
  - external
    - female Q52.79
    - male Q55.8
  - internal
    - female Q52.8
    - male Q55.8
- glottis Q31.8
- gullet Q39.0
  - with tracheoesophageal fistula Q39.1
- heart valve NEC Q24.8
  - pulmonary Q22.0
  - tricuspid Q22.4
- hymen Q52.3
  - acquired (postinfective) N89.6
- ileum Q41.2
- intestine (small) Q41.9
  - large Q42.9
    - specified NEC Q42.8
- iris, filtration angle Q15.0
- jejunum Q41.1
- lacrimal apparatus Q10.4
- larynx Q31.8
- meatus urinarius Q64.33
- mitral valve Q23.2
  - in hypoplastic left heart syndrome Q23.4
- nares (anterior) (posterior) Q30.0
- nasopharynx Q34.8
- nose, nostril Q30.0
  - acquired J34.89
- organ or site NEC Q89.8
- osseous meatus (ear) Q16.1
- oviduct (congenital) Q50.6
  - acquired N97.1
- parotid duct Q38.4
  - acquired K11.8
- pulmonary (artery) Q25.5
  - valve Q22.0
- pulmonic Q22.0
- pupil Q13.2
- rectum Q42.1
  - with fistula Q42.0
- salivary duct Q38.4
  - acquired K11.8
- sublingual duct Q38.4
  - acquired K11.8
- submandibular duct Q38.4
  - acquired K11.8

Atresia, atretic *(continued)*
- submaxillary duct Q38.4
  - acquired K11.8
- thyroid cartilage Q31.8
- trachea Q32.1
- tricuspid valve Q22.4
- ureter Q62.10
  - pelvic junction Q62.11
  - vesical orifice Q62.12
- ureteropelvic junction Q62.11
- ureterovesical orifice Q62.12
- urethra (valvular) Q64.39
  - stricture Q64.32
- urinary tract NEC Q64.8
- uterus Q51.818
  - acquired N85.8
- vagina (congenital) Q52.4
  - acquired (postinfectional) (senile) N89.5
- vas deferens Q55.3
- vascular NEC Q27.8
  - cerebral Q28.3
  - digestive system Q27.8
  - lower limb Q27.8
  - specified site NEC Q27.8
  - upper limb Q27.8
- vein NEC Q27.8
  - digestive system Q27.8
  - great Q26.8
  - lower limb Q27.8
  - portal Q26.5
  - pulmonary Q26.4
    - partial Q26.3
    - total Q26.2
  - specified site NEC Q27.8
  - upper limb Q27.8
- vena cava (inferior) (superior) Q26.8
- vesicourethral orifice Q64.31
- vulva Q52.79
  - acquired N90.5

Atrichia, atrichosis *—see* Alopecia

Atrophia *—see also* Atrophy
- cutis senilis L90.8
  - due to radiation L57.8
- gyrata of choroid and retina H31.23
- senilis R54
  - dermatological L90.8
    - due to radiation (nonionizing) (solar) L57.8
- unguium L60.3
  - congenita Q84.6

Atrophie blanche (en plaque) (de Milian) L95.0

Atrophoderma, atrophodermia (of) L90.9
- diffusum (idiopathic) L90.4
- maculatum L90.8
  - et striatum L90.8
    - due to syphilis A52.79
  - syphilitic A51.39
- neuriticum L90.8
- Pasini and Pierini L90.3
- pigmentosum Q82.1
- reticulatum symmetricum faciei L66.4
- senile L90.8
  - due to radiation (nonionizing) (solar) L57.8
- vermiculata (cheeks) L66.4

Atrophy, atrophic (of)
- adrenal (capsule) (gland) E27.49
  - primary (autoimmune) E27.1
- alveolar process or ridge (edentulous) K08.20
- anal sphincter (disuse) N81.84
- appendix K38.8
- arteriosclerotic *—see* Arteriosclerosis
- bile duct (common) (hepatic) K83.8

Atrophy, atrophic *(continued)*
- bladder N32.89
  - neurogenic N31.8
- blanche (en plaque) (of Milian) L95.0
- bone (senile) NEC *—see also* Disorder, bone, specified type NEC
  - due to
    - tabes dorsalis (neurogenic) A52.11
- brain (cortex) (progressive) G31.9
  - frontotemporal circumscribed G31.01 *[F02.80]*
    - with behavioral disturbance G31.01 *[F02.81]*
  - senile NEC G31.1
- breast N64.2
  - obstetric *—see* Disorder, breast, specified type NEC
- buccal cavity K13.79
- cardiac *—see* Degeneration, myocardial
- cartilage (infectional) (joint) *—see* Disorder, cartilage, specified NEC
- cerebellar *—see* Atrophy, brain
- cerebral *—see* Atrophy, brain
- cervix (mucosa) (senile) (uteri) N88.8
  - menopausal N95.8
- Charcot-Marie-Tooth G60.0
- choroid (central) (macular) (myopic) (retina) H31.10-
  - diffuse secondary H31.12-
  - gyrate H31.23
  - senile H31.11-
- ciliary body *—see* Atrophy, iris
- conjunctiva (senile) H11.89
- corpus cavernosum N48.89
- cortical *—see* Atrophy, brain
- cystic duct K82.8
- Déjérine-Thomas G23.8
- disuse NEC *—see* Atrophy, muscle
- Duchenne-Aran G12.21
- ear H93.8-
- edentulous alveolar ridge K08.20
- endometrium (senile) N85.8
  - cervix N88.8
- enteric K63.89
- epididymis N50.89
- eyeball *—see* Disorder, globe, degenerated condition, atrophy
- eyelid (senile) *—see* Disorder, eyelid, degenerative
- facial (skin) L90.9
- fallopian tube (senile) N83.32-
  - with ovary N83.33-
- fascioscapulohumeral (Landouzy-Déjérine) G71.02
- fatty, thymus (gland) E32.8
- gallbladder K82.8
- gastric K29.40
  - with bleeding K29.41
- gastrointestinal K63.89
- glandular I89.8
- globe H44.52-
- gum *-see* Recession, gingival
- hair L67.8
- heart (brown) *—see* Degeneration, myocardial
- hemifacial Q67.4
  - Romberg G51.8
- infantile E41
  - paralysis, acute *—see* Poliomyelitis, paralytic
- intestine K63.89
- iris (essential) (progressive) H21.26-
  - specified NEC H21.29

Atrophy, atrophic *(continued)*
- kidney (senile) (terminal) *(see also* Sclerosis, renal) N26.1
  - congenital or infantile Q60.5
    - bilateral Q60.4
    - unilateral Q60.3
  - hydronephrotic *—see* Hydronephrosis
- lacrimal gland (primary) H04.14-
  - secondary H04.15-
- Landouzy-Déjérine G71.02
- laryngitis, infective J37.0
- larynx J38.7
- Leber's optic (hereditary) H47.22
- lip K13.0
- liver (yellow) K72.90
  - with coma K72.91
  - acute, subacute K72.00
    - with coma K72.01
  - chronic K72.10
    - with coma K72.11
- lung (senile) J98.4
- macular (dermatological) L90.8
  - syphilitic, skin A51.39
    - striated A52.79
- mandible (edentulous) K08.20
  - minimal K08.21
  - moderate K08.22
  - severe K08.23
- maxilla K08.20
  - minimal K08.24
  - moderate K08.25
  - severe K08.26
- muscle, muscular (diffuse) (general) (idiopathic) (primary) M62.50
  - ankle M62.57-
  - Duchenne-Aran G12.21
  - foot M62.57-
  - forearm M62.53-
  - hand M62.54-
  - infantile spinal G12.0
  - lower leg M62.56-
  - multiple sites M62.59
  - myelopathic *—see* Atrophy, muscle, spinal
  - myotonic G71.11
  - neuritic G58.9
  - neuropathic (peroneal) (progressive) G60.0
  - pelvic (disuse) N81.84
  - peroneal G60.0
  - progressive (bulbar) G12.21
    - adult G12.1
    - infantile (spinal) G12.0
    - spinal G12.25
      - adult G12.1
      - infantile G12.0
  - pseudohypertrophic G71.02
  - shoulder region M62.51-
  - specified site NEC M62.58
  - spinal G12.9
    - adult form G12.1
    - Aran-Duchenne G12.21
    - childhood form, type II G12.1
    - distal G12.1
    - hereditary NEC G12.1
    - infantile, type I (Werdnig-Hoffmann) G12.0
    - juvenile form, type III (Kugelberg- Welander) G12.1
    - progressive G12.25
    - scapuloperoneal form G12.1
    - specified NEC G12.8
  - syphilitic A52.78
  - thigh M62.55-
  - upper arm M62.52-
- myocardium *—see* Degeneration, myocardial

Atrophy, atrophic *(continued)*
- myometrium (senile) N85.8
  - cervix N88.8
- myopathic NEC *—see* Atrophy, muscle
- myotonia G71.11
- nail L60.3
- nasopharynx J31.1
- nerve *—see also* Disorder, nerve
  - abducens *—see* Strabismus, paralytic, sixth nerve
  - accessory G52.8
  - acoustic or auditory H93.3
  - cranial G52.9
    - eighth (auditory) H93.3
    - eleventh (accessory) G52.8
    - fifth (trigeminal) G50.8
    - first (olfactory) G52.0
    - fourth (trochlear) *—see* Strabismus, paralytic, fourth nerve
    - second (optic) H47.20
    - sixth (abducens) *—see* Strabismus, paralytic, sixth nerve
    - tenth (pneumogastric) (vagus) G52.2
    - third (oculomotor) *—see* Strabismus, paralytic, third nerve
    - twelfth (hypoglossal) G52.3
  - hypoglossal G52.3
  - oculomotor *—see* Strabismus, paralytic, third nerve
  - olfactory G52.0
  - optic (papillomacular bundle)
    - syphilitic (late) A52.15
      - congenital A50.44
  - pneumogastric G52.2
  - trigeminal G50.8
  - trochlear *—see* Strabismus, paralytic, fourth nerve
  - vagus (pneumogastric) G52.2
- neurogenic, bone, tabetic A52.11
- nutritional E43
  - with marasmus E41
- old age R54
- olivopontocerebellar G23.8
- optic (nerve) H47.20
  - glaucomatous H47.23-
  - hereditary H47.22
  - primary H47.21-
  - specified type NEC H47.29-
  - syphilitic (late) A52.15
    - congenital A50.44
- orbit H05.31-
- ovary (senile) N83.31-
  - with fallopian tube N83.33-
- oviduct (senile) *—see* Atrophy, fallopian tube
- palsy, diffuse (progressive) G12.22
- pancreas (duct) (senile) K86.89
- parotid gland K11.0
- pelvic muscle N81.84
- penis N48.89
- pharynx J39.2
- pluriglandular E31.8
  - autoimmune E31.0
- polyarthritis M15.9
- prostate N42.89
- pseudohypertrophic (muscle) G71.02
- renal (*see also* Sclerosis, renal) N26.1
- retina, retinal (postinfectional) H35.89
- rhinitis J31.0
- salivary gland K11.0
- scar L90.5

Atrophy, atrophic *(continued)*
- sclerosis, lobar (of brain) G31.09 *[F02.80]*
  - with behavioral disturbance G31.09 *[F02.81]*
- scrotum N50.89
- seminal vesicle N50.89
- senile R54
  - due to radiation (nonionizing) (solar) L57.8
- skin (patches) (spots) L90.9
  - degenerative (senile) L90.8
  - due to radiation (nonionizing) (solar) L57.8
  - senile L90.8
- spermatic cord N50.89
- spinal (acute) (cord) G95.89
  - muscular *—see* Atrophy, muscle, spinal
  - paralysis G12.20
    - acute *—see* Poliomyelitis, paralytic
    - meaning progressive muscular atrophy G12.25
- spine (column) *—see* Spondylopathy, specified NEC
- spleen (senile) D73.0
- stomach K29.40
  - with bleeding K29.41
- striate (skin) L90.6
  - syphilitic A52.79
- subcutaneous L90.9
- sublingual gland K11.0
- submandibular gland K11.0
- submaxillary gland K11.0
- Sudeck's *—see* Algoneurodystrophy
- suprarenal (capsule) (gland) E27.49
  - primary E27.1
- systemic affecting central nervous system
  - in
    - myxedema E03.9 *[G13.2]*
    - neoplastic disease (*see also* Neoplasm) D49.9 *[G13.1]*
    - specified disease NEC G13.8
- tarso-orbital fascia, congenital Q10.3
- testis N50.0
- thenar, partial *—see* Syndrome, carpal tunnel
- thymus (fatty) E32.8
- thyroid (gland) (acquired) E03.4
  - with cretinism E03.1
  - congenital (with myxedema) E03.1
- tongue (senile) K14.8
  - papillae K14.4
- trachea J39.8
- tunica vaginalis N50.89
- turbinate J34.89
- tympanic membrane (nonflaccid) H73.82-
  - flaccid H73.81-
- upper respiratory tract J39.8
- uterus, uterine (senile) N85.8
  - cervix N88.8
  - due to radiation (intended effect) N85.8
    - adverse effect or misadventure N99.89
- vagina (senile) N95.2
- vas deferens N50.89
- vascular I99.8
- vertebra (senile) *—see* Spondylopathy, specified NEC
- vulva (senile) N90.5
- Werdnig-Hoffmann G12.0
- yellow *—see* Failure, hepatic

Attack, attacks
- with alteration of consciousness (with automatisms) *—see* Epilepsy, localization-related, symptomatic, with complex partial seizures
- Adams-Stokes I45.9
- akinetic *—see* Epilepsy, generalized, specified NEC
- angina *—see* Angina
- atonic *—see* Epilepsy, generalized, specified NEC
- benign shuddering G25.83
- cataleptic *—see* Catalepsy
- sp
- coronary *—see* Infarct, myocardium
- cyanotic, newborn P28.2
- drop NEC R55
- epileptic *—see* Epilepsy
- heart *—see* infarct, myocardium
- hysterical F44.9
- jacksonian *—see* Epilepsy, localization-related, symptomatic, with simple partial seizures
- myocardium, myocardial *—see* Infarct, myocardium
- myoclonic *—see* Epilepsy, generalized, specified NEC
- panic F41.0
- psychomotor *—see* Epilepsy, localization-related, symptomatic, with complex partial seizures
- salaam *—see* Epilepsy, spasms
- schizophreniform, brief F23
- shuddering, benign G25.83
- Stokes-Adams I45.9
- syncope R55
- transient ischemic (TIA) G45.9
  - specified NEC G45.8
- unconsciousness R55
  - hysterical F44.89
- vasomotor R55
- vasovagal (paroxysmal) (idiopathic) R55
- without alteration of consciousness *—see* Epilepsy, localization-related, symptomatic, with simple partial seizures

Attention (to)
- artificial
  - opening (of) Z43.9
    - digestive tract NEC Z43.4
      - colon Z43.3
      - ilium Z43.2
      - stomach Z43.1
    - specified NEC Z43.8
    - trachea Z43.0
    - urinary tract NEC Z43.6
      - cystostomy Z43.5
      - nephrostomy Z43.6
      - ureterostomy Z43.6
      - urethrostomy Z43.6
  - vagina Z43.7
- colostomy Z43.3
- cystostomy Z43.5
- deficit disorder or syndrome F98.8
  - with hyperactivity *—see* Disorder, attention-deficit hyperactivity
- gastrostomy Z43.1
- ileostomy Z43.2
- jejunostomy Z43.4
- nephrostomy Z43.6
- surgical dressings Z48.01
- sutures Z48.02
- tracheostomy Z43.0

Attention *(continued)*
- ureterostomy Z43.6
- urethrostomy Z43.6

Attrition
- gum *-see* Recession, gingival
- tooth, teeth (excessive) (hard tissues) K03.0

Atypical, atypism *—see also* condition
- cells (on cytological smear) (endocervical) (endometrial) (glandular)
  - cervix R87.619
  - vagina R87.629
- cervical N87.9
- endometrium N85.9
  - hyperplasia N85.00
- parenting situation Z62.9

Auditory *—see* condition

Aujeszky's disease B33.8

Aurantiasis, cutis E67.1

Auricle, auricular *—see also* condition
- cervical Q18.2

Auriculotemporal syndrome G50.8

Austin Flint murmur (aortic insufficiency) I35.1

Australian
- Q fever A78
- X disease A83.4

Autism, autistic (childhood) (infantile) F84.0
- atypical F84.9
- spectrum disorder F84.0

Autodigestion R68.89

Autoerythrocyte sensitization (syndrome) D69.2

Autographism L50.3

Autoimmune
- disease (systemic) M35.9
- inhibitors to clotting factors D68.311
- lymphoproliferative syndrome [ALPS] D89.82
- thyroiditis E06.3

Autointoxication R68.89

Automatism G93.89
- with temporal sclerosis G93.81
- epileptic *—see* Epilepsy, localization-related, symptomatic, with complex partial seizures
- paroxysmal, idiopathic *—see* Epilepsy, localization-related, symptomatic, with complex partial seizures

Autonomic, autonomous
- bladder (neurogenic) N31.2
- hysteria seizure F44.5

Autosensitivity, erythrocyte D69.2

Autosensitization, cutaneous L30.2

Autosome *—see* condition by chromosome involved

Autotopagnosia R48.1

Autotoxemia R68.89

Autumn *—see* condition

Avellis' syndrome G46.8

Aversion
oral R63.39
newborn P92.-
nonorganic origin F98.2
sexual F52.1

Aviator's
disease or sickness *—see* Effect, adverse, high altitude
ear T70.0

Avitaminosis (multiple) (*see also* Deficiency, vitamin) E56.9
B E53.9
with
beriberi E51.11
pellagra E52
B2 E53.0
B6 E53.1
B12 E53.8
D E55.9
with rickets E55.0
G E53.0
K E56.1
nicotinic acid E52

AVNRT (atrioventricular nodal re-entrant tachycardia) I47.1

AVRT (atrioventricular nodal re-entrant tachycardia) I47.1

Avulsion (traumatic)
blood vessel *—see* Injury, blood vessel
bone *—see* Fracture, by site
cartilage *—see also* Dislocation, by site
symphyseal (inner), complicating delivery O71.6
external site other than limb *—see* Wound, open, by site
eye S05.7-
head (intracranial)
external site NEC S08.89
scalp S08.0
internal organ or site *—see* Injury, by site
joint *—see also* Dislocation, by site
capsule *—see* Sprain, by site
kidney S37.06-
ligament *—see* Sprain, by site
limb *—see also* Amputation, traumatic, by site
skin and subcutaneous tissue *—see* Wound, open, by site
muscle *—see* Injury, muscle
nerve (root) *—see* Injury, nerve
scalp S08.0
skin and subcutaneous tissue *—see* Wound, open, by site
spleen S36.032
symphyseal cartilage (inner), complicating delivery O71.6
tendon *—see* Injury, muscle
tooth S03.2

Awareness of heart beat R00.2

Axenfeld's
anomaly or syndrome Q15.0
degeneration (calcareous) Q13.4

Axilla, axillary *—see also* condition
breast Q83.1

Axonotmesis *—see* Injury, nerve

Ayerza's disease or syndrome (pulmonary artery sclerosis with pulmonary hypertension) I27.0

Azoospermia (organic) N46.01
due to
drug therapy N46.021
efferent duct obstruction N46.023
infection N46.022
radiation N46.024
specified cause NEC N46.029
systemic disease N46.025

Azotemia R79.89
meaning uremia N19

Aztec ear Q17.3

Azygos
continuation inferior vena cava Q26.8
lobe (lung) Q33.1

B

Baastrup's disease *—see* Kissing spine

Babesiosis B60.00
due to
Babesia
divergens B60.03
duncani B60.02
KO-1 B60.09
microti B60.01
MO-1 B60.03
species
unspecified B60.00
venatorum B60.09
specified NEC B60.09

Babington's disease (familial hemorrhagic telangiectasia) I78.0

Babinski's syndrome A52.79

Baby
crying constantly R68.11
floppy (syndrome) P94.2

Bacillary *—see* condition

Bacilluria R82.71

Bacillus *—see also* Infection, bacillus
abortus infection A23.1
anthracis infection A22.9
coli infection *—see also* Escherichia coli B96.20
Flexner's A03.1
mallei infection A24.0
Shiga's A03.0
suipestifer infection *—see* Infection, salmonella

Back *—see* condition

Backache (postural) M54.9
sacroiliac M53.3
specified NEC M54.89

Backflow *—see* Reflux

Backward reading (dyslexia) F81.0

Bacteremia R78.81
with sepsis *—see* Sepsis

Bactericholia *—see* Cholecystitis, acute

Bacterid, bacteride (pustular) L40.3

Bacterium, bacteria, bacterial
agent NEC, as cause of disease classified elsewhere B96.89
in blood *—see* Bacteremia
in urine *—see* Bacteriuria

Bacteriuria, bacteruria R82.71
asymptomatic R82.71

Bacteroides
fragilis, as cause of disease classified elsewhere B96.6

Bad
heart *—see* Disease, heart
trip
due to drug abuse *—see* Abuse, drug, hallucinogen
due to drug dependence *—see* Dependence, drug, hallucinogen

Baelz's disease (cheilitis glandularis apostematosa) K13.0

Baerensprung's disease (eczema marginatum) B35.6

Bagasse disease or pneumonitis J67.1

Bagassosis J67.1

Baker's cyst *—see* Cyst, Baker's

Bakwin-Krida syndrome (metaphyseal dysplasia) Q78.5

Balancing side interference M26.56

Balanitis (circinata) (erosiva) (gangrenosa) (phagedenic) (vulgaris) N48.1
amebic A06.82
candidal B37.42
due to Haemophilus ducreyi A57
gonococcal (acute) (chronic) A54.23
xerotica obliterans N48.0

Balanoposthitis N47.6
gonococcal (acute) (chronic) A54.23
ulcerative (specific) A63.8

Balanorrhagia *—see* Balanitis

Balantidiasis, balantidiosis A07.0

Bald tongue K14.4

Baldness *—see also* Alopecia
male-pattern *—see* Alopecia, androgenic

Balkan grippe A78

Balloon disease *—see* Effect, adverse, high altitude

Balo's disease (concentric sclerosis) G37.5

Bamberger-Marie disease *—see* Osteoarthropathy, hypertrophic, specified type NEC

Bancroft's filariasis B74.0

Band(s)
adhesive *—see* Adhesions, peritoneum
anomalous or congenital *—see also* Anomaly, by site
heart (atrial) (ventricular) Q24.8
intestine Q43.3
omentum Q43.3
cervix N88.1
constricting, congenital Q79.8
gallbladder (congenital) Q44.1
intestinal (adhesive) *—see* Adhesions, peritoneum
obstructive
intestine K56.50
complete K56.52
incomplete K56.51
partial K56.51
peritoneum K56.50
complete K56.52
incomplete K56.51
partial K56.51
periappendiceal, congenital Q43.3
peritoneal (adhesive) *—see* Adhesions, peritoneum
uterus N73.6
internal N85.6
vagina N89.5

Bandemia D72.825

Bandl's ring (contraction), **complicating delivery** O62.4

Bangkok hemorrhagic fever A91

Bang's disease (brucella abortus) A23.1

Bankruptcy, anxiety concerning Z59.89

Bannister's disease T78.3
hereditary D84.1

Banti's disease or syndrome (with cirrhosis) (with portal hypertension) K76.6

Bar, median, prostate *—see* Enlargement, enlarged, prostate

Barcoo disease or rot *—see* Ulcer, skin

Barlow's disease E54

Barodontalgia T70.29

Baron Münchausen syndrome *—see* Disorder, factitious

Barosinusitis T70.1

Barotitis T70.0

Barotrauma T70.29
odontalgia T70.29
otitic T70.0
sinus T70.1

Barraquer (-Simons) **disease or syndrome** (progressive lipodystrophy) E88.1

Barré-Guillain disease or syndrome G61.0

Barré-Liéou syndrome (posterior cervical sympathetic) M53.0

Barrel chest M95.4

Barrett's
disease *—see* Barrett's, esophagus
esophagus K22.70
with dysplasia K22.719
high grade K22.711
low grade K22.710
without dysplasia K22.70
syndrome *—see* Barrett's, esophagus
ulcer K22.10
with bleeding K22.11
without bleeding K22.10

Bársony (-Polgár) (-Teschendorf) syndrome (corkscrew esophagus) K22.4

Bartholinitis (suppurating) N75.8
gonococcal (acute) (chronic) (with abscess) A54.1

Barth syndrome E78.71

Bartonellosis A44.9
cutaneous A44.1
mucocutaneous A44.1
specified NEC A44.8
systemic A44.0

Barton's fracture S52.56-

Bartter's syndrome E26.81

Basal *—see* condition

Basan's (hidrotic) **ectodermal dysplasia** Q82.4

Baseball finger *—see* Dislocation, finger

Basedow's disease (exophthalmic goiter) *—see* Hyperthyroidism, with, goiter

Basic *—see* condition

Basilar *—see* condition

Bason's (hidrotic) **ectodermal dysplasia** Q82.4

Basopenia —*see* Agranulocytosis

Basophilia D72.824

Basophilism (cortico-adrenal) (Cushing's) (pituitary) E24.0

Bassen-Kornzweig disease or syndrome E78.6

Bat ear Q17.5

Bateman's
- disease B08.1
- purpura (senile) D69.2

Bathing cramp T75.1

Bathophobia F40.248

Batten (-Mayou) **disease** E75.4
- retina E75.4 *[H36]*

Batten-Steinert syndrome G71.11

Battered —*see* Maltreatment

Battey Mycobacterium infection A31.0

Battle exhaustion F43.0

Battledore placenta O43.19-

Baumgarten-Cruveilhier cirrhosis, disease or syndrome K74.69

Bauxite fibrosis (of lung) J63.1

Bayle's disease (general paresis) A52.17

Bazin's disease (primary) (tuberculous) A18.4

Beach ear —*see* Swimmer's, ear

Beaded hair (congenital) Q84.1

Béal conjunctivitis or syndrome B30.2

Beard's disease (neurasthenia) F48.8

Beat(s)
- atrial, premature I49.1
- ectopic I49.49
- elbow —*see* Bursitis, elbow
- escaped, heart I49.49
- hand —*see* Bursitis, hand
- knee —*see* Bursitis, knee
- premature I49.40
  - atrial I49.1
  - auricular I49.1
  - supraventricular I49.1

Beau's
- disease or syndrome —*see* Degeneration, myocardial
- lines (transverse furrows on fingernails) L60.4

Bechterev's syndrome —*see* Spondylitis, ankylosing

Beck's syndrome (anterior spinal artery occlusion) I65.8

Becker's
- cardiomyopathy I42.8
- disease
  - idiopathic mural endomyocardial disease I42.3
  - myotonia congenita, recessive form G71.12
- dystrophy G71.01
- pigmented hairy nevus D22.5

Beckwith-Wiedemann syndrome Q87.3

Bed confinement status Z74.01

Bed sore —*see* Ulcer, pressure, by site

Bedbug bite(s) —*see* Bite(s), by site, superficial, insect

Bedclothes, asphyxiation or suffocation by —*see* Asphyxia, traumatic, due to, mechanical, trapped

Bednar's
- aphthae K12.0
- tumor —*see* Neoplasm, malignant, by site

Bedridden Z74.01

Bedsore —*see* Ulcer, pressure, by site

Bedwetting —*see* Enuresis

Bee sting (with allergic or anaphylactic shock) —*see* Toxicity, venom, arthropod, bee

Beer drinker's heart (disease) I42.6

Begbie's disease (exophthalmic goiter) —*see* Hyperthyroidism, with, goiter

Behavior
- antisocial
  - adult Z72.811
  - child or adolescent Z72.810
- disorder, disturbance —*see* Disorder, conduct
- disruptive —*see* Disorder, conduct
- drug seeking Z76.5
- inexplicable R46.2
- marked evasiveness R46.5
- obsessive-compulsive R46.81
- overactivity R46.3
- poor responsiveness R46.4
- self-damaging(life-style) Z72.89
- sleep-incompatible Z72.821
- slowness R46.4
- specified NEC R46.89
- strange (and inexplicable) R46.2
- suspiciousness R46.5
- type A pattern Z73.1
- undue concern or preoccupation with stressful events R46.6
- verbosity and circumstantial detail obscuring reason for contact R46.7

Behçet's disease or syndrome M35.2

Behr's disease —*see* Degeneration, macula

Beigel's disease or morbus (white piedra) B36.2

Bejel A65

Bekhterev's syndrome —*see* Spondylitis, ankylosing

Belching —*see* Eructation

Bell's
- mania F30.8
- palsy, paralysis G51.0
  - infant or newborn P11.3
- spasm G51.3-

Bence Jones albuminuria or proteinuria NEC R80.3

Bends T70.3

Benedikt's paralysis or syndrome G46.3

Benign —*see also* condition
- prostatic hyperplasia —*see* Hyperplasia, prostate

Bennett's fracture (displaced) S62.21-

Benson's disease —*see* Deposit, crystalline

Bent
- back (hysterical) F44.4
- nose M95.0
  - congenital Q67.4

Bereavement (uncomplicated) Z63.4

Bergeron's disease (hysterical chorea) F44.4

Berger's disease —*see* Nephropathy, IgA

Beriberi (dry) E51.11
- heart (disease) E51.12
- polyneuropathy E51.11
- wet E51.12
  - involving circulatory system E51.11

Berlin's disease or edema (traumatic) S05.8X-

Berlock (berloque) **dermatitis** L56.2

Bernard-Horner syndrome G90.2

Bernard-Soulier disease or thrombopathia D69.1

Bernhardt (-Roth) **disease** —*see* Mononeuropathy, lower limb, meralgia paresthetica

Bernheim's syndrome —*see* Failure, heart, right

Bertielliasis B71.8

Berylliosis (lung) J63.2

Besnier-Boeck (-Schaumann) **disease** —*see* Sarcoidosis

Besnier's
- lupus pernio D86.3
- prurigo L20.0

Bestiality F65.89

Best's disease H35.50

Beta-mercaptolactate-cysteine disulfiduria E72.09

Betalipoproteinemia, broad or floating E78.2

Betting and gambling Z72.6
- pathological (compulsive) F63.0

Bezoar T18.9
- intestine T18.3
- stomach T18.2

Bezold's abscess —*see* Mastoiditis, acute

Bianchi's syndrome R48.8

Bicornate or bicornis uterus Q51.3
- in pregnancy or childbirth O34.00
  - causing obstructed labor O65.5

Bicuspid aortic valve Q23.1

Biedl-Bardet syndrome Q87.89

Bielschowsky (-Jansky) **disease** E75.4

Biermer's (pernicious) **anemia or disease** D51.0

Biett's disease L93.0

Bifid (congenital)
- apex, heart Q24.8
- clitoris Q52.6
- kidney Q63.8
- nose Q30.2
- patella Q74.1
- scrotum Q55.29
- toe NEC Q74.2
- tongue Q38.3
- ureter Q62.8
- uterus Q51.3
- uvula Q35.7

Biforis uterus (suprasimplex) Q51.3

Bifurcation (congenital)
- gallbladder Q44.1
- kidney pelvis Q63.8
- renal pelvis Q63.8
- rib Q76.6
- tongue, congenital Q38.3
- trachea Q32.1
- ureter Q62.8
- urethra Q64.74
- vertebra Q76.49

Big spleen syndrome D73.1

Bigeminal pulse R00.8

Bilateral —*see* condition

Bile
- duct —*see* condition
- pigments in urine R82.2

Bilharziasis —*see also* Schistosomiasis
- chyluria B65.0
- cutaneous B65.3
- galacturia B65.0
- hematochyluria B65.0
- intestinal B65.1
- lipemia B65.9
- lipuria B65.0
- oriental B65.2
- piarhemia B65.9
- pulmonary NOS B65.9 *[J99]*
  - pneumonia B65.9 *[J17]*
- tropical hematuria B65.0
- vesical B65.0

Biliary —*see* condition

Bilirubin metabolism disorder E80.7
- specified NEC E80.6

Bilirubinemia, familial nonhemolytic E80.4

Bilirubinuria R82.2

Biliuria R82.2

Bilocular stomach K31.2

Binswanger's disease I67.3

Biparta, bipartite
- carpal scaphoid Q74.0
- patella Q74.1
- vagina Q52.10

Bird
- face Q75.8
- fancier's disease or lung J67.2

Birt-Hogg-Dube syndrome Q87.89

Birth
- complications in mother —*see* Delivery, complicated
- compression during NOS P15.9
- defect —*see* Anomaly

Birth
- immature (less than 37 completed weeks) —*see* Preterm, newborn
  - extremely (less than 28 completed weeks) —*see* Immaturity, extreme
- inattention, at or after —*see* Maltreatment, child, neglect
- injury NOS P15.9
  - basal ganglia P11.1
  - brachial plexus NEC P14.3
  - brain (compression) (pressure) P11.2
  - central nervous system NOS P11.9
  - cerebellum P11.1
  - cerebral hemorrhage P10.1
  - external genitalia P15.5
  - eye P15.3
  - face P15.4

Birth *(continued)*
- injury *(continued)*
  - fracture
    - bone P13.9
      - specified NEC P13.8
    - clavicle P13.4
    - femur P13.2
    - humerus P13.3
    - long bone, except femur P13.3
    - radius and ulna P13.3
    - skull P13.0
    - spine P11.5
    - tibia and fibula P13.3
  - intracranial P11.2
    - laceration or hemorrhage P10.9
      - specified NEC P10.8
  - intraventricular hemorrhage P10.2
  - laceration
    - brain P10.1
    - by scalpel P15.8
    - peripheral nerve P14.9
  - liver P15.0
  - meninges
    - brain P11.1
    - spinal cord P11.5
  - nerve
    - brachial plexus P14.3
    - cranial NEC (except facial) P11.4
    - facial P11.3
    - peripheral P14.9
    - phrenic (paralysis) P14.2
  - paralysis
    - facial nerve P11.3
    - spinal P11.5
  - penis P15.5
  - rupture
    - spinal cord P11.5
  - scalp P12.9
  - scalpel wound P15.8
  - scrotum P15.5
  - skull NEC P13.1
    - fracture P13.0
  - specified type NEC P15.8
  - spinal cord P11.5
  - spine P11.5
  - spleen P15.1
  - sternomastoid (hematoma) P15.2
  - subarachnoid hemorrhage P10.3
  - subcutaneous fat necrosis P15.6
  - subdural hemorrhage P10.0
  - tentorial tear P10.4
  - testes P15.5
  - vulva P15.5
- lack of care, at or after *—see* Maltreatment, child, neglect
- neglect, at or after *—see* Maltreatment, child, neglect
- palsy or paralysis, newborn, NOS (birth injury) P14.9
- premature (infant) *—see* Preterm, newborn
- shock, newborn P96.89
- trauma *—see* Birth, injury
- weight
  - low (2499 grams or less) *—see* Low, birthweight
    - extremely (999 grams or less) *—see* Low, birthweight, extreme
  - 4000 grams to 4499 grams P08.1
  - 4500 grams or more P08.0

Birthmark Q82.5

Bisalbuminemia E88.09

Biskra's button B55.1

Bite(s) (animal) (human)
- abdomen, abdominal
  - wall S31.159
    - with penetration into peritoneal cavity S31.659
    - epigastric region S31.152
      - with penetration into peritoneal cavity S31.652
    - left
      - lower quadrant S31.154
        - with penetration into peritoneal cavity S31.654
      - upper quadrant S31.151
        - with penetration into peritoneal cavity S31.651
    - periumbilic region S31.155
      - with penetration into peritoneal cavity S31.655
    - right
      - lower quadrant S31.153
        - with penetration into peritoneal cavity S31.653
      - upper quadrant S31.150
        - with penetration into peritoneal cavity S31.650
    - superficial NEC S30.871
      - insect S30.861
- alveolar (process) *—see* Bite, oral cavity
- amphibian (venomous) *—see* Venom, bite, amphibian
- animal *—see also* Bite, by site
  - venomous *—see* Venom
- ankle S91.05-
  - superficial NEC S90.57-
    - insect S90.56-
- antecubital space *—see* Bite, elbow
- anus S31.835
  - superficial NEC S30.877
    - insect S30.867
- arm (upper) S41.15-
  - lower *—see* Bite, forearm
  - superficial NEC S40.87-
    - insect S40.86-
- arthropod NEC *—see* Venom, bite, arthropod
- auditory canal (external) (meatus) *—see* Bite, ear
- auricle, ear *—see* Bite, ear
- axilla *—see* Bite, arm
- back *—see also* Bite, thorax, back
  - lower S31.050
    - with penetration into retroperitoneal space S31.051
    - superficial NEC S30.870
      - insect S30.860
- bedbug *—see* Bite(s), by site, superficial, insect
- breast S21.05-
  - superficial NEC S20.17-
    - insect S20.16-
- brow *—see* Bite, head, specified site NEC
- buttock S31.805
  - left S31.825
  - right S31.815
  - superficial NEC S30.870
    - insect S30.860
- calf *—see* Bite, leg
- canaliculus lacrimalis *—see* Bite, eyelid
- canthus, eye *—see* Bite, eyelid
- centipede *—see* Toxicity, venom, arthropod, centipede
- cheek (external) S01.45-
  - superficial NEC S00.87
    - insect S00.86
  - internal *—see* Bite, oral cavity
- chest wall *—see* Bite, thorax
- chigger B88.0
- chin *—see* Bite, head, specified site NEC
- clitoris *—see* Bite, vulva
- costal region *—see* Bite, thorax
- digit(s)
  - hand *—see* Bite, finger
  - toe *—see* Bite, toe
- ear (canal) (external) S01.35-
  - superficial NEC S00.47-
    - insect S00.46-
- elbow S51.05-
  - superficial NEC S50.37-
    - insect S50.36-
- epididymis *—see* Bite, testis
- epigastric region *—see* Bite, abdomen
- epiglottis *—see* Bite, neck, specified site NEC
- esophagus, cervical S11.25
  - superficial NEC S10.17
    - insect S10.16
- eyebrow *—see* Bite, eyelid
- eyelid S01.15-
  - superficial NEC S00.27-
    - insect S00.26-
- face NEC *—see* Bite, head, specified site NEC
- finger(s) S61.259
  - with
    - damage to nail S61.359
  - index S61.258
    - with
      - damage to nail S61.358
    - left S61.251
      - with
        - damage to nail S61.351
    - right S61.250
      - with
        - damage to nail S61.350
    - superficial NEC S60.478
      - insect S60.46-
  - little S61.25-
    - with
      - damage to nail S61.35-
    - superficial NEC S60.47-
      - insect S60.46-
  - middle S61.25-
    - with
      - damage to nail S61.35-
    - superficial NEC S60.47-
      - insect S60.46-
  - ring S61.25-
    - with
      - damage to nail S61.35-
    - superficial NEC S60.47-
      - insect S60.46-
  - superficial NEC S60.479
    - insect S60.469
  - thumb *—see* Bite, thumb
- flank *—see* Bite, abdomen, wall
- flea *—see* Bite, by site, superficial, insect
- foot (except toe(s) alone) S91.35-
  - superficial NEC S90.87-
    - insect S90.86-
  - toe *—see* Bite, toe
- forearm S51.85-
  - elbow only *—see* Bite, elbow
  - superficial NEC S50.87-
    - insect S50.86-
- forehead *—see* Bite, head, specified site NEC
- genital organs, external
  - female S31.552
    - superficial NEC S30.876
      - insect S30.866
    - vagina and vulva *—see* Bite, vulva
  - male S31.551
    - penis *—see* Bite, penis
    - scrotum *—see* Bite, scrotum
    - superficial NEC S30.875
      - insect S30.865
    - testes *—see* Bite, testis
- groin *—see* Bite, abdomen, wall
- gum *—see* Bite, oral cavity
- hand S61.45-
  - finger *—see* Bite, finger
  - superficial NEC S60.57-
    - insect S60.56-
  - thumb *—see* Bite, thumb
- head S01.95
  - cheek *—see* Bite, cheek
  - ear *—see* Bite, ear
  - eyelid *—see* Bite, eyelid
  - lip *—see* Bite, lip
  - nose *—see* Bite, nose
  - oral cavity *—see* Bite, oral cavity
  - scalp *—see* Bite, scalp
  - specified site NEC S01.85
    - superficial NEC S00.87
      - insect S00.86
  - superficial NEC S00.97
    - insect S00.96
  - temporomandibular area *—see* Bite, cheek
- heel *—see* Bite, foot
- hip S71.05-
  - superficial NEC S70.27-
    - insect S70.26-
- hymen S31.45
- hypochondrium *—see* Bite, abdomen, wall
- hypogastric region *—see* Bite, abdomen, wall
- inguinal region *—see* Bite, abdomen, wall
- insect *—see* Bite, by site, superficial, insect
- instep *—see* Bite, foot
- interscapular region *—see* Bite, thorax, back
- jaw *—see* Bite, head, specified site NEC
- knee S81.05-
  - superficial NEC S80.27-
    - insect S80.26-
- labium (majus) (minus) *—see* Bite, vulva
- lacrimal duct *—see* Bite, eyelid
- larynx S11.015
  - superficial NEC S10.17
    - insect S10.16
- leg (lower) S81.85-
  - ankle *—see* Bite, ankle
  - foot *—see* Bite, foot
  - knee *—see* Bite, knee
  - superficial NEC S80.87-
    - insect S80.86-
  - toe *—see* Bite, toe
  - upper *—see* Bite, thigh
- lip S01.551
  - superficial NEC S00.571
    - insect S00.561
- lizard (venomous) *—see* Venom, bite, reptile
- loin *—see* Bite, abdomen, wall
- lower back *—see* Bite, back, lower
- lumbar region *—see* Bite, back, lower
- malar region *—see* Bite, head, specified site NEC
- mammary *—see* Bite, breast
- marine animals (venomous) *—see* Toxicity, venom, marine animal
- mastoid region *—see* Bite, head, specified site NEC
- mouth *—see* Bite, oral cavity

Bite *(continued)*
- nail
  - finger *—see* Bite, finger
  - toe *—see* Bite, toe
- nape *—see* Bite, neck, specified site NEC
- nasal (septum) (sinus) *—see* Bite, nose
- nasopharynx *—see* Bite, head, specified site NEC
- neck S11.95
  - involving
    - cervical esophagus *—see* Bite, esophagus, cervical
    - larynx *—see* Bite, larynx
    - pharynx *—see* Bite, pharynx
    - thyroid gland S11.15
    - trachea *—see* Bite, trachea
  - specified site NEC S11.85
    - superficial NEC S10.87
      - insect S10.86
  - superficial NEC S10.97
    - insect S10.96
  - throat S11.85
    - superficial NEC S10.17
      - insect S10.16
- nose (septum) (sinus) S01.25
  - superficial NEC S00.37
    - insect S00.36
- occipital region *—see* Bite, scalp
- oral cavity S01.552
  - superficial NEC S00.572
    - insect S00.562
- orbital region *—see* Bite, eyelid
- palate *—see* Bite, oral cavity
- palm *—see* Bite, hand
- parietal region *—see* Bite, scalp
- pelvis S31.050
  - with penetration into retroperitoneal space S31.051
  - superficial NEC S30.870
    - insect S30.860
- penis S31.25
  - superficial NEC S30.872
    - insect S30.862
- perineum
  - female *—see* Bite, vulva
  - male *—see* Bite, pelvis
- periocular area (with or without lacrimal passages) *—see* Bite, eyelid
- phalanges
  - finger *—see* Bite, finger
  - toe *—see* Bite, toe
- pharynx S11.25
  - superficial NEC S10.17
    - insect S10.16
- pinna *—see* Bite, ear
- poisonous *—see* Venom
- popliteal space *—see* Bite, knee
- prepuce *—see* Bite, penis
- pubic region *—see* Bite, abdomen, wall
- rectovaginal septum *—see* Bite, vulva
- red bug B88.0
- reptile NEC *—see also* Venom, bite, reptile
  - nonvenomous *—see* Bite, by site
  - snake *—see* Venom, bite, snake
- sacral region *—see* Bite, back, lower
- sacroiliac region *—see* Bite, back, lower
- salivary gland *—see* Bite, oral cavity
- scalp S01.05
  - superficial NEC S00.07
    - insect S00.06
- scapular region *—see* Bite, shoulder
- scrotum S31.35
  - superficial NEC S30.873
    - insect S30.863
- sea-snake (venomous) *—see* Toxicity, venom, snake, sea snake
- shin *—see* Bite, leg
- shoulder S41.05-
  - superficial NEC S40.27-
    - insect S40.26-
- snake *—see also* Venom, bite, snake
  - nonvenomous *—see* Bite, by site
- spermatic cord *—see* Bite, testis
- spider (venomous) *—see* Toxicity, venom, spider
  - nonvenomous *—see* Bite, by site, superficial, insect
- sternal region *—see* Bite, thorax, front
- submaxillary region *—see* Bite, head, specified site NEC
- submental region *—see* Bite, head, specified site NEC
- subungual
  - finger(s) *—see* Bite, finger
  - toe *—see* Bite, toe
- superficial *—see* Bite, by site, superficial
- supraclavicular fossa S11.85
- supraorbital *—see* Bite, head, specified site NEC
- temple, temporal region *—see* Bite, head, specified site NEC
- temporomandibular area *—see* Bite, cheek
- testis S31.35
  - superficial NEC S30.873
    - insect S30.863
- thigh S71.15-
  - superficial NEC S70.37-
    - insect S70.36-
- thorax, thoracic (wall) S21.95
  - back S21.25-
    - with penetration into thoracic cavity S21.45-
  - breast *—see* Bite, breast
  - front S21.15-
    - with penetration into thoracic cavity S21.35-
  - superficial NEC S20.97
    - back S20.47-
    - front S20.37-
    - insect S20.96
      - back S20.46-
      - front S20.36-
- throat *—see* Bite, neck, throat
- thumb S61.05-
  - with
    - damage to nail S61.15-
  - superficial NEC S60.37-
    - insect S60.36-
- thyroid S11.15
  - superficial NEC S10.87
    - insect S10.86
- toe(s) S91.15-
  - with
    - damage to nail S91.25-
  - great S91.15-
    - with
      - damage to nail S91.25-
  - lesser S91.15-
    - with
      - damage to nail S91.25-
  - superficial NEC S90.47-
    - great S90.47-
    - insect S90.46-
      - great S90.46-
- tongue S01.552
- trachea S11.025
  - superficial NEC S10.17
    - insect S10.16
- tunica vaginalis *—see* Bite, testis
- tympanum, tympanic membrane *—see* Bite, ear
- umbilical region S31.155
- uvula *—see* Bite, oral cavity
- vagina *—see* Bite, vulva
- venomous *—see* Venom
- vocal cords S11.035
  - superficial NEC S10.17
    - insect S10.16
- vulva S31.45
  - superficial NEC S30.874
    - insect S30.864
- wrist S61.55-
  - superficial NEC S60.87-
    - insect S60.86-

Biting, cheek or lip K13.1

Biventricular failure (heart) I50.82

Björck (-Thorson) syndrome (malignant carcinoid) E34.0

Black
- death A20.9
- eye S00.1-
- hairy tongue K14.3
- heel (foot) S90.3-
- lung (disease) J60
- palm (hand) S60.22-

Blackfan-Diamond anemia or syndrome (congenital hypoplastic anemia) D61.01

Blackhead L70.0

Blackout R55

Bladder *—see* condition

Blast (air) (hydraulic) (immersion) (underwater)
- blindness S05.8X-
- injury
  - abdomen or thorax *—see* Injury, by site
  - ear (acoustic nerve trauma) *—see* Injury, nerve, acoustic, specified type NEC
  - syndrome NEC T70.8

Blastoma *—see* Neoplasm, malignant, by site
- pulmonary *—see* Neoplasm, lung, malignant

Blastomycosis, blastomycotic B40.9
- Brazilian *—see* Paracoccidioidomycosis
- cutaneous B40.3
- disseminated B40.7
- European *—see* Cryptococcosis
- generalized B40.7
- keloidal B48.0
- North American B40.9
- primary pulmonary B40.0
- pulmonary B40.2
  - acute B40.0
  - chronic B40.1
- skin B40.3
- South American *—see* Paracoccidioidomycosis
- specified NEC B40.89

Bleb(s) R23.8
- emphysematous (lung) (solitary) J43.9
- endophthalmitis H59.43
- filtering (vitreous), after glaucoma surgery Z98.83
- inflammed (infected), postprocedural H59.40
  - stage 1 H59.41
  - stage 2 H59.42
  - stage 3 H59.43
- lung (ruptured) J43.9
  - congenital *—see* Atelectasis
  - newborn P25.8
- subpleural (emphysematous) J43.9

Blebitis, postprocedural H59.40
- stage 1 H59.41
- stage 2 H59.42
- stage 3 H59.43

Bleeder (familial) (hereditary) *—see* Hemophilia

Bleeding *—see also* Hemorrhage
- anal K62.5
- anovulatory N97.0
- atonic, following delivery O72.1
- capillary I78.8
  - puerperal O72.2
- contact (postcoital) N93.0
- due to uterine subinvolution N85.3
- ear *—see* Otorrhagia
- excessive, associated with menopausal onset N92.4
- familial *—see* Defect, coagulation
- following intercourse N93.0
- gastrointestinal K92.2
- hemorrhoids *—see* Hemorrhoids
- intermenstrual (regular) N92.3
  - irregular N92.1
- intraoperative *—see* Complication, intraoperative, hemorrhage
- irregular N92.6
- menopausal N92.4
- newborn, intraventricular *—see* Newborn, affected by, hemorrhage, intraventricular
- nipple N64.59
- nose R04.0
- ovulation N92.3
- perimenopausal N92.4
- pre-pubertal vaginal N93.1
- postclimacteric N95.0
- postcoital N93.0
- postmenopausal N95.0
- postoperative *—see* Complication, postprocedural, hemorrhage
- preclimacteric N92.4
- puberty (excessive, with onset of menstrual periods) N92.2
- rectum, rectal K62.5
  - newborn P54.2
- tendencies *—see* Defect, coagulation
- throat R04.1
- tooth socket (post-extraction) K91.840
- umbilical stump P51.9
- uterus, uterine NEC N93.9
  - climacteric N92.4
  - dysfunctional or functional N93.8
  - menopausal N92.4
  - preclimacteric or premenopausal N92.4
  - unrelated to menstrual cycle N93.9
- vagina, vaginal (abnormal) N93.9
  - dysfunctional or functional N93.8
  - newborn P54.6
  - pre-pubertal N93.1
- vicarious N94.89

Blennorrhagia, blennorrhagic *—see* Gonorrhea

Block, blocked *(continued)*
foramen Magendie (acquired) G91.1
congenital Q03.1
with spina bifida *—see* Spina bifida, by site, with hydrocephalus
heart I45.9
bundle branch I45.4
bilateral I45.2
complete (atrioventricular) I44.2
congenital Q24.6
first degree (atrioventricular) I44.0
second degree (atrioventricular) I44.1
specified type NEC I45.5
third degree (atrioventricular) I44.2
hepatic vein I82.0
intraventricular (nonspecific) I45.4
bundle branch
bilateral I45.2
kidney N28.9
postcystoscopic or postprocedural N99.0
Mobitz (types I and II) I44.1
myocardial *—see* Block, heart
nodal I45.5
organ or site, congenital NEC *—see* Atresia, by site
portal (vein) I81
second degree (types I and II) I44.1
sinoatrial I45.5
sinoauricular I45.5
third degree I44.2
trifascicular I45.3
tubal N97.1
vein NOS I82.90
Wenckebach (types I and II) I44.1

Blockage *—see* Obstruction

Blocq's disease F44.4

Blood
constituents, abnormal R78.9
disease D75.9
donor *—see* Donor, blood
dyscrasia D75.9
with
abortion *—see* Abortion, by type, complicated by, hemorrhage
ectopic pregnancy O08.1
molar pregnancy O08.1
following ectopic or molar pregnancy O08.1
newborn P61.9
puerperal, postpartum O72.3
flukes NEC *—see* Schistosomiasis
in
feces K92.1
occult R19.5
urine *—see* Hematuria
mole O02.0
occult in feces R19.5
pressure
decreased, due to shock following injury T79.4
examination only Z01.30
fluctuating I99.8
high *—see* Hypertension
borderline R03.0
incidental reading, without diagnosis of hypertension R03.0
low *—see also* Hypotension
incidental reading, without diagnosis of hypotension R03.1
spitting *—see* Hemoptysis

Blood *(continued)*
staining cornea *—see* Pigmentation, cornea, stromal
transfusion
reaction or complication *—see* Complications, transfusion
type
A (Rh positive) Z67.10
Rh negative Z67.11
AB (Rh positive) Z67.30
Rh negative Z67.31
B (Rh positive) Z67.20
Rh negative Z67.21
O (Rh positive) Z67.40
Rh negative Z67.41
Rh (positive) Z67.90
negative Z67.91
vessel rupture *—see* Hemorrhage
vomiting *—see* Hematemesis

Blood-forming organs, disease D75.9

Bloodgood's disease *—see* Mastopathy, cystic

Bloom (-Machacek) (-Torre) syndrome Q82.8

Blount disease or osteochondrosis M92.51-

Blue
baby Q24.9
diaper syndrome E72.09
dome cyst (breast) *—see* Cyst, breast
dot cataract Q12.0
nevus D22.9
sclera Q13.5
with fragility of bone and deafness Q78.0
toe syndrome I75.02-

Blueness *—see* Cyanosis

Blues, postpartal O90.6
baby O90.6

Blurring, visual H53.8

Blushing (abnormal) (excessive) R23.2

BMI *—see* Body, mass index

Boarder, hospital NEC Z76.4
accompanying sick person Z76.3
healthy infant or child Z76.2
foundling Z76.1

Bockhart's impetigo L01.02

Bodechtel-Guttman disease (subacute sclerosing panencephalitis) A81.1

Boder-Sedgwick syndrome (ataxia-telangiectasia) G11.3

Body, bodies
Aschoff's *—see* Myocarditis, rheumatic
asteroid, vitreous *—see* Deposit, crystalline
cytoid (retina) *—see* Occlusion, artery, retina
drusen (degenerative) (macula) (retinal) *—see also* Degeneration, macula, drusen
optic disc *—see* Drusen, optic disc
foreign *—see* Foreign body
loose
joint, except knee *—see* Loose, body, joint
knee M23.4-
sheath, tendon *—see* Disorder, tendon, specified type NEC

Body, bodies *(continued)*
mass index (BMI)
adult
19.9 or less Z68.1
20.0-20.9 Z68.20
21.0-21.9 Z68.21
22.0-22.9 Z68.22
23.0-23.9 Z68.23
24.0-24.9 Z68.24
25.0-25.9 Z68.25
26.0-26.9 Z68.26
27.0-27.9 Z68.27
28.0-28.9 Z68.28
29.0-29.9 Z68.29
30.0-30.9 Z68.30
31.0-31.9 Z68.31
32.0-32.9 Z68.32
33.0-33.9 Z68.33
34.0-34.9 Z68.34
35.0-35.9 Z68.35
36.0-36.9 Z68.36
37.0-37.9 Z68.37
38.0-38.9 Z68.38
39.0-39.9 Z68.39
40.0-44.9 Z68.41
45.0-49.9 Z68.42
50.0-59.9 Z68.43
60.0-69.9 Z68.44
70 and over Z68.45
pediatric
5th percentile to less than 85th percentile for age Z68.52
85th percentile to less than 95th percentile for age Z68.53
greater than or equal to ninety-fifth percentile for age Z68.54
less than fifth percentile for age Z68.51
Mooser's A75.2
rice *—see also* Loose, body, joint
knee M23.4-
rocking F98.4

Boeck's
disease or sarcoid *—see* Sarcoidosis
lupoid (miliary) D86.3

Boerhaave's syndrome (spontaneous esophageal rupture) K22.3

Boggy
cervix N88.8
uterus N85.8

Boil *—see also* Furuncle, by site
Aleppo B55.1
Baghdad B55.1
Delhi B55.1
lacrimal
gland *—see* Dacryoadenitis
passages (duct) (sac) *—see* Inflammation, lacrimal, passages, acute
Natal B55.1
orbit, orbital *—see* Abscess, orbit
tropical B55.1

Bold hives *—see* Urticaria

Bombé, iris *—see* Membrane, pupillary

Bone *—see* condition

Bonnevie-Ullrich syndrome (*see also* Turner's syndrome) Q87.19

Bonnier's syndrome *—see* subcategory H81.8

Bonvale dam fever T73.3

Bony block of joint *—see* Ankylosis

BOOP (bronchiolitis obliterans organized pneumonia) J84.89

Borderline
diabetes mellitus R73.03
hypertension R03.0
osteopenia M85.8-
pelvis, with obstruction during labor O65.1
personality F60.3

Borna disease A83.9

Bornholm disease B33.0

Boston exanthem A88.0

Botalli, ductus (patent) (persistent) Q25.0

Bothriocephalus latus infestation B70.0

Botulism (foodborne intoxication) A05.1
infant A48.51
non-foodborne A48.52
wound A48.52

Bouba *—see* Yaws

Bouchard's nodes (with arthropathy) M15.2

Bouffée délirante F23

Bouillaud's disease or syndrome (rheumatic heart disease) I01.9

Bourneville's disease Q85.1

Boutonniere deformity (finger) *—see* Deformity, finger, boutonniere

Bouveret (-Hoffmann) syndrome (paroxysmal tachycardia) I47.9

Bovine heart *—see* Hypertrophy, cardiac

Bowel *—see* condition

Bowen's
dermatosis (precancerous) *—see* Neoplasm, skin, in situ
disease *—see* Neoplasm, skin, in situ
epithelioma *—see* Neoplasm, skin, in situ
type
epidermoid carcinoma-in-situ *—see* Neoplasm, skin, in situ
intraepidermal squamous cell carcinoma *—see* Neoplasm, skin, in situ

Bowing
femur *—see also* Deformity, limb, specified type NEC, thigh
congenital Q68.3
fibula *—see also* Deformity, limb, specified type NEC, lower leg
congenital Q68.4
forearm *—see* Deformity, limb, specified type NEC, forearm
leg(s), long bones, congenital Q68.5
radius *—see* Deformity, limb, specified type NEC, forearm
tibia *—see also* Deformity, limb, specified type NEC, lower leg
congenital Q68.4

Bowleg(s) (acquired) M21.16-
congenital Q68.5
rachitic E64.3

Boyd's dysentery A03.2

Brachial *—see* condition

Brachycardia R00.1

Brachycephaly Q75.0

Bradley's disease A08.19

Bradyarrhythmia, cardiac I49.8

Bradycardia (sinoatrial) (sinus) (vagal) R00.1
  neonatal P29.12
  reflex G90.09
  tachycardia syndrome I49.5

Bradykinesia R25.8

Bradypnea R06.89

Bradytachycardia I49.5

Brailsford's disease or osteochondrosis *—see* Osteochondrosis, juvenile, radius

Brain *—see also* condition
  death G93.82
  syndrome *—see* Syndrome, brain

Branched-chain amino-acid disorder E71.2

Branchial *—see* condition
  cartilage, congenital Q18.2

Branchiogenic remnant (in neck) Q18.0

Brandt's syndrome (acrodermatitis enteropathica) E83.2

Brash (water) R12

Bravais-jacksonian epilepsy *—see* Epilepsy, localization-related, symptomatic, with simple partial seizures

Braxton Hicks contractions *—see* False, labor

Brazilian leishmaniasis B55.2

BRBPR K62.5

Break, retina (without detachment) H33.30-
  with retinal detachment *—see* Detachment, retina
  horseshoe tear H33.31-
  multiple H33.33-
  round hole H33.32-

Breakdown
  device, graft or implant *—see also* Complications, by site and type, mechanical T85.618
    arterial graft NEC *—see* Complication, cardiovascular device, mechanical, vascular
    breast (implant) T85.41
    catheter NEC T85.618
      cystostomy T83.010
      dialysis (renal) T82.41
        intraperitoneal T85.611
      Hopkins T83.018
      ileostomy T83.018
      infusion NEC T82.514
        cranial T85.610
        epidural T85.610
        intrathecal T85.610
        spinal T85.610
        subarachnoid T85.610
        subdural T85.610
      nephrostomy T83.012
      urethral indwelling T83.011
      urinary NEC T83.018
      urostomy T83.018
    electronic (electrode) (pulse generator) (stimulator)
      bone T84.310
      cardiac T82.119
        electrode T82.110
        pulse generator T82.111
        specified type NEC T82.118

Breakdown *(continued)*
  device, graft or implant *(continued)*
    electronic *(continued)*
      nervous system *—see* Complication, prosthetic device, mechanical, electronic nervous system stimulator
      urinary *—see* Complication, genitourinary, device, urinary, mechanical
    fixation, internal (orthopedic) NEC *—see* Complication, fixation device, mechanical
    gastrointestinal *—see* Complications, prosthetic device, mechanical, gastrointestinal device
    genital NEC T83.418
      intrauterine contraceptive device T83.31
      penile prosthesis (cylinder) (implanted) (pump) (resevoir) T83.410
      testicular prosthesis T83.411
    heart NEC *—see* Complication, cardiovascular device, mechanical
    intrathecal infusion pump T85.615
    joint prosthesis *—see* Complications..., joint prosthesis,internal, mechanical, by site
    nervous system, specified device NEC T85.615
    ocular NEC *—see* Complications, prosthetic device, mechanical, ocular device
    orthopedic NEC *—see* Complication, orthopedic, device, mechanical
    specified NEC T85.618
    subcutaneous device pocket
      nervous system prosthetic device, implant, or graft T85.890
      other internal prosthetic device, implant or graft T85.898
    sutures, permanent T85.612
      used in bone repair *—see* Complications, fixation device, internal (orthopedic), mechanical
    urinary NEC T83.118
      graft T83.21
      sphincter, implanted T83.111
      stent (ileal conduit) (nephroureteral) T83.113
        ureteral indwelling T83.112
    vascular NEC *—see* Complication, cardiovascular device, mechanical
    ventricular intracranial shunt T85.01
  nervous F48.8
  perineum O90.1
  respirator J95.850
    specified NEC J95.859
    ventilator J95.850
    specified NEC J95.859

Breast *—see also* condition
  buds E30.1
    in newborn P96.89
  dense R92.2
  nodule (*see also* Lump, breast) N63.0

Breath
  foul R19.6
  holder, child R06.89
  holding spell R06.89
  shortness R06.02

Breathing
  labored *—see* Hyperventilation
  mouth R06.5
    causing malocclusion M26.5
  periodic R06.3
    high altitude G47.32

Breathlessness R06.81

Breda's disease *—see* Yaws

Breech presentation (mother) O32.1
  causing obstructed labor O64.1
  footling O32.8
    causing obstructed labor O64.8
  incomplete O32.8
    causing obstructed labor O64.8

Breisky's disease N90.4

Brennemann's syndrome I88.0

Brenner
  tumor (benign) D27.9
    borderline malignancy D39.1-
    malignant C56
    proliferating D39.1-

Bretonneau's disease or angina A36.0

Breus' mole O02.0

Brevicollis Q76.49

Brickmakers' anemia B76.9 *[D63.8]*

Bridge, myocardial Q24.5

Bright red blood per rectum (BRBPR) K62.5

Bright's disease *—see also* Nephritis
  arteriosclerotic *—see* Hypertension, kidney

Brill (-Zinsser) disease (recrudescent typhus) A75.1

Brill-Symmers' disease C82.90

Brion-Kayser disease *—see* Fever, parathyroid

Briquet's disorder or syndrome F45.0

Brissaud's
  infantilism or dwarfism E23.0
  motor-verbal tic F95.2

Brittle
  bones disease Q78.0
  nails L60.3
    congenital Q84.6

Broad *—see also* condition
  beta disease E78.2
  ligament laceration syndrome N83.8

Broad- or floating-betalipoproteinemia E78.2

Brock's syndrome (atelectasis due to enlarged lymph nodes) J98.19

Brocq-Duhring disease (dermatitis herpetiformis) L13.0

Brodie's abscess or disease M86.8X-

Broken
  arches *—see also* Deformity, limb, flat foot
  arm (meaning upper limb) *—see* Fracture, arm
  back *—see* Fracture, vertebra
  bone *—see* Fracture

Broken *(continued)*
  implant or internal device *—see* Complications, by site and type, mechanical
  leg (meaning lower limb) *—see* Fracture, leg
  nose S02.2
  tooth, teeth *—see* Fracture, tooth

Bromhidrosis, bromidrosis L75.0

Bromidism, bromism G92.8
  due to
    correct substance properly administered *—see* Table of Drugs and Chemicals, by drug, adverse effect
    overdose or wrong substance given or taken *—see* Table of Drugs and Chemicals, by drug, poisoning
  chronic (dependence) F13.20

Bromidrosiphobia F40.298

Bronchi, bronchial *—see* condition

Bronchiectasis (cylindrical) (diffuse) (fusiform) (localized) (saccular) J47.9
  with
    acute
      bronchitis J47.0
      lower respiratory infection J47.0
    exacerbation (acute) J47.1
  congenital Q33.4
  tuberculous NEC *—see* Tuberculosis, pulmonary

Bronchiolectasis *—see* Bronchiectasis

Bronchiolitis (acute) (infective) (subacute) J21.9
  with
    bronchospasm or obstruction J21.9
    influenza, flu or grippe *—see* Influenza, with, respiratory manifestations NEC
  chemical (chronic) J68.4
    acute J68.0
  chronic (fibrosing) (obliterative) J44.9
  due to
    external agent *—see* Bronchitis, acute, due to
    human metapneumovirus J21.1
    respiratory syncytial virus (RSV) J21.0
    specified organism NEC J21.8
  fibrosa obliterans J44.9
  influenzal *—see* Influenza, with, respiratory manifestations NEC
  obliterans J42
    with organizing pneumonia (BOOP) J84.89
  obliterative (chronic) (subacute) J44.9
    due to fumes or vapors J68.4
    due to chemicals, gases, fumes or vapors (inhalation) J68.4
  respiratory, interstitial lung disease J84.115

Bronchitis (diffuse) (fibrinous) (hypostatic) (infective) (membranous) J40
  with
    influenza, flu or grippe *—see* Influenza, with, respiratory manifestations NEC
    obstruction (airway) (lung) J44.9

- **Bronchitis** *(continued)*
  - with *(continued)*
    - tracheitis (15 years of age and above) J40
      - acute or subacute J20.9
      - chronic J42
      - under 15 years of age J20.9
  - acute or subacute (with bronchospasm or obstruction) J20.9
    - with
      - bronchiectasis J47.0
      - chronic obstructive pulmonary disease J44.0
    - chemical (due to gases, fumes or vapors) J68.0
    - due to
      - fumes or vapors J68.0
      - Haemophilus influenzae J20.1
      - Mycoplasma pneumoniae J20.0
      - radiation J70.0
      - specified organism NEC J20.8
      - Streptococcus J20.2
      - virus
        - coxsackie J20.3
        - echovirus J20.7
        - parainfluenzae J20.4
        - respiratory syncytial (RSV) J20.5
        - rhinovirus J20.6
    - viral NEC J20.8
  - allergic (acute) J45.909
    - with
      - exacerbation (acute) J45.901
      - status asthmaticus J45.902
  - arachidic T17.528
  - aspiration (due to food and vomit) J69.0
  - asthmatic J45.9
    - chronic J44.9
      - with
        - acute lower respiratory infection J44.0
        - exacerbation (acute) J44.1
  - capillary —*see* Pneumonia, broncho
  - caseous (tuberculous) A15.5
  - Castellani's A69.8
  - catarrhal (15 years of age and above) J40
    - acute —*see* Bronchitis, acute
    - chronic J41.0
    - under 15 years of age J20.9
  - chemical (acute) (subacute) J68.0
    - chronic J68.4
    - due to fumes or vapors J68.0
      - chronic J68.4
  - chronic J42
    - with
      - airways obstruction J44.9
      - tracheitis (chronic) J42
    - asthmatic (obstructive) J44.9
    - catarrhal J41.0
    - chemical (due to fumes or vapors) J68.4
    - due to
      - chemicals, gases, fumes or vapors (inhalation) J68.4
      - radiation J70.1
      - tobacco smoking J41.0
    - emphysematous J44.9
    - mucopurulent J41.1
    - non-obstructive J41.0
    - obliterans J44.9
    - obstructive J44.9
    - purulent J41.1
    - simple J41.0
  - croupous —*see* Bronchitis, acute
  - due to gases, fumes or vapors (chemical) J68.0
  - emphysematous (obstructive) J44.9
  - exudative —*see* Bronchitis, acute

- **Bronchitis** *(continued)*
  - fetid J41.1
  - grippal —*see* Influenza, with, respiratory manifestations NEC
  - in those under 15 years age —*see* Bronchitis, acute
    - chronic —*see* Bronchitis, chronic
  - influenzal —*see* Influenza, with, respiratory manifestations NEC
  - mixed simple and mucopurulent J41.8
  - moulder's J62.8
  - mucopurulent (chronic) (recurrent) J41.1
    - acute or subacute J20.9
    - simple (mixed) J41.8
  - obliterans (chronic) J44.9
  - obstructive (chronic) (diffuse) J443.9
  - pituitous J41.1
  - pneumococcal, acute or subacute J20.2
  - pseudomembranous, acute or subacute —*see* Bronchitis, acute
  - purulent (chronic) (recurrent) J41.1
    - acute or subacute —*see* Bronchitis, acute
  - putrid J41.1
  - senile (chronic) J42
  - simple and mucopurulent (mixed) J41.8
  - smokers' J41.0
  - spirochetal NEC A69.8
  - subacute —*see* Bronchitis, acute
  - suppurative (chronic) J41.1
    - acute or subacute —*see* Bronchitis, acute
  - tuberculous A15.5
  - under 15 years of age —*see* Bronchitis, acute
    - chronic —*see* Bronchitis, chronic
  - viral NEC, acute or subacute —*see also* Bronchitis, acute J20.8
- **Bronchoalveolitis** J18.0
- **Bronchoaspergillosis** B44.1
- **Bronchocele meaning goiter** E04.0
- **Broncholithiasis** J98.09
  - tuberculous NEC A15.5
- **Bronchomalacia** J98.09
  - congenital Q32.2
- **Bronchomycosis NOS** B49 *[J99]*
  - candidal B37.1
- **Bronchopleuropneumonia** —*see* Pneumonia, broncho
- **Bronchopneumonia** —*see* Pneumonia, broncho
- **Bronchopneumonitis** —*see* Pneumonia, broncho
- **Bronchopulmonary** —*see* condition
- **Bronchopulmonitis** —*see* Pneumonia, broncho
- **Bronchorrhagia** (*see* Hemoptysis)
- **Bronchorrhea** J98.09
  - acute J20.9
  - chronic (infective) (purulent) J42
- **Bronchospasm** (acute) J98.01
  - with
    - bronchiolitis, acute J21.9
    - bronchitis, acute (conditions in J20) —*see* Bronchitis, acute
  - due to external agent —*see* condition, respiratory, acute, due to
  - exercise induced J45.990
- **Bronchospirochetosis** A69.8
  - Castellani A69.8
- **Bronchostenosis** J98.09
- **Bronchus** —*see* condition
- **Brontophobia** F40.220
- **Bronze baby syndrome** P83.88
- **Brooke's tumor** —*see* Neoplasm, skin, benign
- **Brown enamel of teeth** (hereditary) K00.5
- **Brown's sheath syndrome** H50.61-
- **Brown-Séquard disease, paralysis or syndrome** G83.81
- **Bruce sepsis** A23.0
- **Brucellosis** (infection) A23.9
  - abortus A23.1
  - canis A23.3
  - dermatitis A23.9
  - melitensis A23.0
  - mixed A23.8
  - sepsis A23.9
    - melitensis A23.0
    - specified NEC A23.8
  - suis A23.2
- **Bruck-de Lange disease** Q87.19
- **Bruck's disease** —*see* Deformity, limb
- **BRUE (brief resolved unexplained event)** R68.13
- **Brugsch's syndrome** Q82.8
- **Bruise** (skin surface intact) —*see also* Contusion
  - with
    - open wound —*see* Wound, open
  - internal organ —*see* Injury, by site
  - newborn P54.5
  - scalp, due to birth injury, newborn P12.3
  - umbilical cord O69.5
- **Bruit** (arterial) R09.89
  - cardiac R01.1
- **Brush burn** —*see* Abrasion, by site
- **Bruton's X-linked agammaglobulinemia** D80.0
- **Bruxism**
  - psychogenic F45.8
  - sleep related G47.63
- **Bubbly lung syndrome** P27.0
- **Bubo** I88.8
  - blennorrhagic (gonococcal) A54.89
  - chancroidal A57
  - climatic A55
  - due to Haemophilus ducreyi A57
  - gonococcal A54.89
  - indolent (nonspecific) I88.8
  - inguinal (nonspecific) I88.8
    - chancroidal A57
    - climatic A55
    - due to H. ducreyi A57
    - infective I88.8
  - scrofulous (tuberculous) A18.2
  - soft chancre A57
  - suppurating —*see* Lymphadenitis, acute
  - syphilitic (primary) A51.0
    - congenital A50.07
  - tropical A55
  - virulent (chancroidal) A57
- **Bubonic plague** A20.0
- **Bubonocele** —*see* Hernia, inguinal
- **Buccal** —*see* condition
- **Buchanan's disease or osteochondrosis** M91.0
- **Buchem's syndrome** (hyperostosis corticalis) M85.2
- **Bucket-handle fracture or tear** (semilunar cartilage) —*see* Tear, meniscus
- **Budd-Chiari syndrome** (hepatic vein thrombosis) I82.0
- **Budgerigar fancier's disease or lung** J67.2
- **Buds**
  - breast E30.1
    - in newborn P96.89
- **Buerger's disease** (thromboangiitis obliterans) I73.1
- **Bulbar** —*see* condition
- **Bulbus cordis** (left ventricle) (persistent) Q21.8
- **Bulimia** (nervosa) F50.2
  - atypical F50.9
  - normal weight F50.9
- **Bulky**
  - stools R19.5
  - uterus N85.2
- **Bulla** (e) R23.8
  - lung (emphysematous) (solitary) J43.9
    - newborn P25.8
- **Bullet wound** —*see also* Wound, open
  - fracture - code as Fracture, by site
  - internal organ —*see* Injury, by site
- **Bundle**
  - branch block (complete) (false) (incomplete) —*see* Block, bundle-branch
  - of His —*see* condition
- **Bunion** M21.61-
  - tailor's M21.62-
- **Bunionette** M21.62-
- **Buphthalmia, buphthalmos** (congenital) Q15.0
- **Burdwan fever** B55.0
- **Bürger-Grütz disease or syndrome** E78.3
- **Buried**
  - penis (congenital) Q55.64
    - acquired N48.83
  - roots K08.3
- **Burke's syndrome** K86.89
- **Burkitt**
  - cell leukemia C91.0-
  - lymphoma (malignant) C83.7-
    - small noncleaved, diffuse C83.7-
    - spleen C83.77
    - undifferentiated C83.7-
  - tumor C83.7-
  - type
    - acute lymphoblastic leukemia C91.0-
    - undifferentiated C83.7-
- **Burn** (electricity) (flame) (hot gas, liquid or hot object) (radiation) (steam) (thermal) T30.0
  - abdomen, abdominal (muscle) (wall) T21.02
    - first degree T21.12
    - second degree T21.22
    - third degree T21.32
  - above elbow T22.039
    - first degree T22.139
    - left T22.032
      - first degree T22.132
      - second degree T22.232
      - third degree T22.332

Burn *(continued)*
above elbow *(continued)*
right T22.031
first degree T22.131
second degree T22.231
third degree T22.331
second degree T22.239
third degree T22.339
acid (caustic) (external) (internal) —*see* Corrosion, by site
alimentary tract NEC T28.2
esophagus T28.1
mouth T28.0
pharynx T28.0
alkaline (caustic) (external) (internal) —*see* Corrosion, by site
ankle T25.019
first degree T25.119
left T25.012
first degree T25.112
second degree T25.212
third degree T25.312
multiple with foot —*see* Burn, lower, limb, multiple, ankle and foot
right T25.011
first degree T25.111
second degree T25.211
third degree T25.311
second degree T25.219
third degree T25.319
anus —*see* Burn, buttock
arm (lower) (upper) —*see* Burn, upper, limb
axilla T22.049
first degree T22.149
left T22.042
first degree T22.142
second degree T22.242
third degree T22.342
right T22.041
first degree T22.141
second degree T22.241
third degree T22.341
second degree T22.249
third degree T22.349
back (lower) T21.04
first degree T21.14
second degree T21.24
third degree T21.34
upper T21.03
first degree T21.13
second degree T21.23
third degree T21.33
blisters - code as Burn, second degree, by site
breast(s) —*see* Burn, chest wall
buttock(s) T21.05
first degree T21.15
second degree T21.25
third degree T21.35
calf T24.039
first degree T24.139
left T24.032
first degree T24.132
second degree T24.232
third degree T24.332
right T24.031
first degree T24.131
second degree T24.231
third degree T24.331
second degree T24.239
third degree T24.339
canthus (eye) —*see* Burn, eyelid
caustic acid or alkaline —*see* Corrosion, by site
cervix T28.3
cheek T20.06
first degree T20.16
second degree T20.26
third degree T20.36

Burn *(continued)*
chemical (acids) (alkalines) (caustics) (external) (internal) —*see* Corrosion, by site
chest wall T21.01
first degree T21.11
second degree T21.21
third degree T21.31
chin T20.03
first degree T20.13
second degree T20.23
third degree T20.33
colon T28.2
conjunctiva (and cornea) —*see* Burn, cornea
cornea (and conjunctiva) T26.1-
chemical —*see* Corrosion, cornea
corrosion (external) (internal) —*see* Corrosion, by site
deep necrosis of underlying tissue - code as Burn, third degree, by site
dorsum of hand T23.069
first degree T23.169
left T23.062
first degree T23.162
second degree T23.262
third degree T23.362
right T23.061
first degree T23.161
second degree T23.261
third degree T23.361
second degree T23.269
third degree T23.369
due to ingested chemical agent —*see* Corrosion, by site
ear (auricle) (external) (canal) T20.01
first degree T20.11
second degree T20.21
third degree T20.31
elbow T22.029
first degree T22.129
left T22.022
first degree T22.122
second degree T22.222
third degree T22.322
right T22.021
first degree T22.121
second degree T22.221
third degree T22.321
second degree T22.229
third degree T22.329
epidermal loss - code as Burn, second degree, by site
erythema, erythematous - code as Burn, first degree, by site
esophagus T28.1
extent (percentage of body surface)
less than 10 percent T31.0
10-19 percent T31.10
with 0-9 percent third degree burns T31.10
with 10-19 percent third degree burns T31.11
20-29 percent T31.20
with 0-9 percent third degree burns T31.20
with 10-19 percent third degree burns T31.21
with 20-29 percent third degree burns T31.22
30-39 percent T31.30
with 0-9 percent third degree burns T31.30
with 10-19 percent third degree burns T31.31
with 20-29 percent third degree burns T31.32
with 30-39 percent third degree burns T31.33

Burn *(continued)*
extent *(continued)*
40-49 percent T31.40
with 0-9 percent third degree burns T31.40
with 10-19 percent third degree burns T31.41
with 20-29 percent third degree burns T31.42
with 30-39 percent third degree burns T31.43
with 40-49 percent third degree burns T31.44
50-59 percent T31.50
with 0-9 percent third degree burns T31.50
with 10-19 percent third degree burns T31.51
with 20-29 percent third degree burns T31.52
with 30-39 percent third degree burns T31.53
with 40-49 percent third degree burns T31.54
with 50-59 percent third degree burns T31.55
60-69 percent T31.60
with 0-9 percent third degree burns T31.60
with 10-19 percent third degree burns T31.61
with 20-29 percent third degree burns T31.62
with 30-39 percent third degree burns T31.63
with 40-49 percent third degree burns T31.64
with 50-59 percent third degree burns T31.65
with 60-69 percent third degree burns T31.66
70-79 percent T31.70
with 0-9 percent third degree burns T31.70
with 10-19 percent third degree burns T31.71
with 20-29 percent third degree burns T31.72
with 30-39 percent third degree burns T31.73
with 40-49 percent third degree burns T31.74
with 50-59 percent third degree burns T31.75
with 60-69 percent third degree burns T31.76
with 70-79 percent third degree burns T31.77
80-89 percent T31.80
with 0-9 percent third degree burns T31.80
with 10-19 percent third degree burns T31.81
with 20-29 percent third degree burns T31.82
with 30-39 percent third degree burns T31.83
with 40-49 percent third degree burns T31.84
with 50-59 percent third degree burns T31.85
with 60-69 percent third degree burns T31.86
with 70-79 percent third degree burns T31.87
with 80-89 percent third degree burns T31.88

Burn *(continued)*
extent *(continued)*
90 percent or more T31.90
with 0-9 percent third degree burns T31.90
with 10-19 percent third degree burns T31.91
with 20-29 percent third degree burns T31.92
with 30-39 percent third degree burns T31.93
with 40-49 percent third degree burns T31.94
with 50-59 percent third degree burns T31.95
with 60-69 percent third degree burns T31.96
with 70-79 percent third degree burns T31.97
with 80-89 percent third degree burns T31.98
with 90 percent or more third degree burns T31.99
extremity —*see* Burn, limb
eye(s) and adnexa T26.4-
with resulting rupture and destruction of eyeball T26.2-
conjunctival sac —*see* Burn, cornea
cornea —*see* Burn, cornea
lid —*see* Burn, eyelid
periocular area —*see* Burn, eyelid
specified site NEC T26.3-
eyeball —*see* Burn, eye
eyelid(s) T26.0-
chemical —*see* Corrosion, eyelid
face —*see* Burn, head
finger T23.029
first degree T23.129
left T23.022
first degree T23.122
second degree T23.222
third degree T23.322
multiple sites (without thumb) T23.039
with thumb T23.049
first degree T23.149
left T23.042
first degree T23.142
second degree T23.242
third degree T23.342
right T23.041
first degree T23.141
second degree T23.241
third degree T23.341
second degree T23.249
third degree T23.349
first degree T23.139
left T23.032
first degree T23.132
second degree T23.232
third degree T23.332
right T23.031
first degree T23.131
second degree T23.231
third degree T23.331
second degree T23.239
third degree T23.339
right T23.021
first degree T23.121
second degree T23.221
third degree T23.321
second degree T23.229
third degree T23.329
flank —*see* Burn, abdominal wall
foot T25.029
first degree T25.129
left T25.022
first degree T25.122
second degree T25.222
third degree T25.322

Burn *(continued)*
- foot *(continued)*
  - multiple with ankle —*see* Burn, lower, limb, multiple, ankle and foot
  - right T25.021
    - first degree T25.121
    - second degree T25.221
    - third degree T25.321
  - second degree T25.229
  - third degree T25.329
- forearm T22.019
  - first degree T22.119
  - left T22.012
    - first degree T22.112
    - second degree T22.212
    - third degree T22.312
  - right T22.011
    - first degree T22.111
    - second degree T22.211
    - third degree T22.311
  - second degree T22.219
  - third degree T22.319
- forehead T20.06
  - first degree T20.16
  - second degree T20.26
  - third degree T20.36
- fourth degree - code as Burn, third degree, by site
- friction —*see* Burn, by site
- from swallowing caustic or corrosive substance NEC —*see* Corrosion, by site
- full thickness skin loss - code as Burn, third degree, by site
- gastrointestinal tract NEC T28.2
  - from swallowing caustic or corrosive substance T28.7
- genital organs
  - external
    - female T21.07
      - first degree T21.17
      - second degree T21.27
      - third degree T21.37
    - male T21.06
      - first degree T21.16
      - second degree T21.26
      - third degree T21.36
  - internal T28.3
    - from caustic or corrosive substance T28.8
- groin —*see* Burn, abdominal wall
- hand(s) T23.009
  - back —*see* Burn, dorsum of hand
  - finger —*see* Burn, finger
  - first degree T23.109
  - left T23.002
    - first degree T23.102
    - second degree T23.202
    - third degree T23.302
  - multiple sites with wrist T23.099
    - first degree T23.199
    - left T23.092
      - first degree T23.192
      - second degree T23.292
      - third degree T23.392
    - right T23.091
      - first degree T23.191
      - second degree T23.291
      - third degree T23.391
    - second degree T23.299
    - third degree T23.399
  - palm —*see* Burn, palm
  - right T23.001
    - first degree T23.101
    - second degree T23.201
    - third degree T23.301
  - second degree T23.209
  - third degree T23.309
  - thumb —*see* Burn, thumb

Burn *(continued)*
- head (and face) (and neck) T20.00
  - cheek —*see* Burn, cheek
  - chin —*see* Burn, chin
  - ear —*see* Burn, ear
  - eye(s) only —*see* Burn, eye
  - first degree T20.10
  - forehead —*see* Burn, forehead
  - lip —*see* Burn, lip
  - multiple sites T20.09
    - first degree T20.19
    - second degree T20.29
    - third degree T20.39
  - neck —*see* Burn, neck
  - nose —*see* Burn, nose
  - scalp —*see* Burn, scalp
  - second degree T20.20
  - third degree T20.30
- hip(s) —*see* Burn, thigh
- inhalation —*see* Burn, respiratory tract
  - caustic or corrosive substance (fumes) —*see* Corrosion, respiratory tract
- internal organ(s) T28.40
  - alimentary tract T28.2
    - esophagus T28.1
  - eardrum T28.41
  - esophagus T28.1
  - from caustic or corrosive substance (swallowing) NEC —*see* Corrosion, by site
  - genitourinary T28.3
  - mouth T28.0
  - pharynx T28.0
  - respiratory tract —*see* Burn, respiratory tract
  - specified organ NEC T28.49
- interscapular region —*see* Burn, back, upper
- intestine (large) (small) T28.2
- knee T24.029
  - first degree T24.129
  - left T24.022
    - first degree T24.122
    - second degree T24.222
    - third degree T24.322
  - right T24.021
    - first degree T24.121
    - second degree T24.221
    - third degree T24.321
  - second degree T24.229
  - third degree T24.329
- labium (majus) (minus) —*see* Burn, genital organs, external, female
- lacrimal apparatus, duct, gland or sac —*see* Burn, eye, specified site NEC
- larynx T27.0
  - with lung T27.1
- leg(s) (lower) (upper) —*see* Burn, lower, limb
- lightning —*see* Burn, by site
- limb(s)
  - lower (except ankle or foot alone) —*see* Burn, lower, limb
  - upper —*see* Burn, upper limb
- lip(s) T20.02
  - first degree T20.12
  - second degree T20.22
  - third degree T20.32
- lower
  - back —*see* Burn, back
  - limb T24.009
    - ankle —*see* Burn, ankle
    - calf —*see* Burn, calf
    - first degree T24.109
    - foot —*see* Burn, foot
    - hip —*see* Burn, thigh

Burn *(continued)*
- lower *(continued)*
  - limb *(continued)*
    - knee —*see* Burn, knee
    - left T24.002
      - first degree T24.102
      - second degree T24.202
      - third degree T24.302
    - multiple sites, except ankle and foot T24.099
      - ankle and foot T25.099
        - first degree T25.199
        - left T25.092
          - first degree T25.192
          - second degree T25.292
          - third degree T25.392
        - right T25.091
          - first degree T25.191
          - second degree T25.291
          - third degree T25.391
        - second degree T25.299
        - third degree T25.399
      - first degree T24.199
      - left T24.092
        - first degree T24.192
        - second degree T24.292
        - third degree T24.392
      - right T24.091
        - first degree T24.191
        - second degree T24.291
        - third degree T24.391
      - second degree T24.299
      - third degree T24.399
    - right T24.001
      - first degree T24.101
      - second degree T24.201
      - third degree T24.301
    - second degree T24.209
    - thigh —*see* Burn, thigh
    - third degree T24.309
    - toe —*see* Burn, toe
- lung (with larynx and trachea) T27.1
- mouth T28.0
- neck T20.07
  - first degree T20.17
  - second degree T20.27
  - third degree T20.37
- nose (septum) T20.04
  - first degree T20.14
  - second degree T20.24
  - third degree T20.34
- ocular adnexa —*see* Burn, eye
- orbit region —*see* Burn, eyelid
- palm T23.059
  - first degree T23.159
  - left T23.052
    - first degree T23.152
    - second degree T23.252
    - third degree T23.352
  - right T23.051
    - first degree T23.151
    - second degree T23.251
    - third degree T23.351
  - second degree T23.259
  - third degree T23.359
- partial thickness - code as Burn, by site, second degree
- pelvis —*see* Burn, trunk
- penis —*see* Burn, genital organs, external, male
- perineum
  - female —*see* Burn, genital organs, external, female
  - male —*see* Burn, genital organs, external, male
- periocular area —*see* Burn, eyelid
- pharynx T28.0
- rectum T28.2

Burn *(continued)*
- respiratory tract T27.3
  - larynx —*see* Burn, larynx
  - specified part NEC T27.2
  - trachea —*see* Burn, trachea
- sac, lacrimal —*see* Burn, eye, specified site NEC
- scalp T20.05
  - first degree T20.15
  - second degree T20.25
  - third degree T20.35
- scapular region T22.069
  - first degree T22.169
  - left T22.062
    - first degree T22.162
    - second degree T22.262
    - third degree T22.362
  - right T22.061
    - first degree T22.161
    - second degree T22.261
    - third degree T22.361
  - second degree T22.269
  - third degree T22.369
- sclera —*see* Burn, eye, specified site NEC
- scrotum —*see* Burn, genital organs, external, male
- shoulder T22.059
  - first degree T22.159
  - left T22.052
    - first degree T22.152
    - second degree T22.252
    - third degree T22.352
  - right T22.051
    - first degree T22.151
    - second degree T22.251
    - third degree T22.351
  - second degree T22.259
  - third degree T22.359
- stomach T28.2
- temple —*see* Burn, head
- testis —*see* Burn, genital organs, external, male
- thigh T24.019
  - first degree T24.119
  - left T24.012
    - first degree T24.112
    - second degree T24.212
    - third degree T24.312
  - right T24.011
    - first degree T24.111
    - second degree T24.211
    - third degree T24.311
  - second degree T24.219
  - third degree T24.319
- thorax (external) —*see* Burn, trunk
- throat (meaning pharynx) T28.0
- thumb(s) T23.019
  - first degree T23.119
  - left T23.012
    - first degree T23.112
    - second degree T23.212
    - third degree T23.312
  - multiple sites with fingers T23.049
    - first degree T23.149
    - left T23.042
      - first degree T23.142
      - second degree T23.242
      - third degree T23.342
    - right T23.041
      - first degree T23.141
      - second degree T23.241
      - third degree T23.341
    - second degree T23.249
    - third degree T23.349
  - right T23.011
    - first degree T23.111
    - second degree T23.211
    - third degree T23.311

- **Burn** *(continued)*
  - thumb(s) *(continued)*
    - second degree T23.219
    - third degree T23.319
  - toe T25.039
    - first degree T25.139
    - left T25.032
      - first degree T25.132
      - second degree T25.232
      - third degree T25.332
    - right T25.031
      - first degree T25.131
      - second degree T25.231
      - third degree T25.331
    - second degree T25.239
    - third degree T25.339
  - tongue T28.0
  - tonsil(s) T28.0
  - trachea T27.0
    - with lung T27.1
  - trunk T21.00
    - abdominal wall —*see* Burn, abdominal wall
    - anus —*see* Burn, buttock
    - axilla —*see* Burn, upper limb
    - back —*see* Burn, back
    - breast —*see* Burn, chest wall
    - buttock —*see* Burn, buttock
    - chest wall —*see* Burn, chest wall
    - first degree T21.10
    - flank —*see* Burn, abdominal wall
    - genital
      - female —*see* Burn, genital organs, external, female
      - male —*see* Burn, genital organs, external, male
    - groin —*see* Burn, abdominal wall
    - interscapular region —*see* Burn, back, upper
    - labia —*see* Burn, genital organs, external, female
    - lower back —*see* Burn, back
    - penis —*see* Burn, genital organs, external, male
    - perineum
      - female —*see* Burn, genital organs, external, female
      - male —*see* Burn, genital organs, external, male
    - scapula region —*see* Burn, scapular region
    - scrotum —*see* Burn, genital organs, external, male
    - second degree T21.20
    - specified site NEC T21.09
      - first degree T21.19
      - second degree T21.29
      - third degree T21.39
    - testes —*see* Burn, genital organs, external, male
    - third degree T21.30
    - upper back —*see* Burn, back, upper
    - vulva —*see* Burn, genital organs, external, female
  - unspecified site with extent of body surface involved specified
    - less than 10 percent T31.0
    - 10-19 percent (0-9 percent third degree) T31.10
      - with 10-19 percent third degree T31.11
    - 20-29 percent (0-9 percent third degree) T31.20
      - with
        - 10-19 percent third degree T31.21
        - 20-29 percent third degree T31.22
    - 30-39 percent (0-9 percent third degree) T31.30
      - with
        - 10-19 percent third degree T31.31
        - 20-29 percent third degree T31.32
        - 30-39 percent third degree T31.33
    - 40-49 percent (0-9 percent third degree) T31.40
      - with
        - 10-19 percent third degree T31.41
        - 20-29 percent third degree T31.42
        - 30-39 percent third degree T31.43
        - 40-49 percent third degree T31.44
    - 50-59 percent (0-9 percent third degree) T31.50
      - with
        - 10-19 percent third degree T31.51
        - 20-29 percent third degree T31.52
        - 30-39 percent third degree T31.53
        - 40-49 percent third degree T31.54
        - 50-59 percent third degree T31.55
    - 60-69 percent (0-9 percent third degree) T31.60
      - with
        - 10-19 percent third degree T31.61
        - 20-29 percent third degree T31.62
        - 30-39 percent third degree T31.63
        - 40-49 percent third degree T31.64
        - 50-59 percent third degree T31.65
        - 60-69 percent third degree T31.66
    - 70-79 percent (0-9 percent third degree) T31.70
      - with
        - 10-19 percent third degree T31.71
        - 20-29 percent third degree T31.72
        - 30-39 percent third degree T31.73
        - 40-49 percent third degree T31.74
        - 50-59 percent third degree T31.75
        - 60-69 percent third degree T31.76
        - 70-79 percent third degree T31.77
    - 80-89 percent (0-9 percent third degree) T31.80
      - with
        - 10-19 percent third degree T31.81
        - 20-29 percent third degree T31.82
        - 30-39 percent third degree T31.83
        - 40-49 percent third degree T31.84
        - 50-59 percent third degree T31.85
        - 60-69 percent third degree T31.86
        - 70-79 percent third degree T31.87
        - 80-89 percent third degree T31.88
    - 90 percent or more (0-9 percent third degree) T31.90
      - with
        - 10-19 percent third degree T31.91
        - 20-29 percent third degree T31.92
        - 30-39 percent third degree T31.93
        - 40-49 percent third degree T31.94
        - 50-59 percent third degree T31.95
        - 60-69 percent third degree T31.96
        - 70-79 percent third degree T31.97
        - 80-89 percent third degree T31.98
        - 90-99 percent third degree T31.99
  - upper limb T22.00
    - above elbow —*see* Burn, above elbow
    - axilla —*see* Burn, axilla
    - elbow —*see* Burn, elbow
    - first degree T22.10
    - forearm —*see* Burn, forearm
    - hand —*see* Burn, hand
    - interscapular region —*see* Burn, back, upper
    - multiple sites T22.099
      - first degree T22.199
      - left T22.092
        - first degree T22.192
        - second degree T22.292
        - third degree T22.392
      - right T22.091
        - first degree T22.191
        - second degree T22.291
        - third degree T22.391
      - second degree T22.299
      - third degree T22.399
    - scapular region —*see* Burn, scapular region
    - second degree T22.20
    - shoulder —*see* Burn, shoulder
    - third degree T22.30
    - wrist —*see* Burn, wrist
  - uterus T28.3
  - vagina T28.3
  - vulva —*see* Burn, genital organs, external, female
  - wrist T23.079
    - first degree T23.179
    - left T23.072
      - first degree T23.172
      - second degree T23.272
      - third degree T23.372
    - multiple sites with hand T23.099
      - first degree T23.199
      - left T23.092
        - first degree T23.192
        - second degree T23.292
        - third degree T23.392
      - right T23.091
        - first degree T23.191
        - second degree T23.291
        - third degree T23.391
      - second degree T23.299
      - third degree T23.399
    - right T23.071
      - first degree T23.171
      - second degree T23.271
      - third degree T23.371
    - second degree T23.279
    - third degree T23.379
- **Burnett's syndrome** E83.52
- **Burning**
  - feet syndrome E53.9
  - sensation R20.8
  - tongue K14.6
- **Burn-out** (state) Z73.0
- **Burns' disease or osteochondrosis** —*see* Osteochondrosis, juvenile, ulna
- **Bursa** —*see* condition
- **Bursitis** M71.9
  - Achilles —*see* Tendinitis, Achilles
  - adhesive —*see* Bursitis, specified NEC
  - ankle —*see* Enthesopathy, lower limb, ankle, specified type NEC
  - calcaneal —*see* Enthesopathy, foot, specified type NEC
  - collateral ligament, tibial —*see* Bursitis, tibial collateral
  - due to use, overuse, pressure —*see also* Disorder, soft tissue, due to use, specified type NEC
    - specified NEC —*see* Disorder, soft tissue, due to use, specified NEC
  - Duplay's M75.0
  - elbow NEC M70.3-
    - olecranon M70.2-
  - finger —*see* Disorder, soft tissue, due to use, specified type NEC, hand
  - foot —*see* Enthesopathy, foot, specified type NEC
  - gonococcal A54.49
  - gouty —*see* Gout
  - hand M70.1-
  - hip NEC M70.7-
    - trochanteric M70.6-
  - infective NEC M71.10
    - abscess —*see* Abscess, bursa
    - ankle M71.17-
    - elbow M71.12-
    - foot M71.17-
    - hand M71.14-
    - hip M71.15-
    - knee M71.16-
    - multiple sites M71.19
    - shoulder M71.11-
    - specified site NEC M71.18
    - wrist M71.13-
  - ischial —*see* Bursitis, hip
  - knee NEC M70.5-
    - prepatellar M70.4-
  - occupational NEC —*see also* Disorder, soft tissue, due to, use
  - olecranon —*see* Bursitis, elbow, olecranon
  - pharyngeal J39.1
  - popliteal —*see* Bursitis, knee
  - prepatellar M70.4-
  - radiohumeral M70.3-
  - rheumatoid M06.20
    - ankle M06.27-
    - elbow M06.22-

Bursitis *(continued)*
- rheumatoid *(continued)*
  - foot joint M06.27-
  - hand joint M06.24-
  - hip M06.25-
  - knee M06.26-
  - multiple site M06.29
  - shoulder M06.21-
  - vertebra M06.28
  - wrist M06.23-
- scapulohumeral *—see* Bursitis, shoulder
- semimembranous muscle (knee) *—see* Bursitis, knee
- shoulder M75.5-
  - adhesive *—see* Capsulitis, adhesive
- specified NEC M71.50
  - ankle M71.57-
  - due to use, overuse or pressure *—see* Disorder, soft tissue, due to, use
  - elbow M71.52-
  - foot M71.57-
  - hand M71.54-
  - hip M71.55-
  - knee M71.56-
  - shoulder *—see* Bursitis, shoulder
  - specified site NEC M71.58
  - tibial collateral M76.4-
  - wrist M71.53-
- subacromial *—see* Bursitis, shoulder
- subcoracoid *—see* Bursitis, shoulder
- subdeltoid *—see* Bursitis, shoulder
- syphilitic A52.78
- Thornwaldt, Tornwaldt J39.2
- tibial collateral M76.4-
- toe *—see* Enthesopathy, foot, specified type NEC
- trochanteric (area) *—see* Bursitis, hip, trochanteric
- wrist *—see* Bursitis, hand

Bursopathy M71.9
- specified type NEC M71.80
  - ankle M71.87-
  - elbow M71.82-
  - foot M71.87-
  - hand M71.84-
  - hip M71.85-
  - knee M71.86-
  - multiple sites M71.89
  - shoulder M71.81-
  - specified site NEC M71.88
  - wrist M71.83-

Burst stitches or sutures (complication of surgery) T81.31
- external operation wound T81.31
- internal operation wound T81.32

Buruli ulcer A31.1

Bury's disease L95.1

Buschke's
- disease *—see* Cryptococcosis by site
- scleredema *—see* Sclerosis, systemic

Busse-Buschke disease *—see* Cryptococcosis by site

Buttock *—see* condition

Button
- Biskra B55.1
- Delhi B55.1
- oriental B55.1

Buttonhole deformity (finger) *—see* Deformity, finger, boutonniere

Bwamba fever A92.8

Byssinosis J66.0

Bywaters' syndrome T79.5

C

Cachexia R64
- cancerous R64
- cardiac *—see* Disease, heart
- dehydration E86.0
- due to malnutrition R64
- exophthalmic *—see* Hyperthyroidism
- heart *—see* Disease, heart
- hypophyseal E23.0
- hypopituitary E23.0
- lead *—see* Poisoning, lead
- malignant R64
- marsh *—see* Malaria
- nervous F48.8
- old age R54
- paludal *—see* Malaria
- pituitary E23.0
- pulmonary R64
- renal N28.9
- saturnine *—see* Poisoning, lead
- senile R54
- Simmonds' E23.0
- splenica D73.0
- strumipriva E03.4
- tuberculous NEC *—see* Tuberculosis

CADASIL (cerebral autosomal dominant arteriopathy with subcortical infarcts and leukoencephalopathy) I67.850

Café, au lait spots L81.3

Caffeine-induced
- anxiety disorder F15.980
- sleep disorder F15.982

Caffey's syndrome Q78.8

Caisson disease T70.3

Cake kidney Q63.1

Caked breast (puerperal, postpartum) O92.79

Calabar swelling B74.3

Calcaneal spur *—see* Spur, bone, calcaneal

Calcaneo-apophysitis M92.8

Calcareous *—see* condition

Calcicosis J62.8

Calciferol (vitamin D) **deficiency** E55.9
- with rickets E55.0

Calcification
- adrenal (capsule) (gland) E27.49
  - tuberculous E35 *[B90.8]*
- aorta I70.0
- artery (annular) *—see* Arteriosclerosis
- auricle (ear) *—see* Disorder, pinna, specified type NEC
- basal ganglia G23.8
- bladder N32.89
  - due to Schistosoma hematobium B65.0
- brain (cortex) *—see* Calcification, cerebral
- bronchus J98.09
- bursa M71.40
  - ankle M71.47-
  - elbow M71.42-
  - foot M71.47-
  - hand M71.44-
  - hip M71.45-

Calcification *(continued)*
- bursa *(continued)*
  - knee M71.46-
  - multiple sites M71.49
  - shoulder M75.3-
  - specified site NEC M71.48
  - wrist M71.43-
- cardiac *—see* Degeneration, myocardial
- cerebral (cortex) G93.89
  - artery I67.2
- cervix (uteri) N88.8
- choroid plexus G93.89
- conjunctiva *—see* Concretion, conjunctiva
- corpora cavernosa (penis) N48.89
- cortex (brain) *—see* Calcification, cerebral
- dental pulp (nodular) K04.2
- dentinal papilla K00.4
- fallopian tube N83.8
- falx cerebri G96.198
- gallbladder K82.8
- general E83.59
- heart *—see also* Degeneration, myocardial
  - valve *—see* Endocarditis
- idiopathic infantile arterial (IIAC) Q28.8
- intervertebral cartilage or disc (postinfective) *—see* Disorder, disc, specified NEC
- intracranial *—see* Calcification, cerebral
- joint *—see* Disorder, joint, specified type NEC
- kidney N28.89
  - tuberculous N29 *[B90.1]*
- larynx (senile) J38.7
- lens *—see* Cataract, specified NEC
- lung (active) (postinfectional) J98.4
  - tuberculous B90.9
- lymph gland or node (postinfectional) I89.8
  - tuberculous (*see also* Tuberculosis, lymph gland) B90.8
- mammographic R92.1
- massive (paraplegic) *—see* Myositis, ossificans, in, quadriplegia
- medial *—see* Arteriosclerosis, extremities
- meninges (cerebral) (spinal) G96.198
- metastatic E83.59
- Mönckeberg's *—see* Arteriosclerosis, extremities
- muscle M61.9
  - due to burns *—see* Myositis, ossificans, in, burns
  - paralytic *—see* Myositis, ossificans, in, quadriplegia
  - specified type NEC M61.40
    - ankle M61.47-
    - foot M61.47-
    - forearm M61.43-
    - hand M61.44-
    - lower leg M61.46-
    - multiple sites M61.49
    - pelvic region M61.45-
    - shoulder region M61.41-
    - specified site NEC M61.48
    - thigh M61.45-
    - upper arm M61.42-
- myocardium, myocardial *—see* Degeneration, myocardial
- ovary N83.8
- pancreas K86.89
- penis N48.89
- periarticular *—see* Disorder, joint, specified type NEC

Calcification *(continued)*
- pericardium *—see also* Pericarditis I31.1
- pineal gland E34.8
- pleura J94.8
  - postinfectional J94.8
  - tuberculous NEC B90.9
- pulpal (dental) (nodular) K04.2
- sclera H15.89
- spleen D73.89
- subcutaneous L94.2
- suprarenal (capsule) (gland) E27.49
- tendon (sheath) *—see also* Tenosynovitis, specified type NEC
  - with bursitis, synovitis or tenosynovitis *—see* Tendinitis, calcific
- trachea J39.8
- ureter N28.89
- uterus N85.8
- vitreous *—see* Deposit, crystalline

Calcified *—see* Calcification

Calcinosis (interstitial) (tumoral) (universalis) E83.59
- with Raynaud's phenomenon, esophageal dysfunction, sclerodactyly, telangiectasia (CREST syndrome) M34.1
- circumscripta (skin) L94.2
- cutis L94.2

Calciphylaxis *—see also* Calcification, by site E83.59

Calcium
- deposits *—see* Calcification, by site
- metabolism disorder E83.50
- salts or soaps in vitreous *—see* Deposit, crystalline

Calciuria R82.994

Calculi *—see* Calculus

Calculosis, intrahepatic *—see* Calculus, bile duct

Calculus, calculi, calculous
- ampulla of Vater *—see* Calculus, bile duct
- anuria (impacted) (recurrent) *—see also* Calculus, urinary N20.9
- appendix K38.1
- bile duct (common) (hepatic) K80.50
  - with
    - calculus of gallbladder *—see* Calculus, gallbladder and bile duct
    - cholangitis K80.30
      - with
        - cholecystitis *—see* Calculus, bile duct, with cholecystitis
        - obstruction K80.31
      - acute K80.32
        - with
          - chronic cholangitis K80.36
            - with obstruction K80.37
          - obstruction K80.33
      - chronic K80.34
        - with
          - acute cholangitis K80.36
            - with obstruction K80.37
          - obstruction K80.35
    - cholecystitis (with cholangitis) K80.40
      - with obstruction K80.41

- **Calculus, calculi, calculous** *(continued)*
  - bile duct *(continued)*
    - with *(continued)*
      - cholecystitis *(continued)*
        - acute K80.42
          - with
            - chronic cholecystitis K80.46
              - with obstruction K80.47
            - obstruction K80.43
        - chronic K80.44
          - with
            - acute cholecystitis K80.46
              - with obstruction K80.47
            - obstruction K80.45
      - obstruction K80.51
  - biliary —*see also* Calculus, gallbladder
    - specified NEC K80.80
      - with obstruction K80.81
  - bilirubin, multiple —*see* Calculus, gallbladder
  - bladder (encysted) (impacted) (urinary) (diverticulum) N21.0
  - bronchus J98.09
  - calyx (kidney) (renal) —*see* Calculus, kidney
  - cholesterol (pure) (solitary) —*see* Calculus, gallbladder
  - common duct (bile) —*see* Calculus, bile duct
  - conjunctiva —*see* Concretion, conjunctiva
  - cystic N21.0
    - duct —*see* Calculus, gallbladder
  - dental (subgingival) (supragingival) K03.6
  - diverticulum
    - bladder N21.0
    - kidney N20.0
  - epididymis N50.89
  - gallbladder K80.20
    - with
      - bile duct calculus —*see* Calculus, gallbladder and bile duct
      - cholecystitis K80.10
        - with obstruction K80.11
        - acute K80.00
          - with
            - chronic cholecystitis K80.12
              - with obstruction K80.13
            - obstruction K80.01
        - chronic K80.10
          - with
            - acute cholecystitis K80.12
              - with obstruction K80.13
            - obstruction K80.11
        - specified NEC K80.18
          - with obstruction K80.19
      - obstruction K80.21
  - gallbladder and bile duct K80.70
    - with
      - cholecystitis K80.60
        - with obstruction K80.61
        - acute K80.62
          - with
            - chronic cholecystitis K80.66
              - with obstruction K80.67
            - obstruction K80.63

- **Calculus, calculi, calculous** *(continued)*
  - gallbladder and bile duct *(continued)*
    - with *(continued)*
      - cholecystitis *(continued)*
        - chronic K80.64
          - with
            - acute cholecystitis K80.66
              - with obstruction K80.67
            - obstruction K80.65
      - obstruction K80.71
  - hepatic (duct) —*see* Calculus, bile duct
  - hepatobiliary K80.80
    - with obstruction K80.81
  - ileal conduit N21.8
  - intestinal (impaction) (obstruction) K56.49
  - kidney (impacted) (multiple) (pelvis) (recurrent) (staghorn) N20.0
    - with calculus, ureter N20.2
    - congenital Q63.8
  - lacrimal passages —*see* Dacryolith
  - liver (impacted) —*see* Calculus, bile duct
  - lung J98.4
  - mammographic R92.1
  - nephritic (impacted) (recurrent) —*see* Calculus, kidney
  - nose J34.89
  - pancreas (duct) K86.89
  - parotid duct or gland K11.5
  - pelvis, encysted —*see* Calculus, kidney
  - prostate N42.0
  - pulmonary J98.4
  - pyelitis (impacted) (recurrent) N20.0
    - with hydronephrosis N13.6
  - pyelonephritis (impacted) (recurrent) N20
    - with hydronephrosis N13.6
  - renal (impacted) (recurrent) —*see* Calculus, kidney
  - salivary (duct) (gland) K11.5
  - seminal vesicle N50.89
  - staghorn —*see* Calculus, kidney
  - Stensen's duct K11.5
  - stomach K31.89
  - sublingual duct or gland K11.5
    - congenital Q38.4
  - submandibular duct, gland or region K11.5
  - submaxillary duct, gland or region K11.5
  - suburethral N21.8
  - tonsil J35.8
  - tooth, teeth (subgingival) (supragingival) K03.6
  - tunica vaginalis N50.89
  - ureter (impacted) (recurrent) N20.1
    - with calculus, kidney N20.2
      - with hydronephrosis N13.2
        - with infection N13.6
  - ureteropelvic junction N20.1
  - urethra (impacted) N21.1
  - urinary (duct) (impacted) (passage) (tract) N20.9
    - with hydronephrosis N13.2
      - with infection N13.6
    - in (due to)
    - lower N21.9
      - specified NEC N21.8
  - vagina N89.8
  - vesical (impacted) N21.0
  - Wharton's duct K11.5
  - xanthine E79.8 *[N22]*

Calicectasis N28.89

Caliectasis N28.89

- **California**
  - disease B38.9
  - encephalitis A83.5

Caligo cornea —*see* Opacity, cornea, central

Callositas, callosity (infected) L84

- **Callus** (infected) L84
  - bone —*see* Osteophyte
    - excessive, following fracture - code as Sequelae of fracture

CALME (childhood asymmetric labium majus enlargement) N90.61

Calorie deficiency or malnutrition (*see also* Malnutrition) E46

Calvé-Perthes disease —*see* Legg-Calvé-Perthes disease

Calvé's disease —*see* Osteochondrosis, juvenile, spine

Calvities —*see* Alopecia, androgenic

Cameroon fever —*see* Malaria

Camptocormia (hysterical) F44.4

Camurati-Engelmann syndrome Q78.3

- **Canal** —*see also* condition
  - atrioventricular common Q21.2

- **Canaliculitis** (lacrimal) (acute) (subacute) H04.33-
  - Actinomyces A42.89
  - chronic H04.42-

Canavan's disease E75.29

- **Canceled procedure** (surgical) Z53.9
  - because of
    - contraindication Z53.09
      - smoking Z53.01
    - left against medical advice (AMA) Z53.29
    - patient's decision Z53.20
      - for reasons of belief or group pressure Z53.1
      - specified reason NEC Z53.29
    - specified reason NEC Z53.8

- **Cancer** —*see also* Neoplasm, by site, malignant
  - bile duct type liver C22.1
  - blood —*see* Leukemia
  - breast (*see also* Neoplasm, breast, malignant) C50.91-
  - hepatocellular C22.0
  - lung (*see also* Neoplasm, lung, malignant) C34.90-
  - ovarian (*see also* Neoplasm, ovary, malignant) C56.9-
  - unspecified site (primary) C80.1

Cancer (o)phobia F45.29

Cancerous —*see* Neoplasm, malignant, by site

Cancrum oris A69.0

- **Candidiasis, candidal** B37.9
  - balanitis B37.42
  - bronchitis B37.1
  - cheilitis B37.83
  - congenital P37.5
  - cystitis B37.41
  - disseminated B37.7
  - endocarditis B37.6
  - enteritis B37.82
  - esophagitis B37.81
  - intertrigo B37.2
  - lung B37.1
  - meningitis B37.5
  - mouth B37.0
  - nails B37.2
  - neonatal P37.5
  - onychia B37.2

- **Candidiasis, candidal** *(continued)*
  - oral B37.0
  - osteomyelitis B37.89
  - otitis externa B37.84
  - paronychia B37.2
  - perionyxis B37.2
  - pneumonia B37.1
  - proctitis B37.82
  - pulmonary B37.1
  - pyelonephritis B37.49
  - sepsis B37.7
  - skin B37.2
  - specified site NEC B37.89
  - stomatitis B37.0
  - systemic B37.7
  - urethritis B37.41
  - urogenital site NEC B37.49
  - vagina B37.3
  - vulva B37.3
  - vulvovaginitis B37.3

Candidid L30.2

Candidosis —*see* Candidiasis

Candiru infection or infestation B88.8

- **Canities** (premature) L67.1
  - congenital Q84.2

- **Canker** (mouth) (sore) K12.0
  - rash A38.9

Cannabinosis J66.2

- **Cannabis induced**
  - anxiety disorder F12.980
  - psychotic disorder F12.959
  - sleep disorder F12.988

Canton fever A75.9

Cantrell's syndrome Q87.89

- **Capillariasis** (intestinal) B81.1
  - hepatic B83.8

Capillary —*see* condition

Caplan's syndrome —*see* Rheumatoid, lung

Capsule —*see* condition

- **Capsulitis** (joint) —*see also* Enthesopathy
  - adhesive (shoulder) M75.0-
  - hepatic K65.8
  - labyrinthine —*see* Otosclerosis, specified NEC
  - thyroid E06.9

- **Caput**
  - crepitus Q75.8
  - medusae I86.8
  - succedaneum P12.81

Car sickness T75.3

Carapata (disease) A68.0

Carate —*see* Pinta

Carbon lung J60

- **Carbuncle** L02.93
  - abdominal wall L02.231
  - anus K61.0
  - auditory canal, external —*see* Abscess, ear, external
  - auricle ear —*see* Abscess, ear, external
  - axilla L02.43-
  - back (any part) L02.232
  - breast N61.1
  - buttock L02.33
  - cheek (external) L02.03
  - chest wall L02.233
  - chin L02.03
  - corpus cavernosum N48.21
  - ear (any part) (external) (middle) —*see* Abscess, ear, external

Carbuncle *(continued)*
  external auditory canal *—see* Abscess, ear, external
  eyelid *—see* Abscess, eyelid
  face NEC L02.03
  femoral (region) *—see* Carbuncle, lower limb
  finger *—see* Carbuncle, hand
  flank L02.231
  foot L02.63-
  forehead L02.03
  genital *—see* Abscess, genital
  gluteal (region) L02.33
  groin L02.234
  hand L02.53-
  head NEC L02.831
  heel *—see* Carbuncle, foot
  hip *—see* Carbuncle, lower limb
  kidney *—see* Abscess, kidney
  knee *—see* Carbuncle, lower limb
  labium (majus) (minus) N76.4
  lacrimal
    gland *—see* Dacryoadenitis
    passages (duct) (sac) *—see* Inflammation, lacrimal, passages, acute
  leg *—see* Carbuncle, lower limb
  lower limb L02.43-
  malignant A22.0
  navel L02.236
  neck L02.13
  nose (external) (septum) J34.0
  orbit, orbital *—see* Abscess, orbit
  palmar (space) *—see* Carbuncle, hand
  partes posteriores L02.33
  pectoral region L02.233
  penis N48.21
  perineum L02.235
  pinna *—see* Abscess, ear, external
  popliteal *—see* Carbuncle, lower limb
  scalp L02.831
  seminal vesicle N49.0
  shoulder *—see* Carbuncle, upper limb
  specified site NEC L02.838
  temple (region) L02.03
  thumb *—see* Carbuncle, hand
  toe *—see* Carbuncle, foot
  trunk L02.239
    abdominal wall L02.231
    back L02.232
    chest wall L02.233
    groin L02.234
    perineum L02.235
    umbilicus L02.236
  umbilicus L02.236
  upper limb L02.43-
  urethra N34.0
  vulva N76.4

Carbunculus *—see* Carbuncle

Carcinoid (tumor) *—see* Tumor, carcinoid

Carcinoidosis E34.0

Carcinoma (malignant) *—see also* Neoplasm, by site, malignant
  acidophil
    specified site *—see* Neoplasm, malignant, by site
    unspecified site C75.1
  acidophil-basophil, mixed
    specified site *—see* Neoplasm, malignant, by site
    unspecified site C75.1
  adnexal (skin) *—see* Neoplasm, skin, malignant
  adrenal cortical C74.0-

Carcinoma *(continued)*
  alveolar *—see* Neoplasm, lung, malignant
    cell *—see* Neoplasm, lung, malignant
  ameloblastic C41.1
    upper jaw (bone) C41.0
  apocrine
    breast *—see* Neoplasm, breast, malignant
    specified site NEC *—see* Neoplasm, skin, malignant
    unspecified site C44.99
  basal cell (pigmented) (*see also* Neoplasm, skin, malignant) C44.91
    fibro-epithelial *—see* Neoplasm, skin, malignant
    morphea *—see* Neoplasm, skin, malignant
    multicentric *—see* Neoplasm, skin, malignant
  basaloid
  basal-squamous cell, mixed *—see* Neoplasm, skin, malignant
  basophil
    specified site *—see* Neoplasm, malignant, by site
    unspecified site C75.1
  basophil-acidophil, mixed
    specified site *—see* Neoplasm, malignant, by site
    unspecified site C75.1
  basosquamous *—see* Neoplasm, skin, malignant
  bile duct
    with hepatocellular, mixed C22.0
    liver C22.1
    specified site NEC *—see* Neoplasm, malignant, by site
    unspecified site C22.1
  branchial or branchiogenic C10.4
  bronchial or bronchogenic *—see* Neoplasm, lung, malignant
  bronchiolar *—see* Neoplasm, lung, malignant
  bronchioloalveolar *—see* Neoplasm, lung, malignant
  C cell
    specified site *—see* Neoplasm, malignant, by site
    unspecified site C73
  ceruminous C44.29-
  cervix uteri
    in situ D06.9
      endocervix D06.0
      exocervix D06.1
      specified site NEC D06.7
  chorionic
    specified site *—see* Neoplasm, malignant, by site
    unspecified site
      female C58
      male C62.90
  chromophobe
    specified site *—see* Neoplasm, malignant, by site
    unspecified site C75.1
  cloacogenic
    specified site *—see* Neoplasm, malignant, by site
    unspecified site C21.2
  diffuse type
    specified site *—see* Neoplasm, malignant, by site
    unspecified site C16.9
  duct (cell)
    with Paget's disease *—see* Neoplasm, breast, malignant

Carcinoma *(continued)*
  duct (cell) *(continued)*
    infiltrating
      with lobular carcinoma (in situ)
        specified site *—see* Neoplasm, malignant, by site
        unspecified site (female) C50.91-
          male C50.92-
      specified site *—see* Neoplasm, malignant, by site
      unspecified site (female) C50.91-
        male C50.92-
  ductal
    with lobular
      specified site *—see* Neoplasm, malignant, by site
      unspecified site (female) C50.91-
        male C50.92-
  ductular, infiltrating
    specified site *—see* Neoplasm, malignant, by site
    unspecified site (female) C50.91-
      male C50.92-
  embryonal
    liver C22.7
  endometrioid
    specified site *—see* Neoplasm, malignant, by site
    unspecified site
      female C56.9
      male C61
  eosinophil
    specified site *—see* Neoplasm, malignant, by site
    unspecified site C75.1
  epidermoid *—see also* Neoplasm, skin malignant
    in situ, Bowen's type *—see* Neoplasm, skin, in situ
  fibroepithelial, basal cell *—see* Neoplasm, skin, malignant
  follicular
    with papillary (mixed) C73
    moderately differentiated C73
    pure follicle C73
    specified site *—see* Neoplasm, malignant, by site
    trabecular C73
    unspecified site C73
    well differentiated C73
  generalized, with unspecified primary site C80.0
  glycogen-rich *—see* Neoplasm, breast, malignant
  granulosa cell C56-
  hepatic cell C22.0
  hepatocellular C22.0
    with bile duct, mixed C22.0
    fibrolamellar C22.0
  hepatocholangiolitic C22.0
  Hurthle cell C73
  in
    adenomatous polyposis coli C18.9
    pleomorphic adenoma *—see* Neoplasm, salivary glands, malignant
    situ *—see* Carcinoma-in-situ

Carcinoma *(continued)*
  infiltrating
    duct
      with lobular
        specified site *—see* Neoplasm, malignant, by site
        unspecified site (female) C50.91-
          male C50.92-
      with Paget's disease *—see* Neoplasm, breast, malignant
      specified site *—see* Neoplasm, malignant
      unspecified site (female) C50.91-
        male C50.92-
    ductular
      specified site *—see* Neoplasm, malignant
      unspecified site (female) C50.91-
        male C50.92-
    lobular
      specified site *—see* Neoplasm, malignant
      unspecified site (female) C50.91-
        male C50.92-
  inflammatory
    specified site *—see* Neoplasm, malignant
    unspecified site (female) C50.91-
      male C50.92-
  intestinal type
    specified site *—see* Neoplasm, malignant, by site
    unspecified site C16.9
  intracystic
    noninfiltrating *—see* Neoplasm, in situ, by site
  intraductal (noninfiltrating)
    with Paget's disease *—see* Neoplasm, breast, malignant
    breast D05.1-
    papillary
      with invasion
        specified site *—see* Neoplasm, malignant, by site
        unspecified site (female) C50.91-
          male C50.92-
      breast D05.1-
      specified site NEC *—see* Neoplasm, in situ, by site
      unspecified site (female) D05.1-
    specified site NEC *—see* Neoplasm, in situ, by site
    unspecified site (female) D05.1-
  intraepidermal *—see* Neoplasm, in situ
    squamous cell, Bowen's type *—see* Neoplasm, skin, in situ
  intraepithelial *—see* Neoplasm, in situ, by site
    squamous cell *—see* Neoplasm, in situ, by site
  intraosseous C41.1
    upper jaw (bone) C41.0
  islet cell
    with exocrine, mixed
      specified site *—see* Neoplasm, malignant, by site
      unspecified site C25.9
    pancreas C25.4

Carcinoma *(continued)*
- islet cell *(continued)*
  - specified site NEC *—see* Neoplasm, malignant, by site
  - unspecified site C25.4
- juvenile, breast *—see* Neoplasm, breast, malignant
- large cell
  - small cell
    - specified site *—see* Neoplasm, malignant, by site
    - unspecified site C34.90
- Leydig cell (testis)
  - specified site *—see* Neoplasm, malignant, by site
  - unspecified site
    - female C56.9
    - male C62.90
- lipid-rich (female) C50.91-
  - male C50.92-
- liver cell C22.0
- liver NEC C22.7
- lobular (infiltrating)
  - with intraductal
    - specified site *—see* Neoplasm, malignant, by site
    - unspecified site (female) C50.91-
      - male C50.92-
  - noninfiltrating
    - breast D05.0-
    - specified site NEC *—see* Neoplasm, in situ, by site
    - unspecified site D05.0-
  - specified site *—see* Neoplasm, malignant, by site
  - unspecified site (female) C50.91-
    - male C50.92-
- medullary
  - with
    - amyloid stroma
      - specified site *—see* Neoplasm, malignant, by site
      - unspecified site C73
    - lymphoid stroma
      - specified site *—see* Neoplasm, malignant, by site
      - unspecified site (female) C50.91-
        - male C50.92-
- Merkel cell C4A.9
  - anal margin C4A.51
  - anal skin C4A.51
  - canthus C4A.1-
  - ear and external auricular canal C4A.2-
  - external auricular canal C4A.2-
  - eyelid, including canthus C4A.1-
  - face C4A.30
    - specified NEC C4A.39
  - hip C4A.7-
  - lip C4A.0
  - lower limb, including hip C4A.7-
  - neck C4A.4
  - nodal presentation C7B.1
  - nose C4A.31
  - overlapping sites C4A.8
  - perianal skin C4A.51
  - scalp C4A.4
  - secondary C7B.1
  - shoulder C4A.6-
  - skin of breast C4A.52
  - trunk NEC C4A.59
  - upper limb, including shoulder C4A.6-
  - visceral metastatic C7B.1
- metastatic *—see* Neoplasm, secondary, by site

Carcinoma *(continued)*
- metatypical *—see* Neoplasm, skin, malignant
- morphea, basal cell *—see* Neoplasm, skin, malignant
- mucoid
  - cell
    - specified site *—see* Neoplasm, malignant, by site
    - unspecified site C75.1
- neuroendocrine *—see also* Tumor, neuroendocrine
  - high grade, any site C7A.1
  - poorly differentiated, any site C7A.1
- nonencapsulated sclerosing C73
- noninfiltrating
  - intracystic *—see* Neoplasm, in situ, by site
  - intraductal
    - breast D05.1-
    - papillary
      - breast D05.1-
      - specified site NEC *—see* Neoplasm, in situ, by site
      - unspecified site D05.1-
    - specified site *—see* Neoplasm, in situ, by site
    - unspecified site D05.1-
  - lobular
    - breast D05.0-
    - specified site NEC *—see* Neoplasm, in situ, by site
    - unspecified site (female) D05.0-
- oat cell
  - specified site *—see* Neoplasm, malignant, by site
  - unspecified site C34.90
- odontogenic C41.1
  - upper jaw (bone) C41.0
- papillary
  - with follicular (mixed) C73
  - follicular variant C73
  - intraductal (noninfiltrating)
    - with invasion
      - specified site *—see* Neoplasm, malignant, by site
      - unspecified site (female) C50.91-
        - male C50.92-
    - breast D05.1-
    - specified site NEC *—see* Neoplasm, in situ, by site
    - unspecified site D05.1-
  - serous
    - specified site *—see* Neoplasm, malignant, by site
    - surface
      - specified site *—see* Neoplasm, malignant, by site
      - unspecified site C56.9
    - unspecified site C56.9
- papillocystic
  - specified site *—see* Neoplasm, malignant, by site
  - unspecified site C56.9
- parafollicular cell
  - specified site *—see* Neoplasm, malignant, by site
  - unspecified site C73
- pilomatrix *—see* Neoplasm, skin, malignant
- pseudomucinous
  - specified site *—see* Neoplasm, malignant, by site
  - unspecified site C56.9

Carcinoma *(continued)*
- renal cell C64-
- Schmincke *—see* Neoplasm, nasopharynx, malignant
- Schneiderian
  - specified site *—see* Neoplasm, malignant, by site
  - unspecified site C30.0
- sebaceous *—see* Neoplasm, skin, malignant
- secondary *—see also* Neoplasm, secondary, by site
  - Merkel cell C7B.1
- secretory, breast *—see* Neoplasm, breast, malignant
- serous
  - papillary
    - specified site *—see* Neoplasm, malignant, by site
    - unspecified site C56.9
  - surface, papillary
    - specified site *—see* Neoplasm, malignant, by site
    - unspecified site C56.9
- Sertoli cell
  - specified site *—see* Neoplasm, malignant, by site
  - unspecified site C62.90
    - female C56.9
    - male C62.90
- skin appendage *—see* Neoplasm, skin, malignant
- small cell
  - fusiform cell
    - specified site *—see* Neoplasm, malignant, by site
    - unspecified site C34.90
  - intermediate cell
    - specified site *—see* Neoplasm, malignant, by site
    - unspecified site C34.90
  - large cell
    - specified site *—see* Neoplasm, malignant, by site
    - unspecified site C34.90
- solid
  - with amyloid stroma
    - specified site *—see* Neoplasm, malignant, by site
    - unspecified site C73
  - microinvasive
    - specified site *—see* Neoplasm, malignant, by site
    - unspecified site C53.9
- sweat gland *—see* Neoplasm, skin, malignant
- theca cell C56.-
- thymic C37
- unspecified site (primary) C80.1
- water-clear cell C75.0

Carcinoma-in-situ *—see also* Neoplasm, in situ, by site
- breast NOS D05.9-
  - specified type NEC D05.8-
- epidermoid *—see also* Neoplasm, in situ, by site
  - with questionable stromal invasion
    - cervix D06.9
    - specified site NEC *—see* Neoplasm, in situ, by site
    - unspecified site D06.9
  - Bowen's type *—see* Neoplasm, skin, in situ
- intraductal
  - breast D05.1-
  - specified site NEC *—see* Neoplasm, in situ, by site
  - unspecified site D05.1-

Carcinoma-in-situ *(continued)*
- lobular
  - with
    - infiltrating duct
      - breast (female) C50.91-
        - male C50.92-
      - specified site NEC *—see* Neoplasm, malignant
      - unspecified site (female) C50.91-
        - male C50.92-
    - intraductal
      - breast D05.8-
      - specified site NEC *—see* Neoplasm, in situ, by site
      - unspecified site (female) D05.8-
  - breast D05.0-
  - specified site NEC *—see* Neoplasm, in situ, by site
  - unspecified site D05.0-
- squamous cell *—see also* Neoplasm, in situ, by site
  - with questionable stromal invasion
    - cervix D06.9
    - specified site NEC *—see* Neoplasm, in situ, by site
    - unspecified site D06.9

Carcinomaphobia F45.29

Carcinomatosis C80.0
- peritonei C78.6
- unspecified site (primary) (secondary) C80.0

Carcinosarcoma *—see* Neoplasm, malignant, by site
- embryonal *—see* Neoplasm, malignant, by site

Cardia, cardial *—see* condition

Cardiac *—see also* condition
- death, sudden *—see* Arrest, cardiac
- pacemaker
  - in situ Z95.0
    - management or adjustment Z45.018
- tamponade I31.4

Cardialgia *—see* Pain, precordial

Cardiectasis *—see* Hypertrophy, cardiac

Cardiochalasia K21.9

Cardiomalacia I51.5

Cardiomegalia glycogenica diffusa E74.02 *[I43]*

Cardiomegaly *—see also* Hypertrophy, cardiac
- congenital Q24.8
- glycogen E74.02 *[I43]*
- idiopathic I51.7

Cardiomyoliposis I51.5

Cardiomyopathy (familial) (idiopathic) I42.9
- alcoholic I42.6
- amyloid E85.4 *[I43]*
  - transthyretin-related (ATTR) familial E85.4 *[I43]*
- arteriosclerotic *—see* Disease, heart, ischemic, atherosclerotic
- beriberi E51.12
- cobalt-beer I42.6
- congenital I42.4
- congestive I42.0
- constrictive NOS I42.5
- dilated I42.0
- due to
  - alcohol I42.6
  - beriberi E51.12
  - cardiac glycogenosis E74.02 *[I43]*
  - drugs I42.7

Cardiomyopathy *(continued)*
- due to *(continued)*
  - external agents NEC I42.7
  - Friedreich's ataxia G11.11
  - myotonia atrophica G71.11 *[I43]*
  - progressive muscular dystrophy G71.09 *[I43]*
- glycogen storage E74.02 *[I43]*
- hypertensive —*see* Hypertension, heart
- hypertrophic (nonobstructive) I42.2
  - obstructive I42.1
    - congenital Q24.8
- in
  - Chagas' disease (chronic) B57.2
    - acute B57.0
  - sarcoidosis D86.85
- ischemic I25.5
- metabolic E88.9 *[I43]*
  - thyrotoxic E05.90 *[I43]*
    - with thyroid storm E05.91 *[I43]*
- newborn I42.8
  - congenital I42.4
- non-ischemic (*see also* by cause) I42.8
- nutritional E63.9 *[I43]*
  - beriberi E51.12
- obscure of Africa I42.8
- peripartum O90.3
- postpartum O90.3
- restrictive NEC I42.5
- rheumatic I09.0
- secondary I42.9
- specified NEC I42.8
- stress induced I51.81
- takotsubo I51.81
- thyrotoxic E05.90 *[I43]*
  - with thyroid storm E05.91 *[I43]*
- toxic NEC I42.7
- transthyretin-related (ATTR) familial amyloid E85.4
- tuberculous A18.84
- viral B33.24

Cardionephritis —*see* Hypertension, cardiorenal

Cardionephropathy —*see* Hypertension, cardiorenal

Cardionephrosis —*see* Hypertension, cardiorenal

Cardiopathia nigra I27.0

Cardiopathy —*see also* Disease, heart I51.9
- idiopathic I42.9
- mucopolysaccharidosis E76.3 *[I52]*

Cardiopericarditis —*see* Pericarditis

Cardiophobia F45.29

Cardiorenal —*see* condition

Cardiorrhexis —*see* Infarct, myocardium

Cardiosclerosis —*see* Disease, heart, ischemic, atherosclerotic

Cardiosis —*see* Disease, heart

Cardiospasm (esophagus) (reflex) (stomach) K22.0
- congenital Q39.5
  - with megaesophagus Q39.5

Cardiostenosis —*see* Disease, heart

Cardiosymphysis I31.0

Cardiovascular —*see* condition

Carditis (acute) (bacterial) (chronic) (subacute) I51.89
- meningococcal A39.50
- rheumatic —*see* Disease, heart, rheumatic
- rheumatoid —*see* Rheumatoid, carditis
- viral B33.20

Care (of) (for) (following)
- child (routine) Z76.2
- family member (handicapped) (sick)
  - creating problem for family Z63.6
  - provided away from home for holiday relief Z75.5
  - unavailable, due to
    - absence (person rendering care) (sufferer) Z74.2
    - inability (any reason) of person rendering care Z74.2
- foundling Z76.1
- holiday relief Z75.5
- improper —*see* Maltreatment
- lack of (at or after birth) (infant) —*see* Maltreatment, child, neglect
- lactating mother Z39.1
- palliative Z51.5
- postpartum
  - immediately after delivery Z39.0
  - routine follow-up Z39.2
- respite Z75.5
- unavailable, due to
  - absence of person rendering care Z74.2
  - inability (any reason) of person rendering care Z74.2
- well-baby Z76.2

Caries
- bone NEC A18.03
- dental (dentino enamel junction) (early in childhood) (of dentine) (pre-eruptive) (recurrent) (to the pulp) K02.9
  - arrested (coronal) (root) K02.3
  - chewing surface
    - limited to enamel K02.51
    - penetrating into dentin K02.52
    - penetrating into pulp K02.53
  - coronal surface
    - chewing surface
      - limited to enamel K02.51
      - penetrating into dentin K02.52
      - penetrating into pulp K02.53
    - pit and fissure surface
      - limited to enamel K02.51
      - penetrating into dentin K02.52
      - penetrating into pulp K02.53
    - smooth surface
      - limited to enamel K02.61
      - penetrating into dentin K02.62
      - penetrating into pulp K02.63
  - pit and fissure surface
    - limited to enamel K02.51
    - penetrating into dentin K02.52
    - penetrating into pulp K02.53
  - primary, cervical origin K02.52
  - root K02.7
  - smooth surface
    - limited to enamel K02.61
    - penetrating into dentin K02.62
    - penetrating into pulp K02.63
- external meatus —*see* Disorder, ear, external, specified type NEC
- hip (tuberculous) A18.02
- initial (tooth)
  - chewing surface K02.51
  - pit and fissure surface K02.51
  - smooth surface K02.61
- knee (tuberculous) A18.02
- labyrinth —*see* subcategory H83.8
- limb NEC (tuberculous) A18.03
- mastoid process (chronic) —*see* Mastoiditis, chronic
  - tuberculous A18.03
- middle ear —*see* subcategory H74.8
- nose (tuberculous) A18.03
- orbit (tuberculous) A18.03
- ossicles, ear —*see* Abnormal, ear ossicles
- petrous bone —*see* Petrositis
- root (dental) (tooth) K02.7
- sacrum (tuberculous) A18.01
- spine, spinal (column) (tuberculous) A18.01
- syphilitic A52.77
  - congenital (early) A50.02 *[M90.80]*
- tooth, teeth —*see* Caries, dental
- tuberculous A18.03
- vertebra (column) (tuberculous) A18.01

Carious teeth —*see* Caries, dental

Carneous mole O02.0

Carnitine insufficiency E71.40

Carotenemia (dietary) E67.1

Carotenosis (cutis) (skin) E67.1

Carotid body or sinus syndrome G90.01

Carotidynia G90.01

Carpal tunnel syndrome —*see* Syndrome, carpal tunnel

Carpenter's syndrome Q87.0

Carpopedal spasm —*see* Tetany

Carr-Barr-Plunkett syndrome Q97.1

Carrier (suspected) of
- amebiasis Z22.1
- bacterial disease NEC Z22.39
  - diphtheria Z22.2
  - intestinal infectious NEC Z22.1
    - typhoid Z22.0
  - meningococcal Z22.31
  - sexually transmitted Z22.4
  - specified NEC Z22.39
  - staphylococcal (Methicillin susceptible) Z22.321
    - Methicillin resistant Z22.322
  - streptococcal Z22.338
    - group B Z22.330
      - complicating pregnancy or delivery O99.82-
  - typhoid Z22.0
- cholera Z22.1
- diphtheria Z22.2
- gastrointestinal pathogens NEC Z22.1
- genetic Z14.8
  - cystic fibrosis Z14.1
  - hemophilia A (asymptomatic) Z14.01
    - symptomatic Z14.02
- gestational, pregnant Z33.1
- gonorrhea Z22.4
- HAA (hepatitis Australian-antigen) B18.8
- HB (c)(s)-AG B18.1
- hepatitis (viral) B18.9
  - Australia-antigen (HAA) B18.8
  - B surface antigen (HBsAg) B18.1
    - with acute delta-(super) infection B17.0
  - C B18.2
  - specified NEC B18.8
- human T-cell lymphotropic virus type-1(HTLV-1) infection Z22.6
- infectious organism Z22.9
  - specified NEC Z22.8
- meningococci Z22.31
- Salmonella typhosa Z22.0
- serum hepatitis —*see* Carrier, hepatitis
- staphylococci (Methicillin susceptible) Z22.321
  - Methicillin resistant Z22.322
- streptococci Z22.338
  - group B Z22.330
    - complicating pregnancy or delivery O99.82-
- syphilis Z22.4
- typhoid Z22.0
- venereal disease NEC Z22.4

Carrion's disease A44.0

Carter's relapsing fever (Asiatic) A68.1

Cartilage —*see* condition

Caruncle (inflamed)
- conjunctiva (acute) —*see* Conjunctivitis, acute
- labium (majus) (minus) N90.89
- lacrimal —*see* Inflammation, lacrimal, passages
- myrtiform N89.8
- urethral (benign) N36.2

Cascade stomach K31.2

Caseation lymphatic gland (tuberculous) A18.2

Cassidy (-Scholte) **syndrome** (malignant carcinoid) E34.0

Castellani's disease A69.8

Castration, traumatic, male S38.231

Casts in urine R82.998

Cat
- cry syndrome Q93.4
- ear Q17.3
- eye syndrome Q92.8

Catabolism, senile R54

Catalepsy (hysterical) F44.2
- schizophrenic F20.2

Cataplexy (idiopathic) —*see* - Narcolepsy

Cataract (cortical) (immature) (incipient) H26.9
- with
  - neovascularization —*see* Cataract, complicated
- age-related —*see* Cataract, senile
- anterior
  - and posterior axial embryonal Q12.0
  - pyramidal Q12.0
- associated with
  - galactosemia E74.21 *[H28]*
  - myotonic disorders G71.19 *[H28]*
- blue Q12.0
- central Q12.0
- cerulean Q12.0
- complicated H26.20
  - with
    - neovascularization H26.21-
    - ocular disorder H26.22-
    - glaucomatous flecks H26.23-

Cataract *(continued)*
- congenital Q12.0
- coraliform Q12.0
- coronary Q12.0
- crystalline Q12.0
- diabetic *—see* Diabetes, cataract
- drug-induced H26.3-
- due to
  - ocular disorder *—see* Cataract, complicated
  - radiation H26.8
- electric H26.8
- extraction status Z98.4-
- glass-blower's H26.8
- heat ray H26.8
- heterochromic *—see* Cataract, complicated
- hypermature *—see* Cataract, senile, morgagnian type
- in (due to)
  - chronic iridocyclitis *—see* Cataract, complicated
  - diabetes *—see* Diabetes, cataract
  - endocrine disease E34.9 *[H28]*
  - eye disease *—see* Cataract, complicated
  - hypoparathyroidism E20.9 *[H28]*
  - malnutrition-dehydration E46 *[H28]*
  - metabolic disease E88.9 *[H28]*
  - myotonic disorders G71.19 *[H28]*
  - nutritional disease E63.9 *[H28]*
- infantile *—see* Cataract, presenile
- irradiational *—see* Cataract, specified NEC
- juvenile *—see* Cataract, presenile
- malnutrition-dehydration E46 *[H28]*
- morgagnian *—see* Cataract, senile, morgagnian type
- myotonic G71.19 *[H28]*
- myxedema E03.9 *[H28]*
- nuclear
  - embryonal Q12.0
  - sclerosis *—see* Cataract, senile, nuclear
- presenile H26.00-
  - combined forms H26.06-
  - cortical H26.01-
  - lamellar *—see* Cataract, presenile, cortical
  - nuclear H26.03-
  - specified NEC H26.09
  - subcapsular polar (anterior) H26.04-
    - posterior H26.05-
  - zonular *—see* Cataract, presenile, cortical
- secondary H26.40
  - Soemmering's ring H26.41-
  - specified NEC H26.49-
  - to eye disease *—see* Cataract, complicated
- senile H25.9
  - brunescens *—see* Cataract, senile, nuclear
  - combined forms H25.81-
  - coronary *—see* Cataract, senile, incipient
  - cortical H25.01-
  - hypermature *—see* Cataract, senile, morgagnian type
  - incipient (mature) (total) H25.09-
    - cortical *—see* Cataract, senile, cortical
    - subcapsular *—see* Cataract, senile, subcapsular
  - morgagnian type (hypermature) H25.2-

Cataract *(continued)*
- senile *(continued)*
  - nuclear (sclerosis) H25.1-
  - polar subcapsular (anterior) (posterior) *—see* Cataract, senile, incipient
  - punctate *—see* Cataract, senile, incipient
  - specified NEC H25.89
  - subcapsular polar (anterior) H25.03-
    - posterior H25.04-
- snowflake *—see* Diabetes, cataract
- specified NEC H26.8
- toxic *—see* Cataract, drug-induced
- traumatic H26.10-
  - localized H26.11-
  - partially resolved H26.12-
  - total H26.13-
- zonular (perinuclear) Q12.0

Cataracta *—see also* Cataract
- brunescens *—see* Cataract, senile, nuclear
- centralis pulverulenta Q12.0
- cerulea Q12.0
- complicata *—see* Cataract, complicated
- congenita Q12.0
- coralliformis Q12.0
- coronaria Q12.0
- diabetic *—see* Diabetes, cataract
- membranacea
  - accreta *—see* Cataract, secondary
  - congenita Q12.0
- nigra *—see* Cataract, senile, nuclear
- sunflower *—see* Cataract, complicated

Catarrh, catarrhal (acute) (febrile) (infectious) (inflammation) *—see also* condition J00
- bronchial *—see* Bronchitis
- chest *—see* Bronchitis
- chronic J31.0
- due to congenital syphilis A50.03
- enteric *—see* Enteritis
- eustachian H68.009
- fauces *—see* Pharyngitis
- gastrointestinal *—see* Enteritis
- gingivitis K05.00
  - nonplaque induced K05.01
  - plaque induced K05.00
- hay *—see* Fever, hay
- intestinal *—see* Enteritis
- larynx, chronic J37.0
- liver B15.9
  - with hepatic coma B15.0
- lung *—see* Bronchitis
- middle ear, chronic *—see* Otitis, media, nonsuppurative, chronic, serous
- mouth K12.1
- nasal (chronic) *—see* Rhinitis
- nasobronchial J31.1
- nasopharyngeal (chronic) J31.1
  - acute J00
- pulmonary *—see* Bronchitis
- spring (eye) (vernal) *—see* Conjunctivitis, acute, atopic
- summer (hay) *—see* Fever, hay
- throat J31.2
- tubotympanal *—see also* Otitis, media, nonsuppurative
  - chronic *—see* Otitis, media, nonsuppurative, chronic, serous

Catatonia (schizophrenic) F20.2

Catatonic
- disorder due to known physiologic condition F06.1
- schizophrenia F20.2
- stupor R40.1

Cat-scratch *—see also* Abrasion
- disease or fever A28.1

Cauda equina *—see* condition

Cauliflower ear M95.1-

Causalgia (upper limb) G56.4-
- lower limb G57.7-

Cause
- external, general effects T75.89

Caustic burn *—see* Corrosion, by site

Cavare's disease (familial periodic paralysis) G72.3

Cave-in, injury
- crushing (severe) *—see* Crush
- suffocation *—see* Asphyxia, traumatic, due to low oxygen, due to cave-in

Cavernitis (penis) N48.29

Cavernositis N48.29

Cavernous *—see* condition

Cavitation of lung *—see also* Tuberculosis, pulmonary
- nontuberculous J98.4

Cavities, dental *—see* Caries, dental

Cavity
- lung *—see* Cavitation of lung
- optic papilla Q14.2
- pulmonary *—see* Cavitation of lung

Cavovarus foot, congenital Q66.1-

Cavus foot (congenital) Q66.7-
- acquired *—see* Deformity, limb, foot, specified NEC

Cazenave's disease L10.2

CDKL5 (Cyclin-Dependent Kinase-Like 5 Deficiency Disorder) G40.42

Cecitis K52.9
- with perforation, peritonitis, or rupture K65.8

Cecoureterocele Q62.32

Cecum *—see* condition

Celiac
- artery compression syndrome I77.4
- disease (with steatorrhea) K90.0
- infantilism K90.0

Cell(s), cellular *—see also* condition
- in urine R82.998

Cellulitis (diffuse) (phlegmonous) (septic) (suppurative) L03.90
- abdominal wall L03.311
- anaerobic A48.0
- ankle *—see* Cellulitis, lower limb
- anus K61.0
- arm *—see* Cellulitis, upper limb
- auricle (ear) *—see* Cellulitis, ear
- axilla L03.11-
- back (any part) L03.312
- breast (acute) (nonpuerperal) (subacute) N61.0
  - nipple N61.0
- broad ligament
  - acute N73.0
- buttock L03.317
- cervical (meaning neck) L03.221
- cervix (uteri) *—see* Cervicitis
- cheek (external) L03.211
  - internal K12.2
- chest wall L03.313

Cellulitis *(continued)*
- chronic L03.90
- clostridial A48.0
- corpus cavernosum N48.22
- digit
  - finger *—see* Cellulitis, finger
  - toe *—see* Cellulitis, toe
- Douglas' cul-de-sac or pouch
  - acute N73.0
- drainage site (following operation) T81.49
- ear (external) H60.1-
- eosinophilic (granulomatous) L98.3
- erysipelatous *—see* Erysipelas
- external auditory canal *—see* Cellulitis, ear
- eyelid *—see* Abscess, eyelid
- face NEC L03.211
- finger (intrathecal) (periosteal) (subcutaneous) (subcuticular) L03.01-
- foot *—see* Cellulitis, lower limb
- gangrenous *—see* Gangrene
- genital organ NEC
  - female (external) N76.4
  - male N49.9
    - multiple sites N49.8
    - specified NEC N49.8
- gluteal (region) L03.317
- gonococcal A54.89
- groin L03.314
- hand *—see* Cellulitis, upper limb
- head NEC L03.811
  - face (any part, except ear, eye and nose) L03.211
- heel *—see* Cellulitis, lower limb
- hip *—see* Cellulitis, lower limb
- jaw (region) L03.211
- knee *—see* Cellulitis, lower limb
- labium (majus) (minus) *—see* Vulvitis
- lacrimal passages *—see* Inflammation, lacrimal, passages
- larynx J38.7
- leg *—see* Cellulitis, lower limb
- lip K13.0
- lower limb L03.11-
  - toe *—see* Cellulitis, toe
- mouth (floor) K12.2
- multiple sites, so stated L03.90
- nasopharynx J39.1
- navel L03.316
  - newborn P38.9
    - with mild hemorrhage P38.1
    - without hemorrhage P38.9
- neck (region) L03.221
- nipple (acute) (nonpuerperal) (subacute) N61.0
- nose (septum) (external) J34.0
- orbit, orbital H05.01-
- palate (soft) K12.2
- pectoral (region) L03.313
- pelvis, pelvic (chronic)
  - female *—see also* Disease, pelvis, inflammatory N73.2
    - acute N73.0
  - following ectopic or molar pregnancy O08.0
  - male K65.0
- penis N48.22
- perineal, perineum L03.315
- periorbital L03.213
- perirectal K61.1
- peritonsillar J36
- periurethral N34.0
- periuterine (*see also* Disease pelvis, inflammatory) N73.2
  - acute N73.0
- pharynx J39.1
- preseptal L03.213
- rectum K61.1

Cellulitis *(continued)*
- retroperitoneal K68.9
- round ligament
  - acute N73.0
- scalp (any part) L03.811
- scrotum N49.2
- seminal vesicle N49.0
- shoulder —*see* Cellulitis, upper limb
- specified site NEC L03.818
- submandibular (region) (space) (triangle) K12.2
  - gland K11.3
- submaxillary (region) K12.2
  - gland K11.3
- thigh —*see* Cellulitis, lower limb
- thumb (intrathecal) (periosteal) (subcutaneous) (subcuticular) —*see* Cellulitis, finger
- toe (intrathecal) (periosteal) (subcutaneous) (subcuticular) L03.03-
- tonsil J36
- trunk L03.319
  - abdominal wall L03.311
  - back (any part) L03.312
  - buttock L03.317
  - chest wall L03.313
  - groin L03.314
  - perineal, perineum L03.315
  - umbilicus L03.316
- tuberculous (primary) A18.4
- umbilicus L03.316
- upper limb L03.11-
  - axilla —*see* Cellulitis, axilla
  - finger —*see* Cellulitis, finger
  - thumb —*see* Cellulitis, finger
- vaccinal T88.0
- vocal cord J38.3
- vulva —*see* Vulvitis
- wrist —*see* Cellulitis, upper limb

Cementoblastoma, benign —*see* Cyst, calcifying odontogenic

Cementoma —*see* Cyst, calcifying odontogenic

Cementoperiostitis —*see* Periodontitis

Cementosis K03.4

Central auditory processing disorder H93.25

Central pain syndrome G89.0

Cephalematocele, cephalhematocele
- newborn P52.8
  - birth injury P10.8
- traumatic —*see* Hematoma, brain

Cephalematoma, cephalhematoma (calcified)
- newborn (birth injury) P12.0
- traumatic —*see* Hematoma, brain

Cephalgia, cephalalgia —*see also* Headache
- histamine G44.009
  - intractable G44.001
  - not intractable G44.009
- trigeminal autonomic (TAC) NEC G44.099
  - intractable G44.091
  - not intractable G44.099

Cephalic —*see* condition

Cephalitis —*see* Encephalitis

Cephalocele —*see* Encephalocele

Cephalomenia N94.89

Cephalopelvic —*see* condition

Cerclage (with cervical incompetence) **in pregnancy** —*see* Incompetence, cervix, in pregnancy

Cerebellitis —*see* Encephalitis

Cerebellum, cerebellar —*see* condition

Cerebral —*see* condition

Cerebritis —*see* Encephalitis

Cerebro-hepato-renal syndrome Q87.89

Cerebromalacia —*see* Softening, brain
- sequelae of cerebrovascular disease I69.398

Cerebroside lipidosis E75.22

Cerebrospasticity (congenital) G80.1

Cerebrospinal —*see* condition

Cerebrum —*see* condition

Ceroid-lipofuscinosis, neuronal E75.4

Cerumen (accumulation) (impacted) H61.2-

Cervical —*see also* condition
- auricle Q18.2
- dysplasia in pregnancy —*see* Abnormal, cervix, in pregnancy or childbirth
- erosion in pregnancy —*see* Abnormal, cervix, in pregnancy or childbirth
- fibrosis in pregnancy —*see* Abnormal, cervix, in pregnancy or childbirth
- fusion syndrome Q76.1
- rib Q76.5
- shortening (complicating pregnancy) O26.87-

Cervicalgia M54.2

Cervicitis (acute) (chronic) (nonvenereal) (senile (atrophic)) (subacute) (with ulceration) N72
- with
  - abortion —*see* Abortion, by type complicated by genital tract and pelvic infection
  - ectopic pregnancy O08.0
  - molar pregnancy O08.0
- chlamydial A56.09
- gonococcal A54.03
- herpesviral A60.03
- puerperal (postpartum) O86.11
- syphilitic A52.76
- trichomonal A59.09
- tuberculous A18.16

Cervicocolpitis (emphysematosa) (*see also* Cervicitis) N72

Cervix —*see* condition

Cesarean delivery, previous, affecting management of pregnancy O34.219
- classical (vertical) scar O34.212
- isthmocele O34.22
- low transverse scar O34.211
- mid-transverse T incision O34.218
- scar
  - defect (isthmocele) O34.22
  - specified type NEC O34.218

Céstan (-Chenais) **paralysis or syndrome** G46.3

Céstan-Raymond syndrome I65.8

Cestode infestation B71.9
- specified type NEC B71.8

Cestodiasis B71.9

Chabert's disease A22.9

Chacaleh E53.8

Chafing L30.4

Chagas' (-Mazza) **disease** (chronic) B57.2
- with
  - cardiovascular involvement NEC B57.2
  - digestive system involvement B57.30
    - megacolon B57.32
    - megaesophagus B57.31
    - other specified B57.39
  - megacolon B57.32
  - megaesophagus B57.31
  - myocarditis B57.2
  - nervous system involvement B57.40
    - meningitis B57.41
    - meningoencephalitis B57.42
    - other specified B57.49
  - specified organ involvement NEC B57.5
- acute (with) B57.1
  - cardiovascular NEC B57.0
  - myocarditis B57.0

Chagres fever B50.9

Chairridden Z74.09

Chalasia (cardiac sphincter) K21.9

Chalazion H00.19
- left H00.16
  - lower H00.15
  - upper H00.14
- right H00.13
  - lower H00.12
  - upper H00.11

Chalcosis —*see also* Disorder, globe, degenerative, chalcosis
- cornea —*see* Deposit, cornea
- crystalline lens —*see* Cataract, complicated
- retina H35.89

Chalicosis (pulmonum) J62.8

Chancre (any genital site) (hard) (hunterian) (mixed) (primary) (seronegative) (seropositive) (syphilitic) A51.0
- congenital A50.07
- conjunctiva NEC A51.2
- Ducrey's A57
- extragenital A51.2
- eyelid A51.2
- lip A51.2
- nipple A51.2
- Nisbet's A57
- of
  - carate A67.0
  - pinta A67.0
  - yaws A66.0
- palate, soft A51.2
- phagedenic A57
- simple A57
- soft A57
  - bubo A57
  - palate A51.2
- urethra A51.0
- yaws A66.0

Chancroid (anus) (genital) (penis) (perineum) (rectum) (urethra) (vulva) A57

Chandler's disease (osteochondritis dissecans, hip) —*see* Osteochondritis, dissecans, hip

Change(s) (in) (of) —*see also* Removal
- arteriosclerotic —*see* Arteriosclerosis
- bone —*see also* Disorder, bone
  - diabetic —*see* Diabetes, bone change

Change(s) *(continued)*
- bowel habit R19.4
- cardiorenal (vascular) —*see* Hypertension, cardiorenal
- cardiovascular —*see* Disease, cardiovascular
- circulatory I99.9
- cognitive (mild) (organic) R41.89
- color, tooth, teeth
  - during formation K00.8
  - posteruptive K03.7
- contraceptive device Z30.433
- corneal membrane H18.30
  - Bowman's membrane fold or rupture H18.31-
  - Descemet's membrane
    - fold H18.32-
    - rupture H18.33-
- coronary —*see* Disease, heart, ischemic
- degenerative, spine or vertebra —*see* Spondylosis
- dental pulp, regressive K04.2
- dressing (nonsurgical) Z48.00
  - surgical Z48.01
- heart —*see* Disease, heart
- hip joint —*see* Derangement, joint, hip
- hyperplastic larynx J38.7
- hypertrophic
  - nasal sinus J34.89
  - turbinate, nasal J34.3
  - upper respiratory tract J39.8
- indwelling catheter Z46.6
- inflammatory —*see also* Inflammation
  - sacroiliac M46.1
- job, anxiety concerning Z56.1
- joint —*see* Derangement, joint
- life —*see* Menopause
- mental status R41.82
- minimal (glomerular) (*see also* N00-N07 with fourth character .0) N05.0
- myocardium, myocardial —*see* Degeneration, myocardial
- of life —*see* Menopause
- pacemaker Z45.018
  - pulse generator Z45.010
- personality (enduring) F68.8
  - due to (secondary to)
    - general medical condition F07.0
  - secondary (nonspecific) F60.89
- regressive, dental pulp K04.2
- renal —*see* Disease, renal
- retina H35.9
  - myopic (*see also* Myopia, degenerative) H44.2-
- sacroiliac joint M53.3
- senile (*see also* condition) R54
- sensory R20.8
- skin R23.9
  - acute, due to ultraviolet radiation L56.9
    - specified NEC L56.8
  - chronic, due to nonionizing radiation L57.9
    - specified NEC L57.8
  - cyanosis R23.0
  - flushing R23.2
  - pallor R23.1
  - petechiae R23.3
  - specified change NEC R23.8
  - swelling —*see* Mass, localized
  - texture R23.4
- trophic
  - arm —*see* Mononeuropathy, upper limb
  - leg —*see* Mononeuropathy, lower limb
- vascular I99.9
- vasomotor I73.9

Change *(continued)*
voice R49.9
psychogenic F44.4
specified NEC R49.8
Changing sleep-work schedule, affecting sleep G47.26
Changuinola fever A93.1
Chapping skin T69.8
Charcot-Marie-Tooth disease, paralysis or syndrome G60.0
Charcot's
arthropathy *—see* Arthropathy, neuropathic
cirrhosis K74.3
disease (tabetic arthropathy) A52.16
joint (disease) (tabetic) A52.16
diabetic *—see* Diabetes, with, arthropathy
syringomyelic G95.0
syndrome (intermittent claudication) I73.9
CHARGE association Q89.8
Charley-horse (quadriceps) M62.831
traumatic (quadriceps) S76.11-
Charlouis' disease *—see* Yaws
Cheadle's disease E54
Checking (of)
cardiac pacemaker (battery) (electrode(s)) Z45.018
pulse generator Z45.010
implantable subdermal contraceptive Z30.46
intrauterine contraceptive device Z30.431
wound Z48.0-
due to injury - code to Injury, by site, using appropriate seventh character for subsequent encounter
Check-up *—see* Examination
Chédiak-Higashi (-Steinbrinck) **syndrome** (congenital gigantism of peroxidase granules) E70.330
Cheek *—see* condition
Cheese itch B88.0
Cheese-washer's lung J67.8
Cheese-worker's lung J67.8
Cheilitis (acute) (angular) (catarrhal) (chronic) (exfoliative) (gangrenous) (glandular) (infectional) (suppurative) (ulcerative) (vesicular) K13.0
actinic (due to sun) L56.8
other than from sun L59.8
candidal B37.83
Cheilodynia K13.0
Cheiloschisis *—see* Cleft, lip
Cheilosis (angular) K13.0
with pellagra E52
due to
vitamin B2(riboflavin) deficiency E53.0
Cheiromegaly M79.89
Cheiropompholyx L30.1
Cheloid *—see* Keloid
Chemical burn *—see* Corrosion, by site
Chemodectoma *—see* Paraganglioma, nonchromaffin
Chemosis, conjunctiva *—see* Edema, conjunctiva
Chemotherapy (session) (for)
cancer Z51.11
neoplasm Z51.11
Cherubism M27.8
Chest *—see* condition
Cheyne-Stokes breathing (respiration) R06.3
Chiari's
disease or syndrome (hepatic vein thrombosis) I82.0
malformation
type I G93.5
type II *—see* Spina bifida
net Q24.8
Chicago disease B40.9
Chickenpox *—see* Varicella
Chiclero ulcer or sore B55.1
Chigger (infestation) B88.0
Chignon (disease) B36.8
newborn (from vacuum extraction) (birth injury) P12.1
Chilaiditi's syndrome (subphrenic displacement, colon) Q43.3
Chilblain(s) (lupus) T69.1
Child
custody dispute Z65.3
Childbirth *—see* Delivery
Childhood
cerebral X-linked adrenoleukodystrophy E71.520
period of rapid growth Z00.2
Chill(s) R68.83
with fever R50.9
congestive in malarial regions B54
without fever R68.83
Chilomastigiasis A07.8
Chimera 46,XX/46,XY Q99.0
Chin *—see* condition
Chinese dysentery A03.9
Chionophobia F40.228
Chitral fever A93.1
Chlamydia, chlamydial A74.9
cervicitis A56.09
conjunctivitis A74.0
cystitis A56.01
endometritis A56.11
epididymitis A56.19
female
pelvic inflammatory disease A56.11
pelviperitonitis A56.11
orchitis A56.19
peritonitis A74.81
pharyngitis A56.4
proctitis A56.3
psittaci (infection) A70
salpingitis A56.11
sexually-transmitted infection NEC A56.8
specified NEC A74.89
urethritis A56.01
vulvovaginitis A56.02
Chlamydiosis *—see* Chlamydia
Chloasma (skin) (idiopathic) (symptomatic) L81.1
eyelid H02.719
hyperthyroid E05.90 *[H02.719]*
with thyroid storm E05.91 *[H02.719]*
left H02.716
lower H02.715
upper H02.714
right H02.713
lower H02.712
upper H02.711
Chloroma C92.3-
Chlorosis D50.9
Egyptian B76.9 *[D63.8]*
miner's B76.9 *[D63.8]*
Chlorotic anemia D50.8
Chocolate cyst (ovary) N80.1
Choked
disc or disk *—see* Papilledema
on food, phlegm, or vomitus NOS *—see* Foreign body, by site
while vomiting NOS *—see* Foreign body, by site
Chokes (resulting from bends) T70.3
Choking sensation R09.89
Cholangiectasis K83.8
Cholangiocarcinoma
with hepatocellular carcinoma, combined C22.0
liver C22.1
specified site NEC *—see* Neoplasm, malignant, by site
unspecified site C22.1
Cholangiohepatitis K83.8
due to fluke infestation B66.1
Cholangiohepatoma C22.0
Cholangiolitis (acute) (chronic) (extrahepatic) (gangrenous) (intrahepatic) K83.09
paratyphoidal *—see* Fever, paratyphoid
typhoidal A01.09
Cholangioma D13.4
malignant *—see* Cholangiocarcinoma
Cholangitis (ascending) (primary) (recurrent) (sclerosing) (secondary) (stenosing) (suppurative) K83.09
with calculus, bile duct *—see* Calculus, bile duct, with cholangitis
chronic nonsuppurative destructive K74.3
primary K83.09
sclerosing K83.01
sclerosing K83.09
Cholecystectasia K82.8
Cholecystitis K81.9
with
calculus, stones in
bile duct (common) (hepatic) *—see* Calculus, bile duct, with cholecystitis
cystic duct *—see* Calculus, gallbladder, with cholecystitis
gallbladder *—see* Calculus, gallbladder, with cholecystitis
choledocholithiasis *—see* Calculus, bile duct, with cholecystitis
cholelithiasis *—see* Calculus, gallbladder, with cholecystitis
gangrene of gallbladder K82.A1
perforation of gallbladder K82.A2
acute (emphysematous) (gangrenous) (suppurative) K81.0
with
calculus, stones in
cystic duct *—see* Calculus, gallbladder, with cholecystitis, acute
gallbladder *—see* Calculus, gallbladder, with cholecystitis, acute
choledocholithiasis *—see* Calculus, bile duct, with cholecystitis, acute
cholelithiasis *—see* Calculus, gallbladder, with cholecystitis, acute
chronic cholecystitis K81.2
Cholecystitis *(continued)*
acute *(continued)*
with *(continued)*
chronic cholecystitis *(continued)*
with gallbladder calculus K80.12
with obstruction K80.13
chronic K81.1
with acute cholecystitis K81.2
with gallbladder calculus K80.12
with obstruction K80.13
emphysematous (acute) *—see* Cholecystitis, acute
gangrenous *—see* Cholecystitis, acute
paratyphoidal, current A01.4
suppurative *—see* Cholecystitis, acute
typhoidal A01.09
Cholecystolithiasis *—see* Calculus, gallbladder
Choledochitis (suppurative) K83.09
Choledocholith *—see* Calculus, bile duct
Choledocholithiasis (common duct) (hepatic duct) *—see* Calculus, bile duct
cystic *—see* Calculus, gallbladder
typhoidal A01.09
Cholelithiasis (cystic duct) (gallbladder) (impacted) (multiple) *—see* Calculus, gallbladder
bile duct (common) (hepatic) *—see* Calculus, bile duct
hepatic duct *—see* Calculus, bile duct
specified NEC K80.80
with obstruction K80.81
Cholemia *—see also* Jaundice
familial (simple) (congenital) E80.4
Gilbert's E80.4
Choleperitoneum, choleperitonitis K65.3
Cholera (Asiatic) (epidemic) (malignant) A00.9
antimonial *—see* Poisoning, antimony
classical A00.0
due to Vibrio cholerae 01 A00.9
biovar cholerae A00.0
biovar eltor A00.1
el tor A00.1
el tor A00.1
Cholerine *—see* Cholera
Cholestasis NEC K83.1
with hepatocyte injury K71.0
due to total parenteral nutrition (TPN) K76.89
pure K71.0
Cholesteatoma (ear) (middle) (with reaction) H71.9-
attic H71.0-
external ear (canal) H60.4-
mastoid H71.2-
postmastoidectomy cavity (recurrent) *—see* Complications, postmastoidectomy, recurrent cholesteatoma
recurrent (postmastoidectomy) *—see* Complications, postmastoidectomy, recurrent cholesteatoma
tympanum H71.1-
Cholesteatosis, diffuse H71.3-
Cholesteremia E78.00

Cholesterin in vitreous —*see* Deposit, crystalline

Cholesterol
- deposit
  - retina H35.89
  - vitreous —*see* Deposit, crystalline
- elevated (high) E78.00
  - with elevated (high) triglycerides E78.2
  - screening for Z13.220
- imbibition of gallbladder K82.4

Cholesterolemia (essential) (pure) E78.00
- familial E78.01
- hereditary E78.01

Cholesterolosis, cholesterosis (gallbladder) K82.4
- cerebrotendinous E75.5

Cholocolic fistula K82.3

Choluria R82.2

Chondritis M94.8X9
- aurical H61.03-
- costal (Tietze's) M94.0
- external ear H61.03-
- patella, posttraumatic —*see* Chondromalacia, patella
- pinna H61.03-
- purulent M94.8X-
- tuberculous NEC A18.02
  - intervertebral A18.01

Chondroblastoma —*see also* Neoplasm, bone, benign
- malignant —*see* Neoplasm, bone, malignant

Chondrocalcinosis M11.20
- ankle M11.27-
- elbow M11.22-
- familial M11.10
  - ankle M11.17-
  - elbow M11.12-
  - foot joint M11.17-
  - hand joint M11.14-
  - hip M11.15-
  - knee M11.16-
  - multiple site M11.19
  - shoulder M11.11-
  - vertebrae M11.18
  - wrist M11.13-
- foot joint M11.27-
- hand joint M11.24-
- hip M11.25-
- knee M11.26-
- multiple site M11.29
- shoulder M11.21-
- vertebrae M11.28
- specified type NEC M11.20
  - ankle M11.27-
  - elbow M11.22-
  - foot joint M11.27-
  - hand joint M11.24-
  - hip M11.25-
  - knee M11.26-
  - multiple site M11.29
  - shoulder M11.21-
  - vertebrae M11.28
  - wrist M11.23-
- wrist M11.23-

Chondrodermatitis nodularis helicis or anthelicis —*see* Perichondritis, ear

Chondrodysplasia Q78.9
- with hemangioma Q78.4
- calcificans congenita Q77.3
- fetalis Q77.4
- metaphyseal (Jansen's) (McKusick's) (Schmid's) Q78.8
- punctata Q77.3

Chondrodystrophy, chondrodystrophia (familial) (fetalis) (hypoplastic) Q78.9
- calcificans congenita Q77.3
- myotonic (congenital) G71.13
- punctata Q77.3

Chondroectodermal dysplasia Q77.6

Chondrogenesis imperfecta Q77.4

Chondrolysis M94.35-

Chondroma —*see also* Neoplasm, cartilage, benign
- juxtacortical —*see* Neoplasm, bone, benign
- periosteal —*see* Neoplasm, bone, benign

Chondromalacia (systemic) M94.20
- acromioclavicular joint M94.21-
- ankle M94.27-
- elbow M94.22-
- foot joint M94.27-
- glenohumeral joint M94.21-
- hand joint M94.24-
- hip M94.25-
- knee M94.26-
  - patella M22.4-
- multiple sites M94.29
- patella M22.4-
- rib M94.28
- sacroiliac joint M94.259
- shoulder M94.21-
- sternoclavicular joint M94.21-
- vertebral joint M94.28
- wrist M94.23-

Chondromatosis —*see also* Neoplasm, cartilage, uncertain behavior
- internal Q78.4

Chondromyxosarcoma —*see* Neoplasm, cartilage, malignant

Chondro-osteodysplasia (Morquio-Brailsford type) E76.219

Chondro-osteodystrophy E76.29

Chondro-osteoma —*see* Neoplasm, bone, benign

Chondropathia tuberosa M94.0

Chondrosarcoma —*see* Neoplasm, cartilage, malignant
- juxtacortical —*see* Neoplasm, bone, malignant
- mesenchymal —*see* Neoplasm, connective tissue, malignant
- myxoid —*see* Neoplasm, cartilage, malignant

Chordee (nonvenereal) N48.89
- congenital Q54.4
- gonococcal A54.09

Chorditis (fibrinous) (nodosa) (tuberosa) J38.2

Chordoma —*see* Neoplasm, vertebral (column), malignant

Chorea (chronic) (gravis) (posthemiplegic) (senile) (spasmodic) G25.5
- with
  - heart involvement I02.0
    - active or acute (conditions in I01-) I02.0
    - rheumatic I02.9
      - with valvular disorder I02.0
  - rheumatic heart disease (chronic) (inactive) (quiescent) - code to rheumatic heart condition involved

Chorea *(continued)*
- drug-induced G25.4
- habit F95.8
- hereditary G10
- Huntington's G10
- hysterical F44.4
- minor I02.9
  - with heart involvement I02.0
- progressive G25.5
  - hereditary G10
- rheumatic (chronic) I02.9
  - with heart involvement I02.0
- Sydenham's I02.9
  - with heart involvement —*see* Chorea, with rheumatic heart disease
  - nonrheumatic G25.5

Choreoathetosis (paroxysmal) G25.5

Chorioadenoma (destruens) D39.2

Chorioamnionitis O41.12-

Chorioangioma D26.7

Choriocarcinoma —*see* Neoplasm, malignant, by site
- combined with
  - embryonal carcinoma —*see* Neoplasm, malignant, by site
  - other germ cell elements —*see* Neoplasm, malignant, by site
  - teratoma —*see* Neoplasm, malignant, by site
- specified site —*see* Neoplasm, malignant, by site
- unspecified site
  - female C58
  - male C62.90

Chorioencephalitis (acute) (lymphocytic) (serous) A87.2

Chorioepithelioma —*see* Choriocarcinoma

Choriomeningitis (acute) (lymphocytic) (serous) A87.2

Chorionepithelioma —*see* Choriocarcinoma

Chorioretinitis —*see also* Inflammation, chorioretinal
- disseminated —*see also* Inflammation, chorioretinal, disseminated
  - in neurosyphilis A52.19
- Egyptian B76.9 *[D63.8]*
- focal —*see also* Inflammation, chorioretinal, focal
- histoplasmic B39.9 *[H32]*
- in (due to)
  - histoplasmosis B39.9 *[H32]*
  - syphilis (secondary) A51.43
    - late A52.71
  - toxoplasmosis (acquired) B58.01
    - congenital (active) P37.1 *[H32]*
  - tuberculosis A18.53
- juxtapapillary, juxtapapillaris —*see* Inflammation, chorioretinal, focal, juxtapapillary
- leprous A30.9 *[H32]*
- miner's B76.9 *[D63.8]*
- progressive myopia (degeneration) (*see also* Myopia, degenerative) H44.2-
- syphilitic (secondary) A51.43
  - congenital (early) A50.01 *[H32]*
    - late A50.32
  - late A52.71
- tuberculous A18.53

Chorioretinopathy, central serous H35.71-

Choroid —*see* condition

Choroideremia H31.21

Choroiditis —*see* Chorioretinitis

Choroidopathy —*see* Disorder, choroid

Choroidoretinitis —*see* Chorioretinitis

Choroidoretinopathy, central serous —*see* Chorioretinopathy, central serous

Christian-Weber disease M35.6

Christmas disease D67

Chromaffinoma —*see also* Neoplasm, benign, by site
- malignant —*see* Neoplasm, malignant, by site

Chromatopsia —*see* Deficiency, color vision

Chromhidrosis, chromidrosis L75.1

Chromoblastomycosis —*see* Chromomycosis

Chromoconversion R82.91

Chromomycosis B43.9
- brain abscess B43.1
- cerebral B43.1
- cutaneous B43.0
- skin B43.0
- specified NEC B43.8
- subcutaneous abscess or cyst B43.2

Chromophytosis B36.0

Chromosome —*see* condition by chromosome involved
- D (1) —*see* condition, chromosome 13
- E (3) —*see* condition, chromosome 18
- G —*see* condition, chromosome 21

Chromotrichomycosis B36.8

Chronic —*see* condition
- fracture —*see* Fracture, pathological

Churg-Strauss syndrome M30.1

Chyle cyst, mesentery I89.8

Chylocele (nonfilarial) I89.8
- filarial (*see also* Infestation, filarial) B74.9 *[N51]*
- tunica vaginalis N50.89
  - filarial (*see also* Infestation, filarial) B74.9 *[N51]*

Chylomicronemia (fasting) (with hyperprebetalipoproteinemia) E78.3

Chylopericardium I31.3
- acute I30.9

Chylothorax (nonfilarial) J94.0
- filarial (*see also* Infestation, filarial) B74.9 *[J91.8]*

Chylous —*see* condition

Chyluria (nonfilarial) R82.0
- due to
  - bilharziasis B65.0
  - Brugia (malayi) B74.1
    - timori B74.2
  - schistosomiasis (bilharziasis) B65.0
  - Wuchereria (bancrofti) B74.0
- filarial —*see* Infestation, filarial

Cicatricial (deformity) —*see* Cicatrix

Cicatrix (adherent) (contracted) (painful) (vicious) (*see also* Scar) L90.5
- adenoid (and tonsil) J35.8
- alveolar process M26.79
- anus K62.89
- auricle —*see* Disorder, pinna, specified type NEC
- bile duct (common) (hepatic) K83.8
- bladder N32.89
- bone —*see* Disorder, bone, specified type NEC
- brain G93.89
- cervix (postoperative) (postpartal) N88.1
- common duct K83.8
- cornea H17.9
  - tuberculous A18.59
- duodenum (bulb), obstructive K31.5
- esophagus K22.2
- eyelid —*see* Disorder, eyelid function
- hypopharynx J39.2
- lacrimal passages —*see* Obstruction, lacrimal
- larynx J38.7
- lung J98.4
- middle ear H74.8
- mouth K13.79
- muscle M62.89
  - with contracture —*see* Contraction, muscle NEC
- nasopharynx J39.2
- palate (soft) K13.79
- penis N48.89
- pharynx J39.2
- prostate N42.89
- rectum K62.89
- retina —*see* Scar, chorioretinal
- semilunar cartilage —*see* Derangement, meniscus
- seminal vesicle N50.89
- skin L90.5
  - infected L08.89
  - postinfective L90.5
  - tuberculous B90.8
- specified site NEC L90.5
- throat J39.2
- tongue K14.8
- tonsil (and adenoid) J35.8
- trachea J39.8
- tuberculous NEC B90.9
- urethra N36.8
- uterus N85.8
- vagina N89.8
  - postoperative N99.2
- vocal cord J38.3
- wrist, constricting (annular) L90.5

CIDP (chronic inflammatory demyelinating polyneuropathy) G61.81

CIN —*see* Neoplasia, intraepithelial, cervix

CINCA (chronic infantile neurological, cutaneous and articular syndrome) M04.2

Cinchonism —*see* Deafness, ototoxic
- correct substance properly administered —*see* Table of Drugs and Chemicals, by drug, adverse effect
- overdose or wrong substance given or taken —*see* Table of Drugs and Chemicals, by drug, poisoning

Circle of Willis —*see* condition

Circular —*see* condition

Circulating anticoagulants (*see also* Disorder, hemorrhagic) D68.318
- due to drugs (*see also* Disorder, hemorrhagic) D68.32
- following childbirth O72.3

Circulation
- collateral, any site I99.8
- defective (lower extremity) I99.9
  - congenital Q28.9
- embryonic Q28.9
- failure (peripheral) R57.9
  - newborn P29.89
- fetal, persistent P29.38
- heart, incomplete Q28.9

Circulatory system —*see* condition

Circulus senilis (cornea) —*see* Degeneration, cornea, senile

Circumcision (in absence of medical indication) (ritual) (routine) Z41.2

Circumscribed —*see* condition

Circumvallate placenta O43.11-

Cirrhosis, cirrhotic (hepatic) (liver) K74.60
- alcoholic K70.30
  - with ascites K70.31
- atrophic —*see* Cirrhosis, liver
- Baumgarten-Cruveilhier K74.69
- biliary (cholangiolitic) (cholangitic) (hypertrophic) (obstructive) (pericholangiolitic) K74.5
  - due to
    - Clonorchiasis B66.1
    - flukes B66.3
  - primary K74.3
  - secondary K74.4
- cardiac (of liver) K76.1
- Charcot's K74.3
- cholangiolitic, cholangitic, cholostatic (primary) K74.3
- congestive K76.1
- Cruveilhier-Baumgarten K74.69
- cryptogenic (liver) K74.69
- due to
  - hepatolenticular degeneration E83.01
  - Wilson's disease E83.01
  - xanthomatosis E78.2
- fatty K76.0
  - alcoholic K70.0
- Hanot's (hypertrophic) K74.3
- hepatic —*see* Cirrhosis, liver
- hypertrophic K74.3
- Indian childhood K74.69
- kidney —*see* Sclerosis, renal
- Laennec's K70.30
  - with ascites K70.31
  - alcoholic K70.30
    - with ascites K70.31
  - nonalcoholic K74.69
- liver K74.60
  - alcoholic K70.30
    - with ascites K70.31
    - fatty K70.0
  - congenital P78.81
  - syphilitic A52.74
- lung (chronic) J84.10
- macronodular K74.69
  - alcoholic K70.30
    - with ascites K70.31
- micronodular K74.69
  - alcoholic K70.30
    - with ascites K70.31
- mixed type K74.69
- monolobular K74.3
- nephritis —*see* Sclerosis, renal
- nutritional K74.69
  - alcoholic K70.30
    - with ascites K70.31

Cirrhosis, cirrhotic *(continued)*
- obstructive —*see* Cirrhosis, biliary
- ovarian N83.8
- pancreas (duct) K86.89
- pigmentary E83.110
- portal K74.69
  - alcoholic K70.30
    - with ascites K70.31
- postnecrotic K74.69
  - alcoholic K70.30
    - with ascites K70.31
- pulmonary J84.10
- renal —*see* Sclerosis, renal
- spleen D73.2
- stasis K76.1
- Todd's K74.3
- unilobar K74.3
- xanthomatous (biliary) K74.5
  - due to xanthomatosis (familial) (metabolic) (primary) E78.2

Cistern, subarachnoid R93.0

Citrullinemia E72.23

Citrullinuria E72.23

Civatte's disease or poikiloderma L57.3

Clam digger's itch B65.3

Clammy skin R23.1

Clap —*see* Gonorrhea

Clarke-Hadfield syndrome (pancreatic infantilism) K86.89

Clark's paralysis G80.9

Clastothrix L67.8

Claude Bernard-Horner syndrome G90.2
- traumatic —*see* Injury, nerve, cervical sympathetic

Claude's disease or syndrome G46.3

Claudication (intermittent) I73.9
- cerebral (artery) G45.9
- spinal cord (arteriosclerotic) G95.19
  - syphilitic A52.09
- venous (axillary) I87.8

Claudicatio venosa intermittens I87.8

Claustrophobia F40.240

Clavus (infected) L84

Clawfoot (congenital) Q66.89
- acquired —*see* Deformity, limb, clawfoot

Clawhand (acquired) —*see also* Deformity, limb, clawhand
- congenital Q68.1

Clawtoe (congenital) Q66.89
- acquired —*see* Deformity, toe, specified NEC

Clay eating —*see* Pica

Cleansing of artificial opening —*see* Attention to, artificial, opening

Cleft (congenital) —*see also* Imperfect, closure
- alveolar process M26.79
- branchial (persistent) Q18.2
  - cyst Q18.0
    - fistula Q18.0
    - sinus Q18.0
- cricoid cartilage, posterior Q31.8
- foot Q72.7
- hand Q71.6
- lip (unilateral) Q36.9
  - with cleft palate Q37.9
    - hard Q37.1
      - with soft Q37.5
    - soft Q37.3
      - with hard Q37.5

Cleft *(continued)*
- lip *(continued)*
  - bilateral Q36.0
    - with cleft palate Q37.8
      - hard Q37.0
        - with soft Q37.4
      - soft Q37.2
        - with hard Q37.4
  - median Q36.1
- nose Q30.2
- palate Q35.9
  - with cleft lip (unilateral) Q37.9
    - bilateral Q37.8
  - hard Q35.1
    - with
      - cleft lip (unilateral) Q37.1
        - bilateral Q37.0
      - soft Q35.5
        - with cleft lip (unilateral) Q37.5
          - bilateral Q37.4
  - medial Q35.5
  - soft Q35.3
    - with
      - cleft lip (unilateral) Q37.3
        - bilateral Q37.2
      - hard Q35.5
        - with cleft lip (unilateral) Q37.5
          - bilateral Q37.4
- penis Q55.69
- scrotum Q55.29
- thyroid cartilage Q31.8
- uvula Q35.7

Cleidocranial dysostosis Q74.0

Cleptomania F63.2

Clicking hip (newborn) R29.4

Climacteric (female) —*see also* Menopause
- arthritis (any site) NEC —*see* Arthritis, specified form NEC
- depression (single episode) F32.89
  - recurrent episode F33.8
- melancholia (single episodie) F32.89
  - recurrent episode F33.8
- male (symptoms) (syndrome) NEC N50.89
- paranoid state F22
- polyarthritis NEC —*see* Arthritis, specified form NEC
- symptoms (female) N95.1

Clinical research investigation (clinical trial) (control subject) (normal comparison) (participant) Z00.6

Clitoris —*see* condition

Cloaca (persistent) Q43.7

Clonorchiasis, clonorchis infection (liver) B66.1

Clonus R25.8

Closed bite M26.29

Clostridium (C.) **perfringens, as cause of disease classified elsewhere** B96.7

Closure
- congenital, nose Q30.0
- cranial sutures, premature Q75.0
- defective or imperfect NEC —*see* Imperfect, closure
- fistula, delayed —*see* Fistula
- foramen ovale, imperfect Q21.1
- hymen N89.6
- interauricular septum, defective Q21.1
- interventricular septum, defective Q21.0

Closure *(continued)*
- lacrimal duct *—see also* Stenosis, lacrimal, duct
  - congenital Q10.5
- nose (congenital) Q30.0
  - acquired M95.0
- of artificial opening *—see* Attention to, artificial, opening
- primary angle, without glaucoma damage H40.06-
- vagina N89.5
- valve *—see* Endocarditis
- vulva N90.5

Clot (blood) *—see also* Embolism
- artery (obstruction) (occlusion) *—see* Embolism
- bladder N32.89
- brain (intradural or extradural) *—see* Occlusion, artery, cerebral
- circulation I74.9
- heart *—see also* Infarct, myocardium
  - not resulting in infarction I51.3
- vein *—see* Thrombosis

Clouded state R40.1
- epileptic *—see* Epilepsy, specified NEC
- paroxysmal *—see* Epilepsy, specified NEC

Cloudy antrum, antra J32.0

Clouston's (hidrotic) **ectodermal dysplasia** Q82.4

Clubbed nail pachydermoperiostosis M89.40 *[L62]*

Clubbing of finger(s) (nails) R68.3

Clubfinger R68.3
- congenital Q68.1

Clubfoot (congenital) Q66.89
- acquired *—see* Deformity, limb, clubfoot
- equinovarus Q66.0-
- paralytic *—see* Deformity, limb, clubfoot

Clubhand (congenital) (radial) Q71.4-
- acquired *—see* Deformity, limb, clubhand

Clubnail R68.3
- congenital Q84.6

Clump, kidney Q63.1

Clumsiness, clumsy child syndrome F82

Cluttering F80.81

Clutton's joints A50.51 *[M12.80]*

Coagulation, intravascular (diffuse) (disseminated) *—see also* Defibrination syndrome
- complicating abortion *—see* Abortion, by type, complicated by, intravascular coagulation
- following ectopic or molar pregnancy O08.1

Coagulopathy *—see also* Defect, coagulation
- consumption D65
- intravascular D65
  - newborn P60

Coalition
- calcaneo-scaphoid Q66.89
- tarsal Q66.89

Coalminer's
- elbow *—see* Bursitis, elbow, olecranon
- lung or pneumoconiosis J60

Coalworker's lung or pneumoconiosis J60

Coarctation
- aorta (preductal) (postductal) Q25.1
- pulmonary artery Q25.71

Coated tongue K14.3

Coats' disease (exudative retinopathy) *—see* Retinopathy, exudative

Cocaine-induced
- anxiety disorder F14.980
- bipolar and related disorder F14.94
- depressive disorder F14.94
- obsessive-compulsive and related disorder F14.988
- psychotic disorder F14.959
- sleep disorder F14.982
- sexual dysfunction F14.981

Cocainism *—see* Disorder, cocaine use

Coccidioidomycosis B38.9
- cutaneous B38.3
- disseminated B38.7
- generalized B38.7
- meninges B38.4
- prostate B38.81
- pulmonary B38.2
  - acute B38.0
  - chronic B38.1
- skin B38.3
- specified NEC B38.89

Coccidioidosis *—see* Coccidioidomycosis

Coccidiosis (intestinal) A07.3

Coccydynia, coccygodynia M53.3

Coccyx *—see* condition

Cochin-China diarrhea K90.1

Cockayne's syndrome Q87.19

Cocked up toe *—see* Deformity, toe, specified NEC

Cock's peculiar tumor L72.3

Codman's tumor *—see* Neoplasm, bone, benign

Coenurosis B71.8

Coffee-worker's lung J67.8

Cogan's syndrome H16.32-
- oculomotor apraxia H51.8

Coitus, painful (female) N94.10
- male N53.12
- psychogenic F52.6

Cold J00
- with influenza, flu, or grippe *—see* Influenza, with, respiratory manifestations NEC
- agglutinin disease or hemoglobinuria (chronic) D59.12
- bronchial *—see* Bronchitis
- chest *—see* Bronchitis
- common (head) J00
- effects of T69.9
  - specified effect NEC T69.8
- excessive, effects of T69.9
  - specified effect NEC T69.8
- exhaustion from T69.8
- exposure to T69.9
  - specified effect NEC T69.8
- head J00
- injury syndrome (newborn) P80.0
- on lung *—see* Bronchitis
- rose J30.1
- sensitivity, auto-immune D59.12
- symptoms J00
- virus J00

Coldsore B00.1

Colibacillosis A49.8
- as the cause of other disease (*see also* Escherichia coli) B96.20
- generalized A41.50

Colic (bilious) (infantile) (intestinal) (recurrent) (spasmodic) R10.83
- abdomen R10.83
  - psychogenic F45.8
- appendix, appendicular K38.8
- bile duct *—see* Calculus, bile duct
- biliary *—see* Calculus, bile duct
- common duct *—see* Calculus, bile duct
- cystic duct *—see* Calculus, gallbladder
- Devonshire NEC *—see* Poisoning, lead
- gallbladder *—see* Calculus, gallbladder
- gallstone *—see* Calculus, gallbladder
  - gallbladder or cystic duct *—see* Calculus, gallbladder
- hepatic (duct) *—see* Calculus, bile duct
- hysterical F45.8
- kidney N23
- lead NEC *—see* Poisoning, lead
- mucous K58.9
  - with diarrhea K58.0
  - psychogenic F54
- nephritic N23
- painter's NEC *—see* Poisoning, lead
- pancreas K86.89
- psychogenic F45.8
- renal N23
- saturnine NEC *—see* Poisoning, lead
- ureter N23
- urethral N36.8
  - due to calculus N21.1
- uterus NEC N94.89
  - menstrual *—see* Dysmenorrhea
- worm NOS B83.9

Colicystitis *—see* Cystitis

Colitis (acute) (catarrhal) (chronic) (noninfective) (hemorrhagic) (*see also* Enteritis) K52.9
- allergic K52.29
  - with
    - food protein-induced enterocolitis syndrome K52.21
    - proctocolitis K52.29
- amebic (acute) (*see also* Amebiasis) A06.0
  - nondysenteric A06.2
- anthrax A22.2
- bacillary *—see* Infection, Shigella
- balantidial A07.0
- Clostridium difficile
  - not specified as recurrent A04.72
  - recurrent A04.71
- coccidial A07.3
- collagenous K52.831
- cystica superficialis K52.89
- dietary counseling and surveillance (for) Z71.3
- dietetic (*see also* Colitis, allergic) K52.29
- drug-induced K52.1
- due to radiation K52.0
- eosinophilic K52.82
- food hypersensitivity (*see also* Colitis, allergic) K52.29
- giardial A07.1
- granulomatous *—see* Enteritis, regional, large intestine

Colitis *(continued)*
- indeterminate, so stated K52.3
- infectious *—see* Enteritis, infectious
- ischemic K55.9
  - acute (subacute) (*see also* Ischemia, intestine, acute) K55.039
  - chronic K55.1
  - due to mesenteric artery insufficiency K55.1
  - fulminant (acute) (*see also* Ischemia, intestine, acute) K55.039
- left sided K51.50
  - with
    - abscess K51.514
    - complication K51.519
      - specified NEC K51.518
    - fistula K51.513
    - obstruction K51.512
    - rectal bleeding K51.511
- lymphocytic K52.832
- membranous
  - psychogenic F54
- microscopic K52.839
  - specified NEC K52.838
- mucous *—see* Syndrome, irritable, bowel
  - psychogenic F54
- noninfective K52.9
  - specified NEC K52.89
- polyposa *—see* Polyp, colon, inflammatory
- protozoal A07.9
- pseudomembranous
  - not specified as recurrent A04.72
  - recurrent A04.71
- pseudomucinous *—see* Syndrome, irritable, bowel
- regional *—see* Enteritis, regional, large intestine
  - infectious A09
- segmental *—see* Enteritis, regional, large intestine
- septic *—see* Enteritis, infectious
- spastic K58.9
  - with diarrhea K58.0
  - psychogenic F54
- staphylococcal A04.8
  - foodborne A05.0
- subacute ischemic (*see also* Ischemia, intestine, acute) K55.039
- thromboulcerative (*see also* Ischemia, intestine, acute) K55.039
- toxic NEC K52.1
  - due to Clostridium difficile
    - not specified as recurrent A04.72
    - recurrent A04.71
- transmural *—see* Enteritis, regional, large intestine
- trichomonal A07.8
- tuberculous (ulcerative) A18.32
- ulcerative (chronic) K51.90
  - with
    - complication K51.919
      - abscess K51.914
      - fistula K51.913
      - obstruction K51.912
      - rectal bleeding K51.911
      - specified complication NEC K51.918
  - enterocolitis *—see* Enterocolitis, ulcerative
  - ileocolitis *—see* Ileocolitis, ulcerative
  - mucosal proctocolitis *—see* Proctocolitis, mucosal

Colitis *(continued)*
- ulcerative *(continued)*
  - proctitis —*see* Proctitis, ulcerative
  - pseudopolyposis —*see* Polyp, colon, inflammatory
  - psychogenic F54
  - rectosigmoiditis —*see* Rectosigmoiditis, ulcerative
  - specified type NEC K51.80
    - with
      - complication K51.819
        - abscess K51.814
        - fistula K51.813
        - obstruction K51.812
        - rectal bleeding K51.811
        - specified complication NEC K51.818

Collagenosis, collagen disease (nonvascular) (vascular) M35.9
- cardiovascular I42.8
- reactive perforating L87.1
- specified NEC M35.89

Collapse R55
- adrenal E27.2
- cardiorespiratory R57.0
- cardiovascular R57.0
  - newborn P29.89
- circulatory (peripheral) R57.9
  - during or after labor and delivery O75.1
  - following ectopic or molar pregnancy O08.3
  - newborn P29.89
- during or
  - after labor and delivery O75.1
  - resulting from a procedure, not elsewhere classified T81.10
- external ear canal —*see* Stenosis, external ear canal
- general R55
- heart —*see* Disease, heart
- heat T67.1
- hysterical F44.89
- labyrinth, membranous (congenital) Q16.5
- lung (massive) (*see also* Atelectasis) J98.19
  - pressure due to anesthesia (general) (local) or other sedation T88.2
    - during labor and delivery O74.1
    - in pregnancy O29.02-
    - postpartum, puerperal O89.09
- myocardial —*see* Disease, heart
- nervous F48.8
- neurocirculatory F45.8
- nose M95.0
- postoperative T81.10
- pulmonary (*see also* Atelectasis) J98.19
  - newborn —*see* Atelectasis
- trachea J39.8
- tracheobronchial J98.09
- valvular —*see* Endocarditis
- vascular (peripheral) R57.9
  - during or after labor and delivery O75.1
  - following ectopic or molar pregnancy O08.3
  - newborn P29.89
- vertebra M48.50-
  - cervical region M48.52-
  - cervicothoracic region M48.53-
  - in (due to)
    - metastasis —*see* Collapse, vertebra, in, specified disease NEC

Collapse *(continued)*
- vertebra *(continued)*
  - in *(continued)*
    - osteoporosis (*see also* Osteoporosis) M80.88
      - cervical region M80.88
      - cervicothoracic region M80.88
      - lumbar region M80.88
      - lumbosacral region M80.88
      - multiple sites M80.88
      - occipito-atlanto-axial region M80.88
      - sacrococcygeal region M80.88
      - thoracic region M80.88
      - thoracolumbar region M80.88
    - specified disease NEC M48.50-
      - cervical region M48.52-
      - cervicothoracic region M48.53-
      - lumbar region M48.56-
      - lumbosacral region M48.57-
      - occipito-atlanto-axial region M48.51-
      - sacrococcygeal region M48.58-
      - thoracic region M48.54-
      - thoracolumbar region M48.55-
  - lumbar region M48.56-
  - lumbosacral region M48.57-
  - occipito-atlanto-axial region M48.51-
  - sacrococcygeal region M48.58-
  - thoracic region M48.54-
  - thoracolumbar region M48.55-

Collateral —*see also* condition
- circulation (venous) I87.8
- dilation, veins I87.8

Colles' fracture S52.53-

Collet (-Sicard) **syndrome** G52.7

Collier's asthma or lung J60

Collodion baby Q80.2

Colloid nodule (of thyroid) (cystic) E04.1

Coloboma (iris) Q13.0
- eyelid Q10.3
- fundus Q14.8
- lens Q12.2
- optic disc (congenital) Q14.2
  - acquired H47.31-

Coloenteritis —*see* Enteritis

Colon —*see* condition

Colonization
- MRSA (Methicillin resistant Staphylococcus aureus) Z22.322
- MSSA (Methicillin susceptible Staphylococcus aureus) Z22.321
- status —*see* Carrier (suspected) of

Coloptosis K63.4

Color blindness —*see* Deficiency, color vision

Colostomy
- attention to Z43.3
- fitting or adjustment Z46.89
- malfunctioning K94.03
- status Z93.3

Colpitis (acute) —*see* Vaginitis

Colpocele N81.5

Colpocystitis —*see* Vaginitis

Colpospasm N94.2

Column, spinal, vertebral —*see* condition

Coma R40.20
- with
  - motor response (none) R40.231
    - abnormal R40.233
    - abnormal extensor posturing to pain or noxious stimuli (<2 years of age) R40.232
    - abnormal flexure posturing to pain or noxious stimuli (0-5 years of age) R40.233
    - extension R40.232
    - extensor posturing to pain or noxious stimuli (2-5 years of age) R40.232
    - flexion/decorticate posturing (<2 years of age) R40.233
    - flexion withdrawal R40.234
    - localizes pain (2-5 years of age) R40.235
    - normal or spontaneous movement (<2 years of age) R40.236
    - obeys commands (2-5 years of age) R40.236
    - score of
      - 1 R40.231
      - 2 R40.232
      - 3 R40.233
      - 4 R40.234
      - 5 R40.235
      - 6 R40.236
    - withdraws from pain or noxious stimuli (0-5 years of age) R40.234
    - withdraws to touch (<2 years of age) R40.235
  - opening of eyes (never) R40.211
    - in response to pain R40.212
      - sound R40.213
    - score of
      - 1 R40.211
      - 2 R40.212
      - 3 R40.213
      - 4 R40.214
    - spontaneous R40.214
  - verbal response (none) R40.221
    - confused conversation R40.224
    - cooing or babbling or crying appropriately (<2 years of age) R40.225
    - inappropriate crying or screaming (<2 years of age) R40.223
    - inappropriate words (2-5 years of age) R40.224
    - incomprehensible sounds (2-5 years of age) R40.222
    - incomprehensible words R40.222
    - irritable cries (<2 years of age) R40.224
    - moans/grunts to pain; restless (<2 years of age) R40.222
    - oriented R40.225
    - score of
      - 1 R40.221
      - 2 R40.222
      - 3 R40.223
      - 4 R40.224
      - 5 R40.225
    - screaming (2-5 years of age) R40.223
    - uses appropriate words (2-5 years of age) R40.225
- eclamptic —*see* Eclampsia
- epileptic —*see* Epilepsy
- Glasgow, scale score —*see* Glasgow coma scale
- hepatic —*see* Failure, hepatic, by type, with coma

Coma *(continued)*
- hyperglycemic (diabetic) —*see* Diabetes, by type, with hyperosmolarity, with coma
- hyperosmolar (diabetic) —*see* Diabetes, by type, with hyperosmolarity, with coma
- hypoglycemic (diabetic) —*see* Diabetes, by type, with hypoglycemia, with coma
  - nondiabetic E15
- in diabetes —*see* Diabetes, coma
- insulin-induced —*see* Coma, hypoglycemic
- ketoacidotic (diabetic) —*see* Diabetes, by type, with ketoacidosis, with coma
- myxedematous E03.5
- newborn P91.5
- persistent vegetative state R40.3
- specified NEC, without documented Glasgow coma scale score, or with partial Glasgow coma scale score reported R40.244

Comatose —*see* Coma

Combat fatigue F43.0

Combined —*see* condition

Comedo, comedones (giant) L70.0

Comedocarcinoma —*see also* Neoplasm, breast, malignant
- noninfiltrating
  - breast D05.8-
  - specified site —*see* Neoplasm, in situ, by site
  - unspecified site D05.8-

Comedomastitis —*see* Ectasia, mammary duct

Comminuted fracture - code as Fracture, closed

Common
- arterial trunk Q20.0
- atrioventricular canal Q21.2
- atrium Q21.1
- cold (head) J00
- truncus (arteriosus) Q20.0
- variable immunodeficiency —*see* Immunodeficiency, common variable
- ventricle Q20.4

Commotio, commotion (current)
- brain —*see* Injury, intracranial, concussion
- cerebri —*see* Injury, intracranial, concussion
- retinae S05.8X-
- spinal cord —*see* Injury, spinal cord, by region
- spinalis —*see* Injury, spinal cord, by region

Communication
- between
  - base of aorta and pulmonary artery Q21.4
  - left ventricle and right atrium Q20.5
  - pericardial sac and pleural sac Q34.8
  - pulmonary artery and pulmonary vein, congenital Q25.72
- congenital between uterus and digestive or urinary tract Q51.7

Compartment syndrome (deep) (posterior) (traumatic) T79.A0
- abdomen T79.A3
- lower extremity (hip, buttock, thigh, leg, foot, toes) T79.A2
- nontraumatic
  - abdomen M79.A3

Compartment syndrome *(continued)*
nontraumatic *(continued)*
lower extremity (hip, buttock, thigh, leg, foot, toes) M79.A2-
specified site NEC M79.A9
upper extremity (shoulder, arm, forearm, wrist, hand, fingers) M79.A1-
specified site NEC T79.A9
upper extremity (shoulder, arm, forearm, wrist, hand, fingers) T79.A1

Compensation
failure *—see* Disease, heart
neurosis, psychoneurosis *—see* Disorder, factitious

Complaint *—see also* Disease
bowel, functional K59.9
psychogenic F45.8
intestine, functional K59.9
psychogenic F45.8
kidney *—see* Disease, renal
miners' J60

Complete *—see* condition

Complex
Addison-Schilder E71.528
cardiorenal *—see* Hypertension, cardiorenal
Costen's M26.69
disseminated mycobacterium avium- intracellulare (DMAC) A31.2
Eisenmenger's (ventricular septal defect) I27.83
hypersexual F52.8
jumped process, spine *—see* Dislocation, vertebra
primary, tuberculous A15.7
Schilder-Addison E71.528
subluxation (vertebral) M99.19
abdomen M99.19
acromioclavicular M99.17
cervical region M99.11
cervicothoracic M99.11
costochondral M99.18
costovertebral M99.18
head region M99.10
hip M99.15
lower extremity M99.16
lumbar region M99.13
lumbosacral M99.13
occipitocervical M99.10
pelvic region M99.15
pubic M99.15
rib cage M99.18
sacral region M99.14
sacrococcygeal M99.14
sacroiliac M99.14
specified NEC M99.19
sternochondral M99.18
sternoclavicular M99.17
thoracic region M99.12
thoracolumbar M99.12
upper extremity M99.17
Taussig-Bing (transposition, aorta and overriding pulmonary artery) Q20.1

Complication(s) (from) (of)
accidental puncture or laceration during a procedure (of) *—see* Complications, intraoperative (intraprocedural), puncture or laceration
amputation stump (surgical) (late) NEC T87.9
dehiscence T87.81
infection or inflammation T87.40
lower limb T87.4-
upper limb T87.4-

Complication(s) *(continued)*
amputation stump *(continued)*
necrosis T87.50
amputation stump (surgical)
lower limb T87.5-
upper limb T87.5-
neuroma T87.30
lower limb T87.3-
upper limb T87.3-
specified type NEC T87.89
anastomosis (and bypass) *—see also* Complications, prosthetic device or implant
intestinal (internal) NEC K91.89
involving urinary tract N99.89
urinary tract (involving intestinal tract) N99.89
vascular *—see* Complications, cardiovascular device or implant
anesthesia, anesthetic (*see also* Anesthesia, complication) T88.59
general, unintended awareness during procedure T88.53
unintended awareness under general anesthesia during procedure T88.53
brain, postpartum, puerperal O89.2
cardiac
in
labor and delivery O74.2
pregnancy O29.19-
postpartum, puerperal O89.1
central nervous system
in
labor and delivery O74.3
pregnancy O29.29-
postpartum, puerperal O89.2
difficult or failed intubation T88.4
in pregnancy O29.6-
failed sedation (conscious) (moderate) during procedure T88.52
hyperthermia, malignant T88.3
hypothermia T88.51
intubation failure T88.4
malignant hyperthermia T88.3
pulmonary
in
labor and delivery O74.1
pregnancy NEC O29.09-
postpartum, puerperal O89.09
shock T88.2
spinal and epidural
in
labor and delivery NEC O74.6
headache O74.5
pregnancy NEC O29.5X-
postpartum, puerperal NEC O89.5
headache O89.4
anti-reflux device *—see* Complications, esophageal anti-reflux device
aortic (bifurcation) graft *—see* Complications, graft, vascular
aortocoronary (bypass) graft *—see* Complications, coronary artery (bypass) graft
aortofemoral (bypass) graft *—see* Complications, extremity artery (bypass) graft
arteriovenous
fistula, surgically created T82.9
embolism T82.818
fibrosis T82.828
hemorrhage T82.838
infection or inflammation T82.7
mechanical
breakdown T82.510

Complication *(continued)*
arteriovenous *(continued)*
fistula, surgically created *(continued)*
mechanical *(continued)*
displacement T82.520
leakage T82.530
malposition T82.520
obstruction T82.590
perforation T82.590
protrusion T82.590
pain T82.848
specified type NEC T82.898
stenosis T82.858
thrombosis T82.868
shunt, surgically created T82.9
embolism T82.818
fibrosis T82.828
hemorrhage T82.838
infection or inflammation T82.7
mechanical
breakdown T82.511
displacement T82.521
leakage T82.531
malposition T82.521
obstruction T82.591
perforation T82.591
protrusion T82.591
pain T82.848
specified type NEC T82.898
stenosis T82.858
thrombosis T82.868
arthroplasty *—see* Complications, joint prosthesis
artificial
fertilization or insemination N98.9
attempted introduction (of)
embryo in embryo transfer N98.3
ovum following in vitro fertilization N98.2
hyperstimulation of ovaries N98.1
infection N98.0
specified NEC N98.8
heart T82.9
embolism T82.817
fibrosis T82.827
hemorrhage T82.837
infection or inflammation T82.7
mechanical
breakdown T82.512
displacement T82.522
leakage T82.532
malposition T82.522
obstruction T82.592
perforation T82.592
protrusion T82.592
pain T82.847
specified type NEC T82.897
stenosis T82.857
thrombosis T82.867
opening
cecostomy *—see* Complications, colostomy
colostomy *—see* Complications, colostomy
cystostomy *—see* Complications, cystostomy
enterostomy *—see* Complications, enterostomy
gastrostomy *—see* Complications, gastrostomy
ileostomy *—see* Complications, enterostomy
jejunostomy *—see* Complications, enterostomy
nephrostomy *—see* Complications, stoma, urinary tract

Complication *(continued)*
artificial *(continued)*
opening *(continued)*
tracheostomy *—see* Complications, tracheostomy
ureterostomy *—see* Complications, stoma, urinary tract
urethrostomy *—see* Complications, stoma, urinary tract
balloon implant or device
gastrointestinal T85.9
embolism T85.818
fibrosis T85.828
hemorrhage T85.838
infection and inflammation T85.79
pain T85.848
specified type NEC T85.898
stenosis T85.858
thrombosis T85.868
vascular (counterpulsation) T82.9
embolism T82.818
fibrosis T82.828
hemorrhage T82.838
infection or inflammation T82.7
mechanical
breakdown T82.513
displacement T82.523
leakage T82.533
malposition T82.523
obstruction T82.593
perforation T82.593
protrusion T82.593
pain T82.848
specified type NEC T82.898
stenosis T82.858
thrombosis T82.868
bariatric procedure
gastric band procedure K95.09
infection K95.01
specified procedure NEC K95.89
infection K95.81
bile duct implant (prosthetic) T85.9
embolism T85.818
fibrosis T85.828
hemorrhage T85.838
infection and inflammation T85.79
mechanical
breakdown T85.510
displacement T85.520
malfunction T85.510
malposition T85.520
obstruction T85.590
perforation T85.590
protrusion T85.590
specified NEC T85.590
pain T85.848
specified type NEC T85.898
stenosis T85.858
thrombosis T85.868
bladder device (auxiliary) *—see* Complications, genitourinary, device or implant, urinary system
bleeding (postoperative) *—see* Complication, postoperative, hemorrhage
intraoperative *—see* Complication, intraoperative, hemorrhage
blood vessel graft *—see* Complications, graft, vascular
bone
device NEC T84.9
embolism T84.81
fibrosis T84.82

Complication *(continued)*
bone *(continued)*
device NEC *(continued)*
hemorrhage T84.83
infection or inflammation T84.7
mechanical
breakdown T84.318
displacement T84.328
malposition T84.328
obstruction T84.398
perforation T84.398
protrusion T84.398
pain T84.84
specified type NEC T84.89
stenosis T84.85
thrombosis T84.86
graft *—see* Complications, graft, bone
growth stimulator (electrode) *—see* Complications, electronic stimulator device, bone
marrow transplant *—see* Complications, transplant, bone, marrow
brain neurostimulator (electrode) *—see* Complications, electronic stimulator device, brain
breast implant (prosthetic) T85.9
capsular contracture T85.44
embolism T85.818
fibrosis T85.828
hemorrhage T85.838
infection and inflammation T85.79
mechanical
breakdown T85.41
displacement T85.42
leakage T85.43
malposition T85.42
obstruction T85.49
perforation T85.49
protrusion T85.49
specified NEC T85.49
pain T85.848
specified type NEC T85.898
stenosis T85.858
thrombosis T85.868
bypass *—see also* Complications, prosthetic device or implant
aortocoronary *—see* Complications, coronary artery (bypass) graft
arterial *—see also* Complications, graft, vascular
extremity *—see* Complications, extremity artery (bypass) graft
cardiac *—see also* Disease, heart
device, implant or graft T82.9
embolism T82.817
fibrosis T82.827
hemorrhage T82.837
infection or inflammation T82.7
valve prosthesis T82.6
mechanical
breakdown T82.519
specified device NEC T82.518
displacement T82.529
specified device NEC T82.528
leakage T82.539
specified device NEC T82.538
malposition T82.529
specified device NEC T82.528
obstruction T82.599
specified device NEC T82.598
perforation T82.599
specified device NEC T82.598

Complication *(continued)*
cardiac *—see also* Disease, heart *(continued)*
device, implant or graft *(continued)*
mechanical *(continued)*
protrusion T82.599
specified device NEC T82.598
pain T82.847
specified type NEC T82.897
stenosis T82.857
thrombosis T82.867
cardiovascular device, graft or implant T82.9
aortic graft *—see* Complications, graft, vascular
arteriovenous
fistula, artificial *—see* Complication, arteriovenous, fistula, surgically created
shunt *—see* Complication, arteriovenous, shunt, surgically created
artificial heart *—see* Complication, artificial, heart
balloon (counterpulsation) device *—see* Complication, balloon implant, vascular
carotid artery graft *—see* Complications, graft, vascular
coronary bypass graft *—see* Complication, coronary artery (bypass) graft
dialysis catheter (vascular) *—see* Complication, catheter, dialysis
electronic T82.9
electrode T82.9
embolism T82.817
fibrosis T82.827
hemorrhage T82.837
infection T82.7
mechanical
breakdown T82.110
displacement T82.120
leakage T82.190
obstruction T82.190
perforation T82.190
protrusion T82.190
specified type NEC T82.190
pain T82.847
specified NEC T82.897
stenosis T82.857
thrombosis T82.867
embolism T82.817
fibrosis T82.827
hemorrhage T82.837
infection T82.7
mechanical
breakdown T82.119
displacement T82.129
leakage T82.199
obstruction T82.199
perforation T82.199
protrusion T82.199
specified type NEC T82.199
pain T82.847
pulse generator T82.9
embolism T82.817
fibrosis T82.827
hemorrhage T82.837
infection T82.7
mechanical
breakdown T82.111
displacement T82.121
leakage T82.191
obstruction T82.191
perforation T82.191
protrusion T82.191
specified type NEC T82.191

Complication *(continued)*
cardiovascular device, graft or implant *(continued)*
electronic *(continued)*
pulse generator *(continued)*
pain T82.847
specified NEC T82.897
stenosis T82.857
thrombosis T82.867
specified condition NEC T82.897
specified device NEC T82.9
embolism T82.817
fibrosis T82.827
hemorrhage T82.837
infection T82.7
mechanical
breakdown T82.118
displacement T82.128
leakage T82.198
obstruction T82.198
perforation T82.198
protrusion T82.198
specified type NEC T82.198
pain T82.847
specified NEC T82.897
stenosis T82.857
thrombosis T82.867
stenosis T82.857
thrombosis T82.867
extremity artery graft *—see* Complication, extremity artery (bypass) graft
femoral artery graft *—see* Complication, extremity artery (bypass) graft
heart-lung transplant *—see* Complication, transplant, heart, with lung
heart
transplant *—see* Complication, transplant, heart
valve *—see* Complication, prosthetic device, heart valve
graft *—see* Complication, heart, valve, graft
infection or inflammation T82.7
umbrella device *—see* Complication, umbrella device, vascular
vascular graft (or anastomosis) *—see* Complication, graft, vascular
carotid artery (bypass) graft *—see* Complications, graft, vascular
catheter (device) NEC *—see also* Complications, prosthetic device or implant
cranial infusion
infection and inflammation T85.735
mechanical
breakdown T85.610
displacement T85.620
leakage T85.630
malfunction T85.690
malposition T85.620
obstruction T85.690
perforation T85.690
protrusion T85.690
specified NEC T85.690
cystostomy T83.9
embolism T83.81
fibrosis T83.82
hemorrhage T83.83
infection and inflammation T83.510
mechanical
breakdown T83.010
displacement T83.020

Complication *(continued)*
catheter (device) NEC *(continued)*
cystostomy *(continued)*
mechanical *(continued)*
leakage T83.030
malposition T83.020
obstruction T83.090
perforation T83.090
protrusion T83.090
specified NEC T83.090
pain T83.84
specified type NEC T83.89
stenosis T83.85
thrombosis T83.86
dialysis (vascular) T82.9
embolism T82.818
fibrosis T82.828
hemorrhage T82.838
infection and inflammation T82.7
intraperitoneal *—see* Complications, catheter, intraperitoneal
mechanical
breakdown T82.41
displacement T82.42
leakage T82.43
malposition T82.42
obstruction T82.49
perforation T82.49
protrusion T82.49
pain T82.848
specified type NEC T82.898
stenosis T82.858
thrombosis T82.868
epidural infusion T85.9
embolism T85.810
fibrosis T85.820
hemorrhage T85.830
infection and inflammation T85.735
mechanical
breakdown T85.610
displacement T85.620
leakage T85.630
malfunction T85.610
malposition T85.620
obstruction T85.690
perforation T85.690
protrusion T85.690
specified NEC T85.690
pain T85.840
specified type NEC T85.890
stenosis T85.850
thrombosis T85.860
intraperitoneal dialysis T85.9
embolism T85.818
fibrosis T85.828
hemorrhage T85.838
infection and inflammation T85.735
mechanical
breakdown T85.611
displacement T85.621
leakage T85.631
malfunction T85.611
malposition T85.621
obstruction T85.691
perforation T85.691
protrusion T85.691
specified NEC T85.691
pain T85.848
specified type NEC T85.898
stenosis T85.858
thrombosis T85.868
intrathecal infusion
infection and inflammation T85.735
mechanical
breakdown T85.610
displacement T85.620
leakage T85.630

Complication *(continued)*
- catheter (device) NEC *(continued)*
  - intrathecal infusion *(continued)*
    - mechanical *(continued)*
      - malfunction T85.690
      - malposition T85.620
      - obstruction T85.690
      - perforation T85.690
      - protrusion T85.690
      - specified NEC T85.690
  - intravenous infusion T82.9
    - embolism T82.818
    - fibrosis T82.828
    - hemorrhage T82.838
    - infection or inflammation T82.7
    - mechanical
      - breakdown T82.514
      - displacement T82.524
      - leakage T82.534
      - malposition T82.524
      - obstruction T82.594
      - perforation T82.594
      - protrusion T82.594
    - pain T82.848
    - specified type NEC T82.898
    - stenosis T82.858
    - thrombosis T82.868
  - spinal infusion
    - infection and inflammation T85.735
    - mechanical
      - breakdown T85.610
      - displacement T85.620
      - leakage T85.630
      - malfunction T85.690
      - malposition T85.620
      - obstruction T85.690
      - perforation T85.690
      - protrusion T85.690
      - specified NEC T85.690
  - subarachnoid infusion
    - infection and inflammation T85.735
    - mechanical
      - breakdown T85.610
      - displacement T85.620
      - leakage T85.630
      - malfunction T85.690
      - malposition T85.620
      - obstruction T85.690
      - perforation T85.690
      - protrusion T85.690
      - specified NEC T85.690
  - subdural infusion T85.9
    - embolism T85.810
    - fibrosis T85.820
    - hemorrhage T85.830
    - infection and inflammation T85.735
    - mechanical
      - breakdown T85.610
      - displacement T85.620
      - leakage T85.630
      - malfunction T85.610
      - malposition T85.620
      - obstruction T85.690
      - perforation T85.690
      - protrusion T85.690
      - specified NEC T85.690
    - pain T85.840
    - specified type NEC T85.890
    - stenosis T85.850
    - thrombosis T85.860
  - urethral T83.9
    - displacement T83.028
    - embolism T83.81
    - fibrosis T83.82
    - hemorrhage T83.83
    - indwelling
      - breakdown T83.011
      - displacement T83.021

Complication *(continued)*
- catheter (device) NEC *(continued)*
  - urethral *(continued)*
    - indwelling *(continued)*
      - infection and inflammation T83.511
      - leakage T83.031
      - specified complication NEC T83.091
    - infection and inflammation T83.511
    - leakage T83.038
    - malposition T83.028
    - mechanical
      - breakdown T83.011
    - obstruction (mechanical) T83.091
    - pain T83.84
    - perforation T83.091
    - protrusion T83.091
    - specified type NEC T83.091
    - stenosis T83.85
    - thrombosis T83.86
  - urinary NEC
    - breakdown T83.018
    - displacement T83.028
    - infection and inflammation T83.518
    - leakage T83.038
    - specified complication NEC T83.098
- cecostomy (stoma) —*see* Complications, colostomy
- cesarean delivery wound NEC O90.89
  - disruption O90.0
  - hematoma O90.2
  - infection (following delivery) O86.00
- chemotherapy (antineoplastic) NEC T88.7
- chimeric antigen receptor (CAR-T) cell therapy T80.82
- chin implant (prosthetic) —*see* Complication, prosthetic device or implant, specified NEC
- circulatory system I99.8
  - intraoperative I97.88
  - postprocedural I97.89
    - following cardiac surgery (*see also* Infarct, myocardium, associated with revascularization procedure) I97.19-
      - postcardiotomy syndrome I97.0
    - hypertension I97.3
    - lymphedema after mastectomy I97.2
    - postcardiotomy syndrome I97.0
    - seroma —*see* Complications, postprocedural, seroma (of), mastoid process
    - specified NEC I97.89
- colostomy (stoma) K94.00
  - hemorrhage K94.01
  - infection K94.02
  - malfunction K94.03
  - mechanical K94.03
  - specified complication NEC K94.09
- contraceptive device, intrauterine —*see* Complications, intrauterine, contraceptive device
- cord (umbilical) —*see* Complications, umbilical cord
- corneal graft —*see* Complications, graft, cornea
- coronary artery (bypass) graft T82.9

Complication *(continued)*
- coronary artery (bypass) graft *(continued)*
  - atherosclerosis —*see* Arteriosclerosis, coronary (artery)
  - embolism T82.818
  - fibrosis T82.828
  - hemorrhage T82.838
  - infection and inflammation T82.7
  - mechanical
    - breakdown T82.211
    - displacement T82.212
    - leakage T82.213
    - malposition T82.212
    - obstruction T82.218
    - perforation T82.218
    - protrusion T82.218
    - specified NEC T82.218
  - pain T82.848
  - specified type NEC T82.898
  - stenosis T82.858
  - thrombosis T82.868
- counterpulsation device (balloon), intra- aortic —*see* Complications, balloon implant, vascular
- cystostomy (stoma) N99.518
  - catheter —*see* Complications, catheter, cystostomy
  - hemorrhage N99.510
  - infection N99.511
  - malfunction N99.512
  - specified type NEC N99.518
- delivery (*see also* Complications, obstetric) O75.9
  - procedure (instrumental) (manual) (surgical) O75.4
  - specified NEC O75.89
- dialysis (peritoneal) (renal) —*see also* Complications, infusion
  - catheter (vascular) —*see* Complication, catheter, dialysis
    - peritoneal, intraperitoneal —*see* Complications, catheter, intraperitoneal
- dorsal column (spinal) neurostimulator —*see* Complications, electronic stimulator device, spinal cord
- drug NEC T88.7
- ear procedure —*see also* Disorder, ear
  - intraoperative H95.88
    - hematoma —*see* Complications, intraoperative, hemorrhage (hematoma) (of), ear
    - hemorrhage —*see* Complications, intraoperative, hemorrhage (hematoma) (of), ear
    - laceration —*see* Complications, intraoperative, puncture or laceration..., ear
    - specified NEC H95.88
  - postoperative H95.89
    - external ear canal stenosis H95.81-
    - hematoma —*see* Complications, postprocedural, hematoma (of), ear
    - hemorrhage —*see* Complications, postprocedural, hemorrhage (of), ear
    - postmastoidectomy —*see* Complications, postmastoidectomy

Complication *(continued)*
- ear procedure *(continued)*
  - postoperative *(continued)*
    - specified NEC H95.89
    - seroma — *see* Complications, postprocedural, seroma (of), mastoid process
- ectopic pregnancy O08.9
  - damage to pelvic organs O08.6
  - embolism O08.2
  - genital infection O08.0
  - hemorrhage (delayed) (excessive) O08.1
  - metabolic disorder O08.5
  - renal failure O08.4
  - shock O08.3
  - specified type NEC O08.0
  - venous complication NEC O08.7
- electronic stimulator device
  - bladder (urinary) —*see* Complications, electronic stimulator device, urinary
  - bone T84.9
    - breakdown T84.310
    - displacement T84.320
    - embolism T84.81
    - fibrosis T84.82
    - hemorrhage T84.83
    - infection or inflammation T84.7
    - malfunction T84.310
    - malposition T84.320
    - mechanical NEC T84.390
    - obstruction T84.390
    - pain T84.84
    - perforation T84.390
    - protrusion T84.390
    - specified type NEC T84.89
    - stenosis T84.85
    - thrombosis T84.86
  - brain T85.9
    - embolism T85.810
    - fibrosis T85.820
    - hemorrhage T85.830
    - infection and inflammation T85.731
    - mechanical
      - breakdown T85.110
      - displacement T85.120
      - leakage T85.190
      - malposition T85.120
      - obstruction T85.190
      - perforation T85.190
      - protrusion T85.190
      - specified NEC T85.190
    - pain T85.840
    - specified type NEC T85.890
    - stenosis T85.850
    - thrombosis T85.860
  - cardiac (defibrillator) (pacemaker) —*see* Complications, cardiovascular device or implant, electronic
  - generator (brain) (gastric) (peripheral) (sacral) (spinal)
    - breakdown T85.113
    - displacement T85.123
    - leakage T85.193
    - malposition T85.123
    - obstruction T85.193
    - perforation T85.193
    - protrusion T85.193
    - specified NEC T85.193
  - muscle T84.9
    - breakdown T84.418
    - displacement T84.428
    - embolism T84.81
    - fibrosis T84.82
    - hemorrhage T84.83

Complication *(continued)*
- electronic stimulator device *(continued)*
  - muscle *(continued)*
    - infection or inflammation T84.7
    - mechanical NEC T84.498
    - pain T84.84
    - specified type NEC T84.89
    - stenosis T84.85
    - thrombosis T84.86
  - nervous system T85.9
    - brain *—see* Complications, electronic stimulator device, brain
    - cranial nerve *—see* Complications, electronic stimulator device, peripheral nerve
    - embolism T85.810
    - fibrosis T85.820
    - gastric nerve *—see* Complications, electronic stimulator device, peripheral nerve
    - hemorrhage T85.830
    - infection and inflammation T85.738
    - mechanical
      - breakdown T85.118
      - displacement T85.128
      - leakage T85.199
      - malposition T85.128
      - obstruction T85.199
      - perforation T85.199
      - protrusion T85.199
      - specified NEC T85.199
    - pain T85.840
    - peripheral nerve *—see* Complications, electronic stimulator device, peripheral nerve
    - sacral nerve *—see* Complications, electronic stimulator device, peripheral nerve
    - specified type NEC T85.890
    - spinal cord *—see* Complications, electronic stimulator device, spinal cord
    - stenosis T85.850
    - thrombosis T85.860
    - vagal nerve *—see* Complications, electronic stimulator device, peripheral nerve
  - peripheral nerve T85.9
    - embolism T85.810
    - fibrosis T85.820
    - hemorrhage T85.830
    - infection and inflammation T85.732
    - mechanical
      - breakdown T85.111
      - displacement T85.121
      - leakage T85.191
      - malposition T85.121
      - obstruction T85.191
      - perforation T85.191
      - protrusion T85.191
      - specified NEC T85.191
    - pain T85.840
    - specified type NEC T85.890
    - stenosis T85.850
    - thrombosis T85.860
  - spinal cord T85.9
    - embolism T85.810
    - fibrosis T85.820
    - hemorrhage T85.830

Complication *(continued)*
- electronic stimulator device *(continued)*
  - spinal cord *(continued)*
    - infection and inflammation T85.733
    - mechanical
      - breakdown T85.112
      - displacement T85.122
      - leakage T85.192
      - malposition T85.122
      - obstruction T85.192
      - perforation T85.192
      - protrusion T85.192
      - specified NEC T85.192
    - pain T85.840
    - specified type NEC T85.890
    - stenosis T85.850
    - thrombosis T85.860
  - urinary T83.9
    - embolism T83.81
    - fibrosis T83.82
    - hemorrhage T83.83
    - infection and inflammation T83.598
    - mechanical
      - breakdown T83.110
      - displacement T83.120
      - malposition T83.120
      - perforation T83.190
      - protrusion T83.190
      - specified NEC T83.190
    - pain T83.84
    - specified type NEC T83.89
    - stenosis T83.85
    - thrombosis T83.86
- electroshock therapy T88.9
  - specified NEC T88.8
- endocrine E34.9
  - postprocedural
    - adrenal hypofunction E89.6
    - hypoinsulinemia E89.1
    - hypoparathyroidism E89.2
    - hypopituitarism E89.3
    - hypothyroidism E89.0
    - ovarian failure E89.40
      - asymptomatic E89.40
      - symptomatic E89.41
    - specified NEC E89.89
    - testicular hypofunction E89.5
- endodontic treatment NEC M27.59
- enterostomy (stoma) K94.10
  - hemorrhage K94.11
  - infection K94.12
  - malfunction K94.13
  - mechanical K94.13
  - specified complication NEC K94.19
- episiotomy, disruption O90.1
- esophageal anti-reflux device T85.9
  - embolism T85.818
  - fibrosis T85.828
  - hemorrhage T85.838
  - infection and inflammation T85.79
  - mechanical
    - breakdown T85.511
    - displacement T85.521
    - malfunction T85.511
    - malposition T85.521
    - obstruction T85.591
    - perforation T85.591
    - protrusion T85.591
    - specified NEC T85.591
  - pain T85.848
  - specified type NEC T85.898
  - stenosis T85.858
  - thrombosis T85.868
- esophagostomy K94.30
  - hemorrhage K94.31

Complication *(continued)*
- esophagostomy *(continued)*
  - infection K94.32
  - malfunction K94.33
  - mechanical K94.33
  - specified complication NEC K94.39
- extracorporeal circulation T80.90
- extremity artery (bypass) graft T82.9
  - arteriosclerosis *—see* Arteriosclerosis, extremities, bypass graft
  - embolism T82.818
  - fibrosis T82.828
  - hemorrhage T82.838
  - infection and inflammation T82.7
  - mechanical
    - breakdown T82.318
      - femoral artery T82.312
    - displacement T82.328
      - femoral artery T82.322
    - leakage T82.338
      - femoral artery T82.332
    - malposition T82.328
      - femoral artery T82.322
    - obstruction T82.398
      - femoral artery T82.392
    - perforation T82.398
      - femoral artery T82.392
    - protrusion T82.398
      - femoral artery T82.392
  - pain T82.848
  - specified type NEC T82.898
  - stenosis T82.858
  - thrombosis T82.868
- eye H57.9
  - corneal graft *—see* Complications, graft, cornea
  - implant (prosthetic) T85.9
    - embolism T85.818
    - fibrosis T85.828
    - hemorrhage T85.838
    - infection and inflammation T85.79
    - mechanical
      - breakdown T85.318
      - displacement T85.328
      - leakage T85.398
      - malposition T85.328
      - obstruction T85.398
      - perforation T85.398
      - protrusion T85.398
      - specified NEC T85.398
    - pain T85.848
    - specified type NEC T85.898
    - stenosis T85.858
    - thrombosis T85.868
  - intraocular lens *—see* Complications, intraocular lens
  - orbital prosthesis *—see* Complications, orbital prosthesis
- female genital N94.9
  - device, implant or graft NEC *—see* Complications, genitourinary, device or implant, genital tract
- femoral artery (bypass) graft *—see* Complication, extremity artery (bypass) graft
- fixation device, internal (orthopedic) T84.9
  - infection and inflammation T84.60
    - arm T84.61-
      - humerus T84.61-
      - radius T84.61-
      - ulna T84.61-

Complication *(continued)*
- fixation device, internal *(continued)*
  - infection and inflammation *(continued)*
    - leg T84.629
      - femur T84.62-
      - fibula T84.62-
      - tibia T84.62-
    - specified site NEC T84.69
    - spine T84.63
  - mechanical
    - breakdown
      - limb T84.119
        - carpal T84.210
        - femur T84.11-
        - fibula T84.11-
        - humerus T84.11-
        - metacarpal T84.210
        - metatarsal T84.213
        - phalanx
          - foot T84.213
          - hand T84.210
        - radius T84.11-
        - tarsal T84.213
        - tibia T84.11-
        - ulna T84.11-
      - specified bone NEC T84.218
      - spine T84.216
    - displacement
      - limb T84.129
        - carpal T84.220
        - femur T84.12-
        - fibula T84.12-
        - humerus T84.12-
        - metacarpal T84.220
        - metatarsal T84.223
        - phalanx
          - foot T84.223
          - hand T84.220
        - radius T84.12-
        - tarsal T84.223
        - tibia T84.12-
        - ulna T84.12-
      - specified bone NEC T84.228
      - spine T84.226
    - malposition *—see* Complications, fixation device, internal, mechanical, displacement
    - obstruction *—see* Complications, fixation device, internal, mechanical, specified type NEC
    - perforation *—see* Complications, fixation device, internal, mechanical, specified type NEC
    - protrusion *—see* Complications, fixation device, internal, mechanical, specified type NEC
    - specified type NEC
      - limb T84.199
        - carpal T84.290
        - femur T84.19-
        - fibula T84.19-
        - humerus T84.19-
        - metacarpal T84.290
        - metatarsal T84.293
        - phalanx
          - foot T84.293
          - hand T84.290
        - radius T84.19-
        - tarsal T84.293
        - tibia T84.19-
        - ulna T84.19-
      - specified bone NEC T84.298
      - vertebra T84.296

Complication *(continued)*
fixation device, internal *(continued)*
specified type NEC T84.89
embolism T84.81
fibrosis T84.82
hemorrhage T84.83
pain T84.84
specified complication NEC T84.89
stenosis T84.85
thrombosis T84.86
following
acute myocardial infarction NEC I23.8
aneurysm (false) (of cardiac wall) (of heart wall) (ruptured) I23.3
angina I23.7
atrial
septal defect I23.1
thrombosis I23.6
cardiac wall rupture I23.3
chordae tendinae rupture I23.4
defect
septal
atrial (heart) I23.1
ventricular (heart) I23.2
hemopericardium I23.0
papillary muscle rupture I23.5
rupture
cardiac wall I23.3
with hemopericardium I23.0
chordae tendineae I23.4
papillary muscle I23.5
specified NEC I23.8
thrombosis
atrium I23.6
auricular appendage I23.6
ventricle (heart) I23.6
ventricular
septal defect I23.2
thrombosis I23.6
ectopic or molar pregnancy O08.9
cardiac arrest O08.81
sepsis O08.82
specified type NEC O08.89
urinary tract infection O08.83
termination of pregnancy *—see* Abortion
gastrointestinal K92.9
bile duct prosthesis *—see* Complications, bile duct implant
esophageal anti-reflux device *—see* Complications, esophageal anti-reflux device
postoperative
colostomy *—see* Complications, colostomy
dumping syndrome K91.1
enterostomy *—see* Complications, enterostomy
gastrostomy *—see* Complications, gastrostomy
malabsorption NEC K91.2
obstruction (*see also* Obstruction, intestine, postoperative) K91.30
postcholecystectomy syndrome K91.5
specified NEC K91.89
vomiting after GI surgery K91.0
prosthetic device or implant
bile duct prosthesis *—see* Complications, bile duct implant

Complication *(continued)*
gastrointestinal *(continued)*
prosthetic device or implant *(continued)*
esophageal anti-reflux device *—see* Complications, esophageal anti-reflux device
specified type NEC
embolism T85.818
fibrosis T85.828
hemorrhage T85.838
mechanical
breakdown T85.518
displacement T85.528
malfunction T85.518
malposition T85.528
obstruction T85.598
perforation T85.598
protrusion T85.598
specified NEC T85.598
pain T85.848
specified complication NEC T85.898
stenosis T85.858
thrombosis T85.868
gastrostomy (stoma) K94.20
hemorrhage K94.21
infection K94.22
malfunction K94.23
mechanical K94.23
specified complication NEC K94.29
genitourinary
device or implant T83.9
genital tract T83.9
infection or inflammation T83.69
intrauterine contraceptive device *—see* Complications, intrauterine, contraceptive device
mechanical *—see* Complications, by device, mechanical
mesh *—see* Complications, prosthetic device or implant, mesh
penile prosthesis *—see* Complications, prosthetic device, penile
specified type NEC T83.89
embolism T83.81
fibrosis T83.82
hemorrhage T83.83
pain T83.84
specified complication NEC T83.89
stenosis T83.85
thrombosis T83.86
vaginal mesh *—see* Complications, prosthetic device or implant mesh
urinary system T83.9
cystostomy catheter *—see* Complication, catheter, cystostomy
electronic stimulator *—see* Complications, electronic stimulator device, urinary
indwelling urethral catheter *—see* Complications, catheter, urethral, indwelling
infection or inflammation T83.598
indwelling urethral catheter T83.511

Complication *(continued)*
genitourinary *(continued)*
device or implant *(continued)*
urinary system *(continued)*
kidney transplant *—see* Complication, transplant, kidney
organ graft *—see* Complication, graft, urinary organ
specified type NEC T83.89
embolism T83.81
fibrosis T83.82
hemorrhage T83.83
mechanical T83.198
breakdown T83.118
displacement T83.128
malfunction T83.118
malposition T83.128
obstruction T83.198
perforation T83.198
protrusion T83.198
specified NEC T83.198
sphincter implant *—see* Complications, implant, urinary sphincter
sphincter, implanted T83.191
stent (ileal conduit) (nephroureteral) T83.193
pain T83.84
specified complication NEC T83.89
stenosis T83.85
thrombosis T83.86
ureteral indwelling T83.192
postprocedural
pelvic peritoneal adhesions N99.4
renal failure N99.0
specified NEC N99.89
stoma *—see* Complications, stoma, urinary tract
urethral stricture *—see* Stricture, urethra, postprocedural
vaginal
adhesions N99.2
vault prolapse N99.3
graft (bypass) (patch) *—see also* Complications, prosthetic device or implant
aorta *—see* Complications, graft, vascular
arterial *—see* Complication, graft, vascular
bone T86.839
failure T86.831
infection T86.832
mechanical T84.318
breakdown T84.318
displacement T84.328
protrusion T84.398
specified type NEC T84.398
rejection T86.830
specified type NEC T86.838
carotid artery *—see* Complications, graft, vascular
cornea T86.849-
failure T86.841-
infection T86.842-
mechanical T85.398
breakdown T85.318
displacement T85.328
protrusion T85.398
specified type NEC T85.398-
rejection T86.840-
retroprosthetic membrane T85.398
specified type NEC T86.848-

Complication *(continued)*
graft *(continued)*
femoral artery (bypass) *—see* Complication, extremity artery (bypass) graft
genital organ or tract *—see* Complications, genitourinary, device or implant, genital tract
muscle T84.9
breakdown T84.410
displacement T84.420
embolism T84.81
fibrosis T84.82
hemorrhage T84.83
infection and inflammation T84.7
mechanical NEC T84.490
pain T84.84
specified type NEC T84.89
stenosis T84.85
thrombosis T84.86
nerve *—see* Complication, prosthetic device or implant, specified NEC
skin *—see* Complications, prosthetic device or implant, skin graft
tendon T84.9
breakdown T84.410
displacement T84.420
embolism T84.81
fibrosis T84.82
hemorrhage T84.83
infection and inflammation T84.7
mechanical NEC T84.490
pain T84.84
specified type NEC T84.89
stenosis T84.85
thrombosis T84.86
urinary organ T83.9
embolism T83.81
fibrosis T83.82
hemorrhage T83.83
infection and inflammation T83.598
indwelling urethral catheter T83.511
mechanical
breakdown T83.21
displacement T83.22
erosion T83.24
exposure T83.25
leakage T83.23
malposition T83.22
obstruction T83.29
perforation T83.29
protrusion T83.29
specified NEC T83.29
pain T83.84
specified type NEC T83.89
stenosis T83.85
thrombosis T83.86
vascular T82.9
embolism T82.818
femoral artery *—see* Complication, extremity artery (bypass) graft
fibrosis T82.828
hemorrhage T82.838
mechanical
breakdown T82.319
aorta (bifurcation) T82.310
carotid artery T82.311
specified vessel NEC T82.318

- **Complication** *(continued)*
  - graft *(continued)*
    - vascular *(continued)*
      - mechanical *(continued)*
        - displacement T82.329
          - aorta (bifurcation) T82.320
          - carotid artery T82.321
          - specified vessel NEC T82.328
        - leakage T82.339
          - aorta (bifurcation) T82.330
          - carotid artery T82.331
          - specified vessel NEC T82.338
        - malposition T82.329
          - aorta (bifurcation) T82.320
          - carotid artery T82.321
          - specified vessel NEC T82.328
        - obstruction T82.399
          - aorta (bifurcation) T82.390
          - carotid artery T82.391
          - specified vessel NEC T82.398
        - perforation T82.399
          - aorta (bifurcation) T82.390
          - carotid artery T82.391
          - specified vessel NEC T82.398
        - protrusion T82.399
          - aorta (bifurcation) T82.390
          - carotid artery T82.391
          - specified vessel NEC T82.398
      - pain T82.848
      - specified complication NEC T82.898
      - stenosis T82.858
      - thrombosis T82.868
  - heart I51.9
    - assist device
      - infection and inflammation T82.7
    - following acute myocardial infarction *—see* Complications, following, acute myocardial infarction
    - postoperative *—see* Complications, circulatory system
    - transplant *—see* Complication, transplant, heart
      - and lung(s) *—see* Complications, transplant, heart, with lung
    - valve
      - graft (biological) T82.9
        - embolism T82.817
        - fibrosis T82.827
        - hemorrhage T82.837
        - infection and inflammation T82.7
        - mechanical T82.228
          - breakdown T82.221
          - displacement T82.222
          - leakage T82.223
          - malposition T82.222
          - obstruction T82.228
          - perforation T82.228
          - protrusion T82.228
        - pain T82.847
        - specified type NEC T82.897
        - stenosis T82.857
        - thrombosis T82.867
      - prosthesis T82.9
        - embolism T82.817

- **Complication** *(continued)*
  - heart *(continued)*
    - valve *(continued)*
      - prosthesis *(continued)*
        - fibrosis T82.827
        - hemorrhage T82.837
        - infection or inflammation T82.6
        - mechanical T82.09
          - breakdown T82.01
          - displacement T82.02
          - leakage T82.03
          - malposition T82.02
          - obstruction T82.09
          - perforation T82.09
          - protrusion T82.09
        - pain T82.847
        - specified type NEC T82.897
          - mechanical T82.09
        - stenosis T82.857
        - thrombosis T82.867
  - hematoma
    - intraoperative *—see* Complication, intraoperative, hemorrhage
    - postprocedural *—see* Complication, postprocedural, hematoma
  - hemodialysis *—see* Complications, dialysis
  - hemorrhage
    - intraoperative *—see* Complication, intraoperative, hemorrhage
    - postprocedural *—see* Complication, postprocedural, hemorrhage
  - IEC (immune effector cellular) therapy T80.82
  - ileostomy (stoma) *—see* Complications, enterostomy
  - immune effector cellular (IEC) therapy T80.82
  - immunization (procedure) *—see* Complications, vaccination
  - implant *—see also* Complications, by site and type
    - urinary sphincter T83.9
      - embolism T83.81
      - fibrosis T83.82
      - hemorrhage T83.83
      - infection and inflammation T83.591
      - mechanical
        - breakdown T83.111
        - displacement T83.121
        - leakage T83.191
        - malposition T83.121
        - obstruction T83.191
        - perforation T83.191
        - protrusion T83.191
        - specified NEC T83.191
      - pain T83.84
      - specified type NEC T83.89
      - stenosis T83.85
      - thrombosis T83.86
  - infusion (procedure) T80.90
    - air embolism T80.0
    - blood *—see* Complications, transfusion
    - catheter *—see* Complications, catheter
    - infection T80.29
    - pump *—see* Complications, cardiovascular, device or implant
    - sepsis T80.29
    - serum reaction (*see also* Reaction, serum) T80.69

- **Complication** *(continued)*
  - infusion *(continued)*
    - serum reaction *(continued)*
      - anaphylactic shock (*see also* Shock, anaphylactic) T80.59
    - specified type NEC T80.89
  - inhalation therapy NEC T81.81
  - injection (procedure) T80.90
    - drug reaction *—see* Reaction, drug
    - infection T80.29
    - sepsis T80.29
    - serum (prophylactic) (therapeutic) *—see* Complications, vaccination
    - specified type NEC T80.89
    - vaccine (any) *—see* Complications, vaccination
  - inoculation (any) *—see* Complications, vaccination
  - insulin pump
    - infection and inflammation T85.72
    - mechanical
      - breakdown T85.614
      - displacement T85.624
      - leakage T85.633
      - malposition T85.624
      - obstruction T85.694
      - perforation T85.694
      - protrusion T85.694
      - specified NEC T85.694
  - intestinal pouch NEC K91.858
  - intraocular lens (prosthetic) T85.9
    - embolism T85.818
    - fibrosis T85.828
    - hemorrhage T85.838
    - infection and inflammation T85.79
    - mechanical
      - breakdown T85.21
      - displacement T85.22
      - malposition T85.22
      - obstruction T85.29
      - perforation T85.29
      - protrusion T85.29
      - specified NEC T85.29
    - pain T85.848
    - specified type NEC T85.898
    - stenosis T85.858
    - thrombosis T85.868
  - intraoperative (intraprocedural)
    - cardiac arrest *—see also* Infarct, myocardium, associated with revascularization procedure
      - during cardiac surgery I97.710
      - during other surgery I97.711
    - cardiac functional disturbance NEC *—see also* Infarct, myocardium, associated with revascularization procedure
      - during cardiac surgery I97.790
      - during other surgery I97.791
    - hemorrhage (hematoma) (of)
      - circulatory system organ or structure
        - during cardiac bypass I97.411
        - during cardiac catheterization I97.410
        - during other circulatory system procedure I97.418
        - during other procedure I97.42
      - digestive system organ
        - during procedure on digestive system K91.61
        - during procedure on other organ K91.62

- **Complication** *(continued)*
  - intraoperative *(continued)*
    - hemorrhage *(continued)*
      - ear
        - during procedure on ear and mastoid process H95.21
        - during procedure on other organ H95.22
      - endocrine system organ or structure
        - during procedure on endocrine system organ or structure E36.01
        - during procedure on other organ E36.02
      - eye and adnexa
        - during ophthalmic procedure H59.11-
        - during other procedure H59.12-
      - genitourinary organ or structure
        - during procedure on genitourinary organ or structure N99.61
        - during procedure on other organ N99.62
      - mastoid process
        - during procedure on ear and mastoid process H95.21
        - during procedure on other organ H95.22
      - musculoskeletal structure
        - during musculoskeletal surgery M96.810
        - during non-orthopedic surgery M96.811
        - during orthopedic surgery M96.810
      - nervous system
        - during a nervous system procedure G97.31
        - during other procedure G97.32
      - respiratory system
        - during other procedure J95.62
        - during procedure on respiratory system organ or structure J95.61
      - skin and subcutaneous tissue
        - during a dermatologic procedure L76.01
        - during a procedure on other organ L76.02
      - spleen
        - during a procedure on other organ D78.02
        - during a procedure on the spleen D78.01
    - puncture or laceration (accidental) (unintentional) (of)
      - brain
        - during a nervous system procedure G97.48
        - during other procedure G97.49
      - circulatory system organ or structure
        - during circulatory system procedure I97.51
        - during other procedure I97.52
      - digestive system
        - during procedure on digestive system K91.71
        - during procedure on other organ K91.72
      - ear
        - during procedure on ear and mastoid process H95.31
        - during procedure on other organ H95.32

- **Complication** *(continued)*
  - intraoperative *(continued)*
    - puncture or laceration *(continued)*
      - endocrine system organ or structure
        - during procedure on endocrine system organ or structure E36.11
        - during procedure on other organ E36.12
      - eye and adnexa
        - during ophthalmic procedure H59.21-
        - during other procedure H59.22-
      - genitourinary organ or structure
        - during procedure on genitourinary organ or structure N99.71
        - during procedure on other organ N99.72
      - mastoid process
        - during procedure on ear and mastoid process H95.31
        - during procedure on other organ H95.32
      - musculoskeletal structure
        - during musculoskeletal surgery M96.820
        - during non-orthopedic surgery M96.821
        - during orthopedic surgery M96.820
      - nervous system
        - during a nervous system procedure G97.48
        - during other procedure G97.49
      - respiratory system
        - during other procedure J95.72
        - during procedure on respiratory system organ or structure J95.71
      - skin and subcutaneous tissue
        - during a dermatologic procedure L76.11
        - during a procedure on other organ L76.12
      - spleen
        - during a procedure on other organ D78.12
        - during a procedure on the spleen D78.11
    - specified NEC
      - circulatory system I97.88
      - digestive system K91.81
      - ear H95.88
      - endocrine system E36.8
      - eye and adnexa H59.88
      - genitourinary system N99.81
      - mastoid process H95.88
      - musculoskeletal structure M96.89
      - nervous system G97.81
      - respiratory system J95.88
      - skin and subcutaneous tissue L76.81
      - spleen D78.81
  - intraperitoneal catheter (dialysis) (infusion) *—see* Complication(s), catheter, intraperitoneal dialysis
  - intrathecal infusion pump
    - infection and inflammation T85.738
    - mechanical
      - breakdown T85.615
      - displacement T85.625
      - leakage T85.635
      - malfunction T85.695
      - malposition T85.625

- **Complication** *(continued)*
  - intrathecal infusion pump *(continued)*
    - mechanical *(continued)*
      - obstruction T85.695
      - perforation T85.695
      - protrusion T85.695
      - specified NEC T85.695
  - intrauterine
    - contraceptive device
      - embolism T83.81
      - fibrosis T83.82
      - hemorrhage T83.83
      - infection and inflammation T83.69
      - mechanical
        - breakdown T83.31
        - displacement T83.32
        - malposition T83.32
        - obstruction T83.39
        - perforation T83.39
        - protrusion T83.39
        - specified NEC T83.39
      - pain T83.84
      - specified type NEC T83.89
      - stenosis T83.85
      - thrombosis T83.86
    - procedure (fetal), to newborn P96.5
  - jejunostomy (stoma) *—see* Complications, enterostomy
  - joint prosthesis, internal T84.9
    - breakage (fracture) T84.01-
    - dislocation T84.02-
    - fracture T84.01-
    - infection or inflammation T84.50
      - hip T84.5-
      - knee T84.5-
      - specified joint NEC T84.59
    - instability T84.02-
    - malposition *—see* Complications, joint prosthesis, mechanical, displacement
    - mechanical
      - breakage, broken T84.01-
      - dislocation T84.02-
      - fracture T84.01-
      - instability T84.02-
      - leakage *—see* Complications, joint prosthesis, mechanical, specified NEC
      - loosening T84.039
        - hip T84.03-
        - knee T84.03-
        - specified joint NEC T84.038
      - obstruction *—see* Complications, joint prosthesis, mechanical, specified NEC
      - perforation *—see* Complications, joint prosthesis, mechanical, specified NEC
      - osteolysis T84.059
        - hip T84.05-
        - knee T84.05-
        - other specified joint T84.058
      - periprosthetic osteolysis T84.059
      - protrusion *—see* Complications, joint prosthesis, mechanical, specified NEC
      - specified complication NEC T84.099
        - hip T84.09-
        - knee T84.09-
        - other specified joint T84.098
      - subluxation T84.02-

- **Complication** *(continued)*
  - joint prosthesis, internal *(continued)*
    - mechanical *(continued)*
      - wear of articular bearing surface T84.069
        - hip T84.06-
        - knee T84.06-
        - other specified joint T84.068
    - specified joint NEC T84.89
      - embolism T84.81
      - fibrosis T84.82
      - hemorrhage T84.83
      - pain T84.84
      - specified complication NEC T84.89
      - stenosis T84.85
      - thrombosis T84.86
    - subluxation T84.02-
  - kidney transplant *—see* Complications, transplant, kidney
  - labor O75.9
    - specified NEC O75.89
  - liver transplant (immune or nonimmune) *—see* Complications, transplant, liver
  - lumbar puncture G97.1
    - cerebrospinal fluid leak G97.0
    - headache or reaction G97.1
  - lung transplant *—see* Complications, transplant, lung
    - and heart *—see* Complications, transplant, lung, with heart
  - male genital N50.9
    - device, implant or graft *—see* Complications, genitourinary, device or implant, genital tract
    - postprocedural or postoperative *—see* Complications, genitourinary, postprocedural
    - specified NEC N99.89
  - mastoid (process) procedure
    - intraoperative H95.88
      - hematoma *—see* Complications, intraoperative, hemorrhage (hematoma) (of), mastoid process
      - hemorrhage *—see* Complications, intraoperative, hemorrhage (hematoma) (of), mastoid process
      - laceration *—see* Complications, intraoperative, puncture or laceration..., mastoid process
      - specified NEC H95.88
    - postmastoidectomy *—see* Complications, postmastoidectomy
    - postoperative H95.89
      - external ear canal stenosis H95.81-
      - hematoma *—see* Complications..., postprocedural, hematoma (of), mastoid process
      - hemorrhage *—see* Complications..., postprocedural, hemorrhage (of), mastoid process
      - postmastoidectomy *—see* Complications, postmastoidectomy

- **Complication** *(continued)*
  - mastoid *(continued)*
    - postoperative *(continued)*
      - seroma *—see* Complications, postprocedureal, seroma (of), mastoid process
      - specified NEC H95.89
  - mastoidectomy cavity *—see* Complications, postmastoidectomy
  - mechanical *—see* Complications, by site and type, mechanical
  - medical procedures (*see also* Complication(s), intraoperative) T88.9
  - metabolic E88.9
    - postoperative E89.89
      - specified NEC E89.89
  - molar pregnancy NOS O08.9
    - damage to pelvic organs O08.6
    - embolism O08.2
    - genital infection O08.0
    - hemorrhage (delayed) (excessive) O08.1
    - metabolic disorder O08.5
    - renal failure O08.4
    - shock O08.3
    - specified type NEC O08.0
    - venous complication NEC O08.7
  - musculoskeletal system *—see also* Complication, intraoperative (intraprocedural), by site
    - device, implant or graft NEC *—see* Complications, orthopedic, device or implant
    - internal fixation (nail) (plate) (rod) *—see* Complications, fixation device, internal
    - joint prosthesis *—see* Complications, joint prosthesis
    - postoperative (postprocedural) M96.89
      - with osteoporosis *—see* Osteoporosis
      - fracture following insertion of device *—see* Fracture, following insertion of orthopedic implant, joint prosthesis or bone plate
      - joint instability after prosthesis removal M96.89
      - lordosis M96.4
      - postlaminectomy syndrome NEC M96.1
        - kyphosis M96.3
      - pseudarthrosis M96.0
      - specified complication NEC M96.89
    - post radiation M96.89
      - kyphosis M96.2
      - scoliosis M96.5
      - specified complication NEC M96.89
  - nephrostomy (stoma) *—see* Complications, stoma, urinary tract, external NEC
  - nervous system G98.8
    - central G96.9
    - device, implant or graft *—see also* Complication, prosthetic device or implant, specified NEC
      - electronic stimulator (electrode(s)) *—see* Complications, electronic stimulator device
      - specified NEC
        - infection and inflammation T85.738

Complication *(continued)*
- nervous system *(continued)*
  - device, implant or graft *(continued)*
    - specified *(continued)*
      - mechanical T85.695
        - breakdown T85.615
        - displacement T85.625
        - leakage T85.635
        - malfunction T85.695
        - malposition T85.625
        - obstruction T85.695
        - perforation T85.695
        - protrusion T85.695
        - specified NEC T85.695
    - ventricular shunt *—see* Complications, ventricular shunt
  - electronic stimulator (electrode(s)) *—see* Complications, electronic stimulator device
  - postprocedural G97.82
    - intracranial hypotension G97.2
    - specified NEC G97.82
    - spinal fluid leak G97.0
- newborn, due to intrauterine (fetal) procedure P96.5
- nonabsorbable (permanent) sutures *—see* Complication, sutures, permanent
- obstetric O75.9
  - procedure (instrumental) (manual) (surgical) specified NEC O75.4
  - specified NEC O75.89
  - surgical wound NEC O90.89
    - hematoma O90.2
    - infection O86.00
- ocular lens implant *—see* Complications, intraocular lens
- ophthalmologic
  - postprocedural bleb *—see* Blebitis
- orbital prosthesis T85.9
  - embolism T85.818
  - fibrosis T85.828
  - hemorrhage T85.838
  - infection and inflammation T85.79
  - mechanical
    - breakdown T85.31-
    - displacement T85.32-
    - malposition T85.32-
    - obstruction T85.39-
    - perforation T85.39-
    - protrusion T85.39-
    - specified NEC T85.39-
  - pain T85.848
  - specified type NEC T85.898
  - stenosis T85.858
  - thrombosis T85.868
- organ or tissue transplant (partial) (total) *—see* Complications, transplant
- orthopedic *—see also* Disorder, soft tissue
  - device or implant T84.9
    - bone
      - device or implant *—see* Complication, bone, device NEC
      - graft *—see* Complication, graft, bone
    - breakdown T84.418
    - displacement T84.428
    - electronic bone stimulator *—see* Complications, electronic stimulator device, bone

Complication *(continued)*
- orthopedic *(continued)*
  - device or implant *(continued)*
    - embolism T84.81
    - fibrosis T84.82
    - fixation device *—see* Complication, fixation device, internal
    - hemorrhage T84.83
    - infection or inflammation T84.7
    - joint prosthesis *—see* Complication, joint prosthesis, internal
    - malfunction T84.418
    - malposition T84.428
    - mechanical NEC T84.498
    - muscle graft *—see* Complications, graft, muscle
    - obstruction T84.498
    - pain T84.84
    - perforation T84.498
    - protrusion T84.498
    - specified complication NEC T84.89
    - stenosis T84.85
    - tendon graft *—see* Complications, graft, tendon
    - thrombosis T84.86
  - fracture (following insertion of device) *—see* Fracture, following insertion of orthopedic implant, joint prosthesis or bone plate
  - postprocedural M96.89
    - fracture *—see* Fracture, following insertion of orthopedic implant, joint prosthesis or bone plate
    - postlaminectomy syndrome NEC M96.1
      - kyphosis M96.3
      - lordosis M96.4
    - postradiation
      - kyphosis M96.2
      - scoliosis M96.5
    - pseudarthrosis post-fusion M96.0
    - specified type NEC M96.89
- pacemaker (cardiac) *—see* Complications, cardiovascular device or implant, electronic
- pancreas transplant *—see* Complications, transplant, pancreas
- penile prosthesis (implant) *—see* Complications, prosthetic device, penile
- perfusion NEC T80.90
- perineal repair (obstetrical) NEC O90.89
  - disruption O90.1
  - hematoma O90.2
  - infection (following delivery) O86.09
- phototherapy T88.9
  - specified NEC T88.8
- postmastoidectomy NEC H95.19-
  - cyst, mucosal H95.13-
  - granulation H95.12-
  - inflammation, chronic H95.11-
  - recurrent cholesteatoma H95.0-
- postoperative *—see* Complications, postprocedural
  - circulatory *—see* Complications, circulatory system
  - ear *—see* Complications, ear

Complication *(continued)*
- postoperative *(continued)*
  - endocrine *—see* Complications, endocrine
  - eye *—see* Complications, eye
  - lumbar puncture G97.1
    - cerebrospinal fluid leak G97.0
  - nervous system (central) (peripheral) *—see* Complications, nervous system
  - respiratory system *—see* Complications, respiratory system
- postprocedural *—see also* Complications, surgical procedure
  - cardiac arrest *—see also* Infarct, myocardium, associated with revascularization procedure
    - following cardiac surgery I97.120
    - following other surgery I97.121
  - cardiac functional disturbance NEC *—see also* Infarct, myocardium, associated with revascularization procedure
    - following cardiac surgery I97.190
    - following other surgery I97.191
  - cardiac insufficiency
    - following cardiac surgery I97.110
    - following other surgery I97.111
  - chorioretinal scars following retinal surgery H59.81-
  - following cataract surgery
    - cataract (lens) fragments H59.02-
    - cystoid macular edema H59.03-
    - specified NEC H59.09-
    - vitreous (touch) syndrome H59.01-
  - heart failure
    - following cardiac surgery I97.130
    - following other surgery I97.131
  - hematoma (of)
    - circulatory system organ or structure
      - following cardiac bypass I97.631
      - following cardiac catheterization I97.630
      - following other circulatory system procedure I97.638
      - following other procedure I97.621
    - digestive system
      - following procedure on digestive system K91.870
      - following procedure on other organ K91.871
    - ear
      - following other procedure H95.52
      - following procedure on ear and mastoid process H95.51
    - endocrine system
      - following endocrine system procedure E89.820
      - following other procedure E89.821
    - eye and adnexa
      - following ophthalmic procedure H59.33-

Complication *(continued)*
- postprocedural *(continued)*
  - hematoma *(continued)*
    - eye and adnexa *(continued)*
      - following other procedure H59.34-
    - genitourinary organ or structure
      - following procedure on genitourinary organ or structure N99.840
      - following procedure on other organ N99.841
    - mastoid process
      - following other procedure H95.52
      - following procedure on ear and mastoid process H95.51
    - musculoskeletal structure
      - following musculoskeletal surgery M96.840
      - following non-orthopedic surgery M96.841
      - following orthopedic surgery M96.840
    - nervous system
      - following nervous system procedure G97.61
      - following other procedure G97.62
    - respiratory system
      - following other procedure J95.861
      - following procedure on respiratory system organ or structure J95.860
    - skin and subcutaneous tissue
      - following dematologic procedure L76.31
      - following procedure on other organ L76.32
    - spleen
      - following procedure on other organ D78.32
      - following procedure on the spleen D78.31
  - hemorrhage (of)
    - circulatory system organ or structure
      - following cardiac bypass I97.611
      - following cardiac catheterization I97.610
      - following other circulatory system procedure I97.618
      - following other procedure I97.620
    - digestive system
      - following procedure on digestive system K91.840
      - following procedure on other organ K91.841
    - ear
      - following other procedure H95.42
      - following procedure on ear and mastoid process H95.41
    - endocrine system
      - following endocrine system procedure E89.810
      - following other procedure E89.811
    - eye and adnexa
      - following ophthalmic procedure H59.31-
      - following other procedure H59.32-

Complication *(continued)*
- postprocedural *(continued)*
  - hemorrhage *(continued)*
    - genitourinary organ or structure
      - following procedure on genitourinary organ or structure N99.820
      - following procedure on other organ N99.821
    - mastoid process
      - following other procedure H95.42
      - following procedure on ear and mastoid process H95.41
    - musculoskeletal structure
      - following musculoskeletal surgery M96.830
      - following non-orthopedic surgery M96.831
      - following orthopedic surgery M96.830
    - nervous system
      - following nervous system procedure G97.51
      - following other procedure G97.52
    - respiratory system
      - following other procedure J95.831
      - following procedure on respiratory system organ or structure J95.830
    - skin and subcutaneous tissue
      - following dermatologic procedure L76.21
      - following a procedure on other organ L76.22
    - spleen
      - following procedure on other organ D78.22
      - following procedure on the spleen D78.21
  - seroma (of)
    - circulatory system organ or structure
      - following cardiac bypass I97.641
      - following cardiac catheterization I97.640
      - following other circulatory system procedure I97.648
      - following other procedure I97.622
    - digestive system
      - following procedure on digestive system K91.872
      - following procedure on other organ K91.873
    - ear
      - following other procedure H95.54
      - following procedure on ear and mastoid process H95.53
    - endocrine system
      - following endocrine system procedure E89.822
      - following other procedure E89.823
    - eye and adnexa
      - following ophthalmic procedure H59.35-
      - following other procedure H59.36-
    - genitourinary organ or structure
      - following procedure on genitourinary organ or structure N99.842

Complication *(continued)*
- postprocedural *(continued)*
  - seroma *(continued)*
    - genitourinary organ or structure *(continued)*
      - following procedure on other organ N99.843
    - mastoid process
      - following other procedure H95.54
      - following procedure on ear and mastoid process H95.53
    - musculoskeletal structure
      - following musculoskeletal surgery M96.842
      - following non-orthopedic surgery M96.843
      - following orthopedic surgery M96.842
    - nervous system
      - following nervous system procedure G97.63
      - following other procedure G97.64
    - respiratory system
      - following other procedure J95.863
      - following procedure on respiratory system organ or structure J95.862
    - skin and subcutaneous tissue
      - following dematologic procedure L76.33
      - following procedure on other organ L76.34
    - spleen
      - following procedure on other organ D78.34
      - following procedure on the spleen D78.33
  - specified NEC
    - circulatory system I97.89
    - digestive K91.89
    - ear H95.89
    - endocrine E89.89
    - eye and adnexa H59.89
    - genitourinary N99.89
    - mastoid process H95.89
    - metabolic E89.89
    - musculoskeletal structure M96.89
    - nervous system G97.82
    - respiratory system J95.89
    - skin and subcutaneous tissue L76.82
    - spleen D78.89
- pregnancy NEC —*see* Pregnancy, complicated by
- prosthetic device or implant T85.9
  - bile duct —*see* Complications, bile duct implant
  - breast —*see* Complications, breast implant
  - bulking agent
    - ureteral
      - erosion T83.714
      - exposure T83.724
    - urethral
      - erosion T83.713
      - exposure T83.723
  - cardiac and vascular NEC —*see* Complications, cardiovascular device or implant
  - corneal transplant —*see* Complications, graft, cornea
  - electronic nervous system stimulator —*see* Complications, electronic stimulator device

Complication *(continued)*
- prosthetic device or implant *(continued)*
  - epidural infusion catheter —*see* Complications, catheter, epidural
  - esophageal anti-reflux device —*see* Complications, esophageal anti-reflux device
  - genital organ or tract —*see* Complications, genitourinary, device or implant, genital tract
    - specified NEC T83.79
  - heart valve —*see* Complications, heart, valve, prosthesis
  - infection or inflammation T85.79
    - intestine transplant T86.892
    - liver transplant T86.43
    - lung transplant T86.812
    - pancreas transplant T86.892
    - skin graft T86.822
  - intraocular lens —*see* Complications, intraocular lens
  - intraperitoneal (dialysis) catheter —*see* Complication(s), catheter, intraperitoneal dialysis
  - joint —*see* Complications, joint prosthesis, internal
  - mechanical NEC T85.698
    - dialysis catheter (vascular) —*see also* Complication, catheter, dialysis, mechanical
      - peritoneal —*see* Complication(s), catheter, intraperitoneal, dialysis
    - gastrointestinal device T85.598
    - ocular device T85.398
    - subdural (infusion) catheter T85.690
    - suture, permanent T85.692
      - that for bone repair —*see* Complications, fixation device, internal (orthopedic), mechanical
    - ventricular shunt
      - breakdown T85.01
      - displacement T85.02
      - leakage T85.03
      - malposition T85.02
      - obstruction T85.09
      - perforation T85.09
      - protrusion T85.09
      - specified NEC T85.09
  - mesh
    - erosion (to surrounding organ or tissue) T83.718
      - vaginal (into pelvic floor muscles) T83.711
      - urethral (into pelvic floor muscles) T83.712
    - exposure (into surrounding organ or tissue) T83.728
      - vaginal (into vagina) (through vaginal wall) T83.721
      - urethral (through urethral wall) T83.722
  - orbital —*see* Complications, orbital prosthesis
  - penile T83.9
    - embolism T83.81
    - fibrosis T83.82
    - hemorrhage T83.83
    - infection and inflammation T83.61

Complication *(continued)*
- prosthetic device or implant *(continued)*
  - penile *(continued)*
    - mechanical
      - breakdown T83.410
      - displacement T83.420
      - leakage T83.490
      - malposition T83.420
      - obstruction T83.490
      - perforation T83.490
      - protrusion T83.490
      - specified NEC T83.490
    - pain T83.848
    - specified type NEC T83.89
    - stenosis T83.85
    - thrombosis T83.86
  - prosthetic materials NEC
    - erosion (to surrounding organ or tissue) T83.718
    - exposure (into surrounding organ or tissue) T83.728
  - skin graft T86.829
    - artificial skin or decellularized allodermis
      - embolism T85.818
      - fibrosis T85.828
      - hemorrhage T85.838
      - infection and inflammation T85.79
      - mechanical
        - breakdown T85.613
        - displacement T85.623
      - malfunction T85.613
        - malposition T85.623
        - obstruction T85.693
        - perforation T85.693
        - protrusion T85.693
        - specified NEC T85.693
      - pain T85.848
      - specified type NEC T85.898
      - stenosis T85.858
      - thrombosis T85.868
    - failure T86.821
    - infection T86.822
    - rejection T86.820
    - specified NEC T86.828
  - sling
    - urethral (female) (male)
      - erosion T83.712
      - exposure T83.722
  - specified NEC T85.9
    - embolism T85.818
    - fibrosis T85.828
    - hemorrhage T85.838
    - infection and inflammation T85.79
    - mechanical
      - breakdown T85.618
      - displacement T85.628
      - leakage T85.638
      - malfunction T85.618
      - malposition T85.628
      - obstruction T85.698
      - perforation T85.698
      - protrusion T85.698
      - specified NEC T85.698
    - pain T85.848
    - specified type NEC T85.898
    - stenosis T85.858
    - thrombosis T85.868
  - subdural infusion catheter —*see* Complications, catheter, subdural
  - sutures —*see* Complications, sutures
  - urinary organ or tract NEC —*see* Complications, genitourinary, device or implant, urinary system

Complication *(continued)*
- prosthetic device or implant *(continued)*
  - vascular —*see* Complications, cardiovascular device or implant
  - ventricular shunt —*see* Complications, ventricular shunt (device)
- puerperium —*see* Puerperal
- puncture, spinal G97.1
  - cerebrospinal fluid leak G97.0
  - headache or reaction G97.1
- pyelogram N99.89
- radiation
  - kyphosis M96.2
  - scoliosis M96.5
- reattached
  - extremity (infection) (rejection)
    - lower T87.1X-
    - upper T87.0X-
  - specified body part NEC T87.2
- reconstructed breast
  - asymmetry between native and reconstructed breast N65.1
  - deformity N65.0
  - disproportion between native and reconstructed breast N65.1
  - excess tissue N65.0
  - misshappen N65.0
- reimplant NEC —*see also* Complications, prosthetic device or implant
  - limb (infection) (rejection) —*see* Complications, reattached, extremity
  - organ (partial) (total) —*see* Complications, transplant
  - prosthetic device NEC —*see* Complications, prosthetic device
- renal N28.9
  - allograft —*see* Complications, transplant, kidney
  - dialysis —*see* Complications, dialysis
- respirator
  - mechancial J95.850
    - specified NEC J95.859
- respiratory system J98.9
  - device, implant or graft —*see* Complication, prosthetic device or implant, specified NEC
  - lung transplant —*see* Complications, prosthetic device or implant, lung transplant
  - postoperative J95.89
    - air leak J95.812
    - Mendelson's syndrome (chemical pneumonitis) J95.4
    - pneumothorax J95.811
    - pulmonary insufficiency (acute) (after nonthoracic surgery) J95.2
      - chronic J95.3
      - following thoracic surgery J95.1
    - respiratory failure (acute) J95.821
      - acute and chronic J95.822
    - specified NEC J95.89
    - subglottic stenosis J95.5
    - tracheostomy complication —*see* Complications, tracheostomy
  - therapy T81.89
- sedation during labor and delivery O74.9
  - cardiac O74.2
  - central nervous system O74.3
  - pulmonary NEC O74.1

Complication *(continued)*
- sedation during labor and delivery *(continued)*
- shunt —*see also* Complications, prosthetic device or implant
  - arteriovenous —*see* Complications, arteriovenous, shunt
  - ventricular (communicating) —*see* Complications, ventricular shunt
- skin
  - graft T86.829
    - failure T86.821
    - infection T86.822
    - rejection T86.820
    - specified type NEC T86.828
- spinal
  - anesthesia —*see* Complications, anesthesia, spinal
  - catheter (epidural) (subdural) —*see* Complications, catheter
  - puncture or tap G97.1
    - cerebrospinal fluid leak G97.0
    - headache or reaction G97.1
- stent
  - bile duct —*see* Complications, bile duct prosthesis
  - ureteral indwelling
    - breakdown T83.112
    - displacement T83.122
    - leakage T83.192
    - malposition T83.122
    - obstruction T83.192
    - perforation T83.192
    - protrusion T83.192
    - specified NEC T83.192
  - urinary NEC (ileal conduit) (nephroureteral) T83.193
    - embolism T83.81
    - fibrosis T83.82
    - hemorrhage T83.83
    - infection and inflammation T83.593
    - mechanical
      - breakdown T83.113
      - displacement T83.123
      - leakage T83.193
      - malposition T83.123
      - obstruction T83.193
      - perforation T83.193
      - protrusion T83.193
      - specified NEC T83.193
    - pain T83.84
    - specified type NEC T83.89
    - stenosis T83.85
    - thrombosis T83.86
  - vascular
    - end stent stenosis —*see* Restenosis, stent
    - in stent stenosis —*see* Restenosis, stent
- stoma
  - digestive tract
    - colostomy —*see* Complications, colostomy
    - enterostomy —*see* Complications, enterostomy
    - esophagostomy —*see* Complications, esophagostomy
    - gastrostomy —*see* Complications, gastrostomy
  - urinary tract N99.528
    - continent N99.538
      - hemorrhage N99.530
      - herniation N99.533
      - infection N99.531
      - malfunction N99.532
      - specified type NEC N99.538

Complication *(continued)*
- stoma *(continued)*
  - urinary tract *(continued)*
    - continent *(continued)*
      - stenosis N99.534
    - cystostomy —*see* Complications, cystostomy
    - external NOS N99.528
    - hemorrhage N99.520
    - herniation N99.523
    - incontinent N99.528
      - hemorrhage N99.520
      - herniation N99.523
      - infection N99.521
      - malfunction N99.522
      - specified type NEC N99.528
      - stenosis N99.524
    - infection N99.521
    - malfunction N99.522
    - specified type NEC N99.528
  - stenosis N99.524
- stomach banding —*see* Complication(s), bariatric procedure
- stomach stapling —*see* Complication(s), bariatric procedure
- surgical material, nonabsorbable —*see* Complication, suture, permanent
- surgical procedure (on) T81.9
  - amputation stump (late) —*see* Complications, amputation stump
  - cardiac —*see* Complications, circulatory system
  - cholesteatoma, recurrent —*see* Complications, postmastoidectomy, recurrent cholesteatoma
  - circulatory (early) —*see* Complications, circulatory system
  - digestive system —*see* Complications, gastrointestinal
  - dumping syndrome (postgastrectomy) K91.1
  - ear —*see* Complications, ear
  - elephantiasis or lymphedema I97.89
    - postmastectomy I97.2
  - emphysema (surgical) T81.82
  - endocrine —*see* Complications, endocrine
  - eye —*see* Complications, eye
  - fistula (persistent postoperative) T81.83
  - foreign body inadvertently left in wound (sponge) (suture) (swab) —*see* Foreign body, accidentally left during a procedure
  - gastrointestinal —*see* Complications, gastrointestinal
  - genitourinary NEC N99.89
  - hematoma
    - intraoperative —*see* Complication, intraoperative, hemorrhage
    - postprocedural —*see* Complication, postprocedural, hematoma
  - hemorrhage
    - intraoperative —*see* Complication, intraoperative, hemorrhage

Complication *(continued)*
- surgical procedure *(continued)*
  - hemorrhage *(continued)*
    - postprocedural —*see* Complication, postprocedural, hemorrhage
  - hepatic failure K91.82
  - hyperglycemia (postpancreatectomy) E89.1
  - hypoinsulinemia (postpancreatectomy) E89.1
  - hypoparathyroidism (postparathyroidectomy) E89.2
  - hypopituitarism (posthypophysectomy) E89.3
  - hypothyroidism (post-thyroidectomy) E89.0
  - intestinal obstruction (*see also* Obstruction, intestine, postoperative) K91.30
  - intracranial hypotension following ventricular shunting (ventriculostomy) G97.2
  - lymphedema I97.89
    - postmastectomy I97.2
  - malabsorption (postsurgical) NEC K91.2
    - osteoporosis —*see* Osteoporosis, postsurgical malabsorption
  - mastoidectomy cavity NEC —*see* Complications, postmastoidectomy
  - metabolic E89.89
    - specified NEC E89.89
  - musculoskeletal —*see* Complications, musculoskeletal system
  - nervous system (central) (peripheral) —*see* Complications, nervous system
  - ovarian failure E89.40
    - asymptomatic E89.40
    - symptomatic E89.41
  - peripheral vascular —*see* Complications, surgical procedure, vascular
  - postcardiotomy syndrome I97.0
  - postcholecystectomy syndrome K91.5
  - postcommissurotomy syndrome I97.0
  - postgastrectomy dumping syndrome K91.1
  - postlaminectomy syndrome NEC M96.1
    - kyphosis M96.3
  - postmastectomy lymphedema syndrome I97.2
  - postmastoidectomy cholesteatoma —*see* Complications, postmastoidectomy, recurrent cholesteatoma
  - postvagotomy syndrome K91.1
  - postvalvulotomy syndrome I97.0
  - pulmonary insufficiency (acute) J95.2
    - chronic J95.3
    - following thoracic surgery J95.1
  - reattached body part —*see* Complications, reattached
  - respiratory —*see* Complications, respiratory system
  - shock (hypovolemic) T81.19
  - spleen (postoperative) D78.89
    - intraoperative D78.81

Complication *(continued)*
- surgical procedure *(continued)*
  - stitch abscess T81.41
  - subglottic stenosis (postsurgical) J95.5
  - testicular hypofunction E89.5
  - transplant —*see* Complications, organ or tissue transplant
  - urinary NEC N99.89
  - vaginal vault prolapse (posthysterectomy) N99.3
  - vascular (peripheral)
    - artery T81.719
      - mesenteric T81.710
      - renal T81.711
      - specified NEC T81.718
    - vein T81.72
  - wound infection T81.49
- suture, permanent (wire) NEC T85.9
  - with repair of bone —*see* Complications, fixation device, internal
  - embolism T85.818
  - fibrosis T85.828
  - hemorrhage T85.838
  - infection and inflammation T85.79
  - mechanical
    - breakdown T85.612
    - displacement T85.622
    - malfunction T85.612
    - malposition T85.622
    - obstruction T85.692
    - perforation T85.692
    - protrusion T85.692
    - specified NEC T85.692
  - pain T85.848
  - specified type NEC T85.898
  - stenosis T85.858
  - thrombosis T85.868
- tracheostomy J95.00
  - granuloma J95.09
  - hemorrhage J95.01
  - infection J95.02
  - malfunction J95.03
  - mechanical J95.03
  - obstruction J95.03
  - specified type NEC J95.09
  - tracheo-esophageal fistula J95.04
- transfusion (blood) (lymphocytes) (plasma) T80.92
  - air emblism T80.0
  - circulatory overload E87.71
  - febrile nonhemolytic transfusion reaction R50.84
  - hemolysis T80.89
  - hemochromatosis E83.111
  - hemolytic reaction (antigen unspecified) T80.919
  - incompatibility reaction (antigen unspecified) T80.919
    - ABO T80.30
      - delayed serologic (DSTR) T80.39
      - hemolytic transfusion reaction (HTR) (unspecified time after transfusion) T80.319
        - acute (AHTR) (less than 24 hours after transfusion) T80.310
        - delayed (DHTR) (24 hours or more after transfusion) T80.311
      - specified NEC T80.39
    - acute (antigen unspecified) T80.910
    - delayed (antigen unspecified) T80.911

Complication *(continued)*
- transfusion *(continued)*
  - incompatibility reaction *(continued)*
    - delayed serologic (DSTR) T80.89
    - Non-ABO (minor antigens (Duffy) (K) (Kell) (Kidd) (Lewis) (M) (N) (P) (S)) T80.A0
      - delayed serologic (DSTR) T80.A9
      - hemolytic transfusion reaction (HTR) (unspecified time after transfusion) T80.A19
        - acute (AHTR) (less than 24 hours after transfusion) T80.A10
        - delayed (DHTR) (24 hours or more after transfusion) T80.A11
      - specified NEC T80.A9
    - Rh (antigens (C) (c) (D) (E) (e)) (factor) T80.40
      - delayed serologic (DSTR) T80.49
      - hemolytic transfusion reaction (HTR) (unspecified time after transfusion) T80.419
      - hemolytic transfusion acute (AHTR) (less than 24 hours after transfusion) T80.410
        - delayed (DHTR) (24 hours or more after transfusion) T80.411
      - specified NEC T80.49
  - infection T80.29
    - acute T80.22
  - reaction NEC T80.89
  - sepsis T80.29
  - shock T80.89
- transplant T86.90
  - bone T86.839
    - failure T86.831
    - infection T86.832
    - rejection T86.830
    - specified type NEC T86.838
  - bone marrow T86.00
    - failure T86.02
    - infection T86.03
    - rejection T86.01
    - specified type NEC T86.09
  - cornea T86.849-
    - failure T86.841-
    - infection T86.842-
    - rejection T86.840-
    - specified type NEC T86.848-
  - failure T86.92
  - heart T86.20
    - with lung T86.30
    - cardiac allograft vasculopathy T86.290
      - failure T86.32
      - infection T86.33
      - rejection T86.31
      - specified type NEC T86.39
    - failure T86.22
    - infection T86.23
    - rejection T86.21
    - specified type NEC T86.298
  - infection T86.93
  - intestine T86.859
    - failure T86.851
    - infection T86.852
    - rejection T86.850
    - specified type NEC T86.858

Complication *(continued)*
- transplant *(continued)*
  - kidney T86.10
    - failure T86.12
    - infection T86.13
    - rejection T86.11
    - specified type NEC T86.19
  - liver T86.40
    - failure T86.42
    - infection T86.43
    - rejection T86.41
    - specified type NEC T86.49
  - lung T86.819
    - with heart T86.30
      - failure T86.32
      - infection T86.33
      - rejection T86.31
      - specified type NEC T86.39
    - failure T86.811
    - infection T86.812
    - rejection T86.810
    - specified type NEC T86.818
  - malignant neoplasm C80.2
  - pancreas T86.899
    - failure T86.891
    - infection T86.892
    - rejection T86.890
    - specified type NEC T86.898
  - peripheral blood stem cells T86.5
  - post-transplant
    - lymphoproliferative disorder (PTLD) D47.Z1
  - rejection T86.91
  - skin T86.829
    - failure T86.821
    - infection T86.822
    - rejection T86.820
    - specified type NEC T86.828
  - specified
    - tissue T86.899
      - failure T86.891
      - infection T86.892
      - rejection T86.890
      - specified type NEC T86.898
    - type NEC T86.99
  - stem cell (from peripheral blood) (from umbilical cord) T86.5
  - umbilical cord stem cells T86.5
- trauma (early) T79.9
  - specified NEC T79.8
- ultrasound therapy NEC T88.9
- umbilical cord NEC
  - complicating delivery O69.9
    - specified NEC O69.89
- umbrella device, vascular T82.9
  - embolism T82.818
  - fibrosis T82.828
  - hemorrhage T82.838
  - infection or inflammation T82.7
  - mechanical
    - breakdown T82.515
    - displacement T82.525
    - leakage T82.535
    - malposition T82.525
    - obstruction T82.595
    - perforation T82.595
    - protrusion T82.595
  - pain T82.848
  - specified type NEC T82.898
  - stenosis T82.858
  - thrombosis T82.868
- urethral catheter —*see* Complications, catheter, urethral, indwelling
- vaccination T88.1
  - anaphylaxis NEC T80.52
  - arthropathy —*see* Arthropathy, postimmunization

Complication *(continued)*
- vaccination *(continued)*
  - cellulitis T88.0
  - encephalitis or encephalomyelitis G04.02
  - infection (general) (local) NEC T88.0
  - meningitis G03.8
  - myelitis G04.02
  - protein sickness T80.62
  - rash T88.1
  - reaction (allergic) T88.1
    - serum T80.62
  - sepsis T88.0
  - serum intoxication, sickness, rash, or other serum reaction NEC T80.62
    - anaphylactic shock T80.52
  - shock (allergic) (anaphylactic) T80.52
  - vaccinia (generalized) (localized) T88.1
- vas deferens device or implant —*see* Complications, genitourinary, device or implant, genital tract
- vascular I99.9
  - device or implant T82.9
    - embolism T82.818
    - fibrosis T82.828
    - hemorrhage T82.838
    - infection or inflammation T82.7
    - mechanical
      - breakdown T82.519
        - specified device NEC T82.518
      - displacement T82.529
        - specified device NEC T82.528
      - leakage T82.539
        - specified device NEC T82.538
      - malposition T82.529
        - specified device NEC T82.528
      - obstruction T82.599
        - specified device NEC T82.598
      - perforation T82.599
        - specified device NEC T82.598
      - protrusion T82.599
        - specified device NEC T82.598
    - pain T82.848
    - specified type NEC T82.898
    - stenosis T82.858
    - thrombosis T82.868
  - dialysis catheter —*see* Complication, catheter, dialysis
  - following infusion, therapeutic injection or transfusion T80.1
  - graft T82.9
    - embolism T82.818
    - fibrosis T82.828
    - hemorrhage T82.838
    - mechanical
      - breakdown T82.319
        - aorta (bifurcation) T82.310
        - carotid artery T82.311
        - specified vessel NEC T82.318
      - displacement T82.329
        - aorta (bifurcation) T82.320
        - carotid artery T82.321
        - specified vessel NEC T82.328

Complication *(continued)*
vascular *(continued)*
graft *(continued)*
mechanical *(continued)*
leakage T82.339
aorta (bifurcation) T82.330
carotid artery T82.331
specified vessel NEC T82.338
malposition T82.329
aorta (bifurcation) T82.320
carotid artery T82.321
specified vessel NEC T82.328
obstruction T82.399
aorta (bifurcation) T82.390
carotid artery T82.391
specified vessel NEC T82.398
perforation T82.399
aorta (bifurcation) T82.390
carotid artery T82.391
specified vessel NEC T82.398
protrusion T82.399
aorta (bifurcation) T82.390
carotid artery T82.391
specified vessel NEC T82.398
pain T82.848
specified complication NEC T82.898
stenosis T82.858
thrombosis T82.868
postoperative —*see* Complications, postoperative, circulatory
vena cava device (filter) (sieve) (umbrella) —*see* Complications, umbrella device, vascular
ventilation therapy NEC T81.81
ventilator
mechanical J95.850
specified NEC J95.859
ventricular (communicating) shunt (device) T85.9
embolism T85.810
fibrosis T85.820
hemorrhage T85.830
infection and inflammation T85.730
mechanical
breakdown T85.01
displacement T85.02
leakage T85.03
malposition T85.02
obstruction T85.09
perforation T85.09
protrusion T85.09
specified NEC T85.09
pain T85.840
specified type NEC T85.890
stenosis T85.850
thrombosis T85.860
wire suture, permanent (implanted) —*see* Complications, suture, permanent

Compressed air disease T70.3

Compression
with injury - code by Nature of injury
artery I77.1
celiac, syndrome I77.4
brachial plexus G54.0
brain (stem) G93.5
due to
contusion (diffuse) (*see also* Injury, intracranial, diffuse) S06.A0
with herniation S06.A1
focal (*see also* Injury, intracranial, focal) S06.A0
with herniation S06.A1
injury NEC (*see also* Injury, intracranial, diffuse) S06.A0
nontraumatic G93.5
traumatic (*see also* Injury, intracranial, diffuse) S06.A0
with herniation S06.A1
bronchus J98.09
cauda equina G83.4
celiac (artery) (axis) I77.4
cerebral —*see* Compression, brain
cervical plexus G54.2
cord
spinal —*see* Compression, spinal
umbilical —*see* Compression, umbilical cord
cranial nerve G52.9
eighth H93.3
eleventh G52.8
fifth G50.8
first G52.0
fourth —*see* Strabismus, paralytic, fourth nerve
ninth G52.1
second —*see* Disorder, nerve, optic
seventh G51.8
sixth —*see* Strabismus, paralytic, sixth nerve
tenth G52.2
third —*see* Strabismus, paralytic, third nerve
twelfth G52.3
diver's squeeze T70.3
during birth (newborn) P15.9
esophagus K22.2
eustachian tube —*see* Obstruction, eustachian tube, cartilaginous
facies Q67.1
fracture
nontraumatic NOS —*see* Collapse, vertebra
pathological —*see* Fracture, pathological
traumatic —*see* Fracture, traumatic
heart —*see* Disease, heart
intestine —*see* Obstruction, intestine
laryngeal nerve, recurrent G52.2
with paralysis of vocal cords and larynx J38.00
bilateral J38.02
unilateral J38.01
lumbosacral plexus G54.1
lung J98.4
lymphatic vessel I89.0
medulla —*see* Compression, brain
nerve (*see also* Disorder, nerve) G58.9
arm NEC —*see* Mononeuropathy, upper limb
axillary G54.0
cranial —*see* Compression, cranial nerve
leg NEC —*see* Mononeuropathy, lower limb
median (in carpal tunnel) —*see* Syndrome, carpal tunnel
optic —*see* Disorder, nerve, optic
plantar —*see* Lesion, nerve, plantar
posterior tibial (in tarsal tunnel) —*see* Syndrome, tarsal tunnel
root or plexus NOS (in) G54.9
intervertebral disc disorder NEC —*see* Disorder, disc, with, radiculopathy
with myelopathy —*see* Disorder, disc, with, myelopathy
neoplastic disease —*see also* Neoplasm D49.9 *[G55]*
spondylosis —*see* Spondylosis, with radiculopathy
sciatic (acute) —*see* Lesion, nerve, sciatic
sympathetic G90.8
traumatic —*see* Injury, nerve
ulnar —*see* Lesion, nerve, ulnar
upper extremity NEC —*see* Mononeuropathy, upper limb
spinal (cord) G95.20
by displacement of intervertebral disc NEC —*see also* Disorder, disc, with, myelopathy
nerve root NOS G54.9
due to displacement of intervertebral disc NEC —*see* Disorder, disc, with, radiculopathy
with myelopathy —*see* Disorder, disc, with, myelopathy
specified NEC G95.29
spondylogenic (cervical) (lumbar, lumbosacral) (thoracic) —*see* Spondylosis, with myelopathy NEC
anterior —*see* Syndrome, anterior, spinal artery, compression
traumatic —*see* Injury, spinal cord, by region
subcostal nerve (syndrome) —*see* Mononeuropathy, upper limb, specified NEC
sympathetic nerve NEC G90.8
syndrome T79.5
trachea J39.8
ulnar nerve (by scar tissue) —*see* Lesion, nerve, ulnar
umbilical cord
complicating delivery O69.2
cord around neck O69.1
prolapse O69.0
specified NEC O69.2
ureter N13.5
vein I87.1
vena cava (inferior) (superior) I87.1

Compulsion, compulsive
gambling F63.0
neurosis F42.8
personality F60.5
states F42.8
swearing F42.8
in Gilles de la Tourette's syndrome F95.2
tics and spasms F95.9

Concato's disease (pericardial polyserositis) A19.9
nontubercular I31.1
pleural —*see* Pleurisy, with effusion

Concavity chest wall M95.4

Concealed penis Q55.64

Concern (normal) about sick person in family Z63.6

Concrescence (teeth) K00.2

Concretio cordis I31.1
rheumatic I09.2

Concretion —*see also* Calculus
appendicular K38.1
canaliculus —*see* Dacryolith
clitoris N90.89
conjunctiva H11.12-
eyelid —*see* Disorder, eyelid, specified type NEC
lacrimal passages —*see* Dacryolith
prepuce (male) N47.8
salivary gland (any) K11.5
seminal vesicle N50.89
tonsil J35.8

Concussion (brain) (cerebral) (current) S06.0X9
with
loss of consciousness of 30 minutes or less S06.0X1
loss of consciousness of unspecified duration S06.0X9
blast (air) (hydraulic) (immersion) (underwater)
abdomen or thorax —*see* Injury, blast, by site
ear with acoustic nerve injury —*see* Injury, nerve, acoustic, specified type NEC
cauda equina S34.3
conus medullaris S34.02
ocular S05.8X-
spinal (cord)
cervical S14.0
lumbar S34.01
sacral S34.02
thoracic S24.0
syndrome F07.81
without loss of consciousness S06.0X0

Condition —*see also* Disease
post COVID-19 U09.9

Conditions arising in the perinatal period —*see* Newborn, affected by

Conduct disorder —*see* Disorder, conduct

Condyloma A63.0
acuminatum A63.0
gonorrheal A54.09
latum A51.31
syphilitic A51.31
congenital A50.07
venereal, syphilitic A51.31

Conflagration —*see also* Burn
asphyxia (by inhalation of gases, fumes or vapors) (*see also* Table of Drugs and Chemicals) T59.9-

Conflict (with) —*see also* Discord
family Z73.9
marital Z63.0
involving divorce or estrangement Z63.5
parent-child Z62.820
parent-adopted child Z62.821
parent-biological child Z62.820
parent-foster child Z62.822
social role NEC Z73.5

Confluent —*see* condition

Confusion, confused R41.0
- epileptic F05
- mental state (psychogenic) F44.89
- psychogenic F44.89
- reactive (from emotional stress, psychological trauma) F44.89

Confusional arousals G47.51

Congelation T69.9

Congenital —*see also* condition
- aortic septum Q25.49
- intrinsic factor deficiency D51.0
- malformation —*see* Anomaly

Congestion, congestive
- bladder N32.89
- bowel K63.89
- brain G93.89
- breast N64.59
- bronchial J98.09
- catarrhal J31.0
- chest R09.89
- chill, malarial —*see* Malaria
- circulatory NEC I99.8
- duodenum K31.89
- eye —*see* Hyperemia, conjunctiva
- facial, due to birth injury P15.4
- general R68.89
- glottis J37.0
- heart —*see* Failure, heart, congestive
- hepatic K76.1
- hypostatic (lung) —*see* Edema, lung
- intestine K63.89
- kidney N28.89
- labyrinth —*see* subcategory H83.8
- larynx J37.0
- liver K76.1
- lung R09.89
  - active or acute —*see* Pneumonia
- malaria, malarial —*see* Malaria
- nasal R09.81
- nose R09.81
- orbit, orbital —*see also* Exophthalmos
  - inflammatory (chronic) —*see* Inflammation, orbit
- ovary N83.8
- pancreas K86.89
- pelvic, female N94.89
- pleural J94.8
- prostate (active) N42.1
- pulmonary —*see* Congestion, lung
- renal N28.89
- retina H35.81
- seminal vesicle N50.1
- spinal cord G95.19
- spleen (chronic) D73.2
- stomach K31.89
- trachea —*see* Tracheitis
- urethra N36.8
- uterus N85.8
  - with subinvolution N85.3
- venous (passive) I87.8
- viscera R68.89

Congestive —*see* Congestion

Conical
- cervix (hypertrophic elongation) N88.4
- cornea —*see* Keratoconus
- teeth K00.2

Conjoined twins Q89.4

Conjugal maladjustment Z63.0
- involving divorce or estrangement Z63.5

Conjunctiva —*see* condition

Conjunctivitis (staphylococcal) (streptococcal) **NOS** H10.9
- Acanthamoeba B60.12
- acute H10.3-
  - atopic H10.1-
  - mucopurulent H10.02-
    - follicular H10.01-
  - chemical (*see also* Corrosion, cornea) H10.21-
  - pseudomembranous H10.22-
  - serous except viral H10.23-
    - viral —*see* Conjunctivitis, viral
  - toxic H10.21-
- adenoviral (acute) (follicular) B30.1
- allergic (acute) —*see* Conjunctivitis, acute, atopic
  - chronic H10.45
    - vernal H10.44
- anaphylactic —*see* Conjunctivitis, acute, atopic
- Apollo B30.3
- atopic (acute) —*see* Conjunctivitis, acute, atopic
- Béal's B30.2
- blennorrhagic (gonococcal) (neonatorum) A54.31
- chemical (acute) (*see also* Corrosion, cornea) H10.21-
- chlamydial A74.0
  - due to trachoma A71.1
  - neonatal P39.1
- chronic (nodosa) (petrificans) (phlyctenular) H10.40-
  - allergic H10.45
    - vernal H10.44
  - follicular H10.43-
  - giant papillary H10.41-
  - simple H10.42-
  - vernal H10.44
- coxsackievirus 24 B30.3
- diphtheritic A36.86
- due to
  - dust —*see* Conjunctivitis, acute, atopic
  - filariasis B74.9
  - mucocutaneous leishmaniasis B55.2
- enterovirus type 70 (hemorrhagic) B30.3
- epidemic (viral) B30.9
  - hemorrhagic B30.3
- gonococcal (neonatorum) A54.31
- granular (trachomatous) A71.1
  - sequelae (late effect) B94.0
- hemorrhagic (acute) (epidemic) B30.3
- herpes zoster B02.31
- in (due to)
  - Acanthamoeba B60.12
  - adenovirus (acute) (follicular) B30.1
  - Chlamydia A74.0
  - coxsackievirus 24 B30.3
  - diphtheria A36.86
  - enterovirus type 70 (hemorrhagic) B30.3
  - filariasis B74.9
  - gonococci A54.31
  - herpes (simplex) virus B00.53
    - zoster B02.31
  - infectious disease NEC B99
  - meningococci A39.89
  - mucocutaneous leishmaniasis B55.2
  - rosacea H10.82-
  - syphilis (late) A52.71
  - zoster B02.31

Conjunctivitis *(continued)*
- inclusion A74.0
- infantile P39.1
  - gonococcal A54.31
- Koch-Weeks' —*see* Conjunctivitis, acute, mucopurulent
- light —*see* Conjunctivitis, acute, atopic
- ligneous —*see* Blepharoconjunctivitis, ligneous
- meningococcal A39.89
- mucopurulent —*see* Conjunctivitis, acute, mucopurulent
- neonatal P39.1
  - gonococcal A54.31
- Newcastle B30.8
- of Béal B30.2
- parasitic
  - filariasis B74.9
  - mucocutaneous leishmaniasis B55.2
- Parinaud's H10.89
- petrificans H10.89
- rosacea H10.82-
- specified NEC H10.89
- swimming-pool B30.1
- trachomatous A71.1
  - acute A71.0
  - sequelae (late effect) B94.0
- traumatic NEC H10.89
- tuberculous A18.59
- tularemic A21.1
- tularensis A21.1
- viral B30.9
  - due to
    - adenovirus B30.1
    - enterovirus B30.3
  - specified NEC B30.8

Conjunctivochalasis H11.82-

Connective tissue —*see* condition

Conn's syndrome E26.01

Conradi (-Hunermann) **disease** Q77.3

Consanguinity Z84.3
- counseling Z71.89

Conscious simulation (of illness) Z76.5

Consecutive —*see* condition

Consolidation lung (base) —*see* Pneumonia, lobar

Constipation (atonic) (neurogenic) (simple) (spastic) K59.00
- chronic K59.09
  - idiopathic K59.04
- drug-induced K59.03
- functional K59.04
- outlet dysfunction K59.02
- psychogenic F45.8
- slow transit K59.01
- specified NEC K59.09

Constitutional —*see also* condition
- substandard F60.7

Constitutionally substandard F60.7

Constriction —*see also* Stricture
- auditory canal —*see* Stenosis, external ear canal
- bronchial J98.09
- duodenum K31.5
- esophagus K22.2
- external
  - abdomen, abdominal (wall) S30.841
  - alveolar process S00.542
  - ankle S90.54-
  - antecubital space —*see* Constriction, external, forearm

Constriction *(continued)*
- external *(continued)*
  - arm (upper) S40.84-
  - auricle —*see* Constriction, external, ear
  - axilla —*see* Constriction, external, arm
  - back, lower S30.840
  - breast S20.14-
  - brow S00.84
  - buttock S30.840
  - calf —*see* Constriction, external, leg
  - canthus —*see* Constriction, external, eyelid
  - cheek S00.84
    - internal S00.542
  - chest wall —*see* Constriction, external, thorax
  - chin S00.84
  - clitoris S30.844
  - costal region —*see* Constriction, external, thorax
  - digit(s)
    - foot —*see* Constriction, external, toe
    - hand —*see* Constriction, external, finger
  - ear S00.44-
  - elbow S50.34-
  - epididymis S30.843
  - epigastric region S30.841
  - esophagus, cervical S10.14
  - eyebrow —*see* Constriction, external, eyelid
  - eyelid S00.24-
  - face S00.84
  - finger(s) S60.44-
    - index S60.44-
    - little S60.44-
    - middle S60.44-
    - ring S60.44-
  - flank S30.841
  - foot (except toe(s) alone) S90.84-
    - toe —*see* Constriction, external, toe
  - forearm S50.84-
    - elbow only —*see* Constriction, external, elbow
  - forehead S00.84
  - genital organs, external
    - female S30.846
    - male S30.845
  - groin S30.841
  - gum S00.542
  - hand S60.54-
  - head S00.94
    - ear —*see* Constriction, external, ear
    - eyelid —*see* Constriction, external, eyelid
    - lip S00.541
    - nose S00.34
    - oral cavity S00.542
    - scalp S00.04
    - specified site NEC S00.84
  - heel —*see* Constriction, external, foot
  - hip S70.24-
  - inguinal region S30.841
  - interscapular region S20.449
  - jaw S00.84
  - knee S80.24-
  - labium (majus) (minus) S30.844
  - larynx S10.14
  - leg (lower) S80.84-
    - knee —*see* Constriction, external, knee
    - upper —*see* Constriction, external, thigh

Constriction *(continued)*
- external *(continued)*
  - lip S00.541
  - lower back S30.840
  - lumbar region S30.840
  - malar region S00.84
  - mammary —*see* Constriction, external, breast
  - mastoid region S00.84
  - mouth S00.542
  - nail
    - finger —*see* Constriction, external, finger
    - toe —*see* Constriction, external, toe
  - nasal S00.34
  - neck S10.94
    - specified site NEC S10.84
    - throat S10.14
  - nose S00.34
  - occipital region S00.04
  - oral cavity S00.542
  - orbital region —*see* Constriction, external, eyelid
  - palate S00.542
  - palm —*see* Constriction, external, hand
  - parietal region S00.04
  - pelvis S30.840
  - penis S30.842
  - perineum
    - female S30.844
    - male S30.840
  - periocular area —*see* Constriction, external, eyelid
  - phalanges
    - finger —*see* Constriction, external, finger
    - toe —*see* Constriction, external, toe
  - pharynx S10.14
  - pinna —*see* Constriction, external, ear
  - popliteal space —*see* Constriction, external, knee
  - prepuce S30.842
  - pubic region S30.840
  - pudendum
    - female S30.846
    - male S30.845
  - sacral region S30.840
  - scalp S00.04
  - scapular region —*see* Constriction, external, shoulder
  - scrotum S30.843
  - shin —*see* Constriction, external, leg
  - shoulder S40.24-
  - sternal region S20.349
  - submaxillary region S00.84
  - submental region S00.84
  - subungual
    - finger(s) —*see* Constriction, external, finger
    - toe(s) —*see* Constriction, external, toe
  - supraclavicular fossa S10.84
  - supraorbital S00.84
  - temple S00.84
  - temporal region S00.84
  - testis S30.843
  - thigh S70.34-
  - thorax, thoracic (wall) S20.94
    - back S20.44-
    - front S20.34-
  - throat S10.14
  - thumb S60.34-
  - toe(s) (lesser) S90.44-
    - great S90.44-
  - tongue S00.542

Constriction *(continued)*
- external *(continued)*
  - trachea S10.14
  - tunica vaginalis S30.843
  - uvula S00.542
  - vagina S30.844
  - vulva S30.844
  - wrist S60.84-
- gallbladder —*see* Obstruction, gallbladder
- intestine —*see* Obstruction, intestine
- larynx J38.6
  - congenital Q31.8
    - specified NEC Q31.8
    - subglottic Q31.1
- organ or site, congenital NEC —*see* Atresia, by site
- prepuce (acquired) (congenital) N47.1
- pylorus (adult hypertrophic) K31.1
  - congenital or infantile Q40.0
  - newborn Q40.0
- ring dystocia (uterus) O62.4
- spastic —*see also* Spasm
  - ureter N13.5
- ureter N13.5
  - with infection N13.6
- urethra —*see* Stricture, urethra
- visual field (peripheral) (functional) —*see* Defect, visual field

Constrictive —*see* condition

Consultation
- medical —*see* Counseling, medical
- religious Z71.81
- specified reason NEC Z71.89
- spiritual Z71.81
- without complaint or sickness Z71.9
  - feared complaint unfounded Z71.1
  - specified reason NEC Z71.89

Consumption —*see* Tuberculosis

Contact (with) —*see also* Exposure (to)
- acariasis Z20.7
- AIDS virus Z20.6
- air pollution Z77.110
- algae and algae toxins Z77.121
- algae bloom Z77.121
- anthrax Z20.810
- aromatic amines Z77.020
- aromatic (hazardous) compounds NEC Z77.028
- aromatic dyes NOS Z77.028
- arsenic Z77.010
- asbestos Z77.090
- bacterial disease NEC Z20.818
- benzene Z77.021
- blue-green algae bloom Z77.121
- body fluids (potentially hazardous) Z77.21
- brown tide Z77.121
- chemicals (chiefly nonmedicinal) (hazardous) NEC Z77.098
- cholera Z20.09
- chromium compounds Z77.018
- communicable disease Z20.9
  - bacterial NEC Z20.818
  - specified NEC Z20.89
  - viral NEC Z20.828
  - Zika virus Z20.821
- coronavirus (disease) (novel) 2019 Z20.822
- COVID-19 Z20.822
- cyanobacteria bloom Z77.121
- dyes Z77.098
- Escherichia coli (E. coli) Z20.01
- fiberglass —*see* Table of Drugs and Chemicals, fiberglass
- German measles Z20.4
- gonorrhea Z20.2
- hazardous metals NEC Z77.018

Contact *(continued)*
- hazardous substances NEC Z77.29
- hazards in the physical environment NEC Z77.128
- hazards to health NEC Z77.9
- HIV Z20.6
- HTLV-III/LAV Z20.6
- human immunodeficiency virus (HIV) Z20.6
- infection Z20.9
  - specified NEC Z20.89
- infestation (parasitic) NEC Z20.7
- intestinal infectious disease NEC Z20.09
  - Escherichia coli (E. coli) Z20.01
- lead Z77.011
- meningococcus Z20.811
- mold (toxic) Z77.120
- nickel dust Z77.018
- noise Z77.122
- parasitic disease Z20.7
- pediculosis Z20.7
- pfiesteria piscicida Z77.121
- poliomyelitis Z20.89
- pollution
  - air Z77.110
  - environmental NEC Z77.118
  - soil Z77.112
  - water Z77.111
- polycyclic aromatic hydrocarbons Z77.028
- positive maternal group B streptococcus P00.82
- rabies Z20.3
- radiation, naturally occurring NEC Z77.123
- radon Z77.123
- red tide (Florida) Z77.121
- rubella Z20.4
- SARS-CoV-2 Z20.822
- sexually-transmitted disease Z20.2
- smallpox (laboratory) Z20.89
- syphilis Z20.2
- tuberculosis Z20.1
- uranium Z77.012
- varicella Z20.820
- venereal disease Z20.2
- viral disease NEC Z20.828
- viral hepatitis Z20.5
- water pollution Z77.111
- Zika virus Z20.821

Contamination, food —*see* Intoxication, foodborne

Contraception, contraceptive
- advice Z30.09
- counseling Z30.09
- device (intrauterine) (in situ) Z97.5
  - causing menorrhagia T83.83
  - checking Z30.431
  - complications —*see* Complications, intrauterine, contraceptive device
  - in place Z97.5
  - initial prescription Z30.014
  - reinsertion Z30.433
  - removal Z30.432
  - replacement Z30.433
- emergency (postcoital) Z30.012
- initial prescription Z30.019
  - barrier Z30.018
  - diaphragm Z30.018
  - injectable Z30.013
  - intrauterine device Z30.014
  - pills Z30.011
  - postcoital (emergency) Z30.012
  - specified type NEC Z30.018
  - subdermal implantable Z30.017
  - transdermal patch hormonal Z30.016
  - vaginal ring hormonal Z30.015

Contraception, contraceptive *(continued)*
- maintenance Z30.40
  - barrier Z30.49
  - diaphragm Z30.49
  - examination Z30.8
  - injectable Z30.42
  - intrauterine device Z30.431
  - pills Z30.41
  - specified type NEC Z30.49
  - subdermal implantable Z30.46
  - transdermal patch hormonal Z30.45
  - vaginal ring hormonal Z30.44
- management Z30.9
  - specified NEC Z30.8
- postcoital (emergency) Z30.012
- prescription Z30.019
  - repeat Z30.40
- sterilization Z30.2
- surveillance (drug) —*see* Contraception, maintenance

Contraction(s), contracture, contracted
- Achilles tendon —*see also* Short, tendon, Achilles
  - congenital Q66.89
- amputation stump (surgical) (flexion) (late) (next proximal joint) T87.89
- anus K59.89
- bile duct (common) (hepatic) K83.8
- bladder N32.89
  - neck or sphincter N32.0
- bowel, cecum, colon or intestine, any part —*see* Obstruction, intestine
- Braxton Hicks —*see* False, labor
- breast implant, capsular T85.44
- bronchial J98.09
- burn (old) —*see* Cicatrix
- cervix —*see* Stricture, cervix
- cicatricial —*see* Cicatrix
- conjunctiva, trachomatous, active A71.1
  - sequelae (late effect) B94.0
- Dupuytren's M72.0
- eyelid —*see* Disorder, eyelid function
- fascia (lata) (postural) M72.8
  - Dupuytren's M72.0
  - palmar M72.0
  - plantar M72.2
- finger NEC —*see also* Deformity, finger
  - congenital Q68.1
  - joint —*see* Contraction, joint, hand
- flaccid —*see* Contraction, paralytic
- gallbladder K82.0
- heart valve —*see* Endocarditis
- hip —*see* Contraction, joint, hip
- hourglass
  - bladder N32.89
    - congenital Q64.79
  - gallbladder K82.0
    - congenital Q44.1
  - stomach K31.89
    - congenital Q40.2
    - psychogenic F45.8
  - uterus (complicating delivery) O62.4
- hysterical F44.4
- internal os —*see* Stricture, cervix
- joint (abduction) (acquired) (adduction) (flexion) (rotation) M24.50
  - ankle M24.57-
  - congenital NEC Q68.8
    - hip Q65.89

Contraction(s), contracture, contracted *(continued)*
joint *(continued)*
elbow M24.52-
foot joint M24.57-
hand joint M24.54-
hip M24.55-
congenital Q65.89
hysterical F44.4
knee M24.56-
shoulder M24.51-
specified site NEC M24.59
wrist M24.53-
kidney (granular) (secondary) N26.9
congenital Q63.8
hydronephritic *—see* Hydronephrosis
Page N26.2
pyelonephritic *—see* Pyelitis, chronic
tuberculous A18.11
ligament *—see also* Disorder, ligament
congenital Q79.8
muscle (postinfective) (postural) NEC M62.40
with contracture of joint *—see* Contraction, joint
ankle M62.47-
congenital Q79.8
sternocleidomastoid Q68.0
extraocular *—see* Strabismus
eye (extrinsic) *—see* Strabismus
foot M62.47-
forearm M62.43-
hand M62.44-
hysterical F44.4
ischemic (Volkmann's) T79.6
lower leg M62.46-
multiple sites M62.49
pelvic region M62.45-
posttraumatic *—see* Strabismus, paralytic
psychogenic F45.8
conversion reaction F44.4
shoulder region M62.41-
specified site NEC M62.48
thigh M62.45-
upper arm M62.42-
neck *—see* Torticollis
ocular muscle *—see* Strabismus
organ or site, congenital NEC *—see* Atresia, by site
outlet (pelvis) *—see* Contraction, pelvis
palmar fascia M72.0
paralytic
joint *—see* Contraction, joint
muscle *—see also* Contraction, muscle NEC
ocular *—see* Strabismus, paralytic
pelvis (acquired) (general) M95.5
with disproportion (fetopelvic) O33.1
causing obstructed labor O65.1
inlet O33.2
mid-cavity O33.3
outlet O33.3
plantar fascia M72.2
premature
atrium I49.1
auriculoventricular I49.49
heart I49.49
junctional I49.2
supraventricular I49.1
ventricular I49.3
prostate N42.89

Contraction(s), contracture, contracted *(continued)*
pylorus NEC *—see also* Pylorospasm
psychogenic F45.8
rectum, rectal (sphincter) K59.89
ring (Bandl's) (complicating delivery) O62.4
scar *—see* Cicatrix
spine *—see* Dorsopathy, deforming
sternocleidomastoid (muscle), congenital Q68.0
stomach K31.89
hourglass K31.89
congenital Q40.2
psychogenic F45.8
psychogenic F45.8
tendon (sheath) M62.40
with contracture of joint *—see* Contraction, joint
Achilles *—see* Short, tendon, Achilles
ankle M62.47-
Achilles *—see* Short, tendon, Achilles
foot M62.47-
forearm M62.43-
hand M62.44-
lower leg M62.46-
multiple sites M62.49
neck M62.48
pelvic region M62.45-
shoulder region M62.41-
specified site NEC M62.48
thigh M62.45-
thorax M62.48
trunk M62.48
upper arm M62.42-
toe *—see* Deformity, toe, specified NEC

Contraction(s), contracture,
ureterovesical orifice (postinfectional) N13.5
with infection N13.6
urethra *—see also* Stricture, urethra
orifice N32.0
uterus N85.8
abnormal NEC O62.9
clonic (complicating delivery) O62.4
dyscoordinate (complicating delivery) O62.4
hourglass (complicating delivery) O62.4
hypertonic O62.4
hypotonic NEC O62.2
inadequate
primary O62.0
secondary O62.1
incoordinate (complicating delivery) O62.4
poor O62.2
tetanic (complicating delivery) O62.4
vagina (outlet) N89.5
vesical N32.89
neck or urethral orifice N32.0
visual field *—see* Defect, visual field, generalized
Volkmann's (ischemic) T79.6

Contusion (skin surface intact) T14.8
abdomen, abdominal (muscle) (wall) S30.1
adnexa, eye NEC S05.8X-
adrenal gland S37.812
alveolar process S00.532
ankle S90.0-
antecubital space *—see* Contusion, forearm
anus S30.3

Contusion *(continued)*
arm (upper) S40.02-
lower (with elbow) *—see* Contusion, forearm
auditory canal *—see* Contusion, ear
auricle *—see* Contusion, ear
axilla *—see* Contusion, arm, upper
back *—see also* Contusion, thorax, back
lower S30.0
bile duct S36.13
bladder S37.22
bone NEC T14.8
brain (diffuse) *—see* Injury, intracranial, diffuse
focal *—see* Injury, intracranial, focal
brainstem S06.38-
breast S20.0-
broad ligament S37.892
brow S00.83
buttock S30.0
canthus, eye S00.1-
cauda equina S34.3
cerebellar, traumatic S06.37-
cerebral S06.33-
left side S06.32-
right side S06.31-
cheek S00.83
internal S00.532
chest (wall) *—see* Contusion, thorax
chin S00.83
clitoris S30.23
colon *—see* Injury, intestine, large, contusion
common bile duct S36.13
conjunctiva S05.1-
with foreign body (in conjunctival sac) *—see* Foreign body, conjunctival sac
conus medullaris (spine) S34.139
cornea *—see* Contusion, eyeball
with foreign body *—see* Foreign body, cornea
corpus cavernosum S30.21
cortex (brain) (cerebral) *—see* Injury, intracranial, diffuse
focal *—see* Injury, intracranial, focal
costal region *—see* Contusion, thorax
cystic duct S36.13
diaphragm S27.802
duodenum S36.420
ear S00.43-
elbow S50.0-
with forearm *—see* Contusion, forearm
epididymis S30.22
epigastric region S30.1
epiglottis S10.0
esophagus (thoracic) S27.812
cervical S10.0
eyeball S05.1-
eyebrow S00.1-
eyelid (and periocular area) S00.1-
face NEC S00.83
fallopian tube S37.529
bilateral S37.522
unilateral S37.521
femoral triangle S30.1
finger(s) S60.00
with damage to nail (matrix) S60.10
index S60.02-
with damage to nail S60.12-
little S60.05-
with damage to nail S60.15-
middle S60.03-
with damage to nail S60.13-
ring S60.04-
with damage to nail S60.14-
thumb *—see* Contusion, thumb

Contusion *(continued)*
flank S30.1
foot (except toe(s) alone) S90.3-
toe *—see* Contusion, toe
forearm S50.1-
elbow only *—see* Contusion, elbow
forehead S00.83
gallbladder S36.122
genital organs, external
female S30.202
male S30.201
globe (eye) *—see* Contusion, eyeball
groin S30.1
gum S00.532
hand S60.22-
finger(s) *—see* Contusion, finger
wrist *—see* Contusion, wrist
head S00.93
ear *—see* Contusion, ear
eyelid *—see* Contusion, eyelid
lip S00.531
nose S00.33
oral cavity S00.532
scalp S00.03
specified part NEC S00.83
heart (*see also* Injury, heart) S26.91
heel *—see* Contusion, foot
hepatic duct S36.13
hip S70.0-
ileum S36.428
iliac region S30.1
inguinal region S30.1
interscapular region S20.229
intra-abdominal organ S36.92
colon *—see* Injury, intestine, large, contusion
liver S36.112
pancreas *—see* Contusion, pancreas
rectum S36.62
small intestine *—see* Injury, intestine, small, contusion
specified organ NEC S36.892
spleen *—see* Contusion, spleen
stomach S36.32
iris (eye) *—see* Contusion, eyeball
jaw S00.83
jejunum S36.428
kidney S37.01-
major (greater than 2 cm) S37.02-
minor (less than 2 cm) S37.01-
knee S80.0-
labium (majus) (minus) S30.23
lacrimal apparatus, gland or sac S05.8X-
larynx S10.0
leg (lower) S80.1-
knee *—see* Contusion, knee
lens *—see* Contusion, eyeball
lip S00.531
liver S36.112
lower back S30.0
lumbar region S30.0
lung S27.329
bilateral S27.322
unilateral S27.321
malar region S00.83
mastoid region S00.83
membrane, brain *—see* Injury, intracranial, diffuse
focal *—see* Injury, intracranial, focal
mesentery S36.892
mesosalpinx S37.892
mouth S00.532
muscle *—see* Contusion, by site
nail
finger *—see* Contusion, finger, with damage to nail
toe *—see* Contusion, toe, with damage to nail

Corrosion *(continued)*
- calf *(continued)*
  - left T24.432
    - first degree T24.532 sickle-cell D57.00
    - second degree T24.632
    - third degree T24.732
  - right T24.431
    - first degree T24.531
    - second degree T24.631
    - third degree T24.731
  - second degree T24.639
  - third degree T24.739
- canthus (eye) —*see* Corrosion, eyelid
- cervix T28.8
- cheek T20.46
  - first degree T20.56
  - second degree T20.66
  - third degree T20.76
- chest wall T21.41
  - first degree T21.51
  - second degree T21.61
  - third degree T21.71
- chin T20.43
  - first degree T20.53
  - second degree T20.63
  - third degree T20.73
- colon T28.7
- conjunctiva (and cornea) —*see* Corrosion, cornea
- cornea (and conjunctiva) T26.6-
- deep necrosis of underlying tissue - code as Corrosion, third degree, by site
- dorsum of hand T23.469
  - first degree T23.569
  - left T23.462
    - first degree T23.562
    - second degree T23.662
    - third degree T23.762
  - right T23.461
    - first degree T23.561
    - second degree T23.661
    - third degree T23.761
  - second degree T23.669
  - third degree T23.769
- ear (auricle) (external) (canal) T20.41
  - drum T28.91
  - first degree T20.51
  - second degree T20.61
  - third degree T20.71
- elbow T22.429
  - first degree T22.529
  - left T22.422
    - first degree T22.522
    - second degree T22.622
    - third degree T22.722
  - right T22.421
    - first degree T22.521
    - second degree T22.621
    - third degree T22.721
  - second degree T22.629
  - third degree T22.729
- entire body —*see* Corrosion, multiple body regions
- epidermal loss - code as Corrosion, second degree, by site
- epiglottis T27.4
- erythema, erythematous - code as Corrosion, first degree, by site
- esophagus T28.6
- extent (percentage of body surface)
  - less than 10 percent T32.0
  - 10-19 percent (0-9 percent third degree) T32.10
    - with 10-19 percent third degree T32.11

Corrosion *(continued)*
- extent *(continued)*
  - 20-29 percent (0-9 percent third degree) T32.20
    - with
      - 10-19 percent third degree T32.21
      - 20-29 percent third degree T32.22
  - 30-39 percent (0-9 percent third degree) T32.30
    - with
      - 10-19 percent third degree T32.31
      - 20-29 percent third degree T32.32
      - 30-39 percent third degree T32.33
  - 40-49 percent (0-9 percent third degree) T32.40
    - with
      - 10-19 percent third degree T32.41
      - 20-29 percent third degree T32.42
      - 30-39 percent third degree T32.43
      - 40-49 percent third degree T32.44
  - 50-59 percent (0-9 percent third degree) T32.50
    - with
      - 10-19 percent third degree T32.51
      - 20-29 percent third degree T32.52
      - 30-39 percent third degree T32.53
      - 40-49 percent third degree T32.54
      - 50-59 percent third degree T32.55
  - 60-69 percent (0-9 percent third degree) T32.60
    - with
      - 10-19 percent third degree T32.61
      - 20-29 percent third degree T32.62
      - 30-39 percent third degree T32.63
      - 40-49 percent third degree T32.64
      - 50-59 percent third degree T32.65
      - 60-69 percent third degree T32.66
  - 70-79 percent (0-9 percent third degree) T32.70
    - with
      - 10-19 percent third degree T32.71
      - 20-29 percent third degree T32.72
      - 30-39 percent third degree T32.73
      - 40-49 percent third degree T32.74
      - 50-59 percent third degree T32.75
      - 60-69 percent third degree T32.76
      - 70-79 percent third degree T32.77
  - 80-89 percent (0-9 percent third degree) T32.80
    - with
      - 10-19 percent third degree T32.81
      - 20-29 percent third degree T32.82

Corrosion *(continued)*
- extent *(continued)*
  - 80-89 percent *(continued)*
    - with *(continued)*
      - 30-39 percent third degree T32.83
      - 40-49 percent third degree T32.84
      - 50-59 percent third degree T32.85
      - 60-69 percent third degree T32.86
      - 70-79 percent third degree T32.87
      - 80-89 percent third degree T32.88
  - 90 percent or more (0-9 percent third degree) T32.90
    - with
      - 10-19 percent third degree T32.91
      - 20-29 percent third degree T32.92
      - 30-39 percent third degree T32.93
      - 40-49 percent third degree T32.94
      - 50-59 percent third degree T32.95
      - 60-69 percent third degree T32.96
      - 70-79 percent third degree T32.97
      - 80-89 percent third degree T32.98
      - 90-99 percent third degree T32.99
- extremity —*see* Corrosion, limb
- eye(s) and adnexa T26.9-
  - with resulting rupture and destruction of eyeball T26.7-
  - conjunctival sac —*see* Corrosion, cornea
  - cornea —*see* Corrosion, cornea
  - lid —*see* Corrosion, eyelid
  - periocular area —*see* Corrosion eyelid
  - specified site NEC T26.8-
- eyeball —*see* Corrosion, eye
- eyelid(s) T26.5-
- face —*see* Corrosion, head
- finger T23.429
  - first degree T23.529
  - left T23.422
    - first degree T23.522
    - second degree T23.622
    - third degree T23.722
  - multiple sites (without thumb) T23.439
    - with thumb T23.449
      - first degree T23.549
      - left T23.442
        - first degree T23.542
        - second degree T23.642
        - third degree T23.742
      - right T23.441
        - first degree T23.541
        - second degree T23.641
        - third degree T23.741
      - second degree T23.649
      - third degree T23.749
    - first degree T23.539
    - left T23.432
      - first degree T23.532
      - second degree T23.632
      - third degree T23.732
    - right T23.431
      - first degree T23.531
      - second degree T23.631
      - third degree T23.731

Corrosion *(continued)*
- finger *(continued)*
  - multiple sites *(continued)*
    - second degree T23.639
    - third degree T23.739
  - right T23.421
    - first degree T23.521
    - second degree T23.621
    - third degree T23.721
  - second degree T23.629
  - third degree T23.729
- flank —*see* Corrosion, abdomen
- foot T25.429
  - first degree T25.529
  - left T25.422
    - first degree T25.522
    - second degree T25.622
    - third degree T25.722
  - multiple with ankle —*see* Corrosion, lower, limb, multiple, ankle and foot
  - right T25.421
    - first degree T25.521
    - second degree T25.621
    - third degree T25.721
  - second degree T25.629
  - third degree T25.729
- forearm T22.419
  - first degree T22.519
  - left T22.412
    - first degree T22.512
    - second degree T22.612
    - third degree T22.712
  - right T22.411
    - first degree T22.511
    - second degree T22.611
    - third degree T22.711
  - second degree T22.619
  - third degree T22.719
- forehead T20.46
  - first degree T20.56
  - second degree T20.66
  - third degree T20.76
- fourth degree - code as Corrosion, third degree, by site
- full thickness skin loss - code as Corrosion, third degree, by site
- gastrointestinal tract NEC T28.7
- genital organs
  - external
    - female T21.47
      - first degree T21.57
      - second degree T21.67
      - third degree T21.77
    - male T21.46
      - first degree T21.56
      - second degree T21.66
      - third degree T21.76
  - internal T28.8
- groin —*see* Corrosion, abdominal wall
- hand(s) T23.409
  - back —*see* Corrosion, dorsum of hand
  - finger —*see* Corrosion, finger
  - first degree T23.509
  - left T23.402
    - first degree T23.502
    - second degree T23.602
    - third degree T23.702
  - multiple sites with wrist T23.499
    - first degree T23.599
    - left T23.492
      - first degree T23.592
      - second degree T23.692
      - third degree T23.792
    - right T23.491
      - first degree T23.591
      - second degree T23.691
      - third degree T23.791
    - second degree T23.699
    - third degree T23.799

Corrosion *(continued)*
hand(s) *(continued)*
palm —*see* Corrosion, palm
right T23.401
first degree T23.501
second degree T23.601
third degree T23.701
second degree T23.609
third degree T23.709
thumb —*see* Corrosion, thumb
head (and face) (and neck) T20.40
cheek —*see* Corrosion, cheek
chin —*see* Corrosion, chin
ear —*see* Corrosion, ear
eye(s) only —*see* Corrosion, eye
first degree T20.50
forehead —*see* Corrosion, forehead
lip —*see* Corrosion, lip
multiple sites T20.49
first degree T20.59
second degree T20.69
third degree T20.79
neck —*see* Corrosion, neck
nose —*see* Corrosion, nose
scalp —*see* Corrosion, scalp
second degree T20.60
third degree T20.70
hip(s) —*see* Corrosion, lower, limb
inhalation —*see* Corrosion, respiratory tract
internal organ(s) (*see also* Corrosion, by site) T28.90
alimentary tract T28.7
esophagus T28.6
esophagus T28.6
genitourinary T28.8
mouth T28.5
pharynx T28.5
specified organ NEC T28.99
interscapular region —*see* Corrosion, back, upper
intestine (large) (small) T28.7
knee T24.429
first degree T24.529
left T24.422
first degree T24.522
second degree T24.622
third degree T24.722
right T24.421
first degree T24.521
second degree T24.621
third degree T24.721
second degree T24.629
third degree T24.729
labium (majus) (minus) —*see* Corrosion, genital organs, external, female
lacrimal apparatus, duct, gland or sac —*see* Corrosion, eye, specified site NEC
larynx T27.4
with lung T27.5
leg(s) (meaning lower limb(s)) —*see* Corrosion, lower limb
limb(s)
lower —*see* Corrosion, lower, limb
upper —*see* Corrosion, upper limb
lip(s) T20.42
first degree T20.52
second degree T20.62
third degree T20.72
lower
back —*see* Corrosion, back
limb T24.409
ankle —*see* Corrosion, ankle
calf —*see* Corrosion, calf
first degree T24.509
foot —*see* Corrosion, foot

Corrosion *(continued)*
lower *(continued)*
limb *(continued)*
knee —*see* Corrosion, knee
left T24.402
first degree T24.502
second degree T24.602
third degree T24.702
multiple sites, except ankle and foot T24.499
ankle and foot T25.499
first degree T25.599
left T25.492
first degree T25.592
second degree T25.692
third degree T25.792
right T25.491
first degree T25.591
second degree T25.691
third degree T25.791
second degree T25.699
third degree T25.799
first degree T24.599
left T24.492
first degree T24.592
second degree T24.692
third degree T24.792
right T24.491
first degree T24.591
second degree T24.691
third degree T24.791
second degree T24.699
third degree T24.799
right T24.401
first degree T24.501
second degree T24.601
third degree T24.701
second degree T24.609
hip —*see* Corrosion, thigh
thigh —*see* Corrosion, thigh
third degree T24.709
lung (with larynx and trachea) T27.5
mouth T28.5
neck T20.47
first degree T20.57
second degree T20.67
third degree T20.77
nose (septum) T20.44
first degree T20.54
second degree T20.64
third degree T20.74
ocular adnexa —*see* Corrosion, eye
orbit region —*see* Corrosion, eyelid
palm T23.459
first degree T23.559
left T23.452
first degree T23.552
second degree T23.652
third degree T23.752
right T23.451
first degree T23.551
second degree T23.651
third degree T23.751
second degree T23.659
third degree T23.759
partial thickness - code as Corrosion, unspecified degree, by site
pelvis —*see* Corrosion, trunk
penis —*see* Corrosion, genital organs, external, male
perineum
female —*see* Corrosion, genital organs, external, female
male —*see* Corrosion, genital organs, external, male
periocular area —*see* Corrosion, eyelid
pharynx T28.5
rectum T28.7

Corrosion *(continued)*
respiratory tract T27.7
larynx —*see* Corrosion, larynx
specified part NEC T27.6
trachea —*see* Corrosion, larynx
sac, lacrimal —*see* Corrosion, eye, specified site NEC
scalp T20.45
first degree T20.55
second degree T20.65
third degree T20.75
scapular region T22.469
first degree T22.569
left T22.462
first degree T22.562
second degree T22.662
third degree T22.762
right T22.461
first degree T22.561
second degree T22.661
third degree T22.761
second degree T22.669
third degree T22.769
sclera —*see* Corrosion, eye, specified site NEC
scrotum —*see* Corrosion, genital organs, external, male
shoulder T22.459
first degree T22.559
left T22.452
first degree T22.552
second degree T22.652
third degree T22.752
right T22.451
first degree T22.551
second degree T22.651
third degree T22.751
second degree T22.659
third degree T22.759
stomach T28.7
temple —*see* Corrosion, head
testis —*see* Corrosion, genital organs, external, male
thigh T24.419
first degree T24.519
left T24.412
first degree T24.512
second degree T24.612
third degree T24.712
right T24.411
first degree T24.511
second degree T24.611
third degree T24.711
second degree T24.619
third degree T24.719
thorax (external) —*see* Corrosion, trunk
throat (meaning pharynx) T28.5
thumb(s) T23.419
first degree T23.519
left T23.412
first degree T23.512
second degree T23.612
third degree T23.712
multiple sites with fingers T23.449
first degree T23.549
left T23.442
first degree T23.542
second degree T23.642
third degree T23.742
right T23.441
first degree T23.541
second degree T23.641
third degree T23.741
second degree T23.649
third degree T23.749
right T23.411
first degree T23.511
second degree T23.611
third degree T23.711
second degree T23.619

Corrosion *(continued)*
thumb(s) *(continued)*
third degree T23.719
toe T25.439
first degree T25.539
left T25.432
first degree T25.532
second degree T25.632
third degree T25.732
right T25.431
first degree T25.531
second degree T25.631
third degree T25.731
second degree T25.639
third degree T25.739
tongue T28.5
tonsil(s) T28.5
total body —*see* Corrosion, multiple body regions
trachea T27.4
with lung T27.5
trunk T21.40
abdominal wall —*see* Corrosion, abdominal wall
anus —*see* Corrosion, buttock
axilla —*see* Corrosion, upper limb
back —*see* Corrosion, back
breast —*see* Corrosion, chest wall
buttock —*see* Corrosion, buttock
chest wall —*see* Corrosion, chest wall
first degree T21.50
flank —*see* Corrosion, abdominal wall
genital
female —*see* Corrosion, genital organs, external, female
male —*see* Corrosion, genital organs, external, male
groin —*see* Corrosion, abdominal wall
interscapular region —*see* Corrosion, back, upper
labia —*see* Corrosion, genital organs, external, female
lower back —*see* Corrosion, back
penis —*see* Corrosion, genital organs, external, male
perineum
female —*see* Corrosion, genital organs, external, female
male —*see* Corrosion, genital organs, external, male
scapular region —*see* Corrosion, upper limb
scrotum —*see* Corrosion, genital organs, external, male
second degree T21.60
shoulder —*see* Corrosion, upper limb
specified site NEC T21.49
first degree T21.59
second degree T21.69
third degree T21.79
testes —*see* Corrosion, genital organs, external, male
third degree T21.70
upper back —*see* Corrosion, back, upper
vagina T28.8
vulva —*see* Corrosion, genital organs, external, female
unspecified site with extent of body surface involved specified
less than 10 percent T32.0
10-19 percent (0-9 percent third degree) T32.10
with 10-19 percent third degree T32.11

Corrosion *(continued)*
unspecified site with extent of body surface involved specified *(continued)*
20-29 percent (0-9 percent third degree) T32.20
with
10-19 percent third degree T32.21
20-29 percent third degree T32.22
30-39 percent (0-9 percent third degree) T32.30
with
10-19 percent third degree T32.31
20-29 percent third degree T32.32
30-39 percent third degree T32.33
40-49 percent (0-9 percent third degree) T32.40
with
10-19 percent third degree T32.41
20-29 percent third degree T32.42
30-39 percent third degree T32.43
40-49 percent third degree T32.44
50-59 percent (0-9 percent third degree) T32.50
with
10-19 percent third degree T32.51
20-29 percent third degree T32.52
30-39 percent third degree T32.53
40-49 percent third degree T32.54
50-59 percent third degree T32.55
60-69 percent (0-9 percent third degree) T32.60
with
10-19 percent third degree T32.61
20-29 percent third degree T32.62
30-39 percent third degree T32.63
40-49 percent third degree T32.64
50-59 percent third degree T32.65
60-69 percent third degree T32.66
70-79 percent (0-9 percent third degree) T32.70
with
10-19 percent third degree T32.71
20-29 percent third degree T32.72
30-39 percent third degree T32.73
40-49 percent third degree T32.74
50-59 percent third degree T32.75
60-69 percent third degree T32.76
70-79 percent third degree T32.77
80-89 percent (0-9 percent third degree) T32.80
with
10-19 percent third degree T32.81

Corrosion *(continued)*
unspecified site with extent of body surface involved specified *(continued)*
80-89 percent *(continued)*
with *(continued)*
20-29 percent third degree T32.82
30-39 percent third degree T32.83
40-49 percent third degree T32.84
50-59 percent third degree T32.85
60-69 percent third degree T32.86
70-79 percent third degree T32.87
80-89 percent third degree T32.88
90 percent or more (0-9 percent third degree) T32.90
with
10-19 percent third degree T32.91
20-29 percent third degree T32.92
30-39 percent third degree T32.93
40-49 percent third degree T32.94
50-59 percent third degree T32.95
60-69 percent third degree T32.96
70-79 percent third degree T32.97
80-89 percent third degree T32.98
90-99 percent third degree T32.99
upper limb (axilla) (scapular region) T22.40
above elbow *—see* Corrosion, above elbow
axilla *—see* Corrosion, axilla
elbow *—see* Corrosion, elbow
first degree T22.50
forearm *—see* Corrosion, forearm
hand *—see* Corrosion, hand
interscapular region *—see* Corrosion, back, upper
multiple sites T22.499
first degree T22.599
left T22.492
first degree T22.592
second degree T22.692
third degree T22.792
right T22.491
first degree T22.591
second degree T22.691
third degree T22.791
second degree T22.699
third degree T22.799
scapular region *—see* Corrosion, scapular region
second degree T22.60
shoulder *—see* Corrosion, shoulder
third degree T22.70
wrist *—see* Corrosion, hand
uterus T28.8
vagina T28.8
vulva *—see* Corrosion, genital organs, external, female
wrist T23.479
first degree T23.579
left T23.472
first degree T23.572
second degree T23.672
third degree T23.772

Corrosion *(continued)*
wrist *(continued)*
multiple sites with hand T23.499
first degree T23.599
left T23.492
first degree T23.592
second degree T23.692
third degree T23.792
right T23.491
first degree T23.591
second degree T23.691
third degree T23.791
second degree T23.699
third degree T23.799
right T23.471
first degree T23.571
second degree T23.671
third degree T23.771
second degree T23.679
third degree T23.779

Corrosive burn *—see* Corrosion

Corsican fever *—see* Malaria

Cortical *—see* condition

Cortico-adrenal *—see* condition

Coryza (acute) J00
with grippe or influenza *—see* Influenza, with, respiratory manifestations NEC
syphilitic
congenital (chronic) A50.05

Costen's syndrome or complex M26.69

Costiveness *—see* Constipation

Costochondritis M94.0

Cotard's syndrome F22

Cot death R99

Cotia virus B08.8

Cotton wool spots (retinal) H35.81

Cotungo's disease *—see* Sciatica

Cough (affected) (epidemic) (nervous) R05.9
with hemorrhage *—see* Hemoptysis
acute R05.1
bronchial R05.8
with grippe or influenza *—see* Influenza, with, respiratory manifestations NEC
chronic R05.3
functional F45.8
hysterical F45.8
laryngeal, spasmodic R05.8
paroxysmal, due to Bordetella pertussis (without pneumonia) A37.00
with pneumonia A37.01
persistent R05.3
psychogenic F45.8
refractory R05.3
specified NEC R05.8
smokers' J41.0
subacute R05.2
syncope R05.4
tea taster's B49
unexplained R05.3

Counseling (for) Z71.9
abuse NEC
perpetrator Z69.82
victim Z69.81
alcohol abuser Z71.41
family Z71.42
child abuse
nonparental
perpetrator Z69.021
victim Z69.020

Counseling *(continued)*
child abuse *(continued)*
parental
perpetrator Z69.011
victim Z69.010
consanguinity Z71.89
contraceptive Z30.09
dietary Z71.3
drug abuser Z71.51
family member Z71.52
exercise Z71.82
family Z71.89
fertility preservation (prior to cancer therapy) (prior to removal of gonads) Z31.62
for non-attending third party Z71.0
related to sexual behavior or orientation Z70.2
genetic
nonprocreative Z71.83
procreative NEC Z31.5
gestational carrier Z31.7
health (advice) (education) (instruction) *—see* Counseling, medical
risk for travel (international) Z71.84
human immunodeficiency virus (HIV) Z71.7
immunization safety Z71.85
impotence Z70.1
insulin pump use Z46.81
medical (for) Z71.9
boarding school resident Z59.3
consanguinity Z71.89
feared complaint and no disease found Z71.1
human immunodeficiency virus (HIV) Z71.7
institutional resident Z59.3
on behalf of another Z71.0
related to sexual behavior or orientation Z70.2
person living alone Z60.2
specified reason NEC Z71.89
natural family planning
procreative Z31.61
to avoid pregnancy Z30.02
perpetrator (of)
abuse NEC Z69.82
child abuse
non-parental Z69.021
parental Z69.011
rape NEC Z69.82
spousal abuse Z69.12
procreative NEC Z31.69
fertility preservation (prior to cancer therapy) (prior to removal of gonads) Z31.62
using natural family planning Z31.61
promiscuity Z70.1
rape victim Z69.81
religious Z71.81
safety for travel (international) Z71.84
sex, sexual (related to) Z70.9
attitude(s) Z70.0
behavior or orientation Z70.1
combined concerns Z70.3
non-responsiveness Z70.1
on behalf of third party Z70.2
specified reason NEC Z70.8
specified reason NEC Z71.89
spiritual Z71.81
spousal abuse (perpetrator) Z69.12
victim Z69.11
substance abuse Z71.89
alcohol Z71.41
drug Z71.51
tobacco Z71.6
tobacco use Z71.6

Counseling *(continued)*
- travel (international) Z71.84
- use (of)
  - insulin pump Z46.81
- vaccine product safety Z71.85
- victim (of)
  - abuse Z69.81
  - child abuse
    - by parent Z69.010
    - non-parental Z69.020
  - rape NEC Z69.81

Coupled rhythm R00.8

Couvelaire syndrome or uterus (complicating delivery) O45.8X-

COVID-19 U07.1
- condition post U09.9
- contact (with) Z20.822
- exposure (to) Z20.822
- history of (personal) Z86.16
- long (haul) U09.9
- pneumonia J12.82
- screening Z11.52
- sequelae (post acute) U09.9

Cowperitis *—see* Urethritis

Cowper's gland *—see* condition

Cowpox B08.010
- due to vaccination T88.1

Coxa
- magna M91.4-
- plana M91.2-
- valga (acquired) *—see also* Deformity, limb, specified type NEC, thigh
  - congenital Q65.81
  - sequelae (late effect) of rickets E64.3
- vara (acquired) *—see also* Deformity, limb, specified type NEC, thigh
  - congenital Q65.82
  - sequelae (late effect) of rickets E64.3

Coxalgia, coxalgic (nontuberculous) *—see also* Pain, joint, hip
- tuberculous A18.02

Coxitis *—see* Monoarthritis, hip

Coxsackie (virus) (infection) B34.1
- as cause of disease classified elsewhere B97.11
- carditis B33.20
- central nervous system NEC A88.8
- endocarditis B33.21
- enteritis A08.39
- meningitis (aseptic) A87.0
- myocarditis B33.22
- pericarditis B33.23
- pharyngitis B08.5
- pleurodynia B33.0
- specific disease NEC B33.8

Crabs, meaning pubic lice B85.3

Crack baby P04.41

Cracked nipple N64.0
- associated with
  - lactation O92.13
  - pregnancy O92.11-
  - puerperium O92.12

Cracked tooth K03.81

Cradle cap L21.0

Craft neurosis F48.8

Cramp(s) R25.2
- abdominal *—see* Pain, abdominal
- bathing T75.1
- colic R10.83
  - psychogenic F45.8
- due to immersion T75.1
- fireman T67.2
- heat T67.2
- immersion T75.1
- intestinal *—see* Pain, abdominal
  - psychogenic F45.8
- leg, sleep related G47.62
- limb (lower) (upper) NEC R25.2
  - sleep related G47.62
- linotypist's F48.8
  - organic G25.89
- muscle (limb) (general) R25.2
  - due to immersion T75.1
  - psychogenic F45.8
- occupational (hand) F48.8
  - organic G25.89
- salt-depletion E87.1
- sleep related, leg G47.62
- stoker's T67.2
- swimmer's T75.1
- telegrapher's F48.8
  - organic G25.89
- typist's F48.8
  - organic G25.89
- uterus N94.89
  - menstrual *—see* Dysmenorrhea
- writer's F48.8
  - organic G25.89

Cranial *—see* condition

Craniocleidodysostosis Q74.0

Craniofenestria (skull) Q75.8

Craniolacunia (skull) Q75.8

Craniopagus Q89.4

Craniopathy, metabolic M85.2

Craniopharyngeal *—see* condition

Craniopharyngioma D44.4

Craniorachischisis (totalis) Q00.1

Cranioschisis Q75.8

Craniostenosis Q75.0

Craniosynostosis Q75.0

Craniotabes (cause unknown) M83.8
- neonatal P96.3
- rachitic E64.3
- syphilitic A50.56

Cranium *—see* condition

Craw-craw *—see* Onchocerciasis

Creaking joint *—see* Derangement, joint, specified type NEC

Creeping
- eruption B76.9
- palsy or paralysis G12.22

Crenated tongue K14.8

Creotoxism A05.9

Crepitus
- caput Q75.8
- joint *—see* Derangement, joint, specified type NEC

Crescent or conus choroid, congenital Q14.3

CREST syndrome M34.1

Cretin, cretinism (congenital) (endemic) (nongoitrous) (sporadic) E00.9
- pelvis
  - with disproportion (fetopelvic) O33.0
    - causing obstructed labor O65.0
- type
  - hypothyroid E00.1
  - mixed E00.2
  - myxedematous E00.1
  - neurological E00.0

Creutzfeldt-Jakob disease or syndrome (with dementia) A81.00
- familial A81.09
- iatrogenic A81.09
- specified NEC A81.09
- sporadic A81.09
- variant (vCJD) A81.01

Crib death R99

Cribriform hymen Q52.3

Cri-du-chat syndrome Q93.4

Crigler-Najjar disease or syndrome E80.5

Crime, victim of Z65.4

Crimean hemorrhagic fever A98.0

Criminalism F60.2

Crisis
- abdomen R10.0
- acute reaction F43.0
- addisonian E27.2
- adrenal (cortical) E27.2
- celiac K90.0
- Dietl's N13.8
- emotional *—see also* Disorder, adjustment
  - acute reaction to stress F43.0
  - specific to childhood and adolescence F93.8
- glaucomatocyclitic *—see* Glaucoma, secondary, inflammation
- heart *—see* Failure, heart
- nitritoid I95.2
  - correct substance properly administered *—see* Table of Drugs and Chemicals, by drug, adverse effect
  - overdose or wrong substance given or taken *—see* Table of Drugs and Chemicals, by drug, poisoning
- oculogyric H51.8
  - psychogenic F45.8
- Pel's (tabetic) A52.11
- psychosexual identity F64.2
- renal N28.0
- sickle-cell D57.00
  - with
    - acute chest syndrome D57.01
    - cerebral vascular involvement D57.03
    - crisis (painful) D57.00
      - with complication specified NEC D57.09
    - splenic sequestration D57.02
    - vasoocclusive pain D57.00
- state (acute reaction) F43.0
- tabetic A52.11
- thyroid *—see* Thyrotoxicosis with thyroid storm
- thyrotoxic *—see* Thyrotoxicosis with thyroid storm

Crocq's disease (acrocyanosis) I73.89

Crohn's disease *—see* Enteritis, regional

Crooked septum, nasal J34.2

Cross syndrome E70.328

Crossbite (anterior) (posterior) M26.24

Cross-eye *—see* Strabismus, convergent concomitant

Croup, croupous (catarrhal) (infectious) (inflammatory) (nondiphtheritic) J05.0
- bronchial J20.9
- diphtheritic A36.2
- false J38.5
- spasmodic J38.5
  - diphtheritic A36.2
- stridulous J38.5
  - diphtheritic A36.2

Crouzon's disease Q75.1

Crowding, tooth, teeth, fully erupted M26.31

CRST syndrome M34.1

Cruchet's disease A85.8

Cruelty in children *—see also* Disorder, conduct

Crural ulcer *—see* Ulcer, lower limb

Crush, crushed, crushing T14.8
- abdomen S38.1
- ankle S97.0-
- arm (upper) (and shoulder) S47.-
- axilla *—see* Crush, arm
- back, lower S38.1
- buttock S38.1
- cheek S07.0
- chest S28.0
- cranium S07.1
- ear S07.0
- elbow S57.0-
- extremity
  - lower
    - ankle *—see* Crush, ankle
    - below knee *—see* Crush, leg
    - foot *—see* Crush, foot
    - hip *—see* Crush, hip
    - knee *—see* Crush, knee
    - thigh *—see* Crush, thigh
    - toe *—see* Crush, toe
  - upper
    - below elbow S67.9-
    - elbow *—see* Crush, elbow
    - finger *—see* Crush, finger
    - forearm *—see* Crush, forearm
    - hand *—see* Crush, hand
    - thumb *—see* Crush, thumb
    - upper arm *—see* Crush, arm
    - wrist *—see* Crush, wrist
- face S07.0
- finger(s) S67.1-
  - with hand (and wrist) *—see* Crush, hand, specified site NEC
  - index S67.19-
  - little S67.19-
  - middle S67.19-
  - ring S67.19-
  - thumb *—see* Crush, thumb
- foot S97.8-
  - toe *—see* Crush, toe
- forearm S57.8-
- genitalia, external
  - female S38.002
    - vagina S38.03
    - vulva S38.03
  - male S38.001
    - penis S38.01
    - scrotum S38.02
    - testis S38.02
- hand (except fingers alone) S67.2-
  - with wrist S67.4-
- head S07.9
  - specified NEC S07.8
- heel *—see* Crush, foot
- hip S77.0-
  - with thigh S77.2-
- internal organ (abdomen, chest, or pelvis) NEC T14.8
- knee S87.0-
- labium (majus) (minus) S38.03
- larynx S17.0
- leg (lower) S87.8-
  - knee *—see* Crush, knee
- lip S07.0
- lower
  - back S38.1
  - leg *—see* Crush, leg
- neck S17.9

Cyst *(continued)*

- bursa, bursal NEC M71.30
  - with rupture —*see* Rupture, synovium
  - ankle M71.37-
  - elbow M71.32-
  - foot M71.37-
  - hand M71.34-
  - hip M71.35-
  - multiple sites M71.39
  - pharyngeal J39.2
  - popliteal space —*see* Cyst, Baker's
  - shoulder M71.31-
  - specified site NEC M71.38
  - wrist M71.33-
- calcifying odontogenic D16.5
  - upper jaw (bone) (maxilla) D16.4
- canal of Nuck (female) N94.89
  - congenital Q52.4
- canthus —*see* Cyst, conjunctiva
- carcinomatous —*see* Neoplasm, malignant, by site
- cauda equina G95.89
- cavum septi pellucidi —*see* Cyst, brain
- celomic (pericardium) Q24.8
- cerebellopontine (angle) —*see* Cyst, brain
- cerebellum —*see* Cyst, brain
- cerebral —*see* Cyst, brain
- cervical lateral Q18.0
- cervix NEC N88.8
  - embryonic Q51.6
  - nabothian N88.8
- chiasmal optic NEC —*see* Disorder, optic, chiasm
- chocolate (ovary) N80.1
- choledochus, congenital Q44.4
- chorion O41.8X-
- choroid plexus G93.0
  - congenital Q04.6
- ciliary body —*see* Cyst, iris
- clitoris N90.7
- colon K63.89
- common (bile) duct K83.5
- congenital NEC Q89.8
  - adrenal gland Q89.1
  - epiglottis Q31.8
  - esophagus Q39.8
  - fallopian tube Q50.4
  - kidney Q61.00
    - more than one (multiple) Q61.02
      - specified as polycystic Q61.3
        - adult type Q61.2
        - infantile type NEC Q61.19
          - collecting duct dilation Q61.11
    - solitary Q61.01
  - larynx Q31.8
  - liver Q44.6
  - lung Q33.0
  - mediastinum Q34.1
  - ovary Q50.1
  - oviduct Q50.4
  - periurethral (tissue) Q64.79
  - prepuce Q55.69
  - salivary gland (any) Q38.4
  - sublingual Q38.6
  - submaxillary gland Q38.6
  - thymus (gland) Q89.2
  - tongue Q38.3
  - ureterovesical orifice Q62.8
  - vulva Q52.79
- conjunctiva H11.44-
- cornea H18.89-
- corpora quadrigemina G93.0

Cyst *(continued)*

- corpus
  - albicans N83.29-
  - luteum (hemorrhagic) (ruptured) N83.1-
- Cowper's gland (benign) (infected) N36.8
- cranial meninges G93.0
- craniobuccal pouch E23.6
- craniopharyngeal pouch E23.6
- cystic duct K82.8
- Cysticercus —*see* Cysticercosis
- Dandy-Walker Q03.1
  - with spina bifida —*see* Spina bifida
- dental (root) K04.8
  - developmental K09.0
  - eruption K09.0
  - primordial K09.0
- dentigerous (mandible) (maxilla) K09.0
- dermoid —*see* Neoplasm, benign, by site
  - with malignant transformation C56.-
  - implantation
    - external area or site (skin) NEC L72.0
    - iris —*see* Cyst, iris, implantation
    - vagina N89.8
    - vulva N90.7
  - mouth K09.8
  - oral soft tissue K09.8
  - sacrococcygeal —*see* Cyst, pilonidal
- developmental K09.1
  - odontogenic K09.0
  - oral region (nonodontogenic) K09.1
  - ovary, ovarian Q50.1
- dura (cerebral) G93.0
  - spinal G96.198
- ear (external) Q18.1
- echinococcal —*see* Echinococcus
- embryonic
  - cervix uteri Q51.6
  - fallopian tube Q50.4
  - vagina Q52.4
- endometrium, endometrial (uterus) N85.8
  - ectopic —*see* Endometriosis
- enterogenous Q43.8
- epidermal, epidermoid (inclusion) (*see also* Cyst, skin) L72.0
  - mouth K09.8
  - oral soft tissue K09.8
- epididymis N50.3
- epiglottis J38.7
- epiphysis cerebri E34.8
- epithelial (inclusion) L72.0
- epoophoron Q50.5
- eruption K09.0
- esophagus K22.89
- ethmoid sinus J34.1
- external female genital organs NEC N90.7
- eye NEC H57.89
  - congenital Q15.8
- eyelid (sebaceous) H02.829
  - infected —*see* Hordeolum
  - left H02.826
    - lower H02.825
    - upper H02.824
  - right H02.823
    - lower H02.822
    - upper H02.821
- fallopian tube N83.8
  - congenital Q50.4
- fimbrial (twisted) Q50.4
- fissural (oral region) K09.1

Cyst *(continued)*

- follicle (graafian) (hemorrhagic) N83.0-
  - nabothian N88.8
- follicular (atretic) (hemorrhagic) (ovarian) N83.0-
  - dentigerous K09.0
  - odontogenic K09.0
  - skin L72.9
    - specified NEC L72.8
- frontal sinus J34.1
- gallbladder K82.8
- ganglion —*see* Ganglion
- Gartner's duct Q52.4
- gingiva K09.0
- gland of Moll —*see* Cyst, eyelid
- globulomaxillary K09.1
- graafian follicle (hemorrhagic) N83.0-
- granulosal lutein (hemorrhagic) N83.1-
- hemangiomatous D18.00
  - intra-abdominal D18.03
  - intracranial D18.02
  - skin D18.01
  - specified site NEC D18.09
- hemorrhagic M27.49
- hydatid (*see also* Echinococcus) B67.90
  - brain B67.99 *[G94]*
  - liver (*see also* Cyst, liver, hydatid) B67.8
  - lung NEC B67.99 *[J99]*
  - Morgagni
    - female Q50.5
    - male (epididymal) Q55.4
      - testicular Q55.29
  - specified site NEC B67.99
- hymen N89.8
  - embryonic Q52.4
- hypopharynx J39.2
- hypophysis, hypophyseal (duct) (recurrent) E23.6
  - cerebri E23.6
- implantation (dermoid)
  - external area or site (skin) NEC L72.0
  - iris —*see* Cyst, iris, implantation
  - vagina N89.8
  - vulva N90.7
- incisive canal K09.1
- inclusion (epidermal) (epithelial) (epidermoid) (squamous) L72.0
  - not of skin - code under Cyst, by site
- intestine (large) (small) K63.89
- intracranial —*see* Cyst, brain
- intraligamentous —*see also* Disorder, ligament
  - knee —*see* Derangement, knee
- intrasellar E23.6
- iris H21.309
  - exudative H21.31-
  - idiopathic H21.30-
  - implantation H21.32-
  - parasitic H21.33-
  - pars plana (primary) H21.34-
    - exudative H21.35-
- jaw (bone) M27.40
  - aneurysmal M27.49
  - developmental (odontogenic) K09.0
  - fissural K09.1
  - hemorrhagic M27.49
  - traumatic M27.49
- joint NEC —*see* Disorder, joint, specified type NEC
- kidney (acquired) N28.1
  - calyceal —*see* Hydronephrosis
  - congenital Q61.00

Cyst *(continued)*

- kidney *(continued)*
  - more than one (multiple) Q61.02
    - specified as polycystic Q61.3
      - adult type (autosomal dominant) Q61.2
      - infantile type (autosomal recessive) NEC Q61.19
        - collecting duct dilation Q61.11
  - pyelogenic —*see* Hydronephrosis
  - simple N28.1
  - solitary (single) Q61.01
    - acquired N28.1
- labium (majus) (minus) N90.7
  - sebaceous N90.7
- lacrimal —*see also* Disorder, lacrimal system, specified NEC
  - gland H04.13-
  - passages or sac —*see* Disorder, lacrimal system, specified NEC
- larynx J38.7
- lateral periodontal K09.0
- lens H27.8
  - congenital Q12.8
- lip (gland) K13.0
- liver (idiopathic) (simple) K76.89
  - congenital Q44.6
  - hydatid B67.8
    - granulosus B67.0
    - multilocularis B67.5
- lung J98.4
  - congenital Q33.0
  - giant bullous J43.9
- lutein N83.1-
- lymphangiomatous D18.1
- lymphoepithelial, oral soft tissue K09.8
- macula —*see* Degeneration, macula, hole
- malignant —*see* Neoplasm, malignant, by site
- mammary gland —*see* Cyst, breast
- mandible M27.40
  - dentigerous K09.0
  - radicular K04.8
- maxilla M27.40
  - dentigerous K09.0
  - radicular K04.8
- medial, face and neck Q18.8
- median
  - anterior maxillary K09.1
  - palatal K09.1
- mediastinum, congenital Q34.1
- meibomian (gland) —*see* Chalazion
  - infected —*see* Hordeolum
- membrane, brain G93.0
- meninges (cerebral) G93.0
  - spinal G96.198
- meniscus, knee —*see* Derangement, knee, meniscus, cystic
- mesentery, mesenteric K66.8
  - chyle I89.8
- mesonephric duct
  - female Q50.5
  - male Q55.4
- milk N64.89
- Morgagni (hydatid)
  - female Q50.5
  - male (epididymal) Q55.4
    - testicular Q55.29
- mouth K09.8
- Müllerian duct Q50.4
  - appendix testis Q55.29
  - cervix Q51.6
  - fallopian tube Q50.4
  - female Q50.4
  - male Q55.29

Cyst *(continued)*
- Müllerian duct *(continued)*
  - prostatic utricle Q55.4
  - vagina (embryonal) Q52.4
- multilocular (ovary) D39.10
  - benign —*see* Neoplasm, benign, by site
- myometrium N85.8
- nabothian (follicle) (ruptured) N88.8
- nasoalveolar K09.1
- nasolabial K09.1
- nasopalatine (anterior) (duct) K09.1
- nasopharynx J39.2
- neoplastic —*see* Neoplasm, uncertain behavior, by site
  - benign —*see* Neoplasm, benign, by site
- nerve root
  - cervical G96.191
  - lumbar G96.191
  - sacral G96.191
  - thoracic G96.191
- nervous system NEC G96.89
- neuroenteric (congenital) Q06.8
- nipple —*see* Cyst, breast
- nose (turbinates) J34.1
  - sinus J34.1
- odontogenic, developmental K09.0
- omentum (lesser) K66.8
  - congenital Q45.8
- ora serrata —*see* Cyst, retina, ora serrata
- oral
  - region K09.9
    - developmental (nonodontogenic) K09.1
    - specified NEC K09.8
  - soft tissue K09.9
    - specified NEC K09.8
- orbit H05.81-
- ovary, ovarian (twisted) N83.20-
  - adherent N83.20-
  - chocolate N80.1
  - corpus
    - albicans N83.29-
    - luteum (hemorrhagic) N83.1-
  - dermoid D27.9
  - developmental Q50.1
  - due to failure of involution NEC N83.20-
  - endometrial N80.1
  - follicular (graafian) (hemorrhagic) N83.0-
  - hemorrhagic N83.20-
  - in pregnancy or childbirth O34.8-
    - with obstructed labor O65.5
  - multilocular D39.10
  - pseudomucinous D27.9
  - retention N83.29-
  - serous N83.20-
  - specified NEC N83.29-
  - theca lutein (hemorrhagic) N83.1-
  - tuberculous A18.18
- oviduct N83.8
- palate (median) (fissural) K09.1
- palatine papilla (jaw) K09.1
- pancreas, pancreatic (hemorrhagic) (true) K86.2
  - congenital Q45.2
  - false K86.3
- paralabral
  - hip M24.85-
  - shoulder S43.43-
- paramesonephric duct Q50.4
  - female Q50.4
  - male Q55.29
- paranephric N28.1

Cyst *(continued)*
- paraphysis, cerebri, congenital Q04.6
- parasitic B89
- parathyroid (gland) E21.4
- paratubal N83.8
- paraurethral duct N36.8
- paroophoron Q50.5
- parotid gland K11.6
- parovarian Q50.5
- pelvis, female N94.89
  - in pregnancy or childbirth O34.8-
    - causing obstructed labor O65.5
- penis (sebaceous) N48.89
- periapical K04.8
- pericardial (congenital) Q24.8
  - acquired (secondary) I31.8
- pericoronal K09.0
- perineural G96.191
- periodontal K04.8
  - lateral K09.0
- peripelvic (lymphatic) N28.1
- peritoneum K66.8
  - chylous I89.8
- periventricular, acquired, newborn P91.1
- pharynx (wall) J39.2
- pilar L72.11
- pilonidal (infected) (rectum) L05.91
  - with abscess L05.01
  - malignant C44.59-
- pituitary (duct) (gland) E23.6
- placenta O43.19-
- pleura J94.8
- popliteal —*see* Cyst, Baker's
- porencephalic Q04.6
  - acquired G93.0
- postanal (infected) —*see* Cyst, pilonidal
- postmastoidectomy cavity (mucosal) —*see* Complications, postmastoidectomy, cyst
- preauricular Q18.1
- prepuce N47.4
  - congenital Q55.69
- primordial (jaw) K09.0
- prostate N42.83
- pseudomucinous (ovary) D27.9
- pupillary, miotic H21.27-
- radicular (residual) K04.8
- radiculodental K04.8
- ranular K11.8
- Rathke's pouch E23.6
- rectum (epithelium) (mucous) K62.89
- renal —*see* Cyst, kidney
- residual (radicular) K04.8
- retention (ovary) N83.29-
  - salivary gland K11.6
- retina H33.19-
  - ora serrata H33.11-
  - parasitic H33.12-
- retroperitoneal K68.9
- sacrococcygeal (dermoid) —*see* Cyst, pilonidal
- salivary gland or duct (mucous extravasation or retention) K11.6
- Sampson's N80.1
- sclera H15.89
- scrotum L72.9
  - sebaceous L72.3
- sebaceous (duct) (gland) L72.3
  - breast —*see* Dysplasia, mammary, specified type NEC
  - eyelid —*see* Cyst, eyelid
  - genital organ NEC
    - female N94.89
    - male N50.89
  - scrotum L72.3

Cyst *(continued)*
- semilunar cartilage (knee) (multiple) —*see* Derangement, knee, meniscus, cystic
- seminal vesicle N50.89
- serous (ovary) N83.20-
- sinus (accessory) (nasal) J34.1
- Skene's gland N36.8
- skin L72.9
  - breast —*see* Dysplasia, mammary, specified type NEC
  - epidermal, epidermoid L72.0
  - epithelial L72.0
  - eyelid —*see* Cyst, eyelid
  - genital organ NEC
    - female N90.7
    - male N50.89
  - inclusion L72.0
  - scrotum L72.9
  - sebaceous L72.3
  - sweat gland or duct L74.8
- solitary
  - bone —*see* Cyst, bone, solitary
  - jaw M27.40
  - kidney N28.1
- spermatic cord N50.89
- sphenoid sinus J34.1
- spinal meninges G96.198
- spleen NEC D73.4
  - congenital Q89.09
  - hydatid (*see also* Echinococcus) B67.99 *[D77]*
- Stafne's M27.0
- subarachnoid intrasellar R93.0
- subcutaneous, pheomycotic (chromomycotic) B43.2
- subdural (cerebral) G93.0
  - spinal cord G96.198
- sublingual gland K11.6
- submandibular gland K11.6
- submaxillary gland K11.6
- suburethral N36.8
- suprarenal gland E27.8
- suprasellar —*see* Cyst, brain
- sweat gland or duct L74.8
- synovial —*see also* Cyst, bursa
  - ruptured —*see* Rupture, synovium
- Tarlov G96.191
- tarsal —*see* Chalazion
- tendon (sheath) —*see* Disorder, tendon, specified type NEC
- testis N44.2
  - tunica albuginea N44.1
- theca lutein (ovary) N83.1-
- Thornwaldt's J39.2
- thymus (gland) E32.8
- thyroglossal duct (infected) (persistent) Q89.2
- thyrolingual duct (infected) (persistent) Q89.2
- thyroid (gland) E04.1
- tongue K14.8
- tonsil J35.8
- tooth —*see* Cyst, dental
- Tornwaldt's J39.2
- trichilemmal (proliferating) L72.12
- trichodermal L72.12
- tubal (fallopian) N83.8
  - inflammatory —*see* Salpingitis, chronic
- tubo-ovarian N83.8
  - inflammatory N70.13
- tunica
  - albuginea testis N44.1
  - vaginalis N50.89
- turbinate (nose) J34.1
- Tyson's gland N48.89
- urachus, congenital Q64.4
- ureter N28.89

Cyst *(continued)*
- ureterovesical orifice N28.89
- urethra, urethral (gland) N36.8
- uterine ligament N83.8
- uterus (body) (corpus) (recurrent) N85.8
  - embryonic Q51.818
    - cervix Q51.6
- vagina, vaginal (implantation) (inclusion) (squamous cell) (wall) N89.8
  - embryonic Q52.4
- vallecula, vallecular (epiglottis) J38.7
- vesical (orifice) N32.89
- vitreous body H43.89
- vulva (implantation) (inclusion) N90.7
  - congenital Q52.79
  - sebaceous gland N90.7
- vulvovaginal gland N90.7
- wolffian
  - female Q50.5
  - male Q55.4

Cystadenocarcinoma —*see* Neoplasm, malignant, by site
- bile duct C22.1
- endometrioid —*see* Neoplasm, malignant, by site
  - specified site —*see* Neoplasm, malignant, by site
  - unspecified site
    - female C56.9
    - male C61
- mucinous
  - papillary
    - specified site —*see* Neoplasm, malignant, by site
    - unspecified site C56.9
  - specified site —*see* Neoplasm, malignant, by site
  - unspecified site C56.9
- papillary
  - mucinous
    - specified site —*see* Neoplasm, malignant, by site
    - unspecified site C56.9
  - pseudomucinous
    - specified site —*see* Neoplasm, malignant, by site
    - unspecified site C56.9
  - serous
    - specified site —*see* Neoplasm, malignant, by site
    - unspecified site C56.9
  - specified site —*see* Neoplasm, malignant, by site
  - unspecified site C56.9
- pseudomucinous
  - papillary
    - specified site —*see* Neoplasm, malignant, by site
    - unspecified site C56.9
  - specified site —*see* Neoplasm, malignant, by site
  - unspecified site C56.9
- serous
  - papillary
    - specified site —*see* Neoplasm, malignant, by site
    - unspecified site C56.9
  - specified site —*see* Neoplasm, malignant, by site
  - unspecified site C56.9

Cystadenofibroma
- clear cell —*see* Neoplasm, benign, by site
- endometrioid D27.9
  - borderline malignancy D39.1-
  - malignant C56.-

Cystadenofibroma *(continued)*
- mucinous
  - specified site —*see* Neoplasm, benign, by site
  - unspecified site D27.9
- serous
  - specified site —*see* Neoplasm, benign, by site
  - unspecified site D27.9
- specified site —*see* Neoplasm, benign, by site
- unspecified site D27.9

Cystadenoma —*see also* Neoplasm, benign, by site
- bile duct D13.4
- endometrioid —*see* Neoplasm, benign, by site
  - borderline malignancy —*see* Neoplasm, uncertain behavior, by site
- malignant —*see* Neoplasm, malignant, by site
- mucinous
  - borderline malignancy
    - ovary C56.-
    - specified site NEC —*see* Neoplasm, uncertain behavior, by site
    - unspecified site C56.9
  - papillary
    - borderline malignancy
      - ovary C56.-
      - specified site NEC —*see* Neoplasm, uncertain behavior, by site
      - unspecified site C56.9
    - specified site —*see* Neoplasm, benign, by site
    - unspecified site D27.9
  - specified site —*see* Neoplasm, benign, by site
  - unspecified site D27.9
- papillary
  - borderline malignancy
    - ovary C56.-
    - specified site NEC —*see* Neoplasm, uncertain behavior, by site
    - unspecified site C56.9
  - lymphomatosum
    - specified site —*see* Neoplasm, benign, by site
    - unspecified site D11.9
  - mucinous
    - borderline malignancy
      - ovary C56.-
      - specified site NEC —*see* Neoplasm, uncertain behavior, by site
      - unspecified site C56.9
    - specified site —*see* Neoplasm, benign, by site
    - unspecified site D27.9
  - pseudomucinous
    - borderline malignancy
      - ovary C56.-
      - specified site NEC —*see* Neoplasm, uncertain behavior, by site
      - unspecified site C56.9
    - specified site —*see* Neoplasm, benign, by site
    - unspecified site D27.9
  - serous
    - borderline malignancy
      - ovary C56.-
      - specified site NEC —*see* Neoplasm, uncertain behavior, by site
      - unspecified site C56.9

Cystadenoma *(continued)*
- papillary *(continued)*
  - serous *(continued)*
    - specified site —*see* Neoplasm, benign, by site
    - unspecified site D27.9
  - specified site —*see* Neoplasm, benign, by site
  - unspecified site D27.9
- pseudomucinous
  - borderline malignancy
    - ovary C56.-
    - specified site NEC —*see* Neoplasm, uncertain behavior, by site
    - unspecified site C56.9
  - papillary
    - borderline malignancy
      - ovary C56.-
      - specified site NEC —*see* Neoplasm, uncertain behavior, by site
      - unspecified site C56.9
    - specified site —*see* Neoplasm, benign, by site
    - unspecified site D27.9
  - specified site —*see* Neoplasm, benign, by site
  - unspecified site D27.9
- serous
  - borderline malignancy
    - ovary C56.-
    - specified site NEC —*see* Neoplasm, uncertain behavior, by site
    - unspecified site C56.9
  - papillary
    - borderline malignancy
      - ovary C56.-
      - specified site NEC —*see* Neoplasm, uncertain behavior, by site
      - unspecified site C56.9
    - specified site —*see* Neoplasm, benign, by site
    - unspecified site D27.9
  - specified site —*see* Neoplasm, benign, by site
  - unspecified site D27.9

Cystathionine synthase deficiency E72.11

Cystathioninemia E72.19

Cystathioninuria E72.19

Cystic —*see also* condition
- breast (chronic) —*see* Mastopathy, cystic
- corpora lutea (hemorrhagic) N83.1-
- duct —*see* condition
- eyeball (congenital) Q11.0
- fibrosis —*see* Fibrosis, cystic
- kidney (congenital) Q61.9
  - adult type Q61.2
  - infantile type NEC Q61.19
    - collecting duct dilatation Q61.11
  - medullary Q61.5
- liver, congenital Q44.6
- lung disease J98.4
  - congenital Q33.0
- mastitis, chronic —*see* Mastopathy, cystic
- medullary, kidney Q61.5
- meniscus —*see* Derangement, knee, meniscus, cystic
- ovary N83.20-

Cysticercosis, cysticerciasis B69.9
- with
  - epileptiform fits B69.0
  - myositis B69.81

Cysticercosis, cysticerciasis *(continued)*
- brain B69.0
- central nervous system B69.0
- cerebral B69.0
- ocular B69.1
- specified NEC B69.89

Cysticercus cellulose infestation —*see* Cysticercosis

Cystinosis (malignant) E72.04

Cystinuria E72.01

Cystitis (exudative) (hemorrhagic) (septic) (suppurative) N30.90
- with
  - fibrosis —*see* Cystitis, chronic, interstitial
  - hematuria N30.91
  - leukoplakia —*see* Cystitis, chronic, interstitial
  - malakoplakia —*see* Cystitis, chronic, interstitial
  - metaplasia —*see* Cystitis, chronic, interstitial
  - prostatitis N41.3
- acute N30.00
  - with hematuria N30.01
  - of trigone N30.30
    - with hematuria N30.31
- allergic —*see* Cystitis, specified type NEC
- amebic A06.81
- bilharzial B65.9 *[N33]*
- blennorrhagic (gonococcal) A54.01
- bullous —*see* Cystitis, specified type NEC
- calculous N21.0
- chlamydial A56.01
- chronic N30.20
  - with hematuria N30.21
  - interstitial N30.10
    - with hematuria N30.11
  - of trigone N30.30
    - with hematuria N30.31
  - specified NEC N30.20
    - with hematuria N30.21
- cystic (a) —*see* Cystitis, specified type NEC
- diphtheritic A36.85
- echinococcal
  - granulosus B67.39
  - multilocularis B67.69
- emphysematous —*see* Cystitis, specified type NEC
- encysted —*see* Cystitis, specified type NEC
- eosinophilic —*see* Cystitis, specified type NEC
- follicular —*see* Cystitis, of trigone
- gangrenous —*see* Cystitis, specified type NEC
- glandularis —*see* Cystitis, specified type NEC
- gonococcal A54.01
- incrusted —*see* Cystitis, specified type NEC
- interstitial (chronic) —*see* Cystitis, chronic, interstitial
- irradiation N30.40
  - with hematuria N30.41
- irritation —*see* Cystitis, specified type NEC
- malignant —*see* Cystitis, specified type NEC
- of trigone N30.30
  - with hematuria N30.31
- panmural —*see* Cystitis, chronic, interstitial
- polyposa —*see* Cystitis, specified type NEC

Cystitis *(continued)*
- prostatic N41.3
- puerperal (postpartum) O86.22
- radiation —*see* Cystitis, irradiation
- specified type NEC N30.80
  - with hematuria N30.81
- subacute —*see* Cystitis, chronic
- submucous —*see* Cystitis, chronic, interstitial
- syphilitic (late) A52.76
- trichomonal A59.03
- tuberculous A18.12
- ulcerative —*see* Cystitis, chronic, interstitial

Cystocele (-urethrocele)
- female N81.10
  - with prolapse of uterus —*see* Prolapse, uterus
  - lateral N81.12
  - midline N81.11
  - paravaginal N81.12
- in pregnancy or childbirth O34.8-
  - causing obstructed labor O65.5
- male N32.89

Cystolithiasis N21.0

Cystoma —*see also* Neoplasm, benign, by site
- endometrial, ovary N80.1
- mucinous
  - specified site —*see* Neoplasm, benign, by site
  - unspecified site D27.9
- serous
  - specified site —*see* Neoplasm, benign, by site
  - unspecified site D27.9
- simple (ovary) N83.29-

Cystoplegia N31.2

Cystoptosis N32.89

Cystopyelitis —*see* Pyelonephritis

Cystorrhagia N32.89

Cystosarcoma phyllodes D48.6-
- benign D24-
- malignant —*see* Neoplasm, breast, malignant

Cystostomy
- attention to Z43.5
- complication —*see* Complications, cystostomy
- status Z93.50
  - appendico-vesicostomy Z93.52
  - cutaneous Z93.51
  - specified NEC Z93.59

Cystourethritis —*see* Urethritis

Cystourethrocele —*see also* Cystocele
- female N81.10
  - with uterine prolapse —*see* Prolapse, uterus
  - lateral N81.12
  - midline N81.11
  - paravaginal N81.12
- male N32.89

Cytomegalic inclusion disease
- congenital P35.1

Cytomegalovirus infection B25.9

Cytomycosis (reticuloendothelial) B39.4

Cytopenia D75.9
- refractory
  - with multilineage dysplasia D46.A
    - and ring sideroblasts (RCMD RS) D46.B

Czerny's disease (periodic hydrarthrosis of the knee) —*see* Effusion, joint, knee

D

Daae (-Finsen) **disease** (epidemic pleurodynia) B33.0

Da Costa's syndrome F45.8

Dabney's grip B33.0

Dacryoadenitis, dacryadenitis H04.00-
  acute H04.01-
  chronic H04.02-

Dacryocystitis H04.30-
  acute H04.32-
  chronic H04.41-
  neonatal P39.1
  phlegmonous H04.31-
  syphilitic A52.71
    congenital (early) A50.01
  trachomatous, active A71.1
    sequelae (late effect) B94.0

Dacryocystoblenorrhea —*see* Inflammation, lacrimal, passages, chronic

Dacryocystocele —*see* Disorder, lacrimal system, changes

Dacryolith, dacryolithiasis H04.51-

Dacryoma —*see* Disorder, lacrimal system, changes

Dacryopericystitis —*see* Dacryocystitis

Dacryops H04.11-

Dacryostenosis —*see also* Stenosis, lacrimal
  congenital Q10.5

Dactylitis
  bone —*see* Osteomyelitis
  sickle-cell D57.00
    Hb C D57.219
    Hb SS D57.00
    specified NEC D57.819
  skin L08.9
  syphilitic A52.77
  tuberculous A18.03

Dactylolysis spontanea (ainhum) L94.6

Dactylosymphysis Q70.9
  fingers —*see* Syndactylism, complex, fingers
  toes —*see* Syndactylism, complex, toes

Damage
  arteriosclerotic —*see* Arteriosclerosis
  brain (nontraumatic) G93.9
    anoxic, hypoxic G93.1
      resulting from a procedure G97.82
    child NEC G80.9
    due to birth injury P11.2
  cardiorenal (vascular) —*see* Hypertension, cardiorenal
  cerebral NEC —*see* Damage, brain
  coccyx, complicating delivery O71.6
  coronary —*see* Disease, heart, ischemic
  deep tissue, pressure-induced —*see also* L89 with final character .6
  eye, birth injury P15.3
  liver (nontraumatic) K76.9
    alcoholic K70.9
    due to drugs —*see* Disease, liver, toxic
    toxic —*see* Disease, liver, toxic

Damage *(continued)*
  lung
    dabbing (related) U07.0
    electronic cigarette (related) U07.0
    vaping (associated) (device) (product) (use) U07.0
  medication T88.7
  organ
    dabbing (related) U07.0
    electronic cigarette (related) U07.0
    vaping (associated) (device) (product) (use) U07.0
  pelvic
    joint or ligament, during delivery O71.6
    organ NEC
      during delivery O71.5
      following ectopic or molar pregnancy O08.6
  renal —*see* Disease, renal
  subendocardium, subendocardial —*see* Degeneration, myocardial
  vascular I99.9

Dana-Putnam syndrome (subacute combined sclerosis with pernicious anemia) —*see* Degeneration, combined

Danbolt (-Cross) **syndrome** (acrodermatitis enteropathica) E83.2

Dandruff L21.0

Dandy-Walker syndrome Q03.1
  with spina bifida —*see* Spina bifida

Danlos' syndrome (*see also* Syndrome, Ehlers-Danlos) Q79.60

Darier (-White) disease (congenital) Q82.8
  meaning erythema annulare centrifugum L53.1

Darier-Roussy sarcoid D86.3

Darling's disease or histoplasmosis B39.4

Darwin's tubercle Q17.8

Dawson's (inclusion body) **encephalitis** A81.1

De Beurmann (-Gougerot) **disease** B42.1

De la Tourette's syndrome F95.2

De Lange's syndrome Q87.19

De Morgan's spots (senile angiomas) I78.1

De Quervain's
  disease (tendon sheath) M65.4
  syndrome E34.51
  thyroiditis (subacute granulomatous thyroiditis) E06.1

De Toni-Fanconi (-Debré) **syndrome** E72.09
  with cystinosis E72.04

Dead
  fetus, retained (mother) O36.4
    early pregnancy O02.1
  labyrinth H83.2
  ovum, retained O02.0

Deaf nonspeaking NEC H91.3

Deafmutism (acquired) (congenital) **NEC** H91.3
  hysterical F44.6
  syphilitic, congenital (*see also* subcategory H94.8) A50.09

Deafness (acquired) (complete) (hereditary) (partial) H91.9-

Deafness *(continued)*
  with blue sclera and fragility of bone Q78.0
  auditory fatigue —*see* Deafness, specified type NEC
  aviation T70.0
    nerve injury —*see* Injury, nerve, acoustic, specified type NEC
  boilermaker's —*see* subcategory H83.3
  central —*see* Deafness, sensorineural
  conductive H90.2
    and sensorineural
      mixed H90.8
        bilateral H90.6
    bilateral H90.0
    unilateral H90.1-
      with restricted hearing on the contralateral side H90.A-
  congenital H90.5
    with blue sclera and fragility of bone Q78.0
  due to toxic agents —*see* Deafness, ototoxic
  emotional (hysterical) F44.6
  functional (hysterical) F44.6
  high frequency H91.9-
  hysterical F44.6
  low frequency H91.9-
  mental R48.8
  mixed conductive and sensorineural H90.8
    bilateral H90.6
    unilateral H90.7-
  nerve —*see* Deafness, sensorineural
  neural —*see* Deafness, sensorineural
  noise-induced —*see also* subcategory H83.3
    nerve injury —*see* Injury, nerve, acoustic, specified type NEC
  nonspeaking H91.3
  ototoxic H91.0
  perceptive —*see* Deafness, sensorineural
  psychogenic (hysterical) F44.6
  sensorineural H90.5
    and conductive
      mixed H90.8
        bilateral H90.6
    bilateral H90.3
    unilateral H90.4-
      with restricted hearing on the contralateral side H90.A-
  sensory —*see* Deafness, sensorineural
  specified type NEC H91.8
  sudden (idiopathic) H91.2-
  syphilitic A52.15
  transient ischemic H93.01-
  traumatic —*see* Injury, nerve, acoustic, specified type NEC
  word (developmental) H93.25

Death (cause unknown) (of) (unexplained) (unspecified cause) R99
  brain G93.82
  cardiac (sudden) (with successful resuscitation) - code to underlying disease
    family history of Z82.41
    personal history of Z86.74
  family member (assumed) Z63.4

Debility (chronic) (general) (nervous) R53.81
  congenital or neonatal NOS P96.9
  nervous R53.81

Debility *(continued)*
  old age R54
  senile R54

Débove's disease (splenomegaly) R16.1

Decalcification
  bone —*see* Osteoporosis
  teeth K03.89

Decapsulation, kidney N28.89

Decay
  dental —*see* Caries, dental
  senile R54
  tooth, teeth —*see* Caries, dental

Deciduitis (acute)
  following ectopic or molar pregnancy O08.0

Decline (general) —*see* Debility
  cognitive, age-associated R41.81

Decompensation
  cardiac (acute) (chronic) —*see* Disease, heart
  cardiovascular —*see* Disease, cardiovascular
  heart —*see* Disease, heart
  hepatic —*see* Failure, hepatic
  myocardial (acute) (chronic) —*see* Disease, heart
  respiratory J98.8

Decompression sickness T70.3

Decrease (d)
  absolute neutrophile count —*see* Neutropenia
  blood
    platelets —*see* Thrombocytopenia
    pressure R03.1
      due to shock following
        injury T79.4
        operation T81.19
  estrogen E28.39
    postablative E89.40
      asymptomatic E89.40
      symptomatic E89.41
  fragility of erythrocytes D58.8
  function
    lipase (pancreatic) K90.3
    ovary in hypopituitarism E23.0
    parenchyma of pancreas K86.89
    pituitary (gland) (anterior) (lobe) E23.0
      posterior (lobe) E23.0
  functional activity R68.89
  glucose R73.09
  hematocrit R71.0
  hemoglobin R71.0
  leukocytes D72.819
    specified NEC D72.818
  libido R68.82
  lymphocytes D72.810
  platelets D69.6
  respiration, due to shock following injury T79.4
  sexual desire R68.82
  tear secretion NEC —*see* Syndrome, dry eye
  tolerance
    fat K90.49
    glucose R73.09
    pancreatic K90.3
    salt and water E87.8
  vision NEC H54.7
  white blood cell count D72.819
    specified NEC D72.818

Decubitus (ulcer) —*see* Ulcer, pressure, by site
  cervix N86

Deepening acetabulum —*see* Derangement, joint, specified type NEC, hip

Defect, defective Q89.9
- 3-beta-hydroxysteroid dehydrogenase E25.0
- 11-hydroxylase E25.0
- 21-hydroxylase E25.0
- abdominal wall, congenital Q79.59
- antibody immunodeficiency D80.9
- aorticopulmonary septum Q21.4
- atrial septal (ostium secundum type) Q21.1
  - following acute myocardial infarction (current complication) I23.1
  - ostium primum type Q21.2
- atrioventricular
  - canal Q21.2
  - septum Q21.2
- auricular septal Q21.1
- bilirubin excretion NEC E80.6
- biosynthesis, androgen (testicular) E29.1
- bulbar septum Q21.0
- catalase E80.3
- cell membrane receptor complex (CR3) D71
- circulation I99.9
  - congenital Q28.9
  - newborn Q28.9
- coagulation (factor) (*see also* Deficiency, factor) D68.9
  - with
    - ectopic pregnancy O08.1
    - molar pregnancy O08.1
  - acquired D68.4
  - antepartum with hemorrhage —*see* Hemorrhage, antepartum, with coagulation defect
  - due to
    - liver disease D68.4
    - vitamin K deficiency D68.4
  - hereditary NEC D68.2
  - intrapartum O67.0
  - newborn, transient P61.6
  - postpartum O99.13
    - with hemorrhage O72.3
  - specified type NEC D68.8
- complement system D84.1
- conduction (heart) I45.9
  - bone —*see* Deafness, conductive
- congenital, organ or site not listed —*see* Anomaly, by site
- coronary sinus Q21.1
- cushion, endocardial Q21.2
- degradation, glycoprotein E77.1
- dental bridge, crown, fillings —*see* Defect, dental restoration
- dental restoration K08.50
  - specified NEC K08.59
- dentin (hereditary) K00.5
- Descemet's membrane, congenital Q13.89
- developmental —*see also* Anomaly
  - cauda equina Q06.3
- diaphragm
  - with elevation, eventration or hernia —*see* Hernia, diaphragm
  - congenital Q79.1
    - with hernia Q79.0
    - gross (with hernia) Q79.0
- ectodermal, congenital Q82.9
- Eisenmenger's Q21.8
- enzyme
  - catalase E80.3
  - peroxidase E80.3
- esophagus, congenital Q39.9

Defect, defective *(continued)*
- extensor retinaculum M62.89
- fibrin polymerization D68.2
- filling
  - bladder R93.41
  - kidney R93.42-
  - renal pelvis R93.41
  - stomach R93.3
  - ureter R93.41
  - urinary organs, specified NEC R93.49
- GABA (gamma aminobutyric acid) metabolic E72.81
- Gerbode Q21.0
- glucose transport, blood-brain barrier E74.810
- glycoprotein degradation E77.1
- Hageman (factor) D68.2
- hearing —*see* Deafness
- high grade F70
- interatrial septal Q21.1
- interauricular septal Q21.1
- interventricular septal Q21.0
  - with dextroposition of aorta, pulmonary stenosis and hypertrophy of right ventricle Q21.3
  - in tetralogy of Fallot Q21.3
- learning (specific) —*see* Disorder, learning
- lymphocyte function antigen-1(LFA-1) D84.0
- lysosomal enzyme, post-translational modification E77.0
- major osseous M89.70
  - ankle M89.77-
  - carpus M89.74-
  - clavicle M89.71-
  - femur M89.75-
  - fibula M89.76-
  - fingers M89.74-
  - foot M89.77-
  - forearm M89.73-
  - hand M89.74-
  - humerus M89.72-
  - lower leg M89.76-
  - metacarpus M89.74-
  - metatarsus M89.77-
  - multiple sites M89.79
  - pelvic region M89.75-
  - pelvis M89.75-
  - radius M89.73-
  - scapula M89.71-
  - shoulder region M89.71-
  - specified NEC M89.78
  - tarsus M89.77-
  - thigh M89.75-
  - tibia M89.76-
  - toes M89.77-
  - ulna M89.73-
- mental —*see* Disability, intellectual
- modification, lysosomal enzymes, post-translational E77.0
- obstructive, congenital
  - renal pelvis Q62.39
  - ureter Q62.39
    - atresia —*see* Atresia, ureter
    - cecoureterocele Q62.32
    - megaureter Q62.2
    - orthotopic ureterocele Q62.31
- osseous, major M89.70
  - ankle M89.77-
  - carpus M89.74-
  - clavicle M89.71-
  - femur M89.75-
  - fibula M89.76-
  - fingers M89.74-
  - foot M89.77-
  - forearm M89.73-
  - hand M89.74-
  - humerus M89.72-

Defect, defective *(continued)*
- osseous, major *(continued)*
  - lower leg M89.76-
  - metacarpus M89.74-
  - metatarsus M89.77-
  - multiple sites M89.9
  - pelvic region M89.75-
  - pelvis M89.75-
  - radius M89.73-
  - scapula M89.71-
  - shoulder region M89.71-
  - specified NEC M89.78
  - tarsus M89.77-
  - thigh M89.75-
  - tibia M89.76-
  - toes M89.77-
  - ulna M89.73-
- osteochondral NEC (*see also* Deformity) M95.8
- ostium
  - primum Q21.2
  - secundum Q21.1
- peroxidase E80.3
- placental blood supply —*see* Insufficiency, placental
- platelets, qualitative D69.1
  - constitutional D68.0
- postural NEC, spine —*see* Dorsopathy, deforming
- reduction
  - limb Q73.8
    - lower Q72.9-
      - absence —*see* Agenesis, leg
        - foot —*see* Agenesis, foot
      - longitudinal
        - femur Q72.4-
        - fibula Q72.6-
        - tibia Q72.5-
      - specified type NEC Q72.89-
      - split foot Q72.7-
    - specified type NEC Q73.8
    - upper Q71.9-
      - absence —*see* Agenesis, arm
        - forearm —*see* Agenesis, forearm
        - hand —*see* Agenesis, hand
      - lobster-claw hand Q71.6-
      - longitudinal
        - radius Q71.4-
        - ulna Q71.5-
      - specified type NEC Q71.89-
- renal pelvis Q63.8
  - obstructive Q62.39
- respiratory system, congenital Q34.9
- restoration, dental K08.50
  - specified NEC K08.59
- retinal nerve bundle fibers H35.89
- septal (heart) NOS Q21.9
  - acquired (atrial) (auricular) (ventricular) (old) I51.0
  - atrial Q21.1
    - concurrent with acute myocardial infarction —*see* Infarct, myocardium
    - following acute myocardial infarction (current complication) I23.1
  - ventricular (*see also* Defect, ventricular septal) Q21.0
- sinus venosus Q21.1
- speech —*see* disorder speech
  - developmental F80.9
  - specified NEC R47.89
- Taussig-Bing (aortic transposition and overriding pulmonary artery) Q20.1

Defect, defective *(continued)*
- teeth, wedge K03.1
- vascular (local) I99.9
  - congenital Q27.9
- ventricular septal Q21.0
  - concurrent with acute myocardial infarction —*see* Infarct, myocardium
  - following acute myocardial infarction (current complication) I23.2
  - in tetralogy of Fallot Q21.3
- vision NEC H54.7
- visual field H53.40
  - bilateral
    - heteronymous H53.47
    - homonymous H53.46-
  - generalized contraction H53.48-
  - localized
    - arcuate H53.43-
    - scotoma (central area) H53.41-
      - blind spot area H53.42-
    - sector H53.43-
    - specified type NEC H53.45-
- voice R49.9
  - specified NEC R49.8
- wedge, tooth, teeth (abrasion) K03.1

Deferentitis N49.1
- gonorrheal (acute) (chronic) A54.23

Defibrination (syndrome) D65
- antepartum —*see* Hemorrhage, antepartum, with coagulation defect, disseminated intravascular coagulation
- following ectopic or molar pregnancy O08.1
- intrapartum O67.0
- newborn P60
- postpartum O72.3

Deficiency, deficient
- 3-beta hydroxysteroid dehydrogenase E25.0
- 5-alpha reductase (with male pseudohermaphroditism) E29.1
- 11-hydroxylase E25.0
- 21-hydroxylase E25.0
- AADC (aromatic L-amino acid decarboxylase) E70.81
- abdominal muscle syndrome Q79.4
- accelerator globulin (Ac G) (blood) D68.2
- AC globulin (congenital) (hereditary) D68.2
  - acquired D68.4
- acid phosphatase E83.39
- acid sphingomyelinase (ASMD) E75.249
  - type
    - A E75.240
    - A/B E75.244
    - B E75.241
- activating factor (blood) D68.2
- ADA2 (adenosine deaminase 2) D81.32
- adenosine deaminase (ADA) D81.30
  - with severe combined immunodeficiency (SCID) D81.32
  - partial (type 1) D81.39
  - specified NEC D81.39
  - type 1 (without SCID) (without severe combined immunodeficiency) D81.39
  - type 2 D81.32
- aldolase (hereditary) E74.19
- alpha-1-antitrypsin E88.01
- amino-acids E72.9

Deficiency, deficient *(continued)*
anemia —*see* Anemia
aneurin E51.9
antibody with
hyperimmunoglobulinemia D80.6
near-normal immunoglobins D80.6
antidiuretic hormone E23.2
anti-hemophilic
factor (A) D66
B D67
C D68.1
globulin (AHG) NEC D66
antithrombin (antithrombin III) D68.59
aromatic L-amino acid decarboxylase (AADC) E70.81
ascorbic acid E54
attention (disorder) (syndrome) F98.8
with hyperactivity —*see* Disorder, attention-deficit hyperactivity
autoprothrombin
I D68.2
II D67
C D68.2
beta-glucuronidase E76.29
biotin E53.8
biotin-dependent carboxylase D81.819
biotinidase D81.810
brancher enzyme (amylopectinosis) E74.03
calciferol E55.9
with
adult osteomalacia M83.8
rickets —*see* Rickets
calcium (dietary) E58
calorie, severe E43
with marasmus E41
and kwashiorkor E42
cardiac —*see* Insufficiency, myocardial
carnitine E71.40
due to
hemodialysis E71.43
inborn errors of metabolism E71.42
Valproic acid therapy E71.43
iatrogenic E71.43
muscle palmityltransferase E71.314
primary E71.41
secondary E71.448
carotene E50.9
central nervous system G96.89
ceruloplasmin (Wilson) E83.01
choline E53.8
Christmas factor D67
chromium E61.4
chronic neurovisceral acid sphingomyelinase E75.244
chronic visceral acid sphingomyelinase E75.241
clotting (blood) (*see also* Deficiency, coagulation factor) D68.9
clotting factor NEC (hereditary) (*see also* Deficiency, factor) D68.2
coagulation NOS D68.9
with
ectopic pregnancy O08.1
molar pregnancy O08.1
acquired (any) D68.4
antepartum hemorrhage —*see* Hemorrhage, antepartum, with coagulation defect

Deficiency, deficient *(continued)*
coagulation *(continued)*
clotting factor NEC (*see also* Deficiency, factor) D68.2
due to
hyperprothrombinemia D68.4
liver disease D68.4
vitamin K deficiency D68.4
newborn, transient P61.6
postpartum O72.3
specified NEC D68.8
cognitive F09
color vision H53.50
achromatopsia H53.51
acquired H53.52
deuteranomaly H53.53
protanomaly H53.54
specified type NEC H53.59
tritanomaly H53.55
combined glucocorticoid and mineralocorticoid E27.49
contact factor D68.2
copper (nutritional) E61.0
corticoadrenal E27.40
primary E27.1
craniofacial axis Q75.0
cyanocobalamin E53.8
C1 esterase inhibitor (C1-INH)D84.1
debrancher enzyme (limit dextrinosis) E74.03
dehydrogenase
long chain/very long chain acyl CoA E71.310
medium chain acyl CoA E71.311
short chain acyl CoA E71.312
diet E63.9
dihydropyrimidine dehydrogenase (DPD) E88.89
disaccharidase E73.9
edema —*see* Malnutrition, severe
endocrine E34.9
energy-supply —*see* Malnutrition
enzymes, circulating NEC E88.09
ergosterol E55.9
with
adult osteomalacia M83.8
rickets —*see* Rickets
essential fatty acid (EFA) E63.0
eye movements
saccadic H55.81
smooth pursuit H55.82
factor —*see also* Deficiency, coagulation
Hageman D68.2
I (congenital) (hereditary) D68.2
II (congenital) (hereditary) D68.2
IX (congenital) (functional) (hereditary) (with functional defect) D67
multiple (congenital) D68.8
acquired D68.4
V (congenital) (hereditary) D68.2
VII (congenital) (hereditary) D68.2
VIII (congenital) (functional) (hereditary) (with functional defect) D66
with vascular defect D68.0
X (congenital) (hereditary) D68.2
XI (congenital) (hereditary) D68.1
XII (congenital) (hereditary) D68.2
XIII (congenital) (hereditary) D68.2
femoral, proximal focal (congenital) —*see* Defect, reduction, lower limb, longitudinal, femur
fibrin-stabilizing factor (congenital) (hereditary) D68.2
acquired D68.4
fibrinase D68.2
fibrinogen (congenital) (hereditary) D68.2
acquired D65

Deficiency, deficient *(continued)*
folate E53.8
folic acid E53.8
foreskin N47.3
fructokinase E74.11
fructose 1,6-diphosphatase E74.19
fructose-1-phosphate aldolase E74.19
GABA (gamma aminobutyric acid) transaminase E72.81
GABA-T (gamma aminobutyric acid transaminase) E72.81
galactokinase E74.29
galactose-1-phosphate uridyl transferase E74.29
gammaglobulin in blood D80.1
hereditary D80.0
glass factor D68.2
glucocorticoid E27.49
mineralocorticoid E27.49
glucose-6-phosphatase E74.01
glucose-6-phosphate dehydrogenase
anemia D55.0
without anemia D75.A
glucose transporter protein type 1 E74.810
glucuronyl transferase E80.5
Glut1 E74.810
glycogen synthetase E74.09
gonadotropin (isolated) E23.0
growth hormone (idiopathic) (isolated) E23.0
Hageman factor D68.2
hemoglobin D64.9
hepatophosphorylase E74.09
homogentisate 1,2-dioxygenase E70.29
hormone
anterior pituitary (partial) NEC E23.0
growth E23.0
growth (isolated) E23.0
pituitary E23.0
testicular E29.1
hypoxanthine-(guanine)-phosphoribosyltransferase (HG-PRT) (total H-PRT) E79.1
immunity D84.9
cell-mediated D84.89
with thrombocytopenia and eczema D82.0
combined D81.9
humoral D80.9
IgA (secretory) D80.2
IgG D80.3
IgM D80.4
immuno —*see* Immunodeficiency
immunoglobulin, selective
A (IgA) D80.2
G (IgG) (subclasses) D80.3
M (IgM) D80.4
infantile neurovisceral acid sphingomyelinase E75.240
inositol (B complex) E53.8
intrinsic
factor (congenital) D51.0
sphincter N36.42
with urethral hypermobility N36.43
iodine E61.8
congenital syndrome —*see* Syndrome, iodine-deficiency, congenital
iron E61.1
anemia D50.9
kalium E87.6
kappa-light chain D80.8
labile factor (congenital) (hereditary) D68.2
acquired D68.4

Deficiency, deficient *(continued)*
lacrimal fluid (acquired) —*see also* Syndrome, dry eye
congenital Q10.6
lactase
congenital E73.0
secondary E73.1
Laki-Lorand factor D68.2
lecithin cholesterol acyltransferase E78.6
lipocaic K86.89
lipoprotein (familial) (high density) E78.6
liver phosphorylase E74.09
lysosomal alpha-1, 4 glucosidase E74.02
magnesium E61.2
major histocompatibility complex
class I D81.6
class II D81.7
manganese E61.3
menadione (vitamin K) E56.1
newborn P53
mental (familial) (hereditary) —*see* Disability, intellectual
methylenetetrahydrofolate reductase (MTHFR) E72.12
mevalonate kinase M04.1
mineral NEC E61.8
mineralocorticoid E27.49
with glucocorticoid E27.49
molybdenum (nutritional) E61.5
moral F60.2
multiple nutrient elements E61.7
multiple sulfatase (MSD) E75.26
muscle
carnitine (palmityltransferase) E71.314
phosphofructokinase E74.09
myoadenylate deaminase E79.2
myocardial —*see* Insufficiency, myocardial
myophosphorylase E74.04
NADH diaphorase or reductase (congenital) D74.0
NADH-methemoglobin reductase (congenital) D74.0
natrium E87.1
niacin (amide) (-tryptophan) E52
nicotinamide E52
nicotinic acid E52
number of teeth —*see* Anodontia
nutrient element E61.9
multiple E61.7
specified NEC E61.8
nutrition, nutritional E63.9
sequelae —*see* Sequelae, nutritional deficiency
specified NEC E63.8
of interleukin 1 receptor antagonist [DIRA] M04.8
ornithine transcarbamylase E72.4
ovarian E28.39
oxygen —*see* Anoxia
pantothenic acid E53.8
parathyroid (gland) E20.9
perineum (female) N81.89
phenylalanine hydroxylase E70.1
phosphoenolpyruvate carboxykinase E74.4
phosphofructokinase E74.19
phosphomannomutuse E74.818
phosphomannose isomerase E74.818
phosphomannosyl mutase E74.818
phosphorylase kinase, liver E74.09
pituitary hormone (isolated) E23.0
plasma thromboplastin
antecedent (PTA) D68.1
component (PTC) D67

Deficiency, deficient *(continued)*
- plasminogen (type 1) (type 2) E88.02
- platelet NEC D69.1
  - constitutional D68.0
- polyglandular E31.8
  - autoimmune E31.0
- potassium (K) E87.6
- prepuce N47.3
- proaccelerin (congenital) (hereditary) D68.2
  - acquired D68.4
- proconvertin factor (congenital) (hereditary) D68.2
  - acquired D68.4
- protein (*see also* Malnutrition) E46
  - anemia D53.0
  - C D68.59
  - S D68.59
- prothrombin (congenital) (heredItary) D68.2
  - acquired D68.4
- Prower factor D68.2
- pseudocholinesterase E88.09
- PTA (plasma thromboplastin antecedent) D68.1
- PTC (plasma thromboplastin component) D67
- purine nucleoside phosphorylase (PNP) D81.5
- pyracin (alpha) (beta) E53.1
- pyridoxal E53.1
- pyridoxamine E53.1
- pyridoxine (derivatives) E53.1
- pyruvate
  - carboxylase E74.4
  - dehydrogenase E74.4
- riboflavin (vitamin B2) E53.0
- salt E87.1
- secretion
  - ovary E28.39
  - salivary gland (any) K11.7
  - urine R34
- selenium (dietary) E59
- serum antitrypsin, familial E88.01
- short stature homeobox gene (SHOX)
  - with
    - dyschondrosteosis Q78.8
    - short stature (idiopathic) E34.3
    - Turner's syndrome Q96.9
- sodium (Na) E87.1
- SPCA(factor VII) D68.2
- sphincter, intrinsic N36.42
  - with urethral hypermobility N36.43
- stable factor (congenital) (hereditary) D68.2
  - acquired D68.4
- Stuart-Prower (factor X) D68.2
- succinic semialdehyde dehydrogenase E72.81
- sucrase E74.39
- sulfatase E75.26
- sulfite oxidase E72.19
- thiamin, thiaminic (chloride) E51.9
  - beriberi (dry) E51.11
    - wet E51.12
- thrombokinase D68.2
  - newborn P53
- thyroid (gland) —*see* Hypothyroidism
- tocopherol E56.0
- tooth bud K00.0
- transcobalamine II (anemia) D51.2
- vanadium E61.6
- vascular I99.9
- vasopressin E23.2
- vertical ridge K06.8
- viosterol —*see* Deficiency, calciferol

Deficiency, deficient *(continued)*
- vitamin (multiple) NOS E56.9
  - A E50.9
    - with
      - Bitot's spot (corneal) E50.1
      - follicular keratosis E50.8
      - keratomalacia E50.4
      - manifestations NEC E50.8
      - night blindness E50.5
      - scar of cornea, xerophthalmic E50.6
      - xeroderma E50.8
      - xerophthalmia E50.7
      - xerosis
        - conjunctival E50.0
          - and Bitot's spot E50.1
        - cornea E50.2
          - and ulceration E50.3
    - sequelae E64.1
  - B (complex) NOS E53.9
    - with
      - beriberi (dry) E51.11
        - wet E51.12
      - pellagra E52
  - B1 NOS E51.9
    - beriberi (dry) E51.11
      - with circulatory system manifestations E51.11
      - wet E51.12
  - B12 E53.8
  - B2 (riboflavin) E53.0
  - B6 E53.1
  - C E54
    - sequelae E64.2
  - D E55.9
    - with
      - adult osteomalacia M83.8
      - rickets —*see* Rickets
    - 25-hydroxylase E83.32
  - E E56.0
  - folic acid E53.8
  - G E53.0
  - group B E53.9
    - specified NEC E53.8
  - H (biotin) E53.8
  - K E56.1
    - of newborn P53
  - nicotinic E52
  - P E56.8
  - PP (pellagra-preventing) E52
  - specified NEC E56.8
  - thiamin E51.9
    - beriberi —*see* Beriberi
- zinc, dietary E60

Deficit —*see also* Deficiency
- attention and concentration R41.840
  - disorder —*see* Attention, deficit
  - following
    - cerebral infarction I69.310
    - cerebrovascular disease I69.910
      - specified disease NEC I69.810
    - nontraumatic
      - intracerebral hemorrhage I69.110
      - specified intracranial hemorrhage NEC I69.210
      - subarachnoid hemorrhage I69.010
- cognitive
  - communication R41.841
  - emotional
    - following
      - cerebral infarction I69.315
      - cerebrovascular disease I69.915
        - specified disease NEC I69.815

Deficit *(continued)*
- cognitive *(continued)*
  - emotional *(continued)*
    - following *(continued)*
      - nontraumantic
        - intracerebral hemorrhage I69.115
        - specified intracranial hemorrhage NEC I69.215
        - subarachnoid hemorrhage I69.015
  - following
    - cerebral infarction I69.319
    - cerebrovascular disease I69.919
      - specified disease NEC I69.819
    - nontraumatic
      - intracerebral hemorrhage I69.119
      - specified intracranial hemorrhage NEC I69.219
      - subarachnoid hemorrhage I69.019
  - social
    - following
      - cerebral infarction I69.315
      - cerebrovascular disease I69.915
        - specified disease NEC I69.815
      - nontraumatic
        - intracerebral hemorrhage I69.115
        - specified intracranial hemorrhage NEC I69.215
        - subarachnoid hemorrhage I69.015
- cognitive NEC R41.89
  - following
    - cerebral infarction I69.318
    - cerebrovascular disease I69.918
      - specified disease NEC I69.818
    - nontraumatic
      - intracerebral hemorrhage I69.118
      - specified intracaranial hemorrhage NEC I69.218
      - subarachnoid hemorrhage I69.018
- concentration R41.840
- executive function R41.844
  - following
    - cerebral infarction I69.314
    - cerebrovascular disease I69.914
      - specified disease NEC I69.814
    - nontraumatic
      - intracerebral hemorrhage I69.114
      - specified intracranial hemorrhage NEC I69.214
      - subarachnoid hemorrhage I69.014
- frontal lobe R41.844
  - following
    - cerebral infarction I69.314
    - cerebrovascular disease I69.914
      - specified disease NEC I69.814
    - nontraumatic
      - intracerebral hemorrhage I69.114
      - specified intracranial hemorrhage NEC I69.214
      - subarachnoid hemorrhage I69.014

Deficit *(continued)*
- memory
  - following
    - cerebral infarction I69.311
    - cerebrovascular disease I69.911
      - specified disease NEC I69.811
    - nontraumatic
      - intracerebral hemorrhage I69.111
      - specified intracranial hemorrhage NEC I69.211
      - subarachnoid hemorrhage I69.011
- neurologic NEC R29.818
  - ischemic
    - reversible (RIND) I63.9
      - prolonged (PRIND) I63.9
- oxygen R09.02
- prolonged reversible ischemic neurologic (PRIND) I63.9
- psychomotor R41.843
  - following
    - cerebral infarction I69.313
    - cerebrovascular disease I69.913
      - specified disease NEC I69.813
    - nontraumatic
      - intracerebral hemorrhage I69.113
      - specified intracranial hemorrhage NEC I69.213
      - subarachnoid hemorrhage I69.013
- visuospatial R41.842
  - following
    - cerebral infarction I69.312
    - cerebrovascular disease I69.912
      - specified disease NEC I69.812
    - nontraumatic
      - intracerebral hemorrhage I69.112
      - specified intracranial hemorrhage NEC I69.212
      - subarachnoid hemorrhage I69.012

Deflection
- radius —*see* Deformity, limb, specified type NEC, forearm
- septum (acquired) (nasal) (nose) J34.2
- spine —*see* Curvature, spine
- turbinate (nose) J34.2

Defluvium
- capillorum —*see* Alopecia
- ciliorum —*see* Madarosis
- unguium L60.8

Deformity Q89.9
- abdomen, congenital Q89.9
- abdominal wall
  - acquired M95.8
  - congenital Q79.59
- acquired (unspecified site) M95.9
- adrenal gland Q89.1
- alimentary tract, congenital Q45.9
  - upper Q40.9
- ankle (joint) (acquired) —*see also* Deformity, limb, lower leg
  - abduction —*see* Contraction, joint, ankle
  - congenital Q68.8
  - contraction —*see* Contraction, joint, ankle
  - specified type NEC —*see* Deformity, limb, foot, specified NEC

Deformity *(continued)*
- anus (acquired) K62.89
  - congenital Q43.9
- aorta (arch) (congenital) Q25.40
  - acquired I77.89
- aortic
  - arch, acquired I77.89
  - cusp or valve (congenital) Q23.8
    - acquired (*see also* Endocarditis, aortic) I35.8
- arm (acquired) (upper) —*see also* Deformity, limb, upper arm
  - congenital Q68.8
  - forearm —*see* Deformity, limb, forearm
- artery (congenital) (peripheral) NOS Q27.9
  - acquired I77.89
  - coronary (acquired) I25.9
    - congenital Q24.5
  - umbilical Q27.0
- atrial septal Q21.1
- auditory canal (external) (congenital) —*see also* Malformation, ear, external
  - acquired —*see* Disorder, ear, external, specified type NEC
- auricle
  - ear (congenital) —*see also* Malformation, ear, external
    - acquired —*see* Disorder, pinna, deformity
- back —*see* Dorsopathy, deforming
- bile duct (common) (congenital) (hepatic) Q44.5
  - acquired K83.8
- biliary duct or passage (congenital) Q44.5
  - acquired K83.8
- bladder (neck) (trigone) (sphincter) (acquired) N32.89
  - congenital Q64.79
- bone (acquired) NOS M95.9
  - congenital Q79.9
  - turbinate M95.0
- brain (congenital) Q04.9
  - acquired G93.89
  - reduction Q04.3
- breast (acquired) N64.89
  - congenital Q83.9
  - reconstructed N65.0
- bronchus (congenital) Q32.4
  - acquired NEC J98.09
- bursa, congenital Q79.9
- canaliculi (lacrimalis) (acquired) —*see also* Disorder, lacrimal system, changes
  - congenital Q10.6
- canthus, acquired —*see* Disorder, eyelid, specified type NEC
- capillary (acquired) I78.8
- cardiovascular system, congenital Q28.9
- caruncle, lacrimal (acquired) —*see also* Disorder, lacrimal system, changes
  - congenital Q10.6
- cascade, stomach K31.2
- cecum (congenital) Q43.9
  - acquired K63.89
- cerebral, acquired G93.89
  - congenital Q04.9
- cervix (uterus) (acquired) NEC N88.8
  - congenital Q51.9
- cheek (acquired) M95.2
  - congenital Q18.9

Deformity *(continued)*
- chest (acquired) (wall) M95.4
  - congenital Q67.8
  - sequelae (late effect) of rickets E64.3
- chin (acquired) M95.2
  - congenital Q18.9
- choroid (congenital) Q14.3
  - acquired H31.8
  - plexus Q07.8
    - acquired G96.198
- cicatricial —*see* Cicatrix
- cilia, acquired —*see* Disorder, eyelid, specified type NEC
- clavicle (acquired) M95.8
  - congenital Q68.8
- clitoris (congenital) Q52.6
  - acquired N90.89
- clubfoot —*see* Clubfoot
- coccyx (acquired) M43.8
- colon (congenital) Q43.9
  - acquired K63.89
- concha (ear), congenital —*see also* Malformation, ear, external
  - acquired —*see* Disorder, pinna, deformity
- cornea (acquired) H18.70
  - congenital Q13.4
  - descemetocele —*see* Descemetocele
  - ectasia —*see* Ectasia, cornea
  - specified NEC H18.79-
  - staphyloma —*see* Staphyloma, cornea
- coronary artery (acquired) I25.9
  - congenital Q24.5
- cranium (acquired) —*see* Deformity, skull
- cricoid cartilage (congenital) Q31.8
  - acquired J38.7
- cystic duct (congenital) Q44.5
  - acquired K82.8
- Dandy-Walker Q03.1
  - with spina bifida —*see* Spina bifida
- diaphragm (congenital) Q79.1
  - acquired J98.6
- digestive organ NOS Q45.9
- ductus arteriosus Q25.0
- duodenal bulb K31.89
- duodenum (congenital) Q43.9
  - acquired K31.89
- dura —*see* Deformity, meninges
- ear (acquired) —*see also* Disorder, pinna, deformity
  - congenital (external) Q17.9
    - internal Q16.5
    - middle Q16.4
      - ossicles Q16.3
    - ossicles Q16.3
- ectodermal (congenital) NEC Q84.9
- ejaculatory duct (congenital) Q55.4
  - acquired N50.89
- elbow (joint) (acquired) —*see also* Deformity, limb, upper arm
  - congenital Q68.8
  - contraction —*see* Contraction, joint, elbow
- endocrine gland NEC Q89.2
- epididymis (congenital) Q55.4
  - acquired N50.89
- epiglottis (congenital) Q31.8
  - acquired J38.7
- esophagus (congenital) Q39.9
  - acquired K22.89
- eustachian tube (congenital) NEC Q17.8

Deformity *(continued)*
- eye, congenital Q15.9
- eyebrow (congenital) Q18.8
- eyelid (acquired) —*see also* Disorder, eyelid, specified type NEC
  - congenital Q10.3
- face (acquired) M95.2
  - congenital Q18.9
- fallopian tube, acquired N83.8
- femur (acquired) —*see* Deformity, limb, specified type NEC, thigh
- fetal
  - with fetopelvic disproportion O33.7
  - causing obstructed labor O66.3
- finger (acquired) M20.00-
  - boutonniere M20.02-
  - congenital Q68.1
  - flexion contracture —*see* Contraction, joint, hand
  - mallet finger M20.01-
  - specified NEC M20.09-
  - swan-neck M20.03-
- flexion (joint) (acquired) (*see also* Deformity, limb, flexion) M21.20
  - congenital NOS Q74.9
    - hip Q65.89
- foot (acquired) —*see also* Deformity, limb, lower leg
  - cavovarus (congenital) Q66.1-
  - congenital NOS Q66.9-
    - specified type NEC Q66.89
  - specified type NEC —*see* Deformity, limb, foot, specified NEC
  - valgus (congenital) Q66.6
    - acquired —*see* Deformity, valgus, ankle
  - varus (congenital) NEC Q66.3-
    - acquired —*see* Deformity, varus, ankle
- forearm (acquired) —*see also* Deformity, limb, forearm
  - congenital Q68.8
- forehead (acquired) M95.2
  - congenital Q75.8
- frontal bone (acquired) M95.2
  - congenital Q75.8
- gallbladder (congenital) Q44.1
  - acquired K82.8
- gastrointestinal tract (congenital) NOS Q45.9
  - acquired K63.89
- genitalia, genital organ(s) or system NEC
  - female (congenital) Q52.9
    - acquired N94.89
    - external Q52.70
  - male (congenital) Q55.9
    - acquired N50.89
- globe (eye) (congenital) Q15.8
  - acquired H44.89
- gum, acquired NEC K06.8
- hand (acquired) —*see* Deformity, limb, hand
  - congenital Q68.1
- head (acquired) M95.2
  - congenital Q75.8
- heart (congenital) Q24.9
  - septum Q21.9
    - auricular Q21.1
    - ventricular Q21.0

Deformity *(continued)*
- heart *(continued)*
  - septum *(continued)*
  - valve (congenital) NEC Q24.8
    - acquired —*see* Endocarditis
- heel (acquired) —*see* Deformity, foot
- hepatic duct (congenital) Q44.5
  - acquired K83.8
- hip (joint) (acquired) —*see also* Deformity, limb, thigh
  - congenital Q65.9
  - due to (previous) juvenile osteochondrosis —*see* Coxa, plana
  - flexion —*see* Contraction, joint, hip
- hourglass —*see* Contraction, hourglass
- humerus (acquired) M21.82-
  - congenital Q74.0
- hypophyseal (congenital) Q89.2
- ileocecal (coil) (valve) (acquired) K63.89
  - congenital Q43.9
- ileum (congenital) Q43.9
  - acquired K63.89
- ilium (acquired) M95.5
  - congenital Q74.2
- integument (congenital) Q84.9
- intervertebral cartilage or disc (acquired) —*see* Disorder, disc, specified NEC
- intestine (large) (small) (congenital) NOS Q43.9
  - acquired K63.89
- intrinsic minus or plus (hand) —*see* Deformity, limb, specified type NEC, forearm
- iris (acquired) H21.89
  - congenital Q13.2
- ischium (acquired) M95.5
  - congenital Q74.2
- jaw (acquired) (congenital) M26.9
- joint (acquired) NEC M21.90
  - congenital Q68.8
  - elbow M21.92-
  - hand M21.94-
  - hip M21.95-
  - knee M21.96-
  - shoulder M21.92-
  - wrist M21.93-
- kidney(s) (calyx) (pelvis) (congenital) Q63.9
  - acquired N28.89
  - artery (congenital) Q27.2
    - acquired I77.89
- Klippel-Feil (brevicollis) Q76.1
- knee (acquired) NEC —*see also* Deformity, limb, lower leg
  - congenital Q68.2
- labium (majus) (minus) (congenital) Q52.79
  - acquired N90.89
- lacrimal passages or duct (congenital) NEC Q10.6
  - acquired —*see* Disorder, lacrimal system, changes
- larynx (muscle) (congenital) Q31.8
  - acquired J38.7
  - web (glottic) Q31.0
- leg (upper) (acquired) NEC —*see also* Deformity, limb, thigh
  - congenital Q68.8

Deformity *(continued)*
- leg *(continued)*
  - lower leg *—see* Deformity, limb, lower leg
- lens (acquired) H27.8
  - congenital Q12.9
- lid (fold) (acquired) *—see also* Disorder, eyelid, specified type NEC
  - congenital Q10.3
- ligament (acquired) *—see* Disorder, ligament
  - congenital Q79.9
- limb (acquired) M21.90
  - clawfoot M21.53-
  - clawhand M21.51-
  - clubfoot M21.54-
  - clubhand M21.52-
  - congenital, except reduction deformity Q74.9
  - flat foot M21.4-
  - flexion M21.20
    - ankle M21.27-
    - elbow M21.22-
    - finger M21.24-
    - hip M21.25-
    - knee M21.26-
    - shoulder M21.21-
    - toe M21.27-
    - wrist M21.23-
  - foot
    - claw *—see* Deformity, limb, clawfoot
    - club *—see* Deformity, limb, clubfoot
    - drop M21.37-
    - flat *—see* Deformity, limb, flat foot
    - specified NEC M21.6X-
  - forearm M21.93-
  - hand M21.94-
  - lower leg M21.96-
  - specified type NEC M21.80
    - forearm M21.83-
    - lower leg M21.86-
    - thigh M21.85-
    - upper arm M21.82-
  - thigh M21.95-
  - unequal length M21.70
    - short site is
      - femur M21.75-
      - fibula M21.76-
      - humerus M21.72-
      - radius M21.73-
      - tibia M21.76-
      - ulna M21.73-
  - upper arm M21.92-
  - valgus *—see* Deformity, valgus
  - varus *—see* Deformity, varus
  - wrist drop M21.33-
- lip (acquired) NEC K13.0
  - congenital Q38.0
- liver (congenital) Q44.7
  - acquired K76.89
- lumbosacral (congenital) (joint) (region) Q76.49
  - acquired M43.8
  - kyphosis *—see* Kyphosis, congenital
  - lordosis *—see* Lordosis, congenital
- lung (congenital) Q33.9
  - acquired J98.4
- lymphatic system, congenital Q89.9
- Madelung's (radius) Q74.0
- mandible (acquired) (congenital) M26.9
- maxilla (acquired) (congenital) M26.9

Deformity *(continued)*
- meninges or membrane (congenital) Q07.9
  - cerebral Q04.8
    - acquired G96.198
  - spinal cord (congenital) Q06.-
    - acquired G96.198
- metacarpus (acquired) *—see* Deformity, limb, forearm
  - congenital Q74.0
- metatarsus (acquired) *—see* Deformity, foot
  - congenital Q66.9-
- middle ear (congenital) Q16.4
  - ossicles Q16.3
- mitral (leaflets) (valve) I05.8
  - parachute Q23.2
  - stenosis, congenital Q23.2
- mouth (acquired) K13.79
  - congenital Q38.6
- multiple, congenital NEC Q89.7
- muscle (acquired) M62.89
  - congenital Q79.9
    - sternocleidomastoid Q68.0
- musculoskeletal system (acquired) M95.9
  - congenital Q79.9
  - specified NEC M95.8
- nail (acquired) L60.8
  - congenital Q84.6
- nasal *—see* Deformity, nose
- neck (acquired) M95.3
  - congenital Q18.9
    - sternocleidomastoid Q68.0
- nervous system (congenital) Q07.9
- nipple (congenital) Q83.9
  - acquired N64.89
- nose (acquired) (cartilage) M95.0
  - bone (turbinate) M95.0
  - congenital Q30.9
    - bent or squashed Q67.4
  - saddle M95.0
    - syphilitic A50.57
  - septum (acquired) J34.2
    - congenital Q30.8
  - sinus (wall) (congenital) Q30.8
    - acquired M95.0
  - syphilitic (congenital) A50.57
    - late A52.73
- ocular muscle (congenital) Q10.3
  - acquired *—see* Strabismus, mechanical
- opticociliary vessels (congenital) Q13.2
- orbit (eye) (acquired) H05.30
  - atrophy *—see* Atrophy, orbit
  - congenital Q10.7
  - due to
    - bone disease NEC H05.32-
    - trauma or surgery H05.33-
  - enlargement *—see* Enlargement, orbit
  - exostosis *—see* Exostosis, orbit
- organ of Corti (congenital) Q16.5
- ovary (congenital) Q50.39
  - acquired N83.8
- oviduct, acquired N83.8
- palate (congenital) Q38.5
  - acquired M27.8
  - cleft (congenital) *—see* Cleft, palate
- pancreas (congenital) Q45.3
  - acquired K86.89
- parathyroid (gland) Q89.2
- parotid (gland) (congenital) Q38.4
  - acquired K11.8
- patella (acquired) *—see* Disorder, patella, specified NEC

Deformity *(continued)*
- pelvis, pelvic (acquired) (bony) M95.5
  - with disproportion (fetopelvic) O33.0
    - causing obstructed labor O65.0
  - congenital Q74.2
  - rachitic sequelae (late effect) E64.3
- penis (glans) (congenital) Q55.69
  - acquired N48.89
- pericardium (congenital) Q24.8
  - acquired *—see* Pericarditis
- pharynx (congenital) Q38.8
  - acquired J39.2
- pinna, acquired *—see also* Disorder, pinna, deformity
  - congenital Q17.9
- pituitary (congenital) Q89.2
- posture *—see* Dorsopathy, deforming
- prepuce (congenital) Q55.69
  - acquired N47.8
- prostate (congenital) Q55.4
  - acquired N42.89
- pupil (congenital) Q13.2
  - acquired *—see* Abnormality, pupillary
- pylorus (congenital) Q40.3
  - acquired K31.89
- rachitic (acquired), old or healed E64.3
- radius (acquired) *—see also* Deformity, limb, forearm
  - congenital Q68.8
- rectum (congenital) Q43.9
  - acquired K62.89
- reduction (extremity) (limb), congenital (*see also* condition and site) Q73.8
  - brain Q04.3
  - lower *—see* Defect, reduction, lower limb
  - upper *—see* Defect, reduction, upper limb
- renal *—see* Deformity, kidney
- respiratory system (congenital) Q34.9
- rib (acquired) M95.4
  - congenital Q76.6
    - cervical Q76.5
- rotation (joint) (acquired) *—see* Deformity, limb, specified site NEC
  - congenital Q74.9
  - hip *—see* Deformity, limb, specified type NEC, thigh
    - congenital Q65.89
- sacroiliac joint (congenital) Q74.2
  - acquired *—see* subcategory M43.8
- sacrum (acquired) *—see* subcategory M43.8
- saddle
  - back *—see* Lordosis
  - nose M95.0
    - syphilitic A50.57
- salivary gland or duct (congenital) Q38.4
  - acquired K11.8
- scapula (acquired) M95.8
  - congenital Q68.8
- scrotum (congenital) *—see also* Malformation, testis and scrotum
  - acquired N50.89
- seminal vesicles (congenital) Q55.4
  - acquired N50.89
- septum, nasal (acquired) J34.2

Deformity *(continued)*
- shoulder (joint) (acquired) *—see* Deformity, limb, upper arm
  - congenital Q74.0
  - contraction *—see* Contraction, joint, shoulder
- sigmoid (flexure) (congenital) Q43.9
  - acquired K63.89
- skin (congenital) Q82.9
- skull (acquired) M95.2
  - congenital Q75.8
    - with
      - anencephaly Q00.0
      - encephalocele *—see* Encephalocele
      - hydrocephalus Q03.9
        - with spina bifida *—see* Spina bifida, by site, with hydrocephalus
      - microcephaly Q02
- soft parts, organs or tissues (of pelvis)
  - in pregnancy or childbirth NEC O34.8-
    - causing obstructed labor O65.5
- spermatic cord (congenital) Q55.4
  - acquired N50.89
    - torsion *—see* Torsion, spermatic cord
- spinal *—see* Dorsopathy, deforming
  - column (acquired) *—see* Dorsopathy, deforming
    - congenital Q67.5
  - cord (congenital) Q06.9
    - acquired G95.89
  - nerve root (congenital) Q07.9
- spine (acquired) *—see also* Dorsopathy, deforming
  - congenital Q67.5
  - rachitic E64.3
  - specified NEC *—see* Dorsopathy, deforming, specified NEC
- spleen
  - acquired D73.89
  - congenital Q89.09
- Sprengel's (congenital) Q74.0
- sternocleidomastoid (muscle), congenital Q68.0
- sternum (acquired) M95.4
  - congenital NEC Q76.7
- stomach (congenital) Q40.3
  - acquired K31.89
- submandibular gland (congenital) Q38.4
- submaxillary gland (congenital) Q38.4
  - acquired K11.8
- talipes *—see* Talipes
- testis (congenital) *—see also* Malformation, testis and scrotum
  - acquired N44.8
    - torsion *—see* Torsion, testis
- thigh (acquired) *—see also* Deformity, limb, thigh
  - congenital NEC Q68.8
- thorax (acquired) (wall) M95.4
  - congenital Q67.8
  - sequelae of rickets E64.3
- thumb (acquired) *—see also* Deformity, finger
  - congenital NEC Q68.1
- thymus (tissue) (congenital) Q89.2
- thyroid (gland) (congenital) Q89.2
  - cartilage Q31.8
    - acquired J38.7
- tibia (acquired) *—see also* Deformity, limb, specified type NEC, lower leg

Deformity *(continued)*
- tibia *(continued)*
  - congenital NEC Q68.8
  - saber (syphilitic) A50.56
- toe (acquired) M20.6-
  - congenital Q66.9-
  - hallux rigidus M20.2-
  - hallux valgus M20.1-
  - hallux varus M20.3-
  - hammer toe M20.4-
  - specified NEC M20.5X-
- tongue (congenital) Q38.3
  - acquired K14.8
- tooth, teeth K00.2
- trachea (rings) (congenital) Q32.1
  - acquired J39.8
- transverse aortic arch (congenital) Q25.49
- tricuspid (leaflets) (valve) I07.8
  - atresia or stenosis Q22.4
  - Ebstein's Q22.5
- trunk (acquired) M95.8
  - congenital Q89.9
- ulna (acquired) *—see also* Deformity, limb, forearm
  - congenital NEC Q68.8
- urachus, congenital Q64.4
- ureter (opening) (congenital) Q62.8
  - acquired N28.89
- urethra (congenital) Q64.79
  - acquired N36.8
- urinary tract (congenital) Q64.9
  - urachus Q64.4
- uterus (congenital) Q51.9
  - acquired N85.8
- uvula (congenital) Q38.5
- vagina (acquired) N89.8
  - congenital Q52.4
- valgus NEC M21.00
  - ankle M21.07-
  - elbow M21.02-
  - hip M21.05-
  - knee M21.06-
- valve, valvular (congenital) (heart) Q24.8
  - acquired *—see* Endocarditis
- varus NEC M21.10
  - ankle M21.17-
  - elbow M21.12-
  - hip M21.15
  - knee M21.16-
  - tibia *—see* Osteochondrosis, juvenile, tibia
- vas deferens (congenital) Q55.4
  - acquired N50.89
- vein (congenital) Q27.9
  - great Q26.9
- vertebra *—see* Dorsopathy, deforming
- vertical talus (congenital) Q66.80
  - left foot Q66.82
  - right foot Q66.81
- vesicourethral orifice (acquired) N32.89
  - congenital NEC Q64.79
- vessels of optic papilla (congenital) Q14.2
- visual field (contraction) *—see* Defect, visual field
- vitreous body, acquired H43.89
- vulva (congenital) Q52.79
  - acquired N90.89
- wrist (joint) (acquired) *—see also* Deformity, limb, forearm
  - congenital Q68.8
  - contraction *—see* Contraction, joint, wrist

Degeneration, degenerative
- adrenal (capsule) (fatty) (gland) (hyaline) (infectional) E27.8
- amyloid (*see also* Amyloidosis) E85.9
- anterior cornua, spinal cord G12.29
- anterior labral S43.49-
- aorta, aortic I70.0
  - fatty I77.89
- aortic valve (heart) *—see* Endocarditis, aortic
- arteriovascular *—see* Arteriosclerosis
- artery, arterial (atheromatous) (calcareous) *—see also* Arteriosclerosis
  - cerebral, amyloid E85.4 *[I68.0]*
  - medial *—see* Arteriosclerosis, extremities
- articular cartilage NEC *—see* Derangement, joint, articular cartilage, by site
- atheromatous *—see* Arteriosclerosis
- basal nuclei or ganglia G23.9
  - specified NEC G23.8
- bone NEC *—see* Disorder, bone, specified type NEC
- brachial plexus G54.0
- brain (cortical) (progressive) G31.9
  - alcoholic G31.2
  - arteriosclerotic I67.2
  - childhood G31.9
    - specified NEC G31.89
  - cystic G31.89
    - congenital Q04.6
  - in
    - alcoholism G31.2
    - beriberi E51.2
    - cerebrovascular disease I67.9
    - congenital hydrocephalus Q03.9
      - with spina bifida *—see also* Spina bifida
    - Fabry-Anderson disease E75.21
    - Gaucher's disease E75.22
    - Hunter's syndrome E76.1
    - lipidosis
      - cerebral E75.4
      - generalized E75.6
    - mucopolysaccharidosis *—see* Mucopolysaccharidosis
    - myxedema E03.9 *[G32.89]*
    - neoplastic disease (*see also* Neoplasm) D49.6 *[G32.89]*
    - Niemann-Pick disease E75.249 *[G32.89]*
    - sphingolipidosis E75.3 *[G32.89]*
    - vitamin B12 deficiency E53.8 *[G32.89]*
  - senile NEC G31.1
- breast N64.89
- Bruch's membrane *—see* Degeneration, choroid
- capillaries (fatty) I78.8
  - amyloid E85.89 *[I79.8]*
- cardiac *—see also* Degeneration, myocardial
  - valve, valvular *—see* Endocarditis
- cardiorenal *—see* Hypertension, cardiorenal
- cardiovascular *—see also* Disease, cardiovascular
  - renal *—see* Hypertension, cardiorenal
- cerebellar NOS G31.9
  - alcoholic G31.2
  - primary (hereditary) (sporadic) G11.9

Degeneration, degenerative *(continued)*
- cerebral *—see* Degeneration, brain
- cerebrovascular I67.9
  - due to hypertension I67.4
- cervical plexus G54.2
- cervix N88.8
  - due to radiation (intended effect) N88.8
    - adverse effect or misadventure N99.89
- chamber angle H21.21-
- changes, spine or vertebra *—see* Spondylosis
- chorioretinal *—see also* Degeneration, choroid
  - hereditary H31.20
- choroid (colloid) (drusen) H31.10-
  - atrophy *—see* Atrophy, choroidal
  - hereditary *—see* Dystrophy, choroidal, hereditary
- ciliary body H21.22-
- cochlear H83.8
- combined (spinal cord) (subacute) E53.8 *[G32.0]*
  - with anemia (pernicious) D51.0 *[G32.0]*
    - due to dietary vitamin B12 deficiency D51.3 *[G32.0]*
  - in (due to)
    - vitamin B12 deficiency E53.8 *[G32.0]*
      - anemia D51.9 *[G32.0]*
- conjunctiva H11.10
  - concretions *—see* Concretion, conjunctiva
  - deposits *—see* Deposit, conjunctiva
  - pigmentations *—see* Pigmentation, conjunctiva
  - pinguecula *—see* Pinguecula
  - xerosis *—see* Xerosis, conjunctiva
- cornea H18.40
  - calcerous H18.43
    - band keratopathy H18.42-
  - familial, hereditary *—see* Dystrophy, cornea
  - hyaline (of old scars) H18.49
  - keratomalacia *—see* Keratomalacia
  - nodular H18.45-
  - peripheral H18.46-
  - senile H18.41-
  - specified type NEC H18.49
- cortical (cerebellar) (parenchymatous) G31.89
  - alcoholic G31.2
  - diffuse, due to arteriopathy I67.2
- corticobasal G31.85
- cutis L98.8
  - amyloid E85.4 *[L99]*
- dental pulp K04.2
- disc disease *—see* Degeneration, intervertebral disc NEC
- dorsolateral (spinal cord) *—see* Degeneration, combined
- extrapyramidal G25.9
- eye, macular *—see also* Degeneration, macula
  - congenital or hereditary *—see* Dystrophy, retina
- facet joints *—see* Spondylosis
- fatty
  - liver NEC K76.0
    - alcoholic K70.0
- grey matter (brain) (Alpers') G31.81
- heart *—see also* Degeneration, myocardial
  - amyloid E85.4 *[I43]*

Degeneration, degenerative *(continued)*
- heart *(continued)*
  - atheromatous *—see* Disease, heart, ischemic, atherosclerotic
  - ischemic *—see* Disease, heart, ischemic
- hepatolenticular (Wilson's) E83.01
- hepatorenal K76.7
- hyaline (diffuse) (generalized)
  - localized *—see* Degeneration, by site
- infrapatellar fat pad M79.4
- intervertebral disc NOS
  - with
    - myelopathy *—see* Disorder, disc, with, myelopathy
    - radiculitis or radiculopathy *—see* Disorder, disc, with, radiculopathy
  - cervical, cervicothoracic *—see* Disorder, disc, cervical, degeneration
    - with
      - myelopathy *—see* Disorder, disc, cervical, with myelopathy
      - neuritis, radiculitis or radiculopathy *—see* Disorder, disc, cervical, with neuritis
  - lumbar region M51.36
    - with
      - myelopathy M51.06
      - neuritis, radiculitis, radiculopathy or sciatica M51.16
  - lumbosacral region M51.37
    - with
      - neuritis, radiculitis, radiculopathy or sciatica M51.17
  - sacrococcygeal region M53.3
  - thoracic region M51.34
    - with
      - myelopathy M51.04
      - neuritis, radiculitis, radiculopathy M51.14
  - thoracolumbar region M51.35
    - with
      - myelopathy M51.05
      - neuritis, radiculitis, radiculopathy M51.15
- intestine, amyloid E85.4
- iris (pigmentary) H21.23-
- ischemic *—see* Ischemia
- joint disease *—see* Osteoarthritis
- kidney N28.89
  - amyloid E85.4 *[N29]*
  - cystic, congenital Q61.9
  - fatty N28.89
  - polycystic Q61.3
    - adult type (autosomal dominant) Q61.2
    - infantile type (autosomal recessive) NEC Q61.19
      - collecting duct dilatation Q61.11
- Kuhnt-Junius (*see also* Degeneration, macula) H35.32-
- lens *—see* Cataract
- lenticular (familial) (progressive) (Wilson's) (with cirrhosis of liver) E83.01
- liver (diffuse) NEC K76.89
  - amyloid E85.4 *[K77]*
  - cystic K76.89
    - congenital Q44.6
  - fatty NEC K76.0
    - alcoholic K70.0

Degeneration, degenerative *(continued)*
- liver *(continued)*
  - hypertrophic K76.89
  - parenchymatous, acute or subacute K72.00
    - with coma K72.01
  - pigmentary K76.89
  - toxic (acute) K71.9
- lung J98.4
- lymph gland I89.8
  - hyaline I89.8
- macula, macular (acquired) (age-related) (senile) H35.30
  - angioid streaks H35.33
  - atrophic age-related H35.31-
  - congenital or hereditary —*see* Dystrophy, retina
  - cystoid H35.35-
  - dry age-related H35.31-
  - drusen H35.36-
  - exudative H35.32-
  - hole H35.34-
  - nonexudative H35.31-
  - puckering H35.37-
  - toxic H35.38-
  - wet age-related H35.32-
- membranous labyrinth, congenital (causing impairment of hearing) Q16.5
- meniscus —*see* Derangement, meniscus
- mitral —*see* Insufficiency, mitral
- Mönckeberg's —*see* Arteriosclerosis, extremities
- motor centers, senile G31.1
- multi-system G90.3
- mural —*see* Degeneration, myocardial
- muscle (fatty) (fibrous) (hyaline) (progressive) M62.89
  - heart —*see* Degeneration, myocardial
- myelin, central nervous system G37.9
- myocardial, myocardium (fatty) (hyaline) (senile) I51.5
  - with rheumatic fever (conditions in I00) I09.0
    - active, acute or subacute I01.2
      - with chorea I02.0
    - inactive or quiescent (with chorea) I09.0
  - hypertensive —*see* Hypertension, heart
  - rheumatic —*see* Degeneration, myocardial, with rheumatic fever
  - syphilitic A52.06
- nasal sinus (mucosa) J32.9
  - frontal J32.1
  - maxillary J32.0
- nerve —*see* Disorder, nerve
- nervous system G31.9
  - alcoholic G31.2
  - amyloid E85.4 *[G99.8]*
  - autonomic G90.9
  - fatty G31.89
  - specified NEC G31.89
- nipple N64.89
- olivopontocerebellar (hereditary) (familial) G23.8
- osseous labyrinth —*see* subcategory H83.8
- ovary N83.8
  - cystic N83.20-
  - microcystic N83.20-
- pallidal pigmentary (progressive) G23.0
- pancreas K86.89
  - tuberculous A18.83

Degeneration, degenerative *(continued)*
- penis N48.89
- pigmentary (diffuse) (general)
  - localized —*see* Degeneration, by site
  - pallidal (progressive) G23.0
- pineal gland E34.8
- pituitary (gland) E23.6
- popliteal fat pad M79.4
- posterolateral (spinal cord) —*see* Degeneration, combined
- pulmonary valve (heart) I37.8
- pulp (tooth) K04.2
- pupillary margin H21.24-
- renal —*see* Degeneration, kidney
- retina H35.9
  - hereditary (cerebroretinal) (congenital) (juvenile) (macula) (peripheral) (pigmentary) —*see* Dystrophy, retina
  - Kuhnt-Junius (*see also* Degeneration, macula) H35.32-
  - macula (cystic) (exudative) (hole) (nonexudative) (pseudohole) (senile) (toxic) —*see* Degeneration, macula
  - peripheral H35.40
    - lattice H35.41-
    - microcystoid H35.42-
    - paving stone H35.43-
    - secondary
      - pigmentary H35.45-
      - vitreoretinal H35.46-
    - senile reticular H35.44-
  - pigmentary (primary) —*see also* Dystrophy, retina
    - secondary —*see* Degeneration, retina, peripheral, secondary
  - posterior pole —*see* Degeneration, macula
- saccule, congenital (causing impairment of hearing) Q16.5
- senile R54
  - brain G31.1
  - cardiac, heart or myocardium —*see* Degeneration, myocardial
  - motor centers G31.1
  - vascular —*see* Arteriosclerosis
- sinus (cystic) —*see also* Sinusitis
  - polypoid J33.1
- skin L98.8
  - amyloid E85.4 *[L99]*
  - colloid L98.8
- spinal (cord) G31.89
  - amyloid E85.4 *[G32.89]*
  - combined (subacute) —*see* Degeneration, combined
  - dorsolateral —*see* Degeneration, combined
  - familial NEC G31.89
  - fatty G31.89
  - funicular —*see* Degeneration, combined
  - posterolateral —*see* Degeneration, combined
  - subacute combined —*see* Degeneration, combined
  - tuberculous A17.81
- spleen D73.0
  - amyloid E85.4 *[D77]*
- stomach K31.89
- striatonigral G23.2
- suprarenal (capsule) (gland) E27.8
- synovial membrane (pulpy) —*see* Disorder, synovium, specified type NEC
- tapetoretinal —*see* Dystrophy, retina

Degeneration, degenerative *(continued)*
- thymus (gland) E32.8
  - fatty E32.8
- thyroid (gland) E07.89
- tricuspid (heart) (valve) I07.9
- tuberculous NEC —*see* Tuberculosis
- turbinate J34.89
- uterus (cystic) N85.8
- vascular (senile) —*see* Arteriosclerosis
  - hypertensive —*see* Hypertension
- vitreoretinal, secondary —*see* Degeneration, retina, peripheral, secondary, vitreoretinal
- vitreous (body) H43.81-
- Wallerian —*see* Disorder, nerve
- Wilson's hepatolenticular E83.01

Deglutition
- paralysis R13.0
  - hysterical F44.4
- pneumonia J69.0

Degos' disease I77.89

Dehiscence (of)
- amputation stump T87.81
- cesarean wound O90.0
- closure of
  - cornea T81.31
  - craniotomy T81.32
  - fascia (muscular) (superficial) T81.32
  - internal organ or tissue T81.32
  - laceration (external) (internal) T81.33
  - ligament T81.32
  - mucosa T81.31
  - muscle or muscle flap T81.32
  - ribs or rib cage T81.32
  - skin and subcutaneous tissue (full-thickness) (superficial) T81.31
  - skull T81.32
  - sternum (sternotomy) T81.32
  - tendon T81.32
  - traumatic laceration (external) (internal) T81.33
- episiotomy O90.1
- operation wound NEC T81.31
  - external operation wound (superficial) T81.31
  - internal operation wound (deep) T81.32
- perineal wound (postpartum) O90.1
- traumatic injury wound repair T81.33
- wound T81.30
  - traumatic repair T81.33

Dehydration E86.0
- newborn P74.1

Déjérine-Roussy syndrome G89.0

Déjérine-Sottas disease or neuropathy (hypertrophic) G60.0

Déjérine-Thomas atrophy G23.8

Delay, delayed
- any plane in pelvis
  - complicating delivery O66.9
- birth or delivery NOS O63.9
- closure, ductus arteriosus (Botalli) P29.38
- coagulation —*see* Defect, coagulation
- conduction (cardiac) (ventricular) I45.9
- delivery, second twin, triplet, etc O63.2
- development R62.50
  - global F88
  - intellectual (specific) F81.9

Delay, delayed *(continued)*
- development *(continued)*
  - language F80.9
    - due to hearing loss F80.4
  - learning F81.9
  - pervasive F84.9
  - physiological R62.50
    - specified stage NEC R62.0
  - reading F81.0
  - sexual E30.0
  - speech F80.9
    - due to hearing loss F80.4
  - spelling F81.81
- ejaculation F52.32
- gastric emptying K30
- menarche E30.0
- menstruation (cause unknown) N91.0
- milestone R62.0
- passage of meconium (newborn) P76.0
- primary respiration P28.9
- puberty (constitutional) E30.0
- separation of umbilical cord P96.82
- sexual maturation, female E30.0
- sleep phase syndrome G47.21
- union, fracture —*see* Fracture, by site
- vaccination Z28.9

Deletion(s)
- autosome Q93.9
  - identified by fluorescence in situ hybridization (FISH) Q93.89
  - identified by in situ hybridization (ISH) Q93.89
- chromosome
  - with complex rearrangements NEC Q93.7
  - part of NEC Q93.59
  - seen only at prometaphase Q93.89
  - short arm
    - 4 Q93.3
    - 5p Q93.4
    - 22q11.2 Q93.81
  - specified NEC Q93.89
- long arm chromosome 18 or 21 Q93.89
  - with complex rearrangements NEC Q93.7
- microdeletions NEC Q93.88

Delhi boil or button B55.1

Delinquency (juvenile) (neurotic) F91.8
- group Z72.810

Delinquent immunization status Z28.3

Delirium, delirious (acute or subacute) (not alcohol- or drug-induced) (with dementia) R41.0
- alcoholic (acute) (tremens) (withdrawal) F10.921
  - with intoxication F10.921
    - in
      - abuse F10.121
      - dependence F10.221
- due to (secondary to)
  - alcohol
    - intoxication F10.921
      - in
        - abuse F10.121
        - dependence F10.221
    - withdrawal F10.231
  - amphetamine intoxication F15.921
    - in
      - abuse F15.121
      - dependence F15.221
  - anxiolytic
    - intoxication F13.921
      - in
        - abuse F13.121
        - dependence F13.221
    - withdrawal F13.231

Delirium, delirious *(continued)*
- due to *(continued)*
  - cannabis intoxication (acute) F12.921
    - in
      - abuse F12.121
      - dependence F12.221
  - cocaine intoxication (acute) F14.921
    - in
      - abuse F14.121
      - dependence F14.221
  - general medical condition F05
  - hallucinogen intoxication F16.921
    - in
      - abuse F16.121
      - dependence F16.221
  - hypnotic
    - intoxication F13.921
      - in
        - abuse F13.121
        - dependence F13.221
    - withdrawal F13.231
  - inhalant intoxication (acute) F18.921
    - in
      - abuse F18.121
      - dependence F18.221
  - multiple etiologies F05
  - opioid intoxication (acute) F11.921
    - in
      - abuse F11.121
      - dependence F11.221
  - other (or unknown) substance F19.921
  - phencyclidine intoxication (acute) F16.921
    - in
      - abuse F16.121
      - dependence F16.221
  - psychoactive substance NEC intoxication (acute) F19.921
    - in
      - abuse F19.121
      - dependence F19.221
  - sedative
    - intoxication F13.921
      - in
        - abuse F13.121
        - dependence F13.221
    - withdrawal F13.231
  - unknown etiology R41.0
- exhaustion F43.0
- hysterical F44.89
- postprocedural (postoperative) F05
- puerperal F05
- thyroid —*see* Thyrotoxicosis with thyroid storm
- traumatic —*see* Injury, intracranial
- tremens (alcohol-induced) F10.231
  - sedative-induced F13.231

Delivery (childbirth) (labor)
- arrested active phase O62.1
- cesarean (for)
  - abnormal
    - pelvis (bony) (deformity) (major) NEC with disproportion (fetopelvic) O33.0
      - with obstructed labor O65.0
    - presentation or position O32.9
  - abruptio placentae (*see also* Abruptio placentae) O45.9-
  - acromion presentation O32.2
  - atony, uterus O62.2
  - breech presentation O32.1
    - incomplete O32.8
  - brow presentation O32.3

Delivery *(continued)*
- cesarean *(continued)*
  - cephalopelvic disproportion O33.9
  - cerclage O34.3-
  - chin presentation O32.3
  - cicatrix of cervix O34.4-
  - contracted pelvis (general)
    - inlet O33.2
    - outlet O33.3
  - cord presentation or prolapse O69.0
  - cystocele O34.8-
  - deformity (acquired) (congenital)
    - pelvic organs or tissues NEC O34.8-
    - pelvis (bony) NEC O33.0
  - disproportion NOS O33.9
  - eclampsia —*see* Eclampsia
  - face presentation O32.3
  - failed
    - forceps O66.5
    - induction of labor O61.9
      - instrumental O61.1
      - mechanical O61.1
      - medical O61.0
      - specified NEC O61.8
      - surgical O61.1
    - trial of labor NOS O66.40
      - following previous cesarean delivery O66.41
    - vacuum extraction O66.5
    - ventouse O66.5
  - fetal-maternal hemorrhage O43.01-
  - hemorrhage (intrapartum) O67.9
    - with coagulation defect O67.0
    - specified cause NEC O67.8
  - high head at term O32.4
  - hydrocephalic fetus O33.6
  - incarceration of uterus O34.51-
  - incoordinate uterine action O62.4
  - increased size, fetus O33.5
  - inertia, uterus O62.2
    - primary O62.0
    - secondary O62.1
  - isthmocele O34.22
  - lateroversion, uterus O34.59-
  - mal lie O32.9
  - malposition
    - fetus O32.9
    - pelvic organs or tissues NEC O34.8-
    - uterus NEC O34.59-
  - malpresentation NOS O32.9
  - oblique presentation O32.2
  - occurring after 37 completed weeks of gestation but before 39 completed weeks gestation due to (spontaneous) onset of labor O75.82
  - oversize fetus O33.5
  - pelvic tumor NEC O34.8-
  - placenta previa O44.0-
    - complete O44.0-
      - with hemorrhage O44.1-
  - placental insufficiency O36.51-
  - planned, occurring after 37 completed weeks of gestation but before 39 completed weeks gestation due to (spontaneous) onset of labor O75.82
  - polyp, cervix O34.4-
    - causing obstructed labor O65.5
  - poor dilatation, cervix O62.0
  - pre-eclampsia O14.94
    - mild O14.04
    - moderate O14.04

Delivery *(continued)*
- cesarean *(continued)*
  - pre-eclampsia *(continued)*
    - severe O14.14
      - with hemolysis, elevated liver enzymes and low platelet count (HELLP) O14.24
  - previous
    - cesarean delivery O34.219
      - classical (vertical) O34.212
      - isthmocele O34.22
      - low transverse scar O34.211
      - mid-transverse T incision O34.218
      - scar
        - defect (isthmocele) O34.22
        - specified type NEC O34.218
    - surgery (to)
      - cervix O34.4-
      - gynecological NEC O34.8-
      - rectum O34.7-
      - uterus O34.29
      - vagina O34.6-
  - prolapse
    - arm or hand O32.2
    - uterus O34.52-
  - prolonged labor NOS O63.9
  - rectocele O34.8-
  - retroversion
    - uterus O34.53-
  - rigid
    - cervix O34.4-
    - pelvic floor O34.8-
    - perineum O34.7-
    - vagina O34.6-
    - vulva O34.7-
  - sacculation, pregnant uterus O34.59-
  - scar(s)
    - cervix O34.4-
    - cesarean delivery O34.219
      - classical (vertical) O34.212
      - isthmocele O34.22
      - low transverse O34.211
      - mid-transverse T incision O34.218
      - scar
        - defect (isthmocele) O34.22
        - specified type NEC O34.218
    - defect (isthmocele) O34.22
    - transmural uterine O34.29
    - uterus O34.29
  - Shirodkar suture in situ O34.3-
  - shoulder presentation O32.2
  - stenosis or stricture, cervix O34.4-
  - streptococcus group B (GBS) carrier state O99.824
  - transmural uterine scar O34.29
  - transverse presentation or lie O32.2
  - tumor, pelvic organs or tissues NEC O34.8-
    - cervix O34.4-
  - umbilical cord presentation or prolapse O69.0
  - without indication O82
- completely normal case O80
- complicated O75.9
  - by
    - abnormal, abnormality (of)
      - forces of labor O62.9
        - specified type NEC O62.8
      - glucose O99.814

Delivery *(continued)*
- complicated *(continued)*
  - by *(continued)*
    - abnormal, abnormality *(continued)*
      - uterine contractions NOS O62.9
    - abruptio placentae (*see also* Abruptio placentae) O45.9-
    - abuse
      - physical O9A.32
      - psychological O9A.52
      - sexual O9A.42
    - adherent placenta O72.0
      - without hemorrhage O73.0
    - alcohol use O99.314
    - anemia (pre-existing) O99.02
    - anesthetic death O74.8
    - annular detachment of cervix O71.3
    - atony, uterus O62.2
    - attempted vacuum extraction and forceps O66.5
    - Bandl's ring O62.4
    - bariatric surgery status O99.844
    - biliary tract disorder O26.62
    - bleeding —*see* Delivery, complicated by, hemorrhage
    - blood disorder NEC O99.12
    - cervical dystocia (hypotonic) O62.2
      - primary O62.0
      - secondary O62.1
    - circulatory system disorder O99.42
    - compression of cord (umbilical) NEC O69.2
    - condition NEC O99.892
    - contraction, contracted ring O62.4
    - cord (umbilical)
      - around neck
        - with compression O69.1
        - without compression O69.81
      - bruising O69.5
      - complication O69.9
        - specified NEC O69.89
      - compression NEC O69.2
      - entanglement O69.2
        - without compression O69.82
      - hematoma O69.5
      - presentation O69.0
      - prolapse O69.0
      - short O69.3
      - thrombosis (vessels) O69.5
      - vascular lesion O69.5
    - Couvelaire uterus O45.8X-
    - damage to (injury to) NEC
      - perineum O71.82
      - periurethral tissue O71.82
      - vulva O71.82
    - delay following rupture of membranes (spontaneous) —*see* Pregnancy, complicated by, premature rupture of membranes
    - depressed fetal heart tones O76
    - diabetes O24.92
      - gestational
        - diabetes O24.429
          - diet controlled O24.420
          - insulin (and diet) controlled O24.424
          - oral drug controlled (antidiabetic) (hypoglycemic) O24.425

Delivery *(continued)*
complicated *(continued)*
by *(continued)*
diabetes *(continued)*
gestational *(continued)*
edema O12.04
with proteinuria O12.24
proteinuria O12.14
pre-existing O24.32
specified NEC O24.82
type 1 O24.02
type 2 O24.12
diastasis recti (abdominis) O71.89
dilatation
bladder O66.8
cervix incomplete, poor or slow O62.0
disease NEC O99.892
disruptio uteri —*see* Delivery, complicated by, rupture, uterus
drug use O99.324
dysfunction, uterus NOS O62.9
hypertonic O62.4
hypotonic O62.2
primary O62.0
secondary O62.1
incoordinate O62.4
eclampsia O15.1
embolism (pulmonary) —*see* Embolism, obstetric
endocrine, nutritional or metabolic disease NEC O99.284
failed
attempted vaginal birth after previous cesarean delivery O66.41
induction of labor O61.9
instrumental O61.1
mechanical O61.1
medical O61.0
specified NEC O61.8
surgical O61.1
trial of labor O66.40
female genital mutilation O65.5
fetal
abnormal acid-base balance O68
acidemia O68
acidosis O68
alkalosis O68
death, early O02.1
deformity O66.3
heart rate or rhythm (abnormal) (non-reassuring) O76
hypoxia O77.8
stress O77.9
due to drug administration O77.1
electrocardiographic evidence of O77.8
specified NEC O77.8
ultrasound evidence of O77.8
fever during labor O75.2
gastric banding status O99.844
gastric bypass status O99.844
gastrointestinal disease NEC O99.62
gestational
diabetes O24.429
diet controlled O24.420
insulin (and diet) controlled O24.424
oral drug controlled (antidiabetic) (hypoglycemic) O24.425

Delivery *(continued)*
complicated *(continued)*
by *(continued)*
gestational *(continued)*
edema O12.04
with proteinuria O12.14
proteinuria O12.14
gonorrhea O98.22
hematoma O71.7
ischial spine O71.7
pelvic O71.7
vagina O71.7
vulva or perineum O71.7
hemorrhage (uterine) O67.9
associated with
afibrinogenemia O67.0
coagulation defect O67.0
hyperfibrinolysis O67.0
hypofibrinogenemia O67.0
due to
low implantation of placenta O44.5-
low-lying placenta O44.5-
placenta previa O44.1-
marginal O44.3-
partial O44.3-
premature separation of placenta (normally implanted) (*see also* Abruptio placentae) O45.9-
retained placenta O72.0
uterine leiomyoma O67.8
placenta NEC O67.8
postpartum NEC (atonic) (immediate) O72.1
with retained or trapped placenta O72.0
delayed O72.2
secondary O72.2
third stage O72.0
hourglass contraction, uterus O62.4
hypertension, hypertensive (pre-existing) —*see* Hypertension, complicated by, childbirth (labor)
hypotension O26.5-
incomplete dilatation (cervix) O62.0
incoordinate uterus contractions O62.4
inertia, uterus O62.2
during latent phase of labor O62.0
primary O62.0
secondary O62.1
infection (maternal) O98.92
carrier state NEC O99.834
gonorrhea O98.22
human immunodeficiency virus (HIV) O98.72
sexually transmitted NEC O98.32
specified NEC O98.82
syphilis O98.12
tuberculosis O98.02
viral hepatitis O98.42
viral NEC O98.52
injury (to mother) (*see also* Delivery, complicated by, damage to) O71.9
nonobstetric O9A.22
caused by abuse —*see* Delivery, complicated by, abuse
intrauterine fetal death, early O02.1
inversion, uterus O71.2

Delivery *(continued)*
complicated *(continued)*
by *(continued)*
laceration (perineal) O70.9
anus (sphincter) O70.4
with third degree laceration (*see also* Delivery, complicated, by, laceration, perineum, third degree) O70.20
with mucosa O70.3
without third degree laceration O70.4
bladder (urinary) O71.5
bowel O71.5
cervix (uteri) O71.3
fourchette O70.0
hymen O70.0
labia O70.0
pelvic
floor O70.1
organ NEC O71.5
perineum, perineal O70.9
first degree O70.0
fourth degree O70.3
muscles O70.1
second degree O70.1
skin O70.0
slight O70.0
third degree O70.20
with
both external anal sphincter (EAS) and internal anal sphincter (IAS) torm (IIIc) O70.23
less than 50% of external anal sphincter (EAS) thickness torn (IIIa) O70.21
more than 50% of external anal sphincter (EAS) thickness torn (IIIb) O70.22
IIIa O70.21
IIIb O70.22
IIIc O70.23
peritoneum (pelvic) O71.5
rectovaginal (septum) (without perineal laceration) O71.4
with perineum (*see also* Delivery, complicated, by, laceration, perineum, third degree) O70.20
with anal or rectal mucosa O70.3
specified NEC O71.89
sphincter ani —*see* Delivery, complicated, by, laceration, anus (sphincter)
urethra O71.5
uterus O71.81
before labor O71.81
vagina, vaginal (deep) (high) (without perineal laceration) O71.4
with perineum O70.0
muscles, with perineum O70.1
vulva O70.0
liver disorder O26.62
malignancy O9A.12
malnutrition O25.2
malposition, malpresentation
placenta O44.0-
with hemorrhage O44.1-

Delivery *(continued)*
complicated *(continued)*
by *(continued)*
malposition, malpresentation *(continued)*
uterus or cervix O65.5
without obstruction (*see also* Delivery, complicated by, obstruction) O32.9
breech O32.1
compound O32.6
face (brow) (chin) O32.3
footling O32.8
high head O32.4
oblique O32.2
specified NEC O32.8
transverse O32.2
unstable lie O32.0
meconium in amniotic fluid O77.0
mental disorder NEC O99.344
metrorrhexis —*see* Delivery, complicated by, rupture, uterus
nervous system disorder O99.354
obesity (pre-existing) O99.214
obesity surgery status O99.844
obstetric trauma O71.9
specified NEC O71.89
obstructed labor
due to
breech (complete) (frank) presentation O64.1
incomplete O64.8
brow presentation O64.3
buttock presentation O64.1
chin presentation O64.2
compound presentation O64.5
contracted pelvis O65.1
deep transverse arrest O64.0
deformed pelvis O65.0
dystocia (fetal) O66.9
due to
conjoined twins O66.3
fetal
abnormality NEC O66.3
ascites O66.3
hydrops O66.3
meningomyelocele O66.3
sacral teratoma O66.3
tumor O66.3
hydrocephalic fetus O66.3
shoulder O66.0
face presentation O64.2
fetopelvic disproportion O65.4
footling presentation O64.8
impacted shoulders O66.0
incomplete rotation of fetal head O64.0
large fetus O66.2
locked twins O66.1
malposition O64.9
specified NEC O64.8
malpresentation O64.9
specified NEC O64.8
multiple fetuses NEC O66.6
pelvic
abnormality (maternal) O65.9
organ O65.5
specified NEC O65.8

Dementia *(continued)*
  paralytica, paralytic *(continued)*
    with behavioral disturbance A52.17 *[F02.81]*
    juvenilis A50.45
  paretic A52.17
  praecox *—see* Schizophrenia
  presenile F03
    Alzheimer's type *—see* Disease, Alzheimer's, early onset
  primary degenerative F03
  progressive, syphilitic A52.17
  senile F03
    with acute confusional state F05
    Alzheimer's type *—see* Disease, Alzheimer's, late onset
    depressed or paranoid type F03
  vascular (acute onset) (mixed) (multi-infarct) (subcortical) F01.50
    with behavioral disturbance F01.51

Demineralization, bone *—see* Osteoporosis

Demodex folliculorum (infestation) B88.0

Demophobia F40.248

Demoralization R45.3

Demyelination, demyelinization
  central nervous system G37.9
    specified NEC G37.8
  corpus callosum (central) G37.1
  disseminated, acute G36.9
    specified NEC G36.8
  global G35
  in optic neuritis G36.0

Dengue (classical) (fever) A90
  hemorrhagic A91
  sandfly A93.1

Dennie-Marfan syphilitic syndrome A50.45

Dens evaginatus, in dente or invaginatus K00.2

Dense breasts R92.2

Density
  increased, bone (disseminated) (generalized) (spotted) *—see* Disorder, bone, density and structure, specified type NEC
  lung (nodular) J98.4

Dental *—see also* condition
  examination Z01.20
    with abnormal findings Z01.21
  restoration
    aesthetically inadequate or displeasing K08.56
    defective K08.50
      specified NEC K08.59
    failure of marginal integrity K08.51
    failure of periodontal anatomical integrity K08.54

Dentia praecox K00.6

Denticles (pulp) K04.2

Dentigerous cyst K09.0

Dentin
  irregular (in pulp) K04.3
  opalescent K00.5
  secondary (in pulp) K04.3
  sensitive K03.89

Dentinogenesis imperfecta K00.5

Dentinoma *—see* Cyst, calcifying odontogenic

Dentition (syndrome) K00.7
  delayed K00.6
  difficult K00.7
  precocious K00.6

Dentition *(continued)*
  premature K00.6
  retarded K00.6

Dependence (on) (syndrome) F19.20
  with remission F19.21
  alcohol (ethyl) (methyl) (without remission) F10.20
    with
      amnestic disorder, persisting F10.26
      anxiety disorder F10.280
      dementia, persisting F10.27
      intoxication F10.229
        with delirium F10.221
        uncomplicated F10.220
      mood disorder F10.24
      psychotic disorder F10.259
        with
          delusions F10.250
          hallucinations F10.251
      remission F10.21
      sexual dysfunction F10.281
      sleep disorder F10.282
      specified disorder NEC F10.288
      withdrawal F10.239
        with
          delirium F10.231
          perceptual disturbance F10.232
        uncomplicated F10.230
    counseling and surveillance Z71.41
    in remission F10.21
  amobarbital *—see* Dependence, drug, sedative
  amphetamine(s) (type) *—see* Dependence, drug, stimulant NEC
  amytal (sodium) *—see* Dependence, drug, sedative
  analgesic NEC F55.8
  anesthetic (agent) (gas) (general) (local) NEC *—see* Dependence, drug, psychoactive NEC
  anxiolytic NEC *—see* Dependence, drug, sedative
  barbital(s) *—see* Dependence, drug, sedative
  barbiturate(s) (compounds) (drugs classifiable to T42) *—see* Dependence, drug, sedative
  benzedrine *—see* Dependence, drug, stimulant NEC
  bhang *—see* Dependence, drug, cannabis
  bromide(s) NEC *—see* Dependence, drug, sedative
  caffeine *—see* Dependence, drug, stimulant NEC
  cannabis (sativa) (indica) (resin) (derivatives) (type) *—see* Dependence, drug, cannabis
  chloral (betaine) (hydrate) *—see* Dependence, drug, sedative
  chlordiazepoxide *—see* Dependence, drug, sedative
  coca (leaf) (derivatives) *—see* Dependence, drug, cocaine
  cocaine *—see* Dependence, drug, cocaine
  codeine *—see* Dependence, drug, opioid
  combinations of drugs F19.20
  dagga *—see* Dependence, drug, cannabis
  demerol *—see* Dependence, drug, opioid
  dexamphetamine *—see* Dependence, drug, stimulant NEC

Dependence *(continued)*
  dexedrine *—see* Dependence, drug, stimulant NEC
  dextromethorphan *—see* Dependence, drug, opioid
  dextromoramide *—see* Dependence, drug, opioid
  dextro-nor-pseudo-ephedrine *—see* Dependence, drug, stimulant NEC
  dextrorphan *—see* Dependence, drug, opioid
  diazepam *—see* Dependence, drug, sedative
  dilaudid *—see* Dependence, drug, opioid
  D-lysergic acid diethylamide *—see* Dependence, drug, hallucinogen
  drug NEC F19.20
    with sleep disorder F19.282
    cannabis F12.20
      with
        anxiety disorder F12.280
        intoxication F12.229
          with
            delirium F12.221
            perceptual disturbance F12.222
          uncomplicated F12.220
        other specified disorder F12.288
        psychosis F12.259
          delusions F12.250
          hallucinations F12.251
        unspecified disorder F12.29
        withdrawal F12.23
      in remission F12.21
    cocaine F14.20
      with
        anxiety disorder F14.280
        intoxication F14.229
          with
            delirium F14.221
            perceptual disturbance F14.222
          uncomplicated F14.220
        mood disorder F14.24
        other specified disorder F14.288
        psychosis F14.259
          delusions F14.250
          hallucinations F14.251
        sexual dysfunction F14.281
        sleep disorder F14.282
        unspecified disorder F14.29
        withdrawal F14.23
      in remission F14.21
      withdrawal symptoms in newborn P96.1
    counseling and surveillance Z71.51
    hallucinogen F16.20
      with
        anxiety disorder F16.280
        flashbacks F16.283
        intoxication F16.229
          with delirium F16.221
          uncomplicated F16.220
        mood disorder F16.24
        other specified disorder F16.288
        perception disorder, persisting F16.283
        psychosis F16.259
          delusions F16.250
          hallucinations F16.251
        unspecified disorder F16.29
      in remission F16.21
    in remission F19.21
    inhalant F18.20

Dependence *(continued)*
  drug NEC *(continued)*
    inhalant *(continued)*
      with
        anxiety disorder F18.280
        dementia, persisting F18.27
        intoxication F18.229
          with delirium F18.221
          uncomplicated F18.220
        mood disorder F18.24
        other specified disorder F18.288
        psychosis F18.259
          delusions F18.250
          hallucinations F18.251
        unspecified disorder F18.29
      in remission F18.21
    nicotine F17.200
      with disorder F17.209
        in remission F17.201
        specified disorder NEC F17.208
        withdrawal F17.203
      chewing tobacco F17.220
        with disorder F17.229
          in remission F17.221
          specified disorder NEC F17.228
          withdrawal F17.223
      cigarettes F17.210
        with disorder F17.219
          in remission F17.211
          specified disorder NEC F17.218
          withdrawal F17.213
      specified product NEC F17.290
        with disorder F17.299
          remission F17.291
          specified disorder NEC F17.298
          withdrawal F17.293
    opioid F11.20
      with
        intoxication F11.229
          with
            delirium F11.221
            perceptual disturbance F11.222
          uncomplicated F11.220
        mood disorder F11.24
        other specified disorder F11.288
        psychosis F11.259
          delusions F11.250
          hallucinations F11.251
        sexual dysfunction F11.281
        sleep disorder F11.282
        unspecified disorder F11.29
        withdrawal F11.23
      in remission F11.21
    psychoactive NEC F19.20
      with
        amnestic disorder F19.26
        anxiety disorder F19.280
        dementia F19.27
        intoxication F19.229
          with
            delirium F19.221
            perceptual disturbance F19.222
          uncomplicated F19.220
        mood disorder F19.24
        other specified disorder F19.288
        psychosis F19.259
          delusions F19.250
          hallucinations F19.251
        sexual dysfunction F19.281
        sleep disorder F19.282

Dependence *(continued)*
- drug NEC *(continued)*
  - psychoactive NEC *(continued)*
    - with *(continued)*
      - unspecified disorder F19.29
      - withdrawal F19.239
        - with
          - delirium F19.231
          - perceptual disturbance F19.232
        - uncomplicated F19.230
  - sedative, hypnotic or anxiolytic F13.20
    - with
      - amnestic disorder F13.26
      - anxiety disorder F13.280
      - dementia, persisting F13.27
      - intoxication F13.229
        - with delirium F13.221
        - uncomplicated F13.220
      - mood disorder F13.24
      - other specified disorder F13.288
      - psychosis F13.259
        - delusions F13.250
        - hallucinations F13.251
      - sexual dysfunction F13.281
      - sleep disorder F13.282
      - unspecified disorder F13.29
      - withdrawal F13.239
        - with
          - delirium F13.231
          - perceptual disturbance F13.232
        - uncomplicated F13.230
    - in remission F13.21
  - stimulant NEC F15.20
    - with
      - anxiety disorder F15.280
      - intoxication F15.229
        - with
          - delirium F15.221
          - perceptual disturbance F15.222
        - uncomplicated F15.220
      - mood disorder F15.24
      - other specified disorder F15.288
      - psychosis F15.259
        - delusions F15.250
        - hallucinations F15.251
      - sexual dysfunction F15.281
      - sleep disorder F15.282
      - unspecified disorder F15.29
      - withdrawal F15.23
    - in remission F15.21
- ethyl
  - alcohol (without remission) F10.20
    - with remission F10.21
  - bromide —*see* Dependence, drug, sedative
  - carbamate F19.20
  - chloride F19.20
  - morphine —*see* Dependence, drug, opioid
- ganja —*see* Dependence, drug, cannabis
- glue (airplane) (sniffing) —*see* Dependence, drug, inhalant
- glutethimide —*see* Dependence, drug, sedative
- hallucinogenics —*see* Dependence, drug, hallucinogen
- hashish —*see* Dependence, drug, cannabis
- hemp —*see* Dependence, drug, cannabis

Dependence *(continued)*
- heroin (salt) (any) —*see* Dependence, drug, opioid
- hypnotic NEC —*see* Dependence, drug, sedative
- Indian hemp —*see* Dependence, drug, cannabis
- inhalants —*see* Dependence, drug, inhalant
- khat —*see* Dependence, drug, stimulant NEC
- laudanum —*see* Dependence, drug, opioid
- LSD(-25) (derivatives) —*see* Dependence, drug, hallucinogen
- luminal —*see* Dependence, drug, sedative
- lysergic acid —*see* Dependence, drug, hallucinogen
- maconha —*see* Dependence, drug, cannabis
- marihuana —*see* Dependence, drug, cannabis
- meprobamate —*see* Dependence, drug, sedative
- mescaline —*see* Dependence, drug, hallucinogen
- methadone —*see* Dependence, drug, opioid
- methamphetamine(s) —*see* Dependence, drug, stimulant NEC
- methaqualone —*see* Dependence, drug, sedative
- methyl
  - alcohol (without remission) F10.20
    - with remission F10.21
  - bromide —*see* Dependence, drug, sedative
  - morphine —*see* Dependence, drug, opioid
  - phenidate —*see* Dependence, drug, stimulant NEC
  - sulfonal —*see* Dependence, drug, sedative
- morphine (sulfate) (sulfite) (type) —*see* Dependence, drug, opioid
- narcotic (drug) NEC —*see* Dependence, drug, opioid
- nembutal —*see* Dependence, drug, sedative
- neraval —*see* Dependence, drug, sedative
- neravan —*see* Dependence, drug, sedative
- neurobarb —*see* Dependence, drug, sedative
- nicotine —*see* Dependence, drug, nicotine
- nitrous oxide F19.20
- nonbarbiturate sedatives and tranquilizers with similar effect —*see* Dependence, drug, sedative
- on
  - artificial heart (fully implantable) (mechanical) Z95.812
  - aspirator Z99.0
  - care provider (because of) Z74.9
    - impaired mobility Z74.09
    - need for
      - assistance with personal care Z74.1
      - continuous supervision Z74.3
    - no other household member able to render care Z74.2
    - specified reason NEC Z74.8

Dependence *(continued)*
- on *(continued)*
  - machine Z99.89
    - enabling NEC Z99.89
    - specified type NEC Z99.89
  - renal dialysis (hemodialysis) (peritoneal) Z99.2
  - respirator Z99.11
  - ventilator Z99.11
  - wheelchair Z99.3
- opiate —*see* Dependence, drug, opioid
- opioids —*see* Dependence, drug, opioid
- opium (alkaloids) (derivatives) (tincture) —*see* Dependence, drug, opioid
- oxygen (long-term) (supplemental) Z99.81
- paraldehyde —*see* Dependence, drug, sedative
- paregoric —*see* Dependence, drug, opioid
- PCP (phencyclidine) (or related substance) —*see* Dependence, drug, hallucinogen
- pentobarbital —*see* Dependence, drug, sedative
- pentobarbitone (sodium) —*see* Dependence, drug, sedative
- pentothal —*see* Dependence, drug, sedative
- peyote —*see* Dependence, drug, hallucinogen
- phencyclidine (PCP) (or related substance) —*see* Dependence, drug, hallucinogen
- phenmetrazine —*see* Dependence, drug, stimulant NEC
- phenobarbital —*see* Dependence, drug, sedative
- polysubstance F19.20
- psilocibin, psilocin, psilocyn, psilocyline —*see* Dependence, drug, hallucinogen
- psychostimulant NEC —*see* Dependence, drug, stimulant NEC
- secobarbital —*see* Dependence, drug, sedative
- seconal —*see* Dependence, drug, sedative
- sedative NEC —*see* Dependence, drug, sedative
- specified drug NEC —*see* Dependence, drug
- stimulant NEC —*see* Dependence, drug, stimulant NEC
- substance NEC —*see* Dependence, drug
- supplemental oxygen Z99.81
- tobacco —*see* Dependence, drug, nicotine
  - counseling and surveillance Z71.6
- tranquilizer NEC —*see* Dependence, drug, sedative
- vitamin B6 E53.1
- volatile solvents —*see* Dependence, drug, inhalant

Dependency
- care-provider Z74.9
- passive F60.7
- reactions (persistent) F60.7

Depersonalization (in neurotic state) (neurotic) (syndrome) F48.1

Depletion
- extracellular fluid E86.9
- plasma E86.1
- potassium E87.6
  - nephropathy N25.89

Depletion *(continued)*
- salt or sodium E87.1
  - causing heat exhaustion or prostration T67.4
  - nephropathy N28.9
- volume NOS E86.9

Deployment (current) (military) **status** Z56.82
- in theater or in support of military war, peacekeeping and humanitarian operations Z56.82
- personal history of Z91.82
  - military war, peacekeeping and humanitarian deployment (current or past conflict) Z91.82
- returned from Z91.82

Depolarization, premature I49.40
- atrial I49.1
- junctional I49.2
- specified NEC I49.49
- ventricular I49.3

Deposit
- bone in Boeck's sarcoid D86.89
- calcareous, calcium —*see* Calcification
- cholesterol
  - retina H35.89
  - vitreous (body) (humor) —*see* Deposit, crystalline
- conjunctiva H11.11-
- cornea H18.00-
  - argentous H18.02-
  - due to metabolic disorder H18.03-
  - Kayser-Fleischer ring H18.04-
  - pigmentation —*see* Pigmentation, cornea
- crystalline, vitreous (body) (humor) H43.2-
- hemosiderin in old scars of cornea —*see* Pigmentation, cornea, stromal
- metallic in lens —*see* Cataract, specified NEC
- skin R23.8
- tooth, teeth (betel) (black) (green) (materia alba) (orange) (tobacco) K03.6
- urate, kidney —*see* Calculus, kidney

Depraved appetite —*see* Pica

Depressed
- HDL cholesterol E78.6

Depression (acute) (mental) F32.A
- agitated (single episode) F32.2
- anaclitic —*see* Disorder, adjustment
- anxiety F41.8
  - persistent F34.1
- arches —*see also* Deformity, limb, flat foot
- atypical (single episode) F32.89
  - recurrent episode F33.8
- basal metabolic rate R94.8
- bone marrow D75.89
- central nervous system R09.2
- cerebral R29.818
  - newborn P91.4
- cerebrovascular I67.9
- chest wall M95.4
- climacteric (single episode) F32.89
  - recurrent episode F33.8
- endogenous (without psychotic symptoms) F33.2
  - with psychotic symptoms F33.3
- functional activity R68.89
- hysterical F44.89

Depression *(continued)*
- involutional (single episode) F32.89
  - recurrent episode F33.8
- major F32.9
  - with psychotic symptoms F32.3
  - recurrent —*see* Disorder, depressive, recurrent
- manic-depressive —*see* Disorder, depressive, recurrent
- masked (single episode) F32.89
- medullary G93.89
- menopausal (single episode) F32.89
  - recurrent episode F33.8
- metatarsus —*see* Depression, arches
- monopolar F33.9
- nervous F34.1
- neurotic F34.1
- nose M95.0
- postnatal NOS F53.0
- postpartum NOS F53.0
- post-psychotic of schizophrenia F32.89
- post-schizophrenic F32.89
- psychogenic (reactive) (single episode) F32.9
- psychoneurotic F34.1
- psychotic (single episode) F32.3
  - recurrent F33.3
- reactive (psychogenic) (single episode) F32.9
  - psychotic (single episode) F32.3
- recurrent —*see* Disorder, depressive, recurrent
- respiratory center G93.89
- seasonal —*see* Disorder, depressive, recurrent
- senile F03
- severe, single episode F32.2
- situational F43.21
- skull Q67.4
- specified NEC (single episode) F32.89
- sternum M95.4
- visual field —*see* Defect, visual field
- vital (recurrent) (without psychotic symptoms) F33.2
  - with psychotic symptoms F33.3
  - single episode F32.2

Deprivation
- cultural Z60.3
- effects NOS T73.9
  - specified NEC T73.8
- emotional NEC Z65.8
  - affecting infant or child —*see* Maltreatment, child, psychological
- food T73.0
- protein —*see* Malnutrition
- sleep Z72.820
- social Z60.4
  - affecting infant or child —*see* Maltreatment, child, psychological
- specified NEC T73.8
- vitamins —*see* Deficiency, vitamin
- water T73.1

Derangement
- ankle (internal) —*see* Derangement, joint, ankle
- cartilage (articular) NEC —*see* Derangement, joint, articular cartilage, by site
  - recurrent —*see* Dislocation, recurrent
- cruciate ligament, anterior, current injury —*see* Sprain, knee, cruciate, anterior
- elbow (internal) —*see* Derangement, joint, elbow
- hip (joint) (internal) (old) —*see* Derangement, joint, hip
- joint (internal) M24.9
  - ankylosis —*see* Ankylosis
  - articular cartilage M24.10
    - ankle M24.17-
    - elbow M24.12-
    - foot M24.17-
    - hand M24.14-
    - hip M24.15-
    - knee NEC M23.9-
    - loose body —*see* Loose, body
    - shoulder M24.11-
    - specified site NEC M24.19
    - wrist M24.13-
  - contracture —*see* Contraction, joint
  - current injury —*see also* Dislocation
    - knee, meniscus or cartilage —*see* Tear, meniscus
  - dislocation
    - pathological —*see* Dislocation, pathological
    - recurrent —*see* Dislocation, recurrent
  - knee —*see* Derangement, knee
  - ligament —*see* Disorder, ligament
  - loose body —*see* Loose, body
  - recurrent —*see* Dislocation, recurrent
  - specified type NEC M24.80
    - ankle M24.87-
    - elbow M24.82-
    - foot joint M24.87-
    - hand joint M24.84-
    - hip M24.85-
    - shoulder M24.81-
    - specified site NEC M24.89
    - wrist M24.83-
  - temporomandibular M26.69
- knee (recurrent) M23.9-
  - ligament disruption, spontaneous M23.60-
    - anterior cruciate M23.61-
    - capsular M23.67-
    - instability, chronic M23.5-
    - lateral collateral M23.64-
    - medial collateral M23.63-
    - posterior cruciate M23.62-
  - loose body M23.4-
  - meniscus M23.30-
    - cystic M23.00-
      - lateral M23.002
        - anterior horn M23.04-
        - posterior horn M23.05-
        - specified NEC M23.06-
      - medial M23.005
        - anterior horn M23.01-
        - posterior horn M23.02-
        - specified NEC M23.03-
    - degenerate —*see* Derangement, knee, meniscus, specified NEC
    - detached —*see* Derangement, knee, meniscus, specified NEC
    - due to old tear or injury M23.20-
      - lateral M23.20-
        - anterior horn M23.24-
        - posterior horn M23.25-
        - specified NEC M23.26-
      - medial M23.20-

Derangement *(continued)*
- knee *(continued)*
  - meniscus *(continued)*
    - due to old tear or injury *(continued)*
      - medial *(continued)*
        - anterior horn M23.21-
        - posterior horn M23.22-
        - specified NEC M23.23-
    - retained —*see* Derangement, knee, meniscus, specified NEC
    - specified NEC M23.30-
      - lateral M23.30-
        - anterior horn M23.34-
        - posterior horn M23.35-
        - specified NEC M23.36-
      - medial M23.30-
        - anterior horn M23.31-
        - posterior horn M23.32-
        - specified NEC M23.33-
  - old M23.8X-
  - specified NEC —*see* subcategory M23.8
- low back NEC —*see* Dorsopathy, specified NEC
- meniscus —*see* Derangement, knee, meniscus
- mental —*see* Psychosis
- patella, specified NEC —*see* Disorder, patella, derangement NEC
- semilunar cartilage (knee) —*see* Derangement, knee, meniscus, specified NEC
- shoulder (internal) —*see* Derangement, joint, shoulder

Dercum's disease E88.2

Derealization (neurotic) F48.1

Dermal —*see* condition

Dermaphytid —*see* Dermatophytosis

Dermatitis (eczematous) L30.9
- ab igne L59.0
- acarine B88.0
- actinic (due to sun) L57.8
  - other than from sun L59.8
- allergic —*see* Dermatitis, contact, allergic
- ambustionis, due to burn or scald —*see* Burn
- amebic A06.7
- ammonia L22
- arsenical (ingested) L27.8
- artefacta L98.1
  - psychogenic F54
- atopic L20.9
  - psychogenic F54
  - specified NEC L20.89
- autoimmune progesterone L30.8
- berlock, berloque L56.2
- blastomycotic B40.3
- blister beetle L24.89
- bullous, bullosa L13.9
  - mucosynechial, atrophic L12.1
  - seasonal L30.8
  - specified NEC L13.8
- calorica L59.0
  - due to burn or scald —*see* Burn
- caterpillar L24.89
- cercarial B65.3
- combustionis L59.0
  - due to burn or scald —*see* Burn
- congelationis T69.1
- contact (occupational) L25.9
  - allergic L23.9
    - due to
      - adhesives L23.1
      - cement L23.5
      - chemical products NEC L23.5

Dermatitis *(continued)*
- contact *(continued)*
  - allergic *(continued)*
    - due to *(continued)*
      - chromium L23.0
      - cosmetics L23.2
      - dander (cat) (dog) L23.81
      - drugs in contact with skin L23.3
      - dyes L23.4
      - food in contact with skin L23.6
      - hair (cat) (dog) L23.81
      - insecticide L23.5
      - metals L23.0
      - nickel L23.0
      - plants, non-food L23.7
      - plastic L23.5
      - rubber L23.5
      - specified agent NEC L23.89
  - due to
    - cement L25.3
    - chemical products NEC L25.3
    - cosmetics L25.0
    - dander (cat) (dog) L23.81
    - drugs in contact with skin L25.1
    - dyes L25.2
    - food in contact with skin L25.4
    - hair (cat) (dog) L23.81
    - plants, non-food L25.5
    - specified agent NEC L25.8
  - irritant L24.9
    - due to
      - body fluids L24.A0
        - incontinence (dual) (fecal) (urinary) L24.A2
        - saliva L24.A1
        - specified NEC L24.A9
      - cement L24.5
      - chemical products NEC L24.5
      - cosmetics L24.3
      - detergents L24.0
      - drugs in contact with skin L24.4
      - food in contact with skin L24.6
      - oils and greases L24.1
      - plants, non-food L24.7
      - solvents L24.2
      - specified agent NEC L24.89
    - related to
      - colostomy L24.B3
      - endotracheal tube L24.A9
      - enterocutaneous fistula L24.B3
      - gastrostomy L24.B1
      - ileostomy L24.B3
      - jejunostomy L24.B1
      - saliva or spit fistula L24.B1
      - stoma or fistula L24.B0
        - digestive L24.B1
        - fecal or urinary L24.B3
        - respiratory L24.B2
      - tracheostomy L24.B2
- contusiformis L52
- desquamative L30.8
- diabetic —*see* E08-E13 with .620
- diaper L22
- diphtheritica A36.3
- dry skin L85.3
- due to
  - acetone (contact) (irritant) L24.2
  - acids (contact) (irritant) L24.5
  - adhesive(s) (allergic) (contact) (plaster) L23.1
    - irritant L24.5
  - alcohol (irritant) (skin contact) (substances in category T51) L24.2
    - taken internally L27.8

Dermatitis *(continued)*
- due to *(continued)*
  - alkalis (contact) (irritant) L24.5
  - arsenic (ingested) L27.8
  - carbon disulfide (contact) (irritant) L24.2
  - caustics (contact) (irritant) L24.5
  - cement (contact) L25.3
  - cereal (ingested) L27.2
  - chemical(s) NEC L25.3
    - taken internally L27.8
  - chlorocompounds L24.2
  - chromium (contact) (irritant) L24.81
  - coffee (ingested) L27.2
  - cold weather L30.8
  - cosmetics (contact) L25.0
    - allergic L23.2
    - irritant L24.3
  - cyclohexanes L24.2
  - dander (cat) (dog) L23.81
  - Demodex species B88.0
  - Dermanyssus gallinae B88.0
  - detergents (contact) (irritant) L24.0
  - dichromate L24.81
  - drugs and medicaments (generalized) (internal use) L27.0
    - external *—see* Dermatitis, due to, drugs, in contact with skin
    - in contact with skin L25.1
      - allergic L23.3
      - irritant L24.4
    - localized skin eruption L27.1
    - specified substance *—see* Table of Drugs and Chemicals
  - dyes (contact) L25.2
    - allergic L23.4
    - irritant L24.89
  - epidermophytosis *—see* Dermatophytosis
  - esters L24.2
  - external irritant NEC L24.9
  - fish (ingested) L27.2
  - flour (ingested) L27.2
  - food (ingested) L27.2
    - in contact with skin L25.4
  - fruit (ingested) L27.2
  - furs (allergic) (contact) L23.81
  - glues *—see* Dermatitis, due to, adhesives
  - glycols L24.2
  - greases NEC (contact) (irritant) L24.1
  - hair (cat) (dog) L23.81
  - hot
    - objects and materials *—see* Burn
    - weather or places L59.0
  - hydrocarbons L24.2
  - infrared rays L59.8
  - ingestion, ingested substance L27.9
    - chemical NEC L27.8
    - drugs and medicaments *—see* Dermatitis, due to, drugs
    - food L27.2
    - specified NEC L27.8
  - insecticide in contact with skin L24.5
  - internal agent L27.9
    - drugs and medicaments (generalized) *—see* Dermatitis, due to, drugs
    - food L27.2
  - irradiation *—see* Dermatitis, due to, radioactive substance
  - ketones L24.2
  - lacquer tree (allergic) (contact) L23.7
  - light (sun) NEC L57.8
    - acute L56.8
    - other L59.8
  - Liponyssoides sanguineus B88.0

Dermatitis *(continued)*
- due to *(continued)*
  - low temperature L30.8
  - meat (ingested) L27.2
  - metals, metal salts (contact) (irritant) L24.81
  - milk (ingested) L27.2
  - nickel (contact) (irritant) L24.81
  - nylon (contact) (irritant) L24.5
  - oils NEC (contact) (irritant) L24.1
  - paint solvent (contact) (irritant) L24.2
  - petroleum products (contact) (irritant) (substances in T52.0) L24.2
  - plants NEC (contact) L25.5
    - allergic L23.7
    - irritant L24.7
  - plasters (adhesive) (any) (allergic) (contact) L23.1
    - irritant L24.5
  - plastic (contact) L25.3
  - preservatives (contact) *—see* Dermatitis, due to, chemical, in contact with skin
  - primrose (allergic) (contact) L23.7
  - primula (allergic) (contact) L23.7
  - radiation L59.8
    - nonionizing (chronic exposure) L57.8
    - sun NEC L57.8
      - acute L56.8
  - radioactive substance L58.9
    - acute L58.0
    - chronic L58.1
  - radium L58.9
    - acute L58.0
    - chronic L58.1
  - ragweed (allergic) (contact) L23.7
  - Rhus (allergic) (contact) (diversiloba) (radicans) (toxicodendron) (venenata) (verniciflua) L23.7
  - rubber (contact) L24.5
  - Senecio jacobaea (allergic) (contact) L23.7
  - solvents (contact) (irritant) (substances in categories T52) L24.2
  - specified agent NEC (contact) L25.8
    - allergic L23.89
    - irritant L24.89
  - sunshine NEC L57.8
    - acute L56.8
  - tetrachlorethylene (contact) (irritant) L24.2
  - toluene (contact) (irritant) L24.2
  - turpentine (contact) L24.2
  - ultraviolet rays (sun NEC) (chronic exposure) L57.8
    - acute L56.8
  - vaccine or vaccination L27.0
    - specified substance *—see* Table of Drugs and Chemicals
  - varicose veins *—see* Varix, leg, with, inflammation
  - X-rays L58.9
    - acute L58.0
    - chronic L58.1
- dyshydrotic L30.1
- dysmenorrheica N94.6
- escharotica *—see* Burn
- exfoliative, exfoliativa (generalized) L26
  - neonatorum L00

Dermatitis *(continued)*
- eyelid (*see also* Dermatosis, eyelid) H01.9
  - allergic H01.119
    - left H01.116
      - lower H01.115
      - upper H01.114
    - right H01.113
      - lower H01.112
      - upper H01.111
  - contact *—see* Dermatitis, eyelid, allergic
  - due to
    - Demodex species B88.0
    - herpes (zoster) B02.39
      - simplex B00.59
  - eczematous H01.139
    - left H01.136
      - lower H01.135
      - upper H01.134
    - right H01.133
      - lower H01.132
      - upper H01.131
  - specified NEC H01.8
- facta, factitia, factitial L98.1
  - psychogenic F54
- flexural NEC L20.82
- friction L30.4
- fungus B36.9
  - specified type NEC B36.8
- gangrenosa, gangrenous infantum L08.0
- harvest mite B88.0
- heat L59.0
- herpesviral, vesicular (ear) (lip) B00.1
- herpetiformis (bullous) (erythematous) (pustular) (vesicular) L13.0
  - juvenile L12.2
  - senile L12.0
- hiemalis L30.8
- hypostatic, hypostatica *—see* Varix, leg, with, inflammation
- infectious eczematoid L30.3
- infective L30.3
- irritant *—see* Dermatitis, contact, irritant
- Jacquet's (diaper dermatitis) L22
- Leptus B88.0
- lichenified NEC L28.0
- medicamentosa (generalized) (internal use) *—see* Dermatitis, due to drugs
- mite B88.0
- multiformis L13.0
  - juvenile L12.2
- napkin L22
- neurotica L13.0
- nummular L30.0
- papillaris capillitii L73.0
- pellagrous E52
- perioral L71.0
- photocontact L56.2
- polymorpha dolorosa L13.0
- pruriginosa L13.0
- pruritic NEC L30.8
- psychogenic F54
- purulent L08.0
- pustular
  - contagious B08.02
  - subcorneal L13.1
- pyococcal L08.0
- pyogenica L08.0
- repens L40.2
- Ritter's (exfoliativa) L00
- Schamberg's L81.7
- schistosome B65.3
- seasonal bullous L30.8
- seborrheic L21.9
  - infantile L21.1
  - specified NEC L21.8

Dermatitis *(continued)*
- sensitization NOS L23.9
- septic L08.0
- solare L57.8
- specified NEC L30.8
- stasis I87.2
  - with
    - varicose ulcer *—see* Varix, leg, with ulcer, with inflammation
    - Varicose veins *—see* Varix, leg, with, inflammation
  - due to postthrombotic syndrome *—see* Syndrome, postthrombotic
- suppurative L08.0
- traumatic NEC L30.4
- trophoneurotica L13.0
- ultraviolet (sun) (chronic exposure) L57.8
  - acute L56.8
- varicose *—see* Varix, leg, with, inflammation
- vegetans L10.1
- verrucosa B43.0
- vesicular, herpesviral B00.1

Dermatoarthritis, lipoid E78.81

Dermatochalasis, eyelid H02.839
- left H02.836
  - lower H02.835
  - upper H02.834
- right H02.833
  - lower H02.832
  - upper H02.831

Dermatofibroma (lenticulare) *—see* Neoplasm, skin, benign
- protuberans *—see* Neoplasm, skin, uncertain behavior

Dermatofibrosarcoma (pigmented) (protuberans) *—see* Neoplasm, skin, malignant

Dermatographia L50.3

Dermatolysis (exfoliativa) (congenital) Q82.8
- acquired L57.4
- eyelids *—see* Blepharochalasis
- palpebrarum *—see* Blepharochalasis
- senile L57.4

Dermatomegaly NEC Q82.8

Dermatomucosomyositis M33.10
- with
  - myopathy M33.12
  - respiratory involvement M33.11
  - specified organ involvement NEC M33.19

Dermatomycosis B36.9
- furfuracea B36.0
- specified type NEC B36.8

Dermatomyositis (acute) (chronic) *—see also* Dermatopolymyositis
- adult (*see also* Dematomyositis, specified NEC) M33.10
- in (due to) neoplastic disease (*see also* Neoplasm) D49.9 *[M36.0]*
- juvenile M33.00
  - with
    - myopathy M33.02
    - respiratory involvement M33.01
    - specified organ involvement NEC M33.09
  - without myopathy M33.03

Dermatomyositis *(continued)*
- specified NEC M33.10
  - with
    - myopathy M33.12
    - respiratory involvement M33.11
    - specified organ involvement NEC M33.19
  - without myopathy M33.13

Dermatoneuritis of children *—see* Poisoning, mercury

Dermatophilosis A48.8

Dermatophytid L30.2

Dermatophytide *—see* Dermatophytosis

Dermatophytosis (epidermophyton) (infection) (Microsporum) (tinea) (Trichophyton) B35.9
- beard B35.0
- body B35.4
- capitis B35.0
- corporis B35.4
- deep-seated B35.8
- disseminated B35.8
- foot B35.3
- granulomatous B35.8
- groin B35.6
- hand B35.2
- nail B35.1
- perianal (area) B35.6
- scalp B35.0
- specified NEC B35.8

Dermatopolymyositis M33.90
- with
  - myopathy M33.92
  - respiratory involvement M33.91
  - specified organ involvement NEC M33.99
- without myopathy M33.93
- in neoplastic disease (*see also* Neoplasm) D49.9 *[M36.0]*
- juvenile M33.00
  - with
    - myopathy M33.02
    - respiratory involvement M33.01
    - specified organ involvement NEC M33.09
- specified NEC M33.10
  - myopathy M33.12
  - respiratory involvement M33.11
  - specified organ involvement NEC M33.19

Dermatopolyneuritis *—see* Poisoning, mercury

Dermatorrhexis (*see also* Syndrome, Ehlers-Danlos) Q79.60
- acquired L57.4

Dermatosclerosis *—see also* Scleroderma
- localized L94.0

Dermatosis L98.9
- Andrews' L08.89
- Bowen's *—see* Neoplasm, skin, in situ
- bullous L13.9
  - specified NEC L13.8
- exfoliativa L26
- eyelid (noninfectious) (*see also* Dermatitis, eyelid) H01.9
  - discoid lupus erythematosus *—see* Lupus, erythematosus, eyelid
  - xeroderma *—see* Xeroderma, acquired, eyelid
- factitial L98.1
- febrile neutrophilic L98.2
- gonococcal A54.89

Dermatosis *(continued)*
- herpetiformis L13.0
  - juvenile L12.2
- linear IgA L13.8
- menstrual NEC L98.8
- neutrophilic, febrile L98.2
- occupational *—see* Dermatitis, contact
- papulosa nigra L82.1
- pigmentary L81.9
  - progressive L81.7
  - Schamberg's L81.7
- psychogenic F54
- purpuric, pigmented L81.7
- pustular, subcorneal L13.1
- transient acantholytic L11.1

Dermographia, dermographism L50.3

Dermoid (cyst) *—see also* Neoplasm, benign, by site
- with malignant transformation C56-
- due to radiation (nonionizing) L57.8

Dermopathy
- infiltrative with thyrotoxicosis *—see* Thyrotoxicosis
- nephrogenic fibrosing L90.8

Dermophytosis *—see* Dermatophytosis

Descemetocele H18.73-

Descemet's membrane *—see* condition

Descending *—see* condition

Descensus uteri *—see* Prolapse, uterus

Desert
- rheumatism B38.0
- sore *—see* Ulcer, skin

Desertion (newborn) *—see* Maltreatment

Desmoid (extra-abdominal) (tumor) *—see* Neoplasm, connective tissue, uncertain behavior
- abdominal D48.1

Despondency F32.A

Desquamation, skin R23.4

Destruction, destructive *—see also* Damage
- articular facet *—see also* Derangement, joint, specified type NEC
  - knee M23.8X-
  - vertebra *—see* Spondylosis
- bone *—see also* Disorder, bone, specified type NEC
  - syphilitic A52.77
- joint *—see also* Derangement, joint, specified type NEC
  - sacroiliac M53.3
- rectal sphincter K62.89
- septum (nasal) J34.89
- tuberculous NEC *—see* Tuberculosis
- tympanum, tympanic membrane (nontraumatic) *—see* Disorder, tympanic membrane, specified NEC
- vertebral disc *—see* Degeneration, intervertebral disc

Destructiveness *—see also* Disorder, conduct
- adjustment reaction *—see* Disorder, adjustment

Desultory labor O62.2

Detachment
- cartilage *—see* Sprain

Detachment *(continued)*
- cervix, annular N88.8
  - complicating delivery O71.3
- choroid (old) (postinfectional) (simple) (spontaneous) H31.40-
  - hemorrhagic H31.41-
  - serous H31.42-
- ligament *—see* Sprain
- meniscus (knee) *—see also* Derangement, knee, meniscus, specified NEC
  - current injury *—see* Tear, meniscus
  - due to old tear or injury *—see* Derangement, knee, meniscus, due to old tear
- retina (without retinal break) (serous) H33.2-
  - with retinal:
    - break H33.00-
      - giant H33.03-
      - multiple H33.02-
      - single H33.01-
    - dialysis H33.04-
  - pigment epithelium *—see* Degeneration, retina, separation of layers, pigment epithelium detachment
  - rhegmatogenous *—see* Detachment, retina, with retinal, break
  - specified NEC H33.8
  - total H33.05-
  - traction H33.4-
- vitreous (body) H43.81

Detergent asthma J69.8

Deterioration
- epileptic F06.8
- general physical R53.81
- heart, cardiac *—see* Degeneration, myocardial
- mental *—see* Psychosis
- myocardial, myocardium *—see* Degeneration, myocardial
- senile (simple) R54

Deuteranomaly (anomalous trichromat) H53.53

Deuteranopia (complete) (incomplete) H53.53

Development
- abnormal, bone Q79.9
- arrested R62.50
  - bone *—see* Arrest, development or growth, bone
  - child R62.50
  - due to malnutrition E45
- defective, congenital *—see also* Anomaly, by site
  - cauda equina Q06.3
  - left ventricle Q24.8
    - in hypoplastic left heart syndrome Q23.4
  - valve Q24.8
    - pulmonary Q22.3
- delayed *—see also* Delay, development R62.50
  - arithmetical skills F81.2
  - language (skills) (expressive) F80.1
  - learning skill F81.9
  - mixed skills F88
  - motor coordination F82
  - reading F81.0
  - specified learning skill NEC F81.89
  - speech F80.9
  - spelling F81.81
  - written expression F81.81

Development *(continued)*
- imperfect, congenital *—see also* Anomaly, by site
  - heart Q24.9
  - lungs Q33.6
- incomplete
  - bronchial tree Q32.4
  - organ or site not listed *—see* Hypoplasia, by site
  - respiratory system Q34.9
- sexual, precocious NEC E30.1
- tardy, mental (*see also* Disability, intellectual) F79

Developmental *—see* condition
- testing, infant or child *—see* Examination, child

Devergie's disease (pityriasis rubra pilaris) L44.0

Deviation (in)
- conjugate palsy (eye) (spastic) H51.0
- esophagus (acquired) K22.89
- eye, skew H51.8
- midline (jaw) (teeth) (dental arch) M26.29
  - specified site NEC *—see* Malposition
- nasal septum J34.2
  - congenital Q67.4
- opening and closing of the mandible M26.53
- organ or site, congenital NEC *—see* Malposition, congenital
- septum (nasal) (acquired) J34.2
  - congenital Q67.4
- sexual F65.9
  - bestiality F65.89
  - erotomania F52.8
  - exhibitionism F65.2
  - fetishism, fetishistic F65.0
    - transvestism F65.1
  - frotteurism F65.81
  - masochism F65.51
  - multiple F65.89
  - necrophilia F65.89
  - nymphomania F52.8
  - pederosis F65.4
  - pedophilia F65.4
  - sadism, sadomasochism F65.52
  - satyriasis F52.8
  - specified type NEC F65.89
  - transvestism F64.1
  - voyeurism F65.3
- teeth, midline M26.29
- trachea J39.8
- ureter, congenital Q62.61

Device
- cerebral ventricle (communicating) in situ Z98.2
- contraceptive *—see* Contraceptive, device
- drainage, cerebrospinal fluid, in situ Z98.2

Devic's disease G36.0

Devil's
- grip B33.0
- pinches (purpura simplex) D69.2

Devitalized tooth K04.99

Devonshire colic *—see* Poisoning, lead

Dextraposition, aorta Q20.3
- in tetralogy of Fallot Q21.3

Dextrinosis, limit (debrancher enzyme deficiency) E74.03

Dextrocardia (true) Q24.0
- with
  - complete transposition of viscera Q89.3
  - situs inversus Q89.3

Dextrotransposition, aorta Q20.3
d-glycericacidemia E72.59
Dhat syndrome F48.8
Dhobi itch B35.6
Di George's syndrome D82.1
Di Guglielmo's disease C94.0-
Diabetes, diabetic (mellitus) (sugar) E11.9
with
amyotrophy E11.44
arthropathy NEC E11.618
autonomic (poly)neuropathy E11.43
cataract E11.36
Charcot's joints E11.610
chronic kidney disease E11.22
circulatory complication NEC E11.59
coma due to
hyperosmolarity E11.01
hypoglycemia E11.641
ketoacidosis E11.11
complication E11.8
specified NEC E11.69
dermatitis E11.620
foot ulcer E11.621
gangrene E11.52
gastroparalysis E11.43
gastroparesis E11.43
glomerulonephrosis, intracapillary E11.21
glomerulosclerosis, intercapillary E11.21
hyperglycemia E11.65
hyperosmolarity E11.00
with coma E11.01
hypoglycemia E11.649
with coma E11.641
ketoacidosis E11.10
with coma E11.11
kidney complications NEC E11.29
Kimmelsteil-Wilson disease E11.21
loss of protective sensation (LOPS) —*see* Diabetes, by type, with neuropathy
mononeuropathy E11.41
myasthenia E11.44
necrobiosis lipoidica E11.620
nephropathy E11.21
neuralgia E11.42
neurologic complication NEC E11.49
neuropathic arthropathy E11.610
neuropathy E11.40
ophthalmic complication NEC E11.39
oral complication NEC E11.638
osteomyelitis E11.69
periodontal disease E11.630
peripheral angiopathy E11.51
with gangrene E11.52
polyneuropathy E11.42
renal complication NEC E11.29
renal tubular degeneration E11.29
retinopathy E11.319
with macular edema E11.311
resolved following treatment E11.37
nonproliferative E11.329
with macular edema E11.321
mild E11.329
with macular edema E11.321
moderate E11.339
with macular edema E11.331

Diabetes, diabetic *(continued)*
with *(continued)*
retinopathy *(continued)*
nonproliferative *(continued)*
severe E11.349
with macular edema E11.341
with
combined traction retinal detachment and rhegmatogenous retinal detachment E11.354
macular edema E11.351
stable proliferative diabetic retinopathy E11.355
traction retinal detachment involving the macula E11.352
traction retinal detachment no involving the macula E11.353
proliferative E11.359
with
combined traction retinal detachment and rhegmatogenous retinal detachment E11.354
macular edema E11.351
stable proliferative diabetic retinopathy E11.355
traction retinal detachment involving the macula E11.352
traction retinal detachement not involving the macula E11.353
skin complication NEC E11.628
skin ulcer NEC E11.622
brittle —*see* Diabetes, type 1
bronzed E83.110
complicating pregnancy —*see* Pregnancy, complicated by, diabetes
dietary counseling and surveillance Z71.3
due to
autoimmune process —*see* Diabetes, type 1
immune mediated pancreatic islet beta-cell destruction —*see* Diabetes, type 1
due to drug or chemical E09.9
with
amyotrophy E09.44
arthropathy NEC E09.618
autonomic (poly)neuropathy E09.43
cataract E09.36
Charcot's joints E09.610
chronic kidney disease E09.22
circulatory complication NEC E09.59
complication E09.8
specified NEC E09.69
dermatitis E09.620
foot ulcer E09.621
gangrene E09.52
gastroparalysis E09.43
gastroparesis E09.43
glomerulonephrosis, intracapillary E09.21
glomerulosclerosis, intercapillary E09.21
hyperglycemia E09.65
hyperosmolarity E09.00
with coma E09.01

Diabetes, diabetic *(continued)*
due to drug or chemical *(continued)*
with *(continued)*
hypoglycemia E09.649
with coma E09.641
ketoacidosis E09.10
with coma E09.11
kidney complications NEC E09.29
Kimmelsteil-Wilson disease E09.21
mononeuropathy E09.41
myasthenia E09.44
necrobiosis lipoidica E09.620
nephropathy E09.21
neuralgia E09.42
neurologic complication NEC E09.49
neuropathic arthropathy E09.610
neuropathy E09.40
ophthalmic complication NEC E09.39
oral complication NEC E09.638
periodontal disease E09.630
peripheral angiopathy E09.51
with gangrene E09.52
polyneuropathy E09.42
renal complication NEC E09.29
renal tubular degeneration E09.29
retinopathy E09.319
with macular edema E09.311
resolved following treatment E09.37
nonproliferative E09.329
with macular edema E09.321
mild E09.329
with macular edema E09.321
moderate E09.339
with macular edema E09.331
severe E09.349
with macular edema E09.341
proliferative E09.359
with
combined traction retinal detachment and rhegmatogenous retinal detachment E09.354
macular edema E09.351
stable proliferative diabetic retinopathy E09.355
traction retinal detachment involving the macula E09.352
traction retinal detachment not involving the macula E09.353
skin complication NEC E09.628
skin ulcer NEC E09.622
due to underlying condition E08.9
with
amyotrophy E08.44
arthropathy NEC E08.618

Diabetes, diabetic *(continued)*
due to underlying condition *(continued)*
with *(continued)*
autonomic (poly)neuropathy E08.43
cataract E08.36
Charcot's joints E08.610
chronic kidney disease E08.22
circulatory complication NEC E08.59
complication E08.8
specified NEC E08.69
dermatitis E08.620
foot ulcer E08.621
gangrene E08.52
gastroparalysis E08.43
gastroparesis E08.43
glomerulonephrosis, intracapillary E08.21
glomerulosclerosis, intercapillary E08.21
hyperglycemia E08.65
hyperosmolarity E08.00
with coma E08.01
hypoglycemia E08.649
with coma E08.641
ketoacidosis E08.10
with coma E08.11
kidney complications NEC E08.29
Kimmelsteil-WIlson disease E08.21
mononeuropathy E08.41
myasthenia E08.44
necrobiosis lipoidica E08.620
nephropathy E08.21
neuralgia E08.42
neurologic complication NEC E08.49
neuropathic arthropathy E08.610
neuropathy E08.40
ophthalmic complication NEC E08.39
oral complication NEC E08.638
periodontal disease E08.630
peripheral angiopathy E08.51
with gangrene E08.52
polyneuropathy E08.42
renal complication NEC E08.29
renal tubular degeneration E08.29
retinopathy E08.319
with macular edema E08.311
resolved following treatment E08.37
nonproliferative E08.329
with macular edema E08.321
mild E08.329
with macular edema E08.321
moderate E08.339
with macular edema E08.331
severe E08.349
with macular edema E08.341
proliferative E08.359
with
combined traction retinal detachment and rhegmatogenous retinal detachment E08.354
macular edema E08.351

Diabetes, diabetic *(continued)*
due to underlying condition *(continued)*
with *(continued)*
retinopathy *(continued)*
proliferative *(continued)*
with *(continued)*
stable proliferative diabetic retinopathy E08.355
traction retinal detachment involving the macula E08.352
traction retinal detachment not involving the macula E08.353
skin complication NEC E08.628
skin ulcer NEC E08.622
gestational (in pregnancy) O24.419
affecting newborn P70.0
diet controlled O24.410
in childbirth O24.429
diet controlled O24.420
insulin (and diet) controlled O24.424
oral drug controlled (antidiabetic) (hypoglycemic) O24.425
oral drug controlled (antidiabetic) (hypoglycemic) O24.415
insulin (and diet) controlled O24.414
puerperal O24.439
diet controlled O24.430
insulin (and diet) controlled O24.434
oral drug controlled (antidiabetic) (hypoglycemic) O24.435
hepatogenous E13.9
idiopathic *—see* Diabetes, type 1
inadequately controlled - code to Diabetes, by type, with hyperglycemia
insipidus E23.2
nephrogenic N25.1
pituitary E23.2
vasopressin resistant N25.1
insulin dependent - code to type of diabetes
juvenile-onset *—see* Diabetes, type 1
ketosis-prone *—see* Diabetes, type 1
latent R73.03
neonatal (transient) P70.2
non-insulin dependent - code to type of diabetes
out of control - code to Diabetes, by type, with hyperglycemia
phosphate E83.39
poorly controlled - code to Diabetes, by type, with hyperglycemia
postpancreatectomy *—see* Diabetes, specified type NEC
postprocedural *—see* Diabetes, specified type NEC
secondary diabetes mellitus NEC *—see* Diabetes, specified type NEC
specified type NEC E13.9
with
amyotrophy E13.44
arthropathy NEC E13.618
autonomic (poly)neuropathy E13.43
cataract E13.36
Charcot's joints E13.610

Diabetes, diabetic *(continued)*
specified type *(continued)*
with *(continued)*
chronic kidney disease E13.22
circulatory complication NEC E13.59
complication E13.8
specified NEC E13.69
dermatitis E13.620
foot ulcer E13.621
gangrene E13.52
gastroparalysis E13.43
gastroparesis E13.43
glomerulonephrosis, intracapillary E13.21
glomerulosclerosis, intercapillary E13.21
hyperglycemia E13.65
hyperosmolarity E13.00
with coma E13.01
hypoglycemia E13.649
with coma E13.641
ketoacidosis E13.10
with coma E13.11
kidney complications NEC E13.29
Kimmelsteil-Wilson disease E13.21
mononeuropathy E13.41
myasthenia E13.44
necrobiosis lipoidica E13.620
nephropathy E13.21
neuralgia E13.42
neurologic complication NEC E13.49
neuropathic arthropathy E13.610
neuropathy E13.40
ophthalmic complication NEC E13.39
oral complication NEC E13.638
periodontal disease E13.630
peripheral angiopathy E13.51
with gangrene E13.52
polyneuropathy E13.42
renal complication NEC E13.29
renal tubular degeneration E13.29
retinopathy E13.319
with macular edema E13.311
resolved following treatment E13.37
nonproliferative E13.329
with macular edema E13.321
mild E13.329
with macular edema E13.321
moderate E13.339
with macular edema E13.331
severe E13.349
with macular edema E13.341
proliferative E13.359
with
combined traction retinal detachment and rhegmatogenous retinal detachment E13.354
macular edema E13.351
stable proliferative diabetic retinopathy E13.355

Diabetes, diabetic *(continued)*
specified type *(continued)*
with *(continued)*
retinopathy *(continued)*
proliferative *(continued)*
with *(continued)*
traction retinal detachment involving the macula E13.352
traction retinal detachment not involving the macula E13.353
skin complication NEC E13.628
skin ulcer NEC E13.622
steroid-induced *—see* Diabetes, due to, drug or chemical
type 1 E10.9
with
amyotrophy E10.44
arthropathy NEC E10.618
autonomic (poly)neuropathy E10.43
cataract E10.36
Charcot's joints E10.610
chronic kidney disease E10.22
circulatory complication NEC E10.59
coma due to
hypoglycemia E10.641
ketoacidosis E10.11
complication E10.8
specified NEC E10.69
dermatitis E10.620
foot ulcer E10.621
gangrene E10.52
gastroparalysis E10.43
gastroparesis E10.43
glomerulonephrosis, intracapillary E10.21
glomerulosclerosis, intercapillary E10.21
hyperglycemia E10.65
hypoglycemia E10.649
with coma E10.641
ketoacidosis E10.10
with coma E10.11
kidney complications NEC E10.29
Kimmelsteil-Wilson disease E10.21
mononeuropathy E10.41
myasthenia E10.44
necrobiosis lipoidica E10.620
nephropathy E10.21
neuralgia E10.42
neurologic complication NEC E10.49
neuropathic arthropathy E10.610
neuropathy E10.40
ophthalmic complication NEC E10.39
oral complication NEC E10.638
osteomyelitis E10.69
periodontal disease E10.630
peripheral angiopathy E10.51
with gangrene E10.52
polyneuropathy E10.42
renal complication NEC E10.29
renal tubular degeneration E10.29
retinopathy E10.319
with macular edema E10.311
resolved following treatment E10.37

Diabetes, diabetic *(continued)*
type 1 *(continued)*
with *(continued)*
retinopathy *(continued)*
nonproliferative E10.329
with macular edema E10.321
mild E10.329
with macular edema E10.321
moderate E10.339
with macular edema E10.331
severe E10.349
with macular edema E10.341
proliferative E10.359
with
combined traction retinal detachment and rhegmatogenous retinal detachment E10.354
with
macular edema E10.351
stable proliferative diabetic retinopathy E10.355
traction retinal detachment involving the macula E10.352
traction retinal detachment not involving the macula E10.353
skin complication NEC E10.628
skin ulcer NEC E10.622
type 2 E11.9
with
amyotrophy E11.44
arthropathy NEC E11.618
autonomic (poly)neuropathy E11.43
cataract E11.36
Charcot's joints E11.610
chronic kidney disease E11.22
circulatory complication NEC E11.59
coma due to
hyperosmolarity E11.01
hypoglycemia E11.641
ketoacidosis E11.11
complication E11.8
specified NEC E11.69
dermatitis E11.620
foot ulcer E11.621
gangrene E11.52
gastroparalysis E11.43
gastroparesis E11.43
glomerulonephrosis, intracapillary E11.21
glomerulosclerosis, intercapillary E11.21
hyperglycemia E11.65
hyperosmolarity E11.00
with coma E11.01
hypoglycemia E11.649
with coma E11.641
ketoacidosis E11.10
with coma E11.11
kidney complications NEC E11.29
Kimmelsteil-Wilson disease E11.21
mononeuropathy E11.41
myasthenia E11.44

Diabetes, diabetic *(continued)*
- type 2 *(continued)*
  - with *(continued)*
    - necrobiosis lipoidica E11.620
    - nephropathy E11.21
    - neuralgia E11.42
    - neurologic complication NEC E11.49
    - neuropathic arthropathy E11.610
    - neuropathy E11.40
    - ophthalmic complication NEC E11.39
    - oral complication NEC E11.638
    - osteomyelitis E11.69
    - periodontal disease E11.630
    - peripheral angiopathy E11.51
      - with gangrene E11.52
    - polyneuropathy E11.42
    - renal complication NEC E11.29
    - renal tubular degeneration E11.29
    - retinopathy E11.319
      - with macular edema E11.311
      - resolved following treatment E11.37
      - nonproliferative E11.329
        - with macular edema E11.321
        - mild E11.329
          - with macular edema E11.321
        - moderate E11.339
          - with macular edema E11.331
        - severe E11.349
          - with macular edema E11.341
      - proliferative E11.359
        - with
          - combined traction retinal detachment and rhegmatogenous retinal detachment E11.354
          - macular edema E11.351
          - stable proliferative diabetic retinopathy E11.355
          - traction retinal detachment involving the macula E11.352
          - traction retinal detachment not involving the macula E11.353
    - skin complication NEC E11.628
    - skin ulcer NEC E11.622
- uncontrolled
- meaning
- hyperglycemia *—see* Diabetes, by type, with, hyperglycemia
- hypoglycemia *—see* Diabetes, by type, with, hypoglycemia

Diacyclothrombopathia D69.1

Diagnosis deferred R69

Dialysis (intermittent) (treatment)
- noncompliance (with) Z91.15
- renal (hemodialysis) (peritoneal), status Z99.2
- retina, retinal *—see* Detachment, retina, with retinal, dialysis

Diamond-Blackfan anemia (congenital hypoplastic) D61.01

Diamond-Gardener syndrome (autoerythrocyte sensitization) D69.2

Diaper rash L22

Diaphoresis (excessive) R61

Diaphragm *—see* condition

Diaphragmalgia R07.1

Diaphragmatitis, diaphragmitis J98.6

Diaphysial aclasis Q78.6

Diaphysitis *—see* Osteomyelitis, specified type NEC

Diarrhea, diarrheal (disease) (infantile) (inflammatory) R19.7
- achlorhydric K31.83
- allergic K52.29
  - due to
    - colitis *—see* Colitis, allergic
    - enteritis *—see* Enteritis, allergic
- amebic (*see also* Amebiasis) A06.0
  - with abscess *—see* Abscess, amebic
  - acute A06.0
  - chronic A06.1
  - nondysenteric A06.2
- bacillary *—see* Dysentery, bacillary
- balantidial A07.0
- cachectic NEC K52.89
- Chilomastix A07.8
- choleriformis A00.1
- chronic (noninfectious) K52.9
- coccidial A07.3
- Cochin-China K90.1
  - strongyloidiasis B78.0
- Dientamoeba A07.8
- dietetic (*see also* Diarrhea, allergic) K52.29
- drug-induced K52.1
- due to
  - bacteria A04.9
    - specified NEC A04.8
  - Campylobacter A04.5
  - Capillaria philippinensis B81.1
  - Clostridium difficile
    - not specified as recurrent A04.72
    - recurrent A04.71
  - Clostridium perfringens (C) (F) A04.8
  - Cryptosporidium A07.2
  - drugs K52.1
  - Escherichia coli A04.4
    - enteroaggregative A04.4
    - enterohemorrhagic A04.3
    - enteroinvasive A04.2
    - enteropathogenic A04.0
    - enterotoxigenic A04.1
    - specified NEC A04.4
  - food hypersensitivity (*see also* Diarrhea, allergic) K52.29
  - Necator americanus B76.1
  - S. japonicum B65.2
  - specified organism NEC A08.8
    - bacterial A04.8
    - viral A08.39
  - Staphylococcus A04.8
  - Trichuris trichiuria B79
  - virus *—see* Enteritis, viral
  - Yersinia enterocolitica A04.6
- dysenteric A09
- endemic A09
- epidemic A09
- flagellate A07.9
- Flexner's (ulcerative) A03.1
- functional K59.1
  - following gastrointestinal surgery K91.89
  - psychogenic F45.8

Diarrhea, diarrheal *(continued)*
- Giardia lamblia A07.1
- giardial A07.1
- hill K90.1
- infectious A09
- malarial *—see* Malaria
- mite B88.0
- mycotic NEC B49
- neonatal (noninfectious) P78.3
- nervous F45.8
- neurogenic K59.1
- noninfectious K52.9
- postgastrectomy K91.1
- postvagotomy K91.1
- protozoal A07.9
  - specified NEC A07.8
- psychogenic F45.8
- specified
  - bacterium NEC A04.8
  - virus NEC A08.39
- strongyloidiasis B78.0
- toxic K52.1
- trichomonal A07.8
- tropical K90.1
- tuberculous A18.32
- viral *—see* Enteritis, viral

Diastasis
- cranial bones M84.88
  - congenital NEC Q75.8
- joint (traumatic) *—see* Dislocation
- muscle M62.00
  - ankle M62.07-
  - congenital Q79.8
  - foot M62.07-
  - forearm M62.03-
  - hand M62.04-
  - lower leg M62.06-
  - pelvic region M62.05-
  - shoulder region M62.01-
  - specified site NEC M62.08
  - thigh M62.05-
  - upper arm M62.02-
- recti (abdomen)
  - complicating delivery O71.89
  - congenital Q79.59

Diastema, tooth, teeth, fully erupted M26.32

Diastematomyelia Q06.2

Diataxia, cerebral G80.4

Diathesis
- allergic *—see* History, allergy
- bleeding (familial) D69.9
- cystine (familial) E72.00
- gouty *—see* Gout
- hemorrhagic (familial) D69.9
  - newborn NEC P53
- spasmophilic R29.0

Diaz's disease or osteochondrosis (juvenile) (talus) *—see* Osteochondrosis, juvenile, tarsus

Dibothriocephalus, dibothriocephaliasis (latus) (infection) (infestation) B70.0
- larval B70.1

Dicephalus, dicephaly Q89.4

Dichotomy, teeth K00.2

Dichromat, dichromatopsia (congenital) *—see* Deficiency, color vision

Dichuchwa A65

Dicroceliasis B66.2

Didelphia, didelphys *—see* Double uterus

Didymytis N45.1
- with orchitis N45.3

Dietary
- inadequacy or deficiency E63.9
- surveillance and counseling Z71.3

Dietl's crisis N13.8

Dieulafoy lesion (hemorrhagic)
- duodenum K31.82
- esophagus K22.89
- intestine (colon) K63.81
- stomach K31.82

Difficult, difficulty (in)
- acculturation Z60.3
- feeding R63.30
  - newborn P92.9
    - breast P92.5
    - specified NEC P92.8
  - nonorganic (infant or child) F98.29
  - specified NEC R63.39
- intubation, in anesthesia T88.4
- mechanical, gastroduodenal stoma K91.89
  - causing obstruction (*see also* Obstruction, intestine, postoperative) K91.30
- micturition
  - need to immediately re-void R39.191
  - position dependent R39.192
  - specified NEC R39.198
- reading (developmental) F81.0
  - secondary to emotional disorders F93.9
- spelling (specific) F81.81
  - with reading disorder F81.89
  - due to inadequate teaching Z55.8
- swallowing *—see* Dysphagia
- walking R26.2
- work
  - conditions NEC Z56.5
  - schedule Z56.3

Diffuse *—see* condition

DiGeorge's syndrome (thymic hypoplasia) D82.1

Digestive *—see* condition

Dihydropyrimidine dehydrogenase disease (DPD) E88.89

Diktyoma *—see* Neoplasm, malignant, by site

Dilaceration, tooth K00.4

Dilatation
- anus K59.89
  - venule *—see* Hemorrhoids
- aorta (focal) (general) *—see* Ectasia, aorta
  - with aneuysm *—see* Aneurysm, aorta
  - congenital Q25.44
- artery *—see* Aneurysm
- bladder (sphincter) N32.89
  - congenital Q64.79
- blood vessel I99.8
- bronchial J47.9
  - with
    - exacerbation (acute) J47.1
    - lower respiratory infection J47.0
- calyx N28.89
  - due to obstruction *—see* Hydronephrosis
- capillaries I78.8
- cardiac (acute) (chronic) *—see also* Hypertrophy, cardiac
  - congenital Q24.8
    - valve NEC Q24.8
      - pulmonary Q22.3
  - valve *—see* Endocarditis

Dilatation *(continued)*
- cavum septi pellucidi Q06.8
- cervix (uteri) *—see also* Incompetency, cervix
  - incomplete, poor, slow
    - complicating delivery O62.0
- colon K59.39
  - congenital Q43.1
  - psychogenic F45.8
  - toxic K59.31
- common duct (acquired) K83.8
  - congenital Q44.5
- cystic duct (acquired) K82.8
  - congenital Q44.5
- duct, mammary *—see* Ectasia, mammary duct
- duodenum K59.89
- esophagus K22.89
  - congenital Q39.5
  - due to achalasia K22.0
- eustachian tube, congenital Q17.8
- gallbladder K82.8
- gastric *—see* Dilatation, stomach
- heart (acute) (chronic) *—see also* Hypertrophy, cardiac
  - congenital Q24.8
  - valve *—see* Endocarditis
- ileum K59.89
  - psychogenic F45.8
- jejunum K59.89
  - psychogenic F45.8
- kidney (calyx) (collecting structures) (cystic) (parenchyma) (pelvis) (idiopathic) N28.89
  - due to obstruction *—see* Hydronephrosis
- lacrimal passages or duct *—see* Disorder, lacrimal system, changes
- lymphatic vessel I89.0
- mammary duct *—see* Ectasia, mammary duct
- Meckel's diverticulum (congenital) Q43.0
  - malignant *—see* Table of Neoplasms, small intestine, malignant
- myocardium (acute) (chronic) *—see* Hypertrophy, cardiac
- organ or site, congenital NEC *—see* Distortion
- pancreatic duct K86.89
- pericardium *—see* Pericarditis
- pharynx J39.2
- prostate N42.89
- pulmonary
  - artery (idiopathic) I28.8
  - valve, congenital Q22.3
- pupil H57.04
- rectum K59.39
- saccule, congenital Q16.5
- salivary gland (duct) K11.8
- sphincter ani K62.89
- stomach K31.89
  - acute K31.0
  - psychogenic F45.8
- submaxillary duct K11.8
- trachea, congenital Q32.1
- ureter (idiopathic) N28.82
  - congenital Q62.2
  - due to obstruction N13.4
- urethra (acquired) N36.8
- vasomotor I73.9
- vein I86.8
- ventricular, ventricle (acute) (chronic) *—see also* Hypertrophy, cardiac
  - cerebral, congenital Q04.8
- venule NEC I86.8
- vesical orifice N32.89

Dilated, dilation *—see* Dilatation

Diminished, diminution
- hearing (acuity) *—see* Deafness
- sense or sensation (cold) (heat) (tactile) (vibratory) R20.8
- vision NEC H54.7
- vital capacity R94.2

Diminuta taenia B71.0

Dimitri-Sturge-Weber disease Q85.8

Dimple
- congenital sacral Q82.6
- parasacral Q82.6
- pilonidal or postanal *—see* Cyst, pilonidal

Dioctophyme renalis (infection) (infestation) B83.8

Dipetalonemiasis B74.4

Diphallus Q55.69

Diphtheria, diphtheritic (gangrenous) (hemorrhagic) A36.9
- carrier (suspected) Z22.2
- cutaneous A36.3
- faucial A36.0
- infection of wound A36.3
- laryngeal A36.2
- myocarditis A36.81
- nasal, anterior A36.89
- nasopharyngeal A36.1
- neurological complication A36.89
- pharyngeal A36.0
- specified site NEC A36.89
- tonsillar A36.0

Diphyllobothriasis (intestine) B70.0
- larval B70.1

Diplacusis H93.22-

Diplegia (upper limbs) G83.0
- congenital (cerebral) G80.8
- facial G51.0
- lower limbs G82.20
- spastic G80.1

Diplococcus, diplococcal *—see* condition

Diplopia H53.2

Dipsomania F10.20
- with
  - psychosis *—see* Psychosis, alcoholic
  - remission F10.21

Dipylidiasis B71.1

DIRA (deficiency of interleukin 1 receptor antagonist) M04.8

Direction, teeth, abnormal, fully erupted M26.30

Dirofilariasis B74.8

Dirt-eating child F98.3

Disability, disabilities
- heart *—see* Disease, heart
- intellectual F79
  - with
    - autistic features F84.9
    - pathogenic CHAMP1 (genetic) (variant) F78.A9
    - pathogenic HNRNPH2 (genetic) (variant) F78.A9
    - pathogenic SATB2 (genetic) (variant) F78.A9
    - pathogenic SETBP1 (genetic) (variant) F78.A9
    - pathogenic STXBP1 (genetic) (variant) F78.A9
    - pathogenic SYNGAP1 (genetic) (variant) F78.A1
  - autosomal dominant F78.A9

Disability, disabilities *(continued)*
- intellectual *(continued)*
  - autosomal recessive F78.A9
  - genetic related F78.A9
    - with
      - pathogenic CHAMP1 (variant) F78.A9
      - pathogenic HNRNPH2 (variant) F78.A9
      - pathogenic SATB2 (variant) F78.A9
      - pathogenic SETBP1 (variant) F78.A9
      - pathogenic STXBP1 (variant) F78.A9
      - pathogenic SYNGAP1 (variant) F78.A1
      - specified NEC F78.A9
      - SYNGAP1-related F78.A1
    - in
      - autosomal dominant mental retardation F78.A9
      - autosomal recessive mental retardation F78.A9
      - SATB2-associated syndrome F78.A9
      - SETBP1 disorder F78.A9
      - STXBP1 encephalopathy with epilepsy (*see also* Encephalopathy; and *see also* Epilepsy) F78.A9
      - X-linked mental retardation (syndromic) (Bain type) F78.A9
  - mild (I.Q.50-69) F70
  - moderate (I.Q.35-49) F71
  - profound (I.Q. under 20) F73
  - severe (I.Q.20-34) F72
  - specified level NEC F78.A9
  - SYNGAP1-related F78.A1
  - X-linked (syndromic) (Bain type) F78.A9
- knowledge acquisition F81.9
- learning F81.9
- limiting activities Z73.6
- spelling, specific F81.81

Disappearance of family member Z63.4

Disarticulation *—see* Amputation
- meaning traumatic amputation *—see* Amputation, traumatic

Discharge (from)
- abnormal finding in *—see* Abnormal, specimen
- breast (female) (male) N64.52
- diencephalic autonomic idiopathic *—see* Epilepsy, specified NEC
- ear *—see also* Otorrhea
  - blood *—see* Otorrhagia
- excessive urine R35.89
- nipple N64.52
- penile R36.9
- postnasal R09.82
- prison, anxiety concerning Z65.2
- urethral R36.9
  - without blood R36.0
  - hematospermia R36.1
- vaginal N89.8

Discitis, diskitis M46.40
- cervical region M46.42
- cervicothoracic region M46.43
- lumbar region M46.46
- lumbosacral region M46.47
- multiple sites M46.49
- occipito-atlanto-axial region M46.41

Discitis, diskitis *(continued)*
- pyogenic *—see* Infection, intervertebral disc, pyogenic
- sacrococcygeal region M46.48
- thoracic region M46.44
- thoracolumbar region M46.45

Discoid
- meniscus (congenital) Q68.6
- semilunar cartilage (congenital) *—see* Derangement, knee, meniscus, specified NEC

Discoloration
- nails L60.8
- teeth (posteruptive) K03.7
  - during formation K00.8

Discomfort
- chest R07.89
- visual H53.14-

Discontinuity, ossicles, ear H74.2-

Discord (with)
- boss Z56.4
- classmates Z55.4
- counselor Z64.4
- employer Z56.4
- family Z63.8
- fellow employees Z56.4
- in-laws Z63.1
- landlord Z59.2
- lodgers Z59.2
- neighbors Z59.2
- probation officer Z64.4
- social worker Z64.4
- teachers Z55.4
- workmates Z56.4

Discordant connection
- atrioventricular (congenital) Q20.5
- ventriculoarterial Q20.3

Discrepancy
- centric occlusion maximum intercuspation M26.55
- leg length (acquired) *—see* Deformity, limb, unequal length
  - congenital *—see* Defect, reduction, lower limb
- uterine size date O26.84-

Discrimination
- ethnic Z60.5
- political Z60.5
- racial Z60.5
- religious Z60.5
- sex Z60.5

Disease, diseased *—see also* Syndrome
- absorbent system I87.8
- acid-peptic K30
- Acosta's T70.29
- Adams-Stokes (-Morgagni) (syncope with heart block) I45.9
- Addison's anemia (pernicious) D51.0
- adenoids (and tonsils) J35.9
- adrenal (capsule) (cortex) (gland) (medullary) E27.9
  - hyperfunction E27.0
  - specified NEC E27.8
- ainhum L94.6
- airway
  - obstructive, chronic J44.9
    - due to
      - cotton dust J66.0
      - specific organic dusts NEC J66.8
  - reactive *—see* Asthma
- akamushi (scrub typhus) A75.3
- Albers-Schönberg (marble bones) Q78.2
- Albert's *—see* Tendinitis, Achilles

Disease, diseased *(continued)*
- alimentary canal K63.9
- alligator-skin Q80.9
  - acquired L85.0
- alpha heavy chain C88.3
- alpine T70.29
- altitude T70.20
- alveolar ridge
  - edentulous K06.9
    - specified NEC K06.8
- alveoli, teeth K08.9
- Alzheimer's G30.9 *[F02.80]*
  - with behavioral disturbance G30.9 *[F02.81]*
  - early onset G30.0 *[F02.80]*
    - with behavioral disturbance G30.0 *[F02.81]*
  - late onset G30.1 *[F02.80]*
    - with behavioral disturbance G30.1 *[F02.81]*
  - specified NEC G30.8 *[F02.80]*
    - with behavioral disturbance G30.8 *[F02.81]*
- amyloid —*see* Amyloidosis
- Andersen's (glycogenosis IV) E74.09
- Andes T70.29
- Andrews'(bacterid) L08.89
- angiospastic I73.9
  - cerebral G45.9
  - vein I87.8
- anterior
  - chamber H21.9
  - horn cell G12.29
- antiglomerular basement membrane (anti- GBM) antibody M31.0
  - tubulo-interstitial nephritis N12
- antral —*see* Sinusitis, maxillary
- anus K62.9
  - specified NEC K62.89
- aorta (nonsyphilitic) I77.9
  - syphilitic NEC A52.02
- aortic (heart) (valve) I35.9
  - rheumatic I06.9
- Apollo B30.3
- aponeuroses —*see* Enthesopathy
- appendix K38.9
  - specified NEC K38.8
- aqueous (chamber) H21.9
- Arnold-Chiari —*see* Arnold-Chiari disease
- arterial I77.9
  - occlusive —*see* Occlusion, by site
    - due to stricture or stenosis I77.1
  - peripheral I73.9
- arteriocardiorenal —*see* Hypertension, cardiorenal
- arteriolar (generalized) (obliterative) I77.9
- arteriorenal —*see* Hypertension, kidney
- arteriosclerotic —*see also* Arteriosclerosis
  - cardiovascular —*see* Disease, heart, ischemic, atherosclerotic
  - coronary (artery) —*see* Disease, heart, ischemic, atherosclerotic
  - heart —*see* Disease, heart, ischemic, atherosclerotic
- artery I77.9
  - cerebral I67.9
  - coronary I25.10
    - with angina pectoris —*see* Arteriosclerosis, coronary (artery)
  - peripheral I73.9

Disease, diseased *(continued)*
- arthropod-borne NOS (viral) A94
  - specified type NEC A93.8
- atticoantral, chronic H66.20
  - left H66.22
    - with right H66.23
  - right H66.21
    - with left H66.23
- auditory canal —*see* Disorder, ear, external
- auricle, ear NEC —*see* Disorder, pinna
- Australian X A83.4
- autoimmune (systemic) NOS M35.9
  - hemolytic D59.10
    - cold type (primary) (secondary) (symptomatic) D59.12
    - drug-induced D59.0
    - mixed type (primary) (secondary) (symptomatic) D59.13
    - warm type (primary) (secondary) (symptomatic) D59.11
  - thyroid E06.3
- autoinflammatory M04.9
  - NOD2-associated M04.8
  - specified type NEC M04.8
- aviator's —*see* Effect, adverse, high altitude
- Ayerza's (pulmonary artery sclerosis with pulmonary hypertension) I27.0
- Babington's (familial hemorrhagic telangiectasia) I78.0
- bacterial A49.9
  - specified NEC A48.8
  - zoonotic A28.9
    - specified type NEC A28.8
- Baelz's (cheilitis glandularis apostematosa) K13.0
- bagasse J67.1
- balloon —*see* Effect, adverse, high altitude
- Bang's (brucella abortus) A23.1
- Bannister's T78.3
- barometer makers' —*see* Poisoning, mercury
- Barraquer (-Simons') (progressive lipodystrophy) E88.1
- Barrett's —*see* Barrett's, esophagus
- Bartholin's gland N75.9
- basal ganglia G25.9
  - degenerative G23.9
    - specified NEC G23.8
  - specified NEC G25.89
- Basedow's (exophthalmic goiter) —*see* Hyperthyroidism, with, goiter (diffuse)
- Bateman's B08.1
- Batten-Steinert G71.11
- Battey A31.0
- Beard's (neurasthenia) F48.8
- Becker
  - idiopathic mural endomyocardial I42.3
  - myotonia congenita G71.12
- Begbie's (exophthalmic goiter) —*see* Hyperthyroidism, with, goiter (diffuse)
- behavioral, organic F07.9
- Beigel's (white piedra) B36.2
- Benson's —*see* Deposit, crystalline
- Bernard-Soulier (thrombopathy) D69.1
- Bernhardt (-Roth) —*see* Mononeuropathy, lower limb, meralgia paresthetica

Disease, diseased *(continued)*
- Biermer's (pernicious anemia) D51.0
- bile duct (common) (hepatic) K83.9
  - with calculus, stones —*see* Calculus, bile duct
  - specified NEC K83.8
- biliary (tract) K83.9
  - specified NEC K83.8
- Billroth's —*see* Spina bifida
- bird fancier's J67.2
- black lung J60
- bladder N32.9
  - in (due to)
    - schistosomiasis (bilharziasis) B65.0 *[N33]*
  - specified NEC N32.89
- bleeder's D66
- blood D75.9
  - forming organs D75.9
  - vessel I99.9
- Bloodgood's —*see* Mastopathy, cystic
- Blount M92.51-
- Bodechtel-Guttmann (subacute sclerosing panencephalitis) A81.1
- bone —*see also* Disorder, bone
  - aluminum M83.4
  - fibrocystic NEC
    - jaw M27.49
- bone-marrow D75.9
- Borna A83.9
- Bornholm (epidemic pleurodynia) B33.0
- Bouchard's (myopathic dilatation of the stomach) K31.0
- Bouillaud's (rheumatic heart disease) I01.9
- Bourneville (-Brissaud) (tuberous sclerosis) Q85.1
- Bouveret (-Hoffmann) (paroxysmal tachycardia) I47.9
- bowel K63.9
  - functional K59.9
    - psychogenic F45.8
- brain G93.9
  - arterial, artery I67.9
  - arteriosclerotic I67.2
  - congenital Q04.9
  - degenerative —*see* Degeneration, brain
  - inflammatory —*see* Encephalitis
  - organic G93.9
    - arteriosclerotic I67.2
  - parasitic NEC B71.9 *[G94]*
  - senile NEC G31.1
  - specified NEC G93.89
- breast —*see also* Disorder, breast N64.9
  - cystic (chronic) —*see* Mastopathy, cystic
  - fibrocystic —*see* Mastopathy, cystic
  - Paget's
    - female, unspecified side C50.91-
    - male, unspecified side C50.92-
  - specified NEC N64.89
- Breda's —*see* Yaws
- Bretonneau's (diphtheritic malignant angina) A36.0
- Bright's —*see* Nephritis
  - arteriosclerotic —*see* Hypertension, kidney
- Brill's (recrudescent typhus) A75.1

Disease, diseased *(continued)*
- Brill-Zinsser (recrudescent typhus) A75.1
- Brion-Kayser —*see* Fever, paratyphoid
- broad
  - beta E78.2
  - ligament (noninflammatory) N83.9
    - inflammatory —*see* Disease, pelvis, inflammatory
    - specified NEC N83.8
- Brocq-Duhring (dermatitis herpetiformis) L13.0
- Brocq's
  - meaning
    - dermatitis herpetiformis L13.0
    - prurigo L28.2
- bronchopulmonary J98.4
- bronchus NEC J98.09
- bronze Addison's E27.1
  - tuberculous A18.7
- budgerigar fancier's J67.2
- bullous L13.9
  - chronic of childhood L12.2
  - specified NEC L13.8
- Buerger's (thromboangiitis obliterans) I73.1
- Bürger-Grütz (essential familial hyperlipemia) E78.3
- bursa —*see* Bursopathy
- caisson T70.3
- California —*see* Coccidioidomycosis
- capillaries I78.9
  - specified NEC I78.8
- Carapata A68.0
- cardiac —*see* Disease, heart
- cardiopulmonary, chronic I27.9
- cardiorenal (hepatic) (hypertensive) (vascular) —*see* Hypertension, cardiorenal
- cardiovascular (atherosclerotic) I25.10
  - with angina pectoris —*see* Arteriosclerosis, coronary (artery),
  - congenital Q28.9
  - newborn P29.9
    - specified NEC P29.89
  - hypertensive —*see* Hypertension, heart
  - renal (hypertensive) —*see* Hypertension, cardiorenal
  - syphilitic (asymptomatic) A52.00
- cartilage —*see* Disorder, cartilage
- Castellani's A69.8
- Castleman (unicentric) (multicentric) D47.Z2
  - HHV-8-associated (*see also* Herpesvirus, human, 8) D47.Z2
- cat-scratch A28.1
- Cavare's (familial periodic paralysis) G72.3
- cecum K63.9
- celiac (adult) (infantile) (with steatorrhea) K90.0
- cellular tissue L98.9
- central core G71.29
- cerebellar, cerebellum —*see* Disease, brain
- cerebral —*see also* Disease, brain
  - degenerative —*see* Degeneration, brain
- cerebrospinal G96.9
- cerebrovascular I67.9
  - acute I67.89
    - embolic I63.4-
    - thrombotic I63.3-

Disease, diseased *(continued)*
- cerebrovascular *(continued)*
  - arteriosclerotic I67.2
  - hereditary NEC I67.858
  - specified NEC I67.89
- cervix (uteri) (noninflammatory) N88.9
  - inflammatory *—see* Cervicitis
  - specified NEC N88.8
- Chabert's A22.9
- Chandler's (osteochondritis dissecans, hip) *—see* Osteochondritis, dissecans, hip
- Charlouis *—see* Yaws
- Chédiak-Steinbrinck (-Higashi) (congenital gigantism of peroxidase granules) E70.330
- chest J98.9
- Chiari's (hepatic vein thrombosis) I82.0
- Chicago B40.9
- Chignon B36.8
- chigo, chigoe B88.1
- childhood granulomatous D71
- Chinese liver fluke B66.1
- chlamydial A74.9
  - specified NEC A74.89
- cholecystic K82.9
- choroid H31.9
  - specified NEC H31.8
- Christmas D67
- chronic bullous of childhood L12.2
- chylomicron retention E78.3
- ciliary body H21.9
  - specified NEC H21.89
- circulatory (system) NEC I99.8
  - newborn P29.9
  - syphilitic A52.00
    - congenital A50.54
- coagulation factor deficiency (congenital) *—see* Defect, coagulation
- coccidioidal *—see* Coccidioidomycosis
- cold
  - agglutinin or hemoglobinuria D59.12
    - paroxysmal D59.6
  - hemagglutinin (chronic) D59.12
- collagen NOS (nonvascular) (vascular) M35.9
  - specified NEC M35.89
- colon K63.9
  - functional K59.9
    - congenital Q43.2
  - ischemic (*see also* Ischemia, intestine, acute) K55.039
- colonic inflammatory bowel, unclassified (IBDU) K52.3
- combined system *—see* Degeneration, combined
- compressed air T70.3
- Concato's (pericardial polyserositis) A19.9
  - nontubercular I31.1
  - pleural *—see* Pleurisy, with effusion
- conjunctiva H11.9
  - chlamydial A74.0
  - specified NEC H11.89
  - viral B30.9
    - specified NEC B30.8
- connective tissue, systemic (diffuse) M35.9
  - in (due to)
    - hypogammaglobulinemia D80.1 *[M36.8]*
    - ochronosis E70.29 *[M36.8]*
  - specified NEC M35.89
- Conor and Bruch's (boutonneuse fever) A77.1
- Cooper's *—see* Mastopathy, cystic
- Cori's (glycogenosis III) E74.03
- corkhandler's or corkworker's J67.3
- cornea H18.9
  - specified NEC H18.89-
- coronary (artery) *—see* Disease, heart, ischemic, atherosclerotic
  - congenital Q24.5
  - ostial, syphilitic (aortic) (mitral) (pulmonary) A52.03
- corpus cavernosum N48.9
  - specified NEC N48.89
- Cotugno's *—see* Sciatica
- COVID-19 U07.1
- coxsackie (virus) NEC B34.1
- cranial nerve NOS G52.9
- Creutzfeldt-Jakob *—see* Creutzfeldt-Jakob disease or syndrome
- Crocq's (acrocyanosis) I73.89
- Crohn's *—see* Enteritis, regional
- Curschmann G71.11
- cystic
  - breast (chronic) *—see* Mastopathy, cystic
  - kidney, congenital Q61.9
  - liver, congenital Q44.6
  - lung J98.4
    - congenital Q33.0
- cytomegalic inclusion (generalized) B25.9
  - with pneumonia B25.0
  - congenital P35.1
- cytomegaloviral B25.9
  - specified NEC B25.8
- Czerny's (periodic hydrarthrosis of the knee) *—see* Effusion, joint, knee
- Daae (-Finsen) (epidemic pleurodynia) B33.0
- Darling's *—see* Histoplasmosis capsulati
- Débove's (splenomegaly) R16.1
- deer fly *—see* Tularemia
- Degos' I77.89
- demyelinating, demyelinizating (nervous system) G37.9
  - multiple sclerosis G35
  - specified NEC G37.8
- dense deposit (*see also* N00-N07 with fourth character .6) N05.6
- deposition, hydroxyapatite *— see* Disease, hydroxyapatite deposition
- de Quervain's (tendon sheath) M65.4
  - thyroid (subacute granulomatous thyroiditis) E06.1
- Devergie's (pityriasis rubra pilaris) L44.0
- Devic's G36.0
- diaphorase deficiency D74.0
- diaphragm J98.6
- diarrheal, infectious NEC A09
- digestive system K92.9
  - specified NEC K92.89
- disc, degenerative *—see* Degeneration, intervertebral disc
- discogenic *—see also* Displacement, intervertebral disc NEC
  - with myelopathy *—see* Disorder, disc, with, myelopathy
- diverticular *—see* Diverticula
- Dubois (thymus) A50.59 *[E35]*
- Duchenne-Griesinger G71.01
- Duchenne's
  - muscular dystrophy G71.01
  - pseudohypertrophy, muscles G71.01
- ductless glands E34.9
- Duhring's (dermatitis herpetiformis) L13.0
- duodenum K31.9
  - specified NEC K31.89
- Dupré's (meningism) R29.1
- Dupuytren's (muscle contracture) M72.0
- Durand-Nicholas-Favre (climatic bubo) A55
- Duroziez's (congenital mitral stenosis) Q23.2
- ear *—see* Disorder, ear
- Eberth's *—see* Fever, typhoid
- Ebola (virus) A98.4
- Ebstein's heart Q22.5
- Echinococcus *—see* Echinococcus
- echovirus NEC B34.1
- Eddowes'(brittle bones and blue sclera) Q78.0
- edentulous (alveolar) ridge K06.9
  - specified NEC K06.8
- Edsall's T67.2
- Eichstedt's (pityriasis versicolor) B36.0
- Eisenmenger's (irreversible) I27.83
- Ellis-van Creveld (chondroectodermal dysplasia) Q77.6
- end stage renal (ESRD) N18.6
  - due to hypertension I12.0
- endocrine glands or system NEC E34.9
- endomyocardial (eosinophilic) I42.3
- English (rickets) E55.0
- enteroviral, enterovirus NEC B34.1
  - central nervous system NEC A88.8
- epidemic B99.9
  - specified NEC B99.8
- epididymis N50.9
- Erb (-Landouzy) G71.02
- Erdheim-Chester (ECD) E88.89
- esophagus K22.9
  - functional K22.4
  - psychogenic F45.8
  - specified NEC K22.89
- Eulenburg's (congenital paramyotonia) G71.19
- eustachian tube *—see* Disorder, eustachian tube
- external
  - auditory canal *—see* Disorder, ear, external
  - ear *—see* Disorder, ear, external
- extrapyramidal G25.9
  - specified NEC G25.89
- eye H57.9
  - anterior chamber H21.9
  - inflammatory NEC H57.89
  - muscle (external) *—see* Strabismus
  - specified NEC H57.89
  - syphilitic *—see* Oculopathy, syphilitic
- eyeball H44.9
  - specified NEC H44.89
- eyelid *—see* Disorder, eyelid
  - specified NEC *—see* Disorder, eyelid, specified type NEC
- eyeworm of Africa B74.3
- facial nerve (seventh) G51.9
  - newborn (birth injury) P11.3
- Fahr (of brain) G23.8
- Fahr Volhard (of kidney) I12.-
- fallopian tube (noninflammatory) N83.9
  - inflammatory *—see* Salpingo-oophoritis
  - specified NEC N83.8
- familial periodic paralysis G72.3
- Fanconi's (congenital pancytopenia) D61.09
- fascia NEC *—see also* Disorder, muscle
  - inflammatory *—see* Myositis
  - specified NEC M62.89
- Fauchard's (periodontitis) *—see* Periodontitis
- Favre-Durand-Nicolas (climatic bubo) A55
- Fede's K14.0
- Feer's *—see* Poisoning, mercury
- female pelvic inflammatory *—see also* Disease, pelvis, inflammatory N73.9
  - syphilitic (secondary) A51.42
  - tuberculous A18.17
- Fernels'(aortic aneurysm) I71.9
- fibrocaseous of lung *—see* Tuberculosis, pulmonary
- fibrocystic *—see* Fibrocystic disease
- Fiedler's (leptospiral jaundice) A27.0
- fifth B08.3
- file-cutter's *—see* Poisoning, lead
- fish-skin Q80.9
  - acquired L85.0
- Flajani (-Basedow) (exophthalmic goiter) *—see* Hyperthyroidism, with, goiter (diffuse)
- flax-dresser's J66.1
- fluke *—see* Infestation, fluke
- foot and mouth B08.8
- foot process N04.9
- Forbes'(glycogenosis III) E74.03
- Fordyce-Fox (apocrine miliaria) L75.2
- Fordyce's (ectopic sebaceous glands) (mouth) Q38.6
- Forestier's (rhizomelic pseudopolyarthritis) M35.3
  - meaning ankylosing hyperostosis *—see* Hyperostosis, ankylosing
- Fothergill's
  - neuralgia *—see* Neuralgia, trigeminal
  - scarlatina anginosa A38.9
- Fournier (gangrene) N49.3
  - female N76.89
- fourth B08.8
- Fox (-Fordyce) (apocrine miliaria) L75.2
- Francis' *—see* Tularemia
- Franklin C88.2
- Frei's (climatic bubo) A55
- Friedreich's
  - combined systemic or ataxia G11.11
  - myoclonia G25.3
- frontal sinus *—see* Sinusitis, frontal
- fungus NEC B49
- Gaisböck's (polycythemia hypertonica) D75.1
- gallbladder K82.9
  - calculus *—see* Calculus, gallbladder
  - cholecystitis *—see* Cholecystitis
  - cholesterolosis K82.4
  - fistula *—see* Fistula, gallbladder
  - hydrops K82.1
  - obstruction *—see* Obstruction, gallbladder

Disease, diseased *(continued)*
- gallbladder *(continued)*
  - perforation K82.2
  - specified NEC K82.8
- gamma heavy chain C88.2
- Gamna's (siderotic splenomegaly) D73.2
- Gamstorp's (adynamia episodica hereditaria) G72.3
- Gandy-Nanta (siderotic splenomegaly) D73.2
- ganister J62.8
- gastric *—see* Disease, stomach
- gastroesophageal reflux (GERD) K21.9
  - with esophagitis (without bleeding) K21.00
    - with bleeding K21.01
- gastrointestinal (tract) K92.9
  - amyloid E85.4
  - functional K59.9
    - psychogenic F45.8
  - specified NEC K92.89
- Gee (-Herter) (-Heubner) (-Thaysen) (nontropical sprue) K90.0
- genital organs
  - female N94.9
  - male N50.9
- Gerhardt's (erythromelalgia) I73.81
- Gibert's (pityriasis rosea) L42
- Gierke's (glycogenosis I) E74.01
- Gilles de la Tourette's (motor-verbal tic) F95.2
- gingiva K06.9
  - plaque induced K05.00
  - specified NEC K06.8
- gland (lymph) I89.9
- Glanzmann's (hereditary hemorrhagic thrombasthenia) D69.1
- glass-blower's (cataract) *—see* Cataract, specified NEC
  - salivary gland hypertrophy K11.1
- Glisson's *—see* Rickets
- globe H44.9
  - specified NEC H44.89
- glomerular *—see also* Glomerulonephritis
  - with edema *—see* Nephrosis
  - acute *—see* Nephritis, acute
  - chronic *—see* Nephritis, chronic
  - minimal change N05.0
  - rapidly progressive N01.9
- glycogen storage E74.00
  - Andersen's E74.09
  - Cori's E74.03
  - Forbes' E74.03
  - generalized E74.00
  - glucose-6-phosphatase deficiency E74.01
  - heart E74.02 *[I43]*
  - hepatorenal E74.09
  - Hers' E74.09
  - liver and kidney E74.09
  - McArdle's E74.04
  - muscle phosphofructokinase E74.09
  - myocardium E74.02 *[I43]*
  - Pompe's E74.02
  - Tauri's E74.09
  - type 0 E74.09
  - type I E74.01
  - type II E74.02
  - type III E74.03

Disease, diseased *(continued)*
- glycogen storage *(continued)*
  - type IV E74.09
  - type V E74.04
  - type VI-XI E74.09
  - Von Gierke's E74.01
- Goldstein's (familial hemorrhagic telangiectasia) I78.0
- gonococcal NOS A54.9
- graft-versus-host (GVH) D89.813
  - acute D89.810
  - acute on chronic D89.812
  - chronic D89.811
- grainhandler's J67.8
- granulomatous (childhood) (chronic) D71
- Graves'(exophthalmic goiter) *—see* Hyperthyroidism, with, goiter (diffuse)
- Griesinger's *—see* Ancylostomiasis
- Grisel's M43.6
- Gruby's (tinea tonsurans) B35.0
- Guillain-Barré G61.0
- Guinon's (motor-verbal tic) F95.2
- gum K06.9
- gynecological N94.9
- H (Hartnup's) E72.02
- Haff *—see* Poisoning, mercury
- Hageman (congenital factor XII deficiency) D68.2
- hair (color) (shaft) L67.9
  - follicles L73.9
    - specified NEC L73.8
- Hamman's (spontaneous mediastinal emphysema) J98.2
- hand, foot and mouth B08.4
- Hansen's *—see* Leprosy
- Hantavirus, with pulmonary manifestations B33.4
  - with renal manifestations A98.5
- Harada's H30.81-
- Hartnup (pellagra-cerebellar ataxia-renal aminoaciduria) E72.02
- Hart's (pellagra-cerebellar ataxia-renal aminoaciduria) E72.02
- Hashimoto's (struma lymphomatosa) E06.3
- Hb *—see* Disease, hemoglobin
- heart (organic) I51.9
  - with
    - pulmonary edema (acute) *—see also* Failure, ventricular, left I50.1
    - rheumatic fever (conditions in I00)
      - active I01.9
        - with chorea I02.0
        - specified NEC I01.8
      - inactive or quiescent (with chorea) I09.9
        - specified NEC I09.89
  - amyloid E85.4 *[I43]*
  - aortic (valve) I35.9
  - arteriosclerotic or sclerotic (senile) *—see* Disease, heart, ischemic, atherosclerotic
  - artery, arterial *—see* Disease, heart, ischemic, atherosclerotic
  - beer drinkers' I42.6
  - beriberi (wet) E51.12
  - black I27.0
  - congenital Q24.9
    - cyanotic Q24.9
    - specified NEC Q24.8
  - coronary *—see* Disease, heart, ischemic
  - cryptogenic I51.9
  - fibroid *—see* Myocarditis
  - functional I51.89
    - psychogenic F45.8

Disease, diseased *(continued)*
- heart *(continued)*
  - glycogen storage E74.02 *[I43]*
  - gonococcal A54.83
  - hypertensive *—see* Hypertension, heart
  - hyperthyroid *—see also* Hyperthyroidism E05.90 *[I43]*
    - with thyroid storm E05.91 *[I43]*
  - ischemic (chronic or with a stated duration of over 4 weeks) I25.9
    - atherosclerotic (of) I25.10
      - with angina pectoris *—see* Arteriosclerosis, coronary (artery)
      - coronary artery bypass graft *—see* Arteriosclerosis, coronary (artery),
    - cardiomyopathy I25.5
    - diagnosed on ECG or other special investigation, but currently presenting no symptoms I25.6
    - silent I25.6
    - specified form NEC I25.89
  - kyphoscoliotic I27.1
  - meningococcal A39.50
    - endocarditis A39.51
    - myocarditis A39.52
    - pericarditis A39.53
  - mitral I05.9
    - specified NEC I05.8
  - muscular *—see* Degeneration, myocardial
  - psychogenic (functional) F45.8
  - pulmonary (chronic) I27.9
    - in schistosomiasis B65.9 *[I52]*
    - specified NEC I27.89
  - rheumatic (chronic) (inactive) (old) (quiescent) (with chorea) I09.9
    - active or acute I01.9
      - with chorea (acute) (rheumatic) (Sydenham's) I02.0
    - specified NEC I09.89
  - senile *—see* Myocarditis
  - syphilitic A52.06
    - aortic A52.03
      - aneurysm A52.01
    - congenital A50.54 *[I52]*
  - thyrotoxic (*see also* Thyrotoxicosis) E05.90 *[I43]*
    - with thyroid storm E05.91 *[I43]*
  - valve, valvular (obstructive) (regurgitant) *—see also* Endocarditis
    - congenital NEC Q24.8
      - pulmonary Q22.3
  - vascular *—see* Disease, cardiovascular
- heavy chain NEC C88.2
  - alpha C88.3
  - gamma C88.2
  - mu C88.2
- Hebra's
  - pityriasis
    - maculata et circinata L42
    - rubra pilaris L44.0
  - prurigo L28.2
- hematopoietic organs D75.9
- hemoglobin or Hb
  - abnormal (mixed) NEC D58.2
    - with thalassemia D56.9
  - AS genotype D57.3
  - Bart's D56.0

Disease, diseased *(continued)*
- hemoglobin or Hb *(continued)*
  - C (Hb-C) D58.2
    - with other abnormal hemoglobin NEC D58.2
    - elliptocytosis D58.1
    - Hb-S D57.2-
    - sickle-cell D57.2-
    - thalassemia D56.8
  - Constant Spring D58.2
  - D(Hb-D) D58.2
  - E(Hb-E) D58.2
  - E-beta thalassemia D56.5
  - elliptocytosis D58.1
  - H(Hb-H) (thalassemia) D56.0
    - with other abnormal hemoglobin NEC D56.9
    - Constant Spring D56.0
  - I thalassemia D56.9
  - M D74.0
  - S or SS D57.1
    - with
      - acute chest syndrome D57.01
      - cerebral vascular involvement D57.03
      - crisis (painful) D57.00
        - with complication specified NEC D57.09
      - splenic sequestration D57.02
      - vasooclusive pain D57.00
    - beta plus D57.44
      - with
        - acute chest syndrome D57.451
        - cerebral vascular involvement D57.453
        - crisis D57.459
          - with specified complication NEC D57.458
        - splenic sequestration D57.452
        - vasooclusive pain D57.459
      - without crisis D57.44
    - beta zero D57.42
      - with
        - acute chest syndrome D57.431
        - cerebral vascular involvement D57.433
        - crisis D57.439
          - with specified complication NEC D57.438
        - splenic sequestration D57.432
        - vasooclusive pain D57.439
      - without crisis D57.42
  - SC D57.2-
  - SD D57.8-
  - SE D57.8-
  - spherocytosis D58.0
  - unstable, hemolytic D58.2
- hemolytic (newborn) P55.9
  - autoimmune D59.10
    - cold type (primary) (secondary) (symptomatic) D59.12
    - mixed type (primary) (secondary) (symptomatic) D59.13
    - warm type (primary) (secondary) (symptomatic) D59.11
  - drug-induced D59.0

Disease, diseased *(continued)*
- hemolytic *(continued)*
  - due to or with
    - incompatibility
      - ABO (blood group) P55.1
      - blood (group) (Duffy) (K) (Kell) (Kidd) (Lewis) (M) (S) NEC P55.8
      - Rh (blood group) (factor) P55.0
    - Rh negative mother P55.0
  - specified type NEC P55.8
  - unstable hemoglobin D58.2
- hemorrhagic D69.9
  - newborn P53
- Henoch (-Schönlein) (purpura nervosa) D69.0
- hepatic *—see* Disease, liver
- hepatobiliary K83.9
  - toxic K71.9
- hepatolenticular E83.01
- heredodegenerative NEC
  - spinal cord G95.89
- herpesviral, disseminated B00.7
- Hers'(glycogenosis VI) E74.09
- Herter (-Gee) (-Heubner) (nontropical sprue) K90.0
- Heubner-Herter (nontropical sprue) K90.0
- high fetal gene or hemoglobin thalassemia D56.9
- Hildenbrand's *—see* Typhus
- hip (joint) M25.9
  - congenital Q65.89
  - suppurative M00.9
  - tuberculous A18.02
- His (-Werner) (trench fever) A79.0
- Hodgson's I71.2
  - ruptured I71.1
- Holla *—see* Spherocytosis
- hookworm B76.9
  - specified NEC B76.8
- host-versus-graft D89.813
  - acute D89.810
  - acute on chronic D89.812
  - chronic D89.811
- human immunodeficiency virus (HIV) B20
- Huntington's G10
  - with dementia G10 *[F02.80]*
- Hutchinson's (cheiropompholyx) *—see* Hutchinson's disease
- hyaline (diffuse) (generalized)
  - membrane (lung) (newborn) P22.0
    - adult J80
- hydatid *—see* Echinococcus
- hydroxyapatite deposition M11.00
  - ankle M11.07-
  - elbow M11.02-
  - foot joint M11.07-
  - hand joint M11.04-
  - hip M11.05-
  - knee M11.06-
  - multiple site M11.09
  - shoulder M11.01-
  - vertebra M11.08
  - wrist M11.03-
- hyperkinetic *—see* Hyperkinesia
- hypertensive *—see* Hypertension
- hypophysis E23.7
- Iceland G93.3
- I-cell E77.0
- immune D89.9
- immunoproliferative (malignant) C88.9
  - small intestinal C88.3
  - specified NEC C88.8
- inclusion B25.9
  - salivary gland B25.9

Disease, diseased *(continued)*
- infectious, infective B99.9
  - congenital P37.9
    - specified NEC P37.8
    - viral P35.9
      - specified type NEC P35.8
  - specified NEC B99.8
- inflammatory
  - penis N48.29
    - abscess N48.21
    - cellulitis N48.22
  - prepuce N47.7
    - balanoposthitis N47.6
  - tubo-ovarian *—see* Salpingo-oophoritis
- intervertebral disc *—see also* Disorder, disc
  - with myelopathy *—see* Disorder, disc, with, myelopathy
  - cervical, cervicothoracic *—see* Disorder, disc, cervical
    - with
      - myelopathy *—see* Disorder, disc, cervical, with myelopathy
      - neuritis, radiculitis or radiculopathy *—see* Disorder, disc, cervical, with neuritis
      - specified NEC *—see* Disorder, disc, cervical, specified type NEC
  - lumbar (with)
    - myelopathy M51.06
    - neuritis, radiculitis, radiculopathy or sciatica M51.16
    - specified NEC M51.86
  - lumbosacral (with)
    - neuritis, radiculitis, radiculopathy or sciatica M51.17
    - specified NEC M51.87
  - specified NEC *—see* Disorder, disc, specified NEC
  - thoracic (with)
    - myelopathy M51.04
    - neuritis, radiculitis or radiculopathy M51.14
    - specified NEC M51.84
  - thoracolumbar (with)
    - myelopathy M51.05
    - neuritis, radiculitis or radiculopathy M51.15
    - specified NEC M51.85
- intestine K63.9
  - functional K59.9
    - psychogenic F45.8
    - specified NEC K59.89
  - organic K63.9
  - protozoal A07.9
  - specified NEC K63.89
- iris H21.9
  - specified NEC H21.89
- iron metabolism or storage E83.10
- island (scrub typhus) A75.3
- itai-itai *—see* Poisoning, cadmium
- Jakob-Creutzfeldt *—see* Creutzfeldt-Jakob disease or syndrome
- jaw M27.9
  - fibrocystic M27.49
  - specified NEC M27.8
- jigger B88.1
- joint *—see also* Disorder, joint
  - Charcot's *—see* Arthropathy, neuropathic (Charcot)
  - degenerative *—see* Osteoarthritis
    - multiple M15.9
    - spine *—see* Spondylosis

Disease, diseased *(continued)*
- joint *(continued)*
  - facet joint (*see also* Spondylosis) M47.819
  - hypertrophic *—see* Osteoarthritis
  - sacroiliac M53.3
  - specified NEC *—see* Disorder, joint, specified type NEC
  - spine NEC *—see* Dorsopathy
  - suppurative *—see* Arthritis, pyogenic or pyemic
- Jourdain's (acute gingivitis) K05.00
  - nonplaque induced K05.01
  - plaque induced K05.00
- Kaschin-Beck (endemic polyarthritis) M12.10
  - ankle M12.17-
  - elbow M12.12-
  - foot joint M12.17-
  - hand joint M12.14-
  - hip M12.15-
  - knee M12.16-
  - multiple site M12.19
  - shoulder M12.11-
  - vertebra M12.18
  - wrist M12.13-
- Katayama B65.2
- Kedani (scrub typhus) A75.3
- Keshan E59
- kidney (functional) (pelvis) N28.9
  - chronic N18.9
    - hypertensive *—see* Hypertension, kidney
    - stage 1 N18.1
    - stage 2(mild) N18.2
    - stage 3(moderate) N18.30
    - stage 3a N18.31
    - stage 3b N18.32
    - stage 4(severe) N18.4
    - stage 5 N18.5
  - complicating pregnancy *—see* Pregnancy, complicated by, renal disease
  - cystic (congenital) Q61.9
  - diabetic *—see* E08-E13 with .22
  - fibrocystic (congenital) Q61.8
  - hypertensive *—see* Hypertension, kidney
  - in (due to)
    - schistosomiasis (bilharziasis) B65.9 *[N29]*
  - multicystic Q61.4
  - polycystic Q61.3
    - adult type Q61.2
    - childhood type NEC Q61.19
      - collecting duct dilatation Q61.11
- Kimmelstiel (-Wilson) (intercapillary polycystic (congenital) glomerulosclerosis) *—see* E08-E13 with .21
- Kimura D21.9
  - specified site (*see* Neoplasm, connective tissue benign)
- Kinnier Wilson's (hepatolenticular degeneration) E83.01
- kissing *—see* Mononucleosis, infectious
- Klebs' (*see also* Glomerulonephritis) N05.-
- Klippel-Feil (brevicollis) Q76.1
- Köhler-Pellegrini-Stieda (calcification, knee joint) *—see* Bursitis, tibial collateral
- Kok Q89.8
- König's (osteochondritis dissecans) *—see* Osteochondritis, dissecans
- Korsakoff's (nonalcoholic) F04
  - alcoholic F10.96
    - with dependence F10.26

Disease, diseased *(continued)*
- Kostmann's (infantile genetic agranulocytosis) D70.0
- kuru A81.81
- Kyasanur Forest A98.2
- labyrinth, ear *—see* Disorder, ear, inner
- lacrimal system *—see* Disorder, lacrimal system
- Lafora's *—see* Epilepsy, generalized, idiopathic
- Lancereaux-Mathieu (leptospiral jaundice) A27.0
- Landry's G61.0
- Larrey-Weil (leptospiral jaundice) A27.0
- larynx J38.7
- legionnaires' A48.1
  - nonpneumonic A48.2
- Lenegre's I44.2
- lens H27.9
  - specified NEC H27.8
- Lev's (acquired complete heart block) I44.2
- Lewy body (dementia) G31.83 *[F02.80]*
  - with behavioral disturbance G31.83 *[F02.81]*
- Lichtheim's (subacute combined sclerosis with pernicious anemia) D51.0
- Lightwood's (renal tubular acidosis) N25.89
- Lignac's (cystinosis) E72.04
- lip K13.0
- lipid-storage E75.6
  - specified NEC E75.5
- Lipschütz's N76.6
- liver (chronic) (organic) K76.9
  - alcoholic (chronic) K70.9
    - acute *—see* Disease, liver, alcoholic, hepatitis
    - cirrhosis K70.30
      - with ascites K70.31
    - failure K70.40
      - with coma K70.41
    - fatty liver K70.0
    - fibrosis K70.2
    - hepatitis K70.10
      - with ascites K70.11
    - sclerosis K70.2
  - cystic, congenital Q44.6
  - drug-induced (idiosyncratic) (toxic) (predictable) (unpredictable) *—see* Disease, liver, toxic
  - end stage K72.10
    - with coma K72.11
    - due to hepatitis *—see* Hepatitis
  - fatty, nonalcoholic (NAFLD) K76.0
    - alcoholic K70.0
  - fibrocystic (congenital) Q44.6
  - fluke
    - Chinese B66.1
    - oriental B66.1
    - sheep B66.3
  - gestational alloimmune (GALD) P78.84
  - glycogen storage E74.09 *[K77]*
  - in (due to)
    - schistosomiasis (bilharziasis) B65.9 *[K77]*
  - inflammatory K75.9
    - alcoholic K70.1
    - specified NEC K75.89
  - polycystic (congenital) Q44.6

Disease, diseased *(continued)*
- liver *(continued)*
  - toxic K71.9
    - with
      - cholestasis K71.0
      - cirrhosis (liver) K71.7
      - fibrosis (liver) K71.7
      - focal nodular hyperplasia K71.8
      - hepatic granuloma K71.8
      - hepatic necrosis K71.10
        - with coma K71.11
      - hepatitis NEC K71.6
        - acute K71.2
        - chronic
          - active K71.50
            - with ascites K71.51
          - lobular K71.4
          - persistent K71.3
        - lupoid K71.50
          - with ascites K71.51
      - peliosis hepatis K71.8
      - veno-occlusive disease (VOD) of liver K71.8
  - veno-occlusive K76.5
- Lobo's (keloid blastomycosis) B48.0
- Lobstein's (brittle bones and blue sclera) Q78.0
- Ludwig's (submaxillary cellulitis) K12.2
- lumbosacral region M53.87
- lung J98.4
  - black J60
  - congenital Q33.9
  - cystic J98.4
    - congenital Q33.0
  - dabbing (related) U07.0
  - electronic cigarette (related) U07.0
  - fibroid (chronic) —*see* Fibrosis, lung
  - fluke B66.4
    - oriental B66.4
  - in
    - amyloidosis E85.4 *[J99]*
    - sarcoidosis D86.0
    - Sjögren's syndrome M35.02
    - systemic
      - lupus erythematosus M32.13
      - sclerosis M34.81
  - interstitial J84.9
    - with progressive fibrotic phenotype, in diseases classified elsewhere J84.170
    - of childhood, specified NEC J84.848
    - respiratory bronchiolitis J84.115
    - specified NEC J84.89
  - obstructive (chronic) J44.9
    - with
      - acute
        - bronchitis J44.0
        - exacerbation NEC J44.1
        - lower respiratory infection J44.0
      - alveolitis, allergic J67.9
      - asthma J44.9
      - bronchiectasis J47.9
        - with
          - exacerbation (acute) J47.1
          - lower respiratory infection J47.0
      - bronchitis J44.9
        - with
          - exacerbation (acute) J44.1
          - lower respiratory infection J44.0

Disease, diseased *(continued)*
- lung *(continued)*
  - obstructive *(continued)*
    - with *(continued)*
      - emphysema J43.9
      - hypersensitivity pneumonitis J67.9
    - decompensated J44.1
      - with
        - exacerbation (acute) J44.1
  - polycystic J98.4
    - congenital Q33.0
  - rheumatoid (diffuse) (interstitial) —*see* Rheumatoid, lung
  - vaping (associated) (device) (product) (use) U07.0
- Lutembacher's (atrial septal defect with mitral stenosis) Q21.1
- Lyme A69.20
- lymphatic (gland) (system) (channel) (vessel) I89.9
- lymphoproliferative D47.9
  - specified NEC D47.Z9
  - T-gamma D47.Z9
  - X-linked D82.3
- Magitot's M27.2
- malarial —*see* Malaria
- malignant —*see also* Neoplasm, malignant, by site
- Manson's B65.1
- maple bark J67.6
- maple-syrup-urine E71.0
- Marburg (virus) A98.3
- Marion's (bladder neck obstruction) N32.0
- Marsh's (exophthalmic goiter) —*see* Hyperthyroidism, with, goiter (diffuse)
- mastoid (process) —*see* Disorder, ear, middle
- Mathieu's (leptospiral jaundice) A27.0
- Maxcy's A75.2
- McArdle (-Schmid-Pearson) (glycogenosis V) E74.04
- mediastinum J98.59
- medullary center (idiopathic) (respiratory) G93.89
- Meige's (chronic hereditary edema) Q82.0
- meningococcal —*see* Infection, meningococcal
- mental F99
  - organic F09
- mesenchymal M35.9
- mesenteric embolic (*see also* Ischemia, intestine, acute) K55.039
- metabolic, metabolism E88.9
  - bilirubin E80.7
- metal-polisher's J62.8
- metastatic (*see also* Neoplasm, secondary, by site) C794.9
- microvascular - code to condition
- microvillus
  - atrophy Q43.8
  - inclusion (MVD) Q43.8
- middle ear —*see* Disorder, ear, middle
- Mikulicz'(dryness of mouth, absent or decreased lacrimation) K11.8
- Milroy's (chronic hereditary edema) Q82.0
- Minamata —*see* Poisoning, mercury
- minicore G71.29
- Minor's G95.19
- Minot's (hemorrhagic disease, newborn) P53

Disease, diseased *(continued)*
- Minot-von Willebrand-Jürgens (angiohemophilia) D68.0
- Mitchell's (erythromelalgia) I73.81
- mitral (valve) I05.9
  - nonrheumatic I34.9
- mixed connective tissue M35.1
- moldy hay J67.0
- Monge's T70.29
- Morgagni-Adams-Stokes (syncope with heart block) I45.9
- Morgagni's (syndrome) (hyperostosis frontalis interna) M85.2
- Morton's (with metatarsalgia) —*see* Lesion, nerve, plantar
- Morvan's G60.8
- motor neuron (bulbar) (mixed type) (spinal) G12.20
  - amyotrophic lateral sclerosis G12.21
  - familial G12.24
  - progressive bulbar palsy G12.22
  - specified NEC G12.29
- moyamoya I67.5
- mu heavy chain disease C88.2
- multicore G71.29
- multiminicore G71.29
- muscle —*see also* Disorder, muscle
  - inflammatory —*see* Myositis
  - ocular (external) —*see* Strabismus
- musculoskeletal system, soft tissue —*see also* Disorder, soft tissue
  - specified NEC —*see* Disorder, soft tissue, specified type NEC
- mushroom workers' J67.5
- mycotic B49
- myelodysplastic, not classified (*see also* Syndrome, myelodysplasia) C94.6
- myeloproliferative, not classified C94.6
  - chronic D47.1
- myocardium, myocardial (*see also* Degeneration, myocardial) I51.5
  - primary (idiopathic) I42.9
- myoneural G70.9
- Naegeli's D69.1
- nails L60.9
  - specified NEC L60.8
- Nairobi (sheep virus) A93.8
- nasal J34.9
- nemaline body G71.21
- nerve —*see* Disorder, nerve
- nervous system G98.8
  - autonomic G90.9
  - central G96.9
    - specified NEC G96.89
  - congenital Q07.9
  - parasympathetic G90.9
  - specified NEC G98.8
  - sympathetic G90.9
  - vegetative G90.9
- neuromuscular system G70.9
- Newcastle B30.8
- Nicolas (-Durand)-Favre (climatic bubo) A55
- nipple N64.9
  - Paget's C50.01-
    - female C50.01-
    - male C50.02-
- Nishimoto (-Takeuchi) I67.5
- nonarthropod-borne NOS (viral) B34.9
  - enterovirus NEC B34.1
- nonautoimmune hemolytic D59.4
  - drug-induced D59.2
- Nonne-Milroy-Meige (chronic hereditary edema) Q82.0
- nose J34.9

Disease, diseased *(continued)*
- nucleus pulposus —*see* Disorder, disc
- nutritional E63.9
- oast-house-urine E72.19
- ocular
  - herpesviral B00.50
  - zoster B02.30
- obliterative vascular I77.1
- Ohara's —*see* Tularemia
- Opitz's (congestive splenomegaly) D73.2
- Oppenheim-Urbach (necrobiosis lipoidica diabeticorum) —*see* E08-E13 with .620
- optic nerve NEC —*see* Disorder, nerve, optic
- orbit —*see* Disorder, orbit
- organ
  - dabbing (related) U07.0
  - electronic cigarette (related) U07.0
  - vaping (associated) (device) (product) (use) U07.0
- Oriental liver fluke B66.1
- Oriental lung fluke B66.4
- Ormond's N13.5
- Oropouche virus A93.0
- Osler-Rendu (familial hemorrhagic telangiectasia) I78.0
- osteofibrocystic E21.0
- Otto's M24.7
- outer ear —*see* Disorder, ear, external
- ovary (noninflammatory) N83.9
  - cystic N83.20-
  - inflammatory —*see* Salpingo-oophoritis
  - polycystic E28.2
  - specified NEC N83.8
- Owren's (congenital) —*see* Defect, coagulation
- pancreas K86.9
  - cystic K86.2
  - fibrocystic E84.9
  - specified NEC K86.89
- panvalvular I08.9
  - specified NEC I08.8
- parametrium (noninflammatory) N83.9
- parasitic B89
  - cerebral NEC B71.9 *[G94]*
  - intestinal NOS B82.9
  - mouth B37.0
  - skin NOS B88.9
  - specified type —*see* Infestation
  - tongue B37.0
- parathyroid (gland) E21.5
  - specified NEC E21.4
- Parkinson's G20
- parodontal K05.6
- Parrot's (syphilitic osteochondritis) A50.02
- Parry's (exophthalmic goiter) —*see* Hyperthyroidism, with, goiter (diffuse)
- Parson's (exophthalmic goiter) —*see* Hyperthyroidism, with, goiter (diffuse)
- Paxton's (white piedra) B36.2
- pearl-worker's —*see* Osteomyelitis, specified type NEC
- Pellegrini-Stieda (calcification, knee joint) —*see* Bursitis, tibial collateral
- pelvis, pelvic
  - female NOS N94.9
    - specified NEC N94.89
  - gonococcal (acute) (chronic) A54.24

- pelvis, pelvic *(continued)*
  - inflammatory (female) N73.9
    - acute N73.0
    - chlamydial A56.11
    - chronic N73.1
    - specified NEC N73.8
    - syphilitic (secondary) A51.42
      - late A52.76
    - tuberculous A18.17
  - organ, female N94.9
  - peritoneum, female NEC N94.89
- penis N48.9
  - inflammatory N48.29
    - abscess N48.21
    - cellulitis N48.22
  - specified NEC N48.89
- periapical tissues NOS K04.90
- periodontal K05.6
  - specified NEC K05.5
- periosteum *—see* Disorder, bone, specified type NEC
- peripheral
  - arterial I73.9
  - autonomic nervous system G90.9
  - nerves *—see* Polyneuropathy
  - vascular NOS I73.9
- peritoneum K66.9
  - pelvic, female NEC N94.89
  - specified NEC K66.8
- persistent mucosal (middle ear) H66.20
  - left H66.22
    - with right H66.23
  - right H66.21
    - with left H66.23
- Petit's *—see* Hernia, abdomen, specified site NEC
- pharynx J39.2
  - specified NEC J39.2
- Phocas' *—see* Mastopathy, cystic
- photochromogenic (acid-fast bacilli) (pulmonary) A31.0
  - nonpulmonary A31.9
- Pick's G31.01 *[F02.80]*
  - with behavioral disturbance G31.01 *[F02.81]*
  - brain G31.01 *[F02.80]*
    - with behavioral disturbance G31.01 *[F02.81]*
  - of pericardium (pericardial pseudocirrhosis of liver) I31.1
- pigeon fancier's J67.2
- pineal gland E34.8
- pink *—see* Poisoning, mercury
- Pinkus' (lichen nitidus) L44.1
- pinworm B80
- Piry virus A93.8
- pituitary (gland) E23.7
- pituitary-snuff-taker's J67.8
- pleura (cavity) J94.9
  - specified NEC J94.8
- pneumatic drill (hammer) T75.21
- Pollitzer's (hidradenitis suppurativa) L73.2
- polycystic
  - kidney or renal Q61.3
    - adult type Q61.2
    - childhood type NEC Q61.19
      - collecting duct dilatation Q61.11
  - liver or hepatic Q44.6
  - lung or pulmonary J98.4
    - congenital Q33.0
  - ovary, ovaries E28.2
  - spleen Q89.09
- polyethylene T84.05-
- Pompe's (glycogenosis II) E74.02
- Posadas-Wernicke B38.9
- Potain's (pulmonary edema) *—see* Edema, lung

- prepuce N47.8
  - inflammatory N47.7
    - balanoposthitis N47.6
- Pringle's (tuberous sclerosis) Q85.1
- prion, central nervous system A81.9
  - specified NEC A81.89
- prostate N42.9
  - specified NEC N42.89
- protozoal B64
  - acanthamebiasis *—see* Acanthamebiasis
  - African trypanosomiasis *—see* African trypanosomiasis
  - babesiosis (*see also* Babesiosis) B60.00
  - Chagas disease *—see* Chagas disease
  - intestine, intestinal A07.9
  - leishmaniasis *—see* Leishmaniasis
  - malaria *—see* Malaria
  - naegleriasis B60.2
  - pneumocystosis B59
  - specified organism NEC B60.8
  - toxoplasmosis *—see* Toxoplasmosis
- pseudo-Hurler's E77.0
- psychiatric F99
- psychotic *—see* Psychosis
- Puente's (simple glandular cheilitis) K13.0
- puerperal (*see also* Puerperal) O90.89
- pulmonary *—see also* Disease, lung
  - artery I28.9
  - chronic obstructive J44.9
    - with
      - acute bronchitis J44.0
      - exacerbation (acute) J44.1
      - lower respiratory infection (acute) J44.0
    - decompensated J44.1
      - with
        - exacerbation (acute) J44.1
  - heart I27.9
    - specified NEC I27.89
  - hypertensive (vascular) (*see also* Hypertension, pulmonary) I27.20
    - primary (idiopathic) I27.0
  - valve I37.9
    - rheumatic I09.89
- pulp (dental) NOS K04.90
- pulseless M31.4
- Putnam's (subacute combined sclerosis with pernicious anemia) D51.0
- Pyle (-Cohn) (metaphyseal dysplasia) Q78.5
- ragpicker's or ragsorter's A22.1
- Raynaud's *—see* Raynaud's disease
- reactive airway *—see* Asthma
- Reclus' (cystic) *—see* Mastopathy, cystic
- rectum K62.9
  - specified NEC K62.89
- Refsum's (heredopathia atactica polyneuritiformis) G60.1
- renal (functional) (pelvis) (*see also* Disease, kidney) N28.9
  - with
    - edema *—see* Nephrosis
    - glomerular lesion *—see* Glomerulonephritis
      - with edema *—see* Nephrosis
    - interstitial nephritis N12
  - acute N28.9
  - chronic (*see also* Disease, kidney, chronic) N18.9
  - cystic, congenital Q61.9

- renal *(continued)*
  - diabetic *—see* E08-E13 with .22
  - end-stage (failure) N18.6
    - due to hypertension I12.0
  - fibrocystic (congenital) Q61.8
  - hypertensive *—see* Hypertension, kidney
  - lupus M32.14
  - phosphate-losing (tubular) N25.0
  - polycystic (congenital) Q61.3
    - adult type Q61.2
    - childhood type NEC Q61.19
      - collecting duct dilatation Q61.11
  - rapidly progressive N01.9
  - subacute N01.9
- Rendu-Osler-Weber (familial hemorrhagic telangiectasia) I78.0
- renovascular (arteriosclerotic) *—see* Hypertension, kidney
- respiratory (tract) J98.9
  - acute or subacute NOS J06.9
    - due to
      - chemicals, gases, fumes or vapors (inhalation) J68.3
      - external agent J70.9
        - specified NEC J70.8
      - radiation J70.0
      - smoke inhalation J70.5
    - noninfectious J39.8
  - chronic NOS J98.9
    - due to
      - chemicals, gases, fumes or vapors J68.4
      - external agent J70.9
        - specified NEC J70.8
      - radiation J70.1
    - newborn P27.9
      - specified NEC P27.8
  - due to
    - chemicals, gases, fumes or vapors J68.9
      - acute or subacute NEC J68.3
      - chronic J68.4
    - external agent J70.9
      - specified NEC J70.8
  - newborn P28.9
    - specified type NEC P28.89
  - upper J39.9
    - acute or subacute J06.9
    - noninfectious NEC J39.8
    - specified NEC J39.8
    - streptococcal J06.9
- retina, retinal H35.9
  - Batten's or Batten-Mayou E75.4 *[H36]*
  - specified NEC H35.89
- rheumatoid *—see* Arthritis, rheumatoid
- rickettsial NOS A79.9
  - specified type NEC A79.89
- Riga (-Fede) (cachectic aphthae) K14.0
- Riggs' (compound periodontitis) *—see* Periodontitis
- Ritter's L00
- Rivalta's (cervicofacial actinomycosis) A42.2
- Robles' (onchocerciasis) B73.01
- rod body G71.21
- Roger's (congenital interventricular septal defect) Q21.0
- Rosenthal's (factor XI deficiency) D68.1
- Rossbach's (hyperchlorhydria) K31.89
  - psychogenic F45.8
- Ross River B33.1
- Rotes Quérol *—see* Hyperostosis, ankylosing

- Roth (-Bernhardt) *—see* Mononeuropathy, lower limb, meralgia paresthetica
- Runeberg's (progressive pernicious anemia) D51.0
- sacroiliac NEC M53.3
- salivary gland or duct K11.9
  - inclusion B25.9
  - specified NEC K11.8
  - virus B25.9
- sandworm B76.9
- Schimmelbusch's *—see* Mastopathy, cystic
- Schmorl's *—see* Schmorl's disease or nodes
- Schönlein (-Henoch) (purpura rheumatica) D69.0
- Schottmüller's *—see* Fever, paratyphoid
- Schultz's (agranulocytosis) *—see* Agranulocytosis
- Schwalbe-Ziehen-Oppenheim G24.1
- Schwartz-Jampel G71.13
- sclera H15.9
  - specified NEC H15.89
- scrofulous (tuberculous) A18.2
- scrotum N50.9
- sebaceous glands L73.9
- semilunar cartilage, cystic *—see also* Derangement, knee, meniscus, cystic
- seminal vesicle N50.9
- serum NEC (*see also* Reaction, serum) T80.69
- sexually transmitted A64
  - anogenital
    - herpesviral infection *—see* Herpes, anogenital
    - warts A63.0
  - chancroid A57
  - chlamydial infection *—see* Chlamydia
  - gonorrhea *—see* Gonorrhea
  - granuloma inguinale A58
  - specified organism NEC A63.8
  - syphilis *—see* Syphilis
  - trichomoniasis *—see* Trichomoniasis
- Sézary C84.1-
- shimamushi (scrub typhus) A75.3
- shipyard B30.0
- sickle-cell D57.1
  - with
    - acute chest syndrome D57.01
    - cerebral vascular involvement D57.03
    - crisis (painful) D57.00
      - with complication specified NEC D57.09
    - splenic sequestration D57.02
    - vasoocclusive pain D57.00
  - elliptocytosis D57.8-
  - Hb-C D57.20
    - with
      - acute chest syndrome D57.211
      - cerebral vascular involvement D57.213
      - crisis D57.219
        - with specified complication NEC D57.218
      - splenic sequestration D57.212
      - vasoocclusive pain D57.219
    - without crisis D57.20
  - Hb-SD D57.80
    - with
      - acute chest syndrome D57.811

Disease, diseased *(continued)*
- sickle-cell *(continued)*
  - Hb-SD *(continued)*
    - with *(continued)*
      - cerebral vascular involvement D57.813
      - crisis D57.819
        - with complication
          - specified NEC D57.818
      - splenic sequestration D57.812
      - vasoocclusive pain D57.819
    - without crisis D57.80
  - Hb-SE D57.80
    - with
      - acute chest syndrome D57.811
      - cerebral vascular involvement D57.813
      - crisis D57.819
        - with complication
          - specified NEC D57.818
      - splenic sequestration D57.812
      - vasoocclusive pain D57.819
    - without crisis D57.80
  - specified NEC D57.80
    - with
      - acute chest syndrome D57.811
      - cerebral vascular involvement D57.813
      - crisis D57.819
        - with complication
          - specified NEC D57.818
      - splenic sequestration D57.812
      - vasoocclusive pain D57.819
    - without crisis D57.80
  - spherocytosis D57.80
    - with
      - acute chest syndrome D57.811
      - cerebral vascular involvement D57.813
      - crisis D57.819
        - with complication
          - specified NEC D57.818
      - splenic sequestration D57.812
      - vasoocclusive pain D57.819
    - without crisis D57.80
  - thalassemia D57.40
    - with
      - acute chest syndrome D57.411
      - cerebral vascular involvement D57.413
      - crisis D57.419
        - with specified complication NEC D57.418
      - splenic sequestration D57.412
      - vasoocclusive pain D57.419
    - beta plus D57.44
      - with
        - acute chest syndrome D57.451
        - cerebral vascular involvement D57.453
        - crisis D57.459
          - with specified complication NEC D57.458
        - splenic sequestration D57.452

Disease, diseased *(continued)*
sickle-cell *(continued)*
thalassemia *(continued)*
beta plus *(continued)*
with *(continued)*

        - vasoocclusive pain D57.459
      - without crisis D57.44
    - beta zero D57.42
      - with
        - acute chest syndrome D57.431
        - cerebral vascular involvement D57.433
        - crisis D57.439
          - with specified complication NEC D57.438
        - splenic sequestration D57.432
        - vasoocclusive pain D57.439
      - without crisis D57.42
- silo-filler's J68.8
  - bronchitis J68.0
  - pneumonitis J68.0
  - pulmonary edema J68.1
- simian B B00.4
- Simons'(progressive lipodystrophy) E88.1
- sin nombre virus B33.4
- sinus —*see* Sinusitis
- Sirkari's B55.0
- sixth B08.20
  - due to human herpesvirus 6 B08.21
  - due to human herpesvirus 7 B08.22
- skin L98.9
  - due to metabolic disorder NEC E88.9 *[L99]*
  - specified NEC L98.8
- slim (HIV) B20
- small vessel I73.9
- Sneddon-Wilkinson (subcorneal pustular dermatosis) L13.1
- South African creeping B88.0
- spinal (cord) G95.9
  - congenital Q06.9
  - specified NEC G95.89
- spine —*see also* Spondylopathy
  - joint —*see* Dorsopathy
  - tuberculous A18.01
- spinocerebellar (hereditary) G11.9
  - specified NEC G11.8
- spleen D73.9
  - amyloid E85.4 *[D77]*
  - organic D73.9
  - polycystic Q89.09
  - postinfectional D73.89
- sponge-diver's —*see* Toxicity, venom, marine animal, sea anemone
- Startle Q89.8
- Steinert's G71.11
- Sticker's (erythema infectiosum) B08.3
- Stieda's (calcification, knee joint) —*see* Bursitis, tibial collateral
- Stokes'(exophthalmic goiter) —*see* Hyperthyroidism, with, goiter (diffuse)
- Stokes-Adams (syncope with heart block) I45.9
- stomach K31.9
  - functional, psychogenic F45.8
  - specified NEC K31.89
- stonemason's J62.8
- storage
  - glycogen —*see* Disease, glycogen storage

Disease, diseased *(continued)*
storage *(continued)*

  - mucopolysaccharide —*see* Mucopolysaccharidosis
- striatopallidal system NEC G25.89
- Stuart-Prower (congenital factor X deficiency) D68.2
- Stuart's (congenital factor X deficiency) D68.2
- subcutaneous tissue —*see* Disease, skin
- supporting structures of teeth K08.9
  - specified NEC K08.89
- suprarenal (capsule) (gland) E27.9
  - hyperfunction E27.0
  - specified NEC E27.8
- sweat glands L74.9
  - specified NEC L74.8
- Sweeley-Klionsky E75.21
- Swift (-Feer) —*see* Poisoning, mercury
- swimming-pool granuloma A31.1
- Sylvest's (epidemic pleurodynia) B33.0
- sympathetic nervous system G90.9
- synovium —*see* Disorder, synovium
- syphilitic —*see* Syphilis
- systemic tissue mast cell D47.02
- tanapox (virus) B08.71
- Tangier E78.6
- Tarral-Besnier (pityriasis rubra pilaris) L44.0
- Tauri's E74.09
- tear duct —*see* Disorder, lacrimal system
- tendon, tendinous —*see also* Disorder, tendon
  - nodular —*see* Trigger finger
- terminal vessel I73.9
- testis N50.9
- thalassemia Hb-S —*see* Disease, sickle-cell, thalassemia
- Thaysen-Gee (nontropical sprue) K90.0
- Thomsen G71.12
- throat J39.2
  - septic J02.0
- thromboembolic —*see* Embolism
- thymus (gland) E32.9
  - specified NEC E32.8
- thyroid (gland) E07.9
  - heart (*see also* Hyperthyroidism) E05.90 *[I43]*
    - with thyroid storm E05.91 *[I43]*
  - specified NEC E07.89
- Tietze's M94.0
- tongue K14.9
  - specified NEC K14.8
- tonsils, tonsillar (and adenoids) J35.9
- tooth, teeth K08.9
  - hard tissues K03.9
    - specified NEC K03.89
  - pulp NEC K04.99
  - specified NEC K08.89
- Tourette's F95.2
- trachea NEC J39.8
- tricuspid I07.9
  - nonrheumatic I36.9
- triglyceride-storage E75.5
- trophoblastic —*see* Mole, hydatidiform
- tsutsugamushi A75.3
- tube (fallopian) (noninflammatory) N83.9
  - inflammatory —*see* Salpingitis
  - specified NEC N83.8

Disease, diseased *(continued)*

- tuberculous NEC —*see* Tuberculosis
- tubo-ovarian (noninflammatory) N83.9
  - inflammatory —*see* Salpingo-oophoritis
  - specified NEC N83.8
- tubotympanic, chronic —*see* Otitis, media, suppurative, chronic, tubotympanic
- tubulo-interstitial N15.9
  - specified NEC N15.8
- tympanum —*see* Disorder, tympanic membrane
- Uhl's Q24.8
- Underwood's (sclerema neonatorum) P83.0
- Unverricht (-Lundborg) —*see* Epilepsy, generalized, idiopathic
- Urbach-Oppenheim (necrobiosis lipoidica diabeticorum) —*see* E08-E13 with .620
- ureter N28.9
  - in (due to)
    - schistosomiasis (bilharziasis) B65.0 *[N29]*
- urethra N36.9
  - specified NEC N36.8
- urinary (tract) N39.9
  - bladder N32.9
    - specified NEC N32.89
  - specified NEC N39.8
- uterus (noninflammatory) N85.9
  - infective —*see* Endometritis
  - inflammatory —*see* Endometritis
  - specified NEC N85.8
- uveal tract (anterior) H21.9
  - posterior H31.9
- vagabond's B85.1
- vagina, vaginal (noninflammatory) N89.9
  - inflammatory NEC N76.89
  - specified NEC N89.8
- valve, valvular I38
  - multiple I08.9
    - specified NEC I08.8
- van Creveld-von Gierke (glycogenosis I) E74.01
- vas deferens N50.9
- vascular I99.9
  - arteriosclerotic —*see* Arteriosclerosis
  - ciliary body NEC —*see* Disorder, iris, vascular
  - hypertensive —*see* Hypertension
  - iris NEC —*see* Disorder, iris, vascular
  - obliterative I77.1
    - peripheral I73.9
  - occlusive I99.8
  - peripheral (occlusive) I73.9
    - in diabetes mellitus —*see* E08-E13 with .51
- vasomotor I73.9
- vasospastic I73.9
- vein I87.9
- venereal (*see also* Disease, sexually transmitted) A64
  - chlamydial NEC A56.8
    - anus A56.3
    - genitourinary NOS A56.2
    - pharynx A56.4
    - rectum A56.3
  - fifth A55
  - sixth A55
  - specified nature or type NEC A63.8

Disease, diseased *(continued)*
- vertebra, vertebral —*see also* Spondylopathy
  - disc —*see* Disorder, disc
- vibration —*see* Vibration, adverse effects
- viral, virus (*see also* Disease, by type of virus) B34.9
  - arbovirus NOS A94
  - arthropod-borne NOS A94
  - congenital P35.9
    - specified NEC P35.8
  - Hanta (with renal manifestations) (Dobrava) (Puumala) (Seoul) A98.5
    - with pulmonary manifestations (Andes) (Bayou) (Bermejo) (Black Creek Canal) (Choclo) (Juquitiba) (Laguna negra) (Lechiguanas) (New York) (Oran) (Sin nombre) B33.4
  - Hantaan (Korean hemorrhagic fever) A98.5
  - human immunodeficiency (HIV) B20
  - Kunjin A83.4
  - nonarthropod-borne NOS B34.9
  - Powassan A84.81
  - Rocio (encephalitis) A83.6
  - Sin nombre (Hantavirus) (cardio)-pulmonary syndrome) B33.4
  - Tahyna B33.8
  - vesicular stomatitis A93.8
- vitreous H43.9
  - specified NEC H43.89
- vocal cord J38.3
- Volkmann's, acquired T79.6
- von Eulenburg's (congenital paramyotonia) G71.19
- von Gierke's (glycogenosis I) E74.01
- von Graefe's —*see* Strabismus, paralytic, ophthalmoplegia, progressive
- von Willebrand (-Jürgens) (angiohemophilia) D68.0
- Vrolik's (osteogenesis imperfecta) Q78.0
- vulva (noninflammatory) N90.9
  - inflammatory NEC N76.89
  - specified NEC N90.89
- Wallgren's (obstruction of splenic vein with collateral circulation) I87.8
- Wassilieff's (leptospiral jaundice) A27.0
- wasting NEC R64
  - due to malnutrition E43
    - with marasmus E41
- Waterhouse-Friderichsen A39.1
- Wegner's (syphilitic osteochondritis) A50.02
- Weil's (leptospiral jaundice of lung) A27.0
- Weir Mitchell's (erythromelalgia) I73.81
- Werdnig-Hoffmann G12.0
- Wermer's E31.21
- Werner-His (trench fever) A79.0
- Werner-Schultz (neutropenic splenomegaly) D73.81
- Wernicke-Posadas B38.9
- whipworm B79
- white blood cells D72.9
  - specified NEC D72.89
- white matter R90.82
- white-spot, meaning lichen sclerosus et atrophicus L90.0
  - penis N48.0
  - vulva N90.4
- Wilkie's K55.1

Disease, diseased *(continued)*
- Wilkinson-Sneddon (subcorneal pustular dermatosis) L13.1
- Willis' —*see* Diabetes
- Wilson's (hepatolenticular degeneration) E83.01
- woolsorter's A22.1
- yaba monkey tumor B08.72
- yaba pox (virus) B08.72
- Zika virus A92.5
  - congenital P35.4
- zoonotic, bacterial A28.9
  - specified type NEC A28.8

Disfigurement (due to scar) L90.5

Disgerminoma —*see* Dysgerminoma

DISH (diffuse idiopathic skeletal hyperostosis) —*see* Hyperostosis, ankylosing

Disinsertion, retina —*see* Detachment, retina

Dislocatable hip, congenital Q65.6

Dislocation (articular)
- with fracture —*see* Fracture
- acromioclavicular (joint) S43.10-
  - with displacement
    - 100%-200% S43.12-
    - more than 200% S43.13-
  - inferior S43.14-
  - posterior S43.15-
- ankle S93.0-
- astragalus —*see* Dislocation, ankle
- atlantoaxial S13.121
- atlantooccipital S13.111
- atloidooccipital S13.111
- breast bone S23.29
- capsule, joint - code by site under Dislocation
- carpal (bone) —*see* Dislocation, wrist
- carpometacarpal (joint) NEC S63.05-
  - thumb S63.04-
- cartilage (joint) - code by site under Dislocation
- cervical spine (vertebra) —*see* Dislocation, vertebra, cervical
- chronic —*see* Dislocation, recurrent
- clavicle —*see* Dislocation, acromioclavicular joint
- coccyx S33.2
- congenital NEC Q68.8
- coracoid —*see* Dislocation, shoulder
- costal cartilage S23.29
- costochondral S23.29
- cricoarytenoid articulation S13.29
- cricothyroid articulation S13.29
- dorsal vertebra —*see* Dislocation, vertebra, thoracic
- ear ossicle —*see* Discontinuity, ossicles, ear
- elbow S53.10-
  - congenital Q68.8
  - pathological —*see* Dislocation, pathological NEC, elbow
  - radial head alone —*see* Dislocation, radial head
  - recurrent —*see* Dislocation, recurrent, elbow
  - traumatic S53.10-
    - anterior S53.11-
    - lateral S53.14-
    - medial S53.13-
    - posterior S53.12-
    - specified type NEC S53.19-
- eye, nontraumatic —*see* Luxation, globe

Dislocation *(continued)*
- eyeball, nontraumatic —*see* Luxation, globe
- femur
  - distal end —*see* Dislocation, knee
  - proximal end —*see* Dislocation, hip
- fibula
  - distal end —*see* Dislocation, ankle
  - proximal end —*see* Dislocation, knee
- finger S63.25-
  - index S63.25-
  - interphalangeal S63.27-
    - distal S63.29-
      - index S63.29-
      - little S63.29-
      - middle S63.29-
      - ring S63.29-
    - index S63.27-
    - little S63.27-
    - middle S63.27-
    - proximal S63.28-
      - index S63.28-
      - little S63.28-
      - middle S63.28-
      - ring S63.28-
    - ring S63.27-
  - little S63.25-
  - metacarpophalangeal S63.26-
    - index S63.26-
    - little S63.26-
    - middle S63.26-
    - ring S63.26-
  - middle S63.25-
  - recurrent —*see* Dislocation, recurrent, finger
  - ring S63.25-
  - thumb —*see* Dislocation, thumb
- foot S93.30-
  - recurrent —*see* Dislocation, recurrent, foot
  - specified site NEC S93.33-
  - tarsal joint S93.31-
  - tarsometatarsal joint S93.32-
  - toe —*see* Dislocation, toe
- fracture —*see* Fracture
- glenohumeral (joint) —*see* Dislocation, shoulder
- glenoid —*see* Dislocation, shoulder
- habitual —*see* Dislocation, recurrent
- hip S73.00-
  - anterior S73.03-
    - obturator S73.02-
  - central S73.04-
  - congenital (total) Q65.2
    - bilateral Q65.1
    - partial Q65.5
      - bilateral Q65.4
      - unilateral Q65.3-
    - unilateral Q65.0-
  - developmental M24.85-
  - pathological —*see* Dislocation, pathological NEC, hip
  - posterior S73.01-
  - recurrent —*see* Dislocation, recurrent, hip
- humerus, proximal end —*see* Dislocation, shoulder
- incomplete —*see* Subluxation, by site
- incus —*see* Discontinuity, ossicles, ear
- infracoracoid —*see* Dislocation, shoulder
- innominate (pubic junction) (sacral junction) S33.39
  - acetabulum —*see* Dislocation, hip

Dislocation *(continued)*
- interphalangeal (joint(s))
  - finger S63.279
    - distal S63.29-
      - index S63.29-
      - little S63.29-
      - middle S63.29-
      - ring S63.29-
    - index S63.27-
    - little S63.27-
    - middle S63.27-
    - proximal S63.28-
      - index S63.28-
      - little S63.28-
      - middle S63.28-
      - ring S63.28-
    - ring S63.27-
  - foot or toe —*see* Dislocation, toe
  - thumb S63.12-
- jaw (cartilage) (meniscus) S03.0-
- joint prosthesis —*see* Complications, joint prosthesis, mechanical, displacement, by site
- knee S83.106
  - cap —*see* Dislocation, patella
  - congenital Q68.2
  - old M23.8X-
  - patella —*see* Dislocation, patella
  - pathological —*see* Dislocation, pathological NEC, knee
  - proximal tibia
    - anteriorly S83.11-
    - laterally S83.14-
    - medially S83.13-
    - posteriorly S83.12-
  - recurrent —*see also* Derangement, knee, specified NEC
  - specified type NEC S83.19-
- lacrimal gland H04.16-
- lens (complete) H27.10
  - anterior H27.12-
  - congenital Q12.1
  - ocular implant —*see* Complications, intraocular lens
  - partial H27.11-
  - posterior H27.13-
  - traumatic S05.8X-
- ligament - code by site under Dislocation
- lumbar (vertebra) —*see* Dislocation, vertebra, lumbar
- lumbosacral (vertebra) —*see also* Dislocation, vertebra, lumbar
  - congenital Q76.49
- mandible S03.0-
- meniscus (knee) —*see* Tear, meniscus
  - other sites - code by site under Dislocation
- metacarpal (bone)
  - distal end —*see* Dislocation, finger
  - proximal end S63.06-
- metacarpophalangeal (joint)
  - finger S63.26-
    - index S63.26-
    - little S63.26-
    - middle S63.26-
    - ring S63.26-
  - thumb S63.11-
- metatarsal (bone) —*see* Dislocation, foot
- metatarsophalangeal (joint(s)) —*see* Dislocation, toe
- midcarpal (joint) S63.03-
- midtarsal (joint) —*see* Dislocation, foot
- neck S13.20
  - specified site NEC S13.29
  - vertebra —*see* Dislocation, vertebra, cervical
- nose (septal cartilage) S03.1

Dislocation *(continued)*
- occipitoatloid S13.111
- old —*see* Derangement, joint, specified type NEC
- ossicles, ear —*see* Discontinuity, ossicles, ear
- partial —*see* Subluxation, by site
- patella S83.006
  - congenital Q74.1
  - lateral S83.01-
  - recurrent (nontraumatic) M22.0-
    - incomplete M22.1-
  - specified type NEC S83.09-
- pathological NEC M24.30
  - ankle M24.37-
  - elbow M24.32-
  - foot joint M24.37-
  - hand joint M24.34-
  - hip M24.35-
  - knee M24.36-
  - lumbosacral joint —*see* subcategory M53.2
  - pelvic region —*see* Dislocation, pathological, hip
  - sacroiliac —*see* subcategory M53.2
  - shoulder M24.31-
  - specified site NEC M24.39
  - wrist M24.33-
- pelvis NEC S33.30
  - specified NEC S33.39
- phalanx
  - finger or hand —*see* Dislocation, finger
  - foot or toe —*see* Dislocation, toe
- prosthesis, internal —*see* Complications, prosthetic device, by site, mechanical
- radial head S53.006
  - anterior S53.01-
  - posterior S53.02-
  - specified type NEC S53.09-
- radiocarpal (joint) S63.02-
- radiohumeral (joint) —*see* Dislocation, radial head
- radioulnar (joint)
  - distal S63.01-
  - proximal —*see* Dislocation, elbow
- radius
  - distal end —*see* Dislocation, wrist
  - proximal end —*see* Dislocation, radial head
- recurrent M24.40
  - ankle M24.47-
  - elbow M24.42-
  - finger M24.44-
  - foot joint M24.47-
  - hand joint M24.44-
  - hip M24.45-
  - knee M24.46-
    - patella —*see* Dislocation, patella, recurrent
  - patella —*see* Dislocation, patella, recurrent
  - sacroiliac —*see* subcategory M53.2
  - shoulder M24.41-
  - specified site NEC M24.49
  - toe M24.47-
  - vertebra (*see also* subcategory) M43.5
    - atlantoaxial M43.4
      - with myelopathy M43.3
  - wrist M24.43-
- rib (cartilage) S23.29
- sacrococcygeal S33.2
- sacroiliac (joint) (ligament) S33.2
  - congenital Q74.2
  - recurrent M53.2

Dislocation *(continued)*
- sacrum S33.2
- scaphoid (bone) (hand) (wrist) —*see* Dislocation, wrist
  - foot —*see* Dislocation, foot
- scapula —*see* Dislocation, shoulder, girdle, scapula
- semilunar cartilage, knee —*see* Tear, meniscus
- septal cartilage (nose) S03.1
- septum (nasal) (old) J34.2
- sesamoid bone - code by site under Dislocation
- shoulder (blade) (ligament) (joint) (traumatic) S43.006
  - acromioclavicular —*see* Dislocation, acromioclavicular
  - chronic —*see* Dislocation, recurrent, shoulder
  - congenital Q68.8
  - girdle S43.30-
    - scapula S43.31-
    - specified site NEC S43.39-
  - humerus S43.00-
    - anterior S43.01-
    - inferior S43.03-
    - posterior S43.02-
  - pathological —*see* Dislocation, pathological NEC, shoulder
  - recurrent —*see* Dislocation, recurrent, shoulder
  - specified type NEC S43.08-
- spine
  - cervical —*see* Dislocation, vertebra, cervical
  - congenital Q76.49
  - due to birth trauma P11.5
  - lumbar —*see* Dislocation, vertebra, lumbar
  - thoracic —*see* Dislocation, vertebra, thoracic
- spontaneous —*see* Dislocation, pathological
- sternoclavicular (joint) S43.206
  - anterior S43.21-
  - posterior S43.22-
- sternum S23.29
- subglenoid —*see* Dislocation, shoulder
- symphysis pubis S33.4
- talus —*see* Dislocation, ankle
- tarsal (bone(s)) (joint(s)) —*see* Dislocation, foot
- tarsometatarsal (joint(s)) —*see* Dislocation, foot
- temporomandibular (joint) S03.0-
- thigh, proximal end —*see* Dislocation, hip
- thorax S23.20
  - specified site NEC S23.29
  - vertebra —*see* Dislocation, vertebra
- thumb S63.10-
  - interphalangeal joint —*see* Dislocation, interphalangeal (joint), thumb
  - metacarpophalangeal joint —*see* Dislocation, metacarpophalangeal (joint), thumb
- thyroid cartilage S13.29
- tibia
  - distal end —*see* Dislocation, ankle
  - proximal end —*see* Dislocation, knee
- tibiofibular (joint)
  - distal —*see* Dislocation, ankle
  - superior —*see* Dislocation, knee

Dislocation *(continued)*
- toe(s) S93.106
  - great S93.10-
    - interphalangeal joint S93.11-
    - metatarsophalangeal joint S93.12-
  - interphalangeal joint S93.119
  - lesser S93.106
    - interphalangeal joint S93.11-
    - metatarsophalangeal joint S93.12-
  - metatarsophalangeal joint S93.12-
- tooth S03.2
- trachea S23.29
- ulna
  - distal end S63.07-
  - proximal end —*see* Dislocation, elbow
- ulnohumeral (joint) —*see* Dislocation, elbow
- vertebra (articular process) (body) (traumatic)
  - cervical S13.101
    - atlantoaxial joint S13.121
    - atlantooccipital joint S13.111
    - atloidooccipital joint S13.111
    - joint between
      - C0 and C1 S13.111
      - C1 and C2 S13.121
      - C2 and C3 S13.131
      - C3 and C4 S13.141
      - C4 and C5 S13.151
      - C5and C6 S13.161
      - C6and C7 S13.171
      - C7and T1 S13.181
    - occipitoatloid joint S13.111
  - congenital Q76.49
  - lumbar S33.101
    - joint between
      - L1and L2 S33.111
      - L2and L3 S33.121
      - L3 and L4 S33.131
      - L4and L5 S33.141
  - nontraumatic —*see* Displacement, intervertebral disc
  - partial —*see* Subluxation, by site
  - recurrent NEC —*see* subcategory M43.5
  - thoracic S23.101
    - joint between
      - T1 and T2 S23.111
      - T2 and T3 S23.121
      - T3 and T4 S23.123
      - T4 and T5 S23.131
      - T5 and T6 S23.133
      - T6 and T7 S23.141
      - T7 and T8 S23.143
      - T8 and T9 S23.151
      - T9 and T10 S23.153
      - T10 and T11 S23.161
      - T11 and T12 S23.163
      - T12 and L1 S23.171
- wrist (carpal bone) S63.006
  - carpometacarpal joint —*see* Dislocation, carpometacarpal (joint)
  - distal radioulnar joint —*see* Dislocation, radioulnar (joint), distal
  - metacarpal bone, proximal —*see* Dislocation, metacarpal (bone), proximal end
  - midcarpal —*see* Dislocation, midcarpal (joint)
  - radiocarpal joint —*see* Dislocation, radiocarpal (joint)
  - recurrent —*see* Dislocation, recurrent, wrist

Dislocation *(continued)*
- wrist *(continued)*
  - specified site NEC S63.09-
  - ulna —*see* Dislocation, ulna, distal end
- xiphoid cartilage S23.29

Disorder (of) —*see also* Disease
- acantholytic L11.9
  - specified NEC L11.8
- acute
  - psychotic —*see* Psychosis, acute
  - stress F43.0
- adjustment (grief) F43.20
  - with
    - anxiety F43.22
      - with depressed mood F43.23
    - conduct disturbance F43.24
      - with emotional disturbance F43.25
    - depressed mood F43.21
      - with anxiety F43.23
    - other specified symptom F43.29
- adrenal (capsule) (gland) (medullary) E27.9
  - specified NEC E27.8
- adrenogenital E25.9
  - drug-induced E25.8
  - iatrogenic E25.8
  - idiopathic E25.8
- adult personality (and behavior) F69
  - specified NEC F68.8
- affective (mood) —*see* Disorder, mood
- aggressive, unsocialized F91.1
- alcohol-related F10.99
  - with
    - amnestic disorder, persisting F10.96
    - anxiety disorder F10.980
    - dementia, persisting F10.97
    - intoxication F10.929
      - with delirium F10.921
      - uncomplicated F10.920
    - mood disorder F10.94
    - other specified F10.988
    - psychotic disorder F10.959
      - with
        - delusions F10.950
        - hallucinations F10.951
    - sexual dysfunction F10.981
    - sleep disorder F10.982
- alcohol use
  - mild F10.10
    - with
      - alcohol-induced
        - anxiety disorder F10.180
        - bipolar and related disorder F10.14
        - depressive disorder F10.14
        - psychotic disorder F10.159
        - sexual dysfunction F10.181
        - sleep disorder F10.182
      - alcohol intoxication F10.129
        - delirium F10.121
    - in remission (early) (sustained) F10.11

Disorder *(continued)*
- alcohol use *(continued)*
  - moderate or severe F10.20
    - with
      - alcohol-induced
        - anxiety disorder F10.280
        - bipolar and related disorder F10.24
        - depressive disorder F10.24
        - major neurocognitive disorder, amnestic-confabulatory type F10.26
        - major neurocognitive disorder, nonamnestic-confabulatory type F10.27
        - mild neurocognitive disorder F10.288
        - psychotic disorder F10.259
        - sexual dysfunction F10.281
        - sleep disorder F10.282
      - alcohol intoxication F10.229
        - delirium F10.221
    - in remission (early) (sustained) F10.21
- allergic —*see* Allergy
- alveolar NEC J84.09
- amino-acid
  - cystathioninuria E72.19
  - cystinosis E72.04
  - cystinuria E72.01
  - glycinuria E72.09
  - homocystinuria E72.11
  - metabolism —*see* Disturbance, metabolism, amino-acid
    - specified NEC E72.89
  - neonatal, transitory P74.8
  - renal transport NEC E72.09
  - transport NEC E72.09
- amnesic, amnestic
  - alcohol-induced F10.96
    - with dependence F10.26
  - due to (secondary to) general medical condition F04
  - psychoactive NEC-induced F19.96
    - with
      - abuse F19.16
      - dependence F19.26
  - sedative, hypnotic or anxiolytic-induced F13.96
    - with dependence F13.26
- amphetamine-type substance use
  - mild F15.10
    - in remission (early) (sustained) F15.11
  - moderate F15.20
    - in remission (early) (sustained) F15.21
  - severe 15.20
    - in remission (early) (sustained) F15.21
- use
  - mild F15.10
    - with
      - amphetamine (or other stimulant) -induced
        - anxiety disorder F15.180
        - bipolar and related disorder F15.14
        - depressive disorder F15.14
        - obsessive-compulsive and related disorder F15.188

Disorder *(continued)*
- use *(continued)*
  - mild *(continued)*
    - with *(continued)*
      - amphetamine *(continued)*
        - psychotic disorder F15.159
        - sexual dysfunction F15.181
      - amphetamine, cocaine, or other stimulant intoxication
        - with perceptual disturbances F15.122
        - without perceptual disturbances F15.129
      - intoxication delirium F15.121
    - in remission (early) (sustained) F15.11
  - moderate or severe
    - with
      - amphetamine (or other stimulant) -induced
        - anxiety disorder F15.280
        - bipolar and related disorder F15.14
        - depressive disorder F15.24
        - obsessive-compulsive and related disorder F15.288
        - psychotic disorder F15.259
        - sexual dysfunction F15.281
      - amphetamine, cocaine, or other stimulant intoxication
        - with perceptual disturbances F15.222
        - without perceptual disturbances F15.229
      - intoxication delirium F15.221
- anaerobic glycolysis with anemia D55.29
- anxiety F41.9
  - due to (secondary to)
    - alcohol F10.980
      - in
        - abuse F10.980
        - dependence F10.280
    - amphetamine F15.980
      - in
        - abuse F15.180
        - dependence F15.280
    - anxiolytic F13.980
      - in
        - abuse F13.180
        - dependence F13.280
    - caffeine F15.980
      - in
        - abuse F15.180
        - dependence F15.280
    - cannabis F12.980
      - in
        - abuse F12.180
        - dependence F12.280
    - cocaine F14.980
      - in
        - abuse F14.180
        - dependence F14.180
    - general medical condition F06.4
    - hallucinogen F16.980
      - in
        - abuse F16.180
        - dependence F16.280

Disorder *(continued)*
- anxiety *(continued)*
  - due to *(continued)*
    - hypnotic F13.980
      - in
        - abuse F13.180
        - dependence F13.280
    - inhalant F18.980
      - in
        - abuse F18.180
        - dependence F18.280
    - phencyclidine F16.980
      - in
        - abuse F16.180
        - dependence F16.280
    - psychoactive substance NEC F19.980
      - in
        - abuse F19.180
        - dependence F19.280
    - sedative F13.980
      - in
        - abuse F13.180
        - dependence F13.280
    - volatile solvents F18.980
      - in
        - abuse F18.180
        - dependence F18.280
  - generalized F41.1
  - illness F45.21
  - mixed
    - with depression (mild) F41.8
    - specified NEC F41.3
  - organic F06.4
  - phobic F40.9
    - of childhood F40.8
  - specified NEC F41.8
- aortic valve —*see* Endocarditis, aortic
- aromatic amino-acid metabolism E70.9
  - specified NEC E70.89
- arteriole NEC I77.89
- artery NEC I77.89
- articulation —*see* Disorder, joint
- attachment (childhood)
  - disinhibited F94.2
  - reactive F94.1
- attention-deficit hyperactivity (adolescent) (adult) (child) F90.0
  - combined
    - presentation F90.2
    - type F90.2
  - hyperactive
    - impulsive presentation F90.1
    - type F90.1
  - inattentive
    - presentation F90.0
    - type F90.0
  - specified type NEC F90.8
- attention-deficit without hyperactivity (adolescent) (adult) (child) F98.8
- auditory processing (central) H93.25
- autistic F84.0
- autoimmune D89.89
- autonomic nervous system G90.9
  - specified NEC G90.8
- autism spectrum F84.0
- avoidant
  - child or adolescent F40.10
  - restrictive food intake F50.82
- balance
  - acid-base E87.8
    - mixed E87.4
  - electrolyte E87.8
  - fluid NEC E87.8
- behavioral (disruptive) —*see* Disorder, conduct

Disorder *(continued)*
- beta-amino-acid metabolism E72.89
- bile acid and cholesterol metabolism E78.70
  - Barth syndrome E78.71
  - other specified E78.79
  - Smith-Lemli-Opitz syndrome E78.72
- bilirubin excretion E80.6
- binge eating F50.81
- binocular
  - movement H51.9
    - convergence
      - excess H51.12
      - insufficiency H51.11
    - internuclear ophthalmoplegia —*see* Ophthalmoplegia, internuclear
    - palsy of conjugate gaze H51.0
    - specified type NEC H51.8
  - vision NEC —*see* Disorder, vision, binocular
- bipolar (I) (type 1) F31.9
  - and related due to a known physiological condition
    - with
      - manic features F06.33
      - manic- or hypomanic-like episodes F06.33
      - mixed features F06.34
  - current (or most recent) episode
    - depressed F31.9
      - with psychotic features F31.5
      - without psychotic features F31.30
        - mild F31.31
        - moderate F31.32
        - severe (without psychotic features) F31.4
          - with psychotic features F31.5
    - hypomanic F31.0
    - manic F31.9
      - with psychotic features F31.2
      - without psychotic features F31.10
        - mild F31.11
        - moderate F31.12
        - severe (without psychotic features) F31.13
          - with psychotic features F31.2
    - mixed F31.60
      - mild F31.61
      - moderate F31.62
      - severe (without psychotic features) F31.63
        - with psychotic features F31.64
    - severe depression (without psychotic features) F31.4
      - with psychotic features F31.5
  - in remission (currently) F31.70
    - in full remission
      - most recent episode
        - depressed F31.76
        - hypomanic F31.72
        - manic F31.74
        - mixed F31.78
    - in partial remission
      - most recent episode
        - depressed F31.75
        - hypomanic F31.71
        - manic F31.73
        - mixed F31.77

- **Disorder** *(continued)*
  - bipolar *(continued)*
    - specified NEC F31.89
    - II (type 2) F31.81
    - organic F06.30
    - single manic episode F30.9
      - mild F30.11
      - moderate F30.12
      - severe (without psychotic symptoms) F30.13
        - with psychotic symptoms F30.2
  - bladder N32.9
    - functional NEC N31.9
    - in schistosomiasis B65.0 *[N33]*
    - specified NEC N32.89
  - bleeding D68.9
  - blood D75.9
    - in congenital early syphilis A50.09 *[D77]*
  - body dysmorphic F45.22
  - bone M89.9
    - continuity M84.9
      - specified type NEC M84.80
        - ankle M84.87-
        - fibula M84.86-
        - foot M84.87-
        - hand M84.84-
        - humerus M84.82-
        - neck M84.88
        - pelvis M84.859
        - radius M84.83-
        - rib M84.88
        - shoulder M84.81-
        - skull M84.88
        - thigh M84.85-
        - tibia M84.86-
        - ulna M84.83-
        - vertebra M84.88
    - density and structure M85.9
      - cyst *—see also* Cyst, bone, specified type NEC
        - aneurysmal *—see* Cyst, bone, aneurysmal
        - solitary *—see* Cyst, bone, solitary
      - diffuse idiopathic skeletal hyperostosis *—see* Hyperostosis, ankylosing
      - fibrous dysplasia (monostotic) *—see* Dysplasia, fibrous, bone
      - fluorosis *—see* Fluorosis, skeletal
      - hyperostosis of skull M85.2
      - osteitis condensans *—see* Osteitis, condensans
      - specified type NEC M85.8-
        - ankle M85.87-
        - foot M85.87-
        - forearm M85.83-
        - hand M85.84-
        - lower leg M85.86-
        - multiple sites M85.89
        - neck M85.88
        - rib M85.88
        - shoulder M85.81-
        - skull M85.88
        - thigh M85.85-
        - upper arm M85.82-
        - vertebra M85.88
    - development and growth NEC M89.20
      - carpus M89.24-
      - clavicle M89.21-
      - femur M89.25-
      - fibula M89.26-
      - finger M89.24-
      - humerus M89.22-
      - ilium M89.259
      - ischium M89.259

- **Disorder** *(continued)*
  - bone *(continued)*
    - development and growth NEC *(continued)*
      - metacarpus M89.24-
      - metatarsus M89.27-
      - multiple sites M89.29
      - neck M89.28
      - radius M89.23-
      - rib M89.28
      - scapula M89.21-
      - skull M89.28
      - tarsus M89.27-
      - tibia M89.26-
      - toe M89.27-
      - ulna M89.23-
      - vertebra M89.28
    - specified type NEC M89.8X-
  - brachial plexus G54.0
  - branched-chain amino-acid metabolism E71.2
    - specified NEC E71.19
  - breast N64.9
    - agalactia *—see* Agalactia
    - associated with
      - lactation O92.70
        - specified NEC O92.79
      - pregnancy O92.20
        - specified NEC O92.29
      - puerperium O92.20
        - specified NEC O92.29
    - cracked nipple *—see* Cracked nipple
    - galactorrhea *—see* Galactorrhea
    - hypogalactia O92.4
    - lactation disorder NEC O92.79
    - mastitis *—see* Mastitis
    - nipple infection *—see* Infection, nipple
    - retracted nipple *—see* Retraction, nipple
    - specified type NEC N64.89
  - Briquet's F45.0
  - bullous, in diseases classified elsewhere L14
  - caffeine use
    - mild
      - with
        - caffeine-induced
          - anxiety disorder F15.180
          - sleep disorder F15.182
    - moderate or severe
      - with
        - caffeine-induced
          - anxiety disorder F15.280
          - sleep disorder F15.282
  - cannabis use
    - mild F12.10
      - with
        - cannabis-induced
          - anxiety disorder F12.180
          - psychotic disorder F12.159
          - sleep disorder F12.188
        - cannabis intoxication
          - delirium F12.121
          - with perceptual disturbances F12.122
          - without perceptual disturbances F12.129
      - in remission (early) (sustained) F12.11
    - moderate or severe F12.20
      - with
        - cannabis-induced
          - anxiety disorder F12.280
          - psychotic disorder F12.259
          - sleep disorder F12.288
        - cannabis intoxication
          - with perceptual disturbances F12.222
          - without perceptual disturbances F12.229

- **Disorder** *(continued)*
  - cannabis use *(continued)*
    - moderate or severe *(continued)*
      - with *(continued)*
        - delirium F12.221
      - in remission (early) (sustained) F12.21
  - carbohydrate
    - absorption, intestinal NEC E74.39
    - metabolism (congenital) E74.9
      - specified NEC E74.89
  - cardiac, functional I51.89
  - carnitine metabolism E71.40
  - cartilage M94.9
    - articular NEC *—see* Derangement, joint, articular cartilage
      - chondrocalcinosis *—see* Chondrocalcinosis
    - specified type NEC M94.8X-
      - articular *—see* Derangement, joint, articular cartilage
      - multiple sites M94.8X0
  - catatonia (due to known physiological condition) (with another mental disorder) F06.1
  - catatonic
    - due to (secondary to) known physiological condition F06.1
    - organic F06.1
  - central auditory processing H93.25
  - cervical
    - region NEC M53.82
    - root (nerve) NEC G54.2
  - character NOS F60.9
  - childhood disintegrative NEC F84.3
  - cholesterol and bile acid metabolism E78.70
    - Barth syndrome E78.71
    - other specified E78.79
    - Smith-Lemli-Opitz syndrome E78.72
  - choroid H31.9
    - atrophy *—see* Atrophy, choroid
    - degeneration *—see* Degeneration, choroid
    - detachment *—see* Detachment, choroid
    - dystrophy *—see* Dystrophy, choroid
    - hemorrhage *—see* Hemorrhage, choroid
    - rupture *—see* Rupture, choroid
    - scar *—see* Scar, chorioretinal
    - solar retinopathy *—see* Retinopathy, solar
    - specified type NEC H31.8
  - ciliary body *—see* Disorder, iris
    - degeneration *—see* Degeneration, ciliary body
  - coagulation (factor) *(see also* Defect, coagulation) D68.9
    - newborn, transient P61.6
  - cocaine use
    - mild F14.10
      - with
        - amphetamine, cocaine, or other stimulant intoxication
          - with perceptual disturbances F14.122
          - without perceptual disturbances F14.129
        - cocaine-induced
          - anxiety disorder F14.180
          - bipolar and related disorder F14.14
          - depressive disorder F14.14

- **Disorder** *(continued)*
  - cocaine use *(continued)*
    - mild *(continued)*
      - with *(continued)*
        - cocaine-induced *(continued)*
          - obsessive-compulsive and related disorder F14.188
          - psychotic disorder F14.159
          - sexual dysfunction F14.181
          - sleep disorder F14.182
        - cocaine intoxication
          - delirium F14.121
      - in remission (early) (sustained) F14.11
    - moderate or severe
      - with
        - amphetamine, cocaine, or other stimulant intoxication
          - with perceptual disturbances F14.222
          - without perceptual disturbances F14.229
        - cocaine-induced
          - anxiety disorder F14.280
          - bipolar and related disorder F14.24
          - depressive disorder F14.24
          - obsessive-compulsive and related disorder F14.288
          - psychotic disorder F14.259
          - sexual dysfunction F14.281
          - sleep disorder F14.282
        - cocaine intoxication
          - delirium F14.221
      - in remission (early) (sustained) F14.21
  - coccyx NEC M53.3
  - cognitive F09
    - due to (secondary to) general medical condition F09
    - persisting R41.89
      - due to
        - alcohol F10.97
          - with dependence F10.27
        - anxiolytics F13.97
          - with dependence F13.27
        - hypnotics F13.97
          - with dependence F13.27
        - sedatives F13.97
          - with dependence F13.27
        - specified substance NEC F19.97
          - with
            - abuse F19.17
            - dependence F19.27
  - communication F80.9
    - social pragmatic F80.82
  - conduct (childhood) F91.9
    - adjustment reaction *—see* Disorder, adjustment
    - adolescent onset type F91.2
    - childhood onset type F91.1
    - compulsive F63.9
    - confined to family context F91.0
    - depressive F91.8
    - group type F91.2
    - hyperkinetic *—see* Disorder, attention-deficit hyperactivity
    - oppositional defiance F91.3
    - socialized F91.2
    - solitary aggressive type F91.1
    - specified NEC F91.8
    - unsocialized (aggressive) F91.1
  - conduction, heart I45.9

Disorder *(continued)*
- congenital glycosylation (CDG) E74.89
- conjunctiva H11.9
  - infection *—see* Conjunctivitis
- connective tissue, localized L94.9
  - specified NEC L94.8
- conversion (functional neurological symptom disorder)
  - with
    - abnormal movement F44.4
    - anesthesia or sensory loss F44.6
    - attacks or seizures F44.5
    - mixed symptoms F44.7
    - special sensory symptoms F44.6
    - speech symptoms F44.4
    - swallowing symptoms F44.4
    - weakness or paralysis F44.4
- convulsive (secondary) *—see* Convulsions
- cornea H18.9
  - deformity *—see* Deformity, cornea
  - degeneration *—see* Degeneration, cornea
  - deposits *—see* Deposit, cornea
  - due to contact lens H18.82-
    - specified as edema *—see* Edema, cornea
  - edema *—see* Edema, cornea
  - keratitis *—see* Keratitis
  - keratoconjunctivitis *—see* Keratoconjunctivitis
  - membrane change *—see* Change, corneal membrane
  - neovascularization *—see* Neovascularization, cornea
  - scar *—see* Opacity, cornea
  - specified type NEC H18.89-
  - ulcer *—see* Ulcer, cornea
- corpus cavernosum N48.9
- cranial nerve *—see* Disorder, nerve, cranial
- Cyclin-Dependent Kinase-Like 5 Deficiency (CDKL5) G40.42
- cyclothymic F34.0
- defiant oppositional F91.3
- delusional (persistent) (systematized) F22
  - induced F24
- depersonalization F48.1
- depressive F32.A
  - due to known physiological condition
  - with
    - depressive features F06.31
    - major depressive-like episode F06.32
    - mixed features F06.34
  - major F32.9
    - with psychotic symptoms F32.3
    - in remission (full) F32.5
      - partial F32.4
    - recurrent F33.9
      - with psychotic features F33.3
    - single episode F32.9
      - mild F32.0
      - moderate F32.1
      - severe (without psychotic symptoms) F32.2
        - with psychotic symptoms F32.3
  - organic F06.31
  - persistent F34.1
  - recurrent F33.9
    - current episode
      - mild F33.0

Disorder *(continued)*
- depressive *(continued)*
  - recurrent *(continued)*
    - current episode *(continued)*
      - moderate F33.1
      - severe (without psychotic symptoms) F33.2
        - with psychotic symptoms F33.3
    - in remission F33.40
      - full F33.42
      - partial F33.41
    - specified NEC F33.8
  - single episode *—see* Episode, depressive
  - specified NEC F32.89
- developmental F89
  - arithmetical skills F81.2
  - coordination (motor) F82
  - expressive writing F81.81
  - language F80.9
    - expressive F80.1
    - mixed receptive and expressive F80.2
    - receptive type F80.2
    - specified NEC F80.89
  - learning F81.9
    - arithmetical F81.2
    - reading F81.0
  - mixed F88
  - motor coordination or function F82
  - pervasive F84.9
    - specified NEC F84.8
  - phonological F80.0
  - reading F81.0
  - scholastic skills *—see also* Disorder, learning
    - mixed F81.89
  - specified NEC F88
  - speech F80.9
    - articulation F80.0
    - specified NEC F80.89
  - written expression F81.81
- diaphragm J98.6
- digestive (system) K92.9
  - newborn P78.9
    - specified NEC P78.89
  - postprocedural *—see* Complication, gastrointestinal
  - psychogenic F45.8
- disc (intervertebral) M51.9
  - with
    - myelopathy
      - cervical region M50.00
      - cervicothoracic region M50.03
      - high cervical region M50.01
      - lumbar region M51.06
      - mid-cervical region M50.020
      - sacrococcygeal region M53.3
      - thoracic region M51.04
      - thoracolumbar region M51.05
    - radiculopathy
      - cervical region M50.10
      - cervicothoracic region M50.13
      - high cervical region M50.11
      - lumbar region M51.16
      - lumbosacral region M51.17
      - mid-cervical region M50.120
      - sacrococcygeal region M53.3
      - thoracic region M51.14
      - thoracolumbar region M51.15

Disorder *(continued)*
- disc *(continued)*
  - cervical M50.90
    - with
      - myelopathy M50.00
        - C2-C3 M50.01
        - C3-C4 M50.01
        - C4-C5 M50.021
        - C5-C6 M50.022
        - C6-C7 M50.023
        - C7-T1 M50.03
        - cervicothoracic region M50.03
        - high cervical region M50.01
        - mid-cervical region M50.020
      - neuritis, radiculitis or radiculopathy M50.10
        - C2-C3 M50.11
        - C3-C4 M50.11
        - C4-C5 M50.121
        - C5-C6 M50.122
        - C6-C7 M50.123
        - C7-T1 M50.13
        - cervicothoracic region M50.13
        - high cervical region M50.11
        - mid-cervical region M50.120
    - C2-C3 M50.91
    - C3-C4 M50.91
    - C4-C5 M50.921
    - C5-C6 M50.922
    - C6-C7 M50.923
    - C7-T1 M50.93
    - cervicothoracic region M50.93
    - degeneration M50.30
      - C2-C3 M50.31
      - C3-C4 M50.31
      - C4-C5 M50.321
      - C5-C6 M50.322
      - C6-C7 M50.323
      - C7-T1 M50.33
      - cervicothoracic region M50.33
      - high cervical region M50.31
      - mid-cervical region M50.320
    - displacement M50.20
      - C2-C3 M50.21
      - C3-C4 M50.21
      - C4-C5 M50.221
      - C5-C6 M50.222
      - C6-C7 M50.223
      - C7-T1 M50.23
      - cervicothoracic region M50.23
      - high cervical region M50.21
      - mid-cervical region M50.220
    - high cervical region M50.91
    - mid-cervical region M50.920
    - specified type NEC M50.80
      - C2-C3 M50.81
      - C3-C4 M50.81
      - C4-C5 M50.821
      - C5-C6 M50.822
      - C6-C7 M50.823
      - C7-T1 M50.83
      - cervicothoracic region M50.83
      - high cervical region M50.81
      - mid-cervical region M50.820
  - specified NEC
    - lumbar region M51.86
    - lumbosacral region M51.87
    - sacrococcygeal region M53.3
    - thoracic region M51.84
    - thoracolumbar region M51.85

Disorder *(continued)*
- disinhibited attachment (childhood) F94.2
- disintegrative, childhood NEC F84.3
- disruptive F91.9
  - mood dysregulation F34.81
  - specified NEC F91.8
- disruptive behavior *—see* Disorder, conduct
- dissocial personality F60.2
- dissociative F44.9
  - affecting
    - motor function F44.4
      - and sensation F44.7
    - sensation F44.6
      - and motor function F44.7
  - brief reactive F43.0
  - due to (secondary to) general medical condition F06.8
  - mixed F44.7
  - organic F06.8
  - other specified NEC F44.89
- double heterozygous sickling *—see* Disease, sickle-cell
- dream anxiety F51.5
- drug induced hemorrhagic D68.32
- drug related F19.99
  - abuse *—see* Abuse, drug
  - dependence *—see* Dependence, drug
- dysmorphic body F45.22
- dysthymic F34.1
- ear H93.9-
  - bleeding *—see* Otorrhagia
  - deafness *—see* Deafness
  - degenerative H93.09-
  - discharge *—see* Otorrhea
  - external H61.9-
    - auditory canal stenosis *—see* Stenosis, external ear canal
    - exostosis *—see* Exostosis, external ear canal
    - impacted cerumen *—see* Impaction, cerumen
    - otitis *—see* Otitis, externa
    - perichondritis *—see* Perichondritis, ear
    - pinna *—see* Disorder, pinna
    - specified type NEC H61.89-
      - in diseases classified elsewhere H62.8X-
  - inner H83.9-
    - vestibular dysfunction *—see* Disorder, vestibular function
  - middle H74.9-
    - adhesive H74.1-
    - ossicle *—see* Abnormal, ear ossicles
    - polyp *—see* Polyp, ear (middle)
    - specified NEC, in diseases classified elsewhere H75.8-
  - postprocedural *—see* Complications, ear, procedure
  - specified NEC, in diseases classified elsewhere H94.8-
- eating (adult) (psychogenic) F50.9
  - anorexia *—see* Anorexia
  - binge F50.81
  - bulimia F50.2
  - child F98.29
    - pica F98.3
    - rumination disorder F98.21
  - pica F50.89
    - childhood F98.3

Disorder *(continued)*
- electrolyte (balance) NEC E87.8
  - with
    - abortion —*see* Abortion by type complicated by specified condition NEC
    - ectopic pregnancy O08.5
    - molar pregnancy O08.5
  - acidosis (metabolic) (respiratory) E87.2
  - alkalosis (metabolic) (respiratory) E87.3
- elimination, transepidermal L87.9
  - specified NEC L87.8
- emotional (persistent) F34.9
  - of childhood F93.9
    - specified NEC F93.8
- endocrine E34.9
  - postprocedural E89.89
    - specified NEC E89.89
- erectile (male) (organic) (*see also* Dysfunction, sexual, male, erectile) N52.9
  - nonorganic F52.21
- erythematous —*see* Erythema
- esophagus K22.9
  - functional K22.4
  - psychogenic F45.8
- eustachian tube H69.9-
  - infection —*see* Salpingitis, eustachian
  - obstruction —*see* Obstruction, eustachian tube
  - patulous —*see* Patulous, eustachian tube
  - specified NEC H69.8-
- exhibitionistic F65.2
- extrapyramidal G25.9
  - in diseases classified elsewhere —*see* category G26
  - specified type NEC G25.89
- eye H57.9
  - postprocedural —*see* Complication, postprocedural, eye
- eyelid H02.9
  - cyst —*see* Cyst, eyelid
  - degenerative H02.70
    - chloasma —*see* Chloasma, eyelid
    - madarosis —*see* Madarosis
    - specified type NEC H02.79
    - vitiligo —*see* Vitiligo, eyelid
    - xanthelasma —*see* Xanthelasma
  - dermatochalasis —*see* Dermatochalasis
  - edema —*see* Edema, eyelid
  - elephantiasis —*see* Elephantiasis, eyelid
  - foreign body, retained —*see* Foreign body, retained, eyelid
  - function H02.59
    - abnormal innervation syndrome —*see* Syndrome, abnormal innervation
    - blepharochalasis —*see* Blepharochalasis
    - blepharoclonus —*see* Blepharoclonus
    - blepharophimosis —*see* Blepharophimosis
    - blepharoptosis —*see* Blepharoptosis
    - lagophthalmos —*see* Lagophthalmos
    - lid retraction —*see* Retraction, lid
  - hypertrichosis —*see* Hypertrichosis, eyelid
  - specified type NEC H02.89

Disorder *(continued)*
- eyelid *(continued)*
  - vascular H02.879
    - left H02.876
      - lower H02.875
      - upper H02.874
    - right H02.873
      - lower H02.872
      - upper H02.871
- factitious
  - by proxy F68.A
  - imposed on another F68.A
  - imposed on self F68.10
    - with predominantly
      - psychological symptoms F68.11
        - with physical symptoms F68.13
      - physical symptoms F68.12
        - with psychological symptoms F68.13
- factor, coagulation —*see* Defect, coagulation
- fatty acid
  - metabolism E71.30
    - specified NEC E71.39
  - oxidation
    - LCAD E71.310
    - MCAD E71.311
    - SCAD E71.312
    - specified deficiency NEC E71.318
- feeding (infant or child) (*see also* Disorder, eating) R63.30
  - or eating disorder F50.9
  - pediatric
    - acute R63.31
    - chronic R63.32
  - specified NEC F50.9
- feigned (with obvious motivation) Z76.5
  - without obvious motivation —*see* Disorder, factitious
- female
  - hypoactive sexual desire F52.0
  - orgasmic F52.31
  - sexual interest/arousal F52.22
- fetishistic F65.0
- fibroblastic M72.9
  - specified NEC M72.8
- fluency
  - adult onset F98.5
  - childhood onset F80.81
  - following
    - cerebral infarction I69.323
    - cerebrovascular disease I69.923
      - specified disease NEC I69.823
    - intracerebral hemorrhage I69.123
    - nontraumatic intracranial hemorrhage NEC I69.223
    - subarachnoid hemorrhage I69.023
  - in conditions classified elsewhere R47.82
- fluid balance E87.8
- follicular (skin) L73.9
  - specified NEC L73.8
- frotteuristic F65.81
- fructose metabolism E74.10
  - essential fructosuria E74.11
  - fructokinase deficiency E74.11
  - fructose-1, 6-diphosphatase deficiency E74.19
  - hereditary fructose intolerance E74.12
  - other specified E74.19
- functional polymorphonuclear neutrophils D71

Disorder *(continued)*
- gallbladder, biliary tract and pancreas in diseases classified elsewhere K87
- gambling F63.0
- gamma aminobutyric acid (GABA) metabolism E72.81
- gamma-glutamyl cycle E72.89
- gastric (functional) K31.9
  - motility K30
  - psychogenic F45.8
  - secretion K30
- gastrointestinal (functional) NOS K92.9
  - newborn P78.9
  - psychogenic F45.8
- gender-identity or -role F64.9
  - childhood F64.2
  - effect on relationship F66
  - of adolescence or adulthood F64.0
    - nontranssexual F64.8
  - specified NEC F64.8
  - uncertainty F66
- genito-pelvic pain penetration F52.6
- genitourinary system
  - female N94.9
  - male N50.9
  - psychogenic F45.8
- globe H44.9
  - degenerated condition H44.50
    - absolute glaucoma H44.51-
    - atrophy H44.52-
    - leucocoria H44.53-
  - degenerative H44.30
    - chalcosis H44.31-
    - myopia (*see also* Myopia, degenerative) H44.2-
    - siderosis H44.32-
    - specified type NEC H44.39-
  - endophthalmitis —*see* Endophthalmitis
  - foreign body, retained —*see* Foreign body, intraocular, old, retained
  - hemophthalmos —*see* Hemophthalmos
  - hypotony H44.40
    - due to
      - ocular fistula H44.42-
      - specified disorder NEC H44.43-
    - flat anterior chamber H44.41-
    - primary H44.44-
  - luxation —*see* Luxation, globe
  - specified type NEC H44.89
- glomerular (in) N05.9
  - amyloidosis E85.4 *[N08]*
  - cryoglobulinemia D89.1 *[N08]*
  - disseminated intravascular coagulation D65 *[N08]*
  - Fabry's disease E75.21 *[N08]*
  - familial lecithin cholesterol acyltransferase deficiency E78.6 *[N08]*
  - Goodpasture's syndrome M31.0
  - hemolytic-uremic syndrome D59.3
  - Henoch (-Schönlein) purpura D69.0 *[N08]*
  - malariae malaria B52.0
  - microscopic polyangiitis M31.7 *[N08]*
  - multiple myeloma C90.0- *[N08]*
  - mumps B26.83
  - schistosomiasis B65.9 *[N08]*
  - sepsis NEC A41.- *[N08]*
    - streptococcal A40.- [N08]
  - sickle-cell disorders D57.- *[N08]*
  - strongyloidiasis B78.9 *[N08]*

Disorder *(continued)*
- glomerular *(continued)*
  - subacute bacterial endocarditis I33.0 *[N08]*
  - syphilis A52.75
  - systemic lupus erythematosus M32.14
  - thrombotic thrombocytopenic purpura M31.19 *[N08]*
  - Waldenström macroglobulinemia C88.0 *[N08]*
  - Wegener's granulomatosis M31.31
- gluconeogenesis E74.4
- glucosaminoglycan metabolism —*see* Disorder, metabolism, glucosaminoglycan
- glucose transport E74.819
  - specified NEC E74.818
- glycine metabolism E72.50
  - d-glycericacidemia E72.59
  - hyperhydroxyprolinemia E72.59
  - hyperoxaluria R82.992
    - primary E72.53
  - hyperprolinemia E72.59
  - non-ketotic hyperglycinemia E72.51
  - oxalosis E72.53
  - oxaluria E72.53
  - sarcosinemia E72.59
  - trimethylaminuria E72.52
- glycoprotein metabolism E77.9
  - specified NEC E77.8
- habit (and impulse) F63.9
  - involving sexual behavior NEC F65.9
  - specified NEC F63.89
- hallucinogen use
  - mild F16.10
    - with
      - hallucinogen-induced
        - anxiety disorder F16.180
        - bipolar and related disorder F16.14
        - depressive disorder F16.14
        - psychotic disorder F16.159
      - hallucinogen intoxication delirium F16.121
      - other hallucinogen intoxication F16.129
    - in remission (early) (sustained) F16.11
  - moderate or severe F16.20
    - with
      - hallucinogen-induced
        - anxiety disorder F16.280
        - bipolar and related disorder F16.24
        - depressive disorder F16.24
        - psychotic disorder F16.259
      - hallucinogen intoxication delirium F16.221
      - other hallucinogen intoxication F16.229
    - in remission (early) (sustained) F16.21
- heart action I49.9
- hematological D75.9
  - newborn (transient) P61.9
    - specified NEC P61.8
- hematopoietic organs D75.9
- hemorrhagic NEC D69.9
  - drug-induced D68.32
  - due to
    - extrinsic circulating anticoagulants D68.32
    - increase in
      - anti-IIa D68.32
      - anti-Xa D68.32

Disorder *(continued)*
- hemorrhagic NEC *(continued)*
  - due to *(continued)*
    - intrinsic
      - circulating anticoagulants D68.318
      - increase in
        - antithrombin D68.318
        - anti-VIIIa D68.318
        - anti-IXa D68.318
        - anti-XIa D68.318
  - following childbirth O72.3
- hemostasis *—see* Defect, coagulation
- histidine metabolism E70.40
  - histidinemia E70.41
  - other specified E70.49
- hoarding F42.3
- hyperkinetic *—see* Disorder, attention-deficit hyperactivity
- hyperleucine-isoleucinemia E71.19
- hypervalinemia E71.19
- hypoactive sexual desire F52.0
- hypochondriacal F45.20
  - body dysmorphic F45.22
  - neurosis F45.21
  - other specified F45.29
- identity
  - dissociative F44.81
  - illness anxiety F45.21
  - of childhood F93.8
- immune mechanism (immunity) D89.9
  - specified type NEC D89.89
- impaired renal tubular function N25.9
  - specified NEC N25.89
- impulse (control) F63.9
- inflammatory
  - pelvic, in diseases classified elsewhere *—see* category N74
  - penis N48.29
    - abscess N48.21
    - cellulitis N48.22
- inhalant use
  - mild F18.10
    - with
      - inhalant-induced
        - anxiety disorder F18.180
        - depressive disorder F18.14
        - major neurocognitive disorder F18.17
        - mild neurocognitive disorder F18.188
        - psychotic disorder F18.159
      - inhalant intoxication F18.129
      - inhalant intoxication delirium F18.121
    - in remission (early) (sustained) F18.11
  - moderate or severe F18.20
    - with
      - inhalant-induced
        - anxiety disorder F18.280
        - depressive disorder F18.24
        - major neurocognitive disorder F18.27
        - mild neurocognitive disorder F18.288
        - psychotic disorder F18.259
      - inhalant intoxication F18.229
      - inhalant intoxication delirium F18.221
    - in remission (early) (sustained) F18.21

Disorder *(continued)*
- integument, newborn P83.9
  - specified NEC P83.88
- intermittent explosive F63.81
- internal secretion pancreas *—see* Increased, secretion, pancreas, endocrine
- intestine, intestinal
  - carbohydrate absorption NEC E74.39
    - postoperative K91.2
  - functional NEC K59.9
    - postoperative K91.89
  - psychogenic F45.8
  - vascular K55.9
    - chronic K55.1
    - specified NEC K55.8
- intraoperative (intraprocedural) *—see* Complications, intraoperative
- involuntary emotional expression (IEED) F48.2
- iris H21.9
  - adhesions *—see* Adhesions, iris
  - atrophy *—see* Atrophy, iris
  - chamber angle recession *—see* Recession, chamber angle
  - cyst *—see* Cyst, iris
  - degeneration *—see* Degeneration, iris
  - in diseases classified elsewhere H22
  - iridodialysis *—see* Iridodialysis
  - iridoschisis *—see* Iridoschisis
  - miotic pupillary cyst *—see* Cyst, pupillary
  - pupillary
    - abnormality *—see* Abnormality, pupillary
    - membrane *—see* Membrane, pupillary
  - specified type NEC H21.89
  - vascular NEC H21.1X-
- iron metabolism E83.10
  - specified NEC E83.19
- isovaleric acidemia E71.110
- jaw, developmental M27.0
  - temporomandibular (*see* Anomaly, dentofacial, temporomandibular joint) M26.60-
- joint M25.9
  - derangement *—see* Derangement, joint
  - effusion *—see* Effusion, joint
  - fistula *—see* Fistula, joint
  - hemarthrosis *—see* Hemarthrosis
  - instability *—see* Instability, joint
  - osteophyte *—see* Osteophyte
  - pain *—see* Pain, joint
  - psychogenic F45.8
  - specified type NEC M25.80
    - ankle M25.87-
    - elbow M25.82-
    - foot joint M25.87-
    - hand joint M25.84-
    - hip M25.85-
    - knee M25.86-
    - shoulder M25.81-
    - wrist M25.83-
  - stiffness *—see* Stiffness, joint
- ketone metabolism E71.32
- kidney N28.9
  - functional (tubular) N25.9
  - in
    - schistosomiasis B65.9 *[N29]*

Disorder *(continued)*
- kidney *(continued)*
  - tubular function N25.9
    - specified NEC N25.89
- lacrimal system H04.9
  - changes H04.69
    - fistula *—see* Fistula, lacrimal
  - gland H04.19
    - atrophy *—see* Atrophy, lacrimal gland
    - cyst *—see* Cyst, lacrimal, gland
    - dacryops *—see* Dacryops
    - dislocation *—see* Dislocation, lacrimal gland
    - dry eye syndrome *—see* Syndrome, dry eye
    - infection *—see* Dacryoadenitis
  - granuloma *—see* Granuloma, lacrimal
  - inflammation *—see* Inflammation, lacrimal
  - obstruction *—see* Obstruction, lacrimal
  - specified NEC H04.89
- lactation NEC O92.79
- language (developmental) F80.9
  - expressive F80.1
  - mixed receptive and expressive F80.2
  - receptive F80.2
- late luteal phase dysphoric N94.89
- learning (specific) F81.9
  - acalculia R48.8
  - alexia R48.0
  - mathematics F81.2
  - reading F81.0
  - specified
    - with impairment in
      - mathematics F81.2
      - reading F81.0
      - written expression F81.81
  - specified NEC F81.89
  - spelling F81.81
  - written expression F81.81
- lens H27.9
  - aphakia *—see* Aphakia
  - cataract *—see* Cataract
  - dislocation *—see* Dislocation, lens
  - specified type NEC H27.8
- ligament M24.20
  - ankle M24.27-
  - attachment, spine *—see* Enthesopathy, spinal
  - elbow M24.22-
  - foot joint M24.27-
  - hand joint M24.24-
  - hip M24.25-
  - knee *—see* Derangement, knee, specified NEC
  - shoulder M24.21-
  - specified site NEC M24.29
  - vertebra M24.28
  - wrist M24.23-
- ligamentous attachments *—see also* Enthesopathy
  - spine *—see* Enthesopathy, spinal
- lipid
  - metabolism, congenital E78.9
  - storage E75.6
    - specified NEC E75.5
- lipoprotein
  - deficiency (familial) E78.6
  - metabolism E78.9
    - specified NEC E78.89
- liver K76.9
  - malarial B54 *[K77]*

Disorder *(continued)*
- low back *—see also* Dorsopathy, specified NEC
- lumbosacral
  - plexus G54.1
  - root (nerve) NEC G54.4
- lung, interstitial, drug-induced J70.4
  - acute J70.2
  - chronic J70.3
  - dabbing (related) U07.0
  - e-cigarette (related) U07.0
  - electronic cigarette (related) U07.0
  - vaping (associated) (device) (product) (related) (use) U07.0
- lymphoproliferative, post-transplant (PTLD) D47.Z1
- lysine and hydroxylysine metabolism E72.3
- male
  - erectile (organic) (*see also* Dysfunction, sexual, male, erectile) N52.9
    - nonorganic F52.21
  - hypoactive sexual desire F52.0
  - orgasmic F52.32
- major neurocognitive *—see* Dementia, in (due to)
- manic F30.9
  - organic F06.33
- mast cell activation *—see* Activation, mast cell
- mastoid *—see also* Disorder, ear, middle
  - postprocedural *—see* Complications, ear, procedure
- meninges, specified type NEC G96.198
- meniscus *—see* Derangement, knee, meniscus
- menopausal N95.9
  - specified NEC N95.8
- menstrual N92.6
  - psychogenic F45.8
  - specified NEC N92.5
- mental (or behavioral) (nonpsychotic) F99
  - due to (secondary to)
    - amphetamine
      - due to drug abuse *—see* Abuse, drug, stimulant
      - due to drug dependence *—see* Dependence, drug, stimulant
    - brain disease, damage and dysfunction F09
    - caffeine use
      - due to drug abuse *—see* Abuse, drug, stimulant
      - due to drug dependence *—see* Dependence, drug, stimulant
    - cannabis use
      - due to drug abuse *—see* Abuse, drug, cannabis
      - due to drug dependence *—see* Dependence, drug, cannabis
    - general medical condition F09
    - sedative or hypnotic use
      - due to drug abuse *—see* Abuse, drug, sedative
      - due to drug dependence *—see* Dependence, drug, sedative
    - tobacco (nicotine) use *—see* Dependence, drug, nicotine

Disorder *(continued)*
- mental *(continued)*
  - following organic brain damage F07.9
    - frontal lobe syndrome F07.0
    - personality change F07.0
    - postconcussional syndrome F07.81
    - specified NEC F07.89
  - infancy, childhood or adolescence F98.9
  - neurotic —*see* Neurosis
  - organic or symptomatic F09
  - presenile, psychotic F03
  - problem NEC
  - psychoneurotic —*see* Neurosis
  - psychotic —*see* Psychosis
  - puerperal F53.0
  - senile, psychotic NEC F03
- metabolic, amino acid, transitory, newborn P74.8
- metabolism NOS E88.9
  - amino-acid E72.9
    - aromatic E70.9
      - albinism —*see* Albinism
      - histidine E70.40
        - histidinemia E70.41
        - other specified E70.49
      - hyperphenylalaninemia E70.1
        - classical phenylketonuria E70.0
      - other specified E70.89
      - tryptophan E70.5
      - tyrosine E70.20
        - hypertyrosinemia E70.21
        - other specified E70.29
    - branched chain E71.2
      - 3-methylglutaconic aciduria E71.111
      - hyperleucine-isoleucinemia E71.19
      - hypervalinemia E71.19
      - isovaleric acidemia E71.110
      - maple syrup urine disease E71.0
      - methylmalonic acidemia E71.120
      - organic aciduria NEC E71.118
      - other specified E71.19
      - proprionate NEC E71.128
      - proprionic acidemia E71.121
    - glycine E72.50
      - d-glycericacidemia E72.59
      - hyperhydroxyprolinemia E72.59
      - hyperoxaluria R82.992
        - primary E72.53
      - hyperprolinemia E72.59
      - non-ketotic hyperglycinemia E72.51
      - other specified E72.59
      - sarcosinemia E72.59
      - trimethylaminuria E72.52
    - hydroxylysine E72.3
    - lysine E72.3
    - ornithine E72.4
    - other specified E72.89
      - beta-amino acid E72.89
      - gamma-glutamyl cycle E72.89
    - straight-chain E72.89
    - sulfur-bearing E72.10
      - homocystinuria E72.11
      - methylenetetrahydrofolate reductase deficiency E72.12
      - other specified E72.19

Disorder *(continued)*
- metabolism NOS *(continued)*
  - bile acid and cholesterol metabolism E78.70
  - bilirubin E80.7
    - specified NEC E80.6
  - calcium E83.50
    - hypercalcemia E83.52
    - hypocalcemia E83.51
    - other specified E83.59
  - carbohydrate E74.9
    - specified NEC E74.89
  - cholesterol and bile acid metabolism E78.70
  - congenital E88.9
  - copper E83.00
    - Wilson's disease E83.01
    - specified type NEC E83.09
  - cystinuria E72.01
  - fructose E74.10
  - galactose E74.20
  - glucosaminoglycan E76.9
    - mucopolysaccharidosis —*see* Mucopolysaccharidosis
    - specified NEC E76.8
  - glutamine E72.89
  - glycine E72.50
  - glycogen storage (hepatorenal) E74.09
  - glycoprotein E77.9
    - specified NEC E77.8
  - glycosaminoglycan E76.9
    - specified NEC E76.8
  - in labor and delivery O75.89
  - iron E83.10
  - isoleucine E71.19
  - leucine E71.19
  - lipoid E78.9
  - lipoprotein E78.9
    - specified NEC E78.89
  - magnesium E83.40
    - hypermagnesemia E83.41
    - hypomagnesemia E83.42
    - other specified E83.49
  - mineral E83.9
    - specified NEC E83.89
  - mitochondrial E88.40
    - MELAS syndrome E88.41
    - MERRF syndrome (myoclonic epilepsy associated with ragged-red fibers) E88.42
    - other specified E88.49
  - ornithine E72.4
  - phosphatases E83.30
  - phosphorus E83.30
    - acid phosphatase deficiency E83.39
    - hypophosphatasia E83.39
    - hypophosphatemia E83.39
      - familial E83.31
    - other specified E83.39
    - pseudovitamin D deficiency E83.32
  - plasma protein NEC E88.09
  - porphyrin —*see* Porphyria
  - postprocedural E89.89
    - specified NEC E89.89
  - purine E79.9
    - specified NEC E79.8
  - pyrimidine E79.9
    - specified NEC E79.8
  - pyruvate E74.4
  - serine E72.89
  - sodium E87.8
  - specified NEC E88.89
  - threonine E72.89
  - valine E71.19
  - zinc E83.2
- methylmalonic acidemia E71.120

Disorder *(continued)*
- micturition NEC (*see also* Difficulty, micturition) R39.198
  - feeling of incomplete emptying R39.14
  - hesitancy R39.11
  - poor stream R39.12
  - psychogenic F45.8
  - split stream R39.13
  - straining R39.16
  - urgency R39.15
- mild neurocognitive G31.84
- mitochondrial metabolism E88.40
- mitral (valve) —*see* Endocarditis, mitral
- mixed
  - anxiety and depressive F41.8
  - of scholastic skills (developmental) F81.89
  - receptive expressive language F80.2
- mood F39
  - bipolar —*see* Disorder, bipolar
  - depressive —*see* Disorder, depressive
  - due to (secondary to)
    - alcohol F10.94
    - amphetamine F15.94
      - in
        - abuse F15.14
        - dependence F15.24
    - anxiolytic F13.94
      - in
        - abuse F13.14
        - dependence F13.24
    - cocaine F14.94
      - in
        - abuse F14.14
        - dependence F14.24
    - general medical condition F06.30
    - hallucinogen F16.94
      - in
        - abuse F16.14
        - dependence F16.24
    - hypnotic F13.94
      - in
        - abuse F13.14
        - dependence F13.24
    - inhalant F18.94
      - in
        - abuse F18.14
        - dependence F18.24
    - opioid F11.94
      - in
        - abuse F11.14
        - dependence F11.24
    - phencyclidine (PCP) F16.94
      - in
        - abuse F16.14
        - dependence F16.24
    - physiological condition F06.30
      - with
        - depressive features F06.31
        - major depressive-like episode F06.32
        - manic features F06.33
        - mixed features F06.34
    - psychoactive substance NEC F19.94
      - in
        - abuse F19.14
        - dependence F19.24
    - sedative F13.94
      - in
        - abuse F13.14
        - dependence F13.24
    - volatile solvents F18.94

Disorder *(continued)*
- mood *(continued)*
  - due to *(continued)*
    - volatile solvents *(continued)*
      - in
        - abuse F18.14
        - dependence F18.24
  - manic episode F30.9
    - with psychotic symptoms F30.2
    - in remission (full) F30.4
      - partial F30.3
    - specified type NEC F30.8
    - without psychotic symptoms F30.10
      - mild F30.11
      - moderate F30.12
      - severe F30.13
  - organic F06.30
    - right hemisphere F07.89
  - persistent F34.9
    - cyclothymia F34.0
    - dysthymia F34.1
    - specified type NEC F34.89
  - recurrent F39
  - right hemisphere organic F07.89
- movement G25.9
  - drug-induced G25.70
    - akathisia G25.71
    - specified NEC G25.79
  - hysterical F44.4
  - in diseases classified elsewhere —*see* category G26
  - periodic limb G47.61
    - sleep related G47.61
  - specified NEC G25.89
  - sleep related NEC G47.69
  - stereotyped F98.4
  - treatment-induced G25.9
- multiple personality F44.81
- muscle M62.9
  - attachment, spine —*see* Enthesopathy, spinal
  - in trichinellosis —*see* Trichinellosis, with muscle disorder
  - psychogenic F45.8
  - specified type NEC M62.89
  - tone, newborn P94.9
    - specified NEC P94.8
- muscular
  - attachments —*see also* Enthesopathy
    - spine —*see* Enthesopathy, spinal
  - urethra N36.44
- musculoskeletal system, soft tissue —*see* Disorder, soft tissue
  - postprocedural M96.89
  - psychogenic F45.8
- myoneural G70.9
  - due to lead G70.1
  - specified NEC G70.89
  - toxic G70.1
- myotonic NEC G71.19
- nail, in diseases classified elsewhere L62
- neck region NEC —*see* Dorsopathy, specified NEC
- neonatal onset multisystemic inflammatory (NOMID) M04.2
- nerve G58.9
  - abducent NEC —*see* Strabismus, paralytic, sixth nerve
  - accessory G52.8
  - acoustic —*see* subcategory H93.3
  - auditory —*see* subcategory H93.3
  - auriculotemporal G50.8
  - axillary G54.0

Disorder *(continued)*
- nerve *(continued)*
  - cerebral *—see* Disorder, nerve, cranial
  - cranial G52.9
    - eighth *—see* subcategory H93.3
    - eleventh G52.8
    - fifth G50.9
    - first G52.0
    - fourth NEC *—see* Strabismus, paralytic, fourth nerve
    - multiple G52.7
    - ninth G52.1
    - second NEC *—see* Disorder, nerve, optic
    - seventh NEC G51.8
    - sixth NEC *—see* Strabismus, paralytic, sixth nerve
    - specified NEC G52.8
    - tenth G52.2
    - third NEC *—see* Strabismus, paralytic, third nerve
    - twelfth G52.3
  - entrapment *—see* Neuropathy, entrapment
  - facial G51.9
    - specified NEC G51.8
  - femoral *—see* Lesion, nerve, femoral
  - glossopharyngeal NEC G52.1
  - hypoglossal G52.3
  - intercostal G58.0
  - lateral
    - cutaneous of thigh *—see* Mononeuropathy, lower limb, meralgia paresthetica
    - popliteal *—see* Lesion, nerve, popliteal
  - lower limb *—see* Mononeuropathy, lower limb
  - medial popliteal *—see* Lesion, nerve, popliteal, medial
  - median NEC *—see* Lesion, nerve, median
  - multiple G58.7
  - oculomotor NEC *—see* Strabismus, paralytic, third nerve
  - olfactory G52.0
  - optic NEC H47.09-
    - hemorrhage into sheath *—see* Hemorrhage, optic nerve
    - ischemic H47.01-
  - peroneal *—see* Lesion, nerve, popliteal
  - phrenic G58.8
  - plantar *—see* Lesion, nerve, plantar
  - pneumogastric G52.2
  - posterior tibial *—see* Syndrome, tarsal tunnel
  - radial *—see* Lesion, nerve, radial
  - recurrent laryngeal G52.2
  - root G54.9
    - cervical G54.2
    - lumbosacral G54.1
    - specified NEC G54.8
    - thoracic G54.3
  - sciatic NEC *—see* Lesion, nerve, sciatic
  - specified NEC G58.8
    - lower limb *—see* Mononeuropathy, lower limb, specified NEC
    - upper limb *—see* Mononeuropathy, upper limb, specified NEC
  - sympathetic G90.9

Disorder *(continued)*
- nerve *(continued)*
  - tibial *—see* Lesion, nerve, popliteal, medial
  - trigeminal G50.9
    - specified NEC G50.8
  - trochlear NEC *—see* Strabismus, paralytic, fourth nerve
  - ulnar *—see* Lesion, nerve, ulnar
  - upper limb *—see* Mononeuropathy, upper limb
  - vagus G52.2
- nervous system G98.8
  - autonomic (peripheral) G90.9
    - specified NEC G90.8
  - central G96.9
    - specified NEC G96.89
  - parasympathetic G90.9
  - specified NEC G98.8
  - sympathetic G90.9
  - vegetative G90.9
- neurocognitive R41.9
  - major
    - with
      - aggressive behavior F01.51
      - combative behavior F01.51
      - violent behavior F01.51
    - due to vascular disease, with behavioral disturbance F01.51
    - in (due to) (other diseases classified elsewhere) (*see also* Dementia, in (due to)) F02.80
      - with
        - aggressive behavior F02.81
        - combative behavior F02.81
        - violent behavior F02.81
      - without behavioral disturbance F01.50
  - mild G31.84
- neurodevelopment F89
  - specified NEC F88
- neurohypophysis NEC E23.3
- neurological NEC R29.818
- neuromuscular G70.9
  - hereditary NEC G71.9
  - specified NEC G70.89
  - toxic G70.1
- neurotic F48.9
  - specified NEC F48.8
- neutrophil, polymorphonuclear D71
- nicotine use *—see* Dependence, drug, nicotine
- nightmare F51.5
- non-rapid eye movement sleep arousal
  - sleep terror type F51.4
  - sleepwalking type F51.3
- nose J34.9
  - specified NEC J34.89
- obsessive-compulsive F42.9
  - and related disorder due to a known physiological condition F06.8
- odontogenesis NOS K00.9
- opioid use
  - with
    - opioid-induced psychotic disorder F11.959
      - with
        - delusions F11.950
        - hallucinations F11.951
  - due to drug abuse *—see* Abuse, drug, opioid
  - due to drug dependence *—see* Dependence, drug, opioid

Disorder *(continued)*
- opioid use *(continued)*
  - mild F11.10
    - with
      - opioid-induced
        - anxiety disorder F11.188
        - depressive disorder F11.14
        - sexual dysfunction F11.181
      - opioid intoxication
        - with perceptual disturbances F11.122
        - delirium F11.121
        - without perceptual disturbances F11.129
    - in remission (early) (sustained) F11.11
  - moderate or severe F11.20
    - with
      - opioid-induced
        - anxiety disorder F11.288
        - anxiety disorder F11.988
        - depressive disorder F11.24
        - depressive disorder F11.94
        - sexual dysfunction F11.281
        - sexual dysfunction F11.981
      - opioid intoxication
        - with perceptual disturbances F11.222
        - delirium F11.221
        - without perceptual disturbances F11.229
    - in remission (early) (sustained) F11.21
- oppositional defiant F91.3
- optic
  - chiasm H47.49
    - due to
      - inflammatory disorder H47.41
      - neoplasm H47.42
      - vascular disorder H47.43
  - disc H47.39-
    - coloboma *—see* Coloboma, optic disc
    - drusen *—see* Drusen, optic disc
    - pseudopapilledema *—see* Pseudopapilledema
  - radiations *—see* Disorder, visual, pathway
  - tracts *—see* Disorder, visual, pathway
- orbit H05.9
  - cyst *—see* Cyst, orbit
  - deformity *—see* Deformity, orbit
  - edema *—see* Edema, orbit
  - enophthalmos *—see* Enophthalmos
  - exophthalmos *—see* Exophthalmos
  - hemorrhage *—see* Hemorrhage, orbit
  - inflammation *—see* Inflammation, orbit
  - myopathy *—see* Myopathy, extraocular muscles
  - retained foreign body *—see* Foreign body, orbit, old
  - specified type NEC H05.89
- organic
  - anxiety F06.4
  - catatonic F06.1
  - delusional F06.2
  - dissociative F06.8

Disorder *(continued)*
- organic *(continued)*
  - emotionally labile (asthenic) F06.8
  - mood (affective) F06.30
  - schizophrenia-like F06.2
- orgasmic (female) F52.31
  - male F52.32
- ornithine metabolism E72.4
- overanxious F41.1
  - of childhood F93.8
- pain
  - with related psychological factors F45.42
  - exclusively related to psychological factors F45.41
  - genito-pelvic penetration disorder F52.6
- pancreatic internal secretion E16.9
  - specified NEC E16.8
- panic F41.0
  - with agoraphobia F40.01
- papulosquamous L44.9
  - in diseases classified elsewhere L45
  - specified NEC L44.8
- paranoid F22
  - induced F24
  - shared F24
- paraphilic F65.9
  - specified NEC F65.89
- parathyroid (gland) E21.5
  - specified NEC E21.4
- parietoalveolar NEC J84.09
- paroxysmal, mixed R56.9
- patella M22.9-
  - chondromalacia *—see* Chondromalacia, patella
  - derangement NEC M22.3X-
  - recurrent
    - dislocation *—see* Dislocation, patella, recurrent
    - subluxation *—see* Dislocation, patella, recurrent, incomplete
  - specified NEC M22.8X-
- patellofemoral M22.2X-
- pedophilic F65.4
- pentose phosphate pathway with anemia D55.1
- perception, due to hallucinogens F16.983
  - in
    - abuse F16.183
    - dependence F16.283
- peripheral nervous system NEC G64
- peroxisomal E71.50
  - biogenesis
    - neonatal adrenoleukodystrophy E71.511
    - specified disorder NEC E71.518
    - Zellweger syndrome E71.510
  - rhizomelic chondrodysplasia punctata E71.540
  - specified form NEC E71.548
    - group 1 E71.518
    - group 2 E71.53
    - group 3 E71.542
  - X-linked adrenoleukodystrophy E71.529
    - adolescent E71.521
    - adrenomyeloneuropathy E71.522
    - childhood E71.520
    - specified form NEC E71.528
  - Zellweger-like syndrome E71.541

Disorder *(continued)*
- persistent
  - (somatoform) pain F45.41
  - affective (mood) F34.9
- personality *—see also* Personality F60.9
  - affective F34.0
  - aggressive F60.3
  - amoral F60.2
  - anankastic F60.5
  - antisocial F60.2
  - anxious F60.6
  - asocial F60.2
  - asthenic F60.7
  - avoidant F60.6
  - borderline F60.3
  - change (secondary) due to general medical condition F07.0
  - compulsive F60.5
  - cyclothymic F34.0
  - dependent (passive) F60.7
  - depressive F34.1
  - dissocial F60.2
  - emotional instability F60.3
  - expansive paranoid F60.0
  - explosive F60.3
  - following organic brain damage F07.9
  - histrionic F60.4
  - hyperthymic F34.0
  - hypothymic F34.1
  - hysterical F60.4
  - immature F60.89
  - inadequate F60.7
  - labile F60.3
  - mixed (nonspecific) F60.89
  - moral deficiency F60.2
  - narcissistic F60.81
  - negativistic F60.89
  - obsessional F60.5
  - obsessive (-compulsive) F60.5
  - organic F07.9
  - overconscientious F60.5
  - paranoid F60.0
  - passive (-dependent) F60.7
  - passive-aggressive F60.89
  - pathological NEC F60.9
  - pseudosocial F60.2
  - psychopathic F60.2
  - schizoid F60.1
  - schizotypal F21
  - self-defeating F60.7
  - specified NEC F60.89
  - type A F60.5
  - unstable (emotional) F60.3
- pervasive, developmental F84.9
- phencyclidine use
  - mild F16.10
    - with
      - phencyclidine-induced
        - anxiety disorder F16.180
        - bipolar and related disorder F16.14
        - depressive disorder F16.14
        - psychotic disorder F16.159
      - phencyclidine intoxication F16.129
      - phencyclidine intoxication delirium F16.121
    - in remission (early) (sustained) F16.11
  - moderate or severe F16.20
    - with
      - phencyclidine-induced
        - anxiety disorder F16.280
        - bipolar and related disorder F16.24

Disorder *(continued)*
- phencyclidine use *(continued)*
  - moderate or severe *(continued)*
    - with *(continued)*
      - phencyclidine-induced *(continued)*
        - depressive disorder F16.24
        - psychotic disorder F16.259
      - phencyclidine intoxication F16.229
      - phencyclidine intoxication delirium F16.221
    - in remission (early) (sustained) F16.21
- phobic anxiety, childhood F40.8
- phosphate-losing tubular N25.0
- pigmentation L81.9
  - choroid, congenital Q14.3
  - diminished melanin formation L81.6
  - iron L81.8
  - specified NEC L81.8
- pinna (noninfective) H61.10-
  - deformity, acquired H61.11-
  - hematoma H61.12-
  - perichondritis *—see* Perichondritis, ear
  - specified type NEC H61.19-
- pituitary gland E23.7
  - iatrogenic (postprocedural) E89.3
  - specified NEC E23.6
- platelets D69.1
- plexus G54.9
  - specified NEC G54.8
- polymorphonuclear neutrophils D71
- porphyrin metabolism *—see* Porphyria
- postconcussional F07.81
- posthallucinogen perception F16.983
  - in
    - abuse F16.183
    - dependence F16.283
- postmenopausal N95.9
  - specified NEC N95.8
- postprocedural (postoperative) *—see* Complications, postprocedural
- post-transplant lymphoproliferative D47.Z1
- post-traumatic stress (PTSD) F43.10
  - acute F43.11
  - chronic F43.12
- premenstrual dysphoric (PMDD) F32.81
- prepuce N47.8
- propionic acidemia E71.121
- prostate N42.9
  - specified NEC N42.89
- psychogenic NOS (*see also* condition) F45.9
  - anxiety F41.8
  - appetite F50.9
  - asthenic F48.8
  - cardiovascular (system) F45.8
  - compulsive F42.8
  - cutaneous F54
  - depressive F32.9
  - digestive (system) F45.8
  - dysmenorrheic F45.8
  - dyspneic F45.8
  - endocrine (system) F54
  - eye NEC F45.8
  - feeding *—see* Disorder, eating
  - functional NEC F45.8
  - gastric F45.8

Disorder *(continued)*
- psychogenic NOS *(continued)*
  - gastrointestinal (system) F45.8
  - genitourinary (system) F45.8
  - heart (function) (rhythm) F45.8
  - hyperventilatory F45.8
  - hypochondriacal *—see* Disorder, hypochondriacal
  - intestinal F45.8
  - joint F45.8
  - learning F81.9
  - limb F45.8
  - lymphatic (system) F45.8
  - menstrual F45.8
  - micturition F45.8
  - monoplegic NEC F44.4
  - motor F44.4
  - muscle F45.8
  - musculoskeletal F45.8
  - neurocirculatory F45.8
  - obsessive F42.8
  - occupational F48.8
  - organ or part of body NEC F45.8
  - paralytic NEC F44.4
  - phobic F40.9
  - physical NEC F45.8
  - rectal F45.8
  - respiratory (system) F45.8
  - rheumatic F45.8
  - sexual (function) F52.9
  - skin (allergic) (eczematous) F54
  - sleep F51.9
  - specified part of body NEC F45.8
  - stomach F45.8
- psychological F99
  - associated with
    - disease classified elsewhere F54
    - sexual
      - development F66
      - relationship F66
    - uncertainty about gender identity F64.9
- psychomotor NEC F44.4
  - hysterical F44.4
- psychoneurotic *—see also* Neurosis
  - mixed NEC F48.8
- psychophysiologic *—see* Disorder, somatoform
- psychosexual F65.9
  - development F66
  - identity of childhood F64.2
- psychosomatic NOS *—see* Disorder, somatoform
  - multiple F45.0
  - undifferentiated F45.1
- psychotic *—see* Psychosis
  - transient (acute) F23
- puberty E30.9
  - specified NEC E30.8
- pulmonary (valve) *—see* Endocarditis, pulmonary
- purine metabolism E79.9
- pyrimidine metabolism E79.9
- pyruvate metabolism E74.4
- reactive attachment (childhood) F94.1
- reading R48.0
  - developmental (specific) F81.0
- receptive language F80.2
- receptor, hormonal, peripheral (*see also* Syndrome, androgen insensitivity) E34.50
- recurrent brief depressive F33.8
- reflex R29.2
- refraction H52.7
  - aniseikonia H52.32
  - anisometropia H52.31
  - astigmatism *—see* Astigmatism

Disorder *(continued)*
- refraction *(continued)*
  - hypermetropia *—see* Hypermetropia
  - myopia *—see* Myopia
  - presbyopia H52.4
  - specified NEC H52.6
- relationship F68.8
  - due to sexual orientation F66
- REM sleep behavior G47.52
- renal function, impaired (tubular) N25.9
- resonance R49.9
  - specified NEC R49.8
- respiratory function, impaired *—see also* Failure, respiration
  - postprocedural *—see* Complication, postoperative, respiratory system
  - psychogenic F45.8
- retina H35.9
  - angioid streaks H35.33
  - changes in vascular appearance H35.01-
  - degeneration *—see* Degeneration, retina
  - dystrophy (hereditary) *—see* Dystrophy, retina
  - edema H35.81
  - hemorrhage *—see* Hemorrhage, retina
  - ischemia H35.82
  - macular degeneration *—see* Degeneration, macula
  - microaneurysms H35.04-
  - microvascular abnormality NEC H35.09
  - neovascularization *—see* Neovascularization, retina
  - retinopathy *—see* Retinopathy
  - separation of layers H35.70
    - central serous chorioretinopathy H35.71-
    - pigment epithelium detachment (serous) H35.72-
      - hemorrhagic H35.73-
  - specified type NEC H35.89
  - telangiectasis *—see* Telangiectasis, retina
  - vasculitis *—see* Vasculitis, retina
- retroperitoneal K68.9
- right hemisphere organic affective F07.89
- rumination (infant or child) F98.21
- sacrum, sacrococcygeal NEC M53.3
- schizoaffective F25.9
  - bipolar type F25.0
  - depressive type F25.1
  - manic type F25.0
  - mixed type F25.0
  - specified NEC F25.8
- schizoid of childhood F84.5
- schizophrenia spectrum and other psychotic disorder F29
  - specified NEC F28
- schizophreniform F20.81
  - brief F23
- schizotypal (personality) F21
- secretion, thyrocalcitonin E07.0
- sedative, hypnotic, or anxiolytic-induced
  - mild F13.10
    - with
      - sedative, hypnotic, or anxiolytic-induced
        - anxiety disorder F13.180
        - bipolar and related disorder F13.14

Disorder *(continued)*
- sedative, hypnotic, or anxiolytic-induced *(continued)*
  - mild *(continued)*
    - with *(continued)*
      - sedative, hypnotic, or anxiolytic-induced *(continued)*
        - depressive disorder F13.14
        - psychotic disorder F13.159
        - sexual dysfunction F13.181
      - sedative, hypnotic, or anxiolytic intoxication F13.129
      - sedative, hypnotic, or anxiolytic intoxication delirium F13.121
    - in remission (early) (sustained) F13.11
  - moderate or severe F13.20
    - with
      - sedative, hypnotic, or anxiolytic-induced
        - anxiety disorder F13.280
        - bipolar and related disorder F13.24
        - depressive disorder F13.24
        - major neurocognitive disorder F13.27
        - mild neurocognitive disorder F13.288
        - psychotic disorder F13.259
        - sexual dysfunction F13.281
      - sedative, hypnotic, or anxiolytic intoxication F13.229
      - sedative, hypnotic, or anxiolytic intoxication delirium F13.221
    - in remission (early) (sustained) F13.21
- seizure (*see also* Epilepsy) G40.909
  - intractable G40.919
    - with status epilepticus G40.911
- semantic pragmatic F80.89
  - with autism F84.0
- sense of smell R43.1
  - psychogenic F45.8
- separation anxiety, of childhood F93.0
- sexual
  - arousal, female F52.22
  - aversion F52.1
  - function, psychogenic F52.9
  - interest/arousal, female F52.22
  - masochism F65.51
  - maturation F66
  - nonorganic F52.9
  - preference (*see also* Deviation, sexual) F65.9
    - fetishistic transvestism F65.1
  - relationship F66
  - sadism F65.52
- shyness, of childhood and adolescence F40.10
- sibling rivalry F93.8
- sickle-cell (sickling) (homozygous) —*see* Disease, sickle-cell
  - heterozygous D57.3
  - specified type NEC D57.8-
  - trait D57.3
- sinus (nasal) J34.9
  - specified NEC J34.89
- skin L98.9
  - atrophic L90.9
    - specified NEC L90.8
  - granulomatous L92.9
    - specified NEC L92.8
  - hypertrophic L91.9
    - specified NEC L91.8
  - infiltrative NEC L98.6
  - newborn P83.9
    - specified NEC P83.88
  - picking F42.4
  - psychogenic (allergic) (eczematous) F54
- sleep G47.9
  - breathing-related —*see* Apnea, sleep
  - circadian rhythm G47.20
    - advance sleep phase type G47.22
    - delayed sleep phase type G47.21
    - due to
      - alcohol
        - abuse F10.182
        - dependence F10.282
        - use F10.982
      - amphetamines
        - abuse F15.182
        - dependence F15.282
        - use F15.982
      - caffeine
        - abuse F15.182
        - dependence F15.282
        - use F15.982
      - cocaine
        - abuse F14.182
        - dependence F14.282
        - use F14.982
      - drug NEC
        - abuse F19.182
        - dependence F19.282
        - use F19.982
      - opioid
        - abuse F11.182
        - dependence F11.282
        - use F11.982
      - psychoactive substance NEC
        - abuse F19.182
        - dependence F19.282
        - use F19.982
      - sedative, hypnotic, or anxiolytic
        - abuse F13.182
        - dependence F13.282
        - use F13.982
      - stimulant NEC
        - abuse F15.182
        - dependence F15.282
        - use F15.982
    - free running type G47.24
    - in conditions classified elsewhere G47.27
    - irregular sleep wake type G47.23
    - jet lag type G47.25
    - non-24-hour sleep-wake type G47.24
    - shift work type G47.26
    - specified NEC G47.29
  - due to
    - alcohol
      - abuse F10.182
      - dependence F10.282
      - use F10.982
    - amphetamine
      - abuse F15.182
      - dependence F15.282
      - use F15.982

Disorder *(continued)*
- sleep *(continued)*
  - due to *(continued)*
    - anxiolytic
      - abuse F13.182
      - dependence F13.282
      - use F13.982
    - caffeine
      - abuse F15.182
      - dependence F15.282
      - use F15.982
    - cocaine
      - abuse F14.182
      - dependence F14.282
      - use F14.982
    - drug NEC
      - abuse F19.182
      - dependence F19.282
      - use F19.982
    - hypnotic
      - abuse F13.182
      - dependence F13.282
      - use F13.982
    - opioid
      - abuse F11.182
      - dependence F11.282
      - use F11.982
    - psychoactive substance NEC
      - abuse F19.182
      - dependence F19.282
      - use F19.982
    - sedative
      - abuse F13.182
      - dependence F13.282
      - use F13.982
    - stimulant NEC
      - abuse F15.182
      - dependence F15.282
      - use F15.982
  - emotional F51.9
  - excessive somnolence —*see* Hypersomnia
  - hypersomnia type —*see* Hypersomnia
  - initiating or maintaining —*see* Insomnia
  - nightmares F51.5
  - nonorganic F51.9
    - specified NEC F51.8
  - parasomnia type G47.50
  - specified NEC G47.8
  - terrors F51.4
  - walking F51.3
- sleep-wake pattern or schedule — (*see also* Disorder, sleep, circadian rhythm) G47.9
  - specified NEC G47.8
- social
  - anxiety (of childhood) F40.10
    - generalized F40.11
  - functioning in childhood F94.9
    - specified NEC F94.8
  - pragmatic F80.82
- soft tissue M79.9
  - ankle M79.9
  - due to use, overuse and pressure M70.90
    - ankle M70.97-
    - bursitis —*see* Bursitis
    - foot M70.97-
    - forearm M70.93-
    - hand M70.94-
    - lower leg M70.96-
    - multiple sites M70.99
    - pelvic region M70.95-
    - shoulder region M70.91-
    - specified site NEC M70.98
    - specified type NEC M70.80
      - ankle M70.87-
      - foot M70.87-
      - forearm M70.83-

Disorder *(continued)*
- soft tissue *(continued)*
  - due to use, overuse and pressure *(continued)*
    - specified type NEC *(continued)*
      - hand M70.84-
      - lower leg M70.86-
      - multiple sites M70.89
      - pelvic region M70.85-
      - shoulder region M70.81-
      - specified site NEC M70.88
      - thigh M70.85-
      - upper arm M70.82-
    - thigh M70.95-
    - upper arm M70.92-
  - foot M79.9
  - forearm M79.9
  - hand M79.9
  - lower leg M79.9
  - multiple sites M79.9
  - occupational —*see* Disorder, soft tissue, due to use, overuse and pressure
  - pelvic region M79.9
  - shoulder region M79.9
  - specified type NEC M79.89
  - thigh M79.9
  - upper arm M79.9
- somatic symptom F45.1
- somatization F45.0
- somatoform F45.9
  - pain (persistent) F45.41
  - somatization (multiple) (long-lasting) F45.0
  - specified NEC F45.8
  - undifferentiated F45.1
- somnolence, excessive —*see* Hypersomnia
- specific
  - arithmetical F81.2
  - developmental, of motor F82
  - reading F81.0
  - speech and language F80.9
  - spelling F81.81
  - written expression F81.81
- speech R47.9
  - articulation (functional) (specific) F80.0
  - developmental F80.9
  - specified NEC R47.89
- speech-sound F80.0
- spelling (specific) F81.81
- spine —*see also* Dorsopathy
  - ligamentous or muscular attachments, peripheral —*see* Enthesopathy, spinal
  - specified NEC —*see* Dorsopathy, specified NEC
- stereotyped, habit or movement F98.4
- stimulant use (other) (unspecified)
  - mild F15.10
    - in remission (early) (sustained) F15.11
  - moderate or severe F15.20
    - in remission (early) (sustained) F15.21
- stomach (functional) —*see* Disorder, gastric
- stress F43.9
  - acute F43.0
  - post-traumatic F43.10
    - acute F43.11
    - chronic F43.12
- substance use (other) (unknown)
  - mild F19.10
    - with substance-induced
      - anxiety disorder F19.180
      - bipolar and related disorder F19.14
      - depressive disorder F19.14

Disorder *(continued)*
- substance use *(continued)*
  - mild *(continued)*
    - with substance-induced *(continued)*
      - major neurocognitive disorder F19.17
      - mild neurocognitive disorder F19.188
      - obsessive-compulsive and related disorder F19.188
      - sexual dysfunction F19.181
    - substance intoxication F19.129
    - substance intoxication delirium F19.121
  - moderate or severe F19.20
    - with substance-induced
      - anxiety disorder F19.280
      - bipolar and related disorder F19.24
      - depressive disorder F19.24
      - major neurocognitive disorder F19.27
      - mild neurocognitive disorder F19.288
      - obsessive-compulsive and related disorder F19.288
      - sexual dysfunction F19.281
    - in remission (early) (sustained) F19.21
    - substance intoxication F19.229
    - substance intoxication delirium F19.221
- sulfur-bearing amino-acid metabolism E72.10
- sweat gland (eccrine) L74.9
  - apocrine L75.9
    - specified NEC L75.8
  - specified NEC L74.8
- synovium M67.90
  - acromioclavicular M67.91-
  - ankle M67.97-
  - elbow M67.92-
  - foot M67.97-
  - forearm M67.93-
  - hand M67.94-
  - hip M67.95-
  - knee M67.96-
  - multiple sites M67.99
  - rupture *—see* Rupture, synovium
  - shoulder M67.91-
  - specified type NEC M67.80
    - acromioclavicular M67.81-
    - ankle M67.87-
    - elbow M67.82-
    - foot M67.87-
    - hand M67.84-
    - hip M67.85-
    - knee M67.86-
    - multiple sites M67.89
    - wrist M67.83-
  - synovitis *—see* Synovitis
  - upper arm M67.92-
  - wrist M67.93-
- temperature regulation, newborn P81.9
  - specified NEC P81.8
- temporomandibular joint M26.60-
- tendon M67.90
  - acromioclavicular M67.91-
  - ankle M67.97-
  - contracture *—see* Contracture, tendon
  - elbow M67.92-
  - foot M67.97-
  - forearm M67.93-
  - hand M67.94-
  - hip M67.95-
  - knee M67.96-

Disorder *(continued)*
- tendon *(continued)*
  - multiple sites M67.99
  - rupture *—see* Rupture, tendon
  - shoulder M67.91-
  - specified type NEC M67.80
    - acromioclavicular M67.81-
    - ankle M67.87-
    - elbow M67.82-
    - foot M67.87-
    - hand M67.84-
    - hip M67.85-
    - knee M67.86-
    - multiple sites M67.89
    - trunk M67.88
    - wrist M67.83-
  - synovitis *—see* Synovitis
  - tendinitis *—see* Tendinitis
  - tenosynovitis *—see* Tenosynovitis
  - trunk M67.98
  - upper arm M67.92-
  - wrist M67.93-
- thoracic root (nerve) NEC G54.3
- thyrocalcitonin hypersecretion E07.0
- thyroid (gland) E07.9
  - function NEC, neonatal, transitory P72.2
  - iodine-deficiency related E01.8
  - specified NEC E07.89
- tic *—see* Tic
- tobacco use
  - chewing tobacco (mild) (moderate) (severe)
    - in remission (early) (sustained) F17.221
  - cigarettes (mild) (moderate) (severe)
    - in remission (early) (sustained) F17.211
  - mild F17.200
    - in remission (early) (sustained) F17.201
  - moderate F17.200
    - in remission (early) (sustained) F17.201
  - severe F17.200
    - in remission (early) (sustained) F17.201
  - specified product NEC (mild) (moderate) (severe)
    - in remission (early) (sustained) F17.291
- tooth K08.9
  - development K00.9
    - specified NEC K00.8
  - eruption K00.6
- Tourette's F95.2
- trance and possession F44.89
- transvestic F65.1
- trauma and stressor-related F43.9
  - other specified F43.8
- tricuspid (valve) *—see* Endocarditis, tricuspid
- tryptophan metabolism E70.5
- tubular, phosphate-losing N25.0
- tubulo-interstitial (in)
  - brucellosis A23.9 *[N16]*
  - cystinosis E72.04
  - diphtheria A36.84
  - glycogen storage disease E74.00 *[N16]*
  - leukemia NEC C95.9- *[N16]*
  - lymphoma NEC C85.9- *[N16]*
  - mixed cryoglobulinemia D89.1 *[N16]*
  - multiple myeloma C90.0- *[N16]*
  - Salmonella infection A02.25
  - sarcoidosis D86.84
  - sepsis A41.9 *[N16]*
    - streptococcal A40.9 *[N16]*

Disorder *(continued)*
- tubulo-interstitial *(continued)*
  - systemic lupus erythematosus M32.15
  - toxoplasmosis B58.83
  - transplant rejection T86.91 *[N16]*
  - Wilson's disease E83.01 *[N16]*
- tubulo-renal function, impaired N25.9
  - specified NEC N25.89
- tympanic membrane H73.9-
  - atrophy *—see* Atrophy, tympanic membrane
  - infection *—see* Myringitis
  - perforation *—see* Perforation, tympanum
  - specified NEC H73.89-
- unsocialized aggressive F91.1
- urea cycle metabolism E72.20
  - argininemia E72.21
  - arginosuccinic aciduria E72.22
  - citrullinemia E72.23
  - ornithine transcarbamylase deficiency E72.4
  - other specified E72.29
- ureter (in) N28.9
  - schistosomiasis B65.0 *[N29]*
  - tuberculosis A18.11
- urethra N36.9
  - specified NEC N36.8
- urinary system N39.9
  - specified NEC N39.8
- valve, heart
  - aortic *—see* Endocarditis, aortic
  - mitral *—see* Endocarditis, mitral
  - pulmonary *—see* Endocarditis, pulmonary
  - rheumatic
    - aortic *—see* Endocarditis, aortic, rheumatic
    - mitral *—see* Endocarditis, mitral
    - pulmonary *—see* Endocarditis, pulmonary, rheumatic
    - tricuspid *—see* Endocarditis, tricuspid
  - tricuspid *—see* Endocarditis, tricuspid
- vestibular function H81.9-
  - specified NEC *—see* subcategory H81.8
    - in diseases classified elsewhere H82.-
  - vertigo *—see* Vertigo
- vision, binocular H53.30
  - abnormal retinal correspondence H53.31
  - diplopia H53.2
  - fusion with defective stereopsis H53.32
  - simultaneous perception H53.33
  - suppression H53.34
- visual
  - cortex
    - blindness H47.619
      - left brain H47.612
      - right brain H47.611
    - due to
      - inflammatory disorder H47.629
        - left brain H47.622
        - right brain H47.621
      - neoplasm H47.639
        - left brain H47.632
        - right brain H47.631
      - vascular disorder H47.649
        - left brain H47.642
        - right brain H47.641
  - pathway H47.9

Disorder *(continued)*
- visual *(continued)*
  - pathway *(continued)*
    - due to
      - inflammatory disorder H47.51-
      - neoplasm H47.52-
      - vascular disorder H47.53-
    - optic chiasm *—see* Disorder, optic, chiasm
- vitreous body H43.9
  - crystalline deposits *—see* Deposit, crystalline
  - degeneration *—see* Degeneration, vitreous
  - hemorrhage *—see* Hemorrhage, vitreous
  - opacities *—see* Opacity, vitreous
  - prolapse *—see* Prolapse, vitreous
  - specified type NEC H43.89
- voice R49.9
  - specified type NEC R49.8
- volatile solvent use
  - due to drug abuse *—see* Abuse, drug, inhalant
  - due to drug dependence *—see* Dependence, drug, inhalant
- voyeuristic F65.3
- white blood cells D72.9
  - specified NEC D72.89
- withdrawing, child or adolescent F40.10

Disorientation R41.0

Displacement, displaced
- acquired traumatic of bone, cartilage, joint, tendon NEC *—see* Dislocation
- adrenal gland (congenital) Q89.1
- appendix, retrocecal (congenital) Q43.8
- auricle (congenital) Q17.4
- bladder (acquired) N32.89
  - congenital Q64.19
- brachial plexus (congenital) Q07.8
- brain stem, caudal (congenital) Q04.8
- canaliculus (lacrimalis), congenital Q10.6
- cardia through esophageal hiatus (congenital) Q40.1
- cerebellum, caudal (congenital) Q04.8
- cervix *—see* Malposition, uterus
- colon (congenital) Q43.3
- device, implant or graft (*see also* Complications, by site and type, mechanical) T85.628
  - arterial graft NEC *—see* Complication, cardiovascular device, mechanical, vascular
  - breast (implant) T85.42
  - catheter NEC T85.628
    - dialysis (renal) T82.42
      - intraperitoneal T85.621
    - infusion NEC T82.524
      - spinal (epidural) (subdural) T85.620
    - urinary
      - cystostomy T83.020
      - Hopkins T83.028
      - ileostomy T83.028
      - indwelling T83.021
      - nephrostomy T83.022
      - specified NEC T83.028
      - urostomy T83.028
  - electronic (electrode) (pulse generator) (stimulator) *—see* Complication, electronic stimulator

Displacement, displaced *(continued)*
- device, implant or graft *(continued)*
  - fixation, internal (orthopedic) NEC *—see* Complication, fixation device, mechanical
  - gastrointestinal *—see* Complications, prosthetic device, mechanical, gastrointestinal device
  - genital NEC T83.428
    - intrauterine contraceptive device (string) T83.32
    - penile prosthesis (cylinder) (implanted) (pump) (resevoir) T83.420
    - testicular prosthesis T83.421
  - heart NEC *—see* Complication, cardiovascular device, mechanical
  - joint prosthesis *—see* Complications, joint prosthesis, mechanical
  - ocular *—see* Complications, prosthetic device, mechanical, ocular device
  - orthopedic NEC *—see* Complication, orthopedic, device or graft, mechanical
  - specified NEC T85.628
  - urinary NEC T83.128
    - graft T83.22
    - sphincter, implanted T83.121
    - stent (ileal conduit) (nephroureteral) T83.123
      - ureteral indwelling T83.122
  - vascular NEC *—see* Complication, cardiovascular device, mechanical
  - ventricular intracranial shunt T85.02
- electronic stimulator
  - bone T84.320
  - cardiac *—see* Complications, cardiac device, electronic
  - nervous system *—see* Complication, prosthetic device, mechanical, electronic nervous system stimulator
  - urinary *—see* Complications, electronic stimulator, urinary
- esophageal mucosa into cardia of stomach, congenital Q39.8
- esophagus (acquired) K22.89
  - congenital Q39.8
- eyeball (acquired) (lateral) (old) *—see* Displacement, globe
  - congenital Q15.8
  - current *—see* Avulsion, eye
- fallopian tube (acquired) N83.4-
  - congenital Q50.6
  - opening (congenital) Q50.6
- gallbladder (congenital) Q44.1
- gastric mucosa (congenital) Q40.2
- globe (acquired) (old) (lateral) H05.21-
  - current *—see* Avulsion, eye
- heart (congenital) Q24.8
  - acquired I51.89
- hymen (upward) (congenital) Q52.4
- intervertebral disc NEC
  - with myelopathy *—see* Disorder, disc, with, myelopathy
  - cervical, cervicothoracic (with) M50.20
    - myelopathy *—see* Disorder, disc, cervical, with myelopathy
    - neuritis, radiculitis or radiculopathy *—see* Disorder, disc, cervical, with neuritis

Displacement, displaced *(continued)*
- intervertebral disc NEC *(continued)*
  - due to trauma *—see* Dislocation, vertebra
  - lumbar region M51.26
    - with
      - myelopathy M51.06
      - neuritis, radiculitis, radiculopathy or sciatica M51.16
  - lumbosacral region M51.27
    - with
      - neuritis, radiculitis, radiculopathy or sciatica M51.17
  - sacrococcygeal region M53.3
  - thoracic region M51.24
    - with
      - myelopathy M51.04
      - neuritis, radiculitis, radiculopathy M51.14
  - thoracolumbar region M51.25
    - with
      - myelopathy M51.05
      - neuritis, radiculitis, radiculopathy M51.15
- intrauterine device (string) T83.32
- kidney (acquired) N28.83
  - congenital Q63.2
- lachrymal, lacrimal apparatus or duct (congenital) Q10.6
- lens, congenital Q12.1
- macula (congenital) Q14.1
- Meckel's diverticulum Q43.0
  - malignant *—see* Table of Neoplasms, small intestine, malignant
- nail (congenital) Q84.6
  - acquired L60.8
- opening of Wharton's duct in mouth Q38.4
- organ or site, congenital NEC *—see* Malposition, congenital
- ovary (acquired) N83.4-
  - congenital Q50.39
  - free in peritoneal cavity (congenital) Q50.39
  - into hernial sac N83.4-
- oviduct (acquired) N83.4-
  - congenital Q50.6
- parathyroid (gland) E21.4
- parotid gland (congenital) Q38.4
- punctum lacrimale (congenital) Q10.6
- sacro-iliac (joint) (congenital) Q74.2
  - current injury S33.2
  - old *—see* subcategory M53.2
- salivary gland (any) (congenital) Q38.4
- spleen (congenital) Q89.09
- stomach, congenital Q40.2
- sublingual duct Q38.4
- tongue (downward) (congenital) Q38.3
- tooth, teeth, fully erupted M26.30
  - horizontal M26.33
  - vertical M26.34
- trachea (congenital) Q32.1
- ureter or ureteric opening or orifice (congenital) Q62.62
- uterine opening of oviducts or fallopian tubes Q50.6
- uterus, uterine *—see* Malposition, uterus
- ventricular septum Q21.0
  - with rudimentary ventricle Q20.4

Disproportion
- between native and reconstructed breast N65.1
- fiber-type G71.20
  - congenital G71.29

Disruptio uteri *—see* Rupture, uterus

Disruption (of)
- ciliary body NEC H21.89
- closure of
  - cornea T81.31
  - craniotomy T81.32
  - fascia (muscular) (superficial) T81.32
  - internal organ or tissue T81.32
  - laceration (external) (internal) T81.33
  - ligament T81.32
  - mucosa T81.31
  - muscle or muscle flap T81.32
  - ribs or rib cage T81.32
  - skin and subcutaneous tissue (full-thickness) (superficial) T81.31
  - skull T81.32
  - sternum (sternotomy) T81.32
  - tendon T81.32
  - traumatic laceration (external) (internal) T81.33
- family Z63.8
  - due to
    - absence of family member due to military deployment Z63.31
    - absence of family member NEC Z63.32
    - alcoholism and drug addiction in family Z63.72
    - bereavement Z63.4
    - death (assumed) or disappearance of family member Z63.4
    - divorce or separation Z63.5
    - drug addiction in family Z63.72
    - return of family member from military deployment (current or past conflict) Z63.71
    - stressful life events NEC Z63.79
- iris NEC H21.89
- ligament(s) *—see also* Sprain
  - knee
    - current injury *—see* Dislocation, knee
    - old (chronic) *—see* Derangement, knee, ligament, instability, chronic
    - spontaneous NEC *—see* Derangement, knee, disruption ligament
- ossicular chain *—see* Discontinuity, ossicles, ear
- pelvic ring (stable) S32.810
  - unstable S32.811
- wound T81.30
  - episiotomy O90.1
  - operation T81.31
    - cesarean O90.0
    - external operation wound (superficial) T81.31
    - internal operation wound (deep) T81.32
  - perineal (obstetric) O90.1
  - traumatic injury repair T81.33
- traumatic injury wound repair T81.33

Dissatisfaction with
- employment Z56.9
- school environment Z55.4

Dissecting *—see* condition

Dissection
- aorta I71.00

Dissection *(continued)*
- aorta *(continued)*
  - abdominal I71.02
  - thoracic I71.01
  - thoracoabdominal I71.03
- artery I77.70
  - basilar (trunk) I77.75
  - carotid I77.71
  - cerebral (nonruptured) I67.0
    - ruptured *—see* Hemorrhage, intracranial, subarachnoid
  - coronary I25.42
  - extremity
    - lower I77.77
    - upper I77.76
  - iliac I77.72
  - precerebral
    - congenital (nonruptured) Q28.1
    - specified site NEC I77.75
  - renal I77.73
  - specified NEC I77.79
  - vertebral I77.74
- precerebral artery, congential (nonruptured) Q28.1
  - Heartland A93.8
- traumatic *—see* Wound, open, by site
- vascular I99.8
- wound *—see* Wound, open

Disseminated *—see* condition

Dissociation
- auriculoventricular or atrioventricular (AV) (any degree) (isorhythmic) I45.89
  - with heart block I44.2
- interference I45.89

Dissociative reaction, state F44.9

Dissolution, vertebra *—see* Osteoporosis

Distension, distention
- abdomen R14.0
- bladder N32.89
- cecum K63.89
- colon K63.89
- gallbladder K82.8
- intestine K63.89
- kidney N28.89
- liver K76.89
- seminal vesicle N50.89
- stomach K31.89
  - acute K31.0
  - psychogenic F45.8
- ureter *—see* Dilatation, ureter
- uterus N85.8

Distoma hepaticum infestation B66.3

Distomiasis B66.9
- bile passages B66.3
- hemic B65.9
- hepatic B66.3
  - due to Clonorchis sinensis B66.1
- intestinal B66.5
- liver B66.3
  - due to Clonorchis sinensis B66.1
- lung B66.4
- pulmonary B66.4

Distomolar (fourth molar) K00.1

Disto-occlusion (Division I) (Division II) M26.212

Distortion(s) (congenital)
- adrenal (gland) Q89.1
- arm NEC Q68.8
- bile duct or passage Q44.5
- bladder Q64.79
- brain Q04.9
- cervix (uteri) Q51.9

Distortion *(continued)*
- chest (wall) Q67.8
  - bones Q76.8
- clavicle Q74.0
- clitoris Q52.6
- coccyx Q76.49
- common duct Q44.5
- coronary Q24.5
- cystic duct Q44.5
- ear (auricle) (external) Q17.3
  - inner Q16.5
  - middle Q16.4
    - ossicles Q16.3
- endocrine NEC Q89.2
- eustachian tube Q17.8
- eye (adnexa) Q15.8
- face bone(s) NEC Q75.8
- fallopian tube Q50.6
- femur NEC Q68.8
- fibula NEC Q68.8
- finger(s) Q68.1
- foot Q66.9-
- genitalia, genital organ(s)
  - female Q52.8
    - external Q52.79
    - internal NEC Q52.8
- gyri Q04.8
- hand bone(s) Q68.1
- heart (auricle) (ventricle) Q24.8
  - valve (cusp) Q24.8
- hepatic duct Q44.5
- humerus NEC Q68.8
- hymen Q52.4
- intrafamilial communications Z63.8
- jaw NEC M26.89
- labium (majus) (minus) Q52.79
- leg NEC Q68.8
- lens Q12.8
- liver Q44.7
- lumbar spine Q76.49
  - with disproportion O33.8
    - causing obstructed labor O65.0
- lumbosacral (joint) (region) Q76.49
  - kyphosis *—see* Kyphosis, congenital
  - lordosis *—see* Lordosis, congenital
- nerve Q07.8
- nose Q30.8
- organ
  - of Corti Q16.5
  - or site not listed *—see* Anomaly, by site
- ossicles, ear Q16.3
- oviduct Q50.6
- pancreas Q45.3
- parathyroid (gland) Q89.2
- pituitary (gland) Q89.2
- radius NEC Q68.8
- sacroiliac joint Q74.2
- sacrum Q76.49
- scapula Q74.0
- shoulder girdle Q74.0
- skull bone(s) NEC Q75.8
  - with
    - anencephalus Q00.0
    - encephalocele *—see* Encephalocele
    - hydrocephalus Q03.9
      - with spina bifida *—see* Spina bifida, with hydrocephalus
    - microcephaly Q02
- spinal cord Q06.8
- spine Q76.49
  - kyphosis *—see* Kyphosis, congenital
  - lordosis *—see* Lordosis, congenital

Distortion *(continued)*
- spleen Q89.09
- sternum NEC Q76.7
- thorax (wall) Q67.8
  - bony Q76.8
- thymus (gland) Q89.2
- thyroid (gland) Q89.2
- tibia NEC Q68.8
- toe(s) Q66.9-
- tongue Q38.3
- trachea (cartilage) Q32.1
- ulna NEC Q68.8
- ureter Q62.8
- urethra Q64.79
  - causing obstruction Q64.39
- uterus Q51.9
- vagina Q52.4
- vertebra Q76.49
  - kyphosis *—see* Kyphosis, congenital
  - lordosis *—see* Lordosis, congenital
- visual *—see also* Disturbance, vision
  - shape and size H53.15
- vulva Q52.79
- wrist (bones) (joint) Q68.8

Distress
- abdomen *—see* Pain, abdominal
- acute respiratory R06.03
  - syndrome (adult) (child) J80
- epigastric R10.13
- fetal P84
  - complicating pregnancy *—see* Stress, fetal
- gastrointestinal (functional) K30
  - psychogenic F45.8
- intestinal (functional) NOS K59.9
  - psychogenic F45.8
- maternal, during labor and delivery O75.0
- relationship, with spouse or intimate partner Z63.0
- respiratory (adult) (child) R06.03
  - newborn P22.9
    - specified NEC P22.8
  - orthopnea R06.01
  - psychogenic F45.8
  - shortness of breath R06.02
  - specified type NEC R06.09

Distribution vessel, atypical Q27.9
- coronary artery Q24.5
- precerebral Q28.1

Districhiasis L68.8

Disturbance(s) *—see also* Disease
- absorption K90.9
  - calcium E58
  - carbohydrate K90.49
  - fat K90.49
    - pancreatic K90.3
  - protein K90.49
  - starch K90.49
  - vitamin *—see* Deficiency, vitamin
- acid-base equilibrium E87.8
  - mixed E87.4
- activity and attention (with hyperkinesis) *—see* Disorder, attention-deficit hyperactivity
- amino acid transport E72.00
- assimilation, food K90.9
- auditory nerve, except deafness *—see* subcategory H93.3
- behavior *—see* Disorder, conduct
- blood clotting (mechanism) (*see also* Defect, coagulation) D68.9
- cerebral
  - nerve *—see* Disorder, nerve, cranial
  - status, newborn P91.9
    - specified NEC P91.88

Disturbance *(continued)*
- circulatory I99.9
- conduct (*see also* Disorder, conduct) F91.9
  - adjustment reaction *—see* Disorder, adjustment
  - compulsive F63.9
  - disruptive F91.9
  - hyperkinetic *—see* Disorder, attention-deficit hyperactivity
  - socialized F91.2
  - specified NEC F91.8
  - unsocialized F91.1
- coordination R27.8
- cranial nerve *—see* Disorder, nerve, cranial
- deep sensibility *—see* Disturbance, sensation
- digestive K30
  - psychogenic F45.8
- electrolyte *—see also* Imbalance, electrolyte
  - newborn, transitory P74.49
    - hyperammonemia P74.6
    - hyperchloremia P74.421
    - hyperchloremic metabolic acidosis P74.421
    - hypochloremia P74.422
    - potassium balance
      - hyperkalemia P74.31
      - hypokalemia P74.32
    - sodium balance
      - hypernatremia P74.21
      - hyponatremia P74.22
    - specified type NEC P74.49
- emotions specific to childhood and adolescence F93.9
  - with
    - anxiety and fearfulness NEC F93.8
    - elective mutism F94.0
    - oppositional disorder F91.3
    - sensitivity (withdrawal) F40.10
    - shyness F40.10
    - social withdrawal F40.10
  - involving relationship problems F93.8
  - mixed F93.8
  - specified NEC F93.8
- endocrine (gland) E34.9
  - neonatal, transitory P72.9
    - specified NEC P72.8
- equilibrium R42
- fructose metabolism E74.10
- gait *—see* Gait
  - hysterical F44.4
  - psychogenic F44.4
- gastrointestinal (functional) K30
  - psychogenic F45.8
- habit, child F98.9
- hearing, except deafness and tinnitus *—see* Abnormal, auditory perception
- heart, functional (conditions in I44-I50)
  - due to presence of (cardiac) prosthesis I97.19-
  - postoperative I97.89
    - cardiac surgery (*see also* Infarct, myocardium, associated with revascularization procedure) I97.19-
- hormones E34.9
- innervation uterus (parasympathetic) (sympathetic) N85.8
- keratinization NEC
  - gingiva K05.10
    - nonplaque induced K05.11
    - plaque induced K05.10

Disturbance *(continued)*
- keratinization NEC *(continued)*
  - lip K13.0
  - oral (mucosa) (soft tissue) K13.29
  - tongue K13.29
- learning (specific) *—see* Disorder, learning
- memory *—see* Amnesia
  - mild, following organic brain damage F06.8
- mental F99
  - associated with diseases classified elsewhere F54
- metabolism E88.9
  - with
    - abortion *—see* Abortion, by type with other specified complication
    - ectopic pregnancy O08.5
    - molar pregnancy O08.5
  - amino-acid E72.9
    - aromatic E70.9
    - branched-chain E71.2
    - straight-chain E72.89
    - sulfur-bearing E72.10
  - ammonia E72.20
  - arginine E72.21
  - arginosuccinic acid E72.22
  - carbohydrate E74.9
  - cholesterol E78.9
  - citrulline E72.23
  - cystathionine E72.19
  - general E88.9
  - glutamine E72.89
  - histidine E70.40
  - homocystine E72.19
  - hydroxylysine E72.3
  - in labor or delivery O75.89
  - iron E83.10
  - lipoid E78.9
  - lysine E72.3
  - methionine E72.19
  - neonatal, transitory P74.9
    - calcium and magnesium P71.9
      - specified type NEC P71.8
    - carbohydrate metabolism P70.9
      - specified type NEC P70.8
    - specified NEC P74.8
  - ornithine E72.4
  - phosphate E83.39
  - sodium NEC E87.8
  - threonine E72.89
  - tryptophan E70.5
  - tyrosine E70.20
  - urea cycle E72.20
- motor R29.2
- nervous, functional R45.0
- neuromuscular mechanism (eye), due to syphilis A52.15
- nutritional E63.9
  - nail L60.3
- ocular motion H51.9
  - psychogenic F45.8
- oculogyric H51.8
  - psychogenic F45.8
- oculomotor H51.9
  - psychogenic F45.8
- olfactory nerve R43.1
- optic nerve NEC *—see* Disorder, nerve, optic
- oral epithelium, including tongue NEC K13.29
- perceptual due to
  - alcohol withdrawal F10.232
  - amphetamine intoxication F15.922
    - in
      - abuse F15.122
      - dependence F15.222

Disturbance *(continued)*
- perceptual due to *(continued)*
  - anxiolytic withdrawal F13.232
  - cannabis intoxication (acute) F12.922
    - in
      - abuse F12.122
      - dependence F12.222
  - cocaine intoxication (acute) F14.922
    - in
      - abuse F14.122
      - dependence F14.222
  - hypnotic withdrawal F13.232
  - opioid intoxication (acute) F19.122
  - phencyclidine intoxication (acute) F16.122
  - sedative withdrawal F13.232
- personality (pattern) (trait) *—see also* Disorder, personality F60.9
  - following organic brain damage F07.9
- polyglandular E31.9
  - specified NEC E31.8
- potassium balance, newborn
  - hyperkalemia P74.31
  - hypokalemia P74.32
- psychogenic F45.9
- psychomotor F44.4
- psychophysical visual H53.16
- pupillary *—see* Anomaly, pupil, function
- reflex R29.2
- rhythm, heart I49.9
- salivary secretion K11.7
- sensation (cold) (heat) (localization) (tactile discrimination) (texture) (vibratory) NEC R20.9
  - hysterical F44.6
  - skin R20.9
    - anesthesia R20.0
    - hyperesthesia R20.3
    - hypoesthesia R20.1
    - paresthesia R20.2
    - specified type NEC R20.8
  - smell R43.9
    - and taste (mixed) R43.8
    - anosmia R43.0
    - parosmia R43.1
    - specified NEC R43.8
  - taste R43.9
    - and smell (mixed) R43.8
    - parageusia R43.2
    - specified NEC R43.8
- sensory *—see* Disturbance, sensation
- situational (transient) *—see also* Disorder, adjustment
  - acute F43.0
- sleep G47.9
  - nonorganic origin F51.9
- smell *—see* Disturbance, sensation, smell
- sociopathic F60.2
- sodium balance, newborn
  - hypernatremia P74.21
  - hyponatremia P74.22
- speech R47.9
  - developmental F80.9
  - specified NEC R47.89
- stomach (functional) K31.9
- sympathetic (nerve) G90.9
- taste *—see* Disturbance, sensation, taste
- temperature
  - regulation, newborn P81.9
    - specified NEC P81.8
  - sense R20.8
    - hysterical F44.6

Disturbance *(continued)*
- tooth
  - eruption K00.6
  - formation K00.4
  - structure, hereditary NEC K00.5
- touch *—see* Disturbance, sensation
- vascular I99.9
  - arteriosclerotic *—see* Arteriosclerosis
- vasomotor I73.9
- vasospastic I73.9
- vision, visual H53.9
  - following
    - cerebral infarction I69.398
    - cerebrovascular disease I69.998
      - specified NEC I69.898
    - intracerebral hemorrhage I69.198
    - nontraumatic intracranial hemorrhage NEC I69.298
    - specified disease NEC I69.898
    - subarachnoid hemorrhage I69.098
  - psychophysical H53.16
  - specified NEC H53.8
  - subjective H53.10
    - day blindness H53.11
    - discomfort H53.14-
    - distortions of shape and size H53.15
    - loss
      - sudden H53.13-
      - transient H53.12-
    - specified type NEC H53.19
- voice R49.9
  - psychogenic F44.4
  - specified NEC R49.8

Diuresis R35.89

Diver's palsy, paralysis or squeeze T70.3

Diverticulitis (acute) K57.92
- bladder *—see* Cystitis
- ileum *—see* Diverticulitis, intestine, small
- intestine K57.92
  - with
    - abscess, perforation K57.80
      - with bleeding K57.81
    - bleeding K57.93
  - congenital Q43.8
  - large K57.32
    - with
      - abscess, perforation K57.20
        - with bleeding K57.21
      - bleeding K57.33
      - small intestine K57.52
        - with
          - abscess, perforation K57.40
            - with bleeding K57.41
          - bleeding K57.53
  - small K57.12
    - with
      - abscess, perforation K57.00
        - with bleeding K57.01
      - bleeding K57.13
      - large intestine K57.52
        - with
          - abscess, perforation K57.40
            - with bleeding K57.41
          - bleeding K57.53

Diverticulosis K57.90
- with bleeding K57.91

Diverticulosis *(continued)*
- large intestine K57.30
  - with
    - bleeding K57.31
    - small intestine K57.50
      - with bleeding K57.51
- small intestine K57.10
  - with
    - bleeding K57.11
    - large intestine K57.50
      - with bleeding K57.51

Diverticulum, diverticula (multiple) K57.90
- appendix (noninflammatory) K38.2
- bladder (sphincter) N32.3
  - congenital Q64.6
- bronchus (congenital) Q32.4
  - acquired J98.09
- calyx, calyceal (kidney) N28.89
- cardia (stomach) K31.4
- cecum *—see* Diverticulosis, intestine, large
  - congenital Q43.8
- colon *—see* Diverticulosis, intestine, large
  - congenital Q43.8
- duodenum *—see* Diverticulosis, intestine, small
  - congenital Q43.8
- epiphrenic (esophagus) K22.5
- esophagus (congenital) Q39.6
  - acquired (epiphrenic) (pulsion) (traction) K22.5
- eustachian tube *—see* Disorder, eustachian tube, specified NEC
- fallopian tube N83.8
- gastric K31.4
- heart (congenital) Q24.8
- ileum *—see* Diverticulosis, intestine, small
- jejunum *—see* Diverticulosis, intestine, small
- kidney (pelvis) (calyces) N28.89
  - with calculus *—see* Calculus, kidney
- Meckel's (displaced) (hypertrophic) Q43.0
  - malignant *—see* Table of Neoplasms, small intestine, malignant
- midthoracic K22.5
- organ or site, congenital NEC *—see* Distortion
- pericardium (congenital) (cyst) Q24.8
  - acquired I31.8
- pharyngoesophageal (congenital) Q39.6
  - acquired K22.5
- pharynx (congenital) Q38.7
- rectosigmoid *—see* Diverticulosis, intestine, large
  - congenital Q43.8
- rectum *—see* Diverticulosis, intestine, large
- Rokitansky's K22.5
- seminal vesicle N50.89
- sigmoid *—see* Diverticulosis, intestine, large
  - congenital Q43.8
- stomach (acquired) K31.4
  - congenital Q40.2
- trachea (acquired) J39.8
- ureter (acquired) N28.89
  - congenital Q62.8
- ureterovesical orifice N28.89
- urethra (acquired) N36.1
  - congenital Q64.79
- ventricle, left (congenital) Q24.8

Diverticulum, diverticula *(continued)*
- vesical N32.3
  - congenital Q64.6
- Zenker's (esophagus) K22.5

Division
- cervix uteri (acquired) N88.8
- glans penis Q55.69
- labia minora (congenital) Q52.79
- ligament (partial or complete) (current) *—see also* Sprain
  - with open wound *—see* Wound, open
- muscle (partial or complete) (current) *—see also* Injury, muscle
  - with open wound *—see* Wound, open
- nerve (traumatic) *—see* Injury, nerve
- spinal cord *—see* Injury, spinal cord, by region
- vein I87.8

Divorce, causing family disruption Z63.5

Dix-Hallpike neurolabyrinthitis *—see* Neuronitis, vestibular

Dizziness R42
- hysterical F44.89
- psychogenic F45.8

DMAC (disseminated mycobacterium avium- intracellulare complex) A31.2

DNR (do not resuscitate) Z66

Doan-Wiseman syndrome (primary splenic neutropenia) *—see* Agranulocytosis

Doehle-Heller aortitis A52.02

Dog bite *—see* Bite

Dohle body panmyelopathic syndrome D72.0

Dolichocephaly Q67.2

Dolichocolon Q43.8

Dolichostenomelia *—see* Syndrome, Marfan's

Donohue's syndrome E34.8

Donor (organ or tissue) Z52.9
- blood (whole) Z52.000
  - autologous Z52.010
  - specified component (lymphocytes) (platelets) NEC Z52.008
    - autologous Z52.018
    - specified donor NEC Z52.098
  - specified donor NEC Z52.090
  - stem cells Z52.001
    - autologous Z52.011
    - specified donor NEC Z52.091
- bone Z52.20
  - autologous Z52.21
  - marrow Z52.3
  - specified type NEC Z52.29
- cornea Z52.5
- egg (Oocyte) Z52.819
  - age 35 and over Z52.812
    - anonymous recipient Z52.812
    - designated recipient Z52.813
  - under age 35 Z52.810
    - anonymous recipient Z52.810
    - designated recipient Z52.811
- kidney Z52.4
- liver Z52.6
- lung Z52.89
- lymphocyte *—see* Donor, blood, specified components NEC

Dysarthria *(continued)*
following *(continued)*
cerebrovascular disease I69.922
specified disease NEC I69.822
intracerebral hemorrhage I69.122
nontraumatic intracranial hemorrhage NEC I69.222
subarachnoid hemorrhage I69.022

Dysautonomia (familial) G90.1

Dysbarism T70.3

Dysbasia R26.2
angiosclerotica intermittens I73.9
hysterical F44.4
lordotica (progressiva) G24.1
nonorganic origin F44.4
psychogenic F44.4

Dysbetalipoproteinemia (familial) E78.2

Dyscalculia R48.8
developmental F81.2

Dyschezia K59.00

Dyschondroplasia (with hemangiomata) Q78.4

Dyschromia (skin) L81.9

Dyscollagenosis M35.9

Dyscranio-pygo-phalangy Q87.0

Dyscrasia
blood (with) D75.9
antepartum hemorrhage *—see* Hemorrhage, antepartum, with coagulation defect
newborn P61.9
specified type NEC P61.8
intrapartum hemorrhage O67.0
puerperal, postpartum O72.3
polyglandular, pluriglandular E31.9

Dysendocrinism E34.9

Dysentery, dysenteric (catarrhal) (diarrhea) (epidemic) (hemorrhagic) (infectious) (sporadic) (tropical) A09
abscess, liver A06.4
amebic (*see also* Amebiasis) A06.0
with abscess *—see* Abscess, amebic
acute A06.0
chronic A06.1
arthritis (*see also* category M01) A09
bacillary (*see also* category M01) A03.9
bacillary A03.9
arthritis (*see also* category M01) A03.9
Boyd A03.2
Flexner A03.1
Schmitz (-Stutzer) A03.0
Shiga (-Kruse) A03.0
Shigella A03.9
boydii A03.2
dysenteriae A03.0
flexneri A03.1
group A A03.0
group B A03.1
group C A03.2
group D A03.3
sonnei A03.3
specified type NEC A03.8
Sonne A03.3
specified type NEC A03.8
balantidial A07.0
Balantidium coli A07.0
Boyd's A03.2
candidal B37.82
Chilomastix A07.8

Dysentery, dysenteric *(continued)*
Chinese A03.9
coccidial A07.3
Dientamoeba (fragilis) A07.8
Embadomonas A07.8
Entamoeba, entamebic *—see* Dysentery, amebic
Flexner-Boyd A03.2
Flexner's A03.1
Giardia lamblia A07.1
Hiss-Russell A03.1
Lamblia A07.1
leishmanial B55.0
malarial *—see* Malaria
metazoal B82.0
monilial B37.82
protozoal A07.9
Salmonella A02.0
schistosomal B65.1
Schmitz (-Stutzer) A03.0
Shiga (-Kruse) A03.0
Shigella NOS *—see* Dysentery, bacillary
Sonne A03.3
strongyloidiasis B78.0
trichomonal A07.8
viral *—see also* Enteritis, viral A08.4

Dysequilibrium R42

Dysesthesia R20.8
hysterical F44.6

Dysfibrinogenemia (congenital) D68.2

Dysfunction
adrenal E27.9
hyperfunction E27.0
autonomic
due to alcohol G31.2
somatoform F45.8
bladder N31.9
neurogenic NOS *—see* Dysfunction, bladder, neuromuscular
neuromuscular NOS N31.9
atonic (motor) (sensory) N31.2
autonomous N31.2
flaccid N31.2
nonreflex N31.2
reflex N31.1
specified NEC N31.8
uninhibited N31.0
bleeding, uterus N93.8
cerebral G93.89
colon K59.9
psychogenic F45.8
colostomy K94.03
cystic duct K82.8
cystostomy (stoma) *—see* Complications, cystostomy
ejaculatory N53.19
anejaculatory orgasm N53.13
painful N53.12
premature F52.4
retarded N53.11
endocrine NOS E34.9
endometrium N85.8
enterostomy K94.13
erectile *—see* Dysfunction, sexual, male, erectile
feeding, pediatric
acute R63.31
chronic R63.32
gallbladder K82.8
gastrostomy (stoma) K94.23
gland, glandular NOS E34.9
meibomian, of eyelid *—see* Dysfunction, meibomian gland
heart I51.89
hemoglobin D75.89
hepatic K76.89

Dysfunction *(continued)*
hypophysis E23.7
hypothalamic NEC E23.3
ileostomy (stoma) K94.13
jejunostomy (stoma) K94.13
kidney *—see* Disease, renal
labyrinthine *—see* subcategory H83.2
left ventricular, following sudden emotional stress I51.81
liver K76.89
male *—see* Dysfunction, sexual, male
meibomian gland, of eyelid H02.889
left H02.886
lower H02.885
upper H02.884
upper and lower eyelids H02.88B
right H02.883
lower H02.882
upper H02.881
upper and lower eyelids H02.88A
orgasmic (female) F52.31
male F52.32
ovary E28.9
specified NEC E28.8
papillary muscle I51.89
parathyroid E21.4
physiological NEC R68.89
psychogenic F59
pineal gland E34.8
pituitary (gland) E23.3
platelets D69.1
polyglandular E31.9
specified NEC E31.8
psychophysiologic F59
psychosexual F52.9
with
dyspareunia F52.6
premature ejaculation F52.4
vaginismus F52.5
pylorus K31.9
rectum K59.9
psychogenic F45.8
reflex (sympathetic) *—see* Syndrome, pain, complex regional I
segmental *—see* Dysfunction, somatic
senile R54
sexual (due to) R37
alcohol F10.981
amphetamine F15.981
in
abuse F15.181
dependence F15.281
anxiolytic F13.981
in
abuse F13.181
dependence F13.281
cocaine F14.981
in
abuse F14.181
dependence F14.281
excessive sexual drive F52.8
failure of genital response (male) F52.21
female F52.22
female N94.9
aversion F52.1
dyspareunia N94.10
psychogenic F52.6
frigidity F52.22
nymphomania F52.8
orgasmic F52.31
psychogenic F52.9
aversion F52.1
dyspareunia F52.6

Dysfunction *(continued)*
sexual *(continued)*
female *(continued)*
psychogenic *(continued)*
frigidity F52.22
nymphomania F52.8
orgasmic F52.31
vaginismus F52.5
vaginismus N94.2
psychogenic F52.5
hypnotic F13.981
in
abuse F13.181
dependence F13.281
inhibited orgasm (female) F52.31
male F52.32
lack
of sexual enjoyment F52.1
or loss of sexual desire F52.0
male N53.9
anejaculatory orgasm N53.13
ejaculatory N53.19
painful N53.12
premature F52.4
retarded N53.11
erectile N52.9
drug induced N52.2
due to
disease classified elsewhere N52.1
drug N52.2
postoperative (postprocedural) N52.39
following
cryotherapy N52.37
interstitial seed therapy N52.36
prostate ablative therapy N52.37
prostatectomy N52.34
radical N52.31
radical cystectomy N52.32
radiation therapy N52.35
ultrasound ablative therapy N52.37
urethral surgery N52.33
psychogenic F52.21
specified cause NEC N52.8
vasculogenic
arterial insufficiency N52.01
with corporo-venous occlusive N52.03
corporo-venous occlusive N52.02
with arterial insufficiency N52.03
impotence *—see* Dysfunction, sexual, male, erectile
psychogenic F52.9
aversion F52.1
erectile F52.21
orgasmic F52.32
premature ejaculation F52.4
satyriasis F52.8
specified type NEC F52.8
specified type NEC N53.8
nonorganic F52.9
specified NEC F52.8
opioid F11.981
in
abuse F11.181
dependence F11.281
orgasmic dysfunction (female) F52.31
male F52.32
premature ejaculation F52.4

Dysfunction *(continued)*
- sexual *(continued)*
  - psychoactive substances NEC F19.981
    - in
      - abuse F19.181
      - dependence F19.281
  - psychogenic F52.9
  - sedative F13.981
    - in
      - abuse F13.181
      - dependence F13.281
  - sexual aversion F52.1
  - vaginismus (nonorganic) (psychogenic) F52.5
- sinoatrial node I49.5
- somatic M99.09
  - abdomen M99.09
  - acromioclavicular M99.07
  - cervical region M99.01
  - cervicothoracic M99.01
  - costochondral M99.08
  - costovertebral M99.08
  - head region M99.00
  - hip M99.05
  - lower extremity M99.06
  - lumbar region M99.03
  - lumbosacral M99.03
  - occipitocervical M99.00
  - pelvic region M99.05
  - pubic M99.05
  - rib cage M99.08
  - sacral region M99.04
  - sacrococcygeal M99.04
  - sacroiliac M99.04
  - specified NEC M99.09
  - sternochondral M99.08
  - sternoclavicular M99.07
  - thoracic region M99.02
  - thoracolumbar M99.02
  - upper extremity M99.07
- somatoform autonomic F45.8
- stomach K31.89
  - psychogenic F45.8
- suprarenal E27.9
  - hyperfunction E27.0
- symbolic R48.9
  - specified type NEC R48.8
- temporomandibular (joint) M26.69
  - joint-pain syndrome M26.62-
- testicular (endocrine) E29.9
  - specified NEC E29.8
- thymus E32.9
- thyroid E07.9
- ureterostomy (stoma) *—see* Complications, stoma, urinary tract
- urethrostomy (stoma) *—see* Complications, stoma, urinary tract
- uterus, complicating delivery O62.9
  - hypertonic O62.4
  - hypotonic O62.2
    - primary O62.0
    - secondary O62.1
- ventricular I51.9
  - with congestive heart failure (*see also* Failure, heart) I50.9
  - left, reversible, following sudden emotional stress I51.81

Dysgenesis
- gonadal (due to chromosomal anomaly) Q96.9
  - pure Q99.1
- renal Q60.5
  - bilateral Q60.4
  - unilateral Q60.3
- reticular D72.0
- tidal platelet D69.3

Dysgerminoma
- specified site *—see* Neoplasm, malignant, by site
- unspecified site
  - female C56.9
  - male C62.90

Dysgeusia R43.2

Dysgraphia R27.8

Dyshidrosis, dysidrosis L30.1

Dyskaryotic cervical smear R87.619

Dyskeratosis L85.8
- cervix *—see* Dysplasia, cervix
- congenital Q82.8
- uterus NEC N85.8

Dyskinesia G24.9
- biliary (cystic duct or gallbladder) K82.8
- drug induced
  - orofacial G24.01
- esophagus K22.4
- hysterical F44.4
- intestinal K59.89
- nonorganic origin F44.4
- orofacial (idiopathic) G24.4
  - drug induced G24.01
- psychogenic F44.4
- subacute, drug induced G24.01
- tardive G24.01
  - neuroleptic induced G24.01
- trachea J39.8
- tracheobronchial J98.09

Dyslalia (developmental) F80.0

Dyslexia R48.0
- developmental F81.0

Dyslipidemia E78.5
- depressed HDL cholesterol E78.6
- elevated fasting triglycerides E78.1

Dysmaturity *—see also* Light for dates
- pulmonary (newborn) (Wilson-Mikity) P27.0

Dysmenorrhea (essential) (exfoliative) N94.6
- congestive (syndrome) N94.6
- primary N94.4
- psychogenic F45.8
- secondary N94.5

Dysmetabolic syndrome X E88.81

Dysmetria R27.8

Dysmorphism (due to)
- alcohol Q86.0
- exogenous cause NEC Q86.8
- hydantoin Q86.1
- warfarin Q86.2

Dysmorphophobia (nondelusional) F45.22
- delusional F22

Dysnomia R47.01

Dysorexia R63.0
- psychogenic F50.89

Dysostosis
- cleidocranial, cleidocranialis Q74.0
- craniofacial Q75.1
- Fairbank's (idiopathic familial generalized osteophytosis) Q78.9
- mandibulofacial (incomplete) Q75.4
- multiplex E76.01
- oculomandibular Q75.5

Dyspareunia (female) N94.10
- deep N94.12
- male N53.12
- nonorganic F52.6
- psychogenic F52.6
- secondary N94.19
- specified NEC N94.19
- superficial (introital) N94.11

Dyspepsia R10.13
- atonic K30
- functional (allergic) (congenital) (gastrointestinal) (occupational) (reflex) K30
- intestinal K59.89
- nervous F45.8
- neurotic F45.8
- psychogenic F45.8

Dysphagia R13.10
- cervical R13.19
- following
  - cerebral infarction I69.391
  - cerebrovascular disease I69.991
    - specified NEC I69.891
  - intracerebral hemorrhage I69.191
  - nontraumatic intracranial hemorrhage NEC I69.291
  - specified disease NEC I69.891
  - subarachnoid hemorrhage I69.091
- functional (hysterical) F45.8
- hysterical F45.8
- nervous (hysterical) F45.8
- neurogenic R13.19
- oral phase R13.11
- oropharyngeal phase R13.12
- pharyngeal phase R13.13
- pharyngoesophageal phase R13.14
- psychogenic F45.8
- sideropenic D50.1
- spastica K22.4
- specified NEC R13.19

Dysphagocytosis, congenital D71

Dysphasia R47.02
- developmental
  - expressive type F80.1
  - receptive type F80.2
- following
  - cerebrovascular disease I69.921
    - cerebral infarction I69.321
    - intracerebral hemorrhage I69.121
    - nontraumatic intracranial hemorrhage NEC I69.221
    - specified disease NEC I69.821
    - subarachnoid hemorrhage I69.021

Dysphonia R49.0
- functional F44.4
- hysterical F44.4
- psychogenic F44.4
- spastica J38.3

Dysphoria
- gender F64.9
  - in
    - adolescence and adulthood F64.0
    - children F64.2
  - postpartal O90.6
  - specified NEC F64.8

Dyspituitarism E23.3

Dysplasia *—see also* Anomaly
- acetabular, congenital Q65.89
- alveolar capillary, with vein misalignment J84.843
- anus (histologically confirmed) (mild) (moderate) K62.82
  - severe D01.3
- arrhythmogenic right ventricular I42.8
- arterial, fibromuscular I77.3
- asphyxiating thoracic (congenital) Q77.2
- brain Q07.9
- bronchopulmonary, perinatal P27.1
- cervix (uteri) N87.9
  - mild N87.0
  - moderate N87.1
  - severe D06.9
- chondroectodermal Q77.6
- colon D12.6
- craniometaphyseal Q78.8
- dentinal K00.5
- diaphyseal, progressive Q78.3
- dystrophic Q77.5
- ectodermal (anhidrotic) (congenital) (hereditary) Q82.4
  - hydrotic Q82.8
- epithelial, uterine cervix *—see* Dysplasia, cervix
- eye (congenital) Q11.2
- fibrous
  - bone NEC (monostotic) M85.00
    - ankle M85.07-
    - foot M85.07-
    - forearm M85.03-
    - hand M85.04-
    - lower leg M85.06-
    - multiple site M85.09
    - neck M85.08
    - rib M85.08
    - shoulder M85.01-
    - skull M85.08
    - specified site NEC M85.08
    - thigh M85.05-
    - toe M85.07-
    - upper arm M85.02-
    - vertebra M85.08
  - diaphyseal, progressive Q78.3
  - jaw M27.8
  - polyostotic Q78.1
- florid osseous *—see also* Cyst, calcifying odontogenic
- high grade, focal D12.6
- hip, congenital Q65.89
- joint, congenital Q74.8
- kidney Q61.4
  - multicystic Q61.4
- leg Q74.2
- lung, congenital (not associated with short gestation) Q33.6
- mammary (gland) (benign) N60.9-
  - cyst (solitary) *—see* Cyst, breast
  - cystic *—see* Mastopathy, cystic
  - duct ectasia *—see* Ectasia, mammary duct
  - fibroadenosis *—see* Fibroadenosis, breast
  - fibrosclerosis *—see* Fibrosclerosis, breast
  - specified type NEC N60.8-
- metaphyseal Q78.5
  - specified NEC N42.39
- muscle Q79.8
- oculodentodigital Q87.0
- periapical (cemental) (cemento-osseous) *—see* Cyst, calcifying odontogenic
- periosteum *—see* Disorder, bone, specified type NEC
- polyostotic fibrous Q78.1
- prostate (*see also* Neoplasia, intraepithelial, prostate) N42.30
  - severe D07.5
  - specified NEC N42.39
- renal Q61.4
  - multicystic Q61.4
- retinal, congenital Q14.1
- right ventricular, arrhythmogenic I42.8
- septo-optic Q04.4
- skin L98.8
- spinal cord Q06.1

Dysplasia *(continued)*
- spondyloepiphyseal Q77.7
- thymic, with immunodeficiency D82.1
- vagina N89.3
  - mild N89.0
  - moderate N89.1
  - severe NEC D07.2
- vulva N90.3
  - mild N90.0
  - moderate N90.1
  - severe NEC D07.1

Dysplasminogenemia E88.02

Dyspnea (nocturnal) (paroxysmal) R06.00
- asthmatic (bronchial) J45.909
  - with
    - exacerbation (acute) J45.901
    - bronchitis J45.909
      - with
        - exacerbation (acute) J45.901
        - status asthmaticus J45.902
      - chronic J44.9
    - status asthmaticus J45.902
  - cardiac *—see* Failure, ventricular, left
- cardiac *—see* Failure, ventricular, left
- functional F45.8
- hyperventilation R06.4
- hysterical F45.8
- newborn P28.89
- orthopnea R06.01
- psychogenic F45.8
- shortness of breath R06.02
- specified type NEC R06.09

Dyspraxia R27.8
- developmental (syndrome) F82

Dysproteinemia E88.09

Dysreflexia, autonomic G90.4

Dysrhythmia
- cardiac I49.9
  - newborn
    - bradycardia P29.12
    - occurring before birth P03.819
      - before onset of labor P03.810
      - during labor P03.811
    - tachycardia P29.11
  - postoperative I97.89
- cerebral or cortical *—see* Epilepsy

Dyssomnia *—see* Disorder, sleep

Dyssynergia
- biliary K83.8
- bladder sphincter N36.44
- cerebellaris myoclonica (Hunt's ataxia) G11.19

Dysthymia F34.1

Dysthyroidism E07.9

Dystocia O66.9
- affecting newborn P03.1
- cervical (hypotonic) O62.2
  - affecting newborn P03.6
  - primary O62.0
  - secondary O62.1
- contraction ring O62.4
- fetal O66.9
  - abnormality NEC O66.3
  - conjoined twins O66.3
  - oversize O66.2
- maternal O66.9
- positional O64.9
- shoulder (girdle) O66.0
  - causing obstructed labor O66.0
- uterine NEC O62.4

Dystonia G24.9
- cervical G24.3
- deformans progressiva G24.1
- drug induced NEC G24.09
  - acute G24.02
  - specified NEC G24.09
- familial G24.1
- idiopathic G24.1
  - familial G24.1
  - nonfamilial G24.2
  - orofacial G24.4
- lenticularis G24.8
- musculorum deformans G24.1
- neuroleptic induced (acute) G24.02
- orofacial (idiopathic) G24.4
- oromandibular G24.4
  - due to drug G24.01
- specified NEC G24.8
- torsion (familial) (idiopathic) G24.1
  - acquired G24.8
  - genetic G24.1
  - symptomatic (nonfamilial) G24.2

Dystonic movements R25.8

Dystrophy, dystrophia
- adiposogenital E23.6
- autosomal recessive, childhood type, muscular dystrophy resembling Duchenne or Becker G71.01
- Becker's type G71.01
- cervical sympathetic G90.2
- choroid (hereditary) H31.20
  - central areolar H31.22
  - choroideremia H31.21
  - gyrate atrophy H31.23
  - specified type NEC H31.29
- cornea (hereditary) H18.50-
  - endothelial H18.51-
  - epithelial H18.52-
  - granular H18.53-
  - lattice H18.54-
  - macular H18.55-
  - specified type NEC H18.59-
- Duchenne's type G71.01
- due to malnutrition E45
- Erb's G71.02
- Fuchs' H18.51-
- Gower's muscular G71.01
- hair L67.8
- infantile neuraxonal G31.89
- Landouzy-Déjérine G71.02
- Leyden-Möbius G71.09
- muscular G71.00
  - autosomal recessive, childhood type, muscular dystrophy resembling Duchenne or Becker G71.01
  - benign (Becker type) G71.01
    - scapuloperoneal with early contractures [Emery-Dreifuss] G71.09
  - congenital (hereditary) (progressive) (with specific morphological abnormalities of the muscle fiber) G71.09
    - myotonic G71.11
  - distal G71.09
  - Duchenne type G71.01
  - Emery-Dreifuss G71.09
  - Erb type G71.02
  - facioscapulohumeral G71.02
  - Gower's G71.01
  - hereditary (progressive) G71.09
  - Landouzy-Déjérine type G71.02
  - limb-girdle G71.09
  - myotonic G71.11
  - progressive (hereditary) G71.09
    - Charcot-Marie (-Tooth) type G60.0

Dystrophy, dystrophia *(continued)*
- muscular *(continued)*
  - pseudohypertrophic (infantile) G71.01
  - scapulohumeral G71.02
  - scapuloperoneal G71.09
  - severe (Duchenne type) G71.01
  - specified type NEC G71.09
- myocardium, myocardial *—see* Degeneration, myocardial
- nail L60.3
  - congenital Q84.6
- nutritional E45
- ocular G71.09
- oculocerebrorenal E72.03
- oculopharyngeal G71.09
- ovarian N83.8
- polyglandular E31.8
- reflex (neuromuscular) (sympathetic) *—see* Syndrome, pain, complex regional I
- retinal (hereditary) H35.50
  - in
    - lipid storage disorders E75.6 *[H36]*
    - systemic lipidoses E75.6 *[H36]*
  - involving
    - pigment epithelium H35.54
    - sensory area H35.53
  - pigmentary H35.52
  - vitreoretinal H35.51
- Salzmann's nodular *—see* Degeneration, cornea, nodular
- scapuloperoneal G71.09
- skin NEC L98.8
- sympathetic (reflex) *—see* Syndrome, pain, complex regional I
  - cervical G90.2
- tapetoretinal H35.54
- thoracic, asphyxiating Q77.2
- unguium L60.3
  - congenital Q84.6
- vitreoretinal H35.51
- vulva N90.4
- yellow (liver) *—see* Failure, hepatic

Dysuria R30.0
- psychogenic F45.8

E

Eales' disease H35.06-

Ear *—see also* condition
- piercing Z41.3
- tropical NEC B36.9 *[H62.40]*
  - in
    - aspergillosis B44.89
    - candidiasis B37.84
    - moniliasis B37.84
- wax (impacted) H61.20
  - left H61.22
    - with right H61.23
  - right H61.21
    - with left H61.23

Earache *—see* subcategory H92.0

Early satiety R68.81

Eaton-Lambert syndrome *—see* Syndrome, Lambert-Eaton

Eberth's disease (typhoid fever) A01.00

Ebola virus disease A98.4

Ebstein's anomaly or syndrome (heart) Q22.5

Eccentro-osteochondrodysplasia E76.29

Ecchondroma *—see* Neoplasm, bone, benign

Ecchondrosis D48.0

Ecchymosis R58
- conjunctiva *—see* Hemorrhage, conjunctiva
- eye (traumatic) *—see* Contusion, eyeball
- eyelid (traumatic) *—see* Contusion, eyelid
- newborn P54.5
- spontaneous R23.3
- traumatic *—see* Contusion

Echinococciasis *—see* Echinococcus

Echinococcosis *—see* Echinococcus

Echinococcus (infection) B67.90
- granulosus B67.4
  - bone B67.2
  - liver B67.0
  - lung B67.1
  - multiple sites B67.32
  - specified site NEC B67.39
  - thyroid B67.31
- liver NOS B67.8
  - granulosus B67.0
  - multilocularis B67.5
- lung NEC B67.99
  - granulosus B67.1
  - multilocularis B67.69
- multilocularis B67.7
  - liver B67.5
  - multiple sites B67.61
  - specified site NEC B67.69
- specified site NEC B67.99
  - granulosus B67.39
  - multilocularis B67.69
- thyroid NEC B67.99
  - granulosus B67.31
  - multilocularis B67.69 *[E35]*

Echinorhynchiasis B83.8

Echinostomiasis B66.8

Echolalia R48.8

Echovirus, as cause of disease classified elsewhere B97.12

Eclampsia, eclamptic (coma) (convulsions) (delirium) (with hypertension) **NEC** O15.9
- complicating
  - labor and delivery O15.1
  - postpartum O15.2
  - pregnancy O15.0-
  - puerperal O15.2

Economic circumstances affecting care Z59.9

Economo's disease A85.8

Ectasia, ectasis
- annuloaortic I35.8
- aorta I77.819
  - with aneurysm *—see* Aneurysm, aorta
  - abdominal I77.811
  - thoracic I77.810
  - thoracoabdominal I77.812
- breast *—see* Ectasia, mammary duct
- capillary I78.8
- cornea H18.71-
- gastric antral vascular (GAVE) K31.819
  - with hemorrhage K31.811
  - without hemorrhage K31.819
- mammary duct N60.4-
- salivary gland (duct) K11.8
- sclera *—see* Sclerectasia

Ecthyma L08.0
- contagiosum B08.02
- gangrenosum L08.0
- infectiosum B08.02

Ectocardia Q24.8

Ectodermal dysplasia (anhidrotic) Q82.4

Ectodermosis erosiva pluriorificialis L51.1

Ectopic, ectopia (congenital)
- abdominal viscera Q45.8
  - due to defect in anterior abdominal wall Q79.59
- ACTH syndrome E24.3
- adrenal gland Q89.1
- anus Q43.5
- atrial beats I49.1
- beats I49.49
  - atrial I49.1
  - ventricular I49.3
- bladder Q64.10
- bone and cartilage in lung Q33.5
- brain Q04.8
- breast tissue Q83.8
- cardiac Q24.8
- cerebral Q04.8
- cordis Q24.8
- endometrium —*see* Endometriosis
- gastric mucosa Q40.2
- gestation —*see* Pregnancy, by site
- heart Q24.8
- hormone secretion NEC E34.2
- kidney (crossed) (pelvis) Q63.2
- lens, lentis Q12.1
- mole —*see* Pregnancy, by site
- organ or site NEC —*see* Malposition, congenital
- pancreas Q45.3
- pregnancy —*see* Pregnancy, ectopic
- pupil —*see* Abnormality, pupillary
- renal Q63.2
- sebaceous glands of mouth Q38.6
- spleen Q89.09
- testis Q53.00
  - bilateral Q53.02
  - unilateral Q53.01
- thyroid Q89.2
- tissue in lung Q33.5
- ureter Q62.63
- ventricular beats I49.3
- vesicae Q64.10

Ectromelia Q73.8
- lower limb —*see* Defect, reduction, limb, lower, specified type NEC
- upper limb —*see* Defect, reduction, limb, upper, specified type NEC

Ectropion H02.109
- cervix N86
  - with cervicitis N72
- congenital Q10.1
- eyelid H02.109
  - cicatricial H02.119
    - left H02.116
      - lower H02.115
      - upper H02.114
    - right H02.113
      - lower H02.112
      - upper H02.111
  - congenital Q10.1
  - left H02.106
    - lower H02.105
    - upper H02.104
  - mechanical H02.129
    - left H02.126
      - lower H02.125
      - upper H02.124
    - right H02.123
      - lower H02.122
      - upper H02.121
  - paralytic H02.159
    - left H02.156
      - lower H02.155
      - upper H02.154

Ectropion *(continued)*
- eyelid *(continued)*
  - paralytic *(continued)*
    - right H02.153
      - lower H02.152
      - upper H02.151
  - right H02.103
    - lower H02.102
    - upper H02.101
  - senile H02.139
    - left H02.136
      - lower H02.135
      - upper H02.134
    - right H02.133
      - lower H02.132
      - upper H02.131
  - spastic H02.149
    - left H02.146
      - lower H02.145
      - upper H02.144
    - right H02.143
      - lower H02.142
      - upper H02.141
- iris H21.89
- lip (acquired) K13.0
  - congenital Q38.0
- urethra N36.8
- uvea H21.89

Eczema (acute) (chronic) (erythematous) (fissum) (rubrum) (squamous) —*see also* Dermatitis L30.9
- contact —*see* Dermatitis, contact
- dyshydrotic L30.1
- external ear —*see* Otitis, externa, acute, eczematoid
- flexural L20.82
- herpeticum B00.0
- hypertrophicum L28.0
- hypostatic —*see* Varix, leg, with, inflammation
- impetiginous L01.1
- infantile (due to any substance) L20.83
  - intertriginous L21.1
  - seborrheic L21.1
- intertriginous NEC L30.4
  - infantile L21.1
- intrinsic (allergic) L20.84
- lichenified NEC L28.0
- marginatum (hebrae) B35.6
- pustular L30.3
- stasis I87.2
  - with varicose veins —*see* Varix, leg, with, inflammation
- vaccination, vaccinatum T88.1
- varicose —*see* Varix, leg, with, inflammation

Eczematid L30.2

Eddowes (-Spurway) **syndrome** Q78.0

Edema, edematous (infectious) (pitting) (toxic) R60.9
- with nephritis —*see* Nephrosis
- allergic T78.3
- amputation stump (surgical) (sequelae (late effect)) T87.89
- angioneurotic (allergic) (any site) (with urticaria) T78.3
  - hereditary D84.1
- angiospastic I73.9
- Berlin's (traumatic) S05.8X-
- brain (cytotoxic) (vasogenic) G93.6
  - due to birth injury P11.0
  - newborn (anoxia or hypoxia) P52.4
    - birth injury P11.0
  - traumatic —*see* Injury, intracranial, cerebral edema

Edema, edematous *(continued)*
- cardiac —*see* Failure, heart, congestive
- cardiovascular —*see* Failure, heart, congestive
- cerebral —*see* Edema, brain
- cerebrospinal —*see* Edema, brain
- cervix (uteri) (acute) N88.8
  - puerperal, postpartum O90.89
- chronic hereditary Q82.0
- circumscribed, acute T78.3
  - hereditary D84.1
- conjunctiva H11.42-
- cornea H18.2-
  - idiopathic H18.22-
  - secondary H18.23-
    - due to contact lens H18.21-
- due to
  - lymphatic obstruction I89.0
  - salt retention E87.0
- epiglottis —*see* Edema, glottis
- essential, acute T78.3
  - hereditary D84.1
- extremities, lower —*see* Edema, legs
- eyelid NEC H02.849
  - left H02.846
    - lower H02.845
    - upper H02.844
  - right H02.843
    - lower H02.842
    - upper H02.841
- familial, hereditary Q82.0
- famine —*see* Malnutrition, severe
- generalized R60.1
- glottis, glottic, glottidis (obstructive) (passive) J38.4
  - allergic T78.3
    - hereditary D84.1
- heart —*see* Failure, heart, congestive
- heat T67.7
- hereditary Q82.0
- inanition —*see* Malnutrition, severe
- intracranial G93.6
- iris H21.89
- joint —*see* Effusion, joint
- larynx —*see* Edema, glottis
- legs R60.0
  - due to venous obstruction I87.1
  - hereditary Q82.0
- localized R60.0
  - due to venous obstruction I87.1
- lower limbs —*see* Edema, legs
- lung J81.1
  - with heart condition or failure —*see* Failure, ventricular, left
  - acute J81.0
  - chemical (acute) J68.1
    - chronic J68.1
  - chronic J81.1
    - due to
      - chemicals, gases, fumes or vapors (inhalation) J68.1
      - external agent J70.9
        - specified NEC J70.8
      - radiation J70.1
  - due to
    - chemicals, fumes or vapors (inhalation) J68.1
    - external agent J70.9
      - specified NEC J70.8
    - high altitude T70.29
    - near drowning T75.1
    - radiation J70.0
  - meaning failure, left ventricle I50.1
- lymphatic I89.0
  - due to mastectomy I97.2
- macula H35.81

Edema, edematous *(continued)*
- macula *(continued)*
  - cystoid, following cataract surgery —*see* Complications, postprocedural, following cataract surgery
  - diabetic —*see* Diabetes, by type, with, retinopathy, with macular edema
- malignant —*see* Gangrene, gas
- Milroy's Q82.0
- nasopharynx J39.2
- newborn P83.30
  - hydrops fetalis —*see* Hydrops, fetalis
  - specified NEC P83.39
- nutritional —*see also* Malnutrition, severe
  - with dyspigmentation, skin and hair E40
- optic disc or nerve —*see* Papilledema
- orbit H05.22-
- pancreas K86.89
- papilla, optic —*see* Papilledema
- penis N48.89
- periodic T78.3
  - hereditary D84.1
- pharynx J39.2
- pulmonary —*see* Edema, lung
- Quincke's T78.3
  - hereditary D84.1
- renal —*see* Nephrosis
- retina H35.81
  - diabetic —*see* Diabetes, by type, with, retinopathy, with macular edema
- salt E87.0
- scrotum N50.89
- seminal vesicle N50.89
- spermatic cord N50.89
- spinal (cord) (vascular) (nontraumatic) G95.19
- starvation —*see* Malnutrition, severe
- stasis —*see* Hypertension, venous, (chronic)
- subglottic —*see* Edema, glottis
- supraglottic —*see* Edema, glottis
- testis N44.8
- tunica vaginalis N50.89
- vas deferens N50.89
- vulva (acute) N90.89

Edentulism —*see* Absence, teeth, acquired

Edsall's disease T67.2

Educational handicap Z55.9
- less than a high school diploma Z55.5
- no general equivalence degree (GED) Z55.5
- specified NEC Z55.8

Edward's syndrome —*see* Trisomy, 18

Effect, adverse
- abnormal gravitational (G) forces or states T75.81
- abuse —*see* Maltreatment
- air pressure T70.9
  - specified NEC T70.8
- altitude (high) —*see* Effect, adverse, high altitude
- anesthesia (*see also* Anesthesia) T88.59
  - in labor and delivery O74.9
  - local, toxic
    - in labor and delivery O74.4
    - in pregnancy NEC O29.3-
    - postpartum, puerperal O89.3

Effect, adverse *(continued)*
- anesthesia *(continued)*
  - postpartum, puerperal O89.9
  - specified NEC T88.59
    - in labor and delivery O74.8
    - postpartum, puerperal O89.8
  - spinal and epidural T88.59
    - headache T88.59
      - in labor and delivery O74.5
      - postpartum, puerperal O89.4
    - specified NEC
      - in labor and delivery O74.6
      - postpartum, puerperal O89.5
- antitoxin —*see* Complications, vaccination
- atmospheric pressure T70.9
  - due to explosion T70.8
  - high T70.3
  - low —*see* Effect, adverse, high altitude
  - specified effect NEC T70.8
- biological, correct substance properly administered —*see* Effect, adverse, drug
- blood (derivatives) (serum) (transfusion) —*see* Complications, transfusion
- chemical substance —*see* Table of Drugs and Chemicals
- cold (temperature) (weather) T69.9
  - chilblains T69.1
  - frostbite —*see* Frostbite
  - specified effect NEC T69.8
- drugs and medicaments T88.7
  - specified drug —*see* Table of Drugs and Chemicals, by drug, adverse effect
  - specified effect - code to condition
- electric current, electricity (shock) T75.4
  - burn —*see* Burn
- exertion (excessive) T73.3
- exposure —*see* Exposure
- external cause NEC T75.89
- foodstuffs T78.1
  - allergic reaction —*see* Allergy, food
    - causing anaphylaxis —*see* Shock, anaphylactic, due to food
  - noxious —*see* Poisoning, food, noxious
- gases, fumes, or vapors T59.9-
  - specified agent —*see* Table of Drugs and Chemicals
- glue (airplane) sniffing
  - due to drug abuse —*see* Abuse, drug, inhalant
  - due to drug dependence —*see* Dependence, drug, inhalant
- heat —*see* Heat
- high altitude NEC T70.29
  - anoxia T70.29
  - on
    - ears T70.0
    - sinuses T70.1
  - polycythemia D75.1
- high pressure fluids T70.4
- hot weather —*see* Heat
- hunger T73.0
- immersion, foot —*see* Immersion
- immunization —*see* Complications, vaccination
- immunological agents —*see* Complications, vaccination
- infrared (radiation) (rays) NOS T66
  - dermatitis or eczema L59.8
- infusion —*see* Complications, infusion
- lack of care of infants —*see* Maltreatment, child

Effect, adverse *(continued)*
- lightning —*see* Lightning
- medical care T88.9
  - specified NEC T88.8
- medicinal substance, correct, properly administered —*see* Effect, adverse, drug
- motion T75.3
- noise, on inner ear —*see* subcategory H83.3
- overheated places —*see* Heat
- psychosocial, of work environment Z56.5
- radiation (diagnostic) (infrared) (natural source) (therapeutic) (ultraviolet) (X-ray) NOS T66
  - dermatitis or eczema —*see* Dermatitis, due to, radiation
  - fibrosis of lung J70.1
  - pneumonitis J70.0
  - pulmonary manifestations
    - acute J70.0
    - chronic J70.1
  - skin L59.9
- radioactive substance NOS
  - dermatitis or eczema —*see* Radiodermatitis
- reduced temperature T69.9
  - immersion foot or hand —*see* Immersion
  - specified effect NEC T69.8
- serum NEC (*see also* Reaction, serum) T80.69
- specified NEC T78.8
  - external cause NEC T75.89
- strangulation —*see* Asphyxia, traumatic
- submersion T75.1
- thirst T73.1
- toxic —*see* Toxicity
- transfusion —*see* Complications, transfusion
- ultraviolet (radiation) (rays) NOS T66
  - burn —*see* Burn
  - dermatitis or eczema —*see* Dermatitis, due to, ultraviolet rays
    - acute L56.8
- vaccine (any) —*see* Complications, vaccination
- vibration —*see* Vibration, adverse effects
- water pressure NEC T70.9
  - specified NEC T70.8
- weightlessness T75.82
- whole blood —*see* Complications, transfusion
- work environment Z56.5

Effect(s) (of) (from) —*see* Effect, adverse NEC

Effects, late —*see* Sequelae

Effluvium
- anagen L65.1
- telogen L65.0

Effort syndrome (psychogenic) F45.8

Effusion
- amniotic fluid —*see* Pregnancy, complicated by, premature rupture of membranes
- brain (serous) G93.6
- bronchial —*see* Bronchitis
- cerebral G93.6
- cerebrospinal —*see also* Meningitis
  - vessel G93.6
- chest —*see* Effusion, pleura
- chylous, chyliform (pleura) J94.0
- intracranial G93.6
- joint M25.40
  - ankle M25.47-

Effusion *(continued)*
- joint *(continued)*
  - elbow M25.42-
  - foot joint M25.47-
  - hand joint M25.44-
  - hip M25.45-
  - knee M25.46-
  - shoulder M25.41-
  - specified joint NEC M25.48
  - wrist M25.43-
- malignant pleural J91.0
- meninges —*see* Meningitis
- pericardium, pericardial (noninflammatory) I31.3
  - acute —*see* Pericarditis, acute
- peritoneal (chronic) R18.8
- pleura, pleurisy, pleuritic, pleuropericardial J90
  - chylous, chyliform J94.0
  - due to systemic lupus erythematosis M32.13
  - in conditions classified elsewhere J91.8
  - influenzal —*see* Influenza, with, respiratory manifestations NEC
  - malignant J91.0
  - newborn P28.89
  - tuberculous NEC A15.6
    - primary (progressive) A15.7
- spinal —*see* Meningitis
- thorax, thoracic —*see* Effusion, pleura

Egg shell nails L60.3
- congenital Q84.6

EGPA (eosinophilic granulomatosis with polyangitis) M30.1

Egyptian splenomegaly B65.1

Ehrlichiosis A77.40
- due to
  - E. chafeensis A77.41
  - E. ewingii A77.49
  - E. muris euclairensis A77.49
  - E. sennetsu A79.81
  - specified organism NEC A77.49

Ehlers-Danlos syndrome (*see also* Syndrome, Ehlers-Danlos) Q79.60

Eichstedt's disease B36.0

Eisenmenger's
- complex or syndrome I27.83
- defect Q21.8

Ejaculation
- delayed F52.32
- painful N53.12
- premature F52.4
- retarded N53.11
- retrograde N53.14
- semen, painful N53.12
  - psychogenic F52.6

Ekbom's syndrome (restless legs) G25.81

Ekman's syndrome (brittle bones and blue sclera) Q78.0

Elastic skin Q82.8
- acquired L57.4

Elastofibroma —*see* Neoplasm, connective tissue, benign

Elastoma (juvenile) Q82.8
- Miescher's L87.2

Elastomyofibrosis I42.4

Elastosis
- actinic, solar L57.8
- atrophicans (senile) L57.4
- perforans serpiginosa L87.2
- senilis L57.4

Elbow —*see* condition

Electric current, electricity, effects (concussion) (fatal) (nonfatal) (shock) T75.4
- burn —*see* Burn

Electric feet syndrome E53.8

Electrocution T75.4
- from electroshock gun (taser) T75.4

Electrolyte imbalance E87.8
- with
  - abortion —*see* Abortion by type, complicated by, electrolyte imbalance
  - ectopic pregnancy O08.5
  - molar pregnancy O08.5

Elephantiasis (nonfilarial) I89.0
- arabicum —*see* Infestation, filarial
- bancroftian B74.0
- congenital (any site) (hereditary) Q82.0
- due to
  - Brugia (malayi) B74.1
    - timori B74.2
  - mastectomy I97.2
  - Wuchereria (bancrofti) B74.0
- eyelid H02.859
  - left H02.856
    - lower H02.855
    - upper H02.854
  - right H02.853
    - lower H02.852
    - upper H02.851
- filarial, filariensis —*see* Infestation, filarial
- glandular I89.0
- graecorum A30.9
- lymphangiectatic I89.0
- lymphatic vessel I89.0
  - due to mastectomy I97.2
- scrotum (nonfilarial) I89.0
- streptococcal I89.0
- surgical I97.89
  - postmastectomy I97.2
- telangiectodes I89.0
- vulva (nonfilarial) N90.89

Elevated, elevation
- alanine transaminase (ALT) R74.01
- ALT (alanine transaminase) R74.01
- antibody titer R76.0
- aspartate transaminase (AST) R74.01
- AST (aspartate transaminase) R74.01
- basal metabolic rate R94.8
- blood pressure —*see also* Hypertension
  - reading (incidental) (isolated) (nonspecific), no diagnosis of hypertension R03.0
- blood sugar R73.9
- body temperature (of unknown origin) R50.9
- C-reactive protein (CRP) R79.82
- cancer antigen 125 [CA 125] R97.1
- carcinoembryonic antigen [CEA] R97.0
- cholesterol E78.00
  - with high triglycerides E78.2
- conjugate, eye H51.0
- diaphragm, congenital Q79.1
- erythrocyte sedimentation rate R70.0
- fasting glucose R73.01
- fasting triglycerides E78.1
- finding on laboratory examination —*see* Findings, abnormal, inconclusive, without diagnosis, by type of exam
- GFR (glomerular filtration rate) —*see* Findings, abnormal, inconclusive, without diagnosis, by type of exam

Elevated, elevation *(continued)*
- glucose tolerance (oral) R73.02
- immunoglobulin level R76.8
- indoleacetic acid R82.5
- lactic acid dehydrogenase (LDH) level R74.02
- leukocytes D72.829
- lipoprotein a (Lp(a)) level E78.41
- liver function
  - study R94.5
  - test R79.89
    - alkaline phosphatase R74.8
    - aminotransferase R74.01
    - bilirubin R17
    - hepatic enzyme R74.8
    - lactate dehydrogenase R74.02
- Lp(a) (lipoprotein(a)) E78.41
- lymphocytes D72.820
- prostate specific antigen [PSA] R97.20
- Rh titer —*see* Complication(s), transfusion, incompatibility reaction, Rh (factor)
- scapula, congenital Q74.0
- sedimentation rate R70.0
- SGOT R74.01
- SGPT R74.01
- transaminase level R74.01
- triglycerides E78.1
  - with high cholesterol E78.2
- troponin R77.8
- tumor associated antigens [TAA] NEC R97.8
- tumor specific antigens [TSA] NEC R97.8
- urine level of
  - catecholamine R82.5
  - indoleacetic acid R82.5
  - 17-ketosteroids R82.5
  - steroids R82.5
  - vanillylmandelic acid (VMA) R82.5
- venous pressure I87.8
- white blood cell count D72.829
  - specified NEC D72.828

Elliptocytosis (congenital) (hereditary) D58.1
- Hb C (disease) D58.1
- hemoglobin disease D58.1
- sickle-cell (disease) D57.8-
  - trait D57.3

Ellison-Zollinger syndrome E16.4

Ellis-van Creveld syndrome (chondroectodermal dysplasia) Q77.6

Elongated, elongation (congenital) —*see also* Distortion
- bone Q79.9
- cervix (uteri) Q51.828
  - acquired N88.4
  - hypertrophic N88.4
- colon Q43.8
- common bile duct Q44.5
- cystic duct Q44.5
- frenulum, penis Q55.69
- labia minora (acquired) N90.69
- ligamentum patellae Q74.1
- petiolus (epiglottidis) Q31.8
- tooth, teeth K00.2
- uvula Q38.6

Eltor cholera A00.1

Emaciation R64
- due to malnutrition E43

Embadomoniasis A07.8

Embedded tooth, teeth K01.0
- root only K08.3

Embolic —*see* condition

Embolism (multiple) (paradoxical) I74.9
- air (any site) (traumatic) T79.0
  - following
    - abortion —*see* Abortion by type complicated by embolism
    - ectopic pregnancy O08.2
    - infusion, therapeutic injection or transfusion T80.0
    - molar pregnancy O08.2
    - procedure NEC
      - artery T81.719
        - mesenteric T81.710
        - renal T81.711
        - specified NEC T81.718
      - vein T81.72
  - in pregnancy, childbirth or puerperium —*see* Embolism, obstetric
- amniotic fluid (pulmonary) —*see also* Embolism, obstetric
  - following
    - abortion —*see* Abortion by type complicated by embolism
    - ectopic pregnancy O08.2
    - molar pregnancy O08.2
- aorta, aortic I74.10
  - abdominal I74.09
    - saddle I74.01
  - bifurcation I74.09
  - saddle I74.01
  - thoracic I74.11
- artery I74.9
  - auditory, internal I65.8
  - basilar —*see* Occlusion, artery, basilar
  - carotid (common) (internal) —*see* Occlusion, artery, carotid
  - cerebellar (anterior inferior) (posterior inferior) (superior) I66.3
  - cerebral —*see* Occlusion, artery, cerebral
  - choroidal (anterior) I65.8
  - communicating posterior I65.8
  - coronary —*see also* Infarct, myocardium
    - not resulting in infarction I24.0
  - extremity I74.4
    - lower I74.3
    - upper I74.2
  - hypophyseal I65.8
  - iliac I74.5
  - limb I74.4
    - lower I74.3
    - upper I74.2
  - mesenteric (with gangrene) (*see also* Ischemia, intestine, acute) K55.059
  - ophthalmic —*see* Occlusion, artery, retina
  - peripheral I74.4
  - pontine I65.8
  - precerebral —*see* Occlusion, artery, precerebral
  - pulmonary —*see* Embolism, pulmonary
  - renal N28.0
  - retinal —*see* Occlusion, artery, retina
  - septic I76
  - specified NEC I74.8
  - vertebral —*see* Occlusion, artery, vertebral
- basilar (artery) I65.1
- blood clot
  - following
    - abortion —*see* Abortion by type complicated by embolism
    - ectopic or molar pregnancy O08.2

Embolism *(continued)*
- blood clot *(continued)*
  - in pregnancy, childbirth or puerperium —*see* Embolism, obstetric
- brain —*see also* Occlusion, artery, cerebral
  - following
    - abortion —*see* Abortion by type complicated by embolism
    - ectopic or molar pregnancy O08.2
  - puerperal, postpartum, childbirth —*see* Embolism, obstetric
- capillary I78.8
- cardiac —*see also* Infarct, myocardium
  - not resulting in infarction I51.3
- carotid (artery) (common) (internal) —*see* Occlusion, artery, carotid
- cavernous sinus (venous) —*see* Embolism, intracranial venous sinus
- cerebral —*see* Occlusion, artery, cerebral
- cholesterol —*see* Atheroembolism
- coronary (artery or vein) (systemic) —*see* Occlusion, coronary
- due to device, implant or graft —*see also* Complications, by site and type, specified NEC
  - arterial graft NEC T82.818
  - breast (implant) T85.818
  - catheter NEC T85.818
    - dialysis (renal) T82.818
      - intraperitoneal T85.818
    - infusion NEC T82.818
      - spinal (epidural) (subdural) T85.810
    - urinary (indwelling) T83.81
  - electronic (electrode) (pulse generator) (stimulator)
    - bone T84.81
    - cardiac T82.817
    - nervous system (brain) (peripheral nerve) (spinal) T85.810
    - urinary T83.81
  - fixation, internal (orthopedic) NEC T84.81
  - gastrointestinal (bile duct) (esophagus) T85.818
  - genital NEC T83.81
  - heart (graft) (valve) T82.817
  - joint prosthesis T84.81
  - ocular (corneal graft) (orbital implant) T85.818
  - orthopedic (bone graft) NEC T86.838
  - specified NEC T85.818
  - urinary (graft) NEC T83.81
  - vascular NEC T82.818
  - ventricular intracranial shunt T85.810
- extremities
  - lower —*see* Embolism, vein, lower extremity
    - arterial I74.3
  - upper I74.2
- eye H34.9
- fat (cerebral) (pulmonary) (systemic) T79.1
  - following
    - abortion —*see* Abortion by type complicated by embolism
    - ectopic or molar pregnancy O08.2
  - complicating delivery —*see* Embolism, obstetric

Embolism *(continued)*
- following
  - abortion —*see* Abortion by type complicated by embolism
  - ectopic or molar pregnancy O08.2
  - infusion, therapeutic injection or transfusion
    - air T80.0
- heart (fatty) —*see also* Infarct, myocardium
  - not resulting in infarction I51.3
- hepatic (vein) I82.0
- in pregnancy, childbirth or puerperium —*see* Embolism, obstetric
- intestine (artery) (vein) (with gangrene) (*see also* Ischemia, intestine, acute) K55.039
- intracranial —*see also* Occlusion, artery, cerebral
  - venous sinus (any) G08
    - nonpyogenic I67.6
- intraspinal venous sinuses or veins G08
  - nonpyogenic G95.19
- kidney (artery) N28.0
- lateral sinus (venous) —*see* Embolism, intracranial, venous sinus
- leg —*see* Embolism, vein, lower extremity
  - arterial I74.3
- longitudinal sinus (venous) —*see* Embolism, intracranial, venous sinus
- lung (massive) —*see* Embolism, pulmonary
- meninges I66.8
- mesenteric (artery) (vein) (with gangrene) (*see also* Ischemia, intestine, acute) K55.059
- obstetric (in) (pulmonary)
  - childbirth O88.22
    - air O88.02
    - amniotic fluid O88.12
    - blood clot O88.22
    - fat O88.82
    - pyemic O88.32
    - septic O88.32
    - specified type NEC O88.82
  - pregnancy O88.21-
    - air O88.01-
    - amniotic fluid O88.11-
    - blood clot O88.21-
    - fat O88.81-
    - pyemic O88.31-
    - septic O88.31-
    - specified type NEC O88.81-
  - puerperal O88.23
    - air O88.03
    - amniotic fluid O88.13
    - blood clot O88.23
    - fat O88.83
    - pyemic O88.33
    - septic O88.33
    - specified type NEC O88.83
- ophthalmic —*see* Occlusion, artery, retina
- penis N48.81
- peripheral artery NOS I74.4
- pituitary E23.6
- popliteal (artery) I74.3
- portal (vein) I81
- postoperative, postprocedural
  - artery T81.719
    - mesenteric T81.710
    - renal T81.711
    - specified NEC T81.718
  - vein T81.72

Embolism *(continued)*
precerebral artery —*see* Occlusion, artery, precerebral
puerperal —*see* Embolism, obstetric
pulmonary (acute) (artery) (vein) I26.99
with acute cor pulmonale I26.09
chronic I27.82
following
abortion —*see* Abortion by type complicated by embolism
ectopic or molar pregnancy O08.2
healed or old Z86.711
in pregnancy, childbirth or puerperium —*see* Embolism, obstetric
multiple subsegmental without acute cor pulmonale I26.94
personal history of Z86.711
saddle I26.92
with acute cor pulmonale I26.02
septic I26.90
with acute cor pulmonale I26.01
single subsegmental without acute cor pulmonale I26.93
subsegmental NOS I26.93
pyemic (multiple) I76
following
abortion —*see* Abortion by type complicated by embolism
ectopic or molar pregnancy O08.2
Hemophilus influenzae A41.3
pneumococcal A40.3
with pneumonia J13
puerperal, postpartum, childbirth (any organism) —*see* Embolism, obstetric
specified organism NEC A41.89
staphylococcal A41.2
streptococcal A40.9
renal (artery) N28.0
vein I82.3
retina, retinal —*see* Occlusion, artery, retina
saddle
abdominal aorta I74.01
pulmonary artery I26.92
with acute cor pulmonale I26.02
septic (arterial) I76
complicating abortion —*see* Abortion, by type, complicated by, embolism
sinus —*see* Embolism, intracranial, venous sinus
soap complicating abortion —*see* Abortion, by type, complicated by, embolism
spinal cord G95.19
pyogenic origin G06.1
spleen, splenic (artery) I74.8
upper extremity I74.2
vein (acute) I82.90
antecubital I82.61-
chronic I82.71-
axillary I82.A1-
chronic I82.A2-
basilic I82.61-
chronic I82.71-
brachial I82.62-
chronic I82.72-
brachiocephalic (innominate) I82.290
chronic I82.291

Embolism *(continued)*
vein *(continued)*
cephalic I82.61-
chronic I82.71-
chronic I82.91
deep (DVT) I82.40-
calf I82.4Z-
chronic I82.5Z-
lower leg I82.4Z-
chronic I82.5Z-
thigh I82.4Y-
chronic I82.5Y-
upper leg I82.4Y
chronic I82.5y-
femoral I82.41-
chronic I82.51-
iliac (iliofemoral) I82.42-
chronic I82.52-
innominate I82.290
chronic I82.291
internal jugular I82.C1-
chronic I82.C2-
lower extremity
deep I82.40-
chronic I82.50-
specified NEC I82.49-
chronic NEC I82.59-
distal
deep I82.4Z-
proximal
deep I82.4Y-
chronic I82.5Y-
superficial I82.81-
popliteal I82.43-
chronic I82.53-
radial I82.62-
chronic I82.72-
renal I82.3
saphenous (greater) (lesser) I82.81-
specified NEC I82.890
chronic NEC I82.891
subclavian I82.B1-
chronic I82.B2-
thoracic NEC I82.290
chronic I82.291
tibial I82.44-
chronic I82.54-
ulnar I82.62-
chronic I82.72-
upper extremity I82.60-
chronic I82.70-
deep I82.62-
chronic I82.72-
superficial I82.61-
chronic I82.71-
vena cava
inferior (acute) I82.220
chronic I82.221
superior (acute) I82.210
chronic I82.211
venous sinus G08
vessels of brain —*see* Occlusion, artery, cerebral

Embolus —*see* Embolism

Embryoma —*see also* Neoplasm, uncertain behavior, by site
benign —*see* Neoplasm, benign, by site
kidney C64.-
liver C22.0
malignant —*see also* Neoplasm, malignant, by site
kidney C64.-
liver C22.0
testis C62.9-
descended (scrotal) C62.1-
undescended C62.0-
testis C62.9-
descended (scrotal) C62.1-
undescended C62.0-

Embryonic
circulation Q28.9
heart Q28.9
vas deferens Q55.4

Embryopathia NOS Q89.9

Embryotoxon Q13.4

Emesis —*see* Vomiting

Emotional lability R45.86

Emotionality, pathological F60.3

Emotogenic disease —*see* Disorder, psychogenic

Emphysema (atrophic) (bullous) (chronic) (interlobular) (lung) (obstructive) (pulmonary) (senile) (vesicular) J43.9
cellular tissue (traumatic) T79.7
surgical T81.82
centrilobular J43.2
compensatory J98.3
congenital (interstitial) P25.0
conjunctiva H11.89
connective tissue (traumatic) T79.7
surgical T81.82
due to chemicals, gases, fumes or vapors J68.4
eyelid(s) —*see* Disorder, eyelid, specified type NEC
surgical T81.82
traumatic T79.7
interstitial J98.2
congenital P25.0
perinatal period P25.0
laminated tissue T79.7
surgical T81.82
mediastinal J98.2
newborn P25.2
orbit, orbital —*see* Disorder, orbit, specified type NEC
panacinar J43.1
panlobular J43.1
specified NEC J43.8
subcutaneous (traumatic) T79.7
nontraumatic J98.2
postprocedural T81.82
surgical T81.82
surgical T81.82
thymus (gland) (congenital) E32.8
traumatic (subcutaneous) T79.7
unilateral J43.0

Empty nest syndrome Z60.0

Empyema (acute) (chest) (double) (pleura) (supradiaphragmatic) (thorax) J86.9
with fistula J86.0
accessory sinus (chronic) —*see* Sinusitis
antrum (chronic) —*see* Sinusitis, maxillary
brain (any part) —*see* Abscess, brain
ethmoidal (chronic) (sinus) —*see* Sinusitis, ethmoidal
extradural —*see* Abscess, extradural
frontal (chronic) (sinus) —*see* Sinusitis, frontal
gallbladder K81.0
mastoid (process) (acute) —*see* Mastoiditis, acute
maxilla, maxillary M27.2
sinus (chronic) —*see* Sinusitis, maxillary
nasal sinus (chronic) —*see* Sinusitis
sinus (accessory) (chronic) (nasal) —*see* Sinusitis
sphenoidal (sinus) (chronic) —*see* Sinusitis, sphenoidal

Empyema *(continued)*
subarachnoid —*see* Abscess, extradural
subdural —*see* Abscess, subdural
tuberculous A15.6
ureter —*see* Ureteritis
ventricular —*see* Abscess, brain

En coup de sabre lesion L94.1

Enamel pearls K00.2

Enameloma K00.2

Enanthema, viral B09

Encephalitis (chronic) (hemorrhagic) (idiopathic) (nonepidemic) (spurious) (subacute) G04.90
acute (*see also* Encephalitis, viral) A86
disseminated G04.00
infectious G04.01
noninfectious G04.81
postimmunization (postvaccination) G04.02
postinfectious G04.01
inclusion body A85.8
necrotizing hemorrhagic G04.30
postimmunization G04.32
postinfectious G04.31
specified NEC G04.39
arboviral, arbovirus NEC A85.2
arthropod-borne NEC (viral) A85.2
Australian A83.4
California (virus) A83.5
Central European (tick-borne) A84.1
Czechoslovakian A84.1
Dawson's (inclusion body) A81.1
diffuse sclerosing A81.1
disseminated, acute G04.00
due to
cat scratch disease A28.1
human immunodeficiency virus (HIV) disease B20 *[G05.3]*
malaria —*see* Malaria
rickettsiosis —*see* Rickettsiosis
smallpox inoculation G04.02
typhus —*see* Typhus
Eastern equine A83.2
endemic (viral) A86
epidemic NEC (viral) A86
equine (acute) (infectious) (viral) A83.9
Eastern A83.2
Venezuelan A92.2
Western A83.1
Far Eastern (tick-borne) A84.0
following vaccination or other immunization procedure G04.02
herpes zoster B02.0
herpesviral B00.4
due to herpesvirus 6 B10.01
due to herpesvirus 7 B10.09
specified NEC B10.09
Ilheus (virus) A83.8
inclusion body A81.1
in (due to)
actinomycosis A42.82
adenovirus A85.1
African trypanosomiasis B56.9 *[G05.3]*
Chagas' disease (chronic) B57.42
cytomegalovirus B25.8
enterovirus A85.0
herpes (simplex) virus B00.4
due to herpesvirus 6 B10.01
due to herpesvirus 7 B10.09
specified NEC B10.09
infectious disease NEC B99 *[G05.3]*

Encephalitis *(continued)*
in *(continued)*
influenza *—see* Influenza, with, encephalopathy
listeriosis A32.12
measles B05.0
mumps B26.2
naegleriasis B60.2
parasitic disease NEC B89 *[G05.3]*
poliovirus A80.9 *[G05.3]*
rubella B06.01
syphilis
congenital A50.42
late A52.14
systemic lupus erythematosus M32.19
toxoplasmosis (acquired) B58.2
congenital P37.1
tuberculosis A17.82
zoster B02.0
infectious (acute) (virus) NEC A86
Japanese (B type) A83.0
La Crosse A83.5
lead *—see* Poisoning, lead
lethargica (acute) (infectious) A85.8
louping ill A84.89
lupus erythematosus, systemic M32.19
lymphatica A87.2
Mengo A85.8
meningococcal A39.81
Murray Valley A83.4
otitic NEC H66.40 *[G05.3]*
parasitic NOS B71.9
periaxial G37.0
periaxialis (concentrica) (diffuse) G37.5
postchickenpox B01.11
postexanthematous NEC B09
postimmunization G04.02
postinfectious NEC G04.01
postmeasles B05.0
postvaccinal G04.02
postvaricella B01.11
postviral NEC A86
Powassan A84.81
Rasmussen G04.81
Rio Bravo A85.8
Russian
autumnal A83.0
spring-summer (taiga) A84.0
saturnine *—see* Poisoning, lead
specified NEC G04.81
St. Louis A83.3
subacute sclerosing A81.1
summer A83.0
suppurative G04.81
tick-borne A84.9
Torula, torular (cryptococcal) B45.1
toxic NEC G92.8
trichinosis B75 *[G05.3]*
type
B A83.0
C A83.3
van Bogaert's A81.1
Venezuelan equine A92.2
Vienna A85.8
viral, virus A86
arthropod-borne NEC A85.2
mosquito-borne A83.9
Australian X disease A83.4
California virus A83.5
Eastern equine A83.2
Japanese (B type) A83.0
Murray Valley A83.4
specified NEC A83.8
St. Louis A83.3
type B A83.0
type C A83.3
Western equine A83.1

Encephalitis *(continued)*
viral, virus *(continued)*
arthropod-borne NEC *(continued)*
tick-borne A84.9
biundulant A84.1
central European A84.1
Czechoslovakian A84.1
diphasic meningoencephalitis A84.1
Far Eastern A84.0
Russian spring-summer (taiga) A84.0
specified NEC A84.89
specified type NEC A85.8
tick-borne, specified NEC A84.89
Western equine A83.1

Encephalocele Q01.9
frontal Q01.0
nasofrontal Q01.1
occipital Q01.2
specified NEC Q01.8

Encephalocystocele *—see* Encephalocele

Encephaloduroarterio-myosynangiosis (EDAMS) I67.5

Encephalomalacia (brain) (cerebellar) (cerebral) *—see* Softening, brain

Encephalomeningitis *—see* Meningoencephalitis

Encephalomeningocele *—see* Encephalocele

Encephalomeningomyelitis *—see* Meningoencephalitis

Encephalomyelitis *—see also* Encephalitis G04.90
acute disseminated G04.00
infectious G04.01
noninfectious G04.81
postimmunization G04.02
postinfectious G04.01
acute necrotizing hemorrhagic G04.30
postimmunization G04.32
postinfectious G04.31
specified NEC G04.39
benign myalgic G93.3
equine A83.9
Eastern A83.2
Venezuelan A92.2
Western A83.1
in diseases classified elsewhere G05.3
myalgic, benign G93.3
postchickenpox B01.11
postinfectious NEC G04.01
postmeasles B05.0
postvaccinal G04.02
postvaricella B01.11
rubella B06.01
specified NEC G04.81
Venezuelan equine A92.2

Encephalomyelocele *—see* Encephalocele

Encephalomyelomeningitis *—see* Meningoencephalitis

Encephalomyelopathy G96.9

Encephalomyeloradiculitis (acute) G61.0

Encephalomyeloradiculoneuritis (acute) (Guillain-Barré) G61.0

Encephalomyeloradiculopathy G96.9

Encephalopathia hyperbilirubinemica, newborn P57.9
due to isoimmunization (conditions in P55) P57.0

Encephalopathy (acute) G93.40
acute necrotizing hemorrhagic G04.30
postimmunization G04.32
postinfectious G04.31
specified NEC G04.39
alcoholic G31.2
anoxic *—see* Damage, brain, anoxic
arteriosclerotic I67.2
centrolobar progressive (Schilder) G37.0
congenital Q07.9
degenerative, in specified disease NEC G32.89
demyelinating callosal G37.1
due to
drugs (*see also* Table of Drugs and Chemicals) G92.8
hepatic *—see* Failure, hepatic
hyperbilirubinemic, newborn P57.9
due to isoimmunization (conditions in P55) P57.0
hypertensive I67.4
hypoglycemic E16.2
hypoxic *—see* Damage, brain, anoxic
hypoxic ischemic P91.60
mild P91.61
moderate P91.62
severe P91.63
in (due to) (with)
birth injury P11.1
hyperinsulinism E16.1 *[G94]*
influenza *—see* Influenza, with, encephalopathy
lack of vitamin (*see also* Deficiency, vitamin) E56.9 *[G32.89]*
neoplastic disease (*see also* Neoplasm) D49.9 *[G13.1]*
serum (*see also* Reaction, serum) T80.69
syphilis A52.17
trauma (postconcussional) F07.81
current injury *—see* Injury, intracranial
vaccination G04.02
lead *—see* Poisoning, lead
metabolic G93.41
drug induced G92.8
toxic G92.8
myoclonic, early, symptomatic *—see* Epilepsy, generalized, specified NEC
necrotizing, subacute (Leigh) G31.82
neonatal P91.819
in diseases classified elsewhere P91.811
pellagrous E52 *[G32.89]*
portosystemic *—see* Failure, hepatic
postcontusional F07.81
current injury *—see* Injury, intracranial, diffuse
posthypoglycemic (coma) E16.1 *[G94]*
postradiation G93.89
saturnine *—see* Poisoning, lead
septic G93.41
specified NEC G93.49
spongioform, subacute (viral) A81.09

Encephalopathy *(continued)*
toxic G92.9
metabolic G92.8
traumatic (postconcussional) F07.81
current injury *—see* Injury, intracranial
vitamin B deficiency NEC E53.9 *[G32.89]*
vitamin B1 E51.2
Wernicke's E51.2

Encephalorrhagia *—see* Hemorrhage, intracranial, intracerebral

Encephalosis, posttraumatic F07.81

Enchondroma *—see also* Neoplasm, bone, benign

Enchondromatosis (cartilaginous) (multiple) Q78.4

Encopresis R15.9
functional F98.1
nonorganic origin F98.1
psychogenic F98.1

Encounter (with health service) (for) Z76.89
adjustment and management (of)
breast implant Z45.81
implanted device NEC Z45.89
myringotomy device (stent) (tube) Z45.82
neurostimulator (brain) (gastric) (peripheral nerve) (sacral nerve) (spinal cord) (vagus nerve) Z45.42
administrative purpose only Z02.9
examination for
adoption Z02.82
armed forces Z02.3
disability determination Z02.71
driving license Z02.4
employment Z02.1
insurance Z02.6
medical certificate NEC Z02.79
paternity testing Z02.81
residential institution admission Z02.2
school admission Z02.0
sports Z02.5
specified reason NEC Z02.89
aftercare *—see* Aftercare
antenatal screening Z36.9
cervical length Z36.86
chromosomal anomalies Z36.0
congenital cardiac abnormalities Z36.83
elevated maternal serum alphafetoprotein level Z36.1
fetal growth retardation Z36.4
fetal lung maturity Z36.84
fetal macrosomia Z36.88
hydrops fetalis Z36.81
intrauterine growth restriction (IUGR)/small-for-dates Z36.4
isoimmunization Z36.5
large-for-dates Z36.88
malformations Z36.3
non-visualized anatomy on a previous scan Z36.2
nuchal translucency Z36.82
raised alphafetoprotein level Z36.1
risk of pre-term labor Z36.86
specified type NEC Z36.89
specified follow-up NEC Z36.2
specified genetic defects NEC Z36.8A
Streptococcus B Z36.85

Encounter *(continued)*
- antenatal screening *(continued)*
  - suspected anomaly Z36.3
  - uncertain dates Z36.87
- assisted reproductive fertility procedure cycle Z31.83
- blood typing Z01.83
  - Rh typing Z01.83
- breast augmentation or reduction Z41.1
- breast implant exchange (different material) (different size) Z45.81
- breast reconstruction following mastectomy Z42.1
- check-up *—see* Examination
- chemotherapy for neoplasm Z51.11
- colonoscopy, screening Z12.11
- counseling *—see* Counseling
- delivery, full-term, uncomplicated O80
  - cesarean, without indication O82
- desensitization to allergens Z51.6
- ear piercing Z41.3
- examination *—see* Examination
- expectant parent(s) (adoptive)
  - pre-birth pediatrician visit Z76.81
- fertility preservation procedure (prior to cancer therapy) (prior to removal of gonads) Z31.84
- fitting (of) *—see* Fitting (and adjustment) (of)
- genetic
  - counseling
    - nonprocreative Z71.83
    - procreative Z31.5
  - testing *—see* Test, genetic
- hearing conservation and treatment Z01.12
- immunotherapy for neoplasm Z51.12
- in vitro fertilization cycle Z31.83
- instruction (in)
  - childbirth Z32.2
  - child care (postpartal) (prenatal) Z32.3
  - natural family planning
    - procreative Z31.61
    - to avoid pregnancy Z30.02
- insulin pump titration Z46.81
- joint prosthesis insertion following prior explantation of joint prosthesis (staged procedure)
  - hip Z47.32
  - knee Z47.33
  - shoulder Z47.31
- laboratory (as part of a general medical examination) Z00.00
  - with abnormal findings Z00.01
- mental health services (for)
  - abuse NEC
    - perpetrator Z69.82
    - victim Z69.81
  - child abuse
    - nonparental
      - perpetrator Z69.021
      - victim Z69.020
    - parental
      - perpetrator Z69.011
      - victim Z69.010
  - child neglect
    - nonparental
      - perpetrator Z69.021
      - victim Z69.020
    - parental
      - perpetrator Z69.011
      - victim Z69.010
  - child psychological abuse
    - nonparental
      - perpetrator Z69.021
      - victim Z69.020

Encounter *(continued)*
- mental health services *(continued)*
  - child psychological abuse *(continued)*
    - parental
      - perpetrator Z69.011
      - victim Z69.010
  - child sexual abuse
    - nonparental
      - perpetrator Z69.021
      - victim Z69.020
    - parental
      - perpetrator Z69.011
      - victim Z69.010
  - non-spousal adult abuse
    - perpetrator Z69.82
    - victim Z69.81
  - spousal or parter
    - abuse
      - perpetrator Z69.12
      - victim Z69.11
    - neglect
      - perpetrator Z69.12
      - victim Z69.11
    - psychological abuse
      - perpetrator Z69.12
      - victim Z69.11
    - violence
      - perpetrator (physical) (sexual) Z69.12
      - victim (physical) Z69.11
        - sexual Z69.81
- observation (for) (ruled out)
  - exposure to (suspected)
    - anthrax Z03.810
    - biological agent NEC Z03.818
- pediatrician visit, by expectant parent(s) (adoptive) Z76.81
- placental sample (taken vaginally) (*see also* Encounter, antenatal screening) Z36.9
- plastic and reconstructive surgery following medical procedure or healed injury NEC Z42.8
- pregnancy
  - supervision of *—see* Pregnancy, supervision of
  - test Z32.00
    - result negative Z32.02
    - result positive Z32.01
- procreative management and counseling for gestational carrier Z31.7
- prophylactic measures Z29.9
  - antivenin Z29.12
  - fluoride administration Z29.3
  - immunotherapy for respiratory syncytial virus (RSV) Z29.11
  - rabies immune globulin Z29.14
  - Rho (D) immune globulin Z29.13
  - specified NEC Z29.8
- radiation therapy (antineoplastic) Z51.0
- radiological (as part of a general medical examination) Z00.00
  - with abnormal findings Z00.01
- reconstructive surgery following medical procedure or healed injury NEC Z42.8
- removal (of) *—see also* Removal
  - artificial
    - arm Z44.00-
      - complete Z44.01-
      - partial Z44.02-
    - eye Z44.2-
    - leg Z44.10-
      - complete Z44.11-
      - partial Z44.12-
  - breast implant Z45.81

Encounter *(continued)*
- removal *(continued)*
  - breast implant *(continued)*
    - tissue expander (with or without synchronous insertion of permanent implant) Z45.81
  - device Z46.9
    - specified NEC Z46.89
  - external
    - fixation device - code to fracture with seventh character D
    - prosthesis, prosthetic device Z44.9
      - breast Z44.3-
      - specified NEC Z44.8
  - implanted device NEC Z45.89
  - insulin pump Z46.81
  - internal fixation device Z47.2
  - myringotomy device (stent) (tube) Z45.82
  - nervous system device NEC Z46.2
    - brain neuropacemaker Z46.2
    - visual substitution device Z46.2
      - implanted Z45.31
  - non-vascular catheter Z46.82
  - orthodontic device Z46.4
  - stent
    - ureteral Z46.6
  - urinary device Z46.6
- repeat cervical smear to confirm findings of recent normal smear following initial abnormal smear Z01.42
- respirator [ventilator] use during power failure Z99.12
- Rh typing Z01.83
- screening *—see* Screening
- specified NEC Z76.89
- sterilization Z30.2
- suspected condition, ruled out
  - amniotic cavity and membrane Z03.71
  - cervical shortening Z03.75
  - fetal anomaly Z03.73
  - fetal growth Z03.74
  - maternal and fetal conditions NEC Z03.79
  - oligohydramnios Z03.71
  - placental problem Z03.72
  - polyhydramnios Z03.71
- suspected exposure (to), ruled out
  - anthrax Z03.810
  - biological agents NEC Z03.818
- termination of pregnancy, elective Z33.2
- testing *—see* Test
- therapeutic drug level monitoring Z51.81
- titration, insulin pump Z46.81
- to determine fetal viability of pregnancy O36.80
- training
  - insulin pump Z46.81
- X-ray of chest (as part of a general medical examination) Z00.00
  - with abnormal findings Z00.01

Encystment *—see* Cyst

Endarteritis (bacterial, subacute) (infective) I77.6
- brain I67.7
- cerebral or cerebrospinal I67.7
- deformans *—see* Arteriosclerosis
- embolic *—see* Embolism
- obliterans *—see also* Arteriosclerosis
  - pulmonary I28.8

Endarteritis *(continued)*
- pulmonary I28.8
- retina *—see* Vasculitis, retina
- senile *—see* Arteriosclerosis
- syphilitic A52.09
  - brain or cerebral A52.04
  - congenital A50.54 *[I79.8]*
- tuberculous A18.89

Endemic *—see* condition

Endocarditis (chronic) (marantic) (nonbacterial) (thrombotic) (valvular) I38
- with rheumatic fever (conditions in I00)
  - active *—see* Endocarditis, acute, rheumatic
  - inactive or quiescent (with chorea) I09.1
- acute or subacute I33.9
  - infective I33.0
  - rheumatic (aortic) (mitral) (pulmonary) (tricuspid) I01.1
    - with chorea (acute) (rheumatic) (Sydenham's) I02.0
- aortic (heart) (nonrheumatic) (valve) I35.8
  - with
    - mitral disease I08.0
      - with tricuspid (valve) disease I08.3
      - active or acute I01.1
        - with chorea (acute) (rheumatic) (Sydenham's) I02.0
    - rheumatic fever (conditions in I00)
      - active *—see* Endocarditis, acute, rheumatic
      - inactive or quiescent (with chorea) I06.9
    - tricuspid (valve) disease I08.2
      - with mitral (valve) disease I08.3
  - acute or subacute I33.9
  - arteriosclerotic I35.8
  - rheumatic I06.9
    - with mitral disease I08.0
      - with tricuspid (valve) disease I08.3
      - active or acute I01.1
        - with chorea (acute) (rheumatic) (Sydenham's) I02.0
    - active or acute I01.1
      - with chorea (acute) (rheumatic) (Sydenham's) I02.0
    - specified NEC I06.8
  - specified cause NEC I35.8
  - syphilitic A52.03
- arteriosclerotic I38
- atypical verrucous (Libman-Sacks) M32.11
- bacterial (acute) (any valve) (subacute) I33.0
- candidal B37.6
- congenital Q24.8
- constrictive I33.0
- Coxiella burnetii A78 *[I39]*
- Coxsackie B33.21
- due to
  - prosthetic cardiac valve T82.6
  - Q fever A78 *[I39]*
  - Serratia marcescens I33.0
  - typhoid (fever) A01.02
- gonococcal A54.83
- infectious or infective (acute) (any valve) (subacute) I33.0

Endocarditis *(continued)*
- lenta (acute) (any valve) (subacute) I33.0
- Libman-Sacks M32.11
- listerial A32.82
- Löffler's I42.3
- malignant (acute) (any valve) (subacute) I33.0
- meningococcal A39.51
- mitral (chronic) (double) (fibroid) (heart) (inactive) (valve) (with chorea) I05.9
  - with
    - aortic (valve) disease I08.0
      - with tricuspid (valve) disease I08.3
      - active or acute I01.1
        - with chorea (acute) (rheumatic) (Sydenham's) I02.0
    - rheumatic fever (conditions in I00)
      - active *—see* Endocarditis, acute, rheumatic
      - inactive or quiescent (with chorea) I05.9
    - tricuspid (valve) disease I08.1
      - with aortic (valve) disease I08.3
  - active or acute I01.1
    - with chorea (acute) (rheumatic) (Sydenham's) I02.0
    - bacterial I33.0
  - arteriosclerotic I34.8
  - nonrheumatic I34.8
    - acute or subacute I33.9
  - specified NEC I05.8
- monilial B37.6
- multiple valves I08.9
  - specified disorders I08.8
- mycotic (acute) (any valve) (subacute) I33.0
- pneumococcal (acute) (any valve) (subacute) I33.0
- pulmonary (chronic) (heart) (valve) I37.8
  - with rheumatic fever (conditions in I00)
    - active *—see* Endocarditis, acute, rheumatic
    - inactive or quiescent (with chorea) I09.89
      - with aortic, mitral or tricuspid disease I08.8
  - acute or subacute I33.9
    - rheumatic I01.1
      - with chorea (acute) (rheumatic) (Sydenham's) I02.0
  - arteriosclerotic I37.8
  - congenital Q22.2
  - rheumatic (chronic) (inactive) (with chorea) I09.89
    - active or acute I01.1
      - with chorea (acute) (rheumatic) (Sydenham's) I02.0
  - syphilitic A52.03
- purulent (acute) (any valve) (subacute) I33.0
- Q fever A78 *[I39]*
- rheumatic (chronic) (inactive) (with chorea) I09.1
  - active or acute (aortic) (mitral) (pulmonary) (tricuspid) I01.1
    - with chorea (acute) (rheumatic) (Sydenham's) I02.0
- rheumatoid *—see* Rheumatoid, carditis
- septic (acute) (any valve) (subacute) I33.0
- streptococcal (acute) (any valve) (subacute) I33.0
- subacute *—see* Endocarditis, acute
- suppurative (acute) (any valve) (subacute) I33.0
- syphilitic A52.03
- toxic I33.9
- tricuspid (chronic) (heart) (inactive) (rheumatic) (valve) (with chorea) I07.9
  - with
    - aortic (valve) disease I08.2
      - mitral (valve) disease I08.3
    - mitral (valve) disease I08.1
      - aortic (valve) disease I08.3
    - rheumatic fever (conditions in I00)
      - active *—see* Endocarditis, acute, rheumatic
      - inactive or quiescent (with chorea) I07.8
  - active or acute I01.1
    - with chorea (acute) (rheumatic) (Sydenham's) I02.0
  - arteriosclerotic I36.8
  - nonrheumatic I36.8
    - acute or subacute I33.9
  - specified cause, except rheumatic I36.8
- tuberculous *—see* Tuberculosis, endocarditis
- typhoid A01.02
- ulcerative (acute) (any valve) (subacute) I33.0
- vegetative (acute) (any valve) (subacute) I33.0
- verrucous (atypical) (nonbacterial) (nonrheumatic) M32.11

Endocardium, endocardial *—see also* condition
- cushion defect Q21.2

Endocervicitis *—see also* Cervicitis
- due to intrauterine (contraceptive) device T83.69
- hyperplastic N72

Endocrine *—see* condition

Endocrinopathy, pluriglandular E31.9

Endodontic
- overfill M27.52
- underfill M27.53

Endodontitis K04.01
- irreversible K04.02
- reversible K04.01

Endomastoiditis *—see* Mastoiditis

Endometrioma N80.9

Endometriosis N80.9
- appendix N80.5
- bladder N80.8
- bowel N80.5
- broad ligament N80.3
- cervix N80.0
- colon N80.5
- cul-de-sac (Douglas') N80.3
- exocervix N80.0
- fallopian tube N80.2
- female genital organ NEC N80.8
- gallbladder N80.8
- in scar of skin N80.6
- internal N80.0
- intestine N80.5
- lung N80.8
- myometrium N80.0
- ovary N80.1
- parametrium N80.3
- pelvic peritoneum N80.3
- peritoneal (pelvic) N80.3
- rectovaginal septum N80.4
- rectum N80.5
- round ligament N80.3
- skin (scar) N80.6
- specified site NEC N80.8
- stromal D39.0
- thorax N80.8
- umbilicus N80.8
- uterus (internal) N80.0
- vagina N80.4
- vulva N80.8

Endometritis (decidual) (nonspecific) (purulent) (senile) (atrophic) (suppurative) N71.9
- with ectopic pregnancy O08.0
- acute N71.0
- blenorrhagic (gonococcal) (acute) (chronic) A54.24
- cervix, cervical (with erosion or ectropion) *—see also* Cervicitis
  - hyperplastic N72
- chlamydial A56.11
- chronic N71.1
- following
  - abortion *—see* Abortion by type complicated by genital infection
  - ectopic or molar pregnancy O08.0
- gonococcal, gonorrheal (acute) (chronic) A54.24
- hyperplastic (*see also* Hyperplasia, endometrial) N85.00-
  - cervix N72
- puerperal, postpartum, childbirth O86.12
- subacute N71.0
- tuberculous A18.17

Endometrium *—see* condition

Endomyocardiopathy, South African I42.3

Endomyocarditis *—see* Endocarditis

Endomyofibrosis I42.3

Endomyometritis *—see* Endometritis

Endopericarditis *—see* Endocarditis

Endoperineuritis *—see* Disorder, nerve

Endophlebitis *—see* Phlebitis

Endophthalmia *—see* Endophthalmitis, purulent

Endophthalmitis (acute) (infective) (metastatic) (subacute) H44.009
- bleb associated H59.4 *—see also* Bleb, inflammed (infected), postprocedural
- gonorrheal A54.39
- in (due to)
  - cysticercosis B69.1
  - onchocerciasis B73.01
  - toxocariasis B83.0
- panuveitis *—see* Panuveitis
- parasitic H44.12-
- purulent H44.00-
  - panophthalmitis *—see* Panophthalmitis
  - vitreous abscess H44.02-
- specified NEC H44.19
- sympathetic *—see* Uveitis, sympathetic

Endosalpingioma D28.2

Endosalpingiosis N94.89

Endosteitis *—see* Osteomyelitis

Endothelioma, bone *—see* Neoplasm, bone, malignant

Endotheliosis (hemorrhagic infectional) D69.8

Endotoxemia - code to condition

Endotrachelitis *—see* Cervicitis

Engelmann (-Camurati) **syndrome** Q78.3

English disease *—see* Rickets

Engman's disease L30.3

Engorgement
- breast N64.59
  - newborn P83.4
  - puerperal, postpartum O92.79
- lung (passive) *—see* Edema, lung
- pulmonary (passive) *—see* Edema, lung
- stomach K31.89
- venous, retina *—see* Occlusion, retina, vein, engorgement

Enlargement, enlarged *—see also* Hypertrophy
- adenoids J35.2
  - with tonsils J35.3
- alveolar ridge K08.89
  - congenital *—see* Anomaly, alveolar
- apertures of diaphragm (congenital) Q79.1
- gingival K06.1
- heart, cardiac *—see* Hypertrophy, cardiac
- labium majus, childhood asymmetric (CALME) N90.61
- lacrimal gland, chronic H04.03-
- liver *—see* Hypertrophy, liver
- lymph gland or node R59.9
  - generalized R59.1
  - localized R59.0
- orbit H05.34-
- organ or site, congenital NEC *—see* Anomaly, by site
- parathyroid (gland) E21.0
- pituitary fossa R93.0
- prostate N40.0
  - with lower urinary tract symptoms (LUTS) N40.1
  - without lower urinary tract symtpoms (LUTS) N40.0
- sella turcica R93.0
- spleen *—see* Splenomegaly
- thymus (gland) (congenital) E32.0
- thyroid (gland) *—see* Goiter
- tongue K14.8
- tonsils J35.1
  - with adenoids J35.3
- uterus N85.2
- vestibular aqueduct A16.5

Enophthalmos H05.40-
- due to
  - orbital tissue atrophy H05.41-
  - trauma or surgery H05.42-

Enostosis M27.8

Entamebic, entamebiasis *—see* Amebiasis

Entanglement
- umbilical cord(s) O69.82
  - with compression O69.2
  - around neck (with compression) O69.81
    - with compression O69.1
    - without compression O69.81
  - of twins in monoamniotic sac O69.2
  - without compression O69.82

Enteralgia *—see* Pain, abdominal

Enteric —*see* condition

Enteritis (acute) (diarrheal) (hemorrhagic) (noninfective) K52.9
- adenovirus A08.2
- aertrycke infection A02.0
- allergic K52.29
  - with
    - eosinophilic gastritis or gastroenteritis K52.81
    - food protein-induced entercolitis syndrome K52.21
    - food protein-induced enteropathy K52.22
    - FPIES K52.21
- amebic (acute) A06.0
  - with abscess —*see* Abscess, amebic
  - chronic A06.1
    - with abscess —*see* Abscess, amebic
    - nondysenteric A06.2
  - nondysenteric A06.2
- astrovirus A08.32
- bacillary NOS A03.9
- bacterial A04.9
  - specified NEC A04.8
- calicivirus A08.31
- candidal B37.82
- Chilomastix A07.8
- choleriformis A00.1
- chronic (noninfectious) K52.9
  - ulcerative —*see* Colitis, ulcerative
- cicatrizing (chronic) —*see* Enteritis, regional, small intestine
- Clostridium
  - botulinum (food poisoning) A05.1
  - difficile
    - not specified as recurrent A04.72
    - recurrent A04.71
- coccidial A07.3
- coxsackie virus A08.39
- dietetic (*see also* Enteritis, allergic) K52.29
- drug-induced K52.1
- due to
  - astrovirus A08.32
  - calicivirus A08.31
  - coxsackie virus A08.39
  - drugs K52.1
  - echovirus A08.39
  - enterovirus NEC A08.39
  - food hypersensitivity (*see also* Enteritis, allergic) K52.29
  - infectious organism (bacterial) (viral) —*see* Enteritis, infectious
  - torovirus A08.39
  - Yersinia enterocolitica A04.6
- echovirus A08.39
- eltor A00.1
- enterovirus NEC A08.39
- eosinophilic K52.81
- epidemic (infectious) A09
- fulminant (*see also* Ischemia, intestine acute) K55.019
- gangrenous —*see* Enteritis, infectious
- giardial A07.1
- infectious NOS A09
  - due to
    - adenovirus A08.2
    - Aerobacter aerogenes A04.8
    - Arizona (bacillus) A02.0
    - bacteria NOS A04.9
      - specified NEC A04.8
    - Campylobacter A04.5
    - Clostridium difficile
      - not specified as recurrent A04.72
      - recurrent A04.71
    - Clostridium perfringens A04.8
    - Enterobacter aerogenes A04.8
    - enterovirus A08.39
    - Escherichia coli A04.4
      - enteroaggregative A04.4
      - enterohemorrhagic A04.3
      - enteroinvasive A04.2
      - enteropathogenic A04.0
      - enterotoxigenic A04.1
      - specified NEC A04.4
    - specified
      - bacteria NEC A04.8
      - virus NEC A08.39
    - Staphylococcus A04.8
    - virus NEC A08.4
      - specified type NEC A08.39
    - Yersinia enterocolitica A04.6
  - specified organism NEC A08.8
- influenzal —*see* Influenza, with, digestive manifestations
- ischemic K55.9
  - acute (*see also* Ischemia, intestine acute) K55.019
  - chronic K55.1
- microsporidial A07.8
- mucomembranous, myxomembranous —*see* Syndrome, irritable bowel
- mucous —*see* Syndrome, irritable bowel
- necroticans A05.2
- necrotizing of newborn —*see* Enterocolitis, necrotizing, in newborn
- neurogenic —*see* Syndrome, irritable bowel
- newborn necrotizing —*see* Enterocolitis, necrotizing, in newborn
- noninfectious K52.9
- norovirus A08.11
- parasitic NEC B82.9
- paratyphoid (fever) —*see* Fever, paratyphoid
- protozoal A07.9
  - specified NEC A07.8
- radiation K52.0
- regional (of) K50.90
  - with
    - complication K50.919
      - abscess K50.914
      - fistula K50.913
      - intestinal obstruction K50.912
      - rectal bleeding K50.911
      - specified complication NEC K50.918
  - colon —*see* Enteritis, regional, large intestine
  - duodenum —*see* Enteritis, regional, small intestine
  - ileum —*see* Enteritis, regional, small intestine
  - jejunum —*see* Enteritis, regional, small intestine
  - large bowel —*see* Enteritis, regional, large intestine
  - large intestine (colon) (rectum) K50.10
    - with
      - complication K50.119
        - abscess K50.114
        - fistula K50.113
        - intestinal obstruction K50.112
        - rectal bleeding K50.111
        - small intestine (duodenum) (ileum) (jejunum) involvement K50.80
          - with
            - complication K50.819
              - abscess K50.814
              - fistula K50.813
              - intestinal obstruction K50.812
              - rectal bleeding K50.811
              - specified complication NEC K50.818
        - specified complication NEC K50.118
  - rectum —*see* Enteritis, regional, large intestine
  - small intestine (duodenum) (ileum) (jejunum) K50.00
    - with
      - complication K50.019
        - abscess K50.014
        - fistula K50.013
        - intestinal obstruction K50.012
        - large intestine (colon) (rectum) involvement K50.80
          - with
            - complication K50.819
              - abscess K50.814
              - fistula K50.813
              - intestinal obstruction K50.812
              - rectal bleeding K50.811
              - specified complication NEC K50.818
        - rectal bleeding K50.011
        - specified complication NEC K50.018
- rotaviral A08.0
- Salmonella, salmonellosis (arizonae) (cholerae-suis) (enteritidis) (typhimurium) A02.0
- segmental —*see* Enteritis, regional
- septic A09
- Shigella —*see* Infection, Shigella
- small round structured NEC A08.19
- spasmodic, spastic —*see* Syndrome, irritable bowel
- staphylococcal A04.8
  - due to food A05.0
- torovirus A08.39
- toxic NEC K52.1
  - due to Clostridium difficile
    - not specified as recurrent A04.72
    - recurrent A04.71
- trichomonal A07.8
- tuberculous A18.32
- typhosa A01.00
- ulcerative (chronic) —*see* Colitis, ulcerative
- viral A08.4
  - adenovirus A08.2
  - enterovirus A08.39
  - Rotavirus A08.0
  - small round structured NEC A08.19
  - specified NEC A08.39
  - virus specified NEC A08.39

Enterobiasis B80

Enterobius vermicularis (infection) (infestation) B80

Enterocele —*see also* Hernia, abdomen
- pelvic, pelvis (acquired) (congenital) N81.5
- vagina, vaginal (acquired) (congenital) NEC N81.5

Enterocolitis (*see also* Enteritis) K52.9
- due to Clostridium difficile
  - not specified as recurrent A04.72
  - recurrent A04.71
- fulminant ischemic (*see also* Ischemia, intestine acute) K55.059
- granulomatous —*see* Enteritis, regional
- hemorrhagic (acute) (*see also* Ischemia, intestine acute) K55.059
  - chronic K55.1
- infectious NEC A09
- ischemic K55.9
- necrotizing K55.30
  - with
    - perforation K55.33
    - pneumatosis K55.32
      - and perforation K55.33
  - due to Clostridium difficile
    - not specified as recurrent A04.72
    - recurrent A04.71
  - in newborn P77.9
    - stage 1 (without pneumatosis, without perforation) P77.1
    - stage 2 (with pneumatosis, without perforation) P77.2
    - stage 3 (with pneumatosis, with perforation) P77.3
  - in non-newborn K55.30
    - stage 1 (without pneumatosis, without perforation) K55.31
    - stage 2 (with pneumatosis, without perforation) K55.32
    - stage 3 (with pneumatosis, with perforation) K55.33
  - without pneumatosis or perforation K55.31
- noninfectious K52.9
  - newborn —*see* Enterocolitis, necrotizing, in newborn
- pseudomembranous (newborn)
  - not specified as recurrent A04.72
  - recurrent A04.71
- radiation K52.0
  - newborn —*see* Enterocolitis, necrotizing, in newborn
- ulcerative (chronic) —*see* Pancolitis, ulcerative (chronic)

Enterogastritis —*see* Enteritis

Enteropathy K63.9
- celiac-gluten-sensitive K90.0
  - non-celiac K90.41
- food protein-induced K52.22
- hemorrhagic, terminal (*see also* Ischemia, intestine, acute) K55.059
- protein-losing K90.49

Enteroperitonitis *—see* Peritonitis

Enteroptosis K63.4

Enterorrhagia K92.2

Enterospasm *—see also* Syndrome, irritable, bowel
- psychogenic F45.8

Enterostenosis (*see also* Obstruction, intestine specified NEC) K56.699

Enterostomy
- complication *—see* Complication, enterostomy
- status Z93.4

Enterovirus, as cause of disease classified elsewhere B97.10
- coxsackievirus B97.11
- echovirus B97.12
- other specified B97.19

Enthesopathy (peripheral) M77.9
- Achilles tendinitis *—see* Tendinitis, Achilles
- ankle and tarsus M77.5-
  - specified type NEC *—see* Enthesopathy, foot, specified type NEC
- anterior tibial syndrome M76.81-
- calcaneal spur *—see* Spur, bone, calcaneal
- elbow region M77.8
  - lateral epicondylitis *—see* Epicondylitis, lateral
  - medial epicondylitis *—see* Epicondylitis, medial
- foot NEC M77.8
  - metatarsalgia *—see* Metatarsalgia
  - specified type NEC M77.5-
- forearm M77.8
- gluteal tendinitis *—see* Tendinitis, gluteal
- hand M77.8
- hip *—see* Enthesopathy, lower limb, specified type NEC
- iliac crest spur *—see* Spur, bone, iliac crest
- iliotibial band syndrome *—see* Syndrome, iliotibial band
- knee *—see* Enthesopathy, lower limb, lower leg, specified type NEC
- lateral epicondylitis *—see* Epicondylitis, lateral
- lower limb (excluding foot) M76.9
  - Achilles tendinitis *—see* Tendinitis, Achilles
  - ankle and tarsus M77.5-
    - specified type NEC *—see* Enthesopathy, foot, specified type NEC
  - anterior tibial syndrome M76.81-
  - gluteal tendinitis *—see* Tendinitis, gluteal
  - iliac crest spur *—see* Spur, bone, iliac crest
  - iliotibial band syndrome *—see* Syndrome, iliotibial band
  - patellar tendinitis *—see* Tendinitis, patellar
  - pelvic region *—see* Enthesopathy, lower limb, specified type NEC
  - peroneal tendinitis *—see* Tendinitis, peroneal
  - posterior tibial syndrome M76.82-
  - psoas tendinitis *—see* Tendinitis, psoas
  - specified type NEC M76.89-
  - tibial collateral bursitis *—see* Bursitis, tibial collateral
- medial epicondylitis *—see* Epicondylitis, medial
- metatarsalgia *—see* Metatarsalgia
- multiple sites M77.8
- patellar tendinitis *—see* Tendinitis, patellar
- pelvis M77.8
- periarthritis of wrist *—see* Periarthritis, wrist
- peroneal tendinitis *—see* Tendinitis, peroneal
- posterior tibial syndrome M76.82-
- psoas tendinitis *—see* Tendinitis, psoas
- shoulder M77.8
- shoulder region *—see* Lesion, shoulder
- specified type NEC M77.8
- spinal M46.00
  - cervical region M46.02
  - cervicothoracic region M46.03
  - lumbar region M46.06
  - lumbosacral region M46.07
  - multiple sites M46.09
  - occipito-atlanto-axial region M46.01
  - sacrococcygeal region M46.08
  - thoracic region M46.04
  - thoracolumbar region M46.05
- tibial collateral bursitis *—see* Bursitis, tibial collateral
- upper arm M77.8
- wrist and carpus NEC M77.8
  - calcaneal spur *—see* Spur, bone, calcaneal
  - periarthritis of wrist *—see* Periarthritis, wrist

Entomophobia F40.218

Entomophthoromycosis B46.8

Entrance, air into vein *—see* Embolism, air

Entrapment, nerve *—see* Neuropathy, entrapment

Entropion (eyelid) (paralytic) H02.009
- cicatricial H02.019
  - left H02.016
    - lower H02.015
    - upper H02.014
  - right H02.013
    - lower H02.012
    - upper H02.011
- congenital Q10.2
- left H02.006
  - lower H02.005
  - upper H02.004
- mechanical H02.029
  - left H02.026
    - lower H02.025
    - upper H02.024
  - right H02.023
    - lower H02.022
    - upper H02.021
- right H02.003
  - lower H02.002
  - upper H02.001
- senile H02.039
  - left H02.036
    - lower H02.035
    - upper H02.034
  - right H02.033
    - lower H02.032
    - upper H02.031
- spastic H02.049
  - left H02.046
    - lower H02.045
    - upper H02.044
  - right H02.043
    - lower H02.042
    - upper H02.041

Enucleated eye (traumatic, current) S05.7-

Enuresis R32
- functional F98.0
- habit disturbance F98.0
- nocturnal N39.44
  - psychogenic F98.0
- nonorganic origin F98.0
- psychogenic F98.0

Eosinopenia *—see* Agranulocytosis

Eosinophilia (allergic) (idiopathic) (secondary) D72.10
- with
  - angiolymphoid hyperplasia (ALHE) D18.01
- familial D71.19
- hereditary D72.19
- in diseases classified elsewhere D72.18
- infiltrative *—see* Eosinophilia, pulmonary
- Löffler's J82.89
- peritoneal *—see* Peritonitis, eosinophilic
- pulmonary NEC J82.89
  - acute J82.82
  - asthmatic J82.83
  - chronic J82.81
- specified NEC D72.19
- tropical (pulmonary) J82.89

Eosinophilia-myalgia syndrome M35.89

Ependymitis (acute) (cerebral) (chronic) (granular) *—see* Encephalomyelitis

Ependymoblastoma
- specified site *—see* Neoplasm, malignant, by site
- unspecified site C71.9

Ependymoma (epithelial) (malignant)
- anaplastic
  - specified site *—see* Neoplasm, malignant, by site
  - unspecified site C71.9
- benign
  - specified site *—see* Neoplasm, benign, by site
  - unspecified site D33.2
- myxopapillary D43.2
  - specified site *—see* Neoplasm, uncertain behavior, by site
  - unspecified site D43.2
- papillary D43.2
  - specified site *—see* Neoplasm, uncertain behavior, by site
  - unspecified site D43.2
- specified site *—see* Neoplasm, malignant, by site
- unspecified site C71.9

Ependymopathy G93.89

Ephelis, ephelides L81.2

Epiblepharon (congenital) Q10.3

Epicanthus, epicanthic fold (eyelid) (congenital) Q10.3

Epicondylitis (elbow)
- lateral M77.1-
- medial M77.0-

Epicystitis *—see* Cystitis

Epidemic *—see* condition

Epidermidalization, cervix *—see* Dysplasia, cervix

Epidermis, epidermal *—see* condition

Epidermodysplasia verruciformis B07.8

Epidermolysis
- bullosa (congenital) Q81.9
  - acquired L12.30
    - drug-induced L12.31
    - specified cause NEC L12.35
  - dystrophica Q81.2
  - letalis Q81.1
  - simplex Q81.0
  - specified NEC Q81.8
- necroticans combustiformis L51.2
  - due to drug *—see* Table of Drugs and Chemicals, by drug

Epidermophytid *—see* Dermatophytosis

Epidermophytosis (infected) *—see* Dermatophytosis

Epididymis *—see* condition

Epididymitis (acute) (nonvenereal) (recurrent) (residual) N45.1
- with orchitis N45.3
- blennorrhagic (gonococcal) A54.23
- caseous (tuberculous) A18.15
- chlamydial A56.19
- filarial (*see also* Infestation, filarial) B74.9 *[N51]*
- gonococcal A54.23
- syphilitic A52.76
- tuberculous A18.15

Epididymo-orchitis (*see also* Epididymitis) N45.3

Epidural *—see* condition

Epigastrium, epigastric *—see* condition

Epigastrocele *—see* Hernia, ventral

Epiglottis *—see* condition

Epiglottitis, epiglottiditis (acute) J05.10
- with obstruction J05.11
- chronic J37.0

Epignathus Q89.4

Epilepsia partialis continua (*see also* Kozhevnikof's epilepsy) G40.1-

Epilepsy, epileptic, epilepsia (attack) (cerebral) (convulsion) (fit) (seizure) G40.909

> Note: the following terms are to be considered equivalent to intractable: pharmacoresistant (pharmacologically resistant), treatment resistant, refractory (medically) and poorly controlled

- with
  - complex partial seizures *—see* Epilepsy, localization-related, symptomatic, with complex partial seizures
  - grand mal seizures on awakening *—see* Epilepsy, generalized, specified NEC
  - myoclonic absences *—see* Epilepsy, generalized, specified NEC
  - myoclonic-astatic seizures *—see* Epilepsy, generalized, specified NEC
  - simple partial seizures *—see* Epilepsy, localization-related, symptomatic, with simple partial seizures
- akinetic *—see* Epilepsy, generalized, specified NEC

Epilepsy, epileptic, epilepsia *(continued)*
- benign childhood with centrotemporal EEG spikes —*see* Epilepsy, localization-related, idiopathic
- benign myoclonic in infancy G40.80-
- Bravais-jacksonian —*see* Epilepsy, localization-related, symptomatic, with simple partial seizures
- childhood
  - with occipital EEG paroxysms —*see* Epilepsy, localization-related, idiopathic
  - absence G40.A09
    - intractable G40.A19
      - with status epilepticus G40.A11
      - without status epilepticus G40.A19
    - not intractable G40.A09
      - with status epilepticus G40.A01
      - without status epilepticus G40.A09
- climacteric —*see* Epilepsy, specified NEC
- cysticercosis B69.0
- deterioration (mental) F06.8
- due to syphilis A52.19
- focal —*see* Epilepsy, localization-related, symptomatic, with simple partial seizures
- generalized
  - idiopathic G40.309
    - intractable G40.319
      - with status epilepticus G40.311
      - without status epilepticus G40.319
    - not intractable G40.309
      - with status epilepticus G40.301
      - without status epilepticus G40.309
  - specified NEC G40.409
    - intractable G40.419
      - with status epilepticus G40.411
      - without status epilepticus G40.419
    - not intractable G40.409
      - with status epilepticus G40.401
      - without status epilepticus G40.409
- impulsive petit mal —*see* Epilepsy, juvenile myoclonic
- intractable G40.919
  - with status epilepticus G40.911
  - without status epilepticus G40.919
- juvenile absence G40.A09
  - intractable G40.A19
    - with status epilepticus G40.A11
    - without status epilepticus G40.A19
  - not intractable G40.A09
    - with status epilepticus G40.A01
    - without status epilepticus G40.A09
- juvenile myoclonic G40.B09
  - intractable G40.B19
    - with status epilepticus G40.B11
    - without status epilepticus G40.B19
  - not intractable G40.B09
    - with status epilepticus G40.B01

Epilepsy, epileptic, epilepsia *(continued)*
- juvenile myoclonic *(continued)*
  - not intractable *(continued)*
    - without status epilepticus G40.B09
- localization-related (focal) (partial)
  - idiopathic G40.009
    - with seizures of localized onset G40.009
      - intractable G40.019
        - with status epilepticus G40.011
        - without status epilepticus G40.019
      - not intractable G40.009
        - with status epilepticus G40.001
        - without status epilepticus G40.009
  - symptomatic
    - with complex partial seizures G40.209
      - intractable G40.219
        - with status epilepticus G40.211
        - without status epilepticus G40.219
      - not intractable G40.209
        - with status epilepticus G40.201
        - without status epilepticus G40.209
    - with simple partial seizures G40.109
      - intractable G40.119
        - with status epilepticus G40.111
        - without status epilepticus G40.119
      - not intractable G40.109
        - with status epilepticus G40.101
        - without status epilepticus G40.109
- myoclonus, myoclonic —*see also* Epilepsy, generalized, specified NEC
  - progressive —*see* Epilepsy, generalized, idiopathic
  - severe, in infancy (SMEI) G40.83-
- not intractable G40.909
  - with status epilepticus G40.901
  - without status epilepticus G40.909
- on awakening —*see* Epilepsy, generalized, specified NEC
- parasitic NOS B71.9 *[G94]*
- partialis continua (*see also* Kozhevnikof's epilepsy) G40.1-
- peripheral —*see* Epilepsy, specified NEC
- polymorphic, in infancy (PMEI) G40.83-
- procursiva —*see* Epilepsy, localization-related, symptomatic, with simple partial seizures
- progressive (familial) myoclonic —*see* Epilepsy, generalized, idiopathic
- reflex —*see* Epilepsy, specified NEC
- related to
  - alcohol G40.509
    - not intractable G40.509
      - with status epilepticus G40.501
      - without status epliepticus G40.509

Epilepsy, epileptic, epilepsia *(continued)*
- related to *(continued)*
  - drugs G40.509
    - not intractable G40.509
      - with status epilepticus G40.501
      - without status epliepticus G40.509
  - external causes G40.509
    - not intractable G40.509
      - with status epilepticus G40.501
      - without status epliepticus G40.509
  - hormonal changes G40.509
    - not intractable G40.509
      - with status epilepticus G40.501
      - without status epliepticus G40.509
  - sleep deprivation G40.509
    - not intractable G40.509
      - with status epilepticus G40.501
      - without status epliepticus G40.509
  - stress G40.509
    - not intractable G40.509
      - with status epilepticus G40.501
      - without status epliepticus G40.509
- somatomotor —*see* Epilepsy, localization-related, symptomatic, with simple partial seizures
- somatosensory —*see* Epilepsy, localization-related, symptomatic, with simple partial seizures
- spasms G40.822
  - intractable G40.824
    - with status epilepticus G40.823
    - without status epilepticus G40.824
  - not intractable G40.822
    - with status epilepticus G40.821
    - without status epilepticus G40.822
- specified NEC G40.802
  - intractable G40.804
    - with status epilepticus G40.803
    - without status epilepticus G40.804
  - not intractable G40.802
    - with status epilepticus G40.801
    - without status epilepticus G40.802
- syndromes
  - generalized
    - idiopathic G40.309
      - intractable G40.319
        - with status epilepticus G40.311
        - without status epilepticus G40.319
      - not intractable G40.309
        - with status epilepticus G40.301
        - without status epilepticus G40.309
    - specified NEC G40.409
      - intractable G40.419
        - with status epilepticus G40.411
        - without status epilepticus G40.419

Epilepsy, epileptic, epilepsia *(continued)*
- syndromes *(continued)*
  - generalized *(continued)*
    - specified NEC *(continued)*
      - not intractable G40.409
        - with status epilepticus G40.401
        - without status epilepticus G40.409
  - localization-related (focal) (partial)
    - idiopathic G40.009
      - with seizures of localized onset G40.009
        - intractable G40.019
          - with status epilepticus G40.011
          - without status epilepticus G40.019
        - not intractable G40.009
          - with status epilepticus G40.001
          - without status epilepticus G40.009
    - symptomatic
      - with complex partial seizures G40.209
        - intractable G40.219
          - with status epilepticus G40.211
          - without status epilepticus G40.219
        - not intractable G40.209
          - with status epilepticus G40.201
          - without status epilepticus G40.209
      - with simple partial seizures G40.109
        - intractable G40.119
          - with status epilepticus G40.111
          - without status epilepticus G40.119
        - not intractable G40.109
          - with status epilepticus G40.101
          - without status epilepticus G40.109
  - specified NEC G40.802
    - intractable G40.804
      - with status epilepticus G40.803
      - without status epilepticus G40.804
    - not intractable G40.802
      - with status epilepticus G40.801
      - without status epilepticus G40.802
- tonic (-clonic) —*see* Epilepsy, generalized, specified NEC
- twilight F05
- uncinate (gyrus) —*see* Epilepsy, localization-related, symptomatic, with complex partial seizures
- Unverricht (-Lundborg) (familial myoclonic) —*see* Epilepsy, generalized, idiopathic
- visceral —*see* Epilepsy, specified NEC
- visual —*see* Epilepsy, specified NEC

Epiloia Q85.1

Epimenorrhea N92.0

Epipharyngitis —*see* Nasopharyngitis

Epiphora H04.20-
- due to
  - excess lacrimation H04.21-
  - insufficient drainage H04.22-

Epiphyseal arrest *—see* Arrest, epiphyseal

Epiphyseolysis, epiphysiolysis *—see* Osteochondropathy

Epiphysitis *—see also* Osteochondropathy
- juvenile M92.9
- syphilitic (congenital) A50.02

Epiplocele *—see* Hernia, abdomen

Epiploitis *—see* Peritonitis

Epiplosarcomphalocele *—see* Hernia, umbilicus

Episcleritis (suppurative) H15.10-
- in (due to)
  - syphilis A52.71
  - tuberculosis A18.51
- nodular H15.12-
- periodica fugax H15.11-
  - angioneurotic *—see* Edema, angioneurotic
- syphilitic (late) A52.71
- tuberculous A18.51

Episode
- affective, mixed F39
- depersonalization (in neurotic state) F48.1
- depressive F32.A
  - major F32.9
    - mild F32.0
    - moderate F32.1
    - severe (without psychotic symptoms) F32.2
      - with psychotic symptoms F32.3
  - recurrent F33.9
    - brief F33.8
  - specified NEC F32.89
- hypomanic F30.8
- manic F30.9
  - with
    - psychotic symptoms F30.2
    - remission (full) F30.4
      - partial F30.3
  - other specified F30.8
  - recurrent F31.89
  - without psychotic symptoms F30.10
    - mild F30.11
    - moderate F30.12
    - severe (without psychotic symptoms) F30.13
      - with psychotic symptoms F30.2
- psychotic F23
  - organic F06.8
- schizophrenic (acute) NEC, brief F23

Epispadias (female) (male) Q64.0

Episplenitis D73.89

Epistaxis (multiple) R04.0
- hereditary I78.0
- vicarious menstruation N94.89

Epithelioma (malignant) *—see also* Neoplasm, malignant, by site
- adenoides cysticum *—see* Neoplasm, skin, benign
- basal cell *—see* Neoplasm, skin, malignant
- benign *—see* Neoplasm, benign, by site
- Bowen's *—see* Neoplasm, skin, in situ

Epithelioma *(continued)*
- calcifying, of Malherbe *—see* Neoplasm, skin, benign
- external site *—see* Neoplasm, skin, malignant
- intraepidermal, Jadassohn *—see* Neoplasm, skin, benign
- squamous cell *—see* Neoplasm, malignant, by site

Epitheliomatosis pigmented Q82.1

Epitheliopathy, multifocal placoid pigment H30.14-

Epithelium, epithelial *—see* condition

Epituberculosis (with atelectasis) (allergic) A15.7

Eponychia Q84.6

Epstein's
- nephrosis or syndrome *—see* Nephrosis
- pearl K09.8

Epulis (gingiva) (fibrous) (giant cell) K06.8

Equinia A24.0

Equinovarus (congenital) (talipes) Q66.0-
- acquired *—see* Deformity, limb, clubfoot

Equivalent
- convulsive (abdominal) *—see* Epilepsy, specified NEC
- epileptic (psychic) *—see* Epilepsy, localization-related, symptomatic, with complex partial seizures

Erb (-Duchenne) **paralysis** (birth injury) (newborn) P14.0

Erb-Goldflam disease or syndrome G70.00
- with exacerbation (acute) G70.01
- in crisis G70.01

Erb's
- disease G71.02
- palsy, paralysis (brachial) (birth) (newborn) P14.0
  - spinal (spastic) syphilitic A52.17
- pseudohypertrophic muscular dystrophy G71.02

Erdheim's syndrome (acromegalic macrospondylitis) E22.0

Erection, painful (persistent) *—see* Priapism

Ergosterol deficiency (vitamin D) E55.9
- with
  - adult osteomalacia M83.8
  - rickets *—see* Rickets

Ergotism *—see also* Poisoning, food, noxious, plant
- from ergot used as drug (migraine therapy) *—see* Table of Drugs and Chemicals

Erosio interdigitalis blastomycetica B37.2

Erosion
- artery I77.2
  - without rupture I77.89
- bone *—see* Disorder, bone, density and structure, specified NEC
- bronchus J98.09
- cartilage (joint) *—see* Disorder, cartilage, specified type NEC
- cervix (uteri) (acquired) (chronic) (congenital) N86
  - with cervicitis N72

Erosion *(continued)*
- cornea (nontraumatic) *—see* Ulcer, cornea
  - recurrent H18.83-
  - traumatic *—see* Abrasion, cornea
- dental (idiopathic) (occupational) (due to diet, drugs or vomiting) K03.2
- duodenum, postpyloric *—see* Ulcer, duodenum
- esophagus K22.10
  - with bleeding K22.11
- gastric *—see* Ulcer, stomach
- gastrojejunal *—see* Ulcer, gastrojejunal
- implanted mesh *—see* Complications, prosthetic device or implant, mesh
- intestine K63.3
- lymphatic vessel I89.8
- pylorus, pyloric (ulcer) *—see* Ulcer, stomach
- spine, aneurysmal A52.09
- stomach *—see* Ulcer, stomach
- subcutaneous device pocket
  - nervous system prosthetic device, implant, or graft T85.890
  - other internal prosthetic device, implant, or graft T85.898
- teeth (idiopathic) (occupational) (due to diet, drugs or vomiting) K03.2
- urethra N36.8
- uterus N85.8

Erotomania F52.8

Error
- metabolism, inborn -- se Disorder, metabolism
- refractive *—see* Disorder, refraction

Eructation R14.2
- nervous or psychogenic F45.8

Eruption
- creeping B76.9
- drug (generalized) (taken internally) L27.0
  - fixed L27.1
  - in contact with skin *—see* Dermatitis, due to drugs
  - localized L27.1
- Hutchinson, summer L56.4
- Kaposi's varicelliform B00.0
- napkin L22
- polymorphous light (sun) L56.4
- recalcitrant pustular L13.8
- ringed R23.8
- skin (nonspecific) R21
  - creeping (meaning hookworm) B76.9
  - due to inoculation/vaccination (generalized) (*see also* Dermatitis, due to, vaccine) L27.0
    - localized L27.1
  - erysipeloid A26.0
  - feigned L98.1
  - Kaposi's varicelliform B00.0
  - lichenoid L28.0
  - meaning dermatitis *—see* Dermatitis
  - toxic NEC L53.0
- tooth, teeth, abnormal (incomplete) (late) (premature) (sequence) K00.6
- vesicular R23.8

Erysipelas (gangrenous) (infantile) (newborn) (phlegmonous) (suppurative) A46
- external ear A46 *[H62.40]*
- puerperal, postpartum O86.89

Erysipeloid A26.9
- cutaneous (Rosenbach's) A26.0
- disseminated A26.8
- sepsis A26.7
- specified NEC A26.8

Erythema, erythematous (infectional) (inflammation) L53.9
- ab igne L59.0
- annulare (centrifugum) (rheumaticum) L53.1
- arthriticum epidemicum A25.1
- brucellum *—see* Brucellosis
- chronic figurate NEC L53.3
- chronicum migrans (Borrelia burgdorferi) A69.20
- diaper L22
- due to
  - chemical NEC L53.0
    - in contact with skin L24.5
  - drug (internal use) *—see* Dermatitis, due to, drugs
- elevatum diutinum L95.1
- endemic E52
- epidemic, arthritic A25.1
- figuratum perstans L53.3
- gluteal L22
- heat - code by site under Burn, first degree
- ichthyosiforme congenitum bullous Q80.3
- in diseases classified elsewhere L54
- induratum (nontuberculous) L52
  - tuberculous A18.4
- infectiosum B08.3
- intertrigo L30.4
- iris L51.9
- marginatum L53.2
  - in (due to) acute rheumatic fever I00
- medicamentosum *—see* Dermatitis, due to, drugs
- migrans A26.0
  - chronicum A69.20
  - tongue K14.1
- multiforme (major) (minor) L51.9
  - bullous, bullosum L51.1
  - conjunctiva L51.1
  - nonbullous L51.0
  - pemphigoides L12.0
  - specified NEC L51.8
- napkin L22
- neonatorum P83.88
  - toxic P83.1
- nodosum L52
  - tuberculous A18.4
- palmar L53.8
- pernio T69.1
- rash, newborn P83.88
- scarlatiniform (recurrent) (exfoliative) L53.8
- solare L55.0
- specified NEC L53.8
- toxic, toxicum NEC L53.0
  - newborn P83.1
- tuberculous (primary) A18.4

Erythematous, erythematosus *—see* condition

Erythermalgia (primary) I73.81

Erythralgia I73.81

Erythrasma L08.1

Erythredema (polyneuropathy) *—see* Poisoning, mercury

Erythremia (acute) C94.0-
- chronic D45
- secondary D75.1

Erythroblastopenia *—see also* Aplasia, red cell D60.9
- congenital D61.01

Erythroblastophthisis D61.09

Erythroblastosis (fetalis) (newborn) P55.9
- due to
  - ABO (antibodies) (incompatibility) (isoimmunization) P55.1
  - Rh (antibodies) (incompatibility) (isoimmunization) P55.0

Erythrocyanosis (crurum) I73.89

Erythrocythemia *—see* Erythremia

Erythrocytosis (megalosplenic) (secondary) D75.1
- familial D75.0
- oval, hereditary *—see* Elliptocytosis
- secondary D75.1
- stress D75.1

Erythroderma (secondary) (*see also* Erythema) L53.9
- bullous ichthyosiform, congenital Q80.3
- desquamativum L21.1
- ichthyosiform, congenital (bullous) Q80.3
- neonatorum P83.88
- psoriaticum L40.8

Erythrodysesthesia, palmar plantar (PPE) L27.1

Erythrogenesis imperfecta D61.09

Erythroleukemia C94.0-

Erythromelalgia I73.81

Erythrophagocytosis D75.89

Erythrophobia F40.298

Erythroplakia, oral epithelium, and tongue K13.29

Erythroplasia (Queyrat) D07.4
- specified site *—see* Neoplasm, skin, in situ
- unspecified site D07.4

Escherichia coli (E. coli), as cause of disease classified elsewhere B96.20
- non-O157 Shiga toxin-producing (with known O group) B96.22
- non-Shiga toxin-producing B96.29
- O157 B96.21
- O157 with confirmation of Shiga toxin when H antigen is unknown, or is not H7 B96.21
- O157:H-(nonmotile) with confirmation of Shiga toxin B96.21
- O157:H7 with or without confirmation of Shiga toxin-production B96.21
- Shiga toxin-producing (with unspecified O group) (STEC) B96.23
- specified NEC B96.29

Esophagismus K22.4

Esophagitis (acute) (alkaline) (chemical) (chronic) (infectional) (necrotic) (peptic) (postoperative) (without bleeding) K20.90
- with bleeding K20.91
- candidal B37.81
- due to gastrointestinal reflux disease (without bleeding) K21.00
  - with bleeding K21.01
- eosinophilic K20.0
- reflux K21.00
- specified NEC (without bleeding) K20.80
  - with bleeding K21.81

Esophagitis *(continued)*
- tuberculous A18.83
- ulcerative K22.10
  - with bleeding K22.11

Esophagocele K22.5

Esophagomalacia K22.89

Esophagospasm K22.4

Esophagostenosis K22.2

Esophagostomiasis B81.8

Esophagotracheal *—see* condition

Esophagus *—see* condition

Esophoria H50.51
- convergence, excess H51.12
- divergence, insufficiency H51.8

Esotropia *—see* Strabismus, convergent concomitant

Espundia B55.2

Essential *—see* condition

Esthesioneuroblastoma C30.0

Esthesioneurocytoma C30.0

Esthesioneuroepithelioma C30.0

Esthiomene A55

Estivo-autumnal malaria (fever) B50.9

Estrangement (marital) Z63.5
- parent-child NEC Z62.890

Estriasis *—see* Myiasis

Ethanolism *—see* Alcoholism

Etherism *—see* Dependence, drug, inhalant

Ethmoid, ethmoidal *—see* condition

Ethmoiditis (chronic) (nonpurulent) (purulent) *—see also* Sinusitis, ethmoidal
- influenzal *—see* Influenza, with, respiratory manifestations NEC
- Woakes' J33.1

Ethylism *—see* Alcoholism

Eulenburg's disease (congenital paramyotonia) G71.19

Eumycetoma B47.0

Eunuchoidism E29.1
- hypogonadotropic E23.0

European blastomycosis *—see* Cryptococcosis

Eustachian *—see* condition

Evaluation (for) (of)
- development state
  - adolescent Z00.3
  - period of
    - delayed growth in childhood Z00.70
      - with abnormal findings Z00.71
    - rapid growth in childhood Z00.2
  - puberty Z00.3
- growth and developmental state (period of rapid growth) Z00.2
  - delayed growth Z00.70
    - with abnormal findings Z00.71
- mental health (status) Z00.8
  - requested by authority Z04.6
- period of
  - delayed growth in childhood Z00.70
    - with abnormal findings Z00.71
  - rapid growth in childhood Z00.2
- suspected condition *—see* Observation

Evans syndrome D69.41

Event
- apparent life threatening in newborn and infact (ALTE) R68.13
- brief resolved unexplained event (BRUE) R68.13

Eventration *—see also* Hernia, ventral
- colon into chest *—see* Hernia, diaphragm
- diaphragm (congenital) Q79.1

Eversion
- bladder N32.89
- cervix (uteri) N86
  - with cervicitis N72
- foot NEC *—see also* Deformity, valgus, ankle
  - congenital Q66.6
- punctum lacrimale (postinfectional) (senile) H04.52-
- ureter (meatus) N28.89
- urethra (meatus) N36.8
- uterus N81.4

Evidence
- cytologic
  - of malignancy on anal smear R85.614
  - of malignancy on cervical smear R87.614
  - of malignancy on vaginal smear R87.624

Evisceration
- birth injury P15.8
- traumatic NEC
  - eye *—see* Enucleated eye

Evulsion *—see* Avulsion

Ewing's sarcoma or tumor *—see* Neoplasm, bone, malignant

Examination (for) (following) (general) (of) (routine) Z00.00
- with abnormal findings Z00.01
- abuse, physical (alleged), ruled out
  - adult Z04.71
  - child Z04.72
- adolescent (development state) Z00.3
- alleged rape or sexual assault (victim), ruled out
  - adult Z04.41
  - child Z04.42
- allergy Z01.82
- annual (adult) (periodic) (physical) Z00.00
  - with abnormal findings Z00.01
  - gynecological Z01.419
    - with abnormal findings Z01.411
- antibody response Z01.84
- blood *—see* Examination, laboratory
- blood pressure Z01.30
  - with abnormal findings Z01.31
- cancer staging *—see* Neoplasm, malignant, by site
- cervical Papanicolaou smear Z12.4
  - as part of routine gynecological examination Z01.419
    - with abnormal findings Z01.411
- child (over 28 days old) Z00.129
  - with abnormal findings Z00.121
  - under 28 days old *—see* Newborn, examination
- clinical research control or normal comparison (control) (participant) Z00.6
- contraceptive (drug) maintenance (routine) Z30.8
  - device (intrauterine) Z30.431
- dental Z01.20
  - with abnormal findings Z01.21
- developmental *—see* Examination, child
- donor (potential) Z00.5

Examination *(continued)*
- ear Z01.10
  - with abnormal findings NEC Z01.118
- eye Z01.00
  - with abnormal findings Z01.01
  - following failed vision screening Z01.020
    - with abnormal findings Z01.021
- following
  - accident NEC Z04.3
    - transport Z04.1
    - work Z04.2
  - assault, alleged, ruled out
    - adult Z04.71
    - child Z04.72
  - motor vehicle accident Z04.1
  - treatment (for) Z09
    - combined NEC Z09
      - fracture Z09
      - malignant neoplasm Z08
    - malignant neoplasm Z08
    - mental disorder Z09
    - specified condition NEC Z09
- follow-up (routine) (following) Z09
  - chemotherapy NEC Z09
    - malignant neoplasm Z08
  - fracture Z09
  - malignant neoplasm Z08
  - postpartum Z39.2
  - psychotherapy Z09
  - radiotherapy NEC Z09
    - malignant neoplasm Z08
  - surgery NEC Z09
    - malignant neoplasm Z08
- forced sexual exploitation Z04.81
- forced labor exploitation Z04.82
- gynecological Z01.419
  - with abnormal findings Z01.411
  - for contraceptive maintenance Z30.8
- health *—see* Examination, medical
- hearing Z01.10
  - with abnormal findings NEC Z01.118
  - following failed hearing screening Z01.110
  - infant or child (over 28 days old) Z00.129
    - with abnormal findings Z00.121
- immunity status testing Z01.84
- laboratory (as part of a general medical examination) Z00.00
  - with abnormal findings Z00.01
  - preprocedural Z01.812
- lactating mother Z39.1
- medical (adult) (for) (of) Z00.00
  - with abnormal findings Z00.01
  - administrative purpose only Z02.9
    - specified NEC Z02.89
  - admission to
    - armed forces Z02.3
    - old age home Z02.2
    - prison Z02.89
    - residential institution Z02.2
    - school Z02.0
      - following illness or medical treatment Z02.0
    - summer camp Z02.89
  - adoption Z02.82
  - blood alcohol or drug level Z02.83
  - camp (summer) Z02.89
  - clinical research, normal subject (control) (participant) Z00.6
  - control subject in clinical research (normal comparison) (participant) Z00.6
  - donor (potential) Z00.5

Examination *(continued)*
- medical *(continued)*
  - driving license Z02.4
  - general (adult) Z00.00
    - with abnormal findings Z00.01
  - immigration Z02.89
  - insurance purposes Z02.6
  - marriage Z02.89
  - medicolegal reasons NEC Z04.89
  - naturalization Z02.89
  - participation in sport Z02.5
  - paternity testing Z02.81
  - population survey Z00.8
  - pre-employment Z02.1
  - pre-operative *—see* Examination, pre-procedural
  - pre-procedural
    - cardiovascular Z01.810
    - respiratory Z01.811
    - specified NEC Z01.818
  - preschool children
    - for admission to school Z02.0
  - prisoners
    - for entrance into prison Z02.89
  - recruitment for armed forces Z02.3
  - specified NEC Z00.8
  - sport competition Z02.5
- medicolegal reason NEC Z04.89
  - following
    - forced sexual exploitation Z04.81
    - forced labor exploitation Z04.82
- newborn *—see* Newborn, examination
- pelvic (annual) (periodic) Z01.419
  - with abnormal findings Z01.411
- period of rapid growth in childhood Z00.2
- periodic (adult) (annual) (routine) Z00.00
  - with abnormal findings Z00.01
- physical (adult) (*see also* Examination, medical) Z00.00
  - sports Z02.5
- postpartum
  - immediately after delivery Z39.0
  - routine follow-up Z39.2
- prenatal (normal pregnancy) (*see also* Pregnancy, normal) Z34.9-
- pre-chemotherapy (antineoplastic) Z01.818
- pre-procedural (pre-operative)
  - cardiovascular Z01.810
  - laboratory Z01.812
  - respiratory Z01.811
  - specified NEC Z01.818
- prior to chemotherapy (antineoplastic) Z01.818
- psychiatric NEC Z00.8
  - follow-up not needing further care Z09
  - requested by authority Z04.6
- radiological (as part of a general medical examination) Z00.00
  - with abnormal findings Z00.01
- repeat cervical smear to confirm findings of recent normal smear following initial abnormal smear Z01.42
- skin (hypersensitivity) Z01.82
- special (*see also* Examination, by type) Z01.89
  - specified type NEC Z01.89
- specified type or reason NEC Z04.89
- teeth Z01.20
  - with abnormal findings Z01.21

Examination *(continued)*
- urine *—see* Examination, laboratory
- vision Z01.00
  - with abnormal findings Z01.01
  - following failed vision screening Z01.020
    - with abnormal findings Z01.021
  - infant or child (over 28 days old) Z00.129
    - with abnormal findings Z00.121

Exanthem, exanthema *—see also* Rash
- with enteroviral vesicular stomatitis B08.4
- Boston A88.0
- epidemic with meningitis A88.0 *[G02]*
- subitum B08.20
  - due to human herpesvirus 6 B08.21
  - due to human herpesvirus 7 B08.22
- viral, virus B09
  - specified type NEC B08.8

Excess, excessive, excessively
- alcohol level in blood R78.0
- androgen (ovarian) E28.1
- attrition, tooth, teeth K03.0
- carotene, carotin (dietary) E67.1
- cold, effects of T69.9
  - specified effect NEC T69.8
- convergence H51.12
- crying
  - in child, adolescent, or adult R45.83
  - in infant R68.11
- development, breast N62
- divergence H51.8
- drinking (alcohol) NEC (without dependence) F10.10
  - habitual (continual) (without remission) F10.20
- eating R63.2
- estrogen E28.0
- fat *—see also* Obesity
  - in heart *—see* Degeneration, myocardial
  - localized E65
- foreskin N47.8
- gas R14.0
- glucagon E16.3
- heat *—see* Heat
- intermaxillary vertical dimension of fully erupted teeth M26.37
- interocclusal distance of fully erupted teeth M26.37
- kalium E87.5
- large
  - colon K59.39
    - congenital Q43.8
  - infant P08.0
  - organ or site, congenital NEC *—see* Anomaly, by site
- long
  - organ or site, congenital NEC *—see* Anomaly, by site
- menstruation (with regular cycle) N92.0
  - with irregular cycle N92.1
- napping Z72.821
- natrium E87.0
- number of teeth K00.1
- nutrient (dietary) NEC R63.2
- potassium (K) E87.5
- salivation K11.7
- secretion *—see also* Hypersecretion
  - milk O92.6
  - sputum R09.3
  - sweat R61

Excess, excessive, excessively *(continued)*
- sexual drive F52.8
- short
  - organ or site, congenital NEC *—see* Anomaly, by site
  - umbilical cord in labor or delivery O69.3
- skin L98.7
  - and subcutaneous tissue L98.7
  - eyelid (acquired) *—see* Blepharochalasis
    - congenital Q10.3
- sodium (Na) E87.0
- spacing of fully erupted teeth M26.32
- sputum R09.3
- sweating R61
- thirst R63.1
  - due to deprivation of water T73.1
- tuberosity of jaw M26.07
- vitamin
  - A (dietary) E67.0
    - administered as drug (prolonged intake) *—see* Table of Drugs and Chemicals, vitamins, adverse effect
    - overdose or wrong substance given or taken *—see* Table of Drugs and Chemicals, vitamins, poisoning
  - D (dietary) E67.3
    - administered as drug (prolonged intake) *—see* Table of Drugs and Chemicals, vitamins, adverse effect
    - overdose or wrong substance given or taken *—see* Table of Drugs and Chemicals, vitamins, poisoning
- weight
  - gain R63.5
  - loss R63.4

Excitability, abnormal, under minor stress (personality disorder) F60.3

Excitation
- anomalous atrioventricular I45.6
- psychogenic F30.8
- reactive (from emotional stress, psychological trauma) F30.8

Excitement
- hypomanic F30.8
- manic F30.9
- mental, reactive (from emotional stress, psychological trauma) F30.8
- state, reactive (from emotional stress, psychological trauma) F30.8

Excoriation (traumatic) *—see also* Abrasion
- neurotic L98.1
- skin picking disorder F42.4

Exfoliation
- due to erythematous conditions according to extent of body surface involved L49.0
  - 10-19 percent of body surface L49.1
  - 20-29 percent of body surface L49.2
  - 30-39 percent of body surface L49.3
  - 40-49 percent of body surface L49.4

Exfoliation *(continued)*
- due to erythematous conditions according to extent of body surface involved L49.0 *(continued)*
  - 50-59 percent of body surface L49.5
  - 60-69 percent of body surface L49.6
  - 70-79 percent of body surface L49.7
  - 80-89 percent of body surface L49.8
  - 90-99 percent of body surface L49.9
  - less than 10 percent of body surface L49.0
- teeth, due to systemic causes K08.0

Exfoliative *—see* condition

Exhaustion, exhaustive (physical NEC) R53.83
- battle F43.0
- cardiac *—see* Failure, heart
- delirium F43.0
- due to
  - cold T69.8
  - excessive exertion T73.3
  - exposure T73.2
  - neurasthenia F48.8
- heart *—see* Failure, heart
- heat (*see also* Heat, exhaustion) T67.5
  - due to
    - salt depletion T67.4
    - water depletion T67.3
- maternal, complicating delivery O75.81
- mental F48.8
- myocardium, myocardial *—see* Failure, heart
- nervous F48.8
- old age R54
- psychogenic F48.8
- psychosis F43.0
- senile R54
- vital NEC Z73.0

Exhibitionism F65.2

Exocervicitis *—see* Cervicitis

Exomphalos Q79.2
- meaning hernia *—see* Hernia, umbilicus

Exophoria H50.52
- convergence, insufficiency H51.11
- divergence, excess H51.8

Exophthalmos H05.2-
- congenital Q15.8
- constant NEC H05.24-
- displacement, globe *—see* Displacement, globe
- due to thyrotoxicosis (hyperthyroidism) *—see* Hyperthyroidism, with, goiter (diffuse)
- dysthyroid *—see* Hyperthyroidism, with, goiter (diffuse)
- goiter *—see* Hyperthyroidism, with, goiter (diffuse)
- intermittent NEC H05.25-
- malignant *—see* Hyperthyroidism, with, goiter (diffuse)
- orbital
  - edema *—see* Edema, orbit
  - hemorrhage *—see* Hemorrhage, orbit
- pulsating NEC H05.26-
- thyrotoxic, thyrotropic *—see* Hyperthyroidism, with, goiter (diffuse)

Exploitation
- labor
  - confirmed
    - adult forced T74.61
    - child forced T74.62
  - suspected
    - adult forced T76.61
    - child forced T76.62
- sexual
  - confirmed
    - adult forced T74.51
    - child forced T74.52
  - suspected
    - adult forced T76.51
    - child forced T76.52

Exostosis —*see also* Disorder, bone
- cartilaginous —*see* Neoplasm, bone, benign
- congenital (multiple) Q78.6
- external ear canal H61.81-
- gonococcal A54.49
- jaw (bone) M27.8
- multiple, congenital Q78.6
- orbit H05.35-
- osteocartilaginous —*see* Neoplasm, bone, benign
- syphilitic A52.77

Exotropia —*see* Strabismus, divergent concomitant

Explanation of
- investigation finding Z71.2
- medication Z71.89

Exposure (to) (*see also* Contact, with) T75.89
- acariasis Z20.7
- AIDS virus Z20.6
- air pollution Z77.110
- algae and algae toxins Z77.121
- algae bloom Z77.121
- anthrax Z20.810
- aromatic amines Z77.020
- aromatic (hazardous) compounds NEC Z77.028
- aromatic dyes NOS Z77.028
- arsenic Z77.010
- asbestos Z77.090
- bacterial disease NEC Z20.818
- benzene Z77.021
- blue-green algae bloom Z77.121
- body fluids (potentially hazardous) Z77.21
- brown tide Z77.121
- chemicals (chiefly nonmedicinal) (hazardous) NEC Z77.098
- cholera Z20.09
- chromium compounds Z77.018
- cold, effects of T69.9
  - specified effect NEC T69.8
- communicable disease Z20.9
  - bacterial NEC Z20.818
  - specified NEC Z20.89
  - viral NEC Z20.828
  - Zika virus Z20.821
- coronavirus (disease) (novel) 2019 Z20.822
- COVID-19 Z20.822
- cyanobacteria bloom Z77.121
- disaster Z65.5
- discrimination Z60.5
- dyes Z77.098
- effects of T73.9
- environmental tobacco smoke (acute) (chronic) Z77.22
- Escherichia coli (E. coli) Z20.01
- exhaustion due to T73.2
- fiberglass —*see* Table of Drugs and Chemicals, fiberglass
- German measles Z20.4
- gonorrhea Z20.2
- hazardous metals NEC Z77.018

Exposure *(continued)*
- hazardous substances NEC Z77.29
- hazards in the physical environment NEC Z77.128
- hazards to health NEC Z77.9
- human immunodeficiency virus (HIV) Z20.6
- human T-lymphotropic virus type-1 (HTLV-1) Z20.89
- implanted
  - mesh —*see* Complications, prosthetic device or implant, mesh
  - prosthetic materials NEC —*see* Complications, prosthetic materials NEC
- infestation (parasitic) NEC Z20.7
- intestinal infectious disease NEC Z20.09
  - Escherichia coli (E. coli) Z20.01
- lead Z77.011
- meningococcus Z20.811
- mold (toxic) Z77.120
- nickel dust Z77.018
- noise Z77.122
- occupational
  - air contaminants NEC Z57.39
  - dust Z57.2
  - environmental tobacco smoke Z57.31
  - extreme temperature Z57.6
  - noise Z57.0
  - radiation Z57.1
  - risk factors Z57.9
    - specified NEC Z57.8
  - toxic agents (gases) (liquids) (solids) (vapors) in agriculture Z57.4
  - toxic agents (gases) (liquids) (solids) (vapors) in industry NEC Z57.5
  - vibration Z57.7
- parasitic disease NEC Z20.7
- pediculosis Z20.7
- persecution Z60.5
- pfiesteria piscicida Z77.121
- poliomyelitis Z20.89
- polycyclic aromatic hydrocarbons Z77.028
- pollution
  - air Z77.110
  - environmental NEC Z77.118
  - soil Z77.112
  - water Z77.111
- prenatal (drugs) (toxic chemicals) —*see* Newborn, affected by, noxious substances transmitted via placenta or breast milk
- rabies Z20.3
- radiation, naturally occurring NEC Z77.123
- radon Z77.123
- red tide (Florida) Z77.121
- rubella Z20.4
- SARS-CoV-2 Z20.822
- second hand tobacco smoke (acute) (chronic) Z77.22
  - in the perinatal period P96.81
- sexually-transmitted disease Z20.2
- smallpox (laboratory) Z20.89
- syphilis Z20.2
- terrorism Z65.4
- torture Z65.4
- tuberculosis Z20.1
- uranium Z77.012
- varicella Z20.820
- venereal disease Z20.2
- viral disease NEC Z20.828
- war Z65.5
- water pollution Z77.111
- Zika virus Z20.821

Exsanguination —*see* Hemorrhage

Exstrophy
- abdominal contents Q45.8
- bladder Q64.10
  - cloacal Q64.12
  - specified type NEC Q64.19
  - supravesical fissure Q64.11

Extensive —*see* condition

Extra (*see also* Accessory marker chromosomes) (normal individual) Q92.61
- in abnormal individual Q92.62
- rib Q76.6
  - cervical Q76.5

Extrasystoles (supraventricular) I49.49
- atrial I49.1
- auricular I49.1
- junctional I49.2
- ventricular I49.3

Extrauterine gestation or pregnancy —*see* Pregnancy, by site

Extravasation
- blood R58
- chyle into mesentery I89.8
- pelvicalyceal N13.8
- pyelosinus N13.8
- urine (from ureter) R39.0
- vesicant agent
  - antineoplastic chemotherapy T80.810
  - other agent NEC T80.818

Extremity —*see* condition, limb

Extrophy —*see* Exstrophy

Extroversion
- bladder Q64.19
- uterus N81.4
  - complicating delivery O71.2
  - postpartal (old) N81.4

Extruded tooth (teeth) M26.34

Extrusion
- breast implant (prosthetic) T85.42
- eye implant (globe) (ball) T85.328
- intervertebral disc —*see* Displacement, intervertebral disc
- ocular lens implant (prosthetic) —*see* Complications, intraocular lens
- vitreous —*see* Prolapse, vitreous

Exudate
- pleural —*see* Effusion, pleura
- retina H35.89
- wound fluids L24.A9

Exudative —*see* condition

Eye, eyeball, eyelid —*see* condition

Eyestrain —*see* Disturbance, vision, subjective

Eyeworm disease of Africa B74.3

F

Faber's syndrome (achlorhydric anemia) D50.9

Fabry (-Anderson) **disease** E75.21

Facet syndrome M47.89-

Faciocephalalgia, autonomic (*see also* Neuropathy, peripheral, autonomic) G90.09

Factor(s)
- psychic, associated with diseases classified elsewhere F54

Factor(s) *(continued)*
- psychological
  - affecting physical conditions F54
  - or behavioral
    - affecting general medical condition F54
    - associated with disorders or diseases classified elsewhere F54

Fahr disease (of brain) G23.8

Fahr Volhard disease (of kidney) I12.-

Failure, failed
- abortion —*see* Abortion, attempted
- aortic (valve) I35.8
  - rheumatic I06.8
- attempted abortion —*see* Abortion, attempted
- biventricular I50.82
  - due to left heart failure I50.814
- bone marrow —*see* Anemia, aplastic
- cardiac —*see* Failure, heart
- cardiorenal (chronic) (*see also* Failure, renal, and Failure, heart) I50.9
  - hypertensive I13.2
- cardiorespiratory (*see also* Failure, heart) R09.2
- cardiovascular (chronic) —*see* Failure, heart
- cerebrovascular I67.9
- cervical dilatation in labor O62.0
- circulation, circulatory (peripheral) R57.9
  - newborn P29.89
- compensation —*see* Disease, heart
- compliance with medical treatment or regimen —*see* Noncompliance
- congestive —*see* Failure, heart, congestive
- dental implant (endosseous) M27.69
  - due to
    - failure of dental prosthesis M27.63
    - lack of attached gingiva M27.62
    - occlusal trauma (poor prosthetic design) M27.62
    - parafunctional habits M27.62
    - periodontal infection (peri-implantitis) M27.62
    - poor oral hygiene M27.62
  - osseointegration M27.61
    - due to
      - complications of systemic disease M27.61
      - poor bone quality M27.61
    - iatrogenic M27.61
  - post-osseointegration
    - biological M27.62
    - due to complications of systemic disease M27.62
    - iatrogenic M27.62
    - mechanical M27.63
  - pre-integration M27.61
  - pre-osseointegration M27.61
  - specified NEC M27.69
- descent of head (at term) of pregnancy (mother) O32.4
- endosseous dental implant —*see* Failure, dental implant
- engagement of head (term of pregnancy) (mother) O32.4
- erection (penile) (*see also* Dysfunction, sexual, male, erectile) N52.9
  - nonorganic F52.21

Failure, failed *(continued)*
- examination(s), anxiety concerning Z55.2
- expansion terminal respiratory units (newborn) (primary) P28.0
- forceps NOS (with subsequent cesarean delivery) O66.5
- gain weight (child over 28 days old) R62.51
  - adult R62.7
  - newborn P92.6
- genital response (male) F52.21
  - female F52.22
- heart (acute) (senile) (sudden) I50.9
  - with
    - acute pulmonary edema *—see* Failure, ventricular, left
    - decompensation I50.9
      - with
        - normal ejection fraction I50.33
        - preserved ejection fraction I50.33
        - reduced ejection fraction I50.23
          - with diastolic dysfunction I50.43
      - combined systolic and diastolic I50.43
      - diastolic I50.33
      - right I50.813
      - systolic I50.23
    - dilatation *—see* Disease, heart
    - hypertension *—see* Hypertension, heart
    - normal ejection fraction *—see* Failure, heart diastolic
    - preserved ejection fraction *—see* Failure, heart diastolic
    - reduced ejection fraction *—see* Failure, heart systolic
  - arteriosclerotic I70.90
  - biventricular I50.82
    - due to left heart failure I50.814
  - combined left-right sided I50.82
    - due to left heart failure I50.814
  - compensated (*see also* Failure, heart, by type as diastolic or systolic, chronic) I50.9
  - complicating
    - anesthesia (general) (local) or other sedation
      - in labor and delivery O74.2
      - in pregnancy O29.12-
      - postpartum, puerperal O89.1
    - delivery (cesarean) (instrumental) O75.4
  - congestive I50.9
    - with rheumatic fever (conditions in I00)
      - active I01.8
      - inactive or quiescent (with chorea) I09.81
    - newborn P29.0
    - rheumatic (chronic) (inactive) (with chorea) I09.81
      - active or acute I01.8
        - with chorea I02.0
  - decompensated (*see also* Failure, heart, by type as diastolic or systolic, acute and chronic) I50.9
  - degenerative *—see* Degeneration, myocardial

Failure, failed *(continued)*
- heart *(continued)*
  - diastolic (congestive) (left ventricular) I50.30
    - acute (congestive) I50.31
      - and (on) chronic (congestive) I50.33
    - chronic (congestive) I50.32
      - and (on) acute (congestive) I50.33
    - combined with systolic (congestive) I50.40
      - acute (congestive) I50.41
        - and (on) chronic (congestive) I50.43
      - chronic (congestive) I50.42
        - and (on) acute (congestive) I50.43
  - due to presence of cardiac prosthesis I97.13-
  - end stage (*see also* Failure, heart, by type as diastolic or systolic, chronic) I50.84
  - following cardiac surgery I97.13-
  - high output NOS I50.83
  - hypertensive *—see* Hypertension, heart
  - left (ventricular) *—see also* Failure, ventricular, left
    - combined diastolic and systolic *—see* Failure, heart, diastolic, combined with systolic
    - diastolic *—see* Failure, heart, diastolic
    - systolic *—see* Failure, heart, systolic
  - low output (syndrome) NOS I50.9
  - newborn P29.0
  - organic *—see* Disease, heart
  - peripartum O90.3
  - postprocedural I97.13-
  - rheumatic (chronic) (inactive) I09.9
  - right (isolated) I50.810
    - acute I50.811
      - and (on) chronic I50.813
    - chronic I50.812
      - and acute I50.813
    - secondary to left heart failure I50.814
  - specified NEC I50.89

Note: heart failure stages A, B, C and D are based on the American College of Cardiology and American Heart Association stages of heart failure, which complement and should not be confused with the New York Heart Association Classification of Heart Failure, into Class I, Class II, Class III and Class IV

- - stage A Z91.89
  - stage B (*see also* Failure, heart, by type as diastolic or systolic) I50.9
  - stage C (*see also* Failure, heart, by type as diastolic or systolic) I50.9
  - stage D (*see also* Failure, heart, by type as diastolic or systolic, chronic) I50.84
  - systolic (congestive) (left ventricular) I50.20
    - acute (congestive) I50.21
      - and (on) chronic (congestive) I50.23
    - chronic (congestive) I50.22
      - and (on) acute (congestive) I50.23

Failure, failed *(continued)*
- hepatic *(continued)*
  - systolic *(continued)*
    - combined with diastolic (congestive) I50.40
      - acute (congestive) I50.41
        - and (on) chronic (congestive) I50.43
      - chronic (congestive) I50.42
        - and (on) acute (congestive) I50.43
  - thyrotoxic (*see also* Thyrotoxicosis) E05.90 *[I43]*
    - with
      - high output (*see also* Thyrotoxicosis) I50.83
      - thyroid storm E05.91 *[I43]*
        - high output (*see also* Thyrotoxicosis) I50.83
  - valvular *—see* Endocarditis
- hepatic K72.90
  - with coma K72.91
  - acute or subacute K72.00
    - with coma K72.01
    - due to drugs K71.10
      - with coma K71.11
  - alcoholic (acute) (chronic) (subacute) K70.40
    - with coma K70.41
  - chronic K72.10
    - with coma K72.11
    - due to drugs (acute) (subacute) (chronic) K71.10
      - with coma K71.11
  - due to drugs (acute) (subacute) (chronic) K71.10
    - with coma K71.11
  - postprocedural K91.82
- hepatorenal K76.7
- induction (of labor) O61.9
  - abortion *—see* Abortion, attempted
  - by
    - oxytocic drugs O61.0
    - prostaglandins O61.0
  - instrumental O61.1
  - mechanical O61.1
  - medical O61.0
  - specified NEC O61.8
  - surgical O61.1
- intubation during anesthesia T88.4
  - in pregnancy O29.6-
  - labor and delivery O74.7
  - postpartum, puerperal O89.6
- involution, thymus (gland) E32.0
- kidney (*see also* Disease, kidney, chronic) N19
  - acute (*see also* Failure, renal, acute) N17.9-
  - diabetic *—see* E08-E13 with .22
- lactation (complete) O92.3
  - partial O92.4
- Leydig's cell, adult E29.1
- liver *—see* Failure, hepatic
- menstruation at puberty N91.0
- mitral I05.8
- myocardial, myocardium (*see also* Failure, heart) I50.9
  - chronic (*see also* Failure, heart, congestive) I50.9
  - congestive (*see also* Failure, heart, congestive) I50.9
- newborn screening *— see* Abnormal, neonatal screening
  - neonatal congenital heart disease P09.5
- orgasm (female) (psychogenic) F52.31
  - male F52.32

Failure, failed *(continued)*
- ovarian (primary) E28.39
  - iatrogenic E89.40
    - asymptomatic E89.40
    - symptomatic E89.41
  - postprocedural (postablative) (postirradiation) (postsurgical) E89.40
    - asymptomatic E89.40
    - symptomatic E89.41
- ovulation causing infertility N97.0
- polyglandular, autoimmune E31.0
- prosthetic joint implant *—see* Complications, joint prosthesis, mechanical, breakdown, by site
- renal N19
  - with
    - tubular necrosis (acute) N17.0
  - acute N17.9
    - with
      - cortical necrosis N17.1
      - medullary necrosis N17.2
      - tubular necrosis N17.0
    - specified NEC N17.8
  - chronic N18.9
    - hypertensive *—see* Hypertension, kidney
  - congenital P96.0
  - end stage (chronic) N18.6
    - due to hypertension I12.0
  - following
    - abortion *—see* Abortion by type complicated by specified condition NEC
    - crushing T79.5
    - ectopic or molar pregnancy O08.4
    - labor and delivery (acute) O90.4
  - hypertensive *—see* Hypertension, kidney
  - postprocedural N99.0
- respiration, respiratory J96.90
  - with
    - hypercarbia J96.92
    - hypercapnia J96.92
    - hypoxia J96.91
  - acute J96.00
    - with
      - hypercarbia J96.02
      - hypercapnia J96.02
      - hypoxia J96.01
  - center G93.89
  - acute and (on) chronic J96.20
    - with
      - hypercarbia J96.22
      - hypercapnia J96.22
      - hypoxia J96.21
  - chronic J96.10
    - with
      - hypercarbia J96.12
      - hypercapnia J96.12
      - hypoxia J96.11
  - newborn P28.5
  - postprocedural (acute) J95.821
    - acute and chronic J95.822
- rotation
  - cecum Q43.3
  - colon Q43.3
  - intestine Q43.3
  - kidney Q63.2
- sedation (conscious) (moderate) during procedure T88.52
  - history of Z92.83

Failure, failed *(continued)*
- segmentation —*see also* Fusion
  - fingers —*see* Syndactylism, complex, fingers
  - vertebra Q76.49
    - with scoliosis Q76.3
- seminiferous tubule, adult E29.1
- senile (general) R54
- sexual arousal (male) F52.21
  - female F52.22
- testicular endocrine function E29.1
- to thrive (child over 28 days old) R62.51
  - adult R62.7
  - newborn P92.6
- transplant T86.92
  - bone T86.831
    - marrow T86.02
  - cornea T86.841-
  - heart T86.22
    - with lung(s) T86.32
  - intestine T86.851
  - kidney T86.12
  - liver T86.42
  - lung(s) T86.811
    - with heart T86.32
  - pancreas T86.891
  - skin (allograft) (autograft) T86.821
  - specified organ or tissue NEC T86.891
  - stem cell (peripheral blood) (umbilical cord) T86.5
- trial of labor (with subsequent cesarean delivery) O66.40
  - following previous cesarean delivery O66.41
- tubal ligation N99.89
- urinary —*see* Disease, kidney, chronic
- vacuum extraction NOS (with subsequent cesarean delivery) O66.5
- vasectomy N99.89
- ventouse NOS (with subsequent cesarean delivery) O66.5
- ventricular (*see also* Failure, heart) I50.9
  - left (*see also* Failure, heart) I50.1
    - with rheumatic fever (conditions in I00)
      - active I01.8
        - with chorea I02.0
      - inactive or quiescent (with chorea) I09.81
    - rheumatic (chronic) (inactive) (with chorea) I09.81
      - active or acute I01.8
        - with chorea I02.0
  - right —*see* Failure, heart, right
- vital centers, newborn P91.88

Fainting (fit) R55

Fallen arches —*see* Deformity, limb, flat foot

Falling, falls (repeated) R29.6
- any organ or part —*see* Prolapse

Fallopian
- insufflation Z31.41
- tube —*see* condition

Fallot's
- pentalogy Q21.8
- tetrad or tetralogy Q21.3
- triad or trilogy Q22.3

False —*see also* condition
- croup J38.5
- joint —*see* Nonunion, fracture

False *(continued)*
- labor (pains) O47.9
  - at or after 37 completed weeks of gestation O47.1
  - before 37 completed weeks of gestation O47.0-
- passage, urethra (prostatic) N36.5
- pregnancy F45.8

Family, familial —*see also* condition
- disruption Z63.8
  - involving divorce or separation Z63.5
- Li-Fraumeni (syndrome) Z15.01
- planning advice Z30.09
- problem Z63.9
  - specified NEC Z63.8
- retinoblastoma C69.2-

Famine (effects of) T73.0
- edema —*see* Malnutrition, severe

Fanconi (-de Toni) (-Debré) **syndrome** E72.09
- with cystinosis E72.04

Fanconi's anemia (congenital pancytopenia) D61.09

Farber's disease or syndrome E75.29

Farcy A24.0

Farmer's
- lung J67.0
- skin L57.8

Farsightedness —*see* Hypermetropia

Fascia —*see* condition

Fasciculation R25.3

Fasciitis M72.9
- diffuse (eosinophilic) M35.4
- infective M72.8
  - necrotizing M72.6
- necrotizing M72.6
- nodular M72.4
- perirenal (with ureteral obstruction) N13.5
  - with infection N13.6
- plantar M72.2
- specified NEC M72.8
- traumatic (old) M72.8
  - current - code by site under Sprain

Fascioliasis B66.3

Fasciolopsis, fasciolopsiasis (intestinal) B66.5

Fascioscapulohumeral myopathy G71.02

Fast pulse R00.0

Fat
- embolism —*see* Embolism, fat
- excessive —*see also* Obesity
  - in heart —*see* Degeneration, myocardial
- in stool R19.5
- localized (pad) E65
  - heart —*see* Degeneration, myocardial
  - knee M79.4
  - retropatellar M79.4
- necrosis
  - breast N64.1
  - mesentery K65.4
  - omentum K65.4
- pad E65
  - knee M79.4

Fatigue R53.83
- auditory deafness —*see* Deafness
- chronic R53.82
- combat F43.0

Fatigue *(continued)*
- general R53.83
  - psychogenic F48.8
- heat (transient) T67.6
- muscle M62.89
- myocardium —*see* Failure, heart
- neoplasm-related R53.0
- nervous, neurosis F48.8
- operational F48.8
- psychogenic (general) F48.8
- senile R54
- voice R49.8

Fatness —*see* Obesity

Fatty —*see also* condition
- apron E65
- degeneration —*see* Degeneration, fatty
- heart (enlarged) —*see* Degeneration, myocardial
- liver NEC K76.0
  - alcoholic K70.0
  - nonalcoholic K76.0
- necrosis —*see* Degeneration, fatty

Fauces —*see* condition

Fauchard's disease (periodontitis) —*see* Periodontitis

Faucitis J02.9

Favism (anemia) D55.0

Favus —*see* Dermatophytosis

Fazio-Londe disease or syndrome G12.1

Fear complex or reaction F40.9

Fear of —*see* Phobia

Feared complaint unfounded Z71.1

Febris, febrile —*see also* Fever
- flava (*see also* Fever, yellow) A95.9
- melitensis A23.0
- pestis —*see* Plague
- recurrens —*see* Fever, relapsing
- rubra A38.9

Fecal
- incontinence R15.9
- smearing R15.1
- soiling R15.1
- urgency R15.2

Fecalith (impaction) K56.41
- appendix K38.1
- congenital P76.8

Fede's disease K14.0

Feeble rapid pulse due to shock following injury T79.4

Feeble-minded F70

Feeding
- difficulties R63.30
- problem (elderly) (infant) R63.39
  - newborn P92.9
    - specified NEC P92.8
  - nonorganic (adult) —*see* Disorder, eating

Feeling (of)
- foreign body in throat R09.89

Feer's disease —*see* Poisoning, mercury

Feet —*see* condition

Feigned illness Z76.5

Feil-Klippel syndrome (brevicollis) Q76.1

Feinmesser's (hidrotic) **ectodermal dysplasia** Q82.4

Felinophobia F40.218

Felon —*see also* Cellulitis, digit
- with lymphangitis —*see* Lymphangitis, acute, digit

Felty's syndrome M05.00
- ankle M05.07-
- elbow M05.02-
- foot joint M05.07-
- hand joint M05.04-
- hip M05.05-
- knee M05.06-
- multiple site M05.09
- shoulder M05.01-
- vertebra —*see* Spondylitis, ankylosing
- wrist M05.03-

Female genital cutting status —*see* Female genital mutilation status (FGM)

Female genital mutilation status (FGM) N90.810
- specified NEC N90.818
- type I (clitorectomy status) N90.811
- type II (clitorectomy with excision of labia minora status) N90.812
- type III (infibulation status) N90.813
- type IV N90.818

Femur, femoral —*see* condition

Fenestration, fenestrated —*see also* Imperfect, closure
- aortico-pulmonary Q21.4
- cusps, heart valve NEC Q24.8
  - pulmonary Q22.3
- pulmonic cusps Q22.3

Fernell's disease (aortic aneurysm) I71.9

Fertile eunuch syndrome E23.0

Fetid
- breath R19.6
- sweat L75.0

Fetishism F65.0
- transvestic F65.1

Fetus, fetal —*see also* condition
- alcohol syndrome (dysmorphic) Q86.0
- compressus O31.0-
- hydantoin syndrome Q86.1
- lung tissue P28.0
- papyraceous O31.0-

Fever (inanition) (of unknown origin) (persistent) (with chills) (with rigor) R50.9
- abortus A23.1
- Aden (dengue) A90
- African tick bite A77.8
- African tick-borne A68.1
- American
  - mountain (tick) A93.2
  - spotted A77.0
- aphthous B08.8
- arbovirus, arboviral A94
  - hemorrhagic A94
  - specified NEC A93.8
- Argentinian hemorrhagic A96.0
- Assam B55.0
- Australian Q A78
- Bangkok hemorrhagic A91
- Barmah forest A92.8
- Bartonella A44.0
- bilious, hemoglobinuric B50.8
- blackwater B50.8
- blister B00.1
- Bolivian hemorrhagic A96.1
- Bonvale dam T73.3
- boutonneuse A77.1
- brain —*see* Encephalitis

Fever *(continued)*
- Brazilian purpuric A48.4
- breakbone A90
- Bullis A77.0
- Bunyamwera A92.8
- Burdwan B55.0
- Bwamba A92.8
- Cameroon *—see* Malaria
- Canton A75.9
- catarrhal (acute) J00
  - chronic J31.0
- cat-scratch A28.1
- Central Asian hemorrhagic A98.0
- cerebral *—see* Encephalitis
- cerebrospinal meningococcal A39.0
- Chagres B50.9
- Chandipura A92.8
- Changuinola A93.1
- Charcot's (biliary) (hepatic) (intermittent) *—see* Calculus, bile duct
- Chikungunya (viral) (hemorrhagic) A92.0
- Chitral A93.1
- Colombo *—see* Fever, paratyphoid
- Colorado tick (virus) A93.2
- congestive (remittent) *—see* Malaria
- Congo virus A98.0
- continued malarial B50.9
- Corsican *—see* Malaria
- Crimean-Congo hemorrhagic A98.0
- Cyprus *—see* Brucellosis
- dandy A90
- deer fly *—see* Tularemia
- dengue (virus) A90
  - hemorrhagic A91
  - sandfly A93.1
- desert B38.0
- drug induced R50.2
- due to
  - conditions classified elsewhere R50.81
  - heat T67.01
- enteric A01.00
- enteroviral exanthematous (Boston exanthem) A88.0
- ephemeral (of unknown origin) R50.9
- epidemic hemorrhagic A98.5
- erysipelatous *—see* Erysipelas
- estivo-autumnal (malarial) B50.9
- famine A75.0
- five day A79.0
- following delivery O86.4
- Fort Bragg A27.89
- gastroenteric A01.00
- gastromalarial *—see* Malaria
- Gibraltar *—see* Brucellosis
- glandular *—see* Mononucleosis, infectious
- Guama (viral) A92.8
- Haverhill A25.1
- hay (allergic) J30.1
  - with asthma (bronchial) J45.909
    - with
      - exacerbation (acute) J45.901
      - status asthmaticus J45.902
  - due to
    - allergen other than pollen J30.89
    - pollen, any plant or tree J30.1
- heat (effects) T67.01
- hematuric, bilious B50.8
- hemoglobinuric (malarial) (bilious) B50.8

Fever *(continued)*
- hemorrhagic (arthropod-borne)
  - NOS A94
  - with renal syndrome A98.5
  - arenaviral A96.9
    - specified NEC A96.8
  - Argentinian A96.0
  - Bangkok A91
  - Bolivian A96.1
  - Central Asian A98.0
  - Chikungunya A92.0
  - Crimean-Congo A98.0
  - dengue (virus) A91
  - epidemic A98.5
  - Junin (virus) A96.0
  - Korean A98.5
  - Kyasanur forest A98.2
  - Machupo (virus) A96.1
  - mite-borne A93.8
  - mosquito-borne A92.8
  - Omsk A98.1
  - Philippine A91
  - Russian A98.5
  - Singapore A91
  - Southeast Asia A91
  - Thailand A91
  - tick-borne NEC A93.8
  - viral A99
    - specified NEC A98.8
- hepatic *—see* Cholecystitis
- herpetic *—see* Herpes
- icterohemorrhagic A27.0
- Indiana A93.8
- infective B99.9
  - specified NEC B99.8
- intermittent (bilious) *—see also* Malaria
  - of unknown origin R50.9
  - pernicious B50.9
- iodide R50.2
- Japanese river A75.3
- jungle *—see also* Malaria
  - yellow A95.0
- Junin (virus) hemorrhagic A96.0
- Katayama B65.2
- kedani A75.3
- Kenya (tick) A77.1
- Kew Garden A79.1
- Korean hemorrhagic A98.5
- Lassa A96.2
- Lone Star A77.0
- Machupo (virus) hemorrhagic A96.1
- malaria, malarial *—see* Malaria
- Malta A23.9
- Marseilles A77.1
- marsh *—see* Malaria
- Mayaro (viral) A92.8
- Mediterranean (*see also* Brucellosis) A23.9
  - familial M04.1
  - tick A77.1
- meningeal *—see* Meningitis
- Meuse A79.0
- Mexican A75.2
- mianeh A68.1
- miasmatic *—see* Malaria
- mosquito-borne (viral) A92.9
  - hemorrhagic A92.8
- mountain (*see also* Brucellosis)
  - meaning Rocky Mountain spotted fever A77.0
  - tick (American) (Colorado) (viral) A93.2
- Mucambo (viral) A92.8
- mud A27.9
- Neapolitan *—see* Brucellosis
- neutropenic D70.9
- newborn P81.9
  - environmental P81.0
- Nine-Mile A78

Fever *(continued)*
- non-exanthematous tick A93.2
- North Asian tick-borne A77.2
- Omsk hemorrhagic A98.1
- O'nyong-nyong (viral) A92.1
- Oropouche (viral) A93.0
- Oroya A44.0
- pacific coast tick A77.8
- paludal *—see* Malaria
- Panama (malarial) B50.9
- Pappataci A93.1
- paratyphoid A01.4
  - A A01.1
  - B A01.2
  - C A01.3
- parrot A70
- periodic (Mediterranean) M04.1
- persistent (of unknown origin) R50.9
- petechial A39.0
- pharyngoconjunctival B30.2
- Philippine hemorrhagic A91
- phlebotomus A93.1
- Piry (virus) A93.8
- Pixuna (viral) A92.8
- Plasmodium ovale B53.0
- polioviral (nonparalytic) A80.4
- Pontiac A48.2
- postimmunization R50.83
- postoperative R50.82
  - due to infection T81.40
- posttransfusion R50.84
- postvaccination R50.83
- presenting with conditions classified elsewhere R50.81
- pretibial A27.89
- puerperal O86.4
- Q A78
- quadrilateral A78
- quartan (malaria) B52.9
- Queensland (coastal) (tick) A77.3
- quintan A79.0
- rabbit *—see* Tularemia
- rat-bite A25.9
  - due to
    - Spirillum A25.0
    - Streptobacillus moniliformis A25.1
- recurrent *—see* Fever, relapsing
- relapsing (Borrelia) A68.9
  - Carter's (Asiatic) A68.1
  - Dutton's (West African) A68.1
  - Koch's A68.9
  - louse-borne A68.0
  - Novy's
    - louse-borne A68.0
    - tick-borne A68.1
  - Obermeyer's (European) A68.0
  - tick-borne A68.1
- remittent (bilious) (congestive) (gastric) *—see* Malaria
- rheumatic (active) (acute) (chronic) (subacute) I00
  - with central nervous system involvement I02.9
  - active with heart involvement *—see* category I01
  - inactive or quiescent with
    - cardiac hypertrophy I09.89
    - carditis I09.9
    - endocarditis I09.1
      - aortic (valve) I06.9
        - with mitral (valve) disease I08.0
      - mitral (valve) I05.9
        - with aortic (valve) disease I08.0
      - pulmonary (valve) I09.89
      - tricuspid (valve) I07.8
    - heart disease NEC I09.89

Fever *(continued)*
- rheumatic *(continued)*
  - inactive or quiescent with *(continued)*
    - heart failure (congestive) (conditions in category I50.) I09.81
    - left ventricular failure (conditions in I50.1-I50.4-) I09.81
    - myocarditis, myocardial degeneration (conditions in I51.4) I09.0
    - pancarditis I09.9
    - pericarditis I09.2
- Rift Valley (viral) A92.4
- Rocky Mountain spotted A77.0
- rose J30.1
- Ross River B33.1
- Russian hemorrhagic A98.5
- San Joaquin (Valley) B38.0
- sandfly A93.1
- Sao Paulo A77.0
- scarlet A38.9
- seven day (leptospirosis) (autumnal) (Japanese) A27.89
  - dengue A90
- shin-bone A79.0
- Singapore hemorrhagic A91
- solar A90
- Songo A98.5
- sore B00.1
- South African tick-bite A68.1
- Southeast Asia hemorrhagic A91
- spinal *—see* Meningitis
- spirillary A25.0
- splenic *—see* Anthrax
- spotted A77.9
  - American A77.0
  - Brazilian A77.0
  - cerebrospinal meningitis A39.0
  - Colombian A77.0
  - due to Rickettsia
    - africae (African tick bite fever) A77.8
    - australis A77.3
    - conorii A77.1
    - parkeri A77.8
    - rickettsii A77.0
    - sibirica A77.2
    - specified type NEC A77.8
  - Ehrlichiosis A77.40
    - due to
      - E. chafeensis A77.41
      - specified organism NEC A77.49
  - Rocky Mountain A77.0
- steroid R50.2
- streptobacillary A25.1
- subtertian B50.9
- Sumatran mite A75.3
- sun A90
- swamp A27.9
- swine A02.8
- sylvatic, yellow A95.0
- Tahyna B33.8
- tertian *—see* Malaria, tertian
- Thailand hemorrhagic A91
- thermic T67.01
- three-day A93.1
- tick
  - American mountain A93.2
  - Colorado A93.2
  - Kemerovo A93.8
  - Mediterranean A77.1
  - mountain A93.2
  - nonexanthematous A93.2
  - Quaranfil A93.8
- tick-bite NEC A93.8
- tick-borne (hemorrhagic) NEC A93.8
- trench A79.0
- tsutsugamushi A75.3

Findings, abnormal, inconclusive, without diagnosis *(continued)*
- sodium (deficiency) E87.1
  - excess E87.0
- specified body fluid NEC R88.8
- stress test R94.39
- thyroid (function) (metabolic rate) (scan) (uptake) R94.6
- transaminase (level) R74.01
- triglycerides E78.9
  - high E78.1
    - with high cholesterol E78.2
- tuberculin skin test (without active tuberculosis) R76.11
- urine R82.90
  - acetone R82.4
  - bacteria R82.71
  - bile R82.2
  - casts or cells R82.998
  - chyle R82.0
  - culture positive R82.79
  - glucose R81
  - hemoglobin R82.3
  - ketone R82.4
  - sugar R81
- vanillylmandelic acid (VMA), elevated R82.5
- vectorcardiogram (VCG) R94.39
- ventriculogram R93.0
- white blood cell (count) (differential) (morphology) D72.9
- xerography R92.8

Finger —*see* condition

Fire, Saint Anthony's —*see* Erysipelas

Fire-setting
- pathological (compulsive) F63.1

Fish hook stomach K31.89

Fishmeal-worker's lung J67.8

Fissure, fissured
- anus, anal K60.2
  - acute K60.0
  - chronic K60.1
  - congenital Q43.8
- ear, lobule, congenital Q17.8
- epiglottis (congenital) Q31.8
- larynx J38.7
  - congenital Q31.8
- lip K13.0
  - congenital —*see* Cleft, lip
- nipple N64.0
  - associated with
    - lactation O92.13
    - pregnancy O92.11-
    - puerperium O92.12
- nose Q30.2
- palate (congenital) —*see* Cleft, palate
- skin R23.4
- spine (congenital) —*see also* Spina bifida
  - with hydrocephalus —*see* Spina bifida, by site, with hydrocephalus
- tongue (acquired) K14.5
  - congenital Q38.3

Fistula (cutaneous) L98.8
- abdomen (wall) K63.2
  - bladder N32.2
  - intestine NEC K63.2
  - ureter N28.89
  - uterus N82.5
- abdominorectal K63.2
- abdominosigmoidal K63.2
- abdominothoracic J86.0
- abdominouterine N82.5
  - congenital Q51.7
- abdominovesical N32.2

Fistula *(continued)*
- accessory sinuses —*see* Sinusitis
- actinomycotic —*see* Actinomycosis
- alveolar antrum —*see* Sinusitis, maxillary
- alveolar process K04.6
- anorectal K60.5
- antrobuccal —*see* Sinusitis, maxillary
- antrum —*see* Sinusitis, maxillary
- anus, anal (recurrent) (infectional) K60.3
  - congenital Q43.6
    - with absence, atresia and stenosis Q42.2
  - tuberculous A18.32
- aorta-duodenal I77.2
- appendix, appendicular K38.3
- arteriovenous (acquired) (nonruptured) I77.0
  - brain I67.1
    - congenital Q28.2
      - ruptured —*see* Fistula, arteriovenous, brain, ruptured
    - ruptured I60.8
      - intracerebral I61.8
      - intraparenchymal I61.8
      - Intraventricular I61.5
      - subarachnoid I60.8
  - cerebral —*see* Fistula, arteriovenous, brain
  - congenital (peripheral) —*see also* Malformation, arteriovenous
    - brain Q28.2
      - ruptured —*see* Fistula, arteriovenous, brain, ruptured
    - coronary Q24.5
    - pulmonary Q25.72
  - coronary I25.41
    - congenital Q24.5
  - pulmonary I28.0
    - congenital Q25.72
  - surgically created (for dialysis) Z99.2
    - complication —*see* Complication, arteriovenous, fistula, surgically created
  - traumatic —*see* Injury, blood vessel
- artery I77.2
- aural (mastoid) —*see* Mastoiditis, chronic
- auricle —*see also* Disorder, pinna, specified type NEC
  - congenital Q18.1
- Bartholin's gland N82.8
- bile duct (common) (hepatic) K83.3
  - with calculus, stones (*see also* Calculus, bile duct) K83.3
- biliary (tract) —*see* Fistula, bile duct
- bladder (sphincter) NEC (*see also* Fistula, vesico-) N32.2
  - into seminal vesicle N32.2
- bone —*see also* Disorder, bone, specified type NEC
  - with osteomyelitis, chronic —*see* Osteomyelitis, chronic, with draining sinus
- brain G93.89
  - arteriovenous (acquired) (*see also* Fistula, arteriovenous, brain) I67.1
    - congenital Q28.2
- branchial (cleft) Q18.0
- branchiogenous Q18.0

Fistula *(continued)*
- breast N61.0
  - puerperal, postpartum or gestational, due to mastitis (purulent) —*see* Mastitis, obstetric, purulent
- bronchial J86.0
- bronchocutaneous, bronchomediastinal, bronchopleural, bronchopleuromediastinal (infective) J86.0
  - tuberculous NEC A15.5
- bronchoesophageal J86.0
  - congenital Q39.2
    - with atresia of esophagus Q39.1
- bronchovisceral J86.0
- buccal cavity (infective) K12.2
- cecosigmoidal K63.2
- cecum K63.2
- cerebrospinal (fluid) G96.08
- cervical, lateral Q18.1
- cervicoaural Q18.1
- cervicosigmoidal N82.4
- cervicovesical N82.1
- cervix N82.8
- chest (wall) J86.0
- cholecystenteric —*see* Fistula, gallbladder
- cholecystocolic —*see* Fistula, gallbladder
- cholecystocolonic —*see* Fistula, gallbladder
- cholecystoduodenal —*see* Fistula, gallbladder
- cholecystogastric —*see* Fistula, gallbladder
- cholecystointestinal —*see* Fistula, gallbladder
- choledochoduodenal —*see* Fistula, bile duct
- cholocolic K82.3
- coccyx —*see* Sinus, pilonidal
- colon K63.2
- colostomy K94.09
- colovesical N32.1
- common duct —*see* Fistula, bile duct
- congenital, site not listed —*see* Anomaly, by site
- coronary, arteriovenous I25.41
  - congenital Q24.5
- costal region J86.0
- cul-de-sac, Douglas' N82.8
- cystic duct —*see also* Fistula, gallbladder
  - congenital Q44.5
- dental K04.6
- diaphragm J86.0
- duodenum K31.6
- ear (external) (canal) —*see* Disorder, ear, external, specified type NEC
- enterocolic K63.2
- enterocutaneous K63.2
- enterouterine N82.4
  - congenital Q51.7
- enterovaginal N82.4
  - congenital Q52.2
  - large intestine N82.3
  - small intestine N82.2
- enterovesical N32.1
- epididymis N50.89
  - tuberculous A18.15
- esophagobronchial J86.0
  - congenital Q39.2
    - with atresia of esophagus Q39.1
- esophagocutaneous K22.89
- esophagopleural-cutaneous J86.0

Fistula *(continued)*
- esophagotracheal J86.0
  - congenital Q39.2
    - with atresia of esophagus Q39.1
- esophagus K22.89
  - congenital Q39.2
    - with atresia of esophagus Q39.1
- ethmoid —*see* Sinusitis, ethmoidal
- eyeball (cornea) (sclera) —*see* Disorder, globe, hypotony
- eyelid H01.8
- fallopian tube, external N82.5
- fecal K63.2
  - congenital Q43.6
- from periapical abscess K04.6
- frontal sinus —*see* Sinusitis, frontal
- gallbladder K82.3
  - with calculus, cholelithiasis, stones —*see* Calculus, gallbladder
- gastric K31.6
- gastrocolic K31.6
  - congenital Q40.2
  - tuberculous A18.32
- gastroenterocolic K31.6
- gastroesophageal K31.6
- gastrojejunal K31.6
- gastrojejunocolic K31.6
- genital tract (female) N82.9
  - specified NEC N82.8
  - to intestine NEC N82.4
  - to skin N82.5
- hepatic artery-portal vein, congenital Q26.6
- hepatopleural J86.0
- hepatopulmonary J86.0
- ileorectal or ileosigmoidal K63.2
- ileovaginal N82.2
- ileovesical N32.1
- ileum K63.2
- in ano K60.3
  - tuberculous A18.32
- inner ear (labyrinth) H83.1
- intestine NEC K63.2
- intestinocolonic (abdominal) K63.2
- intestinoureteral N28.89
- intestinouterine N82.4
- intestinovaginal N82.4
  - large intestine N82.3
  - small intestine N82.2
- intestinovesical N32.1
- ischiorectal (fossa) K61.39
- jejunum K63.2
- joint M25.10
  - ankle M25.17-
  - elbow M25.12-
  - foot joint M25.17-
  - hand joint M25.14-
  - hip M25.15-
  - knee M25.16-
  - shoulder M25.11-
  - specified joint NEC M25.18
  - tuberculous —*see* Tuberculosis, joint
  - vertebrae M25.18
  - wrist M25.13-
- kidney N28.89
- labium (majus) (minus) N82.8
- labyrinth H83.1
- lacrimal (gland) (sac) H04.61-
- lacrimonasal duct —*see* Fistula, lacrimal
- laryngotracheal, congenital Q34.8
- larynx J38.7
- lip K13.0
  - congenital Q38.0
- lumbar, tuberculous A18.01

Flail
  chest S22.5
    newborn (birth injury) P13.8
  joint (paralytic) M25.20
    ankle M25.27-
    elbow M25.22-
    foot joint M25.27-
    hand joint M25.24-
    hip M25.25-
    knee M25.26-
    shoulder M25.21-
    specified joint NEC M25.28
    wrist M25.23-

Flajani's disease —*see* Hyperthyroidism, with, goiter (diffuse)

Flap, liver K71.3

Flashbacks (residual to hallucinogen use) F16.283

Flat
  chamber (eye) —*see* Disorder, globe, hypotony, flat anterior chamber
  chest, congenital Q67.8
  foot (acquired) (fixed type) (painful) (postural) —*see also* Deformity, limb, flat foot
    congenital (rigid) (spastic (everted)) Q66.5-
    rachitic sequelae (late effect) E64.3
  organ or site, congenital NEC —*see* Anomaly, by site
  pelvis M95.5
    with disproportion (fetopelvic) O33.0
      causing obstructed labor O65.0
    congenital Q74.2

Flatau-Schilder disease G37.0

Flatback syndrome M40.30
  lumbar region M40.36
  lumbosacral region M40.37
  thoracolumbar region M40.35

Flattening
  head, femur M89.8X5
  hip —*see* Coxa, plana
  lip (congenital) Q18.8
  nose (congenital) Q67.4
    acquired M95.0

Flatulence R14.3
  psychogenic F45.8

Flatus R14.3
  vaginalis N89.8

Flax-dresser's disease J66.1

Flea bite —*see* Injury, bite, by site, superficial, insect

Flecks, glaucomatous (subcapsular) —*see* Cataract, complicated

Fleischer (-Kayser) **ring** (cornea) H18.04-

Fleshy mole O02.0

Flexibilitas cerea —*see* Catalepsy

Flexion
  amputation stump (surgical) T87.89
  cervix —*see* Malposition, uterus
  contracture, joint —*see* Contraction, joint
  deformity, joint (*see also* Deformity, limb, flexion) M21.20
    hip, congenital Q65.89
  uterus —*see also* Malposition, uterus
    lateral —*see* Lateroversion, uterus

Flexner-Boyd dysentery A03.2

Flexner's dysentery A03.1

Flexure —*see* Flexion

Flint murmur (aortic insufficiency) I35.1

Floater, vitreous —*see* Opacity, vitreous

Floating
  cartilage (joint) —*see also* Loose, body, joint
    knee —*see* Derangement, knee, loose body
  gallbladder, congenital Q44.1
  kidney N28.89
    congenital Q63.8
  spleen D73.89

Flooding N92.0

Floor —*see* condition

Floppy
  baby syndrome (nonspecific) P94.2
  iris syndrome (intraoperative) (IFIS) H21.81
  nonrheumatic mitral valve syndrome I34.1

Flu —*see also* Influenza
  avian (*see also* Influenza, due to, identified novel influenza A virus) J09.X2
  bird (*see also* Influenza, due to, identified novel influenza A virus) J09.X2
  intestinal NEC A08.4
  swine (viruses that normally cause infections in pigs) (*see also* Influenza, due to, identified novel influenza A virus) J09.X2

Fluctuating blood pressure I99.8

Fluid
  abdomen R18.8
  chest J94.8
  heart —*see* Failure, heart, congestive
  joint —*see* Effusion, joint
  loss (acute) E86.9
  lung —*see* Edema, lung
  overload E87.70
    specified NEC E87.79
  peritoneal cavity R18.8
  pleural cavity J94.8
  retention R60.9

Flukes NEC —*see also* Infestation, fluke
  blood NEC —*see* Schistosomiasis
  liver B66.3

Fluor (vaginalis) N89.8
  trichomonal or due to Trichomonas (vaginalis) A59.00

Fluorosis
  dental K00.3
  skeletal M85.10
    ankle M85.17-
    foot M85.17-
    forearm M85.13-
    hand M85.14-
    lower leg M85.16-
    multiple site M85.19
    neck M85.18
    rib M85.18
    shoulder M85.11-
    skull M85.18
    specified site NEC M85.18
    thigh M85.15-
    toe M85.17-
    upper arm M85.12-
    vertebra M85.18

Flush syndrome E34.0

Flushing R23.2
  menopausal N95.1

Flutter
  atrial or auricular I48.92
    atypical I48.4
    type I I48.3
    type II I48.4
    typical I48.3
  heart I49.8
    atrial or auricular I48.92
      atypical I48.4
      type I I48.3
      type II I48.4
      typical I48.3
    ventricular I49.02
  ventricular I49.02

FNHTR (febrile nonhemolytic transfusion reaction) R50.84

Fochier's abscess - code by site under Abscess

Focus, Assmann's —*see* Tuberculosis, pulmonary

Fogo selvagem L10.3

Foix-Alajouanine syndrome G95.19

Fold, folds (anomalous) —*see also* Anomaly, by site
  Descemet's membrane —*see* Change, corneal membrane, Descemet's, fold
  epicanthic Q10.3
  heart Q24.8

Folie à deux F24

Follicle
  cervix (nabothian) (ruptured) N88.8
  graafian, ruptured, with hemorrhage N83.0-
  nabothian N88.8

Follicular —*see* condition

Folliculitis (superficial) L73.9
  abscedens et suffodiens L66.3
  cyst N83.0-
  decalvans L66.2
  deep —*see* Furuncle, by site
  gonococcal (acute) (chronic) A54.01
  keloid, keloidalis L73.0
  pustular L01.02
  ulerythematosa reticulata L66.4

Folliculome lipidique
  specified site —*see* Neoplasm, benign, by site
  unspecified site
    female D27.9
    male D29.20

Følling's disease E70.0

Follow-up —*see* Examination, follow-up

Fong's syndrome (hereditary osteo-onychodysplasia) Q87.2

Food
  allergy L27.2
  asphyxia (from aspiration or inhalation) —*see* Foreign body, by site
  choked on —*see* Foreign body, by site
  deprivation T73.0
    specified kind of food NEC E63.8
  insecurity Z59.41
  intoxication —*see* Poisoning, food
  lack of T73.0
  poisoning —*see* Poisoning, food
  rejection NEC —*see* Disorder, eating

Food (*continued*)
  strangulation or suffocation —*see* Foreign body, by site
  toxemia —*see* Poisoning, food

Foot —*see* condition

Foramen ovale (nonclosure) (patent) (persistent) Q21.1

Forbes' glycogen storage disease E74.03

Fordyce-Fox disease L75.2

Fordyce's disease (mouth) Q38.6

Forearm —*see* condition

Foreclosure on loan Z59.89

Foreign body
  with
    laceration —*see* Laceration, by site, with foreign body
    puncture wound —*see* Puncture, by site, with foreign body
  accidentally left following a procedure T81.509
    aspiration T81.506
      resulting in
        adhesions T81.516
        obstruction T81.526
        perforation T81.536
        specified complication NEC T81.596
    cardiac catheterization T81.505
      resulting in
        acute reaction T81.60
          aseptic peritonitis T81.61
          specified NEC T81.69
  accidentally left following a
    adhesions T81.515
      obstruction T81.525
      perforation T81.535
      specified complication NEC T81.595
    causing
      acute reaction T81.60
        aseptic peritonitis T81.61
        specified complication NEC T81.69
      adhesions T81.519
      aseptic peritonitis T81.61
      obstruction T81.529
      perforation T81.539
      specified complication NEC T81.599
    endoscopy T81.504
      resulting in
        adhesions T81.514
        obstruction T81.524
        perforation T81.534
        specified complication NEC T81.594
    immunization T81.503
      resulting in
        adhesions T81.513
        obstruction T81.523
        perforation T81.533
        specified complication NEC T81.593
    infusion T81.501
      resulting in
        adhesions T81.511
        obstruction T81.521
        perforation T81.531
        specified complication NEC T81.591
    injection T81.503
      resulting in
        adhesions T81.513
        obstruction T81.523
        perforation T81.533
        specified complication NEC T81.593

Foreign body *(continued)*

- accidentally left following a
  - adhesions *(continued)*
    - kidney dialysis T81.502
      - resulting in
        - adhesions T81.512
        - obstruction T81.522
        - perforation T81.532
        - specified complication NEC T81.592
    - packing removal T81.507
      - resulting in
        - acute reaction T81.60
          - aseptic peritonitis T81.61
          - specified NEC T81.69
        - adhesions T81.517
        - obstruction T81.527
        - perforation T81.537
        - specified complication NEC T81.597
    - puncture T81.506
      - resulting in
        - adhesions T81.516
        - obstruction T81.526
        - perforation T81.536
        - specified complication NEC T81.596
    - specified procedure NEC T81.508
      - resulting in
        - acute reaction T81.60
          - aseptic peritonitis T81.61
          - specified NEC T81.69
        - adhesions T81.518
        - obstruction T81.528
        - perforation T81.538
        - specified complication NEC T81.598
    - surgical operation T81.500
      - resulting in
        - acute reaction T81.60
          - aseptic peritonitis T81.61
          - specified NEC T81.69
        - adhesions T81.510
        - obstruction T81.520
        - perforation T81.530
        - specified complication NEC T81.590
    - transfusion T81.501
      - resulting in
        - adhesions T81.511
        - obstruction T81.521
        - perforation T81.531
        - specified complication NEC T81.591
- alimentary tract T18.9
  - anus T18.5
  - colon T18.4
  - esophagus —*see* Foreign body, esophagus
  - mouth T18.0
  - multiple sites T18.8
  - rectosigmoid (junction) T18.5
  - rectum T18.5
  - small intestine T18.3
  - specified site NEC T18.8
  - stomach T18.2
- anterior chamber (eye) S05.5-
- auditory canal —*see* Foreign body, entering through orifice, ear
- bronchus T17.508
  - causing
    - asphyxiation T17.500
      - food (bone) (seed) T17.520
      - gastric contents (vomitus) T17.510
      - specified type NEC T17.590
    - injury NEC T17.508
      - food (bone) (seed) T17.528
      - gastric contents (vomitus) T17.518
      - specified type NEC T17.598

Foreign body *(continued)*

- canthus —*see* Foreign body, conjunctival sac
- ciliary body (eye) S05.5-
- conjunctival sac T15.1-
- cornea T15.0-
- entering through orifice
  - accessory sinus T17.0
  - alimentary canal T18.9
    - multiple parts T18.8
    - specified part NEC T18.8
  - alveolar process T18.0
  - antrum (Highmore's) T17.0
  - anus T18.5
  - appendix T18.4
  - auditory canal —*see* Foreign body, entering through orifice, ear
  - auricle —*see* Foreign body, entering through orifice, ear
  - bladder T19.1
  - bronchioles —*see* Foreign body, respiratory tract, specified site NEC
  - bronchus (main) —*see* Foreign body, bronchus
  - buccal cavity T18.0
  - canthus (inner) —*see* Foreign body, conjunctival sac
  - cecum T18.4
  - cervix (canal) (uteri) T19.3
  - colon T18.4
  - conjunctival sac —*see* Foreign body, conjunctival sac
  - cornea —*see* Foreign body, cornea
  - digestive organ or tract NOS T18.9
    - multiple parts T18.8
    - specified part NEC T18.8
  - duodenum T18.3
  - ear (external) T16.-
  - esophagus —*see* Foreign body, esophagus
  - eye (external) NOS T15.9-
    - conjunctival sac —*see* Foreign body, conjunctival sac
    - cornea —*see* Foreign body, cornea
    - specified part NEC T15.8-
  - eyeball —*see also* Foreign body, entering through orifice, eye, specified part NEC
    - with penetrating wound —*see* Puncture, eyeball
  - eyelid —*see also* Foreign body, conjunctival sac
    - with
      - laceration —*see* Laceration, eyelid, with foreign body
      - puncture —*see* Puncture, eyelid, with foreign body
      - superficial injury —*see* Foreign body, superficial, eyelid
  - gastrointestinal tract T18.9
    - multiple parts T18.8
    - specified part NEC T18.8
  - genitourinary tract T19.9
    - multiple parts T19.8
    - specified part NEC T19.8
  - globe —*see* Foreign body, entering through orifice, eyeball
  - gum T18.0
  - Highmore's antrum T17.0
  - hypopharynx —*see* Foreign body, pharynx
  - ileum T18.3
  - intestine (small) T18.3
    - large T18.4

Foreign body *(continued)*

- entering through orifice *(continued)*
  - lacrimal apparatus (punctum) —*see* Foreign body, entering through orifice, eye, specified part NEC
  - large intestine T18.4
  - larynx —*see* Foreign body, larynx
  - lung —*see* Foreign body, respiratory tract, specified site NEC
  - maxillary sinus T17.0
  - mouth T18.0
  - nasal sinus T17.0
  - nasopharynx —*see* Foreign body, pharynx
  - nose (passage) T17.1
  - nostril T17.1
  - oral cavity T18.0
  - palate T18.0
  - penis T19.4
  - pharynx —*see* Foreign body, pharynx
  - piriform sinus —*see* Foreign body, pharynx
  - rectosigmoid (junction) T18.5
  - rectum T18.5
  - respiratory tract —*see* Foreign body, respiratory tract
  - sinus (accessory) (frontal) (maxillary) (nasal) T17.0
    - piriform —*see* Foreign body, pharynx
  - small intestine T18.3
  - stomach T18.2
  - suffocation by —*see* Foreign body, by site
  - tear ducts or glands —*see* Foreign body, entering through orifice, eye, specified part NEC
  - throat —*see* Foreign body, pharynx
  - tongue T18.0
  - tonsil, tonsillar (fossa) —*see* Foreign body, pharynx
  - trachea —*see* Foreign body, trachea
  - ureter T19.8
  - urethra T19.0
  - uterus (any part) T19.3
  - vagina T19.2
  - vulva T19.2
- esophagus T18.108
  - causing
    - injury NEC T18.108
      - food (bone) (seed) T18.128
      - gastric contents (vomitus) T18.118
      - specified type NEC T18.198
    - tracheal compression T18.100
      - food (bone) (seed) T18.120
      - gastric contents (vomitus) T18.110
      - specified type NEC T18.190
- feeling of, in throat R09.89
- fragment —*see* Retained, foreign body fragments (type of)
- genitourinary tract T19.9
  - bladder T19.1
  - multiple parts T19.8
  - penis T19.4
  - specified site NEC T19.8
  - urethra T19.0
  - uterus T19.3
    - IUD Z97.5
  - vagina T19.2
    - contraceptive device Z97.5
  - vulva T19.2

Foreign body *(continued)*

- granuloma (old) (soft tissue) —*see also* Granuloma, foreign body
  - skin L92.3
- in
  - laceration —*see* Laceration, by site, with foreign body
  - puncture wound —*see* Puncture, by site, with foreign body
  - soft tissue (residual) M79.5
- inadvertently left in operation wound —*see* Foreign body, accidentally left during a procedure
- ingestion, ingested NOS T18.9
- inhalation or inspiration —*see* Foreign body, by site
- internal organ, not entering through a natural orifice - code as specific injury with foreign body
- intraocular S05.5-
  - old, retained (nonmagnetic) H44.70-
    - anterior chamber H44.71-
    - ciliary body H44.72-
    - iris H44.72-
    - lens H44.73-
    - magnetic H44.60-
      - anterior chamber H44.61-
      - ciliary body H44.62-
      - iris H44.62-
      - lens H44.63-
      - posterior wall H44.64-
      - specified site NEC H44.69-
      - vitreous body H44.65-
    - posterior wall H44.74-
    - specified site NEC H44.79-
    - vitreous body H44.75-
- iris —*see* Foreign body, intraocular
- lacrimal punctum —*see* Foreign body, entering through orifice, eye, specified part NEC
- larynx T17.308
  - causing
    - asphyxiation T17.300
      - food (bone) (seed) T17.320
      - gastric contents (vomitus) T17.310
      - specified type NEC T17.390
    - injury NEC T17.308
      - food (bone) (seed) T17.328
      - gastric contents (vomitus) T17.318
      - specified type NEC T17.398
- lens —*see* Foreign body, intraocular
- ocular muscle S05.4-
  - old, retained —*see* Foreign body, orbit, old
- old or residual
  - soft tissue (residual) M79.5
- operation wound, left accidentally —*see* Foreign body, accidentally left during a procedure
- orbit S05.4-
  - old, retained H05.5-
- pharynx T17.208
  - causing
    - asphyxiation T17.200
      - food (bone) (seed) T17.220
      - gastric contents (vomitus) T17.210
      - specified type NEC T17.290
    - injury NEC T17.208
      - food (bone) (seed) T17.228
      - gastric contents (vomitus) T17.218
      - specified type NEC T17.298

Foreign body *(continued)*
- respiratory tract T17.908
  - bronchioles *—see* Foreign body, respiratory tract, specified site NEC
  - bronchus *—see* Foreign body, bronchus
  - causing
    - asphyxiation T17.900
      - food (bone) (seed) T17.920
      - gastric contents (vomitus) T17.910
      - specified type NEC T17.990
    - injury NEC T17.908
      - food (bone) (seed) T17.928
      - gastric contents (vomitus) T17.918
      - specified type NEC T17.998
  - larynx *—see* Foreign body, larynx
  - lung *—see* Foreign body, respiratory tract, specified site NEC
  - multiple parts *—see* Foreign body, respiratory tract, specified site NEC
  - nasal sinus T17.0
  - nasopharynx *—see* Foreign body, pharynx
  - nose T17.1
  - nostril T17.1
  - pharynx *—see* Foreign body, pharynx
  - specified site NEC T17.808
    - causing
      - asphyxiation T17.800
        - food (bone) (seed) T17.820
        - gastric contents (vomitus) T17.810
        - specified type NEC T17.890
      - injury NEC T17.808
        - food (bone) (seed) T17.828
        - gastric contents (vomitus) T17.818
        - specified type NEC T17.898
  - throat *—see* Foreign body, pharynx
  - trachea *—see* Foreign body, trachea
- retained (old) (nonmagnetic) (in)
  - anterior chamber (eye) *—see* Foreign body, intraocular, old, retained, anterior chamber
    - magnetic *—see* Foreign body, intraocular, old, retained, magnetic, anterior chamber
  - ciliary body *—see* Foreign body, intraocular, old, retained, ciliary body
    - magnetic *—see* Foreign body, intraocular, old, retained, magnetic, ciliary body
  - eyelid H02.819
    - left H02.816
      - lower H02.815
      - upper H02.814
    - right H02.813
      - lower H02.812
      - upper H02.811
  - fragments *—see* Retained, foreign body fragments (type of)
  - globe *—see* Foreign body, intraocular, old, retained
    - magnetic *—see* Foreign body, intraocular, old, retained, magnetic

Foreign body *(continued)*
- retained *(continued)*
  - intraocular *—see* Foreign body, intraocular, old, retained
    - magnetic *—see* Foreign body, intraocular, old, retained, magnetic
  - iris *—see* Foreign body, intraocular, old, retained, iris
    - magnetic *—see* Foreign body, intraocular, old, retained, magnetic, iris
  - lens *—see* Foreign body, intraocular, old, retained, lens
    - magnetic *—see* Foreign body, intraocular, old, retained, magnetic, lens
  - muscle *—see* Foreign body, retained, soft tissue
  - orbit *—see* Foreign body, orbit, old
  - posterior wall of globe *—see* Foreign body, intraocular, old, retained, posterior wall
    - magnetic *—see* Foreign body, intraocular, old, retained, magnetic, posterior wall
  - retrobulbar *—see* Foreign body, orbit, old, retrobulbar
  - soft tissue M79.5
  - vitreous *—see* Foreign body, intraocular, old, retained, vitreous body
    - magnetic *—see* Foreign body, intraocular, old, retained, magnetic, vitreous body
- retina S05.5-
- superficial, without open wound
  - abdomen, abdominal (wall) S30.851
  - alveolar process S00.552
  - ankle S90.55-
  - antecubital space *—see* Foreign body, superficial, forearm
  - anus S30.857
  - arm (upper) S40.85-
  - auditory canal *—see* Foreign body, superficial, ear
  - auricle *—see* Foreign body, superficial, ear
  - axilla *—see* Foreign body, superficial, arm
  - back, lower S30.850
  - breast S20.15-
  - brow S00.85
  - buttock S30.850
  - calf *—see* Foreign body, superficial, leg
  - canthus *—see* Foreign body, superficial, eyelid
  - cheek S00.85
    - internal S00.552
  - chest wall *—see* Foreign body, superficial, thorax
  - chin S00.85
  - clitoris S30.854
  - costal region *—see* Foreign body, superficial, thorax
  - digit(s)
    - hand *—see* Foreign body, superficial, finger
    - foot *—see* Foreign body, superficial, toe
  - ear S00.45-
  - elbow S50.35-
  - epididymis S30.853
  - epigastric region S30.851
  - epiglottis S10.15
  - esophagus, cervical S10.15
  - eyebrow *—see* Foreign body, superficial, eyelid

Foreign body *(continued)*
- superficial, without open wound *(continued)*
  - eyelid S00.25-
  - face S00.85
  - finger(s) S60.459
    - index S60.45-
    - little S60.45-
    - middle S60.45-
    - ring S60.45-
  - flank S30.851
  - foot (except toe(s) alone) S90.85-
    - toe *—see* Foreign body, superficial, toe
  - forearm S50.85-
    - elbow only *—see* Foreign body, superficial, elbow
  - forehead S00.85
  - genital organs, external
    - female S30.856
    - male S30.855
  - groin S30.851
  - gum S00.552
  - hand S60.55-
  - head S00.95
    - ear *—see* Foreign body, superficial, ear
    - eyelid *—see* Foreign body, superficial, eyelid
    - lip S00.551
    - nose S00.35
    - oral cavity S00.552
    - scalp S00.05
    - specified site NEC S00.85
  - heel *—see* Foreign body, superficial, foot
  - hip S70.25-
  - inguinal region S30.851
  - interscapular region S20.459
  - jaw S00.85
  - knee S80.25-
  - labium (majus) (minus) S30.854
  - larynx S10.15
  - leg (lower) S80.85-
    - knee *—see* Foreign body, superficial, knee
    - upper *—see* Foreign body, superficial, thigh
  - lip S00.551
  - lower back S30.850
  - lumbar region S30.850
  - malar region S00.85
  - mammary *—see* Foreign body, superficial, breast
  - mastoid region S00.85
  - mouth S00.552
  - nail
    - finger *—see* Foreign body, superficial, finger
    - toe *—see* Foreign body, superficial, toe
  - nape S10.85
  - nasal S00.35
  - neck S10.95
    - specified site NEC S10.85
    - throat S10.15
  - nose S00.35
  - occipital region S00.05
  - oral cavity S00.552
  - orbital region *—see* Foreign body, superficial, eyelid
  - palate S00.552
  - palm *—see* Foreign body, superficial, hand
  - parietal region S00.05
  - pelvis S30.850
  - penis S30.852
  - perineum
    - female S30.854
    - male S30.850

Foreign body *(continued)*
- superficial, without open wound *(continued)*
  - periocular area *—see* Foreign body, superficial, eyelid
  - phalanges
    - finger *—see* Foreign body, superficial, finger
    - toe *—see* Foreign body, superficial, toe
  - pharynx S10.15
  - pinna *—see* Foreign body, superficial, ear
  - popliteal space *—see* Foreign body, superficial, knee
  - prepuce S30.852
  - pubic region S30.850
  - pudendum
    - female S30.856
    - male S30.855
  - sacral region S30.850
  - scalp S00.05
  - scapular region *—see* Foreign body, superficial, shoulder
  - scrotum S30.853
  - shin *—see* Foreign body, superficial, leg
  - shoulder S40.25-
  - sternal region S20.359
  - submaxillary region S00.85
  - submental region S00.85
  - subungual
    - finger(s) *—see* Foreign body, superficial, finger
    - toe(s) *—see* Foreign body, superficial, toe
  - supraclavicular fossa S10.85
  - supraorbital S00.85
  - temple S00.85
  - temporal region S00.85
  - testis S30.853
  - thigh S70.35-
  - thorax, thoracic (wall) S20.95
    - back S20.45-
    - front S20.35-
  - throat S10.15
  - thumb S60.35-
  - toe(s) (lesser) S90.456
    - great S90.45-
  - tongue S00.552
  - trachea S10.15
  - tunica vaginalis S30.853
  - tympanum, tympanic membrane *—see* Foreign body, superficial, ear
  - uvula S00.552
  - vagina S30.854
  - vocal cords S10.15
  - vulva S30.854
  - wrist S60.85-
- swallowed T18.9
- trachea T17.408
  - causing
    - asphyxiation T17.400
      - food (bone) (seed) T17.420
      - gastric contents (vomitus) T17.410
      - specified type NEC T17.490
    - injury NEC T17.408
      - food (bone) (seed) T17.428
      - gastric contents (vomitus) T17.418
      - specified type NEC T17.498
- type of fragment *—see* Retained, foreign body fragments (type of)
- vitreous (humor) S05.5-

Forestier's disease (rhizomelic pseudopolyarthritis) M35.3
- meaning ankylosing hyperostosis —*see* Hyperostosis, ankylosing

Formation
- hyalin in cornea —*see* Degeneration, cornea
- sequestrum in bone (due to infection) —*see* Osteomyelitis, chronic
- valve
  - colon, congenital Q43.8
  - ureter (congenital) Q62.39

Formication R20.2

Fort Bragg fever A27.89

Fossa —*see also* condition
- pyriform —*see* condition

Foster-Kennedy syndrome H47.14-

Fothergill's
- disease (trigeminal neuralgia) —*see also* Neuralgia, trigeminal
- scarlatina anginosa A38.9

Foul breath R19.6

Foundling Z76.1

Fournier disease or gangrene N49.3
- female N76.89

Fourth
- cranial nerve —*see* condition
- molar K00.1

Foville's (peduncular) **disease or syndrome** G46.3

Fox (Fordyce) disease (apocrine miliaria) L75.2

FPIES (food protein-induced enterocolitis syndrome) K52.21

Fracture, burst —*see* Fracture, traumatic, by site

Fracture, chronic —*see* Fracture, pathological, by site

Fracture, insufficiency —*see* Fracture, pathologic, by site

Fracture, nontraumatic, NEC
- atypical
  - femur M84.750-
    - complete
      - oblique M84.759
        - left side M84.758
        - right side M84.757
      - transverse M84.756
        - left side M84.755
        - right side M84.754
    - incomplete M84.753
      - left side M84.752
      - right side M84.751

Fracture, pathological (pathologic) —*see also* Fracture, traumatic M84.40
- ankle M84.47-
- carpus M84.44-
- clavicle M84.41-
- compression (not due to trauma) (*see also* Collapse, vertebra) M48.50-
- dental implant M27.63
- dental restorative material K08.539
  - with loss of material K08.531
  - without loss of material K08.530
- due to
  - neoplastic disease NEC (*see also* Neoplasm) M84.50
    - ankle M84.57-
    - carpus M84.54-
    - clavicle M84.51-

Fracture, pathological *(continued)*
- due to *(continued)*
  - neoplastic disease NEC *(continued)*
    - femur M84.55-
    - fibula M84.56-
    - finger M84.54-
    - hip M84.559
    - humerus M84.52-
    - ilium M84.550
    - ischium M84.550
    - metacarpus M84.54-
    - metatarsus M84.57-
    - neck M84.58
    - pelvis M84.550
    - radius M84.53-
    - rib M84.58
    - scapula M84.51-
    - skull M84.58
    - specified site NEC M84.58
    - tarsus M84.57-
    - tibia M84.56-
    - toe M84.57-
    - ulna M84.53-
    - vertebra M84.58
  - osteoporosis M80.00
    - disuse —*see* Osteoporosis, specified type NEC, with pathological fracture
    - drug-induced —*see* Osteoporosis, drug induced, with pathological fracture
    - idiopathic —*see* Osteoporosis, specified type NEC, with pathological fracture
    - postmenopausal —*see* Osteoporosis, postmenopausal, with pathological fracture
    - postoophorectomy —*see* Osteoporosis, postoophorectomy, with pathological fracture
    - postsurgical malabsorption —*see* Osteoporosis, specified type NEC, with pathological fracture
    - specified cause NEC —*see* Osteoporosis, specified type NEC, with pathological fracture
  - specified disease NEC M84.60
    - ankle M84.67-
    - carpus M84.64-
    - clavicle M84.61-
    - femur M84.65-
    - fibula M84.66-
    - finger M84.64-
    - hip M84.65-
    - humerus M84.62-
    - ilium M84.650
    - ischium M84.650
    - metacarpus M84.64-
    - metatarsus M84.67-
    - neck M84.68
    - radius M84.63-
    - rib M84.68
    - scapula M84.61-
    - skull M84.68
    - tarsus M84.67-
    - tibia M84.66-
    - toe M84.67-
    - ulna M84.63-
    - vertebra M84.68
- femur M84.45-
- fibula M84.46-
- finger M84.44-
- hip M84.459
- humerus M84.42-
- ilium M84.454
- ischium M84.454

Fracture, pathological *(continued)*
- joint prosthesis —*see* Complications, joint prosthesis, mechanical, breakdown, by site
  - periprosthetic —*see* Fracture, pathological, periprosthetic
- metacarpus M84.44-
- metatarsus M84.47-
- neck M84.48
- pelvis M84.454
- periprosthetic M97.9
  - ankle M97.2-
  - elbow M97.4-
  - finger M97.8
  - hip M97.0-
  - knee M97.1-
  - other specified joint M97.8
  - shoulder M97.3-
  - spinal joint M97.8
  - toe joint M97.8
  - wrist joint M97.8
- radius M84.43-
- restorative material (dental) K08.539
  - with loss of material K08.531
  - without loss of material K08.530
- rib M84.48
- scapula M84.41-
- skull M84.48
- tarsus M84.47-
- tibia M84.46-
- toe M84.47-
- ulna M84.43-
- vertebra M84.48

Fracture, traumatic (abduction) (adduction) (separation) (*see also* Fracture, pathological) T14.8
- acetabulum S32.40-
  - column
    - anterior (displaced) (iliopubic) S32.43-
      - nondisplaced S32.436
    - posterior (displaced) (ilioischial) S32.443
      - nondisplaced S32.44-
  - dome (displaced) S32.48-
    - nondisplaced S32.48
  - specified NEC S32.49-
  - transverse (displaced) S32.45-
    - with associated posterior wall fracture (displaced) S32.46-
      - nondisplaced S32.46-
    - nondisplaced S32.45-
  - wall
    - anterior (displaced) S32.41-
      - nondisplaced S32.41-
    - medial (displaced) S32.47-
      - nondisplaced S32.47-
    - posterior (displaced) S32.42-
      - with associated transverse fracture (displaced) S32.46-
        - nondisplaced S32.46-
      - nondisplaced S32.42-
- acromion —*see* Fracture, scapula, acromial process
- ankle S82.899
  - bimalleolar (displaced) S82.84-
    - nondisplaced S82.84-
  - lateral malleolus only (displaced) S82.6-
    - nondisplaced S82.6-
  - medial malleolus (displaced) S82.5-
    - associated with Maisonneuve's fracture —*see* Fracture, Maisonneuve's
    - nondisplaced S82.5-

Fracture, traumatic *(continued)*
- ankle *(continued)*
  - talus —*see* Fracture, tarsal, talus
  - trimalleolar (displaced) S82.85-
    - nondisplaced S82.85-
- arm (upper) —*see also* Fracture, humerus, shaft
  - humerus —*see* Fracture, humerus
  - radius —*see* Fracture, radius
  - ulna —*see* Fracture, ulna
- astragalus —*see* Fracture, tarsal, talus
- atlas —*see* Fracture, neck, cervical vertebra, first
- axis —*see* Fracture, neck, cervical vertebra, second
- back —*see* Fracture, vertebra
- Barton's —*see* Barton's fracture
- base of skull —*see* Fracture, skull, base
- basicervical (basal) (femoral) S72.0
- Bennett's —*see* Bennett's fracture
- bimalleolar —*see* Fracture, ankle, bimalleolar
- blow-out S02.3-
- bone NEC T14.8
  - birth injury P13.9
  - following insertion of orthopedic implant, joint prosthesis or bone plate —*see* Fracture, following insertion of orthopedic implant, joint prosthesis or bone plate
  - in (due to) neoplastic disease NEC —*see* Fracture, pathological, due to, neoplastic disease
  - pathological (cause unknown) —*see* Fracture, pathological
- breast bone —*see* Fracture, sternum
- bucket handle (semilunar cartilage) —*see* Tear, meniscus
- buckle —*see* Fracture, by site, torus
- burst —*see* Fracture, traumatic, by site
- calcaneus —*see* Fracture, tarsal, calcaneus
- carpal bone(s) S62.10-
  - capitate (displaced) S62.13-
    - nondisplaced S62.13-
  - cuneiform —*see* Fracture, carpal bone, triquetrum
  - hamate (body) (displaced) S62.143
    - hook process (displaced) S62.15-
      - nondisplaced S62.15-
    - nondisplaced S62.14-
  - larger multangular —*see* Fracture, carpal bones, trapezium
  - lunate (displaced) S62.12-
    - nondisplaced S62.12-
  - navicular S62.00-
    - distal pole (displaced) S62.01-
      - nondisplaced S62.01-
    - middle third (displaced) S62.02-
      - nondisplaced S62.02-
    - proximal third (displaced) S62.03-
      - nondisplaced S62.03-
    - volar tuberosity —*see* Fracture, carpal bones, navicular, distal pole
  - os magnum —*see* Fracture, carpal bones, capitate

Fracture, traumatic *(continued)*
- carpal bone(s) *(continued)*
  - pisiform (displaced) S62.16-
    - nondisplaced S62.16-
  - semilunar *—see* Fracture, carpal bones, lunate
  - smaller multangular *—see* Fracture, carpal bones, trapezoid
  - trapezium (displaced) S62.17-
    - nondisplaced S62.17-
  - trapezoid (displaced) S62.18-
    - nondisplaced S62.18-
  - triquetrum (displaced) S62.11-
    - nondisplaced S62.11-
  - unciform *—see* Fracture, carpal bones, hamate
- cervical *—see* Fracture, vertebra, cervical
- clavicle S42.00-
  - acromial end (displaced) S42.03-
    - nondisplaced S42.03-
  - birth injury P13.4
  - lateral end *—see* Fracture, clavicle, acromial end
  - shaft (displaced) S42.02-
    - nondisplaced S42.02-
  - sternal end (anterior) (displaced) S42.01-
    - nondisplaced S42.01-
    - posterior S42.01-
- coccyx S32.2
- collapsed *—see* Collapse, vertebra
- collar bone *—see* Fracture, clavicle
- Colles' *—see* Colles' fracture
- coronoid process *—see* Fracture, ulna, upper end, coronoid process
- corpus cavernosum penis S39.840
- costochondral cartilage S23.41
- costochondral, costosternal junction *—see* Fracture, rib
- cranium *—see* Fracture, skull
- cricoid cartilage S12.8
- cuboid (ankle) *—see* Fracture, tarsal, cuboid
- cuneiform
  - foot *—see* Fracture, tarsal, cuneiform
  - wrist *—see* Fracture, carpal, triquetrum
- delayed union *—see* Delay, union, fracture
- dental restorative material K08.539
  - with loss of material K08.531
  - without loss of material K08.530
- due to
  - birth injury *—see* Birth, injury, fracture
  - osteoporosis *—see* Osteoporosis, with fracture
- Dupuytren's *—see* Fracture, ankle, lateral malleolus
- elbow S42.40-
- ethmoid (bone) (sinus) *—see* Fracture, skull, base
- face bone S02.92
- fatigue *—see also* Fracture, stress
  - vertebra M48.40
    - cervical region M48.42
    - cervicothoracic region M48.43
    - lumbar region M48.46
    - lumbosacral region M48.47
    - occipito-atlanto-axial region M48.41
    - sacrococcygeal region M48.48
    - thoracic region M48.44
    - thoracolumbar region M48.45

Fracture, traumatic *(continued)*
- fatigue S72.9-
  - basicervical (basal) S72.0
  - birth injury P13.2
  - capital epiphyseal S79.01-
  - condyles, epicondyles *—see* Fracture, femur, lower end
  - distal end *—see* Fracture, femur, lower end
  - epiphysis
    - head *—see* Fracture, femur, upper end, epiphysis
    - lower *—see* Fracture, femur, lower end, epiphysis
    - upper *—see* Fracture, femur, upper end, epiphysis
  - following insertion of implant, prosthesis or plate M96.66-
  - head *—see* Fracture, femur, upper end, head
  - intertrochanteric *—see* Fracture, femur, trochanteric
  - intratrochanteric *—see* Fracture, femur, trochanteric
  - lower end S72.40-
    - condyle (displaced) S72.41-
      - lateral (displaced) S72.42-
        - nondisplaced S72.42-
      - medial (displaced) S72.43-
        - nondisplaced S72.43-
      - nondisplaced S72.41-
    - epiphysis (displaced) S72.44-
      - nondisplaced S72.44-
    - physeal S79.10-
      - Salter-Harris
        - Type I S79.11-
        - Type II S79.12-
        - Type III S79.13-
        - Type IV S79.14-
      - specified NEC S79.19-
    - specified NEC S72.49-
    - supracondylar (displaced) S72.45-
      - with intracondylar extension (displaced) S72.46-
        - nondisplaced S72.46-
      - nondisplaced S72.45-
    - torus S72.47-
  - neck *—see* Fracture, femur, upper end, neck
  - pertrochanteric *—see* Fracture, femur, trochanteric
  - shaft (lower third) (middle third) (upper third) S72.30-
    - comminuted (displaced) S72.35-
      - nondisplaced S72.35-
    - oblique (displaced) S72.33-
      - nondisplaced S72.33-
    - segmental (displaced) S72.36-
      - nondisplaced S72.36-
    - specified NEC S72.39-
    - spiral (displaced) S72.34-
      - nondisplaced S72.34-
    - transverse (displaced) S72.32-
      - nondisplaced S72.32-
  - specified site NEC S72.8
  - subcapital (displaced) S72.01-
  - subtrochanteric (region) (section) (displaced) S72.2-
    - nondisplaced S72.2-
  - transcervical *—see* Fracture, femur, midcervical
  - transtrochanteric *—see* Fracture, femur, trochanteric
  - trochanteric S72.10-
    - apophyseal (displaced) S72.13-
      - nondisplaced S72.13-

Fracture, traumatic *(continued)*
- fatigue *(continued)*
  - trochanteric *(continued)*
    - greater trochanter (displaced) S72.11-
      - nondisplaced S72.11-
    - intertrochanteric (displaced) S72.14-
      - nondisplaced S72.14-
    - lesser trochanter (displaced) S72.12-
      - nondisplaced S72.12-
  - upper end S72.00-
    - apophyseal (displaced) S72.13-
      - nondisplaced S72.13-
    - cervicotrochanteric *—see* Fracture, femur, upper end, neck, base
    - epiphysis (displaced) S72.02-
      - nondisplaced S72.02-
    - head S72.05-
      - articular (displaced) S72.06-
        - nondisplaced S72.06-
      - specified NEC S72.09-
    - intertrochanteric (displaced) S72.14-
      - nondisplaced S72.14-
    - intracapsular S72.01-
    - midcervical (displaced) S72.03-
      - nondisplaced S72.03-
    - neck S72.00-
      - base (displaced) S72.04-
        - nondisplaced S72.04-
      - specified NEC S72.09-
    - pertrochanteric *—see* Fracture, femur, upper end, trochanteric
    - physeal S79.00-
      - Salter-Harris type I S79.01-
      - specified NEC S79.09-
    - subcapital (displaced) S72.01-
    - subtrochanteric (displaced) S72.2-
      - nondisplaced S72.2-
    - transcervical *—see* Fracture, femur, midcervical
    - trochanteric S72.10-
      - greater (displaced) S72.11-
        - nondisplaced S72.11-
      - lesser (displaced) S72.12-
        - nondisplaced S72.12-
- fibula (shaft) (styloid) S82.40-
  - comminuted (displaced) S82.45-
    - nondisplaced S82.45-
  - following insertion of implant, prosthesis or plate M96.67-
  - involving ankle or malleolus *—see* Fracture, fibula, lateral malleolus
  - lateral malleolus (displaced) S82.6-
    - nondisplaced S82.6-
  - lower end
    - physeal S89.30-
      - Salter-Harris
        - Type I S89.31-
        - Type II S89.32-
      - specified NEC S89.39-
    - specified NEC S82.83-
    - torus S82.82-
  - oblique (displaced) S82.43-
    - nondisplaced S82.43-
  - segmental (displaced) S82.46-
    - nondisplaced S82.46-
  - specified NEC S82.49-
  - spiral (displaced) S82.44-
    - nondisplaced S82.44-

Fracture, traumatic *(continued)*
- fibula *(continued)*
  - transverse (displaced) S82.42-
    - nondisplaced S82.42-
  - upper end
    - physeal S89.20-
      - Salter-Harris
        - Type I S89.21-
        - Type II S89.22-
      - specified NEC S89.29-
    - specified NEC S82.83-
    - torus S82.81-
- finger (except thumb) S62.60-
  - distal phalanx (displaced) S62.63-
    - nondisplaced S62.66-
  - index S62.60-
    - distal phalanx (displaced) S62.63-
      - nondisplaced S62.66-
    - middle phalanx (displaced) S62.62-
      - nondisplaced S62.65-
    - proximal phalanx (displaced) S62.61-
      - nondisplaced S62.64-
  - little S62.60-
    - distal phalanx (displaced) S62.63-
      - nondisplaced S62.66-
    - middle phalanx (displaced) S62.62-
      - nondisplaced S62.65-
    - proximal phalanx (displaced) S62.61-
      - nondisplaced S62.64-
  - middle phalanx (displaced) S62.62-
    - nondisplaced S62.65-
  - middle S62.60-
    - distal phalanx (displaced) S62.63-
      - nondisplaced S62.66-
    - middle phalanx (displaced) S62.62-
      - nondisplaced S62.65-
    - proximal phalanx (displaced) S62.61-
      - nondisplaced S62.64-
  - proximal phalanx (displaced) S62.61-
    - nondisplaced S62.64-
  - ring S62.60-
    - distal phalanx (displaced) S62.63-
      - nondisplaced S62.66-
    - middle phalanx (displaced) S62.62-
      - nondisplaced S62.65-
    - proximal phalanx (displaced) S62.61-
      - nondisplaced S62.64-
  - thumb *—see* Fracture, thumb
- following insertion (intraoperative) (postoperative) of orthopedic implant, joint prosthesis or bone plate M96.69
  - femur M96.66-
  - fibula M96.67-
  - humerus M96.62-
  - pelvis M96.65
  - radius M96.63-
  - specified bone NEC M96.69
  - tibia M96.67-
  - ulna M96.63-
- foot S92.90-
  - astragalus *—see* Fracture, tarsal, talus
  - calcaneus *—see* Fracture, tarsal, calcaneus

Fracture, traumatic *(continued)*
- foot *(continued)*
  - cuboid —*see* Fracture, tarsal, cuboid
  - cuneiform —*see* Fracture, tarsal, cuneiform
  - metatarsal —*see* Fracture, metatarsal
  - navicular —*see* Fracture, tarsal, navicular
  - sesamoid S92.81-
  - specified NEC S92.81-
  - talus —*see* Fracture, tarsal, talus
  - tarsal —*see* Fracture, tarsal
  - toe —*see* Fracture, toe
- forearm S52.9-
  - radius —*see* Fracture, radius
  - ulna —*see* Fracture, ulna
- fossa (anterior) (middle) (posterior) S02.19
- fragility —*see* Fracture, pathological, due to osteoporosis
- frontal (bone) (skull) S02.0
  - sinus S02.19
- glenoid (cavity) (scapula) —*see* Fracture, scapula, glenoid cavity
- greenstick —*see* Fracture, by site
- hallux —*see* Fracture, toe, great
- hand S62.9-
  - carpal —*see* Fracture, carpal bone
  - finger (except thumb) —*see* Fracture, finger
  - metacarpal —*see* Fracture, metacarpal
  - navicular (scaphoid) (hand) —*see* Fracture, carpal bone, navicular
  - thumb —*see* Fracture, thumb
- healed or old
  - with complications - code by Nature of the complication
- heel bone —*see* Fracture, tarsal, calcaneus
- Hill-Sachs S42.29-
- hip —*see* Fracture, femur, neck
- humerus S42.30-
  - anatomical neck —*see* Fracture, humerus, upper end
  - articular process —*see* Fracture, humerus, lower end
  - capitellum —*see* Fracture, humerus, lower end, condyle, lateral
  - distal end —*see* Fracture, humerus, lower end
  - epiphysis
    - lower —*see* Fracture, humerus, lower end, physeal
    - upper —*see* Fracture, humerus, upper end, physeal
  - external condyle —*see* Fracture, humerus, lower end, condyle, lateral
  - following insertion of implant, prosthesis or plate M96.62-
  - great tuberosity —*see* Fracture, humerus, upper end, greater tuberosity
  - intercondylar —*see* Fracture, humerus, lower end
  - internal epicondyle —*see* Fracture, humerus, lower end, epicondyle, medial
  - lesser tuberosity —*see* Fracture, humerus, upper end, lesser tuberosity

Fracture, traumatic *(continued)*
- humerus *(continued)*
  - lower end S42.40-
    - condyle
      - lateral (displaced) S42.45-
        - nondisplaced S42.45-
      - medial (displaced) S42.46-
        - nondisplaced S42.46-
    - epicondyle
      - lateral (displaced) S42.43-
        - nondisplaced S42.43-
      - medial (displaced) S42.44-
        - incarcerated S42.44-
        - nondisplaced S42.44-
    - physeal S49.10-
      - Salter-Harris
        - Type I S49.11-
        - Type II S49.12-
        - Type III S49.13-
        - Type IV S49.14-
      - specified NEC S49.19-
    - specified NEC (displaced) S42.49-
      - nondisplaced S42.49-
    - supracondylar (simple) (displaced) S42.41-
      - with intercondylar fracture - *see* Fracture, humerus, lower end
      - comminuted (displaced) S42.42-
        - nondisplaced S42.42-
      - nondisplaced S42.41-
    - torus S42.48-
    - transcondylar (displaced) S42.47-
      - nondisplaced S42.47-
  - proximal end —*see* Fracture, humerus, upper end
  - shaft S42.30-
    - comminuted (displaced) S42.35-
      - nondisplaced S42.35-
    - greenstick S42.31-
    - oblique (displaced) S42.33-
      - nondisplaced S42.33-
    - segmental (displaced) S42.36-
      - nondisplaced S42.36-
    - specified NEC S42.39-
    - spiral (displaced) S42.34-
      - nondisplaced S42.34-
    - transverse (displaced) S42.32-
      - nondisplaced S42.32-
  - supracondylar —*see* Fracture, humerus, lower end
  - surgical neck —*see* Fracture, humerus, upper end, surgical neck
  - trochlea —*see* Fracture, humerus, lower end, condyle, medial
  - tuberosity —*see* Fracture, humerus, upper end
  - upper end S42.20-
    - anatomical neck —*see* Fracture, humerus, upper end, specified NEC
    - articular head —*see* Fracture, humerus, upper end, specified NEC
    - epiphysis —*see* Fracture, humerus, upper end, physeal
    - greater tuberosity (displaced) S42.25-
      - nondisplaced S42.25-
    - lesser tuberosity (displaced) S42.26-
      - nondisplaced S42.26-

Fracture, traumatic *(continued)*
- humerus *(continued)*
  - upper end *(continued)*
    - physeal S49.00-
      - Salter-Harris
        - Type I S49.01-
        - Type II S49.02-
        - Type III S49.03-
        - Type IV S49.04-
      - specified NEC S49.09-
    - specified NEC (displaced) S42.29-
      - nondisplaced S42.29-
    - surgical neck (displaced) S42.21-
      - four-part S42.24-
      - nondisplaced S42.21-
      - three-part S42.23-
      - two-part (displaced) S42.22-
        - nondisplaced S42.22-
    - torus S42.27-
    - transepiphyseal —*see* Fracture, humerus, upper end, physeal
- hyoid bone S12.8
- ilium S32.30-
  - with disruption of pelvic ring —*see* Disruption, pelvic ring
  - avulsion (displaced) S32.31-
    - nondisplaced S32.31-
  - specified NEC S32.39-
- impaction, impacted - code as Fracture, by site
- innominate bone —*see* Fracture, ilium
- instep —*see* Fracture, foot
- ischium S32.60-
  - with disruption of pelvic ring —*see* Disruption, pelvic ring
  - avulsion (displaced) S32.61-
    - nondisplaced S32.61-
  - specified NEC S32.69-
- jaw (bone) (lower) —*see* Fracture, mandible
  - upper —*see* Fracture, maxilla
- joint prosthesis —*see* Complications, joint prosthesis, mechanical, breakdown, by site
  - periprosthetic —*see* Fracture, traumatic, periprosthetic
- knee cap —*see* Fracture, patella
- larynx S12.8
- late effects —*see* Sequelae, fracture
- leg (lower) S82.9-
  - ankle —*see* Fracture, ankle
  - femur —*see* Fracture, femur
  - fibula —*see* Fracture, fibula
  - malleolus —*see* Fracture, ankle
  - patella —*see* Fracture, patella
  - specified site NEC S82.89-
  - tibia —*see* Fracture, tibia
- lumbar spine —*see* Fracture, vertebra, lumbar
- lumbosacral spine S32.9
- Maisonneuve's (displaced) S82.86-
  - nondisplaced S82.86-
- malar bone —*see also* Fracture, maxilla S02.400
  - left side S02.40B
  - right side S02.40A
- malleolus —*see* Fracture, ankle
- malunion —*see* Fracture, by site
- mandible (lower jaw (bone)) S02.609
  - alveolus S02.67-
  - angle (of jaw) S02.65-
  - body, unspecified S02.600
    - left side S02.602
    - right side S02.601

Fracture, traumatic *(continued)*
- mandible *(continued)*
  - condylar process S02.61-
  - coronoid process S02.63-
  - ramus, unspecified S02.64-
  - specified site NEC S02.69
  - subcondylar process S02.62-
  - symphysis S02.66
- manubrium (sterni) S22.21
  - dissociation from sternum S22.23
- march —*see* Fracture, traumatic, stress, by site
- maxilla, maxillary (bone) (sinus) (superior) (upper jaw) S02.401
  - alveolus S02.42
  - inferior —*see* Fracture, mandible
  - LeFort I S02.411
  - LeFort II S02.412
  - LeFort III S02.413
  - left side S02.40D
  - right side S02.40C
- metacarpal S62.309
  - base (displaced) S62.319
    - nondisplaced S62.349
  - fifth S62.30-
    - base (displaced) S62.31-
      - nondisplaced S62.34-
    - neck (displaced) S62.33-
      - nondisplaced S62.36-
    - shaft (displaced) S62.32-
      - nondisplaced S62.35-
    - specified NEC S62.398
  - first S62.20-
    - base NEC (displaced) S62.23-
      - nondisplaced S62.23-
    - Bennett's —*see* Bennett's fracture
    - neck (displaced) S62.25-
      - nondisplaced S62.25-
    - shaft (displaced) S62.24-
      - nondisplaced S62.24-
    - specified NEC S62.29-
  - fourth S62.30-
    - base (displaced) S62.31-
      - nondisplaced S62.34-
    - neck (displaced) S62.33-
      - nondisplaced S62.36-
    - shaft (displaced) S62.32-
      - nondisplaced S62.35-
    - specified NEC S62.39-
  - neck (displaced) S62.33-
    - nondisplaced S62.36-
  - Rolando's —*see* Rolando's fracture
  - second S62.30-
    - base (displaced) S62.31-
      - nondisplaced S62.34-
    - neck (displaced) S62.33-
      - nondisplaced S62.36-
    - shaft (displaced) S62.32-
      - nondisplaced S62.35-
    - specified NEC S62.39-
  - shaft (displaced) S62.32-
    - nondisplaced S62.35-
  - third S62.30-
    - base (displaced) S62.31-
      - nondisplaced S62.34-
    - neck (displaced) S62.33-
      - nondisplaced S62.36-
    - shaft (displaced) S62.32-
      - nondisplaced S62.35-
    - specified NEC S62.39-
  - specified NEC S62.399
- metaphyseal —*see* Fracture, traumatic, by site, shaft
- metastatic —*see* Fracture, pathological, due to, neoplastic disease —*see also* Neoplasm

Fracture, traumatic *(continued)*
metatarsal bone S92.30-
  fifth (displaced) S92.35-
    nondisplaced S92.35-
  first (displaced) S92.31-
    nondisplaced S92.31-
  fourth (displaced) S92.34-
    nondisplaced S92.34-
  physeal S99.10-
    Salter-Harris
      Type I S99.11-
      Type II S99.12-
      Type III S99.13-
      Type IV S99.14-
    specified NEC S99.19-
  second (displaced) S92.32-
    nondisplaced S92.32-
  third (displaced) S92.33-
    nondisplaced S92.33-
Monteggia's —*see* Monteggia's fracture
multiple
  hand (and wrist) NEC —*see* Fracture, by site
  ribs —*see* Fracture, rib, multiple
nasal (bone(s)) S02.2
navicular (scaphoid) (foot) —*see also* Fracture, tarsal, navicular
  hand —*see* Fracture, carpal, navicular
neck S12.9
  cervical vertebra S12.9
    fifth (displaced) S12.400
      nondisplaced S12.401
      specified type NEC (displaced) S12.490
        nondisplaced S12.491
    first (displaced) S12.000
      burst (stable) S12.01
        unstable S12.02
      lateral mass (displaced) S12.040
        nondisplaced S12.041
      nondisplaced S12.001
      posterior arch (displaced) S12.030
        nondisplaced S12.031
      specified type NEC (displaced) S12.090
        nondisplaced S12.091
    fourth (displaced) S12.300
      nondisplaced S12.301
      specified type NEC (displaced) S12.390
        nondisplaced S12.391
    second (displaced) S12.100
      nondisplaced S12.101
      dens (anterior) (displaced) (type II) S12.110
        nondisplaced S12.112
        posterior S12.111
        specified type NEC (displaced) S12.120
          nondisplaced S12.121
      specified type NEC (displaced) S12.190
        nondisplaced S12.191
    seventh (displaced) S12.600
      nondisplaced S12.601
      specified type NEC (displaced) S12.690
        non displaced S12.691
    sixth (displaced) S12.500
      nondisplaced S12.501
      specified type NEC (displaced) S12.590
        non displaced S12.591

Fracture, traumatic *(continued)*
neck *(continued)*
  cervical vertebra *(continued)*
    third (displaced) S12.200
      nondisplaced S12.201
      specified type NEC (displaced) S12.290
        non displaced S12.291
  hyoid bone S12.8
  larynx S12.8
  specified site NEC S12.8
  thyroid cartilage S12.8
  trachea S12.8
neoplastic NEC —*see* Fracture, pathological, due to, neoplastic disease
neural arch —*see* Fracture, vertebra
newborn —*see* Birth, injury, fracture
nontraumatic —*see* Fracture, pathological
nonunion —*see* Nonunion, fracture
nose, nasal (bone) (septum) S02.2
occiput —*see* Fracture, skull, base, occiput
odontoid process —*see* Fracture, neck, cervical vertebra, second
olecranon (process) (ulna) —*see* Fracture, ulna, upper end, olecranon process
orbit, orbital (bone) (region) S02.85
  floor (blow-out) S02.3-
  roof S02.12-
    wall S02.85
      lateral S02.84-
      medial S02.83-
os
  calcis —*see* Fracture, tarsal, calcaneus
  magnum —*see* Fracture, carpal, capitate
  pubis —*see* Fracture, pubis
palate S02.8-
parietal bone (skull) S02.0
patella S82.00-
  comminuted (displaced) S82.04-
    nondisplaced S82.04-
  longitudinal (displaced) S82.02-
    nondisplaced S82.02-
  osteochondral (displaced) S82.01-
    nondisplaced S82.01-
  specified NEC S82.09-
  transverse (displaced) S82.03-
    nondisplaced S82.03-
pedicle (of vertebral arch) —*see* Fracture, vertebra
pelvis, pelvic (bone) S32.9
  acetabulum —*see* Fracture, acetabulum
  circle —*see* Disruption, pelvic ring
  following insertion of implant, prosthesis or plate M96.65
  ilium —*see* Fracture, ilium
  ischium —*see* Fracture, ischium
  multiple
    with disruption of pelvic ring (circle) —*see* Disruption, pelvic ring
    without disruption of pelvic ring (circle) S32.82
  pubis —*see* Fracture, pubis
  specified site NEC S32.89
  sacrum —*see* Fracture, sacrum
periprosthetic, around internal prosthetic joint M97.9
  ankle M97.2-
  elbow M97.4-
  finger M97.8
  hip M97.0-

Fracture, traumatic *(continued)*
periprosthetic, around internal prosthetic joint *(continued)*
  knee M97.1-
  shoulder M97.3-
  specified joint NEC M97.8
  spine M97.8
  toe M97.8
  wrist M97.8
phalanx
  foot —*see* Fracture, toe
  hand —*see* Fracture, finger
pisiform —*see* Fracture, carpal, pisiform
pond —*see* Fracture, skull
prosthetic device, internal —*see* Complications, prosthetic device, by site, mechanical
pubis S32.50-
  with disruption of pelvic ring —*see* Disruption, pelvic ring
  specified site NEC S32.59-
  superior rim S32.51-
radius S52.9-
  distal end —*see* Fracture, radius, lower end
  following insertion of implant, prosthesis or plate M96.63-
  head —*see* Fracture, radius, upper end, head
  lower end S52.50-
    Barton's —*see* Barton's fracture
    Colles' —*see* Colles' fracture
    extraarticular NEC S52.55-
    intraarticular NEC S52.57-
    physeal S59.20-
      Salter-Harris
        Type I S59.21-
        Type II S59.22-
        Type III S59.23-
        Type IV S59.24-
      specified NEC S59.29-
    Smith's —*see* Smith's fracture
    specified NEC S52.59-
    styloid process (displaced) S52.51-
      nondisplaced S52.51-
    torus S52.52-
  neck —*see* Fracture, radius, upper end
  proximal end —*see* Fracture, radius, upper end
  shaft S52.30-
    bent bone S52.38-
    comminuted (displaced) S52.35-
      nondisplaced S52.35-
    Galeazzi's —*see* Galeazzi's fracture
    greenstick S52.31-
    oblique (displaced) S52.33-
      nondisplaced S52.33-
    segmental (displaced) S52.36-
      nondisplaced S52.36-
    specified NEC S52.39-
    spiral (displaced) S52.34-
      nondisplaced S52.34-
    transverse (displaced) S52.32-
      nondisplaced S52.32-
  upper end S52.10-
    head (displaced) S52.12-
      nondisplaced S52.12-
    neck (displaced) S52.13-
      nondisplaced S52.13-
    specified NEC S52.18-

Fracture, traumatic *(continued)*
radius *(continued)*
  upper end *(continued)*
    physeal S59.10-
      Salter-Harris
        Type I S59.11-
        Type II S59.12-
        Type III S59.13-
        Type IV S59.14-
      specified NEC S59.19-
    torus S52.11-
ramus
  inferior or superior, pubis —*see* Fracture, pubis
  mandible —*see* Fracture, mandible
restorative material (dental) K08.539
  with loss of material K08.531
  without loss of material K08.530
rib S22.3-
  with flail chest —*see* Flail, chest
  multiple S22.4-
    with flail chest —*see* Flail, chest
root, tooth —*see* Fracture, tooth
sacrum S32.10
  specified NEC S32.19
  Type
    1 S32.14
    2 S32.15
    3 S32.16
    4 S32.17
  Zone
    I S32.119
      displaced (minimally) S32.111
        severely S32.112
      nondisplaced S32.110
    II S32.129
      displaced (minimally) S32.121
        severely S32.122
      nondisplaced S32.120
    III S32.139
      displaced (minimally) S32.131
        severely S32.132
      nondisplaced S32.130
scaphoid (hand) —*see also* Fracture, carpal, navicular
  foot —*see* Fracture, tarsal, navicular
scapula S42.10-
  acromial process (displaced) S42.12-
    nondisplaced S42.12-
  body (displaced) S42.11-
    nondisplaced S42.11-
  coracoid process (displaced) S42.13-
    nondisplaced S42.13-
  glenoid cavity (displaced) S42.14-
    nondisplaced S42.14-
  neck (displaced) S42.15-
    nondisplaced S42.15-
  specified NEC S42.19-
semilunar bone, wrist —*see* Fracture, carpal, lunate
sequelae —*see* Sequelae, fracture
sesamoid bone
  hand —*see* Fracture, carpal
  foot S92.81-
  other —*see* Fracture, traumatic, by site
shepherd's —*see* Fracture, tarsal, talus

Fracture, traumatic *(continued)*

- shoulder (girdle) S42.9-
  - blade —*see* Fracture, scapula
- sinus (ethmoid) (frontal) S02.19
- skull S02.91
  - base S02.10-
    - occiput S02.119
      - condyle S02.113
        - type I S02.110
          - left side S02.11B
          - right side S02.11A
        - type II S02.111
          - left side S02.11D
          - right side S02.11C
        - type III S02.112
          - left side S02.11F
          - right side S02.11E
        - specified NEC S02.118
          - left side S02.11H
          - right side S02.11G
    - specified NEC S02.19
  - birth injury P13.0
  - frontal bone S02.0
  - parietal bone S02.0
  - specified site NEC S02.8-
  - temporal bone S02.19
  - vault S02.0
- Smith's —*see* Smith's fracture
- sphenoid (bone) (sinus) S02.19
- spine —*see* Fracture, vertebra
- spinous process —*see* Fracture, vertebra
- spontaneous (cause unknown) —*see* Fracture, pathological
- stave (of thumb) —*see* Fracture, metacarpal, first
- sternum S22.20
  - with flail chest —*see* Flail, chest
  - body S22.22
  - manubrium S22.21
  - xiphoid (process) S22.24
- stress M84.30
  - ankle M84.37-
  - carpus M84.34-
  - clavicle M84.31-
  - femoral neck M84.359
  - femur M84.35-
  - fibula M84.36-
  - finger M84.34-
  - hip M84.359
  - humerus M84.32-
  - ilium M84.350
  - ischium M84.350
  - metacarpus M84.34-
  - metatarsus M84.37-
  - neck —*see* Fracture, fatigue, vertebra
  - pelvis M84.350
  - radius M84.33-
  - rib M84.38
  - scapula M84.31-
  - skull M84.38
  - tarsus M84.37-
  - tibia M84.36-
  - toe M84.37-
  - ulna M84.33-
  - vertebra —*see* Fracture, fatigue, vertebra
- supracondylar, elbow —*see* Fracture, humerus, lower end, supracondylar
- symphysis pubis —*see* Fracture, pubis
- talus (ankle bone) —*see* Fracture, tarsal, talus
- tarsal bone(s) S92.20-
  - astragalus —*see* Fracture, tarsal, talus

Fracture, traumatic *(continued)*

- tarsal bone(s) *(continued)*
  - calcaneus S92.00-
    - anterior process (displaced) S92.02-
      - nondisplaced S92.02-
    - body (displaced) S92.01-
      - nondisplaced S92.01-
    - extraarticular NEC (displaced) S92.05-
      - nondisplaced S92.05-
    - intraarticular (displaced) S92.06-
      - nondisplaced S92.06-
    - physeal S99.00-
      - Salter-Harris
        - Type I S99.01-
        - Type II S99.02-
        - Type III S99.03-
        - Type IV S99.04-
      - specified NEC S99.09-
    - tuberosity (displaced) S92.04-
      - avulsion (displaced) S92.03-
        - nondisplaced S92.03-
      - nondisplaced S92.04-
  - cuboid (displaced) S92.21-
    - nondisplaced S92.21-
  - cuneiform
    - intermediate (displaced) S92.23-
      - nondisplaced S92.23-
    - lateral (displaced) S92.22-
      - nondisplaced S92.22-
    - medial (displaced) S92.24-
      - nondisplaced S92.24-
  - navicular (displaced) S92.25-
    - nondisplaced S92.25-
  - scaphoid —*see* Fracture, tarsal, navicular
  - talus S92.10-
    - avulsion (displaced) S92.15-
      - nondisplaced S92.15-
    - body (displaced) S92.12-
      - nondisplaced S92.12-
    - dome (displaced) S92.14-
      - nondisplaced S92.14-
    - head (displaced) S92.12-
      - nondisplaced S92.12-
    - lateral process (displaced) S92.14-
      - nondisplaced S92.14-
    - neck (displaced) S92.11-
      - nondisplaced S92.11-
    - posterior process (displaced) S92.13-
      - nondisplaced S92.13-
    - specified NEC S92.19-
- temporal bone (styloid) S02.19
- thorax (bony) S22.9
  - with flail chest —*see* Flail, chest
  - rib S22.3-
    - multiple S22.4-
      - with flail chest —*see* Flail, chest
  - sternum S22.20
    - body S22.22
    - manubrium S22.21
    - xiphoid process S22.24
  - vertebra (displaced) S22.009
    - burst (stable) S22.001
      - unstable S22.002
    - eighth S22.069
      - burst (stable) S22.061
        - unstable S22.062
      - specified type NEC S22.068
      - wedge compression S22.060

Fracture, traumatic *(continued)*

- thorax *(continued)*
  - vertebra *(continued)*
    - eleventh S22.089
      - burst (stable) S22.081
        - unstable S22.082
      - specified type NEC S22.088
      - wedge compression S22.080
    - fifth S22.059
      - burst (stable) S22.051
        - unstable S22.052
      - specified type NEC S22.058
      - wedge compression S22.050
    - first S22.019
      - burst (stable) S22.011
        - unstable S22.012
      - specified type NEC S22.018
      - wedge compression S22.010
    - fourth S22.049
      - burst (stable) S22.041
        - unstable S22.042
      - specified type NEC S22.048
      - wedge compression S22.040
    - ninth S22.079
      - burst (stable) S22.071
        - unstable S22.072
      - specified type NEC S22.078
      - wedge compression S22.070
    - nondisplaced S22.001
    - second S22.029
      - burst (stable) S22.021
        - unstable S22.022
      - specified type NEC S22.028
      - wedge compression S22.020
    - seventh S22.069
      - burst (stable) S22.061
        - unstable S22.062
      - specified type NEC S22.068
      - wedge compression S22.060
    - sixth S22.059
      - burst (stable) S22.051
        - unstable S22.052
      - specified type NEC S22.058
      - wedge compression S22.050
    - specified type NEC S22.008
    - tenth S22.079
      - burst (stable) S22.071
        - unstable S22.072
      - specified type NEC S22.078
      - wedge compression S22.070
    - third S22.039
      - burst (stable) S22.031
        - unstable S22.032
      - specified type NEC S22.038
      - wedge compression S22.030
    - twelfth S22.089
      - burst (stable) S22.081
        - unstable S22.082
      - specified type NEC S22.088
      - wedge compression S22.080
    - wedge compression S22.000
- thumb S62.50-
  - distal phalanx (displaced) S62.52-
    - nondisplaced S62.52-
  - proximal phalanx (displaced) S62.51-
    - nondisplaced S62.51-

Fracture, traumatic *(continued)*

- thyroid cartilage S12.8
- tibia (shaft) S82.20-
  - comminuted (displaced) S82.25-
    - nondisplaced S82.25-
  - condyles —*see* Fracture, tibia, upper end
  - distal end —*see* Fracture, tibia, lower end
  - epiphysis
    - lower —*see* Fracture, tibia, lower end
    - upper —*see* Fracture, tibia, upper end
  - following insertion of implant, prosthesis or plate M96.67-
  - head (involving knee joint) —*see* Fracture, tibia, upper end
  - intercondyloid eminence —*see* Fracture, tibia, upper end
  - involving ankle or malleolus —*see* Fracture, ankle, medial malleolus
  - lower end S82.30-
    - physeal S89.10-
      - Salter-Harris
        - Type I S89.11-
        - Type II S89.12-
        - Type III S89.13-
        - Type IV S89.14-
      - specified NEC S89.19-
    - pilon (displaced) S82.87-
      - nondisplaced S82.87-
    - specified NEC S82.39-
    - torus S82.31-
  - malleolus —*see* Fracture, ankle, medial malleolus
  - oblique (displaced) S82.23-
    - nondisplaced S82.23-
  - pilon —*see* Fracture, tibia, lower end, pilon
  - proximal end —*see* Fracture, tibia, upper end
  - segmental (displaced) S82.26-
    - nondisplaced S82.26-
  - specified NEC S82.29-
  - spine —*see* Fracture, tibia, upper end, spine
  - spiral (displaced) S82.24-
    - nondisplaced S82.24-
  - transverse (displaced) S82.22-
    - nondisplaced S82.22-
  - tuberosity —*see* Fracture, tibia, upper end, tuberosity
  - upper end S82.10-
    - bicondylar (displaced) S82.14-
      - nondisplaced S82.14-
    - lateral condyle (displaced) S82.12-
      - nondisplaced S82.12-
    - medial condyle (displaced) S82.13-
      - nondisplaced S82.13-
    - physeal S89.00-
      - Salter-Harris
        - Type I S89.01-
        - Type II S89.02-
        - Type III S89.03-
        - Type IV S89.04-
      - specified NEC S89.09-
    - plateau —*see* Fracture, tibia, upper end, bicondylar
    - spine (displaced) S82.11-
      - nondisplaced S82.11-
    - torus S82.16-
    - specified NEC S82.19-
    - tuberosity (displaced) S82.15-
      - nondisplaced S82.15-

Fracture, traumatic *(continued)*
toe S92.91-
great (displaced) S92.40-
distal phalanx (displaced) S92.42-
nondisplaced S92.42-
nondisplaced S92.40-
proximal phalanx (displaced) S92.41-
nondisplaced S92.41-
specified NEC S92.49-
lesser (displaced) S92.50-
distal phalanx (displaced) S92.53-
nondisplaced S92.53-
middle phalanx (displaced) S92.52-
nondisplaced S92.52-
nondisplaced S92.50-
proximal phalanx (displaced) S92.51-
nondisplaced S92.51-
specified NEC S92.59-
physeal
phalanx S99.20-
Salter-Harris
Type I S99.21-
Type II S99.22-
Type III S99.23-
Type IV S99.24-
specified NEC S99.29-
tooth (root) S02.5
trachea (cartilage) S12.8
transverse process —*see* Fracture, vertebra
trapezium or trapezoid bone —*see* Fracture, carpal
trimalleolar —*see* Fracture, ankle, trimalleolar
triquetrum (cuneiform of carpus) —*see* Fracture, carpal, triquetrum
trochanter —*see* Fracture, femur, trochanteric
tuberosity (external) —*see* Fracture, traumatic, by site
ulna (shaft) S52.20-
bent bone S52.28-
coronoid process —*see* Fracture, ulna, upper end, coronoid process
distal end —*see* Fracture, ulna, lower end
following insertion of implant, prosthesis or plate M96.63-
head S52.60-
lower end S52.60-
physeal S59.00-
Salter-Harris
Type I S59.01-
Type II S59.02-
Type III S59.03-
Type IV S59.04-
specified NEC S59.09-
specified NEC S52.69-
styloid process (displaced) S52.61-
nondisplaced S52.61-
torus S52.62-
proximal end —*see* Fracture, ulna, upper end
shaft S52.20-
comminuted (displaced) S52.25-
nondisplaced S52.25-
greenstick S52.21-
Monteggia's —*see* Monteggia's fracture
oblique (displaced) S52.23-
nondisplaced S52.23-

Fracture, traumatic *(continued)*
ulna *(continued)*
shaft *(continued)*
segmental (displaced) S52.26-
nondisplaced S52.26-
specified NEC S52.29-
spiral (displaced) S52.24-
nondisplaced S52.24-
transverse (displaced) S52.22-
nondisplaced S52.22-
upper end S52.00-
coronoid process (displaced) S52.04-
nondisplaced S52.04-
olecranon process (displaced) S52.02-
with intraarticular extension S52.03-
nondisplaced S52.02-
with intraarticular extension S52.03-
specified NEC S52.09-
torus S52.01-
unciform —*see* Fracture, carpal, hamate
vault of skull S02.0
vertebra, vertebral (arch) (body) (column) (neural arch) (pedicle) (spinous process) (transverse process)
atlas —*see* Fracture, neck, cervical vertebra, first
axis —*see* Fracture, neck, cervical vertebra, second
cervical (teardrop) S12.9
axis —*see* Fracture, neck, cervical vertebra, second
first (atlas) —*see* Fracture, neck, cervical vertebra, first
second (axis) —*see* Fracture, neck, cervical vertebra, second
chronic M84.48
coccyx S32.2
dorsal —*see* Fracture, thorax, vertebra
lumbar S32.009
burst (stable) S32.001
unstable S32.002
fifth S32.059
burst (stable) S32.051
unstable S32.052
specified type NEC S32.058
wedge compression S32.050
first S32.019
burst (stable) S32.011
unstable S32.012
specified type NEC S32.018
wedge compression S32.010
fourth S32.049
burst (stable) S32.041
unstable S32.042
specified type NEC S32.048
wedge compression S32.040
second S32.029
burst (stable) S32.021
unstable S32.022
specified type NEC S32.028
wedge compression S32.020
specified type NEC S32.008
third S32.039
burst (stable) S32.031
unstable S32.032
specified type NEC S32.038
wedge compression S32.030
wedge compression S32.000

Fracture, traumatic *(continued)*
vertebra, vertebral *(continued)*
metastatic —*see* Collapse, vertebra, in, specified disease NEC —*see also* Neoplasm
newborn (birth injury) P11.5
sacrum S32.10
specified NEC S32.19
Type
1 S32.14
2 S32.15
3 S32.16
4 S32.17
Zone
I S32.119
displaced (minimally) S32.111
severely S32.112
nondisplaced S32.110
II S32.129
displaced (minimally) S32.121
severely S32.122
nondisplaced S32.120
III S32.139
displaced (minimally) S32.131
severely S32.132
nondisplaced S32.130
thoracic —*see* Fracture, thorax, vertebra
vertex S02.0
vomer (bone) S02.2
wrist S62.10-
carpal —*see* Fracture, carpal bone
navicular (scaphoid) (hand) —*see* Fracture, carpal, navicular
xiphisternum, xiphoid (process) S22.24
zygoma S02.402
left side S02.40F
right side S02.40E

Fragile, fragility
autosomal site Q95.5
bone, congenital (with blue sclera) Q78.0
capillary (hereditary) D69.8
hair L67.8
nails L60.3
non-sex chromosome site Q95.5
X chromosome Q99.2

Fragilitas
crinium L67.8
ossium (with blue sclerae) (hereditary) Q78.0
unguium L60.3
congenital Q84.6

Fragments, cataract (lens), **following cataract surgery** H59.02-
retained foreign body —*see* Retained, foreign body fragments (type of)

Frailty (frail) R54
mental R41.81

Frambesia, frambesial (tropica) —*see also* Yaws
initial lesion or ulcer A66.0
primary A66.0

Frambeside
gummatous A66.4
of early yaws A66.2

Frambesioma A66.1

Franceschetti-Klein (-Wildervanck) **disease or syndrome** Q75.4

Francis' disease —*see* Tularemia

Franklin disease C88.2

Frank's essential thrombocytopenia D69.3

Fraser's syndrome Q87.0

Freckle(s) L81.2
malignant melanoma in —*see* Melanoma
melanotic (Hutchinson's) —*see* Melanoma, in situ
retinal D49.81

Frederickson's hyperlipoproteinemia, type
I and V E78.3
IIA E78.00
IIB and III E78.2
IV E78.1

Freeman Sheldon syndrome Q87.0

Freezing (*see also* Effect, adverse, cold) T69.9

Freiberg's disease (infraction of metatarsal head or osteochondrosis) —*see* Osteochondrosis, juvenile, metatarsus

Frei's disease A55

Fremitus, friction, cardiac R01.2

Frenum, frenulum
external os Q51.828
tongue (shortening) (congenital) Q38.1

Frequency micturition (nocturnal) R35.0
psychogenic F45.8

Frey's syndrome
auriculotemporal G50.8
hyperhidrosis L74.52

Friction
burn —*see* Burn, by site
fremitus, cardiac R01.2
precordial R01.2
sounds, chest R09.89

Friderichsen-Waterhouse syndrome or disease A39.1

Friedländer's B (bacillus) **NEC** (*see also* condition) A49.8

Friedreich's
ataxia G11.11
combined systemic disease G11.11
facial hemihypertrophy Q67.4
sclerosis (cerebellum) (spinal cord) G11.11

Frigidity F52.22

Fröhlich's syndrome E23.6

Frontal —*see also* condition
lobe syndrome F07.0

Frostbite (superficial) T33.90
with
partial thickness skin loss —*see* Frostbite (superficial), by site
tissue necrosis T34.90
abdominal wall T33.3
with tissue necrosis T34.3
ankle T33.81-
with tissue necrosis T34.81-
arm T33.4-
with tissue necrosis T34.4-
finger(s) —*see* Frostbite, finger
hand —*see* Frostbite, hand
wrist —*see* Frostbite, wrist
ear T33.01-
with tissue necrosis T34.01-
face T33.09
with tissue necrosis T34.09

Frostbite *(continued)*
finger T33.53-
with tissue necrosis T34.53-
foot T33.82-
with tissue necrosis T34.82-
hand T33.52-
with tissue necrosis T34.52-
head T33.09
with tissue necrosis T34.09
ear —*see* Frostbite, ear
nose —*see* Frostbite, nose
hip (and thigh) T33.6-
with tissue necrosis T34.6-
knee T33.7-
with tissue necrosis T34.7-
leg T33.9-
with tissue necrosis T34.9-
ankle —*see* Frostbite, ankle
foot —*see* Frostbite, foot
knee —*see* Frostbite, knee
lower T33.7-
with tissue necrosis T34.7-
thigh —*see* Frostbite, hip
toe —*see* Frostbite, toe
limb
lower T33.99
with tissue necrosis T34.99
upper —*see* Frostbite, arm
neck T33.1
with tissue necrosis T34.1
nose T33.02
with tissue necrosis T34.02
pelvis T33.3
with tissue necrosis T34.3
specified site NEC T33.99
with tissue necrosis T34.99
thigh —*see* Frostbite, hip
thorax T33.2
with tissue necrosis T34.2
toes T33.83-
with tissue necrosis T34.83-
trunk T33.99
with tissue necrosis T34.99
wrist T33.51-
with tissue necrosis T34.51-

Frotteurism F65.81

Frozen —*see also* Effect, adverse, cold T69.9
pelvis (female) N94.89
male K66.8
shoulder —*see* Capsulitis, adhesive

Fructokinase deficiency E74.11

Fructose 1,6 diphosphatase deficiency E74.19

Fructosemia (benign) (essential) E74.12

Fructosuria (benign) (essential) E74.11

Fuchs'
black spot (myopic) (*see also* Myopia, degenerative) H44.2-
dystrophy (corneal endothelium) H18.51-
heterochromic cyclitis —*see* Cyclitis, Fuchs' heterochromic

Fucosidosis E77.1

Fugue R68.89
dissociative F44.1
hysterical (dissociative) F44.1
postictal in epilepsy —*see* Epilepsy
reaction to exceptional stress (transient) F43.0

Fulminant, fulminating —*see* condition

Functional —*see also* condition
bleeding (uterus) N93.8

Functioning, intellectual, borderline R41.83

Fundus —*see* condition

Fungemia NOS B49

Fungus, fungous
cerebral G93.89
disease NOS B49
infection —*see* Infection, fungus

Funiculitis (acute) (chronic) (endemic) N49.1
gonococcal (acute) (chronic) A54.23
tuberculous A18.15

Funnel
breast (acquired) M95.4
congenital Q67.6
sequelae (late effect) of rickets E64.3
chest (acquired) M95.4
congenital Q67.6
sequelae (late effect) of rickets E64.3
pelvis (acquired) M95.5
with disproportion (fetopelvic) O33.3
causing obstructed labor O65.3
congenital Q74.2

FUO (fever of unknown origin) R50.9

Furfur L21.0
microsporon B36.0

Furrier's lung J67.8

Furrowed K14.5
nail(s) (transverse) L60.4
congenital Q84.6
tongue K14.5
congenital Q38.3

Furuncle L02.92
abdominal wall L02.221
ankle —*see* Furuncle, lower limb
anus K61.0
antecubital space —*see* Furuncle, upper limb
arm —*see* Furuncle, upper limb
auditory canal, external —*see* Abscess, ear, external
auricle (ear) —*see* Abscess, ear, external
axilla (region) L02.42-
back (any part) L02.222
breast N61.1
buttock L02.32
cheek (external) L02.02
chest wall L02.223
chin L02.02
corpus cavernosum N48.21
ear, external —*see* Abscess, ear, external
external auditory canal —*see* Abscess, ear, external
eyelid —*see* Abscess, eyelid
face L02.02
femoral (region) —*see* Furuncle, lower limb
finger —*see* Furuncle, hand
flank L02.221
foot L02.62-
forehead L02.02
gluteal (region) L02.32
groin L02.224
hand L02.52-
head L02.821
face L02.02
hip —*see* Furuncle, lower limb
kidney —*see* Abscess, kidney
knee —*see* Furuncle, lower limb
labium (majus) (minus) N76.4

Furuncle *(continued)*
lacrimal
gland —*see* Dacryoadenitis
passages (duct) (sac) —*see* Inflammation, lacrimal, passages, acute
leg (any part) —*see* Furuncle, lower limb
lower limb L02.42-
malignant A22.0
mouth K12.2
navel L02.226
neck L02.12
nose J34.0
orbit, orbital —*see* Abscess, orbit
palmar (space) —*see* Furuncle, hand
partes posteriores L02.32
pectoral region L02.223
penis N48.21
perineum L02.225
pinna —*see* Abscess, ear, external
popliteal —*see* Furuncle, lower limb
prepatellar —*see* Furuncle, lower limb
scalp L02.821
seminal vesicle N49.0
shoulder —*see* Furuncle, upper limb
specified site NEC L02.828
submandibular K12.2
temple (region) L02.02
thumb —*see* Furuncle, hand
toe —*see* Furuncle, foot
trunk L02.229
abdominal wall L02.221
back L02.222
chest wall L02.223
groin L02.224
perineum L02.225
umbilicus L02.226
umbilicus L02.226
upper limb L02.42-
vulva N76.4

Furunculosis —*see* Furuncle

Fused —*see* Fusion, fused

Fusion, fused (congenital)
astragaloscaphoid Q74.2
atria Q21.1
auditory canal Q16.1
auricles, heart Q21.1
binocular with defective stereopsis H53.32
bone Q79.8
cervical spine M43.22
choanal Q30.0
commissure, mitral valve Q23.2
cusps, heart valve NEC Q24.8
mitral Q23.2
pulmonary Q22.1
tricuspid Q22.4
ear ossicles Q16.3
fingers Q70.0-
hymen Q52.3
joint (acquired) —*see also* Ankylosis
congenital Q74.8
kidneys (incomplete) Q63.1
labium (majus) (minus) Q52.5
larynx and trachea Q34.8
limb, congenital Q74.8
lower Q74.2
upper Q74.0
lobes, lung Q33.8
lumbosacral (acquired) M43.27
arthrodesis status Z98.1
congenital Q76.49
postprocedural status Z98.1
nares, nose, nasal, nostril(s) Q30.0

Fusion, fused *(continued)*
organ or site not listed —*see* Anomaly, by site
ossicles Q79.9
auditory Q16.3
pulmonic cusps Q22.1
ribs Q76.6
sacroiliac (joint) (acquired) M43.28
arthrodesis status Z98.1
congenital Q74.2
postprocedural status Z98.1
spine (acquired) NEC M43.20
arthrodesis status Z98.1
cervical region M43.22
cervicothoracic region M43.23
congenital Q76.49
lumbar M43.26
lumbosacral region M43.27
occipito-atlanto-axial region M43.21
postoperative status Z98.1
sacrococcygeal region M43.28
thoracic region M43.24
thoracolumbar region M43.25
sublingual duct with submaxillary duct at opening in mouth Q38.4
testes Q55.1
toes Q70.2-
tooth, teeth K00.2
trachea and esophagus Q39.8
twins Q89.4
vagina Q52.4
ventricles, heart Q21.0
vertebra (arch) —*see* Fusion, spine
vulva Q52.5

Fusospirillosis (mouth) (tongue) (tonsil) A69.1

Fussy baby R68.12

G

Gain in weight (abnormal) (excessive) —*see also* Weight, gain

Gaisböck's disease (polycythemia hypertonica) D75.1

Gait abnormality R26.9
ataxic R26.0
falling R29.6
hysterical (ataxic) (staggering) F44.4
paralytic R26.1
spastic R26.1
specified type NEC R26.89
staggering R26.0
unsteadiness R26.81
walking difficulty NEC R26.2

Galactocele (breast) N64.89
puerperal, postpartum O92.79

Galactokinase deficiency E74.29

Galactophoritis N61.0
gestational, puerperal, postpartum O91.2-

Galactorrhea O92.6
not associated with childbirth N64.3

Galactosemia (classic) (congenital) E74.21

Galactosuria E74.29

Galacturia R82.0
schistosomiasis (bilharziasis) B65.0

GALD (gestational alloimmune liver disease) P78.84

Galeazzi's fracture S52.37-

Galen's vein —*see* condition

Galeophobia F40.218

Gall duct —*see* condition

Gallbladder —*see also* condition
- acute K81.0

Gallop rhythm R00.8

Gallstone (colic) (cystic duct) (gallbladder) (impacted) (multiple) —*see also* Calculus, gallbladder
- with
  - cholecystitis —*see* Calculus, gallbladder, with cholecystitis
- bile duct (common) (hepatic) —*see* Calculus, bile duct
- causing intestinal obstruction K56.3
- specified NEC K80.80
  - with obstruction K80.81

Gambling Z72.6
- pathological (compulsive) F63.0

Gammopathy (of undetermined significance [MGUS]) D47.2
- associated with lymphoplasmacytic dyscrasia D47.2
- monoclonal D47.2
- polyclonal D89.0

Gamna's disease (siderotic splenomegaly) D73.1

Gamophobia F40.298

Gampsodactylia (congenital) Q66.7-

Gamstorp's disease (adynamia episodica hereditaria) G72.3

Gandy-Nanta disease (siderotic splenomegaly) D73.1

Gang
- membership offenses Z72.810

Gangliocytoma D36.10

Ganglioglioma —*see* Neoplasm, uncertain behavior, by site

Ganglion (compound) (diffuse) (joint) (tendon (sheath)) M67.40
- ankle M67.47-
- foot M67.47-
- forearm M67.43-
- hand M67.44-
- lower leg M67.46-
- multiple sites M67.49
- of yaws (early) (late) A66.6
- pelvic region M67.45-
- periosteal —*see* Periostitis
- shoulder region M67.41-
- specified site NEC M67.48
- thigh region M67.45-
- tuberculous A18.09
- upper arm M67.42-
- wrist M67.43-

Ganglioneuroblastoma —*see* Neoplasm, nerve, malignant

Ganglioneuroma D36.10
- malignant —*see* Neoplasm, nerve, malignant

Ganglioneuromatosis D36.10

Ganglionitis
- fifth nerve —*see* Neuralgia, trigeminal
- gasserian (postherpetic) (postzoster) B02.21
- geniculate G51.1
  - newborn (birth injury) P11.3
  - postherpetic, postzoster B02.21
- herpes zoster B02.21
- postherpetic geniculate B02.21

Gangliosidosis E75.10
- GM1 E75.19
- GM2 E75.00
  - other specified E75.09
  - Sandhoff disease E75.01
  - Tay-Sachs disease E75.02
- GM3 E75.19
- mucolipidosis IV E75.11

Gangosa A66.5

Gangrene, gangrenous (connective tissue) (dropsical) (dry) (moist) (skin) (ulcer) —*see also* Necrosis I96
- with diabetes (mellitus) —*see* Diabetes, with, gangrene
- abdomen (wall) I96
- alveolar M27.3
- appendix K35.80
  - with
    - peritonitis, localized —*see also* Appendicitis K35.31
- arteriosclerotic (general) (senile) —*see* Arteriosclerosis, extremities, with, gangrene
- auricle I96
- Bacillus welchii A48.0
- bladder (infectious) —*see* Cystitis, specified type NEC
- bowel, cecum, or colon —*see* Gangrene, intestine
- Clostridium perfringens or welchii A48.0
- cornea H18.89-
- corpora cavernosa N48.29
  - noninfective N48.89
- cutaneous, spreading I96
- decubital —*see* Ulcer, pressure, by site
- diabetic (any site) —*see* Diabetes, with, gangrene
- epidemic —*see* Poisoning, food, noxious, plant
- epididymis (infectional) N45.1
- erysipelas —*see* Erysipelas
- emphysematous —*see* Gangrene, gas
- extremity (lower) (upper) I96
- Fournier N49.3
  - female N76.89
- fusospirochetal A69.0
- gallbladder —*see* Cholecystitis, acute
- gas (bacillus) A48.0
  - following
    - abortion —*see* Abortion by type complicated by infection
    - ectopic or molar pregnancy O08.0
- glossitis K14.0
- hernia —*see* Hernia, by site, with gangrene
- intestine, intestinal (hemorrhagic) (massive) (*see also* Infarct, intestine) K55.069
  - with
    - mesenteric embolism (*see also* Infarct, intestine) K55.069
    - obstruction —*see* Obstruction, intestine
- laryngitis J04.0
- limb (lower) (upper) I96
- lung J85.0
  - spirochetal A69.8
- lymphangitis I89.1

Gangrene, gangrenous *(continued)*
- Meleney's (synergistic) —*see* Ulcer, skin
- mesentery (*see also* Infarct, intestine) K55.069
  - with
    - embolism (*see also* Infarct, intestine) K55.069
    - intestinal obstruction —*see* Obstruction, intestine
- mouth A69.0
- ovary —*see* Oophoritis
- pancreas —*see* Pancreatitis, acute
- penis N48.29
  - noninfective N48.89
- perineum I96
- pharynx —*see also* Pharyngitis
  - Vincent's A69.1
- presenile I73.1
- progressive synergistic —*see* Ulcer, skin
- pulmonary J85.0
- pulpal (dental) K04.1
- quinsy J36
- Raynaud's (symmetric gangrene) I73.01
- retropharyngeal J39.2
- scrotum N49.3
  - noninfective N50.89
- senile (atherosclerotic) —*see* Arteriosclerosis, extremities, with, gangrene
- spermatic cord N49.1
  - noninfective N50.89
- spine I96
- spirochetal NEC A69.8
- spreading cutaneous I96
- stomatitis A69.0
- symmetrical I73.01
- testis (infectional) N45.2
  - noninfective N44.8
- throat —*see also* Pharyngitis
  - diphtheritic A36.0
  - Vincent's A69.1
- thyroid (gland) E07.89
- tooth (pulp) K04.1
- tuberculous NEC —*see* Tuberculosis
- tunica vaginalis N49.1
  - noninfective N50.89
- umbilicus I96
- uterus —*see* Endometritis
- uvulitis K12.2
- vas deferens N49.1
  - noninfective N50.89
- vulva N76.89

Ganister disease J62.8

Ganser's syndrome (hysterical) F44.89

Gardner-Diamond syndrome (autoerythrocyte sensitization) D69.2

Gargoylism E76.01

Garré's disease, osteitis (sclerosing), **osteomyelitis** —*see* Osteomyelitis, specified type NEC

Garrod's pad, knuckle M72.1

Gartner's duct
- cyst Q52.4
- persistent Q50.6

Gas R14.3
- asphyxiation, inhalation, poisoning, suffocation NEC —*see* Table of Drugs and Chemicals
- excessive R14.0
- gangrene A48.0

Gas *(continued)*
- gangrene *(continued)*
  - following
    - abortion —*see* Abortion by type complicated by infection
    - ectopic or molar pregnancy O08.0
- on stomach R14.0
- pains R14.1

Gastralgia —*see also* Pain, abdominal

Gastrectasis K31.0
- psychogenic F45.8

Gastric —*see* condition

Gastrinoma
- malignant
  - pancreas C25.4
  - specified site NEC —*see* Neoplasm, malignant, by site
  - unspecified site C25.4
- specified site —*see* Neoplasm, uncertain behavior
- unspecified site D37.9

Gastritis (simple) K29.70
- with bleeding K29.71
- acute (erosive) K29.00
  - with bleeding K29.01
- alcoholic K29.20
  - with bleeding K29.21
- allergic K29.60
  - with bleeding K29.61
- atrophic (chronic) K29.40
  - with bleeding K29.41
- chronic (antral) (fundal) K29.50
  - with bleeding K29.51
  - atrophic K29.40
    - with bleeding K29.41
  - superficial K29.30
    - with bleeding K29.31
- dietary counseling and surveillance Z71.3
- due to diet deficiency E63.9
- eosinophilic K52.81
- giant hypertrophic K29.60
  - with bleeding K29.61
- granulomatous K29.60
  - with bleeding K29.61
- hypertrophic (mucosa) K29.60
  - with bleeding K29.61
- nervous F54
- spastic K29.60
  - with bleeding K29.61
- specified NEC K29.60
  - with bleeding K29.61
- superficial chronic K29.30
  - with bleeding K29.31
- tuberculous A18.83
- viral NEC A08.4

Gastrocarcinoma —*see* Neoplasm, malignant, stomach

Gastrocolic —*see* condition

Gastrodisciasis, gastrodiscoidiasis B66.8

Gastroduodenitis K29.90
- with bleeding K29.91
- virus, viral A08.4
  - specified type NEC A08.39

Gastrodynia —*see* Pain, abdominal

Gastroenteritis (acute) (chronic) (noninfectious) (*see also* Enteritis) K52.9
- allergic K52.29
  - with
    - eosinophilic gastritis or gastroenteritis K52.81

Gastroenteritis *(continued)*
- allergic *(continued)*
  - with *(continued)*
    - food protein-induced enterocolitis syndrome K52.21
    - food protein-induced enteropathy K52.22
- dietetic (*see also* Gastroenteritis, allergic) K52.29
- drug-induced K52.1
- due to
  - Cryptosporidium A07.2
  - drugs K52.1
  - food poisoning *—see* Intoxication, foodborne
  - radiation K52.0
- eosinophilic K52.81
- epidemic (infectious) A09
- food hypersensitivity (*see also* Gastroenteritis, allergic) K52.29
- infectious *—see* Enteritis, infectious
- influenzal *—see* Influenza, with gastroenteritis
- noninfectious K52.9
  - specified NEC K52.89
- rotaviral A08.0
- Salmonella A02.0
- toxic K52.1
- viral NEC A08.4
  - acute infectious A08.39
    - type Norwalk A08.11
  - infantile (acute) A08.39
  - Norwalk agent A08.11
  - rotaviral A08.0
  - severe of infants A08.39
  - specified type NEC A08.39

Gastroenteropathy (*see also* Gastroenteritis) K52.9
- acute, due to Norwalk agent A08.11
- acute, due to Norovirus A08.11
- infectious A09

Gastroenteroptosis K63.4

Gastroesophageal laceration-hemorrhage syndrome K22.6

Gastrointestinal *—see* condition

Gastrojejunal *—see* condition

Gastrojejunitis (*see also* Enteritis) K52.9

Gastrojejunocolic *—see* condition

Gastroliths K31.89

Gastromalacia K31.89

Gastroparalysis K31.84
- diabetic *—see* Diabetes, gastroparalysis

Gastroparesis K31.84
- diabetic *—see* Diabetes, by type, with gastroparesis

Gastropathy K31.9
- congestive portal (*see also*, Hypertension, portal) K31.89
- erythematous K29.70
- exudative K90.89
- portal hypertensive (*see also*, Hypertension, portal) K31.89

Gastroptosis K31.89

Gastrorrhagia K92.2
- psychogenic F45.8

Gastroschisis (congenital) Q79.3

Gastrospasm (neurogenic) (reflex) K31.89
- neurotic F45.8
- psychogenic F45.8

Gastrostaxis *—see* Gastritis, with bleeding

Gastrostenosis K31.89

Gastrostomy
- attention to Z43.1
- status Z93.1

Gastrosuccorrhea (continuous) (intermittent) K31.89
- neurotic F45.8
- psychogenic F45.8

Gatophobia F40.218

Gaucher's disease or splenomegaly (adult) (infantile) E75.22

Gee (-Herter) (-Thaysen) **disease** (nontropical sprue) K90.0

Gélineau's syndrome G47.419
- with cataplexy G47.411

Gemination, tooth, teeth K00.2

Gemistocytoma
- specified site *—see* Neoplasm, malignant, by site
- unspecified site C71.9

General, generalized *—see* condition

Genetic
- carrier (status)
  - cystic fibrosis Z14.1
  - hemophilia A (asymptomatic) Z14.01
    - symptomatic Z14.02
  - specified NEC Z14.8
- susceptibility to disease NEC Z15.89
  - malignant neoplasm Z15.09
    - breast Z15.01
    - endometrium Z15.04
    - ovary Z15.02
    - prostate Z15.03
    - specified NEC Z15.09
  - multiple endocrine neoplasia Z15.81

Genital *—see* condition

Genito-anorectal syndrome A55

Genitourinary system *—see* condition

Genu
- congenital Q74.1
- extrorsum (acquired) *—see also* Deformity, varus, knee
  - congenital Q74.1
  - sequelae (late effect) of rickets E64.3
- introrsum (acquired) *—see also* Deformity, valgus, knee
  - congenital Q74.1
  - sequelae (late effect) of rickets E64.3
- rachitic (old) E64.3
- recurvatum (acquired) *—see also* Deformity, limb, specified type NEC, lower leg
  - congenital Q68.2
  - sequelae (late effect) of rickets E64.3
- valgum (acquired) (knock-knee) M21.06-
  - congenital Q74.1
  - sequelae (late effect) of rickets E64.3
- varum (acquired) (bowleg) M21.16-
  - congenital Q74.1
  - sequelae (late effect) of rickets E64.3

Geographic tongue K14.1

Geophagia *—see* Pica

Geotrichosis B48.3
- stomatitis B48.3

Gephyrophobia F40.242

Gerbode defect Q21.0

GERD (gastroesophageal reflux disease) K21.9

Gerhardt's
- disease (erythromelalgia) I73.81
- syndrome (vocal cord paralysis) J38.00
  - bilateral J38.02
  - unilateral J38.01

German measles *—see also* Rubella
- exposure to Z20.4

Germinoblastoma (diffuse) C85.9-
- follicular C82.9-

Germinoma *—see* Neoplasm, malignant, by site

Gerontoxon *—see* Degeneration, cornea, senile

Gerstmann-Sträussler-Scheinker syndrome (GSS) A81.82

Gerstmann's syndrome R48.8
- developmental F81.2

Gestation (period) *—see also* Pregnancy
- ectopic *—see* Pregnancy, by site
- multiple O30.9-
  - greater than quadruplets *—see* Pregnancy, multiple (gestation), specified NEC
  - specified NEC *—see* Pregnancy, multiple (gestation), specified NEC

Gestational
- mammary abscess O91.11-
- purulent mastitis O91.11-
- subareolar abscess O91.11-

Ghon tubercle, primary infection A15.7

Ghost
- teeth K00.4
- vessels (cornea) H16.41-

Ghoul hand A66.3

Gianotti-Crosti disease L44.4

Giant
- cell
  - epulis K06.8
  - peripheral granuloma K06.8
- esophagus, congenital Q39.5
- kidney, congenital Q63.3
- urticaria T78.3
  - hereditary D84.1

Giardiasis A07.1

Gibert's disease or pityriasis L42

Giddiness R42
- hysterical F44.89
- psychogenic F45.8

Gierke's disease (glycogenosis I) E74.01

Gigantism (cerebral) (hypophyseal) (pituitary) E22.0
- constitutional E34.4

Gilbert's disease or syndrome E80.4

Gilchrist's disease B40.9

Gilford-Hutchinson disease E34.8

Gilles de la Tourette's disease or syndrome (motor-verbal tic) F95.2

Gingivitis K05.10
- acute (catarrhal) K05.00
  - necrotizing A69.1
  - nonplaque induced K05.01
  - plaque induced K05.00
- chronic (desquamative) (hyperplastic) (simple marginal) (pregnancy associated) (ulcerative) K05.10
  - nonplaque induced K05.11
  - plaque induced K05.10
- expulsiva *—see* Periodontitis
- necrotizing ulcerative (acute) A69.1
- pellagrous E52
  - acute necrotizing A69.1
- Vincent's A69.1

Gingivoglossitis K14.0

Gingivopericementitis *—see* Periodontitis

Gingivosis *—see* Gingivitis, chronic

Gingivostomatitis K05.10
- herpesviral B00.2
- necrotizing ulcerative (acute) A69.1

Gland, glandular *—see* condition

Glanders A24.0

Glanzmann (-Naegeli) **disease or thrombasthenia** D69.1

Glasgow coma scale
- total score
  - 3-8 R40.243
  - 9-12 R40.242
  - 13-15 R40.241

Glass-blower's disease (cataract) *—see* Cataract, specified NEC

Glaucoma H40.9
- with
  - increased episcleral venous pressure H40.81-
  - pseudoexfoliation of lens *—see* Glaucoma, open angle, primary, capsular
- absolute H44.51-
- angle-closure (primary) H40.20-
  - acute (attack) (crisis) H40.21-
  - chronic H40.22-
  - intermittent H40.23-
  - residual stage H40.24-
- borderline H40.00-
- capsular (with pseudoexfoliation of lens) *—see* Glaucoma, open angle, primary, capsular
- childhood Q15.0
- closed angle *—see* Glaucoma, angle-closure
- congenital Q15.0
- corticosteroid-induced *—see* Glaucoma, secondary, drugs
- hypersecretion H40.82-
- in (due to)
  - amyloidosis E85.4 *[H42]*
  - aniridia Q13.1 *[H42]*
  - concussion of globe *—see* Glaucoma, secondary, trauma
  - dislocation of lens *—see* Glaucoma, secondary
  - disorder of lens NEC *—see* Glaucoma, secondary
  - drugs *—see* Glaucoma, secondary, drugs
  - endocrine disease NOS E34.9 *[H42]*
  - eye
    - inflammation *—see* Glaucoma, secondary, inflammation
    - trauma *—see* Glaucoma, secondary, trauma

Glaucoma *(continued)*
- in *(continued)*
  - hypermature cataract *—see* Glaucoma, secondary
  - iridocyclitis *—see* Glaucoma, secondary, inflammation
  - lens disorder *—see* Glaucoma, secondary,
  - Lowe's syndrome E72.03 *[H42]*
  - metabolic disease NOS E88.9 *[H42]*
  - ocular disorders NEC *—see* Glaucoma, secondary
  - onchocerciasis B73.02
  - pupillary block *—see* Glaucoma, secondary
  - retinal vein occlusion *—see* Glaucoma, secondary
  - Rieger's anomaly Q13.81 *[H42]*
  - rubeosis of iris *—see* Glaucoma, secondary
  - tumor of globe *—see* Glaucoma, secondary
- infantile Q15.0
- low tension *—see* Glaucoma, open angle, primary, low-tension
- malignant H40.83-
- narrow angle *—see* Glaucoma, angle-closure
- newborn Q15.0
- noncongestive (chronic) *—see* Glaucoma, open angle
- nonobstructive *—see* Glaucoma, open angle
- obstructive *—see also* Glaucoma, angle-closure
  - due to lens changes *—see* Glaucoma, secondary
- open angle H40.10-
  - primary H40.11-
    - capsular (with pseudoexfoliation of lens) H40.14-
    - low-tension H40.12-
    - pigmentary H40.13-
    - residual stage H40.15-
- phacolytic *—see* Glaucoma, secondary
- pigmentary *—see* Glaucoma, open angle, primary, pigmentary
- postinfectious *—see* Glaucoma, secondary, inflammation
- secondary (to) H40.5-
  - drugs H40.6-
  - inflammation H40.4-
  - trauma H40.3-
- simple (chronic) H40.11-
- simplex H40.11-
- specified type NEC H40.89
- suspect H40.00-
- syphilitic A52.71
- traumatic *—see also* Glaucoma, secondary, trauma
  - newborn (birth injury) P15.3
- tuberculous A18.59

Glaucomatous flecks (subcapsular) *—see* Cataract, complicated

Glazed tongue K14.4

Gleet (gonococcal) A54.01

Glénard's disease K63.4

Glioblastoma (multiforme)
- with sarcomatous component
  - specified site *—see* Neoplasm, malignant, by site
  - unspecified site C71.9
- giant cell
  - specified site *—see* Neoplasm, malignant, by site

Glioblastoma *(continued)*
- giant cell *(continued)*
  - unspecified site C71.9
- specified site *—see* Neoplasm, malignant, by site
- unspecified site C71.9

Glioma (malignant)
- astrocytic
  - specified site *—see* Neoplasm, malignant, by site
  - unspecified site C71.9
- mixed
  - specified site *—see* Neoplasm, malignant, by site
  - unspecified site C71.9
- nose Q30.8
- specified site NEC *—see* Neoplasm, malignant, by site
- subependymal D43.2
  - specified site *—see* Neoplasm, uncertain behavior, by site
  - unspecified site D43.2
- unspecified site C71.9

Gliomatosis cerebri C71.0

Glioneuroma *—see* Neoplasm, uncertain behavior, by site

Gliosarcoma
- specified site *—see* Neoplasm, malignant, by site
- unspecified site C71.9

Gliosis (cerebral) G93.89
- spinal G95.89

Glisson's disease *—see* Rickets

Globinuria R82.3

Globus (hystericus) F45.8

Glomangioma D18.00
- intra-abdominal D18.03
- intracranial D18.02
- skin D18.01
- specified site NEC D18.09

Glomangiomyoma D18.00
- intra-abdominal D18.03
- intracranial D18.02
- skin D18.01
- specified site NEC D18.09

Glomangiosarcoma *—see* Neoplasm, connective tissue, malignant

Glomerular
- disease in syphilis A52.75
- nephritis *—see* Glomerulonephritis

Glomerulitis *—see* Glomerulonephritis

Glomerulonephritis (*see also* Nephritis) N05.9
- with
  - C3
    - glomerulonephritis N05.A
    - glomerulopathy N05.A
      - with dense deposit disease N05.6
  - edema *—see* Nephrosis
  - minimal change N05.0
  - minor glomerular abnormality N05.0
- acute N00.9
- chronic N03.9
- crescentic (diffuse) NEC (*see also* N00-N07 with fourth character .7) N05.7
- dense deposit (*see also* N00-N07 with fourth character .6) N05.6
- diffuse
  - crescentic (*see also* N00-N07 with fourth character .7) N05.7
  - endocapillary proliferative (*see also* N00-N07 with fourth character .4) N05.4

Glomerulonephritis *(continued)*
- diffuse *(continued)*
  - membranous (*see also* N00-N07 with fourth character .2) N05.2
  - mesangial proliferative (*see also* N00-N07 with fourth character .3) N05.3
  - mesangiocapillary (*see also* N00-N07 with fourth character .5) N05.5
  - sclerosing N18.9
- endocapillary proliferative (diffuse) NEC (*see also* N00-N07 with fourth character .4) N05.4
- extracapillary NEC (*see also* N00-N07 with fourth character .7) N05.7
- focal (and segmental) (*see also* N00-N07 with fourth character .1) N05.1
- hypocomplementemic *—see* Glomerulonephritis, membranoproliferative
- IgA *—see* Nephropathy, IgA
- immune complex (circulating) NEC N05.8
- in (due to)
  - amyloidosis E85.4 *[N08]*
  - bilharziasis B65.9 *[N08]*
  - cryoglobulinemia D89.1 *[N08]*
  - defibrination syndrome D65 *[N08]*
  - diabetes mellitus *—see* Diabetes, glomerulosclerosis
  - disseminated intravascular coagulation D65 *[N08]*
  - Fabry (-Anderson) disease E75.21 *[N08]*
  - Goodpasture's syndrome M31.0
  - hemolytic-uremic syndrome D59.3
  - Henoch (-Schönlein) purpura D69.0 *[N08]*
  - lecithin cholesterol acyltransferase deficiency E78.6 *[N08]*
  - microscopic polyangiitis M31.7 *[N08]*
  - multiple myeloma C90.0- *[N08]*
  - Plasmodium malariae B52.0
  - schistosomiasis B65.9 *[N08]*
  - sepsis A41.9 *[N08]*
    - streptococcal A40- *[N08]*
  - sickle-cell disorders D57.- *[N08]*
  - strongyloidiasis B78.9 *[N08]*
  - subacute bacterial endocarditis I33.0 *[N08]*
  - syphilis (late) congenital A50.59 *[N08]*
  - systemic lupus erythematosus M32.14
  - thrombotic thrombocytopenic purpura M31.19 *[N08]*
  - typhoid fever A01.09
  - Waldenström macroglobulinemia C88.0 *[N08]*
  - Wegener's granulomatosis M31.31
- latent or quiescent N03.9
- lobular, lobulonodular *—see* Glomerulonephritis, membranoproliferative
- membranoproliferative (diffuse) (type 1 or 3) (*see also* N00-N07 with fourth character .5) N05.5
  - dense deposit (type 2) NEC (*see also* N00-N07 with fourth character .6) N05.6
- membranous (diffuse) NEC (*see also* N00-N07 with fourth character .2) N05.2

Glomerulonephritis *(continued)*
- mesangial
  - IgA/IgG *—see* Nephropathy, IgA
  - proliferative (diffuse) NEC (*see also* N00-N07 with fourth character .3) N05.3
- mesangiocapillary (diffuse) NEC (*see also* N00-N07 with fourth character .5) N05.5
- necrotic, necrotizing NEC (*see also* N00-N07 with fourth character .8) N05.8
- nodular *—see* Glomerulonephritis, membranoproliferative
- poststreptococcal NEC N05.9
  - acute N00.9
  - chronic N03.9
  - rapidly progressive N01.9
- proliferative NEC (*see also* N00-N07 with fourth character .8) N05.8
  - diffuse (lupus) M32.14
- rapidly progressive N01.9
- sclerosing, diffuse N18.9
- specified pathology NEC (*see also* N00-N07 with fourth character .8) N05.8
- subacute N01.9

Glomerulopathy *—see* Glomerulonephritis

Glomerulosclerosis *—see also* Sclerosis, renal
- intercapillary (nodular) (with diabetes) *—see* Diabetes, glomerulosclerosis
- intracapillary *—see* Diabetes, glomerulosclerosis

Glossagra K14.6

Glossalgia K14.6

Glossitis (chronic superficial) (gangrenous) (Moeller's) K14.0
- areata exfoliativa K14.1
- atrophic K14.4
- benign migratory K14.1
- cortical superficial, sclerotic K14.0
- Hunter's D51.0
- interstitial, sclerous K14.0
- median rhomboid K14.2
- pellagrous E52
- superficial, chronic K14.0

Glossocele K14.8

Glossodynia K14.6
- exfoliativa K14.4

Glossoncus K14.8

Glossopathy K14.9

Glossophytia K14.3

Glossoplegia K14.8

Glossoptosis K14.8

Glossopyrosis K14.6

Glossotrichia K14.3

Glossy skin L90.8

Glottis *—see* condition

Glottitis *—see also* Laryngitis J04.0

Glucagonoma
- pancreas
  - benign D13.7
  - malignant C25.4
  - uncertain behavior D37.8
- specified site NEC
  - benign *—see* Neoplasm, benign, by site
  - malignant *—see* Neoplasm, malignant, by site
  - uncertain behavior *—see* Neoplasm, uncertain behavior, by site

Glucagonoma *(continued)*
- specified site NEC *(continued)*
- unspecified site
  - benign D13.7
  - malignant C25.4
  - uncertain behavior D37.8

Glucoglycinuria E72.51

Glucose-galactose malabsorption E74.39

Glue
- ear *—see* Otitis, media, nonsuppurative, chronic, mucoid
- sniffing (airplane) *—see* Abuse, drug, inhalant
  - dependence *—see* Dependence, drug, inhalant

GLUT1 deficiency syndrome 1, infantile onset E74.810

GLUT1 deficiency syndrome 2, childhood onset E74.810

Glutaric aciduria E72.3

Glycinemia E72.51

Glycinuria (renal) (with ketosis) E72.09

Glycogen
- infiltration *—see* Disease, glycogen storage
- storage disease *—see* Disease, glycogen storage

Glycogenosis (diffuse) (generalized) *—see also* Disease, glycogen storage
- cardiac E74.02 *[I43]*
- diabetic, secondary *—see* Diabetes, glycogenosis, secondary
- pulmonary interstitial J84.842

Glycopenia E16.2

Glycosuria R81
- renal (familial) E74.818

Gnathostoma spinigerum (infection) (infestation)**,** gnathostomiasis (wandering swelling) B83.1

Goiter (plunging) (substernal) E04.9
- with
  - hyperthyroidism (recurrent) *—see* Hyperthyroidism, with, goiter
  - thyrotoxicosis *—see* Hyperthyroidism, with, goiter
- adenomatous *—see* Goiter, nodular
- cancerous C73
- congenital (nontoxic) E03.0
  - diffuse E03.0
  - parenchymatous E03.0
  - transitory, with normal functioning P72.0
- cystic E04.2
  - due to iodine-deficiency E01.1
- due to
  - enzyme defect in synthesis of thyroid hormone E07.1
  - iodine-deficiency (endemic) E01.2
- dyshormonogenetic (familial) E07.1
- endemic (iodine-deficiency) E01.2
  - diffuse E01.0
  - multinodular E01.1
- exophthalmic *—see* Hyperthyroidism, with, goiter
- iodine-deficiency (endemic) E01.2
  - diffuse E01.0
  - multinodular E01.1
  - nodular E01.1
- lingual Q89.2
- lymphadenoid E06.3
- malignant C73

Goiter *(continued)*
- multinodular (cystic) (nontoxic) E04.2
  - toxic or with hyperthyroidism E05.20
    - with thyroid storm E05.21
- neonatal NEC P72.0
- nodular (nontoxic) (due to) E04.9
  - with
    - hyperthyroidism E05.20
      - with thyroid storm E05.21
    - thyrotoxicosis E05.20
      - with thyroid storm E05.21
  - endemic E01.1
  - iodine-deficiency E01.1
  - sporadic E04.9
  - toxic E05.20
    - with thyroid storm E05.21
- nontoxic E04.9
  - diffuse (colloid) E04.0
  - multinodular E04.2
  - simple E04.0
  - specified NEC E04.8
  - uninodular E04.1
- simple E04.0
- toxic *—see* Hyperthyroidism, with, goiter
- uninodular (nontoxic) E04.1
  - toxic or with hyperthyroidism E05.10
    - with thyroid storm E05.11

Goiter-deafness syndrome E07.1

Goldberg syndrome Q89.8

Goldberg-Maxwell syndrome E34.51

Goldblatt's hypertension or kidney I70.1

Goldenhar (-Gorlin) **syndrome** Q87.0

Goldflam-Erb disease or syndrome G70.00
- with exacerbation (acute) G70.01
- in crisis G70.01

Goldscheider's disease Q81.8

Goldstein's disease (familial hemorrhagic telangiectasia) I78.0

Golfer's elbow *—see* Epicondylitis, medial

Gonadoblastoma
- specified site *—see* Neoplasm, uncertain behavior, by site
- unspecified site
  - female D39.10
  - male D40.10

Gonecystitis *—see* Vesiculitis

Gongylonemiasis B83.8

Goniosynechiae *—see* Adhesions, iris, goniosynechiae

Gonococcemia A54.86

Gonococcus, gonococcal (disease) (infection) (*see also* condition) A54.9
- anus A54.6
- bursa, bursitis A54.49
- conjunctiva, conjunctivitis (neonatorum) A54.31
- endocardium A54.83
- eye A54.30
  - conjunctivitis A54.31
  - iridocyclitis A54.32
  - keratitis A54.33
  - newborn A54.31
  - other specified A54.39
- fallopian tubes (acute) (chronic) A54.24

Gonococcus, gonococcal *(continued)*
- genitourinary (organ) (system) (tract) (acute)
  - lower A54.00
    - with abscess (accessory gland) (periurethral) A54.1
  - upper (*see also* condition) A54.29
- heart A54.83
- iridocyclitis A54.32
- joint A54.42
- lymphatic (gland) (node) A54.89
- meninges, meningitis A54.81
- musculoskeletal A54.40
  - arthritis A54.42
  - osteomyelitis A54.43
  - other specified A54.49
  - spondylopathy A54.41
- pelviperitonitis A54.24
- pelvis (acute) (chronic) A54.24
- pharynx A54.5
- proctitis A54.6
- pyosalpinx (acute) (chronic) A54.24
- rectum A54.6
- skin A54.89
- specified site NEC A54.89
- tendon sheath A54.49
- throat A54.5
- urethra (acute) (chronic) A54.01
  - with abscess (accessory gland) (periurethral) A54.1
- vulva (acute) (chronic) A54.02

Gonocytoma
- specified site *—see* Neoplasm, uncertain behavior, by site
- unspecified site
  - female D39.10
  - male D40.10

Gonorrhea (acute) (chronic) A54.9
- Bartholin's gland (acute) (chronic) (purulent) A54.02
  - with abscess (accessory gland) (periurethral) A54.1
- bladder A54.01
- cervix A54.03
- conjunctiva, conjunctivitis (neonatorum) A54.31
- contact Z20.2
- Cowper's gland (with abscess) A54.1
- exposure to Z20.2
- fallopian tube (acute) (chronic) A54.24
- kidney (acute) (chronic) A54.21
- lower genitourinary tract A54.00
  - with abscess (accessory gland) (periurethral) A54.1
- ovary (acute) (chronic) A54.24
- pelvis (acute) (chronic) A54.24
  - female pelvic inflammatory disease A54.24
- penis A54.09
- prostate (acute) (chronic) A54.22
- seminal vesicle (acute) (chronic) A54.23
- specified site not listed (*see also* Gonococcus) A54.89
- spermatic cord (acute) (chronic) A54.23
- urethra A54.01
  - with abscess (accessory gland) (periurethral) A54.1
- vagina A54.02
- vas deferens (acute) (chronic) A54.23
- vulva A54.02

Goodall's disease A08.19

Goodpasture's syndrome M31.0

Gopalan's syndrome (burning feet) E53.0

Gorlin-Chaudry-Moss syndrome Q87.0

Gottron's papules L94.4

Gougerot's syndrome (trisymptomatic) L81.7

Gougerot-Blum syndrome (pigmented purpuric lichenoid dermatitis) L81.7

Gougerot-Carteaud disease or syndrome (confluent reticulate papillomatosis) L83

Gouley's syndrome (constrictive pericarditis) I31.1

Goundou A66.6

Gout, gouty (acute) (attack) (flare) (*see also* Gout, chronic) M10.9
- drug-induced M10.20
  - ankle M10.27-
  - elbow M10.22-
  - foot joint M10.27-
  - hand joint M10.24-
  - hip M10.25-
  - knee M10.26-
  - multiple site M10.29
  - shoulder M10.21-
  - vertebrae M10.28
  - wrist M10.23-
- idiopathic M10.00
  - ankle M10.07-
  - elbow M10.02-
  - foot joint M10.07-
  - hand joint M10.04-
  - hip M10.05-
  - knee M10.06-
  - multiple site M10.09
  - shoulder M10.01-
  - vertebrae M10.08
  - wrist M10.03-
- in (due to) renal impairment M10.30
  - ankle M10.37-
  - elbow M10.32-
  - foot joint M10.37-
  - hand joint M10.34-
  - hip M10.35-
  - knee M10.36-
  - multiple site M10.39
  - shoulder M10.31-
  - vertebrae M10.38
  - wrist M10.33-
- lead-induced M10.10
  - ankle M10.17-
  - elbow M10.12-
  - foot joint M10.17-
  - hand joint M10.14-
  - hip M10.15-
  - knee M10.16-
  - multiple site M10.19
  - shoulder M10.11-
  - vertebrae M10.18
  - wrist M10.13-
- primary *—see* Gout, idiopathic
- saturnine *—see* Gout, lead-induced
- secondary NEC M10.40
  - ankle M10.47-
  - elbow M10.42-
  - foot joint M10.47-
  - hand joint M10.44-
  - hip M10.45-
  - knee M10.46-
  - multiple site M10.49
  - shoulder M10.41-
  - vertebrae M10.48
  - wrist M10.43-

Gout, gouty *(continued)*
- syphilitic (*see also* subcategory M14.8-) A52.77
- tophi —*see* Gout, chronic

Gout, chronic (*see also* Gout, gouty) M1A.9
- drug-induced M1A.20
  - ankle M1A.27-
  - elbow M1A.22-
  - foot joint M1A.27-
  - hand joint M1A.24-
  - hip M1A.25-
  - knee M1A.26-
  - multiple site M1A.29-
  - shoulder M1A.21-
  - vertebrae M1A.28
  - wrist M1A.23-
- idiopathic M1A.00
  - ankle M1A.07-
  - elbow M1A.02-
  - foot joint M1A.07-
  - hand joint M1A.04-
  - hip M1A.05-
  - knee M1A.06-
  - multiple site M1A.09
  - shoulder M1A.01-
  - vertebrae M1A.08
  - wrist M1A.03-
- in (due to) renal impairment M1A.30
  - ankle M1A.37-
  - elbow M1A.32-
  - foot joint M1A.37-
  - hand joint M1A.34-
  - hip M1A.35-
  - knee M1A.36-
  - multiple site M1A.39
  - shoulder M1A.31-
  - vertebrae M1A.38
  - wrist M1A.33-
- lead-induced M1A.10
  - ankle M1A.17-
  - elbow M1A.12-
  - foot joint M1A.17-
  - hand joint M1A.14-
  - hip M1A.15-
  - knee M1A.16-
  - multiple site M1A.19
  - shoulder M1A.11-
  - vertebrae M1A.18
  - wrist M1A.13-
- primary —*see* Gout, chronic, idiopathic
- saturnine —*see* Gout, chronic, lead-induced
- secondary NEC M1A.40
  - ankle M1A.47-
  - elbow M1A.42-
  - foot joint M1A.47-
  - hand joint M1A.44-
  - hip M1A.45-
  - knee M1A.46-
  - multiple site M1A.49
  - shoulder M1A.41-
  - vertebrae M1A.48
  - wrist M1A.43-
- syphilitic (*see also* subcategory M14.8-) A52.77
- tophi M1A.9

Gower's
- muscular dystrophy G71.01
- syndrome (vasovagal attack) R55

Gradenigo's syndrome —*see* Otitis, media, suppurative, acute

Graefe's disease —*see* Strabismus, paralytic, ophthalmoplegia, progressive

Graft-versus-host disease D89.813
- acute D89.810
- acute on chronic D89.812
- chronic D89.811

Grainhandler's disease or lung J67.8

Grain mite (itch) B88.0

Grand mal —*see* Epilepsy, generalized, specified NEC

Grand multipara status only (not pregnant) Z64.1
- pregnant —*see* Pregnancy, complicated by, grand multiparity

Granite worker's lung J62.8

Granular —*see also* condition
- inflammation, pharynx J31.2
- kidney (contracting) —*see* Sclerosis, renal
- liver K74.69

Granulation tissue (abnormal) (excessive) L92.9
- postmastoidectomy cavity —*see* Complications, postmastoidectomy, granulation

Granulocytopenia (primary) (malignant) —*see* Agranulocytosis

Granuloma L92.9
- abdomen K66.8
  - from residual foreign body L92.3
  - pyogenicum L98.0
- actinic L57.5
- annulare (perforating) L92.0
- apical K04.5
- aural —*see* Otitis, externa, specified NEC
- beryllium (skin) L92.3
- bone
  - eosinophilic C96.6
  - from residual foreign body —*see* Osteomyelitis, specified type NEC
  - lung C96.6
- brain (any site) G06.0
  - schistosomiasis B65.9 *[G07]*
- canaliculus lacrimalis —*see* Granuloma, lacrimal
- candidal (cutaneous) B37.2
- cerebral (any site) G06.0
- coccidioidal (primary) (progressive) B38.7
  - lung B38.1
  - meninges B38.4
- colon K63.89
- conjunctiva H11.22-
- dental K04.5
- ear, middle —*see* Cholesteatoma
- eosinophilic C96.6
  - bone C96.6
  - lung C96.6
  - oral mucosa K13.4
  - skin L92.2
- eyelid H01.8
- facial (e) L92.2
- foreign body (in soft tissue) NEC M60.20
  - ankle M60.27-
  - foot M60.27-
  - forearm M60.23-
  - hand M60.24-
  - in operation wound —*see* Foreign body, accidentally left during a procedure
  - lower leg M60.26-
  - pelvic region M60.25-
  - shoulder region M60.21-
  - skin L92.3

Granuloma *(continued)*
- foreign body NEC *(continued)*
  - specified site NEC M60.28
  - subcutaneous tissue L92.3
  - thigh M60.25-
  - upper arm M60.22-
- gangraenescens M31.2
- genito-inguinale A58
- giant cell (central) (reparative) (jaw) M27.1
  - gingiva (peripheral) K06.8
- gland (lymph) I88.8
- hepatic NEC K75.3
  - in (due to)
    - berylliosis J63.2 *[K77]*
    - sarcoidosis D86.89
- Hodgkin C81.9
- ileum K63.89
- infectious B99.9
  - specified NEC B99.8
- inguinale (Donovan) (venereal) A58
- intestine NEC K63.89
- intracranial (any site) G06.0
- intraspinal (any part) G06.1
- iridocyclitis —*see* Iridocyclitis, chronic
- jaw (bone) (central) M27.1
  - reparative giant cell M27.1
- kidney (*see also* Infection, kidney) N15.8
- lacrimal H04.81-
- larynx J38.7
- lethal midline (faciale(e)) M31.2
- liver NEC —*see* Granuloma, hepatic
- lung (infectious) —*see also* Fibrosis, lung
  - coccidioidal B38.1
  - eosinophilic C96.6
- Majocchi's B35.8
- malignant (facial(e)) M31.2
- mandible (central) M27.1
- midline (lethal) M31.2
- monilial (cutaneous) B37.2
- nasal sinus —*see* Sinusitis
- operation wound T81.89
  - foreign body —*see* Foreign body, accidentally left during a procedure
  - stitch T81.89
  - talc —*see* Foreign body, accidentally left during a procedure
- oral mucosa K13.4
- orbit, orbital H05.11-
- paracoccidioidal B41.8
- penis, venereal A58
- periapical K04.5
- peritoneum K66.8
  - due to ova of helminths NOS (*see also* Helminthiasis) B83.9 *[K67]*
- postmastoidectomy cavity —*see* Complications, postmastoidectomy, recurrent cholesteatoma
- prostate N42.89
- pudendi (ulcerating) A58
- pulp, internal (tooth) K03.3
- pyogenic, pyogenicum (of) (skin) L98.0
  - gingiva K06.8
  - maxillary alveolar ridge K04.5
  - oral mucosa K13.4
- rectum K62.89
- reticulohistiocytic D76.3
- rubrum nasi L74.8
- Schistosoma —*see* Schistosomiasis
- septic (skin) L98.0

Granuloma *(continued)*
- silica (skin) L92.3
- sinus (accessory) (infective) (nasal) —*see* Sinusitis
- skin L92.9
  - from residual foreign body L92.3
  - pyogenicum L98.0
- spine
  - syphilitic (epidural) A52.19
  - tuberculous A18.01
- stitch (postoperative) T81.89
- suppurative (skin) L98.0
- swimming pool A31.1
- talc —*see also* Granuloma, foreign body
  - in operation wound —*see* Foreign body, accidentally left during a procedure
- telangiectaticum (skin) L98.0
- tracheostomy J95.09
- trichophyticum B35.8
- tropicum A66.4
- umbilical P83.81
- umbilicus P83.81
- urethra N36.8
- uveitis —*see* Iridocyclitis, chronic
- vagina A58
- venereum A58
- vocal cord J38.3

Granulomatosis L92.9
- with polyangiitis M31.3
- eosinophilic, with polyangiitis [EGPA] M30.1
- lymphoid C83.8-
- miliary (listerial) A32.89
- necrotizing, respiratory M31.30
- progressive septic D71
- specified NEC L92.8
- Wegener's M31.30
  - with renal involvement M31.31

Granulomatous tissue (abnormal) (excessive) L92.9

Granulosis rubra nasi L74.8

Graphite fibrosis (of lung) J63.3

Graphospasm F48.8
- organic G25.89

Grating scapula M89.8X1

Gravel (urinary) —*see* Calculus, urinary

Graves' disease —*see* Hyperthyroidism, with, goiter

Gravis —*see* condition

Grawitz tumor C64.-

Gray syndrome (newborn) P93.0

Grayness, hair (premature) L67.1
- congenital Q84.2

Green sickness D50.8

Greenfield's disease
- meaning
  - concentric sclerosis (encephalitis periaxialis concentrica) G37.5
  - metachromatic leukodystrophy E75.25

Greenstick fracture - code as Fracture, by site

Grey syndrome (newborn) P93.0

Grief F43.21
- prolonged F43.29
- reaction (*see also* Disorder, adjustment) F43.20

Griesinger's disease B76.0

Grinder's lung or pneumoconiosis J62.8

Grinding, teeth
psychogenic F45.8
sleep related G47.63

Grip
Dabney's B33.0
devil's B33.0

Grippe, grippal —*see also* Influenza
Balkan A78
summer, of Italy A93.1

Grisel's disease M43.6

Groin —*see* condition

Grooved tongue K14.5

Ground itch B76.9

Grover's disease or syndrome L11.1

Growing pains, children R29.898

Growth (fungoid) (neoplastic) (new) —*see also* Neoplasm
adenoid (vegetative) J35.8
benign —*see* Neoplasm, benign, by site
malignant —*see* Neoplasm, malignant, by site
rapid, childhood Z00.2
secondary —*see* Neoplasm, secondary, by site

Gruby's disease B35.0

Gubler-Millard paralysis or syndrome G46.3

Guerin-Stern syndrome Q74.3

Guidance, insufficient anterior (occlusal) M26.54

Guillain-Barré disease or syndrome G61.0
sequelae G65.0

Guinea worms (infection) (infestation) B72

Guinon's disease (motor-verbal tic) F95.2

Gull's disease E03.4

Gum —*see* condition

Gumboil K04.7
with sinus K04.6

Gumma (syphilitic) A52.79
artery A52.09
cerebral A52.04
bone A52.77
of yaws (late) A66.6
brain A52.19
cauda equina A52.19
central nervous system A52.3
ciliary body A52.71
congenital A50.59
eyelid A52.71
heart A52.06
intracranial A52.19
iris A52.71
kidney A52.75
larynx A52.73
leptomeninges A52.19
liver A52.74
meninges A52.19
myocardium A52.06
nasopharynx A52.73
neurosyphilitic A52.3
nose A52.73
orbit A52.71
palate (soft) A52.79
penis A52.76
pericardium A52.06
pharynx A52.73
pituitary A52.79
scrofulous (tuberculous) A18.4
skin A52.79
specified site NEC A52.79

Gumma *(continued)*
spinal cord A52.19
tongue A52.79
tonsil A52.73
trachea A52.73
tuberculous A18.4
ulcerative due to yaws A66.4
ureter A52.75
yaws A66.4
bone A66.6

Gunn's syndrome Q07.8

Gunshot wound —*see also* Puncture, open
fracture - code as Fracture, by site
internal organs —*see* Injury, by site

Gynandrism Q56.0

Gynandroblastoma
specified site —*see* Neoplasm, uncertain behavior, by site
unspecified site
female D39.10
male D40.10

Gynecological examination (periodic) (routine) Z01.419
with abnormal findings Z01.411

Gynecomastia N62

Gynephobia F40.291

Gyrate scalp Q82.8

H

H (Hartnup's) **disease** E72.02

Haas' disease or osteochondrosis (juvenile) (head of humerus) —*see* Osteochondrosis, juvenile, humerus

Habit, habituation
bad sleep Z72.821
chorea F95.8
disturbance, child F98.9
drug —*see* Dependence, drug
irregular sleep Z72.821
laxative F55.2
spasm —*see* Tic
tic —*see* Tic

Haemophilus (H.) **influenzae, as cause of disease classified elsewhere** B96.3

Haff disease —*see* Poisoning, mercury

Hageman's factor defect, deficiency or disease D68.2

Haglund's disease or osteochondrosis (juvenile) (os tibiale externum) —*see* Osteochondrosis, juvenile, tarsus

Hailey-Hailey disease Q82.8

Hair —*see also* condition
plucking F63.3
in stereotyped movement disorder F98.4
tourniquet syndrome —*see also* Constriction, external, by site
finger S60.44-
penis S30.842
thumb S60.34-
toe S90.44-

Hairball in stomach T18.2

Hair-pulling, pathological (compulsive) F63.3

Hairy black tongue K14.3

Half vertebra Q76.49

Halitosis R19.6

Hallerman-Streiff syndrome Q87.0

Hallervorden-Spatz disease G23.0

Hallopeau's acrodermatitis or disease L40.2

Hallucination R44.3
auditory R44.0
gustatory R44.2
olfactory R44.2
specified NEC R44.2
tactile R44.2
visual R44.1

Hallucinosis (chronic) F28
alcoholic (acute) F10.951
in
abuse F10.151
dependence F10.251
drug-induced F19.951
cannabis F12.951
cocaine F14.951
hallucinogen F16.151
in
abuse F19.151
cannabis F12.151
cocaine F14.151
hallucinogen F16.151
inhalant F18.151
opioid F11.151
sedative, anxiolytic or hypnotic F13.151
stimulant NEC F15.151
dependence F19.251
cannabis F12.251
cocaine F14.251
hallucinogen F16.251
inhalant F18.251
opioid F11.251
sedative, anxiolytic or hypnotic F13.251
stimulant NEC F15.251
inhalant F18.951
opioid F11.951
sedative, anxiolytic or hypnotic F13.951
stimulant NEC F15.951
organic F06.0

Hallux
deformity (acquired) NEC M20.5X-
limitus M20.5X-
malleus (acquired) NEC M20.3-
rigidus (acquired) M20.2-
congenital Q74.2
sequelae (late effect) of rickets E64.3
valgus (acquired) M20.1-
congenital Q66.6
varus (acquired) M20.3-
congenital Q66.3-

Halo, visual H53.19

Hamartoma, hamartoblastoma Q85.9
epithelial (gingival), odontogenic, central or peripheral —*see* Cyst, calcifying odontogenic

Hamartosis Q85.9

Hamman-Rich syndrome J84.114

Hammer toe (acquired) **NEC** —*see also* Deformity, toe, hammer toe
congenital Q66.89
sequelae (late effect) of rickets E64.3

Hand —*see* condition

Hand-foot syndrome L27.1

Handicap, handicapped
educational Z55.9
specified NEC Z55.8

Hand-Schüller-Christian disease or syndrome C96.5

Hanging (asphyxia) (strangulation) (suffocation) —*see* Asphyxia, traumatic, due to mechanical threat

Hangnail —*see also* Cellulitis, digit
with lymphangitis —*see* Lymphangitis, acute, digit

Hangover (alcohol) F10.129

Hanhart's syndrome Q87.0

Hanot-Chauffard (-Troisier) **syndrome** E83.19

Hanot's cirrhosis or disease K74.3

Hansen's disease —*see* Leprosy

Hantaan virus disease (Korean hemorrhagic fever) A98.5

Hantavirus disease (with renal manifestations) (Dobrava) (Puumala) (Seoul) A98.5
with pulmonary manifestations (Andes) (Bayou) (Bermejo) (Black Creek Canal) (Choclo) (Juquitiba) (Laguna negra) (Lechiguanas) (New York) (Oran) (Sin nombre) B33.4

Happy puppet syndrome Q93.51

Harada's disease or syndrome H30.81-

Hardening
artery —*see* Arteriosclerosis
brain G93.89

Harelip (complete) (incomplete) —*see* Cleft, lip

Harlequin (newborn) Q80.4

Harley's disease D59.6

Harmful use (of)
alcohol F10.10
anxiolytics —*see* Abuse, drug, sedative
cannabinoids —*see* Abuse, drug, cannabis
cocaine —*see* Abuse, drug, cocaine
drug —*see* Abuse, drug
hallucinogens —*see* Abuse, drug, hallucinogen
hypnotics —*see* Abuse, drug, sedative
opioids —*see* Abuse, drug, opioid
PCP (phencyclidine) —*see* Abuse, drug, hallucinogen
sedatives —*see* Abuse, drug, sedative
stimulants NEC —*see* Abuse, drug, stimulant

Harris' lines —*see* Arrest, epiphyseal

Hartnup's disease E72.02

Harvester's lung J67.0

Harvesting ovum for in vitro fertilization Z31.83

Hashimoto's disease or thyroiditis E06.3

Hashitoxicosis (transient) E06.3

Hassal-Henle bodies or warts (cornea) H18.49

Haut mal —*see* Epilepsy, generalized, specified NEC

Haverhill fever A25.1

Hay fever (*see also* Fever, hay) J30.1

Hayem-Widal syndrome D59.8

Haygarth's nodes M15.8

Haymaker's lung J67.0

Hb (abnormal)
Bart's disease D56.0
disease —*see* Disease, hemoglobin
trait —*see* Trait

Head —*see* condition

Headache R51.9
- with
  - orthostatic component NEC R51.0
  - positional component NEC R51.0
- allergic NEC G44.89
- associated with sexual activity G44.82
- cervicogenic G44.86
- chronic daily R51.9
- cluster G44.009
  - chronic G44.029
    - intractable G44.021
    - not intractable G44.029
  - episodic G44.019
    - intractable G44.011
    - not intractable G44.019
  - intractable G44.001
  - not intractable G44.009
- cough (primary) G44.83
- daily chronic R51.9
- drug-induced NEC G44.40
  - intractable G44.41
  - not intractable G44.40
- exertional (primary) G44.84
- histamine G44.009
  - intractable G44.001
  - not intractable G44.009
- hypnic G44.81
- lumbar puncture G97.1
- medication overuse G44.40
  - intractable G44.41
  - not intractable G44.40
- menstrual —*see* Migraine, menstrual
- migraine (type) (*see also* Migraine) G43.909
- nasal septum R51.9
- neuralgiform, short lasting unilateral, with conjunctival injection and tearing (SUNCT) G44.059
  - intractable G44.051
  - not intractable G44.059
- new daily persistent (NDPH) G44.52
- orgasmic G44.82
- periodic syndromes in adults and children G43.C0
  - with refractory migraine G43.C1
  - intractable G43.C1
  - not intractable G43.C0
  - without refractory migraine G43.C0
- postspinal puncture G97.1
- post-traumatic G44.309
  - acute G44.319
    - intractable G44.311
    - not intractable G44.319
  - chronic G44.329
    - intractable G44.321
    - not intractable G44.329
  - intractable G44.301
  - not intractable G44.309
- pre-menstrual —*see* Migraine, menstrual
- preorgasmic G44.82
- primary
  - cough G44.83
  - exertional G44.84
  - stabbing G44.85
  - thunderclap G44.53
- rebound G44.40
  - intractable G44.41
  - not intractable G44.40
- short lasting unilateral neuralgiform, with conjunctival injection and tearing (SUNCT) G44.059
  - intractable G44.051
  - not intractable G44.059
- specified syndrome NEC G44.89
- spinal and epidural anesthesia - induced T88.59
  - in labor and delivery O74.5
  - in pregnancy O29.4-
  - postpartum, puerperal O89.4
- spinal fluid loss (from puncture) G97.1
- stabbing (primary) G44.85
- tension (-type) G44.209
  - chronic G44.229
    - intractable G44.221
    - not intractable G44.229
  - episodic G44.219
    - intractable G44.211
    - not intractable G44.219
  - intractable G44.201
  - not intractable G44.209
- thunderclap (primary) G44.53
- vascular NEC G44.1

Healthy
- infant
  - accompanying sick mother Z76.3
  - receiving care Z76.2
- person accompanying sick person Z76.3

Hearing examination Z01.10
- with abnormal findings NEC Z01.118
- following failed hearing screening Z01.110
- for hearing conservation and treatment Z01.12
- infant or child (over 28 days old) Z00.129
  - with abnormal finding Z00.121

Heart —*see* condition

Heart beat
- abnormality R00.9
  - specified NEC R00.8
- awareness R00.2
- rapid R00.0
- slow R00.1

Heartburn R12
- psychogenic F45.8

Heartland virus disease A93.8

Heat (effects) T67.9
- apoplexy T67.01
- burn (*see also* Burn) L55.9
- collapse T67.1
- cramps T67.2
- dermatitis or eczema L59.0
- edema T67.7
- erythema - code by site under Burn, first degree
- excessive T67.9
  - specified effect NEC T67.8
- exhaustion T67.5
  - anhydrotic T67.3
  - due to
    - salt (and water) depletion T67.4
    - water depletion T67.3
      - with salt depletion T67.4
- fatigue (transient) T67.6
- fever T67.01
- hyperpyrexia T67.01
- prickly L74.0
- prostration —*see* Heat, exhaustion
- pyrexia T67.01
- rash L74.0
- specified effect NEC T67.8
- stroke T67.01
  - exertional T67.02
  - specified NEC T67.09
- sunburn —*see* Sunburn
- syncope T67.1

Heavy-for-dates NEC (infant) (4000g to 4499g) P08.1
- exceptionally (4500g or more) P08.0

Hebephrenia, hebephrenic (schizophrenia) F20.1

Heberden's disease or nodes (with arthropathy) M15.1

Hebra's
- pityriasis L26
- prurigo L28.2

Heel —*see* condition

Heerfordt's disease D86.89

Hegglin's anomaly or syndrome D72.0

Heilmeyer-Schoner disease D45

Heine-Medin disease A80.9

Heinz body anemia, congenital D58.2

Heliophobia F40.228

Heller's disease or syndrome F84.3

HELLP syndrome (hemolysis, elevated liver enzymes and low platelet count) O14.2-
- complicating
  - childbirth O14.24
  - puerperium O14.25

Helminthiasis —*see also* Infestation, helminth
- Ancylostoma B76.0
- intestinal B82.0
  - mixed types (types classifiable to more than one of the titles B65.0-B81.3 and B81.8) B81.4
  - specified type NEC B81.8
- mixed types (intestinal) (types classifiable to more than one of the titles B65.0-B81.3 and B81.8) B81.4
- Necator (americanus) B76.1
- specified type NEC B83.8

Heloma L84

Hemangioblastoma —*see* Neoplasm, connective tissue, uncertain behavior
- malignant —*see* Neoplasm, connective tissue, malignant

Hemangioendothelioma —*see also* Neoplasm, uncertain behavior, by site
- benign D18.00
  - intra-abdominal D18.03
  - intracranial D18.02
  - skin D18.01
  - specified site NEC D18.09
- bone (diffuse) —*see* Neoplasm, bone, malignant
- epithelioid —*see also* Neoplasm, uncertain behavior, by site
  - malignant —*see* Neoplasm, malignant, by site
- malignant —*see* Neoplasm, connective tissue, malignant

Hemangiofibroma —*see* Neoplasm, benign, by site

Hemangiolipoma —*see* Lipoma

Hemangioma D18.00
- arteriovenous D18.00
  - intra-abdominal D18.03
  - intracranial D18.02
  - skin D18.01
  - specified site NEC D18.09
- capillary I78.1
  - intra-abdominal D18.03
  - intracranial D18.02
  - skin D18.01
  - specified site NEC D18.09
- cavernous D18.00
  - intra-abdominal D18.03
  - intracranial D18.02
  - skin D18.01
  - specified site NEC D18.09
- epithelioid D18.00
  - intra-abdominal D18.03
  - intracranial D18.02
  - skin D18.01
  - specified site NEC D18.09
- histiocytoid D18.00
  - intra-abdominal D18.03
  - intracranial D18.02
  - skin D18.01
  - specified site NEC D18.09
- infantile D18.00
  - intra-abdominal D18.03
  - intracranial D18.02
  - skin D18.01
  - specified site NEC D18.09
- intra-abdominal D18.03
- intracranial D18.02
- intramuscular D18.00
  - intra-abdominal D18.03
  - intracranial D18.02
  - skin D18.01
  - specified site NEC D18.09
- intrathoracic structures D18.09
- juvenile D18.00
- malignant —*see* Neoplasm,connective tissue, malignant
- plexiform D18.00
  - intra-abdominal D18.03
  - intracranial D18.02
  - skin D18.01
  - specified site NEC D18.09
- racemose D18.00
  - intra-abdominal D18.03
  - intracranial D18.02
  - skin D18.01
  - specified site NEC D18.09
- sclerosing —*see* Neoplasm,skin, benign
- simplex D18.00
  - intra-abdominal D18.03
  - intracranial D18.02
  - skin D18.01
  - specified site NEC D18.09
- skin D18.01
- specified site NEC D18.09
- venous D18.00
  - intra-abdominal D18.03
  - intracranial D18.02
  - skin D18.01
  - specified site NEC D18.09
- verrucous keratotic D18.00
  - intra-abdominal D18.03
  - intracranial D18.02
  - skin D18.01
  - specified site NEC D18.09

Hemangiomatosis (systemic) I78.8
- involving single site —*see* Hemangioma

Hemangiopericytoma —*see also* Neoplasm, connective tissue, uncertain behavior
- benign —*see* Neoplasm, connective tissue, benign
- malignant —*see* Neoplasm, connective tissue, malignant

Hemangiosarcoma —*see* Neoplasm, connective tissue, malignant

Hemarthrosis (nontraumatic) M25.00
ankle M25.07-
elbow M25.02-
foot joint M25.07-
hand joint M25.04-
hip M25.05-
in hemophilic arthropathy *—see* Arthropathy, hemophilic
knee M25.06-
shoulder M25.01-
specified joint NEC M25.08
traumatic *—see* Sprain, by site
vertebrae M25.08
wrist M25.03-

Hematemesis K92.0
with ulcer - code by site under Ulcer, with hemorrhage K27.4
newborn, neonatal P54.0
due to swallowed maternal blood P78.2

Hematidrosis L74.8

Hematinuria *—see also* Hemoglobinuria
malarial B50.8

Hematobilia K83.8

Hematocele
female NEC N94.89
with ectopic pregnancy O00.90
with intrauterine pregnancy O00.91
ovary N83.8
male N50.1

Hematochezia (*see also* Melena) K92.1

Hematochyluria *—see also* Infestation, filarial
schistosomiasis (bilharziasis) B65.0

Hematocolpos (with hematometra or hematosalpinx) N89.7

Hematocornea *—see* Pigmentation, cornea, stromal

Hematogenous *—see* condition

Hematoma (traumatic) (skin surface intact) *—see also* Contusion
with
injury of internal organs *—see* Injury, by site
open wound *—see* Wound, open
amputation stump (surgical) (late) T87.89
aorta, dissecting I71.00
abdominal I71.02
thoracic I71.01
thoracoabdominal I71.03
aortic intramural *—see* Dissection, aorta
arterial (complicating trauma) *—see* Injury, blood vessel, by site
auricle *—see* Contusion, ear
nontraumatic *—see* Disorder, pinna, hematoma
birth injury NEC P15.8
brain (traumatic)
with
cerebral laceration or contusion (diffuse) *—see* Injury, intracranial, diffuse
focal *—see* Injury, intracranial, focal
cerebellar, traumatic S06.37-
newborn NEC P52.4
birth injury P10.1
intracerebral, traumatic *—see* Injury, intracranial, intracerebral hemorrhage

Hematoma *(continued)*
brain *(continued)*
nontraumatic *—see* Hemorrhage, intracranial
subarachnoid, arachnoid, traumatic *—see* Injury, intracranial, subarachnoid hemorrhage
subdural, traumatic *—see* Injury, intracranial, subdural hemorrhage
breast (nontraumatic) N64.89
broad ligament (nontraumatic) N83.7
traumatic S37.892
cerebellar, traumatic S06.37-
cerebral *—see* Hematoma, brain
cerebrum S06.36-
left S06.35-
right S06.34-
cesarean delivery wound O90.2
complicating delivery (perineal) (pelvic) (vagina) (vulva) O71.7
corpus cavernosum (nontraumatic) N48.89
epididymis (nontraumatic) N50.1
epidural (traumatic) *—see* Injury, intracranial, epidural hemorrhage
spinal *—see* Injury, spinal cord, by region
episiotomy O90.2
face, birth injury P15.4
genital organ NEC (nontraumatic)
female (nonobstetric) N94.89
traumatic S30.202
male N50.1
traumatic S30.201
internal organs *—see* Injury, by site
intracerebral, traumatic *—see* Injury, intracranial, intracerebral hemorrhage
intraoperative *—see* Complications, intraoperative, hemorrhage
labia (nontraumatic) (nonobstetric) N90.89
liver (subcapsular) (nontraumatic) K76.89
birth injury P15.0
mediastinum *—see* Injury, intrathoracic
mesosalpinx (nontraumatic) N83.7
traumatic S37.898
muscle - code by site under Contusion
nontraumatic
muscle M79.81
soft tissue M79.81
obstetrical surgical wound O90.2
orbit, orbital (nontraumatic) *—see also* Hemorrhage, orbit
traumatic *—see* Contusion, orbit
pelvis (female) (nontraumatic) (nonobstetric) N94.89
obstetric O71.7
traumatic *—see* Injury, by site
penis (nontraumatic) N48.89
birth injury P15.5
perianal (nontraumatic) K64.5
perineal S30.23
complicating delivery O71.7
perirenal *—see* Injury, kidney
pinna *—see* Contusion, ear
nontraumatic *—see* Disorder, pinna, hematoma
placenta O43.89-
postoperative (postprocedural) *—see* Complication, postprocedural, hematoma
retroperitoneal (nontraumatic) K66.1
traumatic S36.892

Hematoma *(continued)*
scrotum, superficial S30.22
birth injury P15.5
seminal vesicle (nontraumatic) N50.1
traumatic S37.892
spermatic cord (traumatic) S37.892
nontraumatic N50.1
spinal (cord) (meninges) *—see also* Injury, spinal cord, by region
newborn (birth injury) P11.5
spleen D73.5
intraoperative *—see* Complications, intraoperative, hemorrhage, spleen
postprocedural (postoperative) *—see* Complications, postprocedural, hemorrhage, spleen
sternocleidomastoid, birth injury P15.2
sternomastoid, birth injury P15.2
subarachnoid (traumatic) *—see* Injury, intracranial, subarachnoid hemorrhage
newborn (nontraumatic) P52.5
due to birth injury P10.3
nontraumatic *—see* Hemorrhage, intracranial, subarachnoid
subdural (traumatic) *—see* Injury, intracranial, subdural hemorrhage
newborn (localized) P52.8
birth injury P10.0
nontraumatic *—see* Hemorrhage, intracranial, subdural
superficial, newborn P54.5
testis (nontraumatic) N50.1
birth injury P15.5
tunica vaginalis (nontraumatic) N50.1
umbilical cord, complicating delivery O69.5
uterine ligament (broad) (nontraumatic) N83.7
traumatic S37.892
vagina (ruptured) (nontraumatic) N89.8
complicating delivery O71.7
vas deferens (nontraumatic) N50.1
traumatic S37.892
vitreous *—see* Hemorrhage, vitreous
vulva (nontraumatic) (nonobstetric) N90.89
complicating delivery O71.7
newborn (birth injury) P15.5

Hematometra N85.7
with hematocolpos N89.7

Hematomyelia (central) G95.19
newborn (birth injury) P11.5
traumatic T14.8

Hematomyelitis G04.90

Hematoperitoneum *—see* Hemoperitoneum

Hematophobia F40.230

Hematopneumothorax (*see* Hemothorax)

Hematopoiesis, cyclic D70.4

Hematoporphyria *—see* Porphyria

Hematorachis, hematorrhachis G95.19
newborn (birth injury) P11.5

Hematosalpinx N83.6
with
hematocolpos N89.7
hematometra N85.7
with hematocolpos N89.7
infectional *—see* Salpingitis

Hematospermia R36.1

Hematothorax (see Hemothorax)

Hematuria R31.9
due to sulphonamide, sulfonamide *—see* Table of Drugs and Chemicals, by drug
benign (familial) (of childhood) *—see also* Hematuria, idiopathic
essential microscopic R31.1
endemic (*see also* Schistosomiasis) B65.0
gross R31.0
idiopathic N02.9
with glomerular lesion
C3
glomerulonepritis N02.A
glomerulopathy N02.A
with dense deposit disease N02.6
crescentic (diffuse) glomerulonephritis N02.7
dense deposit disease N02.6
endocapillary proliferative glomerulonephritis N02.4
focal and segmental hyalinosis or sclerosis N02.1
membranoproliferative (diffuse) N02.5
membranous (diffuse) N02.2
mesangial proliferative (diffuse) N02.3
mesangiocapillary (diffuse) N02.5
minor abnormality N02.0
proliferative NEC N02.8
specified pathology NEC N02.8
intermittent *—see* Hematuria, idiopathic
malarial B50.8
microscopic NEC (with symptoms) R31.29
asymptomatic R31.21
benign essential R31.1
paroxysmal *—see also* Hematuria, idiopathic
nocturnal D59.5
persistent *—see* Hematuria, idiopathic
recurrent *—see* Hematuria, idiopathic
tropical (*see also* Schistosomiasis) B65.0
tuberculous A18.13

Hemeralopia (day blindness) H53.11
vitamin A deficiency E50.5

Hemi-akinesia R41.4

Hemianalgesia R20.0

Hemianencephaly Q00.0

Hemianesthesia R20.0

Hemianopia, hemianopsia (heteronymous) H53.47
homonymous H53.46-
syphilitic A52.71

Hemiathetosis R25.8

Hemiatrophy R68.89
cerebellar G31.9
face, facial, progressive (Romberg) G51.8
tongue K14.8

Hemiballism (us) G25.5

Hemicardia Q24.8

Hemicephalus, hemicephaly Q00.0

Hemichorea G25.5

Hemicolitis, left *—see* Colitis, left sided

Hemicrania
congenital malformation Q00.0
continua G44.51

Hemicrania *(continued)*
- meaning migraine (*see also* Migraine) G43.909
- paroxysmal G44.039
  - chronic G44.049
    - intractable G44.041
    - not intractable G44.049
  - episodic G44.039
    - intractable G44.031
    - not intractable G44.039
  - intractable G44.031
  - not intractable G44.039

Hemidystrophy —*see* Hemiatrophy

Hemiectromelia Q73.8

Hemihypalgesia R20.8

Hemihypesthesia R20.1

Hemi-inattention R41.4

Hemimelia Q73.8
- lower limb —*see* Defect, reduction, lower limb, specified type NEC
- upper limb —*see* Defect, reduction, upper limb, specified type NEC

Hemiparalysis —*see* Hemiplegia

Hemiparesis —*see* Hemiplegia

Hemiparesthesia R20.2

Hemiparkinsonism G20

Hemiplegia G81.9-
- alternans facialis G83.89
- ascending NEC G81.90
  - spinal G95.89
- congenital (cerebral) G80.8
  - spastic G80.2
- embolic (current episode) I63.4-
- flaccid G81.0-
- following
  - cerebrovascular disease I69.959
    - cerebral infarction I69.35-
    - intracerebral hemorrhage I69.15-
    - nontraumatic intracranial hemorrhage NEC I69.25-
    - specified disease NEC I69.85-
    - stroke NOS I69.35-
    - subarachnoid hemorrhage I69.05-
- hysterical F44.4
- newborn NEC P91.88
  - birth injury P11.9
- spastic G81.1-
  - congenital G80.2
- thrombotic (current episode) I63.3-

Hemisection, spinal cord —*see* Injury, spinal cord, by region

Hemispasm (facial) R25.2

Hemisporosis B48.8

Hemitremor R25.1

Hemivertebra Q76.49
- failure of segmentation with scoliosis Q76.3
- fusion with scoliosis Q76.3

Hemochromatosis E83.119
- with refractory anemia D46.1
- due to repeated red blood cell transfusion E83.111
- hereditary (primary) E83.110
- neonatal P78.84
- primary E83.110
- specified NEC E83.118

Hemoglobin —*see also* condition
- abnormal (disease) —*see* Disease, hemoglobin
- AS genotype D57.3
- Constant Spring D58.2

Hemoglobin *(continued)*
- E-beta thalassemia D56.5
- fetal, hereditary persistence (HPFH) D56.4
- H Constant Spring D56.0
- low NOS D64.9
- S (Hb S), heterozygous D57.3

Hemoglobinemia D59.9
- due to blood transfusion T80.89
- paroxysmal D59.6
  - nocturnal D59.5

Hemoglobinopathy (mixed) D58.2
- with thalassemia D56.8
- sickle-cell D57.1
  - with thalassemia D57.40
    - with
      - acute chest syndrome D57.411
      - cerebral vascular involvement D57.413
      - crisis (painful) D57.419
        - with specified complication NEC D57.418
      - splenic sequestration D57.412
      - vasoocclusive pain D57.419
    - without crisis D57.40

Hemoglobinuria R82.3
- with anemia, hemolytic, acquired (chronic) NEC D59.6
- cold (paroxysmal) (with Raynaud's syndrome) D59.6
  - agglutinin D59.12
- due to exertion or hemolysis NEC D59.6
- intermittent D59.6
- malarial B50.8
- march D59.6
- nocturnal (paroxysmal) D59.5
- paroxysmal (cold) D59.6
  - nocturnal D59.5

Hemolymphangioma D18.1

Hemolysis
- intravascular
  - with
    - abortion —*see* Abortion, by type, complicated by, hemorrhage
    - ectopic or molar pregnancy O08.1
    - hemorrhage
      - antepartum —*see* Hemorrhage, antepartum, with coagulation defect
      - intrapartum (*see also* Hemorrhage, complicating, delivery) O67.0
  - postpartum O72.3
- neonatal (excessive) P58.9
  - specified NEC P58.8

Hemolytic —*see* condition

Hemopericardium I31.2
- following acute myocardial infarction (current complication) I23.0
- newborn P54.8
- traumatic —*see* Injury, heart, with hemopericardium

Hemoperitoneum K66.1
- infectional K65.9
- traumatic S36.899
  - with open wound —*see* Wound, open, with penetration into peritoneal cavity

Hemophilia (classical) (familial) (hereditary) D66
- A D66
- B D67
- C D68.1

Hemophilia *(continued)*
- acquired D68.311
- autoimmune D68.311

Hemophilia
- calcipriva (*see also* Defect, coagulation) D68.4
- nonfamilial (*see also* Defect, coagulation) D68.4
- secondary D68.311
- vascular D68.0

Hemophthalmos H44.81-

Hemopneumothorax —*see also* Hemothorax
- traumatic S27.2

Hemoptysis R04.2
- newborn P26.9
- tuberculous —*see* Tuberculosis, pulmonary

Hemorrhage, hemorrhagic (concealed) R58
- abdomen R58
- accidental antepartum —*see* Hemorrhage, antepartum
- acute idiopathic pulmonary, in infants R04.81
- adenoid J35.8
- adrenal (capsule) (gland) E27.49
  - medulla E27.8
  - newborn P54.4
- after delivery —*see* Hemorrhage, postpartum
- alveolar
  - lung, newborn P26.8
  - process K08.89
- alveolus K08.89
- amputation stump (surgical) T87.89
- anemia (chronic) D50.0
  - acute D62
- antepartum (with) O46.90
  - with coagulation defect O46.00-
    - afibrinogenemia O46.01-
    - disseminated intravascular coagulation O46.02-
    - hypofibrinogenemia O46.01-
    - specified defect NEC O46.09-
  - before 20 weeks gestation O20.9
    - specified type NEC O20.8
    - threatened abortion O20.0
  - due to
    - abruptio placenta (*see also* Abuptio placentae) O45.9-
    - leiomyoma, uterus —*see* Hemorrhage, antepartum, specified cause NEC
    - placenta previa O44.1-
  - specified cause NEC O46.8X-
- anus (sphincter) K62.5
- apoplexy (stroke) —*see* Hemorrhage, intracranial, intracerebral
- arachnoid —*see* Hemorrhage, intracranial, subarachnoid
- artery R58
  - brain —*see* Hemorrhage, intracranial, intracerebral
- basilar (ganglion) I61.0
- bladder N32.89
- bowel K92.2
  - newborn P54.3
- brain (miliary) (nontraumatic) —*see* Hemorrhage, intracranial, intracerebral
  - due to
    - birth injury P10.1
    - syphilis A52.05
  - epidural or extradural (traumatic) —*see* Injury, intracranial, epidural hemorrhage
  - newborn P52.4
    - birth injury P10.1

Hemorrhage, hemorrhagic *(continued)*
- brain *(continued)*
  - subarachnoid —*see* Hemorrhage, intracranial, subarachnoid
  - subdural —*see* Hemorrhage, intracranial, subdural
- brainstem (nontraumatic) I61.3
  - traumatic S06.38-
- breast N64.59
- bronchial tube —*see* Hemorrhage, lung
- bronchopulmonary —*see* Hemorrhage, lung
- bronchus —*see* Hemorrhage, lung
- bulbar I61.5
- capillary I78.8
  - primary D69.8
- cecum K92.2
- cerebellar, cerebellum (nontraumatic) I61.4
  - newborn P52.6
  - traumatic S06.37-
- cerebral, cerebrum —*see also* Hemorrhage, intracranial, intracerebral
  - newborn (anoxic) P52.4
    - birth injury P10.1
  - lobe I61.1
- cerebromeningeal I61.8
- cerebrospinal —*see* Hemorrhage, intracranial, intracerebral
- cervix (uteri) (stump) NEC N88.8
- chamber, anterior (eye) —*see* Hyphema
- childbirth —*see* Hemorrhage, complicating, delivery
- choroid H31.30-
  - expulsive H31.31-
- ciliary body —*see* Hyphema
- cochlea —*see* subcategory H83.8
- colon K92.2
- complicating
  - abortion —*see* Abortion, by type, complicated by, hemorrhage
  - delivery O67.9
    - associated with coagulation defect (afibrinogenemia) (DIC) (hyperfibrinolysis) O67.0
    - specified cause NEC O67.8
  - surgical procedure —*see* Hemorrhage, intraoperative
- conjunctiva H11.3-
  - newborn P54.8
- cord, newborn (stump) P51.9
- corpus luteum (ruptured) cyst N83.1-
- cortical (brain) I61.1
- cranial —*see* Hemorrhage, intracranial
- cutaneous R23.3
  - due to autosensitivity, erythrocyte D69.2
  - newborn P54.5
- delayed
  - following ectopic or molar pregnancy O08.1
  - postpartum O72.2
- diathesis (familial) D69.9
- disease D69.9
  - newborn P53
  - specified type NEC D69.8
- due to or associated with
  - afibrinogenemia or other coagulation defect (conditions in categories D65-D69)
    - antepartum —*see* Hemorrhage, antepartum, with coagulation defect
    - intrapartum O67.0
  - dental implant M27.61

Hemorrhage, hemorrhagic *(continued)*

- due to or associated with *(continued)*
  - device, implant or graft (*see also* Complications, by site and type, specified NEC) T85.838
    - arterial graft NEC T82.838
    - breast T85.838
    - catheter NEC T85.838
      - dialysis (renal) T82.838
        - intraperitoneal T85.838
      - infusion NEC T82.838
        - spinal (epidural) (subdural) T85.830
      - urinary (indwelling) T83.83
    - electronic (electrode) (pulse generator) (stimulator)
      - bone T84.83
      - cardiac T82.837
      - nervous system (brain) (peripheral nerve) (spinal) T85.830
      - urinary T83.83
    - fixation, internal (orthopedic) NEC T84.83
    - gastrointestinal (bile duct) (esophagus) T85.838
    - genital NEC T83.83
    - heart NEC T82.837
    - joint prosthesis T84.83
    - ocular (corneal graft) (orbital implant) NEC T85.838
    - orthopedic NEC T84.83
      - bone graft T86.838
    - specified NEC T85.838
    - urinary NEC T83.83
    - vascular NEC T82.838
    - ventricular intracranial shunt T85.830
- duodenum, duodenal K92.2
  - ulcer *—see* Ulcer, duodenum, with hemorrhage
- dura mater *—see* Hemorrhage, intracranial, subdural
- endotracheal *—see* Hemorrhage, lung
- epicranial subaponeurotic (massive), birth injury P12.2
- epidural (traumatic) *—see also* Injury, intracranial, epidural hemorrhage
  - nontraumatic I62.1
- esophagus K22.89
  - varix I85.01
    - secondary I85.11
- excessive, following ectopic gestation (subsequent episode) O08.1
- extradural (traumatic) *—see* Injury, intracranial, epidural hemorrhage
  - birth injury P10.8
  - newborn (anoxic) (nontraumatic) P52.8
  - nontraumatic I62.1
- eye NEC H57.89
  - fundus *—see* Hemorrhage, retina
  - lid *—see* Disorder, eyelid, specified type NEC
- fallopian tube N83.6
- fibrinogenolysis *—see* Fibrinolysis
- fibrinolytic (acquired) *—see* Fibrinolysis
- from
  - ear (nontraumatic) *—see* Otorrhagia
  - tracheostomy stoma J95.01
- fundus, eye *—see* Hemorrhage, retina
- funis *—see* Hemorrhage, umbilicus, cord

Hemorrhage, hemorrhagic *(continued)*

- gastric *—see* Hemorrhage, stomach
- gastroenteric K92.2
  - newborn P54.3
- gastrointestinal (tract) K92.2
  - newborn P54.3
- genital organ, male N50.1
- genitourinary (tract) NOS R31.9
- gingiva K06.8
- globe (eye) *—see* Hemophthalmos
- graafian follicle cyst (ruptured) N83.0-
- gum K06.8
- heart I51.89
- hypopharyngeal (throat) R04.1
- intermenstrual (regular) N92.3
  - irregular N92.1
- internal (organs) NEC R58
  - capsule I61.0
  - ear H83.8
  - newborn P54.8
- intestine K92.2
  - newborn P54.3
- intra-abdominal R58
- intra-alveolar (lung), newborn P26.8
- intracerebral (nontraumatic) *—see* Hemorrhage, intracranial, intracerebral
- intracranial (nontraumatic) I62.9
  - birth injury P10.9
  - epidural, nontraumatic I62.1
  - extradural, nontraumatic I62.1
  - newborn P52.9
    - specified NEC P52.8
  - intracerebral (nontraumatic) (in) I61.9
    - brain stem I61.3
    - cerebellum I61.4
    - newborn P52.4
      - birth injury P10.1
    - hemisphere I61.2
      - cortical (superficial) I61.1
      - subcortical (deep) I61.0
    - intraoperative
      - during a nervous system procedure G97.31
      - during other procedure G97.32
    - intraventricular I61.5
    - multiple localized I61.6
    - postprocedural
      - following a nervous system procedure G97.51
      - following other procedure G97.52
    - specified NEC I61.8
    - superficial I61.1
    - traumatic (diffuse) *—see* Injury, intracranial, diffuse
      - focal *—see* Injury, intracranial, focal
  - subarachnoid (nontraumatic) (from) I60.9
    - newborn P52.5
      - birth injury P10.3
    - intracranial (cerebral) artery I60.7
      - anterior communicating I60.2
      - basilar I60.4
      - carotid siphon and bifurcation I60.0-
      - communicating I60.7
        - anterior I60.2
        - posterior I60.3-
      - middle cerebral I60.1-
      - posterior communicating I60.3-

Hemorrhage, hemorrhagic *(continued)*

- intracranial *(continued)*
  - subarachnoid *(continued)*
    - intracranial artery *(continued)*
      - specified artery NEC I60.6
      - vertebral I60.5-
    - specified NEC I60.8
    - traumatic S06.6X-
  - subdural (nontraumatic) I62.00
    - acute I62.01
    - birth injury P10.0
    - chronic I62.03
    - newborn (anoxic) (hypoxic) P52.8
      - birth injury P10.0
    - spinal G95.19
    - subacute I62.02
    - traumatic *—see* Injury, intracranial, subdural hemorrhage
  - traumatic *—see* Injury, intracranial, focal brain injury
- intramedullary NEC G95.19
- intraocular *—see* Hemophthalmos
- intraoperative, intraprocedural *—see* Complication, hemorrhage (hematoma), intraoperative (intraprocedural), by site
- intrapartum *—see* Hemorrhage, complicating, delivery
- intrapelvic
  - female N94.89
  - male K66.1
- intraperitoneal K66.1
- intrapontine I61.3
- intraprocedural *—see* Complication, hemorrhage (hematoma), intraoperative (intraprocedural), by site
- intrauterine N85.7
  - complicating delivery (*see also* Hemorrhage, complicating, delivery) O67.9
  - postpartum *—see* Hemorrhage, postpartum
- intraventricular I61.5
  - newborn (nontraumatic) (*see also* Newborn, affected by, hemorrhage) P52.3
    - due to birth injury P10.2
    - grade
      - 1 P52.0
      - 2 P52.1
      - 3 P52.21
      - 4 P52.22
- intravesical N32.89
- iris (postinfectional) (postinflammatory) (toxic) *—see* Hyphema
- joint (nontraumatic) *—see* Hemarthrosis
- kidney N28.89
- knee (joint) (nontraumatic) *—see* Hemarthrosis, knee
- labyrinth *—see* subcategory H83.8
- lenticular striate artery I61.0
- ligature, vessel *—see* Hemorrhage, postoperative
- liver K76.89
- lung R04.89
  - newborn P26.9
    - massive P26.1
    - specified NEC P26.8
  - tuberculous *—see* Tuberculosis, pulmonary
- massive umbilical, newborn P51.0
- mediastinum *—see* Hemorrhage, lung
- medulla I61.3

Hemorrhage, hemorrhagic *(continued)*

- membrane (brain) I60.8
  - spinal cord *—see* Hemorrhage, spinal cord
- meninges, meningeal (brain) (middle) I60.8
  - spinal cord *—see* Hemorrhage, spinal cord
- mesentery K66.1
- metritis *—see* Endometritis
- mouth K13.79
- mucous membrane NEC R58
  - newborn P54.8
- muscle M62.89
- nail (subungual) L60.8
- nasal turbinate R04.0
  - newborn P54.8
- navel, newborn P51.9
- newborn P54.9
  - specified NEC P54.8
- nipple N64.59
- nose R04.0
  - newborn P54.8
- omentum K66.1
- optic nerve (sheath) H47.02-
- orbit, orbital H05.23-
- ovary NEC N83.8
- oviduct N83.6
- pancreas K86.89
- parathyroid (gland) (spontaneous) E21.4
- parturition *—see* Hemorrhage, complicating, delivery
- penis N48.89
- pericardium, pericarditis I31.2
- peritoneum, peritoneal K66.1
- peritonsillar tissue J35.8
  - due to infection J36
- petechial R23.3
  - due to autosensitivity, erythrocyte D69.2
- pituitary (gland) E23.6
- pleura *—see* Hemorrhage, lung
- polioencephalitis, superior E51.2
- polymyositis *—see* Polymyositis
- pons, pontine I61.3
- posterior fossa (nontraumatic) I61.8
  - newborn P52.6
- postmenopausal N95.0
- postnasal R04.0
- postoperative *—see* Complications, postprocedural, hemorrhage, by site
- postpartum NEC (following delivery of placenta) O72.1
  - delayed or secondary O72.2
  - retained placenta O72.0
  - third stage O72.0
- pregnancy *—see* Hemorrhage, antepartum
- preretinal *—see* Hemorrhage, retina
- prostate N42.1
- puerperal *—see* Hemorrhage, postpartum
  - delayed or secondary O72.2
- pulmonary R04.89
  - newborn P26.9
    - massive P26.1
    - specified NEC P26.8
  - tuberculous *—see* Tuberculosis, pulmonary
- purpura (primary) D69.3
- rectum (sphincter) K62.5
  - newborn P54.2
- recurring, following initial hemorrhage at time of injury T79.2
- renal N28.89
- respiratory passage or tract R04.9
  - specified NEC R04.89

Hemorrhage, hemorrhagic *(continued)*
- retina, retinal (vessels) H35.6-
  - diabetic —*see* Diabetes, retinal, hemorrhage
- retroperitoneal R58
- scalp R58
- scrotum N50.1
- secondary (nontraumatic) R58
  - following initial hemorrhage at time of injury T79.2
- seminal vesicle N50.1
- skin R23.3
  - newborn P54.5
- slipped umbilical ligature P51.8
- spermatic cord N50.1
- spinal (cord) G95.19
  - newborn (birth injury) P11.5
- spleen D73.5
  - intraoperative —*see* Complications, intraoperative, hemorrhage, spleen
  - postprocedural —*see* Complications, postprocedural, hemorrhage, spleen
- stomach K92.2
  - newborn P54.3
  - ulcer —*see* Ulcer, stomach, with hemorrhage
- subarachnoid (nontraumatic) —*see* Hemorrhage, intracranial, subarachnoid
- subconjunctival —*see also* Hemorrhage, conjunctiva
  - birth injury P15.3
- subcortical (brain) I61.0
- subcutaneous R23.3
- subdiaphragmatic R58
- subdural (acute) (nontraumatic) —*see* Hemorrhage, intracranial, subdural
- subependymal
  - newborn P52.0
    - with intraventricular extension P52.1
      - and intracerebral extension P52.22
- subgaleal P12.2
- subhyaloid —*see* Hemorrhage, retina
- subperiosteal —*see* Disorder, bone, specified type NEC
- subretinal —*see* Hemorrhage, retina
- subtentorial —*see* Hemorrhage, intracranial, subdural
- subungual L60.8
- suprarenal (capsule) (gland) E27.49
  - newborn P54.4
- tentorium (traumatic) NEC —*see* Hemorrhage, brain
  - newborn (birth injury) P10.4
- testis N50.1
- third stage (postpartum) O72.0
- thorax —*see* Hemorrhage, lung
- throat R04.1
- thymus (gland) E32.8
- thyroid (cyst) (gland) E07.89
- tongue K14.8
- tonsil J35.8
- trachea —*see* Hemorrhage, lung
- tracheobronchial R04.89
  - newborn P26.0
- traumatic - code to specific injury
  - cerebellar —*see* Hemorrhage, brain
  - intracranial —*see* Hemorrhage, brain
  - recurring or secondary (following initial hemorrhage at time of injury) T79.2

Hemorrhage, hemorrhagic *(continued)*
- tuberculous NEC (*see also* Tuberculosis, pulmonary) A15.0
- tunica vaginalis N50.1
- ulcer - code by site under Ulcer, with hemorrhage K27.4
- umbilicus, umbilical
  - cord
    - after birth, newborn P51.9
    - complicating delivery O69.5
  - newborn P51.9
    - massive P51.0
    - slipped ligature P51.8
  - stump P51.9
- urethra (idiopathic) N36.8
- uterus, uterine (abnormal) N93.9
  - climacteric N92.4
  - complicating delivery —*see* Hemorrhage, complicating, delivery
  - dysfunctional or functional N93.8
  - intermenstrual (regular) N92.3
    - irregular N92.1
  - postmenopausal N95.0
  - postpartum —*see* Hemorrhage, postpartum
  - preclimacteric or premenopausal N92.4
  - prepubertal N93.8
  - pubertal N92.2
- vagina (abnormal) N93.9
  - newborn P54.6
- vas deferens N50.1
- vasa previa O69.4
- ventricular I61.5
- vesical N32.89
- viscera NEC R58
  - newborn P54.8
- vitreous (humor) (intraocular) H43.1-
- vulva N90.89

Hemorrhoids (bleeding) (without mention of degree) K64.9
- 1st degree (grade/stage I) (without prolapse outside of anal canal) K64.0
- 2nd degree (grade/stage II) (that prolapse with straining but retract spontaneously) K64.1
- 3rd degree (grade/stage III) (that prolapse with straining and require manual replacement back inside anal canal) K64.2
- 4th degree (grade/stage IV) (with prolapsed tissue that cannot be manually replaced) K64.3
- complicating
  - pregnancy O22.4
  - puerperium O87.2
- external K64.4
  - with
    - thrombosis K64.5
- internal (without mention of degree) K64.8
- prolapsed K64.8
- skin tags
  - anus K64.4
  - residual K64.4
- specified NEC K64.8
- strangulated (*see also* Hemorrhoids, by degree) K64.8
- thrombosed (*see also* Hemorrhoids, by degree) K64.5
- ulcerated (*see also* Hemorrhoids, by degree) K64.8

Hemosalpinx N83.6
- with
  - hematocolpos N89.7

Hemosalpinx *(continued)*
- with *(continued)*
  - hematometra N85.7
    - with hematocolpos N89.7

Hemosiderosis (dietary) E83.19
- pulmonary, idiopathic E83.1- *[J84.03]*
- transfusion T80.89

Hemothorax (bacterial) (nontuberculous) J94.2
- newborn P54.8
- traumatic S27.1
  - with pneumothorax S27.2
- tuberculous NEC A15.6

Henoch (-Schönlein) **disease or syndrome** (purpura) D69.0

Henpue, henpuye A66.6

Hepar lobatum (syphilitic) A52.74

Hepatalgia K76.89

Hepatitis K75.9
- acute B17.9
  - with coma K72.01
  - with hepatic failure —*see* Failure, hepatic
  - alcoholic —*see* Hepatitis, alcoholic
  - infectious B17.9
  - non-viral K72.0
  - viral B17.9
- alcoholic (acute) (chronic) K70.10
  - with ascites K70.11
- amebic —*see* Abscess, liver, amebic
- anicteric,(viral) —*see* Hepatitis, viral
- antigen-associated (HAA) —*see* Hepatitis, B
- Australia-antigen (positive) —*see* Hepatitis, B
- autoimmune K75.4
- B B19.10
  - with hepatic coma B19.11
  - acute B16.9
    - with
      - delta-agent (coinfection) (without hepatic coma) B16.1
        - with hepatic coma B16.0
      - hepatic coma (without delta-agent coinfection) B16.2
  - chronic B18.1
    - with delta-agent B18.0
- bacterial NEC K75.89
- C (viral) B19.20
  - with hepatic coma B19.21
  - acute B17.10
    - with hepatic coma B17.11
  - chronic B18.2
- catarrhal (acute) B15.9
  - with hepatic coma B15.0
- cholangiolitic K75.89
- cholestatic K75.89
- chronic K73.9
  - active NEC K73.2
  - lobular NEC K73.1
  - persistent NEC K73.0
  - specified NEC K73.8
- cytomegaloviral B25.1
- due to ethanol (acute) (chronic) —*see* Hepatitis, alcoholic
- epidemic B15.9
  - with hepatic coma B15.0
- fulminant NEC (viral) —*see* Hepatitis, viral
- granulomatous NEC K75.3
- herpesviral B00.81

Hepatitis *(continued)*
- history of
  - B Z86.19
  - C Z86.19
- homologous serum —*see* Hepatitis, viral, type B
- in (due to)
  - mumps B26.81
  - toxoplasmosis (acquired) B58.1
    - congenital (active) P37.1 *[K77]*
- infectious, infective B15.9
  - acute (subacute) B17.9
  - chronic B18.9
- inoculation —*see* Hepatitis, viral, type B
- interstitial (chronic) K74.69
- ischemia, ischemic K72.00
- lupoid NEC K75.4
- malignant NEC (with hepatic failure) K72.90
  - with coma K72.91
- neonatal (idiopathic) (toxic) P59.29
- neonatal giant cell P59.29
- newborn P59.29
- postimmunization —*see* Hepatitis, viral, type B
- post-transfusion —*see* Hepatitis, viral, type B
- reactive, nonspecific K75.2
- serum —*see* Hepatitis, viral, type B
- shock K72.00
- specified type NEC
  - with hepatic failure —*see* Failure, hepatic
- syphilitic (late) A52.74
  - congenital (early) A50.08 *[K77]*
    - late A50.59 *[K77]*
  - secondary A51.45
- toxic (*see also* Disease, liver, toxic) K71.6
- tuberculous A18.83
- viral, virus B19.9
  - with hepatic coma B19.0
  - acute B17.9
  - chronic B18.9
    - specified NEC B18.8
    - type
      - B B18.1
        - with delta-agent B18.0
      - C B18.2
  - congenital P35.3
  - coxsackie B33.8 *[K77]*
  - cytomegalic inclusion B25.1
  - in remission, any type - code to Hepatitis, chronic, by type
  - non-A, non-B B17.8
  - specified type NEC (with or without coma) B17.8
  - type
    - A B15.9
      - with hepatic coma B15.0
    - B B19.10
      - with hepatic coma B19.11
      - acute B16.9
        - with
          - delta-agent (coinfection) (without hepatic coma) B16.1
            - with hepatic coma B16.0
          - hepatic coma (without delta-agent coinfection) B16.2
      - chronic B18.1
        - with delta-agent B18.0
    - C B19.20
      - with hepatic coma B19.21
      - acute B17.10
        - with hepatic coma B17.11
      - chronic B18.2

Hepatitis *(continued)*
- viral, virus *(continued)*
  - type *(continued)*
    - E B17.2
    - non-A, non-B B17.8

Hepatization lung (acute) *—see* Pneumonia, lobar

Hepatoblastoma C22.2

Hepatocarcinoma C22.0

Hepatocholangiocarcinoma C22.0

Hepatocholangioma, benign D13.4

Hepatocholangitis K75.89

Hepatolenticular degeneration E83.01

Hepatoma (malignant) C22.0
- benign D13.4
- embryonal C22.0

Hepatomegaly *—see also* Hypertrophy, liver
- with splenomegaly R16.2
- congenital Q44.7
- in mononucleosis
  - gammaherpesviral B27.09
  - infectious specified NEC B27.89

Hepatoptosis K76.89

Hepatorenal syndrome following labor and delivery O90.4

Hepatosis K76.89

Hepatosplenomegaly R16.2
- hyperlipemic (Bürger-Grütz type) E78.3 *[K77]*

Hereditary *—see* condition

Hereditary alpha tryptasemia (syndrome) D89.44

Heredodegeneration, macular *—see* Dystrophy, retina

Heredopathia atactica polyneuritiformis G60.1

Heredosyphilis *—see* Syphilis, congenital

Herlitz' syndrome Q81.1

Hermansky-Pudlak syndrome E70.331

Hermaphrodite, hermaphroditism (true) Q56.0
- 46,XX with streak gonads Q99.1
- 46,XX/46,XY Q99.0
- 46,XY with streak gonads Q99.1
- chimera 46,XX/46,XY Q99.0

Hernia, hernial (acquired) (recurrent) K46.9
- with
  - gangrene *—see* Hernia, by site, with, gangrene
  - incarceration *—see* Hernia, by site, with, obstruction
  - irreducible *—see* Hernia, by site, with, obstruction
  - obstruction *—see* Hernia, by site, with, obstruction
  - strangulation *—see* Hernia, by site, with, obstruction
- abdomen, abdominal K46.9
  - with
    - gangrene (and obstruction) K46.1
    - obstruction K46.0
  - femoral *—see* Hernia, femoral
  - incisional *—see* Hernia, incisional
  - inguinal *—see* Hernia, inguinal

Hernia, hernial *(continued)*
- abdomen, abdominal *(continued)*
  - specified site NEC K45.8
    - with
      - gangrene (and obstruction) K45.1
      - obstruction K45.0
  - umbilical *—see* Hernia, umbilical
  - wall *—see* Hernia, ventral
- appendix *—see* Hernia, abdomen
- bladder (mucosa) (sphincter)
  - congenital (female) (male) Q79.51
  - female *—see* Cystocele
  - male N32.89
- brain, congenital *—see* Encephalocele
- cartilage, vertebra *—see* Displacement, intervertebral disc
- cerebral, congenital *—see also* Encephalocele
  - endaural Q01.8
- ciliary body (traumatic) S05.2-
- colon *—see* Hernia, abdomen
- Cooper's *—see* Hernia, abdomen, specified site NEC
- crural *—see* Hernia, femoral
- diaphragm, diaphragmatic K44.9
  - with
    - gangrene (and obstruction) K44.1
    - obstruction K44.0
  - congenital Q79.0
- direct (inguinal) *—see* Hernia, inguinal
- diverticulum, intestine *—see* Hernia, abdomen
- double (inguinal) *—see* Hernia, inguinal, bilateral
- due to adhesions (with obstruction) K56.50
- epigastric (*see also* Hernia, ventral) K43.9
- esophageal hiatus *—see* Hernia, hiatal
- external (inguinal) *—see* Hernia, inguinal
- fallopian tube N83.4-
- fascia M62.89
- femoral K41.90
  - with
    - gangrene (and obstruction) K41.40
      - not specified as recurrent K41.40
      - recurrent K41.41
    - obstruction K41.30
      - not specified as recurrent K41.30
      - recurrent K41.31
  - bilateral K41.20
    - with
      - gangrene (and obstruction) K41.10
        - not specified as recurrent K41.10
        - recurrent K41.11
      - obstruction K41.00
        - not specified as recurrent K41.00
        - recurrent K41.01
    - not specified as recurrent K41.20
    - recurrent K41.21
  - unilateral K41.90
    - with
      - gangrene (and obstruction) K41.40
        - not specified as recurrent K41.40

Hernia, hernial *(continued)*
- femoral *(continued)*
  - unilateral *(continued)*
    - with *(continued)*
      - gangrene *(continued)*
        - recurrent K41.41
      - obstruction K41.30
        - not specified as recurrent K41.30
        - recurrent K41.31
    - not specified as recurrent K41.90
    - recurrent K41.91
  - not specified as recurrent K41.90
  - recurrent K41.91
- foramen magnum G93.5
  - congenital Q01.8
- funicular (umbilical) *—see also* Hernia, umbilicus
  - spermatic (cord) *—see* Hernia, inguinal
- gastrointestinal tract *—see* Hernia, abdomen
- Hesselbach's *—see* Hernia, femoral, specified site NEC
- hiatal (esophageal) (sliding) K44.9
  - with
    - gangrene (and obstruction) K44.1
    - obstruction K44.0
  - congenital Q40.1
- hypogastric *—see* Hernia, ventral
- incarcerated *—see also* Hernia, by site, with obstruction
  - with gangrene *—see* Hernia, by site, with gangrene
- incisional K43.2
  - with
    - gangrene (and obstruction) K43.1
    - obstruction K43.0
- indirect (inguinal) *—see* Hernia, inguinal
- inguinal (direct) (external) (funicular) (indirect) (internal) (oblique) (scrotal) (sliding) K40.90
  - with
    - gangrene (and obstruction) K40.40
      - not specified as recurrent K40.40
      - recurrent K40.41
    - obstruction K40.30
      - not specified as recurrent K40.30
      - recurrent K40.31
  - not specified as recurrent K40.90
  - recurrent K40.91
  - bilateral K40.20
    - with
      - gangrene (and obstruction) K40.10
        - not specified as recurrent K40.10
        - recurrent K40.11
      - obstruction K40.00
        - not specified as recurrent K40.00
        - recurrent K40.01
    - not specified as recurrent K40.20
    - recurrent K40.21
  - unilateral K40.90
    - with
      - gangrene (and obstruction) K40.40
        - not specified as recurrent K40.40
        - recurrent K40.41

Hernia, hernial *(continued)*
- inguinal *(continued)*
  - unilateral *(continued)*
    - with *(continued)*
      - obstruction K40.30
        - not specified as recurrent K40.30
        - recurrent K40.31
    - not specified as recurrent K40.90
    - recurrent K40.91
- internal *—see also* Hernia, abdomen
  - inguinal *—see* Hernia, inguinal
- interstitial *—see* Hernia, abdomen
- intervertebral cartilage or disc *—see* Displacement, intervertebral disc
- intestine, intestinal *—see* Hernia, by site
- intra-abdominal *—see* Hernia, abdomen
- iris (traumatic) S05.2-
- irreducible *—see also* Hernia, by site, with obstruction
  - with gangrene *—see* Hernia, by site, with gangrene
- ischiatic *—see* Hernia, abdomen, specified site NEC
- ischiorectal *—see* Hernia, abdomen, specified site NEC
- lens (traumatic) S05.2-
- linea (alba) (semilunaris) *—see* Hernia, ventral
- Littre's *—see* Hernia, abdomen
- lumbar *—see* Hernia, abdomen, specified site NEC
- lung (subcutaneous) J98.4
- mediastinum J98.59
- mesenteric (internal) *—see* Hernia, abdomen
- midline *—see* Hernia, ventral
- muscle (sheath) M62.89
- nucleus pulposus *—see* Displacement, intervertebral disc
- oblique (inguinal) *—see* Hernia, inguinal
- obstructive *—see also* Hernia, by site, with obstruction
  - with gangrene *—see* Hernia, by site, with gangrene
- obturator *—see* Hernia, abdomen, specified site NEC
- omental *—see* Hernia, abdomen
- ovary N83.4-
- oviduct N83.4-
- paraesophageal *—see also* Hernia, diaphragm
  - congenital Q40.1
- parastomal K43.5
  - with
    - gangrene (and obstruction) K43.4
    - obstruction K43.3
- paraumbilical *—see* Hernia, umbilicus
- perineal *—see* Hernia, abdomen, specified site NEC
- Petit's *—see* Hernia, abdomen, specified site NEC
- postoperative *—see* Hernia, incisional
- pregnant uterus *—see* Abnormal, uterus in pregnancy or childbirth
- prevesical N32.89
- properitoneal *—see* Hernia, abdomen, specified site NEC
- pudendal *—see* Hernia, abdomen, specified site NEC
- rectovaginal N81.6

Hernia, hernial *(continued)*
- retroperitoneal *—see* Hernia, abdomen, specified site NEC
- Richter's *—see* Hernia, abdomen, with obstruction
- Rieux's, Riex's *—see* Hernia, abdomen, specified site NEC
- sac condition (adhesion) (dropsy) (inflammation) (laceration) (suppuration) - code by site under Hernia
- sciatic *—see* Hernia, abdomen, specified site NEC
- scrotum, scrotal *—see* Hernia, inguinal
- sliding (inguinal) *—see also* Hernia, inguinal
  - hiatus *—see* Hernia, hiatal
- spigelian *—see* Hernia, ventral
- spinal *—see* Spina bifida
- strangulated *—see also* Hernia, by site, with obstruction
  - with gangrene *—see* Hernia, by site, with gangrene
- subxiphoid *—see* Hernia, ventral
- supra-umbilicus *—see* Hernia, ventral
- tendon *—see* Disorder, tendon, specified type NEC
- Treitz's (fossa) *—see* Hernia, abdomen, specified site NEC
- tunica vaginalis Q55.29
- umbilicus, umbilical K42.9
  - with
    - gangrene (and obstruction) K42.1
    - obstruction K42.0
- ureter N28.89
- urethra, congenital Q64.79
- urinary meatus, congenital Q64.79
- uterus N81.4
  - pregnant *—see* Abnormal, uterus in pregnancy or childbirth
- vaginal (anterior) (wall) *—see* Cystocele
- Velpeau's *—see* Hernia, femoral
- ventral K43.9
  - with
    - gangrene (and obstruction) K43.7
    - obstruction K43.6
  - recurrent *—see* Hernia, incisional
  - incisional K43.2
    - with
      - gangrene (and obstruction) K43.1
      - obstruction K43.0
  - specified NEC K43.9
    - with
      - gangrene (and obstruction) K43.7
      - obstruction K43.6
- vesical
  - congenital (female) (male) Q79.51
  - female *—see* Cystocele
  - male N32.89
- vitreous (into wound) S05.2-
  - into anterior chamber *—see* Prolapse, vitreous

Herniation *—see also* Hernia
- brain (stem) G93.5
  - nontraumatic G93.5
  - traumatic S06.A1
    - cerebellar S06.A1
    - subfalcine (cingulate) S06.A1
    - tonsillar S06.A1
    - transtentorial (central) (upward cerebellar) S06.A1
    - uncal S06.A1

Herniation *(continued)*
- cerebral G93.5
  - nontraumatic G93.5
  - traumatic S06.A1
- mediastinum J98.59
- nucleus pulposus *—see* Displacement, intervertebral disc

Herpangina B08.5

Herpes, herpesvirus, herpetic B00.9
- anogenital A60.9
  - perianal skin A60.1
  - rectum A60.1
  - urogenital tract A60.00
    - cervix A60.03
    - male genital organ NEC A60.02
    - penis A60.01
    - specified site NEC A60.09
    - vagina A60.04
    - vulva A60.04
- blepharitis (zoster) B02.39
  - simplex B00.59
- circinatus B35.4
  - bullosus L12.0
- conjunctivitis (simplex) B00.53
  - zoster B02.31
- cornea B02.33
- encephalitis B00.4
  - due to herpesvirus 6 B10.01
  - due to herpesvirus 7 B10.09
  - specified NEC B10.09
- eye (zoster) B02.30
  - simplex B00.50
- eyelid (zoster) B02.39
  - simplex B00.59
- facialis B00.1
- febrilis B00.1
- geniculate ganglionitis B02.21
- genital, genitalis A60.00
  - female A60.09
  - male A60.02
- gestational, gestationis O26.4-
- gingivostomatitis B00.2
- human B00.9
  - 1 *—see* Herpes, simplex
  - 2 *—see* Herpes, simplex
  - 3 *—see* Varicella
  - 4 *—see* Mononucleosis, Epstein-Barr (virus)
  - 5 *—see* Disease, cytomegalic inclusion (generalized)
  - 6
    - encephalitis B10.01
    - specified NEC B10.81
  - 7
    - encephalitis B10.09
    - specified NEC B10.82
  - 8 B10.89
- infection NEC B10.89
  - Kaposi's sarcoma associated B10.89
- iridocyclitis (simplex) B00.51
  - zoster B02.32
- iris (vesicular erythema multiforme) L51.9
- iritis (simplex) B00.51
- Kaposi's sarcoma associated B10.89
- keratitis (simplex) (dendritic) (disciform) (interstitial) B00.52
  - zoster (interstitial) B02.33
- keratoconjunctivitis (simplex) B00.52
  - zoster B02.33
- labialis B00.1
- lip B00.1
- meningitis (simplex) B00.3
  - zoster B02.1
- ophthalmicus (zoster) NEC B02.30
  - simplex B00.50

Herpes, herpesvirus, herpetic *(continued)*
- penis A60.01
- perianal skin A60.1
- pharyngitis, pharyngotonsillitis B00.2
- rectum A60.1
- scrotum A60.02
- sepsis B00.7
- simplex B00.9
  - complicated NEC B00.89
  - congenital P35.2
  - conjunctivitis B00.53
  - external ear B00.1
  - eyelid B00.59
  - hepatitis B00.81
  - keratitis (interstitial) B00.52
  - myleitis B00.82
  - specified complication NEC B00.89
  - visceral B00.89
- stomatitis B00.2
- tonsurans B35.0
- visceral B00.89
- vulva A60.04
- whitlow B00.89
- zoster (*see also* condition) B02.9
  - auricularis B02.21
  - complicated NEC B02.8
  - conjunctivitis B02.31
  - disseminated B02.7
  - encephalitis B02.0
  - eye (lid) B02.39
  - geniculate ganglionitis B02.21
  - keratitis (interstitial) B02.33
  - meningitis B02.1
  - myelitis B02.24
  - neuritis, neuralgia B02.29
  - ophthalmicus NEC B02.30
  - oticus B02.21
  - polyneuropathy B02.23
  - specified complication NEC B02.8
  - trigeminal neuralgia B02.22

Herpesvirus (human) *—see* Herpes

Herpetophobia F40.218

Herrick's anemia *—see* Disease, sickle-cell

Hers' disease E74.09

Herter-Gee syndrome K90.0

Herxheimer's reaction R68.89

Hesitancy
- of micturition R39.11
- urinary R39.11

Hesselbach's hernia *—see* Hernia, femoral, specified site NEC

Heterochromia (congenital) Q13.2
- cataract *—see* Cataract, complicated
- cyclitis (Fuchs) *—see* Cyclitis, Fuchs' heterochromic
- hair L67.1
- iritis *—see* Cyclitis, Fuchs' heterochromic
- retained metallic foreign body (nonmagnetic) *—see* Foreign body, intraocular, old, retained
  - magnetic *—see* Foreign body, intraocular, old, retained, magnetic
- uveitis *—see* Cyclitis, Fuchs' heterochromic

Heterophoria *—see* Strabismus, heterophoria

Heterophyes, heterophyiasis (small intestine) B66.8

Heterotopia, heterotopic *—see also* Malposition, congenital
- cerebralis Q04.8

Heterotropia *—see* Strabismus

Heubner-Herter disease K90.0

Hexadactylism Q69.9

HGSIL (cytology finding) (high grade squamous intraepithelial lesion on cytologic smear) (Pap smear finding)
- anus R85.613
- cervix R87.613
  - biopsy (histology) finding *—see* Neoplasia, intraepithelial, cervix, grade II or grade III
- vagina R87.623
  - biopsy (histology) finding *—see* Neoplasia, intraepithelial, vagina, grade II or grade III

Hibernoma *—see* Lipoma

Hiccup, hiccough R06.6
- epidemic B33.0
- psychogenic F45.8

Hidden penis (congenital) Q55.64
- acquired N48.83

Hidradenitis (axillaris) (suppurative) L73.2

Hidradenoma (nodular) *—see also* Neoplasm, skin, benign
- clear cell *—see* Neoplasm, skin, benign
- papillary *—see* Neoplasm, skin, benign

Hidrocystoma *—see* Neoplasm, skin, benign

High
- altitude effects T70.20
  - anoxia T70.29
  - on
    - ears T70.0
    - sinuses T70.1
  - polycythemia D75.1
- arch
  - foot Q66.7-
  - palate, congenital Q38.5
- arterial tension *—see* Hypertension
- basal metabolic rate R94.8
- blood pressure *—see also* Hypertension
  - borderline R03.0
  - reading (incidental) (isolated) (nonspecific), without diagnosis of hypertension R03.0
- cholesterol E78.00
  - with high triglycerides E78.2
- diaphragm (congenital) Q79.1
- expressed emotional level within family Z63.8
- head at term O32.4
- palate, congenital Q38.5
- risk
  - infant NEC Z76.2
  - sexual behavior (heterosexual) Z72.51
    - bisexual Z72.53
    - homosexual Z72.52
- scrotal testis, testes
  - bilateral Q53.23
  - unilateral Q53.13
- temperature (of unknown origin) R50.9
- thoracic rib Q76.6
- triglycerides E78.1
  - with high cholesterol E78.2

Hildenbrand's disease A75.0

Hilum —*see* condition

Hip —*see* condition

Hippel's disease Q85.8

Hippophobia F40.218

Hippus H57.09

Hirschsprung's disease or megacolon Q43.1

Hirsutism, hirsuties L68.0

Hirudiniasis
- external B88.3
- internal B83.4

Hiss-Russell dysentery A03.1

Histidinemia, histidinuria E70.41

Histiocytoma —*see also* Neoplasm, skin, benign
- fibrous —*see also* Neoplasm, skin, benign
  - atypical —*see* Neoplasm, connective tissue, uncertain behavior
  - malignant —*see* Neoplasm, connective tissue, malignant

Histiocytosis D76.3
- acute differentiated progressive C96.0
- Langerhans' cell NEC C96.6
  - multifocal X
    - multisystemic (disseminated) C96.0
    - unisystemic C96.5
  - pulmonary, adult (adult PLCH) J84.82
  - unifocal (X) C96.6
- lipid, lipoid D76.3
  - essential E75.29
- malignant C96.A
- mononuclear phagocytes NEC D76.1
  - Langerhans' cells C96.6
- non-Langerhans cell D76.3
- polyostotic sclerosing D76.3
- sinus, with massive lymphadenopathy D76.3
- syndrome NEC D76.3
- X NEC C96.6
  - acute (progressive) C96.0
  - chronic C96.6
  - multifocal C96.5
  - multisystemic C96.0
  - unifocal C96.6

Histoplasmosis B39.9
- with pneumonia NEC B39.2
- African B39.5
- American —*see* Histoplasmosis, capsulati
- capsulati B39.4
  - disseminated B39.3
  - generalized B39.3
  - pulmonary B39.2
    - acute B39.0
    - chronic B39.1
- Darling's B39.4
- duboisii B39.5
- lung NEC B39.2

History
- family (of) —*see also* History, personal (of)
  - alcohol abuse Z81.1
  - allergy NEC Z84.89
  - anemia Z83.2
  - arthritis Z82.61
  - asthma Z82.5
  - blindness Z82.1
  - cardiac death (sudden) Z82.41
  - carrier of genetic disease Z84.81
  - chromosomal anomaly Z82.79

History *(continued)*
- family *(continued)*
  - chronic
    - disabling disease NEC Z82.8
    - lower respiratory disease Z82.5
  - colonic polyps Z83.71
  - congenital malformations and deformations Z82.79
    - polycystic kidney Z82.71
  - consanguinity Z84.3
  - deafness Z82.2
  - diabetes mellitus Z83.3
  - disability NEC Z82.8
  - disease or disorder (of)
    - allergic NEC Z84.89
    - behavioral NEC Z81.8
    - blood and blood-forming organs Z83.2
    - cardiovascular NEC Z82.49
    - chronic disabling NEC Z82.8
    - digestive Z83.79
    - ear NEC Z83.52
    - elevated lipoprotein (a) (Lp(a)) Z83.430
    - endocrine NEC Z83.49
    - eye NEC Z83.518
      - glaucoma Z83.511
    - familial hypercholesterolemia Z83.42
    - genitourinary NEC Z84.2
    - glaucoma Z83.511
    - hematological Z83.2
    - immune mechanism Z83.2
    - infectious NEC Z83.1
    - ischemic heart Z82.49
    - kidney Z84.1
    - lipoprotein metabolism Z83.438
    - mental NEC Z81.8
    - metabolic Z83.49
    - musculoskeletal NEC Z82.69
    - neurological NEC Z82.0
    - nutritional Z83.49
    - parasitic NEC Z83.1
    - psychiatric NEC Z81.8
    - respiratory NEC Z83.6
    - skin and subcutaneous tissue NEC Z84.0
    - specified NEC Z84.89
  - drug abuse NEC Z81.3
  - elevated lipoprotein (a) (Lp(a)) Z83.430
  - epilepsy Z82.0
  - familial hypercholesterolemia Z83.42
  - genetic disease carrier Z84.81
  - glaucoma Z83.511
  - hearing loss Z82.2
  - human immunodeficiency virus (HIV) infection Z83.0
  - Huntington's chorea Z82.0
  - hyperlipidemia, familial combined Z83.438
  - intellectual disability Z81.0
  - leukemia Z80.6
  - lipidemia NEC Z83.438
  - malignant neoplasm (of) NOS Z80.9
    - bladder Z80.52
    - breast Z80.3
    - bronchus Z80.1
    - digestive organ Z80.0
    - gastrointestinal tract Z80.0
    - genital organ Z80.49
      - ovary Z80.41
      - prostate Z80.42
      - specified organ NEC Z80.49
      - testis Z80.43

History *(continued)*
- family *(continued)*
  - malignant neoplasm (of) *(continued)*
    - hematopoietic NEC Z80.7
    - intrathoracic organ NEC Z80.2
    - kidney Z80.51
    - lung Z80.1
    - lymphatic NEC Z80.7
    - ovary Z80.41
    - prostate Z80.42
    - respiratory organ NEC Z80.2
    - specified site NEC Z80.8
    - testis Z80.43
    - trachea Z80.1
    - urinary organ or tract Z80.59
      - bladder Z80.52
      - kidney Z80.51
  - mental
    - disorder NEC Z81.8
  - multiple endocrine neoplasia (MEN) syndrome Z83.41
  - osteoporosis Z82.62
  - polycystic kidney Z82.71
  - polyps (colon) Z83.71
  - psychiatric disorder Z81.8
  - psychoactive substance abuse NEC Z81.3
  - respiratory condition NEC Z83.6
    - asthma and other lower respiratory conditions Z82.5
  - self-harmful behavior Z81.8
  - SIDS (sudden infant death syndrome) Z84.82
  - skin condition Z84.0
  - specified condition NEC Z84.89
  - stroke (cerebrovascular) Z82.3
  - substance abuse NEC Z81.4
    - alcohol Z81.1
    - drug NEC Z81.3
    - psychoactive NEC Z81.3
    - tobacco Z81.2
  - sudden
    - cardiac death Z82.41
    - infant death syndrome (SIDS) Z84.82
  - tobacco abuse Z81.2
  - violence, violent behavior Z81.8
  - visual loss Z82.1
- personal (of) —*see also* History, family (of)
  - abuse
    - adult Z91.419
      - forced labor or sexual exploitation Z91.42
      - physical and sexual Z91.410
      - psychological Z91.411
    - childhood Z62.819
      - forced labor or sexual exploitation in childhood Z62.813
      - physical Z62.810
      - psychological Z62.811
      - sexual Z62.810
  - alcohol dependence F10.21
  - allergy (to) Z88.9
    - analgesic agent NEC Z88.6
    - anesthetic Z88.4
    - antibiotic agent NEC Z88.1
    - anti-infective agent NEC Z88.3
    - contrast media Z91.041
    - drugs, medicaments and biological substances Z88.9
      - specified NEC Z88.8
    - food Z91.018
      - additives Z91.02
      - beef Z91.014
      - eggs Z91.012

History *(continued)*
- personal *(continued)*
  - allergy *(continued)*
    - food *(continued)*
      - lamb Z91.014
      - mammalian meats Z91.014
      - milk products Z91.011
      - peanuts Z91.010
      - pork Z91.014
      - red meats Z91.014
      - seafood Z91.013
      - specified food NEC Z91.018
    - insect Z91.038
      - bee Z91.030
    - latex Z91.040
    - medicinal agents Z88.9
      - specified NEC Z88.8
    - narcotic agent NEC Z88.5
    - nonmedicinal agents Z91.048
    - penicillin Z88.0
    - serum Z88.7
    - specified NEC Z91.09
    - sulfonamides Z88.2
    - vaccine Z88.7
  - anaphylactic shock Z87.892
  - anaphylaxis Z87.892
  - behavioral disorders Z86.59
  - benign carcinoid tumor Z86.012
  - benign neoplasm Z86.018
    - carcinoid Z86.012
    - brain Z86.011
    - colonic polyps Z86.010
  - brain injury (traumatic) Z87.820
  - breast implant removal Z98.86
  - calculi, renal Z87.442
  - cancer —*see* History, personal (of), malignant neoplasm (of)
  - cardiac arrest (death), successfully resuscitated Z86.74
  - CAR-T (Chimeric Antigen Receptor T-cell) therapy Z92.850
  - cellular therapy Z92.859
    - specified NEC Z92.858
  - cerebral infarction without residual deficit Z86.73
  - cervical dysplasia Z87.410
  - chemotherapy for neoplastic condition Z92.21
  - childhood abuse —*see* History, personal (of), abuse
  - Chimeric Antigen Receptor T-cell (CAR-T) therapy Z92.850
  - cleft lip (corrected) Z87.730
  - cleft palate (corrected) Z87.730
  - collapsed vertebra (healed) Z87.311
    - due to osteoporosis Z87.310
  - combat and operational stress reaction Z86.51
  - congenital malformation (corrected) Z87.798
    - circulatory system (corrected) Z87.74
    - digestive system (corrected) NEC Z87.738
    - ear (corrected) Z87.721
    - eye (corrected) Z87.720
    - face and neck (corrected) Z87.790
    - genitourinary system (corrected) NEC Z87.718
    - heart (corrected) Z87.74
    - integument (corrected) Z87.76
    - limb(s) (corrected) Z87.76
    - musculoskeletal system (corrected) Z87.76
    - neck (corrected) Z87.790

History *(continued)*
personal *(continued)*
congenital malformation *(continued)*
nervous system (corrected) NEC Z87.728
respiratory system (corrected) Z87.75
sense organs (corrected) NEC Z87.728
specified NEC Z87.798
contraception Z92.0
coronavirus (disease) (novel) 2019 Z86.16
COVID-19 Z86.16
deployment (military) Z91.82
diabetic foot ulcer Z86.31
disease or disorder (of) Z87.898
blood and blood-forming organs Z86.2
circulatory system Z86.79
specified condition NEC Z86.79
connective tissue NEC Z87.39
digestive system Z87.19
colonic polyp Z86.010
peptic ulcer disease Z87.11
specified condition NEC Z87.19
ear Z86.69
endocrine Z86.39
diabetic foot ulcer Z86.31
gestational diabetes Z86.32
specified type NEC Z86.39
eye Z86.69
genital (track) system NEC
female Z87.42
male Z87.438
hematological Z86.2
Hodgkin Z85.71
immune mechanism Z86.2
infectious Z86.19
coronarvirus (disease) (novel) 2019 Z86.16
COVID-19 Z86.16
malaria Z86.13
Methicillin resistant Staphylococcus aureus (MRSA) Z86.14
poliomyelitis Z86.12
SARS-CoV2 Z86.16
specified NEC Z86.19
tuberculosis Z86.11
mental NEC Z86.59
metabolic Z86.39
diabetic foot ulcer Z86.31
gestational diabetes Z86.32
specified type NEC Z86.39
musculoskeletal NEC Z87.39
nervous system Z86.69
nutritional Z86.39
parasitic Z86.19
respiratory system NEC Z87.09
sense organs Z86.69
skin Z87.2
specified site or type NEC Z87.898
subcutaneous tissue Z87.2
trophoblastic Z87.59
urinary system NEC Z87.448
drug dependence *—see* Dependence, drug, by type, in remission
drug therapy
antineoplastic chemotherapy Z92.21
estrogen Z92.23
immunosuppression Z92.25
inhaled steroids Z92.240
monoclonal drug Z92.22

History *(continued)*
personal *(continued)*
drug therapy *(continued)*
specified NEC Z92.29
steroid Z92.241
systemic steroids Z92.241
dysplasia
cervical (mild) (moderate) Z87.410
severe (grade III) Z86.001
prostatic Z87.430
vaginal (mild) (moderate) Z87.411
severe (grade III) Z86.002
vulvar (mild) (moderate) Z87.412
severe (grade III) Z86.002
embolism (venous) Z86.718
pulmonary Z86.711
encephalitis Z86.61
estrogen therapy Z92.23
extracorporeal membrane oxygenation (ECMO) Z92.81
failed moderate sedation Z92.83
failed conscious sedation Z92.83
fall, falling Z91.81
forced labor or sexual exploitation Z91.42
in childhood Z62.813
fracture (healed)
fatigue Z87.312
fragility Z87.310
osteoporosis Z87.310
pathological NEC Z87.311
stress Z87.312
traumatic Z87.81
gene therapy Z92.86
gestational diabetes Z86.32
hepatitis
B Z86.19
C Z86.19
Hodgkin disease Z85.71
hyperthermia, malignant Z88.4
hypospadias (corrected) Z87.710
hysterectomy Z90.710
immunosuppression therapy Z92.25
in situ neoplasm
breast Z86.000
cervix uteri Z86.001
digestive organs, specified NEC Z86.004
esophagus Z86.003
genital organs, specified NEC Z86.002
melanoma Z86.006
middle ear Z86.005
oral cavity Z86.003
respiratory system Z86.005
skin Z86.007
specified NEC Z86.008
stomach Z86.003
infection NEC Z86.19
central nervous system Z86.61
coronarvirus (disease) (novel) 2019 Z86.16
COVID-19 Z86.16
latent tuberculosis Z86.15
Methicillin resistant Staphylococcus aureus (MRSA) Z86.14
SARS-CoV2 Z86.16
urinary (recurrent) (tract) Z87.440
injury NEC Z87.828
in utero procedure during pregnancy Z98.870
in utero procedure while a fetus Z98.871
irradiation Z92.3
kidney stones Z87.442

History *(continued)*
personal *(continued)*
latent tuberculosis infection Z86.15
leukemia Z85.6
lymphoma (non-Hodgkin) Z85.72
malignant melanoma (skin) Z85.820
malignant neoplasm (of) Z85.9
accessory sinuses Z85.22
anus NEC Z85.048
carcinoid Z85.040
bladder Z85.51
bone Z85.830
brain Z85.841
breast Z85.3
bronchus NEC Z85.118
carcinoid Z85.110
carcinoid *—see* History, personal (of), malignant neoplasm, by site, carcinioid
cervix Z85.41
colon NEC Z85.038
carcinoid Z85.030
digestive organ Z85.00
specified NEC Z85.09
endocrine gland NEC Z85.858
epididymis Z85.48
esophagus Z85.01
eye Z85.840
gastrointestinal tract *—see* History, malignant neoplasm, digestive organ
genital organ
female Z85.40
specified NEC Z85.44
male Z85.45
specified NEC Z85.49
hematopoietic NEC Z85.79
intrathoracic organ Z85.20
kidney NEC Z85.528
carcinoid Z85.520
large intestine NEC Z85.038
carcinoid Z85.030
larynx Z85.21
liver Z85.05
lung NEC Z85.118
carcinoid Z85.110
mediastinum Z85.29
Merkel cell Z85.821
middle ear Z85.22
nasal cavities Z85.22
nervous system NEC Z85.848
oral cavity Z85.819
specified site NEC Z85.818
ovary Z85.43
pancreas Z85.07
pharynx Z85.819
specified site NEC Z85.818
pelvis Z85.53
pleura Z85.29
prostate Z85.46
rectosigmoid junction NEC Z85.048
carcinoid Z85.040
rectum NEC Z85.048
carcinoid Z85.040
respiratory organ Z85.20
sinuses, accessory Z85.22
skin NEC Z85.828
melanoma Z85.820
Merkel cell Z85.821
small intestine NEC Z85.068
carcinoid Z85.060
soft tissue Z85.831
specified site NEC Z85.89
stomach NEC Z85.028
carcinoid Z85.020
testis Z85.47

History *(continued)*
personal *(continued)*
malignant neoplasm (of) *(continued)*
thymus NEC Z85.238
carcinoid Z85.230
thyroid Z85.850
tongue Z85.810
trachea Z85.12
ureter Z85.54
urinary organ or tract Z85.50
specified NEC Z85.59
uterus Z85.42
maltreatment Z91.89
medical treatment NEC Z92.89
melanoma Z85.820
in situ Z86.006
malignant (skin) Z85.820
meningitis Z86.61
mental disorder Z86.59
Merkel cell carcinoma (skin) Z85.821
Methicillin resistant Staphylococcus aureus (MRSA) Z86.14
military deployment Z91.82
military war, peacekeeping and humanitarian deployment (current or past conflict) Z91.82
myocardial infarction (old) I25.2
neglect (in)
adult Z91.412
childhood Z62.812
neoplasia
anal intraepithelial, III [AIN] Z86.004
high-grade prostatic intraepithelial, III [HGPIN III] Z86.002
vaginal intraepithelial, III [VAIN III] Z86.002
vulvar intraepithelial, III [VIN III] Z86.002
neoplasm
benign Z86.018
brain Z86.011
colon polyp Z86.010
in situ
breast Z86.000
cervix uteri Z86.001
digestive organs, specified NEC Z86.004
esophagus Z86.003
genital organs, specified NEC Z86.002
melanoma Z86.006
middle ear Z86.005
oral cavity Z86.003
respiratory system Z86.005
skin Z86.007
specified NEC Z86.008
stomach Z86.003
malignant *—see* History of, malignant neoplasm
uncertain behavior Z86.03
nephrotic syndrome Z87.441
nicotine dependence Z87.891
noncompliance with medical treatment or regimen *—see* Noncompliance
nutritional deficiency Z86.39
obstetric complications Z87.59
childbirth Z87.59
pregnancy Z87.59
pre-term labor Z87.51
puerperium Z87.59
osteoporosis fractures Z87.31
parasuicide (attempt) Z91.51
physical trauma NEC Z87.828
self-harm or suicide attempt Z91.51

History *(continued)*
personal *(continued)*
poisoning NEC Z91.89
self-harm or suicide attempt Z91.51
poor personal hygiene Z91.89
pneumonia (recurrent) Z87.01
preterm labor Z87.51
prolonged reversible ischemic neurologic deficit (PRIND) Z86.73
procedure during pregnancy Z98.870
procedure while a fetus Z98.871
prostatic dysplasia Z87.430
psychological
abuse
adult Z91.411
child Z62.811
trauma, specified NEC Z91.49
radiation therapy Z92.3
removal
implant
breast Z98.86
renal calculi Z87.442
respiratory condition NEC Z87.09
retained foreign body fully removed Z87.821
risk factors NEC Z91.89
SARS-CoV2 infection Z86.16
self-harm
nonsuicidal Z91.52
suicidal Z91.51
self-inflicted injury without suicidal intent Z91.52
self-injury
nonsuicidal Z91.52
self-mutilation Z91.52
self-poisoning attempt Z91.51
sex reassignment Z87.890
sleep-wake cycle problem Z72.821
specified NEC Z87.898
steroid therapy (systemic) Z92.241
inhaled Z92.240
stroke without residual deficits Z86.73
substance abuse NEC F10-F19
sudden cardiac arrest Z86.74
sudden cardiac death successfully resuscitated Z86.74
suicidal behavior Z91.51
suicide attempt Z91.51
surgery NEC Z98.890
with uterine scar Z98.891
sex reassignment Z87.890
transplant —*see* Transplant
thrombophlebitis Z86.72
thrombosis (venous) Z86.718
pulmonary Z86.711
tobacco dependence Z87.891
transient ischemic attack (TIA) without residual deficits Z86.73
trauma (physical) NEC Z87.828
psychological NEC Z91.49
self-harm Z91.51
traumatic brain injury Z87.820
tuberculosis, latent infection Z86.15
unhealthy sleep-wake cycle Z72.821
unintended awareness under general anesthesia Z92.84
urinary calculi Z87.442
urinary (recurrent) (tract) infection(s) Z87.440
uterine scar from previous surgery Z98.891
vaginal dysplasia Z87.411

History *(continued)*
personal *(continued)*
venous thrombosis or embolism Z86.718
pulmonary Z86.711
vulvar dysplasia Z87.412

His-Werner disease A79.0

HIV (*see also* Human, immunodeficiency virus) B20
laboratory evidence (nonconclusive) R75
positive, seropositive Z21
nonconclusive test (in infants) R75

Hives (bold) —*see* Urticaria

Hoarseness R49.0

Hobo Z59.00

Hodgkin disease —*see* Lymphoma, Hodgkin

Hodgson's disease I71.2
ruptured I71.1

Hoffa-Kastert disease E88.89

Hoffa's disease E88.89

Hoffmann-Bouveret syndrome I47.9

Hoffmann's syndrome E03.9 *[G73.7]*

Hole (round)
macula H35.34-
retina (without detachment) —*see* Break, retina, round hole
with detachment —*see* Detachment, retina, with retinal, break

Holiday relief care Z75.5

Hollenhorst's plaque —*see* Occlusion, artery, retina

Hollow foot (congenital) Q66.7-
acquired —*see* Deformity, limb, foot, specified NEC

Holoprosencephaly Q04.2

Holt-Oram syndrome Q87.2

Homelessness Z59.00
sheltered Z59.01
unsheltered Z59.02

Homesickness —*see* Disorder, adjustment

Homocysteinemia R79.83

Homocystinemia, homocystinuria E72.11

Homogentisate 1,2-dioxygenase deficiency E70.29

Homologous serum hepatitis (prophylactic) (therapeutic) —*see* Hepatitis, viral, type B

Honeycomb lung J98.4
congenital Q33.0

Hooded
clitoris Q52.6
penis Q55.69

Hookworm (disease) (infection) (infestation) B76.9
with anemia B76.9 *[D63.8]*
specified NEC B76.8

Hordeolum (eyelid) (externum) (recurrent) H00.019
internum H00.029
left H00.026
lower H00.025
upper H00.024
right H00.023
lower H00.022
upper H00.021
left H00.016
lower H00.015
upper H00.014

Hordeolum *(continued)*
right H00.013
lower H00.012
upper H00.011

Horn
cutaneous L85.8
nail L60.2
congenital Q84.6

Horner (-Claude Bernard) **syndrome** G90.2
traumatic —*see* Injury, nerve, cervical sympathetic

Horseshoe kidney (congenital) Q63.1

Horton's headache or neuralgia G44.099
intractable G44.091
not intractable G44.099

Hospital hopper syndrome —*see* Disorder, factitious

Hospitalism in children —*see* Disorder, adjustment

Hostility R45.5
towards child Z62.3

Hot flashes
menopausal N95.1

Hourglass (contracture) —*see also* Contraction, hourglass
stomach K31.89
congenital Q40.2
stricture K31.2

Household, housing circumstance affecting care Z59.9
specified NEC Z59.89

Housemaid's knee —*see* Bursitis, prepatellar

HSCT-TMA (hematopoietic stem cell transplantation-associated thrombotic microangiopathy) M31.11

Hudson (-Stähli) **line** (cornea) —*see* Pigmentation, cornea, anterior

Human
bite (open wound) —*see also* Bite
intact skin surface —*see* Bite, superficial
herpesvirus —*see* Herpes
immunodeficiency virus (HIV)
disease (infection) B20
asymptomatic status Z21
contact Z20.6
counseling Z71.7
dementia B20 *[F02.80]*
with behavioral disturbance B20 *[F02.81]*
exposure to Z20.6
laboratory evidence R75
type-2(HIV 2) as cause of disease classified elsewhere B97.35
papillomavirus (HPV)
DNA test positive
high risk
cervix R87.810
vagina R87.811
low risk
cervix R87.820
vagina R87.821
screening for Z11.51
T-cell lymphotropic virus
type-1(HTLV-I) infection B33.3
as cause of disease classified elsewhere B97.33
carrier Z22.6
type-2(HTLV-II) as cause of disease classified elsewhere B97.34

Humidifier lung or pneumonitis J67.7

Humiliation (experience) **in childhood** Z62.898

Humpback (acquired) —*see* Kyphosis

Hunchback (acquired) —*see* Kyphosis

Hunger T73.0
air, psychogenic F45.8

Hungry bone syndrome E83.81

Hunner's ulcer —*see* Cystitis, chronic, interstitial

Hunter's
glossitis D51.0
syndrome E76.1

Huntington's disease or chorea G10
with dementia G10 *[F02.80]*
with behavioral disturbance G10 *[F02.81]*

Hunt's
disease or syndrome (herpetic geniculate ganglionitis) B02.21
dyssynergia cerebellaris myoclonica G11.19
neuralgia B02.21

Hurler (-Scheie) **disease or syndrome** E76.02

Hurst's disease G36.1

Hurthle cell
adenocarcinoma C73
adenoma D34
carcinoma C73
tumor D34

Hutchinson-Boeck disease or syndrome —*see* Sarcoidosis

Hutchinson-Gilford disease or syndrome E34.8

Hutchinson's
disease, meaning
angioma serpiginosum L81.7
pompholyx (cheiropompholyx) L30.1
prurigo estivalis L56.4
summer eruption or summer prurigo L56.4
melanotic freckle —*see* Melanoma, in situ
malignant melanoma in —*see* Melanoma
teeth or incisors (congenital syphilis) A50.52
triad (congenital syphilis) A50.53

Hyalin plaque, sclera, senile H15.89

Hyaline membrane (disease) (lung) (pulmonary) (newborn) P22.0

Hyalinosis
cutis (et mucosae) E78.89
focal and segmental (glomerular) (*see also* N00-N07 with fourth character .1) N05.1

Hyalitis, hyalosis, asteroid —*see also* Deposit, crystalline
syphilitic (late) A52.71

Hydatid
cyst or tumor —*see* Echinococcus
mole —*see* Hydatidiform mole
Morgagni
female Q50.5
male (epididymal) Q55.4
testicular Q55.29

Hydatidiform mole (benign) (complicating pregnancy) (delivered) (undelivered) O01.9
classical O01.0
complete O01.0
incomplete O01.1
invasive D39.2

Hydatidiform mole *(continued)*
  malignant D39.2
  partial O01.1

Hydatidosis *—see* Echinococcus

Hydradenitis (axillaris) (suppurative) L73.2

Hydradenoma *—see* Hidradenoma

Hydramnios O40.-

Hydrancephaly, hydranencephaly Q04.3
  with spina bifida *—see* Spina bifida, with hydrocephalus

Hydrargyrism NEC *—see* Poisoning, mercury

Hydrarthrosis *—see also* Effusion, joint
  gonococcal A54.42
  intermittent M12.40
    ankle M12.47-
    elbow M12.42-
    foot joint M12.47-
    hand joint M12.44-
    hip M12.45-
    knee M12.46-
    multiple site M12.49
    shoulder M12.41-
    specified joint NEC M12.48
    wrist M12.43-
  of yaws (early) (late) (*see also* subcategory M14.8-) A66.6
  syphilitic (late) A52.77
    congenital A50.55 *[M12.80]*

Hydremia D64.89

Hydrencephalocele (congenital) *—see* Encephalocele

Hydrencephalomeningocele (congenital) *—see* Encephalocele

Hydroa R23.8
  aestivale L56.4
  vacciniforme L56.4

Hydroadenitis (axillaris) (suppurative) L73.2

Hydrocalycosis *—see* Hydronephrosis

Hydrocele (spermatic cord) (testis) (tunica vaginalis) N43.3
  canal of Nuck N94.89
  communicating N43.2
    congenital P83.5
  congenital P83.5
  encysted N43.0
  female NEC N94.89
  infected N43.1
  newborn P83.5
  round ligament N94.89
  specified NEC N43.2
  spinalis *—see* Spina bifida
  vulva N90.89

Hydrocephalus (acquired) (external) (internal) (malignant) (recurrent) G91.9
  aqueduct Sylvius stricture Q03.0
  causing disproportion O33.6
    with obstructed labor O66.3
  communicating G91.0
  congenital (external) (internal) Q03.9
    with spina bifida Q05.4
      cervical Q05.0
      dorsal Q05.1
      lumbar Q05.2
      lumbosacral Q05.2
      sacral Q05.3
      thoracic Q05.1
      thoracolumbar Q05.1
    specified NEC Q03.8

Hydrocephalus *(continued)*
  due to toxoplasmosis (congenital) P37.1
  foramen Magendie block (acquired) G91.1
    congenital (*see also* Hydrocephalus, congenital) Q03.1
  in (due to)
    infectious disease NEC B89 *[G91.4]*
    neoplastic disease NEC (*see also* Neoplasm) G91.4
    parasitic disease B89 *[G91.4]*
  newborn Q03.9
    with spina bifida *—see* Spina bifida, with hydrocephalus
  noncommunicating G91.1
  normal pressure G91.2
    secondary G91.0
  obstructive G91.1
  otitic G93.2
  post-traumatic NEC G91.3
  secondary G91.4
    post-traumatic G91.3
  specified NEC G91.8
  syphilitic, congenital A50.49

Hydrocolpos (congenital) N89.8

Hydrocystoma *—see* Neoplasm, skin, benign

Hydroencephalocele (congenital) *—see* Encephalocele

Hydroencephalomeningocele (congenital) *—see* Encephalocele

Hydrohematopneumothorax *—see* Hemothorax

Hydromeningitis *—see* Meningitis

Hydromeningocele (spinal) *—see also* Spina bifida
  cranial *—see* Encephalocele

Hydrometra N85.8

Hydrometrocolpos N89.8

Hydromicrocephaly Q02

Hydromphalos (since birth) Q45.8

Hydromyelia Q06.4

Hydromyelocele *—see* Spina bifida

Hydronephrosis (atrophic) (early) (functionless) (intermittent) (primary) (secondary) **NEC** N13.30
  with
    infection N13.6
    obstruction (by) (of)
      renal calculus N13.2
        with infection N13.6
      ureteral NEC N13.1
        with infection N13.6
        calculus N13.2
          with infection N13.6
      ureteropelvic junction (congenital) Q62.11
      acquired N13.0
        with infection N13.6
    ureteral stricture NEC N13.1
      with infection N13.6
  congenital Q62.0
    due to acquired occlusion of ureteropelvic junction N13.0
  specified type NEC N13.39
  tuberculous A18.11

Hydropericarditis *—see* Pericarditis

Hydropericardium *—see* Pericarditis

Hydroperitoneum R18.8

Hydrophobia *—see* Rabies

Hydrophthalmos Q15.0

Hydropneumohemothorax *—see* Hemothorax

Hydropneumopericarditis *—see* Pericarditis

Hydropneumopericardium *—see* Pericarditis

Hydropneumothorax J94.8
  traumatic *—see* Injury, intrathoracic, lung
  tuberculous NEC A15.6

Hydrops R60.9
  abdominis R18.8
  articulorum intermittens *—see* Hydrarthrosis, intermittent
  cardiac *—see* Failure, heart, congestive
  causing obstructed labor (mother) O66.3
  endolymphatic H81.0-
  fetal *—see* Pregnancy, complicated by, hydrops, fetalis
  fetalis P83.2
    due to
      ABO isoimmunization P56.0
      alpha thalassemia D56.0
      hemolytic disease P56.90
        specified NEC P56.99
      isoimmunization (ABO) (Rh) P56.0
      other specified nonhemolytic disease NEC P83.2
      Rh incompatibility P56.0
    during pregnancy *—see* Pregnancy, complicated by, hydrops, fetalis
  gallbladder K82.1
  joint *—see* Effusion, joint
  labyrinth H81.0-
  newborn (idiopathic) P83.2
    due to
      ABO isoimmunization P56.0
      alpha thalassemia D56.0
      hemolytic disease P56.90
        specified NEC P56.99
      isoimmunization (ABO) (Rh) P56.0
      Rh incompatibility P56.0
  nutritional *—see* Malnutrition, severe
  pericardium *—see* Pericarditis
  pleura *—see* Hydrothorax
  spermatic cord *—see* Hydrocele

Hydropyonephrosis N13.6

Hydrorachis Q06.4

Hydrorrhea (nasal) J34.89
  pregnancy *—see* Rupture, membranes, premature

Hydrosadenitis (axillaris) (suppurative) L73.2

Hydrosalpinx (fallopian tube) (follicularis) N70.11

Hydrothorax (double) (pleura) J94.8
  chylous (nonfilarial) I89.8
    filarial (*see also* Infestation, filarial) B74.9 *[J91.8]*
  traumatic *—see* Injury, intrathoracic
  tuberculous NEC (non primary) A15.6

Hydroureter (*see also* Hydronephrosis) N13.4
  with infection N13.6
  congenital Q62.39

Hydroureteronephrosis *—see* Hydronephrosis

Hydrourethra N36.8

Hydroxykynureninuria E70.89

Hydroxylysinemia E72.3

Hydroxyprolinemia E72.59

Hygiene, sleep
  abuse Z72.821
  inadequate Z72.821
  poor Z72.821

Hygroma (congenital) (cystic) D18.1
  praepatellare, prepatellar *—see* Bursitis, prepatellar

Hymen *—see* condition

Hymenolepis, hymenolepiasis (diminuta) (infection) (infestation) (nana) B71.0

Hypalgesia R20.8

Hyperacidity (gastric) K31.89
  psychogenic F45.8

Hyperactive, hyperactivity F90.9
  basal cell, uterine cervix *—see* Dysplasia, cervix
  bowel sounds R19.12
  cervix epithelial (basal) *—see* Dysplasia, cervix
  child F90.9
    attention deficit *—see* Disorder, attention-deficit hyperactivity
  detrusor muscle N32.81
  gastrointestinal K31.89
    psychogenic F45.8
  nasal mucous membrane J34.3
  stomach K31.89
  thyroid (gland) *—see* Hyperthyroidism

Hyperacusis H93.23-

Hyperadrenalism E27.5

Hyperadrenocorticism E24.9
  congenital E25.0
  iatrogenic E24.2
    correct substance properly administered *—see* Table of Drugs and Chemicals, by drug, adverse effect
    overdose or wrong substance given or taken *—see* Table of Drugs and Chemicals, by drug, poisoning
  not associated with Cushing's syndrome E27.0
  pituitary-dependent E24.0

Hyperaldosteronism E26.9
  familial (type I) E26.02
  glucocorticoid-remediable E26.02
  primary (due to (bilateral) adrenal hyperplasia) E26.09
  primary NEC E26.09
  secondary E26.1
  specified NEC E26.89

Hyperalgesia R20.8

Hyperalimentation R63.2
  carotene, carotin E67.1
  specified NEC E67.8
  vitamin
    A E67.0
    D E67.3

Hyperaminoaciduria
  arginine E72.21
  cystine E72.01
  lysine E72.3
  ornithine E72.4

Hyperammonemia (congenital) E72.20

Hyperazotemia *—see* Uremia

Hyperbetalipoproteinemia (familial) E78.00
  with prebetalipoproteinemia E78.2

Hyperbicarbonatemia P74.41

Hyperbilirubinemia
  constitutional E80.6
  familial conjugated E80.6
  neonatal (transient) —*see* Jaundice, newborn

Hypercalcemia, hypocalciuric, familial E83.52

Hypercalciuria, idiopathic R82.994

Hypercapnia R06.89
  newborn P84

Hypercarotenemia (dietary) E67.1

Hypercementosis K03.4

Hyperchloremia E87.8

Hyperchlorhydria K31.89
  neurotic F45.8
  psychogenic F45.8

Hypercholesterinemia —*see* Hypercholesterolemia

Hypercholesterolemia (essential) (primary) (pure) E78.00
  with hyperglyceridemia, endogenous E78.2
  dietary counseling and surveillance Z71.3
  familial E78.01
  hereditary E78.01

Hyperchylia gastrica, psychogenic F45.8

Hyperchylomicronemia (familial) (primary) E78.3
  with hyperbetalipoproteinemia E78.3

Hypercoagulable (state) D68.59
  activated protein C resistance D68.51
  antithrombin (III) deficiency D68.59
  factor V Leiden mutation D68.51
  primary NEC D68.59
  protein C deficiency D68.59
  protein S deficiency D68.59
  prothrombin gene mutation D68.52
  secondary D68.69
  specified NEC D68.69

Hypercoagulation (state) D68.59

Hypercorticalism, pituitary-dependent E24.0

Hypercorticosolism —*see* Cushing's, syndrome

Hypercorticosteronism E24.2
  correct substance properly administered —*see* Table of Drugs and Chemicals, by drug, adverse effect
  overdose or wrong substance given or taken —*see* Table of Drugs and Chemicals, by drug, poisoning

Hypercortisonism E24.2
  correct substance properly administered —*see* Table of Drugs and Chemicals, by drug, adverse effect
  overdose or wrong substance given or taken —*see* Table of Drugs and Chemicals, by drug, poisoning

Hyperekplexia Q89.8

Hyperelectrolytemia E87.8

Hyperemesis R11.10
  with nausea R11.2
  gravidarum (mild) O21.0
    with
      carbohydrate depletion O21.1
      dehydration O21.1
      electrolyte imbalance O21.1
      metabolic disturbance O21.1
    severe (with metabolic disturbance) O21.1
  projectile R11.12
  psychogenic F45.8

Hyperemia (acute) (passive) R68.89
  anal mucosa K62.89
  bladder N32.89
  cerebral I67.89
  conjunctiva H11.43-
  ear internal, acute H83.0
  enteric K59.89
  eye —*see* Hyperemia, conjunctiva
  eyelid (active) (passive) —*see* Disorder, eyelid, specified type NEC
  intestine K59.89
  iris —*see* Disorder, iris, vascular
  kidney N28.89
  labyrinth H83.0
  liver (active) K76.89
  lung (passive) —*see* Edema, lung
  pulmonary (passive) —*see* Edema, lung
  renal N28.89
  retina H35.89
  stomach K31.89

Hyperesthesia (body surface) R20.3
  larynx (reflex) J38.7
    hysterical F44.89
  pharynx (reflex) J39.2
    hysterical F44.89

Hyperestrogenism (drug-induced) (iatrogenic) E28.0

Hyperexplexia Q89.8

Hyperfibrinolysis —*see* Fibrinolysis

Hyperfructosemia E74.19

Hyperfunction
  adrenal cortex, not associated with Cushing's syndrome E27.0
    medulla E27.5
      adrenomedullary E27.5
    virilism E25.9
      congenital E25.0
  ovarian E28.8
  pancreas K86.89
  parathyroid (gland) E21.3
  pituitary (gland) (anterior) E22.9
    specified NEC E22.8
  polyglandular E31.1
  testicular E29.0

Hypergammaglobulinemia D89.2
  polyclonal D89.0
  Waldenström D89.0

Hypergastrinemia E16.4

Hyperglobulinemia R77.1

Hyperglycemia, hyperglycemic (transient) R73.9
  coma —*see* Diabetes, by type, with coma
  postpancreatectomy E89.1

Hyperglyceridemia (endogenous) (essential) (familial) (hereditary) (pure) E78.1
  mixed E78.3

Hyperglycinemia (non-ketotic) E72.51

Hypergonadism
  ovarian E28.8
  testicular (primary) (infantile) E29.0

Hyperheparinemia D68.32

Hyperhidrosis, hyperidrosis R61
  focal
    primary L74.519
      axilla L74.510
      face L74.511
      palms L74.512
      soles L74.513
    secondary L74.52
  generalized R61
  localized
    primary L74.519
      axilla L74.510
      face L74.511
      palms L74.512
      soles L74.513
    secondary L74.52
  psychogenic F45.8
  secondary R61
    focal L74.52

Hyperhistidinemia E70.41

Hyperhomocysteinemia E72.11

Hyperhydroxyprolinemia E72.59

Hyperinsulinism (functional) E16.1
  with
    coma (hypoglycemic) E15
    encephalopathy E16.1 *[G94]*
  ectopic E16.1
  therapeutic misadventure (from administration of insulin) T38.3

Hyperkalemia E87.5

Hyperkeratosis (*see also* Keratosis) L85.9
  cervix N88.0
  due to yaws (early) (late) (palmar or plantar) A66.3
  follicularis Q82.8
    penetrans (in cutem) L87.0
  palmoplantaris climacterica L85.1
  pinta A67.1
  senile (with pruritus) L57.0
  universalis congenita Q80.8
  vocal cord J38.3
  vulva N90.4

Hyperkinesia, hyperkinetic (disease) (reaction) (syndrome) (childhood) (adolescence) —*see also* Disorder, attention-deficit hyperactivity
  heart I51.89

Hyperleucine-isoleucinemia E71.19

Hyperlipemia, hyperlipidemia E78.5
  combined E78.2
    familial E78.49
  group
    A E78.00
    B E78.1
    C E78.2
    D E78.3
  mixed E78.2
  specified NEC E78.49

Hyperlipidosis E75.6
  hereditary NEC E75.5

Hyperlipoproteinemia E78.5
  Fredrickson's type
    I E78.3
    IIa E78.00
    IIb E78.2
    III E78.2
    IV E78.1
    V E78.3

Hyperlipoproteinemia *(continued)*
  low-density-lipoprotein-type (LDL) E78.00
  very-low-density-lipoprotein-type (VLDL) E78.1

Hyperlucent lung, unilateral J43.0

Hyperlysinemia E72.3

Hypermagnesemia E83.41
  neonatal P71.8

Hypermenorrhea N92.0

Hypermethioninemia E72.19

Hypermetropia (congenital) H52.0-

Hypermobility, hypermotility
  cecum —*see* Syndrome, irritable bowel
  coccyx —*see* subcategory M53.2
  colon —*see* Syndrome, irritable bowel
    psychogenic F45.8
  ileum K58.9
  intestine (*see also* Syndrome, irritable bowel) K58.9
    psychogenic F45.8
  meniscus (knee) —*see* Derangement, knee, meniscus
  scapula —*see* Instability, joint, shoulder
  stomach K31.89
    psychogenic F45.8
  syndrome M35.7
  urethra N36.41
    with intrinsic sphincter deficiency N36.43

Hypernasality R49.21

Hypernatremia E87.0

Hypernephroma C64.-

Hyperopia —*see* Hypermetropia

Hyperorexia nervosa F50.2

Hyperornithinemia E72.4

Hyperosmia R43.1

Hyperosmolality E87.0

Hyperostosis (monomelic) —*see also* Disorder, bone, density and structure, specified NEC
  ankylosing (spine) M48.10
    cervical region M48.12
    cervicothoracic region M48.13
    lumbar region M48.16
    lumbosacral region M48.17
    multiple sites M48.19
    occipito-atlanto-axial region M48.11
    sacrococcygeal region M48.18
    thoracic region M48.14
    thoracolumbar region M48.15
  cortical (skull) M85.2
    infantile M89.8X-
  frontal, internal of skull M85.2
  interna frontalis M85.2
  skeletal, diffuse idiopathic —*see* Hyperostosis, ankylosing
  skull M85.2
    congenital Q75.8
  vertebral, ankylosing —*see* Hyperostosis, ankylosing

Hyperovarism E28.8

Hyperoxaluria R82.992
  primary E72.53

Hyperparathyroidism E21.3
  primary E21.0
  secondary (renal) N25.81
    non-renal E21.1
  specified NEC E21.2
  tertiary E21.2

Hyperpathia R20.8

Hyperperistalsis R19.2
- psychogenic F45.8

Hyperpermeability, capillary I78.8

Hyperphagia R63.2

Hyperphenylalaninemia NEC E70.1

Hyperphoria (alternating) H50.53

Hyperphosphatemia E83.39

Hyperpiesis, hyperpiesia *—see* Hypertension

Hyperpigmentation *—see also* Pigmentation
- melanin NEC L81.4
- postinflammatory L81.0

Hyperpinealism E34.8

Hyperpituitarism E22.9

Hyperplasia, hyperplastic
- adenoids J35.2
- adrenal (capsule) (cortex) (gland) E27.8
  - with
    - sexual precocity (male) E25.9
      - congenital E25.0
    - virilism, adrenal E25.9
      - congenital E25.0
    - virilization (female) E25.9
      - congenital E25.0
  - congenital E25.0
    - salt-losing E25.0
- adrenomedullary E27.5
- angiolymphoid, eosinophilia (ALHE) D18.01
- appendix (lymphoid) K38.0
- artery, fibromuscular I77.3
- bone *—see also* Hypertrophy, bone
  - marrow D75.89
- breast *—see also* Hypertrophy, breast
  - atypical, atypia N60.9-
    - ductal N60.9-
    - lobular N60.9-
- C-cell, thyroid E07.0
- cementation (tooth) (teeth) K03.4
- cervical gland R59.0
- cervix (uteri) (basal cell) (endometrium) (polypoid) *—see also* Dysplasia, cervix
  - congenital Q51.828
- clitoris, congenital Q52.6
- denture K06.2
- endocervicitis N72
- endometrium, endometrial (adenomatous) (cystic) (glandular) (glandular-cystic) (polypoid) N85.00
  - with atypia N85.02
  - benign N85.01
  - cervix *—see* Dysplasia, cervix
  - complex (without atypia) N85.01
  - simple (without atypia) N85.01
- epithelial L85.9
  - focal, oral, including tongue K13.29
  - nipple N62
  - skin L85.9
  - tongue K13.29
  - vaginal wall N89.3
- erythroid D75.89
- fibromuscular of artery (carotid) (renal) I77.3
- genital
  - female NEC N94.89
  - male N50.89
- gingiva K06.1
- glandularis cystica uteri (interstitialis) (*see also* Hyperplasia, endometrial) N85.00-

Hyperplasia, hyperplastic *(continued)*
- gum K06.1
- hymen, congenital Q52.4
- irritative, edentulous (alveolar) K06.2
- jaw M26.09
  - alveolar M26.79
  - lower M26.03
    - alveolar M26.72
  - upper M26.01
    - alveolar M26.71
- kidney (congenital) Q63.3
- labia N90.69
  - epithelial N90.3
- liver (congenital) Q44.7
  - nodular, focal K76.89
- lymph gland or node R59.9
- mandible, mandibular M26.03
  - alveolar M26.72
  - unilateral condylar M27.8
- maxilla, maxillary M26.01
  - alveolar M26.71
- myometrium, myometrial N85.2
- neuroendocrine cell, of infancy J84.841
- nose
  - lymphoid J34.89
  - polypoid J33.9
- oral mucosa (irritative) K13.6
- organ or site, congenital NEC *—see* Anomaly, by site
- ovary N83.8
- palate, papillary (irritative) K13.6
- pancreatic islet cells E16.9
  - alpha E16.8
    - with excess
      - gastrin E16.4
      - glucagon E16.3
  - beta E16.1
- parathyroid (gland) E21.0
- pharynx (lymphoid) J39.2
- prostate (adenofibromatous) (nodular) N40.0
  - with lower urinary tract symptoms (LUTS) N40.1
  - without lower urinary tract symtpoms (LUTS) N40.0
- renal artery I77.89
- reticulo-endothelial (cell) D75.89
- salivary gland (any) K11.1
- Schimmelbusch's *—see* Mastopathy, cystic
- suprarenal capsule (gland) E27.8
- thymus (gland) (persistent) E32.0
- thyroid (gland) *—see* Goiter
- tonsils (faucial) (infective) (lingual) (lymphoid) J35.1
  - with adenoids J35.3
- unilateral condylar M27.8
- uterus, uterine N85.2
  - endometrium (glandular) (*see also* Hyperplasia, endometrial) N85.00-
- vulva N90.69
  - epithelial N90.3

Hyperpnea *—see* Hyperventilation

Hyperpotassemia E87.5

Hyperprebetalipoproteinemia (familial) E78.1

Hyperprolactinemia E22.1

Hyperprolinemia (type I) (type II) E72.59

Hyperproteinemia E88.09

Hyperprothrombinemia, causing coagulation factor deficiency D68.4

Hyperpyrexia R50.9
- heat (effects) T67.01
- malignant, due to anesthetic T88.3
- rheumatic *—see* Fever, rheumatic
- unknown origin R50.9

Hyper-reflexia R29.2

Hypersalivation K11.7

Hypersecretion
- ACTH (not associated with Cushing's syndrome) E27.0
  - pituitary E24.0
- adrenaline E27.5
- adrenomedullary E27.5
- androgen (testicular) E29.0
  - ovarian (drug-induced) (iatrogenic) E28.1
- calcitonin E07.0
- catecholamine E27.5
- corticoadrenal E24.9
- cortisol E24.9
- epinephrine E27.5
- estrogen E28.0
- gastric K31.89
  - psychogenic F45.8
- gastrin E16.4
- glucagon E16.3
- hormone(s)
  - ACTH (not associated with Cushing's syndrome) E27.0
    - pituitary E24.0
  - antidiuretic E22.2
  - growth E22.0
  - intestinal NEC E34.1
  - ovarian androgen E28.1
  - pituitary E22.9
  - testicular E29.0
  - thyroid stimulating E05.80
    - with thyroid storm E05.81
- insulin *—see* Hyperinsulinism
- lacrimal glands *—see* Epiphora
- medulloadrenal E27.5
- milk O92.6
- ovarian androgens E28.1
- salivary gland (any) K11.7
- thyrocalcitonin E07.0
- upper respiratory J39.8

Hypersegmentation, leukocytic, hereditary D72.0

Hypersensitive, hypersensitiveness, hypersensitivity *—see also* Allergy
- carotid sinus G90.01
- colon *—see* Irritable, colon
- drug T88.7
- gastrointestinal K52.29
  - immediate K52.29
  - psychogenic F45.8
- labyrinth H83.2
- pain R20.8
- pneumonitis *—see* Pneumonitis, allergic
- reaction T78.40
  - upper respiratory tract NEC J39.3

Hypersomnia (organic) G47.10
- due to
  - alcohol
    - abuse F10.182
    - dependence F10.282
    - use F10.982
  - amphetamines
    - abuse F15.182

Hypersomnia *(continued)*
- due to *(continued)*
  - amphetamines *(continued)*
    - dependence F15.282
    - use F15.982
  - caffeine
    - abuse F15.182
    - dependence F15.282
    - use F15.982
  - cocaine
    - abuse F14.182
    - dependence F14.282
    - use F14.982
  - drug NEC
    - abuse F19.182
    - dependence F19.282
    - use F19.982
  - medical condition G47.14
  - mental disorder F51.13
  - opioid
    - abuse F11.182
    - dependence F11.282
    - use F11.982
  - psychoactive substance NEC
    - abuse F19.182
    - dependence F19.282
    - use F19.982
  - sedative, hypnotic, or anxiolytic
    - abuse F13.182
    - dependence F13.282
    - use F13.982
  - stimulant NEC
    - abuse F15.182
    - dependence F15.282
    - use F15.982
- idiopathic G47.11
  - with long sleep time G47.11
  - without long sleep time G47.12
- menstrual related G47.13
- nonorganic origin F51.11
  - specified NEC F51.19
- not due to a substance or known physiological condition F51.11
  - specified NEC F51.19
- primary F51.11
- recurrent G47.13
- specified NEC G47.19

Hypersplenia, hypersplenism D73.1

Hyperstimulation, ovaries (associated with induced ovulation) N98.1

Hypersusceptibility *—see* Allergy

Hypertelorism (ocular) (orbital) Q75.2

Hypertension, hypertensive (accelerated) (benign) (essential) (idiopathic) (malignant) (systemic) I10
- with
  - heart failure (congestive) I11.0
  - heart involvement (conditions in I50.- or I51.4- I51.7, I51.89, I51.9 due to hypertension) *—see* Hypertension, heart
  - kidney involvement *—see* Hypertension, kidney
- benign, intracranial G93.2
- borderline R03.0
- cardiorenal (disease) I13.10
  - with heart failure I13.0
    - with stage 1 through stage 4 chronic kidney disease I13.0
    - with stage 5 or end stage renal disease I13.2
  - without heart failure I13.10
    - with stage 1 through stage 4 chronic kidney disease I13.10

Hypertension, hypertensive *(continued)*
cardiorenal *(continued)*
without heart failure *(continued)*
with stage 5 or end stage renal disease I13.11
cardiovascular
disease (arteriosclerotic) (sclerotic) —*see* Hypertension, heart
renal (disease) —*see* Hypertension, cardiorenal
chronic venous —*see* Hypertension, venous (chronic)
complicating
childbirth (labor) O16.4
pre-existing O10.92
with
heart disease O12.12
with renal disease O10.32
pre-eclampsia O11.4
renal disease O10.22
with heart disease O10.32
essential O10.02
secondary O10.42
pregnancy O16.-
with edema (*see also* Pre-eclampsia) O14.9-
gestational (pregnancy induced) (without proteinuria) O13.-
with proteinuria O14.9-
mild pre-eclampsia O14.0-
moderate pre-eclampsia O14.0-
severe pre-eclampsia O14.1-
with hemolysis, elevated liver enzymes and low platelet count (HELLP) O14.2-
pre-existing O10.91-
with
heart disease O10.11-
with renal disease O10.31-
pre-eclampsia —*see* category O11
renal disease O10.21-
with heart disease O10.31-
essential O10.01-
secondary O10.41-
transient O13.-
puerperium, pre-existing O16.5
pre-existing
with
heart disease O10.13
with renal disease O10.33
pre-eclampsia O11.5
renal disease O10.23
with heart disease O10.33
essential O10.03
pregnancy-induced O13.9
secondary O10.43
crisis I16.9
due to
endocrine disorders I15.2
pheochromocytoma I15.2
renal disorders NEC I15.1
arterial I15.0
renovascular disorders I15.0
specified disease NEC I15.8
emergency I16.1
encephalopathy I67.4

Hypertension, hypertensive *(continued)*
gestational (without significant proteinuria) (pregnancy-induced) (transient) O13.-
with significant proteinuria —*see* Pre-eclampsia
complicating
delivery O13.4
puerperium O13.5
Goldblatt's I70.1
heart (disease) (conditions in I51.4-I51.9 due to hypertension) I11.9
with
heart failure (congestive) I11.0
kidney disease (chronic) —*see* Hypertension, cardiorenal
intracranial, benign G93.2
kidney I12.9
with
heart disease —*see* Hypertension, cardiorenal
stage 5 chronic kidney disease (CKD) or end stage renal disease (ESRD) I12.0
stage 1 through stage 4 chronic kidney disease I12.9
lesser circulation I27.0
maternal O16.-
newborn P29.2
pulmonary (persistent) P29.30
ocular H40.05-
pancreatic duct - code to underlying condition
with chronic pancreatitis K86.1
portal (due to chronic liver disease) (idiopathic) K76.6
gastropathy K31.89
in (due to) schistosomiasis (bilharziasis) B65.9 *[K77]*
postoperative I97.3
psychogenic F45.8
pulmonary I27.20
with
cor pulmonale (chronic) I27.29
acute I26.09
right heart ventricular strain/failure I27.29
acute I26.09
right to left shunt related to congenital heart disease I27.83
unclear multifactorial mechanisms I27.29
arterial (associated) (drug-induced) (toxin-induced) I27.21
chronic thromboembolic I27.24
due to
hematologic disorders I27.29
kyphoscoliotic heart disease I27.1
left heart disease I27.22
lung diseases and hypoxia I27.23
metabolic disorders I27.29
specified systemic disorders NEC I27.29
group 1 (associated) (drug-induced) (toxin-induced) I27.21
group 2 I27.22
group 3 I27.23
group 4 I27.24
group 5 I27.29
of newborn (persistent) P29.30
secondary
arterial I27.21
specified NEC I27.29
primary (idiopathic) I27.0

Hypertension, hypertensive *(continued)*
renal —*see* Hypertension, kidney
renovascular I15.0
secondary NEC I15.9
due to
endocrine disorders I15.2
pheochromocytoma I15.2
renal disorders NEC I15.1
arterial I15.0
renovascular disorders I15.0
specified NEC I15.8
transient R03.0
of pregnancy O13.-
urgency I16.0
venous (chronic)
due to
deep vein thrombosis —*see* Syndrome, postthrombotic
idiopathic I87.309
with
inflammation I87.32-
with ulcer I87.33-
specified complication NEC I87.39-
ulcer I87.31-
with inflammation I87.33-
asymptomatic I87.30-

Hypertensive urgency —*see* Hypertension

Hyperthecosis ovary E28.8

Hyperthermia (of unknown origin) —*see also* Hyperpyrexia
malignant, due to anesthesia T88.3
newborn P81.9
environmental P81.0

Hyperthyroid (recurrent) —*see* Hyperthyroidism

Hyperthyroidism (latent) (pre-adult) (recurrent) E05.90
with
goiter (diffuse) E05.00
with thyroid storm E05.01
nodular (multinodular) E05.20
with thyroid storm E05.21
uninodular E05.10
with thyroid storm E05.11
storm E05.91
due to ectopic thyroid tissue E05.30
with thyroid storm E05.31
neonatal, transitory P72.1
specified NEC E05.80
with thyroid storm E05.81

Hypertony, hypertonia, hypertonicity
bladder N31.8
congenital P94.1
stomach K31.89
psychogenic F45.8
uterus, uterine (contractions) (complicating delivery) O62.4

Hypertrichosis L68.9
congenital Q84.2
eyelid H02.869
left H02.866
lower H02.865
upper H02.864
right H02.863
lower H02.862
upper H02.861
lanuginosa Q84.2
acquired L68.1
localized L68.2
specified NEC L68.8

Hypertriglyceridemia, essential E78.1

Hypertrophy, hypertrophic
adenofibromatous, prostate —*see* Enlargement, enlarged, prostate
adenoids (infective) J35.2
with tonsils J35.3
adrenal cortex E27.8
alveolar process or ridge —*see* Anomaly, alveolar
anal papillae K62.89
artery I77.89
congenital NEC Q27.8
digestive system Q27.8
lower limb Q27.8
specified site NEC Q27.8
upper limb Q27.8
auricular —*see* Hypertrophy, cardiac
Bartholin's gland N75.8
bile duct (common) (hepatic) K83.8
bladder (sphincter) (trigone) N32.89
bone M89.30
carpus M89.34-
clavicle M89.31-
femur M89.35-
fibula M89.36-
finger M89.34-
humerus M89.32-
ilium M89.359
ischium M89.359
metacarpus M89.34-
metatarsus M89.37-
multiple sites M89.39
neck M89.38
radius M89.33-
rib M89.38
scapula M89.31-
skull M89.38
tarsus M89.37-
tibia M89.36-
toe M89.37-
ulna M89.33-
vertebra M89.38
brain G93.89
breast N62
cystic —*see* Mastopathy, cystic
newborn P83.4
pubertal, massive N62
puerperal, postpartum —*see* Disorder, breast, specified type NEC
senile (parenchymatous) N62
cardiac (chronic) (idiopathic) I51.7
with rheumatic fever (conditions in I00)
active I01.8
inactive or quiescent (with chorea) I09.89
congenital NEC Q24.8
fatty —*see* Degeneration, myocardial
hypertensive —*see* Hypertension, heart
rheumatic (with chorea) I09.89
active or acute I01.8
with chorea I02.0
valve —*see* Endocarditis
cartilage —*see* Disorder, cartilage, specified type NEC
cecum —*see* Megacolon
cervix (uteri) N88.8
congenital Q51.828
elongation N88.4
clitoris (cirrhotic) N90.89
congenital Q52.6
colon —*see also* Megacolon
congenital Q43.2
conjunctiva, lymphoid H11.89
corpora cavernosa N48.89
cystic duct K82.8

- **Hypertrophy, hypertrophic** *(continued)*
  - duodenum K31.89
  - endometrium (glandular) (*see also* Hyperplasia, endometrial) N85.00-
    - cervix N88.8
  - epididymis N50.89
  - esophageal hiatus (congenital) Q79.1
    - with hernia —*see* Hernia, hiatal
  - eyelid —*see* Disorder, eyelid, specified type NEC
  - facet joint (*see also* Spondylosis) M47.819
  - fat pad E65
    - knee (infrapatellar) (popliteal) (prepatellar) (retropatellar) M79.4
  - foot (congenital) Q74.2
  - frenulum, frenum (tongue) K14.8
    - lip K13.0
  - gallbladder K82.8
  - gastric mucosa K29.60
    - with bleeding K29.61
  - gland, glandular R59.9
    - generalized R59.1
    - localized R59.0
  - gum (mucous membrane) K06.1
  - heart (idiopathic) —*see also* Hypertrophy, cardiac
    - valve (*see also* Endocarditis) I38
  - hemifacial Q67.4
  - hepatic —*see* Hypertrophy, liver
  - hiatus (esophageal) Q79.1
  - hilus gland R59.0
  - hymen, congenital Q52.4
  - ileum K63.89
  - intestine NEC K63.89
  - jejunum K63.89
  - kidney (compensatory) N28.81
    - congenital Q63.3
  - labium (majus) (minus) N90.60
  - ligament —*see* Disorder, ligament
  - lingual tonsil (infective) J35.1
    - with adenoids J35.3
  - lip K13.0
    - congenital Q18.6
  - liver R16.0
    - acute K76.89
    - congenital Q44.7
    - cirrhotic —*see* Cirrhosis, liver
    - fatty —*see* Fatty, liver
  - lymph, lymphatic gland R59.9
    - generalized R59.1
    - localized R59.0
    - tuberculous —*see* Tuberculosis, lymph gland
  - mammary gland —*see* Hypertrophy, breast
  - Meckel's diverticulum (congenital) Q43.0
    - malignant —*see* Table of Neoplasms, small intestine, malignant
  - median bar —*see* Hyperplasia, prostate
  - meibomian gland —*see* Chalazion
  - meniscus, knee, congenital Q74.1
  - metatarsal head —*see* Hypertrophy, bone, metatarsus
  - metatarsus —*see* Hypertrophy, bone, metatarsus
  - mucous membrane
    - alveolar ridge K06.2
    - gum K06.1
    - nose (turbinate) J34.3
  - muscle M62.89
  - muscular coat, artery I77.89
  - myocardium —*see also* Hypertrophy, cardiac
    - idiopathic I42.2
  - myometrium N85.2
  - nail L60.2
    - congenital Q84.5
  - nasal J34.89
    - alae J34.89
    - bone J34.89
    - cartilage J34.89
    - mucous membrane (septum) J34.3
    - sinus J34.89
    - turbinate J34.3
  - nasopharynx, lymphoid (infectional) (tissue) (wall) J35.2
  - nipple N62
  - organ or site, congenital NEC —*see* Anomaly, by site
  - ovary N83.8
  - palate (hard) M27.8
    - soft K13.79
  - pancreas, congenital Q45.3
  - parathyroid (gland) E21.0
  - parotid gland K11.1
  - penis N48.89
  - pharyngeal tonsil J35.2
  - pharynx J39.2
    - lymphoid (infectional) (tissue) (wall) J35.2
  - pituitary (anterior) (fossa) (gland) E23.6
  - prepuce (congenital) N47.8
    - female N90.89
  - prostate —*see* Enlargement, enlarged, prostate
    - congenital Q55.4
  - pseudomuscular G71.09
  - pylorus (adult) (muscle) (sphincter) K31.1
    - congenital or infantile Q40.0
  - rectal, rectum (sphincter) K62.89
  - rhinitis (turbinate) J31.0
  - salivary gland (any) K11.1
    - congenital Q38.4
  - scaphoid (tarsal) —*see* Hypertrophy, bone, tarsus
  - scar L91.0
  - scrotum N50.89
  - seminal vesicle N50.89
  - sigmoid —*see* Megacolon
  - skin L91.9
    - specified NEC L91.8
  - spermatic cord N50.89
  - spleen —*see* Splenomegaly
  - spondylitis —*see* Spondylosis
  - stomach K31.89
  - sublingual gland K11.1
  - submandibular gland K11.1
  - suprarenal cortex (gland) E27.8
  - synovial NEC M67.20
    - acromioclavicular M67.21-
    - ankle M67.27-
    - elbow M67.22-
    - foot M67.27-
    - hand M67.24-
    - hip M67.25-
    - knee M67.26-
    - multiple sites M67.29
    - specified site NEC M67.28
    - wrist M67.23-
  - tendon —*see* Disorder, tendon, specified type NEC
  - testis N44.8
    - congenital Q55.29
  - thymic, thymus (gland) (congenital) E32.0
  - thyroid (gland) —*see* Goiter
  - toe (congenital) Q74.2
    - acquired —*see also* Deformity, toe, specified NEC
  - tongue K14.8
    - congenital Q38.2
    - papillae (foliate) K14.3
  - tonsils (faucial) (infective) (lingual) (lymphoid) J35.1
    - with adenoids J35.3
  - tunica vaginalis N50.89
  - ureter N28.89
  - urethra N36.8
  - uterus N85.2
    - neck (with elongation) N88.4
    - puerperal O90.89
  - uvula K13.79
  - vagina N89.8
  - vas deferens N50.89
  - vein I87.8
  - ventricle, ventricular (heart) —*see also* Hypertrophy, cardiac
    - congenital Q24.8
    - in tetralogy of Fallot Q21.3
  - verumontanum N36.8
  - vocal cord J38.3
  - vulva N90.60
    - stasis (nonfilarial) N90.69
- **Hypertropia** H50.2-
- **Hypertyrosinemia** E70.21
- **Hyperuricemia** (asymptomatic) E79.0
- **Hyperuricosuria** R82.993
- **Hypervalinemia** E71.19
- **Hyperventilation** (tetany) R06.4
  - hysterical F45.8
  - psychogenic F45.8
  - syndrome F45.8
- **Hypervitaminosis** (dietary) **NEC** E67.8
  - A E67.0
    - administered as drug (prolonged intake) —*see* Table of Drugs and Chemicals, vitamins, adverse effect
    - overdose or wrong substance given or taken —*see* Table of Drugs and Chemicals, vitamins, poisoning
  - B6 E67.2
  - D E67.3
    - administered as drug (prolonged intake) —*see* Table of Drugs and Chemicals, vitamins, adverse effect
    - overdose or wrong substance given or taken —*see* Table of Drugs and Chemicals, vitamins, poisoning
  - K E67.8
    - administered as drug (prolonged intake) —*see* Table of Drugs and Chemicals, vitamins, adverse effect
    - overdose or wrong substance given or taken —*see* Table of Drugs and Chemicals, vitamins, poisoning
- **Hypervolemia** E87.70
  - specified NEC E87.79
- **Hypesthesia** R20.1
  - cornea —*see* Anesthesia, cornea
- **Hyphema** H21.0-
  - traumatic S05.1-
- **Hypoacidity, gastric** K31.89
  - psychogenic F45.8
- **Hypoadrenalism, hypoadrenia** E27.40
  - primary E27.1
  - tuberculous A18.7
- **Hypoadrenocorticism** E27.40
  - pituitary E23.0
  - primary E27.1
- **Hypoalbuminemia** E88.09
- **Hypoaldosteronism** E27.40
- **Hypoalphalipoproteinemia** E78.6
- **Hypobarism** T70.29
- **Hypobaropathy** T70.29
- **Hypobetalipoproteinemia** (familial) E78.6
- **Hypocalcemia** E83.51
  - dietary E58
  - neonatal P71.1
    - due to cow's milk P71.0
  - phosphate-loading (newborn) P71.1
- **Hypochloremia** E87.8
- **Hypochlorhydria** K31.89
  - neurotic F45.8
  - psychogenic F45.8
- **Hypochondria, hypochondriac, hypochondriasis** (reaction) F45.21
  - sleep F51.03
- **Hypochondrogenesis** Q77.0
- **Hypochondroplasia** Q77.4
- **Hypochromasia, blood cells** D50.8
- **Hypocitraturia** R82.991
- **Hypodontia** —*see* Anodontia
- **Hypoeosinophilia** D72.89
- **Hypoesthesia** R20.1
- **Hypofibrinogenemia** D68.8
  - acquired D65
  - congenital (hereditary) D68.2
- **Hypofunction**
  - adrenocortical E27.40
    - drug-induced E27.3
    - postprocedural E89.6
    - primary E27.1
  - adrenomedullary, postprocedural E89.6
  - cerebral R29.818
  - corticoadrenal NEC E27.40
  - intestinal K59.89
  - labyrinth H83.2
  - ovary E28.39
  - pituitary (gland) (anterior) E23.0
  - testicular E29.1
    - postprocedural (postsurgical) (postirradiation) (iatrogenic) E89.5
- **Hypogalactia** O92.4
- **Hypogammaglobulinemia** (*see also* Agammaglobulinemia) D80.1
  - hereditary D80.0
  - nonfamilial D80.1
  - transient, of infancy D80.7
- **Hypogenitalism** (congenital) —*see* Hypogonadism
- **Hypoglossia** Q38.3
- **Hypoglycemia** (spontaneous) E16.2
  - coma E15
    - diabetic —*see* Diabetes, by type, with hypoglycemia, with coma
  - diabetic —*see* Diabetes, hypoglycemia
  - dietary counseling and surveillance Z71.3
  - drug-induced E16.0
    - with coma (nondiabetic) E15
  - due to insulin E16.0
    - with coma (nondiabetic) E15
    - therapeutic misadventure —*see* subcategory T38.3
  - functional, nonhyperinsulinemic E16.1
  - iatrogenic E16.0
    - with coma (nondiabetic) E15

Hypoplasia, hypoplastic *(continued)*
  zonule (ciliary) Q12.8
Hypoplasminogenemia E88.02
Hypopnea, obstructive sleep apnea G47.33
Hypopotassemia E87.6
Hypoproconvertinemia, congenital (hereditary) D68.2
Hypoproteinemia E77.8
Hypoprothrombinemia (congenital) (hereditary) (idiopathic) D68.2
  acquired D68.4
  newborn, transient P61.6
Hypoptyalism K11.7
Hypopyon (eye) (anterior chamber) —*see* Iridocyclitis, acute, hypopyon
Hypopyrexia R68.0
Hyporeflexia R29.2
Hyposecretion
  ACTH E23.0
  antidiuretic hormone E23.2
  ovary E28.39
  salivary gland (any) K11.7
  vasopressin E23.2
Hyposegmentation, leukocytic, hereditary D72.0
Hyposiderinemia D50.9
Hypospadias Q54.9
  balanic Q54.0
  coronal Q54.0
  glandular Q54.0
  penile Q54.1
  penoscrotal Q54.2
  perineal Q54.3
  specified NEC Q54.8
Hypospermatogenesis —*see* Oligospermia
Hyposplenism D73.0
Hypostasis pulmonary, passive —*see* Edema, lung
Hypostatic —*see* condition
Hyposthenuria N28.89
Hypotension (arterial) (constitutional) I95.9
  chronic I95.89
  due to (of) hemodialysis I95.3
  drug-induced I95.2
  iatrogenic I95.89
  idiopathic (permanent) I95.0
  intracranial G96.810
    following
      lumbar cerebrospinal fluid shunting G97.83
      specified procedure NEC G97.84
      ventricular shunting (ventriculostomy) G97.2
    specified NEC G96.819
    spontaneous G96.811
  intra-dialytic I95.3
  maternal, syndrome (following labor and delivery) O26.5-
  neurogenic, orthostatic G90.3
  orthostatic (chronic) I95.1
    due to drugs I95.2
    neurogenic G90.3
  postoperative I95.81
  postural I95.1
  specified NEC I95.89
Hypothermia (accidental) T68
  due to anesthesia, anesthetic T88.51
  low environmental temperature T68
  neonatal P80.9
    environmental (mild) NEC P80.8

Hypothermia *(continued)*
    mild P80.8
    severe (chronic) (cold injury syndrome) P80.0
    specified NEC P80.8
  not associated with low environmental temperature R68.0
Hypothyroidism (acquired) E03.9
  autoimmune —*see* Thyroiditis, autoimmune
  congenital (without goiter) E03.1
    with goiter (diffuse) E03.0
  due to
    exogenous substance NEC E03.2
    iodine-deficiency, acquired E01.8
      subclinical E02
    irradiation therapy E89.0
    medicament NEC E03.2
    P-aminosalicylic acid (PAS) E03.2
    phenylbutazone E03.2
    resorcinol E03.2
    sulfonamide E03.2
    surgery E89.0
    thiourea group drugs E03.2
  iatrogenic NEC E03.2
  iodine-deficiency (acquired) E01.8
    congenital —*see* Syndrome, iodine- deficiency, congenital
    subclinical E02
  neonatal, transitory P72.2
  postinfectious E03.3
  postirradiation E89.0
  postprocedural E89.0
  postsurgical E89.0
  specified NEC E03.8
  subclinical, iodine-deficiency related E02
Hypotonia, hypotonicity, hypotony
  bladder N31.2
  congenital (benign) P94.2
  eye —*see* Disorder, globe, hypotony
Hypotrichosis —*see* Alopecia
Hypotropia H50.2-
Hypoventilation R06.89
  congenital central alveolar G47.35
  sleep related
    idiopathic nonobstructive alveolar G47.34
    in conditions classified elsewhere G47.36
Hypovitaminosis —*see* Deficiency, vitamin
Hypovolemia E86.1
  surgical shock T81.19
  traumatic (shock) T79.4
Hypoxemia R09.02
  newborn P84
  sleep related, in conditions classified elsewhere G47.36
Hypoxia (*see also* Anoxia) R09.02
  cerebral, during a procedure NEC G97.81
    postprocedural NEC G97.82
  intrauterine P84
  myocardial —*see* Insufficiency, coronary
  newborn P84
  sleep-related G47.34
Hypsarhythmia —*see* Epilepsy, generalized, specified NEC
Hysteralgia, pregnant uterus O26.89-
Hysteria, hysterical (conversion) (dissociative state) F44.9
  anxiety F41.8

Hysteria, hysterical *(continued)*
  convulsions F44.5
  psychosis, acute F44.9
Hysteroepilepsy F44.5

I

IBDU (colonic inflammatory bowel disease unclassified) K52.3
ICANS (immune effector cell-associated neurotoxicity syndrome) —*see* Syndrome, immue effector cell-associated neurotoxicity
Ichthyoparasitism due to Vandellia cirrhosa B88.8
Ichthyosis (congenital) Q80.9
  acquired L85.0
  fetalis Q80.4
  hystrix Q80.8
  lamellar Q80.2
  lingual K13.29
  palmaris and plantaris Q82.8
  simplex Q80.0
  vera Q80.8
  vulgaris Q80.0
  X-linked Q80.1
Ichthyotoxism —*see* Poisoning, fish
  bacterial —*see* Intoxication, foodborne
Icteroanemia, hemolytic (acquired) D59.9
  congenital —*see* Spherocytosis
Icterus —*see also* Jaundice
  conjunctiva R17
  newborn P59.9
  gravis, newborn P55.0
  hematogenous (acquired) D59.9
  hemolytic (acquired) D59.9
    congenital —*see* Spherocytosis
  hemorrhagic (acute) (leptospiral) (spirochetal) A27.0
    newborn P53
  infectious B15.9
    with hepatic coma B15.0
    leptospiral A27.0
    spirochetal A27.0
  neonatorum —*see* Jaundice, newborn
  spirochetal A27.0
Ictus solaris, solis T67.01
Ideation
  homicidal R45.850
  suicidal R45.851
Identity disorder (child) F64.9
  gender role F64.2
  psychosexual F64.2
Id reaction (due to bacteria) L30.2
Idioglossia F80.0
Idiopathic —*see* condition
Idiot, idiocy (congenital) F73
  amaurotic (Bielschowsky (-Jansky)) (family) (infantile (late)) (juvenile (late)) (Vogt-Spielmeyer) E75.4
  microcephalic Q02
IgE asthma J45.909
IIAC (idiopathic infantile arterial calcification) Q28.8
Ileitis (chronic) (noninfectious) —*see also* Enteritis K52.9
  backwash —*see* Pancolitis, ulcerative (chronic)
  infectious A09

Ileitis *(continued)*
  regional (ulcerative) —*see* Enteritis, regional, small intestine
  segmental —*see* Enteritis, regional
  terminal (ulcerative) —*see* Enteritis, regional, small intestine
Ileocolitis (*see also* Enteritis) K52.9
  regional —*see* Enteritis, regional
  infectious A09
  ulcerative K51.0-
Ileostomy
  attention to Z43.2
  malfunctioning K94.13
  status Z93.2
    with complication —*see* Complications, enterostomy
Ileotyphus —*see* Typhoid
Ileum —*see* condition
Ileus (bowel) (colon) (inhibitory) (intestine) K56.7
  adynamic K56.0
  due to gallstone (in intestine) K56.3
  duodenal (chronic) K31.5
  gallstone K56.3
  mechanical NEC (*see also* Obstruction, intestine, specified NEC) K56.699
  meconium P76.0
    in cystic fibrosis E84.11
    meaning meconium plug (without cystic fibrosis) P76.0
  myxedema K59.89
  neurogenic K56.0
    Hirschsprung's disease or megacolon Q43.1
  newborn
    due to meconium P76.0
      in cystic fibrosis E84.11
      meaning meconium plug (without cystic fibrosis) P76.0
    transitory P76.1
  obstructive (*see also* Obstruction, intestine, specified NEC) K56.699
  paralytic K56.0
  postoperative K91.89
Iliac —*see* condition
Iliotibial band syndrome M76.3-
Illiteracy Z55.0
Illness (*see also* Disease) R69
  manic-depressive —*see* Disorder, bipolar
Imbalance R26.89
  autonomic G90.8
  constituents of food intake E63.1
  electrolyte E87.8
    with
      abortion —*see* Abortion by type, complicated by, electrolyte imbalance
      molar pregnancy O08.5
    due to hyperemesis gravidarum O21.1
    following ectopic or molar pregnancy O08.5
    neonatal, transitory NEC P74.49
      potassium
        hyperkalemia P74.31
        hypokalemia P74.32
      sodium
        hypernatremia P74.21
        hyponatremia P74.22
  endocrine E34.9
  eye muscle NOS H50.9
  hormone E34.9
  hysterical F44.4

Imbalance *(continued)*
- labyrinth H83.2
- posture R29.3
- protein-energy *—see* Malnutrition
- sympathetic G90.8

Imbecile, imbecility (I.Q.35-49) F71

Imbedding, intrauterine device T83.39

Imbibition, cholesterol (gallbladder) K82.4

Imbrication, teeth,, fully erupted M26.30

Imerslund (-Gräsbeck) **syndrome** D51.1

Immature *—see also* Immaturity
- birth (less than 37 completed weeks) *—see* Preterm, newborn
  - extremely (less than 28 completed weeks) *—see* Immaturity, extreme
- personality F60.89

Immaturity (less than 37 completed weeks) *—see also* Preterm, newborn
- extreme of newborn (less than 28 completed weeks of gestation) (less than 196 completed days of gestation) (unspecified weeks of gestation) P07.20
  - gestational age
    - 23 completed weeks (23 weeks, 0 days through 23 weeks, 6 days) P07.22
    - 24 completed weeks (24 weeks, 0 days through 24 weeks, 6 days) P07.23
    - 25 completed weeks (25 weeks, 0 days through 25 weeks, 6 days) P07.24
    - 26 completed weeks (26 weeks, 0 days through 26 weeks, 6 days) P07.25
    - 27 completed weeks (27 weeks, 0 days through 27 weeks, 6 days) P07.26
    - less than 23 completed weeks P07.21
- fetus or infant light-for-dates *—see* Light-for-dates
- lung, newborn P28.0
- organ or site NEC *—see* Hypoplasia
- pulmonary, newborn P28.0
- reaction F60.89
- sexual (female) (male), after puberty E30.0

Immersion T75.1
- hand T69.01-
- foot T69.02-

Immobile, immobility
- complete, due to severe physical disability or frailty R53.2
- intestine K59.89
- syndrome (paraplegic) M62.3

Immune reconstitution (inflammatory) **syndrome [IRIS]** D89.3

Immunization *—see also* Vaccination
- ABO *—see* Incompatibility, ABO
  - in newborn P55.1
- appropriate for age
  - child (over 28 days old) Z00.129
    - with abnormal findings Z00.121
- complication *—see* Complications, vaccination
- encounter for Z23
- not done (not carried out) Z28.9
  - because (of)
    - acute illness of patient Z28.01
    - allergy to vaccine (or component) Z28.04
    - caregiver refusal Z28.82
    - chronic illness of patient Z28.02
    - contraindication NEC Z28.09
    - delay in delivery of vaccine Z28.83
    - group pressure Z28.1
    - guardian refusal Z28.82
    - immune compromised state of patient Z28.03
    - lack of availability of vaccine Z28.83
    - manufacturer delay of vaccine Z28.83
    - parent refusal Z28.82
    - patient's belief Z28.1
    - patient had disease being vaccinated against Z28.81
    - patient refusal Z28.21
    - religious beliefs of patient Z28.1
    - specified reason NEC Z28.89
      - of patient Z28.29
    - unavailability of vaccine Z28.83
    - unspecified patient reason Z28.20
- Rh factor
  - affecting management of pregnancy NEC O36.09-
    - anti-D antibody O36.01-
  - from transfusion *—see* Complication(s), transfusion, incompatibility reaction, Rh (factor)

Immunocompromised NOS D84.9

Immunocytoma C83.0-

Immunodeficiency D84.9
- with
  - adenosine-deaminase deficiency (*see also* Deficiency, adenosine deaminase) D81.30
  - antibody defects D80.9
    - specified type NEC D80.8
  - hyperimmunoglobulinemia D80.6
  - increased immunoglobulin M (IgM) D80.5
  - major defect D82.9
    - specified type NEC D82.8
  - partial albinism D82.8
  - short-limbed stature D82.2
  - thrombocytopenia and eczema D82.0
- antibody with
  - hyperimmunoglobulinemia D80.6
  - near-normal immunoglobulins D80.6
- autosomal recessive, Swiss type D80.0
- combined D81.9
  - biotin-dependent carboxylase D81.819
    - biotinidase D81.810
    - holocarboxylase synthetase D81.818
    - specified type NEC D81.818
  - severe (SCID) D81.9
    - with
      - low or normal B-cell numbers D81.2
      - low T- and B-cell numbers D81.1
      - reticular dysgenesis D81.0
  - specified type NEC D81.89
- common variable D83.9
  - with
    - abnormalities of B-cell numbers and function D83.0
    - autoantibodies to B- or T-cells D83.2
    - immunoregulatory T-cell disorders D83.1
  - specified type NEC D83.8
- due to
  - conditions classified elsewhere D84.81
  - drugs D84.821
  - external causes D84.822
  - medication (current or past) D84.821
- following hereditary defective response to Epstein-Barr virus (EBV) D82.3
- selective, immunoglobulin
  - A (IgA) D80.2
  - G (IgG) (subclasses) D80.3
  - M (IgM) D80.4
- severe combined (SCID) D81.9
  - due to adenosine deaminase deficiency D81.31
- specified type NEC D84.89
- X-linked, with increased IgM D80.5

Immunodeficient NOS D84.9

Immunosuppressed NOS D84.9

Immunotherapy (encounter for)
- antineoplastic Z51.12

Impaction, impacted
- bowel, colon, rectum (*see also* Impaction, fecal) K56.49
  - by gallstone K56.3
- calculus *—see* Calculus
- cerumen (ear) (external) H61.2-
- cuspid *—see* Impaction, tooth
- dental (same or adjacent tooth) K01.1
- fecal, feces K56.41
- fracture *—see* Fracture, by site
- gallbladder *—see* Calculus, gallbladder
- gallstone(s) *—see* Calculus, gallbladder
  - bile duct (common) (hepatic) *—see* Calculus, bile duct
  - cystic duct *—see* Calculus, gallbladder
  - in intestine, with obstruction (any part) K56.3
- intestine (calculous) NEC *—see also* Impaction, fecal K56.49
  - gallstone, with ileus K56.3
- intrauterine device (IUD) T83.39
- molar *—see* Impaction, tooth
- shoulder, causing obstructed labor O66.0
- tooth, teeth K01.1
- turbinate J34.89

Impaired, impairment (function)
- auditory discrimination *—see* Abnormal, auditory perception
- cognitive, mild, so stated G31.84
- dual sensory Z73.82
- fasting glucose R73.01
- glucose tolerance (oral) R73.02
- hearing *—see* Deafness
- heart *—see* Disease, heart
- kidney N28.9
  - disorder resulting from N25.9
    - specified NEC N25.89
- liver K72.90
  - with coma K72.91
- mastication K08.89
- mild cognitive, so stated G31.84
- mobility
  - ear ossicles *—see* Ankylosis, ear ossicles
  - requiring care provider Z74.09
- myocardium, myocardial *—see* Insufficiency, myocardial
- rectal sphincter R19.8
- renal (acute) (chronic) N28.9
  - disorder resulting from N25.9
    - specified NEC N25.89
- vision NEC H54.7
  - both eyes H54.3

Impediment, speech (*see also* Disorder, speech) R47.9
- psychogenic (childhood) F98.8
- slurring R47.81
- specified NEC R47.89

Impending
- coronary syndrome I20.0
- delirium tremens F10.239
- myocardial infarction I20.0

Imperception auditory (acquired) *—see also* Deafness
- congenital H93.25

Imperfect
- aeration, lung (newborn) NEC *—see* Atelectasis
- closure (congenital)
  - alimentary tract NEC Q45.8
    - lower Q43.8
    - upper Q40.8
  - atrioventricular ostium Q21.2
  - atrium (secundum) Q21.1
  - branchial cleft NOS Q18.2
    - cyst Q18.0
    - fistula Q18.0
    - sinus Q18.0
  - choroid Q14.3
  - cricoid cartilage Q31.8
  - cusps, heart valve NEC Q24.8
    - pulmonary Q22.3
  - ductus
    - arteriosus Q25.0
    - Botalli Q25.0
  - ear drum (causing impairment of hearing) Q16.4
  - esophagus with communication to bronchus or trachea Q39.1
  - eyelid Q10.3
  - foramen
    - botalli Q21.1
    - ovale Q21.1
  - genitalia, genital organ(s) or system
    - female Q52.8
      - external Q52.79
      - internal NEC Q52.8
    - male Q55.8
  - glottis Q31.8
  - interatrial ostium or septum Q21.1
  - interauricular ostium or septum Q21.1
  - interventricular ostium or septum Q21.0
  - larynx Q31.8
  - lip *—see* Cleft, lip
  - nasal septum Q30.3
  - nose Q30.2
  - omphalomesenteric duct Q43.0
  - optic nerve entry Q14.2
  - organ or site not listed *—see* Anomaly, by site
  - ostium
    - interatrial Q21.1
    - interauricular Q21.1
    - interventricular Q21.0
  - palate *—see* Cleft, palate
  - preauricular sinus Q18.1
  - retina Q14.1

Imperfect *(continued)*
- closure *(continued)*
  - roof of orbit Q75.8
  - sclera Q13.5
  - septum
    - aorticopulmonary Q21.4
    - atrial (secundum) Q21.1
    - between aorta and pulmonary artery Q21.4
    - heart Q21.9
    - interatrial (secundum) Q21.1
    - interauricular (secundum) Q21.1
    - interventricular Q21.0
      - in tetralogy of Fallot Q21.3
    - nasal Q30.3
    - ventricular Q21.0
      - with pulmonary stenosis or atresia, dextraposition of aorta, and hypertrophy of right ventricle Q21.3
      - in tetralogy of Fallot Q21.3
  - skull Q75.0
    - with
      - anencephaly Q00.0
      - encephalocele —*see* Encephalocele
      - hydrocephalus Q03.9
        - with spina bifida —*see* Spina bifida, by site, with hydrocephalus
      - microcephaly Q02
  - spine (with meningocele) —*see* Spina bifida
  - trachea Q32.1
  - tympanic membrane (causing impairment of hearing) Q16.4
  - uterus Q51.818
  - vitelline duct Q43.0
- erection —*see* Dysfunction, sexual, male, erectile
- fusion —*see* Imperfect, closure
- inflation, lung (newborn) —*see* Atelectasis
- posture R29.3
- rotation, intestine Q43.3
- septum, ventricular Q21.0

Imperfectly descended testis —*see* Cryptorchid

Imperforate (congenital) —*see also* Atresia
- anus Q42.3
  - with fistula Q42.2
- cervix (uteri) Q51.828
- esophagus Q39.0
  - with tracheoesophageal fistula Q39.1
- hymen Q52.3
- jejunum Q41.1
- pharynx Q38.8
- rectum Q42.1
  - with fistula Q42.0
- urethra Q64.39
- vagina Q52.4

Impervious (congenital) —*see also* Atresia
- anus Q42.3
  - with fistula Q42.2
- bile duct Q44.2
- esophagus Q39.0
  - with tracheoesophageal fistula Q39.1
- intestine (small) Q41.9
  - large Q42.9
    - specified NEC Q42.8
- rectum Q42.1
  - with fistula Q42.0
- ureter —*see* Atresia, ureter
- urethra Q64.39

Impetiginization of dermatoses L01.1

Impetigo (any organism) (any site) (circinate) (contagiosa) (simplex) (vulgaris) L01.00
- Bockhart's L01.02
- bullous, bullosa L01.03
- external ear L01.00 *[H62.40]*
- follicularis L01.02
- furfuracea L30.5
- herpetiformis L40.1
  - nonobstetrical L40.1
- neonatorum L01.03
- nonbullous L01.01
- specified type NEC L01.09
- ulcerative L01.09

Impingement (on teeth)
- joint —*see* Disorder, joint, specified type NEC
- soft tissue
  - anterior M26.81
  - posterior M26.82

Implant, endometrial N80.9

Implantation
- anomalous —*see* Anomaly, by site
  - ureter Q62.63
- cyst
  - external area or site (skin) NEC L72.0
  - iris —*see* Cyst, iris, implantation
  - vagina N89.8
  - vulva N90.7
- dermoid (cyst) —*see* Implantation, cyst

Impotence (sexual) N52.9
- counseling Z70.1
- organic origin (*see also* Dysfunction, sexual, male, erectile) N52.9
- psychogenic F52.21

Impression, basilar Q75.8

Imprisonment, anxiety concerning Z65.1

Improper care (child) (newborn) —*see* Maltreatment

Improperly tied umbilical cord (causing hemorrhage) P51.8

Impulsiveness (impulsive) R45.87

Inability to swallow —*see* Aphagia

Inaccessible, inaccessibility
- health care NEC Z75.3
  - due to
    - waiting period Z75.2
      - for admission to facility elsewhere Z75.1
- other helping agencies Z75.4

Inactive —*see* condition

Inadequate, inadequacy
- aesthetics of dental restoration K08.56
- biologic, constitutional, functional, or social F60.7
- development
  - child R62.50
  - genitalia
    - after puberty NEC E30.0
    - congenital
      - female Q52.8
        - external Q52.79
        - internal Q52.8
      - male Q55.8
  - lungs Q33.6
    - associated with short gestation P28.0
  - organ or site not listed —*see* Anomaly, by site

Inadequate, inadequacy *(continued)*
- diet (causing nutritional deficiency) E63.9
- drinking-water supply Z58.6
- eating habits Z72.4
- environment, household Z59.18
- family support Z63.8
- food (supply) NEC Z59.48
  - hunger effects T73.0
- functional F60.7
- household care, due to
  - family member
    - handicapped or ill Z74.2
    - on vacation Z75.5
    - temporarily away from home Z74.2
  - technical defects in home Z59.1
  - temporary absence from home of person rendering care Z74.2
- housing (heating) (space) Z59.1
- income (financial) Z59.6
- intrafamilial communication Z63.8
- material resources Z59.9
- mental —*see* Disability, intellectual
- parental supervision or control of child Z62.0
- personality F60.7
- pulmonary
  - function R06.89
    - newborn P28.5
  - ventilation, newborn P28.5
- sample of cytologic smear
  - anus R85.615
  - cervix R87.615
  - vagina R87.625
- social F60.7
  - insurance Z59.7
  - skills NEC Z73.4
- supervision of child by parent Z62.0
- teaching affecting education Z55.8
- welfare support Z59.7

Inanition R64
- with edema —*see* Malnutrition, severe
- due to
  - deprivation of food T73.0
  - malnutrition —*see* Malnutrition
- fever R50.9

Inappropriate
- change in quantitative human chorionic gonadotropin (hCG) in early pregnancy O02.81
- diet or eating habits Z72.4
- level of quantitative human chorionic gonadotropin (hCG) for gestational age in early pregnancy O02.81
- secretion
  - antidiuretic hormone (ADH) (excessive) E22.2
    - deficiency E23.2
  - pituitary (posterior) E22.2

Inattention at or after birth —*see* Neglect

Incarceration, incarcerated
- enterocele K46.0
  - gangrenous K46.1
- epiplocele K46.0
  - gangrenous K46.1
- exomphalos K42.0
  - gangrenous K42.1
- hernia —*see also* Hernia, by site, with obstruction
  - with gangrene —*see* Hernia, by site, with gangrene

Incarceration, incarcerated *(continued)*
- iris, in wound —*see* Injury, eye, laceration, with prolapse
- lens, in wound —*see* Injury, eye, laceration, with prolapse
- omphalocele K42.0
- prison, anxiety concerning Z65.1
- rupture —*see* Hernia, by site
- sarcoepiplocele K46.0
  - gangrenous K46.1
- sarcoepiplomphalocele K42.0
  - with gangrene K42.1
- uterus N85.8
  - gravid O34.51-
    - causing obstructed labor O65.5

Incised wound
- external —*see* Laceration
- internal organs —*see* Injury, by site

Incision, incisional
- hernia K43.2
  - with
    - gangrene (and obstruction) K43.1
    - obstruction K43.0
- surgical, complication —*see* Complications, surgical procedure
- traumatic
  - external —*see* Laceration
  - internal organs —*see* Injury, by site

Inclusion
- azurophilic leukocytic D72.0
- blennorrhea (neonatal) (newborn) P39.1
- gallbladder in liver (congenital) Q44.1

Incompatibility
- ABO
  - affecting management of pregnancy O36.11-
    - anti-A sensitization O36.11-
    - anti-B sensitization O36.19-
    - specified NEC O36.19-
  - infusion or transfusion reaction —*see* Complication(s), transfusion, incompatibility reaction, ABO
  - newborn P55.1
- blood (group) (Duffy) (K) (Kell) (Kidd) (Lewis) (M) (S) NEC
  - affecting management of pregnancy O36.11-
    - anti-A sensitization O36.11-
    - anti-B sensitization O36.19-
  - infusion or transfusion reaction T80.89
  - newborn P55.8
- divorce or estrangement Z63.5
- Rh (blood group) (factor) Z31.82
  - affecting management of pregnancy NEC O36.09-
    - anti-D antibody O36.01-
  - infusion or transfusion reaction —*see* Complication(s), transfusion, incompatibility reaction, Rh (factor)
  - newborn P55.0
- rhesus —*see* Incompatibility, Rh

Incompetency, incompetent, incompetence
- annular
  - aortic (valve) —*see* Insufficiency, aortic
  - mitral (valve) I34.0
  - pulmonary valve (heart) I37.1
- aortic (valve) —*see* Insufficiency, aortic

Incompetency, incompetent, incompetence *(continued)*
- cardiac valve *—see* Endocarditis
- cervix, cervical (os) N88.3
  - in pregnancy O34.3-
- chronotropic I45.89
  - with
    - autonomic dysfunction G90.8
    - ischemic heart disease I25.89
    - left ventricular dysfunction I51.89
    - sinus node dysfunction I49.8
- esophagogastric (junction) (sphincter) K22.0
- mitral (valve) *—see* Insufficiency, mitral
- pelvic fundus N81.89
- pubocervical tissue N81.82
- pulmonary valve (heart) I37.1
  - congenital Q22.3
- rectovaginal tissue N81.83
- tricuspid (annular) (valve) *—see* Insufficiency, tricuspid
- valvular *—see* Endocarditis
  - congenital Q24.8
- vein, venous (saphenous) (varicose) *—see* Varix, leg

Incomplete *—see also* condition
- bladder, emptying R33.9
- defecation R15.0
- expansion lungs (newborn) NEC *—see* Atelectasis
- rotation, intestine Q43.3

Inconclusive
- diagnostic imaging due to excess body fat of patient R93.9
- findings on diagnostic imaging of breast NEC R92.8
- mammogram (due to dense breasts) R92.2

Incontinence R32
- anal sphincter R15.9
- coital N39.491
- feces R15.9
  - nonorganic origin F98.1
- insensible (urinary) N39.42
- overflow N39.490
- postural (urinary) N39.492
- psychogenic F45.8
- rectal R15.9
- reflex N39.498
- stress (female) (male) N39.3
  - and urge N39.46
- urethral sphincter R32
- urge N39.41
  - and stress (female) (male) N39.46
- urine (urinary) R32
  - continuous N39.45
  - due to cognitive impairment, or severe physical disability or immobility R39.81
  - functional R39.81
  - insensible N39.42
  - mixed (stress and urge) N39.46
  - nocturnal N39.44
  - nonorganic origin F98.0
  - overflow N39.490
  - post dribbling N39.43
  - postural N39.492
  - reflex N39.498
  - specified NEC N39.498
  - stress (female) (male) N39.3
    - and urge N39.46
  - total N39.498
  - unaware N39.42
  - urge N39.41
    - and stress (female) (male) N39.46

Incontinentia pigmenti Q82.3

Incoordinate, incoordination
- esophageal-pharyngeal (newborn) *—see* Dysphagia
- muscular R27.8
- uterus (action) (contractions) (complicating delivery) O62.4

Increase, increased
- abnormal, in development R63.8
- androgens (ovarian) E28.1
- anticoagulants (antithrombin) (anti-VIIIa) (anti-IXa) (anti-Xa) (anti-XIa) *—see* Circulating anticoagulants
- cold sense R20.8
- estrogen E28.0
- function
  - adrenal
    - cortex *—see* Cushing's, syndrome
    - medulla E27.5
  - pituitary (gland) (anterior) (lobe) E22.9
    - posterior E22.2
- heat sense R20.8
- intracranial pressure (benign) G93.2
- permeability, capillaries I78.8
- pressure, intracranial G93.2
- secretion
  - gastrin E16.4
  - glucagon E16.3
  - pancreas, endocrine E16.9
    - growth hormone-releasing hormone E16.8
    - pancreatic polypeptide E16.8
    - somatostatin E16.8
    - vasoactive-intestinal polypeptide E16.8
- sphericity, lens Q12.4
- splenic activity D73.1
- venous pressure I87.8
  - portal K76.6

Increta placenta O43.22-

Incrustation, cornea, foreign body (lead) (zinc) *—see* Foreign body, cornea

Incyclophoria H50.54

Incyclotropia *—see* Cyclotropia

Indeterminate sex Q56.4

India rubber skin Q82.8

Indigestion (acid) (bilious) (functional) K30
- catarrhal K31.89
- due to decomposed food NOS A05.9
- nervous F45.8
- psychogenic F45.8

Indirect *—see* condition

Induratio penis plastica N48.6

Induration, indurated
- brain G93.89
- breast (fibrous) N64.51
  - puerperal, postpartum O92.29
- broad ligament N83.8
- chancre
  - anus A51.1
  - congenital A50.07
  - extragenital NEC A51.2
- corpora cavernosa (penis) (plastic) N48.6
- liver (chronic) K76.89
- lung (black) (chronic) (fibroid) *—see also* Fibrosis, lung J84.10
  - essential brown J84.03
- penile (plastic) N48.6
- phlebitic *—see* Phlebitis
- skin R23.4

Inebriety (without dependence) *—see* Alcohol, intoxication

Inefficiency, kidney N28.9

Inelasticity, skin R23.4

Inequality, leg (length) (acquired) *—see also* Deformity, limb, unequal length
- congenital *—see* Defect, reduction, lower limb
- lower leg *—see* Deformity, limb, unequal length

Inertia
- bladder (neurogenic) N31.2
- stomach K31.89
  - psychogenic F45.8
- uterus, uterine during labor O62.2
  - during latent phase of labor O62.0
  - primary O62.0
  - secondary O62.1
- vesical (neurogenic) N31.2

Infancy, infantile, infantilism *—see also* condition
- celiac K90.0
- genitalia, genitals (after puberty) E30.0
- Herter's (nontropical sprue) K90.0
- intestinal K90.0
- Lorain E23.0
- pancreatic K86.89
- pelvis M95.5
  - with disproportion (fetopelvic) O33.1
    - causing obstructed labor O65.1
- pituitary E23.0
- renal N25.0
- uterus *—see* Infantile, genitalia

Infant(s) *—see also* Infancy
- excessive crying R68.11
- irritable child R68.12
- lack of care *—see* Neglect
- liveborn (singleton) Z38.2
  - born in hospital Z38.00
    - by cesarean Z38.01
  - born outside hospital Z38.1
  - multiple NEC Z38.8
    - born in hospital Z38.68
      - by cesarean Z38.69
    - born outside hospital Z38.7
  - quadruplet Z38.8
    - born in hospital Z38.63
      - by cesarean Z38.64
    - born outside hospital Z38.7
  - quintuplet Z38.8
    - born in hospital Z38.65
      - by cesarean Z38.66
    - born outside hospital Z38.7
  - triplet Z38.8
    - born in hospital Z38.61
      - by cesarean Z38.62
    - born outside hospital Z38.7
  - twin Z38.5
    - born in hospital Z38.30
      - by cesarean Z38.31
    - born outside hospital Z38.4
- of diabetic mother (syndrome of) P70.1
  - gestational diabetes P70.0

Infantile *—see also* condition
- genitalia, genitals E30.0
- os, uterine E30.0
- penis E30.0
- testis E29.1
- uterus E30.0

Infantilism *—see* Infancy

Infarct, infarction
- adrenal (capsule) (gland) E27.49
- appendices epiploicae (*see also* Infarct, intestine) K55.069

Infarct, infarction *(continued)*
- bowel (*see also* Infarct, intestine) K55.0 069
- brain (stem) *—see* Infarct, cerebral
- breast N64.89
- brewer's (kidney) N28.0
- cardiac *—see* Infarct, myocardium
- cerebellar *—see* Infarct, cerebral
- cerebral (acute) (chronic) *—see also* Occlusion, artery cerebral or precerebral, with infarction I63.9-
  - aborted I63.9
  - cortical I63.9
  - due to
    - cerebral venous thrombosis, nonpyogenic I63.6
    - embolism
      - cerebral arteries I63.4-
      - precerebral arteries I63.1-
    - occlusion NEC
      - cerebral arteries I63.5-
      - precerebral arteries I63.2-
      - small artery I63.81
    - stenosis NEC
      - cerebral arteries I63.5-
      - precerebral arteries I63.2-
      - small artery I63.81
    - thrombosis
      - cerebral artery I63.3-
      - precerebral artery I63.0-
  - intraoperative
    - during cardiac surgery I97.810
    - during other surgery I97.811
  - neonatal P91.82-
  - perinatal (arterial ischemic) P91.82-
  - postprocedural
    - following cardiac surgery I97.820
    - following other surgery I97.821
  - specified NEC I63.89
- colon (acute) (agnogenic) (embolic) (hemorrhagic) (nonocclusive) (nonthrombotic) (occlusive) (segmental) (thrombotic) (with gangrene) (*see also* Infarct, intestine) K55.049
- coronary artery *—see* Infarct, myocardium
- embolic *—see* Embolism
- fallopian tube N83.8
- gallbladder K82.8
- heart *—see* Infarct, myocardium
- hepatic K76.3
- hypophysis (anterior lobe) E23.6
- impending (myocardium) I20.0
- intestine (acute) (agnogenic) (embolic) (hemorrhagic) (nonocclusive) (nonthrombotic) (occlusive) (thrombotic) (with gangrene) K55.069
  - diffuse K55.062
  - focal K55.061
  - large K55.049
    - diffuse K55.042
    - focal K55.041
  - small K55.029
    - diffuse K55.029
    - focal K55.021
- kidney N28.0
- lacunar I63.81
- liver K76.3
- lung (embolic) (thrombotic) *—see* Embolism, pulmonary
- lymph node I89.8
- mesentery, mesenteric (embolic) (thrombotic) (with gangrene) (*see also* Infarct, intestine) K55.069

Infarct, infarction *(continued)*
- muscle (ischemic) M62.20
  - ankle M62.27-
  - foot M62.27-
  - forearm M62.23-
  - hand M62.24-
  - lower leg M62.26-
  - pelvic region M62.25-
  - shoulder region M62.21-
  - specified site NEC M62.28
  - thigh M62.25-
  - upper arm M62.22-
- myocardium, myocardial (acute) (with stated duration of 4 weeks or less) I21.9
  - associated with revascularization procedure I21.A9
  - diagnosed on ECG, but presenting no symptoms I25.2
  - due to
    - demand ischemia I21.A1
    - ischemic imbalance I21.A1
  - healed or old I25.2
  - intraoperative *—see also* Infarct, myocardium, associated with revascularization procedure
    - during cardiac surgery I97.790
    - during other surgery I97.791
  - non-Q wave I21.4
  - non-ST elevation (NSTEMI) I21.4
    - subsequent I22.2
  - nontransmural I21.4
  - past (diagnosed on ECG or other investigation, but currently presenting no symptoms) I25.2
  - postprocedural *—see also* Infarct, myocardium, associated with revascularization procedure
    - following cardiac surgery (*see also* Infarct, myocardium, type 4 or type 5) I97.190
    - following other surgery I97.191
  - Q wave (*see also*, Infarct, myocardium, by site) I21.3
  - secondary to
    - demand ischemia I21.A1
    - ischemic imbalance I21.A1
  - ST elevation (STEMI) I21.3
    - anterior (anteroapical) (anterolateral) (anteroseptal) (Q wave) (wall) I21.09
      - subsequent I22.0
    - inferior (diaphragmatic) (inferolateral) (inferoposterior) (wall) NEC I21.19
      - subsequent I22.1
    - inferoposterior transmural (Q wave) I21.11
    - involving
      - coronary artery of anterior wall NEC I21.09
      - coronary artery of inferior wall NEC I21.19
      - diagonal coronary artery I21.02
      - left anterior descending coronary artery I21.02
      - left circumflex coronary artery I21.21
      - left main coronary artery I21.01
      - oblique marginal coronary artery I21.21
      - right coronary artery I21.11
    - lateral (apical-lateral) (basal-lateral) (high) I21.29
      - subsequent I22.8

Infarct, infarction *(continued)*
- myocardium, myocardial *(continued)*
  - ST elevation *(continued)*
    - posterior (posterobasal) (posterolateral) (posteroseptal) (true) I21.29
      - subsequent I22.8
    - septal I21.29
      - subsequent I22.8
    - specified NEC I21.29
      - subsequent I22.8
    - subsequent I22.9
  - subsequent (recurrent) (reinfarction) I22.9
    - anterior (anteroapical) (anterolateral) (anteroseptal) (wall) I22.0
    - diaphragmatic (wall) I22.1
    - inferior (diaphragmatic) (inferolateral) (inferoposterior) (wall) I22.1
    - lateral (apical-lateral) (basal-lateral) (high) I22.8
    - non-ST elevation (NSTEMI) I22.2
    - posterior (posterobasal) (posterolateral) (posteroseptal) (true) I22.8
    - septal I22.8
    - specified NEC I22.8
    - ST elevation I22.9
      - anterior (anteroapical) (anterolateral) (anteroseptal) (wall) I22.0
      - inferior (diaphragmatic) (inferolateral) (inferoposterior) (wall) I22.1
      - specified NEC I22.8
    - subendocardial I22.2
    - transmural I21.3
      - anterior (anteroapical) (anterolateral) (anteroseptal) (wall) I22.0
    - transmural
      - diaphragmatic (wall) I22.1
      - inferior (diaphragmatic) (inferolateral) (inferoposterior) (wall) I22.1
      - lateral (apical-lateral) (basal-lateral) (high) I22.8
      - posterior (posterobasal) (posterolateral) (posteroseptal) (true) I22.8
      - specified NEC I22.8
    - type 1 (*see also* Infarction, myocardial, subsequent, by site, or by ST elevation or non-ST elevation) I22.9
    - type 2 I21.A1
    - type 3 I21.A9
    - type 4 I21.A9
    - type 5 I21.A9
  - syphilitic A52.06
  - transmural I21.9
    - anterior (anteroapical) (anterolateral) (anteroseptal) (Q wave) (wall) NEC I21.09
    - inferior (diaphragmatic) (inferolateral) (inferoposterior) (Q wave) (wall) NEC I21.19

Infarct, infarction *(continued)*
- myocardium, myocardial *(continued)*
  - transmural *(continued)*
    - inferoposterior (Q wave) I21.11
    - lateral (apical-lateral) (basal-lateral) (high) NEC I21.29
    - posterior (posterobasal) (posterolateral) (posteroseptal) (true) NEC I21.29
    - septal NEC I21.29
    - specified NEC I21.29
  - type 1 (*see also* Infarction, myocardial, by site, or by ST elevation or non-ST elevation) I21.9
  - type 2 I21.A1
  - type 3 I21.A9
  - type 4 (a) (b) (c) I21.A9
  - type 5 I21.A9
- nontransmural I21.4
- omentum (*see also* Infarct, intestine) K55.069
- ovary N83.8
- pancreas K86.89
- papillary muscle *—see* Infarct, myocardium
- parathyroid gland E21.4
- pituitary (gland) E23.6
- placenta O43.81-
- prostate N42.89
- pulmonary (artery) (vein) (hemorrhagic) *—see* Embolism, pulmonary
- renal (embolic) (thrombotic) N28.0
- retina, retinal (artery) *—see* Occlusion, artery, retina
- spinal (cord) (acute) (embolic) (nonembolic) G95.11
- spleen D73.5
  - embolic or thrombotic I74.8
- subendocardial (acute) (nontransmural) I21.4
- suprarenal (capsule) (gland) E27.49
- testis N50.1
- thrombotic *—see also* Thrombosis
  - artery, arterial *—see* Embolism
- thyroid (gland) E07.89
- ventricle (heart) *—see* Infarct, myocardium

Infecting *—see* condition

Infection, infected, infective (opportunistic) B99.9
- with
  - drug resistant organism *—see* Resistance (to), drug *—see also* specific organism
  - lymphangitis *—see* Lymphangitis
  - organ dysfunction (acute) R65.20
    - with septic shock R65.21
- abscess (skin)- code by site under Abscess
- Absidia *—see* Mucormycosis
- Acanthamoeba *—see* Acanthamebiasis
- Acanthocheilonema (perstans) (streptocerca) B74.4
- accessory sinus (chronic) *—see* Sinusitis
- achorion *—see* Dermatophytosis
- Acremonium falciforme B47.0
- acromioclavicular M00.9
- Actinobacillus (actinomycetem-comitans) A28.8
  - mallei A24.0
  - muris A25.1

Infection, infected, infective *(continued)*
- Actinomadura B47.1
- Actinomyces (israelii) (*see also* Actinomycosis) A42.9
- Actinomycetales *—see* Actinomycosis
- actinomycotic NOS *—see* Actinomycosis
- adenoid (and tonsil) J03.90
  - chronic J35.02
- adenovirus NEC
  - as cause of disease classified elsewhere B97.0
  - unspecified nature or site B34.0
- aerogenes capsulatus A48.0
- aertrycke *—see* Infection, salmonella
- alimentary canal NOS *—see* Enteritis, infectious
- Allescheria boydii B48.2
- Alternaria B48.8
- alveolus, alveolar (process) K04.7
- Ameba, amebic (histolytica) *—see* Amebiasis
- amniotic fluid, sac or cavity O41.10-
  - chorioamnionitis O41.12-
  - placentitis O41.14-
- amputation stump (surgical) *—see* Complication, amputation stump, infection
- Ancylostoma (duodenalis) B76.0
- Anisakiasis, Anisakis larvae B81.0
- anthrax *—see* Anthrax
- antrum (chronic) *—see* Sinusitis, maxillary
- anus, anal (papillae) (sphincter) K62.89
- arbovirus (arbor virus) A94
  - specified type NEC A93.8
- artificial insemination N98.0
- Ascaris lumbricoides *—see* Ascariasis
- Ascomycetes B47.0
- Aspergillus (flavus) (fumigatus) (terreus) *—see* Aspergillosis
- atypical
  - acid-fast (bacilli) *—see* Mycobacterium, atypical
  - mycobacteria *—see* Mycobacterium, atypical
  - virus A81.9
    - specified type NEC A81.89
- auditory meatus (external) *—see* Otitis, externa, infective
- auricle (ear) *—see* Otitis, externa, infective
- axillary gland (lymph) L04.2
- Bacillus A49.9
  - abortus A23.1
  - anthracis *—see* Anthrax
  - Ducrey's (any location) A57
  - Flexner's A03.1
  - Friedländer's NEC A49.8
  - gas (gangrene) A48.0
  - mallei A24.0
  - melitensis A23.0
  - paratyphoid, paratyphosus A01.4
    - A A01.1
    - B A01.2
    - C A01.3
  - Shiga (-Kruse) A03.0
  - suipestifer *—see* Infection, salmonella
  - swimming pool A31.1
  - typhosa A01.00
  - welchii *—see* Gangrene, gas

- bacterial NOS A49.9
  - as cause of disease classified elsewhere B96.89
    - Clostridium perfringens [C. perfringens] B96.7
    - Bacteroides fragilis [B. fragilis] B96.6
    - Enterobacter sakazakii B96.89
    - Enterococcus B95.2
    - Escherichia coli [E. coli] —*see also* Escherichia coli B96.20
    - Helicobacter pylori [H.pylori] B96.81
    - Hemophilus influenzae [H. influenzae] B96.3
    - Klebsiella pneumoniae [K. pneumoniae] B96.1
    - Mycoplasma pneumoniae [M. pneumoniae] B96.0
    - Proteus (mirabilis) (morganii) B96.4
    - Pseudomonas (aeruginosa) (mallei) (pseudomallei) B96.5
    - Staphylococcus B95.8
      - aureus (methicillin susceptible) (MSSA) B95.61
        - methicillin resistant (MRSA) B95.62
      - specified NEC B95.7
    - Streptococcus B95.5
      - group A B95.0
      - group B B95.1
      - pneumoniae B95.3
      - specified NEC B95.4
    - Vibrio vulnificus B96.82
  - specified NEC A48.8
- Bacterium
  - paratyphosum A01.4
    - A A01.1
    - B A01.2
    - C A01.3
  - typhosum A01.00
- Bacteroides NEC A49.8
  - fragilis, as cause of disease classified elsewhere B96.6
- Balantidium coli A07.0
- Bartholin's gland N75.8
- Basidiobolus B46.8
- bile duct (common) (hepatic) —*see* Cholangitis
- bladder —*see* Cystitis
- Blastomyces, blastomycotic —*see also* Blastomycosis
  - brasiliensis —*see* Paracoccidioidomycosis
  - dermatitidis —*see* Blastomycosis
  - European —*see* Cryptococcosis
  - Loboi B48.0
  - North American B40.9
  - South American —*see* Paracoccidioidomycosis
- bleb, postprocedure —*see* Blebitis
- bone —*see* Osteomyelitis
- Bordetella —*see* Whooping cough
- Borrelia bergdorfi A69.20
- brain (*see also* Encephalitis) G04.90
  - membranes —*see* Meningitis
  - septic G06.0
    - meninges —*see* Meningitis, bacterial
- branchial cyst Q18.0
- breast —*see* Mastitis
- bronchus —*see* Bronchitis
- Brucella A23.9
  - abortus A23.1

- Brucella *(continued)*
  - canis A23.3
  - melitensis A23.0
  - mixed A23.8
  - specified NEC A23.8
  - suis A23.2
- Brugia (malayi) B74.1
  - timori B74.2
- bursa —*see* Bursitis, infective
- buttocks (skin) L08.9
- Campylobacter, intestinal A04.5
  - as cause of disease classified elsewhere B96.81
- Candida (albicans) (tropicalis) —*see* Candidiasis
- candiru B88.8
- Capillaria (intestinal) B81.1
  - hepatica B83.8
  - philippinensis B81.1
- cartilage —*see* Disorder, cartilage, specified type NEC
- catheter-related bloodstream (CRBSI) T80.211
- cat liver fluke B66.0
- cellulitis - code by site under Cellulitis
- central line-associated T80.219
  - bloodstream (CLABSI) T80.211
  - specified NEC T80.218
- Cephalosporium falciforme B47.0
- cerebrospinal —*see* Meningitis
- cervical gland (lymph) L04.0
- cervix —*see* Cervicitis
- cesarean delivery wound (puerperal) O86.00
- cestodes —*see* Infestation, cestodes
- chest J22
- Chilomastix (intestinal) A07.8
- Chlamydia, chlamydial A74.9
  - anus A56.3
  - genitourinary tract A56.2
    - lower A56.00
    - specified NEC A56.19
  - lymphogranuloma A55
  - pharynx A56.4
  - psittaci A70
  - rectum A56.3
  - sexually transmitted NEC A56.8
- cholera —*see* Cholera
- Cladosporium
  - bantianum (brain abscess) B43.1
  - carrionii B43.0
  - castellanii B36.1
  - trichoides (brain abscess) B43.1
  - werneckii B36.1
- Clonorchis (sinensis) (liver) B66.1
- Clostridium NEC
  - bifermentans A48.0
  - botulinum (food poisoning) A05.1
    - infant A48.51
    - wound A48.52
  - difficile
    - as cause of disease classified elsewhere B96.89
    - foodborne (disease)
      - not specified as recurrent A04.72
      - recurrent A04.71
    - gas gangrene A48.0
    - necrotizing enterocolitis
      - not specified as recurrent A04.72
      - recurrent A04.71
    - sepsis A41.4
  - gas-forming NEC A48.0
  - histolyticum A48.0
  - novyi, causing gas gangrene A48.0

- Clostridium *(continued)*
  - oedematiens A48.0
  - perfringens
    - as cause of disease classified elsewhere B96.7
    - due to food A05.2
    - foodborne (disease) A05.2
    - gas gangrene A48.0
    - sepsis A41.4
  - septicum, causing gas gangrene A48.0
  - sordellii, causing gas gangrene A48.0
  - welchii
    - as cause of disease classified elsewhere B96.7
    - foodborne (disease) A05.2
    - gas gangrene A48.0
    - necrotizing enteritis A05.2
    - sepsis A41.4
- Coccidioides (immitis) —*see* Coccidioidomycosis
- colon —*see* Enteritis, infectious
- colostomy K94.02
- common duct —*see* Cholangitis
- congenital P39.9
  - Candida (albicans) P37.5
  - cytomegalovirus P35.1
  - hepatitis, viral P35.3
  - herpes simplex P35.2
  - infectious or parasitic disease P37.9
    - specified NEC P37.8
  - listeriosis (disseminated) P37.2
  - malaria NEC P37.4
    - falciparum P37.3
  - Plasmodium falciparum P37.3
  - poliomyelitis P35.8
  - rubella P35.0
  - skin P39.4
  - toxoplasmosis (acute) (subacute) (chronic) P37.1
  - tuberculosis P37.0
  - urinary (tract) P39.3
  - vaccinia P35.8
  - virus P35.9
    - specified type NEC P35.8
- Conidiobolus B46.8
- coronavirus-2019 U07.1
- coronavirus NEC B34.2
  - as cause of disease classified elsewhere B97.29
  - severe acute respiratory syndrome (SARS associated) B97.21
- corpus luteum —*see* Salpingo-oophoritis
- Corynebacterium diphtheriae —*see* Diphtheria
- cotia virus B08.8
- COVID-19 (*see also* COVID-19) U07.1
- Coxiella burnetii A78
- coxsackie —*see* Coxsackie
- Cryptococcus neoformans —*see* Cryptococcosis
- Cryptosporidium A07.2
- Cunninghamella —*see* Mucormycosis
- cyst —*see* Cyst
- cystic duct (*see also* Cholecystitis) K81.9
- Cysticercus cellulosae —*see* Cysticercosis
- cytomegalovirus, cytomegaloviral B25.9
  - congenital P35.1
  - maternal, maternal care for (suspected) damage to fetus O35.3

- cytomegalovirus, cytomegaloviral *(continued)*
  - mononucleosis B27.10
    - with
      - complication NEC B27.19
      - meningitis B27.12
      - polyneuropathy B27.11
- delta-agent (acute), in hepatitis B carrier B17.0
- dental (pulpal origin) K04.7
- Deuteromycetes B47.0
- Dicrocoelium dendriticum B66.2
- Dipetalonema (perstans) (streptocerca) B74.4
- diphtherial —*see* Diphtheria
- Diphyllobothrium (adult) (latum) (pacificum) B70.0
  - larval B70.1
- Diplogonoporus (grandis) B71.8
- Dipylidium caninum B67.4
- Dirofilaria B74.8
- Dracunculus medinensis B72
- Drechslera (hawaiiensis) B43.8
- Ducrey Haemophilus (any location) A57
- due to or resulting from
  - artificial insemination N98.0
  - Babesia
    - divergens (-like) strain B60.03
    - duncani (-type) species B60.02
    - microti B60.01
    - species
      - specified NEC B60.09
  - central venous catheter T80.219
    - bloodstream T80.211
    - exit or insertion site T80.212
    - localized T80.212
    - port or reservoir T80.212
    - specified NEC T80.218
    - tunnel T80.212
  - device, implant or graft (*see also* Complications, by site and type, infection or inflammation) T85.79
    - arterial graft NEC T82.7
    - breast (implant) T85.79
    - catheter NEC T85.79
      - dialysis (renal) T82.7
        - central line T80.211
        - intraperitoneal T85.71
      - infusion NEC T82.7
        - cranial T85.735
        - intrathecal T85.735
        - spinal (epidural) (subdural) T85.735
        - subarachnoid T85.735
      - urinary T83.518
        - cystostomy T83.510
        - Hopkins T83.518
        - ileostomy T83.518
        - nephrostomy T83.512
        - specified NEC T83.518
        - urethral indwelling T83.511
        - urostomy T83.518
    - electronic (electrode) (pulse generator) (stimulator)
      - bone T84.7
      - cardiac T82.7
      - nervous system T85.738
        - brain T85.731
        - cranial nerve T85.732
        - gastric nerve T85.732
        - generator pocket T85.734
        - neurostimulator generator T85.734
        - peripheral nerve T85.732
        - sacral nerve T85.732
        - spinal cord T85.733

Infection, infected, infective *(continued)*

- due to or resulting from *(continued)*
  - device, implant or graft *(continued)*
    - electronic *(continued)*
      - nervous system *(continued)*
        - vagal nerve T85.732
      - urinary T83.590
    - fixation, internal (orthopedic) NEC *—see* Complication, fixation device, infection
    - gastrointestinal (bile duct) (esophagus) T85.79
      - neurostimulator electrode (lead) T85.732
    - genital NEC T83.69
    - heart NEC T82.7
      - valve (prosthesis) T82.6
        - graft T82.7
    - joint prosthesis *—see* Complication, joint prosthesis, infection
    - ocular (corneal graft) (orbital implant) NEC T85.79
    - orthopedic NEC T84.7
    - penile (cylinder) (pump) (resevoir) T83.61
    - specified NEC T85.79
    - testicular T83.62
    - urinary NEC T83.598
      - ileal conduit stent T83.593
      - implanted neurostimulation T83.590
      - implanted sphincter T83.591
      - indwelling ureteral stent T83.592
      - nephroureteral stent T83.593
      - specified stent NEC T83.593
    - vascular NEC T82.7
    - ventricular intracranial (communicating) shunt T85.730
  - Hickman catheter T80.219
    - bloodstream T80.211
    - localized T80.212
    - specified NEC T80.218
  - immunization or vaccination T88.0
  - infusion, injection or transfusion NEC T80.29
    - acute T80.22
  - injury NEC - code by site under Wound, open
  - peripherally inserted central catheter (PICC) T80.219
    - bloodstream T80.211
    - localized T80.212
    - specified NEC T80.218
  - portacath (port-a-cath) T80.219
    - bloodstream T80.211
    - localized T80.212
    - specified NEC T80.218
  - protozoa of the order Piroplasmida NEC B60.09
  - pulmonary artery catheter *—see* Infection, due to or resulting from, central venous catheter
  - surgery T81.40
  - Swan Ganz catheter *—see* Infection, due to or resulting from, central venous catheter
  - triple lumen catheter T80.219
    - bloodstream T80.211
    - localized T80.212
    - specified NEC T80.218
  - umbilical venous catheter T80.219
    - bloodstream T80.211
    - localized T80.212
    - specified NEC T80.218
- during labor NEC O75.3

Infection, infected, infective *(continued)*

- ear (middle) *—see also* Otitis media
  - external *—see* Otitis, externa, infective
  - inner *—see* subcategory H83.0
- Eberthella typhosa A01.00
- Echinococcus *—see* Echinococcus
- echovirus
  - as cause of disease classified elsewhere B97.12
  - unspecified nature or site B34.1
- endocardium I33.0
- endocervix *—see* Cervicitis
- Entamoeba *—see* Amebiasis
- enteric *—see* Enteritis, infectious
- Enterobacter sakazakii B96.89
- Enterobius vermicularis B80
- enterostomy K94.12
- enterovirus B34.1
  - as cause of disease classified elsewhere B97.10
    - coxsackievirus B97.11
    - echovirus B97.12
    - specified NEC B97.19
- Entomophthora B46.8
- Epidermophyton *—see* Dermatophytosis
- epididymis *—see* Epididymitis
- episiotomy (puerperal) O86.09
- Erysipelothrix (insidiosa) (rhusiopathiae) *—see* Erysipeloid
- erythema infectiosum B08.3
- Escherichia (E.) coli NEC A49.8
  - as cause of disease classified elsewhere (*see also* Escherichia coli) B96.20
  - congenital P39.8
    - sepsis P36.4
  - generalized A41.51
  - intestinal *—see* Enteritis, infectious, due to, Escherichia coli
- ethmoidal (chronic) (sinus) *—see* Sinusitis, ethmoidal
- eustachian tube (ear) *—see* Salpingitis, eustachian
- external auditory canal (meatus) NEC *—see* Otitis, externa, infective
- eye (purulent) *—see* Endophthalmitis, purulent
- eyelid *—see* Inflammation, eyelid
- fallopian tube *—see* Salpingo-oophoritis
- Fasciola (gigantica) (hepatica) (indica) B66.3
- Fasciolopsis (buski) B66.5
- filarial *—see* Infestation, filarial
- finger (skin) L08.9
  - nail L03.01-
    - fungus B35.1
- fish tapeworm B70.0
  - larval B70.1
- flagellate, intestinal A07.9
- fluke *—see* Infestation, fluke
- focal
  - teeth (pulpal origin) K04.7
  - tonsils J35.01
- Fonsecaea (compactum) (pedrosoi) B43.0
- food *—see* Intoxication, foodborne
- foot (skin) L08.9
  - dermatophytic fungus B35.3
- Francisella tularensis *—see* Tularemia
- frontal (sinus) (chronic) *—see* Sinusitis, frontal
- fungus NOS B49
  - beard B35.0
  - dermatophytic *—see* Dermatophytosis

Infection, infected, infective *(continued)*

- fungus *(continued)*
  - foot B35.3
  - groin B35.6
  - hand B35.2
  - nail B35.1
  - pathogenic to compromised host only B48.8
  - perianal (area) B35.6
  - scalp B35.0
  - skin B36.9
    - foot B35.3
    - hand B35.2
    - toenails B35.1
- Fusarium B48.8
- gallbladder *—see* Cholecystitis
- gas bacillus *—see* Gangrene, gas
- gastrointestinal *—see* Enteritis, infectious
- generalized NEC *—see* Sepsis
- generator pocket, implanted electronic neurostimulator T85.734
- genital organ or tract
  - female *—see* Disease, pelvis, inflammatory
  - male N49.9
    - multiple sites N49.8
    - specified NEC N49.8
- Ghon tubercle, primary A15.7
- Giardia lamblia A07.1
- gingiva (chronic) K05.10
  - acute K05.00
    - nonplaque induced K05.01
    - plaque induced K05.00
  - nonplaque induced K05.11
  - plaque induced K05.10
- glanders A24.0
- glenosporopsis B48.0
- Gnathostoma (spinigerum) B83.1
- Gongylonema B83.8
- gonococcal *—see* Gonococcus
- gram-negative bacilli NOS A49.9
- guinea worm B72
- gum (chronic) K05.10
  - acute K05.00
    - nonplaque induced K05.01
    - plaque induced K05.00
  - nonplaque induced K05.11
  - plaque induced K05.10
- Haemophilus *—see* Infection, Hemophilus
- heart *—see* Carditis
- Helicobacter pylori A04.8
  - as cause of disease classified elsewhere B96.81
- helminths B83.9
  - intestinal B82.0
    - mixed (types classifiable to more than one of the titles B65.0-B81.3 and B81.8) B81.4
    - specified type NEC B81.8
  - specified type NEC B83.8
- Hemophilus
  - aegyptius, systemic A48.4
  - ducrey (any location) A57
  - influenzae NEC A49.2
    - as cause of disease classified elsewhere B96.3
  - generalized A41.3
- herpes (simplex) *—see also* Herpes
  - congenital P35.2
  - disseminated B00.7
  - zoster B02.9
- herpesvirus, herpesviral *—see* Herpes

Infection, infected, infective *(continued)*

- hip (joint) NEC M00.9
  - due to internal joint prosthesis
    - left T84.52
    - right T84.51
  - skin NEC L08.9
- Heterophyes (heterophyes) B66.8
- Histoplasma *—see* Histoplasmosis
  - American B39.4
  - capsulatum B39.4
- hookworm B76.9
- human
  - papilloma virus A63.0
  - T-cell lymphotropic virus type-1(HTLV-1) B33.3
- hydrocele N43.0
- Hymenolepis B71.0
- hypopharynx *—see* Pharyngitis
- inguinal (lymph) glands L04.1
  - due to soft chancre A57
- intervertebral disc, pyogenic M46.30
  - cervical region M46.32
  - cervicothoracic region M46.33
  - lumbar region M46.36
  - lumbosacral region M46.37
  - multiple sites M46.39
  - occipito-atlanto-axial region M46.31
  - sacrococcygeal region M46.38
  - thoracic region M46.34
  - thoracolumbar region M46.35
- intestine, intestinal *—see* Enteritis, infectious
  - specified NEC A08.8
- intra-amniotic affecting newborn NEC P39.2
- intrauterine inflammation O41.12-
- Isospora belli or hominis A07.3
- Japanese B encephalitis A83.0
- jaw (bone) (lower) (upper) M27.2
- joint NEC M00.9
  - due to internal joint prosthesis T84.50
- kidney (cortex) (hematogenous) N15.9
  - with calculus N20.0
    - with hydronephrosis N13.6
  - following ectopic gestation O08.83
  - pelvis and ureter (cystic) N28.85
  - puerperal (postpartum) O86.21
  - specified NEC N15.8
- Klebsiella (K.) pneumoniae NEC A49.8
  - as cause of disease classified elsewhere B96.1
- knee (joint) NEC M00.9
  - joint M00.9
  - due to internal joint prosthesis
    - left T84.54
    - right T84.53
  - skin L08.9
- Koch's *—see* Tuberculosis
- labia (majora) (minora) (acute) *—see* Vulvitis
- lacrimal
  - gland *—see* Dacryoadenitis
  - passages (duct) (sac) *—see* Inflammation, lacrimal, passages
- lancet fluke B66.2
- larynx NEC J38.7
- leg (skin) NOS L08.9
- Legionella pneumophila A48.1
  - nonpneumonic A48.2
- Leishmania *—see also* Leishmaniasis
  - aethiopica B55.1
  - braziliensis B55.2
  - chagasi B55.0

Infection, infected, infective *(continued)*
Leishmania *(continued)*
donovani B55.0
infantum B55.0
major B55.1
mexicana B55.1
tropica B55.1
lentivirus, as cause of disease classified elsewhere B97.31
Leptosphaeria senegalensis B47.0
Leptospira interrogans A27.9
autumnalis A27.89
canicola A27.89
hebdomadis A27.89
icterohaemorrhagiae A27.0
pomona A27.89
specified type NEC A27.89
leptospirochetal NEC *—see* Leptospirosis
Listeria monocytogenes *—see also* Listeriosis
congenital P37.2
Loa loa B74.3
with conjunctival infestation B74.3
eyelid B74.3
Loboa loboi B48.0
local, skin (staphylococcal) (streptococcal) L08.9
abscess - code by site under Abscess
cellulitis - code by site under Cellulitis
specified NEC L08.89
ulcer *—see* Ulcer, skin
Loefflerella mallei A24.0
lung (*see also* Pneumonia) J18.9
atypical Mycobacterium A31.0
spirochetal A69.8
tuberculous *—see* Tuberculosis, pulmonary
virus *—see* Pneumonia, viral
lymph gland *—see also* Lymphadenitis, acute
mesenteric I88.0
lymphoid tissue, base of tongue or posterior pharynx, NEC (chronic) J35.03
Madurella (grisea) (mycetomii) B47.0
major
following ectopic or molar pregnancy O08.0
puerperal, postpartum, childbirth O85
Malassezia furfur B36.0
Malleomyces
mallei A24.0
pseudomallei (whitmori) *—see* Melioidosis
mammary gland N61.0
Mansonella (ozzardi) (perstans) (streptocerca) B74.4
mastoid *—see* Mastoiditis
maxilla, maxillary M27.2
sinus (chronic) *—see* Sinusitis, maxillary
mediastinum J98.51
Medina (worm) B72
meibomian cyst or gland *—see* Hordeolum
meninges *—see* Meningitis, bacterial
meningococcal (*see also* condition) A39.9
adrenals A39.1
brain A39.81
cerebrospinal A39.0
conjunctiva A39.89
endocardium A39.51

Infection, infected, infective *(continued)*
meningococcal *(continued)*
heart A39.50
endocardium A39.51
myocardium A39.52
pericardium A39.53
joint A39.83
meninges A39.0
meningococcemia A39.4
acute A39.2
chronic A39.3
myocardium A39.52
pericardium A39.53
retrobulbar neuritis A39.82
specified site NEC A39.89
mesenteric lymph nodes or glands NEC I88.0
Metagonimus B66.8
metatarsophalangeal M00.9
methicillin
resistant Staphylococcus aureus (MRSA) A49.02
susceptible Staphylococcus aureus (MSSA) A49.01
Microsporum, microsporic *—see* Dermatophytosis
mixed flora (bacterial) NEC A49.8
Monilia *—see* Candidiasis
Monosporium apiospermum B48.2
mouth, parasitic B37.0
Mucor *—see* Mucormycosis
muscle NEC *—see* Myositis, infective
mycelium NOS B49
mycetoma B47.9
actinomycotic NEC B47.1
mycotic NEC B47.0
Mycobacterium, mycobacterial *—see* Mycobacterium
Mycoplasma NEC A49.3
pneumoniae, as cause of disease classified elsewhere B96.0
mycotic NOS B49
pathogenic to compromised host only B48.8
skin NOS B36.9
myocardium NEC I40.0
nail (chronic)
with lymphangitis *—see* Lymphangitis, acute, digit
finger L03.01-
fungus B35.1
ingrowing L60.0
toe L03.03-
fungus B35.1
nasal sinus (chronic) *—see* Sinusitis
nasopharynx *—see* Nasopharyngitis
navel L08.82
Necator americanus B76.1
Neisseria *—see* Gonococcus
Neotestudina rosatii B47.0
newborn P39.9
vintra-amniotic NEC P39.2
skin P39.4
specified type NEC P39.8
nipple N61.0
associated with
lactation O91.03
pregnancy O91.01-
puerperium O91.02
Nocardia *—see* Nocardiosis
obstetrical surgical wound (puerperal) O86.00
incisional site
deep O86.02
superficial O86.01
organ and space site O86.03
surgical site specified NEC O86.09

Infection, infected, infective *(continued)*
Oesophagostomum (apiostomum) B81.8
Oestrus ovis *—see* Myiasis
Oidium albicans B37.9
Onchocerca (volvulus) *—see* Onchocerciasis
oncovirus, as cause of disease classified elsewhere B97.32
operation wound T81.49
Opisthorchis (felineus) (viverrini) B66.0
orbit, orbital *—see* Inflammation, orbit
orthopoxvirus NEC B08.09
ovary *—see* Salpingo-oophoritis
Oxyuris vermicularis B80
pancreas (acute) *—see* Pancreatitis, acute
abscess *—see* Pancreatitis, acute
specified NEC (*see also* Pancreatitis, acute) K85.80
papillomavirus, as cause of disease classified elsewhere B97.7
papovavirus NEC B34.4
Paracoccidioides brasiliensis *—see* Paracoccidioidomycosis
Paragonimus (westermani) B66.4
parainfluenza virus B34.8
parameningococcus NOS A39.9
parapoxvirus B08.60
specified NEC B08.69
parasitic B89
Parastrongylus
cantonensis B83.2
costaricensis B81.3
paratyphoid A01.4
Type A A01.1
Type B A01.2
Type C A01.3
paraurethral ducts N34.2
parotid gland *—see* Sialoadenitis
parvovirus NEC B34.3
as cause of disease classified elsewhere B97.6
Pasteurella NEC A28.0
multocida A28.0
pestis *—see* Plague
pseudotuberculosis A28.0
septica (cat bite) (dog bite) A28.0
tularensis *—see* Tularemia
pelvic, female *—see* Disease, pelvis, inflammatory
Penicillium (marneffei) B48.4
penis (glans) (retention) NEC N48.29
periapical K04.5
peridental, periodontal K05.20
generalized *—see* Periodontitis, aggressive, generalized
localized *—see* Periodontitis, aggressive, localized
perinatal period P39.9
specified type NEC P39.8
perineal repair (puerperal) O86.09
periorbital *—see* Inflammation, orbit
perirectal K62.89
perirenal *—see* Infection, kidney
peritoneal *—see* Peritonitis
periureteral N28.89
Petriellidium boydii B48.2
pharynx *—see also* Pharyngitis
coxsackievirus B08.5
posterior, lymphoid (chronic) J35.03
Phialophora
gougerotii (subcutaneous abscess or cyst) B43.2

Infection, infected, infective *(continued)*
Phialophora *(continued)*
jeanselmei (subcutaneous abscess or cyst) B43.2
verrucosa (skin) B43.0
Piedraia hortae B36.3
pinta A67.9
intermediate A67.1
late A67.2
mixed A67.3
primary A67.0
pinworm B80
pityrosporum furfur B36.0
pleuro-pneumonia-like organism (PPLO) NEC A49.3
as cause of disease classified elsewhere B96.0
pneumococcus, pneumococcal NEC A49.1
as cause of disease classified elsewhere B95.3
generalized (purulent) A40.3
with pneumonia J13
Pneumocystis carinii (pneumonia) B59
Pneumocystis jiroveci (pneumonia) B59
port or reservoir T80.212
postoperative T81.40
postoperative wound T81.49
surgical site
deep incisional T81.42
organ and space T81.43
specified NEC T81.49
superficial incisional T81.41
postprocedural T81.40
postvaccinal T88.0
prepuce NEC N47.7
with penile inflammation N47.6
prion *—see* Disease, prion, central nervous system
prostate (capsule) *—see* Prostatitis
Proteus (mirabilis) (morganii) (vulgaris) NEC A49.8
as cause of disease classified elsewhere B96.4
protozoal NEC B64
intestinal A07.9
specified NEC A07.8
specified NEC B60.8
Pseudoallescheria boydii B48.2
Pseudomonas NEC A49.8
as cause of disease classified elsewhere B96.5
mallei A24.0
pneumonia J15.1
pseudomallei *—see* Melioidosis
puerperal O86.4
genitourinary tract NEC O86.89
major or generalized O85
minor O86.4
specified NEC O86.89
pulmonary *—see* Infection, lung
purulent *—see* Abscess
Pyrenochaeta romeroi B47.0
Q fever A78
rectum (sphincter) K62.89
renal *—see also* Infection, kidney
pelvis and ureter (cystic) N28.85
reovirus, as cause of disease classified elsewhere B97.5
respiratory (tract) NEC J98.8
acute J22
chronic J98.8
influenzal (upper) (acute) *—see* Influenza, with, respiratory manifestations NEC
lower (acute) J22
chronic *—see* Bronchitis, chronic

Infection, infected, infective *(continued)*
respiratory *(continued)*
rhinovirus J00
syncytial virus (RSV) *—see* Infection, virus, respiratory syncytial (RSV)
upper (acute) NOS J06.9
chronic J39.8
streptococcal J06.9
viral NOS J06.9
due to respiratory syncytial virus (RSV) J06.9 *[B97.4]*
resulting from
presence of internal prosthesis, implant, graft *—see* Complications, by site and type, infection
retortamoniasis A07.8
retroperitoneal NEC K68.9
retrovirus B33.3
as cause of disease classified elsewhere B97.30
human
immunodeficiency, type 2(HIV 2) B97.35
T-cell lymphotropic
type I (HTLV-I) B97.33
type II (HTLV-II) B97.34
lentivirus B97.31
oncovirus B97.32
specified NEC B97.39
Rhinosporidium (seeberi) B48.1
rhinovirus
as cause of disease classified elsewhere B97.89
unspecified nature or site B34.8
Rhizopus *—see* Mucormycosis
rickettsial NOS A79.9
roundworm (large) NEC B82.0
Ascariasis (*see also* Ascariasis) B77.9
rubella *—see* Rubella
Saccharomyces *—see* Candidiasis
salivary duct or gland (any) *—see* Sialoadenitis
Salmonella (aertrycke) (arizonae) (callinarum) (cholerae-suis) (enteritidis) (suipestifer) (typhimurium) A02.9
with
(gastro)enteritis A02.0
sepsis A02.1
specified manifestation NEC A02.8
due to food (poisoning) A02.9
hirschfeldii A01.3
localized A02.20
arthritis A02.23
meningitis A02.21
osteomyelitis A02.24
pneumonia A02.22
pyelonephritis A02.25
specified NEC A02.29
paratyphi A01.4
A A01.1
B A01.2
C A01.3
schottmuelleri A01.2
typhi, typhosa *—see* Typhoid
Sarcocystis A07.8
SARS-Cov-2 *—see* Infection, COVID-19
scabies B86
Schistosoma *—see* Infestation, Schistosoma
scrotum (acute) NEC N49.2
seminal vesicle *—see* Vesiculitis
septic
localized, skin *—see* Abscess

Infection, infected, infective *(continued)*
sheep liver fluke B66.3
Shigella A03.9
boydii A03.2
dysenteriae A03.0
flexneri A03.1
group
A A03.0
B A03.1
C A03.2
D A03.3
Schmitz (-Stutzer) A03.0
schmitzii A03.0
shigae A03.0
sonnei A03.3
specified NEC A03.8
shoulder (joint) NEC M00.9
due to internal joint prosthesis T84.59
skin NEC L08.9
sinus (accessory) (chronic) (nasal) *—see also* Sinusitis
pilonidal *—see* Sinus, pilonidal
skin NEC L08.89
Skene's duct or gland *—see* Urethritis
skin (local) (staphylococcal) (streptococcal) L08.9
abscess - code by site under Abscess
cellulitis - code by site under Cellulitis
due to fungus B36.9
specified type NEC B36.8
mycotic B36.9
specified type NEC B36.8
newborn P39.4
ulcer *—see* Ulcer, skin
slow virus A81.9
specified NEC A81.89
Sparganum (mansoni) (proliferum) (baxteri) B70.1
specific *—see also* Syphilis
to perinatal period *—see* Infection, congenital
specified NEC B99.8
spermatic cord NEC N49.1
sphenoidal (sinus) *—see* Sinusitis, sphenoidal
spinal cord NOS *—see also* Myelitis G04.91
abscess G06.1
meninges *—see* Meningitis
streptococcal G04.89
Spirillum A25.0
spirochetal NOS A69.9
lung A69.8
specified NEC A69.8
Spirometra larvae B70.1
spleen D73.89
Sporotrichum, Sporothrix (schenckii) *—see* Sporotrichosis
staphylococcal, unspecified site
aureus (methicillin susceptible) (MSSA) A49.01
methicillin resistant (MRSA) A49.02
as cause of disease classified elsewhere B95.8
aureus (methicillin susceptible) (MSSA) B95.61
methicillin resistant (MRSA) B95.62
specified NEC B95.7
food poisoning A05.0
generalized (purulent) A41.2
pneumonia *—see* Pneumonia, staphylococcal
Stellantchasmus falcatus B66.8

Infection, infected, infective *(continued)*
streptobacillus moniliformis A25.1
streptococcal NEC A49.1
as cause of disease classified elsewhere B95.5
B genitourinary complicating
childbirth O98.82
pregnancy O98.81-
puerperium O98.83
congenital
sepsis P36.10
group B P36.0
specified NEC P36.19
generalized (purulent) A40.9
Streptomyces B47.1
Strongyloides (stercoralis) *—see* Strongyloidiasis
stump (amputation) (surgical) *—see* Complication, amputation stump, infection
subcutaneous tissue, local L08.9
suipestifer *—see* Infection, salmonella
swimming pool bacillus A31.1
Taenia *—see* Infestation, Taenia
Taeniarhynchus saginatus B68.1
tapeworm *—see* Infestation, tapeworm
tendon (sheath) *—see* Tenosynovitis, infective NEC
Ternidens diminutus B81.8
testis *—see* Orchitis
threadworm B80
throat *—see* Pharyngitis
thyroglossal duct K14.8
toe (skin) L08.9
cellulitis L03.03-
fungus B35.1
nail L03.03-
fungus B35.1
tongue NEC K14.0
parasitic B37.0
tonsil (and adenoid) (faucial) (lingual) (pharyngeal) *—see* Tonsillitis
tooth, teeth K04.7
periapical K04.7
peridental, periodontal K05.20
generalized *—see* Periodontitis, aggressive, generalized
localized *—see* Periodontitis, aggressive, localized
pulp K04.01
irreversible K04.02
reversible K04.01
socket M27.3
TORCH *—see* Infection, congenital
without active infection P00.2
Torula histolytica *—see* Cryptococcosis
Toxocara (canis) (cati) (felis) B83.0
Toxoplasma gondii *—see* Toxoplasma
trachea, chronic J42
trematode NEC *—see* Infestation, fluke
trench fever A79.0
Treponema pallidum *—see* Syphilis
Trichinella (spiralis) B75
Trichomonas A59.9
cervix A59.09
intestine A07.8
prostate A59.02
specified site NEC A59.8
urethra A59.03
urogenitalis A59.00
vagina A59.01
vulva A59.01

Infection, infected, infective *(continued)*
Trichophyton, trichophytic *—see* Dermatophytosis
Trichosporon (beigelii) cutaneum B36.2
Trichostrongylus B81.2
Trichuris (trichiura) B79
Trombicula (irritans) B88.0
Trypanosoma
brucei
gambiense B56.0
rhodesiense B56.1
cruzi *—see* Chagas' disease
tubal *—see* Salpingo-oophoritis
tuberculous
latent (LTBI) Z22.7
NEC *—see* Tuberculosis
tubo-ovarian *—see* Salpingo-oophoritis
tunnel T80.212
tunica vaginalis N49.1
tympanic membrane NEC *—see* Myringitis
typhoid (abortive) (ambulant) (bacillus) *—see* Typhoid
typhus A75.9
flea-borne A75.2
mite-borne A75.3
recrudescent A75.1
tick-borne A77.9
African A77.1
North Asian A77.2
umbilicus L08.82
ureter *—see* Ureteritis
urethra *—see* Urethritis
urinary (tract) N39.0
bladder *—see* Cystitis
complicating
pregnancy O23.4-
specified type NEC O23.3-
kidney *—see* Infection, kidney
newborn P39.3
puerperal (postpartum) O86.20
tuberculous A18.13
urethra *—see* Urethritis
uterus, uterine *—see* Endometritis
vaccination T88.0
vaccinia not from vaccination B08.011
vagina (acute) *—see* Vaginitis
varicella B01.9
varicose veins *—see* Varix
vas deferens NEC N49.1
vesical *—see* Cystitis
Vibrio
cholerae A00.0
El Tor A00.1
parahaemolyticus (food poisoning) A05.3
vulnificus
as cause of disease classified elsewhere B96.82
foodborne intoxication A05.5
Vincent's (gum) (mouth) (tonsil) A69.1
virus, viral NOS B34.9
adenovirus
as cause of disease classified elsewhere B97.0
unspecified nature or site B34.0
arborvirus, arbovirus arthropod-borne A94
as cause of disease classified elsewhere B97.89
adenovirus B97.0
coronavirus B97.29
SARS-associated B97.21
coxsackievirus B97.11

Infection, infected, infective *(continued)*
- virus, viral NOS *(continued)*
  - as cause of disease classified elsewhere *(continued)*
    - echovirus B97.12
    - enterovirus B97.10
      - coxsackievirus B97.11
      - echovirus B97.12
      - specified NEC B97.19
    - human
      - immunodeficiency, type 2 (HIV 2) B97.35
      - T-cell lymphotropic,
        - type I (HTLV-I) B97.33
        - type II (HTLV-II) B97.34
      - metapneumovirus B97.81
    - papillomavirus B97.7
    - parvovirus B97.6
    - reovirus B97.5
    - respiratory syncytial (RSV) *—see* Infection, virus, respiratory syncytial (RSV)
    - retrovirus B97.30
      - human
        - immunodeficiency, type 2(HIV 2) B97.35
        - T-cell lymphotropic,
          - type I (HTLV-I) B97.33
          - type II (HTLV-II) B97.34
      - lentivirus B97.31
      - oncovirus B97.32
      - specified NEC B97.39
    - specified NEC B97.89
  - central nervous system A89
    - atypical A81.9
      - specified NEC A81.89
    - enterovirus NEC A88.8
      - meningitis A87.0
    - slow virus A81.9
      - specified NEC A81.89
    - specified NEC A88.8
  - chest J98.8
  - cotia B08.8
  - COVID-19 U07.1
  - coxsackie (*see also* Infection, coxsackie) B34.1
    - as cause of disease classified elsewhere B97.11
  - ECHO
    - as cause of disease classified elsewhere B97.12
    - unspecified nature or site B34.1
  - encephalitis, tick-borne A84.9
  - enterovirus, as cause of disease classified elsewhere B97.10
    - coxsackievirus B97.11
    - echovirus B97.12
    - specified NEC B97.19
  - exanthem NOS B09
  - human papilloma as cause of disease classified elsewhere B97.7
  - human metapneumovirus as cause of disease classified elsewhere B97.81
  - intestine *—see* Enteritis, viral
  - respiratory syncytial (RSV)
    - as cause of disease classified elsewhere B97.4
    - bronchiolitis J21.0
    - bronchitis J20.5
    - bronchopneumonia J12.1
    - otitis media H65.- *[B97.4]*
    - pneumonia J12.1
    - upper respiratory infection J06.9 *[B97.4]*

Infection, infected, infective *(continued)*
- virus, viral NOS *(continued)*
  - rhinovirus
    - as cause of disease classified elsewhere B97.89
    - unspecified nature or site B34.8
  - slow A81.9
    - specified NEC A81.89
  - specified type NEC B33.8
    - as cause of disease classified elsewhere B97.89
    - unspecified nature or site B34.8
  - unspecified nature or site B34.9
  - West Nile *—see* Virus, West Nile
- vulva (acute) *—see* Vulvitis
- West Nile *—see* Virus, West Nile
- whipworm B79
- worms B83.9
  - specified type NEC B83.8
- Wuchereria (bancrofti) B74.0
  - malayi B74.1
- yatapoxvirus B08.70
  - specified NEC B08.79
- yeast (*see also* Candidiasis) B37.9
- yellow fever *—see* Fever, yellow
- Yersinia
  - enterocolitica (intestinal) A04.6
  - pestis *—see* Plague
  - pseudotuberculosis A28.2
- Zeis' gland *—see* Hordeolum
- Zika virus A92.5
  - congenital P35.4
- zoonotic bacterial NOS A28.9
- Zopfia senegalensis B47.0

Infective, infectious *—see* condition

Infertility
- female N97.9
  - age-related N97.8
  - associated with
    - anovulation N97.0
    - cervical (mucus) disease or anomaly N88.3
    - congenital anomaly
      - cervix N88.3
      - fallopian tube N97.1
      - uterus N97.2
      - vagina N97.8
    - dysmucorrhea N88.3
    - fallopian tube disease or anomaly N97.1
    - pituitary-hypothalamic origin E23.0
    - specified origin NEC N97.8
    - Stein-Leventhal syndrome E28.2
    - uterine disease or anomaly N97.2
    - vaginal disease or anomaly N97.8
  - due to
    - cervical anomaly N88.3
    - fallopian tube anomaly N97.1
    - ovarian failure E28.39
    - Stein-Leventhal syndrome E28.2
    - uterine anomaly N97.2
    - vaginal anomaly N97.8
  - nonimplantation N97.2
  - origin
    - cervical N88.3
    - tubal (block) (occlusion) (stenosis) N97.1
    - uterine N97.2
    - vaginal N97.8

Infertility *(continued)*
- male N46.9
  - azoospermia N46.01
    - extratesticular cause N46.029
      - drug therapy N46.021
      - efferent duct obstruction N46.023
      - infection N46.022
      - radiation N46.024
      - specified cause NEC N46.029
      - systemic disease N46.025
  - oligospermia N46.11
    - extratesticular cause N46.129
      - drug therapy N46.121
      - efferent duct obstruction N46.123
      - infection N46.122
      - radiation N46.124
      - specified cause NEC N46.129
      - systemic disease N46.125
  - specified type NEC N46.8

Infestation B88.9
- Acanthocheilonema (perstans) (streptocerca) B74.4
- Acariasis B88.0
  - demodex folliculorum B88.0
  - sarcoptes scabiei B86
  - trombiculae B88.0
- Agamofilaria streptocerca B74.4
- Ancylostoma, ankylostoma (braziliense) (caninum) (ceylanicum) (duodenale) B76.0
  - americanum B76.1
  - new world B76.1
- Anisakis larvae, anisakiasis B81.0
- arthropod NEC B88.2
- Ascaris lumbricoides *—see* Ascariasis
- Balantidium coli A07.0
- beef tapeworm B68.1
- Bothriocephalus (latus) B70.0
  - larval B70.1
- broad tapeworm B70.0
  - larval B70.1
- Brugia (malayi) B74.1
  - timori B74.2
- candiru B88.8
- Capillaria
  - hepatica B83.8
  - philippinensis B81.1
- cat liver fluke B66.0
- cestodes B71.9
  - diphyllobothrium *—see* Infestation, diphyllobothrium
  - dipylidiasis B71.1
  - hymenolepiasis B71.0
  - specified type NEC B71.8
- chigger B88.0
- chigo, chigoe B88.1
- Clonorchis (sinensis) (liver) B66.1
- coccidial A07.3
- crab-lice B85.3
- Cysticercus cellulosae *—see* Cysticercosis
- Demodex (folliculorum) B88.0
- Dermanyssus gallinae B88.0
- Dermatobia (hominis) *—see* Myiasis
- Dibothriocephalus (latus) B70.0
  - larval B70.1
- Dicrocoelium dendriticum B66.2
- Diphyllobothrium (adult) (latum) (intestinal) (pacificum) B70.0
  - larval B70.1
- Diplogonoporus (grandis) B71.8
- Dipylidium caninum B67.4

Infestation *(continued)*
- Distoma hepaticum B66.3
- dog tapeworm B67.4
- Dracunculus medinensis B72
- dragon worm B72
- dwarf tapeworm B71.0
- Echinococcus *—see* Echinococcus
- Echinostomum ilocanum B66.8
- Entamoeba (histolytica) *—see* Infection, Ameba
- Enterobius vermicularis B80
- eyelid
  - in (due to)
    - leishmaniasis B55.1
    - loiasis B74.3
    - onchocerciasis B73.09
    - phthiriasis B85.3
  - parasitic NOS B89
- eyeworm B74.3
- Fasciola (gigantica) (hepatica) (indica) B66.3
- Fasciolopsis (buski) (intestine) B66.5
- filarial B74.9
  - bancroftian B74.0
  - conjunctiva B74.9
  - due to
    - Acanthocheilonema (perstans) (streptocerca) B74.4
    - Brugia (malayi) B74.1
      - timori B74.2
    - Dracunculus medinensis B72
    - guinea worm B72
    - loa loa B74.3
    - Mansonella (ozzardi) (perstans) (streptocerca) B74.4
    - Onchocerca volvulus B73.00
      - eye B73.00
      - eyelid B73.09
    - Wuchereria (bancrofti) B74.0
  - Malayan B74.1
  - ozzardi B74.4
  - specified type NEC B74.8
- fish tapeworm B70.0
  - larval B70.1
- fluke B66.9
  - blood NOS *—see* Schistosomiasis
  - cat liver B66.0
  - intestinal B66.5
  - liver (sheep) B66.3
    - cat B66.0
    - Chinese B66.1
    - due to clonorchiasis B66.1
    - oriental B66.1
  - lancet B66.2
  - lung (oriental) B66.4
  - sheep liver B66.3
  - specified type NEC B66.8
- fly larvae *—see* Myiasis
- Gasterophilus (intestinalis) *—see* Myiasis
- Gastrodiscoides hominis B66.8
- Giardia lamblia A07.1
- Gnathostoma (spinigerum) B83.1
- Gongylonema B83.8
- guinea worm B72
- helminth B83.9
  - angiostrongyliasis B83.2
    - intestinal B81.3
  - gnathostomiasis B83.1
  - hirudiniasis, internal B83.4
  - intestinal B82.0
    - angiostrongyliasis B81.3
    - anisakiasis B81.0
    - ascariasis *—see* Ascariasis
    - capillariasis B81.1
    - cysticercosis *—see* Cysticercosis

Infestation *(continued)*
- helminth *(continued)*
  - intestinal *(continued)*
    - diphyllobothriasis —*see* Infestation, diphyllobothriasis
    - dracunculiasis B72
    - echinococcus —*see* Echinococcosis
    - enterobiasis B80
    - filariasis —*see* Infestation, filarial
    - fluke —*see* Infestation, fluke
    - hookworm —*see* Infestation, hookworm
    - mixed (types classifiable to more than one of the titles B65.0-B81.3 and B81.8) B81.4
    - onchocerciasis —*see* Onchocerciasis
    - schistosomiasis —*see* Infestation, schistosoma
    - specified
      - cestode NEC —*see* Infestation, cestode
      - type NEC B81.8
    - strongyloidiasis —*see* Strongyloidiasis
    - taenia —*see* Infestation, taenia
    - trichinellosis B75
    - trichostrongyliasis B81.2
    - trichuriasis B79
  - specified type NEC B83.8
  - syngamiasis B83.3
  - visceral larva migrans B83.0
- Heterophyes (heterophyes) B66.8
- hookworm B76.9
  - ancylostomiasis B76.0
  - necatoriasis B76.1
  - specified type NEC B76.8
- Hymenolepis (diminuta) (nana) B71.0
- intestinal NEC B82.9
- leeches (aquatic) (land) —*see* Hirudiniasis
- Leishmania —*see* Leishmaniasis
- lice, louse —*see* Infestation, Pediculus
- Linguatula B88.8
- Liponyssoides sanguineus B88.0
- Loa loa B74.3
  - conjunctival B74.3
  - eyelid B74.3
- louse —*see* Infestation, Pediculus
- maggots —*see* Myiasis
- Mansonella (ozzardi) (perstans) (streptocerca) B74.4
- Medina (worm) B72
- Metagonimus (yokogawai) B66.8
- microfilaria streptocerca —*see* Onchocerciasis
  - eye B73.00
  - eyelid B73.09
- mites B88.9
  - scabic B86
- Monilia (albicans) —*see* Candidiasis
- mouth B37.0
- Necator americanus B76.1
- nematode NEC (intestinal) B82.0
  - Ancylostoma B76.0
  - conjunctiva NEC B83.9
  - Enterobius vermicularis B80
  - Gnathostoma spinigerum B83.1
  - physaloptera B80
  - specified NEC B81.8
  - trichostrongylus B81.2
  - trichuris (trichuria) B79
- Oesophagostomum (apiostomum) B81.8

Infestation *(continued)*
- Oestrus ovis (*see also* Myiasis) B87.9
- Onchocerca (volvulus) —*see* Onchocerciasis
- Opisthorchis (felineus) (viverrini) B66.0
- orbit, parasitic NOS B89
- Oxyuris vermicularis B80
- Paragonimus (westermani) B66.4
- parasite, parasitic B89
  - eyelid B89
  - intestinal NOS B82.9
  - mouth B37.0
  - skin B88.9
  - tongue B37.0
- Parastrongylus
  - cantonensis B83.2
  - costaricensis B81.3
- Pediculus B85.2
  - body B85.1
  - capitis (humanus) (any site) B85.0
  - corporis (humanus) (any site) B85.1
  - head B85.0
  - mixed (classifiable to more than one of the titles B85.0-B85.3) B85.4
  - pubis (any site) B85.3
- Pentastoma B88.8
- Phthirus (pubis) (any site) B85.3
  - with any infestation classifiable to B85.0-B85.2 B85.4
- pinworm B80
- pork tapeworm (adult) B68.0
- protozoal NEC B64
  - intestinal A07.9
    - specified NEC A07.8
  - specified NEC B60.8
- pubic, louse B85.3
- rat tapeworm B71.0
- red bug B88.0
- roundworm (large) NEC B82.0
  - Ascariasis (*see also* Ascariasis) B77.9
- sandflea B88.1
- Sarcoptes scabiei B86
- scabies B86
- Schistosoma B65.9
  - bovis B65.8
  - cercariae B65.3
  - haematobium B65.0
  - intercalatum B65.8
  - japonicum B65.2
  - mansoni B65.1
  - mattheei B65.8
  - mekongi B65.8
  - specified type NEC B65.8
  - spindale B65.8
- screw worms —*see* Myiasis
- skin NOS B88.9
- Sparganum (mansoni) (proliferum) (baxteri) B70.1
  - larval B70.1
- specified type NEC B88.8
- Spirometra larvae B70.1
- Stellantchasmus falcatus B66.8
- Strongyloides stercoralis —*see* Strongyloidiasis
- Taenia B68.9
  - diminuta B71.0
  - echinococcus —*see* Echinococcus
  - mediocanellata B68.1
  - nana B71.0
  - saginata B68.1
  - solium (intestinal form) B68.0
    - larval form —*see* Cysticercosis

Infestation *(continued)*
- Taeniarhynchus saginatus B68.1
- tapeworm B71.9
  - beef B68.1
  - broad B70.0
    - larval B70.1
  - dog B67.4
  - dwarf B71.0
  - fish B70.0
    - larval B70.1
  - pork B68.0
  - rat B71.0
- Ternidens diminutus B81.8
- Tetranychus molestissimus B88.0
- threadworm B80
- tongue B37.0
- Toxocara (canis) (cati) (felis) B83.0
- trematode(s) NEC —*see* Infestation, fluke
- Trichinella (spiralis) B75
- Trichocephalus B79
- Trichomonas —*see* Trichomoniasis
- Trichostrongylus B81.2
- Trichuris (trichiura) B79
- Trombicula (irritans) B88.0
- Tunga penetrans B88.1
- Uncinaria americana B76.1
- Vandellia cirrhosa B88.8
- whipworm B79
- worms B83.9
  - intestinal B82.0
- Wuchereria (bancrofti) B74.0

Infiltrate, infiltration
- amyloid (generalized) (localized) —*see* Amyloidosis
- calcareous NEC R89.7
  - localized —*see* Degeneration, by site
- calcium salt R89.7
- cardiac
  - fatty —*see* Degeneration, myocardial
  - glycogenic E74.02 *[I43]*
- corneal —*see* Edema, cornea
- eyelid —*see* Inflammation, eyelid
- glycogen, glycogenic —*see* Disease, glycogen storage
- heart, cardiac
  - fatty —*see* Degeneration, myocardial
  - glycogenic E74.02 *[I43]*
- inflammatory in vitreous H43.89
- kidney N28.89
- leukemic —*see* Leukemia
- liver K76.89
  - fatty —*see* Fatty, liver NEC
  - glycogen (*see also* Disease, glycogen storage) E74.03 *[K77]*
- lung R91.8
  - eosinophilic —*see* Eosinophilia, pulmonary
- lymphatic (*see also* Leukemia, lymphatic) C91.9-
  - gland I88.9
- muscle, fatty M62.89
- myocardium, myocardial
  - fatty —*see* Degeneration, myocardial
  - glycogenic E74.02 *[I43]*
- on chest x-ray R91.8
- pulmonary R91.8
  - with eosinophilia —*see* Eosinophilia, pulmonary
- skin (lymphocytic) L98.6
- thymus (gland) (fatty) E32.8
- urine R39.0
- vesicant agent
  - antineoplastic chemotherapy T80.810
  - other agent NEC T80.818
- vitreous body H43.89

Infirmity R68.89
- senile R54

Inflammation, inflamed, inflammatory (with exudation)
- abducent (nerve) —*see* Strabismus, paralytic, sixth nerve
- accessory sinus (chronic) —*see* Sinusitis
- adrenal (gland) E27.8
- alveoli, teeth M27.3
  - scorbutic E54
- anal canal, anus K62.89
- antrum (chronic) —*see* Sinusitis, maxillary
- appendix —*see* Appendicitis
- arachnoid —*see* Meningitis
- areola N61.0
  - puerperal, postpartum or gestational —*see* Infection, nipple
- areolar tissue NOS L08.9
- artery —*see* Arteritis
- auditory meatus (external) —*see* Otitis, externa
- Bartholin's gland N75.8
- bile duct (common) (hepatic) or passage —*see* Cholangitis
- bladder —*see* Cystitis
- bone —*see* Osteomyelitis
- brain —*see also* Encephalitis
  - membrane —*see* Meningitis
- breast N61.0
  - puerperal, postpartum, gestational —*see* Mastitis, obstetric
- broad ligament —*see* Disease, pelvis, inflammatory
- bronchi —*see* Bronchitis
- catarrhal J00
- cecum —*see* Appendicitis
- cerebral —*see also* Encephalitis
  - membrane —*see* Meningitis
- cerebrospinal
  - meningococcal A39.0
- cervix (uteri) —*see* Cervicitis
- chest J98.8
- chorioretinal H30.9-
  - cyclitis —*see* Cyclitis
  - disseminated H30.10-
    - generalized H30.13-
    - peripheral H30.12-
    - posterior pole H30.11-
  - epitheliopathy —*see* Epitheliopathy
  - focal H30.00-
    - juxtapapillary H30.01-
    - macular H30.04-
    - paramacular —*see* Inflammation, chorioretinal, focal, macular
    - peripheral H30.03-
    - posterior pole H30.02-
  - specified type NEC H30.89-
- choroid —*see* Inflammation, chorioretinal
- chronic, postmastoidectomy cavity —*see* Complications, postmastoidectomy, inflammation
- colon —*see* Enteritis
- connective tissue (diffuse) NEC —*see* Disorder, soft tissue, specified type NEC
- cornea —*see* Keratitis
- corpora cavernosa N48.29
- cranial nerve —*see* Disorder, nerve, cranial
- Douglas' cul-de-sac or pouch (chronic) N73.0

Inflammation, inflamed, inflammatory *(continued)*
- due to device, implant or graft —*see also* Complications, by site and type, infection or inflammation
  - arterial graft T82.7
  - breast (implant) T85.79
  - catheter T85.79
    - dialysis (renal) T82.7
      - intraperitoneal T85.71
    - infusion T82.7
      - cranial T85.735
      - intrathecal T85.735
      - spinal (epidural) (subdural) T85.735
      - subarachnoid T85.735
    - urinary T83.51
      - cystostomy T83.510
      - Hopkins T83.518
      - ileostomy T83.518
      - nephrostomy T83.512
      - specified NEC T83.518
      - urethral indwelling T83.511
      - urostomy T83.518
  - electronic (electrode) (pulse generator) (stimulator)
    - bone T84.7
    - cardiac T82.7
    - nervous system T85.738
      - brain T85.731
      - cranial nerve T85.732
      - gastric nerve T85.732
      - neurostimulator generator T85.734
      - peripheral nerve T85.732
      - sacral nerve T85.732
      - spinal cord T85.733
      - vagal nerve T85.732
    - urinary T83.590
  - fixation, internal (orthopedic) NEC —*see* Complication, fixation device, infection
  - gastrointestinal (bile duct) (esophagus) T85.79
    - neurostimulator electrode (lead) T85.732
  - genital NEC T83.69
  - heart NEC T82.7
    - valve (prosthesis) T82.6
      - graft T82.7
  - joint prosthesis —*see* Complication, joint prosthesis, infection
  - ocular (corneal graft) (orbital implant) NEC T85.79
  - orthopedic NEC T84.7
  - penile (cylinder) (pump) (resevoir) T83.61
  - specified NEC T85.79
  - testicular T83.62
  - urinary NEC T83.598
    - ileal conduit stent T83.593
    - implanted neurostimulation T83.590
    - implanted sphincter T83.591
    - indwelling ureteral stent T83.592
    - nephroureteral stent T83.593
    - specified stent NEC T83.593
  - vascular NEC T82.7
  - ventricular intracranial (communicating) shunt T85.730
- duodenum K29.80
  - with bleeding K29.81
- dura mater —*see* Meningitis
- ear (middle) —*see also* Otitis, media
  - external —*see* Otitis, externa
  - inner —*see* subcategory H83.0

Inflammation, inflamed, inflammatory *(continued)*
- epididymis —*see* Epididymitis
- esophagus —*see* Esophagitis
- ethmoidal (sinus) (chronic) —*see* Sinusitis, ethmoidal
- eustachian tube (catarrhal) —*see* Salpingitis, eustachian
- eyelid H01.9
  - abscess —*see* Abscess, eyelid
  - blepharitis —*see* Blepharitis
  - chalazion —*see* Chalazion
  - dermatosis (noninfectious) —*see* Dermatosis, eyelid
  - hordeolum —*see* Hordeolum
  - specified NEC H01.8
- fallopian tube —*see* Salpingo-oophoritis
- fascia —*see* Myositis
- follicular, pharynx J31.2
- frontal (sinus) (chronic) —*see* Sinusitis, frontal
- gallbladder —*see* Cholecystitis
- gastric —*see* Gastritis
- gastrointestinal —*see* Enteritis
- genital organ (internal) (diffuse)
  - female —*see* Disease, pelvis, inflammatory
  - male N49.9
    - multiple sites N49.8
    - specified NEC N49.8
- gland (lymph) —*see* Lymphadenitis
- glottis —*see* Laryngitis
- granular, pharynx J31.2
- gum K05.10
  - nonplaque induced K05.11
  - plaque induced K05.10
- heart —*see* Carditis
- hepatic duct —*see* Cholangitis
- ileoanal (internal) pouch K91.850
- ileum —*see also* Enteritis
  - regional or terminal —*see* Enteritis, regional
- intestine (any part) —*see* Enteritis
- intestinal pouch K91.850
- jaw (acute) (bone) (chronic) (lower) (suppurative) (upper) M27.2
- joint NEC —*see* Arthritis
  - sacroiliac M46.1
- kidney —*see* Nephritis
- knee (joint) M13.169
  - tuberculous A18.02
- labium (majus) (minus) —*see* Vulvitis
- lacrimal
  - gland —*see* Dacryoadenitis
  - passages (duct) (sac) —*see also* Dacryocystitis
    - canaliculitis —*see* Canaliculitis, lacrimal
- larynx —*see* Laryngitis
- leg NOS L08.9
- lip K13.0
- liver (capsule) —*see also* Hepatitis
  - chronic K73.9
  - suppurative K75.0
- lung (acute) —*see also* Pneumonia
  - chronic J98.4
- lymph gland or node —*see* Lymphadenitis
- lymphatic vessel —*see* Lymphangitis
- maxilla, maxillary M27.2
  - sinus (chronic) —*see* Sinusitis, maxillary
- membranes of brain or spinal cord —*see* Meningitis
- meninges —*see* Meningitis
- mouth K12.1
- muscle —*see* Myositis
- myocardium —*see* Myocarditis

Inflammation, inflamed, inflammatory *(continued)*
- nasal sinus (chronic) —*see* Sinusitis
- nasopharynx —*see* Nasopharyngitis
- navel L08.82
- nerve NEC —*see* Neuritis
- nipple N61.0
  - puerperal, postpartum or gestational —*see* Infection, nipple
- nose —*see* Rhinitis
- oculomotor (nerve) —*see* Strabismus, paralytic, third nerve
- optic nerve —*see* Neuritis, optic
- orbit (chronic) H05.10
  - acute H05.00
    - abscess —*see* Abscess, orbit
    - cellulitis —*see* Cellulitis, orbit
    - osteomyelitis —*see* Osteomyelitis, orbit
    - periostitis —*see* Periostitis, orbital
    - tenonitis —*see* Tenonitis, eye
  - granuloma —*see* Granuloma, orbit
  - myositis —*see* Myositis, orbital
- ovary —*see* Salpingo-oophoritis
- oviduct —*see* Salpingo-oophoritis
- pancreas (acute) —*see* Pancreatitis
- parametrium N73.0
- parotid region L08.9
- pelvis, female —*see* Disease, pelvis, inflammatory
- penis (corpora cavernosa) N48.29
- perianal K62.89
- pericardium —*see* Pericarditis
- perineum (female) (male) L08.9
- perirectal K62.89
- peritoneum —*see* Peritonitis
- periuterine —*see* Disease, pelvis, inflammatory
- perivesical —*see* Cystitis
- petrous bone (acute) (chronic) —*see* Petrositis
- pharynx (acute) —*see* Pharyngitis
- pia mater —*see* Meningitis
- pleura —*see* Pleurisy
- polyp, colon (*see also* Polyp, colon, inflammatory) K51.40
- prostate —*see also* Prostatitis
  - specified type NEC N41.8
- rectosigmoid —*see* Rectosigmoiditis
- rectum (*see also* Proctitis) K62.89
- respiratory, upper (*see also* Infection, respiratory, upper) J06.9
  - acute, due to radiation J70.0
  - chronic, due to external agent —*see* condition, respiratory, chronic, due to
  - due to
    - chemicals, gases, fumes or vapors (inhalation) J68.2
    - radiation J70.1
- retina —*see* Chorioretinitis
- retrocecal —*see* Appendicitis
- retroperitoneal —*see* Peritonitis
- salivary duct or gland (any) (suppurative) —*see* Sialoadenitis
- scorbutic, alveoli, teeth E54
- scrotum N49.2
- seminal vesicle —*see* Vesiculitis
- sigmoid —*see* Enteritis
- sinus —*see* Sinusitis
- Skene's duct or gland —*see* Urethritis
- skin L08.9

Inflammation, inflamed, inflammatory *(continued)*
- spermatic cord N49.1
- sphenoidal (sinus) —*see* Sinusitis, sphenoidal
- spinal
  - cord —*see* Encephalitis
  - membrane —*see* Meningitis
  - nerve —*see* Disorder, nerve
- spine —*see* Spondylopathy, inflammatory
- spleen (capsule) D73.89
- stomach —*see* Gastritis
- subcutaneous tissue L08.9
- suprarenal (gland) E27.8
- synovial —*see* Tenosynovitis
- tendon (sheath) NEC —*see* Tenosynovitis
- testis —*see* Orchitis
- throat (acute) —*see* Pharyngitis
- thymus (gland) E32.8
- thyroid (gland) —*see* Thyroiditis
- tongue K14.0
- tonsil —*see* Tonsillitis
- trachea —*see* Tracheitis
- trochlear (nerve) —*see* Strabismus, paralytic, fourth nerve
- tubal —*see* Salpingo-oophoritis
- tuberculous NEC —*see* Tuberculosis
- tubo-ovarian —*see* Salpingo-oophoritis
- tunica vaginalis N49.1
- tympanic membrane —*see* Tympanitis
- umbilicus, umbilical L08.82
- uterine ligament —*see* Disease, pelvis, inflammatory
- uterus (catarrhal) —*see* Endometritis
- uveal tract (anterior) NOS —*see also* Iridocyclitis
  - posterior —*see* Chorioretinitis
- vagina —*see* Vaginitis
- vas deferens N49.1
- vein —*see also* Phlebitis
  - intracranial or intraspinal (septic) G08
  - thrombotic I80.9
    - leg —*see* Phlebitis, leg
    - lower extremity —*see* Phlebitis, leg
- vocal cord J38.3
- vulva —*see* Vulvitis
- Wharton's duct (suppurative) —*see* Sialoadenitis

Inflation, lung, imperfect (newborn) —*see* Atelectasis

Influenza (bronchial) (epidemic) (respiratory (upper)) (unidentified influenza virus) J11.1
- with
  - digestive manifestations J11.2
  - encephalopathy J11.81
  - enteritis J11.2
  - gastroenteritis J11.2
  - gastrointestinal manifestations J11.2
  - laryngitis J11.1
  - myocarditis J11.82
  - otitis media J11.83
  - pharyngitis J11.1
  - pneumonia J11.00
    - specified type J11.08
  - respiratory manifestations NEC J11.1
  - specified manifestation NEC J11.89
- A (non-novel) J10-

Influenza *(continued)*
- A/H5N1 (*see also* Influenza, due to, identified novel influenza A virus) J09.X2
- avian (*see also* Influenza, due to, identified novel influenza A virus) J09.X2
- B J10-
- bird (*see also* Influenza, due to, identified novel influenza A virus) J09.X2
- C J10-
- due to
  - avian (*see also* Influenza, due to, identified novel influenza A virus) J09.X2
  - identified influenza virus NEC J10.1
    - with
      - digestive manifestations J10.2
      - encephalopathy J10.81
      - enteritis J10.2
      - gastroenteritis J10.2
      - gastrointestinal manifestations J10.2
      - laryngitis J10.1
      - myocarditis J10.82
      - otitis media J10.83
      - pharyngitis J10.1
      - pneumonia (unspecified type) J10.00
        - with same identified influenza virus J10.01
        - specified type NEC J10.08
      - respiratory manifestations NEC J10.1
      - specified manifestation NEC J10.89
  - identified novel influenza A virus J09.X2
    - with
      - digestive manifestations J09.X3
      - encephalopathy J09.X9
      - enteritis J09.X3
      - gastroenteritis J09.X3
      - gastrointestinal manifestations J09.X3
      - laryngitis J09.X2
      - myocarditis J09.X9
      - otitis media J09.X9
      - pharyngitis J09.X2
      - pneumonia J09.X1
      - respiratory manifestations NEC J09.X2
      - specified manifestation NEC J09.X9
      - upper respiratory symptoms J09.X2
- novel (2009) H1N1 influenza (*see also* Influenza, due to, identified novel influenza A virus) NEC J10.1
- novel influenza A/H1N1 (*see also* Influenza, due to, identified novel influenza A virus) NEC J10.1
- of other animal origin, not bird or swine (*see also* Influenza, due to, identified novel influenza A virus) J09.X2
- swine (viruses that normally cause infections in pigs) (*see also* Influenza, due to, identified novel influenza A virus) J09.X2

Influenza-like disease *—see* Influenza

Influenzal *—see* Influenza

Infraction, Freiberg's (metatarsal head) *—see* Osteochondrosis, juvenile, metatarsus

Infraeruption of tooth (teeth) M26.34

Infusion complication, misadventure, or reaction *—see* Complications, infusion

Ingestion
- chemical *—see* Table of Drugs and Chemicals, by substance, poisoning
- drug or medicament
  - correct substance properly administered *—see* Table of Drugs and Chemicals, by drug, adverse effect
  - overdose or wrong substance given or taken *—see* Table of Drugs and Chemicals, by drug, poisoning
- foreign body *—see* Foreign body, alimentary tract
- multiple drug *—see* Table of Drugs and Chemicals, multiple
- tularemia A21.3

Ingrowing
- hair (beard) L73.1
- nail (finger) (toe) L60.0

Inguinal *—see also* condition
- testicle Q53.9
  - bilateral Q53.212
  - unilateral Q53.112

Inhalant-induced
- anxiety disorder F18.980
- depressive disorder F18.94
- major neurocognitive disorder F18.97
- mild neurocognitive disorder F18.988
- psychotic disorder F18.959

Inhalation
- anthrax A22.1
- flame T27.3
- food or foreign body *—see* Foreign body, by site
- gases, fumes, or vapors T59.9-
  - specified agent NEC *—see* Table of Drugs and Chemicals, by substance T59.89-
- liquid or vomitus *—see* Asphyxia
- meconium (newborn) P24.00
  - with
    - pneumonia (pneumonitis) P24.01
    - with respiratory symptoms P24.01
- mucus *—see* Asphyxia, mucus
- oil or gasoline (causing suffocation) *—see* Foreign body, by site
- smoke T59.81-
  - with respiratory conditions J70.5
    - due to chemicals, gases, fumes and vapors J68.9
- steam (*see also* Burn, respiratory tract) T59.9-
- stomach contents or secretions *—see* Foreign body, by site
  - due to anesthesia (general) (local) or other sedation T88.59
    - in labor and delivery O74.0
    - in pregnancy O29.01-
    - postpartum, puerperal O89.01

Inhibition, orgasm
- female F52.31
- male F52.32

Inhibitor, systemic lupus erythematosus (presence of) D68.62

Iniencephalus, iniencephaly Q00.2

Injection, traumatic jet (air) (industrial) (water) (paint or dye) T70.4

Injury (*see also* specified injury type) T14.90
- abdomen, abdominal S39.91
  - blood vessel *—see* Injury, blood vessel, abdomen
  - cavity *—see* Injury, intra-abdominal
  - contusion S30.1
  - internal *—see* Injury, intra-abdominal
  - intra-abdominal organ *—see* Injury, intra-abdominal
  - nerve *—see* Injury, nerve, abdomen
  - open *—see* Wound, open, abdomen
  - specified NEC S39.81
  - superficial *—see* Injury, superficial, abdomen
- Achilles tendon S86.00-
  - laceration S86.02-
  - specified type NEC S86.09-
  - strain S86.01-
- acoustic, resulting in deafness *—see* Injury, nerve, acoustic
- adrenal (gland) S37.819
  - contusion S37.812
  - laceration S37.813
  - specified type NEC S37.818
- alveolar (process) S09.93
- ankle S99.91-
  - contusion *—see* Contusion, ankle
  - dislocation *—see* Dislocation, ankle
  - fracture *—see* Fracture, ankle
  - nerve *—see* Injury, nerve, ankle
  - open *—see* Wound, open, ankle
  - specified type NEC S99.81-
  - sprain *—see* Sprain, ankle
  - superficial *—see* Injury, superficial, ankle
- anterior chamber, eye *—see* Injury, eye, specified site NEC
- anus *—see* Injury, abdomen
- aorta (thoracic) S25.00
  - abdominal S35.00
    - laceration (minor) (superficial) S35.01
      - major S35.02
    - specified type NEC S35.09
  - laceration (minor) (superficial) S25.01
    - major S25.02
  - specified type NEC S25.09
- arm (upper) S49.9-
  - blood vessel *—see* Injury, blood vessel, arm
  - contusion *—see* Contusion, arm, upper
  - fracture *—see* Fracture, humerus
  - lower *—see* Injury, forearm
  - muscle *—see* Injury, muscle, shoulder
  - nerve *—see* Injury, nerve, arm
  - open *—see* Wound, open, arm
  - specified type NEC S49.8-
  - superficial *—see* Injury, superficial, arm

Injury *(continued)*
- artery (complicating trauma) *—see also* Injury, blood vessel, by site
  - cerebral or meningeal *—see* Injury, intracranial
- auditory canal (external) (meatus) S09.91
- auricle, auris, ear S09.91
- axilla *—see* Injury, shoulder
- back *—see* Injury, back, lower
- bile duct S36.13
- birth *—see also* Birth, injury P15.9
- bladder (sphincter) S37.20
  - at delivery O71.5
  - contusion S37.22
  - laceration S37.23
  - obstetrical trauma O71.5
  - specified type NEC S37.29
- blast (air) (hydraulic) (immersion) (underwater) NEC T14.8
  - acoustic nerve trauma *—see* Injury, nerve, acoustic
  - bladder *—see* Injury, bladder
  - brain *—see* Concussion
  - colon *—see* Injury, intestine, large, blast injury
  - ear (primary) S09.31-
    - secondary S09.39-
  - generalized T70.8
  - lung *—see* Injury, intrathoracic, lung, blast injury
  - multiple body organs T70.8
  - peritoneum S36.81
  - rectum S36.61
  - retroperitoneum S36.898
  - small intestine S36.419
    - duodenum S36.410
    - specified site NEC S36.418
  - specified
    - intra-abdominal organ NEC S36.898
    - pelvic organ NEC S37.899
- blood vessel NEC T14.8
  - abdomen S35.9-
    - aorta *—see* Injury, aorta, abdominal
    - celiac artery *—see* Injury, blood vessel, celiac artery
    - iliac vessel *—see* Injury, blood vessel, iliac
    - laceration S35.91
    - mesenteric vessel *—see* Injury, mesenteric
    - portal vein *—see* Injury, blood vessel, portal vein
    - renal vessel *—see* Injury, blood vessel, renal
    - specified vessel NEC S35.8X-
    - splenic vessel *—see* Injury, blood vessel, splenic
    - vena cava *—see* Injury, vena cava, inferior
  - ankle *—see* Injury, blood vessel, foot
  - aorta (abdominal) (thoracic) *—see* Injury, aorta
  - arm (upper) NEC S45.90-
    - forearm *—see* Injury, blood vessel, forearm
    - laceration S45.91-
    - specified
      - site NEC S45.80-
        - laceration S45.81-
        - specified type NEC S45.89-
      - type NEC S45.99-
    - superficial vein S45.30-
      - laceration S45.31-
      - specified type NEC S45.39-

Influenza–Injury

Injury *(continued)*
- blood vessel NEC *(continued)*
  - axillary
    - artery S45.00-
      - laceration S45.01-
      - specified type NEC S45.09-
    - vein S45.20-
      - laceration S45.21-
      - specified type NEC S45.29-
  - azygos vein —*see* Injury, blood vessel, thoracic, specified site NEC
  - brachial
    - artery S45.10-
      - laceration S45.11-
      - specified type NEC S45.19-
    - vein S45.20-
      - laceration S45.219
      - specified type NEC S45.29-
  - carotid artery (common) (external) (internal, extracranial) S15.00-
    - internal, intracranial S06.8-
    - laceration (minor) (superficial) S15.01-
      - major S15.02-
    - specified type NEC S15.09-
  - celiac artery S35.219
    - branch S35.299
      - laceration (minor) (superficial) S35.291
        - major S35.292
      - specified NEC S35.298
    - laceration (minor) (superficial) S35.211
      - major S35.212
    - specified type NEC S35.218
  - cerebral —*see* Injury, intracranial
  - deep plantar —*see* Injury, blood vessel, plantar artery
  - digital (hand) —*see* Injury, blood vessel, finger
  - dorsal
    - artery (foot) S95.00-
      - laceration S95.01-
      - specified type NEC S95.09-
    - vein (foot) S95.20-
      - laceration S95.21-
      - specified type NEC S95.29-
  - due to accidental laceration during procedure —*see* Laceration, accidental complicating surgery
  - extremity —*see* Injury, blood vessel, limb
  - femoral
    - artery (common) (superficial) S75.00-
      - laceration (minor) (superficial) S75.01-
        - major S75.02-
      - specified type NEC S75.09-
    - vein (hip level) (thigh level) S75.10-
      - laceration (minor) (superficial) S75.11-
        - major S75.12-
      - specified type NEC S75.19-
  - finger S65.50-
    - index S65.50-
      - laceration S65.51-
      - specified type NEC S65.59-
    - laceration S65.51-
    - little S65.50-
      - laceration S65.51-
      - specified type NEC S65.59-
    - middle S65.50-
      - laceration S65.51-
      - specified type NEC S65.59-
    - specified type NEC S65.59-

Injury *(continued)*
- blood vessel NEC *(continued)*
  - finger *(continued)*
    - thumb —*see* Injury, blood vessel, thumb
  - foot S95.90-
    - dorsal
      - artery —*see* Injury, blood vessel, dorsal, artery
      - vein —*see* Injury, blood vessel, dorsal, vein
    - laceration S95.91-
    - plantar artery —*see* Injury, blood vessel, plantar artery
    - specified
      - site NEC S95.80-
        - laceration S95.81-
        - specified type NEC S95.89-
      - specified type NEC S95.99-
  - forearm S55.90-
    - laceration S55.91-
    - radial artery —*see* Injury, blood vessel, radial artery
    - specified
      - site NEC S55.80-
        - laceration S55.81-
        - specified type NEC S55.89-
      - type NEC S55.99-
    - ulnar artery —*see* Injury, blood vessel, ulnar artery
    - vein S55.20-
      - laceration S55.21-
      - specified type NEC S55.29-
  - gastric
    - artery —*see* Injury, mesenteric, artery, branch
    - vein —*see* Injury, blood vessel, abdomen
  - gastroduodenal artery —*see* Injury, mesenteric, artery, branch
  - greater saphenous vein (lower leg level) S85.30-
    - hip (and thigh) level S75.20-
      - laceration (minor) (superficial) S75.21-
        - major S75.22-
      - specified type NEC S75.29-
    - laceration S85.31-
    - specified type NEC S85.39-
  - hand (level) S65.90-
    - finger —*see* Injury, blood vessel, finger
    - laceration S65.91-
    - palmar arch —*see* Injury, blood vessel, palmar arch
    - radial artery —*see* Injury, blood vessel, radial artery, hand
    - specified
      - site NEC S65.80-
        - laceration S65.81-
        - specified type NEC S65.89-
      - type NEC S65.99-
    - thumb —*see* Injury, blood vessel, thumb
    - ulnar artery —*see* Injury, blood vessel, ulnar artery, hand
  - head S09.0
    - intracranial —*see* Injury, intracranial
    - multiple S09.0
  - hepatic
    - artery —*see* Injury, mesenteric, artery
    - vein —*see* Injury, vena cava, inferior

Injury *(continued)*
- blood vessel NEC *(continued)*
  - hip S75.90-
    - femoral artery —*see* Injury, blood vessel, femoral, artery
    - femoral vein —*see* Injury, blood vessel, femoral, vein
    - greater saphenous vein —*see* Injury, blood vessel, greater saphenous, hip level
    - laceration S75.91-
    - specified
      - site NEC S75.80-
        - laceration S75.81-
        - specified type NEC S75.89-
      - type NEC S75.99-
  - hypogastric (artery) (vein) —*see* Injury, blood vessel, iliac
  - iliac S35.5-
    - artery S35.51-
    - specified vessel NEC S35.5-
    - uterine vessel —*see* Injury, blood vessel, uterine
    - vein S35.51-
  - innominate —*see* Injury, blood vessel, thoracic, innominate
  - intercostal (artery) (vein) —*see* Injury, blood vessel, thoracic, intercostal
  - jugular vein (external) S15.20-
    - internal S15.30-
      - laceration (minor) (superficial) S15.31-
        - major S15.32-
      - specified type NEC S15.39-
    - laceration (minor) (superficial) S15.21-
      - major S15.22-
    - specified type NEC S15.29-
  - leg (level) (lower) S85.90-
    - greater saphenous —*see* Injury, blood vessel, greater saphenous
    - laceration S85.91-
    - lesser saphenous —*see* Injury, blood vessel, lesser saphenous
    - peroneal artery —*see* Injury, blood vessel, peroneal artery
    - popliteal
      - artery —*see* Injury, blood vessel, popliteal, artery
      - vein —*see* Injury, blood vessel, popliteal, vein
    - specified
      - site NEC S85.80-
        - laceration S85.81-
        - specified type NEC S85.89-
      - type NEC S85.99-
    - thigh —*see* Injury, blood vessel, hip
    - tibial artery —*see* Injury, blood vessel, tibial artery
  - lesser saphenous vein (lower leg level) S85.40-
    - laceration S85.41-
    - specified type NEC S85.49-
  - limb
    - lower —*see* Injury, blood vessel, leg
    - upper —*see* Injury, blood vessel, arm
  - lower back —*see* Injury, blood vessel, abdomen
    - specified NEC —*see* Injury, blood vessel, abdomen, specified, site NEC

Injury *(continued)*
- blood vessel NEC *(continued)*
  - mammary (artery) (vein) —*see* Injury, blood vessel, thoracic, specified site NEC
  - mesenteric (inferior) (superior)
    - artery —*see* Injury, mesenteric, artery
    - vein —*see* Injury, mesenteric, vein
  - neck S15.9
    - specified site NEC S15.8
  - ovarian (artery) (vein) —*see* subcategory S35.8
  - palmar arch (superficial) S65.20-
    - deep S65.30-
      - laceration S65.31-
      - specified type NEC S65.39-
    - laceration S65.21-
    - specified type NEC S65.29-
  - pelvis —*see* Injury, blood vessel, abdomen
    - specified NEC —*see* Injury, blood vessel, abdomen, specified, site NEC
  - peroneal artery S85.20-
    - laceration S85.21-
    - specified type NEC S85.29-
  - plantar artery (deep) (foot) S95.10-
    - laceration S95.11-
    - specified type NEC S95.19-
  - popliteal
    - artery S85.00-
      - laceration S85.01-
      - specified type NEC S85.09-
    - vein S85.50-
      - laceration S85.51-
      - specified type NEC S85.59-
  - portal vein S35.319
    - laceration S35.311
    - specified type NEC S35.318
  - precerebral —*see* Injury, blood vessel, neck
  - pulmonary (artery) (vein) —*see* Injury, blood vessel, thoracic, pulmonary
  - radial artery (forearm level) S55.10-
    - hand and wrist (level) S65.10-
      - laceration S65.11-
      - specified type NEC S65.19-
    - laceration S55.11-
    - specified type NEC S55.19-
  - renal
    - artery S35.40-
      - laceration S35.41-
      - specified NEC S35.49-
    - vein S35.40-
      - laceration S35.41-
      - specified NEC S35.49-
  - saphenous vein (greater) (lower leg level) —*see* Injury, blood vessel, greater saphenous
    - hip and thigh level —*see* Injury, blood vessel, greater saphenous, hip level
    - lesser —*see* Injury, blood vessel, lesser saphenous
  - shoulder
    - specified NEC —*see* Injury, blood vessel, arm, specified site NEC
    - superficial vein —*see* Injury, blood vessel, arm, superficial vein
  - specified NEC T14.8
  - splenic
    - artery —*see* Injury, blood vessel, celiac artery, branch

Injury *(continued)*
- blood vessel NEC *(continued)*
  - splenic *(continued)*
    - vein S35.329
      - laceration S35.321
      - specified NEC S35.328
  - subclavian —*see* Injury, blood vessel, thoracic, innominate
  - thigh —*see* Injury, blood vessel, hip
  - thoracic S25.90
    - aorta S25.00
      - laceration (minor) (superficial) S25.01
        - major S25.02
      - specified type NEC S25.09
    - azygos vein —*see* Injury, blood vessel, thoracic, specified, site NEC
    - innominate
      - artery S25.10-
        - laceration (minor) (superficial) S25.11-
          - major S25.12-
        - specified type NEC S25.19-
      - vein S25.30-
        - laceration (minor) (superficial) S25.31-
          - major S25.32-
        - specified type NEC S25.39-
    - intercostal S25.50-
      - laceration S25.51-
      - specified type NEC S25.59-
    - laceration S25.91
    - mammary vessel —*see* Injury, blood vessel, thoracic, specified, site NEC
    - pulmonary S25.40-
      - laceration (minor) (superficial) S25.41-
        - major S25.42-
      - specified type NEC S25.49-
    - specified
      - site NEC S25.80-
        - laceration S25.81-
        - specified type NEC S25.89-
      - type NEC S25.99
    - subclavian —*see* Injury, blood vessel, thoracic, innominate
    - vena cava (superior) S25.20
      - laceration (minor) (superficial) S25.21
        - major S25.22
      - specified type NEC S25.29
  - thumb S65.40-
    - laceration S65.41-
    - specified type NEC S65.49-
  - tibial artery S85.10-
    - anterior S85.13-
      - laceration S85.14-
      - specified injury NEC S85.15-
    - laceration S85.11-
    - posterior S85.16-
      - laceration S85.17-
      - specified injury NEC S85.18-
    - specified injury NEC S85.12-
  - ulnar artery (forearm level) S55.00-
    - hand and wrist (level) S65.00-
      - laceration S65.01-
      - specified type NEC S65.09-
    - laceration S55.01-
    - specified type NEC S55.09-

Injury *(continued)*
- blood vessel NEC *(continued)*
  - upper arm (level) —*see* Injury, blood vessel, arm
    - superficial vein —*see* Injury, blood vessel, arm, superficial vein
  - uterine S35.5-
    - artery S35.53-
    - vein S35.53-
  - vena cava —*see* Injury, vena cava
  - vertebral artery S15.10-
    - laceration (minor) (superficial) S15.11-
      - major S15.12-
    - specified type NEC S15.19-
  - wrist (level) —*see* Injury, blood vessel, hand
- brachial plexus S14.3
  - newborn P14.3
- brain (traumatic) S06.9-
  - diffuse (axonal) S06.2X-
  - focal S06.30-
- brainstem S06.38-
- breast NOS S29.9
- broad ligament —*see* Injury, pelvic organ, specified site NEC
- bronchus, bronchi —*see* Injury, intrathoracic, bronchus
- brow S09.90
- buttock S39.92
- canthus, eye S05.90
- cardiac plexus —*see* Injury, nerve, thorax, sympathetic
- cauda equina S34.3
- cavernous sinus —*see* Injury, intracranial
- cecum —*see* Injury, colon
- celiac ganglion or plexus —*see* Injury, nerve, lumbosacral, sympathetic
- cerebellum —*see* Injury, intracranial
- cerebral —*see* Injury, intracranial
- cervix (uteri) —*see* Injury, uterus
- cheek (wall) S09.93
- chest —*see* Injury, thorax
- childbirth (newborn) —*see also* Birth, injury
  - maternal NEC O71.9
- chin S09.93
- choroid (eye) —*see* Injury, eye, specified site NEC
- clitoris S39.94
- coccyx —*see also* Injury, back, lower
  - complicating delivery O71.6
- colon —*see* Injury, intestine, large
- common bile duct —*see* Injury, liver
- conjunctiva (superficial) —*see* Injury, eye, conjunctiva
- conus medullaris —*see* Injury, spinal, sacral
- cord
  - spermatic (pelvic region) S37.898
    - scrotal region S39.848
  - spinal —*see* Injury, spinal cord, by region
- cornea —*see* Injury, eye, specified site NEC
  - abrasion —*see* Injury, eye, cornea, abrasion
- cortex (cerebral) —*see also* Injury, intracranial
  - visual —*see* Injury, nerve, optic
- costal region NEC S29.9
- costochondral NEC S29.9

Injury *(continued)*
- cranial
  - cavity —*see* Injury, intracranial
  - nerve —*see* Injury, nerve, cranial
- crushing —*see* Crush
- cutaneous sensory nerve
- cystic duct —*see* Injury, liver
- deep tissue —*see* Contusion, by site
  - meaning pressure ulcer —*see* Ulcer, pressure L89 with final character .6
- delivery (newborn) P15.9
  - maternal NEC O71.9
- Descemet's membrane —*see* Injury, eyeball, penetrating
- diaphragm —*see* Injury, intrathoracic, diaphragm
- duodenum —*see* Injury, intestine, small, duodenum
- ear (auricle) (external) (canal) S09.91
  - abrasion —*see* Abrasion, ear
  - bite —*see* Bite, ear
  - blister —*see* Blister, ear
  - bruise —*see* Contusion, ear
  - contusion —*see* Contusion, ear
  - external constriction —*see* Constriction, external, ear
  - hematoma —*see* Hematoma, ear
  - inner —*see* Injury, ear, middle
  - laceration —*see* Laceration, ear
  - middle S09.30-
    - blast —*see* Injury, blast, ear
    - specified NEC S09.39-
  - puncture —*see* Puncture, ear
  - superficial —*see* Injury, superficial, ear
- eighth cranial nerve (acoustic or auditory) —*see* Injury, nerve, acoustic
- elbow S59.90-
  - contusion —*see* Contusion, elbow
  - dislocation —*see* Dislocation, elbow
  - fracture —*see* Fracture, ulna, upper end
  - open —*see* Wound, open, elbow
  - specified NEC S59.80-
  - sprain —*see* Sprain, elbow
  - superficial —*see* Injury, superficial, elbow
- eleventh cranial nerve (accessory) —*see* Injury, nerve, accessory
- epididymis S39.94
- epigastric region S39.91
- epiglottis NEC S19.89
- esophageal plexus —*see* Injury, nerve, thorax, sympathetic
- esophagus (thoracic part) —*see also* Injury, intrathoracic, esophagus
  - cervical NEC S19.85
- eustachian tube S09.30-
- eye S05.9-
  - avulsion S05.7-
  - ball —*see* Injury, eyeball
  - conjunctiva S05.0-
  - cornea
    - abrasion S05.0-
    - laceration S05.3-
      - with prolapse S05.2-
  - lacrimal apparatus S05.8X-
  - orbit penetration S05.4-
  - specified site NEC S05.8X-

Injury *(continued)*
- eyeball S05.8X-
  - contusion S05.1-
  - penetrating S05.6-
    - with
      - foreign body S05.5-
      - prolapse or loss of intraocular tissue S05.2-
    - without prolapse or loss of intraocular tissue S05.3-
  - specified type NEC S05.8-
- eyebrow S09.93
- eyelid S09.93
  - abrasion —*see* Abrasion, eyelid
  - contusion —*see* Contusion, eyelid
  - open —*see* Wound, open, eyelid
- face S09.93
- fallopian tube S37.509
  - bilateral S37.502
    - blast injury S37.512
    - contusion S37.522
    - laceration S37.532
    - specified type NEC S37.592
  - blast injury (primary) S37.519
    - bilateral S37.512
    - secondary —*see* Injury, fallopian tube, specified type NEC
    - unilateral S37.511
  - contusion S37.529
    - bilateral S37.522
    - unilateral S37.521
  - laceration S37.539
    - bilateral S37.532
    - unilateral S37.531
  - specified type NEC S37.599
    - bilateral S37.592
    - unilateral S37.591
  - unilateral S37.501
    - blast injury S37.511
    - contusion S37.521
    - laceration S37.531
    - specified type NEC S37.591
- fascia —*see* Injury, muscle
- fifth cranial nerve (trigeminal) —*see* Injury, nerve, trigeminal
- finger (nail) S69.9-
  - blood vessel —*see* Injury, blood vessel, finger
  - contusion —*see* Contusion, finger
  - dislocation —*see* Dislocation, finger
  - fracture —*see* Fracture, finger
  - muscle —*see* Injury, muscle, finger
  - nerve —*see* Injury, nerve, digital, finger
  - open —*see* Wound, open, finger
  - specified NEC S69.8-
  - sprain —*see* Sprain, finger
  - superficial —*see* Injury, superficial, finger
- first cranial nerve (olfactory) —*see* Injury, nerve, olfactory
- flank —*see* Injury, abdomen
- foot S99.92-
  - blood vessel —*see* Injury, blood vessel, foot
  - contusion —*see* Contusion, foot
  - dislocation —*see* Dislocation, foot
  - fracture —*see* Fracture, foot
  - muscle —*see* Injury, muscle, foot
  - open —*see* Wound, open, foot
  - specified type NEC S99.82-
  - sprain —*see* Sprain, foot
  - superficial —*see* Injury, superficial, foot

Injury *(continued)*
- forceps NOS P15.9
- forearm S59.91-
  - blood vessel —*see* Injury, blood vessel, forearm
  - contusion —*see* Contusion, forearm
  - fracture —*see* Fracture, forearm
  - muscle —*see* Injury, muscle, forearm
  - nerve —*see* Injury, nerve, forearm
  - open —*see* Wound, open, forearm
  - specified NEC S59.81-
  - superficial —*see* Injury, superficial, forearm
- forehead S09.90
- fourth cranial nerve (trochlear) —*see* Injury, nerve, trochlear
- gallbladder S36.129
  - contusion S36.122
  - laceration S36.123
  - specified NEC S36.128
- ganglion
  - celiac, coeliac —*see* Injury, nerve, lumbosacral, sympathetic
  - gasserian —*see* Injury, nerve, trigeminal
  - stellate —*see* Injury, nerve, thorax, sympathetic
  - thoracic sympathetic —*see* Injury, nerve, thorax, sympathetic
- gasserian ganglion —*see* Injury, nerve, trigeminal
- gastric artery —*see* Injury, blood vessel, celiac artery, branch
- gastroduodenal artery —*see* Injury, blood vessel, celiac artery, branch
- gastrointestinal tract —*see* Injury, intra-abdominal
  - with open wound into abdominal cavity —*see* Wound, open, with penetration into peritoneal cavity
  - colon —*see* Injury, intestine, large
  - rectum —*see* Injury, intestine, large, rectum
    - with open wound into abdominal cavity S36.61
  - specified site NEC —*see* Injury, intra-abdominal, specified, site NEC
  - stomach —*see* Injury, stomach
  - small intestine —*see* Injury, intestine, small
- genital organ(s)
  - external S39.94
    - specified NEC S39.848
  - internal S37.90
    - fallopian tube —*see* Injury, fallopian tube
    - ovary —*see* Injury, ovary
    - prostate —*see* Injury, prostate
    - seminal vesicle —*see* Injury, pelvis, organ, specified site NEC
    - uterus —*see* Injury, uterus
    - vas deferens —*see* Injury, pelvis, organ, specified site NEC
  - obstetrical trauma O71.9
- gland
  - lacrimal laceration —*see* Injury, eye, specified site NEC
  - salivary S09.93
  - thyroid NEC S19.84

Injury *(continued)*
- globe (eye) S05.90
  - specified NEC S05.8X-
- groin —*see* Injury, abdomen
- gum S09.90
- hand S69.9-
  - blood vessel —*see* Injury, blood vessel, hand
  - contusion —*see* Contusion, hand
  - fracture —*see* Fracture, hand
  - muscle —*see* Injury, muscle, hand
  - nerve —*see* Injury, nerve, hand
  - open —*see* Wound, open, hand
  - specified NEC S69.8-
  - sprain —*see* Sprain, hand
  - superficial —*see* Injury, superficial, hand
- head S09.90
  - with loss of consciousness S06.9-
  - specified NEC S09.8
- heart (traumatic) S26.90
  - with hemopericardium S26.00
    - contusion S26.01
    - laceration (mild) S26.020
      - moderate S26.021
      - major S26.022
    - specified type NEC S26.09
  - contusion S26.91
  - laceration S26.92
  - nontraumatic (acute) (chronic) (non-ischemic) I5A
  - specified type NEC S26.99
  - without hemopericardium S26.10
    - contusion S26.11
    - laceration S26.12
    - specified type NEC S26.19
- heel —*see* Injury, foot
- hepatic
  - artery —*see* Injury, blood vessel, celiac artery, branch
  - duct —*see* Injury, liver
  - vein —*see* Injury, vena cava, inferior
- hip S79.91-
  - blood vessel —*see* Injury, blood vessel, hip
  - contusion —*see* Contusion, hip
  - dislocation —*see* Dislocation, hip
  - fracture —*see* Fracture, femur, neck
  - muscle —*see* Injury, muscle, hip
  - nerve —*see* Injury, nerve, hip
  - open —*see* Wound, open, hip
  - sprain —*see* Sprain, hip
  - superficial —*see* Injury, superficial, hip
  - specified NEC S79.81-
- hymen S39.94
- hypogastric
  - blood vessel —*see* Injury, blood vessel, iliac
  - plexus —*see* Injury, nerve, lumbosacral, sympathetic
- ileum —*see* Injury, intestine, small
- iliac region S39.91
- instrumental (during surgery) —*see* Laceration, accidental complicating surgery
  - birth injury —*see* Birth, injury
  - nonsurgical —*see* Injury, by site
  - obstetrical O71.9
    - bladder O71.5
    - cervix O71.3
    - high vaginal O71.4
    - perineal NOS O70.9
    - urethra O71.5

Injury *(continued)*
- instrumental *(continued)*
  - obstetrical *(continued)*
    - uterus O71.5
      - with rupture or perforation O71.1
- internal T14.8
  - aorta —*see* Injury, aorta
  - bladder (sphincter) —*see* Injury, bladder
    - with
      - ectopic or molar pregnancy O08.6
    - following ectopic or molar pregnancy O08.6
    - obstetrical trauma O71.5
  - bronchus, bronchi —*see* Injury, intrathoracic, bronchus
  - cecum —*see* Injury, intestine, large
  - cervix (uteri) —*see also* Injury, uterus
    - with ectopic or molar pregnancy O08.6
    - following ectopic or molar pregnancy O08.6
    - obstetrical trauma O71.3
  - chest —*see* Injury, intrathoracic
  - gastrointestinal tract —*see* Injury, intra-abdominal
  - heart —*see* Injury, heart
  - intestine NEC —*see* Injury, intestine
  - intrauterine —*see* Injury, uterus
  - mesentery —*see* Injury, intra-abdominal, specified, site NEC
  - pelvis, pelvic (organ) S37.90
    - following ectopic or molar pregnancy (subsequent episode) O08.6
    - obstetrical trauma NEC O71.5
      - rupture or perforation O71.1
    - specified NEC S39.83
  - rectum —*see* Injury, intestine, large, rectum
  - stomach —*see* Injury, stomach
  - ureter —*see* Injury, ureter
  - urethra (sphincter) following ectopic or molar pregnancy O08.6
  - uterus —*see* Injury, uterus
- interscapular area —*see* Injury, thorax
- intestine
  - large S36.509
    - ascending (right) S36.500
      - blast injury (primary) S36.510
        - secondary S36.590
      - contusion S36.520
      - laceration S36.530
      - specified type NEC S36.590
    - blast injury (primary) S36.519
      - ascending (right) S36.510
      - descending (left) S36.512
      - rectum S36.61
      - sigmoid S36.513
      - specified site NEC S36.518
      - transverse S36.511
    - contusion S36.529
      - ascending (right) S36.520
      - descending (left) S36.522
      - rectum S36.62
      - sigmoid S36.523
      - specified site NEC S36.528
      - transverse S36.521
    - descending (left) S36.502
      - blast injury (primary) S36.512
        - secondary S36.592

Injury *(continued)*
- intestine *(continued)*
  - large *(continued)*
    - descending *(continued)*
      - contusion S36.522
      - laceration S36.532
      - specified type NEC S36.592
    - laceration S36.539
      - ascending (right) S36.530
      - descending (left) S36.532
      - rectum S36.63
      - sigmoid S36.533
      - specified site NEC S36.538
      - transverse S36.531
    - rectum S36.60
      - blast injury (primary) S36.61
        - secondary S36.69
      - contusion S36.62
      - laceration S36.63
      - specified type NEC S36.69
    - sigmoid S36.503
      - blast injury (primary) S36.513
        - secondary S36.593
      - contusion S36.523
      - laceration S36.533
      - specified type NEC S36.593
    - specified
      - site NEC S36.508
        - blast injury (primary) S36.518
          - secondary S36.598
        - contusion S36.528
        - laceration S36.538
        - specified type NEC S36.598
      - type NEC S36.599
        - ascending (right) S36.590
        - descending (left) S36.592
        - rectum S36.69
        - sigmoid S36.593
        - specified site NEC S36.598
        - transverse S36.591
    - transverse S36.501
      - blast injury (primary) S36.511
        - secondary S36.591
      - contusion S36.521
      - laceration S36.531
      - specified type NEC S36.591
  - small S36.409
    - blast injury (primary) S36.419
      - duodenum S36.410
      - secondary S36.499
        - duodenum S36.490
        - specified site NEC S36.498
      - specified site NEC S36.418
    - contusion S36.429
      - duodenum S36.420
      - specified site NEC S36.428
    - duodenum S36.400
      - blast injury (primary) S36.410
        - secondary S36.490
      - contusion S36.420
      - laceration S36.430
      - specified NEC S36.490
    - laceration S36.439
      - duodenum S36.430
      - specified site NEC S36.438
    - specified
      - type NEC S36.499
        - duodenum S36.490
        - specified site NEC S36.498
      - site NEC S36.408

Injury *(continued)*
- intra-abdominal S36.90
  - adrenal gland —*see* Injury, adrenal gland
  - bladder —*see* Injury, bladder
  - colon —*see* Injury, intestine, large
  - contusion S36.92
  - fallopian tube —*see* Injury, fallopian tube
  - gallbladder —*see* Injury, gallbladder
  - intestine —*see* Injury, intestine
  - laceration S36.93
  - liver —*see* Injury, liver
  - kidney —*see* Injury, kidney
  - ovary —*see* Injury, ovary
  - pancreas —*see* Injury, pancreas
  - pelvic NOS S37.90
  - peritoneum —*see* Injury, intra-abdominal, specified, site NEC
  - prostate —*see* Injury, prostate
  - rectum —*see* Injury, intestine, large, rectum
  - retroperitoneum —*see* Injury, intra-abdominal, specified, site NEC
  - seminal vesicle —*see* Injury, pelvis, organ, specified site NEC
  - small intestine —*see* Injury, intestine, small
  - specified
    - site NEC S36.899
      - contusion S36.892
      - laceration S36.893
      - specified type NEC S36.898
    - type NEC S36.99
    - pelvic S37.90
      - specified
        - site NEC S37.899
          - specified type NEC S37.898
        - type NEC S37.99
  - spleen —*see* Injury, spleen
  - stomach —*see* Injury, stomach
  - ureter —*see* Injury, ureter
  - urethra —*see* Injury, urethra
  - uterus —*see* Injury, uterus
  - vas deferens —*see* Injury, pelvis, organ, specified site NEC
- intracranial (traumatic) (*see also*, if applicable, Compression, brain, traumatic) S06.9-
  - cerebellar hemorrhage, traumatic —*see* Injury, intracranial, focal
  - cerebral edema, traumatic S06.1X-
    - diffuse S06.1X-
    - focal S06.1X-
  - diffuse (axonal) S06.2X-
  - epidural hemorrhage (traumatic) S06.4X-
  - focal brain injury S06.30-
    - contusion —*see* Contusion, cerebral
    - laceration —*see* Laceration, cerebral
  - intracerebral hemorrhage, traumatic S06.36-
    - left side S06.35-
    - right side S06.34-
  - subarachnoid hemorrhage, traumatic S06.6X-
  - subdural hemorrhage, traumatic S06.5X-
- intraocular —*see* Injury, eyeball, penetrating

Injury *(continued)*
- intrathoracic S27.9
  - bronchus S27.409
    - bilateral S27.402
    - blast injury (primary) S27.419
      - bilateral S27.412
      - secondary —*see* Injury, intrathoracic, bronchus, specified type NEC
      - unilateral S27.411
    - contusion S27.429
      - bilateral S27.422
      - unilateral S27.421
    - laceration S27.439
      - bilateral S27.432
      - unilateral S27.431
    - specified type NEC S27.499
      - bilateral S27.492
      - unilateral S27.491
    - unilateral S27.401
  - diaphragm S27.809
    - contusion S27.802
    - laceration S27.803
    - specified type NEC S27.808
  - esophagus (thoracic) S27.819
    - contusion S27.812
    - laceration S27.813
    - specified type NEC S27.818
  - heart —*see* Injury, heart
  - hemopneumothorax S27.2
  - hemothorax S27.1
  - lung S27.309
    - aspiration J69.0
    - bilateral S27.302
    - blast injury (primary) S27.319
      - bilateral S27.312
      - secondary —*see* Injury, intrathoracic, lung, specified type NEC
      - unilateral S27.311
    - contusion S27.329
      - bilateral S27.322
      - unilateral S27.321
    - laceration S27.339
      - bilateral S27.332
      - unilateral S27.331
    - specified type NEC S27.399
      - bilateral S27.392
      - unilateral S27.391
    - unilateral S27.301
  - pleura S27.60
    - laceration S27.63
    - specified type NEC S27.69
  - pneumothorax S27.0
  - specified organ NEC S27.899
    - contusion S27.892
    - laceration S27.893
    - specified type NEC S27.898
  - thoracic duct —*see* Injury, intrathoracic, specified organ NEC
  - thymus gland —*see* Injury, intrathoracic, specified organ NEC
  - trachea, thoracic S27.50
    - blast (primary) S27.51
    - contusion S27.52
    - laceration S27.53
    - specified type NEC S27.59
- iris —*see* Injury, eye, specified site NEC
  - penetrating —*see* Injury, eyeball, penetrating
- jaw S09.93
- jejunum —*see* Injury, intestine, small
- joint NOS T14.8
  - old or residual —*see* Disorder, joint, specified type NEC
- kidney S37.00-
  - acute (nontraumatic) N17.9

Injury *(continued)*
- kidney *(continued)*
  - contusion —*see* Contusion, kidney
  - laceration —*see* Laceration, kidney
  - specified NEC S37.09-
- knee S89.9-
  - contusion —*see* Contusion, knee
  - dislocation —*see* Dislocation, knee
  - meniscus (lateral) (medial) —*see* Sprain, knee, specified site NEC
    - old injury or tear —*see* Derangement, knee, meniscus, due to old injury
  - open —*see* Wound, open, knee
  - specified NEC S89.8-
  - sprain —*see* Sprain, knee
  - superficial —*see* Injury, superficial, knee
- labium (majus) (minus) S39.94
- labyrinth, ear S09.30-
- lacrimal apparatus, duct, gland, or sac —*see* Injury, eye, specified site NEC
- larynx NEC S19.81
- leg (lower) S89.9-
  - blood vessel —*see* Injury, blood vessel, leg
  - contusion —*see* Contusion, leg
  - fracture —*see* Fracture, leg
  - muscle —*see* Injury, muscle, leg
  - nerve —*see* Injury, nerve, leg
  - open —*see* Wound, open, leg
  - specified NEC S89.8-
  - superficial —*see* Injury, superficial, leg
- lens, eye —*see* Injury, eye, specified site NEC
  - penetrating —*see* Injury, eyeball, penetrating
- limb NEC T14.8
- lip S09.93
- liver S36.119
  - contusion S36.112
  - laceration S36.113
    - major (stellate) S36.116
    - minor S36.114
    - moderate S36.115
  - specified NEC S36.118
- lower back S39.92
  - specified NEC S39.82
- lumbar, lumbosacral (region) S39.92
  - plexus —*see* Injury, lumbosacral plexus
- lumbosacral plexus S34.4
- lung —*see also* Injury, intrathoracic, lung
  - aspiration J69.0
  - dabbing (related) U07.0
  - electronic cigarette (related) U07.0
  - EVALI - [e-cigarette, or vaping product use associated] U07.0
  - transfusion-related (TRALI) J95.84
  - vaping (associated) (device) (product) (use) V07.0
- lymphatic thoracic duct —*see* Injury, intrathoracic, specified organ NEC
- malar region S09.93
- mastoid region S09.90
- maxilla S09.93
- mediastinum —*see* Injury, intrathoracic, specified organ NEC
- membrane, brain —*see* Injury, intracranial

Injury *(continued)*
- meningeal artery —*see* Injury, intracranial, subdural hemorrhage
- meninges (cerebral) —*see* Injury, intracranial
- mesenteric
  - artery
    - branch S35.299
      - laceration (minor) (superficial) S35.291
        - major S35.292
      - specified NEC S35.298
    - inferior S35.239
      - laceration (minor) (superficial) S35.231
        - major S35.232
      - specified NEC S35.238
    - superior S35.229
      - laceration (minor) (superficial) S35.221
        - major S35.222
      - specified NEC S35.228
  - plexus (inferior) (superior) —*see* Injury, nerve, lumbosacral, sympathetic
  - vein
    - inferior S35.349
      - laceration S35.341
      - specified NEC S35.348
    - superior S35.339
      - laceration S35.331
      - specified NEC S35.338
- mesentery —*see* Injury, intra-abdominal, specified site NEC
- mesosalpinx —*see* Injury, pelvic organ, specified site NEC
- middle ear S09.30-
- midthoracic region NOS S29.9
- mouth S09.93
- multiple NOS T07
- muscle (and fascia) (and tendon)
  - abdomen S39.001
    - laceration S39.021
    - specified type NEC S39.091
    - strain S39.011
  - abductor
    - thumb, forearm level —*see* Injury, muscle, thumb, abductor
  - adductor
    - thigh S76.20-
      - laceration S76.22-
      - specified type NEC S76.29-
      - strain S76.21-
  - ankle —*see* Injury, muscle, foot
  - anterior muscle group, at leg level (lower) S86.20-
    - laceration S86.22-
    - specified type NEC S86.29-
    - strain S86.21-
  - arm (upper) —*see* Injury, muscle, shoulder
  - biceps (parts NEC) S46.20-
    - laceration S46.22-
    - long head S46.10-
      - laceration S46.12-
      - strain S46.11-
      - specified type NEC S46.19-
    - specified type NEC S46.29-
    - strain S46.21-
  - extensor
    - finger(s) (other than thumb) —*see* Injury, muscle, finger by site, extensor
    - forearm level, specified NEC —*see* Injury, muscle, forearm, extensor
    - thumb —*see* Injury, muscle, thumb, extensor

Injury *(continued)*
- muscle *(continued)*
  - extensor *(continued)*
    - toe (large) (ankle level) (foot level) —*see* Injury, muscle, toe, extensor
  - finger
    - extensor (forearm level) S56.40-
      - hand level S66.309
        - laceration S66.329
        - specified type NEC S66.399
        - strain S66.319
      - laceration S56.429
      - specified type NEC S56.499
      - strain S56.419
    - flexor (forearm level) S56.10-
      - hand level S66.109
        - laceration S66.129
        - specified type NEC S66.199
        - strain S66.119
      - laceration S56.129
      - specified type NEC S56.199
      - strain S56.119
    - intrinsic S66.509
      - laceration S66.529
      - specified type NEC S66.599
      - strain S66.519
    - index
      - extensor (forearm level)
        - hand level S66.308
          - laceration S66.32-
          - specified type NEC S66.39-
          - strain S66.31-
        - specified type NEC S56.492-
      - flexor (forearm level)
        - hand level S66.108
          - laceration S66.12-
          - specified type NEC S66.19-
          - strain S66.11-
        - specified type NEC S56.19-
        - strain S56.11-
      - intrinsic S66.50-
        - laceration S66.52-
        - specified type NEC S66.59-
        - strain S66.51-
    - little
      - extensor (forearm level)
        - hand level S66.30-
          - laceration S66.32-
          - specified type NEC S66.39-
          - strain S66.31-
        - laceration S56.42-
        - specified type NEC S56.49-
        - strain S56.41-
      - flexor (forearm level)
        - hand level S66.10-
          - laceration S66.12-
          - specified type NEC S66.19-
          - strain S66.11-
        - laceration S56.12-
        - specified type NEC S56.19-
        - strain S56.11-
      - intrinsic S66.50-
        - laceration S66.52-
        - specified type NEC S66.59-
        - strain S66.51-

Injury *(continued)*
- muscle *(continued)*
  - finger *(continued)*
    - middle
      - extensor (forearm level)
        - hand level S66.30-
          - laceration S66.32-
          - specified type NEC S66.39-
          - strain S66.31-
        - laceration S56.42-
        - specified type NEC S56.49-
        - strain S56.41-
      - flexor (forearm level)
        - hand level S66.10-
          - laceration S66.12-
          - specified type NEC S66.19-
          - strain S66.11-
        - laceration S56.12-
        - specified type NEC S56.19-
        - strain S56.11-
      - intrinsic S66.50-
        - laceration S66.52-
        - specified type NEC S66.59-
        - strain S66.51-
    - ring
      - extensor (forearm level)
        - hand level S66.30-
          - laceration S66.32-
          - specified type NEC S66.39-
          - strain S66.31-
        - laceration S56.42-
        - specified type NEC S56.49-
        - strain S56.41-
      - flexor (forearm level)
        - hand level S66.10-
          - laceration S66.12-
          - specified type NEC S66.19-
          - strain S66.11-
        - laceration S56.12-
        - specified type NEC S56.19-
        - strain S56.11-
      - intrinsic S66.50-
        - laceration S66.52-
        - specified type NEC S66.59-
        - strain S66.51-
  - flexor
    - finger(s) (other than thumb) —*see* Injury, muscle, finger
    - forearm level, specified NEC —*see* Injury, muscle, forearm, flexor
    - thumb —*see* Injury, muscle, thumb, flexor
    - toe (long) (ankle level) (foot level) —*see* Injury, muscle, toe, flexor
  - foot S96.90-
    - intrinsic S96.20-
      - laceration S96.22-
      - specified type NEC S96.29-
      - strain S96.21-
    - laceration S96.92-
    - long extensor, toe —*see* Injury, muscle, toe, extensor
    - long flexor, toe —*see* Injury, muscle, toe, flexor

Injury *(continued)*
- muscle *(continued)*
  - foot *(continued)*
    - specified
      - site NEC S96.80-
        - laceration S96.82-
        - specified type NEC S96.89-
        - strain S96.81-
      - type NEC S96.99-
    - strain S96.91-
  - forearm (level) S56.90-
    - extensor S56.50-
      - laceration S56.52-
      - specified type NEC S56.59-
      - strain S56.51-
    - flexor S56.20-
      - laceration S56.22-
      - specified type NEC S56.29-
      - strain S56.21-
    - laceration S56.92-
    - specified S56.99-
      - site NEC S56.80-
        - laceration S56.82-
        - strain S56.81-
      - type NEC S56.89-
    - strain S56.91-
  - hand (level) S66.90-
    - laceration S66.92-
    - specified
      - site NEC S66.80-
        - laceration S66.82-
        - specified type NEC S66.89-
        - strain S66.81-
      - type NEC S66.99-
    - strain S66.91-
  - head S09.10
    - laceration S09.12
    - specified type NEC S09.19
    - strain S09.11
  - hip NEC S76.00-
    - laceration S76.02-
    - specified type NEC S76.09-
    - strain S76.01-
  - intrinsic
    - ankle and foot level —*see* Injury, muscle, foot, intrinsic
    - finger (other than thumb) —*see* Injury, muscle, finger by site, intrinsic
    - foot (level) —*see* Injury, muscle, foot, intrinsic
    - thumb —*see* Injury, muscle, thumb, intrinsic
  - leg (level) (lower) S86.90-
    - Achilles tendon —*see* Injury, Achilles tendon
    - anterior muscle group —*see* Injury, muscle, anterior muscle group
    - laceration S86.92-
    - peroneal muscle group —*see* Injury, muscle, peroneal muscle group
    - posterior muscle group —*see* Injury, muscle, posterior muscle group, leg level
    - specified
      - site NEC S86.80-
        - laceration S86.82-
        - specified type NEC S86.89-
        - strain S86.81-
      - type NEC S86.99-
    - strain S86.91-
  - long
    - extensor toe, at ankle and foot level —*see* Injury, muscle, toe, extensor

Injury *(continued)*
- muscle *(continued)*
  - long *(continued)*
    - flexor, toe, at ankle and foot level —*see* Injury, muscle, toe, flexor
    - head, biceps —*see* Injury, muscle, biceps, long head
  - lower back S39.002
    - laceration S39.022
    - specified type NEC S39.092
    - strain S39.012
  - neck (level) S16.9
    - laceration S16.2
    - specified type NEC S16.8
    - strain S16.1
  - pelvis S39.003
    - laceration S39.023
    - specified type NEC S39.093
    - strain S39.013
  - peroneal muscle group, at leg level (lower) S86.30-
    - laceration S86.32-
    - specified type NEC S86.39-
    - strain S86.31-
  - posterior muscle (group)
    - leg level (lower) S86.10-
      - laceration S86.12-
      - specified type NEC S86.19-
      - strain S86.11-
    - thigh level S76.30-
      - laceration S76.32-
      - specified type NEC S76.39-
      - strain S76.31-
  - quadriceps (thigh) S76.10-
    - laceration S76.12-
    - specified type NEC S76.19-
    - strain S76.11-
  - shoulder S46.90-
    - laceration S46.92-
    - rotator cuff —*see* Injury, rotator cuff
    - specified site NEC S46.80-
      - laceration S46.82-
      - strain S46.81-
      - specified type NEC S46.89-
    - strain S46.91-
    - specified type NEC S46.99-
  - thigh NEC (level) S76.90-
    - adductor —*see* Injury, muscle, adductor, thigh
    - laceration S76.92-
    - posterior muscle (group) —*see* Injury, muscle, posterior muscle, thigh level
    - quadriceps —*see* Injury, muscle, quadriceps
    - specified
      - site NEC S76.80-
        - laceration S76.82-
        - specified type NEC S76.89-
        - strain S76.81-
      - type NEC S76.99-
    - strain S76.91-
  - thorax (level) S29.009
    - back wall S29.002
    - front wall S29.001
    - laceration S29.029
      - back wall S29.022
      - front wall S29.021
    - specified type NEC S29.099
      - back wall S29.092
      - front wall S29.091
    - strain S29.019
      - back wall S29.012
      - front wall S29.011

- **Injury** *(continued)*
  - nerve NEC *(continued)*
    - pneumogastric *—see* Injury, nerve, vagus
    - radial (forearm level) S54.2-
      - hand (level) S64.2-
      - upper arm (level) S44.2-
      - wrist (level) *—see* Injury, nerve, radial, hand
    - root *—see* Injury, nerve, spinal, root
    - sacral plexus *—see* Injury, lumbosacral plexus
    - sacral spinal
      - peripheral S34.6
      - root S34.22
      - sympathetic S34.5
    - sciatic (hip level) (thigh level) S74.0-
    - second cranial (optic) *—see* Injury, nerve, optic
    - seventh cranial (facial) *—see* Injury, nerve, facial
    - shoulder *—see* Injury, nerve, arm
    - sixth cranial (abducent) *—see* Injury, nerve, abducens
    - spinal
      - plexus *—see* Injury, nerve, plexus, spinal
      - root
        - cervical S14.2
        - dorsal S24.2
        - lumbar S34.21
        - sacral S34.22
        - thoracic *—see* Injury, nerve, spinal, root, dorsal
    - splanchnic *—see* Injury, nerve, lumbosacral, sympathetic
    - sympathetic NEC *—see* Injury, nerve, lumbosacral, sympathetic
      - cervical *—see* Injury, nerve, cervical sympathetic
    - tenth cranial (pneumogastric or vagus) *—see* Injury, nerve, vagus
    - thigh (level) *—see* Injury, nerve, hip
      - cutaneous sensory *—see* Injury, nerve, cutaneous sensory, hip
      - femoral *—see* Injury, nerve, femoral
      - sciatic *—see* Injury, nerve, sciatic
      - specified NEC *—see* Injury, nerve, hip
    - third cranial (oculomotor) *—see* Injury, nerve, oculomotor
    - thorax S24.9
      - peripheral S24.3
      - specified site NEC S24.8
      - sympathetic S24.4
    - thumb, digital *—see* Injury, nerve, digital, thumb
    - tibial (lower leg level) (posterior) S84.0-
    - toe *—see* Injury, nerve, ankle
    - trigeminal S04.3-
      - contusion S04.3-
      - laceration S04.3-
      - specified type NEC S04.3-
    - trochlear S04.2-
      - contusion S04.2-
      - laceration S04.2-
      - specified type NEC S04.2-
    - twelfth cranial (hypoglossal) *—see* Injury, nerve, hypoglossal
    - ulnar (forearm level) S54.0-
      - arm (upper) (level) S44.0-
      - hand (level) S64.0-

- **Injury** *(continued)*
  - nerve NEC *(continued)*
    - ulnar *(continued)*
      - wrist (level) *—see* Injury, nerve, ulnar, hand
    - vagus S04.89-
      - specified type NEC S04.89-
    - wrist (level) *—see* Injury, nerve, hand
  - ninth cranial nerve (glossopharyngeal) *—see* Injury, nerve, glossopharyngeal
  - nose (septum) S09.92
  - obstetrical O71.9
    - specified NEC O71.89
  - occipital (region) (scalp) S09.90
    - lobe *—see* Injury, intracranial
  - optic chiasm S04.02
  - optic radiation S04.03-
  - optic tract and pathways S04.03-
  - orbit, orbital (region) *—see* Injury, eye
    - penetrating (with foreign body) *—see* Injury, eye, orbit, penetrating
    - specified NEC *—see* Injury, eye, specified site NEC
  - ovary, ovarian S37.409
    - bilateral S37.402
      - contusion S37.422
      - laceration S37.432
      - specified type NEC S37.492
    - blood vessel *—see* Injury, blood vessel, ovarian
    - contusion S37.429
      - bilateral S37.422
      - unilateral S37.421
    - laceration S37.439
      - bilateral S37.432
      - unilateral S37.431
    - specified type NEC S37.499
      - bilateral S37.492
      - unilateral S37.491
    - unilateral S37.401
      - contusion S37.421
      - laceration S37.431
      - specified type NEC S37.491
  - palate (hard) (soft) S09.93
  - pancreas S36.209
    - body S36.201
      - contusion S36.221
      - laceration S36.231
        - major S36.261
        - minor S36.241
        - moderate S36.251
      - specified type NEC S36.291
    - contusion S36.229
    - head S36.200
      - contusion S36.220
      - laceration S36.230
        - major S36.260
        - minor S36.240
        - moderate S36.250
      - specified type NEC S36.290
    - laceration S36.239
      - major S36.269
      - minor S36.249
      - moderate S36.259
    - specified type NEC S36.299
    - tail S36.202
      - contusion S36.222
      - laceration S36.232
        - major S36.262
        - minor S36.242
        - moderate S36.252
      - specified type NEC S36.292
  - parietal (region) (scalp) S09.90
    - lobe *—see* Injury, intracranial
  - patellar ligament (tendon) S76.10-
    - laceration S76.12-
    - specified NEC S76.19-

- **Injury** *(continued)*
  - patellar ligament *(continued)*
    - strain S76.11-
  - pelvis, pelvic (floor) S39.93
    - complicating delivery O70.1
    - joint or ligament, complicating delivery O71.6
    - organ S37.90
      - with ectopic or molar pregnancy O08.6
      - complication of abortion *—see* Abortion
      - contusion S37.92
      - following ectopic or molar pregnancy O08.6
      - laceration S37.93
      - obstetrical trauma NEC O71.5
      - specified
        - site NEC S37.899
          - contusion S37.892
          - laceration S37.893
          - specified type NEC S37.898
        - type NEC S37.99
    - specified NEC S39.83
  - penis S39.94
  - perineum S39.94
  - peritoneum S36.81
    - laceration S36.893
  - periurethral tissue *—see* Injury, urethra
    - complicating delivery O71.82
  - phalanges
    - foot *—see* Injury, foot
    - hand *—see* Injury, hand
  - pharynx NEC S19.85
  - pleura *—see* Injury, intrathoracic, pleura
  - plexus
    - brachial *—see* Injury, brachial plexus
    - cardiac *—see* Injury, nerve, thorax, sympathetic
    - celiac, coeliac *—see* Injury, nerve, lumbosacral, sympathetic
    - esophageal *—see* Injury, nerve, thorax, sympathetic
    - hypogastric *—see* Injury, nerve, lumbosacral, sympathetic
    - lumbar, lumbosacral *—see* Injury, lumbosacral plexus
    - mesenteric *—see* Injury, nerve, lumbosacral, sympathetic
    - pulmonary *—see* Injury, nerve, thorax, sympathetic
  - postcardiac surgery (syndrome) I97.0
  - prepuce S39.94
  - pressure
    - injury *—see* Ulcer, pressure, by site
  - prostate S37.829
    - contusion S37.822
    - laceration S37.823
    - specified type NEC S37.828
  - pubic region S39.94
  - pudendum S39.94
  - pulmonary plexus *—see* Injury, nerve, thorax, sympathetic
  - rectovaginal septum NEC S39.83
  - rectum *—see* Injury, intestine, large, rectum
  - retina *—see* Injury, eye, specified site NEC
    - penetrating *—see* Injury, eyeball, penetrating
  - retroperitoneal *—see* Injury, intra-abdominal, specified site NEC
  - rotator cuff (muscle(s)) (tendon(s)) S46.00-

- **Injury** *(continued)*
  - rotator cuff *(continued)*
    - laceration S46.02-
    - specified type NEC S46.09-
    - strain S46.01-
  - round ligament *—see* Injury, pelvic organ, specified site NEC
  - sacral plexus *—see* Injury, lumbosacral plexus
  - salivary duct or gland S09.93
  - scalp S09.90
    - newborn (birth injury) P12.9
      - due to monitoring (electrode) (sampling incision) P12.4
      - specified NEC P12.89
        - caput succedaneum P12.81
  - scapular region *—see* Injury, shoulder
  - sclera *—see* Injury, eye, specified site NEC
    - penetrating *—see* Injury, eyeball, penetrating
  - scrotum S39.94
  - second cranial nerve (optic) *—see* Injury, nerve, optic
  - self-inflicted, without suicidal intent R45.88
  - seminal vesicle *—see* Injury, pelvic organ, specified site NEC
  - seventh cranial nerve (facial) *—see* Injury, nerve, facial
  - shoulder S49.9-
    - blood vessel *—see* Injury, blood vessel, arm
    - contusion *—see* Contusion, shoulder
    - dislocation *—see* Dislocation, shoulder
    - fracture *—see* Fracture, shoulder
  - shoulder S49.9-
    - muscle *—see* Injury, muscle, shoulder
    - nerve *—see* Injury, nerve, shoulder
    - open *—see* Wound, open, shoulder
    - specified type NEC S49.8-
    - sprain *—see* Sprain, shoulder girdle
    - superficial *—see* Injury, superficial, shoulder
  - sinus
    - cavernous *—see* Injury, intracranial
    - nasal S09.92
  - sixth cranial nerve (abducent) *—see* Injury, nerve, abducens
  - skeleton, birth injury P13.9
    - specified part NEC P13.8
  - skin NEC T14.8
    - surface intact *—see* Injury, superficial
  - skull NEC S09.90
  - specified NEC T14.8
  - spermatic cord (pelvic region) S37.898
    - scrotal region S39.848
  - spinal (cord)
    - cervical (neck) S14.109
      - anterior cord syndrome S14.139
        - C1 level S14.131
        - C2 level S14.132
        - C3 level S14.133
        - C4 level S14.134
        - C5 level S14.135
        - C6 level S14.136
        - C7 level S14.137
        - C8 level S14.138

Injury *(continued)*
- spinal *(continued)*
  - cervical *(continued)*
    - Brown-Séquard syndrome S14.149
      - C1 level S14.141
      - C2 level S14.142
      - C3 level S14.143
      - C4 level S14.144
      - C5 level S14.145
      - C6 level S14.146
      - C7 level S14.147
      - C8 level S14.148
    - C1 level S14.101
    - C2 level S14.102
    - C3 level S14.103
    - C4 level S14.104
    - C5 level S14.105
    - C6 level S14.106
    - C7 level S14.107
    - C8 level S14.108
    - central cord syndrome S14.129
      - C1 level S14.121
      - C2 level S14.122
      - C3 level S14.123
      - C4 level S14.124
      - C5 level S14.125
      - C6 level S14.126
      - C7 level S14.127
      - C8 level S14.128
    - complete lesion S14.119
      - C1 level S14.111
      - C2 level S14.112
      - C3 level S14.113
      - C4 level S14.114
      - C5 level S14.115
      - C6 level S14.116
      - C7 level S14.117
      - C8 level S14.118
    - concussion S14.0
    - edema S14.0
    - incomplete lesion specified NEC S14.159
      - C1 level S14.151
      - C2 level S14.152
      - C3 level S14.153
      - C4 level S14.154
      - C5 level S14.155
      - C6 level S14.156
      - C7 level S14.157
      - C8 level S14.158
    - posterior cord syndrome S14.159
      - C1 level S14.151
      - C2 level S14.152
      - C3 level S14.153
      - C4 level S14.154
      - C5 level S14.155
      - C6 level S14.156
      - C7 level S14.157
      - C8 level S14.158
  - dorsal —*see* Injury, spinal, thoracic
  - lumbar S34.109
    - complete lesion S34.119
      - L1 level S34.111
      - L2 level S34.112
      - L3 level S34.113
      - L4 level S34.114
      - L5 level S34.115
    - concussion S34.01
    - edema S34.01
    - incomplete lesion S34.129
      - L1 level S34.121
      - L2 level S34.122
      - L3 level S34.123
      - L4 level S34.124
      - L5 level S34.125
    - L1 level S34.101
    - L2 level S34.102
    - L3 level S34.103

Injury *(continued)*
- spinal *(continued)*
  - lumbar *(continued)*
    - L4 level S34.104
    - L5 level S34.105
  - nerve root NEC
    - cervical —*see* Injury, nerve, spinal, root, cervical
    - dorsal —*see* Injury, nerve, spinal, root, dorsal
    - lumbar S34.21
    - sacral S34.22
    - thoracic —*see* Injury, nerve, spinal, root, dorsal
  - plexus
    - brachial —*see* Injury, brachial plexus
    - lumbosacral —*see* Injury, lumbosacral plexus
  - sacral S34.139
    - complete lesion S34.131
    - incomplete lesion S34.132
  - thoracic S24.109
    - anterior cord syndrome S24.139
      - T1 level S24.131
      - T2-T6 level S24.132
      - T7-T10 level S24.133
      - T11-T12 level S24.134
    - Brown-Séquard syndrome S24.149
      - T1 level S24.141
      - T2-T6 level S24.142
      - T7-T10 level S24.143
      - T11-T12 level S24.144
    - complete lesion S24.119
      - T1 level S24.111
      - T2-T6 level S24.112
      - T7-T10 level S24.113
      - T11-T12 level S24.114
    - concussion S24.0
    - edema S24.0
    - incomplete lesion specified NEC S24.159
      - T1 level S24.151
      - T2-T6 level S24.152
      - T7-T10 level S24.153
      - T11-T12 level S24.154
    - posterior cord syndrome S24.159
      - T1 level S24.151
      - T2-T6 level S24.152
      - T7-T10 level S24.153
      - T11-T12 level S24.154
    - T1 level S24.101
    - T2-T6 level S24.102
    - T7-T10 level S24.103
    - T11-T12 level S24.104
- splanchnic nerve —*see* Injury, nerve, lumbosacral, sympathetic
- spleen S36.00
  - contusion S36.029
    - major S36.021
    - minor S36.020
  - laceration S36.039
    - major (massive) (stellate) S36.032
    - moderate S36.031
    - superficial (capsular) (minor) S36.030
  - specified type NEC S36.09
- splenic artery —*see* Injury, blood vessel, celiac artery, branch
- stellate ganglion —*see* Injury, nerve, thorax, sympathetic
- sternal region S29.9
- stomach S36.30
  - contusion S36.32
  - laceration S36.33
  - specified type NEC S36.39

Injury *(continued)*
- subconjunctival —*see* Injury, eye, conjunctiva
- subcutaneous NEC T14.8
- submaxillary region S09.93
- submental region S09.93
- subungual
  - fingers —*see* Injury, hand
  - toes —*see* Injury, foot
- superficial NEC T14.8
  - abdomen, abdominal (wall) S30.92
    - abrasion S30.811
    - bite S30.871
      - insect S30.861
    - contusion S30.1
    - external constriction S30.841
    - foreign body S30.851
  - abrasion —*see* Abrasion, by site
  - adnexa, eye NEC —*see* Injury, eye, specified site NEC
  - alveolar process —*see* Injury, superficial, oral cavity
  - ankle S90.91-
    - abrasion —*see* Abrasion, ankle
    - blister —*see* Blister, ankle
    - bite —*see* Bite, ankle
    - contusion —*see* Contusion, ankle
    - external constriction —*see* Constriction, external, ankle
    - foreign body —*see* Foreign body, superficial, ankle
  - anus S30.98
  - arm (upper) S40.92-
    - abrasion —*see* Abrasion, arm
    - bite —*see* Bite, superficial, arm
    - blister —*see* Blister, arm (upper)
    - contusion —*see* Contusion, arm
    - external constriction —*see* Constriction, external, arm
    - foreign body —*see* Foreign body, superficial, arm
  - auditory canal (external) (meatus) —*see* Injury, superficial, ear
  - auricle —*see* Injury, superficial, ear
  - axilla —*see* Injury, superficial, arm
  - back —*see also* Injury, superficial, thorax, back
    - lower S30.91
      - abrasion S30.810
      - contusion S30.0
      - external constriction S30.840
      - superficial
        - bite NEC S30.870
          - insect S30.860
        - foreign body S30.850
  - bite NEC —*see* Bite, superficial NEC, by site
  - blister —*see* Blister, by site
  - breast S20.10-
    - abrasion —*see* Abrasion, breast
    - bite —*see* Bite, superficial, breast
    - contusion —*see* Contusion, breast
    - external constriction —*see* Constriction, external, breast
    - foreign body —*see* Foreign body, superficial, breast

Injury *(continued)*
- superficial NEC *(continued)*
  - brow —*see* Injury, superficial, head, specified NEC
  - buttock S30.91
  - calf —*see* Injury, superficial, leg
  - canthus, eye —*see* Injury, superficial, periocular area
  - cheek (external) —*see* Injury, superficial, head, specified NEC
    - internal —*see* Injury, superficial, oral cavity
  - chest wall —*see* Injury, superficial, thorax
  - chin —*see* Injury, superficial, head NEC
  - clitoris S30.95
  - conjunctiva —*see* Injury, eye, conjunctiva
    - with foreign body (in conjunctival sac) —*see* Foreign body, conjunctival sac
  - contusion —*see* Contusion, by site
  - costal region —*see* Injury, superficial, thorax
  - digit(s)
    - hand —*see* Injury, superficial, finger
  - ear (auricle) (canal) (external) S00.40-
    - abrasion —*see* Abrasion, ear
    - bite —*see* Bite, superficial, ear
    - contusion —*see* Contusion, ear
    - external constriction —*see* Constriction, external, ear
    - foreign body —*see* Foreign body, superficial, ear
  - elbow S50.90-
    - abrasion —*see* Abrasion, elbow
    - bite —*see* Bite, superficial, elbow
    - blister —*see* Blister, elbow
    - contusion —*see* Contusion, elbow
    - external constriction —*see* Constriction, external, elbow
    - foreign body —*see* Foreign body, superficial, elbow
  - epididymis S30.94
  - epigastric region S30.92
  - epiglottis —*see* Injury, superficial, throat
  - esophagus
    - cervical —*see* Injury, superficial, throat
  - external constriction —*see* Constriction, external, by site
  - extremity NEC T14.8
  - eyeball NEC —*see* Injury, eye, specified site NEC
  - eyebrow —*see* Injury, superficial, periocular area
  - eyelid S00.20-
    - abrasion —*see* Abrasion, eyelid
    - bite —*see* Bite, superficial, eyelid
    - contusion —*see* Contusion, eyelid
    - external constriction —*see* Constriction, external, eyelid
    - foreign body —*see* Foreign body, superficial, eyelid

Injury *(continued)*
- superficial NEC *(continued)*
  - face NEC —*see* Injury, superficial, head, specified NEC
  - finger(s) S60.949
    - abrasion —*see* Abrasion, finger
    - bite —*see* Bite, superficial, finger
    - blister —*see* Blister, finger
    - contusion —*see* Contusion, finger
    - external constriction —*see* Constriction, external, finger
    - foreign body —*see* Foreign body, superficial, finger
    - insect bite —*see* Bite, by site, superficial, insect
    - index S60.94-
    - little S60.94-
    - middle S60.94-
    - ring S60.94-
  - flank S30.92
  - foot S90.92-
    - abrasion —*see* Abrasion, foot
    - bite —*see* Bite, foot
    - blister —*see* Blister, foot
    - contusion —*see* Contusion, foot
    - external constriction —*see* Constriction, external, foot
    - foreign body —*see* Foreign body, superficial, foot
  - forearm S50.91-
    - abrasion —*see* Abrasion, forearm
    - bite —*see* Bite, forearm, superficial
    - blister —*see* Blister, forearm
    - contusion —*see* Contusion, forearm
    - elbow only —*see* Injury, superficial, elbow
    - external constriction —*see* Constriction, external, forearm
    - foreign body —*see* Foreign body, superficial, forearm
  - forehead —*see* Injury, superficial, head NEC
  - foreign body —*see* Foreign body, superficial
  - genital organs, external
    - female S30.97
    - male S30.96
  - globe (eye) —*see* Injury, eye, specified site NEC
  - groin S30.92
  - gum —*see* Injury, superficial, oral cavity
  - hand S60.92-
    - abrasion —*see* Abrasion, hand
    - bite —*see* Bite, superficial, hand
    - contusion —*see* Contusion, hand
    - external constriction —*see* Constriction, external, hand
    - foreign body —*see* Foreign body, superficial, hand
  - head S00.90
    - ear —*see* Injury, superficial, ear
    - eyelid —*see* Injury, superficial, eyelid
    - nose S00.30
    - oral cavity S00.502
    - scalp S00.00

Injury *(continued)*
- superficial NEC *(continued)*
  - head *(continued)*
    - specified site NEC S00.80
  - heel —*see* Injury, superficial, foot
  - hip S70.91-
    - abrasion —*see* Abrasion, hip
    - bite —*see* Bite, superficial, hip
    - blister —*see* Blister, hip
    - contusion —*see* Contusion, hip
    - external constriction —*see* Constriction, external, hip
    - foreign body —*see* Foreign body, superficial, hip
  - iliac region —*see* Injury, superficial, abdomen
  - inguinal region —*see* Injury, superficial, abdomen
  - insect bite —*see* Bite, by site, superficial, insect
  - interscapular region —*see* Injury, superficial, thorax, back
  - jaw —*see* Injury, superficial, head, specified NEC
  - knee S80.91-
    - abrasion —*see* Abrasion, knee
    - bite —*see* Bite, superficial, knee
    - blister —*see* Blister, knee
    - contusion —*see* Contusion, knee
    - external constriction —*see* Constriction, external, knee
    - foreign body —*see* Foreign body, superficial, knee
  - labium (majus) (minus) S30.95
  - lacrimal (apparatus) (gland) (sac) —*see* Injury, eye, specified site NEC
  - larynx —*see* Injury, superficial, throat
  - leg (lower) S80.92-
    - abrasion —*see* Abrasion, leg
    - bite —*see* Bite, superficial, leg
    - contusion —*see* Contusion, leg
    - external constriction —*see* Constriction, external, leg
    - foreign body —*see* Foreign body, superficial, leg
    - knee —*see* Injury, superficial, knee
  - limb NEC T14.8
  - lip S00.501
  - lower back S30.91
  - lumbar region S30.91
  - malar region —*see* Injury, superficial, head, specified NEC
  - mammary —*see* Injury, superficial, breast
  - mastoid region —*see* Injury, superficial, head, specified NEC
  - mouth —*see* Injury, superficial, oral cavity
  - muscle NEC T14.8
  - nail NEC T14.8
    - finger —*see* Injury, superficial, finger
    - toe —*see* Injury, superficial, toe
  - nasal (septum) —*see* Injury, superficial, nose
  - neck S10.90
    - specified site NEC S10.80
  - nose (septum) S00.30
  - occipital region —*see* Injury, superficial, scalp

Injury *(continued)*
- superficial NEC *(continued)*
  - oral cavity S00.502
  - orbital region —*see* Injury, superficial, periocular area
  - palate —*see* Injury, superficial, oral cavity
  - palm —*see* Injury, superficial, hand
  - parietal region —*see* Injury, superficial, scalp
  - pelvis S30.91
    - girdle —*see* Injury, superficial, hip
  - penis S30.93
  - perineum
    - female S30.95
    - male S30.91
  - periocular area S00.20-
    - abrasion —*see* Abrasion, eyelid
    - bite —*see* Bite, superficial, eyelid
    - contusion —*see* Contusion, eyelid
    - external constriction —*see* Constriction, external, eyelid
    - foreign body —*see* Foreign body, superficial, eyelid
  - phalanges
    - finger —*see* Injury, superficial, finger
    - toe —*see* Injury, superficial, toe
  - pharynx —*see* Injury, superficial, throat
  - pinna —*see* Injury, superficial, ear
  - popliteal space —*see* Injury, superficial, knee
  - prepuce S30.93
  - pubic region S30.91
  - pudendum
    - female S30.97
    - male S30.96
  - sacral region S30.91
  - scalp S00.00
  - scapular region —*see* Injury, superficial, shoulder
  - sclera —*see* Injury, eye, specified site NEC
  - scrotum S30.94
  - shin —*see* Injury, superficial, leg
  - shoulder S40.91-
    - abrasion —*see* Abrasion, shoulder
    - bite —*see* Bite, superficial, shoulder
    - blister —*see* Blister, shoulder
    - contusion —*see* Contusion, shoulder
    - external constriction —*see* Constriction, external, shoulder
    - foreign body —*see* Foreign body, superficial, shoulder
  - skin NEC T14.8
  - sternal region —*see* Injury, superficial, thorax, front
  - subconjunctival —*see* Injury, eye, specified site NEC
  - subcutaneous NEC T14.8
  - submaxillary region —*see* Injury, superficial, head, specified NEC
  - submental region —*see* Injury, superficial, head, specified NEC

Injury *(continued)*
- superficial NEC *(continued)*
  - subungual
    - finger(s) —*see* Injury, superficial, finger
    - toe(s) —*see* Injury, superficial, toe
  - supraclavicular fossa —*see* Injury, superficial, neck
  - supraorbital —*see* Injury, superficial, head, specified NEC
  - temple —*see* Injury, superficial, head, specified NEC
  - temporal region —*see* Injury, superficial, head, specified NEC
  - testis S30.94
  - thigh S70.92-
    - abrasion —*see* Abrasion, thigh
    - bite —*see* Bite, superficial, thigh
    - blister —*see* Blister, thigh
    - contusion —*see* Contusion, thigh
    - external constriction —*see* Constriction, external, thigh
    - foreign body —*see* Foreign body, superficial, thigh
  - thorax, thoracic (wall) S20.90
    - abrasion —*see* Abrasion, thorax
    - back S20.40-
    - bite —*see* Bite, thorax, superficial
    - blister —*see* Blister, thorax
    - contusion —*see* Contusion, thorax
    - external constriction —*see* Constriction, external, thorax
    - foreign body —*see* Foreign body, superficial, thorax
    - front S20.30-
  - throat S10.10
    - abrasion S10.11
    - bite S10.17
      - insect S10.16
    - blister S10.12
    - contusion S10.0
    - external constriction S10.14
    - foreign body S10.15
  - thumb S60.93-
    - abrasion —*see* Abrasion, thumb
    - bite —*see* Bite, superficial, thumb
    - blister —*see* Blister, thumb
    - contusion —*see* Contusion, thumb
    - external constriction —*see* Constriction, external, thumb
    - foreign body —*see* Foreign body, superficial, thumb
    - insect bite —*see* Bite, by site, superficial, insect
    - specified type NEC S60.39-
  - toe(s) S90.93-
    - abrasion —*see* Abrasion, toe
    - bite —*see* Bite, toe
    - blister —*see* Blister, toe
    - contusion —*see* Contusion, toe
    - external constriction —*see* Constriction, external, toe
    - foreign body —*see* Foreign body, superficial, toe
    - great S90.93-

Injury *(continued)*
- superficial NEC *(continued)*
  - tongue —*see* Injury, superficial, oral cavity
  - tooth, teeth —*see* Injury, superficial, oral cavity
  - trachea S10.10
  - tunica vaginalis S30.94
  - tympanum, tympanic membrane —*see* Injury, superficial, ear
  - uvula —*see* Injury, superficial, oral cavity
  - vagina S30.95
  - vocal cords —*see* Injury, superficial, throat
  - vulva S30.95
  - wrist S60.91-
- supraclavicular region —*see* Injury, neck
- supraorbital S09.93
- suprarenal gland (multiple) —*see* Injury, adrenal
- surgical complication (external or internal site) —*see* Laceration, accidental complicating surgery
- temple S09.90
- temporal region S09.90
- tendon —*see also* Injury, muscle, by site
  - abdomen —*see* Injury, muscle, abdomen
  - Achilles —*see* Injury, Achilles tendon
  - lower back —*see* Injury, muscle, lower back
  - pelvic organs —*see* Injury, muscle, pelvis
- tenth cranial nerve (pneumogastric or vagus) —*see* Injury, nerve, vagus
- testis S39.94
- thigh S79.92-
  - blood vessel —*see* Injury, blood vessel, hip
  - contusion —*see* Contusion, thigh
  - fracture —*see* Fracture, femur
  - muscle —*see* Injury, muscle, thigh
  - nerve —*see* Injury, nerve, thigh
  - open —*see* Wound, open, thigh
  - specified NEC S79.82-
  - superficial —*see* Injury, superficial, thigh
- third cranial nerve (oculomotor) —*see* Injury, nerve, oculomotor
- thorax, thoracic S29.9
  - blood vessel —*see* Injury, blood vessel, thorax
  - cavity —*see* Injury, intrathoracic
  - dislocation —*see* Dislocation, thorax
  - external (wall) S29.9
    - contusion —*see* Contusion, thorax
    - nerve —*see* Injury, nerve, thorax
    - open —*see* Wound, open, thorax
    - specified NEC S29.8
    - sprain —*see* Sprain, thorax
    - superficial —*see* Injury, superficial, thorax
  - fracture —*see* Fracture, thorax
  - internal —*see* Injury, intrathoracic
  - intrathoracic organ —*see* Injury, intrathoracic
  - sympathetic ganglion —*see* Injury, nerve, thorax, sympathetic
- throat (*see also* Injury, neck) S19.9

Injury *(continued)*
- thumb S69.9-
  - blood vessel —*see* Injury, blood vessel, thumb
  - contusion —*see* Contusion, thumb
  - dislocation —*see* Dislocation, thumb
  - fracture —*see* Fracture, thumb
  - muscle —*see* Injury, muscle, thumb
  - nerve —*see* Injury, nerve, digital, thumb
  - open —*see* Wound, open, thumb
  - specified NEC S69.8-
  - sprain —*see* Sprain, thumb
  - superficial —*see* Injury, superficial, thumb
- thymus (gland) —*see* Injury, intrathoracic, specified organ NEC
- thyroid (gland) NEC S19.84
- toe S99.92-
  - contusion —*see* Contusion, toe
  - dislocation —*see* Dislocation, toe
  - fracture —*see* Fracture, toe
  - muscle —*see* Injury, muscle, toe
  - open —*see* Wound, open, toe
  - specified type NEC S99.82-
  - sprain —*see* Sprain, toe
  - superficial —*see* Injury, superficial, toe
- tongue S09.93
- tonsil S09.93
- tooth S09.93
- trachea (cervical) NEC S19.82
  - thoracic —*see* Injury, intrathoracic, trachea, thoracic
- transfusion-related acute lung (TRALI) J95.84
- tunica vaginalis S39.94
- twelfth cranial nerve (hypoglossal) —*see* Injury, nerve, hypoglossal
- ureter S37.10
  - contusion S37.12
  - laceration S37.13
  - specified type NEC S37.19
- urethra (sphincter) S37.30
  - at delivery O71.5
  - contusion S37.32
  - laceration S37.33
  - specified type NEC S37.39
- urinary organ S37.90
  - contusion S37.92
  - laceration S37.93
  - specified
    - site NEC S37.899
      - contusion S37.892
      - laceration S37.893
      - specified type NEC S37.898
    - type NEC S37.99
- uterus, uterine S37.60
  - with ectopic or molar pregnancy O08.6
  - blood vessel —*see* Injury, blood vessel, iliac
  - contusion S37.62
  - laceration S37.63
    - cervix at delivery O71.3
  - rupture associated with obstetrics —*see* Rupture, uterus
  - specified type NEC S37.69
- uvula S09.93
- vagina S39.93
  - abrasion S30.814
  - bite S31.45
    - insect S30.864
    - superficial NEC S30.874
  - contusion S30.23
  - crush S38.03

Injury *(continued)*
- vagina *(continued)*
  - during delivery —*see* Laceration, vagina, during delivery
  - external constriction S30.844
  - insect bite S30.864
  - laceration S31.41
    - with foreign body S31.42
  - open wound S31.40
  - puncture S31.43
    - with foreign body S31.44
  - superficial S30.95
    - foreign body S30.854
- vas deferens —*see* Injury, pelvic organ, specified site NEC
- vascular NEC T14.8
- vein —*see* Injury, blood vessel
- vena cava (superior) S25.20
  - inferior S35.10
    - laceration (minor) (superficial) S35.11
      - major S35.12
    - specified type NEC S35.19
  - laceration (minor) (superficial) S25.21
    - major S25.22
  - specified type NEC S25.29
- vesical (sphincter) —*see* Injury, bladder
- visual cortex S04.04-
- vitreous (humor) S05.90
  - specified NEC S05.8X-
- vocal cord NEC S19.83
- vulva S39.94
  - abrasion S30.814
  - bite S31.45
    - insect S30.864
    - superficial NEC S30.874
  - contusion S30.23
  - crush S38.03
  - during delivery —*see* Laceration, perineum, female, during delivery
  - external constriction S30.844
  - insect bite S30.864
  - laceration S31.41
    - with foreign body S31.42
  - open wound S31.40
  - puncture S31.43
    - with foreign body S31.44
  - superficial S30.95
    - foreign body S30.854
- whiplash (cervical spine) S13.4
- wrist S69.9-
  - blood vessel —*see* Injury, blood vessel, hand
  - contusion —*see* Contusion, wrist
  - dislocation —*see* Dislocation, wrist
  - fracture —*see* Fracture, wrist
  - muscle —*see* Injury, muscle, hand
  - nerve —*see* Injury, nerve, hand
  - open —*see* Wound, open, wrist
  - specified NEC S69.8-
  - sprain —*see* Sprain, wrist
  - superficial —*see* Injury, superficial, wrist

Inoculation —*see also* Vaccination
- complication or reaction —*see* Complications, vaccination

Insanity, insane —*see also* Psychosis
- adolescent —*see* Schizophrenia
- confusional F28
  - acute or subacute F05
- delusional F22
- senile F03

Insect
- bite —*see* Bite, by site, superficial, insect
- venomous, poisoning NEC (by) —*see* Venom, arthropod

Insecurity, food Z59.41

Insensitivity
- adrenocorticotropin hormone (ACTH) E27.49
- androgen E34.50
  - complete E34.51
  - partial E34.52

Insertion
- cord (umbilical) lateral or velamentous O43.12-
- intrauterine contraceptive device (encounter for) —*see* Intrauterine contraceptive device

Insolation (sunstroke) T67.01

Insomnia (organic) G47.00
- adjustment F51.02
- adjustment disorder F51.02
- behavioral, of childhood Z73.819
  - combined type Z73.812
  - limit setting type Z73.811
  - sleep-onset association type Z73.810
- childhood Z73.819
- chronic F51.04
  - somatized tension F51.04
- conditioned F51.04
- due to
  - alcohol
    - abuse F10.182
    - dependence F10.282
    - use F10.982
  - amphetamines
    - abuse F15.182
    - dependence F15.282
    - use F15.982
  - anxiety disorder F51.05
  - caffeine
    - abuse F15.182
    - dependence F15.282
    - use F15.982
  - cocaine
    - abuse F14.182
    - dependence F14.282
    - use F14.982
  - depression F51.05
  - drug NEC
    - abuse F19.182
    - dependence F19.282
    - use F19.982
  - medical condition G47.01
  - mental disorder NEC F51.05
  - opioid
    - abuse F11.182
    - dependence F11.282
    - use F11.982
  - psychoactive substance NEC
    - abuse F19.182
    - dependence F19.282
    - use F19.982
  - sedative, hypnotic, or anxiolytic
    - abuse F13.182
    - dependence F13.282
    - use F13.982
  - stimulant NEC
    - abuse F15.182
    - dependence F15.282
    - use F15.982
- fatal familial (FFI) A81.83
- idiopathic F51.01
- learned F51.3
- nonorganic origin F51.01

Insomnia *(continued)*
- not due to a substance or known physiological condition F51.01
  - specified NEC F51.09
- paradoxical F51.03
- primary F51.01
- psychiatric F51.05
- psychophysiologic F51.04
- related to psychopathology F51.05
- short-term F51.02
- specified NEC G47.09
- stress-related F51.02
- transient F51.02
- without objective findings F51.02

Inspiration
- food or foreign body *—see* Foreign body, by site
- mucus *—see* Asphyxia, mucus

Inspissated bile syndrome (newborn) P59.1

Instability
- emotional (excessive) F60.3
- housing
  - housed Z59.819
    - with risk of homelessness Z59.811
    - homelessness in past 12 months Z59.812
- joint (post-traumatic) M25.30
  - ankle M25.37-
  - due to old ligament injury *—see* Disorder, ligament
  - elbow M25.32-
  - flail *—see* Flail, joint
  - foot M25.37-
  - hand M25.34-
  - hip M25.35-
  - knee M25.36-
  - lumbosacral M53.2
  - prosthesis *—see* Complications, joint prosthesis, mechanical, displacement, by site
  - sacroiliac M53.2
  - secondary to
    - old ligament injury *—see* Disorder, ligament
    - removal of joint prosthesis M96.89
  - shoulder (region) M25.31-
  - specified site NEC M25.39
  - spine M53.2
  - wrist M25.33-
- knee (chronic) M23.5-
- lumbosacral M53.2
- nervous F48.8
- personality (emotional) F60.3
- spine *—see* Instability, joint, spine
- vasomotor R55

Institutional syndrome (childhood) F94.2

Institutionalization, affecting child Z62.22
- disinhibited attachment F94.2

Insufficiency, insufficient
- accommodation, old age H52.4
- adrenal (gland) E27.40
  - primary E27.1
- adrenocortical E27.40
  - drug-induced E27.3
  - iatrogenic E27.3
  - primary E27.1
- anatomic crown height K08.89
- anterior (occlusal) guidance M26.54
- anus K62.89
- aortic (valve) I35.1
  - with
    - mitral (valve) disease I08.0
      - with tricuspid (valve) disease I08.3
    - stenosis I35.2
    - tricuspid (valve) disease I08.2
      - with mitral (valve) disease I08.3
  - congenital Q23.1
  - rheumatic I06.1
    - with
      - mitral (valve) disease I08.0
        - with tricuspid (valve) disease I08.3
      - stenosis I06.2
        - with mitral (valve) disease I08.0
          - with tricuspid (valve) disease I08.3
      - tricuspid (valve) disease I08.2
        - with mitral (valve) disease I08.3
  - specified cause NEC I35.1
  - syphilitic A52.03
- arterial I77.1
  - basilar G45.0
  - carotid (hemispheric) G45.1
  - cerebral I67.81
  - coronary (acute or subacute) I24.8
  - mesenteric K55.1
  - peripheral I73.9
  - precerebral (multiple) (bilateral) G45.2
  - vertebral G45.0
- arteriovenous I99.8
- biliary K83.8
- cardiac *—see also* Insufficiency, myocardial
  - due to presence of (cardiac) prosthesis I97.11-
  - postprocedural I97.11-
- cardiorenal, hypertensive I13.2
- cardiovascular *—see* Disease, cardiovascular
- cerebrovascular (acute) I67.81
  - with transient focal neurological signs and symptoms G45.8
- circulatory NEC I99.8
  - newborn P29.89
- clinical crown height K08.89
- convergence H51.11
- coronary (acute or subacute) I24.8
  - chronic or with a stated duration of over 4 weeks I25.89
- corticoadrenal E27.40
  - primary E27.1
- dietary E63.9
- divergence H51.8
- food T73.0
- gastroesophageal K22.89
- gonadal
  - ovary E28.39
  - testis E29.1
- heart *—see also* Insufficiency, myocardial
  - newborn P29.0
  - valve *—see* Endocarditis
- hepatic *—see* Failure, hepatic
- idiopathic autonomic G90.09
- interocclusal distance of fully erupted teeth (ridge) M26.36
- kidney N28.9
  - acute N28.9
  - chronic N18.9
- lacrimal (secretion) H04.12-
  - passages *—see* Stenosis, lacrimal
- liver *—see* Failure, hepatic
- lung *—see* Insufficiency, pulmonary
- mental (congenital) *—see* Disability, intellectual
- mesenteric K55.1
- mitral (valve) I34.0
  - with
    - aortic valve disease I08.0
      - with tricuspid (valve) disease I08.3
    - obstruction or stenosis I05.2
      - with aortic valve disease I08.0
    - tricuspid (valve) disease I08.1
      - with aortic (valve) disease I08.3
  - congenital Q23.3
  - rheumatic I05.1
    - with
      - aortic valve disease I08.0
        - with tricuspid (valve) disease I08.3
      - obstruction or stenosis I05.2
        - with aortic valve disease I08.0
          - with tricuspid (valve) disease I08.3
      - tricuspid (valve) disease I08.1
        - with aortic (valve) disease I08.3
    - active or acute I01.1
      - with chorea, rheumatic (Sydenham's) I02.0
  - specified cause, except rheumatic I34.0
- muscle *—see also* Disease, muscle
  - heart *—see* Insufficiency, myocardial
  - ocular NEC H50.9
- myocardial, myocardium (with arteriosclerosis) (*see also* Failure, heart) I50.9
  - with
    - rheumatic fever (conditions in I00) I09.0
      - active, acute or subacute I01.2
        - with chorea I02.0
      - inactive or quiescent (with chorea) I09.0
  - congenital Q24.8
  - hypertensive *—see* Hypertension, heart
  - newborn P29.0
  - rheumatic I09.0
    - active, acute, or subacute I01.2
  - syphilitic A52.06
- nourishment T73.0
- pancreatic K86.89
  - exocrine K86.81
- parathyroid (gland) E20.9
- peripheral vascular (arterial) I73.9
- pituitary E23.0
- placental (mother) O36.51-
- platelets D69.6
- prenatal care affecting management of pregnancy O09.3-
- progressive pluriglandular E31.0
- pulmonary J98.4
  - acute, following surgery (nonthoracic) J95.2
    - thoracic J95.1
  - chronic, following surgery J95.3
  - following
    - shock J98.4
    - trauma J98.4
  - newborn P28.89
  - valve I37.1
    - with stenosis I37.2
    - congenital Q22.2
    - rheumatic I09.89
      - with aortic, mitral or tricuspid (valve) disease I08.8
- pyloric K31.89
- renal (acute) N28.9
  - chronic N18.9
- respiratory R06.89
  - newborn P28.5
- rotation *—see* Malrotation
- sleep syndrome F51.12
- social insurance Z59.7
- suprarenal E27.40
  - primary E27.1
- tarso-orbital fascia, congenital Q10.3
- testis E29.1
- thyroid (gland) (acquired) E03.9
  - congenital E03.1
- tricuspid (valve) (rheumatic) I07.1
  - with
    - aortic (valve) disease I08.2
      - with mitral (valve) disease I08.3
    - mitral (valve) disease I08.1
      - with aortic (valve) disease I08.3
    - obstruction or stenosis I07.2
      - with aortic (valve) disease I08.2
        - with mitral (valve) disease I08.3
  - congenital Q22.8
  - nonrheumatic I36.1
    - with stenosis I36.2
- urethral sphincter R32
- valve, valvular (heart) I38
  - aortic *—see* Insufficiency, aortic (valve)
  - congenital Q24.8
  - mitral *—see* Insufficiency, mitral (valve)
  - pulmonary *—see* Insufficiency, pulmonary valve
  - tricuspid *—see* Insufficiency, tricuspid (valve)
- vascular I99.8
  - intestine K55.9
    - acute (*see also* Ischemia, intestine, acute) K55.059
  - mesenteric K55.1
  - peripheral I73.9
  - renal *—see* Hypertension, kidney
- velopharyngeal
  - acquired K13.79
  - congenital Q38.8
- venous (chronic) (peripheral) I87.2
- ventricular *—see* Insufficiency, myocardial
- welfare support Z59.7

Insufflation, fallopian Z31.41

Insular *—see* condition

Insulinoma
- pancreas
  - benign D13.7
  - malignant C25.4
  - uncertain behavior D37.8
- specified site
  - benign *—see* Neoplasm, by site, benign
  - malignant *—see* Neoplasm, by site, malignant

Insulinoma *(continued)*
specified site *(continued)*
uncertain behavior —*see* Neoplasm, by site, uncertain behavior
unspecified site
benign D13.7
malignant C25.4
uncertain behavior D37.8

Insuloma —*see* Insulinoma

Interference
balancing side M26.56
non-working side M26.56

Intermenstrual —*see* condition

Intermittent —*see* condition

Internal —*see* condition

Interrogation
cardiac defibrillator (automatic) (implantable) Z45.02
cardiac pacemaker Z45.018
cardiac (event) (loop) recorder Z45.09
infusion pump (implanted) (intrathecal) Z45.1
neurostimulator Z46.2

Interruption
aortic arch Q25.21
bundle of His I44.30
phase-shift, sleep cycle —*see* Disorder, sleep, circadian rhythm
sleep phase-shift, or 24 hour sleep-wake cycle —*see* Disorder, sleep, circadian rhythm

Interstitial —*see* condition

Intertrigo L30.4
labialis K13.0

Intervertebral disc —*see* condition

Intestine, intestinal —*see* condition

Intolerance
carbohydrate K90.49
disaccharide, hereditary E73.0
fat NEC K90.49
pancreatic K90.3
food K90.49
dietary counseling and surveillance Z71.3
fructose E74.10
hereditary E74.12
glucose (-galactose) E74.39
gluten K90.41
lactose E73.9
specified NEC E73.8
lysine E72.3
milk NEC K90.49
lactose E73.9
protein K90.49
starch NEC K90.49
sucrose (-isomaltose) E74.31

Intoxicated NEC (without dependence) —*see* Alcohol, intoxication

Intoxication
acid E87.2
alcoholic (acute) (without dependence) —*see* Alcohol, intoxication
alimentary canal K52.1
amphetamine (without dependence) —*see also* Abuse, drug, stimulant, with intoxication
with dependence —*see* Dependence, drug, stimulant, with intoxication

Intoxication *(continued)*
amphetamine *(continued)*
stimulant NEC F15.10
with
anxiety disorder F15.180
intoxication F15.129
with
delirium F15.121
perceptual disturbance F15.122
anxiolytic (acute) (without dependence) —*see* Abuse, drug, sedative, with intoxication
with dependence —*see* Dependence, drug, sedative, with intoxication
caffeine F15.929
with
abuse —*see* Abuse, drug, cannabis, with intoxication
dependence —*see* Dependence, drug, cannabis, with intoxication
cannabinoids (acute) (without dependence) —*see* Use, cannabis, with intoxication
with
abuse —*see* Abuse, drug, cannabis, with intoxication
dependence —*see* Dependence, drug, cannabis, with intoxication
chemical —*see* Table of Drugs and Chemicals
via placenta or breast milk —*see* - Absorption, chemical, through placenta
cocaine (acute) (without dependence) —*see* Abuse, drug, cocaine, with intoxication
with dependence —*see* Dependence, drug, cocaine, with intoxication
drug
acute (without dependence) —*see* Abuse, drug, by type with intoxication
with dependence —*see* Dependence, drug, by type with intoxication
addictive
via placenta or breast milk —*see* Absorption, drug, addictive, through placenta
newborn P93.8
gray baby syndrome P93.0
overdose or wrong substance given or taken —*see* Table of Drugs and Chemicals, by drug, poisoning
enteric K52.1
foodborne A05.9
bacterial A05.9
classical (Clostridium botulinum) A05.1
due to
Bacillus cereus A05.4
bacterium A05.9
specified NEC A05.8
Clostridium
botulinum A05.1
perfringens A05.2
welchii A05.2

Intoxication *(continued)*
foodborne *(continued)*
due to *(continued)*
Salmonella A02.9
with
(gastro)enteritis A02.0
localized infection(s) A02.20
arthritis A02.23
meningitis A02.21
osteomyelitis A02.24
pneumonia A02.22
pyelonephritis A02.25
specified NEC A02.29
sepsis A02.1
specified manifestation NEC A02.8
Staphylococcus A05.0
Vibrio
parahaemolyticus A05.3
vulnificus A05.5
enterotoxin, staphylococcal A05.0
noxious —*see* Poisoning, food, noxious
gastrointestinal K52.1
hallucinogenic (without dependence) —*see* Abuse, drug, hallucinogen, with intoxication
with dependence —*see* Dependence, drug, hallucinogen, with intoxication
hypnotic (acute) (without dependence) —*see* Abuse, drug, sedative, with intoxication
with dependence —*see* Dependence, drug, sedative, with intoxication
inhalant (acute) (without dependence) —*see* Abuse, drug, inhalant, with intoxication
with dependence —*see* Dependence, drug, inhalant, with intoxication
meaning
inebriation F10
poisoning —*see* Table of Drugs and Chemicals
methyl alcohol (acute) (without dependence) —*see* Alcohol, intoxication
opioid (acute) (without dependence) —*see* Abuse, drug, opioid, with intoxication
with dependence —*see* Dependence, drug, opioid, with intoxication
pathologic NEC (without dependence) —*see* Alcohol, intoxication
phencyclidine (without dependence) —*see* Abuse, drug, hallucinogen, with intoxication
with dependence —*see* Dependence, drug, hallucinogen, with intoxication
potassium (K) E87.5
psychoactive substance NEC (without dependence) —*see* Abuse, drug, psychoactive NEC, with intoxication
with dependence —*see* Dependence, drug, psychoactive NEC, with intoxication

Intoxication *(continued)*
sedative (acute) (without dependence) —*see* Abuse, drug, sedative, with intoxication
with dependence —*see* Dependence, drug, sedative, with intoxication
serum (*see also* Reaction, serum) T80.69
uremic —*see* Uremia
volatile solvents (acute) (without dependence) —*see* Abuse, drug, inhalant, with intoxication
with dependence —*see* Dependence, drug, inhalant, with intoxication
water E87.79

Intraabdominal testis, testes
bilateral Q53.211
unilateral Q53.111

Intracranial —*see* condition

Intrahepatic gallbladder Q44.1

Intraligamentous —*see* condition

Intrathoracic —*see also* condition
kidney Q63.2

Intrauterine contraceptive device
checking Z30.431
insertion Z30.430
immediately following removal Z30.433
in situ Z97.5
management Z30.431
reinsertion Z30.433
removal Z30.432
replacement Z30.433
retention in pregnancy O26.3-

Intraventricular —*see* condition

Intrinsic deformity —*see* Deformity

Intubation, difficult or failed T88.4

Intumescence, lens (eye) (cataract) —*see* Cataract

Intussusception (bowel) (colon) (enteric) (ileocecal) (ileocolic) (intestine) (rectum) K56.1
appendix K38.8
congenital Q43.8
ureter (with obstruction) N13.5

Invagination (bowel, colon, intestine or rectum) K56.1

Inversion
albumin-globulin (A-G) ratio E88.09
bladder N32.89
cecum —*see* Intussusception
cervix N88.8
chromosome in normal individual Q95.1
circadian rhythm —*see* Disorder, sleep, circadian rhythm
nipple N64.59
congenital Q83.8
gestational —*see* Retraction, nipple
puerperal, postpartum —*see* Retraction, nipple
nyctohemeral rhythm —*see* Disorder, sleep, circadian rhythm
optic papilla Q14.2
organ or site, congenital NEC —*see* Anomaly, by site
sleep rhythm —*see* Disorder, sleep, circadian rhythm
testis (congenital) Q55.29
uterus (chronic) (postinfectional) (postpartal, old) N85.5
postpartum O71.2

Inversion *(continued)*
vagina (posthysterectomy) N99.3
ventricular Q20.5

Investigation (*see also* Examination) Z04.9
clinical research subject (control) (normal comparison) (participant) Z00.6

Involuntary movement, abnormal R25.9

Involution, involutional —*see also* condition
breast, cystic —*see* Dysplasia, mammary, specified type NEC
depression (single episode) F32.89
recurrent episode F33.9
melancholia (single episode) F32.89
recurrent episode F33.8
ovary, senile —*see* Atrophy, ovary
thymus failure E32.8

I.Q.
under 20 F73
20-34 F72
35-49 F71
50-69 F70

IRDS (type I) P22.0
type II P22.1

Irideremia Q13.1

Iridis rubeosis —*see* Disorder, iris, vascular

Iridochoroiditis (panuveitis) —*see* Panuveitis

Iridocyclitis H20.9
acute H20.0-
hypopyon H20.05-
primary H20.01-
recurrent H20.02-
secondary (noninfectious) H20.04-
infectious H20.03-
chronic H20.1-
due to allergy —*see* Iridocyclitis, acute, secondary
endogenous —*see* Iridocyclitis, acute, primary
Fuchs' —*see* Cyclitis, Fuchs' heterochromic
gonococcal A54.32
granulomatous —*see* Iridocyclitis, chronic
herpes, herpetic (simplex) B00.51
zoster B02.32
hypopyon —*see* Iridocyclitis, acute, hypopyon
in (due to)
ankylosing spondylitis M45.9
gonococcal infection A54.32
herpes (simplex) virus B00.51
zoster B02.32
infectious disease NOS B99
parasitic disease NOS B89 *[H22]*
sarcoidosis D86.83
syphilis A51.43
tuberculosis A18.54
zoster B02.32
lens-induced H20.2-
nongranulomatous —*see* Iridocyclitis, acute
recurrent —*see* Iridocyclitis, acute, recurrent

Iridocyclitis *(continued)*
rheumatic —*see* Iridocyclitis, chronic
subacute —*see* Iridocyclitis, acute
sympathetic —*see* Uveitis, sympathetic
syphilitic (secondary) A51.43
tuberculous (chronic) A18.54
Vogt-Koyanagi H20.82-

Iridocyclochoroiditis (panuveitis) —*see* Panuveitis

Iridodialysis H21.53-

Iridodonesis H21.89

Iridoplegia (complete) (partial) (reflex) H57.09

Iridoschisis H21.25-

Iris —*see also* condition
bombé —*see* Membrane, pupillary

Iritis —*see also* Iridocyclitis
chronic —*see* Iridocyclitis, chronic
diabetic —*see* E08-E13 with .39
due to
herpes simplex B00.51
leprosy A30.9 *[H22]*
gonococcal A54.32
gouty (*see also* Gout, by type) M10.9 *[H22]*
granulomatous —*see* Iridocyclitis, chronic
lens induced —*see* Iridocyclitis, lens-induced
papulosa (syphilitic) A52.71
rheumatic —*see* Iridocyclitis, chronic
syphilitic (secondary) A51.43
congenital (early) A50.01
late A52.71
tuberculous A18.54

Iron —*see* condition

Iron-miner's lung J63.4

Irradiated enamel (tooth, teeth) K03.89

Irradiation effects, adverse T66

Irreducible, irreducibility —*see* condition

Irregular, irregularity
action, heart I49.9
alveolar process K08.89
bleeding N92.6
breathing R06.89
contour of cornea (acquired) —*see* Deformity, cornea
congenital Q13.4
contour, reconstructed breast N65.0
dentin (in pulp) K04.3
eye movements H55.89
nystagmus —*see* Nystagmus
deficient
saccadic H55.81
smooth H55.82
labor O62.2
menstruation (cause unknown) N92.6
periods N92.6
prostate N42.9
pupil —*see* Abnormality, pupillary
reconstructed breast N65.0
respiratory R06.89

Irregular, irregularity *(continued)*
septum (nasal) J34.2
shape, organ or site, congenital NEC —*see* Distortion
sleep-wake pattern (rhythm) G47.23

Irritable, irritability R45.4
bladder N32.89
bowel (syndrome) K58.9
with
constipation K58.1
diarrhea K58.0
mixed K58.2
psychogenic F45.8
specified NEC K58.8
bronchial —*see* Bronchitis
cerebral, in newborn P91.3
colon (*see also* Irritable, bowel) K58.9
with diarrhea K58.0
psychogenic F45.8
duodenum K59.89
heart (psychogenic) F45.8
hip —*see* Derangement, joint, specified type NEC, hip
ileum K59.89
infant R68.12
jejunum K59.89
rectum K59.89
stomach K31.89
psychogenic F45.8
sympathetic G90.8
urethra N36.8

Irritation
anus K62.89
axillary nerve G54.0
bladder N32.89
brachial plexus G54.0
bronchial —*see* Bronchitis
cervical plexus G54.2
cervix —*see* Cervicitis
choroid, sympathetic —*see* Endophthalmitis
cranial nerve —*see* Disorder, nerve, cranial
gastric K31.89
psychogenic F45.8
globe, sympathetic —*see* Uveitis, sympathetic
labyrinth —*see* subcategory H83.2
lumbosacral plexus G54.1
meninges (traumatic) —*see* Injury, intracranial
nontraumatic —*see* Meningismus
nerve —*see* Disorder, nerve
nervous R45.0
penis N48.89
perineum NEC L29.3
peripheral autonomic nervous system G90.8
peritoneum —*see* Peritonitis
pharynx J39.2
plantar nerve —*see* Lesion, nerve, plantar
spinal (cord) (traumatic) —*see also* Injury, spinal cord, by region
nerve G58.9
root NEC —*see* Radiculopathy
nontraumatic —*see* Myelopathy
stomach K31.89
psychogenic F45.8
sympathetic nerve NEC G90.8
ulnar nerve —*see* Lesion, nerve, ulnar
vagina N89.8

Ischemia, ischemic I99.8
brain —*see* Ischemia, cerebral
bowel (transient)
acute (*see also* Ischemia, intestine, acute) K55.019
diffuse K55.012
focal K55.011
chronic K55.1
due to mesenteric artery insufficiency K55.1
cardiac (*see* Disease, heart, ischemic)
cardiomyopathy I25.5
cerebral (chronic) (generalized) I67.82
arteriosclerotic I67.2
intermittent G45.9
newborn P91.0
recurrent focal G45.8
transient G45.9
colon chronic (due to mesenteric artery insufficiency) K55.1
coronary —*see* Disease, heart, ischemic
demand (coronary) (*see also* Angina) I24.8
with myocardial infarction I21.A1
resulting in myocardial infarction I21.A1
heart (chronic or with a stated duration of over 4 weeks) I25.9
acute or with a stated duration of 4 weeks or less I24.9
subacute I24.9
infarction, muscle —*see* Infarct, muscle
intestine (large) (small) (transient) K55.9
acute K55.059
diffuse K55.052
focal K55.051
large K55.039
diffuse K55.032
focal K55.031
small K55.019
diffuse K55.012
focal K55.011
chronic K55.1
due to mesenteric artery insufficiency K55.1
kidney N28.0
limb, critical —*see* Arteriosclerosis, with critical limb ischemia
limb-threatening, chronic —*see* Arteriosclerosis, with critical limb ischemia
mesenteric, acute (*see also* Ischemia, intestine, acute) K55.059
muscle, traumatic T79.6
myocardium, myocardial (chronic or with a stated duration of over 4 weeks) I25.9
acute, without myocardial infarction I51.3
silent (asymptomatic) I25.6
transient of newborn P29.4
renal N28.0
retina, retinal —*see* Occlusion, artery, retina
small bowel
acute K55.019
diffuse K55.012
focal K55.011

Ischemia, ischemic *(continued)*
small bowel *(continued)*
chronic K55.1
due to mesenteric artery insufficiency K55.1
spinal cord G95.11
subendocardial *—see* Insufficiency, coronary
supply (coronary) (*see also* Angina) I25.9
due to vasospasm I20.1

Ischial spine *—see* condition

Ischialgia *—see* Sciatica

Ischiopagus Q89.4

Ischium, ischial *—see* condition

Ischuria R34

Iselin's disease or osteochondrosis *—see* Osteochondrosis, juvenile, metatarsus

Islands of
parotid tissue in
lymph nodes Q38.6
neck structures Q38.6
submaxillary glands in
fascia Q38.6
lymph nodes Q38.6
neck muscles Q38.6

Islet cell tumor, pancreas D13.7

Isoimmunization NEC *—see also* Incompatibility
affecting management of pregnancy (ABO) (with hydrops fetalis) O36.11-
anti-A sensitization O36.11-
anti-B sensitization O36.19-
anti-c sensitization O36.09-
anti-C sensitization O36.09-
anti-e sensitization O36.09-
anti-E sensitization O36.09-
Rh NEC O36.09-
anti-D antibody O36.01-
specified NEC O36.19-
newborn P55.9
with
hydrops fetalis P56.0
kernicterus P57.0
ABO (blood groups) P55.1
Rhesus (Rh) factor P55.0
specified type NEC P55.8

Isolation, isolated
dwelling Z59.89
family Z63.79
social Z60.4

Isoleucinosis E71.19

Isomerism atrial appendages (with asplenia or polysplenia) Q20.6

Isosporiasis, isosporosis A07.3

Isovaleric acidemia E71.110

Issue of
medical certificate Z02.79
for disability determination Z02.71
repeat prescription (appliance) (glasses) (medicinal substance, medicament, medicine) Z76.0
contraception *—see* Contraception

Itch, itching *—see also* Pruritus
baker's L23.6
barber's B35.0
bricklayer's L24.5
cheese B88.0
clam digger's B65.3
coolie B76.9
copra B88.0
dew B76.9

Itch, itching *(continued)*
dhobi B35.6
filarial *—see* Infestation, filarial
grain B88.0
grocer's B88.0
ground B76.9
harvest B88.0
jock B35.6
Malabar B35.5
beard B35.0
foot B35.3
scalp B35.0
meaning scabies B86
Norwegian B86
perianal L29.0
poultrymen's B88.0
sarcoptic B86
scabies B86
scrub B88.0
straw B88.0
swimmer's B65.3
water B76.9
winter L29.8

Ivemark's syndrome (asplenia with congenital heart disease) Q89.01

Ivory bones Q78.2

Ixodiasis NEC B88.8

J

Jaccoud's syndrome *—see* Arthropathy, postrheumatic, chronic

Jackson's
membrane Q43.3
paralysis or syndrome G83.89
veil Q43.3

Jacquet's dermatitis (diaper dermatitis) L22

Jadassohn-Pellizari's disease or anetoderma L90.2

Jadassohn's
blue nevus *—see* Nevus
intraepidermal epithelioma *—see* Neoplasm, skin, benign

Jaffe-Lichtenstein (-Uehlinger) **syndrome** *—see* Dysplasia, fibrous, bone NEC

Jakob-Creutzfeldt disease or syndrome *—see* Creutzfeldt-Jakob disease or syndrome

Jaksch-Luzet disease D64.89

Jamaican
neuropathy G92.8
paraplegic tropical ataxic-spastic syndrome G92.8

Janet's disease F48.8

Janiceps Q89.4

Jansky-Bielschowsky amaurotic idiocy E75.4

Japanese
B-type encephalitis A83.0
river fever A75.3

Jaundice (yellow) R17
acholuric (familial) (splenomegalic) *—see also* Spherocytosis
acquired D59.8
breast-milk (inhibitor) P59.3
catarrhal (acute) B15.9
with hepatic coma B15.0
cholestatic (benign) R17

Jaundice *(continued)*
due to or associated with
delayed conjugation P59.8
associated with (due to) preterm delivery P59.0
preterm delivery P59.0
epidemic (catarrhal) B15.9
with hepatic coma B15.0
leptospiral A27.0
spirochetal A27.0
familial nonhemolytic (congenital) (Gilbert) E80.4
Crigler-Najjar E80.5
febrile (acute) B15.9
with hepatic coma B15.0
leptospiral A27.0
spirochetal A27.0
hematogenous D59.9
hemolytic (acquired) D59.9
congenital *—see* Spherocytosis
hemorrhagic (acute) (leptospiral) (spirochetal) A27.0
infectious (acute) (subacute) B15.9
with hepatic coma B15.0
leptospiral A27.0
spirochetal A27.0
leptospiral (hemorrhagic) A27.0
malignant (without coma) K72.90
with coma K72.91
newborn P59.9
due to or associated with
ABO
antibodies P55.1
incompatibility, maternal/fetal P55.1
isoimmunization P55.1
absence or deficiency of enzyme system for bilirubin conjugation (congenital) P59.8
bleeding P58.1
breast milk inhibitors to conjugation P59.3
associated with preterm delivery P59.0
bruising P58.0
Crigler-Najjar syndrome E80.5
delayed conjugation P59.8
associated with preterm delivery P59.0
drugs or toxins
given to newborn P58.42
transmitted from mother P58.41
excessive hemolysis P58.9
due to
bleeding P58.1
bruising P58.0
drugs or toxins
given to newborn P58.42
transmitted from mother P58.41
infection P58.2
polycythemia P58.3
swallowed maternal blood P58.5
specified type NEC P58.8
galactosemia E74.21
Gilbert syndrome E80.4
hemolytic disease P55.9
ABO isoimmunization P55.1

Jaundice *(continued)*
newborn *(continued)*
due to or associated with *(continued)*
hemolytic disease *(continued)*
Rh isoimmunization P55.0
specified NEC P55.8
hepatocellular damage P59.20
specified NEC P59.29
hereditary hemolytic anemia P58.8
hypothyroidism, congenital E03.1
incompatibility, maternal/fetal NOS P55.9
infection P58.2
inspissated bile syndrome P59.1
isoimmunization NOS P55.9
mucoviscidosis E84.9
polycythemia P58.3
preterm delivery P59.0
Rh
antibodies P55.0
incompatibility, maternal/fetal P55.0
isoimmunization P55.0
specified cause NEC P59.8
swallowed maternal blood P58.5
spherocytosis (congenital) D58.0
neonatal *—see* Jaundice, newborn
nonhemolytic congenital familial (Gilbert) E80.4
nuclear, newborn (*see also* Kernicterus of newborn) P57.9
obstructive (*see also* Obstruction, bile duct) K83.1
post-immunization *—see* Hepatitis, viral, type, B
post-transfusion *—see* Hepatitis, viral, type, B
regurgitation (*see also* Obstruction, bile duct) K83.1
serum (homologous) (prophylactic) (therapeutic) *—see* Hepatitis, viral, type, B
spirochetal (hemorrhagic) A27.0
symptomatic R17
newborn P59.9

Jaw *—see* condition

Jaw-winking phenomenon or syndrome Q07.8

Jealousy
alcoholic F10.988
childhood F93.8
sibling F93.8

Jejunitis *—see* Enteritis

Jejunostomy status Z93.4

Jejunum, jejunal *—see* condition

Jensen's disease *—see* Inflammation, chorioretinal, focal, juxtapapillary

Jerks, myoclonic G25.3

Jervell-Lange-Nielsen syndrome I45.81

Jeune's disease Q77.2

Jigger disease B88.1

Job's syndrome (chronic granulomatous disease) D71

Joint *—see also* condition
mice *—see* Loose, body, joint
knee M23.4-

Jordan's anomaly or syndrome D72.0

Joseph-Diamond-Blackfan anemia (congenital hypoplastic) D61.01

Jungle yellow fever A95.0

Jüngling's disease *—see* Sarcoidosis

Juvenile *—see* condition

K

Kahler's disease C90.0-

Kakke E51.11

Kala-azar B55.0

Kallmann's syndrome E23.0

Kanner's syndrome (autism) *—see* Psychosis, childhood

Kaposi's
- dermatosis (xeroderma pigmentosum) Q82.1
- lichen ruber L44.0
  - acuminatus L44.0
- sarcoma
  - colon C46.4
  - connective tissue C46.1
  - gastrointestinal organ C46.4
  - lung C46.5-
  - lymph node (multiple) C46.3
  - palate (hard) (soft) C46.2
  - rectum C46.4
  - skin (multiple sites) C46.0
  - specified site NEC C46.7
  - stomach C46.4
  - unspecified site C46.9
- varicelliform eruption B00.0
  - vaccinia T88.1

Kartagener's syndrome or triad (sinusitis, bronchiectasis, situs inversus) Q89.3

Karyotype
- with abnormality except iso (Xq) Q96.2
- 45,X Q96.0
- 46,X
  - iso (Xq) Q96.1
- 46,XX Q98.3
  - with streak gonads Q50.32
  - hermaphrodite (true) Q99.1
  - male Q98.3
- 46,XY
  - with streak gonads Q56.1
  - female Q97.3
  - hermaphrodite (true) Q99.1
- 47,XXX Q97.0
- 47,XXY Q98.0
- 47,XYY Q98.5

Kaschin-Beck disease *—see* Disease, Kaschin-Beck

Katayama's disease or fever B65.2

Kawasaki's syndrome M30.3

Kayser-Fleischer ring (cornea) (pseudosclerosis) H18.04-

Kaznelson's syndrome (congenital hypoplastic anemia) D61.01

Kearns-Sayre syndrome H49.81-

Kedani fever A75.3

Kelis L91.0

Kelly (-Patterson) **syndrome** (sideropenic dysphagia) D50.1

Keloid, cheloid L91.0
- acne L73.0
- Addison's L94.0
- cornea *—see* Opacity, cornea
- Hawkin's L91.0
- scar L91.0

Keloma L91.0

Kenya fever A77.1

Keratectasia *—see also* Ectasia, cornea
- congenital Q13.4

Keratinization of alveolar ridge mucosa
- excessive K13.23
- minimal K13.22

Keratinized residual ridge mucosa
- excessive K13.23
- minimal K13.22

Keratitis (nodular) (nonulcerative) (simple) (zonular) H16.9
- with ulceration (central) (marginal) (perforated) (ring) *—see* Ulcer, cornea
- actinic *—see* Photokeratitis
- arborescens (herpes simplex) B00.52
- areolar H16.11-
- bullosa H16.8
- deep H16.309
  - specified type NEC H16.399
- dendritic (a) (herpes simplex) B00.52
- disciform (is) (herpes simplex) B00.52
  - varicella B01.81
- filamentary H16.12-
- gonococcal (congenital or prenatal) A54.33
- herpes, herpetic (simplex) B00.52
  - zoster B02.33
- in (due to)
  - acanthamebiasis B60.13
  - adenovirus B30.0
  - exanthema (*see also* Exanthem) B09
  - herpes (simplex) virus B00.52
  - measles B05.81
  - syphilis A50.31
  - tuberculosis A18.52
  - zoster B02.33
- interstitial (nonsyphilitic) H16.30-
  - diffuse H16.32-
  - herpes, herpetic (simplex) B00.52
    - zoster B02.33
  - sclerosing H16.33-
  - specified type NEC H16.39-
  - syphilitic (congenital) (late) A50.31
  - tuberculous A18.52
- macular H16.11-
- nummular H16.11-
- oyster shuckers' H16.8
- parenchymatous *—see* Keratitis, interstitial
- petrificans H16.8
- postmeasles B05.81
- punctata
  - leprosa A30.9 *[H16.14-]*
  - syphilitic (profunda) A50.31
- punctate H16.14-
- purulent H16.8
- rosacea L71.8
- sclerosing H16.33-
- specified type NEC H16.8

Keratitis *(continued)*
- stellate H16.11-
- striate H16.11-
- superficial H16.10-
  - with conjunctivitis *—see* Keratoconjunctivitis
  - due to light *—see* Photokeratitis
- suppurative H16.8
- syphilitic (congenital) (prenatal) A50.31
- trachomatous A71.1
  - sequelae B94.0
- tuberculous A18.52
- vesicular H16.8
- xerotic (*see also* Keratomlacia) H16.8
  - vitamin A deficiency E50.4

Keratoacanthoma L85.8

Keratocele *—see* Descemetocele

Keratoconjunctivitis H16.20-
- Acanthamoeba B60.13
- adenoviral B30.0
- epidemic B30.0
- exposure H16.21-
- herpes, herpetic (simplex) B00.52
  - zoster B02.33
- in exanthema (*see also* Exanthem) B09
- infectious B30.0
- lagophthalmic *—see* Keratoconjunctivitis, specified type NEC
- neurotrophic H16.23-
- phlyctenular H16.25-
- postmeasles B05.81
- shipyard B30.0
- sicca (Sjogren's) M35.0-
  - not Sjogren's H16.22-
- specified type NEC H16.29-
- tuberculous (phlyctenular) A18.52
- vernal H16.26-

Keratoconus H18.60-
- congenital Q13.4
- stable H18.61-
- unstable H18.62-

Keratocyst (dental) (odontogenic) *—see* Cyst, calcifying odontogenic

Keratoderma, keratodermia (congenital) (palmaris et plantaris) (symmetrical) Q82.8
- acquired L85.1
  - in diseases classified elsewhere L86
- climactericum L85.1
- gonococcal A54.89
- gonorrheal A54.89
- punctata L85.2
- Reiter's *—see* Reiter's disease

Keratodermatocele *—see* Descemetocele

Keratoglobus H18.79
- congenital Q15.8
  - with glaucoma Q15.0

Keratohemia *—see* Pigmentation, cornea, stromal

Keratoiritis *—see also* Iridocyclitis
- syphilitic A50.39
- tuberculous A18.54

Keratoma L57.0
- palmaris and plantaris hereditarium Q82.8
- senile L57.0

Keratomalacia H18.44-
- vitamin A deficiency E50.4

Keratomegaly Q13.4

Keratomycosis B49
- nigrans, nigricans (palmaris) B36.1

Keratopathy H18.9
- band H18.42-
- bullous H18.1-
- bullous (aphakic), following cataract surgery H59.01-

Keratoscleritis, tuberculous A18.52

Keratosis L57.0
- actinic L57.0
- arsenical L85.8
- congenital, specified NEC Q80.8
- female genital NEC N94.89
- follicularis Q82.8
  - acquired L11.0
  - congenita Q82.8
  - et parafollicularis in cutem penetrans L87.0
  - spinulosa (decalvans) Q82.8
  - vitamin A deficiency E50.8
- gonococcal A54.89
- male genital (external) N50.89
- nigricans L83
- obturans, external ear (canal) *—see* Cholesteatoma, external ear
- palmaris et plantaris (inherited) (symmetrical) Q82.8
  - acquired L85.1
- penile N48.89
- pharynx J39.2
- pilaris, acquired L85.8
- punctata (palmaris et plantaris) L85.2
- scrotal N50.89
- seborrheic L82.1
  - inflamed L82.0
- senile L57.0
- solar L57.0
- tonsillaris J35.8
- vagina N89.4
- vegetans Q82.8
- vitamin A deficiency E50.8
- vocal cord J38.3

Kerato-uveitis *—see* Iridocyclitis

Kerunoparalysis T75.09

Kerion (celsi) B35.0

Kernicterus of newborn (not due to isoimmunization) P57.9
- due to isoimmunization (conditions in P55.0-P55.9) P57.0
- specified type NEC P57.8

Keshan disease E59

Ketoacidosis E87.2
- diabetic *—see* Diabetes, by type, with ketoacidosis

Ketonuria R82.4

Ketosis NEC E88.89
- diabetic *—see* Diabetes, by type, with ketoacidosis

Kew Garden fever A79.1

Kidney *—see* condition

Kienböck's disease *—see also* Osteochondrosis, juvenile, hand, carpal lunate
- adult M93.1

Kimmelstiel (-Wilson) **disease** *—see* Diabetes, Kimmelstiel (-Wilson) disease

Kimura disease D21.9
- specified site —*see* Neoplasm, connective tissue benign

Kink, kinking
- artery I77.1
- hair (acquired) L67.8
- ileum or intestine —*see* Obstruction, intestine
- Lane's —*see* Obstruction, intestine
- organ or site, congenital NEC —*see* Anomaly, by site
- ureter (pelvic junction) N13.5
  - with
    - hydronephrosis N13.1
      - with infection N13.6
    - pyelonephritis (chronic) N11.1
  - congenital Q62.39
- vein(s) I87.8
  - caval I87.1
  - peripheral I87.1

Kinnier Wilson's disease (hepatolenticular degeneration) E83.01

Kissing spine M48.20
- cervical region M48.22
- cervicothoracic region M48.23
- lumbar region M48.26
- lumbosacral region M48.27
- occipito-atlanto-axial region M48.21
- thoracic region M48.24
- thoracolumbar region M48.25

Klatskin's tumor C24.0

Klauder's disease A26.8

Klebs' disease (*see also* Glomerulonephritis) N05.-

Klebsiella (K.) **pneumoniae, as cause of disease classified elsewhere** B96.1

Klein (e)**-Levin syndrome** G47.13

Kleptomania F63.2

Klinefelter's syndrome Q98.4
- karyotype 47,XXY Q98.0
- male with more than two X chromosomes Q98.1

Klippel-Feil deficiency, disease, or syndrome (brevicollis) Q76.1

Klippel's disease I67.2

Klippel-Trenaunay (-Weber) **syndrome** Q87.2

Klumpke (-Déjerine) palsy, paralysis (birth) (newborn) P14.1

Knee —*see* condition

Knock knee (acquired) M21.06-
- congenital Q74.1

Knot(s)
- intestinal, syndrome (volvulus) K56.2
- surfer S89.8-
- umbilical cord (true) O69.2

Knotting (of)
- hair L67.8
- intestine K56.2

Knuckle pad (Garrod's) M72.1

Koch's
- infection —*see* Tuberculosis
- relapsing fever A68.9

Koch-Weeks' conjunctivitis —*see* Conjunctivitis, acute, mucopurulent

Köebner's syndrome Q81.8

Köenig's disease (osteochondritis dissecans) —*see* Osteochondritis, dissecans

Köhler-Pellegrini-Steida disease or syndrome (calcification, knee joint) —*see* Bursitis, tibial collateral

Köhler's disease
- patellar —*see* Osteochondrosis, juvenile, patella
- tarsal navicular —*see* Osteochondrosis, juvenile, tarsus

Koilonychia L60.3
- congenital Q84.6

Kojevnikov's, epilepsy —*see* Kozhevnikof's epilepsy

Koplik's spots B05.9

Kopp's asthma E32.8

Korsakoff's (Wernicke) disease, psychosis or syndrome (alcoholic) F10.96
- with dependence F10.26
- drug-induced
  - due to drug abuse —*see* Abuse, drug, by type, with amnestic disorder
  - due to drug dependence —*see* Dependence, drug, by type, with amnestic disorder
- nonalcoholic F04

Korsakov's disease, psychosis or syndrome —*see* Korsakoff's disease

Korsakow's disease, psychosis or syndrome —*see* Korsakoff's disease

Kostmann's disease or syndrome (infantile genetic agranulocytosis) —*see* Agranulocytosis

Kozhevnikof's epilepsy G40.109
- intractable G40.119
  - with status epilepticus G40.111
  - without status epilepticus G40.119
- not intractable G40.109
  - with status epilepticus G40.101
  - without status epilepticus G40.109

Krabbe's
- disease E75.23
- syndrome, congenital muscle hypoplasia Q79.8

Kraepelin-Morel disease —*see* Schizophrenia

Kraft-Weber-Dimitri disease Q85.8

Kraurosis
- ani K62.89
- penis N48.0
- vagina N89.8
- vulva N90.4

Kreotoxism A05.9

Krukenberg's
- spindle —*see* Pigmentation, cornea, posterior
- tumor C79.6-

Kufs' disease E75.4

Kugelberg-Welander disease G12.1

Kuhnt-Junius degeneration (*see also* Degeneration, macula) H35.32 -

Kümmell's disease or spondylitis —*see* Spondylopathy, traumatic

Kupffer cell sarcoma C22.3

Kuru A81.81

Kussmaul's
- disease M30.0
- respiration E87.2
  - in diabetic acidosis —*see* Diabetes, by type, with ketoacidosis

Kwashiorkor E40
- marasmic, marasmus type E42

Kyasanur Forest disease A98.2

Kyphoscoliosis, kyphoscoliotic (acquired) (*see also* Scoliosis) M41.9
- congenital Q67.5
- heart (disease) I27.1
- sequelae of rickets E64.3
- tuberculous A18.01

Kyphosis, kyphotic (acquired) M40.209
- cervical region M40.202
- cervicothoracic region M40.203
- congenital Q76.419
  - cervical region Q76.412
  - cervicothoracic region Q76.413
  - occipito-atlanto-axial region Q76.411
  - thoracic region Q76.414
  - thoracolumbar region Q76.415
- Morquio-Brailsford type (spinal) (*see also* subcategory M49.8) E76.219
- postlaminectomy M96.3
- postradiation therapy M96.2
- postural (adolescent) M40.00
  - cervicothoracic region M40.03
  - thoracic region M40.04
  - thoracolumbar region M40.05
- secondary NEC M40.10
  - cervical region M40.12
  - cervicothoracic region M40.13
  - thoracic region M40.14
  - thoracolumbar region M40.15
- sequelae of rickets E64.3
- specified type NEC M40.299
  - cervical region M40.292
  - cervicothoracic region M40.293
  - thoracic region M40.294
  - thoracolumbar region M40.295
- syphilitic, congenital A50.56
- thoracic region M40.204
- thoracolumbar region M40.205
- tuberculous A18.01

Kyrle disease L87.0

L

Labia, labium —*see* condition

Labile
- blood pressure R09.89
- vasomotor system I73.9

Labioglossal paralysis G12.29

Labium leporinum —*see* Cleft, lip

Labor —*see* Delivery

Labored breathing —*see* Hyperventilation

Labyrinthitis (circumscribed) (destructive) (diffuse) (inner ear) (latent) (purulent) (suppurative) —*see also* subcategory H83.0
- syphilitic A52.79

Laceration
- with abortion —*see* Abortion, by type, complicated by laceration of pelvic organs
- abdomen, abdominal
  - wall S31.119

Laceration *(continued)*
- abdomen, abdominal *(continued)*
  - wall *(continued)*
    - with
      - foreign body S31.129
      - penetration into peritoneal cavity S31.619
        - with foreign body S31.629
    - epigastric region S31.112
      - with
        - foreign body S31.122
        - penetration into peritoneal cavity S31.612
          - with foreign body S31.622
    - left
      - lower quadrant S31.114
        - with
          - foreign body S31.124
          - penetration into peritoneal cavity S31.614
            - with foreign body S31.624
      - upper quadrant S31.111
        - with
          - foreign body S31.121
          - penetration into peritoneal cavity S31.611
            - with foreign body S31.621
    - periumbilic region S31.115
      - with
        - foreign body S31.125
        - penetration into peritoneal cavity S31.615
          - with foreign body S31.625
    - right
      - lower quadrant S31.113
        - with
          - foreign body S31.123
          - penetration into peritoneal cavity S31.613
            - with foreign body S31.623
      - upper quadrant S31.110
        - with
          - foreign body S31.120
          - penetration into peritoneal cavity S31.610
            - with foreign body S31.620
- accidental, complicating surgery —*see* Complications, surgical, accidental puncture or laceration
- Achilles tendon S86.02-
- adrenal gland S37.813
- alveolar (process) —*see* Laceration, oral cavity
- ankle S91.01-
  - with
    - foreign body S91.02-
- antecubital space —*see* Laceration, elbow
- anus (sphincter) S31.831
  - with
    - ectopic or molar pregnancy O08.6
    - foreign body S31.832
  - complicating delivery —*see* Delivery, complicated, by, laceration, anus (sphincter)

Laceration *(continued)*
- anus *(continued)*
  - following ectopic or molar pregnancy O08.6
  - nontraumatic, nonpuerperal —*see* Fissure, anus
- arm (upper) S41.11-
  - with foreign body S41.12-
  - lower —*see* Laceration, forearm
- auditory canal (external) (meatus) —*see* Laceration, ear
- auricle, ear —*see* Laceration, ear
- axilla —*see* Laceration, arm
- back —*see also* Laceration, thorax, back
  - lower S31.010
    - with
      - foreign body S31.020
        - with penetration into retroperitoneal space S31.021
      - penetration into retroperitoneal space S31.011
- bile duct S36.13
- bladder S37.23
  - with ectopic or molar pregnancy O08.6
  - following ectopic or molar pregnancy O08.6
  - obstetrical trauma O71.5
- blood vessel —*see* Injury, blood vessel
- bowel —*see also* Laceration, intestine
  - with ectopic or molar pregnancy O08.6
  - complicating abortion —*see* Abortion, by type, complicated by, specified condition NEC
  - following ectopic or molar pregnancy O08.6
  - obstetrical trauma O71.5
- brain (any part) (cortex) (diffuse) (membrane) —*see also* Injury, intracranial, diffuse
  - during birth P10.8
    - with hemorrhage P10.1
  - focal —*see* Injury, intracranial, focal brain injury
- brainstem S06.38-
- breast S21.01-
  - with foreign body S21.02-
- broad ligament S37.893
  - with ectopic or molar pregnancy O08.6
  - following ectopic or molar pregnancy O08.6
  - laceration syndrome N83.8
  - obstetrical trauma O71.6
  - syndrome (laceration) N83.8
- buttock S31.801
  - with foreign body S31.802
  - left S31.821
    - with foreign body S31.822
  - right S31.811
    - with foreign body S31.812
- calf —*see* Laceration, leg
- canaliculus lacrimalis —*see* Laceration, eyelid
- canthus, eye —*see* Laceration, eyelid
- capsule, joint —*see* Sprain
- causing eversion of cervix uteri (old) N86
- central (perineal), complicating delivery O70.9
- cerebellum, traumatic S06.37-

Laceration *(continued)*
- cerebral S06.33-
  - left side S06.32-
  - during birth P10.8
    - with hemorrhage P10.1
  - right side S06.31-
- cervix (uteri)
  - with ectopic or molar pregnancy O08.6
  - following ectopic or molar pregnancy O08.6
  - nonpuerperal, nontraumatic N88.1
  - obstetrical trauma (current) O71.3
  - old (postpartal) N88.1
  - traumatic S37.63
- cheek (external) S01.41-
  - with foreign body S01.42-
  - internal —*see* Laceration, oral cavity
- chest wall —*see* Laceration, thorax
- chin —*see* Laceration, head, specified site NEC
- chordae tendinae NEC I51.1
  - concurrent with acute myocardial infarction —*see* Infarct, myocardium
  - following acute myocardial infarction (current complication) I23.4
- clitoris —*see* Laceration, vulva
- colon —*see* Laceration, intestine, large, colon
- common bile duct S36.13
- cortex (cerebral) —*see* Injury, intracranial, diffuse
- costal region —*see* Laceration, thorax
- cystic duct S36.13
- diaphragm S27.803
- digit(s)
  - hand —*see* Laceration, finger
  - foot —*see* Laceration, toe
- duodenum S36.430
- ear (canal) (external) S01.31-
  - with foreign body S01.32-
  - drum S09.2-
- elbow S51.01-
  - with
    - foreign body S51.02-
- epididymis —*see* Laceration, testis
- epigastric region —*see* Laceration, abdomen, wall, epigastric region
- esophagus K22.89
  - traumatic
    - cervical S11.21
      - with foreign body S11.22
    - thoracic S27.813
- eye (ball) S05.3-
  - with prolapse or loss of intraocular tissue S05.2-
  - penetrating S05.6-
- eyebrow —*see* Laceration, eyelid
- eyelid S01.11-
  - with foreign body S01.12-
- face NEC —*see* Laceration, head, specified site NEC
- fallopian tube S37.539
  - bilateral S37.532
  - unilateral S37.531
- finger(s) S61.219
  - with
    - damage to nail S61.319
      - with
        - foreign body S61.329
    - foreign body S61.229
  - index S61.218
    - with
      - damage to nail S61.318
        - with
          - foreign body S61.328
      - foreign body S61.228

Laceration *(continued)*
- finger(s) *(continued)*
  - index *(continued)*
    - left S61.211
      - with
        - damage to nail S61.311
          - with
            - foreign body S61.321
        - foreign body S61.221
    - right S61.210
      - with
        - damage to nail S61.310
          - with
            - foreign body S61.320
        - foreign body S61.220
  - little S61.218
    - with
      - damage to nail S61.318
        - with
          - foreign body S61.328
      - foreign body S61.228
    - left S61.217
      - with
        - damage to nail S61.317
          - with
            - foreign body S61.327
        - foreign body S61.227
    - right S61.216
      - with
        - damage to nail S61.316
          - with
            - foreign body S61.326
        - foreign body S61.226
  - middle S61.218
    - with
      - damage to nail S61.318
        - with
          - foreign body S61.328
      - foreign body S61.228
    - left S61.213
      - with
        - damage to nail S61.313
          - with
            - foreign body S61.323
        - foreign body S61.223
    - right S61.212
      - with
        - damage to nail S61.312
          - with
            - foreign body S61.322
        - foreign body S61.222
  - ring S61.218
    - with
      - damage to nail S61.318
        - with
          - foreign body S61.328
      - foreign body S61.228
    - left S61.215
      - with
        - damage to nail S61.315
          - with
            - foreign body S61.325
        - foreign body S61.225
    - right S61.214
      - with
        - damage to nail S61.314
          - with
            - foreign body S61.324
        - foreign body S61.224
- flank S31.119
  - with foreign body S31.129
- foot (except toe(s) alone) S91.319
  - with foreign body S91.329

Laceration *(continued)*
- foot *(continued)*
  - left S91.312
    - with foreign body S91.322
  - right S91.311
    - with foreign body S91.321
  - toe —*see* Laceration, toe
- forearm S51.819
  - with
    - foreign body S51.829
  - elbow only —*see* Laceration, elbow
  - left S51.812
    - with
      - foreign body S51.822
  - right S51.811
    - with
      - foreign body S51.821
- forehead S01.81
  - with foreign body S01.82
- fourchette O70.0
  - with ectopic or molar pregnancy O08.6
  - complicating delivery O70.0
  - following ectopic or molar pregnancy O08.6
- gallbladder S36.123
- genital organs, external
  - female S31.512
    - with foreign body S31.522
    - vagina —*see* Laceration, vagina
    - vulva —*see* Laceration, vulva
  - male S31.511
    - with foreign body S31.521
    - penis —*see* Laceration, penis
    - scrotum —*see* Laceration, scrotum
    - testis —*see* Laceration, testis
- groin —*see* Laceration, abdomen, wall
- gum —*see* Laceration, oral cavity
- hand S61.419
  - with
    - foreign body S61.429
  - finger —*see* Laceration, finger
  - left S61.412
    - with
      - foreign body S61.422
  - right S61.411
    - with
      - foreign body S61.421
  - thumb —*see* Laceration, thumb
- head S01.91
  - with foreign body S01.92
  - cheek —*see* Laceration, cheek
  - ear —*see* Laceration, ear
  - eyelid —*see* Laceration, eyelid
  - lip —*see* Laceration, lip
  - nose —*see* Laceration, nose
  - oral cavity —*see* Laceration, oral cavity
  - scalp S01.01
    - with foreign body S01.02
  - specified site NEC S01.81
    - with foreign body S01.82
  - temporomandibular area —*see* Laceration, cheek
- heart —*see* Injury, heart, laceration
- heel —*see* Laceration, foot
- hepatic duct S36.13
- hip S71.019
  - with foreign body S71.029
  - left S71.012
    - with foreign body S71.022
  - right S71.011
    - with foreign body S71.021
- hymen —*see* Laceration, vagina

Laceration *(continued)*
- hypochondrium —*see* Laceration, abdomen, wall
- hypogastric region —*see* Laceration, abdomen, wall
- ileum S36.438
- inguinal region —*see* Laceration, abdomen, wall
- instep —*see* Laceration, foot
- internal organ —*see* Injury, by site
- interscapular region —*see* Laceration, thorax, back
- intestine
  - large
    - colon S36.539
      - ascending S36.530
      - descending S36.532
      - sigmoid S36.533
      - specified site NEC S36.538
    - rectum S36.63
      - transverse S36.531
  - small S36.439
    - duodenum S36.430
    - specified site NEC S36.438
- intra-abdominal organ S36.93
  - intestine —*see* Laceration, intestine
  - liver —*see* Laceration, liver
  - pancreas —*see* Laceration, pancreas
  - peritoneum S36.81
  - specified site NEC S36.893
  - spleen —*see* Laceration, spleen
  - stomach —*see* Laceration, stomach
- intracranial NEC —*see also* Injury, intracranial, diffuse
  - birth injury P10.9
- jaw —*see* Laceration, head, specified site NEC
- jejunum S36.438
- joint capsule —*see* Sprain, by site
- kidney S37.03-
  - major (greater than 3 cm) (massive) (stellate) S37.06-
  - minor (less than 1 cm) S37.04-
  - moderate (1 to 3 cm) S37.05-
  - multiple S37.06-
- knee S81.01-
  - with foreign body S81.02-
- labium (majus) (minus) —*see* Laceration, vulva
- lacrimal duct —*see* Laceration, eyelid
- large intestine —*see* Laceration, intestine, large
- larynx S11.011
  - with foreign body S11.012
- leg (lower) S81.819
  - with foreign body S81.829
  - foot —*see* Laceration, foot
  - knee —*see* Laceration, knee
  - left S81.812
    - with foreign body S81.822
  - right S81.811
    - with foreign body S81.821
  - upper —*see* Laceration, thigh
- ligament —*see* Sprain
- lip S01.511
  - with foreign body S01.521
- liver S36.113
  - major (stellate) S36.116
  - minor S36.114
  - moderate S36.115
- loin —*see* Laceration, abdomen, wall
- lower back —*see* Laceration, back, lower
- lumbar region —*see* Laceration, back, lower

Laceration *(continued)*
- lung S27.339
  - bilateral S27.332
  - unilateral S27.331
- malar region —*see* Laceration, head, specified site NEC
- mammary —*see* Laceration, breast
- mastoid region —*see* Laceration, head, specified site NEC
- meninges —*see* Injury, intracranial, diffuse
- meniscus —*see* Tear, meniscus
- mesentery S36.893
- mesosalpinx S37.893
- mouth —*see* Laceration, oral cavity
- muscle —*see* Injury, muscle, by site, laceration
- nail
  - finger —*see* Laceration, finger, with damage to nail
  - toe —*see* Laceration, toe, with damage to nail
- nasal (septum) (sinus) —*see* Laceration, nose
- nasopharynx —*see* Laceration, head, specified site NEC
- neck S11.91
  - with foreign body S11.92
  - involving
    - cervical esophagus S11.21
      - with foreign body S11.22
    - larynx —*see* Laceration, larynx
    - pharynx —*see* Laceration, pharynx
    - thyroid gland —*see* Laceration, thyroid gland
    - trachea —*see* Laceration, trachea
  - specified site NEC S11.81
    - with foreign body S11.82
- nerve —*see* Injury, nerve
- nose (septum) (sinus) S01.21
  - with foreign body S01.22
- ocular NOS S05.3-
  - adnexa NOS S01.11-
- oral cavity S01.512
  - with foreign body S01.522
- orbit (eye) —*see* Wound, open, ocular, orbit
- ovary S37.439
  - bilateral S37.432
  - unilateral S37.431
- palate —*see* Laceration, oral cavity
- palm —*see* Laceration, hand
- pancreas S36.239
  - body S36.231
    - major S36.261
    - minor S36.241
    - moderate S36.251
  - head S36.230
    - major S36.260
    - minor S36.240
    - moderate S36.250
  - major S36.269
  - minor S36.249
  - moderate S36.259
  - tail S36.232
    - major S36.262
    - minor S36.242
    - moderate S36.252
- pelvic S31.010
  - with
    - foreign body S31.020
      - penetration into retroperitoneal cavity S31.021
    - penetration into retroperitoneal cavity S31.011
  - floor —*see also* Laceration, back, lower

Laceration *(continued)*
- pelvic *(continued)*
  - floor *(continued)*
    - with ectopic or molar pregnancy O08.6
    - complicating delivery O70.1
    - following ectopic or molar pregnancy O08.6
    - old (postpartal) N81.89
  - organ S37.93
    - with ectopic or molar pregnancy O08.6
    - adrenal gland S37.813
    - bladder S37.23
    - fallopian tube —*see* Laceration, fallopian tube
    - following ectopic or molar pregnancy O08.6
    - kidney —*see* Laceration, kidney
    - obstetrical trauma O71.5
    - ovary —*see* Laceration, ovary
    - prostate S37.823
    - specified site NEC S37.893
    - ureter S37.13
    - urethra S37.33
    - uterus S37.63
- penis S31.21
  - with foreign body S31.22
- perineum
  - female S31.41
    - with
      - ectopic or molar pregnancy O08.6
      - foreign body S31.42
    - during delivery O70.9
      - first degree O70.0
      - fourth degree O70.3
      - second degree O70.1
      - third degree (*see also* Delivery, complicated, by, laceraton, perineum, third degree) O70.20
    - old (postpartal) N81.89
    - postpartal N81.89
    - secondary (postpartal) O90.1
  - male S31.119
    - with foreign body S31.129
- periocular area (with or without lacrimal passages) —*see* Laceration, eyelid
- peritoneum S36.893
- periumbilic region —*see* Laceration, abdomen, wall, periumbilic
- periurethral tissue —*see* Laceration, urethra
- phalanges
  - finger —*see* Laceration, finger
  - toe —*see* Laceration, toe
- pharynx S11.21
  - with foreign body S11.22
- pinna —*see* Laceration, ear
- popliteal space —*see* Laceration, knee
- prepuce —*see* Laceration, penis
- prostate S37.823
- pubic region S31.119
  - with foreign body S31.129
- pudendum —*see* Laceration, genital organs, external
- rectovaginal septum —*see* Laceration, vagina
- rectum S36.63
- retroperitoneum S36.893
- round ligament S37.893
- sacral region —*see* Laceration, back, lower
- sacroiliac region —*see* Laceration, back, lower

Laceration *(continued)*
- salivary gland —*see* Laceration, oral cavity
- scalp S01.01
  - with foreign body S01.02
- scapular region —*see* Laceration, shoulder
- scrotum S31.31
  - with foreign body S31.32
- seminal vesicle S37.893
- shin —*see* Laceration, leg
- shoulder S41.019
  - with foreign body S41.029
  - left S41.012
    - with foreign body S41.022
  - right S41.011
    - with foreign body S41.021
- small intestine —*see* Laceration, intestine, small
- spermatic cord —*see* Laceration, testis
- spinal cord (meninges) —*see also* Injury, spinal cord, by region
  - due to injury at birth P11.5
  - newborn (birth injury) P11.5
- spleen S36.039
  - major (massive) (stellate) S36.032
  - moderate S36.031
  - superficial (minor) S36.030
- sternal region —*see* Laceration, thorax, front
- stomach S36.33
- submaxillary region —*see* Laceration, head, specified site NEC
- submental region —*see* Laceration, head, specified site NEC
- subungual
  - finger(s) —*see* Laceration, finger, with damage to nail
  - toe(s) —*see* Laceration, toe, with damage to nail
- suprarenal gland —*see* Laceration, adrenal gland
- temple, temporal region —*see* Laceration, head, specified site NEC
- temporomandibular area —*see* Laceration, cheek
- tendon —*see* Injury, muscle, by site, laceration
  - Achilles S86.02-
- tentorium cerebelli —*see* Injury, intracranial, diffuse
- testis S31.31
  - with foreign body S31.32
- thigh S71.11-
  - with foreign body S71.12-
- thorax, thoracic (wall) S21.91
  - with foreign body S21.92
    - back S21.22-
      - with penetration into thoracic cavity S21.42-
    - front S21.12-
      - with penetration into thoracic cavity S21.32-
  - back S21.21-
    - with
      - foreign body S21.22-
        - with penetration into thoracic cavity S21.42-
      - penetration into thoracic cavity S21.41-
  - breast —*see* Laceration, breast
  - front S21.11-
    - with
      - foreign body S21.12-
        - with penetration into thoracic cavity S21.32-
      - penetration into thoracic cavity S21.31-

Laceration *(continued)*
- thumb S61.019
  - with
    - damage to nail S61.119
      - with
        - foreign body S61.129
    - foreign body S61.029
  - left S61.012
    - with
      - damage to nail S61.112
        - with
          - foreign body S61.122
      - foreign body S61.022
  - right S61.011
    - with
      - damage to nail S61.111
        - with
          - foreign body S61.121
      - foreign body S61.021
- thyroid gland S11.11
  - with foreign body S11.12
- toe(s) S91.119
  - with
    - damage to nail S91.219
      - with
        - foreign body S91.229
    - foreign body S91.129
  - great S91.113
    - with
      - damage to nail S91.213
        - with
          - foreign body S91.223
      - foreign body S91.123
    - left S91.112
      - with
        - damage to nail S91.212
          - with
            - foreign body S91.222
        - foreign body S91.122
    - right S91.111
      - with
        - damage to nail S91.211
          - with
            - foreign body S91.221
        - foreign body S91.121
  - lesser S91.116
    - with
      - damage to nail S91.216
        - with
          - foreign body S91.226
      - foreign body S91.126
    - left S91.115
      - with
        - damage to nail S91.215
          - with
            - foreign body S91.225
        - foreign body S91.125
    - right S91.114
      - with
        - damage to nail S91.214
          - with
            - foreign body S91.224
        - foreign body S91.124
- tongue *—see* Laceration, oral cavity
- trachea S11.021
  - with foreign body S11.022
- tunica vaginalis *—see* Laceration, testis
- tympanum, tympanic membrane *—see* Laceration, ear, drum
- umbilical region S31.115
  - with foreign body S31.125
- ureter S37.13
- urethra S37.33
  - with or following ectopic or molar pregnancy O08.6
  - obstetrical trauma O71.5
- urinary organ NEC S37.893
- uterus S37.63
  - with ectopic or molar pregnancy O08.6

Laceration *(continued)*
- uterus *(continued)*
  - following ectopic or molar pregnancy O08.6
  - nonpuerperal, nontraumatic N85.8
  - obstetrical trauma NEC O71.81
  - old (postpartal) N85.8
- uvula *—see* Laceration, oral cavity
- vagina S31.41
  - with
    - ectopic or molar pregnancy O08.6
    - foreign body S31.42
  - during delivery O71.4
    - with perineal laceration *—see* Laceration, perineum, female, during delivery
  - following ectopic or molar pregnancy O08.6
  - nonpuerperal, nontraumatic N89.8
  - old (postpartal) N89.8
- vas deferens S37.893
- vesical *—see* Laceration, bladder
- vocal cords S11.031
  - with foreign body S11.032
- vulva S31.41
  - with
    - ectopic or molar pregnancy O08.6
    - foreign body S31.42
  - complicating delivery O70.0
  - following ectopic or molar pregnancy O08.6
  - nonpuerperal, nontraumatic N90.89
  - old (postpartal) N90.89
- wrist S61.519
  - with
    - foreign body S61.529
  - left S61.512
    - with
      - foreign body S61.522
  - right S61.511
    - with
      - foreign body S61.521

Lack of
- achievement in school Z55.3
- adequate
  - food Z59.48
  - intermaxillary vertical dimension of fully erupted teeth M26.36
  - sleep Z72.820
- appetite (*see* Anorexia) R63.0
- awareness R41.9
- care
  - in home Z74.2
  - of infant (at or after birth) T76.02
    - confirmed T74.02
- cognitive functions R41.9
- coordination R27.9
  - ataxia R27.0
  - specified type NEC R27.8
- development (physiological) R62.50
  - failure to thrive (child over 28 days old) R62.51
    - adult R62.7
    - newborn P92.6
  - short stature R62.52
  - specified type NEC R62.59
- energy R53.83
- financial resources Z59.6
- food Z59.48
- growth R62.52
- heating Z59.1

Lack of *(continued)*
- housing (permanent) (temporary) Z59.00
  - adequate Z59.1
- learning experiences in childhood Z62.898
- leisure time (affecting life-style) Z73.2
- material resources Z59.9
- memory *—see also* Amnesia
  - mild, following organic brain damage F06.8
- ovulation N97.0
- parental supervision or control of child Z62.0
- person able to render necessary care Z74.2
- physical exercise Z72.3
- play experience in childhood Z62.898
- posterior occlusal support M26.57
- relaxation (affecting life-style) Z73.2
- safe drinking water Z58.6
- sexual
  - desire F52.0
  - enjoyment F52.1
- shelter Z59.02
- sleep (adequate) Z72.820
- supervision of child by parent Z62.0
- support, posterior occlusal M26.57
- water T73.1
  - safe drinking Z58.6

Lacrimal *—see* condition

Lacrimation, abnormal *—see* Epiphora

Lacrimonasal duct *—see* condition

Lactation, lactating (breast) (puerperal, postpartum)
- associated
  - cracked nipple O92.13
  - retracted nipple O92.03
- defective O92.4
- disorder NEC O92.79
- excessive O92.6
- failed (complete) O92.3
  - partial O92.4
- mastitis NEC *—see* Mastitis, obstetric
- mother (care and/or examination) Z39.1
- nonpuerperal N64.3

Lacticemia, excessive E87.2

Lacunar skull Q75.8

Laennec's cirrhosis K70.30
- with ascites K70.31
- nonalcoholic K74.69

Lafora's disease *—see* Epilepsy, generalized, idiopathic

Lag, lid (nervous) — *see* Retraction, lid

Lagophthalmos (eyelid) (nervous) H02.209
- bilateral, upper and lower eyelids H02.20C
- cicatricial H02.219
  - bilateral, upper and lower eyelids H02.21C
  - left H02.216
    - lower H02.215
    - upper H02.214
    - upper and lower eyelids H02.21B
  - right H02.213
    - lower H02.212
    - upper H02.211
    - upper and lower eyelids H02.21A

Lagophthalmos *(continued)*
- keratoconjunctivitis *—see* Keratoconjunctivitis
- left H02.206
  - lower H02.205
  - upper H02.204
  - upper and lower eyelids H02.20B
- mechanical H02.229
  - bilateral, upper and lower eyelids H02.22C
  - left H02.226
    - lower H02.225
    - upper H02.224
    - upper and lower eyelids H02.22B
  - right H02.223
    - lower H02.222
    - upper H02.221
    - upper and lower eyelids H02.22A
- paralytic H02.239
  - bilateral, upper and lower eyelids H02.23C
  - left H02.236
    - lower H02.235
    - upper H02.234
    - upper and lower eyelids H02.23B
  - right H02.233
    - lower H02.232
    - upper H02.231
    - upper and lower eyelids H02.23A
- right H02.203
  - lower H02.202
  - upper H02.201
  - upper and lower eyelids H02.20A

Laki-Lorand factor deficiency *—see* Defect, coagulation, specified type NEC

Lalling F80.0

Lambert-Eaton syndrome *—see* Syndrome, Lambert-Eaton

Lambliasis, lambliosis A07.1

Landau-Kleffner syndrome *—see* Epilepsy, specified NEC

Landouzy-Déjérine dystrophy or facioscapulohumeral atrophy G71.02

Landouzy's disease (icterohemorrhagic leptospirosis) A27.0

Landry-Guillain-Barré, syndrome or paralysis G61.0

Landry's disease or paralysis G61.0

Lane's
- band Q43.3
- kink *—see* Obstruction, intestine
- syndrome K90.2

Langdon Down syndrome *—see* Trisomy, 21

Lapsed immunization schedule status Z28.3

Large
- baby (regardless of gestational age) (4000g to 4499g) P08.1
- ear, congenital Q17.1
- physiological cup Q14.2
- stature R68.89

Large-for-dates NEC (infant) (4000g to 4499g) P08.1
- affecting management of pregnancy O36.6-

- **Large-for-dates NEC** *(continued)*
  - exceptionally (4500g or more) P08.0
- **Larsen-Johansson disease orosteochondrosis** —*see* Osteochondrosis, juvenile, patella
- **Larsen's syndrome** (flattened facies and multiple congenital dislocations) Q74.8
- **Larva migrans**
  - cutaneous B76.9
    - Ancylostoma B76.0
  - visceral B83.0
- **Laryngeal** —*see* condition
- **Laryngismus** (stridulus) J38.5
  - congenital P28.89
  - diphtheritic A36.2
- **Laryngitis** (acute) (edematous) (fibrinous) (infective) (infiltrative) (malignant) (membranous) (phlegmonous) (pneumococcal) (pseudomembranous) (septic) (subglottic) (suppurative) (ulcerative) J04.0
  - with
    - influenza, flu, or grippe —*see* Influenza, with, laryngitis
    - tracheitis (acute) —*see* Laryngotracheitis
  - atrophic J37.0
  - catarrhal J37.0
  - chronic J37.0
    - with tracheitis (chronic) J37.1
  - diphtheritic A36.2
  - due to external agent —*see* Inflammation, respiratory, upper, due to
  - Hemophilus influenzae J04.0
  - H. influenzae J04.0
  - hypertrophic J37.0
  - influenzal —*see* Influenza, with, respiratory manifestations NEC
  - obstructive J05.0
  - sicca J37.0
  - spasmodic J05.0
    - acute J04.0
  - streptococcal J04.0
  - stridulous J05.0
  - syphilitic (late) A52.73
    - congenital A50.59 *[J99]*
      - early A50.03 *[J99]*
  - tuberculous A15.5
  - Vincent's A69.1
- **Laryngocele** (congenital) (ventricular) Q31.3
- **Laryngofissure** J38.7
  - congenital Q31.8
- **Laryngomalacia** (congenital) Q31.5
- **Laryngopharyngitis** (acute) J06.0
  - chronic J37.0
  - due to external agent —*see* Inflammation, respiratory, upper, due to
- **Laryngoplegia** J38.00
  - bilateral J38.02
  - unilateral J38.01
- **Laryngoptosis** J38.7
- **Laryngospasm** J38.5
- **Laryngostenosis** J38.6
- **Laryngotracheitis** (acute) (Infectional) (infective) (viral) J04.2
  - atrophic J37.1
  - catarrhal J37.1
  - chronic J37.1
  - diphtheritic A36.2
  - due to external agent —*see* Inflammation, respiratory, upper, due to
  - Hemophilus influenzae J04.2
  - hypertrophic J37.1
  - influenzal —*see* Influenza, with, respiratory manifestations NEC
  - pachydermic J38.7
  - sicca J37.1
  - spasmodic J38.5
    - acute J05.0
  - streptococcal J04.2
  - stridulous J38.5
  - syphilitic (late) A52.73
    - congenital A50.59 *[J99]*
      - early A50.03 *[J99]*
  - tuberculous A15.5
  - Vincent's A69.1
- **Laryngotracheobronchitis** —*see* Bronchitis
- **Larynx, laryngeal** —*see* condition
- **Lassa fever** A96.2
- **Lassitude** —*see* Weakness
- **Late**
  - talker R62.0
  - walker R62.0
- **Late effect**(s) —*see* Sequelae
- **Latent** —*see* condition
- **LTBI (latent tuberculosis infection)** Z22.7
- **Laterocession** —*see* Lateroversion
- **Lateroflexion** —*see* Lateroversion
- **Lateroversion**
  - cervix —*see* Lateroversion, uterus
  - uterus, uterine (cervix) (postinfectional) (postpartal, old) N85.4
    - congenital Q51.818
    - in pregnancy or childbirth O34.59-
- **Lathyrism** —*see* Poisoning, food, noxious, plant
- **Launois' syndrome** (pituitary gigantism) E22.0
- **Launois-Bensaude adenolipomatosis** E88.89
- **Laurence-Moon** (-Bardet)-**Biedl syndrome** Q87.89
- **Lax, laxity** —*see also* Relaxation
  - ligament (ous) —*see also* Disorder, ligament
    - familial M35.7
    - knee —*see* Derangement, knee
  - skin (acquired) L57.4
    - congenital Q82.8
- **Laxative habit** F55.2
- **Lazy leukocyte syndrome** D70.8
- **Lead miner's lung** J63.6
- **Leak, leakage**
  - air NEC J93.82
    - postprocedural J95.812
  - amniotic fluid —*see* Rupture, membranes, premature
  - blood (microscopic), fetal, into maternal circulation affecting management of pregnancy —*see* Pregnancy, complicated by
  - cerebrospinal fluid G96.00
    - cranial
      - postoperative G96.08
      - specified NEC G96.08
      - spontaneous G96.01
      - traumatic G96.08
    - from spinal (lumbar) puncture G97.0
    - spinal
      - postoperative G96.09
      - post-traumatic G96.09
      - specified NEC G96.09
      - spontaneous G96.02
    - spontaneous
      - from
        - skull base G96.01
        - spine G96.02
  - CSF —*see* Leak, cerebrospinal fluid
  - device, implant or graft —*see also* Complications, by site and type, mechanical
    - arterial graft NEC —*see* Complication, cardiovascular device, mechanical, vascular
    - breast (implant) T85.43
    - catheter NEC T85.638
      - urinary T83.038
        - cystostomy T83.030
        - Hopkins T83.038
        - ileostomy T83.038
        - indwelling T83.031
        - nephrostomy T83.032
        - specified NEC T83.038
        - urostomy T83.038
      - dialysis (renal) T82.43
        - intraperitoneal T85.631
      - infusion NEC T82.534
        - spinal (epidural) (subdural) T85.630
    - gastrointestinal —*see* Complications, prosthetic device, mechanical, gastrointestinal device
    - genital NEC T83.498
      - penile prosthesis (cylinder) (implanted) (pump) (resevoir) T83.490
      - testicular prosthesis T83.491
    - heart NEC —*see* Complication, cardiovascular device, mechanical
    - joint prosthesis —*see* Complications, joint prosthesis, mechanical, specified NEC, by site
    - ocular NEC —*see* Complications, prosthetic device, mechanical, ocular device
    - orthopedic NEC —*see* Complication, orthopedic, device, mechanical
    - persistent air J93.82
    - specified NEC T85.638
    - urinary NEC —*see also* Complication, genitourinary, device, urinary, mechanical
      - graft T83.23
    - vascular NEC —*see* Complication, cardiovascular device, mechanical
    - ventricular intracranial shunt T85.03
  - urine —*see* Incontinence
- **Leaky heart** —*see* Endocarditis
- **Learning defect** (specific) F81.9
- **Leather bottle stomach** C16.9
- **Leber's**
  - congenital amaurosis H35.50
  - optic atrophy (hereditary) H47.22
- **Lederer's anemia** D59.19
- **Leeches** (external) —*see* Hirudiniasis
- **Leg** —*see* condition
- **Legg** (-Calvé)-**Perthes disease, syndrome or osteochondrosis** M91.1-
- **Legionellosis** A48.1
  - nonpneumonic A48.2
- **Legionnaires'**
  - disease A48.1
    - nonpneumonic A48.2
  - pneumonia A48.1
- **Leigh's disease** G31.82
- **Leiner's disease** L21.1
- **Leiofibromyoma** —*see* Leiomyoma
- **Leiomyoblastoma** —*see* Neoplasm, connective tissue, benign
- **Leiomyofibroma** —*see also* Neoplasm, connective tissue, benign
  - uterus (cervix) (corpus) D25.9
- **Leiomyoma** —*see also* Neoplasm, connective tissue, benign
  - bizarre —*see* Neoplasm, connective tissue, benign
  - cellular —*see* Neoplasm, connective tissue, benign
  - epithelioid —*see* Neoplasm, connective tissue, benign
  - uterus (cervix) (corpus) D25.9
    - intramural D25.1
    - submucous D25.0
    - subserosal D25.2
  - vascular —*see* Neoplasm, connective tissue, benign
- **Leiomyoma, leiomyomatosis** (intravascular) —*see* Neoplasm, connective tissue, uncertain behavior
- **Leiomyosarcoma** —*see also* Neoplasm, connective tissue, malignant
  - epithelioid —*see* Neoplasm, connective tissue, malignant
  - myxoid —*see* Neoplasm, connective tissue, malignant
- **Leishmaniasis** B55.9
  - American (mucocutaneous) B55.2
    - cutaneous B55.1
  - Asian Desert B55.1
  - Brazilian B55.2
  - cutaneous (any type) B55.1
  - dermal —*see also* Leishmaniasis, cutaneous
    - post-kala-azar B55.0
  - eyelid B55.1
  - infantile B55.0
  - Mediterranean B55.0
  - mucocutaneous (American) (New World) B55.2
  - naso-oral B55.2
  - nasopharyngeal B55.2
  - old world B55.1
  - tegumentaria diffusa B55.1
  - visceral B55.0
- **Leishmanoid, dermal** —*see also* Leishmaniasis, cutaneous
  - post-kala-azar B55.0
- **Lenegre's disease** I44.2
- **Lengthening, leg** —*see* Deformity, limb, unequal length
- **Lennert's lymphoma** —*see* Lymphoma, Lennert's

Lennox-Gastaut syndrome G40.812
- intractable G40.814
  - with status epilepticus G40.813
  - without status epilepticus G40.814
- not intractable G40.812
  - with status epilepticus G40.811
  - without status epilepticus G40.812

Lens *—see* condition

Lenticonus (anterior) (posterior) (congenital) Q12.8

Lenticular degeneration, progressive E83.01

Lentiglobus (posterior) (congenital) Q12.8

Lentigo (congenital) L81.4
- maligna *—see also* Melanoma, in situ
  - melanoma *—see* Melanoma

Lentivirus, as cause of disease classified elsewhere B97.31

Leontiasis
- ossium M85.2
- syphilitic (late) A52.78
  - congenital A50.59

Lepothrix A48.8

Lepra *—see* Leprosy

Leprechaunism E34.8

Leprosy A30.-
- with muscle disorder A30.9 *[M63.80]*
  - ankle A30.9 *[M63.87-]*
  - foot A30.9 *[M63.87-]*
  - forearm A30.9 *[M63.83-]*
  - hand A30.9 *[M63.84-]*
  - lower leg A30.9 *[M63.86-]*
  - multiple sites A30.9 *[M63.89]*
  - pelvic region A30.9 *[M63.85-]*
  - shoulder region A30.9 *[M63.81-]*
  - specified site NEC A30.9 *[M63.88]*
  - thigh A30.9 *[M63.85-]*
  - upper arm A30.9 *[M63.82-]*
- anesthetic A30.9
- BB A30.3
- BL A30.4
- borderline (infiltrated) (neuritic) A30.3
  - lepromatous A30.4
  - tuberculoid A30.2
- BT A30.2
- dimorphous (infiltrated) (neuritic) A30.3
- I A30.0
- indeterminate (macular) (neuritic) A30.0
- lepromatous (diffuse) (infiltrated) (macular) (neuritic) (nodular) A30.5
- LL A30.5
- macular (early) (neuritic) (simple) A30.9
- maculoanesthetic A30.9
- mixed A30.3
- neural A30.9
- nodular A30.5
- primary neuritic A30.3
- specified type NEC A30.8
- TT A30.1
- tuberculoid (major) (minor) A30.1

Leptocytosis, hereditary D56.9

Leptomeningitis (chronic) (circumscribed) (hemorrhagic) (nonsuppurative) *—see* Meningitis

Leptomeningopathy G96.198

Leptospiral *—see* condition

Leptospirochetal *—see* condition

Leptospirosis A27.9
- canicola A27.89
- due to Leptospira interrogans serovar icterohaemorrhagiae A27.0
- icterohemorrhagica A27.0
- pomona A27.89
- Weil's disease A27.0

Leptus dermatitis B88.0

Leriche's syndrome (aortic bifurcation occlusion) I74.09

Leri's pleonosteosis Q78.8

Leri-Weill syndrome Q77.8

Lermoyez' syndrome *—see* Vertigo, peripheral NEC

Lesch-Nyhan syndrome E79.1

Leser-Trélat disease L82.1
- inflamed L82.0

Lesion(s) (nontraumatic)
- abducens nerve *—see* Strabismus, paralytic, sixth nerve
- alveolar process K08.9
- angiocentric immunoproliferative D47.Z9
- anorectal K62.9
- aortic (valve) I35.9
- auditory nerve *—see* subcategory H93.3
- basal ganglion G25.9
- bile duct *—see* Disease, bile duct
- biomechanical M99.9
  - specified type NEC M99.89
    - abdomen M99.89
    - acromioclavicular M99.87
    - cervical region M99.81
    - cervicothoracic M99.81
    - costochondral M99.88
    - costovertebral M99.88
    - head region M99.80
    - hip M99.85
    - lower extremity M99.86
    - lumbar region M99.83
    - lumbosacral M99.83
    - occipitocervical M99.80
    - pelvic region M99.85
    - pubic M99.85
    - rib cage M99.88
    - sacral region M99.84
    - sacrococcygeal M99.84
    - sacroiliac M99.84
    - specified NEC M99.89
    - sternochondral M99.88
    - sternoclavicular M99.87
    - thoracic region M99.82
    - thoracolumbar M99.82
    - upper extremity M99.87
- bladder N32.9
- bone *—see* Disorder, bone
- brachial plexus G54.0
- brain G93.9
  - congenital Q04.9
  - vascular I67.9
    - degenerative I67.9
    - hypertensive I67.4
- buccal cavity K13.79
- calcified *—see* Calcification
- canthus *—see* Disorder, eyelid
- carate *—see* Pinta, lesions
- cardia K31.9
- cardiac (*see also* Disease, heart) I51.9
  - congenital Q24.9
  - valvular *—see* Endocarditis
- cauda equina G83.4
- cecum K63.9
- cerebral *—see* Lesion, brain

Lesion *(continued)*
- cerebrovascular I67.9
  - degenerative I67.9
  - hypertensive I67.4
- cervical (nerve) root NEC G54.2
- chiasmal *—see* Disorder, optic, chiasm
- chorda tympani G51.8
- coin, lung R91.1
- colon K63.9
- combined periodontic - endodontic K05.5
- congenital *—see* Anomaly, by site
- conjunctiva H11.9
- conus medullaris *—see* Injury, conus medullaris
- coronary artery *—see* Ischemia, heart
- cranial nerve G52.9
  - eighth *—see* Disorder, ear
  - eleventh G52.9
  - fifth G50.9
  - first G52.0
  - fourth *—see* Strabismus, paralytic, fourth nerve
  - seventh G51.9
  - sixth *—see* Strabismus, paralytic, sixth nerve
  - tenth G52.2
  - twelfth G52.3
- cystic *—see* Cyst
- degenerative *—see* Degeneration
- duodenum K31.9
- edentulous (alveolar) ridge, associated with trauma, due to traumatic occlusion K06.2
- en coup de sabre L94.1
- eyelid *—see* Disorder, eyelid
- gasserian ganglion G50.8
- gastric K31.9
- gastroduodenal K31.9
- gastrointestinal K63.9
- gingiva, associated with trauma K06.2
- glomerular
  - focal and segmental (*see also* N00-N07 with fourth character .1) N05.1
  - minimal change (*see also* N00-N07 with fourth character .0) N05.0
- heart (organic) *—see* Disease, heart
- hyperchromic, due to pinta (carate) A67.1
- hyperkeratotic *—see* Hyperkeratosis
- hypothalamic E23.7
- ileocecal K63.9
- ileum K63.9
- iliohypogastric nerve G57.8-
- inflammatory *—see* Inflammation
- intestine K63.9
- intracerebral *—see* Lesion, brain
- intrachiasmal (optic) *—see* Disorder, optic, chiasm
- intracranial, space-occupying R90.0
- joint *—see* Disorder, joint
  - sacroiliac (old) M53.3
- keratotic *—see* Keratosis
- kidney *—see* Disease, renal
- laryngeal nerve (recurrent) G52.2
- lip K13.0
- liver K76.9
- lumbosacral
  - plexus G54.1
  - root (nerve) NEC G54.4
- lung (coin) R91.1
- maxillary sinus J32.0
- mitral I05.9

Lesion *(continued)*
- Morel-Lavallée *—see* Hematoma, by site
- motor cortex NEC G93.89
- mouth K13.79
- nerve G58.9
  - femoral G57.2-
  - median G56.1-
    - carpal tunnel syndrome *—see* Syndrome, carpal tunnel
  - plantar G57.6-
  - popliteal (lateral) G57.3-
    - medial G57.4-
  - radial G56.3-
  - sciatic G57.0-
  - spinal *—see* Injury, nerve, spinal
  - ulnar G56.2-
- nervous system, congenital Q07.9
- nonallopathic *—see* Lesion, biomechanical
- nose (internal) J34.89
- obstructive *—see* Obstruction
- obturator nerve G57.8-
- oral mucosa K13.70
- organ or site NEC *—see* Disease, by site
- osteolytic *—see* Osteolysis
- peptic K27.9
- periodontal, due to traumatic occlusion K05.5
- pharynx J39.2
- pigment, pigmented (skin) L81.9
- pinta *—see* Pinta, lesions
- polypoid *—see* Polyp
- prechiasmal (optic) *—see* Disorder, optic, chiasm
- primary (*see also* Syphilis, primary) A51.0
  - carate A67.0
  - pinta A67.0
  - yaws A66.0
- pulmonary J98.4
  - valve I37.9
- pylorus K31.9
- rectosigmoid K63.9
- retina, retinal H35.9
- sacroiliac (joint) (old) M53.3
- salivary gland K11.9
  - benign lymphoepithelial K11.8
- saphenous nerve G57.8-
- sciatic nerve G57.0-
- secondary *—see* Syphilis, secondary
- shoulder (region) M75.9-
  - specified NEC M75.8-
- sigmoid K63.9
- sinus (accessory) (nasal) J34.89
- skin L98.9
  - suppurative L08.0
- SLAP S43.43-
- spinal cord G95.9
  - congenital Q06.9
- spleen D73.89
- stomach K31.9
- superior glenoid labrum S43.43-
- syphilitic *—see* Syphilis
- tertiary *—see* Syphilis, tertiary
- thoracic root (nerve) NEC G54.3
- tonsillar fossa J35.9
- tooth, teeth K08.9
  - white spot
    - chewing surface K02.51
    - pit and fissure surface K02.51
    - smooth surface K02.61
- traumatic *—see* specific type of injury by site
- tricuspid (valve) I07.9
  - nonrheumatic I36.9

Lesion *(continued)*
- trigeminal nerve G50.9
- ulcerated or ulcerative —*see* Ulcer, skin
- uterus N85.9
- vagina N89.8
- vagus nerve G52.2
- valvular —*see* Endocarditis
- vascular I99.9
  - affecting central nervous system I67.9
  - following trauma NEC T14.8
  - umbilical cord, complicating delivery O69.5
- vulva N90.89
- warty —*see* Verruca
- white spot (tooth)
  - chewing surface K02.51
  - pit and fissure surface K02.51
  - smooth surface K02.61

Lethargic —*see* condition

Less than a high school diploma Z55.5

Lethargy R53.83

Letterer-Siwe's disease C96.0

Leukemia, leukemic C95.9-
- acute basophilic C94.8-
- acute bilineal C95.0-
- acute erythroid C94.0-
- acute lymphoblastic C91.0-
- acute megakaryoblastic C94.2-
- acute megakaryocytic C94.2-
- acute mixed lineage C95.0-
- acute monoblastic (monoblastic/monocytic) C93.0-
- acute monocytic (monoblastic/monocytic) C93.0-
- acute myeloblastic (minimal differentiation) (with maturation) C92.0-
- acute myeloid, NOS C92.0-
  - with
    - 11q23-abnormality C92.6-
    - dysplasia of remaining hematopoesis and/or myelodysplastic disease in its history C92.A-
    - multilineage dysplasia C92.A-
    - variation of MLL-gene C92.6-
  - M6 (a)(b) C94.0-
  - M7 C94.2-
- acute myelomonocytic C92.5-
- acute promyelocytic C92.4-
- adult T-cell (HTLV-1-associated) (acute variant) (chronic variant) (lymphomatoid variant) (smouldering variant) C91.5-
- aggressive NK-cell C94.8-
- AML (1/ETO) (M0) (M1) (M2) (without a FAB classification) C92.0-
- AML M3 C92.4-
- AML M4 (Eo with inv (16) or t (16;16)) C92.5-
- AML M5 C93.0-
- AML M5a C93.0-
- AML M5b C93.0-
- AML Me with t (15;17) and variants C92.4-
- atypical chronic myeloid, BCR/ABL-negative C92.2-
- biphenotypic acute C95.0-
- blast cell C95.0-
- Burkitt-type, mature B-cell C91.A-
- chronic eosinophilic (*see also* Syndrome, hypereosinophilic, myeloid) C94.8-
- chronic lymphocytic, of B-cell type C91.1-

Leukemia, leukemic *(continued)*
- chronic monocytic C93.1-
- chronic myelogenous (Philadelphia chromosome (Ph1) positive) (t (9;22)) (q34;q11) (with crisis of blast cells) C92.1-
- chronic myeloid, BCR/ABL-positive C92.1-
  - atypical, BCR/ABL-negative C92.2-
- chronic myelomonocytic C93.1-
- chronic neutrophilic D47.1
- CMML (-1) (-2) (with eosinophilia) C93.1-
- granulocytic (*see also* Category C92) C92.9-
- hairy cell C91.4-
- juvenile myelomonocytic C93.3-
- lymphoid C91.9-
  - specified NEC C91.Z-
- mast cell C94.3-
- mature B-cell, Burkitt-type C91.A-
- monocytic (subacute) C93.9-
  - specified NEC C93.Z-
- myelogenous (*see also* Category C92) C92.9-
- myeloid C92.9-
  - specified NEC C92.Z-
- plasma cell C90.1-
- plasmacytic C90.1-
- prolymphocytic
  - of B-cell type C91.3-
  - of T-cell type C91.6-
- specified NEC C94.8-
- stem cell, of unclear lineage C95.0-
- subacute lymphocytic C91.9-
- T-cell large granular lymphocytic C91.Z-
- unspecified cell type C95.9-
  - acute C95.0-
  - chronic C95.1-

Leukemoid reaction (*see also* Reaction, leukemoid) D72.823-

Leukoaraiosis (hypertensive) I67.81

Leukoariosis —*see* Leukoaraiosis

Leukocoria —*see* Disorder, globe, degenerated condition, leucocoria

Leukocytopenia D72.819

Leukocytosis D72.829
- eosinophilic D72.19

Leukoderma, leukodermia NEC L81.5
- syphilitic A51.39
  - late A52.79

Leukodystrophy E75.29

Leukoedema, oral epithelium K13.29

Leukoencephalitis G04.81
- acute (subacute) hemorrhagic G36.1
  - postimmunization or postvaccinal G04.02
- postinfectious G04.01
- subacute sclerosing A81.1
- van Bogaert's (sclerosing) A81.1

Leukoencephalopathy (*see also* Encephalopathy) G93.49
- Binswanger's I67.3
- heroin vapor G92.8
- metachromatic E75.25
- multifocal (progressive) A81.2
- postimmunization and postvaccinal G04.02
- progressive multifocal A81.2
- reversible, posterior G93.6
- van Bogaert's (sclerosing) A81.1
- vascular, progressive I67.3

Leukoerythroblastosis D75.9

Leukokeratosis —*see also* Leukoplakia
- mouth K13.21
- nicotina palati K13.24
- oral mucosa K13.21
- tongue K13.21
- vocal cord J38.3

Leukokraurosis vulva (e) N90.4

Leukoma (cornea) —*see also* Opacity, cornea
- adherent H17.0-
- interfering with central vision —*see* Opacity, cornea, central

Leukomalacia, cerebral, newborn P91.2
- periventricular P91.2

Leukomelanopathy, hereditary D72.0

Leukonychia (punctata) (striata) L60.8
- congenital Q84.4

Leukopathia unguium L60.8
- congenital Q84.4

Leukopenia D72.819
- basophilic D72.818
- chemotherapy (cancer) induced D70.1
- congenital D70.0
- cyclic D70.0
- drug induced NEC D70.2
  - due to cytoreductive cancer chemotherapy D70.1
- eosinophilic D72.818
- familial D70.0
- infantile genetic D70.0
- malignant D70.9
- periodic D70.0
- transitory neonatal P61.5

Leukopenic —*see* condition

Leukoplakia
- anus K62.89
- bladder (postinfectional) N32.89
- buccal K13.21
- cervix (uteri) N88.0
- esophagus K22.89
- gingiva K13.21
- hairy (oral mucosa) (tongue) K13.3
- kidney (pelvis) N28.89
- larynx J38.7
- lip K13.21
- mouth K13.21
- oral epithelium, including tongue (mucosa) K13.21
- palate K13.21
- pelvis (kidney) N28.89
- penis (infectional) N48.0
- rectum K62.89
- syphilitic (late) A52.79
- tongue K13.21
- ureter (postinfectional) N28.89
- urethra (postinfectional) N36.8
- uterus N85.8
- vagina N89.4
- vocal cord J38.3
- vulva N90.4

Leukorrhea N89.8
- due to Trichomonas (vaginalis) A59.00
- trichomonal A59.00

Leukosarcoma C85.9-

Levocardia (isolated) Q24.1
- with situs inversus Q89.3

Levotransposition Q20.5

Lev's disease or syndrome (acquired complete heart block) I44.2

Levulosuria —*see* Fructosuria

Levurid L30.2

Lewy body (ies) (dementia) (disease) G31.83

Leyden-Moebius dystrophy G71.09

Leydig cell
- carcinoma
  - specified site —*see* Neoplasm, malignant, by site
  - unspecified site
    - female C56.9
    - male C62.9-
- tumor
  - benign
    - specified site —*see* Neoplasm, benign, by site
    - unspecified site
      - female D27.-
      - male D29.2-
  - malignant
    - specified site —*see* Neoplasm, malignant, by site
    - unspecified site
      - female C56.-
      - male C62.9-
  - specified site —*see* Neoplasm, uncertain behavior, by site
  - unspecified site
    - female D39.1-
    - male D40.1-

Leydig-Sertoli cell tumor
- specified site —*see* Neoplasm, benign, by site
- unspecified site
  - female D27.-
  - male D29.2-

LGSIL (Low grade squamous intraepithelial lesion on cytologic smear of)
- anus R85.612
- cervix R87.612
- vagina R87.622

Liar, pathologic F60.2

Libido
- decreased R68.82

Libman-Sacks disease M32.11

Lice (infestation) B85.2
- body (Pediculus corporis) B85.1
- crab B85.3
- head (Pediculus capitis) B85.0
- mixed (classifiable to more than one of the titles B85.0-B85.3) B85.4
- pubic (Phthirus pubis) B85.3

Lichen L28.0
- albus L90.0
  - penis N48.0
  - vulva N90.4
- amyloidosis E85.4 *[L99]*
- atrophicus L90.0
  - penis N48.0
  - vulva N90.4
- congenital Q82.8
- myxedematosus L98.5
- nitidus L44.1
- pilaris Q82.8
  - acquired L85.8
- planopilaris L66.1
- planus (chronicus) L43.9
  - annularis L43.8
  - bullous L43.1
  - follicular L66.1
  - hypertrophic L43.0
  - moniliformis L44.3

Lichen *(continued)*
- planus *(continued)*
  - of Wilson L43.9
  - specified NEC L43.8
  - subacute (active) L43.3
  - tropicus L43.3
- ruber
  - acuminatus L44.0
  - moniliformis L44.3
  - planus L43.9
- sclerosus (et atrophicus) L90.0
  - penis N48.0
  - vulva N90.4
- scrofulosus (primary) (tuberculous) A18.4
- simplex (chronicus) (circumscriptus) L28.0
- striatus L44.2
- urticatus L28.2

Lichenification L28.0

Lichenoides tuberculosis (primary) A18.4

Lichtheim's disease or syndrome D51.0

Lien migrans D73.89

Ligament —*see* condition

Light
- for gestational age —*see* Light for dates
- headedness R42

Light-for-dates (infant) P05.00
- with weight of
  - 499 grams or less P05.01
  - 500-749 grams P05.02
  - 750-999 grams P05.03
  - 1000-1249 grams P05.04
  - 1250-1499 grams P05.05
  - 1500-1749 grams P05.06
  - 1750-1999 grams P05.07
  - 2000-2499 grams P05.08
  - 2500 grams and over P05.09
- and small-for-dates —*see* Small for dates
- affecting management of pregnancy O36.59-
- specified NEC P05.09

Lightning (effects) (stroke) (struck by) T75.00
- burn —*see* Burn
- foot E53.8
- shock T75.01
- specified effect NEC T75.09

Lightwood-Albright syndrome N25.89

Lightwood's disease or syndrome (renal tubular acidosis) N25.89

Lignac (-de Toni) (-Fanconi) (-Debré) **disease or syndrome** E72.09
- with cystinosis E72.04

Ligneous thyroiditis E06.5

Likoff's syndrome I20.8

Limb —*see* condition

Limbic epilepsy personality syndrome F07.0

Limitation, limited
- activities due to disability Z73.6
- cardiac reserve —*see* Disease, heart
- eye muscle duction, traumatic —*see* Strabismus, mechanical
- mandibular range of motion M26.52

Lindau (-von Hippel) **disease** Q85.8

Line(s)
- Beau's L60.4
- Harris' —*see* Arrest, epiphyseal
- Hudson's (cornea) —*see* Pigmentation, cornea, anterior
- Stähli's (cornea) —*see* Pigmentation, cornea, anterior

Linea corneae senilis —*see* Change, cornea, senile

Lingua
- geographica K14.1
- nigra (villosa) K14.3
- plicata K14.5
- tylosis K13.29

Lingual —*see* condition

Linguatulosis B88.8

Linitis (gastric) **plastica** C16.9

Lip —*see* condition

Lipedema —*see* Edema

Lipemia —*see also* Hyperlipidemia
- retina, retinalis E78.3

Lipidosis E75.6
- cerebral (infantile) (juvenile) (late) E75.4
- cerebroretinal E75.4
- cerebroside E75.22
- cholesterol (cerebral) E75.5
- glycolipid E75.21
- hepatosplenomegalic E78.3
- sphingomyelin —*see* Niemann-Pick disease or syndrome
- sulfatide E75.29

Lipoadenoma —*see* Neoplasm, benign, by site

Lipoblastoma —*see* Lipoma

Lipoblastomatosis —*see* Lipoma

Lipochondrodystrophy E76.01

Lipodermatosclerosis —*see* Varix, leg, with, inflammation
- ulcerated —*see* Varix, leg, with, ulcer, with inflammation by site

Lipochrome histiocytosis (familial) D71

Lipodystrophia progressiva E88.1

Lipodystrophy (progressive) E88.1
- insulin E88.1
- intestinal K90.81
- mesenteric K65.4

Lipofibroma —*see* Lipoma

Lipofuscinosis, neuronal (with ceroidosis) E75.4

Lipogranuloma, sclerosing L92.8

Lipogranulomatosis E78.89

Lipoid —*see also* condition
- histiocytosis D76.3
  - essential E75.29
- nephrosis N04.9
- proteinosis of Urbach E78.89

Lipoidemia —*see* Hyperlipidemia

Lipoidosis —*see* Lipidosis

Lipoma D17.9
- fetal D17.9
  - fat cell D17.9
- infiltrating D17.9
- intramuscular D17.9
- pleomorphic D17.9
- site classification
  - arms (skin) (subcutaneous) D17.2-
  - connective tissue D17.30
    - intra-abdominal D17.5
    - intrathoracic D17.4

Lipoma *(continued)*
- site classification *(continued)*
  - connective tissue *(continued)*
    - peritoneum D17.79
    - retroperitoneum D17.79
    - specified site NEC D17.39
    - spermatic cord D17.6
  - face (skin) (subcutaneous) D17.0
  - genitourinary organ NEC D17.72
  - head (skin) (subcutaneous) D17.0
  - intra-abdominal D17.5
  - intrathoracic D17.4
  - kidney D17.71
  - legs (skin) (subcutaneous) D17.2-
  - neck (skin) (subcutaneous) D17.0
  - peritoneum D17.79
  - retroperitoneum D17.79
  - skin D17.30
    - specified site NEC D17.39
  - specified site NEC D17.79
  - spermatic cord D17.6
  - subcutaneous D17.30
    - specified site NEC D17.39
  - trunk (skin) (subcutaneous) D17.1
  - unspecified D17.9
- spindle cell D17.9

Lipomatosis E88.2
- dolorosa (Dercum) E88.2
- fetal —*see* Lipoma
- Launois-Bensaude E88.89

Lipomyoma —*see* Lipoma

Lipomyxoma —*see* Lipoma

Lipomyxosarcoma —*see* Neoplasm, connective tissue, malignant

Lipoprotein metabolism disorder E78.9

Lipoproteinemia E78.5
- broad-beta E78.2
- floating-beta E78.2
- hyper-pre-beta E78.1

Liposarcoma —*see also* Neoplasm, connective tissue, malignant
- dedifferentiated —*see* Neoplasm, connective tissue, malignant
- differentiated type —*see* Neoplasm, connective tissue, malignant
- embryonal —*see* Neoplasm, connective tissue, malignant
- mixed type —*see* Neoplasm, connective tissue, malignant
- myxoid —*see* Neoplasm, connective tissue, malignant
- pleomorphic —*see* Neoplasm, connective tissue, malignant
- round cell —*see* Neoplasm, connective tissue, malignant
- well differentiated type —*see* Neoplasm, connective tissue, malignant

Liposynovitis prepatellaris E88.89

Lipping, cervix N86

Lipschütz disease or ulcer N76.6

Lipuria R82.0
- schistosomiasis (bilharziasis) B65.0

Lisping F80.0

Lissauer's paralysis A52.17

Lissencephalia, lissencephaly Q04.3

Listeriosis, listerellosis A32.9
- congenital (disseminated) P37.2
- cutaneous A32.0

Listeriosis, listerellosis *(continued)*
- neonatal, newborn (disseminated) P37.2
- oculoglandular A32.81
- specified NEC A32.89

Lithemia E79.0

Lithiasis —*see* Calculus

Lithosis J62.8

Lithuria R82.998

Litigation, anxiety concerning Z65.3

Little leaguer's elbow —*see* Epicondylitis, medial

Little's disease G80.9

Littre's
- gland —*see* condition
- hernia —*see* Hernia, abdomen

Littritis —*see* Urethritis

Livedo (annularis) (racemosa) (reticularis) R23.1

Liver —*see* condition

Living alone (problems with) Z60.2
- with handicapped person Z74.2

Living in a shelter (motel) (scattered site housing) (temporary or transitional living situation) Z59.01

Lloyd's syndrome —*see* Adenomatosis, endocrine

Loa loa, loaiasis, loasis B74.3

Lobar —*see* condition

Lobomycosis B48.0

Lobo's disease B48.0

Lobotomy syndrome F07.0

Lobstein (-Ekman) **disease or syndrome** Q78.0

Lobster-claw hand Q71.6-

Lobulation (congenital) —*see also* Anomaly, by site
- kidney, Q63.1
- liver, abnormal Q44.7
- spleen Q89.09

Lobule, lobular —*see* condition

Local, localized —*see* condition

Locked-in state G83.5

Locked twins causing obstructed labor O66.1

Locking
- joint —*see* Derangement, joint, specified type NEC
  - knee —*see* Derangement, knee

Lockjaw —*see* Tetanus

Löffler's
- endocarditis I42.3
- eosinophilia J82.89
- pneumonia J82.89
- syndrome (eosinophilic pneumonitis) J82.89

Loiasis (with conjunctival infestation) (eyelid) B74.3

Lone Star fever A77.0

Long
- COVID (-19) (*see also* COVID-19) U09.9
- labor O63.9
  - first stage O63.0
  - second stage O63.1
- QT syndrome I45.81

Long-term (current) (prophylactic)
drug therapy (use of)
agents affecting estrogen receptors and estrogen levels NEC Z79.818
anastrozole (Arimidex) Z79.811
antibiotics Z79.2
short-term use - omit code
anticoagulants Z79.01
anti-inflammatory, non-steroidal (NSAID) Z79.1
antiplatelet Z79.02
antithrombotics Z79.02
aromatase inhibitors Z79.811
aspirin Z79.82
birth control pill or patch Z79.3
bisphosphonates Z79.83
contraceptive, oral Z79.3
drug, specified NEC Z79.899
estrogen receptor downregulators Z79.818
Evista Z79.810
exemestane (Aromasin) Z79.811
Fareston Z79.810
fulvestrant (Faslodex) Z79.818
gonadotropin-releasing hormone (GnRH) agonist Z79.818
goserelin acetate (Zoladex) Z79.818
hormone replacement Z79.890
insulin Z79.4
letrozole (Femara) Z79.811
leuprolide acetate (leuprorelin) (Lupron) Z79.818
megestrol acetate (Megace) Z79.818
methadone for pain management Z79.891
Nolvadex Z79.810
non-insulin antidiabetic drug, injectable Z79.899
non-steroidal anti-inflammatories (NSAID) Z79.1
opiate analgesic Z79.891
oral
antidiabetic Z79.84
contraceptive Z79.3
hypoglycemic Z79.84
raloxifene (Evista) Z79.810
selective estrogen receptor modulators (SERMs) Z79.810
steroids
inhaled Z79.51
systemic Z79.52
tamoxifen (Nolvadex) Z79.810
toremifene (Fareston) Z79.810

Longitudinal stripes or grooves, nails L60.8
congenital Q84.6

Loop
intestine *—see* Volvulus
vascular on papilla (optic) Q14.2

Loose *—see also* condition
body
joint M24.00
ankle M24.07-
elbow M24.02-
hand M24.04-
hip M24.05-
knee M23.4-
shoulder (region) M24.01-
specified site NEC M24.08
vertebra M24.08
toe M24.07-
wrist M24.03-
knee M23.4-
sheath, tendon *—see* Disorder, tendon, specified type NEC
cartilage *—see* Loose, body, joint

Loose *(continued)*
skin and subcutaneous tissue (following bariatric surgery weight loss) (following dietary weight loss) L98.7
tooth, teeth K08.89

Loosening
aseptic
joint prosthesis *—see* Complications, joint prosthesis, mechanical, loosening, by site
epiphysis *—see* Osteochondropathy
mechanical
joint prosthesis *—see* Complications, joint prosthesis, mechanical, loosening, by site

Looser-Milkman (-Debray) **syndrome** M83.8

Lop ear (deformity) Q17.3

Lorain (-Levi) **short stature syndrome** E23.0

Lordosis M40.50
acquired *—see* Lordosis, specified type NEC
congenital Q76.429
lumbar region Q76.426
lumbosacral region Q76.427
sacral region Q76.428
sacrococcygeal region Q76.428
thoracolumbar region Q76.425
lumbar region M40.56
lumbosacral region M40.57
postsurgical M96.4
postural *—see* Lordosis, specified type NEC
rachitic (late effect) (sequelae) E64.3
sequelae of rickets E64.3
specified type NEC M40.40
lumbar region M40.46
lumbosacral region M40.47
thoracolumbar region M40.45
thoracolumbar region M40.55
tuberculous A18.01

Loss (of)
appetite (*see* Anorexia) R63.0
hysterical F50.89
nonorganic origin F50.89
psychogenic F50.89
blood *—see* Hemorrhage
bone *—see* Loss, substance of, bone
control, sphincter, rectum R15.9
nonorganic origin F98.1
consciousness, transient R55
traumatic *—see* Injury, intracranial
elasticity, skin R23.4
family (member) in childhood Z62.898
fluid (acute) E86.9
function of labyrinth H83.2
hair, nonscarring *—see* Alopecia
hearing *—see also* Deafness
central NOS H90.5
conductive H90.2
bilateral H90.0
unilateral
with
restricted hearing on the contralateral side H90.A1-
unrestricted hearing on the contralateral side H90.1-

Loss *(continued)*
hearing *(continued)*
mixed conductive and sensorineural hearing loss H90.8
bilateral H90.6
unilateral
with
restricted hearing on the contralateral side H90.A3-
unrestricted hearing on the contralateral side H90.7-
neural NOS H90.5
perceptive NOS H90.5
sensorineural NOS H90.5
bilateral H90.3
unilateral
with
restricted hearing on the contralateral side H90.A2-
unrestricted hearing on the contralateral side H90.4-
sensory NOS H90.5
height R29.890
limb or member, traumatic, current *—see* Amputation, traumatic
love relationship in childhood Z62.898
memory *—see also* Amnesia
mild, following organic brain damage F06.8
mind *—see* Psychosis
occlusal vertical dimension of fully erupted teeth M26.37
organ or part *—see* Absence, by site, acquired
ossicles, ear (partial) H74.32-
parent in childhood Z63.4
pregnancy, recurrent N96
care in current pregnancy O26.2-
without current pregnancy N96
recurrent pregnancy *—see* Loss, pregnancy, recurrent
self-esteem, in childhood Z62.898
sense of
smell *—see* Disturbance, sensation, smell
taste *—see* Disturbance, sensation, taste
touch R20.8
sensory R44.9
dissociative F44.6
sexual desire F52.0
sight (acquired) (complete) (congenital) *—see* Blindness
substance of
bone *—see* Disorder, bone, density and structure, specified NEC
horizontal alveolar K06.3
cartilage *—see* Disorder, cartilage, specified type NEC
auricle (ear) *—see* Disorder, pinna, specified type NEC
vitreous (humor) H15.89
tooth, teeth *—see* Absence, teeth, acquired
vision, visual H54.7
both eyes H54.3
one eye H54.60
left (normal vision on right) H54.62
right (normal vision on left) H54.61

Loss *(continued)*
vision *(continued)*
specified as blindness *—see* Blindness
subjective
sudden H53.13-
transient H53.12-
vitreous *—see* Prolapse, vitreous
voice *—see* Aphonia
weight (abnormal) (cause unknown) R63.4

Louis-Bar syndrome (ataxia-telangiectasia) G11.3

Louping ill (encephalitis) A84.89

Louse, lousiness *—see* Lice

Low
achiever, school Z55.3
back syndrome M54.50
basal metabolic rate R94.8
birthweight (2499 grams or less) P07.10
with weight of
1000-1249 grams P07.14
1250-1499 grams P07.15
1500-1749 grams P07.16
1750-1999 grams P07.17
2000-2499 grams P07.18
extreme (999 grams or less) P07.00
with weight of
499 grams or less P07.01
500-749 grams P07.02
750-999 grams P07.03
for gestational age *—see* Light for dates
blood pressure *—see also* Hypotension
reading (incidental) (isolated) (nonspecific) R03.1
cardiac reserve *—see* Disease, heart
function *—see also* Hypofunction
kidney N28.9
hematocrit D64.9
hemoglobin D64.9
income Z59.6
level of literacy Z55.0
lying
kidney N28.89
organ or site, congenital *—see* Malposition, congenital
output syndrome (cardiac) *—see* Failure, heart
platelets (blood) *—see* Thrombocytopenia
reserve, kidney N28.89
salt syndrome E87.1
self esteem R45.81
set ears Q17.4
vision H54.2X-
one eye (other eye normal) H54.50
left (normal vision on right) H54.52A-
other eye blind *—see* Blindness
right (normal vision on left) H54.511-

Low-density-lipoprotein-type (LDL) **hyperlipoproteinemia** E78.00

Lowe's syndrome E72.03

Lown-Ganong-Levine syndrome I45.6

LSD reaction (acute) (without dependence) F16.90
with dependence F16.20

L-shaped kidney Q63.8

- **Ludwig's angina or disease** K12.2
- **Lues** (venerea), **luetic** —*see* Syphilis
- **Luetscher's syndrome** (dehydration) E86.0
- **Lumbago, lumbalgia** M54.50
  - with sciatica M54.4-
    - due to intervertebral disc disorder M51.17
  - due to displacement, intervertebral disc M51.27
    - with sciatica M51.17
- **Lumbar** —*see* condition
- **Lumbarization, vertebra, congenital** Q76.49
- **Lumbermen's itch** B88.0
- **Lump** —*see also* Mass
  - breast N63.0
    - axillary tail
      - left N63.32
      - right N63.31
    - left
      - lower inner quadrant N63.24
      - lower outer quadrant N63.23
      - overlapping quadrants N63.25
      - unspecified quadrant N63.20
      - upper inner quadrant N63.22
      - upper outer quadrant N63.21
    - right
      - lower inner quadrant N63.14
      - lower outer quadrant N63.13
      - overlapping quadrants N63.15
      - unspecified quadrant N63.10
      - upper inner quadrant N63.12
      - upper outer quadrant N63.11
    - subareolar
      - left N63.42
      - right N63.41
- **Lunacy** —*see* Psychosis
- **Lung** —*see* condition
- **Lupoid** (miliary) **of Boeck** D86.3
- **Lupus**
  - anticoagulant D68.62
    - with
      - hemorrhagic disorder D68.312
      - hypercoagulable state D68.62
    - finding without diagnosis R76.0
  - discoid (local) L93.0
  - erythematosus (discoid) (local) L93.0
    - disseminated —*see* Lupus, erythematosus, systemic
    - eyelid H01.129
      - left H01.126
        - lower H01.125
        - upper H01.124
      - right H01.123
        - lower H01.122
        - upper H01.121
    - profundus L93.2
    - specified NEC L93.2
    - subacute cutaneous L93.1
    - systemic M32.9
      - with organ or system involvement M32.10
        - endocarditis M32.11
        - lung M32.13
        - pericarditis M32.12
        - renal (glomerular) M32.14
          - tubulo-interstitial M32.15
        - specified organ or system NEC M32.19
      - drug-induced M32.0
      - inhibitor (presence of) D68.62
        - with
          - hemorrhagic disorder D68.312
          - hypercoagulable state D68.62

- **Lupus** *(continued)*
  - erythematosus *(continued)*
    - systemic *(continued)*
      - inhibitor *(continued)*
        - finding without diagnosis R76.0
      - specified NEC M32.8
  - exedens A18.4
  - hydralazine M32.0
    - correct substance properly administered —*see* Table of Drugs and Chemicals, by drug, adverse effect
    - overdose or wrong substance given or taken —*see* Table of Drugs and Chemicals, by drug, poisoning
  - nephritis (chronic) M32.14
  - nontuberculous, not disseminated L93.0
  - panniculitis L93.2
  - pernio (Besnier) D86.3
  - systemic —*see* Lupus, erythematosus, systemic
  - tuberculous A18.4
    - eyelid A18.4
  - vulgaris A18.4
    - eyelid A18.4
- **Luteinoma** D27.-
- **Lutembacher's disease or syndrome** (atrial septal defect with mitral stenosis) Q21.1
- **Luteoma** D27.-
- **Lutz** (-Splendore-de Almeida) **disease** —*see* Paracoccidioidomycosis
- **Luxation** —*see also* Dislocation
  - eyeball (nontraumatic) —*see* Luxation, globe
    - birth injury P15.3
  - globe, nontraumatic H44.82-
  - lacrimal gland —*see* Dislocation, lacrimal gland
  - lens (old) (partial) (spontaneous)
    - congenital Q12.1
      - syphilitic A50.39
- **Lycanthropy** F22
- **Lyell's syndrome** L51.2
  - due to drug L51.2
    - correct substance properly administered —*see* Table of Drugs and Chemicals, by drug, adverse effect
    - overdose or wrong substance given or taken —*see* Table of Drugs and Chemicals, by drug, poisoning
- **Lyme disease** A69.20
- **Lymph**
  - gland or node —*see* condition
  - scrotum —*see* Infestation, filarial
- **Lymphadenitis** I88.9
  - with ectopic or molar pregnancy O08.0
  - acute L04.9
    - axilla L04.2
    - face L04.0
    - head L04.0
    - hip L04.3
    - limb
      - lower L04.3
      - upper L04.2
    - neck L04.0
    - shoulder L04.2
    - specified site NEC L04.8
    - trunk L04.1

- **Lymphadenitis** *(continued)*
  - anthracosis (occupational) J60
  - any site, except mesenteric I88.9
    - chronic I88.1
    - subacute I88.1
  - breast
    - gestational —*see* Mastitis, obstetric
    - puerperal, postpartum (nonpurulent) O91.22
  - chancroidal (congenital) A57
  - chronic I88.1
    - mesenteric I88.0
  - due to
    - Brugia (malayi) B74.1
      - timori B74.2
    - chlamydial lymphogranuloma A55
    - diphtheria (toxin) A36.89
    - lymphogranuloma venereum A55
    - Wuchereria bancrofti B74.0
  - following ectopic or molar pregnancy O08.0
  - gonorrheal A54.89
  - infective —*see* Lymphadenitis, acute
  - mesenteric (acute) (chronic) (nonspecific) (subacute) I88.0
    - due to Salmonella typhi A01.09
    - tuberculous A18.39
  - mycobacterial A31.8
  - purulent —*see* Lymphadenitis, acute
  - pyogenic —*see* Lymphadenitis, acute
  - regional, nonbacterial I88.8
  - septic —*see* Lymphadenitis, acute
  - subacute, unspecified site I88.1
  - suppurative —*see* Lymphadenitis, acute
  - syphilitic (early) (secondary) A51.49
    - late A52.79
  - tuberculous —*see* Tuberculosis, lymph gland
  - venereal (chlamydial) A55
- **Lymphadenoid goiter** E06.3
- **Lymphadenopathy** (generalized) R59.1
  - angioimmunoblastic, with dysproteinemia (AILD) C86.5
  - due to toxoplasmosis (acquired) B58.89
    - congenital (acute) (subacute) (chronic) P37.1
  - localized R59.0
  - syphilitic (early) (secondary) A51.49
- **Lymphadenosis** R59.1
- **Lymphangiectasis** I89.0
  - conjunctiva H11.89
  - postinfectional I89.0
  - scrotum I89.0
- **Lymphangiectatic elephantiasis, nonfilarial** I89.0
- **Lymphangioendothelioma** D18.1
  - malignant —*see* Neoplasm, connective tissue, malignant
- **Lymphangioleiomyomatosis** J84.81
- **Lymphangioma** D18.1
  - capillary D18.1
  - cavernous D18.1
  - cystic D18.1
  - malignant —*see* Neoplasm, connective tissue, malignant
- **Lymphangiomyoma** D18.1
- **Lymphangiomyomatosis** J84.81
- **Lymphangiosarcoma** —*see* Neoplasm, connective tissue, malignant

- **Lymphangitis** I89.1
  - with
    - abscess - code by site under Abscess
    - cellulitis - code by site under Cellulitis
    - ectopic or molar pregnancy O08.0
  - acute L03.91
    - abdominal wall L03.321
    - ankle —*see* Lymphangitis, acute, lower limb
    - arm —*see* Lymphangitis, acute, upper limb
    - auricle (ear) —*see* Lymphangitis, acute, ear
    - axilla L03.12-
    - back (any part) L03.322
    - buttock L03.327
    - cervical (meaning neck) L03.222
    - cheek (external) L03.212
    - chest wall L03.323
    - digit
      - finger —*see* Lymphangitis, acute, finger
      - toe —*see* Lymphangitis, acute, toe
    - ear (external) H60.1-
    - external auditory canal —*see* Lymphangitis, acute, ear
    - eyelid —*see* Abscess, eyelid
    - face NEC L03.212
    - finger (intrathecal) (periosteal) (subcutaneous) (subcuticular) L03.02-
    - foot —*see* Lymphangitis, acute, lower limb
    - gluteal (region) L03.327
    - groin L03.324
    - hand —*see* Lymphangitis, acute, upper limb
    - head NEC L03.891
      - face (any part, except ear, eye and nose) L03.212
    - heel —*see* Lymphangitis, acute, lower limb
    - hip —*see* Lymphangitis, acute, lower limb
    - jaw (region) L03.212
    - knee —*see* Lymphangitis, acute, lower limb
    - leg —*see* Lymphangitis, acute, lower limb
    - lower limb L03.12-
      - toe —*see* Lymphangitis, acute, toe
    - navel L03.326
    - neck (region) L03.222
    - orbit, orbital —*see* Cellulitis, orbit
    - pectoral (region) L03.323
    - perineal, perineum L03.325
    - scalp (any part) L03.891
    - shoulder —*see* Lymphangitis, acute, upper limb
    - specified site NEC L03.898
    - thigh —*see* Lymphangitis, acute, lower limb
    - thumb (intrathecal) (periosteal) (subcutaneous) (subcuticular) —*see* Lymphangitis, acute, finger
    - toe (intrathecal) (periosteal) (subcutaneous) (subcuticular) L03.04-
    - trunk L03.329
      - abdominal wall L03.321
      - back (any part) L03.322
      - buttock L03.327
      - chest wall L03.323
      - groin L03.324
      - perineal, perineum L03.325
      - umbilicus L03.326

Lymphangitis *(continued)*
acute *(continued)*
umbilicus L03.326
upper limb L03.12-
axilla —*see* Lymphangitis, acute, axilla
finger —*see* Lymphangitis, acute, finger
thumb —*see* Lymphangitis, acute, finger
wrist —*see* Lymphangitis, acute, upper limb
breast
gestational —*see* Mastitis, obstetric
chancroidal A57
chronic (any site) I89.1
due to
Brugia (malayi) B74.1
timori B74.2
Wuchereria bancrofti B74.0
following ectopic or molar pregnancy O08.89
penis
acute N48.29
gonococcal (acute) (chronic) A54.09
puerperal, postpartum, childbirth O86.89
strumous, tuberculous A18.2
subacute (any site) I89.1
tuberculous —*see* Tuberculosis, lymph gland

Lymphatic (vessel) —*see* condition

Lymphatism E32.8

Lymphectasia I89.0

Lymphedema (acquired) —*see also* Elephantiasis
congenital Q82.0
hereditary (chronic) (idiopathic) Q82.0
postmastectomy I97.2
praecox I89.0
secondary I89.0
surgical NEC I97.89
postmastectomy (syndrome) I97.2

Lymphoblastic —*see* condition

Lymphoblastoma (diffuse) —*see* Lymphoma, lymphoblastic (diffuse)
giant follicular —*see* Lymphoma, lymphoblastic (diffuse)
macrofollicular —*see* Lymphoma, lymphoblastic (diffuse)

Lymphocele I89.8

Lymphocytic
chorioencephalitis (acute) (serous) A87.2
choriomeningitis (acute) (serous) A87.2
meningoencephalitis A87.2

Lymphocytoma, benign cutis L98.8

Lymphocytopenia D72.810

Lymphocytosis (symptomatic) D72.820
infectious (acute) B33.8

Lymphoepithelioma —*see* Neoplasm, malignant, by site

Lymphogranuloma (malignant) —*see also* Lymphoma, Hodgkin
chlamydial A55
inguinale A55
venereum (any site) (chlamydial) (with stricture of rectum) A55

Lymphogranulomatosis (malignant) —*see also* Lymphoma, Hodgkin
benign (Boeck's sarcoid) (Schaumann's) D86.1

Lymphohistiocytosis, hemophagocytic (familial) D76.1

Lymphoid —*see* condition

Lymphoma (of) (malignant) C85.90
adult T-cell (HTLV-1-associated) (acute variant) (chronic variant) (lymphomatoid variant) (smouldering variant) C91.5-
anaplastic large cell
ALK-negative C84.7-
ALK-positive C84.6-
breast implant associated (BIA-ALCL) C84.7A
CD30-positive C84.6-
primary cutaneous C86.6
angioimmunoblastic T-cell C86.5
BALT C88.4
B-cell C85.1-
B-precursor C83.5-
blastic NK-cell C86.4
blastic plasmacytoid dendritic cell neoplasm (BPDCN) C86.4
blastic plasmacytoid dendritic cell neoplasm (BPDCN) C86.4
bronchial-associated lymphoid tissue [BALT-lymphoma] C88.4
Burkitt (atypical) C83.7-
Burkitt-like C83.7-
centrocytic C83.1-
cutaneous follicle center C82.6-
cutaneous T-cell C84.A-
diffuse follicle center C82.5-
diffuse large cell C83.3-
anaplastic C83.3-
B-cell C83.3-
diffuse large cell C83.3-
CD30-positive C83.3-
centroblastic C83.3-
immunoblastic C83.3-
plasmablastic C83.3-
subtype not specified C83.3-
T-cell rich C83.3-
enteropathy-type (associated) (intestinal) T-cell C86.2
extranodal NK/T-cell, nasal type C86.0
extranodal marginal zone B-cell lymphoma of mucosa-associated lymphoid tissue [MALT-lymphoma] C88.4
follicular C82.9-
grade
I C82.0-
II C82.1-
III C82.2-
IIIa C82.3-
IIIb C82.4-
specified NEC C82.8-
hepatosplenic T-cell (alpha-beta) (gamma-delta) C86.1
histiocytic C85.9-
true C96.A
Hodgkin C81.9
lymphocyte-rich (classical) C81.4-
lymphocyte depleted (classical) C81.3-
mixed cellularity (classical) C81.2-
nodular sclerosis (classical) C81.1-
specified NEC (classical) C81.7-
nodular
lymphocyte predominant C81.0-
sclerosis (classical) C81.1-

Lymphoma *(continued)*
intravascular large B-cell C83.8-
Lennert's C84.4-
lymphoblastic B-cell C83.5-
lymphoblastic (diffuse) C83.5-
lymphoblastic T-cell C83.5-
lymphoepithelioid C84.4-
lymphoplasmacytic C83.0-
with IgM-production C88.0
MALT C88.4
mantle cell C83.1-
mature T-cell NEC C84.4-
mature T/NK-cell C84.9-
specified NEC C84.Z-
mediastinal (thymic) large B-cell C85.2-
Mediterranean C88.3
mucosa-associated lymphoid tissue [MALT-lymphoma] C88.4
NK/T cell C84.9-
nodal marginal zone C83.0-
non-follicular (diffuse) C83.9-
specified NEC C83.8-
non-Hodgkin (*see also* Lymphoma, by type) C85.9-
specified NEC C85.8-
non-leukemic variant of B-CLL C83.0-
peripheral T-cell, not classified C84.4-
primary cutaneous
anaplastic large cell C86.6
CD30-positive large T-cell C86.6
primary effusion B-cell C83.8-
SALT C88.4
skin-associated lymphoid tissue [SALT-lymphoma] C88.4
small cell B-cell C83.0-
splenic marginal zone C83.0-
subcutaneous panniculitis-like T-cell C86.3
T-precursor C83.5-
true histiocytic C96.A

Lymphomatosis —*see* Lymphoma

Lymphopathia venereum, veneris A55

Lymphopenia D72.810

Lymphoplasmacytic leukemia —*see* Leukemia, chronic lymphocytic, B-cell type

Lymphoproliferation, X-linked disease D82.3

Lymphoreticulosis, benign (of inoculation) A28.1

Lymphorrhea I89.8

Lymphosarcoma (diffuse) (*see also* Lymphoma) C85.9-

Lymphostasis I89.8

Lypemania —*see* Melancholia

Lysine and hydroxylysine metabolism disorder E72.3

Lyssa —*see* Rabies

M

Macacus ear Q17.3

Maceration, wet feet, tropical (syndrome) T69.02-

MacLeod's syndrome J43.0

Macrocephalia, macrocephaly Q75.3

Macrocheilia, macrochilia (congenital) Q18.6

Macrocolon (*see also* Megacolon) Q43.1

Macrocornea Q15.8
with glaucoma Q15.0

Macrocytic —*see* condition

Macrocytosis D75.89

Macrodactylia, macrodactylism (fingers) (thumbs) Q74.0
toes Q74.2

Macrodontia K00.2

Macrogenia M26.05

Macrogenitosomia (adrenal) (male) (praecox) E25.9
congenital E25.0

Macroglobulinemia (idiopathic) (primary) C88.0
monoclonal (essential) D47.2
Waldenström C88.0

Macroglossia (congenital) Q38.2
acquired K14.8

Macrognathia, macrognathism (congenital) (mandibular) (maxillary) M26.09

Macrogyria (congenital) Q04.8

Macrohydrocephalus —*see* Hydrocephalus

Macromastia —*see* Hypertrophy, breast

Macrophthalmos Q11.3
in congenital glaucoma Q15.0

Macropsia H53.15

Macrosigmoid K59.39
congenital Q43.2

Macrospondylitis, acromegalic E22.0

Macrostomia (congenital) Q18.4

Macrotia (external ear) (congenital) Q17.1

Macula
cornea, corneal —*see* Opacity, cornea
degeneration (atrophic) (exudative) (senile) —*see also* Degeneration, macula
hereditary —*see* Dystrophy, retina

Maculae ceruleae B85.1

Maculopathy, toxic —*see* Degeneration, macula, toxic

Madarosis (eyelid) H02.729
left H02.726
lower H02.725
upper H02.724
right H02.723
lower H02.722
upper H02.721

Madelung's
deformity (radius) Q74.0
disease
radial deformity Q74.0
symmetrical lipomas, neck E88.89

Madness —*see* Psychosis

Madura
foot B47.9
actinomycotic B47.1
mycotic B47.0

Maduromycosis B47.0

Maffucci's syndrome Q78.4

Magnesium metabolism disorder *—see* Disorder, metabolism, magnesium

Main en griffe (acquired) *—see also* Deformity, limb, clawhand
  congenital Q74.0

Maintenance (encounter for)
  antineoplastic chemotherapy Z51.11
  antineoplastic radiation therapy Z51.0
  methadone F11.20

Majocchi's
  disease L81.7
  granuloma B35.8

Major *—see* condition

Malabar itch (any site) B35.5

Malabsorption K90.9
  calcium K90.89
  carbohydrate K90.49
  disaccharide E73.9
  fat K90.49
  galactose E74.20
  glucose (-galactose) E74.39
  intestinal K90.9
    specified NEC K90.89
  isomaltose E74.31
  lactose E73.9
  methionine E72.19
  monosaccharide E74.39
  postgastrectomy K91.2
  postsurgical K91.2
  protein K90.49
  starch K90.49
  sucrose E74.39
  syndrome K90.9
    postsurgical K91.2

Malacia, bone (adult) M83.9
  juvenile *—see* Rickets

Malacoplakia
  bladder N32.89
  pelvis (kidney) N28.89
  ureter N28.89
  urethra N36.8

Malacosteon, juvenile *—see* Rickets

Maladaptation *—see* Maladjustment

Maladie de Roger Q21.0

Maladjustment
  conjugal Z63.0
    involving divorce or estrangement Z63.5
  educational Z55.4
  family Z63.9
  marital Z63.0
    involving divorce or estrangement Z63.5
  occupational NEC Z56.89
  simple, adult *—see* Disorder, adjustment
  situational *—see* Disorder, adjustment
  social Z60.9
    due to
      acculturation difficulty Z60.3
      discrimination and persecution (perceived) Z60.5
      exclusion and isolation Z60.4
      life-cycle (phase of life) transition Z60.0
      rejection Z60.4
      specified reason NEC Z60.8

Malaise R53.81

Malakoplakia *—see* Malacoplakia

Malaria, malarial (fever) B54
  with
    blackwater fever B50.8
      hemoglobinuric (bilious) B50.8
    hemoglobinuria B50.8
  accidentally induced (therapeutically) - code by type under Malaria
  algid B50.9
  cerebral B50.0 *[G94]*
  clinically diagnosed (without parasitological confirmation) B54
  congenital NEC P37.4
    falciparum P37.3
  congestion, congestive B54
  continued (fever) B50.9
  estivo-autumnal B50.9
  falciparum B50.9
    with complications NEC B50.8
      cerebral B50.0 *[G94]*
    severe B50.8
  hemorrhagic B54
  malariae B52.9
    with
      complications NEC B52.8
      glomerular disorder B52.0
  malignant (tertian) *—see* Malaria, falciparum
  mixed infections - code to first listed type in B50-B53
  ovale B53.0
  parasitologically confirmed NEC B53.8
  pernicious, acute *—see* Malaria, falciparum
  Plasmodium (P.)
    falciparum NEC *—see* Malaria, falciparum
    malariae NEC B52.9
      with Plasmodium
        falciparum (and or vivax) *—see* Malaria, falciparum
        vivax *—see also* Malaria, vivax
          and falciparum *—see* Malaria, falciparum
    ovale B53.0
      with Plasmodium malariae *—see also* Malaria, malariae
        and vivax *—see also* Malaria, vivax
          and falciparum *—see* Malaria, falciparum
    simian B53.1
      with Plasmodium malariae *—see also* Malaria, malariae
        and vivax *—see also* Malaria, vivax
          and falciparum *—see* Malaria, falciparum
    vivax NEC B51.9
      with Plasmodium falciparum *—see* Malaria, falciparum
  quartan *—see* Malaria, malariae
  quotidian *—see* Malaria, falciparum
  recurrent B54
  remittent B54
  specified type NEC (parasitologically confirmed) B53.8
  spleen B54
  subtertian (fever) *—see* Malaria, falciparum
  tertian (benign) *—see also* Malaria, vivax
    malignant B50.9

Malaria, malarial *(continued)*
  tropical B50.9
  typhoid B54
  vivax B51.9
    with
      complications NEC B51.8
      ruptured spleen B51.0

Malassimilation K90.9

Malassez's disease (cystic) N50.89

Mal de los pintos *—see* Pinta

Mal de mer T75.3

Maldescent, testis Q53.9
  bilateral Q53.20
    abdominal Q53.211
    perineal Q53.22
  unilateral Q53.10
    abdominal Q53.111
    perineal Q53.12

Maldevelopment *—see also* Anomaly
  brain Q07.9
  colon Q43.9
  hip Q74.2
    congenital dislocation Q65.2
      bilateral Q65.1
      unilateral Q65.0-
  mastoid process Q75.8
  middle ear Q16.4
    except ossicles Q16.4
    ossicles Q16.3
  ossicles Q16.3
  spine Q76.49
  toe Q74.2

Male type pelvis Q74.2
  with disproportion (fetopelvic) O33.3
    causing obstructed labor O65.3

Malformation (congenital) *—see also* Anomaly
  adrenal gland Q89.1
  affecting multiple systems with skeletal changes NEC Q87.5
  alimentary tract Q45.9
    specified type NEC Q45.8
    upper Q40.9
      specified type NEC Q40.8
  aorta Q25.40
    absence Q25.41
    aneurysm, congenital Q25.43
    aplasia Q25.41
    atresia Q25.29
      aortic arch Q25.21
    coarctation (preductal) (postductal) Q25.1
    dilatation, congenital Q25.44
    hypoplasia Q25.42
    patent ductus arteriosus Q25.0
    specified type NEC Q25.49
    stenosis Q25.1
      supravalvular Q25.3
  aortic valve Q23.9
    specified NEC Q23.8
  arteriovenous, aneurysmatic (congenital) Q27.30
    brain Q28.2
      ruptured I60.8
        intracerebral I61.8
        intraparenchymal I61.8
        intraventricular I61.5
        subarachnoid I60.8
    cerebral (*see* also Malformation, arteriovenous, brain) Q28.2
    peripheral Q27.30
      digestive system *—see* Angiodysplasia
        congenital Q27.33
      lower limb Q27.32

Malformation *(continued)*
  arteriovenous, aneurysmatic *(continued)*
    peripheral *(continued)*
      other specified site Q27.39
      renal vessel Q27.34
      upper limb Q27.31
    precerebral vessels (nonruptured) Q28.0
  auricle
    ear (congenital) Q17.3
      acquired H61.119
        left H61.112
          with right H61.113
        right H61.111
          with left H61.113
  bile duct Q44.5
  bladder Q64.79
    aplasia Q64.5
    diverticulum Q64.6
    exstrophy *—see* Exstrophy, bladder
    neck obstruction Q64.31
  bone Q79.9
    face Q75.9
      specified type NEC Q75.8
    skull Q75.9
      specified type NEC Q75.8
  brain (multiple) Q04.9
    arteriovenous Q28.2
    specified type NEC Q04.8
  branchial cleft Q18.2
  breast Q83.9
    specified type NEC Q83.8
  broad ligament Q50.6
  bronchus Q32.4
  bursa Q79.9
  cardiac
    chambers Q20.9
      specified type NEC Q20.8
    septum Q21.9
      specified type NEC Q21.8
  cerebral Q04.9
    vessels Q28.3
  cervix uteri Q51.9
    specified type NEC Q51.828
  Chiari
    Type I G93.5
    Type II Q07.01
  choroid (congenital) Q14.3
    plexus Q07.8
  circulatory system Q28.9
  cochlea Q16.5
  cornea Q13.4
  coronary vessels Q24.5
  corpus callosum (congenital) Q04.0
  diaphragm Q79.1
  digestive system NEC, specified type NEC Q45.8
  dura Q07.9
    brain Q04.9
    spinal Q06.9
  ear Q17.9
    causing impairment of hearing Q16.9
    external Q17.9
      accessory auricle Q17.0
      causing impairment of hearing Q16.9
        absence of
          auditory canal Q16.1
          auricle Q16.0
      macrotia Q17.1
      microtia Q17.2
      misplacement Q17.4
      misshapen NEC Q17.3
      prominence Q17.5
      specified type NEC Q17.8

- **Malformation** *(continued)*
  - ear *(continued)*
    - inner Q16.5
    - middle Q16.4
      - absence of eustachian tube Q16.2
      - ossicles (fusion) Q16.3
    - ossicles Q16.3
    - specified type NEC Q17.8
  - epididymis Q55.4
  - esophagus Q39.9
    - specified type NEC Q39.8
  - eye Q15.9
    - lid Q10.3
    - specified NEC Q15.8
  - fallopian tube Q50.6
  - genital organ —*see* Anomaly, genitalia
  - great
    - artery Q25.9
      - aorta —*see* Malformation, aorta
      - pulmonary artery —*see* Malformation, pulmonary, artery
      - specified type NEC Q25.8
    - vein Q26.9
      - anomalous
        - portal venous connection Q26.5
        - pulmonary venous connection Q26.4
          - partial Q26.3
          - total Q26.2
      - persistent left superior vena cava Q26.1
      - portal vein-hepatic artery fistula Q26.6
      - specified type NEC Q26.8
      - vena cava stenosis, congenital Q26.0
  - gum Q38.6
  - hair Q84.2
  - heart Q24.9
    - specified type NEC Q24.8
  - integument Q84.9
    - specified type NEC Q84.8
  - internal ear Q16.5
  - intestine Q43.9
    - specified type NEC Q43.8
  - iris Q13.2
  - joint Q74.9
    - ankle Q74.2
    - lumbosacral Q76.49
    - sacroiliac Q74.2
    - specified type NEC Q74.8
  - kidney Q63.9
    - accessory Q63.0
    - giant Q63.3
    - horseshoe Q63.1
    - hydronephrosis Q62.0
    - malposition Q63.2
    - specified type NEC Q63.8
  - lacrimal apparatus Q10.6
  - lip Q38.0
  - lingual Q38.3
  - liver Q44.7
  - lung Q33.9
  - meninges or membrane (congenital) Q07.9
    - cerebral Q04.8
    - spinal (cord) Q06.9
  - middle ear Q16.4
    - ossicles Q16.3
  - mitral valve Q23.9
    - specified NEC Q23.8
  - Mondini's (congenital) (malformation, cochlea) Q16.5
  - mouth (congenital) Q38.6
  - multiple types NEC Q89.7
  - musculoskeletal system Q79.9

- **Malformation** *(continued)*
  - myocardium Q24.8
  - nail Q84.6
  - nervous system (central) Q07.9
  - nose Q30.9
    - specified type NEC Q30.8
  - optic disc Q14.2
  - orbit Q10.7
  - ovary Q50.39
  - palate Q38.5
  - parathyroid gland Q89.2
  - pelvic organs or tissues NEC
    - in pregnancy or childbirth O34.8-
      - causing obstructed labor O65.5
  - penis Q55.69
    - aplasia Q55.5
    - curvature (lateral) Q55.61
    - hypoplasia Q55.62
  - pericardium Q24.8
  - peripheral vascular system Q27.9
    - specified type NEC Q27.8
  - pharynx Q38.8
  - precerebral vessels Q28.1
  - prostate Q55.4
  - pulmonary
    - arteriovenous Q25.72
    - artery Q25.9
      - atresia Q25.5
      - specified type NEC Q25.79
      - stenosis Q25.6
    - valve Q22.3
  - renal artery Q27.2
  - respiratory system Q34.9
  - retina Q14.1
  - scrotum —*see* Malformation, testis and scrotum
  - seminal vesicles Q55.4
  - sense organs NEC Q07.9
  - skin Q82.9
  - specified NEC Q89.8
  - spinal
    - cord Q06.9
    - nerve root Q07.8
  - spine Q76.49
    - kyphosis —*see* Kyphosis, congenital
    - lordosis —*see* Lordosis, congenital
  - spleen Q89.09
  - stomach Q40.3
    - specified type NEC Q40.2
  - teeth, tooth K00.9
  - tendon Q79.9
  - testis and scrotum Q55.20
    - aplasia Q55.0
    - hypoplasia Q55.1
    - polyorchism Q55.21
    - retractile testis Q55.22
    - scrotal transposition Q55.23
    - specified NEC Q55.29
  - throat Q38.8
  - thorax, bony Q76.9
  - thyroid gland Q89.2
  - tongue (congenital) Q38.3
    - hypertrophy Q38.2
    - tie Q38.1
  - trachea Q32.1
  - tricuspid valve Q22.9
    - specified type NEC Q22.8
  - umbilical cord NEC (complicating delivery) O69.89
  - umbilicus Q89.9
  - ureter Q62.8
    - agenesis Q62.4
    - duplication Q62.5
    - malposition —*see* Malposition, congenital, ureter

- **Malformation** *(continued)*
  - ureter *(continued)*
    - obstructive defect —*see* Defect, obstructive, ureter
    - vesico-uretero-renal reflux Q62.7
  - urethra Q64.79
    - aplasia Q64.5
    - duplication Q64.74
    - posterior valves Q64.2
    - prolapse Q64.71
    - stricture Q64.32
  - urinary system Q64.9
  - uterus Q51.9
    - specified type NEC Q51.818
  - vagina Q52.4
  - vascular system, peripheral Q27.9
  - vas deferens Q55.4
    - atresia Q55.3
  - venous —*see* Anomaly, vein(s)
  - vulva Q52.70

- **Malfunction** —*see also* Dysfunction
  - cardiac electronic device T82.119
    - electrode T82.110
    - pulse generator T82.111
    - specified type NEC T82.118
  - catheter device NEC T85.618
    - cystostomy T83.010
    - dialysis (renal) (vascular) T82.41
      - intraperitoneal T85.611
    - infusion NEC T82.514
      - cranial T85.610
      - epidural T85.610
      - intrathecal T85.610
      - spinal T85.610
      - subarachnoid T85.610
      - subdural T85.610
    - urinary (*see also* Breakdown, device, catheter), T83.018
  - colostomy K94.03
    - valve K94.03
  - cystostomy (stoma) N99.512
    - catheter T83.010
  - enteric stoma K94.13
  - enterostomy K94.13
  - esophagostomy K94.33
  - gastroenteric K31.89
  - gastrostomy K94.23
  - ileostomy K94.13
    - valve K94.13
  - intrathecal infusion pump T85.615
  - jejunostomy K94.13
  - nervous system device, implant or graft, specified NEC T85.615
  - pacemaker —*see* Malfunction, cardiac electronic device
  - prosthetic device, internal —*see* Complications, prosthetic device, by site, mechanical
  - tracheostomy J95.03
  - urinary device NEC —*see* Complication, genitourinary, device, urinary, mechanical
  - valve
    - colostomy K94.03
    - heart T82.09
    - ileostomy K94.13
  - vascular graft or shunt NEC —*see* Complication, cardiovascular device, mechanical, vascular
  - ventricular (communicating shunt) T85.01

- **Malherbe's tumor** —*see* Neoplasm, skin, benign

- **Malibu disease** L98.8

- **Malignancy** —*see also* Neoplasm, malignant, by site
  - unspecified site (primary) C80.1

- **Malignant** —*see* condition

- **Malingerer, malingering** Z76.5

- **Mallet finger** (acquired) —*see* Deformity, finger, mallet finger
  - congenital Q74.0
  - sequelae of rickets E64.3

- **Malleus** A24.0

- **Mallory's bodies** R89.7

- **Mallory-Weiss syndrome** K22.6

- **Malnutrition** E46
  - degree
    - first E44.1
    - mild (protein) E44.1
    - moderate (protein) E44.0
    - second E44.0
    - severe (protein-energy) E43
      - intermediate form E42
        - with
          - kwashiorkor (and marasmus) E42
          - marasmus E41
    - third E43
  - following gastrointestinal surgery K91.2
  - intrauterine
    - light-for-dates —*see* Light for dates
    - small-for-dates —*see* Small for dates
  - lack of care, or neglect (child) (infant) T76.02
    - confirmed T74.02
  - malignant E40
  - protein E46
    - calorie E46
      - mild E44.1
      - moderate E44.0
      - severe E43
        - intermediate form E42
          - with
            - kwashiorkor (and marasmus) E42
            - marasmus E41
    - energy E46
      - mild E44.1
      - moderate E44.0
      - severe E43
        - intermediate form E42
          - with
            - kwashiorkor (and marasmus) E42
            - marasmus E41
  - severe (protein-energy) E43
    - with
      - kwashiorkor (and marasmus) E42
      - marasmus E41

- **Malocclusion** (teeth) M26.4
  - Angle's M26.219
    - class I M26.211
    - class II M26.212
    - class III M26.213
  - due to
    - abnormal swallowing M26.59
    - mouth breathing M26.59
    - tongue, lip or finger habits M26.59
  - temporomandibular (joint) M26.69

- **Malposition**
  - cervix —*see* Malposition, uterus
  - congenital
    - adrenal (gland) Q89.1
    - alimentary tract Q45.8
      - lower Q43.8
      - upper Q40.8
    - aorta Q25.49
    - appendix Q43.8
    - arterial trunk Q20.0

Malposition *(continued)*
- congenital *(continued)*
  - artery (peripheral) Q27.8
    - coronary Q24.5
    - digestive system Q27.8
    - lower limb Q27.8
    - pulmonary Q25.79
    - specified site NEC Q27.8
    - upper limb Q27.8
  - auditory canal Q17.8
    - causing impairment of hearing Q16.9
  - auricle (ear) Q17.4
    - causing impairment of hearing Q16.9
    - cervical Q18.2
  - biliary duct or passage Q44.5
  - bladder (mucosa) —*see* Exstrophy, bladder
  - brachial plexus Q07.8
  - brain tissue Q04.8
  - breast Q83.8
  - bronchus Q32.4
  - cecum Q43.8
  - clavicle Q74.0
  - colon Q43.8
  - digestive organ or tract NEC Q45.8
    - lower Q43.8
    - upper Q40.8
  - ear (auricle) (external) Q17.4
    - ossicles Q16.3
  - endocrine (gland) NEC Q89.2
  - epiglottis Q31.8
  - eustachian tube Q17.8
  - eye Q15.8
  - facial features Q18.8
  - fallopian tube Q50.6
  - finger(s) Q68.1
    - supernumerary Q69.0
  - foot Q66.9-
  - gallbladder Q44.1
  - gastrointestinal tract Q45.8
  - genitalia, genital organ(s) or tract
    - female Q52.8
      - external Q52.79
      - internal NEC Q52.8
    - male Q55.8
  - glottis Q31.8
  - hand Q68.1
  - heart Q24.8
    - dextrocardia Q24.0
      - with complete transposition of viscera Q89.3
  - hepatic duct Q44.5
  - hip (joint) Q65.89
  - intestine (large) (small) Q43.8
    - with anomalous adhesions, fixation or malrotation Q43.3
  - joint NEC Q68.8
  - kidney Q63.2
  - larynx Q31.8
  - limb Q68.8
    - lower Q68.8
    - upper Q68.8
  - liver Q44.7
  - lung (lobe) Q33.8
  - nail(s) Q84.6
  - nerve Q07.8
  - nervous system NEC Q07.8
  - nose, nasal (septum) Q30.8
  - organ or site not listed —*see* Anomaly, by site
  - ovary Q50.39
  - pancreas Q45.3
  - parathyroid (gland) Q89.2
  - patella Q74.1
  - peripheral vascular system Q27.8
  - pituitary (gland) Q89.2
  - respiratory organ or system NEC Q34.8
  - rib (cage) Q76.6
    - supernumerary in cervical region Q76.5
  - scapula Q74.0
  - shoulder Q74.0
  - spinal cord Q06.8
  - spleen Q89.09
  - sternum NEC Q76.7
  - stomach Q40.2
  - symphysis pubis Q74.2
  - thymus (gland) Q89.2
  - thyroid (gland) (tissue) Q89.2
    - cartilage Q31.8
  - toe(s) Q66.9-
    - supernumerary Q69.2
  - tongue Q38.3
  - trachea Q32.1
  - ureter Q62.60
    - deviation Q62.61
    - displacement Q62.62
    - ectopia Q62.63
    - specified type NEC Q62.69
  - uterus Q51.818
  - vein(s) (peripheral) Q27.8
    - great Q26.8
  - vena cava (inferior) (superior) Q26.8
- device, implant or graft (*see also* Complications, by site and type, mechanical) T85.628
  - arterial graft NEC —*see* Complication, cardiovascular device, mechanical, vascular
  - breast (implant) T85.42
  - catheter NEC T85.628
    - cystostomy T83.020
    - dialysis (renal) T82.42
      - intraperitoneal T85.621
    - infusion NEC T82.524
      - spinal (epidural) (subdural) T85.620
    - urinary (*see also* Displacement, device, catheter, urinary), T83.028
  - electronic (electrode) (pulse generator) (stimulator)
    - bone T84.320
    - cardiac T82.129
      - electrode T82.120
      - pulse generator T82.121
      - specified type NEC T82.128
    - nervous system —*see* Complication, prosthetic device, mechanical, electronic nervous system stimulator
    - urinary —*see* Complication, genitourinary, device, urinary, mechanical
  - fixation, internal (orthopedic) NEC —*see* Complication, fixation device, mechanical
  - gastrointestinal —*see* Complications, prosthetic device, mechanical, gastrointestinal device
  - genital NEC T83.428
    - intrauterine contraceptive device (string) T83.32
    - penile prosthesis (cylinder) (implanted) (pump) (resevoir) T83.420
    - testicular prosthesis T83.421
  - heart NEC —*see* Complication, cardiovascular device, mechanical
  - joint prosthesis —*see* Complication, joint prosthesis, mechanical
  - ocular NEC —*see* Complications, prosthetic device, mechanical, ocular device
  - orthopedic NEC —*see* Complication, orthopedic, device, mechanical
  - specified NEC T85.628
  - urinary NEC —*see also* Complication, genitourinary, device, urinary, mechanical
    - graft T83.22
  - vascular NEC —*see* Complication, cardiovascular device, mechanical
  - ventricular intracranial shunt T85.02
- fetus —*see* Pregnancy, complicated by (management affected by), presentation, fetal
- gallbladder K82.8
- gastrointestinal tract, congenital Q45.8
- heart, congenital NEC Q24.8
- joint prosthesis —*see* Complications, joint prosthesis, mechanical, displacement, by site
- stomach K31.89.
  - congenital Q40.2
- tooth, teeth, fully erupted M26.30
- uterus (acute) (acquired) (adherent) (asymptomatic) (postinfectional) (postpartal, old) N85.4
  - anteflexion or anteversion N85.4
    - congenital Q51.818
  - flexion N85.4
    - lateral —*see* Lateroversion, uterus
  - inversion N85.5
  - lateral (flexion) (version) —*see* Lateroversion, uterus
    - in pregnancy or childbirth —*see* subcategory O34.5
  - retroflexion or retroversion —*see* Retroversion, uterus

Malposture R29.3

Malrotation
- cecum Q43.3
- colon Q43.3
- intestine Q43.3
- kidney Q63.2

Maltreatment
- adult
  - abandonment
    - confirmed T74.01
    - suspected T76.01
  - bullying
    - confirmed T74.31
    - suspected T76.31
  - confirmed T74.91
  - history of Z91.419
  - intimidation (through social media)
    - confirmed T74.31
    - suspected T76.31
  - neglect
    - confirmed T74.01
    - suspected T76.01
  - physical abuse
    - confirmed T74.11
    - suspected T76.11
  - psychological abuse
    - confirmed T74.31
    - suspected T76.31
    - history of Z91.411
  - sexual abuse
    - confirmed T74.21
    - suspected T76.21
  - suspected T76.91
- child
  - abandonment
    - confirmed T74.02
    - suspected T76.02
  - bullying
    - confirmed T74.32
    - suspected T76.32
  - confirmed T74.92
  - history of —*see* History, personal (of), abuse
  - intimidation (through social media)
    - confirmed T74.32
    - suspected T76.32
  - neglect
    - confirmed T74.02
    - history of —*see* History, personal (of), abuse
    - suspected T76.02
  - physical abuse
    - confirmed T74.12
    - history of —*see* History, personal (of), abuse
    - suspected T76.12
  - psychological abuse
    - confirmed T74.32
    - history of —*see* History, personal (of), abuse
    - suspected T76.32
  - sexual abuse
    - confirmed T74.22
    - history of —*see* History, personal (of), abuse
    - suspected T76.22
  - suspected T76.92
- personal history of Z91.89

Malta fever —*see* Brucellosis

Maltworker's lung J67.4

Malunion, fracture —*see* Fracture, by site

Mammillitis N61.0
- puerperal, postpartum O91.02

Mammitis —*see* Mastitis

Mammogram (examination) Z12.39
- routine Z12.31

Mammoplasia N62

Management (of)
- bone conduction hearing device (implanted) Z45.320
- cardiac pacemaker NEC Z45.018
- cerebrospinal fluid drainage device Z45.41
- cochlear device (implanted) Z45.321
- contraceptive Z30.9
  - specified NEC Z30.8
- implanted device Z45.9
  - specified NEC Z45.89
- infusion pump Z45.1
- procreative Z31.9
  - male factor infertility in female Z31.81
  - specified NEC Z31.89
- prosthesis (external) (*see also* Fitting) Z44.9
  - implanted Z45.9
    - specified NEC Z45.89
- renal dialysis catheter Z49.01
- vascular access device Z45.2

Mangled —*see* specified injury by site

Mania (monopolar) *—see also* Disorder, mood, manic episode
- with psychotic symptoms F30.2
- without psychotic symptoms F30.10
  - mild F30.11
  - moderate F30.12
  - severe F30.13
- Bell's F30.8
- chronic (recurrent) F31.89
- hysterical F44.89
- puerperal F30.8
- recurrent F31.89

Manic depression F31.9

Manic-depressive insanity, psychosis, or syndrome *—see* Disorder, bipolar

Mannosidosis E77.1

Mansonelliasis, mansonellosis B74.4

Manson's
- disease B65.1
- schistosomiasis B65.1

Manual *—see* condition

Maple-bark-stripper's lung (disease) J67.6

Maple-syrup-urine disease E71.0

Marable's syndrome (celiac artery compression) I77.4

Marasmus E41
- due to malnutrition E41
- intestinal E41
- nutritional E41
- senile R54
- tuberculous NEC *—see* Tuberculosis

Marble
- bones Q78.2
- skin R23.8

Marburg virus disease A98.3

March
- fracture *—see* Fracture, traumatic, stress, by site
- hemoglobinuria D59.6

Marchesani (-Weill) **syndrome** Q87.0

Marchiafava (-Bignami) **syndrome or disease** G37.1

Marchiafava-Micheli syndrome D59.5

Marcus Gunn's syndrome Q07.8

Marfan's syndrome *—see* Syndrome, Marfan's

Marie-Bamberger disease *—see* Osteoarthropathy, hypertrophic, specified NEC

Marie-Charcot-Tooth neuropathic muscular atrophy G60.0

Marie's
- cerebellar ataxia (late-onset) G11.2
- disease or syndrome (acromegaly) E22.0

Marie-Strümpell arthritis, disease or spondylitis *—see* Spondylitis, ankylosing

Marion's disease (bladder neck obstruction) N32.0

Marital conflict Z63.0

Mark
- port wine Q82.5
- raspberry Q82.5

Mark *(continued)*
- strawberry Q82.5
- stretch L90.6
- tattoo L81.8

Marker heterochromatin *—see* Extra, marker chromosomes

Maroteaux-Lamy syndrome (mild) (severe) E76.29

Marrow (bone)
- arrest D61.9
- poor function D75.89

Marseilles fever A77.1

Marsh fever *—see* Malaria

Marshall's (hidrotic) **ectodermal dysplasia** Q82.4

Marsh's disease (exophthalmic goiter) E05.00
- with storm E05.01

Masculinization (female) **with adrenal hyperplasia** E25.9
- congenital E25.0

Masculinovoblastoma D27.-

Masochism (sexual) F65.51

Mason's lung J62.8

Mass
- abdominal R19.00
  - epigastric R19.06
  - generalized R19.07
  - left lower quadrant R19.04
  - left upper quadrant R19.02
  - periumbilic R19.05
  - right lower quadrant R19.03
  - right upper quadrant R19.01
  - specified site NEC R19.09
- breast (*see also* Lump, breast) N63.0
- chest R22.2
- cystic *—see* Cyst
- ear H93.8-
- head R22.0
- intra-abdominal (diffuse) (generalized) *—see* Mass, abdominal
- kidney N28.89
- liver R16.0
- localized (skin) R22.9
  - chest R22.2
  - head R22.0
  - limb
    - lower R22.4-
    - upper R22.3-
  - neck R22.1
  - trunk R22.2
- lung R91.8
- malignant *—see* Neoplasm, malignant, by site
- neck R22.1
- pelvic (diffuse) (generalized) *—see* Mass, abdominal
- specified organ NEC *—see* Disease, by site
- splenic R16.1
- substernal thyroid *—see* Goiter
- superficial (localized) R22.9
- umbilical (diffuse) (generalized) R19.09

Massive *—see* condition

Mast cell
- disease, systemic tissue D47.02
- neoplasm
  - malignant C96.20
    - specified type NEC C96.29
  - of uncertain behavior NEC D47.09
- leukemia C94.3-

Mast cell *(continued)*
- sarcoma C96.22
- tumor D47.09

Mastalgia N64.4

Masters-Allen syndrome N83.8

Mastitis (acute) (diffuse) (nonpuerperal) (subacute) N61.0
- with abscess N61.1
- chronic (cystic) *—see* Mastopathy, cystic
- cystic (Schimmelbusch's type) *—see* Mastopathy, cystic
- fibrocystic *—see* Mastopathy, cystic
- granulomatous N61.2-
- infective N61.0
  - newborn P39.0
- interstitial, gestational or puerperal *—see* Mastitis, obstetric
- neonatal (noninfective) P83.4
  - infective P39.0
- obstetric (interstitial) (nonpurulent)
  - associated with
    - lactation O91.23
    - pregnancy O91.21-
    - puerperium O91.22
  - purulent
    - associated with
      - lactation O91.13
      - pregnancy O91.11-
      - puerperium O91.12
- periductal *—see* Ectasia, mammary duct
- phlegmonous *—see* Mastopathy, cystic
- plasma cell *—see* Ectasia, mammary duct
- without abscess N61.0

Mastocytoma (extracutaneous) D47.09
- malignant C96.29
- solitary D47.01

Mastocytosis D47.09
- aggressive systemic C96.21
- cutaneous (diffuse) (maculopapular) D47.01
  - congenital Q82.2
  - of neonatal onset Q82.2
  - of newborn onset Q82.2
- indolent systemic D47.02
- isolated bone marrow D47.02
- malignant C96.29
- systemic (indolent) (smoldering)
  - with an associated hematological non-mast cell lineage disease (SM-AHNMD) D47.02

Mastodynia N64.4

Mastoid *—see* condition

Mastoidalgia *—see* subcategory H92.0

Mastoiditis (coalescent) (hemorrhagic) (suppurative) H70.9-
- acute, subacute H70.00-
  - complicated NEC H70.09-
  - subperiosteal H70.01-
- chronic (necrotic) (recurrent) H70.1-
- in (due to)
  - infectious disease NEC B99 *[H75.0-]*
  - parasitic disease NEC B89 *[H75.0-]*
  - tuberculosis A18.03
- petrositis *—see* Petrositis
- postauricular fistula *—see* Fistula, postauricular
- specified NEC H70.89-
- tuberculous A18.03

Mastopathy, mastopathia N64.9
- chronica cystica *—see* Mastopathy, cystic
- cystic (chronic) (diffuse) N60.1-
  - with epithelial proliferation N60.3-
- diffuse cystic *—see* Mastopathy, cystic
- estrogenic, oestrogenica N64.89
- ovarian origin N64.89

Mastoplasia, mastoplastia N62

Masturbation (excessive) F98.8

Maternal care (for) *—see* Pregnancy (complicated by) (management affected by)

Matheiu's disease (leptospiral jaundice) A27.0

Mauclaire's disease or osteochondrosis *—see* Osteochondrosis, juvenile, hand, metacarpal

Maxcy's disease A75.2

Maxilla, maxillary *—see* condition

May (-Hegglin) **anomaly or syndrome** D72.0

McArdle (-Schmid) (-Pearson) **disease** (glycogen storage) E74.04

McCune-Albright syndrome Q78.1

McQuarrie's syndrome (idiopathic familial hypoglycemia) E16.2

Meadow's syndrome Q86.1

Measles (black) (hemorrhagic) (suppressed) B05.9
- with
  - complications NEC B05.89
  - encephalitis B05.0
  - intestinal complications B05.4
  - keratitis (keratoconjunctivitis) B05.81
  - meningitis B05.1
  - otitis media B05.3
  - pneumonia B05.2
- French *—see* Rubella
- German *—see* Rubella
- Liberty *—see* Rubella

Meatitis, urethral *—see* Urethritis

Meatus, meatal *—see* condition

Meat-wrappers' asthma J68.9

Meckel-Gruber syndrome Q61.9

Meckel's diverticulitis, diverticulum (displaced) (hypertrophic) Q43.0
- malignant *—see* Table of Neoplasms, small intestine, malignant

Meconium
- ileus, newborn P76.0
  - in cystic fibrosis E84.11
  - meaning meconium plug (without cystic fibrosis) P76.0
- obstruction, newborn P76.0
  - due to fecaliths P76.0
  - in mucoviscidosis E84.11
- peritonitis P78.0
- plug syndrome (newborn) NEC P76.0

Median *—see also* condition
- arcuate ligament syndrome I77.4
- bar (prostate) (vesical orifice) *—see* Hyperplasia, prostate
- rhomboid glossitis K14.2

Mediastinal shift R93.89

Mediastinitis (acute) (chronic) J98.51
- syphilitic A52.73
- tuberculous A15.8

Mediastinopericarditis —*see also* Pericarditis
- acute I30.9
- adhesive I31.0
- chronic I31.8
  - rheumatic I09.2

Mediastinum, mediastinal —*see* condition

Medicine poisoning —*see* Table of Drugs and Chemicals, by drug, poisoning

Mediterranean
- fever —*see* Brucellosis
  - familial M04.1
  - tick A77.1
- kala-azar B55.0
- leishmaniasis B55.0
- tick fever A77.1

Medulla —*see* condition

Medullary cystic kidney Q61.5

Medullated fibers
- optic (nerve) Q14.8
- retina Q14.1

Medulloblastoma
- desmoplastic C71.6
- specified site —*see* Neoplasm, malignant, by site
- unspecified site C71.6

Medulloepithelioma —*see also* Neoplasm, malignant, by site
- teratoid —*see* Neoplasm, malignant, by site

Medullomyoblastoma
- specified site —*see* Neoplasm, malignant, by site
- unspecified site C71.6

Meekeren-Ehlers-Danlos syndrome (*see also* Syndrome, Ehlers-Danlos) Q79.69

Megacolon (acquired) (functional) (not Hirschsprung's disease) (in) K59.39
- Chagas' disease B57.32
- congenital, congenitum (aganglionic) Q43.1
- Hirschsprung's (disease) Q43.1
- toxic NEC K59.31
  - due to Clostridium difficile
    - not specified as recurrent A04.72
    - recurrent A04.71

Megaesophagus (functional) K22.0
- congenital Q39.5
- in (due to) Chagas' disease B57.31

Megalencephaly Q04.5

Megalerythema (epidemic) B08.3

Megaloappendix Q43.8

Megalocephalus, megalocephaly NEC Q75.3

Megalocornea Q15.8
- with glaucoma Q15.0

Megalocytic anemia D53.1

Megalodactylia (fingers) (thumbs) (congenital) Q74.0
- toes Q74.2

Megaloduodenum Q43.8

Megaloesophagus (functional) K22.0
- congenital Q39.5

Megalogastria (acquired) K31.89
- congenital Q40.2

Megalophthalmos Q11.3

Megalopsia H53.15

Megalosplenia —*see* Splenomegaly

Megaloureter N28.82
- congenital Q62.2

Megarectum K62.89

Megasigmoid K59.39
- congenital Q43.2

Megaureter N28.82
- congenital Q62.2

Megavitamin-B6 syndrome E67.2

Megrim —*see* Migraine

Meibomian
- cyst, infected —*see* Hordeolum
- gland —*see* condition
- sty, stye —*see* Hordeolum

Meibomitis —*see* Hordeolum

Meige-Milroy disease (chronic hereditary edema) Q82.0

Meige's syndrome Q82.0

Melalgia, nutritional E53.8

Melancholia F32.A
- climacteric (single episode) F32.89
  - recurrent episode F33.8
- hypochondriac F45.29
- intermittent (single episode) F32.89
  - recurrent episode F33.8
- involutional (single episode) F32.89
  - recurrent episode F33.8
- menopausal (single episode) F32.89
  - recurrent episode F33.8
- puerperal F32.89
- reactive (emotional stress or trauma) F32.3
- recurrent F33.9
- senile F03
- stuporous (single episode) F32.89
  - recurrent episode F33.8

Melanemia R79.89

Melanoameloblastoma —*see* Neoplasm, bone, benign

Melanoblastoma —*see* Melanoma

Melanocarcinoma —*see* Melanoma

Melanocytoma, eyeball D31.9-

Melanocytosis, neurocutaneous Q82.8

Melanoderma, melanodermia L81.4

Melanodontia, infantile K03.89

Melanodontoclasia K03.89

Melanoepithelioma —*see* Melanoma

Melanoma (malignant) C43.9
- acral lentiginous, malignant —*see* Melanoma, skin, by site
- amelanotic —*see* Melanoma, skin, by site
- balloon cell —*see* Melanoma, skin, by site
- benign —*see* Nevus
- desmoplastic, malignant —*see* Melanoma, skin, by site
- epithelioid cell —*see* Melanoma, skin, by site
  - with spindle cell, mixed —*see* Melanoma, skin, by site
- in
  - giant pigmented nevus —*see* Melanoma, skin, by site
  - Hutchinson's melanotic freckle —*see* Melanoma, skin, by site

Melanoma *(continued)*
- in *(continued)*
  - junctional nevus —*see* Melanoma, skin, by site
  - precancerous melanosis —*see* Melanoma, skin, by site
- in situ D03.9
  - abdominal wall D03.59
  - ala nasi D03.39
  - ankle D03.7-
  - anus, anal (margin) (skin) D03.51
  - arm D03.6-
  - auditory canal D03.2-
  - auricle (ear) D03.2-
  - auricular canal (external) D03.2-
  - axilla, axillary fold D03.59
  - back D03.59
  - breast D03.52
  - brow D03.39
  - buttock D03.59
  - canthus (eye) D03.1-
  - cheek (external) D03.39
  - chest wall D03.59
  - chin D03.39
  - choroid D03.8
  - conjunctiva D03.8
  - ear (external) D03.2-
  - external meatus (ear) D03.2-
  - eye D03.8
  - eyebrow D03.39
  - eyelid (lower) (upper) D03.1-
  - face D03.30
    - specified NEC D03.39
  - female genital organ (external) NEC D03.8
  - finger D03.6-
  - flank D03.59
  - foot D03.7-
  - forearm D03.6-
  - forehead D03.39
  - foreskin D03.8
  - gluteal region D03.59
  - groin D03.59
  - hand D03.6-
  - heel D03.7-
  - helix D03.2-
  - hip D03.7-
  - interscapular region D03.59
  - iris D03.8
  - jaw D03.39
  - knee D03.7-
  - labium (majus) (minus) D03.8
  - lacrimal gland D03.8
  - leg D03.7-
  - lip (lower) (upper) D03.0
  - lower limb NEC D03.7-
  - male genital organ (external) NEC D03.8
  - nail D03.9
    - finger D03.6-
    - toe D03.7-
  - neck D03.4
  - nose (external) D03.39
  - orbit D03.8
  - penis D03.8
  - perianal skin D03.51
  - perineum D03.51
  - pinna D03.2-
  - popliteal fossa or space D03.7-
  - prepuce D03.8
  - pudendum D03.8
  - retina D03.8
  - retrobulbar D03.8
  - scalp D03.4
  - scrotum D03.8
  - shoulder D03.6-
  - specified site NEC D03.8
  - submammary fold D03.52

Melanoma *(continued)*
- in situ *(continued)*
  - temple D03.39
  - thigh D03.7-
  - toe D03.7-
  - trunk NEC D03.59
  - umbilicus D03.59
  - upper limb NEC D03.6-
  - vulva D03.8
- juvenile —*see* Nevus
- malignant, of soft parts except skin —*see* Neoplasm, connective tissue, malignant
- metastatic
  - breast C79.81
  - genital organ C79.82
  - specified site NEC C79.89
- neurotropic, malignant —*see* Melanoma, skin, by site
- nodular —*see* Melanoma, skin, by site
- regressing, malignant —*see* Melanoma, skin, by site
- skin C43.9
  - abdominal wall C43.59
  - ala nasi C43.31
  - ankle C43.7-
  - anus, anal (skin) C43.51
  - arm C43.6-
  - auditory canal (external) C43.2-
  - auricle (ear) C43.2-
  - auricular canal (external) C43.2-
  - axilla, axillary fold C43.59
  - back C43.59
  - breast (female) (male) C43.52
  - brow C43.39
  - buttock C43.59
  - canthus (eye) C43.1-
  - cheek (external) C43.39
  - chest wall C43.59
  - chin C43.39
  - ear (external) C43.2-
  - elbow C43.6-
  - external meatus (ear) C43.2-
  - eyebrow C43.39
  - eyelid (lower) (upper) C43.1-
  - face C43.30
    - specified NEC C43.39
  - female genital organ (external) NEC C51.9
  - finger C43.6-
  - flank C43.59
  - foot C43.7-
  - forearm C43.6-
  - forehead C43.39
  - foreskin C60.0
  - glabella C43.39
  - gluteal region C43.59
  - groin C43.59
  - hand C43.6-
  - heel C43.7-
  - helix C43.2-
  - hip C43.7-
  - interscapular region C43.59
  - jaw (external) C43.39
  - knee C43.7-
  - labium C51.9
    - majus C51.0
    - minus C51.1
  - leg C43.7-
  - lip (lower) (upper) C43.0
  - lower limb NEC C43.7-
  - male genital organ (external) NEC C63.9
  - nail
    - finger C43.6-
    - toe C43.7-
  - nasolabial groove C43.39
  - nates C43.59
  - neck C43.4

Melanoma *(continued)*
- skin *(continued)*
  - nose (external) C43.31
  - overlapping site C43.8
  - palpebra C43.1-
  - penis C60.9
  - perianal skin C43.51
  - perineum C43.51
  - pinna C43.2-
  - popliteal fossa or space C43.7-
  - prepuce C60.0
  - pudendum C51.9
  - scalp C43.4
  - scrotum C63.2
  - shoulder C43.6-
  - skin NEC C43.9
  - submammary fold C43.52
  - temple C43.39
  - thigh C43.7-
  - toe C43.7-
  - trunk NEC C43.59
  - umbilicus C43.59
  - upper limb NEC C43.6-
  - vulva C51.9
    - overlapping sites C51.8
- spindle cell
  - with epithelioid, mixed —*see* Melanoma, skin, by site
  - type A C69.4-
  - type B C69.4-
- superficial spreading —*see* Melanoma, skin, by site

Melanosarcoma —*see also* Melanoma
- epithelioid cell —*see* Melanoma

Melanosis L81.4
- addisonian E27.1
  - tuberculous A18.7
- adrenal E27.1
- colon K63.89
- conjunctiva —*see* Pigmentation, conjunctiva
  - congenital Q13.89
- cornea (presenile) (senile) —*see also* Pigmentation, cornea
  - congenital Q13.4
- eye NEC H57.89
  - congenital Q15.8
- lenticularis progressiva Q82.1
- liver K76.89
- precancerous —*see also* Melanoma, in situ
  - malignant melanoma in —*see* Melanoma
- Riehl's L81.4
- sclera H15.89
  - congenital Q13.89
- suprarenal E27.1
- tar L81.4
- toxic L81.4

Melanuria R82.998

MELAS syndrome E88.41

Melasma L81.1
- adrenal (gland) E27.1
- suprarenal (gland) E27.1

Melena K92.1
- with ulcer - code by site under Ulcer, with hemorrhage K27.4
- due to swallowed maternal blood P78.2
- newborn, neonatal P54.1
  - due to swallowed maternal blood P78.2

Meleney's
- gangrene (cutaneous) —*see* Ulcer, skin
- ulcer (chronic undermining) —*see* Ulcer, skin

Melioidosis A24.9
- acute A24.1
- chronic A24.2
- fulminating A24.1
- pneumonia A24.1
- pulmonary (chronic) A24.2
  - acute A24.1
  - subacute A24.2
- sepsis A24.1
- specified NEC A24.3
- subacute A24.2

Melitensis, febris A23.0

Melkersson (-Rosenthal) **syndrome** G51.2

Mellitus, diabetes —*see* Diabetes

Melorheostosis (bone) —*see* Disorder, bone, density and structure, specified NEC

Meloschisis Q18.4

Melotia Q17.4

Membrana
- capsularis lentis posterior Q13.89
- epipapillaris Q14.2

Membranacea placenta O43.19-

Membranaceous uterus N85.8

Membrane(s), membranous —*see also* condition
- cyclitic —*see* Membrane, pupillary
- folds, congenital —*see* Web
- Jackson's Q43.3
- over face of newborn P28.9
- premature rupture —*see* Rupture, membranes, premature
- pupillary H21.4-
  - persistent Q13.89
- retained (with hemorrhage) (complicating delivery) O72.2
  - without hemorrhage O73.1
- secondary cataract —*see* Cataract, secondary
- unruptured (causing asphyxia) —*see* Asphyxia, newborn
- vitreous —*see* Opacity, vitreous, membranes and strands

Membranitis —*see* Chorioamnionitis

Memory disturbance, lack or loss —*see also* Amnesia
- mild, following organic brain damage F06.8

Menadione deficiency E56.1

Menarche
- delayed E30.0
- precocious E30.1

Mendacity, pathologic F60.2

Mendelson's syndrome (due to anesthesia) J95.4
- in labor and delivery O74.0
- in pregnancy O29.01-
- obstetric O74.0
- postpartum, puerperal O89.01

Ménétrier's disease or syndrome K29.60
- with bleeding K29.61

Ménière's disease, syndrome or vertigo H81.0-

Meninges, meningeal —*see* condition

Meningioma —*see also* Neoplasm, meninges, benign
- angioblastic —*see* Neoplasm, meninges, benign
- angiomatous —*see* Neoplasm, meninges, benign
- atypical —*see* Neoplasm, meninges, uncertain behavior
- endotheliomatous —*see* Neoplasm, meninges, benign
- fibroblastic —*see* Neoplasm, meninges, benign
- fibrous —*see* Neoplasm, meninges, benign
- hemangioblastic —*see* Neoplasm, meninges, benign
- hemangiopericytic —*see* Neoplasm, meninges, benign
- malignant —*see* Neoplasm, meninges, malignant
- meningiothelial —*see* Neoplasm, meninges, benign
- meningotheliomatous —*see* Neoplasm, meninges, benign
- mixed —*see* Neoplasm, meninges, benign
- multiple —*see* Neoplasm, meninges, uncertain behavior
- papillary —*see* Neoplasm, meninges, uncertain behavior
- psammomatous —*see* Neoplasm, meninges, benign
- syncytial —*see* Neoplasm, meninges, benign
- transitional —*see* Neoplasm, meninges, benign

Meningiomatosis (diffuse) —*see* Neoplasm, meninges, uncertain behavior

Meningism —*see* Meningismus

Meningismus (infectional) (pneumococcal) R29.1
- due to serum or vaccine R29.1
- influenzal —*see* Influenza, with, manifestations NEC

Meningitis (basal) (basic) (brain) (cerebral) (cervical) (congestive) (diffuse) (hemorrhagic) (infantile) (membranous) (metastatic) (nonspecific) (pontine) (progressive) (simple) (spinal) (subacute) (sympathetic) (toxic) G03.9
- abacterial G03.0
- actinomycotic A42.81
- adenoviral A87.1
- arbovirus A87.8
- aseptic (acute) G03.0
- bacterial G00.9
  - Escherichia coli (E. coli) G00.8
  - Friedländer (bacillus) G00.8
  - gram-negative G00.9
  - H. influenzae G00.0
  - Klebsiella G00.8
  - pneumococcal G00.1
  - specified organism NEC G00.8
  - staphylococcal G00.3
  - streptococcal (acute) G00.2
- benign recurrent (Mollaret) G03.2
- candidal B37.5
- caseous (tuberculous) A17.0
- cerebrospinal A39.0
- chronic NEC G03.1
- clear cerebrospinal fluid NEC G03.0
- coxsackievirus A87.0
- cryptococcal B45.1
- diplococcal (gram positive) A39.0
- echovirus A87.0
- enteroviral A87.0
- eosinophilic B83.2
- epidemic NEC A39.0
- Escherichia coli (E. coli) G00.8
- fibrinopurulent G00.9
  - specified organism NEC G00.8
- Friedländer (bacillus) G00.8
- gonococcal A54.81
- gram-negative cocci G00.9
- gram-positive cocci G00.9
- Haemophilus (influenzae) G00.0
- H. influenzae G00.0
- in (due to)
  - adenovirus A87.1
  - African trypanosomiasis B56.9 *[G02]*
  - anthrax A22.8
  - bacterial disease NEC A48.8 *[G01]*
  - Chagas' disease (chronic) B57.41
  - chickenpox B01.0
  - coccidioidomycosis B38.4
  - Diplococcus pneumoniae G00.1
  - enterovirus A87.0
  - herpes (simplex) virus B00.3
    - zoster B02.1
  - infectious mononucleosis B27.92
  - leptospirosis A27.81
  - Listeria monocytogenes A32.11
  - Lyme disease A69.21
  - measles B05.1
  - mumps (virus) B26.1
  - neurosyphilis (late) A52.13
  - parasitic disease NEC B89 *[G02]*
  - poliovirus A80.9 *[G02]*
  - preventive immunization, inoculation or vaccination G03.8
  - rubella B06.02
  - Salmonella infection A02.21
  - specified cause NEC G03.8
  - Streptococcal pneumoniae G00.1
  - typhoid fever A01.01
  - varicella B01.0
  - viral disease NEC A87.8
  - whooping cough A37.90
  - zoster B02.1
- infectious G00.9
- influenzal (H. influenzae) G00.0
- Klebsiella G00.8
- leptospiral (aseptic) A27.81
- lymphocytic (acute) (benign) (serous) A87.2
- meningococcal A39.0
- Mima polymorpha G00.8
- Mollaret (benign recurrent) G03.2
- monilial B37.5
- mycotic NEC B49 *[G02]*
- Neisseria A39.0
- nonbacterial G03.0
- nonpyogenic NEC G03.0
- ossificans G96.198
- pneumococcal streptococcus pneumoniae G00.1
- poliovirus A80.9 *[G02]*
- postmeasles B05.1
- purulent G00.9
  - specified organism NEC G00.8
- pyogenic G00.9
  - specified organism NEC G00.8
- Salmonella (arizonae) (Cholerae-Suis) (enteritidis) (typhimurium) A02.21
- septic G00.9
  - specified organism NEC G00.8
- serosa circumscripta NEC G03.0
- serous NEC G93.2
- specified organism NEC G00.8
- sporotrichosis B42.81
- staphylococcal G00.3

Meningitis *(continued)*
- sterile G03.0
- Streptococcal (acute) G00.2
  - pneumoniae G00.1
- suppurative G00.9
  - specified organism NEC G00.8
- syphilitic (late) (tertiary) A52.13
  - acute A51.41
  - congenital A50.41
  - secondary A51.41
- Torula histolytica (cryptococcal) B45.1
- traumatic (complication of injury) T79.8
- tuberculous A17.0
- typhoid A01.01
- viral NEC A87.9
- Yersinia pestis A20.3

Meningocele (spinal) —*see also* Spina bifida
- with hydrocephalus —*see* Spina bifida, by site, with hydrocephalus
- acquired (traumatic) G96.198
- cerebral —*see* Encephalocele

Meningocerebritis —*see* Meningoencephalitis

Meningococcemia A39.4
- acute A39.2
- chronic A39.3

Meningococcus, meningococcal —*see also* condition A39.9
- adrenalitis, hemorrhagic A39.1
- carrier (suspected) of Z22.31
- meningitis (cerebrospinal) A39.0

Meningoencephalitis (*see also* Encephalitis) G04.90
- acute NEC (*see also* Encephalitis, viral) A86
- bacterial NEC G04.2
- California A83.5
- diphasic A84.1
- eosinophilic B83.2
- epidemic A39.81
- herpesviral, herpetic B00.4
  - due to herpesvirus 6 B10.01
  - due to herpesvirus 7 B10.09
  - specified NEC B10.09
- in (due to)
  - blastomycosis NEC B40.81
  - diseases classified elsewhere G05.3
  - free-living amebae B60.2
  - Hemophilus influenzae (H .influenzae) G00.0
  - herpes B00.4
    - due to herpesvirus 6 B10.01
    - due to herpesvirus 7 B10.09
    - specified NEC B10.09
  - H. influenzae G00.0
  - Lyme disease A69.22
  - mercury —*see* subcategory T56.1
  - mumps B26.2
  - Naegleria (amebae) (organisms) (fowleri) B60.2
  - Parastrongylus cantonensis B83.2
  - toxoplasmosis (acquired) B58.2
    - congenital P37.1
- infectious (acute) (viral) A86
- influenzal (H. influenzae) G00.0
- Listeria monocytogenes A32.12
- lymphocytic (serous) A87.2
- mumps B26.2
- parasitic NEC B89 *[G05.3]*
- pneumococcal G04.2
- primary amebic B60.2
- specific (syphilitic) A52.14

Meningoencephalitis *(continued)*
- specified organism NEC G04.81
- staphylococcal G04.2
- streptococcal G04.2
- syphilitic A52.14
- toxic NEC G92.8
  - due to mercury —*see* subcategory T56.1
- tuberculous A17.82
- virus NEC A86

Meningoencephalocele —*see also* Encephalocele
- syphilitic A52.19
  - congenital A50.49

Meningoencephalomyelitis —*see also* Meningoencephalitis
- acute NEC (viral) A86
  - disseminated G04.00
    - postimmunization or postvaccination G04.02
    - postinfectious G04.01
- due to
  - actinomycosis A42.82
  - Torula B45.1
  - Toxoplasma or toxoplasmosis (acquired) B58.2
    - congenital P37.1
- postimmunization or postvaccination G04.02

Meningoencephalomyelopathy G96.9

Meningoencephalopathy G96.9

Meningomyelitis —*see also* Meningoencephalitis
- bacterial NEC G04.2
- blastomycotic NEC B40.81
- cryptococcal B45.1
- in diseases classified elsewhere G05.4
- meningococcal A39.81
- syphilitic A52.14
- tuberculous A17.82

Meningomyelocele —*see also* Spina bifida
- syphilitic A52.19

Meningomyeloneuritis —*see* Meningoencephalitis

Meningoradiculitis —*see* Meningitis

Meningovascular —*see* condition

Menkes' disease or syndrome E83.09
- meaning maple-syrup-urine disease E71.0

Menometrorrhagia N92.1

Menopause, menopausal
- (asymptomatic) (state) Z78.0
- arthritis (any site) NEC —*see* Arthritis, specified form NEC
- bleeding N92.4
- depression (single episode) F32.89
  - agitated (single episode) F32.2
    - recurrent episode F33.9
  - psychotic (single episode) F32.89
    - recurrent episode F33.8
  - recurrent episode F33.9
- melancholia (single episode) F32.89
  - recurrent episode F33.8
- paranoid state F22
- premature E28.319
  - asymptomatic E28.319
    - postirradiation E89.40
    - postsurgical E89.40

Menopause, menopausal *(continued)*
- premature *(continued)*
  - symptomatic E28.310
    - postirradiation E89.41
    - postsurgical E89.41
- psychosis NEC F28
- symptomatic N95.1
- toxic polyarthritis NEC —*see* Arthritis, specified form NEC

Menorrhagia (primary) N92.0
- climacteric N92.4
  - menopausal N92.4
- menopausal N92.4
- perimenopausal N92.4
- postclimacteric N95.0
- postmenopausal N95.0
- preclimacteric or premenopausal N92.4
- pubertal (menses retained) N92.2

Menostaxis N92.0

Menses, retention N94.89

Menstrual —*see* Menstruation

Menstruation
- absent —*see* Amenorrhea
- anovulatory N97.0
- cycle, irregular N92.6
- delayed N91.0
- disorder N93.9
  - psychogenic F45.8
- during pregnancy O20.8
- excessive (with regular cycle) N92.0
  - with irregular cycle N92.1
  - at puberty N92.2
- frequent N92.0
- infrequent —*see* Oligomenorrhea
- irregular N92.6
  - specified NEC N92.5
- latent N92.5
- membranous N92.5
- painful (*see also* Dysmenorrhea) N94.6
  - primary N94.4
  - psychogenic F45.8
  - secondary N94.5
- passage of clots N92.0
- precocious E30.1
- protracted N92.5
- rare —*see* Oligomenorrhea
- retained N94.89
- retrograde N92.5
- scanty —*see* Oligomenorrhea
- suppression N94.89
- vicarious (nasal) N94.89

Mental —*see also* condition
- deficiency —*see* Disability, intellectual
- deterioration —*see* Psychosis
- disorder —*see* Disorder, mental
- exhaustion F48.8
- insufficiency (congenital) —*see* Disability, intellectual
- observation without need for further medical care Z03.89
- retardation —*see* Disability, intellectual
- subnormality —*see* Disability, intellectuall
- upset —*see* Disorder, mental

Meralgia paresthetica G57.1-

Mercurial —*see* condition

Mercurialism —*see* subcategory T56.1

MERRF syndrome (myoclonic epilepsy associated with ragged-red fiber) E88.42

Merkel cell tumor —*see* Carcinoma, Merkel cell

Merocele —*see* Hernia, femoral

Meromelia
- lower limb —*see* Defect, reduction, lower limb
  - intercalary
    - femur —*see* Defect, reduction, lower limb, specified type NEC
    - tibiofibular (complete) (incomplete) —*see* Defect, reduction, lower limb
- upper limb —*see* Defect, reduction, upper limb
  - intercalary, humeral, radioulnar —*see* Agenesis, arm, with hand present

Merzbacher-Pelizaeus disease E75.29

Mesaortitis —*see* Aortitis

Mesarteritis —*see* Arteritis

Mesencephalitis —*see* Encephalitis

Mesenchymoma —*see also* Neoplasm, connective tissue, uncertain behavior
- benign —*see* Neoplasm, connective tissue, benign
- malignant —*see* Neoplasm, connective tissue, malignant

Mesenteritis
- retractile K65.4
- sclerosing K65.4

Mesentery, mesenteric —*see* condition

Mesiodens, mesiodentes K00.1

Mesio-occlusion M26.213

Mesocolon —*see* condition

Mesonephroma (malignant) —*see* Neoplasm, malignant, by site
- benign —*see* Neoplasm, benign, by site

Mesophlebitis —*see* Phlebitis

Mesostromal dysgenesia Q13.89

Mesothelioma (malignant) C45.9
- benign
  - mesentery D19.1
  - mesocolon D19.1
  - omentum D19.1
  - peritoneum D19.1
  - pleura D19.0
  - specified site NEC D19.7
  - unspecified site D19.9
- biphasic C45.9
  - benign
    - mesentery D19.1
    - mesocolon D19.1
    - omentum D19.1
    - peritoneum D19.1
    - pleura D19.0
    - specified site NEC D19.7
    - unspecified site D19.9
- cystic D48.4
- epithelioid C45.9
  - benign
    - mesentery D19.1
    - mesocolon D19.1
    - omentum D19.1
    - peritoneum D19.1
    - pleura D19.0
    - specified site NEC D19.7
    - unspecified site D19.9

Mesothelioma *(continued)*
- fibrous C45.9
  - benign
    - mesentery D19.1
    - mesocolon D19.1
    - omentum D19.1
    - peritoneum D19.1
    - pleura D19.0
    - specified site NEC D19.7
    - unspecified site D19.9
- site classification
  - liver C45.7
  - lung C45.7
  - mediastinum C45.7
  - mesentery C45.1
  - mesocolon C45.1
  - omentum C45.1
  - pericardium C45.2
  - peritoneum C45.1
  - pleura C45.0
    - parietal C45.0
  - retroperitoneum C45.7
  - specified site NEC C45.7
  - unspecified C45.9

Metabolic syndrome E88.81

Metagonimiasis B66.8

Metagonimus infestation (intestine) B66.8

Metal
- pigmentation L81.8
- polisher's disease J62.8

Metamorphopsia H53.15

Metaplasia
- apocrine (breast) *—see* Dysplasia, mammary, specified type NEC
- cervix (squamous) *—see* Dysplasia, cervix
- endometrium (squamous) (uterus) N85.8
- esophagus K22.7-
- gastric intestinal K31.A0
  - with dysplasia K31.A29
    - high grade K31.A22
    - low grade K31.A21
  - indefinite for dysplasia K31.A0
  - without dysplasia K31.A19
    - involving
      - antrum K31.A11
      - body (corpus) K31.A12
      - cardia K31.A14
      - fundus K31.A13
      - multiple sites K31.A15
- kidney (pelvis) (squamous) N28.89
- myelogenous D73.1
- myeloid (agnogenic) (megakaryocytic) D73.1
- spleen D73.1
- squamous cell, bladder N32.89

Metastasis, metastatic
- abscess *—see* Abscess
- calcification E83.59
- cancer
  - from specified site *—see* Neoplasm, malignant, by site
  - to specified site *—see* Neoplasm, secondary, by site
- deposits (in) *—see* Neoplasm, secondary, by site
- disease (*see also* Neoplasm, secondary, by site) C79.9
- spread (to) *—see* Neoplasm, secondary, by site

Metastrongyliasis B83.8

Metatarsalgia M77.4-
- anterior G57.6-
- Morton's G57.6-

Metatarsus, metatarsal *—see also* condition
- adductus, congenital Q66.22-
- valgus (abductus), congenital Q66.6
- varus (congenital) Q66.22-
  - primus Q66.21-

Methadone use *—see* Use, opioid

Methemoglobinemia D74.9
- acquired (with sulfhemoglobinemia) D74.8
- congenital D74.0
- enzymatic (congenital) D74.0
- Hb M disease D74.0
- hereditary D74.0
- toxic D74.8

Methemoglobinuria *—see* Hemoglobinuria

Methioninemia E72.19

Methylmalonic acidemia E71.120

Metritis (catarrhal) (hemorrhagic) (septic) (suppurative) *—see also* Endometritis
- cervical *—see* Cervicitis

Metropathia hemorrhagica N93.8

Metroperitonitis *—see* Peritonitis, pelvic, female

Metrorrhagia N92.1
- climacteric N92.4
- menopausal N92.4
- perimenopausal N92.4
- postpartum NEC (atonic) (following delivery of placenta) O72.1
  - delayed or secondary O72.2
- preclimacteric or premenopausal N92.4
- psychogenic F45.8

Metrorrhexis *—see* Rupture, uterus

Metrosalpingitis N70.91

Metrostaxis N93.8

Metrovaginitis *—see* Endometritis

Meyer-Schwickerath and Weyers syndrome Q87.0

Meynert's amentia (nonalcoholic) F04
- alcoholic F10.96
  - with dependence F10.26

Mibelli's disease (porokeratosis) Q82.8

Mice, joint *—see* Loose, body, joint
- knee M23.4-

Micrencephalon, micrencephaly Q02

Microalbuminuria R80.9

Microaneurysm, retinal *— see also* Disorder, retina, microaneurysms
- diabetic *—see* E08-E13 with .31

Microangiopathy (peripheral) I73.9
- thrombotic M31.10
  - hematopoietic stem cell transplantation-associated [HSCT-TMA} M31.10

Microcalcifications, breast R92.0

Microcephalus, microcephalic, microcephaly Q02
- due to toxoplasmosis (congenital) P37.1

Microcheilia Q18.7

Microcolon (congenital) Q43.8

Microcornea (congenital) Q13.4

Microcytic *—see* condition

Microdeletions NEC Q93.88

Microdontia K00.2

Microdrepanocytosis D57.40
- with
  - acute chest syndrome D57.411
  - cerebral vascular involvement D57.413
  - crisis (painful) D57.419
    - with specified complication NEC D57.418
  - splenic sequestration D57.412
  - vasoocclusive pain D57.419

Microembolism
- atherothrombotic *—see* Atheroembolism
- retinal *—see* Occlusion, artery, retina

Microencephalon Q02

Microfilaria streptocerca infestation *—see* Onchocerciasis

Microgastria (congenital) Q40.2

Microgenia M26.06

Microgenitalia, congenital
- female Q52.8
- male Q55.8

Microglioma *—see* Lymphoma, non-Hodgkin, specified NEC

Microglossia (congenital) Q38.3

Micrognathia, micrognathism (congenital) (mandibular) (maxillary) M26.09

Microgyria (congenital) Q04.3

Microinfarct of heart *—see* Insufficiency, coronary

Microlentia (congenital) Q12.8

Microlithiasis, alveolar, pulmonary J84.02

Micromastia N64.82

Micromyelia (congenital) Q06.8

Micropenis Q55.62

Microphakia (congenital) Q12.8

Microphthalmos, microphthalmia (congenital) Q11.2
- due to toxoplasmosis P37.1

Micropsia H53.15

Microscopic polyangiitis (polyarteritis) M31.7

Microsporidiosis B60.8
- intestinal A07.8

Microsporon furfur infestation B36.0

Microsporosis *—see also* Dermatophytosis
- nigra B36.1

Microstomia (congenital) Q18.5

Microtia (congenital) (external ear) Q17.2

Microtropia H50.40

Microvillus inclusion disease (MVD) (MVID) Q43.8

Micturition
- disorder NEC (*see also* Difficulty, micturition) R39.198
  - psychogenic F45.8
- frequency R35.0
  - psychogenic F45.8
- hesitancy R39.11
- incomplete emptying R39.14
- nocturnal R35.1
- painful R30.9
  - dysuria R30.0
  - psychogenic F45.8
  - tenesmus R30.1

Micturition *(continued)*
- poor stream R39.12
- position dependent R39.192
- split stream R39.13
- straining R39.16
- urgency R39.15

Mid plane *—see* condition

Middle
- ear *—see* condition
- lobe (right) syndrome J98.19

Miescher's elastoma L87.2

Mietens' syndrome Q87.2

Migraine (idiopathic) G43.909
- with refractory migraine G43.919
  - with status migrainosus G43.911
  - without status migrainosus G43.919
- with aura (acute-onset) (prolonged) (typical) (without headache) G43.109
  - with refractory migraine G43.119
    - with status migrainosus G43.111
    - without status migrainosus G43.119
  - intractable G43.119
    - with status migrainosus G43.111
    - without status migrainosus G43.119
  - not intractable G43.109
    - with status migrainosus G43.101
    - without status migrainosus G43.109
  - persistent G43.509
    - with cerebral infarction G43.609
      - with refractory migraine G43.619
        - with status migrainosus G43.611
        - without status migrainosus G43.619
      - intractable G43.619
        - with status migrainosus G43.611
        - without status migrainosus G43.619
      - not intractable G43.609
        - with status migrainosus G43.601
        - without status migrainosus G43.609
      - without refractory migraine G43.609
        - with status migrainosus G43.601
        - without status migrainosus G43.609
    - without cerebral infarction G43.509
      - with refractory migraine G43.519
        - with status migrainosus G43.511
        - without status migrainosus G43.519
      - intractable G43.519
        - with status migrainosus G43.511
        - without status migrainosus G43.519
      - not intractable G43.509
        - with status migrainosus G43.501
        - without status migrainosus G43.509

Migraine *(continued)*
- with aura *(continued)*
  - persistent *(continued)*
    - without cerebral infarction *(continued)*
      - without refractory migraine G43.509
        - with status migrainosus G43.501
        - without status migrainosus G43.509
  - without mention of refractory migraine G43.109
    - with status migrainosus G43.101
    - without status migrainosus G43.109
- abdominal G43.D0
  - with refractory migraine G43.D1
  - intractable G43.D1
  - not intractable G43.D0
  - without refractory migraine G43.D0
- basilar *—see* Migraine, with aura
- classical *—see* Migraine, with aura
- common *—see* Migraine, without aura
- complicated G43.109
- equivalents *—see* Migraine, with aura
- familiar *—see* Migraine, hemiplegic
- hemiplegic G43.409
  - with refractory migraine G43.419
    - with status migrainosus G43.411
    - without status migrainosus G43.419
  - intractable G43.419
    - with status migrainosus G43.411
    - without status migrainosus G43.419
  - not intractable G43.409
    - with status migrainosus G43.401
    - without status migrainosus G43.409
  - without refractory migraine G43.409
    - with status migrainosus G43.401
    - without status migrainosus G43.409
- intractable G43.919
  - with status migrainosus G43.911
  - without status migrainosus G43.919
- menstrual G43.829
  - with refractory migraine G43.839
    - with status migrainosus G43.831
    - without status migrainosus G43.839
  - intractable G43.839
    - with status migrainosus G43.831
    - without status migrainosus G43.839
  - not intractable G43.829
    - with status migrainosus G43.821
    - without status migrainosus G43.829
  - without refractory migraine G43.829
    - with status migrainosus G43.821

Migraine *(continued)*
- menstrual *(continued)*
  - without refractory migraine *(continued)*
    - without status migrainosus G43.829
- menstrually related *—see* Migraine, menstrual
- not intractable G43.909
  - with status migrainosus G43.901
  - without status migrainosus G43.919
- ophthalmoplegic G43.B0
  - with refractory migraine G43.B1
  - intractable G43.B1
  - not intractable G43.B0
  - without refractory migraine G43.B0
- persistent aura (with, without) cerebral infarction *—see* Migraine, with aura, persistent
- preceded or accompanied by transient focal neurological phenomena *—see* Migraine, with aura
- pre-menstrual *—see* Migraine, menstrual
- pure menstrual *—see* Migraine, menstrual
- retinal *—see* Migraine, with aura
- specified NEC G43.809
  - intractable G43.819
    - with status migrainosus G43.811
    - without status migrainosus G43.819
  - not intractable G43.809
    - with status migrainosus G43.801
    - without status migrainosus G43.809
- sporadic *—see* Migraine, hemiplegic
- transformed *—see* Migraine, without aura, chronic
- triggered seizures *—see* Migraine, with aura
- without aura G43.009
  - with refractory migraine G43.019
    - with status migrainosus G43.011
    - without status migrainosus G43.019
  - chronic G43.709
    - with refractory migraine G43.719
      - with status migrainosus G43.711
      - without status migrainosus G43.719
    - intractable
      - with status migrainosus G43.711
      - without status migrainosus G43.719
    - not intractable
      - with status migrainosus G43.701
      - without status migrainosus G43.709
    - without refractory migraine G43.709
      - with status migrainosus G43.701
      - without status migrainosus G43.709
  - intractable
    - with status migrainosus G43.011

Migraine *(continued)*
- without aura *(continued)*
  - intractable *(continued)*
    - without status migrainosus G43.019
  - not intractable
    - with status migrainosus G43.001
    - without status migrainosus G43.009
  - without mention of refractory migraine G43.009
    - with status migrainosus G43.001
    - without status migrainosus G43.009
- without refractory migraine G43.909
  - with status migrainosus G43.901
  - without status migrainosus G43.919

Migrant, social Z59.00

Migration, anxiety concerning Z60.3

Migratory, migrating *—see also* condition
- person Z59.00
- testis Q55.29

Mikity-Wilson disease or syndrome P27.0

Mikulicz' disease or syndrome K11.8

Miliaria L74.3
- alba L74.1
- apocrine L75.2
- crystallina L74.1
- profunda L74.2
- rubra L74.0
- tropicalis L74.2

Miliary *—see* condition

Milium L72.0
- colloid L57.8

Milk
- crust L21.0
- excessive secretion O92.6
- poisoning *—see* Poisoning, food, noxious
- retention O92.79
- sickness *—see* Poisoning, food, noxious
- spots I31.0

Milk-alkali disease or syndrome E83.52

Milk-leg (deep vessels) (nonpuerperal) *—see* Embolism, vein, lower extremity
- complicating pregnancy O22.3-
- puerperal, postpartum, childbirth O87.1

Milkman's disease or syndrome M83.8

Milky urine *—see* Chyluria

Millard-Gubler (-Foville) **paralysis or syndrome** G46.3

Millar's asthma J38.5

Miller Fisher syndrome G61.0

Mills' disease *—see* Hemiplegia

Millstone maker's pneumoconiosis J62.8

Milroy's disease (chronic hereditary edema) Q82.0

Minamata disease T56.1

Miners' asthma or lung J60

Minkowski-Chauffard syndrome *—see* Spherocytosis

Minor *—see* condition

Minor's disease (hematomyelia) G95.19

Minot's disease (hemorrhagic disease), **newborn** P53

Minot-von Willebrand-Jurgens disease or syndrome (angiohemophilia) D68.0

Minus (and plus) hand (intrinsic) *—see* Deformity, limb, specified type NEC, forearm

Miosis (pupil) H57.03

Mirizzi's syndrome (hepatic duct stenosis) K83.1

Mirror writing F81.0

MIS-A M35.81

MIS-C M35.81

Misadventure (of) (prophylactic) (therapeutic) (*see also* Complications) T88.9
- administration of insulin (by accident) T38.3
- infusion *—see* Complications, infusion
- local applications (of fomentations, plasters, etc.) T88.9
  - burn or scald *—see* Burn
  - specified NEC T88.8
- medical care (early) (late) T88.9
  - adverse effect of drugs or chemicals *—see* Table of Drugs and Chemicals
  - burn or scald *—see* Burn
  - specified NEC T88.8
- specified NEC T88.8
- surgical procedure (early) (late) *—see* Complications, surgical procedure
- transfusion *—see* Complications, transfusion
- vaccination or other immunological procedure *—see* Complications, vaccination

Miscarriage O03.9

Misdirection, aqueous H40.83-

Misperception, sleep state F51.02

Misplaced, misplacement
- ear Q17.4
- kidney (acquired) N28.89
  - congenital Q63.2
- organ or site, congenital NEC *—see* Malposition, congenital

Missed
- abortion O02.1
- delivery O36.4

Missing *—see also* Absence
- string of intrauterine contraceptive device T83.32

Misuse of drugs F19.99

Mitchell's disease (erythromelalgia) I73.81

Mite(s) (infestation) B88.9
- diarrhea B88.0
- grain (itch) B88.0
- hair follicle (itch) B88.0
- in sputum B88.0

Mitral *—see* condition

Mittelschmerz N94.0

Mixed *—see* condition

MMN (multifocal motor neuropathy) G61.82

MNGIE (Mitochondrial Neurogastrointestinal Encephalopathy) **syndrome** E88.49

Mobile, mobility
- cecum Q43.3
- excessive —*see* Hypermobility
- gallbladder, congenital Q44.1
- kidney N28.89
- organ or site, congenital NEC —*see* Malposition, congenital

Mobitz heart block (atrioventricular) I44.1

Moebius, Möbius
- disease (ophthalmoplegic migraine) —*see* Migraine, ophthalmoplegic
- syndrome Q87.0
  - congenital oculofacial paralysis (with other anomalies) Q87.0
  - ophthalmoplegic migraine —*see* Migraine, ophthalmoplegic

Moeller's glossitis K14.0

Mohr's syndrome (Types I and II) Q87.0

Mola destruens D39.2

Molar pregnancy O02.0

Molarization of premolars K00.2

Molding, head (during birth) - omit code

Mole (pigmented) —*see also* Nevus
- blood O02.0
- Breus' O02.0
- cancerous —*see* Melanoma
- carneous O02.0
- destructive D39.2
- fleshy O02.0
- hydatid, hydatidiform (benign) (complicating pregnancy) (delivered) (undelivered) O01.9
  - classical O01.0
  - complete O01.0
  - incomplete O01.1
  - invasive D39.2
  - malignant D39.2
  - partial O01.1
- intrauterine O02.0
- invasive (hydatidiform) D39.2
- malignant
  - meaning
    - malignant hydatidiform mole D39.2
    - melanoma —*see* Melanoma
- nonhydatidiform O02.0
- nonpigmented —*see* Nevus
- pregnancy NEC O02.0
- skin —*see* Nevus
- tubal O00.10-
  - with intrauterine pregnancy O00.11-
- vesicular —*see* Mole, hydatidiform

Molimen, molimina (menstrual) N94.3

Molluscum contagiosum (epitheliale) B08.1

Mönckeberg's arteriosclerosis, disease, or sclerosis —*see* Arteriosclerosis, extremities

Mondini's malformation (cochlea) Q16.5

Mondor's disease I80.8

Monge's disease T70.29

Monilethrix (congenital) Q84.1

Moniliasis (*see also* Candidiasis) B37.9
- neonatal P37.5

Monitoring (encounter for)
- therapeutic drug level Z51.81

Monkey malaria B53.1

Monkeypox B04

Monoarthritis M13.10
- ankle M13.17-
- elbow M13.12-
- foot joint M13.17-
- hand joint M13.14-
- hip M13.15-
- knee M13.16-
- shoulder M13.11-
- wrist M13.13-

Monoblastic —*see* condition

Monochromat (ism), monochromatopsia (acquired) (congenital) H53.51

Monocytic —*see* condition

Monocytopenia D72.818

Monocytosis (symptomatic) D72.821

Monomania —*see* Psychosis

Mononeuritis G58.9
- cranial nerve —*see* Disorder, nerve, cranial
- femoral nerve G57.2-
- lateral
  - cutaneous nerve of thigh G57.1-
  - popliteal nerve G57.3-
- lower limb G57.9-
  - specified nerve NEC G57.8-
- medial popliteal nerve G57.4-
- median nerve G56.1-
- multiplex G58.7
- plantar nerve G57.6-
- posterior tibial nerve G57.5-
- radial nerve G56.3-
- sciatic nerve G57.0-
- specified NEC G58.8
- tibial nerve G57.4-
- ulnar nerve G56.2-
- upper limb G56.9-
  - specified nerve NEC G56.8-
- vestibular —*see* subcategory H93.3

Mononeuropathy G58.9
- carpal tunnel syndrome —*see* Syndrome, carpal tunnel
- diabetic NEC —*see* E08-E13 with .41
- femoral nerve —*see* Lesion, nerve, femoral
- ilioinguinal nerve G57.8-
- in diseases classified elsewhere —*see* category G59
- intercostal G58.0
- lower limb G57.9-
  - causalgia —*see* Causalgia, lower limb
  - femoral nerve —*see* Lesion, nerve, femoral
  - meralgia paresthetica G57.1-
  - plantar nerve —*see* Lesion, nerve, plantar
  - popliteal nerve —*see* Lesion, nerve, popliteal
  - sciatic nerve —*see* Lesion, nerve, sciatic
  - specified NEC G57.8-

Mononeuropathy *(continued)*
- lower limb *(continued)*
  - tarsal tunnel syndrome —*see* Syndrome, tarsal tunnel
- median nerve —*see* Lesion, nerve, median
- multiplex G58.7
- obturator nerve G57.8-
- popliteal nerve —*see* Lesion, nerve, popliteal
- radial nerve —*see* Lesion, nerve, radial
- saphenous nerve G57.8-
- specified NEC G58.8
- tarsal tunnel syndrome —*see* Syndrome, tarsal tunnel
- tuberculous A17.83
- ulnar nerve —*see* Lesion, nerve, ulnar
- upper limb G56.9-
  - carpal tunnel syndrome —*see* Syndrome, carpal tunnel
  - causalgia —*see* Causalgia
  - median nerve —*see* Lesion, nerve, median
  - radial nerve —*see* Lesion, nerve, radial
  - specified site NEC G56.8-
  - ulnar nerve —*see* Lesion, nerve, ulnar

Mononucleosis, infectious B27.90
- with
  - complication NEC B27.99
  - meningitis B27.92
  - polyneuropathy B27.91
- cytomegaloviral B27.10
  - with
    - complication NEC B27.19
    - meningitis B27.12
    - polyneuropathy B27.11
- Epstein-Barr (virus) B27.00
  - with
    - complication NEC B27.09
    - meningitis B27.02
    - polyneuropathy B27.01
- gammaherpesviral B27.00
  - with
    - complication NEC B27.09
    - meningitis B27.02
    - polyneuropathy B27.01
- specified NEC B27.80
  - with
    - complication NEC B27.89
    - meningitis B27.82
    - polyneuropathy B27.81

Monoplegia G83.3-
- congenital (cerebral) G80.8
  - spastic G80.1
- embolic (current episode) I63.4-
- following
  - cerebrovascular disease
    - cerebral infarction
      - lower limb I69.34-
      - upper limb I69.33-
    - intracerebral hemorrhage
      - lower limb I69.14-
      - upper limb I69.13-
    - lower limb I69.94-
    - nontraumatic intracranial hemorrhage NEC
      - lower limb I69.24-
      - upper limb I69.23-
    - specified disease NEC
      - lower limb I69.84-
      - upper limb I69.83-
    - stroke NOS
      - lower limb I69.34-
      - upper limb I69.33-

Monoplegia *(continued)*
- following *(continued)*
  - cerebrovascular disease *(continued)*
    - subarachnoid hemorrhage
      - lower limb I69.04-
      - upper limb I69.03-
    - upper limb I69.93-
- hysterical (transient) F44.4
- lower limb G83.1-
- psychogenic (conversion reaction) F44.4
- thrombotic (current episode) I63.3-
- transient R29.818
- upper limb G83.2-

Monorchism, monorchidism Q55.0

Monosomy (*see also* Deletion, chromosome) Q93.9
- specified NEC Q93.89
- whole chromosome
  - meiotic nondisjunction Q93.0
  - mitotic nondisjunction Q93.1
  - mosaicism Q93.1
- X Q96.9

Monster, monstrosity (single) Q89.7
- acephalic Q00.0
- twin Q89.4

Monteggia's fracture (-dislocation) S52.27-

Mooren's ulcer (cornea) —*see* Ulcer, cornea, Mooren's

Moore's syndrome —*see* Epilepsy, specified NEC

Mooser-Neill reaction A75.2

Mooser's bodies A75.2

Morbidity not stated or unknown R69

Morbilli —*see* Measles

Morbus —*see also* Disease
- angelicus, anglorum E55.0
- Beigel B36.2
- caducus —*see* Epilepsy
- celiacus K90.0
- comitialis —*see* Epilepsy
- cordis (*see also* Disease, heart) I51.9
  - valvulorum —*see* Endocarditis
- coxae senilis M16.9
  - tuberculous A18.02
- hemorrhagicus neonatorum P53
- maculosus neonatorum P54.5

Morel (-Stewart) (-Morgagni) **syndrome** M85.2

Morel-Kraepelin disease —*see* Schizophrenia

Morel-Moore syndrome M85.2

Morgagni's
- cyst, organ, hydatid, or appendage
  - female Q50.5
  - male (epididymal) Q55.4
    - testicular Q55.29
- syndrome M85.2

Morgagni-Stokes-Adams syndrome I45.9

Morgagni-Stewart-Morel syndrome M85.2

Morgagni-Turner (-Albright) **syndrome** Q96.9

Moria F07.0

Moron (I.Q.50-69) F70

Morphea L94.0

Morphinism (without remission) F11.20
- with remission F11.21

Morphinomania (without remission) F11.20
- with remission F11.21

Morquio (-Ullrich) (-Brailsford) **disease or syndrome** —*see* Mucopolysaccharidosis

Mortification (dry) (moist) —*see* Gangrene

Morton's metatarsalgia (neuralgia) (neuroma) (syndrome) G57.6-

Morvan's disease or syndrome G60.8

Mosaicism, mosaic (autosomal) (chromosomal)
- 45,X/other cell lines NEC with abnormal sex chromosome Q96.4
- 45,X/46,XX Q96.3
- sex chromosome
  - female Q97.8
  - lines with various numbers of X chromosomes Q97.2
  - male Q98.7
- XY Q96.3

Moschowitz' disease M31.19

Mother yaw A66.0

Motion sickness (from travel, any vehicle) (from roundabouts or swings) T75.3

Mottled, mottling, teeth (enamel) (endemic) (nonendemic) K00.3

Mounier-Kuhn syndrome Q32.4
- with bronchiectasis J47.9
  - exacerbation (acute) J47.1
  - lower respiratory infection J47.0
- acquired J98.09
  - with bronchiectasis J47.9
    - with
      - exacerbation (acute) J47.1
      - lower respiratory infection J47.0

Mountain
- sickness T70.29
  - with polycythemia, acquired (acute) D75.1
- tick fever A93.2

Mouse, joint —*see* Loose, body, joint
- knee M23.4-

Mouth —*see* condition

Movable
- coccyx —*see* subcategory M53.2
- kidney N28.89
  - congenital Q63.8
- spleen D73.89

Movements, dystonic R25.8

Moyamoya disease I67.5

MRSA (Methicillin resistant Staphylococcus aureus)
- infection A49.02
  - as the cause of diseases classified elsewhere B95.62
- sepsis A41.02

MSD (multiple sulfatase deficiency) E75.26

MSSA (Methicillin susceptible Staphylococcus aureus)
- infection A49.01
  - as the cause of diseases classified elsewhere B95.61
- sepsis A41.01

Mucha-Habermann disease L41.0

Mucinosis (cutaneous) (focal) (papular) (reticular erythematous) (skin) L98.5
- oral K13.79

Mucocele
- appendix K38.8
- buccal cavity K13.79
- gallbladder K82.1
- lacrimal sac, chronic H04.43-
- nasal sinus J34.1
- nose J34.1
- salivary gland (any) K11.6
- sinus (accessory) (nasal) J34.1
- turbinate (bone) (middle) (nasal) J34.1
- uterus N85.8

Mucolipidosis
- I E77.1
- II, III E77.0
- IV E75.11

Mucopolysaccharidosis E76.3
- beta-gluduronidase deficiency E76.29
- cardiopathy E76.3 *[I52]*
- Hunter's syndrome E76.1
- Hurler's syndrome E76.01
- Hurler-Scheie syndrome E76.02
- Maroteaux-Lamy syndrome E76.29
- Morquio syndrome E76.219
  - A E76.210
  - B E76.211
  - classic E76.210
- Sanfilippo syndrome E76.22
- Scheie's syndrome E76.03
- specified NEC E76.29
- type
  - I
    - Hurler's syndrome E76.01
    - Hurler-Scheie syndrome E76.02
    - Scheie's syndrome E76.03
  - II E76.1
  - III E76.22
  - IV E76.219
  - IVA E76.210
  - IVB E76.211
  - VI E76.29
  - VII E76.29

Mucormycosis B46.5
- cutaneous B46.3
- disseminated B46.4
- gastrointestinal B46.2
- generalized B46.4
- pulmonary B46.0
- rhinocerebral B46.1
- skin B46.3
- subcutaneous B46.3

Mucositis (ulcerative) K12.30
- due to drugs NEC K12.32
- gastrointestinal K92.81
- mouth (oral) (oropharyngeal) K12.30
  - due to antineoplastic therapy K12.31
  - due to drugs NEC K12.32
  - due to radiation K12.33
  - specified NEC K12.39
  - viral K12.39
- nasal J34.81
- oral cavity —*see* Mucositis, mouth
- oral soft tissues —*see* Mucositis, mouth
- vagina and vulva N76.81

Mucositis necroticans agranulocytica —*see* Agranulocytosis

Mucous —*see also* condition
- patches (syphilitic) A51.39
  - congenital A50.07

Mucoviscidosis E84.9
- with meconium obstruction E84.11

Mucus
- asphyxia or suffocation —*see* Asphyxia, mucus
- in stool R19.5
- plug —*see* Asphyxia, mucus

Muguet B37.0

Mulberry molars (congenital syphilis) A50.52

Müllerian mixed tumor
- specified site —*see* Neoplasm, malignant, by site
- unspecified site C54.9

Multicystic kidney (development) Q61.4

Multiparity (grand) Z64.1
- affecting management of pregnancy, labor and delivery (supervision only) O09.4-
- requiring contraceptive management —*see* Contraception

Multipartita placenta O43.19-

Multiple, multiplex —*see also* condition
- digits (congenital) Q69.9
- endocrine neoplasia —*see* Neoplasia, endocrine, multiple (MEN)
- personality F44.81

Multisystem inflammatory syndrome (in adult) (in children) M35.81

Mumps B26.9
- arthritis B26.85
- complication NEC B26.89
- encephalitis B26.2
- hepatitis B26.81
- meningitis (aseptic) B26.1
- meningoencephalitis B26.2
- myocarditis B26.82
- oophoritis B26.89
- orchitis B26.0
- pancreatitis B26.3
- polyneuropathy B26.84

Mumu —*see also* Infestation, filarial B74.9 *[N51]*

Münchhausen's syndrome —*see* Disorder, factitious

Münchmeyer's syndrome —*see* Myositis, ossificans, progressiva

Mural —*see* condition

Murmur (cardiac) (heart) (organic) R01.1
- abdominal R19.15
- aortic (valve) —*see* Endocarditis, aortic
- benign R01.0
- diastolic —*see* Endocarditis
- Flint I35.1
- functional R01.0
- Graham Steell I37.1
- innocent R01.0
- mitral (valve) —*see* Insufficiency, mitral
- nonorganic R01.0
- presystolic, mitral —*see* Insufficiency, mitral
- pulmonic (valve) I37.8
- systolic R01.1

Murmur *(continued)*
- tricuspid (valve) I07.9
- valvular —*see* Endocarditis

Murri's disease (intermittent hemoglobinuria) D59.6

Muscle, muscular —*see also* condition
- carnitine (palmityltransferase) deficiency E71.314

Musculoneuralgia —*see* Neuralgia

Mushroom-workers'(pickers') **disease or lung** J67.5

Mushrooming hip —*see* Derangement, joint, specified NEC, hip

Mutation(s)
- factor V Leiden D68.51
- surfactant, of lung J84.83
- prothrombin gene D68.52

Mutism —*see also* Aphasia
- deaf (acquired) (congenital) NEC H91.3
- elective (adjustment reaction) (childhood) F94.0
- hysterical F44.4
- selective (childhood) F94.0

MVD (microvillus inclusion disease) Q43.8

MVID (microvillus inclusion disease) Q43.8

Myalgia M79.10
- auxiliary muscles, head and neck M79.12
- epidemic (cervical) B33.0
- mastication muscle M79.11
- site specified NEC M79.18
- traumatic NEC T14.8

Myasthenia G70.9
- congenital G70.2
- cordis —*see* Failure, heart
- developmental G70.2
- gravis G70.00
  - with exacerbation (acute) G70.01
  - in crisis G70.01
  - neonatal, transient P94.0
  - pseudoparalytica G70.00
    - with exacerbation (acute) G70.01
    - in crisis G70.01
- stomach, psychogenic F45.8
- syndrome
  - in
    - diabetes mellitus —*see* E08-E13 with .44
    - neoplastic disease (*see also* Neoplasm) D49.9 *[G73.3]*
    - pernicious anemia D51.0 *[G73.3]*
    - thyrotoxicosis E05.90 *[G73.3]*
      - with thyroid storm E05.91 *[G73.3]*

Myasthenic M62.81

Mycelium infection B49

Mycetismus —*see* Poisoning, food, noxious, mushroom

Mycetoma B47.9
- actinomycotic B47.1
- bone (mycotic) B47.9 *[M90.80]*
- eumycotic B47.0
- foot B47.9
  - actinomycotic B47.1
  - mycotic B47.0
- madurae NEC B47.9
  - mycotic B47.0

Mycetoma *(continued)*
- maduromycotic B47.0
- mycotic B47.0
- nocardial B47.1

Mycobacteriosis *—see* Mycobacterium

Mycobacterium, mycobacterial (infection) A31.9
- anonymous A31.9
- atypical A31.9
  - cutaneous A31.1
  - pulmonary A31.0
    - tuberculous *—see* Tuberculosis, pulmonary
  - specified site NEC A31.8
- avium (intracellulare complex) A31.0
- balnei A31.1
- Battey A31.0
- chelonei A31.8
- cutaneous A31.1
- extrapulmonary systemic A31.8
- fortuitum A31.8
- intracellulare (Battey bacillus) A31.0
- kansasii (yellow bacillus) A31.0
- kakaferifu A31.8
- kasongo A31.8
- leprae (*see also* Leprosy) A30.9
- luciflavum A31.1
- marinum (M. balnei) A31.1
- nonspecific *—see* Mycobacterium, atypical
- pulmonary (atypical) A31.0
  - tuberculous *—see* Tuberculosis, pulmonary
- scrofulaceum A31.8
- simiae A31.8
- systemic, extrapulmonary A31.8
- szulgai A31.8
- terrae A31.8
- triviale A31.8
- tuberculosis (human, bovine) *—see* Tuberculosis
- ulcerans A31.1
- xenopi A31.8

Mycoplasma (M.) **pneumoniae, as cause of disease classified elsewhere** B96.0

Mycosis, mycotic B49
- cutaneous NEC B36.9
- ear B36.9
  - in
    - aspergillosis B44.89
    - candidiasis B37.84
    - moniliasis B37.84
- fungoides (extranodal) (solid organ) C84.0-
- mouth B37.0
- nails B35.1
- opportunistic B48.8
- skin NEC B36.9
- specified NEC B48.8
- stomatitis B37.0
- vagina, vaginitis (candidal) B37.3

Mydriasis (pupil) H57.04

Myelatelia Q06.1

Myelinolysis, pontine, central G37.2

Myelitis (acute) (ascending) (childhood) (chronic) (descending) (diffuse) (disseminated) (idiopathic) (pressure) (progressive) (spinal cord) (subacute) (*see also* Encephalitis) G04.91
- flaccid G04.82
- herpes simplex B00.82
- herpes zoster B02.24
- in diseases classified elsewhere G05.4

Myelitis *(continued)*
- necrotizing, subacute G37.4
- optic neuritis in G36.0
- postchickenpox B01.12
- postherpetic B02.24
- postimmunization G04.02
- postinfectious NEC G04.89
- postvaccinal G04.02
- specified NEC G04.89
- syphilitic (transverse) A52.14
- toxic G92.9
- transverse (in demyelinating diseases of central nervous system) G37.3
- tuberculous A17.82
- varicella B01.12

Myeloblastic *—see* condition

Myeloblastoma
- granular cell *—see also* Neoplasm, connective tissue
  - malignant *—see* Neoplasm, connective tissue, malignant
- tongue D10.1

Myelocele *—see* Spina bifida

Myelocystocele *—see* Spina bifida

Myelocytic *—see* condition

Myelodysplasia D46.9
- specified NEC D46.Z
- spinal cord (congenital) Q06.1

Myelodysplastic syndrome (*see also*, Syndrome, myelodysplastic) D46.9
- with
  - 5q deletion D46.C
  - isolated del (5q) chromosomal abnormality D46.C
- specified NEC D46.Z

Myeloencephalitis *—see* Encephalitis

Myelofibrosis D75.81
- with myeloid metaplasia D47.4
- acute C94.4-
- idiopathic (chronic) D47.4
- primary D47.1
- secondary D75.81
  - in myeloproliferative disease D47.4

Myelogenous *—see* condition

Myeloid *—see* condition

Myelokathexis D70.9

Myeloleukodystrophy E75.29

Myelolipoma *—see* Lipoma

Myeloma (multiple) C90.0-
- monostotic C90.3
  - plasma cell C90.0-
- plasma cell C90.0-
- solitary (*see also* Plasmacytoma, solitary) C90.3-

Myelomalacia G95.89

Myelomatosis C90.0-

Myelomeningitis *—see* Meningoencephalitis

Myelomeningocele (spinal cord) *—see* Spina bifida

Myelo-osteo-musculodysplasia hereditaria Q79.8

Myelopathic
- anemia D64.89
- muscle atrophy *—see* Atrophy, muscle, spinal
- pain syndrome G89.0

Myelopathy (spinal cord) G95.9
- drug-induced G95.89
- in (due to)
  - degeneration or displacement, intervertebral disc NEC *—see* Disorder, disc, with, myelopathy
  - infection *—see* Encephalitis
  - intervertebral disc disorder *—see also* Disorder, disc, with, myelopathy
  - mercury *—see* subcategory T56.1
  - neoplastic disease (*see also* Neoplasm) D49.9 *[G99.2]*
  - pernicious anemia D51.0 *[G99.2]*
  - spondylosis *—see* Spondylosis, with myelopathy NEC
- necrotic (subacute) (vascular) G95.19
- radiation-induced G95.89
- spondylogenic NEC *—see* Spondylosis, with myelopathy NEC
- toxic G95.89
- transverse, acute G37.3
- vascular G95.19
- vitamin B12 E53.8 *[G32.0]*

Myelophthisis D61.82

Myeloradiculitis G04.91

Myeloradiculodysplasia (spinal) Q06.1

Myelosarcoma C92.3-

Myelosclerosis D75.89
- with myeloid metaplasia D47.4
- disseminated, of nervous system G35
- megakaryocytic D47.4
  - with myeloid metaplasia D47.4

Myelosis
- acute C92.0-
- aleukemic C92.9-
- chronic D47.1
- erythremic (acute) C94.0-
- megakaryocytic C94.2-
- nonleukemic D72.828
- subacute C92.9-

Myiasis (cavernous) B87.9
- aural B87.4
- creeping B87.0
- cutaneous B87.0
- dermal B87.0
- ear (external) (middle) B87.4
- eye B87.2
- genitourinary B87.81
- intestinal B87.82
- laryngeal B87.3
- nasopharyngeal B87.3
- ocular B87.2
- orbit B87.2
- skin B87.0
- specified site NEC B87.89
- traumatic B87.1
- wound B87.1

Myoadenoma, prostate *—see* Hyperplasia, prostate

Myoblastoma
- granular cell *—see also* Neoplasm, connective tissue, benign
  - malignant *—see* Neoplasm, connective tissue, malignant
- tongue D10.1

Myocardial *—see* condition

Myocardiopathy (congestive) (constrictive) (familial) (hypertrophic nonobstructive) (idiopathic) (infiltrative) (obstructive) (primary) (restrictive) (sporadic) (*see also* Cardiomyopathy) I42.9

Myocardiopathy *(continued)*
- alcoholic I42.6
- cobalt-beer I42.6
- glycogen storage E74.02 *[I43]*
- hypertrophic obstructive I42.1
- in (due to)
  - beriberi E51.12
  - cardiac glycogenosis E74.02 *[I43]*
  - Friedreich's ataxia G11.11 *[I43]*
  - myotonia atrophica G71.11 *[I43]*
  - progressive muscular dystrophy G71.09 *[I43]*
- obscure (African) I42.8
- secondary I42.9
- thyrotoxic E05.90 *[I43]*
  - with storm E05.91 *[I43]*
- toxic NEC I42.7

Myocarditis (with arteriosclerosis) (chronic) (fibroid) (interstitial) (old) (progressive) (senile) I51.4
- with
  - rheumatic fever (conditions in I00) I09.0
    - active *—see* Myocarditis, acute, rheumatic
    - inactive or quiescent (with chorea) I09.0
- active I40.9
  - rheumatic I01.2
    - with chorea (acute) (rheumatic) (Sydenham's) I02.0
- acute or subacute (interstitial) I40.9
  - due to
    - streptococcus (beta-hemolytic) I01.2
  - idiopathic I40.1
  - rheumatic I01.2
    - with chorea (acute) (rheumatic) (Sydenham's) I02.0
  - specified NEC I40.8
- aseptic of newborn B33.22
- bacterial (acute) I40.0
- Coxsackie (virus) B33.22
- diphtheritic A36.81
- eosinophilic I40.1
- epidemic of newborn (Coxsackie) B33.22
- Fiedler's (acute) (isolated) I40.1
- giant cell (acute) (subacute) I40.1
- gonococcal A54.83
- granulomatous (idiopathic) (isolated) (nonspecific) I40.1
- hypertensive *—see* Hypertension, heart
- idiopathic (granulomatous) I40.1
- in (due to)
  - diphtheria A36.81
  - epidemic louse-borne typhus A75.0 *[I41]*
  - Lyme disease A69.29
  - sarcoidosis D86.85
  - scarlet fever A38.1
  - toxoplasmosis (acquired) B58.81
  - typhoid A01.02
  - typhus NEC A75.9 *[I41]*
- infective I40.0
- influenzal *—see* Influenza, with, myocarditis
- isolated (acute) I40.1
- meningococcal A39.52
- mumps B26.82
- nonrheumatic, active I40.9
- parenchymatous I40.9
- pneumococcal I40.0

Myocarditis *(continued)*
- rheumatic (chronic) (inactive) (with chorea) I09.0
  - active or acute I01.2
    - with chorea (acute) (rheumatic) (Sydenham's) I02.0
- rheumatoid *—see* Rheumatoid, carditis
- septic I40.0
- staphylococcal I40.0
- suppurative I40.0
- syphilitic (chronic) A52.06
- toxic I40.8
  - rheumatic *—see* Myocarditis, acute, rheumatic
- tuberculous A18.84
- typhoid A01.02
- valvular *—see* Endocarditis
- virus, viral I40.0
  - of newborn (Coxsackie) B33.22

Myocardium, myocardial *—see* condition

Myocardosis *—see* Cardiomyopathy

Myoclonus, myoclonic, myoclonia (familial) (essential) (multifocal) (simplex) G25.3
- drug-induced G25.3
- epilepsy (*see also* Epilepsy, generalized, specified NEC) G40.4-
  - familial (progressive) G25.3
- epileptica G40.409
  - with status epilepticus G40.401
- facial G51.3-
- familial progressive G25.3
- Friedreich's G25.3
- jerks G25.3
- massive G25.3
- palatal G25.3
- pharyngeal G25.3

Myocytolysis I51.5

Myodiastasis *—see* Diastasis, muscle

Myoendocarditis *—see* Endocarditis

Myoepithelioma *—see* Neoplasm, benign, by site

Myofasciitis (acute) *—see* Myositis

Myofibroma *—see also* Neoplasm, connective tissue, benign
- uterus (cervix) (corpus) *—see* Leiomyoma

Myofibromatosis D48.1
- infantile Q89.8

Myofibrosis M62.89
- heart *—see* Myocarditis
- scapulohumeral *—see* Lesion, shoulder, specified NEC

Myofibrositis M79.7
- scapulohumeral *—see* Lesion, shoulder, specified NEC

Myoglobulinuria, myoglobinuria (primary) R82.1

Myokymia, facial G51.4

Myolipoma *—see* Lipoma

Myoma *—see also* Neoplasm, connective tissue, benign
- malignant *—see* Neoplasm, connective tissue, malignant
- prostate D29.1
- uterus (cervix) (corpus) *—see* Leiomyoma

Myomalacia M62.89

Myometritis *—see* Endometritis

Myometrium *—see* condition

Myonecrosis, clostridial A48.0

Myopathy G72.9
- acute
  - necrotizing G72.81
  - quadriplegic G72.81
- alcoholic G72.1
- benign congenital G71.20
- central core G71.29
- centronuclear G71.228
  - autosomal (dominant) (recessive) G71.228
  - other specified NEC G71.228
- congenital (benign) G71.20
- critical illness G72.81
- distal G71.09
- drug-induced G72.0
- endocrine NEC E34.9 *[G73.7]*
- extraocular muscles H05.82-
- facioscapulohumeral G71.02
- hereditary G71.9
  - specified NEC G71.8
- hyaline body G71.29
- immune NEC G72.49
- in (due to)
  - Addison's disease E27.1 *[G73.7]*
  - alcohol G72.1
  - amyloidosis E85.0 *[G73.7]*
  - cretinism E00.9 *[G73.7]*
  - Cushing's syndrome E24.9 *[G73.7]*
  - drugs G72.0
  - endocrine disease NEC E34.9 *[G73.7]*
  - giant cell arteritis M31.6 *[G73.7]*
  - glycogen storage disease E74.00 *[G73.7]*
  - hyperadrenocorticism E24.9 *[G73.7]*
  - hyperparathyroidism NEC E21.3 *[G73.7]*
  - hypoparathyroidism E20.9 *[G73.7]*
  - hypopituitarism E23.0 *[G73.7]*
  - hypothyroidism E03.9 *[G73.7]*
  - infectious disease NEC B99 *[G73.7]*
  - lipid storage disease E75.6 *[G73.7]*
  - metabolic disease NEC E88.9 *[G73.7]*
  - myxedema E03.9 *[G73.7]*
  - parasitic disease NEC B89 *[G73.7]*
  - polyarteritis nodosa M30.0 *[G73.7]*
  - rheumatoid arthritis *—see* Rheumatoid, myopathy
  - sarcoidosis D86.87
  - scleroderma M34.82
  - sicca syndrome M35.03
  - Sjögren's syndrome M35.03
  - systemic lupus erythematosus M32.19
  - thyrotoxicosis (hyperthyroidism) E05.90 *[G73.7]*
    - with thyroid storm E05.91 *[G73.7]*
  - toxic agent NEC G72.2
- inflammatory NEC G72.49
- intensive care (ICU) G72.81
- limb-girdle G71.09
- mitochondrial NEC G71.3
- myosin storage G71.29
- myotubular (centronuclear) G71.220
  - X-linked G71.220
- mytonic, proximal (PROMM) G71.11
- nemaline G71.21
- ocular G71.09
- oculopharyngeal G71.09
- of critical illness G72.81
- primary G71.9
  - specified NEC G71.8
- progressive NEC G72.89
- proximal myotonic (PROMM) G71.11
- rod (body) G71.21
- scapulohumeral G71.02
- specified NEC G72.89
- toxic G72.2

Myopericarditis *—see also* Pericarditis
- chronic rheumatic I09.2

Myopia (axial) (congenital) H52.1-
- degenerative (malignant) H44.20
  - with
    - choroidal neovascularization H44.2A-
    - foveoschisis H44.2D-
    - macular hole H44.2B-
    - retinal detachment H44.2C-
    - specified maculopathy NEC H44.2E-
  - bilateral H44.23
  - left eye H44.22
  - right eye H44.21
- malignant (*see also* Myopia, degenerative) H44.2-
- pernicious (*see also* Myopia, degenerative) H44.2-
- progressive high (degenerative) (*see also* Myopia, degenerative) H44.2-

Myosarcoma *—see* Neoplasm, connective tissue, malignant

Myosis (pupil) H57.03
- stromal (endolymphatic) D39.0

Myositis M60.9
- clostridial A48.0
- due to posture *—see* Myositis, specified type NEC
- epidemic B33.0
- fibrosa or fibrous (chronic), Volkmann's T79.6
- foreign body granuloma *—see* Granuloma, foreign body
- in (due to)
  - bilharziasis B65.9 *[M63.8-]*
  - cysticercosis B69.81
  - leprosy A30.9 *[M63.8-]*
  - mycosis B49 *[M63.8-]*
  - sarcoidosis D86.87
  - schistosomiasis B65.9 *[M63.8-]*
  - syphilis
    - late A52.78
    - secondary A51.49
  - toxoplasmosis (acquired) B58.82
  - trichinellosis B75 *[M63.8-]*
  - tuberculosis A18.09
- inclusion body [IBM] G72.41
- infective M60.009
  - arm M60.002
    - left M60.001
    - right M60.000
  - leg M60.005
    - left M60.004
    - right M60.003
  - lower limb M60.005
    - ankle M60.07-
    - foot M60.07-
    - lower leg M60.06-
    - thigh M60.05-
    - toe M60.07-
  - multiple sites M60.09
  - specified site NEC M60.08
  - upper limb M60.002
    - finger M60.04-
    - forearm M60.03-
    - hand M60.04-
    - shoulder region M60.01-
    - upper arm M60.02-
- interstitial M60.10
  - ankle M60.17-
  - foot M60.17-
  - forearm M60.13-
  - hand M60.14-
  - lower leg M60.16-
  - multiple sites M60.19
  - shoulder region M60.11-
  - specified site NEC M60.18
  - thigh M60.15-
  - upper arm M60.12-
- mycotic B49 *[M63.8-]*
- orbital, chronic H05.12-
- ossificans or ossifying (circumscripta) *—see also* Ossification, muscle, specified NEC
  - in (due to)
    - burns M61.30
      - ankle M61.37-
      - foot M61.37-
      - forearm M61.33-
      - hand M61.34-
      - lower leg M61.36-
      - multiple sites M61.39
      - pelvic region M61.35-
      - shoulder region M61.31-
      - specified site NEC M61.38
      - thigh M61.35-
      - upper arm M61.32-
    - quadriplegia or paraplegia M61.20
      - ankle M61.27-
      - foot M61.27-
      - forearm M61.23-
      - hand M61.24-
      - lower leg M61.26-
      - multiple sites M61.29
      - pelvic region M61.25-
      - shoulder region M61.21-
      - specified site NEC M61.28
      - thigh M61.25-
      - upper arm M61.22-
  - progressiva M61.10
    - ankle M61.17-
    - finger M61.14-
    - foot M61.17-
    - forearm M61.13-
    - hand M61.14-
    - lower leg M61.16-
    - multiple sites M61.19
    - pelvic region M61.15-
    - shoulder region M61.11-
    - specified site NEC M61.18
    - thigh M61.15-
    - toe M61.17-
    - upper arm M61.12-
  - traumatica M61.00
    - ankle M61.07-
    - foot M61.07-
    - forearm M61.03-
    - hand M61.04-
    - lower leg M61.06-
    - multiple sites M61.09
    - pelvic region M61.05-
    - shoulder region M61.01-
    - specified site NEC M61.08
    - thigh M61.05-
    - upper arm M61.02-
- purulent *—see* Myositis, infective
- specified type NEC M60.80
  - ankle M60.87-
  - foot M60.87-
  - forearm M60.83-

Myositis *(continued)*
- specified type *(continued)*
  - hand M60.84-
  - lower leg M60.86-
  - multiple sites M60.89
  - pelvic region M60.85-
  - shoulder region M60.81-
  - specified site NEC M60.88
  - thigh M60.85-
  - upper arm M60.82-
- suppurative *—see* Myositis, infective
- traumatic (old) *—see* Myositis, specified type NEC

Myospasia impulsiva F95.2

Myotonia (acquisita) (intermittens) M62.89
- atrophica G71.11
- chondrodystrophic G71.13
- congenita (acetazolamide responsive) (dominant) (recessive) G71.12
- drug-induced G71.14
- dystrophica G71.11
- fluctuans G71.19
- levior G71.12
- permanens G71.19
- symptomatic G71.19

Myotonic pupil *—see* Anomaly, pupil, function, tonic pupil

Myriapodiasis B88.2

Myringitis H73.2-
- with otitis media *—see* Otitis, media
- acute H73.00-
  - bullous H73.01-
  - specified NEC H73.09-
- bullous *—see* Myringitis, acute, bullous
- chronic H73.1-

Mysophobia F40.228

Mytilotoxism *—see* Poisoning, fish

Myxadenitis labialis K13.0

Myxedema (adult) (idiocy) (infantile) (juvenile) (*see also* Hypothyroidism) E03.9
- circumscribed E05.90
  - with storm E05.91
- coma E03.5
- congenital E00.1
- cutis L98.5
- localized (pretibial) E05.90
  - with storm E05.91
- papular L98.5

Myxochondrosarcoma *—see* Neoplasm, cartilage, malignant

Myxofibroma *—see* Neoplasm, connective tissue, benign
- odontogenic *—see* Cyst, calcifying odontogenic

Myxofibrosarcoma *—see* Neoplasm, connective tissue, malignant

Myxolipoma D17.9

Myxoliposarcoma *—see* Neoplasm, connective tissue, malignant

Myxoma *—see also* Neoplasm, connective tissue, benign
- nerve sheath *—see* Neoplasm, nerve, benign
- odontogenic *—see* Cyst, calcifying odontogenic

Myxosarcoma *—see* Neoplasm, connective tissue, malignant

N

Naegeli's
- disease Q82.8
- leukemia, monocytic C93.1-

Naegleriasis (with meningoencephalitis) B60.2

Naffziger's syndrome G54.0

Naga sore *—see* Ulcer, skin

Nägele's pelvis M95.5
- with disproportion (fetopelvic) O33.0
  - causing obstructed labor O65.0

Nail *—see also* condition
- biting F98.8
- patella syndrome Q87.2

Nanism, nanosomia *—see* Dwarfism

Nanophyetiasis B66.8

Nanukayami A27.89

Napkin rash L22

Narcolepsy G47.419
- with cataplexy G47.411
- in conditions classified elsewhere G47.429
  - with cataplexy G47.421

Narcosis R06.89

Narcotism *—see* Dependence

NARP (Neuropathy, Ataxia and Retinitis pigmentosa) **syndrome** E88.49

Narrow
- anterior chamber angle H40.03-
- gingival width (of periodontal soft tissue) K05.5
- pelvis *—see* Contraction, pelvis

Narrowing *—see also* Stenosis
- artery I77.1
  - auditory, internal I65.8
  - basilar *—see* Occlusion, artery, basilar
  - carotid *—see* Occlusion, artery, carotid
  - cerebellar *—see* Occlusion, artery, cerebellar
  - cerebral *—see* Occlusion artery, cerebral
  - choroidal *—see* Occlusion, artery, precerebral, specified NEC
  - communicating posterior *—see* Occlusion, artery, precerebral, specified NEC
  - coronary *—see also* Disease, heart, ischemic, atherosclerotic
    - congenital Q24.5
      - syphilitic A50.54 *[I52]*
    - due to syphilis NEC A52.06
  - hypophyseal *—see* Occlusion, artery, precerebral, specified NEC
  - pontine *—see* Occlusion, artery, precerebral, specified NEC
  - precerebral *—see* Occlusion, artery, precerebral
  - vertebral *—see* Occlusion, artery, vertebral
- auditory canal (external) *—see* Stenosis, external ear canal
- eustachian tube *—see* Obstruction, eustachian tube
- eyelid *—see* Disorder, eyelid function
- larynx J38.6

Narrowing *(continued)*
- mesenteric artery (*see also* Ischemia, intestine, acute) K55.059
- palate M26.89
- palpebral fissure *—see* Disorder, eyelid function
- ureter N13.5
  - with infection N13.6
- urethra *—see* Stricture, urethra

Narrowness, abnormal, eyelid Q10.3

Nasal *—see* condition

Nasolachrymal, nasolacrimal *—see* condition

Nasopharyngeal *—see also* condition
- pituitary gland Q89.2
- torticollis M43.6

Nasopharyngitis (acute) (infective) (streptococcal) (subacute) J00
- chronic (suppurative) (ulcerative) J31.1

Nasopharynx, nasopharyngeal *—see* condition

Natal tooth, teeth K00.6

Nausea (without vomiting) R11.0
- with vomiting R11.2
- gravidarum *—see* Hyperemesis, gravidarum
- marina T75.3
- navalis T75.3

Navel *—see* condition

Neapolitan fever *—see* Brucellosis

Near drowning T75.1

Nearsightedness *—see* Myopia

Near-syncope R55

Nebula, cornea *—see* Opacity, cornea

Necator americanus infestation B76.1

Necatoriasis B76.1

Neck *—see* condition

Necrobiosis R68.89
- lipoidica NEC L92.1
  - with diabetes *—see* E08-E13 with .620

Necrolysis, toxic epidermal L51.2
- due to drug
  - correct substance properly administered *—see* Table of Drugs and Chemicals, by drug, adverse effect
  - overdose or wrong substance given or taken *—see* Table of Drugs and Chemicals, by drug, poisoning

Necrophilia F65.89

Necrosis, necrotic (ischemic) *—see also* Gangrene
- adrenal (capsule) (gland) E27.49
- amputation stump (surgical) (late) T87.50
  - arm T87.5-
  - leg T87.5-
- antrum J32.0
- aorta (hyaline) *—see also* Aneurysm, aorta
  - cystic medial *—see* Dissection, aorta
- artery I77.5
- bladder (aseptic) (sphincter) N32.89

Necrosis, necrotic *(continued)*
- bone *—see also* Osteonecrosis M87.9
  - aseptic or avascular *—see* Osteonecrosis
    - idiopathic M87.00
  - ethmoid J32.2
  - jaw M27.2
  - tuberculous *—see* Tuberculosis, bone
- brain I67.89
- breast (aseptic) (fat) (segmental) N64.1
- bronchus J98.09
- central nervous system NEC I67.89
- cerebellar I67.89
- cerebral I67.89
- colon (*see also* Infarct, intestine) K55.049
- cornea H18.89-
- cortical (acute) (renal) N17.1
- cystic medial (aorta) *—see* Dissection, aorta
- dental pulp K04.1
- esophagus K22.89
- ethmoid (bone) J32.2
- eyelid *—see* Disorder, eyelid, degenerative
- fat, fatty (generalized) *—see also* Disorder, soft tissue, specified type NEC
  - abdominal wall K65.4
  - breast (aseptic) (segmental) N64.1
  - localized *—see* Degeneration, by site, fatty
  - mesentery K65.4
  - omentum K65.4
  - pancreas K86.89
  - peritoneum K65.4
  - skin (subcutaneous), newborn P83.0
  - subcutaneous, due to birth injury P15.6
- gallbladder *—see* Cholecystitis, acute
- heart *—see* Infarct, myocardium
- hip, aseptic or avascular *—see* Osteonecrosis, by type, femur
- intestine (acute) (hemorrhagic) (massive) (*see also* Infarct, intestine) K55.069
- jaw M27.2
- kidney (bilateral) N28.0
  - acute N17.9
  - cortical (acute) (bilateral) N17.1
    - with ectopic or molar pregnancy O08.4
  - medullary (bilateral) (in acute renal failure) (papillary) N17.2
  - papillary (bilateral) (in acute renal failure) N17.2
  - tubular N17.0
    - with ectopic or molar pregnancy O08.4
    - complicating
      - abortion *—see* Abortion, by type, complicated by, tubular necrosis
      - ectopic or molar pregnancy O08.4
      - pregnancy *—see* Pregnancy, complicated by, diseases of, specified type or system NEC
    - following ectopic or molar pregnancy O08.4
    - traumatic T79.5

Necrosis, necrotic *(continued)*
- larynx J38.7
- liver (with hepatic failure) (cell) —*see* Failure, hepatic
  - hemorrhagic, central K76.2
- lung J85.0
- lymphatic gland —*see* Lymphadenitis, acute
- mammary gland (fat) (segmental) N64.1
- mastoid (chronic) —*see* Mastoiditis, chronic
- medullary (acute) (renal) N17.2
- mesentery (*see also* Infarct, intestine) K55.069
  - fat K65.4
- mitral valve —*see* Insufficiency, mitral
- myocardium, myocardial —*see* Infarct, myocardium
- nose J34.0
- omentum (with mesenteric infarction) (*see also* Infarct, intestine) K55.069
  - fat K65.4
- orbit, orbital —*see* Osteomyelitis, orbit
- ossicles, ear —*see* Abnormal, ear ossicles
- ovary N70.92
- pancreas (aseptic) (duct) (fat) K86.89
  - acute (infective) —*see* Pancreatitis, acute
  - infective —*see* Pancreatitis, acute
- papillary (acute) (renal) N17.2
- perineum N90.89
- peritoneum (with mesenteric infarction) (*see also* Infarct, intestine) K55.069
  - fat K65.4
- pharynx J02.9
  - in granulocytopenia —*see* Neutropenia
  - Vincent's A69.1
- phosphorus —*see* subcategory T54.2
- pituitary (gland) E23.0
  - postpartum O99.285
  - Sheehan O99.285
- pressure —*see* Ulcer, pressure, by site
- pulmonary J85.0
- pulp (dental) K04.1
- radiation —*see* Necrosis, by site
- radium —*see* Necrosis, by site
- renal —*see* Necrosis, kidney
- sclera H15.89
- scrotum N50.89
- skin or subcutaneous tissue NEC I96
- spine, spinal (column) —*see also* Osteonecrosis, by type, vertebra
  - cord G95.19
- spleen D73.5
- stomach K31.89
- stomatitis (ulcerative) A69.0
- subcutaneous fat, newborn P83.88
- subendocardial (acute) I21.4
  - chronic I25.89
- suprarenal (capsule) (gland) E27.49
- testis N50.89
- thymus (gland) E32.8
- tonsil J35.8
- trachea J39.8
- tuberculous NEC —*see* Tuberculosis
- tubular (acute) (anoxic) (renal) (toxic) N17.0
  - postprocedural N99.0
- vagina N89.8
- vertebra —*see also* Osteonecrosis, by type, vertebra
  - tuberculous A18.01
- vulva N90.89
- X-ray —*see* Necrosis, by site

Necrospermia —*see* Infertility, male

Need (for)
- care provider because (of)
  - assistance with personal care Z74.1
  - continuous supervision required Z74.3
  - impaired mobility Z74.09
  - no other household member able to render care Z74.2
  - specified reason NEC Z74.8
- immunization —*see* Vaccination
- vaccination —*see* Vaccination

Neglect
- adult
  - confirmed T74.01
  - history of Z91.412
  - suspected T76.01
- child (childhood)
  - confirmed T74.02
  - history of Z62.812
  - suspected T76.02
- emotional, in childhood Z62.898
- hemispatial R41.4
- left-sided R41.4
- sensory R41.4
- visuospatial R41.4

Neisserian infection NEC —*see* Gonococcus

Nelaton's syndrome G60.8

Nelson's syndrome E24.1

Nematodiasis (intestinal) B82.0
- Ancylostoma B76.0

Neonatal —*see also* Newborn
- acne L70.4
- bradycardia P29.12
- tachycardia P29.11
- screening, abnormal findings on — *see* Abnormal, neonatal screening
- tooth, teeth K00.6

Neonatorum —*see* condition

Neoplasia
- endocrine, multiple (MEN) E31.20
  - type I E31.21
  - type IIA E31.22
  - type IIB E31.23
- intraepithelial (histologically confirmed)
  - anal (AIN) (histologically confirmed) K62.82
    - grade I K62.82
    - grade II K62.82
    - severe D01.3
  - cervical glandular (histologically confirmed) D06.9
  - cervix (uteri) (CIN) (histologically confirmed) N87.9
    - glandular D06.9
    - grade I N87.0
    - grade II N87.1
    - grade III (severe dysplasia) (*see also* Carcinoma, cervix uteri, in situ) D06.9
  - prostate (histologically confirmed) (PIN) N42.31
    - grade I N42.31
    - grade II N42.31
    - grade III (severe dysplasia) D07.5
  - vagina (histologically confirmed) (VAIN) N89.3
    - grade I N89.0
    - grade II N89.1
    - grade III (severe dysplasia) D07.2
  - vulva (histologically confirmed) (VIN) N90.3
    - grade I N90.0
    - grade II N90.1
    - grade III (severe dysplasia) D07.1

Neoplasm, neoplastic —*see also* Table of Neoplasms
- lipomatous, benign —*see* Lipoma
- malignant mast cell C96.20
  - specified type NEC C96.29
- mast cell, of uncertain behavior NEC D47.09

Neovascularization
- ciliary body —*see* Disorder, iris, vascular
- cornea H16.40-
  - deep H16.44-
  - ghost vessels —*see* Ghost, vessels
  - localized H16.43-
  - pannus —*see* Pannus
- iris —*see* Disorder, iris, vascular
- retina H35.05-

Nephralgia N23

Nephritis, nephritic (albuminuric) (azotemic) (congenital) (disseminated) (epithelial) (familial) (focal) (granulomatous) (hemorrhagic) (infantile) (nonsuppurative, excretory) (uremic) N05.9
- with
  - C3
    - glomerulonephritis N05.A
    - glomerulopathy N05.A
      - with dense deposit disease N05.6
  - dense deposit disease N05.6
  - diffuse
    - crescentic glomerulonephritis N05.7
    - endocapillary proliferative glomerulonephritis N05.4
    - membranous glomerulonephritis N05.2
    - mesangial proliferative glomerulonephritis N05.3
    - mesangiocapillary glomerulonephritis N05.5
  - edema —*see* Nephrosis
  - focal and segmental glomerular lesions N05.1
  - foot process disease N04.9
  - glomerular lesion
    - diffuse sclerosing N05.8
    - hypocomplementemic —*see* Nephritis, membranoproliferative
    - IgA —*see* Nephropathy, IgA
    - lobular, lobulonodular —*see* Nephritis, membranoproliferative
    - nodular —*see* Nephritis, membranoproliferative
  - lesion of
    - glomerulonephritis, proliferative N05.8
    - renal necrosis N05.9
  - minor glomerular abnormality N05.0
  - specified morphological changes NEC N05.8
- acute N00.9
  - with
    - C3
      - glomerulonephritis N00.A
      - glomerulopathy N00.A
        - with dense deposit disease N00.6
    - dense deposit disease N00.6
    - diffuse
      - crescentic glomerulonephritis N00.7
      - endocapillary proliferative glomerulonephritis N00.4
      - membranous glomerulonephritis N00.2
      - mesangial proliferative glomerulonephritis N00.3
      - mesangiocapillary glomerulonephritis N00.5
    - focal and segmental glomerular lesions N00.1
    - minor glomerular abnormality N00.0
    - specified morphological changes NEC N00.8
- amyloid E85.4 *[N08]*
- antiglomerular basement membrane (anti-GBM) antibody NEC
  - in Goodpasture's syndrome M31.0
- antitubular basement membrane (tubulo-interstitial) NEC N12
  - toxic —*see* Nephropathy, toxic
- arteriolar —*see* Hypertension, kidney
- arteriosclerotic —*see* Hypertension, kidney
- ascending —*see* Nephritis, tubulo-interstitial
- atrophic N03.9
- Balkan (endemic) N15.0
- calculous, calculus —*see* Calculus, kidney
- cardiac —*see* Hypertension, kidney
- cardiovascular —*see* Hypertension, kidney
- chronic N03.9
  - with
    - C3
      - glomerulonephritis N03.A
      - glomerulopathy N03.A
        - with dense deposit disease N03.6
    - dense deposit disease N03.6
    - diffuse
      - crescentic glomerulonephritis N03.7
      - endocapillary proliferative glomerulonephritis N03.4
      - membranous glomerulonephritis N03.2
      - mesangial proliferative glomerulonephritis N03.3
      - mesangiocapillary glomerulonephritis N03.5
    - focal and segmental glomerular lesions N03.1
    - minor glomerular abnormality N03.0
    - specified morphological changes NEC N03.8

Nephritis, nephritic *(continued)*
- chronic *(continued)*
  - arteriosclerotic —*see* Hypertension, kidney
- cirrhotic N26.9
- complicating pregnancy O26.83-
- croupous N00.9
- degenerative —*see* Nephrosis
- diffuse sclerosing N05.8
- due to
  - diabetes mellitus —*see* E08-E13 with .21
  - subacute bacterial endocarditis I33.0
  - systemic lupus erythematosus (chronic) M32.14
  - typhoid fever A01.09
- gonococcal (acute) (chronic) A54.21
- hypocomplementemic —*see* Nephritis, membranoproliferative
- IgA —*see* Nephropathy, IgA
- immune complex (circulating) NEC N05.8
- infective —*see* Nephritis, tubulo-interstitial
- interstitial —*see* Nephritis, tubulo-interstitial
- lead N14.3
- membranoproliferative (diffuse) (type 1 or 3) (*see also* N00-N07 with fourth character .5) N05.5
  - type 2 (*see also* N00-N07 with fourth character .6) N05.6
- minimal change N05.0
- necrotic, necrotizing NEC (*see also* N00-N07 with fourth character .8) N05.8
- nephrotic —*see* Nephrosis
- nodular —*see* Nephritis, membranoproliferative
- polycystic Q61.3
  - adult type Q61.2
  - autosomal
    - dominant Q61.2
    - recessive NEC Q61.19
  - childhood type NEC Q61.19
  - infantile type NEC Q61.19
- poststreptococcal N05.9
  - acute N00.9
  - chronic N03.9
  - rapidly progressive N01.9
- proliferative NEC (*see also* N00-N07 with fourth character .8) N05.8
- purulent —*see* Nephritis, tubulo-interstitial
- rapidly progressive N01.9
  - with
    - C3
      - glomerulonephritis N01.A
      - glomerulopathy N01.A
        - with dense deposit disease N01.6
    - dense deposit disease N01.6
    - diffuse
      - crescentic glomerulonephritis N01.7
      - endocapillary proliferative glomerulonephritis N01.4
      - membranous glomerulonephritis N01.2
      - mesangial proliferative glomerulonephritis N01.3
      - mesangiocapillary glomerulonephritis N01.5
    - focal and segmental glomerular lesions N01.1
    - minor glomerular abnormality N01.0
    - specified morphological changes NEC N01.8
- salt losing or wasting NEC N28.89

Nephritis, nephritic *(continued)*
- saturnine N14.3
- sclerosing, diffuse N05.8
- septic —*see* Nephritis, tubulo-interstitial
- specified pathology NEC (*see also* N00-N07 with fourth character .8) N05.8
- subacute N01.9
- suppurative —*see* Nephritis, tubulo-interstitial
- syphilitic (late) A52.75
  - congenital A50.59 *[N08]*
  - early (secondary) A51.44
- toxic —*see* Nephropathy, toxic
- tubal, tubular —*see* Nephritis, tubulo-interstitial
- tuberculous A18.11
- tubulo-interstitial (in) N12
  - acute (infectious) N10
  - chronic (infectious) N11.9
    - nonobstructive N11.8
      - reflux-associated N11.0
    - obstructive N11.1
    - specified NEC N11.8
  - due to
    - brucellosis A23.9 *[N16]*
    - cryoglobulinemia D89.1 *[N16]*
    - glycogen storage disease E74.00 *[N16]*
  - Sjögren's syndrome M35.04
- vascular —*see* Hypertension, kidney
- war N00.9

Nephroblastoma (epithelial) (mesenchymal) C64-

Nephrocalcinosis E83.59 *[N29]*

Nephrocystitis, pustular —*see* Nephritis, tubulo-interstitial

Nephrolithiasis (congenital) (pelvis) (recurrent) —*see also* Calculus, kidney

Nephroma C64-
- mesoblastic D41.0-

Nephronephritis —*see* Nephrosis

Nephronophthisis Q61.5

Nephropathia epidemica A98.5

Nephropathy —*see also* Nephritis N28.9
- with
  - edema —*see* Nephrosis
  - glomerular lesion —*see* Glomerulonephritis
- amyloid, hereditary E85.0
- analgesic N14.0
  - with medullary necrosis, acute N17.2
- Balkan (endemic) N15.0
- chemical —*see* Nephropathy, toxic
- diabetic —*see* E08-E13 with .21
- drug-induced N14.2
  - specified NEC N14.1
- focal and segmental hyalinosis or sclerosis N02.1
- heavy metal-induced N14.3
- hereditary NEC N07.9
  - with
    - C3
      - glomerulonephritis N07.A
      - glomerulopathy N07.A
        - with dense deposit disease N07.6
    - dense deposit disease N07.6
    - diffuse
      - crescentic glomerulonephritis N07.7
      - endocapillary proliferative glomerulonephritis N07.4

Nephropathy *(continued)*
- hereditary NEC *(continued)*
  - with *(continued)*
    - diffuse *(continued)*
      - membranous glomerulonephritis N07.2
      - mesangial proliferative glomerulonephritis N07.3
      - mesangiocapillary glomerulonephritis N07.5
    - focal and segmental glomerular lesions N07.1
    - minor glomerular abnormality N07.0
    - specified morphological changes NEC N07.8
- hypercalcemic N25.89
- hypertensive —*see* Hypertension, kidney
- hypokalemic (vacuolar) N25.89
- IgA N02.8
  - with glomerular lesion N02.9
    - focal and segmental hyalinosis or sclerosis N02.1
    - membranoproliferative (diffuse) N02.5
    - membranous (diffuse) N02.2
    - mesangial proliferative (diffuse) N02.3
    - mesangiocapillary (diffuse) N02.5
    - proliferative NEC N02.8
    - specified pathology NEC N02.8
- lead N14.3
- membranoproliferative (diffuse) N02.5
- membranous (diffuse) N02.2
- mesangial (IgA/IgG) —*see* Nephropathy, IgA
  - proliferative (diffuse) N02.3
- mesangiocapillary (diffuse) N02.5
- obstructive N13.8
- phenacetin N17.2
- phosphate-losing N25.0
- potassium depletion N25.89
- pregnancy-related O26.83-
- proliferative NEC (*see also* N00-N07 with fourth character .8) N05.8
- protein-losing N25.89
- saturnine N14.3
- sickle-cell D57.- *[N08]*
- toxic NEC N14.4
  - due to
    - drugs N14.2
      - analgesic N14.0
      - specified NEC N14.1
    - heavy metals N14.3
- vasomotor N17.0
- water-losing N25.89

Nephroptosis N28.83

Nephropyosis —*see* Abscess, kidney

Nephrorrhagia N28.89

Nephrosclerosis (arteriolar) (arteriosclerotic) (chronic) (hyaline) —*see also* Hypertension, kidney
- hyperplastic —*see* Hypertension, kidney
- senile N26.9

Nephrosis, nephrotic (Epstein's) (syndrome) (congenital) N04.9
- with
  - foot process disease N04.9
  - glomerular lesion N04.1
  - hypocomplementemic N04.5
- acute N04.9
- anoxic —*see* Nephrosis, tubular
- chemical —*see* Nephrosis, tubular
- cholemic K76.7
- diabetic —*see* E08-E13 with .21

Nephrosis, nephrotic *(continued)*
- Finnish type (congenital) Q89.8
- hemoglobin N10
- hemoglobinuric —*see* Nephrosis, tubular
- in
  - amyloidosis E85.4 *[N08]*
  - diabetes mellitus —*see* E08-E13 with .21
  - epidemic hemorrhagic fever A98.5
  - malaria (malariae) B52.0
- ischemic —*see* Nephrosis, tubular
- lipoid N04.9
- lower nephron —*see* Nephrosis, tubular
- malarial (malariae) B52.0
- minimal change N04.0
- myoglobin N10
- necrotizing —*see* Nephrosis, tubular
- osmotic (sucrose) N25.89
- radiation N04.9
- syphilitic (late) A52.75
- toxic —*see* Nephrosis, tubular
- tubular (acute) N17.0
  - postprocedural N99.0
  - radiation N04.9

Nephrosonephritis, hemorrhagic (endemic) A98.5

Nephrostomy
- attention to Z43.6
- status Z93.6

Nerve —*see also* condition
- injury —*see* Injury, nerve, by body site

Nerves R45.0

Nervous (*see also* condition) R45.0
- heart F45.8
- stomach F45.8
- tension R45.0

Nervousness R45.0

Nesidioblastoma
- pancreas D13.7
- specified site NEC —*see* Neoplasm, benign, by site
- unspecified site D13.7

Nettleship's syndrome —*see* Urticaria pigmentosa

Neumann's disease or syndrome L10.1

Neuralgia, neuralgic (acute) M79.2
- accessory (nerve) G52.8
- acoustic (nerve) H93.3
- auditory (nerve) H93.3
- ciliary G44.009
  - intractable G44.001
  - not intractable G44.009
- cranial
  - nerve —*see also* Disorder, nerve, cranial
    - fifth or trigeminal —*see* Neuralgia, trigeminal
  - postherpetic, postzoster B02.29
- ear —*see* subcategory H92.0
- facialis vera G51.1
- Fothergill's —*see* Neuralgia, trigeminal
- glossopharyngeal (nerve) G52.1
- Horton's G44.099
  - intractable G44.091
  - not intractable G44.099
- Hunt's B02.21
- hypoglossal (nerve) G52.3
- infraorbital —*see* Neuralgia, trigeminal
- malarial —*see* Malaria
- migrainous G44.009
  - intractable G44.001
  - not intractable G44.009

Neuralgia, neuralgic *(continued)*
- Morton's G57.6-
- nerve, cranial —*see* Disorder, nerve, cranial
- nose G52.0
- occipital M54.81
- olfactory G52.0
- penis N48.9
- perineum R10.2
- postherpetic NEC B02.29
  - trigeminal B02.22
- pubic region R10.2
- scrotum R10.2
- Sluder's G44.89
- specified nerve NEC G58.8
- spermatic cord R10.2
- sphenopalatine (ganglion) G90.09
- trifacial —*see* Neuralgia, trigeminal
- trigeminal G50.0
  - postherpetic, postzoster B02.22
- vagus (nerve) G52.2
- writer's F48.8
  - organic G25.89

Neurapraxia —*see* Injury, nerve

Neurasthenia F48.8
- cardiac F45.8
- gastric F45.8
- heart F45.8

Neurilemmoma —*see also* Neoplasm, nerve, benign
- acoustic (nerve) D33.3
- malignant —*see also* Neoplasm, nerve, malignant
  - acoustic (nerve) C72.4-

Neurilemmosarcoma —*see* Neoplasm, nerve, malignant

Neurinoma —*see* Neoplasm, nerve, benign

Neurinomatosis —*see* Neoplasm, nerve, uncertain behavior

Neuritis (rheumatoid) M79.2
- abducens (nerve) —*see* Strabismus, paralytic, sixth nerve
- accessory (nerve) G52.8
- acoustic (nerve) (*see also* subcategory) H93.3
  - in (due to)
    - infectious disease NEC B99 *[H94.0-]*
    - parasitic disease NEC B89 *[H94.0-]*
  - syphilitic A52.15
- alcoholic G62.1
  - with psychosis —*see* Psychosis, alcoholic
- amyloid, any site E85.4 *[G63]*
- auditory (nerve) —*see* subcategory H93.3
- brachial —*see* Radiculopathy
  - due to displacement, intervertebral disc —*see* Disorder, disc, cervical, with neuritis
- cranial nerve
  - due to Lyme disease A69.22
  - eighth or acoustic or auditory H93.3
  - eleventh or accessory G52.8
  - fifth or trigeminal G51.0
  - first or olfactory G52.0
  - fourth or trochlear —*see* Strabismus, paralytic, fourth nerve
  - second or optic —*see* Neuritis, optic
  - seventh or facial G51.8
    - newborn (birth injury) P11.3
  - sixth or abducent —*see* Strabismus, paralytic, sixth nerve

Neuritis *(continued)*
- cranial nerve *(continued)*
  - tenth or vagus G52.2
  - third or oculomotor —*see* Strabismus, paralytic, third nerve
  - twelfth or hypoglossal G52.3
- Déjérine-Sottas G60.0
- diabetic (mononeuropathy) —*see* E08-E13 with .41
  - polyneuropathy —*see* E08-E13 with .42
- due to
  - beriberi E51.11
  - displacement, prolapse or rupture, intervertebral disc —*see* Disorder, disc, with, radiculopathy
  - herniation, nucleus pulposus M51.9 *[G55]*
- endemic E51.11
- facial G51.8
  - newborn (birth injury) P11.3
- general —*see* Polyneuropathy
- geniculate ganglion G51.1
  - due to herpes (zoster) B02.21
- gouty (*see also* Gout, by type) M10.9 *[G63]*
- hypoglossal (nerve) G52.3
- ilioinguinal (nerve) G57.9-
- infectious (multiple) NEC G61.0
- interstitial hypertrophic progressive G60.0
- lumbar M54.16
- lumbosacral M54.17
- multiple —*see also* Polyneuropathy
  - endemic E51.11
  - infective, acute G61.0
- multiplex endemica E51.11
- nerve root —*see* Radiculopathy
- oculomotor (nerve) —*see* Strabismus, paralytic, third nerve
- olfactory nerve G52.0
- optic (nerve) (hereditary) (sympathetic) H46.9
  - with demyelination G36.0
  - in myelitis G36.0
  - nutritional H46.2
  - papillitis —*see* Papillitis, optic
  - retrobulbar H46.1-
  - specified type NEC H46.8
  - toxic H46.3
- peripheral (nerve) G62.9
  - multiple —*see* Polyneuropathy
  - single —*see* Mononeuritis
- pneumogastric (nerve) G52.2
- postherpetic, postzoster B02.29
- progressive hypertrophic interstitial G60.0
- retrobulbar —*see also* Neuritis, optic, retrobulbar
  - in (due to)
    - late syphilis A52.15
    - meningococcal infection A39.82
  - meningococcal A39.82
  - syphilitic A52.15
- sciatic (nerve) —*see also* Sciatica
  - due to displacement of intervertebral disc —*see* Disorder, disc, with, radiculopathy
- serum (*see also* Reaction, serum) T80.69
- shoulder-girdle G54.5
- specified nerve NEC G58.8
- spinal (nerve) root —*see* Radiculopathy
- syphilitic A52.15
- thenar (median) G56.1-
- thoracic M54.14
- toxic NEC G62.2

Neuritis *(continued)*
- trochlear (nerve) —*see* Strabismus, paralytic, fourth nerve
- vagus (nerve) G52.2

Neuroastrocytoma —*see* Neoplasm, uncertain behavior, by site

Neuroavitaminosis E56.9 *[G99.8]*

Neuroblastoma
- olfactory C30.0
- specified site —*see* Neoplasm, malignant, by site
- unspecified site C74.90

Neurochorioretinitis —*see* Chorioretinitis

Neurocirculatory asthenia F45.8

Neurocysticercosis B69.0

Neurocytoma —*see* Neoplasm, benign, by site

Neurodermatitis (circumscribed) (circumscripta) (local) L28.0
- atopic L20.81
- diffuse (Brocq) L20.81
- disseminated L20.81

Neuroencephalomyelopathy, optic G36.0

Neuroepithelioma —*see also* Neoplasm, malignant, by site
- olfactory C30.0

Neurofibroma —*see also* Neoplasm, nerve, benign
- melanotic —*see* Neoplasm, nerve, benign
- multiple —*see* Neurofibromatosis
- plexiform —*see* Neoplasm, nerve, benign

Neurofibromatosis (multiple) (nonmalignant) Q85.00
- acoustic Q85.02
- malignant —*see* Neoplasm, nerve, malignant
- specified NEC Q85.09
- type 1 (von Recklinghausen) Q85.01
- type 2 Q85.02

Neurofibrosarcoma —*see* Neoplasm, nerve, malignant

Neurogenic —*see also* condition
- bladder (*see also* Dysfunction bladder, neuromuscular) N31.9
  - cauda equina syndrome G83.4
- bowel NEC K59.2
- heart F45.8

Neuroglioma —*see* Neoplasm, uncertain behavior, by site

Neurolabyrinthitis (of Dix and Hallpike) —*see* Neuronitis, vestibular

Neurolathyrism —*see* Poisoning, food, noxious, plant

Neuroleprosy A30.9

Neuroma —*see also* Neoplasm, nerve, benign
- acoustic (nerve) D33.3
- amputation (stump) (traumatic) (surgical complication) (late) T87.3-
  - arm T87.3-
  - leg T87.3-
- digital (toe) G57.6-
- interdigital G58.8
  - lower limb (toe) G57.8-
  - upper limb G56.8-
- intermetatarsal G57.8-
- Morton's G57.6-

Neuroma *(continued)*
- nonneoplastic
  - arm G56.9-
  - leg G57.9-
  - lower extremity G57.9-
  - upper extremity G56.9-
- optic (nerve) D33.3
- plantar G57.6-
- plexiform —*see* Neoplasm, nerve, benign
- surgical (nonneoplastic)
  - arm G56.9-
  - leg G57.9-
  - lower extremity G57.9-
  - upper extremity G56.9-

Neuromyalgia —*see* Neuralgia

Neuromyasthenia (epidemic) (postinfectious) G93.3

Neuromyelitis G36.9
- ascending G61.0
- optica G36.0

Neuromyopathy G70.9
- paraneoplastic D49.9 *[G13.0]*

Neuromyotonia (Isaacs) G71.19

Neuronevus —*see* Nevus

Neuronitis G58.9
- ascending (acute) G57.2-
- vestibular H81.2-

Neuroparalytic —*see* condition

Neuropathy, neuropathic G62.9
- acute motor G62.81
- alcoholic G62.1
  - with psychosis —*see* Psychosis, alcoholic
- arm G56.9-
- autonomic, peripheral —*see* Neuropathy, peripheral, autonomic
- axillary G56.9-
- bladder N31.9
  - atonic (motor) (sensory) N31.2
  - autonomous N31.2
  - flaccid N31.2
  - nonreflex N31.2
  - reflex N31.1
  - uninhibited N31.0
- brachial plexus G54.0
- cervical plexus G54.2
- chronic
  - progressive segmentally demyelinating G62.89
  - relapsing demyelinating G62.89
- Déjérine-Sottas G60.0
- diabetic —*see* E08-E13 with .40
  - mononeuropathy —*see* E08-E13 with .41
  - polyneuropathy —*see* E08-E13 with .42
- entrapment G58.9
  - iliohypogastric nerve G57.8-
  - ilioinguinal nerve G57.8-
  - lateral cutaneous nerve of thigh G57.1-
  - median nerve G56.0-
  - obturator nerve G57.8-
  - peroneal nerve G57.3-
  - posterior tibial nerve G57.5-
  - saphenous nerve G57.8-
  - ulnar nerve G56.2-
- facial nerve G51.9
- hereditary G60.9
  - motor and sensory (types I-IV) G60.0
  - sensory G60.8
  - specified NEC G60.8
- hypertrophic G60.0
  - Charcot-Marie-Tooth G60.0

Neuropathy, neuropathic *(continued)*
- hypertrophic *(continued)*
  - -Sottas G60.0
  - interstitial progressive G60.0
  - of infancy G60.0
  - Refsum G60.1
- idiopathic G60.9
  - progressive G60.3
  - specified NEC G60.8
- in association with hereditary ataxia G60.2
- intercostal G58.0
- ischemic —*see* Disorder, nerve
- Jamaica (ginger) G62.2
- leg NEC G57.9-
- lower extremity G57.9-
- lumbar plexus G54.1
- median nerve G56.1-
- motor and sensory —*see also* Polyneuropathy
  - hereditary (types I-IV) G60.0
- multifocal motor (MMN) G61.82
- multiple (acute) (chronic) —*see* Polyneuropathy
- optic (nerve) —*see also* Neuritis, optic
  - ischemic H47.01-
- paraneoplastic (sensorial) (Denny Brown) D49.9 *[G13.0]*
- peripheral (nerve) (*see also* Polyneuropathy) G62.9
  - autonomic G90.9
    - idiopathic G90.09
    - in (due to)
      - amyloidosis E85.4 *[G99.0]*
      - diabetes mellitus —*see* E08-E13 with .43
      - endocrine disease NEC E34.9 *[G99.0]*
      - gout M10.00 *[G99.0]*
      - hyperthyroidism E05.90 *[G99.0]*
        - with thyroid storm E05.91 *[G99.0]*
      - metabolic disease NEC E88.9 *[G99.0]*
  - idiopathic G60.9
    - progressive G60.3
  - in (due to)
    - antitetanus serum G62.0
    - arsenic G62.2
    - drugs NEC G62.0
    - lead G62.2
    - organophosphate compounds G62.2
    - toxic agent NEC G62.2
- plantar nerves G57.6-
- progressive
  - hypertrophic interstitial G60.0
  - inflammatory G62.81
- radicular NEC —*see* Radiculopathy
- sacral plexus G54.1
- sciatic G57.0-
- serum G61.1
- toxic NEC G62.2
- trigeminal sensory G50.8
- ulnar nerve G56.2-
- uremic N18.9 *[G63]*
- vitamin B12 E53.8 *[G63]*
  - with anemia (pernicious) D51.0 *[G63]*
    - due to dietary deficiency D51.3 *[G63]*

Neurophthisis —*see also* Disorder, nerve
- peripheral, diabetic —*see* E08-E13 with .42

Neuroretinitis —*see* Chorioretinitis

Neuroretinopathy, hereditary optic H47.22

Neurosarcoma —*see* Neoplasm, nerve, malignant

Neurosclerosis —*see* Disorder, nerve

Neurosis, neurotic F48.9
- anankastic F42.8
- anxiety (state) F41.1
  - panic type F41.0
- asthenic F48.8
- bladder F45.8
- cardiac (reflex) F45.8
- cardiovascular F45.8
- character F60.9
- colon F45.8
- compensation F68.10
- compulsive, compulsion F42.8
- conversion F44.9
- craft F48.8
- cutaneous F45.8
- depersonalization F48.1
- depressive (reaction) (type) F34.1
- environmental F48.8
- excoriation L98.1
- fatigue F48.8
- functional —*see* Disorder, somatoform
- gastric F45.8
- gastrointestinal F45.8
- heart F45.8
- hypochondriacal F45.21
- hysterical F44.9
- incoordination F45.8
  - larynx F45.8
  - vocal cord F45.8
- intestine F45.8
- larynx (sensory) F45.8
  - hysterical F44.4
- mixed NEC F48.8
- musculoskeletal F45.8
- obsessional F42.8
- obsessive-compulsive F42.8
- occupational F48.8
- ocular NEC F45.8
- organ —*see* Disorder, somatoform
- pharynx F45.8
- phobic F40.9
- posttraumatic (situational) F43.10
  - acute F43.11
  - chronic F43.12
- psychasthenic (type) F48.8
- railroad F48.8
- rectum F45.8
- respiratory F45.8
- rumination F45.8
- sexual F65.9
- situational F48.8
- social F40.10
  - generalized F40.11
- specified type NEC F48.8
- state F48.9
  - with depersonalization episode F48.1
- stomach F45.8
- traumatic F43.10
  - acute F43.11
  - chronic F43.12
- vasomotor F45.8
- visceral F45.8
- war F48.8

Neurospongioblastosis diffusa Q85.1

Neurosyphilis (arrested) (early) (gumma) (late) (latent) (recurrent) (relapse) A52.3
- with ataxia (cerebellar) (locomotor) (spastic) (spinal) A52.19
- aneurysm (cerebral) A52.05
- arachnoid (adhesive) A52.13
- arteritis (any artery) (cerebral) A52.04
- asymptomatic A52.2
- congenital A50.40
- dura (mater) A52.13
- general paresis A52.17
- hemorrhagic A52.05
- juvenile (asymptomatic) (meningeal) A50.40
- leptomeninges (aseptic) A52.13
- meningeal, meninges (adhesive) A52.13
- meningitis A52.13
- meningovascular (diffuse) A52.13
- optic atrophy A52.15
- parenchymatous (degenerative) A52.19
- paresis, paretic A52.17
  - juvenile A50.45
- remission in (sustained) A52.3
- serological (without symptoms) A52.2
- specified nature or site NEC A52.19
- tabes, tabetic (dorsalis) A52.11
  - juvenile A50.45
- taboparesis A52.17
  - juvenile A50.45
- thrombosis (cerebral) A52.05
- vascular (cerebral) NEC A52.05

Neurothekeoma —*see* Neoplasm, nerve, benign

Neurotic —*see* Neurosis

Neurotoxemia —*see* Toxemia

Neutroclusion M26.211

Neutropenia, neutropenic (chronic) (genetic) (idiopathic) (immune) (infantile) (malignant) (pernicious) (splenic) D70.9
- congenital (primary) D70.0
- cyclic D70.4
- cytoreductive cancer chemotherapy sequela D70.1
- drug-induced D70.2
  - due to cytoreductive cancer chemotherapy D70.1
- due to infection D70.3
- fever D70.9
- neonatal, transitory (isoimmune) (maternal transfer) P61.5
- periodic D70.4
- secondary (cyclic) (periodic) (splenic) D70.4
  - drug-induced D70.2
    - due to cytoreductive cancer chemotherapy D70.1
- toxic D70.8

Neutrophilia, hereditary giant D72.0

Nevocarcinoma —*see* Melanoma

Nevus D22.9
- achromic —*see* Neoplasm, skin, benign
- amelanotic —*see* Neoplasm, skin, benign
- angiomatous D18.00
  - intra-abdominal D18.03
  - intracranial D18.02
  - skin D18.01
  - specified site NEC D18.09
- araneus I78.1
- balloon cell —*see* Neoplasm, skin, benign
- bathing trunk D48.5
- blue —*see* Neoplasm, skin, benign
  - cellular —*see* Neoplasm, skin, benign
  - giant —*see* Neoplasm, skin, benign

Nevus *(continued)*
- blue *(continued)*
  - Jadassohn's —*see* Neoplasm, skin, benign
  - malignant —*see* Melanoma
- capillary D18.00
  - intra-abdominal D18.03
  - intracranial D18.02
  - skin D18.01
  - specified site NEC D18.09
- cavernous D18.00
  - intra-abdominal D18.03
  - intracranial D18.02
  - skin D18.01
  - specified site NEC D18.09
- cellular —*see* Neoplasm, skin, benign
  - blue —*see* Neoplasm, skin, benign
- choroid D31.3-
- comedonicus Q82.5
- conjunctiva D31.0-
- dermal —*see* Neoplasm, skin, benign
  - with epidermal nevus —*see* Neoplasm, skin, benign
- dysplastic —*see* Neoplasm, skin, benign
- eye D31.9-
- flammeus Q82.5
- hemangiomatous D18.00
  - intra-abdominal D18.03
  - intracranial D18.02
  - skin D18.01
  - specified site NEC D18.09
- iris D31.4-
- lacrimal gland D31.5-
- lymphatic D18.1
- magnocellular
  - specified site —*see* Neoplasm, benign, by site
  - unspecified site D31.40
- malignant —*see* Melanoma
- meaning hemangioma D18.00
  - intra-abdominal D18.03
  - intracranial D18.02
  - skin D18.01
  - specified site NEC D18.09
- mouth (mucosa) D10.30
  - specified site NEC D10.39
  - white sponge Q38.6
- multiplex Q85.1
- non-neoplastic I78.1
- oral mucosa D10.30
  - specified site NEC D10.39
  - white sponge Q38.6
- orbit D31.6-
- pigmented
  - giant (*see also* Neoplasm, skin, uncertain behavior) D48.5
    - malignant melanoma in —*see* Melanoma
- portwine Q82.5
- retina D31.2-
- retrobulbar D31.6-
- sanguineous Q82.5
- senile I78.1
- skin D22.9
  - abdominal wall D22.5
  - ala nasi D22.39
  - ankle D22.7-
  - anus, anal D22.5
  - arm D22.6-
  - auditory canal (external) D22.2-
  - auricle (ear) D22.2-
  - auricular canal (external) D22.2-
  - axilla, axillary fold D22.5
  - back D22.5
  - breast D22.5
  - brow D22.39
  - buttock D22.5
  - canthus (eye) D22.1-

Nevus *(continued)*
- skin *(continued)*
  - cheek (external) D22.39
  - chest wall D22.5
  - chin D22.39
  - ear (external) D22.2-
  - external meatus (ear) D22.2-
  - eyebrow D22.39
  - eyelid (lower) (upper) D22.1-
  - face D22.30
    - specified NEC D22.39
  - female genital organ (external) NEC D28.0
  - finger D22.6-
  - flank D22.5
  - foot D22.7-
  - forearm D22.6-
  - forehead D22.39
  - foreskin D29.0
  - genital organ (external) NEC
    - female D28.0
    - male D29.9
  - gluteal region D22.5
  - groin D22.5
  - hand D22.6-
  - heel D22.7-
  - helix D22.2-
  - hip D22.7-
  - interscapular region D22.5
  - jaw D22.39
  - knee D22.7-
  - labium (majus) (minus) D28.0
  - leg D22.7-
  - lip (lower) (upper) D22.0
  - lower limb D22.7-
  - male genital organ (external) D29.9
  - nail D22.9
    - finger D22.6-
    - toe D22.7-
  - nasolabial groove D22.39
  - nates D22.5
  - neck D22.4
  - nose (external) D22.39
  - palpebra D22.1-
  - penis D29.0
  - perianal skin D22.5
  - perineum D22.5
  - pinna D22.2-
  - popliteal fossa or space D22.7-
  - prepuce D29.0
  - pudendum D28.0
  - scalp D22.4
  - scrotum D29.4
  - shoulder D22.6-
  - submammary fold D22.5
  - temple D22.39
  - thigh D22.7-
  - toe D22.7-
  - trunk NEC D22.5
  - umbilicus D22.5
  - upper limb D22.6-
  - vulva D28.0
- specified site NEC —*see* Neoplasm, by site, benign
- spider I78.1
- stellar I78.1
- strawberry Q82.5
- Sutton's benign D22.9
- unius lateris Q82.5
- Unna's Q82.5
- vascular Q82.5
- verrucous Q82.5

Newborn (infant) (liveborn) (singleton) Z38.2
- acne L70.4
- abstinence syndrome P96.1
- affected by
  - abnormalities of membranes P02.9
    - specified NEC P02.8
  - abruptio placenta P02.1

Newborn *(continued)*
- affected by *(continued)*
  - amino-acid metabolic disorder, transitory P74.8
  - amniocentesis (while in utero) P00.6
  - amnionitis P02.78
  - apparent life threatening event (ALTE) R68.13
  - bleeding (into)
    - cerebral cortex P52.22
    - germinal matrix P52.0
    - ventricles P52.1
  - breech delivery P03.0
  - cardiac arrest P29.81
  - cardiomyopathy I42.8
    - congenital I42.4
  - cerebral ischemia P91.0
  - Cesarean delivery P03.4
  - chemotherapy agents P04.11
  - chorioamnionitis P02.78
  - cocaine (crack) P04.41
  - complications of labor and delivery P03.9
    - specified NEC P03.89
  - compression of umbilical cord NEC P02.5
  - contracted pelvis P03.1
  - cyanosis P28.2
  - delivery P03.9
    - Cesarean P03.4
    - forceps P03.2
    - vacuum extractor P03.3
  - drugs of addiction P04.40
    - cocaine P04.41
    - hallucinogens P04.42
    - specified drug NEC P04.49
  - environmental chemicals P04.6
  - entanglement (knot) in umbilical cord P02.5
  - fetal (intrauterine)
    - growth retardation P05.9
    - inflammatory response syndrome (FIRS) P02.70
    - malnutrition not light or small for gestational age P05.2
  - FIRS (fetal inflammatory response syndrome) P02.70
  - forceps delivery P03.2
  - heart rate abnormalities
    - bradycardia P29.12
    - intrauterine P03.819
      - before onset of labor P03.810
      - during labor P03.811
    - tachycardia P29.11
  - hemorrhage (antepartum) P02.1
    - cerebellar (nontraumatic) P52.6
    - intracerebral (nontraumatic) P52.4
    - intracranial (nontraumatic) P52.9
      - specified NEC P52.8
    - intraventricular (nontraumatic) P52.3
      - grade 1 P52.0
      - grade 2 P52.1
      - grade 3 P52.21
      - grade 4 P52.22
    - posterior fossa (nontraumatic) P52.6
    - subarachnoid (nontraumatic) P52.5
    - subependymal P52.0
      - with intracerebral extension P52.22
      - with intraventricular extension P52.1
        - with enlargment of ventricles P52.21
      - without intraventricular extension P52.0

Newborn *(continued)*
- affected by *(continued)*
  - hypoxic ischemic encephalopathy [HIE] P91.60
    - mild P91.61
    - moderate P91.62
    - severe P91.63
  - induction of labor P03.89
  - intestinal perforation P78.0
  - intrauterine (fetal) blood loss P50.9
    - due to (from)
      - cut end of co-twin cord P50.5
      - hemorrhage into
        - co-twin P50.3
        - maternal circulation P50.4
      - placenta P50.2
      - ruptured cord blood P50.1
      - vasa previa P50.0
    - specified NEC P50.8
  - intrauterine (fetal) hemorrhage P50.9
  - intrauterine (in utero) procedure P96.5
  - malpresentation (malposition) NEC P03.1
  - maternal (complication of) (use of)
    - alcohol P04.3
    - amphetamines P04.16
    - analgesia (maternal) P04.0
    - anesthesia (maternal) P04.0
    - anticonvulsants P04.13
    - antidepressants P04.15
    - antineoplastic chemotherapy P04.11
    - anxiolytics P04.1A
    - blood loss P02.1
    - cannabis P04.81
    - circulatory disease P00.3
    - condition P00.9
      - specified NEC P00.89
    - cytotoxic drugs P04.12
    - delivery P03.9
      - Cesarean P03.4
      - forceps P03.2
      - vacuum extractor P03.3
    - diabetes mellitus (pre-existing) P70.1
    - disorder P00.9
      - specified NEC P00.89
    - drugs (addictive) (illegal) NEC P04.49
    - ectopic pregnancy P01.4
    - gestational diabetes P70.0
    - group B streptococcus (GBS) colonization (positive) P00.82
    - hemorrhage P02.1
    - hypertensive disorder P00.0
    - incompetent cervix P01.0
    - infectious disease P00.2
    - injury P00.5
    - labor and delivery P03.9
    - malpresentation before labor P01.7
    - maternal death P01.6
    - medical procedure P00.7
    - medication P04.19
      - specified type NEC P04.18
    - multiple pregnancy P01.5
    - nutritional disorder P00.4
    - oligohydramnios P01.2
    - opiates P04.14
      - administered for procedures during pregnancy or labor and delivery P04.0
    - parasitic disease P00.2
    - periodontal disease P00.81

Newborn *(continued)*
- affected by *(continued)*
  - maternal *(continued)*
    - placenta previa P02.0
    - polyhydramnios P01.3
    - precipitate delivery P03.5
    - pregnancy P01.9
      - specified P01.8
    - premature rupture of membranes P01.1
    - renal disease P00.1
    - respiratory disease P00.3
    - sedative-hypnotics P04.17
    - surgical procedure P00.6
    - tranquilizers administered for procedures during pregnancy or labor and delivery P04.0
    - urinary tract disease P00.1
    - uterine contraction (abnormal) P03.6
  - meconium peritonitis P78.0
  - medication (legal) (maternal use) (prescribed) P04.19
  - membrane abnormalities P02.9
    - specified NEC P02.8
  - membranitis P02.78
  - methamphetamine(s) P04.49
  - mixed metabolic and respiratory acidosis P84
  - neonatal abstinence syndrome P96.1
  - noxious substances transmitted via placenta or breast milk P04.9
    - cannabis P04.81
    - specified NEC P04.89
  - nutritional supplements P04.5
  - placenta previa P02.0
  - placental
    - abnormality (functional) (morphological) P02.20
      - specified NEC P02.29
    - dysfunction P02.29
    - infarction P02.29
    - insufficiency P02.29
    - separation NEC P02.1
    - transfusion syndromes P02.3
  - placentitis P02.78
  - precipitate delivery P03.5
  - prolapsed cord P02.4
  - respiratory arrest P28.81
  - slow intrauterine growth P05.9
  - tobacco P04.2
  - twin to twin transplacental transfusion P02.3
  - umbilical cord (tightly) around neck P02.5
  - umbilical cord condition P02.60
    - short cord P02.69
    - specified NEC P02.69
  - uterine contractions (abnormal) P03.6
  - vasa previa P02.69
    - from intrauterine blood loss P50.0
- apnea P28.4
  - primary P28.3
  - obstructive P28.4
  - sleep (central) (obstructive) (primary) P28.3
- born in hospital Z38.00
  - by cesarean Z38.01
- born outside hospital Z38.1
- breast buds P96.89
- breast engorgement P83.4
- check-up —*see* Newborn, examination
- convulsion P90
- dehydration P74.1
- examination
  - 8 to 28 days old Z00.111
  - under 8 days old Z00.110

Newborn *(continued)*
- fever P81.9
  - environmentally-induced P81.0
- hyperbilirubinemia P59.9
  - of prematurity P59.0
- hypernatremia P74.21
- hyponatremia P74.22
- infection P39.9
  - candidal P37.5
  - specified NEC P39.8
  - urinary tract P39.3
- jaundice P59.9
  - due to
    - breast milk inhibitor P59.3
    - hepatocellular damage P59.20
      - specified NEC P59.29
    - preterm delivery P59.0
  - of prematurity P59.0
  - specified NEC P59.8
- late metabolic acidosis P74.0
- mastitis P39.0
  - infective P39.0
  - noninfective P83.4
- multiple born NEC Z38.8
  - born in hospital Z38.68
    - by cesarean Z38.69
  - born outside hospital Z38.7
- omphalitis P38.9
  - with mild hemorrhage P38.1
  - without hemorrhage P38.9
- post-term P08.21
- prolonged gestation (over 42 completed weeks) P08.22
- quadruplet Z38.8
  - born in hospital Z38.63
    - by cesarean Z38.64
  - born outside hospital Z38.7
- quintuplet Z38.8
  - born in hospital Z38.65
    - by cesarean Z38.66
  - born outside hospital Z38.7
- seizure P90
- sepsis (congenital) P36.9
  - due to
    - anaerobes NEC P36.5
    - Escherichia coli P36.4
    - Staphylococcus P36.30
      - aureus P36.2
      - specified NEC P36.39
    - Streptococcus P36.10
      - group B P36.0
      - specified NEC P36.19
  - specified NEC P36.8
- triplet Z38.8
  - born in hospital Z38.61
    - by cesarean Z38.62
  - born outside hospital Z38.7
- twin Z38.5
  - born in hospital Z38.30
    - by cesarean Z38.31
  - born outside hospital Z38.4
- vomiting P92.09
  - bilious P92.01
- weight check Z00.111

Newcastle conjunctivitis or disease B30.8

Nezelof's syndrome (pure alymphocytosis) D81.4

Niacin (amide) **deficiency** E52

Nicolas (-Durand)**-Favre disease** A55

Nicotine —*see* Tobacco

Nicotinic acid deficiency E52

Niemann-Pick disease or syndrome E75.249
- specified NEC E75.248
- type
  - A E75.240
  - A/B E75.244

Niemann-Pick disease or syndrome *(continued)*
- type *(continued)*
  - B E75.241
  - C E75.242
  - D E75.243

Night
- blindness —*see* Blindness, night
- sweats R61
- terrors (child) F51.4

Nightmares (REM sleep type) F51.5

NIHSS (National Institutes of Health Stroke Scale) score R29.7-

Nipple —*see* condition

Nisbet's chancre A57

Nishimoto (-Takeuchi) **disease** I67.5

Nitritoid crisis or reaction —*see* Crisis, nitritoid

Nitrosohemoglobinemia D74.8

Njovera A65

No general equivalence degree (GED) Z55.5

Nocardiosis, nocardiasis A43.9
- cutaneous A43.1
- lung A43.0
- pneumonia A43.0
- pulmonary A43.0
- specified site NEC A43.8

Nocturia R35.1
- psychogenic F45.8

Nocturnal —*see* condition

Nodal rhythm I49.8

Node(s) —*see also* Nodule
- Bouchard's (with arthropathy) M15.2
- Haygarth's M15.8
- Heberden's (with arthropathy) M15.1
- larynx J38.7
- lymph —*see* condition
- milker's B08.03
- Osler's I33.0
- Schmorl's —*see* Schmorl's disease
- singer's J38.2
- teacher's J38.2
- tuberculous —*see* Tuberculosis, lymph gland
- vocal cord J38.2

Nodule(s), nodular
- actinomycotic —*see* Actinomycosis
- breast NEC (*see also* Lump, breast) N63.0
- colloid (cystic), thyroid E04.1
- cutaneous —*see* Swelling, localized
- endometrial (stromal) D26.1
- Haygarth's M15.8
- inflammatory —*see* Inflammation
- juxta-articular
  - syphilitic A52.77
  - yaws A66.7
- larynx J38.7
- lung, solitary (subsegmental branch of the bronchial tree) R91.1
  - multiple R91.8
- milker's B08.03
- prostate N40.2
  - with lower urinary tract symptoms (LUTS) N40.3
  - without lower urinary tract symtpoms (LUTS) N40.2
- pulmonary, solitary (subsegmental branch of the bronchial tree) R91.1
- retrocardiac R09.89
- rheumatoid M06.30
  - ankle M06.37-

Nodule(s), nodular *(continued)*
- rheumatoid *(continued)*
  - elbow M06.32-
  - foot joint M06.37-
  - hand joint M06.34-
  - hip M06.35-
  - knee M06.36-
  - multiple site M06.39
  - shoulder M06.31-
  - vertebra M06.38
  - wrist M06.33-
- scrotum (inflammatory) N49.2
- singer's J38.2
- solitary, lung (subsegmental branch of the bronchial tree) R91.1
  - multiple R91.8
- subcutaneous —*see* Swelling, localized
- teacher's J38.2
- thyroid (cold) (gland) (nontoxic) E04.1
  - with thyrotoxicosis E05.20
    - with thyroid storm E05.21
  - toxic or with hyperthyroidism E05.20
    - with thyroid storm E05.21
- vocal cord J38.2

Noma (gangrenous) (hospital) (infective) A69.0
- auricle I96
- mouth A69.0
- pudendi N76.89
- vulvae N76.89

Nomad, nomadism Z59.00

NOMID (neonatal onset multisystemic inflammatory disorder) M04.2

Nonadherence to medical treatment Z91.19

Nonautoimmune hemolytic anemia D59.4
- drug-induced D59.2

Nonclosure —*see also* Imperfect, closure
- ductus arteriosus (Botallo's) Q25.0
- foramen
  - botalli Q21.1
  - ovale Q21.1

Noncompliance Z91.19
- with
  - dietary regimen Z91.11
  - dialysis Z91.15
  - medical treatment Z91.19
  - medication regimen NEC Z91.14
    - underdosing (*see also* Table of Drugs and Chemicals, categories T36-T50, with final character 6) Z91.14
      - intentional NEC Z91.128
        - due to financial hardship of patient Z91.120
      - unintentional NEC Z91.138
        - due to patient's age related debility Z91.130
  - renal dialysis Z91.15

Nondescent (congenital) —*see also* Malposition, congenital
- cecum Q43.3
- colon Q43.3
- testicle Q53.9
  - bilateral Q53.20
    - abdominal Q53.211
    - perineal Q53.22
  - unilateral Q53.10
    - abdominal Q53.111
    - perineal Q53.12

Nondevelopment
- brain Q02
  - part of Q04.3
- heart Q24.8
- organ or site, congenital NEC —*see* Hypoplasia

Nonengagement
- head NEC O32.4
  - in labor, causing obstructed labor O64.8

Nonexanthematous tick fever A93.2

Nonexpansion, lung (newborn) P28.0

Nonfunctioning
- cystic duct (*see also* Disease, gallbladder) K82.8
- gallbladder (*see also* Disease, gallbladder) K82.8
- kidney N28.9
- labyrinth H83.2

Non-Hodgkin lymphoma NEC —*see* Lymphoma, non-Hodgkin

Non-working side interference M26.56

Nonimplantation, ovum N97.2

Noninsufflation, fallopian tube N97.1

Non-ketotic hyperglycinemia E72.51

Nonne-Milroy syndrome Q82.0

Nonovulation N97.0

Nonpatent fallopian tube N97.1

Non-palpable testicle(s)
- bilateral R39.84
- unilateral R39.83

Nonpneumatization, lung NEC P28.0

Nonrotation —*see* Malrotation

Nonsecretion, urine —*see* Anuria

Nonunion
- fracture —*see* Fracture, by site
- joint, following fusion or arthrodesis M96.0
- organ or site, congenital NEC —*see* Imperfect, closure
- symphysis pubis, congenital Q74.2

Nonvisualization, gallbladder R93.2

Nonvital, nonvitalized tooth K04.99

Noonan's syndrome Q87.19

Normocytic anemia (infectional) **due to blood loss** (chronic) D50.0
- acute D62

Norrie's disease (congenital) Q15.8

North American blastomycosis B40.9

Norwegian itch B86

Nose, nasal —*see* condition

Nosebleed R04.0

Nose-picking F98.8

Nosomania F45.21

Nosophobia F45.22

Nostalgia F43.20

Notch of iris Q13.2

Notching nose, congenital (tip) Q30.2

Nothnagel's
- syndrome —*see* Strabismus, paralytic, third nerve
- vasomotor acroparesthesia I73.89

Novy's relapsing fever A68.9
- louse-borne A68.0
- tick-borne A68.1

Noxious
- foodstuffs, poisoning by —*see* Poisoning, food, noxious, plant
- substances transmitted through placenta or breast milk P04.9

Nucleus pulposus —*see* condition

Numbness R20.0

Nuns' knee —*see* Bursitis, prepatellar

Nursemaid's elbow S53.03-

Nutcracker esophagus K22.4

Nutmeg liver K76.1

Nutrient element deficiency E61.9
- specified NEC E61.8

Nutrition deficient or insufficient (*see also* Malnutrition) E46
- due to
  - insufficient food T73.0
  - lack of
    - care (child) T76.02
      - adult T76.01
    - food T73.0

Nutritional stunting E45

Nyctalopia (night blindness) —*see* Blindness, night

Nycturia R35.1
- psychogenic F45.8

Nymphomania F52.8

Nystagmus H55.00
- benign paroxysmal —*see* Vertigo, benign paroxysmal
- central positional H81.4
- congenital H55.01
- dissociated H55.04
- latent H55.02
- miners' H55.09
- positional
  - benign paroxysmal H81.4
  - central H81.4
- specified form NEC H55.09
- visual deprivation H55.03

O

Obermeyer's relapsing fever (European) A68.0

Obesity E66.9
- with alveolar hypoventilation E66.2
- adrenal E27.8
- complicating
  - childbirth O99.214
  - pregnancy O99.21-
  - puerperium O99.215
- constitutional E66.8
- dietary counseling and surveillance Z71.3
- drug-induced E66.1
- due to
  - drug E66.1
  - excess calories E66.09
    - morbid E66.01
    - severe E66.01
- endocrine E66.8
- endogenous E66.8
- exogenous E66.09
- familial E66.8
- glandular E66.8
- hypothyroid —*see* Hypothyroidism
- hypoventilation syndrome (OHS) E66.2
- morbid E66.01
  - with
    - alveolar hypoventilation E66.2
    - obesity hypoventilation syndrome (OHS) E66.2
  - due to excess calories E66.01

Obesity *(continued)*
- nutritional E66.09
- pituitary E23.6
- severe E66.01
- specified type NEC E66.8

Oblique —*see* condition

Obliteration
- appendix (lumen) K38.8
- artery I77.1
- bile duct (noncalculous) K83.1
- common duct (noncalculous) K83.1
- cystic duct —*see* Obstruction, gallbladder
- disease, arteriolar I77.1
- endometrium N85.8
- eye, anterior chamber —*see* Disorder, globe, hypotony
- fallopian tube N97.1
- lymphatic vessel I89.0
  - due to mastectomy I97.2
- organ or site, congenital NEC —*see* Atresia, by site
- ureter N13.5
  - with infection N13.6
- urethra —*see* Stricture, urethra
- vein I87.8
- vestibule (oral) K08.89

Observation (following) (for) (without need for further medical care) Z04.9
- accident NEC Z04.3
  - at work Z04.2
  - transport Z04.1
- adverse effect of drug Z03.6
- alleged rape or sexual assault (victim), ruled out
  - adult Z04.41
  - child Z04.42
- criminal assault Z04.89
- development state
  - adolescent Z00.3
  - period of rapid growth in childhood Z00.2
  - puberty Z00.3
- disease, specified NEC Z03.89
- following work accident Z04.2
- forced sexual exploitation Z04.81
- forced labor exploitation Z04.82
- growth and development state —*see* Observation, development state
- injuries (accidental) NEC —*see also* Observation, accident
- newborn (for)
  - suspected condition, related to exposure from the mother or birth process —*see* Newborn, affected by, maternal
  - ruled out Z05.9
    - cardiac Z05.0
    - connective tissue Z05.73
    - gastrointestinal Z05.5
    - genetic Z05.41
    - genitourinary Z05.6
    - immunologic Z05.43
    - infectious Z05.1
    - metabolic Z05.42
    - mesculoskeletal Z05.72
    - neurological Z05.2
    - respiratory Z05.3
    - skin and subcutaneous tissue Z05.71
    - specified condition NEC Z05.8
- postpartum
  - immediately after delivery Z39.0
  - routine follow-up Z39.2
- pregnancy (normal) (without complication) Z34.9-
  - high risk O09.9-

Observation *(continued)*
- suicide attempt, alleged NEC Z03.89
  - self-poisoning Z03.6
- suspected, ruled out —*see also* Suspected condition, ruled out
  - abuse, physical
    - adult Z04.71
    - child Z04.72
  - accident at work Z04.2
  - adult battering victim Z04.71
  - child battering victim Z04.72
  - condition NEC Z03.89
    - newborn (*see also* Observation, newborn (for), suspected condition, ruled out) Z05.9
  - drug poisoning or adverse effect Z03.6
  - exposure (to)
    - anthrax Z03.810
    - biological agent NEC Z03.818
  - foreign body
    - aspirated (inhaled) Z03.822
    - ingested Z03.821
    - inserted (injected), in (eye) (orifice) (skin) Z03.823
  - inflicted injury NEC Z04.89
  - suicide attempt, alleged Z03.89
    - self-poisoning Z03.6
  - toxic effects from ingested substance (drug) (poison) Z03.6
- toxic effects from ingested substance (drug) (poison) Z03.6

Obsession, obsessional state F42.8
- mixed thoughts and acts F42.2

Obsessive-compulsive neurosis or reaction F42.8

Obstetric embolism, septic —*see* Embolism, obstetric, septic

Obstetrical trauma (complicating delivery) O71.9
- with or following ectopic or molar pregnancy O08.6
- specified type NEC O71.89

Obstipation —*see* Constipation

Obstruction, obstructed, obstructive
- airway J98.8
  - with
    - allergic alveolitis J67.9
    - asthma J45.909
      - with
        - exacerbation (acute) J45.901
        - status asthmaticus J45.902
    - bronchiectasis J47.9
      - with
        - exacerbation (acute) J47.1
        - lower respiratory infection J47.0
    - bronchitis (chronic) J44.9
    - emphysema J43.9
  - chronic J44.9
    - with
      - allergic alveolitis —*see* Pneumonitis, hypersensitivity
      - bronchiectasis J47.9
        - with
          - exacerbation (acute) J47.1
          - lower respiratory infection J47.0

Obstruction, obstructed, obstructive *(continued)*
- due to
  - foreign body —*see* Foreign body, by site, causing asphyxia
  - inhalation of fumes or vapors J68.9
  - laryngospasm J38.5
- ampulla of Vater K83.1
- aortic (heart) (valve) —*see* Stenosis, aortic
- aortoiliac I74.09
- aqueduct of Sylvius G91.1
  - congenital Q03.0
    - with spina bifida —*see* Spina bifida, by site, with hydrocephalus
- Arnold-Chiari —*see* Arnold-Chiari disease
- artery (*see also* Atherosclerosis, artery) I70.9
  - basilar (complete) (partial) —*see* Occlusion, artery, basilar
  - carotid (complete) (partial) —*see* Occlusion, artery, carotid
  - cerebellar —*see* Occlusion, artery, cerebellar
  - cerebral (anterior) (middle) (posterior) —*see* Occlusion, artery, cerebral
  - precerebral —*see* Occlusion, artery, precerebral
  - renal N28.0
  - retinal NEC —*see* Occlusion, artery, retina
  - stent —*see* Restenosis, stent
  - vertebral (complete) (partial) —*see* Occlusion, artery, vertebral
- band (intestinal) (*see also* Obstruction, intestine, specified NEC) K56.699
- bile duct or passage (common) (hepatic) (noncalculous) K83.1
  - with calculus K80.51
  - congenital (causing jaundice) Q44.3
- biliary (duct) (tract) K83.1
  - gallbladder K82.0
- bladder-neck (acquired) N32.0
  - congenital Q64.31
  - due to hyperplasia (hypertrophy) of prostate —*see* Hyperplasia, prostate
- bowel —*see* Obstruction, intestine
- bronchus J98.09
- canal, ear —*see* Stenosis, external ear canal
- cardia K22.2
- caval veins (inferior) (superior) I87.1
- cecum —*see* Obstruction, intestine
- circulatory I99.8
- colon —*see* Obstruction, intestine
- common duct (noncalculous) K83.1
- coronary (artery) —*see* Occlusion, coronary
- cystic duct —*see also* Obstruction, gallbladder
  - with calculus K80.21
- device, implant or graft (*see also* Complications, by site and type, mechanical) T85.698
  - arterial graft NEC —*see* Complication, cardiovascular device, mechanical, vascular
  - catheter NEC T85.628
    - cystostomy T83.090
    - dialysis (renal) T82.49
      - intraperitoneal T85.691
    - Hopkins T83.098
    - ileostomy T83.098

- **Obstruction, obstructed, obstructive** *(continued)*
  - device, implant or graft *(continued)*
    - catheter NEC *(continued)*
      - infusion NEC T82.594
        - spinal (epidural) (subdural) T85.690
      - nephrostomy T83.092
      - urethral indwelling T83.091
      - urinary T83.098
      - urostomy T83.098
    - due to infection T85.79
    - gastrointestinal *—see* Complications, prosthetic device, mechanical, gastrointestinal device
    - genital NEC T83.498
      - intrauterine contraceptive device T83.39
      - penile prosthesis (cylinder) (implanted) (pump) (resevoir) T83.490
      - testicular prosthesis T83.491
    - heart NEC *—see* Complication, cardiovascular device, mechanical
    - joint prosthesis *—see* Complications, joint prosthesis, mechanical, specified NEC, by site
    - orthopedic NEC *—see* Complication, orthopedic, device, mechanical
    - specified NEC T85.628
    - urinary NEC *—see also* Complication, genitourinary, device, urinary, mechanical
      - graft T83.29
    - vascular NEC *—see* Complication, cardiovascular device, mechanical
    - ventricular intracranial shunt T85.09
  - due to foreign body accidentally left in operative wound T81.529
  - duodenum K31.5
  - ejaculatory duct N50.89
  - esophagus K22.2
  - eustachian tube (complete) (partial) H68.10-
    - cartilagenous (extrinsic) H68.13-
      - intrinsic H68.12-
    - osseous H68.11-
  - fallopian tube (bilateral) N97.1
  - fecal K56.41
    - with hernia *—see* Hernia, by site, with obstruction
  - foramen of Monro (congenital) Q03.8
    - with spina bifida *—see* Spina bifida, by site, with hydrocephalus
  - foreign body *—see* Foreign body
  - gallbladder K82.0
    - with calculus, stones K80.21
    - congenital Q44.1
  - gastric outlet K31.1
  - gastrointestinal *—see* Obstruction, intestine
  - hepatic K76.89
    - duct (noncalculous) K83.1
  - hepatobiliary K83.1
  - ileum *—see* Obstruction, intestine
  - iliofemoral (artery) I74.5
  - intestine K56.609
    - complete K56.601
    - incomplete K56.600
    - partial K56.600

- **Obstruction, obstructed, obstructive** *(continued)*
  - intestine *(continued)*
    - with
      - adhesions (intestinal) (peritoneal) K56.50
      - complete K56.52
      - incomplete K56.51
      - partial K56.51
    - adynamic K56.0
    - by gallstone K56.3
    - congenital (small) Q41.9
      - large Q42.9
        - specified part NEC Q42.8
    - neurogenic K56.0
      - Hirschsprung's disease or megacolon Q43.1
    - newborn P76.9
      - due to
        - fecaliths P76.8
        - inspissated milk P76.2
        - meconium (plug) P76.0
          - in mucoviscidosis E84.11
      - specified NEC P76.8
    - postoperative K91.30
      - complete K91.32
      - incomplete K91.31
      - partial K91.31
    - reflex K56.0
    - specified NEC K56.699
      - complete K56.691
      - incomplete K56.690
      - partial K56.690
    - volvulus K56.2
  - intracardiac ball valve prosthesis T82.09
  - jejunum *—see* Obstruction, intestine
  - joint prosthesis *—see* Complications, joint prosthesis, mechanical, specified NEC, by site
  - kidney (calices) (*see also* Hydronephrosis) N28.89
  - labor *—see* Delivery
  - lacrimal (passages) (duct)
    - by
      - dacryolith *—see* Dacryolith
      - stenosis *—see* Stenosis, lacrimal
    - congenital Q10.5
    - neonatal H04.53-
  - lacrimonasal duct *—see* Obstruction, lacrimal
  - lacteal, with steatorrhea K90.2
  - laryngitis *—see* Laryngitis
  - larynx NEC J38.6
    - congenital Q31.8
  - lung J98.4
    - disease, chronic J44.9
  - lymphatic I89.0
  - meconium (plug)
    - newborn P76.0
      - due to fecaliths P76.0
      - in mucoviscidosis E84.11
  - mitral *—see* Stenosis, mitral
  - nasal J34.89
  - nasolacrimal duct *—see also* Obstruction, lacrimal
    - congenital Q10.5
  - nasopharynx J39.2
  - nose J34.89
  - organ or site, congenital NEC *—see* Atresia, by site
  - pancreatic duct K86.89
  - parotid duct or gland K11.8
  - pelviureteral junction N13.5
    - with hydronephrosis N13.0
    - congenital Q62.39
  - pharynx J39.2

- **Obstruction, obstructed, obstructive** *(continued)*
  - portal (circulation) (vein) I81
  - prostate *—see also* Hyperplasia, prostate
    - valve (urinary) N32.0
  - pulmonary valve (heart) I37.0
  - pyelonephritis (chronic) N11.1
  - pylorus
    - adult K31.1
    - congenital or infantile Q40.0
  - rectosigmoid *—see* Obstruction, intestine
  - rectum K62.4
  - renal (*see also* Hydronephrosis) N28.89
    - outflow N13.8
    - pelvis, congenital Q62.39
  - respiratory J98.8
    - chronic J44.9
  - retinal (vessels) H34.9
  - salivary duct (any) K11.8
    - with calculus K11.5
  - sigmoid *—see* Obstruction, intestine
  - sinus (accessory) (nasal) J34.89
  - Stensen's duct K11.8
  - stomach NEC K31.89
    - acute K31.0
    - congenital Q40.2
    - due to pylorospasm K31.3
  - submandibular duct K11.8
  - submaxillary gland K11.8
    - with calculus K11.5
  - thoracic duct I89.0
  - thrombotic *—see* Thrombosis
  - trachea J39.8
  - tracheostomy airway J95.03
  - tricuspid (valve) *—see* Stenosis, tricuspid
  - upper respiratory, congenital Q34.8
  - ureter (functional) (pelvic junction) NEC N13.5
    - with
      - hydronephrosis N13.1
        - with infection N13.6
        - congenital Q62.39
      - pyelonephritis (chronic) N11.1
    - congenital Q62.39
    - due to calculus *—see* Calculus, ureter
  - urethra NEC N36.8
    - congenital Q64.39
  - urinary (moderate) N13.9
    - due to hyperplasia (hypertrophy) of prostate *—see* Hyperplasia, prostate
    - organ or tract (lower) N13.9
    - prostatic valve N32.0
    - specified NEC N13.8
  - uropathy N13.9
  - uterus N85.8
  - vagina N89.5
  - valvular *—see* Endocarditis
  - vein, venous I87.1
    - caval (inferior) (superior) I87.1
    - thrombotic *—see* Thrombosis
  - vena cava (inferior) (superior) I87.1
  - vesical NEC N32.0
  - vesicourethral orifice N32.0
    - congenital Q64.31
  - vessel NEC I99.8
    - stent *—see* Restenosis, stent
- **Obturator** *—see* condition
- **Occlusal wear, teeth** K03.0
- **Occlusio pupillae** *—see* Membrane, pupillary
- **Occlusion, occluded**
  - anus K62.4
    - congenital Q42.3
      - with fistula Q42.2
  - aortoiliac (chronic) I74.09
  - aqueduct of Sylvius G91.1
    - congenital Q03.0
      - with spina bifida *—see* Spina bifida, by site, with hydrocephalus
  - artery (*see also* Atherosclerosis, artery) I70.9
    - auditory, internal I65.8
    - basilar I65.1
      - with
        - infarction I63.22
          - due to
            - embolism I63.12
            - thrombosis I63.02
    - brain or cerebral I66.9
      - with infarction (due to) I63.5-
        - embolism I63.4-
        - thrombosis I63.3-
    - carotid I65.2-
      - with
        - infarction I63.23-
          - due to
            - embolism I63.13-
            - thrombosis I63.03-
    - cerebellar (anterior inferior) (posterior inferior) (superior) I66.3
      - with infarction I63.54-
        - due to
          - embolism I63.44-
          - thrombosis I63.34-
    - cerebral I66.9
      - with infarction I63.50
        - due to
          - embolism I63.40
            - specified NEC I63.49
          - thrombosis I63.30
            - specified NEC I63.39
      - anterior I66.1-
        - with infarction I63.52-
          - due to
            - embolism I63.42-
            - thrombosis I63.32-
      - middle I66.0-
        - with infarction I63.51-
          - due to
            - embolism I63.41-
            - thrombosis I63.31-
      - posterior I66.2-
        - with infarction I63.53-
          - due to
            - embolism I63.43-
            - thrombosis I63.33-
      - specified NEC I66.8
        - with infarction I63.59
          - due to
            - embolism I63.4-
            - thrombosis I63.3-
    - choroidal (anterior) *—see* Occlusion, artery, precerebral, specified NEC
    - communicating posterior *—see* Occlusion, artery, precerebral, specified NEC
    - complete
      - coronary I25.82
      - extremities I70.92
    - coronary (acute) (thrombotic) (without myocardial infarction) I24.0
      - with myocardial infarction *— see* Infarction, myocardium
      - chronic total I25.82
      - complete I25.82
      - healed or old I25.2
      - total (chronic) I25.82

Occlusion, occluded *(continued)*
- artery *(continued)*
  - hypophyseal *—see* Occlusion, artery, precerebral, specified NEC
  - iliac I74.5
  - lower extremities due to stenosis or stricture I77.1
  - mesenteric (embolic) (thrombotic) (*see also* Infarct, intestine) K55.069
  - perforating *—see* Occlusion, artery, cerebral, specified NEC
  - peripheral I77.9
    - thrombotic or embolic I74.4
  - pontine *—see* Occlusion, artery, precerebral, specified NEC
  - precerebral I65.9
    - with infarction I63.20
      - specified NEC I63.29
      - due to
        - embolism I63.10
          - specified NEC I63.19
        - thrombosis I63.09
          - specified NEC I63.09
    - basilar *—see* Occlusion, artery, basilar
    - carotid *—see* Occlusion, artery, carotid
    - puerperal O88.23
    - specified NEC I65.8
      - with infarction I63.29
        - due to
          - embolism I63.19
          - thrombosis I63.09
    - vertebral *—see* Occlusion, artery, vertebral
  - renal N28.0
  - retinal
    - central H34.1-
    - partial H34.21-
    - branch H34.23-
    - transient H34.0-
  - spinal *—see* Occlusion, artery, precerebral, vertebral
  - total (chronic)
    - coronary I25.82
    - extremities I70.92
  - vertebral I65.0-
    - with
      - infarction I63.21-
        - due to
          - embolism I63.11-
          - thrombosis I63.01-
- basilar artery *—see* Occlusion, artery, basilar
- bile duct (common) (hepatic) (noncalculous) K83.1
- bowel *—see* Obstruction, intestine
- carotid (artery) (common) (internal) *—see* Occlusion, artery, carotid
- centric (of teeth) M26.59
  - maximum intercuspation discrepancy M26.55
- cerebellar (artery) *—see* Occlusion, artery, cerebellar
- cerebral (artery) *—see* Occlusion, artery, cerebral
- cerebrovascular *—see also* Occlusion, artery, cerebral
  - with infarction I63.5-
- cervical canal *—see* Stricture, cervix
- cervix (uteri) *—see* Stricture, cervix
- choanal Q30.0
- choroidal (artery) *—see* Occlusion, artery, precerebral, specified NEC
- colon *—see* Obstruction, intestine
- communicating posterior artery *—see* Occlusion, artery, precerebral, specified NEC
- coronary (artery) (vein) (thrombotic) *—see also* Infarct, myocardium
  - chronic total I25.82
  - healed or old I25.2
  - not resulting in infarction I24.0
  - total (chronic) I25.82
- cystic duct *—see* Obstruction, gallbladder
- embolic *—see* Embolism
- fallopian tube N97.1
  - congenital Q50.6
- gallbladder *—see also* Obstruction, gallbladder
  - congenital (causing jaundice) Q44.1
- gingiva, traumatic K06.2
- hymen N89.6
  - congenital Q52.3
- hypophyseal (artery) *—see* Occlusion, artery, precerebral, specified NEC
- iliac artery I74.5
- intestine *—see* Obstruction, intestine
- lacrimal passages *—see* Obstruction, lacrimal
- lung J98.4
- lymph or lymphatic channel I89.0
- mammary duct N64.89
- mesenteric artery (embolic) (thrombotic) (*see also* Infarct, intestine) K55.069
- nose J34.89
  - congenital Q30.0
- organ or site, congenital NEC *—see* Atresia, by site
- oviduct N97.1
  - congenital Q50.6
- peripheral arteries
  - due to stricture or stenosis I77.1
  - upper extremity I74.2
- pontine (artery) *—see* Occlusion, artery, precerebral, specified NEC
- posterior lingual, of mandibular teeth M26.29
- precerebral artery *—see* Occlusion, artery, precerebral
- punctum lacrimale *—see* Obstruction, lacrimal
- pupil *—see* Membrane, pupillary
- pylorus, adult (*see also* Stricture, pylorus) K31.1
- renal artery N28.0
- retina, retinal
  - artery *—see* Occlusion, artery, retinal
  - vein (central) H34.81-
    - engorgement H34.82-
    - tributary H34.83-
  - vessels H34.9
- spinal artery *—see* Occlusion, artery, precerebral, vertebral
- teeth (mandibular) (posterior lingual) M26.29
- thoracic duct I89.0
- thrombotic *—see* Thrombosis, artery
- traumatic
  - edentulous (alveolar) ridge K06.2
  - gingiva K06.2
  - periodontal K05.5
- tubal N97.1
- ureter (complete) (partial) N13.5
  - congenital Q62.10
- ureteropelvic junction N13.5
  - congenital Q62.11
- ureterovesical orifice N13.5
  - congenital Q62.12
- urethra *—see* Stricture, urethra
- uterus N85.8
- vagina N89.5
- vascular NEC I99.8
- vein *—see* Thrombosis
  - retinal *—see* Occlusion, retinal, vein
- vena cava (inferior) (superior) *—see* Embolism, vena cava
- ventricle (brain) NEC G91.1
- vertebral (artery) *—see* Occlusion, artery, vertebral
- vessel (blood) I99.8
- vulva N90.5

Occult
- blood in feces (stools) R19.5

Occupational
- problems NEC Z56.89

Ochlophobia *—see* Agoraphobia

Ochronosis (endogenous) E70.29

Ocular muscle *—see* condition

Oculogyric crisis or disturbance H51.8
- psychogenic F45.8

Oculomotor syndrome H51.9

Oculopathy
- syphilitic NEC A52.71
  - congenital
    - early A50.01
    - late A50.30
  - early (secondary) A51.43
  - late A52.71

Oddi's sphincter spasm K83.4

Odontalgia K08.89

Odontoameloblastoma *—see* Cyst, calcifying odontogenic

Odontoclasia K03.89

Odontodysplasia, regional K00.4

Odontogenesis imperfecta K00.5

Odontoma (ameloblastic) (complex) (compound) (fibroameloblastic) *—see* Cyst, calcifying odontogenic

Odontomyelitis (closed) (open) K04.01
- irreversible K04.02
- reversible K04.01

Odontorrhagia K08.89

Odontosarcoma, ameloblastic C41.1
- upper jaw (bone) C41.0

Oestriasis *—see* Myiasis

Oguchi's disease H53.63

Ohara's disease *—see* Tularemia

OHS (obesity hypoventilation syndrome) E66.2

Oidiomycosis *—see* Candidiasis

Oidium albicans infection *—see* Candidiasis

Old age (without mention of debility) R54
- dementia F03

Old (previous) **myocardial infarction** I25.2

Olfactory *—see* condition

Oligemia *—see* Anemia

Oligoastrocytoma
- specified site *—see* Neoplasm, malignant, by site
- unspecified site C71.9

Oligocythemia D64.9

Oligodendroblastoma
- specified site *—see* Neoplasm, malignant
- unspecified site C71.9

Oligodendroglioma
- anaplastic type
  - specified site *—see* Neoplasm, malignant, by site
  - unspecified site C71.9
- specified site *—see* Neoplasm, malignant, by site
- unspecified site C71.9

Oligodontia *—see* Anodontia

Oligoencephalon Q02

Oligohidrosis L74.4

Oligohydramnios O41.0-

Oligohydrosis L74.4

Oligomenorrhea N91.5
- primary N91.3
- secondary N91.4

Oligophrenia *—see also* Disability, intellectual
- phenylpyruvic E70.0

Oligospermia N46.11
- due to
  - drug therapy N46.121
  - efferent duct obstruction N46.123
  - infection N46.122
  - radiation N46.124
  - specified cause NEC N46.129
  - systemic disease N46.125

Oligotrichia *—see* Alopecia

Oliguria R34
- with, complicating or following ectopic or molar pregnancy O08.4
- postprocedural N99.0

Ollier's disease Q78.4

Omentitis *—see* Peritonitis

Omenotocele *—see* Hernia, abdomen, specified site NEC

Omentum, omental *—see* condition

Omphalitis (congenital) (newborn) P38.9
- with mild hemorrhage P38.1
- without hemorrhage P38.9
- not of newborn L08.82
- tetanus A33

Omphalocele Q79.2

Omphalomesenteric duct, persistent Q43.0

Omphalorrhagia, newborn P51.9

Omsk hemorrhagic fever A98.1

Onanism (excessive) F98.8

Onchocerciasis, onchocercosis B73.1
- with
  - eye disease B73.00
    - endophthalmitis B73.01
    - eyelid B73.09
    - glaucoma B73.02
    - specified NEC B73.09
  - eye NEC B73.00
  - eyelid B73.09

Oncocytoma —*see* Neoplasm, benign, by site

Oncovirus, as cause of disease classified elsewhere B97.32

Ondine's curse —*see* Apnea, sleep

Oneirophrenia F23

Onychauxis L60.2
  congenital Q84.5

Onychia —*see also* Cellulitis, digit
  with lymphangitis —*see* Lymphangitis, acute, digit
  candidal B37.2
  dermatophytic B35.1

Onychitis —*see also* Cellulitis, digit
  with lymphangitis —*see* Lymphangitis, acute, digit

Onychocryptosis L60.0

Onychodystrophy L60.3
  congenital Q84.6

Onychogryphosis, onychogryposis L60.2

Onycholysis L60.1

Onychomadesis L60.8

Onychomalacia L60.3

Onychomycosis (finger) (toe) B35.1

Onycho-osteodysplasia Q87.2

Onychophagia F98.8

Onychophosis L60.8

Onychoptosis L60.8

Onychorrhexis L60.3
  congenital Q84.6

Onychoschizia L60.3

Onyxis (finger) (toe) L60.0

Onyxitis —*see also* Cellulitis, digit
  with lymphangitis —*see* Lymphangitis, acute, digit

Oophoritis (cystic) (infectional) (interstitial) N70.92
  with salpingitis N70.93
  acute N70.02
    with salpingitis N70.03
  chronic N70.12
    with salpingitis N70.13
  complicating abortion —*see* Abortion, by type, complicated by, oophoritis

Oophorocele N83.4-

Opacity, opacities
  cornea H17.-
    central H17.1-
    congenital Q13.3
    degenerative —*see* Degeneration, cornea
    hereditary —*see* Dystrophy, cornea
    inflammatory —*see* Keratitis
    minor H17.81-
    peripheral H17.82-
  cornea
    sequelae of trachoma (healed) B94.0
    specified NEC H17.89
  enamel (teeth) (fluoride) (nonfluoride) K00.3
  lens —*see* Cataract
  snowball —*see* Deposit, crystalline
  vitreous (humor) NEC H43.39-
    congenital Q14.0
    membranes and strands H43.31-

Opalescent dentin (hereditary) K00.5

Open, opening
  abnormal, organ or site, congenital —*see* Imperfect, closure
  angle with
    borderline
      findings
        high risk H40.02-
        low risk H40.01-
      intraocular pressure H40.00-
    cupping of discs H40.01-
    glaucoma (primary) —*see* Glaucoma, open angle
  bite
    anterior M26.220
    posterior M26.221
  false —*see* Imperfect, closure
  margin on tooth restoration K08.51
  restoration margins of tooth K08.51
  wound —*see* Wound, open

Operational fatigue F48.8

Operative —*see* condition

Operculitis —*see* Periodontitis

Operculum —*see* Break, retina

Ophiasis L63.2

Ophthalmia (*see also* Conjunctivitis) H10.9
  actinic rays —*see* Photokeratitis
  allergic (acute) —*see* Conjunctivitis, acute, atopic
  blennorrhagic (gonococcal) (neonatorum) A54.31
  diphtheritic A36.86
  Egyptian A71.1
  electrica —*see* Photokeratitis
  gonococcal (neonatorum) A54.31
  metastatic —*see* Endophthalmitis, purulent
  migraine —*see* Migraine, ophthalmoplegic
  neonatorum, newborn P39.1
    gonococcal A54.31
  nodosa H16.24-
  purulent —*see* Conjunctivitis, acute, mucopurulent
  spring —*see* Conjunctivitis, acute, atopic
  sympathetic —*see* Uveitis, sympathetic

Ophthalmitis —*see* Ophthalmia

Ophthalmocele (congenital) Q15.8

Ophthalmoneuromyelitis G36.0

Ophthalmoplegia —*see also* Strabismus, paralytic
  anterior internuclear —*see* Ophthalmoplegia, internuclear
  ataxia-areflexia G61.0
  diabetic —*see* E08-E13 with .39
  exophthalmic E05.00
    with thyroid storm E05.01
  external H49.88-
    progressive H49.4-
      with pigmentary retinopathy —*see* Kearns-Sayre syndrome
    total H49.3-
  internal (complete) (total) H52.51-
  internuclear H51.2-
  migraine —*see* Migraine, ophthalmoplegic
  Parinaud's H49.88-
  progressive external —*see* Ophthalmoplegia, external, progressive
  supranuclear, progressive G23.1
  total (external) —*see* Ophthalmoplegia, external, total

Opioid(s)
  abuse —*see* Abuse, drug, opioids
  dependence —*see* Dependence, drug, opioids
  induced, without use disorder
    anxiety disorder F11.988
    delirium F11.921
    depressive disorder F11.94
    sexual dysfunction F11.981
    sleep disorder F11.982

Opisthognathism M26.09

Opisthorchiasis (felineus) (viverrini) B66.0

Opitz' disease D73.2

Opiumism —*see* Dependence, drug, opioid

Oppenheim's disease G70.2

Oppenheim-Urbach disease (necrobiosis lipoidica diabeticorum) —*see* E08-E13 with .620

Optic nerve —*see* condition

Orbit —*see* condition

Orchioblastoma C62.9-

Orchitis (gangrenous) (nonspecific) (septic) (suppurative) N45.2
  blennorrhagic (gonococcal) (acute) (chronic) A54.23
  chlamydial A56.19
  filarial —*see also* Infestation, filarial B74.9 *[N51]*
  gonococcal (acute) (chronic) A54.23
  mumps B26.0
  syphilitic A52.76
  tuberculous A18.15

Orf (virus disease) B08.02

Organic —*see also* condition
  brain syndrome F09
  heart —*see* Disease, heart
  mental disorder F09
  psychosis F09

Orgasm
  anejaculatory N53.13

Oriental
  bilharziasis B65.2
  schistosomiasis B65.2

Orifice —*see* condition

Origin of both great vessels from right ventricle Q20.1

Ormond's disease (with ureteral obstruction) N13.5
  with infection N13.6

Ornithine metabolism disorder E72.4

Ornithinemia (Type I) (Type II) E72.4

Ornithosis A70

Orotaciduria, oroticaciduria (congenital) (hereditary) (pyrimidine deficiency) E79.8
  anemia D53.0

Orthodontics
  adjustment Z46.4
  fitting Z46.4

Orthopnea R06.01

Orthopoxvirus B08.09

Os, uterus —*see* condition

Osgood-Schlatter disease or osteochondrosis M92.52-

Osler (-Weber)-**Rendu disease** I78.0

Osler's nodes I33.0

Osmidrosis L75.0

Osseous —*see* condition

Ossification
  artery —*see* Arteriosclerosis
  auricle (ear) —*see* Disorder, pinna, specified type NEC
  bronchial J98.09
  cardiac —*see* Degeneration, myocardial
  cartilage (senile) —*see* Disorder, cartilage, specified type NEC
  coronary (artery) —*see* Disease, heart, ischemic, atherosclerotic
  diaphragm J98.6
  ear, middle —*see* Otosclerosis
  falx cerebri G96.198
  fontanel, premature Q75.0
  heart —*see also* Degeneration, myocardial
    valve —*see* Endocarditis
  larynx J38.7
  ligament —*see* Disorder, tendon, specified type NEC
    posterior longitudinal —*see* Spondylopathy, specified NEC
  meninges (cerebral) (spinal) G96.198
  multiple, eccentric centers —*see* Disorder, bone, development or growth
  muscle —*see also* Calcification, muscle
    due to burns —*see* Myositis, ossificans, in, burns
    paralytic —*see* Myositis, ossificans, in, quadriplegia
    progressive —*see* Myositis, ossificans, progressiva
    specified NEC M61.50
      ankle M61.57-
      foot M61.57-
      forearm M61.53-
      hand M61.54-
      lower leg M61.56-
      multiple sites M61.59
      pelvic region M61.55-
      shoulder region M61.51-
      specified site NEC M61.58
      thigh M61.55-
      upper arm M61.52-
    traumatic —*see* Myositis, ossificans, traumatica
  myocardium, myocardial —*see* Degeneration, myocardial
  penis N48.89
  periarticular —*see* Disorder, joint, specified type NEC
  pinna —*see* Disorder, pinna, specified type NEC
  rider's bone —*see* Ossification, muscle, specified NEC
  sclera H15.89
  subperiosteal, post-traumatic M89.8X-
  tendon —*see* Disorder, tendon, specified type NEC
  trachea J39.8
  tympanic membrane —*see* Disorder, tympanic membrane, specified NEC
  vitreous (humor) —*see* Deposit, crystalline

Osteitis —*see also* Osteomyelitis
  alveolar M27.3
  condensans M85.30
    ankle M85.37-
    foot M85.37-

Osteitis *(continued)*
- condensans *(continued)*
  - forearm M85.33-
  - hand M85.34-
  - lower leg M85.36-
  - multiple site M85.39
  - neck M85.38
  - rib M85.38
  - shoulder M85.31-
  - skull M85.38
  - specified site NEC M85.38
  - thigh M85.35-
  - toe M85.37-
  - upper arm M85.32-
  - vertebra M85.38
- deformans M88.9
  - malignant neoplasm of bone C41.9 *[M90.60]*
  - neoplastic disease (*see also* Neoplasm) D49.9 *[M90.60]*
    - carpus D49.9 *[M90.64-]*
    - clavicle D49.9 *[M90.61-]*
    - femur D49.9 *[M90.65-]*
    - fibula D49.9 *[M90.66-]*
    - finger D49.9 *[M90.64-]*
    - humerus D49.9 *[M90.62-]*
    - ilium D49.9 *[M90.65-]*
    - ischium D49.9 *[M90.65-]*
    - metacarpus D49.9 *[M90.64-]*
    - metatarsus D49.9 *[M90.67-]*
    - multiple sites D49.9 *[M90.69]*
    - neck D49.9 *[M90.68]*
    - radius D49.9 *[M90.63-]*
    - rib D49.9 *[M90.68]*
    - scapula D49.9 *[M90.61-]*
    - skull D49.9 *[M90.68]*
    - tarsus D49.9 *[M90.67-]*
    - tibia D49.9 *[M90.66-]*
    - toe D49.9 *[M90.67-]*
    - ulna D49.9 *[M90.63-]*
    - vertebra D49.9 *[M90.68]*
  - skull M88.0
  - specified NEC *—see* Paget's disease, bone, by site
  - vertebra M88.1
- due to yaws A66.6
- fibrosa NEC *—see* Cyst, bone, by site
  - circumscripta *—see* Dysplasia, fibrous, bone NEC
  - cystica (generalisata) E21.0
  - disseminata Q78.1
  - osteoplastica E21.0
- fragilitans Q78.0
- Garr's (sclerosing) *—see* Osteomyelitis, specified type NEC
- jaw (acute) (chronic) (lower) (suppurative) (upper) M27.2
- parathyroid E21.0
- petrous bone (acute) (chronic) *—see* Petrositis
- sclerotic, nonsuppurative *—see* Osteomyelitis, specified type NEC
- tuberculosa A18.09
  - cystica D86.89
  - multiplex cystoides D86.89

Osteoarthritis M19.90
- ankle M19.07-
- elbow M19.02-
- foot joint M19.07-
- generalized (multiple joints) M15.9
  - erosive M15.4
  - primary M15.0
  - specified NEC M15.8
- hand joint M19.04-
  - first carpometacarpal joint M18.9
- hip M16.1-
  - bilateral M16.0
  - due to hip dysplasia (unilateral) M16.3-
    - bilateral M16.2
- interphalangeal
  - distal (Heberden) M15.1
  - proximal (Bouchard) M15.2
- knee M17.1-
  - bilateral M17.0
- post-traumatic NEC M19.92
  - ankle M19.17-
  - elbow M19.12-
  - foot joint M19.17-
  - hand joint M19.14-
    - first carpometacarpal joint M18.3-
      - bilateral M18.2
  - hip M16.5-
    - bilateral M16.4
  - knee M17.3-
    - bilateral M17.2
  - shoulder M19.11-
  - specified site NEC M19.19
  - wrist M19.13-
- primary M19.91
  - ankle M19.07-
  - elbow M19.02-
  - foot joint M19.07-
  - hand joint M19.04-
    - first carpometacarpal joint M18.1-
      - bilateral M18.0
  - hip M16.1-
    - bilateral M16.0
  - knee M17.1-
    - bilateral M17.0
  - multiple sites M15.9
  - shoulder M19.01-
  - spine *—see* Spondylosis
  - wrist M19.03-
- secondary M19.93
  - ankle M19.27-
  - elbow M19.22-
  - foot joint M19.27-
  - hand joint M19.24-
    - first carpometacarpal joint M18.5-
      - bilateral M18.4
  - hip M16.7
    - bilateral M16.6
  - knee M17.5
    - bilateral M17.4
  - multiple M15.3
  - shoulder M19.21-
  - specified site NEC M19.29
  - spine *—see* Spondylosis
  - wrist M19.23-
- shoulder M19.01-
- specified site NEC M19.09
- spine *—see* Spondylosis
- wrist M19.03-

Osteoarthropathy (hypertrophic) M19.90
- ankle *—see* Osteoarthritis, primary, ankle
- elbow *—see* Osteoarthritis, primary, elbow
- foot joint *—see* Osteoarthritis, primary, foot
- hand joint *—see* Osteoarthritis, primary, hand joint
- knee joint *—see* Osteoarthritis, primary, knee
- multiple site *—see* Osteoarthritis, primary, multiple joint
- pulmonary *—see also* Osteoarthropathy, specified type NEC
  - hypertrophic *—see* Osteoarthropathy, hypertrophic, specified type NEC
- secondary hypertrophic *—see* Osteoarthropathy, specified type NEC
- shoulder *—see* Osteoarthritis, primary, shoulder
- specified joint NEC *—see* Osteoarthritis, primary, specified joint NEC
- specified type NEC M89.40
  - carpus M89.44-
  - clavicle M89.41-
  - femur M89.45-
  - fibula M89.46-
  - finger M89.44-
  - humerus M89.42-
  - ilium M89.459
  - ischium M89.459
  - metacarpus M89.44-
  - metatarsus M89.47-
  - multiple sites M89.49
  - neck M89.48
  - radius M89.43-
  - rib M89.48
  - scapula M89.41-
  - skull M89.48
  - tarsus M89.47-
  - tibia M89.46-
  - toe M89.47-
  - ulna M89.43-
  - vertebra M89.48
- secondary *—see* Osteoarthropathy, specified type NEC
- spine *—see* Spondylosis
- wrist *—see* Osteoarthritis, primary, wrist

Osteoarthrosis (degenerative) (hypertrophic) (joint) *—see also* Osteoarthritis
- deformans alkaptonurica E70.29 *[M36.8]*
- erosive M15.4
- generalized M15.9
  - primary M15.0
- polyarticular M15.9
- spine *—see* Spondylosis

Osteoblastoma *—see* Neoplasm, bone, benign
- aggressive *—see* Neoplasm, bone, uncertain behavior

Osteochondroarthrosis deformans endemica *—see* Disease, Kaschin-Beck

Osteochondritis *—see also* Osteochondropathy, by site
- Brailsford's *—see* Osteochondrosis, juvenile, radius
- dissecans M93.20
  - ankle M93.27-
  - elbow M93.22-
  - foot M93.27-
  - hand M93.24-
  - hip M93.25-
  - knee M93.26-
  - multiple sites M93.29
  - shoulder joint M93.21-
  - specified site NEC M93.28
  - wrist M93.23-
- juvenile M92.9
  - patellar *—see* Osteochondrosis, juvenile, patella
- syphilitic (congenital) (early) A50.02 *[M90.80]*
  - ankle A50.02 *[M90.87-]*
  - elbow A50.02 *[M90.82-]*
  - foot A50.02 *[M90.87-]*
  - forearm A50.02 *[M90.83-]*
  - hand A50.02 *[M90.84-]*
  - hip A50.02 *[M90.85-]*
  - knee A50.02 *[M90.86-]*
  - multiple sites A50.02 *[M90.89]*
  - shoulder joint A50.02 *[M90.81-]*
  - specified site NEC A50.02 *[M90.88]*

Osteochondrodysplasia Q78.9
- with defects of growth of tubular bones and spine Q77.9
  - specified NEC Q77.8
- specified NEC Q78.8

Osteochondrodystrophy E78.9

Osteochondrolysis *—see* Osteochondritis, dissecans

Osteochondroma *—see* Neoplasm, bone, benign

Osteochondromatosis D48.0
- syndrome Q78.4

Osteochondromyxosarcoma *—see* Neoplasm, bone, malignant

Osteochondropathy M93.90
- ankle M93.97-
- elbow M93.92-
- foot M93.97-
- hand M93.94-
- hip M93.95-
- Kienböck's disease of adults M93.1
- knee M93.96-
- multiple joints M93.99
- osteochondritis dissecans *—see* Osteochondritis, dissecans
- osteochondrosis *—see* Osteochondrosis
- shoulder region M93.91-
- slipped upper femoral epiphysis *—see* Slipped, epiphysis, upper femoral
- specified joint NEC M93.98
- specified type NEC M93.80
  - ankle M93.87-
  - elbow M93.82-
  - foot M93.87-
  - hand M93.84-
  - hip M93.85-
  - knee M93.86-
  - multiple joints M93.89
  - shoulder region M93.81-
  - specified joint NEC M93.88
  - wrist M93.83-
- syphilitic, congenital
  - early A50.02 *[M90.80]*
  - late A50.56 *[M90.80]*
- wrist M93.93-

Osteochondrosarcoma *—see* Neoplasm, bone, malignant

Osteochondrosis *—see also* Osteochondropathy, by site
- acetabulum (juvenile) M91.0
- adult *—see* Osteochondropathy, specified type NEC, by site
- astragalus (juvenile) *—see* Osteochondrosis, juvenile, tarsus
- Blount M92.51-
- Buchanan's M91.0
- Burns' *—see* Osteochondrosis, juvenile, ulna
- calcaneus (juvenile) *—see* Osteochondrosis, juvenile, tarsus
- capitular epiphysis (femur) (juvenile) *—see* Legg-Calvé-Perthes disease

Osteochondrosis *(continued)*
- carpal (juvenile) (lunate) (scaphoid) *—see* Osteochondrosis, juvenile, hand, carpal lunate
  - adult M93.1
- coxae juvenilis *—see* Legg-Calvé-Perthes disease
- deformans juvenilis, coxae *—see* Legg-Calvé-Perthes disease
- Diaz's *—see* Osteochondrosis, juvenile, tarsus
- dissecans (knee) (shoulder) *—see* Osteochondritis, dissecans
- femoral capital epiphysis (juvenile) *—see* Legg-Calvé-Perthes disease
- femur (head), juvenile *—see* Legg-Calvé-Perthes disease
- fibula (juvenile) *—see* Osteochondrosis, juvenile, fibula
- foot NEC (juvenile) M92.8
- Freiberg's *—see* Osteochondrosis, juvenile, metatarsus
- Haas' (juvenile) *—see* Osteochondrosis, juvenile, humerus
- Haglund's *—see* Osteochondrosis, juvenile, tarsus
- hip (juvenile) *—see* Legg-Calvé-Perthes disease
- humerus (capitulum) (head) (juvenile) *—see* Osteochondrosis, juvenile, humerus
- ilium, iliac crest (juvenile) M91.0
- ischiopubic synchondrosis M91.0
- Iselin's *—see* Osteochondrosis, juvenile, metatarsus
- juvenile, juvenilis M92.9
  - after congenital dislocation of hip reduction *—see* Osteochondrosis, juvenile, hip, specified NEC
  - arm *—see* Osteochondrosis, juvenile, upper limb NEC
  - capitular epiphysis (femur) *—see* Legg-Calvé-Perthes disease
  - clavicle, sternal epiphysis *—see* Osteochondrosis, juvenile, upper limb NEC
  - coxae *—see* Legg-Calvé-Perthes disease
  - deformans M92.9
  - fibula M92.50-
  - foot NEC M92.8
  - hand M92.20-
    - carpal lunate M92.21-
    - metacarpal head M92.22-
    - specified site NEC M92.29-
  - head of femur *—see* Legg-Calvé-Perthes disease
  - hip and pelvis M91.9-
    - coxa plana *—see* Coxa, plana
    - femoral head *—see* Legg-Calvé-Perthes disease
    - pelvis M91.0
    - pseudocoxalgia *—see* Pseudocoxalgia
    - specified NEC M91.8-
  - humerus M92.0-
  - limb
    - lower NEC M92.8
    - upper NEC *—see* Osteochondrosis, juvenile, upper limb NEC
  - medial cuneiform bone *—see* Osteochondrosis, juvenile, tarsus
  - metatarsus M92.7-
  - patella M92.4-
  - radius M92.1-
  - specified
    - site NEC M92.8
    - type NEC M92.8
      - tibia and fibula M92.59-
  - spine M42.00
    - cervical region M42.02
    - cervicothoracic region M42.03
    - lumbar region M42.06
    - lumbosacral region M42.07
    - multiple sites M42.09
    - occipito-atlanto-axial region M42.01
    - sacrococcygeal region M42.08
    - thoracic region M42.04
    - thoracolumbar region M42.05
  - tarsus M92.6-
  - tibia M92.50-
    - proximal M92.51-
    - tubercle M92.52-
  - ulna M92.1-
  - upper limb NEC M92.3-
  - vertebra (body) (epiphyseal plates) (Calvé's) (Scheuermann's) *—see* Osteochondrosis, juvenile, spine
- Kienböck's *—see* Osteochondrosis, juvenile, hand, carpal lunate
  - adult M93.1
- Köhler's
  - patellar *—see* Osteochondrosis, juvenile, patella
  - tarsal navicular *—see* Osteochondrosis, juvenile, tarsus
- Legg-Perthes (-Calvé) (-Waldenström) *—see* Legg-Calvé-Perthes disease
- limb
  - lower NEC (juvenile) M92.8
    - tibia and fibula M92.59-
  - upper NEC (juvenile) *—see* Osteochondrosis, juvenile, upper limb NEC
- lunate bone (carpal) (juvenile) *—see also* Osteochondrosis, juvenile, hand, carpal lunate
  - adult M93.1
- Mauclaire's *—see* Osteochondrosis, juvenile, hand, metacarpal
- metacarpal (head) (juvenile) *—see* Osteochondrosis, juvenile, hand, metacarpal
- metatarsus (fifth) (head) (juvenile) (second) *—see* Osteochondrosis, juvenile, metatarsus
- navicular (juvenile) *—see* Osteochondrosis, juvenile, tarsus
- os
  - calcis (juvenile) *—see* Osteochondrosis, juvenile, tarsus
  - tibiale externum (juvenile) *—see* Osteochondrosis, juvenile, tarsus
- Osgood-Schlatter M92.52-
- Panner's *—see* Osteochondrosis, juvenile, humerus
- patellar center (juvenile) (primary) (secondary) *—see* Osteochondrosis, juvenile, patella
- pelvis (juvenile) M91.0
- Pierson's M91.0
- radius (head) (juvenile) *—see* Osteochondrosis, juvenile, radius
- Scheuermann's *—see* Osteochondrosis, juvenile, spine
- Sever's *—see* Osteochondrosis, juvenile, tarsus
- Sinding-Larsen *—see* Osteochondrosis, juvenile, patella
- spine M42.9
  - adult M42.10
    - cervical region M42.12
    - cervicothoracic region M42.13
    - lumbar region M42.16
    - lumbosacral region M42.17
    - multiple sites M42.19
    - occipito-atlanto-axial region M42.11
    - sacrococcygeal region M42.18
    - thoracic region M42.14
    - thoracolumbar region M42.15
  - juvenile *—see* Osteochondrosis, juvenile, spine
- symphysis pubis (juvenile) M91.0
- syphilitic (congenital) A50.02
- talus (juvenile) *—see* Osteochondrosis, juvenile, tarsus
- tarsus (navicular) (juvenile) *—see* Osteochondrosis, juvenile, tarsus
- tibia (proximal) (tubercle) (juvenile) *—see* Osteochondrosis, juvenile, tibia
- tuberculous *—see* Tuberculosis, bone
- ulna (lower) (juvenile) *—see* Osteochondrosis, juvenile, ulna
- van Neck's M91.0
- vertebral *—see* Osteochondrosis, spine

Osteoclastoma D48.0
- malignant *—see* Neoplasm, bone, malignant

Osteodynia *—see* Disorder, bone, specified type NEC

Osteodystrophy Q78.9
- azotemic N25.0
- congenital Q78.9
- parathyroid, secondary E21.1
- renal N25.0

Osteofibroma *—see* Neoplasm, bone, benign

Osteofibrosarcoma *—see* Neoplasm, bone, malignant

Osteogenesis imperfecta Q78.0

Osteogenic *—see* condition

Osteolysis M89.50
- carpus M89.54-
- clavicle M89.51-
- femur M89.55-
- fibula M89.56-
- finger M89.54-
- humerus M89.52-
- ilium M89.559
- ischium M89.559
- joint prosthesis (periprosthetic) *—see* Complications, joint prosthesis, mechanical, periprosthetic, osteolysis, by site
- metacarpus M89.54-
- metatarsus M89.57-
- multiple sites M89.59
- neck M89.58
- periprosthetic *—see* Complications, joint prosthesis, mechanical, periprosthetic, osteolysis, by site
- radius M89.53-
- rib M89.58
- scapula M89.51-
- skull M89.58
- tarsus M89.57-
- tibia M89.56-
- toe M89.57-
- ulna M89.53-
- vertebra M89.58

Osteoma *—see also* Neoplasm, bone, benign
- osteoid *—see also* Neoplasm, bone, benign
  - giant *—see* Neoplasm, bone, benign

Osteomalacia M83.9
- adult M83.9
  - drug-induced NEC M83.5
  - due to
    - malabsorption (postsurgical) M83.2
    - malnutrition M83.3
  - specified NEC M83.8
- aluminium-induced M83.4
- infantile *—see* Rickets
- juvenile *—see* Rickets
- oncogenic E83.89
- pelvis M83.8
- puerperal M83.0
- senile M83.1
- vitamin-D-resistant in adults E83.31 *[M90.8-]*
  - carpus E83.31 *[M90.84-]*
  - clavicle E83.31 *[M90.81-]*
  - femur E83.31 *[M90.85-]*
  - fibula E83.31 *[M90.86-]*
  - finger E83.31 *[M90.84-]*
  - humerus E83.31 *[M90.82-]*
  - ilium E83.31 *[M90.859]*
  - ischium E83.31 *[M90.859]*
  - metacarpus E83.31 *[M90.84-]*
  - metatarsus E83.31 *[M90.87-]*
  - multiple sites E83.31 *[M90.89]*
  - neck E83.31 *[M90.88]*
  - radius E83.31 *[M90.83-]*
  - rib E83.31 *[M90.88]*
  - scapula E83.31 *[M90.819]*
  - skull E83.31 *[M90.88]*
  - tarsus E83.31 *[M90.879]*
  - tibia E83.31 *[M90.869]*
  - toe E83.31 *[M90.879]*
  - ulna E83.31 *[M90.839]*
  - vertebra E83.31 *[M90.88]*

Osteomyelitis (general) (infective) (localized) (neonatal) (purulent) (septic) (staphylococcal) (streptococcal) (suppurative) (with periostitis) M86.9
- acute M86.10
  - carpus M86.14-
  - clavicle M86.11-
  - femur M86.15-
  - fibula M86.16-
  - finger M86.14-
  - hematogenous M86.00
    - carpus M86.04-
    - clavicle M86.01-
    - femur M86.05-
    - fibula M86.06-
    - finger M86.04-
    - humerus M86.02-
    - ilium M86.08
    - ischium M86.08
    - mandible M27.2
    - metacarpus M86.04-
    - metatarsus M86.07-
    - multiple sites M86.09
    - neck M86.08
    - orbit H05.02-
    - petrous bone *—see* Petrositis
    - radius M86.03-
    - rib M86.08
    - scapula M86.01-
    - skull M86.08
    - tarsus M86.07-
    - tibia M86.06-
    - toe M86.07-

Osteomyelitis *(continued)*
- acute *(continued)*
  - hematogenous *(continued)*
    - ulna M86.03-
    - vertebra *—see* Osteomyelitis, vertebra
  - humerus M86.12-
  - ilium M86.18
  - ischium M86.18
  - mandible M27.2
  - metacarpus M86.14-
  - metatarsus M86.17-
  - multiple sites M86.19
  - neck M86.18
  - orbit H05.02-
  - petrous bone *—see* Petrositis
  - radius M86.13-
  - rib M86.18
  - scapula M86.11-
  - skull M86.18
  - tarsus M86.17-
  - tibia M86.16-
  - toe M86.17-
  - ulna M86.13-
  - vertebra *—see* Osteomyelitis, vertebra
- chronic (or old) M86.60
  - with draining sinus M86.40
    - carpus M86.44-
    - clavicle M86.41-
    - femur M86.45-
    - fibula M86.46-
    - finger M86.44-
    - humerus M86.42-
    - ilium M86.459
    - ischium M86.459
    - mandible M27.2
    - metacarpus M86.44-
    - metatarsus M86.47-
    - multiple sites M86.49
    - neck M86.48
    - orbit H05.02-
    - petrous bone *—see* Petrositis
    - radius M86.43-
    - rib M86.48
    - scapula M86.41-
    - skull M86.48
    - tarsus M86.47-
    - tibia M86.46-
    - toe M86.47-
    - ulna M86.43-
    - vertebra *—see* Osteomyelitis, vertebra
  - carpus M86.64-
  - clavicle M86.61-
  - femur M86.65-
  - fibula M86.66-
  - finger M86.64-
  - hematogenous NEC M86.50
    - carpus M86.54-
    - clavicle M86.51-
    - femur M86.55-
    - fibula M86.56-
    - finger M86.54-
    - humerus M86.52-
    - ilium M86.559
    - ischium M86.559
    - mandible M27.2
    - metacarpus M86.54-
    - metatarsus M86.57-
    - multifocal M86.30
      - carpus M86.34-
      - clavicle M86.31-
      - femur M86.35-
      - fibula M86.36-
      - finger M86.34-
      - humerus M86.32-
      - ilium M86.359
      - ischium M86.359
      - metacarpus M86.34-

Osteomyelitis *(continued)*
- chronic *(continued)*
  - hematogenous NEC *(continued)*
    - multifocal *(continued)*
      - metatarsus M86.37-
      - multiple sites M86.39
      - neck M86.38
      - radius M86.33-
      - rib M86.38
      - scapula M86.31-
      - skull M86.38
      - tarsus M86.37-
      - tibia M86.36-
      - toe M86.37-
      - ulna M86.33-
      - vertebra *—see* Osteomyelitis, vertebra
    - multiple sites M86.59
    - neck M86.58
    - orbit H05.02-
    - petrous bone *—see* Petrositis
    - radius M86.53-
    - rib M86.58
    - scapula M86.51-
    - skull M86.58
    - tarsus M86.57-
    - tibia M86.56-
    - toe M86.57-
    - ulna M86.53-
    - vertebra *—see* Osteomyelitis, vertebra
  - humerus M86.62-
  - ilium M86.659
  - ischium M86.659
  - mandible M27.2
  - metacarpus M86.64-
  - metatarsus M86.67-
  - multifocal *—see* Osteomyelitis, chronic, hematogenous, multifocal
  - multiple sites M86.69
  - neck M86.68
  - orbit H05.02-
  - petrous bone *—see* Petrositis
  - radius M86.63-
  - rib M86.68
  - scapula M86.61-
  - skull M86.68
  - tarsus M86.67-
  - tibia M86.66-
  - toe M86.67-
  - ulna M86.63-
  - vertebra *—see* Osteomyelitis, vertebra
- echinococcal B67.2
- Garr's *—see* Osteomyelitis, specified type NEC
- in diabetes mellitus *—see* E08-E13 with .69
- jaw (acute) (chronic) (lower) (neonatal) (suppurative) (upper) M27.2
- nonsuppurating *—see* Osteomyelitis, specified type NEC
- orbit H05.02-
- petrous bone *—see* Petrositis
- Salmonella (arizonae) (cholerae-suis) (enteritidis) (typhimurium) A02.24
- sclerosing, nonsuppurative *—see* Osteomyelitis, specified type NEC
- specified type NEC (*see also* subcategory) M86.8X-
  - mandible M27.2
  - orbit H05.02-
  - petrous bone *—see* Petrositis
  - vertebra *—see* Osteomyelitis, vertebra

Osteomyelitis *(continued)*
- subacute M86.20
  - carpus M86.24-
  - clavicle M86.21-
  - femur M86.25-
  - fibula M86.26-
  - finger M86.24-
  - humerus M86.22-
  - mandible M27.2
  - metacarpus M86.24-
  - metatarsus M86.27-
  - multiple sites M86.29
  - neck M86.28
  - orbit H05.02-
  - petrous bone *—see* Petrositis
  - radius M86.23-
  - rib M86.28
  - scapula M86.21-
  - skull M86.28
  - tarsus M86.27-
  - tibia M86.26-
  - toe M86.27-
  - ulna M86.23-
  - vertebra *—see* Osteomyelitis, vertebra
- syphilitic A52.77
  - congenital (early) A50.02 *[M90.80]*
- tuberculous *—see* Tuberculosis, bone
- typhoid A01.05
- vertebra M46.20
  - cervical region M46.22
  - cervicothoracic region M46.23
  - lumbar region M46.26
  - lumbosacral region M46.27
  - occipito-atlanto-axial region M46.21
  - sacrococcygeal region M46.28
  - thoracic region M46.24
  - thoracolumbar region M46.25

Osteomyelofibrosis D47.4

Osteomyelosclerosis D75.89

Osteonecrosis M87.9
- due to
  - drugs *—see* Osteonecrosis, secondary, due to, drugs
  - trauma *—see* Osteonecrosis, secondary, due to, trauma
- idiopathic aseptic M87.00
  - ankle M87.07-
  - carpus M87.03-
  - clavicle M87.01-
  - femur M87.05-
  - fibula M87.06-
  - finger M87.04-
  - humerus M87.02-
  - ilium M87.050
  - ischium M87.050
  - metacarpus M87.04-
  - metatarsus M87.07-
  - multiple sites M87.09
  - neck M87.08
  - pelvis M87.050
  - radius M87.03-
  - rib M87.08
  - scapula M87.01-
  - skull M87.08
  - tarsus M87.07-
  - tibia M87.06-
  - toe M87.07-
  - ulna M87.03-
  - vertebra M87.08
- secondary NEC M87.30
  - carpus M87.33-
  - clavicle M87.31-
  - due to
    - drugs M87.10
      - carpus M87.13-
      - clavicle M87.11-

Osteonecrosis *(continued)*
- secondary NEC *(continued)*
  - due to *(continued)*
    - drugs *(continued)*
      - femur M87.15-
      - fibula M87.16-
      - finger M87.14-
      - humerus M87.12-
      - ilium M87.159
      - ischium M87.159
      - jaw M87.180
      - metacarpus M87.14-
      - metatarsus M87.17-
      - multiple sites M87.19
      - neck M87.18
      - radius M87.13-
      - rib M87.18
      - scapula M87.11-
      - skull M87.18
      - tarsus M87.17-
      - tibia M87.16-
      - toe M87.17-
      - ulna M87.13-
      - vertebra M87.18
    - hemoglobinopathy NEC D58.2 *[M90.50]*
      - carpus D58.2 *[M90.54-]*
      - clavicle D58.2 *[M90.51-]*
      - femur D58.2 *[M90.55-]*
      - fibula D58.2 *[M90.56-]*
      - finger D58.2 *[M90.54-]*
      - humerus D58.2 *[M90.52-]*
      - ilium D58.2 *[M90.55-]*
      - ischium D58.2 *[M90.55-]*
      - metacarpus D58.2 *[M90.54-]*
      - metatarsus D58.2 *[M90.57-]*
      - multiple sites D58.2 *[M90.58]*
      - neck D58.2 *[M90.58]*
      - radius D58.2 *[M90.53-]*
      - rib D58.2 *[M90.58]*
      - scapula D58.2 *[M90.51-]*
      - skull D58.2 *[M90.58]*
      - tarsus D58.2 *[M90.57-]*
      - tibia D58.2 *[M90.56-]*
      - toe D58.2 *[M90.57-]*
      - ulna D58.2 *[M90.53-]*
      - vertebra D58.2 *[M90.58]*
    - trauma (previous) M87.20
      - carpus M87.23-
      - clavicle M87.21-
      - femur M87.25-
      - fibula M87.26-
      - finger M87.24-
      - humerus M87.22-
      - ilium M87.25-
      - ischium M87.25-
      - metacarpus M87.24-
      - metatarsus M87.27-
      - multiple sites M87.29
      - neck M87.28
      - radius M87.23-
      - rib M87.28
      - scapula M87.21-
      - skull M87.28
      - tarsus M87.27-
      - tibia M87.26-
      - toe M87.27-
      - ulna M87.23-
      - vertebra M87.28
  - femur M87.35-
  - fibula M87.36-
  - finger M87.34-
  - humerus M87.32-
  - ilium M87.350
  - in
    - caisson disease T70.3 *[M90.50]*
      - carpus T70.3 *[M90.54-]*
      - clavicle T70.3 *[M90.51-]*
      - femur T70.3 *[M90.55-]*

Osteonecrosis *(continued)*
secondary NEC *(continued)*
in *(continued)*
caisson disease *(continued)*
fibula T70.3 *[M90.56-]*
finger T70.3 *[M90.54-]*
humerus T70.3 *[M90.52-]*
ilium T70.3 *[M90.55-]*
ischium T70.3 *[M90.55-]*
metacarpus T70.3 *[M90.54-]*
metatarsus T70.3 *[M90.57-]*
multiple sites T70.3 *[M90.59]*
neck T70.3 *[M90.58]*
radius T70.3 *[M90.53-]*
rib T70.3 *[M90.58]*
scapula T70.3 *[M90.51-]*
skull T70.3 *[M90.58]*
tarsus T70.3 *[M90.57-]*
tibia T70.3 *[M90.56-]*
toe T70.3 *[M90.57-]*
ulna T70.3 *[M90.53-]*
vertebra T70.3 *[M90.58]*
ischium M87.350
metacarpus M87.34-
metatarsus M87.37-
multiple site M87.39
neck M87.38
radius M87.33-
rib M87.38
scapula M87.319
skull M87.38
tarsus M87.379
tibia M87.366
toe M87.379
ulna M87.33-
vertebra M87.38
specified type NEC M87.80
carpus M87.83-
clavicle M87.81-
femur M87.85-
fibula M87.86-
finger M87.84-
humerus M87.82-
ilium M87.85-
ischium M87.85-
metacarpus M87.84-
metatarsus M87.87-
multiple sites M87.89
neck M87.88
radius M87.83-
rib M87.88
scapula M87.81-
skull M87.88
tarsus M87.87-
tibia M87.86-
toe M87.87-
ulna M87.83-
vertebra M87.88

Osteo-onycho-arthro-dysplasia Q87.2

Osteo-onychodysplasia, hereditary Q87.2

Osteopathia condensans disseminata Q78.8

Osteopathy —*see also* Osteomyelitis, Osteonecrosis, Osteoporosis
after poliomyelitis M89.60
carpus M89.64-
clavicle M89.61-
femur M89.65-
fibula M89.66-
finger M89.64-
humerus M89.62-
ilium M89.659
ischium M89.659
metacarpus M89.64-
metatarsus M89.67-
multiple sites M89.69

Osteopathy *(continued)*
after poliomyelitis *(continued)*
neck M89.68
radius M89.63-
rib M89.68
scapula M89.61-
skull M89.68
tarsus M89.67-
tibia M89.66-
toe M89.67-
ulna M89.63-
vertebra M89.68
in (due to)
renal osteodystrophy N25.0
specified diseases classified elsewhere M90.8

Osteopenia M85.8-
borderline M85.8-

Osteoperiostitis —*see* Osteomyelitis, specified type NEC

Osteopetrosis (familial) Q78.2

Osteophyte M25.70
ankle M25.77-
elbow M25.72-
foot joint M25.77-
hand joint M25.74-
hip M25.75-
knee M25.76-
shoulder M25.71-
spine M25.78
vertebrae M25.78
wrist M25.73-

Osteopoikilosis Q78.8

Osteoporosis (female) (male) M81.0
with current pathological fracture M80.00
age-related M81.0
with current pathologic fracture M80.00
carpus M80.04-
clavicle M80.01-
fibula M80.06-
finger M80.04-
humerus M80.02-
ilium M80.05-
ischium M80.05-
metacarpus M80.04-
metatarsus M80.07-
pelvis M80.05-
radius M80.03-
scapula M80.01-
specified site NEC M80.0A
tarsus M80.07-
tibia M80.06-
toe M80.07-
ulna M80.03-
vertebra M80.08
disuse M81.8
with current pathological fracture M80.80
carpus M80.84-
clavicle M80.81-
fibula M80.86-
finger M80.84-
humerus M80.82-
ilium M80.85-
ischium M80.85-
metacarpus M80.84-
metatarsus M80.87-
pelvis M80.85-
radius M80.83-
scapula M80.81-
specified site NEC M80.8A
tarsus M80.87-
tibia M80.86-
toe M80.87-
ulna M80.83-
vertebra M80.88

Osteoporosis *(continued)*
drug-induced —*see* Osteoporosis, specified type NEC
idiopathic —*see* Osteoporosis, specified type NEC
involutional —*see* Osteoporosis, age-related
Lequesne M81.6
localized M81.6
postmenopausal M81.0
with pathological fracture M80.00
carpus M80.04-
clavicle M80.01-
fibula M80.06-
finger M80.04-
humerus M80.02-
ilium M80.05-
ischium M80.05-
metacarpus M80.04-
metatarsus M80.07-
pelvis M80.05-
radius M80.03-
scapula M80.01-
specified site NEC M80.0A
tarsus M80.07-
tibia M80.06-
toe M80.07-
ulna M80.03-
vertebra M80.08
postoophorectomy —*see* Osteoporosis, specified type NEC
postsurgical malabsorption —*see* Osteoporosis, specified type NEC
post-traumatic —*see* Osteoporosis, specified type NEC
senile —*see* Osteoporosis, age-related
specified type NEC M81.8
with pathological fracture M80.80
carpus M80.84-
clavicle M80.81-
fibula M80.86-
finger M80.84-
humerus M80.82-
ilium M80.85-
ischium M80.85-
metacarpus M80.84-
metatarsus M80.87-
pelvis M80.85-
radius M80.83-
scapula M80.81-
specified site NEC M80.8A
tarsus M80.87-
tibia M80.86-
toe M80.87-
ulna M80.83-
vertebra M80.88

Osteopsathyrosis (idiopathica) Q78.0

Osteoradionecrosis, jaw (acute) (chronic) (lower) (suppurative) (upper) M27.2

Osteosarcoma (any form) —*see* Neoplasm, bone, malignant

Osteosclerosis Q78.2
acquired M85.8-
congenita Q77.4
fragilitas (generalisata) Q78.2
myelofibrosis D75.81

Osteosclerotic anemia D64.89

Osteosis
cutis L94.2
renal fibrocystic N25.0

Österreicher-Turner syndrome Q87.2

Ostium
atrioventriculare commune Q21.2
primum (arteriosum) (defect) (persistent) Q21.2
secundum (arteriosum) (defect) (patent) (persistent) Q21.1

Ostrum-Furst syndrome Q75.8

Otalgia —*see* subcategory H92.0

Otitis (acute) H66.90
with effusion —*see also* Otitis, media, nonsuppurative
purulent —*see* Otitis, media, suppurative
adhesive H74.1
chronic —*see also* Otitis, media, chronic
with effusion —*see also* Otitis, media, nonsuppurative, chronic
externa H60.9-
abscess —*see* Abscess, ear, external
acute (noninfective) H60.50-
actinic H60.51-
chemical H60.52-
contact H60.53-
eczematoid H60.54-
infective —*see* Otitis, externa, infective
reactive H60.55-
specified NEC H60.59-
cellulitis —*see* Cellulitis, ear
chronic H60.6-
diffuse —*see* Otitis, externa, infective, diffuse
hemorrhagic —*see* Otitis, externa, infective, hemorrhagic
in (due to)
aspergillosis B44.89
candidiasis B37.84
erysipelas A46 *[H62.40]*
herpes (simplex) virus infection B00.1
zoster B02.8
impetigo L01.00 *[H62.40]*
infectious disease NEC B99 *[H62.4-]*
mycosis NEC B36.9 *[H62.40]*
parasitic disease NEC B89 *[H62.40]*
viral disease NEC B34.9 *[H62.40]*
zoster B02.8
infective NEC H60.39-
abscess —*see* Abscess, ear, external
cellulitis —*see* Cellulitis, ear
diffuse H60.31-
hemorrhagic H60.32-
swimmer's ear —*see* Swimmer's, ear
malignant H60.2-
mycotic NEC B36.9 *[H62.40]*
in
aspergillosis B44.89
candidiasis B37.84
moniliasis B37.84
necrotizing —*see* Otitis, externa, malignant
Pseudomonas aeruginosa —*see* Otitis, externa, malignant
reactive —*see* Otitis, externa, acute, reactive
specified NEC —*see* subcategory H60.8
tropical NEC B36.9 *[H62.40]*
in
aspergillosis B44.89
candidiasis B37.84
moniliasis B37.84
insidiosa —*see* Otosclerosis
interna —*see* subcategory H83.0
media (hemorrhagic) (staphylococcal) (streptococcal) H66.9-

Otitis *(continued)*
- media *(continued)*
  - with effusion (nonpurulent) —*see* Otitis, media, nonsuppurative
  - acute, subacute H66.90
    - allergic —*see* Otitis, media, nonsuppurative, acute, allergic
    - exudative —*see* Otitis, media, suppurative, acute
    - mucoid —*see* Otitis, media, nonsuppurative, acute
    - necrotizing —*see also* Otitis, media, suppurative, acute
      - in
        - measles B05.3
        - scarlet fever A38.0
    - nonsuppurative NEC —*see* Otitis, media, nonsuppurative, acute
    - purulent —*see* Otitis, media, suppurative, acute
    - sanguinous —*see* Otitis, media, nonsuppurative, acute
    - secretory —*see* Otitis, media, nonsuppurative, acute, serous
    - seromucinous —*see* Otitis, media, nonsuppurative, acute
    - serous —*see* Otitis, media, nonsuppurative, acute, serous
    - suppurative —*see* Otitis, media, suppurative, acute
  - allergic —*see* Otitis, media, nonsuppurative
  - catarrhal —*see* Otitis, media, nonsuppurative
  - chronic H66.90
    - with effusion (nonpurulent) —*see* Otitis, media, nonsuppurative, chronic
    - allergic —*see* Otitis, media, nonsuppurative, chronic, allergic
    - benign suppurative —*see* Otitis, media, suppurative, chronic, tubotympanic
    - catarrhal —*see* Otitis, media, nonsuppurative, chronic, serous
    - exudative —*see* Otitis, media, nonsuppurative, chronic
    - mucinous —*see* Otitis, media, nonsuppurative, chronic, mucoid
    - mucoid —*see* Otitis, media, nonsuppurative, chronic, mucoid
    - nonsuppurative NEC —*see* Otitis, media, nonsuppurative, chronic
    - purulent —*see* Otitis, media, suppurative, chronic
    - secretory —*see* Otitis, media, nonsuppurative, chronic, mucoid
    - seromucinous —*see* Otitis, media, nonsuppurative, chronic
    - serous —*see* Otitis, media, nonsuppurative, chronic, serous
    - suppurative —*see* Otitis, media, suppurative, chronic
    - transudative —*see* Otitis, media, nonsuppurative, chronic, mucoid

Otitis *(continued)*
- media *(continued)*
  - exudative —*see* Otitis, media, suppurative
  - in (due to) (with)
    - influenza —*see* Influenza, with, otitis media
    - measles B05.3
    - scarlet fever A38.0
    - tuberculosis A18.6
    - viral disease NEC B34.- *[H67.-]*
  - mucoid —*see* Otitis, media, nonsuppurative
  - nonsuppurative H65.9-
    - acute or subacute NEC H65.19-
      - allergic H65.11-
        - recurrent H65.11-
      - recurrent H65.19-
      - secretory —*see* Otitis, media, nonsuppurative, serous
      - serous H65.0-
        - recurrent H65.0-
    - chronic H65.49-
      - allergic H65.41-
      - mucoid H65.3-
      - serous H65.2-
  - postmeasles B05.3
  - purulent —*see* Otitis, media, suppurative
  - secretory —*see* Otitis, media, nonsuppurative
  - seromucinous —*see* Otitis, media, nonsuppurative
  - serous —*see* Otitis, media, nonsuppurative
  - suppurative H66.4-
    - acute H66.00-
      - with rupture of ear drum H66.01-
      - recurrent H66.00-
        - with rupture of ear drum H66.01-
    - chronic (*see also* subcategory) H66.3
      - atticoantral H66.2-
      - benign —*see* Otitis, media, suppurative, chronic, tubotympanic
      - tubotympanic H66.1-
  - transudative —*see* Otitis, media, nonsuppurative
  - tuberculous A18.6

Otocephaly Q18.2

Otolith syndrome —*see* subcategory H81.8

Otomycosis (diffuse) **NEC** B36.9 *[H62.40]*
- in
  - aspergillosis B44.89
  - candidiasis B37.84
  - moniliasis B37.84

Otoporosis —*see* Otosclerosis

Otorrhagia (nontraumatic) H92.2-
- traumatic - code by Type of injury

Otorrhea H92.1-
- cerebrospinal (fluid) G96.01
  - postoperative G96.08
  - specified NEC G96.08
  - spontaneous G96.01
  - traumatic G96.08

Otosclerosis (general) H80.9-
- cochlear (endosteal) H80.2-
- involving
  - otic capsule —*see* Otosclerosis, cochlear

Otosclerosis *(continued)*
- involving *(continued)*
  - oval window
    - nonobliterative H80.0-
    - obliterative H80.1-
  - round window —*see* Otosclerosis, cochlear
- nonobliterative —*see* Otosclerosis, involving, oval window, nonobliterative
- obliterative —*see* Otosclerosis, involving, oval window, obliterative
- specified NEC H80.8-

Otospongiosis —*see* Otosclerosis

Otto's disease or pelvis M24.7

Outcome of delivery Z37.9
- multiple births Z37.9
  - all liveborn Z37.50
    - quadruplets Z37.52
    - quintuplets Z37.53
    - sextuplets Z37.54
    - specified number NEC Z37.59
    - triplets Z37.51
  - all stillborn Z37.7
  - some liveborn Z37.60
    - quadruplets Z37.62
    - quintuplets Z37.63
    - sextuplets Z37.64
    - specified number NEC Z37.69
    - triplets Z37.61
- single NEC Z37.9
  - liveborn Z37.0
  - stillborn Z37.1
- twins NEC Z37.9
  - both liveborn Z37.2
  - both stillborn Z37.4
  - one liveborn, one stillborn Z37.3

Outlet —*see* condition

Ovalocytosis (congenital) (hereditary) —*see* Elliptocytosis

Ovarian —*see* Condition

Ovariocele N83.4-

Ovaritis (cystic) —*see* Oophoritis

Ovary, ovarian —*see also* condition
- resistant syndrome E28.39
- vein syndrome N13.8

Overactive —*see also* Hyperfunction
- adrenal cortex NEC E27.0
- bladder N32.81
- hypothalamus E23.3
- thyroid —*see* Hyperthyroidism

Overactivity R46.3
- child —*see* Disorder, attention-deficit hyperactivity

Overbite (deep) (excessive) (horizontal) (vertical) M26.29

Overbreathing —*see* Hyperventilation

Overconscientious personality F60.5

Overdevelopment —*see* Hypertrophy

Overdistension —*see* Distension

Overdose, overdosage (drug) —*see* Table of Drugs and Chemicals, by drug, poisoning

Overeating R63.2
- nonorganic origin F50.89
- psychogenic F50.89

Overexertion (effects) (exhaustion) T73.3

Overexposure (effects) T73.9
- exhaustion T73.2

Overfeeding —*see* Overeating
- newborn P92.4

Overfill, endodontic M27.52

Overgrowth, bone —*see* Hypertrophy, bone

Overhanging of dental restorative material (unrepairable) K08.52

Overheated (places) (effects) —*see* Heat

Overjet (excessive horizontal) M26.23

Overlaid, overlying (suffocation) —*see* Asphyxia, traumatic, due to mechanical threat

Overlap, excessive horizontal (teeth) M26.23

Overlapping toe (acquired) —*see also* Deformity, toe, specified NEC
- congenital (fifth toe) Q66.89

Overload
- circulatory, due to transfusion (blood) (blood components) (TACO) E87.71
- fluid E87.70
  - due to transfusion (blood) (blood components) E87.71
  - specified NEC E87.79
- iron, due to repeated red blood cell transfusions E83.111
- potassium (K) E87.5
- sodium (Na) E87.0

Overnutrition —*see* Hyperalimentation

Overproduction —*see also* Hypersecretion
- ACTH E27.0
- catecholamine E27.5
- growth hormone E22.0

Overprotection, child by parent Z62.1

Overriding
- aorta Q25.49
- finger (acquired) —*see* Deformity, finger
  - congenital Q68.1
- toe (acquired) —*see also* Deformity, toe, specified NEC
  - congenital Q66.89

Overstrained R53.83
- heart —*see* Hypertrophy, cardiac

Overuse, muscle NEC M70.8-

Overweight E66.3

Overworked R53.83

Oviduct —*see* condition

Ovotestis Q56.0

Ovulation (cycle)
- failure or lack of N97.0
- pain N94.0

Ovum —*see* condition

Owren's disease or syndrome (parahemophilia) D68.2

Ox heart —*see* Hypertrophy, cardiac

Oxalosis E72.53

Oxaluria E72.53

Oxycephaly, oxycephalic Q75.0
- syphilitic, congenital A50.02

Oxyuriasis B80

Oxyuris vermicularis (infestation) B80

Ozena J31.0

P

- **Pachyderma, pachydermia** L85.9
  - larynx (verrucosa) J38.7
- **Pachydermatocele** (congenital) Q82.8
- **Pachydermoperiostosis** *—see also* Osteoarthropathy, hypertrophic, specified type NEC
  - clubbed nail M89.40 *[L62]*
- **Pachygyria** Q04.3
- **Pachymeningitis** (adhesive) (basal) (brain) (cervical) (chronic) (circumscribed) (external) (fibrous) (hemorrhagic) (hypertrophic) (internal) (purulent) (spinal) (suppurative) *—see* Meningitis
- **Pachyonychia** (congenital) Q84.5
- **Pacinian tumor** *—see* Neoplasm, skin, benign
- **Pad, knuckle or Garrod's** M72.1
- **Paget-Schroetter syndrome** I82.890
- **Paget's disease**
  - with infiltrating duct carcinoma *—see* Neoplasm, breast, malignant
  - bone M88.9
    - carpus M88.84-
    - clavicle M88.81-
    - femur M88.85-
    - fibula M88.86-
    - finger M88.84-
    - humerus M88.82-
    - ilium M88.85-
    - in neoplastic disease *—see* Osteitis, deformans, in neoplastic disease
    - ischium M88.85-
    - metacarpus M88.84-
    - metatarsus M88.87-
    - multiple sites M88.89
    - neck M88.88
    - radius M88.83-
    - rib M88.88
    - scapula M88.81-
    - skull M88.0
    - specified NEC M88.88
    - tarsus M88.87-
    - tibia M88.86-
    - toe M88.87-
    - ulna M88.83-
    - vertebra M88.1
  - breast (female) C50.01-
    - male C50.02-
  - extramammary *—see also* Neoplasm, skin, malignant
    - anus C21.0
      - margin C44.590
      - skin C44.590
  - intraductal carcinoma *—see* Neoplasm, breast, malignant
  - malignant *—see* Neoplasm, skin, malignant
    - breast (female) C50.01-
      - male C50.02-
    - unspecified site (female) C50.01-
      - male C50.02-
  - mammary *—see* Paget's disease, breast
  - nipple *—see* Paget's disease, breast
  - osteitis deformans *—see* Paget's disease, bone
- **Pain**(s) (*see also* Painful) R52
  - abdominal R10.9
    - colic R10.83
    - generalized R10.84
      - with acute abdomen R10.0
    - lower R10.30
      - left quadrant R10.32
      - pelvic or perineal R10.2
      - periumbilical R10.33
      - right quadrant R10.31
    - rebound *—see* Tenderness, abdominal, rebound
    - severe with abdominal rigidity R10.0
    - tenderness *—see* Tenderness, abdominal
    - upper R10.10
      - epigastric R10.13
      - left quadrant R10.12
      - right quadrant R10.11
  - acute R52
    - due to trauma G89.11
    - neoplasm related G89.3
    - postprocedural NEC G89.18
    - post-thoracotomy G89.12
    - specified by site - code to Pain, by site
  - adnexa (uteri) R10.2
  - anginoid *—see* Pain, precordial
  - anus K62.89
  - arm *—see* Pain, limb, upper
  - axillary (axilla) M79.62-
  - back (postural) M54.9
  - bladder R39.89
    - associated with micturition *—see* Micturition, painful
    - chronic R39.82
  - bone *—see* Disorder, bone, specified type NEC
  - breast N64.4
  - broad ligament R10.2
  - cancer associated (acute) (chronic) G89.3
  - cecum *—see* Pain, abdominal
  - cervicobrachial M53.1
  - chest (central) R07.9
    - anterior wall R07.89
    - atypical R07.89
    - ischemic I20.9
    - musculoskeletal R07.89
    - non-cardiac R07.89
    - on breathing R07.1
    - pleurodynia R07.81
    - precordial R07.2
    - wall (anterior) R07.89
  - chronic G89.29
    - associated with significant psychosocial dysfunction G89.4
    - due to trauma G89.21
    - neoplasm related G89.3
    - postoperative NEC G89.28
    - postprocedural NEC G89.28
    - post-thoracotomy G89.22
    - specified NEC G89.29
  - coccyx M53.3
  - colon *—see* Pain, abdominal
  - coronary *—see* Angina
  - costochondral R07.1
  - diaphragm R07.1
  - due to cancer G89.3
  - due to device, implant or graft (*see also* Complications, by site and type, specified NEC) T85.848
    - arterial graft NEC T82.848
    - breast (implant) T85.848
    - catheter NEC T85.848
      - dialysis (renal) T82.848
        - intraperitoneal T85.848

Pain(s) *(continued)*

- due to device, implant or graft *(continued)*
  - catheter NEC *(continued)*
    - infusion NEC T82.848
      - spinal (epidural) (subdural) T85.840
    - urinary (indwelling) T83.84
  - electronic (electrode) (pulse generator) (stimulator)
    - bone T84.84
    - cardiac T82.847
    - nervous system (brain) (peripheral nerve) (spinal) T85.840
    - urinary T83.84
  - fixation, internal (orthopedic) NEC T84.84
  - gastrointestinal (bile duct) (esophagus) T85.848
  - genital NEC T83.84
  - heart NEC T82.847
  - infusion NEC T85.848
  - joint prosthesis T84.84
  - ocular (corneal graft) (orbital implant) NEC T85.848
  - orthopedic NEC T84.84
  - specified NEC T85.848
  - urinary NEC T83.84
  - vascular NEC T82.848
  - ventricular intracranial shunt T85.840
- due to malignancy (primary) (secondary) G89.3
- ear *—see* subcategory H92.0
- epigastric, epigastrium R10.13
- eye *—see* Pain, ocular
- face, facial R51.9
  - atypical G50.1
- female genital organs NEC N94.89
- finger *—see* Pain, limb, upper
- flank *—see* Pain, abdominal
- foot *—see* Pain, limb, lower
- gallbladder K82.9
- gas (intestinal) R14.1
- gastric *—see* Pain, abdominal
- generalized NOS R52
- genital organ
  - female N94.89
  - male N50.89
- groin *—see* Pain, abdominal, lower
- hand *—see* Pain, limb, upper
- head *—see* Headache
- heart *—see* Pain, precordial
- infra-orbital *—see* Neuralgia, trigeminal
- intercostal R07.82
- intermenstrual N94.0
- jaw R68.84
- joint M25.50
  - ankle M25.57-
  - elbow M25.52-
  - finger M25.54-
  - foot M25.57-
  - hand M25.54-
  - hip M25.55-
  - knee M25.56-
  - shoulder M25.51-
  - specified site NEC M25.59
  - toe M25.57-
  - wrist M25.53-
- kidney N23
- laryngeal R07.0
- leg *—see* Pain, limb, lower
- limb M79.609
  - lower M79.60-
    - foot M79.67-
    - lower leg M79.66-
    - thigh M79.65-
    - toe M79.67-

Pain(s) *(continued)*

- limb *(continued)*
  - upper M79.60-
    - axilla M79.62-
    - finger M79.64-
    - forearm M79.63-
    - hand M79.64-
    - upper arm M79.62-
- loin M54.50
- low back M54.50
  - specified NEC M54.59
  - vertebral end plate M54.51
  - vertebrogenic M54.51
- lumbar region M54.50
  - vertebral end plate M54.51
  - vertebrogenic M54.51
- mandibular R68.84
- mastoid *—see* subcategory H92.0
- maxilla R68.84
- menstrual (*see also* Dysmenorrhea) N94.6
- metacarpophalangeal (joint) *—see* Pain, joint, hand
- metatarsophalangeal (joint) *—see* Pain, joint, foot
- mouth K13.79
- muscle *—see* Myalgia
- musculoskeletal (*see also* Pain, by site) M79.18
- myofascial M79.18
- nasal J34.89
- nasopharynx J39.2
- neck NEC M54.2
- nerve NEC *—see* Neuralgia
- neuromuscular *—see* Neuralgia
- nose J34.89
- ocular H57.1-
- ophthalmic *—see* Pain, ocular
- orbital region *—see* Pain, ocular
- ovary N94.89
- over heart *—see* Pain, precordial
- ovulation N94.0
- pelvic (female) R10.2
- penis N48.89
- pericardial *—see* Pain, precordial
- perineal, perineum R10.2
- pharynx J39.2
- pleura, pleural, pleuritic R07.81
- postoperative NOS G89.18
- postprocedural NOS G89.18
- post-thoracotomy G89.12
- precordial (region) R07.2
- premenstrual N94.3
- psychogenic (persistent) (any site) F45.41
- radicular (spinal) *—see* Radiculopathy
- rectum K62.89
- respiration R07.1
- retrosternal R07.2
- rheumatoid, muscular *—see* Myalgia
- rib R07.81
- root (spinal) *—see* Radiculopathy
- round ligament (stretch) R10.2
- sacroiliac M53.3
- sciatic *—see* Sciatica
- scrotum N50.82
- seminal vesicle N50.89
- shoulder M25.51-
- spermatic cord N50.89
- spinal root *—see* Radiculopathy
- spine M54.9
  - cervical M54.2
  - low back M54.50
    - with sciatica M54.4-
  - thoracic M54.6
- stomach *—see* Pain, abdominal
- substernal R07.2
- temporomandibular (joint) M26.62-
- testis N50.81-

Panophthalmitis H44.01-

Pansinusitis (chronic) (hyperplastic) (nonpurulent) (purulent) J32.4
  acute J01.40
    recurrent J01.41
  tuberculous A15.8

Panuveitis (sympathetic) H44.11-

Panvalvular disease I08.9
  specified NEC I08.8

PAPA (pyogenic arthritis, pyoderma gangrenosum, and acne syndrome) M04.8

Papanicolaou smear, cervix Z12.4
  as part of routine gynecological examination Z01.419
    with abnormal findings Z01.411
  for suspected neoplasm Z12.4
  nonspecific abnormal finding R87.619
  routine Z01.419
    with abnormal findings Z01.411

Papilledema (choked disc) H47.10
  associated with
    decreased ocular pressure H47.12
    increased intracranial pressure H47.11
    retinal disorder H47.13
  Foster-Kennedy syndrome H47.14-

Papillitis H46.00
  anus K62.89
  chronic lingual K14.4
  necrotizing, kidney N17.2
  optic H46.0-
  rectum K62.89
  renal, necrotizing N17.2
  tongue K14.0

Papilloma —*see also* Neoplasm, benign, by site
  basal cell L82.1
    inflamed L82.0
  acuminatum (female) (male) (anogenital) A63.0
  benign pinta (primary) A67.0
  bladder (urinary) (transitional cell) D41.4
  choroid plexus (lateral ventricle) (third ventricle) D33.0
    anaplastic C71.5
    fourth ventricle D33.1
    malignant C71.5
  renal pelvis (transitional cell) D41.1-
    benign D30.1-
  Schneiderian
    specified site —*see* Neoplasm, benign, by site
    unspecified site D14.0
  serous surface
    borderline malignancy
      specified site —*see* Neoplasm, uncertain behavior, by site
      unspecified site D39.10
    specified site —*see* Neoplasm, benign, by site
    unspecified site D27.9
  transitional (cell)
    bladder (urinary) D41.4
    inverted type —*see* Neoplasm, uncertain behavior, by site
    renal pelvis D41.1-
    ureter D41.2-
  ureter (transitional cell) D41.2-
    benign D30.2-
  urothelial —*see* Neoplasm, uncertain behavior, by site
  villous —*see* Neoplasm, uncertain behavior, by site

Papilloma *(continued)*
  villous *(continued)*
    adenocarcinoma in —*see* Neoplasm, malignant, by site
    in situ —*see* Neoplasm, in situ
  yaws, plantar or palmar A66.1

Papillomata, multiple, of yaws A66.1

Papillomatosis —*see also* Neoplasm, benign, by site
  confluent and reticulated L83
  cystic, breast —*see* Mastopathy, cystic
  ductal, breast —*see* Mastopathy, cystic
  intraductal (diffuse) —*see* Neoplasm, benign, by site
  subareolar duct D24-

Papillomavirus, as cause of disease classified elsewhere B97.7

Papillon-Léage and Psaume syndrome Q87.0

Papule(s) R23.8
  carate (primary) A67.0
  fibrous, of nose D22.39
  Gottron's L94.4
  pinta (primary) A67.0

Papulosis
  lymphomatoid C86.6
  malignant I77.89

Papyraceous fetus O31.0-

Para-albuminemia E88.09

Paracephalus Q89.7

Parachute mitral valve Q23.2

Paracoccidioidomycosis B41.9
  disseminated B41.7
  generalized B41.7
  mucocutaneous-lymphangitic B41.8
  pulmonary B41.0
  specified NEC B41.8
  visceral B41.8

Paradentosis K05.4

Paraffinoma T88.8

Paraganglioma D44.7
  adrenal D35.0-
    malignant C74.1-
  aortic body D44.7
    malignant C75.5
  carotid body D44.6
    malignant C75.4
  chromaffin —*see also* Neoplasm, benign, by site
    malignant —*see* Neoplasm, malignant, by site
  extra-adrenal D44.7
    malignant C75.5
      specified site —*see* Neoplasm, malignant, by site
      unspecified site C75.5
    specified site —*see* Neoplasm, uncertain behavior, by site
    unspecified site D44.7
  gangliocytic D13.2
    specified site —*see* Neoplasm, benign, by site
    unspecified site D13.2
  glomus jugulare D44.7
    malignant C75.5
  jugular D44.7
  malignant C75.5
    specified site —*see* Neoplasm, malignant, by site
    unspecified site C75.5

Paraganglioma *(continued)*
  nonchromaffin D44.7
    malignant C75.5
      specified site —*see* Neoplasm, malignant, by site
      unspecified site C75.5
    specified site —*see* Neoplasm, uncertain behavior, by site
    unspecified site D44.7
  parasympathetic D44.7
    specified site —*see* Neoplasm, uncertain behavior, by site
    unspecified site D44.7
  specified site —*see* Neoplasm, uncertain behavior, by site
  sympathetic D44.7
    specified site —*see* Neoplasm, uncertain behavior, by site
    unspecified site D44.7
  unspecified site D44.7

Parageusia R43.2
  psychogenic F45.8

Paragonimiasis B66.4

Paragranuloma, Hodgkin —*see* Lymphoma, Hodgkin, specified NEC

Parahemophilia (*see also* Defect, coagulation) D68.2

Parakeratosis R23.4
  variegata L41.0

Paralysis, paralytic (complete) (incomplete) G83.9
  with
    syphilis A52.17
  abducens, abducent (nerve) —*see* Strabismus, paralytic, sixth nerve
  abductor, lower extremity G57.9-
  accessory nerve G52.8
  accommodation —*see also* Paresis, of accommodation
    hysterical F44.89
  acoustic nerve (except Deafness) —*see* subcategory H93.3
  agitans (*see also* Parkinsonism) G20
    arteriosclerotic G21.4
  alternating (oculomotor) G83.89
  amyotrophic G12.21
  ankle G57.9-
  anus (sphincter) K62.89
  arm —*see* Monoplegia, upper limb
  ascending (spinal), acute G61.0
  association G12.29
  asthenic bulbar G70.00
    with exacerbation (acute) G70.01
    in crisis G70.01
  ataxic (hereditary) G11.9
    general (syphilitic) A52.17
  atrophic G58.9
    infantile, acute —*see* Poliomyelitis, paralytic
    progressive G12.22
    spinal (acute) —*see* Poliomyelitis, paralytic
  axillary G54.0
  Babinski-Nageotte's G83.89
  Bell's G51.0
    newborn P11.3
  Benedikt's G46.3
  birth injury P14.9
    spinal cord P11.5
  bladder (neurogenic) (sphincter) N31.2
  bowel, colon or intestine K56.0
  brachial plexus G54.0
    birth injury P14.3
    newborn (birth injury) P14.3

Paralysis, paralytic *(continued)*
  brain G83.9
    diplegia G83.0
    triplegia G83.89
  bronchial J98.09
  Brown-Séquard G83.81
  bulbar (chronic) (progressive) G12.22
    infantile —*see* Poliomyelitis, paralytic
    poliomyelitic —*see* Poliomyelitis, paralytic
    pseudo G12.29
  bulbospinal G70.00
    with exacerbation (acute) G70.01
    in crisis G70.01
  cardiac (*see also* Failure, heart) I50.9
  cerebrocerebellar, diplegic G80.1
  cervical
    plexus G54.2
    sympathetic G90.09
  Céstan-Chenais G46.3
  Charcot-Marie-Tooth type G60.0
  Clark's G80.9
  colon K56.0
  compressed air T70.3
  compression
    arm G56.9-
    leg G57.9-
    lower extremity G57.9-
    upper extremity G56.9-
  congenital (cerebral) —*see* Palsy, cerebral
  conjugate movement (gaze) (of eye) H51.0
    cortical (nuclear) (supranuclear) H51.0
  cordis —*see* Failure, heart
  cranial or cerebral nerve G52.9
  creeping G12.22
  crossed leg G83.89
  crutch —*see* Injury, brachial plexus
  deglutition R13.0
    hysterical F44.4
  dementia A52.17
  descending (spinal) NEC G12.29
  diaphragm (flaccid) J98.6
    due to accidental dissection of phrenic nerve during procedure —*see* Puncture, accidental complicating surgery
  digestive organs NEC K59.89
  diplegic —*see* Diplegia
  divergence (nuclear) H51.8
  diver's T70.3
  Duchenne's
    birth injury P14.0
    due to or associated with
      motor neuron disease G12.22
      muscular dystrophy G71.01
  due to intracranial or spinal birth injury —*see* Palsy, cerebral
  embolic (current episode) I63.4-
  Erb (-Duchenne) (birth) (newborn) P14.0
  Erb's syphilitic spastic spinal A52.17
  esophagus K22.89
  eye muscle (extrinsic) H49.9
    intrinsic —*see also* Paresis, of accommodation
  facial (nerve) G51.0
    birth injury P11.3
    congenital P11.3
    following operation NEC —*see* Puncture, accidental complicating surgery
    newborn (birth injury) P11.3
  familial (recurrent) (periodic) G72.3
    spastic G11.4

Paralysis, paralytic *(continued)*
- fauces J39.2
- finger G56.9-
- gait R26.1
- gastric nerve (nondiabetic) G52.2
- gaze, conjugate H51.0
- general (progressive) (syphilitic) A52.17
  - juvenile A50.45
- glottis J38.00
  - bilateral J38.02
  - unilateral J38.01
- gluteal G54.1
- Gubler (-Millard) G46.3
- hand *—see* Monoplegia, upper limb
- heart *—see* Arrest, cardiac
- hemiplegic *—see* Hemiplegia
- hyperkalemic periodic (familial) G72.3
- hypoglossal (nerve) G52.3
- hypokalemic periodic G72.3
- hysterical F44.4
- ileus K56.0
- infantile (*see also* Poliomyelitis, paralytic) A80.30
  - bulbar *—see* Poliomyelitis, paralytic
  - cerebral *—see* Palsy, cerebral
  - spastic *—see* Palsy, cerebral, spastic
- infective *—see* Poliomyelitis, paralytic
- inferior nuclear G83.9
- internuclear *—see* Ophthalmoplegia, internuclear
- intestine K56.0
- iris H57.09
  - due to diphtheria (toxin) A36.89
- ischemic, Volkmann's (complicating trauma) T79.6
- Jackson's G83.89
- jake *—see* Poisoning, food, noxious, plant
- Jamaica ginger (jake) G62.2
- juvenile general A50.45
- Klumpke (-Déjérine) (birth) (newborn) P14.1
- labioglossal (laryngeal) (pharyngeal) G12.29
- Landry's G61.0
- laryngeal nerve (recurrent) (superior) (unilateral) J38.00
  - bilateral J38.02
  - unilateral J38.01
- larynx J38.00
  - bilateral J38.02
  - due to diphtheria (toxin) A36.2
  - unilateral J38.01
- lateral G12.23
- lead *—see* subcategory T56.0
- left side *—see* Hemiplegia
- leg G83.1-
  - both *—see* Paraplegia
  - crossed G83.89
  - hysterical F44.4
  - psychogenic F44.4
  - transient or transitory R29.818
    - traumatic NEC *—see* Injury, nerve, leg
- levator palpebrae superioris *—see* Blepharoptosis, paralytic
- limb *—see* Monoplegia
- lip K13.0
- Lissauer's A52.17
- lower limb *—see* Monoplegia, lower limb
  - both *—see* Paraplegia
- lung J98.4
- median nerve G56.1-
- medullary (tegmental) G83.89

Paralysis, paralytic *(continued)*
- mesencephalic NEC G83.89
  - tegmental G83.89
- middle alternating G83.89
- Millard-Gubler-Foville G46.3
- monoplegic *—see* Monoplegia
- motor G83.9
- muscle, muscular NEC G72.89
  - due to nerve lesion G58.9
  - eye (extrinsic) H49.9
    - intrinsic *—see* Paresis, of accommodation
    - oblique *—see* Strabismus, paralytic, fourth nerve
  - iris sphincter H21.9
  - ischemic (Volkmann's) (complicating trauma) T79.6
  - progressive G12.21
  - progressive, spinal G12.25
  - pseudohypertrophic G71.02
  - spinal progressive G12.25
- musculocutaneous nerve G56.9-
- musculospiral G56.9-
- nerve *—see also* Disorder, nerve
  - abducent *—see* Strabismus, paralytic, sixth nerve
  - accessory G52.8
  - auditory (except Deafness) *—see* subcategory H93.3
  - birth injury P14.9
  - cranial or cerebral G52.9
  - facial G51.0
    - birth injury P11.3
    - congenital P11.3
    - newborn (birth injury) P11.3
  - fourth or trochlear *—see* Strabismus, paralytic, fourth nerve
  - newborn (birth injury) P14.9
  - oculomotor *—see* Strabismus, paralytic, third nerve
  - phrenic (birth injury) P14.2
  - radial G56.3-
  - seventh or facial G51.0
    - newborn (birth injury) P11.3
  - sixth or abducent *—see* Strabismus, paralytic, sixth nerve
  - syphilitic A52.15
  - third or oculomotor *—see* Strabismus, paralytic, third nerve
  - trigeminal G50.9
  - trochlear *—see* Strabismus, paralytic, fourth nerve
  - ulnar G56.2-
- normokalemic periodic G72.3
- ocular H49.9
  - alternating G83.89
- oculofacial, congenital (Moebius) Q87.0
- oculomotor (external bilateral) (nerve) *—see* Strabismus, paralytic, third nerve
- palate (soft) K13.79
- paratrigeminal G50.9
- periodic (familial) (hyperkalemic) (hypokalemic) (myotonic) (normokalemic) (potassium sensitive) (secondary) G72.3
- peripheral autonomic nervous system *—see* Neuropathy, peripheral, autonomic
- peroneal (nerve) G57.3-
- pharynx J39.2
- phrenic nerve G56.8-
- plantar nerve(s) G57.6-
- pneumogastric nerve G52.2
- poliomyelitis (current) *—see* Poliomyelitis, paralytic

Paralysis, paralytic *(continued)*
- popliteal nerve G57.3-
- postepileptic transitory G83.84
- progressive (atrophic) (bulbar) (spinal) G12.22
  - general A52.17
  - infantile acute *—see* Poliomyelitis, paralytic
  - supranuclear G23.1
- pseudobulbar G12.29
- pseudohypertrophic (muscle) G71.09
- psychogenic F44.4
- quadriceps G57.9-
- quadriplegic *—see* Tetraplegia
- radial nerve G56.3-
- rectus muscle (eye) H49.9
- recurrent isolated sleep G47.53
- respiratory (muscle) (system) (tract) R06.81
  - center NEC G93.89
  - congenital P28.89
  - newborn P28.89
- right side *—see* Hemiplegia
- saturnine *—see* subcategory T56.0
- sciatic nerve G57.0-
- senile G83.9
- shaking *—see* Parkinsonism
- shoulder G56.9-
- sleep, recurrent isolated G47.53
- spastic G83.9
  - cerebral *—see* Palsy, cerebral, spastic
  - congenital (cerebral) *—see* Palsy, cerebral, spastic
  - familial G11.4
  - hereditary G11.4
  - quadriplegic G80.0
  - syphilitic (spinal) A52.17
- sphincter, bladder *—see* Paralysis, bladder
- spinal (cord) G83.9
  - accessory nerve G52.8
  - acute *—see* Poliomyelitis, paralytic
  - ascending acute G61.0
  - atrophic (acute) *—see also* Poliomyelitis, paralytic
    - spastic, syphilitic A52.17
  - congenital NEC *—see* Palsy, cerebral
  - infantile *—see* Poliomyelitis, paralytic
  - hereditary G95.89
  - progressive G12.21
    - muscle G12.25
  - sequelae NEC G83.89
- sternomastoid G52.8
- stomach K31.84
  - diabetic *—see* Diabetes, by type, with gastroparesis
  - nerve G52.2
    - diabetic *—see* Diabetes, by type, with gastroparesis
- stroke *—see* Infarct, brain
- subcapsularis G56.8-
- supranuclear (progressive) G23.1
- sympathetic G90.8
  - cervical G90.09
  - nervous system *—see* Neuropathy, peripheral, autonomic
- syndrome G83.9
  - specified NEC G83.89
- syphilitic spastic spinal (Erb's) A52.17
- thigh G57.9-
- throat J39.2
  - diphtheritic A36.0
  - muscle J39.2

Paralysis, paralytic *(continued)*
- thrombotic (current episode) I63.3-
- thumb G56.9-
- tick *—see* Toxicity, venom, arthropod, specified NEC
- Todd's (postepileptic transitory paralysis) G83.84
- toe G57.6-
- tongue K14.8
- transient R29.5
  - arm or leg NEC R29.818
    - traumatic NEC *—see* Injury, nerve
- trapezius G52.8
- traumatic, transient NEC *—see* Injury, nerve
- trembling *—see* Parkinsonism
- triceps brachii G56.9-
- trigeminal nerve G50.9
- trochlear (nerve) *—see* Strabismus, paralytic, fourth nerve
- ulnar nerve G56.2-
- upper limb *—see* Monoplegia, upper limb
- uremic N18.9 *[G99.8]*
- uveoparotitic D86.89
- uvula K13.79
  - postdiphtheritic A36.0
- vagus nerve G52.2
- vasomotor NEC G90.8
- velum palati K13.79
- vesical *—see* Paralysis, bladder
- vestibular nerve (except Vertigo) *—see* subcategory H93.3
- vocal cords J38.00
  - bilateral J38.02
  - unilateral J38.01
- Volkmann's (complicating trauma) T79.6
- wasting G12.29
- Weber's G46.3
- wrist G56.9-

Paramedial urethrovesical orifice Q64.79

Paramenia N92.6

Parametritis (*see also* Disease, pelvis, inflammatory) N73.2
- acute N73.0
- complicating abortion *—see* Abortion, by type, complicated by, parametritis

Parametrium, parametric *—see* condition

Paramnesia *—see* Amnesia

Paramolar K00.1

Paramyloidosis E85.89

Paramyoclonus multiplex G25.3

Paramyotonia (congenita) G71.19

Parangi *—see* Yaws

Paranoia (querulans) F22
- senile F03

Paranoid
- dementia (senile) F03
  - praecox *—see* Schizophrenia
- personality F60.0
- psychosis (climacteric) (involutional) (menopausal) F22
  - psychogenic (acute) F23
  - senile F03
- reaction (acute) F23
  - chronic F22
- schizophrenia F20.0
- state (climacteric) (involutional) (menopausal) (simple) F22
  - senile F03
- tendencies F60.0

Paranoid *(continued)*
- traits F60.0
- trends F60.0
- type, psychopathic personality F60.0

Paraparesis *—see* Paraplegia

Paraphasia R47.02

Paraphilia F65.9

Paraphimosis (congenital) N47.2
- chancroidal A57

Paraphrenia, paraphrenic (late) F22
- schizophrenia F20.0

Paraplegia (lower) G82.20
- ataxic *—see* Degeneration, combined, spinal cord
- complete G82.21
- congenital (cerebral) G80.8
  - spastic G80.1
- familial spastic G11.4
- functional (hysterical) F44.4
- hereditary, spastic G11.4
- hysterical F44.4
- incomplete G82.22
- Pott's A18.01
- psychogenic F44.4
- spastic
  - Erb's spinal, syphilitic A52.17
  - hereditary G11.4
  - tropical G04.1
- syphilitic (spastic) A52.17
- traumatic
  - current injury - code to injury with seventh character A
  - sequela of previous injury - code to injury with seventh character S
- tropical spastic G04.1

Parapoxvirus B08.60
- specified NEC B08.69

Paraproteinemia D89.2
- benign (familial) D89.2
- monoclonal D47.2
- secondary to malignant disease D47.2

Parapsoriasis L41.9
- en plaques L41.4
- guttata L41.1
- large plaque L41.4
- retiform, retiformis L41.5
- small plaque L41.3
- specified NEC L41.8
- varioliformis (acuta) L41.0

Parasitic *—see also* condition
- disease NEC B89
- stomatitis B37.0
- sycosis (beard) (scalp) B35.0
- twin Q89.4

Parasitism B89
- intestinal B82.9
- skin B88.9
- specified *—see* Infestation

Parasitophobia F40.218

Parasomnia G47.50
- due to
  - alcohol
    - abuse F10.182
    - dependence F10.282
    - use F10.982
  - amphetamines
    - abuse F15.182
    - dependence F15.282
    - use F15.982
  - caffeine
    - abuse F15.182
    - dependence F15.282
    - use F15.982

Parasomnia *(continued)*
- due to *(continued)*
  - cocaine
    - abuse F14.182
    - dependence F14.282
    - use F14.982
  - drug NEC
    - abuse F19.182
    - dependence F19.282
    - use F19.982
  - opioid
    - abuse F11.182
    - dependence F11.282
    - use F11.982
  - psychoactive substance NEC
    - abuse F19.182
    - dependence F19.282
    - use F19.982
  - sedative, hypnotic, or anxiolytic
    - abuse F13.182
    - dependence F13.282
    - use F13.982
  - stimulant NEC
    - abuse F15.182
    - dependence F15.282
    - use F15.982
- in conditions classified elsewhere G47.54
- nonorganic origin F51.8
- organic G47.50
- specified NEC G47.59

Paraspadias Q54.9

Paraspasmus facialis G51.8

Parasuicide (attempt)
- history of (personal) Z91.51
  - in family Z81.8

Parathyroid gland *—see* condition

Parathyroid tetany E20.9

Paratrachoma A74.0

Paratyphilitis *—see* Appendicitis

Paratyphoid (fever) *—see* Fever, paratyphoid

Paratyphus *—see* Fever, paratyphoid

Paraurethral duct Q64.79

Paraurethritis *—see also* Urethritis
- gonococcal (acute) (chronic) (with abscess) A54.1

Paravaccinia NEC B08.04

Paravaginitis *—see* Vaginitis

Parencephalitis *—see also* Encephalitis
- sequelae G09

Parent-child conflict *—see* Conflict, parent-child
- estrangement NEC Z62.890

Paresis *—see also* Paralysis
- accommodation *—see* Paresis, of accommodation
- Bernhardt's G57.1-
- bladder (sphincter) *—see also* Paralysis, bladder
  - tabetic A52.17
- bowel, colon or intestine K56.0
- extrinsic muscle, eye H49.9
- general (progressive) (syphilitic) A52.17
  - juvenile A50.45
- heart *—see* Failure, heart
- insane (syphilitic) A52.17
- juvenile (general) A50.45
- of accommodation H52.52-
- peripheral progressive (idiopathic) G60.3
- pseudohypertrophic G71.09
- senile G83.9

Paresis *(continued)*
- syphilitic (general) A52.17
  - congenital A50.45
- vesical NEC N31.2

Paresthesia (*see also* Disturbance, sensation, skin) R20.2
- Bernhardt G57.1-

Paretic *—see* condition

Parinaud's
- conjunctivitis H10.89
- oculoglandular syndrome H10.89
- ophthalmoplegia H49.88-

Parkinsonism (idiopathic) (primary) G20
- with neurogenic orthostatic hypotension (symptomatic) G90.3
- arteriosclerotic G21.4
- dementia G31.83 *[F02.80]*
  - with behavioral disturbance G31.83 *[F02.81]*
- due to
  - drugs NEC G21.19
    - neuroleptic G21.11
- medication-induced NEC G21.19
- neuroleptic induced G21.11
- postencephalitic G21.3
- secondary G21.9
  - due to
    - arteriosclerosis G21.4
    - drugs NEC G21.19
      - neuroleptic G21.11
    - encephalitis G21.3
    - external agents NEC G21.2
    - syphilis A52.19
  - specified NEC G21.8
- syphilitic A52.19
- treatment-induced NEC G21.19
- vascular G21.4

Parkinson's disease, syndrome or tremor *—see* Parkinsonism

Parodontitis *—see* Periodontitis

Parodontosis K05.4

Paronychia *—see also* Cellulitis, digit
- with lymphangitis *—see* Lymphangitis, acute, digit
- candidal (chronic) B37.2
- tuberculous (primary) A18.4

Parorexia (psychogenic) F50.89

Parosmia R43.1
- psychogenic F45.8

Parotid gland *—see* condition

Parotitis, parotiditis (allergic) (nonspecific toxic) (purulent) (septic) (suppurative) *—see also* Sialoadenitis
- epidemic *—see* Mumps
- infectious *—see* Mumps
- postoperative K91.89
- surgical K91.89

Parrot fever A70

Parrot's disease (early congenital syphilitic pseudoparalysis) A50.02

Parry-Romberg syndrome G51.8

Parry's disease or syndrome E05.00
- with thyroid storm E05.01

Pars planitis *—see* Cyclitis

Parsonage (-Aldren)-**Turner syndrome** G54.5

Parson's disease (exophthalmic goiter) E05.00
- with thyroid storm E05.01

Particolored infant Q82.8

Parturition *—see* Delivery

Parulis K04.7
- with sinus K04.6

Parvovirus, as cause of disease classified elsewhere B97.6

Pasini and Pierini's atrophoderma L90.3

Passage
- false, urethra N36.5
- meconium (newborn) during delivery P03.82
- of sounds or bougies *—see* Attention to, artificial, opening

Passive *—see* condition
- smoking Z77.22

Past due on rent or mortgage Z59.81-

Pasteurella septica A28.0

Pasteurellosis *—see* Infection, Pasteurella

PAT (paroxysmal atrial tachycardia) I47.1

Patau's syndrome *—see* Trisomy, 13

Patches
- mucous (syphilitic) A51.39
  - congenital A50.07
- smokers' (mouth) K13.24

Patellar *—see* condition

Patent *—see also* Imperfect, closure
- canal of Nuck Q52.4
- cervix N88.3
- ductus arteriosus or Botallo's Q25.0
- foramen
  - botalli Q21.1
  - ovale Q21.1
- interauricular septum Q21.1
- interventricular septum Q21.0
- omphalomesenteric duct Q43.0
- os (uteri) *—see* Patent, cervix
- ostium secundum Q21.1
- urachus Q64.4
- vitelline duct Q43.0

Paterson (-Brown) (-Kelly) **syndrome or web** D50.1

Pathologic, pathological *—see also* condition
- asphyxia R09.01
- fire-setting F63.1
- gambling F63.0
- ovum O02.0
- resorption, tooth K03.3
- stealing F63.2

Pathology (of) *—see* Disease
- periradicular, associated with previous endodontic treatment NEC M27.59

Pattern, sleep-wake, irregular G47.23

Patulous *—see also* Imperfect, closure (congenital)
- alimentary tract Q45.8
  - lower Q43.8
  - upper Q40.8
- eustachian tube H69.0-

Pause, sinoatrial I49.5

Paxton's disease B36.2

Pearl(s)
- enamel K00.2
- Epstein's K09.8

Pearl-worker's disease *—see* Osteomyelitis, specified type NEC

Pectenosis K62.4

Pectoral *—see* condition

Pectus
- carinatum (congenital) Q67.7
  - acquired M95.4
  - rachitic sequelae (late effect) E64.3
- excavatum (congenital) Q67.6
  - acquired M95.4
  - rachitic sequelae (late effect) E64.3
- recurvatum (congenital) Q67.6

Pedatrophia E41

Pederosis F65.4

Pediatric inflammatory multisystem syndrome M35.81

Pediculosis (infestation) B85.2
- capitis (head-louse) (any site) B85.0
- corporis (body-louse) (any site) B85.1
- eyelid B85.0
- mixed (classifiable to more than one of the titles B85.0-B85.3) B85.4
- pubis (pubic louse) (any site) B85.3
- vestimenti B85.1
- vulvae B85.3

Pediculus (infestation) *—see* Pediculosis

Pedophilia F65.4

Peg-shaped teeth K00.2

Pelade *—see* Alopecia, areata

Pelger-Huët anomaly or syndrome D72.0

Peliosis (rheumatica) D69.0
- hepatis K76.4
  - with toxic liver disease K71.8

Pelizaeus-Merzbacher disease E75.29

Pellagra (alcoholic) (with polyneuropathy) E52

Pellagra-cerebellar-ataxia-renal aminoaciduria syndrome E72.02

Pellegrini (-Stieda) **disease or syndrome** *—see* Bursitis, tibial collateral

Pellizzi's syndrome E34.8

Pel's crisis A52.11

Pelvic *—see also* condition
- examination (periodic) (routine) Z01.419
  - with abnormal findings Z01.411
- kidney, congenital Q63.2

Pelviolithiasis *—see* Calculus, kidney

Pelviperitonitis *—see also* Peritonitis, pelvic
- gonococcal A54.24
- puerperal O85

Pelvis *—see* condition or type

Pemphigoid L12.9
- benign, mucous membrane L12.1
- bullous L12.0
- cicatricial L12.1
- juvenile L12.2
- ocular L12.1
- specified NEC L12.8

Pemphigus L10.9
- benign familial (chronic) Q82.8
- Brazilian L10.3
- circinatus L13.0

Pemphigus *(continued)*
- conjunctiva L12.1
- drug-induced L10.5
- erythematosus L10.4
- foliaceous L10.2
- gangrenous *—see* Gangrene
- neonatorum L01.03
- ocular L12.1
- paraneoplastic L10.81
- specified NEC L10.89
- syphilitic (congenital) A50.06
- vegetans L10.1
- vulgaris L10.0
- wildfire L10.3

Pendred's syndrome E07.1

Pendulous
- abdomen, in pregnancy *—see* Pregnancy, complicated by, abnormal, pelvic organs or tissues NEC
- breast N64.89

Penetrating wound *—see also* Puncture
- with internal injury *—see* Injury, by site
- eyeball *—see* Puncture, eyeball
- orbit (with or without foreign body) *—see* Puncture, orbit
- uterus by instrument with or following ectopic or molar pregnancy O08.6

Penicillosis B48.4

Penis *—see* condition

Penitis N48.29

Pentalogy of Fallot Q21.8

Pentasomy X syndrome Q97.1

Pentosuria (essential) E74.89

Percreta placenta O43.23-

Peregrinating patient *—see* Disorder, factitious

Perforation, perforated (nontraumatic) (of)
- accidental during procedure (blood vessel) (nerve) (organ) *—see* Complication, accidental puncture or laceration
- antrum *—see* Sinusitis, maxillary
- appendix K35.32
  - with localized peritonitis K35.32
- atrial septum, multiple Q21.1
- attic, ear *—see* Perforation, tympanum, attic
- bile duct (common) (hepatic) K83.2
  - cystic K82.2
- bladder (urinary)
  - with or following ectopic or molar pregnancy O08.6
  - obstetrical trauma O71.5
  - traumatic S37.29
    - at delivery O71.5
- bowel K63.1
  - with or following ectopic or molar pregnancy O08.6
  - newborn P78.0
  - obstetrical trauma O71.5
  - traumatic *—see* Laceration, intestine
- broad ligament N83.8
  - with or following ectopic or molar pregnancy O08.6
  - obstetrical trauma O71.6

Perforation, perforated *(continued)*
- by
  - device, implant or graft (*see also* Complications, by site and type, mechanical) T85.628
    - arterial graft NEC *—see* Complication, cardiovascular device, mechanical, vascular
    - breast (implant) T85.49
    - catheter NEC T85.698
      - cystostomy T83.090
      - dialysis (renal) T82.49
        - intraperitoneal T85.691
      - infusion NEC T82.594
        - spinal (epidural) (subdural) T85.690
      - urinary (*see also* Complications, catheter, urinary) T83.098
    - electronic (electrode) (pulse generator) (stimulator)
      - bone T84.390
      - cardiac T82.199
        - electrode T82.190
        - pulse generator T82.191
        - specified type NEC T82.198
      - nervous system *—see* Complication, prosthetic device, mechanical, electronic nervous system stimulator
      - urinary *—see* Complication, genitourinary, device, urinary, mechanical
    - fixation, internal (orthopedic) NEC *—see* Complication, fixation device, mechanical
    - gastrointestinal *—see* Complications, prosthetic device, mechanical, gastrointestinal device
    - genital NEC T83.498
      - intrauterine contraceptive device T83.39
      - penile prosthesis T83.490
    - heart NEC *—see* Complication, cardiovascular device, mechanical
    - joint prosthesis *—see* Complications, joint prosthesis, mechanical, specified NEC, by site
    - ocular NEC *—see* Complications, prosthetic device, mechanical, ocular device
    - orthopedic NEC *—see* Complication, orthopedic, device, mechanical
    - specified NEC T85.628
    - urinary NEC *—see also* Complication, genitourinary, device, urinary, mechanical
      - graft T83.29
    - vascular NEC *—see* Complication, cardiovascular device, mechanical
    - ventricular intracranial shunt T85.09
  - foreign body left accidentally in operative wound T81.539
  - instrument (any) during a procedure, accidental *—see* Puncture, accidental complicating surgery
- cecum K35.32
  - with localized peritonitis K35.32

Perforation, perforated *(continued)*
- cervix (uteri) N88.8
  - with or following ectopic or molar pregnancy O08.6
  - obstetrical trauma O71.3
- colon K63.1
  - newborn P78.0
  - obstetrical trauma O71.5
  - traumatic *—see* Laceration, intestine, large
- common duct (bile) K83.2
- cornea (due to ulceration) *—see* Ulcer, cornea, perforated
- cystic duct K82.2
- diverticulum (intestine) K57.80
  - with bleeding K57.81
  - large intestine K57.20
    - with
      - bleeding K57.21
      - small intestine K57.40
        - with bleeding K57.41
  - small intestine K57.00
    - with
      - bleeding K57.01
      - large intestine K57.40
        - with bleeding K57.41
- ear drum *—see* Perforation, tympanum
- esophagus K22.3
- ethmoidal sinus *—see* Sinusitis, ethmoidal
- frontal sinus *—see* Sinusitis, frontal
- gallbladder K82.2
- heart valve *—see* Endocarditis
- ileum K63.1
  - newborn P78.0
  - obstetrical trauma O71.5
  - traumatic *—see* Laceration, intestine, small
- instrumental, surgical (accidental) (blood vessel) (nerve) (organ) *—see* Puncture, accidental complicating surgery
- intestine NEC K63.1
  - with ectopic or molar pregnancy O08.6
  - newborn P78.0
  - obstetrical trauma O71.5
  - traumatic *—see* Laceration, intestine
  - ulcerative NEC K63.1
    - newborn P78.0
- jejunum, jejunal K63.1
  - obstetrical trauma O71.5
  - traumatic *—see* Laceration, intestine, small
  - ulcer *—see* Ulcer, gastrojejunal, with perforation
- joint prosthesis *—see* Complications, joint prosthesis, mechanical, specified NEC, by site
- mastoid (antrum) (cell) *—see* Disorder, mastoid, specified NEC
- maxillary sinus *—see* Sinusitis, maxillary
- membrana tympani *—see* Perforation, tympanum
- nasal
  - septum J34.89
    - congenital Q30.3
    - syphilitic A52.73
  - sinus J34.89
    - congenital Q30.8
    - due to sinusitis *—see* Sinusitis
- palate (*see also* Cleft, palate) Q35.9
  - syphilitic A52.79
- palatine vault (*see also* Cleft, palate, hard) Q35.1
  - syphilitic A52.79
    - congenital A50.59

Perforation, perforated *(continued)*
- pars flaccida (ear drum) —*see* Perforation, tympanum, attic
- pelvic
  - floor S31.030
    - with
      - ectopic or molar pregnancy O08.6
      - penetration into retroperitoneal space S31.031
      - retained foreign body S31.040
        - with penetration into retroperitoneal space S31.041
    - following ectopic or molar pregnancy O08.6
    - obstetrical trauma O70.1
  - organ S37.99
    - adrenal gland S37.818
    - bladder —*see* Perforation, bladder
    - fallopian tube S37.599
      - bilateral S37.592
      - unilateral S37.591
    - kidney S37.09-
    - obstetrical trauma O71.5
    - ovary S37.499
      - bilateral S37.492
      - unilateral S37.491
    - prostate S37.828
    - specified organ NEC S37.898
    - ureter —*see* Perforation, ureter
    - urethra —*see* Perforation, urethra
    - uterus —*see* Perforation, uterus
- perineum —*see* Laceration, perineum
- pharynx J39.2
- rectum K63.1
  - newborn P78.0
  - obstetrical trauma O71.5
  - traumatic S36.63
- root canal space due to endodontic treatment M27.51
- sigmoid K63.1
  - newborn P78.0
  - obstetrical trauma O71.5
  - traumatic S36.533
- sinus (accessory) (chronic) (nasal) J34.89
- sphenoidal sinus —*see* Sinusitis, sphenoidal
- surgical (accidental) (by instrument) (blood vessel) (nerve) (organ) —*see* Puncture, accidental complicating surgery
- traumatic
  - external —*see* Puncture
  - eye —*see* Puncture, eyeball
  - internal organ —*see* Injury, by site
- tympanum, tympanic (membrane) (persistent post-traumatic) (postinflammatory) H72.9-
  - attic H72.1-
    - multiple —*see* Perforation, tympanum, multiple
    - total —*see* Perforation, tympanum, total
  - central H72.0-
    - multiple —*see* Perforation, tympanum, multiple
    - total —*see* Perforation, tympanum, total
  - marginal NEC —*see* subcategory H72.2
  - multiple H72.81-

Perforation, perforated *(continued)*
- tympanum, tympanic *(continued)*
  - pars flaccida —*see* Perforation, tympanum, attic
  - total H72.82-
  - traumatic, current episode S09.2-
- typhoid, gastrointestinal —*see* Typhoid
- ulcer —*see* Ulcer, by site, with perforation
- ureter N28.89
  - traumatic S37.19
- urethra N36.8
  - with ectopic or molar pregnancy O08.6
  - following ectopic or molar pregnancy O08.6
  - obstetrical trauma O71.5
  - traumatic S37.39
    - at delivery O71.5
- uterus
  - with ectopic or molar pregnancy O08.6
  - by intrauterine contraceptive device T83.39
  - following ectopic or molar pregnancy O08.6
  - obstetrical trauma O71.1
  - traumatic S37.69
    - obstetric O71.1
- uvula K13.79
  - syphilitic A52.79
- vagina
  - obstetrical trauma O71.4
  - other trauma —*see* Puncture, vagina

Periadenitis mucosa necrotica recurrens K12.0

Periappendicitis (acute) —*see* Appendicitis

Periarteritis nodosa (disseminated) (infectious) (necrotizing) M30.0

Periarthritis (joint) —*see also* Enthesopathy
- Duplay's M75.0-
- gonococcal A54.42
- humeroscapularis —*see* Capsulitis, adhesive
- scapulohumeral —*see* Capsulitis, adhesive
- shoulder —*see* Capsulitis, adhesive
- wrist M77.2-

Periarthrosis (angioneural) —*see* Enthesopathy

Pericapsulitis, adhesive (shoulder) —*see* Capsulitis, adhesive

Pericarditis (with decompensation) (with effusion) I31.9
- with rheumatic fever (conditions in I00)
  - active —*see* Pericarditis, rheumatic
  - inactive or quiescent I09.2
- acute (hemorrhagic) (nonrheumatic) (Sicca) I30.9
  - with chorea (acute) (rheumatic) (Sydenham's) I02.0
  - benign I30.8
  - nonspecific I30.0
  - rheumatic I01.0
    - with chorea (acute) (Sydenham's) I02.0
- adhesive or adherent (chronic) (external) (internal) I31.0
  - acute —*see* Pericarditis, acute
  - rheumatic I09.2

Pericarditis *(continued)*
- bacterial (acute) (subacute) (with serous or seropurulent effusion) I30.1
- calcareous I31.1
- cholesterol (chronic) I31.8
  - acute I30.9
- chronic (nonrheumatic) I31.9
  - rheumatic I09.2
- constrictive (chronic) I31.1
- coxsackie B33.23
- fibrinocaseous (tuberculous) A18.84
- fibrinopurulent I30.1
- fibrinous I30.8
- fibrous I31.0
- gonococcal A54.83
- idiopathic I30.0
- in systemic lupus erythematosus M32.12
- infective I30.1
- meningococcal A39.53
- neoplastic (chronic) I31.8
  - acute I30.9
- obliterans, obliterating I31.0
- plastic I31.0
- pneumococcal I30.1
- postinfarction I24.1
- purulent I30.1
- rheumatic (active) (acute) (with effusion) (with pneumonia) I01.0
  - with chorea (acute) (rheumatic) (Sydenham's) I02.0
  - chronic or inactive (with chorea) I09.2
- rheumatoid —*see* Rheumatoid, carditis
- septic I30.1
- serofibrinous I30.8
- staphylococcal I30.1
- streptococcal I30.1
- suppurative I30.1
- syphilitic A52.06
- tuberculous A18.84
- uremic N18.9 *[I32]*
- viral I30.1

Pericardium, pericardial —*see* condition

Pericellulitis —*see* Cellulitis

Pericementitis (chronic) (suppurative) —*see also* Periodontitis
- acute K05.20
  - generalized —*see* Periodontitis, aggressive, generalized
  - localized —*see* Periodontitis, aggressive, localized

Perichondritis
- auricle —*see* Perichondritis, ear
- bronchus J98.09
- ear (external) H61.00-
  - acute H61.01-
  - chronic H61.02-
- external auditory canal —*see* Perichondritis, ear
- larynx J38.7
  - syphilitic A52.73
  - typhoid A01.09
- nose J34.89
- pinna —*see* Perichondritis, ear
- trachea J39.8

Periclasia K05.4

Pericoronitis —*see* Periodontitis

Pericystitis N30.90
- with hematuria N30.91

Peridiverticulitis (intestine) K57.92
- cecum —*see* Diverticulitis, intestine, large
- colon —*see* Diverticulitis, intestine, large
- duodenum —*see* Diverticulitis, intestine, small
- intestine —*see* Diverticulitis, intestine
- jejunum —*see* Diverticulitis, intestine, small
- rectosigmoid —*see* Diverticulitis, intestine, large
- rectum —*see* Diverticulitis, intestine, large
- sigmoid —*see* Diverticulitis, intestine, large

Periendocarditis —*see* Endocarditis

Periepididymitis N45.1

Perifolliculitis L01.02
- abscedens, caput, scalp L66.3
- capitis, abscedens (et suffodiens) L66.3
- superficial pustular L01.02

Perihepatitis K65.8

Perilabyrinthitis (acute) —*see* subcategory H83.0

Perimeningitis —*see* Meningitis

Perimetritis —*see* Endometritis

Perimetrosalpingitis —*see* Salpingo-oophoritis

Perineocele N81.81

Perinephric, perinephritic —*see* condition

Perinephritis —*see also* Infection, kidney
- purulent —*see* Abscess, kidney

Perineum, perineal —*see* condition

Perineuritis NEC —*see* Neuralgia

Periodic —*see* condition

Periodontitis (chronic) (complex) (compound) (local) (simplex) K05.30
- acute K05.20
  - generalized K05.229
    - moderate K05.222
    - severe K05.223
    - slight K05.221
  - localized K05.219
    - moderate K05.212
    - severe K05.213
    - slight K05.211
- apical K04.5
  - acute (pulpal origin) K04.4
- generalized K05.329
  - moderate K05.322
  - severe K05.323
  - slight K05.321
- localized K05.319
  - moderate K05.312
  - severe K05.313
  - slight K05.311

Periodontoclasia K05.4

Periodontosis (juvenile) K05.4

Periods —*see also* Menstruation
- heavy N92.0
- irregular N92.6
- shortened intervals (irregular) N92.1

Perionychia —*see also* Cellulitis, digit
- with lymphangitis —*see* Lymphangitis, acute, digit

Personality *(continued)*
  expansive paranoid F60.0
  explosive F60.3
  fanatic F60.0
  haltlose type F60.89
  histrionic F60.4
  hyperthymic F34.0
  hypothymic F34.1
  hysterical F60.4
  immature F60.89
  inadequate F60.7
  labile (emotional) F60.3
  mixed (nonspecific) F60.89
  morally defective F60.2
  multiple F44.81
  narcissistic F60.81
  obsessional F60.5
  obsessive (-compulsive) F60.5
  organic F07.0
  overconscientious F60.5
  paranoid F60.0
  passive (-dependent) F60.7
  passive-aggressive F60.89
  pathologic F60.9
  pattern defect or disturbance F60.9
  pseudopsychopathic (organic) F07.0
  pseudoretarded (organic) F07.0
  psychoinfantile F60.4
  psychoneurotic NEC F60.89
  psychopathic F60.2
  querulant F60.0
  sadistic F60.89
  schizoid F60.1
  self-defeating F60.89
  sensitive paranoid F60.0
  sociopathic (amoral) (antisocial) (asocial) (dissocial) F60.2
  specified NEC F60.89
  type A Z73.1
  unstable (emotional) F60.3

Perthes' disease *—see* Legg-Calvé-Perthes disease

Pertussis (*see also* Whooping cough) A37.90

Perversion, perverted
  appetite F50.89
    psychogenic F50.89
  function
    pituitary gland E23.2
      posterior lobe E22.2
  sense of smell and taste R43.8
    psychogenic F45.8
  sexual *—see* Deviation, sexual

Pervious, congenital *—see also* Imperfect, closure
  ductus arteriosus Q25.0

Pes (congenital) *—see also* Talipes
  acquired *—see also* Deformity, limb, foot, specified NEC
    planus *—see* Deformity, limb, flat foot
  adductus Q66.89
  cavus Q66.7-
  deformity NEC, acquired *—see* Deformity, limb, foot, specified NEC
  planus (acquired) (any degree) *—see also* Deformity, limb, flat foot
    rachitic sequelae (late effect) E64.3
  valgus Q66.6

Pest, pestis *—see* Plague

Petechia, petechiae R23.3
  newborn P54.5

Petechial typhus A75.9

Peter's anomaly Q13.4

Petit mal seizure *—see* Epilepsy, childhood, absence

Petit's hernia *—see* Hernia, abdomen, specified site NEC

Petrellidosis B48.2

Petrositis H70.20-
  acute H70.21-
  chronic H70.22-

Peutz-Jeghers disease or syndrome Q85.8

Peyronie's disease N48.6

PFAPA (periodic fever, aphthous stomatitis, pharyngitis, and adenopathy syndrome) M04.8

Pfeiffer's disease *—see* Mononucleosis, infectious

Phagedena (dry) (moist) (sloughing) *—see also* Gangrene
  geometric L88
  penis N48.29
  tropical *—see* Ulcer, skin
  vulva N76.6

Phagedenic *—see* condition

Phakoma H35.89

Phakomatosis (*see also* specific eponymous syndromes) Q85.9
  Bourneville's Q85.1
  specified NEC Q85.8

Phantom limb syndrome (without pain) G54.7
  with pain G54.6

Pharyngeal pouch syndrome D82.1

Pharyngitis (acute) (catarrhal)(gangrenous) (infective) (malignant) (membranous) (phlegmonous) (pseudomembranous) (simple) (subacute) (suppurative) (ulcerative) (viral) J02.9
  with influenza, flu, or grippe *—see* Influenza, with, pharyngitis
  aphthous B08.5
  atrophic J31.2
  chlamydial A56.4
  chronic (atrophic) (granular) (hypertrophic) J31.2
  coxsackievirus B08.5
  diphtheritic A36.0
  enteroviral vesicular B08.5
  follicular (chronic) J31.2
  fusospirochetal A69.1
  gonococcal A54.5
  granular (chronic) J31.2
  herpesviral B00.2
  hypertrophic J31.2
  infectional, chronic J31.2
  influenzal *—see* Influenza, with, respiratory manifestations NEC
  lymphonodular, acute (enteroviral) B08.8
  pneumococcal J02.8
  purulent J02.9
  putrid J02.9
  septic J02.0
  sicca J31.2
  specified organism NEC J02.8
  staphylococcal J02.8
  streptococcal J02.0
  syphilitic, congenital (early) A50.03
  tuberculous A15.8
  vesicular, enteroviral B08.5
  viral NEC J02.8

Pharyngoconjunctivitis, viral B30.2

Pharyngolaryngitis (acute) J06.0
  chronic J37.0

Pharyngoplegia J39.2

Pharyngotonsillitis, herpesviral B00.2

Pharyngotracheitis, chronic J42

Pharynx, pharyngeal *—see* condition

Phencyclidine-induced
  anxiety disorder F16.980
  bipolar and related disorder F16.94
  depressive disorder F16.94
  psychotic disorder F16.959

Phenomenon
  Arthus' *—see* Arthus' phenomenon
  jaw-winking Q07.8
  lupus erythematosus (LE) cell M32.9
  Raynaud's (secondary) I73.00
    with gangrene I73.01
  vasomotor R55
  vasospastic I73.9
  vasovagal R55
  Wenckebach's I44.1

Phenylketonuria E70.1
  classical E70.0
  maternal E70.1

Pheochromoblastoma
  specified site *—see* Neoplasm, malignant, by site
  unspecified site C74.10

Pheochromocytoma
  malignant
    specified site *—see* Neoplasm, malignant, by site
    unspecified site C74.10
  specified site *—see* Neoplasm, benign, by site
  unspecified site D35.00

Pheohyphomycosis *—see* Chromomycosis

Pheomycosis *—see* Chromomycosis

Phimosis (congenital) (due to infection) N47.1
  chancroidal A57

Phlebectasia *—see also* Varix
  congenital Q27.4

Phlebitis (infective) (pyemic) (septic) (suppurative) I80.9
  antepartum *—see* Thrombophlebitis, antepartum
  blue *—see* Phlebitis, leg, deep
  breast, superficial I80.8
  calf muscular vein (NOS) I80.25-
  cavernous (venous) sinus *—see* Phlebitis, intracranial (venous) sinus
  cerebral (venous) sinus *—see* Phlebitis, intracranial (venous) sinus
  chest wall, superficial I80.8
  cranial (venous) sinus *—see* Phlebitis, intracranial (venous) sinus
  deep (vessels) *—see* Phlebitis, leg, deep
  due to implanted device *—see* Complications, by site and type, specified NEC
  during or resulting from a procedure T81.72
  femoral vein (superficial) I80.1-
  femoropopliteal vein I80.0-
  gastrocnemial vein I80.25-

Phlebitis *(continued)*
  gestational *—see* Phlebopathy, gestational
  hepatic veins I80.8
  iliac vein (common) (external) (internal) I80.21-
  iliofemoral *—see* Phlebitis, femoral vein
  intracranial (venous) sinus (any) G08
    nonpyogenic I67.6
  intraspinal venous sinuses and veins G08
    nonpyogenic G95.19
  lateral (venous) sinus *—see* Phlebitis, intracranial (venous) sinus
  leg I80.3
    antepartum *—see* Thrombophlebitis, antepartum
    deep (vessels) NEC I80.20-
      iliac I80.21-
      popliteal vein I80.22-
      specified vessel NEC I80.29-
      tibial vein (anterior) (posterior) I80.23-
    femoral vein (superficial) I80.1-
    superficial (vessels) I80.0-
  longitudinal sinus *—see* Phlebitis, intracranial (venous) sinus
  lower limb *—see* Phlebitis, leg
  migrans, migrating (superficial) I82.1
  pelvic
    with ectopic or molar pregnancy O08.0
    following ectopic or molar pregnancy O08.0
    puerperal, postpartum O87.1
  peroneal vein I80.24-
  popliteal vein *—see* Phlebitis, leg, deep, popliteal
  portal (vein) K75.1
  postoperative T81.72
  pregnancy *—see* Thrombophlebitis, antepartum
  puerperal, postpartum, childbirth O87.0
    deep O87.1
    pelvic O87.1
    superficial O87.0
  retina *—see* Vasculitis, retina
  saphenous (accessory) (great) (long) (small) *—see* Phlebitis, leg, superficial
  sinus (meninges) *—see* Phlebitis, intracranial (venous) sinus
  soleal vein I80.25-
  specified site NEC I80.8
  syphilitic A52.09
  tibial vein *—see* Phlebitis, leg, deep, tibial
  ulcerative I80.9
    leg *—see* Phlebitis, leg
  umbilicus I80.8
  uterus (septic) *—see* Endometritis
  varicose (leg) (lower limb) *—see* Varix, leg, with, inflammation

Phlebofibrosis I87.8

Phleboliths I87.8

Phlebopathy,
  gestational O22.9-
  puerperal O87.9

Phlebosclerosis I87.8

Phlebothrombosis *—see also* Thrombosis
  antepartum *—see* Thrombophlebitis, antepartum

Phlebothrombosis *(continued)*
pregnancy *—see* Thrombophlebitis, antepartum
puerperal *—see* Thrombophlebitis, puerperal

Phlebotomus fever A93.1

Phlegmasia
alba dolens O87.1
nonpuerperal *—see* Phlebitis, femoral vein
cerulea dolens *—see* Phlebitis, leg, deep

Phlegmon *—see* Abscess

Phlegmonous *—see* condition

Phlyctenulosis (allergic) (keratoconjunctivitis) (nontuberculous) *—see also* Keratoconjunctivitis
cornea *—see* Keratoconjunctivitis
tuberculous A18.52

Phobia, phobic F40.9
animal F40.218
spiders F40.210
examination F40.298
reaction F40.9
simple F40.298
social F40.10
generalized F40.11
specific (isolated) F40.298
animal F40.218
spiders F40.210
blood F40.230
injection F40.231
injury F40.233
men F40.290
natural environment F40.228
thunderstorms F40.220
situational F40.248
bridges F40.242
closed in spaces F40.240
flying F40.243
heights F40.241
specified focus NEC F40.298
transfusion F40.231
women F40.291
specified NEC F40.8
medical care NEC F40.232
state F40.9

Phocas' disease *—see* Mastopathy, cystic

Phocomelia Q73.1
lower limb *—see* Agenesis, leg, with foot present
upper limb *—see* Agenesis, arm, with hand present

Phoria H50.50

Phosphate-losing tubular disorder N25.0

Phosphatemia E83.39

Phosphaturia E83.39

Photodermatitis (sun) L56.8
chronic L57.8
due to drug L56.8
light other than sun L59.8

Photokeratitis H16.13-

Photophobia H53.14-

Photophthalmia *—see* Photokeratitis

Photopsia H53.19

Photoretinitis *—see* Retinopathy, solar

Photosensitivity, photosensitization (sun) **skin** L56.8
light other than sun L59.8

Phrenitis *—see* Encephalitis

Phrynoderma (vitamin A deficiency) E50.8

Phthiriasis (pubis) B85.3
with any infestation classifiable to B85.0-B85.2 *[B85.4]*

Phthirus infestation *—see* Phthiriasis

Phthisis *—see also* Tuberculosis
bulbi (infectional) *—see* Disorder, globe, degenerated condition, atrophy
eyeball (due to infection) *—see* Disorder, globe, degenerated condition, atrophy

Phycomycosis *—see* Zygomycosis

Physalopteriasis B81.8

Physical restraint status Z78.1

Phytobezoar T18.9
intestine T18.3
stomach T18.2

Pian *—see* Yaws

Pianoma A66.1

Pica F50.89
in adults F50.89
infant or child F98.3

Picking, nose F98.8

Pick-Niemann disease *—see* Niemann-Pick disease or syndrome

Pick's
cerebral atrophy G31.01 *[F02.80]*
with behavioral disturbance G31.01 *[F02.81]*
disease or syndrome (brain) G31.01 *[F02.80]*
with behavioral disturbance G31.01 *[F02.81]*
brain G31.01 *[F02.80]*
with behavioral disturbance G31.01 *[F02.81]*
pericardium (pericardial pseudocirrhosis of liver) I31.1
syndrome
brain G31.01 *[F02.80]*
with behavioral disturbance G31.01 *[F02.81]*
of heart (pericardial pseudocirrhosis of liver) I31.1

Pickwickian syndrome E66.2

Piebaldism E70.39

Piedra (beard) (scalp) B36.8
black B36.3
white B36.2

Pierre Robin deformity or syndrome Q87.0

Pierson's disease or osteochondrosis M91.0

Pig-bel A05.2

Pigeon
breast or chest (acquired) M95.4
congenital Q67.7
rachitic sequelae (late effect) E64.3
breeder's disease or lung J67.2
fancier's disease or lung J67.2
toe *—see* Deformity, toe, specified NEC

Pigmentation (abnormal) (anomaly) L81.9
conjunctiva H11.13-
cornea (anterior) H18.01-
posterior H18.05-
stromal H18.06-

Pigmentation *(continued)*
diminished melanin formation NEC L81.6
iron L81.8
lids, congenital Q82.8
limbus corneae *—see* Pigmentation, cornea
metals L81.8
optic papilla, congenital Q14.2
retina, congenital (grouped) (nevoid) Q14.1
scrotum, congenital Q82.8
tattoo L81.8

Piles (*see also* Hemorrhoids) K64.9

Pili
annulati or torti (congenital) Q84.1
incarnati L73.1

Pill roller hand (intrinsic) *—see* Parkinsonism

Pilomatrixoma *—see* Neoplasm, skin, benign
malignant *—see* Neoplasm, skin, malignant

Pilonidal *—see* condition

Pimple R23.8

PIMS M35.81

PIN *—see* Neoplasia, intraepithelial, prostate

Pinched nerve *—see* Neuropathy, entrapment

Pindborg tumor *—see* Cyst, calcifying odontogenic

Pineal body or gland *—see* condition

Pinealoblastoma C75.3

Pinealoma D44.5
malignant C75.3

Pineoblastoma C75.3

Pineocytoma D44.5

Pinguecula H11.15-

Pingueculitis H10.81-

Pinhole meatus (*see also* Stricture, urethra) N35.919

Pink
disease *—see* subcategory T56.1
eye *—see* Conjunctivitis, acute, mucopurulent

Pinkus' disease (lichen nitidus) L44.1

Pinpoint
meatus *—see* Stricture, urethra
os (uteri) *—see* Stricture, cervix

Pins and needles R20.2

Pinta A67.9
cardiovascular lesions A67.2
chancre (primary) A67.0
erythematous plaques A67.1
hyperchromic lesions A67.1
hyperkeratosis A67.1
lesions A67.9
cardiovascular A67.2
hyperchromic A67.1
intermediate A67.1
late A67.2
mixed A67.3
primary A67.0
skin (achromic) (cicatricial) (dyschromic) A67.2
hyperchromic A67.1

Pinta *(continued)*
lesions *(continued)*
skin *(continued)*
mixed (achromic and hyperchromic) A67.3
papule (primary) A67.0
skin lesions (achromic) (cicatricial) (dyschromic) A67.2
hyperchromic A67.1
mixed (achromic and hyperchromic) A67.3
vitiligo A67.2

Pintids A67.1

Pinworm (disease) (infection) (infestation) B80

Piroplasmosis (*see also* Babesiosis) B60.00
specified NEC B60.09

Pistol wound *—see* Gunshot wound

Pitchers' elbow *—see* Derangement, joint, specified type NEC, elbow

Pithecoid pelvis Q74.2
with disproportion (fetopelvic) O33.0
causing obstructed labor O65.0

Pithiatism F48.8

Pitted *—see* Pitting

Pitting (*see also* Edema) R60.9
lip R60.0
nail L60.8
teeth K00.4

Pituitary gland *—see* condition

Pituitary-snuff-taker's disease J67.8

Pityriasis (capitis) L21.0
alba L30.5
circinata (et maculata) L42
furfuracea L21.0
Hebra's L26
lichenoides L41.0
chronica L41.1
et varioliformis (acuta) L41.0
maculata (et circinata) L30.5
nigra B36.1
pilaris, Hebra's L44.0
rosea L42
rotunda L44.8
rubra (Hebra) pilaris L44.0
simplex L30.5
specified type NEC L30.5
streptogenes L30.5
versicolor (scrotal) B36.0

Placenta, placental *—see* Pregnancy, complicated by (care of) (management affected by), specified condition

Placentitis O41.14-

Plagiocephaly Q67.3

Plague A20.9
abortive A20.8
ambulatory A20.8
asymptomatic A20.8
bubonic A20.0
cellulocutaneous A20.1
cutaneobubonic A20.1
lymphatic gland A20.0
meningitis A20.3
pharyngeal A20.8
pneumonic (primary) (secondary) A20.2
pulmonary, pulmonic A20.2
septicemic A20.7
tonsillar A20.8
septicemic A20.7

Planning, family
contraception Z30.9
procreation Z31.69

Plaque(s)
  artery, arterial —*see* Arteriosclerosis
  calcareous —*see* Calcification
  coronary, lipid rich I25.83
  epicardial I31.8
  erythematous, of pinta A67.1
  Hollenhorst's —*see* Occlusion, artery, retina
  lipid rich, coronary I25.83
  pleural (without asbestos) J92.9
    with asbestos J92.0
  tongue K13.29
Plasmacytoma C90.3-
  extramedullary C90.2-
  medullary C90.0-
  solitary C90.3-
Plasmacytopenia D72.818
Plasmacytosis D72.822
Plaster ulcer —*see* Ulcer, pressure, by site
Plateau iris syndrome (post-iridectomy) (postprocedural) (without glaucoma) H21.82
  with glaucoma H40.22-
Platybasia Q75.8
Platyonychia (congenital) Q84.6
  acquired L60.8
Platypelloid pelvis M95.5
  with disproportion (fetopelvic) O33.0
    causing obstructed labor O65.0
  congenital Q74.2
Platyspondylisis Q76.49
Plaut (-Vincent) **disease** (*see also* Vincent's) A69.1
Plethora R23.2
  newborn P61.1
Pleura, pleural —*see* condition
Pleuralgia R07.81
Pleurisy (acute) (adhesive) (chronic) (costal) (diaphragmatic) (double) (dry) (fibrinous) (fibrous) (interlobar) (latent) (plastic) (primary) (residual) (sicca) (sterile) (subacute) (unresolved) R09.1
  with
    adherent pleura J86.0
    effusion J90
      chylous, chyliform J94.0
      tuberculous (non primary) A15.6
        primary (progressive) A15.7
    tuberculosis —*see* Pleurisy, tuberculous (non primary)
  encysted —*see* Pleurisy, with effusion
  exudative —*see* Pleurisy, with effusion
  fibrinopurulent, fibropurulent —*see* Pyothorax
  hemorrhagic —*see* Hemothorax
  pneumococcal J90
  purulent —*see* Pyothorax
  septic —*see* Pyothorax
  serofibrinous —*see* Pleurisy, with effusion
  seropurulent —*see* Pyothorax
  serous —*see* Pleurisy, with effusion
  staphylococcal J86.9
  streptococcal J90
  suppurative —*see* Pyothorax
  traumatic (post) (current) —*see* Injury, intrathoracic, pleura
  tuberculous (with effusion) (non primary) A15.6
    primary (progressive) A15.7
Pleuritis sicca —*see* Pleurisy
Pleurobronchopneumonia —*see* Pneumonia, broncho-
Pleurodynia R07.81
  epidemic B33.0
  viral B33.0
Pleuropericarditis —*see also* Pericarditis
  acute I30.9
Pleuropneumonia (acute) (bilateral) (double) (septic) (*see also* Pneumonia) J18.8
  chronic —*see* Fibrosis, lung
Pleuro-pneumonia-like-organism (PPLO), **as cause of disease classified elsewhere** B96.0
Pleurorrhea —*see* Pleurisy, with effusion
Plexitis, brachial G54.0
Plica
  polonica B85.0
  syndrome, knee M67.5-
  tonsil J35.8
Plicated tongue K14.5
Plug
  bronchus NEC J98.09
  meconium (newborn) NEC
    syndrome P76.0
  mucus —*see* Asphyxia, mucus
Plumbism —*see* subcategory T56.0
Plummer's disease E05.20
  with thyroid storm E05.21
Plummer-Vinson syndrome D50.1
Pluricarential syndrome of infancy E40
Plus (and minus) hand (intrinsic) —*see* Deformity, limb, specified type NEC, forearm
PMEI (polymorphic epilepsy in infancy) G40.83-
Pneumathemia —*see* Air, embolism
Pneumatic hammer (drill) **syndrome** T75.21
Pneumatocele (lung) J98.4
  intracranial G93.89
  tension J44.9
Pneumatosis
  cystoides intestinalis K63.89
  intestinalis K63.89
  peritonei K66.8
Pneumaturia R39.89
Pneumoblastoma —*see* Neoplasm, lung, malignant
Pneumocephalus G93.89
Pneumococcemia A40.3
Pneumococcus, pneumococcal —*see* condition
Pneumoconiosis (due to) (inhalation of) J64
  with tuberculosis (any type in A15) J65
  aluminum J63.0
  asbestos J61
  bagasse, bagassosis J67.1
  bauxite J63.1
  beryllium J63.2
  coal miners' (simple) J60
  coalworkers' (simple) J60
  collier's J60
  cotton dust J66.0
  diatomite (diatomaceous earth) J62.8
  dust
    inorganic NEC J63.6
    lime J62.8
    marble J62.8
    organic NEC J66.8
Pneumoconiosis *(continued)*
  fumes or vapors (from silo) J68.9
  graphite J63.3
  grinder's J62.8
  kaolin J62.8
  mica J62.8
  millstone maker's J62.8
  mineral fibers NEC J61
  miner's J60
  moldy hay J67.0
  potter's J62.8
  rheumatoid —*see* Rheumatoid, lung
  sandblaster's J62.8
  silica, silicate NEC J62.8
    with carbon J60
  stonemason's J62.8
  talc (dust) J62.0
Pneumocystis carinii pneumonia B59
Pneumocystis jiroveci (pneumonia) B59
Pneumocystosis (with pneumonia) B59
Pneumohemopericardium I31.2
Pneumohemothorax J94.2
  traumatic S27.2
Pneumohydropericardium —*see* Pericarditis
Pneumohydrothorax —*see* Hydrothorax
Pneumomediastinum J98.2
  congenital or perinatal P25.2
Pneumomycosis B49 *[J99]*
Pneumonia (acute) (double) (migratory) (purulent) (septic) (unresolved) J18.9
  with
    lung abscess J85.1
      due to specified organism —*see* Pneumonia, in (due to)
    influenza —*see* Influenza, with, pneumonia
  2019 (novel) coronavirus J12.82
  adenoviral J12.0
  adynamic J18.2
  alba A50.04
  allergic (*see also* Pneumonitis, hypersensitivity) J82.89
  alveolar —*see* Pneumonia, lobar
  anaerobes J15.8
  anthrax A22.1
  apex, apical —*see* Pneumonia, lobar
  Ascaris B77.81
  aspiration J69.0
    due to
      aspiration of microorganisms
        bacterial J15.9
        viral J12.9
      food (regurgitated) J69.0
      gastric secretions J69.0
      milk (regurgitated) J69.0
      oils, essences J69.1
      solids, liquids NEC J69.8
      vomitus J69.0
    newborn P24.81
      amniotic fluid (clear) P24.11
      blood P24.21
      liquor (amnii) P24.11
      meconium P24.01
      milk P24.31
      mucus P24.11
      food (regurgitated) P24.31
      specified NEC P24.81
      stomach contents P24.31
    postprocedural J95.4
  atypical NEC J18.9
Pneumonia *(continued)*
  bacillus J15.9
    specified NEC J15.8
  bacterial J15.9
    specified NEC J15.8
  Bacteroides (fragilis) (oralis) (melaninogenicus) J15.8
  basal, basic, basilar —*see* Pneumonia, by type
  bronchiolitis obliterans organized (BOOP) J84.89
  broncho-, bronchial (confluent) (croupous) (diffuse) (disseminated) (hemorrhagic) (involving lobes) (lobar) (terminal) J18.0
    allergic (*see also* Pneumonitis, hypersensitivity) J82.89
    aspiration —*see* Pneumonia, aspiration
    bacterial J15.9
      specified NEC J15.8
    chronic —*see* Fibrosis, lung
    diplococcal J13
    Eaton's agent J15.7
    Escherichia coli (E. coli) J15.5
    Friedländer's bacillus J15.0
    Hemophilus influenzae J14
    hypostatic J18.2
    inhalation —*see also* Pneumonia, aspiration
      due to fumes or vapors (chemical) J68.0
      of oils or essences J69.1
    Klebsiella (pneumoniae) J15.0
    lipid, lipoid J69.1
      endogenous J84.89
    Mycoplasma (pneumoniae) J15.7
    pleuro-pneumonia-like-organisms (PPLO) J15.7
    pneumococcal J13
    Proteus J15.6
    Pseudomonas J15.1
    Serratia marcescens J15.6
    specified organism NEC J16.8
    staphylococcal —*see* Pneumonia, staphylococcal
    streptococcal NEC J15.4
      group B J15.3
      pneumoniae J13
    viral, virus —*see* Pneumonia, viral
  Butyrivibrio (fibriosolvens) J15.8
  Candida B37.1
  caseous —*see* Tuberculosis, pulmonary
  catarrhal —*see* Pneumonia, broncho
  chlamydial J16.0
    congenital P23.1
  cholesterol J84.89
  cirrhotic (chronic) —*see* Fibrosis, lung
  Clostridium (haemolyticum) (novyi) J15.8
  confluent —*see* Pneumonia, broncho
  congenital (infective) P23.9
    due to
      bacterium NEC P23.6
      Chlamydia P23.1
      Escherichia coli P23.4
      Haemophilus influenzae P23.6
      infective organism NEC P23.8
      Klebsiella pneumoniae P23.6
      Mycoplasma P23.6
      Pseudomonas P23.5
      Staphylococcus P23.2
      Streptococcus (except group B) P23.6

Pneumonia *(continued)*
- congenital *(continued)*
  - due to *(continued)*
    - Streptococcus *(continued)*
      - group B P23.3
    - viral agent P23.0
  - specified NEC P23.8
- coronavirus (novel) (disease) 2019 J12.82
- COVID-19 J12.82
- croupous —*see* Pneumonia, lobar
- cryptogenic organizing J84.116
- cytomegalic inclusion B25.0
- cytomegaloviral B25.0
- deglutition —*see* Pneumonia, aspiration
- desquamative interstitial J84.117
- diffuse —*see* Pneumonia, broncho
- diplococcal, diplococcus (broncho-) (lobar) J13
- disseminated (focal) —*see* Pneumonia, broncho
- Eaton's agent J15.7
- embolic, embolism —*see* Embolism, pulmonary
- Enterobacter J15.6
- eosinophilic J82.81
  - acute J82.82
  - chronic J82.81
- Escherichia coli (E. coli) J15.5
- Eubacterium J15.8
- fibrinous —*see* Pneumonia, lobar
- fibroid, fibrous (chronic) —*see* Fibrosis, lung
- Friedländer's bacillus J15.0
- Fusobacterium (nucleatum) J15.8
- gangrenous J85.0
- giant cell (measles) B05.2
- gonococcal A54.84
- gram-negative bacteria NEC J15.6
  - anaerobic J15.8
- Hemophilus influenzae (broncho) (lobar) J14
- human metapneumovirus J12.3
- hypostatic (broncho) (lobar) J18.2
- in (due to)
  - actinomycosis A42.0
  - adenovirus J12.0
  - anthrax A22.1
  - ascariasis B77.81
  - aspergillosis B44.9
  - Bacillus anthracis A22.1
  - Bacterium anitratum J15.6
  - candidiasis B37.1
  - chickenpox B01.2
  - Chlamydia J16.0
    - neonatal P23.1
  - coccidioidomycosis B38.2
    - acute B38.0
    - chronic B38.1
  - cytomegalovirus disease B25.0
  - Diplococcus (pneumoniae) J13
  - Eaton's agent J15.7
  - Enterobacter J15.6
  - Escherichia coli (E. coli) J15.5
  - Friedländer's bacillus J15.0
  - fumes and vapors (chemical) (inhalation) J68.0
  - gonorrhea A54.84
  - Hemophilus influenzae (H. influenzae) J14
  - Herellea J15.6
  - histoplasmosis B39.2
    - acute B39.0
    - chronic B39.1
  - human metapneumovirus J12.3
  - Klebsiella (pneumoniae) J15.0
  - measles B05.2
  - Mycoplasma (pneumoniae) J15.7
  - nocardiosis, nocardiasis A43.0
  - ornithosis A70

Pneumonia *(continued)*
- in *(continued)*
  - parainfluenza virus J12.2
  - pleuro-pneumonia-like-organism (PPLO) J15.7
  - pneumococcus J13
  - pneumocystosis (Pneumocystis carinii) (Pneumocystis jiroveci) B59
  - Proteus J15.6
  - Pseudomonas NEC J15.1
    - pseudomallei A24.1
  - psittacosis A70
  - Q fever A78
  - respiratory syncytial virus (RSV) J12.1
  - rheumatic fever I00 *[J17]*
  - rubella B06.81
  - Salmonella (infection) A02.22
    - typhi A01.03
  - schistosomiasis B65.9 *[J17]*
  - Serratia marcescens J15.6
  - specified
    - bacterium NEC J15.8
    - organism NEC J16.8
  - spirochetal NEC A69.8
  - Staphylococcus J15.20
    - aureus (methicillin susceptible) (MSSA) J15.211
      - methicillin resistant (MRSA) J15.212
    - specified NEC J15.29
  - Streptococcus J15.4
    - group B J15.3
    - pneumoniae J13
    - specified NEC J15.4
  - toxoplasmosis B58.3
  - tularemia A21.2
  - typhoid (fever) A01.03
  - varicella B01.2
  - virus —*see* Pneumonia, viral
  - whooping cough A37.91
    - due to
      - Bordetella parapertussis A37.11
      - Bordetella pertussis A37.01
      - specified NEC A37.81
  - Yersinia pestis A20.2
- inhalation of food or vomit —*see* Pneumonia, aspiration
- interstitial J84.9
  - chronic J84.111
  - desquamative J84.117
  - due to
    - collagen vascular disease J84.178
    - known underlying cause J84.178
  - idiopathic NOS J84.111
  - in disease classified elsewhere J84.178
  - lymphocytic (due to collagen vascular disease) (in diseases classified elsewhere) J84.178
  - lymphoid J84.2
  - non-specific J84.89
    - due to
      - collagen vascular disease J84.178
      - known underlying cause J84.178
    - idiopathic J84.113
    - in diseases classified elsewhere J84.178
  - plasma cell B59
  - pseudomonas J15.1
  - usual J84.112
    - due to collagen vascular disease J84.178
    - idiopathic J84.112

Pneumonia *(continued)*
- interstitial *(continued)*
  - usual *(continued)*
    - in diseases classified elsewhere J84.178
- Klebsiella (pneumoniae) J15.0
- lipid, lipoid (exogenous) J69.1
  - endogenous J84.89
- lobar (disseminated) (double) (interstitial) J18.1
  - bacterial J15.9
    - specified NEC J15.8
  - chronic —*see* Fibrosis, lung
  - Escherichia coli (E. coli) J15.5
  - Friedländer's bacillus J15.0
  - Hemophilus influenzae J14
  - hypostatic J18.2
  - Klebsiella (pneumoniae) J15.0
  - pneumococcal J13
  - Proteus J15.6
  - Pseudomonas J15.1
  - specified organism NEC J16.8
  - staphylococcal —*see* Pneumonia, staphylococcal
  - streptococcal NEC J15.4
  - Streptococcus pneumoniae J13
  - viral, virus —*see* Pneumonia, viral
- lobular —*see* Pneumonia, broncho
- Löffler's J82.89
- lymphoid interstitial J84.2
- massive —*see* Pneumonia, lobar
- meconium P24.01
- MRSA (Methicillin resistant Staphylococcus aureus) J15.212
- MSSA (methicillin susceptible Staphylococcus aureus) J15.211
- multilobar —*see* Pneumonia, by type
- Mycoplasma (pneumoniae) J15.7
- necrotic J85.0
- neonatal P23.9
  - aspiration —*see* Aspiration, by substance, with pneumonia
- nitrogen dioxide J68.0
- organizing J84.89
  - due to
    - collagen vascular disease J84.178
    - known underlying cause J84.178
  - in diseases classified elsewhere J84.178
- orthostatic J18.2
- parainfluenza virus J12.2
- parenchymatous —*see* Fibrosis, lung
- passive J18.2
- patchy —*see* Pneumonia, broncho
- Peptococcus J15.8
- Peptostreptococcus J15.8
- plasma cell (of infants) B59
- pleurolobar —*see* Pneumonia, lobar
- pleuro-pneumonia-like organism (PPLO) J15.7
- pneumococcal (broncho) (lobar) J13
- Pneumocystis (carinii) (jiroveci) B59
- postinfectional NEC B99 *[J17]*
- postmeasles B05.2
- Proteus J15.6
- Pseudomonas J15.1
- psittacosis A70
- radiation J70.0
- respiratory syncytial virus (RSV) J12.1
- resulting from a procedure J95.89
- rheumatic I00 *[J17]*

Pneumonia *(continued)*
- Salmonella (arizonae) (choleraesuis) (enteritidis) (typhimurium) A02.22
  - typhi A01.03
  - typhoid fever A01.03
- SARS-associated coronavirus J12.81
- SARS-CoV-2 J12.82
- segmented, segmental —*see* Pneumonia, broncho-
- Serratia marcescens J15.6
- specified NEC J18.8
  - bacterium NEC J15.8
  - organism NEC J16.8
  - virus NEC J12.89
- spirochetal NEC A69.8
- staphylococcal (broncho) (lobar) J15.20
  - aureus (methicillin susceptible) (MSSA) J15.211
    - methicillin resistant (MRSA) J15.212
  - specified NEC J15.29
- static, stasis J18.2
- streptococcal NEC (broncho) (lobar) J15.4
  - group
    - A J15.4
    - B J15.3
    - specified NEC J15.4
- Streptococcus pneumoniae J13
- syphilitic, congenital (early) A50.04
- traumatic (complication) (early) (secondary) T79.8
- tuberculous (any) —*see* Tuberculosis, pulmonary
- tularemic A21.2
- varicella B01.2
- Veillonella J15.8
- ventilator associated J95.851
- viral, virus (broncho) (interstitial) (lobar) J12.9
  - adenoviral J12.0
  - congenital P23.0
  - human metapneumovirus J12.3
  - parainfluenza J12.2
  - respiratory syncytial (RSV) J12.1
  - SARS-associated coronavirus J12.81
  - specified NEC J12.89
- white (congenital) A50.04

Pneumonic —*see* condition

Pneumonitis (acute) (primary) —*see also* Pneumonia
- air-conditioner J67.7
- allergic (due to) J67.9
  - organic dust NEC J67.8
  - red cedar dust J67.8
  - sequoiosis J67.8
  - wood dust J67.8
- aspiration J69.0
  - due to
    - anesthesia J95.4
      - during
        - labor and delivery O74.0
        - pregnancy O29.01-
        - puerperium O89.01
    - fumes or gases J68.0
  - obstetric O74.0
- chemical (due to gases, fumes or vapors) (inhalation) J68.0
  - due to anesthesia J95.4
- cholesterol J84.89
- crack (cocaine) J68.0
- chronic —*see* Fibrosis, lung
- congenital rubella P35.0

Pneumonitis *(continued)*
- due to
  - beryllium J68.0
  - cadmium J68.0
  - crack (cocaine) J68.0
  - detergent J69.8
  - fluorocarbon-polymer J68.0
  - food, vomit (aspiration) J69.0
  - fumes or vapors J68.0
  - gases, fumes or vapors (inhalation) J68.0
  - inhalation
    - blood J69.8
    - essences J69.1
    - food (regurgitated), milk, vomit J69.0
    - oils, essences J69.1
    - saliva J69.0
    - solids, liquids NEC J69.8
  - manganese J68.0
  - nitrogen dioxide J68.0
  - oils, essences J69.1
  - solids, liquids NEC J69.8
  - toxoplasmosis (acquired) B58.3
    - congenital P37.1
  - vanadium J68.0
  - ventilator J95.851
- eosinophilic J82.81
  - acute J82.82
  - chronic J82.81
- hypersensitivity J67.9
  - air conditioner lung J67.7
  - bagassosis J67.1
  - bird fancier's lung J67.2
  - farmer's lung J67.0
  - maltworker's lung J67.4
  - maple bark-stripper's lung J67.6
  - mushroom worker's lung J67.5
  - specified organic dust NEC J67.8
  - suberosis J67.3
- interstitial (chronic) J84.89
  - acute J84.114
  - lymphoid J84.2
  - non-specific J84.89
    - idiopathic J84.113
- lymphoid, interstitial J84.2
- meconium P24.01
- postanesthetic J95.4
  - correct substance properly administered —*see* Table of Drugs and Chemicals, by drug, adverse effect
  - in labor and delivery O74.0
  - in pregnancy O29.01-
  - obstetric O74.0
  - overdose or wrong substance given or taken (by accident) —*see* Table of Drugs and Chemicals, by drug, poisoning
  - postpartum, puerperal O89.01
- postoperative J95.4
  - obstetric O74.0
- radiation J70.0
- rubella, congenital P35.0
- ventilation (air-conditioning) J67.7
- ventilator associated J95.851
- wood-dust J67.8

Pneumonoconiosis —*see* Pneumoconiosis

Pneumoparotid K11.8

Pneumopathy NEC J98.4
- alveolar J84.09
- due to organic dust NEC J66.8
- parietoalveolar J84.09

Pneumopericarditis —*see also* Pericarditis
- acute I30.9

Pneumopericardium —*see also* Pericarditis
- congenital P25.3
- newborn P25.3
- traumatic (post) —*see* Injury, heart

Pneumophagia (psychogenic) F45.8

Pneumopleurisy, pneumopleuritis (*see also* Pneumonia) J18.8

Pneumopyopericardium I30.1

Pneumopyothorax —*see* Pyopneumothorax
- with fistula J86.0

Pneumorrhagia —*see also* Hemorrhage, lung
- tuberculous —*see* Tuberculosis, pulmonary

Pneumothorax NOS J93.9
- acute J93.83
- chronic J93.81
- congenital P25.1
- perinatal period P25.1
- postprocedural J95.811
- specified NEC J93.83
- spontaneous NOS J93.83
  - newborn P25.1
  - primary J93.11
  - secondary J93.12
  - tension J93.0
- tense valvular, infectional J93.0
- tension (spontaneous) J93.0
- traumatic S27.0
  - with hemothorax S27.2
- tuberculous —*see* Tuberculosis, pulmonary

Podagra (*see also* Gout) M10.9

Podencephalus Q01.9

Poikilocytosis R71.8

Poikiloderma L81.6
- Civatte's L57.3
- congenital Q82.8
- vasculare atrophicans L94.5

Poikilodermatomyositis M33.10
- with
  - myopathy M33.12
  - respiratory involvement M33.11
  - specified organ involvement NEC M33.19

Pointed ear (congenital) Q17.3

Poison ivy, oak, sumac or other plant dermatitis (allergic) (contact) L23.7

Poisoning (acute) —*see also* Table of Drugs and Chemicals
- algae and toxins T65.82-
- Bacillus B (aertrycke) (cholerae (suis)) (paratyphosus) (suipestifer) A02.9
  - botulinus A05.1
- bacterial toxins A05.9
- berries, noxious —*see* Poisoning, food, noxious, berries
- botulism A05.1
- ciguatera fish T61.0-
- Clostridium botulinum A05.1
- death-cap (Amanita phalloides) (Amanita verna) —*see* Poisoning, food, noxious, mushrooms
- drug —*see* Table of Drugs and Chemicals, by drug, poisoning
- epidemic, fish (noxious) —*see* Poisoning, seafood
  - bacterial A05.9
- fava bean D55.0

Poisoning *(continued)*
- fish (noxious) T61.9-
  - bacterial —*see* Intoxication, foodborne, by agent
  - ciguatera fish —*see* Poisoning, ciguatera fish
  - scombroid fish —*see* Poisoning, scombroid fish
  - specified type NEC T61.77-
- food NEC A05.9
  - bacterial —*see* Intoxication, foodborne, by agent
  - due to
    - Bacillus (aertrycke) (choleraesuis) (paratyphosus) (suipestifer) A02.9
      - botulinus A05.1
    - Clostridium (perfringens) (Welchii) A05.2
    - salmonella (aertrycke) (callinarum) (choleraesuis) (enteritidis) (paratyphi) (suipestifer) A02.9
      - with
        - gastroenteritis A02.0
        - sepsis A02.1
    - staphylococcus A05.0
    - Vibrio
      - parahaemolyticus A05.3
      - vulnificus A05.5
  - noxious or naturally toxic T62.9-
    - berries —*see* subcategory T62.1-
    - fish —*see* Poisoning, seafood
    - mushrooms —*see* subcategory T62.0X-
    - plants NEC —*see* subcategory T62.2X-
    - seafood —*see* Poisoning, seafood
    - specified NEC T62.8X-
- ichthyotoxism —*see* Poisoning, seafood
- kreotoxism, food A05.9
- latex T65.81-
- lead T56.0-
- mushroom —*see* Poisoning, food, noxious, mushroom
- mussels —*see also* Poisoning, shellfish
  - bacterial —*see* Intoxication, foodborne, by agent
- nicotine (tobacco) T65.2-
- noxious foodstuffs —*see* Poisoning, food, noxious
- plants, noxious —*see* Poisoning, food, noxious, plants NEC
- ptomaine —*see* Poisoning, food
- radiation J70.0
- Salmonella (arizonae) (cholerae-suis) (enteritidis) (typhimurium) A02.9
- scombroid fish T61.1-
- seafood (noxious) T61.9-
  - bacterial —*see* Intoxication, foodborne, by agent
  - fish —*see* Poisoning, fish
  - shellfish —*see* Poisoning, shellfish
  - specified NEC —*see* subcategory T61.8X-
- shellfish (amnesic) (azaspiracid) (diarrheic) (neurotoxic) (noxious) (paralytic) T61.78-
  - bacterial —*see* Intoxication, foodborne, by agent
  - ciguatera mollusk —*see* Poisoning, ciguatera fish

Poisoning *(continued)*
- specified substance NEC T65.891
- Staphylococcus, food A05.0
- tobacco (nicotine) T65.2-
- water E87.79

Poker spine —*see* Spondylitis, ankylosing

Poland syndrome Q79.8

Polioencephalitis (acute) (bulbar) A80.9
- inferior G12.22
- influenzal —*see* Influenza, with, encephalopathy
- superior hemorrhagic (acute) (Wernicke's) E51.2
- Wernicke's E51.2

Polioencephalomyelitis (acute) (anterior) A80.9
- with beriberi E51.2

Polioencephalopathy, superior hemorrhagic E51.2
- with
  - beriberi E51.11
  - pellagra E52

Poliomeningoencephalitis —*see* Meningoencephalitis

Poliomyelitis (acute) (anterior) (epidemic) A80.9
- with paralysis (bulbar) —*see* Poliomyelitis, paralytic
- abortive A80.4
- ascending (progressive) —*see* Poliomyelitis, paralytic
- bulbar (paralytic) —*see* Poliomyelitis, paralytic
- congenital P35.8
- nonepidemic A80.9
- nonparalytic A80.4
- paralytic A80.30
  - specified NEC A80.39
  - vaccine-associated A80.0
  - wild virus
    - imported A80.1
    - indigenous A80.2
- spinal, acute A80.9

Poliosis (eyebrow) (eyelashes) L67.1
- circumscripta, acquired L67.1

Pollakiuria R35.0
- psychogenic F45.8

Pollinosis J30.1

Pollitzer's disease L73.2

Polyadenitis —*see also* Lymphadenitis
- malignant A20.0

Polyalgia M79.89

Polyangiitis M30.0
- microscopic M31.7
- overlap syndrome M30.8

Polyarteritis
- microscopic M31.7
- nodosa M30.0
  - with lung involvement M30.1
  - juvenile M30.2
  - related condition NEC M30.8

Polyarthralgia —*see* Pain, joint

Polyarthritis, polyarthropathy (*see also* Arthritis) M13.0
- due to or associated with other specified conditions —*see* Arthritis
- epidemic (Australian) (with exanthema) B33.1
- infective —*see* Arthritis, pyogenic or pyemic

Polyarthritis, polyarthropathy *(continued)*
- inflammatory M06.4
- juvenile (chronic) (seronegative) M08.3
- migratory M13.8-
- rheumatic, acute *—see* Fever, rheumatic

Polyarthrosis M15.9
- post-traumatic M15.3
- primary M15.0
- specified NEC M15.8

Polycarential syndrome of infancy E40

Polychondritis (atrophic) (chronic) *—see also* Disorder, cartilage, specified type NEC
- relapsing M94.1

Polycoria Q13.2

Polycystic (disease)
- degeneration, kidney Q61.3
  - autosomal dominant (adult type) Q61.2
  - autosomal recessive (infantile type) NEC Q61.19
- kidney Q61.3
  - autosomal
    - dominant Q61.2
    - recessive NEC Q61.19
  - autosomal dominant (adult type) Q61.2
  - autosomal recessive (childhood type) NEC Q61.19
  - infantile type NEC Q61.19
- liver Q44.6
- lung J98.4
  - congenital Q33.0
- ovary, ovaries E28.2
- spleen Q89.09

Polycythemia (secondary) D75.1
- acquired D75.1
- benign (familial) D75.0
- due to
  - donor twin P61.1
  - erythropoietin D75.1
  - fall in plasma volume D75.1
  - high altitude D75.1
  - maternal-fetal transfusion P61.1
  - stress D75.1
- emotional D75.1
- erythropoietin D75.1
- familial (benign) D75.0
- Gaisböck's (hypertonica) D75.1
- high altitude D75.1
- hypertonica D75.1
- hypoxemic D75.1
- neonatorum P61.1
- nephrogenous D75.1
- relative D75.1
- secondary D75.1
- spurious D75.1
- stress D75.1
- vera D45

Polycytosis cryptogenica D75.1

Polydactylism, polydactyly Q69.9
- toes Q69.2

Polydipsia R63.1

Polydystrophy, pseudo-Hurler E77.0

Polyembryoma *—see* Neoplasm, malignant, by site

Polyglandular
- deficiency E31.0
- dyscrasia E31.9
- dysfunction E31.9
- syndrome E31.8

Polyhydramnios O40.-

Polymastia Q83.1

Polymenorrhea N92.0

Polymyalgia M35.3
- arteritica, giant cell M31.5
- rheumatica M35.3
  - with giant cell arteritis M31.5

Polymyositis (acute) (chronic) (hemorrhagic) M33.20
- with
  - myopathy M33.22
  - respiratory involvement M33.21
  - skin involvement *—see* Dermatopolymyositis
  - specified organ involvement NEC M33.29
- ossificans (generalisata) (progressiva) *—see* Myositis, ossificans, progressiva

Polyneuritis, polyneuritic *—see also* Polyneuropathy
- acute (post-)infective G61.0
- alcoholic G62.1
- cranialis G52.7
- demyelinating, chronic inflammatory (CIDP) G61.81
- diabetic *—see* Diabetes, polyneuropathy
- diphtheritic A36.83
- due to lack of vitamin NEC E56.9 *[G63]*
- endemic E51.11
- erythredema *—see* subcategory T56.1
- febrile, acute G61.0
- hereditary ataxic G60.1
- idiopathic, acute G61.0
- infective (acute) G61.0
- inflammatory, chronic demyelinating (CIDP) G61.81
- nutritional E63.9 *[G63]*
- postinfective (acute) G61.0
- specified NEC G62.89

Polyneuropathy (peripheral) G62.9
- alcoholic G62.1
- amyloid (Portuguese) E85.1 *[G63]*
  - transthyretin-related (ATTR) familial E85.1 *[G63]*
- arsenical G62.2
- critical illness G62.81
- demyelinating, chronic inflammatory (CIDP) G61.81
- diabetic *—see* Diabetes, polyneuropathy
- drug-induced G62.0
- hereditary G60.9
  - specified NEC G60.8
- idiopathic G60.9
  - progressive G60.3
- in (due to)
  - alcohol G62.1
    - sequelae G65.2
  - amyloidosis, familial (Portuguese) E85.1 *[G63]*
  - antitetanus serum G61.1
  - arsenic G62.2
    - sequelae G65.2
  - avitaminosis NEC E56.9 *[G63]*
  - beriberi E51.11
  - collagen vascular disease NEC M35.9 *[G63]*
  - deficiency (of)
    - B (-complex) vitamins E53.9 *[G63]*
    - vitamin B6 E53.1 *[G63]*
  - diabetes *—see* Diabetes, polyneuropathy

Polyneuropathy *(continued)*
- in *(continued)*
  - diphtheria A36.83
  - drug or medicament G62.0
    - correct substance properly administered *—see* Table of Drugs and Chemicals, by drug, adverse effect
    - overdose or wrong substance given or taken *—see* Table of Drugs and Chemicals, by drug, poisoning
  - endocrine disease NEC E34.9 *[G63]*
  - herpes zoster B02.23
  - hypoglycemia E16.2 *[G63]*
  - infectious
    - disease NEC B99 *[G63]*
    - mononucleosis B27.91
  - lack of vitamin NEC E56.9 *[G63]*
  - lead G62.2
    - sequelae G65.2
  - leprosy A30.9 *[G63]*
  - Lyme disease A69.22
  - metabolic disease NEC E88.9 *[G63]*
  - microscopic polyangiitis M31.7 *[G63]*
  - mumps B26.84
  - neoplastic disease (*see also* Neoplasm) D49.9 *[G63]*
  - nutritional deficiency NEC E63.9 *[G63]*
  - organophosphate compounds G62.2
    - sequelae G65.2
  - parasitic disease NEC B89 *[G63]*
  - pellagra E52 *[G63]*
  - polyarteritis nodosa M30.0
  - porphyria E80.20 *[G63]*
  - radiation G62.82
  - rheumatoid arthritis *—see* Rheumatoid, polyneuropathy
  - sarcoidosis D86.89
  - serum G61.1
  - syphilis (late) A52.15
    - congenital A50.43
  - systemic
    - connective tissue disorder M35.9 *[G63]*
    - lupus erythematosus M32.19
  - toxic agent NEC G62.2
    - sequelae G65.2
  - transthyretin-related (ATTR) familial amyloid E85.1
- inflammatory G61.9
  - chronic demyelinating (CIDP) G61.81
  - sequelae G65.1
  - specified NEC G61.89
- lead G62.2
  - sequelae G65.2
- nutritional NEC E63.9 *[G63]*
- postherpetic (zoster) B02.23
- progressive G60.3
- radiation-induced G62.82
- sensory (hereditary) (idiopathic) G60.8
- specified NEC G62.89
- syphilitic (late) A52.15
  - congenital A50.43
- triorthocresyl phosphate G62.2
  - sequelae G65.2
- tuberculosis A17.89
- uremia N18.9 *[G63]*

Polyneuropathy *(continued)*
- syphilitic *(continued)*
  - vitamin B12 deficiency E53.8 *[G63]*
    - with anemia (pernicious) D51.0 *[G63]*
      - due to dietary deficiency D51.3 *[G63]*
- zoster B02.23

Polyopia H53.8

Polyorchism, polyorchidism Q55.21

Polyosteoarthritis (*see also* Osteoarthritis, generalized) M15.9-
- post-traumatic M15.3
- specified NEC M15.8

Polyostotic fibrous dysplasia Q78.1

Polyotia Q17.0

Polyp, polypus
- accessory sinus J33.8
- adenocarcinoma in *—see* Neoplasm, malignant, by site
- adenocarcinoma in situ in *—see* Neoplasm, in situ, by site
- adenoid tissue J33.0
- adenomatous *—see also* Neoplasm, benign, by site
  - adenocarcinoma in *—see* Neoplasm, malignant, by site
  - adenocarcinoma in situ in *—see* Neoplasm, in situ, by site
  - carcinoma in *—see* Neoplasm, malignant, by site
  - carcinoma in situ in *—see* Neoplasm, in situ, by site
  - multiple *—see* Neoplasm, benign
    - adenocarcinoma in *—see* Neoplasm, malignant, by site
    - adenocarcinoma in situ in *—see* Neoplasm, in situ, by site
- antrum J33.8
- anus, anal (canal) K62.0
- Bartholin's gland N84.3
- bladder D41.4
- carcinoma in *—see* Neoplasm, malignant, by site
- carcinoma in situ in *—see* Neoplasm, in situ, by site
- cecum D12.0
- cervix (uteri) N84.1
  - in pregnancy or childbirth *—see* Pregnancy, complicated by, abnormal, cervix
  - mucous N84.1
  - nonneoplastic N84.1
- choanal J33.0
- cholesterol K82.4
- clitoris N84.3
- colon K63.5
  - adenomatous D12.6
    - ascending D12.2
    - cecum D12.0
    - descending D12.4
    - sigmoid D12.5
    - transverse D12.3
  - ascending K63.5
  - cecum K63.5
  - descending K63.5
  - hyperplastic, (any site) K63.5
  - inflammatory K51.40
    - with
      - abscess K51.414
      - complication K51.419
        - specified NEC K51.418
      - fistula K51.413
      - intestinal obstruction K51.412
      - rectal bleeding K51.411

Polyp, polypus *(continued)*
- colon *(continued)*
  - sigmoid K63.5
  - transverse K63.5
- corpus uteri N84.0
- dental K04.01
  - irreversible K04.02
  - reversible K04.01
- duodenum K31.7
- ear (middle) H74.4-
- endometrium N84.0
- esophageal K22.81
- esophagogastric junction K22.82
- ethmoidal (sinus) J33.8
- fallopian tube N84.8
- female genital tract N84.9
  - specified NEC N84.8
- frontal (sinus) J33.8
- gallbladder K82.4
- gingiva, gum K06.8
- labia, labium (majus) (minus) N84.3
- larynx (mucous) J38.1
  - adenomatous D14.1
- malignant *—see* Neoplasm, malignant, by site
- maxillary (sinus) J33.8
- middle ear *—see* Polyp, ear (middle)
- myometrium N84.0
- nares
  - anterior J33.9
  - posterior J33.0
- nasal (mucous) J33.9
  - cavity J33.0
  - septum J33.0
- nasopharyngeal J33.0
- nose (mucous) J33.9
- oviduct N84.8
- pharynx J39.2
- placenta O90.89
- prostate *—see* Enlargement, enlarged, prostate
- pudenda, pudendum N84.3
- pulpal (dental) K04.01
  - irreversible K04.02
  - reversible K04.01
- rectum (nonadenomatous) K62.1
  - adenomatous *—see* Polyp, adenomatous
- septum (nasal) J33.0
- sinus (accessory) (ethmoidal) (frontal) (maxillary) (sphenoidal) J33.8
- sphenoidal (sinus) J33.8
- stomach K31.7
  - adenomatous D13.1
- tube, fallopian N84.8
- turbinate, mucous membrane J33.8
- umbilical, newborn P83.6
- ureter N28.89
- urethra N36.2
- uterus (body) (corpus) (mucous) N84.0
  - cervix N84.1
  - in pregnancy or childbirth *—see* Pregnancy, complicated by, tumor, uterus
- vagina N84.2
- vocal cord (mucous) J38.1
- vulva N84.3

Polyphagia R63.2

Polyploidy Q92.7

Polypoid *—see* condition

Polyposis *—see also* Polyp
- coli (adenomatous) D12.6
  - adenocarcinoma in C18.9
  - adenocarcinoma in situ in *—see* Neoplasm, in situ, by site
  - carcinoma in C18.9

Polyposis *(continued)*
- colon (adenomatous) D12.6
- familial D12.6
  - adenocarcinoma in situ in *—see* Neoplasm, in situ, by site
- intestinal (adenomatous) D12.6
- malignant lymphomatous C83.1-
- multiple, adenomatous (*see also* Neoplasm, benign) D36.9

Polyradiculitis *—see* Polyneuropathy

Polyradiculoneuropathy (acute) (postinfective) (segmentally demyelinating) G61.0

Polyserositis
- due to pericarditis I31.1
- pericardial I31.1
- periodic, familial E85.0
- tuberculous A19.9
  - acute A19.1
  - chronic A19.8

Polysplenia syndrome Q89.09

Polysyndactyly (*see also* Syndactylism, syndactyly) Q70.4

Polytrichia L68.3

Polyunguia Q84.6

Polyuria R35.89
- nocturnal R35.81
- psychogenic F45.8
- specified NEC R35.89

Pompe's disease (glycogen storage) E74.02

Pompholyx L30.1

Poncet's disease (tuberculous rheumatism) A18.09

Pond fracture *—see* Fracture, skull

Ponos B55.0

Pons, pontine *—see* condition

Poor
- aesthetic of existing restoration of tooth K08.56
- contractions, labor O62.2
- gingival margin to tooth restoration K08.51
- personal hygiene R46.0
- prenatal care, affecting management of pregnancy *—see* Pregnancy, complicated by, insufficient, prenatal care
- sucking reflex (newborn) R29.2
- urinary stream R39.12
- vision NEC H54.7

Poradenitis, nostras inguinalis or venerea A55

Porencephaly (congenital) (developmental) (true) Q04.6
- acquired G93.0
- nondevelopmental G93.0
- traumatic (post) F07.89

Porocephaliasis B88.8

Porokeratosis Q82.8

Poroma, eccrine *—see* Neoplasm, skin, benign

Porphyria (South African) E80.20
- acquired E80.20
- acute intermittent (hepatic) (Swedish) E80.21
- cutanea tarda (hereditary) (symptomatic) E80.1
- due to drugs E80.20
  - correct substance properly administered *—see* Table of Drugs and Chemicals, by drug, adverse effect

Porphyria *(continued)*
- due to drugs *(continued)*
  - overdose or wrong substance given or taken *—see* Table of Drugs and Chemicals, by drug, poisoning
- erythropoietic (congenital) (hereditary) E80.0
- hepatocutaneous type E80.1
- secondary E80.20
- toxic NEC E80.20
- variegata E80.20

Porphyrinuria *—see* Porphyria

Porphyruria *—see* Porphyria

Portal *—see* condition

Port wine nevus, mark, or stain Q82.5

Posadas-Wernicke disease B38.9

Positive
- culture (nonspecific)
  - blood R78.81
  - bronchial washings R84.5
  - cerebrospinal fluid R83.5
  - cervix uteri R87.5
  - nasal secretions R84.5
  - nipple discharge R89.5
  - nose R84.5
    - staphylococcus (Methicillin susceptible) Z22.321
      - Methicillin resistant Z22.322
  - peritoneal fluid R85.5
  - pleural fluid R84.5
  - prostatic secretions R86.5
  - saliva R85.5
  - seminal fluid R86.5
  - sputum R84.5
  - synovial fluid R89.5
  - throat scrapings R84.5
  - urine R82.79
  - vagina R87.5
  - vulva R87.5
  - wound secretions R89.5
- PPD (skin test) R76.11
- serology for syphilis A53.0
  - false R76.8
  - with signs or symptoms - code as Syphilis, by site and stage
- skin test, tuberculin (without active tuberculosis) R76.11
- test, human immunodeficiency virus (HIV) R75
- VDRL A53.0
  - with signs or symptoms - code by site and stage under Syphilis A53.9
- Wassermann reaction A53.0

Postcardiotomy syndrome I97.0

Postcaval ureter Q62.62

Postcholecystectomy syndrome K91.5

Postclimacteric bleeding N95.0

Postcommissurotomy syndrome I97.0

Postconcussional syndrome F07.81

Postcontusional syndrome F07.81

Postcricoid region *—see* condition

Post COVID-19 condition, unspecified U09.9

Post-dates (40-42 weeks) (pregnancy) (mother) O48.0
- more than 42 weeks gestation O48.1

Postencephalitic syndrome F07.89

Posterior *—see* condition

Posterolateral sclerosis (spinal cord) *—see* Degeneration, combined

Postexanthematous *—see* condition

Postfebrile *—see* condition

Postgastrectomy dumping syndrome K91.1

Posthemiplegic chorea *—see* Monoplegia

Posthemorrhagic anemia (chronic) D50.0
- acute D62
- newborn P61.3

Postherpetic neuralgia (zoster) B02.29
- trigeminal B02.22

Posthitis N47.7

Postimmunization complication or reaction *—see* Complications, vaccination

Postinfectious *—see* condition

Postlaminectomy syndrome NEC M96.1

Postleukotomy syndrome F07.0

Postmastectomy lymphedema (syndrome) I97.2

Postmaturity, postmature (over 42 weeks)
- maternal (over 42 weeks gestation) O48.1
- newborn P08.22

Postmeasles complication NEC *— see also* condition B05.89

Postmenopausal
- endometrium (atrophic) N95.8
  - suppurative (*see also* Endometritis) N71.9
- osteoporosis *—see* Osteoporosis, postmenopausal

Postnasal drip R09.82
- due to
  - allergic rhinitis *—see* Rhinitis, allergic
  - common cold J00
  - gastroesophageal reflux *—see* Reflux, gastroesophageal
  - nasopharyngitis *—see* Nasopharyngitis
  - other know condition - code to condition
  - sinusitis *—see* Sinusitis

Postnatal *—see* condition

Postoperative (postprocedural) *—see* Complication, postoperative
- pneumothorax, therapeutic Z98.3
- state NEC Z98.890

Postpancreatectomy hyperglycemia E89.1

Postpartum *—see* Puerperal

Postphlebitic syndrome *—see* Syndrome, postthrombotic

Postpoliomyelitic *—see also* condition
- osteopathy *—see* Osteopathy, after poliomyelitis

Postpolio (myelitic) **syndrome** G14

Postprocedural *—see also* Postoperative
- hypoinsulinemia E89.1

Postschizophrenic depression F32.89

Postsurgery status —*see also* Status (post)
- pneumothorax, therapeutic Z98.3

Post-term (40-42 weeks) (pregnancy) (mother) O48.0
- infant P08.21
- more than 42 weeks gestation (mother) O48.1

Post-traumatic brain syndrome, nonpsychotic F07.81

Post-typhoid abscess A01.09

Postures, hysterical F44.2

Postvaccinal reaction or complication —*see* Complications, vaccination

Postvalvulotomy syndrome I97.0

Potain's
- disease (pulmonary edema) —*see* Edema, lung
- syndrome (gastrectasis with dyspepsia) K31.0

Potter's
- asthma J62.8
- facies Q60.6
- lung J62.8
- syndrome (with renal agenesis) Q60.6

Pott's
- curvature (spinal) A18.01
- disease or paraplegia A18.01
- spinal curvature A18.01
- tumor, puffy —*see* Osteomyelitis, specified type NEC

Pouch
- bronchus Q32.4
- Douglas' —*see* condition
- esophagus, esophageal, congenital Q39.6
  - acquired K22.5
- gastric K31.4
- Hartmann's K82.8
- pharynx, pharyngeal (congenital) Q38.7

Pouchitis K91.850

Poultrymen's itch B88.0

Poverty NEC Z59.6
- extreme Z59.5

Poxvirus NEC B08.8

Prader-Willi syndrome Q87.11

Prader-Willi-like syndrome Q87.19

Preauricular appendage or tag Q17.0

Prebetalipoproteinemia (acquired) (essential) (familial) (hereditary) (primary) (secondary) E78.1
- with chylomicronemia E78.3

Precipitate labor or delivery O62.3

Preclimacteric bleeding (menorrhagia) N92.4

Precocious
- adrenarche E30.1
- menarche E30.1
- menstruation E30.1
- pubarche E30.1
- puberty E30.1
  - central E22.8
- sexual development NEC E30.1
- thelarche E30.8

Precocity, sexual (constitutional) (cryptogenic) (female) (idiopathic) (male) E30.1
- with adrenal hyperplasia E25.9
- congenital E25.0

Precordial pain R07.2

Predeciduous teeth K00.2

Prediabetes, prediabetic R73.03
- complicating
  - pregnancy —*see* Pregnancy, complicated by, diseases of, specified type or system NEC
  - puerperium O99.893

Predislocation status of hip at birth Q65.6

Pre-eclampsia O14.9-
- with pre-existing hypertension —*see* Hypertension, complicating pregnancy, pre-existing, with, pre-eclampsia
- complicating
  - childbirth O14.94
  - puerperium O14.95
- mild O14.0-
  - complicating
    - childbirth O14.04
    - puerperium O14.05
- moderate O14.0-
  - complicating
    - childbirth O14.04
    - puerperium O14.05
- severe O14.1-
  - with hemolysis, elevated liver enzymes and low platelet count (HELLP) O14.2-
    - complicating
      - childbirth O14.24
      - puerperium O14.25
  - complicating
    - childbirth O14.14
    - puerperium O14.15

Pre-eruptive color change, teeth, tooth K00.8

Pre-excitation atrioventricular conduction I45.6

Preglaucoma H40.00-

Pregnancy (single) (uterine) —*see also* Delivery and Puerperal Z33.1

> Note: The Tabular must be reviewed for assignment of the appropriate character indicating the trimester of the pregnancy
> Note: The Tabular must be reviewed for assignment of appropriate seventh character for multiple gestation codes in Chapter 15

- abdominal (ectopic) O00.00
  - with intrauterine pregnancy O00.01
  - with viable fetus O36.7-
- ampullar O00.10-
  - with intrauterine pregnancy O00.11-
- biochemical O02.81
- broad ligament O00.80
  - with intrauterine pregnancy O00.81
- cervical O00.80
  - with intrauterine pregnancy O00.81
- chemical O02.81
- complicated NOS O26.9-

Pregnancy *(continued)*
- complicated by (care of) (management affected by)
  - abnormal, abnormality
    - cervix O34.4-
      - causing obstructed labor O65.5
    - cord (umbilical) O69.9
    - fetal heart rate or rhythm O36.83-
    - findings on antenatal screening of mother O28.9
      - biochemical O28.1
      - cytological O28.2
      - chromosomal O28.5
      - genetic O28.5
      - hematological O28.0
      - radiological O28.4
      - specified NEC O28.8
      - ultrasonic O28.3
    - glucose (tolerance) NEC O99.810
    - pelvic organs O34.9-
      - specified NEC O34.8-
        - causing obstructed labor O65.5
    - pelvis (bony) (major) NEC O33.0
    - perineum O34.7-
    - position
      - placenta O44.0
        - with hemorrhage O44.1-
      - uterus O34.59-
    - uterus O34.59-
      - causing obstructed labor O65.5
      - congenital O34.0-
    - vagina O34.6-
      - causing obstructed labor O65.5
    - vulva O34.7-
      - causing obstructed labor O65.5
  - abruptio placentae —*see* Abruptio placentae
  - abscess or cellulitis
    - bladder O23.1-
    - breast O91.11-
    - genital organ or tract O23.9-
  - abuse
    - physical O9A.31-
    - psychological O9A.51-
    - sexual O9A.41-
  - adverse effect anesthesia O29.9-
    - aspiration pneumonitis O29.01-
    - cardiac arrest O29.11-
    - cardiac complication NEC O29.19-
    - cardiac failure O29.12-
    - central nervous system complication NEC O29.29-
    - cerebral anoxia O29.21-
    - failed or difficult intubation O29.6-
    - inhalation of stomach contents or secretions NOS O29.01-
    - local, toxic reaction O29.3X
    - Mendelson's syndrome O29.01-
    - pressure collapse of lung O29.02-
    - pulmonary complications NEC O29.09-
    - specified NEC O29.8X-
    - spinal and epidural type NEC O29.5X
      - induced headache O29.4-

Pregnancy *(continued)*
- complicated by *(continued)*
  - albuminuria (*see also* Proteinuria, gestational) O12.1-
  - alcohol use O99.31-
  - amnionitis O41.12-
  - anaphylactoid syndrome of pregnancy O88.01-
  - anemia (conditions in D50-D64) (pre-existing) O99.01-
    - complicating the puerperium O99.03
  - antepartum hemorrhage O46.9-
    - with coagulation defect —*see* Hemorrhage, antepartum, with coagulation defect
    - specified NEC O46.8X-
  - appendicitis O99.61-
  - atrophy (yellow) (acute) liver (subacute) O26.61-
  - bariatric surgery status O99.84-
  - bicornis or bicornuate uterus O34.0-
  - biliary tract problems O26.61-
  - breech presentation O32.1
  - cardiovascular diseases (conditions in I00-I09, I20-I52, I70-I99) O99.41-
  - cerebrovascular disorders (conditions in I60-I69) O99.41-
  - cervical shortening O26.87-
  - cervicitis O23.51-
  - cesarean scar defect (isthmocele) O34.22
  - chloasma (gravidarum) O26.89-
  - cholestasis (intrahepatic) O26.61-
  - cholecystitis O99.61-
  - chorioamnionitis O41.12-
  - circulatory system disorder (conditions in I00-I09, I20-I99, O99.41-)
  - compound presentation O32.6
  - conjoined twins O30.02-
  - connective system disorders (conditions in M00-M99) O99.891
  - contracted pelvis (general) O33.1
    - inlet O33.2
    - outlet O33.3
  - convulsions (eclamptic) (uremic) (*see also* Eclampsia) O15.9-
  - cracked nipple O92.11-
  - cystitis O23.1-
  - cystocele O34.8-
  - death of fetus (near term) O36.4
    - early pregnancy O02.1
    - of one fetus or more in multiple gestation O31.2-
  - deciduitis O41.14-
  - decreased fetal movement O36.81-
  - dental problems O99.61-
  - diabetes (mellitus) O24.91-
    - gestational (pregnancy induced) —*see* Diabetes, gestational
    - pre-existing O24.31-
      - specified NEC O24.81-
      - type 1 O24.01-
      - type 2 O24.11-
  - digestive system disorders (conditions in K00-K93) O99.61-
  - diseases of —*see* Pregnancy, complicated by, specified body system disease
    - biliary tract O26.61-

Pregnancy *(continued)*
- complicated by *(continued)*
  - diseases of *(continued)*
    - blood NEC (conditions in D65-D77) O99.11-
    - liver O26.61-
    - specified NEC O99.891
  - disorders of *—see* Pregnancy, complicated by, specified body system disorder
    - amniotic fluid and membranes O41.9-
      - specified NEC O41.8X-
    - biliary tract O26.61-
    - ear and mastoid process (conditions in H60-H95) O99.891
    - eye and adnexa (conditions in H00-H59) O99.891
    - liver O26.61-
    - skin (conditions in L00-L99) O99.71-
    - specified NEC O99.891
  - displacement, uterus NEC O34.59-
    - causing obstructed labor O65.5
  - disproportion (due to) O33.9
    - fetal (ascites) (hydrops) (meningomyelocele) (sacral teratoma) (tumor) deformities NEC O33.7
    - generally contracted pelvis O33.1
    - hydrocephalic fetus O33.6
    - inlet contraction of pelvis O33.2
    - mixed maternal and fetal origin O33.4
    - specified NEC O33.8
  - double uterus O34.0-
    - causing obstructed labor O65.5
  - drug use (conditions in F11-F19) O99.32-
  - eclampsia, eclamptic (coma) (convulsions) (delirium) (nephritis) (uremia) (*see also* Eclampsia) O15.-
  - ectopic pregnancy *—see* Pregnancy, ectopic
  - edema O12.0-
    - with
      - gestational hypertension, mild (*see also* Pre-eclampsia) O14.0-
      - proteinuria O12.2-
  - effusion, amniotic fluid *—see* Pregnancy, complicated by, premature rupture of membranes
  - elderly
    - multigravida O09.52-
    - primigravida O09.51-
  - embolism (*see also* Embolism, obstetric, pregnancy) O88.-
  - endocrine diseases NEC O99.28-
  - endometritis O86.12
  - excessive weight gain O26.0-
  - exhaustion O26.81-
    - during labor and delivery O75.81
  - face presentation O32.3
  - failed induction of labor O61.9
    - instrumental O61.1
    - mechanical O61.1
    - medical O61.0
    - specified NEC O61.8
    - surgical O61.1
  - failed or difficult intubation for anesthesia O29.6-

Pregnancy *(continued)*
complicated by *(continued)*

  - false labor (pains) O47.9
    - at or after 37 completed weeks of pregnancy O47.1
    - before 37 completed weeks of pregnancy O47.0-
  - fatigue O26.81-
    - during labor and delivery O75.81
  - fatty metamorphosis of liver O26.61-
  - female genital mutilation O34.8- *[N90.81-]*
  - fetal (maternal care for)
    - abnormality or damage O35.9
      - acid-base balance O68
      - specified type NEC O35.8
    - acidemia O68
    - acidosis O68
    - alkalosis O68
    - anemia and thrombocytopenia O36.82-
    - anencephaly O35.0
    - bradycardia O36.83-
    - chromosomal abnormality (conditions in Q90-Q99) O35.1
    - conjoined twins O30.02-
    - damage from
      - amniocentesis O35.7
      - biopsy procedures O35.7
      - drug addiction O35.5
      - hematological investigation O35.7
      - intrauterine contraceptive device O35.7
      - maternal
        - alcohol addiction O35.4
        - cytomegalovirus infection O35.3
        - disease NEC O35.8
        - drug addiction O35.5
        - listeriosis O35.8
        - rubella O35.3
        - toxoplasmosis O35.8
        - viral infection O35.3
      - medical procedure NEC O35.7
      - radiation O35.6
    - death (near term) O36.4
      - early pregnancy O02.1
    - decreased movement O36.81-
    - depressed heart rate tones O36.83-
    - disproportion due to deformity (fetal) O33.7
    - excessive growth (large for dates) O36.6-
    - growth retardation O36.59-
      - light for dates O36.59-
      - small for dates O36.59-
    - heart rate irregularity (abnormal variability) (bradycardia) (decelerations) (tachycardia) O36.83-
    - hereditary disease O35.2
    - hydrocephalus O35.0
    - intrauterine death O36.4
    - non-reassuring heart rate or rhythm O36.83-
    - poor growth O36.59-
      - light for dates O36.59-
      - small for dates O36.59-
    - problem O36.9-
      - specified NEC O36.89-
    - reduction (elective) O31.3-
    - selective termination O31.3-
    - spina bifida O35.0
    - thrombocytopenia O36.82-

Pregnancy *(continued)*
complicated by *(continued)*

  - fibroid (tumor) (uterus) O34.1-
  - fissure of nipple O92.11-
  - gallstones O99.61-
  - gastric banding status O99.84-
  - gastric bypass status O99.84-
  - genital herpes (asymptomatic) (history of) (inactive) O98.3-
  - genital tract infection O23.9-
  - glomerular diseases (conditions in N00-N07) O26.83-
    - with hypertension,
      - pre-existing *—see* Hypertension, complicating, pregnancy, pre-existing, with, renal disease
  - gonorrhea O98.21-
  - grand multiparity O09.4
  - habitual aborter *—see* Pregnancy, complicated by, recurrent pregnancy loss
  - HELLP syndrome (hemolysis, elevated liver enzymes and low platelet count) O14.2-
  - hemorrhage
    - antepartum *—see* Hemorrhage, antepartum
    - before 20 completed weeks gestation O20.9
      - specified NEC O20.8
    - due to premature separation, placenta (*see also* Abruptio placentae) O45.9-
    - early O20.9
      - specified NEC O20.8
    - threatened abortion O20.0
  - hemorrhoids O22.4-
  - hepatitis (viral) O98.41-
  - herniation of uterus O34.59-
  - high
    - head at term O32.4
    - risk *—see* Supervision (of) (for), high-risk
  - history of in utero procedure during previous pregnancy O09.82-
  - HIV O98.71-
  - human immunodeficiency virus (HIV) disease O98.71-
  - hydatidiform mole (*see also* Mole, hydatidiform) O01.9-
  - hydramnios O40.-
  - hydrocephalic fetus (disproportion) O33.6
  - hydrops
    - amnii O40.-
    - fetalis O36.2-
      - associated with isoimmunization (*see also* Pregnancy, complicated by, isoimmunization) O36.11-
  - hydrorrhea O42.90
  - hyperemesis (gravidarum) (mild) (*see also* Hyperemesis, gravidarum) O21.0-
  - hypertension *—see* Hypertension, complicating pregnancy
  - hypertensive
    - heart and renal disease, pre-existing *—see* Hypertension, complicating, pregnancy, pre-existing, with, heart disease, with renal disease

Pregnancy *(continued)*
complicated by *(continued)*

  - hypertensive *(continued)*
    - heart disease, pre-existing *—see* Hypertension, complicating, pregnancy, pre-existing, with, heart disease
    - renal disease, pre-existing *—see* Hypertension, complicating, pregnancy, pre-existing, with, renal disease
  - hypotension O26.5-
  - immune disorders NEC (conditions in D80-D89) O99.11-
  - incarceration, uterus O34.51-
  - incompetent cervix O34.3-
  - inconclusive fetal viability O36.80
  - infection(s) O98.91-
    - amniotic fluid or sac O41.10-
    - bladder O23.1-
    - carrier state NEC O99.830
      - streptococcus B O99.820
    - genital organ or tract O23.9-
      - specified NEC O23.59-
    - genitourinary tract O23.9-
    - gonorrhea O98.21-
    - hepatitis (viral) O98.41-
    - HIV O98.71-
    - human immunodeficiency virus (HIV) O98.71-
    - intrauterine O41.12
    - kidney O23.0-
    - nipple O91.01-
    - parasitic disease O98.91-
      - specified NEC O98.81-
    - protozoal disease O98.61-
    - sexually transmitted NEC O98.31-
    - specified type NEC O98.81-
    - syphilis O98.11-
    - tuberculosis O98.01-
    - urethra O23.2-
    - urinary (tract) O23.4-
      - specified NEC O23.3-
    - viral disease O98.51-
  - inflammation
    - intrauterine O41.12
  - injury or poisoning (conditions in S00-T88) O9A.21-
    - due to abuse
      - physical O9A.31-
      - psychological O9A.51-
      - sexual O9A.41-
  - insufficient
    - prenatal care O09.3-
    - weight gain O26.1-
  - insulin resistance O26.89
  - intrauterine fetal death (near term) O36.4
    - early pregnancy O02.1
    - multiple gestation (one fetus or more) O31.2-
  - isoimmunization O36.11-
    - anti-A sensitization O36.11-
    - anti-B sensitization O36.19-
    - Rh O36.09-
      - anti-D antibody O36.01-
    - specified NEC O36.19-
  - laceration of uterus NEC O71.81
  - malformation
    - placenta, placental (vessel) O43.10-
      - specified NEC O43.19-
    - uterus (congenital) O34.0-
  - malnutrition (conditions in E40-E46) O25.1-

Pregnancy *(continued)*
- cornual O00.80
  - with intrauterine pregnancy O00.81
- ectopic (ruptured) O00.90
  - with intrauterine pregnancy O00.91
  - abdominal O00.00
    - with
      - intrauterine pregnancy O00.01
      - viable fetus O36.7-
  - cervical O00.80
    - with intrauterine pregnancy O00.81
  - complicated (by) O08.9
    - afibrinogenemia O08.1
    - cardiac arrest O08.81
    - chemical damage of pelvic organ(s) O08.6
    - circulatory collapse O08.3
    - defibrination syndrome O08.1
    - electrolyte imbalance O08.5
    - embolism (amniotic fluid) (blood clot) (pulmonary) (septic) O08.2
    - endometritis O08.0
    - genital tract and pelvic infection O08.0
    - hemorrhage (delayed) (excessive) O08.1
    - infection
      - genital tract or pelvic O08.0
      - kidney 008.83
      - urinary tract O08.83
    - intravascular coagulation O08.1
    - laceration of pelvic organ(s) O08.6
    - metabolic disorder O08.5
    - oliguria O08.4
    - oophoritis O08.0
    - parametritis O08.0
    - pelvic peritonitis O08.0
    - perforation of pelvic organ(s) O08.6
    - renal failure or shutdown O08.4
    - salpingitis or salpingo-oophoritis O08.0
    - sepsis O08.82
    - shock O08.83
      - septic O08.82
    - specified condition NEC O08.89
    - tubular necrosis (renal) O08.4
    - uremia O08.4
    - urinary infection O08.83
    - venous complication NEC O08.7
      - embolism O08.2
  - cornual O00.80
    - with intrauterine pregnancy O00.81
  - intraligamentous O00.80
    - with intrauterine pregnancy O00.81
  - mural O00.80
    - with intrauterine pregnancy O00.81
  - ovarian O00.20-
    - with intrauterine pregnancy O00.21-
  - specified site NEC O00.80
    - with intrauterine pregnancy O00.81
  - tubal (ruptured) O00.10-
    - with intrauterine pregnancy O00.11-
- examination (normal) Z34.9-
  - high-risk —*see* Pregnancy, supervision of, high-risk
  - first Z34.0-
  - specified Z34.8-
- extrauterine —*see* Pregnancy, ectopic
- fallopian O00.10-
  - with intrauterine pregnancy O00.11-
- false F45.8
- gestational carrier Z33.3
- heptachorionic, hepta-amniotic (septuplets) O30.83-
- hexachorionic, hexa-amniotic (septuplets) O30.83-
- hidden O09.3-
- high-risk —*see* Pregnancy, supervision of, high-risk
- incidental finding Z33.1
- interstitial O00.80
  - with intrauterine pregnancy O00.81
- intraligamentous O00.80
  - with intrauterine pregnancy O00.81
- intramural O00.80
  - with intrauterine pregnancy O00.81
- intraperitoneal O00.00
  - with intrauterine pregnancy O00.01
- isthmian O00.10-
  - with intrauterine pregnancy O00.11-
- mesometric (mural) O00.80
  - with intrauterine pregnancy O00.81
- molar NEC O02.0
  - complicated (by) O08.9
    - afibrinogenemia O08.1
    - cardiac arrest O08.81
    - chemical damage of pelvic organ(s) O08.6
    - circulatory collapse O08.3
    - defibrination syndrome O08.1
    - electrolyte imbalance O08.5
    - embolism (amniotic fluid) (blood clot) (pulmonary) (septic) O08.2
    - endometritis O08.0
    - genital tract and pelvic infection O08.0
    - hemorrhage (delayed) (excessive) O08.1
    - infection
      - genital tract or pelvic O08.0
      - kidney O08.83
      - urinary tract O08.83
    - intravascular coagulation O08.1
    - laceration of pelvic organ(s) O08.6
    - metabolic disorder O08.5
    - oliguria O08.4
    - oophoritis O08.0
    - parametritis O08.0
    - pelvic peritonitis O08.0
    - perforation of pelvic organ(s) O08.6
    - renal failure or shutdown O08.4
    - salpingitis or salpingo-oophoritis O08.0
    - sepsis O08.82
    - shock O08.3
      - septic O08.82
    - specified condition NEC O08.89
    - tubular necrosis (renal) O08.4
    - uremia O08.4
    - urinary infection O08.83
    - venous complication NEC O08.7
      - embolism O08.2
  - hydatidiform (*see also* Mole, hydatidiform) O01.9-
- multiple (gestation) O30.9-
  - greater than quadruplets —*see* Pregnancy, multiple (gestation), specified NEC
  - specified NEC O30.80-
    - with
      - two or more monoamniotic fetuses O30.82-
      - two or more monochorionic fetuses O30.81-
    - number of chorions and amnions are both equal to the number of fetuses O30.83-
    - two or more monoamniotic fetuses O30.82-
    - two or more monochorionic fetuses O30.81-
    - unable to determine number of placenta and number of amniotic sacs O30.89-
    - unspecified number of placenta and unspecified number of amniotic sacs O30.80-
- mural O00.80
  - with intrauterine pregnancy O00.81
- normal (supervision of) Z34.9-
  - high-risk —*see* Pregnancy, supervision of, high-risk
  - first Z34.0-
  - specified Z34.8-
- ovarian O00.20-
  - with intrauterine pregnancy O00.21-
- pentachorionic, penta-amniotic (quintuplets) O30.83-
- postmature (40 to 42 weeks) O48.0
  - more than 42 weeks gestation O48.1
- post-term (40 to 42 weeks) O48.0
- prenatal care only Z34.9-
  - high-risk —*see* Pregnancy, supervision of, high-risk
  - first Z34.0-
  - specified Z34.8-
- prolonged (more than 42 weeks gestation) O48.1
- quadruplet O30.20-
  - with
    - two or more monoamniotic fetuses O30.22-
    - two or more monochorionic fetuses O30.21-
  - quadrachorionic/quadra-amniotic O30.23-
  - two or more monoamniotic fetuses O30.22-
  - two or more monochorionic fetuses O30.21-
  - unable to determine number of placenta and number of amniotic sacs O30.29-
  - unspecified number of placenta and unspecified number of amniotic sacs O30.20-
- quintuplet —*see* Pregnancy, multiple (gestation), specified NEC
- sextuplet —*see* Pregnancy, multiple (gestation), specified NEC
- supervision of
  - concealed pregnancy O09.3-
  - elderly mother
    - multigravida O09.52-
    - primigravida O09.51-
  - hidden pregnancy O09.3-
  - high-risk O09.9-
    - due to (history of)
      - ectopic pregnancy O09.1-
      - elderly —*see* Pregnancy, supervision, elderly mother
      - grand multiparity O09.4
      - infertility O09.0-
      - insufficient prenatal care O09.3-
      - in utero procedure during previous pregnancy O09.82-
      - in vitro fertilization O09.81-
      - molar pregnancy O09.A-
      - multiple previous pregnancies O09.4-
      - older mother —*see* Pregnancy, supervision of, elderly mother
      - poor reproductive or obstetric history NEC O09.29-
      - pre-term labor O09.21-
      - previous
        - neonatal death O09.29-
      - social problems O09.7-
      - specified NEC O09.89-
      - very young mother —*see* Pregnancy, supervision, young mother
    - resulting from in vitro fertilization O09.81-
  - normal Z34.9-
    - first Z34.0-
    - specified NEC Z34.8-
  - young mother
    - multigravida O09.62-
    - primigravida O09.61-
- triplet O30.10-
  - with
    - two or more monoamniotic fetuses O30.12-
    - two or more monochorionic fetuses O30.11-
  - trichorionic/triamniotic O30.13-
  - two or more monoamniotic fetuses O30.12-
  - two or more monochorionic fetuses O30.11-
  - unable to determine number of placenta and number of amniotic sacs O30.19-
  - unspecified number of placenta and unspecified number of amniotic sacs O30.10-
- tubal (with abortion) (with rupture) O00.10-
  - with intrauterine pregnancy O00.11-
- twin O30.00-
  - conjoined O30.02-
  - dichorionic/diamniotic (two placenta, two amniotic sacs) O30.04-
  - monochorionic/diamniotic (one placenta, two amniotic sacs) O30.03-
  - monochorionic/monoamniotic (one placenta, one amniotic sac) O30.01-

Pregnancy *(continued)*
- twin *(continued)*
  - unable to determine number of placenta and number of amniotic sacs O30.09-
  - unspecified number of placenta and unspecified number of amniotic sacs O30.00-
- unwanted Z64.0
- weeks of gestation
  - 8 weeks Z3A.08
  - 9 weeks Z3A.09
  - 10 weeks Z3A.10
  - 11 weeks Z3A.11
  - 12 weeks Z3A.12
  - 13 weeks Z3A.13
  - 14 weeks Z3A.14
  - 15 weeks Z3A.15
  - 16 weeks Z3A.16
  - 17 weeks Z3A.17
  - 18 weeks Z3A.18
  - 19 weeks Z3A.19
  - 20 weeks Z3A.20
  - 21 weeks Z3A.21
  - 22 weeks Z3A.22
  - 23 weeks Z3A.23
  - 24 weeks Z3A.24
  - 25 weeks Z3A.25
  - 26 weeks Z3A.26
  - 27 weeks Z3A.27
  - 28 weeks Z3A.28
  - 29 weeks Z3A.29
  - 30 weeks Z3A.30
  - 31 weeks Z3A.31
  - 32 weeks Z3A.32
  - 33 weeks Z3A.33
  - 34 weeks Z3A.34
  - 35 weeks Z3A.35
  - 36 weeks Z3A.36
  - 37 weeks Z3A.37
  - 38 weeks Z3A.38
  - 39 weeks Z3A.39
  - 40 weeks Z3A.40
  - 41 weeks Z3A.41
  - 42 weeks Z3A.42
  - greater than 42 weeks Z3A.49
  - less than 8 weeks Z3A.01
  - not specified Z3A.00

Preiser's disease *—see* Osteonecrosis, secondary, due to, trauma, metacarpus

Pre-kwashiorkor *—see* Malnutrition, severe

Preleukemia (syndrome) D46.9

Preluxation, hip, congenital Q65.6

Premature *—see also* condition
- adrenarche E27.0
- aging E34.8
- beats I49.40
  - atrial I49.1
  - auricular I49.1
  - supraventricular I49.1
- birth NEC *—see* Preterm, newborn
- closure, foramen ovale Q21.8
- contraction
  - atrial I49.1
  - atrioventricular I49.2
  - auricular I49.1
  - auriculoventricular I49.49
  - heart (extrasystole) I49.49
  - junctional I49.2
  - ventricular I49.3
- delivery (*see also* Pregnancy, complicated by, preterm labor) O60.10
- ejaculation F52.4
- infant NEC *—see* Preterm, newborn
  - light-for-dates *—see* Light for dates
- labor *—see* Pregnancy, complicated by, preterm labor
- lungs P28.0
- menopause E28.319
  - asymptomatic E28.319
  - symptomatic E28.310
- newborn
  - extreme (less than 28 completed weeks) *—see* Immaturity, extreme
  - less than 37 completed weeks *—see* Preterm, newborn
- puberty E30.1
- rupture membranes or amnion *—see* Pregnancy, complicated by, premature rupture of membranes
- senility E34.8
- thelarche E30.8
- ventricular systole I49.3

Prematurity NEC (less than 37 completed weeks) *—see* Preterm, newborn
- extreme (less than 28 completed weeks) *—see* Immaturity, extreme

Premenstrual
- dysphoric disorder (PMDD) F32.81
- tension (syndrome) N94.3

Premolarization, cuspids K00.2

Prenatal
- care, normal pregnancy *—see* Pregnancy, normal
- screening of mother (*see also* Encounter, antenatal screening) Z36.9
- teeth K00.6

Preparatory care for subsequent treatment NEC
- for dialysis Z49.01
  - peritoneal Z49.02

Prepartum *—see* condition

Preponderance, left or right ventricular I51.7

Prepuce *—see* condition

PRES (posterior reversible encephalopathy syndrome) I67.83

Presbycardia R54

Presbycusis, presbyacusia H91.1-

Presbyesophagus K22.89

Presbyophrenia F03

Presbyopia H52.4

Prescription of contraceptives (initial) Z30.019
- barrier Z30.018
- diaphragm Z30.018
- emergency (postcoital) Z30.012
- implantable subdermal Z30.017
- injectable Z30.013
- intrauterine contraceptive device Z30.014
- pills Z30.011
- postcoital (emergency) Z30.012
- repeat Z30.40
  - barrier Z30.49
  - diaphragm Z30.49
  - implantable subdermal Z30.46
  - injectable Z30.42
  - pills Z30.41
  - specified type NEC Z30.49
  - transdermal patch hormonal Z30.45
  - vaginal ring hormonal Z30.44
- specified type NEC Z30.018
  - transdermal patch hormonal Z30.016
  - vaginal ring hormonal Z30.015

Presence (of)
- ankle-joint implant (functional) (prosthesis) Z96.66-
- aortocoronary (bypass) graft Z95.1
- arterial-venous shunt (dialysis) Z99.2
- artificial
  - eye (globe) Z97.0
  - heart (fully implantable) (mechanical) Z95.812
    - valve Z95.2
  - larynx Z96.3
  - lens (intraocular) Z96.1
  - limb (complete) (partial) Z97.1-
    - arm Z97.1-
      - bilateral Z97.15
    - leg Z97.1-
      - bilateral Z97.16
- audiological implant (functional) Z96.29
- bladder implant (functional) Z96.0
- bone
  - conduction hearing device Z96.29
  - implant (functional) NEC Z96.7
  - joint (prosthesis) *—see* Presence, joint implant
- cardiac
  - defibrillator (functional) (with synchronous cardiac pacemaker) Z95.810
  - implant or graft Z95.9
    - specified type NEC Z95.818
  - pacemaker Z95.0
  - resynchronization therapy
    - defibrillator Z95.810
    - pacemaker Z95.0
- cardioverter-defibrillator (ICD) Z95.810
- cerebrospinal fluid drainage device Z98.2
- cochlear implant (functional) Z96.21
- contact lens (es) Z97.3
- coronary artery graft or prosthesis Z95.5
- CRT-D (cardiac resynchronization therapy defibrillator) Z95.810
- CRT-P (cardiac resynchronization therapy pacemaker) Z95.0
- CSF shunt Z98.2
- dental prosthesis device Z97.2
- dentures Z97.2
- device (external) NEC Z97.8
  - cardiac NEC Z95.818
  - heart assist Z95.811
  - implanted (functional) Z96.9
    - specified NEC Z96.89
  - prosthetic Z97.8
- ear implant Z96.20
  - cochlear implant Z96.21
  - myringotomy tube Z96.22
  - specified type NEC Z96.29
- elbow-joint implant (functional) (prosthesis) Z96.62-
- endocrine implant (functional) NEC Z96.49
- eustachian tube stent or device (functional) Z96.29
- external hearing-aid or device Z97.4
- finger-joint implant (functional) (prosthetic) Z96.69-
- functional implant Z96.9
  - specified NEC Z96.89
- graft
  - cardiac NEC Z95.818
  - vascular NEC Z95.828
- hearing-aid or device (external) Z97.4
  - implant (bone) (cochlear) (functional) Z96.21
- heart assist device Z95.811
- heart valve implant (functional) Z95.2
  - prosthetic Z95.2
  - specified type NEC Z95.4
  - xenogenic Z95.3
- hip-joint implant (functional) (prosthesis) Z96.64-
- ICD (cardioverter-defibrillator) Z95.810
- implanted device (artificial) (functional) (prosthetic) Z96.9
  - automatic cardiac defibrillator (with synchronous cardiac pacemaker) Z95.810
  - cardiac pacemaker Z95.0
  - cochlear Z96.21
  - dental Z96.5
  - heart Z95.812
  - heart valve Z95.2
    - prosthetic Z95.2
    - specified NEC Z95.4
    - xenogenic Z95.3
  - insulin pump Z96.41
  - intraocular lens Z96.1
  - joint Z96.60
    - ankle Z96.66-
    - elbow Z96.62-
    - finger Z96.69-
    - hip Z96.64-
    - knee Z96.65-
    - shoulder Z96.61-
    - specified NEC Z96.698
    - wrist Z96.63-
  - larynx Z96.3
  - myringotomy tube Z96.22
  - otological Z96.20
    - cochlear Z96.21
    - eustachian stent Z96.29
    - myringotomy Z96.22
    - specified NEC Z96.29
    - stapes Z96.29
  - skin Z96.81
  - skull plate Z96.7
  - specified NEC Z96.89
  - urogenital Z96.0
- insulin pump (functional) Z96.41
- intestinal bypass or anastomosis Z98.0
- intraocular lens (functional) Z96.1
- intrauterine contraceptive device (IUD) Z97.5
- intravascular implant (functional) (prosthetic) NEC Z95.9
  - coronary artery Z95.5
  - defibrillator (with synchronous cardiac pacemaker) Z95.810
  - peripheral vessel (with angioplasty) Z95.820
- joint implant (prosthetic) (any) Z96.60
  - ankle *—see* Presence, ankle joint implant
  - elbow *—see* Presence, elbow joint implant
  - finger *—see* Presence, finger joint implant
  - hip *—see* Presence, hip joint implant
  - knee *—see* Presence, knee joint implant

Problem *(continued)*
- life-style Z72.9
  - gambling Z72.6
  - high-risk sexual behavior (heterosexual) Z72.51
    - bisexual Z72.53
    - homosexual Z72.52
  - inappropriate eating habits Z72.4
  - self-damaging behavior NEC Z72.89
  - specified NEC Z72.89
  - tobacco use Z72.0
- literacy Z55.9
  - low level Z55.0
  - specified NEC Z55.8
- living alone Z60.2
- lodgers Z59.2
- loss of love relationship in childhood Z62.898
- marital Z63.0
  - involving
    - divorce Z63.5
    - estrangement Z63.5
    - gender identity F66
- mastication K08.89
- medical
  - care, within family Z63.6
  - facilities Z75.9
    - specified NEC Z75.8
- mental F48.9
- multiparity Z64.1
- negative life events in childhood Z62.9
  - altered pattern of family relationships Z62.898
  - frightening experience Z62.898
  - loss of
    - love relationship Z62.898
    - self-esteem Z62.898
  - physical abuse (alleged) *—see* Maltreatment, child
  - removal from home Z62.29
  - specified event NEC Z62.898
- neighbor Z59.2
- neurological NEC R29.818
- new step-parent affecting child Z62.898
- none (feared complaint unfounded) Z71.1
- occupational NEC Z56.89
- parent-child *—see* Conflict, parent-child
- personal hygiene Z91.89
- personality F69
- phase-of-life transition, adjustment Z60.0
- presence of sick or disabled person in family or household Z63.79
  - needing care Z63.6
- primary support group (family) Z63.9
  - specified NEC Z63.8
- probation officer Z64.4
- psychiatric F99
- psychosexual (development) F66
- psychosocial Z65.9
  - religious or spiritual Z65.8
  - specified NEC Z65.8
- relationship Z63.9
  - childhood F93.8
- release from prison Z65.2
  - religious or spiritual Z65.8
- removal from home affecting child Z62.29
- seeking and accepting known hazardous and harmful
  - behavioral or psychological interventions Z65.8
  - chemical, nutritional or physical interventions Z65.8
- sexual function (nonorganic) F52.9

Problem *(continued)*
- sight H54.7
- sleep disorder, child F51.9
- smell *—see* Disturbance, sensation, smell
- social
  - environment Z60.9
    - specified NEC Z60.8
  - exclusion and rejection Z60.4
  - worker Z64.4
- speech R47.9
  - developmental F80.9
  - specified NEC R47.89
- swallowing *—see* Dysphagia
- taste *—see* Disturbance, sensation, taste
- tic, child F95.0
- underachievement in school Z55.3
- unemployment Z56.0
  - threatened Z56.2
- unwanted pregnancy Z64.0
- upbringing Z62.9
  - specified NEC Z62.898
- urinary N39.9
- voice production R47.89
- work schedule (stressful) Z56.3

Procedure (surgical)
- converted
  - arthroscopic to open Z53.33
  - laparoscopic to open Z53.31
  - specified procedure NEC to open Z53.39
  - thoracoscopic to open Z53.32
- for purpose other than remedying health state Z41.9
  - specified NEC Z41.8
- not done Z53.9
  - because of
    - administrative reasons Z53.8
    - contraindication Z53.09
      - smoking Z53.01
    - patient's decision Z53.20
      - for reasons of belief or group pressure Z53.1
      - left against medical advice (AMA) Z53.29
      - left without being seen Z53.21
      - specified reason NEC Z53.29
    - specified reason NEC Z53.8

Procidentia (uteri) N81.3

Proctalgia K62.89
- fugax K59.4
- spasmodic K59.4

Proctitis K62.89
- amebic (acute) A06.0
- chlamydial A56.3
- gonococcal A54.6
- granulomatous *—see* Enteritis, regional, large intestine
- herpetic A60.1
- radiation K62.7
- tuberculous A18.32
- ulcerative (chronic) K51.20
  - with
    - complication K51.219
      - abscess K51.214
      - fistula K51.213
      - obstruction K51.212
      - rectal bleeding K51.211
      - specified NEC K51.218

Proctocele
- female (without uterine prolapse) N81.6
  - with uterine prolapse N81.2
    - complete N81.3
- male K62.3

Proctocolitis
- allergic K52.29
- food-induced eosinophilic K52.29
- food protein-induced K52.29
- mild protein-induced K52.29
- mucosal *—see* Rectosigmoiditis, ulcerative

Proctoptosis K62.3

Proctorrhagia K62.5

Proctosigmoiditis K63.89
- ulcerative (chronic) *—see* Rectosigmoiditis, ulcerative

Proctospasm K59.4
- psychogenic F45.8

Profichet's disease *—see* Disorder, soft tissue, specified type NEC

Progeria E34.8

Prognathism (mandibular) (maxillary) M26.19

Progonoma (melanotic) *—see* Neoplasm, benign, by site

Progressive *—see* condition

Prolactinoma
- specified site *—see* Neoplasm, benign, by site
- unspecified site D35.2

Prolapse, prolapsed
- anus, anal (canal) (sphincter) K62.2
- arm or hand O32.2
  - causing obstructed labor O64.4
- bladder (mucosa) (sphincter) (acquired)
  - congenital Q79.4
  - female *—see* Cystocele
  - male N32.89
- breast implant (prosthetic) T85.49
- cecostomy K94.09
- cecum K63.4
- cervix, cervical (hypertrophied) N81.2
  - anterior lip, obstructing labor O65.5
  - congenital Q51.828
  - postpartal, old N81.2
  - stump N81.85
- ciliary body (traumatic) *—see* Laceration, eye (ball), with prolapse or loss of interocular tissue
- colon (pedunculated) K63.4
- colostomy K94.09
- disc (intervertebral) *—see* Displacement, intervertebral disc
- eye implant (orbital) T85.398
  - lens (ocular) *—see* Complications, intraocular lens
- fallopian tube N83.4-
- gastric (mucosa) K31.89
- genital, female N81.9
  - specified NEC N81.89
- globe, nontraumatic *—see* Luxation, globe
- ileostomy bud K94.19
- intervertebral disc *—see* Displacement, intervertebral disc
- intestine (small) K63.4
- iris (traumatic) *—see* Laceration, eye (ball), with prolapse or loss of interocular tissue
  - nontraumatic H21.89
- kidney N28.83
  - congenital Q63.2
- laryngeal muscles or ventricle J38.7
- liver K76.89

Prolapse, prolapsed *(continued)*
- meatus urinarius N36.8
- mitral (valve) I34.1
- ocular lens implant *—see* Complications, intraocular lens
- organ or site, congenital NEC *—see* Malposition, congenital
- ovary N83.4-
- pelvic floor, female N81.89
- perineum, female N81.89
- rectum (mucosa) (sphincter) K62.3
  - due to trichuris trichuria B79
- spleen D73.89
- stomach K31.89
- umbilical cord
  - complicating delivery O69.0
- urachus, congenital Q64.4
- ureter N28.89
  - with obstruction N13.5
    - with infection N13.6
- ureterovesical orifice N28.89
- urethra (acquired) (infected) (mucosa) N36.8
  - congenital Q64.71
- urinary meatus N36.8
  - congenital Q64.72
- uterovaginal N81.4
  - complete N81.3
  - incomplete N81.2
- uterus (with prolapse of vagina) N81.4
  - complete N81.3
  - congenital Q51.818
  - first degree N81.2
  - in pregnancy or childbirth *—see* Pregnancy, complicated by, abnormal, uterus
  - incomplete N81.2
  - postpartal (old) N81.4
  - second degree N81.2
  - third degree N81.3
- uveal (traumatic) *—see* Laceration, eye (ball), with prolapse or loss of interocular tissue
- vagina (anterior) (wall) *—see* Cystocele
  - with prolapse of uterus N81.4
    - complete N81.3
    - incomplete N81.2
  - posterior wall N81.6
  - posthysterectomy N99.3
- vitreous (humor) H43.0-
  - in wound *—see* Laceration, eye (ball), with prolapse or loss of interocular tissue
- womb *—see* Prolapse, uterus

Prolapsus, female N81.9
- specified NEC N81.89

Proliferation(s)
- primary cutaneous CD30-positive large T-cell C86.6
- prostate, atypical small acinar N42.32

Proliferative *—see* condition

Prolonged, prolongation (of)
- bleeding (time) (idiopathic) R79.1
- coagulation (time) R79.1
- gestation (over 42 completed weeks)
  - mother O48.1
  - newborn P08.22
- interval I44.0
- labor O63.9
  - first stage O63.0
  - second stage O63.1
- partial thromboplastin time (PTT) R79.1
- pregnancy (more than 42 weeks gestation) O48.1
- prothrombin time R79.1

Prolonged, prolongation *(continued)*
- QT interval R94.31
- uterine contractions in labor O62.4

Prominence, prominent
- auricle (congenital) (ear) Q17.5
- ischial spine or sacral promontory
  - with disproportion (fetopelvic) O33.0
    - causing obstructed labor O65.0
- nose (congenital) acquired M95.0

Promiscuity —*see* High, risk, sexual behavior

Pronation
- ankle —*see* Deformity, limb, foot, specified NEC
- foot —*see also* Deformity, limb, foot, specified NEC
  - congenital Q74.2

Prophylactic
- administration of
  - antibiotics, long-term Z79.2
    - short-term use - omit code
  - drug (*see also* Long-term (current) drug therapy (use of)) Z79.899-
- medication Z79.899
- organ removal (for neoplasia management) Z40.00
  - breast Z40.01
  - fallopian tube(s) Z40.03
    - with ovary(s) Z40.02
  - ovary(s) Z40.02
  - specified site NEC Z40.09
- surgery Z40.9
  - for risk factors related to malignant neoplasm —*see* Prophylactic, organ removal
  - specified NEC Z40.8
- vaccination Z23

Propionic acidemia E71.121

Proptosis (ocular) —*see also* Exophthalmos
- thyroid —*see* Hyperthyroidism, with goiter

Prosecution, anxiety concerning Z65.3

Prosopagnosia R48.3

Prostadynia N42.81

Prostate, prostatic —*see* condition

Prostatism —*see* Hyperplasia, prostate

Prostatitis (congestive) (suppurative) (with cystitis) N41.9
- acute N41.0
- cavitary N41.8
- chronic N41.1
- diverticular N41.8
- due to Trichomonas (vaginalis) A59.02
- fibrous N41.1
- gonococcal (acute) (chronic) A54.22
- granulomatous N41.4
- hypertrophic N41.1
- subacute N41.1
- trichomonal A59.02
- tuberculous A18.14

Prostatocystitis N41.3

Prostatorrhea N42.89

Prostatosis N42.82

Prostration R53.83
- heat —*see also* Heat, exhaustion
  - anhydrotic T67.3
  - due to
    - salt (and water) depletion T67.4
    - water depletion T67.3
- nervous F48.8
- senile R54

Protanomaly (anomalous trichromat) H53.54

Protanopia (complete) (incomplete) H53.54

Protection (against) (from) —*see* Prophylactic

Protein
- deficiency NEC —*see* Malnutrition
- malnutrition —*see* Malnutrition
- sickness (*see also* Reaction, serum) T80.69

Proteinemia R77.9

Proteinosis
- alveolar (pulmonary) J84.01
- lipid or lipoid (of Urbach) E78.89

Proteinuria R80.9
- Bence Jones R80.3
- complicating pregnancy —*see* Proteinuria, gestational
- gestational
  - complicating
    - childbirth O12.14
    - pregnancy O12.1-
      - with edema O12.2-
    - puerperium O12.15
- idiopathic R80.0
- isolated R80.0
  - with glomerular lesion N06.9
    - C3
      - glomerulonephritis N06.A
      - glomerulopathy N06.A
        - with dense deposit disease N06.6
    - dense deposit disease N06.6
    - diffuse
      - crescentic glomerulonephritis N06.7
      - endocapillary proliferative glomerulonephritis N06.4
      - mesangiocapillary glomerulonephritis N06.5
    - focal and segmental hyalinosis or sclerosis N06.1
    - membranous (diffuse) N06.2
    - mesangial proliferative (diffuse) N06.3
    - minimal change N06.0
    - specified pathology NEC N06.8
- orthostatic R80.2
  - with glomerular lesion —*see* Proteinuria, isolated, with glomerular lesion
- persistent R80.1
  - with glomerular lesion —*see* Proteinuria, isolated, with glomerular lesion
- postural R80.2
  - with glomerular lesion —*see* Proteinuria, isolated, with glomerular lesion
- pre-eclamptic —*see* Pre-eclampsia
- puerperal O12.15
- specified type NEC R80.8

Proteolysis, pathologic D65

Proteus (mirabilis) (morganii), **as cause of disease classified elsewhere** B96.4

Prothrombin gene mutation D68.52

Protoporphyria, erythropoietic E80.0

Protozoal —*see also* condition
- disease B64
  - specified NEC B60.8

Protrusion, protrusio
- acetabuli M24.7
- acetabulum (into pelvis) M24.7
- device, implant or graft (*see also* Complications, by site and type, mechanical) T85.698
  - arterial graft NEC —*see* Complication, cardiovascular device, mechanical, vascular
  - breast (implant) T85.49
  - catheter NEC T85.698
    - cystostomy T83.090
    - dialysis (renal) T82.49
      - intraperitoneal T85.691
    - infusion NEC T82.594
      - spinal (epidural) (subdural) T85.690
    - urinary (*see also* Complications, catheter, urinary), T83.098
  - electronic (electrode) (pulse generator) (stimulator)
    - bone T84.390
    - nervous system —*see* Complication, prosthetic device, mechanical, electronic nervous system stimulator
  - fixation, internal (orthopedic) NEC —*see* Complication, fixation device, mechanical
  - gastrointestinal —*see* Complications, prosthetic device, mechanical, gastrointestinal device
  - genital NEC T83.498
    - intrauterine contraceptive device T83.39
    - penile prosthesis (cylinder) (implanted) (pump) (resevoir) T83.490
    - testicular prosthesis T83.491
  - heart NEC —*see* Complication, cardiovascular device, mechanical
  - joint prosthesis —*see* Complications, joint prosthesis, mechanical, specified NEC, by site
  - ocular NEC —*see* Complications, prosthetic device, mechanical, ocular device
  - orthopedic NEC —*see* Complication, orthopedic, device, mechanical
  - specified NEC T85.628
  - urinary NEC —*see also* Complication, genitourinary, device, urinary, mechanical
    - graft T83.29
  - vascular NEC —*see* Complication, cardiovascular device, mechanical
  - ventricular intracranial shunt T85.09
- intervertebral disc —*see* Displacement, intervertebral disc
- joint prosthesis —*see* Complications, joint prosthesis, mechanical, specified NEC, by site
- nucleus pulposus —*see* Displacement, intervertebral disc

Prune belly (syndrome) Q79.4

Prurigo (ferox) (gravis) (Hebrae) (Hebra's) (mitis) (simplex) L28.2
- Besnier's L20.0
- estivalis L56.4
- nodularis L28.1
- psychogenic F45.8

Pruritus, pruritic (essential) L29.9
- ani, anus L29.0
  - psychogenic F45.8
- anogenital L29.3
  - psychogenic F45.8
- due to onchocerca volvulus B73.1
- gravidarum —*see* Pregnancy, complicated by, specified pregnancy-related condition NEC
- hiemalis L29.8
- neurogenic (any site) F45.8
- perianal L29.0
- psychogenic (any site) F45.8
- scroti, scrotum L29.1
  - psychogenic F45.8
- senile, senilis L29.8
- specified NEC L29.8
  - psychogenic F45.8
- Trichomonas A59.9
- vulva, vulvae L29.2
  - psychogenic F45.8

Pseudarthrosis, pseudoarthrosis (bone) —*see* Nonunion, fracture
- clavicle, congenital Q74.0
- joint, following fusion or arthrodesis M96.0

Pseudoaneurysm —*see* Aneurysm

Pseudoangioma I81

Pseudoangina (pectoris) —*see* Angina

Pseudoarteriosus Q28.8

Pseudoarthrosis —*see* Pseudarthrosis

Pseudobulbar affect (PBA) F48.2

Pseudochromhidrosis L67.8

Pseudocirrhosis, liver, pericardial I31.1

Pseudocowpox B08.03

Pseudocoxalgia M91.3-

Pseudocroup J38.5

Pseudo-Cushing's syndrome, alcohol-induced E24.4

Pseudocyesis F45.8

Pseudocyst
- lung J98.4
- pancreas K86.3
- retina —*see* Cyst, retina

Pseudoelephantiasis neuroarthritica Q82.0

Pseudoexfoliation, capsule (lens) —*see* Cataract, specified NEC

Pseudofolliculitis barbae L73.1

Pseudoglioma H44.89

Pseudohemophilia (Bernuth's) (hereditary) (type B) D68.0
- Type A D69.8
- vascular D69.8

Pseudohermaphroditism Q56.3
- adrenal E25.8
- female Q56.2
  - with adrenocortical disorder E25.8
  - without adrenocortical disorder Q56.2
  - adrenal (congenital) E25.0
  - unspecified E25.9

Pseudohermaphroditism *(continued)*
male Q56.1
with
adrenocortical disorder E25.8
androgen resistance E34.51
cleft scrotum Q56.1
feminizing testis E34.51
5-alpha-reductase deficiency E29.1
without gonadal disorder Q56.1
adrenal E25.8
unspecified E25.9

Pseudo-Hurler's polydystrophy E77.0

Pseudohydrocephalus G93.2

Pseudohypertrophic muscular dystrophy (Erb's) G71.02

Pseudohypertrophy, muscle G71.09

Pseudohypoparathyroidism E20.1

Pseudoinsomnia F51.03

Pseudoleukemia, infantile D64.89

Pseudomembranous *—see* condition

Pseudomenses (newborn) P54.6

Pseudomenstruation (newborn) P54.6

Pseudomeningocele (cerebral) (infective) (post-traumatic) G96.198
postprocedural (spinal) G97.82

Pseudomonas
aeruginosa, as cause of disease classified elsewhere B96.5
mallei infection A24.0
as cause of disease classified elsewhere B96.5
pseudomallei, as cause of disease classified elsewhere B96.5

Pseudomyotonia G71.19

Pseudomyxoma peritonei C78.6

Pseudoneuritis, optic (nerve) (disc) (papilla)**, congenital** Q14.2

Pseudo-obstruction intestine (acute) (chronic) (idiopathic) (intermittent secondary) (primary) K59.89
colonic K59.81

Pseudopapilledema H47.33-
congenital Q14.2

Pseudoparalysis
arm or leg R29.818
atonic, congenital P94.2

Pseudopelade L66.0

Pseudophakia Z96.1

Pseudopolyarthritis, rhizomelic M35.3

Pseudopolycythemia D75.1

Pseudopseudohypoparathyroidism E20.1

Pseudopterygium H11.81-

Pseudoptosis (eyelid) *—see* Blepharochalasis

Pseudopuberty, precocious
female heterosexual E25.8
male isosexual E25.8

Pseudorickets (renal) N25.0

Pseudorubella B08.20

Pseudosclerema, newborn P83.88

Pseudosclerosis (brain)
of Westphal (Strümpell) E83.01
Jakob's *—see* Creutzfeldt-Jakob disease or syndrome
spastic *—see* Creutzfeldt-Jakob disease or syndrome

Pseudotetanus *—see* Convulsions

Pseudotetany R29.0
hysterical F44.5

Pseudotruncus arteriosus Q25.49

Pseudotuberculosis A28.2
enterocolitis A04.8
pasteurella (infection) A28.0

Pseudotumor G93.2
cerebri G93.2
orbital H05.11-

Pseudoxanthoma elasticum Q82.8

Psilosis (sprue) (tropical) K90.1
nontropical K90.0

Psittacosis A70

Psoitis M60.88

Psoriasis L40.9
arthropathic L40.50
arthritis mutilans L40.52
distal interphalangeal L40.51
juvenile L40.54
other specified L40.59
spondylitis L40.53
buccal K13.29
flexural L40.8
guttate L40.4
mouth K13.29
nummular L40.0
plaque L40.0
psychogenic F54
pustular (generalized) L40.1
palmaris et plantaris L40.3
specified NEC L40.8
vulgaris L40.0

Psychasthenia F48.8

Psychiatric disorder or problem F99

Psychogenic *—see also* condition
factors associated with physical conditions F54

Psychological and behavioral factors affecting medical condition F59

Psychoneurosis, psychoneurotic *—see also* Neurosis
anxiety (state) F41.1
depersonalization F48.1
hypochondriacal F45.21
hysteria F44.9
neurasthenic F48.8
personality NEC F60.89

Psychopathy, psychopathic
affectionless F94.2
autistic F84.5
constitution, post-traumatic F07.81
personality *—see* Disorder, personality
sexual *—see* Deviation, sexual
state F60.2

Psychosexual identity disorder of childhood F64.2

Psychosis, psychotic F29
acute (transient) F23
hysterical F44.9
affective *—see* Disorder, mood
alcoholic F10.959
with
abuse F10.159
anxiety disorder F10.980
with
abuse F10.180
dependence F10.280
delirium tremens F10.231
delusions F10.950
with
abuse F10.150
dependence F10.250

Psychosis, psychotic *(continued)*
alcoholic *(continued)*
with *(continued)*
dementia F10.97
with dependence F10.27
dependence F10.259
hallucinosis F10.951
with
abuse F10.151
dependence F10.251
mood disorder F10.94
with
abuse F10.14
dependence F10.24
paranoia F10.950
with
abuse F10.150
dependence F10.250
persisting amnesia F10.96
with dependence F10.26
amnestic confabulatory F10.96
with dependence F10.26
delirium tremens F10.231
Korsakoff's, Korsakov's, Korsakow's F10.26
paranoid type F10.950
with
abuse F10.150
dependence F10.250
anergastic *—see* Psychosis, organic
arteriosclerotic (simple type) (uncomplicated) F01.50
with behavioral disturbance F01.51
childhood F84.0
atypical F84.8
climacteric *—see* Psychosis, involutional
confusional F29
acute or subacute F05
reactive F23
cycloid F23
depressive *—see* Disorder, depressive
disintegrative (childhood) F84.3
drug-induced *—see* F11-F19 with .x59
paranoid and hallucinatory states *—see* F11-F19 with .x50 or .x51
due to or associated with
addiction, drug *—see* F11-F19 with .x59
dependence
alcohol F10.259
drug *—see* F11-F19 with .x59
epilepsy F06.8
Huntington's chorea F06.8
ischemia, cerebrovascular (generalized) F06.8
multiple sclerosis F06.8
physical disease F06.8
presenile dementia F03
senile dementia F03
vascular disease (arteriosclerotic) (cerebral) F01.50
with behavioral disturbance F01.51
epileptic F06.8
episode F23
due to or associated with physical condition F06.8
exhaustive F43.0
hallucinatory, chronic F28
hypomanic F30.8
hysterical (acute) F44.9
induced F24
infantile F84.0
atypical F84.8
infective (acute) (subacute) F05

Psychosis, psychotic *(continued)*
involutional F28
depressive *—see* Disorder, depressive
melancholic *—see* Disorder, depressive
paranoid (state) F22
Korsakoff's, Korsakov's, Korsakow's (nonalcoholic) F04
alcoholic F10.96
in dependence F10.26
induced by other psychoactive substance *—see* categories F11-F19 with .x5x
mania, manic (single episode) F30.2
recurrent type F31.89
manic-depressive *—see* Disorder, bipolar
menopausal *—see* Psychosis, involutional
mixed schizophrenic and affective F25.8
multi-infarct (cerebrovascular) F01.50
with behavioral disturbance F01.51
nonorganic F29
specified NEC F28
organic F09
due to or associated with
arteriosclerosis (cerebral) *—see* Psychosis, arteriosclerotic
cerebrovascular disease, arteriosclerotic *—see* Psychosis, arteriosclerotic
childbirth *—see* Psychosis, puerperal
Creutzfeldt-Jakob disease or syndrome *—see* Creutzfeldt-Jakob disease or syndrome
dependence, alcohol F10.259
disease
alcoholic liver F10.259
brain, arteriosclerotic *—see* Psychosis, arteriosclerotic
cerebrovascular F01.50
with behavioral disturbance F01.51
Creutzfeldt-Jakob *—see* Creutzfeldt-Jakob disease or syndrome
endocrine or metabolic F06.8
acute or subacute F05
liver, alcoholic F10.259
epilepsy transient (acute) F05
infection
brain (intracranial) F06.8
acute or subacute F05
intoxication
alcoholic (acute) F10.259
drug F11-F19 with .x59
ischemia, cerebrovascular (generalized) *—see* Psychosis, arteriosclerotic
puerperium *—see* Psychosis, puerperal
trauma, brain (birth) (from electric current) (surgical) F06.8
acute or subacute F05
infective F06.8
acute or subacute F05
post-traumatic F06.8
acute or subacute F05
paranoiac F22

Psychosis, psychotic *(continued)*
- paranoid (climacteric) (involutional) (menopausal) F22
  - psychogenic (acute) F23
  - schizophrenic F20.0
  - senile F03
- postpartum (NOS) F53.1
- presbyophrenic (type) F03
- presenile F03
- psychogenic (paranoid) F23
  - depressive (NOS) F32.3
- puerperal F53
  - specified type *—see* Psychosis, by type
- reactive (brief) (transient) (emotional stress) (psychological trauma) F23
  - depressive F32.3
    - recurrent F33.3
  - excitative type F30.8
- schizoaffective F25.9
  - depressive type F25.1
  - manic type F25.0
- schizophrenia, schizophrenic *—see* Schizophrenia
- schizophrenia-like, in epilepsy F06.2
- schizophreniform F20.81
  - affective type F25.9
  - brief F23
  - confusional type F23
  - mixed type F25.0
- senile NEC F03
  - depressed or paranoid type F03
  - simple deterioration F03
  - specified type - code to condition
- shared F24
- situational (reactive) F23
- symbiotic (childhood) F84.3
- symptomatic F09

Psychosomatic *—see* Disorder, psychosomatic

Psychosyndrome, organic F07.9

Psychotic episode due to or associated with physical condition F06.8

Pterygium (eye) H11.00-
- amyloid H11.01-
- central H11.02-
- colli Q18.3
- double H11.03-
- peripheral
  - progressive H11.05-
  - stationary H11.04-
- recurrent H11.06-

Ptilosis (eyelid) *—see* Madarosis

Ptomaine (poisoning) *—see* Poisoning, food

Ptosis *—see also* Blepharoptosis
- adiposa (false) *—see* Blepharoptosis
- breast N64.81
- brow H57.81-
- cecum K63.4
- colon K63.4
- congenital (eyelid) Q10.0
  - specified site NEC *—see* Anomaly, by site
- eyebrow H57.81-
- eyelid *—see* Blepharoptosis
  - congenital Q10.0
- gastric K31.89
- intestine K63.4
- kidney N28.83
- liver K76.89
- renal N28.83
- splanchnic K63.4
- spleen D73.89
- stomach K31.89
- viscera K63.4

PTP D69.51

Ptyalism (periodic) K11.7
- hysterical F45.8
- pregnancy *—see* Pregnancy, complicated by, specified pregnancy-related condition NEC
- psychogenic F45.8

Ptyalolithiasis K11.5

Pubarche, precocious E30.1

Pubertas praecox E30.1

Puberty (development state) Z00.3
- bleeding (excessive) N92.2
- delayed E30.0
- precocious (constitutional) (cryptogenic) (idiopathic) E30.1
  - central E22.8
  - due to
    - ovarian hyperfunction E28.1
      - estrogen E28.0
    - testicular hyperfunction E29.0
- premature E30.1
  - due to
    - adrenal cortical hyperfunction E25.8
    - pineal tumor E34.8
    - pituitary (anterior) hyperfunction E22.8

Puckering, macula *—see* Degeneration, macula, puckering

Pudenda, pudendum *—see* condition

Puente's disease (simple glandular cheilitis) K13.0

Puerperal, puerperium (complicated by, complications)
- abnormal glucose (tolerance test) O99.815
- abscess
  - areola O91.02
    - associated with lactation O91.03
  - Bartholin's gland O86.19
  - breast O91.12
    - associated with lactation O91.13
  - cervix (uteri) O86.11
  - genital organ NEC O86.19
  - kidney O86.21
  - mammary O91.12
    - associated with lactation O91.13
  - nipple O91.02
    - associated with lactation O91.03
  - peritoneum O85
  - subareolar O91.12
    - associated with lactation O91.13
  - urinary tract *—see* Puerperal, infection, urinary
  - uterus O86.12
  - vagina (wall) O86.13
  - vaginorectal O86.13
  - vulvovaginal gland O86.13
- adnexitis O86.19
- afibrinogenemia, or other coagulation defect O72.3
- albuminuria (acute) (subacute) *—see* Proteinuria, gestational
- alcohol use O99.315
- anemia O90.81
  - pre-existing (pre-pregnancy) O99.03
- anesthetic death O89.8
- apoplexy O99.43
- bariatric surgery status O99.845
- blood disorder NEC O99.13

Puerperal, puerperium *(continued)*
- blood dyscrasia O72.3
- cardiomyopathy O90.3
- cerebrovascular disorder (conditions in I60-I69) O99.43
- cervicitis O86.11
- circulatory system disorder O99.43
- coagulopathy (any) O99.13
  - with hemorrhage O72.3
- complications O90.9
  - specified NEC O90.89
- convulsions *—see* Eclampsia
- cystitis O86.22
- cystopyelitis O86.29
- delirium NEC F05
- diabetes O24.93
  - gestational *—see* Puerperal, gestational diabetes
  - pre-existing O24.33
    - specified NEC O24.83
    - type 1 O24.03
    - type 2 O24.13
- digestive system disorder O99.63
- disease O90.9
  - breast NEC O92.29
  - cerebrovascular (acute) O99.43
  - nonobstetric NEC O99.893
  - tubo-ovarian O86.19
  - Valsuani's O99.03
- disorder O90.9
  - biliary tract O26.63
  - lactation O92.70
  - liver O26.63
  - nonobstetric NEC O99.893
- disruption
  - cesarean wound O90.0
  - episiotomy wound O90.1
  - perineal laceration wound O90.1
- drug use O99.325
- eclampsia (with pre-existing hypertension) O15.2
- embolism (pulmonary) (blood clot) *—see* Embolism, obstetric, puerperal
- endocrine, nutritional or metabolic disease NEC O99.285
- endophlebitis *—see* Puerperal, phlebitis
- endotrachelitis O86.11
- failure
  - lactation (complete) O92.3
    - partial O92.4
  - renal, acute O90.4
- fever (of unknown origin) O86.4
  - septic O85
- fissure, nipple O92.12
  - associated with lactation O92.13
- fistula
  - breast (due to mastitis) O91.12
    - associated with lactation O91.13
  - nipple O91.02
    - associated with lactation O91.03
- galactophoritis O91.22
  - associated with lactation O91.23
- galactorrhea O92.6
- gastric banding status O99.845
- gastric bypass status O99.845
- gastrointestinal disease NEC O99.63
- gestational
  - diabetes O24.439
    - diet controlled O24.430
    - insulin (and diet) controlled O24.434
    - oral drug controlled (antidiabetic) (hypoglycemic) O24.435

Puerperal, puerperium *(continued)*
- gestational *(continued)*
  - edema O12.05
    - with proteinuria O12.25
  - proteinuria O12.15
- gonorrhea O98.23
- hematoma, subdural O99.43
- hemiplegia, cerebral O99.355
  - due to cerbrovascular disorder O99.43
- hemorrhage O72.1
  - brain O99.43
  - bulbar O99.43
  - cerebellar O99.43
  - cerebral O99.43
  - cortical O99.43
  - delayed or secondary O72.2
  - extradural O99.43
  - internal capsule O99.43
  - intracranial O99.43
  - intrapontine O99.43
  - meningeal O99.43
  - pontine O99.43
  - retained placenta O72.0
  - subarachnoid O99.43
  - subcortical O99.43
  - subdural O99.43
  - third stage O72.0
  - uterine, delayed O72.2
  - ventricular O99.43
- hemorrhoids O87.2
- hepatorenal syndrome O90.4
- hypertension *—see* Hypertension, complicating, puerperium
- hypertrophy, breast O92.29
- induration breast (fibrous) O92.29
- infection O86.4
  - cervix O86.11
  - generalized O85
  - genital tract NEC O86.19
    - obstetric surgical wound O86.09
  - kidney (bacillus coli) O86.21
  - maternal O98.93
    - carrier state NEC O99.835
    - gonorrhea O98.23
    - human immunodeficiency virus (HIV) O98.73
    - protozoal O98.63
    - sexually transmitted NEC O98.33
    - specified NEC O98.83
    - streptococcus group B (GBS) carrier state O99.825
    - syphilis O98.13
    - tuberculosis O98.03
    - viral hepatitis O98.43
    - viral NEC O98.53
  - nipple O91.02
    - associated with lactation O91.03
  - peritoneum O85
  - renal O86.21
  - specified NEC O86.89
  - urinary (asymptomatic) (tract) NEC O86.20
    - bladder O86.22
    - kidney O86.21
    - specified site NEC O86.29
    - urethra O86.22
  - vagina O86.13
  - vein *—see* Puerperal, phlebitis
- ischemia, cerebral O99.43
- lymphangitis O86.89
  - breast O91.22
    - associated with lactation O91.23
- malignancy O9A.13
- malnutrition O25.3
- mammillitis O91.02
  - associated with lactation O91.03

Puerperal, puerperium *(continued)*
- mammitis O91.22
  - associated with lactation O91.23
- mania F30.8
- mastitis O91.22
  - associated with lactation O91.23
  - purulent O91.12
    - associated with lactation O91.13
- melancholia —*see* Disorder, depressive
- mental disorder NEC O99.345
- metroperitonitis O85
- metrorrhagia —*see* Hemorrhage, postpartum
- metrosalpingitis O86.19
- metrovaginitis O86.13
- milk leg O87.1
- monoplegia, cerebral O99.43
- mood disturbance O90.6
- necrosis, liver (acute) (subacute) (conditions in subcategory K72.0) O26.63
  - with renal failure O90.4
- nervous system disorder O99.355
- neuritis O90.89
- obesity (pre-existing prior to pregnancy) O99.215
- obesity surgery status O99.845
- occlusion, precerebral artery O99.43
- paralysis
  - bladder (sphincter) O90.89
  - cerebral O99.43
- paralytic stroke O99.43
- parametritis O85
- paravaginitis O86.13
- pelviperitonitis O85
- perimetritis O86.12
- perimetrosalpingitis O86.19
- perinephritis O86.21
- periphlebitis —*see* Puerperal phlebitis
- peritoneal infection O85
- peritonitis (pelvic) O85
- perivaginitis O86.13
- phlebitis O87.0
  - deep O87.1
  - pelvic O87.1
  - superficial O87.0
- phlebothrombosis, deep O87.1
- phlegmasia alba dolens O87.1
- placental polyp O90.89
- pneumonia, embolic —*see* Embolism, obstetric, puerperal
- pre-eclampsia (NOS) —*see* Pre-eclampsia
- psychosis F53.1
- pyelitis O86.21
- pyelocystitis O86.29
- pyelonephritis O86.21
- pyelonephrosis O86.21
- pyemia O85
- pyocystitis O86.29
- pyohemia O85
- pyometra O86.12
- pyonephritis O86.21
- pyosalpingitis O86.19
- pyrexia (of unknown origin) O86.4
- renal
  - disease NEC O90.89
  - failure O90.4
- respiratory disease NEC O99.53
- retention
  - decidua —*see* Retention, decidua
  - placenta O72.0
  - secundines —*see* Retention, secundines
- retrated nipple O92.02
- salpingo-ovaritis O86.19
- salpingoperitonitis O85
- secondary perineal tear O90.1

Puerperal, puerperium *(continued)*
- sepsis (pelvic) O85
- sepsis O85
- septic thrombophlebitis O86.81
- skin disorder NEC O99.73
- specified condition NEC O99.893
- stroke O99.43
- subinvolution (uterus) O90.89
- subluxation of symphysis (pubis) O26.73
- suppuration —*see* Puerperal, abscess
- tetanus A34
- thelitis O91.02
  - associated with lactation O91.03
- thrombocytopenia O72.3
- thrombophlebitis (superficial) O87.0
  - deep O87.1
  - pelvic O87.1
  - septic O86.81
- thrombosis (venous) —*see* Thrombosis, puerperal
- thyroiditis O90.5
- toxemia (eclamptic) (pre-eclamptic) (with convulsions) O15.2
- trauma, non-obstetric O9A.23
  - caused by abuse (physical) (suspected) O9A.33
    - confirmed O9A.33
    - psychological (suspected) O9A.53
      - confirmed O9A.53
    - sexual (suspected) O9A.43
      - confirmed O9A.43
- uremia (due to renal failure) O90.4
- urethritis O86.22
- vaginitis O86.13
- varicose veins (legs) O87.4
  - vulva or perineum O87.8
- venous O87.9
- vulvitis O86.19
- vulvovaginitis O86.13
- white leg O87.1

Puerperium —*see* Puerperal

Pulmolithiasis J98.4

Pulmonary —*see* condition

Pulpitis (acute) (anachoretic) (chronic) (hyperplastic) (putrescent) (suppurative) (ulcerative) K04.01
- irreversible K04.02
- reversible K04.01

Pulpless tooth K04.99

Pulse
- alternating R00.8
- bigeminal R00.8
- fast R00.0
- feeble, rapid due to shock following injury T79.4
- rapid R00.0
- weak R09.89

Pulsus alternans or trigeminus R00.8

Punch drunk F07.81

Punctum lacrimale occlusion —*see* Obstruction, lacrimal

Puncture
- abdomen, abdominal
  - wall S31.139
    - with
      - foreign body S31.149
      - penetration into peritoneal cavity S31.639
        - with foreign body S31.649

Puncture *(continued)*
- abdomen, abdominal *(continued)*
  - wall S31.139
    - epigastric region S31.132
      - with
        - foreign body S31.142
        - penetration into
          - peritoneal cavity S31.632
          - with foreign body S31.642
    - left
      - lower quadrant S31.134
        - with
          - foreign body S31.144
          - penetration into
            - peritoneal cavity S31.634
            - with foreign body S31.644
      - upper quadrant S31.131
        - with
          - foreign body S31.141
          - penetration into
            - peritoneal cavity S31.631
            - with foreign body S31.641
    - periumbilic region S31.135
      - with
        - foreign body S31.145
        - penetration into
          - peritoneal cavity S31.635
          - with foreign body S31.645
    - right
      - lower quadrant S31.133
        - with
          - foreign body S31.143
          - penetration into
            - peritoneal cavity S31.633
            - with foreign body S31.643
      - upper quadrant S31.130
        - with
          - foreign body S31.140
          - penetration into
            - peritoneal cavity S31.630
            - with foreign body S31.640
- accidental, complicating surgery —*see* Complication, accidental puncture or laceration
- alveolar (process) —*see* Puncture, oral cavity
- ankle S91.039
  - with
    - foreign body S91.049
  - left S91.032
    - with
      - foreign body S91.042
  - right S91.031
    - with
      - foreign body S91.041
- anus S31.833
  - with foreign body S31.834
- arm (upper) S41.139
  - with foreign body S41.149
  - left S41.132
    - with foreign body S41.142
  - lower —*see* Puncture, forearm
  - right S41.131
    - with foreign body S41.141
- auditory canal (external) (meatus) —*see* Puncture, ear
- auricle, ear —*see* Puncture, ear
- axilla —*see* Puncture, arm

Puncture *(continued)*
- back —*see also* Puncture, thorax, back
  - lower S31.030
    - with
      - foreign body S31.040
        - with penetration into retroperitoneal space S31.041
      - penetration into retroperitoneal space S31.031
- bladder (traumatic) S37.29
  - nontraumatic N32.89
- breast S21.039
  - with foreign body S21.049
  - left S21.032
    - with foreign body S21.042
  - right S21.031
    - with foreign body S21.041
- buttock S31.803
  - with foreign body S31.804
  - left S31.823
    - with foreign body S31.824
  - right S31.813
    - with foreign body S31.814
- by
  - device, implant or graft —*see* Complications, by site and type, mechanical
  - foreign body left accidentally in operative wound T81.539
  - instrument (any) during a procedure, accidental —*see* Puncture, accidental complicating surgery
- calf —*see* Puncture, leg
- canaliculus lacrimalis —*see* Puncture, eyelid
- canthus, eye —*see* Puncture, eyelid
- cervical esophagus S11.23
  - with foreign body S11.24
- cheek (external) S01.439
  - with foreign body S01.449
  - left S01.432
    - with foreign body S01.442
  - right S01.431
    - with foreign body S01.441
  - internal —*see* Puncture, oral cavity
- chest wall —*see* Puncture, thorax
- chin —*see* Puncture, head, specified site NEC
- clitoris —*see* Puncture, vulva
- costal region —*see* Puncture, thorax
- digit(s)
  - hand —*see* Puncture, finger
  - foot —*see* Puncture, toe
- ear (canal) (external) S01.339
  - with foreign body S01.349
  - left S01.332
    - with foreign body S01.342
  - right S01.331
    - with foreign body S01.341
  - drum S09.2-
- elbow S51.039
  - with
    - foreign body S51.049
  - left S51.032
    - with
      - foreign body S51.042
  - right S51.031
    - with
      - foreign body S51.041
- epididymis —*see* Puncture, testis
- epigastric region —*see* Puncture, abdomen, wall, epigastric
- epiglottis S11.83
  - with foreign body S11.84

Pyemia, pyemic *(continued)*
- puerperal, postpartum, childbirth O85
- specified organism NEC A41.89
- tuberculous *—see* Tuberculosis, miliary

Pygopagus Q89.4

Pyknoepilepsy (idiopathic) *—see* Pyknolepsy

Pyknolepsy G40.A09
- intractable G40.A19
  - with status epilepticus G40.A11
  - without status epilepticus G40.A19
- not intractable G40.A09
  - with status epilepticus G40.A01
  - without status epilepticus G40.A09

Pylephlebitis K75.1

Pyle's syndrome Q78.5

Pylethrombophlebitis K75.1

Pylethrombosis K75.1

Pyloritis K29.90
- with bleeding K29.91

Pylorospasm (reflex) **NEC** K31.3
- congenital or infantile Q40.0
- newborn Q40.0
- neurotic F45.8
- psychogenic F45.8

Pylorus, pyloric *—see* condition

Pyoarthrosis *—see* Arthritis, pyogenic or pyemic

Pyocele
- mastoid *—see* Mastoiditis, acute
- sinus (accessory) *—see* Sinusitis
- turbinate (bone) J32.9
- urethra (*see also* Urethritis) N34.0

Pyocolpos *—see* Vaginitis

Pyocystitis N30.80
- with hematuria N30.81

Pyoderma, pyodermia L08.0
- gangrenosum L88
- newborn P39.4
- phagedenic L88
- vegetans L08.81

Pyodermatitis L08.0
- vegetans L08.81

Pyogenic *—see* condition

Pyohydronephrosis N13.6

Pyometra, pyometrium, pyometritis *—see* Endometritis

Pyomyositis (tropical) *—see* Myositis, infective

Pyonephritis N12

Pyonephrosis N13.6
- tuberculous A18.11

Pyo-oophoritis *—see* Salpingo-oophoritis

Pyo-ovarium *—see* Salpingo-oophoritis

Pyopericarditis, pyopericardium I30.1

Pyophlebitis *—see* Phlebitis

Pyopneumopericardium I30.1

Pyopneumothorax (infective) J86.9
- with fistula J86.0
- tuberculous NEC A15.6

Pyosalpinx, pyosalpingitis *—see also* Salpingo-oophoritis

Pyothorax J86.9
- with fistula J86.0
- tuberculous NEC A15.6

Pyoureter N28.89
- tuberculous A18.11

Pyramidopallidonigral syndrome G20

Pyrexia (of unknown origin) R50.9
- atmospheric T67.01
- during labor NEC O75.2
- heat T67.01
- newborn P81.9
  - environmentally-induced P81.0
- persistent R50.9
- puerperal O86.4

Pyroglobulinemia NEC E88.09

Pyromania F63.1

Pyrosis R12

Pyuria (bacterial) (sterile) R82.81

Q

Q fever A78
- with pneumonia A78

Quadricuspid aortic valve Q23.8

Quadrilateral fever A78

Quadriparesis *—see* Quadriplegia
- meaning muscle weakness M62.81

Quadriplegia G82.50
- complete
  - C1-C4 level G82.51
  - C5-C7 level G82.53
- congenital (cerebral) (spinal) G80.8
  - spastic G80.0
- embolic (current episode) I63.4-
- functional R53.2
- incomplete
  - C1-C4 level G82.52
  - C5-C7 level G82.54
- thrombotic (current episode) I63.3-
- traumatic -- code to injury with seventh character S
  - current episode *—see* Injury, spinal (cord), cervical

Quadruplet, pregnancy *—see* Pregnancy, quadruplet

Quarrelsomeness F60.3

Queensland fever A77.3

Quervain's disease M65.4
- thyroid E06.1

Queyrat's erythroplasia D07.4
- penis D07.4
- specified site *—see* Neoplasm, skin, in situ
- unspecified site D07.4

Quincke's disease or edema T78.3
- hereditary D84.1

Quinsy (gangrenous) J36

Quintan fever A79.0

Quintuplet, pregnancy *—see* Pregnancy, quintuplet

R

Rabbit fever *—see* Tularemia

Rabies A82.9
- contact Z20.3
- exposure to Z20.3
- inoculation reaction *—see* Complications, vaccination
- sylvatic A82.0
- urban A82.1

Rachischisis *—see* Spina bifida

Rachitic *—see also* condition
- deformities of spine (late effect) (sequelae) E64.3
- pelvis (late effect) (sequelae) E64.3
  - with disproportion (fetopelvic) O33.0
    - causing obstructed labor O65.0

Rachitis, rachitism (acute) (tarda) *—see also* Rickets
- renalis N25.0
- sequelae E64.3

Radial nerve *—see* condition

Radiation
- burn *—see* Burn
- effects NOS T66
- sickness NOS T66
- therapy, encounter for Z51.0

Radiculitis (pressure) (vertebrogenic) *—see* Radiculopathy

Radiculomyelitis *—see also* Encephalitis
- toxic, due to
  - Clostridium tetani A35
  - Corynebacterium diphtheriae A36.82

Radiculopathy M54.10
- cervical region M54.12
- cervicothoracic region M54.13
- due to
  - disc disorder
    - C3 M50.11
    - C4 M50.11
    - C5 M50.121
    - C6 M50.122
    - C7 M50.123
    - C8 M50.13
  - displacement of intervertebral disc *—see* Disorder, disc, with, radiculopathy
- leg M54.1-
- lumbar region M54.16
- lumbosacral region M54.17
- occipito-atlanto-axial region M54.11
- postherpetic B02.29
- sacrococcygeal region M54.18
- syphilitic A52.11
- thoracic region (with visceral pain) M54.14
- thoracolumbar region M54.15

Radiodermal burns (acute, chronic, or occupational) *—see* Burn

Radiodermatitis L58.9
- acute L58.0
- chronic L58.1

Radiotherapy session Z51.0

RAEB (refractory anemia with excess blasts) D46.2-

Rage, meaning rabies *—see* Rabies

Ragpicker's disease A22.1

Ragsorter's disease A22.1

Raillietiniasis B71.8

Railroad neurosis F48.8

Railway spine F48.8

Raised *—see also* Elevated
- antibody titer R76.0

Rake teeth, tooth M26.39

Rales R09.89

Ramifying renal pelvis Q63.8

Ramsay-Hunt disease or syndrome (*see also* Hunt's disease) B02.21
- meaning dyssynergia cerebellaris myoclonica G11.19

Ranula K11.6
- congenital Q38.4

Rape
- adult
  - confirmed T74.21
  - suspected T76.21
- alleged, observation or examination, ruled out
  - adult Z04.41
  - child Z04.42
- child
  - confirmed T74.22
  - suspected T76.22

Rapid
- feeble pulse, due to shock, following injury T79.4
- heart (beat) R00.0
  - psychogenic F45.8
- second stage (delivery) O62.3
- time-zone change syndrome G47.25

Rarefaction, bone *—see* Disorder, bone, density and structure, specified NEC

Rash (toxic) R21
- canker A38.9
- diaper L22
- drug (internal use) L27.0
  - contact (*see also* Dermatitis, due to, drugs, external) L25.1
- following immunization T88.1
- food *—see* Dermatitis, due to, food
- heat L74.0
- napkin (psoriasiform) L22
- nettle *—see* Urticaria
- pustular L08.0
- rose R21
  - epidemic B06.9
- scarlet A38.9
- serum (*see also* Reaction, serum) T80.69
- wandering tongue K14.1

Rasmussen aneurysm *—see* Tuberculosis, pulmonary

Rasmussen encephalitis G04.81

Rat-bite fever A25.9
- due to Streptobacillus moniliformis A25.1
- spirochetal (morsus muris) A25.0

Rathke's pouch tumor D44.3

Raymond (-Céstan) **syndrome** I65.8

Raynaud's disease, phenomenon or syndrome (secondary) I73.00
- with gangrene (symmetric) I73.01

RDS (newborn) (type I) P22.0
- type II P22.1

Reaction *—see also* Disorder
- adaptation *—see* Disorder, adjustment
- adjustment (anxiety) (conduct disorder) (depressiveness) (distress) *—see* Disorder, adjustment
  - with
    - mutism, elective (child) (adolescent) F94.0
- adverse
  - food (any) (ingested) NEC T78.1
    - anaphylactic *—see* Shock, anaphylactic, due to food
- affective *—see* Disorder, mood
- allergic *—see* Allergy
- anaphylactic *—see* Shock, anaphylactic
- anaphylactoid *—see* Shock, anaphylactic

Reaction *(continued)*
- anesthesia *—see* Anesthesia, complication
- antitoxin (prophylactic) (therapeutic) *—see* Complications, vaccination
- anxiety F41.1
- Arthus *—see* Arthus' phenomenon
- asthenic F48.8
- combat and operational stress F43.0
- compulsive F42.8
- conversion F44.9
- crisis, acute F43.0
- deoxyribonuclease (DNA) (DNase) hypersensitivity D69.2
- depressive (single episode) F32.9
  - affective (single episode) F31.4
    - recurrent episode F33.9
  - neurotic F34.1
  - psychoneurotic F34.1
  - psychotic F32.3
  - recurrent *—see* Disorder, depressive, recurrent
- dissociative F44.9
- drug NEC T88.7
  - addictive *—see* Dependence, drug
    - transmitted via placenta or breast milk *—see* Absorption, drug, addictive, through placenta
  - allergic *—see* Allergy, drug
  - lichenoid L43.2
  - newborn P93.8
    - gray baby syndrome P93.0
  - overdose or poisoning (by accident) *—see* Table of Drugs and Chemicals, by drug, poisoning
  - photoallergic L56.1
  - phototoxic L56.0
  - withdrawal *—see* Dependence, by drug, with, withdrawal
    - infant of dependent mother P96.1
    - newborn P96.1
  - wrong substance given or taken (by accident) *—see* Table of Drugs and Chemicals, by drug, poisoning
- fear F40.9
  - child (abnormal) F93.8
- febrile nonhemolytic transfusion (FNHTR) R50.84
- fluid loss, cerebrospinal G97.1
- foreign
  - body NEC *—see* Granuloma, foreign body
    - in operative wound (inadvertently left) *—see* Foreign body, accidentally left during a procedure
  - substance accidentally left during a procedure (chemical) (powder) (talc) T81.60
    - aseptic peritonitis T81.61
    - body or object (instrument) (sponge) (swab) *—see* Foreign body, accidentally left during a procedure
    - specified reaction NEC T81.69
- grief *—see* Disorder, adjustment
- Herxheimer's R68.89
- hyperkinetic *—see* Hyperkinesia
- hypochondriacal F45.20
- hypoglycemic, due to insulin E16.0
  - with coma (diabetic) *—see* Diabetes, coma
    - nondiabetic E15
  - therapeutic misadventure *—see* subcategory T38.3

Reaction *(continued)*
- hypomanic F30.8
- hysterical F44.9
- immunization *—see* Complications, vaccination
- incompatibility
  - ABO blood group (infusion) (transfusion) *—see* Complication(s), transfusion, incompatibility reaction, ABO
    - delayed serologic T80.39
  - minor blood group (Duffy) (E) (K) (Kell) (Kidd) (Lewis) (M) (N) (P) (S) T80.89
  - Rh (factor) (infusion) (transfusion) *—see* Complication(s), transfusion, incompatibility reaction, Rh (factor)
- inflammatory *—see* Infection
- infusion *—see* Complications, infusion
- inoculation (immune serum) *—see* Complications, vaccination
- insulin T38.3-
- involutional psychotic *—see* Disorder, depressive
- leukemoid D72.823
  - basophilic D72.823
  - lymphocytic D72.823
  - monocytic D72.823
  - myelocytic D72.823
  - neutrophilic D72.823
- LSD (acute)
  - due to drug abuse *—see* Abuse, drug, hallucinogen
  - due to drug dependence *—see* Dependence, drug, hallucinogen
- lumbar puncture G97.1
- manic-depressive *—see* Disorder, bipolar
- neurasthenic F48.8
- neurogenic *—see* Neurosis
- neurotic F48.9
- neurotic-depressive F34.1
- nitritoid *—see* Crisis, nitritoid
- nonspecific
  - to
    - cell mediated immunity measurement of gamma interferon antigen response without active tuberculosis R76.12
    - QuantiFERON-TB test (QFT) without active tuberculosis R76.12
    - tuberculin test (*see also* Reaction, tuberculin skin test) R76.11
- obsessive-compulsive F42.8
- organic, acute or subacute *—see* Delirium
- paranoid (acute) F23
  - chronic F22
  - senile F03
- passive dependency F60.7
- phobic F40.9
- post-traumatic stress, uncomplicated Z73.3
- psychogenic F99
- psychoneurotic *—see also* Neurosis
  - compulsive F42.8
  - depersonalization F48.1
  - depressive F34.1
  - hypochondriacal F45.20
  - neurasthenic F48.8
  - obsessive F42.8
- psychophysiologic *—see* Disorder, somatoform

Reaction *(continued)*
- psychosomatic *—see* Disorder, somatoform
- psychotic *—see* Psychosis
- scarlet fever toxin *—see* Complications, vaccination
- schizophrenic F23
  - acute (brief) (undifferentiated) F23
  - latent F21
  - undifferentiated (acute) (brief) F23
- serological for syphilis *—see* Serology for syphilis
- serum T80.69
  - anaphylactic (immediate) *—see also* Shock, anaphylactic T80.59
  - specified reaction NEC
    - due to
      - administration of blood and blood products T80.61
      - immunization T80.62
      - serum specified NEC T80.69
      - vaccination T80.62
- situational *—see* Disorder, adjustment
- somatization *—see* Disorder, somatoform
- spinal puncture G97.1
  - dural G97.1
- stress (severe) F43.9
  - acute (agitation) ("daze") (disorientation) (disturbance of consciousness) (flight reaction) (fugue) F43.0
  - specified NEC F43.8
- surgical procedure *—see* Complications, surgical procedure
- tetanus antitoxin *—see* Complications, vaccination
- toxic, to local anesthesia T88.59
  - in labor and delivery O74.4
  - in pregnancy O29.3X-
  - postpartum, puerperal O89.3
- toxin-antitoxin *—see* Complications, vaccination
- transfusion (blood) (bone marrow) (lymphocytes) (allergic) *—see* Complications, transfusion
- tuberculin skin test, abnormal R76.11
- vaccination (any) *—see* Complications, vaccination
- withdrawing, child or adolescent F93.8

Reactive airway disease *—see* Asthma

Reactive depression *—see* Reaction, depressive

Rearrangement
- chromosomal
  - balanced (in) Q95.9
    - abnormal individual (autosomal) Q95.2
    - non-sex (autosomal) chromosomes Q95.2
    - sex/non-sex chromosomes Q95.3
  - specified NEC Q95.8

Recalcitrant patient *—see* Noncompliance

Recanalization, thrombus *—see* Thrombosis

Recession, receding
- chamber angle (eye) H21.55-
- chin M26.09
- gingival (postinfective) (postoperative)
  - generalized K06.020
    - minimal K06.021
    - moderate K06.022
    - severe K06.023
  - localized K06.010
    - minimal K06.011
    - moderate K06.012
    - severe K06.013

Recklinghausen disease Q85.01
- bones E21.0

Reclus' disease (cystic) *—see* Mastopathy, cystic

Recrudescent typhus (fever) A75.1

Recruitment, auditory H93.21-

Rectalgia K62.89

Rectitis K62.89

Rectocele
- female (without uterine prolapse) N81.6
  - with uterine prolapse N81.4
    - incomplete N81.2
- in pregnancy *—see* Pregnancy, complicated by, abnormal, pelvic organs or tissues NEC
- male K62.3

Rectosigmoid junction *—see* condition

Rectosigmoiditis K63.89
- ulcerative (chronic) K51.30
  - with
    - complication K51.319
      - abscess K51.314
      - fistula K51.313
      - obstruction K51.312
      - rectal bleeding K51.311
      - specified NEC K51.318

Rectourethral *—see* condition

Rectovaginal *—see* condition

Rectovesical *—see* condition

Rectum, rectal *—see* condition

Recurrent *—see* condition
- pregnancy loss *—see* Loss (of), pregnancy, recurrent

Red bugs B88.0

Red-cedar lung or pneumonitis J67.8

Red tide (*see also* Table of Drugs and Chemicals) T65.82-

Reduced
- mobility Z74.09
- ventilatory or vital capacity R94.2

Redundant, redundancy
- anus (congenital) Q43.8
- clitoris N90.89
- colon (congenital) Q43.8
- foreskin (congenital) N47.8
- intestine (congenital) Q43.8
- labia N90.69
- organ or site, congenital NEC *—see* Accessory
- panniculus (abdominal) E65
- prepuce (congenital) N47.8
- pylorus K31.89
- rectum (congenital) Q43.8
- scrotum N50.89
- sigmoid (congenital) Q43.8

- **Redundant, redundancy** *(continued)*
  - skin L98.7
    - and subcutaneous tissue L98.7
    - of face L57.4
      - eyelids —*see* Blepharochalasis
  - stomach K31.89
- **Reduplication** —*see* Duplication
- **Reflex** R29.2
  - hyperactive gag J39.2
  - pupillary, abnormal —*see* Anomaly, pupil, function
  - vasoconstriction I73.9
  - vasovagal R55
- **Reflux** K21.9
  - acid K21.9
  - esophageal K21.9
    - with esophagitis (without bleeding) K21.00
      - with bleeding K21.01
    - newborn P78.83
  - gastroesophageal K21.9
    - with esophagitis (without bleeding) K21.00
      - with bleeding K21.01
  - mitral —*see* Insufficiency, mitral
  - ureteral —*see* Reflux, vesicoureteral
  - vesicoureteral (with scarring) N13.70
    - with
      - nephropathy N13.729
        - with hydroureter N13.739
          - bilateral N13.732
          - unilateral N13.731
        - bilateral N13.722
        - unilateral N13.721
        - without hydroureter N13.729
          - bilateral N13.722
          - unilateral N13.721
      - pyelonephritis (chronic) N11.0
    - congenital Q62.7
    - without nephropathy N13.71
- **Reforming, artificial openings** —*see* Attention to, artificial, opening
- **Refractive error** —*see* Disorder, refraction
- **Refsum's disease or syndrome** G60.1
- **Refusal of**
  - food, psychogenic F50.89
  - treatment (because of) Z53.20
    - left against medical advice (AMA) Z53.29
    - left without being seen Z53.21
    - patient's decision NEC Z53.29
    - reasons of belief or group pressure Z53.9
- **Regional** —*see* condition
- **Regurgitation** R11.10
  - aortic (valve) —*see* Insufficiency, aortic
  - food —*see also* Vomiting
    - with reswallowing —*see* Rumination
    - newborn P92.1
  - gastric contents —*see* Vomiting
  - heart —*see* Endocarditis
  - mitral (valve) —*see* Insufficiency, mitral
    - congenital Q23.3
  - myocardial —*see* Endocarditis
  - pulmonary (valve) (heart) I37.1
    - congenital Q22.2
    - syphilitic A52.03
  - tricuspid —*see* Insufficiency, tricuspid
  - valve, valvular —*see* Endocarditis
    - congenital Q24.8
- **Regurgitation** *(continued)*
  - vesicoureteral —*see* Reflux, vesicoureteral
- **Reifenstein syndrome** E34.52
- **Reinsertion**
  - implantable subdermal contraceptive Z30.46
  - intrauterine contraceptive device Z30.433
- **Reiter's disease, syndrome, or urethritis** M02.30
  - ankle M02.37-
  - elbow M02.32-
  - foot joint M02.37-
  - hand joint M02.34-
  - hip M02.35-
  - knee M02.36-
  - multiple site M02.39
  - shoulder M02.31-
  - vertebra M02.38
  - wrist M02.33-
- **Reichmann's disease or syndrome** K31.89
- **Rejection**
  - food, psychogenic F50.89
  - transplant T86.91
    - bone T86.830
      - marrow T86.01
    - cornea T86.840-
    - heart T86.21
      - with lung(s) T86.31
    - intestine T86.850
    - kidney T86.11
    - liver T86.41
    - lung(s) T86.810
      - with heart T86.31
    - organ (immune or nonimmune cause) T86.91
    - pancreas T86.890
    - skin (allograft) (autograft) T86.820
    - specified NEC T86.890
    - stem cell (peripheral blood) (umbilical cord) T86.5
- **Relapsing fever** A68.9
  - Carter's (Asiatic) A68.1
  - Dutton's (West African) A68.1
  - Koch's A68.9
  - louse-borne (epidemic) A68.0
  - Novy's (American) A68.1
  - Obermeyers's (European) A68.0
  - Spirillum A68.9
  - tick-borne (endemic) A68.1
- **Relationship**
  - occlusal
    - open anterior M26.220
    - open posterior M26.221
- **Relaxation**
  - anus (sphincter) K62.89
    - psychogenic F45.8
  - arch (foot) —*see also* Deformity, limb, flat foot
  - back ligaments —*see* Instability, joint, spine
  - bladder (sphincter) N31.2
  - cardioesophageal K21.9
  - cervix —*see* Incompetency, cervix
  - diaphragm J98.6
  - joint (capsule) (ligament) (paralytic) —*see* Flail, joint
    - congenital NEC Q74.8
  - lumbosacral (joint) —*see* subcategory M53.2
  - pelvic floor N81.89
  - perineum N81.89
  - posture R29.3
  - rectum (sphincter) K62.89
  - sacroiliac (joint) —*see* subcategory M53.2
- **Relaxation** *(continued)*
  - scrotum N50.89
  - urethra (sphincter) N36.44
  - vesical N31.2
- **Release from prison, anxiety concerning** Z65.2
- **Remains**
  - canal of Cloquet Q14.0
  - capsule (opaque) Q14.8
- **Remittent fever** (malarial) B54
- **Remnant**
  - canal of Cloquet Q14.0
  - capsule (opaque) Q14.8
  - cervix, cervical stump (acquired) (postoperative) N88.8
  - cystic duct, postcholecystectomy K91.5
  - fingernail L60.8
    - congenital Q84.6
  - meniscus, knee —*see* Derangement, knee, meniscus, specified NEC
  - thyroglossal duct Q89.2
  - tonsil J35.8
    - infected (chronic) J35.01
  - urachus Q64.4
- **Removal** (from) (of)
  - artificial
    - arm Z44.00-
      - complete Z44.01-
      - partial Z44.02-
    - eye Z44.2-
    - leg Z44.10-
      - complete Z44.11-
      - partial Z44.12-
  - breast implant Z45.81
  - cardiac pulse generator (battery) (end-of-life) Z45.010
  - catheter (urinary) (indwelling) Z46.6
    - from artificial opening —*see* Attention to, artificial, opening
    - non-vascular Z46.82
    - vascular NEC Z45.2
  - drains Z48.03
  - device Z46.9
    - contraceptive Z30.432
      - implantable subdermal Z30.46
    - implanted NEC Z45.89
    - specified NEC Z46.89
  - dressing (nonsurgical) Z48.00
    - surgical Z48.01
  - external
    - fixation device - code to fracture with seventh character D
    - prosthesis, prosthetic device Z44.9
      - breast Z44.3-
      - specified NEC Z44.8
  - home in childhood (to foster home or institution) Z62.29
  - ileostomy Z43.2
  - insulin pump Z46.81
  - myringotomy device (stent) (tube) Z45.82
  - nervous system device NEC Z46.2
    - brain neuropacemaker Z46.2
    - visual substitution device Z46.2
      - implanted Z45.31
  - non-vascular catheter Z46.82
  - orthodontic device Z46.4
  - organ, prophylactic (for neoplasia management) —*see* Prophylactic, organ removal
  - staples Z48.02
  - stent
    - ureteral Z46.6
  - suture Z48.02
  - urinary device Z46.6
- **Removal** *(continued)*
  - vascular access device or catheter Z45.2
- **Ren**
  - arcuatus Q63.1
  - mobile, mobilis N28.89
    - congenital Q63.8
  - unguliformis Q63.1
- **Renal** —*see* condition
- **Rendu-Osler-Weber disease or syndrome** I78.0
- **Reninoma** D41.0-
- **Renon-Delille syndrome** E23.3
- **Reovirus, as cause of disease classified elsewhere** B97.5
- **Repeated falls NEC** R29.6
- **Replaced chromosome by dicentric ring** Q93.2
- **Replacement by artificial or mechanical device or prosthesis of**
  - bladder Z96.0
  - blood vessel NEC Z95.828
  - bone NEC Z96.7
  - cochlea Z96.21
  - coronary artery Z95.5
  - eustachian tube Z96.29
  - eye globe Z97.0
  - heart Z95.812
    - valve Z95.2
      - prosthetic Z95.2
      - specified NEC Z95.4
      - xenogenic Z95.3
  - intestine Z96.89
  - joint Z96.60
    - hip —*see* Presence, hip joint implant
    - knee —*see* Presence, knee joint implant
    - specified site NEC Z96.698
  - larynx Z96.3
  - lens Z96.1
  - limb(s) —*see* Presence, artificial, limb
  - mandible NEC (for tooth root implant(s)) Z96.5
  - organ NEC Z96.89
  - peripheral vessel NEC Z95.828
  - stapes Z96.29
  - teeth Z97.2
  - tendon Z96.7
  - tissue NEC Z96.89
  - tooth root(s) Z96.5
  - vessel NEC Z95.828
    - coronary (artery) Z95.5
- **Request for expert evidence** Z04.89
- **Reserve, decreased or low**
  - cardiac —*see* Disease, heart
  - kidney N28.89
- **Residing**
  - in place not meant for human habitation (abandoned building) (car) (park) (sidewalk) Z59.02
  - on the street Z59.02
- **Residual** —*see also* condition
  - ovary syndrome N99.83
  - state, schizophrenic F20.5
  - urine R39.198
- **Resistance, resistant** (to)
  - activated protein C D68.51
  - complicating pregnancy O26.89
  - insulin E88.81

Resistance, resistant *(continued)*
- organism(s)
  - to
    - drug Z16.30
      - aminoglycosides Z16.29
      - amoxicillin Z16.11
      - ampicillin Z16.11
      - antibiotic(s) Z16.20
        - multiple Z16.24
        - specified NEC Z16.29
      - antifungal Z16.32
      - antimicrobial (single) Z16.30
        - multiple Z16.35
        - specified NEC Z16.39
      - antimycobacterial (single) Z16.341
        - multiple Z16.342
      - antiparasitic Z16.31
      - antiviral Z16.33
      - beta lactam antibiotics Z16.10
        - specified NEC Z16.19
      - cephalosporins Z16.19
      - extended beta lactamase (ESBL) Z16.12
      - fluoroquinolones Z16.23
      - macrolides Z16.29
      - methicillin *—see* MRSA
      - multiple drugs (MDRO)
        - antibiotics Z16.24
        - antimicrobial Z16.35
        - antimycobacterials Z16.342
      - penicillins Z16.11
      - quinine (and related compounds) Z16.31
      - quinolones Z16.23
      - sulfonamides Z16.29
      - tetracyclines Z16.29
      - tuberculostatics (single) Z16.341
        - multiple Z16.342
      - vancomycin Z16.21
        - related antibiotics Z16.22
- thyroid hormone E07.89

Resorption
- dental (roots) K03.3
  - alveoli M26.79
- teeth (external) (internal) (pathological) (roots) K03.3

Respiration
- Cheyne-Stokes R06.3
- decreased due to shock, following injury T79.4
- disorder of, psychogenic F45.8
- insufficient, or poor R06.89
  - newborn P28.5
- painful R07.1
- sighing, psychogenic F45.8

Respiratory *—see also* condition
- distress syndrome (newborn) (type I) P22.0
  - type II P22.1
- syncytial virus, as cause of disease classified elsewhere (*see also* Virus, respiratory syncytial (RSV)) B97.4

Respite care Z75.5

Response (drug)
- photoallergic L56.1
- phototoxic L56.0

Restenosis
- stent
  - vascular
    - end stent
      - adjacent to stent *—see* Arteriosclerosis

Restenosis *(continued)*
- stent *(continued)*
  - vascular *(continued)*
    - end stent *(continued)*
      - within the stent
        - coronary T82.855
        - peripheral T82.856
    - in stent
      - coronary vessel T82.855
      - peripheral vessel T82.856

Restless legs (syndrome) G25.81

Restlessness R45.1

Restriction of housing space Z59.1

Restoration (of)
- dental
  - aesthetically inadequate or displeasing K08.56
  - defective K08.50
    - specified NEC K08.59
  - failure of marginal integrity K08.51
  - failure of periodontal anatomical intergrity K08.54
- organ continuity from previous sterilization (tuboplasty) (vasoplasty) Z31.0
  - aftercare Z31.42
- tooth (existing)
  - contours biologically incompatible with oral health K08.54
  - open margins K08.51
  - overhanging K08.52
  - poor aesthetic K08.56
  - poor gingival margins K08.51
- unsatisfactory, of tooth K08.50
  - specified NEC K08.59

Restorative material (dental)
- allergy to K08.55
- fractured K08.539
  - with loss of material K08.531
  - without loss of material K08.530
- unrepairable overhanging of K08.52

Rests, ovarian, in fallopian tube Q50.6

Restzustand (schizophrenic) F20.5

Retained *—see also* Retention
- cholelithiasis following cholecystectomy K91.86
- foreign body fragments (type of) Z18.9
  - acrylics Z18.2
  - animal quill(s) or spines Z18.31
  - cement Z18.83
  - concrete Z18.83
  - crystalline Z18.83
  - depleted isotope Z18.09
  - depleted uranium Z18.01
  - diethylhexyl phthalates Z18.2
  - glass Z18.81
  - isocyanate Z18.2
  - magnetic metal Z18.11
  - metal Z18.10
  - nonmagnectic metal Z18.12
  - nontherapeutic radioactive Z18.09
  - organic NEC Z18.39
  - plastic Z18.2
  - quill(s) (animal) Z18.31
  - radioactive (nontherapeutic) NEC Z18.09
  - specified NEC Z18.89
  - spine(s) (animal) Z18.31
  - stone Z18.83
  - tooth (teeth) Z18.32
  - wood Z18.33
- fragments (type of) Z18.9
  - acrylics Z18.2

Retained *(continued)*
- fragments *(continued)*
  - animal quill(s) or spines Z18.31
  - cement Z18.83
  - concrete Z18.83
  - crystalline Z18.83
  - depleted isotope Z18.09
  - depleted uranium Z18.01
  - diethylhexyl phthalates Z18.2
  - glass Z18.81
  - isocyanate Z18.2
  - magnetic metal Z18.11
  - metal Z18.10
  - nonmagnectic metal Z18.12
  - nontherapeutic radioactive Z18.09
  - organic NEC Z18.39
  - plastic Z18.2
  - quill(s) (animal) Z18.31
  - radioactive (nontherapeutic) NEC Z18.09
  - specified NEC Z18.89
  - spine(s) (animal) Z18.31
  - stone Z18.83
  - tooth (teeth) Z18.32
  - wood Z18.33
- gallstones, following cholecystectomy K91.86

Retardation
- development, developmental, specific *—see* Disorder, developmental
- endochondral bone growth *—see* Disorder, bone, development or growth
- growth R62.50
  - due to malnutrition E45
- mental *—see* Disability, intellectual
- motor function, specific F82
- physical (child) R62.52
  - due to malnutrition E45
- reading (specific) F81.0
- spelling (specific) (without reading disorder) F81.81

Retching *—see* Vomiting

Retention *—see also* Retained
- bladder *—see* Retention, urine
- carbon dioxide E87.2
- cholelithiasis following cholecystectomy K91.86
- cyst *—see* Cyst
- dead
  - fetus (at or near term) (mother) O36.4
    - early fetal death O02.1
  - ovum O02.0
- decidua (fragments) (following delivery) (with hemorrhage) O72.2
  - without hemorrhage O73.1
- deciduous tooth K00.6
- dental root K08.3
- fecal *—see* Constipation
- fetus
  - dead O36.4
    - early O02.1
- fluid R60.9
- foreign body *—see also* Foreign body, retained
  - current trauma - code as Foreign body, by site or type
- gallstones, following cholecystectomy K91.86
- gastric K31.89
- intrauterine contraceptive device, in pregnancy *—see* Pregnancy, complicated by, retention, intrauterine device

Retention *(continued)*
- membranes (complicating delivery) (with hemorrhage) O72.2
  - with abortion *—see* Abortion, by type
  - without hemorrhage O73.1
- meniscus *—see* Derangement, meniscus
- menses N94.89
- milk (puerperal, postpartum) O92.79
- nitrogen, extrarenal R39.2
- ovary syndrome N99.83
- placenta (total) (with hemorrhage) O72.0
  - without hemorrhage O73.0
  - portions or fragments (with hemorrhage) O72.2
    - without hemorrhage O73.1
- products of conception
  - early pregnancy (dead fetus) O02.1
  - following
    - delivery (with hemorrhage) O72.2
      - without hemorrhage O73.1
- secundines (following delivery) (with hemorrhage) O72.0
  - without hemorrhage O73.0
  - complicating puerperium (delayed hemorrhage) O72.2
  - partial O72.2
    - without hemorrhage O73.1
- smegma, clitoris N90.89
- urine R33.9
  - due to hyperplasia (hypertrophy) of prostate *—see* Hyperplasia, prostate
  - drug-induced R33.0
  - organic R33.8
    - drug-induced R33.0
  - psychogenic F45.8
  - specified NEC R33.8
- water (in tissues) *—see* Edema

Reticular erythematous mucinosis L98.5

Reticulation, dust *—see* Pneumoconiosis

Reticulocytosis R70.1

Reticuloendotheliosis
- acute infantile C96.0
- leukemic C91.4-
- nonlipid C96.0

Reticulohistiocytoma (giant-cell) D76.3

Reticuloid, actinic L57.1

Reticulosis (skin)
- acute of infancy C96.0
- hemophagocytic, familial D76.1
- histiocytic medullary C96.A
- lipomelanotic I89.8
- malignant (midline) C86.0
- polymorphic C86.0
- Sézary *—see* Sézary disease

Retina, retinal *—see also* condition
- dark area D49.81

Retinitis *—see also* Inflammation, chorioretinal
- albuminurica N18.9 *[H32]*
- diabetic *—see* Diabetes, retinitis
- disciformis *—see* Degeneration, macula
- focal *—see* Inflammation, chorioretinal, focal
- gravidarum *—see* Pregnancy, complicated by, specified pregnancy-related condition NEC

- **Retinitis** *(continued)*
  - juxtapapillaris *—see* Inflammation, chorioretinal, focal, juxtapapillary
  - luetic *—see* Retinitis, syphilitic
  - pigmentosa H35.52
  - proliferans *—see* Disorder, globe, degenerative, specified type NEC
  - proliferating *—see* Disorder, globe, degenerative, specified type NEC
  - renal N18.9 *[H32]*
  - syphilitic (early) (secondary) A51.43
    - central, recurrent A52.71
    - congenital (early) A50.01 *[H32]*
    - late A52.71
  - tuberculous A18.53
- **Retinoblastoma** C69.2-
  - differentiated C69.2-
  - undifferentiated C69.2-
- **Retinochoroiditis** *—see also* Inflammation, chorioretinal
  - disseminated *—see* Inflammation, chorioretinal, disseminated
    - syphilitic A52.71
  - focal *—see* Inflammation, chorioretinal
  - juxtapapillaris *—see* Inflammation, chorioretinal, focal, juxtapapillary
- **Retinopathy** (background) H35.00
  - arteriosclerotic I70.8 *[H35.0-]*
  - atherosclerotic I70.8 *[H35.0-]*
  - central serous *—see* Chorioretinopathy, central serous
  - Coats H35.02-
  - diabetic *—see* Diabetes, retinopathy
  - exudative H35.02-
  - hypertensive H35.03-
  - in (due to)
    - diabetes *—see* Diabetes, retinopathy
    - sickle-cell disorders D57.- H36
  - of prematurity H35.10-
    - stage 0 H35.11-
    - stage 1 H35.12-
    - stage 2 H35.13-
    - stage 3 H35.14-
    - stage 4 H35.15-
    - stage 5 H35.16-
  - pigmentary, congenital *—see* Dystrophy, retina
  - proliferative NEC H35.2-
    - diabetic *—see* Diabetes, retinopathy, proliferative
    - sickle-cell D57.- *[H36]*
  - solar H31.02-
- **Retinoschisis** H33.10-
  - congenital Q14.1
  - specified type NEC H33.19-
- **Retortamoniasis** A07.8
- **Retractile testis** Q55.22
- **Retraction**
  - cervix *—see* Retroversion, uterus
  - drum (membrane) *—see* Disorder, tympanic membrane, specified NEC
  - finger *—see* Deformity, finger
  - lid H02.539
    - left H02.536
      - lower H02.535
      - upper H02.534
    - right H02.533
      - lower H02.532
      - upper H02.531
- **Retraction** *(continued)*
  - lung J98.4
  - mediastinum J98.59
  - nipple N64.53
    - associated with
      - lactation O92.03
      - pregnancy O92.01-
      - puerperium O92.02
    - congenital Q83.8
  - palmar fascia M72.0
  - pleura *—see* Pleurisy
  - ring, uterus (Bandl's) (pathological) O62.4
  - sternum (congenital) Q76.7
    - acquired M95.4
  - uterus *—see* Retroversion, uterus
  - valve (heart) *—see* Endocarditis
- **Retrobulbar** *—see* condition
- **Retrocecal** *—see* condition
- **Retrocession** *—see* Retroversion
- **Retrodisplacement** *—see* Retroversion
- **Retroflection, retroflexion** *—see* Retroversion
- **Retrognathia, retrognathism** (mandibular) (maxillary) M26.19
- **Retrograde menstruation** N92.5
- **Retroperineal** *—see* condition
- **Retroperitoneal** *—see* condition
- **Retroperitonitis** K68.9
- **Retropharyngeal** *—see* condition
- **Retroplacental** *—see* condition
- **Retroposition** *—see* Retroversion
- **Retroprosthetic membrane** T85.398
- **Retrosternal thyroid** (congenital) Q89.2
- **Retroversion, retroverted**
  - cervix *—see* Retroversion, uterus
  - female NEC *—see* Retroversion, uterus
  - iris H21.89
  - testis (congenital) Q55.29
  - uterus (acquired) (acute) (any degree) (asymptomatic) (cervix) (postinfectional) (postpartal, old) N85.4
    - congenital Q51.818
    - in pregnancy O34.53-
- **Retrovirus, as cause of disease classified elsewhere** B97.30
  - human
    - immunodeficiency, type 2 (HIV 2) B97.35
    - T-cell lymphotropic
      - type I (HTLV-I) B97.33
      - type II (HTLV-II) B97.34
  - lentivirus B97.31
  - oncovirus B97.32
  - specified NEC B97.39
- **Retrusion, premaxilla** (developmental) M26.09
- **Rett's disease or syndrome** F84.2
- **Reverse peristalsis** R19.2
- **Reye's syndrome** G93.7
- **Rh** (factor)
  - hemolytic disease (newborn) P55.0
  - incompatibility, immunization or sensitization
    - affecting management of pregnancy NEC O36.09-
      - anti-D antibody O36.01-
- **Rh** *(continued)*
  - incompatibility, immunization or sensitization *(continued)*
    - newborn P55.0
    - transfusion reaction *—see* Complication(s), transfusion, incompatibility reaction, Rh (factor)
  - negative mother affecting newborn P55.0
  - titer elevated *—see* Complication(s), transfusion, incompatibility reaction, Rh (factor)
  - transfusion reaction *—see* Complication(s), transfusion, incompatibility reaction, Rh (factor)
- **Rhabdomyolysis** (idiopathic) **NEC** M62.82
  - traumatic T79.6
- **Rhabdomyoma** *—see also* Neoplasm, connective tissue, benign
  - adult *—see* Neoplasm, connective tissue, benign
  - fetal *—see* Neoplasm, connective tissue, benign
  - glycogenic *—see* Neoplasm, connective tissue, benign
- **Rhabdomyosarcoma** (any type) *—see* Neoplasm, connective tissue, malignant
- **Rhabdosarcoma** *—see* Rhabdomyosarcoma
- **Rhesus** (factor) **incompatibility** *—see* Rh, incompatibility
- **Rheumatic** (acute) (subacute)
  - adherent pericardium I09.2
  - chronic I09.89
  - coronary arteritis I01.8
  - degeneration, myocardium I09.0
  - fever (acute) *—see* Fever, rheumatic
  - heart *—see* Disease, heart, rheumatic
  - myocardial degeneration *—see* Degeneration, myocardium
  - myocarditis (chronic) (inactive) (with chorea) I09.0
    - active or acute I01.2
      - with chorea (acute) (rheumatic) (Sydenham's) I02.0
  - pancarditis, acute I01.8
    - with chorea (acute (rheumatic) Sydenham's) I02.0
  - pericarditis (active) (acute) (with effusion) (with pneumonia) I01.0
    - with chorea (acute) (rheumatic) (Sydenham's) I02.0
    - chronic or inactive I09.2
  - pneumonia I00 *[J17]*
  - torticollis M43.6
  - typhoid fever A01.09
- **Rheumatism** (articular) (neuralgic) (nonarticular) M79.0
  - gout *—see* Arthritis, rheumatoid
  - intercostal, meaning Tietze's disease M94.0
  - palindromic (any site) M12.30
    - ankle M12.37-
    - elbow M12.32-
    - foot joint M12.37-
    - hand joint M12.34-
    - hip M12.35-
    - knee M12.36-
    - multiple site M12.39
- **Rheumatism** *(continued)*
  - palindromic *(continued)*
    - shoulder M12.31-
    - specified joint NEC M12.38
    - vertebrae M12.38
    - wrist M12.33-
  - sciatic M54.4-
- **Rheumatoid** *—see also* condition
  - arthritis *—see also* Arthritis, rheumatoid
    - with involvement of organs NEC M05.60
      - ankle M05.67-
      - elbow M05.62-
      - foot joint M05.67-
      - hand joint M05.64-
      - hip M05.65-
      - knee M05.66-
      - multiple site M05.69
      - shoulder M05.61-
      - vertebra *—see* Spondylitis, ankylosing
      - wrist M05.63-
    - seronegative *—see* Arthritis, rheumatoid, seronegative
    - seropositive *—see* Arthritis, rheumatoid, seropositive
  - carditis M05.30
    - ankle M05.37-
    - elbow M05.32-
    - foot joint M05.37-
    - hand joint M05.34-
    - hip M05.35-
    - knee M05.36-
    - multiple site M05.39
    - shoulder M05.31-
    - vertebra *—see* Spondylitis, ankylosing
    - wrist M05.33-
  - endocarditis *—see* Rheumatoid, carditis
  - lung (disease) M05.10
    - ankle M05.17-
    - elbow M05.12-
    - foot joint M05.17-
    - hand joint M05.14-
    - hip M05.15-
    - knee M05.16-
    - multiple site M05.19
    - shoulder M05.11-
    - vertebra *—see* Spondylitis, ankylosing
    - wrist M05.13-
  - myocarditis *—see* Rheumatoid, carditis
  - myopathy M05.40
    - ankle M05.47-
    - elbow M05.42-
    - foot joint M05.47-
    - hand joint M05.44-
    - hip M05.45-
    - knee M05.46-
    - multiple site M05.49
    - shoulder M05.41-
    - vertebra *—see* Spondylitis, ankylosing
    - wrist M05.43-
  - pericarditis *—see* Rheumatoid, carditis
  - polyarthritis *—see* Arthritis, rheumatoid
  - polyneuropathy M05.50
    - ankle M05.57-
    - elbow M05.52-
    - foot joint M05.57-
    - hand joint M05.54-
    - hip M05.55-
    - knee M05.56-
    - multiple site M05.59
    - shoulder M05.51-

Rheumatoid *(continued)*
  polyneuropathy *(continued)*
    vertebra *—see* Spondylitis, ankylosing
    wrist M05.53-
  vasculitis M05.20
    ankle M05.27-
    elbow M05.22-
    foot joint M05.27-
    hand joint M05.24-
    hip M05.25-
    knee M05.26-
    multiple site M05.29
    shoulder M05.21-
    vertebra *—see* Spondylitis, ankylosing
    wrist M05.23-

Rhinitis (atrophic) (catarrhal) (chronic) (croupous) (fibrinous) (granulomatous) (hyperplastic) (hypertrophic) (membranous) (obstructive) (purulent) (suppurative) (ulcerative) J31.0
  with
    sore throat *—see* Nasopharyngitis
  acute J00
  allergic J30.9
    with asthma J45.909
      with
        exacerbation (acute) J45.901
        status asthmaticus J45.902
    due to
      food J30.5
      pollen J30.1
    nonseasonal J30.89
    perennial J30.89
    seasonal NEC J30.2
    specified NEC J30.89
  infective J00
  pneumococcal J00
  syphilitic A52.73
    congenital A50.05 *[J99]*
  tuberculous A15.8
  vasomotor J30.0

Rhinoantritis (chronic) *—see* Sinusitis, maxillary

Rhinodacryolith *—see* Dacryolith

Rhinolith (nasal sinus) J34.89

Rhinomegaly J34.89

Rhinopharyngitis (acute) (subacute) *—see also* Nasopharyngitis
  chronic J31.1
  destructive ulcerating A66.5
  mutilans A66.5

Rhinophyma L71.1

Rhinorrhea J34.89
  cerebrospinal (fluid) G96.01
    postoperative G96.08
    specified NEC G96.08
    spontaneous G96.01
    traumatic G96.08
  paroxysmal *—see* Rhinitis, allergic
  spasmodic *—see* Rhinitis, allergic

Rhinosalpingitis *—see* Salpingitis, eustachian

Rhinoscleroma A48.8

Rhinosporidiosis B48.1

Rhinovirus infection NEC B34.8

Rhizomelic chondrodysplasia punctata E71.540

Rhythm
  atrioventricular nodal I49.8
  disorder I49.9
    coronary sinus I49.8
    ectopic I49.8

Rhythm *(continued)*
  disorder *(continued)*
    nodal I49.8
  escape I49.9
  heart, abnormal I49.9
  idioventricular I44.2
  nodal I49.8
  sleep, inversion G47.2-
    nonorganic origin *—see* Disorder, sleep, circadian rhythm, psychogenic

Rhytidosis facialis L98.8

Rib *—see also* condition
  cervical Q76.5

Riboflavin deficiency E53.0

Rice bodies *—see also* Loose, body, joint
  knee M23.4-

Richter syndrome *—see* Leukemia, chronic lymphocytic, B-cell type

Richter's hernia *—see* Hernia, abdomen, with obstruction

Ricinism *—see* Poisoning, food, noxious, plant

Rickets (active) (acute) (adolescent) (chest wall) (congenital) (current) (infantile) (intestinal) E55.0
  adult *—see* Osteomalacia
  celiac K90.0
  hypophosphatemic with nephrotic-glycosuric dwarfism E72.09
  inactive E64.3
  kidney N25.0
  renal N25.0
  sequelae, any E64.3
  vitamin-D-resistant E83.31 *[M90.80]*

Rickettsia 364D/R. philipii (Pacific Coast tick fever) A77.8

Rickettsial disease A79.9
  specified type NEC A79.89

Rickettsialpox (Rickettsia akari) A79.1

Rickettsiosis A79.9
  due to
    Ehrlichia sennetsu A79.81
    Neorickettsia sennetsu A79.81
    Rickettsia akari (rickettsialpox) A79.1
  specified type NEC A79.89
  tick-borne A77.9
  vesicular A79.1

Rider's bone *—see* Ossification, muscle, specified NEC

Ridge, alveolus *—see also* condition
  flabby K06.8

Ridged ear, congenital Q17.3

Riedel's
  lobe, liver Q44.7
  struma, thyroiditis or disease E06.5

Rieger's anomaly or syndrome Q13.81

Riehl's melanosis L81.4

Rietti-Greppi-Micheli anemia D56.9

Rieux's hernia *—see* Hernia, abdomen, specified site NEC

Riga (-Fede) **disease** K14.0

Riggs' disease *—see* Periodontitis

Right aortic arch Q25.47

Right middle lobe syndrome J98.11

Rigid, rigidity *—see also* condition
  abdominal R19.30
    with severe abdominal pain R10.0
    epigastric R19.36
    generalized R19.37
    left lower quadrant R19.34
    left upper quadrant R19.32
    periumbilic R19.35
    right lower quadrant R19.33
    right upper quadrant R19.31
  articular, multiple, congenital Q68.8
  cervix (uteri) in pregnancy *—see* Pregnancy, complicated by, abnormal, cervix
  hymen (acquired) (congenital) N89.6
  nuchal R29.1
  pelvic floor in pregnancy *—see* Pregnancy, complicated by, abnormal, pelvic organs or tissues NEC
  perineum or vulva in pregnancy *—see* Pregnancy, complicated by, abnormal, vulva
  spine *—see* Dorsopathy, specified NEC
  vagina in pregnancy *—see* Pregnancy, complicated by, abnormal, vagina

Rigors R68.89
  with fever R50.9

Riley-Day syndrome G90.1

RIND (reversible ischemic neurologic deficit) I63.9

Ring(s)
  aorta (vascular) Q25.45
  Bandl's O62.4
  contraction, complicating delivery O62.4
  esophageal, lower (muscular) K22.2
  Fleischer's (cornea) H18.04-
  hymenal, tight (acquired) (congenital) N89.6
  Kayser-Fleischer (cornea) H18.04-
  retraction, uterus, pathological O62.4
  Schatzki's (esophagus) (lower) K22.2
    congenital Q39.3
  Soemmerring's *—see* Cataract, secondary
  vascular (congenital) Q25.8
    aorta Q25.45

Ringed hair (congenital) Q84.1

Ringworm B35.9
  beard B35.0
  black dot B35.0
  body B35.4
  Burmese B35.5
  corporeal B35.4
  foot B35.3
  groin B35.6
  hand B35.2
  honeycomb B35.0
  nails B35.1
  perianal (area) B35.6
  scalp B35.0
  specified NEC B35.8
  Tokelau B35.5

Rise, venous pressure I87.8

Rising, PSA following treatment for malignant neoplasm of prostate R97.21

Risk
  for
    dental caries Z91.849
      high Z91.843
      low Z91.841
      moderate Z91.842
    homelessness, imminent Z59.811
  suicidal
    meaning personal history of attempted suicide Z91.51
    meaning suicidal ideation *—see* Ideation, suicidal

Ritter's disease L00

Rivalry, sibling Z62.891

Rivalta's disease A42.2

River blindness B73.01

Robert's pelvis Q74.2
  with disproportion (fetopelvic) O33.0
    causing obstructed labor O65.0

Robin (-Pierre) **syndrome** Q87.0

Robinow-Silvermann-Smith syndrome Q87.19

Robinson's (hidrotic) **ectodermal dysplasia or syndrome** Q82.4

Robles' disease B73.01

Rocky Mountain (spotted) **fever** A77.0

Roetheln *—see* Rubella

Roger's disease Q21.0

Rokitansky-Aschoff sinuses (gallbladder) K82.8

Rolando's fracture (displaced) S62.22-
  nondisplaced S62.22-

Romano-Ward (prolonged QT interval) **syndrome** I45.81

Romberg's disease or syndrome G51.8

Roof, mouth *—see* condition

Rosacea L71.9
  acne L71.9
  keratitis L71.8
  specified NEC L71.8

Rosary, rachitic E55.0

Rose
  cold J30.1
  fever J30.1
  rash R21
    epidemic B06.9

Rosenbach's erysipeloid A26.0

Rosenthal's disease or syndrome D68.1

Roseola B09
  infantum B08.20
    due to human herpesvirus 6 B08.21
    due to human herpesvirus 7 B08.22

Rossbach's disease K31.89
  psychogenic F45.8

Ross River disease or fever B33.1

Rostan's asthma (cardiac) *—see* Failure, ventricular, left

Rotation
  anomalous, incomplete or insufficient, intestine Q43.3
  cecum (congenital) Q43.3
  colon (congenital) Q43.3
  spine, incomplete or insufficient *—see* Dorsopathy, deforming, specified NEC

Rupture, ruptured *(continued)*
- operation wound —*see* Disruption, wound, operation
- ovary, ovarian N83.8
  - corpus luteum cyst N83.1-
  - follicle (graafian) N83.0-
- oviduct (nonobstetric) (nontraumatic) N83.8
  - due to pregnancy O00.10-
    - with intrauterine pregnancy O00.11-
- pancreas (nontraumatic) K86.89
  - traumatic S36.299
- papillary muscle NEC I51.2
  - following acute myocardial infarction (current complication) I23.5
- pelvic
  - floor, complicating delivery O70.1
  - organ NEC, obstetrical trauma O71.5
- perineum (nonobstetric) (nontraumatic) N90.89
  - complicating delivery —*see* Delivery, complicated, by, laceration, anus (sphincter)
- postoperative wound —*see* Disruption, wound, operation
- prostate (traumatic) S37.828
- pulmonary
  - artery I28.8
  - valve (heart) I37.8
  - vein I28.8
  - vessel I28.8
- pus tube —*see* Salpingitis
- pyosalpinx —*see* Salpingitis
- rectum (nontraumatic) K63.1
  - traumatic S36.69
- retina, retinal (traumatic) (without detachment) —*see also* Break, retina
  - with detachment —*see* Detachment, retina, with retinal, break
- rotator cuff (nontraumatic) M75.10-
  - complete M75.12-
  - incomplete M75.11-
- sclera —*see* Injury, eye, laceration
- sigmoid (nontraumatic) K63.1
  - traumatic S36.593
- spinal cord —*see also* Injury, spinal cord, by region
  - due to injury at birth P11.5
  - newborn (birth injury) P11.5
- spleen (traumatic) S36.09
  - birth injury P15.1
  - congenital (birth injury) P15.1
  - due to P. vivax malaria B51.0
  - nontraumatic D73.5
  - spontaneous D73.5
- splenic vein R58
  - traumatic —*see* Injury, blood vessel, splenic vein
- stomach (nontraumatic) (spontaneous) K31.89
  - traumatic S36.39
- supraspinatus (complete) (incomplete) (nontraumatic) —*see* Tear, rotator cuff
- symphysis pubis
  - obstetric O71.6
  - traumatic S33.4
- synovium (cyst) M66.10
  - ankle M66.17-
  - elbow M66.12-
  - finger M66.14-
  - foot M66.17-
  - forearm M66.13-
  - hand M66.14-

Rupture, ruptured *(continued)*
- synovium (cyst) *(continued)*
  - pelvic region M66.15-
  - shoulder region M66.11-
  - specified site NEC M66.18
  - thigh M66.15-
  - toe M66.17-
  - upper arm M66.12-
  - wrist M66.13-
- tendon (traumatic) —*see* Strain
  - nontraumatic (spontaneous) M66.9
    - ankle M66.87-
    - extensor M66.20
      - ankle M66.27-
      - foot M66.27-
      - forearm M66.23-
      - hand M66.24-
      - lower leg M66.26-
      - multiple sites M66.29
      - pelvic region M66.25-
      - shoulder region M66.21-
      - specified site NEC M66.28
      - thigh M66.25-
      - upper arm M66.22-
    - flexor M66.30
      - ankle M66.37-
      - foot M66.37-
      - forearm M66.33-
      - hand M66.34-
      - lower leg M66.36-
      - multiple sites M66.39
      - pelvic region M66.35-
      - shoulder region M66.31-
      - specified site NEC M66.38
      - thigh M66.35-
      - upper arm M66.32-
    - foot M66.87-
    - forearm M66.83-
    - hand M66.84-
    - lower leg M66.86-
    - multiple sites M66.89
    - pelvic region M66.85-
    - shoulder region M66.81-
    - specified
      - site NEC M66.88
      - tendon M66.80
    - thigh M66.85-
    - upper arm M66.82-
- thoracic duct I89.8
- tonsil J35.8
- traumatic
  - aorta —*see* Injury, aorta, laceration, major
  - diaphragm —*see* Injury, intrathoracic, diaphragm
  - external site —*see* Wound, open, by site
  - eye —*see* Injury, eye, laceration
  - internal organ —*see* Injury, by site
  - intervertebral disc
    - cervical S13.0
    - lumbar S33.0
    - thoracic S23.0
  - kidney S37.06-
  - ligament —*see also* Sprain
    - ankle —*see* Sprain, ankle
    - carpus —*see* Rupture, traumatic, ligament, wrist
    - collateral (hand) —*see* Rupture, traumatic, ligament, finger, collateral
    - finger (metacarpophalangeal) (interphalangeal) S63.40-
      - collateral S63.41-
        - index S63.41-
        - little S63.41-
        - middle S63.41-
        - ring S63.41-
      - index S63.40-

Rupture, ruptured *(continued)*
- traumatic *(continued)*
  - ligament *(continued)*
    - finger *(continued)*
      - little S63.40-
      - middle S63.40-
      - palmar S63.42-
        - index S63.42-
        - little S63.42-
        - middle S63.42-
        - ring S63.42-
      - ring S63.40-
      - specified site NEC S63.499
        - index S63.49-
        - little S63.49-
        - middle S63.49-
        - ring S63.49-
      - volar plate S63.43-
        - index S63.43-
        - little S63.43-
        - middle S63.43-
        - ring S63.43-
    - foot —*see* Sprain, foot
    - radial collateral S53.2-
    - radiocarpal —*see* Rupture, traumatic, ligament, wrist, radiocarpal
    - ulnar collateral S53.3-
    - ulnocarpal —*see* Rupture, traumatic, ligament, wrist, ulnocarpal
    - wrist S63.30-
      - collateral S63.31-
      - radiocarpal S63.32-
      - specified site NEC S63.39-
      - ulnocarpal (palmar) S63.33-
  - liver S36.116
  - membrana tympani —*see* Rupture, ear drum, traumatic
  - muscle or tendon —*see* Strain
  - myocardium —*see* Injury, heart
  - pancreas S36.299
  - rectum S36.69
  - sigmoid S36.593
  - spleen S36.09
  - stomach S36.39
  - symphysis pubis S33.4
  - tympanum, tympanic (membrane) —*see* Rupture, ear drum, traumatic
  - ureter S37.19
  - uterus S37.69
  - vagina —*see* Injury, vagina
  - vena cava —*see* Injury, vena cava, laceration, major
- tricuspid (heart) (valve) I07.8
- tube, tubal (nonobstetric) (nontraumatic) N83.8
  - abscess —*see* Salpingitis
  - due to pregnancy O00.10-
    - with intrauterine pregnancy O00.11-
- tympanum, tympanic (membrane) (nontraumatic) (*see also* Perforation, tympanic membrane) H72.9-
  - traumatic —*see* Rupture, ear drum, traumatic
- umbilical cord, complicating delivery O69.89
- ureter (traumatic) S37.19
  - nontraumatic N28.89
- urethra (nontraumatic) N36.8
  - with ectopic or molar pregnancy O08.6
  - following ectopic or molar pregnancy O08.6
  - obstetrical trauma O71.5
  - traumatic S37.39

Rupture, ruptured *(continued)*
- uterosacral ligament (nonobstetric) (nontraumatic) N83.8
- uterus (traumatic) S37.69
  - before labor O71.0-
  - during or after labor O71.1
  - nonpuerperal, nontraumatic N85.8
  - pregnant (during labor) O71.1
    - before labor O71.0-
- vagina —*see* Injury, vagina
- valve, valvular (heart) —*see* Endocarditis
- varicose vein —*see* Varix
- varix —*see* Varix
- vena cava R58
  - traumatic —*see* Injury, vena cava, laceration, major
- vesical (urinary) N32.89
- vessel (blood) R58
  - pulmonary I28.8
  - traumatic —*see* Injury, blood vessel
- viscus R19.8
- vulva complicating delivery O70.0

Russell-Silver syndrome Q87.19

Russian spring-summer type encephalitis A84.0

Rust's disease (tuberculous cervical spondylitis) A18.01

Ruvalcaba-Myhre-Smith syndrome E71.440

Rytand-Lipsitch syndrome I44.2

S

Saber, sabre shin or tibia (syphilitic) A50.56 *[M90.8-]*

Sac lacrimal —*see* condition

Saccharomyces infection B37.9

Saccharopinuria E72.3

Saccular —*see* condition

Sacculation
- aorta (nonsyphilitic) —*see* Aneurysm, aorta
- bladder N32.3
- intralaryngeal (congenital) (ventricular) Q31.3
- larynx (congenital) (ventricular) Q31.3
- organ or site, congenital —*see* Distortion
- pregnant uterus —*see* Pregnancy, complicated by, abnormal, uterus
- ureter N28.89
- urethra N36.1
- vesical N32.3

Sachs' amaurotic familial idiocy or disease E75.02

Sachs-Tay disease E75.02

Sacks-Libman disease M32.11

Sacralgia M53.3

Sacralization Q76.49

Sacrodynia M53.3

Sacroiliac joint —*see* condition

Sacroiliitis NEC M46.1

Sacrum —*see* condition

Saddle
- back —*see* Lordosis
- embolus
  - abdominal aorta I74.01
  - pulmonary artery I26.92
    - with acute cor pulmonale I26.02

Saddle *(continued)*
- injury - code to condition
- nose M95.0
  - due to syphilis A50.57

Sadism (sexual) F65.52

Sadness, postpartal O90.6

Sadomasochism F65.50

Saemisch's ulcer (cornea) *—see* Ulcer, cornea, central

Sagging
- skin and subcutaneous tissue (following bariatric surgery weight loss) (following dietary weight loss) L98.7

Sahib disease B55.0

Sailors' skin L57.8

Saint
- Anthony's fire *—see* Erysipelas
- triad *—see* Hernia, diaphragm
- Vitus' dance *—see* Chorea, Sydenham's

Salaam
- attack(s) *—see* Epilepsy, spasms
- tic R25.8

Salicylism
- abuse F55.8
- overdose or wrong substance given *—see* Table of Drugs and Chemicals, by drug, poisoning

Salivary duct or gland *—see* condition

Salivation, excessive K11.7

Salmonella *—see* Infection, Salmonella

Salmonellosis A02.0

Salpingitis (catarrhal) (fallopian tube) (nodular) (pseudofollicular) (purulent) (septic) N70.91
- with oophoritis N70.93
- acute N70.01
  - with oophoritis N70.03
- chlamydial A56.11
- chronic N70.11
  - with oophoritis N70.13
- complicating abortion *—see* Abortion, by type, complicated by, salpingitis
- ear *—see* Salpingitis, eustachian
- eustachian (tube) H68.00-
  - acute H68.01-
  - chronic H68.02-
- follicularis N70.11
  - with oophoritis N70.13
- gonococcal (acute) (chronic) A54.24
- interstitial, chronic N70.11
  - with oophoritis N70.13
- isthmica nodosa N70.11
  - with oophoritis N70.13
- specific (gonococcal) (acute) (chronic) A54.24
- tuberculous (acute) (chronic) A18.17
- venereal (gonococcal) (acute) (chronic) A54.24

Salpingocele N83.4-

Salpingo-oophoritis (catarrhal) (purulent) (ruptured) (septic) (suppurative) N70.93
- acute N70.03
  - with ectopic or molar pregnancy O08.0
  - following ectopic or molar pregnancy O08.0
  - gonococcal A54.24

Salpingo-oophoritis *(continued)*
- chronic N70.13
- following ectopic or molar pregnancy O08.0
- gonococcal (acute) (chronic) A54.24
- puerperal O86.19
- specific (gonococcal) (acute) (chronic) A54.24
- subacute N70.03
- tuberculous (acute) (chronic) A18.17
- venereal (gonococcal) (acute) (chronic) A54.24

Salpingo-ovaritis *—see* Salpingo-oophoritis

Salpingoperitonitis *—see* Salpingo-oophoritis

Salzmann's nodular dystrophy *—see* Degeneration, cornea, nodular

Sampson's cyst or tumor N80.1

San Joaquin (Valley) **fever** B38.0

Sandblaster's asthma, lung or pneumoconiosis J62.8

Sander's disease (paranoia) F22

Sandfly fever A93.1

Sandhoff's disease E75.01

Sanfilippo (Type B) (Type C) (Type D) **syndrome** E76.22

Sanger-Brown ataxia G11.2

Sao Paulo fever or typhus A77.0

Saponification, mesenteric K65.8

Sarcocele (benign)
- syphilitic A52.76
  - congenital A50.59

Sarcocystosis A07.8

Sarcoepiplocele *—see* Hernia

Sarcoepiplomphalocele Q79.2

Sarcoid *—see also* Sarcoidosis
- arthropathy D86.86
- Boeck's D86.9
- Darier-Roussy D86.3
- iridocyclitis D86.83
- meningitis D86.81
- myocarditis D86.85
- myositis D86.87
- pyelonephritis D86.84
- Spiegler-Fendt L08.89

Sarcoidosis D86.9
- with
  - cranial nerve palsies D86.82
  - hepatic granuloma D86.89
  - polyarthritis D86.86
  - tubulo-interstitial nephropathy D86.84
- combined sites NEC D86.89
- lung D86.0
  - and lymph nodes D86.2
- lymph nodes D86.1
  - and lung D86.2
- meninges D86.81
- skin D86.3
- specified type NEC D86.89

Sarcoma (of) *—see also* Neoplasm, connective tissue, malignant
- alveolar soft part *—see* Neoplasm, connective tissue, malignant
- ameloblastic C41.1
  - upper jaw (bone) C41.0
- botryoid *—see* Neoplasm, connective tissue, malignant
- botryoides *—see* Neoplasm, connective tissue, malignant

Sarcoma *(continued)*
- cerebellar C71.6
  - circumscribed (arachnoidal) C71.6
- circumscribed (arachnoidal) cerebellar C71.6
- clear cell *—see also* Neoplasm, connective tissue, malignant
  - kidney C64.-
- dendritic cells (accessory cells) C96.4
- embryonal *—see* Neoplasm, connective tissue, malignant
- endometrial (stromal) C54.1
  - isthmus C54.0
- epithelioid (cell) *—see* Neoplasm, connective tissue, malignant
- Ewing's *—see* Neoplasm, bone, malignant
- follicular dendritic cell C96.4
- germinoblastic (diffuse) *—see* Lymphoma, diffuse large cell
  - follicular *—see* Lymphoma, follicular, specified NEC
- giant cell (except of bone) *—see also* Neoplasm, connective tissue, malignant
  - bone *—see* Neoplasm, bone, malignant
- glomoid *—see* Neoplasm, connective tissue, malignant
- granulocytic C92.3-
- hemangioendothelial *—see* Neoplasm, connective tissue, malignant
- hemorrhagic, multiple *—see* Sarcoma, Kaposi's
- histiocytic C96.A
- Hodgkin *—see* Lymphoma, Hodgkin
- immunoblastic (diffuse) *—see* Lymphoma, diffuse large cell
- interdigitating dendritic cell C96.4
- Kaposi's
  - colon C46.4
  - connective tissue C46.1
  - gastrointestinal organ C46.4
  - lung C46.5-
  - lymph node(s) C46.3
  - palate (hard) (soft) C46.2
  - rectum C46.4
  - skin C46.0
  - specified site NEC C46.7
  - stomach C46.4
  - unspecified site C46.9
- Kupffer cell C22.3
- Langerhans cell C96.4
- leptomeningeal *—see* Neoplasm, meninges, malignant
- liver NEC C22.4
- lymphangioendothelial *—see* Neoplasm, connective tissue, malignant
- lymphoblastic *—see* Lymphoma, lymphoblastic (diffuse)
- lymphocytic *—see* Lymphoma, small cell B-cell
- mast cell C96.22
- melanotic *—see* Melanoma
- meningeal *—see* Neoplasm, meninges, malignant
- meningothelial *—see* Neoplasm, meninges, malignant
- mesenchymal *—see also* Neoplasm, connective tissue, malignant
  - mixed *—see* Neoplasm, connective tissue, malignant
- mesothelial *—see* Mesothelioma

Sarcoma *(continued)*
- monstrocellular
  - specified site *—see* Neoplasm, malignant, by site
  - unspecified site C71.9
- myeloid C92.3-
- neurogenic *—see* Neoplasm, nerve, malignant
- odontogenic C41.1
  - upper jaw (bone) C41.0
- osteoblastic *—see* Neoplasm, bone, malignant
- osteogenic *—see also* Neoplasm, bone, malignant
  - juxtacortical *—see* Neoplasm, bone, malignant
  - periosteal *—see* Neoplasm, bone, malignant
- periosteal *—see also* Neoplasm, bone, malignant
  - osteogenic *—see* Neoplasm, bone, malignant
- pleomorphic cell *—see* Neoplasm, connective tissue, malignant
- reticulum cell (diffuse) *—see* Lymphoma, diffuse large cell
  - nodular *—see* Lymphoma, follicular
  - pleomorphic cell type *—see* Lymphoma, diffuse large cell
- rhabdoid *—see* Neoplasm, malignant, by site
- round cell *—see* Neoplasm, connective tissue, malignant
- small cell *—see* Neoplasm, connective tissue, malignant
- soft tissue *—see* Neoplasm, connective tissue, malignant
- spindle cell *—see* Neoplasm, connective tissue, malignant
- stromal (endometrial) C54.1
  - isthmus C54.0
- synovial *—see also* Neoplasm, connective tissue, malignant
  - biphasic *—see* Neoplasm, connective tissue, malignant
  - epithelioid cell *—see* Neoplasm, connective tissue, malignant
  - spindle cell *—see* Neoplasm, connective tissue, malignant

Sarcomatosis
- meningeal *—see* Neoplasm, meninges, malignant
- specified site NEC *—see* Neoplasm, connective tissue, malignant
- unspecified site C80.1

Sarcopenia (age-related) M62.84

Sarcosinemia E72.59

Sarcosporidiosis (intestinal) A07.8

SARS-CoV-2 *— see also* COVID-19
- sequelae (post acute) U09.9

Satiety, early R68.81

Saturnine *—see* condition

Saturnism
- overdose or wrong substance given or taken *—see* Table of Drugs and Chemicals, by drug, poisoning

Satyriasis F52.8

Sauriasis *—see* Ichthyosis

SBE (subacute bacterial endocarditis) I33.0

Scabs R23.4

Scabies (any site) B86

Scaglietti-Dagnini syndrome E22.0

Scald *—see* Burn

Scalenus anticus (anterior) **syndrome** G54.0

Scales R23.4

Scaling, skin R23.4

Scalp *—see* condition

Scapegoating affecting child Z62.3

Scaphocephaly Q75.0

Scapulalgia M89.8X1

Scapulohumeral myopathy G71.02

Scar, scarring (*see also* Cicatrix) L90.5
- adherent L90.5
- atrophic L90.5
- cervix
  - in pregnancy or childbirth *—see* Pregnancy, complicated by, abnormal cervix
- cheloid L91.0
- chorioretinal H31.00-
  - posterior pole macula H31.01-
  - postsurgical H59.81-
  - solar retinopathy H31.02-
  - specified type NEC H31.09-
- choroid *—see* Scar, chorioretinal
- conjunctiva H11.24-
- cornea H17.9
  - xerophthalmic *—see also* Opacity, cornea
    - vitamin A deficiency E50.6
- defect (isthmocele) O34.22
- duodenum, obstructive K31.5
- hypertrophic L91.0
- keloid L91.0
- labia N90.89
- lung (base) J98.4
- macula *—see* Scar, chorioretinal, posterior pole
- muscle M62.89
- myocardium, myocardial I25.2
- painful L90.5
- posterior pole (eye) *—see* Scar, chorioretinal, posterior pole
- retina *—see* Scar, chorioretinal
- trachea J39.8
- transmural uterine, in pregnancy O34.29
- uterus N85.8
  - in pregnancy O34.29
- vagina N89.8
  - postoperative N99.2
- vulva N90.89

Scarabiasis B88.2

Scarlatina (anginosa) (maligna) A38.9
- myocarditis (acute) A38.1
  - old *—see* Myocarditis
- otitis media A38.0
- ulcerosa A38.8

Scarlet fever (albuminuria) (angina) A38.9

Schamberg's disease (progressive pigmentary dermatosis) L81.7

Schatzki's ring (acquired) (esophagus) (lower) K22.2
- congenital Q39.3

Schaufenster krankheit I20.8

Schaumann's
- benign lymphogranulomatosis D86.1
- disease or syndrome *—see* Sarcoidosis

Scheie's syndrome E76.03

Schenck's disease B42.1

Scheuermann's disease or osteochondrosis *—see* Osteochondrosis, juvenile, spine

Schilder (-Flatau) **disease** G37.0

Schilling-type monocytic leukemia C93.0-

Schimmelbusch's disease, cystic mastitis, or hyperplasia *—see* Mastopathy, cystic

Schistosoma infestation *—see* Infestation, Schistosoma

Schistosomiasis B65.9
- with muscle disorder B65.9 *[M63.80]*
  - ankle B65.9 *[M63.87-]*
  - foot B65.9 *[M63.87-]*
  - forearm B65.9 *[M63.83-]*
  - hand B65.9 *[M63.84-]*
  - lower leg B65.9 *[M63.86-]*
  - multiple sites B65.9 *[M63.89]*
  - pelvic region B65.9 *[M63.85-]*
  - shoulder region B65.9 *[M63.81-]*
  - specified site NEC B65.9 *[M63.88]*
  - thigh B65.9 *[M63.85-]*
  - upper arm B65.9 *[M63.82-]*
- Asiatic B65.2
- bladder B65.0
- chestermani B65.8
- colon B65.1
- cutaneous B65.3
- due to
  - S. haematobium B65.0
  - S. japonicum B65.2
  - S. mansoni B65.1
  - S. mattheii B65.8
- Eastern B65.2
- genitourinary tract B65.0
- intestinal B65.1
- lung NEC B65.9 *[J99]*
  - pneumonia B65.9 *[J17]*
- Manson's (intestinal) B65.1
- oriental B65.2
- pulmonary NEC B65.9 *[J99]*
  - pneumonia B65.9
- Schistosoma
  - haematobium B65.0
  - japonicum B65.2
  - mansoni B65.1
- specified type NEC B65.8
- urinary B65.0
- vesical B65.0

Schizencephaly Q04.6

Schizoaffective psychosis F25.9

Schizodontia K00.2

Schizoid personality F60.1

Schizophrenia, schizophrenic F20.9
- acute (brief) (undifferentiated) F23
- atypical (form) F20.3
- borderline F21
- catalepsy F20.2
- catatonic (type) (excited) (withdrawn) F20.2
- cenesthopathic, cenesthesiopathic F20.89
- childhood type F84.5
- chronic undifferentiated F20.9
- cyclic F25.0
- disorganized (type) F20.1
- flexibilitas cerea F20.2
- hebephrenic (type) F20.1
- incipient F21
- latent F21
- negative type F20.5
- paranoid (type) F20.0
- paraphrenic F20.0
- post-psychotic depression F32.89
- prepsychotic F21
- prodromal F21

Schizophrenia, schizophrenic *(continued)*
- pseudoneurotic F21
- pseudopsychopathic F21
- reaction F23
- residual (state) (type) F20.5
- restzustand F20.5
- schizoaffective (type) *—see* Psychosis, schizoaffective
- simple (type) F20.89
- simplex F20.89
- specified type NEC F20.89
- spectrum and other psychotic disorder F29
  - specified NEC F28
- stupor F20.2
- syndrome of childhood F84.5
- undifferentiated (type) F20.3
  - chronic F20.5

Schizothymia (persistent) F60.1

Schlatter-Osgood disease or osteochondrosis M92.52-

Schlatter's tibia *—see* Osteochondrosis, juvenile, tibia

Schmidt's syndrome (polyglandular, autoimmune) E31.0

Schmincke's carcinoma or tumor *—see* Neoplasm, nasopharynx, malignant

Schmitz (-Stutzer) **dysentery** A03.0

Schmorl's disease or nodes
- lumbar region M51.46
- lumbosacral region M51.47
- sacrococcygeal region M53.3
- thoracic region M51.44
- thoracolumbar region M51.45

Schneiderian
- papilloma *—see* Neoplasm, nasopharynx, benign
  - specified site *—see* Neoplasm, benign, by site
  - unspecified site D14.0
- specified site *—see* Neoplasm, malignant, by site
  - unspecified site C30.0

Scholte's syndrome (malignant carcinoid) E34.0

Scholz (-Bielchowsky-Henneberg) **disease or syndrome** E75.25

Schönlein (-Henoch) **disease or purpura** (primary) (rheumatic) D69.0

Schottmuller's disease A01.4

Schroeder's syndrome (endocrine hypertensive) E27.0

Schüller-Christian disease or syndrome C96.5

Schultze's type acroparesthesia, simple I73.89

Schultz's disease or syndrome *—see* Agranulocytosis

Schwalbe-Ziehen-Oppenheim disease G24.1

Schwannoma *—see also* Neoplasm, nerve, benign
- malignant *—see also* Neoplasm, nerve, malignant
  - with rhabdomyoblastic differentiation *—see* Neoplasm, nerve, malignant
- melanocytic *—see* Neoplasm, nerve, benign
- pigmented *—see* Neoplasm, nerve, benign

Schwannomatosis Q85.03

Schwartz (-Jampel) **syndrome** G71.13

Schwartz-Bartter syndrome E22.2

Schweniger-Buzzi anetoderma L90.1

Sciatic *—see* condition

Sciatica (infective) M54.3
- with lumbago M54.4-
  - due to intervertebral disc disorder *—see* Disorder, disc, with, radiculopathy
- due to displacement of intervertebral disc (with lumbago) *—see* Disorder, disc, with, radiculopathy
- wallet M54.3-

Scimitar syndrome Q26.8

Sclera *—see* condition

Sclerectasia H15.84-

Scleredema
- adultorum *—see* Sclerosis, systemic
- Buschke's *—see* Sclerosis, systemic
- newborn P83.0

Sclerema (adiposum) (edematosum) (neonatorum) (newborn) P83.0
- adultorum *—see* Sclerosis, systemic

Scleriasis *—see* Scleroderma

Scleritis H15.00-
- with corneal involvement H15.04-
- anterior H15.01-
- brawny H15.02-
- in (due to) zoster B02.34
- posterior H15.03-
- specified type NEC H15.09-
- syphilitic A52.71
- tuberculous (nodular) A18.51

Sclerochoroiditis H31.8

Scleroconjunctivitis *—see* Scleritis

Sclerocystic ovary syndrome E28.2

Sclerodactyly, sclerodactylia L94.3

Scleroderma, sclerodermia (acrosclerotic) (diffuse) (generalized) (progressive) (pulmonary) (*see also* Sclerosis, systemic) M34.9-
- circumscribed L94.0
- linear L94.1
- localized L94.0
- newborn P83.88
- systemic M34.9

Sclerokeratitis H16.8
- tuberculous A18.52

Scleroma nasi A48.8

Scleromalacia (perforans) H15.05-

Scleromyxedema L98.5

Sclérose en plaques G35

Sclerosis, sclerotic
- adrenal (gland) E27.8
- Alzheimer's *—see* Disease, Alzheimer's
- amyotrophic (lateral) G12.21
- aorta, aortic I70.0
  - valve *—see* Endocarditis, aortic
- artery, arterial, arteriolar, arteriovascular *—see* Arteriosclerosis
- ascending multiple G35
- brain (generalized) (lobular) G37.9
  - artery, arterial I67.2

Sclerosis, sclerotic *(continued)*
- brain *(continued)*
  - diffuse G37.0
  - disseminated G35
  - insular G35
  - Krabbe's E75.23
  - miliary G35
  - multiple G35
  - presenile (Alzheimer's) *—see* Disease, Alzheimer's, early onset
  - senile (arteriosclerotic) I67.2
  - stem, multiple G35
  - tuberous Q85.1
- bulbar, multiple G35
- bundle of His I44.39
- cardiac *—see* Disease, heart, ischemic, atherosclerotic
- cardiorenal *—see* Hypertension, cardiorenal
- cardiovascular *—see also* Disease, cardiovascular
  - renal *—see* Hypertension, cardiorenal
- cerebellar *—see* Sclerosis, brain
- cerebral *—see* Sclerosis, brain
- cerebrospinal (disseminated) (multiple) G35
- cerebrovascular I67.2
- choroid *—see* Degeneration, choroid
- combined (spinal cord) *—see also* Degeneration, combined
  - multiple G35
- concentric (Balo) G37.5
- cornea *—see* Opacity, cornea
- coronary (artery) I25.10
  - with angina pectoris *—see* Arteriosclerosis, coronary (artery),
- corpus cavernosum
  - female N90.89
  - male N48.6
- diffuse (brain) (spinal cord) G37.0
- disseminated G35
- dorsal G35
- dorsolateral (spinal cord) *—see* Degeneration, combined
- endometrium N85.5
- extrapyramidal G25.9
- eye, nuclear (senile) *—see* Cataract, senile, nuclear
- focal and segmental (glomerular) (*see also* N00-N07 with fourth character .1) N05.1
- Friedreich's (spinal cord) G11.11
- funicular (spermatic cord) N50.89
- general (vascular) *—see* Arteriosclerosis
- gland (lymphatic) I89.8
- hepatic K74.1
  - alcoholic K70.2
- hereditary
  - cerebellar G11.9
  - spinal (Friedreich's ataxia) G11.11
- hippocampal G93.81
- insular G35
- kidney *—see* Sclerosis, renal
- larynx J38.7
- lateral (amyotrophic) (descending) (spinal) G12.21
  - primary G12.23
- lens, senile nuclear *—see* Cataract, senile, nuclear
- liver K74.1
  - with fibrosis K74.2
    - alcoholic K70.2
  - alcoholic K70.2
  - cardiac K76.1
- lung *—see* Fibrosis, lung
- mastoid *—see* Mastoiditis, chronic
- mesial temporal G93.81
- mitral I05.8
- Mönckeberg's (medial) *—see* Arteriosclerosis, extremities
- multiple (brain stem) (cerebral) (generalized) (spinal cord) G35
- myocardium, myocardial *—see* Disease, heart, ischemic, atherosclerotic
- nuclear (senile), eye *—see* Cataract, senile, nuclear
- ovary N83.8
- pancreas K86.89
- penis N48.6
- peripheral arteries *—see* Arteriosclerosis, extremities
- plaques G35
- pluriglandular E31.8
- polyglandular E31.8
- posterolateral (spinal cord) *—see* Degeneration, combined
- presenile (Alzheimer's) *—see* Disease, Alzheimer's, early onset
- primary, lateral G12.23
- progressive, systemic M34.0
- pulmonary *—see* Fibrosis, lung
  - artery I27.0
  - valve (heart) *—see* Endocarditis, pulmonary
- renal N26.9
  - with
    - cystine storage disease E72.09
    - hypertensive heart disease (conditions in I11) *—see* Hypertension, cardiorenal
  - arteriolar (hyaline) (hyperplastic) *—see* Hypertension, kidney
- retina (senile) (vascular) H35.00
- senile (vascular) *—see* Arteriosclerosis
- spinal (cord) (progressive) G95.89
  - ascending G61.0
  - combined *—see also* Degeneration, combined
    - multiple G35
    - syphilitic A52.11
  - disseminated G35
  - dorsolateral *—see* Degeneration, combined
  - hereditary (Friedreich's) (mixed form) G11.11
  - lateral (amyotrophic) G12.21
    - progressive G12.23
  - multiple G35
  - posterior (syphilitic) A52.11
- stomach K31.89
- subendocardial, congenital I42.4
- systemic M34.9
  - with
    - lung involvement M34.81
    - myopathy M34.82
    - polyneuropathy M34.83
  - drug-induced M34.2
  - due to chemicals NEC M34.2
  - progressive M34.0
  - specified NEC M34.89
- temporal (mesial) G93.81
- tricuspid (heart) (valve) I07.8
- tuberous (brain) Q85.1
- tympanic membrane *—see* Disorder, tympanic membrane, specified NEC
- valve, valvular (heart) *—see* Endocarditis
- vascular *—see* Arteriosclerosis
- vein I87.8

Scoliosis (acquired) (postural) M41.9
- adolescent (idiopathic) *—see* Scoliosis, idiopathic, adolescent
- congenital Q67.5
  - due to bony malformation Q76.3
  - failure of segmentation (hemivertebra) Q76.3
  - hemivertebra fusion Q76.3
  - postural Q67.5
- degenerative M41.8-
- idiopathic M41.20
  - adolescent M41.129
    - cervical region M41.122
    - cervicothoracic region M41.123
    - lumbar region M41.126
    - lumbosacral region M41.127
    - thoracic region M41.124
    - thoracolumbar region M41.125
  - cervical region M41.22
  - cervicothoracic region M41.23
  - infantile M41.00
    - cervical region M41.02
    - cervicothoracic region M41.03
    - lumbar region M41.06
    - lumbosacral region M41.07
    - sacrococcygeal region M41.08
    - thoracic region M41.04
    - thoracolumbar region M41.05
  - juvenile M41.119
    - cervical region M41.112
    - cervicothoracic region M41.113
    - lumbar region M41.116
    - lumbosacral region M41.117
    - thoracic region M41.114
    - thoracolumbar region M41.115
  - lumbar region M41.26
  - lumbosacral region M41.27
  - thoracic region M41.24
  - thoracolumbar region M41.25
- infantile *—see* Scoliosis, idiopathic, infantile
- neuromuscular M41.40
  - cervical region M41.42
  - cervicothoracic region M41.43
  - lumbar region M41.46
  - lumbosacral region M41.47
  - occipito-atlanto-axial region M41.41
  - thoracic region M41.44
  - thoracolumbar region M41.45
- paralytic *—see* Scoliosis, neuromuscular
- postradiation therapy M96.5
- rachitic (late effect or sequelae) E64.3 *[M49.80]*
  - cervical region E64.3 *[M49.82]*
  - cervicothoracic region E64.3 *[M49.83]*
  - lumbar region E64.3 *[M49.86]*
  - lumbosacral region E64.3 *[M49.87]*
  - multiple sites E64.3 *[M49.89]*
  - occipito-atlanto-axial region E64.3 *[M49.81]*
  - sacrococcygeal region E64.3 *[M49.88]*
  - thoracic region E64.3 *[M49.84]*
  - thoracolumbar region E64.3 *[M49.85]*
- sciatic M54.4-
- secondary (to) NEC M41.50
  - cerebral palsy, Friedreich's ataxia, poliomyelitis, neuromuscular disorders *—see* Scoliosis, neuromuscular
  - cervical region M41.52
  - cervicothoracic region M41.53
  - lumbar region M41.56
  - lumbosacral region M41.57
  - thoracic region M41.54
  - thoracolumbar region M41.55
- specified form NEC M41.80
  - cervical region M41.82
  - cervicothoracic region M41.83
  - lumbar region M41.86
  - lumbosacral region M41.87
  - thoracic region M41.84
  - thoracolumbar region M41.85
- thoracogenic M41.30
  - thoracic region M41.34
  - thoracolumbar region M41.35
- tuberculous A18.01

Scoliotic pelvis
- with disproportion (fetopelvic) O33.0
  - causing obstructed labor O65.0

Scorbutus, scorbutic *—see also* Scurvy
- anemia D53.2

Score, NIHSS (National Institutes of Health Stoke Scale) R29.7-

Scotoma (arcuate) (Bjerrum) (central) (ring) *—see also* Defect, visual field, localized, scotoma
- scintillating H53.19

Scratch *—see* Abrasion

Scratchy throat R09.89

Screening (for) Z13.9
- alcoholism Z13.39
- anemia Z13.0
- anomaly, congenital Z13.89
- antenatal, of mother (*see also* Encounter, antenatal screening) Z36.9
- arterial hypertension Z13.6
- arthropod-borne viral disease NEC Z11.59
- autism Z13.41
- bacteriuria, asymptomatic Z13.89
- behavioral disorder Z13.30
  - specified NEC Z13.39
- brain injury, traumatic Z13.850
- bronchitis, chronic Z13.83
- brucellosis Z11.2
- cardiovascular disorder Z13.6
- cataract Z13.5
- chlamydial diseases Z11.8
- cholera Z11.0
- chromosomal abnormalities (nonprocreative) NEC Z13.79
- colonoscopy Z12.11
- congenital
  - dislocation of hip Z13.89
  - eye disorder Z13.5
  - malformation or deformation Z13.89
- contamination NEC Z13.88
- coronavirus (disease) (novel) 2019 Z11.52
- COVID-19 Z11.52
- cystic fibrosis Z13.228
- dengue fever Z11.59
- dental disorder Z13.84
- depression (adult) (adolescent) (child) Z13.31
  - maternal Z13.32
  - perinatal Z13.32
- developmental
  - delays Z13.40
    - global (milestones) Z13.42
    - specified NEC Z13.49
  - handicap Z13.42
    - in early childhood Z13.42
- diabetes mellitus Z13.1
- diphtheria Z11.2
- disability, intellectual Z13.39

- **Sepsis** *(continued)*
  - Shigella (*see also* Dysentery, bacillary) A03.9
  - specified organism NEC A41.89
  - Staphylococcus, staphylococcal A41.2
    - aureus (methicillin susceptible) (MSSA) A41.01
      - methicillin resistant (MRSA) A41.02
    - coagulase-negative A41.1
    - specified NEC A41.1
  - Streptococcus, streptococcal A40.9
    - agalactiae A40.1
    - group
      - A A40.0
      - B A40.1
      - D A41.81
    - neonatal P36.10
      - group B P36.0
      - specified NEC P36.19
    - pneumoniae A40.3
    - pyogenes A40.0
    - specified NEC A40.8
  - tracheostomy stoma J95.02
  - tularemic A21.7
  - umbilical, umbilical cord (newborn) —*see* Sepsis, newborn
  - Yersinia pestis A20.7
- **Septate** —*see* Septum
- **Septic** —*see* condition
  - arm —*see* Cellulitis, upper limb
    - with lymphangitis —*see* Lymphangitis, acute, upper limb
  - embolus —*see* Embolism
  - finger —*see* Cellulitis, digit
    - with lymphangitis —*see* Lymphangitis, acute, digit
  - foot —*see* Cellulitis, lower limb
    - with lymphangitis —*see* Lymphangitis, acute, lower limb
  - gallbladder (acute) K81.0
  - hand —*see* Cellulitis, upper limb
    - with lymphangitis —*see* Lymphangitis, acute, upper limb
  - joint —*see* Arthritis, pyogenic or pyemic
  - leg —*see* Cellulitis, lower limb
    - with lymphangitis —*see* Lymphangitis, acute, lower limb
  - nail —*see also* Cellulitis, digit
    - with lymphangitis —*see* Lymphangitis, acute, digit
  - sore —*see also* Abscess
    - throat J02.0
      - streptococcal J02.0
  - spleen (acute) D73.89
  - teeth, tooth (pulpal origin) K04.4
  - throat —*see* Pharyngitis
  - thrombus —*see* Thrombosis
  - toe —*see* Cellulitis, digit
    - with lymphangitis —*see* Lymphangitis, acute, digit
  - tonsils, chronic J35.01
    - with adenoiditis J35.03
  - uterus —*see* Endometritis
- **Septicemia** A41.9
  - meaning sepsis —*see* Sepsis
- **Septum, septate** (congenital) —*see also* Anomaly, by site
  - anal Q42.3
    - with fistula Q42.2
  - aqueduct of Sylvius Q03.0
    - with spina bifida —*see* Spina bifida, by site, with hydrocephalus
- **Septum, septate** *(continued)*
  - uterus Q51.28
    - complete Q51.21
    - partial Q51.22
    - specified NEC Q51.28
  - vagina Q52.10
    - in pregnancy —*see* Pregnancy, complicated by, abnormal vagina
      - causing obstructed labor O65.5
    - longitudinal Q52.129
      - microperforate
        - left side Q52.124
        - right side Q52.123
      - nonobstruction Q52.120
      - obstructing Q52.129
        - left side Q52.122
        - right side Q52.1221
    - transverse Q52.11
- **Sequelae** (of) —*see also* condition
  - abscess, intracranial or intraspinal (conditions in G06) G09
  - amputation -- code to injury with seventh character S
  - burn and corrosion -- code to injury with seventh character S
  - calcium deficiency E64.8
  - cerebrovascular disease —*see* Sequelae, disease, cerebrovascular
  - childbirth O94
  - contusion -- code to injury with seventh character S
  - corrosion —*see* Sequelae, burn and corrosion
  - COVID-19 (post acute) U09.9
  - crushing injury -- code to injury with seventh character S
  - disease
    - cerebrovascular I69.90
      - alteration of sensation I69.998
      - aphasia I69.920
      - apraxia I69.990
      - ataxia I69.993
      - cognitive deficits I69.91
      - disturbance of vision I69.998
      - dysarthria I69.922
      - dysphagia I69.991
      - dysphasia I69.921
      - facial droop I69.992
      - facial weakness I69.992
      - fluency disorder I69.923
      - hemiplegia I69.95-
      - hemorrhage
        - intracerebral —*see* Sequelae, hemorrhage, intracerebral
        - intracranial, nontraumatic NEC —*see* Sequelae, hemorrhage, intracranial, nontraumatic
        - subarachnoid —*see* Sequelae, hemorrhage, subarachnoid
      - language deficit I69.928
      - monoplegia
        - lower limb I69.94-
        - upper limb I69.93-
      - paralytic syndrome I69.96-
      - specified effect NEC I69.998
      - specified type NEC I69.80
        - alteration of sensation I69.898
        - aphasia I69.820
        - apraxia I69.890
        - ataxia I69.893
        - cognitive deficits I69.81
        - disturbance of vision I69.898
        - dysarthria I69.822
- **Sequelae** *(continued)*
  - disease *(continued)*
    - cerebrovascular *(continued)*
      - specified type *(continued)*
        - dysphagia I69.891
        - dysphasia I69.821
        - facial droop I69.892
        - facial weakness I69.892
        - fluency disorder I69.823
        - hemiplegia I69.85-
        - language deficit I69.828
        - monoplegia
          - lower limb I69.84-
          - upper limb I69.83-
        - paralytic syndrome I69.86-
        - specified effect NEC I69.898
      - speech deficit I69.928
        - speech deficit I69.828
      - stroke NOS —*see* Sequelae, stroke NOS
  - dislocation -- code to injury with seventh character S
  - encephalitis or encephalomyelitis (conditions in G04) G09
    - in infectious disease NEC B94.8
    - viral B94.1
  - external cause -- code to injury with seventh character S
  - foreign body entering natural orifice -- code to injury with seventh character S
  - fracture -- code to injury with seventh character S
  - frostbite -- code to injury with seventh character S
  - Hansen's disease B92
  - hemorrhage
    - intracerebral I69.10
      - alteration of sensation I69.198
      - aphasia I69.120
      - apraxia I69.190
      - ataxia I69.193
      - cognitive deficits I69.11
      - disturbance of vision I69.198
      - dysarthria I69.122
      - dysphagia I69.191
      - dysphasia I69.121
      - facial droop I69.192
      - facial weakness I69.192
      - fluency disorder I69.123
      - hemiplegia I69.15-
      - language deficit NEC I69.128
      - monoplegia
        - lower limb I69.14-
        - upper limb I69.13-
      - paralytic syndrome I69.16-
      - specified effect NEC I69.198
      - speech deficit NEC I69.128
    - intracranial, nontraumatic NEC I69.20
      - alteration of sensation I69.298
      - aphasia I69.220
      - apraxia I69.290
      - ataxia I69.293
      - cognitive deficits I69.21
      - disturbance of vision I69.298
      - dysarthria I69.222
      - dysphagia I69.291
      - dysphasia I69.221
      - facial droop I69.292
      - facial weakness I69.292
      - fluency disorder I69.223
      - hemiplegia I69.25-
      - language deficit NEC I69.228
      - monoplegia
        - lower limb I69.24-
        - upper limb I69.23-
      - paralytic syndrome I69.26-
      - specified effect NEC I69.298
      - speech deficit NEC I69.228
- **Sequelae** *(continued)*
  - hemorrhage *(continued)*
    - subarachnoid I69.00
      - alteration of sensation I69.098
      - aphasia I69.020
      - apraxia I69.090
      - ataxia I69.093
      - cognitive deficits —*see* subcategory I69.01-
      - disturbance of vision I69.098
      - dysarthria I69.022
      - dysphagia I69.091
      - dysphasia I69.021
      - facial droop I69.092
      - facial weakness I69.092
      - fluency disorder I69.023
      - hemiplegia I69.05-
      - language deficit NEC I69.028
      - monoplegia
        - lower limb I69.04-
        - upper limb I69.03-
      - paralytic syndrome I69.06-
      - specified effect NEC I69.098
      - speech deficit NEC I69.028
  - hepatitis, viral B94.2
  - hyperalimentation E68
  - infarction
    - cerebral I69.30
      - alteration of sensation I69.398
      - aphasia I69.320
      - apraxia I69.390
      - ataxia I69.393
      - cognitive deficits I69.31
      - disturbance of vision I69.398
      - dysarthria I69.322
      - dysphagia I69.391
      - dysphasia I69.321
      - facial droop I69.392
      - facial weakness I69.392
      - fluency disorder I69.323
      - hemiplegia I69.35-
      - language deficit NEC I69.328
      - monoplegia
        - lower limb I69.34-
        - upper limb I69.33-
      - paralytic syndrome I69.36-
      - specified effect NEC I69.398
      - speech deficit NEC I69.328
  - infection, pyogenic, intracranial or intraspinal G09
  - infectious disease B94.9
    - specified NEC B94.8
  - injury -- code to injury with seventh character S
  - leprosy B92
  - meningitis
    - bacterial (conditions in G00) G09
    - other or unspecified cause (conditions in G03) G09
  - muscle (and tendon) injury - code to injury with seventh character S
  - myelitis —*see* Sequelae, encephalitis
  - niacin deficiency E64.8
  - nutritional deficiency E64.9
    - specified NEC E64.8
  - obstetrical condition O94
  - parasitic disease B94.9
  - phlebitis or thrombophlebitis of intracranial or intraspinal venous sinuses and veins (conditions in G08) G09
  - poisoning -- code to poisoning with seventh character S
    - nonmedicinal substance —*see* Sequelae, toxic effect, nonmedicinal substance
  - poliomyelitis (acute) B91
  - pregnancy O94
  - protein-energy malnutrition E64.0

Sequelae *(continued)*
puerperium O94
rickets E64.3
SARS-CoV-2 (post acute) U09.9
selenium deficiency E64.8
sprain and strain - code to injury with seventh character S
stroke NOS I69.30
alteration in sensation I69.398
aphasia I69.320
apraxia I69.390
ataxia I69.393
cognitive deficits I69.31
disturbance of vision I69.398
dysarthria I69.322
dysphagia I69.391
dysphasia I69.321
facial droop I69.392
facial weakness I69.392
hemiplegia I69.35-
language deficit NEC I69.328
monoplegia
lower limb I69.34-
upper limb I69.33-
paralytic syndrome I69.36-
specified effect NEC I69.398
speech deficit NEC I69.328
tendon and muscle injury - code to injury with seventh character S
thiamine deficiency E64.8
trachoma B94.0
tuberculosis B90.9
bones and joints B90.2
central nervous system B90.0
genitourinary B90.1
pulmonary (respiratory) B90.9
specified organs NEC B90.8
viral
encephalitis B94.1
hepatitis B94.2
vitamin deficiency NEC E64.8
A E64.1
B E64.8
C E64.2
wound, open - code to injury with seventh character S

Sequestration *—see also* Sequestrum
disc *—see* Displacement, intervertebral disc
lung, congenital Q33.2

Sequestrum
bone *—see* Osteomyelitis, chronic
dental M27.2
jaw bone M27.2
orbit *—see* Osteomyelitis, orbit
sinus (accessory) (nasal) *—see* Sinusitis

Sequoiosis lung or pneumonitis J67.8

Serology for syphilis
doubtful
with signs or symptoms - code by site and stage under Syphilis
follow-up of latent syphilis *—see* Syphilis, latent
negative, with signs or symptoms - code by site and stage under Syphilis
positive A53.0
with signs or symptoms - code by site and stage under Syphilis
reactivated A53.0

Seroma *—see also* Hematoma
postprocedural *—see* Complication, postprocedural, seroma
traumatic, secondary and recurrent T79.2

Seropurulent *—see* condition

Serositis, multiple K65.8
pericardial I31.1
peritoneal K65.8

Serous *—see* condition

Sertoli cell
adenoma
specified site *—see* Neoplasm, benign, by site
unspecified site
female D27.9
male D29.20
carcinoma
specified site *—see* Neoplasm, malignant, by site
unspecified site (male) C62.9-
female C56.9
tumor
with lipid storage
specified site *—see* Neoplasm, benign, by site
unspecified site
female D27.9
male D29.20
specified site *—see* Neoplasm, benign, by site
unspecified site
female D27.9
male D29.20

Sertoli-Leydig cell tumor *—see* Neoplasm, benign, by site
specified site *—see* Neoplasm, benign, by site
unspecified site
female D27.9
male D29.20

Serum
allergy, allergic reaction (*see also* Reaction, serum) T80.69
shock (*see also* Shock, anaphylactic) T80.59
arthritis (*see also* Reaction, serum) T80.69
complication or reaction NEC (*see also* Reaction, serum) T80.69
disease NEC (*see also* Reaction, serum) T80.69
hepatitis *—see also* Hepatitis, viral, type B
carrier (suspected) of B18.1
intoxication (*see also* Reaction, serum) T80.69
neuritis (*see also* Reaction, serum) T80.69
neuropathy G61.1
poisoning NEC (*see also* Reaction, serum) T80.69
rash NEC (*see also* Reaction, serum) T80.69
reaction NEC (*see also* Reaction, serum) T80.69
sickness NEC (*see also* Reaction, serum) T80.69
urticaria (*see also* Reaction, serum) T80.69

Sesamoiditis M25.8-

Sever's disease or osteochondrosis *—see* Osteochondrosis, juvenile, tarsus

Severe sepsis R65.20
with septic shock R65.21

Sex
chromosome mosaics Q97.8
lines with various numbers of X chromosomes Q97.2
education Z70.8
reassignment surgery status Z87.890

Sextuplet pregnancy *—see* Pregnancy, sextuplet

Sexual
function, disorder of (psychogenic) F52.9
immaturity (female) (male) E30.0
impotence (psychogenic) organic origin NEC *—see* Dysfunction, sexual, male
precocity (constitutional) (cryptogenic) (female) (idiopathic) (male) E30.1

Sexuality, pathologic *—see* Deviation, sexual

Sézary disease C84.1-

Shadow, lung R91.8

Shaking palsy or paralysis *—see* Parkinsonism

Shallowness, acetabulum *—see* Derangement, joint, specified type NEC, hip

Shaver's disease J63.1

Sheath (tendon) *—see* condition

Sheathing, retinal vessels H35.01-

Shedding
nail L60.8
premature, primary (deciduous) teeth K00.6

Sheehan's disease or syndrome E23.0

Shelf, rectal K62.89

Shell teeth K00.5

Shellshock (current) F43.0
lasting state *—see* Disorder, post-traumatic stress

Shield kidney Q63.1

Shift
auditory threshold (temporary) H93.24-
mediastinal R93.89

Shifting sleep-work schedule (affecting sleep) G47.26

Shiga (-Kruse) **dysentery** A03.0

Shiga's bacillus A03.0

Shigella (dysentery) *—see* Dysentery, bacillary

Shigellosis A03.9
Group A A03.0
Group B A03.1
Group C A03.2
Group D A03.3

Shin splints S86.89

Shingles *—see* Herpes, zoster

Shipyard disease or eye B30.0

Shirodkar suture, in pregnancy *—see* Pregnancy, complicated by, incompetent cervix

Shock R57.9
with ectopic or molar pregnancy O08.3
adrenal (cortical) (Addisonian) E27.2
adverse food reaction (anaphylactic) *—see* Shock, anaphylactic, due to food
allergic *—see* Shock, anaphylactic
anaphylactic T78.2
chemical *—see* Table of Drugs and Chemicals

Shock *(continued)*
anaphylactic *(continued)*
due to drug or medicinal substance
correct substance properly administered T88.6
overdose or wrong substance given or taken (by accident) *—see* Table of Drugs and Chemicals, by drug, poisoning
due to food (nonpoisonous) T78.00
additives T78.06
dairy products T78.07
eggs T78.08
fish T78.03
shellfish T78.02
fruit T78.04
milk T78.07
nuts T78.05
multiple types T78.05
peanuts T78.01
peanuts T78.01
seeds T78.05
specified type NEC T78.09
vegetable T78.04
following sting(s) *—see* Venom
immunization T80.52
serum T80.59
blood and blood products T80.51
immunization T80.52
specified NEC T80.59
vaccination T80.52
anaphylactoid *—see* Shock, anaphylactic
anesthetic
correct substance properly administered T88.2
overdose or wrong substance given or taken *—see* Table of Drugs and Chemicals, by drug, poisoning
specified anesthetic *—see* Table of Drugs and Chemicals, by drug, poisoning
cardiogenic R57.0
chemical substance *—see* Table of Drugs and Chemicals
complicating ectopic or molar pregnancy O08.3
culture *—see* Disorder, adjustment
drug
due to correct substance properly administered T88.6
overdose or wrong substance given or taken (by accident) *—see* Table of Drugs and Chemicals, by drug, poisoning
during or after labor and delivery O75.1
electric T75.4
(taser) T75.4
endotoxic R65.21
postprocedural (resulting from a procedure, not elsewhere classified) T81.12
following
ectopic or molar pregnancy O08.3
injury (immediate) (delayed) T79.4
labor and delivery O75.1
food (anaphylactic) *—see* Shock, anaphylactic, due to food
from electroshock gun (taser) T75.4

Shock *(continued)*
  gram-negative R65.21
    postprocedural (resulting from a procedure, not elsewhere classified) T81.12
  hematologic R57.8
  hemorrhagic R57.8
    surgery (intraoperative) (postoperative) T81.19
    trauma T79.4
  hypovolemic R57.1
    surgical T81.19
    traumatic T79.4
  insulin E15
    therapeutic misadventure *—see* subcategory T38.3
  kidney N17.0
    traumatic (following crushing) T79.5
  lightning T75.01
  liver K72.00
  lung J80
  obstetric O75.1
    with ectopic or molar pregnancy O08.3
    following ectopic or molar pregnancy O08.3
  pleural (surgical) T81.19
    due to trauma T79.4
  postprocedural (postoperative) T81.10
    with ectopic or molar pregnancy O08.3
    cardiogenic T81.11
    endotoxic T81.12
    following ectopic or molar pregnancy O08.3
    gram-negative T81.12
    hypovolemic T81.19
    septic T81.12
    specified type NEC T81.19
  psychic F43.0
  septic (due to severe sepsis) R65.21
  specified NEC R57.8
  surgical T81.10
  taser gun (taser) T75.4
  therapeutic misadventure NEC T81.10
  thyroxin
    overdose or wrong substance given or taken *—see* Table of Drugs and Chemicals, by drug, poisoning
  toxic, syndrome A48.3
  transfusion *—see* Complications, transfusion
  traumatic (immediate) (delayed) T79.4

Shoemaker's chest M95.4

Short, shortening, shortness
  arm (acquired) *—see also* Deformity, limb, unequal length
    congenital Q71.81-
    forearm *—see* Deformity, limb, unequal length
  bowel syndrome K91.2
  breath R06.02
  cervical (complicating pregnancy) O26.87-
    non-gravid uterus N88.3
  common bile duct, congenital Q44.5
  cord (umbilical), complicating delivery O69.3
  cystic duct, congenital Q44.5
  esophagus (congenital) Q39.8
  femur (acquired) *—see* Deformity, limb, unequal length, femur

Short, shortening, shortness *(continued)*
  femur *(continued)*
    congenital *—see* Defect, reduction, lower limb, longitudinal, femur
  frenum, frenulum, linguae (congenital) Q38.1
  hip (acquired) *—see also* Deformity, limb, unequal length
    congenital Q65.89
  leg (acquired) *—see also* Deformity, limb, unequal length
    congenital Q72.81-
    lower leg *—see also* Deformity, limb, unequal length
  limbed stature, with immunodeficiency D82.2
  lower limb (acquired) *—see also* Deformity, limb, unequal length
    congenital Q72.81-
  organ or site, congenital NEC *—see* Distortion
  palate, congenital Q38.5
  radius (acquired) *—see also* Deformity, limb, unequal length
    congenital *—see* Defect, reduction, upper limb, longitudinal, radius
  rib syndrome Q77.2
  stature (child) (hereditary) (idiopathic) NEC R62.52
    constitutional E34.3
    due to endocrine disorder E34.3
    Laron-type E34.3
  tendon *—see also* Contraction, tendon
    with contracture of joint *—see* Contraction, joint
    Achilles (acquired) M67.0-
      congenital Q66.89
    congenital Q79.8
  thigh (acquired) *—see also* Deformity, limb, unequal length, femur
    congenital *—sese* Defect, reduction, lower limb, longitudinal, femur
  tibialis anterior (tendon) *—see* Contraction, tendon
  umbilical cord
    complicating delivery O69.3
  upper limb, congenital *—see* Defect, reduction, upper limb, specified type NEC
  urethra N36.8
  uvula, congenital Q38.5
  vagina (congenital) Q52.4

Shortsightedness *—see* Myopia

Shoshin (acute fulminating beriberi) E51.11

Shoulder *—see* condition

Shovel-shaped incisors K00.2

Shower, thromboembolic *—see* Embolism

Shunt
  arterial-venous (dialysis) Z99.2
  arteriovenous, pulmonary (acquired) I28.0
    congenital Q25.72
  cerebral ventricle (communicating) in situ Z98.2
  surgical, prosthetic, with complications *—see* Complications, cardiovascular, device or implant

Shutdown, renal N28.9

Shy-Drager syndrome G90.3

Sialadenitis, sialadenosis (any gland) (chronic) (periodic) (suppurative) *—see* Sialoadenitis

Sialectasia K11.8

Sialidosis E77.1

Sialitis, silitis (any gland) (chronic) (suppurative) *—see* Sialoadenitis

Sialoadenitis (any gland) (periodic) (suppurative) K11.20
  acute K11.21
    recurrent K11.22
  chronic K11.23

Sialoadenopathy K11.9

Sialoangitis *—see* Sialoadenitis

Sialodochitis (fibrinosa) *—see* Sialoadenitis

Sialodocholithiasis K11.5

Sialolithiasis K11.5

Sialometaplasia, necrotizing K11.8

Sialorrhea *—see also* Ptyalism
  periodic *—see* Sialoadenitis

Sialosis K11.7

Siamese twin Q89.4

Sibling rivalry Z62.891

Sicard's syndrome G52.7

Sicca syndrome *— see* Syndrome, Sjögren

Sick R69
  or handicapped person in family Z63.79
    needing care at home Z63.6
  sinus (syndrome) I49.5

Sick-euthyroid syndrome E07.81

Sickle-cell
  anemia *—see* Disease, sickle-cell
  beta plus *—see* Disease, sickle-cell, thalassemia, beta plus
  beta zero *—see* Disease, sickle-cell, thalassemia, beta zero
  trait D57.3

Sicklemia *—see also* Disease, sickle-cell
  trait D57.3

Sickness
  air (travel) T75.3
  airplane T75.3
  alpine T70.29
  altitude T70.20
  Andes T70.29
  aviator's T70.29
  balloon T70.29
  car T75.3
  compressed air T70.3
  decompression T70.3
  green D50.8
  milk *—see* Poisoning, food, noxious
  motion T75.3
  mountain T70.29
    acute D75.1
  protein (*see also* Reaction, serum) T80.69
  radiation T66
  roundabout (motion) T75.3
  sea T75.3
  serum NEC (*see also* Reaction, serum) T80.69

Sickness *(continued)*
  sleeping (African) B56.9
    by Trypanosoma B56.9
      brucei
        gambiense B56.0
        rhodesiense B56.1
    East African B56.1
    Gambian B56.0
    Rhodesian B56.1
    West African B56.0
  swing (motion) T75.3
  train (railway) (travel) T75.3
  travel (any vehicle) T75.3

Sideropenia *—see* Anemia, iron deficiency

Siderosilicosis J62.8

Siderosis (lung) J63.4
  brain G93.89
  eye (globe) *—see* Disorder, globe, degenerative, siderosis

Siemens' syndrome (ectodermal dysplasia) Q82.8

Sighing R06.89
  psychogenic F45.8

Sigmoid *—see also* condition
  flexure *—see* condition
  kidney Q63.1

Sigmoiditis (*see also* Enteritis) K52.9
  infectious A09
  noninfectious K52.9

Silfversköld's syndrome Q78.9

Silicosiderosis J62.8

Silicosis, silicotic (simple) (complicated) J62.8
  with tuberculosis J65

Silicotuberculosis J65

Silo-fillers' disease J68.8
  bronchitis J68.0
  pneumonitis J68.0
  pulmonary edema J68.1

Silver's syndrome Q87.19

Simian malaria B53.1

Simmonds' cachexia or disease E23.0

Simons' disease or syndrome (progressive lipodystrophy) E88.1

Simple, simplex *—see* condition

Simulation, conscious (of illness) Z76.5

Simultanagnosia (asimultagnosia) R48.3

Sin Nombre virus disease (Hantavirus) (cardio)-**pulmonary syndrome)** B33.4

Sinding-Larsen disease or osteochondrosis *—see* Osteochondrosis, juvenile, patella

Singapore hemorrhagic fever A91

Singer's node or nodule J38.2

Single
  atrium Q21.2
  coronary artery Q24.5
  umbilical artery Q27.0
  ventricle Q20.4

Singultus R06.6
  epidemicus B33.0

Sinus *—see also* Fistula
  abdominal K63.89
  arrest I45.5
  arrhythmia I49.8
  bradycardia R00.1
  branchial cleft (internal) (external) Q18.0

- **Sinus** *(continued)*
  - coccygeal *—see* Sinus, pilonidal
  - dental K04.6
  - dermal (congenital) Q06.8
    - with abscess Q06.8
    - coccygeal, pilonidal *—see* Sinus, coccygeal
  - infected, skin NEC L08.89
  - marginal, ruptured or bleeding *—see* Hemorrhage, antepartum, specified cause NEC
  - medial, face and neck Q18.8
  - pause I45.5
  - pericranii Q01.9
  - pilonidal (infected) (rectum) L05.92
    - with abscess L05.02
  - preauricular Q18.1
  - rectovaginal N82.3
  - Rokitansky-Aschoff (gallbladder) K82.8
  - sacrococcygeal (dermoid) (infected) *—see* Sinus, pilonidal
  - tachycardia R00.0
    - paroxysmal I47.1
  - tarsi syndrome M25.57-
  - testis N50.89
  - tract (postinfective) *—see* Fistula
  - urachus Q64.4
- **Sinusitis** (accessory) (chronic) (hyperplastic) (nasal) (nonpurulent) (purulent) J32.9
  - acute J01.90
    - ethmoidal J01.20
      - recurrent J01.21
    - frontal J01.10
      - recurrent J01.11
    - involving more than one sinus, other than pansinusitis J01.80
      - recurrent J01.81
    - maxillary J01.00
      - recurrent J01.01
    - pansinusitis J01.40
      - recurrent J01.41
    - recurrent J01.91
    - specified NEC J01.80
      - recurrent J01.81
    - sphenoidal J01.30
      - recurrent J01.31
  - allergic *—see* Rhinitis, allergic
  - due to high altitude T70.1
  - ethmoidal J32.2
    - acute J01.20
      - recurrent J01.21
  - frontal J32.1
    - acute J01.10
      - recurrent J01.11
  - influenzal *—see* Influenza, with, respiratory manifestations NEC
  - involving more than one sinus but not pansinusitis J32.8
    - acute J01.80
      - recurrent J01.81
  - maxillary J32.0
    - acute J01.00
      - recurrent J01.01
  - sphenoidal J32.3
    - acute J01.30
      - recurrent J01.31
  - tuberculous, any sinus A15.8
- **Sinusitis-bronchiectasis-situs inversus** (syndrome) (triad) Q89.3
- **Sipple's syndrome** E31.22
- **Sirenomelia** (syndrome) Q87.2
- **Siriasis** T67.01
- **Sirkari's disease** B55.0
- **Siti** A65
- **Situation, psychiatric** F99
- **Situational**
  - disturbance (transient) *—see* Disorder, adjustment
    - acute F43.0
  - maladjustment *—see* Disorder, adjustment
  - reaction *—see* Disorder, adjustment
    - acute F43.0
- **Situs inversus or transversus** (abdominalis) (thoracis) Q89.3
- **Sixth disease** B08.20
  - due to human herpesvirus 6 B08.21
  - due to human herpesvirus 7 B08.22
- **Sjögren-Larsson syndrome** Q87.19
- **Sjögren's syndrome or disease** *—see* Syndrome, Sjögren
- **Skeletal** *—see* condition
- **Skene's gland** *—see* condition
- **Skenitis** *—see* Urethritis
- **Skerljevo** A65
- **Skevas-Zerfus disease** *—see* Toxicity, venom, marine animal, sea anemone
- **Skin** *—see also* condition
  - clammy R23.1
  - donor *—see* Donor, skin
  - dry L85.3
  - hidebound M35.9
- **Slate-dressers' or slate-miners' lung** J62.8
- **Sleep**
  - apnea *—see* Apnea, sleep
  - deprivation Z72.820
  - disorder or disturbance G47.9
    - child F51.9
    - nonorganic origin F51.9
    - specified NEC G47.8
  - disturbance G47.9
    - nonorganic origin F51.9
  - drunkenness F51.9
  - rhythm inversion G47.2-
  - terrors F51.4
  - walking F51.3
    - hysterical F44.89
- **Sleep hygiene**
  - abuse Z72.821
  - inadequate Z72.821
  - poor Z72.821
- **Sleeping sickness** *—see* Sickness, sleeping
- **Sleeplessness** *—see* Insomnia
  - menopausal N95.1
- **Sleep-wake schedule disorder** G47.20
- **Slim disease** (in HIV infection) B20
- **Slipped, slipping**
  - epiphysis (traumatic) *—see also* Osteochondropathy, specified type NEC
    - capital femoral (traumatic)
      - acute (on chronic) S79.01-
    - current traumatic - code as Fracture, by site
    - upper femoral (nontraumatic) M93.00-
      - acute M93.01-
        - on chronic M93.03-
      - chronic M93.02-
  - intervertebral disc *—see* Displacement, intervertebral disc
  - ligature, umbilical P51.8
  - patella *—see* Disorder, patella, derangement NEC
  - rib M89.8X8
  - sacroiliac joint *—see* subcategory M53.2
- **Slipped, slipping** *(continued)*
  - tendon *—see* Disorder, tendon
  - ulnar nerve, nontraumatic *—see* Lesion, nerve, ulnar
  - vertebra NEC *—see* Spondylolisthesis
- **Slocumb's syndrome** E27.0
- **Sloughing** (multiple) (phagedena) (skin) *—see also* Gangrene
  - abscess *—see* Abscess
  - appendix K38.8
  - sfascia *—see* Disorder, soft tissue, specified type NEC
  - scrotum N50.89
  - tendon *—see* Disorder, tendon
  - transplanted organ *—see* Rejection, transplant
  - ulcer *—see* Ulcer, skin
- **Slow**
  - feeding, newborn P92.2
  - flow syndrome, coronary I20.8
  - heart (beat) R00.1
- **Slowing, urinary stream** R39.198
- **Sluder's neuralgia** (syndrome) G44.89
- **Slurred, slurring speech** R47.81
- **Small** (ness)
  - for gestational age *—see* Small for dates
  - introitus, vagina N89.6
  - kidney (unknown cause) N27.9
    - bilateral N27.1
    - unilateral N27.0
  - ovary (congenital) Q50.39
  - pelvis
    - with disproportion (fetopelvic) O33.1
      - causing obstructed labor O65.1
  - uterus N85.8
  - white kidney N03.9
- **Small-and-light-for-dates** *—see* Small for dates
- **Small-for-dates** (infant) P05.10
  - with weight of
    - 499 grams or less P05.11
    - 500-749 grams P05.12
    - 750-999 grams P05.13
    - 1000-1249 grams P05.14
    - 1250-1499 grams P05.15
    - 1500-1749 grams P05.16
    - 1750-1999 grams P05.17
    - 2000-2499 grams P05.18
    - 2500 grams and over P05.19
  - specified NEC P05.19
- **Smallpox** B03
- **Smearing, fecal** R15.1
- **SMEI** (severe myoclonic epilepsy in infancy) G40.83-
- **Smith-Lemli-Opitz syndrome** E78.72
- **Smith's fracture** S52.54-
- **Smoker** *—see* Dependence, drug, nicotine
- **Smoker's**
  - bronchitis J41.0
  - cough J41.0
  - palate K13.24
  - throat J31.2
  - tongue K13.24
- **Smoking**
  - passive Z77.22
- **Smothering spells** R06.81
- **Snaggle teeth, tooth** M26.39
- **Snapping**
  - finger *—see* Trigger finger
  - hip *—see* Derangement, joint, specified type NEC, hip
    - involving the iliotiblial band M76.3-
  - knee *—see* Derangement, knee
    - involving the iliotiblial band M76.3-
- **Sneddon-Wilkinson disease or syndrome** (sub-corneal pustular dermatosis) L13.1
- **Sneezing** (intractable) R06.7
- **Sniffing**
  - cocaine
    - abuse *—see* Abuse, drug, cocaine
    - dependence *—see* Dependence, drug, cocaine
  - gasoline
    - abuse *—see* Abuse, drug, inhalant
    - dependence *—see* Dependence, drug, inhalant
  - glue (airplane)
    - abuse *—see* Abuse, drug, inhalant
    - drug dependence *—see* Dependence, drug, inhalant
- **Sniffles**
  - newborn P28.89
- **Snoring** R06.83
- **Snow blindness** *—see* Photokeratitis
- **Snuffles** (non-syphilitic) R06.5
  - newborn P28.89
  - syphilitic (infant) A50.05 *[J99]*
- **Social**
  - exclusion Z60.4
    - due to discrimination or persecution (perceived) Z60.5
  - migrant Z59.00
    - acculturation difficulty Z60.3
  - rejection Z60.4
    - due to discrimination or persecution Z60.5
  - role conflict NEC Z73.5
  - skills inadequacy NEC Z73.4
  - transplantation Z60.3
- **Sodoku** A25.0
- **Soemmerring's ring** *—see* Cataract, secondary
- **Soft** *—see also* condition
  - nails L60.3
- **Softening**
  - bone *—see* Osteomalacia
  - brain (necrotic) (progressive) G93.89
    - congenital Q04.8
    - embolic I63.4-
    - hemorrhagic *—see* Hemorrhage, intracranial, intracerebral
    - occlusive I63.5-
    - thrombotic I63.3-
  - cartilage M94.2-
    - patella M22.4-
  - cerebellar *—see* Softening, brain
  - cerebral *—see* Softening, brain
  - cerebrospinal *—see* Softening, brain
  - myocardial, heart *—see* Degeneration, myocardial
  - spinal cord G95.89
  - stomach K31.89
- **Soldier's**
  - heart F45.8
  - patches I31.0

- **Solitary**
  - cyst, kidney N28.1
  - kidney, congenital Q60.0
- **Solvent abuse** —*see* Abuse, drug, inhalant
  - dependence —*see* Dependence, drug, inhalant
- **Somatization reaction, somatic reaction** —*see* Disorder, somatoform
- **Somnambulism** F51.3
  - hysterical F44.89
- **Somnolence** R40.0
  - nonorganic origin F51.11
- **Sonne dysentery** A03.3
- **Soor** B37.0
- **Sore**
  - bed —*see* Ulcer, pressure, by site
  - chiclero B55.1
  - Delhi B55.1
  - desert —*see* Ulcer, skin
  - eye H57.1-
  - Lahore B55.1
  - mouth K13.79
    - canker K12.0
  - muscle M79.10
  - Naga —*see* Ulcer, skin
  - of skin —*see* Ulcer, skin
  - oriental B55.1
  - pressure —*see* Ulcer, pressure, by site
  - skin L98.9
  - soft A57
  - throat (acute) —*see also* Pharyngitis
    - with influenza, flu, or grippe —*see* Influenza, with, respiratory manifestations NEC
    - chronic J31.2
    - coxsackie (virus) B08.5
    - diphtheritic A36.0
    - herpesviral B00.2
    - influenzal —*see* Influenza, with, respiratory manifestations NEC
    - septic J02.0
    - streptococcal (ulcerative) J02.0
    - viral NEC J02.8
      - coxsackie B08.5
  - tropical —*see* Ulcer, skin
  - veldt —*see* Ulcer, skin
- **Soto's syndrome** (cerebral gigantism) Q87.3
- **South African cardiomyopathy syndrome** I42.8
- **Southeast Asian hemorrhagic fever** A91
- **Spacing**
  - abnormal, tooth, teeth, fully erupted M26.30
  - excessive, tooth, fully erupted M26.32
- **Spade-like hand** (congenital) Q68.1
- **Spading nail** L60.8
  - congenital Q84.6
- **Spanish collar** N47.1
- **Sparganosis** B70.1
- **Spasm**(s), **spastic, spasticity** (*see also* condition) R25.2
  - accommodation —*see* Spasm, of accommodation
  - ampulla of Vater K83.4
  - anus, ani (sphincter) (reflex) K59.4
    - psychogenic F45.8

Spasm(s), **spastic, spasticity** *(continued)*

  - artery I73.9
    - cerebral G45.9
  - Bell's G51.3-
  - bladder (sphincter, external or internal) N32.89
    - psychogenic F45.8
  - bronchus, bronchiole J98.01
  - cardia K22.0
  - cardiac I20.1
  - carpopedal —*see* Tetany
  - cerebral (arteries) (vascular) G45.9
  - cervix, complicating delivery O62.4
  - ciliary body (of accommodation) —*see* Spasm, of accommodation
  - colon (*see also* Irritable, bowel) K58.9
    - with diarrhea K58.0
    - psychogenic F45.8
  - common duct K83.8
  - compulsive —*see* Tic
  - conjugate H51.8
  - coronary (artery) I20.1
  - diaphragm (reflex) R06.6
    - epidemic B33.0
    - psychogenic F45.8
  - duodenum K59.89
  - epidemic diaphragmatic (transient) B33.0
  - esophagus (diffuse) K22.4
    - psychogenic F45.8
  - facial G51.3-
  - fallopian tube N83.8
  - gastrointestinal (tract) K31.89
    - psychogenic F45.8
  - glottis J38.5
    - hysterical F44.4
    - psychogenic F45.8
      - conversion reaction F44.4
    - reflex through recurrent laryngeal nerve J38.5
  - habit —*see* Tic
  - heart I20.1
  - hemifacial (clonic) G51.3-
  - hourglass —*see* Contraction, hourglass
  - hysterical F44.4
  - infantile —*see* Epilepsy, spasms
  - inferior oblique, eye H51.8
  - intestinal (*see also* Syndrome, irritable bowel) K58.9
    - psychogenic F45.8
  - larynx, laryngeal J38.5
    - hysterical F44.4
    - psychogenic F45.8
      - conversion reaction F44.4
  - levator palpebrae superioris —*see* Disorder, eyelid function
  - muscle NEC M62.838
    - back M62.830
  - nerve, trigeminal G51.0
  - nervous F45.8
  - nodding F98.4
  - occupational F48.8
  - oculogyric H51.8
    - psychogenic F45.8
  - of accommodation H52.53-
  - ophthalmic artery —*see* Occlusion, artery, retina
  - perineal, female N94.89
  - peroneo-extensor —*see also* Deformity, limb, flat foot
  - pharynx (reflex) J39.2
    - hysterical F45.8
    - psychogenic F45.8
  - psychogenic F45.8

Spasm(s), **spastic, spasticity** *(continued)*

  - pylorus NEC K31.3
    - adult hypertrophic K31.89
    - congenital or infantile Q40.0
    - psychogenic F45.8
  - rectum (sphincter) K59.4
    - psychogenic F45.8
  - retinal (artery) —*see* Occlusion, artery, retina
  - sigmoid (*see also* Syndrome, irritable bowel) K58.9
    - psychogenic F45.8
  - sphincter of Oddi K83.4
  - stomach K31.89
    - neurotic F45.8
  - throat J39.2
    - hysterical F45.8
    - psychogenic F45.8
  - tic F95.9
    - chronic F95.1
    - transient of childhood F95.0
  - tongue K14.8
  - torsion (progressive) G24.1
  - trigeminal nerve —*see* Neuralgia, trigeminal
  - ureter N13.5
  - urethra (sphincter) N35.919
  - uterus N85.8
    - complicating labor O62.4
  - vagina N94.2
    - psychogenic F52.5
  - vascular I73.9
  - vasomotor I73.9
  - vein NEC I87.8
  - viscera —*see* Pain, abdominal
- **Spasmodic** —*see* condition
- **Spasmophilia** —*see* Tetany
- **Spasmus nutans** F98.4
- **Spastic, spasticity** —*see also* Spasm
  - child (cerebral) (congenital) (paralysis) G80.1
- **Speaker's throat** R49.8
- **Specific, specified** —*see* condition
- **Speech**
  - defect, disorder, disturbance, impediment —*see* Disorder, speech R47.9
    - psychogenic, in childhood and adolescence F98.8
    - slurring R47.81
    - specified NEC R47.89
- **Spencer's disease** A08.19
- **Spens' syndrome** (syncope with heart block) I45.9
- **Sperm counts** (fertility testing) Z31.41
  - postvasectomy Z30.8
    - reversal Z31.42
- **Spermatic cord** —*see* condition
- **Spermatocele** N43.40
  - congenital Q55.4
  - multiple N43.42
  - single N43.41
- **Spermatocystitis** N49.0
- **Spermatocytoma** C62.9-
  - specified site —*see* Neoplasm, malignant, by site
- **Spermatorrhea** N50.89
- **Sphacelus** —*see* Gangrene
- **Sphenoidal** —*see* condition
- **Sphenoiditis** (chronic) —*see* Sinusitis, sphenoidal
- **Sphenopalatine ganglion neuralgia** G90.09
- **Sphericity, increased, lens** (congenital) Q12.4
- **Spherocytosis** (congenital) (familial) (hereditary) D58.0
  - hemoglobin disease D58.0
  - sickle-cell (disease) D57.8-
- **Spherophakia** Q12.4
- **Sphincter** —*see* condition
- **Sphincteritis, sphincter of Oddi** —*see* Cholangitis
- **Sphingolipidosis** E75.3
  - specified NEC E75.29
- **Sphingomyelinosis** E75.3
- **Spicule tooth** K00.2
- **Spider**
  - bite —*see* Toxicity, venom, spider
    - nonvenomous —*see* Bite, by site, superficial, insect
  - fingers —*see* Syndrome, Marfan's
  - nevus I78.1
  - toes —*see* Syndrome, Marfan's
  - vascular I78.1
- **Spiegler-Fendt**
  - benign lymphocytoma L98.8
  - sarcoid L08.89
- **Spielmeyer-Vogt disease** E75.4
- **Spina bifida** (aperta) Q05.9
  - with hydrocephalus NEC Q05.4
  - cervical Q05.5
    - with hydrocephalus Q05.0
  - dorsal Q05.6
    - with hydrocephalus Q05.1
  - lumbar Q05.7
    - with hydrocephalus Q05.2
  - lumbosacral Q05.7
    - with hydrocephalus Q05.2
  - occulta Q76.0
  - sacral Q05.8
    - with hydrocephalus Q05.3
  - thoracic Q05.6
    - with hydrocephalus Q05.1
  - thoracolumbar Q05.6
    - with hydrocephalus Q05.1
- **Spindle, Krukenberg's** —*see* Pigmentation, cornea, posterior
- **Spine, spinal** —*see* condition
- **Spiradenoma** (eccrine) —*see* Neoplasm, skin, benign
- **Spirillosis** A25.0
- **Spirillum**
  - minus A25.0
  - obermeieri infection A68.0
- **Spirochetal** —*see* condition
- **Spirochetosis** A69.9
  - arthritic, arthritica A69.9
  - bronchopulmonary A69.8
  - icterohemorrhagic A27.0
  - lung A69.8
- **Spirometrosis** B70.1
- **Spitting blood** —*see* Hemoptysis
- **Splanchnoptosis** K63.4
- **Spleen, splenic** —*see* condition
- **Splenectasis** —*see* Splenomegaly
- **Splenitis** (interstitial) (malignant) (nonspecific) D73.89
  - malarial (*see also* Malaria) B54 *[D77]*
  - tuberculous A18.85
- **Splenocele** D73.89

Splenomegaly, splenomegalia (Bengal) (cryptogenic) (idiopathic) (tropical) R16.1
- with hepatomegaly R16.2
- cirrhotic D73.2
- congenital Q89.09
- congestive, chronic D73.2
- Egyptian B65.1
- Gaucher's E75.22
- malarial (*see also* Malaria) B54 *[D77]*
- neutropenic D73.81
- Niemann-Pick —*see* Niemann-Pick disease or syndrome
- siderotic D73.2
- syphilitic A52.79
  - congenital (early) A50.08 *[D77]*

Splenopathy D73.9

Splenoptosis D73.89

Splenosis D73.89

Splinter —*see* Foreign body, superficial, by site

Split, splitting
- foot Q72.7-
- hand Q71.6
- heart sounds R01.2
- lip, congenital —*see* Cleft, lip
- nails L60.3
- urinary stream R39.13

Spondylarthrosis —*see* Spondylosis

Spondylitis (chronic) —*see also* Spondylopathy, inflammatory
- ankylopoietica —*see* Spondylitis, ankylosing
- ankylosing (chronic) M45.9
  - with lung involvement M45.9 *[J99]*
  - cervical region M45.2
  - cervicothoracic region M45.3
  - juvenile M08.1
  - lumbar region M45.6
  - lumbosacral region M45.7
  - multiple sites M45.0
  - occipito-atlanto-axial region M45.1
  - sacrococcygeal region M45.8
  - thoracic region M45.4
  - thoracolumbar region M45.5
- atrophic (ligamentous) —*see* Spondylitis, ankylosing
- deformans (chronic) —*see* Spondylosis
- gonococcal A54.41
- gouty (*see also* Gout, by type, vertebrae) M10.08
- in (due to)
  - brucellosis A23.9 *[M49.80]*
    - cervical region A23.9 *[M49.82]*
    - cervicothoracic region A23.9 *[M49.83]*
    - lumbar region A23.9 *[M49.86]*
    - lumbosacral region A23.9 *[M49.87]*
    - multiple sites A23.9 *[M49.89]*
    - occipito-atlanto-axial region A23.9 *[M49.81]*
    - sacrococcygeal region A23.9 *[M49.88]*
    - thoracic region A23.9 *[M49.84]*
    - thoracolumbar region A23.9 *[M49.85]*
  - enterobacteria (*see also* subcategory M49.8) A04.9
  - tuberculosis A18.01
- infectious NEC —*see* Spondylopathy, infective
- juvenile ankylosing (chronic) M08.1

Spondylitis *(continued)*
- Kümmell's —*see* Spondylopathy, traumatic
- Marie-Strümpell —*see* Spondylitis, ankylosing
- muscularis —*see* Spondylopathy, specified NEC
- psoriatic L40.53
- rheumatoid —*see* Spondylitis, ankylosing
- rhizomelica —*see* Spondylitis, ankylosing
- sacroiliac NEC M46.1
- senescent, senile —*see* Spondylosis
- traumatic (chronic) or post-traumatic —*see* Spondylopathy, traumatic
- tuberculous A18.01
- typhosa A01.05

Spondyloarthritis
- axial —*see also* Spondlyitis, ankylosing
  - non-radiographic M45.A0
    - cervical M45.A2
    - cervicothoracic M45.A3
    - lumbar M45.A6
    - lumbosacral M45.A7
    - multiple sites M45.AB
    - occipito-atlanto-axial region M45.A1
    - sacral and sacrococcygeal M45.A8
    - thoracic M45.A4
    - thoracolumbar M45.A5

Spondylolisthesis (acquired) (degenerative) M43.10
- with disproportion (fetopelvic) O33.0
  - causing obstructed labor O65.0
- cervical region M43.12
- cervicothoracic region M43.13
- congenital Q76.2
- lumbar region M43.16
- lumbosacral region M43.17
- multiple sites M43.19
- occipito-atlanto-axial region M43.11
- sacrococcygeal region M43.18
- thoracic region M43.14
- thoracolumbar region M43.15
- traumatic (old) M43.10
  - acute
    - fifth cervical (displaced) S12.430
      - nondisplaced S12.431
      - specified type NEC (displaced) S12.450
        - nondisplaced S12.451
      - type III S12.44
    - fourth cervical (displaced) S12.330
      - nondisplaced S12.331
      - specified type NEC (displaced) S12.350
        - nondisplaced S12.351
      - type III S12.34
    - second cervical (displaced) S12.130
      - nondisplaced S12.131
      - specified type NEC (displaced) S12.150
        - nondisplaced S12.151
      - type III S12.14
    - seventh cervical (displaced) S12.630
      - nondisplaced S12.631
      - specified type NEC (displaced) S12.650
        - nondisplaced S12.651
      - type III S12.64

Spondylolisthesis *(continued)*
- traumatic *(continued)*
  - acute *(continued)*
    - sixth cervical (displaced) S12.530
      - nondisplaced S12.531
      - specified type NEC (displaced) S12.550
        - nondisplaced S12.551
      - type III S12.54
    - third cervical (displaced) S12.230
      - nondisplaced S12.231
      - specified type NEC (displaced) S12.250
        - nondisplaced S12.251
      - type III S12.24

Spondylolysis (acquired) M43.00
- cervical region M43.02
- cervicothoracic region M43.03
- congenital Q76.2
- lumbar region M43.06
- lumbosacral region M43.07
  - with disproportion (fetopelvic) O33.0
    - causing obstructed labor O65.8
- multiple sites M43.09
- occipito-atlanto-axial region M43.01
- sacrococcygeal region M43.08
- thoracic region M43.04
- thoracolumbar region M43.05

Spondylopathy M48.9
- infective NEC M46.50
  - cervical region M46.52
  - cervicothoracic region M46.53
  - lumbar region M46.56
  - lumbosacral region M46.57
  - multiple sites M46.59
  - occipito-atlanto-axial region M46.51
  - sacrococcygeal region M46.58
  - thoracic region M46.54
  - thoracolumbar region M46.55
- inflammatory M46.90
  - cervical region M46.92
  - cervicothoracic region M46.93
  - lumbar region M46.96
  - lumbosacral region M46.97
  - multiple sites M46.99
  - occipito-atlanto-axial region M46.91
  - sacrococcygeal region M46.98
  - specified type NEC M46.80
    - cervical region M46.82
    - cervicothoracic region M46.83
    - lumbar region M46.86
    - lumbosacral region M46.87
    - multiple sites M46.89
    - occipito-atlanto-axial region M46.81
    - sacrococcygeal region M46.88
    - thoracic region M46.84
    - thoracolumbar region M46.85
  - thoracic region M46.94
  - thoracolumbar region M46.95
- neuropathic, in
  - syringomyelia and syringobulbia G95.0
  - tabes dorsalis A52.11
- specified NEC M48.8
- traumatic M48.30
  - cervical region M48.32
  - cervicothoracic region M48.33
  - lumbar region M48.36
  - lumbosacral region M48.37
  - occipito-atlanto-axial region M48.31
  - sacrococcygeal region M48.38
  - thoracic region M48.34
  - thoracolumbar region M48.35

Spondylosis M47.9
- with
  - disproportion (fetopelvic) O33.0
    - causing obstructed labor O65.0
  - myelopathy NEC M47.10
    - cervical region M47.12
    - cervicothoracic region M47.13
    - lumbar region M47.16
    - occipito-atlanto-axial region M47.11
    - thoracic region M47.14
    - thoracolumbar region M47.15
  - radiculopathy M47.20
    - cervical region M47.22
    - cervicothoracic region M47.23
    - lumbar region M47.26
    - lumbosacral region M47.27
    - occipito-atlanto-axial region M47.21
    - sacrococcygeal region M47.28
    - thoracic region M47.24
    - thoracolumbar region M47.25
- specified NEC M47.899
  - cervical region M47.892
  - cervicothoracic region M47.893
  - facet joint (*see* also Spondylosis) M47.819
  - lumbar region M47.896
  - lumbosacral region M47.897
  - occipito-atlanto-axial region M47.891
  - sacrococcygeal region M47.898
  - thoracic region M47.894
  - thoracolumbar region M47.895
- traumatic —*see* Spondylopathy, traumatic
- without myelopathy or radiculopathy M47.819
  - cervical region M47.812
  - cervicothoracic region M47.813
  - lumbar region M47.816
  - lumbosacral region M47.817
  - occipito-atlanto-axial region M47.811
  - sacrococcygeal region M47.818
  - thoracic region M47.814
  - thoracolumbar region M47.815

Sponge
- inadvertently left in operation wound —*see* Foreign body, accidentally left during a procedure
- kidney (medullary) Q61.5

Sponge-diver's disease —*see* Toxicity, venom, marine animal, sea anemone

Spongioblastoma (any type) —*see* Neoplasm, malignant, by site
- specified site —*see* Neoplasm, malignant, by site
- unspecified site C71.9

Spongioneuroblastoma —*see* Neoplasm, malignant, by site

Spontaneous —*see also* condition
- fracture (cause unknown) —*see* Fracture, pathological

Spoon nail L60.3
- congenital Q84.6

Sporadic —*see* condition

Sporothrix schenckii infection —*see* Sporotrichosis

Sporotrichosis B42.9
- arthritis B42.82
- disseminated B42.7
- generalized B42.7
- lymphocutaneous (fixed) (progressive) B42.1
- pulmonary B42.0
- specified NEC B42.89

Spots, spotting (in) (of)
- Bitot's —*see also* Pigmentation, conjunctiva
  - in the young child E50.1
  - vitamin A deficiency E50.1
- café, au lait L81.3
- Cayenne pepper I78.1
- cotton wool, retina —*see* Occlusion, artery, retina
- de Morgan's (senile angiomas) I78.1
- Fuchs' black (myopic) (*see also* Myopia, degenerative) H44.2-
- intermenstrual (regular) N92.0
  - irregular N92.1
- Koplik's B05.9
- liver L81.4
- pregnancy O26.85-
- purpuric R23.3
- ruby I78.1

Spotted fever —*see* Fever, spotted A77.9

Sprain (joint) (ligament)
- acromioclavicular joint or ligament S43.5-
- ankle S93.40-
  - calcaneofibular ligament S93.41-
  - deltoid ligament S93.42-
  - internal collateral ligament —*see* Sprain, ankle, specified ligament NEC
  - specified ligament NEC S93.49-
  - talofibular ligament —*see* Sprain, ankle, specified ligament NEC
  - tibiofibular ligament S93.43-
- anterior longitudinal, cervical S13.4
- atlas, atlanto-axial, atlanto-occipital S13.4
- breast bone —*see* Sprain, sternum
- calcaneofibular —*see* Sprain, ankle
- carpal —*see* Sprain, wrist
- carpometacarpal —*see* Sprain, hand, specified site NEC
- cartilage
  - costal S23.41
  - semilunar (knee) —*see* Sprain, knee, specified site NEC
    - with current tear —*see* Tear, meniscus
  - thyroid region S13.5
  - xiphoid —*see* Sprain, sternum
- cervical, cervicodorsal, cervicothoracic S13.4
- chondrosternal S23.421
- coracoclavicular S43.8-
- coracohumeral S43.41-
- coronary, knee —*see* Sprain, knee, specified site NEC
- costal cartilage S23.41
- cricoarytenoid articulation or ligament S13.5
- cricothyroid articulation S13.5
- cruciate, knee —*see* Sprain, knee, cruciate
- deltoid, ankle —*see* Sprain, ankle
- dorsal (spine) S23.3
- elbow S53.40-
  - radial collateral ligament S53.43-
  - radiohumeral S53.41-
  - rupture
    - radial collateral ligament —*see* Rupture, traumatic, ligament, radial collateral
    - ulnar collateral ligament —*see* Rupture, traumatic, ligament, ulnar collateral
  - specified type NEC S53.49-
  - ulnar collateral ligament S53.44-
  - ulnohumeral S53.42-

Sprain *(continued)*
- femur, head —*see* Sprain, hip
- fibular collateral, knee —*see* Sprain, knee, collateral
- fibulocalcaneal —*see* Sprain, ankle
- finger(s) S63.61-
  - index S63.61-
  - interphalangeal (joint) S63.63-
    - index S63.63-
    - little S63.63-
    - middle S63.63-
    - ring S63.63-
  - little S63.61-
  - middle S63.61-
  - ring S63.61-
  - metacarpophalangeal (joint) S63.65-
  - specified site NEC S63.69-
    - index S63.69-
    - little S63.69-
    - middle S63.69-
    - ring S63.69-
- foot S93.60-
  - specified ligament NEC S93.69-
  - tarsal ligament S93.61-
  - tarsometatarsal ligament S93.62-
  - toe —*see* Sprain, toe
- hand S63.9-
  - finger —*see* Sprain, finger
  - specified site NEC S63.8
  - thumb —*see* Sprain, thumb
- head S03.9
- hip S73.10-
  - iliofemoral ligament S73.11-
  - ischiocapsular (ligament) S73.12-
  - specified NEC S73.19-
- iliofemoral —*see* Sprain, hip
- innominate
  - acetabulum —*see* Sprain, hip
  - sacral junction S33.6
- internal
  - collateral, ankle —*see* Sprain, ankle
  - semilunar cartilage —*see* Sprain, knee, specified site NEC
- interphalangeal
  - finger —*see* Sprain, finger, interphalangeal (joint)
  - toe —*see* Sprain, toe, interphalangeal joint
- ischiocapsular —*see* Sprain, hip
- ischiofemoral —*see* Sprain, hip
- jaw (articular disc) (cartilage) (meniscus) S03.4-
  - old M26.69
- knee S83.9-
  - collateral ligament S83.40-
    - lateral (fibular) S83.42-
    - medial (tibial) S83.41-
  - cruciate ligament S83.50-
    - anterior S83.51-
    - posterior S83.52-
  - lateral (fibular) collateral ligament S83.42-
  - medial (tibial) collateral ligament S83.41-
  - patellar ligament S76.11-
  - specified site NEC S83.8X-
  - superior tibiofibular joint (ligament) S83.6-
- lateral collateral, knee —*see* Sprain, knee, collateral
- lumbar (spine) S33.5
- lumbosacral S33.9
- mandible (articular disc) S03.4-
  - old M26.69
- medial collateral, knee —*see* Sprain, knee, collateral

Sprain *(continued)*
- meniscus
  - jaw S03.4-
    - old M26.69
  - knee —*see* Sprain, knee, specified site NEC
    - with current tear —*see* Tear, meniscus
      - old —*see* Derangement, knee, meniscus, due to old tear
  - mandible S03.4-
    - old M26.69
- metacarpal (distal) (proximal) —*see* Sprain, hand, specified site NEC
- metacarpophalangeal —*see* Sprain, finger, metacarpophalangeal (joint)
- metatarsophalangeal —*see* Sprain, toe, metatarsophalangeal joint
- midcarpal —*see* Sprain, hand, specified site NEC
- midtarsal —*see* Sprain, foot, specified site NEC
- neck S13.9
  - anterior longitudinal cervical ligament S13.4
  - atlanto-axial joint S13.4
  - atlanto-occipital joint S13.4
  - cervical spine S13.4
  - cricoarytenoid ligament S13.5
  - cricothyroid ligament S13.5
  - specified site NEC S13.8
  - thyroid region (cartilage) S13.5
- nose S03.8
- orbicular, hip —*see* Sprain, hip
- patella —*see* Sprain, knee, specified site NEC
- patellar ligament S76.11-
- pelvis NEC S33.8
- phalanx
  - finger —*see* Sprain, finger
  - toe —*see* Sprain, toe
- pubofemoral —*see* Sprain, hip
- radiocarpal —*see* Sprain, wrist
- radiohumeral —*see* Sprain, elbow
- radius, collateral —*see* Rupture, traumatic, ligament, radial collateral
- rib (cage) S23.41
- rotator cuff (capsule) S43.42-
- sacroiliac (region)
  - chronic or old —*see* subcategory M53.2
  - joint S33.6
- scaphoid (hand) —*see* Sprain, hand, specified site NEC
- scapula (r) —*see* Sprain, shoulder girdle, specified site NEC
- semilunar cartilage (knee) —*see* Sprain, knee, specified site NEC
  - with current tear —*see* Tear, meniscus
    - old —*see* Derangement, knee, meniscus, due to old tear
- shoulder joint S43.40-
  - acromioclavicular joint (ligament) —*see* Sprain, acromioclavicular joint
  - blade —*see* Sprain, shoulder, girdle, specified site NEC
  - coracoclavicular joint (ligament) —*see* Sprain, coracoclavicular joint
  - coracohumeral ligament —*see* Sprain, coracohumeral joint
  - girdle S43.9-
    - specified site NEC S43.8-

Sprain *(continued)*
- shoulder joint *(continued)*
  - rotator cuff —*see* Sprain, rotator cuff
  - specified site NEC S43.49-
  - sternoclavicular joint (ligament) —*see* Sprain, sternoclavicular joint
- spine
  - cervical S13.4
  - lumbar S33.5
  - thoracic S23.3
- sternoclavicular joint S43.6-
- sternum S23.429
  - chondrosternal joint S23.421
  - specified site NEC S23.428
  - sternoclavicular (joint) (ligament) S23.420
- symphysis
  - jaw S03.4-
    - old M26.69
  - mandibular S03.4-
    - old M26.69
- talofibular —*see* Sprain, ankle
- tarsal —*see* Sprain, foot, specified site NEC
- tarsometatarsal —*see* Sprain, foot, specified site NEC
- temporomandibular S03.4-
  - old M26.69
- thorax S23.9
  - ribs S23.41
  - specified site NEC S23.8
  - spine S23.3
  - sternum —*see* Sprain, sternum
- thumb S63.60-
  - interphalangeal (joint) S63.62-
  - metacarpophalangeal (joint) S63.64-
  - specified site NEC S63.68-
- thyroid cartilage or region S13.5
- tibia (proximal end) —*see* Sprain, knee, specified site NEC
- tibial collateral, knee —*see* Sprain, knee, collateral
- tibiofibular
  - distal —*see* Sprain, ankle
  - superior —*see* Sprain, knee, specified site NEC
- toe(s) S93.50-
  - great S93.50-
  - interphalangeal joint S93.51-
    - great S93.51-
    - lesser S93.51-
  - lesser S93.50-
  - metatarsophalangeal joint S93.52-
    - great S93.52-
    - lesser S93.52-
- ulna, collateral —*see* Rupture, traumatic, ligament, ulnar collateral
- ulnohumeral —*see* Sprain, elbow
- wrist S63.50-
  - carpal S63.51-
  - radiocarpal S63.52-
  - specified site NEC S63.59-
- xiphoid cartilage —*see* Sprain, sternum

Sprengel's deformity (congenital) Q74.0

Sprue (tropical) K90.1
- celiac K90.0
- idiopathic K90.49
- meaning thrush B37.0
- nontropical K90.0

Spur, bone —*see also* Enthesopathy
- calcaneal M77.3-
- iliac crest M76.2-
- nose (septum) J34.89

Spurway's syndrome Q78.0
Sputum
abnormal (amount) (color) (odor) (purulent) R09.3
blood-stained R04.2
excessive (cause unknown) R09.3
Squamous —*see also* condition
epithelium in
cervical canal (congenital) Q51.828
uterine mucosa (congenital) Q51.818
Squashed nose M95.0
congenital Q67.4
Squeeze, diver's T70.3
Squint —*see also* Strabismus
accommodative —*see* Strabismus, convergent concomitant
SSADHD (succinic semialdehyde dehydrogenase deficiency) E72.81
St. Hubert's disease A82.9
Stab —*see also* Laceration
internal organs —*see* Injury, by site
Stafne's cyst or cavity M27.0
Staggering gait R26.0
hysterical F44.4
Staghorn calculus —*see* Calculus, kidney
Stähli's line (cornea) (pigment) —*see* Pigmentation, cornea, anterior
Stain, staining
meconium (newborn) P96.83
port wine Q82.5
tooth, teeth (hard tissues) (extrinsic) K03.6
due to
accretions K03.6
deposits (betel) (black) (green) (materia alba) (orange) (soft) (tobacco) K03.6
metals (copper) (silver) K03.7
nicotine K03.6
pulpal bleeding K03.7
tobacco K03.6
intrinsic K00.8
Stammering (*see also* Disorder, fluency) F80.81
Standstill
auricular I45.5
cardiac —*see* Arrest, cardiac
sinoatrial I45.5
ventricular —*see* Arrest, cardiac
Stannosis J63.5
Stanton's disease —*see* Melioidosis
Staphylitis (acute) (catarrhal) (chronic) (gangrenous) (membranous) (suppurative) (ulcerative) K12.2
Staphylococcal scalded skin syndrome L00
Staphylococcemia A41.2
Staphylococcus, staphylococcal —*see also* condition
as cause of disease classified elsewhere B95.8
aureus (methicillin susceptible) (MSSA) B95.61
methicillin resistant (MRSA) B95.62
specified NEC, as cause of disease classified elsewhere B95.7
Staphyloma (sclera)
cornea H18.72-
equatorial H15.81-
localized (anterior) H15.82-

Staphyloma *(continued)*
posticum H15.83-
ring H15.85-
Stargardt's disease —*see* Dystrophy, retina
Starvation (inanition) (due to lack of food) T73.0
edema —*see* Malnutrition, severe
Stasis
bile (noncalculous) K83.1
bronchus J98.09
with infection —*see* Bronchitis
cardiac —*see* Failure, heart, congestive
cecum K59.89
colon K59.89
dermatitis I87.2
with
varicose ulcer —*see* Varix, leg, with ulcer, with inflammation
varicose veins —*see* Varix, leg, with inflammation
due to postthrombotic syndrome —*see* Syndrome, postthombotic
duodenal K31.5
eczema —*see* Varix, leg, with, inflammation
edema —*see* Hypertension, venous (chronic), idiopathic
foot T69.0-
ileocecal coil K59.89
ileum K59.89
intestinal K59.89
jejunum K59.89
kidney N19
liver (cirrhotic) K76.1
lymphatic I89.8
pneumonia J18.2
pulmonary —*see* Edema, lung
rectal K59.89
renal N19
tubular N17.0
ulcer —*see* Varix, leg, with, ulcer
without varicose veins I87.2
urine —*see* Retention, urine
venous I87.8
State (of)
affective and paranoid, mixed, organic psychotic F06.8
agitated R45.1
acute reaction to stress F43.0
anxiety (neurotic) F41.1
apprehension F41.1
burn-out Z73.0
climacteric, female Z78.0
symptomatic N95.1
compulsive F42.8
mixed with obsessional thoughts F42.2
confusional (psychogenic) F44.89
acute —*see also* Delirium
with
arteriosclerotic dementia F01.50
with behavioral disturbance F01.51
senility or dementia F05
alcoholic F10.231
epileptic F05
reactive (from emotional stress, psychological trauma) F44.89
subacute —*see* Delirium
convulsive —*see* Convulsions
crisis F43.0
depressive F32.A
neurotic F34.1
dissociative F44.9
emotional shock (stress) R45.7

State *(continued)*
hypercoagulation —*see* Hypercoagulable
locked-in G83.5
menopausal Z78.0
symptomatic N95.1
neurotic F48.9
with depersonalization F48.1
obsessional F42.8
oneiroid (schizophrenia-like) F23
organic
hallucinatory (nonalcoholic) F06.0
paranoid (-hallucinatory) F06.2
panic F41.0
paranoid F22
climacteric F22
involutional F22
menopausal F22
organic F06.2
senile F03
simple F22
persistent vegetative R40.3
phobic F40.9
postleukotomy F07.0
pregnant
gestational carrier Z33.3
incidental Z33.1
psychogenic, twilight F44.89
psychopathic (constitutional) F60.2
psychotic, organic —*see also* Psychosis, organic
mixed paranoid and affective F06.8
senile or presenile F03
transient NEC F06.8
with
hallucinations F06.0
depression F06.31
residual schizophrenic F20.5
restlessness R45.1
stress (emotional) R45.7
tension (mental) F48.9
specified NEC F48.8
transient organic psychotic NEC F06.8
depressive type F06.31
hallucinatory type F06.0
twilight
epileptic F05
psychogenic F44.89
vegetative, persistent R40.3
vital exhaustion Z73.0
withdrawal, —*see* Withdrawal, state
Status (post) —*see also* Presence (of)
absence, epileptic —*see* Epilepsy, by type, with status epilepticus
administration of tPA (rtPA) in a different facility within the last 24 hours prior to admission to current facility Z92.82
adrenalectomy (unilateral) (bilateral) E89.6
anastomosis Z98.0
angioplasty (peripheral) Z98.62
with implant Z95.820
coronary artery Z98.61
with implant Z95.5
anginosus I20.9
aortocoronary bypass Z95.1
arthrodesis Z98.1
artificial opening (of) Z93.9
gastrointestinal tract Z93.4
specified NEC Z93.8
urinary tract Z93.6
vagina Z93.8
asthmaticus —*see* Asthma, by type, with status asthmaticus
awaiting organ transplant Z76.82

Status *(continued)*
bariatric surgery Z98.84
bed confinement Z74.01
bleb, filtering (vitreous), after glaucoma surgery Z98.83
breast implant Z98.82
removal Z98.86
cataract extraction Z98.4-
cholecystectomy Z90.49
clitorectomy N90.811
with excision of labia minora N90.812
colectomy (complete) (partial) Z90.49
colonization —*see* Carrier (suspected) of
colostomy Z93.3
convulsivus idiopathicus —*see* Epilepsy, by type, with status epilepticus
coronary artery angioplasty —*see* Status, angioplasty, coronary artery
coronary artery bypass graft Z95.1
cystectomy (urinary bladder) Z90.6
cystostomy Z93.50
appendico-vesicostomy Z93.52
cutaneous Z93.51
specified NEC Z93.59
delinquent immunization Z28.3
dental Z98.818
crown Z98.811
fillings Z98.811
restoration Z98.811
sealant Z98.810
specified NEC Z98.818
deployment (current) (military) Z56.82
dialysis (hemodialysis) (peritoneal) Z99.2
do not resuscitate (DNR) Z66
donor —*see* Donor
embedded fragments —*see* Retained, foreign body fragments (type of)
embedded splinter —*see* Retained, foreign body fragments (type of)
enterostomy Z93.4
epileptic, epilepticus (*see also* Epilepsy, by type, with status epilepticus) G40.901
estrogen receptor
negative Z17.1
positive Z17.0
female genital cutting —*see* Female genital mutilation status
female genital mutilation —*see* Female genital mutilation status
filtering (vitreous) bleb after glaucoma surgery Z98.83
gastrectomy (complete) (partial) Z90.3
gastric banding Z98.84
gastric bypass for obesity Z98.84
gastrostomy Z93.1
human immunodeficiency virus (HIV) infection, asymptomatic Z21
hysterectomy (complete) (total) Z90.710
partial (with remaining cervial stump) Z90.711
ileostomy Z93.2
implant
breast Z98.82
infibulation N90.813
intestinal bypass Z98.0
jejunostomy Z93.4
laryngectomy Z90.02
lapsed immunization schedule Z28.3

Status *(continued)*
- lymphaticus E32.8
- malignancy
  - castrate resistant prostate Z19.2
  - hormone resistant Z19.2
  - hormone sensitive Z19.1
- marmoratus G80.3
- mastectomy (unilateral) (bilateral) Z90.1-
- military deployment status (current) Z56.82
  - in theater or in support of military war, peacekeeping and humanitarian operations Z56.82
- nephrectomy (unilateral) (bilateral) Z90.5
- nephrostomy Z93.6
- obesity surgery Z98.84
- oophorectomy
  - bilateral Z90.722
  - unilateral Z90.721
- organ replacement
  - by artificial or mechanical device or prosthesis of
    - artery Z95.828
    - bladder Z96.0
    - blood vessel Z95.828
    - breast Z97.8
    - eye globe Z97.0
    - heart Z95.812
      - valve Z95.2
    - intestine Z97.8
    - joint Z96.60
      - hip *—see* Presence, hip joint implant
      - knee *—see* Presence, knee joint implant
      - specified site NEC Z96.698
    - kidney Z97.8
    - larynx Z96.3
    - lens Z96.1
    - limbs *—see* Presence, artificial, limb
    - liver Z97.8
    - lung Z97.8
    - pancreas Z97.8
  - by organ transplant (heterologous)(homologous) *—see* Transplant
- pacemaker
  - brain Z96.89
  - cardiac Z95.0
  - specified NEC Z96.89
- pancreatectomy Z90.410
  - complete Z90.410
  - partial Z90.411
  - total Z90.410
- physical restraint Z78.1
- pneumonectomy (complete) (partial) Z90.2
- pneumothorax, therapeutic Z98.3
- postcommotio cerebri F07.81
- postoperative (postprocedural) NEC Z98.890
  - breast implant Z98.82
  - dental Z98.818
    - crown Z98.811
    - fillings Z98.811
    - restoration Z98.811
    - sealant Z98.810
    - specified NEC Z98.818
  - pneumothorax, therapeutic Z98.3
  - uterine scar Z98.891
- postpartum (routine follow-up) Z39.2
  - care immediately after delivery Z39.0

Status *(continued)*
- postsurgical (postprocedural) NEC Z98.890
  - pneumothorax, therapeutic Z98.3
- pregnancy, incidental Z33.1
- prosthesis coronary angioplasty Z95.5
- pseudophakia Z96.1
- renal dialysis (hemodialysis) (peritoneal) Z99.2
- retained foreign body *—see* Retained, foreign body fragments (type of)
- reversed jejunal transposition (for bypass) Z98.0
- salpingo-oophorectomy
  - bilateral Z90.722
  - unilateral Z90.721
- sex reassignment surgery status Z87.890
- shunt
  - arteriovenous (for dialysis) Z99.2
  - cerebrospinal fluid Z98.2
  - ventricular (communicating) (for drainage) Z98.2
- splenectomy Z90.81
- thymicolymphaticus E32.8
- thymicus E32.8
- thymolymphaticus E32.8
- thyroidectomy (hypothyroidism) E89.0
- tooth (teeth) extraction (*see also* Absence, teeth, acquired) K08.409
- tPA (rtPA) administration in a different facility within the last 24 hours prior to admission to current facility Z92.82
- tracheostomy Z93.0
- transplant *—see* Transplant
  - organ removed Z98.85
- tubal ligation Z98.51
- underimmunization Z28.3
- ureterostomy Z93.6
- urethrostomy Z93.6
- vagina, artificial Z93.8
- vasectomy Z98.52
- wheelchair confinement Z99.3

Stealing
- child problem F91.8
  - in company with others Z72.810
- pathological (compulsive) F63.2

Steam burn *—see* Burn

Steatocystoma multiplex L72.2

Steatohepatitis (nonalcoholic) (NASH) K75.81

Steatoma L72.3
- eyelid (cystic) *—see* Dermatosis, eyelid
  - infected *—see* Hordeolum

Steatorrhea (chronic) K90.4
- with lacteal obstruction K90.2
- idiopathic (adult) (infantile) K90.9
- pancreatic K90.3
- primary K90.0
- tropical K90.1

Steatosis E88.89
- heart *—see* Degeneration, myocardial
- kidney N28.89
- liver NEC K76.0

Steele-Richardson-Olszewski disease or syndrome G23.1

Steinbrocker's syndrome G90.8

Steinert's disease G71.11

Stein-Leventhal syndrome E28.2

Stein's syndrome E28.2

STEMI (*see also* Infarct, myocardium ST elevation) I21.3

Stenocardia I20.8

Stenocephaly Q75.8

Stenosis, stenotic (cicatricial) *—see also* Stricture
- ampulla of Vater K83.1
- anus, anal (canal) (sphincter) K62.4
  - and rectum K62.4
  - congenital Q42.3
    - with fistula Q42.2
- aorta (ascending) (supraventricular) (congenital) Q25.1
  - arteriosclerotic I70.0
  - calcified I70.0
  - supravalvular Q25.3
- aortic (valve) I35.0
  - with insufficiency I35.2
  - congenital Q23.0
  - rheumatic I06.0
    - with
      - incompetency, insufficiency or regurgitation I06.2
        - with mitral (valve) disease I08.0
          - with tricuspid (valve) disease I08.3
      - mitral (valve) disease I08.0
        - with tricuspid (valve) disease I08.3
      - tricuspid (valve) disease I08.2
        - with mitral (valve) disease I08.3
  - specified cause NEC I35.0
  - syphilitic A52.03
- aqueduct of Sylvius (congenital) Q03.0
  - with spina bifida *—see* Spina bifida, by site, with hydrocephalus
  - acquired G91.1
- artery NEC (*see also* Arteriosclerosis) I77.1
  - celiac I77.4
  - cerebral *—see* Occlusion, artery, cerebral
  - extremities *—see* Arteriosclerosis, extremities
  - precerebral *—see* Occlusion, artery, precerebral
  - pulmonary (congenital) Q25.6
    - acquired I28.8
  - renal I70.1
  - stent
    - coronary T82.855
    - peripheral T82.856
- bile duct (common) (hepatic) K83.1
  - congenital Q44.3
- bladder-neck (acquired) N32.0
  - congenital Q64.31
- brain G93.89
- bronchus J98.09
  - congenital Q32.3
  - syphilitic A52.72
- cardia (stomach) K22.2
  - congenital Q39.3
- cardiovascular *—see* Disease, cardiovascular
- caudal M48.08
- cervix, cervical (canal) N88.2
  - congenital Q51.828
  - in pregnancy or childbirth *—see* Pregnancy, complicated by, abnormal cervix

Stenosis, stenotic *(continued)*
- colon *—see also* Obstruction, intestine
  - congenital Q42.9
    - specified NEC Q42.8
- colostomy K94.03
- common (bile) duct K83.1
  - congenital Q44.3
- coronary (artery) *—see* Disease, heart, ischemic, atherosclerotic
- cystic duct *—see* Obstruction, gallbladder
- due to presence of device, implant or graft (*see also* Complications, by site and type, specified NEC) T85.858
  - arterial graft NEC T82.858
  - breast (implant) T85.858
  - catheter T85.858
    - dialysis (renal) T82.858
      - intraperitoneal T85.858
    - infusion NEC T82.858
      - spinal (epidural) (subdural) T85.850
    - urinary (indwelling) T83.85
  - fixation, internal (orthopedic) NEC T84.85
  - gastrointestinal (bile duct) (esophagus) T85.858
  - genital NEC T83.85
  - heart NEC T82.857
  - joint prosthesis T84.85
  - ocular (corneal graft) (orbital implant) NEC T85.858
  - orthopedic NEC T84.85
  - specified NEC T85.858
  - urinary NEC T83.85
  - vascular NEC T82.858
  - ventricular intracranial shunt T85.850
- duodenum K31.5
  - congenital Q41.0
- ejaculatory duct NEC N50.89
- endocervical os *—see* Stenosis, cervix
- enterostomy K94.13
- esophagus K22.2
  - congenital Q39.3
  - syphilitic A52.79
    - congenital A50.59 *[K23]*
- eustachian tube *—see* Obstruction, eustachian tube
- external ear canal (acquired) H61.30-
  - congenital Q16.1
  - due to
    - inflammation H61.32-
    - trauma H61.31-
  - postprocedural H95.81-
  - specified cause NEC H61.39-
- gallbladder *—see* Obstruction, gallbladder
- glottis J38.6
- heart valve (*see also* Endocarditis) I38
  - aortic *— see* Stenosis, aortic
  - congenital Q24.8
  - mitral *— see* Stenosis, mitral
  - pulmonary *— see* Stenosis, pulmonary, valve
  - tricuspid *— see* Stenosis, tricuspid Q22.4
- hepatic duct K83.1
- hymen N89.6
- hypertrophic subaortic (idiopathic) I42.1
- ileum (*see also* Obstruction, intestine, specified NEC) K56.699
  - congenital Q41.2
- infundibulum cardia Q24.3

Stenosis, stenotic *(continued)*
intervertebral foramina *—see also* Lesion, biomechanical, specified NEC
connective tissue M99.79
abdomen M99.79
cervical region M99.71
cervicothoracic M99.71
head region M99.70
lumbar region M99.73
lumbosacral M99.73
occipitocervical M99.70
sacral region M99.74
sacrococcygeal M99.74
sacroiliac M99.74
specified NEC M99.79
thoracic region M99.72
thoracolumbar M99.72
disc M99.79
abdomen M99.79
cervical region M99.71
cervicothoracic M99.71
head region M99.70
lower extremity M99.76
lumbar region M99.73
lumbosacral M99.73
occipitocervical M99.70
pelvic M99.75
rib cage M99.78
sacral region M99.74
sacrococcygeal M99.74
sacroiliac M99.74
specified NEC M99.79
thoracic region M99.72
thoracolumbar M99.72
upper extremity M99.77
osseous M99.69
abdomen M99.69
cervical region M99.61
cervicothoracic M99.61
head region M99.60
lower extremity M99.66
lumbar region M99.63
lumbosacral M99.63
occipitocervical M99.60
pelvic M99.65
rib cage M99.68
sacral region M99.64
sacrococcygeal M99.64
sacroiliac M99.64
specified NEC M99.69
thoracic region M99.62
thoracolumbar M99.62
upper extremity M99.67
subluxation *—see* Stenosis, intervertebral foramina, Vosseous
intestine *—see also* Obstruction, intestine
congenital (small) Q41.9
large Q42.9
specified NEC Q42.8
specified NEC Q41.8
jejunum (*see also* Obstruction, intestine, specified NEC) K56.699
congenital Q41.1
lacrimal (passage)
canaliculi H04.54-
congenital Q10.5
duct H04.55-
punctum H04.56-
sac H04.57-
lacrimonasal duct *—see* Stenosis, lacrimal, duct
congenital Q10.5
larynx J38.6
congenital NEC Q31.8
subglottic Q31.1
syphilitic A52.73
congenital A50.59 *[J99]*

Stenosis, stenotic *(continued)*
mitral (chronic) (inactive) (valve) I05.0
with
aortic valve disease I08.0
incompetency, insufficiency or regurgitation I05.2
active or acute I01.1
with rheumatic or Sydenham's chorea I02.0
congenital Q23.2
specified cause, except rheumatic I34.2
syphilitic A52.03
myocardium, myocardial *—see also* Degeneration, myocardial
hypertrophic subaortic (idiopathic) I42.1
nares (anterior) (posterior) J34.89
congenital Q30.0
nasal duct *—see also* Stenosis, lacrimal, duct
congenital Q10.5
nasolacrimal duct *—see also* Stenosis, lacrimal, duct
congenital Q10.5
neural canal *—see also* Lesion, biomechanical, specified NEC
connective tissue M99.49
abdomen M99.49
cervical region M99.41
cervicothoracic M99.41
head region M99.40
lower extremity M99.46
lumbar region M99.43
lumbosacral M99.43
occipitocervical M99.40
pelvic M99.45
rib cage M99.48
sacral region M99.44
sacrococcygeal M99.44
sacroiliac M99.44
specified NEC M99.49
thoracic region M99.42
thoracolumbar M99.42
upper extremity M99.47
intervertebral disc M99.59
abdomen M99.59
cervical region M99.51
cervicothoracic M99.51
head region M99.50
lower extremity M99.56
lumbar region M99.53
lumbosacral M99.53
occipitocervical M99.50
pelvic M99.55
rib cage M99.58
sacral region M99.54
sacrococcygeal M99.54
sacroiliac M99.54
specified NEC M99.59
thoracic region M99.52
thoracolumbar M99.52
upper extremity M99.57
osseous M99.39
abdomen M99.39
cervical region M99.31
cervicothoracic M99.31
head region M99.30
lower extremity M99.36
lumbar region M99.33
lumbosacral M99.33
pelvic M99.35
rib cage M99.38
occipitocervical M99.30
sacral region M99.34
sacrococcygeal M99.34
sacroiliac M99.34
specified NEC M99.39
thoracic region M99.32
thoracolumbar M99.32

Stenosis, stenotic *(continued)*
neural canal *(continued)*
osseous *(continued)*
upper extremity M99.37
subluxation M99.29
cervical region M99.21
cervicothoracic M99.21
head region M99.20
lower extremity M99.26
lumbar region M99.23
lumbosacral M99.23
occipitocervical M99.20
pelvic M99.25
rib cage M99.28
sacral region M99.24
sacrococcygeal M99.24
sacroiliac M99.24
specified NEC M99.29
thoracic region M99.22
thoracolumbar M99.22
upper extremity M99.27
organ or site, congenital NEC *—see* Atresia, by site
papilla of Vater K83.1
pulmonary (artery) (congenital) Q25.6
with ventricular septal defect, transposition of aorta, and hypertrophy of right ventricle Q21.3
acquired I28.8
in tetralogy of Fallot Q21.3
infundibular Q24.3
subvalvular Q24.3
supravalvular Q25.6
valve I37.0
with insufficiency I37.2
congenital Q22.1
rheumatic I09.89
with aortic, mitral or tricuspid (valve) disease I08.8
vein, acquired I28.8
vessel NEC I28.8
pulmonic (congenital) Q22.1
infundibular Q24.3
subvalvular Q24.3
pylorus (hypertrophic) (acquired) K31.1
adult K31.1
congenital Q40.0
infantile Q40.0
rectum (sphincter) *—see* Stricture, rectum
renal artery I70.1
congenital Q27.1
salivary duct (any) K11.8
sphincter of Oddi K83.1
spinal M48.00
cervical region M48.02
cervicothoracic region M48.03
lumbar region (NOS) (without neurogenic claudication) M48.061
with neurogenic claudication M48.062
lumbosacral region M48.07
occipito-atlanto-axial region M48.01
sacrococcygeal region M48.08
thoracic region M48.04
thoracolumbar region M48.05
stent
vascular
end stent
adjacent to stent —see Arteriosclerosis
within the stent
coronary T82.855
peripheral T82.856

Stenosis, stenotic *(continued)*
stent *(continued)*
vascular *(continued)*
in stent
coronary vessel T82.855
peripheral vessel T82.856
stomach, hourglass K31.2
subaortic (congenital) Q24.4
hypertrophic (idiopathic) I42.1
subglottic J38.6
congenital Q31.1
postprocedural J95.5
trachea J39.8
congenital Q32.1
syphilitic A52.73
tuberculous NEC A15.5
tracheostomy J95.03
tricuspid (valve) I07.0
with
aortic (valve) disease I08.2
incompetency, insufficiency or regurgitation I07.2
with aortic (valve) disease I08.2
with mitral (valve) disease I08.3
mitral (valve) disease I08.1
with aortic (valve) disease I08.3
congenital Q22.4
nonrheumatic I36.0
with insufficiency I36.2
tubal N97.1
ureter *—see* Atresia, ureter
ureteropelvic junction, congenital Q62.11
ureterovesical orifice, congenital Q62.12
urethra (valve) *—see also* Stricture, urethra
congenital Q64.32
urinary meatus, congenital Q64.33
vagina N89.5
congenital Q52.4
in pregnancy *—see* Pregnancy, complicated by, abnormal vagina
causing obstructed labor O65.5
valve (cardiac) (heart) (*see also* Endocarditis) I38
congenital Q24.8
aortic Q23.0
mitral Q23.2
pulmonary Q22.1
tricuspid Q22.4
vena cava (inferior) (superior) I87.1
congenital Q26.0
vesicourethral orifice Q64.31
vulva N90.5

Stent jail T82.897

Stercolith (impaction) K56.41
appendix K38.1

Stercoraceous, stercoral ulcer K63.3
anus or rectum K62.6

Stereotypies NEC F98.4

Sterility *—see* Infertility

Sterilization *—see* Encounter (for), sterilization

Sternalgia *—see* Angina

Sternopagus Q89.4

Sternum bifidum Q76.7

Steroid
- effects (adverse) (adrenocortical) (iatrogenic)
  - cushingoid E24.2
    - correct substance properly administered *—see* Table of Drugs and Chemicals, by drug, adverse effect
    - overdose or wrong substance given or taken *—see* Table of Drugs and Chemicals, by drug, poisoning
  - diabetes *—see* category E09
    - correct substance properly administered *—see* Table of Drugs and Chemicals, by drug, adverse effect
    - overdose or wrong substance given or taken *—see* Table of Drugs and Chemicals, by drug, poisoning
  - fever R50.2
  - insufficiency E27.3
    - correct substance properly administered *—see* Table of Drugs and Chemicals, by drug, adverse effect
    - overdose or wrong substance given or taken *—see* Table of Drugs and Chemicals, by drug, poisoning
- responder H40.04-

Stevens-Johnson disease or syndrome L51.1
- toxic epidermal necrolysis overlap L51.3

Stewart-Morel syndrome M85.2

Sticker's disease B08.3

Sticky eye *—see* Conjunctivitis, acute, mucopurulent

Stieda's disease *—see* Bursitis, tibial collateral

Stiff neck *—see* Torticollis

Stiff-man syndrome G25.82

Stiffness, joint NEC M25.60-
- ankle M25.67-
- ankylosis *—see* Ankylosis, joint
- contracture *—see* Contraction, joint
- elbow M25.62-
- foot M25.67-
- hand M25.64-
- hip M25.65-
- knee M25.66-
- shoulder M25.61-
- specified site NEC M25.69
- wrist M25.63-

Stigmata congenital syphilis A50.59

Stillbirth P95

Still-Felty syndrome *—see* Felty's syndrome

Still's disease or syndrome (juvenile) M08.20
- adult-onset M06.1
- ankle M08.27-
- elbow M08.22-
- foot joint M08.27-
- hand joint M08.24-
- hip M08.25-
- knee M08.26-
- multiple site M08.29
- shoulder M08.21-
- specified site NEC M08.2A

Still's disease or syndrome *(continued)*
- vertebra M08.28
- wrist M08.23-

Stimulation, ovary E28.1

Sting (venomous) (with allergic or anaphylactic shock) *—see* Table of Drugs and Chemicals, by animal or substance, poisoning

Stippled epiphyses Q78.8

Stitch
- abscess T81.41
- burst (in operation wound) *—see* Disruption, wound, operation

Stokes-Adams disease or syndrome I45.9

Stokes' disease E05.00
- with thyroid storm E05.01

Stokvis (-Talma) **disease** D74.8

Stoma malfunction
- colostomy K94.03
- enterostomy K94.13
- gastrostomy K94.23
- ileostomy K94.13
- tracheostomy J95.03

Stomach *—see* condition

Stomatitis (denture) (ulcerative) K12.1
- angular K13.0
  - due to dietary or vitamin deficiency E53.0
- aphthous K12.0
- bovine B08.61
- candidal B37.0
- catarrhal K12.1
- diphtheritic A36.89
- due to
  - dietary deficiency E53.0
  - thrush B37.0
  - vitamin deficiency
    - B group NEC E53.9
    - B2(riboflavin) E53.0
- epidemic B08.8
- epizootic B08.8
- follicular K12.1
- gangrenous A69.0
- Geotrichum B48.3
- herpesviral, herpetic B00.2
- herpetiformis K12.0
- malignant K12.1
- membranous acute K12.1
- monilial B37.0
- mycotic B37.0
- necrotizing ulcerative A69.0
- parasitic B37.0
- septic K12.1
- spirochetal A69.1
- suppurative (acute) K12.2
- ulceromembranous A69.1
- vesicular K12.1
  - with exanthem (enteroviral) B08.4
  - virus disease A93.8
- Vincent's A69.1

Stomatocytosis D58.8

Stomatomycosis B37.0

Stomatorrhagia K13.79

Stone(s) *—see also* Calculus
- bladder (diverticulum) N21.0
- cystine E72.09
- heart syndrome I50.1
- kidney N20.0
- prostate N42.0
- pulpal (dental) K04.2
- renal N20.0
- salivary gland or duct (any) K11.5
- urethra (impacted) N21.1

Stone *(continued)*
- urinary (duct) (impacted) (passage) N20.9
  - bladder (diverticulum) N21.0
  - lower tract N21.9
  - specified NEC N21.8
- xanthine E79.8 *[N22]*

Stonecutter's lung J62.8

Stonemason's asthma, disease, lung or pneumoconiosis J62.8

Stoppage
- heart *—see* Arrest, cardiac
- urine *—see* Retention, urine

Storm, thyroid *—see* Thyrotoxicosis

Strabismus (congenital) (nonparalytic) H50.9
- concomitant H50.40
  - convergent *—see* Strabismus, convergent concomitant
  - divergent *—see* Strabismus, divergent concomitant
- convergent concomitant H50.00
  - accommodative component H50.43
  - alternating H50.05
    - with
      - A pattern H50.06
      - specified nonconcomitances NEC H50.08
      - V pattern H50.07
  - monocular H50.01-
    - with
      - A pattern H50.02-
      - specified nonconcomitances NEC H50.04-
      - V pattern H50.03-
    - intermittent H50.31-
      - alternating H50.32
- cyclotropia H50.41
- divergent concomitant H50.10
  - alternating H50.15
    - with
      - A pattern H50.16
      - specified noncomitances NEC H50.18
      - V pattern H50.17
  - monocular H50.11-
    - with
      - A pattern H50.12-
      - specified noncomitances NEC H50.14-
      - V pattern H50.13-
    - intermittent H50.33
      - alternating H50.34
- Duane's syndrome H50.81-
- due to adhesions, scars H50.69
- heterophoria H50.50
  - alternating H50.55
  - cyclophoria H50.54
  - esophoria H50.51
  - exophoria H50.52
  - vertical H50.53
- heterotropia H50.40
  - intermittent H50.30
- hypertropia H50.2-
- hypotropia *—see* Hypertropia
- latent H50.50
- mechanical H50.60
  - Brown's sheath syndrome H50.61-
  - specified type NEC H50.69
- monofixation syndrome H50.42
- paralytic H49.9
  - abducens nerve H49.2-
  - fourth nerve H49.1-
  - Kearns-Sayre syndrome H49.81-
  - ophthalmoplegia (external)
    - progressive H49.4-
      - with pigmentary retinopathy H49.81-
    - total H49.3-

Strabismus *(continued)*
- paralytic *(continued)*
  - sixth nerve H49.2-
  - specified type NEC H49.88-
  - third nerve H49.0-
  - trochlear nerve H49.1-
- specified type NEC H50.89
- vertical H50.2-

Strain
- back S39.012
- cervical S16.1
- eye NEC *—see* Disturbance, vision, subjective
- heart *—see* Disease, heart
- low back S39.012
- mental NOS Z73.3
  - work-related Z56.6
- muscle (tendon) *—see* Injury, muscle, by site, strain
- neck S16.1
- postural *—see also* Disorder, soft tissue, due to use
- physical NOS Z73.3
  - work-related Z56.6
- psychological NEC Z73.3
- tendon *—see* Injury, muscle, by site, strain

Straining, on urination R39.16

Strand, vitreous *—see* Opacity, vitreous, membranes and strands

Strangulation, strangulated *—see also* Asphyxia, traumatic
- appendix K38.8
- bladder-neck N32.0
- bowel or colon K56.2
- food or foreign body *—see* Foreign body, by site
- hemorrhoids *—see* Hemorrhoids, with complication
- hernia *—see also* Hernia, by site, with obstruction
  - with gangrene *—see* Hernia, by site, with gangrene
- intestine (large) (small) K56.2
  - with hernia *—see also* Hernia, by site, with obstruction
    - with gangrene *—see* Hernia, by site, with gangrene
- mesentery K56.2
- mucus *—see* Asphyxia, mucus
- omentum K56.2
- organ or site, congenital NEC *—see* Atresia, by site
- ovary *—see* Torsion, ovary
- penis N48.89
  - foreign body T19.4
- rupture *—see* Hernia, by site, with obstruction
- stomach due to hernia *—see also* Hernia, by site, with obstruction
  - with gangrene *—see* Hernia, by site, with gangrene
- vesicourethral orifice N32.0

Strangury R30.0

Straw itch B88.0

Strawberry
- gallbladder K82.4
- mark Q82.5
- tongue (red) (white) K14.3

Streak(s)
- macula, angioid H35.33
- ovarian Q50.32

Strephosymbolia F81.0
- secondary to organic lesion R48.8

Streptobacillary fever A25.1

Streptobacillosis A25.1

Streptobacillus moniliformis A25.1

- **Streptococcus, streptococcal** —*see also* condition
  - as cause of disease classified elsewhere B95.5
  - group
    - A, as cause of disease classified elsewhere B95.0
    - B, as cause of disease classified elsewhere B95.1
    - D, as cause of disease classified elsewhere B95.2
  - pneumoniae, as cause of disease classified elsewhere B95.3
  - specified NEC, as cause of disease classified elsewhere B95.4
- **Streptomycosis** B47.1
- **Streptotrichosis** A48.8
- **Stress** F43.9
  - family —*see* Disruption, family
  - fetal P84
    - complicating pregnancy O77.9
      - due to drug administration O77.1
  - mental NEC Z73.3
    - work-related Z56.6
  - physical NEC Z73.3
    - work-related Z56.6
  - polycythemia D75.1
  - reaction (*see also* Reaction, stress) F43.9
  - work schedule Z56.3
- **Stretching, nerve** —*see* Injury, nerve
- **Striae albicantes, atrophicae or distensae** (cutis) L90.6
- **Stricture** —*see also* Stenosis
  - ampulla of Vater K83.1
  - anus (sphincter) K62.4
    - congenital Q42.3
      - with fistula Q42.2
    - infantile Q42.3
      - with fistula Q42.2
  - aorta (ascending) (congenital) Q25.1
    - arteriosclerotic I70.0
    - calcified I70.0
    - supravalvular, congenital Q25.3
  - aortic (valve) —*see* Stenosis, aortic
  - aqueduct of Sylvius (congenital) Q03.0
    - with spina bifida —*see* Spina bifida, by site, with hydrocephalus
    - acquired G91.1
  - artery I77.1
    - basilar —*see* Occlusion, artery, basilar
    - carotid —*see* Occlusion, artery, carotid
    - celiac I77.4
    - congenital (peripheral) Q27.8
      - cerebral Q28.3
      - coronary Q24.5
      - digestive system Q27.8
      - lower limb Q27.8
      - retinal Q14.1
      - specified site NEC Q27.8
      - umbilical Q27.0
      - upper limb Q27.8
    - coronary —*see* Disease, heart, ischemic, atherosclerotic
      - congenital Q24.5
    - precerebral —*see* Occlusion, artery, precerebral
    - pulmonary (congenital) Q25.6
      - acquired I28.8
    - renal I70.1
    - vertebral —*see* Occlusion, artery, vertebral

Stricture *(continued)*

  - auditory canal (external) (congenital)
    - acquired —*see* Stenosis, external ear canal
  - bile duct (common) (hepatic) K83.1
    - congenital Q44.3
    - postoperative K91.89
  - bladder N32.89
    - neck N32.0
  - bowel —*see* Obstruction, intestine
  - brain G93.89
  - bronchus J98.09
    - congenital Q32.3
    - syphilitic A52.72
  - cardia (stomach) K22.2
    - congenital Q39.3
  - cardiac —*see also* Disease, heart
    - orifice (stomach) K22.2
  - cecum —*see* Obstruction, intestine
  - cervix, cervical (canal) N88.2
    - congenital Q51.828
    - in pregnancy —*see* Pregnancy, complicated by, abnormal cervix
      - causing obstructed labor O65.5
  - colon —*see also* Obstruction, intestine
    - congenital Q42.9
      - specified NEC Q42.8
  - colostomy K94.03
  - common (bile) duct K83.1
  - coronary (artery) —*see* Disease, heart, ischemic, atherosclerotic
  - cystic duct —*see* Obstruction, gallbladder
  - digestive organs NEC, congenital Q45.8
  - duodenum K31.5
    - congenital Q41.0
  - ear canal (external) (congenital) Q16.1
    - acquired —*see* Stricture, auditory canal, acquired
  - ejaculatory duct N50.89
  - enterostomy K94.13
  - esophagus K22.2
    - congenital Q39.3
    - syphilitic A52.79
      - congenital A50.59 *[K23]*
  - eustachian tube —*see also* Obstruction, eustachian tube
    - congenital Q17.8
  - fallopian tube N97.1
    - gonococcal A54.24
    - tuberculous A18.17
  - gallbladder —*see* Obstruction, gallbladder
  - glottis J38.6
  - heart —*see also* Disease, heart
    - valve (*see also* Endocarditis) I38
      - aortic Q23.0
      - mitral Q23.2
      - pulmonary Q22.1
      - tricuspid Q22.4
  - hepatic duct K83.1
  - hourglass, of stomach K31.2
  - hymen N89.6
  - hypopharynx J39.2
  - ileum (*see also* Obstruction, intestine, specified NEC) K56.699
    - congenital Q41.2
  - intestine —*see also* Obstruction, intestine
    - congenital (small) Q41.9
      - large Q42.9
        - specified NEC Q42.8
      - specified NEC Q41.8
    - ischemic K55.1

Stricture *(continued)*

  - jejunum (*see also* Obstruction, intestine, specified NEC) K56.699
    - congenital Q41.1
  - lacrimal passages —*see also* Stenosis, lacrimal
    - congenital Q10.5
  - larynx J38.6
    - congenital NEC Q31.8
      - subglottic Q31.1
    - syphilitic A52.73
      - congenital A50.59 *[J99]*
  - meatus
    - ear (congenital) Q16.1
      - acquired —*see* Stricture, auditory canal, acquired
    - osseous (ear) (congenital) Q16.1
      - acquired —*see* Stricture, auditory canal, acquired
    - urinarius —*see also* Stricture, urethra
      - congenital Q64.33
  - mitral (valve) —*see* Stenosis, mitral
  - myocardium, myocardial I51.5
    - hypertrophic subaortic (idiopathic) I42.1
  - nares (anterior) (posterior) J34.89
    - congenital Q30.0
  - nasal duct —*see also* Stenosis, lacrimal, duct
    - congenital Q10.5
  - nasolacrimal duct —*see also* Stenosis, lacrimal, duct
    - congenital Q10.5
  - nasopharynx J39.2
    - syphilitic A52.73
  - nose J34.89
    - congenital Q30.0
  - nostril (anterior) (posterior) J34.89
    - congenital Q30.0
    - syphilitic A52.73
      - congenital A50.59 *[J99]*
  - organ or site, congenital NEC —*see* Atresia, by site
  - os uteri —*see* Stricture, cervix
  - osseous meatus (ear) (congenital) Q16.1
    - acquired —*see* Stricture, auditory canal, acquired
  - oviduct —*see* Stricture, fallopian tube
  - pelviureteric junction (congenital) Q62.11
    - acquired, with hydronephrosis N13.0
  - penis, by foreign body T19.4
  - pharynx J39.2
  - prostate N42.89
  - pulmonary, pulmonic
    - artery (congenital) Q25.6
      - acquired I28.8
      - noncongenital I28.8
    - infundibulum (congenital) Q24.3
    - valve I37.0
      - congenital Q22.1
    - vein, acquired I28.8
    - vessel NEC I28.8
  - punctum lacrimale —*see also* Stenosis, lacrimal, punctum
    - congenital Q10.5
  - pylorus (hypertrophic) K31.1
    - adult K31.1
    - congenital Q40.0
    - infantile Q40.0
  - rectosigmoid (*see also* Obstruction, intestine, specified NEC) K56.699

Stricture *(continued)*

  - rectum (sphincter) K62.4
    - congenital Q42.1
      - with fistula Q42.0
    - due to
      - chlamydial lymphogranuloma A55
      - irradiation K91.89
      - lymphogranuloma venereum A55
    - gonococcal A54.6
    - inflammatory (chlamydial) A55
    - syphilitic A52.74
    - tuberculous A18.32
  - renal artery I70.1
    - congenital Q27.1
  - salivary duct or gland (any) K11.8
  - sigmoid (flexure) —*see* Obstruction, intestine
  - spermatic cord N50.89
  - stoma (following) (of)
    - colostomy K94.03
    - enterostomy K94.13
    - gastrostomy K94.23
    - ileostomy K94.13
    - tracheostomy J95.03
  - stomach K31.89
    - congenital Q40.2
    - hourglass K31.2
  - subaortic Q24.4
    - hypertrophic (acquired) (idiopathic) I42.1
  - subglottic J38.6
  - syphilitic NEC A52.79
  - trachea J39.8
    - congenital Q32.1
    - syphilitic A52.73
    - tuberculous NEC A15.5
  - tracheostomy J95.03
  - tricuspid (valve) —*see* Stenosis, tricuspid
  - tunica vaginalis N50.89
  - ureter (postoperative) N13.5
    - with
      - hydronephrosis N13.1
        - with infection N13.6
      - pyelonephritis (chronic) N11.1
    - congenital —*see* Atresia, ureter
    - tuberculous A18.11
  - ureteropelvic junction (congenital) Q62.11
    - acquired, with hydronephrosis N13.0
  - ureterovesical orifice N13.5
    - with infection N13.6
  - urethra (organic) (spasmodic) (*see also* Stricture, urethra, male) N35.919
    - associated with schistosomiasis B65.0 *[N37]*
    - congenital Q64.39
      - valvular (posterior) Q64.2
    - due to
      - infection —*see* Stricture, urethra, postinfective
      - trauma —*see* Stricture, urethra, post-traumatic
    - female N35.92
    - gonococcal, gonorrheal A54.01
    - infective NEC —*see* Stricture, urethra, postinfective
    - late effect (sequelae) of injury —*see* Stricture, urethra, post-traumatic
    - male N35.919
      - anterior urethra N35.914
      - bulbous urethra N35.912
      - meatal N35.911
      - membranous urethra N35.913
      - overlapping site N35.916

Stricture *(continued)*
urethra *(continued)*
postcatheterization —*see* Stricture, urethra, postprocedural
postinfective NEC
female N35.12
male N35.119
anterior urethra N35.114
bulbous urethra N35.112
meatal N35.111
membranous urethra N35.113
overlapping sites N35.116
postobstetric N35.021
postoperative —*see* Stricture, urethra, postprocedural
postprocedural
female N99.12
male N99.114
anterior bulbous urethra N99.113
bulbous urethra N99.111
fossa navicularis N99.115
meatal N99.110
membranous urethra N99.112
overlapping sites N99.116
post-traumatic
female N35.028
due to childbirth N35.021
male N35.014
anterior urethra N35.013
bulbous urethra N35.011
meatal N35.010
membranous urethra N35.012
overlapping sites N35.016
sequela (late effect) of
childbirth N35.021
injury —*see* Stricture, urethra, post-traumatic
specified cause NEC
female N35.82
male N35.819
anterior urethra N35.814
bulbous urethra N35.812
meatal N35.811
membranous urethra N35.813
overlapping site N35.816
syphilitic A52.76
traumatic —*see* Stricture, urethra, post-traumatic
valvular (posterior), congenital Q64.2
urinary meatus —*see* Stricture, urethra
uterus, uterine (synechiae) N85.6
os (external) (internal) —*see* Stricture, cervix
vagina (outlet) —*see* Stenosis, vagina
valve (cardiac) (heart) —*see also* Endocarditis
congenital
aortic Q23.0
mitral Q23.2
pulmonary Q22.1
tricuspid Q22.4
vas deferens N50.89
congenital Q55.4
vein I87.1
vena cava (inferior) (superior) NEC I87.1
congenital Q26.0
vesicourethral orifice N32.0
congenital Q64.31
vulva (acquired) N90.5

Stridor R06.1
congenital (larynx) P28.89

Stridulous —*see* condition

Stroke (apoplectic) (brain) (embolic) (ischemic) (paralytic) (thrombotic) I63.9
cerebral, perinatal P91.82-
cryptogenic (*see also* Infarction, cerebral) I63.9
epileptic —*see* Epilepsy
heat T67.01
exertional T67.02
specified NEC T67.09
in evolution I63.9
intraoperative
during cardiac surgery I97.810
during other surgery I97.811
ischemic, perinatal arterial P91.82-
lightning —*see* Lightning
meaning
cerebral hemorrhage - code to Hemorrhage, intracranial
cerebral infarction - code to Infarction, cerebral
neonatal P91.82-
postprocedural
following cardiac surgery I97.820
following other surgery I97.821
sun T67.01
specified NEC T67.09
unspecified (NOS) I63.9

Stromatosis, endometrial D39.0

Strongyloidiasis, strongyloidosis B78.9
cutaneous B78.1
disseminated B78.7
intestinal B78.0

Strophulus pruriginosus L28.2

Struck by lightning —*see* Lightning

Struma —*see also* Goiter
Hashimoto E06.3
lymphomatosa E06.3
nodosa (simplex) E04.9
endemic E01.2
multinodular E01.1
multinodular E04.2
iodine-deficiency related E01.1
toxic or with hyperthyroidism E05.20
with thyroid storm E05.21
multinodular E05.20
with thyroid storm E05.21
uninodular E05.10
with thyroid storm E05.11
toxicosa E05.20
with thyroid storm E05.21
multinodular E05.20
with thyroid storm E05.21
uninodular E05.10
with thyroid storm E05.11
uninodular E04.1
ovarii D27.-
Riedel's E06.5

Strumipriva cachexia E03.4

Strümpell-Marie spine —*see* Spondylitis, ankylosing

Strümpell-Westphal pseudosclerosis E83.01

Stuart deficiency disease (factor X) D68.2

Stuart-Prower factor deficiency (factor X) D68.2

Student's elbow —*see* Bursitis, elbow, olecranon

Stump —*see* Amputation

Stunting, nutritional E45

Stupor (catatonic) R40.1
depressive (single episode) F32.89
recurrent episode F33.8
dissociative F44.2
manic F30.2
manic-depressive F31.89
psychogenic (anergic) F44.2
reaction to exceptional stress (transient) F43.0

Sturge (-Weber) (-Dimitri) (-Kalischer) **disease or syndrome** Q85.8

Stuttering F80.81
adult onset F98.5
childhood onset F80.81
following cerebrovascular disease —*see* Disorder, fluency. following cerebrovascular disease
in conditions classified elsewhere R47.82

Sty, stye (external) (internal) (meibomian) (zeisian) —*see* Hordeolum

Subacidity, gastric K31.89
psychogenic F45.8

Subacute —*see* condition

Subarachnoid —*see* condition

Subcortical —*see* condition

Subcostal syndrome, nerve compression —*see* Mononeuropathy, upper limb, specified site NEC

Subcutaneous, subcuticular —*see* condition

Subdural —*see* condition

Subendocardium —*see* condition

Subependymoma
specified site —*see* Neoplasm, uncertain behavior, by site
unspecified site D43.2

Suberosis J67.3

Subglossitis —*see* Glossitis

Subhemophilia D66

Subinvolution
breast (postlactational) (postpuerperal) N64.89
puerperal O90.89
uterus (chronic) (nonpuerperal) N85.3
puerperal O90.89

Sublingual —*see* condition

Sublinguitis —*see* Sialoadenitis

Subluxatable hip Q65.6

Subluxation —*see also* Dislocation
acromioclavicular S43.11-
ankle S93.0-
atlantoaxial, recurrent M43.4
with myelopathy M43.3
carpometacarpal (joint) NEC S63.05-
thumb S63.04-
complex, vertebral —*see* Complex, subluxation
congenital —*see also* Malposition, congenital
hip —*see* Dislocation, hip, congenital, partial
joint (excluding hip)
lower limb Q68.8
shoulder Q68.8
upper limb Q68.8
elbow (traumatic) S53.10-
anterior S53.11-
lateral S53.14-

Subluxation *(continued)*
elbow *(continued)*
medial S53.13-
posterior S53.12-
specified type NEC S53.19-
finger S63.20-
index S63.20-
interphalangeal S63.22-
distal S63.24-
index S63.24-
little S63.24-
middle S63.24-
ring S63.24-
index S63.22-
little S63.22-
middle S63.22-
proximal S63.23-
index S63.23-
little S63.23-
middle S63.23-
ring S63.23-
ring S63.22-
little S63.20-
metacarpophalangeal S63.21-
index S63.21-
little S63.21-
middle S63.21-
ring S63.21-
middle S63.20-
ring S63.20-
foot S93.30-
specified site NEC S93.33-
tarsal joint S93.31-
tarsometatarsal joint S93.32-
toe —*see* Subluxation, toe
hip S73.00-
anterior S73.03-
obturator S73.02-
central S73.04-
posterior S73.01-
interphalangeal (joint)
finger S63.22-
distal joint S63.24-
index S63.24-
little S63.24-
middle S63.24-
ring S63.24-
index S63.22-
little S63.22-
middle S63.22-
proximal joint S63.23-
index S63.23-
little S63.23-
middle S63.23-
ring S63.23-
ring S63.22-
thumb S63.12-
toe S93.13-
great S93.13-
lesser S93.13-
joint prosthesis —*see* Complications, joint prosthesis, mechanical, displacement, by site
knee S83.10-
cap —*see* Subluxation, patella
patella —*see* Subluxation, patella
proximal tibia
anteriorly S83.11-
laterally S83.14-
medially S83.13-
posteriorly S83.12-
specified type NEC S83.19-
lens —*see* Dislocation, lens, partial
ligament, traumatic —*see* Sprain, by site
metacarpal (bone)
proximal end S63.06-

Subluxation *(continued)*
- metacarpophalangeal (joint)
  - finger S63.21-
    - index S63.21-
    - little S63.21-
    - middle S63.21-
    - ring S63.21-
  - thumb S63.11-
- metatarsophalangeal joint S93.14-
  - great toe S93.14-
  - lesser toe S93.14-
- midcarpal (joint) S63.03-
- patella S83.00-
  - lateral S83.01-
  - recurrent (nontraumatic) —*see* Dislocation, patella, recurrent, incomplete
  - specified type NEC S83.09-
- pathological —*see* Dislocation, pathological
- radial head S53.00-
  - anterior S53.01-
  - nursemaid's elbow S53.03-
  - posterior S53.02-
  - specified type NEC S53.09-
- radiocarpal (joint) S63.02-
- radioulnar (joint)
  - distal S63.01-
  - proximal —*see* Subluxation, elbow
- shoulder
  - congenital Q68.8
  - girdle S43.30-
    - scapula S43.31-
    - specified site NEC S43.39-
  - traumatic S43.00-
    - anterior S43.01-
    - inferior S43.03-
    - posterior S43.02-
    - specified type NEC S43.08-
- sternoclavicular (joint) S43.20-
  - anterior S43.21-
  - posterior S43.22-
- symphysis (pubis)
- thumb S63.103
  - interphalangeal joint —*see* Subluxation, interphalangeal (joint), thumb
  - metacarpophalangeal joint —*see* Subluxation, metacarpophalangeal (joint), thumb
- toe(s) S93.10-
  - great S93.10-
    - interphalangeal joint S93.13-
    - metatarsophalangeal joint S93.14-
  - interphalangeal joint S93.13-
  - lesser S93.10-
    - interphalangeal joint S93.13-
    - metatarsophalangeal joint S93.14-
  - metatarsophalangeal joint S93.149
- ulna
  - distal end S63.07-
  - proximal end —*see* Subluxation, elbow
- ulnohumeral joint —*see* Subluxation, elbow
- vertebral
  - recurrent NEC —*see* subcategory M43.5
  - traumatic
    - cervical S13.100
      - atlantoaxial joint S13.120
      - atlantooccipital joint S13.110
      - atloidooccipital joint S13.110

Subluxation *(continued)*
- vertebral *(continued)*
  - traumatic *(continued)*
    - cervical *(continued)*
      - joint between
        - C0 and C1 S13.110
        - C1 and C2 S13.120
        - C2 and C3 S13.130
        - C3 and C4 S13.140
        - C4 and C5 S13.150
        - C5 and C6 S13.160
        - C6 and C7 S13.170
        - C7 and T1 S13.180
      - occipitoatloid joint S13.110
    - lumbar S33.100
      - joint between
        - L1 and L2 S33.110
        - L2 and L3 S33.120
        - L3 and L4 S33.130
        - L4 and L5 S33.140
    - thoracic S23.100
      - joint between
        - T1 and T2 S23.110
        - T2 and T3 S23.120
        - T3 and T4 S23.122
        - T4 and T5 S23.130
        - T5 and T6 S23.132
        - T6 and T7 S23.140
        - T7 and T8 S23.142
        - T8 and T9 S23.150
        - T9 and T10 S23.152
        - T10 and T11 S23.160
        - T11 and T12 S23.162
        - T12 and L1 S23.170
- wrist (carpal bone) S63.00-
  - carpometacarpal joint —*see* Subluxation, carpometacarpal (joint)
  - distal radioulnar joint —*see* Subluxation, radioulnar (joint), distal
  - metacarpal bone, proximal —*see* Subluxation, metacarpal (bone), proximal end
  - midcarpal —*see* Subluxation, midcarpal (joint)
  - radiocarpal joint —*see* Subluxation, radiocarpal (joint)
  - recurrent —*see* Dislocation, recurrent, wrist
  - specified site NEC S63.09-
  - ulna —*see* Subluxation, ulna, distal end

Submaxillary —*see* condition

Submersion (fatal) (nonfatal) T75.1

Submucous —*see* condition

Subnormal, subnormality
- accommodation (old age) H52.4
- mental —*see* Disability, intellectual
- temperature (accidental) T68

Subphrenic —*see* condition

Subscapular nerve —*see* condition

Subseptus uterus Q51.28

Subsiding appendicitis K36

Substance (other psychoactive) -induced
- anxiety disorder F19.980
- bipolar and related disorder F19.94
- delirium F19.921
- depressive disorder F19.94
- major neurocognitive disorder F19.97
- mild neurocognitive disorder F19.988
- obsessive-compulsive and related disorder F19.988
- psychotic disorder F19.959

Substance *(continued)*
- sexual dysfunction F19.981
- sleep disorder F19.982

Substernal thyroid E04.9
- congenital Q89.2

Substitution disorder F44.9

Subtentorial —*see* condition

Subthyroidism (acquired) —*see also* Hypothyroidism
- congenital E03.1

Succenturiate placenta O43.19-

Sucking thumb, child (excessive) F98.8

Sudamen, sudamina L74.1

Sudanese kala-azar B55.0

Sudden
- heart failure —*see* Failure, heart
- hearing loss —*see* Deafness, sudden

Sudeck's atrophy, disease, or syndrome —*see* Algoneurodystrophy

Suffocation —*see* Asphyxia, traumatic

Sugar
- blood
  - high (transient) R73.9
  - low (transient) E16.2
- in urine R81

Suicide, suicidal (attempted) T14.91
- by poisoning —*see* Table of Drugs and Chemicals
- history of (personal) Z91.51
  - in family Z81.8
- ideation —*see* Ideation, suicidal
- risk
  - meaning personal history of attempted suicide Z91.51
  - meaning suicidal ideation —*see* Ideation, suicidal
- tendencies
  - meaning personal history of attempted suicide Z91.51
  - meaning suicidal ideation —*see* Ideation, suicidal
- trauma —*see* nature of injury by site

Suipestifer infection —*see* Infection, salmonella

Sulfhemoglobinemia, sulphemoglobinemia (acquired) (with methemoglobinemia) D74.8

Sumatran mite fever A75.3

Summer —*see* condition

Sunburn L55.9
- due to
  - tanning bed (acute) L56.8
    - chronic L57.8
  - ultraviolet radiation (acute) L56.8
    - chronic L57.8
- first degree L55.0
- second degree L55.1
- third degree L55.2

SUNCT (short lasting unilateral neuralgiform headache with conjunctival injection and tearing) G44.059
- intractable G44.051
- not intractable G44.059

Sundowning F05

Sunken acetabulum —*see* Derangement, joint, specified type NEC, hip

Sunstroke T67.01
- specified NEC T67.09

Superfecundation —*see* Pregnancy, multiple

Superfetation —*see* Pregnancy, multiple

Superinvolution (uterus) N85.8

Supernumerary (congenital)
- aortic cusps Q23.8
- auditory ossicles Q16.3
- bone Q79.8
- breast Q83.1
- carpal bones Q74.0
- cusps, heart valve NEC Q24.8
  - aortic Q23.8
  - mitral Q23.2
  - pulmonary Q22.3
- digit(s) Q69.9
- ear (lobule) Q17.0
- fallopian tube Q50.6
- finger Q69.0
- hymen Q52.4
- kidney Q63.0
- lacrimonasal duct Q10.6
- lobule (ear) Q17.0
- mitral cusps Q23.2
- muscle Q79.8
- nipple(s) Q83.3
- organ or site not listed —*see* Accessory
- ossicles, auditory Q16.3
- ovary Q50.31
- oviduct Q50.6
- pulmonary, pulmonic cusps Q22.3
- rib Q76.6
  - cervical or first (syndrome) Q76.5
- roots (of teeth) K00.2
- spleen Q89.09
- tarsal bones Q74.2
- teeth K00.1
- testis Q55.29
- thumb Q69.1
- toe Q69.2
- uterus Q51.28
- vagina Q52.1
- vertebra Q76.49

Supervision (of)
- contraceptive —*see* Prescription, contraceptives
- dietary (for) Z71.3
  - allergy (food) Z71.3
  - colitis Z71.3
  - diabetes mellitus Z71.3
  - food allergy or intolerance Z71.3
  - gastritis Z71.3
  - hypercholesterolemia Z71.3
  - hypoglycemia Z71.3
  - intolerance (food) Z71.3
  - obesity Z71.3
  - specified NEC Z71.3
- healthy infant or child Z76.2
  - foundling Z76.1
- high-risk pregnancy —*see* Pregnancy, complicated by, high, risk
- lactation Z39.1
- pregnancy —*see* Pregnancy, supervision of

Supplemental teeth K00.1

Suppression
- binocular vision H53.34
- lactation O92.5
- menstruation N94.89
- ovarian secretion E28.39
- renal N28.9
- urine, urinary secretion R34

Suppuration, suppurative *—see also* condition
- accessory sinus (chronic) *—see* Sinusitis
- adrenal gland
- antrum (chronic) *—see* Sinusitis, maxillary
- bladder *—see* Cystitis
- brain G06.0
  - sequelae G09
- breast N61.1
  - puerperal, postpartum or gestational *—see* Mastitis, obstetric, purulent
- dental periosteum M27.3
- ear (middle) *—see also* Otitis, media
  - external NEC *—see* Otitis, externa, infective
  - internal *—see* subcategory H83.0
- ethmoidal (chronic) (sinus) *—see* Sinusitis, ethmoidal
- fallopian tube *—see* Salpingo-oophoritis
- frontal (chronic) (sinus) *—see* Sinusitis, frontal
- gallbladder (acute) K81.0
- gum K05.20
  - generalized *—see* Periodontitis, aggressive, generalized
  - localized *—see* Periodontitis, aggressive, localized
- intracranial G06.0
- joint *—see* Arthritis, pyogenic or pyemic
- labyrinthine *—see* subcategory H83.0
- lung *—see* Abscess, lung
- mammary gland N61.1
  - puerperal, postpartum O91.12
    - associated with lactation O91.13
- maxilla, maxillary M27.2
  - sinus (chronic) *—see* Sinusitis, maxillary
- muscle *—see* Myositis, infective
- nasal sinus (chronic) *—see* Sinusitis
- pancreas, acute (*see also* Pancreatitis, acute) K85.80
- parotid gland *—see* Sialoadenitis
- pelvis, pelvic
  - female *—see* Disease, pelvis, inflammatory
  - male K65.0
- pericranial *—see* Osteomyelitis
- salivary duct or gland (any) *—see* Sialoadenitis
- sinus (accessory) (chronic) (nasal) *—see* Sinusitis
- sphenoidal sinus (chronic) *—see* Sinusitis, sphenoidal
- thymus (gland) E32.1
- thyroid (gland) E06.0
- tonsil *—see* Tonsillitis
- uterus *—see* Endometritis

Supraeruption of tooth (teeth) M26.34

Supraglottitis J04.30
- with obstruction J04.31

Suprarenal (gland) *—see* condition

Suprascapular nerve *—see* condition

Suprasellar *—see* condition

Surfer's knots or nodules S89.8-

Surgical
- emphysema T81.82

Surgical *(continued)*
- procedures, complication or misadventure *—see* Complications, surgical procedures
- shock T81.10

Surveillance (of) (for) *—see also* Observation
- alcohol abuse Z71.41
- contraceptive *—see* Prescription, contraceptives
- dietary Z71.3
- drug abuse Z71.51

Susceptibility to disease, genetic Z15.89
- malignant neoplasm Z15.09
  - breast Z15.01
  - endometrium Z15.04
  - ovary Z15.02
  - prostate Z15.03
  - specified NEC Z15.09
- multiple endocrine neoplasia Z15.81

Suspected condition, ruled out *— see also* Observation, suspected
- amniotic cavity and membrane Z03.71
- cervical shortening Z03.75
- fetal anomaly Z03.73
- fetal growth Z03.74
- maternal and fetal conditions NEC Z03.79
- newborn (*see also* Observation, newborn, suspected condition ruled out) Z05.9
- oligohydramnios Z03.71
- placental problem Z03.72
- polyhydramnios Z03.71

Suspended uterus
- in pregnancy or childbirth *—see* Pregnancy, complicated by, abnormal uterus

Sutton's nevus D22.9

Suture
- burst (in operation wound) T81.31
  - external operation wound T81.31
  - internal operation wound T81.32
- inadvertently left in operation wound *—see* Foreign body, accidentally left during a procedure
- removal Z48.02

Swab inadvertently left in operation wound *—see* Foreign body, accidentally left during a procedure

Swallowed, swallowing
- difficulty *—see* Dysphagia
- foreign body *—see* Foreign body, alimentary tract

Swan-neck deformity (finger) *—see* Deformity, finger, swan-neck

Swearing, compulsive F42.8
- in Gilles de la Tourette's syndrome F95.2

Sweat, sweats
- fetid L75.0
- night R61

Sweating, excessive R61

Sweeley-Klionsky disease E75.21

Sweet's disease or dermatosis L98.2

Swelling (of) R60.9
- abdomen, abdominal (not referable to any particular organ) *—see* Mass, abdominal
- ankle *—see* Effusion, joint, ankle
- arm M79.89
  - forearm M79.89

Swelling *(continued)*
- breast (*see also* Lump, breast) N63.0
- Calabar B74.3
- cervical gland R59.0
- chest, localized R22.2
- ear H93.8-
- extremity (lower) (upper) *—see* Disorder, soft tissue, specified type NEC
- finger M79.89
- foot M79.89
- glands R59.9
  - generalized R59.1
  - localized R59.0
- hand M79.89
- head (localized) R22.0
- inflammatory *—see* Inflammation
- intra-abdominal *—see* Mass, abdominal
- joint *—see* Effusion, joint
- leg M79.89
  - lower M79.89
- limb *—see* Disorder, soft tissue, specified type NEC
- localized (skin) R22.9
  - chest R22.2
  - head R22.0
  - limb
    - lower *—see* Mass, localized, limb, lower
    - upper *—see* Mass, localized, limb, upper
  - neck R22.1
  - trunk R22.2
- neck (localized) R22.1
- pelvic *—see* Mass, abdominal
- scrotum N50.89
- splenic *—see* Splenomegaly
- testis N50.89
- toe M79.89
- umbilical R19.09
- wandering, due to Gnathostoma (spinigerum) B83.1
- white *—see* Tuberculosis, arthritis

Swift (-Feer) **disease**
- overdose or wrong substance given or taken *—see* Table of Drugs and Chemicals, by drug, poisoning

Swimmer's
- cramp T75.1
- ear H60.33-
- itch B65.3

Swimming in the head R42

Swollen *—see* Swelling

Swyer syndrome Q99.1

Sycosis L73.8
- barbae (not parasitic) L73.8
- contagiosa (mycotic) B35.0
- lupoides L73.8
- mycotic B35.0
- parasitic B35.0
- vulgaris L73.8

Sydenham's chorea *—see* Chorea, Sydenham's

Sylvatic yellow fever A95.0

Sylvest's disease B33.0

Symblepharon H11.23-
- congenital Q10.3

Symond's syndrome G93.2

Sympathetic *—see* condition

Sympatheticotonia G90.8

Sympathicoblastoma
- specified site *—see* Neoplasm, malignant, by site
- unspecified site C74.90

Sympathogonioma *—see* Sympathicoblastoma

Symphalangy (fingers) (toes) Q70.9

Symptoms NEC R68.89
- breast NEC N64.59
- cold J00
- development NEC R63.8
- factitious, self-induced *—see* Disorder, factitious
- genital organs, female R10.2
- involving
  - abdomen NEC R19.8
  - appearance NEC R46.89
  - awareness R41.9
    - altered mental status R41.82
    - amnesia *—see* Amnesia
    - borderline intellectual functioning R41.83
    - coma *—see* Coma
    - disorientation R41.0
    - neurologic neglect syndrome R41.4
    - senile cognitive decline R41.81
    - specified symptom NEC R41.89
  - behavior NEC R46.89
  - cardiovascular system NEC R09.89
  - chest NEC R09.89
  - circulatory system NEC R09.89
  - cognitive functions R41.9
    - altered mental status R41.82
    - amnesia *—see* Amnesia
    - borderline intellectual functioning R41.83
    - coma *—see* Coma
    - disorientation R41.0
    - neurologic neglect syndrome R41.4
    - senile cognitive decline R41.81
    - specified symptom NEC R41.89
  - development NEC R62.50
  - digestive system NEC R19.8
  - emotional state NEC R45.89
    - emotional lability R45.86
  - food and fluid intake R63.8
  - general perceptions and sensations R44.9
    - specified NEC R44.8
  - musculoskeletal system R29.91
    - specified NEC R29.898
  - nervous system R29.90
    - specified NEC R29.818
  - pelvis NEC R19.8
  - respiratory system NEC R09.89
  - skin and integument R23.9
  - urinary system R39.9
- menopausal N95.1
- metabolism NEC R63.8
- neurotic F48.8
- of infancy R68.19
- pelvis NEC, female R10.2
- skin and integument NEC R23.9
- subcutaneous tissue NEC R23.9
- viral cold J00

Sympus Q74.2

Syncephalus Q89.4

Synchondrosis
- abnormal (congenital) Q78.8
- ischiopubic M91.0

Synchysis (scintillans) (senile) (vitreous body) H43.89

Syncope (near) (pre-) R55
- anginosa I20.8
- bradycardia R00.1
- cardiac R55

Syncope *(continued)*
  carotid sinus G90.01
  due to spinal (lumbar) puncture G97.1
  heart R55
  heat T67.1
  laryngeal R05.4
  psychogenic F48.8
  tussive R05.8
  vasoconstriction R55
  vasodepressor R55
  vasomotor R55
  vasovagal R55

Syndactylism, syndactyly Q70.9
  complex (with synostosis)
    fingers Q70.0-
    toes Q70.2-
  simple (without synostosis)
    fingers Q70.1-
    toes Q70.3-

Syndrome —*see also* Disease
  5q minus NOS D46.C
  48, XXXX Q97.1
  49, XXXXX Q97.1
  abdominal
    acute R10.0
    muscle deficiency Q79.4
  abnormal innervation H02.519
    left H02.516
      lower H02.515
      upper H02.514
    right H02.513
      lower H02.512
      upper H02.511
  abstinence, neonatal P96.1
  acid pulmonary aspiration, obstetric O74.0
  acquired immunodeficiency —*see* Human, immunodeficiency virus (HIV) disease
  acute abdominal R10.0
  acute respiratory distress (adult) (child) J80
    idiopathic J84.114
  Adair-Dighton Q78.0
  Adams-Stokes (-Morgagni) I45.9
  adiposogenital E23.6
  adrenal
    hemorrhage (meningococcal) A39.1
    meningococcic A39.1
  adrenocortical —*see* Cushing's, syndrome
  adrenogenital E25.9
    congenital, associated with enzyme deficiency E25.0
  afferent loop NEC K91.89
  Alagille's Q44.7
  alcohol withdrawal (without convulsions) —*see* Dependence, alcohol, with, withdrawal
  Alder's D72.0
  Aldrich (-Wiskott) D82.0
  alien hand R41.4
  Alport Q87.81
  alveolar hypoventilation E66.2
  alveolocapillary block J84.10
  amnesic, amnestic (confabulatory) (due to) —*see* Disorder, amnesic
  amyostatic (Wilson's disease) E83.01
  androgen insensitivity E34.50
    complete E34.51
    partial E34.52
  androgen resistance (*see also* Syndrome, androgen insensitivity) E34.50
  Angelman Q93.51
  anginal —*see* Angina
  ankyloglossia superior Q38.1

Syndrome *(continued)*
  anterior
    chest wall R07.89
    cord G83.82
    spinal artery G95.19
      compression M47.019
        cervical region M47.012
        cervicothoracic region M47.013
        lumbar region M47.016
        occipito-atlanto-axial region M47.011
        thoracic region M47.014
        thoracolumbar region M47.015
    tibial M76.81-
  antibody deficiency D80.9
    agammaglobulinemic D80.1
      hereditary D80.0
    congenital D80.0
    hypogammaglobulinemic D80.1
      hereditary D80.0
  anticardiolipin (-antibody) D68.61
  antidepressant discontinuation T43.205
  antiphospholipid (-antibody) D68.61
  aortic
    arch M31.4
    bifurcation I74.09
  aortomesenteric duodenum occlusion K31.5
  apical ballooning (transient left ventricular) I51.81
  arcuate ligament I77.4
  argentaffin, argintaffinoma E34.0
  Arnold-Chiari —*see* Arnold-Chiari disease
  Arrillaga-Ayerza I27.0
  arterial tortuosity Q87.82
  arteriovenous steal T82.898-
  Asherman's N85.6
  aspiration, of newborn —*see* Aspiration, by substance, with pneumonia
    meconium P24.01
  ataxia-telangiectasia G11.3
  auriculotemporal G50.8
  autoerythrocyte sensitization (Gardner-Diamond) D69.2
  autoimmune polyglandular E31.0
  autoimmune lymphoproliferative [ALPS] D89.82
  autoinflammatory M04.9
    specified type NEC M04.8
  autosomal —*see* Abnormal, autosomes
  Avellis' G46.8
  Ayerza (-Arrillaga) I27.0
  Babinski-Nageotte G83.89
  Bakwin-Krida Q78.5
  bare lymphocyte D81.6
  Barré-Guillain G61.0
  Barré-Liéou M53.0
  Barrett's —*see* Barrett's, esophagus
  Barsony-Polgar K22.4
  Barsony-Teschendorf K22.4
  Barth E78.71
  Bartter's E26.81
  basal cell nevus Q87.89
  Basedow's E05.00
    with thyroid storm E05.01
  basilar artery G45.0
  Batten-Steinert G71.11
  battered
    baby or child —*see* Maltreatment, child, physical abuse
    spouse —*see* Maltreatment, adult, physical abuse
  Beals Q87.40
  Beau's I51.5

Syndrome *(continued)*
  Beck's I65.8
  Benedikt's G46.3
  Béquez César (-Steinbrinck-Chédiak-Higashi) E70.330
  Bernhardt-Roth —*see* Meralgia paresthetica
  Bernheim's —*see* Failure, heart, right
  big spleen D73.1
  bilateral polycystic ovarian E28.2
  Bing-Horton's —*see* Horton's headache
  Birt-Hogg-Dube syndrome Q87.89
  Björck (-Thorsen) E34.0
  black
    lung J60
    widow spider bite —*see* Toxicity, venom, spider, black widow
  Blackfan-Diamond D61.01
  Blau M04.8
  blind loop K90.2
    congenital Q43.8
    postsurgical K91.2
  blue sclera Q78.0
  blue toe I75.02-
  Boder-Sedgewick G11.3
  Boerhaave's K22.3
  Borjeson Forssman Lehmann Q89.8
  Bouillaud's I01.9
  Bourneville (-Pringle) Q85.1
  Bouveret (-Hoffman) I47.9
  brachial plexus G54.0
  bradycardia-tachycardia I49.5
  brain (nonpsychotic) F09
    with psychosis, psychotic reaction F09
    acute or subacute —*see* Delirium
    congenital —*see* Disability, intellectual
    organic F09
      post-traumatic (nonpsychotic) F07.81
      psychotic F09
    personality change F07.0
    postcontusional F07.81
    post-traumatic, nonpsychotic F07.81
    psycho-organic F09
    psychotic F06.8
  brain stem stroke G46.3
  Brandt's (acrodermatitis enteropathica) E83.2
  broad ligament laceration N83.8
  Brock's J98.11
  bronze baby P83.88
  Brown-Sequard G83.81
  Brugada I49.8
  bubbly lung P27.0
  Buchem's M85.2
  Budd-Chiari I82.0
  bulbar (progressive) G12.22
  Bürger-Grütz E78.3
  Burke's K86.89
  Burnett's (milk-alkali) E83.52
  burning feet E53.9
  Bywaters' T79.5
  Call-Fleming I67.841
  carbohydrate-deficient glycoprotein (CDGS) E77.8
  carcinogenic thrombophlebitis I82.1
  carcinoid E34.0
  cardiac asthma I50.1
  cardiacos negros I27.0
  cardiofaciocutaneous Q87.89
  cardiopulmonary-obesity E66.2
  cardiorenal —*see* Hypertension, cardiorenal

Syndrome *(continued)*
  cardiorespiratory distress (idiopathic), newborn P22.0
  cardiovascular renal —*see* Hypertension, cardiorenal
  carotid
    artery (hemispheric) (internal) G45.1
    body G90.01
    sinus G90.01
  carpal tunnel G56.0-
  Cassidy (-Scholte) E34.0
  cat cry Q93.4
  cat eye Q92.8
  cauda equina G83.4
  causalgia —*see* Causalgia
  celiac K90.0
    artery compression I77.4
    axis I77.4
  central pain G89.0
  cerebellar
    hereditary G11.9
    stroke G46.4
  cerebellomedullary malformation —*see* Spina bifida
  cerebral
    artery
      anterior G46.1
      middle G46.0
      posterior G46.2
    gigantism E22.0
  cervical (root) M53.1
    disc —*see* Disorder, disc, cervical, with neuritis
    fusion Q76.1
    posterior, sympathicus M53.0
    rib Q76.5
    sympathetic paralysis G90.2
  cervicobrachial (diffuse) M53.1
  cervicocranial M53.0
  cervicodorsal outlet G54.2
  cervicothoracic outlet G54.0
  Céstan (-Raymond) I65.8
  Charcot's (angina cruris) (intermittent claudication) I73.9
  Charcot-Weiss-Baker G90.09
  CHARGE Q89.8
  Chédiak-Higashi (-Steinbrinck) E70.330
  chest wall R07.1
  Chiari's (hepatic vein thrombosis) I82.0
  Chilaiditi's Q43.3
  child maltreatment —*see* Maltreatment, child
  chondrocostal junction M94.0
  chondroectodermal dysplasia Q77.6
  chromosome 4 short arm deletion Q93.3
  chromosome 5 short arm deletion Q93.4
  chronic
    infantile neurological, cutaneous and articular (CINCA) M04.2
    pain G89.4
      personality F68.8
  Churg-Strauss M30.1
  Clarke-Hadfield K86.89
  Clerambault's automatism G93.89
  Clouston's (hidrotic ectodermal dysplasia) Q82.4
  clumsiness, clumsy child F82
  cluster headache G44.009
    intractable G44.001
    not intractable G44.009
  Coffin-Lowry Q89.8
  cold injury (newborn) P80.0
  combined immunity deficiency D81.9

Syndrome *(continued)*
Gouley's I31.1
Gower's R55
gray or grey (newborn) P93.0
platelet D69.1
Gubler-Millard G46.3
Guillain-Barré (-Strohl) G61.0
gustatory sweating G50.8
Hadfield-Clarke K86.89
hair tourniquet *—see* Constriction, external, by site
Hamman's J98.19
hand-foot L27.1
hand-shoulder G90.8
hantavirus (cardio)-pulmonary (HPS) (HCPS) B33.4
happy puppet Q93.51
Harada's H30.81-
Hayem-Faber D50.9
headache NEC G44.89
complicated NEC G44.59
Heberden's I20.8
Hedinger's E34.0
Hegglin's D72.0
HELLP (hemolysis, elevated liver enzymes and low platelet count) O14.2-
complicating
childbirth O14.24
puerperium O14.25
hemolytic-uremic D59.3
hemophagocytic, infection-associated D76.2
Henoch-Schönlein D69.0
hepatic flexure K59.89
hepatopulmonary K76.81
hepatorenal K76.7
following delivery O90.4
postoperative or postprocedural K91.83
postpartum, puerperal O90.4
hepatourologic K76.7
hereditary alpha tryptasemia D89.44
Herter (-Gee) (nontropical sprue) K90.0
Heubner-Herter K90.0
Heyd's K76.7
Hilger's G90.09
histamine-like (fish poisoning) *—see* Poisoning, fish
histiocytic D76.3
histiocytosis NEC D76.3
HIV infection, acute B20
Hoffmann-Werdnig G12.0
Hollander-Simons E88.1
Hoppe-Goldflam G70.00
with exacerbation (acute) G70.01
in crisis G70.01
Horner's G90.2
hungry bone E83.81
hunterian glossitis D51.0
Hutchinson's triad A50.53
hyperabduction G54.0
hyperammonemia-hyperornithinemia-homocitrullinemia E72.4
hypereosinophilic (HES) D72.119
idiopathic (IHES) D72.110
lymphocytic variant (LHES) D72.111
myeloid D72.118
specified NEC D72.118
hyperimmunoglobulin D M04.1
hyperimmunoglobulin E (IgE) D82.4
hyperkalemic E87.5
hyperkinetic *—see* Hyperkinesia
hypermobility M35.7
hypernatremia E87.0
hyperosmolarity E87.0
hyperperfusion G97.82

Syndrome *(continued)*
hypersplenic D73.1
hypertransfusion, newborn P61.1
hyperventilation F45.8
hyperviscosity (of serum)
polycythemic D75.1
sclerothymic D58.8
hypoglycemic (familial) (neonatal) E16.2
hypokalemic E87.6
hyponatremic E87.1
hypopituitarism E23.0
hypoplastic left-heart Q23.4
hypopotassemia E87.6
hyposmolality E87.1
hypotension, maternal O26.5-
hypothenar hammer I73.89
hypoventilation, obesity (OHS) E66.2
ICF (intravascular coagulation-fibrinolysis) D65
idiopathic
cardiorespiratory distress, newborn P22.0
nephrotic (infantile) N04.9
iliotibial band M76.3-
immobility, immobilization (paraplegic) M62.3
immune effector cell-associated neurotoxicity (ICANS) G92.00
grade
1 G92.01
2 G92.02
3 G92.03
4 G92.04
5 G92.05
unspecified G92.00
immune reconstitution D89.3
immune reconstitution inflammatory [IRIS] D89.3
immunity deficiency, combined D81.9
immunodeficiency
acquired *—see* Human, immunodeficiency virus (HIV) disease
combined D81.9
impending coronary I20.0
impingement, shoulder M75.4-
inappropriate secretion of antidiuretic hormone E22.2
infant
of diabetic mother P70.1
gestational diabetes P70.0
infantilism (pituitary) E23.0
inferior vena cava I87.1
inspissated bile (newborn) P59.1
institutional (childhood) F94.2
insufficient sleep F51.12
intermediate coronary (artery) I20.0
interspinous ligament *—see* Spondylopathy, specified NEC
intestinal
carcinoid E34.0
knot K56.2
intravascular coagulation-fibrinolysis (ICF) D65
iodine-deficiency, congenital E00.9
type
mixed E00.2
myxedematous E00.1
neurological E00.0
IRDS (idiopathic respiratory distress, newborn) P22.0
irritable
bowel K58.9
with
constipation K58.1
diarrhea K58.0
mixed K58.2
psychogenic F45.8
specified NEC K58.8
heart (psychogenic) F45.8

Syndrome *(continued)*
irritable *(continued)*
weakness F48.8
ischemic
bowel (transient) K55.9
chronic K55.1
due to mesenteric artery insufficiency K55.1
steal T82.898
IVC (intravascular coagulopathy) D65
Ivemark's Q89.01
Jaccoud's *—see* Arthropathy, postrheumatic, chronic
Jackson's G83.89
Jakob-Creutzfeldt *—see* Creutzfeldt-Jakob disease or syndrome
jaw-winking Q07.8
Jervell-Lange-Nielsen I45.81
jet lag G47.25
Job's D71
Joseph-Diamond-Blackfan D61.01
jugular foramen G52.7
Kabuki Q89.8
Kanner's (autism) F84.0
Kartagener's Q89.3
Kelly's D50.1
Kimmelsteil-Wilson *—see* Diabetes, specified type, with Kimmelsteil-Wilson disease
Klein (e)-Levine G47.13
Klippel-Feil (brevicollis) Q76.1
Köhler-Pellegrini-Steida *—see* Bursitis, tibial collateral
König's K59.89
Korsakoff (-Wernicke) (nonalcoholic) F04
alcoholic F10.26
Kostmann's D70.0
Krabbe's congenital muscle hypoplasia Q79.8
labyrinthine H83.2
lacunar NEC G46.7
Lambert-Eaton G70.80
in
neoplastic disease G73.1
specified disease NEC G70.81
Landau-Kleffner *—see* Epilepsy, specified NEC
Larsen's Q74.8
lateral
cutaneous nerve of thigh G57.1-
medullary G46.4
Launois' E22.0
lazy
leukocyte D70.8
posture M62.3
Lemiere I80.8
Lennox-Gastaut G40.812
intractable G40.814
with status epilepticus G40.813
without status epilepticus G40.814
not intractable G40.812
with status epilepticus G40.811
without status epilepticus G40.812
lenticular, progressive E83.01
Leopold-Levi's E05.90
Lev's I44.2
Li-Fraumeni Z15.01
Lichtheim's D51.0
Lightwood's N25.89
Lignac (de Toni) (-Fanconi) (-Debré) E72.09
with cystinosis E72.04
Likoff's I20.8
limbic epilepsy personality F07.0
liver-kidney K76.7
lobotomy F07.0

Syndrome *(continued)*
Loffler's J82.89
long arm 18 or 21 deletion Q93.89
long QT I45.81
Louis-Barré G11.3
low
atmospheric pressure T70.29
back M54.50
output (cardiac) I50.9
lower radicular, newborn (birth injury) P14.8
Luetscher's (dehydration) E86.0
Lupus anticoagulant D68.62
Lutembacher's Q21.1
macrophage activation D76.1
due to infection D76.2
magnesium-deficiency R29.0
Majeed M04.8
Mal de Debarquement R42
malabsorption K90.9
postsurgical K91.2
malformation, congenital, due to
alcohol Q86.0
exogenous cause NEC Q86.8
hydantoin Q86.1
warfarin Q86.2
malignant
carcinoid E34.0
neuroleptic G21.0
Mallory-Weiss K22.6
mandibulofacial dysostosis Q75.4
manic-depressive *—see* Disorder, bipolar
maple-syrup-urine E71.0
Marable's I77.4
Marfan's Q87.40
with
cardiovascular manifestations Q87.418
aortic dilation Q87.410
ocular manifestations Q87.42
skeletal manifestations Q87.43
Marie's (acromegaly) E22.0
mast cell activation *—see* Activation, mast cell
maternal hypotension *—see* Syndrome, hypotension, maternal
May (-Hegglin) D72.0
McArdle (-Schmidt) (-Pearson) E74.04
McQuarrie's E16.2
meconium plug (newborn) P76.0
median arcuate ligament I77.4
Meekeren-Ehlers-Danlos Q79.6
megavitamin-B6 E67.2
Meige G24.4
MELAS E88.41
Mendelson's O74.0
MERRF (myoclonic epilepsy associated with ragged-red fibers) E88.42
mesenteric
artery (superior) K55.1
vascular insufficiency K55.1
metabolic E88.81
metastatic carcinoid E34.0
micrognathia-glossoptosis Q87.0
midbrain NEC G93.89
middle lobe (lung) J98.19
middle radicular G54.0
migraine (*see also* Migraine) G43.909-
Mikulicz' K11.8
milk-alkali E83.52
Millard-Gubler G46.3
Miller-Dieker Q93.88
Miller-Fisher G61.0
Minkowski-Chauffard D58.0
Mirizzi's K83.1

Syndrome *(continued)*
- MNGIE (Mitochondrial Neurogastrointestinal Encephalopathy) E88.49
- Möbius, ophthalmoplegic migraine —*see* Migraine, ophthalmoplegic
- monofixation H50.42
- Morel-Moore M85.2
- Morel-Morgagni M85.2
- Morgagni (-Morel) (-Stewart) M85.2
- Morgagni-Adams-Stokes I45.9
- Mounier-Kuhn Q32.4
  - with bronchiectasis J47.9
    - with
      - exacerbation (acute) J47.1
      - lower respiratory infection J47.0
  - acquired J98.09
    - with bronchiectasis J47.9
      - with
        - exacerbation (acute) J47.1
        - lower respiratory infection J47.0
- Muckle-Wells M04.2
- mucocutaneous lymph node (acute febrile) (MCLS) M30.3
- multiple endocrine neoplasia (MEN) —*see* Neoplasia, endocrine, multiple (MEN)
- multiple operations —*see* Disorder, factitious
- multisystem inflammatory (in adults) (in children) M35.81
- myasthenic G70.9
  - in
    - diabetes mellitus —*see* Diabetes, amyotrophy
    - endocrine disease NEC E34.9 *[G73.3]*
    - neoplastic disease (*see also* Neoplasm) D49.9 *[G73.3]*
    - thyrotoxicosis (hyperthyroidism) E05.90 *[G73.3]*
      - with thyroid storm E05.91 *[G73.3]*
- myelodysplastic D46.9
  - with
    - 5q deletion D46.C
    - isolated del (5q) chromosomal abnormality D46.C
    - multilineage dysplasia D46.A
      - with ringed sideroblasts D46.B
  - lesions, low grade D46.20
  - specified NEC D46.Z
- myeloid hypereosinophilic D72.118
- myelopathic pain G89.0
- myeloproliferative (chronic) D47.1
- myofascial pain M79.18
- Naffziger's G54.0
- nail patella Q87.2
- NARP (Neuropathy, Ataxia and Retinitis pigmentosa) E88.49
- neonatal abstinence P96.1
- nephritic —*see also* Nephritis
  - with edema —*see* Nephrosis
  - acute N00.9
  - chronic N03.9
  - rapidly progressive N01.9
- nephrotic (congenital) (*see also* Nephrosis) N04.9
  - with
    - C3
      - glomerulonephritis N04.A
      - glomerulopathy N04.A
        - with dense deposit disease N04.6

Syndrome *(continued)*
- nephrotic *(continued)*
  - with *(continued)*
    - dense deposit disease N04.6
    - diffuse
      - crescentic glomerulonephritis N04.7
      - endocapillary proliferative glomerulonephritis N04.4
      - membranous glomerulonephritis N04.2
      - mesangial proliferative glomerulonephritis N04.3
      - mesangiocapillary glomerulonephritis N04.5
    - focal and segmental glomerular lesions N04.1
    - minor glomerular abnormality N04.0
    - specified morphological changes NEC N04.8
  - diabetic —*see* Diabetes, nephrosis
- neurologic neglect R41.4
- Nezelof's D81.4
- Nonne-Milroy-Meige Q82.0
- Nothnagel's vasomotor acroparesthesia I73.89
- obesity hypoventilation (OHS) E66.2
- oculomotor H51.9
- Ogilvie K59.81
- ophthalmoplegia-cerebellar ataxia —*see* Strabismus, paralytic, third nerve
- oral allergy T78.1
- oral-facial-digital Q87.0
- organic
  - affective F06.30
  - amnesic (not alcohol- or drug-induced) F04
  - brain F09
  - depressive F06.31
  - hallucinosis F06.0
  - personality F07.0
- Ormond's N13.5
- oro-facial-digital Q87.0
- os trigonum Q68.8
- Osler-Weber-Rendu I78.0
- osteoporosis-osteomalacia M83.8
- Osterreicher-Turner Q87.2
- otolith —*see* subcategory H81.8
- oto-palatal-digital Q87.0
- outlet (thoracic) G54.0
- ovary
  - polycystic E28.2
  - resistant E28.39
  - sclerocystic E28.2
- Owren's D68.2
- Paget-Schroetter I82.890
- pain —*see also* Pain
  - complex regional I G90.50
    - lower limb G90.52-
    - specified site NEC G90.59
    - upper limb G90.51-
  - complex regional II —*see* Causalgia
- painful
  - bruising D69.2
  - feet E53.8
  - prostate N42.81
- paralysis agitans —*see* Parkinsonism
- paralytic G83.9
  - specified NEC G83.89
- Parinaud's H51.0
- parkinsonian —*see* Parkinsonism
- Parkinson's —*see* Parkinsonism
- paroxysmal facial pain G50.0
- Parry's E05.00
  - with thyroid storm E05.01
- Parsonage (-Aldren)-Turner G54.5

Syndrome *(continued)*
- patella clunk M25.86-
- Paterson (-Brown) (-Kelly) D50.1
- pectoral girdle I77.89
- pectoralis minor I77.89
- pediatric autoimmune neuropsychiatric disorders associated with streptococcal infections (PANDAS) D89.89
- Pelger-Huet D72.0
- pellagra-cerebellar ataxia-renal aminoaciduria E72.02
- pellagroid E52
- Pellegrini-Stieda —*see* Bursitis, tibial collateral
- pelvic congestion-fibrosis, female N94.89
- penta X Q97.1
- peptic ulcer —*see* Ulcer, peptic
- perabduction I77.89
- periodic fever M04.1
- periodic fever, aphthous stomatitis, pharyngitis, and adenopathy [PFAPA] M04.8
- periodic headache, in adults and children —*see* Headache, periodic syndromes in adults and children
- periurethral fibrosis N13.5
- phantom limb (without pain) G54.7
  - with pain G54.6
- pharyngeal pouch D82.1
- Pick's *see* Disease, Pick's
- Pickwickian E66.2
- PIE (pulmonary infiltration with eosinophilia) (*see also* Eosinophilia, pulmonary) J82.89
- pigmentary pallidal degeneration (progressive) G23.0
- pineal E34.8
- pituitary E22.0
- plantar fascia M72.2
- placental transfusion —*see* Pregnancy, complicated by, placental transfusion syndromes
- plateau iris (post-iridectomy) (postprocedural) H21.82
- Plummer-Vinson D50.1
- pluricarential of infancy E40
- plurideficiency E40
- pluriglandular (compensatory) E31.8
  - autoimmune E31.0
- pneumatic hammer T75.21
- polyangiitis overlap M30.8
- polycarential of infancy E40
- polyglandular E31.8
  - autoimmune E31.0
- polysplenia Q89.09
- pontine NEC G93.89
- popliteal
  - artery entrapment I77.89
  - web Q87.89
- postcardiac injury
  - postcardiotomy I97.0
  - postmyocardial infarction I24.1
- postcardiotomy I97.0
- post chemoembolization - code to associated conditions
- postcholecystectomy K91.5
- postcommissurotomy I97.0
- postconcussional F07.81
- postcontusional F07.81
- post-COVID (-19) U09.9
- postencephalitic F07.89
- post endometrial ablation N99.85
- posterior
  - cervical sympathetic M53.0
  - cord G83.83
  - fossa compression G93.5
  - reversible encephalopathy (PRES) I67.83
- postgastrectomy (dumping) K91.1

Syndrome *(continued)*
- postgastric surgery K91.1
- postinfarction I24.1
- postlaminectomy NEC M96.1
- postleukotomy F07.0
- postmastectomy lymphedema I97.2
- postmyocardial infarction I24.1
- postoperative NEC T81.9
  - blind loop K90.2
- postpartum panhypopituitary (Sheehan) E23.0
- postpolio (myelitic) G14
- postthrombotic I87.009
  - with
    - inflammation I87.02-
      - with ulcer I87.03-
    - specified complication NEC I87.09-
    - ulcer I87.01-
      - with inflammation I87.03-
  - asymptomatic I87.00-
- postvagotomy K91.1
- postvalvulotomy I97.0
- postviral NEC G93.3
  - fatigue G93.3
- Potain's K31.0
- potassium intoxication E87.5
- Prader-Willi Q87.11
- Prader-Willi-like Q87.19
- precerebral artery (multiple) (bilateral) G45.2
- preinfarction I20.0
- preleukemic D46.9
- premature senility E34.8
- premenstrual dysphoric F32.81
- premenstrual tension N94.3
- Prinzmetal-Massumi R07.1
- prune belly Q79.4
- pseudocarpal tunnel (sublimis) —*see* Syndrome, carpal tunnel
- pseudoparalytica G70.00
  - with exacerbation (acute) G70.01
  - in crisis G70.01
- pseudo -Turner's Q87.19
- psycho-organic (nonpsychotic severity) F07.9
  - acute or subacute F05
  - depressive type F06.31
  - hallucinatory type F06.0
  - nonpsychotic severity F07.0
  - specified NEC F07.89
- pulmonary
  - arteriosclerosis I27.0
  - dysmaturity (Wilson-Mikity) P27.0
  - hypoperfusion (idiopathic) P22.0
  - renal (hemorrhagic) (Goodpasture's) M31.0
- pure
  - motor lacunar G46.5
  - sensory lacunar G46.6
- Putnam-Dana D51.0
- pyogenic arthritis, pyoderma gangrenosum, and acne [PAPA] M04.8
- pyramidopallidonigral G20
- pyriformis —*see* Lesion, nerve, sciatic
- QT interval prolongation I45.81
- radicular NEC —*see* Radiculopathy
  - upper limbs, newborn (birth injury) P14.3
- rapid time-zone change G47.25
- Rasmussen G04.81
- Raymond (-Céstan) I65.8
- Raynaud's I73.00
  - with gangrene I73.01
- RDS (respiratory distress syndrome, newborn) P22.0
- reactive airways dysfunction J68.3

Syndrome *(continued)*
Refsum's G60.1
Reifenstein E34.52
renal glomerulohyalinosis-diabetic —*see* Diabetes, nephrosis
Rendu-Osler-Weber I78.0
residual ovary N99.83
resistant ovary E28.39
respiratory
  distress
    acute J80
      adult J80
      child J80
      idiopathic J84.114
    newborn (idiopathic) (type I) P22.0
      type II P22.1
restless legs G25.81
retinoblastoma (familial) C69.2
retroperitoneal fibrosis N13.5
retroviral seroconversion (acute) Z21
Reye's G93.7
Richter —*see* Leukemia, chronic lymphocytic, B-cell type
Ridley's I50.1
right
  heart, hypoplastic Q22.6
  ventricular obstruction —*see* Failure, heart, right
Romano-Ward (prolonged QT interval) I45.81
rotator cuff, shoulder (*see also* Tear, rotator cuff) M75.10-
Rotes Quérol —*see* Hyperostosis, ankylosing
Roth —*see* Meralgia paresthetica
rubella (congenital) P35.0
Ruvalcaba-Myhre-Smith E71.440
Rytand-Lipsitch I44.2
salt
  depletion E87.1
    due to heat NEC T67.8
      causing heat exhaustion or prostration T67.4
  low E87.1
salt-losing N28.89
SATB2-associated Q87.89
Scaglietti-Dagnini E22.0
scalenus anticus (anterior) G54.0
scapulocostal —*see* Mononeuropathy, upper limb, specified site NEC
scapuloperoneal G71.09
schizophrenic, of childhood NEC F84.5
Schnitzler D47.2
Scholte's E34.0
Schroeder's E27.0
Schüller-Christian C96.5
Schwachman's —*see* Syndrome, Shwachman's
Schwartz (-Jampel) G71.13
Schwartz-Bartter E22.2
scimitar Q26.8
sclerocystic ovary E28.2
Seitelberger's G31.89
septicemic adrenal hemorrhage A39.1
seroconversion, retroviral (acute) Z21
serous meningitis G93.2
severe acute respiratory (SARS) J12.81
  coronavirus 2019 (*see* also COVID-19) U07.1
    pneumonia J12.82
shaken infant T74.4
shock (traumatic) T79.4
  kidney N17.0
    following crush injury T79.5
  toxic A48.3
shock-lung J80

Syndrome *(continued)*
Shone's — code to specific anomalies
short
  bowel K91.2
  rib Q77.2
shoulder-hand —*see* Algoneurodystrophy
Shwachman's D70.4
sicca —*see* Syndrome, Sjögren
sick
  cell E87.1
  sinus I49.5
sick-euthyroid E07.81
sideropenic D50.1
Siemens' ectodermal dysplasia Q82.4
Silfverskjöld's Q78.9
Simons' E88.1
sinus tarsi M25.57-
sinusitis-bronchiectasis-situs inversus Q89.3
Sipple's E31.22
sirenomelia Q87.2
Sjögren M35.00
  with
    central nervous system involvement M35.07
    dental involvement M35.0C
    gastrointestinal involvement M35.08
    glomerular disease M35.0A
    inflammatory arthritis M35.05
    keratoconjunctivitis M35.01
    lung involvement M35.02
    myopathy M35.03
    peripheral nervous system involvement M35.06
    renal tubular acidosis M35.04
    specified organ involvement, NEC M35.09
    tubulo-interstitial nephropathy M35.04
    vasculitis M35.0B
Slocumb's E27.0
slow flow, coronary I20.8
Sluder's G44.89
Smith-Magenis Q93.88
Sneddon-Wilkinson L13.1
Sotos' Q87.3
South African cardiomyopathy I42.8
spasmodic
  upward movement, eyes H51.8
  winking F95.8
Spen's I45.9
splenic
  agenesis Q89.01
  flexure K59.89
  neutropenia D73.81
Spurway's Q78.0
staphylococcal scalded skin L00
steal
  arteriovenous T82.898-
  ischemic T82.898-
  subclavian G45.8
Stein-Leventhal E28.2
Stein's E28.2
Stevens-Johnson syndrome L51.1
  toxic epidermal necrolysis overlap L51.3
Stewart-Morel M85.2
Stickler Q89.8
stiff baby Q89.8
stiff man G25.82
Still-Felty —*see* Felty's syndrome
Stokes (-Adams) I45.9
stone heart I50.1
straight back, congenital Q76.49
subclavian steal G45.8
subcoracoid-pectoralis minor G54.0
subcostal nerve compression I77.89
subphrenic interposition Q43.3

Syndrome *(continued)*
superior
  cerebellar artery I63.89
  mesenteric artery K55.1
  semi-circular canal dehiscence H83.8X-
  vena cava I87.1
supine hypotensive (maternal) —*see* Syndrome, hypotension, maternal
suprarenal cortical E27.0
supraspinatus (*see also* Tear, rotator cuff) M75.10-
Susac G93.49
swallowed blood P78.2
sweat retention L74.0
Swyer Q99.1
Symond's G93.2
sympathetic
  cervical paralysis G90.2
  pelvic, female N94.89
systemic inflammatory response (SIRS), of non-infectious origin (without organ dysfunction) R65.10
  with acute organ dysfunction R65.11
tachycardia-bradycardia I49.5
takotsubo I51.81
TAR (thrombocytopenia with absent radius) Q87.2
tarsal tunnel G57.5-
teething K00.7
tegmental G93.89
telangiectasic-pigmentation-cataract Q82.8
temporal pyramidal apex —*see* Otitis, media, suppurative, acute
temporomandibular joint-pain-dysfunction M26.62-
Terry's (*see also* Myopia, degenerative) H44.2-
testicular feminization (*see also* Syndrome, androgen insensitivity) E34.51
thalamic pain (hyperesthetic) G89.0
thoracic outlet (compression) G54.0
Thorson-Björck E34.0
thrombocytopenia with absent radius (TAR) Q87.2
thyroid-adrenocortical insufficiency E31.0
tibial
  anterior M76.81-
  posterior M76.82-
Tietze's M94.0
time-zone (rapid) G47.25
Toni-Fanconi E72.09
  with cystinosis E72.04
Touraine's Q79.8
tourniquet —*see* Constriction, external, by site
toxic shock A48.3
transient left ventricular apical ballooning I51.81
traumatic vasospastic T75.22
Treacher Collins Q75.4
triple X, female Q97.0
trisomy Q92.9
  13 Q91.7
    meiotic nondisjunction Q91.4
    mitotic nondisjunction Q91.5
    mosaicism Q91.5
    translocation Q91.6
  18 Q91.3
    meiotic nondisjunction Q91.0
    mitotic nondisjunction Q91.1
    mosaicism Q91.1
    translocation Q91.2
  20 (q)(p) Q92.8

Syndrome *(continued)*
trisomy *(continued)*
  21 Q90.9
    meiotic nondisjunction Q90.0
    mitotic nondisjunction Q90.1
    mosaicism Q90.1
    translocation Q90.2
  22 Q92.8
tropical wet feet T69.0-
Trousseau's I82.1
tumor lysis (following antineoplastic chemotherapy) (spontaneous) NEC E88.3
tumor necrosis factor receptor associated periodic (TRAPS) M04.1
Twiddler's (due to)
  automatic implantable defibrillator T82.198
  cardiac pacemaker T82.198
Unverricht (-Lundborg) —*see* Epilepsy, generalized, idiopathic
upward gaze H51.8
uremia, chronic (*see also* Disease, kidney, chronic) N18.9
urethral N34.3
urethro-oculo-articular —*see* Reiter's disease
urohepatic K76.7
vago-hypoglossal G52.7
vascular NEC in cerebrovascular disease G46.8
vasoconstriction, reversible cerebrovascular I67.841
vasomotor I73.9
vasospastic (traumatic) T75.22
vasovagal R55
van Buchem's M85.2
van der Hoeve's Q78.0
VATER Q87.2
velo-cardio-facial Q93.81
vena cava (inferior) (superior) (obstruction) I87.1
vertebral
  artery G45.0
    compression —*see* Syndrome, anterior, spinal artery, compression
  steal G45.0
vertebro-basilar artery G45.0
vertebrogenic (pain) (*see also*, Pain, vertebrogenic) M54.89
vertiginous —*see* Disorder, vestibular function
Vinson-Plummer D50.1
virus B34.9
visceral larva migrans B83.0
visual disorientation H53.8
vitamin B6 deficiency E53.1
vitreal corneal H59.01-
vitreous (touch) H59.01-
Vogt-Koyanagi H20.82-
Volkmann's T79.6
von Schroetter's I82.890
von Willebrand (-Jürgen) D68.0
Waldenström-Kjellberg D50.1
Wallenberg's G46.3
water retention E87.79
Waterhouse (-Friderichsen) A39.1
Weber-Gubler G46.3
Weber-Leyden G46.3
Weber's G46.3
Wegener's M31.30
  with
    kidney involvement M31.31
    lung involvement M31.30
      with kidney involvement M31.31
Weingarten's (tropical eosinophilia) J82.89

Syndrome *(continued)*
- Weiss-Baker G90.09
- Werdnig-Hoffman G12.0
- Wermer's E31.21
- Werner's E34.8
- Wernicke-Korsakoff (nonalcoholic) F04
  - alcoholic F10.26
- West's *—see* Epilepsy, spasms
- Westphal-Strümpell E83.01
- wet
  - feet (maceration) (tropical) T69.0-
  - lung, newborn P22.1
- whiplash S13.4
- whistling face Q87.0
- Wilkie's K55.1
- Wilkinson-Sneddon L13.1
- Willebrand (-Jürgens) D68.0
- Williams Q93.82
- Wilson's (hepatolenticular degeneration) E83.01
- Wiskott-Aldrich D82.0
- withdrawal *—see* Withdrawal, state
  - drug
    - infant of dependent mother P96.1
    - therapeutic use, newborn P96.2
- Woakes' (ethmoiditis) J33.1
- Wright's (hyperabduction) G54.0
- X I20.9
- XXXX Q97.1
- XXXXX Q97.1
- XXXXY Q98.1
- XXY Q98.0
- Yao M04.8
- yellow nail L60.5
- Zahorsky's B08.5
- Zellweger syndrome E71.510
- Zellweger-like syndrome E71.541

Synechia (anterior) (iris) (posterior) (pupil) *—see also* Adhesions, iris
- intra-uterine (traumatic) N85.6

Synesthesia R20.8

Syngamiasis, syngamosis B83.3

Synodontia K00.2

Synorchidism, synorchism Q55.1

Synostosis (congenital) Q78.8
- astragalo-scaphoid Q74.2
- radioulnar Q74.0

Synovial sarcoma *—see* Neoplasm, connective tissue, malignant

Synovioma (malignant) *—see also* Neoplasm, connective tissue, malignant
- benign *—see* Neoplasm, connective tissue, benign

Synoviosarcoma *—see* Neoplasm, connective tissue, malignant

Synovitis (*see also* Tenosynovitis) M65.9
- crepitant
  - hand M70.0-
  - wrist M70.03-
- gonococcal A54.49
- gouty *—see* Gout,
- in (due to)
  - crystals M65.8-
  - gonorrhea A54.49
  - syphilis (late) A52.78
  - use, overuse, pressure *—see* Disorder, soft tissue, due to use
- infective NEC *—see* Tenosynovitis, infective NEC

Synovitis *(continued)*
- specified NEC *—see* Tenosynovitis, specified type NEC
- syphilitic A52.78
  - congenital (early) A50.02
- toxic *—see* Synovitis, transient
- transient M67.3-
  - ankle M67.37-
  - elbow M67.32-
  - foot joint M67.37-
  - hand joint M67.34-
  - hip M67.35-
  - knee M67.36-
  - multiple site M67.39
  - pelvic region M67.35-
  - shoulder M67.31-
  - specified joint NEC M67.38
  - wrist M67.33-
- traumatic, current *—see* Sprain
- tuberculous *—see* Tuberculosis, synovitis
- villonodular (pigmented) M12.2-
  - ankle M12.27-
  - elbow M12.22-
  - foot joint M12.27-
  - hand joint M12.24-
  - hip M12.25-
  - knee M12.26-
  - multiple site M12.29
  - pelvic region M12.25-
  - shoulder M12.21-
  - specified joint NEC M12.28
  - vertebrae M12.28
  - wrist M12.23-

Syphilid A51.39
- congenital A50.06
- newborn A50.06
- tubercular (late) A52.79

Syphilis, syphilitic (acquired) A53.9
- abdomen (late) A52.79
- acoustic nerve A52.15
- adenopathy (secondary) A51.49
- adrenal (gland) (with cortical hypofunction) A52.79
- age under 2 years NOS *—see also* Syphilis, congenital, early
  - acquired A51.9
- alopecia (secondary) A51.32
- anemia (late) A52.79 *[D63.8]*
- aneurysm (aorta) (ruptured) A52.01
  - central nervous system A52.05
  - congenital A50.54 *[I79.0]*
- anus (late) A52.74
  - primary A51.1
  - secondary A51.39
- aorta (arch) (abdominal) (thoracic) A52.02
  - aneurysm A52.01
- aortic (insufficiency) (regurgitation) (stenosis) A52.03
  - aneurysm A52.01
- arachnoid (adhesive) (cerebral) (spinal) A52.13
- asymptomatic *—see* Syphilis, latent
- ataxia (locomotor) A52.11
- atrophoderma maculatum A51.39
- auricular fibrillation A52.06
- bladder (late) A52.76
- bone A52.77
  - secondary A51.46
- brain A52.17
- breast (late) A52.79
- bronchus (late) A52.72
- bubo (primary) A51.0
- bulbar palsy A52.19
- bursa (late) A52.78
- cardiac decompensation A52.06
- cardiovascular A52.00

Syphilis, syphilitic *(continued)*
- central nervous system (late) (recurrent) (relapse) (tertiary) A52.3
  - with
    - ataxia A52.11
    - general paralysis A52.17
      - juvenile A50.45
    - paresis (general) A52.17
      - juvenile A50.45
    - tabes (dorsalis) A52.11
      - juvenile A50.45
    - taboparesis A52.17
      - juvenile A50.45
  - aneurysm A52.05
  - congenital A50.40
  - juvenile A50.40
  - remission in (sustained) A52.3
  - serology doubtful, negative, or positive A52.3
  - specified nature or site NEC A52.19
  - vascular A52.05
- cerebral A52.17
  - meningovascular A52.13
  - nerves (multiple palsies) A52.15
  - sclerosis A52.17
  - thrombosis A52.05
- cerebrospinal (tabetic type) A52.12
- cerebrovascular A52.05
- cervix (late) A52.76
- chancre (multiple) A51.0
  - extragenital A51.2
  - Rollet's A51.0
- Charcot's joint A52.16
- chorioretinitis A51.43
  - congenital A50.01
  - late A52.71
  - prenatal A50.01
- choroiditis *—see* Syphilitic chorioretinitis
- choroidoretinitis *—see* Syphilitic chorioretinitis
- ciliary body (secondary) A51.43
  - late A52.71
- colon (late) A52.74
- combined spinal sclerosis A52.11
- condyloma (latum) A51.31
- congenital A50.9
  - with
    - paresis (general) A50.45
    - tabes (dorsalis) A50.45
    - taboparesis A50.45
  - chorioretinitis, choroiditis A50.01 *[H32]*
  - early, or less than 2 years after birth NEC A50.2
    - with manifestations *—see* Syphilis, congenital, early, symptomatic
    - latent (without manifestations) A50.1
      - negative spinal fluid test A50.1
      - serology positive A50.1
    - symptomatic A50.09
      - cutaneous A50.06
      - mucocutaneous A50.07
      - oculopathy A50.01
      - osteochondropathy A50.02
      - pharyngitis A50.03
      - pneumonia A50.04
      - rhinitis A50.05
      - visceral A50.08
  - interstitial keratitis A50.31
  - juvenile neurosyphilis A50.45
  - late, or 2 years or more after birth NEC A50.7
    - chorioretinitis, choroiditis A50.32

Syphilis, syphilitic *(continued)*
- congenital *(continued)*
  - late, or 2 years or more after birth *(continued)*
    - interstitial keratitis A50.31
    - juvenile neurosyphilis A50.45
    - latent (without manifestations) A50.6
      - negative spinal fluid test A50.6
      - serology positive A50.6
    - symptomatic or with manifestations NEC A50.59
      - arthropathy A50.55
      - cardiovascular A50.54
      - Clutton's joints A50.51
      - Hutchinson's teeth A50.52
      - Hutchinson's triad A50.53
      - osteochondropathy A50.56
      - saddle nose A50.57
- conjugal A53.9
  - tabes A52.11
- conjunctiva (late) A52.71
- contact Z20.2
- cord bladder A52.19
- cornea, late A52.71
- coronary (artery) (sclerosis) A52.06
- coryza, congenital A50.05
- cranial nerve A52.15
  - multiple palsies A52.15
- cutaneous *—see* Syphilis, skin
- dacryocystitis (late) A52.71
- degeneration, spinal cord A52.12
- dementia paralytica A52.17
  - juvenilis A50.45
- destruction of bone A52.77
- dilatation, aorta A52.01
- due to blood transfusion A53.9
- dura mater A52.13
- ear A52.79
  - inner A52.79
    - nerve (eighth) A52.15
    - neurorecurrence A52.15
- early A51.9
  - cardiovascular A52.00
  - central nervous system A52.3
  - latent (without manifestations) (less than 2 years after infection) A51.5
    - negative spinal fluid test A51.5
    - serological relapse after treatment A51.5
    - serology positive A51.5
  - relapse (treated, untreated) A51.9
  - skin A51.39
  - symptomatic A51.9
    - extragenital chancre A51.2
    - primary, except extragenital chancre A51.0
    - secondary (*see also* Syphilis, secondary) A51.39
      - relapse (treated, untreated) A51.49
  - ulcer A51.39
- eighth nerve (neuritis) A52.15
- endemic A65
- endocarditis A52.03
  - aortic A52.03
  - pulmonary A52.03
- epididymis (late) A52.76
- epiglottis (late) A52.73
- epiphysitis (congenital) (early) A50.02
- episcleritis (late) A52.71
- esophagus A52.79
- eustachian tube A52.73
- exposure to Z20.2
- eye A52.71
- eyelid (late) (with gumma) A52.71
- fallopian tube (late) A52.76

Syphilis, syphilitic *(continued)*
- fracture A52.77
- gallbladder (late) A52.74
- gastric (polyposis) (late) A52.74
- general A53.9
  - paralysis A52.17
    - juvenile A50.45
- genital (primary) A51.0
- glaucoma A52.71
- gumma NEC A52.79
  - cardiovascular system A52.00
  - central nervous system A52.3
  - congenital A50.59
- heart (block) (decompensation) (disease) (failure) A52.06 *[I52]*
  - valve NEC A52.03
- hemianesthesia A52.19
- hemianopsia A52.71
- hemiparesis A52.17
- hemiplegia A52.17
- hepatic artery A52.09
- hepatis A52.74
- hepatomegaly, congenital A50.08
- hereditaria tarda —*see* Syphilis, congenital, late
- hereditary —*see* Syphilis, congenital
- Hutchinson's teeth A50.52
- hyalitis A52.71
- inactive —*see* Syphilis, latent
- infantum —*see* Syphilis, congenital
- inherited —*see* Syphilis, congenital
- internal ear A52.79
- intestine (late) A52.74
- iris, iritis (secondary) A51.43
  - late A52.71
- joint (late) A52.77
- keratitis (congenital) (interstitial) (late) A50.31
- kidney (late) A52.75
- lacrimal passages (late) A52.71
- larynx (late) A52.73
- late A52.9
  - cardiovascular A52.00
  - central nervous system A52.3
  - kidney A52.75
  - latent or 2 years or more after infection (without manifestations) A52.8
    - negative spinal fluid test A52.8
    - serology positive A52.8
  - paresis A52.17
  - specified site NEC A52.79
  - symptomatic or with manifestations A52.79
  - tabes A52.11
- latent A53.0
  - with signs or symptoms - code by site and stage under Syphilis
  - central nervous system A52.2
  - date of infection unspecified A53.0
  - early, or less than 2 years after infection A51.5
  - follow-up of latent syphilis A53.0
    - date of infection unspecified A53.0
    - late, or 2 years or more after infection A52.8
  - late, or 2 years or more after infection A52.8
  - positive serology (only finding) A53.0
    - date of infection unspecified A53.0
    - early, or less than 2 years after infection A51.5
    - late, or 2 years or more after infection A52.8

Syphilis, syphilitic *(continued)*
- lens (late) A52.71
- leukoderma A51.39
  - late A52.79
- lienitis A52.79
- lip A51.39
  - chancre (primary) A51.2
  - late A52.79
- Lissauer's paralysis A52.17
- liver A52.74
- locomotor ataxia A52.11
- lung A52.72
- lymph gland (early) (secondary) A51.49
  - late A52.79
- lymphadenitis (secondary) A51.49
- macular atrophy of skin A51.39
  - striated A52.79
- mediastinum (late) A52.73
- meninges (adhesive) (brain) (spinal cord) A52.13
- meningitis A52.13
  - acute (secondary) A51.41
  - congenital A50.41
- meningoencephalitis A52.14
- meningovascular A52.13
  - congenital A50.41
- mesarteritis A52.09
  - brain A52.04
- middle ear A52.77
- mitral stenosis A52.03
- monoplegia A52.17
- mouth (secondary) A51.39
  - late A52.79
- mucocutaneous (secondary) A51.39
  - late A52.79
- mucous
  - membrane (secondary) A51.39
    - late A52.79
  - patches A51.39
    - congenital A50.07
- mulberry molars A50.52
- muscle A52.78
- myocardium A52.06
- nasal sinus (late) A52.73
- neonatorum —*see* Syphilis, congenital
- nephrotic syndrome (secondary) A51.44
- nerve palsy (any cranial nerve) A52.15
  - multiple A52.15
- nervous system, central A52.3
- neuritis A52.15
  - acoustic A52.15
- neurorecidive of retina A52.19
- neuroretinitis A52.19
- newborn —*see* Syphilis, congenital
- nodular superficial (late) A52.79
- nonvenereal A65
- nose (late) A52.73
  - saddle back deformity A50.57
- occlusive arterial disease A52.09
- oculopathy A52.71
- ophthalmic (late) A52.71
- optic nerve (atrophy) (neuritis) (papilla) A52.15
- orbit (late) A52.71
- organic A53.9
- osseous (late) A52.77
- osteochondritis (congenital) (early) A50.02 *[M90.80]*
- osteoporosis A52.77
- ovary (late) A52.76
- oviduct (late) A52.76
- palate (late) A52.79
- pancreas (late) A52.74
- paralysis A52.17
  - general A52.17
    - juvenile A50.45

Syphilis, syphilitic *(continued)*
- paresis (general) A52.17
  - juvenile A50.45
- paresthesia A52.19
- Parkinson's disease or syndrome A52.19
- paroxysmal tachycardia A52.06
- pemphigus (congenital) A50.06
- penis (chancre) A51.0
  - late A52.76
- pericardium A52.06
- perichondritis, larynx (late) A52.73
- periosteum (late) A52.77
  - congenital (early) A50.02 *[M90.80]*
  - early (secondary) A51.46
- peripheral nerve A52.79
- petrous bone (late) A52.77
- pharynx (late) A52.73
  - secondary A51.39
- pituitary (gland) A52.79
- pleura (late) A52.73
- pneumonia, white A50.04
- pontine lesion A52.17
- portal vein A52.09
- primary A51.0
  - anal A51.1
  - and secondary —*see* Syphilis, secondary
  - central nervous system A52.3
  - extragenital chancre NEC A51.2
  - fingers A51.2
  - genital A51.0
  - lip A51.2
  - specified site NEC A51.2
  - tonsils A51.2
- prostate (late) A52.76
- ptosis (eyelid) A52.71
- pulmonary (late) A52.72
  - artery A52.09
- pyelonephritis (late) A52.75
- recently acquired, symptomatic A51.9
- rectum (late) A52.74
- respiratory tract (late) A52.73
- retina, late A52.71
- retrobulbar neuritis A52.15
- salpingitis A52.76
- sclera (late) A52.71
- sclerosis
  - cerebral A52.17
  - coronary A52.06
  - multiple A52.11
- scotoma (central) A52.71
- scrotum (late) A52.76
- secondary (and primary) A51.49
  - adenopathy A51.49
  - anus A51.39
  - bone A51.46
  - chorioretinitis, choroiditis A51.43
  - hepatitis A51.45
  - liver A51.45
  - lymphadenitis A51.49
  - meningitis (acute) A51.41
  - mouth A51.39
  - mucous membranes A51.39
  - periosteum, periostitis A51.46
  - pharynx A51.39
  - relapse (treated, untreated) A51.49
  - skin A51.39
  - specified form NEC A51.49
  - tonsil A51.39
  - ulcer A51.39
  - viscera NEC A51.49
  - vulva A51.39
- seminal vesicle (late) A52.76
- seronegative with signs or symptoms - code by site and stage under Syphilis

Syphilis, syphilitic *(continued)*
- seropositive
  - with signs or symptoms - code by site and stage under Syphilis
  - follow-up of latent syphilis —*see* Syphilis, latent
  - only finding —*see* Syphilis, latent
- seventh nerve (paralysis) A52.15
- sinus, sinusitis (late) A52.73
- skeletal system A52.77
- skin (with ulceration) (early) (secondary) A51.39
  - late or tertiary A52.79
- small intestine A52.74
- spastic spinal paralysis A52.17
- spermatic cord (late) A52.76
- spinal (cord) A52.12
- spleen A52.79
- splenomegaly A52.79
- spondylitis A52.77
- staphyloma A52.71
- stigmata (congenital) A50.59
- stomach A52.74
- synovium A52.78
- tabes dorsalis (late) A52.11
  - juvenile A50.45
- tabetic type A52.11
  - juvenile A50.45
- taboparesis A52.17
  - juvenile A50.45
- tachycardia A52.06
- tendon (late) A52.78
- tertiary A52.9
  - with symptoms NEC A52.79
  - cardiovascular A52.00
  - central nervous system A52.3
  - multiple NEC A52.79
  - specified site NEC A52.79
- testis A52.76
- thorax A52.73
- throat A52.73
- thymus (gland) (late) A52.79
- thyroid (late) A52.79
- tongue (late) A52.79
- tonsil (lingual) (late) A52.73
  - primary A51.2
  - secondary A51.39
- trachea (late) A52.73
- tunica vaginalis (late) A52.76
- ulcer (any site) (early) (secondary) A51.39
  - late A52.79
  - perforating A52.79
    - foot A52.11
- urethra (late) A52.76
- urogenital (late) A52.76
- uterus (late) A52.76
- uveal tract (secondary) A51.43
  - late A52.71
- uveitis (secondary) A51.43
  - late A52.71
- uvula (late) (perforated) A52.79
- vagina A51.0
  - late A52.76
- valvulitis NEC A52.03
- vascular A52.00
  - brain (cerebral) A52.05
- ventriculi A52.74
- vesicae urinariae (late) A52.76
- viscera (abdominal) (late) A52.74
  - secondary A51.49
- vitreous (opacities) (late) A52.71
  - hemorrhage A52.71
- vulva A51.0
  - late A52.76
  - secondary A51.39

Syphiloma A52.79
- cardiovascular system A52.00
- central nervous system A52.3
- circulatory system A52.00
- congenital A50.59

Syphilophobia F45.29

Syringadenoma —*see also* Neoplasm, skin, benign
- papillary —*see* Neoplasm, skin, benign

Syringobulbia G95.0

Syringocystadenoma —*see* Neoplasm, skin, benign
- papillary —*see* Neoplasm, skin, benign

Syringoma —*see also* Neoplasm, skin, benign
- chondroid —*see* Neoplasm, skin, benign

Syringomyelia G95.0

Syringomyelitis —*see* Encephalitis

Syringomyelocele —*see* Spina bifida

Syringopontia G95.0

System, systemic —*see also* condition
- disease, combined —*see* Degeneration, combined
- inflammatory response syndrome (SIRS) of non-infectious origin (without organ dysfunction) R65.10
  - with acute organ dysfunction R65.11
- lupus erythematosus M32.9
  - inhibitor present D68.62

T

Tabacism, tabacosis, tabagism —*see also* Poisoning, tobacco
- meaning dependence (without remission) F17.200
  - with
    - disorder F17.299
      - in remission F17.211
      - specified disorder NEC F17.298
      - withdrawal F17.203

Tabardillo A75.9
- flea-borne A75.2
- louse-borne A75.0

Tabes, tabetic A52.10
- with
  - central nervous system syphilis A52.10
  - Charcot's joint A52.16
  - cord bladder A52.19
  - crisis, viscera (any) A52.19
  - paralysis, general A52.17
  - paresis (general) A52.17
  - perforating ulcer (foot) A52.19
- arthropathy (Charcot) A52.16
- bladder A52.19
- bone A52.11
- cerebrospinal A52.12
- congenital A50.45
- conjugal A52.10
- dorsalis A52.11
  - juvenile A50.49
- juvenile A50.49
- latent A52.19
- mesenterica A18.39
- paralysis, insane, general A52.17
- spasmodic A52.17
- syphilis (cerebrospinal) A52.12

Taboparalysis A52.17

Taboparesis (remission) A52.17
- juvenile A50.45

TAC (trigeminal autonomic cephalgia) **NEC** G44.099
- intractable G44.091
- not intractable G44.099

Tache noir S60.22-

Tachyalimentation K91.2

Tachyarrhythmia, tachyrhythmia —*see* Tachycardia

Tachycardia R00.0
- atrial (paroxysmal) I47.1
- auricular I47.1
- AV nodal re-entry (re-entrant) I47.1
- junctional (paroxysmal) I47.1
- newborn P29.11
- nodal (paroxysmal) I47.1
- non-paroxysmal AV nodal I45.89
- paroxysmal (sustained) (nonsustained) I47.9
  - with sinus bradycardia I49.5
  - atrial (PAT) I47.1
  - atrioventricular (AV) (re-entrant) I47.1
    - psychogenic F54
  - junctional I47.1
    - ectopic I47.1
  - nodal I47.1
  - psychogenic (atrial) (supraventricular) (ventricular) F54
  - supraventricular (sustained) I47.1
    - psychogenic F54
  - ventricular I47.2
    - psychogenic F54
- psychogenic F45.8
- sick sinus I49.5
- sinoauricular NOS R00.0
  - paroxysmal I47.1
- sinus [sinusal] NOS R00.0
  - paroxysmal I47.1
- supraventricular I47.1
- ventricular (paroxysmal) (sustained) I47.2
  - psychogenic F54

Tachygastria K31.89

Tachypnea R06.82
- hysterical F45.8
- newborn (idiopathic) (transitory) P22.1
- psychogenic F45.8
- transitory, of newborn P22.1

Taenia (infection) (infestation) B68.9
- diminuta B71.0
- echinococcal infestation B67.90
- mediocanellata B68.1
- nana B71.0
- saginata B68.1
- solium (intestinal form) B68.0
  - larval form —*see* Cysticercosis

Taeniasis (intestine) —*see* Taenia

TACO (transfusion associated circulatory overload) E87.71

Tag (hypertrophied skin) (infected) L91.8
- adenoid J35.8
- anus K64.4
- hemorrhoidal K64.4
- hymen N89.8
- perineal N90.89
- preauricular Q17.0
- sentinel K64.4

Tag *(continued)*
- skin L91.8
  - accessory (congenital) Q82.8
  - anus K64.4
  - congenital Q82.8
  - preauricular Q17.0
- tonsil J35.8
- urethra, urethral N36.8
- vulva N90.89

Tahyna fever B33.8

Takahara's disease E80.3

Takayasu's disease or syndrome M31.4

Talaromycosis B48.4

Talcosis (pulmonary) J62.0

Talipes (congenital) Q66.89
- acquired, planus —*see* Deformity, limb, flat foot
- asymmetric Q66.89
- calcaneovalgus Q66.4-
- calcaneovarus Q66.1-
- calcaneus Q66.89
- cavus Q66.7-
- equinovalgus Q66.6
- equinovarus Q66.0-
- equinus Q66.89
- percavus Q66.7-
- planovalgus Q66.6
- planus (acquired) (any degree) —*see also* Deformity, limb, flat foot
  - congenital Q66.5-
  - due to rickets (sequelae) E64.3
- valgus Q66.6
- varus Q66.3-

Tall stature, constitutional E34.4

Talma's disease M62.89

Talon noir S90.3-
- hand S60.22-
- heel S90.3-
- toe S90.1-

Tamponade, heart I31.4

Tanapox (virus disease) B08.71

Tangier disease E78.6

Tantrum, child problem F91.8

Tapeworm (infection) (infestation) —*see* Infestation, tapeworm

Tapia's syndrome G52.7

TAR (thrombocytopenia with absent radius) **syndrome** Q87.2

Tarral-Besnier disease L44.0

Tarsal tunnel syndrome —*see* Syndrome, tarsal tunnel

Tarsalgia —*see* Pain, limb, lower

Tarsitis (eyelid) H01.8
- syphilitic A52.71
- tuberculous A18.4

Tartar (teeth) (dental calculus) K03.6

Tattoo (mark) L81.8

Tauri's disease E74.09

Taurodontism K00.2

Taussig-Bing syndrome Q20.1

Taybi's syndrome Q87.2

Tay-Sachs amaurotic familial idiocy or disease E75.02

TBI (traumatic brain injury) S06.9

Teacher's node or nodule J38.2

Tear, torn (traumatic) —*see also* Laceration
- with abortion —*see* Abortion
- annular fibrosis M51.35

Tear, torn *(continued)*
- anus, anal (sphincter) S31.831
  - complicating delivery
    - with third degree perineal laceration (*see also* Delivery, complicated, by, laceration, perineum, third degree) O70.20
      - with mucosa O70.3
    - without third degree perineal laceration O70.4
  - nontraumatic (healed) (old) K62.81
- articular cartilage, old —*see* Derangement, joint, articular cartilage, by site
- bladder
  - with ectopic or molar pregnancy O08.6
  - following ectopic or molar pregnancy O08.6
  - obstetrical O71.5
  - traumatic —*see* Injury, bladder
- bowel
  - with ectopic or molar pregnancy O08.6
  - following ectopic or molar pregnancy O08.6
  - obstetrical trauma O71.5
- broad ligament
  - with ectopic or molar pregnancy O08.6
- broad ligament
  - following ectopic or molar pregnancy O08.6
  - obstetrical trauma O71.6
- bucket handle (knee) (meniscus) —*see* Tear, meniscus
- capsule, joint —*see* Sprain
- cartilage —*see also* Sprain
  - articular, old —*see* Derangement, joint, articular cartilage, by site
- cervix
  - with ectopic or molar pregnancy O08.6
  - following ectopic or molar pregnancy O08.6
  - obstetrical trauma (current) O71.3
  - old N88.1
  - traumatic —*see* Injury, uterus
- dural G97.41
  - nontraumatic G96.11
- internal organ —*see* Injury, by site
- knee cartilage
  - articular (current) S83.3-
  - old —*see* Derangement, knee, meniscus, due to old tear
- ligament —*see* Sprain
- meniscus (knee) (current injury) S83.209
  - bucket-handle S83.20-
  - lateral
    - bucket-handle S83.25-
    - complex S83.27-
    - peripheral S83.26-
    - specified type NEC S83.28-
  - medial
    - bucket-handle S83.21-
    - complex S83.23-
    - peripheral S83.22-
    - specified type NEC S83.24-
  - old —*see* Derangement, knee, meniscus, due to old tear
  - site other than knee - code as Sprain
  - specified type NEC S83.20-
- muscle —*see* Strain

Tear, torn *(continued)*
- pelvic
  - floor, complicating delivery O70.1
  - organ NEC, obstetrical trauma O71.5
    - with ectopic or molar pregnancy O08.6
    - following ectopic or molar pregnancy O08.6
- perineal, secondary O90.1
- periurethral tissue, obstetrical trauma O71.82
  - with ectopic or molar pregnancy O08.6
  - following ectopic or molar pregnancy O08.6
- rectovaginal septum —*see* Laceration, vagina
- retina, retinal (without detachment) (horseshoe) —*see also* Break, retina, horseshoe
  - with detachment —*see* Detachment, retina, with retinal, break
- rotator cuff (nontraumatic) M75.10-
  - complete M75.12-
  - incomplete M75.11-
  - traumatic S46.01-
    - capsule S43.42-
- semilunar cartilage, knee —*see* Tear, meniscus
- supraspinatus (complete) (incomplete) (nontraumatic) (*see also* Tear, rotator cuff) M75.10-
- tendon —*see* Strain
- tentorial, at birth P10.4
- umbilical cord
  - complicating delivery O69.89
- urethra
  - with ectopic or molar pregnancy O08.6
  - following ectopic or molar pregnancy O08.6
  - obstetrical trauma O71.5
- uterus —*see* Injury, uterus
- vagina —*see* Laceration, vagina
- vessel, from catheter —*see* Puncture, accidental complicating surgery
- vulva, complicating delivery O70.0

Tear-stone —*see* Dacryolith

Teeth —*see also* condition
- grinding
  - psychogenic F45.8
  - sleep related G47.63

Teething (syndrome) K00.7

Telangiectasia, telangiectasis (verrucous) I78.1
- ataxic (cerebellar) (Louis-Bar) G11.3
- familial I78.0
- hemorrhagic, hereditary (congenital) (senile) I78.0
- hereditary, hemorrhagic (congenital) (senile) I78.0
- juxtafoveal H35.07-
- macular H35.07-
- macularis eruptiva perstans D47.01
- parafoveal H35.07-
- retinal (idiopathic) (juxtafoveal) (macular) (parafoveal) H35.07-
- spider I78.1

Telephone scatologia F65.89

Telescoped bowel or intestine K56.1
- congenital Q43.8

Temperature
- body, high (of unknown origin) R50.9
- cold, trauma from T69.9
  - newborn P80.0
  - specified effect NEC T69.8

Temple —*see* condition

Temporal —*see* condition

Temporomandibular joint pain-dysfunction syndrome M26.62-

Temporosphenoidal —*see* condition

Tendency
- bleeding —*see* Defect, coagulation
- suicide
  - meaning personal history of attempted suicide Z91.51
  - meaning suicidal ideation —*see* Ideation, suicidal
- to fall R29.6

Tenderness, abdominal R10.819
- epigastric R10.816
- generalized R10.817
- left lower quadrant R10.814
- left upper quadrant R10.812
- periumbilic R10.815
- right lower quadrant R10.813
- right upper quadrant R10.811
- rebound R10.829
  - epigastric R10.826
  - generalized R10.827
  - left lower quadrant R10.824
  - left upper quadrant R10.822
  - periumbilic R10.825
  - right lower quadrant R10.823
  - right upper quadrant R10.821

Tendinitis, tendonitis —*see also* Enthesopathy
- Achilles M76.6-
- adhesive —*see* Tenosynovitis, specified type NEC
  - shoulder —*see* Capsulitis, adhesive
- bicipital M75.2-
- calcific M65.2-
  - ankle M65.27-
  - foot M65.27-
  - forearm M65.23-
  - hand M65.24-
  - lower leg M65.26-
  - multiple sites M65.29
  - pelvic region M65.25-
  - shoulder M75.3-
  - specified site NEC M65.28
  - thigh M65.25-
  - upper arm M65.22-
- due to use, overuse, pressure —*see also* Disorder, soft tissue, due to use
  - specified NEC —*see* Disorder, soft tissue, due to use, specified NEC
- gluteal M76.0-
- patellar M76.5-
- peroneal M76.7-
- psoas M76.1-
- tibial (posterior) M76.82-
  - anterior M76.81-
- trochanteric —*see* Bursitis, hip, trochanteric

Tendon —*see* condition

Tendosynovitis —*see* Tenosynovitis

Tenesmus (rectal) R19.8
- vesical R30.1

Tennis elbow —*see* Epicondylitis, lateral

Tenonitis —*see also* Tenosynovitis
- eye (capsule) H05.04-

Tenontosynovitis —*see* Tenosynovitis

Tenontothecitis —*see* Tenosynovitis

Tenophyte —*see* Disorder, synovium, specified type NEC

Tenosynovitis (*see also* Synovitis) M65.9
- adhesive —*see* Tenosynovitis, specified type NEC
  - shoulder —*see* Capsulitis, adhesive
- bicipital (calcifying) —*see* Tendinitis, bicipital
- gonococcal A54.49
- in (due to)
  - crystals M65.8-
  - gonorrhea A54.49
  - syphilis (late) A52.78
  - use, overuse, pressure —*see also* Disorder, soft tissue, due to use
    - specified NEC —*see* Disorder, soft tissue, due to use, specified NEC
- infective NEC M65.1-
  - ankle M65.17-
  - foot M65.17-
  - forearm M65.13-
  - hand M65.14-
  - lower leg M65.16-
  - multiple sites M65.19
  - pelvic region M65.15-
  - shoulder region M65.11-
  - specified site NEC M65.18
  - thigh M65.15-
  - upper arm M65.12-
- radial styloid M65.4
- shoulder region M65.81-
  - adhesive —*see* Capsulitis, adhesive
- specified type NEC M65.88
  - ankle M65.87-
  - foot M65.87-
  - forearm M65.83-
  - hand M65.84-
  - lower leg M65.86-
  - multiple sites M65.89
  - pelvic region M65.85-
  - shoulder region M65.81-
  - specified site NEC M65.88
  - thigh M65.85-
  - upper arm M65.82-
- tuberculous —*see* Tuberculosis, tenosynovitis

Tenovaginitis —*see* Tenosynovitis

Tension
- arterial, high —*see also* Hypertension
  - without diagnosis of hypertension R03.0
- headache G44.209
  - intractable G44.201
  - not intractable G44.209
- nervous R45.0
- pneumothorax J93.0
- premenstrual N94.3
- state (mental) F48.9

Tentorium —*see* condition

Teratencephalus Q89.8

Teratism Q89.7

Teratoblastoma (malignant) —*see* Neoplasm, malignant, by site

Teratocarcinoma —*see also* Neoplasm, malignant, by site
- liver C22.7

Teratoma (solid) —*see also* Neoplasm, uncertain behavior, by site
- with embryonal carcinoma, mixed —*see* Neoplasm, malignant, by site
- with malignant transformation —*see* Neoplasm, malignant, by site
- adult (cystic) —*see* Neoplasm, benign, by site
- benign —*see* Neoplasm, benign, by site
- combined with choriocarcinoma —*see* Neoplasm, malignant, by site
- cystic (adult) —*see* Neoplasm, benign, by site
- differentiated —*see* Neoplasm, benign, by site
- embryonal —*see also* Neoplasm, malignant, by site
  - liver C22.7
- immature —*see* Neoplasm, malignant, by site
- liver C22.7
  - adult, benign, cystic, differentiated type or mature D13.4
- malignant —*see also* Neoplasm, malignant, by site
  - anaplastic —*see* Neoplasm, malignant, by site
  - intermediate —*see* Neoplasm, malignant, by site
  - specified site —*see* Neoplasm, malignant, by site
  - unspecified site C62.90
  - undifferentiated —*see* Neoplasm, malignant, by site
- mature —*see* Neoplasm, uncertain behavior, by site
  - malignant —*see* Neoplasm, by site, malignant, by site
- ovary D27.-
  - embryonal, immature or malignant C56-
- solid —*see* Neoplasm, uncertain behavior, by site
- testis C62.9-
  - adult, benign, cystic, differentiated type or mature D29.2-
  - scrotal C62.1-
  - undescended C62.0-

Termination
- anomalous —*see also* Malposition, congenital
  - right pulmonary vein Q26.3
- pregnancy, elective Z33.2

Ternidens diminutus infestation B81.8

Ternidensiasis B81.8

Terror(s) night (child) F51.4

Terrorism, victim of Z65.4

Terry's syndrome (*see also* Myopia, degenerative) H44.2-

Tertiary —*see* condition

Test, tests, testing (for)
- adequacy (for dialysis)
  - hemodialysis Z49.31
  - peritoneal Z49.32

Test, tests, testing *(continued)*
- blood-alcohol Z02.83
  - positive *—see* Findings, abnormal, in blood
- blood-drug Z02.83
  - positive *—see* Findings, abnormal, in blood
- blood pressure Z01.30
  - abnormal reading *—see* Blood, pressure
- blood typing Z01.83
  - Rh typing Z01.83
- cardiac pulse generator (battery) Z45.010
- fertility Z31.41
- genetic
  - disease carrier status for procreative management
    - female Z31.430
    - male Z31.440
  - male partner of patient with recurrent pregnancy loss Z31.441
  - procreative management NEC
    - female Z31.438
    - male Z31.448
- hearing Z01.10
  - with abnormal findings NEC Z01.118
  - infant or child (over 28 days old) Z00.129
    - with abnormal findings Z00.121
- HIV (human immunodeficiency virus)
  - nonconclusive (in infants) R75
  - positive Z21
  - seropositive Z21
- immunity status Z01.84
- intelligence NEC Z01.89
- laboratory (as part of a general medical examination) Z00.00
  - with abnormal finding Z00.01
  - for medicolegal reason NEC Z04.89
- male partner of patient with recurrent pregnancy loss Z31.441
- Mantoux (for tuberculosis) Z11.1
  - abnormal result R76.11
- pregnancy, positive first pregnancy *—see* Pregnancy, normal, first
- procreative Z31.49
  - fertility Z31.41
- skin, diagnostic
  - allergy Z01.82
    - special screening examination *—see* Screening, by name of disease
  - Mantoux Z11.1
  - tuberculin Z11.1
- specified NEC Z01.89
- tuberculin Z11.1
  - abnormal result R76.11
- vision Z01.00
  - with abnormal findings Z01.01
  - following failed vision screening Z01.020
    - with abnormal findings Z01.021
  - infant or child (over 28 days old) Z00.129
    - with abnormal findings Z00.121
- Wassermann Z11.3
  - positive *—see* Serology for syphilis, positive

Testicle, testicular, testis *—see also* condition
- feminization syndrome (*see also* Syndrome, androgen insensitivity) E34.51
- migrans Q55.29

Tetanus, tetanic (cephalic) (convulsions) A35
- with
  - abortion A34
  - ectopic or molar pregnancy O08.0
- following ectopic or molar pregnancy O08.0
- inoculation reaction (due to serum) *—see* Complications, vaccination
- neonatorum A33
- obstetrical A34
- puerperal, postpartum, childbirth A34

Tetany (due to) R29.0
- alkalosis E87.3
- associated with rickets E55.0
- convulsions R29.0
  - hysterical F44.5
- functional (hysterical) F44.5
- hyperkinetic R29.0
  - hysterical F44.5
- hyperpnea R06.4
  - hysterical F44.5
  - psychogenic F45.8
- hyperventilation (*see also* Hyperventilation) R06.4
  - hysterical F44.5
- neonatal (without calcium or magnesium deficiency) P71.3
- parathyroid (gland) E20.9
- parathyroprival E89.2
- post- (para)thyroidectomy E89.2
- postoperative E89.2
- pseudotetany R29.0
- psychogenic (conversion reaction) F44.5

Tetralogy of Fallot Q21.3

Tetraplegia (chronic) (*see also* Quadriplegia) G82.50

Thailand hemorrhagic fever A91

Thalassanemia *—see* Thalassemia

Thalassemia (anemia) (disease) D56.9
- with other hemoglobinopathy D56.8
- alpha (major) (severe) (triple gene defect) D56.0
  - minor D56.3
  - silent carrier D56.3
  - trait D56.3
- beta (severe) D56.1
  - homozygous D56.1
  - major D56.1
  - minor D56.3
  - trait D56.3
- delta-beta (homozygous) D56.2
  - minor D56.3
  - trait D56.3
- dominant D56.8
- hemoglobin
  - C D56.8
  - E-beta D56.5
- intermedia D56.1
- major D56.1
- minor D56.3
- mixed D56.8
- sickle-cell *—see* Disease, sickle-cell, thalassemia

Thalassemia *(continued)*
- specified type NEC D56.8
- trait D56.3
- variants D56.8

Thanatophoric dwarfism or short stature Q77.1

Thaysen-Gee disease (nontropical sprue) K90.0

Thaysen's disease K90.0

Thecoma D27-
- luteinized D27-
- malignant C56-

Thelarche, premature E30.8

Thelaziasis B83.8

Thelitis N61.0
- puerperal, postpartum or gestational *—see* Infection, nipple

Therapeutic *—see* condition

Therapy
- drug, long-term (current) (prophylactic)
  - agents affecting estrogen receptors and estrogen levels NEC Z79.818
  - anastrozole (Arimidex) Z79.811
  - antibiotics Z79.2
    - short-term use - omit code
  - anticoagulants Z79.01
  - anti-inflammatory Z79.1
  - antiplatelet Z79.02
  - antithrombotics Z79.02
  - aromatase inhibitors Z79.811
  - aspirin Z79.82
  - birth control pill or patch Z79.3
  - bisphosphonates Z79.83
  - contraceptive, oral Z79.3
  - drug, specified NEC Z79.899
  - estrogen receptor downregulators Z79.818
  - Evista Z79.810
  - exemestane (Aromasin) Z79.811
  - Fareston Z79.810
  - fulvestrant (Faslodex) Z79.818
  - gonadotropin-releasing hormone (GnRH) agonist Z79.818
  - goserelin acetate (Zoladex) Z79.818
  - hormone replacement Z79.890
  - insulin Z79.4
  - letrozole (Femara) Z79.811
  - leuprolide acetate (leuprorelin) (Lupron) Z79.818
  - megestrol acetate (Megace) Z79.818
  - methadone
    - for pain management Z79.891
    - maintenance therapy F11.20
  - Nolvadex Z79.810
  - opiate analgesic Z79.891
  - oral contraceptive Z79.3
  - raloxifene (Evista) Z79.810
  - selective estrogen receptor modulators (SERMs) Z79.810
  - short term - omit code
  - steroids
    - inhaled Z79.51
    - systemic Z79.52
  - tamoxifen (Nolvadex) Z79.810
  - toremifene (Fareston) Z79.810

Thermic *—see* condition

Thermography (abnormal) (*see also* Abnormal, diagnostic imaging) R93.89
- breast R92.8

Thermoplegia T67.01

Thesaurismosis, glycogen *—see* Disease, glycogen storage

Thiamin deficiency E51.9
- specified NEC E51.8

Thiaminic deficiency with beriberi E51.11

Thibierge-Weissenbach syndrome *—see* Sclerosis, systemic

Thickening
- bone *—see* Hypertrophy, bone
- breast N64.59
- endometrium R93.89
- epidermal L85.9
  - specified NEC L85.8
- hymen N89.6
- larynx J38.7
- nail L60.2
  - congenital Q84.5
- periosteal *—see* Hypertrophy, bone
- pleura J92.9
  - with asbestos J92.0
- skin R23.4
- subepiglottic J38.7
- tongue K14.8
- valve, heart *—see* Endocarditis

Thigh *—see* condition

Thinning vertebra *—see* Spondylopathy, specified NEC

Thirst, excessive R63.1
- due to deprivation of water T73.1

Thomsen disease G71.12

Thoracic *—see also* condition
- kidney Q63.2
- outlet syndrome G54.0

Thoracogastroschisis (congenital) Q79.8

Thoracopagus Q89.4

Thorax *—see* condition

Thorn's syndrome N28.89

Thorson-Björck syndrome E34.0

Threadworm (infection) (infestation) B80

Threatened
- abortion O20.0
  - with subsequent abortion O03.9
- job loss, anxiety concerning Z56.2
- labor (without delivery) O47.9
  - at or after 37 completed weeks of gestation O47.1
  - before 37 completed weeks of gestation O47.0-
- loss of job, anxiety concerning Z56.2
- miscarriage O20.0
- unemployment, anxiety concerning Z56.2

Three-day fever A93.1

Threshers' lung J67.0

Thrix annulata (congenital) Q84.1

Throat *—see* condition

Thrombasthenia (Glanzmann) (hemorrhagic) (hereditary) D69.1

Thromboangiitis I73.1
- obliterans (general) I73.1
  - cerebral I67.89
  - vessels
    - brain I67.89
    - spinal cord I67.89

Thromboarteritis *—see* Arteritis

Thromboasthenia (Glanzmann) (hemorrhagic) (hereditary) D69.1

Thrombocytasthenia (Glanzmann) D69.1

Thrombocythemia (hemorrhagic) (*see also* Thrombocytosis) D75.839
- essential D47.3
- idiopathic D47.3
- primary D47.3

Thrombocytopathy (dystrophic) (granulopenic) D69.1

Thrombocytopenia, thrombocytopenic D69.6
- with absent radius (TAR) Q87.2
- congenital D69.42
- dilutional D69.59
- due to
  - drugs D69.59
  - extracorporeal circulation of blood D69.59
  - (massive) blood transfusion D69.59
  - platelet alloimmunization D69.59
- essential D69.3
- heparin induced (HIT) D75.82
- hereditary D69.42
- idiopathic D69.3
- neonatal, transitory P61.0
  - due to
    - exchange transfusion P61.0
    - idiopathic maternal thrombocytopenia P61.0
    - isoimmunization P61.0
- primary NEC D69.49
  - idiopathic D69.3
- puerperal, postpartum O72.3
- secondary D69.59
- transient neonatal P61.0

Thrombocytosis D75.839
- essential D47.3
- idiopathic D47.3
- primary D47.3
- reactive D75.838
- secondary D75.838
- specified NEC D75.838

Thromboembolism *—see* Embolism

Thrombopathy (Bernard-Soulier) D69.1
- constitutional D68.0
- Willebrand-Jurgens D68.0

Thrombopenia *—see* Thrombocytopenia

Thrombophilia D68.59
- primary NEC D68.59
- secondary NEC D68.69
- specified NEC D68.69

Thrombophlebitis I80.9
- antepartum O22.2-
  - deep O22.3-
  - superficial O22.2-
- calf muscular vein (NOS) I80.25-
- cavernous (venous) sinus G08
  - complicating pregnancy O22.5-
  - nonpyogenic I67.6
- cerebral (sinus) (vein) G08
  - nonpyogenic I67.6
  - sequelae G09
- due to implanted device *—see* Complications, by site and type, specified NEC
- during or resulting from a procedure NEC T81.72
- femoral vein (superficial) I80.1-
- femoropopliteal vein I80.0-

Thrombophlebitis *(continued)*
- gastrocnemial vein I80.25
- hepatic (vein) I80.8
- idiopathic, recurrent I82.1
- iliac vein (common) (external) (internal) I80.21-
- iliofemoral I80.1-
- intracranial venous sinus (any) G08
  - nonpyogenic I67.6
  - sequelae G09
- intraspinal venous sinuses and veins G08
  - nonpyogenic G95.19
- lateral (venous) sinus G08
  - nonpyogenic I67.6
- leg I80.3
  - superficial I80.0-
- longitudinal (venous) sinus G08
  - nonpyogenic I67.6
- lower extremity I80.299
- migrans, migrating I82.1
- pelvic
  - with ectopic or molar pregnancy O08.0
  - following ectopic or molar pregnancy O08.0
  - puerperal O87.1
- peroneal vein I80.24-
- popliteal vein *—see* Phlebitis, leg, deep, popliteal
- portal (vein) K75.1
- postoperative T81.72
- pregnancy *—see* Thrombophlebitis, antepartum
- puerperal, postpartum, childbirth O87.0
  - deep O87.1
  - pelvic O87.1
  - septic O86.81
  - superficial O87.0
- saphenous (greater) (lesser) I80.0-
- sinus (intracranial) G08
  - nonpyogenic I67.6
- soleal vein I80.25-
- specified site NEC I80.8
- tibial vein (anterior) (posterior) I80.23-

Thrombosis, thrombotic (bland) (multiple) (progressive) (silent) (vessel) I82.90
- anal K64.5
- antepartum *—see* Thrombophlebitis, antepartum
- aorta, aortic I74.10
  - abdominal I74.09
    - saddle I74.01
  - bifurcation I74.09
  - saddle I74.01
  - specified site NEC I74.19
  - terminal I74.09
  - thoracic I74.11
  - valve *—see* Endocarditis, aortic
- apoplexy I63.3-
- artery, arteries (postinfectional) I74.9
  - auditory, internal *—see* Occlusion, artery, precerebral, specified NEC
  - basilar *—see* Occlusion, artery, basilar
  - carotid (common) (internal) *—see* Occlusion, artery, carotid
  - cerebellar (anterior inferior) (posterior inferior) (superior) *—see* Occlusion, artery, cerebellar
  - cerebral *—see* Occlusion, artery, cerebral

Thrombosis, thrombotic *(continued)*
- artery, arteries (continued)
  - choroidal (anterior) *—see* Occlusion, artery, precerebral, specified NEC
  - communicating, posterior *—see* Occlusion, artery, precerebral, specified NEC
  - coronary *—see also* Infarct, myocardium
    - not resulting in infarction I24.0
  - hepatic I74.8
  - hypophyseal *—see* Occlusion, artery, precerebral, specified NEC
  - iliac I74.5
  - limb I74.4
    - lower I74.3
    - upper I74.2
  - meningeal, anterior or posterior *—see* Occlusion, artery, cerebral, specified NEC
  - mesenteric (with gangrene) (*see also* Infarct, intestine) K55.069
  - ophthalmic *—see* Occlusion, artery, retina
  - pontine *—see* Occlusion, artery, precerebral, specified NEC
  - precerebral *—see* Occlusion, artery, precerebral
  - pulmonary (iatrogenic) *—see* Embolism, pulmonary
  - renal N28.0
  - retinal *—see* Occlusion, artery, retina
  - spinal, anterior or posterior G95.11
  - traumatic NEC T14.8
  - vertebral *—see* Occlusion, artery, vertebral
- atrium, auricular *—see also* Infarct, myocardium
  - following acute myocardial infarction (current complication) I23.6
  - not resulting in infarction I51.3
  - old I51.3
- basilar (artery) *—see* Occlusion, artery, basilar
- brain (artery) (stem) *—see also* Occlusion, artery, cerebral
  - due to syphilis A52.05
  - puerperal O99.43
  - sinus *—see* Thrombosis, intracranial venous sinus
- capillary I78.8
- cardiac *—see also* Infarct, myocardium
  - not resulting in infarction I51.3
  - old I51.3
  - valve *—see* Endocarditis
- carotid (artery) (common) (internal) *—see* Occlusion, artery, carotid
- cavernous (venous) sinus *—see* Thrombosis, intracranial venous sinus
- cerebellar artery (anterior inferior) (posterior inferior) (superior) I66.3
- cerebral (artery) *—see* Occlusion, artery, cerebral
- cerebrovenous sinus *—see also* Thrombosis, intracranial venous sinus
  - puerperium O87.3
- chronic I82.91

Thrombosis, thrombotic *(continued)*
- coronary (artery) (vein) *—see also* Infarct, myocardium
  - not resulting in infarction I24.0
- corpus cavernosum N48.89
- cortical I66.9
- deep *—see* Embolism, vein, lower extremity
- due to device, implant or graft (*see also* Complications, by site and type, specified NEC) T85.868
  - arterial graft NEC T82.868
  - breast (implant) T85.868
  - catheter NEC T85.868
    - dialysis (renal) T82.868
      - intraperitoneal T85.868
    - infusion NEC T82.868
      - spinal (epidural) (subdural) T85.860
    - urinary (indwelling) T83.86
  - electronic (electrode) (pulse generator) (stimulator)
    - bone T84.86
    - cardiac T82.867
    - nervous system (brain) (peripheral nerve) (spinal) T85.860
    - urinary T83.86
  - fixation, internal (orthopedic) NEC T84.86
  - gastrointestinal (bile duct) (esophagus) T85.868
  - genital NEC T83.86
  - heart T82.867
  - joint prosthesis T84.86
  - ocular (corneal graft) (orbital implant) NEC T85.868
  - orthopedic NEC T84.86
  - specified NEC T85.868
  - urinary NEC T83.86
  - vascular NEC T82.868
  - ventricular intracranial shunt T85.860
- during the puerperium *—see* Thrombosis, puerperal
- endocardial *—see also* Infarct, myocardium
  - not resulting in infarction I51.3
- eye *—see* Occlusion, retina
- genital organ
  - female NEC N94.89
    - pregnancy *—see* Thrombophlebitis, antepartum
  - male N50.1
- gestational *—see* Phlebopathy, gestational
- heart (chamber) *—see also* Infarct, myocardium
  - not resulting in infarction I51.3
  - old I51.3
- hepatic (vein) I82.0
  - artery I74.8
- history (of) Z86.718
- intestine (with gangrene (*see also* Infarct, intestine)) K55.069
- intracardiac NEC (apical) (atrial) (auricular) (ventricular) (old) I51.3
- intracranial (arterial) I66.9
  - venous sinus (any) G08
    - nonpyogenic origin I67.6
    - puerperium O87.3
- intramural *—see also* Infarct, myocardium
  - not resulting in infarction I51.3
  - old I51.3
- intraspinal venous sinuses and veins G08
  - nonpyogenic G95.19

Thrombosis, thrombotic *(continued)*
- kidney (artery) N28.0
- lateral (venous) sinus *—see* Thrombosis, intracranial venous sinus
- leg *—see* Thrombosis, vein, lower extremity
  - arterial I74.3
- liver (venous) I82.0
  - artery I74.8
  - portal vein I81
- longitudinal (venous) sinus *—see* Thrombosis, intracranial venous sinus
- lower limb *—see* Thrombosis, vein, lower extremity
- lung (iatrogenic) (postoperative) *—see* Embolism, pulmonary
- meninges (brain) (arterial) I66.8
- mesenteric (artery) (with gangrene) (*see also* Infarct, intestine) K55.069
  - vein (inferior) (superior) K55.0-
- mitral I34.8
- mural *—see also* Infarct, myocardium
  - due to syphilis A52.06
  - not resulting in infarction I51.3
  - old I51.3
- omentum (with gangrene) (*see also* Infarct, intestine) K55.069
- ophthalmic *—see* Occlusion, retina
- pampiniform plexus (male) N50.1
- parietal *—see also* Infarct, myocardium
  - not resulting in infarction I24.0
- penis, superficial vein N48.81
- perianal venous K64.5
- peripheral arteries I74.4
  - upper I74.2
- personal history (of) Z86.718
- portal I81
  - due to syphilis A52.09
- precerebral artery *—see* Occlusion, artery, precerebral
- puerperal, postpartum O87.0
  - brain (artery) O99.43
    - venous (sinus) O87.3
  - cardiac O99.43
  - cerebral (artery) O99.43
    - venous (sinus) O87.3
  - superficial O87.0
- pulmonary (artery) (iatrogenic) (postoperative) (vein) *—see* Embolism, pulmonary
- renal (artery) N28.0
  - vein I82.3
- resulting from presence of device, implant or graft *—see* Complications, by site and type, specified NEC
- retina, retinal *—see* Occlusion, retina
- scrotum N50.1
- seminal vesicle N50.1
- sigmoid (venous) sinus *—see* Thrombosis, intracranial venous sinus
- sinus, intracranial (any) *—see* Thrombosis, intracranial venous sinus
- specified site NEC I82.890
  - chronic I82.891
- spermatic cord N50.1
- spinal cord (arterial) G95.11
  - due to syphilis A52.09
  - pyogenic origin G06.1
- spleen, splenic D73.5
  - artery I74.8

Thrombosis, thrombotic *(continued)*
- testis N50.1
- tumor *—see* Neoplasm, unspecified behavior, by site
- traumatic NEC T14.8
- tricuspid I07.8
- tunica vaginalis N50.1
- umbilical cord (vessels), complicating delivery O69.5
- vas deferens N50.1
- vein (acute) I82.90
  - antecubital I82.61-
    - chronic I82.71-
  - axillary I82.A1-
    - chronic I82.A2-
  - basilic I82.61-
    - chronic I82.71-
  - brachial I82.62-
    - chronic I82.72-
  - brachiocephalic (innominate) I82.290
    - chronic I82.291
  - cerebral, nonpyogenic I67.6
  - cephalic I82.61-
    - chronic I82.71-
  - chronic I82.91
  - deep (DVT) I82.40-
    - calf I82.4Z-
      - chronic I82.5Z-
    - lower leg I82.4Z-
      - chronic I82.5Z-
    - thigh I82.4Y-
      - chronic I82.5Y-
    - upper leg I82.4Y-
      - chronic I82.5Y-
  - femoral I82.41-
    - chronic I82.51-
  - iliac (iliofemoral) I82.42-
    - chronic I82.52-
  - innominate I82.290
    - chronic I82.291
  - internal jugular I82.C1-
    - chronic I82.C2-
  - lower extremity
    - deep I82.40-
      - chronic I82.50-
      - specified NEC I82.49-
        - chronic NEC I82.59-
    - distal
      - deep I82.4Z-
    - proximal
      - deep I82.4Y-
        - chronic I82.5Y-
    - superficial I82.81-
  - perianal K64.5
  - popliteal I82.43-
    - chronic I82.53-
  - radial I82.62-
    - chronic I82.72-
  - renal I82.3
  - saphenous (greater) (lesser) I82.81-
  - specified NEC I82.890
    - chronic NEC I82.891
  - subclavian I82.B1-
    - chronic I82.B2-
  - thoracic NEC I82.290
    - chronic I82.291
  - tibial I82.44-
    - chronic I82.54-
  - ulnar I82.62-
    - chronic I82.72-
  - upper extremity I82.60-
    - chronic I82.70-
    - deep I82.62-
      - chronic I82.72-
    - superficial I82.61-
      - chronic I82.71-
- vena cava
  - inferior I82.220
    - chronic I82.221

Thrombosis, thrombotic *(continued)*
- vena cava *(continued)*
  - superior I82.210
    - chronic I82.211
- venous, perianal K64.5
- ventricle *—see also* Infarct, myocardium
  - following acute myocardial infarction (current complication) I23.6
  - not resulting in infarction I24.0
  - old I51.3

Thrombus *—see* Thrombosis

Thrush *—see also* Candidiasis
- oral B37.0
  - newborn P37.5
- vaginal B37.3

Thumb *—see also* condition
- sucking (child problem) F98.8

Thymitis E32.8

Thymoma *—see also* Neoplasm, thymus, by type
- malignant C37
- metaplastic C37
- microscopic D15.0
- sclerosing C37
- type A C37
- type AB C37
- type B1 C37
- type B2 C37
- type B3 C37

Thymus, thymic (gland) *—see* condition

Thyrocele *—see* Goiter

Thyroglossal *—see also* condition
- cyst Q89.2
- duct, persistent Q89.2

Thyroid (gland) (body) *—see also* condition
- hormone resistance E07.89
- lingual Q89.2
- nodule (cystic) (nontoxic) (single) E04.1

Thyroiditis E06.9
- acute (nonsuppurative) (pyogenic) (suppurative) E06.0
- autoimmune E06.3
- chronic (nonspecific) (sclerosing) E06.5
  - with thyrotoxicosis, transient E06.2
  - fibrous E06.5
  - lymphadenoid E06.3
  - lymphocytic E06.3
  - lymphoid E06.3
- de Quervain's E06.1
- drug-induced E06.4
- fibrous (chronic) E06.5
- giant-cell (follicular) E06.1
- granulomatous (de Quervain) (subacute) E06.1
- Hashimoto's (struma lymphomatosa) E06.3
- iatrogenic E06.4
- ligneous E06.5
- lymphocytic (chronic) E06.3
- lymphoid E06.3
- lymphomatous E06.3
- nonsuppurative E06.1
- postpartum, puerperal O90.5
- pseudotuberculous E06.1
- pyogenic E06.0
- radiation E06.4
- Riedel's E06.5
- subacute (granulomatous) E06.1
- suppurative E06.0
- tuberculous A18.81

Thyroiditis *(continued)*
- viral E06.1
- woody E06.5

Thyrolingual duct, persistent Q89.2

Thyromegaly E01.0

Thyrotoxic
- crisis *—see* Thyrotoxicosis
- heart disease or failure (*see also* Thyrotoxicosis) E05.90 *[I43]*
  - with thyroid storm E05.91 *[I43]*
- storm *—see* Thyrotoxicosis

Thyrotoxicosis (recurrent) E05.90
- with
  - goiter (diffuse) E05.00
    - with thyroid storm E05.01
    - adenomatous uninodular E05.10
      - with thyroid storm E05.11
    - multinodular E05.20
      - with thyroid storm E05.21
    - nodular E05.20
      - with thyroid storm E05.21
    - uninodular E05.10
      - with thyroid storm E05.11
  - infiltrative
    - dermopathy E05.00
      - with thyroid storm E05.01
    - ophthalmopathy E05.00
      - with thyroid storm E05.01
  - single thyroid nodule E05.10
    - with thyroid storm E05.11
  - thyroid storm E05.91
- due to
  - ectopic thyroid nodule or tissue E05.30
    - with thyroid storm E05.31
  - ingestion of (excessive) thyroid material E05.40
    - with thyroid storm E05.41
  - overproduction of thyroid-stimulating hormone E05.80
    - with thyroid storm E05.81
  - specified cause NEC E05.80
    - with thyroid storm E05.81
- factitia E05.40
  - with thyroid storm E05.41
- heart (*see also* Failure, heart, high-output) E05.90 *[I43]*
  - with thyroid storm (*see* also Failure, heart, high-output) E05.91 *[I43]*
  - failure (*see* also Failure, heart, high-output) E05.90 *[I43]*
- neonatal (transient) P72.1
- transient with chronic thyroiditis E06.2

Tibia vara M92.51-

Tic (disorder) F95.9
- breathing F95.8
- child problem F95.0
- compulsive F95.1
- de la Tourette F95.2
- degenerative (generalized) (localized) G25.69
  - facial G25.69
- disorder
  - chronic
    - motor F95.1
    - vocal F95.1
  - combined vocal and multiple motor F95.2
  - transient F95.0
- douloureux G50.0
  - atypical G50.1
  - postherpetic, postzoster B02.22
- drug-induced G25.61
- eyelid F95.8

Tic *(continued)*
habit F95.9
chronic F95.1
transient of childhood F95.0
lid, transient of childhood F95.0
motor-verbal F95.2
occupational F48.8
orbicularis F95.8
transient of childhood F95.0
organic origin G25.69
postchoreic G25.69
provisional F95.0
psychogenic, compulsive F95.1
salaam R25.8
spasm (motor or vocal) F95.9
chronic F95.1
transient of childhood F95.0
specified NEC F95.8

Tick-borne *—see* condition

Tietze's disease or syndrome M94.0

Tight, tightness
anus K62.89
chest R07.89
fascia (lata) M62.89
foreskin (congenital) N47.1
hymen, hymenal ring N89.6
introitus (acquired) (congenital) N89.6
rectal sphincter K62.89
tendon *—see* Short, tendon
urethral sphincter N35.919

Tilting vertebra *—see* Dorsopathy, deforming, specified NEC

Timidity, child F93.8

Tin-miner's lung J63.5

Tinea (intersecta) (tarsi) B35.9
amiantacea L44.8
asbestina B35.0
barbae B35.0
beard B35.0
black dot B35.0
blanca B36.2
capitis B35.0
corporis B35.4
cruris B35.6
flava B36.0
foot B35.3
furfuracea B36.0
imbricata (Tokelau) B35.5
kerion B35.0
manuum B35.2
microsporic *—see* Dermatophytosis
nigra B36.1
nodosa *—see* Piedra
pedis B35.3
scalp B35.0
specified NEC B35.8
sycosis B35.0
tonsurans B35.0
trichophytic *—see* Dermatophytosis
unguium B35.1
versicolor B36.0

Tingling sensation (skin) R20.2

Tinnitus NOS H93.1-
audible H93.1-
aurium H93.1-
pulsatile H93.A-
subjective H93.1-

Tipped tooth (teeth) M26.33

Tipping
pelvis M95.5
with disproportion (fetopelvic) O33.0
causing obstructed labor O65.0
tooth (teeth), fully erupted M26.33

Tiredness R53.83

Tissue *—see* condition

Tobacco (nicotine)
abuse, *—see* Tobacco, use
dependence *—see* Dependence, drug, nicotine
harmful use Z72.0
heart *—see* Tobacco, toxic effect
maternal use, affecting newborn P04.2
toxic effect *—see* Table of Drugs and Chemicals, by substance, poisoning
chewing tobacco *—see* Table of Drugs and Chemicals, by substance, poisoning
cigarettes *—see* Table of Drugs and Chemicals, by substance, poisoning
use Z72.0
complicating
childbirth O99.334
pregnancy O99.33-
puerperium O99.335
counseling and surveillance Z71.6
history Z87.891
withdrawal state (*see also* Dependence, drug, nicotine) F17.203

Tocopherol deficiency E56.0

Todd's
cirrhosis K74.3
paralysis (postepileptic) (transitory) G83.84

Toe *—see* condition

Toilet, artificial opening *—see* Attention to, artificial, opening

Tokelau (ringworm) B35.5

Tollwut *—see* Rabies

Tommaselli's disease R31.9
correct substance properly administered *—see* Table of Drugs and Chemicals, by drug, adverse effect
overdose or wrong substance given or taken *—see* Table of Drugs and Chemicals, by drug, poisoning

Tongue *—see also* condition
tie Q38.1

Tonic pupil *—see* Anomaly, pupil, function, tonic pupil

Toni-Fanconi syndrome (cystinosis) E72.09
with cystinosis E72.04

Tonsil *—see* condition

Tonsillitis (acute) (catarrhal) (croupous) (follicular) (gangrenous) (infective) (lacunar) (lingual) (malignant) (membranous) (parenchymatous) (phlegmonous) (pseudomembranous) (purulent) (septic) (subacute) (suppurative) (toxic) (ulcerative) (vesicular) (viral) J03.90
chronic J35.01
with adenoiditis J35.03
diphtheritic A36.0
hypertrophic J35.01
with adenoiditis J35.03
recurrent J03.91
specified organism NEC J03.80
recurrent J03.81
staphylococcal J03.80
recurrent J03.81

Tonsillitis *(continued)*
streptococcal J03.00
recurrent J03.01
tuberculous A15.8
Vincent's A69.1

Tooth, teeth *—see* condition

Toothache K08.89

Topagnosis R20.8

Tophi *—see* Gout, chronic

TORCH infection *—see* Infection, congenital
without active infection P00.2

Torn *—see* Tear

Tornwaldt's cyst or disease J39.2

Torsion
accessory tube *—see* Torsion, fallopian tube
adnexa (female) *—see* Torsion, fallopian tube
aorta, acquired I77.1
appendix epididymis N44.04
appendix testis N44.03
bile duct (common) (hepatic) K83.8
congenital Q44.5
bowel, colon or intestine K56.2
cervix *—see* Malposition, uterus
cystic duct K82.8
dystonia *—see* Dystonia, torsion
epididymis (appendix) N44.04
fallopian tube N83.52-
with ovary N83.53
gallbladder K82.8
congenital Q44.1
hydatid of Morgagni
female N83.52-
male N44.03
kidney (pedicle) (leading to infarction) N28.0
Meckel's diverticulum (congenital) Q43.0
malignant *—see* Table of Neoplasms, small intestine, malignant
mesentery K56.2
omentum K56.2
organ or site, congenital NEC *—see* Anomaly, by site
ovary (pedicle) N83.51-
with fallopian tube N83.53
congenital Q50.2
oviduct *—see* Torsion, fallopian tube
penis (acquired) N48.82
congenital Q55.63
spasm *—see* Dystonia, torsion
spermatic cord N44.02
extravaginal N44.01
intravaginal N44.02
spleen D73.5
testis, testicle N44.00
appendix N44.03
tibia *—see* Deformity, limb, specified type NEC, lower leg
uterus *—see* Malposition, uterus

Torticollis (intermittent) (spastic) M43.6
congenital (sternomastoid) Q68.0
due to birth injury P15.8
hysterical F44.4
ocular R29.891
psychogenic F45.8
conversion reaction F44.4
rheumatic M43.6
rheumatoid M06.88
spasmodic G24.3
traumatic, current S13.4

Tortipelvis G24.1

Tortuous
aortic arch Q25.46
artery I77.1
organ or site, congenital NEC *—see* Distortion
retinal vessel, congenital Q14.1
ureter N13.8
urethra N36.8
vein *—see* Varix

Torture, victim of Z65.4

Torula, torular (histolytica) (infection) *—see* Cryptococcosis

Torulosis *—see* Cryptococcosis

Torus (mandibularis) (palatinus) M27.0
fracture *—see* Fracture, by site, torus

Touraine's syndrome Q79.8

Tourette's syndrome F95.2

Tourniquet syndrome *—see* Constriction, external, by site

Tower skull Q75.0
with exophthalmos Q87.0

Toxemia R68.89
bacterial *—see* Sepsis
burn *—see* Burn
eclamptic (with pre-existing hypertension) *—see* Eclampsia
erysipelatous *—see* Erysipelas
fatigue R68.89
food *—see* Poisoning, food
gastrointestinal K52.1
intestinal K52.1
kidney *—see* Uremia
malarial *—see* Malaria
myocardial *—see* Myocarditis, toxic
of pregnancy *—see* Pre-eclampsia
pre-eclamptic *—see* Pre-eclampsia
small intestine K52.1
staphylococcal, due to food A05.0
stasis R68.89
uremic *—see* Uremia
urinary *—see* Uremia

Toxemica cerebropathia psychica (nonalcoholic) F04
alcoholic *—see* Alcohol, amnestic disorder

Toxic (poisoning) (*see also* condition) T65.91
effect *—see* Table of Drugs and Chemicals, by substance, poisoning
shock syndrome A48.3
thyroid (gland) *—see* Thyrotoxicosis

Toxicemia *—see* Toxemia

Toxicity *—see* Table of Drugs and Chemicals, by substance, poisoning
fava bean D55.0
food, noxious *—see* Poisoning, food
from drug or nonmedicinal substance *—see* Table of Drugs and Chemicals, by drug

Toxicosis *—see also* Toxemia
capillary, hemorrhagic D69.0

Toxinfection, gastrointestinal K52.1

Toxocariasis B83.0

Toxoplasma, toxoplasmosis (acquired) B58.9
- with
  - hepatitis B58.1
  - meningoencephalitis B58.2
  - ocular involvement B58.00
  - other organ involvement B58.89
  - pneumonia, pneumonitis B58.3
- congenital (acute) (subacute) (chronic) P37.1
- maternal, manifest toxoplasmosis in infant (acute) (subacute) (chronic) P37.1

tPA (rtPA) **administation in a different facility within the last 24 hours prior to admission to current facility** Z92.82

Trabeculation, bladder N32.89

Trachea —*see* condition

Tracheitis (catarrhal) (infantile) (membranous) (plastic) (septal) (suppurative) (viral) J04.10
- with
  - bronchitis (15 years of age and above) J40
    - acute or subacute —*see* Bronchitis, acute
    - chronic J42
    - tuberculous NEC A15.5
    - under 15 years of age J20.9
  - laryngitis (acute) J04.2
    - chronic J37.1
    - tuberculous NEC A15.5
- acute J04.10
  - with obstruction J04.11
- chronic J42
  - with
    - bronchitis (chronic) J42
    - laryngitis (chronic) J37.1
- diphtheritic (membranous) A36.89
- due to external agent —*see* Inflammation, respiratory, upper, due to
- syphilitic A52.73
- tuberculous A15.5

Trachelitis (nonvenereal) —*see* Cervicitis

Tracheobronchial —*see* condition

Tracheobronchitis (15 years of age and above) —*see also* Bronchitis
- due to
  - Bordetella bronchiseptica A37.80
    - with pneumonia A37.81
  - Francisella tularensis A21.8

Tracheobronchomegaly Q32.4
- with bronchiectasis J47.9
  - with
    - exacerbation (acute) J47.1
    - lower respiratory infection J47.0
- acquired J98.09
  - with bronchiectasis J47.9
    - with
      - exacerbation (acute) J47.1
      - lower respiratory infection J47.0

Tracheobronchopneumonitis —*see* Pneumonia, broncho-

Tracheocele (external) (internal) J39.8
- congenital Q32.1

Tracheomalacia J39.8
- congenital Q32.0

Tracheopharyngitis (acute) J06.9
- chronic J42
- due to external agent —*see* Inflammation, respiratory, upper, due to

Tracheostenosis J39.8

Tracheostomy
- complication —*see* Complication, tracheostomy
- status Z93.0
  - attention to Z43.0
  - malfunctioning J95.03

Trachoma, trachomatous A71.9
- active (stage) A71.1
- contraction of conjunctiva A71.1
- dubium A71.0
- initial (stage) A71.0
- healed or sequelae B94.0
- pannus A71.1
- Türck's J37.0

Traction, vitreomacular H43.82-

Train sickness T75.3

Trait(s)
- Hb-S D57.3
- hemoglobin
  - abnormal NEC D58.2
    - with thalassemia D56.3
  - C —*see* Disease, hemoglobin C
  - S (Hb-S) D57.3
- Lepore D56.3
- personality, accentuated Z73.1
- sickle-cell D57.3
  - with elliptocytosis or spherocytosis D57.3
- type A personality Z73.1

Tramp Z59.00

Trance R41.89
- hysterical F44.89

Transaminasemia R74.01

Transection
- abdomen (partial) S38.3
- aorta (incomplete) —*see also* Injury, aorta
  - complete —*see* Injury, aorta, laceration, major
- carotid artery (incomplete) —*see also* Injury, blood vessel, carotid, laceration
  - complete —*see* Injury, blood vessel, carotid, laceration, major
- celiac artery (incomplete) S35.211
  - branch (incomplete) S35.291
    - complete S35.292
  - complete S35.212
- innominate
  - artery (incomplete) —*see also* Injury, blood vessel, thoracic, innominate, artery, laceration
    - complete —*see* Injury, blood vessel, thoracic, innominate, artery, laceration, major
  - vein (incomplete) —*see also* Injury, blood vessel, thoracic, innominate, vein, laceration
    - complete —*see* Injury, blood vessel, thoracic, innominate, vein, laceration, major
- jugular vein (external) (incomplete) —*see also* Injury, blood vessel, jugular vein, laceration
  - complete —*see* Injury, blood vessel, jugular vein, laceration, major

Transection *(continued)*
- jugular vein *(continued)*
  - internal (incomplete) —*see also* Injury, blood vessel, jugular vein, internal, laceration
    - complete —*see* Injury, blood vessel, jugular vein, internal, laceration, major
- mesenteric artery (incomplete) —*see also* Injury, mesenteric, artery, laceration
  - complete —*see* Injury, mesenteric artery, laceration, major
- pulmonary vessel (incomplete) —*see also* Injury, blood vessel, thoracic, pulmonary, laceration
  - complete —*see* Injury, blood vessel, thoracic, pulmonary, laceration, major
- subclavian —*see* Transection, innominate
- vena cava (incomplete) —*see also* Injury, vena cava
  - complete —*see* Injury, vena cava, laceration, major
- vertebral artery (incomplete) —*see also* Injury, blood vessel, vertebral, laceration
  - complete —*see* Injury, blood vessel, vertebral, laceration, major

Transfusion
- associated (red blood cell) hemochromatosis E83.111
- blood
  - ABO incompatible —*see* Complication(s), transfusion, incompatibility reaction, ABO
  - minor blood group (Duffy) (E) (K) (Kell) (Kidd) (Lewis) (M) (N) (P) (S) T80.89
  - reaction or complication —*see* Complications, transfusion
- fetomaternal (mother) —*see* Pregnancy, complicated by, placenta, transfusion syndrome
- maternofetal (mother) —*see* Pregnancy, complicated by, placenta, transfusion syndrome
- placental (syndrome) (mother) —*see* Pregnancy, complicated by, placenta, transfusion syndrome
- reaction (adverse) —*see* Complications, transfusion
- related acute lung injury (TRALI) J95.84
- twin-to-twin —*see* Pregnancy, complicated by, placenta, transfusion syndrome, fetus to fetus

Transient (meaning homeless) —*see also* condition Z59.00

Translocation
- balanced autosomal Q95.9
  - in normal individual Q95.0
- chromosomes NEC Q99.8
  - balanced and insertion in normal individual Q95.0
- Down syndrome Q90.2
- trisomy
  - 13 Q91.6
  - 18 Q91.2
  - 21 Q90.2

Translucency, iris —*see* Degeneration, iris

Transmission of chemical substances through the placenta —*see* Absorption, chemical, through placenta

Transparency, lung, unilateral J43.0

Transplant (ed) (status) Z94.9
- awaiting organ Z76.82
- bone Z94.6
  - marrow Z94.81
- candidate Z76.82
- complication —*see* Complication, transplant
- cornea Z94.7
- heart Z94.1
  - and lung(s) Z94.3
  - valve Z95.2
    - prosthetic Z95.2
    - specified NEC Z95.4
    - xenogenic Z95.3
- intestine Z94.82
- kidney Z94.0
- liver Z94.4
- lung(s) Z94.2
  - and heart Z94.3
- organ (failure) (infection) (rejection) Z94.9
  - removal status Z98.85
- pancreas Z94.83
- skin Z94.5
- social Z60.3
- specified organ or tissue NEC Z94.89
- stem cells Z94.84
- tissue Z94.9

Transplants, ovarian, endometrial N80.1

Transposed —*see* Transposition

Transposition (congenital) —*see also* Malposition, congenital
- abdominal viscera Q89.3
- aorta (dextra) Q20.3
- appendix Q43.8
- colon Q43.8
- corrected Q20.5
- great vessels (complete) (partial) Q20.3
- heart Q24.0
  - with complete transposition of viscera Q89.3
- intestine (large) (small) Q43.8
- reversed jejunal (for bypass) (status) Z98.0
- scrotum Q55.23
- stomach Q40.2
  - with general transposition of viscera Q89.3
- tooth, teeth, fully erupted M26.30
- vessels, great (complete) (partial) Q20.3
- viscera (abdominal) (thoracic) Q89.3

Transsexualism F64.0

Transverse —*see also* condition
- arrest (deep), in labor O64.0
- lie (mother) O32.2
  - causing obstructed labor O64.8

Transvestism, transvestitism (dual-role) F64.1
- fetishistic F65.1

Trapped placenta (with hemorrhage) O72.0
- without hemorrhage O73.0

TRAPS (tumor necrosis factor receptor associated periodic syndrome) M04.1

Trauma, traumatism —*see also* Injury
acoustic —*see* subcategory H83.3
birth —*see* Birth, injury
complicating ectopic or molar pregnancy O08.6
during delivery O71.9
following ectopic or molar pregnancy O08.6
obstetric O71.9
specified NEC O71.89
occlusal
primary K08.81
secondary K08.82

Traumatic —*see also* condition
brain injury S06.9

Treacher Collins syndrome Q75.4

Treitz's hernia —*see* Hernia, abdomen, specified site NEC

Trematode infestation —*see* Infestation, fluke

Trematodiasis —*see* Infestation, fluke

Trembling paralysis —*see* Parkinsonism

Tremor(s) R25.1
drug induced G25.1
essential (benign) G25.0
familial G25.0
hereditary G25.0
hysterical F44.4
intention G25.2
medication induced postural G25.1
mercurial —*see* subcategory T56.1
Parkinson's —*see* Parkinsonism
psychogenic (conversion reaction) F44.4
senilis R54
specified type NEC G25.2

Trench
fever A79.0
foot —*see* Immersion, foot
mouth A69.1

Treponema pallidum infection —*see* Syphilis

Treponematosis
due to
T. pallidum —*see* Syphilis
T. pertenue —*see* Yaws

Triad
Hutchinson's (congenital syphilis) A50.53
Kartagener's Q89.3
Saint's —*see* Hernia, diaphragm

Trichiasis (eyelid) H02.059
with entropion —*see* Entropion
left H02.056
lower H02.055
upper H02.054
right H02.053
lower H02.052
upper H02.051

Trichinella spiralis (infection) (infestation) B75

Trichinellosis, trichiniasis, trichinelliasis, trichinosis B75
with muscle disorder B75 *[M63.80]*
ankle B75 *[M63.87-]*
foot B75 *[M63.87-]*
forearm B75 *[M63.83-]*
hand B75 *[M63.84-]*

Trichinellosis, trichiniasis, trichinelliasis, trichinosis *(continued)*
with muscle disorder *(continued)*
lower leg B75 *[M63.86-]*
multiple sites B75 *[M63.89]*
pelvic region B75 *[M63.85-]*
shoulder region B75 *[M63.81-]*
specified site NEC B75 *[M63.88]*
thigh B75 *[M63.85-]*
upper arm B75 *[M63.82-]*

Trichobezoar T18.9
intestine T18.3
stomach T18.2

Trichocephaliasis, trichocephalosis B79

Trichocephalus infestation B79

Trichoclasis L67.8

Trichoepithelioma —*see also* Neoplasm, skin, benign
malignant —*see* Neoplasm, skin, malignant

Trichofolliculoma —*see* Neoplasm, skin, benign

Tricholemmoma —*see* Neoplasm, skin, benign

Trichomoniasis A59.9
bladder A59.03
cervix A59.09
intestinal A07.8
prostate A59.02
seminal vesicles A59.09
specified site NEC A59.8
urethra A59.03
urogenitalis A59.00
vagina A59.01
vulva A59.01

Trichomycosis
axillaris A48.8
nodosa, nodularis B36.8

Trichonodosis L67.8

Trichophytid, trichophyton infection —*see* Dermatophytosis

Trichophytobezoar T18.9
intestine T18.3
stomach T18.2

Trichophytosis —*see* Dermatophytosis

Trichoptilosis L67.8

Trichorrhexis (nodosa) (invaginata) L67.0

Trichosis axillaris A48.8

Trichosporosis nodosa B36.2

Trichostasis spinulosa (congenital) Q84.1

Trichostrongyliasis, trichostrongylosis (small intestine) B81.2

Trichostrongylus infection B81.2

Trichotillomania F63.3

Trichromat, trichromatopsia, anomalous (congenital) H53.55

Trichuriasis B79

Trichuris trichiura (infection) (infestation) (any site) B79

Tricuspid (valve) —*see* condition

Trifid —*see also* Accessory
kidney (pelvis) Q63.8
tongue Q38.3

Trigeminal neuralgia —*see* Neuralgia, trigeminal

Trigeminy R00.8

Trigger finger (acquired) M65.30
congenital Q74.0
index finger M65.32-
little finger M65.35-
middle finger M65.33-
ring finger M65.34-
thumb M65.31-

Trigonitis (bladder) (chronic) (pseudomembranous) N30.30
with hematuria N30.31

Trigonocephaly Q75.0

Trilocular heart —*see* Cor triloculare

Trimethylaminuria E72.52

Tripartite placenta O43.19-

Triphalangeal thumb Q74.0

Triple —*see also* Accessory
kidneys Q63.0
uteri Q51.818
X, female Q97.0

Triple I O41.12-

Triplegia G83.89
congenital G80.8

Triplet (newborn) —*see also* Newborn, triplet
complicating pregnancy —*see* Pregnancy, triplet

Triplication —*see* Accessory

Triploidy Q92.7

Trismus R25.2
neonatorum A33
newborn A33

Trisomy (syndrome) Q92.9
autosomes Q92.9
chromosome specified NEC Q92.8
partial Q92.2
due to unbalanced translocation Q92.5
whole (nonsex chromosome)
meiotic nondisjunction Q92.0
mitotic nondisjunction Q92.1
mosaicism Q92.1
specified NEC Q92.8
due to
dicentrics —*see* Extra, marker chromosomes
extra rings —*see* Extra, marker chromosomes
isochromosomes —*see* Extra, marker chromosomes
specified NEC Q92.8
whole chromosome Q92.9
meiotic nondisjunction Q92.0
mitotic nondisjunction Q92.1
mosaicism Q92.1
partial Q92.9
specified NEC Q92.8
13 (partial) Q91.7
meiotic nondisjunction Q91.4
mitotic nondisjunction Q91.5
mosaicism Q91.5
translocation Q91.6
18 (partial) Q91.3
meiotic nondisjunction Q91.0
mitotic nondisjunction Q91.1
mosaicism Q91.1
translocation Q91.2
20 Q92.8
21 (partial) Q90.9
meiotic nondisjunction Q90.0
mitotic nondisjunction Q90.1
mosaicism Q90.1
translocation Q90.2
22 Q92.8

Tritanomaly, tritanopia H53.55

Trombiculosis, trombiculiasis, trombidiosis B88.0

Trophedema (congenital) (hereditary) Q82.0

Trophoblastic disease (*see also* Mole, hydatidiform) O01.9

Tropholymphedema Q82.0

Trophoneurosis NEC G96.89
disseminated M34.9

Tropical —*see* condition

Trouble —*see also* Disease
heart —*see* Disease, heart
kidney —*see* Disease, renal
nervous R45.0
sinus —*see* Sinusitis

Trousseau's syndrome (thrombophlebitis migrans) I82.1

Truancy, childhood
from school Z72.810

Truncus
arteriosus (persistent) Q20.0
communis Q20.0

Trunk —*see* condition

Trypanosomiasis
African B56.9
by Trypanosoma brucei
gambiense B56.0
rhodesiense B56.1
American —*see* Chagas' disease
Brazilian —*see* Chagas' disease
by Trypanosoma
brucei gambiense B56.0
brucei rhodesiense B56.1
cruzi —*see* Chagas' disease
gambiensis, Gambian B56.0
rhodesiensis, Rhodesian B56.1
South American —*see* Chagas' disease
where
African trypanosomiasis is prevalent B56.9
Chagas' disease is prevalent B57.2

Tryptasemia, hereditary alpha D89.44

T-shaped incisors K00.2

Tsutsugamushi (disease) (fever) A75.3

Tube, tubal, tubular —*see* condition

Tubercle —*see also* Tuberculosis
brain, solitary A17.81
Darwin's Q17.8
Ghon, primary infection A15.7

Tuberculid, tuberculide (indurating, subcutaneous) (lichenoid) (miliary) (papulonecrotic) (primary) (skin) A18.4

Tuberculoma —*see also* Tuberculosis
brain A17.81
meninges (cerebral) (spinal) A17.1
spinal cord A17.81

Tuberculosis, tubercular, tuberculous (calcification) (calcified) (caseous) (chromogenic acid-fast bacilli) (degeneration) (fibrocaseous) (fistula) (interstitial) (isolated circumscribed lesions) (necrosis) (parenchymatous) (ulcerative) A15.9
with pneumoconiosis (any condition in J60-J64) J65

Tuberculosis, tubercular, tuberculous *(continued)*
- mediastinitis *(continued)*
  - primary (progressive) A15.7
- mediastinum A15.8
  - primary (progressive) A15.7
- medulla A17.81
- melanosis, Addisonian A18.7
- meninges, meningitis (basilar) (cerebral) (cerebrospinal) (spinal) A17.0
- meningoencephalitis A17.82
- mesentery, mesenteric (gland or node) A18.39
- miliary A19.9
  - acute A19.2
    - multiple sites A19.1
    - single specified site A19.0
  - chronic A19.8
  - specified NEC A19.8
- millstone makers' J65
- miner's J65
- molder's J65
- mouth A18.83
- multiple A19.9
  - acute A19.1
  - chronic A19.8
- muscle A18.09
- myelitis A17.82
- myocardium, myocarditis A18.84
- nasal (passage) (sinus) A15.8
- nasopharynx A15.8
- neck gland A18.2
- nephritis A18.11
- nerve (mononeuropathy) A17.83
- nervous system A17.9
- nose (septum) A15.8
- ocular A18.50
- omentum A18.31
- oophoritis (acute) (chronic) A18.17
- optic (nerve trunk) (papilla) A18.59
- orbit A18.59
- orchitis A18.15
- organ, specified NEC A18.89
- osseous —*see* Tuberculosis, bone
- osteitis —*see* Tuberculosis, bone
- osteomyelitis —*see* Tuberculosis, bone
- otitis media A18.6
- ovary, ovaritis (acute) (chronic) A18.17
- oviduct (acute) (chronic) A18.17
- pachymeningitis A17.0
- palate (soft) A18.83
- pancreas A18.83
- papulonecrotic (a) (primary) A18.4
- parathyroid glands A18.82
- paronychia (primary) A18.4
- parotid gland or region A18.83
- pelvis (bony) A18.03
- penis A18.15
- peribronchitis A15.5
- pericardium, pericarditis A18.84
- perichondritis, larynx A15.5
- periostitis —*see* Tuberculosis, bone
- perirectal fistula A18.32
- peritoneum NEC A18.31
- peritonitis A18.31
- pharynx, pharyngitis A15.8
- phlyctenulosis (keratoconjunctivitis) A18.52
- phthisis NEC —*see* Tuberculosis, pulmonary
- pituitary gland A18.82
- pleura, pleural, pleurisy, pleuritis (fibrinous) (obliterative) (purulent) (simple plastic) (with effusion) A15.6

Tuberculosis, tubercular, tuberculous *(continued)*
- pleura, pleural, pleurisy, pleuritis *(continued)*
  - primary (progressive) A15.7
- pneumonia, pneumonic —*see* Tuberculosis, pulmonary
- pneumothorax (spontaneous) (tense valvular) —*see* Tuberculosis, pulmonary
- polyneuropathy A17.89
- polyserositis A19.9
  - acute A19.1
  - chronic A19.8
- potter's J65
- prepuce A18.15
- primary (complex) A15.7
- proctitis A18.32
- prostate, prostatitis A18.14
- pulmonalis —*see* Tuberculosis, pulmonary
- pulmonary (cavitated) (fibrotic) (infiltrative) (nodular) A15.0
  - childhood type or first infection A15.7
  - primary (complex) A15.7
- pyelitis A18.11
- pyelonephritis A18.11
- pyemia —*see* Tuberculosis, miliary
- pyonephrosis A18.11
- pyopneumothorax A15.6
- pyothorax A15.6
- rectum (fistula) (with abscess) A18.32
- reinfection stage —*see* Tuberculosis, pulmonary
- renal A18.11
- renis A18.11
- respiratory A15.9
  - primary A15.7
  - specified site NEC A15.8
- retina, retinitis A18.53
- retroperitoneal (lymph gland or node) A18.39
- rheumatism NEC A18.09
- rhinitis A15.8
- sacroiliac (joint) A18.01
- sacrum A18.01
- salivary gland A18.83
- salpingitis (acute) (chronic) A18.17
- sandblaster's J65
- sclera A18.51
- scoliosis A18.01
- scrofulous A18.2
- scrotum A18.15
- seminal tract or vesicle A18.15
- senile A15.9
- septic —*see* Tuberculosis, miliary
- shoulder (joint) A18.02
  - blade A18.03
- sigmoid A18.32
- sinus (any nasal) A15.8
  - bone A18.03
  - epididymis A18.15
- skeletal NEC A18.03
- skin (any site) (primary) A18.4
- small intestine A18.32
- soft palate A18.83
- spermatic cord A18.15
- spine, spinal (column) A18.01
  - cord A17.81
  - medulla A17.81
  - membrane A17.0
  - meninges A17.0
- spleen, splenitis A18.85
- spondylitis A18.01
- sternoclavicular joint A18.02
- stomach A18.83
- stonemason's J65

Tuberculosis, tubercular, tuberculous *(continued)*
- subcutaneous tissue (cellular) (primary) A18.4
- subcutis (primary) A18.4
- subdeltoid bursa A18.83
- submaxillary (region) A18.83
- supraclavicular gland A18.2
- suprarenal (capsule) (gland) A18.7
- swelling, joint (*see also* category M01) (*see also* Tuberculosis, joint) A18.02
- symphysis pubis A18.02
- synovitis A18.09
  - articular A18.02
  - spine or vertebra A18.01
- systemic —*see* Tuberculosis, miliary
- tarsitis A18.4
- tendon (sheath) —*see* Tuberculosis, tenosynovitis
- tenosynovitis A18.09
  - spine or vertebra A18.01
- testis A18.15
- throat A15.8
- thymus gland A18.82
- thyroid gland A18.81
- tongue A18.83
- tonsil, tonsillitis A15.8
- trachea, tracheal A15.5
  - lymph gland or node A15.4
    - primary (progressive) A15.7
- tracheobronchial A15.5
  - lymph gland or node A15.4
    - primary (progressive) A15.7
- tubal (acute) (chronic) A18.17
- tunica vaginalis A18.15
- ulcer (skin) (primary) A18.4
  - bowel or intestine A18.32
  - specified NEC - code under Tuberculosis, by site
- unspecified site A15.9
- ureter A18.11
- urethra, urethral (gland) A18.13
- urinary organ or tract A18.13
- uterus A18.17
- uveal tract A18.54
- uvula A18.83
- vagina A18.18
- vas deferens A18.15
- verruca, verrucosa (cutis) (primary) A18.4
- vertebra (column) A18.01
- vesiculitis A18.15
- vulva A18.18
- wrist (joint) A18.02

Tuberculum
- Carabelli —*see* Note at K00.2
- occlusal —*see* Note at K00.2
- paramolare K00.2

Tuberosity, enitre maxillary M26.07

Tuberous sclerosis (brain) Q85.1

Tubo-ovarian —*see* condition

Tuboplasty, after previous sterilization Z31.0
- aftercare Z31.42

Tubotympanitis, catarrhal (chronic) —*see* Otitis, media, nonsuppurative, chronic, serous

Tularemia A21.9
- with
  - conjunctivitis A21.1
  - pneumonia A21.2
- abdominal A21.3
- bronchopneumonic A21.2
- conjunctivitis A21.1

Tularemia *(continued)*
- cryptogenic A21.3
- enteric A21.3
- gastrointestinal A21.3
- generalized A21.7
- ingestion A21.3
- intestinal A21.3
- oculoglandular A21.1
- ophthalmic A21.1
- pneumonia (any), pneumonic A21.2
- pulmonary A21.2
- sepsis A21.7
- specified NEC A21.8
- typhoidal A21.7
- ulceroglandular A21.0

Tularensis conjunctivitis A21.1

Tumefaction —*see also* Swelling
- liver —*see* Hypertrophy, liver

Tumor —*see also* Neoplasm, unspecified behavior, by site
- acinar cell —*see* Neoplasm, uncertain behavior, by site
- acinic cell —*see* Neoplasm, uncertain behavior, by site
- adenocarcinoid —*see* Neoplasm, malignant, by site
- adenomatoid —*see also* Neoplasm, benign, by site
  - odontogenic —*see* Cyst, calcifying odontogenic
- adnexal (skin) —*see* Neoplasm, skin, benign, by site
- adrenal
  - cortical (benign) D35.0-
    - malignant C74.0-
  - rest —*see* Neoplasm, benign, by site
- alpha-cell
  - malignant
    - pancreas C25.4
    - specified site NEC —*see* Neoplasm, malignant, by site
    - unspecified site C25.4
  - pancreas D13.7
  - specified site NEC —*see* Neoplasm, benign, by site
  - unspecified site D13.7
- aneurysmal —*see* Aneurysm
- aortic body D44.7
  - malignant C75.5
- Askin's —*see* Neoplasm, connective tissue, malignant
- basal cell (*see also* Neoplasm, skin, uncertain behavior) D48.5
- Bednar —*see* Neoplasm, skin, malignant
- benign (unclassified) —*see* Neoplasm, benign, by site
- beta-cell
  - malignant
    - pancreas C25.4
    - specified site NEC —*see* Neoplasm, malignant, by site
    - unspecified site C25.4
  - pancreas D13.7
  - specified site NEC —*see* Neoplasm, benign, by site
  - unspecified site D13.7
- Brenner D27.9
  - borderline malignancy D39.1-
  - malignant C56-
  - proliferating D39.1-
- bronchial alveolar, intravascular D38.1
- Brooke's —*see* Neoplasm, skin, benign
- brown fat —*see* Lipoma

Tumor *(continued)*
- Burkitt —*see* Lymphoma, Burkitt
- calcifying epithelial odontogenic —*see* Cyst, calcifying odontogenic
- carcinoid D3A.00
  - benign D3A.00
    - appendix D3A.020
    - ascending colon D3A.022
    - bronchus (lung) D3A.090
    - cecum D3A.021
    - colon D3A.029
    - descending colon D3A.024
    - duodenum D3A.010
    - foregut NOS D3A.094
    - hindgut NOS D3A.096
    - ileum D3A.012
    - jejunum D3A.011
    - kidney D3A.093
    - large intestine D3A.029
    - lung (bronchus) D3A.090
    - midgut NOS D3A.095
    - rectum D3A.026
    - sigmoid colon D3A.025
    - small intestine D3A.019
    - specified NEC D3A.098
    - stomach D3A.092
    - thymus D3A.091
    - transverse colon D3A.023
  - malignant C7A.00
    - appendix C7A.020
    - ascending colon C7A.022
    - bronchus (lung) C7A.090
    - cecum C7A.021
    - colon C7A.029
    - descending colon C7A.024
    - duodenum C7A.010
    - foregut NOS C7A.094
    - hindgut NOS C7A.096
    - ileum C7A.012
    - jejunum C7A.011
    - kidney C7A.093
    - large intestine C7A.029
    - lung (bronchus) C7A.090
    - midgut NOS C7A.095
    - rectum C7A.026
    - sigmoid colon C7A.025
    - small intestine C7A.019
    - specified NEC C7A.098
    - stomach C7A.092
    - thymus C7A.091
    - transverse colon C7A.023
  - mesentary metastasis C7B.04
  - secondary C7B.00
    - bone C7B.03
    - distant lymph nodes C7B.01
    - liver C7B.02
    - peritoneum C7B.04
    - specified NEC C7B.09
- carotid body D44.6
  - malignant C75.4
- cells —*see also* Neoplasm, unspecified behavior, by site
  - benign —*see* Neoplasm, benign, by site
  - malignant —*see* Neoplasm, malignant, by site
  - uncertain whether benign or malignant —*see* Neoplasm, uncertain behavior, by site
- cervix, in pregnancy or childbirth —*see* Pregnancy, complicated by, tumor, cervix
- chondromatous giant cell —*see* Neoplasm, bone, benign
- chromaffin —*see also* Neoplasm, benign, by site
  - malignant —*see* Neoplasm, malignant, by site
- Cock's peculiar L72.3

Tumor *(continued)*

- Codman's —*see* Neoplasm, bone, benign
- dentigerous, mixed —*see* Cyst, calcifying odontogenic
- dermoid —*see* Neoplasm, benign, by site
  - with malignant transformation C56-
- desmoid (extra-abdominal) —*see also* Neoplasm, connective tissue, uncertain behavior
  - abdominal —*see* Neoplasm, connective tissue, uncertain behavior
- embolus —*see* Neoplasm, secondary, by site
- embryonal (mixed) —*see also* Neoplasm, uncertain behavior, by site
  - liver C22.7
- endodermal sinus
  - specified site —*see* Neoplasm, malignant, by site
  - unspecified site
    - female C56.-
    - male C62.90
- epithelial
  - benign —*see* Neoplasm, benign, by site
  - malignant —*see* Neoplasm, malignant, by site
- Ewing's —*see* Neoplasm, bone, malignant, by site
- fatty —*see* Lipoma
- fibroid —*see* Leiomyoma
- G cell
  - malignant
    - pancreas C25.4
    - specified site NEC —*see* Neoplasm, malignant, by site
    - unspecified site C25.4
  - specified site —*see* Neoplasm, uncertain behavior, by site
  - unspecified site D37.8
- germ cell —*see also* Neoplasm, malignant, by site
  - mixed —*see* Neoplasm, malignant, by site
- ghost cell, odontogenic —*see* Cyst, calcifying odontogenic
- giant cell —*see also* Neoplasm, uncertain behavior, by site
  - bone D48.0
    - malignant —*see* Neoplasm, bone, malignant
  - chondromatous —*see* Neoplasm, bone, benign
  - malignant —*see* Neoplasm, malignant, by site
  - soft parts —*see* Neoplasm, connective tissue, uncertain behavior
    - malignant —*see* Neoplasm, connective tissue, malignant
- glomus D18.00
  - intra-abdominal D18.03
  - intracranial D18.02
  - jugulare D44.7
    - malignant C75.5
  - skin D18.01
  - specified site NEC D18.09
- gonadal stromal —*see* Neoplasm, uncertain behavior, by site
- granular cell —*see also* Neoplasm, connective tissue, benign
  - malignant —*see* Neoplasm, connective tissue, malignant

Tumor *(continued)*

- granulosa cell D39.1-
  - juvenile D39.1-
  - malignant C56-
- granulosa cell-theca cell D39.1-
  - malignant C56-
- Grawitz's C64-
- hemorrhoidal —*see* Hemorrhoids
- hilar cell D27-
- hilus cell D27-
- Hurthle cell (benign) D34
  - malignant C73
- hydatid —*see* Echinococcus
- hypernephroid —*see also* Neoplasm, uncertain behavior, by site
- interstitial cell —*see also* Neoplasm, uncertain behavior, by site
  - benign —*see* Neoplasm, benign, by site
  - malignant —*see* Neoplasm, malignant, by site
- intravascular bronchial alveolar D38.1
- islet cell —*see* Neoplasm, benign, by site
  - malignant —*see* Neoplasm, malignant, by site
    - pancreas C25.4
    - specified site NEC —*see* Neoplasm, malignant, by site
    - unspecified site C25.4
  - pancreas D13.7
  - specified site NEC —*see* Neoplasm, benign, by site
  - unspecified site D13.7
- juxtaglomerular D41.0-
- Klatskin's C24.0
- Krukenberg's C79.6-
- Leydig cell —*see* Neoplasm, uncertain behavior, by site
  - benign —*see* Neoplasm, benign, by site
    - specified site —*see* Neoplasm, benign, by site
    - unspecified site
      - female D27.9
      - male D29.20
  - malignant —*see* Neoplasm, malignant, by site
    - specified site —*see* Neoplasm, malignant, by site
    - unspecified site
      - female C56.9
      - male C62.90
  - specified site —*see* Neoplasm, uncertain behavior, by site
  - unspecified site
    - female D39.10
    - male D40.10
- lipid cell, ovary D27-
- lipoid cell, ovary D27-
- malignant (*see also* Neoplasm, malignant, by site) C80.1
  - fusiform cell (type) C80.1
  - giant cell (type) C80.1
  - localized, plasma cell —*see* Plasmacytoma, solitary
  - mixed NEC C80.1
  - small cell (type) C80.1
  - spindle cell (type) C80.1
  - unclassified C80.1
- mast cell D47.09
- melanotic, neuroectodermal —*see* Neoplasm, benign, by site
- Merkel cell —*see* Carcinoma, Merkel cell
- mesenchymal
  - malignant —*see* Neoplasm, connective tissue, malignant

Tumor *(continued)*

- mesenchymal *(continued)*
  - mixed —*see* Neoplasm, connective tissue, uncertain behavior
- mesodermal, mixed —*see also* Neoplasm, malignant, by site
  - liver C22.4
- mesonephric —*see also* Neoplasm, uncertain behavior, by site
  - malignant —*see* Neoplasm, malignant, by site
- metastatic
  - from specified site —*see* Neoplasm, malignant, by site
  - of specified site —*see* Neoplasm, malignant, by site
  - to specified site —*see* Neoplasm, secondary, by site
- mixed NEC —*see also* Neoplasm, benign, by site
  - malignant —*see* Neoplasm, malignant, by site
- mucinous of low malignant potential
  - specified site —*see* Neoplasm, malignant, by site
  - unspecified site C56.9
- mucocarcinoid
  - specified site —*see* Neoplasm, malignant, by site
  - unspecified site C18.1
- mucoepidermoid —*see* Neoplasm, uncertain behavior, by site
- Müllerian, mixed
  - specified site —*see* Neoplasm, malignant, by site
  - unspecified site C54.9
- myoepithelial —*see* Neoplasm, benign, by site
- neuroectodermal (peripheral) —*see* Neoplasm, malignant, by site
  - primitive
    - specified site —*see* Neoplasm, malignant, by site
    - unspecified site C71.9
- neuroendocrine D3A.8
  - malignant poorly differentiated C7A.1
  - secondary NEC C7B.8
  - specified NEC C7A.8
- neurogenic olfactory C30.0
- nonencapsulated sclerosing C73
- odontogenic (adenomatoid) (benign) (calcifying epithelial) (keratocystic) (squamous) —*see* Cyst, calcifying odontogenic
  - malignant C41.1
    - upper jaw (bone) C41.0
- ovarian stromal D39.1-
- ovary, in pregnancy —*see* Pregnancy, complicated by
- pacinian —*see* Neoplasm, skin, benign
- Pancoast's —*see* Pancoast's syndrome
- papillary —*see also* Papilloma
  - cystic D37.9
  - mucinous of low malignant potential C56-
    - specified site —*see* Neoplasm, malignant, by site
    - unspecified site C56.9
  - serous of low malignant potential
    - specified site —*see* Neoplasm, malignant, by site
    - unspecified site C56.9
- pelvic, in pregnancy or childbirth —*see* Pregnancy, complicated by

Tumor *(continued)*
- phantom F45.8
- phyllodes D48.6-
  - benign D24-
  - malignant *—see* Neoplasm, breast, malignant
- Pindborg *—see* Cyst, calcifying odontogenic
- placental site trophoblastic D39.2
- plasma cell (malignant) (localized) *—see* Plasmacytoma, solitary
- polyvesicular vitelline
  - specified site *—see* Neoplasm, malignant, by site
  - unspecified site
    - female C56.9
    - male C62.90
- Pott's puffy *—see* Osteomyelitis, specified NEC
- Rathke's pouch D44.3
- retinal anlage *—see* Neoplasm, benign, by site
- salivary gland type, mixed *—see* Neoplasm, salivary gland, benign
  - malignant *—see* Neoplasm, salivary gland, malignant
- Sampson's N80.1
- Schmincke's *—see* Neoplasm, nasopharynx, malignant
- sclerosing stromal D27-
- sebaceous *—see* Cyst, sebaceous
- secondary *—see* Neoplasm, secondary, by site
  - carcinoid C7B.00
    - bone C7B.03
    - distant lymph nodes C7B.01
    - liver C7B.02
    - peritoneum C7B.04
    - specified NEC C7B.09
  - neuroendocrine NEC C7B.8
- serous of low malignant potential
  - specified site *—see* Neoplasm, malignant, by site
  - unspecified site C56.9
- Sertoli cell *—see* Neoplasm, benign, by site
  - with lipid storage
    - specified site *—see* Neoplasm, benign, by site
    - unspecified site
      - female D27.9
      - male D29.20
  - specified site *—see* Neoplasm, benign, by site
  - unspecified site
    - female D27.9
    - male D29.20
- Sertoli-Leydig cell *—see* Neoplasm, benign, by site
  - specified site *—see* Neoplasm, benign, by site
  - unspecified site
    - female D27.9
    - male D29.20
- sex cord (-stromal) *—see* Neoplasm, uncertain behavior, by site
  - with annular tubules D39.1-
- skin appendage *—see* Neoplasm, skin, benign
- smooth muscle *—see* Neoplasm, connective tissue, uncertain behavior
- soft tissue
  - benign *—see* Neoplasm, connective tissue, benign
  - malignant *—see* Neoplasm, connective tissue, malignant
- sternomastoid (congenital) Q68.0

Tumor *(continued)*
- stromal
  - endometrial D39.0
  - gastric D48.1
    - benign D21.4
    - malignant C16.9
    - uncertain behavior D48.1
  - gastrointestinal C49.A-
    - benign D21.4
    - esophagus C49.A1
    - malignant C49.A0
      - colon C49.A4
      - duodenum C49.A3
      - esophagus C49.A1
      - ileum C49.A3
      - jejunum C49.A3
      - Meckel diverticulum C49.A3
      - large intestine C49.A4
      - omentum C49.A9
      - peritoneum C49.A9
      - rectum C49.A5
      - small intestine C49.A3
      - specified site NEC C49.A9
      - stomach C49.A2
    - rectum C49.A5
    - small intestine C49.A3
    - specified site NEC C49.A9
    - stomach C49.A2
    - uncertain behavior D48.1
  - intestine
    - benign D21.4
    - malignant
      - large C49.A4
      - small C49.A3
    - uncertain behavior D48.1
  - ovarian D39.1-
  - stomach C49.A2
    - benign D21.4
    - malignant C49.A2
    - uncertain behavior D48.1
- testicular D40.10
- sweat gland *—see also* Neoplasm, skin, uncertain behavior
  - benign *—see* Neoplasm, skin, benign
  - malignant *—see* Neoplasm, skin, malignant
- syphilitic, brain A52.17
- testicular stromal D40.1-
- theca cell D27.-
- theca cell-granulosa cell D39.1-
- Triton, malignant *—see* Neoplasm, nerve, malignant
- trophoblastic, placental site D39.2
- turban D23.4
- uterus (body), in pregnancy or childbirth *—see* Pregnancy, complicated by, tumor, uterus
- vagina, in pregnancy or childbirth *—see* Pregnancy, complicated by
- varicose *—see* Varix
- von Recklinghausen's *—see* Neurofibromatosis
- vulva or perineum, in pregnancy or childbirth *—see* Pregnancy, complicated by
  - causing obstructed labor O65.5
- Warthin's *—see* Neoplasm, salivary gland, benign
- Wilms' C64-
- yolk sac *—see* Neoplasm, malignant, by site
  - specified site *—see* Neoplasm, malignant, by site

Tumor *(continued)*
- yolk sac *(continued)*
  - unspecified site
    - female C56.9
    - male C62.90

Tumor lysis syndrome (following antineoplastic chemotherapy) (spontaneous) **NEC** E88.3

Tumorlet *—see* Neoplasm, uncertain behavior, by site

Tungiasis B88.1

Tunica vasculosa lentis Q12.2

Turban tumor D23.4

Türck's trachoma J37.0

Turner-Kieser syndrome Q87.2

Turner-like syndrome Q87.19

Turner's
- hypoplasia (tooth) K00.4
- syndrome Q96.9
  - specified NEC Q96.8
- tooth K00.4

Turner-Ullrich syndrome Q96.9

Tussis convulsiva *—see* Whooping cough

Twiddler's syndrome (due to)
- automatic implantable defibrillator T82.198
- cardiac pacemaker T82.198

Twilight state
- epileptic F05
- psychogenic F44.89

Twin (newborn) *—see also* Newborn, twin
- conjoined Q89.4
- pregnancy *—see* Pregnancy, twin

Twinning, teeth K00.2

Twist, twisted
- bowel, colon or intestine K56.2
- hair (congenital) Q84.1
- mesentery K56.2
- omentum K56.2
- organ or site, congenital NEC *—see* Anomaly, by site
- ovarian pedicle *—see* Torsion, ovary

Twitching R25.3

Tylosis (acquired) L84
- buccalis K13.29
- linguae K13.29
- palmaris et plantaris (congenital) (inherited) Q82.8
  - acquired L85.1

Tympanism R14.0

Tympanites (abdominal) (intestinal) R14.0

Tympanitis *—see* Myringitis

Tympanosclerosis *—see* subcategory H74.0

Tympanum *—see* condition

Tympany
- abdomen R14.0
- chest R09.89

Type A behavior pattern Z73.1

Typhlitis *—see* Appendicitis

Typhoenteritis *—see* Typhoid

Typhoid (abortive) (ambulant) (any site) (clinical) (fever) (hemorrhagic) (infection) (intermittent) (malignant) (rheumatic) (Widal negative) A01.00
- with pneumonia A01.03
- abdominal A01.09

Typhoid *(continued)*
- arthritis A01.04
- carrier (suspected) of Z22.0
- cholecystitis (current) A01.09
- endocarditis A01.02
- heart involvement A01.02
- inoculation reaction *—see* Complications, vaccination
- meningitis A01.01
- mesenteric lymph nodes A01.09
- myocarditis A01.02
- osteomyelitis A01.05
- perichondritis, larynx A01.09
- pneumonia A01.03
- spine A01.05
- specified NEC A01.09
- ulcer (perforating) A01.09

Typhomalaria (fever) *—see* Malaria

Typhomania A01.00

Typhoperitonitis A01.09

Typhus (fever) A75.9
- abdominal, abdominalis *—see* Typhoid
- African tick A77.1
- amarillic A95.9
- brain A75.9 *[G94]*
- cerebral A75.9 *[G94]*
- classical A75.0
- due to Rickettsia
  - prowazekii A75.0
    - recrudescent A75.1
  - tsutsugamushi A75.3
  - typhi A75.2
- endemic (flea-borne) A75.2
- epidemic (louse-borne) A75.0
- exanthematic NEC A75.0
- exanthematicus SAI A75.0
  - brillii SAI A75.1
  - mexicanus SAI A75.2
  - typhus murinus A75.2
- flea-borne A75.2
- India tick A77.1
- Kenya (tick) A77.1
- louse-borne A75.0
- Mexican A75.2
- mite-borne A75.3
- murine A75.2
- North Asian tick-borne A77.2
- Orientia Tsutsugamushi (scrub typhus) A75.3
- petechial A75.9
- Queensland tick A77.3
- rat A75.2
- recrudescent A75.1
- recurrens *—see* Fever, relapsing
- Sao Paulo A77.0
- scrub (China) (India) (Malaysia) (New Guinea) A75.3
- shop (of Malaysia) A75.2
- Siberian tick A77.2
- tick-borne A77.9
- tropical (mite-borne) A75.3

Tyrosinemia E70.21
- newborn, transitory P74.5

Tyrosinosis E70.21

Tyrosinuria E70.29

U

Uhl's anomaly or disease Q24.8

Ulcer, ulcerated, ulcerating, ulceration, ulcerative
- alveolar process M27.3
- amebic (intestine) A06.1
  - skin A06.7
- anastomotic *—see* Ulcer, gastrojejunal

Ulcer, ulcerated, ulcerating, ulceration, ulcerative *(continued)*
- anorectal K62.6
- antral *—see* Ulcer, stomach
- anus (sphincter) (solitary) K62.6
- aorta *—see* Aneurysm
- aphthous (oral) (recurrent) K12.0
  - genital organ(s)
    - female N76.6
    - male N50.89
- artery I77.2
- atrophic *—see* Ulcer, skin
  - decubitus *—see* Ulcer, pressure, by site
- back L98.429
  - with
    - bone involvement without evidence of necrosis L98.426
    - bone necrosis L98.424
    - exposed fat layer L98.422
    - muscle involvement without evidence of necrosis L98.425
    - muscle necrosis L98.423
    - skin breakdown only L98.421
    - specified severity NEC L98.428
- Barrett's (esophagus) K22.10
  - with bleeding K22.11
- bile duct (common) (hepatic) K83.8
- bladder (solitary) (sphincter) NEC N32.89
  - bilharzial B65.9 *[N33]*
  - in schistosomiasis (bilharzial) B65.9 *[N33]*
  - submucosal *—see* Cystitis, interstitial
  - tuberculous A18.12
- bleeding K27.4
- bone *—see* Osteomyelitis, specified type NEC
- bowel *—see* Ulcer, intestine
- breast N61.1
- bronchus J98.09
- buccal (cavity) (traumatic) K12.1
- Buruli A31.1
- buttock L98.419
  - with
    - bone involvement without evidence of necrosis L98.416
    - bone necrosis L98.414
    - exposed fat layer L98.412
    - muscle involvement without evidence of necrosis L98.415
    - muscle necrosis L98.413
    - skin breakdown only L98.411
    - specified severity NEC L98.418
- cancerous *—see* Neoplasm, malignant, by site
- cardia K22.10
  - with bleeding K22.11
- cardioesophageal (peptic) K22.10
  - with bleeding K22.11
- cecum *—see* Ulcer, intestine
- cervix (uteri) (decubitus) (trophic) N86
  - with cervicitis N72
- chancroidal A57
- chiclero B55.1
- chronic (cause unknown) *—see* Ulcer, skin
- Cochin-China B55.1
- colon *—see* Ulcer, intestine
- conjunctiva H10.89
- cornea H16.00-

Ulcer, ulcerated, ulcerating, ulceration, ulcerative *(continued)*
- cornea *(continued)*
  - with hypopyon H16.03-
  - central H16.01-
  - dendritic (herpes simplex) B00.52
  - marginal H16.04-
  - Mooren's H16.05-
  - mycotic H16.06-
  - perforated H16.07-
  - ring H16.02-
  - tuberculous (phlyctenular) A18.52
- corpus cavernosum (chronic) N48.5
- crural *—see* Ulcer, lower limb
- Curling's *—see* Ulcer, peptic, acute
- Cushing's *—see* Ulcer, peptic, acute
- cystic duct K82.8
- cystitis (interstitial) *—see* Cystitis, interstitial
- decubitus *—see* Ulcer, pressure, by site
- dendritic, cornea (herpes simplex) B00.52
- diabetes, diabetic *—see* Diabetes, ulcer
- Dieulafoy's K25.0
- due to
  - infection NEC *—see* Ulcer, skin
  - radiation NEC L59.8
  - trophic disturbance (any region) *—see* Ulcer, skin
  - X-ray L58.1
- duodenum, duodenal (eroded) (peptic) K26.9
  - with
    - hemorrhage K26.4
      - and perforation K26.6
    - perforation K26.5
  - acute K26.3
    - with
      - hemorrhage K26.0
        - and perforation K26.2
      - perforation K26.1
  - chronic K26.7
    - with
      - hemorrhage K26.4
        - and perforation K26.6
      - perforation K26.5
- dysenteric A09
- elusive *—see* Cystitis, interstitial
- endocarditis (acute) (chronic) (subacute) I28.8
- epiglottis J38.7
- esophagus (peptic) K22.10
  - with bleeding K22.11
  - due to
    - aspirin K22.10
      - with bleeding K22.11
    - gastrointestinal reflux disease (without bleeding) K21.00
      - with bleeding K21.01
    - ingestion of chemical or medicament K22.10
      - with bleeding K22.11
  - fungal K22.10
    - with bleeding K22.11
  - infective K22.10
    - with bleeding K22.11
  - varicose *—see* Varix, esophagus
- eyelid (region) H01.8
- fauces J39.2
- Fenwick (-Hunner) (solitary) *—see* Cystitis, interstitial

Ulcer, ulcerated, ulcerating, ulceration, ulcerative *(continued)*
- fistulous *—see* Ulcer, skin
- foot (indolent) (trophic) *—see* Ulcer, lower limb
- frambesial, initial A66.0
- frenum (tongue) K14.0
- gallbladder or duct K82.8
- gangrenous *—see* Gangrene
- gastric *—see* Ulcer, stomach
- gastrocolic *—see* Ulcer, gastrojejunal
- gastroduodenal *—see* Ulcer, peptic
- gastroesophageal *—see* Ulcer, stomach
- gastrointestinal *—see* Ulcer, gastrojejunal
- gastrojejunal (peptic) K28.9
  - with
    - hemorrhage K28.4
      - and perforation K28.6
    - perforation K28.5
  - acute K28.3
    - with
      - hemorrhage K28.0
        - and perforation K28.2
      - perforation K28.1
  - chronic K28.7
    - with
      - hemorrhage K28.4
        - and perforation K28.6
      - perforation K28.5
- gastrojejunocolic *—see* Ulcer, gastrojejunal
- gingiva K06.8
- gingivitis K05.10
  - nonplaque induced K05.11
  - plaque induced K05.10
- glottis J38.7
- granuloma of pudenda A58
- gum K06.8
- gumma, due to yaws A66.4
- heel *—see* Ulcer, lower limb
- hemorrhoid (*see also* Hemorrhoids, by degree) K64.8
- Hunner's *—see* Cystitis, interstitial
- hypopharynx J39.2
- hypopyon (chronic) (subacute) *—see* Ulcer, cornea, with hypopyon
- hypostaticum *—see* Ulcer, varicose
- ileum *—see* Ulcer, intestine
- intestine, intestinal K63.3
  - with perforation K63.1
  - amebic A06.1
  - duodenal *—see* Ulcer, duodenum
  - granulocytopenic (with hemorrhage) *—see* Neutropenia
  - marginal *—see* Ulcer, gastrojejunal
  - perforating K63.1
    - newborn P78.0
  - primary, small intestine K63.3
  - rectum K62.6
  - stercoraceous, stercoral K63.3
  - tuberculous A18.32
  - typhoid (fever) *—see* Typhoid
  - varicose I86.8
- jejunum, jejunal *—see* Ulcer, gastrojejunal
- keratitis *—see* Ulcer, cornea
- knee *—see* Ulcer, lower limb
- labium (majus) (minus) N76.6
- laryngitis *—see* Laryngitis
- larynx (aphthous) (contact) J38.7
  - diphtheritic A36.2
- leg *—see* Ulcer, lower limb

Ulcer, ulcerated, ulcerating, ulceration, ulcerative *(continued)*
- lip K13.0
- Lipschütz's N76.6
- lower limb (atrophic) (chronic) (neurogenic) (perforating) (pyogenic) (trophic) (tropical) L97.909
  - with
    - bone involvement without evidence of necrosis L97.906
    - bone necrosis L97.904
    - exposed fat layer L97.902
    - muscle involvement without evidence of necrosis L97.905
    - muscle necrosis L97.903
    - skin breakdown only L97.901
    - specified severity NEC L97.908
  - ankle L97.309
    - with
      - bone involvement without evidence of necrosis L97.306
      - bone necrosis L97.304
      - exposed fat layer L97.302
      - muscle involvement without evidence of necrosis L97.305
      - muscle necrosis L97.303
      - skin breakdown only L97.301
      - specified severity NEC L97.308
    - left L97.329
      - with
        - bone involvement without evidence of necrosis L97.326
        - bone necrosis L97.324
        - exposed fat layer L97.322
        - muscle involvement without evidence of necrosis L97.325
        - muscle necrosis L97.323
        - skin breakdown only L97.321
        - specified severity NEC L97.328
    - right L97.319
      - with
        - bone involvement without evidence of necrosis L97.316
        - bone necrosis L97.314
        - exposed fat layer L97.312
        - muscle involvement without evidence of necrosis L97.315
        - muscle necrosis L97.313
        - skin breakdown only L97.311
        - specified severity NEC L97.318
  - calf L97.209
    - with
      - bone involvement without evidence of necrosis L97.206
      - bone necrosis L97.204
      - exposed fat layer L97.202
      - muscle involvement without evidence of necrosis L97.205
      - muscle necrosis L97.203

Ulcer, ulcerated, ulcerating, ulceration, ulcerative *(continued)*
- lower limb *(continued)*
  - calf *(continued)*
    - with *(continued)*
      - skin breakdown only L97.201
      - specified severity NEC L97.208
    - left L97.229
      - with
        - bone involvement without evidence of necrosis L97.226
        - bone necrosis L97.224
        - exposed fat layer L97.222
        - muscle involvement without evidence of necrosis L97.225
        - muscle necrosis L97.223
        - skin breakdown only L97.221
        - specified severity NEC L97.228
    - right L97.219
      - with
        - bone involvement without evidence of necrosis L97.216
        - bone necrosis L97.214
        - exposed fat layer L97.212
        - muscle involvement without evidence of necrosis L97.215
        - muscle necrosis L97.213
        - skin breakdown only L97.211
        - specified severity NEC L97.218
  - decubitus —*see* Ulcer, pressure, by site
  - foot specified NEC L97.509
    - with
      - bone involvement without evidence of necrosis L97.506
      - bone necrosis L97.504
      - exposed fat layer L97.502
      - muscle involvement without evidence of necrosis L97.505
      - muscle necrosis L97.503
      - skin breakdown only L97.501
      - specified severity NEC L97.508
    - left L97.529
      - with
        - bone involvement without evidence of necrosis L97.526
        - bone necrosis L97.524
        - exposed fat layer L97.522
        - muscle involvement without evidence of necrosis L97.525
        - muscle necrosis L97.523
        - skin breakdown only L97.521
        - specified severity NEC L97.528
    - right L97.519
      - with
        - bone involvement without evidence of necrosis L97.516

Ulcer, ulcerated, ulcerating, ulceration, ulcerative *(continued)*
- lower limb *(continued)*
  - foot specified NEC *(continued)*
    - right *(continued)*
      - with *(continued)*
        - bone necrosis L97.514
        - exposed fat layer L97.512
        - muscle involvement without evidence of necrosis L97.515
        - muscle necrosis L97.513
        - skin breakdown only L97.511
        - specified severity NEC L97.518
  - heel L97.409
    - with
      - bone involvement without evidence of necrosis L97.406
      - bone necrosis L97.404
      - exposed fat layer L97.402
      - muscle involvement without evidence of necrosis L97.405
      - muscle necrosis L97.403
      - skin breakdown only L97.401
      - specified severity NEC L97.408
    - left L97.429
      - with
        - bone involvement without evidence of necrosis L97.426
        - bone necrosis L97.424
        - exposed fat layer L97.422
        - muscle involvement without evidence of necrosis L97.425
        - muscle necrosis L97.423
        - skin breakdown only L97.421
        - specified severity NEC L97.428
    - right L97.419
      - with
        - bone involvement without evidence of necrosis L97.416
        - bone necrosis L97.414
        - exposed fat layer L97.412
        - muscle involvement without evidence of necrosis L97.415
        - muscle necrosis L97.413
        - skin breakdown only L97.411
        - specified severity NEC L97.418
  - left L97.929
    - with
      - bone involvement without evidence of necrosis L97.926
      - bone necrosis L97.924
      - exposed fat layer L97.922
      - muscle involvement without evidence of necrosis L97.925
      - muscle necrosis L97.923
      - skin breakdown only L97.921
      - specified severity NEC L97.928

Ulcer, ulcerated, ulcerating, ulceration, ulcerative *(continued)*
- lower limb *(continued)*
  - lower leg NOS L97.909
    - with
      - bone involvement without evidence of necrosis L97.906
      - bone necrosis L97.904
      - exposed fat layer L97.902
      - muscle involvement without evidence of necrosis L97.905
      - muscle necrosis L97.903
      - skin breakdown only L97.901
      - specified severity NEC L97.908
    - left L97.929
      - with
        - bone involvement without evidence of necrosis L97.926
        - bone necrosis L97.924
        - exposed fat layer L97.922
        - muscle involvement without evidence of necrosis L97.925
        - muscle necrosis L97.923
        - skin breakdown only L97.921
        - specified severity NEC L97.928
    - right L97.919
      - with
        - bone involvement without evidence of necrosis L97.916
        - bone necrosis L97.914
        - exposed fat layer L97.912
        - muscle involvement without evidence of necrosis L97.915
        - muscle necrosis L97.913
        - skin breakdown only L97.911
        - specified severity NEC L97.918
    - specified site NEC L97.809
      - with
        - bone involvement without evidence of necrosis L97.806
        - bone necrosis L97.804
        - exposed fat layer L97.802
        - muscle involvement without evidence of necrosis L97.805
        - muscle necrosis L97.803
        - skin breakdown only L97.801
        - specified severity NEC L97.808
      - left L97.829
        - with
          - bone involvement without evidence of necrosis L97.826
          - bone necrosis L97.824
          - exposed fat layer L97.822
          - muscle involvement without evidence of necrosis L97.825

Ulcer, ulcerated, ulcerating, ulceration, ulcerative *(continued)*
- lower limb *(continued)*
  - lower leg NOS *(continued)*
    - specified site NEC *(continued)*
      - left *(continued)*
        - with *(continued)*
          - muscle necrosis L97.823
          - skin breakdown only L97.821
          - specified severity NEC L97.828
      - right L97.819
        - with
          - bone involvement without evidence of necrosis L97.816
          - bone necrosis L97.814
          - exposed fat layer L97.812
          - muscle involvement without evidence of necrosis L97.815
          - muscle necrosis L97.813
          - skin breakdown only L97.811
          - specified severity NEC L97.818
  - midfoot L97.409
    - with
      - bone involvement without evidence of necrosis L97.406
      - bone necrosis L97.404
      - exposed fat layer L97.402
      - muscle involvement without evidence of necrosis L97.405
      - muscle necrosis L97.403
      - skin breakdown only L97.401
      - specified severity NEC L97.408
    - left L97.429
      - with
        - bone involvement without evidence of necrosis L97.426
        - bone necrosis L97.424
        - exposed fat layer L97.422
        - muscle involvement without evidence of necrosis L97.425
        - muscle necrosis L97.423
        - skin breakdown only L97.421
        - specified severity NEC L97.428
    - right L97.419
      - with
        - bone involvement without evidence of necrosis L97.416
        - bone necrosis L97.414
        - exposed fat layer L97.412
        - muscle involvement without evidence of necrosis L97.415
        - muscle necrosis L97.413
        - skin breakdown only L97.411

Ulcer, ulcerated, ulcerating, ulceration, ulcerative *(continued)*
lower limb *(continued)*
midfoot *(continued)*
right *(continued)*
with *(continued)*
specified severity NEC L97.418
right L97.919
with
bone involvement without evidence of necrosis L97.916
bone necrosis L97.914
exposed fat layer L97.912
muscle involvement without evidence of necrosis L97.915
muscle necrosis L97.913
skin breakdown only L97.911
specified severity NEC L97.918
thigh L97.109
with
bone involvement without evidence of necrosis L97.106
bone necrosis L97.104
exposed fat layer L97.102
muscle involvement without evidence of necrosis L97.105
muscle necrosis L97.103
skin breakdown only L97.101
specified severity NEC L97.108
left L97.129
with
bone involvement without evidence of necrosis L97.126
bone necrosis L97.124
exposed fat layer L97.122
muscle involvement without evidence of necrosis L97.125
muscle necrosis L97.123
skin breakdown only L97.121
specified severity NEC L97.128
right L97.119
with
bone involvement without evidence of necrosis L97.116
bone necrosis L97.114
exposed fat layer L97.112
muscle involvement without evidence of necrosis L97.115
muscle necrosis L97.113
skin breakdown only L97.111
specified severity NEC L97.118
toe L97.509
with
bone involvement without evidence of necrosis L97.506
bone necrosis L97.504
exposed fat layer L97.502

Ulcer, ulcerated, ulcerating, ulceration, ulcerative *(continued)*
lower limb *(continued)*
toe *(continued)*
with *(continued)*
muscle involvement without evidence of necrosis L97.505
muscle necrosis L97.503
skin breakdown only L97.501
specified severity NEC L97.508
left L97.529
with
bone involvement without evidence of necrosis L97.526
bone necrosis L97.524
exposed fat layer L97.522
muscle involvement without evidence of necrosis L97.525
muscle necrosis L97.523
skin breakdown only L97.521
specified severity NEC L97.528
right L97.519
with
bone involvement without evidence of necrosis L97.516
bone necrosis L97.514
exposed fat layer L97.512
muscle involvement without evidence of necrosis L97.515
muscle necrosis L97.513
skin breakdown only L97.511
specified severity NEC L97.518
leprous A30.1
syphilitic A52.19
varicose —*see* Varix, leg, with, ulcer
luetic —*see* Ulcer, syphilitic
lung J98.4
tuberculous —*see* Tuberculosis, pulmonary
malignant —*see* Neoplasm, malignant, by site
marginal NEC —*see* Ulcer, gastrojejunal
meatus (urinarius) N34.2
Meckel's diverticulum Q43.0
malignant —*see* Table of Neoplasms, small intestine, malignant
Meleney's (chronic undermining) —*see* Ulcer, skin
Mooren's (cornea) —*see* Ulcer, cornea, Mooren's
mycobacterial (skin) A31.1
nasopharynx J39.2
neck, uterus N86
neurogenic NEC —*see* Ulcer, skin
nose, nasal (passage) (infective) (septum) J34.0
skin —*see* Ulcer, skin
spirochetal A69.8
varicose (bleeding) I86.8
oral mucosa (traumatic) K12.1

Ulcer, ulcerated, ulcerating, ulceration, ulcerative *(continued)*
palate (soft) K12.1
penis (chronic) N48.5
peptic (site unspecified) K27.9
with
hemorrhage K27.4
and perforation K27.6
perforation K27.5
acute K27.3
with
hemorrhage K27.0
and perforation K27.2
perforation K27.1
chronic K27.7
with
hemorrhage K27.4
and perforation K27.6
perforation K27.5
esophagus K22.10
with bleeding K22.11
newborn P78.82
perforating K27.5
skin —*see* Ulcer, skin
peritonsillar J35.8
phagedenic (tropical) —*see* Ulcer, skin
pharynx J39.2
phlebitis —*see* Phlebitis
plaster —*see* Ulcer, pressure, by site
popliteal space —*see* Ulcer, lower limb
postpyloric —*see* Ulcer, duodenum
prepuce N47.7
prepyloric —*see* Ulcer, stomach
pressure (pressure area) L89.9-
ankle L89.5-
back L89.1-
buttock L89.3-
coccyx L89.15-
contiguous site of back, buttock, hip L89.4-
elbow L89.0-
face L89.81-
head L89.81-
heel L89.6-
hip L89.2-
sacral region (tailbone) L89.15-
specified site NEC L89.89-
stage 1 (healing) (pre-ulcer skin changes limited to persistent focal edema)
ankle L89.5-
back L89.1-
buttock L89.3-
coccyx L89.15-
contiguous site of back, buttock, hip L89.4-
elbow L89.0-
face L89.81-
head L89.81-
heel L89.6-
hip L89.2-
sacral region (tailbone) L89.15-
specified site NEC L89.89-
stage 2 (healing) (abrasion, blister, partial thickness skin loss involving epidermis and/ or dermis)
ankle L89.5-
back L89.1-
buttock L89.3-
coccyx L89.15-
contiguous site of back, buttock, hip L89.4-
elbow L89.0-
face L89.81-

Ulcer, ulcerated, ulcerating, ulceration, ulcerative *(continued)*
pressure *(continued)*
stage 2 *(continued)*
head L89.81-
heel L89.6-
hip L89.2-
sacral region (tailbone) L89.15-
specified site NEC L89.89-
stage 3 (healing) (full thickness skin loss involving damage or necrosis of subcutaneous tissue)
ankle L89.5-
back L89.1-
buttock L89.3-
coccyx L89.15-
contiguous site of back, buttock, hip L89.4-
elbow L89.0-
face L89.81-
head L89.81-
heel L89.6-
hip L89.2-
sacral region (tailbone) L89.15-
specified site NEC L89.89-
stage 4 (healing) (necrosis of soft tissues through to underlying muscle, tendon, or bone)
ankle L89.5-
back L89.1-
buttock L89.3-
coccyx L89.15-
contiguous site of back, buttock, hip L89.4-
elbow L89.0-
face L89.81-
head L89.81-
heel L89.6-
hip L89.2-
sacral region (tailbone) L89.15-
specified site NEC L89.89-
unspecified stage
ankle L89.5-
back L89.1-
buttock L89.3-
coccyx L89.15-
contiguous site of back, buttock, hip L89.4-
elbow L89.0-
face L89.81-
head L89.81-
heel L89.6-
hip L89.2-
sacral region (tailbone) L89.15-
specified site NEC L89.89-
unstageable
ankle L89.5-
back L89.1-
buttock L89.3-
coccyx L89.15-
contiguous site of back, buttock, hip L89.4-
elbow L89.0-
face L89.81-
head L89.81-
heel L89.6-
hip L89.2-
sacral region (tailbone) L89.15-
specified site NEC L89.89-
primary of intestine K63.3
with perforation K63.1
prostate N41.9

Ulcer, ulcerated, ulcerating, ulceration, ulcerative *(continued)*
- pyloric —*see* Ulcer, stomach
- rectosigmoid K63.3
  - with perforation K63.1
- rectum (sphincter) (solitary) K62.6
  - stercoraceous, stercoral K62.6
- retina —*see* Inflammation, chorioretinal
- rodent —*see also* Neoplasm, skin, malignant
- sclera —*see* Scleritis
- scrofulous (tuberculous) A18.2
- scrotum N50.89
  - tuberculous A18.15
  - varicose I86.1
- seminal vesicle N50.89
- sigmoid —*see* Ulcer, intestine
- skin (atrophic) (chronic) (neurogenic) (non-healing) (perforating) (pyogenic) (trophic) (tropical) L98.499
  - with gangrene —*see* Gangrene
  - amebic A06.7
  - back —*see* Ulcer, back
  - buttock —*see* Ulcer, buttock
  - decubitus —*see* Ulcer, pressure
  - lower limb —*see* Ulcer, lower limb
  - mycobacterial A31.1
  - specified site NEC L98.499
    - with
      - bone involvement without evidence of necrosis L98.496
      - bone necrosis L98.494
      - exposed fat layer L98.492
      - muscle involvement without evidence of necrosis L98.495
      - muscle necrosis L98.493
      - skin breakdown only L98.491
      - specified severity NEC L98.498
  - tuberculous (primary) A18.4
  - varicose —*see* Ulcer, varicose
- sloughing —*see* Ulcer, skin
- solitary, anus or rectum (sphincter) K62.6
- sore throat J02.9
  - streptococcal J02.0
- spermatic cord N50.89
- spine (tuberculous) A18.01
- stasis (venous) —*see* Varix, leg, with, ulcer
  - without varicose veins I87.2
- stercoraceous, stercoral K63.3
  - with perforation K63.1
  - anus or rectum K62.6
- stoma, stomal —*see* Ulcer, gastrojejunal
- stomach (eroded) (peptic) (round) K25.9
  - with
    - hemorrhage K25.4
      - and perforation K25.6
    - perforation K25.5
  - acute K25.3
    - with
      - hemorrhage K25.0
        - and perforation K25.2
      - perforation K25.1
  - chronic K25.7
    - with
      - hemorrhage K25.4
        - and perforation K25.6
      - perforation K25.5
- stomal —*see* Ulcer, gastrojejunal

Ulcer, ulcerated, ulcerating, ulceration, ulcerative *(continued)*
- stomatitis K12.1
- stress —*see* Ulcer, peptic
- strumous (tuberculous) A18.2
- submucosal, bladder —*see* Cystitis, interstitial
- syphilitic (any site) (early) (secondary) A51.39
  - late A52.79
    - perforating A52.79
      - foot A52.11
- testis N50.89
- thigh —*see* Ulcer, lower limb
- throat J39.2
  - diphtheritic A36.0
- toe —*see* Ulcer, lower limb
- tongue (traumatic) K14.0
- tonsil J35.8
  - diphtheritic A36.0
- trachea J39.8
- trophic —*see* Ulcer, skin
- tropical —*see* Ulcer, skin
- tuberculous —*see* Tuberculosis, ulcer
- tunica vaginalis N50.89
- turbinate J34.89
- typhoid (perforating) —*see* Typhoid
- unspecified site —*see* Ulcer, skin
- urethra (meatus) —*see* Urethritis
- uterus N85.8
  - cervix N86
    - with cervicitis N72
  - neck N86
    - with cervicitis N72
- vagina N76.5
  - in Behçet's disease M35.2 *[N77.0]*
  - pessary N89.8
- valve, heart I33.0
- varicose (lower limb, any part) —*see also* Varix, leg, with, ulcer
  - broad ligament I86.2
  - esophagus —*see* Varix, esophagus
  - inflamed or infected —*see* Varix, leg, with ulcer, with inflammation
  - nasal septum I86.8
  - perineum I86.3
  - scrotum I86.1
  - specified site NEC I86.8
  - sublingual I86.0
  - vulva I86.3
- vas deferens N50.89
- vulva (acute) (infectional) N76.6
  - in (due to)
    - Behçet's disease M35.2 *[N77.0]*
    - herpesviral (herpes simplex) infection A60.04
    - tuberculosis A18.18
- vulvobuccal, recurring N76.6
- X-ray L58.1
- yaws A66.4

Ulcerosa scarlatina A38.8

Ulcus —*see also* Ulcer
- cutis tuberculosum A18.4
- duodeni —*see* Ulcer, duodenum
- durum (syphilitic) A51.0
  - extragenital A51.2
- gastrojejunale —*see* Ulcer, gastrojejunal
- hypostaticum —*see* Ulcer, varicose
- molle (cutis) (skin) A57
- serpens corneae —*see* Ulcer, cornea, central
- ventriculi —*see* Ulcer, stomach

Ulegyria Q04.8

Ulerythema
- ophryogenes, congenital Q84.2
- sycosiforme L73.8

Ullrich (-Bonnevie) (-Turner) **syndrome** (*see also* Turner's syndrome) Q87.19

Ullrich-Feichtiger syndrome Q87.0

Ulnar —*see* condition

Ulorrhagia, ulorrhea K06.8

Umbilicus, umbilical —*see* condition

Unacceptable
- contours of tooth K08.54
- morphology of tooth K08.54

Unavailability (of)
- bed at medical facility Z75.1
- health service-related agencies Z75.4
- medical facilities (at) Z75.3
  - due to
    - investigation by social service agency Z75.2
    - lack of services at home Z75.0
    - remoteness from facility Z75.3
    - waiting list Z75.1
  - home Z75.0
  - outpatient clinic Z75.3
- schooling Z55.1
- social service agencies Z75.4

Uncinaria americana infestation B76.1

Uncinariasis B76.9

Uncongenial work Z56.5

Unconscious (ness) —*see* Coma

Under observation —*see* Observation

Underachievement in school Z55.3

Underdevelopment —*see also* Undeveloped
- nose Q30.1
- sexual E30.0

Underdosing (*see also* Tables of Drugs and Chemicals, categories T36-T50, with final character 6) Z91.14
- intentional NEC Z91.128
  - due to financial hardship of patient Z91.120
- unintentional NEC Z91.138
  - due to patient's age related debility Z91.130

Underfeeding, newborn P92.3

Underfill, endodontic M27.53

Underimmunization status Z28.3

Undernourishment —*see* Malnutrition

Undernutrition —*see* Malnutrition

Underweight R63.6
- for gestational age —*see* Light for dates

Underwood's disease P83.0

Undescended —*see also* Malposition, congenital
- cecum Q43.3
- colon Q43.3
- testicle —*see* Cryptorchid

Undeveloped, undevelopment —*see also* Hypoplasia
- brain (congenital) Q02

Undeveloped, undevelopment *(continued)*
- cerebral (congenital) Q02
- heart Q24.8
- lung Q33.6
- testis E29.1
- uterus E30.0

Undiagnosed (disease) R69

Undulant fever —*see* Brucellosis

Unemployment, anxiety concerning Z56.0
- threatened Z56.2

Unequal length (acquired) (limb) —*see also* Deformity, limb, unequal length
- leg —*see also* Deformity, limb, unequal length
  - congenital Q72.9-

Unextracted dental root K08.3

Unguis incarnatus L60.0

Unhappiness R45.2

Unicornate uterus Q51.4
- in pregnancy or childbirth O34.00

Unilateral —*see also* condition
- development, breast N64.89
- organ or site, congenital NEC —*see* Agenesis, by site

Unilocular heart Q20.8

Union, abnormal —*see also* Fusion
- larynx and trachea Q34.8

Universal mesentery Q43.3

Unrepairable overhanging of dental restorative materials K08.52

Unsatisfactory
- restoration of tooth K08.50
  - specified NEC K08.59
- sample of cytologic smear
  - anus R85.615
  - cervix R87.615
  - vagina R87.625
- surroundings Z59.1
  - work Z56.5

Unsoundness of mind —*see* Psychosis

Unstable
- back NEC —*see* Instability, joint, spine
- hip (congenital) Q65.6
  - acquired —*see* Derangement, joint, specified type NEC, hip
- joint —*see* Instability, joint
  - secondary to removal of joint prosthesis M96.89
- lie (mother) O32.0
- lumbosacral joint (congenital) —*see* subcategory M53.2
- sacroiliac —*see* subcategory M53.2
- spine NEC —*see* Instability, joint, spine

Unsteadiness on feet R26.81

Untruthfulness, child problem F91.8

Unverricht (-Lundborg) **disease or epilepsy** —*see* Epilepsy, generalized, idiopathic

Unwanted
- multiple moves in the last 12 months Z59.81-
- pregnancy Z64.0

Upbringing, institutional Z62.22
- away from parents NEC Z62.29
- in care of non-parental family member Z62.21
- in foster care Z62.21

Upbringing, institutional *(continued)*
- in orphanage or group home Z62.22
- in welfare custody Z62.21

Upper respiratory *—see* condition

Upset
- gastric K30
- gastrointestinal K30
  - psychogenic F45.8
- intestinal (large) (small) K59.9
  - psychogenic F45.8
- menstruation N93.9
- mental F48.9
- stomach K30
  - psychogenic F45.8

Urachus *—see also* condition
- patent or persistent Q64.4

Urbach-Oppenheim disease (necrobiosis lipoidica diabeticorum) *—see* E08-E13 with .620

Urbach's lipoid proteinosis E78.89

Urbach-Wiethe disease E78.89

Urban yellow fever A95.1

Urea
- blood, high *—see* Uremia
- cycle metabolism disorder *—see* Disorder, urea cycle metabolism

Uremia, uremic N19
- with
  - ectopic or molar pregnancy O08.4
  - polyneuropathy N18.9 *[G63]*
- chronic NOS (*see also* Disease, kidney, chronic) N18.9
  - due to hypertension *—see* Hypertensive, kidney
- complicating
  - ectopic or molar pregnancy O08.4
- congenital P96.0
- extrarenal R39.2
- following ectopic or molar pregnancy O08.4
- newborn P96.0
- prerenal R39.2

Ureter, ureteral *—see* condition

Ureteralgia N23

Ureterectasis *—see* Hydroureter

Ureteritis N28.89
- cystica N28.86
- due to calculus N20.1
  - with calculus, kidney N20.2
    - with hydronephrosis N13.2
- gonococcal (acute) (chronic) A54.21
- nonspecific N28.89

Ureterocele N28.89
- congenital (orthotopic) Q62.31
  - ectopic Q62.32

Ureterolith, ureterolithiasis *—see* Calculus, ureter

Ureterostomy
- attention to Z43.6
- status Z93.6

Urethra, urethral *—see* condition

Urethralgia R39.89

Urethritis (anterior) (posterior) N34.2
- calculous N21.1
- candidal B37.41
- chlamydial A56.01
- diplococcal (gonococcal) A54.01

Urethritis *(continued)*
- diplococcal *(continued)*
  - with abscess (accessory gland) (periurethral) A54.1
- gonococcal A54.01
  - with abscess (accessory gland) (periurethral) A54.1
- nongonococcal N34.1
  - Reiter's *—see* Reiter's disease
- nonspecific N34.1
- nonvenereal N34.1
- postmenopausal N34.2
- puerperal O86.22
- Reiter's *—see* Reiter's disease
- specified NEC N34.2
- trichomonal or due to Trichomonas (vaginalis) A59.03

Urethrocele N81.0
- with
  - cystocele *—see* Cystocele
  - prolapse of uterus *—see* Prolapse, uterus

Urethrolithiasis (with colic or infection) N21.1

Urethrorectal *—see* condition

Urethrorrhagia N36.8

Urethrorrhea R36.9

Urethrostomy
- attention to Z43.6
- status Z93.6

Urethrotrigonitis *—see* Trigonitis

Urethrovaginal *—see* condition

Urgency
- fecal R15.2
- hypertensive *—see* Hypertension
- urinary R39.15

Urhidrosis, uridrosis L74.8

Uric acid in blood (increased) E79.0

Uricacidemia (asymptomatic) E79.0

Uricemia (asymptomatic) E79.0

Uricosuria R82.998

Urinary *—see* condition

Urination
- frequent R35.0
- painful R30.9

Urine
- blood in *—see* Hematuria
- discharge, excessive R35.89
- enuresis, nonorganic origin F98.0
- extravasation R39.0
- frequency R35.0
- incontinence R32
  - nonorganic origin F98.0
- intermittent stream R39.198
- pus in N39.0
- retention or stasis R33.9
  - organic R33.8
    - drug-induced R33.0
  - psychogenic F45.8
- secretion
  - deficient R34
  - excessive R35.89
  - frequency R35.0
- stream
  - intermittent R39.198
  - slowing R39.198
  - splitting R39.13
  - weak R39.12

Urinemia *—see* Uremia

Urinoma, urethra N36.8

Uroarthritis, infectious (Reiter's) *—see* Reiter's disease

Urodialysis R34

Urolithiasis *—see* Calculus, urinary

Uronephrosis *—see* Hydronephrosis

Uropathy N39.9
- obstructive N13.9
  - specified NEC N13.8
- reflux N13.9
  - specified NEC N13.8
- vesicoureteral reflux-associated *—see* Reflux, vesicoureteral

Urosepsis - code to condition

Urticaria L50.9
- with angioneurotic edema T78.3
  - hereditary D84.1
- allergic L50.0
- cholinergic L50.5
- chronic L50.8
- cold, familial L50.2
- contact L50.6
- dermatographic L50.3
- due to
  - cold or heat L50.2
  - drugs L50.0
  - food L50.0
  - inhalants L50.0
  - plants L50.6
  - serum (*see also* Reaction, serum) T80.69
- factitial L50.3
- familial cold M04.2
- giant T78.3
  - hereditary D84.1
- gigantea T78.3
- idiopathic L50.1
- larynx T78.3
  - hereditary D84.1
- neonatorum P83.88
- nonallergic L50.1
- papulosa (Hebra) L28.2
- pigmentosa D47.01
  - congenital Q82.2
  - of neonatal onset Q82.2
  - of newborn onset Q82.2
- recurrent periodic L50.8
- serum (*see also* Reaction, serum) T80.69
- solar L56.3
- specified type NEC L50.8
- thermal (cold) (heat) L50.2
- vibratory L50.4
- xanthelasmoidea *—see* Urticaria pigmentosa

Use (of)
- alcohol Z72.89
  - with
    - intoxication F10.929
    - sleep disorder F10.982
    - withdrawal F10.939
      - with
        - perceptual disturbance F10.932
      - delirium F10.931
      - uncomplicated F10.930
  - harmful *—see* Abuse, alcohol
- amphetamines *—see* Use, stimulant NEC
- caffeine *—see* Use, stimulant NEC
- cannabis F12.90
  - with
    - anxiety disorder F12.980
    - intoxication F12.929
      - with
        - delirium F12.921
        - perceptual disturbance F12.922
      - uncomplicated F12.920
    - other specified disorder F12.988
    - psychosis F12.959
      - delusions F12.950
      - hallucinations F12.951
    - unspecified disorder F12.99
    - withdrawal F12.93

Use *(continued)*
- cocaine F14.90
  - with
    - anxiety disorder F14.980
    - intoxication F14.929
      - with
        - delirium F14.921
        - perceptual disturbance F14.922
      - uncomplicated F14.920
    - other specified disorder F14.988
    - psychosis F14.959
      - delusions F14.950
      - hallucinations F14.951
    - sexual dysfunction F14.981
    - sleep disorder F14.982
    - unspecified disorder F14.99
    - withdrawal F14.93
  - harmful *—see* Abuse, drug, cocaine
- drug(s) NEC F19.90
  - with sleep disorder F19.982
  - harmful *—see* Abuse, drug, by type
- hallucinogen NEC F16.90
  - with
    - anxiety disorder F16.980
    - intoxication F16.929
      - with
        - delirium F16.921
      - uncomplicated F16.920
    - mood disorder F16.94
    - other specified disorder F16.988
    - perception disorder (flashbacks) F16.983
    - psychosis F16.959
      - delusions F16.950
      - hallucinations F16.951
    - unspecified disorder F16.99
  - harmful *—see* Abuse, drug, hallucinogen NEC
- inhalants F18.90
  - with
    - anxiety disorder F18.980
    - intoxication F18.929
      - with delirium F18.921
      - uncomplicated F18.920
    - mood disorder F18.94
    - other specified disorder F18.988
    - persisting dementia F18.97
    - psychosis F18.959
      - delusions F18.950
      - hallucinations F18.951
    - unspecified disorder F18.99
  - harmful *—see* Abuse, drug, inhalant
- methadone *—see* Use, opioid
- nonprescribed drugs F19.90
  - harmful *—see* Abuse, non-psychoactive substance
- opioid F11.90
  - with
    - disorder F11.99
      - mood F11.94
      - sleep F11.982
      - specified type NEC F11.988
    - intoxication F11.929
      - with
        - delirium F11.921
        - perceptual disturbance F11.922
      - uncomplicated F11.920
    - withdrawal F11.93
  - harmful *—see* Abuse, drug, opioid
- patent medicines F19.90
  - harmful *—see* Abuse, non-psychoactive substance

Use *(continued)*
- psychoactive drug NEC F19.90
  - with
    - anxiety disorder F19.980
    - intoxication F19.929
      - with
        - delirium F19.921
        - perceptual disturbance F19.922
      - uncomplicated F19.920
    - mood disorder F19.94
    - other specified disorder F19.988
    - persisting
      - amnestic disorder F19.96
      - dementia F19.97
    - psychosis F19.959
      - delusions F19.950
      - hallucinations F19.951
    - sexual dysfunction F19.981
    - sleep disorder F19.982
    - unspecified disorder F19.99
    - withdrawal F19.939
      - with
        - delirium F19.931
        - perceptual disturbance F19.932
      - uncomplicated F19.930
  - harmful —*see* Abuse, drug NEC, psychoactive NEC
- sedative, hypnotic, or anxiolytic F13.90
  - with
    - anxiety disorder F13.980
    - intoxication F13.929
      - with
        - delirium F13.921
      - uncomplicated F13.920
    - other specified disorder F13.988
    - persisting
      - amnestic disorder F13.96
      - dementia F13.97
    - psychosis F13.959
      - delusions F13.950
      - hallucinations F13.951
    - sexual dysfunction F13.981
    - sleep disorder F13.982
    - unspecified disorder F13.99
  - harmful —*see* Abuse, drug, sedative, hypnotic, or anxiolytic
- stimulant NEC F15.90
  - with
    - anxiety disorder F15.980
    - intoxication F15.929
      - with
        - delirium F15.921
        - perceptual disturbance F15.922
      - uncomplicated F15.920
    - mood disorder F15.94
    - other specified disorder F15.988
    - psychosis F15.959
      - delusions F15.950
      - hallucinations F15.951
    - sexual dysfunction F15.981
    - sleep disorder F15.982
    - unspecified disorder F15.99
    - withdrawal F15.93
  - harmful —*see* Abuse, drug, stimulant NEC
- volatile solvents (*see also* Use, inhalant) F18.90
  - harmful —*see* Abuse, drug, inhalant
- tobacco Z72.0
  - with dependence —*see* Dependence, drug, nicotine

Usher-Senear disease or syndrome L10.4

Uta B55.1

Uteromegaly N85.2

Uterovaginal —*see* condition

Uterovesical —*see* condition

Uveal —*see* condition

Uveitis (anterior) —*see also* Iridocyclitis
- acute —*see* Iridocyclitis, acute
- chronic —*see* Iridocyclitis, chronic
- due to toxoplasmosis (acquired) B58.09
  - congenital P37.1
- granulomatous —*see* Iridocyclitis, chronic
- heterochromic —*see* Cyclitis, Fuchs' heterochromic
- lens-induced —*see* Iridocyclitis, lens-induced
- posterior —*see* Chorioretinitis
- sympathetic H44.13-
- syphilitic (secondary) A51.43
  - congenital (early) A50.01
  - late A52.71
- tuberculous A18.54

Uveoencephalitis —*see* Inflammation, chorioretinal

Uveokeratitis —*see* Iridocyclitis

Uveoparotitis D86.89

Uvula —*see* condition

Uvulitis (acute) (catarrhal) (chronic) (membranous) (suppurative) (ulcerative) K12.2

V

Vaccination (prophylactic)
- complication or reaction —*see* Complications, vaccination
- delayed Z28.9
- encounter for Z23
- not done —*see* Immunization, not done, because (of)

Vaccinia (generalized) (localized) T88.1
- congenital P35.8
- without vaccination B08.011

Vacuum, in sinus (accessory) (nasal) J34.89

Vagabond, vagabondage Z59.00

Vagabond's disease B85.1

Vagina, vaginal —*see* condition

Vaginalitis (tunica) (testis) N49.1

Vaginismus (reflex) N94.2
- functional F52.5
- nonorganic F52.5
- psychogenic F52.5
- secondary N94.2

Vaginitis (acute) (circumscribed) (diffuse) (emphysematous) (nonvenereal) (ulcerative) N76.0
- with ectopic or molar pregnancy O08.0
- amebic A06.82
- atrophic, postmenopausal N95.2
- bacterial N76.0
- blennorrhagic (gonococcal) A54.02
- candidal B37.3
- chlamydial A56.02
- chronic N76.1
- due to Trichomonas (vaginalis) A59.01

Vaginitis *(continued)*
- following ectopic or molar pregnancy O08.0
- gonococcal A54.02
  - with abscess (accessory gland) (periurethral) A54.1
- granuloma A58
- in (due to)
  - candidiasis B37.3
  - herpesviral (herpes simplex) infection A60.04
  - pinworm infection B80 *[N77.1]*
- monilial B37.3
- mycotic (candidal) B37.3
- postmenopausal atrophic N95.2
- puerperal (postpartum) O86.13
- senile (atrophic) N95.2
- subacute or chronic N76.1
- syphilitic (early) A51.0
  - late A52.76
- trichomonal A59.01
- tuberculous A18.18

Vaginosis —*see* Vaginitis

Vagotonia G52.2

Vagrancy Z59.00

VAIN —*see* Neoplasia, intraepithelial, vagina

Vallecula —*see* condition

Valley fever B38.0

Valsuani's disease —*see* Anemia, obstetric

Valve, valvular (formation) —*see also* condition
- cerebral ventricle (communicating) in situ Z98.2
- cervix, internal os Q51.828
- congenital NEC —*see* Atresia, by site
- ureter (pelvic junction) (vesical orifice) Q62.39
- urethra (congenital) (posterior) Q64.2

Valvulitis (chronic) —*see* Endocarditis

Valvulopathy —*see* Endocarditis

Van Bogaert's leukoencephalopathy (sclerosing) (subacute) A81.1

Van Bogaert-Scherer-Epstein disease or syndrome E75.5

Van Buchem's syndrome M85.2

Van Creveld-von Gierke disease E74.01

Van der Hoeve (-de Kleyn) **syndrome** Q78.0

Van der Woude's syndrome Q38.0

Van Neck's disease or osteochondrosis M91.0

Vanishing lung J44.9

Vapor asphyxia or suffocation T59.9
- specified agent —*see* Table of Drugs and Chemicals

Variance, lethal ball, prosthetic heart valve T82.09

Variants, thalassemic D56.8

Variations in hair color L67.1

Varicella B01.9
- with
  - complications NEC B01.89
  - encephalitis B01.11
  - encephalomyelitis B01.11
  - meningitis B01.0

Varicella *(continued)*
- with *(continued)*
  - myelitis B01.12
  - pneumonia B01.2
- congenital P35.8

Varices —*see* Varix

Varicocele (scrotum) (thrombosed) I86.1
- ovary I86.2
- perineum I86.3
- spermatic cord (ulcerated) I86.1

Varicose
- aneurysm (ruptured) I77.0
- dermatitis —*see* Varix, leg, with, inflammation
- eczema —*see* Varix, leg, with, inflammation
- phlebitis —*see* Varix, with, inflammation
- tumor —*see* Varix
- ulcer (lower limb, any part) —*see also* Varix, leg, with, ulcer
  - anus (*see also* Hemorrhoids) K64.8
  - esophagus —*see* Varix, esophagus
  - inflamed or infected —*see* Varix, leg, with ulcer, with inflammation
  - nasal septum I86.8
  - perineum I86.3
  - scrotum I86.1
  - specified site NEC I86.8
- vein —*see* Varix
- vessel —*see* Varix, leg

Varicosis, varicosities, varicosity —*see* Varix

Variola (major) (minor) B03

Varioloid B03

Varix (lower limb) (ruptured) I83.90
- with
  - bleeding I83.899
  - edema I83.899
  - inflammation I83.10
    - with ulcer (venous) I83.209
  - pain I83.819
  - rupture I83.899
  - specified complication NEC I83.899
  - stasis dermatitis I83.10
    - with ulcer (venous) I83.209
  - swelling I83.899
  - ulcer I83.0-
    - with inflammation I83.2-
- aneurysmal I77.0
- asymptomatic I83.9-
- bladder I86.2
- broad ligament I86.2
- complicating
  - childbirth (lower extremity) O87.4
    - anus or rectum O87.2
    - genital (vagina, vulva or perineum) O87.8
  - pregnancy (lower extremity) O22.0-
    - anus or rectum O22.4-
    - genital (vagina, vulva or perineum) O22.1-
  - puerperium (lower extremity) O87.4
    - anus or rectum O87.2
    - genital (vagina, vulva, perineum) O87.8
- congenital (any site) Q27.8
- esophagus (idiopathic) (primary) (ulcerated) I85.00
  - bleeding I85.01

Varix *(continued)*
- esophagus *(continued)*
  - congenital Q27.8
  - in (due to)
    - alcoholic liver disease I85.10
      - bleeding I85.11
    - cirrhosis of liver I85.10
      - bleeding I85.11
    - portal hypertension I85.10
      - bleeding I85.11
    - schistosomiasis I85.10
      - bleeding I85.11
    - toxic liver disease I85.10
      - bleeding I85.11
  - secondary I85.10
    - bleeding I85.11
- gastric I86.4
- inflamed or infected I83.10
  - ulcerated I83.209
- labia (majora) I86.3
- leg (asymptomatic) I83.9-
  - with
    - edema I83.899
    - inflammation I83.10
      - with ulcer *—see* Varix, leg, with, ulcer, with inflammation by site
    - pain I83.819
    - specified complication NEC I83.899
    - swelling I83.899
    - ulcer I83.0-
      - with inflammation I83.2-
      - ankle I83.003
        - with inflammation I83.203
      - calf I83.002
        - with inflammation I83.202
      - foot NEC I83.005
        - with inflammation I83.205
      - heel I83.004
        - with inflammation I83.204
      - lower leg NEC I83.008
        - with inflammation I83.208
      - midfoot I83.004
        - with inflammation I83.204
      - thigh I83.001
        - with inflammation I83.201
  - bilateral (asymptomatic) I83.93
    - with
      - edema I83.893
      - pain I83.813
      - specified complication NEC I83.893
      - swelling I83.893
      - ulcer I83.0-
        - with inflammation I83.209
  - left (asymptomatic) I83.92
    - with
      - edema I83.892
      - pain I83.812
      - specified complication NEC I83.892
      - swelling I83.892
      - inflammation I83.12
        - with ulcer *—see* Varix, leg, with, ulcer, with inflammation by site
      - ulcer I83.029
        - with inflammation I83.229
        - ankle I83.023

Varix *(continued)*
- leg *(continued)*
  - left *(continued)*
    - with *(continued)*
      - ulcer *(continued)*
        - ankle *(continued)*
          - with inflammation I83.223
        - calf I83.022
          - with inflammation I83.222
        - foot NEC I83.025
          - with inflammation I83.225
        - heel I83.024
          - with inflammation I83.224
        - lower leg NEC I83.028
          - with inflammation I83.228
        - midfoot I83.024
          - with inflammation I83.224
        - thigh I83.021
          - with inflammation I83.221
  - right (asymptomatic) I83.91
    - with
      - edema I83.891
      - pain I83.811
      - specified complication NEC I83.891
      - swelling I83.891
      - inflammation I83.11
        - with ulcer *—see* Varix, leg, with, ulcer, with inflammation by site
      - ulcer I83.019
        - with inflammation I83.219
        - ankle I83.013
          - with inflammation I83.213
        - calf I83.012
          - with inflammation I83.212
        - foot NEC I83.015
          - with inflammation I83.215
        - heel I83.014
          - with inflammation I83.214
        - lower leg NEC I83.018
          - with inflammation I83.218
        - midfoot I83.014
          - with inflammation I83.214
        - thigh I83.011
          - with inflammation I83.211
- nasal septum I86.8
- orbit I86.8
  - congenital Q27.8
- ovary I86.2
- papillary I78.1
- pelvis I86.2
- perineum I86.3
- pharynx I86.8
- placenta O43.89-
- renal papilla I86.8
- retina H35.09
- scrotum (ulcerated) I86.1
- sigmoid colon I86.8
- specified site NEC I86.8
- spinal (cord) (vessels) I86.8
- spleen, splenic (vein) (with phlebolith) I86.8
- stomach I86.4
- sublingual I86.0
- ulcerated I83.009

Varix *(continued)*
- ulcerated *(continued)*
  - inflamed or infected I83.209
- uterine ligament I86.2
- vagina I86.8
- vocal cord I86.8
- vulva I86.3

Vas deferens *—see* condition

Vas deferentitis N49.1

Vasa previa O69.4
- hemorrhage from, affecting newborn P50.0

Vascular *—see also* condition
- loop on optic papilla Q14.2
- spasm I73.9
- spider I78.1

Vascularization, cornea *—see* Neovascularization, cornea

Vasculitis I77.6
- allergic D69.0
- cryoglobulinemic D89.1
- disseminated I77.6
- hypocomplementemic M31.8
- kidney I77.89
- leukocytoclastic M31.0
- livedoid L95.0
- nodular L95.8
- retina H35.06-
- rheumatic *—see* Fever, rheumatic
- rheumatoid *—see* Rheumatoid, vasculitis
- skin (limited to) L95.9
  - specified NEC L95.8
- systemic M31.8

Vasculopathy, necrotizing M31.9
- cardiac allograft T86.290
- specified NEC M31.8

Vasitis (nodosa) N49.1
- tuberculous A18.15

Vasodilation I73.9

Vasomotor *—see* condition

Vasoplasty, after previous sterilization Z31.0
- aftercare Z31.42

Vasospasm (vasoconstriction) I73.9
- cerebral (cerebrovascular) (artery) I67.848
  - reversible I67.841
- coronary I20.1
- nerve
  - arm *—see* Mononeuropathy, upper limb
  - brachial plexus G54.0
  - cervical plexus G54.2
  - leg *—see* Mononeuropathy, lower limb
- peripheral NOS I73.9
- retina (artery) *—see* Occlusion, artery, retina

Vasospastic *—see* condition

Vasovagal attack (paroxysmal) R55
- psychogenic F45.8

VATER syndrome Q87.2

Vater's ampulla *—see* condition

Vegetation, vegetative
- adenoid (nasal fossa) J35.8
- endocarditis (acute) (any valve) (subacute) I33.0
- heart (mycotic) (valve) I33.0

Veil
- Jackson's Q43.3

Vein, venous *—see* condition

Veldt sore *—see* Ulcer, skin

Velpeau's hernia *—see* Hernia, femoral

Venereal
- bubo A55
- disease A64
- granuloma inguinale A58
- lymphogranuloma (Durand-Nicolas-Favre) A55

Venofibrosis I87.8

Venom, venomous *—see* Table of Drugs and Chemicals, by animal or substance, poisoning

Venous *—see* condition

Ventilator lung, newborn P27.8

Ventral *—see* condition

Ventricle, ventricular *—see also* condition
- escape I49.3
- inversion Q20.5

Ventriculitis (cerebral) (*see also* Encephalitis) G04.90

Ventriculostomy status Z98.2

Vernet's syndrome G52.7

Verneuil's disease (syphilitic bursitis) A52.78

Verruca (due to HPV) (filiformis) (simplex) (viral) (vulgaris) B07.9
- acuminata A63.0
- necrogenica (primary) (tuberculosa) A18.4
- plana B07.8
- plantaris B07.0
- seborrheica L82.1
  - inflamed L82.0
- senile (seborrheic) L82.1
  - inflamed L82.0
- tuberculosa (primary) A18.4
- venereal A63.0

Verrucosities *—see* Verruca

Verruga peruana, peruviana A44.1

Version
- cervix *—see* Malposition, uterus
- uterus (postinfectional) (postpartal, old) *—see* Malposition, uterus

Vertebra, vertebral *—see* condition

Vertical talus (congenital) Q66.80
- left foot Q66.82
- right foot Q66.81

Vertigo R42
- auditory *—see* Vertigo, aural
- aural H81.31-
- benign paroxysmal (positional) H81.1-
- central (origin) H81.4
- cerebral H81.4
- Dix and Hallpike (epidemic) *—see* Neuronitis, vestibular
- due to infrasound T75.23
- epidemic A88.1
  - Dix and Hallpike *—see* Neuronitis, vestibular
  - Pedersen's *—see* Neuronitis, vestibular
  - vestibular neuronitis *—see* Neuronitis, vestibular
- hysterical F44.89
- infrasound *—see* subcategory T75.23
- labyrinthine H81.0
- laryngeal R05.4
- malignant positional H81.4
- Ménière's *—see* subcategory H81.0
- menopausal N95.1
- otogenic *—see* Vertigo, aural

W

Waldenström-Kjellberg syndrome D50.1

Waldenström
- hypergammaglobulinemia D89.0
- syndrome or macroglobulinemia C88.0

Walking
- difficulty R26.2
  - psychogenic F44.4
- sleep F51.3
  - hysterical F44.89

Wall, abdominal —*see* condition

Wallenberg's disease or syndrome G46.3

Wallgren's disease I87.8

Wandering
- gallbladder, congenital Q44.1
- in diseases classified elsewhere Z91.83
- kidney, congenital Q63.8
- organ or site, congenital NEC —*see* Malposition, congenital, by site
- pacemaker (heart) I49.8
- spleen D73.89

War neurosis F48.8

Wart (due to HPV) (filiform) (infectious) (viral) B07.9
- anogenital region (venereal) A63.0
- common B07.8
- external genital organs (venereal) A63.0
- flat B07.8
- Hassal-Henle's (of cornea) H18.49
- Peruvian A44.1
- plantar B07.0
- prosector (tuberculous) A18.4
- seborrheic L82.1
  - inflamed L82.0
- senile (seborrheic) L82.1
  - inflamed L82.0
- tuberculous A18.4
- venereal A63.0

Warthin's tumor —*see* Neoplasm, salivary gland, benign

Wassilieff's disease A27.0

Wasting
- disease R64
  - due to malnutrition E43
    - with marasmus E41
- extreme (due to malnutrition) E43
  - with marasmus E41
- muscle NEC —*see* Atrophy, muscle

Water
- clefts (senile cataract) —*see* Cataract, senile, incipient
- deprivation of T73.1
- intoxication E87.79
- itch B76.9
- lack of T73.1
  - safe drinking Z58.6
- loading E87.70
- on
  - brain —*see* Hydrocephalus
  - chest J94.8
- poisoning E87.79

Waterbrash R12

Waterhouse (-Friderichsen) **syndrome or disease** (meningococcal) A39.1

Water-losing nephritis N25.89

Watermelon stomach K31.819
- with hemorrhage K31.811
- without hemorrhage K31.819

Watsoniasis B66.8

Wax in ear —*see* Impaction, cerumen

Weak, weakening, weakness (generalized) R53.1
- arches (acquired) —*see also* Deformity, limb, flat foot
- bladder (sphincter) R32
- facial R29.810
  - following
    - cerebrovascular disease I69.992
    - cerebral infarction I69.392
    - intracerebral hemorrhage I69.192
    - nontraumatic intracranial hemorrhage NEC I69.292
    - specified disease NEC I69.892
    - stroke I69.392
    - subarachnoid hemorrhage I69.092
- foot (double) —*see also* Weak, arches
- heart, cardiac —*see* Failure, heart
- mind F70
- muscle M62.81
- myocardium —*see* Failure, heart
- newborn P96.89
- pelvic fundus N81.89
- pubocervical tissue N81.82
- senile R54
- rectovaginal tissue N81.83
- urinary stream R39.12
- valvular —*see* Endocarditis

Wear, worn (with normal or routine use)
- articular bearing surface of internal joint prosthesis —*see* Complications, joint prosthesis, mechanical, wear of articular bearing surfaces, by site
- device, implant or graft —*see* Complications, by site, mechanical complication
- tooth, teeth (approximal) (hard tissues) (interproximal) (occlusal) K03.0

Weather, weathered
- effects of
  - cold T69.9
    - specified effect NEC T69.8
  - hot —*see* Heat
- skin L57.8

Weaver's syndrome Q87.3

Web, webbed (congenital)
- duodenal Q43.8
- esophagus Q39.4
- fingers Q70.1-
- larynx (glottic) (subglottic) Q31.0
- neck (pterygium colli) Q18.3
- Paterson-Kelly D50.1
- popliteal syndrome Q87.89
- toes Q70.3-

Weber-Christian disease M35.6

Weber-Cockayne syndrome (epidermolysis bullosa) Q81.8

Weber-Gubler syndrome G46.3

Weber-Leyden syndrome G46.3

Weber-Osler syndrome I78.0

Weber's paralysis or syndrome G46.3

Wedge-shaped or wedging vertebra —*see* Collapse, vertebra NEC

Wegener's granulomatosis or syndrome M31.30
- with
  - kidney involvement M31.31
  - lung involvement M31.30
    - with kidney involvement M31.31

Wegner's disease A50.02

Weight
- 1000-2499 grams at birth (low) —*see* Low, birthweight
- 999 grams or less at birth (extremely low) —*see* Low, birthweight, extreme
- and length below 10th percentile for gestational age P05.1-
- below but length above 10th percentile for gestational age P05.0-
- gain (abnormal) (excessive) R63.5
  - in pregnancy —*see* Pregnancy, complicated by, excessive weight gain
    - low —*see* Pregnancy, complicated by, insufficient, weight gain
- loss (abnormal) (cause unknown) R63.4

Weightlessness (effect of) T75.82

Weil (l)-Marchesani syndrome Q87.19

Weil's disease A27.0

Weingarten's syndrome J82.89

Weir Mitchell's disease I73.81

Weiss-Baker syndrome G90.09

Wells' disease L98.3

Wen —*see* Cyst, sebaceous

Wenckebach's block or phenomenon I44.1

Werdnig-Hoffmann syndrome (muscular atrophy) G12.0

Werlhof's disease D69.3

Wermer's disease or syndrome E31.21

Werner-His disease A79.0

Werner's disease or syndrome E34.8

Wernicke-Korsakoff's syndrome or psychosis (alcoholic) F10.96
- with dependence F10.26
- drug-induced
  - due to drug abuse —*see* Abuse, drug, by type, with amnestic disorder
  - due to drug dependence —*see* Dependence, drug, by type, with amnestic disorder
- nonalcoholic F04

Wernicke-Posadas disease B38.9

Wernicke's
- developmental aphasia F80.2
- disease or syndrome E51.2
- encephalopathy E51.2
- polioencephalitis, superior E51.2

West African fever B50.8

Westphal-Strümpell syndrome E83.01

West's syndrome —*see* Epilepsy, spasms

Wet
- feet, tropical (maceration) (syndrome) —*see* Immersion, foot
- lung (syndrome), newborn P22.1

Wharton's duct —*see* condition

Wheal —*see* Urticaria

Wheezing R06.2

Whiplash injury S13.4

Whipple's disease (*see also* subcategory M14.8-) K90.81

Whipworm (disease) (infection) (infestation) B79

Whistling face Q87.0

White —*see also* condition
- kidney, small N03.9
- leg, puerperal, postpartum, childbirth O87.1
- mouth B37.0
- patches of mouth K13.29
- spot lesions, teeth
  - chewing surface K02.51
  - pit and fissure surface K02.51
  - smooth surface K02.61

Whitehead L70.0

Whitlow —*see also* Cellulitis, digit
- with lymphangitis —*see* Lymphangitis, acute, digit
- herpesviral B00.89

Whitmore's disease or fever —*see* Melioidosis

Whooping cough A37.90
- with pneumonia A37.91
  - due to Bordetella
    - bronchiseptica A37.81
    - parapertussis A37.11
    - pertussis A37.01
  - specified organism NEC A37.81
- due to
  - Bordetella
    - bronchiseptica A37.80
      - with pneumonia A37.81
    - parapertussis A37.10
      - with pneumonia A37.11
    - pertussis A37.00
      - with pneumonia A37.01
    - specified NEC A37.80
      - with pneumonia A37.81

Wichman's asthma J38.5

Wide cranial sutures, newborn P96.3

Widening aorta —*see* Ectasia, aorta
- with aneurysm —*see* Aneurysm, aorta

Wilkie's disease or syndrome K55.1

Wilkinson-Sneddon disease or syndrome L13.1

Willebrand (-Jürgens) **thrombopathy** D68.0

Willige-Hunt disease or syndrome G23.1

Williams syndrome Q93.82

Wilms' tumor C64-

Wilson-Mikity syndrome P27.0

Wilson's
- disease or syndrome E83.01
- hepatolenticular degeneration E83.01
- lichen ruber L43.9

Window —*see also* Imperfect, closure
aorticopulmonary Q21.4

Winter —*see* condition

Wiskott-Aldrich syndrome D82.0

Withdrawal state —*see also* Dependence, drug by type, with withdrawal
alcohol
with perceptual disturbances F10.232
without perceptual disturbances F10.239
caffeine F15.93
cannabis F12.23
newborn
correct therapeutic substance properly administered P96.2
infant of dependent mother P96.1
therapeutic substance, neonatal P96.2

Witts' anemia D50.8

Witzelsucht F07.0

Woakes' ethmoiditis or syndrome J33.1

Wolff-Hirschorn syndrome Q93.3

Wolff-Parkinson-White syndrome I45.6

Wolhynian fever A79.0

Wolman's disease E75.5

Wood lung or pneumonitis J67.8

Woolly, wooly hair (congenital) (nevus) Q84.1

Woolsorter's disease A22.1

Word
blindness (congenital) (developmental) F81.0
deafness (congenital) (developmental) H93.25

Worm(s) (infection) (infestation) —*see also* Infestation, helminth
guinea B72
in intestine NEC B82.0

Worm-eaten soles A66.3

Worn out —*see* Exhaustion
cardiac
defibrillator (with synchronous cardiac pacemaker) Z45.02
pacemaker
battery Z45.010
lead Z45.018
device, implant or graft —*see* Complications, by site, mechanical

Worried well Z71.1

Worries R45.82

Wound check Z48.0-
due to injury - code to Injury, by site, using appropriate seventh character for subsequent encounter

Wound, open T14.8-
abdomen, abdominal
wall S31.109
with penetration into peritoneal cavity S31.609
bite —*see* Bite, abdomen, wall
epigastric region S31.102
with penetration into peritoneal cavity S31.602

Wound, open *(continued)*
abdomen, abdominal *(continued)*
wall *(continued)*
epigastric region *(continued)*
bite —*see* Bite, abdomen, wall, epigastric region
laceration —*see* Laceration, abdomen, wall, epigastric region
puncture —*see* Puncture, abdomen, wall, epigastric region
laceration —*see* Laceration, abdomen, wall
left
lower quadrant S31.104
with penetration into peritoneal cavity S31.604
bite —*see* Bite, abdomen, wall, left, lower quadrant
laceration —*see* Laceration, abdomen, wall, left, lower quadrant
puncture —*see* Puncture, abdomen, wall, left, lower quadrant
upper quadrant S31.101
with penetration into peritoneal cavity S31.601
bite —*see* Bite, abdomen, wall, left, upper quadrant
laceration —*see* Laceration, abdomen, wall, left, upper quadrant
puncture —*see* Puncture, abdomen, wall, left, upper quadrant
periumbilic region S31.105
with penetration into peritoneal cavity S31.605
bite —*see* Bite, abdomen, wall, periumbilic region
laceration —*see* Laceration, abdomen, wall, periumbilic region
puncture —*see* Puncture, abdomen, wall, periumbilic region
puncture —*see* Puncture, abdomen, wall
right
lower quadrant S31.103
with penetration into peritoneal cavity S31.603
bite —*see* Bite, abdomen, wall, right, lower quadrant
laceration —*see* Laceration, abdomen, wall, right, lower quadrant
puncture —*see* Puncture, abdomen, wall, right, lower quadrant
upper quadrant S31.100
with penetration into peritoneal cavity S31.600
bite —*see* Bite, abdomen, wall, right, upper quadrant

Wound, open *(continued)*
abdomen, abdominal *(continued)*
wall *(continued)*
right *(continued)*
upper quadrant *(continued)*
laceration —*see* Laceration, abdomen, wall, right, upper quadrant
puncture —*see* Puncture, abdomen, wall, right, upper quadrant
alveolar (process) —*see* Wound, open, oral cavity
ankle S91.00-
bite —*see* Bite, ankle
laceration —*see* Laceration, ankle
puncture —*see* Puncture, ankle
antecubital space —*see* Wound, open, elbow
anterior chamber, eye —*see* Wound, open, ocular
anus S31.839
bite S31.835
laceration —*see* Laceration, anus
puncture —*see* Puncture, anus
arm (upper) S41.10-
with amputation —*see* Amputation, traumatic, arm
bite —*see* Bite, arm
forearm —*see* Wound, open, forearm
laceration —*see* Laceration, arm
puncture —*see* Puncture, arm
auditory canal (external) (meatus) —*see* Wound, open, ear
auricle, ear —*see* Wound, open, ear
axilla —*see* Wound, open, arm
back —*see also* Wound, open, thorax, back
lower S31.000
with penetration into retroperitoneal space S31.001
bite —*see* Bite, back, lower
laceration —*see* Laceration, back, lower
puncture —*see* Puncture, back, lower
bite —*see* Bite
blood vessel —*see* Injury, blood vessel
breast S21.00-
with amputation —*see* Amputation, traumatic, breast
bite —*see* Bite, breast
laceration —*see* Laceration, breast
puncture —*see* Puncture, breast
buttock S31.809
bite —*see* Bite, buttock
laceration —*see* Laceration, buttock
left S31.829
puncture —*see* Puncture, buttock
right S31.819
calf —*see* Wound, open, leg
canaliculus lacrimalis —*see* Wound, open, eyelid
canthus, eye —*see* Wound, open, eyelid
cervical esophagus S11.20
bite S11.25
laceration —*see* Laceration, esophagus, traumatic, cervical
puncture —*see* Puncture, cervical esophagus

Wound, open *(continued)*
cheek (external) S01.40-
bite —*see* Bite, cheek
laceration —*see* Laceration, cheek
puncture —*see* Puncture, cheek
internal —*see* Wound, open, oral cavity
chest wall —*see* Wound, open, thorax
chin —*see* Wound, open, head, specified site NEC
choroid —*see* Wound, open, ocular
ciliary body (eye) —*see* Wound, open, ocular
clitoris S31.40
with amputation —*see* Amputation, traumatic, clitoris
bite S31.45
laceration —*see* Laceration, vulva
puncture —*see* Puncture, vulva
conjunctiva —*see* Wound, open, ocular
cornea —*see* Wound, open, ocular
costal region —*see* Wound, open, thorax
Descemet's membrane —*see* Wound, open, ocular
digit(s)
foot —*see* Wound, open, toe
hand —*see* Wound, open, finger
ear (canal) (external) S01.30-
with amputation —*see* Amputation, traumatic, ear
bite —*see* Bite, ear
laceration —*see* Laceration, ear
puncture —*see* Puncture, ear
drum S09.2-
elbow S51.00-
bite —*see* Bite, elbow
laceration —*see* Laceration, elbow
puncture —*see* Puncture, elbow
epididymis —*see* Wound, open, testis
epigastric region S31.102
with penetration into peritoneal cavity S31.602
bite —*see* Bite, abdomen, wall, epigastric region
laceration —*see* Laceration, abdomen, wall, epigastric region
puncture —*see* Puncture, abdomen, wall, epigastric region
epiglottis —*see* Wound, open, neck, specified site NEC
esophagus (thoracic) S27.819
cervical —*see* Wound, open, cervical esophagus
laceration S27.813
specified type NEC S27.818
eye —*see* Wound, open, ocular
eyeball —*see* Wound, open, ocular
eyebrow —*see* Wound, open, eyelid
eyelid S01.10-
bite —*see* Bite, eyelid
laceration —*see* Laceration, eyelid
puncture —*see* Puncture, eyelid
face NEC —*see* Wound, open, head, specified site NEC
finger(s) S61.209

Wound, open *(continued)*
- finger *(continued)*
  - with
    - amputation *—see* Amputation, traumatic, finger
    - damage to nail S61.309
  - bite *—see* Bite, finger
  - index S61.208
    - with
      - damage to nail S61.308
    - left S61.201
      - with
        - damage to nail S61.301
    - right S61.200
      - with
        - damage to nail S61.300
  - laceration *—see* Laceration, finger
  - little S61.208
    - with
      - damage to nail S61.308
    - left S61.207
      - with damage to nail S61.307
    - right S61.206
      - with damage to nail S61.306
  - middle S61.208
    - with
      - damage to nail S61.308
    - left S61.203
      - with damage to nail S61.303
    - right S61.202
      - with damage to nail S61.302
  - puncture *—see* Puncture, finger
  - ring S61.208
    - with
      - damage to nail S61.308
    - left S61.205
      - with damage to nail S61.305
    - right S61.204
      - with damage to nail S61.304
- flank *—see* Wound, open, abdomen, wall
- foot (except toe(s) alone) S91.30-
  - with amputation *—see* Amputation, traumatic, foot
  - bite *—see* Bite, foot
  - laceration *—see* Laceration, foot
  - puncture *—see* Puncture, foot
  - toe *—see* Wound, open, toe
- forearm S51.80-
  - with
    - amputation *—see* Amputation, traumatic, forearm
  - bite *—see* Bite, forearm
  - elbow only *—see* Wound, open, elbow
  - laceration *—see* Laceration, forearm
  - puncture *—see* Puncture, forearm
- forehead *—see* Wound, open, head, specified site NEC
- genital organs, external
  - with amputation *—see* Amputation, traumatic, genital organs
  - bite *—see* Bite, genital organ
  - female S31.502
    - vagina S31.40
    - vulva S31.40
  - laceration *—see* Laceration, genital organ
  - male S31.501

Wound, open *(continued)*
- genital organs, external *(continued)*
  - male *(continued)*
    - penis S31.20
    - scrotum S31.30
    - testes S31.30
  - puncture *—see* Puncture, genital organ
- globe (eye) *—see* Wound, open, ocular
- groin *—see* Wound, open, abdomen, wall
- gum *—see* Wound, open, oral cavity
- hand S61.40-
  - with
    - amputation *—see* Amputation, traumatic, hand
  - bite *—see* Bite, hand
  - finger(s) *—see* Wound, open, finger
  - laceration *—see* Laceration, hand
  - puncture *—see* Puncture, hand
  - thumb *—see* Wound, open, thumb
- head S01.90
  - bite *—see* Bite, head
  - cheek *—see* Wound, open, cheek
  - ear *—see* Wound, open, ear
  - eyelid *—see* Wound, open, eyelid
  - laceration *—see* Laceration, head
  - lip *—see* Wound, open, lip
  - nose S01.20
  - oral cavity *—see* Wound, open, oral cavity
  - puncture *—see* Puncture, head
  - scalp *—see* Wound, open, scalp
  - specified site NEC S01.80
  - temporomandibular area *—see* Wound, open, cheek
- heel *—see* Wound, open, foot
- hip S71.00-
  - with amputation *—see* Amputation, traumatic, hip
  - bite *—see* Bite, hip
  - laceration *—see* Laceration, hip
  - puncture *—see* Puncture, hip
- hymen S31.40
  - bite *—see* Bite, vulva
  - laceration *—see* Laceration, vagina
  - puncture *—see* Puncture, vagina
- hypochondrium S31.109
  - bite *—see* Bite, hypochondrium
  - laceration *—see* Laceration, hypochondrium
  - puncture *—see* Puncture, hypochondrium
- hypogastric region S31.109
  - bite *—see* Bite, hypogastric region
  - laceration *—see* Laceration, hypogastric region
  - puncture *—see* Puncture, hypogastric region
- iliac (region) *—see* Wound, open, inguinal region
- inguinal region S31.109
  - bite *—see* Bite, abdomen, wall, lower quadrant
  - laceration *—see* Laceration, inguinal region
  - puncture *—see* Puncture, inguinal region
- instep *—see* Wound, open, foot

Wound, open *(continued)*
- interscapular region *—see* Wound, open, thorax, back
- intraocular *—see* Wound, open, ocular
- iris *—see* Wound, open, ocular
- jaw *—see* Wound, open, head, specified site NEC
- knee S81.00-
  - bite *—see* Bite, knee
  - laceration *—see* Laceration, knee
  - puncture *—see* Puncture, knee
- labium (majus) (minus) *—see* Wound, open, vulva
- laceration *—see* Laceration, by site
- lacrimal duct *—see* Wound, open, eyelid
- larynx S11.019
  - bite *—see* Bite, larynx
  - laceration *—see* Laceration, larynx
  - puncture *—see* Puncture, larynx
- left
  - lower quadrant S31.104
    - with penetration into peritoneal cavity S31.604
    - bite *—see* Bite, abdomen, wall, left, lower quadrant
    - laceration *—see* Laceration, abdomen, wall, left, lower quadrant
    - puncture *—see* Puncture, abdomen, wall, left, lower quadrant
  - upper quadrant S31.101
    - with penetration into peritoneal cavity S31.601
    - bite *—see* Bite, abdomen, wall, left, upper quadrant
    - laceration *—see* Laceration, abdomen, wall, left, upper quadrant
    - puncture *—see* Puncture, abdomen, wall, left, upper quadrant
- leg (lower) S81.80-
  - with amputation *—see* Amputation, traumatic, leg
  - ankle *—see* Wound, open, ankle
  - bite *—see* Bite, leg
  - foot *—see* Wound, open, foot
  - knee *—see* Wound, open, knee
  - laceration *—see* Laceration, leg
  - puncture *—see* Puncture, leg
  - toe *—see* Wound, open, toe
  - upper *—see* Wound, open, thigh
- lip S01.501
  - bite *—see* Bite, lip
  - laceration *—see* Laceration, lip
  - puncture *—see* Puncture, lip
- loin S31.109
  - bite *—see* Bite, abdomen, wall
  - laceration *—see* Laceration, loin
  - puncture *—see* Puncture, loin
- lower back *—see* Wound, open, back, lower
- lumbar region *—see* Wound, open, back, lower
- malar region *—see* Wound, open, head, specified site NEC
- mammary *—see* Wound, open, breast
- mastoid region *—see* Wound, open, head, specified site NEC

Wound, open *(continued)*
- mouth *—see* Wound, open, oral cavity
- nail
  - finger *—see* Wound, open, finger, with damage to nail
  - toe *—see* Wound, open, toe, with damage to nail
- nape (neck) *—see* Wound, open, neck
- nasal (septum) (sinus) *—see* Wound, open, nose
- nasopharynx *—see* Wound, open, head, specified site NEC
- neck S11.90
  - bite *—see* Bite, neck
  - involving
    - cervical esophagus S11.20
    - larynx *—see* Wound, open, larynx
    - pharynx S11.20
    - thyroid S11.10
    - trachea (cervical) S11.029
      - bite *—see* Bite, trachea
      - laceration S11.021
        - with foreign body S11.022
      - puncture S11.023
        - with foreign body S11.024
  - laceration *—see* Laceration, neck
  - puncture *—see* Puncture, neck
  - specified site NEC S11.80
    - specified type NEC S11.89
- nose (septum) (sinus) S01.20
  - with amputation *—see* Amputation, traumatic, nose
  - bite *—see* Bite, nose
  - laceration *—see* Laceration, nose
  - puncture *—see* Puncture, nose
- ocular S05.90
  - avulsion (traumatic enucleation) S05.7-
  - eyeball S05.6-
    - with foreign body S05.5-
  - eyelid *—see* Wound, open, eyelid
  - laceration and rupture S05.3-
    - with prolapse or loss of intraocular tissue S05.2-
  - orbit (penetrating) (with or without foreign body) S05.4-
  - periocular area *—see* Wound, open, eyelid
  - specified NEC S05.8X-
- oral cavity S01.502
  - bite S01.552
  - laceration *—see* Laceration, oral cavity
  - puncture *—see* Puncture, oral cavity
- orbit *—see* Wound, open, ocular, orbit
- palate *—see* Wound, open, oral cavity
- palm *—see* Wound, open, hand
- pelvis, pelvic *—see also* Wound, open, back, lower
  - girdle *—see* Wound, open, hip
- penetrating *—see* Puncture, by site
- penis S31.20
  - with amputation *—see* Amputation, traumatic, penis
  - bite S31.25
  - laceration *—see* Laceration, penis
  - puncture *—see* Puncture, penis

Wound, open *(continued)*
- perineum
  - bite —*see* Bite, perineum
  - female S31.502
  - laceration —*see* Laceration, perineum
  - male S31.501
  - puncture —*see* Puncture, perineum
- periocular area (with or without lacrimal passages) —*see* Wound, open, eyelid
- periumbilic region S31.105
  - with penetration into peritoneal cavity S31.605
  - bite —*see* Bite, abdomen, wall, periumbilic region
  - laceration —*see* Laceration, abdomen, wall, periumbilic region
  - puncture —*see* Puncture, abdomen, wall, periumbilic region
- phalanges
  - finger —*see* Wound, open, finger
  - toe —*see* Wound, open, toe
- pharynx S11.20
- pinna —*see* Wound, open, ear
- popliteal space —*see* Wound, open, knee
- prepuce —*see* Wound, open, penis
- pubic region —*see* Wound, open, back, lower
- pudendum —*see* Wound, open, genital organs, external
- puncture wound —*see* Puncture
- rectovaginal septum —*see* Wound, open, vagina
- right
  - lower quadrant S31.103
    - with penetration into peritoneal cavity S31.603
    - bite —*see* Bite, abdomen, wall, right, lower quadrant
    - laceration —*see* Laceration, abdomen, wall, right, lower quadrant
    - puncture —*see* Puncture, abdomen, wall, right, lower quadrant
  - upper quadrant S31.100
    - with penetration into peritoneal cavity S31.600
    - bite —*see* Bite, abdomen, wall, right, upper quadrant
    - laceration —*see* Laceration, abdomen, wall, right, upper quadrant
    - puncture —*see* Puncture, abdomen, wall, right, upper quadrant
- sacral region —*see* Wound, open, back, lower
- sacroiliac region —*see* Wound, open, back, lower
- salivary gland —*see* Wound, open, oral cavity
- scalp S01.00
  - bite S01.05
  - laceration —*see* Laceration, scalp
  - puncture —*see* Puncture, scalp
- scalpel, newborn (birth injury) P15.8
- scapular region —*see* Wound, open, shoulder
- sclera —*see* Wound, open, ocular
- scrotum S31.30

Wound, open *(continued)*
- scrotum *(continued)*
  - with amputation —*see* Amputation, traumatic, scrotum
  - bite S31.35
  - laceration —*see* Laceration, scrotum
  - puncture —*see* Puncture, scrotum
- shin —*see* Wound, open, leg
- shoulder S41.00-
  - with amputation —*see* Amputation, traumatic, arm
  - bite —*see* Bite, shoulder
  - laceration —*see* Laceration, shoulder
  - puncture —*see* Puncture, shoulder
- skin NOS T14.8
- spermatic cord —*see* Wound, open, testis
- sternal region —*see* Wound, open, thorax, front wall
- submaxillary region —*see* Wound, open, head, specified site NEC
- submental region —*see* Wound, open, head, specified site NEC
- subungual
  - finger(s) —*see* Wound, open, finger
  - toe(s) —*see* Wound, open, toe
- supraclavicular region —*see* Wound, open, neck, specified site NEC
- temple, temporal region —*see* Wound, open, head, specified site NEC
- temporomandibular area —*see* Wound, open, cheek
- testis S31.30
  - with amputation —*see* Amputation, traumatic, testes
  - bite S31.35
  - laceration —*see* Laceration, testis
  - puncture —*see* Puncture, testis
- thigh S71.10-
  - with amputation —*see* Amputation, traumatic, hip
  - bite —*see* Bite, thigh
  - laceration —*see* Laceration, thigh
  - puncture —*see* Puncture, thigh
- thorax, thoracic (wall) S21.90
  - back S21.20-
    - with penetration S21.40
  - bite —*see* Bite, thorax
  - breast —*see* Wound, open, breast
  - front S21.10-
    - with penetration S21.30
  - laceration —*see* Laceration, thorax
  - puncture —*see* Puncture, thorax
- throat —*see* Wound, open, neck
- thumb S61.009
  - with
    - amputation —*see* Amputation, traumatic, thumb
    - damage to nail S61.109
  - bite —*see* Bite, thumb
  - laceration —*see* Laceration, thumb
  - left S61.002
    - with
      - damage to nail S61.102
  - puncture —*see* Puncture, thumb
  - right S61.001

Wound, open *(continued)*
- thumb *(continued)*
  - right *(continued)*
    - with
      - damage to nail S61.101
- thyroid (gland) —*see* Wound, open, neck, thyroid
- toe(s) S91.109
  - with
    - amputation —*see* Amputation, traumatic, toe
    - damage to nail S91.209
  - bite —*see* Bite, toe
  - great S91.103
    - with
    - damage to nail S91.203
    - left S91.102
      - with
        - damage to nail S91.202
    - right S91.101
      - with
        - damage to nail S91.201
  - laceration —*see* Laceration, toe
  - lesser S91.106
    - with
      - damage to nail S91.206
    - left S91.105
      - with
        - damage to nail S91.205
    - right S91.104
      - with
        - damage to nail S91.204
  - puncture —*see* Puncture, toe
- tongue —*see* Wound, open, oral cavity
- trachea (cervical region) —*see* Wound, open, neck, trachea
- tunica vaginalis —*see* Wound, open, testis
- tympanum, tympanic membrane S09.2-
  - laceration —*see* Laceration, ear, drum
  - puncture —*see* Puncture, tympanum
- umbilical region —*see* Wound, open, abdomen, wall, periumbilic region
- uvula —*see* Wound, open, oral cavity
- vagina S31.40
  - bite S31.45
  - laceration —*see* Laceration, vagina
  - puncture —*see* Puncture, vagina
- vocal cord S11.039
  - bite —*see* Bite, vocal cord
  - laceration S11.031
    - with foreign body S11.032
  - puncture S11.033
    - with foreign body S11.034
- vitreous (humor) —*see* Wound, open, ocular
- vulva S31.40
  - with amputation —*see* Amputation, traumatic, vulva
  - bite S31.45
  - laceration —*see* Laceration, vulva
  - puncture —*see* Puncture, vulva
- wrist S61.50-
  - bite —*see* Bite, wrist
  - laceration —*see* Laceration, wrist
  - puncture —*see* Puncture, wrist

Wound, superficial —*see* Injury —*see also* specified injury type

Wright's syndrome G54.0

Wrist —*see* condition

Wrong drug (by accident) (given in error) —*see* Table of Drugs and Chemicals, by drug, poisoning

Wry neck —*see* Torticollis

Wuchereria (bancrofti) **infestation** B74.0

Wuchereriasis B74.0

Wuchernde Struma Langhans C73

X

Xanthelasma (eyelid) (palpebrarum) H02.60
- left H02.66
  - lower H02.65
  - upper H02.64
- right H02.63
  - lower H02.62
  - upper H02.61

Xanthelasmatosis (essential) E78.2

Xanthinuria, hereditary E79.8

Xanthoastrocytoma
- specified site —*see* Neoplasm, malignant, by site
- unspecified site C71.9

Xanthofibroma —*see* Neoplasm, connective tissue, benign

Xanthogranuloma D76.3

Xanthoma(s), xanthomatosis (primary) (familial) (hereditary) E75.5
- with
  - hyperlipoproteinemia
    - Type I E78.3
    - Type III E78.2
    - Type IV E78.1
    - Type V E78.3
- bone (generalisata) C96.5
- cerebrotendinous E75.5
- cutaneotendinous E75.5
- disseminatum (skin) E78.2
- eruptive E78.2
- hypercholesterinemic E78.00
- hypercholesterolemic E78.00
- hyperlipidemic E78.5
- joint E75.5
- multiple (skin) E78.2
- tendon (sheath) E75.5
- tubo-eruptive E78.2
- tuberosum E78.2
- tuberous E78.2
- verrucous, oral mucosa K13.4

Xanthosis R23.8

Xenophobia F40.10

Xeroderma —*see also* Ichthyosis
- acquired L85.0
  - eyelid H01.149
    - left H01.146
      - lower H01.145
      - upper H01.144
    - right H01.143
      - lower H01.142
      - upper H01.141
- pigmentosum Q82.1
- vitamin A deficiency E50.8

Xerophthalmia (vitamin A deficiency) E50.7
- unrelated to vitamin A deficiency —*see* Keratoconjunctivitis

Xerosis
- conjunctiva H11.14-
  - with Bitot's spots —*see also* Pigmentation, conjunctiva
    - vitamin A deficiency E50.1
  - vitamin A deficiency E50.0

Y

Z

Neoplasm Table Guidance

The Neoplasm Table gives the code numbers for neoplasms by anatomical site. For each site there are six possible code numbers according to whether the neoplasm in question is malignant, benign, in situ, of uncertain behavior, or of unspecified nature. The description of the neoplasm will often indicate which of the six columns is appropriate; e.g., malignant melanoma of skin, benign fibroadenoma of breast, carcinoma in situ of cervix uteri.

Where such descriptors are not present, the remainder of the Index should be consulted where guidance is given to the appropriate column for each morphological (histological) variety listed; e.g., Mesonephroma—see Neoplasm, malignant; Embryoma—see also Neoplasm, uncertain behavior; Disease, Bowen's—see Neoplasm, skin, in situ. However, the guidance in the Index can be overridden if one of the descriptors mentioned above is present; e.g., malignant adenoma of colon is coded to C18.9 and not to D12.6 as the adjective "malignant" overrides the Index entry "Adenoma—see also Neoplasm, benign."

Codes listed with a dash -, following the code have a required additional character for laterality. The tabular must be reviewed for the complete code.

	Malignant Primary	Malignant Secondary	Ca in situ	Benign	Uncertain Behavior	Unspecified Behavior
Neoplasm, neoplastic	C80.1	C79.9	D09.9	D36.9	D48.9	D49.9
A						
abdomen, abdominal	C76.2	C79.8-	D09.8	D36.7	D48.7	D49.89
cavity	C76.2	C79.8-	D09.8	D36.7	D48.7	D49.89
organ	C76.2	C79.8-	D09.8	D36.7	D48.7	D49.89
viscera	C76.2	C79.8-	D09.8	D36.7	D48.7	D49.89
wall—see also Neoplasm, abdomen, wall, skin	C44.509	C79.2	D04.5	D23.5	D48.5	D49.2
connective tissue	C49.4	C79.8-	-	D21.4	D48.1	D49.2
skin	C44.509					
basal cell carcinoma	C44.519	-	-	-	-	-
specified type NEC	C44.599	-	-	-	-	-
squamous cell carcinoma	C44.529	-	-	-	-	-
abdominopelvic	C76.8	C79.8-	-	D36.7	D48.7	D49.89
accessory sinus—see Neoplasm, sinus						
acoustic nerve	C72.4-	C79.49	-	D33.3	D43.3	D49.7
adenoid (pharynx) (tissue)	C11.1	C79.89	D00.08	D10.6	D37.05	D49.0
adipose tissue —see also Neoplasm, connective tissue	C49.4	C79.89	-	D21.9	D48.1	D49.2
adnexa (uterine)	C57.4	C79.89	D07.39	D28.7	D39.8	D49.59
adrenal	C74.9-	C79.7-	D09.3	D35.0-	D44.1-	D49.7
capsule	C74.9-	C79.7-	D09.3	D35.0-	D44.1-	D49.7
cortex	C74.0-	C79.7-	D09.3	D35.0-	D44.1-	D49.7
gland	C74.9-	C79.7-	D09.3	D35.0-	D44.1-	D49.7
medulla	C74.1-	C79.7-	D09.3	D35.0-	D44.1-	D49.7
ala nasi (external)—see also Neoplasm, skin, nose	C44.301	C79.2	D04.39	D23.39	D48.5	D49.2
alimentary canal or tract NEC	C26.9	C78.80	D01.9	D13.9	D37.9	D49.0
alveolar	C03.9	C79.89	D00.03	D10.39	D37.09	D49.0
mucosa	C03.9	C79.89	D00.03	D10.39	D37.09	D49.0
lower	C03.1	C79.89	D00.03	D10.39	D37.09	D49.0
upper	C03.0	C79.89	D00.03	D10.39	D37.09	D49.0
ridge or process	C41.1	C79.51	-	D16.5	D48.0	D49.2
carcinoma	C03.9	C79.8-	-	-	-	-
lower	C03.1	C79.8-	-	-	-	-
upper	C03.0	C79.8-	-	-	-	-
lower	C41.1	C79.51	-	D16.5-	D48.0	D49.2
mucosa	C03.9	C79.89	D00.03	D10.39	D37.09	D49.0
lower	C03.1	C79.89	D00.03	D10.39	D37.09	D49.0
upper	C03.0	C79.89	D00.03	D10.39	D37.09	D49.0
upper	C41.0	C79.51	-	D16.4-	D48.0	D49.2
sulcus	C06.1	C79.89	D00.02	D10.39	D37.09	D49.0
alveolus	C03.9	C79.89	D00.03	D10.39	D37.09	D49.0
lower	C03.1	C79.89	D00.03	D10.39	D37.09	D49.0
upper	C03.0	C79.89	D00.03	D10.39	D37.09	D49.0
ampulla of Vater	C24.1	C78.89	D01.5	D13.5	D37.6	D49.0
ankle NEC	C76.5-	C79.89	D04.7-	D36.7	D48.7	D49.89
anorectum, anorectal (junction)	C21.8	C78.5	D01.3	D12.9	D37.8	D49.0
antecubital fossa or space	C76.4-	C79.89	D04.6-	D36.7	D48.7	D49.89
antrum (Highmore) (maxillary)	C31.0	C78.39	D02.3	D14.0	D38.5	D49.1
pyloric	C16.3	C78.89	D00.2	D13.1	D37.1	D49.0
tympanicum	C30.1	C78.39	D02.3	D14.0	D38.5	D49.1
anus, anal	C21.0	C78.5	D01.3	D12.9	D37.8	D49.0
canal	C21.1	C78.5	D01.3	D12.9	D37.8	D49.0
cloacogenic zone	C21.2	C78.5	D01.3	D12.9	D37.8	D49.0
margin—see also Neoplasm, anus, skin	C44.500	C79.2	D04.5	D23.5	D48.5	D49.2
overlapping lesion with rectosigmoid junction or rectum	C21.8	-	-	-	-	-
skin	C44.500	C79.2	D04.5	D23.5	D48.5	D49.2
basal cell carcinoma	C44.510	-	-	-	-	-
specified type NEC	C44.590	-	-	-	-	-
squamous cell carcinoma	C44.520	-	-	-	-	-
sphincter	C21.1	C78.5	D01.3	D12.9	D37.8	D49.0
aorta (thoracic)	C49.3	C79.89	-	D21.3	D48.1	D49.2
abdominal	C49.4	C79.89	-	D21.4	D48.1	D49.2
aortic body	C75.5	C79.89	-	D35.6	D44.7	D49.7
aponeurosis	C49.9	C79.89	-	D21.9	D48.1	D49.2
palmar	C49.1-	C79.89	-	D21.1-	D48.1	D49.2
plantar	C49.2-	C79.89	-	D21.2-	D48.1	D49.2
appendix	C18.1	C78.5	D01.0	D12.1	D37.3	D49.0
arachnoid	C70.9	C79.49	-	D32.9	D42.9	D49.7
cerebral	C70.0	C79.32	-	D32.0	D42.0	D49.7
spinal	C70.1	C79.49	-	D32.1	D42.1	D49.7
areola	C50.0-	C79.81	D05.-	D24.-	D48.6-	D49.3
arm NEC	C76.4-	C79.89	D04.6-	D36.7	D48.7	D49.89
artery—see Neoplasm, connective tissue						
aryepiglottic fold	C13.1	C79.89	D00.08	D10.7	D37.05	D49.0
hypopharyngeal aspect	C13.1	C79.89	D00.08	D10.7	D37.05	D49.0
laryngeal aspect	C32.1	C78.39	D02.0	D14.1	D38.0	D49.1
marginal zone	C13.1	C79.89	D00.08	D10.7	D37.05	D49.0
arytenoid (cartilage)	C32.3	C78.39	D02.0	D14.1	D38.0	D49.1
fold—see Neoplasm, aryepiglottic						
associated with transplanted organ	C80.2	-	-	-	-	-
atlas	C41.2	C79.51	-	D16.6	D48.0	D49.2
atrium, cardiac	C38.0	C79.89	-	D15.1	D48.7	D49.89
auditory						
canal (external) (skin)	C44.20-	C79.2	D04.2-	D23.2-	D48.5	D49.2
internal	C30.1	C78.39	D02.3	D14.0	D38.5	D49.1
nerve	C72.4-	C79.49	-	D33.3	D43.3	D49.7
tube	C30.1	C78.39	D02.3	D14.0	D38.5	D49.1
opening	C11.2	C79.89	D00.08	D10.6	D37.05	D49.0

	Malignant Primary	Malignant Secondary	Ca in situ	Benign	Uncertain Behavior	Unspecified Behavior
auricle, ear—see also Neoplasm, skin, ear	C44.20-	C79.2	D04.2-	D23.2-	D48.5	D49.2
auricular canal (external)—see also Neoplasm, skin, ear	C44.20-	C79.2	D04.2-	D23.2-	D48.5	D49.2
internal	C30.1	C78.39	D02.3	D14.0	D38.5	D49.2
autonomic nerve or nervous system NEC (see Neoplasm, nerve, peripheral)						
axilla, axillary	C76.1	C79.89	D09.8	D36.7	D48.7	D49.89
fold—see also Neoplasm, skin, trunk	C44.509	C79.2	D04.5	D23.5	D48.5	D49.2
B						
back NEC	C76.8	C79.89	D04.5	D36.7	D48.7	D49.89
Bartholin's gland	C51.0	C79.82	D07.1	D28.0	D39.8	D49.59
basal ganglia	C71.0	C79.31	-	D33.0	D43.0	D49.6
basis pedunculi	C71.7	C79.31	-	D33.1	D43.1	D49.6
bile or biliary (tract)	C24.9	C78.89	D01.5	D13.5	D37.6	D49.0
canaliculi (biliferi) (intrahepatic)	C22.1	C78.7	D01.5	D13.4	D37.6	D49.0
canals, interlobular	C22.1	C78.89	D01.5	D13.4	D37.6	D49.0
duct or passage (common) (cystic) (extrahepatic)	C24.0	C78.89	D01.5	D13.5	D37.6	D49.0
interlobular	C22.1	C78.89	D01.5	D13.4	D37.6	D49.0
intrahepatic	C22.1	C78.7	D01.5	D13.4	D37.6	D49.0
and extrahepatic	C24.8	C78.89	D01.5	D13.5	D37.6	D49.0
bladder (urinary)	C67.9	C79.11	D09.0	D30.3	D41.4	D49.4
dome	C67.1	C79.11	D09.0	D30.3	D41.4	D49.4
neck	C67.5	C79.11	D09.0	D30.3	D41.4	D49.4
orifice	C67.9	C79.11	D09.0	D30.3	D41.4	D49.4
ureteric	C67.6	C79.11	D09.0	D30.3	D41.4	D49.4
urethral	C67.5	C79.11	D09.0	D30.3	D41.4	D49.4
overlapping lesion	C67.8	-	-	-	-	-
sphincter	C67.8	C79.11	D09.0	D30.3	D41.4	D49.4
trigone	C67.0	C79.11	D09.0	D30.3	D41.4	D49.4
urachus	C67.7	C79.11	D09.0	D30.3	D41.4	D49.4
wall	C67.9	C79.11	D09.0	D30.3	D41.4	D49.4
anterior	C67.3	C79.11	D09.0	D30.3	D41.4	D49.4
lateral	C67.2	C79.11	D09.0	D30.3	D41.4	D49.4
posterior	C67.4	C79.11	D09.0	D30.3	D41.4	D49.4
blood vessel—see Neoplasm, connective tissue						
bone (periosteum)	C41.9	C79.51	-	D16.9	D48.0	D49.2
acetabulum	C41.4	C79.51	-	D16.8	D48.0	D49.2
ankle	C40.3-	C79.51	-	D16.3-	-	-
arm NEC	C40.0-	C79.51	-	D16.0-	-	-
astragalus	C40.3-	C79.51	-	D16.3-	-	-
atlas	C41.2	C79.51	-	D16.6	D48.0	D49.2
axis	C41.2	C79.51	-	D16.6	D48.0	D49.2
back NEC	C41.2	C79.51	-	D16.6	D48.0	D49.2
calcaneus	C40.3-	C79.51	-	D16.3-	-	-
calvarium	C41.0	C79.51	-	D16.4	D48.0	D49.2
carpus (any)	C40.1-	C79.51	-	D16.1-	-	-
cartilage NEC	C41.9	C79.51	-	D16.9	D48.0	D49.2
bone — *continued*						
clavicle	C41.3	C79.51	-	D16.7	D48.0	D49.2
clivus	C41.0	C79.51	-	D16.4	D48.0	D49.2
coccygeal vertebra	C41.4	C79.51	-	D16.8	D48.0	D49.2
coccyx	C41.4	C79.51	-	D16.8	D48.0	D49.2
costal cartilage	C41.3	C79.51	-	D16.7	D48.0	D49.2
costovertebral joint	C41.3	C79.51	-	D16.7	D48.0	D49.2
cranial	C41.0	C79.51	-	D16.4	D48.0	D49.2
cuboid	C40.3-	C79.51	-	D16.3-	-	-
cuneiform	C41.9	C79.51	-	D16.9	D48.0	D49.2
elbow	C40.0-	C79.51	-	D16.0-	-	-
ethmoid (labyrinth)	C41.0	C79.51	-	D16.4	D48.0	D49.2
face	C41.0	C79.51	-	D16.4	D48.0	D49.2
femur (any part)	C40.2-	C79.51	-	D16.2-	-	-
fibula (any part)	C40.2-	C79.51	-	D16.2-	-	-
finger (any)	C40.1-	C79.51	-	D16.1-	-	-
foot	C40.3-	C79.51	-	D16.3-	-	-
forearm	C40.0-	C79.51	-	D16.0-	-	-
frontal	C41.0	C79.51	-	D16.4	D48.0	D49.2
hand	C40.1-	C79.51	-	D16.1-	-	-
heel	C40.3-	C79.51	-	D16.3-	-	-
hip	C41.4	C79.51	-	D16.8	D48.0	D49.2
humerus (any part)	C40.0-	C79.51	-	D16.0-	-	-
hyoid	C41.0	C79.51	-	D16.4	D48.0	D49.2
ilium	C41.4	C79.51	-	D16.8	D48.0	D49.2
innominate	C41.4	C79.51	-	D16.8	D48.0	D49.2
intervertebral cartilage or disc	C41.2	C79.51	-	D16.6	D48.0	D49.2
ischium	C41.4	C79.51	-	D16.8	D48.0	D49.2
jaw (lower)	C41.1	C79.51	-	D16.5	D48.0	D49.2
knee	C40.2-	C79.51	-	D16.2-	-	-
leg NEC	C40.2-	C79.51	-	D16.2-	-	-
limb NEC	C40.9-	C79.51	-	D16.9	-	-
lower (long bones)	C40.2-	C79.51	-	D16.2-	-	-
short bones	C40.3-	C79.51	-	D16.3-	-	-
upper (long bones)	C40.0-	C79.51	-	D16.0-	-	-
short bones	C40.1-	C79.51	-	D16.1-	-	-
malar	C41.0	C79.51	-	D16.4	D48.0	D49.2
mandible	C41.1	C79.51	-	D16.5	D48.0	D49.2
marrow NEC (any bone)	C96.9	C79.52	-	-	D47.9	D49.89
mastoid	C41.0	C79.51	-	D16.4	D48.0	D49.2
maxilla, maxillary (superior)	C41.0	C79.51	-	D16.4	D48.0	D49.2
inferior	C41.1	C79.51	-	D16.4	D48.0	D49.2
metacarpus (any)	C40.1-	C79.51	-	D16.1-	-	-
metatarsus (any)	C40.3-	C79.51	-	D16.3-	-	-
navicular						
ankle	C40.3-	C79.51	-	-	-	-
hand	C40.1-	C79.51	-	-	-	-
nose, nasal	C41.0	C79.51	-	D16.4	D48.0	D49.2
occipital	C41.0	C79.51	-	D16.4	D48.0	D49.2
orbit	C41.0	C79.51	-	D16.4	D48.0	D49.2

	Malignant Primary	Malignant Secondary	Ca in situ	Benign	Uncertain Behavior	Unspecified Behavior
bone — *continued*						
overlapping sites	C40.8-	-	-	-	-	-
parietal	C41.0	C79.51	-	D16.4	D48.0	D49.2
patella	C40.2-	C79.51	-	-	-	-
pelvic	C41.4	C79.51	-	D16.8	D48.0	D49.2
phalanges						
foot	C40.3-	C79.51	-	-	-	-
hand	C40.1-	C79.51	-	-	-	-
pubic	C41.4	C79.51	-	D16.8	D48.0	D49.2
radius (any part)	C40.0-	C79.51	-	D16.0-	-	-
rib	C41.3	C79.51	-	D16.7	D48.0	D49.2
sacral vertebra	C41.4	C79.51	-	D16.8	D48.0	D49.2
sacrum	C41.4	C79.51	-	D16.8	D48.0	D49.2
scaphoid	-	-	-	-	-	-
of ankle	C40.3-	C79.51	-	-	-	-
of hand	C40.1-	C79.51	-	-	-	-
scapula (any part)	C40.0-	C79.51	-	D16.0-	-	-
sella turcica	C41.0	C79.51	-	D16.4	D48.0	D49.2
shoulder	C40.0-	C79.51	-	D16.0-	-	-
skull	C41.0	C79.51	-	D16.4	D48.0	D49.2
sphenoid	C41.0	C79.51	-	D16.4	D48.0	D49.2
spine, spinal (column)	C41.2	C79.51	-	D16.6	D48.0	D49.2
coccyx	C41.4	C79.51	-	D16.8	D48.0	D49.2
sacrum	C41.4	C79.51	-	D16.8	D48.0	D49.2
sternum	C41.3	C79.51	-	D16.7	D48.0	D49.2
tarsus (any)	C40.3-	C79.51	-	-	-	-
temporal	C41.0	C79.51	-	D16.4	D48.0	D49.2
thumb	C40.1-	C79.51	-	-	-	-
tibia (any part)	C40.2-	C79.51	-	-	-	-
toe (any)	C40.3-	C79.51	-	-	-	-
trapezium	C40.1-	C79.51	-	-	-	-
trapezoid	C40.1-	C79.51	-	-	-	-
turbinate	C41.0	C79.51	-	D16.4	D48.0	D49.2
ulna (any part)	C40.0-	C79.51	-	D16.0-	-	-
unciform	C40.1-	C79.51	-	-	-	-
vertebra (column)	C41.2	C79.51	-	D16.6	D48.0	D49.2
coccyx	C41.4	C79.51	-	D16.8	D48.0	D49.2
sacrum	C41.4	C79.51	-	D16.8	D48.0	D49.2
vomer	C41.0	C79.51	-	D16.4	D48.0	D49.2
wrist	C40.1-	C79.51	-	-	-	-
xiphoid process	C41.3	C79.51	-	D16.7	D48.0	D49.2
zygomatic	C41.0	C79.51	-	D16.4	D48.0	D49.2
book-leaf (mouth)	C06.89	C79.89	D00.00	D10.39	D37.09	D49.0
bowel—see Neoplasm, intestine						
brachial plexus	C47.1-	C79.89	-	D36.12	D48.2	D49.2
brain NEC	C71.9	C79.31	-	D33.2	D43.2	D49.6
basal ganglia	C71.0	C79.31	-	D33.0	D43.0	D49.6
cerebellopontine angle	C71.6	C79.31	-	D33.1	D43.1	D49.6
cerebellum NOS	C71.6	C79.31	-	D33.1	D43.1	D49.6
cerebrum	C71.0	C79.31	-	D33.0	D43.0	D49.6
choroid plexus	C71.7	C79.31	-	D33.1	D43.1	D49.6
corpus callosum	C71.8	C79.31	-	D33.2	D43.2	D49.6

	Malignant Primary	Malignant Secondary	Ca in situ	Benign	Uncertain Behavior	Unspecified Behavior
brain NEC — *continued*						
corpus striatum	C71.0	C79.31	-	D33.0	D43.0	D49.6
cortex (cerebral)	C71.0	C79.31	-	D33.0	D43.0	D49.6
frontal lobe	C71.1	C79.31	-	D33.0	D43.0	D49.6
globus pallidus	C71.0	C79.31	-	D33.0	D43.0	D49.6
hippocampus	C71.2	C79.31	-	D33.0	D43.0	D49.6
hypothalamus	C71.0	C79.31	-	D33.0	D43.0	D49.6
internal capsule	C71.0	C79.31	-	D33.0	D43.0	D49.6
medulla oblongata	C71.7	C79.31	-	D33.1	D43.1	D49.6
meninges	C70.0	C79.32	-	D32.0	D42.0	D49.7
midbrain	C71.7	C79.31	-	D33.1	D43.1	D49.6
occipital lobe	C71.4	C79.31	-	D33.0	D43.0	D49.6
overlapping lesion	C71.8	C79.31	-	-	-	-
parietal lobe	C71.3	C79.31	-	D33.0	D43.0	D49.6
peduncle	C71.7	C79.31	-	D33.1	D43.1	D49.6
pons	C71.7	C79.31	-	D33.1	D43.1	D49.6
stem	C71.7	C79.31	-	D33.1	D43.1	D49.6
tapetum	C71.8	C79.31	-	D33.2	D43.2	D49.6
temporal lobe	C71.2	C79.31	-	D33.0	D43.0	D49.6
thalamus	C71.0	C79.31	-	D33.0	D43.0	D49.6
uncus	C71.2	C79.31	-	D33.0	D43.0	D49.6
ventricle (floor)	C71.5	C79.31	-	D33.0	D43.0	D49.6
fourth	C71.7	C79.31	-	D33.1	D43.1	D49.6
branchial (cleft) (cyst) (vestiges)	C10.4	C79.89	D00.08	D10.5	D37.05	D49.0
breast (connective tissue) (glandular tissue) (soft parts)	C50.9-	C79.81	D05.-	D24.-	D48.6-	D49.3
areola	C50.0-	C79.81	D05.-	D24.-	D48.6-	D49.3
axillary tail	C50.6-	C79.81	D05.-	D24.-	D48.6-	D49.3
central portion	C50.1-	C79.81	D05.-	D24.-	D48.6-	D49.3
inner	C50.8-	C79.81	D05.-	D24.-	D48.6-	D49.3
lower	C50.8-	C79.81	D05.-	D24.-	D48.6-	D49.3
lower-inner quadrant	C50.3-	C79.81	D05.-	D24.-	D48.6-	D49.3
lower-outer quadrant	C50.5-	C79.81	D05.-	D24.-	D48.6-	D49.3
mastectomy site (skin)—see also Neoplasm, breast, skin	C44.501	C79.2	-	-	-	-
specified as breast tissue	C50.8-	C79.81	-	-	-	-
midline	C50.8-	C79.81	D05.-	D24.-	D48.6-	D49.3
nipple	C50.0-	C79.81	D05.-	D24.-	D48.6-	D49.3
outer	C50.8-	C79.81	D05.-	D24.-	D48.6-	D49.3
overlapping lesion	C50.8-	-	-	-	-	-
skin	C44.501	C79.2	D04.5	D23.5	D48.5	D49.2
basal cell carcinoma	C44.511	-	-	-	-	-
specified type NEC	C44.591	-	-	-	-	-
squamous cell carcinoma	C44.521	-	-	-	-	-
tail (axillary)	C50.6-	C79.81	D05.-	D24.-	D48.6-	D49.3
upper	C50.8-	C79.81	D05.-	D24.-	D48.6-	D49.3
upper-inner quadrant	C50.2-	C79.81	D05.-	D24.-	D48.6-	D49.3
upper-outer quadrant	C50.4-	C79.81	D05.-	D24.-	D48.6-	D49.3
broad ligament	C57.1-	C79.82	D07.39	D28.2	D39.8	D49.59

	Malignant Primary	Malignant Secondary	Ca in situ	Benign	Uncertain Behavior	Unspecified Behavior
bronchiogenic, bronchogenic (lung)	C34.9-	C78.0-	D02.2-	D14.3-	D38.1	D49.1
bronchiole	C34.9-	C78.0-	D02.2-	D14.3-	D38.1	D49.1
bronchus	C34.9-	C78.0-	D02.2-	D14.3-	D38.1	D49.1
carina	C34.0-	C78.0-	D02.2-	D14.3-	D38.1	D49.1
lower lobe of lung	C34.3-	C78.0-	D02.2-	D14.3-	D38.1	D49.1
main	C34.0-	C78.0-	D02.2-	D14.3-	D38.1	D49.1
middle lobe of lung	C34.2	C78.0-	D02.21	D14.31	D38.1	D49.1
overlapping lesion	C34.8-	-	-	-	-	-
upper lobe of lung	C34.1-	C78.0-	D02.2-	D14.3-	D38.1	D49.1
brow	C44.309	C79.2	D04.39	D23.39	D48.5	D49.2
basal cell carcinoma	C44.319	-	-	-	-	-
specified type NEC	C44.399	-	-	-	-	-
squamous cell carcinoma	C44.329	-	-	-	-	-
buccal (cavity)	C06.9	C79.89	D00.00	D10.39	D37.09	D49.0
commissure	C06.0	C79.89	D00.02	D10.39	D37.09	D49.0
groove (lower) (upper)	C06.1	C79.89	D00.02	D10.39	D37.09	D49.0
mucosa	C06.0	C79.89	D00.02	D10.39	D37.09	D49.0
sulcus (lower) (upper)	C06.1	C79.89	D00.02	D10.39	D37.09	D49.0
bulbourethral gland	C68.0	C79.19	D09.19	D30.4	D41.3	D49.59
bursa—see Neoplasm, connective tissue						
buttock NEC	C76.3	C79.89	D04.5	D36.7	D48.7	D49.89
C						
calf	C76.5-	C79.89	D04.7-	D36.7	D48.7	D49.89
calvarium	C41.0	C79.51	-	D16.4	D48.0	D49.2
calyx, renal	C65.-	C79.0-	D09.19	D30.1-	D41.1-	D49.51-
canal						
anal	C21.1	C78.5	D01.3	D12.9	D37.8	D49.0
auditory (external)—see also Neoplasm, skin, ear	C44.20-	C79.2	D04.2-	D23.2-	D48.5	D49.2
auricular (external)—see also Neoplasm, skin, ear	C44.20-	C79.2	D04.2-	D23.2-	D48.5	D49.2
canaliculi, biliary (biliferi) (intrahepatic)	C22.1	C78.7	D01.5	D13.4	D37.6	D49.0
canthus (eye) (inner) (outer)	C44.10-	C79.2	D04.1-	D23.1-	D48.5	D49.2
basal cell carcinoma	C44.11-	-	-	-	-	-
sebaceous cell	C44.13-	-	-	-	-	-
specified type NEC	C44.19-	-	-	-	-	-
squamous cell carcinoma	C44.12-	-	-	-	-	-
capillary—see Neoplasm, connective tissue						
caput coli	C18.0	C78.5	D01.0	D12.0	D37.4	D49.0
carcinoid—see Tumor, carcinoid						
cardia (gastric)	C16.0	C78.89	D00.2	D13.1	D37.1	D49.0
cardiac orifice (stomach)	C16.0	C78.89	D00.2	D13.1	D37.1	D49.0
cardio-esophageal junction	C16.0	C78.89	D00.2	D13.1	D37.1	D49.0
cardio-esophagus	C16.0	C78.89	D00.2	D13.1	D37.1	D49.0
carina (bronchus)	C34.0-	C78.0-	D02.2-	D14.3-	D38.1	D49.1
carotid (artery)	C49.0	C79.89	-	D21.0	D48.1	D49.2
body	C75.4	C79.89	-	D35.5	D44.6	D49.7
carpus (any bone)	C40.1-	C79.51	-	D16.1-	-	-
cartilage (articular) (joint) NEC—see also Neoplasm, bone	C41.9	C79.51	-	D16.9	D48.0	D49.2
arytenoid	C32.3	C78.39	D02.0	D14.1	D38.0	D49.1
cartilage NEC — *continued*						
auricular	C49.0	C79.89	-	D21.0	D48.1	D49.2
bronchi	C34.0-	C78.39	-	D14.3-	D38.1	D49.1
costal	C41.3	C79.51	-	D16.7	D48.0	D49.2
cricoid	C32.3	C78.39	D02.0	D14.1	D38.0	D49.1
cuneiform	C32.3	C78.39	D02.0	D14.1	D38.0	D49.1
ear (external)	C49.0	C79.89	-	D21.0	D48.1	D49.2
ensiform	C41.3	C79.51	-	D16.7	D48.0	D49.2
epiglottis	C32.1	C78.39	D02.0	D14.1	D38.0	D49.1
anterior surface	C10.1	C79.89	D00.08	D10.5	D37.05	D49.0
eyelid	C49.0	C79.89	-	D21.0	D48.1	D49.2
intervertebral	C41.2	C79.51	-	D16.6	D48.0	D49.2
larynx, laryngeal	C32.3	C78.39	D02.0	D14.1	D38.0	D49.1
nose, nasal	C30.0	C78.39	D02.3	D14.0	D38.5	D49.1
pinna	C49.0	C79.89	-	D21.0	D48.1	D49.2
rib	C41.3	C79.51	-	D16.7	D48.0	D49.2
semilunar (knee)	C40.2-	C79.51	-	D16.2-	D48.0	D49.2
thyroid	C32.3	C78.39	D02.0	D14.1	D38.0	D49.1
trachea	C33	C78.39	D02.1	D14.2	D38.1	D49.1
cauda equina	C72.1	C79.49	-	D33.4	D43.4	D49.7
cavity						
buccal	C06.9	C79.89	D00.00	D10.30	D37.09	D49.0
nasal	C30.0	C78.39	D02.3	D14.0	D38.5	D49.1
oral	C06.9	C79.89	D00.00	D10.30	D37.09	D49.0
peritoneal	C48.2	C78.6	-	D20.1	D48.4	D49.0
tympanic	C30.1	C78.39	D02.3	D14.0	D38.5	D49.1
cecum	C18.0	C78.5	D01.0	D12.0	D37.4	D49.0
central nervous system	C72.9	C79.40	-	-	-	-
cerebellopontine (angle)	C71.6	C79.31	-	D33.1	D43.1	D49.6
cerebellum, cerebellar	C71.6	C79.31	-	D33.1	D43.1	D49.6
cerebrum, cerebral (cortex) (hemisphere) (white matter)	C71.0	C79.31	-	D33.0	D43.0	D49.6
meninges	C70.0	C79.32	-	D32.0	D42.0	D49.7
peduncle	C71.7	C79.31	-	D33.1	D43.1	D49.6
ventricle	C71.5	C79.31	-	D33.0	D43.0	D49.6
fourth	C71.7	C79.31	-	D33.1	D43.1	D49.6
cervical region	C76.0	C79.89	D09.8	D36.7	D48.7	D49.89
cervix (cervical) (uteri) (uterus)	C53.9	C79.82	D06.9	D26.0	D39.0	D49.59
canal	C53.0	C79.82	D06.0	D26.0	D39.0	D49.59
endocervix (canal) (gland)	C53.0	C79.82	D06.0	D26.0	D39.0	D49.59
exocervix	C53.1	C79.82	D06.1	D26.0	D39.0	D49.59
external os	C53.1	C79.82	D06.1	D26.0	D39.0	D49.59
internal os	C53.0	C79.82	D06.0	D26.0	D39.0	D49.59
nabothian gland	C53.0	C79.82	D06.0	D26.0	D39.0	D49.59
overlapping lesion	C53.8	-	-	-	-	-
squamocolumnar junction	C53.8	C79.82	D06.7	D26.0	D39.0	D49.59
stump	C53.8	C79.82	D06.7	D26.0	D39.0	D49.59
cheek	C76.0	C79.89	D09.8	D36.7	D48.7	D49.89
external	C44.309	C79.2	D04.39	D23.39	D48.5	D49.2
basal cell carcinoma	C44.319	-	-	-	-	-
specified type NEC	C44.399	-	-	-	-	-
squamous cell carcinoma	C44.329	-	-	-	-	-

	Malignant Primary	Malignant Secondary	Ca in situ	Benign	Uncertain Behavior	Unspecified Behavior
cheek — *continued*						
inner aspect	C06.0	C79.89	D00.02	D10.39	D37.09	D49.0
internal	C06.0	C79.89	D00.02	D10.39	D37.09	D49.0
mucosa	C06.0	C79.89	D00.02	D10.39	D37.09	D49.0
chest (wall) NEC	C76.1	C79.89	D09.8	D36.7	D48.7	D49.89
chiasma opticum	C72.3-	C79.49	-	D33.3	D43.3	D49.7
chin	C44.309	C79.2	D04.39	D23.39	D48.5	D49.2
basal cell carcinoma	C44.319	-	-	-	-	-
specified type NEC	C44.399	-	-	-	-	-
squamous cell carcinoma	C44.329	-	-	-	-	-
choana	C11.3	C79.89	D00.08	D10.6	D37.05	D49.0
cholangiole	C22.1	C78.89	D01.5	D13.4	D37.6	D49.0
choledochal duct	C24.0	C78.89	D01.5	D13.5	D37.6	D49.0
choroid	C69.3-	C79.49	D09.2-	D31.3-	D48.7	D49.81
plexus	C71.5	C79.31	-	D33.0	D43.0	D49.6
ciliary body	C69.4-	C79.49	D09.2-	D31.4-	D48.7	D49.89
clavicle	C41.3	C79.51	-	D16.7	D48.0	D49.2
clitoris	C51.2	C79.82	D07.1	D28.0	D39.8	D49.59
clivus	C41.0	C79.51	-	D16.4-	D48.0	D49.2
cloacogenic zone	C21.2	C78.5	D01.3	D12.9	D37.8	D49.0
coccygeal						
body or glomus	C49.5	C79.89	-	D21.5	D48.1	D49.2
vertebra	C41.4	C79.51	-	D16.8	D48.0	D49.2
coccyx	C41.4	C79.51	-	D16.8	D48.0	D49.2
colon—see also Neoplasm, intestine, large	C18.9	C78.5	-	-	-	-
with rectum	C19	C78.5	D01.1	D12.7	D37.5	D49.0
column, spinal—see Neoplasm, spine						
columnella—see also Neoplasm, skin, face	C44.390	C79.2	D04.39	D23.39	D48.5	D49.2
commissure						
labial, lip	C00.6	C79.89	D00.01	D10.39	D37.01	D49.0
laryngeal	C32.0	C78.39	D02.0	D14.1	D38.0	D49.1
common (bile) duct	C24.0	C78.89	D01.5	D13.5	D37.6	D49.0
concha—see also Neoplasm, skin, ear	C44.20-	C79.2	D04.2-	D23.2-	D48.5	D49.2
nose	C30.0	C78.39	D02.3	D14.0	D38.5	D49.1
conjunctiva	C69.0-	C79.49	D09.2-	D31.0-	D48.7	D49.89
connective tissue NEC	C49.9	C79.89	-	D21.9	D48.1	D49.2
Note: For neoplasms of connective tissue (blood vessel, bursa, fascia, ligament, muscle, peripheral nerves, sympathetic and parasympathetic nerves and ganglia, synovia, tendon, etc.) or of morphological types that indicate connective tissue, code according to the list under "Neoplasm, connective tissue". For sites that do not appear in this list, code to neoplasm of that site; e.g., fibrosarcoma, pancreas (C25.9)						

	Malignant Primary	Malignant Secondary	Ca in situ	Benign	Uncertain Behavior	Unspecified Behavior
connective tissue NEC — *continued*						
Note: Morphological types that indicate connective tissue appear in their proper place in the alphabetic index with the instruction "see Neoplasm, connective tissue …."						
abdomen	C49.4	C79.89	-	D21.4	D48.1	D49.2
abdominal wall	C49.4	C79.89	-	D21.4	D48.1	D49.2
ankle	C49.2-	C79.89	-	D21.2-	D48.1	D49.2
antecubital fossa or space	C49.1-	C79.89	-	D21.1-	D48.1	D49.2
arm	C49.1-	C79.89	-	D21.1-	D48.1	D49.2
auricle (ear)	C49.0	C79.89	-	D21.0	D48.1	D49.2
axilla	C49.3	C79.89	-	D21.3	D48.1	D49.2
back	C49.6	C79.89	-	D21.6	D48.1	D49.2
breast—see Neoplasm, breast						
buttock	C49.5	C79.89	-	D21.5	D48.1	D49.2
calf	C49.2-	C79.89	-	D21.2-	D48.1	D49.2
cervical region	C49.0	C79.89	-	D21.0	D48.1	D49.2
cheek	C49.0	C79.89	-	D21.0	D48.1	D49.2
chest (wall)	C49.3	C79.89	-	D21.3	D48.1	D49.2
chin	C49.0	C79.89	-	D21.0	D48.1	D49.2
diaphragm	C49.3	C79.89	-	D21.3	D48.1	D49.2
ear (external)	C49.0	C79.89	-	D21.0	D48.1	D49.2
elbow	C49.1-	C79.89	-	D21.1-	D48.1	D49.2
extrarectal	C49.5	C79.89	-	D21.5	D48.1	D49.2
extremity	C49.9	C79.89	-	D21.9	D48.1	D49.2
lower	C49.2-	C79.89	-	D21.2-	D48.1	D49.2
upper	C49.1-	C79.89	-	D21.1-	D48.1	D49.2
eyelid	C49.0	C79.89	-	D21.0	D48.1	D49.2
face	C49.0	C79.89	-	D21.0	D48.1	D49.2
finger	C49.1-	C79.89	-	D21.1-	D48.1	D49.2
flank	C49.6	C79.89	-	D21.6	D48.1	D49.2
foot	C49.2-	C79.89	-	D21.2-	D48.1	D49.2
forearm	C49.1-	C79.89	-	D21.1-	D48.1	D49.2
forehead	C49.0	C79.89	-	D21.0	D48.1	D49.2
gastric	C49.4	C79.89	-	D21.4	D48.1	D49.2
gastrointestinal	C49.4	C79.89	-	D21.4	D48.1	D49.2
gluteal region	C49.5	C79.89	-	D21.5	D48.1	D49.2
great vessels NEC	C49.3	C79.89	-	D21.3	D48.1	D49.2
groin	C49.5	C79.89	-	D21.5	D48.1	D49.2
hand	C49.1-	C79.89	-	D21.1-	D48.1	D49.2
head	C49.0	C79.89	-	D21.0	D48.1	D49.2
heel	C49.2-	C79.89	-	D21.2-	D48.1	D49.2
hip	C49.2-	C79.89	-	D21.2-	D48.1	D49.2
hypochondrium	C49.4	C79.89	-	D21.4	D48.1	D49.2
iliopsoas muscle	C49.5	C79.89	-	D21.5	D48.1	D49.2
infraclavicular region	C49.3	C79.89	-	D21.3	D48.1	D49.2
inguinal (canal) (region)	C49.5	C79.89	-	D21.5	D48.1	D49.2
intestinal	C49.4	C79.89	-	D21.4	D48.1	D49.2
intrathoracic	C49.3	C79.89	-	D21.3	D48.1	D49.2
ischiorectal fossa	C49.5	C79.89	-	D21.5	D48.1	D49.2

	Malignant Primary	Malignant Secondary	Ca in situ	Benign	Uncertain Behavior	Unspecified Behavior
connective tissue NEC — *continued*						
jaw	C03.9	C79.89	D00.03	D10.39	D48.1	D49.0
knee	C49.2-	C79.89	-	D21.2-	D48.1	D49.2
leg	C49.2-	C79.89	-	D21.2-	D48.1	D49.2
limb NEC	C49.9	C79.89	-	D21.9	D48.1	D49.2
lower	C49.2-	C79.89	-	D21.2-	D48.1	D49.2
upper	C49.1-	C79.89	-	D21.1-	D48.1	D49.2
nates	C49.5	C79.89	-	D21.5	D48.1	D49.2
neck	C49.0	C79.89	-	D21.0	D48.1	D49.2
orbit	C69.6-	C79.49	D09.2-	D31.6-	D48.1	D49.89
overlapping lesion	C49.8	-	-	-	-	-
pararectal	C49.5	C79.89	-	D21.5	D48.1	D49.2
para-urethral	C49.5	C79.89	-	D21.5	D48.1	D49.2
paravaginal	C49.5	C79.89	-	D21.5	D48.1	D49.2
pelvis (floor)	C49.5	C79.89	-	D21.5	D48.1	D49.2
pelvo-abdominal	C49.8	C79.89	-	D21.6	D48.1	D49.2
perineum	C49.5	C79.89	-	D21.5	D48.1	D49.2
perirectal (tissue)	C49.5	C79.89	-	D21.5	D48.1	D49.2
periurethral (tissue)	C49.5	C79.89	-	D21.5	D48.1	D49.2
popliteal fossa or space	C49.2-	C79.89	-	D21.2-	D48.1	D49.2
presacral	C49.5	C79.89	-	D21.5	D48.1	D49.2
psoas muscle	C49.4	C79.89	-	D21.4	D48.1	D49.2
pterygoid fossa	C49.0	C79.89	-	D21.0	D48.1	D49.2
rectovaginal septum or wall	C49.5	C79.89	-	D21.5	D48.1	D49.2
rectovesical	C49.5	C79.89	-	D21.5	D48.1	D49.2
retroperitoneum	C48.0	C78.6	-	D20.0	D48.3	D49.0
sacrococcygeal region	C49.5	C79.89	-	D21.5	D48.1	D49.2
scalp	C49.0	C79.89	-	D21.0	D48.1	D49.2
scapular region	C49.3	C79.89	-	D21.3	D48.1	D49.2
shoulder	C49.1-	C79.89	-	D21.1-	D48.1	D49.2
skin (dermis) NEC—see also Neoplasm, skin, by site	C44.90	C79.2	D04.9	D23.9	D48.5	D49.2
stomach	C49.4	C79.89	-	D21.4	D48.1	D49.2
submental	C49.0	C79.89	-	D21.0	D48.1	D49.2
supraclavicular region	C49.0	C79.89	-	D21.0	D48.1	D49.2
temple	C49.0	C79.89	-	D21.0	D48.1	D49.2
temporal region	C49.0	C79.89	-	D21.0	D48.1	D49.2
thigh	C49.2-	C79.89	-	D21.2-	D48.1	D49.2
thoracic (duct) (wall)	C49.3	C79.89	-	D21.3	D48.1	D49.2
thorax	C49.3	C79.89	-	D21.3	D48.1	D49.2
thumb	C49.1-	C79.89	-	D21.1-	D48.1	D49.2
toe	C49.2-	C79.89	-	D21.2-	D48.1	D49.2
trunk	C49.6	C79.89	-	D21.6	D48.1	D49.2
umbilicus	C49.4	C79.89	-	D21.4	D48.1	D49.2
vesicorectal	C49.5	C79.89	-	D21.5	D48.1	D49.2
wrist	C49.1-	C79.89	-	D21.1-	D48.1	D49.2
conus medullaris	C72.0	C79.49	-	D33.4	D43.4	D49.7
cord (true) (vocal)	C32.0	C78.39	D02.0	D14.1	D38.0	D49.1
false	C32.1	C78.39	D02.0	D14.1	D38.0	D49.1
spermatic	C63.1-	C79.82	D07.69	D29.8	D40.8	D49.59

	Malignant Primary	Malignant Secondary	Ca in situ	Benign	Uncertain Behavior	Unspecified Behavior
cord (true) (vocal) — *continued*						
spinal (cervical) (lumbar) (thoracic)	C72.0	C79.49	-	D33.4	D43.4	D49.7
cornea (limbus)	C69.1-	C79.49	D09.2-	D31.1-	D48.7	D49.89
corpus						
albicans	C56.-	C79.6-	D07.39	D27.-	D39.1-	D49.59
callosum, brain	C71.0	C79.31	-	D33.2	D43.2	D49.6
cavernosum	C60.2	C79.82	D07.4	D29.0	D40.8	D49.59
gastric	C16.2	C78.89	D00.2	D13.1	D37.1	D49.0
overlapping sites	C54.8	-	-	-	-	-
penis	C60.2	C79.82	D07.4	D29.0	D40.8	D49.59
striatum, cerebrum	C71.0	C79.31	-	D33.0	D43.0	D49.6
uteri	C54.9	C79.82	D07.0	D26.1	D39.0	D49.59
isthmus	C54.0	C79.82	D07.0	D26.1	D39.0	D49.59
cortex						
adrenal	C74.0-	C79.7-	D09.3	D35.0-	D44.1-	D49.7
cerebral	C71.0	C79.31	-	D33.0	D43.0	D49.6
costal cartilage	C41.3	C79.51	-	D16.7	D48.0	D49.2
costovertebral joint	C41.3	C79.51	-	D16.7	D48.0	D49.2
Cowper's gland	C68.0	C79.19	D09.19	D30.4	D41.3	D49.59
cranial (fossa, any)	C71.9	C79.31	-	D33.2	D43.2	D49.6
meninges	C70.0	C79.32	-	D32.0	D42.0	D49.7
nerve	C72.50	C79.49	-	D33.3	D43.3	D49.7
specified NEC	C72.59	C79.49	-	D33.3	D43.3	D49.7
craniobuccal pouch	C75.2	C79.89	D09.3	D35.2	D44.3	D49.7
craniopharyngeal (duct) (pouch)	C75.2	C79.89	D09.3	D35.3	D44.4	D49.7
cricoid	C13.0	C79.89	D00.08	D10.7	D37.05	D49.0
cartilage	C32.3	C78.39	D02.0	D14.1	D38.0	D49.1
cricopharynx	C13.0	C79.89	D00.08	D10.7	D37.05	D49.0
crypt of Morgagni	C21.8	C78.5	D01.3	D12.9	D37.8	D49.0
crystalline lens	C69.4-	C79.49	D09.2-	D31.4-	D48.7	D49.89
cul-de-sac (Douglas')	C48.1	C78.6	-	D20.1	D48.4	D49.0
cuneiform cartilage	C32.3	C78.39	D02.0	D14.1	D38.0	D49.1
cutaneous—see Neoplasm, skin						
cutis—see Neoplasm, skin						
cystic (bile) duct (common)	C24.0	C78.89	D01.5	D13.5	D37.6	D49.0
D						
dermis—see Neoplasm, skin						
diaphragm	C49.3	C79.89	-	D21.3	D48.1	D49.2
digestive organs, system, tube, or tract NEC	C26.9	C78.89	D01.9	D13.9	D37.9	D49.0
disc, intervertebral	C41.2	C79.51	-	D16.6	D48.0	D49.2
disease, generalized	C80.0	-	-	-	-	-
disseminated	C80.0	-	-	-	-	-
Douglas' cul-de-sac or pouch	C48.1	C78.6	-	D20.1	D48.4	D49.0
duodenojejunal junction	C17.8	C78.4	D01.49	D13.39	D37.2	D49.0
duodenum	C17.0	C78.4	D01.49	D13.2	D37.2	D49.0
dura (cranial) (mater)	C70.9	C79.49	-	D32.9	D42.9	D49.7
cerebral	C70.0	C79.32	-	D32.0	D42.0	D49.7
spinal	C70.1	C79.49	-	D32.1	D42.1	D49.7

	Malignant Primary	Malignant Secondary	Ca in situ	Benign	Uncertain Behavior	Unspecified Behavior
E						
ear (external)—see also Neoplasm, skin, ear	C44.20-	C79.2	D04.2-	D23.2-	D48.5	D49.2
auricle or auris—see also Neoplasm, skin, ear	C44.20-	C79.2	D04.2-	D23.2-	D48.5	D49.2
canal, external—see also Neoplasm, skin, ear	C44.20-	C79.2	D04.2-	D23.2-	D48.5	D49.2
cartilage	C49.0	C79.89	-	D21.0	D48.1	D49.2
external meatus—see also Neoplasm, skin, ear	C44.20-	C79.2	D04.2-	D23.2-	D48.5	D49.2
inner	C30.1	C78.39	D02.3	D14.0	D38.5	D49.1
lobule—see also Neoplasm, skin, ear	C44.20-	C79.2	D04.2-	D23.2-	D48.5	D49.2
middle	C30.1	C78.39	D02.3	D14.0	D38.5	D49.1
overlapping lesion with accessory sinuses	C31.8	-	-	-	-	-
skin	C44.20-	C79.2	D04.2-	D23.2-	D48.5	D49.2
basal cell carcinoma	C44.21-	-	-	-	-	-
specified type NEC	C44.29-	-	-	-	-	-
squamous cell carcinoma	C44.22-	-	-	-	-	-
earlobe	C44.20-	C79.2	D04.2-	D23.2-	D48.5	D49.2
basal cell carcinoma	C44.21-	-	-	-	-	-
specified type NEC	C44.29-	-	-	-	-	-
squamous cell carcinoma	C44.22-	-	-	-	-	-
ejaculatory duct	C63.7	C79.82	D07.69	D29.8	D40.8	D49.59
elbow NEC	C76.4-	C79.89	D04.6-	D36.7	D48.7	D49.89
endocardium	C38.0	C79.89	-	D15.1	D48.7	D49.89
endocervix (canal) (gland)	C53.0	C79.82	D06.0	D26.0	D39.0	D49.59
endocrine gland NEC	C75.9	C79.89	D09.3	D35.9	D44.9	D49.7
pluriglandular	C75.8	C79.89	D09.3	D35.7	D44.9	D49.7
endometrium (gland) (stroma)	C54.1	C79.82	D07.0	D26.1	D39.0	D49.59
ensiform cartilage	C41.3	C79.51	-	D16.7	D48.0	D49.2
enteric—see Neoplasm, intestine						
ependyma (brain)	C71.5	C79.31	-	D33.0	D43.0	D49.6
fourth ventricle	C71.7	C79.31	-	D33.1	D43.1	D49.6
epicardium	C38.0	C79.89	-	D15.1	D48.7	D49.89
epididymis	C63.0-	C79.82	D07.69	D29.3-	D40.8	D49.59
epidural	C72.9	C79.49	-	D33.9	D43.9	D49.7
epiglottis	C32.1	C78.39	D02.0	D14.1	D38.0	D49.1
anterior aspect or surface	C10.1	C79.89	D00.08	D10.5	D37.05	D49.0
cartilage	C32.3	C78.39	D02.0	D14.1	D38.0	D49.1
free border (margin)	C10.1	C79.89	D00.08	D10.5	D37.05	D49.0
junctional region	C10.8	C79.89	D00.08	D10.5	D37.05	D49.0
posterior (laryngeal) surface	C32.1	C78.39	D02.0	D14.1	D38.0	D49.1
suprahyoid portion	C32.1	C78.39	D02.0	D14.1	D38.0	D49.1
esophagogastric junction	C16.0	C78.89	D00.2	D13.1	D37.1	D49.0
esophagus	C15.9	C78.89	D00.1	D13.0	D37.8	D49.0
abdominal	C15.5	C78.89	D00.1	D13.0	D37.8	D49.0
cervical	C15.3	C78.89	D00.1	D13.0	D37.8	D49.0
distal (third)	C15.5	C78.89	D00.1	D13.0	D37.8	D49.0
lower (third)	C15.5	C78.89	D00.1	D13.0	D37.8	D49.0
esophagus — *continued*						
middle (third)	C15.4	C78.89	D00.1	D13.0	D37.8	D49.0
overlapping lesion	C15.8	-	-	-	-	-
proximal (third)	C15.3	C78.89	D00.1	D13.0	D37.8	D49.0
thoracic	C15.4	C78.89	D00.1	D13.0	D37.8	D49.0
upper (third)	C15.3	C78.89	D00.1	D13.0	D37.8	D49.0
ethmoid (sinus)	C31.1	C78.39	D02.3	D14.0	D38.5	D49.1
bone or labyrinth	C41.0	C79.51	-	D16.4-	D48.0	D49.2
eustachian tube	C30.1	C78.39	D02.3	D14.0	D38.5	D49.1
exocervix	C53.1	C79.82	D06.1	D26.0	D39.0	D49.59
external						
meatus (ear)—see also Neoplasm, skin, ear	C44.20-	C79.2	D04.2-	D23.2-	D48.5	D49.2
os, cervix uteri	C53.1	C79.82	D06.1	D26.0	D39.0	D49.59
extradural	C72.9	C79.49	-	D33.9	D43.9	D49.7
extrahepatic (bile) duct	C24.0	C78.89	D01.5	D13.5	D37.6	D49.0
overlapping lesion with gallbladder	C24.8	-	-	-	-	-
extraocular muscle	C69.6-	C79.49	D09.2-	D31.6-	D48.7	D49.89
extrarectal	C76.3	C79.89	D09.8	D36.7	D48.7	D49.89
extremity	C76.8	C79.89	D04.8	D36.7	D48.7	D49.89
lower	C76.5-	C79.89	D04.7-	D36.7	D48.7	D49.89
upper	C76.4-	C79.89	D04.6-	D36.7	D48.7	D49.89
eye NEC	C69.9-	C79.49	D09.2-	D31.9	D48.7	D49.89
overlapping sites	C69.8-	-	-	-	-	-
eyeball	C69.9-	C79.49	D09.2-	D31.9-	D48.7	D49.89
eyebrow	C44.309	C79.2	D04.39	D23.39	D48.5	D49.2
basal cell carcinoma	C44.319	-	-	-	-	-
specified type NEC	C44.399	-	-	-	-	-
squamous cell carcinoma	C44.329	-	-	-	-	-
eyelid (lower) (skin) (upper)	C44.10-	-	-	-	-	-
basal cell carcinoma	C44.11-	-	-	-	-	-
sebaceous cell	C44.13-	-	-	-	-	-
specified type NEC	C44.19-	-	-	-	-	-
squamous cell carcinoma	C44.12-	-	-	-	-	-
cartilage	C49.0	C79.89	-	D21.0	D48.1	D49.2
F						
face NEC	C76.0	C79.89	D04.39	D36.7	D48.7	D49.89
fallopian tube (accessory)	C57.0-	C79.82	D07.39	D28.2	D39.8	D49.59
falx (cerebella) (cerebri)	C70.0	C79.32	-	D32.0	D42.0	D49.7
fascia—see also Neoplasm, connective tissue						
palmar	C49.1-	C79.89	-	D21.1-	D48.1	D49.2
plantar	C49.2-	C79.89	-	D21.2-	D48.1	D49.2
fatty tissue—see Neoplasm, connective tissue						
fauces, faucial NEC	C10.9	C79.89	D00.08	D10.5	D37.05	D49.0
pillars	C09.1	C79.89	D00.08	D10.5	D37.05	D49.0
tonsil	C09.9	C79.89	D00.08	D10.4	D37.05	D49.0
femur (any part)	C40.2-	-	-	D16.2-	-	-
fetal membrane	C58	C79.82	D07.0	D26.7	D39.2	D49.59
fibrous tissue—see Neoplasm, connective tissue						

	Malignant Primary	Malignant Secondary	Ca in situ	Benign	Uncertain Behavior	Unspecified Behavior
fibula (any part)	C40.2-	C79.51	-	D16.2-	-	-
filum terminale	C72.0	C79.49	-	D33.4	D43.4	D49.7
finger NEC	C76.4-	C79.89	D04.6-	D36.7	D48.7	D49.89
flank NEC	C76.8	C79.89	D04.5	D36.7	D48.7	D49.89
follicle, nabothian	C53.0	C79.82	D06.0	D26.0	D39.0	D49.59
foot NEC	C76.5-	C79.89	D04.7-	D36.7	D48.7	D49.89
forearm NEC	C76.4-	C79.89	D04.6-	D36.7	D48.7	D49.89
forehead (skin)	C44.309	C79.2	D04.39	D23.39	D48.5	D49.2
basal cell carcinoma	C44.319	-	-	-	-	-
specified type NEC	C44.399	-	-	-	-	-
squamous cell carcinoma	C44.329	-	-	-	-	-
foreskin	C60.0	C79.82	D07.4	D29.0	D40.8	D49.59
fornix						
pharyngeal	C11.3	C79.89	D00.08	D10.6	D37.05	D49.0
vagina	C52	C79.82	D07.2	D28.1	D39.8	D49.59
fossa (of)						
anterior (cranial)	C71.9	C79.31	-	D33.2	D43.2	D49.6
cranial	C71.9	C79.31	-	D33.2	D43.2	D49.6
ischiorectal	C76.3	C79.89	D09.8	D36.7	D48.7	D49.89
middle (cranial)	C71.9	C79.31	-	D33.2	D43.2	D49.6
piriform	C12	C79.89	D00.08	D10.7	D37.05	D49.0
pituitary	C75.1	C79.89	D09.3	D35.2	D44.3	D49.7
posterior (cranial)	C71.9	C79.31	-	D33.2	D43.2	D49.6
pterygoid	C49.0	C79.89	-	D21.0	D48.1	D49.2
pyriform	C12	C79.89	D00.08	D10.7	D37.05	D49.0
Rosenmuller	C11.2	C79.89	D00.08	D10.6	D37.05	D49.0
tonsillar	C09.0	C79.89	D00.08	D10.5	D37.05	D49.0
fourchette	C51.9	C79.82	D07.1	D28.0	D39.8	D49.59
frenulum						
labii—see Neoplasm, lip, internal						
linguae	C02.2	C79.89	D00.07	D10.1	D37.02	D49.0
frontal						
bone	C41.0	C79.51	-	D16.4	D48.0	D49.2
lobe, brain	C71.1	C79.31	-	D33.0	D43.0	D49.6
pole	C71.1	C79.31	-	D33.0	D43.0	D49.6
sinus	C31.2	C78.39	D02.3	D14.0	D38.5	D49.1
fundus						
stomach	C16.1	C78.89	D00.2	D13.1	D37.1	D49.0
uterus	C54.3	C79.82	D07.0	D26.1	D39.0	D49.59
G						
gall duct (extrahepatic)	C24.0	C78.89	D01.5	D13.5	D37.6	D49.0
intrahepatic	C22.1	C78.7	D01.5	D13.4	D37.6	D49.0
gallbladder	C23	C78.89	D01.5	D13.5	D37.6	D49.0
overlapping lesion with extrahepatic bile ducts	C24.8	-	-	-	-	-
ganglia—see also Neoplasm, nerve, peripheral	C47.9	C79.89	-	D36.10	D48.2	D49.2
basal	C71.0	C79.31	-	D33.0	D43.0	D49.6
cranial nerve	C72.50	C79.49	-	D33.3	D43.3	D49.7
Gartner's duct	C52	C79.82	D07.2	D28.1	D39.8	D49.59
gastric—see Neoplasm, stomach						
gastrocolic	C26.9	C78.89	D01.9	D13.9	D37.9	D49.0

	Malignant Primary	Malignant Secondary	Ca in situ	Benign	Uncertain Behavior	Unspecified Behavior
gastroesophageal junction	C16.0	C78.89	D00.2	D13.1	D37.1	D49.0
gastrointestinal (tract) NEC	C26.9	C78.89	D01.9	D13.9	D37.9	D49.0
generalized	C80.0	-	-	-	-	-
genital organ or tract						
female NEC	C57.9	C79.82	D07.30	D28.9	D39.9	D49.59
overlapping lesion	C57.8	-	-	-	-	-
specified site NEC	C57.7	C79.82	D07.39	D28.7	D39.8	D49.59
male NEC	C63.9	C79.82	D07.60	D29.9	D40.9	D49.59
overlapping lesion	C63.8	-	-	-	-	-
specified site NEC	C63.7	C79.82	D07.69	D29.8	D40.8	D49.59
genitourinary tract						
female	C57.9	C79.82	D07.30	D28.9	D39.9	D49.59
male	C63.9	C79.82	D07.60	D29.9	D40.9	D49.59
gingiva (alveolar) (marginal)	C03.9	C79.89	D00.03	D10.39	D37.09	D49.0
lower	C03.1	C79.89	D00.03	D10.39	D37.09	D49.0
mandibular	C03.1	C79.89	D00.03	D10.39	D37.09	D49.0
maxillary	C03.0	C79.89	D00.03	D10.39	D37.09	D49.0
upper	C03.0	C79.89	D00.03	D10.39	D37.09	D49.0
gland, glandular (lymphatic) (system)—see also Neoplasm, lymph gland						
endocrine NEC	C75.9	C79.89	D09.3	D35.9	D44.9	D49.7
salivary—see Neoplasm, salivary gland						
glans penis	C60.1	C79.82	D07.4	D29.0	D40.8	D49.59
globus pallidus	C71.0	C79.31	-	D33.0	D43.0	D49.6
glomus						
coccygeal	C49.5	C79.89	-	D21.5	D48.1	D49.2
jugularis	C75.5	C79.89	-	D35.6	D44.7	D49.7
glosso-epiglottic fold(s)	C10.1	C79.89	D00.08	D10.5	D37.05	D49.0
glossopalatine fold	C09.1	C79.89	D00.08	D10.5	D37.05	D49.0
glossopharyngeal sulcus	C09.0	C79.89	D00.08	D10.5	D37.05	D49.0
glottis	C32.0	C78.39	D02.0	D14.1	D38.0	D49.1
gluteal region	C76.3	C79.89	D04.5	D36.7	D48.7	D49.89
great vessels NEC	C49.3	C79.89	-	D21.3	D48.1	D49.2
groin NEC	C76.3	C79.89	D04.5	D36.7	D48.7	D49.89
gum	C03.9	C79.89	D00.03	D10.39	D37.09	D49.0
lower	C03.1	C79.89	D00.03	D10.39	D37.09	D49.0
upper	C03.0	C79.89	D00.03	D10.39	D37.09	D49.0
H						
hand NEC	C76.4-	C79.89	D04.6-	D36.7	D48.7	D49.89
head NEC	C76.0	C79.89	D04.4	D36.7	D48.7	D49.89
heart	C38.0	C79.89	-	D15.1	D48.7	D49.89
heel NEC	C76.5-	C79.89	D04.7-	D36.7	D48.7	D49.89
helix—see also Neoplasm, skin, ear	C44.20-	C79.2	D04.2-	D23.2-	D48.5	D49.2
hematopoietic, hemopoietic tissue NEC	C96.9	-	-	-	-	-
specified NEC	C96.Z	-	-	-	-	-
hemisphere, cerebral	C71.0	C79.31	-	D33.0	D43.0	D49.6
hemorrhoidal zone	C21.1	C78.5	D01.3	D12.9	D37.8	D49.0
hepatic—see also Index to disease, by histology	C22.9	C78.7	D01.5	D13.4	D37.6	D49.0

	Malignant Primary	Malignant Secondary	Ca in situ	Benign	Uncertain Behavior	Unspecified Behavior
hepatic — *continued*						
duct (bile)	C24.0	C78.89	D01.5	D13.5	D37.6	D49.0
flexure (colon)	C18.3	C78.5	D01.0	D12.3	D37.4	D49.0
primary	C22.8	C78.7	D01.5	D13.4	D37.6	D49.0
hepatobiliary	C24.9	C78.89	D01.5	D13.5	D37.6	D49.0
hepatoblastoma	C22.2	C78.7	D01.5	D13.4	D37.6	D49.0
hepatoma	C22.0	C78.7	D01.5	D13.4	D37.6	D49.0
hilus of lung	C34.0-	C78.0-	D02.2-	D14.3-	D38.1	D49.1
hip NEC	C76.5-	C79.89	D04.7-	D36.7	D48.7	D49.89
hippocampus, brain	C71.2	C79.31	-	D33.0	D43.0	D49.6
humerus (any part)	C40.0-	C79.51	-	D16.0-	-	-
hymen	C52	C79.82	D07.2	D28.1	D39.8	D49.59
hypopharynx, hypopharyngeal NEC	C13.9	C79.89	D00.08	D10.7	D37.05	D49.0
overlapping lesion	C13.8	-	-	-	-	-
postcricoid region	C13.0	C79.89	D00.08	D10.7	D37.05	D49.0
posterior wall	C13.2	C79.89	D00.08	D10.7	D37.05	D49.0
pyriform fossa (sinus)	C12	C79.89	D00.08	D10.7	D37.05	D49.0
hypophysis	C75.1	C79.89	D09.3	D35.2	D44.3	D49.7
hypothalamus	C71.0	C79.31	-	D33.0	D43.0	D49.6
I						
ileocecum, ileocecal (coil) (junction) (valve)	C18.0	C78.5	D01.0	D12.0	D37.4	D49.0
ileum	C17.2	C78.4	D01.49	D13.39	D37.2	D49.0
ilium	C41.4	C79.51	-	D16.8	D48.0	D49.2
immunoproliferative NEC	C88.9	-	-	-	-	-
infraclavicular (region)	C76.1	C79.89	D04.5	D36.7	D48.7	D49.89
inguinal (region)	C76.3	C79.89	D04.5	D36.7	D48.7	D49.89
insula	C71.0	C79.31	-	D33.0	D43.0	D49.6
insular tissue (pancreas)	C25.4	C78.89	D01.7	D13.7	D37.8	D49.0
brain	C71.0	C79.31	-	D33.0	D43.0	D49.6
interarytenoid fold	C13.1	C79.89	D00.08	D10.7	D37.05	D49.0
hypopharyngeal aspect	C13.1	C79.89	D00.08	D10.7	D37.05	D49.0
laryngeal aspect	C32.1	C78.39	D02.0	D14.1	D38.0	D49.1
marginal zone	C13.1	C79.89	D00.08	D10.7	D37.05	D49.0
interdental papillae	C03.9	C79.89	D00.03	D10.39	D37.09	D49.0
lower	C03.1	C79.89	D00.03	D10.39	D37.09	D49.0
upper	C03.0	C79.89	D00.03	D10.39	D37.09	D49.0
internal						
capsule	C71.0	C79.31	-	D33.0	D43.0	D49.6
os (cervix)	C53.0	C79.82	D06.0	D26.0	D39.0	D49.59
intervertebral cartilage or disc	C41.2	C79.51	-	D16.6	D48.0	D49.2
intestine, intestinal	C26.0	C78.80	D01.40	D13.9	D37.8	D49.0
large	C18.9	C78.5	D01.0	D12.6	D37.4	D49.0
appendix	C18.1	C78.5	D01.0	D12.1	D37.3	D49.0
caput coli	C18.0	C78.5	D01.0	D12.0	D37.4	D49.0
cecum	C18.0	C78.5	D01.0	D12.0	D37.4	D49.0
colon	C18.9	C78.5	D01.0	D12.6	D37.4	D49.0
and rectum	C19	C78.5	D01.1	D12.7	D37.5	D49.0
ascending	C18.2	C78.5	D01.0	D12.2	D37.4	D49.0
caput	C18.0	C78.5	D01.0	D12.0	D37.4	D49.0

	Malignant Primary	Malignant Secondary	Ca in situ	Benign	Uncertain Behavior	Unspecified Behavior
intestine, intestinal, large, colon — *continued*						
descending	C18.6	C78.5	D01.0	D12.4	D37.4	D49.0
distal	C18.6	C78.5	D01.0	D12.4	D37.4	D49.0
left	C18.6	C78.5	D01.0	D12.4	D37.4	D49.0
overlapping lesion	C18.8	-	-	-	-	-
pelvic	C18.7	C78.5	D01.0	D12.5	D37.4	D49.0
right	C18.2	C78.5	D01.0	D12.2	D37.4	D49.0
sigmoid (flexure)	C18.7	C78.5	D01.0	D12.5	D37.4	D49.0
transverse	C18.4	C78.5	D01.0	D12.3	D37.4	D49.0
hepatic flexure	C18.3	C78.5	D01.0	D12.3	D37.4	D49.0
ileocecum, ileocecal (coil) (valve)	C18.0	C78.5	D01.0	D12.0	D37.4	D49.0
overlapping lesion	C18.8	-	-	-	-	-
sigmoid flexure (lower) (upper)	C18.7	C78.5	D01.0	D12.5	D37.4	D49.0
splenic flexure	C18.5	C78.5	D01.0	D12.3	D37.4	D49.0
small	C17.9	C78.4	D01.40	D13.30	D37.2	D49.0
duodenum	C17.0	C78.4	D01.49	D13.2	D37.2	D49.0
ileum	C17.2	C78.4	D01.49	D13.39	D37.2	D49.0
jejunum	C17.1	C78.4	D01.49	D13.39	D37.2	D49.0
overlapping lesion	C17.8	-	-	-	-	-
tract NEC	C26.0	C78.89	D01.40	D13.9	D37.8	D49.0
intra-abdominal	C76.2	C79.89	D09.8	D36.7	D48.7	D49.89
intracranial NEC	C71.9	C79.31	-	D33.2	D43.2	D49.6
intrahepatic (bile) duct	C22.1	C78.7	D01.5	D13.4	D37.6	D49.0
intraocular	C69.9-	C79.49	D09.2-	D31.9-	D48.7	D49.89
intraorbital	C69.6-	C79.49	D09.2-	D31.6-	D48.7	D49.89
intrasellar	C75.1	C79.89	D09.3	D35.2	D44.3	D49.7
intrathoracic (cavity) (organs)	C76.1	C79.89	D09.8	D15.9	D48.7	D49.89
specified NEC	C76.1	C79.89	D09.8	D15.7	-	-
iris	C69.4-	C79.49	D09.2-	D31.4-	D48.7	D49.89
ischiorectal (fossa)	C76.3	C79.89	D09.8	D36.7	D48.7	D49.89
ischium	C41.4	C79.51	-	D16.8	D48.0	D49.2
island of Reil	C71.0	C79.31	-	D33.0	D43.0	D49.6
islands or islets of Langerhans	C25.4	C78.89	D01.7	D13.7	D37.8	D49.0
isthmus uteri	C54.0	C79.82	D07.0	D26.1	D39.0	D49.59
J						
jaw	C76.0	C79.89	D09.8	D36.7	D48.7	D49.89
bone	C41.1	C79.51	-	D16.5	D48.0	D49.2
lower	C41.1	C79.51	-	D16.5	-	-
upper	C41.0	C79.51	-	D16.4	-	-
carcinoma (any type) (lower) (upper)	C76.0	C79.89	-	-	-	-
skin—see also Neoplasm, skin, face	C44.309	C79.2	D04.39	D23.39	D48.5	D49.2
soft tissues	C03.9	C79.89	D00.03	D10.39	D37.09	D49.0
lower	C03.1	C79.89	D00.03	D10.39	D37.09	D49.0
upper	C03.0	C79.89	D00.03	D10.39	D37.09	D49.0
jejunum	C17.1	C78.4	D01.49	D13.39	D37.2	D49.0
joint NEC—see also Neoplasm, bone	C41.9	C79.51	-	D16.9	D48.0	D49.2

	Malignant Primary	Malignant Secondary	Ca in situ	Benign	Uncertain Behavior	Unspecified Behavior
joint NEC — *continued*						
acromioclavicular	C40.0-	C79.51	-	D16.0-	-	-
bursa or synovial membrane—see Neoplasm, connective tissue						
costovertebral	C41.3	C79.51	-	D16.7	D48.0	D49.2
sternocostal	C41.3	C79.51	-	D16.7	D48.0	D49.2
temporomandibular	C41.1	C79.51	-	D16.5	D48.0	D49.2
junction						
anorectal	C21.8	C78.5	D01.3	D12.9	D37.8	D49.0
cardioesophageal	C16.0	C78.89	D00.2	D13.1	D37.1	D49.0
esophagogastric	C16.0	C78.89	D00.2	D13.1	D37.1	D49.0
gastroesophageal	C16.0	C78.89	D00.2	D13.1	D37.1	D49.0
hard and soft palate	C05.9	C79.89	D00.00	D10.39	D37.09	D49.0
ileocecal	C18.0	C78.5	D01.0	D12.0	D37.4	D49.0
pelvirectal	C19	C78.5	D01.1	D12.7	D37.5	D49.0
pelviureteric	C65.-	C79.0-	D09.19	D30.1-	D41.1-	D49.59
rectosigmoid	C19	C78.5	D01.1	D12.7	D37.5	D49.0
squamocolumnar, of cervix	C53.8	C79.82	D06.7	D26.0	D39.0	D49.59
K						
Kaposi's sarcoma—see Kaposi's, sarcoma						
kidney (parenchymal)	C64.-	C79.0-	D09.19	D30.0-	D41.0-	D49.51-
calyx	C65.-	C79.0-	D09.19	D30.1-	D41.1-	D49.51-
hilus	C65.-	C79.0-	D09.19	D30.1-	D41.1-	D49.51-
pelvis	C65.-	C79.0-	D09.19	D30.1-	D41.1-	D49.51-
knee NEC	C76.5-	C79.89	D04.7-	D36.7	D48.7	D49.89
L						
labia (skin)	C51.9	C79.82	D07.1	D28.0	D39.8	D49.59
majora	C51.0	C79.82	D07.1	D28.0	D39.8	D49.59
minora	C51.1	C79.82	D07.1	D28.0	D39.8	D49.59
labial—see also Neoplasm, lip	C00.9	C79.89	D00.01	D10.0	D37.01	D49.0
sulcus (lower) (upper)	C06.1	C79.89	D00.02	D10.39	D37.09	D49.0
labium (skin)	C51.9	C79.82	D07.1	D28.0	D39.8	D49.59
majus	C51.0	C79.82	D07.1	D28.0	D39.8	D49.59
minus	C51.1	C79.82	D07.1	D28.0	D39.8	D49.59
lacrimal						
canaliculi	C69.5-	C79.49	D09.2-	D31.5-	D48.7	D49.89
duct (nasal)	C69.5-	C79.49	D09.2-	D31.5-	D48.7	D49.89
gland	C69.5-	C79.49	D09.2-	D31.5-	D48.7	D49.89
punctum	C69.5-	C79.49	D09.2-	D31.5-	D48.7	D49.89
sac	C69.5-	C79.49	D09.2-	D31.5-	D48.7	D49.89
Langerhans, islands or islets	C25.4	C78.89	D01.7	D13.7	D37.8	D49.0
laryngopharynx	C13.9	C79.89	D00.08	D10.7	D37.05	D49.0
larynx, laryngeal NEC	C32.9	C78.39	D02.0	D14.1	D38.0	D49.1
aryepiglottic fold	C32.1	C78.39	D02.0	D14.1	D38.0	D49.1
cartilage (arytenoid) (cricoid) (cuneiform) (thyroid)	C32.3	C78.39	D02.0	D14.1	D38.0	D49.1
commissure (anterior) (posterior)	C32.0	C78.39	D02.0	D14.1	D38.0	D49.1

	Malignant Primary	Malignant Secondary	Ca in situ	Benign	Uncertain Behavior	Unspecified Behavior
larynx, laryngeal NEC — *continued*						
extrinsic NEC	C32.1	C78.39	D02.0	D14.1	D38.0	D49.1
meaning hypopharynx	C13.9	C79.89	D00.08	D10.7	D37.05	D49.0
interarytenoid fold	C32.1	C78.39	D02.0	D14.1	D38.0	D49.1
intrinsic	C32.0	C78.39	D02.0	D14.1	D38.0	D49.1
overlapping lesion	C32.8	-	-	-	-	-
ventricular band	C32.1	C78.39	D02.0	D14.1	D38.0	D49.1
leg NEC	C76.5-	C79.89	D04.7-	D36.7	D48.7	D49.89
lens, crystalline	C69.4-	C79.49	D09.2-	D31.4-	D48.7	D49.89
lid (lower) (upper)	C44.10-	C79.2	D04.1-	D23.1-	D48.5	D49.2
basal cell carcinoma	C44.11-	-	-	-	-	-
sebaceous cell	C44.13-	-	-	-	-	-
specified type NEC	C44.19-	-	-	-	-	-
squamous cell carcinoma	C44.12-	-	-	-	-	-
ligament—see also Neoplasm, connective tissue						
broad	C57.1-	C79.82	D07.39	D28.2	D39.8	D49.59
Mackenrodt's	C57.7	C79.82	D07.39	D28.7	D39.8	D49.59
non-uterine—see Neoplasm, connective tissue						
round	C57.2-	C79.82	-	D28.2	D39.8	D49.59
sacro-uterine	C57.3	C79.82	-	D28.2	D39.8	D49.59
uterine	C57.3	C79.82	-	D28.2	D39.8	D49.59
utero-ovarian	C57.7	C79.82	D07.39	D28.2	D39.8	D49.59
uterosacral	C57.3	C79.82	-	D28.2	D39.8	D49.59
limb	C76.8	C79.89	D04.8	D36.7	D48.7	D49.89
lower	C76.5-	C79.89	D04.7-	D36.7	D48.7	D49.89
upper	C76.4-	C79.89	D04.6-	D36.7	D48.7	D49.89
limbus of cornea	C69.1-	C79.49	D09.2-	D31.1-	D48.7	D49.89
lingual NEC—see also Neoplasm, tongue	C02.9	C79.89	D00.07	D10.1	D37.02	D49.0
lingula, lung	C34.1-	C78.0-	D02.2-	D14.3-	D38.1	D49.1
lip	C00.9	C79.89	D00.01	D10.0	D37.01	D49.0
buccal aspect—see Neoplasm, lip, internal						
commissure	C00.6	C79.89	D00.01	D10.0	D37.01	D49.0
external	C00.2	C79.89	D00.01	D10.0	D37.01	D49.0
lower	C00.1	C79.89	D00.01	D10.0	D37.01	D49.0
upper	C00.0	C79.89	D00.01	D10.0	D37.01	D49.0
frenulum—see Neoplasm, lip, internal						
inner aspect—see Neoplasm, lip, internal						
internal	C00.5	C79.89	D00.01	D10.0	D37.01	D49.0
lower	C00.4	C79.89	D00.01	D10.0	D37.01	D49.0
upper	C00.3	C79.89	D00.01	D10.0	D37.01	D49.0
lipstick area	C00.2	C79.89	D00.01	D10.0	D37.01	D49.0
lower	C00.1	C79.89	D00.01	D10.0	D37.01	D49.0
upper	C00.0	C79.89	D00.01	D10.0	D37.01	D49.0
lower	C00.1	C79.89	D00.01	D10.0	D37.01	D49.0
internal	C00.4	C79.89	D00.01	D10.0	D37.01	D49.0

	Malignant Primary	Malignant Secondary	Ca in situ	Benign	Uncertain Behavior	Unspecified Behavior
lip — *continued*						
mucosa—see Neoplasm, lip, intervnal						
oral aspect—see Neoplasm, lip, internal						
overlapping lesion	C00.8	-	-	-	-	-
with oral cavity or pharynx	C14.8	-	-	-	-	-
skin (commissure) (lower) (upper)	C44.00	C79.2	D04.0	D23.0	D48.5	D49.2
basal cell carcinoma	C44.01	-	-	-	-	-
specified type NEC	C44.09	-	-	-	-	-
squamous cell carcinoma	C44.02	-	-	-	-	-
upper	C00.0	C79.89	D00.01	D10.0	D37.01	D49.0
internal	C00.3	C79.89	D00.01	D10.0	D37.01	D49.0
vermilion border	C00.2	C79.89	D00.01	D10.0	D37.01	D49.0
lower	C00.1	C79.89	D00.01	D10.0	D37.01	D49.0
upper	C00.0	C79.89	D00.01	D10.0	D37.01	D49.0
lipomatous—see Lipoma, by site						
liver—see also Index to disease, by histology	C22.9	C78.7	D01.5	D13.4	D37.6	D49.0
primary	C22.8	C78.7	D01.5	D13.4	D37.6	D49.0
lumbosacral plexus	C47.5	C79.89	-	D36.16	D48.2	D49.2
lung	C34.9-	C78.0-	D02.2-	D14.3-	D38.1	D49.1
azygos lobe	C34.1-	C78.0-	D02.2-	D14.3-	D38.1	D49.1
carina	C34.0-	C78.0-	D02.2-	D14.3-	D38.1	D49.1
hilus	C34.0-	C78.0-	D02.2-	D14.3-	D38.1	D49.1
linqula	C34.1-	C78.0-	D02.2-	D14.3-	D38.1	D49.1
lobe NEC	C34.9-	C78.0-	D02.2-	D14.3-	D38.1	D49.1
lower lobe	C34.3-	C78.0-	D02.2-	D14.3-	D38.1	D49.1
main bronchus	C34.0-	C78.0-	D02.2-	D14.3-	D38.1	D49.1
mesothelioma—see Mesothelioma						
middle lobe	C34.2	C78.0-	D02.21	D14.31	D38.1	D49.1
overlapping lesion	C34.8-	-	-	-	-	-
upper lobe	C34.1-	C78.0-	D02.2-	D14.3-	D38.1	D49.1
lymph, lymphatic channel NEC	C49.9	C79.89	-	D21.9	D48.1	D49.2
gland (secondary)	-	C77.9	-	D36.0	D48.7	D49.89
abdominal	-	C77.2	-	D36.0	D48.7	D49.89
aortic	-	C77.2	-	D36.0	D48.7	D49.89
arm	-	C77.3	-	D36.0	D48.7	D49.89
auricular (anterior) (posterior)	-	C77.0	-	D36.0	D48.7	D49.89
axilla, axillary	-	C77.3	-	D36.0	D48.7	D49.89
brachial	-	C77.3	-	D36.0	D48.7	D49.89
bronchial	-	C77.1	-	D36.0	D48.7	D49.89
bronchopulmonary	-	C77.1	-	D36.0	D48.7	D49.89
celiac	-	C77.2	-	D36.0	D48.7	D49.89
cervical	-	C77.0	-	D36.0	D48.7	D49.89
cervicofacial	-	C77.0	-	D36.0	D48.7	D49.89
Cloquet	-	C77.4	-	D36.0	D48.7	D49.89
colic	-	C77.2	-	D36.0	D48.7	D49.89
common duct	-	C77.2	-	D36.0	D48.7	D49.89

	Malignant Primary	Malignant Secondary	Ca in situ	Benign	Uncertain Behavior	Unspecified Behavior
lymph, lymphatic channel NEC, gland — *continued*						
cubital	-	C77.3	-	D36.0	D48.7	D49.89
diaphragmatic	-	C77.1	-	D36.0	D48.7	D49.89
epigastric, inferior	-	C77.1	-	D36.0	D48.7	D49.89
epitrochlear	-	C77.3	-	D36.0	D48.7	D49.89
esophageal	-	C77.1	-	D36.0	D48.7	D49.89
face	-	C77.0	-	D36.0	D48.7	D49.89
femoral	-	C77.4	-	D36.0	D48.7	D49.89
gastric	-	C77.2	-	D36.0	D48.7	D49.89
groin	-	C77.4	-	D36.0	D48.7	D49.89
head	-	C77.0	-	D36.0	D48.7	D49.89
hepatic	-	C77.2	-	D36.0	D48.7	D49.89
hilar (pulmonary)	-	C77.1	-	D36.0	D48.7	D49.89
splenic	-	C77.2	-	D36.0	D48.7	D49.89
hypogastric	-	C77.5	-	D36.0	D48.7	D49.89
ileocolic	-	C77.2	-	D36.0	D48.7	D49.89
iliac	-	C77.5	-	D36.0	D48.7	D49.89
infraclavicular	-	C77.3	-	D36.0	D48.7	D49.89
inguina, inguinal	-	C77.4	-	D36.0	D48.7	D49.89
innominate	-	C77.1	-	D36.0	D48.7	D49.89
intercostal	-	C77.1	-	D36.0	D48.7	D49.89
intestinal	-	C77.2	-	D36.0	D48.7	D49.89
intrabdominal	-	C77.2	-	D36.0	D48.7	D49.89
intrapelvic	-	C77.5	-	D36.0	D48.7	D49.89
intrathoracic	-	C77.1	-	D36.0	D48.7	D49.89
jugular	-	C77.0	-	D36.0	D48.7	D49.89
leg	-	C77.4	-	D36.0	D48.7	D49.89
limb						
lower	-	C77.4	-	D36.0	D48.7	D49.89
upper	-	C77.3	-	D36.0	D48.7	D49.89
lower limb	-	C77.4	-	D36.0	D48.7	D49.89
lumbar	-	C77.2	-	D36.0	D48.7	D49.89
mandibular	-	C77.0	-	D36.0	D48.7	D49.89
mediastinal	-	C77.1	-	D36.0	D48.7	D49.89
mesenteric (inferior) (superior)	-	C77.2	-	D36.0	D48.7	D49.89
midcolic	-	C77.2	-	D36.0	D48.7	D49.89
multiple sites in categories C77.0 - C77.5	-	C77.8	-	D36.0	D48.7	D49.89
neck	-	C77.0	-	D36.0	D48.7	D49.89
obturator	-	C77.5	-	D36.0	D48.7	D49.89
occipital	-	C77.0	-	D36.0	D48.7	D49.89
pancreatic	-	C77.2	-	D36.0	D48.7	D49.89
para-aortic	-	C77.2	-	D36.0	D48.7	D49.89
paracervical	-	C77.5	-	D36.0	D48.7	D49.89
parametrial	-	C77.5	-	D36.0	D48.7	D49.89
parasternal	-	C77.1	-	D36.0	D48.7	D49.89
parotid	-	C77.0	-	D36.0	D48.7	D49.89
pectoral	-	C77.3	-	D36.0	D48.7	D49.89
pelvic	-	C77.5	-	D36.0	D48.7	D49.89
peri-aortic	-	C77.2	-	D36.0	D48.7	D49.89
peripancreatic	-	C77.2	-	D36.0	D48.7	D49.89

	Malignant Primary	Malignant Secondary	Ca in situ	Benign	Uncertain Behavior	Unspecified Behavior
lymph, lymphatic channel NEC, gland — *continued*						
popliteal	-	C77.4	-	D36.0	D48.7	D49.89
porta hepatis	-	C77.2	-	D36.0	D48.7	D49.89
portal	-	C77.2	-	D36.0	D48.7	D49.89
preauricular	-	C77.0	-	D36.0	D48.7	D49.89
prelaryngeal	-	C77.0	-	D36.0	D48.7	D49.89
presymphysial	-	C77.5	-	D36.0	D48.7	D49.89
pretracheal	-	C77.0	-	D36.0	D48.7	D49.89
primary (any site) NEC	C96.9	-	-	-	-	-
pulmonary (hiler)	-	C77.1	-	D36.0	D48.7	D49.89
pyloric	-	C77.2	-	D36.0	D48.7	D49.89
retroperitoneal	-	C77.2	-	D36.0	D48.7	D49.89
retropharyngeal	-	C77.0	-	D36.0	D48.7	D49.89
Rosenmuller's	-	C77.4	-	D36.0	D48.7	D49.89
sacral	-	C77.5	-	D36.0	D48.7	D49.89
scalene	-	C77.0	-	D36.0	D48.7	D49.89
site NEC	-	C77.9	-	D36.0	D48.7	D49.89
splenic (hilar)	-	C77.2	-	D36.0	D48.7	D49.89
subclavicular	-	C77.3	-	D36.0	D48.7	D49.89
subinguinal	-	C77.4	-	D36.0	D48.7	D49.89
sublingual	-	C77.0	-	D36.0	D48.7	D49.89
submandibular	-	C77.0	-	D36.0	D48.7	D49.89
submaxillary	-	C77.0	-	D36.0	D48.7	D49.89
submental	-	C77.0	-	D36.0	D48.7	D49.89
subscapular	-	C77.3	-	D36.0	D48.7	D49.89
supraclavicular	-	C77.0	-	D36.0	D48.7	D49.89
thoracic	-	C77.1	-	D36.0	D48.7	D49.89
tibial	-	C77.4	-	D36.0	D48.7	D49.89
tracheal	-	C77.1	-	D36.0	D48.7	D49.89
tracheobronchial	-	C77.1	-	D36.0	D48.7	D49.89
upper limb	-	C77.3	-	D36.0	D48.7	D49.89
Virchow's	-	C77.0	-	D36.0	D48.7	D49.89
node—see also Neoplasm, lymph gland						
primary NEC	C96.9	-	-	-	-	-
vessel—see also Neoplasm, connective tissue	C49.9	C79.89	-	D21.9	D48.1	D49.2
M						
Mackenrodt's ligament	C57.7	C79.82	D07.39	D28.7	D39.8	D49.59
malar	C41.0	C79.51	-	D16.4	D48.0	D49.2
region—see Neoplasm, cheek						
mammary gland—see Neoplasm, breast						
mandible	C41.1	C79.51	-	D16.5	D48.0	D49.2
alveolar						
mucosa (carcinoma)	C03.1	C79.89	D00.03	D10.39	D37.09	D49.0
ridge or process	C41.1	C79.51	-	D16.5	D48.0	D49.2
marrow (bone) NEC	C96.9	C79.52	-	-	D47.9	D49.89
mastectomy site (skin)—see also Neoplasm, breast, skin	C44.501	C79.2	-	-	-	-
specified as breast tissue	C50.8-	C79.81	-	-	-	-
mastoid (air cells) (antrum) (cavity)	C30.1	C78.39	D02.3	D14.0	D38.5	D49.1
bone or process	C41.0	C79.51	-	D16.4	D48.0	D49.2
maxilla, maxillary (superior)	C41.0	C79.51	-	D16.4	D48.0	D49.2
alveolar						
mucosa	C03.0	C79.89	D00.03	D10.39	D37.09	D49.0
ridge or process (carcinoma)	C41.0	C79.51	-	D16.4	D48.0	D49.2
antrum	C31.0	C78.39	D02.3	D14.0	D38.5	D49.1
carcinoma	C03.0	C79.51	-	-	-	-
inferior—see Neoplasm, mandible						
sinus	C31.0	C78.39	D02.3	D14.0	D38.5	D49.1
meatus external (ear)—see also Neoplasm, skin, ear	C44.20-	C79.2	D04.2-	D23.2-	D48.5	D49.2
Meckel diverticulum, malignant	C17.3	C78.4	D01.49	D13.39	D37.2	D49.0
mediastinum, mediastinal	C38.3	C78.1	-	D15.2	D38.3	D49.89
anterior	C38.1	C78.1	-	D15.2	D38.3	D49.89
posterior	C38.2	C78.1	-	D15.2	D38.3	D49.89
medulla						
adrenal	C74.1-	C79.7-	D09.3	D35.0-	D44.1-	D49.7
oblongata	C71.7	C79.31	-	D33.1	D43.1	D49.6
meibomian gland	C44.10-	C79.2	D04.1-	D23.1-	D48.5	D49.2
basal cell carcinoma	C44.11-	-	-	-	-	-
sebaceous cell	C44.13-	-	-	-	-	-
specified type NEC	C44.19-	-	-	-	-	-
squamous cell carcinoma	C44.12-	-	-	-	-	-
melanoma—see Melanoma						
meninges	C70.9	C79.49	-	D32.9	D42.9	D49.7
brain	C70.0	C79.32	-	D32.0	D42.0	D49.7
cerebral	C70.0	C79.32	-	D32.0	D42.0	D49.7
crainial	C70.0	C79.32	-	D32.0	D42.0	D49.7
intracranial	C70.0	C79.32	-	D32.0	D42.0	D49.7
spinal (cord)	C70.1	C79.49	-	D32.1	D42.1	D49.7
meniscus, knee joint (lateral) (medial)	C40.2-	C79.51	-	D16.2-	D48.0	D49.2
Merkel cell—see Carcinoma, Merkel cell						
mesentery, mesenteric	C48.1	C78.6	-	D20.1	D48.4	D49.0
mesoappendix	C48.1	C78.6	-	D20.1	D48.4	D49.0
mesocolon	C48.1	C78.6	-	D20.1	D48.4	D49.0
mesopharynx—see Neoplasm, oropharynx						
mesosalpinx	C57.1-	C79.82	D07.39	D28.2	D39.8	D49.59
mesothelial tissue—see Mesothelioma						
mesothelioma—see Mesothelioma						
mesovarium	C57.1-	C79.82	D07.39	D28.2	D39.8	D49.59
metacarpus (any bone)	C40.1-	C79.51	-	D16.1-	-	-
metastatic NEC—see also Neoplasm, by site, secondary	-	C79.9	-	-	-	-
metatarsus (any bone)	C40.3-	C79.51	-	D16.3-	-	-
midbrain	C71.7	C79.31	-	D33.1	D43.1	D49.6

	Malignant Primary	Malignant Secondary	Ca in situ	Benign	Uncertain Behavior	Unspecified Behavior
milk duct—see Neoplasm, breast						
mons						
pubis	C51.9	C79.82	D07.1	D28.0	D39.8	D49.59
veneris	C51.9	C79.82	D07.1	D28.0	D39.8	D49.59
motor tract	C72.9	C79.49	-	D33.9	D43.9	D49.7
brain	C71.9	C79.31	-	D33.2	D43.2	D49.6
cauda equina	C72.1	C79.49	-	D33.4	D43.4	D49.7
spinal	C72.0	C79.49	-	D33.4	D43.4	D49.7
mouth	C06.9	C79.89	D00.00	D10.30	D37.09	D49.0
book-leaf	C06.89	C79.89	-	-	-	-
floor	C04.9	C79.89	D00.06	D10.2	D37.09	D49.0
anterior portion	C04.0	C79.89	D00.06	D10.2	D37.09	D49.0
lateral portion	C04.1	C79.89	D00.06	D10.2	D37.09	D49.0
overlapping lesion	C04.8	-	-	-	-	-
overlapping NEC	C06.80	-	-	-	-	-
roof	C05.9	C79.89	D00.00	D10.39	D37.09	D49.0
specified part NEC	C06.89	C79.89	D00.00	D10.39	D37.09	D49.0
vestibule	C06.1	C79.89	D00.00	D10.39	D37.09	D49.0
mucosa						
alveolar (ridge or process)	C03.9	C79.89	D00.03	D10.39	D37.09	D49.0
lower	C03.1	C79.89	D00.03	D10.39	D37.09	D49.0
upper	C03.0	C79.89	D00.03	D10.39	D37.09	D49.0
buccal	C06.0	C79.89	D00.02	D10.39	D37.09	D49.0
cheek	C06.0	C79.89	D00.02	D10.39	D37.09	D49.0
lip—see Neoplasm, lip, internal						
nasal	C30.0	C78.39	D02.3	D14.0	D38.5	D49.1
oral	C06.0	C79.89	D00.02	D10.39	D37.09	D49.0
Mullerian duct						
female	C57.7	C79.82	D07.39	D28.7	D39.8	D49.59
male	C63.7	C79.82	D07.69	D29.8	D40.8	D49.59
muscle—see also Neoplasm, connective tissue						
extraocular	C69.6-	C79.49	D09.2-	D31.6-	D48.7	D49.89
myocardium	C38.0	C79.89	-	D15.1	D48.7	D49.89
myometrium	C54.2	C79.82	D07.0	D26.1	D39.0	D49.59
myopericardium	C38.0	C79.89	-	D15.1	D48.7	D49.89
N						
nabothian gland (follicle)	C53.0	C79.82	D06.0	D26.0	D39.0	D49.59
nail—see also Neoplasm, skin, limb	C44.90	C79.2	D04.9	D23.9	D48.5	D49.2
finger—see also Neoplasm, skin, limb, upper	C44.60-	C79.2	D04.6-	D23.6-	D48.5	D49.2
toe—see also Neoplasm, skin, limb, lower	C44.70-	C79.2	D04.7-	D23.7-	D48.5	D49.2
nares, naris (anterior) (posterior)	C30.0	C78.39	D02.3	D14.0	D38.5	D49.1
nasal—see Neoplasm, nose						
nasolabial groove—see also Neoplasm, skin, face	C44.309	C79.2	D04.39	D23.39	D48.5	D49.2
nasolacrimal duct	C69.5-	C79.49	D09.2-	D31.5-	D48.7	D49.89
nasopharynx, nasopharyngeal	C11.9	C79.89	D00.08	D10.6	D37.05	D49.0
floor	C11.3	C79.89	D00.08	D10.6	D37.05	D49.0
overlapping lesion	C11.8	-	-	-	-	-
roof	C11.0	C79.89	D00.08	D10.6	D37.05	D49.0
wall	C11.9	C79.89	D00.08	D10.6	D37.05	D49.0
anterior	C11.3	C79.89	D00.08	D10.6	D37.05	D49.0
lateral	C11.2	C79.89	D00.08	D10.6	D37.05	D49.0
posterior	C11.1	C79.89	D00.08	D10.6	D37.05	D49.0
superior	C11.0	C79.89	D00.08	D10.6	D37.05	D49.0
nates—see also Neoplasm, skin, trunk	C44.509	C79.2	D04.5	D23.5	D48.5	D49.2
neck NEC	C76.0	C79.89	D09.8	D36.7	D48.7	D49.89
skin	C44.40	-	-	-	-	-
basal cell carcinoma	C44.41	-	-	-	-	-
specified type NEC	C44.49	-	-	-	-	-
squamous cell carcinoma	C44.42	-	-	-	-	-
nerve (ganglion)	C47.9	C79.89	-	D36.10	D48.2	D49.2
abducens	C72.59	C79.49	-	D33.3	D43.3	D49.7
accessory (spinal)	C72.59	C79.49	-	D33.3	D43.3	D49.7
acoustic	C72.4-	C79.49	-	D33.3	D43.3	D49.7
auditory	C72.4-	C79.49	-	D33.3	D43.3	D49.7
autonomic NEC—see also Neoplasm, nerve, peripheral	C47.9	C79.89	-	D36.10	D48.2	D49.2
brachial	C47.1-	C79.89	-	D36.12	D48.2	D49.2
cranial	C72.50	C79.49	-	D33.3	D43.3	D49.7
specified NEC	C72.59	C79.49	-	D33.3	D43.3	D49.7
facial	C72.59	C79.49	-	D33.3	D43.3	D49.7
femoral	C47.2-	C79.89	-	D36.13	D48.2	D49.2
ganglion NEC—see also Neoplasm, nerve, peripheral	C47.9	C79.89	-	D36.10	D48.2	D49.2
glossopharyngeal	C72.59	C79.49	-	D33.3	D43.3	D49.7
hypoglossal	C72.59	C79.49	-	D33.3	D43.3	D49.7
intercostal	C47.3	C79.89	-	D36.14	D48.2	D49.2
lumbar	C47.6	C79.89	-	D36.17	D48.2	D49.2
median	C47.1-	C79.89	-	D36.12	D48.2	D49.2
obturator	C47.2-	C79.89	-	D36.13	D48.2	D49.2
oculomotor	C72.59	C79.49	-	D33.3	D43.3	D49.7
olfactory	C47.2-	C79.49	-	D33.3	D43.3	D49.7
optic	C72.3-	C79.49	-	D33.3	D43.3	D49.7
parasympathetic NEC	C47.9	C79.89	-	D36.10	D48.2	D49.2
peripheral NEC	C47.9	C79.89	-	D36.10	D48.2	D49.2
abdomen	C47.4	C79.89	-	D36.15	D48.2	D49.2
abdominal wall	C47.4	C79.89	-	D36.15	D48.2	D49.2
ankle	C47.2-	C79.89	-	D36.13	D48.2	D49.2
antecubital fossa or space	C47.1-	C79.89	-	D36.12	D48.2	D49.2
arm	C47.1-	C79.89	-	D36.12	D48.2	D49.2
auricle (ear)	C47.0	C79.89	-	D36.11	D48.2	D49.2
axilla	C47.3	C79.89	-	D36.12	D48.2	D49.2
back	C47.6	C79.89	-	D36.17	D48.2	D49.2
buttock	C47.5	C79.89	-	D36.16	D48.2	D49.2

	Malignant Primary	Malignant Secondary	Ca in situ	Benign	Uncertain Behavior	Unspecified Behavior
nerve (ganglion), peripheral NEC — *continued*						
calf	C47.2-	C79.89	-	D36.13	D48.2	D49.2
cervical region	C47.0	C79.89	-	D36.11	D48.2	D49.2
cheek	C47.0	C79.89	-	D36.11	D48.2	D49.2
chest (wall)	C47.3	C79.89	-	D36.14	D48.2	D49.2
chin	C47.0	C79.89	-	D36.11	D48.2	D49.2
ear (external)	C47.0	C79.89	-	D36.11	D48.2	D49.2
elbow	C47.1-	C79.89	-	D36.12	D48.2	D49.2
extrarectal	C47.5	C79.89	-	D36.16	D48.2	D49.2
extremity	C47.9	C79.89	-	D36.10	D48.2	D49.2
lower	C47.2-	C79.89	-	D36.13	D48.2	D49.2
upper	C47.1-	C79.89	-	D36.12	D48.2	D49.2
eyelid	C47.0	C79.89	-	D36.11	D48.2	D49.2
face	C47.0	C79.89	-	D36.11	D48.2	D49.2
finger	C47.1-	C79.89	-	D36.12	D48.2	D49.2
flank	C47.6	C79.89	-	D36.17	D48.2	D49.2
foot	C47.2-	C79.89	-	D36.13	D48.2	D49.2
forearm	C47.1-	C79.89	-	D36.12	D48.2	D49.2
forehead	C47.0	C79.89	-	D36.11	D48.2	D49.2
gluteal region	C47.5	C79.89	-	D36.16	D48.2	D49.2
groin	C47.5	C79.89	-	D36.16	D48.2	D49.2
hand	C47.1-	C79.89	-	D36.12	D48.2	D49.2
head	C47.0	C79.89	-	D36.11	D48.2	D49.2
heel	C47.2-	C79.89	-	D36.13	D48.2	D49.2
hip	C47.2-	C79.89	-	D36.13	D48.2	D49.2
infraclavicular region	C47.3	C79.89	-	D36.14	D48.2	D49.2
inguinal (canal) (region)	C47.5	C79.89	-	D36.16	D48.2	D49.2
intrathoracic	C47.3	C79.89	-	D36.14	D48.2	D49.2
ischiorectal fossa	C47.5	C79.89	-	D36.16	D48.2	D49.2
knee	C47.2-	C79.89	-	D36.13	D48.2	D49.2
leg	C47.2-	C79.89	-	D36.13	D48.2	D49.2
limb NEC	C47.9	C79.89	-	D36.10	D48.2	D49.2
lower	C47.2-	C79.89	-	D36.13	D48.2	D49.2
upper	C47.1-	C79.89	-	D36.12	D48.2	D49.2
nates	C47.5	C79.89	-	D36.16	D48.2	D49.2
neck	C47.0	C79.89	-	D36.11	D48.2	D49.2
orbit	C69.6-	C79.49	-	D31.6-	D48.7	D49.2
pararectal	C47.5	C79.89	-	D36.16	D48.2	D49.2
paraurethral	C47.5	C79.89	-	D36.16	D48.2	D49.2
paravaginal	C47.5	C79.89	-	D36.16	D48.2	D49.2
pelvis (floor)	C47.5	C79.89	-	D36.16	D48.2	D49.2
pelvoabdominal	C47.8	C79.89	-	D36.17	D48.2	D49.2
perineum	C47.5	C79.89	-	D36.16	D48.2	D49.2
perirectal (tissue)	C47.5	C79.89	-	D36.16	D48.2	D49.2
periurethral (tissue)	C47.5	C79.89	-	D36.16	D48.2	D49.2
popliteal fossa or space	C47.2-	C79.89	-	D36.13	D48.2	D49.2
presacral	C47.5	C79.89	-	D36.16	D48.2	D49.2
pterygoid fossa	C47.0	C79.89	-	D36.11	D48.2	D49.2
rectovaginal septum or wall	C47.5	C79.89	-	D36.16	D48.2	D49.2
rectovesical	C47.5	C79.89	-	D36.16	D48.2	D49.2
sacrococcygeal region	C47.5	C79.89	-	D36.16	D48.2	D49.2
nerve (ganglion), peripheral NEC — *continued*						
scalp	C47.0	C79.89	-	D36.11	D48.2	D49.2
scapular region	C47.3	C79.89	-	D36.14	D48.2	D49.2
shoulder	C47.1-	C79.89	-	D36.12	D48.2	D49.2
submental	C47.0	C79.89	-	D36.11	D48.2	D49.2
supraclavicular region	C47.0	C79.89	-	D36.11	D48.2	D49.2
temple	C47.0	C79.89	-	D36.11	D48.2	D49.2
temporal region	C47.0	C79.89	-	D36.11	D48.2	D49.2
thigh	C47.2-	C79.89	-	D36.13	D48.2	D49.2
thoracic (duct) (wall)	C47.3	C79.89	-	D36.14	D48.2	D49.2
thorax	C47.3	C79.89	-	D36.14	D48.2	D49.2
thumb	C47.1-	C79.89	-	D36.12	D48.2	D49.2
toe	C47.2-	C79.89	-	D36.13	D48.2	D49.2
trunk	C47.6	C79.89	-	D36.17	D48.2	D49.2
umbilicus	C47.4	C79.89	-	D36.15	D48.2	D49.2
vesicorectal	C47.5	C79.89	-	D36.16	D48.2	D49.2
wrist	C47.1-	C79.89	-	D36.12	D48.2	D49.2
radial	C47.1-	C79.89	-	D36.12	D48.2	D49.2
sacral	C47.5	C79.89	-	D36.16	D48.2	D49.2
sciatic	C47.2-	C79.89	-	D36.13	D48.2	D49.2
spinal NEC	C47.9	C79.89	-	D36.10	D48.2	D49.2
accessory	C72.59	C79.49	-	D33.3	D43.3	D49.7
sympathetic NEC—see also Neoplasm, nerve, peripheral	C47.9	C79.89	-	D36.10	D48.2	D49.2
trigeminal	C72.59	C79.49	-	D33.3	D43.3	D49.7
trochlear	C72.59	C79.49	-	D33.3	D43.3	D49.7
ulnar	C47.1-	C79.89	-	D36.12	D48.2	D49.2
vagus	C72.59	C79.49	-	D33.3	D43.3	D49.7
nervous system (central)	C72.9	C79.40	-	D33.9	D43.9	D49.7
autonomic—see Neoplasm, nerve, peripheral						
parasympathetic—see Neoplasm, nerve, peripheral						
specified site NEC	-	C79.49	-	D33.7	D43.8	-
sympathetic—see Neoplasm, nerve, peripheral						
nevus—see Nevus						
nipple	C50.0-	C79.81	D05.-	D24.-	-	-
nose, nasal	C76.0	C79.89	D09.8	D36.7	D48.7	D49.89
ala (external) (nasi)—see also Neoplasm, nose, skin	C44.301	C79.2	D04.39	D23.39	D48.5	D49.2
bone	C41.0	C79.51	-	D16.4	D48.0	D49.2
cartilage	C30.0	C78.39	D02.3	D14.0	D38.5	D49.1
cavity	C30.0	C78.39	D02.3	D14.0	D38.5	D49.1
choana	C11.3	C79.89	D00.08	D10.6	D37.05	D49.0
external (skin)—see also Neoplasm, nose, skin	C44.301	C79.2	D04.39	D23.39	D48.5	D49.2
fossa	C30.0	C78.39	D02.3	D14.0	D38.5	D49.1
internal	C30.0	C78.39	D02.3	D14.0	D38.5	D49.1
mucosa	C30.0	C78.39	D02.3	D14.0	D38.5	D49.1
septum	C30.0	C78.39	D02.3	D14.0	D38.5	D49.1

	Malignant Primary	Malignant Secondary	Ca in situ	Benign	Uncertain Behavior	Unspecified Behavior
nose, nasal, septum — *continued*						
posterior margin	C11.3	C79.89	D00.08	D10.6	D37.05	D49.0
sinus—see Neoplasm, sinus						
skin	C44.301	C79.2	D04.39	D23.39	D48.5	D49.2
basal cell carcinoma	C44.311	-	-	-	-	-
specified type NEC	C44.391	-	-	-	-	-
squamous cell carcinoma	C44.321	-	-	-	-	-
turbinate (mucosa)	C30.0	C78.39	D02.3	D14.0	D38.5	D49.1
bone	C41.0	C79.51	-	D16.4	D48.0	D49.2
vestibule	C30.0	C78.39	D02.3	D14.0	D38.5	D49.1
nostril	C30.0	C78.39	D02.3	D14.0	D38.5	D49.1
nucleus pulposus	C41.2	C79.51	-	D16.6	D48.0	D49.2
O						
occipital						
bone	C41.0	C79.51	-	D16.4	D48.0	D49.2
lobe or pole, brain	C71.4	C79.31	-	D33.0	D43.0	D49.6
odontogenic—see Neoplasm, jaw bone						
olfactory nerve or bulb	C72.2-	C79.49	-	D33.3	D43.3	D49.7
olive (brain)	C71.7	C79.31	-	D33.1	D43.1	D49.6
omentum	C48.1	C78.6	-	D20.1	D48.4	D49.0
operculum (brain)	C71.0	C79.31	-	D33.0	D43.0	D49.6
optic nerve, chiasm, or tract	C72.3-	C79.49	-	D33.3	D43.3	D49.7
oral (cavity)	C06.9	C79.89	D00.00	D10.30	D37.09	D49.0
ill-defined	C14.8	C79.89	D00.00	D10.30	D37.09	D49.0
mucosa	C06.0	C79.89	D00.02	D10.39	D37.09	D49.0
orbit	C69.6-	C79.49	D09.2-	D31.6-	D48.7	D49.89
autonomic nerve	C69.6-	C79.49	-	D31.6-	D48.7	D49.2
bone	C41.0	C79.51	-	D16.4	D48.0	D49.2
eye	C69.6-	C79.49	D09.2-	D31.6-	D48.7	D49.89
peripheral nerves	C69.6-	C79.49	-	D31.6-	D48.7	D49.2
soft parts	C69.6-	C79.49	D09.2-	D31.6-	D48.7	D49.89
organ of Zuckerkandl	C75.5	C79.89	-	D35.6	D44.7	D49.7
oropharynx	C10.9	C79.89	D00.08	D10.5	D37.05	D49.0
branchial cleft (vestige)	C10.4	C79.89	D00.08	D10.5	D37.05	D49.0
junctional region	C10.8	C79.89	D00.08	D10.5	D37.05	D49.0
lateral wall	C10.2	C79.89	D00.08	D10.5	D37.05	D49.0
overlapping lesion	C10.8	-	-	-	-	-
pillars or fauces	C09.1	C79.89	D00.08	D10.5	D37.05	D49.0
posterior wall	C10.3	C79.89	D00.08	D10.5	D37.05	D49.0
vallecula	C10.0	C79.89	D00.08	D10.5	D37.05	D49.0
os						
external	C53.1	C79.82	D06.1	D26.0	D39.0	D49.59
internal	C53.0	C79.82	D06.0	D26.0	D39.0	D49.59
ovary	C56.-	C79.6-	D07.39	D27.-	D39.1-	D49.59
oviduct	C57.0-	C79.82	D07.39	D28.2	D39.8	D49.59
P						
palate	C05.9	C79.89	D00.00	D10.39	D37.09	D49.0
hard	C05.0	C79.89	D00.05	D10.39	D37.09	D49.0
junction of hard and soft palate	C05.9	C79.89	D00.00	D10.39	D37.09	D49.0

	Malignant Primary	Malignant Secondary	Ca in situ	Benign	Uncertain Behavior	Unspecified Behavior
palate — *continued*						
overlapping lesions	C05.8	-	-	-	-	-
soft	C05.1	C79.89	D00.04	D10.39	D37.09	D49.0
nasopharyngeal surface	C11.3	C79.89	D00.08	D10.6	D37.05	D49.0
posterior surface	C11.3	C79.89	D00.08	D10.6	D37.05	D49.0
superior surface	C11.3	C79.89	D00.08	D10.6	D37.05	D49.0
palatoglossal arch	C09.1	C79.89	D00.00	D10.5	D37.09	D49.0
palatopharyngeal arch	C09.1	C79.89	D00.00	D10.5	D37.09	D49.0
pallium	C71.0	C79.31	-	D33.0	D43.0	D49.6
palpebra	C44.10-	C79.2	D04.1-	D23.1-	D48.5	D49.2
basal cell carcinoma	C44.11-	-	-	-	-	-
sebaceous cell	C44.13-	-	-	-	-	-
specified type NEC	C44.19-	-	-	-	-	-
squamous cell carcinoma	C44.12-	-	-	-	-	-
pancreas	C25.9	C78.89	D01.7	D13.6	D37.8	D49.0
body	C25.1	C78.89	D01.7	D13.6	D37.8	D49.0
duct (of Santorini) (of Wirsung)	C25.3	C78.89	D01.7	D13.6	D37.8	D49.0
ectopic tissue	C25.7	C78.89	-	D13.6	D37.8	D49.0
head	C25.0	C78.89	D01.7	D13.6	D37.8	D49.0
islet cells	C25.4	C78.89	D01.7	D13.7	D37.8	D49.0
neck	C25.7	C78.89	D01.7	D13.6	D37.8	D49.0
overlapping lesion	C25.8	-	-	-	-	-
tail	C25.2	C78.89	D01.7	D13.6	D37.8	D49.0
para-aortic body	C75.5	C79.89	-	D35.6	D44.7	D49.7
paraganglion NEC	C75.5	C79.89	-	D35.6	D44.7	D49.7
parametrium	C57.3	C79.82	-	D28.2	D39.8	D49.59
paranephric	C48.0	C78.6	-	D20.0	D48.3	D49.0
pararectal	C76.3	C79.89	-	D36.7	D48.7	D49.89
parasagittal (region)	C76.0	C79.89	D09.8	D36.7	D48.7	D49.89
parasellar	C72.9	C79.49	-	D33.9	D43.8	D49.7
parathyroid (gland)	C75.0	C79.89	D09.3	D35.1	D44.2	D49.7
paraurethral	C76.3	C79.89	-	D36.7	D48.7	D49.89
gland	C68.1	C79.19	D09.19	D30.8	D41.8	D49.59
paravaginal	C76.3	C79.89	-	D36.7	D48.7	D49.89
parenchyma, kidney	C64.-	C79.0-	D09.19	D30.0-	D41.0-	D49.51-
parietal						
bone	C41.0	C79.51	-	D16.4	D48.0	D49.2
lobe, brain	C71.3	C79.31	-	D33.0	D43.0	D49.6
paroophoron	C57.1-	C79.82	D07.39	D28.2	D39.8	D49.59
parotid (duct) (gland)	C07	C79.89	D00.00	D11.0	D37.030	D49.0
parovarium	C57.1-	C79.82	D07.39	D28.2	D39.8	D49.59
patella	C40.20	C79.51	-	-	-	-
peduncle, cerebral	C71.7	C79.31	-	D33.1	D43.1	D49.6
pelvirectal junction	C19	C78.5	D01.1	D12.7	D37.5	D49.0
pelvis, pelvic	C76.3	C79.89	D09.8	D36.7	D48.7	D49.89
bone	C41.4	C79.51	-	D16.8	D48.0	D49.2
floor	C76.3	C79.89	D09.8	D36.7	D48.7	D49.89
renal	C65.-	C79.0-	D09.19	D30.1-	D41.1-	D49.51-
viscera	C76.3	C79.89	D09.8	D36.7	D48.7	D49.89
wall	C76.3	C79.89	D09.8	D36.7	D48.7	D49.89
pelvo-abdominal	C76.8	C79.89	D09.8	D36.7	D48.7	D49.89

	Malignant Primary	Malignant Secondary	Ca in situ	Benign	Uncertain Behavior	Unspecified Behavior
penis	C60.9	C79.82	D07.4	D29.0	D40.8	D49.59
body	C60.2	C79.82	D07.4	D29.0	D40.8	D49.59
corpus (cavernosum)	C60.2	C79.82	D07.4	D29.0	D40.8	D49.59
glans	C60.1	C79.82	D07.4	D29.0	D40.8	D49.59
overlapping sites	C60.8	-	-	-	-	-
skin NEC	C60.9	C79.82	D07.4	D29.0	D40.8	D49.59
periadrenal (tissue)	C48.0	C78.6	-	D20.0	D48.3	D49.0
perianal (skin)—see also Neoplasm, anus, skin	C44.500	C79.2	D04.5	D23.5	D48.5	D49.2
pericardium	C38.0	C79.89	-	D15.1	D48.7	D49.89
perinephric	C48.0	C78.6	-	D20.0	D48.3	D49.0
perineum	C76.3	C79.89	D09.8	D36.7	D48.7	D49.89
periodontal tissue NEC	C03.9	C79.89	D00.03	D10.39	D37.09	D49.0
periosteum—see Neoplasm, bone						
peripancreatic	C48.0	C78.6	-	D20.0	D48.3	D49.0
peripheral nerve NEC	C47.9	C79.89	-	D36.10	D48.2	D49.2
perirectal (tissue)	C76.3	C79.89	-	D36.7	D48.7	D49.89
perirenal (tissue)	C48.0	C78.6	-	D20.0	D48.3	D49.0
peritoneum, peritoneal (cavity)	C48.2	C78.6	-	D20.1	D48.4	D49.0
benign mesothelial tissue—see Mesothelioma, benign						
overlapping lesion	C48.8	-	-	-	-	-
with digestive organs	C26.9	-	-	-	-	-
parietal	C48.1	C78.6	-	D20.1	D48.4	D49.0
pelvic	C48.1	C78.6	-	D20.1	D48.4	D49.0
specified part NEC	C48.1	C78.6	-	D20.1	D48.4	D49.0
peritonsillar (tissue)	C76.0	C79.89	D09.8	D36.7	D48.7	D49.89
periurethral tissue	C76.3	C79.89	-	D36.7	D48.7	D49.89
phalanges						
foot	C40.3-	C79.51	-	D16.3-	-	-
hand	C40.1-	C79.51	-	D16.1-	-	-
pharynx, pharyngeal	C14.0	C79.89	D00.08	D10.9	D37.05	D49.0
bursa	C11.1	C79.89	D00.08	D10.6	D37.05	D49.0
fornix	C11.3	C79.89	D00.08	D10.6	D37.05	D49.0
recess	C11.2	C79.89	D00.08	D10.6	D37.05	D49.0
region	C14.0	C79.89	D00.08	D10.9	D37.05	D49.0
tonsil	C11.1	C79.89	D00.08	D10.6	D37.05	D49.0
wall (lateral) (posterior)	C14.0	C79.89	D00.08	D10.9	D37.05	D49.0
pia mater	C70.9	C79.40	-	D32.9	D42.9	D49.7
cerebral	C70.0	C79.32	-	D32.0	D42.0	D49.7
cranial	C70.0	C79.32	-	D32.0	D42.0	D49.7
spinal	C70.1	C79.49	-	D32.1	D42.1	D49.7
pillars of fauces	C09.1	C79.89	D00.08	D10.5	D37.05	D49.0
pineal (body) (gland)	C75.3	C79.89	D09.3	D35.4	D44.5	D49.7
pinna (ear) NEC—see also Neoplasm, skin, ear	C44.20-	C79.2	D04.2-	D23.2-	D48.5	D49.2
piriform fossa or sinus	C12	C79.89	D00.08	D10.7	D37.05	D49.0
pituitary (body) (fossa) (gland) (lobe)	C75.1	C79.89	D09.3	D35.2	D44.3	D49.7
placenta	C58	C79.82	D07.0	D26.7	D39.2	D49.59

	Malignant Primary	Malignant Secondary	Ca in situ	Benign	Uncertain Behavior	Unspecified Behavior
pleura, pleural (cavity)	C38.4	C78.2	-	D19.0	D38.2	D49.1
overlapping lesion with heart or mediastinum	C38.8	-	-	-	-	-
parietal	C38.4	C78.2	-	D19.0	D38.2	D49.1
visceral	C38.4	C78.2	-	D19.0	D38.2	D49.1
plexus						
brachial	C47.1-	C79.89	-	D36.12	D48.2	D49.2
cervical	C47.0	C79.89	-	D36.11	D48.2	D49.2
choroid	C71.5	C79.31	-	D33.0	D43.0	D49.6
lumbosacral	C47.5	C79.89	-	D36.16	D48.2	D49.2
sacral	C47.5	C79.89	-	D36.16	D48.2	D49.2
pluriendocrine	C75.8	C79.89	D09.3	D35.7	D44.9	D49.7
pole						
frontal	C71.1	C79.31	-	D33.0	D43.0	D49.6
occipital	C71.4	C79.31	-	D33.0	D43.0	D49.6
pons (varolii)	C71.7	C79.31	-	D33.1	D43.1	D49.6
popliteal fossa or space	C76.5-	C79.89	D04.7-	D36.7	D48.7	D49.89
postcricoid (region)	C13.0	C79.89	D00.08	D10.7	D37.05	D49.0
posterior fossa (cranial)	C71.9	C79.31	-	D33.2	D43.2	D49.6
postnasal space	C11.9	C79.89	D00.08	D10.6	D37.05	D49.0
prepuce	C60.0	C79.82	D07.4	D29.0	D40.8	D49.59
prepylorus	C16.4	C78.89	D00.2	D13.1	D37.1	D49.0
presacral (region)	C76.3	C79.89	-	D36.7	D48.7	D49.89
prostate (gland)	C61	C79.82	D07.5	D29.1	D40.0	D49.59
utricle	C68.0	C79.19	D09.19	D30.4	D41.3	D49.59
pterygoid fossa	C49.0	C79.89	-	D21.0	D48.1	D49.2
pubic bone	C41.4	C79.51	-	D16.8	D48.0	D49.2
pudenda, pudendum (femaie)	C51.9	C79.82	D07.1	D28.0	D39.8	D49.59
pulmonary—see also Neoplasm, lung	C34.9-	C78.0-	D02.2-	D14.3-	D38.1	D49.1
putamen	C71.0	C79.31	-	D33.0	D43.0	D49.6
pyloric						
antrum	C16.3	C78.89	D00.2	D13.1	D37.1	D49.0
canal	C16.4	C78.89	D00.2	D13.1	D37.1	D49.0
pylorus	C16.4	C78.89	D00.2	D13.1	D37.1	D49.0
pyramid (brain)	C71.7	C79.31	-	D33.1	D43.1	D49.6
pyriform fossa or sinus	C12	C79.89	D00.08	D10.7	D37.05	D49.0
R						
radius (any part)	C40.0-	C79.51	-	D16.0-	-	-
Rathke's pouch	C75.1	C79.89	D09.3	D35.2	D44.3	D49.7
rectosigmoid (junction)	C19	C78.5	D01.1	D12.7	D37.5	D49.0
overlapping lesion with anus or rectum	C21.8	-	-	-	-	-
rectouterine pouch	C48.1	C78.6	-	D20.1	D48.4	D49.0
rectovaginal septum or wall	C76.3	C79.89	D09.8	D36.7	D48.7	D49.89
rectovesical septum	C76.3	C79.89	D09.8	D36.7	D48.7	D49.89
rectum (ampulla)	C20	C78.5	D01.2	D12.8	D37.5	D49.0
and colon	C19	C78.5	D01.1	D12.7	D37.5	D49.0
overlapping lesion with anus or rectosigmoid junction	C21.8	-	-	-	-	-

	Malignant Primary	Malignant Secondary	Ca in situ	Benign	Uncertain Behavior	Unspecified Behavior
renal	C64.-	C79.0-	D09.19	D30.0-	D41.0-	D49.51-
calyx	C65.-	C79.0-	D09.19	D30.1-	D41.1-	D49.51-
hilus	C65.-	C79.0-	D09.19	D30.1-	D41.1-	D49.51-
parenchyma	C64.-	C79.0-	D09.19	D30.0-	D41.0-	D49.51-
pelvis	C65.-	C79.0-	D09.19	D30.1-	D41.1-	D49.51-
respiratory						
organs or system NEC	C39.9	C78.30	D02.4	D14.4	D38.6	D49.1
tract NEC	C39.9	C78.30	D02.4	D14.4	D38.5	D49.1
upper	C39.0	C78.30	D02.4	D14.4	D38.5	D49.1
retina	C69.2-	C79.49	D09.2-	D31.2-	D48.7	D49.81
retrobulbar	C69.6-	C79.49	-	D31.6-	D48.7	D49.89
retrocecal	C48.0	C78.6	-	D20.0	D48.3	D49.0
retromolar (area) (triangle) (trigone)	C06.2	C79.89	D00.00	D10.39	D37.09	D49.0
retro-orbital	C76.0	C79.89	D09.8	D36.7	D48.7	D49.89
retroperitoneal (space) (tissue)	C48.0	C78.6	-	D20.0	D48.3	D49.0
retroperitoneum	C48.0	C78.6	-	D20.0	D48.3	D49.0
retropharyngeal	C14.0	C79.89	D00.08	D10.9	D37.05	D49.0
retrovesical (septum)	C76.3	C79.89	D09.8	D36.7	D48.7	D49.89
rhinencephalon	C71.0	C79.31	-	D33.0	D43.0	D49.6
rib	C41.3	C79.51	-	D16.7	D48.0	D49.2
Rosenmuller's fossa	C11.2	C79.89	D00.08	D10.6	D37.05	D49.0
round ligament	C57.2-	C79.82	-	D28.2	D39.8	D49.59
S						
sacrococcyx, sacrococcygeal	C41.4	C79.51		D16.8	D48.0	D49.2
region	C76.3	C79.89	D09.8	D36.7	D48.7	D49.89
sacrouterine ligament	C57.3	C79.82	-	D28.2	D39.8	D49.59
sacrum, sacral (vertebra)	C41.4	C79.51	-	D16.8	D48.0	D49.2
salivary gland or duct (major)	C08.9	C79.89	D00.00	D11.9	D37.039	D49.0
minor NEC	C06.9	C79.89	D00.00	D10.39	D37.04	D49.0
overlapping lesion	C08.9	-	-	-	-	-
parotid	C07	C79.89	D00.00	D11.0	D37.030	D49.0
pluriglandular	C08.9	C79.89	D00.00	D11.9	D37.039	D49.0
sublingual	C08.1	C79.89	D00.00	D11.7	D37.031	D49.0
submandibular	C08.0	C79.89	D00.00	D11.7	D37.032	D49.0
submaxillary	C08.0	C79.89	D00.00	D11.7	D37.032	D49.0
salpinx (uterine)	C57.0-	C79.82	D07.39	D28.2	D39.8	D49.59
Santorini's duct	C25.3	C78.89	D01.7	D13.6	D37.8	D49.0
scalp	C44.40	C79.2	D04.4	D23.4	D48.5	D49.2
basal cell carcinoma	C44.41	-	-	-	-	-
specified type NEC	C44.49	-	-	-	-	-
squamous cell carcinoma	C44.42	-	-	-	-	-
scapula (any part)	C40.0-	C79.51	-	D16.0-	-	-
scapular region	C76.1	C79.89	D09.8	D36.7	D48.7	D49.89
scar NEC—see *also* Neoplasm, skin, by site	C44.90	C79.2	D04.9	D23.9	D48.5	D49.2
sciatic nerve	C47.2-	C79.89	-	D36.13	D48.2	D49.2
sclera	C69.4-	C79.49	D09.2-	D31.4-	D48.7	D49.89
scrotum (skin)	C63.2	C79.82	D07.61	D29.4	D40.8	D49.59
sebaceous gland—see Neoplasm, skin						
sella turcica	C75.1	C79.89	D09.3	D35.2	D44.3	D49.7
bone	C41.0	C79.51	-	D16.4	D48.0	D49.2
semilunar cartilage (knee)	C40.2-	C79.51	-	D16.2-	D48.0	D49.2
seminal vesicle	C63.7	C79.82	D07.69	D29.8	D40.8	D49.59
septum						
nasal	C30.0	C78.39	D02.3	D14.0	D38.5	D49.1
posterior margin	C11.3	C79.89	D00.08	D10.6	D37.05	D49.0
rectovaginal	C76.3	C79.89	D09.8	D36.7	D48.7	D49.89
rectovesical	C76.3	C79.89	D09.8	D36.7	D48.7	D49.89
urethrovaginal	C57.9	C79.82	D07.30	D28.9	D39.9	D49.59
vesicovaginal	C57.9	C79.82	D07.30	D28.9	D39.9	D49.59
shoulder NEC	C76.4-	C79.89	D04.6-	D36.7	D48.7	D49.89
sigmoid flexure (lower) (upper)	C18.7	C78.5	D01.0	D12.5	D37.4	D49.0
sinus (accessory)	C31.9	C78.39	D02.3	D14.0	D38.5	D49.1
bone (any)	C41.0	C79.51	-	D16.4	D48.0	D49.2
ethmoidal	C31.1	C78.39	D02.3	D14.0	D38.5	D49.1
frontal	C31.2	C78.39	D02.3	D14.0	D38.5	D49.1
maxillary	C31.0	C78.39	D02.3	D14.0	D38.5	D49.1
nasal, paranasal NEC	C31.9	C78.39	D02.3	D14.0	D38.5	D49.1
overlapping lesion	C31.8	-	-	-	-	-
pyriform	C12	C79.89	D00.08	D10.7	D37.05	D49.0
sphenoid	C31.3	C78.39	D02.3	D14.0	D38.5	D49.1
skeleton, skeletal NEC	C41.9	C79.51	-	D16.9	D48.0	D49.2
Skene's gland	C68.1	C79.19	D09.19	D30.8	D41.8	D49.59
skin NOS	C44.90	C79.2	D04.9	D23.9	D48.5	D49.2
abdominal wall	C44.509	C79.2	D04.5	D23.5	D48.5	D49.2
basal cell carcinoma	C44.519	-	-	-	-	-
specified type NEC	C44.599	-	-	-	-	-
squamous cell carcinoma	C44.529	-	-	-	-	-
ala nasi—see also Neoplasm, nose, skin	C44.301	C79.2	D04.39	D23.39	D48.5	D49.2
ankle—see also Neoplasm, skin, limb, lower	C44.70-	C79.2	D04.7-	D23.7-	D48.5	D49.2
antecubital space—see also Neoplasm, skin, limb, upper	C44.60-	C79.2	D04.6-	D23.6-	D48.5	D49.2
anus	C44.500	C79.2	D04.5	D23.5	D48.5	D49.2
basal cell carcinoma	C44.510	-	-	-	-	-
specified type NEC	C44.590	-	-	-	-	-
squamous cell carcinoma	C44.520	-	-	-	-	-
arm—see also Neoplasm, skin, limb, upper	C44.60-	C79.2	D04.6-	D23.6-	D48.5	D49.2
auditory canal (external)—see also Neoplasm, skin, ear	C44.20-	C79.2	D04.2-	D23.2-	D48.5	D49.2
auricle (ear)—see also Neoplasm, skin, ear	C44.20-	C79.2	D04.2-	D23.2-	D48.5	D49.2
auricular canal (external)—see also Neoplasm, skin, ear	C44.20-	C79.2	D04.2-	D23.2-	D48.5	D49.2
axilla, axillary fold—see also Neoplasm, skin, trunk	C44.509	C79.2	D04.5	D23.5	D48.5	D49.2

	Malignant Primary	Malignant Secondary	Ca in situ	Benign	Uncertain Behavior	Unspecified Behavior
skin NOS — *continued*						
back—see also Neoplasm, skin, trunk	C44.509	C79.2	D04.5	D23.5	D48.5	D49.2
basal cell carcinoma	C44.91					
breast	C44.501	C79.2	D04.5	D23.5	D48.5	D49.2
basal cell carcinoma	C44.511	-	-	-	-	-
specified type NEC	C44.591	-	-	-	-	-
squamous cell carcinoma	C44.521	-	-	-	-	-
brow—see also Neoplasm, skin, face	C44.309	C79.2	D04.39	D23.39	D48.5	D49.2
buttock—see also Neoplasm, skin, trunk	C44.509	C79.2	D04.5	D23.5	D48.5	D49.2
calf—see also Neoplasm, skin, limb, lower	C44.70-	C79.2	D04.7-	D23.7-	D48.5	D49.2
canthus (eye) (inner) (outer)	C44.10-	C79.2	D04.1-	D23.1-	D48.5	D49.2
basal cell carcinoma	C44.11-	-	-	-	-	-
sebaceous cell	C44.13-	-	-	-	-	-
specified type NEC	C44.19-	-	-	-	-	-
squamous cell carcinoma	C44.12-	-	-	-	-	-
cervical region—see also Neoplasm, skin, neck	C44.40	C79.2	D04.4	D23.4	D48.5	D49.2
cheek (external) —see also Neoplasm, skin, face	C44.309	C79.2	D04.39	D23.39	D48.5	D49.2
chest (wall)—see also Neoplasm, skin, trunk	C44.509	C79.2	D04.5	D23.5	D48.5	D49.2
chin—see also Neoplasm, skin, face	C44.309	C79.2	D04.39	D23.39	D48.5	D49.2
clavicular area—see also Neoplasm, skin, trunk	C44.509	C79.2	D04.5	D23.5	D48.5	D49.2
clitoris	C51.2	C79.82	D07.1	D28.0	D39.8	D49.59
columnella—see also Neoplasm, skin, face	C44.309	C79.2	D04.39	D23.39	D48.5	D49.2
concha—see also Neoplasm, skin, ear	C44.20-	C79.2	D04.2-	D23.2-	D48.5	D49.2
ear (external)	C44.20-	C79.2	D04.2-	D23.2-	D48.5	D49.2
basal cell carcinoma	C44.21-	-	-	-	-	-
specified type NEC	C44.29-	-	-	-	-	-
squamous cell carcinoma	C44.22-	-	-	-	-	-
elbow—see also Neoplasm, skin, limb, upper	C44.60-	C79.2	D04.6-	D23.6-	D48.5	D49.2
eyebrow—see also Neoplasm, skin, face	C44.309	C79.2	D04.39	D23.39	D48.5	D49.2
eyelid	C44.10-	C79.2	D04.1-	D23.1-	D48.5	D49.2
basal cell carcinoma	C44.11-	-	-	-	-	-
sebaceous cell	C44.13-	-	-	-	-	-
specified type NEC	C44.19-	-	-	-	-	-
squamous cell carcinoma	C44.12-	-	-	-	-	-
face NOS	C44.300	C79.2	D04.30	D23.30	D48.5	D49.2
basal cell carcinoma	C44.310	-	-	-	-	-
specified type NEC	C44.390	-	-	-	-	-

	Malignant Primary	Malignant Secondary	Ca in situ	Benign	Uncertain Behavior	Unspecified Behavior
skin NOS, face NOS — *continued*						
squamous cell carcinoma	C44.320	-	-	-	-	-
female genital organs (external)	C51.9	C79.82	D07.1	D28.0	D39.8	D49.59
clitoris	C51.2	C79.82	D07.1	D28.0	D39.8	D49.59
labium NEC	C51.9	C79.82	D07.1	D28.0	D39.8	D49.59
majus	C51.0	C79.82	D07.1	D28.0	D39.8	D49.59
minus	C51.1	C79.82	D07.1	D28.0	D39.8	D49.59
pudendum	C51.9	C79.82	D07.1	D28.0	D39.8	D49.59
vulva	C51.9	C79.82	D07.1	D28.0	D39.8	D49.59
finger—see also Neoplasm, skin, limb, upper	C44.60-	C79.2	D04.6-	D23.6-	D48.5	D49.2
flank—see also Neoplasm, skin, trunk	C44.509	C79.2	D04.5	D23.5	D48.5	D49.2
foot—see also Neoplasm, skin, limb, lower	C44.70-	C79.2	D04.7-	D23.7-	D48.5	D49.2
forearm—see also Neoplasm, skin, limb, upper	C44.60-	C79.2	D04.6-	D23.6-	D48.5	D49.2
forehead—see also *Neoplasm, skin, face*	C44.309	C79.2	D04.39	D23.39	D48.5	D49.2
glabella—see also Neoplasm, skin, face	C44.309	C79.2	D04.39	D23.39	D48.5	D49.2
gluteal region—see also Neoplasm, skin, trunk	C44.509	C79.2	D04.5	D23.5	D48.5	D49.2
groin—see also Neoplasm, skin, trunk	C44.509	C79.2	D04.5	D23.5	D48.5	D49.2
hand—see also Neoplasm, skin, limb, upper	C44.60-	C79.2	D04.6-	D23.6-	D48.5	D49.2
head NEC—see also Neoplasm, skin, scalp	C44.40	C79.2	D04.4	D23.4	D48.5	D49.2
heel—see also Neoplasm, skin, limb, lower	C44.70-	C79.2	D04.7-	D23.7-	D48.5	D49.2
helix—see also Neoplasm, skin, ear	C44.20-	C79.2	D04.2-	D23.2-	D48.5	D49.2
hip—see also Neoplasm, skin, limb, lower	C44.70-	C79.2	D04.7-	D23.7-	D48.5	D49.2
infraclavicular region—see also Neoplasm, skin, trunk	C44.509	C79.2	D04.5	D23.5	D48.5	D49.2
inguinal region—see also Neoplasm, skin, trunk	C44.509	C79.2	D04.5	D23.5	D48.5	D49.2
jaw—see also Neoplasm, skin, face	C44.309	C79.2	D04.39	D23.39	D48.5	D49.2
Kaposi's sarcoma —see Kaposi's, sarcoma, skin						
knee—see also Neoplasm, skin, limb, lower	C44.70-	C79.2	D04.7-	D23.7-	D48.5	D49.2
labia						
majora	C51.0	C79.82	D07.1	D28.0	D39.8	D49.59
minora	C51.1	C79.82	D07.1	D28.0	D39.8	D49.59
leg—see also Neoplasm, skin, limb, lower	C44.70-	C79.2	D04.7-	D23.7-	D48.5	D49.2
lid (lower) (upper)	C44.10-	C79.2	D04.1-	D23.1-	D48.5	D49.2
basal cell carcinoma	C44.11-	-	-	-	-	-

	Malignant Primary	Malignant Secondary	Ca in situ	Benign	Uncertain Behavior	Unspecified Behavior
skin NOS, lid (lower) (upper) — *continued*						
sebaceous cell	C44.13-	-	-	-	-	-
specified type NEC	C44.19-	-	-	-	-	-
squamous cell carcinoma	C44.12-	-	-	-	-	-
limb NEC	C44.90	C79.2	D04.9	D23.9	D48.5	D49.2
basal cell carcinoma	C44.91					
lower	C44.70-	C79.2	D04.7-	D23.7-	D48.5	D49.2
basal cell carcinoma	C44.71-	-	-	-	-	-
specified type NEC	C44.79-	-	-	-	-	-
squamous cell carcinoma	C44.72-	-	-	-	-	-
upper	C44.60-	C79.2	D04.6-	D23.6-	D48.5	D49.2
basal cell carcinoma	C44.61-	-	-	-	-	-
specified type NEC	C44.69-	-	-	-	-	-
squamous cell carcinoma	C44.62-	-	-	-	-	-
lip (lower) (upper)	C44.00	C79.2	D04.0	D23.0	D48.5	D49.2
basal cell carcinoma	C44.01	-	-	-	-	-
specified type NEC	C44.09	-	-	-	-	-
squamous cell carcinoma	C44.02	-	-	-	-	-
male genital organs	C63.9	C79.82	D07.60	D29.9	D40.8	D49.59
penis	C60.9	C79.82	D07.4	D29.0	D40.8	D49.59
prepuce	C60.0	C79.82	D07.4	D29.0	D40.8	D49.59
scrotum	C63.2	C79.82	D07.61	D29.4	D40.8	D49.59
mastectomy site (skin)—see also Neoplasm, skin, breast	C44.501	C79.2	-	-	-	-
specified as breast tissue	C50.8-	C79.81	-	-	-	-
meatus, acoustic (external)—see also Neoplasm, skin, ear	C44.20-	C79.2	D04.2-	D23.2-	D48.5	D49.2
melanotic—see Melanoma						
Merkel cell—see Carcinoma, Merkel cell						
nates—see also Neoplasm, skin, trunk	C44.509	C79.2	D04.5	D23.5	D48.5	D49.2
neck	C44.40	C79.2	D04.4	D23.4	D48.5	D49.2
basal cell carcinoma	C44.41	-	-	-	-	-
specified type NEC	C44.49	-	-	-	-	-
squamous cell carcinoma	C44.42	-	-	-	-	-
nevus—see Nevus, skin						
nose (external)—see also Neoplasm, nose, skin	C44.301	C79.2	D04.39	D23.39	D48.5	D49.2
overlapping lesion	C44.80	-	-	-	-	-
basal cell carcinoma	C44.81	-	-	-	-	-
specified type NEC	C44.89	-	-	-	-	-
squamous cell carcinoma	C44.82	-	-	-	-	-
palm—see also Neoplasm, skin, limb, upper	C44.60-	C79.2	D04.6-	D23.6-	D48.5	D49.2
palpebra	C44.10-	C79.2	D04.1-	D23.1-	D48.5	D49.2
basal cell carcinoma	C44.11-	-	-	-	-	-
sebaceous cell	C44.13-	-	-	-	-	-

	Malignant Primary	Malignant Secondary	Ca in situ	Benign	Uncertain Behavior	Unspecified Behavior
skin NOS, palpebra — *continued*						
specified type NEC	C44.19-	-	-	-	-	-
squamous cell carcinoma	C44.12-	-	-	-	-	-
penis NEC	C60.9	C79.82	D07.4	D29.0	D40.8	D49.59
perianal—see also Neoplasm, skin, anus	C44.500	C79.2	D04.5	D23.5	D48.5	D49.2
perineum—see also Neoplasm, skin, anus	C44.500	C79.2	D04.5	D23.5	D48.5	D49.2
pinna—see also Neoplasm, skin, ear	C44.20-	C79.2	D04.2-	D23.2-	D48.5	D49.2
plantar—see also Neoplasm, skin, limb, lower	C44.70-	C79.2	D04.7-	D23.7-	D48.5	D49.2
popliteal fossa or space—see also Neoplasm, skin, limb, lower	C44.70-	C79.2	D04.7-	D23.7-	D48.5	D49.2
prepuce	C60.0	C79.82	D07.4	D29.0	D40.8	D49.59
pubes—see also Neoplasm, skin, trunk	C44.509	C79.2	D04.5	D23.5	D48.5	D49.2
sacrococcygeal region—see also Neoplasm, skin, trunk	C44.509	C79.2	D04.5	D23.5	D48.5	D49.2
scalp	C44.40	C79.2	D04.4	D23.4	D48.5	D49.2
basal cell carcinoma	C44.41	-	-	-	-	-
specified type NEC	C44.49	-	-	-	-	-
squamous cell carcinoma	C44.42	-	-	-	-	-
scapular region—see also Neoplasm, skin, trunk	C44.509	C79.2	D04.5	D23.5	D48.5	D49.2
scrotum	C63.2	C79.82	D07.61	D29.4	D40.8	D49.59
shoulder—see also Neoplasm, skin, limb, upper	C44.60-	C79.2	D04.6-	D23.6-	D48.5	D49.2
sole (foot)—see also Neoplasm, skin, limb, lower	C44.70-	C79.2	D04.7-	D23.7-	D48.5	D49.2
specified sites NEC	C44.80	C79.2	D04.8	D23.9	D48.5	D49.2
basal cell carcinoma	C44.81	-	-	-	-	-
specified type NEC	C44.89	-	-	-	-	-
squamous cell carcinoma	C44.82	-	-	-	-	-
specified type NEC	C44.99	-	-	-	-	-
squamous cell carcinoma	C44.92	-	-	-	-	-
submammary fold—see also Neoplasm, skin, trunk	C44.509	C79.2	D04.5	D23.5	D48.5	D49.2
supraclavicular region—see also Neoplasm, skin, neck	C44.40	C79.2	D04.4	D23.4	D48.5	D49.2
temple—see also Neoplasm, skin, face	C44.309	C79.2	D04.39	D23.39	D48.5	D49.2
thigh—see also Neoplasm, skin, limb, lower	C44.70-	C79.2	D04.7-	D23.7-	D48.5	D49.2
thoracic wall—see also Neoplasm, skin, trunk	C44.509	C79.2	D04.5	D23.5	D48.5	D49.2
thumb—see also Neoplasm, skin, limb, upper	C44.60-	C79.2	D04.6-	D23.6-	D48.5	D49.2

	Malignant Primary	Malignant Secondary	Ca in situ	Benign	Uncertain Behavior	Unspecified Behavior
skin NOS — *continued*						
toe—see also Neoplasm, skin, limb, lower	C44.70-	C79.2	D04.7-	D23.7-	D48.5	D49.2
tragus—see also Neoplasm, skin, ear	C44.20-	C79.2	D04.2-	D23.2-	D48.5	D49.2
trunk	C44.509	C79.2	D04.5	D23.5	D48.5	D49.2
basal cell carcinoma	C44.519	-	-	-	-	-
specified type NEC	C44.599	-	-	-	-	-
squamous cell carcinoma	C44.529	-	-	-	-	-
umbilicus—see also Neoplasm, skin, trunk	C44.509	C79.2	D04.5	D23.5	D48.5	D49.2
vulva	C51.9	C79.82	D07.1	D28.0	D39.8	D49.59
overlapping lesion	C51.8	-	-	-	-	-
wrist—see also Neoplasm, skin, limb, upper	C44.60-	C79.2	D04.6-	D23.6-	D48.5	D49.2
skull	C41.0	C79.51	-	D16.4	D48.0	D49.2
soft parts or tissues—see Neoplasm, connective tissue						
specified site NEC	C76.8	C79.89	D09.8	D36.7	D48.7	D49.89
spermatic cord	C63.1-	C79.82	D07.69	D29.8	D40.8	D49.59
sphenoid	C31.3	C78.39	D02.3	D14.0	D38.5	D49.1
bone	C41.0	C79.51	-	D16.4	D48.0	D49.2
sinus	C31.3	C78.39	D02.3	D14.0	D38.5	D49.1
sphincter						
anal	C21.1	C78.5	D01.3	D12.9	D37.8	D49.0
of Oddi	C24.0	C78.89	D01.5	D13.5	D37.6	D49.0
spine, spinal (column)	C41.2	C79.51	-	D16.6	D48.0	D49.2
bulb	C71.7	C79.31	-	D33.1	D43.1	D49.6
coccyx	C41.4	C79.51	-	D16.8	D48.0	D49.2
cord (cervical) (lumbar) (sacral) (thoracic)	C72.0	C79.49	-	D33.4	D43.4	D49.7
dura mater	C70.1	C79.49	-	D32.1	D42.1	D49.7
lumbosacral	C41.2	C79.51	-	D16.6	D48.0	D49.2
marrow NEC	C96.9	C79.52	-	-	D47.9	D49.89
membrane	C70.1	C79.49	-	D32.1	D42.1	D49.7
meninges	C70.1	C79.49	-	D32.1	D42.1	D49.7
nerve (root)	C47.9	C79.89	-	D36.10	D48.2	D49.2
pia mater	C70.1	C79.49	-	D32.1	D42.1	D49.7
root	C47.9	C79.89	-	D36.10	D48.2	D49.2
sacrum	C41.4	C79.51	-	D16.8	D48.0	D49.2
spleen, splenic NEC	C26.1	C78.89	D01.7	D13.9	D37.8	D49.0
flexure (colon)	C18.5	C78.5	D01.0	D12.3	D37.4	D49.0
stem, brain	C71.7	C79.31	-	D33.1	D43.1	D49.6
Stensen's duct	C07	C79.89	D00.00	D11.0	D37.030	D49.0
sternum	C41.3	C79.51	-	D16.7	D48.0	D49.2
stomach	C16.9	C78.89	D00.2	D13.1	D37.1	D49.0
antrum (pyloric)	C16.3	C78.89	D00.2	D13.1	D37.1	D49.0
body	C16.2	C78.89	D00.2	D13.1	D37.1	D49.0
cardia	C16.0	C78.89	D00.2	D13.1	D37.1	D49.0
cardiac orifice	C16.0	C78.89	D00.2	D13.1	D37.1	D49.0
corpus	C16.2	C78.89	D00.2	D13.1	D37.1	D49.0
fundus	C16.1	C78.89	D00.2	D13.1	D37.1	D49.0

	Malignant Primary	Malignant Secondary	Ca in situ	Benign	Uncertain Behavior	Unspecified Behavior
stomach — *continued*						
greater curvature NEC	C16.6	C78.89	D00.2	D13.1	D37.1	D49.0
lesser curvature NEC	C16.5	C78.89	D00.2	D13.1	D37.1	D49.0
overlapping lesion	C16.8	-	-	-	-	-
prepylorus	C16.4	C78.89	D00.2	D13.1	D37.1	D49.0
pylorus	C16.4	C78.89	D00.2	D13.1	D37.1	D49.0
wall NEC	C16.9	C78.89	D00.2	D13.1	D37.1	D49.0
anterior NEC	C16.8	C78.89	D00.2	D13.1	D37.1	D49.0
posterior NEC	C16.8	C78.89	D00.2	D13.1	D37.1	D49.0
stroma, endometrial	C54.1	C79.82	D07.0	D26.1	D39.0	D49.59
stump, cervical	C53.8	C79.82	D06.7	D26.0	D39.0	D49.59
subcutaneous (nodule) (tissue) NEC—see Neoplasm, connective tissue						
subdural	C70.9	C79.32	-	D32.9	D42.9	D49.7
subglottis, subglottic	C32.2	C78.39	D02.0	D14.1	D38.0	D49.1
sublingual	C04.9	C79.89	D00.06	D10.2	D37.09	D49.0
gland or duct	C08.1	C79.89	D00.00	D11.7	D37.031	D49.0
submandibular gland	C08.0	C79.89	D00.00	D11.7	D37.032	D49.0
submaxillary gland or duct	C08.0	C79.89	D00.00	D11.7	D37.032	D49.0
submental	C76.0	C79.89	D09.8	D36.7	D48.7	D49.89
subpleural	C34.9-	C78.0-	D02.2-	D14.3-	D38.1	D49.1
substernal	C38.1	C78.1	-	D15.2	D38.3	D49.89
sudoriferous, sudoriparous gland, site unspecified	C44.90	C79.2	D04.9	D23.9	D48.5	D49.2
specified site—see Neoplasm, skin						
supraclavicular region	C76.0	C79.89	D09.8	D36.7	D48.7	D49.89
supraglottis	C32.1	C78.39	D02.0	D14.1	D38.0	D49.1
suprarenal	C74.9-	C79.7-	D09.3	D35.0-	D44.1-	D49.7
capsule	C74.9-	C79.7-	D09.3	D35.0-	D44.1-	D49.7
cortex	C74.0-	C79.7-	D09.3	D35.0-	D44.1-	D49.7
gland	C74.9-	C79.7-	D09.3	D35.0-	D44.1-	D49.7
medulla	C74.1-	C79.7-	D09.3	D35.0-	D44.1-	D49.7
suprasellar (region)	C71.9	C79.31	-	D33.2	D43.2	D49.6
supratentorial (brain) NEC	C71.0	C79.31	-	D33.0	D43.0	D49.6
sweat gland (apocrine) (eccrine), site unspecified	C44.90	C79.2	D04.9	D23.9	D48.5	D49.2
specified site—see Neoplasm, skin						
sympathetic nerve or nervous system NEC	C47.9	C79.89	-	D36.10	D48.2	D49.2
symphysis pubis	C41.4	C79.51	-	D16.8	D48.0	D49.2
synovial membrane—see Neoplasm, connective tissue						
T						
tapetum, brain	C71.8	C79.31	-	D33.2	D43.2	D49.6
tarsus (any bone)	C40.3-	C79.51	-	D16.3-	-	-
temple (skin)—see also Neoplasm, skin, face	C44.309	C79.2	D04.39	D23.39	D48.5	D49.2
temporal						
bone	C41.0	C79.51	-	D16.4	D48.0	D49.2

	Malignant Primary	Malignant Secondary	Ca in situ	Benign	Uncertain Behavior	Unspecified Behavior
temporal — *continued*						
lobe or pole	C71.2	C79.31	-	D33.0	D43.0	D49.6
region	C76.0	C79.89	D09.8	D36.7	D48.7	D49.89
skin—see also Neoplasm, skin, face	C44.309	C79.2	D04.39	D23.39	D48.5	D49.2
tendon (sheath)—see Neoplasm, connective tissue						
tentorium (cerebelli)	C70.0	C79.32	-	D32.0	D42.0	D49.7
testis, testes	C62.9-	C79.82	D07.69	D29.2-	D40.1-	D49.59
descended	C62.1-	C79.82	D07.69	D29.2-	D40.1-	D49.59
ectopic	C62.0-	C79.82	D07.69	D29.2-	D40.1-	D49.59
retained	C62.0-	C79.82	D07.69	D29.2-	D40.1-	D49.59
scrotal	C62.1-	C79.82	D07.69	D29.2-	D40.1-	D49.59
undescended	C62.0-	C79.82	D07.69	D29.2-	D40.1-	D49.59
unspecified whether descended or undescended	C62.9-	C79.82	D07.69	D29.2-	D40.1-	D49.59
thalamus	C71.0	C79.31	-	D33.0	D43.0	D49.6
thigh NEC	C76.5-	C79.89	D04.7-	D36.7	D48.7	D49.89
thorax, thoracic (cavity) (organs NEC)	C76.1	C79.89	D09.8	D36.7	D48.7	D49.89
duct	C49.3	C79.89	-	D21.3	D48.1	D49.2
wall NEC	C76.1	C79.89	D09.8	D36.7	D48.7	D49.89
throat	C14.0	C79.89	D00.08	D10.9	D37.05	D49.0
thumb NEC	C76.4-	C79.89	D04.6-	D36.7	D48.7	D49.89
thymus (gland)	C37	C79.89	D09.3	D15.0	D38.4	D49.89
thyroglossal duct	C73	C79.89	D09.3	D34	D44.0	D49.7
thyroid (gland)	C73	C79.89	D09.3	D34	D44.0	D49.7
cartilage	C32.3	C78.39	D02.0	D14.1	D38.0	D49.1
tibia (any part)	C40.2-	C79.51	-	D16.2-	-	-
toe NEC	C76.5-	C79.89	D04.7-	D36.7	D48.7	D49.89
tongue	C02.9	C79.89	D00.07	D10.1	D37.02	D49.0
anterior (two-thirds) NEC	C02.3	C79.89	D00.07	D10.1	D37.02	D49.0
dorsal surface	C02.0	C79.89	D00.07	D10.1	D37.02	D49.0
ventral surface	C02.2	C79.89	D00.07	D10.1	D37.02	D49.0
base (dorsal surface)	C01	C79.89	D00.07	D10.1	D37.02	D49.0
border (lateral)	C02.1	C79.89	D00.07	D10.1	D37.02	D49.0
dorsal surface NEC	C02.0	C79.89	D00.07	D10.1	D37.02	D49.0
fixed part NEC	C01	C79.89	D00.07	D10.1	D37.02	D49.0
foreamen cecum	C02.0	C79.89	D00.07	D10.1	D37.02	D49.0
frenulum linguae	C02.2	C79.89	D00.07	D10.1	D37.02	D49.0
junctional zone	C02.8	C79.89	D00.07	D10.1	D37.02	D49.0
margin (lateral)	C02.1	C79.89	D00.07	D10.1	D37.02	D49.0
midline NEC	C02.0	C79.89	D00.07	D10.1	D37.02	D49.0
mobile part NEC	C02.3	C79.89	D00.07	D10.1	D37.02	D49.0
overlapping lesion	C02.8	-	-	-	-	-
posterior (third)	C01	C79.89	D00.07	D10.1	D37.02	D49.0
root	C01	C79.89	D00.07	D10.1	D37.02	D49.0
surface (dorsal)	C02.0	C79.89	D00.07	D10.1	D37.02	D49.0
base	C01	C79.89	D00.07	D10.1	D37.02	D49.0
ventral	C02.2	C79.89	D00.07	D10.1	D37.02	D49.0
tip	C02.1	C79.89	D00.07	D10.1	D37.02	D49.0
tonsil	C02.4	C79.89	D00.07	D10.1	D37.02	D49.0
tonsil	C09.9	C79.89	D00.08	D10.4	D37.05	D49.0
fauces, faucial	C09.9	C79.89	D00.08	D10.4	D37.05	D49.0
lingual	C02.4	C79.89	D00.07	D10.1	D37.02	D49.0
overlapping sites	C09.8	-	-	-	-	-
palatine	C09.9	C79.89	D00.08	D10.4	D37.05	D49.0
pharyngeal	C11.1	C79.89	D00.08	D10.6	D37.05	D49.0
pillar (anterior) (posterior)	C09.1	C79.89	D00.08	D10.5	D37.05	D49.0
tonsillar fossa	C09.0	C79.89	D00.08	D10.5	D37.05	D49.0
tooth socket NEC	C03.9	C79.89	D00.03	D10.39	D37.09	D49.0
trachea (cartilage) (mucosa)	C33	C78.39	D02.1	D14.2	D38.1	D49.1
overlapping lesion with bronchus or lung	C34.8-	-	-	-	-	-
tracheobronchial	C34.8-	C78.39	D02.1	D14.2	D38.1	D49.1
overlapping lesion with lung	C34.8-	-	-	-	-	-
tragus—see also Neoplasm, skin, ear	C44.20-	C79.2	D04.2-	D23.2-	D48.5	D49.2
trunk NEC	C76.8	C79.89	D04.5	D36.7	D48.7	D49.89
tubo-ovarian	C57.8	C79.82	D07.39	D28.7	D39.8	D49.59
tunica vaginalis	C63.7	C79.82	D07.69	D29.8	D40.8	D49.59
turbinate (bone)	C41.0	C79.51	-	D16.4	D48.0	D49.2
nasal	C30.0	C78.39	D02.3	D14.0	D38.5	D49.1
tympanic cavity	C30.1	C78.39	D02.3	D14.0	D38.5	D49.1
U						
ulna (any part)	C40.0-	C79.51	-	D16.0-	-	-
umbilicus, umbilical—see also Neoplasm, skin, trunk	C44.509	C79.2	D04.5	D23.5	D48.5	D49.2
uncus, brain	C71.2	C79.31	-	D33.0	D43.0	D49.6
unknown site or unspecified	C80.1	C79.9	D09.9	D36.9	D48.9	D49.9
urachus	C67.7	C79.11	D09.0	D30.3	D41.4	D49.4
ureter, ureteral	C66.-	C79.19	D09.19	D30.2-	D41.2-	D49.59
orifice (bladder)	C67.6	C79.11	D09.0	D30.3	D41.4	D49.4
ureter-bladder (junction)	C67.6	C79.11	D09.0	D30.3	D41.4	D49.4
urethra, urethral (gland)	C68.0	C79.19	D09.19	D30.4	D41.3	D49.59
orifice, internal	C67.5	C79.11	D09.0	D30.3	D41.4	D49.4
urethrovaginal (septum)	C57.9	C79.82	D07.30	D28.9	D39.8	D49.59
urinary organ or system	C68.9	C79.10	D09.10	D30.9	D41.9	D49.59
bladder—see Neoplasm, bladder						
overlapping lesion	C68.8	-	-	-	-	-
specified sites NEC	C68.8	C79.19	D09.19	D30.8	D41.8	D49.59
utero-ovarian	C57.8	C79.82	D07.39	D28.7	D39.8	D49.59
ligament	C57.1	C79.82	D07.39	D28.2	D39.8	D49.59
uterosacral ligament	C57.3	C79.82	-	D28.2	D39.8	D49.59
uterus, uteri, uterine	C55	C79.82	D07.0	D26.9	D39.0	D49.59
adnexa NEC	C57.4	C79.82	D07.39	D28.7	D39.8	D49.59
body	C54.9	C79.82	D07.0	D26.1	D39.0	D49.59
cervix	C53.9	C79.82	D06.9	D26.0	D39.0	D49.59
cornu	C54.9	C79.82	D07.0	D26.1	D39.0	D49.59
corpus	C54.9	C79.82	D07.0	D26.1	D39.0	D49.59
endocervix (canal) (gland)	C53.0	C79.82	D06.0	D26.0	D39.0	D49.59
endometrium	C54.1	C79.82	D07.0	D26.1	D39.0	D49.59
exocervix	C53.1	C79.82	D06.1	D26.0	D39.0	D49.59

	Malignant Primary	Malignant Secondary	Ca in situ	Benign	Uncertain Behavior	Unspecified Behavior
uterus, uteri, uterine — *continued*						
external os	C53.1	C79.82	D06.1	D26.0	D39.0	D49.59
fundus	C54.3	C79.82	D07.0	D26.1	D39.0	D49.59
internal os	C53.0	C79.82	D06.0	D26.0	D39.0	D49.59
isthmus	C54.0	C79.82	D07.0	D26.1	D39.0	D49.59
ligament	C57.3	C79.82	-	D28.2	D39.8	D49.59
broad	C57.1	C79.82	D07.39	D28.2	D39.8	D49.59
round	C57.2	C79.82	-	D28.2	D39.8	D49.59
lower segment	C54.0	C79.82	D07.0	D26.1	D39.0	D49.59
myometrium	C54.2	C79.82	D07.0	D26.1	D39.0	D49.59
overlapping sites	C54.8	-	-	-	-	-
squamocolumnar junction	C53.8	C79.82	D06.7	D26.0	D39.0	D49.59
tube	C57.0-	C79.82	D07.39	D28.2	D39.8	D49.59
utricle, prostatic	C68.0	C79.19	D09.19	D30.4	D41.3	D49.59
uveal tract	C69.4-	C79.49	D09.2-	D31.4-	D48.7	D49.89
uvula	C05.2	C79.89	D00.04	D10.39	D37.09	D49.0
V						
vagina, vaginal (fornix) (vault) (wall)	C52	C79.82	D07.2	D28.1	D39.8	D49.59
vaginovesical	C57.9	C79.82	D07.30	D28.9	D39.9	D49.59
septum	C57.9	C79.82	D07.30	D28.9	D39.9	D49.59
vallecula (epigiottis)	C10.0	C79.89	D00.08	D10.5	D37.05	D49.0
vas deferens	C63.1-	C79.82	D07.69	D29.8	D40.8	D49.59
vascular—see Neoplasm, connective tissue						
Vater's ampulla	C24.1	C78.89	D01.5	D13.5	D37.6	D49.0
vein, venous—see Neoplasm, connective tissue						
vena cava (abdominal) (inferior)	C49.4	C79.89	-	D21.4	D48.1	D49.2
superior	C49.3	C79.89	-	D21.3	D48.1	D49.2
ventricle (cerebral) (floor) (lateral) (third)	C71.5	C79.31	-	D33.0	D43.0	D49.6
cardiac (left) (right)	C38.0	C79.89	-	D15.1	D48.7	D49.89
fourth	C71.7	C79.31	-	D33.1	D43.1	D49.6
ventricular band of larynx	C32.1	C78.39	D02.0	D14.1	D38.0	D49.1
ventriculus—see Neoplasm, stomach						
vermillion border—see Neoplasm, lip						
vermis, cerebellum	C71.6	C79.31	-	D33.1	D43.1	D49.6
vertebra (column)	C41.2	C79.51	-	D16.6	D48.0	D49.2
coccyx	C41.4	C79.51	-	D16.8	D48.0	D49.2
marrow NEC	C96.9	C79.52	-	-	D47.9	D49.89
sacrum	C41.4	C79.51	-	D16.8	D48.0	D49.2
vesical—see Neoplasm, bladder						
vesicle, seminal	C63.7	C79.82	D07.69	D29.8	D40.8	D49.59
vesicocervical tissue	C57.9	C79.82	D07.30	D28.9	D39.9	D49.59
vesicorectal	C76.3	C79.82	D09.8	D36.7	D48.7	D49.89
vesicovaginal	C57.9	C79.82	D07.30	D28.9	D39.9	D49.59
septum	C57.9	C79.82	D07.30	D28.9	D39.8	D49.59
vessel (blood)—see Neoplasm, connective tissue						
vestibular gland, greater	C51.0	C79.82	D07.1	D28.0	D39.8	D49.59
vestibule						
mouth	C06.1	C79.89	D00.00	D10.39	D37.09	D49.0
nose	C30.0	C78.39	D02.3	D14.0	D38.5	D49.1
Virchow's gland	C77.0	C77.0	-	D36.0	D48.7	D49.89
viscera NEC	C76.8	C79.89	D09.8	D36.7	D48.7	D49.89
vocal cords (true)	C32.0	C78.39	D02.0	D14.1	D38.0	D49.1
false	C32.1	C78.39	D02.0	D14.1	D38.0	D49.1
vomer	C41.0	C79.51	-	D16.4	D48.0	D49.2
vulva	C51.9	C79.82	D07.1	D28.0	D39.8	D49.59
vulvovaginal gland	C51.0	C79.82	D07.1	D28.0	D39.8	D49.59
W						
Waldeyer's ring	C14.2	C79.89	D00.08	D10.9	D37.05	D49.0
Wharton's duct	C08.0	C79.89	D00.00	D11.7	D37.032	D49.0
white matter (central) (cerebral)	C71.0	C79.31	-	D33.0	D43.0	D49.6
windpipe	C33	C78.39	D02.1	D14.2	D38.1	D49.1
Wirsung's duct	C25.3	C78.89	D01.7	D13.6	D37.8	D49.0
wolffian (body) (duct)						
female	C57.7	C79.82	D07.39	D28.7	D39.8	D49.59
male	C63.7	C79.82	D07.69	D29.8	D40.8	D49.59
womb—see Neoplasm, uterus						
wrist NEC	C76.4-	C79.89	D04.6-	D36.7	D48.7	D49.89
X						
xiphoid process	C41.3	C79.51	-	D16.7	D48.0	D49.2
Z						
Zuckerkandl organ	C75.5	C79.89	-	D35.6	D44.7	D49.7

Substance	Poisoning, Accidental (unintentional)	Poisoning, Intentional self-harm	Poisoning, Assault	Poisoning, Undetermined	Adverse effect	Underdosing
1-propanol	T51.3X1	T51.3X2	T51.3X3	T51.3X4	—	—
2-propanol	T51.2X1	T51.2X2	T51.2X3	T51.2X4	—	—
2,4-D (dichlorophenoxyacetic acid)	T60.3X1	T60.3X2	T60.3X3	T60.3X4	—	—
2,4-toluene diisocyanate	T65.0X1	T65.0X2	T65.0X3	T65.0X4	—	—
2,4,5-T (trichlorophenoxyacetic acid)	T60.1X1	T60.1X2	T60.1X3	T60.1X4	—	—
3,4-methylenedioxymethamphetamine	T43.641	T43.642	T43.643	T43.644	—	—
14-hydroxydihydromorphinone	T40.2X1	T40.2X2	T40.2X3	T40.2X4	T40.2X5	T40.2X6
A						
ABOB	T37.5X1	T37.5X2	T37.5X3	T37.5X4	T37.5X5	T37.5X6
Abrine	T62.2X1	T62.2X2	T62.2X3	T62.2X4	—	—
Abrus (seed)	T62.2X1	T62.2X2	T62.2X3	T62.2X4	—	—
Absinthe	T51.0X1	T51.0X2	T51.0X3	T51.0X4	—	—
beverage	T51.0X1	T51.0X2	T51.0X3	T51.0X4	—	—
Acaricide	T60.8X1	T60.8X2	T60.8X3	T60.8X4	—	—
Acebutolol	T44.7X1	T44.7X2	T44.7X3	T44.7X4	T44.7X5	T44.7X6
Acecarbromal	T42.6X1	T42.6X2	T42.6X3	T42.6X4	T42.6X5	T42.6X6
Aceclidine	T44.1X1	T44.1X2	T44.1X3	T44.1X4	T44.1X5	T44.1X6
Acedapsone	T37.0X1	T37.0X2	T37.0X3	T37.0X4	T37.0X5	T37.0X6
Acefylline piperazine	T48.6X1	T48.6X2	T48.6X3	T48.6X4	T48.6X5	T48.6X6
Acemorphan	T40.2X1	T40.2X2	T40.2X3	T40.2X4	T40.2X5	T40.2X6
Acenocoumarin	T45.511	T45.512	T45.513	T45.514	T45.515	T45.516
Acenocoumarol	T45.511	T45.512	T45.513	T45.514	T45.515	T45.516
Acepifylline	T48.6X1	T48.6X2	T48.6X3	T48.6X4	T48.6X5	T48.6X6
Acepromazine	T43.3X1	T43.3X2	T43.3X3	T43.3X4	T43.3X5	T43.3X6
Acesulfamethoxypyridazine	T37.0X1	T37.0X2	T37.0X3	T37.0X4	T37.0X5	T37.0X6
Acetal	T52.8X1	T52.8X2	T52.8X3	T52.8X4	—	—
Acetaldehyde (vapor)	T52.8X1	T52.8X2	T52.8X3	T52.8X4	—	—
liquid	T65.891	T65.892	T65.893	T65.894	—	—
P-Acetamidophenol	T39.1X1	T39.1X2	T39.1X3	T39.1X4	T39.1X5	T39.1X6
Acetaminophen	T39.1X1	T39.1X2	T39.1X3	T39.1X4	T39.1X5	T39.1X6
Acetaminosalol	T39.1X1	T39.1X2	T39.1X3	T39.1X4	T39.1X5	T39.1X6
Acetanilide	T39.1X1	T39.1X2	T39.1X3	T39.1X4	T39.1X5	T39.1X6
Acetarsol	T37.3X1	T37.3X2	T37.3X3	T37.3X4	T37.3X5	T37.3X6
Acetazolamide	T50.2X1	T50.2X2	T50.2X3	T50.2X4	T50.2X5	T50.2X6
Acetiamine	T45.2X1	T45.2X2	T45.2X3	T45.2X4	T45.2X5	T45.2X6
Acetic						
acid	T54.2X1	T54.2X2	T54.2X3	T54.2X4	—	—
with sodium acetate (ointment)	T49.3X1	T49.3X2	T49.3X3	T49.3X4	T49.3X5	T49.3X6
ester (solvent) (vapor)	T52.8X1	T52.8X2	T52.8X3	T52.8X4	—	—
irrigating solution	T50.3X1	T50.3X2	T50.3X3	T50.3X4	T50.3X5	T50.3X6
medicinal (lotion)	T49.2X1	T49.2X2	T49.2X3	T49.2X4	T49.2X5	T49.2X6
anhydride	T65.891	T65.892	T65.893	T65.894	—	—
ether (vapor)	T52.8X1	T52.8X2	T52.8X3	T52.8X4	—	—
Acetohexamide	T38.3X1	T38.3X2	T38.3X3	T38.3X4	T38.3X5	T38.3X6
Acetohydroxamic acid	T50.991	T50.992	T50.993	T50.994	T50.995	T50.996
Acetomenaphthone	T45.7X1	T45.7X2	T45.7X3	T45.7X4	T45.7X5	T45.7X6
Acetomorphine	T40.1X1	T40.1X2	T40.1X3	T40.1X4	—	—
Acetone (oils)	T52.4X1	T52.4X2	T52.4X3	T52.4X4	—	—
chlorinated	T52.4X1	T52.4X2	T52.4X3	T52.4X4	—	—
vapor	T52.4X1	T52.4X2	T52.4X3	T52.4X4	—	—
Acetonitrile	T52.8X1	T52.8X2	T52.8X3	T52.8X4	—	—
Acetophenazine	T43.3X1	T43.3X2	T43.3X3	T43.3X4	T43.3X5	T43.3X6
Acetophenetedin	T39.1X1	T39.1X2	T39.1X3	T39.1X4	T39.1X5	T39.1X6
Acetophenone	T52.4X1	T52.4X2	T52.4X3	T52.4X4	—	—
Acetorphine	T40.2X1	T40.2X2	T40.2X3	T40.2X4	—	—
Acetosulfone (sodium)	T37.1X1	T37.1X2	T37.1X3	T37.1X4	T37.1X5	T37.1X6
Acetrizoate (sodium)	T50.8X1	T50.8X2	T50.8X3	T50.8X4	T50.8X5	T50.8X6
Acetrizoic acid	T50.8X1	T50.8X2	T50.8X3	T50.8X4	T50.8X5	T50.8X6
Acetyl						
bromide	T53.6X1	T53.6X2	T53.6X3	T53.6X4	—	—
chloride	T53.6X1	T53.6X2	T53.6X3	T53.6X4	—	—
Acetylcarbromal	T42.6X1	T42.6X2	T42.6X3	T42.6X4	T42.6X5	T42.6X6
Acetylcholine						
chloride	T44.1X1	T44.1X2	T44.1X3	T44.1X4	T44.1X5	T44.1X6
derivative	T44.1X1	T44.1X2	T44.1X3	T44.1X4	T44.1X5	T44.1X6
Acetylcysteine	T48.4X1	T48.4X2	T48.4X3	T48.4X4	T48.4X5	T48.4X6
Acetyldigitoxin	T46.0X1	T46.0X2	T46.0X3	T46.0X4	T46.0X5	T46.0X6
Acetyldigoxin	T46.0X1	T46.0X2	T46.0X3	T46.0X4	T46.0X5	T46.0X6
Acetyldihydrocodeine	T40.2X1	T40.2X2	T40.2X3	T40.2X4	—	—
Acetyldihydroco-deinone	T40.2X1	T40.2X2	T40.2X3	T40.2X4	—	—
Acetylene (gas)	T59.891	T59.892	T59.893	T59.894	—	—
dichloride	T53.6X1	T53.6X2	T53.6X3	T53.6X4	—	—
incomplete combustion of	T58.11	T58.12	T58.13	T58.14	—	—
industrial	T59.891	T59.892	T59.893	T59.894	—	—
tetrachloride	T53.6X1	T53.6X2	T53.6X3	T53.6X4	—	—
vapor	T53.6X1	T53.6X2	T53.6X3	T53.6X4	—	—
Acetylpheneturide	T42.6X1	T42.6X2	T42.6X3	T42.6X4	T42.6X5	T42.6X6
Acetylphenylhydra-zine	T39.8X1	T39.8X2	T39.8X3	T39.8X4	T39.8X5	T39.8X6
Acetylsalicylic acid (salts)	T39.011	T39.012	T39.013	T39.014	T39.015	T39.016
enteric coated	T39.011	T39.012	T39.013	T39.014	T39.015	T39.016
Acetylsulfamethoxypyridazine	T37.0X1	T37.0X2	T37.0X3	T37.0X4	T37.0X5	T37.0X6
Achromycin	T36.4X1	T36.4X2	T36.4X3	T36.4X4	T36.4X5	T36.4X6
ophthalmic preparation	T49.5X1	T49.5X2	T49.5X3	T49.5X4	T49.5X5	T49.5X6
topical NEC	T49.0X1	T49.0X2	T49.0X3	T49.0X4	T49.0X5	T49.0X6
Aciclovir	T37.5X1	T37.5X2	T37.5X3	T37.5X4	T37.5X5	T37.5X6
Acid (corrosive) NEC	T54.2X1	T54.2X2	T54.2X3	T54.2X4	—	—
Acidifying agent NEC	T50.901	T50.902	T50.903	T50.904	T50.905	T50.906

Substance	Poisoning, Accidental (unintentional)	Poisoning, Intentional self-harm	Poisoning, Assault	Poisoning, Undetermined	Adverse effect	Underdosing
Acipimox	T46.6X1	T46.6X2	T46.6X3	T46.6X4	T46.6X5	T46.6X6
Acitretin	T50.991	T50.992	T50.993	T50.994	T50.995	T50.996
Aclarubicin	T45.1X1	T45.1X2	T45.1X3	T45.1X4	T45.1X5	T45.1X6
Aclatonium napadisilate	T48.1X1	T48.1X2	T48.1X3	T48.1X4	T48.1X5	T48.1X6
Aconite (wild)	T46.991	T46.992	T46.993	T46.994	T46.995	T46.996
Aconitine	T46.991	T46.992	T46.993	T46.994	T46.995	T46.996
Aconitum ferox	T46.991	T46.992	T46.993	T46.994	T46.995	T46.996
Acridine	T65.6X1	T65.6X2	T65.6X3	T65.6X4	—	—
vapor	T59.891	T59.892	T59.893	T59.894	—	—
Acriflavine	T37.91	T37.92	T37.93	T37.94	T37.95	T37.96
Acriflavinium chloride	T49.0X1	T49.0X2	T49.0X3	T49.0X4	T49.0X5	T49.0X6
Acrinol	T49.0X1	T49.0X2	T49.0X3	T49.0X4	T49.0X5	T49.0X6
Acrisorcin	T49.0X1	T49.0X2	T49.0X3	T49.0X4	T49.0X5	T49.0X6
Acrivastine	T45.0X1	T45.0X2	T45.0X3	T45.0X4	T45.0X5	T45.0X6
Acrolein (gas)	T59.891	T59.892	T59.893	T59.894	—	—
liquid	T54.1X1	T54.1X2	T54.1X3	T54.1X4	—	—
Acrylamide	T65.891	T65.892	T65.893	T65.894	—	—
Acrylic resin	T49.3X1	T49.3X2	T49.3X3	T49.3X4	T49.3X5	T49.3X6
Acrylonitrile	T65.891	T65.892	T65.893	T65.894	—	—
Actaea spicata	T62.2X1	T62.2X2	T62.2X3	T62.2X4	—	—
berry	T62.1X1	T62.1X2	T62.1X3	T62.1X4	—	—
Acterol	T37.3X1	T37.3X2	T37.3X3	T37.3X4	T37.3X5	T37.3X6
ACTH	T38.811	T38.812	T38.813	T38.814	T38.815	T38.816
Actinomycin C	T45.1X1	T45.1X2	T45.1X3	T45.1X4	T45.1X5	T45.1X6
Actinomycin D	T45.1X1	T45.1X2	T45.1X3	T45.1X4	T45.1X5	T45.1X6
Activated charcoal—see also Charcoal, medicinal	T47.6X1	T47.6X2	T47.6X3	T47.6X4	T47.6X5	T47.6X6
Acyclovir	T37.5X1	T37.5X2	T37.5X3	T37.5X4	T37.5X5	T37.5X6
Adenine	T45.2X1	T45.2X2	T45.2X3	T45.2X4	T45.2X5	T45.2X6
arabinoside	T37.5X1	T37.5X2	T37.5X3	T37.5X4	T37.5X5	T37.5X6
Adenosine (phosphate)	T46.2X1	T46.2X2	T46.2X3	T46.2X4	T46.2X5	T46.2X6
ADH	T38.891	T38.892	T38.893	T38.894	T38.895	T38.896
Adhesive NEC	T65.891	T65.892	T65.893	T65.894	—	—
Adicillin	T36.0X1	T36.0X2	T36.0X3	T36.0X4	T36.0X5	T36.0X6
Adiphenine	T44.3X1	T44.3X2	T44.3X3	T44.3X4	T44.3X5	T44.3X6
Adipiodone	T50.8X1	T50.8X2	T50.8X3	T50.8X4	T50.8X5	T50.8X6
Adjunct, pharmaceutical	T50.901	T50.902	T50.903	T50.904	T50.905	T50.906
Adrenal (extract, cortex or medulla) (glucocorticoids) (hormones) (mineralocorticoids)	T38.0X1	T38.0X2	T38.0X3	T38.0X4	T38.0X5	T38.0X6
ENT agent	T49.6X1	T49.6X2	T49.6X3	T49.6X4	T49.6X5	T49.6X6
ophthalmic preparation	T49.5X1	T49.5X2	T49.5X3	T49.5X4	T49.5X5	T49.5X6
topical NEC	T49.0X1	T49.0X2	T49.0X3	T49.0X4	T49.0X5	T49.0X6
Adrenaline	T44.5X1	T44.5X2	T44.5X3	T44.5X4	T44.5X5	T44.5X6
Adrenalin—see Adrenaline						
Adrenergic NEC	T44.901	T44.902	T44.903	T44.904	T44.905	T44.906
blocking agent NEC	T44.8X1	T44.8X2	T44.8X3	T44.8X4	T44.8X5	T44.8X6
beta, heart	T44.7X1	T44.7X2	T44.7X3	T44.7X4	T44.7X5	T44.7X6
specified NEC	T44.991	T44.992	T44.993	T44.994	T44.995	T44.996

Substance	Poisoning, Accidental (unintentional)	Poisoning, Intentional self-harm	Poisoning, Assault	Poisoning, Undetermined	Adverse effect	Underdosing
Adrenochrome						
(mono) semicarbazone	T46.991	T46.992	T46.993	T46.994	T46.995	T46.996
derivative	T46.991	T46.992	T46.993	T46.994	T46.995	T46.996
Adrenocorticotrophic hormone	T38.811	T38.812	T38.813	T38.814	T38.815	T38.816
Adrenocorticotro-phin	T38.811	T38.812	T38.813	T38.814	T38.815	T38.816
Adriamycin	T45.1X1	T45.1X2	T45.1X3	T45.1X4	T45.1X5	T45.1X6
Aerosol spray NEC	T65.91	T65.92	T65.93	T65.94	—	—
Aerosporin	T36.8X1	T36.8X2	T36.8X3	T36.8X4	T36.8X5	T36.8X6
ENT agent	T49.6X1	T49.6X2	T49.6X3	T49.6X4	T49.6X5	T49.6X6
ophthalmic preparation	T49.5X1	T49.5X2	T49.5X3	T49.5X4	T49.5X5	T49.5X6
topical NEC	T49.0X1	T49.0X2	T49.0X3	T49.0X4	T49.0X5	T49.0X6
Aethusa cynapium	T62.2X1	T62.2X2	T62.2X3	T62.2X4	—	—
Afghanistan black	T40.711	T40.712	T40.713	T40.714	T40.715	T40.716
Aflatoxin	T64.01	T64.02	T64.03	T64.04	—	—
Afloqualone	T42.8X1	T42.8X2	T42.8X3	T42.8X4	T42.8X5	T42.8X6
African boxwood	T62.2X1	T62.2X2	T62.2X3	T62.2X4	—	—
Agar	T47.4X1	T47.4X2	T47.4X3	T47.4X4	T47.4X5	T47.4X6
Agonist						
predominantly						
alpha-adrenoreceptor	T44.4X1	T44.4X2	T44.4X3	T44.4X4	T44.4X5	T44.4X6
beta-adrenoreceptor	T44.5X1	T44.5X2	T44.5X3	T44.5X4	T44.5X5	T44.5X6
Agricultural agent NEC	T65.91	T65.92	T65.93	T65.94	—	—
Agrypnal	T42.3X1	T42.3X2	T42.3X3	T42.3X4	T42.3X5	T42.3X6
AHLG	T50.Z11	T50.Z12	T50.Z13	T50.Z14	T50.Z15	T50.Z16
Air contaminant (s), source/type NOS	T65.91	T65.92	T65.93	T65.94	—	—
Ajmaline	T46.2X1	T46.2X2	T46.2X3	T46.2X4	T46.2X5	T46.2X6
Akee	T62.1X1	T62.1X2	T62.1X3	T62.1X4	—	—
Akrinol	T49.0X1	T49.0X2	T49.0X3	T49.0X4	T49.0X5	T49.0X6
Akritoin	T37.8X1	T37.8X2	T37.8X3	T37.8X4	T37.8X5	T37.8X6
Alacepril	T46.4X1	T46.4X2	T46.4X3	T46.4X4	T46.4X5	T46.4X6
Alantolactone	T37.4X1	T37.4X2	T37.4X3	T37.4X4	T37.4X5	T37.4X6
Albamycin	T36.8X1	T36.8X2	T36.8X3	T36.8X4	T36.8X5	T36.8X6
Albendazole	T37.4X1	T37.4X2	T37.4X3	T37.4X4	T37.4X5	T37.4X6
Albumin						
bovine	T45.8X1	T45.8X2	T45.8X3	T45.8X4	T45.8X5	T45.8X6
human serum	T45.8X1	T45.8X2	T45.8X3	T45.8X4	T45.8X5	T45.8X6
salt-poor	T45.8X1	T45.8X2	T45.8X3	T45.8X4	T45.8X5	T45.8X6
normal human serum	T45.8X1	T45.8X2	T45.8X3	T45.8X4	T45.8X5	T45.8X6
Albuterol	T48.6X1	T48.6X2	T48.6X3	T48.6X4	T48.6X5	T48.6X6
Albutoin	T42.0X1	T42.0X2	T42.0X3	T42.0X4	T42.0X5	T42.0X6
Alclometasone	T49.0X1	T49.0X2	T49.0X3	T49.0X4	T49.0X5	T49.0X6
Alcohol	T51.91	T51.92	T51.93	T51.94	—	—
absolute	T51.0X1	T51.0X2	T51.0X3	T51.0X4	—	—
beverage	T51.0X1	T51.0X2	T51.0X3	T51.0X4	—	—
allyl	T51.8X1	T51.8X2	T51.8X3	T51.8X4	—	—
amyl	T51.3X1	T51.3X2	T51.3X3	T51.3X4	—	—
antifreeze	T51.1X1	T51.1X2	T51.1X3	T51.1X4	—	—
beverage	T51.0X1	T51.0X2	T51.0X3	T51.0X4	—	—
butyl	T51.3X1	T51.3X2	T51.3X3	T51.3X4	—	—

Substance	Poisoning, Accidental (unintentional)	Poisoning, Intentional self-harm	Poisoning, Assault	Poisoning, Undetermined	Adverse effect	Underdosing
Alcohol — *Continued*						
dehydrated	T51.0X1	T51.0X2	T51.0X3	T51.0X4	—	—
beverage	T51.0X1	T51.0X2	T51.0X3	T51.0X4	—	—
denatured	T51.0X1	T51.0X2	T51.0X3	T51.0X4	—	—
deterrent NEC	T50.6X1	T50.6X2	T50.6X3	T50.6X4	T50.6X5	T50.6X6
diagnostic (gastric function)	T50.8X1	T50.8X2	T50.8X3	T50.8X4	T50.8X5	T50.8X6
ethyl	T51.0X1	T51.0X2	T51.0X3	T51.0X4	—	—
beverage	T51.0X1	T51.0X2	T51.0X3	T51.0X4	—	—
grain	T51.0X1	T51.0X2	T51.0X3	T51.0X4	—	—
beverage	T51.0X1	T51.0X2	T51.0X3	T51.0X4	—	—
industrial	T51.0X1	T51.0X2	T51.0X3	T51.0X4	—	—
isopropyl	T51.2X1	T51.2X2	T51.2X3	T51.2X4	—	—
methyl	T51.1X1	T51.1X2	T51.1X3	T51.1X4	—	—
preparation for consumption	T51.0X1	T51.0X2	T51.0X3	T51.0X4	—	—
propyl	T51.3X1	T51.3X2	T51.3X3	T51.3X4	—	—
secondary	T51.2X1	T51.2X2	T51.2X3	T51.2X4	—	—
radiator	T51.1X1	T51.1X2	T51.1X3	T51.1X4	—	—
rubbing	T51.2X1	T51.2X2	T51.2X3	T51.2X4	—	—
specified type NEC	T51.8X1	T51.8X2	T51.8X3	T51.8X4	—	—
surgical	T51.0X1	T51.0X2	T51.0X3	T51.0X4	—	—
vapor (from any type of Alcohol)	T59.891	T59.892	T59.893	T59.894	—	—
wood	T51.1X1	T51.1X2	T51.1X3	T51.1X4	—	—
Alcuronium (chloride)	T48.1X1	T48.1X2	T48.1X3	T48.1X4	T48.1X5	T48.1X6
Aldactone	T50.0X1	T50.0X2	T50.0X3	T50.0X4	T50.0X5	T50.0X6
Aldesulfone sodium	T37.1X1	T37.1X2	T37.1X3	T37.1X4	T37.1X5	T37.1X6
Aldicarb	T60.0X1	T60.0X2	T60.0X3	T60.0X4	—	—
Aldomet	T46.5X1	T46.5X2	T46.5X3	T46.5X4	T46.5X5	T46.5X6
Aldosterone	T50.0X1	T50.0X2	T50.0X3	T50.0X4	T50.0X5	T50.0X6
Aldrin (dust)	T60.1X1	T60.1X2	T60.1X3	T60.1X4	—	—
Aleve—see Naproxen						
Alexitol sodium	T47.1X1	T47.1X2	T47.1X3	T47.1X4	T47.1X5	T47.1X6
Alfacalcidol	T45.2X1	T45.2X2	T45.2X3	T45.2X4	T45.2X5	T45.2X6
Alfadolone	T41.1X1	T41.1X2	T41.1X3	T41.1X4	T41.1X5	T41.1X6
Alfaxalone	T41.1X1	T41.1X2	T41.1X3	T41.1X4	T41.1X5	T41.1X6
Alfentanil	T40.411	T40.412	T40.413	T40.414	T40.415	T40.416
Alfuzosin (hydrochloride)	T44.8X1	T44.8X2	T44.8X3	T44.8X4	T44.8X5	T44.8X6
Algae (harmful) (toxin)	T65.821	T65.822	T65.823	T65.824	—	—
Algeldrate	T47.1X1	T47.1X2	T47.1X3	T47.1X4	T47.1X5	T47.1X6
Algin	T47.8X1	T47.8X2	T47.8X3	T47.8X4	T47.8X5	T47.8X6
Alglucerase	T45.3X1	T45.3X2	T45.3X3	T45.3X4	T45.3X5	T45.3X6
Alidase	T45.3X1	T45.3X2	T45.3X3	T45.3X4	T45.3X5	T45.3X6
Alimemazine	T43.3X1	T43.3X2	T43.3X3	T43.3X4	T43.3X5	T43.3X6
Aliphatic thiocyanates	T65.0X1	T65.0X2	T65.0X3	T65.0X4	—	—
Alizapride	T45.0X1	T45.0X2	T45.0X3	T45.0X4	T45.0X5	T45.0X6
Alkali (caustic)	T54.3X1	T54.3X2	T54.3X3	T54.3X4	—	—
Alkaline antiseptic solution (aromatic)	T49.6X1	T49.6X2	T49.6X3	T49.6X4	T49.6X5	T49.6X6

Substance	Poisoning, Accidental (unintentional)	Poisoning, Intentional self-harm	Poisoning, Assault	Poisoning, Undetermined	Adverse effect	Underdosing
Alkalinizing agents (medicinal)	T50.901	T50.902	T50.903	T50.904	T50.905	T50.906
Alkalizing agent NEC	T50.901	T50.902	T50.903	T50.904	T50.905	T50.906
Alka-seltzer	T39.011	T39.012	T39.013	T39.014	T39.015	T39.016
Alkavervir	T46.5X1	T46.5X2	T46.5X3	T46.5X4	T46.5X5	T46.5X6
Alkonium (bromide)	T49.0X1	T49.0X2	T49.0X3	T49.0X4	T49.0X5	T49.0X6
Alkylating drug NEC	T45.1X1	T45.1X2	T45.1X3	T45.1X4	T45.1X5	T45.1X6
antimyeloprolifera-tive	T45.1X1	T45.1X2	T45.1X3	T45.1X4	T45.1X5	T45.1X6
lymphatic	T45.1X1	T45.1X2	T45.1X3	T45.1X4	T45.1X5	T45.1X6
Alkylisocyanate	T65.0X1	T65.0X2	T65.0X3	T65.0X4	—	—
Allantoin	T49.4X1	T49.4X2	T49.4X3	T49.4X4	T49.4X5	T49.4X6
Allegron	T43.011	T43.012	T43.013	T43.014	T43.015	T43.016
Allethrin	T49.0X1	T49.0X2	T49.0X3	T49.0X4	T49.0X5	T49.0X6
Allobarbital	T42.3X1	T42.3X2	T42.3X3	T42.3X4	T42.3X5	T42.3X6
Allopurinol	T50.4X1	T50.4X2	T50.4X3	T50.4X4	T50.4X5	T50.4X6
Allyl						
Alcohol	T51.8X1	T51.8X2	T51.8X3	T51.8X4	—	—
disulfide	T46.6X1	T46.6X2	T46.6X3	T46.6X4	T46.6X5	T46.6X6
Allylestrenol	T38.5X1	T38.5X2	T38.5X3	T38.5X4	T38.5X5	T38.5X6
Allylisopropyl-acetylurea	T42.6X1	T42.6X2	T42.6X3	T42.6X4	T42.6X5	T42.6X6
Allylisopropyl-malonylurea	T42.3X1	T42.3X2	T42.3X3	T42.3X4	T42.3X5	T42.3X6
Allylthiourea	T49.3X1	T49.3X2	T49.3X3	T49.3X4	T49.3X5	T49.3X6
Allyltribromide	T42.6X1	T42.6X2	T42.6X3	T42.6X4	T42.6X5	T42.6X6
Allypropymal	T42.3X1	T42.3X2	T42.3X3	T42.3X4	T42.3X5	T42.3X6
Almagate	T47.1X1	T47.1X2	T47.1X3	T47.1X4	T47.1X5	T47.1X6
Almasilate	T47.1X1	T47.1X2	T47.1X3	T47.1X4	T47.1X5	T47.1X6
Almitrine	T50.7X1	T50.7X2	T50.7X3	T50.7X4	T50.7X5	T50.7X6
Aloes	T47.2X1	T47.2X2	T47.2X3	T47.2X4	T47.2X5	T47.2X6
Aloglutamol	T47.1X1	T47.1X2	T47.1X3	T47.1X4	T47.1X5	T47.1X6
Aloin	T47.2X1	T47.2X2	T47.2X3	T47.2X4	T47.2X5	T47.2X6
Aloxidone	T42.2X1	T42.2X2	T42.2X3	T42.2X4	T42.2X5	T42.2X6
Alpha						
acetyldigoxin	T46.0X1	T46.0X2	T46.0X3	T46.0X4	T46.0X5	T46.0X6
adrenergic blocking drug	T44.6X1	T44.6X2	T44.6X3	T44.6X4	T44.6X5	T44.6X6
amylase	T45.3X1	T45.3X2	T45.3X3	T45.3X4	T45.3X5	T45.3X6
tocoferol (acetate)	T45.2X1	T45.2X2	T45.2X3	T45.2X4	T45.2X5	T45.2X6
tocopherol	T45.2X1	T45.2X2	T45.2X3	T45.2X4	T45.2X5	T45.2X6
Alphadolone	T41.1X1	T41.1X2	T41.1X3	T41.1X4	T41.1X5	T41.1X6
Alphaprodine	T40.491	T40.492	T40.493	T40.494	T40.495	T40.496
Alphaxalone	T41.1X1	T41.1X2	T41.1X3	T41.1X4	T41.1X5	T41.1X6
Alprazolam	T42.4X1	T42.4X2	T42.4X3	T42.4X4	T42.4X5	T42.4X6
Alprenolol	T44.7X1	T44.7X2	T44.7X3	T44.7X4	T44.7X5	T44.7X6
Alprostadil	T46.7X1	T46.7X2	T46.7X3	T46.7X4	T46.7X5	T46.7X6
Alsactide	T38.811	T38.812	T38.813	T38.814	T38.815	T38.816
Alseroxylon	T46.5X1	T46.5X2	T46.5X3	T46.5X4	T46.5X5	T46.5X6
Alteplase	T45.611	T45.612	T45.613	T45.614	T45.615	T45.616
Altizide	T50.2X1	T50.2X2	T50.2X3	T50.2X4	T50.2X5	T50.2X6

Substance	Poisoning, Accidental (unintentional)	Poisoning, Intentional self-harm	Poisoning, Assault	Poisoning, Undetermined	Adverse effect	Underdosing
Altretamine	T45.1X1	T45.1X2	T45.1X3	T45.1X4	T45.1X5	T45.1X6
Alum (medicinal)	T49.4X1	T49.4X2	T49.4X3	T49.4X4	T49.4X5	T49.4X6
nonmedicinal (ammonium) (potassium)	T56.891	T56.892	T56.893	T56.894	—	—
Aluminium, aluminum						
acetate	T49.2X1	T49.2X2	T49.2X3	T49.2X4	T49.2X5	T49.2X6
solution	T49.0X1	T49.0X2	T49.0X3	T49.0X4	T49.0X5	T49.0X6
aspirin	T39.011	T39.012	T39.013	T39.014	T39.015	T39.016
bis (acetylsalicylate)	T39.011	T39.012	T39.013	T39.014	T39.015	T39.016
carbonate (gel, basic)	T47.1X1	T47.1X2	T47.1X3	T47.1X4	T47.1X5	T47.1X6
chlorhydroxide-complex	T47.1X1	T47.1X2	T47.1X3	T47.1X4	T47.1X5	T47.1X6
chloride	T49.2X1	T49.2X2	T49.2X3	T49.2X4	T49.2X5	T49.2X6
clofibrate	T46.6X1	T46.6X2	T46.6X3	T46.6X4	T46.6X5	T46.6X6
diacetate	T49.2X1	T49.2X2	T49.2X3	T49.2X4	T49.2X5	T49.2X6
glycinate	T47.1X1	T47.1X2	T47.1X3	T47.1X4	T47.1X5	T47.1X6
hydroxide (gel)	T47.1X1	T47.1X2	T47.1X3	T47.1X4	T47.1X5	T47.1X6
hydroxide-magnesium carb. gel	T47.1X1	T47.1X2	T47.1X3	T47.1X4	T47.1X5	T47.1X6
magnesium silicate	T47.1X1	T47.1X2	T47.1X3	T47.1X4	T47.1X5	T47.1X6
nicotinate	T46.7X1	T46.7X2	T46.7X3	T46.7X4	T46.7X5	T46.7X6
ointment (surgical) (topical)	T49.3X1	T49.3X2	T49.3X3	T49.3X4	T49.3X5	T49.3X6
phosphate	T47.1X1	T47.1X2	T47.1X3	T47.1X4	T47.1X5	T47.1X6
salicylate	T39.091	T39.092	T39.093	T39.094	T39.095	T39.096
silicate	T47.1X1	T47.1X2	T47.1X3	T47.1X4	T47.1X5	T47.1X6
sodium silicate	T47.1X1	T47.1X2	T47.1X3	T47.1X4	T47.1X5	T47.1X6
subacetate	T49.2X1	T49.2X2	T49.2X3	T49.2X4	T49.2X5	T49.2X6
sulfate	T49.0X1	T49.0X2	T49.0X3	T49.0X4	T49.0X5	T49.0X6
tannate	T47.6X1	T47.6X2	T47.6X3	T47.6X4	T47.6X5	T47.6X6
topical NEC	T49.3X1	T49.3X2	T49.3X3	T49.3X4	T49.3X5	T49.3X6
Alurate	T42.3X1	T42.3X2	T42.3X3	T42.3X4	T42.3X5	T42.3X6
Alverine	T44.3X1	T44.3X2	T44.3X3	T44.3X4	T44.3X5	T44.3X6
Alvodine	T40.2X1	T40.2X2	T40.2X3	T40.2X4	T40.2X5	T40.2X6
Amanita phalloides	T62.0X1	T62.0X2	T62.0X3	T62.0X4	—	—
Amanitine	T62.0X1	T62.0X2	T62.0X3	T62.0X4	—	—
Amantadine	T42.8X1	T42.8X2	T42.8X3	T42.8X4	T42.8X5	T42.8X6
Ambazone	T49.6X1	T49.6X2	T49.6X3	T49.6X4	T49.6X5	T49.6X6
Ambenonium (chloride)	T44.0X1	T44.0X2	T44.0X3	T44.0X4	T44.0X5	T44.0X6
Ambroxol	T48.4X1	T48.4X2	T48.4X3	T48.4X4	T48.4X5	T48.4X6
Ambuphylline	T48.6X1	T48.6X2	T48.6X3	T48.6X4	T48.6X5	T48.6X6
Ambutonium bromide	T44.3X1	T44.3X2	T44.3X3	T44.3X4	T44.3X5	T44.3X6
Amcinonide	T49.0X1	T49.0X2	T49.0X3	T49.0X4	T49.0X5	T49.0X6
Amdinocilline	T36.0X1	T36.0X2	T36.0X3	T36.0X4	T36.0X5	T36.0X6
Ametazole	T50.8X1	T50.8X2	T50.8X3	T50.8X4	T50.8X5	T50.8X6
Amethocaine	T41.3X1	T41.3X2	T41.3X3	T41.3X4	T41.3X5	T41.3X6
regional	T41.3X1	T41.3X2	T41.3X3	T41.3X4	T41.3X5	T41.3X6
spinal	T41.3X1	T41.3X2	T41.3X3	T41.3X4	T41.3X5	T41.3X6
Amethopterin	T45.1X1	T45.1X2	T45.1X3	T45.1X4	T45.1X5	T45.1X6
Amezinium metilsulfate	T44.991	T44.992	T44.993	T44.994	T44.995	T44.996

Substance	Poisoning, Accidental (unintentional)	Poisoning, Intentional self-harm	Poisoning, Assault	Poisoning, Undetermined	Adverse effect	Underdosing
Amfebutamone	T43.291	T43.292	T43.293	T43.294	T43.295	T43.296
Amfepramone	T50.5X1	T50.5X2	T50.5X3	T50.5X4	T50.5X5	T50.5X6
Amfetamine	T43.621	T43.622	T43.623	T43.624	T43.625	T43.626
Amfetaminil	T43.621	T43.622	T43.623	T43.624	T43.625	T43.626
Amfomycin	T36.8X1	T36.8X2	T36.8X3	T36.8X4	T36.8X5	T36.8X6
Amidefrine mesilate	T48.5X1	T48.5X2	T48.5X3	T48.5X4	T48.5X5	T48.5X6
Amidone	T40.3X1	T40.3X2	T40.3X3	T40.3X4	T40.3X5	T40.3X6
Amidopyrine	T39.2X1	T39.2X2	T39.2X3	T39.2X4	T39.2X5	T39.2X6
Amidotrizoate	T50.8X1	T50.8X2	T50.8X3	T50.8X4	T50.8X5	T50.8X6
Amiflamine	T43.1X1	T43.1X2	T43.1X3	T43.1X4	T43.1X5	T43.1X6
Amikacin	T36.5X1	T36.5X2	T36.5X3	T36.5X4	T36.5X5	T36.5X6
Amikhelline	T46.3X1	T46.3X2	T46.3X3	T46.3X4	T46.3X5	T46.3X6
Amiloride	T50.2X1	T50.2X2	T50.2X3	T50.2X4	T50.2X5	T50.2X6
Aminacrine	T49.0X1	T49.0X2	T49.0X3	T49.0X4	T49.0X5	T49.0X6
Amineptine	T43.011	T43.012	T43.013	T43.014	T43.015	T43.016
Aminitrozole	T37.3X1	T37.3X2	T37.3X3	T37.3X4	T37.3X5	T37.3X6
Amino acids	T50.3X1	T50.3X2	T50.3X3	T50.3X4	T50.3X5	T50.3X6
Aminoacetic acid (derivatives)	T50.3X1	T50.3X2	T50.3X3	T50.3X4	T50.3X5	T50.3X6
Aminoacridine	T49.0X1	T49.0X2	T49.0X3	T49.0X4	T49.0X5	T49.0X6
Aminobenzoic acid(-p)	T49.3X1	T49.3X2	T49.3X3	T49.3X4	T49.3X5	T49.3X6
4-Aminobutyric acid	T43.8X1	T43.8X2	T43.8X3	T43.8X4	T43.8X5	T43.8X6
Aminocaproic acid	T45.621	T45.622	T45.623	T45.624	T45.625	T45.626
Aminoethyl-isothiourium	T45.8X1	T45.8X2	T45.8X3	T45.8X4	T45.8X5	T45.8X6
Aminofenazone	T39.2X1	T39.2X2	T39.2X3	T39.2X4	T39.2X5	T39.2X6
Aminoglutethimide	T45.1X1	T45.1X2	T45.1X3	T45.1X4	T45.1X5	T45.1X6
Aminohippuric acid	T50.8X1	T50.8X2	T50.8X3	T50.8X4	T50.8X5	T50.8X6
Aminomethylbenzoic acid	T45.691	T45.692	T45.693	T45.694	T45.695	T45.696
Aminometradine	T50.2X1	T50.2X2	T50.2X3	T50.2X4	T50.2X5	T50.2X6
Aminopentamide	T44.3X1	T44.3X2	T44.3X3	T44.3X4	T44.3X5	T44.3X6
Aminophenazone	T39.2X1	T39.2X2	T39.2X3	T39.2X4	T39.2X5	T39.2X6
Aminophenol	T54.0X1	T54.0X2	T54.0X3	T54.0X4	—	—
4-Aminophenol derivatives	T39.1X1	T39.1X2	T39.1X3	T39.1X4	T39.1X5	T39.1X6
Aminophenylpyri-done	T43.591	T43.592	T43.593	T43.594	T43.595	T43.596
Aminophylline	T48.6X1	T48.6X2	T48.6X3	T48.6X4	T48.6X5	T48.6X6
Aminopterin sodium	T45.1X1	T45.1X2	T45.1X3	T45.1X4	T45.1X5	T45.1X6
Aminopyrine	T39.2X1	T39.2X2	T39.2X3	T39.2X4	T39.2X5	T39.2X6
8-Aminoquinoline drugs	T37.2X1	T37.2X2	T37.2X3	T37.2X4	T37.2X5	T37.2X6
Aminorex	T50.5X1	T50.5X2	T50.5X3	T50.5X4	T50.5X5	T50.5X6
Aminosalicylic acid	T37.1X1	T37.1X2	T37.1X3	T37.1X4	T37.1X5	T37.1X6
Aminosalylum	T37.1X1	T37.1X2	T37.1X3	T37.1X4	T37.1X5	T37.1X6
Amiodarone	T46.2X1	T46.2X2	T46.2X3	T46.2X4	T46.2X5	T46.2X6
Amiphenazole	T50.7X1	T50.7X2	T50.7X3	T50.7X4	T50.7X5	T50.7X6
Amiquinsin	T46.5X1	T46.5X2	T46.5X3	T46.5X4	T46.5X5	T46.5X6
Amisometradine	T50.2X1	T50.2X2	T50.2X3	T50.2X4	T50.2X5	T50.2X6
Amisulpride	T43.591	T43.592	T43.593	T43.594	T43.595	T43.596
Amitriptyline	T43.011	T43.012	T43.013	T43.014	T43.015	T43.016
Amitriptylinoxide	T43.011	T43.012	T43.013	T43.014	T43.015	T43.016

Substance	Poisoning, Accidental (unintentional)	Poisoning, Intentional self-harm	Poisoning, Assault	Poisoning, Undetermined	Adverse effect	Underdosing
Amlexanox	T48.6X1	T48.6X2	T48.6X3	T48.6X4	T48.6X5	T48.6X6
Ammonia (fumes) (gas) (vapor)	T59.891	T59.892	T59.893	T59.894	—	—
aromatic spirit	T48.991	T48.992	T48.993	T48.994	T48.995	T48.996
liquid (household)	T54.3X1	T54.3X2	T54.3X3	T54.3X4	—	—
Ammoniated mercury	T49.0X1	T49.0X2	T49.0X3	T49.0X4	T49.0X5	T49.0X6
Ammonium						
acid tartrate	T49.5X1	T49.5X2	T49.5X3	T49.5X4	T49.5X5	T49.5X6
bromide	T42.6X1	T42.6X2	T42.6X3	T42.6X4	T42.6X5	T42.6X6
carbonate	T54.3X1	T54.3X2	T54.3X3	T54.3X4	—	—
chloride	T50.991	T50.992	T50.993	T50.994	T50.995	T50.996
expectorant	T48.4X1	T48.4X2	T48.4X3	T48.4X4	T48.4X5	T48.4X6
compounds (household) NEC	T54.3X1	T54.3X2	T54.3X3	T54.3X4	—	—
fumes (any usage)	T59.891	T59.892	T59.893	T59.894	—	—
industrial	T54.3X1	T54.3X2	T54.3X3	T54.3X4	—	—
ichthyosulronate	T49.4X1	T49.4X2	T49.4X3	T49.4X4	T49.4X5	T49.4X6
mandelate	T37.91	T37.92	T37.93	T37.94	T37.95	T37.96
sulfamate	T60.3X1	T60.3X2	T60.3X3	T60.3X4	—	—
sulfonate resin	T47.8X1	T47.8X2	T47.8X3	T47.8X4	T47.8X5	T47.8X6
Amobarbital (sodium)	T42.3X1	T42.3X2	T42.3X3	T42.3X4	T42.3X5	T42.3X6
Amodiaquine	T37.2X1	T37.2X2	T37.2X3	T37.2X4	T37.2X5	T37.2X6
Amopyroquin(e)	T37.2X1	T37.2X2	T37.2X3	T37.2X4	T37.2X5	T37.2X6
Amoxapine	T43.011	T43.012	T43.013	T43.014	T43.015	T43.016
Amoxicillin	T36.0X1	T36.0X2	T36.0X3	T36.0X4	T36.0X5	T36.0X6
Amperozide	T43.591	T43.592	T43.593	T43.594	T43.595	T43.596
Amphenidone	T43.591	T43.592	T43.593	T43.594	T43.595	T43.596
Amphetamine NEC	T43.621	T43.622	T43.623	T43.624	T43.625	T43.626
Amphomycin	T36.8X1	T36.8X2	T36.8X3	T36.8X4	T36.8X5	T36.8X6
Amphotalide	T37.4X1	T37.4X2	T37.4X3	T37.4X4	T37.4X5	T37.4X6
Amphotericin B	T36.7X1	T36.7X2	T36.7X3	T36.7X4	T36.7X5	T36.7X6
topical	T49.0X1	T49.0X2	T49.0X3	T49.0X4	T49.0X5	T49.0X6
Ampicillin	T36.0X1	T36.0X2	T36.0X3	T36.0X4	T36.0X5	T36.0X6
Amprotropine	T44.3X1	T44.3X2	T44.3X3	T44.3X4	T44.3X5	T44.3X6
Amsacrine	T45.1X1	T45.1X2	T45.1X3	T45.1X4	T45.1X5	T45.1X6
Amygdaline	T62.2X1	T62.2X2	T62.2X3	T62.2X4	—	—
Amyl						
acetate	T52.8X1	T52.8X2	T52.8X3	T52.8X4	—	—
vapor	T59.891	T59.892	T59.893	T59.894	—	—
alcohol	T51.3X1	T51.3X2	T51.3X3	T51.3X4	—	—
chloride	T53.6X1	T53.6X2	T53.6X3	T53.6X4	—	—
formate	T52.8X1	T52.8X2	T52.8X3	T52.8X4	—	—
nitrite	T46.3X1	T46.3X2	T46.3X3	T46.3X4	T46.3X5	T46.3X6
propionate	T65.891	T65.892	T65.893	T65.894	—	—
Amylase	T47.5X1	T47.5X2	T47.5X3	T47.5X4	T47.5X5	T47.5X6
Amyleine, regional	T41.3X1	T41.3X2	T41.3X3	T41.3X4	T41.3X5	T41.3X6
Amylene						
dichloride	T53.6X1	T53.6X2	T53.6X3	T53.6X4	—	—
hydrate	T51.3X1	T51.3X2	T51.3X3	T51.3X4	—	—
Amylmetacresol	T49.6X1	T49.6X2	T49.6X3	T49.6X4	T49.6X5	T49.6X6
Amylobarbitone	T42.3X1	T42.3X2	T42.3X3	T42.3X4	T42.3X5	T42.3X6
Amylocaine, regional	T41.3X1	T41.3X2	T41.3X3	T41.3X4	T41.3X5	T41.3X6
infiltration (subcutaneous)	T41.3X1	T41.3X2	T41.3X3	T41.3X4	T41.3X5	T41.3X6
nerve block (peripheral) (plexus)	T41.3X1	T41.3X2	T41.3X3	T41.3X4	T41.3X5	T41.3X6
spinal	T41.3X1	T41.3X2	T41.3X3	T41.3X4	T41.3X5	T41.3X6
topical (surface)	T41.3X1	T41.3X2	T41.3X3	T41.3X4	T41.3X5	T41.3X6
Amylopectin	T47.6X1	T47.6X2	T47.6X3	T47.6X4	T47.6X5	T47.6X6
Amytal (sodium)	T42.3X1	T42.3X2	T42.3X3	T42.3X4	T42.3X5	T42.3X6
Anabolic steroid	T38.7X1	T38.7X2	T38.7X3	T38.7X4	T38.7X5	T38.7X6
Analeptic NEC	T50.7X1	T50.7X2	T50.7X3	T50.7X4	T50.7X5	T50.7X6
Analgesic	T39.91	T39.92	T39.93	T39.94	T39.95	T39.96
anti-inflammatory NEC	T39.91	T39.92	T39.93	T39.94	T39.95	T39.96
propionic acid derivative	T39.311	T39.312	T39.313	T39.314	T39.315	T39.316
antirheumatic NEC	T39.4X1	T39.4X2	T39.4X3	T39.4X4	T39.4X5	T39.4X6
aromatic NEC	T39.1X1	T39.1X2	T39.1X3	T39.1X4	T39.1X5	T39.1X6
narcotic NEC	T40.601	T40.602	T40.603	T40.604	T40.605	T40.606
combination	T40.601	T40.602	T40.603	T40.604	T40.605	T40.606
obstetric	T40.601	T40.602	T40.603	T40.604	T40.605	T40.606
non-narcotic NEC	T39.91	T39.92	T39.93	T39.94	T39.95	T39.96
combination	T39.91	T39.92	T39.93	T39.94	T39.95	T39.96
pyrazole	T39.2X1	T39.2X2	T39.2X3	T39.2X4	T39.2X5	T39.2X6
specified NEC	T39.8X1	T39.8X2	T39.8X3	T39.8X4	T39.8X5	T39.8X6
Analgin	T39.2X1	T39.2X2	T39.2X3	T39.2X4	T39.2X5	T39.2X6
Anamirta cocculus	T62.1X1	T62.1X2	T62.1X3	T62.1X4	—	—
Ancillin	T36.0X1	T36.0X2	T36.0X3	T36.0X4	T36.0X5	T36.0X6
Ancrod	T45.691	T45.692	T45.693	T45.694	T45.695	T45.696
Androgen	T38.7X1	T38.7X2	T38.7X3	T38.7X4	T38.7X5	T38.7X6
Androgen-estrogen mixture	T38.7X1	T38.7X2	T38.7X3	T38.7X4	T38.7X5	T38.7X6
Androstalone	T38.7X1	T38.7X2	T38.7X3	T38.7X4	T38.7X5	T38.7X6
Androstanolone	T38.7X1	T38.7X2	T38.7X3	T38.7X4	T38.7X5	T38.7X6
Androsterone	T38.7X1	T38.7X2	T38.7X3	T38.7X4	T38.7X5	T38.7X6
Anemone pulsatilla	T62.2X1	T62.2X2	T62.2X3	T62.2X4	—	—
Anesthesia						
caudal	T41.3X1	T41.3X2	T41.3X3	T41.3X4	T41.3X5	T41.3X6
endotracheal	T41.0X1	T41.0X2	T41.0X3	T41.0X4	T41.0X5	T41.0X6
epidural	T41.3X1	T41.3X2	T41.3X3	T41.3X4	T41.3X5	T41.3X6
inhalation	T41.0X1	T41.0X2	T41.0X3	T41.0X4	T41.0X5	T41.0X6
local	T41.3X1	T41.3X2	T41.3X3	T41.3X4	T41.3X5	T41.3X6
mucosal	T41.3X1	T41.3X2	T41.3X3	T41.3X4	T41.3X5	T41.3X6
muscle relaxation	T48.1X1	T48.1X2	T48.1X3	T48.1X4	T48.1X5	T48.1X6
nerve blocking	T41.3X1	T41.3X2	T41.3X3	T41.3X4	T41.3X5	T41.3X6
plexus blocking	T41.3X1	T41.3X2	T41.3X3	T41.3X4	T41.3X5	T41.3X6
potentiated	T41.201	T41.202	T41.203	T41.204	T41.205	T41.206
rectal	T41.201	T41.202	T41.203	T41.204	T41.205	T41.206
general	T41.201	T41.202	T41.203	T41.204	T41.205	T41.206
local	T41.3X1	T41.3X2	T41.3X3	T41.3X4	T41.3X5	T41.3X6
regional	T41.3X1	T41.3X2	T41.3X3	T41.3X4	T41.3X5	T41.3X6
surface	T41.3X1	T41.3X2	T41.3X3	T41.3X4	T41.3X5	T41.3X6

Substance	Poisoning, Accidental (unintentional)	Poisoning, Intentional self-harm	Poisoning, Assault	Poisoning, Undetermined	Adverse effect	Underdosing
Anesthetic NEC —see also Anesthesia	T41.41	T41.42	T41.43	T41.44	T41.45	T41.46
with muscle relaxant	T41.201	T41.202	T41.203	T41.204	T41.205	T41.206
general	T41.201	T41.202	T41.203	T41.204	T41.205	T41.206
local	T41.3X1	T41.3X2	T41.3X3	T41.3X4	T41.3X5	T41.3X6
gaseous NEC	T41.0X1	T41.0X2	T41.0X3	T41.0X4	T41.0X5	T41.0X6
general NEC	T41.201	T41.202	T41.203	T41.204	T41.205	T41.206
halogenated hydrocarbon derivatives NEC	T41.0X1	T41.0X2	T41.0X3	T41.0X4	T41.0X5	T41.0X6
infiltration NEC	T41.3X1	T41.3X2	T41.3X3	T41.3X4	T41.3X5	T41.3X6
intravenous NEC	T41.1X1	T41.1X2	T41.1X3	T41.1X4	T41.1X5	T41.1X6
local NEC	T41.3X1	T41.3X2	T41.3X3	T41.3X4	T41.3X5	T41.3X6
rectal	T41.201	T41.202	T41.203	T41.204	T41.205	T41.206
general	T41.201	T41.202	T41.203	T41.204	T41.205	T41.206
local	T41.3X1	T41.3X2	T41.3X3	T41.3X4	T41.3X5	T41.3X6
regional NEC	T41.3X1	T41.3X2	T41.3X3	T41.3X4	T41.3X5	T41.3X6
spinal NEC	T41.3X1	T41.3X2	T41.3X3	T41.3X4	T41.3X5	T41.3X6
thiobarbiturate	T41.1X1	T41.1X2	T41.1X3	T41.1X4	T41.1X5	T41.1X6
topical	T41.3X1	T41.3X2	T41.3X3	T41.3X4	T41.3X5	T41.3X6
Aneurine	T45.2X1	T45.2X2	T45.2X3	T45.2X4	T45.2X5	T45.2X6
Angio-Conray	T50.8X1	T50.8X2	T50.8X3	T50.8X4	T50.8X5	T50.8X6
Angiotensin	T44.5X1	T44.5X2	T44.5X3	T44.5X4	T44.5X5	T44.5X6
Angiotensinamide	T44.991	T44.992	T44.993	T44.994	T44.995	T44.996
Anhydrohydroxy-progesterone	T38.5X1	T38.5X2	T38.5X3	T38.5X4	T38.5X5	T38.5X6
Anhydron	T50.2X1	T50.2X2	T50.2X3	T50.2X4	T50.2X5	T50.2X6
Anileridine	T40.491	T40.492	T40.493	T40.494	T40.495	T40.496
Aniline (dye) (liquid)	T65.3X1	T65.3X2	T65.3X3	T65.3X4	—	—
analgesic	T39.1X1	T39.1X2	T39.1X3	T39.1X4	T39.1X5	T39.1X6
derivatives, therapeutic NEC	T39.1X1	T39.1X2	T39.1X3	T39.1X4	T39.1X5	T39.1X6
vapor	T65.3X1	T65.3X2	T65.3X3	T65.3X4	—	—
Aniscoropine	T44.3X1	T44.3X2	T44.3X3	T44.3X4	T44.3X5	T44.3X6
Anise oil	T47.5X1	T47.5X2	T47.5X3	T47.5X4	T47.5X5	T47.5X6
Anisidine	T65.3X1	T65.3X2	T65.3X3	T65.3X4	—	—
Anisindione	T45.511	T45.512	T45.513	T45.514	T45.515	T45.516
Anisotropine methyl-bromide	T44.3X1	T44.3X2	T44.3X3	T44.3X4	T44.3X5	T44.3X6
Anistreplase	T45.611	T45.612	T45.613	T45.614	T45.615	T45.616
Anorexiant (central)	T50.5X1	T50.5X2	T50.5X3	T50.5X4	T50.5X5	T50.5X6
Anorexic agents	T50.5X1	T50.5X2	T50.5X3	T50.5X4	T50.5X5	T50.5X6
Ansamycin	T36.6X1	T36.6X2	T36.6X3	T36.6X4	T36.6X5	T36.6X6
Ant (bite) (sting)	T63.421	T63.422	T63.423	T63.424	—	—
Ant poison—see Insecticide						
Antabuse	T50.6X1	T50.6X2	T50.6X3	T50.6X4	T50.6X5	T50.6X6
Antacid NEC	T47.1X1	T47.1X2	T47.1X3	T47.1X4	T47.1X5	T47.1X6
Antagonist						
Aldosterone	T50.0X1	T50.0X2	T50.0X3	T50.0X4	T50.0X5	T50.0X6
alpha-adrenoreceptor	T44.6X1	T44.6X2	T44.6X3	T44.6X4	T44.6X5	T44.6X6
anticoagulant	T45.7X1	T45.7X2	T45.7X3	T45.7X4	T45.7X5	T45.7X6
Antagonist — *Continued*						
beta-adrenoreceptor	T44.7X1	T44.7X2	T44.7X3	T44.7X4	T44.7X5	T44.7X6
extrapyramidal NEC	T44.3X1	T44.3X2	T44.3X3	T44.3X4	T44.3X5	T44.3X6
folic acid	T45.1X1	T45.1X2	T45.1X3	T45.1X4	T45.1X5	T45.1X6
H2 receptor	T47.0X1	T47.0X2	T47.0X3	T47.0X4	T47.0X5	T47.0X6
heavy metal	T45.8X1	T45.8X2	T45.8X3	T45.8X4	T45.8X5	T45.8X6
narcotic analgesic	T50.7X1	T50.7X2	T50.7X3	T50.7X4	T50.7X5	T50.7X6
opiate	T50.7X1	T50.7X2	T50.7X3	T50.7X4	T50.7X5	T50.7X6
pyrimidine	T45.1X1	T45.1X2	T45.1X3	T45.1X4	T45.1X5	T45.1X6
serotonin	T46.5X1	T46.5X2	T46.5X3	T46.5X4	T46.5X5	T46.5X6
Antazolin(e)	T45.0X1	T45.0X2	T45.0X3	T45.0X4	T45.0X5	T45.0X6
Anterior pituitary hormone NEC	T38.811	T38.812	T38.813	T38.814	T38.815	T38.816
Anthelmintic NEC	T37.4X1	T37.4X2	T37.4X3	T37.4X4	T37.4X5	T37.4X6
Anthiolimine	T37.4X1	T37.4X2	T37.4X3	T37.4X4	T37.4X5	T37.4X6
Anthralin	T49.4X1	T49.4X2	T49.4X3	T49.4X4	T49.4X5	T49.4X6
Anthramycin	T45.1X1	T45.1X2	T45.1X3	T45.1X4	T45.1X5	T45.1X6
Antiadrenergic NEC	T44.8X1	T44.8X2	T44.8X3	T44.8X4	T44.8X5	T44.8X6
Antiallergic NEC	T45.0X1	T45.0X2	T45.0X3	T45.0X4	T45.0X5	T45.0X6
Anti-anemic (drug) (preparation)	T45.8X1	T45.8X2	T45.8X3	T45.8X4	T45.8X5	T45.8X6
Antiandrogen NEC	T38.6X1	T38.6X2	T38.6X3	T38.6X4	T38.6X5	T38.6X6
Antianxiety drug NEC	T43.501	T43.502	T43.503	T43.504	T43.505	T43.506
Antiaris toxicaria	T65.891	T65.892	T65.893	T65.894	—	—
Antiarteriosclerotic drug	T46.6X1	T46.6X2	T46.6X3	T46.6X4	T46.6X5	T46.6X6
Antiasthmatic drug NEC	T48.6X1	T48.6X2	T48.6X3	T48.6X4	T48.6X5	T48.6X6
Antibiotic NEC	T36.91	T36.92	T36.93	T36.94	T36.95	T36.96
aminoglycoside	T36.5X1	T36.5X2	T36.5X3	T36.5X4	T36.5X5	T36.5X6
anticancer	T45.1X1	T45.1X2	T45.1X3	T45.1X4	T45.1X5	T45.1X6
antifungal	T36.7X1	T36.7X2	T36.7X3	T36.7X4	T36.7X5	T36.7X6
antimycobacterial	T36.5X1	T36.5X2	T36.5X3	T36.5X4	T36.5X5	T36.5X6
antineoplastic	T45.1X1	T45.1X2	T45.1X3	T45.1X4	T45.1X5	T45.1X6
cephalosporin (group)	T36.1X1	T36.1X2	T36.1X3	T36.1X4	T36.1X5	T36.1X6
chloramphenicol (group)	T36.2X1	T36.2X2	T36.2X3	T36.2X4	T36.2X5	T36.2X6
ENT	T49.6X1	T49.6X2	T49.6X3	T49.6X4	T49.6X5	T49.6X6
eye	T49.5X1	T49.5X2	T49.5X3	T49.5X4	T49.5X5	T49.5X6
fungicidal (local)	T49.0X1	T49.0X2	T49.0X3	T49.0X4	T49.0X5	T49.0X6
intestinal	T36.8X1	T36.8X2	T36.8X3	T36.8X4	T36.8X5	T36.8X6
b-lactam NEC	T36.1X1	T36.1X2	T36.1X3	T36.1X4	T36.1X5	T36.1X6
local	T49.0X1	T49.0X2	T49.0X3	T49.0X4	T49.0X5	T49.0X6
macrolides	T36.3X1	T36.3X2	T36.3X3	T36.3X4	T36.3X5	T36.3X6
polypeptide	T36.8X1	T36.8X2	T36.8X3	T36.8X4	T36.8X5	T36.8X6
specified NEC	T36.8X1	T36.8X2	T36.8X3	T36.8X4	T36.8X5	T36.8X6
tetracycline (group)	T36.4X1	T36.4X2	T36.4X3	T36.4X4	T36.4X5	T36.4X6
throat	T49.6X1	T49.6X2	T49.6X3	T49.6X4	T49.6X5	T49.6X6
Anticancer agents NEC	T45.1X1	T45.1X2	T45.1X3	T45.1X4	T45.1X5	T45.1X6
Anticholesterolemic drug NEC	T46.6X1	T46.6X2	T46.6X3	T46.6X4	T46.6X5	T46.6X6
Anticholinergic NEC	T44.3X1	T44.3X2	T44.3X3	T44.3X4	T44.3X5	T44.3X6

Substance	Poisoning, Accidental (unintentional)	Poisoning, Intentional self-harm	Poisoning, Assault	Poisoning, Undetermined	Adverse effect	Underdosing
Anticholinesterase	T44.0X1	T44.0X2	T44.0X3	T44.0X4	T44.0X5	T44.0X6
organophosphorus	T44.0X1	T44.0X2	T44.0X3	T44.0X4	T44.0X5	T44.0X6
insecticide	T60.0X1	T60.0X2	T60.0X3	T60.0X4	—	—
nerve gas	T59.891	T59.892	T59.893	T59.894	—	—
reversible	T44.0X1	T44.0X2	T44.0X3	T44.0X4	T44.0X5	T44.0X6
ophthalmological	T49.5X1	T49.5X2	T49.5X3	T49.5X4	T49.5X5	T49.5X6
Anticoagulant NEC	T45.511	T45.512	T45.513	T45.514	T45.515	T45.516
Antagonist	T45.7X1	T45.7X2	T45.7X3	T45.7X4	T45.7X5	T45.7X6
Anti-common-cold drug NEC	T48.5X1	T48.5X2	T48.5X3	T48.5X4	T48.5X5	T48.5X6
Anticonvulsant	T42.71	T42.72	T42.73	T42.74	T42.75	T42.76
barbiturate	T42.3X1	T42.3X2	T42.3X3	T42.3X4	T42.3X5	T42.3X6
combination (with barbiturate)	T42.3X1	T42.3X2	T42.3X3	T42.3X4	T42.3X5	T42.3X6
hydantoin	T42.0X1	T42.0X2	T42.0X3	T42.0X4	T42.0X5	T42.0X6
hypnotic NEC	T42.6X1	T42.6X2	T42.6X3	T42.6X4	T42.6X5	T42.6X6
oxazolidinedione	T42.2X1	T42.2X2	T42.2X3	T42.2X4	T42.2X5	T42.2X6
pyrimidinedione	T42.6X1	T42.6X2	T42.6X3	T42.6X4	T42.6X5	T42.6X6
specified NEC	T42.6X1	T42.6X2	T42.6X3	T42.6X4	T42.6X5	T42.6X6
succinimide	T42.2X1	T42.2X2	T42.2X3	T42.2X4	T42.2X5	T42.2X6
Anti-D immuno-globulin (human)	T50.Z11	T50.Z12	T50.Z13	T50.Z14	T50.Z15	T50.Z16
Antidepressant	T43.201	T43.202	T43.203	T43.204	T43.205	T43.206
monoamine oxidase inhibitor	T43.1X1	T43.1X2	T43.1X3	T43.1X4	T43.1X5	T43.1X6
selective serotonin norepinephrine reuptake inhibitor	T43.211	T43.212	T43.213	T43.214	T43.215	T43.216
selective serotonin reuptake inhibitor	T43.221	T43.222	T43.223	T43.224	T43.225	T43.226
specified NEC	T43.291	T43.292	T43.293	T43.294	T43.295	T43.296
tetracyclic	T43.021	T43.022	T43.023	T43.024	T43.025	T43.026
triazolopyridine	T43.211	T43.212	T43.213	T43.214	T43.215	T43.216
tricyclic	T43.011	T43.012	T43.013	T43.014	T43.015	T43.016
Antidiabetic NEC	T38.3X1	T38.3X2	T38.3X3	T38.3X4	T38.3X5	T38.3X6
biguanide	T38.3X1	T38.3X2	T38.3X3	T38.3X4	T38.3X5	T38.3X6
and sulfonyl combined	T38.3X1	T38.3X2	T38.3X3	T38.3X4	T38.3X5	T38.3X6
combined	T38.3X1	T38.3X2	T38.3X3	T38.3X4	T38.3X5	T38.3X6
sulfonylurea	T38.3X1	T38.3X2	T38.3X3	T38.3X4	T38.3X5	T38.3X6
Antidiarrheal drug NEC	T47.6X1	T47.6X2	T47.6X3	T47.6X4	T47.6X5	T47.6X6
absorbent	T47.6X1	T47.6X2	T47.6X3	T47.6X4	T47.6X5	T47.6X6
Antidiphtheria serum	T50.Z11	T50.Z12	T50.Z13	T50.Z14	T50.Z15	T50.Z16
Antidiuretic hormone	T38.891	T38.892	T38.893	T38.894	T38.895	T38.896
Antidote NEC	T50.6X1	T50.6X2	T50.6X3	T50.6X4	T50.6X5	T50.6X6
heavy metal	T45.8X1	T45.8X2	T45.8X3	T45.8X4	T45.8X5	T45.8X6
Antidysrhythmic NEC	T46.2X1	T46.2X2	T46.2X3	T46.2X4	T46.2X5	T46.2X6
Antiemetic drug	T45.0X1	T45.0X2	T45.0X3	T45.0X4	T45.0X5	T45.0X6
Antiepilepsy agent	T42.71	T42.72	T42.73	T42.74	T42.75	T42.76
combination	T42.5X1	T42.5X2	T42.5X3	T42.5X4	T42.5X5	T42.5X6
mixed	T42.5X1	T42.5X2	T42.5X3	T42.5X4	T42.5X5	T42.5X6
specified, NEC	T42.6X1	T42.6X2	T42.6X3	T42.6X4	T42.6X5	T42.6X6

Substance	Poisoning, Accidental (unintentional)	Poisoning, Intentional self-harm	Poisoning, Assault	Poisoning, Undetermined	Adverse effect	Underdosing
Antiestrogen NEC	T38.6X1	T38.6X2	T38.6X3	T38.6X4	T38.6X5	T38.6X6
Antifertility pill	T38.4X1	T38.4X2	T38.4X3	T38.4X4	T38.4X5	T38.4X6
Antifibrinolytic drug	T45.621	T45.622	T45.623	T45.624	T45.625	T45.626
Antifilarial drug	T37.4X1	T37.4X2	T37.4X3	T37.4X4	T37.4X5	T37.4X6
Antiflatulent	T47.5X1	T47.5X2	T47.5X3	T47.5X4	T47.5X5	T47.5X6
Antifreeze	T65.91	T65.92	T65.93	T65.94	—	—
alcohol	T51.1X1	T51.1X2	T51.1X3	T51.1X4	—	—
ethylene glycol	T51.8X1	T51.8X2	T51.8X3	T51.8X4	—	—
Antifungal						
antibiotic (systemic)	T36.7X1	T36.7X2	T36.7X3	T36.7X4	T36.7X5	T36.7X6
anti-infective NEC	T37.91	T37.92	T37.93	T37.94	T37.95	T37.96
disinfectant, local	T49.0X1	T49.0X2	T49.0X3	T49.0X4	T49.0X5	T49.0X6
nonmedicinal (spray)	T60.3X1	T60.3X2	T60.3X3	T60.3X4	—	—
topical	T49.0X1	T49.0X2	T49.0X3	T49.0X4	T49.0X5	T49.0X6
Anti-gastric-secretion drug NEC	T47.1X1	T47.1X2	T47.1X3	T47.1X4	T47.1X5	T47.1X6
Antigonadotrophin NEC	T38.6X1	T38.6X2	T38.6X3	T38.6X4	T38.6X5	T38.6X6
Antihallucinogen	T43.501	T43.502	T43.503	T43.504	T43.505	T43.506
Antihelmintics	T37.4X1	T37.4X2	T37.4X3	T37.4X4	T37.4X5	T37.4X6
Antihemophilic						
factor	T45.8X1	T45.8X2	T45.8X3	T45.8X4	T45.8X5	T45.8X6
fraction	T45.8X1	T45.8X2	T45.8X3	T45.8X4	T45.8X5	T45.8X6
globulin concentrate	T45.7X1	T45.7X2	T45.7X3	T45.7X4	T45.7X5	T45.7X6
human plasma	T45.8X1	T45.8X2	T45.8X3	T45.8X4	T45.8X5	T45.8X6
plasma, dried	T45.7X1	T45.7X2	T45.7X3	T45.7X4	T45.7X5	T45.7X6
Antihemorrhoidal preparation	T49.2X1	T49.2X2	T49.2X3	T49.2X4	T49.2X5	T49.2X6
Antiheparin drug	T45.7X1	T45.7X2	T45.7X3	T45.7X4	T45.7X5	T45.7X6
Antihistamine	T45.0X1	T45.0X2	T45.0X3	T45.0X4	T45.0X5	T45.0X6
Antihookworm drug	T37.4X1	T37.4X2	T37.4X3	T37.4X4	T37.4X5	T37.4X6
Anti-human lymphocytic globulin	T50.Z11	T50.Z12	T50.Z13	T50.Z14	T50.Z15	T50.Z16
Antihyperlipidemic drug	T46.6X1	T46.6X2	T46.6X3	T46.6X4	T46.6X5	T46.6X6
Antihypertensive drug NEC	T46.5X1	T46.5X2	T46.5X3	T46.5X4	T46.5X5	T46.5X6
Anti-infective NEC	T37.91	T37.92	T37.93	T37.94	T37.95	T37.96
anthelmintic	T37.4X1	T37.4X2	T37.4X3	T37.4X4	T37.4X5	T37.4X6
antibiotics	T36.91	T36.92	T36.93	T36.94	T36.95	T36.96
specified NEC	T36.8X1	T36.8X2	T36.8X3	T36.8X4	T36.8X5	T36.8X6
antimalarial	T37.2X1	T37.2X2	T37.2X3	T37.2X4	T37.2X5	T37.2X6
antimycobacterial NEC	T37.1X1	T37.1X2	T37.1X3	T37.1X4	T37.1X5	T37.1X6
antibiotics	T36.5X1	T36.5X2	T36.5X3	T36.5X4	T36.5X5	T36.5X6
antiprotozoal NEC	T37.3X1	T37.3X2	T37.3X3	T37.3X4	T37.3X5	T37.3X6
blood	T37.2X1	T37.2X2	T37.2X3	T37.2X4	T37.2X5	T37.2X6
antiviral	T37.5X1	T37.5X2	T37.5X3	T37.5X4	T37.5X5	T37.5X6
arsenical	T37.8X1	T37.8X2	T37.8X3	T37.8X4	T37.8X5	T37.8X6
bismuth, local	T49.0X1	T49.0X2	T49.0X3	T49.0X4	T49.0X5	T49.0X6
ENT	T49.6X1	T49.6X2	T49.6X3	T49.6X4	T49.6X5	T49.6X6
eye NEC	T49.5X1	T49.5X2	T49.5X3	T49.5X4	T49.5X5	T49.5X6
heavy metals NEC	T37.8X1	T37.8X2	T37.8X3	T37.8X4	T37.8X5	T37.8X6

Substance	Poisoning, Accidental (unintentional)	Poisoning, Intentional self-harm	Poisoning, Assault	Poisoning, Undetermined	Adverse effect	Underdosing
Anti-infective NEC — *Continued*						
local NEC	T49.0X1	T49.0X2	T49.0X3	T49.0X4	T49.0X5	T49.0X6
specified NEC	T49.0X1	T49.0X2	T49.0X3	T49.0X4	T49.0X5	T49.0X6
mixed	T37.91	T37.92	T37.93	T37.94	T37.95	T37.96
ophthalmic preparation	T49.5X1	T49.5X2	T49.5X3	T49.5X4	T49.5X5	T49.5X6
topical NEC	T49.0X1	T49.0X2	T49.0X3	T49.0X4	T49.0X5	T49.0X6
Anti-inflammatory drug NEC	T39.391	T39.392	T39.393	T39.394	T39.395	T39.396
local	T49.0X1	T49.0X2	T49.0X3	T49.0X4	T49.0X5	T49.0X6
nonsteroidal NEC	T39.391	T39.392	T39.393	T39.394	T39.395	T39.396
propionic acid derivative	T39.311	T39.312	T39.313	T39.314	T39.315	T39.316
specified NEC	T39.391	T39.392	T39.393	T39.394	T39.395	T39.396
Antikaluretic	T50.3X1	T50.3X2	T50.3X3	T50.3X4	T50.3X5	T50.3X6
Antiknock (tetraethyl lead)	T56.0X1	T56.0X2	T56.0X3	T56.0X4	—	—
Antilipemic drug NEC	T46.6X1	T46.6X2	T46.6X3	T46.6X4	T46.6X5	T46.6X6
Antimalarial	T37.2X1	T37.2X2	T37.2X3	T37.2X4	T37.2X5	T37.2X6
prophylactic NEC	T37.2X1	T37.2X2	T37.2X3	T37.2X4	T37.2X5	T37.2X6
pyrimidine derivative	T37.2X1	T37.2X2	T37.2X3	T37.2X4	T37.2X5	T37.2X6
Antimetabolite	T45.1X1	T45.1X2	T45.1X3	T45.1X4	T45.1X5	T45.1X6
Antimitotic agent	T45.1X1	T45.1X2	T45.1X3	T45.1X4	T45.1X5	T45.1X6
Antimony (compounds) (vapor)NEC	T56.891	T56.892	T56.893	T56.894	—	—
anti-infectives	T37.8X1	T37.8X2	T37.8X3	T37.8X4	T37.8X5	T37.8X6
dimercaptosuccinate	T37.3X1	T37.3X2	T37.3X3	T37.3X4	T37.3X5	T37.3X6
hydride	T56.891	T56.892	T56.893	T56.894	—	—
pesticide (vapor)	T60.8X1	T60.8X2	T60.8X3	T60.8X4	—	—
potassium (sodium) tartrate	T37.8X1	T37.8X2	T37.8X3	T37.8X4	T37.8X5	T37.8X6
sodium dimercaptosuccinate	T37.3X1	T37.3X2	T37.3X3	T37.3X4	T37.3X5	T37.3X6
tartrated	T37.8X1	T37.8X2	T37.8X3	T37.8X4	T37.8X5	T37.8X6
Antimuscarinic NEC	T44.3X1	T44.3X2	T44.3X3	T44.3X4	T44.3X5	T44.3X6
Antimycobacterial drug NEC	T37.1X1	T37.1X2	T37.1X3	T37.1X4	T37.1X5	T37.1X6
antibiotics	T36.5X1	T36.5X2	T36.5X3	T36.5X4	T36.5X5	T36.5X6
combination	T37.1X1	T37.1X2	T37.1X3	T37.1X4	T37.1X5	T37.1X6
Antinausea drug	T45.0X1	T45.0X2	T45.0X3	T45.0X4	T45.0X5	T45.0X6
Antinematode drug	T37.4X1	T37.4X2	T37.4X3	T37.4X4	T37.4X5	T37.4X6
Antineoplastic NEC	T45.1X1	T45.1X2	T45.1X3	T45.1X4	T45.1X5	T45.1X6
alkaloidal	T45.1X1	T45.1X2	T45.1X3	T45.1X4	T45.1X5	T45.1X6
antibiotics	T45.1X1	T45.1X2	T45.1X3	T45.1X4	T45.1X5	T45.1X6
combination	T45.1X1	T45.1X2	T45.1X3	T45.1X4	T45.1X5	T45.1X6
estrogen	T38.5X1	T38.5X2	T38.5X3	T38.5X4	T38.5X5	T38.5X6
steroid	T38.7X1	T38.7X2	T38.7X3	T38.7X4	T38.7X5	T38.7X6
Antiparasitic drug (systemic)	T37.91	T37.92	T37.93	T37.94	T37.95	T37.96
local	T49.0X1	T49.0X2	T49.0X3	T49.0X4	T49.0X5	T49.0X6
specified NEC	T37.8X1	T37.8X2	T37.8X3	T37.8X4	T37.8X5	T37.8X6
Antiparkinsonism drug NEC	T42.8X1	T42.8X2	T42.8X3	T42.8X4	T42.8X5	T42.8X6
Antiperspirant NEC	T49.2X1	T49.2X2	T49.2X3	T49.2X4	T49.2X5	T49.2X6
Antiphlogistic NEC	T39.4X1	T39.4X2	T39.4X3	T39.4X4	T39.4X5	T39.4X6
Antiplatyhelmintic drug	T37.4X1	T37.4X2	T37.4X3	T37.4X4	T37.4X5	T37.4X6
Antiprotozoal drug NEC	T37.3X1	T37.3X2	T37.3X3	T37.3X4	T37.3X5	T37.3X6
blood	T37.2X1	T37.2X2	T37.2X3	T37.2X4	T37.2X5	T37.2X6
local	T49.0X1	T49.0X2	T49.0X3	T49.0X4	T49.0X5	T49.0X6
Antipruritic drug NEC	T49.1X1	T49.1X2	T49.1X3	T49.1X4	T49.1X5	T49.1X6
Antipsychotic drug	T43.501	T43.502	T43.503	T43.504	T43.505	T43.506
specified NEC	T43.591	T43.592	T43.593	T43.594	T43.595	T43.596
Antipyretic	T39.91	T39.92	T39.93	T39.94	T39.95	T39.96
specified NEC	T39.8X1	T39.8X2	T39.8X3	T39.8X4	T39.8X5	T39.8X6
Antipyrine	T39.2X1	T39.2X2	T39.2X3	T39.2X4	T39.2X5	T39.2X6
Antirabies hyperimmune serum	T50.Z11	T50.Z12	T50.Z13	T50.Z14	T50.Z15	T50.Z16
Antirheumatic NEC	T39.4X1	T39.4X2	T39.4X3	T39.4X4	T39.4X5	T39.4X6
Antirigidity drug NEC	T42.8X1	T42.8X2	T42.8X3	T42.8X4	T42.8X5	T42.8X6
Antischistosomal drug	T37.4X1	T37.4X2	T37.4X3	T37.4X4	T37.4X5	T37.4X6
Antiscorpion sera	T50.Z11	T50.Z12	T50.Z13	T50.Z14	T50.Z15	T50.Z16
Antiseborrheics	T49.4X1	T49.4X2	T49.4X3	T49.4X4	T49.4X5	T49.4X6
Antiseptics (external) (medicinal)	T49.0X1	T49.0X2	T49.0X3	T49.0X4	T49.0X5	T49.0X6
Antistine	T45.0X1	T45.0X2	T45.0X3	T45.0X4	T45.0X5	T45.0X6
Antitapeworm drug	T37.4X1	T37.4X2	T37.4X3	T37.4X4	T37.4X5	T37.4X6
Antitetanus immunoglobulin	T50.Z11	T50.Z12	T50.Z13	T50.Z14	T50.Z15	T50.Z16
Antithrombotic	T45.521	T45.522	T45.523	T45.524	T45.525	T45.526
Antithyroid drug NEC	T38.2X1	T38.2X2	T38.2X3	T38.2X4	T38.2X5	T38.2X6
Antitoxin	T50.Z11	T50.Z12	T50.Z13	T50.Z14	T50.Z15	T50.Z16
diphtheria	T50.Z11	T50.Z12	T50.Z13	T50.Z14	T50.Z15	T50.Z16
gas gangrene	T50.Z11	T50.Z12	T50.Z13	T50.Z14	T50.Z15	T50.Z16
tetanus	T50.Z11	T50.Z12	T50.Z13	T50.Z14	T50.Z15	T50.Z16
Antitrichomonal drug	T37.3X1	T37.3X2	T37.3X3	T37.3X4	T37.3X5	T37.3X6
Antituberculars	T37.1X1	T37.1X2	T37.1X3	T37.1X4	T37.1X5	T37.1X6
antibiotics	T36.5X1	T36.5X2	T36.5X3	T36.5X4	T36.5X5	T36.5X6
Antitussive NEC	T48.3X1	T48.3X2	T48.3X3	T48.3X4	T48.3X5	T48.3X6
codeine mixture	T40.2X1	T40.2X2	T40.2X3	T40.2X4	T40.2X5	T40.2X6
opiate	T40.2X1	T40.2X2	T40.2X3	T40.2X4	T40.2X5	T40.2X6
Antivaricose drug	T46.8X1	T46.8X2	T46.8X3	T46.8X4	T46.8X5	T46.8X6
Antivenin, antivenom (sera)	T50.Z11	T50.Z12	T50.Z13	T50.Z14	T50.Z15	T50.Z16
crotaline	T50.Z11	T50.Z12	T50.Z13	T50.Z14	T50.Z15	T50.Z16
spider bite	T50.Z11	T50.Z12	T50.Z13	T50.Z14	T50.Z15	T50.Z16
Antivertigo drug	T45.0X1	T45.0X2	T45.0X3	T45.0X4	T45.0X5	T45.0X6
Antiviral drug NEC	T37.5X1	T37.5X2	T37.5X3	T37.5X4	T37.5X5	T37.5X6
eye	T49.5X1	T49.5X2	T49.5X3	T49.5X4	T49.5X5	T49.5X6
Antiwhipworm drug	T37.4X1	T37.4X2	T37.4X3	T37.4X4	T37.4X5	T37.4X6
Antrol—see also by specific chemical substance	T60.91	T60.92	T60.93	T60.94	—	—
fungicide	T60.91	T60.92	T60.93	T60.94	—	—
ANTU (alpha naphthylthiourea)	T60.4X1	T60.4X2	T60.4X3	T60.4X4	—	—
Apalcillin	T36.0X1	T36.0X2	T36.0X3	T36.0X4	T36.0X5	T36.0X6

Substance	Poisoning, Accidental (unintentional)	Poisoning, Intentional self-harm	Poisoning, Assault	Poisoning, Undetermined	Adverse effect	Underdosing
APC	T48.5X1	T48.5X2	T48.5X3	T48.5X4	T48.5X5	T48.5X6
Aplonidine	T44.4X1	T44.4X2	T44.4X3	T44.4X4	T44.4X5	T44.4X6
Apomorphine	T47.7X1	T47.7X2	T47.7X3	T47.7X4	T47.7X5	T47.7X6
Appetite depressants, central	T50.5X1	T50.5X2	T50.5X3	T50.5X4	T50.5X5	T50.5X6
Apraclonidine (hydrochloride)	T44.4X1	T44.4X2	T44.4X3	T44.4X4	T44.4X5	T44.4X6
Apresoline	T46.5X1	T46.5X2	T46.5X3	T46.5X4	T46.5X5	T46.5X6
Aprindine	T46.2X1	T46.2X2	T46.2X3	T46.2X4	T46.2X5	T46.2X6
Aprobarbital	T42.3X1	T42.3X2	T42.3X3	T42.3X4	T42.3X5	T42.3X6
Apronalide	T42.6X1	T42.6X2	T42.6X3	T42.6X4	T42.6X5	T42.6X6
Aprotinin	T45.621	T45.622	T45.623	T45.624	T45.625	T45.626
Aptocaine	T41.3X1	T41.3X2	T41.3X3	T41.3X4	T41.3X5	T41.3X6
Aqua fortis	T54.2X1	T54.2X2	T54.2X3	T54.2X4	—	—
Ara-A	T37.5X1	T37.5X2	T37.5X3	T37.5X4	T37.5X5	T37.5X6
Ara-C	T45.1X1	T45.1X2	T45.1X3	T45.1X4	T45.1X5	T45.1X6
Arachis oil	T49.3X1	T49.3X2	T49.3X3	T49.3X4	T49.3X5	T49.3X6
cathartic	T47.4X1	T47.4X2	T47.4X3	T47.4X4	T47.4X5	T47.4X6
Aralen	T37.2X1	T37.2X2	T37.2X3	T37.2X4	T37.2X5	T37.2X6
Arecoline	T44.1X1	T44.1X2	T44.1X3	T44.1X4	T44.1X5	T44.1X6
Arginine	T50.991	T50.992	T50.993	T50.994	T50.995	T50.996
glutamate	T50.991	T50.992	T50.993	T50.994	T50.995	T50.996
Argyrol	T49.0X1	T49.0X2	T49.0X3	T49.0X4	T49.0X5	T49.0X6
ENT agent	T49.6X1	T49.6X2	T49.6X3	T49.6X4	T49.6X5	T49.6X6
ophthalmic preparation	T49.5X1	T49.5X2	T49.5X3	T49.5X4	T49.5X5	T49.5X6
Aristocort	T38.0X1	T38.0X2	T38.0X3	T38.0X4	T38.0X5	T38.0X6
ENT agent	T49.6X1	T49.6X2	T49.6X3	T49.6X4	T49.6X5	T49.6X6
ophthalmic preparation	T49.5X1	T49.5X2	T49.5X3	T49.5X4	T49.5X5	T49.5X6
topical NEC	T49.0X1	T49.0X2	T49.0X3	T49.0X4	T49.0X5	T49.0X6
Aromatics, corrosive	T54.1X1	T54.1X2	T54.1X3	T54.1X4	—	—
disinfectants	T54.1X1	T54.1X2	T54.1X3	T54.1X4	—	—
Arsenate of lead	T57.0X1	T57.0X2	T57.0X3	T57.0X4	—	—
herbicide	T57.0X1	T57.0X2	T57.0X3	T57.0X4	—	—
Arsenic, arsenicals (compounds) (dust) (vapor) NEC	T57.0X1	T57.0X2	T57.0X3	T57.0X4	—	—
anti-infectives	T37.8X1	T37.8X2	T37.8X3	T37.8X4	T37.8X5	T37.8X6
pesticide (dust) (fumes)	T57.0X1	T57.0X2	T57.0X3	T57.0X4	—	—
Arsine (gas)	T57.0X1	T57.0X2	T57.0X3	T57.0X4	—	—
Arsphenamine (silver)	T37.8X1	T37.8X2	T37.8X3	T37.8X4	T37.8X5	T37.8X6
Arsthinol	T37.3X1	T37.3X2	T37.3X3	T37.3X4	T37.3X5	T37.3X6
Artane	T44.3X1	T44.3X2	T44.3X3	T44.3X4	T44.3X5	T44.3X6
Arthropod (venomous) NEC	T63.481	T63.482	T63.483	T63.484	—	—
Articaine	T41.3X1	T41.3X2	T41.3X3	T41.3X4	T41.3X5	T41.3X6
Asbestos	T57.8X1	T57.8X2	T57.8X3	T57.8X4	—	—
Ascaridole	T37.4X1	T37.4X2	T37.4X3	T37.4X4	T37.4X5	T37.4X6
Ascorbic acid	T45.2X1	T45.2X2	T45.2X3	T45.2X4	T45.2X5	T45.2X6
Asiaticoside	T49.0X1	T49.0X2	T49.0X3	T49.0X4	T49.0X5	T49.0X6
Asparaginase	T45.1X1	T45.1X2	T45.1X3	T45.1X4	T45.1X5	T45.1X6
Aspidium (oleoresin)	T37.4X1	T37.4X2	T37.4X3	T37.4X4	T37.4X5	T37.4X6

Substance	Poisoning, Accidental (unintentional)	Poisoning, Intentional self-harm	Poisoning, Assault	Poisoning, Undetermined	Adverse effect	Underdosing
Aspirin (aluminum) (soluble)	T39.011	T39.012	T39.013	T39.014	T39.015	T39.016
Aspoxicillin	T36.0X1	T36.0X2	T36.0X3	T36.0X4	T36.0X5	T36.0X6
Astemizole	T45.0X1	T45.0X2	T45.0X3	T45.0X4	T45.0X5	T45.0X6
Astringent (local)	T49.2X1	T49.2X2	T49.2X3	T49.2X4	T49.2X5	T49.2X6
specified NEC	T49.2X1	T49.2X2	T49.2X3	T49.2X4	T49.2X5	T49.2X6
Astromicin	T36.5X1	T36.5X2	T36.5X3	T36.5X4	T36.5X5	T36.5X6
Ataractic drug NEC	T43.501	T43.502	T43.503	T43.504	T43.505	T43.506
Atenolol	T44.7X1	T44.7X2	T44.7X3	T44.7X4	T44.7X5	T44.7X6
Atonia drug, intestinal	T47.4X1	T47.4X2	T47.4X3	T47.4X4	T47.4X5	T47.4X6
Atophan	T50.4X1	T50.4X2	T50.4X3	T50.4X4	T50.4X5	T50.4X6
Atracurium besilate	T48.1X1	T48.1X2	T48.1X3	T48.1X4	T48.1X5	T48.1X6
Atropine	T44.3X1	T44.3X2	T44.3X3	T44.3X4	T44.3X5	T44.3X6
derivative	T44.3X1	T44.3X2	T44.3X3	T44.3X4	T44.3X5	T44.3X6
methonitrate	T44.3X1	T44.3X2	T44.3X3	T44.3X4	T44.3X5	T44.3X6
Attapulgite	T47.6X1	T47.6X2	T47.6X3	T47.6X4	T47.6X5	T47.6X6
Auramine	T65.891	T65.892	T65.893	T65.894	—	—
dye	T65.6X1	T65.6X2	T65.6X3	T65.6X4	—	—
fungicide	T60.3X1	T60.3X2	T60.3X3	T60.3X4	—	—
Auranofin	T39.4X1	T39.4X2	T39.4X3	T39.4X4	T39.4X5	T39.4X6
Aurantiin	T46.991	T46.992	T46.993	T46.994	T46.995	T46.996
Aureomycin	T36.4X1	T36.4X2	T36.4X3	T36.4X4	T36.4X5	T36.4X6
ophthalmic preparation	T49.5X1	T49.5X2	T49.5X3	T49.5X4	T49.5X5	T49.5X6
topical NEC	T49.0X1	T49.0X2	T49.0X3	T49.0X4	T49.0X5	T49.0X6
Aurothioglucose	T39.4X1	T39.4X2	T39.4X3	T39.4X4	T39.4X5	T39.4X6
Aurothioglycanide	T39.4X1	T39.4X2	T39.4X3	T39.4X4	T39.4X5	T39.4X6
Aurothiomalate sodium	T39.4X1	T39.4X2	T39.4X3	T39.4X4	T39.4X5	T39.4X6
Aurotioprol	T39.4X1	T39.4X2	T39.4X3	T39.4X4	T39.4X5	T39.4X6
Automobile fuel	T52.0X1	T52.0X2	T52.0X3	T52.0X4	—	—
Autonomic nervous system agent NEC	T44.901	T44.902	T44.903	T44.904	T44.905	T44.906
Avlosulfon	T37.1X1	T37.1X2	T37.1X3	T37.1X4	T37.1X5	T37.1X6
Avomine	T42.6X1	T42.6X2	T42.6X3	T42.6X4	T42.6X5	T42.6X6
Axerophthol	T45.2X1	T45.2X2	T45.2X3	T45.2X4	T45.2X5	T45.2X6
Azacitidine	T45.1X1	T45.1X2	T45.1X3	T45.1X4	T45.1X5	T45.1X6
Azacyclonol	T43.591	T43.592	T43.593	T43.594	T43.595	T43.596
Azadirachta	T60.2X1	T60.2X2	T60.2X3	T60.2X4	—	—
Azanidazole	T37.3X1	T37.3X2	T37.3X3	T37.3X4	T37.3X5	T37.3X6
Azapetine	T46.7X1	T46.7X2	T46.7X3	T46.7X4	T46.7X5	T46.7X6
Azapropazone	T39.2X1	T39.2X2	T39.2X3	T39.2X4	T39.2X5	T39.2X6
Azaribine	T45.1X1	T45.1X2	T45.1X3	T45.1X4	T45.1X5	T45.1X6
Azaserine	T45.1X1	T45.1X2	T45.1X3	T45.1X4	T45.1X5	T45.1X6
Azatadine	T45.0X1	T45.0X2	T45.0X3	T45.0X4	T45.0X5	T45.0X6
Azatepa	T45.1X1	T45.1X2	T45.1X3	T45.1X4	T45.1X5	T45.1X6
Azathioprine	T45.1X1	T45.1X2	T45.1X3	T45.1X4	T45.1X5	T45.1X6
Azelaic acid	T49.0X1	T49.0X2	T49.0X3	T49.0X4	T49.0X5	T49.0X6
Azelastine	T45.0X1	T45.0X2	T45.0X3	T45.0X4	T45.0X5	T45.0X6
Azidocillin	T36.0X1	T36.0X2	T36.0X3	T36.0X4	T36.0X5	T36.0X6
Azidothymidine	T37.5X1	T37.5X2	T37.5X3	T37.5X4	T37.5X5	T37.5X6

Substance	Poisoning, Accidental (unintentional)	Poisoning, Intentional self-harm	Poisoning, Assault	Poisoning, Undetermined	Adverse effect	Underdosing
Azinphos (ethyl) (methyl)	T60.0X1	T60.0X2	T60.0X3	T60.0X4	—	—
Aziridine (chelating)	T54.1X1	T54.1X2	T54.1X3	T54.1X4	—	—
Azithromycin	T36.3X1	T36.3X2	T36.3X3	T36.3X4	T36.3X5	T36.3X6
Azlocillin	T36.0X1	T36.0X2	T36.0X3	T36.0X4	T36.0X5	T36.0X6
Azobenzene smoke	T65.3X1	T65.3X2	T65.3X3	T65.3X4	—	—
acaricide	T60.8X1	T60.8X2	T60.8X3	T60.8X4	—	—
Azosulfamide	T37.0X1	T37.0X2	T37.0X3	T37.0X4	T37.0X5	T37.0X6
AZT	T37.5X1	T37.5X2	T37.5X3	T37.5X4	T37.5X5	T37.5X6
Aztreonam	T36.1X1	T36.1X2	T36.1X3	T36.1X4	T36.1X5	T36.1X6
Azulfidine	T37.0X1	T37.0X2	T37.0X3	T37.0X4	T37.0X5	T37.0X6
Azuresin	T50.8X1	T50.8X2	T50.8X3	T50.8X4	T50.8X5	T50.8X6
B						
Bacampicillin	T36.0X1	T36.0X2	T36.0X3	T36.0X4	T36.0X5	T36.0X6
Bacillus						
lactobacillus	T47.8X1	T47.8X2	T47.8X3	T47.8X4	T47.8X5	T47.8X6
subtilis	T47.6X1	T47.6X2	T47.6X3	T47.6X4	T47.6X5	T47.6X6
Bacimycin	T49.0X1	T49.0X2	T49.0X3	T49.0X4	T49.0X5	T49.0X6
ophthalmic preparation	T49.5X1	T49.5X2	T49.5X3	T49.5X4	T49.5X5	T49.5X6
Bacitracin zinc	T49.0X1	T49.0X2	T49.0X3	T49.0X4	T49.0X5	T49.0X6
with neomycin	T49.0X1	T49.0X2	T49.0X3	T49.0X4	T49.0X5	T49.0X6
ENT agent	T49.6X1	T49.6X2	T49.6X3	T49.6X4	T49.6X5	T49.6X6
ophthalmic preparation	T49.5X1	T49.5X2	T49.5X3	T49.5X4	T49.5X5	T49.5X6
topical NEC	T49.0X1	T49.0X2	T49.0X3	T49.0X4	T49.0X5	T49.0X6
Baclofen	T42.8X1	T42.8X2	T42.8X3	T42.8X4	T42.8X5	T42.8X6
Baking soda	T50.991	T50.992	T50.993	T50.994	T50.995	T50.996
BAL	T45.8X1	T45.8X2	T45.8X3	T45.8X4	T45.8X5	T45.8X6
Bambuterol	T48.6X1	T48.6X2	T48.6X3	T48.6X4	T48.6X5	T48.6X6
Bamethan (sulfate)	T46.7X1	T46.7X2	T46.7X3	T46.7X4	T46.7X5	T46.7X6
Bamifylline	T48.6X1	T48.6X2	T48.6X3	T48.6X4	T48.6X5	T48.6X6
Bamipine	T45.0X1	T45.0X2	T45.0X3	T45.0X4	T45.0X5	T45.0X6
Baneberry—see Actauseea spicata						
Banewort—see Belladonna						
Barbenyl	T42.3X1	T42.3X2	T42.3X3	T42.3X4	T42.3X5	T42.3X6
Barbexaclone	T42.6X1	T42.6X2	T42.6X3	T42.6X4	T42.6X5	T42.6X6
Barbital	T42.3X1	T42.3X2	T42.3X3	T42.3X4	T42.3X5	T42.3X6
sodium	T42.3X1	T42.3X2	T42.3X3	T42.3X4	T42.3X5	T42.3X6
Barbitone	T42.3X1	T42.3X2	T42.3X3	T42.3X4	T42.3X5	T42.3X6
Barbiturate NEC	T42.3X1	T42.3X2	T42.3X3	T42.3X4	T42.3X5	T42.3X6
with tranquilizer	T42.3X1	T42.3X2	T42.3X3	T42.3X4	T42.3X5	T42.3X6
anesthetic (intravenous)	T41.1X1	T41.1X2	T41.1X3	T41.1X4	T41.1X5	T41.1X6
Barium (carbonate) (chloride) (sulfite)	T57.8X1	T57.8X2	T57.8X3	T57.8X4	—	—
diagnostic agent	T50.8X1	T50.8X2	T50.8X3	T50.8X4	T50.8X5	T50.8X6
pesticide	T60.4X1	T60.4X2	T60.4X3	T60.4X4	—	—
rodenticide	T60.4X1	T60.4X2	T60.4X3	T60.4X4	—	—
sulfate (medicinal)	T50.8X1	T50.8X2	T50.8X3	T50.8X4	T50.8X5	T50.8X6
Barrier cream	T49.3X1	T49.3X2	T49.3X3	T49.3X4	T49.3X5	T49.3X6
Basic fuchsin	T49.0X1	T49.0X2	T49.0X3	T49.0X4	T49.0X5	T49.0X6

Substance	Poisoning, Accidental (unintentional)	Poisoning, Intentional self-harm	Poisoning, Assault	Poisoning, Undetermined	Adverse effect	Underdosing
Battery acid or fluid	T54.2X1	T54.2X2	T54.2X3	T54.2X4	—	—
Bay rum	T51.8X1	T51.8X2	T51.8X3	T51.8X4	—	—
BCG (vaccine)	T50.A91	T50.A92	T50.A93	T50.A94	T50.A95	T50.A96
BCNU	T45.1X1	T45.1X2	T45.1X3	T45.1X4	T45.1X5	T45.1X6
Bearsfoot	T62.2X1	T62.2X2	T62.2X3	T62.2X4	—	—
Beclamide	T42.6X1	T42.6X2	T42.6X3	T42.6X4	T42.6X5	T42.6X6
Beclomethasone	T44.5X1	T44.5X2	T44.5X3	T44.5X4	T44.5X5	T44.5X6
Bee (sting) (venom)	T63.441	T63.442	T63.443	T63.444	—	—
Befunolol	T49.5X1	T49.5X2	T49.5X3	T49.5X4	T49.5X5	T49.5X6
Bekanamycin	T36.5X1	T36.5X2	T36.5X3	T36.5X4	T36.5X5	T36.5X6
Belladonna—see also Nightshade						
alkaloids	T44.3X1	T44.3X2	T44.3X3	T44.3X4	T44.3X5	T44.3X6
extract	T44.3X1	T44.3X2	T44.3X3	T44.3X4	T44.3X5	T44.3X6
herb	T44.3X1	T44.3X2	T44.3X3	T44.3X4	T44.3X5	T44.3X6
Bemegride	T50.7X1	T50.7X2	T50.7X3	T50.7X4	T50.7X5	T50.7X6
Benactyzine	T44.3X1	T44.3X2	T44.3X3	T44.3X4	T44.3X5	T44.3X6
Benadryl	T45.0X1	T45.0X2	T45.0X3	T45.0X4	T45.0X5	T45.0X6
Benaprizine	T44.3X1	T44.3X2	T44.3X3	T44.3X4	T44.3X5	T44.3X6
Benazepril	T46.4X1	T46.4X2	T46.4X3	T46.4X4	T46.4X5	T46.4X6
Bencyclane	T46.7X1	T46.7X2	T46.7X3	T46.7X4	T46.7X5	T46.7X6
Bendazol	T46.3X1	T46.3X2	T46.3X3	T46.3X4	T46.3X5	T46.3X6
Bendrofluazide	T50.2X1	T50.2X2	T50.2X3	T50.2X4	T50.2X5	T50.2X6
Bendroflumethiazide	T50.2X1	T50.2X2	T50.2X3	T50.2X4	T50.2X5	T50.2X6
Benemid	T50.4X1	T50.4X2	T50.4X3	T50.4X4	T50.4X5	T50.4X6
Benethamine penicillin	T36.0X1	T36.0X2	T36.0X3	T36.0X4	T36.0X5	T36.0X6
Benexate	T47.1X1	T47.1X2	T47.1X3	T47.1X4	T47.1X5	T47.1X6
Benfluorex	T46.6X1	T46.6X2	T46.6X3	T46.6X4	T46.6X5	T46.6X6
Benfotiamine	T45.2X1	T45.2X2	T45.2X3	T45.2X4	T45.2X5	T45.2X6
Benisone	T49.0X1	T49.0X2	T49.0X3	T49.0X4	T49.0X5	T49.0X6
Benomyl	T60.0X1	T60.0X2	T60.0X3	T60.0X4	—	—
Benoquin	T49.8X1	T49.8X2	T49.8X3	T49.8X4	T49.8X5	T49.8X6
Benoxinate	T41.3X1	T41.3X2	T41.3X3	T41.3X4	T41.3X5	T41.3X6
Benperidol	T43.4X1	T43.4X2	T43.4X3	T43.4X4	T43.4X5	T43.4X6
Benproperine	T48.3X1	T48.3X2	T48.3X3	T48.3X4	T48.3X5	T48.3X6
Benserazide	T42.8X1	T42.8X2	T42.8X3	T42.8X4	T42.8X5	T42.8X6
Bentazepam	T42.4X1	T42.4X2	T42.4X3	T42.4X4	T42.4X5	T42.4X6
Bentiromide	T50.8X1	T50.8X2	T50.8X3	T50.8X4	T50.8X5	T50.8X6
Bentonite	T49.3X1	T49.3X2	T49.3X3	T49.3X4	T49.3X5	T49.3X6
Benzalbutyramide	T46.6X1	T46.6X2	T46.6X3	T46.6X4	T46.6X5	T46.6X6
Benzalkonium (chloride)	T49.0X1	T49.0X2	T49.0X3	T49.0X4	T49.0X5	T49.0X6
ophthalmic preparation	T49.5X1	T49.5X2	T49.5X3	T49.5X4	T49.5X5	T49.5X6
Benzamidosali cylate (calcium)	T37.1X1	T37.1X2	T37.1X3	T37.1X4	T37.1X5	T37.1X6
Benzamine	T41.3X1	T41.3X2	T41.3X3	T41.3X4	T41.3X5	T41.3X6
lactate	T49.1X1	T49.1X2	T49.1X3	T49.1X4	T49.1X5	T49.1X6
Benzamphetamine	T50.5X1	T50.5X2	T50.5X3	T50.5X4	T50.5X5	T50.5X6
Benzapril hydrochloride	T46.5X1	T46.5X2	T46.5X3	T46.5X4	T46.5X5	T46.5X6
Benzathine benzylpenicillin	T36.0X1	T36.0X2	T36.0X3	T36.0X4	T36.0X5	T36.0X6
Benzathine penicillin	T36.0X1	T36.0X2	T36.0X3	T36.0X4	T36.0X5	T36.0X6

Substance	Poisoning, Accidental (unintentional)	Poisoning, Intentional self-harm	Poisoning, Assault	Poisoning, Undetermined	Adverse effect	Underdosing
Benzatropine	T42.8X1	T42.8X2	T42.8X3	T42.8X4	T42.8X5	T42.8X6
Benzbromarone	T50.4X1	T50.4X2	T50.4X3	T50.4X4	T50.4X5	T50.4X6
Benzcarbimine	T45.1X1	T45.1X2	T45.1X3	T45.1X4	T45.1X5	T45.1X6
Benzedrex	T44.991	T44.992	T44.993	T44.994	T44.995	T44.996
Benzedrine (amphetamine)	T43.621	T43.622	T43.623	T43.624	T43.625	T43.626
Benzenamine	T65.3X1	T65.3X2	T65.3X3	T65.3X4	—	—
Benzene	T52.1X1	T52.1X2	T52.1X3	T52.1X4	—	—
homologues (acetyl) (dimethyl) (methyl) (solvent)	T52.2X1	T52.2X2	T52.2X3	T52.2X4	—	—
Benzethonium (chloride)	T49.0X1	T49.0X2	T49.0X3	T49.0X4	T49.0X5	T49.0X6
Benzfetamine	T50.5X1	T50.5X2	T50.5X3	T50.5X4	T50.5X5	T50.5X6
Benzhexol	T44.3X1	T44.3X2	T44.3X3	T44.3X4	T44.3X5	T44.3X6
Benzhydramine (chloride)	T45.0X1	T45.0X2	T45.0X3	T45.0X4	T45.0X5	T45.0X6
Benzidine	T65.891	T65.892	T65.893	T65.894	—	—
Benzilonium bromide	T44.3X1	T44.3X2	T44.3X3	T44.3X4	T44.3X5	T44.3X6
Benzimidazole	T60.3X1	T60.3X2	T60.3X3	T60.3X4	—	—
Benzin(e)—see Ligroin						
Benziodarone	T46.3X1	T46.3X2	T46.3X3	T46.3X4	T46.3X5	T46.3X6
Benznidazole	T37.3X1	T37.3X2	T37.3X3	T37.3X4	T37.3X5	T37.3X6
Benzocaine	T41.3X1	T41.3X2	T41.3X3	T41.3X4	T41.3X5	T41.3X6
Benzodiapin	T42.4X1	T42.4X2	T42.4X3	T42.4X4	T42.4X5	T42.4X6
Benzodiazepine NEC	T42.4X1	T42.4X2	T42.4X3	T42.4X4	T42.4X5	T42.4X6
Benzoic acid	T49.0X1	T49.0X2	T49.0X3	T49.0X4	T49.0X5	T49.0X6
with salicylic acid	T49.0X1	T49.0X2	T49.0X3	T49.0X4	T49.0X5	T49.0X6
Benzoin (tincture)	T48.5X1	T48.5X2	T48.5X3	T48.5X4	T48.5X5	T48.5X6
Benzol (benzene)	T52.1X1	T52.1X2	T52.1X3	T52.1X4	—	—
vapor	T52.0X1	T52.0X2	T52.0X3	T52.0X4	—	—
Benzomorphan	T40.2X1	T40.2X2	T40.2X3	T40.2X4	T40.2X5	T40.2X6
Benzonatate	T48.3X1	T48.3X2	T48.3X3	T48.3X4	T48.3X5	T48.3X6
Benzophenones	T49.3X1	T49.3X2	T49.3X3	T49.3X4	T49.3X5	T49.3X6
Benzopyrone	T46.991	T46.992	T46.993	T46.994	T46.995	T46.996
Benzothiadiazides	T50.2X1	T50.2X2	T50.2X3	T50.2X4	T50.2X5	T50.2X6
Benzoxonium chloride	T49.0X1	T49.0X2	T49.0X3	T49.0X4	T49.0X5	T49.0X6
Benzoyl peroxide	T49.0X1	T49.0X2	T49.0X3	T49.0X4	T49.0X5	T49.0X6
Benzoylpas calcium	T37.1X1	T37.1X2	T37.1X3	T37.1X4	T37.1X5	T37.1X6
Benzperidin	T43.591	T43.592	T43.593	T43.594	T43.595	T43.596
Benzperidol	T43.591	T43.592	T43.593	T43.594	T43.595	T43.596
Benzphetamine	T50.5X1	T50.5X2	T50.5X3	T50.5X4	T50.5X5	T50.5X6
Benzpyrinium bromide	T44.1X1	T44.1X2	T44.1X3	T44.1X4	T44.1X5	T44.1X6
Benzquinamide	T45.0X1	T45.0X2	T45.0X3	T45.0X4	T45.0X5	T45.0X6
Benzthiazide	T50.2X1	T50.2X2	T50.2X3	T50.2X4	T50.2X5	T50.2X6
Benztropine						
anticholinergic	T44.3X1	T44.3X2	T44.3X3	T44.3X4	T44.3X5	T44.3X6
antiparkinson	T42.8X1	T42.8X2	T42.8X3	T42.8X4	T42.8X5	T42.8X6
Benzydamine	T49.0X1	T49.0X2	T49.0X3	T49.0X4	T49.0X5	T49.0X6
Benzyl						
acetate	T52.8X1	T52.8X2	T52.8X3	T52.8X4	—	—
alcohol	T49.0X1	T49.0X2	T49.0X3	T49.0X4	T49.0X5	T49.0X6
Benzyl — *Continued*						
benzoate	T49.0X1	T49.0X2	T49.0X3	T49.0X4	T49.0X5	T49.0X6
Benzoic acid	T49.0X1	T49.0X2	T49.0X3	T49.0X4	T49.0X5	T49.0X6
morphine	T40.2X1	T40.2X2	T40.2X3	T40.2X4	—	—
nicotinate	T46.6X1	T46.6X2	T46.6X3	T46.6X4	T46.6X5	T46.6X6
penicillin	T36.0X1	T36.0X2	T36.0X3	T36.0X4	T36.0X5	T36.0X6
Benzylhydrochl-orthia-zide	T50.2X1	T50.2X2	T50.2X3	T50.2X4	T50.2X5	T50.2X6
Benzylpenicillin	T36.0X1	T36.0X2	T36.0X3	T36.0X4	T36.0X5	T36.0X6
Benzylthiouracil	T38.2X1	T38.2X2	T38.2X3	T38.2X4	T38.2X5	T38.2X6
Bephenium hydroxy-naphthoate	T37.4X1	T37.4X2	T37.4X3	T37.4X4	T37.4X5	T37.4X6
Bepridil	T46.1X1	T46.1X2	T46.1X3	T46.1X4	T46.1X5	T46.1X6
Bergamot oil	T65.891	T65.892	T65.893	T65.894	—	—
Bergapten	T50.991	T50.992	T50.993	T50.994	T50.995	T50.996
Berries, poisonous	T62.1X1	T62.1X2	T62.1X3	T62.1X4	—	—
Beryllium (compounds)	T56.7X1	T56.7X2	T56.7X3	T56.7X4	—	—
b-acetyldigoxin	T46.0X1	T46.0X2	T46.0X3	T46.0X4	T46.0X5	T46.0X6
beta adrenergic blocking agent, heart	T44.7X1	T44.7X2	T44.7X3	T44.7X4	T44.7X5	T44.7X6
b-benzalbutyramide	T46.6X1	T46.6X2	T46.6X3	T46.6X4	T46.6X5	T46.6X6
Betacarotene	T45.2X1	T45.2X2	T45.2X3	T45.2X4	T45.2X5	T45.2X6
b-eucaine	T49.1X1	T49.1X2	T49.1X3	T49.1X4	T49.1X5	T49.1X6
Beta-Chlor	T42.6X1	T42.6X2	T42.6X3	T42.6X4	T42.6X5	T42.6X6
b-galactosidase	T47.5X1	T47.5X2	T47.5X3	T47.5X4	T47.5X5	T47.5X6
Betahistine	T46.7X1	T46.7X2	T46.7X3	T46.7X4	T46.7X5	T46.7X6
Betaine	T47.5X1	T47.5X2	T47.5X3	T47.5X4	T47.5X5	T47.5X6
Betamethasone	T49.0X1	T49.0X2	T49.0X3	T49.0X4	T49.0X5	T49.0X6
topical	T49.0X1	T49.0X2	T49.0X3	T49.0X4	T49.0X5	T49.0X6
Betamicin	T36.8X1	T36.8X2	T36.8X3	T36.8X4	T36.8X5	T36.8X6
Betanidine	T46.5X1	T46.5X2	T46.5X3	T46.5X4	T46.5X5	T46.5X6
b-sitosterol(s)	T46.6X1	T46.6X2	T46.6X3	T46.6X4	T46.6X5	T46.6X6
Betaxolol	T44.7X1	T44.7X2	T44.7X3	T44.7X4	T44.7X5	T44.7X6
Betazole	T50.8X1	T50.8X2	T50.8X3	T50.8X4	T50.8X5	T50.8X6
Bethanechol	T44.1X1	T44.1X2	T44.1X3	T44.1X4	T44.1X5	T44.1X6
chloride	T44.1X1	T44.1X2	T44.1X3	T44.1X4	T44.1X5	T44.1X6
Bethanidine	T46.5X1	T46.5X2	T46.5X3	T46.5X4	T46.5X5	T46.5X6
Betoxycaine	T41.3X1	T41.3X2	T41.3X3	T41.3X4	T41.3X5	T41.3X6
Betula oil	T49.3X1	T49.3X2	T49.3X3	T49.3X4	T49.3X5	T49.3X6
Bevantolol	T44.7X1	T44.7X2	T44.7X3	T44.7X4	T44.7X5	T44.7X6
Bevonium metilsulfate	T44.3X1	T44.3X2	T44.3X3	T44.3X4	T44.3X5	T44.3X6
Bezafibrate	T46.6X1	T46.6X2	T46.6X3	T46.6X4	T46.6X5	T46.6X6
Bezitramide	T40.491	T40.492	T40.493	T40.494	T40.495	T40.496
BHA	T50.991	T50.992	T50.993	T50.994	T50.995	T50.996
Bhang	T40.711	T40.712	T40.713	T40.714	T40.715	T40.716
BHC (medicinal)	T49.0X1	T49.0X2	T49.0X3	T49.0X4	T49.0X5	T49.0X6
nonmedicinal (vapor)	T53.6X1	T53.6X2	T53.6X3	T53.6X4	—	—
Bialamicol	T37.3X1	T37.3X2	T37.3X3	T37.3X4	T37.3X5	T37.3X6
Bibenzonium bromide	T48.3X1	T48.3X2	T48.3X3	T48.3X4	T48.3X5	T48.3X6
Bibrocathol	T49.5X1	T49.5X2	T49.5X3	T49.5X4	T49.5X5	T49.5X6
Bichloride of mercury—see Mercury, chloride						

Substance	Poisoning, Accidental (unintentional)	Poisoning, Intentional self-harm	Poisoning, Assault	Poisoning, Undetermined	Adverse effect	Underdosing
Bichromates (calcium) (potassium) (sodium) (crystals)	T57.8X1	T57.8X2	T57.8X3	T57.8X4	—	—
fumes	T56.2X1	T56.2X2	T56.2X3	T56.2X4	—	—
Biclotymol	T49.6X1	T49.6X2	T49.6X3	T49.6X4	T49.6X5	T49.6X6
Bicucculine	T50.7X1	T50.7X2	T50.7X3	T50.7X4	T50.7X5	T50.7X6
Bifemelane	T43.291	T43.292	T43.293	T43.294	T43.295	T43.296
Biguanide derivatives, oral	T38.3X1	T38.3X2	T38.3X3	T38.3X4	T38.3X5	T38.3X6
Bile salts	T47.5X1	T47.5X2	T47.5X3	T47.5X4	T47.5X5	T47.5X6
Biligrafin	T50.8X1	T50.8X2	T50.8X3	T50.8X4	T50.8X5	T50.8X6
Bilopaque	T50.8X1	T50.8X2	T50.8X3	T50.8X4	T50.8X5	T50.8X6
Binifibrate	T46.6X1	T46.6X2	T46.6X3	T46.6X4	T46.6X5	T46.6X6
Binitrobenzol	T65.3X1	T65.3X2	T65.3X3	T65.3X4	—	—
Bioflavonoid(s)	T46.991	T46.992	T46.993	T46.994	T46.995	T46.996
Biological substance NEC	T50.901	T50.902	T50.903	T50.904	T50.905	T50.906
Biotin	T45.2X1	T45.2X2	T45.2X3	T45.2X4	T45.2X5	T45.2X6
Biperiden	T44.3X1	T44.3X2	T44.3X3	T44.3X4	T44.3X5	T44.3X6
Bisacodyl	T47.2X1	T47.2X2	T47.2X3	T47.2X4	T47.2X5	T47.2X6
Bisbentiamine	T45.2X1	T45.2X2	T45.2X3	T45.2X4	T45.2X5	T45.2X6
Bisbutiamine	T45.2X1	T45.2X2	T45.2X3	T45.2X4	T45.2X5	T45.2X6
Bisdequalinium (salts) (diacetate)	T49.6X1	T49.6X2	T49.6X3	T49.6X4	T49.6X5	T49.6X6
Bishydroxycoumarin	T45.511	T45.512	T45.513	T45.514	T45.515	T45.516
Bismarsen	T37.8X1	T37.8X2	T37.8X3	T37.8X4	T37.8X5	T37.8X6
Bismuth salts	T47.6X1	T47.6X2	T47.6X3	T47.6X4	T47.6X5	T47.6X6
aluminate	T47.1X1	T47.1X2	T47.1X3	T47.1X4	T47.1X5	T47.1X6
anti-infectives	T37.8X1	T37.8X2	T37.8X3	T37.8X4	T37.8X5	T37.8X6
formic iodide	T49.0X1	T49.0X2	T49.0X3	T49.0X4	T49.0X5	T49.0X6
glycolylarsenate	T49.0X1	T49.0X2	T49.0X3	T49.0X4	T49.0X5	T49.0X6
nonmedicinal (compounds) NEC	T65.91	T65.92	T65.93	T65.94	—	—
subcarbonate	T47.6X1	T47.6X2	T47.6X3	T47.6X4	T47.6X5	T47.6X6
subsalicylate	T37.8X1	T37.8X2	T37.8X3	T37.8X4	T37.8X5	T37.8X6
sulfarsphenamine	T37.8X1	T37.8X2	T37.8X3	T37.8X4	T37.8X5	T37.8X6
Bisoprolol	T44.7X1	T44.7X2	T44.7X3	T44.7X4	T44.7X5	T44.7X6
Bisoxatin	T47.2X1	T47.2X2	T47.2X3	T47.2X4	T47.2X5	T47.2X6
Bisulepin (hydrochloride)	T45.0X1	T45.0X2	T45.0X3	T45.0X4	T45.0X5	T45.0X6
Bithionol	T37.8X1	T37.8X2	T37.8X3	T37.8X4	T37.8X5	T37.8X6
anthelminthic	T37.4X1	T37.4X2	T37.4X3	T37.4X4	T37.4X5	T37.4X6
Bitolterol	T48.6X1	T48.6X2	T48.6X3	T48.6X4	T48.6X5	T48.6X6
Bitoscanate	T37.4X1	T37.4X2	T37.4X3	T37.4X4	T37.4X5	T37.4X6
Bitter almond oil	T62.8X1	T62.8X2	T62.8X3	T62.8X4	—	—
Bittersweet	T62.2X1	T62.2X2	T62.2X3	T62.2X4	—	—
Black						
flag	T60.91	T60.92	T60.93	T60.94	—	—
henbane	T62.2X1	T62.2X2	T62.2X3	T62.2X4	—	—
leaf (40)	T60.91	T60.92	T60.93	T60.94	—	—
widow spider (bite)	T63.311	T63.312	T63.313	T63.314	—	—
antivenin	T50.Z11	T50.Z12	T50.Z13	T50.Z14	T50.Z15	T50.Z16

Substance	Poisoning, Accidental (unintentional)	Poisoning, Intentional self-harm	Poisoning, Assault	Poisoning, Undetermined	Adverse effect	Underdosing
Blast furnace gas (carbon monoxide from)	T58.8X1	T58.8X2	T58.8X3	T58.8X4	—	—
Bleach	T54.91	T54.92	T54.93	T54.94	—	—
Bleaching agent (medicinal)	T49.4X1	T49.4X2	T49.4X3	T49.4X4	T49.4X5	T49.4X6
Bleomycin	T45.1X1	T45.1X2	T45.1X3	T45.1X4	T45.1X5	T45.1X6
Blockain	T41.3X1	T41.3X2	T41.3X3	T41.3X4	T41.3X5	T41.3X6
infiltration (subcutaneous)	T41.3X1	T41.3X2	T41.3X3	T41.3X4	T41.3X5	T41.3X6
nerve block (peripheral) (plexus)	T41.3X1	T41.3X2	T41.3X3	T41.3X4	T41.3X5	T41.3X6
topical (surface)	T41.3X1	T41.3X2	T41.3X3	T41.3X4	T41.3X5	T41.3X6
Blockers, calcium channel	T46.1X1	T46.1X2	T46.1X3	T46.1X4	T46.1X5	T46.1X6
Blood (derivatives) (natural) (plasma) (whole)	T45.8X1	T45.8X2	T45.8X3	T45.8X4	T45.8X5	T45.8X6
dried	T45.8X1	T45.8X2	T45.8X3	T45.8X4	T45.8X5	T45.8X6
drug affecting NEC	T45.91	T45.92	T45.93	T45.94	T45.95	T45.96
expander NEC	T45.8X1	T45.8X2	T45.8X3	T45.8X4	T45.8X5	T45.8X6
fraction NEC	T45.8X1	T45.8X2	T45.8X3	T45.8X4	T45.8X5	T45.8X6
substitute (macromolecular)	T45.8X1	T45.8X2	T45.8X3	T45.8X4	T45.8X5	T45.8X6
Blue velvet	T40.2X1	T40.2X2	T40.2X3	T40.2X4	—	—
Bone meal	T62.8X1	T62.8X2	T62.8X3	T62.8X4	—	—
Bonine	T45.0X1	T45.0X2	T45.0X3	T45.0X4	T45.0X5	T45.0X6
Bopindolol	T44.7X1	T44.7X2	T44.7X3	T44.7X4	T44.7X5	T44.7X6
Boracic acid	T49.0X1	T49.0X2	T49.0X3	T49.0X4	T49.0X5	T49.0X6
ENT agent	T49.6X1	T49.6X2	T49.6X3	T49.6X4	T49.6X5	T49.6X6
ophthalmic preparation	T49.5X1	T49.5X2	T49.5X3	T49.5X4	T49.5X5	T49.5X6
Borane complex	T57.8X1	T57.8X2	T57.8X3	T57.8X4	—	—
Borate (s)	T57.8X1	T57.8X2	T57.8X3	T57.8X4	—	—
buffer	T50.991	T50.992	T50.993	T50.994	T50.995	T50.996
cleanser	T54.91	T54.92	T54.93	T54.94	—	—
sodium	T57.8X1	T57.8X2	T57.8X3	T57.8X4	—	—
Borax (cleanser)	T54.91	T54.92	T54.93	T54.94	—	—
Bordeaux mixture	T60.3X1	T60.3X2	T60.3X3	T60.3X4	—	—
Boric acid	T49.0X1	T49.0X2	T49.0X3	T49.0X4	T49.0X5	T49.0X6
ENT agent	T49.6X1	T49.6X2	T49.6X3	T49.6X4	T49.6X5	T49.6X6
ophthalmic preparation	T49.5X1	T49.5X2	T49.5X3	T49.5X4	T49.5X5	T49.5X6
Bornaprine	T44.3X1	T44.3X2	T44.3X3	T44.3X4	T44.3X5	T44.3X6
Boron	T57.8X1	T57.8X2	T57.8X3	T57.8X4	—	—
hydride NEC	T57.8X1	T57.8X2	T57.8X3	T57.8X4	—	—
fumes or gas	T57.8X1	T57.8X2	T57.8X3	T57.8X4	—	—
trifluoride	T59.891	T59.892	T59.893	T59.894	—	—
Botox	T48.291	T48.292	T48.293	T48.294	T48.295	T48.296
Botulinus anti-toxin (type A, B)	T50.Z11	T50.Z12	T50.Z13	T50.Z14	T50.Z15	T50.Z16
Brake fluid vapor	T59.891	T59.892	T59.893	T59.894	—	—
Brallobarbital	T42.3X1	T42.3X2	T42.3X3	T42.3X4	T42.3X5	T42.3X6
Bran (wheat)	T47.4X1	T47.4X2	T47.4X3	T47.4X4	T47.4X5	T47.4X6
Brass (fumes)	T56.891	T56.892	T56.893	T56.894	—	—

Substance	Poisoning, Accidental (unintentional)	Poisoning, Intentional self-harm	Poisoning, Assault	Poisoning, Undetermined	Adverse effect	Underdosing
Brasso	T52.0X1	T52.0X2	T52.0X3	T52.0X4	—	—
Bretylium tosilate	T46.2X1	T46.2X2	T46.2X3	T46.2X4	T46.2X5	T46.2X6
Brevital (sodium)	T41.1X1	T41.1X2	T41.1X3	T41.1X4	T41.1X5	T41.1X6
Brinase	T45.3X1	T45.3X2	T45.3X3	T45.3X4	T45.3X5	T45.3X6
British antilewisite	T45.8X1	T45.8X2	T45.8X3	T45.8X4	T45.8X5	T45.8X6
Brodifacoum	T60.4X1	T60.4X2	T60.4X3	T60.4X4	—	—
Bromal (hydrate)	T42.6X1	T42.6X2	T42.6X3	T42.6X4	T42.6X5	T42.6X6
Bromazepam	T42.4X1	T42.4X2	T42.4X3	T42.4X4	T42.4X5	T42.4X6
Bromazine	T45.0X1	T45.0X2	T45.0X3	T45.0X4	T45.0X5	T45.0X6
Brombenzylcyanide	T59.3X1	T59.3X2	T59.3X3	T59.3X4	—	—
Bromelains	T45.3X1	T45.3X2	T45.3X3	T45.3X4	T45.3X5	T45.3X6
Bromethalin	T60.4X1	T60.4X2	T60.4X3	T60.4X4	—	—
Bromhexine	T48.4X1	T48.4X2	T48.4X3	T48.4X4	T48.4X5	T48.4X6
Bromide salts	T42.6X1	T42.6X2	T42.6X3	T42.6X4	T42.6X5	T42.6X6
Bromindione	T45.511	T45.512	T45.513	T45.514	T45.515	T45.516
Bromine						
compounds (medicinal)	T42.6X1	T42.6X2	T42.6X3	T42.6X4	T42.6X5	T42.6X6
sedative	T42.6X1	T42.6X2	T42.6X3	T42.6X4	T42.6X5	T42.6X6
vapor	T59.891	T59.892	T59.893	T59.894	—	—
Bromisoval	T42.6X1	T42.6X2	T42.6X3	T42.6X4	T42.6X5	T42.6X6
Bromisovalum	T42.6X1	T42.6X2	T42.6X3	T42.6X4	T42.6X5	T42.6X6
Bromobenzylcyanide	T59.3X1	T59.3X2	T59.3X3	T59.3X4	—	—
Bromochloro-salicylanilide	T49.0X1	T49.0X2	T49.0X3	T49.0X4	T49.0X5	T49.0X6
Bromocriptine	T42.8X1	T42.8X2	T42.8X3	T42.8X4	T42.8X5	T42.8X6
Bromodiphenhydramine	T45.0X1	T45.0X2	T45.0X3	T45.0X4	T45.0X5	T45.0X6
Bromoform	T42.6X1	T42.6X2	T42.6X3	T42.6X4	T42.6X5	T42.6X6
Bromophenol blue reagent	T50.991	T50.992	T50.993	T50.994	T50.995	T50.996
Bromopride	T47.8X1	T47.8X2	T47.8X3	T47.8X4	T47.8X5	T47.8X6
Bromosalicyl chloranitide	T49.0X1	T49.0X2	T49.0X3	T49.0X4	T49.0X5	T49.0X6
Bromosalicyl hydroxamic acid	T37.1X1	T37.1X2	T37.1X3	T37.1X4	T37.1X5	T37.1X6
Bromo-seltzer	T39.1X1	T39.1X2	T39.1X3	T39.1X4	T39.1X5	T39.1X6
Bromoxynil	T60.3X1	T60.3X2	T60.3X3	T60.3X4	—	—
Bromperidol	T43.4X1	T43.4X2	T43.4X3	T43.4X4	T43.4X5	T43.4X6
Brompheniramine	T45.0X1	T45.0X2	T45.0X3	T45.0X4	T45.0X5	T45.0X6
Bromsulfophthalein	T50.8X1	T50.8X2	T50.8X3	T50.8X4	T50.8X5	T50.8X6
Bromural	T42.6X1	T42.6X2	T42.6X3	T42.6X4	T42.6X5	T42.6X6
Bromvaletone	T42.6X1	T42.6X2	T42.6X3	T42.6X4	T42.6X5	T42.6X6
Bronchodilator NEC	T48.6X1	T48.6X2	T48.6X3	T48.6X4	T48.6X5	T48.6X6
Brotizolam	T42.4X1	T42.4X2	T42.4X3	T42.4X4	T42.4X5	T42.4X6
Brovincamine	T46.7X1	T46.7X2	T46.7X3	T46.7X4	T46.7X5	T46.7X6
Brown recluse spider (bite) (venom)	T63.331	T63.332	T63.333	T63.334	—	—
Brown spider (bite) (venom)	T63.391	T63.392	T63.393	T63.394	—	—
Broxaterol	T48.6X1	T48.6X2	T48.6X3	T48.6X4	T48.6X5	T48.6X6
Broxuridine	T45.1X1	T45.1X2	T45.1X3	T45.1X4	T45.1X5	T45.1X6

Substance	Poisoning, Accidental (unintentional)	Poisoning, Intentional self-harm	Poisoning, Assault	Poisoning, Undetermined	Adverse effect	Underdosing
Broxyquinoline	T37.8X1	T37.8X2	T37.8X3	T37.8X4	T37.8X5	T37.8X6
Bruceine	T48.291	T48.292	T48.293	T48.294	T48.295	T48.296
Brucia	T62.2X1	T62.2X2	T62.2X3	T62.2X4	—	—
Brucine	T65.1X1	T65.1X2	T65.1X3	T65.1X4	—	—
Brunswick green—see Copper						
Bruten—see Ibuprofen						
Bryonia	T47.2X1	T47.2X2	T47.2X3	T47.2X4	T47.2X5	T47.2X6
Buclizine	T45.0X1	T45.0X2	T45.0X3	T45.0X4	T45.0X5	T45.0X6
Buclosamide	T49.0X1	T49.0X2	T49.0X3	T49.0X4	T49.0X5	T49.0X6
Budesonide	T44.5X1	T44.5X2	T44.5X3	T44.5X4	T44.5X5	T44.5X6
Budralazine	T46.5X1	T46.5X2	T46.5X3	T46.5X4	T46.5X5	T46.5X6
Bufferin	T39.011	T39.012	T39.013	T39.014	T39.015	T39.016
Buflomedil	T46.7X1	T46.7X2	T46.7X3	T46.7X4	T46.7X5	T46.7X6
Buformin	T38.3X1	T38.3X2	T38.3X3	T38.3X4	T38.3X5	T38.3X6
Bufotenine	T40.991	T40.992	T40.993	T40.994	—	—
Bufrolin	T48.6X1	T48.6X2	T48.6X3	T48.6X4	T48.6X5	T48.6X6
Bufylline	T48.6X1	T48.6X2	T48.6X3	T48.6X4	T48.6X5	T48.6X6
Bulk filler	T50.5X1	T50.5X2	T50.5X3	T50.5X4	T50.5X5	T50.5X6
cathartic	T47.4X1	T47.4X2	T47.4X3	T47.4X4	T47.4X5	T47.4X6
Bumetanide	T50.1X1	T50.1X2	T50.1X3	T50.1X4	T50.1X5	T50.1X6
Bunaftine	T46.2X1	T46.2X2	T46.2X3	T46.2X4	T46.2X5	T46.2X6
Bunamiodyl	T50.8X1	T50.8X2	T50.8X3	T50.8X4	T50.8X5	T50.8X6
Bunazosin	T44.6X1	T44.6X2	T44.6X3	T44.6X4	T44.6X5	T44.6X6
Bunitrolol	T44.7X1	T44.7X2	T44.7X3	T44.7X4	T44.7X5	T44.7X6
Buphenine	T46.7X1	T46.7X2	T46.7X3	T46.7X4	T46.7X5	T46.7X6
Bupivacaine	T41.3X1	T41.3X2	T41.3X3	T41.3X4	T41.3X5	T41.3X6
infiltration (subcutaneous)	T41.3X1	T41.3X2	T41.3X3	T41.3X4	T41.3X5	T41.3X6
nerve block (peripheral) (plexus)	T41.3X1	T41.3X2	T41.3X3	T41.3X4	T41.3X5	T41.3X6
spinal	T41.3X1	T41.3X2	T41.3X3	T41.3X4	T41.3X5	T41.3X6
Bupranolol	T44.7X1	T44.7X2	T44.7X3	T44.7X4	T44.7X5	T44.7X6
Buprenorphine	T40.491	T40.492	T40.493	T40.494	T40.495	T40.496
Bupropion	T43.291	T43.292	T43.293	T43.294	T43.295	T43.296
Burimamide	T47.1X1	T47.1X2	T47.1X3	T47.1X4	T47.1X5	T47.1X6
Buserelin	T38.891	T38.892	T38.893	T38.894	T38.895	T38.896
Buspirone	T43.591	T43.592	T43.593	T43.594	T43.595	T43.596
Busulfan, busulphan	T45.1X1	T45.1X2	T45.1X3	T45.1X4	T45.1X5	T45.1X6
Butabarbital (sodium)	T42.3X1	T42.3X2	T42.3X3	T42.3X4	T42.3X5	T42.3X6
Butabarbitone	T42.3X1	T42.3X2	T42.3X3	T42.3X4	T42.3X5	T42.3X6
Butabarpal	T42.3X1	T42.3X2	T42.3X3	T42.3X4	T42.3X5	T42.3X6
Butacaine	T41.3X1	T41.3X2	T41.3X3	T41.3X4	T41.3X5	T41.3X6
Butalamine	T46.7X1	T46.7X2	T46.7X3	T46.7X4	T46.7X5	T46.7X6
Butalbital	T42.3X1	T42.3X2	T42.3X3	T42.3X4	T42.3X5	T42.3X6
Butallylonal	T42.3X1	T42.3X2	T42.3X3	T42.3X4	T42.3X5	T42.3X6
Butamben	T41.3X1	T41.3X2	T41.3X3	T41.3X4	T41.3X5	T41.3X6
Butamirate	T48.3X1	T48.3X2	T48.3X3	T48.3X4	T48.3X5	T48.3X6

Substance	Poisoning, Accidental (unintentional)	Poisoning, Intentional self-harm	Poisoning, Assault	Poisoning, Undetermined	Adverse effect	Underdosing
Butane (distributed in mobile container)	T59.891	T59.892	T59.893	T59.894	—	—
distributed through pipes	T59.891	T59.892	T59.893	T59.894	—	—
incomplete combustion	T58.11	T58.12	T58.13	T58.14	—	—
Butanilicaine	T41.3X1	T41.3X2	T41.3X3	T41.3X4	T41.3X5	T41.3X6
Butanol	T51.3X1	T51.3X2	T51.3X3	T51.3X4	—	—
Butanone, 2-butanone	T52.4X1	T52.4X2	T52.4X3	T52.4X4	—	—
Butantrone	T49.4X1	T49.4X2	T49.4X3	T49.4X4	T49.4X5	T49.4X6
Butaperazine	T43.3X1	T43.3X2	T43.3X3	T43.3X4	T43.3X5	T43.3X6
Butazolidin	T39.2X1	T39.2X2	T39.2X3	T39.2X4	T39.2X5	T39.2X6
Butetamate	T48.6X1	T48.6X2	T48.6X3	T48.6X4	T48.6X5	T48.6X6
Butethal	T42.3X1	T42.3X2	T42.3X3	T42.3X4	T42.3X5	T42.3X6
Butethamate	T44.3X1	T44.3X2	T44.3X3	T44.3X4	T44.3X5	T44.3X6
Buthalitone (sodium)	T41.1X1	T41.1X2	T41.1X3	T41.1X4	T41.1X5	T41.1X6
Butisol (sodium)	T42.3X1	T42.3X2	T42.3X3	T42.3X4	T42.3X5	T42.3X6
Butizide	T50.2X1	T50.2X2	T50.2X3	T50.2X4	T50.2X5	T50.2X6
Butobarbital	T42.3X1	T42.3X2	T42.3X3	T42.3X4	T42.3X5	T42.3X6
sodium	T42.3X1	T42.3X2	T42.3X3	T42.3X4	T42.3X5	T42.3X6
Butobarbitone	T42.3X1	T42.3X2	T42.3X3	T42.3X4	T42.3X5	T42.3X6
Butoconazole (nitrate)	T49.0X1	T49.0X2	T49.0X3	T49.0X4	T49.0X5	T49.0X6
Butorphanol	T40.491	T40.492	T40.493	T40.494	T40.495	T40.496
Butriptyline	T43.011	T43.012	T43.013	T43.014	T43.015	T43.016
Butropium bromide	T44.3X1	T44.3X2	T44.3X3	T44.3X4	T44.3X5	T44.3X6
Butter of antimony—see Antimony						
Buttercups	T62.2X1	T62.2X2	T62.2X3	T62.2X4	—	—
Butyl						
acetate (secondary)	T52.8X1	T52.8X2	T52.8X3	T52.8X4	—	—
alcohol	T51.3X1	T51.3X2	T51.3X3	T51.3X4	—	—
aminobenzoate	T41.3X1	T41.3X2	T41.3X3	T41.3X4	T41.3X5	T41.3X6
butyrate	T52.8X1	T52.8X2	T52.8X3	T52.8X4	—	—
carbinol	T51.3X1	T51.3X2	T51.3X3	T51.3X4	—	—
carbitol	T52.3X1	T52.3X2	T52.3X3	T52.3X4	—	—
cellosolve	T52.3X1	T52.3X2	T52.3X3	T52.3X4	—	—
chloral (hydrate)	T42.6X1	T42.6X2	T42.6X3	T42.6X4	T42.6X5	T42.6X6
formate	T52.8X1	T52.8X2	T52.8X3	T52.8X4	—	—
lactate	T52.8X1	T52.8X2	T52.8X3	T52.8X4	—	—
propionate	T52.8X1	T52.8X2	T52.8X3	T52.8X4	—	—
scopolamine bromide	T44.3X1	T44.3X2	T44.3X3	T44.3X4	T44.3X5	T44.3X6
thiobarbital sodium	T41.1X1	T41.1X2	T41.1X3	T41.1X4	T41.1X5	T41.1X6
Butylated hydroxy-anisole	T50.991	T50.992	T50.993	T50.994	T50.995	T50.996
Butylchloral hydrate	T42.6X1	T42.6X2	T42.6X3	T42.6X4	T42.6X5	T42.6X6
Butyltoluene	T52.2X1	T52.2X2	T52.2X3	T52.2X4	—	—
Butyn	T41.3X1	T41.3X2	T41.3X3	T41.3X4	T41.3X5	T41.3X6
Butyrophenone (-based tranquilizers)	T43.4X1	T43.4X2	T43.4X3	T43.4X4	T43.4X5	T43.4X6
C						
Cabergoline	T42.8X1	T42.8X2	T42.8X3	T42.8X4	T42.8X5	T42.8X6
Cacodyl, cacodylic acid	T57.0X1	T57.0X2	T57.0X3	T57.0X4	—	—
Cactinomycin	T45.1X1	T45.1X2	T45.1X3	T45.1X4	T45.1X5	T45.1X6
Cade oil	T49.4X1	T49.4X2	T49.4X3	T49.4X4	T49.4X5	T49.4X6
Cadexomer iodine	T49.0X1	T49.0X2	T49.0X3	T49.0X4	T49.0X5	T49.0X6
Cadmium (chloride) (fumes) (oxide)	T56.3X1	T56.3X2	T56.3X3	T56.3X4	—	—
sulfide (medicinal) NEC	T49.4X1	T49.4X2	T49.4X3	T49.4X4	T49.4X5	T49.4X6
Cadralazine	T46.5X1	T46.5X2	T46.5X3	T46.5X4	T46.5X5	T46.5X6
Caffeine	T43.611	T43.612	T43.613	T43.614	T43.615	T43.616
Calabar bean	T62.2X1	T62.2X2	T62.2X3	T62.2X4	—	—
Caladium seguinum	T62.2X1	T62.2X2	T62.2X3	T62.2X4	—	—
Calamine (lotion)	T49.3X1	T49.3X2	T49.3X3	T49.3X4	T49.3X5	T49.3X6
Calcifediol	T45.2X1	T45.2X2	T45.2X3	T45.2X4	T45.2X5	T45.2X6
Calciferol	T45.2X1	T45.2X2	T45.2X3	T45.2X4	T45.2X5	T45.2X6
Calcitonin	T50.991	T50.992	T50.993	T50.994	T50.995	T50.996
Calcitriol	T45.2X1	T45.2X2	T45.2X3	T45.2X4	T45.2X5	T45.2X6
Calcium	T50.3X1	T50.3X2	T50.3X3	T50.3X4	T50.3X5	T50.3X6
actylsalicylate	T39.011	T39.012	T39.013	T39.014	T39.015	T39.016
benzamidosalicylate	T37.1X1	T37.1X2	T37.1X3	T37.1X4	T37.1X5	T37.1X6
bromide	T42.6X1	T42.6X2	T42.6X3	T42.6X4	T42.6X5	T42.6X6
bromolactobionate	T42.6X1	T42.6X2	T42.6X3	T42.6X4	T42.6X5	T42.6X6
carbaspirin	T39.011	T39.012	T39.013	T39.014	T39.015	T39.016
carbimide	T50.6X1	T50.6X2	T50.6X3	T50.6X4	T50.6X5	T50.6X6
carbonate	T47.1X1	T47.1X2	T47.1X3	T47.1X4	T47.1X5	T47.1X6
chloride	T50.991	T50.992	T50.993	T50.994	T50.995	T50.996
anhydrous	T50.991	T50.992	T50.993	T50.994	T50.995	T50.996
cyanide	T57.8X1	T57.8X2	T57.8X3	T57.8X4	—	—
dioctyl sulfosuccinate	T47.4X1	T47.4X2	T47.4X3	T47.4X4	T47.4X5	T47.4X6
disodium edathamil	T45.8X1	T45.8X2	T45.8X3	T45.8X4	T45.8X5	T45.8X6
disodium edetate	T45.8X1	T45.8X2	T45.8X3	T45.8X4	T45.8X5	T45.8X6
dobesilate	T46.991	T46.992	T46.993	T46.994	T46.995	T46.996
EDTA	T45.8X1	T45.8X2	T45.8X3	T45.8X4	T45.8X5	T45.8X6
ferrous citrate	T45.4X1	T45.4X2	T45.4X3	T45.4X4	T45.4X5	T45.4X6
folinate	T45.8X1	T45.8X2	T45.8X3	T45.8X4	T45.8X5	T45.8X6
glubionate	T50.3X1	T50.3X2	T50.3X3	T50.3X4	T50.3X5	T50.3X6
gluconate	T50.3X1	T50.3X2	T50.3X3	T50.3X4	T50.3X5	T50.3X6
gluconoga-lactogluconate	T50.3X1	T50.3X2	T50.3X3	T50.3X4	T50.3X5	T50.3X6
hydrate, hydroxide	T54.3X1	T54.3X2	T54.3X3	T54.3X4	—	—
hypochlorite	T54.3X1	T54.3X2	T54.3X3	T54.3X4	—	—
iodide	T48.4X1	T48.4X2	T48.4X3	T48.4X4	T48.4X5	T48.4X6
ipodate	T50.8X1	T50.8X2	T50.8X3	T50.8X4	T50.8X5	T50.8X6
lactate	T50.3X1	T50.3X2	T50.3X3	T50.3X4	T50.3X5	T50.3X6
leucovorin	T45.8X1	T45.8X2	T45.8X3	T45.8X4	T45.8X5	T45.8X6
mandelate	T37.91	T37.92	T37.93	T37.94	T37.95	T37.96
oxide	T54.3X1	T54.3X2	T54.3X3	T54.3X4	—	—
pantothenate	T45.2X1	T45.2X2	T45.2X3	T45.2X4	T45.2X5	T45.2X6
phosphate	T50.3X1	T50.3X2	T50.3X3	T50.3X4	T50.3X5	T50.3X6
salicylate	T39.091	T39.092	T39.093	T39.094	T39.095	T39.096
salts	T50.3X1	T50.3X2	T50.3X3	T50.3X4	T50.3X5	T50.3X6
Calculus-dissolving drug	T50.991	T50.992	T50.993	T50.994	T50.995	T50.996
Calomel	T49.0X1	T49.0X2	T49.0X3	T49.0X4	T49.0X5	T49.0X6
Caloric agent	T50.3X1	T50.3X2	T50.3X3	T50.3X4	T50.3X5	T50.3X6

Substance	Poisoning, Accidental (unintentional)	Poisoning, Intentional self-harm	Poisoning, Assault	Poisoning, Undetermined	Adverse effect	Underdosing
Calusterone	T38.7X1	T38.7X2	T38.7X3	T38.7X4	T38.7X5	T38.7X6
Camazepam	T42.4X1	T42.4X2	T42.4X3	T42.4X4	T42.4X5	T42.4X6
Camomile	T49.0X1	T49.0X2	T49.0X3	T49.0X4	T49.0X5	T49.0X6
Camoquin	T37.2X1	T37.2X2	T37.2X3	T37.2X4	T37.2X5	T37.2X6
Camphor						
insecticide	T60.2X1	T60.2X2	T60.2X3	T60.2X4	—	—
medicinal	T49.8X1	T49.8X2	T49.8X3	T49.8X4	T49.8X5	T49.8X6
Camylofin	T44.3X1	T44.3X2	T44.3X3	T44.3X4	T44.3X5	T44.3X6
Cancer chemotherapy drug regimen	T45.1X1	T45.1X2	T45.1X3	T45.1X4	T45.1X5	T45.1X6
Candeptin	T49.0X1	T49.0X2	T49.0X3	T49.0X4	T49.0X5	T49.0X6
Candicidin	T49.0X1	T49.0X2	T49.0X3	T49.0X4	T49.0X5	T49.0X6
Cannabinoids, synthetic	T40.721	T40.722	T40.723	T40.724	T40.725	T40.726
Cannabinol	T40.711	T40.712	T40.713	T40.714	T40.715	T40.716
Cannabis (derivatives)	T40.711	T40.712	T40.713	T40.714	T40.715	T40.716
Canned heat	T51.1X1	T51.1X2	T51.1X3	T51.1X4	—	—
Canrenoic acid	T50.0X1	T50.0X2	T50.0X3	T50.0X4	T50.0X5	T50.0X6
Canrenone	T50.0X1	T50.0X2	T50.0X3	T50.0X4	T50.0X5	T50.0X6
Cantharides, cantharidin, cantharis	T49.8X1	T49.8X2	T49.8X3	T49.8X4	T49.8X5	T49.8X6
Canthaxanthin	T50.991	T50.992	T50.993	T50.994	T50.995	T50.996
Capillary-active drug NEC	T46.901	T46.902	T46.903	T46.904	T46.905	T46.906
Capreomycin	T36.8X1	T36.8X2	T36.8X3	T36.8X4	T36.8X5	T36.8X6
Capsicum	T49.4X1	T49.4X2	T49.4X3	T49.4X4	T49.4X5	T49.4X6
Captafol	T60.3X1	T60.3X2	T60.3X3	T60.3X4	—	—
Captan	T60.3X1	T60.3X2	T60.3X3	T60.3X4	—	—
Captodiame, captodiamine	T43.591	T43.592	T43.593	T43.594	T43.595	T43.596
Captopril	T46.4X1	T46.4X2	T46.4X3	T46.4X4	T46.4X5	T46.4X6
Caramiphen	T44.3X1	T44.3X2	T44.3X3	T44.3X4	T44.3X5	T44.3X6
Carazolol	T44.7X1	T44.7X2	T44.7X3	T44.7X4	T44.7X5	T44.7X6
Carbachol	T44.1X1	T44.1X2	T44.1X3	T44.1X4	T44.1X5	T44.1X6
Carbacrylamine (resin)	T50.3X1	T50.3X2	T50.3X3	T50.3X4	T50.3X5	T50.3X6
Carbamate (insecticide)	T60.0X1	T60.0X2	T60.0X3	T60.0X4	—	—
Carbamate (sedative)	T42.6X1	T42.6X2	T42.6X3	T42.6X4	T42.6X5	T42.6X6
herbicide	T60.0X1	T60.0X2	T60.0X3	T60.0X4	—	—
insecticide	T60.0X1	T60.0X2	T60.0X3	T60.0X4	—	—
Carbamazepine	T42.1X1	T42.1X2	T42.1X3	T42.1X4	T42.1X5	T42.1X6
Carbamide	T47.3X1	T47.3X2	T47.3X3	T47.3X4	T47.3X5	T47.3X6
peroxide	T49.0X1	T49.0X2	T49.0X3	T49.0X4	T49.0X5	T49.0X6
topical	T49.8X1	T49.8X2	T49.8X3	T49.8X4	T49.8X5	T49.8X6
Carbamylcholine chloride	T44.1X1	T44.1X2	T44.1X3	T44.1X4	T44.1X5	T44.1X6
Carbaril	T60.0X1	T60.0X2	T60.0X3	T60.0X4	—	—
Carbarsone	T37.3X1	T37.3X2	T37.3X3	T37.3X4	T37.3X5	T37.3X6
Carbaryl	T60.0X1	T60.0X2	T60.0X3	T60.0X4	—	—
Carbaspirin	T39.011	T39.012	T39.013	T39.014	T39.015	T39.016
Carbazochrome (salicylate) (sodium sulfonate)	T49.4X1	T49.4X2	T49.4X3	T49.4X4	T49.4X5	T49.4X6
Carbenicillin	T36.0X1	T36.0X2	T36.0X3	T36.0X4	T36.0X5	T36.0X6
Carbenoxolone	T47.1X1	T47.1X2	T47.1X3	T47.1X4	T47.1X5	T47.1X6
Carbetapentane	T48.3X1	T48.3X2	T48.3X3	T48.3X4	T48.3X5	T48.3X6
Carbethyl salicylate	T39.091	T39.092	T39.093	T39.094	T39.095	T39.096
Carbidopa (with levodopa)	T42.8X1	T42.8X2	T42.8X3	T42.8X4	T42.8X5	T42.8X6
Carbimazole	T38.2X1	T38.2X2	T38.2X3	T38.2X4	T38.2X5	T38.2X6
Carbinol	T51.1X1	T51.1X2	T51.1X3	T51.1X4	—	—
Carbinoxamine	T45.0X1	T45.0X2	T45.0X3	T45.0X4	T45.0X5	T45.0X6
Carbiphene	T39.8X1	T39.8X2	T39.8X3	T39.8X4	T39.8X5	T39.8X6
Carbitol	T52.3X1	T52.3X2	T52.3X3	T52.3X4	—	—
Carbo medicinalis	T47.6X1	T47.6X2	T47.6X3	T47.6X4	T47.6X5	T47.6X6
Carbocaine	T41.3X1	T41.3X2	T41.3X3	T41.3X4	T41.3X5	T41.3X6
infiltration (subcutaneous)	T41.3X1	T41.3X2	T41.3X3	T41.3X4	T41.3X5	T41.3X6
nerve block (peripheral) (plexus)	T41.3X1	T41.3X2	T41.3X3	T41.3X4	T41.3X5	T41.3X6
topical (surface)	T41.3X1	T41.3X2	T41.3X3	T41.3X4	T41.3X5	T41.3X6
Carbocisteine	T48.4X1	T48.4X2	T48.4X3	T48.4X4	T48.4X5	T48.4X6
Carbocromen	T46.3X1	T46.3X2	T46.3X3	T46.3X4	T46.3X5	T46.3X6
Carbol fuchsin	T49.0X1	T49.0X2	T49.0X3	T49.0X4	T49.0X5	T49.0X6
Carbolic acid—see also Phenol	T54.0X1	T54.0X2	T54.0X3	T54.0X4	—	—
Carbolonium (bromide)	T48.1X1	T48.1X2	T48.1X3	T48.1X4	T48.1X5	T48.1X6
Carbomycin	T36.8X1	T36.8X2	T36.8X3	T36.8X4	T36.8X5	T36.8X6
Carbon						
bisulfide (liquid)	T65.4X1	T65.4X2	T65.4X3	T65.4X4	—	—
vapor	T65.4X1	T65.4X2	T65.4X3	T65.4X4	—	—
dioxide (gas)	T59.7X1	T59.7X2	T59.7X3	T59.7X4	—	—
medicinal	T41.5X1	T41.5X2	T41.5X3	T41.5X4	T41.5X5	T41.5X6
nonmedicinal	T59.7X1	T59.7X2	T59.7X3	T59.7X4	—	—
snow	T49.4X1	T49.4X2	T49.4X3	T49.4X4	T49.4X5	T49.4X6
disulfide (liquid)	T65.4X1	T65.4X2	T65.4X3	T65.4X4	—	—
vapor	T65.4X1	T65.4X2	T65.4X3	T65.4X4	—	—
monoxide (from incomplete combustion)	T58.91	T58.92	T58.93	T58.94	—	—
blast furnace gas	T58.8X1	T58.8X2	T58.8X3	T58.8X4	—	—
butane (distributed in mobile container)	T58.11	T58.12	T58.13	T58.14	—	—
distributed through pipes	T58.11	T58.12	T58.13	T58.14	—	—
charcoal fumes	T58.2X1	T58.2X2	T58.2X3	T58.2X4	—	—
coal	T58.2X1	T58.2X2	T58.2X3	T58.2X4	—	—
coke (in domestic stoves, fireplaces)	T58.2X1	T58.2X2	T58.2X3	T58.2X4	—	—
gas (piped)	T58.11	T58.12	T58.13	T58.14	—	—
solid (in domestic stoves, fireplaces)	T58.2X1	T58.2X2	T58.2X3	T58.2X4	—	—
exhaust gas (motor) not in transit	T58.01	T58.02	T58.03	T58.04	—	—
combustion engine, any not in watercraft	T58.01	T58.02	T58.03	T58.04	—	—
farm tractor, not in transit	T58.01	T58.02	T58.03	T58.04	—	—

Substance	Poisoning, Accidental (unintentional)	Poisoning, Intentional self-harm	Poisoning, Assault	Poisoning, Undetermined	Adverse effect	Underdosing
Carbon — *Continued*						
gas engine	T58.01	T58.02	T58.03	T58.04	—	—
motor pump	T58.01	T58.02	T58.03	T58.04	—	—
motor vehicle, not in transit	T58.01	T58.02	T58.03	T58.04	—	—
fuel (in domestic use)	T58.2X1	T58.2X2	T58.2X3	T58.2X4	—	—
gas (piped)	T58.11	T58.12	T58.13	T58.14	—	—
in mobile container	T58.11	T58.12	T58.13	T58.14	—	—
piped (natural)	T58.11	T58.12	T58.13	T58.14	—	—
utility	T58.11	T58.12	T58.13	T58.14	—	—
in mobile container	T58.11	T58.12	T58.13	T58.14	—	—
illuminating gas	T58.11	T58.12	T58.13	T58.14	—	—
industrial fuels or gases, any	T58.8X1	T58.8X2	T58.8X3	T58.8X4	—	—
kerosene (in domestic stoves, fireplaces)	T58.2X1	T58.2X2	T58.2X3	T58.2X4	—	—
kiln gas or vapor	T58.8X1	T58.8X2	T58.8X3	T58.8X4	—	—
motor exhaust gas, not in transit	T58.01	T58.02	T58.03	T58.04	—	—
piped gas (manufactured) (natural)	T58.11	T58.12	T58.13	T58.14	—	—
producer gas	T58.8X1	T58.8X2	T58.8X3	T58.8X4	—	—
propane (distributed in mobile container)	T58.11	T58.12	T58.13	T58.14	—	—
distributed through pipes	T58.11	T58.12	T58.13	T58.14	—	—
specified source NEC	T58.8X1	T58.8X2	T58.8X3	T58.8X4	—	—
stove gas	T58.11	T58.12	T58.13	T58.14	—	—
piped	T58.11	T58.12	T58.13	T58.14	—	—
utility gas	T58.11	T58.12	T58.13	T58.14	—	—
piped	T58.11	T58.12	T58.13	T58.14	—	—
water gas	T58.11	T58.12	T58.13	T58.14	—	—
wood (in domestic stoves, fireplaces)	T58.2X1	T58.2X2	T58.2X3	T58.2X4	—	—
tetrachloride (vapor) NEC	T53.0X1	T53.0X2	T53.0X3	T53.0X4	—	—
liquid (cleansing agent) NEC	T53.0X1	T53.0X2	T53.0X3	T53.0X4	—	—
solvent	T53.0X1	T53.0X2	T53.0X3	T53.0X4	—	—
Carbonic acid gas	T59.7X1	T59.7X2	T59.7X3	T59.7X4	—	—
anhydrase inhibitor NEC	T50.2X1	T50.2X2	T50.2X3	T50.2X4	T50.2X5	T50.2X6
Carbophenothion	T60.0X1	T60.0X2	T60.0X3	T60.0X4	—	—
Carboplatin	T45.1X1	T45.1X2	T45.1X3	T45.1X4	T45.1X5	T45.1X6
Carboprost	T48.0X1	T48.0X2	T48.0X3	T48.0X4	T48.0X5	T48.0X6
Carboquone	T45.1X1	T45.1X2	T45.1X3	T45.1X4	T45.1X5	T45.1X6
Carbowax	T49.3X1	T49.3X2	T49.3X3	T49.3X4	T49.3X5	T49.3X6
Carboxymethyl-cellulose	T47.4X1	T47.4X2	T47.4X3	T47.4X4	T47.4X5	T47.4X6
S-Carboxymethyl-cysteine	T48.4X1	T48.4X2	T48.4X3	T48.4X4	T48.4X5	T48.4X6
Carbrital	T42.3X1	T42.3X2	T42.3X3	T42.3X4	T42.3X5	T42.3X6
Carbromal	T42.6X1	T42.6X2	T42.6X3	T42.6X4	T42.6X5	T42.6X6
Carbutamide	T38.3X1	T38.3X2	T38.3X3	T38.3X4	T38.3X5	T38.3X6
Carbuterol	T48.6X1	T48.6X2	T48.6X3	T48.6X4	T48.6X5	T48.6X6
Cardiac						
depressants	T46.2X1	T46.2X2	T46.2X3	T46.2X4	T46.2X5	T46.2X6
rhythm regulator	T46.2X1	T46.2X2	T46.2X3	T46.2X4	T46.2X5	T46.2X6
specified NEC	T46.2X1	T46.2X2	T46.2X3	T46.2X4	T46.2X5	T46.2X6
Cardiografin	T50.8X1	T50.8X2	T50.8X3	T50.8X4	T50.8X5	T50.8X6
Cardio-green	T50.8X1	T50.8X2	T50.8X3	T50.8X4	T50.8X5	T50.8X6
Cardiotonic (glycoside)NEC	T46.0X1	T46.0X2	T46.0X3	T46.0X4	T46.0X5	T46.0X6
Cardiovascular drug NEC	T46.901	T46.902	T46.903	T46.904	T46.905	T46.906
Cardrase	T50.2X1	T50.2X2	T50.2X3	T50.2X4	T50.2X5	T50.2X6
Carfecillin	T36.0X1	T36.0X2	T36.0X3	T36.0X4	T36.0X5	T36.0X6
Carfenazine	T43.3X1	T43.3X2	T43.3X3	T43.3X4	T43.3X5	T43.3X6
Carfusin	T49.0X1	T49.0X2	T49.0X3	T49.0X4	T49.0X5	T49.0X6
Carindacillin	T36.0X1	T36.0X2	T36.0X3	T36.0X4	T36.0X5	T36.0X6
Carisoprodol	T42.8X1	T42.8X2	T42.8X3	T42.8X4	T42.8X5	T42.8X6
Carmellose	T47.4X1	T47.4X2	T47.4X3	T47.4X4	T47.4X5	T47.4X6
Carminative	T47.5X1	T47.5X2	T47.5X3	T47.5X4	T47.5X5	T47.5X6
Carmofur	T45.1X1	T45.1X2	T45.1X3	T45.1X4	T45.1X5	T45.1X6
Carmustine	T45.1X1	T45.1X2	T45.1X3	T45.1X4	T45.1X5	T45.1X6
Carotene	T45.2X1	T45.2X2	T45.2X3	T45.2X4	T45.2X5	T45.2X6
Carphenazine	T43.3X1	T43.3X2	T43.3X3	T43.3X4	T43.3X5	T43.3X6
Carpipramine	T42.4X1	T42.4X2	T42.4X3	T42.4X4	T42.4X5	T42.4X6
Carprofen	T39.311	T39.312	T39.313	T39.314	T39.315	T39.316
Carpronium chloride	T44.3X1	T44.3X2	T44.3X3	T44.3X4	T44.3X5	T44.3X6
Carrageenan	T47.8X1	T47.8X2	T47.8X3	T47.8X4	T47.8X5	T47.8X6
Carteolol	T44.7X1	T44.7X2	T44.7X3	T44.7X4	T44.7X5	T44.7X6
Carter's Little Pills	T47.2X1	T47.2X2	T47.2X3	T47.2X4	T47.2X5	T47.2X6
Cascara (sagrada)	T47.2X1	T47.2X2	T47.2X3	T47.2X4	T47.2X5	T47.2X6
Cassava	T62.2X1	T62.2X2	T62.2X3	T62.2X4	—	—
Castellani's paint	T49.0X1	T49.0X2	T49.0X3	T49.0X4	T49.0X5	T49.0X6
Castor						
bean	T62.2X1	T62.2X2	T62.2X3	T62.2X4	—	—
oil	T47.2X1	T47.2X2	T47.2X3	T47.2X4	T47.2X5	T47.2X6
Catalase	T45.3X1	T45.3X2	T45.3X3	T45.3X4	T45.3X5	T45.3X6
Caterpillar (sting)	T63.431	T63.432	T63.433	T63.434	—	—
Catha (edulis) (tea)	T43.691	T43.692	T43.693	T43.694	—	—
Cathartic NEC	T47.4X1	T47.4X2	T47.4X3	T47.4X4	T47.4X5	T47.4X6
anthacene derivative	T47.2X1	T47.2X2	T47.2X3	T47.2X4	T47.2X5	T47.2X6
bulk	T47.4X1	T47.4X2	T47.4X3	T47.4X4	T47.4X5	T47.4X6
contact	T47.2X1	T47.2X2	T47.2X3	T47.2X4	T47.2X5	T47.2X6
emollient NEC	T47.4X1	T47.4X2	T47.4X3	T47.4X4	T47.4X5	T47.4X6
irritant NEC	T47.2X1	T47.2X2	T47.2X3	T47.2X4	T47.2X5	T47.2X6
mucilage	T47.4X1	T47.4X2	T47.4X3	T47.4X4	T47.4X5	T47.4X6
saline	T47.3X1	T47.3X2	T47.3X3	T47.3X4	T47.3X5	T47.3X6
vegetable	T47.2X1	T47.2X2	T47.2X3	T47.2X4	T47.2X5	T47.2X6
Cathine	T50.5X1	T50.5X2	T50.5X3	T50.5X4	T50.5X5	T50.5X6
Cathomycin	T36.8X1	T36.8X2	T36.8X3	T36.8X4	T36.8X5	T36.8X6

Substance	Poisoning, Accidental (unintentional)	Poisoning, Intentional self-harm	Poisoning, Assault	Poisoning, Undetermined	Adverse effect	Underdosing
Cation exchange resin	T50.3X1	T50.3X2	T50.3X3	T50.3X4	T50.3X5	T50.3X6
Caustic(s) NEC	T54.91	T54.92	T54.93	T54.94	—	—
alkali	T54.3X1	T54.3X2	T54.3X3	T54.3X4	—	—
hydroxide	T54.3X1	T54.3X2	T54.3X3	T54.3X4	—	—
potash	T54.3X1	T54.3X2	T54.3X3	T54.3X4	—	—
soda	T54.3X1	T54.3X2	T54.3X3	T54.3X4	—	—
specified NEC	T54.91	T54.92	T54.93	T54.94	—	—
Ceepryn	T49.0X1	T49.0X2	T49.0X3	T49.0X4	T49.0X5	T49.0X6
ENT agent	T49.6X1	T49.6X2	T49.6X3	T49.6X4	T49.6X5	T49.6X6
lozenges	T49.6X1	T49.6X2	T49.6X3	T49.6X4	T49.6X5	T49.6X6
Cefacetrile	T36.1X1	T36.1X2	T36.1X3	T36.1X4	T36.1X5	T36.1X6
Cefaclor	T36.1X1	T36.1X2	T36.1X3	T36.1X4	T36.1X5	T36.1X6
Cefadroxil	T36.1X1	T36.1X2	T36.1X3	T36.1X4	T36.1X5	T36.1X6
Cefalexin	T36.1X1	T36.1X2	T36.1X3	T36.1X4	T36.1X5	T36.1X6
Cefaloglycin	T36.1X1	T36.1X2	T36.1X3	T36.1X4	T36.1X5	T36.1X6
Cefaloridine	T36.1X1	T36.1X2	T36.1X3	T36.1X4	T36.1X5	T36.1X6
Cefalosporins	T36.1X1	T36.1X2	T36.1X3	T36.1X4	T36.1X5	T36.1X6
Cefalotin	T36.1X1	T36.1X2	T36.1X3	T36.1X4	T36.1X5	T36.1X6
Cefamandole	T36.1X1	T36.1X2	T36.1X3	T36.1X4	T36.1X5	T36.1X6
Cefamycin antibiotic	T36.1X1	T36.1X2	T36.1X3	T36.1X4	T36.1X5	T36.1X6
Cefapirin	T36.1X1	T36.1X2	T36.1X3	T36.1X4	T36.1X5	T36.1X6
Cefatrizine	T36.1X1	T36.1X2	T36.1X3	T36.1X4	T36.1X5	T36.1X6
Cefazedone	T36.1X1	T36.1X2	T36.1X3	T36.1X4	T36.1X5	T36.1X6
Cefazolin	T36.1X1	T36.1X2	T36.1X3	T36.1X4	T36.1X5	T36.1X6
Cefbuperazone	T36.1X1	T36.1X2	T36.1X3	T36.1X4	T36.1X5	T36.1X6
Cefetamet	T36.1X1	T36.1X2	T36.1X3	T36.1X4	T36.1X5	T36.1X6
Cefixime	T36.1X1	T36.1X2	T36.1X3	T36.1X4	T36.1X5	T36.1X6
Cefmenoxime	T36.1X1	T36.1X2	T36.1X3	T36.1X4	T36.1X5	T36.1X6
Cefmetazole	T36.1X1	T36.1X2	T36.1X3	T36.1X4	T36.1X5	T36.1X6
Cefminox	T36.1X1	T36.1X2	T36.1X3	T36.1X4	T36.1X5	T36.1X6
Cefonicid	T36.1X1	T36.1X2	T36.1X3	T36.1X4	T36.1X5	T36.1X6
Cefoperazone	T36.1X1	T36.1X2	T36.1X3	T36.1X4	T36.1X5	T36.1X6
Ceforanide	T36.1X1	T36.1X2	T36.1X3	T36.1X4	T36.1X5	T36.1X6
Cefotaxime	T36.1X1	T36.1X2	T36.1X3	T36.1X4	T36.1X5	T36.1X6
Cefotetan	T36.1X1	T36.1X2	T36.1X3	T36.1X4	T36.1X5	T36.1X6
Cefotiam	T36.1X1	T36.1X2	T36.1X3	T36.1X4	T36.1X5	T36.1X6
Cefoxitin	T36.1X1	T36.1X2	T36.1X3	T36.1X4	T36.1X5	T36.1X6
Cefpimizole	T36.1X1	T36.1X2	T36.1X3	T36.1X4	T36.1X5	T36.1X6
Cefpiramide	T36.1X1	T36.1X2	T36.1X3	T36.1X4	T36.1X5	T36.1X6
Cefradine	T36.1X1	T36.1X2	T36.1X3	T36.1X4	T36.1X5	T36.1X6
Cefroxadine	T36.1X1	T36.1X2	T36.1X3	T36.1X4	T36.1X5	T36.1X6
Cefsulodin	T36.1X1	T36.1X2	T36.1X3	T36.1X4	T36.1X5	T36.1X6
Ceftazidime	T36.1X1	T36.1X2	T36.1X3	T36.1X4	T36.1X5	T36.1X6
Cefteram	T36.1X1	T36.1X2	T36.1X3	T36.1X4	T36.1X5	T36.1X6
Ceftezole	T36.1X1	T36.1X2	T36.1X3	T36.1X4	T36.1X5	T36.1X6
Ceftizoxime	T36.1X1	T36.1X2	T36.1X3	T36.1X4	T36.1X5	T36.1X6
Ceftriaxone	T36.1X1	T36.1X2	T36.1X3	T36.1X4	T36.1X5	T36.1X6
Cefuroxime	T36.1X1	T36.1X2	T36.1X3	T36.1X4	T36.1X5	T36.1X6
Cefuzonam	T36.1X1	T36.1X2	T36.1X3	T36.1X4	T36.1X5	T36.1X6
Celestone	T38.0X1	T38.0X2	T38.0X3	T38.0X4	T38.0X5	T38.0X6
topical	T49.0X1	T49.0X2	T49.0X3	T49.0X4	T49.0X5	T49.0X6

Substance	Poisoning, Accidental (unintentional)	Poisoning, Intentional self-harm	Poisoning, Assault	Poisoning, Undetermined	Adverse effect	Underdosing
Celiprolol	T44.7X1	T44.7X2	T44.7X3	T44.7X4	T44.7X5	T44.7X6
Cell stimulants and proliferants	T49.8X1	T49.8X2	T49.8X3	T49.8X4	T49.8X5	T49.8X6
Cellosolve	T52.91	T52.92	T52.93	T52.94	—	—
Cellulose						
cathartic	T47.4X1	T47.4X2	T47.4X3	T47.4X4	T47.4X5	T47.4X6
hydroxyethyl	T47.4X1	T47.4X2	T47.4X3	T47.4X4	T47.4X5	T47.4X6
nitrates (topical)	T49.3X1	T49.3X2	T49.3X3	T49.3X4	T49.3X5	T49.3X6
oxidized	T49.4X1	T49.4X2	T49.4X3	T49.4X4	T49.4X5	T49.4X6
Centipede (bite)	T63.411	T63.412	T63.413	T63.414	—	—
Central nervous system						
depressants	T42.71	T42.72	T42.73	T42.74	T42.75	T42.76
anesthetic (general) NEC	T41.201	T41.202	T41.203	T41.204	T41.205	T41.206
gases NEC	T41.0X1	T41.0X2	T41.0X3	T41.0X4	T41.0X5	T41.0X6
intravenous	T41.1X1	T41.1X2	T41.1X3	T41.1X4	T41.1X5	T41.1X6
barbiturates	T42.3X1	T42.3X2	T42.3X3	T42.3X4	T42.3X5	T42.3X6
benzodiazepines	T42.4X1	T42.4X2	T42.4X3	T42.4X4	T42.4X5	T42.4X6
bromides	T42.6X1	T42.6X2	T42.6X3	T42.6X4	T42.6X5	T42.6X6
cannabis sativa	T40.711	T40.712	T40.713	T40.714	T40.715	T40.716
chloral hydrate	T42.6X1	T42.6X2	T42.6X3	T42.6X4	T42.6X5	T42.6X6
ethanol	T51.0X1	T51.0X2	T51.0X3	T51.0X4	—	—
hallucinogenics	T40.901	T40.902	T40.903	T40.904	T40.905	T40.906
hypnotics	T42.71	T42.72	T42.73	T42.74	T42.75	T42.76
specified NEC	T42.6X1	T42.6X2	T42.6X3	T42.6X4	T42.6X5	T42.6X6
muscle relaxants	T42.8X1	T42.8X2	T42.8X3	T42.8X4	T42.8X5	T42.8X6
paraldehyde	T42.6X1	T42.6X2	T42.6X3	T42.6X4	T42.6X5	T42.6X6
sedatives; sedative-hypnotics	T42.71	T42.72	T42.73	T42.74	T42.75	T42.76
mixed NEC	T42.6X1	T42.6X2	T42.6X3	T42.6X4	T42.6X5	T42.6X6
specified NEC	T42.6X1	T42.6X2	T42.6X3	T42.6X4	T42.6X5	T42.6X6
muscle-tone depressants	T42.8X1	T42.8X2	T42.8X3	T42.8X4	T42.8X5	T42.8X6
stimulants	T43.601	T43.602	T43.603	T43.604	T43.605	T43.606
amphetamines	T43.621	T43.622	T43.623	T43.624	T43.625	T43.626
analeptics	T50.7X1	T50.7X2	T50.7X3	T50.7X4	T50.7X5	T50.7X6
antidepressants	T43.201	T43.202	T43.203	T43.204	T43.205	T43.206
opiate antagonists	T50.7X1	T50.7X2	T50.7X3	T50.7X4	T50.7X5	T50.7X6
specified NEC	T43.691	T43.692	T43.693	T43.694	T43.695	T43.696
Cephalexin	T36.1X1	T36.1X2	T36.1X3	T36.1X4	T36.1X5	T36.1X6
Cephaloglycin	T36.1X1	T36.1X2	T36.1X3	T36.1X4	T36.1X5	T36.1X6
Cephaloridine	T36.1X1	T36.1X2	T36.1X3	T36.1X4	T36.1X5	T36.1X6
Cephalosporins	T36.1X1	T36.1X2	T36.1X3	T36.1X4	T36.1X5	T36.1X6
N(adicillin)	T36.0X1	T36.0X2	T36.0X3	T36.0X4	T36.0X5	T36.0X6
Cephalothin	T36.1X1	T36.1X2	T36.1X3	T36.1X4	T36.1X5	T36.1X6
Cephalotin	T36.1X1	T36.1X2	T36.1X3	T36.1X4	T36.1X5	T36.1X6
Cephradine	T36.1X1	T36.1X2	T36.1X3	T36.1X4	T36.1X5	T36.1X6
Cerbera (odallam)	T62.2X1	T62.2X2	T62.2X3	T62.2X4	—	—
Cerberin	T46.0X1	T46.0X2	T46.0X3	T46.0X4	T46.0X5	T46.0X6
Cerebral stimulants	T43.601	T43.602	T43.603	T43.604	T43.605	T43.606
psychotherapeutic	T43.601	T43.602	T43.603	T43.604	T43.605	T43.606
specified NEC	T43.691	T43.692	T43.693	T43.694	T43.695	T43.696

Substance	Poisoning, Accidental (unintentional)	Poisoning, Intentional self-harm	Poisoning, Assault	Poisoning, Undetermined	Adverse effect	Underdosing
Cerium oxalate	T45.0X1	T45.0X2	T45.0X3	T45.0X4	T45.0X5	T45.0X6
Cerous oxalate	T45.0X1	T45.0X2	T45.0X3	T45.0X4	T45.0X5	T45.0X6
Ceruletide	T50.8X1	T50.8X2	T50.8X3	T50.8X4	T50.8X5	T50.8X6
Cetalkonium (chloride)	T49.0X1	T49.0X2	T49.0X3	T49.0X4	T49.0X5	T49.0X6
Cethexonium chloride	T49.0X1	T49.0X2	T49.0X3	T49.0X4	T49.0X5	T49.0X6
Cetiedil	T46.7X1	T46.7X2	T46.7X3	T46.7X4	T46.7X5	T46.7X6
Cetirizine	T45.0X1	T45.0X2	T45.0X3	T45.0X4	T45.0X5	T45.0X6
Cetomacrogol	T50.991	T50.992	T50.993	T50.994	T50.995	T50.996
Cetotiamine	T45.2X1	T45.2X2	T45.2X3	T45.2X4	T45.2X5	T45.2X6
Cetoxime	T45.0X1	T45.0X2	T45.0X3	T45.0X4	T45.0X5	T45.0X6
Cetraxate	T47.1X1	T47.1X2	T47.1X3	T47.1X4	T47.1X5	T47.1X6
Cetrimide	T49.0X1	T49.0X2	T49.0X3	T49.0X4	T49.0X5	T49.0X6
Cetrimonium (bromide)	T49.0X1	T49.0X2	T49.0X3	T49.0X4	T49.0X5	T49.0X6
Cetylpyridinium chloride	T49.0X1	T49.0X2	T49.0X3	T49.0X4	T49.0X5	T49.0X6
ENT agent	T49.6X1	T49.6X2	T49.6X3	T49.6X4	T49.6X5	T49.6X6
lozenges	T49.6X1	T49.6X2	T49.6X3	T49.6X4	T49.6X5	T49.6X6
Cevadilla—see Sabadilla						
Cevitamic acid	T45.2X1	T45.2X2	T45.2X3	T45.2X4	T45.2X5	T45.2X6
Chalk, precipitated	T47.1X1	T47.1X2	T47.1X3	T47.1X4	T47.1X5	T47.1X6
Chamomile	T49.0X1	T49.0X2	T49.0X3	T49.0X4	T49.0X5	T49.0X6
Ch'an su	T46.0X1	T46.0X2	T46.0X3	T46.0X4	T46.0X5	T46.0X6
Charcoal	T47.6X1	T47.6X2	T47.6X3	T47.6X4	T47.6X5	T47.6X6
activated—see also Charcoal, medicinal	T47.6X1	T47.6X2	T47.6X3	T47.6X4	T47.6X5	T47.6X6
fumes (Carbon monoxide)	T58.2X1	T58.2X2	T58.2X3	T58.2X4	—	—
industrial	T58.8X1	T58.8X2	T58.8X3	T58.8X4	—	—
medicinal (activated)	T47.6X1	T47.6X2	T47.6X3	T47.6X4	T47.6X5	T47.6X6
antidiarrheal	T47.6X1	T47.6X2	T47.6X3	T47.6X4	T47.6X5	T47.6X6
poison control	T47.8X1	T47.8X2	T47.8X3	T47.8X4	T47.8X5	T47.8X6
specified use other than for diarrhea	T47.8X1	T47.8X2	T47.8X3	T47.8X4	T47.8X5	T47.8X6
topical	T49.8X1	T49.8X2	T49.8X3	T49.8X4	T49.8X5	T49.8X6
Chaulmosulfone	T37.1X1	T37.1X2	T37.1X3	T37.1X4	T37.1X5	T37.1X6
Chelating agent NEC	T50.6X1	T50.6X2	T50.6X3	T50.6X4	T50.6X5	T50.6X6
Chelidonium majus	T62.2X1	T62.2X2	T62.2X3	T62.2X4	—	—
Chemical substance NEC	T65.91	T65.92	T65.93	T65.94	—	—
Chenodeoxycholic acid	T47.5X1	T47.5X2	T47.5X3	T47.5X4	T47.5X5	T47.5X6
Chenodiol	T47.5X1	T47.5X2	T47.5X3	T47.5X4	T47.5X5	T47.5X6
Chenopodium	T37.4X1	T37.4X2	T37.4X3	T37.4X4	T37.4X5	T37.4X6
Cherry laurel	T62.2X1	T62.2X2	T62.2X3	T62.2X4	—	—
Chinidin(e)	T46.2X1	T46.2X2	T46.2X3	T46.2X4	T46.2X5	T46.2X6
Chiniofon	T37.8X1	T37.8X2	T37.8X3	T37.8X4	T37.8X5	T37.8X6
Chlophedianol	T48.3X1	T48.3X2	T48.3X3	T48.3X4	T48.3X5	T48.3X6
Chloral	T42.6X1	T42.6X2	T42.6X3	T42.6X4	T42.6X5	T42.6X6
derivative	T42.6X1	T42.6X2	T42.6X3	T42.6X4	T42.6X5	T42.6X6
hydrate	T42.6X1	T42.6X2	T42.6X3	T42.6X4	T42.6X5	T42.6X6
Chloralamide	T42.6X1	T42.6X2	T42.6X3	T42.6X4	T42.6X5	T42.6X6
Chloralodol	T42.6X1	T42.6X2	T42.6X3	T42.6X4	T42.6X5	T42.6X6
Chloralose	T60.4X1	T60.4X2	T60.4X3	T60.4X4	—	—

Substance	Poisoning, Accidental (unintentional)	Poisoning, Intentional self-harm	Poisoning, Assault	Poisoning, Undetermined	Adverse effect	Underdosing
Chlorambucil	T45.1X1	T45.1X2	T45.1X3	T45.1X4	T45.1X5	T45.1X6
Chloramine	T57.8X1	T57.8X2	T57.8X3	T57.8X4	—	—
T	T49.0X1	T49.0X2	T49.0X3	T49.0X4	T49.0X5	T49.0X6
topical	T49.0X1	T49.0X2	T49.0X3	T49.0X4	T49.0X5	T49.0X6
Chloramphenicol	T36.2X1	T36.2X2	T36.2X3	T36.2X4	T36.2X5	T36.2X6
ENT agent	T49.6X1	T49.6X2	T49.6X3	T49.6X4	T49.6X5	T49.6X6
ophthalmic preparation	T49.5X1	T49.5X2	T49.5X3	T49.5X4	T49.5X5	T49.5X6
topical NEC	T49.0X1	T49.0X2	T49.0X3	T49.0X4	T49.0X5	T49.0X6
Chlorate (potassium) (sodium) NEC	T60.3X1	T60.3X2	T60.3X3	T60.3X4	—	—
herbicide	T60.3X1	T60.3X2	T60.3X3	T60.3X4	—	—
Chlorazanil	T50.2X1	T50.2X2	T50.2X3	T50.2X4	T50.2X5	T50.2X6
Chlorbenzene, chlorbenzol	T53.7X1	T53.7X2	T53.7X3	T53.7X4	—	—
Chlorbenzoxamine	T44.3X1	T44.3X2	T44.3X3	T44.3X4	T44.3X5	T44.3X6
Chlorbutol	T42.6X1	T42.6X2	T42.6X3	T42.6X4	T42.6X5	T42.6X6
Chlorcyclizine	T45.0X1	T45.0X2	T45.0X3	T45.0X4	T45.0X5	T45.0X6
Chlordan(e) (dust)	T60.1X1	T60.1X2	T60.1X3	T60.1X4	—	—
Chlordantoin	T49.0X1	T49.0X2	T49.0X3	T49.0X4	T49.0X5	T49.0X6
Chlordiazepoxide	T42.4X1	T42.4X2	T42.4X3	T42.4X4	T42.4X5	T42.4X6
Chlordiethyl benzamide	T49.3X1	T49.3X2	T49.3X3	T49.3X4	T49.3X5	T49.3X6
Chloresium	T49.8X1	T49.8X2	T49.8X3	T49.8X4	T49.8X5	T49.8X6
Chlorethiazol	T42.6X1	T42.6X2	T42.6X3	T42.6X4	T42.6X5	T42.6X6
Chlorethyl—see Ethyl chloride						
Chloretone	T42.6X1	T42.6X2	T42.6X3	T42.6X4	T42.6X5	T42.6X6
Chlorex	T53.6X1	T53.6X2	T53.6X3	T53.6X4	—	—
insecticide	T60.1X1	T60.1X2	T60.1X3	T60.1X4	—	—
Chlorfenvinphos	T60.0X1	T60.0X2	T60.0X3	T60.0X4	—	—
Chlorhexadol	T42.6X1	T42.6X2	T42.6X3	T42.6X4	T42.6X5	T42.6X6
Chlorhexamide	T45.1X1	T45.1X2	T45.1X3	T45.1X4	T45.1X5	T45.1X6
Chlorhexidine	T49.0X1	T49.0X2	T49.0X3	T49.0X4	T49.0X5	T49.0X6
Chlorhydro-xyquinolin	T49.0X1	T49.0X2	T49.0X3	T49.0X4	T49.0X5	T49.0X6
Chloride of lime (bleach)	T54.3X1	T54.3X2	T54.3X3	T54.3X4	—	—
Chlorimipramine	T43.011	T43.012	T43.013	T43.014	T43.015	T43.016
Chlorinated						
camphene	T53.6X1	T53.6X2	T53.6X3	T53.6X4	—	—
diphenyl	T53.7X1	T53.7X2	T53.7X3	T53.7X4	—	—
hydrocarbons NEC	T53.91	T53.92	T53.93	T53.94	—	—
solvents	T53.91	T53.92	T53.93	T53.94	—	—
lime (bleach)	T54.3X1	T54.3X2	T54.3X3	T54.3X4	—	—
and boric acid solution	T49.0X1	T49.0X2	T49.0X3	T49.0X4	T49.0X5	T49.0X6
naphthalene (insecticide)	T60.1X1	T60.1X2	T60.1X3	T60.1X4	—	—
industrial (non-pesticide)	T53.7X1	T53.7X2	T53.7X3	T53.7X4	—	—
pesticide NEC	T60.8X1	T60.8X2	T60.8X3	T60.8X4	—	—
soda—see also sodium hypochlorite						
solution	T49.0X1	T49.0X2	T49.0X3	T49.0X4	T49.0X5	T49.0X6

Substance	Poisoning, Accidental (unintentional)	Poisoning, Intentional self-harm	Poisoning, Assault	Poisoning, Undetermined	Adverse effect	Underdosing
Chlorine (fumes) (gas)	T59.4X1	T59.4X2	T59.4X3	T59.4X4	—	—
bleach	T54.3X1	T54.3X2	T54.3X3	T54.3X4	—	—
compound gas NEC	T59.4X1	T59.4X2	T59.4X3	T59.4X4	—	—
disinfectant	T59.4X1	T59.4X2	T59.4X3	T59.4X4	—	—
releasing agents NEC	T59.4X1	T59.4X2	T59.4X3	T59.4X4	—	—
Chlorisondamine chloride	T46.991	T46.992	T46.993	T46.994	T46.995	T46.996
Chlormadinone	T38.5X1	T38.5X2	T38.5X3	T38.5X4	T38.5X5	T38.5X6
Chlormephos	T60.0X1	T60.0X2	T60.0X3	T60.0X4	—	—
Chlormerodrin	T50.2X1	T50.2X2	T50.2X3	T50.2X4	T50.2X5	T50.2X6
Chlormethiazole	T42.6X1	T42.6X2	T42.6X3	T42.6X4	T42.6X5	T42.6X6
Chlormethine	T45.1X1	T45.1X2	T45.1X3	T45.1X4	T45.1X5	T45.1X6
Chlormethyle-necycline	T36.4X1	T36.4X2	T36.4X3	T36.4X4	T36.4X5	T36.4X6
Chlormezanone	T42.6X1	T42.6X2	T42.6X3	T42.6X4	T42.6X5	T42.6X6
Chloroacetic acid	T60.3X1	T60.3X2	T60.3X3	T60.3X4	—	—
Chloroacetone	T59.3X1	T59.3X2	T59.3X3	T59.3X4	—	—
Chloroacetophenone	T59.3X1	T59.3X2	T59.3X3	T59.3X4	—	—
Chloroaniline	T53.7X1	T53.7X2	T53.7X3	T53.7X4	—	—
Chlorobenzene, chlorobenzol	T53.7X1	T53.7X2	T53.7X3	T53.7X4	—	—
Chlorobromo methane (fire extinguisher)	T53.6X1	T53.6X2	T53.6X3	T53.6X4	—	—
Chlorobutanol	T49.0X1	T49.0X2	T49.0X3	T49.0X4	T49.0X5	T49.0X6
Chlorocresol	T49.0X1	T49.0X2	T49.0X3	T49.0X4	T49.0X5	T49.0X6
Chlorodehydro-methyltestosterone	T38.7X1	T38.7X2	T38.7X3	T38.7X4	T38.7X5	T38.7X6
Chlorodinitro-benzene	T53.7X1	T53.7X2	T53.7X3	T53.7X4	—	—
dust or vapor	T53.7X1	T53.7X2	T53.7X3	T53.7X4	—	—
Chlorodiphenyl	T53.7X1	T53.7X2	T53.7X3	T53.7X4	—	—
Chloroethane—see Ethyl chloride						
Chloroethylene	T53.6X1	T53.6X2	T53.6X3	T53.6X4	—	—
Chlorofluorocarbons	T53.5X1	T53.5X2	T53.5X3	T53.5X4	—	—
Chloroform (fumes) (vapor)	T53.1X1	T53.1X2	T53.1X3	T53.1X4	—	—
anesthetic	T41.0X1	T41.0X2	T41.0X3	T41.0X4	T41.0X5	T41.0X6
solvent	T53.1X1	T53.1X2	T53.1X3	T53.1X4	—	—
water, concentrated	T41.0X1	T41.0X2	T41.0X3	T41.0X4	T41.0X5	T41.0X6
Chloroguanide	T37.2X1	T37.2X2	T37.2X3	T37.2X4	T37.2X5	T37.2X6
Chloromycetin	T36.2X1	T36.2X2	T36.2X3	T36.2X4	T36.2X5	T36.2X6
ENT agent	T49.6X1	T49.6X2	T49.6X3	T49.6X4	T49.6X5	T49.6X6
ophthalmic preparation	T49.5X1	T49.5X2	T49.5X3	T49.5X4	T49.5X5	T49.5X6
otic solution	T49.6X1	T49.6X2	T49.6X3	T49.6X4	T49.6X5	T49.6X6
topical NEC	T49.0X1	T49.0X2	T49.0X3	T49.0X4	T49.0X5	T49.0X6
Chloronitrobenzene	T53.7X1	T53.7X2	T53.7X3	T53.7X4	—	—
dust or vapor	T53.7X1	T53.7X2	T53.7X3	T53.7X4	—	—
Chlorophacinone	T60.4X1	T60.4X2	T60.4X3	T60.4X4	—	—
Chlorophenol	T53.7X1	T53.7X2	T53.7X3	T53.7X4	—	—
Chlorophenothane	T60.1X1	T60.1X2	T60.1X3	T60.1X4	—	—
Chlorophyll	T50.991	T50.992	T50.993	T50.994	T50.995	T50.996
Chloropicrin (fumes)	T53.6X1	T53.6X2	T53.6X3	T53.6X4	—	—
fumigant	T60.8X1	T60.8X2	T60.8X3	T60.8X4	—	—

Substance	Poisoning, Accidental (unintentional)	Poisoning, Intentional self-harm	Poisoning, Assault	Poisoning, Undetermined	Adverse effect	Underdosing
Chloropicrin — *Continued*						
fungicide	T60.3X1	T60.3X2	T60.3X3	T60.3X4	—	—
pesticide	T60.8X1	T60.8X2	T60.8X3	T60.8X4	—	—
Chloroprocaine	T41.3X1	T41.3X2	T41.3X3	T41.3X4	T41.3X5	T41.3X6
infiltration (subcutaneous)	T41.3X1	T41.3X2	T41.3X3	T41.3X4	T41.3X5	T41.3X6
nerve block (peripheral) (plexus)	T41.3X1	T41.3X2	T41.3X3	T41.3X4	T41.3X5	T41.3X6
spinal	T41.3X1	T41.3X2	T41.3X3	T41.3X4	T41.3X5	T41.3X6
Chloroptic	T49.5X1	T49.5X2	T49.5X3	T49.5X4	T49.5X5	T49.5X6
Chloropurine	T45.1X1	T45.1X2	T45.1X3	T45.1X4	T45.1X5	T45.1X6
Chloropyramine	T45.0X1	T45.0X2	T45.0X3	T45.0X4	T45.0X5	T45.0X6
Chloropyrifos	T60.0X1	T60.0X2	T60.0X3	T60.0X4	—	—
Chloropyrilene	T45.0X1	T45.0X2	T45.0X3	T45.0X4	T45.0X5	T45.0X6
Chloroquine	T37.2X1	T37.2X2	T37.2X3	T37.2X4	T37.2X5	T37.2X6
Chlorothalonil	T60.3X1	T60.3X2	T60.3X3	T60.3X4	—	—
Chlorothen	T45.0X1	T45.0X2	T45.0X3	T45.0X4	T45.0X5	T45.0X6
Chlorothiazide	T50.2X1	T50.2X2	T50.2X3	T50.2X4	T50.2X5	T50.2X6
Chlorothymol	T49.4X1	T49.4X2	T49.4X3	T49.4X4	T49.4X5	T49.4X6
Chlorotrianisene	T38.5X1	T38.5X2	T38.5X3	T38.5X4	T38.5X5	T38.5X6
Chlorovinyldichloro-arsine, not in war	T57.0X1	T57.0X2	T57.0X3	T57.0X4	—	—
Chloroxine	T49.4X1	T49.4X2	T49.4X3	T49.4X4	T49.4X5	T49.4X6
Chloroxylenol	T49.0X1	T49.0X2	T49.0X3	T49.0X4	T49.0X5	T49.0X6
Chlorphenamine	T45.0X1	T45.0X2	T45.0X3	T45.0X4	T45.0X5	T45.0X6
Chlorphenesin	T42.8X1	T42.8X2	T42.8X3	T42.8X4	T42.8X5	T42.8X6
topical (antifungal)	T49.0X1	T49.0X2	T49.0X3	T49.0X4	T49.0X5	T49.0X6
Chlorpheniramine	T45.0X1	T45.0X2	T45.0X3	T45.0X4	T45.0X5	T45.0X6
Chlorphenoxamine	T45.0X1	T45.0X2	T45.0X3	T45.0X4	T45.0X5	T45.0X6
Chlorphentermine	T50.5X1	T50.5X2	T50.5X3	T50.5X4	T50.5X5	T50.5X6
Chlorprocaine—see Chloroprocaine						
Chlorproguanil	T37.2X1	T37.2X2	T37.2X3	T37.2X4	T37.2X5	T37.2X6
Chlorpromazine	T43.3X1	T43.3X2	T43.3X3	T43.3X4	T43.3X5	T43.3X6
Chlorpropamide	T38.3X1	T38.3X2	T38.3X3	T38.3X4	T38.3X5	T38.3X6
Chlorprothixene	T43.4X1	T43.4X2	T43.4X3	T43.4X4	T43.4X5	T43.4X6
Chlorquinaldol	T49.0X1	T49.0X2	T49.0X3	T49.0X4	T49.0X5	T49.0X6
Chlorquinol	T49.0X1	T49.0X2	T49.0X3	T49.0X4	T49.0X5	T49.0X6
Chlortalidone	T50.2X1	T50.2X2	T50.2X3	T50.2X4	T50.2X5	T50.2X6
Chlortetracycline	T36.4X1	T36.4X2	T36.4X3	T36.4X4	T36.4X5	T36.4X6
Chlorthalidone	T50.2X1	T50.2X2	T50.2X3	T50.2X4	T50.2X5	T50.2X6
Chlorthiophos	T60.0X1	T60.0X2	T60.0X3	T60.0X4	—	—
Chlortrianisene	T38.5X1	T38.5X2	T38.5X3	T38.5X4	T38.5X5	T38.5X6
Chlor-Trimeton	T45.0X1	T45.0X2	T45.0X3	T45.0X4	T45.0X5	T45.0X6
Chlorthion	T60.0X1	T60.0X2	T60.0X3	T60.0X4	—	—
Chlorzoxazone	T42.8X1	T42.8X2	T42.8X3	T42.8X4	T42.8X5	T42.8X6
Choke damp	T59.7X1	T59.7X2	T59.7X3	T59.7X4	—	—
Cholagogues	T47.5X1	T47.5X2	T47.5X3	T47.5X4	T47.5X5	T47.5X6
Cholebrine	T50.8X1	T50.8X2	T50.8X3	T50.8X4	T50.8X5	T50.8X6
Cholecalciferol	T45.2X1	T45.2X2	T45.2X3	T45.2X4	T45.2X5	T45.2X6

Substance	Poisoning, Accidental (unintentional)	Poisoning, Intentional self-harm	Poisoning, Assault	Poisoning, Undetermined	Adverse effect	Underdosing
Cholecystokinin	T50.8X1	T50.8X2	T50.8X3	T50.8X4	T50.8X5	T50.8X6
Cholera vaccine	T50.A91	T50.A92	T50.A93	T50.A94	T50.A95	T50.A96
Choleretic	T47.5X1	T47.5X2	T47.5X3	T47.5X4	T47.5X5	T47.5X6
Cholesterol-lowering agents	T46.6X1	T46.6X2	T46.6X3	T46.6X4	T46.6X5	T46.6X6
Cholestyramine (resin)	T46.6X1	T46.6X2	T46.6X3	T46.6X4	T46.6X5	T46.6X6
Cholic acid	T47.5X1	T47.5X2	T47.5X3	T47.5X4	T47.5X5	T47.5X6
Choline	T48.6X1	T48.6X2	T48.6X3	T48.6X4	T48.6X5	T48.6X6
chloride	T50.991	T50.992	T50.993	T50.994	T50.995	T50.996
dihydrogen citrate	T50.991	T50.992	T50.993	T50.994	T50.995	T50.996
salicylate	T39.091	T39.092	T39.093	T39.094	T39.095	T39.096
theophyllinate	T48.6X1	T48.6X2	T48.6X3	T48.6X4	T48.6X5	T48.6X6
Cholinergic (drug) NEC	T44.1X1	T44.1X2	T44.1X3	T44.1X4	T44.1X5	T44.1X6
muscle tone enhancer	T44.1X1	T44.1X2	T44.1X3	T44.1X4	T44.1X5	T44.1X6
organophosphorus	T44.0X1	T44.0X2	T44.0X3	T44.0X4	T44.0X5	T44.0X6
insecticide	T60.0X1	T60.0X2	T60.0X3	T60.0X4	—	—
nerve gas	T59.891	T59.892	T59.893	T59.894	—	—
trimethyl ammonium propanediol	T44.1X1	T44.1X2	T44.1X3	T44.1X4	T44.1X5	T44.1X6
Cholinesterase reactivator	T50.6X1	T50.6X2	T50.6X3	T50.6X4	T50.6X5	T50.6X6
Cholografin	T50.8X1	T50.8X2	T50.8X3	T50.8X4	T50.8X5	T50.8X6
Chorionic gonadotropin	T38.891	T38.892	T38.893	T38.894	T38.895	T38.896
Chromate	T56.2X1	T56.2X2	T56.2X3	T56.2X4	—	—
dust or mist	T56.2X1	T56.2X2	T56.2X3	T56.2X4	—	—
lead—see also lead	T56.0X1	T56.0X2	T56.0X3	T56.0X4	—	—
paint	T56.0X1	T56.0X2	T56.0X3	T56.0X4	—	—
Chromic						
acid	T56.2X1	T56.2X2	T56.2X3	T56.2X4	—	—
dust or mist	T56.2X1	T56.2X2	T56.2X3	T56.2X4	—	—
phosphate 32P	T45.1X1	T45.1X2	T45.1X3	T45.1X4	T45.1X5	T45.1X6
Chromium	T56.2X1	T56.2X2	T56.2X3	T56.2X4	—	—
compounds—see Chromate						
sesquioxide	T50.8X1	T50.8X2	T50.8X3	T50.8X4	T50.8X5	T50.8X6
Chromomycin A3	T45.1X1	T45.1X2	T45.1X3	T45.1X4	T45.1X5	T45.1X6
Chromonar	T46.3X1	T46.3X2	T46.3X3	T46.3X4	T46.3X5	T46.3X6
Chromyl chloride	T56.2X1	T56.2X2	T56.2X3	T56.2X4	—	—
Chrysarobin	T49.4X1	T49.4X2	T49.4X3	T49.4X4	T49.4X5	T49.4X6
Chrysazin	T47.2X1	T47.2X2	T47.2X3	T47.2X4	T47.2X5	T47.2X6
Chymar	T45.3X1	T45.3X2	T45.3X3	T45.3X4	T45.3X5	T45.3X6
ophthalmic preparation	T49.5X1	T49.5X2	T49.5X3	T49.5X4	T49.5X5	T49.5X6
Chymopapain	T45.3X1	T45.3X2	T45.3X3	T45.3X4	T45.3X5	T45.3X6
Chymotrypsin	T45.3X1	T45.3X2	T45.3X3	T45.3X4	T45.3X5	T45.3X6
ophthalmic preparation	T49.5X1	T49.5X2	T49.5X3	T49.5X4	T49.5X5	T49.5X6
Cianidanol	T50.991	T50.992	T50.993	T50.994	T50.995	T50.996
Cianopramine	T43.011	T43.012	T43.013	T43.014	T43.015	T43.016
Cibenzoline	T46.2X1	T46.2X2	T46.2X3	T46.2X4	T46.2X5	T46.2X6
Ciclacillin	T36.0X1	T36.0X2	T36.0X3	T36.0X4	T36.0X5	T36.0X6
Ciclobarbital—see Hexobarbital						
Ciclonicate	T46.7X1	T46.7X2	T46.7X3	T46.7X4	T46.7X5	T46.7X6
Ciclopirox (olamine)	T49.0X1	T49.0X2	T49.0X3	T49.0X4	T49.0X5	T49.0X6
Ciclosporin	T45.1X1	T45.1X2	T45.1X3	T45.1X4	T45.1X5	T45.1X6
Cicuta maculata or virosa	T62.2X1	T62.2X2	T62.2X3	T62.2X4	—	—
Cicutoxin	T62.2X1	T62.2X2	T62.2X3	T62.2X4	—	—
Cigarette lighter fluid	T52.0X1	T52.0X2	T52.0X3	T52.0X4	—	—
Cigarettes (tobacco)	T65.221	T65.222	T65.223	T65.224	—	—
Ciguatoxin	T61.01	T61.02	T61.03	T61.04	—	—
Cilazapril	T46.4X1	T46.4X2	T46.4X3	T46.4X4	T46.4X5	T46.4X6
Cimetidine	T47.0X1	T47.0X2	T47.0X3	T47.0X4	T47.0X5	T47.0X6
Cimetropium bromide	T44.3X1	T44.3X2	T44.3X3	T44.3X4	T44.3X5	T44.3X6
Cinchocaine	T41.3X1	T41.3X2	T41.3X3	T41.3X4	T41.3X5	T41.3X6
topical (surface)	T41.3X1	T41.3X2	T41.3X3	T41.3X4	T41.3X5	T41.3X6
Cinchona	T37.2X1	T37.2X2	T37.2X3	T37.2X4	T37.2X5	T37.2X6
Cinchonine alkaloids	T37.2X1	T37.2X2	T37.2X3	T37.2X4	T37.2X5	T37.2X6
Cinchophen	T50.4X1	T50.4X2	T50.4X3	T50.4X4	T50.4X5	T50.4X6
Cinepazide	T46.7X1	T46.7X2	T46.7X3	T46.7X4	T46.7X5	T46.7X6
Cinnamedrine	T48.5X1	T48.5X2	T48.5X3	T48.5X4	T48.5X5	T48.5X6
Cinnarizine	T45.0X1	T45.0X2	T45.0X3	T45.0X4	T45.0X5	T45.0X6
Cinoxacin	T37.8X1	T37.8X2	T37.8X3	T37.8X4	T37.8X5	T37.8X6
Ciprofibrate	T46.6X1	T46.6X2	T46.6X3	T46.6X4	T46.6X5	T46.6X6
Ciprofloxacin	T36.8X1	T36.8X2	T36.8X3	T36.8X4	T36.8X5	T36.8X6
Cisapride	T47.8X1	T47.8X2	T47.8X3	T47.8X4	T47.8X5	T47.8X6
Cisplatin	T45.1X1	T45.1X2	T45.1X3	T45.1X4	T45.1X5	T45.1X6
Citalopram	T43.221	T43.222	T43.223	T43.224	T43.225	T43.226
Citanest	T41.3X1	T41.3X2	T41.3X3	T41.3X4	T41.3X5	T41.3X6
infiltration (subcutaneous)	T41.3X1	T41.3X2	T41.3X3	T41.3X4	T41.3X5	T41.3X6
nerve block (peripheral) (plexus)	T41.3X1	T41.3X2	T41.3X3	T41.3X4	T41.3X5	T41.3X6
Citric acid	T47.5X1	T47.5X2	T47.5X3	T47.5X4	T47.5X5	T47.5X6
Citrovorum (factor)	T45.8X1	T45.8X2	T45.8X3	T45.8X4	T45.8X5	T45.8X6
Claviceps purpurea	T62.2X1	T62.2X2	T62.2X3	T62.2X4	—	—
Clavulanic acid	T36.1X1	T36.1X2	T36.1X3	T36.1X4	T36.1X5	T36.1X6
Cleaner, cleansing agent, type not specified	T65.891	T65.892	T65.893	T65.894	—	—
of paint or varnish	T52.91	T52.92	T52.93	T52.94	—	—
specified type NEC	T65.891	T65.892	T65.893	T65.894	—	—
Clebopride	T47.8X1	T47.8X2	T47.8X3	T47.8X4	T47.8X5	T47.8X6
Clefamide	T37.3X1	T37.3X2	T37.3X3	T37.3X4	T37.3X5	T37.3X6
Clemastine	T45.0X1	T45.0X2	T45.0X3	T45.0X4	T45.0X5	T45.0X6
Clematis vitalba	T62.2X1	T62.2X2	T62.2X3	T62.2X4	—	—
Clemizole	T45.0X1	T45.0X2	T45.0X3	T45.0X4	T45.0X5	T45.0X6
penicillin	T36.0X1	T36.0X2	T36.0X3	T36.0X4	T36.0X5	T36.0X6
Clenbuterol	T48.6X1	T48.6X2	T48.6X3	T48.6X4	T48.6X5	T48.6X6
Clidinium bromide	T44.3X1	T44.3X2	T44.3X3	T44.3X4	T44.3X5	T44.3X6
Clindamycin	T36.8X1	T36.8X2	T36.8X3	T36.8X4	T36.8X5	T36.8X6
Clinofibrate	T46.6X1	T46.6X2	T46.6X3	T46.6X4	T46.6X5	T46.6X6
Clioquinol	T37.8X1	T37.8X2	T37.8X3	T37.8X4	T37.8X5	T37.8X6
Cliradon	T40.2X1	T40.2X2	T40.2X3	T40.2X4	—	—

Substance	Poisoning, Accidental (unintentional)	Poisoning, Intentional self-harm	Poisoning, Assault	Poisoning, Undetermined	Adverse effect	Underdosing
Clobazam	T42.4X1	T42.4X2	T42.4X3	T42.4X4	T42.4X5	T42.4X6
Clobenzorex	T50.5X1	T50.5X2	T50.5X3	T50.5X4	T50.5X5	T50.5X6
Clobetasol	T49.0X1	T49.0X2	T49.0X3	T49.0X4	T49.0X5	T49.0X6
Clobetasone	T49.0X1	T49.0X2	T49.0X3	T49.0X4	T49.0X5	T49.0X6
Clobutinol	T48.3X1	T48.3X2	T48.3X3	T48.3X4	T48.3X5	T48.3X6
Clocortolone	T38.0X1	T38.0X2	T38.0X3	T38.0X4	T38.0X5	T38.0X6
Clodantoin	T49.0X1	T49.0X2	T49.0X3	T49.0X4	T49.0X5	T49.0X6
Clodronic acid	T50.991	T50.992	T50.993	T50.994	T50.995	T50.996
Clofazimine	T37.1X1	T37.1X2	T37.1X3	T37.1X4	T37.1X5	T37.1X6
Clofedanol	T48.3X1	T48.3X2	T48.3X3	T48.3X4	T48.3X5	T48.3X6
Clofenamide	T50.2X1	T50.2X2	T50.2X3	T50.2X4	T50.2X5	T50.2X6
Clofenotane	T49.0X1	T49.0X2	T49.0X3	T49.0X4	T49.0X5	T49.0X6
Clofezone	T39.2X1	T39.2X2	T39.2X3	T39.2X4	T39.2X5	T39.2X6
Clofibrate	T46.6X1	T46.6X2	T46.6X3	T46.6X4	T46.6X5	T46.6X6
Clofibride	T46.6X1	T46.6X2	T46.6X3	T46.6X4	T46.6X5	T46.6X6
Cloforex	T50.5X1	T50.5X2	T50.5X3	T50.5X4	T50.5X5	T50.5X6
Clomethiazole	T42.6X1	T42.6X2	T42.6X3	T42.6X4	T42.6X5	T42.6X6
Clometocillin	T36.0X1	T36.0X2	T36.0X3	T36.0X4	T36.0X5	T36.0X6
Clomifene	T38.5X1	T38.5X2	T38.5X3	T38.5X4	T38.5X5	T38.5X6
Clomiphene	T38.5X1	T38.5X2	T38.5X3	T38.5X4	T38.5X5	T38.5X6
Clomipramine	T43.011	T43.012	T43.013	T43.014	T43.015	T43.016
Clomocycline	T36.4X1	T36.4X2	T36.4X3	T36.4X4	T36.4X5	T36.4X6
Clonazepam	T42.4X1	T42.4X2	T42.4X3	T42.4X4	T42.4X5	T42.4X6
Clonidine	T46.5X1	T46.5X2	T46.5X3	T46.5X4	T46.5X5	T46.5X6
Clonixin	T39.8X1	T39.8X2	T39.8X3	T39.8X4	T39.8X5	T39.8X6
Clopamide	T50.2X1	T50.2X2	T50.2X3	T50.2X4	T50.2X5	T50.2X6
Clopenthixol	T43.4X1	T43.4X2	T43.4X3	T43.4X4	T43.4X5	T43.4X6
Cloperastine	T48.3X1	T48.3X2	T48.3X3	T48.3X4	T48.3X5	T48.3X6
Clophedianol	T48.3X1	T48.3X2	T48.3X3	T48.3X4	T48.3X5	T48.3X6
Cloponone	T36.2X1	T36.2X2	T36.2X3	T36.2X4	T36.2X5	T36.2X6
Cloprednol	T38.0X1	T38.0X2	T38.0X3	T38.0X4	T38.0X5	T38.0X6
Cloral betaine	T42.6X1	T42.6X2	T42.6X3	T42.6X4	T42.6X5	T42.6X6
Cloramfenicol	T36.2X1	T36.2X2	T36.2X3	T36.2X4	T36.2X5	T36.2X6
Clorazepate (dipotassium)	T42.4X1	T42.4X2	T42.4X3	T42.4X4	T42.4X5	T42.4X6
Clorexolone	T50.2X1	T50.2X2	T50.2X3	T50.2X4	T50.2X5	T50.2X6
Clorfenamine	T45.0X1	T45.0X2	T45.0X3	T45.0X4	T45.0X5	T45.0X6
Clorgiline	T43.1X1	T43.1X2	T43.1X3	T43.1X4	T43.1X5	T43.1X6
Clorotepine	T44.3X1	T44.3X2	T44.3X3	T44.3X4	T44.3X5	T44.3X6
Clorox (bleach)	T54.91	T54.92	T54.93	T54.94	—	—
Clorprenaline	T48.6X1	T48.6X2	T48.6X3	T48.6X4	T48.6X5	T48.6X6
Clortermine	T50.5X1	T50.5X2	T50.5X3	T50.5X4	T50.5X5	T50.5X6
Clotiapine	T43.591	T43.592	T43.593	T43.594	T43.595	T43.596
Clotiazepam	T42.4X1	T42.4X2	T42.4X3	T42.4X4	T42.4X5	T42.4X6
Clotibric acid	T46.6X1	T46.6X2	T46.6X3	T46.6X4	T46.6X5	T46.6X6
Clotrimazole	T49.0X1	T49.0X2	T49.0X3	T49.0X4	T49.0X5	T49.0X6
Cloxacillin	T36.0X1	T36.0X2	T36.0X3	T36.0X4	T36.0X5	T36.0X6
Cloxazolam	T42.4X1	T42.4X2	T42.4X3	T42.4X4	T42.4X5	T42.4X6
Cloxiquine	T49.0X1	T49.0X2	T49.0X3	T49.0X4	T49.0X5	T49.0X6
Clozapine	T42.4X1	T42.4X2	T42.4X3	T42.4X4	T42.4X5	T42.4X6

Substance	Poisoning, Accidental (unintentional)	Poisoning, Intentional self-harm	Poisoning, Assault	Poisoning, Undetermined	Adverse effect	Underdosing
Coagulant NEC	T45.7X1	T45.7X2	T45.7X3	T45.7X4	T45.7X5	T45.7X6
Coal (carbon monoxide from)—see also Carbon, monoxide, coal	T58.2X1	T58.2X2	T58.2X3	T58.2X4	—	—
oil—see Kerosene						
tar	T49.1X1	T49.1X2	T49.1X3	T49.1X4	T49.1X5	T49.1X6
fumes	T59.891	T59.892	T59.893	T59.894	—	—
medicinal (ointment)	T49.4X1	T49.4X2	T49.4X3	T49.4X4	T49.4X5	T49.4X6
analgesics NEC	T39.2X1	T39.2X2	T39.2X3	T39.2X4	T39.2X5	T39.2X6
naphtha (solvent)	T52.0X1	T52.0X2	T52.0X3	T52.0X4	—	—
Cobalamine	T45.2X1	T45.2X2	T45.2X3	T45.2X4	T45.2X5	T45.2X6
Cobalt (nonmedicinal) (fumes) (industrial)	T56.891	T56.892	T56.893	T56.894	—	—
medicinal (trace) (chloride)	T45.8X1	T45.8X2	T45.8X3	T45.8X4	T45.8X5	T45.8X6
Cobra (venom)	T63.041	T63.042	T63.043	T63.044	—	—
Coca (leaf)	T40.5X1	T40.5X2	T40.5X3	T40.5X4	T40.5X5	T40.5X6
Cocaine	T40.5X1	T40.5X2	T40.5X3	T40.5X4	T40.5X5	T40.5X6
topical anesthetic	T41.3X1	T41.3X2	T41.3X3	T41.3X4	T41.3X5	T41.3X6
Cocarboxylase	T45.3X1	T45.3X2	T45.3X3	T45.3X4	T45.3X5	T45.3X6
Coccidioidin	T50.8X1	T50.8X2	T50.8X3	T50.8X4	T50.8X5	T50.8X6
Cocculus indicus	T62.1X1	T62.1X2	T62.1X3	T62.1X4	—	—
Cochineal	T65.6X1	T65.6X2	T65.6X3	T65.6X4	—	—
medicinal products	T50.991	T50.992	T50.993	T50.994	T50.995	T50.996
Codeine	T40.2X1	T40.2X2	T40.2X3	T40.2X4	T40.2X5	T40.2X6
Cod-liver oil	T45.2X1	T45.2X2	T45.2X3	T45.2X4	T45.2X5	T45.2X6
Coenzyme A	T50.991	T50.992	T50.993	T50.994	T50.995	T50.996
Coffee	T62.8X1	T62.8X2	T62.8X3	T62.8X4	—	—
Cogalactoiso-merase	T50.991	T50.992	T50.993	T50.994	T50.995	T50.996
Cogentin	T44.3X1	T44.3X2	T44.3X3	T44.3X4	T44.3X5	T44.3X6
Coke fumes or gas (carbon monoxide)	T58.2X1	T58.2X2	T58.2X3	T58.2X4	—	—
industrial use	T58.8X1	T58.8X2	T58.8X3	T58.8X4	—	—
Colace	T47.4X1	T47.4X2	T47.4X3	T47.4X4	T47.4X5	T47.4X6
Colaspase	T45.1X1	T45.1X2	T45.1X3	T45.1X4	T45.1X5	T45.1X6
Colchicine	T50.4X1	T50.4X2	T50.4X3	T50.4X4	T50.4X5	T50.4X6
Colchicum	T62.2X1	T62.2X2	T62.2X3	T62.2X4	—	—
Cold cream	T49.3X1	T49.3X2	T49.3X3	T49.3X4	T49.3X5	T49.3X6
Colecalciferol	T45.2X1	T45.2X2	T45.2X3	T45.2X4	T45.2X5	T45.2X6
Colestipol	T46.6X1	T46.6X2	T46.6X3	T46.6X4	T46.6X5	T46.6X6
Colestyramine	T46.6X1	T46.6X2	T46.6X3	T46.6X4	T46.6X5	T46.6X6
Colimycin	T36.8X1	T36.8X2	T36.8X3	T36.8X4	T36.8X5	T36.8X6
Colistimethate	T36.8X1	T36.8X2	T36.8X3	T36.8X4	T36.8X5	T36.8X6
Colistin	T36.8X1	T36.8X2	T36.8X3	T36.8X4	T36.8X5	T36.8X6
sulfate (eye preparation)	T49.5X1	T49.5X2	T49.5X3	T49.5X4	T49.5X5	T49.5X6
Collagen	T50.991	T50.992	T50.993	T50.994	T50.995	T50.996
Collagenase	T49.4X1	T49.4X2	T49.4X3	T49.4X4	T49.4X5	T49.4X6
Collodion	T49.3X1	T49.3X2	T49.3X3	T49.3X4	T49.3X5	T49.3X6
Colocynth	T47.2X1	T47.2X2	T47.2X3	T47.2X4	T47.2X5	T47.2X6
Colophony adhesive	T49.3X1	T49.3X2	T49.3X3	T49.3X4	T49.3X5	T49.3X6
Colorant—see also Dye	T50.991	T50.992	T50.993	T50.994	T50.995	T50.996

Substance	Poisoning, Accidental (unintentional)	Poisoning, Intentional self-harm	Poisoning, Assault	Poisoning, Undetermined	Adverse effect	Underdosing
Coloring matter—see Dye(s)						
Combustion gas (after combustion)—see Carbon, monoxide						
prior to combustion	T59.891	T59.892	T59.893	T59.894	—	—
Compazine	T43.3X1	T43.3X2	T43.3X3	T43.3X4	T43.3X5	T43.3X6
Compound						
42 (warfarin)	T60.4X1	T60.4X2	T60.4X3	T60.4X4	—	—
269 (endrin)	T60.1X1	T60.1X2	T60.1X3	T60.1X4	—	—
497 (dieldrin)	T60.1X1	T60.1X2	T60.1X3	T60.1X4	—	—
1080 (sodium fluoroacetate)	T60.4X1	T60.4X2	T60.4X3	T60.4X4	—	—
3422 (parathion)	T60.0X1	T60.0X2	T60.0X3	T60.0X4	—	—
3911 (phorate)	T60.0X1	T60.0X2	T60.0X3	T60.0X4	—	—
3956 (toxaphene)	T60.1X1	T60.1X2	T60.1X3	T60.1X4	—	—
4049 (malathion)	T60.0X1	T60.0X2	T60.0X3	T60.0X4	—	—
4069 (malathion)	T60.0X1	T60.0X2	T60.0X3	T60.0X4	—	—
4124 (dicapthon)	T60.0X1	T60.0X2	T60.0X3	T60.0X4	—	—
E (cortisone)	T38.0X1	T38.0X2	T38.0X3	T38.0X4	T38.0X5	T38.0X6
F (hydrocortisone)	T38.0X1	T38.0X2	T38.0X3	T38.0X4	T38.0X5	T38.0X6
Congener, avwnabolic	T38.7X1	T38.7X2	T38.7X3	T38.7X4	T38.7X5	T38.7X6
Congo red	T50.8X1	T50.8X2	T50.8X3	T50.8X4	T50.8X5	T50.8X6
Coniine, conine	T62.2X1	T62.2X2	T62.2X3	T62.2X4	—	—
Conium (maculatum)	T62.2X1	T62.2X2	T62.2X3	T62.2X4	—	—
Conjugated estrogenic substances	T38.5X1	T38.5X2	T38.5X3	T38.5X4	T38.5X5	T38.5X6
Contac	T48.5X1	T48.5X2	T48.5X3	T48.5X4	T48.5X5	T48.5X6
Contact lens solution	T49.5X1	T49.5X2	T49.5X3	T49.5X4	T49.5X5	T49.5X6
Contraceptive (oral)	T38.4X1	T38.4X2	T38.4X3	T38.4X4	T38.4X5	T38.4X6
vaginal	T49.8X1	T49.8X2	T49.8X3	T49.8X4	T49.8X5	T49.8X6
Contrast medium, radiography	T50.8X1	T50.8X2	T50.8X3	T50.8X4	T50.8X5	T50.8X6
Convallaria glycosides	T46.0X1	T46.0X2	T46.0X3	T46.0X4	T46.0X5	T46.0X6
Convallaria majalis	T62.2X1	T62.2X2	T62.2X3	T62.2X4	—	—
berry	T62.1X1	T62.1X2	T62.1X3	T62.1X4	—	—
Copper (dust) (fumes) (nonmedicinal) NEC	T56.4X1	T56.4X2	T56.4X3	T56.4X4	—	—
arsenate, arsenite	T57.0X1	T57.0X2	T57.0X3	T57.0X4	—	—
insecticide	T60.2X1	T60.2X2	T60.2X3	T60.2X4	—	—
emetic	T47.7X1	T47.7X2	T47.7X3	T47.7X4	T47.7X5	T47.7X6
fungicide	T60.3X1	T60.3X2	T60.3X3	T60.3X4	—	—
gluconate	T49.0X1	T49.0X2	T49.0X3	T49.0X4	T49.0X5	T49.0X6
insecticide	T60.2X1	T60.2X2	T60.2X3	T60.2X4	—	—
medicinal (trace)	T45.8X1	T45.8X2	T45.8X3	T45.8X4	T45.8X5	T45.8X6
oleate	T49.0X1	T49.0X2	T49.0X3	T49.0X4	T49.0X5	T49.0X6
sulfate	T56.4X1	T56.4X2	T56.4X3	T56.4X4	—	—
cupric	T56.4X1	T56.4X2	T56.4X3	T56.4X4	—	—
fungicide	T60.3X1	T60.3X2	T60.3X3	T60.3X4	—	—
medicinal						
ear	T49.6X1	T49.6X2	T49.6X3	T49.6X4	T49.6X5	T49.6X6
emetic	T47.7X1	T47.7X2	T47.7X3	T47.7X4	T47.7X5	T47.7X6
Copper NEC — *Continued*						
eye	T49.5X1	T49.5X2	T49.5X3	T49.5X4	T49.5X5	T49.5X6
cuprous	T56.4X1	T56.4X2	T56.4X3	T56.4X4	—	—
fungicide	T60.3X1	T60.3X2	T60.3X3	T60.3X4	—	—
medicinal						
ear	T49.6X1	T49.6X2	T49.6X3	T49.6X4	T49.6X5	T49.6X6
emetic	T47.7X1	T47.7X2	T47.7X3	T47.7X4	T47.7X5	T47.7X6
eye	T49.5X1	T49.5X2	T49.5X3	T49.5X4	T49.5X5	T49.5X6
Copperhead snake (bite) (venom)	T63.061	T63.062	T63.063	T63.064	—	—
Coral (sting)	T63.691	T63.692	T63.693	T63.694	—	—
snake (bite) (venom)	T63.021	T63.022	T63.023	T63.024	—	—
Corbadrine	T49.6X1	T49.6X2	T49.6X3	T49.6X4	T49.6X5	T49.6X6
Cordite	T65.891	T65.892	T65.893	T65.894	—	—
vapor	T59.891	T59.892	T59.893	T59.894	—	—
Cordran	T49.0X1	T49.0X2	T49.0X3	T49.0X4	T49.0X5	T49.0X6
Corn cures	T49.4X1	T49.4X2	T49.4X3	T49.4X4	T49.4X5	T49.4X6
Corn starch	T49.3X1	T49.3X2	T49.3X3	T49.3X4	T49.3X5	T49.3X6
Cornhusker's lotion	T49.3X1	T49.3X2	T49.3X3	T49.3X4	T49.3X5	T49.3X6
Coronary vasodilator NEC	T46.3X1	T46.3X2	T46.3X3	T46.3X4	T46.3X5	T46.3X6
Corrosive NEC	T54.91	T54.92	T54.93	T54.94	—	—
acid NEC	T54.2X1	T54.2X2	T54.2X3	T54.2X4	—	—
aromatics	T54.1X1	T54.1X2	T54.1X3	T54.1X4	—	—
disinfectant	T54.1X1	T54.1X2	T54.1X3	T54.1X4	—	—
fumes NEC	T54.91	T54.92	T54.93	T54.94	—	—
specified NEC	T54.91	T54.92	T54.93	T54.94	—	—
sublimate	T56.1X1	T56.1X2	T56.1X3	T56.1X4	—	—
Cortate	T38.0X1	T38.0X2	T38.0X3	T38.0X4	T38.0X5	T38.0X6
Cort-Dome	T38.0X1	T38.0X2	T38.0X3	T38.0X4	T38.0X5	T38.0X6
ENT agent	T49.6X1	T49.6X2	T49.6X3	T49.6X4	T49.6X5	T49.6X6
ophthalmic preparation	T49.5X1	T49.5X2	T49.5X3	T49.5X4	T49.5X5	T49.5X6
topical NEC	T49.0X1	T49.0X2	T49.0X3	T49.0X4	T49.0X5	T49.0X6
Cortef	T38.0X1	T38.0X2	T38.0X3	T38.0X4	T38.0X5	T38.0X6
ENT agent	T49.6X1	T49.6X2	T49.6X3	T49.6X4	T49.6X5	T49.6X6
ophthalmic preparation	T49.5X1	T49.5X2	T49.5X3	T49.5X4	T49.5X5	T49.5X6
topical NEC	T49.0X1	T49.0X2	T49.0X3	T49.0X4	T49.0X5	T49.0X6
Corticosteroid	T38.0X1	T38.0X2	T38.0X3	T38.0X4	T38.0X5	T38.0X6
ENT agent	T49.6X1	T49.6X2	T49.6X3	T49.6X4	T49.6X5	T49.6X6
mineral	T50.0X1	T50.0X2	T50.0X3	T50.0X4	T50.0X5	T50.0X6
ophthalmic	T49.5X1	T49.5X2	T49.5X3	T49.5X4	T49.5X5	T49.5X6
topical NEC	T49.0X1	T49.0X2	T49.0X3	T49.0X4	T49.0X5	T49.0X6
Corticotropin	T38.811	T38.812	T38.813	T38.814	T38.815	T38.816
Cortisol	T49.0X1	T49.0X2	T49.0X3	T49.0X4	T49.0X5	T49.0X6
ENT agent	T49.6X1	T49.6X2	T49.6X3	T49.6X4	T49.6X5	T49.6X6
ophthalmic preparation	T49.5X1	T49.5X2	T49.5X3	T49.5X4	T49.5X5	T49.5X6
topical NEC	T49.0X1	T49.0X2	T49.0X3	T49.0X4	T49.0X5	T49.0X6
Cortisone (acetate)	T38.0X1	T38.0X2	T38.0X3	T38.0X4	T38.0X5	T38.0X6
ENT agent	T49.6X1	T49.6X2	T49.6X3	T49.6X4	T49.6X5	T49.6X6

Substance	Poisoning, Accidental (unintentional)	Poisoning, Intentional self-harm	Poisoning, Assault	Poisoning, Undetermined	Adverse effect	Underdosing
Cortisone — *Continued*						
ophthalmic preparation	T49.5X1	T49.5X2	T49.5X3	T49.5X4	T49.5X5	T49.5X6
topical NEC	T49.0X1	T49.0X2	T49.0X3	T49.0X4	T49.0X5	T49.0X6
Cortivazol	T38.0X1	T38.0X2	T38.0X3	T38.0X4	T38.0X5	T38.0X6
Cortogen	T38.0X1	T38.0X2	T38.0X3	T38.0X4	T38.0X5	T38.0X6
ENT agent	T49.6X1	T49.6X2	T49.6X3	T49.6X4	T49.6X5	T49.6X6
ophthalmic preparation	T49.5X1	T49.5X2	T49.5X3	T49.5X4	T49.5X5	T49.5X6
Cortone	T38.0X1	T38.0X2	T38.0X3	T38.0X4	T38.0X5	T38.0X6
ENT agent	T49.6X1	T49.6X2	T49.6X3	T49.6X4	T49.6X5	T49.6X6
ophthalmic preparation	T49.5X1	T49.5X2	T49.5X3	T49.5X4	T49.5X5	T49.5X6
Cortril	T38.0X1	T38.0X2	T38.0X3	T38.0X4	T38.0X5	T38.0X6
ENT agent	T49.6X1	T49.6X2	T49.6X3	T49.6X4	T49.6X5	T49.6X6
ophthalmic preparation	T49.5X1	T49.5X2	T49.5X3	T49.5X4	T49.5X5	T49.5X6
topical NEC	T49.0X1	T49.0X2	T49.0X3	T49.0X4	T49.0X5	T49.0X6
Corynebacterium parvum	T45.1X1	T45.1X2	T45.1X3	T45.1X4	T45.1X5	T45.1X6
Cosmetic preparation	T49.8X1	T49.8X2	T49.8X3	T49.8X4	T49.8X5	T49.8X6
Cosmetics	T49.8X1	T49.8X2	T49.8X3	T49.8X4	T49.8X5	T49.8X6
Cosyntropin	T38.811	T38.812	T38.813	T38.814	T38.815	T38.816
Cotarnine	T45.7X1	T45.7X2	T45.7X3	T45.7X4	T45.7X5	T45.7X6
Co-trimoxazole	T36.8X1	T36.8X2	T36.8X3	T36.8X4	T36.8X5	T36.8X6
Cottonseed oil	T49.3X1	T49.3X2	T49.3X3	T49.3X4	T49.3X5	T49.3X6
Cough mixture (syrup)	T48.4X1	T48.4X2	T48.4X3	T48.4X4	T48.4X5	T48.4X6
containing opiates	T40.2X1	T40.2X2	T40.2X3	T40.2X4	T40.2X5	T40.2X6
expectorants	T48.4X1	T48.4X2	T48.4X3	T48.4X4	T48.4X5	T48.4X6
Coumadin	T45.511	T45.512	T45.513	T45.514	T45.515	T45.516
rodenticide	T60.4X1	T60.4X2	T60.4X3	T60.4X4	—	—
Coumaphos	T60.0X1	T60.0X2	T60.0X3	T60.0X4	—	—
Coumarin	T45.511	T45.512	T45.513	T45.514	T45.515	T45.516
Coumetarol	T45.511	T45.512	T45.513	T45.514	T45.515	T45.516
Cowbane	T62.2X1	T62.2X2	T62.2X3	T62.2X4	—	—
Cozyme	T45.2X1	T45.2X2	T45.2X3	T45.2X4	T45.2X5	T45.2X6
Crack	T40.5X1	T40.5X2	T40.5X3	T40.5X4	—	—
Crataegus extract	T46.0X1	T46.0X2	T46.0X3	T46.0X4	T46.0X5	T46.0X6
Creolin	T54.1X1	T54.1X2	T54.1X3	T54.1X4	—	—
disinfectant	T54.1X1	T54.1X2	T54.1X3	T54.1X4	—	—
Creosol (compound)	T49.0X1	T49.0X2	T49.0X3	T49.0X4	T49.0X5	T49.0X6
Creosote (coal tar) (beechwood)	T49.0X1	T49.0X2	T49.0X3	T49.0X4	T49.0X5	T49.0X6
medicinal (expectorant)	T48.4X1	T48.4X2	T48.4X3	T48.4X4	T48.4X5	T48.4X6
syrup	T48.4X1	T48.4X2	T48.4X3	T48.4X4	T48.4X5	T48.4X6
Cresol(s)	T49.0X1	T49.0X2	T49.0X3	T49.0X4	T49.0X5	T49.0X6
and soap solution	T49.0X1	T49.0X2	T49.0X3	T49.0X4	T49.0X5	T49.0X6
Cresyl acetate	T49.0X1	T49.0X2	T49.0X3	T49.0X4	T49.0X5	T49.0X6
Cresylic acid	T49.0X1	T49.0X2	T49.0X3	T49.0X4	T49.0X5	T49.0X6
Crimidine	T60.4X1	T60.4X2	T60.4X3	T60.4X4	—	—
Croconazole	T37.8X1	T37.8X2	T37.8X3	T37.8X4	T37.8X5	T37.8X6
Cromoglicic acid	T48.6X1	T48.6X2	T48.6X3	T48.6X4	T48.6X5	T48.6X6
Cromolyn	T48.6X1	T48.6X2	T48.6X3	T48.6X4	T48.6X5	T48.6X6
Cromonar	T46.3X1	T46.3X2	T46.3X3	T46.3X4	T46.3X5	T46.3X6
Cropropamide	T39.8X1	T39.8X2	T39.8X3	T39.8X4	T39.8X5	T39.8X6
Cropropamide — *Continued*						
with crotethamide	T50.7X1	T50.7X2	T50.7X3	T50.7X4	T50.7X5	T50.7X6
Crotamiton	T49.0X1	T49.0X2	T49.0X3	T49.0X4	T49.0X5	T49.0X6
Crotethamide	T39.8X1	T39.8X2	T39.8X3	T39.8X4	T39.8X5	T39.8X6
with cropropamide	T50.7X1	T50.7X2	T50.7X3	T50.7X4	T50.7X5	T50.7X6
Croton (oil)	T47.2X1	T47.2X2	T47.2X3	T47.2X4	T47.2X5	T47.2X6
chloral	T42.6X1	T42.6X2	T42.6X3	T42.6X4	T42.6X5	T42.6X6
Crude oil	T52.0X1	T52.0X2	T52.0X3	T52.0X4	—	—
Cryogenine	T39.8X1	T39.8X2	T39.8X3	T39.8X4	T39.8X5	T39.8X6
Cryolite (vapor)	T60.1X1	T60.1X2	T60.1X3	T60.1X4	—	—
insecticide	T60.1X1	T60.1X2	T60.1X3	T60.1X4	—	—
Cryptenamine (tannates)	T46.5X1	T46.5X2	T46.5X3	T46.5X4	T46.5X5	T46.5X6
Crystal violet	T49.0X1	T49.0X2	T49.0X3	T49.0X4	T49.0X5	T49.0X6
Cuckoopint	T62.2X1	T62.2X2	T62.2X3	T62.2X4	—	—
Cumetharol	T45.511	T45.512	T45.513	T45.514	T45.515	T45.516
Cupric						
acetate	T60.3X1	T60.3X2	T60.3X3	T60.3X4	—	—
acetoarsenite	T57.0X1	T57.0X2	T57.0X3	T57.0X4	—	—
arsenate	T57.0X1	T57.0X2	T57.0X3	T57.0X4	—	—
gluconate	T49.0X1	T49.0X2	T49.0X3	T49.0X4	T49.0X5	T49.0X6
oleate	T49.0X1	T49.0X2	T49.0X3	T49.0X4	T49.0X5	T49.0X6
sulfate	T56.4X1	T56.4X2	T56.4X3	T56.4X4	—	—
Cuprous sulfate—see also Copper sulfate	T56.4X1	T56.4X2	T56.4X3	T56.4X4	—	—
Curare, curarine	T48.1X1	T48.1X2	T48.1X3	T48.1X4	T48.1X5	T48.1X6
Cyamemazine	T43.3X1	T43.3X2	T43.3X3	T43.3X4	T43.3X5	T43.3X6
Cyamopsis tetragono-loba	T46.6X1	T46.6X2	T46.6X3	T46.6X4	T46.6X5	T46.6X6
Cyanacetyl hydrazide	T37.1X1	T37.1X2	T37.1X3	T37.1X4	T37.1X5	T37.1X6
Cyanic acid (gas)	T59.891	T59.892	T59.893	T59.894	—	—
Cyanide(s) (compounds) (potassium) (sodium) NEC	T65.0X1	T65.0X2	T65.0X3	T65.0X4	—	—
dust or gas (inhalation) NEC	T57.3X1	T57.3X2	T57.3X3	T57.3X4	—	—
fumigant	T65.0X1	T65.0X2	T65.0X3	T65.0X4	—	—
hydrogen	T57.3X1	T57.3X2	T57.3X3	T57.3X4	—	—
mercuric—see *Mercury*						
pesticide (dust) (fumes)	T65.0X1	T65.0X2	T65.0X3	T65.0X4	—	—
Cyanoacrylate adhesive	T49.3X1	T49.3X2	T49.3X3	T49.3X4	T49.3X5	T49.3X6
Cyanocobalamin	T45.8X1	T45.8X2	T45.8X3	T45.8X4	T45.8X5	T45.8X6
Cyanogen (chloride) (gas) NEC	T59.891	T59.892	T59.893	T59.894	—	—
Cyclacillin	T36.0X1	T36.0X2	T36.0X3	T36.0X4	T36.0X5	T36.0X6
Cyclaine	T41.3X1	T41.3X2	T41.3X3	T41.3X4	T41.3X5	T41.3X6
Cyclamate	T50.991	T50.992	T50.993	T50.994	T50.995	T50.996
Cyclamen europaeum	T62.2X1	T62.2X2	T62.2X3	T62.2X4	—	—
Cyclandelate	T46.7X1	T46.7X2	T46.7X3	T46.7X4	T46.7X5	T46.7X6
Cyclazocine	T50.7X1	T50.7X2	T50.7X3	T50.7X4	T50.7X5	T50.7X6
Cyclizine	T45.0X1	T45.0X2	T45.0X3	T45.0X4	T45.0X5	T45.0X6
Cyclobarbital	T42.3X1	T42.3X2	T42.3X3	T42.3X4	T42.3X5	T42.3X6

Substance	Poisoning, Accidental (unintentional)	Poisoning, Intentional self-harm	Poisoning, Assault	Poisoning, Undetermined	Adverse effect	Underdosing
Cyclobarbitone	T42.3X1	T42.3X2	T42.3X3	T42.3X4	T42.3X5	T42.3X6
Cyclobenzaprine	T48.1X1	T48.1X2	T48.1X3	T48.1X4	T48.1X5	T48.1X6
Cyclodrine	T44.3X1	T44.3X2	T44.3X3	T44.3X4	T44.3X5	T44.3X6
Cycloguanil embonate	T37.2X1	T37.2X2	T37.2X3	T37.2X4	T37.2X5	T37.2X6
Cyclohexane	T52.8X1	T52.8X2	T52.8X3	T52.8X4	—	—
Cyclohexanol	T51.8X1	T51.8X2	T51.8X3	T51.8X4	—	—
Cyclohexanone	T52.4X1	T52.4X2	T52.4X3	T52.4X4	—	—
Cycloheximide	T60.3X1	T60.3X2	T60.3X3	T60.3X4	—	—
Cyclohexyl acetate	T52.8X1	T52.8X2	T52.8X3	T52.8X4	—	—
Cycloleucin	T45.1X1	T45.1X2	T45.1X3	T45.1X4	T45.1X5	T45.1X6
Cyclomethycaine	T41.3X1	T41.3X2	T41.3X3	T41.3X4	T41.3X5	T41.3X6
Cyclopentamine	T44.4X1	T44.4X2	T44.4X3	T44.4X4	T44.4X5	T44.4X6
Cyclopenthiazide	T50.2X1	T50.2X2	T50.2X3	T50.2X4	T50.2X5	T50.2X6
Cyclopentolate	T44.3X1	T44.3X2	T44.3X3	T44.3X4	T44.3X5	T44.3X6
Cyclophosphamide	T45.1X1	T45.1X2	T45.1X3	T45.1X4	T45.1X5	T45.1X6
Cycloplegic drug	T49.5X1	T49.5X2	T49.5X3	T49.5X4	T49.5X5	T49.5X6
Cyclopropane	T41.291	T41.292	T41.293	T41.294	T41.295	T41.296
Cyclopyrabital	T39.8X1	T39.8X2	T39.8X3	T39.8X4	T39.8X5	T39.8X6
Cycloserine	T37.1X1	T37.1X2	T37.1X3	T37.1X4	T37.1X5	T37.1X6
Cyclosporin	T45.1X1	T45.1X2	T45.1X3	T45.1X4	T45.1X5	T45.1X6
Cyclothiazide	T50.2X1	T50.2X2	T50.2X3	T50.2X4	T50.2X5	T50.2X6
Cycrimine	T44.3X1	T44.3X2	T44.3X3	T44.3X4	T44.3X5	T44.3X6
Cyhalothrin	T60.1X1	T60.1X2	T60.1X3	T60.1X4	—	—
Cymarin	T46.0X1	T46.0X2	T46.0X3	T46.0X4	T46.0X5	T46.0X6
Cypermethrin	T60.1X1	T60.1X2	T60.1X3	T60.1X4	—	—
Cyphenothrin	T60.2X1	T60.2X2	T60.2X3	T60.2X4	—	—
Cyproheptadine	T45.0X1	T45.0X2	T45.0X3	T45.0X4	T45.0X5	T45.0X6
Cyproterone	T38.6X1	T38.6X2	T38.6X3	T38.6X4	T38.6X5	T38.6X6
Cysteamine	T50.6X1	T50.6X2	T50.6X3	T50.6X4	T50.6X5	T50.6X6
Cytarabine	T45.1X1	T45.1X2	T45.1X3	T45.1X4	T45.1X5	T45.1X6
Cytisus						
laburnum	T62.2X1	T62.2X2	T62.2X3	T62.2X4	—	—
scoparius	T62.2X1	T62.2X2	T62.2X3	T62.2X4	—	—
Cytochrome C	T47.5X1	T47.5X2	T47.5X3	T47.5X4	T47.5X5	T47.5X6
Cytomel	T38.1X1	T38.1X2	T38.1X3	T38.1X4	T38.1X5	T38.1X6
Cytosine arabinoside	T45.1X1	T45.1X2	T45.1X3	T45.1X4	T45.1X5	T45.1X6
Cytoxan	T45.1X1	T45.1X2	T45.1X3	T45.1X4	T45.1X5	T45.1X6
Cytozyme	T45.7X1	T45.7X2	T45.7X3	T45.7X4	T45.7X5	T45.7X6
2,4-D	T60.3X1	T60.3X2	T60.3X3	T60.3X4	—	—
D						
Dacarbazine	T45.1X1	T45.1X2	T45.1X3	T45.1X4	T45.1X5	T45.1X6
Dactinomycin	T45.1X1	T45.1X2	T45.1X3	T45.1X4	T45.1X5	T45.1X6
DADPS	T37.1X1	T37.1X2	T37.1X3	T37.1X4	T37.1X5	T37.1X6
Dakin's solution	T49.0X1	T49.0X2	T49.0X3	T49.0X4	T49.0X5	T49.0X6
Dalapon (sodium)	T60.3X1	T60.3X2	T60.3X3	T60.3X4	—	—
Dalmane	T42.4X1	T42.4X2	T42.4X3	T42.4X4	T42.4X5	T42.4X6
Danazol	T38.6X1	T38.6X2	T38.6X3	T38.6X4	T38.6X5	T38.6X6
Danilone	T45.511	T45.512	T45.513	T45.514	T45.515	T45.516
Danthron	T47.2X1	T47.2X2	T47.2X3	T47.2X4	T47.2X5	T47.2X6
Dantrolene	T42.8X1	T42.8X2	T42.8X3	T42.8X4	T42.8X5	T42.8X6

Substance	Poisoning, Accidental (unintentional)	Poisoning, Intentional self-harm	Poisoning, Assault	Poisoning, Undetermined	Adverse effect	Underdosing
Dantron	T47.2X1	T47.2X2	T47.2X3	T47.2X4	T47.2X5	T47.2X6
Daphne (gnidium) (mezereum)	T62.2X1	T62.2X2	T62.2X3	T62.2X4	—	—
berry	T62.1X1	T62.1X2	T62.1X3	T62.1X4	—	—
Dapsone	T37.1X1	T37.1X2	T37.1X3	T37.1X4	T37.1X5	T37.1X6
Daraprim	T37.2X1	T37.2X2	T37.2X3	T37.2X4	T37.2X5	T37.2X6
Darnel	T62.2X1	T62.2X2	T62.2X3	T62.2X4	—	—
Darvon	T39.8X1	T39.8X2	T39.8X3	T39.8X4	T39.8X5	T39.8X6
Daunomycin	T45.1X1	T45.1X2	T45.1X3	T45.1X4	T45.1X5	T45.1X6
Daunorubicin	T45.1X1	T45.1X2	T45.1X3	T45.1X4	T45.1X5	T45.1X6
DBI	T38.3X1	T38.3X2	T38.3X3	T38.3X4	T38.3X5	T38.3X6
D-Con	T60.91	T60.92	T60.93	T60.94	—	—
insecticide	T60.2X1	T60.2X2	T60.2X3	T60.2X4	—	—
rodenticide	T60.4X1	T60.4X2	T60.4X3	T60.4X4	—	—
DDAVP	T38.891	T38.892	T38.893	T38.894	T38.895	T38.896
DDE (bis (chlorophenyl)-dichloroethylene)	T60.2X1	T60.2X2	T60.2X3	T60.2X4	—	—
DDS	T37.1X1	T37.1X2	T37.1X3	T37.1X4	T37.1X5	T37.1X6
DDT (dust)	T60.1X1	T60.1X2	T60.1X3	T60.1X4	—	—
Deadly nightshade—see also Belladonna	T62.2X1	T62.2X2	T62.2X3	T62.2X4	—	—
berry	T62.1X1	T62.1X2	T62.1X3	T62.1X4	—	—
Deamino-D-arginine vasopressin	T38.891	T38.892	T38.893	T38.894	T38.895	T38.896
Deanol (aceglumate)	T50.991	T50.992	T50.993	T50.994	T50.995	T50.996
Debrisoquine	T46.5X1	T46.5X2	T46.5X3	T46.5X4	T46.5X5	T46.5X6
Decaborane	T57.8X1	T57.8X2	T57.8X3	T57.8X4	—	—
fumes	T59.891	T59.892	T59.893	T59.894	—	—
Decadron	T38.0X1	T38.0X2	T38.0X3	T38.0X4	T38.0X5	T38.0X6
ENT agent	T49.6X1	T49.6X2	T49.6X3	T49.6X4	T49.6X5	T49.6X6
ophthalmic preparation	T49.5X1	T49.5X2	T49.5X3	T49.5X4	T49.5X5	T49.5X6
topical NEC	T49.0X1	T49.0X2	T49.0X3	T49.0X4	T49.0X5	T49.0X6
Decahydro-naphthalene	T52.8X1	T52.8X2	T52.8X3	T52.8X4	—	—
Decalin	T52.8X1	T52.8X2	T52.8X3	T52.8X4	—	—
Decamethonium (bromide)	T48.1X1	T48.1X2	T48.1X3	T48.1X4	T48.1X5	T48.1X6
Decholin	T47.5X1	T47.5X2	T47.5X3	T47.5X4	T47.5X5	T47.5X6
Declomycin	T36.4X1	T36.4X2	T36.4X3	T36.4X4	T36.4X5	T36.4X6
Decongestant, nasal (mucosa)	T48.5X1	T48.5X2	T48.5X3	T48.5X4	T48.5X5	T48.5X6
combination	T48.5X1	T48.5X2	T48.5X3	T48.5X4	T48.5X5	T48.5X6
Deet	T60.8X1	T60.8X2	T60.8X3	T60.8X4	—	—
Deferoxamine	T45.8X1	T45.8X2	T45.8X3	T45.8X4	T45.8X5	T45.8X6
Deflazacort	T38.0X1	T38.0X2	T38.0X3	T38.0X4	T38.0X5	T38.0X6
Deglycyrrhizinized extract of licorice	T48.4X1	T48.4X2	T48.4X3	T48.4X4	T48.4X5	T48.4X6
Dehydrocholic acid	T47.5X1	T47.5X2	T47.5X3	T47.5X4	T47.5X5	T47.5X6
Dehydroemetine	T37.3X1	T37.3X2	T37.3X3	T37.3X4	T37.3X5	T37.3X6
Dekalin	T52.8X1	T52.8X2	T52.8X3	T52.8X4	—	—
Delalutin	T38.5X1	T38.5X2	T38.5X3	T38.5X4	T38.5X5	T38.5X6
Delorazepam	T42.4X1	T42.4X2	T42.4X3	T42.4X4	T42.4X5	T42.4X6
Delphinium	T62.2X1	T62.2X2	T62.2X3	T62.2X4	—	—

Substance	Poisoning, Accidental (unintentional)	Poisoning, Intentional self-harm	Poisoning, Assault	Poisoning, Undetermined	Adverse effect	Underdosing
Deltamethrin	T60.1X1	T60.1X2	T60.1X3	T60.1X4	—	—
Deltasone	T38.0X1	T38.0X2	T38.0X3	T38.0X4	T38.0X5	T38.0X6
Deltra	T38.0X1	T38.0X2	T38.0X3	T38.0X4	T38.0X5	T38.0X6
Delvinal	T42.3X1	T42.3X2	T42.3X3	T42.3X4	T42.3X5	T42.3X6
Demecarium (bromide)	T49.5X1	T49.5X2	T49.5X3	T49.5X4	T49.5X5	T49.5X6
Demeclocycline	T36.4X1	T36.4X2	T36.4X3	T36.4X4	T36.4X5	T36.4X6
Demecolcine	T45.1X1	T45.1X2	T45.1X3	T45.1X4	T45.1X5	T45.1X6
Demegestone	T38.5X1	T38.5X2	T38.5X3	T38.5X4	T38.5X5	T38.5X6
Demelanizing agents	T49.8X1	T49.8X2	T49.8X3	T49.8X4	T49.8X5	T49.8X6
Demephion -O and -S	T60.0X1	T60.0X2	T60.0X3	T60.0X4	—	—
Demerol	T40.2X1	T40.2X2	T40.2X3	T40.2X4	T40.2X5	T40.2X6
Demethylchlor-tetracycline	T36.4X1	T36.4X2	T36.4X3	T36.4X4	T36.4X5	T36.4X6
Demethyltetracycline	T36.4X1	T36.4X2	T36.4X3	T36.4X4	T36.4X5	T36.4X6
Demeton -O and -S	T60.0X1	T60.0X2	T60.0X3	T60.0X4	—	—
Demulcent (external)	T49.3X1	T49.3X2	T49.3X3	T49.3X4	T49.3X5	T49.3X6
specified NEC	T49.3X1	T49.3X2	T49.3X3	T49.3X4	T49.3X5	T49.3X6
Demulen	T38.4X1	T38.4X2	T38.4X3	T38.4X4	T38.4X5	T38.4X6
Denatured alcohol	T51.0X1	T51.0X2	T51.0X3	T51.0X4	—	—
Dendrid	T49.5X1	T49.5X2	T49.5X3	T49.5X4	T49.5X5	T49.5X6
Dental drug, topical application NEC	T49.7X1	T49.7X2	T49.7X3	T49.7X4	T49.7X5	T49.7X6
Dentifrice	T49.7X1	T49.7X2	T49.7X3	T49.7X4	T49.7X5	T49.7X6
Deodorant spray (feminine hygiene)	T49.8X1	T49.8X2	T49.8X3	T49.8X4	T49.8X5	T49.8X6
Deoxycortone	T50.0X1	T50.0X2	T50.0X3	T50.0X4	T50.0X5	T50.0X6
2-Deoxy-5-fluorouridine	T45.1X1	T45.1X2	T45.1X3	T45.1X4	T45.1X5	T45.1X6
5-Deoxy-5-fluorouridine	T45.1X1	T45.1X2	T45.1X3	T45.1X4	T45.1X5	T45.1X6
Deoxyribonuclease (pancreatic)	T45.3X1	T45.3X2	T45.3X3	T45.3X4	T45.3X5	T45.3X6
Depilatory	T49.4X1	T49.4X2	T49.4X3	T49.4X4	T49.4X5	T49.4X6
Deprenalin	T42.8X1	T42.8X2	T42.8X3	T42.8X4	T42.8X5	T42.8X6
Deprenyl	T42.8X1	T42.8X2	T42.8X3	T42.8X4	T42.8X5	T42.8X6
Depressant, appetite	T50.5X1	T50.5X2	T50.5X3	T50.5X4	T50.5X5	T50.5X6
Depressant						
appetite (central)	T50.5X1	T50.5X2	T50.5X3	T50.5X4	T50.5X5	T50.5X6
cardiac	T46.2X1	T46.2X2	T46.2X3	T46.2X4	T46.2X5	T46.2X6
central nervous system (anesthetic)—see also Central nervous system, depressants	T42.71	T42.72	T42.73	T42.74	T42.75	T42.76
general anesthetic	T41.201	T41.202	T41.203	T41.204	T41.205	T41.206
muscle tone	T42.8X1	T42.8X2	T42.8X3	T42.8X4	T42.8X5	T42.8X6
muscle tone, central	T42.8X1	T42.8X2	T42.8X3	T42.8X4	T42.8X5	T42.8X6
psychotherapeutic	T43.501	T43.502	T43.503	T43.504	T43.505	T43.506
Deptropine	T45.0X1	T45.0X2	T45.0X3	T45.0X4	T45.0X5	T45.0X6
Dequalinium (chloride)	T49.0X1	T49.0X2	T49.0X3	T49.0X4	T49.0X5	T49.0X6
Derris root	T60.2X1	T60.2X2	T60.2X3	T60.2X4	—	—
Deserpidine	T46.5X1	T46.5X2	T46.5X3	T46.5X4	T46.5X5	T46.5X6
Desferrioxamine	T45.8X1	T45.8X2	T45.8X3	T45.8X4	T45.8X5	T45.8X6
Desipramine	T43.011	T43.012	T43.013	T43.014	T43.015	T43.016
Deslanoside	T46.0X1	T46.0X2	T46.0X3	T46.0X4	T46.0X5	T46.0X6
Desloughing agent	T49.4X1	T49.4X2	T49.4X3	T49.4X4	T49.4X5	T49.4X6
Desmethy-limipramine	T43.011	T43.012	T43.013	T43.014	T43.015	T43.016
Desmopressin	T38.891	T38.892	T38.893	T38.894	T38.895	T38.896
Desocodeine	T40.2X1	T40.2X2	T40.2X3	T40.2X4	T40.2X5	T40.2X6
Desogestrel	T38.5X1	T38.5X2	T38.5X3	T38.5X4	T38.5X5	T38.5X6
Desomorphine	T40.2X1	T40.2X2	T40.2X3	T40.2X4	—	—
Desonide	T49.0X1	T49.0X2	T49.0X3	T49.0X4	T49.0X5	T49.0X6
Desoximetasone	T49.0X1	T49.0X2	T49.0X3	T49.0X4	T49.0X5	T49.0X6
Desoxycorticosteroid	T50.0X1	T50.0X2	T50.0X3	T50.0X4	T50.0X5	T50.0X6
Desoxycortone	T50.0X1	T50.0X2	T50.0X3	T50.0X4	T50.0X5	T50.0X6
Desoxyephedrine	T43.621	T43.622	T43.623	T43.624	T43.625	T43.626
Detaxtran	T46.6X1	T46.6X2	T46.6X3	T46.6X4	T46.6X5	T46.6X6
Detergent	T49.2X1	T49.2X2	T49.2X3	T49.2X4	T49.2X5	T49.2X6
external medication	T49.2X1	T49.2X2	T49.2X3	T49.2X4	T49.2X5	T49.2X6
local	T49.2X1	T49.2X2	T49.2X3	T49.2X4	T49.2X5	T49.2X6
medicinal	T49.2X1	T49.2X2	T49.2X3	T49.2X4	T49.2X5	T49.2X6
nonmedicinal	T55.1X1	T55.1X2	T55.1X3	T55.1X4	—	—
specified NEC	T55.1X1	T55.1X2	T55.1X3	T55.1X4	—	—
Deterrent, alcohol	T50.6X1	T50.6X2	T50.6X3	T50.6X4	T50.6X5	T50.6X6
Detoxifying agent	T50.6X1	T50.6X2	T50.6X3	T50.6X4	T50.6X5	T50.6X6
Detrothyronine	T38.1X1	T38.1X2	T38.1X3	T38.1X4	T38.1X5	T38.1X6
Dettol (external medication)	T49.0X1	T49.0X2	T49.0X3	T49.0X4	T49.0X5	T49.0X6
Dexamethasone	T38.0X1	T38.0X2	T38.0X3	T38.0X4	T38.0X5	T38.0X6
ENT agent	T49.6X1	T49.6X2	T49.6X3	T49.6X4	T49.6X5	T49.6X6
ophthalmic preparation	T49.5X1	T49.5X2	T49.5X3	T49.5X4	T49.5X5	T49.5X6
topical NEC	T49.0X1	T49.0X2	T49.0X3	T49.0X4	T49.0X5	T49.0X6
Dexamfetamine	T43.621	T43.622	T43.623	T43.624	T43.625	T43.626
Dexamphetamine	T43.621	T43.622	T43.623	T43.624	T43.625	T43.626
Dexbrom-pheniramine	T45.0X1	T45.0X2	T45.0X3	T45.0X4	T45.0X5	T45.0X6
Dexchlorpheniramine	T45.0X1	T45.0X2	T45.0X3	T45.0X4	T45.0X5	T45.0X6
Dexedrine	T43.621	T43.622	T43.623	T43.624	T43.625	T43.626
Dexetimide	T44.3X1	T44.3X2	T44.3X3	T44.3X4	T44.3X5	T44.3X6
Dexfenfluramine	T50.5X1	T50.5X2	T50.5X3	T50.5X4	T50.5X5	T50.5X6
Dexpanthenol	T45.2X1	T45.2X2	T45.2X3	T45.2X4	T45.2X5	T45.2X6
Dextran (40) (70) (150)	T45.8X1	T45.8X2	T45.8X3	T45.8X4	T45.8X5	T45.8X6
Dextriferron	T45.4X1	T45.4X2	T45.4X3	T45.4X4	T45.4X5	T45.4X6
Dextro calcium pantothenate	T45.2X1	T45.2X2	T45.2X3	T45.2X4	T45.2X5	T45.2X6
Dextro pantothenyl alcohol	T45.2X1	T45.2X2	T45.2X3	T45.2X4	T45.2X5	T45.2X6
Dextroamphetamine	T43.621	T43.622	T43.623	T43.624	T43.625	T43.626
Dextromethorphan	T48.3X1	T48.3X2	T48.3X3	T48.3X4	T48.3X5	T48.3X6
Dextromoramide	T40.491	T40.492	T40.493	T40.494	—	—
topical	T49.8X1	T49.8X2	T49.8X3	T49.8X4	T49.8X5	T49.8X6
Dextropropoxyphene	T40.491	T40.492	T40.493	T40.494	T40.495	T40.496
Dextrorphan	T40.2X1	T40.2X2	T40.2X3	T40.2X4	T40.2X5	T40.2X6
Dextrose	T50.3X1	T50.3X2	T50.3X3	T50.3X4	T50.3X5	T50.3X6
concentrated solution, intravenous	T46.8X1	T46.8X2	T46.8X3	T46.8X4	T46.8X5	T46.8X6
Dextrothyroxin	T38.1X1	T38.1X2	T38.1X3	T38.1X4	T38.1X5	T38.1X6

Substance	Poisoning, Accidental (unintentional)	Poisoning, Intentional self-harm	Poisoning, Assault	Poisoning, Undetermined	Adverse effect	Underdosing
Dextrothyroxine sodium	T38.1X1	T38.1X2	T38.1X3	T38.1X4	T38.1X5	T38.1X6
DFP	T44.0X1	T44.0X2	T44.0X3	T44.0X4	T44.0X5	T44.0X6
DHE	T37.3X1	T37.3X2	T37.3X3	T37.3X4	T37.3X5	T37.3X6
45	T46.5X1	T46.5X2	T46.5X3	T46.5X4	T46.5X5	T46.5X6
Diabinese	T38.3X1	T38.3X2	T38.3X3	T38.3X4	T38.3X5	T38.3X6
Diacetone alcohol	T52.4X1	T52.4X2	T52.4X3	T52.4X4	—	—
Diacetyl monoxime	T50.991	T50.992	T50.993	T50.994	—	—
Diacetylmorphine	T40.1X1	T40.1X2	T40.1X3	T40.1X4	—	—
Diachylon plaster	T49.4X1	T49.4X2	T49.4X3	T49.4X4	T49.4X5	T49.4X6
Diaethylst-ilboestrolum	T38.5X1	T38.5X2	T38.5X3	T38.5X4	T38.5X5	T38.5X6
Diagnostic agent NEC	T50.8X1	T50.8X2	T50.8X3	T50.8X4	T50.8X5	T50.8X6
Dial (soap)	T49.2X1	T49.2X2	T49.2X3	T49.2X4	T49.2X5	T49.2X6
sedative	T42.3X1	T42.3X2	T42.3X3	T42.3X4	T42.3X5	T42.3X6
Dialkyl carbonate	T52.91	T52.92	T52.93	T52.94	—	—
Diallylbarbituric acid	T42.3X1	T42.3X2	T42.3X3	T42.3X4	T42.3X5	T42.3X6
Diallymal	T42.3X1	T42.3X2	T42.3X3	T42.3X4	T42.3X5	T42.3X6
Dialysis solution (intraperitoneal)	T50.3X1	T50.3X2	T50.3X3	T50.3X4	T50.3X5	T50.3X6
Diaminodi-phenylsulfone	T37.1X1	T37.1X2	T37.1X3	T37.1X4	T37.1X5	T37.1X6
Diamorphine	T40.1X1	T40.1X2	T40.1X3	T40.1X4	—	—
Diamox	T50.2X1	T50.2X2	T50.2X3	T50.2X4	T50.2X5	T50.2X6
Diamthazole	T49.0X1	T49.0X2	T49.0X3	T49.0X4	T49.0X5	T49.0X6
Dianthone	T47.2X1	T47.2X2	T47.2X3	T47.2X4	T47.2X5	T47.2X6
Diaphenylsulfone	T37.0X1	T37.0X2	T37.0X3	T37.0X4	T37.0X5	T37.0X6
Diasone (sodium)	T37.1X1	T37.1X2	T37.1X3	T37.1X4	T37.1X5	T37.1X6
Diastase	T47.5X1	T47.5X2	T47.5X3	T47.5X4	T47.5X5	T47.5X6
Diatrizoate	T50.8X1	T50.8X2	T50.8X3	T50.8X4	T50.8X5	T50.8X6
Diazepam	T42.4X1	T42.4X2	T42.4X3	T42.4X4	T42.4X5	T42.4X6
Diazinon	T60.0X1	T60.0X2	T60.0X3	T60.0X4	—	—
Diazomethane (gas)	T59.891	T59.892	T59.893	T59.894	—	—
Diazoxide	T46.5X1	T46.5X2	T46.5X3	T46.5X4	T46.5X5	T46.5X6
Dibekacin	T36.5X1	T36.5X2	T36.5X3	T36.5X4	T36.5X5	T36.5X6
Dibenamine	T44.6X1	T44.6X2	T44.6X3	T44.6X4	T44.6X5	T44.6X6
Dibenzepin	T43.011	T43.012	T43.013	T43.014	T43.015	T43.016
Dibenzheptropine	T45.0X1	T45.0X2	T45.0X3	T45.0X4	T45.0X5	T45.0X6
Dibenzyline	T44.6X1	T44.6X2	T44.6X3	T44.6X4	T44.6X5	T44.6X6
Diborane (gas)	T59.891	T59.892	T59.893	T59.894	—	—
Dibromoch-loropropane	T60.8X1	T60.8X2	T60.8X3	T60.8X4	—	—
Dibromodulcitol	T45.1X1	T45.1X2	T45.1X3	T45.1X4	T45.1X5	T45.1X6
Dibromoethane	T53.6X1	T53.6X2	T53.6X3	T53.6X4	—	—
Dibromomannitol	T45.1X1	T45.1X2	T45.1X3	T45.1X4	T45.1X5	T45.1X6
Dibromopropamidine isethionate	T49.0X1	T49.0X2	T49.0X3	T49.0X4	T49.0X5	T49.0X6
Dibrompropamidine	T49.0X1	T49.0X2	T49.0X3	T49.0X4	T49.0X5	T49.0X6
Dibucaine	T41.3X1	T41.3X2	T41.3X3	T41.3X4	T41.3X5	T41.3X6
topical (surface)	T41.3X1	T41.3X2	T41.3X3	T41.3X4	T41.3X5	T41.3X6
Dibunate sodium	T48.3X1	T48.3X2	T48.3X3	T48.3X4	T48.3X5	T48.3X6
Dibutoline sulfate	T44.3X1	T44.3X2	T44.3X3	T44.3X4	T44.3X5	T44.3X6
Dicamba	T60.3X1	T60.3X2	T60.3X3	T60.3X4	—	—
Dicapthon	T60.0X1	T60.0X2	T60.0X3	T60.0X4	—	—
Dichlobenil	T60.3X1	T60.3X2	T60.3X3	T60.3X4	—	—
Dichlone	T60.3X1	T60.3X2	T60.3X3	T60.3X4	—	—
Dichloralphenozone	T42.6X1	T42.6X2	T42.6X3	T42.6X4	T42.6X5	T42.6X6
Dichlorbenzidine	T65.3X1	T65.3X2	T65.3X3	T65.3X4	—	—
Dichlorhydrin	T52.8X1	T52.8X2	T52.8X3	T52.8X4	—	—
Dichlorhydroxy-quinoline	T37.8X1	T37.8X2	T37.8X3	T37.8X4	T37.8X5	T37.8X6
Dichlorobenzene	T53.7X1	T53.7X2	T53.7X3	T53.7X4	—	—
Dichlorobenzyl alcohol	T49.6X1	T49.6X2	T49.6X3	T49.6X4	T49.6X5	T49.6X6
Dichlorodifluoro-methane	T53.5X1	T53.5X2	T53.5X3	T53.5X4	—	—
Dichloroethane	T52.8X1	T52.8X2	T52.8X3	T52.8X4	—	—
Sym-Dichloroethyl ether	T53.6X1	T53.6X2	T53.6X3	T53.6X4	—	—
Dichloroethyl sulfide, not in war	T59.891	T59.892	T59.893	T59.894	—	—
Dichloroethylene	T53.6X1	T53.6X2	T53.6X3	T53.6X4	—	—
Dichloroformoxine, not in war	T59.891	T59.892	T59.893	T59.894	—	—
Dichlorohydrin, alpha-dichlorohydrin	T52.8X1	T52.8X2	T52.8X3	T52.8X4	—	—
Dichloromethane (solvent)	T53.4X1	T53.4X2	T53.4X3	T53.4X4	—	—
vapor	T53.4X1	T53.4X2	T53.4X3	T53.4X4	—	—
Dichloronaphtho-quinone	T60.3X1	T60.3X2	T60.3X3	T60.3X4	—	—
Dichlorophen	T37.4X1	T37.4X2	T37.4X3	T37.4X4	T37.4X5	T37.4X6
2,4-Dichlorophenoxy-acetic acid	T60.3X1	T60.3X2	T60.3X3	T60.3X4	—	—
Dichloropropene	T60.3X1	T60.3X2	T60.3X3	T60.3X4	—	—
Dichloropropionic acid	T60.3X1	T60.3X2	T60.3X3	T60.3X4	—	—
Dichlorphenamide	T50.2X1	T50.2X2	T50.2X3	T50.2X4	T50.2X5	T50.2X6
Dichlorvos	T60.0X1	T60.0X2	T60.0X3	T60.0X4	—	—
Diclofenac	T39.391	T39.392	T39.393	T39.394	T39.395	T39.396
Diclofenamide	T50.2X1	T50.2X2	T50.2X3	T50.2X4	T50.2X5	T50.2X6
Diclofensine	T43.291	T43.292	T43.293	T43.294	T43.295	T43.296
Diclonixine	T39.8X1	T39.8X2	T39.8X3	T39.8X4	T39.8X5	T39.8X6
Dicloxacillin	T36.0X1	T36.0X2	T36.0X3	T36.0X4	T36.0X5	T36.0X6
Dicophane	T49.0X1	T49.0X2	T49.0X3	T49.0X4	T49.0X5	T49.0X6
Dicoumarol, dicoumarin, dicumarol	T45.511	T45.512	T45.513	T45.514	T45.515	T45.516
Dicrotophos	T60.0X1	T60.0X2	T60.0X3	T60.0X4	—	—
Dicyanogen (gas)	T65.0X1	T65.0X2	T65.0X3	T65.0X4	—	—
Dicyclomine	T44.3X1	T44.3X2	T44.3X3	T44.3X4	T44.3X5	T44.3X6
Dicycloverine	T44.3X1	T44.3X2	T44.3X3	T44.3X4	T44.3X5	T44.3X6
Dideoxycytidine	T37.5X1	T37.5X2	T37.5X3	T37.5X4	T37.5X5	T37.5X6
Dideoxyinosine	T37.5X1	T37.5X2	T37.5X3	T37.5X4	T37.5X5	T37.5X6
Dieldrin (vapor)	T60.1X1	T60.1X2	T60.1X3	T60.1X4	—	—
Diemal	T42.3X1	T42.3X2	T42.3X3	T42.3X4	T42.3X5	T42.3X6
Dienestrol	T38.5X1	T38.5X2	T38.5X3	T38.5X4	T38.5X5	T38.5X6
Dienoestrol	T38.5X1	T38.5X2	T38.5X3	T38.5X4	T38.5X5	T38.5X6
Dietetic drug NEC	T50.901	T50.902	T50.903	T50.904	T50.905	T50.906
Diethazine	T42.8X1	T42.8X2	T42.8X3	T42.8X4	T42.8X5	T42.8X6

Substance	Poisoning, Accidental (unintentional)	Poisoning, Intentional self-harm	Poisoning, Assault	Poisoning, Undetermined	Adverse effect	Underdosing
Diethyl						
barbituric acid	T42.3X1	T42.3X2	T42.3X3	T42.3X4	T42.3X5	T42.3X6
carbamazine	T37.4X1	T37.4X2	T37.4X3	T37.4X4	T37.4X5	T37.4X6
carbinol	T51.3X1	T51.3X2	T51.3X3	T51.3X4	—	—
carbonate	T52.8X1	T52.8X2	T52.8X3	T52.8X4	—	—
ether (vapor)—see also ether	T41.0X1	T41.0X2	T41.0X3	T41.0X4	T41.0X5	T41.0X6
oxide	T52.8X1	T52.8X2	T52.8X3	T52.8X4	—	—
propion	T50.5X1	T50.5X2	T50.5X3	T50.5X4	T50.5X5	T50.5X6
stilbestrol	T38.5X1	T38.5X2	T38.5X3	T38.5X4	T38.5X5	T38.5X6
toluamide (nonmedicinal)	T60.8X1	T60.8X2	T60.8X3	T60.8X4	—	—
medicinal	T49.3X1	T49.3X2	T49.3X3	T49.3X4	T49.3X5	T49.3X6
Diethylcarbamazine	T37.4X1	T37.4X2	T37.4X3	T37.4X4	T37.4X5	T37.4X6
Diethylene						
dioxide	T52.8X1	T52.8X2	T52.8X3	T52.8X4	—	—
glycol (monoacetate) (monobutyl ether) (monoethyl ether)	T52.3X1	T52.3X2	T52.3X3	T52.3X4	—	—
Diethylhexy-lphthalate	T65.891	T65.892	T65.893	T65.894	—	—
Diethylpropion	T50.5X1	T50.5X2	T50.5X3	T50.5X4	T50.5X5	T50.5X6
Diethylstilbestrol	T38.5X1	T38.5X2	T38.5X3	T38.5X4	T38.5X5	T38.5X6
Diethylstilboestrol	T38.5X1	T38.5X2	T38.5X3	T38.5X4	T38.5X5	T38.5X6
Diethylsulfone-diethylmethane	T42.6X1	T42.6X2	T42.6X3	T42.6X4	T42.6X5	T42.6X6
Diethyltoluamide	T49.0X1	T49.0X2	T49.0X3	T49.0X4	T49.0X5	T49.0X6
Diethyltryptamine (DET)	T40.991	T40.992	T40.993	T40.994	—	—
Difebarbamate	T42.3X1	T42.3X2	T42.3X3	T42.3X4	T42.3X5	T42.3X6
Difencloxazine	T40.2X1	T40.2X2	T40.2X3	T40.2X4	T40.2X5	T40.2X6
Difenidol	T45.0X1	T45.0X2	T45.0X3	T45.0X4	T45.0X5	T45.0X6
Difenoxin	T47.6X1	T47.6X2	T47.6X3	T47.6X4	T47.6X5	T47.6X6
Difetarsone	T37.3X1	T37.3X2	T37.3X3	T37.3X4	T37.3X5	T37.3X6
Diffusin	T45.3X1	T45.3X2	T45.3X3	T45.3X4	T45.3X5	T45.3X6
Diflorasone	T49.0X1	T49.0X2	T49.0X3	T49.0X4	T49.0X5	T49.0X6
Diflos	T44.0X1	T44.0X2	T44.0X3	T44.0X4	T44.0X5	T44.0X6
Diflubenzuron	T60.1X1	T60.1X2	T60.1X3	T60.1X4	—	—
Diflucortolone	T49.0X1	T49.0X2	T49.0X3	T49.0X4	T49.0X5	T49.0X6
Diflunisal	T39.091	T39.092	T39.093	T39.094	T39.095	T39.096
Difluoromethyldopa	T42.8X1	T42.8X2	T42.8X3	T42.8X4	T42.8X5	T42.8X6
Difluorophate	T44.0X1	T44.0X2	T44.0X3	T44.0X4	T44.0X5	T44.0X6
Digestant NEC	T47.5X1	T47.5X2	T47.5X3	T47.5X4	T47.5X5	T47.5X6
Digitalin(e)	T46.0X1	T46.0X2	T46.0X3	T46.0X4	T46.0X5	T46.0X6
Digitalis (leaf) (glycoside)	T46.0X1	T46.0X2	T46.0X3	T46.0X4	T46.0X5	T46.0X6
lanata	T46.0X1	T46.0X2	T46.0X3	T46.0X4	T46.0X5	T46.0X6
purpurea	T46.0X1	T46.0X2	T46.0X3	T46.0X4	T46.0X5	T46.0X6
Digitoxin	T46.0X1	T46.0X2	T46.0X3	T46.0X4	T46.0X5	T46.0X6
Digitoxose	T46.0X1	T46.0X2	T46.0X3	T46.0X4	T46.0X5	T46.0X6
Digoxin	T46.0X1	T46.0X2	T46.0X3	T46.0X4	T46.0X5	T46.0X6
Digoxine	T46.0X1	T46.0X2	T46.0X3	T46.0X4	T46.0X5	T46.0X6
Dihydralazine	T46.5X1	T46.5X2	T46.5X3	T46.5X4	T46.5X5	T46.5X6
Dihydrazine	T46.5X1	T46.5X2	T46.5X3	T46.5X4	T46.5X5	T46.5X6
Dihydrocodeine	T40.2X1	T40.2X2	T40.2X3	T40.2X4	T40.2X5	T40.2X6
Dihydrocodeinone	T40.2X1	T40.2X2	T40.2X3	T40.2X4	T40.2X5	T40.2X6
Dihydroergocornine	T46.7X1	T46.7X2	T46.7X3	T46.7X4	T46.7X5	T46.7X6
Dihydroergocristine (mesilate)	T46.7X1	T46.7X2	T46.7X3	T46.7X4	T46.7X5	T46.7X6
Dihydroergokryptine	T46.7X1	T46.7X2	T46.7X3	T46.7X4	T46.7X5	T46.7X6
Dihydroergotamine	T46.5X1	T46.5X2	T46.5X3	T46.5X4	T46.5X5	T46.5X6
Dihydroergotoxine	T46.7X1	T46.7X2	T46.7X3	T46.7X4	T46.7X5	T46.7X6
mesilate	T46.7X1	T46.7X2	T46.7X3	T46.7X4	T46.7X5	T46.7X6
Dihydrohydroxy-codeinone	T40.2X1	T40.2X2	T40.2X3	T40.2X4	T40.2X5	T40.2X6
Dihydrohydroxy-morphinone	T40.2X1	T40.2X2	T40.2X3	T40.2X4	T40.2X5	T40.2X6
Dihydroisocodeine	T40.2X1	T40.2X2	T40.2X3	T40.2X4	T40.2X5	T40.2X6
Dihydromorphine	T40.2X1	T40.2X2	T40.2X3	T40.2X4	—	—
Dihydromorphinone	T40.2X1	T40.2X2	T40.2X3	T40.2X4	T40.2X5	T40.2X6
Dihydrostreptomycin	T36.5X1	T36.5X2	T36.5X3	T36.5X4	T36.5X5	T36.5X6
Dihydrotachysterol	T45.2X1	T45.2X2	T45.2X3	T45.2X4	T45.2X5	T45.2X6
Dihydroxyaluminum aminoacetate	T47.1X1	T47.1X2	T47.1X3	T47.1X4	T47.1X5	T47.1X6
Dihydroxyaluminum sodium carbonate	T47.1X1	T47.1X2	T47.1X3	T47.1X4	T47.1X5	T47.1X6
Dihydroxyanthra-quinone	T47.2X1	T47.2X2	T47.2X3	T47.2X4	T47.2X5	T47.2X6
Dihydroxycodeinone	T40.2X1	T40.2X2	T40.2X3	T40.2X4	T40.2X5	T40.2X6
Dihydroxypropyl theophylline	T50.2X1	T50.2X2	T50.2X3	T50.2X4	T50.2X5	T50.2X6
Diiodohydroxyquin	T37.8X1	T37.8X2	T37.8X3	T37.8X4	T37.8X5	T37.8X6
topical	T49.0X1	T49.0X2	T49.0X3	T49.0X4	T49.0X5	T49.0X6
Diiodo-hydroxyquinoline	T37.8X1	T37.8X2	T37.8X3	T37.8X4	T37.8X5	T37.8X6
Diiodotyrosine	T38.2X1	T38.2X2	T38.2X3	T38.2X4	T38.2X5	T38.2X6
Diisopromine	T44.3X1	T44.3X2	T44.3X3	T44.3X4	T44.3X5	T44.3X6
Diisopropylamine	T46.3X1	T46.3X2	T46.3X3	T46.3X4	T46.3X5	T46.3X6
Diisopropyl-fluorophos-phonate	T44.0X1	T44.0X2	T44.0X3	T44.0X4	T44.0X5	T44.0X6
Dilantin	T42.0X1	T42.0X2	T42.0X3	T42.0X4	T42.0X5	T42.0X6
Dilaudid	T40.2X1	T40.2X2	T40.2X3	T40.2X4	T40.2X5	T40.2X6
Dilazep	T46.3X1	T46.3X2	T46.3X3	T46.3X4	T46.3X5	T46.3X6
Dill	T47.5X1	T47.5X2	T47.5X3	T47.5X4	T47.5X5	T47.5X6
Diloxanide	T37.3X1	T37.3X2	T37.3X3	T37.3X4	T37.3X5	T37.3X6
Diltiazem	T46.1X1	T46.1X2	T46.1X3	T46.1X4	T46.1X5	T46.1X6
Dimazole	T49.0X1	T49.0X2	T49.0X3	T49.0X4	T49.0X5	T49.0X6
Dimefline	T50.7X1	T50.7X2	T50.7X3	T50.7X4	T50.7X5	T50.7X6
Dimefox	T60.0X1	T60.0X2	T60.0X3	T60.0X4	—	—
Dimemorfan	T48.3X1	T48.3X2	T48.3X3	T48.3X4	T48.3X5	T48.3X6
Dimenhydrinate	T45.0X1	T45.0X2	T45.0X3	T45.0X4	T45.0X5	T45.0X6
Dimercaprol (British anti-lewisite)	T45.8X1	T45.8X2	T45.8X3	T45.8X4	T45.8X5	T45.8X6
Dimercaptopropanol	T45.8X1	T45.8X2	T45.8X3	T45.8X4	T45.8X5	T45.8X6
Dimestrol	T38.5X1	T38.5X2	T38.5X3	T38.5X4	T38.5X5	T38.5X6
Dimetane	T45.0X1	T45.0X2	T45.0X3	T45.0X4	T45.0X5	T45.0X6
Dimethicone	T47.1X1	T47.1X2	T47.1X3	T47.1X4	T47.1X5	T47.1X6
Dimethindene	T45.0X1	T45.0X2	T45.0X3	T45.0X4	T45.0X5	T45.0X6

Substance	Poisoning, Accidental (unintentional)	Poisoning, Intentional self-harm	Poisoning, Assault	Poisoning, Undetermined	Adverse effect	Underdosing
Dimethisoquin	T49.1X1	T49.1X2	T49.1X3	T49.1X4	T49.1X5	T49.1X6
Dimethisterone	T38.5X1	T38.5X2	T38.5X3	T38.5X4	T38.5X5	T38.5X6
Dimethoate	T60.0X1	T60.0X2	T60.0X3	T60.0X4	—	—
Dimethocaine	T41.3X1	T41.3X2	T41.3X3	T41.3X4	T41.3X5	T41.3X6
Dimethoxanate	T48.3X1	T48.3X2	T48.3X3	T48.3X4	T48.3X5	T48.3X6
Dimethyl						
arsine, arsinic acid	T57.0X1	T57.0X2	T57.0X3	T57.0X4	—	—
carbinol	T51.2X1	T51.2X2	T51.2X3	T51.2X4	—	—
carbonate	T52.8X1	T52.8X2	T52.8X3	T52.8X4	—	—
diguanide	T38.3X1	T38.3X2	T38.3X3	T38.3X4	T38.3X5	T38.3X6
ketone	T52.4X1	T52.4X2	T52.4X3	T52.4X4	—	—
vapor	T52.4X1	T52.4X2	T52.4X3	T52.4X4	—	—
meperidine	T40.2X1	T40.2X2	T40.2X3	T40.2X4	T40.2X5	T40.2X6
parathion	T60.0X1	T60.0X2	T60.0X3	T60.0X4	—	—
phthlate	T49.3X1	T49.3X2	T49.3X3	T49.3X4	T49.3X5	T49.3X6
polysiloxane	T47.8X1	T47.8X2	T47.8X3	T47.8X4	T47.8X5	T47.8X6
sulfate (fumes)	T59.891	T59.892	T59.893	T59.894	—	—
liquid	T65.891	T65.892	T65.893	T65.894	—	—
sulfoxide (nonmedicinal)	T52.8X1	T52.8X2	T52.8X3	T52.8X4	—	—
medicinal	T49.4X1	T49.4X2	T49.4X3	T49.4X4	T49.4X5	T49.4X6
tryptamine	T40.991	T40.992	T40.993	T40.994	—	—
tubocurarine	T48.1X1	T48.1X2	T48.1X3	T48.1X4	T48.1X5	T48.1X6
Dimethylamine sulfate	T49.4X1	T49.4X2	T49.4X3	T49.4X4	T49.4X5	T49.4X6
Dimethylformamide	T52.8X1	T52.8X2	T52.8X3	T52.8X4	—	—
Dimethyltubocurarinium chloride	T48.1X1	T48.1X2	T48.1X3	T48.1X4	T48.1X5	T48.1X6
Dimeticone	T47.1X1	T47.1X2	T47.1X3	T47.1X4	T47.1X5	T47.1X6
Dimetilan	T60.0X1	T60.0X2	T60.0X3	T60.0X4	—	—
Dimetindene	T45.0X1	T45.0X2	T45.0X3	T45.0X4	T45.0X5	T45.0X6
Dimetotiazine	T43.3X1	T43.3X2	T43.3X3	T43.3X4	T43.3X5	T43.3X6
Dimorpholamine	T50.7X1	T50.7X2	T50.7X3	T50.7X4	T50.7X5	T50.7X6
Dimoxyline	T46.3X1	T46.3X2	T46.3X3	T46.3X4	T46.3X5	T46.3X6
Dinitrobenzene	T65.3X1	T65.3X2	T65.3X3	T65.3X4	—	—
vapor	T59.891	T59.892	T59.893	T59.894	—	—
Dinitrobenzol	T65.3X1	T65.3X2	T65.3X3	T65.3X4	—	—
vapor	T59.891	T59.892	T59.893	T59.894	—	—
Dinitrobutylphenol	T65.3X1	T65.3X2	T65.3X3	T65.3X4	—	—
Dinitro (-ortho-)cresol (pesticide) (spray)	T65.3X1	T65.3X2	T65.3X3	T65.3X4	—	—
Dinitro-cyclohexylphenol	T65.3X1	T65.3X2	T65.3X3	T65.3X4	—	—
Dinitrophenol	T65.3X1	T65.3X2	T65.3X3	T65.3X4	—	—
Dinoprost	T48.0X1	T48.0X2	T48.0X3	T48.0X4	T48.0X5	T48.0X6
Dinoprostone	T48.0X1	T48.0X2	T48.0X3	T48.0X4	T48.0X5	T48.0X6
Dinoseb	T60.3X1	T60.3X2	T60.3X3	T60.3X4	—	—
Dioctyl sulfosuccinate (calcium) (sodium)	T47.4X1	T47.4X2	T47.4X3	T47.4X4	T47.4X5	T47.4X6
Diodone	T50.8X1	T50.8X2	T50.8X3	T50.8X4	T50.8X5	T50.8X6
Diodoquin	T37.8X1	T37.8X2	T37.8X3	T37.8X4	T37.8X5	T37.8X6
Dionin	T40.2X1	T40.2X2	T40.2X3	T40.2X4	T40.2X5	T40.2X6
Diosmin	T46.991	T46.992	T46.993	T46.994	T46.995	T46.996
Dioxane	T52.8X1	T52.8X2	T52.8X3	T52.8X4	—	—
Dioxathion	T60.0X1	T60.0X2	T60.0X3	T60.0X4	—	—
Dioxin	T53.7X1	T53.7X2	T53.7X3	T53.7X4	—	—
Dioxopromethazine	T43.3X1	T43.3X2	T43.3X3	T43.3X4	T43.3X5	T43.3X6
Dioxyline	T46.3X1	T46.3X2	T46.3X3	T46.3X4	T46.3X5	T46.3X6
Dipentene	T52.8X1	T52.8X2	T52.8X3	T52.8X4	—	—
Diperodon	T41.3X1	T41.3X2	T41.3X3	T41.3X4	T41.3X5	T41.3X6
Diphacinone	T60.4X1	T60.4X2	T60.4X3	T60.4X4	—	—
Diphemanil	T44.3X1	T44.3X2	T44.3X3	T44.3X4	T44.3X5	T44.3X6
metilsulfate	T44.3X1	T44.3X2	T44.3X3	T44.3X4	T44.3X5	T44.3X6
Diphenadione	T45.511	T45.512	T45.513	T45.514	T45.515	T45.516
rodenticide	T60.4X1	T60.4X2	T60.4X3	T60.4X4	—	—
Diphenhydramine	T45.0X1	T45.0X2	T45.0X3	T45.0X4	T45.0X5	T45.0X6
Diphenidol	T45.0X1	T45.0X2	T45.0X3	T45.0X4	T45.0X5	T45.0X6
Diphenoxylate	T47.6X1	T47.6X2	T47.6X3	T47.6X4	T47.6X5	T47.6X6
Diphenylamine	T65.3X1	T65.3X2	T65.3X3	T65.3X4	—	—
Diphenylbutazone	T39.2X1	T39.2X2	T39.2X3	T39.2X4	T39.2X5	T39.2X6
Diphenyl-chloroarsine, not in war	T57.0X1	T57.0X2	T57.0X3	T57.0X4	—	—
Diphenylhydantoin	T42.0X1	T42.0X2	T42.0X3	T42.0X4	T42.0X5	T42.0X6
Diphenylmethane dye	T52.1X1	T52.1X2	T52.1X3	T52.1X4	—	—
Diphenylpyraline	T45.0X1	T45.0X2	T45.0X3	T45.0X4	T45.0X5	T45.0X6
Diphtheria						
antitoxin	T50.Z11	T50.Z12	T50.Z13	T50.Z14	T50.Z15	T50.Z16
toxoid	T50.A91	T50.A92	T50.A93	T50.A94	T50.A95	T50.A96
with tetanus toxoid	T50.A21	T50.A22	T50.A23	T50.A24	T50.A25	T50.A26
with pertussis component	T50.A11	T50.A12	T50.A13	T50.A14	T50.A15	T50.A16
vaccine	T50.A91	T50.A92	T50.A93	T50.A94	T50.A95	T50.A96
combination						
including pertussis	T50.A11	T50.A12	T50.A13	T50.A14	T50.A15	T50.A16
without pertussis	T50.A21	T50.A22	T50.A23	T50.A24	T50.A25	T50.A26
Diphylline	T50.2X1	T50.2X2	T50.2X3	T50.2X4	T50.2X5	T50.2X6
Dipipanone	T40.491	T40.492	T40.493	T40.494	—	—
Dipivefrine	T49.5X1	T49.5X2	T49.5X3	T49.5X4	T49.5X5	T49.5X6
Diplovax	T50.B91	T50.B92	T50.B93	T50.B94	T50.B95	T50.B96
Diprophylline	T50.2X1	T50.2X2	T50.2X3	T50.2X4	T50.2X5	T50.2X6
Dipropyline	T48.291	T48.292	T48.293	T48.294	T48.295	T48.296
Dipyridamole	T46.3X1	T46.3X2	T46.3X3	T46.3X4	T46.3X5	T46.3X6
Dipyrone	T39.2X1	T39.2X2	T39.2X3	T39.2X4	T39.2X5	T39.2X6
Diquat (dibromide)	T60.3X1	T60.3X2	T60.3X3	T60.3X4	—	—
Disinfectant	T65.891	T65.892	T65.893	T65.894	—	—
alkaline	T54.3X1	T54.3X2	T54.3X3	T54.3X4	—	—
aromatic	T54.1X1	T54.1X2	T54.1X3	T54.1X4	—	—
intestinal	T37.8X1	T37.8X2	T37.8X3	T37.8X4	T37.8X5	T37.8X6
Disipal	T42.8X1	T42.8X2	T42.8X3	T42.8X4	T42.8X5	T42.8X6
Disodium edetate	T50.6X1	T50.6X2	T50.6X3	T50.6X4	T50.6X5	T50.6X6
Disoprofol	T41.291	T41.292	T41.293	T41.294	T41.295	T41.296
Disopyramide	T46.2X1	T46.2X2	T46.2X3	T46.2X4	T46.2X5	T46.2X6
Distigmine (bromide)	T44.0X1	T44.0X2	T44.0X3	T44.0X4	T44.0X5	T44.0X6
Disulfamide	T50.2X1	T50.2X2	T50.2X3	T50.2X4	T50.2X5	T50.2X6

Substance	Poisoning, Accidental (unintentional)	Poisoning, Intentional self-harm	Poisoning, Assault	Poisoning, Undetermined	Adverse effect	Underdosing
Disulfanilamide	T37.0X1	T37.0X2	T37.0X3	T37.0X4	T37.0X5	T37.0X6
Disulfiram	T50.6X1	T50.6X2	T50.6X3	T50.6X4	T50.6X5	T50.6X6
Disulfoton	T60.0X1	T60.0X2	T60.0X3	T60.0X4	—	—
Dithiazanine iodide	T37.4X1	T37.4X2	T37.4X3	T37.4X4	T37.4X5	T37.4X6
Dithiocarbamate	T60.0X1	T60.0X2	T60.0X3	T60.0X4	—	—
Dithranol	T49.4X1	T49.4X2	T49.4X3	T49.4X4	T49.4X5	T49.4X6
Diucardin	T50.2X1	T50.2X2	T50.2X3	T50.2X4	T50.2X5	T50.2X6
Diupres	T50.2X1	T50.2X2	T50.2X3	T50.2X4	T50.2X5	T50.2X6
Diuretic NEC	T50.2X1	T50.2X2	T50.2X3	T50.2X4	T50.2X5	T50.2X6
benzothiadiazine	T50.2X1	T50.2X2	T50.2X3	T50.2X4	T50.2X5	T50.2X6
carbonic acid anhydrase inhibitors	T50.2X1	T50.2X2	T50.2X3	T50.2X4	T50.2X5	T50.2X6
furfuryl NEC	T50.2X1	T50.2X2	T50.2X3	T50.2X4	T50.2X5	T50.2X6
loop (high-ceiling)	T50.1X1	T50.1X2	T50.1X3	T50.1X4	T50.1X5	T50.1X6
mercurial NEC	T50.2X1	T50.2X2	T50.2X3	T50.2X4	T50.2X5	T50.2X6
osmotic	T50.2X1	T50.2X2	T50.2X3	T50.2X4	T50.2X5	T50.2X6
purine NEC	T50.2X1	T50.2X2	T50.2X3	T50.2X4	T50.2X5	T50.2X6
saluretic NEC	T50.2X1	T50.2X2	T50.2X3	T50.2X4	T50.2X5	T50.2X6
sulfonamide	T50.2X1	T50.2X2	T50.2X3	T50.2X4	T50.2X5	T50.2X6
thiazide NEC	T50.2X1	T50.2X2	T50.2X3	T50.2X4	T50.2X5	T50.2X6
xanthine	T50.2X1	T50.2X2	T50.2X3	T50.2X4	T50.2X5	T50.2X6
Diurgin	T50.2X1	T50.2X2	T50.2X3	T50.2X4	T50.2X5	T50.2X6
Diuril	T50.2X1	T50.2X2	T50.2X3	T50.2X4	T50.2X5	T50.2X6
Diuron	T60.3X1	T60.3X2	T60.3X3	T60.3X4	—	—
Divalproex	T42.6X1	T42.6X2	T42.6X3	T42.6X4	T42.6X5	T42.6X6
Divinyl ether	T41.0X1	T41.0X2	T41.0X3	T41.0X4	T41.0X5	T41.0X6
Dixanthogen	T49.0X1	T49.0X2	T49.0X3	T49.0X4	T49.0X5	T49.0X6
Dixyrazine	T43.3X1	T43.3X2	T43.3X3	T43.3X4	T43.3X5	T43.3X6
D-lysergic acid diethylamide	T40.8X1	T40.8X2	T40.8X3	T40.8X4	—	—
DMCT	T36.4X1	T36.4X2	T36.4X3	T36.4X4	T36.4X5	T36.4X6
DMSO—see Dimethyl sulfoxide						
DNBP	T60.3X1	T60.3X2	T60.3X3	T60.3X4	—	—
DNOC	T65.3X1	T65.3X2	T65.3X3	T65.3X4	—	—
Dobutamine	T44.5X1	T44.5X2	T44.5X3	T44.5X4	T44.5X5	T44.5X6
DOCA	T38.0X1	T38.0X2	T38.0X3	T38.0X4	T38.0X5	T38.0X6
Docusate sodium	T47.4X1	T47.4X2	T47.4X3	T47.4X4	T47.4X5	T47.4X6
Dodicin	T49.0X1	T49.0X2	T49.0X3	T49.0X4	T49.0X5	T49.0X6
Dofamium chloride	T49.0X1	T49.0X2	T49.0X3	T49.0X4	T49.0X5	T49.0X6
Dolophine	T40.3X1	T40.3X2	T40.3X3	T40.3X4	T40.3X5	T40.3X6
Doloxene	T39.8X1	T39.8X2	T39.8X3	T39.8X4	T39.8X5	T39.8X6
Domestic gas (after combustion)—see Gas, utility						
prior to combustion	T59.891	T59.892	T59.893	T59.894	—	—
Domiodol	T48.4X1	T48.4X2	T48.4X3	T48.4X4	T48.4X5	T48.4X6
Domiphen (bromide)	T49.0X1	T49.0X2	T49.0X3	T49.0X4	T49.0X5	T49.0X6
Domperidone	T45.0X1	T45.0X2	T45.0X3	T45.0X4	T45.0X5	T45.0X6
Dopa	T42.8X1	T42.8X2	T42.8X3	T42.8X4	T42.8X5	T42.8X6
Dopamine	T44.991	T44.992	T44.993	T44.994	T44.995	T44.996
Doriden	T42.6X1	T42.6X2	T42.6X3	T42.6X4	T42.6X5	T42.6X6

Substance	Poisoning, Accidental (unintentional)	Poisoning, Intentional self-harm	Poisoning, Assault	Poisoning, Undetermined	Adverse effect	Underdosing
Dormiral	T42.3X1	T42.3X2	T42.3X3	T42.3X4	T42.3X5	T42.3X6
Dormison	T42.6X1	T42.6X2	T42.6X3	T42.6X4	T42.6X5	T42.6X6
Dornase	T48.4X1	T48.4X2	T48.4X3	T48.4X4	T48.4X5	T48.4X6
Dorsacaine	T41.3X1	T41.3X2	T41.3X3	T41.3X4	T41.3X5	T41.3X6
Dosulepin	T43.011	T43.012	T43.013	T43.014	T43.015	T43.016
Dothiepin	T43.011	T43.012	T43.013	T43.014	T43.015	T43.016
Doxantrazole	T48.6X1	T48.6X2	T48.6X3	T48.6X4	T48.6X5	T48.6X6
Doxapram	T50.7X1	T50.7X2	T50.7X3	T50.7X4	T50.7X5	T50.7X6
Doxazosin	T44.6X1	T44.6X2	T44.6X3	T44.6X4	T44.6X5	T44.6X6
Doxepin	T43.011	T43.012	T43.013	T43.014	T43.015	T43.016
Doxifluridine	T45.1X1	T45.1X2	T45.1X3	T45.1X4	T45.1X5	T45.1X6
Doxorubicin	T45.1X1	T45.1X2	T45.1X3	T45.1X4	T45.1X5	T45.1X6
Doxycycline	T36.4X1	T36.4X2	T36.4X3	T36.4X4	T36.4X5	T36.4X6
Doxylamine	T45.0X1	T45.0X2	T45.0X3	T45.0X4	T45.0X5	T45.0X6
Dramamine	T45.0X1	T45.0X2	T45.0X3	T45.0X4	T45.0X5	T45.0X6
Drano (drain cleaner)	T54.3X1	T54.3X2	T54.3X3	T54.3X4	—	—
Dressing, live pulp	T49.7X1	T49.7X2	T49.7X3	T49.7X4	T49.7X5	T49.7X6
Drocode	T40.2X1	T40.2X2	T40.2X3	T40.2X4	T40.2X5	T40.2X6
Dromoran	T40.2X1	T40.2X2	T40.2X3	T40.2X4	T40.2X5	T40.2X6
Dromostanolone	T38.7X1	T38.7X2	T38.7X3	T38.7X4	T38.7X5	T38.7X6
Dronabinol	T40.711	T40.712	T40.713	T40.714	T40.715	T40.716
Droperidol	T43.591	T43.592	T43.593	T43.594	T43.595	T43.596
Dropropizine	T48.3X1	T48.3X2	T48.3X3	T48.3X4	T48.3X5	T48.3X6
Drostanolone	T38.7X1	T38.7X2	T38.7X3	T38.7X4	T38.7X5	T38.7X6
Drotaverine	T44.3X1	T44.3X2	T44.3X3	T44.3X4	T44.3X5	T44.3X6
Drotrecogin alfa	T45.511	T45.512	T45.513	T45.514	T45.515	T45.516
Drug NEC	T50.901	T50.902	T50.903	T50.904	T50.905	T50.906
specified NEC	T50.991	T50.992	T50.993	T50.994	T50.995	T50.996
DTIC	T45.1X1	T45.1X2	T45.1X3	T45.1X4	T45.1X5	T45.1X6
Duboisine	T44.3X1	T44.3X2	T44.3X3	T44.3X4	T44.3X5	T44.3X6
Dulcolax	T47.2X1	T47.2X2	T47.2X3	T47.2X4	T47.2X5	T47.2X6
Duponol (C) (EP)	T49.2X1	T49.2X2	T49.2X3	T49.2X4	T49.2X5	T49.2X6
Durabolin	T38.7X1	T38.7X2	T38.7X3	T38.7X4	T38.7X5	T38.7X6
Dyclone	T41.3X1	T41.3X2	T41.3X3	T41.3X4	T41.3X5	T41.3X6
Dyclonine	T41.3X1	T41.3X2	T41.3X3	T41.3X4	T41.3X5	T41.3X6
Dydrogesterone	T38.5X1	T38.5X2	T38.5X3	T38.5X4	T38.5X5	T38.5X6
Dye NEC	T65.6X1	T65.6X2	T65.6X3	T65.6X4	—	—
antiseptic	T49.0X1	T49.0X2	T49.0X3	T49.0X4	T49.0X5	T49.0X6
diagnostic agents	T50.8X1	T50.8X2	T50.8X3	T50.8X4	T50.8X5	T50.8X6
pharmaceutical NEC	T50.901	T50.902	T50.903	T50.904	T50.905	T50.906
Dyflos	T44.0X1	T44.0X2	T44.0X3	T44.0X4	T44.0X5	T44.0X6
Dymelor	T38.3X1	T38.3X2	T38.3X3	T38.3X4	T38.3X5	T38.3X6
Dynamite	T65.3X1	T65.3X2	T65.3X3	T65.3X4	—	—
fumes	T59.891	T59.892	T59.893	T59.894	—	—
Dyphylline	T44.3X1	T44.3X2	T44.3X3	T44.3X4	T44.3X5	T44.3X6
E						
Ear drug NEC	T49.6X1	T49.6X2	T49.6X3	T49.6X4	T49.6X5	T49.6X6
Ear preparations	T49.6X1	T49.6X2	T49.6X3	T49.6X4	T49.6X5	T49.6X6
Echothiophate, echothiopate, ecothiopate	T49.5X1	T49.5X2	T49.5X3	T49.5X4	T49.5X5	T49.5X6

Substance	Poisoning, Accidental (unintentional)	Poisoning, Intentional self-harm	Poisoning, Assault	Poisoning, Undetermined	Adverse effect	Underdosing
Econazole	T49.0X1	T49.0X2	T49.0X3	T49.0X4	T49.0X5	T49.0X6
Ecothiopate iodide	T49.5X1	T49.5X2	T49.5X3	T49.5X4	T49.5X5	T49.5X6
Ecstasy	T43.641	T43.642	T43.643	T43.644	—	—
Ectylurea	T42.6X1	T42.6X2	T42.6X3	T42.6X4	T42.6X5	T42.6X6
Edathamil disodium	T45.8X1	T45.8X2	T45.8X3	T45.8X4	T45.8X5	T45.8X6
Edecrin	T50.1X1	T50.1X2	T50.1X3	T50.1X4	T50.1X5	T50.1X6
Edetate, disodium (calcium)	T45.8X1	T45.8X2	T45.8X3	T45.8X4	T45.8X5	T45.8X6
Edoxudine	T49.5X1	T49.5X2	T49.5X3	T49.5X4	T49.5X5	T49.5X6
Edrophonium	T44.0X1	T44.0X2	T44.0X3	T44.0X4	T44.0X5	T44.0X6
chloride	T44.0X1	T44.0X2	T44.0X3	T44.0X4	T44.0X5	T44.0X6
EDTA	T50.6X1	T50.6X2	T50.6X3	T50.6X4	T50.6X5	T50.6X6
Eflornithine	T37.2X1	T37.2X2	T37.2X3	T37.2X4	T37.2X5	T37.2X6
Efloxate	T46.3X1	T46.3X2	T46.3X3	T46.3X4	T46.3X5	T46.3X6
Elase	T49.8X1	T49.8X2	T49.8X3	T49.8X4	T49.8X5	T49.8X6
Elastase	T47.5X1	T47.5X2	T47.5X3	T47.5X4	T47.5X5	T47.5X6
Elaterium	T47.2X1	T47.2X2	T47.2X3	T47.2X4	T47.2X5	T47.2X6
Elcatonin	T50.991	T50.992	T50.993	T50.994	T50.995	T50.996
Elder	T62.2X1	T62.2X2	T62.2X3	T62.2X4	—	—
berry,(unripe)	T62.1X1	T62.1X2	T62.1X3	T62.1X4	—	—
Electrolyte balance drug	T50.3X1	T50.3X2	T50.3X3	T50.3X4	T50.3X5	T50.3X6
Electrolytes NEC	T50.3X1	T50.3X2	T50.3X3	T50.3X4	T50.3X5	T50.3X6
Electrolytic agent NEC	T50.3X1	T50.3X2	T50.3X3	T50.3X4	T50.3X5	T50.3X6
Elemental diet	T50.901	T50.902	T50.903	T50.904	T50.905	T50.906
Elliptinium acetate	T45.1X1	T45.1X2	T45.1X3	T45.1X4	T45.1X5	T45.1X6
Embramine	T45.0X1	T45.0X2	T45.0X3	T45.0X4	T45.0X5	T45.0X6
Emepronium (salts)	T44.3X1	T44.3X2	T44.3X3	T44.3X4	T44.3X5	T44.3X6
bromide	T44.3X1	T44.3X2	T44.3X3	T44.3X4	T44.3X5	T44.3X6
Emetic NEC	T47.7X1	T47.7X2	T47.7X3	T47.7X4	T47.7X5	T47.7X6
Emetine	T37.3X1	T37.3X2	T37.3X3	T37.3X4	T37.3X5	T37.3X6
Emollient NEC	T49.3X1	T49.3X2	T49.3X3	T49.3X4	T49.3X5	T49.3X6
Emorfazone	T39.8X1	T39.8X2	T39.8X3	T39.8X4	T39.8X5	T39.8X6
Emylcamate	T43.591	T43.592	T43.593	T43.594	T43.595	T43.596
Enalapril	T46.4X1	T46.4X2	T46.4X3	T46.4X4	T46.4X5	T46.4X6
Enalaprilat	T46.4X1	T46.4X2	T46.4X3	T46.4X4	T46.4X5	T46.4X6
Encainide	T46.2X1	T46.2X2	T46.2X3	T46.2X4	T46.2X5	T46.2X6
Endocaine	T41.3X1	T41.3X2	T41.3X3	T41.3X4	T41.3X5	T41.3X6
Endosulfan	T60.2X1	T60.2X2	T60.2X3	T60.2X4	—	—
Endothall	T60.3X1	T60.3X2	T60.3X3	T60.3X4	—	—
Endralazine	T46.5X1	T46.5X2	T46.5X3	T46.5X4	T46.5X5	T46.5X6
Endrin	T60.1X1	T60.1X2	T60.1X3	T60.1X4	—	—
Enflurane	T41.0X1	T41.0X2	T41.0X3	T41.0X4	T41.0X5	T41.0X6
Enhexymal	T42.3X1	T42.3X2	T42.3X3	T42.3X4	T42.3X5	T42.3X6
Enocitabine	T45.1X1	T45.1X2	T45.1X3	T45.1X4	T45.1X5	T45.1X6
Enovid	T38.4X1	T38.4X2	T38.4X3	T38.4X4	T38.4X5	T38.4X6
Enoxacin	T36.8X1	T36.8X2	T36.8X3	T36.8X4	T36.8X5	T36.8X6
Enoxaparin (sodium)	T45.511	T45.512	T45.513	T45.514	T45.515	T45.516
Enpiprazole	T43.591	T43.592	T43.593	T43.594	T43.595	T43.596
Enprofylline	T48.6X1	T48.6X2	T48.6X3	T48.6X4	T48.6X5	T48.6X6
Enprostil	T47.1X1	T47.1X2	T47.1X3	T47.1X4	T47.1X5	T47.1X6

Substance	Poisoning, Accidental (unintentional)	Poisoning, Intentional self-harm	Poisoning, Assault	Poisoning, Undetermined	Adverse effect	Underdosing
ENT preparations (anti-infectives)	T49.6X1	T49.6X2	T49.6X3	T49.6X4	T49.6X5	T49.6X6
Enterogastrone	T38.891	T38.892	T38.893	T38.894	T38.895	T38.896
Enviomycin	T36.8X1	T36.8X2	T36.8X3	T36.8X4	T36.8X5	T36.8X6
Enzodase	T45.3X1	T45.3X2	T45.3X3	T45.3X4	T45.3X5	T45.3X6
Enzyme NEC	T45.3X1	T45.3X2	T45.3X3	T45.3X4	T45.3X5	T45.3X6
depolymerizing	T49.8X1	T49.8X2	T49.8X3	T49.8X4	T49.8X5	T49.8X6
fibrolytic	T45.3X1	T45.3X2	T45.3X3	T45.3X4	T45.3X5	T45.3X6
gastric	T47.5X1	T47.5X2	T47.5X3	T47.5X4	T47.5X5	T47.5X6
intestinal	T47.5X1	T47.5X2	T47.5X3	T47.5X4	T47.5X5	T47.5X6
local action	T49.4X1	T49.4X2	T49.4X3	T49.4X4	T49.4X5	T49.4X6
proteolytic	T49.4X1	T49.4X2	T49.4X3	T49.4X4	T49.4X5	T49.4X6
thrombolytic	T45.3X1	T45.3X2	T45.3X3	T45.3X4	T45.3X5	T45.3X6
EPAB	T41.3X1	T41.3X2	T41.3X3	T41.3X4	T41.3X5	T41.3X6
Epanutin	T42.0X1	T42.0X2	T42.0X3	T42.0X4	T42.0X5	T42.0X6
Ephedra	T44.991	T44.992	T44.993	T44.994	T44.995	T44.996
Ephedrine	T44.991	T44.992	T44.993	T44.994	T44.995	T44.996
Epichlorhydrin, epichlorohydrin	T52.8X1	T52.8X2	T52.8X3	T52.8X4	—	—
Epicillin	T36.0X1	T36.0X2	T36.0X3	T36.0X4	T36.0X5	T36.0X6
Epiestriol	T38.5X1	T38.5X2	T38.5X3	T38.5X4	T38.5X5	T38.5X6
Epilim—see Sodium valproate						
Epimestrol	T38.5X1	T38.5X2	T38.5X3	T38.5X4	T38.5X5	T38.5X6
Epinephrine	T44.5X1	T44.5X2	T44.5X3	T44.5X4	T44.5X5	T44.5X6
Epirubicin	T45.1X1	T45.1X2	T45.1X3	T45.1X4	T45.1X5	T45.1X6
Epitiostanol	T38.7X1	T38.7X2	T38.7X3	T38.7X4	T38.7X5	T38.7X6
Epitizide	T50.2X1	T50.2X2	T50.2X3	T50.2X4	T50.2X5	T50.2X6
EPN	T60.0X1	T60.0X2	T60.0X3	T60.0X4	—	—
EPO	T45.8X1	T45.8X2	T45.8X3	T45.8X4	T45.8X5	T45.8X6
Epoetin alpha	T45.8X1	T45.8X2	T45.8X3	T45.8X4	T45.8X5	T45.8X6
Epomediol	T50.991	T50.992	T50.993	T50.994	T50.995	T50.996
Epoprostenol	T45.521	T45.522	T45.523	T45.524	T45.525	T45.526
Epoxy resin	T65.891	T65.892	T65.893	T65.894	—	—
Eprazinone	T48.4X1	T48.4X2	T48.4X3	T48.4X4	T48.4X5	T48.4X6
Epsilon amino-caproic acid	T45.621	T45.622	T45.623	T45.624	T45.625	T45.626
Epsom salt	T47.3X1	T47.3X2	T47.3X3	T47.3X4	T47.3X5	T47.3X6
Eptazocine	T40.491	T40.492	T40.493	T40.494	T40.495	T40.496
Equanil	T43.591	T43.592	T43.593	T43.594	T43.595	T43.596
Equisetum	T62.2X1	T62.2X2	T62.2X3	T62.2X4	—	—
diuretic	T50.2X1	T50.2X2	T50.2X3	T50.2X4	T50.2X5	T50.2X6
Ergobasine	T48.0X1	T48.0X2	T48.0X3	T48.0X4	T48.0X5	T48.0X6
Ergocalciferol	T45.2X1	T45.2X2	T45.2X3	T45.2X4	T45.2X5	T45.2X6
Ergoloid mesylates	T46.7X1	T46.7X2	T46.7X3	T46.7X4	T46.7X5	T46.7X6
Ergometrine	T48.0X1	T48.0X2	T48.0X3	T48.0X4	T48.0X5	T48.0X6
Ergonovine	T48.0X1	T48.0X2	T48.0X3	T48.0X4	T48.0X5	T48.0X6
Ergot NEC	T64.81	T64.82	T64.83	T64.84	—	—
derivative	T48.0X1	T48.0X2	T48.0X3	T48.0X4	T48.0X5	T48.0X6
medicinal (alkaloids)	T48.0X1	T48.0X2	T48.0X3	T48.0X4	T48.0X5	T48.0X6
prepared	T48.0X1	T48.0X2	T48.0X3	T48.0X4	T48.0X5	T48.0X6

Substance	Poisoning, Accidental (unintentional)	Poisoning, Intentional self-harm	Poisoning, Assault	Poisoning, Undetermined	Adverse effect	Underdosing
Ergotamine	T46.5X1	T46.5X2	T46.5X3	T46.5X4	T46.5X5	T46.5X6
Ergotocine	T48.0X1	T48.0X2	T48.0X3	T48.0X4	T48.0X5	T48.0X6
Ergotrate	T48.0X1	T48.0X2	T48.0X3	T48.0X4	T48.0X5	T48.0X6
Eritrityl tetranitrate	T46.3X1	T46.3X2	T46.3X3	T46.3X4	T46.3X5	T46.3X6
Erythrityl tetranitrate	T46.3X1	T46.3X2	T46.3X3	T46.3X4	T46.3X5	T46.3X6
Erythrol tetranitrate	T46.3X1	T46.3X2	T46.3X3	T46.3X4	T46.3X5	T46.3X6
Erythromycin (salts)	T36.3X1	T36.3X2	T36.3X3	T36.3X4	T36.3X5	T36.3X6
ophthalmic preparation	T49.5X1	T49.5X2	T49.5X3	T49.5X4	T49.5X5	T49.5X6
topical NEC	T49.0X1	T49.0X2	T49.0X3	T49.0X4	T49.0X5	T49.0X6
Erythropoietin	T45.8X1	T45.8X2	T45.8X3	T45.8X4	T45.8X5	T45.8X6
human	T45.8X1	T45.8X2	T45.8X3	T45.8X4	T45.8X5	T45.8X6
Escin	T46.991	T46.992	T46.993	T46.994	T46.995	T46.996
Esculin	T45.2X1	T45.2X2	T45.2X3	T45.2X4	T45.2X5	T45.2X6
Esculoside	T45.2X1	T45.2X2	T45.2X3	T45.2X4	T45.2X5	T45.2X6
ESDT (ether-soluble tar distillate)	T49.1X1	T49.1X2	T49.1X3	T49.1X4	T49.1X5	T49.1X6
Eserine	T49.5X1	T49.5X2	T49.5X3	T49.5X4	T49.5X5	T49.5X6
Esflurbiprofen	T39.311	T39.312	T39.313	T39.314	T39.315	T39.316
Eskabarb	T42.3X1	T42.3X2	T42.3X3	T42.3X4	T42.3X5	T42.3X6
Eskalith	T43.8X1	T43.8X2	T43.8X3	T43.8X4	T43.8X5	T43.8X6
Esmolol	T44.7X1	T44.7X2	T44.7X3	T44.7X4	T44.7X5	T44.7X6
Estanozolol	T38.7X1	T38.7X2	T38.7X3	T38.7X4	T38.7X5	T38.7X6
Estazolam	T42.4X1	T42.4X2	T42.4X3	T42.4X4	T42.4X5	T42.4X6
Estradiol	T38.5X1	T38.5X2	T38.5X3	T38.5X4	T38.5X5	T38.5X6
with testosterone	T38.7X1	T38.7X2	T38.7X3	T38.7X4	T38.7X5	T38.7X6
benzoate	T38.5X1	T38.5X2	T38.5X3	T38.5X4	T38.5X5	T38.5X6
Estramustine	T45.1X1	T45.1X2	T45.1X3	T45.1X4	T45.1X5	T45.1X6
Estriol	T38.5X1	T38.5X2	T38.5X3	T38.5X4	T38.5X5	T38.5X6
Estrogen	T38.5X1	T38.5X2	T38.5X3	T38.5X4	T38.5X5	T38.5X6
with progesterone	T38.5X1	T38.5X2	T38.5X3	T38.5X4	T38.5X5	T38.5X6
conjugated	T38.5X1	T38.5X2	T38.5X3	T38.5X4	T38.5X5	T38.5X6
Estrone	T38.5X1	T38.5X2	T38.5X3	T38.5X4	T38.5X5	T38.5X6
Estropipate	T38.5X1	T38.5X2	T38.5X3	T38.5X4	T38.5X5	T38.5X6
Etacrynate sodium	T50.1X1	T50.1X2	T50.1X3	T50.1X4	T50.1X5	T50.1X6
Etacrynic acid	T50.1X1	T50.1X2	T50.1X3	T50.1X4	T50.1X5	T50.1X6
Etafedrine	T48.6X1	T48.6X2	T48.6X3	T48.6X4	T48.6X5	T48.6X6
Etafenone	T46.3X1	T46.3X2	T46.3X3	T46.3X4	T46.3X5	T46.3X6
Etambutol	T37.1X1	T37.1X2	T37.1X3	T37.1X4	T37.1X5	T37.1X6
Etamiphyllin	T48.6X1	T48.6X2	T48.6X3	T48.6X4	T48.6X5	T48.6X6
Etamivan	T50.7X1	T50.7X2	T50.7X3	T50.7X4	T50.7X5	T50.7X6
Etamsylate	T45.7X1	T45.7X2	T45.7X3	T45.7X4	T45.7X5	T45.7X6
Etebenecid	T50.4X1	T50.4X2	T50.4X3	T50.4X4	T50.4X5	T50.4X6
Ethacridine	T49.0X1	T49.0X2	T49.0X3	T49.0X4	T49.0X5	T49.0X6
Ethacrynic acid	T50.1X1	T50.1X2	T50.1X3	T50.1X4	T50.1X5	T50.1X6
Ethadione	T42.2X1	T42.2X2	T42.2X3	T42.2X4	T42.2X5	T42.2X6
Ethambutol	T37.1X1	T37.1X2	T37.1X3	T37.1X4	T37.1X5	T37.1X6
Ethamide	T50.2X1	T50.2X2	T50.2X3	T50.2X4	T50.2X5	T50.2X6
Ethamivan	T50.7X1	T50.7X2	T50.7X3	T50.7X4	T50.7X5	T50.7X6
Ethamsylate	T45.7X1	T45.7X2	T45.7X3	T45.7X4	T45.7X5	T45.7X6

Substance	Poisoning, Accidental (unintentional)	Poisoning, Intentional self-harm	Poisoning, Assault	Poisoning, Undetermined	Adverse effect	Underdosing
Ethanol	T51.0X1	T51.0X2	T51.0X3	T51.0X4	—	—
beverage	T51.0X1	T51.0X2	T51.0X3	T51.0X4	—	—
Ethanolamine oleate	T46.8X1	T46.8X2	T46.8X3	T46.8X4	T46.8X5	T46.8X6
Ethaverine	T44.3X1	T44.3X2	T44.3X3	T44.3X4	T44.3X5	T44.3X6
Ethchlorvynol	T42.6X1	T42.6X2	T42.6X3	T42.6X4	T42.6X5	T42.6X6
Ethebenecid	T50.4X1	T50.4X2	T50.4X3	T50.4X4	T50.4X5	T50.4X6
Ether (vapor)	T41.0X1	T41.0X2	T41.0X3	T41.0X4	T41.0X5	T41.0X6
anesthetic	T41.0X1	T41.0X2	T41.0X3	T41.0X4	T41.0X5	T41.0X6
divinyl	T41.0X1	T41.0X2	T41.0X3	T41.0X4	T41.0X5	T41.0X6
ethyl (medicinal)	T41.0X1	T41.0X2	T41.0X3	T41.0X4	T41.0X5	T41.0X6
nonmedicinal	T52.8X1	T52.8X2	T52.8X3	T52.8X4	—	—
petroleum—see Ligroin						
solvent	T52.8X1	T52.8X2	T52.8X3	T52.8X4	—	—
Ethiazide	T50.2X1	T50.2X2	T50.2X3	T50.2X4	T50.2X5	T50.2X6
Ethidium chloride (vapor)	T59.891	T59.892	T59.893	T59.894	—	—
Ethinamate	T42.6X1	T42.6X2	T42.6X3	T42.6X4	T42.6X5	T42.6X6
Ethinylestradiol, ethinyloestradiol	T38.5X1	T38.5X2	T38.5X3	T38.5X4	T38.5X5	T38.5X6
with						
levonorgestrel	T38.4X1	T38.4X2	T38.4X3	T38.4X4	T38.4X5	T38.4X6
norethisterone	T38.4X1	T38.4X2	T38.4X3	T38.4X4	T38.4X5	T38.4X6
Ethiodized oil (131 I)	T50.8X1	T50.8X2	T50.8X3	T50.8X4	T50.8X5	T50.8X6
Ethion	T60.0X1	T60.0X2	T60.0X3	T60.0X4	—	—
Ethionamide	T37.1X1	T37.1X2	T37.1X3	T37.1X4	T37.1X5	T37.1X6
Ethioniamide	T37.1X1	T37.1X2	T37.1X3	T37.1X4	T37.1X5	T37.1X6
Ethisterone	T38.5X1	T38.5X2	T38.5X3	T38.5X4	T38.5X5	T38.5X6
Ethobral	T42.3X1	T42.3X2	T42.3X3	T42.3X4	T42.3X5	T42.3X6
Ethocaine (infiltration) (topical)	T41.3X1	T41.3X2	T41.3X3	T41.3X4	T41.3X5	T41.3X6
nerve block (peripheral) (plexus)	T41.3X1	T41.3X2	T41.3X3	T41.3X4	T41.3X5	T41.3X6
spinal	T41.3X1	T41.3X2	T41.3X3	T41.3X4	T41.3X5	T41.3X6
Ethoheptazine	T40.491	T40.492	T40.493	T40.494	T40.495	T40.496
Ethopropazine	T44.3X1	T44.3X2	T44.3X3	T44.3X4	T44.3X5	T44.3X6
Ethosuximide	T42.2X1	T42.2X2	T42.2X3	T42.2X4	T42.2X5	T42.2X6
Ethotoin	T42.0X1	T42.0X2	T42.0X3	T42.0X4	T42.0X5	T42.0X6
Ethoxazene	T37.91	T37.92	T37.93	T37.94	T37.95	T37.96
Ethoxazorutoside	T46.991	T46.992	T46.993	T46.994	T46.995	T46.996
2-Ethoxyethanol	T52.3X1	T52.3X2	T52.3X3	T52.3X4	—	—
Ethoxzolamide	T50.2X1	T50.2X2	T50.2X3	T50.2X4	T50.2X5	T50.2X6
Ethyl						
acetate	T52.8X1	T52.8X2	T52.8X3	T52.8X4	—	—
alcohol	T51.0X1	T51.0X2	T51.0X3	T51.0X4	—	—
beverage	T51.0X1	T51.0X2	T51.0X3	T51.0X4	—	—
aldehyde (vapor)	T59.891	T59.892	T59.893	T59.894	—	—
liquid	T52.8X1	T52.8X2	T52.8X3	T52.8X4	—	—
aminobenzoate	T41.3X1	T41.3X2	T41.3X3	T41.3X4	T41.3X5	T41.3X6
aminophenothiazine	T43.3X1	T43.3X2	T43.3X3	T43.3X4	T43.3X5	T43.3X6
benzoate	T52.8X1	T52.8X2	T52.8X3	T52.8X4	—	—

Substance	Poisoning, Accidental (unintentional)	Poisoning, Intentional self-harm	Poisoning, Assault	Poisoning, Undetermined	Adverse effect	Underdosing
Ethyl — *Continued*						
biscoumacetate	T45.511	T45.512	T45.513	T45.514	T45.515	T45.516
bromide (anesthetic)	T41.0X1	T41.0X2	T41.0X3	T41.0X4	T41.0X5	T41.0X6
carbamate	T45.1X1	T45.1X2	T45.1X3	T45.1X4	T45.1X5	T45.1X6
carbinol	T51.3X1	T51.3X2	T51.3X3	T51.3X4	—	—
carbonate	T52.8X1	T52.8X2	T52.8X3	T52.8X4	—	—
chaulmoograte	T37.1X1	T37.1X2	T37.1X3	T37.1X4	T37.1X5	T37.1X6
chloride (anesthetic)	T41.0X1	T41.0X2	T41.0X3	T41.0X4	T41.0X5	T41.0X6
anesthetic (local)	T41.3X1	T41.3X2	T41.3X3	T41.3X4	T41.3X5	T41.3X6
inhaled	T41.0X1	T41.0X2	T41.0X3	T41.0X4	T41.0X5	T41.0X6
local	T49.4X1	T49.4X2	T49.4X3	T49.4X4	T49.4X5	T49.4X6
solvent	T53.6X1	T53.6X2	T53.6X3	T53.6X4	—	—
dibunate	T48.3X1	T48.3X2	T48.3X3	T48.3X4	T48.3X5	T48.3X6
dichloroarsine (vapor)	T57.0X1	T57.0X2	T57.0X3	T57.0X4	—	—
estranol	T38.7X1	T38.7X2	T38.7X3	T38.7X4	T38.7X5	T38.7X6
ether—see also ether	T52.8X1	T52.8X2	T52.8X3	T52.8X4	—	—
formate NEC (solvent)	T52.0X1	T52.0X2	T52.0X3	T52.0X4	—	—
fumarate	T49.4X1	T49.4X2	T49.4X3	T49.4X4	T49.4X5	T49.4X6
hydroxyisobutyrate NEC (solvent)	T52.8X1	T52.8X2	T52.8X3	T52.8X4	—	—
iodoacetate	T59.3X1	T59.3X2	T59.3X3	T59.3X4	—	—
lactate NEC (solvent)	T52.8X1	T52.8X2	T52.8X3	T52.8X4	—	—
loflazepate	T42.4X1	T42.4X2	T42.4X3	T42.4X4	T42.4X5	T42.4X6
mercuric chloride	T56.1X1	T56.1X2	T56.1X3	T56.1X4	—	—
methylcarbinol	T51.8X1	T51.8X2	T51.8X3	T51.8X4	—	—
morphine	T40.2X1	T40.2X2	T40.2X3	T40.2X4	T40.2X5	T40.2X6
noradrenaline	T48.6X1	T48.6X2	T48.6X3	T48.6X4	T48.6X5	T48.6X6
oxybutyrate NEC (solvent)	T52.8X1	T52.8X2	T52.8X3	T52.8X4	—	—
Ethylene (gas)	T59.891	T59.892	T59.893	T59.894	—	—
anesthetic (general)	T41.0X1	T41.0X2	T41.0X3	T41.0X4	T41.0X5	T41.0X6
chlorohydrin	T52.8X1	T52.8X2	T52.8X3	T52.8X4	—	—
vapor	T53.6X1	T53.6X2	T53.6X3	T53.6X4	—	—
dichloride	T52.8X1	T52.8X2	T52.8X3	T52.8X4	—	—
vapor	T53.6X1	T53.6X2	T53.6X3	T53.6X4	—	—
dinitrate	T52.3X1	T52.3X2	T52.3X3	T52.3X4	—	—
glycol(s)	T52.8X1	T52.8X2	T52.8X3	T52.8X4	—	—
dinitrate	T52.3X1	T52.3X2	T52.3X3	T52.3X4	—	—
monobutyl ether	T52.3X1	T52.3X2	T52.3X3	T52.3X4	—	—
imine	T54.1X1	T54.1X2	T54.1X3	T54.1X4	—	—
oxide (fumigant) (nonmedicinal)	T59.891	T59.892	T59.893	T59.894	—	—
medicinal	T49.0X1	T49.0X2	T49.0X3	T49.0X4	T49.0X5	T49.0X6
Ethylenediamine theophylline	T48.6X1	T48.6X2	T48.6X3	T48.6X4	T48.6X5	T48.6X6
Ethylenediaminetetra-acetic acid	T50.6X1	T50.6X2	T50.6X3	T50.6X4	T50.6X5	T50.6X6
Ethylen-edinitrilotetra-acetate	T50.6X1	T50.6X2	T50.6X3	T50.6X4	T50.6X5	T50.6X6
Ethylestrenol	T38.7X1	T38.7X2	T38.7X3	T38.7X4	T38.7X5	T38.7X6
Ethylhydro-xycellulose	T47.4X1	T47.4X2	T47.4X3	T47.4X4	T47.4X5	T47.4X6
Ethylidene						
chloride NEC	T53.6X1	T53.6X2	T53.6X3	T53.6X4	—	—
diacetate	T60.3X1	T60.3X2	T60.3X3	T60.3X4	—	—
dicoumarin	T45.511	T45.512	T45.513	T45.514	T45.515	T45.516
dicoumarol	T45.511	T45.512	T45.513	T45.514	T45.515	T45.516
diethyl ether	T52.0X1	T52.0X2	T52.0X3	T52.0X4	—	—
Ethylmorphine	T40.2X1	T40.2X2	T40.2X3	T40.2X4	T40.2X5	T40.2X6
Ethylnorepinephrine	T48.6X1	T48.6X2	T48.6X3	T48.6X4	T48.6X5	T48.6X6
Ethylparachloro-phenoxyisobutyrate	T46.6X1	T46.6X2	T46.6X3	T46.6X4	T46.6X5	T46.6X6
Ethynodiol	T38.4X1	T38.4X2	T38.4X3	T38.4X4	T38.4X5	T38.4X6
with mestranol diacetate	T38.4X1	T38.4X2	T38.4X3	T38.4X4	T38.4X5	T38.4X6
Etidocaine	T41.3X1	T41.3X2	T41.3X3	T41.3X4	T41.3X5	T41.3X6
infiltration (subcutaneous)	T41.3X1	T41.3X2	T41.3X3	T41.3X4	T41.3X5	T41.3X6
nerve (peripheral) (plexus)	T41.3X1	T41.3X2	T41.3X3	T41.3X4	T41.3X5	T41.3X6
Etidronate	T50.991	T50.992	T50.993	T50.994	T50.995	T50.996
Etidronic acid (disodium salt)	T50.991	T50.992	T50.993	T50.994	T50.995	T50.996
Etifoxine	T42.6X1	T42.6X2	T42.6X3	T42.6X4	T42.6X5	T42.6X6
Etilefrine	T44.4X1	T44.4X2	T44.4X3	T44.4X4	T44.4X5	T44.4X6
Etilfen	T42.3X1	T42.3X2	T42.3X3	T42.3X4	T42.3X5	T42.3X6
Etinodiol	T38.4X1	T38.4X2	T38.4X3	T38.4X4	T38.4X5	T38.4X6
Etiroxate	T46.6X1	T46.6X2	T46.6X3	T46.6X4	T46.6X5	T46.6X6
Etizolam	T42.4X1	T42.4X2	T42.4X3	T42.4X4	T42.4X5	T42.4X6
Etodolac	T39.391	T39.392	T39.393	T39.394	T39.395	T39.396
Etofamide	T37.3X1	T37.3X2	T37.3X3	T37.3X4	T37.3X5	T37.3X6
Etofibrate	T46.6X1	T46.6X2	T46.6X3	T46.6X4	T46.6X5	T46.6X6
Etofylline	T46.7X1	T46.7X2	T46.7X3	T46.7X4	T46.7X5	T46.7X6
clofibrate	T46.6X1	T46.6X2	T46.6X3	T46.6X4	T46.6X5	T46.6X6
Etoglucid	T45.1X1	T45.1X2	T45.1X3	T45.1X4	T45.1X5	T45.1X6
Etomidate	T41.1X1	T41.1X2	T41.1X3	T41.1X4	T41.1X5	T41.1X6
Etomide	T39.8X1	T39.8X2	T39.8X3	T39.8X4	T39.8X5	T39.8X6
Etomidoline	T44.3X1	T44.3X2	T44.3X3	T44.3X4	T44.3X5	T44.3X6
Etoposide	T45.1X1	T45.1X2	T45.1X3	T45.1X4	T45.1X5	T45.1X6
Etorphine	T40.2X1	T40.2X2	T40.2X3	T40.2X4	T40.2X5	T40.2X6
Etoval	T42.3X1	T42.3X2	T42.3X3	T42.3X4	T42.3X5	T42.3X6
Etozolin	T50.1X1	T50.1X2	T50.1X3	T50.1X4	T50.1X5	T50.1X6
Etretinate	T50.991	T50.992	T50.993	T50.994	T50.995	T50.996
Etryptamine	T43.691	T43.692	T43.693	T43.694	T43.695	T43.696
Etybenzatropine	T44.3X1	T44.3X2	T44.3X3	T44.3X4	T44.3X5	T44.3X6
Etynodiol	T38.4X1	T38.4X2	T38.4X3	T38.4X4	T38.4X5	T38.4X6
Eucaine	T41.3X1	T41.3X2	T41.3X3	T41.3X4	T41.3X5	T41.3X6
Eucalyptus oil	T49.7X1	T49.7X2	T49.7X3	T49.7X4	T49.7X5	T49.7X6
Eucatropine	T49.5X1	T49.5X2	T49.5X3	T49.5X4	T49.5X5	T49.5X6
Eucodal	T40.2X1	T40.2X2	T40.2X3	T40.2X4	T40.2X5	T40.2X6
Euneryl	T42.3X1	T42.3X2	T42.3X3	T42.3X4	T42.3X5	T42.3X6
Euphthalmine	T44.3X1	T44.3X2	T44.3X3	T44.3X4	T44.3X5	T44.3X6

Substance	Poisoning, Accidental (unintentional)	Poisoning, Intentional self-harm	Poisoning, Assault	Poisoning, Undetermined	Adverse effect	Underdosing
Eurax	T49.0X1	T49.0X2	T49.0X3	T49.0X4	T49.0X5	T49.0X6
Euresol	T49.4X1	T49.4X2	T49.4X3	T49.4X4	T49.4X5	T49.4X6
Euthroid	T38.1X1	T38.1X2	T38.1X3	T38.1X4	T38.1X5	T38.1X6
Evans blue	T50.8X1	T50.8X2	T50.8X3	T50.8X4	T50.8X5	T50.8X6
Evipal	T42.3X1	T42.3X2	T42.3X3	T42.3X4	T42.3X5	T42.3X6
sodium	T41.1X1	T41.1X2	T41.1X3	T41.1X4	T41.1X5	T41.1X6
Evipan	T42.3X1	T42.3X2	T42.3X3	T42.3X4	T42.3X5	T42.3X6
sodium	T41.1X1	T41.1X2	T41.1X3	T41.1X4	T41.1X5	T41.1X6
Exalamide	T49.0X1	T49.0X2	T49.0X3	T49.0X4	T49.0X5	T49.0X6
Exalgin	T39.1X1	T39.1X2	T39.1X3	T39.1X4	T39.1X5	T39.1X6
Excipients, pharmaceutical	T50.901	T50.902	T50.903	T50.904	T50.905	T50.906
Exhaust gas (engine) (motor vehicle)	T58.01	T58.02	T58.03	T58.04	—	—
Ex-Lax (phenolphthalein)	T47.2X1	T47.2X2	T47.2X3	T47.2X4	T47.2X5	T47.2X6
Expectorant NEC	T48.4X1	T48.4X2	T48.4X3	T48.4X4	T48.4X5	T48.4X6
Extended insulin zinc suspension	T38.3X1	T38.3X2	T38.3X3	T38.3X4	T38.3X5	T38.3X6
External medications (skin) (mucous membrane)	T49.91	T49.92	T49.93	T49.94	T49.95	T49.96
dental agent	T49.7X1	T49.7X2	T49.7X3	T49.7X4	T49.7X5	T49.7X6
ENT agent	T49.6X1	T49.6X2	T49.6X3	T49.6X4	T49.6X5	T49.6X6
ophthalmic preparation	T49.5X1	T49.5X2	T49.5X3	T49.5X4	T49.5X5	T49.5X6
specified NEC	T49.8X1	T49.8X2	T49.8X3	T49.8X4	T49.8X5	T49.8X6
Extrapyramidal antagonist NEC	T44.3X1	T44.3X2	T44.3X3	T44.3X4	T44.3X5	T44.3X6
Eye agents (anti-infective)	T49.5X1	T49.5X2	T49.5X3	T49.5X4	T49.5X5	T49.5X6
Eye drug NEC	T49.5X1	T49.5X2	T49.5X3	T49.5X4	T49.5X5	T49.5X6
F						
FAC (fluorouracil + doxorubicin + cyclophosphamide)	T45.1X1	T45.1X2	T45.1X3	T45.1X4	T45.1X5	T45.1X6
Factor						
I (fibrinogen)	T45.8X1	T45.8X2	T45.8X3	T45.8X4	T45.8X5	T45.8X6
III (thromboplastin)	T45.8X1	T45.8X2	T45.8X3	T45.8X4	T45.8X5	T45.8X6
VIII (antihemophilic Factor) (concentrate)	T45.8X1	T45.8X2	T45.8X3	T45.8X4	T45.8X5	T45.8X6
IX complex	T45.7X1	T45.7X2	T45.7X3	T45.7X4	T45.7X5	T45.7X6
human	T45.8X1	T45.8X2	T45.8X3	T45.8X4	T45.8X5	T45.8X6
Famotidine	T47.0X1	T47.0X2	T47.0X3	T47.0X4	T47.0X5	T47.0X6
Fat suspension, intravenous	T50.991	T50.992	T50.993	T50.994	T50.995	T50.996
Fazadinium bromide	T48.1X1	T48.1X2	T48.1X3	T48.1X4	T48.1X5	T48.1X6
Febarbamate	T42.3X1	T42.3X2	T42.3X3	T42.3X4	T42.3X5	T42.3X6
Fecal softener	T47.4X1	T47.4X2	T47.4X3	T47.4X4	T47.4X5	T47.4X6
Fedrilate	T48.3X1	T48.3X2	T48.3X3	T48.3X4	T48.3X5	T48.3X6
Felodipine	T46.1X1	T46.1X2	T46.1X3	T46.1X4	T46.1X5	T46.1X6
Felypressin	T38.891	T38.892	T38.893	T38.894	T38.895	T38.896
Femoxetine	T43.221	T43.222	T43.223	T43.224	T43.225	T43.226
Fenalcomine	T46.3X1	T46.3X2	T46.3X3	T46.3X4	T46.3X5	T46.3X6
Fenamisal	T37.1X1	T37.1X2	T37.1X3	T37.1X4	T37.1X5	T37.1X6

Substance	Poisoning, Accidental (unintentional)	Poisoning, Intentional self-harm	Poisoning, Assault	Poisoning, Undetermined	Adverse effect	Underdosing
Fenazone	T39.2X1	T39.2X2	T39.2X3	T39.2X4	T39.2X5	T39.2X6
Fenbendazole	T37.4X1	T37.4X2	T37.4X3	T37.4X4	T37.4X5	T37.4X6
Fenbutrazate	T50.5X1	T50.5X2	T50.5X3	T50.5X4	T50.5X5	T50.5X6
Fencamfamine	T43.691	T43.692	T43.693	T43.694	T43.695	T43.696
Fendiline	T46.1X1	T46.1X2	T46.1X3	T46.1X4	T46.1X5	T46.1X6
Fenetylline	T43.691	T43.692	T43.693	T43.694	T43.695	T43.696
Fenflumizole	T39.391	T39.392	T39.393	T39.394	T39.395	T39.396
Fenfluramine	T50.5X1	T50.5X2	T50.5X3	T50.5X4	T50.5X5	T50.5X6
Fenobarbital	T42.3X1	T42.3X2	T42.3X3	T42.3X4	T42.3X5	T42.3X6
Fenofibrate	T46.6X1	T46.6X2	T46.6X3	T46.6X4	T46.6X5	T46.6X6
Fenoprofen	T39.311	T39.312	T39.313	T39.314	T39.315	T39.316
Fenoterol	T48.6X1	T48.6X2	T48.6X3	T48.6X4	T48.6X5	T48.6X6
Fenoverine	T44.3X1	T44.3X2	T44.3X3	T44.3X4	T44.3X5	T44.3X6
Fenoxazoline	T48.5X1	T48.5X2	T48.5X3	T48.5X4	T48.5X5	T48.5X6
Fenproporex	T50.5X1	T50.5X2	T50.5X3	T50.5X4	T50.5X5	T50.5X6
Fenquizone	T50.2X1	T50.2X2	T50.2X3	T50.2X4	T50.2X5	T50.2X6
Fentanyl (analogs)	T40.411	T40.412	T40.413	T40.414	T40.415	T40.416
Fentazin	T43.3X1	T43.3X2	T43.3X3	T43.3X4	T43.3X5	T43.3X6
Fenthion	T60.0X1	T60.0X2	T60.0X3	T60.0X4	—	—
Fenticlor	T49.0X1	T49.0X2	T49.0X3	T49.0X4	T49.0X5	T49.0X6
Fenylbutazone	T39.2X1	T39.2X2	T39.2X3	T39.2X4	T39.2X5	T39.2X6
Feprazone	T39.2X1	T39.2X2	T39.2X3	T39.2X4	T39.2X5	T39.2X6
Fer de lance (bite) (venom)	T63.061	T63.062	T63.063	T63.064	—	—
Ferric—see also Iron						
chloride	T45.4X1	T45.4X2	T45.4X3	T45.4X4	T45.4X5	T45.4X6
citrate	T45.4X1	T45.4X2	T45.4X3	T45.4X4	T45.4X5	T45.4X6
hydroxide						
colloidal	T45.4X1	T45.4X2	T45.4X3	T45.4X4	T45.4X5	T45.4X6
polymaltose	T45.4X1	T45.4X2	T45.4X3	T45.4X4	T45.4X5	T45.4X6
pyrophosphate	T45.4X1	T45.4X2	T45.4X3	T45.4X4	T45.4X5	T45.4X6
Ferritin	T45.4X1	T45.4X2	T45.4X3	T45.4X4	T45.4X5	T45.4X6
Ferrocholinate	T45.4X1	T45.4X2	T45.4X3	T45.4X4	T45.4X5	T45.4X6
Ferrodextrane	T45.4X1	T45.4X2	T45.4X3	T45.4X4	T45.4X5	T45.4X6
Ferropolimaler	T45.4X1	T45.4X2	T45.4X3	T45.4X4	T45.4X5	T45.4X6
Ferrous—see also Iron						
phosphate	T45.4X1	T45.4X2	T45.4X3	T45.4X4	T45.4X5	T45.4X6
salt	T45.4X1	T45.4X2	T45.4X3	T45.4X4	T45.4X5	T45.4X6
with folic acid	T45.4X1	T45.4X2	T45.4X3	T45.4X4	T45.4X5	T45.4X6
Ferrous fumerate, gluconate, lactate, salt NEC, sulfate (medicinal)	T45.4X1	T45.4X2	T45.4X3	T45.4X4	T45.4X5	T45.4X6
Ferrovanadium (fumes)	T59.891	T59.892	T59.893	T59.894	—	—
Ferrum—see Iron						
Fertilizers NEC	T65.891	T65.892	T65.893	T65.894	—	—
with herbicide mixture	T60.3X1	T60.3X2	T60.3X3	T60.3X4	—	—
Fetoxilate	T47.6X1	T47.6X2	T47.6X3	T47.6X4	T47.6X5	T47.6X6
Fiber, dietary	T47.4X1	T47.4X2	T47.4X3	T47.4X4	T47.4X5	T47.4X6
Fiberglass	T65.831	T65.832	T65.833	T65.834	—	—
Fibrinogen (human)	T45.8X1	T45.8X2	T45.8X3	T45.8X4	T45.8X5	T45.8X6
Fibrinolysin (human)	T45.691	T45.692	T45.693	T45.694	T45.695	T45.696

Substance	Poisoning, Accidental (unintentional)	Poisoning, Intentional self-harm	Poisoning, Assault	Poisoning, Undetermined	Adverse effect	Underdosing
Fibrinolysis						
affecting drug	T45.601	T45.602	T45.603	T45.604	T45.605	T45.606
inhibitor NEC	T45.621	T45.622	T45.623	T45.624	T45.625	T45.626
Fibrinolytic drug	T45.611	T45.612	T45.613	T45.614	T45.615	T45.616
Filix mas	T37.4X1	T37.4X2	T37.4X3	T37.4X4	T37.4X5	T37.4X6
Filtering cream	T49.3X1	T49.3X2	T49.3X3	T49.3X4	T49.3X5	T49.3X6
Fiorinal	T39.011	T39.012	T39.013	T39.014	T39.015	T39.016
Firedamp	T59.891	T59.892	T59.893	T59.894	—	—
Fish, noxious, nonbacterial	T61.91	T61.92	T61.93	T61.94	—	—
ciguatera	T61.01	T61.02	T61.03	T61.04	—	—
scombroid	T61.11	T61.12	T61.13	T61.14	—	—
shell	T61.781	T61.782	T61.783	T61.784	—	—
specified NEC	T61.771	T61.772	T61.773	T61.774	—	—
Flagyl	T37.3X1	T37.3X2	T37.3X3	T37.3X4	T37.3X5	T37.3X6
Flavine adenine dinucleotide	T45.2X1	T45.2X2	T45.2X3	T45.2X4	T45.2X5	T45.2X6
Flavodic acid	T46.991	T46.992	T46.993	T46.994	T46.995	T46.996
Flavoxate	T44.3X1	T44.3X2	T44.3X3	T44.3X4	T44.3X5	T44.3X6
Flaxedil	T48.1X1	T48.1X2	T48.1X3	T48.1X4	T48.1X5	T48.1X6
Flaxseed (medicinal)	T49.3X1	T49.3X2	T49.3X3	T49.3X4	T49.3X5	T49.3X6
Flecainide	T46.2X1	T46.2X2	T46.2X3	T46.2X4	T46.2X5	T46.2X6
Fleroxacin	T36.8X1	T36.8X2	T36.8X3	T36.8X4	T36.8X5	T36.8X6
Floctafenine	T39.8X1	T39.8X2	T39.8X3	T39.8X4	T39.8X5	T39.8X6
Flomax	T44.6X1	T44.6X2	T44.6X3	T44.6X4	T44.6X5	T44.6X6
Flomoxef	T36.1X1	T36.1X2	T36.1X3	T36.1X4	T36.1X5	T36.1X6
Flopropione	T44.3X1	T44.3X2	T44.3X3	T44.3X4	T44.3X5	T44.3X6
Florantyrone	T47.5X1	T47.5X2	T47.5X3	T47.5X4	T47.5X5	T47.5X6
Floraquin	T37.8X1	T37.8X2	T37.8X3	T37.8X4	T37.8X5	T37.8X6
Florinef	T38.0X1	T38.0X2	T38.0X3	T38.0X4	T38.0X5	T38.0X6
ENT agent	T49.6X1	T49.6X2	T49.6X3	T49.6X4	T49.6X5	T49.6X6
ophthalmic preparation	T49.5X1	T49.5X2	T49.5X3	T49.5X4	T49.5X5	T49.5X6
topical NEC	T49.0X1	T49.0X2	T49.0X3	T49.0X4	T49.0X5	T49.0X6
Flowers of sulfur	T49.4X1	T49.4X2	T49.4X3	T49.4X4	T49.4X5	T49.4X6
Floxuridine	T45.1X1	T45.1X2	T45.1X3	T45.1X4	T45.1X5	T45.1X6
Fluanisone	T43.4X1	T43.4X2	T43.4X3	T43.4X4	T43.4X5	T43.4X6
Flubendazole	T37.4X1	T37.4X2	T37.4X3	T37.4X4	T37.4X5	T37.4X6
Fluclorolone acetonide	T49.0X1	T49.0X2	T49.0X3	T49.0X4	T49.0X5	T49.0X6
Flucloxacillin	T36.0X1	T36.0X2	T36.0X3	T36.0X4	T36.0X5	T36.0X6
Fluconazole	T37.8X1	T37.8X2	T37.8X3	T37.8X4	T37.8X5	T37.8X6
Flucytosine	T37.8X1	T37.8X2	T37.8X3	T37.8X4	T37.8X5	T37.8X6
Fludeoxyglucose (18F)	T50.8X1	T50.8X2	T50.8X3	T50.8X4	T50.8X5	T50.8X6
Fludiazepam	T42.4X1	T42.4X2	T42.4X3	T42.4X4	T42.4X5	T42.4X6
Fludrocortisone	T50.0X1	T50.0X2	T50.0X3	T50.0X4	T50.0X5	T50.0X6
ENT agent	T49.6X1	T49.6X2	T49.6X3	T49.6X4	T49.6X5	T49.6X6
ophthalmic preparation	T49.5X1	T49.5X2	T49.5X3	T49.5X4	T49.5X5	T49.5X6
topical NEC	T49.0X1	T49.0X2	T49.0X3	T49.0X4	T49.0X5	T49.0X6
Fludroxycortide	T49.0X1	T49.0X2	T49.0X3	T49.0X4	T49.0X5	T49.0X6
Flufenamic acid	T39.391	T39.392	T39.393	T39.394	T39.395	T39.396
Fluindione	T45.511	T45.512	T45.513	T45.514	T45.515	T45.516
Flumequine	T37.8X1	T37.8X2	T37.8X3	T37.8X4	T37.8X5	T37.8X6
Flumethasone	T49.0X1	T49.0X2	T49.0X3	T49.0X4	T49.0X5	T49.0X6
Flumethiazide	T50.2X1	T50.2X2	T50.2X3	T50.2X4	T50.2X5	T50.2X6
Flumidin	T37.5X1	T37.5X2	T37.5X3	T37.5X4	T37.5X5	T37.5X6
Flunarizine	T46.7X1	T46.7X2	T46.7X3	T46.7X4	T46.7X5	T46.7X6
Flunidazole	T37.8X1	T37.8X2	T37.8X3	T37.8X4	T37.8X5	T37.8X6
Flunisolide	T48.6X1	T48.6X2	T48.6X3	T48.6X4	T48.6X5	T48.6X6
Flunitrazepam	T42.4X1	T42.4X2	T42.4X3	T42.4X4	T42.4X5	T42.4X6
Fluocinolone (acetonide)	T49.0X1	T49.0X2	T49.0X3	T49.0X4	T49.0X5	T49.0X6
Fluocinonide	T49.0X1	T49.0X2	T49.0X3	T49.0X4	T49.0X5	T49.0X6
Fluocortin (butyl)	T49.0X1	T49.0X2	T49.0X3	T49.0X4	T49.0X5	T49.0X6
Fluocortolone	T49.0X1	T49.0X2	T49.0X3	T49.0X4	T49.0X5	T49.0X6
Fluohydrocortisone	T38.0X1	T38.0X2	T38.0X3	T38.0X4	T38.0X5	T38.0X6
ENT agent	T49.6X1	T49.6X2	T49.6X3	T49.6X4	T49.6X5	T49.6X6
ophthalmic preparation	T49.5X1	T49.5X2	T49.5X3	T49.5X4	T49.5X5	T49.5X6
topical NEC	T49.0X1	T49.0X2	T49.0X3	T49.0X4	T49.0X5	T49.0X6
Fluonid	T49.0X1	T49.0X2	T49.0X3	T49.0X4	T49.0X5	T49.0X6
Fluopromazine	T43.3X1	T43.3X2	T43.3X3	T43.3X4	T43.3X5	T43.3X6
Fluoracetate	T60.8X1	T60.8X2	T60.8X3	T60.8X4	—	—
Fluorescein	T50.8X1	T50.8X2	T50.8X3	T50.8X4	T50.8X5	T50.8X6
Fluorhydrocortisone	T50.0X1	T50.0X2	T50.0X3	T50.0X4	T50.0X5	T50.0X6
Fluoride (nonmedicinal)(pesticide) (sodium) NEC	T60.8X1	T60.8X2	T60.8X3	T60.8X4	—	—
hydrogen—see Hydrofluoric acid						
medicinal NEC	T50.991	T50.992	T50.993	T50.994	T50.995	T50.996
dental use	T49.7X1	T49.7X2	T49.7X3	T49.7X4	T49.7X5	T49.7X6
not pesticide NEC	T54.91	T54.92	T54.93	T54.94	—	—
stannous	T49.7X1	T49.7X2	T49.7X3	T49.7X4	T49.7X5	T49.7X6
Fluorinated corticosteroids	T38.0X1	T38.0X2	T38.0X3	T38.0X4	T38.0X5	T38.0X6
Fluorine (gas)	T59.5X1	T59.5X2	T59.5X3	T59.5X4	—	—
salt—see Fluoride(s)						
Fluoristan	T49.7X1	T49.7X2	T49.7X3	T49.7X4	T49.7X5	T49.7X6
Fluormetholone	T49.0X1	T49.0X2	T49.0X3	T49.0X4	T49.0X5	T49.0X6
Fluoroacetate	T60.8X1	T60.8X2	T60.8X3	T60.8X4	—	—
Fluorocarbon monomer	T53.6X1	T53.6X2	T53.6X3	T53.6X4	—	—
Fluorocytosine	T37.8X1	T37.8X2	T37.8X3	T37.8X4	T37.8X5	T37.8X6
Fluorodeoxyuridine	T45.1X1	T45.1X2	T45.1X3	T45.1X4	T45.1X5	T45.1X6
Fluorometholone	T49.0X1	T49.0X2	T49.0X3	T49.0X4	T49.0X5	T49.0X6
ophthalmic preparation	T49.5X1	T49.5X2	T49.5X3	T49.5X4	T49.5X5	T49.5X6
Fluorophosphate insecticide	T60.0X1	T60.0X2	T60.0X3	T60.0X4	—	—
Fluorosol	T46.3X1	T46.3X2	T46.3X3	T46.3X4	T46.3X5	T46.3X6
Fluorouracil	T45.1X1	T45.1X2	T45.1X3	T45.1X4	T45.1X5	T45.1X6
Fluorphenylalanine	T49.5X1	T49.5X2	T49.5X3	T49.5X4	T49.5X5	T49.5X6
Fluothane	T41.0X1	T41.0X2	T41.0X3	T41.0X4	T41.0X5	T41.0X6
Fluoxetine	T43.221	T43.222	T43.223	T43.224	T43.225	T43.226
Fluoxymesterone	T38.7X1	T38.7X2	T38.7X3	T38.7X4	T38.7X5	T38.7X6
Flupenthixol	T43.4X1	T43.4X2	T43.4X3	T43.4X4	T43.4X5	T43.4X6
Flupentixol	T43.4X1	T43.4X2	T43.4X3	T43.4X4	T43.4X5	T43.4X6

Substance	Poisoning, Accidental (unintentional)	Poisoning, Intentional self-harm	Poisoning, Assault	Poisoning, Undetermined	Adverse effect	Underdosing
Fluphenazine	T43.3X1	T43.3X2	T43.3X3	T43.3X4	T43.3X5	T43.3X6
Fluprednidene	T49.0X1	T49.0X2	T49.0X3	T49.0X4	T49.0X5	T49.0X6
Fluprednisolone	T38.0X1	T38.0X2	T38.0X3	T38.0X4	T38.0X5	T38.0X6
Fluradoline	T39.8X1	T39.8X2	T39.8X3	T39.8X4	T39.8X5	T39.8X6
Flurandrenolide	T49.0X1	T49.0X2	T49.0X3	T49.0X4	T49.0X5	T49.0X6
Flurandrenolone	T49.0X1	T49.0X2	T49.0X3	T49.0X4	T49.0X5	T49.0X6
Flurazepam	T42.4X1	T42.4X2	T42.4X3	T42.4X4	T42.4X5	T42.4X6
Flurbiprofen	T39.311	T39.312	T39.313	T39.314	T39.315	T39.316
Flurobate	T49.0X1	T49.0X2	T49.0X3	T49.0X4	T49.0X5	T49.0X6
Fluroxene	T41.0X1	T41.0X2	T41.0X3	T41.0X4	T41.0X5	T41.0X6
Fluspirilene	T43.591	T43.592	T43.593	T43.594	T43.595	T43.596
Flutamide	T38.6X1	T38.6X2	T38.6X3	T38.6X4	T38.6X5	T38.6X6
Flutazolam	T42.4X1	T42.4X2	T42.4X3	T42.4X4	T42.4X5	T42.4X6
Fluticasone propionate	T38.0X1	T38.0X2	T38.0X3	T38.0X4	T38.0X5	T38.0X6
Flutoprazepam	T42.4X1	T42.4X2	T42.4X3	T42.4X4	T42.4X5	T42.4X6
Flutropium bromide	T48.6X1	T48.6X2	T48.6X3	T48.6X4	T48.6X5	T48.6X6
Fluvoxamine	T43.221	T43.222	T43.223	T43.224	T43.225	T43.226
Folacin	T45.8X1	T45.8X2	T45.8X3	T45.8X4	T45.8X5	T45.8X6
Folic acid	T45.8X1	T45.8X2	T45.8X3	T45.8X4	T45.8X5	T45.8X6
with ferrous salt	T45.2X1	T45.2X2	T45.2X3	T45.2X4	T45.2X5	T45.2X6
antagonist	T45.1X1	T45.1X2	T45.1X3	T45.1X4	T45.1X5	T45.1X6
Folinic acid	T45.8X1	T45.8X2	T45.8X3	T45.8X4	T45.8X5	T45.8X6
Folium stramoniae	T48.6X1	T48.6X2	T48.6X3	T48.6X4	T48.6X5	T48.6X6
Follicle-stimulating hormone, human	T38.811	T38.812	T38.813	T38.814	T38.815	T38.816
Folpet	T60.3X1	T60.3X2	T60.3X3	T60.3X4	—	—
Fominoben	T48.3X1	T48.3X2	T48.3X3	T48.3X4	T48.3X5	T48.3X6
Food, foodstuffs, noxious, nonbacterial, NEC	T62.91	T62.92	T62.93	T62.94	—	—
berries	T62.1X1	T62.1X2	T62.1X3	T62.1X4	—	—
fish—see also Fish	T61.91	T61.92	T61.93	T61.94	—	—
mushrooms	T62.0X1	T62.0X2	T62.0X3	T62.0X4	—	—
plants	T62.2X1	T62.2X2	T62.2X3	T62.2X4	—	—
seafood	T61.91	T61.92	T61.93	T61.94	—	—
specified NEC	T61.8X1	T61.8X2	T61.8X3	T61.8X4	—	—
seeds	T62.2X1	T62.2X2	T62.2X3	T62.2X4	—	—
shellfish	T61.781	T61.782	T61.783	T61.784	—	—
specified NEC	T62.8X1	T62.8X2	T62.8X3	T62.8X4	—	—
Fool's parsley	T62.2X1	T62.2X2	T62.2X3	T62.2X4	—	—
Formaldehyde (solution), gas or vapor	T59.2X1	T59.2X2	T59.2X3	T59.2X4	—	—
fungicide	T60.3X1	T60.3X2	T60.3X3	T60.3X4	—	—
Formalin	T59.2X1	T59.2X2	T59.2X3	T59.2X4	—	—
fungicide	T60.3X1	T60.3X2	T60.3X3	T60.3X4	—	—
vapor	T59.2X1	T59.2X2	T59.2X3	T59.2X4	—	—
Formic acid	T54.2X1	T54.2X2	T54.2X3	T54.2X4	—	—
vapor	T59.891	T59.892	T59.893	T59.894	—	—
Foscarnet sodium	T37.5X1	T37.5X2	T37.5X3	T37.5X4	T37.5X5	T37.5X6
Fosfestrol	T38.5X1	T38.5X2	T38.5X3	T38.5X4	T38.5X5	T38.5X6
Fosfomycin	T36.8X1	T36.8X2	T36.8X3	T36.8X4	T36.8X5	T36.8X6
Fosfonet sodium	T37.5X1	T37.5X2	T37.5X3	T37.5X4	T37.5X5	T37.5X6

Substance	Poisoning, Accidental (unintentional)	Poisoning, Intentional self-harm	Poisoning, Assault	Poisoning, Undetermined	Adverse effect	Underdosing
Fosinopril	T46.4X1	T46.4X2	T46.4X3	T46.4X4	T46.4X5	T46.4X6
sodium	T46.4X1	T46.4X2	T46.4X3	T46.4X4	T46.4X5	T46.4X6
Fowler's solution	T57.0X1	T57.0X2	T57.0X3	T57.0X4	—	—
Foxglove	T62.2X1	T62.2X2	T62.2X3	T62.2X4	—	—
Framycetin	T36.5X1	T36.5X2	T36.5X3	T36.5X4	T36.5X5	T36.5X6
Frangula	T47.2X1	T47.2X2	T47.2X3	T47.2X4	T47.2X5	T47.2X6
extract	T47.2X1	T47.2X2	T47.2X3	T47.2X4	T47.2X5	T47.2X6
Frei antigen	T50.8X1	T50.8X2	T50.8X3	T50.8X4	T50.8X5	T50.8X6
Freon	T53.5X1	T53.5X2	T53.5X3	T53.5X4	—	—
Fructose	T50.3X1	T50.3X2	T50.3X3	T50.3X4	T50.3X5	T50.3X6
Frusemide	T50.1X1	T50.1X2	T50.1X3	T50.1X4	T50.1X5	T50.1X6
FSH	T38.811	T38.812	T38.813	T38.814	T38.815	T38.816
Ftorafur	T45.1X1	T45.1X2	T45.1X3	T45.1X4	T45.1X5	T45.1X6
Fuel						
automobile	T52.0X1	T52.0X2	T52.0X3	T52.0X4	—	—
exhaust gas, not in transit	T58.01	T58.02	T58.03	T58.04	—	—
vapor NEC	T52.0X1	T52.0X2	T52.0X3	T52.0X4	—	—
gas (domestic use)—see also Carbon, monoxide, fuel, utility	T59.891	T59.892	T59.893	T59.894	—	—
utility	T59.891	T59.892	T59.893	T59.894	—	—
in mobile container	T59.891	T59.892	T59.893	T59.894	—	—
incomplete combustion of—see Carbon, monoxide, fuel, utility						
piped (natural)	T59.891	T59.892	T59.893	T59.894	—	—
industrial, incomplete combustion	T58.8X1	T58.8X2	T58.8X3	T58.8X4	—	—
Fugillin	T36.8X1	T36.8X2	T36.8X3	T36.8X4	T36.8X5	T36.8X6
Fulminate of mercury	T56.1X1	T56.1X2	T56.1X3	T56.1X4	—	—
Fulvicin	T36.7X1	T36.7X2	T36.7X3	T36.7X4	T36.7X5	T36.7X6
Fumadil	T36.8X1	T36.8X2	T36.8X3	T36.8X4	T36.8X5	T36.8X6
Fumagillin	T36.8X1	T36.8X2	T36.8X3	T36.8X4	T36.8X5	T36.8X6
Fumaric acid	T49.4X1	T49.4X2	T49.4X3	T49.4X4	T49.4X5	T49.4X6
Fumes (from)	T59.91	T59.92	T59.93	T59.94	—	—
carbon monoxide—see Carbon, monoxide						
charcoal (domestic use)—see Charcoal, fumes						
chloroform—see Chloroform						
coke (in domestic stoves, fireplaces)—see Coke fumes						
corrosive NEC	T54.91	T54.92	T54.93	T54.94	—	—
ether—see ether						
freons	T53.5X1	T53.5X2	T53.5X3	T53.5X4	—	—
hydrocarbons	T59.891	T59.892	T59.893	T59.894	—	—
petroleum (liquefied)	T59.891	T59.892	T59.893	T59.894	—	—
distributed through pipes (pure or mixed with air)	T59.891	T59.892	T59.893	T59.894	—	—

Substance	Poisoning, Accidental (unintentional)	Poisoning, Intentional self-harm	Poisoning, Assault	Poisoning, Undetermined	Adverse effect	Underdosing
Fumes — *Continued*						
lead—see lead						
metal—see Metals, or the specified metal						
nitrogen dioxide	T59.0X1	T59.0X2	T59.0X3	T59.0X4	—	—
pesticides—see Pesticides						
petroleum (liquefied)	T59.891	T59.892	T59.893	T59.894	—	—
distributed through pipes (pure or mixed with air)	T59.891	T59.892	T59.893	T59.894	—	—
polyester	T59.891	T59.892	T59.893	T59.894	—	—
specified source NEC—see also substance specified	T59.891	T59.892	T59.893	T59.894	—	—
sulfur dioxide	T59.1X1	T59.1X2	T59.1X3	T59.1X4	—	—
Fumigant NEC	T60.91	T60.92	T60.93	T60.94	—	—
Fungi, noxious, used as food	T62.0X1	T62.0X2	T62.0X3	T62.0X4	—	—
Fungicide NEC (nonmedicinal)	T60.3X1	T60.3X2	T60.3X3	T60.3X4	—	—
Fungizone	T36.7X1	T36.7X2	T36.7X3	T36.7X4	T36.7X5	T36.7X6
topical	T49.0X1	T49.0X2	T49.0X3	T49.0X4	T49.0X5	T49.0X6
Furacin	T49.0X1	T49.0X2	T49.0X3	T49.0X4	T49.0X5	T49.0X6
Furadantin	T37.91	T37.92	T37.93	T37.94	T37.95	T37.96
Furazolidone	T37.8X1	T37.8X2	T37.8X3	T37.8X4	T37.8X5	T37.8X6
Furazolium chloride	T49.0X1	T49.0X2	T49.0X3	T49.0X4	T49.0X5	T49.0X6
Furfural	T52.8X1	T52.8X2	T52.8X3	T52.8X4	—	—
Furnace (coal burning) (domestic), gas from	T58.2X1	T58.2X2	T58.2X3	T58.2X4	—	—
industrial	T58.8X1	T58.8X2	T58.8X3	T58.8X4	—	—
Furniture polish	T65.891	T65.892	T65.893	T65.894	—	—
Furosemide	T50.1X1	T50.1X2	T50.1X3	T50.1X4	T50.1X5	T50.1X6
Furoxone	T37.91	T37.92	T37.93	T37.94	T37.95	T37.96
Fursultiamine	T45.2X1	T45.2X2	T45.2X3	T45.2X4	T45.2X5	T45.2X6
Fusafungine	T36.8X1	T36.8X2	T36.8X3	T36.8X4	T36.8X5	T36.8X6
Fusel oil (any) (amyl) (butyl) (propyl), vapor	T51.3X1	T51.3X2	T51.3X3	T51.3X4	—	—
Fusidate (ethanolamine) (sodium)	T36.8X1	T36.8X2	T36.8X3	T36.8X4	T36.8X5	T36.8X6
Fusidic acid	T36.8X1	T36.8X2	T36.8X3	T36.8X4	T36.8X5	T36.8X6
Fytic acid, nonasodium	T50.6X1	T50.6X2	T50.6X3	T50.6X4	T50.6X5	T50.6X6
G						
GABA	T43.8X1	T43.8X2	T43.8X3	T43.8X4	T43.8X5	T43.8X6
Gadopentetic acid	T50.8X1	T50.8X2	T50.8X3	T50.8X4	T50.8X5	T50.8X6
Galactose	T50.3X1	T50.3X2	T50.3X3	T50.3X4	T50.3X5	T50.3X6
b-Galactosidase	T47.5X1	T47.5X2	T47.5X3	T47.5X4	T47.5X5	T47.5X6
Galantamine	T44.0X1	T44.0X2	T44.0X3	T44.0X4	T44.0X5	T44.0X6
Gallamine (triethiodide)	T48.1X1	T48.1X2	T48.1X3	T48.1X4	T48.1X5	T48.1X6
Gallium citrate	T50.991	T50.992	T50.993	T50.994	T50.995	T50.996
Gallopamil	T46.1X1	T46.1X2	T46.1X3	T46.1X4	T46.1X5	T46.1X6
Gamboge	T47.2X1	T47.2X2	T47.2X3	T47.2X4	T47.2X5	T47.2X6
Gamimune	T50.Z11	T50.Z12	T50.Z13	T50.Z14	T50.Z15	T50.Z16
Gamma globulin	T50.Z11	T50.Z12	T50.Z13	T50.Z14	T50.Z15	T50.Z16
Gamma-aminobutyric acid	T43.8X1	T43.8X2	T43.8X3	T43.8X4	T43.8X5	T43.8X6
Gamma-benzene hexachloride (medicinal)	T49.0X1	T49,0X2	T49.0X3	T49.0X4	T49.0X5	T49.0X6
nonmedicinal, vapor	T53.6X1	T53.6X2	T53.6X3	T53.6X4	—	—
Gamma-BHC (medicinal)—see also Gamma-benzene hexachloride	T49.0X1	T49.0X2	T49.0X3	T49.0X4	T49.0X5	T49.0X6
Gamulin	T50.Z11	T50.Z12	T50.Z13	T50.Z14	T50.Z15	T50.Z16
Ganciclovir (sodium)	T37.5X1	T37.5X2	T37.5X3	T37.5X4	T37.5X5	T37.5X6
Ganglionic blocking drug NEC	T44.2X1	T44.2X2	T44.2X3	T44.2X4	T44.2X5	T44.2X6
specified NEC	T44.2X1	T44.2X2	T44.2X3	T44.2X4	T44.2X5	T44.2X6
Ganja	T40.711	T40.712	T40.713	T40.714	T40.715	T40.716
Garamycin	T36.5X1	T36.5X2	T36.5X3	T36.5X4	T36.5X5	T36.5X6
ophthalmic preparation	T49.5X1	T49.5X2	T49.5X3	T49.5X4	T49.5X5	T49.5X6
topical NEC	T49.0X1	T49.0X2	T49.0X3	T49.0X4	T49.0X5	T49.0X6
Gardenal	T42.3X1	T42.3X2	T42.3X3	T42.3X4	T42.3X5	T42.3X6
Gardepanyl	T42.3X1	T42.3X2	T42.3X3	T42.3X4	T42.3X5	T42.3X6
Gas NEC	T59.91	T59.92	T59.93	T59.94	—	—
acetylene	T59.891	T59.892	T59.893	T59.894	—	—
incomplete combustion of	T58.11	T58.12	T58.13	T58.14	—	—
air contaminants, source or type not specified	T59.91	T59.92	T59.93	T59.94	—	—
anesthetic	T41.0X1	T41.0X2	T41.0X3	T41.0X4	T41.0X5	T41.0X6
blast furnace	T58.8X1	T58.8X2	T58.8X3	T58.8X4	—	—
butane—see butane						
carbon monoxide—see Carbon, monoxide						
chlorine	T59.4X1	T59.4X2	T59.4X3	T59.4X4	—	—
coal	T58.2X1	T58.2X2	T58.2X3	T58.2X4	—	—
cyanide	T57.3X1	T57.3X2	T57.3X3	T57.3X4	—	—
dicyanogen	T65.0X1	T65.0X2	T65.0X3	T65.0X4	—	—
domestic—see Domestic gas						
exhaust	T58.01	T58.02	T58.03	T58.04	—	—
from utility (for cooking, heating, or lighting) (after combustion)—see Carbon, monoxide, fuel, utility						
prior to combustion	T59.891	T59.892	T59.893	T59.894	—	—
from wood- or coal-burning stove or fireplace	T58.2X1	T58.2X2	T58.2X3	T58.2X4	—	—
fuel (domestic use) (after combustion)—see also Carbon, monoxide, fuel						

Substance	Poisoning, Accidental (unintentional)	Poisoning, Intentional self-harm	Poisoning, Assault	Poisoning, Undetermined	Adverse effect	Underdosing
Gas NEC — *Continued*						
industrial use	T58.8X1	T58.8X2	T58.8X3	T58.8X4	—	—
prior to combustion	T59.891	T59.892	T59.893	T59.894	—	—
utility	T59.891	T59.892	T59.893	T59.894	—	—
in mobile container	T59.891	T59.892	T59.893	T59.894	—	—
incomplete combustion of—see Carbon, monoxide, fuel, utility						
piped (natural)	T59.891	T59.892	T59.893	T59.894	—	—
garage	T58.01	T58.02	T58.03	T58.04	—	—
hydrocarbon NEC	T59.891	T59.892	T59.893	T59.894	—	—
incomplete combustion of—see Carbon, monoxide, fuel, utility						
liquefied—see butane						
piped	T59.891	T59.892	T59.893	T59.894	—	—
hydrocyanic acid	T65.0X1	T65.0X2	T65.0X3	T65.0X4	—	—
illuminating (after combustion)	T58.11	T58.12	T58.13	T58.14	—	—
prior to combustion	T59.891	T59.892	T59.893	T59.894	—	—
incomplete combustion, any—see Carbon, monoxide						
kiln	T58.8X1	T58.8X2	T58.8X3	T58.8X4	—	—
lacrimogenic	T59.3X1	T59.3X2	T59.3X3	T59.3X4	—	—
liquefied petroleum—see butane						
marsh	T59.891	T59.892	T59.893	T59.894	—	—
motor exhaust, not in transit	T58.01	T58.02	T58.03	T58.04	—	—
mustard, not in war	T59.891	T59.892	T59.893	T59.894	—	—
natural	T59.891	T59.892	T59.893	T59.894	—	—
nerve, not in war	T59.91	T59.92	T59.93	T59.94	—	—
oil	T52.0X1	T52.0X2	T52.0X3	T52.0X4	—	—
petroleum (liquefied) (distributed in mobile containers)	T59.891	T59.892	T59.893	T59.894	—	—
piped (pure or mixed with air)	T59.891	T59.892	T59.893	T59.894	—	—
piped (manufactured) (natural) NEC	T59.891	T59.892	T59.893	T59.894	—	—
producer	T58.8X1	T58.8X2	T58.8X3	T58.8X4	—	—
propane—see propane						
refrigerant (chlorofluoro-carbon)	T53.5X1	T53.5X2	T53.5X3	T53.5X4	—	—
not chlorofluoro-carbon	T59.891	T59.892	T59.893	T59.894	—	—
sewer	T59.91	T59.92	T59.93	T59.94	—	—
specified source NEC	T59.91	T59.92	T59.93	T59.94	—	—
stove (after combustion)	T58.11	T58.12	T58.13	T58.14	—	—
prior to combustion	T59.891	T59.892	T59.893	T59.894	—	—
tear	T59.3X1	T59.3X2	T59.3X3	T59.3X4	—	—
therapeutic	T41.5X1	T41.5X2	T41.5X3	T41.5X4	T41.5X5	T41.5X6

Substance	Poisoning, Accidental (unintentional)	Poisoning, Intentional self-harm	Poisoning, Assault	Poisoning, Undetermined	Adverse effect	Underdosing
Gas NEC — *Continued*						
utility (for cooking, heating, or lighting) (piped) NEC	T59.891	T59.892	T59.893	T59.894	—	—
in mobile container	T59.891	T59.892	T59.893	T59.894	—	—
incomplete combustion of—see Carbon, monoxide, fuel, utilty						
piped (natural)	T59.891	T59.892	T59.893	T59.894	—	—
water	T58.11	T58.12	T58.13	T58.14	—	—
incomplete combustion of—see Carbon, monoxide, fuel, utility						
Gaseous substance—see Gas						
Gasoline	T52.0X1	T52.0X2	T52.0X3	T52.0X4	—	—
vapor	T52.0X1	T52.0X2	T52.0X3	T52.0X4	—	—
Gastric enzymes	T47.5X1	T47.5X2	T47.5X3	T47.5X4	T47.5X5	T47.5X6
Gastrografin	T50.8X1	T50.8X2	T50.8X3	T50.8X4	T50.8X5	T50.8X6
Gastrointestinal drug	T47.91	T47.92	T47.93	T47.94	T47.95	T47.96
biological	T47.8X1	T47.8X2	T47.8X3	T47.8X4	T47.8X5	T47.8X6
specified NEC	T47.8X1	T47.8X2	T47.8X3	T47.8X4	T47.8X5	T47.8X6
Gaultheria procumbens	T62.2X1	T62.2X2	T62.2X3	T62.2X4	—	—
Gefarnate	T44.3X1	T44.3X2	T44.3X3	T44.3X4	T44.3X5	T44.3X6
Gelatin (intravenous)	T45.8X1	T45.8X2	T45.8X3	T45.8X4	T45.8X5	T45.8X6
absorbable (sponge)	T45.7X1	T45.7X2	T45.7X3	T45.7X4	T45.7X5	T45.7X6
Gelfilm	T49.8X1	T49.8X2	T49.8X3	T49.8X4	T49.8X5	T49.8X6
Gelfoam	T45.7X1	T45.7X2	T45.7X3	T45.7X4	T45.7X5	T45.7X6
Gelsemine	T50.991	T50.992	T50.993	T50.994	T50.995	T50.996
Gelsemium (sempervirens)	T62.2X1	T62.2X2	T62.2X3	T62.2X4	—	—
Gemeprost	T48.0X1	T48.0X2	T48.0X3	T48.0X4	T48.0X5	T48.0X6
Gemfibrozil	T46.6X1	T46.6X2	T46.6X3	T46.6X4	T46.6X5	T46.6X6
Gemonil	T42.3X1	T42.3X2	T42.3X3	T42.3X4	T42.3X5	T42.3X6
Gentamicin	T36.5X1	T36.5X2	T36.5X3	T36.5X4	T36.5X5	T36.5X6
ophthalmic preparation	T49.5X1	T49.5X2	T49.5X3	T49.5X4	T49.5X5	T49.5X6
topical NEC	T49.0X1	T49.0X2	T49.0X3	T49.0X4	T49.0X5	T49.0X6
Gentian	T47.5X1	T47.5X2	T47.5X3	T47.5X4	T47.5X5	T47.5X6
violet	T49.0X1	T49.0X2	T49.0X3	T49.0X4	T49.0X5	T49.0X6
Gepefrine	T44.4X1	T44.4X2	T44.4X3	T44.4X4	T44.4X5	T44.4X6
Gestonorone caproate	T38.5X1	T38.5X2	T38.5X3	T38.5X4	T38.5X5	T38.5X6
Gexane	T49.0X1	T49.0X2	T49.0X3	T49.0X4	T49.0X5	T49.0X6
Gila monster (venom)	T63.111	T63.112	T63.113	T63.114	—	—
Ginger	T47.5X1	T47.5X2	T47.5X3	T47.5X4	T47.5X5	T47.5X6
Jamaica—see Jamaica, ginger						
Gitalin	T46.0X1	T46.0X2	T46.0X3	T46.0X4	T46.0X5	T46.0X6
amorphous	T46.0X1	T46.0X2	T46.0X3	T46.0X4	T46.0X5	T46.0X6
Gitaloxin	T46.0X1	T46.0X2	T46.0X3	T46.0X4	T46.0X5	T46.0X6
Gitoxin	T46.0X1	T46.0X2	T46.0X3	T46.0X4	T46.0X5	T46.0X6
Glafenine	T39.8X1	T39.8X2	T39.8X3	T39.8X4	T39.8X5	T39.8X6

Substance	Poisoning, Accidental (unintentional)	Poisoning, Intentional self-harm	Poisoning, Assault	Poisoning, Undetermined	Adverse effect	Underdosing
Glandular extract (medicinal) NEC	T50.Z91	T50.Z92	T50.Z93	T50.Z94	T50.Z95	T50.Z96
Glaucarubin	T37.3X1	T37.3X2	T37.3X3	T37.3X4	T37.3X5	T37.3X6
Glibenclamide	T38.3X1	T38.3X2	T38.3X3	T38.3X4	T38.3X5	T38.3X6
Glibornuride	T38.3X1	T38.3X2	T38.3X3	T38.3X4	T38.3X5	T38.3X6
Gliclazide	T38.3X1	T38.3X2	T38.3X3	T38.3X4	T38.3X5	T38.3X6
Glimidine	T38.3X1	T38.3X2	T38.3X3	T38.3X4	T38.3X5	T38.3X6
Glipizide	T38.3X1	T38.3X2	T38.3X3	T38.3X4	T38.3X5	T38.3X6
Gliquidone	T38.3X1	T38.3X2	T38.3X3	T38.3X4	T38.3X5	T38.3X6
Glisolamide	T38.3X1	T38.3X2	T38.3X3	T38.3X4	T38.3X5	T38.3X6
Glisoxepide	T38.3X1	T38.3X2	T38.3X3	T38.3X4	T38.3X5	T38.3X6
Globin zinc insulin	T38.3X1	T38.3X2	T38.3X3	T38.3X4	T38.3X5	T38.3X6
Globulin						
antilymphocytic	T50.Z11	T50.Z12	T50.Z13	T50.Z14	T50.Z15	T50.Z16
antirhesus	T50.Z11	T50.Z12	T50.Z13	T50.Z14	T50.Z15	T50.Z16
antivenin	T50.Z11	T50.Z12	T50.Z13	T50.Z14	T50.Z15	T50.Z16
antiviral	T50.Z11	T50.Z12	T50.Z13	T50.Z14	T50.Z15	T50.Z16
Glucagon	T38.3X1	T38.3X2	T38.3X3	T38.3X4	T38.3X5	T38.3X6
Glucocorticoids	T38.0X1	T38.0X2	T38.0X3	T38.0X4	T38.0X5	T38.0X6
Glucocorticosteroid	T38.0X1	T38.0X2	T38.0X3	T38.0X4	T38.0X5	T38.0X6
Gluconic acid	T50.991	T50.992	T50.993	T50.994	T50.995	T50.996
Glucosamine sulfate	T39.4X1	T39.4X2	T39.4X3	T39.4X4	T39.4X5	T39.4X6
Glucose	T50.3X1	T50.3X2	T50.3X3	T50.3X4	T50.3X5	T50.3X6
with sodium chloride	T50.3X1	T50.3X2	T50.3X3	T50.3X4	T50.3X5	T50.3X6
Glucosulfone sodium	T37.1X1	T37.1X2	T37.1X3	T37.1X4	T37.1X5	T37.1X6
Glucurolactone	T47.8X1	T47.8X2	T47.8X3	T47.8X4	T47.8X5	T47.8X6
Glue NEC	T52.8X1	T52.8X2	T52.8X3	T52.8X4	—	—
Glutamic acid	T47.5X1	T47.5X2	T47.5X3	T47.5X4	T47.5X5	T47.5X6
Glutaral (medicinal)	T49.0X1	T49.0X2	T49.0X3	T49.0X4	T49.0X5	T49.0X6
nonmedicinal	T65.891	T65.892	T65.893	T65.894	—	—
Glutaraldehyde (nonmedicinal)	T65.891	T65.892	T65.893	T65.894	—	—
medicinal	T49.0X1	T49.0X2	T49.0X3	T49.0X4	T49.0X5	T49.0X6
Glutathione	T50.6X1	T50.6X2	T50.6X3	T50.6X4	T50.6X5	T50.6X6
Glutethimide	T42.6X1	T42.6X2	T42.6X3	T42.6X4	T42.6X5	T42.6X6
Glyburide	T38.3X1	T38.3X2	T38.3X3	T38.3X4	T38.3X5	T38.3X6
Glycerin	T47.4X1	T47.4X2	T47.4X3	T47.4X4	T47.4X5	T47.4X6
Glycerol	T47.4X1	T47.4X2	T47.4X3	T47.4X4	T47.4X5	T47.4X6
borax	T49.6X1	T49.6X2	T49.6X3	T49.6X4	T49.6X5	T49.6X6
intravenous	T50.3X1	T50.3X2	T50.3X3	T50.3X4	T50.3X5	T50.3X6
iodinated	T48.4X1	T48.4X2	T48.4X3	T48.4X4	T48.4X5	T48.4X6
Glycerophosphate	T50.991	T50.992	T50.993	T50.994	T50.995	T50.996
Glyceryl						
gualacolate	T48.4X1	T48.4X2	T48.4X3	T48.4X4	T48.4X5	T48.4X6
nitrate	T46.3X1	T46.3X2	T46.3X3	T46.3X4	T46.3X5	T46.3X6
triacetate (topical)	T49.0X1	T49.0X2	T49.0X3	T49.0X4	T49.0X5	T49.0X6
trinitrate	T46.3X1	T46.3X2	T46.3X3	T46.3X4	T46.3X5	T46.3X6
Glycine	T50.3X1	T50.3X2	T50.3X3	T50.3X4	T50.3X5	T50.3X6
Glyclopyramide	T38.3X1	T38.3X2	T38.3X3	T38.3X4	T38.3X5	T38.3X6
Glycobiarsol	T37.3X1	T37.3X2	T37.3X3	T37.3X4	T37.3X5	T37.3X6
Glycols (ether)	T52.3X1	T52.3X2	T52.3X3	T52.3X4	—	—
Glyconiazide	T37.1X1	T37.1X2	T37.1X3	T37.1X4	T37.1X5	T37.1X6
Glycopyrrolate	T44.3X1	T44.3X2	T44.3X3	T44.3X4	T44.3X5	T44.3X6
Glycopyrronium	T44.3X1	T44.3X2	T44.3X3	T44.3X4	T44.3X5	T44.3X6
bromide	T44.3X1	T44.3X2	T44.3X3	T44.3X4	T44.3X5	T44.3X6
Glycoside, cardiac (stimulant)	T46.0X1	T46.0X2	T46.0X3	T46.0X4	T46.0X5	T46.0X6
Glycyclamide	T38.3X1	T38.3X2	T38.3X3	T38.3X4	T38.3X5	T38.3X6
Glycyrrhiza extract	T48.4X1	T48.4X2	T48.4X3	T48.4X4	T48.4X5	T48.4X6
Glycyrrhizic acid	T48.4X1	T48.4X2	T48.4X3	T48.4X4	T48.4X5	T48.4X6
Glycyrrhizinate potassium	T48.4X1	T48.4X2	T48.4X3	T48.4X4	T48.4X5	T48.4X6
Glymidine sodium	T38.3X1	T38.3X2	T38.3X3	T38.3X4	T38.3X5	T38.3X6
Glyphosate	T60.3X1	T60.3X2	T60.3X3	T60.3X4	—	—
Glyphylline	T48.6X1	T48.6X2	T48.6X3	T48.6X4	T48.6X5	T48.6X6
Gold						
colloidal (I98Au)	T45.1X1	T45.1X2	T45.1X3	T45.1X4	T45.1X5	T45.1X6
salts	T39.4X1	T39.4X2	T39.4X3	T39.4X4	T39.4X5	T39.4X6
Golden sulfide of antimony	T56.891	T56.892	T56.893	T56.894	—	—
Goldylocks	T62.2X1	T62.2X2	T62.2X3	T62.2X4	—	—
Gonadal tissue extract	T38.901	T38.902	T38.903	T38.904	T38.905	T38.906
female	T38.5X1	T38.5X2	T38.5X3	T38.5X4	T38.5X5	T38.5X6
male	T38.7X1	T38.7X2	T38.7X3	T38.7X4	T38.7X5	T38.7X6
Gonadorelin	T38.891	T38.892	T38.893	T38.894	T38.895	T38.896
Gonadotropin	T38.891	T38.892	T38.893	T38.894	T38.895	T38.896
chorionic	T38.891	T38.892	T38.893	T38.894	T38.895	T38.896
pituitary	T38.811	T38.812	T38.813	T38.814	T38.815	T38.816
Goserelin	T45.1X1	T45.1X2	T45.1X3	T45.1X4	T45.1X5	T45.1X6
Grain alcohol	T51.0X1	T51.0X2	T51.0X3	T51.0X4	—	—
Gramicidin	T49.0X1	T49.0X2	T49.0X3	T49.0X4	T49.0X5	T49.0X6
Granisetron	T45.0X1	T45.0X2	T45.0X3	T45.0X4	T45.0X5	T45.0X6
Gratiola officinalis	T62.2X1	T62.2X2	T62.2X3	T62.2X4	—	—
Grease	T65.891	T65.892	T65.893	T65.894	—	—
Green hellebore	T62.2X1	T62.2X2	T62.2X3	T62.2X4	—	—
Green soap	T49.2X1	T49.2X2	T49.2X3	T49.2X4	T49.2X5	T49.2X6
Grifulvin	T36.7X1	T36.7X2	T36.7X3	T36.7X4	T36.7X5	T36.7X6
Griseofulvin	T36.7X1	T36.7X2	T36.7X3	T36.7X4	T36.7X5	T36.7X6
Growth hormone	T38.811	T38.812	T38.813	T38.814	T38.815	T38.816
Guaiac reagent	T50.991	T50.992	T50.993	T50.994	T50.995	T50.996
Guaiacol derivatives	T48.4X1	T48.4X2	T48.4X3	T48.4X4	T48.4X5	T48.4X6
Guaifenesin	T48.4X1	T48.4X2	T48.4X3	T48.4X4	T48.4X5	T48.4X6
Guaimesal	T48.4X1	T48.4X2	T48.4X3	T48.4X4	T48.4X5	T48.4X6
Guaiphenesin	T48.4X1	T48.4X2	T48.4X3	T48.4X4	T48.4X5	T48.4X6
Guamecycline	T36.4X1	T36.4X2	T36.4X3	T36.4X4	T36.4X5	T36.4X6
Guanabenz	T46.5X1	T46.5X2	T46.5X3	T46.5X4	T46.5X5	T46.5X6
Guanacline	T46.5X1	T46.5X2	T46.5X3	T46.5X4	T46.5X5	T46.5X6
Guanadrel	T46.5X1	T46.5X2	T46.5X3	T46.5X4	T46.5X5	T46.5X6
Guanatol	T37.2X1	T37.2X2	T37.2X3	T37.2X4	T37.2X5	T37.2X6
Guanethidine	T46.5X1	T46.5X2	T46.5X3	T46.5X4	T46.5X5	T46.5X6
Guanfacine	T46.5X1	T46.5X2	T46.5X3	T46.5X4	T46.5X5	T46.5X6
Guano	T65.891	T65.892	T65.893	T65.894	—	—

Substance	Poisoning, Accidental (unintentional)	Poisoning, Intentional self-harm	Poisoning, Assault	Poisoning, Undetermined	Adverse effect	Underdosing
Guanochlor	T46.5X1	T46.5X2	T46.5X3	T46.5X4	T46.5X5	T46.5X6
Guanoclor	T46.5X1	T46.5X2	T46.5X3	T46.5X4	T46.5X5	T46.5X6
Guanoctine	T46.5X1	T46.5X2	T46.5X3	T46.5X4	T46.5X5	T46.5X6
Guanoxabenz	T46.5X1	T46.5X2	T46.5X3	T46.5X4	T46.5X5	T46.5X6
Guanoxan	T46.5X1	T46.5X2	T46.5X3	T46.5X4	T46.5X5	T46.5X6
Guar gum (medicinal)	T46.6X1	T46.6X2	T46.6X3	T46.6X4	T46.6X5	T46.6X6
H						
Hachimycin	T36.7X1	T36.7X2	T36.7X3	T36.7X4	T36.7X5	T36.7X6
Hair						
dye	T49.4X1	T49.4X2	T49.4X3	T49.4X4	T49.4X5	T49.4X6
preparation NEC	T49.4X1	T49.4X2	T49.4X3	T49.4X4	T49.4X5	T49.4X6
Halazepam	T42.4X1	T42.4X2	T42.4X3	T42.4X4	T42.4X5	T42.4X6
Halcinolone	T49.0X1	T49.0X2	T49.0X3	T49.0X4	T49.0X5	T49.0X6
Halcinonide	T49.0X1	T49.0X2	T49.0X3	T49.0X4	T49.0X5	T49.0X6
Halethazole	T49.0X1	T49.0X2	T49.0X3	T49.0X4	T49.0X5	T49.0X6
Hallucinogen NOS	T40.901	T40.902	T40.903	T40.904	T40.905	T40.906
specified NEC	T40.991	T40.992	T40.993	T40.994	T40.995	T40.996
Halofantrine	T37.2X1	T37.2X2	T37.2X3	T37.2X4	T37.2X5	T37.2X6
Halofenate	T46.6X1	T46.6X2	T46.6X3	T46.6X4	T46.6X5	T46.6X6
Halometasone	T49.0X1	T49.0X2	T49.0X3	T49.0X4	T49.0X5	T49.0X6
Haloperidol	T43.4X1	T43.4X2	T43.4X3	T43.4X4	T43.4X5	T43.4X6
Haloprogin	T49.0X1	T49.0X2	T49.0X3	T49.0X4	T49.0X5	T49.0X6
Halotex	T49.0X1	T49.0X2	T49.0X3	T49.0X4	T49.0X5	T49.0X6
Halothane	T41.0X1	T41.0X2	T41.0X3	T41.0X4	T41.0X5	T41.0X6
Haloxazolam	T42.4X1	T42.4X2	T42.4X3	T42.4X4	T42.4X5	T42.4X6
Halquinols	T49.0X1	T49.0X2	T49.0X3	T49.0X4	T49.0X5	T49.0X6
Hamamelis	T49.2X1	T49.2X2	T49.2X3	T49.2X4	T49.2X5	T49.2X6
Haptendextran	T45.8X1	T45.8X2	T45.8X3	T45.8X4	T45.8X5	T45.8X6
Harmonyl	T46.5X1	T46.5X2	T46.5X3	T46.5X4	T46.5X5	T46.5X6
Hartmann's solution	T50.3X1	T50.3X2	T50.3X3	T50.3X4	T50.3X5	T50.3X6
Hashish	T40.711	T40.712	T40.713	T40.714	T40.715	T40.716
Hawaiian Woodrose seeds	T40.991	T40.992	T40.993	T40.994	—	—
HCB	T60.3X1	T60.3X2	T60.3X3	T60.3X4	—	—
HCH	T53.6X1	T53.6X2	T53.6X3	T53.6X4	—	—
medicinal	T49.0X1	T49.0X2	T49.0X3	T49.0X4	T49.0X5	T49.0X6
HCN	T57.3X1	T57.3X2	T57.3X3	T57.3X4	—	—
Headache cures, drugs, powders NEC	T50.901	T50.902	T50.903	T50.904	T50.905	T50.906
Heavenly Blue (morning glory)	T40.991	T40.992	T40.993	T40.994	—	—
Heavy metal antidote	T45.8X1	T45.8X2	T45.8X3	T45.8X4	T45.8X5	T45.8X6
Hedaquinium	T49.0X1	T49.0X2	T49.0X3	T49.0X4	T49.0X5	T49.0X6
Hedge hyssop	T62.2X1	T62.2X2	T62.2X3	T62.2X4	—	—
Heet	T49.8X1	T49.8X2	T49.8X3	T49.8X4	T49.8X5	T49.8X6
Helenin	T37.4X1	T37.4X2	T37.4X3	T37.4X4	T37.4X5	T37.4X6
Helium (nonmedicinal) NEC	T59.891	T59.892	T59.893	T59.894	—	—
medicinal	T48.991	T48.992	T48.993	T48.994	T48.995	T48.996
Hellebore (black) (green) (white)	T62.2X1	T62.2X2	T62.2X3	T62.2X4	—	—
Hematin	T45.8X1	T45.8X2	T45.8X3	T45.8X4	T45.8X5	T45.8X6
Hematinic preparation	T45.8X1	T45.8X2	T45.8X3	T45.8X4	T45.8X5	T45.8X6
Hematological agent	T45.91	T45.92	T45.93	T45.94	T45.95	T45.96
specified NEC	T45.8X1	T45.8X2	T45.8X3	T45.8X4	T45.8X5	T45.8X6
Hemlock	T62.2X1	T62.2X2	T62.2X3	T62.2X4	—	—
Hemostatic	T45.621	T45.622	T45.623	T45.624	T45.625	T45.626
drug, systemic	T45.621	T45.622	T45.623	T45.624	T45.625	T45.626
Hemostyptic	T49.4X1	T49.4X2	T49.4X3	T49.4X4	T49.4X5	T49.4X6
Henbane	T62.2X1	T62.2X2	T62.2X3	T62.2X4	—	—
Heparin (sodium)	T45.511	T45.512	T45.513	T45.514	T45.515	T45.516
action reverser	T45.7X1	T45.7X2	T45.7X3	T45.7X4	T45.7X5	T45.7X6
Heparin-fraction	T45.511	T45.512	T45.513	T45.514	T45.515	T45.516
Heparinoid (systemic)	T45.511	T45.512	T45.513	T45.514	T45.515	T45.516
Hepatic secretion stimulant	T47.8X1	T47.8X2	T47.8X3	T47.8X4	T47.8X5	T47.8X6
Hepatitis B						
immune globulin	T50.Z11	T50.Z12	T50.Z13	T50.Z14	T50.Z15	T50.Z16
vaccine	T50.B91	T50.B92	T50.B93	T50.B94	T50.B95	T50.B96
Hepronicate	T46.7X1	T46.7X2	T46.7X3	T46.7X4	T46.7X5	T46.7X6
Heptabarb	T42.3X1	T42.3X2	T42.3X3	T42.3X4	T42.3X5	T42.3X6
Heptabarbital	T42.3X1	T42.3X2	T42.3X3	T42.3X4	T42.3X5	T42.3X6
Heptabarbitone	T42.3X1	T42.3X2	T42.3X3	T42.3X4	T42.3X5	T42.3X6
Heptachlor	T60.1X1	T60.1X2	T60.1X3	T60.1X4	—	—
Heptalgin	T40.2X1	T40.2X2	T40.2X3	T40.2X4	T40.2X5	T40.2X6
Heptaminol	T46.3X1	T46.3X2	T46.3X3	T46.3X4	T46.3X5	T46.3X6
Herbicide NEC	T60.3X1	T60.3X2	T60.3X3	T60.3X4	—	—
Heroin	T40.1X1	T40.1X2	T40.1X3	T40.1X4	—	—
Herplex	T49.5X1	T49.5X2	T49.5X3	T49.5X4	T49.5X5	T49.5X6
HES	T45.8X1	T45.8X2	T45.8X3	T45.8X4	T45.8X5	T45.8X6
Hesperidin	T46.991	T46.992	T46.993	T46.994	T46.995	T46.996
Hetacillin	T36.0X1	T36.0X2	T36.0X3	T36.0X4	T36.0X5	T36.0X6
Hetastarch	T45.8X1	T45.8X2	T45.8X3	T45.8X4	T45.8X5	T45.8X6
HETP	T60.0X1	T60.0X2	T60.0X3	T60.0X4	—	—
Hexachlorobenzene (vapor)	T60.3X1	T60.3X2	T60.3X3	T60.3X4	—	—
Hexachlorocyclohexane	T53.6X1	T53.6X2	T53.6X3	T53.6X4	—	—
Hexachlorophene	T49.0X1	T49.0X2	T49.0X3	T49.0X4	T49.0X5	T49.0X6
Hexadiline	T46.3X1	T46.3X2	T46.3X3	T46.3X4	T46.3X5	T46.3X6
Hexadimethrine (bromide)	T45.7X1	T45.7X2	T45.7X3	T45.7X4	T45.7X5	T45.7X6
Hexadylamine	T46.3X1	T46.3X2	T46.3X3	T46.3X4	T46.3X5	T46.3X6
Hexaethyl tetraphosphate	T60.0X1	T60.0X2	T60.0X3	T60.0X4	—	—
Hexafluorenium bromide	T48.1X1	T48.1X2	T48.1X3	T48.1X4	T48.1X5	T48.1X6
Hexafluronium (bromide)	T48.1X1	T48.1X2	T48.1X3	T48.1X4	T48.1X5	T48.1X6
Hexa-germ	T49.2X1	T49.2X2	T49.2X3	T49.2X4	T49.2X5	T49.2X6
Hexahydrobenzol	T52.8X1	T52.8X2	T52.8X3	T52.8X4	—	—
Hexahydrocresol(s)	T51.8X1	T51.8X2	T51.8X3	T51.8X4	—	—
arsenide	T57.0X1	T57.0X2	T57.0X3	T57.0X4	—	—
arseniurated	T57.0X1	T57.0X2	T57.0X3	T57.0X4	—	—
cyanide	T57.3X1	T57.3X2	T57.3X3	T57.3X4	—	—

Substance	Poisoning, Accidental (unintentional)	Poisoning, Intentional self-harm	Poisoning, Assault	Poisoning, Undetermined	Adverse effect	Underdosing
Hexahydrocresol(s) — *Continued*						
gas	T59.891	T59.892	T59.893	T59.894	—	—
Fluoride (liquid)	T57.8X1	T57.8X2	T57.8X3	T57.8X4	—	—
vapor	T59.891	T59.892	T59.893	T59.894	—	—
phophorated	T60.0X1	T60.0X2	T60.0X3	T60.0X4	—	—
sulfate	T57.8X1	T57.8X2	T57.8X3	T57.8X4	—	—
sulfide (gas)	T59.6X1	T59.6X2	T59.6X3	T59.6X4	—	—
arseniurated	T57.0X1	T57.0X2	T57.0X3	T57.0X4	—	—
sulfurated	T57.8X1	T57.8X2	T57.8X3	T57.8X4	—	—
Hexahydrophenol	T51.8X1	T51.8X2	T51.8X3	T51.8X4	—	—
Hexalen	T51.8X1	T51.8X2	T51.8X3	T51.8X4	—	—
Hexamethonium bromide	T44.2X1	T44.2X2	T44.2X3	T44.2X4	T44.2X5	T44.2X6
Hexamethylene	T52.8X1	T52.8X2	T52.8X3	T52.8X4	—	—
Hexamethylmelamine	T45.1X1	T45.1X2	T45.1X3	T45.1X4	T45.1X5	T45.1X6
Hexamidine	T49.0X1	T49.0X2	T49.0X3	T49.0X4	T49.0X5	T49.0X6
Hexamine (mandelate)	T37.8X1	T37.8X2	T37.8X3	T37.8X4	T37.8X5	T37.8X6
Hexanone, 2-hexanone	T52.4X1	T52.4X2	T52.4X3	T52.4X4	—	—
Hexanuorenium	T48.1X1	T48.1X2	T48.1X3	T48.1X4	T48.1X5	T48.1X6
Hexapropymate	T42.6X1	T42.6X2	T42.6X3	T42.6X4	T42.6X5	T42.6X6
Hexasonium iodide	T44.3X1	T44.3X2	T44.3X3	T44.3X4	T44.3X5	T44.3X6
Hexcarbacholine bromide	T48.1X1	T48.1X2	T48.1X3	T48.1X4	T48.1X5	T48.1X6
Hexemal	T42.3X1	T42.3X2	T42.3X3	T42.3X4	T42.3X5	T42.3X6
Hexestrol	T38.5X1	T38.5X2	T38.5X3	T38.5X4	T38.5X5	T38.5X6
Hexethal (sodium)	T42.3X1	T42.3X2	T42.3X3	T42.3X4	T42.3X5	T42.3X6
Hexetidine	T37.8X1	T37.8X2	T37.8X3	T37.8X4	T37.8X5	T37.8X6
Hexobarbital	T42.3X1	T42.3X2	T42.3X3	T42.3X4	T42.3X5	T42.3X6
rectal	T41.291	T41.292	T41.293	T41.294	T41.295	T41.296
sodium	T41.1X1	T41.1X2	T41.1X3	T41.1X4	T41.1X5	T41.1X6
Hexobendine	T46.3X1	T46.3X2	T46.3X3	T46.3X4	T46.3X5	T46.3X6
Hexocyclium	T44.3X1	T44.3X2	T44.3X3	T44.3X4	T44.3X5	T44.3X6
metilsulfate	T44.3X1	T44.3X2	T44.3X3	T44.3X4	T44.3X5	T44.3X6
Hexoestrol	T38.5X1	T38.5X2	T38.5X3	T38.5X4	T38.5X5	T38.5X6
Hexone	T52.4X1	T52.4X2	T52.4X3	T52.4X4	—	—
Hexoprenaline	T48.6X1	T48.6X2	T48.6X3	T48.6X4	T48.6X5	T48.6X6
Hexylcaine	T41.3X1	T41.3X2	T41.3X3	T41.3X4	T41.3X5	T41.3X6
Hexylresorcinol	T52.2X1	T52.2X2	T52.2X3	T52.2X4	—	—
HGH (human growth hormone)	T38.811	T38.812	T38.813	T38.814	T38.815	T38.816
Hinkle's pills	T47.2X1	T47.2X2	T47.2X3	T47.2X4	T47.2X5	T47.2X6
Histalog	T50.8X1	T50.8X2	T50.8X3	T50.8X4	T50.8X5	T50.8X6
Histamine (phosphate)	T50.8X1	T50.8X2	T50.8X3	T50.8X4	T50.8X5	T50.8X6
Histoplasmin	T50.8X1	T50.8X2	T50.8X3	T50.8X4	T50.8X5	T50.8X6
Holly berries	T62.2X1	T62.2X2	T62.2X3	T62.2X4	—	—
Homatropine	T44.3X1	T44.3X2	T44.3X3	T44.3X4	T44.3X5	T44.3X6
methylbromide	T44.3X1	T44.3X2	T44.3X3	T44.3X4	T44.3X5	T44.3X6
Homochlorcyclizine	T45.0X1	T45.0X2	T45.0X3	T45.0X4	T45.0X5	T45.0X6
Homosalate	T49.3X1	T49.3X2	T49.3X3	T49.3X4	T49.3X5	T49.3X6
Homo-tet	T50.Z11	T50.Z12	T50.Z13	T50.Z14	T50.Z15	T50.Z16

Substance	Poisoning, Accidental (unintentional)	Poisoning, Intentional self-harm	Poisoning, Assault	Poisoning, Undetermined	Adverse effect	Underdosing
Hormone	T38.801	T38.802	T38.803	T38.804	T38.805	T38.806
adrenal cortical steroids	T38.0X1	T38.0X2	T38.0X3	T38.0X4	T38.0X5	T38.0X6
androgenic	T38.7X1	T38.7X2	T38.7X3	T38.7X4	T38.7X5	T38.7X6
anterior pituitary NEC	T38.811	T38.812	T38.813	T38.814	T38.815	T38.816
antidiabetic agents	T38.3X1	T38.3X2	T38.3X3	T38.3X4	T38.3X5	T38.3X6
antidiuretic	T38.891	T38.892	T38.893	T38.894	T38.895	T38.896
cancer therapy	T45.1X1	T45.1X2	T45.1X3	T45.1X4	T45.1X5	T45.1X6
follicle stimulating	T38.811	T38.812	T38.813	T38.814	T38.815	T38.816
gonadotropic	T38.891	T38.892	T38.893	T38.894	T38.895	T38.896
pituitary	T38.811	T38.812	T38.813	T38.814	T38.815	T38.816
growth	T38.811	T38.812	T38.813	T38.814	T38.815	T38.816
luteinizing	T38.811	T38.812	T38.813	T38.814	T38.815	T38.816
ovarian	T38.5X1	T38.5X2	T38.5X3	T38.5X4	T38.5X5	T38.5X6
oxytocic	T48.0X1	T48.0X2	T48.0X3	T48.0X4	T48.0X5	T48.0X6
parathyroid (derivatives)	T50.991	T50.992	T50.993	T50.994	T50.995	T50.996
pituitary (posterior) NEC	T38.891	T38.892	T38.893	T38.894	T38.895	T38.896
anterior	T38.811	T38.812	T38.813	T38.814	T38.815	T38.816
specified, NEC	T38.891	T38.892	T38.893	T38.894	T38.895	T38.896
thyroid	T38.1X1	T38.1X2	T38.1X3	T38.1X4	T38.1X5	T38.1X6
Hornet (sting)	T63.451	T63.452	T63.453	T63.454	—	—
Horse anti-human lymphocytic serum	T50.Z11	T50.Z12	T50.Z13	T50.Z14	T50.Z15	T50.Z16
Horticulture agent NEC	T65.91	T65.92	T65.93	T65.94	—	—
with pesticide	T60.91	T60.92	T60.93	T60.94	—	—
Human						
albumin	T45.8X1	T45.8X2	T45.8X3	T45.8X4	T45.8X5	T45.8X6
growth hormone (HGH)	T38.811	T38.812	T38.813	T38.814	T38.815	T38.816
immune serum	T50.Z11	T50.Z12	T50.Z13	T50.Z14	T50.Z15	T50.Z16
Hyaluronidase	T45.3X1	T45.3X2	T45.3X3	T45.3X4	T45.3X5	T45.3X6
Hyazyme	T45.3X1	T45.3X2	T45.3X3	T45.3X4	T45.3X5	T45.3X6
Hycodan	T40.2X1	T40.2X2	T40.2X3	T40.2X4	T40.2X5	T40.2X6
Hydantoin derivative NEC	T42.0X1	T42.0X2	T42.0X3	T42.0X4	T42.0X5	T42.0X6
Hydeltra	T38.0X1	T38.0X2	T38.0X3	T38.0X4	T38.0X5	T38.0X6
Hydergine	T44.6X1	T44.6X2	T44.6X3	T44.6X4	T44.6X5	T44.6X6
Hydrabamine penicillin	T36.0X1	T36.0X2	T36.0X3	T36.0X4	T36.0X5	T36.0X6
Hydralazine	T46.5X1	T46.5X2	T46.5X3	T46.5X4	T46.5X5	T46.5X6
Hydrargaphen	T49.0X1	T49.0X2	T49.0X3	T49.0X4	T49.0X5	T49.0X6
Hydrargyri amino-chloridum	T49.0X1	T49.0X2	T49.0X3	T49.0X4	T49.0X5	T49.0X6
Hydrastine	T48.291	T48.292	T48.293	T48.294	T48.295	T48.296
Hydrazine	T54.1X1	T54.1X2	T54.1X3	T54.1X4	—	—
monoamine oxidase inhibitors	T43.1X1	T43.1X2	T43.1X3	T43.1X4	T43.1X5	T43.1X6
Hydrazoic acid, azides	T54.2X1	T54.2X2	T54.2X3	T54.2X4	—	—
Hydriodic acid	T48.4X1	T48.4X2	T48.4X3	T48.4X4	T48.4X5	T48.4X6
Hydrocarbon gas	T59.891	T59.892	T59.893	T59.894	—	—
incomplete combustion of—see Carbon, monoxide, fuel, utility						

Substance	Poisoning, Accidental (unintentional)	Poisoning, Intentional self-harm	Poisoning, Assault	Poisoning, Undetermined	Adverse effect	Underdosing
Hydrocarbon gas — *Continued*						
liquefied (mobile container)	T59.891	T59.892	T59.893	T59.894	—	—
piped (natural)	T59.891	T59.892	T59.893	T59.894	—	—
Hydrochloric acid (liquid)	T54.2X1	T54.2X2	T54.2X3	T54.2X4	—	—
medicinal (digestant)	T47.5X1	T47.5X2	T47.5X3	T47.5X4	T47.5X5	T47.5X6
vapor	T59.891	T59.892	T59.893	T59.894	—	—
Hydrochlorothiazide	T50.2X1	T50.2X2	T50.2X3	T50.2X4	T50.2X5	T50.2X6
Hydrocodone	T40.2X1	T40.2X2	T40.2X3	T40.2X4	T40.2X5	T40.2X6
Hydrocortisone (derivatives)	T38.0X1	T38.0X2	T38.0X3	T38.0X4	T38.0X5	T38.0X6
aceponate	T49.0X1	T49.0X2	T49.0X3	T49.0X4	T49.0X5	T49.0X6
ENT agent	T49.6X1	T49.6X2	T49.6X3	T49.6X4	T49.6X5	T49.6X6
ophthalmic preparation	T49.5X1	T49.5X2	T49.5X3	T49.5X4	T49.5X5	T49.5X6
topical NEC	T49.0X1	T49.0X2	T49.0X3	T49.0X4	T49.0X5	T49.0X6
Hydrocortone	T38.0X1	T38.0X2	T38.0X3	T38.0X4	T38.0X5	T38.0X6
ENT agent	T49.6X1	T49.6X2	T49.6X3	T49.6X4	T49.6X5	T49.6X6
ophthalmic preparation	T49.5X1	T49.5X2	T49.5X3	T49.5X4	T49.5X5	T49.5X6
topical NEC	T49.0X1	T49.0X2	T49.0X3	T49.0X4	T49.0X5	T49.0X6
Hydrocyanic acid (liquid)	T57.3X1	T57.3X2	T57.3X3	T57.3X4	—	—
gas	T65.0X1	T65.0X2	T65.0X3	T65.0X4	—	—
Hydroflumethiazide	T50.2X1	T50.2X2	T50.2X3	T50.2X4	T50.2X5	T50.2X6
Hydrofluoric acid (liquid)	T54.2X1	T54.2X2	T54.2X3	T54.2X4	—	—
vapor	T59.891	T59.892	T59.893	T59.894	—	—
Hydrogen	T59.891	T59.892	T59.893	T59.894	—	—
arsenide	T57.0X1	T57.0X2	T57.0X3	T57.0X4	—	—
arseniureted	T57.0X1	T57.0X2	T57.0X3	T57.0X4	—	—
chloride	T57.8X1	T57.8X2	T57.8X3	T57.8X4	—	—
cyanide (salts)	T57.3X1	T57.3X2	T57.3X3	T57.3X4	—	—
gas	T57.3X1	T57.3X2	T57.3X3	T57.3X4	—	—
Fluoride	T59.5X1	T59.5X2	T59.5X3	T59.5X4	—	—
vapor	T59.5X1	T59.5X2	T59.5X3	T59.5X4	—	—
peroxide	T49.0X1	T49.0X2	T49.0X3	T49.0X4	T49.0X5	T49.0X6
phosphureted	T57.1X1	T57.1X2	T57.1X3	T57.1X4	—	—
sulfide	T59.6X1	T59.6X2	T59.6X3	T59.6X4	—	—
arseniureted	T57.0X1	T57.0X2	T57.0X3	T57.0X4	—	—
sulfureted	T59.6X1	T59.6X2	T59.6X3	T59.6X4	—	—
Hydromethylpyridine	T46.7X1	T46.7X2	T46.7X3	T46.7X4	T46.7X5	T46.7X6
Hydromorphinol	T40.2X1	T40.2X2	T40.2X3	T40.2X4	—	—
Hydromorphinone	T40.2X1	T40.2X2	T40.2X3	T40.2X4	T40.2X5	T40.2X6
Hydromorphone	T40.2X1	T40.2X2	T40.2X3	T40.2X4	T40.2X5	T40.2X6
Hydromox	T50.2X1	T50.2X2	T50.2X3	T50.2X4	T50.2X5	T50.2X6
Hydrophilic lotion	T49.3X1	T49.3X2	T49.3X3	T49.3X4	T49.3X5	T49.3X6
Hydroquinidine	T46.2X1	T46.2X2	T46.2X3	T46.2X4	T46.2X5	T46.2X6
Hydroquinone	T52.2X1	T52.2X2	T52.2X3	T52.2X4	—	—
vapor	T59.891	T59.892	T59.893	T59.894	—	—
Hydrosulfuric acid (gas)	T59.6X1	T59.6X2	T59.6X3	T59.6X4	—	—

Substance	Poisoning, Accidental (unintentional)	Poisoning, Intentional self-harm	Poisoning, Assault	Poisoning, Undetermined	Adverse effect	Underdosing
Hydrotalcite	T47.1X1	T47.1X2	T47.1X3	T47.1X4	T47.1X5	T47.1X6
Hydrous wool fat	T49.3X1	T49.3X2	T49.3X3	T49.3X4	T49.3X5	T49.3X6
Hydroxide, caustic	T54.3X1	T54.3X2	T54.3X3	T54.3X4	—	—
Hydroxocobalamin	T45.8X1	T45.8X2	T45.8X3	T45.8X4	T45.8X5	T45.8X6
Hydroxyamp-hetamine	T49.5X1	T49.5X2	T49.5X3	T49.5X4	T49.5X5	T49.5X6
Hydroxycarbamide	T45.1X1	T45.1X2	T45.1X3	T45.1X4	T45.1X5	T45.1X6
Hydroxychloroquine	T37.8X1	T37.8X2	T37.8X3	T37.8X4	T37.8X5	T37.8X6
Hydroxydihydro-codeinone	T40.2X1	T40.2X2	T40.2X3	T40.2X4	T40.2X5	T40.2X6
Hydroxyestrone	T38.5X1	T38.5X2	T38.5X3	T38.5X4	T38.5X5	T38.5X6
Hydroxyethyl starch	T45.8X1	T45.8X2	T45.8X3	T45.8X4	T45.8X5	T45.8X6
Hydroxyme-thylpentanone	T52.4X1	T52.4X2	T52.4X3	T52.4X4	—	—
Hydroxyphenamate	T43.591	T43.592	T43.593	T43.594	T43.595	T43.596
Hydroxypheny-lbutazone	T39.2X1	T39.2X2	T39.2X3	T39.2X4	T39.2X5	T39.2X6
Hydroxyprogesterone	T38.5X1	T38.5X2	T38.5X3	T38.5X4	T38.5X5	T38.5X6
caproate	T38.5X1	T38.5X2	T38.5X3	T38.5X4	T38.5X5	T38.5X6
Hydroxyquinoline (derivatives) NEC	T37.8X1	T37.8X2	T37.8X3	T37.8X4	T37.8X5	T37.8X6
Hydroxystilbamidine	T37.3X1	T37.3X2	T37.3X3	T37.3X4	T37.3X5	T37.3X6
Hydroxytoluene (nonmedicinal)	T54.0X1	T54.0X2	T54.0X3	T54.0X4	—	—
medicinal	T49.0X1	T49.0X2	T49.0X3	T49.0X4	T49.0X5	T49.0X6
Hydroxyurea	T45.1X1	T45.1X2	T45.1X3	T45.1X4	T45.1X5	T45.1X6
Hydroxyzine	T43.591	T43.592	T43.593	T43.594	T43.595	T43.596
Hyoscine	T44.3X1	T44.3X2	T44.3X3	T44.3X4	T44.3X5	T44.3X6
Hyoscyamine	T44.3X1	T44.3X2	T44.3X3	T44.3X4	T44.3X5	T44.3X6
Hyoscyamus	T44.3X1	T44.3X2	T44.3X3	T44.3X4	T44.3X5	T44.3X6
dry extract	T44.3X1	T44.3X2	T44.3X3	T44.3X4	T44.3X5	T44.3X6
Hypaque	T50.8X1	T50.8X2	T50.8X3	T50.8X4	T50.8X5	T50.8X6
Hypertussis	T50.Z11	T50.Z12	T50.Z13	T50.Z14	T50.Z15	T50.Z16
Hypnotic	T42.71	T42.72	T42.73	T42.74	T42.75	T42.76
anticonvulsant	T42.71	T42.72	T42.73	T42.74	T42.75	T42.76
specified NEC	T42.6X1	T42.6X2	T42.6X3	T42.6X4	T42.6X5	T42.6X6
Hypochlorite	T49.0X1	T49.0X2	T49.0X3	T49.0X4	T49.0X5	T49.0X6
Hypophysis, posterior	T38.891	T38.892	T38.893	T38.894	T38.895	T38.896
Hypotensive NEC	T46.5X1	T46.5X2	T46.5X3	T46.5X4	T46.5X5	T46.5X6
Hypromellose	T49.5X1	T49.5X2	T49.5X3	T49.5X4	T49.5X5	T49.5X6
I						
Ibacitabine	T37.5X1	T37.5X2	T37.5X3	T37.5X4	T37.5X5	T37.5X6
Ibopamine	T44.991	T44.992	T44.993	T44.994	T44.995	T44.996
Ibufenac	T39.311	T39.312	T39.313	T39.314	T39.315	T39.316
Ibuprofen	T39.311	T39.312	T39.313	T39.314	T39.315	T39.316
Ibuproxam	T39.311	T39.312	T39.313	T39.314	T39.315	T39.316
Ibuterol	T48.6X1	T48.6X2	T48.6X3	T48.6X4	T48.6X5	T48.6X6
Ichthammol	T49.0X1	T49.0X2	T49.0X3	T49.0X4	T49.0X5	T49.0X6
Ichthyol	T49.4X1	T49.4X2	T49.4X3	T49.4X4	T49.4X5	T49.4X6
Idarubicin	T45.1X1	T45.1X2	T45.1X3	T45.1X4	T45.1X5	T45.1X6
Idrocilamide	T42.8X1	T42.8X2	T42.8X3	T42.8X4	T42.8X5	T42.8X6
Ifenprodil	T46.7X1	T46.7X2	T46.7X3	T46.7X4	T46.7X5	T46.7X6

Substance	Poisoning, Accidental (unintentional)	Poisoning, Intentional self-harm	Poisoning, Assault	Poisoning, Undetermined	Adverse effect	Underdosing
Ifosfamide	T45.1X1	T45.1X2	T45.1X3	T45.1X4	T45.1X5	T45.1X6
Iletin	T38.3X1	T38.3X2	T38.3X3	T38.3X4	T38.3X5	T38.3X6
Ilex	T62.2X1	T62.2X2	T62.2X3	T62.2X4	—	—
Illuminating gas (after combustion)	T58.11	T58.12	T58.13	T58.14	—	—
prior to combustion	T59.891	T59.892	T59.893	T59.894	—	—
Ilopan	T45.2X1	T45.2X2	T45.2X3	T45.2X4	T45.2X5	T45.2X6
Iloprost	T46.7X1	T46.7X2	T46.7X3	T46.7X4	T46.7X5	T46.7X6
Ilotycin	T36.3X1	T36.3X2	T36.3X3	T36.3X4	T36.3X5	T36.3X6
ophthalmic preparation	T49.5X1	T49.5X2	T49.5X3	T49.5X4	T49.5X5	T49.5X6
topical NEC	T49.0X1	T49.0X2	T49.0X3	T49.0X4	T49.0X5	T49.0X6
Imidazole-4-carboxamide	T45.1X1	T45.1X2	T45.1X3	T45.1X4	T45.1X5	T45.1X6
Imipenem	T36.0X1	T36.0X2	T36.0X3	T36.0X4	T36.0X5	T36.0X6
Imipramine	T43.011	T43.012	T43.013	T43.014	T43.015	T43.016
Iminostilbene	T42.1X1	T42.1X2	T42.1X3	T42.1X4	T42.1X5	T42.1X6
Immu-G	T50.Z11	T50.Z12	T50.Z13	T50.Z14	T50.Z15	T50.Z16
Immuglobin	T50.Z11	T50.Z12	T50.Z13	T50.Z14	T50.Z15	T50.Z16
Immune						
globulin	T50.Z11	T50.Z12	T50.Z13	T50.Z14	T50.Z15	T50.Z16
serum globulin	T50.Z11	T50.Z12	T50.Z13	T50.Z14	T50.Z15	T50.Z16
Immunoglobin human (intravenous) (normal)	T50.Z11	T50.Z12	T50.Z13	T50.Z14	T50.Z15	T50.Z16
unmodified	T50.Z11	T50.Z12	T50.Z13	T50.Z14	T50.Z15	T50.Z16
Immunosuppressive drug	T45.1X1	T45.1X2	T45.1X3	T45.1X4	T45.1X5	T45.1X6
Immu-tetanus	T50.Z11	T50.Z12	T50.Z13	T50.Z14	T50.Z15	T50.Z16
Indalpine	T43.221	T43.222	T43.223	T43.224	T43.225	T43.226
Indanazoline	T48.5X1	T48.5X2	T48.5X3	T48.5X4	T48.5X5	T48.5X6
Indandione (derivatives)	T45.511	T45.512	T45.513	T45.514	T45.515	T45.516
Indapamide	T46.5X1	T46.5X2	T46.5X3	T46.5X4	T46.5X5	T46.5X6
Indendione (derivatives)	T45.511	T45.512	T45.513	T45.514	T45.515	T45.516
Indenolol	T44.7X1	T44.7X2	T44.7X3	T44.7X4	T44.7X5	T44.7X6
Inderal	T44.7X1	T44.7X2	T44.7X3	T44.7X4	T44.7X5	T44.7X6
Indian						
hemp	T40.711	T40.712	T40.713	T40.714	T40.715	T40.716
tobacco	T62.2X1	T62.2X2	T62.2X3	T62.2X4	—	—
Indigo carmine	T50.8X1	T50.8X2	T50.8X3	T50.8X4	T50.8X5	T50.8X6
Indobufen	T45.521	T45.522	T45.523	T45.524	T45.525	T45.526
Indocin	T39.2X1	T39.2X2	T39.2X3	T39.2X4	T39.2X5	T39.2X6
Indocyanine green	T50.8X1	T50.8X2	T50.8X3	T50.8X4	T50.8X5	T50.8X6
Indometacin	T39.391	T39.392	T39.393	T39.394	T39.395	T39.396
Indomethacin	T39.391	T39.392	T39.393	T39.394	T39.395	T39.396
farnesil	T39.4X1	T39.4X2	T39.4X3	T39.4X4	T39.4X5	T39.4X6
Indoramin	T44.6X1	T44.6X2	T44.6X3	T44.6X4	T44.6X5	T44.6X6
Industrial						
alcohol	T51.0X1	T51.0X2	T51.0X3	T51.0X4	—	—
fumes	T59.891	T59.892	T59.893	T59.894	—	—
solvents (fumes) (vapors)	T52.91	T52.92	T52.93	T52.94	—	—
Influenza vaccine	T50.B91	T50.B92	T50.B93	T50.B94	T50.B95	T50.B96
Ingested substance NEC	T65.91	T65.92	T65.93	T65.94	—	—
INH	T37.1X1	T37.1X2	T37.1X3	T37.1X4	T37.1X5	T37.1X6
Inhalation, gas (noxious)—see Gas						
Inhibitor						
angiotensin-converting enzyme	T46.4X1	T46.4X2	T46.4X3	T46.4X4	T46.4X5	T46.4X6
carbonic anhydrase	T50.2X1	T50.2X2	T50.2X3	T50.2X4	T50.2X5	T50.2X6
fibrinolysis	T45.621	T45.622	T45.623	T45.624	T45.625	T45.626
monoamine oxidase NEC	T43.1X1	T43.1X2	T43.1X3	T43.1X4	T43.1X5	T43.1X6
hydrazine	T43.1X1	T43.1X2	T43.1X3	T43.1X4	T43.1X5	T43.1X6
postsynaptic	T43.8X1	T43.8X2	T43.8X3	T43.8X4	T43.8X5	T43.8X6
prothrombin synthesis	T45.511	T45.512	T45.513	T45.514	T45.515	T45.516
Ink	T65.891	T65.892	T65.893	T65.894	—	—
Inorganic substance NEC	T57.91	T57.92	T57.93	T57.94	—	—
Inosine pranobex	T37.5X1	T37.5X2	T37.5X3	T37.5X4	T37.5X5	T37.5X6
Inositol	T50.991	T50.992	T50.993	T50.994	T50.995	T50.996
nicotinate	T46.7X1	T46.7X2	T46.7X3	T46.7X4	T46.7X5	T46.7X6
Inproquone	T45.1X1	T45.1X2	T45.1X3	T45.1X4	T45.1X5	T45.1X6
Insect (sting), venomous	T63.481	T63.482	T63.483	T63.484	—	—
ant	T63.421	T63.422	T63.423	T63.424	—	—
bee	T63.441	T63.442	T63.443	T63.444	—	—
caterpillar	T63.431	T63.432	T63.433	T63.434	—	—
hornet	T63.451	T63.452	T63.453	T63.454	—	—
wasp	T63.461	T63.462	T63.463	T63.464	—	—
Insecticide NEC	T60.91	T60.92	T60.93	T60.94	—	—
carbamate	T60.0X1	T60.0X2	T60.0X3	T60.0X4	—	—
chlorinated	T60.1X1	T60.1X2	T60.1X3	T60.1X4	—	—
mixed	T60.91	T60.92	T60.93	T60.94	—	—
organochlorine	T60.1X1	T60.1X2	T60.1X3	T60.1X4	—	—
organophosphorus	T60.0X1	T60.0X2	T60.0X3	T60.0X4	—	—
Insular tissue extract	T38.3X1	T38.3X2	T38.3X3	T38.3X4	T38.3X5	T38.3X6
Insulin (amorphous) (globin) (isophane) (Lente) (NPH) (Semilente) (Ultralente)	T38.3X1	T38.3X2	T38.3X3	T38.3X4	T38.3X5	T38.3X6
defalan	T38.3X1	T38.3X2	T38.3X3	T38.3X4	T38.3X5	T38.3X6
human	T38.3X1	T38.3X2	T38.3X3	T38.3X4	T38.3X5	T38.3X6
injection, soluble	T38.3X1	T38.3X2	T38.3X3	T38.3X4	T38.3X5	T38.3X6
biphasic	T38.3X1	T38.3X2	T38.3X3	T38.3X4	T38.3X5	T38.3X6
intermediate acting	T38.3X1	T38.3X2	T38.3X3	T38.3X4	T38.3X5	T38.3X6
protamine zinc	T38.3X1	T38.3X2	T38.3X3	T38.3X4	T38.3X5	T38.3X6
slow acting	T38.3X1	T38.3X2	T38.3X3	T38.3X4	T38.3X5	T38.3X6
zinc						
protamine injection	T38.3X1	T38.3X2	T38.3X3	T38.3X4	T38.3X5	T38.3X6
suspension (amorphous) (crystalline)	T38.3X1	T38.3X2	T38.3X3	T38.3X4	T38.3X5	T38.3X6
Interferon (alpha) (beta) (gamma)	T37.5X1	T37.5X2	T37.5X3	T37.5X4	T37.5X5	T37.5X6
Intestinal motility control drug	T47.6X1	T47.6X2	T47.6X3	T47.6X4	T47.6X5	T47.6X6
biological	T47.8X1	T47.8X2	T47.8X3	T47.8X4	T47.8X5	T47.8X6

Substance	Poisoning, Accidental (unintentional)	Poisoning, Intentional self-harm	Poisoning, Assault	Poisoning, Undetermined	Adverse effect	Underdosing
Intranarcon	T41.1X1	T41.1X2	T41.1X3	T41.1X4	T41.1X5	T41.1X6
Intravenous						
amino acids	T50.991	T50.992	T50.993	T50.994	T50.995	T50.996
fat suspension	T50.991	T50.992	T50.993	T50.994	T50.995	T50.996
Inulin	T50.8X1	T50.8X2	T50.8X3	T50.8X4	T50.8X5	T50.8X6
Invert sugar	T50.3X1	T50.3X2	T50.3X3	T50.3X4	T50.3X5	T50.3X6
Inza—see Naproxen						
Iobenzamic acid	T50.8X1	T50.8X2	T50.8X3	T50.8X4	T50.8X5	T50.8X6
Iocarmic acid	T50.8X1	T50.8X2	T50.8X3	T50.8X4	T50.8X5	T50.8X6
Iocetamic acid	T50.8X1	T50.8X2	T50.8X3	T50.8X4	T50.8X5	T50.8X6
Iodamide	T50.8X1	T50.8X2	T50.8X3	T50.8X4	T50.8X5	T50.8X6
Iodide NEC—see also Iodine	T49.0X1	T49.0X2	T49.0X3	T49.0X4	T49.0X5	T49.0X6
mercury (ointment)	T49.0X1	T49.0X2	T49.0X3	T49.0X4	T49.0X5	T49.0X6
methylate	T49.0X1	T49.0X2	T49.0X3	T49.0X4	T49.0X5	T49.0X6
potassium (expectorant) NEC	T48.4X1	T48.4X2	T48.4X3	T48.4X4	T48.4X5	T48.4X6
Iodinated						
contrast medium	T50.8X1	T50.8X2	T50.8X3	T50.8X4	T50.8X5	T50.8X6
glycerol	T48.4X1	T48.4X2	T48.4X3	T48.4X4	T48.4X5	T48.4X6
human serum albumin (131I)	T50.8X1	T50.8X2	T50.8X3	T50.8X4	T50.8X5	T50.8X6
Iodine (antiseptic, external) (tincture) NEC	T49.0X1	T49.0X2	T49.0X3	T49.0X4	T49.0X5	T49.0X6
125—see also Radiation sickness, and Exposure to radioactivce isotopes	T50.8X1	T50.8X2	T50.8X3	T50.8X4	T50.8X5	T50.8X6
therapeutic	T50.991	T50.992	T50.993	T50.994	T50.995	T50.996
131—see also Radiation sickness, and Exposure to radioactivce isotopes	T50.8X1	T50.8X2	T50.8X3	T50.8X4	T50.8X5	T50.8X6
therapeutic	T38.2X1	T38.2X2	T38.2X3	T38.2X4	T38.2X5	T38.2X6
diagnostic	T50.8X1	T50.8X2	T50.8X3	T50.8X4	T50.8X5	T50.8X6
for thyroid conditions (antithyroid)	T38.2X1	T38.2X2	T38.2X3	T38.2X4	T38.2X5	T38.2X6
solution	T49.0X1	T49.0X2	T49.0X3	T49.0X4	T49.0X5	T49.0X6
vapor	T59.891	T59.892	T59.893	T59.894	—	—
Iodipamide	T50.8X1	T50.8X2	T50.8X3	T50.8X4	T50.8X5	T50.8X6
Iodized (poppy seed) oil	T50.8X1	T50.8X2	T50.8X3	T50.8X4	T50.8X5	T50.8X6
Iodobismitol	T37.8X1	T37.8X2	T37.8X3	T37.8X4	T37.8X5	T37.8X6
Iodochlorhyd-roxyquin	T37.8X1	T37.8X2	T37.8X3	T37.8X4	T37.8X5	T37.8X6
topical	T49.0X1	T49.0X2	T49.0X3	T49.0X4	T49.0X5	T49.0X6
Iodochlorhydroxy-quinoline	T37.8X1	T37.8X2	T37.8X3	T37.8X4	T37.8X5	T37.8X6
Iodocholesterol (131I)	T50.8X1	T50.8X2	T50.8X3	T50.8X4	T50.8X5	T50.8X6
Iodoform	T49.0X1	T49.0X2	T49.0X3	T49.0X4	T49.0X5	T49.0X6
Iodohippuric acid	T50.8X1	T50.8X2	T50.8X3	T50.8X4	T50.8X5	T50.8X6
Iodopanoic acid	T50.8X1	T50.8X2	T50.8X3	T50.8X4	T50.8X5	T50.8X6
Iodophthalein (sodium)	T50.8X1	T50.8X2	T50.8X3	T50.8X4	T50.8X5	T50.8X6
Iodopyracet	T50.8X1	T50.8X2	T50.8X3	T50.8X4	T50.8X5	T50.8X6
Iodoquinol	T37.8X1	T37.8X2	T37.8X3	T37.8X4	T37.8X5	T37.8X6
Iodoxamic acid	T50.8X1	T50.8X2	T50.8X3	T50.8X4	T50.8X5	T50.8X6
Iofendylate	T50.8X1	T50.8X2	T50.8X3	T50.8X4	T50.8X5	T50.8X6
Ioglycamic acid	T50.8X1	T50.8X2	T50.8X3	T50.8X4	T50.8X5	T50.8X6
Iohexol	T50.8X1	T50.8X2	T50.8X3	T50.8X4	T50.8X5	T50.8X6
Ion exchange resin						
anion	T47.8X1	T47.8X2	T47.8X3	T47.8X4	T47.8X5	T47.8X6
cation	T50.3X1	T50.3X2	T50.3X3	T50.3X4	T50.3X5	T50.3X6
cholestyramine	T46.6X1	T46.6X2	T46.6X3	T46.6X4	T46.6X5	T46.6X6
intestinal	T47.8X1	T47.8X2	T47.8X3	T47.8X4	T47.8X5	T47.8X6
Iopamidol	T50.8X1	T50.8X2	T50.8X3	T50.8X4	T50.8X5	T50.8X6
Iopanoic acid	T50.8X1	T50.8X2	T50.8X3	T50.8X4	T50.8X5	T50.8X6
Iophenoic acid	T50.8X1	T50.8X2	T50.8X3	T50.8X4	T50.8X5	T50.8X6
Iopodate, sodium	T50.8X1	T50.8X2	T50.8X3	T50.8X4	T50.8X5	T50.8X6
Iopodic acid	T50.8X1	T50.8X2	T50.8X3	T50.8X4	T50.8X5	T50.8X6
Iopromide	T50.8X1	T50.8X2	T50.8X3	T50.8X4	T50.8X5	T50.8X6
Iopydol	T50.8X1	T50.8X2	T50.8X3	T50.8X4	T50.8X5	T50.8X6
Iotalamic acid	T50.8X1	T50.8X2	T50.8X3	T50.8X4	T50.8X5	T50.8X6
Iothalamate	T50.8X1	T50.8X2	T50.8X3	T50.8X4	T50.8X5	T50.8X6
Iothiouracil	T38.2X1	T38.2X2	T38.2X3	T38.2X4	T38.2X5	T38.2X6
Iotrol	T50.8X1	T50.8X2	T50.8X3	T50.8X4	T50.8X5	T50.8X6
Iotrolan	T50.8X1	T50.8X2	T50.8X3	T50.8X4	T50.8X5	T50.8X6
Iotroxate	T50.8X1	T50.8X2	T50.8X3	T50.8X4	T50.8X5	T50.8X6
Iotroxic acid	T50.8X1	T50.8X2	T50.8X3	T50.8X4	T50.8X5	T50.8X6
Ioversol	T50.8X1	T50.8X2	T50.8X3	T50.8X4	T50.8X5	T50.8X6
Ioxaglate	T50.8X1	T50.8X2	T50.8X3	T50.8X4	T50.8X5	T50.8X6
Ioxaglic acid	T50.8X1	T50.8X2	T50.8X3	T50.8X4	T50.8X5	T50.8X6
Ioxitalamic acid	T50.8X1	T50.8X2	T50.8X3	T50.8X4	T50.8X5	T50.8X6
Ipecac	T47.7X1	T47.7X2	T47.7X3	T47.7X4	T47.7X5	T47.7X6
Ipecacuanha	T48.4X1	T48.4X2	T48.4X3	T48.4X4	T48.4X5	T48.4X6
Ipodate, calcium	T50.8X1	T50.8X2	T50.8X3	T50.8X4	T50.8X5	T50.8X6
Ipral	T42.3X1	T42.3X2	T42.3X3	T42.3X4	T42.3X5	T42.3X6
Ipratropium (bromide)	T48.6X1	T48.6X2	T48.6X3	T48.6X4	T48.6X5	T48.6X6
Ipriflavone	T46.3X1	T46.3X2	T46.3X3	T46.3X4	T46.3X5	T46.3X6
Iprindole	T43.011	T43.012	T43.013	T43.014	T43.015	T43.016
Iproclozide	T43.1X1	T43.1X2	T43.1X3	T43.1X4	T43.1X5	T43.1X6
Iprofenin	T50.8X1	T50.8X2	T50.8X3	T50.8X4	T50.8X5	T50.8X6
Iproheptine	T49.2X1	T49.2X2	T49.2X3	T49.2X4	T49.2X5	T49.2X6
Iproniazid	T43.1X1	T43.1X2	T43.1X3	T43.1X4	T43.1X5	T43.1X6
Iproplatin	T45.1X1	T45.1X2	T45.1X3	T45.1X4	T45.1X5	T45.1X6
Iproveratril	T46.1X1	T46.1X2	T46.1X3	T46.1X4	T46.1X5	T46.1X6
Iron (compounds) (medicinal) NEC	T45.4X1	T45.4X2	T45.4X3	T45.4X4	T45.4X5	T45.4X6
ammonium	T45.4X1	T45.4X2	T45.4X3	T45.4X4	T45.4X5	T45.4X6
dextran injection	T45.4X1	T45.4X2	T45.4X3	T45.4X4	T45.4X5	T45.4X6
nonmedicinal	T56.891	T56.892	T56.893	T56.894	—	—
salts	T45.4X1	T45.4X2	T45.4X3	T45.4X4	T45.4X5	T45.4X6
sorbitex	T45.4X1	T45.4X2	T45.4X3	T45.4X4	T45.4X5	T45.4X6
sorbitol citric acid complex	T45.4X1	T45.4X2	T45.4X3	T45.4X4	T45.4X5	T45.4X6
Irrigating fluid (vaginal)	T49.8X1	T49.8X2	T49.8X3	T49.8X4	T49.8X5	T49.8X6
eye	T49.5X1	T49.5X2	T49.5X3	T49.5X4	T49.5X5	T49.5X6
Isepamicin	T36.5X1	T36.5X2	T36.5X3	T36.5X4	T36.5X5	T36.5X6
Isoaminile (citrate)	T48.3X1	T48.3X2	T48.3X3	T48.3X4	T48.3X5	T48.3X6
Isoamyl nitrite	T46.3X1	T46.3X2	T46.3X3	T46.3X4	T46.3X5	T46.3X6
Isobenzan	T60.1X1	T60.1X2	T60.1X3	T60.1X4	—	—

Substance	Poisoning, Accidental (unintentional)	Poisoning, Intentional self-harm	Poisoning, Assault	Poisoning, Undetermined	Adverse effect	Underdosing
Isobutyl acetate	T52.8X1	T52.8X2	T52.8X3	T52.8X4	—	—
Isocarboxazid	T43.1X1	T43.1X2	T43.1X3	T43.1X4	T43.1X5	T43.1X6
Isoconazole	T49.0X1	T49.0X2	T49.0X3	T49.0X4	T49.0X5	T49.0X6
Isocyanate	T65.0X1	T65.0X2	T65.0X3	T65.0X4	—	—
Isoephedrine	T44.991	T44.992	T44.993	T44.994	T44.995	T44.996
Isoetarine	T48.6X1	T48.6X2	T48.6X3	T48.6X4	T48.6X5	T48.6X6
Isoethadione	T42.2X1	T42.2X2	T42.2X3	T42.2X4	T42.2X5	T42.2X6
Isoetharine	T44.5X1	T44.5X2	T44.5X3	T44.5X4	T44.5X5	T44.5X6
Isoflurane	T41.0X1	T41.0X2	T41.0X3	T41.0X4	T41.0X5	T41.0X6
Isoflurophate	T44.0X1	T44.0X2	T44.0X3	T44.0X4	T44.0X5	T44.0X6
Isomaltose, ferric complex	T45.4X1	T45.4X2	T45.4X3	T45.4X4	T45.4X5	T45.4X6
Isometheptene	T44.3X1	T44.3X2	T44.3X3	T44.3X4	T44.3X5	T44.3X6
Isoniazid	T37.1X1	T37.1X2	T37.1X3	T37.1X4	T37.1X5	T37.1X6
with						
rifampicin	T36.6X1	T36.6X2	T36.6X3	T36.6X4	T36.6X5	T36.6X6
thioacetazone	T37.1X1	T37.1X2	T37.1X3	T37.1X4	T37.1X5	T37.1X6
Isonicotinic acid hydrazide	T37.1X1	T37.1X2	T37.1X3	T37.1X4	T37.1X5	T37.1X6
Isonipecaine	T40.491	T40.492	T40.493	T40.494	T40.495	T40.496
Isopentaquine	T37.2X1	T37.2X2	T37.2X3	T37.2X4	T37.2X5	T37.2X6
Isophane insulin	T38.3X1	T38.3X2	T38.3X3	T38.3X4	T38.3X5	T38.3X6
Isophorone	T65.891	T65.892	T65.893	T65.894	—	—
Isophosphamide	T45.1X1	T45.1X2	T45.1X3	T45.1X4	T45.1X5	T45.1X6
Isopregnenone	T38.5X1	T38.5X2	T38.5X3	T38.5X4	T38.5X5	T38.5X6
Isoprenaline	T48.6X1	T48.6X2	T48.6X3	T48.6X4	T48.6X5	T48.6X6
Isopromethazine	T43.3X1	T43.3X2	T43.3X3	T43.3X4	T43.3X5	T43.3X6
Isopropamide	T44.3X1	T44.3X2	T44.3X3	T44.3X4	T44.3X5	T44.3X6
iodide	T44.3X1	T44.3X2	T44.3X3	T44.3X4	T44.3X5	T44.3X6
Isopropanol	T51.2X1	T51.2X2	T51.2X3	T51.2X4	—	—
Isopropyl						
acetate	T52.8X1	T52.8X2	T52.8X3	T52.8X4	—	—
alcohol	T51.2X1	T51.2X2	T51.2X3	T51.2X4	—	—
medicinal	T49.4X1	T49.4X2	T49.4X3	T49.4X4	T49.4X5	T49.4X6
ether	T52.8X1	T52.8X2	T52.8X3	T52.8X4	—	—
Isopropylamino-phenazone	T39.2X1	T39.2X2	T39.2X3	T39.2X4	T39.2X5	T39.2X6
Isoproterenol	T48.6X1	T48.6X2	T48.6X3	T48.6X4	T48.6X5	T48.6X6
Isosorbide dinitrate	T46.3X1	T46.3X2	T46.3X3	T46.3X4	T46.3X5	T46.3X6
Isothipendyl	T45.0X1	T45.0X2	T45.0X3	T45.0X4	T45.0X5	T45.0X6
Isotretinoin	T50.991	T50.992	T50.993	T50.994	T50.995	T50.996
Isoxazolyl penicillin	T36.0X1	T36.0X2	T36.0X3	T36.0X4	T36.0X5	T36.0X6
Isoxicam	T39.391	T39.392	T39.393	T39.394	T39.395	T39.396
Isoxsuprine	T46.7X1	T46.7X2	T46.7X3	T46.7X4	T46.7X5	T46.7X6
Ispagula	T47.4X1	T47.4X2	T47.4X3	T47.4X4	T47.4X5	T47.4X6
husk	T47.4X1	T47.4X2	T47.4X3	T47.4X4	T47.4X5	T47.4X6
Isradipine	T46.1X1	T46.1X2	T46.1X3	T46.1X4	T46.1X5	T46.1X6
I-thyroxine sodium	T38.1X1	T38.1X2	T38.1X3	T38.1X4	T38.1X5	T38.1X6
Itraconazole	T37.8X1	T37.8X2	T37.8X3	T37.8X4	T37.8X5	T37.8X6
Itramin tosilate	T46.3X1	T46.3X2	T46.3X3	T46.3X4	T46.3X5	T46.3X6
Ivermectin	T37.4X1	T37.4X2	T37.4X3	T37.4X4	T37.4X5	T37.4X6
Izoniazid	T37.1X1	T37.1X2	T37.1X3	T37.1X4	T37.1X5	T37.1X6
with thioacetazone	T37.1X1	T37.1X2	T37.1X3	T37.1X4	T37.1X5	T37.1X6

Substance	Poisoning, Accidental (unintentional)	Poisoning, Intentional self-harm	Poisoning, Assault	Poisoning, Undetermined	Adverse effect	Underdosing
J						
Jalap	T47.2X1	T47.2X2	T47.2X3	T47.2X4	T47.2X5	T47.2X6
Jamaica						
dogwood (bark)	T39.8X1	T39.8X2	T39.8X3	T39.8X4	T39.8X5	T39.8X6
ginger	T65.891	T65.892	T65.893	T65.894	—	—
root	T62.2X1	T62.2X2	T62.2X3	T62.2X4	—	—
Jatropha	T62.2X1	T62.2X2	T62.2X3	T62.2X4	—	—
curcas	T62.2X1	T62.2X2	T62.2X3	T62.2X4	—	—
Jectofer	T45.4X1	T45.4X2	T45.4X3	T45.4X4	T45.4X5	T45.4X6
Jellyfish (sting)	T63.621	T63.622	T63.623	T63.624	—	—
Jequirity (bean)	T62.2X1	T62.2X2	T62.2X3	T62.2X4	—	—
Jimson weed (stramonium)	T62.2X1	T62.2X2	T62.2X3	T62.2X4	—	—
seeds	T62.2X1	T62.2X2	T62.2X3	T62.2X4	—	—
Josamycin	T36.3X1	T36.3X2	T36.3X3	T36.3X4	T36.3X5	T36.3X6
Juniper tar	T49.1X1	T49.1X2	T49.1X3	T49.1X4	T49.1X5	T49.1X6
K						
Kallidinogenase	T46.7X1	T46.7X2	T46.7X3	T46.7X4	T46.7X5	T46.7X6
Kallikrein	T46.7X1	T46.7X2	T46.7X3	T46.7X4	T46.7X5	T46.7X6
Kanamycin	T36.5X1	T36.5X2	T36.5X3	T36.5X4	T36.5X5	T36.5X6
Kantrex	T36.5X1	T36.5X2	T36.5X3	T36.5X4	T36.5X5	T36.5X6
Kaolin	T47.6X1	T47.6X2	T47.6X3	T47.6X4	T47.6X5	T47.6X6
light	T47.6X1	T47.6X2	T47.6X3	T47.6X4	T47.6X5	T47.6X6
Karaya (gum)	T47.4X1	T47.4X2	T47.4X3	T47.4X4	T47.4X5	T47.4X6
Kebuzone	T39.2X1	T39.2X2	T39.2X3	T39.2X4	T39.2X5	T39.2X6
Kelevan	T60.1X1	T60.1X2	T60.1X3	T60.1X4	—	—
Kemithal	T41.1X1	T41.1X2	T41.1X3	T41.1X4	T41.1X5	T41.1X6
Kenacort	T38.0X1	T38.0X2	T38.0X3	T38.0X4	T38.0X5	T38.0X6
Keratolytic drug NEC	T49.4X1	T49.4X2	T49.4X3	T49.4X4	T49.4X5	T49.4X6
anthracene	T49.4X1	T49.4X2	T49.4X3	T49.4X4	T49.4X5	T49.4X6
Keratoplastic NEC	T49.4X1	T49.4X2	T49.4X3	T49.4X4	T49.4X5	T49.4X6
Kerosene, kerosine (fuel) (solvent) NEC	T52.0X1	T52.0X2	T52.0X3	T52.0X4	—	—
insecticide	T52.0X1	T52.0X2	T52.0X3	T52.0X4	—	—
vapor	T52.0X1	T52.0X2	T52.0X3	T52.0X4	—	—
Ketamine	T41.291	T41.292	T41.293	T41.294	T41.295	T41.296
Ketazolam	T42.4X1	T42.4X2	T42.4X3	T42.4X4	T42.4X5	T42.4X6
Ketazon	T39.2X1	T39.2X2	T39.2X3	T39.2X4	T39.2X5	T39.2X6
Ketobemidone	T40.491	T40.492	T40.493	T40.494	—	—
Ketoconazole	T49.0X1	T49.0X2	T49.0X3	T49.0X4	T49.0X5	T49.0X6
Ketols	T52.4X1	T52.4X2	T52.4X3	T52.4X4	—	—
Ketone oils	T52.4X1	T52.4X2	T52.4X3	T52.4X4	—	—
Ketoprofen	T39.311	T39.312	T39.313	T39.314	T39.315	T39.316
Ketorolac	T39.8X1	T39.8X2	T39.8X3	T39.8X4	T39.8X5	T39.8X6
Ketotifen	T45.0X1	T45.0X2	T45.0X3	T45.0X4	T45.0X5	T45.0X6
Khat	T43.691	T43.692	T43.693	T43.694	—	—
Khellin	T46.3X1	T46.3X2	T46.3X3	T46.3X4	T46.3X5	T46.3X6
Khelloside	T46.3X1	T46.3X2	T46.3X3	T46.3X4	T46.3X5	T46.3X6
Kiln gas or vapor (carbon monoxide)	T58.8X1	T58.8X2	T58.8X3	T58.8X4	—	—
Kitasamycin	T36.3X1	T36.3X2	T36.3X3	T36.3X4	T36.3X5	T36.3X6
Konsyl	T47.4X1	T47.4X2	T47.4X3	T47.4X4	T47.4X5	T47.4X6

Substance	Poisoning, Accidental (unintentional)	Poisoning, Intentional self-harm	Poisoning, Assault	Poisoning, Undetermined	Adverse effect	Underdosing
Kosam seed	T62.2X1	T62.2X2	T62.2X3	T62.2X4	—	—
Krait (venom)	T63.091	T63.092	T63.093	T63.094	—	—
Kwell (insecticide)	T60.1X1	T60.1X2	T60.1X3	T60.1X4	—	—
anti-infective (topical)	T49.0X1	T49.0X2	T49.0X3	T49.0X4	T49.0X5	T49.0X6
L						
Labetalol	T44.8X1	T44.8X2	T44.8X3	T44.8X4	T44.8X5	T44.8X6
Laburnum (seeds)	T62.2X1	T62.2X2	T62.2X3	T62.2X4	—	—
leaves	T62.2X1	T62.2X2	T62.2X3	T62.2X4	—	—
Lachesine	T49.5X1	T49.5X2	T49.5X3	T49.5X4	T49.5X5	T49.5X6
Lacidipine	T46.5X1	T46.5X2	T46.5X3	T46.5X4	T46.5X5	T46.5X6
Lacquer	T65.6X1	T65.6X2	T65.6X3	T65.6X4	—	—
Lacrimogenic gas	T59.3X1	T59.3X2	T59.3X3	T59.3X4	—	—
Lactated potassic saline	T50.3X1	T50.3X2	T50.3X3	T50.3X4	T50.3X5	T50.3X6
Lactic acid	T49.8X1	T49.8X2	T49.8X3	T49.8X4	T49.8X5	T49.8X6
Lactobacillus						
acidophilus	T47.6X1	T47.6X2	T47.6X3	T47.6X4	T47.6X5	T47.6X6
compound	T47.6X1	T47.6X2	T47.6X3	T47.6X4	T47.6X5	T47.6X6
bifidus, lyophilized	T47.6X1	T47.6X2	T47.6X3	T47.6X4	T47.6X5	T47.6X6
bulgaricus	T47.6X1	T47.6X2	T47.6X3	T47.6X4	T47.6X5	T47.6X6
sporogenes	T47.6X1	T47.6X2	T47.6X3	T47.6X4	T47.6X5	T47.6X6
Lactoflavin	T45.2X1	T45.2X2	T45.2X3	T45.2X4	T45.2X5	T45.2X6
Lactose (as excipient)	T50.901	T50.902	T50.903	T50.904	T50.905	T50.906
Lactuca (virosa) (extract)	T42.6X1	T42.6X2	T42.6X3	T42.6X4	T42.6X5	T42.6X6
Lactucarium	T42.6X1	T42.6X2	T42.6X3	T42.6X4	T42.6X5	T42.6X6
Lactulose	T47.3X1	T47.3X2	T47.3X3	T47.3X4	T47.3X5	T47.3X6
Laevo—see Levo-						
Lanatosides	T46.0X1	T46.0X2	T46.0X3	T46.0X4	T46.0X5	T46.0X6
Lanolin	T49.3X1	T49.3X2	T49.3X3	T49.3X4	T49.3X5	T49.3X6
Largactil	T43.3X1	T43.3X2	T43.3X3	T43.3X4	T43.3X5	T43.3X6
Larkspur	T62.2X1	T62.2X2	T62.2X3	T62.2X4	—	—
Laroxyl	T43.011	T43.012	T43.013	T43.014	T43.015	T43.016
Lasix	T50.1X1	T50.1X2	T50.1X3	T50.1X4	T50.1X5	T50.1X6
Lassar's paste	T49.4X1	T49.4X2	T49.4X3	T49.4X4	T49.4X5	T49.4X6
Latamoxef	T36.1X1	T36.1X2	T36.1X3	T36.1X4	T36.1X5	T36.1X6
Latex	T65.811	T65.812	T65.813	T65.814	—	—
Lathyrus (seed)	T62.2X1	T62.2X2	T62.2X3	T62.2X4	—	—
Laudanum	T40.0X1	T40.0X2	T40.0X3	T40.0X4	T40.0X5	T40.0X6
Laudexium	T48.1X1	T48.1X2	T48.1X3	T48.1X4	T48.1X5	T48.1X6
Laughing gas	T41.0X1	T41.0X2	T41.0X3	T41.0X4	T41.0X5	T41.0X6
Laurel, black or cherry	T62.2X1	T62.2X2	T62.2X3	T62.2X4	—	—
Laurolinium	T49.0X1	T49.0X2	T49.0X3	T49.0X4	T49.0X5	T49.0X6
Lauryl sulfoacetate	T49.2X1	T49.2X2	T49.2X3	T49.2X4	T49.2X5	T49.2X6
Laxative NEC	T47.4X1	T47.4X2	T47.4X3	T47.4X4	T47.4X5	T47.4X6
osmotic	T47.3X1	T47.3X2	T47.3X3	T47.3X4	T47.3X5	T47.3X6
saline	T47.3X1	T47.3X2	T47.3X3	T47.3X4	T47.3X5	T47.3X6
stimulant	T47.2X1	T47.2X2	T47.2X3	T47.2X4	T47.2X5	T47.2X6
L-dopa	T42.8X1	T42.8X2	T42.8X3	T42.8X4	T42.8X5	T42.8X6
Lead (dust) (fumes) (vapor) NEC	T56.0X1	T56.0X2	T56.0X3	T56.0X4	—	—
acetate	T49.2X1	T49.2X2	T49.2X3	T49.2X4	T49.2X5	T49.2X6
Lead NEC — *Continued*						
alkyl (fuel additive)	T56.0X1	T56.0X2	T56.0X3	T56.0X4	—	—
anti-infectives	T37.8X1	T37.8X2	T37.8X3	T37.8X4	T37.8X5	T37.8X6
antiknock compound (tetraethyl)	T56.0X1	T56.0X2	T56.0X3	T56.0X4	—	—
arsenate, arsenite (dust) (herbicide) (insecticide) (vapor)	T57.0X1	T57.0X2	T57.0X3	T57.0X4	—	—
carbonate	T56.0X1	T56.0X2	T56.0X3	T56.0X4	—	—
paint	T56.0X1	T56.0X2	T56.0X3	T56.0X4	—	—
chromate	T56.0X1	T56.0X2	T56.0X3	T56.0X4	—	—
paint	T56.0X1	T56.0X2	T56.0X3	T56.0X4	—	—
dioxide	T56.0X1	T56.0X2	T56.0X3	T56.0X4	—	—
inorganic	T56.0X1	T56.0X2	T56.0X3	T56.0X4	—	—
iodide	T56.0X1	T56.0X2	T56.0X3	T56.0X4	—	—
pigment (paint)	T56.0X1	T56.0X2	T56.0X3	T56.0X4	—	—
monoxide (dust)	T56.0X1	T56.0X2	T56.0X3	T56.0X4	—	—
paint	T56.0X1	T56.0X2	T56.0X3	T56.0X4	—	—
organic	T56.0X1	T56.0X2	T56.0X3	T56.0X4	—	—
oxide	T56.0X1	T56.0X2	T56.0X3	T56.0X4	—	—
paint	T56.0X1	T56.0X2	T56.0X3	T56.0X4	—	—
paint	T56.0X1	T56.0X2	T56.0X3	T56.0X4	—	—
salts	T56.0X1	T56.0X2	T56.0X3	T56.0X4	—	—
specified compound NEC	T56.0X1	T56.0X2	T56.0X3	T56.0X4	—	—
tetra-ethyl	T56.0X1	T56.0X2	T56.0X3	T56.0X4	—	—
Lebanese red	T40.711	T40.712	T40.713	T40.714	T40.715	T40.716
Lefetamine	T39.8X1	T39.8X2	T39.8X3	T39.8X4	T39.8X5	T39.8X6
Lenperone	T43.4X1	T43.4X2	T43.4X3	T43.4X4	T43.4X5	T43.4X6
Lente lietin (insulin)	T38.3X1	T38.3X2	T38.3X3	T38.3X4	T38.3X5	T38.3X6
Leptazol	T50.7X1	T50.7X2	T50.7X3	T50.7X4	T50.7X5	T50.7X6
Leptophos	T60.0X1	T60.0X2	T60.0X3	T60.0X4	—	—
Leritine	T40.2X1	T40.2X2	T40.2X3	T40.2X4	T40.2X5	T40.2X6
Letosteine	T48.4X1	T48.4X2	T48.4X3	T48.4X4	T48.4X5	T48.4X6
Letter	T38.1X1	T38.1X2	T38.1X3	T38.1X4	T38.1X5	T38.1X6
Lettuce opium	T42.6X1	T42.6X2	T42.6X3	T42.6X4	T42.6X5	T42.6X6
Leucinocaine	T41.3X1	T41.3X2	T41.3X3	T41.3X4	T41.3X5	T41.3X6
Leucocianidol	T46.991	T46.992	T46.993	T46.994	T46.995	T46.996
Leucovorin (factor)	T45.8X1	T45.8X2	T45.8X3	T45.8X4	T45.8X5	T45.8X6
Leukeran	T45.1X1	T45.1X2	T45.1X3	T45.1X4	T45.1X5	T45.1X6
Leuprolide	T38.891	T38.892	T38.893	T38.894	T38.895	T38.896
Levalbuterol	T48.6X1	T48.6X2	T48.6X3	T48.6X4	T48.6X5	T48.6X6
Levallorphan	T50.7X1	T50.7X2	T50.7X3	T50.7X4	T50.7X5	T50.7X6
Levamisole	T37.4X1	T37.4X2	T37.4X3	T37.4X4	T37.4X5	T37.4X6
Levanil	T42.6X1	T42.6X2	T42.6X3	T42.6X4	T42.6X5	T42.6X6
Levarterenol	T44.4X1	T44.4X2	T44.4X3	T44.4X4	T44.4X5	T44.4X6
Levdropropizine	T48.3X1	T48.3X2	T48.3X3	T48.3X4	T48.3X5	T48.3X6
Levobunolol	T49.5X1	T49.5X2	T49.5X3	T49.5X4	T49.5X5	T49.5X6
Levocabastine (hydrochloride)	T45.0X1	T45.0X2	T45.0X3	T45.0X4	T45.0X5	T45.0X6
Levocarnitine	T50.991	T50.992	T50.993	T50.994	T50.995	T50.996

Substance	Poisoning, Accidental (unintentional)	Poisoning, Intentional self-harm	Poisoning, Assault	Poisoning, Undetermined	Adverse effect	Underdosing
Levodopa	T42.8X1	T42.8X2	T42.8X3	T42.8X4	T42.8X5	T42.8X6
with carbidopa	T42.8X1	T42.8X2	T42.8X3	T42.8X4	T42.8X5	T42.8X6
Levo-dromoran	T40.2X1	T40.2X2	T40.2X3	T40.2X4	T40.2X5	T40.2X6
Levoglutamide	T50.991	T50.992	T50.993	T50.994	T50.995	T50.996
Levoid	T38.1X1	T38.1X2	T38.1X3	T38.1X4	T38.1X5	T38.1X6
Levo-iso-methadone	T40.3X1	T40.3X2	T40.3X3	T40.3X4	T40.3X5	T40.3X6
Levomepromazine	T43.3X1	T43.3X2	T43.3X3	T43.3X4	T43.3X5	T43.3X6
Levonordefrin	T49.6X1	T49.6X2	T49.6X3	T49.6X4	T49.6X5	T49.6X6
Levonorgestrel	T38.4X1	T38.4X2	T38.4X3	T38.4X4	T38.4X5	T38.4X6
with ethinylestradiol	T38.5X1	T38.5X2	T38.5X3	T38.5X4	T38.5X5	T38.5X6
Levopromazine	T43.3X1	T43.3X2	T43.3X3	T43.3X4	T43.3X5	T43.3X6
Levoprome	T42.6X1	T42.6X2	T42.6X3	T42.6X4	T42.6X5	T42.6X6
Levopropoxyphene	T40.491	T40.492	T40.493	T40.494	T40.495	T40.496
Levopropylhexedrine	T50.5X1	T50.5X2	T50.5X3	T50.5X4	T50.5X5	T50.5X6
Levoproxyphylline	T48.6X1	T48.6X2	T48.6X3	T48.6X4	T48.6X5	T48.6X6
Levorphanol	T40.491	T40.492	T40.493	T40.494	T40.495	T40.496
Levothyroxine	T38.1X1	T38.1X2	T38.1X3	T38.1X4	T38.1X5	T38.1X6
sodium	T38.1X1	T38.1X2	T38.1X3	T38.1X4	T38.1X5	T38.1X6
Levsin	T44.3X1	T44.3X2	T44.3X3	T44.3X4	T44.3X5	T44.3X6
Levulose	T50.3X1	T50.3X2	T50.3X3	T50.3X4	T50.3X5	T50.3X6
Lewisite (gas), not in war	T57.0X1	T57.0X2	T57.0X3	T57.0X4	—	—
Librium	T42.4X1	T42.4X2	T42.4X3	T42.4X4	T42.4X5	T42.4X6
Lidex	T49.0X1	T49.0X2	T49.0X3	T49.0X4	T49.0X5	T49.0X6
Lidocaine	T41.3X1	T41.3X2	T41.3X3	T41.3X4	T41.3X5	T41.3X6
regional	T41.3X1	T41.3X2	T41.3X3	T41.3X4	T41.3X5	T41.3X6
spinal	T41.3X1	T41.3X2	T41.3X3	T41.3X4	T41.3X5	T41.3X6
Lidofenin	T50.8X1	T50.8X2	T50.8X3	T50.8X4	T50.8X5	T50.8X6
Lidoflazine	T46.1X1	T46.1X2	T46.1X3	T46.1X4	T46.1X5	T46.1X6
Lighter fluid	T52.0X1	T52.0X2	T52.0X3	T52.0X4	—	—
Lignin hemicellulose	T47.6X1	T47.6X2	T47.6X3	T47.6X4	T47.6X5	T47.6X6
Lignocaine	T41.3X1	T41.3X2	T41.3X3	T41.3X4	T41.3X5	T41.3X6
regional	T41.3X1	T41.3X2	T41.3X3	T41.3X4	T41.3X5	T41.3X6
spinal	T41.3X1	T41.3X2	T41.3X3	T41.3X4	T41.3X5	T41.3X6
Ligroin(e) (solvent)	T52.0X1	T52.0X2	T52.0X3	T52.0X4	—	—
vapor	T59.891	T59.892	T59.893	T59.894	—	—
Ligustrum vulgare	T62.2X1	T62.2X2	T62.2X3	T62.2X4	—	—
Lily of the valley	T62.2X1	T62.2X2	T62.2X3	T62.2X4	—	—
Lime (chloride)	T54.3X1	T54.3X2	T54.3X3	T54.3X4	—	—
Limonene	T52.8X1	T52.8X2	T52.8X3	T52.8X4	—	—
Lincomycin	T36.8X1	T36.8X2	T36.8X3	T36.8X4	T36.8X5	T36.8X6
Lindane (insecticide) (nonmedicinal) (vapor)	T53.6X1	T53.6X2	T53.6X3	T53.6X4	—	—
medicinal	T49.0X1	T49.0X2	T49.0X3	T49.0X4	T49.0X5	T49.0X6
Liniments NEC	T49.91	T49.92	T49.93	T49.94	T49.95	T49.96
Linoleic acid	T46.6X1	T46.6X2	T46.6X3	T46.6X4	T46.6X5	T46.6X6
Linolenic acid	T46.6X1	T46.6X2	T46.6X3	T46.6X4	T46.6X5	T46.6X6
Linseed	T47.4X1	T47.4X2	T47.4X3	T47.4X4	T47.4X5	T47.4X6
Liothyronine	T38.1X1	T38.1X2	T38.1X3	T38.1X4	T38.1X5	T38.1X6
Liotrix	T38.1X1	T38.1X2	T38.1X3	T38.1X4	T38.1X5	T38.1X6
Lipancreatin	T47.5X1	T47.5X2	T47.5X3	T47.5X4	T47.5X5	T47.5X6

Substance	Poisoning, Accidental (unintentional)	Poisoning, Intentional self-harm	Poisoning, Assault	Poisoning, Undetermined	Adverse effect	Underdosing
Lipo-alprostadil	T46.7X1	T46.7X2	T46.7X3	T46.7X4	T46.7X5	T46.7X6
Lipo-Lutin	T38.5X1	T38.5X2	T38.5X3	T38.5X4	T38.5X5	T38.5X6
Lipotropic drug NEC	T50.901	T50.902	T50.903	T50.904	T50.905	T50.906
Liquefied petroleum gases	T59.891	T59.892	T59.893	T59.894	—	—
piped (pure or mixed with air)	T59.891	T59.892	T59.893	T59.894	—	—
Liquid						
paraffin	T47.4X1	T47.4X2	T47.4X3	T47.4X4	T47.4X5	T47.4X6
petrolatum	T47.4X1	T47.4X2	T47.4X3	T47.4X4	T47.4X5	T47.4X6
topical	T49.3X1	T49.3X2	T49.3X3	T49.3X4	T49.3X5	T49.3X6
specified NEC	T65.891	T65.892	T65.893	T65.894	—	—
substance	T65.91	T65.92	T65.93	T65.94	—	—
Liquor creosolis compositus	T65.891	T65.892	T65.893	T65.894	—	—
Liquorice	T48.4X1	T48.4X2	T48.4X3	T48.4X4	T48.4X5	T48.4X6
extract	T47.8X1	T47.8X2	T47.8X3	T47.8X4	T47.8X5	T47.8X6
Lisinopril	T46.4X1	T46.4X2	T46.4X3	T46.4X4	T46.4X5	T46.4X6
Lisuride	T42.8X1	T42.8X2	T42.8X3	T42.8X4	T42.8X5	T42.8X6
Lithane	T43.8X1	T43.8X2	T43.8X3	T43.8X4	T43.8X5	T43.8X6
Lithium	T56.891	T56.892	T56.893	T56.894	—	—
gluconate	T43.591	T43.592	T43.593	T43.594	T43.595	T43.596
salts (carbonate)	T43.591	T43.592	T43.593	T43.594	T43.595	T43.596
Lithonate	T43.8X1	T43.8X2	T43.8X3	T43.8X4	T43.8X5	T43.8X6
Liver						
extract	T45.8X1	T45.8X2	T45.8X3	T45.8X4	T45.8X5	T45.8X6
for parenteral use	T45.8X1	T45.8X2	T45.8X3	T45.8X4	T45.8X5	T45.8X6
fraction 1	T45.8X1	T45.8X2	T45.8X3	T45.8X4	T45.8X5	T45.8X6
hydrolysate	T45.8X1	T45.8X2	T45.8X3	T45.8X4	T45.8X5	T45.8X6
Lizard (bite) (venom)	T63.121	T63.122	T63.123	T63.124	—	—
LMD	T45.8X1	T45.8X2	T45.8X3	T45.8X4	T45.8X5	T45.8X6
Lobelia	T62.2X1	T62.2X2	T62.2X3	T62.2X4	—	—
Lobeline	T50.7X1	T50.7X2	T50.7X3	T50.7X4	T50.7X5	T50.7X6
Local action drug NEC	T49.8X1	T49.8X2	T49.8X3	T49.8X4	T49.8X5	T49.8X6
Locorten	T49.0X1	T49.0X2	T49.0X3	T49.0X4	T49.0X5	T49.0X6
Lofepramine	T43.011	T43.012	T43.013	T43.014	T43.015	T43.016
Lolium temulentum	T62.2X1	T62.2X2	T62.2X3	T62.2X4	—	—
Lomotil	T47.6X1	T47.6X2	T47.6X3	T47.6X4	T47.6X5	T47.6X6
Lomustine	T45.1X1	T45.1X2	T45.1X3	T45.1X4	T45.1X5	T45.1X6
Lonidamine	T45.1X1	T45.1X2	T45.1X3	T45.1X4	T45.1X5	T45.1X6
Loperamide	T47.6X1	T47.6X2	T47.6X3	T47.6X4	T47.6X5	T47.6X6
Loprazolam	T42.4X1	T42.4X2	T42.4X3	T42.4X4	T42.4X5	T42.4X6
Lorajmine	T46.2X1	T46.2X2	T46.2X3	T46.2X4	T46.2X5	T46.2X6
Loratidine	T45.0X1	T45.0X2	T45.0X3	T45.0X4	T45.0X5	T45.0X6
Lorazepam	T42.4X1	T42.4X2	T42.4X3	T42.4X4	T42.4X5	T42.4X6
Lorcainide	T46.2X1	T46.2X2	T46.2X3	T46.2X4	T46.2X5	T46.2X6
Lormetazepam	T42.4X1	T42.4X2	T42.4X3	T42.4X4	T42.4X5	T42.4X6
Lotions NEC	T49.91	T49.92	T49.93	T49.94	T49.95	T49.96
Lotusate	T42.3X1	T42.3X2	T42.3X3	T42.3X4	T42.3X5	T42.3X6
Lovastatin	T46.6X1	T46.6X2	T46.6X3	T46.6X4	T46.6X5	T46.6X6
Lowila	T49.2X1	T49.2X2	T49.2X3	T49.2X4	T49.2X5	T49.2X6

Substance	Poisoning, Accidental (unintentional)	Poisoning, Intentional self-harm	Poisoning, Assault	Poisoning, Undetermined	Adverse effect	Underdosing
Loxapine	T43.591	T43.592	T43.593	T43.594	T43.595	T43.596
Lozenges (throat)	T49.6X1	T49.6X2	T49.6X3	T49.6X4	T49.6X5	T49.6X6
LSD	T40.8X1	T40.8X2	T40.8X3	T40.8X4	—	—
L-Tryptophan—see amino acid						
Lubricant, eye	T49.5X1	T49.5X2	T49.5X3	T49.5X4	T49.5X5	T49.5X6
Lubricating oil NEC	T52.0X1	T52.0X2	T52.0X3	T52.0X4	—	—
Lucanthone	T37.4X1	T37.4X2	T37.4X3	T37.4X4	T37.4X5	T37.4X6
Luminal	T42.3X1	T42.3X2	T42.3X3	T42.3X4	T42.3X5	T42.3X6
Lung irritant (gas) NEC	T59.91	T59.92	T59.93	T59.94	—	—
Luteinizing hormone	T38.811	T38.812	T38.813	T38.814	T38.815	T38.816
Lutocylol	T38.5X1	T38.5X2	T38.5X3	T38.5X4	T38.5X5	T38.5X6
Lutromone	T38.5X1	T38.5X2	T38.5X3	T38.5X4	T38.5X5	T38.5X6
Lututrin	T48.291	T48.292	T48.293	T48.294	T48.295	T48.296
Lye (concentrated)	T54.3X1	T54.3X2	T54.3X3	T54.3X4	—	—
Lygranum (skin test)	T50.8X1	T50.8X2	T50.8X3	T50.8X4	T50.8X5	T50.8X6
Lymecycline	T36.4X1	T36.4X2	T36.4X3	T36.4X4	T36.4X5	T36.4X6
Lymphogranuloma venereum antigen	T50.8X1	T50.8X2	T50.8X3	T50.8X4	T50.8X5	T50.8X6
Lynestrenol	T38.4X1	T38.4X2	T38.4X3	T38.4X4	T38.4X5	T38.4X6
Lyovac Sodium Edecrin	T50.1X1	T50.1X2	T50.1X3	T50.1X4	T50.1X5	T50.1X6
Lypressin	T38.891	T38.892	T38.893	T38.894	T38.895	T38.896
Lysergic acid diethylamide	T40.8X1	T40.8X2	T40.8X3	T40.8X4	—	—
Lysergide	T40.8X1	T40.8X2	T40.8X3	T40.8X4	—	—
Lysine vasopressin	T38.891	T38.892	T38.893	T38.894	T38.895	T38.896
Lysol	T54.1X1	T54.1X2	T54.1X3	T54.1X4	—	—
Lysozyme	T49.0X1	T49.0X2	T49.0X3	T49.0X4	T49.0X5	T49.0X6
Lytta (vitatta)	T49.8X1	T49.8X2	T49.8X3	T49.8X4	T49.8X5	T49.8X6
M						
Mace	T59.3X1	T59.3X2	T59.3X3	T59.3X4	—	—
Macrogol	T50.991	T50.992	T50.993	T50.994	T50.995	T50.996
Macrolide						
anabolic drug	T38.7X1	T38.7X2	T38.7X3	T38.7X4	T38.7X5	T38.7X6
antibiotic	T36.3X1	T36.3X2	T36.3X3	T36.3X4	T36.3X5	T36.3X6
Mafenide	T49.0X1	T49.0X2	T49.0X3	T49.0X4	T49.0X5	T49.0X6
Magaldrate	T47.1X1	T47.1X2	T47.1X3	T47.1X4	T47.1X5	T47.1X6
Magic mushroom	T40.991	T40.992	T40.993	T40.994	—	—
Magnamycin	T36.8X1	T36.8X2	T36.8X3	T36.8X4	T36.8X5	T36.8X6
Magnesia magma	T47.1X1	T47.1X2	T47.1X3	T47.1X4	T47.1X5	T47.1X6
Magnesium NEC	T56.891	T56.892	T56.893	T56.894	—	—
carbonate	T47.1X1	T47.1X2	T47.1X3	T47.1X4	T47.1X5	T47.1X6
citrate	T47.4X1	T47.4X2	T47.4X3	T47.4X4	T47.4X5	T47.4X6
hydroxide	T47.1X1	T47.1X2	T47.1X3	T47.1X4	T47.1X5	T47.1X6
oxide	T47.1X1	T47.1X2	T47.1X3	T47.1X4	T47.1X5	T47.1X6
peroxide	T49.0X1	T49.0X2	T49.0X3	T49.0X4	T49.0X5	T49.0X6
salicylate	T39.091	T39.092	T39.093	T39.094	T39.095	T39.096
silicofluoride	T50.3X1	T50.3X2	T50.3X3	T50.3X4	T50.3X5	T50.3X6
sulfate	T47.4X1	T47.4X2	T47.4X3	T47.4X4	T47.4X5	T47.4X6
thiosulfate	T45.0X1	T45.0X2	T45.0X3	T45.0X4	T45.0X5	T45.0X6
trisilicate	T47.1X1	T47.1X2	T47.1X3	T47.1X4	T47.1X5	T47.1X6

Substance	Poisoning, Accidental (unintentional)	Poisoning, Intentional self-harm	Poisoning, Assault	Poisoning, Undetermined	Adverse effect	Underdosing
Malathion (medicinal)	T49.0X1	T49.0X2	T49.0X3	T49.0X4	T49.0X5	T49.0X6
insecticide	T60.0X1	T60.0X2	T60.0X3	T60.0X4	—	—
Male fern extract	T37.4X1	T37.4X2	T37.4X3	T37.4X4	T37.4X5	T37.4X6
M-AMSA	T45.1X1	T45.1X2	T45.1X3	T45.1X4	T45.1X5	T45.1X6
Mandelic acid	T37.8X1	T37.8X2	T37.8X3	T37.8X4	T37.8X5	T37.8X6
Manganese (dioxide) (salts)	T57.2X1	T57.2X2	T57.2X3	T57.2X4	—	—
medicinal	T50.991	T50.992	T50.993	T50.994	T50.995	T50.996
Mannitol	T47.3X1	T47.3X2	T47.3X3	T47.3X4	T47.3X5	T47.3X6
hexanitrate	T46.3X1	T46.3X2	T46.3X3	T46.3X4	T46.3X5	T46.3X6
Mannomustine	T45.1X1	T45.1X2	T45.1X3	T45.1X4	T45.1X5	T45.1X6
MAO inhibitors	T43.1X1	T43.1X2	T43.1X3	T43.1X4	T43.1X5	T43.1X6
Mapharsen	T37.8X1	T37.8X2	T37.8X3	T37.8X4	T37.8X5	T37.8X6
Maphenide	T49.0X1	T49.0X2	T49.0X3	T49.0X4	T49.0X5	T49.0X6
Maprotiline	T43.021	T43.022	T43.023	T43.024	T43.025	T43.026
Marcaine	T41.3X1	T41.3X2	T41.3X3	T41.3X4	T41.3X5	T41.3X6
infiltration (subcutaneous)	T41.3X1	T41.3X2	T41.3X3	T41.3X4	T41.3X5	T41.3X6
nerve block (peripheral) (plexus)	T41.3X1	T41.3X2	T41.3X3	T41.3X4	T41.3X5	T41.3X6
Marezine	T45.0X1	T45.0X2	T45.0X3	T45.0X4	T45.0X5	T45.0X6
Marihuana	T40.711	T40.712	T40.713	T40.714	T40.715	T40.716
Marijuana	T40.711	T40.712	T40.713	T40.714	T40.715	T40.716
Marine (sting)	T63.691	T63.692	T63.693	T63.694	—	—
animals (sting)	T63.691	T63.692	T63.693	T63.694	—	—
plants (sting)	T63.711	T63.712	T63.713	T63.714	—	—
Marplan	T43.1X1	T43.1X2	T43.1X3	T43.1X4	T43.1X5	T43.1X6
Marsh gas	T59.891	T59.892	T59.893	T59.894	—	—
Marsilid	T43.1X1	T43.1X2	T43.1X3	T43.1X4	T43.1X5	T43.1X6
Matulane	T45.1X1	T45.1X2	T45.1X3	T45.1X4	T45.1X5	T45.1X6
Mazindol	T50.5X1	T50.5X2	T50.5X3	T50.5X4	T50.5X5	T50.5X6
MCPA	T60.3X1	T60.3X2	T60.3X3	T60.3X4	—	—
MDMA	T43.641	T43.642	T43.643	T43.644	—	—
Meadow saffron	T62.2X1	T62.2X2	T62.2X3	T62.2X4	—	—
Measles virus vaccine (attenuated)	T50.B91	T50.B92	T50.B93	T50.B94	T50.B95	T50.B96
Meat, noxious	T62.8X1	T62.8X2	T62.8X3	T62.8X4	—	—
Meballymal	T42.3X1	T42.3X2	T42.3X3	T42.3X4	T42.3X5	T42.3X6
Mebanazine	T43.1X1	T43.1X2	T43.1X3	T43.1X4	T43.1X5	T43.1X6
Mebaral	T42.3X1	T42.3X2	T42.3X3	T42.3X4	T42.3X5	T42.3X6
Mebendazole	T37.4X1	T37.4X2	T37.4X3	T37.4X4	T37.4X5	T37.4X6
Mebeverine	T44.3X1	T44.3X2	T44.3X3	T44.3X4	T44.3X5	T44.3X6
Mebhydrolin	T45.0X1	T45.0X2	T45.0X3	T45.0X4	T45.0X5	T45.0X6
Mebumal	T42.3X1	T42.3X2	T42.3X3	T42.3X4	T42.3X5	T42.3X6
Mebutamate	T43.591	T43.592	T43.593	T43.594	T43.595	T43.596
Mecamylamine	T44.2X1	T44.2X2	T44.2X3	T44.2X4	T44.2X5	T44.2X6
Mechlorethamine	T45.1X1	T45.1X2	T45.1X3	T45.1X4	T45.1X5	T45.1X6
Mecillinam	T36.0X1	T36.0X2	T36.0X3	T36.0X4	T36.0X5	T36.0X6
Meclizine (hydrochloride)	T45.0X1	T45.0X2	T45.0X3	T45.0X4	T45.0X5	T45.0X6
Meclocycline	T36.4X1	T36.4X2	T36.4X3	T36.4X4	T36.4X5	T36.4X6

Substance	Poisoning, Accidental (unintentional)	Poisoning, Intentional self-harm	Poisoning, Assault	Poisoning, Undetermined	Adverse effect	Underdosing
Meclofenamate	T39.391	T39.392	T39.393	T39.394	T39.395	T39.396
Meclofenamic acid	T39.391	T39.392	T39.393	T39.394	T39.395	T39.396
Meclofenoxate	T43.691	T43.692	T43.693	T43.694	T43.695	T43.696
Meclozine	T45.0X1	T45.0X2	T45.0X3	T45.0X4	T45.0X5	T45.0X6
Mecobalamin	T45.8X1	T45.8X2	T45.8X3	T45.8X4	T45.8X5	T45.8X6
Mecoprop	T60.3X1	T60.3X2	T60.3X3	T60.3X4	—	—
Mecrilate	T49.3X1	T49.3X2	T49.3X3	T49.3X4	T49.3X5	T49.3X6
Mecysteine	T48.4X1	T48.4X2	T48.4X3	T48.4X4	T48.4X5	T48.4X6
Medazepam	T42.4X1	T42.4X2	T42.4X3	T42.4X4	T42.4X5	T42.4X6
Medicament NEC	T50.901	T50.902	T50.903	T50.904	T50.905	T50.906
Medinal	T42.3X1	T42.3X2	T42.3X3	T42.3X4	T42.3X5	T42.3X6
Medomin	T42.3X1	T42.3X2	T42.3X3	T42.3X4	T42.3X5	T42.3X6
Medrogestone	T38.5X1	T38.5X2	T38.5X3	T38.5X4	T38.5X5	T38.5X6
Medroxalol	T44.8X1	T44.8X2	T44.8X3	T44.8X4	T44.8X5	T44.8X6
Medroxyprogesteron eacetate (depot)	T38.5X1	T38.5X2	T38.5X3	T38.5X4	T38.5X5	T38.5X6
Medrysone	T49.0X1	T49.0X2	T49.0X3	T49.0X4	T49.0X5	T49.0X6
Mefenamic acid	T39.391	T39.392	T39.393	T39.394	T39.395	T39.396
Mefenorex	T50.5X1	T50.5X2	T50.5X3	T50.5X4	T50.5X5	T50.5X6
Mefloquine	T37.2X1	T37.2X2	T37.2X3	T37.2X4	T37.2X5	T37.2X6
Mefruside	T50.2X1	T50.2X2	T50.2X3	T50.2X4	T50.2X5	T50.2X6
Megahallucinogen	T40.901	T40.902	T40.903	T40.904	T40.905	T40.906
Megestrol	T38.5X1	T38.5X2	T38.5X3	T38.5X4	T38.5X5	T38.5X6
Meglumine						
antimoniate	T37.8X1	T37.8X2	T37.8X3	T37.8X4	T37.8X5	T37.8X6
diatrizoate	T50.8X1	T50.8X2	T50.8X3	T50.8X4	T50.8X5	T50.8X6
iodipamide	T50.8X1	T50.8X2	T50.8X3	T50.8X4	T50.8X5	T50.8X6
iotroxate	T50.8X1	T50.8X2	T50.8X3	T50.8X4	T50.8X5	T50.8X6
MEK (methyl ethyl ketone)	T52.4X1	T52.4X2	T52.4X3	T52.4X4	—	—
Meladinin	T49.3X1	T49.3X2	T49.3X3	T49.3X4	T49.3X5	T49.3X6
Meladrazine	T44.3X1	T44.3X2	T44.3X3	T44.3X4	T44.3X5	T44.3X6
Melaleuca alternifolia oil	T49.0X1	T49.0X2	T49.0X3	T49.0X4	T49.0X5	T49.0X6
Melanizing agents	T49.3X1	T49.3X2	T49.3X3	T49.3X4	T49.3X5	T49.3X6
Melanocyte-stimulating hormone	T38.891	T38.892	T38.893	T38.894	T38.895	T38.896
Melarsonyl potassium	T37.3X1	T37.3X2	T37.3X3	T37.3X4	T37.3X5	T37.3X6
Melarsoprol	T37.3X1	T37.3X2	T37.3X3	T37.3X4	T37.3X5	T37.3X6
Melia azedarach	T62.2X1	T62.2X2	T62.2X3	T62.2X4	—	—
Melitracen	T43.011	T43.012	T43.013	T43.014	T43.015	T43.016
Mellaril	T43.3X1	T43.3X2	T43.3X3	T43.3X4	T43.3X5	T43.3X6
Meloxine	T49.3X1	T49.3X2	T49.3X3	T49.3X4	T49.3X5	T49.3X6
Melperone	T43.4X1	T43.4X2	T43.4X3	T43.4X4	T43.4X5	T43.4X6
Melphalan	T45.1X1	T45.1X2	T45.1X3	T45.1X4	T45.1X5	T45.1X6
Memantine	T43.8X1	T43.8X2	T43.8X3	T43.8X4	T43.8X5	T43.8X6
Menadiol	T45.7X1	T45.7X2	T45.7X3	T45.7X4	T45.7X5	T45.7X6
sodium sulfate	T45.7X1	T45.7X2	T45.7X3	T45.7X4	T45.7X5	T45.7X6
Menadione	T45.7X1	T45.7X2	T45.7X3	T45.7X4	T45.7X5	T45.7X6
sodium bisulfite	T45.7X1	T45.7X2	T45.7X3	T45.7X4	T45.7X5	T45.7X6

Substance	Poisoning, Accidental (unintentional)	Poisoning, Intentional self-harm	Poisoning, Assault	Poisoning, Undetermined	Adverse effect	Underdosing
Menaphthone	T45.7X1	T45.7X2	T45.7X3	T45.7X4	T45.7X5	T45.7X6
Menaquinone	T45.7X1	T45.7X2	T45.7X3	T45.7X4	T45.7X5	T45.7X6
Menatetrenone	T45.7X1	T45.7X2	T45.7X3	T45.7X4	T45.7X5	T45.7X6
Meningococcal vaccine	T50.A91	T50.A92	T50.A93	T50.A94	T50.A95	T50.A96
Menningovax (-AC) (-C)	T50.A91	T50.A92	T50.A93	T50.A94	T50.A95	T50.A96
Menotropins	T38.811	T38.812	T38.813	T38.814	T38.815	T38.816
Menthol	T48.5X1	T48.5X2	T48.5X3	T48.5X4	T48.5X5	T48.5X6
Mepacrine	T37.2X1	T37.2X2	T37.2X3	T37.2X4	T37.2X5	T37.2X6
Meparfynol	T42.6X1	T42.6X2	T42.6X3	T42.6X4	T42.6X5	T42.6X6
Mepartricin	T36.7X1	T36.7X2	T36.7X3	T36.7X4	T36.7X5	T36.7X6
Mepazine	T43.3X1	T43.3X2	T43.3X3	T43.3X4	T43.3X5	T43.3X6
Mepenzolate	T44.3X1	T44.3X2	T44.3X3	T44.3X4	T44.3X5	T44.3X6
bromide	T44.3X1	T44.3X2	T44.3X3	T44.3X4	T44.3X5	T44.3X6
Meperidine	T40.491	T40.492	T40.493	T40.494	T40.495	T40.496
Mephebarbital	T42.3X1	T42.3X2	T42.3X3	T42.3X4	T42.3X5	T42.3X6
Mephenamin (e)	T42.8X1	T42.8X2	T42.8X3	T42.8X4	T42.8X5	T42.8X6
Mephenesin	T42.8X1	T42.8X2	T42.8X3	T42.8X4	T42.8X5	T42.8X6
Mephenhydramine	T45.0X1	T45.0X2	T45.0X3	T45.0X4	T45.0X5	T45.0X6
Mephenoxalone	T42.8X1	T42.8X2	T42.8X3	T42.8X4	T42.8X5	T42.8X6
Mephentermine	T44.991	T44.992	T44.993	T44.994	T44.995	T44.996
Mephenytoin	T42.0X1	T42.0X2	T42.0X3	T42.0X4	T42.0X5	T42.0X6
with phenobarbital	T42.3X1	T42.3X2	T42.3X3	T42.3X4	T42.3X5	T42.3X6
Mephobarbital	T42.3X1	T42.3X2	T42.3X3	T42.3X4	T42.3X5	T42.3X6
Mephosfolan	T60.0X1	T60.0X2	T60.0X3	T60.0X4	—	—
Mepindolol	T44.7X1	T44.7X2	T44.7X3	T44.7X4	T44.7X5	T44.7X6
Mepiperphenidol	T44.3X1	T44.3X2	T44.3X3	T44.3X4	T44.3X5	T44.3X6
Mepitiostane	T38.7X1	T38.7X2	T38.7X3	T38.7X4	T38.7X5	T38.7X6
Mepivacaine	T41.3X1	T41.3X2	T41.3X3	T41.3X4	T41.3X5	T41.3X6
epidural	T41.3X1	T41.3X2	T41.3X3	T41.3X4	T41.3X5	T41.3X6
Meprednisone	T38.0X1	T38.0X2	T38.0X3	T38.0X4	T38.0X5	T38.0X6
Meprobam	T43.591	T43.592	T43.593	T43.594	T43.595	T43.596
Meprobamate	T43.591	T43.592	T43.593	T43.594	T43.595	T43.596
Meproscillarin	T46.0X1	T46.0X2	T46.0X3	T46.0X4	T46.0X5	T46.0X6
Meprylcaine	T41.3X1	T41.3X2	T41.3X3	T41.3X4	T41.3X5	T41.3X6
Meptazinol	T39.8X1	T39.8X2	T39.8X3	T39.8X4	T39.8X5	T39.8X6
Mepyramine	T45.0X1	T45.0X2	T45.0X3	T45.0X4	T45.0X5	T45.0X6
Mequitazine	T43.3X1	T43.3X2	T43.3X3	T43.3X4	T43.3X5	T43.3X6
Meralluride	T50.2X1	T50.2X2	T50.2X3	T50.2X4	T50.2X5	T50.2X6
Merbaphen	T50.2X1	T50.2X2	T50.2X3	T50.2X4	T50.2X5	T50.2X6
Merbromin	T49.0X1	T49.0X2	T49.0X3	T49.0X4	T49.0X5	T49.0X6
Mercaptoben-zothiazole salts	T49.0X1	T49.0X2	T49.0X3	T49.0X4	T49.0X5	T49.0X6
Mercaptomerin	T50.2X1	T50.2X2	T50.2X3	T50.2X4	T50.2X5	T50.2X6
Mercaptopurine	T45.1X1	T45.1X2	T45.1X3	T45.1X4	T45.1X5	T45.1X6
Mercumatilin	T50.2X1	T50.2X2	T50.2X3	T50.2X4	T50.2X5	T50.2X6
Mercuramide	T50.2X1	T50.2X2	T50.2X3	T50.2X4	T50.2X5	T50.2X6
Mercurochrome	T49.0X1	T49.0X2	T49.0X3	T49.0X4	T49.0X5	T49.0X6
Mercurophylline	T50.2X1	T50.2X2	T50.2X3	T50.2X4	T50.2X5	T50.2X6

Substance	Poisoning, Accidental (unintentional)	Poisoning, Intentional self-harm	Poisoning, Assault	Poisoning, Undetermined	Adverse effect	Underdosing
Mercury, mercurial, mercuric, mercurous (compounds) (cyanide) (fumes) (nonmedicinal) (vapor) NEC	T56.1X1	T56.1X2	T56.1X3	T56.1X4	—	—
ammoniated	T49.0X1	T49.0X2	T49.0X3	T49.0X4	T49.0X5	T49.0X6
anti-infective						
local	T49.0X1	T49.0X2	T49.0X3	T49.0X4	T49.0X5	T49.0X6
systemic	T37.8X1	T37.8X2	T37.8X3	T37.8X4	T37.8X5	T37.8X6
topical	T49.0X1	T49.0X2	T49.0X3	T49.0X4	T49.0X5	T49.0X6
chloride (ammoniated)	T49.0X1	T49.0X2	T49.0X3	T49.0X4	T49.0X5	T49.0X6
fungicide	T56.1X1	T56.1X2	T56.1X3	T56.1X4	—	—
diuretic NEC	T50.2X1	T50.2X2	T50.2X3	T50.2X4	T50.2X5	T50.2X6
fungicide	T56.1X1	T56.1X2	T56.1X3	T56.1X4	—	—
organic (fungicide)	T56.1X1	T56.1X2	T56.1X3	T56.1X4	—	—
oxide, yellow	T49.0X1	T49.0X2	T49.0X3	T49.0X4	T49.0X5	T49.0X6
Mersalyl	T50.2X1	T50.2X2	T50.2X3	T50.2X4	T50.2X5	T50.2X6
Merthiolate	T49.0X1	T49.0X2	T49.0X3	T49.0X4	T49.0X5	T49.0X6
ophthalmic preparation	T49.5X1	T49.5X2	T49.5X3	T49.5X4	T49.5X5	T49.5X6
Meruvax	T50.B91	T50.B92	T50.B93	T50.B94	T50.B95	T50.B96
Mesalazine	T47.8X1	T47.8X2	T47.8X3	T47.8X4	T47.8X5	T47.8X6
Mescal buttons	T40.991	T40.992	T40.993	T40.994	—	—
Mescaline	T40.991	T40.992	T40.993	T40.994	—	—
Mesna	T48.4X1	T48.4X2	T48.4X3	T48.4X4	T48.4X5	T48.4X6
Mesoglycan	T46.6X1	T46.6X2	T46.6X3	T46.6X4	T46.6X5	T46.6X6
Mesoridazine	T43.3X1	T43.3X2	T43.3X3	T43.3X4	T43.3X5	T43.3X6
Mestanolone	T38.7X1	T38.7X2	T38.7X3	T38.7X4	T38.7X5	T38.7X6
Mesterolone	T38.7X1	T38.7X2	T38.7X3	T38.7X4	T38.7X5	T38.7X6
Mestranol	T38.5X1	T38.5X2	T38.5X3	T38.5X4	T38.5X5	T38.5X6
Mesulergine	T42.8X1	T42.8X2	T42.8X3	T42.8X4	T42.8X5	T42.8X6
Mesulfen	T49.0X1	T49.0X2	T49.0X3	T49.0X4	T49.0X5	T49.0X6
Mesuximide	T42.2X1	T42.2X2	T42.2X3	T42.2X4	T42.2X5	T42.2X6
Metabutethamine	T41.3X1	T41.3X2	T41.3X3	T41.3X4	T41.3X5	T41.3X6
Metactesylacetate	T49.0X1	T49.0X2	T49.0X3	T49.0X4	T49.0X5	T49.0X6
Metacycline	T36.4X1	T36.4X2	T36.4X3	T36.4X4	T36.4X5	T36.4X6
Metaldehyde (snail killer) NEC	T60.8X1	T60.8X2	T60.8X3	T60.8X4	—	—
Metals (heavy) (nonmedicinal)	T56.91	T56.92	T56.93	T56.94	—	—
dust, fumes, or vapor NEC	T56.91	T56.92	T56.93	T56.94	—	—
light NEC	T56.91	T56.92	T56.93	T56.94	—	—
dust, fumes, or vapor NEC	T56.91	T56.92	T56.93	T56.94	—	—
specified NEC	T56.891	T56.892	T56.893	T56.894	—	—
thallium	T56.811	T56.812	T56.813	T56.814	—	—
Metamfetamine	T43.621	T43.622	T43.623	T43.624	T43.625	T43.626
Metamizole sodium	T39.2X1	T39.2X2	T39.2X3	T39.2X4	T39.2X5	T39.2X6
Metampicillin	T36.0X1	T36.0X2	T36.0X3	T36.0X4	T36.0X5	T36.0X6
Metamucil	T47.4X1	T47.4X2	T47.4X3	T47.4X4	T47.4X5	T47.4X6
Metandienone	T38.7X1	T38.7X2	T38.7X3	T38.7X4	T38.7X5	T38.7X6
Metandrostenolone	T38.7X1	T38.7X2	T38.7X3	T38.7X4	T38.7X5	T38.7X6
Metaphen	T49.0X1	T49.0X2	T49.0X3	T49.0X4	T49.0X5	T49.0X6
Metaphos	T60.0X1	T60.0X2	T60.0X3	T60.0X4	—	—
Metapramine	T43.011	T43.012	T43.013	T43.014	T43.015	T43.016
Metaproterenol	T48.291	T48.292	T48.293	T48.294	T48.295	T48.296
Metaraminol	T44.4X1	T44.4X2	T44.4X3	T44.4X4	T44.4X5	T44.4X6
Metaxalone	T42.8X1	T42.8X2	T42.8X3	T42.8X4	T42.8X5	T42.8X6
Metenolone	T38.7X1	T38.7X2	T38.7X3	T38.7X4	T38.7X5	T38.7X6
Metergoline	T42.8X1	T42.8X2	T42.8X3	T42.8X4	T42.8X5	T42.8X6
Metescufylline	T46.991	T46.992	T46.993	T46.994	T46.995	T46.996
Metetoin	T42.0X1	T42.0X2	T42.0X3	T42.0X4	T42.0X5	T42.0X6
Metformin	T38.3X1	T38.3X2	T38.3X3	T38.3X4	T38.3X5	T38.3X6
Methacholine	T44.1X1	T44.1X2	T44.1X3	T44.1X4	T44.1X5	T44.1X6
Methacycline	T36.4X1	T36.4X2	T36.4X3	T36.4X4	T36.4X5	T36.4X6
Methadone	T40.3X1	T40.3X2	T40.3X3	T40.3X4	T40.3X5	T40.3X6
Methallenestril	T38.5X1	T38.5X2	T38.5X3	T38.5X4	T38.5X5	T38.5X6
Methallenoestril	T38.5X1	T38.5X2	T38.5X3	T38.5X4	T38.5X5	T38.5X6
Methamphetamine	T43.621	T43.622	T43.623	T43.624	T43.625	T43.626
Methampyrone	T39.2X1	T39.2X2	T39.2X3	T39.2X4	T39.2X5	T39.2X6
Methandienone	T38.7X1	T38.7X2	T38.7X3	T38.7X4	T38.7X5	T38.7X6
Methandriol	T38.7X1	T38.7X2	T38.7X3	T38.7X4	T38.7X5	T38.7X6
Methandrostenolone	T38.7X1	T38.7X2	T38.7X3	T38.7X4	T38.7X5	T38.7X6
Methane	T59.891	T59.892	T59.893	T59.894	—	—
Methanethiol	T59.891	T59.892	T59.893	T59.894	—	—
Methaniazide	T37.1X1	T37.1X2	T37.1X3	T37.1X4	T37.1X5	T37.1X6
Methanol (vapor)	T51.1X1	T51.1X2	T51.1X3	T51.1X4	—	—
Methantheline	T44.3X1	T44.3X2	T44.3X3	T44.3X4	T44.3X5	T44.3X6
Methanthelinium bromide	T44.3X1	T44.3X2	T44.3X3	T44.3X4	T44.3X5	T44.3X6
Methaphenilene	T45.0X1	T45.0X2	T45.0X3	T45.0X4	T45.0X5	T45.0X6
Methapyrilene	T45.0X1	T45.0X2	T45.0X3	T45.0X4	T45.0X5	T45.0X6
Methaqualone (compound)	T42.6X1	T42.6X2	T42.6X3	T42.6X4	T42.6X5	T42.6X6
Metharbital	T42.3X1	T42.3X2	T42.3X3	T42.3X4	T42.3X5	T42.3X6
Methazolamide	T50.2X1	T50.2X2	T50.2X3	T50.2X4	T50.2X5	T50.2X6
Methdilazine	T43.3X1	T43.3X2	T43.3X3	T43.3X4	T43.3X5	T43.3X6
Methedrine	T43.621	T43.622	T43.623	T43.624	T43.625	T43.626
Methenamine (mandelate)	T37.8X1	T37.8X2	T37.8X3	T37.8X4	T37.8X5	T37.8X6
Methenolone	T38.7X1	T38.7X2	T38.7X3	T38.7X4	T38.7X5	T38.7X6
Methergine	T48.0X1	T48.0X2	T48.0X3	T48.0X4	T48.0X5	T48.0X6
Methetoin	T42.0X1	T42.0X2	T42.0X3	T42.0X4	T42.0X5	T42.0X6
Methiacil	T38.2X1	T38.2X2	T38.2X3	T38.2X4	T38.2X5	T38.2X6
Methicillin	T36.0X1	T36.0X2	T36.0X3	T36.0X4	T36.0X5	T36.0X6
Methimazole	T38.2X1	T38.2X2	T38.2X3	T38.2X4	T38.2X5	T38.2X6
Methiodal sodium	T50.8X1	T50.8X2	T50.8X3	T50.8X4	T50.8X5	T50.8X6
Methionine	T50.991	T50.992	T50.993	T50.994	T50.995	T50.996
Methisazone	T37.5X1	T37.5X2	T37.5X3	T37.5X4	T37.5X5	T37.5X6
Methisoprinol	T37.5X1	T37.5X2	T37.5X3	T37.5X4	T37.5X5	T37.5X6
Methitural	T42.3X1	T42.3X2	T42.3X3	T42.3X4	T42.3X5	T42.3X6
Methixene	T44.3X1	T44.3X2	T44.3X3	T44.3X4	T44.3X5	T44.3X6
Methobarbital, methobarbitone	T42.3X1	T42.3X2	T42.3X3	T42.3X4	T42.3X5	T42.3X6

Substance	Poisoning, Accidental (unintentional)	Poisoning, Intentional self-harm	Poisoning, Assault	Poisoning, Undetermined	Adverse effect	Underdosing
Methocarbamol	T42.8X1	T42.8X2	T42.8X3	T42.8X4	T42.8X5	T42.8X6
skeletal muscle relaxant	T48.1X1	T48.1X2	T48.1X3	T48.1X4	T48.1X5	T48.1X6
Methohexital	T41.1X1	T41.1X2	T41.1X3	T41.1X4	T41.1X5	T41.1X6
Methohexitone	T41.1X1	T41.1X2	T41.1X3	T41.1X4	T41.1X5	T41.1X6
Methoin	T42.0X1	T42.0X2	T42.0X3	T42.0X4	T42.0X5	T42.0X6
Methopholine	T39.8X1	T39.8X2	T39.8X3	T39.8X4	T39.8X5	T39.8X6
Methopromazine	T43.3X1	T43.3X2	T43.3X3	T43.3X4	T43.3X5	T43.3X6
Methorate	T48.3X1	T48.3X2	T48.3X3	T48.3X4	T48.3X5	T48.3X6
Methoserpidine	T46.5X1	T46.5X2	T46.5X3	T46.5X4	T46.5X5	T46.5X6
Methotrexate	T45.1X1	T45.1X2	T45.1X3	T45.1X4	T45.1X5	T45.1X6
Methotrimeprazine	T43.3X1	T43.3X2	T43.3X3	T43.3X4	T43.3X5	T43.3X6
Methoxa-Dome	T49.3X1	T49.3X2	T49.3X3	T49.3X4	T49.3X5	T49.3X6
Methoxamine	T44.4X1	T44.4X2	T44.4X3	T44.4X4	T44.4X5	T44.4X6
Methoxsalen	T50.991	T50.992	T50.993	T50.994	T50.995	T50.996
Methoxyaniline	T65.3X1	T65.3X2	T65.3X3	T65.3X4	—	—
Methoxybenzyl penicillin	T36.0X1	T36.0X2	T36.0X3	T36.0X4	T36.0X5	T36.0X6
Methoxychlor	T53.7X1	T53.7X2	T53.7X3	T53.7X4	—	—
Methoxy-DDT	T53.7X1	T53.7X2	T53.7X3	T53.7X4	—	—
2-Methoxyethanol	T52.3X1	T52.3X2	T52.3X3	T52.3X4	—	—
Methoxyflurane	T41.0X1	T41.0X2	T41.0X3	T41.0X4	T41.0X5	T41.0X6
Methoxyphenamine	T48.6X1	T48.6X2	T48.6X3	T48.6X4	T48.6X5	T48.6X6
Methoxypromazine	T43.3X1	T43.3X2	T43.3X3	T43.3X4	T43.3X5	T43.3X6
5-Methoxypsoralen (5-MOP)	T50.991	T50.992	T50.993	T50.994	T50.995	T50.996
8-Methoxypsoralen (8-MOP)	T50.991	T50.992	T50.993	T50.994	T50.995	T50.996
Methscopolamine bromide	T44.3X1	T44.3X2	T44.3X3	T44.3X4	T44.3X5	T44.3X6
Methsuximide	T42.2X1	T42.2X2	T42.2X3	T42.2X4	T42.2X5	T42.2X6
Methyclothiazide	T50.2X1	T50.2X2	T50.2X3	T50.2X4	T50.2X5	T50.2X6
Methyl						
acetate	T52.4X1	T52.4X2	T52.4X3	T52.4X4	—	—
acetone	T52.4X1	T52.4X2	T52.4X3	T52.4X4	—	—
acrylate	T65.891	T65.892	T65.893	T65.894	—	—
alcohol	T51.1X1	T51.1X2	T51.1X3	T51.1X4	—	—
aminophenol	T65.3X1	T65.3X2	T65.3X3	T65.3X4	—	—
amphetamine	T43.621	T43.622	T43.623	T43.624	T43.625	T43.626
androstanolone	T38.7X1	T38.7X2	T38.7X3	T38.7X4	T38.7X5	T38.7X6
atropine	T44.3X1	T44.3X2	T44.3X3	T44.3X4	T44.3X5	T44.3X6
benzene	T52.2X1	T52.2X2	T52.2X3	T52.2X4	—	—
benzoate	T52.8X1	T52.8X2	T52.8X3	T52.8X4	—	—
benzol	T52.2X1	T52.2X2	T52.2X3	T52.2X4	—	—
bromide (gas)	T59.891	T59.892	T59.893	T59.894	—	—
fumigant	T60.8X1	T60.8X2	T60.8X3	T60.8X4	—	—
butanol	T51.3X1	T51.3X2	T51.3X3	T51.3X4	—	—
carbinol	T51.1X1	T51.1X2	T51.1X3	T51.1X4	—	—
carbonate	T52.8X1	T52.8X2	T52.8X3	T52.8X4	—	—
CCNU	T45.1X1	T45.1X2	T45.1X3	T45.1X4	T45.1X5	T45.1X6
cellosolve	T52.91	T52.92	T52.93	T52.94	—	—
cellulose	T47.4X1	T47.4X2	T47.4X3	T47.4X4	T47.4X5	T47.4X6

Substance	Poisoning, Accidental (unintentional)	Poisoning, Intentional self-harm	Poisoning, Assault	Poisoning, Undetermined	Adverse effect	Underdosing
Methyl — *Continued*						
chloride (gas)	T59.891	T59.892	T59.893	T59.894	—	—
chloroformate	T59.3X1	T59.3X2	T59.3X3	T59.3X4	—	—
cyclohexane	T52.8X1	T52.8X2	T52.8X3	T52.8X4	—	—
cyclohexanol	T51.8X1	T51.8X2	T51.8X3	T51.8X4	—	—
cyclohexanone	T52.8X1	T52.8X2	T52.8X3	T52.8X4	—	—
cyclohexyl acetate	T52.8X1	T52.8X2	T52.8X3	T52.8X4	—	—
demeton	T60.0X1	T60.0X2	T60.0X3	T60.0X4	—	—
dihydromorphinone	T40.2X1	T40.2X2	T40.2X3	T40.2X4	T40.2X5	T40.2X6
ergometrine	T48.0X1	T48.0X2	T48.0X3	T48.0X4	T48.0X5	T48.0X6
ergonovine	T48.0X1	T48.0X2	T48.0X3	T48.0X4	T48.0X5	T48.0X6
ethyl ketone	T52.4X1	T52.4X2	T52.4X3	T52.4X4	—	—
glucamine antimonate	T37.8X1	T37.8X2	T37.8X3	T37.8X4	T37.8X5	T37.8X6
hydrazine	T65.891	T65.892	T65.893	T65.894	—	—
iodide	T65.891	T65.892	T65.893	T65.894	—	—
isobutyl ketone	T52.4X1	T52.4X2	T52.4X3	T52.4X4	—	—
isothiocyanate	T60.3X1	T60.3X2	T60.3X3	T60.3X4	—	—
mercaptan	T59.891	T59.892	T59.893	T59.894	—	—
morphine NEC	T40.2X1	T40.2X2	T40.2X3	T40.2X4	T40.2X5	T40.2X6
nicotinate	T49.4X1	T49.4X2	T49.4X3	T49.4X4	T49.4X5	T49.4X6
paraben	T49.0X1	T49.0X2	T49.0X3	T49.0X4	T49.0X5	T49.0X6
parafynol	T42.6X1	T42.6X2	T42.6X3	T42.6X4	T42.6X5	T42.6X6
parathion	T60.0X1	T60.0X2	T60.0X3	T60.0X4	—	—
peridol	T43.4X1	T43.4X2	T43.4X3	T43.4X4	T43.4X5	T43.4X6
phenidate	T43.631	T43.632	T43.633	T43.634	T43.635	T43.636
prednisolone	T38.0X1	T38.0X2	T38.0X3	T38.0X4	T38.0X5	T38.0X6
ENT agent	T49.6X1	T49.6X2	T49.6X3	T49.6X4	T49.6X5	T49.6X6
ophthalmic preparation	T49.5X1	T49.5X2	T49.5X3	T49.5X4	T49.5X5	T49.5X6
topical NEC	T49.0X1	T49.0X2	T49.0X3	T49.0X4	T49.0X5	T49.0X6
propylcarbinol	T51.3X1	T51.3X2	T51.3X3	T51.3X4	—	—
rosaniline NEC	T49.0X1	T49.0X2	T49.0X3	T49.0X4	T49.0X5	T49.0X6
salicylate	T49.2X1	T49.2X2	T49.2X3	T49.2X4	T49.2X5	T49.2X6
sulfate (fumes)	T59.891	T59.892	T59.893	T59.894	—	—
liquid	T52.8X1	T52.8X2	T52.8X3	T52.8X4	—	—
sulfonal	T42.6X1	T42.6X2	T42.6X3	T42.6X4	T42.6X5	T42.6X6
testosterone	T38.7X1	T38.7X2	T38.7X3	T38.7X4	T38.7X5	T38.7X6
thiouracil	T38.2X1	T38.2X2	T38.2X3	T38.2X4	T38.2X5	T38.2X6
Methylamphetamine	T43.621	T43.622	T43.623	T43.624	T43.625	T43.626
Methylated spirit	T51.1X1	T51.1X2	T51.1X3	T51.1X4	—	—
Methylatropine nitrate	T44.3X1	T44.3X2	T44.3X3	T44.3X4	T44.3X5	T44.3X6
Methylbenactyzium bromide	T44.3X1	T44.3X2	T44.3X3	T44.3X4	T44.3X5	T44.3X6
Methylbenzethonium chloride	T49.0X1	T49.0X2	T49.0X3	T49.0X4	T49.0X5	T49.0X6
Methylcellulose	T47.4X1	T47.4X2	T47.4X3	T47.4X4	T47.4X5	T47.4X6
laxative	T47.4X1	T47.4X2	T47.4X3	T47.4X4	T47.4X5	T47.4X6
Methylchlorophenoxy-acetic acid	T60.3X1	T60.3X2	T60.3X3	T60.3X4	—	—
Methyldopa	T46.5X1	T46.5X2	T46.5X3	T46.5X4	T46.5X5	T46.5X6
Methyldopate	T46.5X1	T46.5X2	T46.5X3	T46.5X4	T46.5X5	T46.5X6

Substance	Poisoning, Accidental (unintentional)	Poisoning, Intentional self-harm	Poisoning, Assault	Poisoning, Undetermined	Adverse effect	Underdosing
Methylene						
blue	T50.6X1	T50.6X2	T50.6X3	T50.6X4	T50.6X5	T50.6X6
chloride or dichloride (solvent) NEC	T53.4X1	T53.4X2	T53.4X3	T53.4X4	—	—
Methylenedioxy-amphetamine	T43.621	T43.622	T43.623	T43.624	T43.625	T43.626
Methylenedioxy-methamphetamine	T43.641	T43.642	T43.643	T43.644	—	—
Methylergometrine	T48.0X1	T48.0X2	T48.0X3	T48.0X4	T48.0X5	T48.0X6
Methylergonovine	T48.0X1	T48.0X2	T48.0X3	T48.0X4	T48.0X5	T48.0X6
Methylestrenolone	T38.5X1	T38.5X2	T38.5X3	T38.5X4	T38.5X5	T38.5X6
Methylethyl cellulose	T50.991	T50.992	T50.993	T50.994	T50.995	T50.996
Methylhexabital	T42.3X1	T42.3X2	T42.3X3	T42.3X4	T42.3X5	T42.3X6
Methylmorphine	T40.2X1	T40.2X2	T40.2X3	T40.2X4	T40.2X5	T40.2X6
Methylparaben (ophthalmic)	T49.5X1	T49.5X2	T49.5X3	T49.5X4	T49.5X5	T49.5X6
Methylparafynol	T42.6X1	T42.6X2	T42.6X3	T42.6X4	T42.6X5	T42.6X6
Methylpentynol, methylpenthynol	T42.6X1	T42.6X2	T42.6X3	T42.6X4	T42.6X5	T42.6X6
Methylphenidate	T43.631	T43.632	T43.633	T43.634	T43.635	T43.636
Methylphenobarbital	T42.3X1	T42.3X2	T42.3X3	T42.3X4	T42.3X5	T42.3X6
Methylpolysiloxane	T47.1X1	T47.1X2	T47.1X3	T47.1X4	T47.1X5	T47.1X6
Methylprednisolone—see Methyl, prednisolone						
Methylrosaniline	T49.0X1	T49.0X2	T49.0X3	T49.0X4	T49.0X5	T49.0X6
Methylrosanilinium chloride	T49.0X1	T49.0X2	T49.0X3	T49.0X4	T49.0X5	T49.0X6
Methyltestosterone	T38.7X1	T38.7X2	T38.7X3	T38.7X4	T38.7X5	T38.7X6
Methylthionine chloride	T50.6X1	T50.6X2	T50.6X3	T50.6X4	T50.6X5	T50.6X6
Methylthioninium chloride	T50.6X1	T50.6X2	T50.6X3	T50.6X4	T50.6X5	T50.6X6
Methylthiouracil	T38.2X1	T38.2X2	T38.2X3	T38.2X4	T38.2X5	T38.2X6
Methyprylon	T42.6X1	T42.6X2	T42.6X3	T42.6X4	T42.6X5	T42.6X6
Methysergide	T46.5X1	T46.5X2	T46.5X3	T46.5X4	T46.5X5	T46.5X6
Metiamide	T47.1X1	T47.1X2	T47.1X3	T47.1X4	T47.1X5	T47.1X6
Meticillin	T36.0X1	T36.0X2	T36.0X3	T36.0X4	T36.0X5	T36.0X6
Meticrane	T50.2X1	T50.2X2	T50.2X3	T50.2X4	T50.2X5	T50.2X6
Metildigoxin	T46.0X1	T46.0X2	T46.0X3	T46.0X4	T46.0X5	T46.0X6
Metipranolol	T49.5X1	T49.5X2	T49.5X3	T49.5X4	T49.5X5	T49.5X6
Metirosine	T46.5X1	T46.5X2	T46.5X3	T46.5X4	T46.5X5	T46.5X6
Metisazone	T37.5X1	T37.5X2	T37.5X3	T37.5X4	T37.5X5	T37.5X6
Metixene	T44.3X1	T44.3X2	T44.3X3	T44.3X4	T44.3X5	T44.3X6
Metizoline	T48.5X1	T48.5X2	T48.5X3	T48.5X4	T48.5X5	T48.5X6
Metoclopramide	T45.0X1	T45.0X2	T45.0X3	T45.0X4	T45.0X5	T45.0X6
Metofenazate	T43.3X1	T43.3X2	T43.3X3	T43.3X4	T43.3X5	T43.3X6
Metofoline	T39.8X1	T39.8X2	T39.8X3	T39.8X4	T39.8X5	T39.8X6
Metolazone	T50.2X1	T50.2X2	T50.2X3	T50.2X4	T50.2X5	T50.2X6
Metopon	T40.2X1	T40.2X2	T40.2X3	T40.2X4	T40.2X5	T40.2X6
Metoprine	T45.1X1	T45.1X2	T45.1X3	T45.1X4	T45.1X5	T45.1X6
Metoprolol	T44.7X1	T44.7X2	T44.7X3	T44.7X4	T44.7X5	T44.7X6
Metrifonate	T60.0X1	T60.0X2	T60.0X3	T60.0X4	—	—
Metrizamide	T50.8X1	T50.8X2	T50.8X3	T50.8X4	T50.8X5	T50.8X6
Metrizoic acid	T50.8X1	T50.8X2	T50.8X3	T50.8X4	T50.8X5	T50.8X6

Substance	Poisoning, Accidental (unintentional)	Poisoning, Intentional self-harm	Poisoning, Assault	Poisoning, Undetermined	Adverse effect	Underdosing
Metronidazole	T37.8X1	T37.8X2	T37.8X3	T37.8X4	T37.8X5	T37.8X6
Metycaine	T41.3X1	T41.3X2	T41.3X3	T41.3X4	T41.3X5	T41.3X6
infiltration (subcutaneous)	T41.3X1	T41.3X2	T41.3X3	T41.3X4	T41.3X5	T41.3X6
nerve block (peripheral) (plexus)	T41.3X1	T41.3X2	T41.3X3	T41.3X4	T41.3X5	T41.3X6
topical (surface)	T41.3X1	T41.3X2	T41.3X3	T41.3X4	T41.3X5	T41.3X6
Metyrapone	T50.8X1	T50.8X2	T50.8X3	T50.8X4	T50.8X5	T50.8X6
Mevinphos	T60.0X1	T60.0X2	T60.0X3	T60.0X4	—	—
Mexazolam	T42.4X1	T42.4X2	T42.4X3	T42.4X4	T42.4X5	T42.4X6
Mexenone	T49.3X1	T49.3X2	T49.3X3	T49.3X4	T49.3X5	T49.3X6
Mexiletine	T46.2X1	T46.2X2	T46.2X3	T46.2X4	T46.2X5	T46.2X6
Mezereon	T62.2X1	T62.2X2	T62.2X3	T62.2X4	—	—
berries	T62.1X1	T62.1X2	T62.1X3	T62.1X4	—	—
Mezlocillin	T36.0X1	T36.0X2	T36.0X3	T36.0X4	T36.0X5	T36.0X6
Mianserin	T43.021	T43.022	T43.023	T43.024	T43.025	T43.026
Micatin	T49.0X1	T49.0X2	T49.0X3	T49.0X4	T49.0X5	T49.0X6
Miconazole	T49.0X1	T49.0X2	T49.0X3	T49.0X4	T49.0X5	T49.0X6
Micronomicin	T36.5X1	T36.5X2	T36.5X3	T36.5X4	T36.5X5	T36.5X6
Midazolam	T42.4X1	T42.4X2	T42.4X3	T42.4X4	T42.4X5	T42.4X6
Midecamycin	T36.3X1	T36.3X2	T36.3X3	T36.3X4	T36.3X5	T36.3X6
Mifepristone	T38.6X1	T38.6X2	T38.6X3	T38.6X4	T38.6X5	T38.6X6
Milk of magnesia	T47.1X1	T47.1X2	T47.1X3	T47.1X4	T47.1X5	T47.1X6
Millipede (tropical) (venomous)	T63.411	T63.412	T63.413	T63.414	—	—
Miltown	T43.591	T43.592	T43.593	T43.594	T43.595	T43.596
Milverine	T44.3X1	T44.3X2	T44.3X3	T44.3X4	T44.3X5	T44.3X6
Minaprine	T43.291	T43.292	T43.293	T43.294	T43.295	T43.296
Minaxolone	T41.291	T41.292	T41.293	T41.294	T41.295	T41.296
Mineral						
acids	T54.2X1	T54.2X2	T54.2X3	T54.2X4	—	—
oil (laxative) (medicinal)	T47.4X1	T47.4X2	T47.4X3	T47.4X4	T47.4X5	T47.4X6
emulsion	T47.2X1	T47.2X2	T47.2X3	T47.2X4	T47.2X5	T47.2X6
nonmedicinal	T52.0X1	T52.0X2	T52.0X3	T52.0X4	—	—
topical	T49.3X1	T49.3X2	T49.3X3	T49.3X4	T49.3X5	T49.3X6
salt NEC	T50.3X1	T50.3X2	T50.3X3	T50.3X4	T50.3X5	T50.3X6
spirits	T52.0X1	T52.0X2	T52.0X3	T52.0X4	—	—
Mineralocorticosteroid	T50.0X1	T50.0X2	T50.0X3	T50.0X4	T50.0X5	T50.0X6
Minocycline	T36.4X1	T36.4X2	T36.4X3	T36.4X4	T36.4X5	T36.4X6
Minoxidil	T46.7X1	T46.7X2	T46.7X3	T46.7X4	T46.7X5	T46.7X6
Miokamycin	T36.3X1	T36.3X2	T36.3X3	T36.3X4	T36.3X5	T36.3X6
Miotic drug	T49.5X1	T49.5X2	T49.5X3	T49.5X4	T49.5X5	T49.5X6
Mipafox	T60.0X1	T60.0X2	T60.0X3	T60.0X4	—	—
Mirex	T60.1X1	T60.1X2	T60.1X3	T60.1X4	—	—
Mirtazapine	T43.021	T43.022	T43.023	T43.024	T43.025	T43.026
Misonidazole	T37.3X1	T37.3X2	T37.3X3	T37.3X4	T37.3X5	T37.3X6
Misoprostol	T47.1X1	T47.1X2	T47.1X3	T47.1X4	T47.1X5	T47.1X6
Mithramycin	T45.1X1	T45.1X2	T45.1X3	T45.1X4	T45.1X5	T45.1X6
Mitobronitol	T45.1X1	T45.1X2	T45.1X3	T45.1X4	T45.1X5	T45.1X6
Mitoguazone	T45.1X1	T45.1X2	T45.1X3	T45.1X4	T45.1X5	T45.1X6

Substance	Poisoning, Accidental (unintentional)	Poisoning, Intentional self-harm	Poisoning, Assault	Poisoning, Undetermined	Adverse effect	Underdosing
Mitolactol	T45.1X1	T45.1X2	T45.1X3	T45.1X4	T45.1X5	T45.1X6
Mitomycin	T45.1X1	T45.1X2	T45.1X3	T45.1X4	T45.1X5	T45.1X6
Mitopodozide	T45.1X1	T45.1X2	T45.1X3	T45.1X4	T45.1X5	T45.1X6
Mitotane	T45.1X1	T45.1X2	T45.1X3	T45.1X4	T45.1X5	T45.1X6
Mitoxantrone	T45.1X1	T45.1X2	T45.1X3	T45.1X4	T45.1X5	T45.1X6
Mivacurium chloride	T48.1X1	T48.1X2	T48.1X3	T48.1X4	T48.1X5	T48.1X6
Miyari bacteria	T47.6X1	T47.6X2	T47.6X3	T47.6X4	T47.6X5	T47.6X6
Moclobemide	T43.1X1	T43.1X2	T43.1X3	T43.1X4	T43.1X5	T43.1X6
Moderil	T46.5X1	T46.5X2	T46.5X3	T46.5X4	T46.5X5	T46.5X6
Mofebutazone	T39.2X1	T39.2X2	T39.2X3	T39.2X4	T39.2X5	T39.2X6
Mogadon—see Nitrazepam						
Molindone	T43.591	T43.592	T43.593	T43.594	T43.595	T43.596
Molsidomine	T46.3X1	T46.3X2	T46.3X3	T46.3X4	T46.3X5	T46.3X6
Mometasone	T49.0X1	T49.0X2	T49.0X3	T49.0X4	T49.0X5	T49.0X6
Monistat	T49.0X1	T49.0X2	T49.0X3	T49.0X4	T49.0X5	T49.0X6
Monkshood	T62.2X1	T62.2X2	T62.2X3	T62.2X4	—	—
Monoamine oxidase inhibitor NEC	T43.1X1	T43.1X2	T43.1X3	T43.1X4	T43.1X5	T43.1X6
hydrazine	T43.1X1	T43.1X2	T43.1X3	T43.1X4	T43.1X5	T43.1X6
Monobenzone	T49.4X1	T49.4X2	T49.4X3	T49.4X4	T49.4X5	T49.4X6
Monochloroacetic acid	T60.3X1	T60.3X2	T60.3X3	T60.3X4	—	—
Monochlorobenzene	T53.7X1	T53.7X2	T53.7X3	T53.7X4	—	—
Monoethanolamine	T46.8X1	T46.8X2	T46.8X3	T46.8X4	T46.8X5	T46.8X6
oleate	T46.8X1	T46.8X2	T46.8X3	T46.8X4	T46.8X5	T46.8X6
Monooctanoin	T50.991	T50.992	T50.993	T50.994	T50.995	T50.996
Monophenylbutazone	T39.2X1	T39.2X2	T39.2X3	T39.2X4	T39.2X5	T39.2X6
Monosodium glutamate	T65.891	T65.892	T65.893	T65.894	—	—
Monosulfiram	T49.0X1	T49.0X2	T49.0X3	T49.0X4	T49.0X5	T49.0X6
Monoxide, carbon—see Carbon, monoxide						
Monoxidine hydrochloride	T46.1X1	T46.1X2	T46.1X3	T46.1X4	T46.1X5	T46.1X6
Monuron	T60.3X1	T60.3X2	T60.3X3	T60.3X4	—	—
Moperone	T43.4X1	T43.4X2	T43.4X3	T43.4X4	T43.4X5	T43.4X6
Mopidamol	T45.1X1	T45.1X2	T45.1X3	T45.1X4	T45.1X5	T45.1X6
MOPP (mechlorethamine + vincristine + prednisone + procarbazine)	T45.1X1	T45.1X2	T45.1X3	T45.1X4	T45.1X5	T45.1X6
Morfin	T40.2X1	T40.2X2	T40.2X3	T40.2X4	T40.2X5	T40.2X6
Morinamide	T37.1X1	T37.1X2	T37.1X3	T37.1X4	T37.1X5	T37.1X6
Morning glory seeds	T40.991	T40.992	T40.993	T40.994	—	—
Moroxydine	T37.5X1	T37.5X2	T37.5X3	T37.5X4	T37.5X5	T37.5X6
Morphazinamide	T37.1X1	T37.1X2	T37.1X3	T37.1X4	T37.1X5	T37.1X6
Morphine	T40.2X1	T40.2X2	T40.2X3	T40.2X4	T40.2X5	T40.2X6
antagonist	T50.7X1	T50.7X2	T50.7X3	T50.7X4	T50.7X5	T50.7X6
Morpholinylethylmorphine	T40.2X1	T40.2X2	T40.2X3	T40.2X4	—	—
Morsuximide	T42.2X1	T42.2X2	T42.2X3	T42.2X4	T42.2X5	T42.2X6
Mosapramine	T43.591	T43.592	T43.593	T43.594	T43.595	T43.596

Substance	Poisoning, Accidental (unintentional)	Poisoning, Intentional self-harm	Poisoning, Assault	Poisoning, Undetermined	Adverse effect	Underdosing
Moth balls—see also Pesticides	T60.2X1	T60.2X2	T60.2X3	T60.2X4	—	—
naphthalene	T60.2X1	T60.2X2	T60.2X3	T60.2X4	—	—
paradichlorobenzene	T60.1X1	T60.1X2	T60.1X3	T60.1X4	—	—
Motor exhaust gas	T58.01	T58.02	T58.03	T58.04	—	—
Mouthwash (antiseptic) (zincchloride)	T49.6X1	T49.6X2	T49.6X3	T49.6X4	T49.6X5	T49.6X6
Moxastine	T45.0X1	T45.0X2	T45.0X3	T45.0X4	T45.0X5	T45.0X6
Moxaverine	T44.3X1	T44.3X2	T44.3X3	T44.3X4	T44.3X5	T44.3X6
Moxisylyte	T46.7X1	T46.7X2	T46.7X3	T46.7X4	T46.7X5	T46.7X6
Mucilage, plant	T47.4X1	T47.4X2	T47.4X3	T47.4X4	T47.4X5	T47.4X6
Mucolytic drug	T48.4X1	T48.4X2	T48.4X3	T48.4X4	T48.4X5	T48.4X6
Mucomyst	T48.4X1	T48.4X2	T48.4X3	T48.4X4	T48.4X5	T48.4X6
Mucous membrane agents (external)	T49.91	T49.92	T49.93	T49.94	T49.95	T49.96
specified NEC	T49.8X1	T49.8X2	T49.8X3	T49.8X4	T49.8X5	T49.8X6
Multiple unspecified drugs, medicaments and biological substances	T50.911	T50.912	T50.913	T50.914	T50.915	T50.916
Mumps						
immune globulin (human)	T50.Z11	T50.Z12	T50.Z13	T50.Z14	T50.Z15	T50.Z16
skin test antigen	T50.8X1	T50.8X2	T50.8X3	T50.8X4	T50.8X5	T50.8X6
vaccine	T50.B91	T50.B92	T50.B93	T50.B94	T50.B95	T50.B96
Mumpsvax	T50.B91	T50.B92	T50.B93	T50.B94	T50.B95	T50.B96
Mupirocin	T49.0X1	T49.0X2	T49.0X3	T49.0X4	T49.0X5	T49.0X6
Muriatic acid—see Hydrochloric acid						
Muromonab-CD3	T45.1X1	T45.1X2	T45.1X3	T45.1X4	T45.1X5	T45.1X6
Muscle-action drug NEC	T48.201	T48.202	T48.203	T48.204	T48.205	T48.206
Muscle affecting agents NEC	T48.201	T48.202	T48.203	T48.204	T48.205	T48.206
oxytocic	T48.0X1	T48.0X2	T48.0X3	T48.0X4	T48.0X5	T48.0X6
relaxants	T48.201	T48.202	T48.203	T48.204	T48.205	T48.206
central nervous system	T42.8X1	T42.8X2	T42.8X3	T42.8X4	T42.8X5	T42.8X6
skeletal	T48.1X1	T48.1X2	T48.1X3	T48.1X4	T48.1X5	T48.1X6
smooth	T44.3X1	T44.3X2	T44.3X3	T44.3X4	T44.3X5	T44.3X6
Muscle relaxant—see Relaxant, muscle						
Muscle-tone depressant, central NEC	T42.8X1	T42.8X2	T42.8X3	T42.8X4	T42.8X5	T42.8X6
specified NEC	T42.8X1	T42.8X2	T42.8X3	T42.8X4	T42.8X5	T42.8X6
Mushroom, noxious	T62.0X1	T62.0X2	T62.0X3	T62.0X4	—	—
Mussel, noxious	T61.781	T61.782	T61.783	T61.784	—	—
Mustard (emetic)	T47.7X1	T47.7X2	T47.7X3	T47.7X4	T47.7X5	T47.7X6
black	T47.7X1	T47.7X2	T47.7X3	T47.7X4	T47.7X5	T47.7X6
gas, not in war	T59.91	T59.92	T59.93	T59.94	—	—
nitrogen	T45.1X1	T45.1X2	T45.1X3	T45.1X4	T45.1X5	T45.1X6
Mustine	T45.1X1	T45.1X2	T45.1X3	T45.1X4	T45.1X5	T45.1X6
M-vac	T45.1X1	T45.1X2	T45.1X3	T45.1X4	T45.1X5	T45.1X6
Mycifradin	T36.5X1	T36.5X2	T36.5X3	T36.5X4	T36.5X5	T36.5X6
topical	T49.0X1	T49.0X2	T49.0X3	T49.0X4	T49.0X5	T49.0X6

Substance	Poisoning, Accidental (unintentional)	Poisoning, Intentional self-harm	Poisoning, Assault	Poisoning, Undetermined	Adverse effect	Underdosing
Mycitracin	T36.8X1	T36.8X2	T36.8X3	T36.8X4	T36.8X5	T36.8X6
ophthalmic preparation	T49.5X1	T49.5X2	T49.5X3	T49.5X4	T49.5X5	T49.5X6
Mycostatin	T36.7X1	T36.7X2	T36.7X3	T36.7X4	T36.7X5	T36.7X6
topical	T49.0X1	T49.0X2	T49.0X3	T49.0X4	T49.0X5	T49.0X6
Mycotoxins	T64.81	T64.82	T64.83	T64.84	—	—
aflatoxin	T64.01	T64.02	T64.03	T64.04	—	—
specified NEC	T64.81	T64.82	T64.83	T64.84	—	—
Mydriacyl	T44.3X1	T44.3X2	T44.3X3	T44.3X4	T44.3X5	T44.3X6
Mydriatic drug	T49.5X1	T49.5X2	T49.5X3	T49.5X4	T49.5X5	T49.5X6
Myelobromal	T45.1X1	T45.1X2	T45.1X3	T45.1X4	T45.1X5	T45.1X6
Myleran	T45.1X1	T45.1X2	T45.1X3	T45.1X4	T45.1X5	T45.1X6
Myochrysin(e)	T39.2X1	T39.2X2	T39.2X3	T39.2X4	T39.2X5	T39.2X6
Myoneural blocking agents	T48.1X1	T48.1X2	T48.1X3	T48.1X4	T48.1X5	T48.1X6
Myralact	T49.0X1	T49.0X2	T49.0X3	T49.0X4	T49.0X5	T49.0X6
Myristica fragrans	T62.2X1	T62.2X2	T62.2X3	T62.2X4	—	—
Myristicin	T65.891	T65.892	T65.893	T65.894	—	—
Mysoline	T42.3X1	T42.3X2	T42.3X3	T42.3X4	T42.3X5	T42.3X6
N						
Nabilone	T40.711	T40.712	T40.713	T40.714	T40.715	T40.716
Nabumetone	T39.391	T39.392	T39.393	T39.394	T39.395	T39.396
Nadolol	T44.7X1	T44.7X2	T44.7X3	T44.7X4	T44.7X5	T44.7X6
Nafcillin	T36.0X1	T36.0X2	T36.0X3	T36.0X4	T36.0X5	T36.0X6
Nafoxidine	T38.6X1	T38.6X2	T38.6X3	T38.6X4	T38.6X5	T38.6X6
Naftazone	T46.991	T46.992	T46.993	T46.994	T46.995	T46.996
Naftidrofuryl (oxalate)	T46.7X1	T46.7X2	T46.7X3	T46.7X4	T46.7X5	T46.7X6
Naftifine	T49.0X1	T49.0X2	T49.0X3	T49.0X4	T49.0X5	T49.0X6
Nail polish remover	T52.91	T52.92	T52.93	T52.94	—	—
Nalbuphine	T40.491	T40.492	T40.493	T40.494	T40.495	T40.496
Naled	T60.0X1	T60.0X2	T60.0X3	T60.0X4	—	—
Nalidixic acid	T37.8X1	T37.8X2	T37.8X3	T37.8X4	T37.8X5	T37.8X6
Nalorphine	T50.7X1	T50.7X2	T50.7X3	T50.7X4	T50.7X5	T50.7X6
Naloxone	T50.7X1	T50.7X2	T50.7X3	T50.7X4	T50.7X5	T50.7X6
Naltrexone	T50.7X1	T50.7X2	T50.7X3	T50.7X4	T50.7X5	T50.7X6
Namenda	T43.8X1	T43.8X2	T43.8X3	T43.8X4	T43.8X5	T43.8X6
Nandrolone	T38.7X1	T38.7X2	T38.7X3	T38.7X4	T38.7X5	T38.7X6
Naphazoline	T48.5X1	T48.5X2	T48.5X3	T48.5X4	T48.5X5	T48.5X6
Naphtha (painters') (petroleum)	T52.0X1	T52.0X2	T52.0X3	T52.0X4	—	—
solvent	T52.0X1	T52.0X2	T52.0X3	T52.0X4	—	—
vapor	T52.0X1	T52.0X2	T52.0X3	T52.0X4	—	—
Naphthalene (non-chlorinated)	T60.2X1	T60.2X2	T60.2X3	T60.2X4	—	—
chlorinated	T60.1X1	T60.1X2	T60.1X3	T60.1X4	—	—
vapor	T60.1X1	T60.1X2	T60.1X3	T60.1X4	—	—
insecticide or moth repellent	T60.2X1	T60.2X2	T60.2X3	T60.2X4	—	—
chlorinated	T60.1X1	T60.1X2	T60.1X3	T60.1X4	—	—
vapor	T60.2X1	T60.2X2	T60.2X3	T60.2X4	—	—
chlorinated	T60.1X1	T60.1X2	T60.1X3	T60.1X4	—	—
Naphthol	T65.891	T65.892	T65.893	T65.894	—	—

Substance	Poisoning, Accidental (unintentional)	Poisoning, Intentional self-harm	Poisoning, Assault	Poisoning, Undetermined	Adverse effect	Underdosing
Naphthylamine	T65.891	T65.892	T65.893	T65.894	—	—
Naphthylthiourea (ANTU)	T60.4X1	T60.4X2	T60.4X3	T60.4X4	—	—
Naprosyn—see Naproxen						
Naproxen	T39.311	T39.312	T39.313	T39.314	T39.315	T39.316
Narcotic (drug)	T40.601	T40.602	T40.603	T40.604	T40.605	T40.606
analgesic NEC	T40.601	T40.602	T40.603	T40.604	T40.605	T40.606
antagonist	T50.7X1	T50.7X2	T50.7X3	T50.7X4	T50.7X5	T50.7X6
specified NEC	T40.691	T40.692	T40.693	T40.694	T40.695	T40.696
synthetic	T40.491	T40.492	T40.493	T40.494	T40.495	T40.496
Narcotine	T48.3X1	T48.3X2	T48.3X3	T48.3X4	T48.3X5	T48.3X6
Nardil	T43.1X1	T43.1X2	T43.1X3	T43.1X4	T43.1X5	T43.1X6
Nasal drug NEC	T49.6X1	T49.6X2	T49.6X3	T49.6X4	T49.6X5	T49.6X6
Natamycin	T49.0X1	T49.0X2	T49.0X3	T49.0X4	T49.0X5	T49.0X6
Natrium cyanide—see Cyanide (s)						
Natural						
blood (product)	T45.8X1	T45.8X2	T45.8X3	T45.8X4	T45.8X5	T45.8X6
gas (piped)	T59.891	T59.892	T59.893	T59.894	—	—
incomplete combustion	T58.11	T58.12	T58.13	T58.14	—	—
Nealbarbital	T42.3X1	T42.3X2	T42.3X3	T42.3X4	T42.3X5	T42.3X6
Nectadon	T48.3X1	T48.3X2	T48.3X3	T48.3X4	T48.3X5	T48.3X6
Nedocromil	T48.6X1	T48.6X2	T48.6X3	T48.6X4	T48.6X5	T48.6X6
Nefopam	T39.8X1	T39.8X2	T39.8X3	T39.8X4	T39.8X5	T39.8X6
Nematocyst (sting)	T63.691	T63.692	T63.693	T63.694	—	—
Nembutal	T42.3X1	T42.3X2	T42.3X3	T42.3X4	T42.3X5	T42.3X6
Nemonapride	T43.591	T43.592	T43.593	T43.594	T43.595	T43.596
Neoarsphenamine	T37.8X1	T37.8X2	T37.8X3	T37.8X4	T37.8X5	T37.8X6
Neocinchophen	T50.4X1	T50.4X2	T50.4X3	T50.4X4	T50.4X5	T50.4X6
Neomycin (derivatives)	T36.5X1	T36.5X2	T36.5X3	T36.5X4	T36.5X5	T36.5X6
with						
bacitracin	T49.0X1	T49.0X2	T49.0X3	T49.0X4	T49.0X5	T49.0X6
neostigmine	T44.0X1	T44.0X2	T44.0X3	T44.0X4	T44.0X5	T44.0X6
ENT agent	T49.6X1	T49.6X2	T49.6X3	T49.6X4	T49.6X5	T49.6X6
ophthalmic preparation	T49.5X1	T49.5X2	T49.5X3	T49.5X4	T49.5X5	T49.5X6
topical NEC	T49.0X1	T49.0X2	T49.0X3	T49.0X4	T49.0X5	T49.0X6
Neonal	T42.3X1	T42.3X2	T42.3X3	T42.3X4	T42.3X5	T42.3X6
Neoprontosil	T37.0X1	T37.0X2	T37.0X3	T37.0X4	T37.0X5	T37.0X6
Neosalvarsan	T37.8X1	T37.8X2	T37.8X3	T37.8X4	T37.8X5	T37.8X6
Neosilversalvarsan	T37.8X1	T37.8X2	T37.8X3	T37.8X4	T37.8X5	T37.8X6
Neosporin	T36.8X1	T36.8X2	T36.8X3	T36.8X4	T36.8X5	T36.8X6
ENT agent	T49.6X1	T49.6X2	T49.6X3	T49.6X4	T49.6X5	T49.6X6
opthalmic preparation	T49.5X1	T49.5X2	T49.5X3	T49.5X4	T49.5X5	T49.5X6
topical NEC	T49.0X1	T49.0X2	T49.0X3	T49.0X4	T49.0X5	T49.0X6
Neostigmine bromide	T44.0X1	T44.0X2	T44.0X3	T44.0X4	T44.0X5	T44.0X6
Neraval	T42.3X1	T42.3X2	T42.3X3	T42.3X4	T42.3X5	T42.3X6
Neravan	T42.3X1	T42.3X2	T42.3X3	T42.3X4	T42.3X5	T42.3X6
Nerium oleander	T62.2X1	T62.2X2	T62.2X3	T62.2X4	—	—
Nerve gas, not in war	T59.91	T59.92	T59.93	T59.94	—	—

Substance	Poisoning, Accidental (unintentional)	Poisoning, Intentional self-harm	Poisoning, Assault	Poisoning, Undetermined	Adverse effect	Underdosing
Nesacaine	T41.3X1	T41.3X2	T41.3X3	T41.3X4	T41.3X5	T41.3X6
infiltration (subcutaneous)	T41.3X1	T41.3X2	T41.3X3	T41.3X4	T41.3X5	T41.3X6
nerve block (peripheral) (plexus)	T41.3X1	T41.3X2	T41.3X3	T41.3X4	T41.3X5	T41.3X6
Netilmicin	T36.5X1	T36.5X2	T36.5X3	T36.5X4	T36.5X5	T36.5X6
Neurobarb	T42.3X1	T42.3X2	T42.3X3	T42.3X4	T42.3X5	T42.3X6
Neuroleptic drug NEC	T43.501	T43.502	T43.503	T43.504	T43.505	T43.506
Neuromuscular blocking drug	T48.1X1	T48.1X2	T48.1X3	T48.1X4	T48.1X5	T48.1X6
Neutral insulin injection	T38.3X1	T38.3X2	T38.3X3	T38.3X4	T38.3X5	T38.3X6
Neutral spirits	T51.0X1	T51.0X2	T51.0X3	T51.0X4	—	—
beverage	T51.0X1	T51.0X2	T51.0X3	T51.0X4	—	—
Niacin	T46.7X1	T46.7X2	T46.7X3	T46.7X4	T46.7X5	T46.7X6
Niacinamide	T45.2X1	T45.2X2	T45.2X3	T45.2X4	T45.2X5	T45.2X6
Nialamide	T43.1X1	T43.1X2	T43.1X3	T43.1X4	T43.1X5	T43.1X6
Niaprazine	T42.6X1	T42.6X2	T42.6X3	T42.6X4	T42.6X5	T42.6X6
Nicametate	T46.7X1	T46.7X2	T46.7X3	T46.7X4	T46.7X5	T46.7X6
Nicardipine	T46.1X1	T46.1X2	T46.1X3	T46.1X4	T46.1X5	T46.1X6
Nicergoline	T46.7X1	T46.7X2	T46.7X3	T46.7X4	T46.7X5	T46.7X6
Nickel (carbonyl) (tetra-carbonyl) (fumes) (vapor)	T56.891	T56.892	T56.893	T56.894	—	—
Nickelocene	T56.891	T56.892	T56.893	T56.894	—	—
Niclosamide	T37.4X1	T37.4X2	T37.4X3	T37.4X4	T37.4X5	T37.4X6
Nicofuranose	T46.7X1	T46.7X2	T46.7X3	T46.7X4	T46.7X5	T46.7X6
Nicomorphine	T40.2X1	T40.2X2	T40.2X3	T40.2X4	—	—
Nicorandil	T46.3X1	T46.3X2	T46.3X3	T46.3X4	T46.3X5	T46.3X6
Nicotiana (plant)	T62.2X1	T62.2X2	T62.2X3	T62.2X4	—	—
Nicotinamide	T45.2X1	T45.2X2	T45.2X3	T45.2X4	T45.2X5	T45.2X6
Nicotine (insecticide) (spray) (sulfate) NEC	T60.2X1	T60.2X2	T60.2X3	T60.2X4	—	—
from tobacco	T65.291	T65.292	T65.293	T65.294	—	—
cigarettes	T65.221	T65.222	T65.223	T65.224	—	—
not insecticide	T65.291	T65.292	T65.293	T65.294	—	—
Nicotinic acid	T46.7X1	T46.7X2	T46.7X3	T46.7X4	T46.7X5	T46.7X6
Nicotinyl alcohol	T46.7X1	T46.7X2	T46.7X3	T46.7X4	T46.7X5	T46.7X6
Nicoumalone	T45.511	T45.512	T45.513	T45.514	T45.515	T45.516
Nifedipine	T46.1X1	T46.1X2	T46.1X3	T46.1X4	T46.1X5	T46.1X6
Nifenazone	T39.2X1	T39.2X2	T39.2X3	T39.2X4	T39.2X5	T39.2X6
Nifuraldezone	T37.91	T37.92	T37.93	T37.94	T37.95	T37.96
Nifuratel	T37.8X1	T37.8X2	T37.8X3	T37.8X4	T37.8X5	T37.8X6
Nifurtimox	T37.3X1	T37.3X2	T37.3X3	T37.3X4	T37.3X5	T37.3X6
Nifurtoinol	T37.8X1	T37.8X2	T37.8X3	T37.8X4	T37.8X5	T37.8X6
Nightshade, deadly (solanum)—see also Belladonna	T62.2X1	T62.2X2	T62.2X3	T62.2X4	—	—
berry	T62.1X1	T62.1X2	T62.1X3	T62.1X4	—	—
Nikethamide	T50.7X1	T50.7X2	T50.7X3	T50.7X4	T50.7X5	T50.7X6
Nilstat	T36.7X1	T36.7X2	T36.7X3	T36.7X4	T36.7X5	T36.7X6
topical	T49.0X1	T49.0X2	T49.0X3	T49.0X4	T49.0X5	T49.0X6
Nilutamide	T38.6X1	T38.6X2	T38.6X3	T38.6X4	T38.6X5	T38.6X6
Nimesulide	T39.391	T39.392	T39.393	T39.394	T39.395	T39.396
Nimetazepam	T42.4X1	T42.4X2	T42.4X3	T42.4X4	T42.4X5	T42.4X6
Nimodipine	T46.1X1	T46.1X2	T46.1X3	T46.1X4	T46.1X5	T46.1X6
Nimorazole	T37.3X1	T37.3X2	T37.3X3	T37.3X4	T37.3X5	T37.3X6
Nimustine	T45.1X1	T45.1X2	T45.1X3	T45.1X4	T45.1X5	T45.1X6
Niridazole	T37.4X1	T37.4X2	T37.4X3	T37.4X4	T37.4X5	T37.4X6
Nisentil	T40.2X1	T40.2X2	T40.2X3	T40.2X4	T40.2X5	T40.2X6
Nisoldipine	T46.1X1	T46.1X2	T46.1X3	T46.1X4	T46.1X5	T46.1X6
Nitramine	T65.3X1	T65.3X2	T65.3X3	T65.3X4	—	—
Nitrate, organic	T46.3X1	T46.3X2	T46.3X3	T46.3X4	T46.3X5	T46.3X6
Nitrazepam	T42.4X1	T42.4X2	T42.4X3	T42.4X4	T42.4X5	T42.4X6
Nitrefazole	T50.6X1	T50.6X2	T50.6X3	T50.6X4	T50.6X5	T50.6X6
Nitrendipine	T46.1X1	T46.1X2	T46.1X3	T46.1X4	T46.1X5	T46.1X6
Nitric						
acid (liquid)	T54.2X1	T54.2X2	T54.2X3	T54.2X4	—	—
vapor	T59.891	T59.892	T59.893	T59.894	—	—
oxide (gas)	T59.0X1	T59.0X2	T59.0X3	T59.0X4	—	—
Nitrimidazine	T37.3X1	T37.3X2	T37.3X3	T37.3X4	T37.3X5	T37.3X6
Nitrite, amyl (medicinal) (vapor)	T46.3X1	T46.3X2	T46.3X3	T46.3X4	T46.3X5	T46.3X6
Nitroaniline	T65.3X1	T65.3X2	T65.3X3	T65.3X4	—	—
vapor	T59.891	T59.892	T59.893	T59.894	—	—
Nitrobenzene, nitrobenzol	T65.3X1	T65.3X2	T65.3X3	T65.3X4	—	—
vapor	T65.3X1	T65.3X2	T65.3X3	T65.3X4	—	—
Nitrocellulose	T65.891	T65.892	T65.893	T65.894	—	—
lacquer	T65.891	T65.892	T65.893	T65.894	—	—
Nitrodiphenyl	T65.3X1	T65.3X2	T65.3X3	T65.3X4	—	—
Nitrofural	T49.0X1	T49.0X2	T49.0X3	T49.0X4	T49.0X5	T49.0X6
Nitrofurantoin	T37.8X1	T37.8X2	T37.8X3	T37.8X4	T37.8X5	T37.8X6
Nitrofurazone	T49.0X1	T49.0X2	T49.0X3	T49.0X4	T49.0X5	T49.0X6
Nitrogen	T59.0X1	T59.0X2	T59.0X3	T59.0X4	—	—
mustard	T45.1X1	T45.1X2	T45.1X3	T45.1X4	T45.1X5	T45.1X6
Nitroglycerin, nitro-glycerol (medicinal)	T46.3X1	T46.3X2	T46.3X3	T46.3X4	T46.3X5	T46.3X6
nonmedicinal	T65.5X1	T65.5X2	T65.5X3	T65.5X4	—	—
fumes	T65.5X1	T65.5X2	T65.5X3	T65.5X4	—	—
Nitroglycol	T52.3X1	T52.3X2	T52.3X3	T52.3X4	—	—
Nitrohydrochloric acid	T54.2X1	T54.2X2	T54.2X3	T54.2X4	—	—
Nitromersol	T49.0X1	T49.0X2	T49.0X3	T49.0X4	T49.0X5	T49.0X6
Nitronaphthalene	T65.891	T65.892	T65.893	T65.894	—	—
Nitrophenol	T54.0X1	T54.0X2	T54.0X3	T54.0X4	—	—
Nitropropane	T52.8X1	T52.8X2	T52.8X3	T52.8X4	—	—
Nitroprusside	T46.5X1	T46.5X2	T46.5X3	T46.5X4	T46.5X5	T46.5X6
Nitrosodimethylamine	T65.3X1	T65.3X2	T65.3X3	T65.3X4	—	—
Nitrothiazol	T37.4X1	T37.4X2	T37.4X3	T37.4X4	T37.4X5	T37.4X6
Nitrotoluene, nitrotoluol	T65.3X1	T65.3X2	T65.3X3	T65.3X4	—	—
vapor	T65.3X1	T65.3X2	T65.3X3	T65.3X4	—	—
Nitrous						
acid (liquid)	T54.2X1	T54.2X2	T54.2X3	T54.2X4	—	—
fumes	T59.891	T59.892	T59.893	T59.894	—	—

Substance	Poisoning, Accidental (unintentional)	Poisoning, Intentional self-harm	Poisoning, Assault	Poisoning, Undetermined	Adverse effect	Underdosing
Nitrous — *Continued*						
ether spirit	T46.3X1	T46.3X2	T46.3X3	T46.3X4	T46.3X5	T46.3X6
oxide	T41.0X1	T41.0X2	T41.0X3	T41.0X4	T41.0X5	T41.0X6
Nitroxoline	T37.8X1	T37.8X2	T37.8X3	T37.8X4	T37.8X5	T37.8X6
Nitrozone	T49.0X1	T49.0X2	T49.0X3	T49.0X4	T49.0X5	T49.0X6
Nizatidine	T47.0X1	T47.0X2	T47.0X3	T47.0X4	T47.0X5	T47.0X6
Nizofenone	T43.8X1	T43.8X2	T43.8X3	T43.8X4	T43.8X5	T43.8X6
Noctec	T42.6X1	T42.6X2	T42.6X3	T42.6X4	T42.6X5	T42.6X6
Noludar	T42.6X1	T42.6X2	T42.6X3	T42.6X4	T42.6X5	T42.6X6
Nomegestrol	T38.5X1	T38.5X2	T38.5X3	T38.5X4	T38.5X5	T38.5X6
Nomifensine	T43.291	T43.292	T43.293	T43.294	T43.295	T43.296
Nonoxinol	T49.8X1	T49.8X2	T49.8X3	T49.8X4	T49.8X5	T49.8X6
Nonylphenoxy (polyethoxy-ethanol)	T49.8X1	T49.8X2	T49.8X3	T49.8X4	T49.8X5	T49.8X6
Noptil	T42.3X1	T42.3X2	T42.3X3	T42.3X4	T42.3X5	T42.3X6
Noradrenaline	T44.4X1	T44.4X2	T44.4X3	T44.4X4	T44.4X5	T44.4X6
Noramidopyrine	T39.2X1	T39.2X2	T39.2X3	T39.2X4	T39.2X5	T39.2X6
methanesulfonate sodium	T39.2X1	T39.2X2	T39.2X3	T39.2X4	T39.2X5	T39.2X6
Norbormide	T60.4X1	T60.4X2	T60.4X3	T60.4X4	—	—
Nordazepam	T42.4X1	T42.4X2	T42.4X3	T42.4X4	T42.4X5	T42.4X6
Norepinephrine	T44.4X1	T44.4X2	T44.4X3	T44.4X4	T44.4X5	T44.4X6
Norethandrolone	T38.7X1	T38.7X2	T38.7X3	T38.7X4	T38.7X5	T38.7X6
Norethindrone	T38.4X1	T38.4X2	T38.4X3	T38.4X4	T38.4X5	T38.4X6
Norethisterone (acetate) (enantate)	T38.4X1	T38.4X2	T38.4X3	T38.4X4	T38.4X5	T38.4X6
with ethinylestradiol	T38.5X1	T38.5X2	T38.5X3	T38.5X4	T38.5X5	T38.5X6
Noretynodrel	T38.5X1	T38.5X2	T38.5X3	T38.5X4	T38.5X5	T38.5X6
Norfenefrine	T44.4X1	T44.4X2	T44.4X3	T44.4X4	T44.4X5	T44.4X6
Norfloxacin	T36.8X1	T36.8X2	T36.8X3	T36.8X4	T36.8X5	T36.8X6
Norgestrel	T38.4X1	T38.4X2	T38.4X3	T38.4X4	T38.4X5	T38.4X6
Norgestrienone	T38.4X1	T38.4X2	T38.4X3	T38.4X4	T38.4X5	T38.4X6
Norlestrin	T38.4X1	T38.4X2	T38.4X3	T38.4X4	T38.4X5	T38.4X6
Norlutin	T38.4X1	T38.4X2	T38.4X3	T38.4X4	T38.4X5	T38.4X6
Normal serum albumin (human), salt-poor	T45.8X1	T45.8X2	T45.8X3	T45.8X4	T45.8X5	T45.8X6
Normethandrone	T38.5X1	T38.5X2	T38.5X3	T38.5X4	T38.5X5	T38.5X6
Normison—see Benzodiazepines						
Normorphine	T40.2X1	T40.2X2	T40.2X3	T40.2X4	—	—
Norpseudoephedrine	T50.5X1	T50.5X2	T50.5X3	T50.5X4	T50.5X5	T50.5X6
Nortestosterone (furanpro pionate)	T38.7X1	T38.7X2	T38.7X3	T38.7X4	T38.7X5	T38.7X6
Nortriptyline	T43.011	T43.012	T43.013	T43.014	T43.015	T43.016
Noscapine	T48.3X1	T48.3X2	T48.3X3	T48.3X4	T48.3X5	T48.3X6
Nose preparations	T49.6X1	T49.6X2	T49.6X3	T49.6X4	T49.6X5	T49.6X6
Novobiocin	T36.5X1	T36.5X2	T36.5X3	T36.5X4	T36.5X5	T36.5X6
Novocain (infiltration) (topical)	T41.3X1	T41.3X2	T41.3X3	T41.3X4	T41.3X5	T41.3X6
nerve block (peripheral) (plexus)	T41.3X1	T41.3X2	T41.3X3	T41.3X4	T41.3X5	T41.3X6
spinal	T41.3X1	T41.3X2	T41.3X3	T41.3X4	T41.3X5	T41.3X6
Noxious foodstuff	T62.91	T62.92	T62.93	T62.94	—	—
specified NEC	T62.8X1	T62.8X2	T62.8X3	T62.8X4	—	—
Noxiptiline	T43.011	T43.012	T43.013	T43.014	T43.015	T43.016
Noxytiolin	T49.0X1	T49.0X2	T49.0X3	T49.0X4	T49.0X5	T49.0X6
NPH lletin (insulin)	T38.3X1	T38.3X2	T38.3X3	T38.3X4	T38.3X5	T38.3X6
Numorphan	T40.2X1	T40.2X2	T40.2X3	T40.2X4	T40.2X5	T40.2X6
Nunol	T42.3X1	T42.3X2	T42.3X3	T42.3X4	T42.3X5	T42.3X6
Nupercaine (spinal anesthetic)	T41.3X1	T41.3X2	T41.3X3	T41.3X4	T41.3X5	T41.3X6
topical (surface)	T41.3X1	T41.3X2	T41.3X3	T41.3X4	T41.3X5	T41.3X6
Nutmeg oil (liniment)	T49.3X1	T49.3X2	T49.3X3	T49.3X4	T49.3X5	T49.3X6
Nutritional supplement	T50.901	T50.902	T50.903	T50.904	T50.905	T50.906
Nux vomica	T65.1X1	T65.1X2	T65.1X3	T65.1X4	—	—
Nydrazid	T37.1X1	T37.1X2	T37.1X3	T37.1X4	T37.1X5	T37.1X6
Nylidrin	T46.7X1	T46.7X2	T46.7X3	T46.7X4	T46.7X5	T46.7X6
Nystatin	T36.7X1	T36.7X2	T36.7X3	T36.7X4	T36.7X5	T36.7X6
topical	T49.0X1	T49.0X2	T49.0X3	T49.0X4	T49.0X5	T49.0X6
Nytol	T45.0X1	T45.0X2	T45.0X3	T45.0X4	T45.0X5	T45.0X6
O						
Obidoxime chloride	T50.6X1	T50.6X2	T50.6X3	T50.6X4	T50.6X5	T50.6X6
Octafonium (chloride)	T49.3X1	T49.3X2	T49.3X3	T49.3X4	T49.3X5	T49.3X6
Octamethyl pyrophos-phoramide	T60.0X1	T60.0X2	T60.0X3	T60.0X4	—	—
Octanoin	T50.991	T50.992	T50.993	T50.994	T50.995	T50.996
Octatropine methyl-bromide	T44.3X1	T44.3X2	T44.3X3	T44.3X4	T44.3X5	T44.3X6
Octotiamine	T45.2X1	T45.2X2	T45.2X3	T45.2X4	T45.2X5	T45.2X6
Octoxinol (9)	T49.8X1	T49.8X2	T49.8X3	T49.8X4	T49.8X5	T49.8X6
Octreotide	T38.991	T38.992	T38.993	T38.994	T38.995	T38.996
Octyl nitrite	T46.3X1	T46.3X2	T46.3X3	T46.3X4	T46.3X5	T46.3X6
Oestradiol	T38.5X1	T38.5X2	T38.5X3	T38.5X4	T38.5X5	T38.5X6
Oestriol	T38.5X1	T38.5X2	T38.5X3	T38.5X4	T38.5X5	T38.5X6
Oestrogen	T38.5X1	T38.5X2	T38.5X3	T38.5X4	T38.5X5	T38.5X6
Oestrone	T38.5X1	T38.5X2	T38.5X3	T38.5X4	T38.5X5	T38.5X6
Ofloxacin	T36.8X1	T36.8X2	T36.8X3	T36.8X4	T36.8X5	T36.8X6
Oil (of)	T65.891	T65.892	T65.893	T65.894	—	—
bitter almond	T62.8X1	T62.8X2	T62.8X3	T62.8X4	—	—
cloves	T49.7X1	T49.7X2	T49.7X3	T49.7X4	T49.7X5	T49.7X6
colors	T65.6X1	T65.6X2	T65.6X3	T65.6X4	—	—
fumes	T59.891	T59.892	T59.893	T59.894	—	—
lubricating	T52.0X1	T52.0X2	T52.0X3	T52.0X4	—	—
Niobe	T52.8X1	T52.8X2	T52.8X3	T52.8X4	—	—
vitriol (liquid)	T54.2X1	T54.2X2	T54.2X3	T54.2X4	—	—
fumes	T54.2X1	T54.2X2	T54.2X3	T54.2X4	—	—
wintergreen (bitter) NEC	T49.3X1	T49.3X2	T49.3X3	T49.3X4	T49.3X5	T49.3X6
Oily preparation (for skin)	T49.3X1	T49.3X2	T49.3X3	T49.3X4	T49.3X5	T49.3X6
Ointment NEC	T49.3X1	T49.3X2	T49.3X3	T49.3X4	T49.3X5	T49.3X6
Olanzapine	T43.591	T43.592	T43.593	T43.594	T43.595	T43.596
Oleander	T62.2X1	T62.2X2	T62.2X3	T62.2X4	—	—
Oleandomycin	T36.3X1	T36.3X2	T36.3X3	T36.3X4	T36.3X5	T36.3X6

Substance	Poisoning, Accidental (unintentional)	Poisoning, Intentional self-harm	Poisoning, Assault	Poisoning, Undetermined	Adverse effect	Underdosing
Oleandrin	T46.0X1	T46.0X2	T46.0X3	T46.0X4	T46.0X5	T46.0X6
Oleic acid	T46.6X1	T46.6X2	T46.6X3	T46.6X4	T46.6X5	T46.6X6
Oleovitamin A	T45.2X1	T45.2X2	T45.2X3	T45.2X4	T45.2X5	T45.2X6
Oleum ricini	T47.2X1	T47.2X2	T47.2X3	T47.2X4	T47.2X5	T47.2X6
Olive oil (medicinal) NEC	T47.4X1	T47.4X2	T47.4X3	T47.4X4	T47.4X5	T47.4X6
Olivomycin	T45.1X1	T45.1X2	T45.1X3	T45.1X4	T45.1X5	T45.1X6
Olsalazine	T47.8X1	T47.8X2	T47.8X3	T47.8X4	T47.8X5	T47.8X6
Omeprazole	T47.1X1	T47.1X2	T47.1X3	T47.1X4	T47.1X5	T47.1X6
OMPA	T60.0X1	T60.0X2	T60.0X3	T60.0X4	—	—
Oncovin	T45.1X1	T45.1X2	T45.1X3	T45.1X4	T45.1X5	T45.1X6
Ondansetron	T45.0X1	T45.0X2	T45.0X3	T45.0X4	T45.0X5	T45.0X6
Ophthaine	T41.3X1	T41.3X2	T41.3X3	T41.3X4	T41.3X5	T41.3X6
Ophthetic	T41.3X1	T41.3X2	T41.3X3	T41.3X4	T41.3X5	T41.3X6
Opiate NEC	T40.601	T40.602	T40.603	T40.604	T40.605	T40.606
antagonists	T50.7X1	T50.7X2	T50.7X3	T50.7X4	T50.7X5	T50.7X6
Opioid NEC	T40.2X1	T40.2X2	T40.2X3	T40.2X4	T40.2X5	T40.2X6
Opipramol	T43.011	T43.012	T43.013	T43.014	T43.015	T43.016
Opium alkaloids (total)	T40.0X1	T40.0X2	T40.0X3	T40.0X4	T40.0X5	T40.0X6
standardized powdered	T40.0X1	T40.0X2	T40.0X3	T40.0X4	T40.0X5	T40.0X6
tincture (camphorated)	T40.0X1	T40.0X2	T40.0X3	T40.0X4	T40.0X5	T40.0X6
Oracon	T38.4X1	T38.4X2	T38.4X3	T38.4X4	T38.4X5	T38.4X6
Oragrafin	T50.8X1	T50.8X2	T50.8X3	T50.8X4	T50.8X5	T50.8X6
Oral contraceptives	T38.4X1	T38.4X2	T38.4X3	T38.4X4	T38.4X5	T38.4X6
Oral rehydration salts	T50.3X1	T50.3X2	T50.3X3	T50.3X4	T50.3X5	T50.3X6
Orazamide	T50.991	T50.992	T50.993	T50.994	T50.995	T50.996
Orciprenaline	T48.291	T48.292	T48.293	T48.294	T48.295	T48.296
Organidin	T48.4X1	T48.4X2	T48.4X3	T48.4X4	T48.4X5	T48.4X6
Organonitrate NEC	T46.3X1	T46.3X2	T46.3X3	T46.3X4	T46.3X5	T46.3X6
Organophosphates	T60.0X1	T60.0X2	T60.0X3	T60.0X4	—	—
Orimune	T50.B91	T50.B92	T50.B93	T50.B94	T50.B95	T50.B96
Orinase	T38.3X1	T38.3X2	T38.3X3	T38.3X4	T38.3X5	T38.3X6
Ormeloxifene	T38.6X1	T38.6X2	T38.6X3	T38.6X4	T38.6X5	T38.6X6
Ornidazole	T37.3X1	T37.3X2	T37.3X3	T37.3X4	T37.3X5	T37.3X6
Ornithine aspartate	T50.991	T50.992	T50.993	T50.994	T50.995	T50.996
Ornoprostil	T47.1X1	T47.1X2	T47.1X3	T47.1X4	T47.1X5	T47.1X6
Orphenadrine (hydrochloride)	T42.8X1	T42.8X2	T42.8X3	T42.8X4	T42.8X5	T42.8X6
Ortal (sodium)	T42.3X1	T42.3X2	T42.3X3	T42.3X4	T42.3X5	T42.3X6
Orthoboric acid	T49.0X1	T49.0X2	T49.0X3	T49.0X4	T49.0X5	T49.0X6
ENT agent	T49.6X1	T49.6X2	T49.6X3	T49.6X4	T49.6X5	T49.6X6
ophthalmic preparation	T49.5X1	T49.5X2	T49.5X3	T49.5X4	T49.5X5	T49.5X6
Orthocaine	T41.3X1	T41.3X2	T41.3X3	T41.3X4	T41.3X5	T41.3X6
Orthodichlorobenzene	T53.7X1	T53.7X2	T53.7X3	T53.7X4	—	—
Ortho-Novum	T38.4X1	T38.4X2	T38.4X3	T38.4X4	T38.4X5	T38.4X6
Orthotolidine (reagent)	T54.2X1	T54.2X2	T54.2X3	T54.2X4	—	—
Osmic acid (liquid)	T54.2X1	T54.2X2	T54.2X3	T54.2X4	—	—
fumes	T54.2X1	T54.2X2	T54.2X3	T54.2X4	—	—
Osmotic diuretics	T50.2X1	T50.2X2	T50.2X3	T50.2X4	T50.2X5	T50.2X6
Otilonium bromide	T44.3X1	T44.3X2	T44.3X3	T44.3X4	T44.3X5	T44.3X6
Otorhinolaryngological drug NEC	T49.6X1	T49.6X2	T49.6X3	T49.6X4	T49.6X5	T49.6X6
Ouabain(e)	T46.0X1	T46.0X2	T46.0X3	T46.0X4	T46.0X5	T46.0X6
Ovarian						
hormone	T38.5X1	T38.5X2	T38.5X3	T38.5X4	T38.5X5	T38.5X6
stimulant	T38.5X1	T38.5X2	T38.5X3	T38.5X4	T38.5X5	T38.5X6
Ovral	T38.4X1	T38.4X2	T38.4X3	T38.4X4	T38.4X5	T38.4X6
Ovulen	T38.4X1	T38.4X2	T38.4X3	T38.4X4	T38.4X5	T38.4X6
Oxacillin	T36.0X1	T36.0X2	T36.0X3	T36.0X4	T36.0X5	T36.0X6
Oxalic acid	T54.2X1	T54.2X2	T54.2X3	T54.2X4	—	—
ammonium salt	T50.991	T50.992	T50.993	T50.994	T50.995	T50.996
Oxamniquine	T37.4X1	T37.4X2	T37.4X3	T37.4X4	T37.4X5	T37.4X6
Oxanamide	T43.591	T43.592	T43.593	T43.594	T43.595	T43.596
Oxandrolone	T38.7X1	T38.7X2	T38.7X3	T38.7X4	T38.7X5	T38.7X6
Oxantel	T37.4X1	T37.4X2	T37.4X3	T37.4X4	T37.4X5	T37.4X6
Oxapium iodide	T44.3X1	T44.3X2	T44.3X3	T44.3X4	T44.3X5	T44.3X6
Oxaprotiline	T43.021	T43.022	T43.023	T43.024	T43.025	T43.026
Oxaprozin	T39.311	T39.312	T39.313	T39.314	T39.315	T39.316
Oxatomide	T45.0X1	T45.0X2	T45.0X3	T45.0X4	T45.0X5	T45.0X6
Oxazepam	T42.4X1	T42.4X2	T42.4X3	T42.4X4	T42.4X5	T42.4X6
Oxazimedrine	T50.5X1	T50.5X2	T50.5X3	T50.5X4	T50.5X5	T50.5X6
Oxazolam	T42.4X1	T42.4X2	T42.4X3	T42.4X4	T42.4X5	T42.4X6
Oxazolidine derivatives	T42.2X1	T42.2X2	T42.2X3	T42.2X4	T42.2X5	T42.2X6
Oxazolidinedione (derivative)	T42.2X1	T42.2X2	T42.2X3	T42.2X4	T42.2X5	T42.2X6
Ox bile extract	T47.5X1	T47.5X2	T47.5X3	T47.5X4	T47.5X5	T47.5X6
Oxcarbazepine	T42.1X1	T42.1X2	T42.1X3	T42.1X4	T42.1X5	T42.1X6
Oxedrine	T44.4X1	T44.4X2	T44.4X3	T44.4X4	T44.4X5	T44.4X6
Oxeladin (citrate)	T48.3X1	T48.3X2	T48.3X3	T48.3X4	T48.3X5	T48.3X6
Oxendolone	T38.5X1	T38.5X2	T38.5X3	T38.5X4	T38.5X5	T38.5X6
Oxetacaine	T41.3X1	T41.3X2	T41.3X3	T41.3X4	T41.3X5	T41.3X6
Oxethazine	T41.3X1	T41.3X2	T41.3X3	T41.3X4	T41.3X5	T41.3X6
Oxetorone	T39.8X1	T39.8X2	T39.8X3	T39.8X4	T39.8X5	T39.8X6
Oxiconazole	T49.0X1	T49.0X2	T49.0X3	T49.0X4	T49.0X5	T49.0X6
Oxidizing agent NEC	T54.91	T54.92	T54.93	T54.94	—	—
Oxipurinol	T50.4X1	T50.4X2	T50.4X3	T50.4X4	T50.4X5	T50.4X6
Oxitriptan	T43.291	T43.292	T43.293	T43.294	T43.295	T43.296
Oxitropium bromide	T48.6X1	T48.6X2	T48.6X3	T48.6X4	T48.6X5	T48.6X6
Oxodipine	T46.1X1	T46.1X2	T46.1X3	T46.1X4	T46.1X5	T46.1X6
Oxolamine	T48.3X1	T48.3X2	T48.3X3	T48.3X4	T48.3X5	T48.3X6
Oxolinic acid	T37.8X1	T37.8X2	T37.8X3	T37.8X4	T37.8X5	T37.8X6
Oxomemazine	T43.3X1	T43.3X2	T43.3X3	T43.3X4	T43.3X5	T43.3X6
Oxophenarsine	T37.3X1	T37.3X2	T37.3X3	T37.3X4	T37.3X5	T37.3X6
Oxprenolol	T44.7X1	T44.7X2	T44.7X3	T44.7X4	T44.7X5	T44.7X6
Oxsoralen	T49.3X1	T49.3X2	T49.3X3	T49.3X4	T49.3X5	T49.3X6
Oxtriphylline	T48.6X1	T48.6X2	T48.6X3	T48.6X4	T48.6X5	T48.6X6
Oxybate sodium	T41.291	T41.292	T41.293	T41.294	T41.295	T41.296
Oxybuprocaine	T41.3X1	T41.3X2	T41.3X3	T41.3X4	T41.3X5	T41.3X6
Oxybutynin	T44.3X1	T44.3X2	T44.3X3	T44.3X4	T44.3X5	T44.3X6
Oxychlorosene	T49.0X1	T49.0X2	T49.0X3	T49.0X4	T49.0X5	T49.0X6

Substance	Poisoning, Accidental (unintentional)	Poisoning, Intentional self-harm	Poisoning, Assault	Poisoning, Undetermined	Adverse effect	Underdosing
Oxycodone	T40.2X1	T40.2X2	T40.2X3	T40.2X4	T40.2X5	T40.2X6
Oxyfedrine	T46.3X1	T46.3X2	T46.3X3	T46.3X4	T46.3X5	T46.3X6
Oxygen	T41.5X1	T41.5X2	T41.5X3	T41.5X4	T41.5X5	T41.5X6
Oxylone	T49.0X1	T49.0X2	T49.0X3	T49.0X4	T49.0X5	T49.0X6
ophthalmic preparation	T49.5X1	T49.5X2	T49.5X3	T49.5X4	T49.5X5	T49.5X6
Oxymesterone	T38.7X1	T38.7X2	T38.7X3	T38.7X4	T38.7X5	T38.7X6
Oxymetazoline	T48.5X1	T48.5X2	T48.5X3	T48.5X4	T48.5X5	T48.5X6
Oxymetholone	T38.7X1	T38.7X2	T38.7X3	T38.7X4	T38.7X5	T38.7X6
Oxymorphone	T40.2X1	T40.2X2	T40.2X3	T40.2X4	T40.2X5	T40.2X6
Oxypertine	T43.591	T43.592	T43.593	T43.594	T43.595	T43.596
Oxyphenbutazone	T39.2X1	T39.2X2	T39.2X3	T39.2X4	T39.2X5	T39.2X6
Oxyphencyclimine	T44.3X1	T44.3X2	T44.3X3	T44.3X4	T44.3X5	T44.3X6
Oxyphenisatine	T47.2X1	T47.2X2	T47.2X3	T47.2X4	T47.2X5	T47.2X6
Oxyphenonium bromide	T44.3X1	T44.3X2	T44.3X3	T44.3X4	T44.3X5	T44.3X6
Oxypolygelatin	T45.8X1	T45.8X2	T45.8X3	T45.8X4	T45.8X5	T45.8X6
Oxyquinoline (derivatives)	T37.8X1	T37.8X2	T37.8X3	T37.8X4	T37.8X5	T37.8X6
Oxytetracycline	T36.4X1	T36.4X2	T36.4X3	T36.4X4	T36.4X5	T36.4X6
Oxytocic drug NEC	T48.0X1	T48.0X2	T48.0X3	T48.0X4	T48.0X5	T48.0X6
Oxytocin (synthetic)	T48.0X1	T48.0X2	T48.0X3	T48.0X4	T48.0X5	T48.0X6
Ozone	T59.891	T59.892	T59.893	T59.894	—	—
P						
PABA	T49.3X1	T49.3X2	T49.3X3	T49.3X4	T49.3X5	T49.3X6
Packed red cells	T45.8X1	T45.8X2	T45.8X3	T45.8X4	T45.8X5	T45.8X6
Padimate	T49.3X1	T49.3X2	T49.3X3	T49.3X4	T49.3X5	T49.3X6
Paint NEC	T65.6X1	T65.6X2	T65.6X3	T65.6X4	—	—
cleaner	T52.91	T52.92	T52.93	T52.94	—	—
fumes NEC	T59.891	T59.892	T59.893	T59.894	—	—
lead (fumes)	T56.0X1	T56.0X2	T56.0X3	T56.0X4	—	—
solvent NEC	T52.8X1	T52.8X2	T52.8X3	T52.8X4	—	—
stripper	T52.8X1	T52.8X2	T52.8X3	T52.8X4	—	—
Palfium	T40.2X1	T40.2X2	T40.2X3	T40.2X4	—	—
Palm kernel oil	T50.991	T50.992	T50.993	T50.994	T50.995	T50.996
Paludrine	T37.2X1	T37.2X2	T37.2X3	T37.2X4	T37.2X5	T37.2X6
PAM (pralidoxime)	T50.6X1	T50.6X2	T50.6X3	T50.6X4	T50.6X5	T50.6X6
Pamaquine (naphthoute)	T37.2X1	T37.2X2	T37.2X3	T37.2X4	T37.2X5	T37.2X6
Panadol	T39.1X1	T39.1X2	T39.1X3	T39.1X4	T39.1X5	T39.1X6
Pancreatic						
digestive secretion stimulant	T47.8X1	T47.8X2	T47.8X3	T47.8X4	T47.8X5	T47.8X6
dornase	T45.3X1	T45.3X2	T45.3X3	T45.3X4	T45.3X5	T45.3X6
Pancreatin	T47.5X1	T47.5X2	T47.5X3	T47.5X4	T47.5X5	T47.5X6
Pancrelipase	T47.5X1	T47.5X2	T47.5X3	T47.5X4	T47.5X5	T47.5X6
Pancuronium (bromide)	T48.1X1	T48.1X2	T48.1X3	T48.1X4	T48.1X5	T48.1X6
Pangamic acid	T45.2X1	T45.2X2	T45.2X3	T45.2X4	T45.2X5	T45.2X6
Panthenol	T45.2X1	T45.2X2	T45.2X3	T45.2X4	T45.2X5	T45.2X6
topical	T49.8X1	T49.8X2	T49.8X3	T49.8X4	T49.8X5	T49.8X6
Pantopon	T40.0X1	T40.0X2	T40.0X3	T40.0X4	T40.0X5	T40.0X6
Pantothenic acid	T45.2X1	T45.2X2	T45.2X3	T45.2X4	T45.2X5	T45.2X6
Panwarfin	T45.511	T45.512	T45.513	T45.514	T45.515	T45.516

Substance	Poisoning, Accidental (unintentional)	Poisoning, Intentional self-harm	Poisoning, Assault	Poisoning, Undetermined	Adverse effect	Underdosing
Papain	T47.5X1	T47.5X2	T47.5X3	T47.5X4	T47.5X5	T47.5X6
digestant	T47.5X1	T47.5X2	T47.5X3	T47.5X4	T47.5X5	T47.5X6
Papaveretum	T40.0X1	T40.0X2	T40.0X3	T40.0X4	T40.0X5	T40.0X6
Papaverine	T44.3X1	T44.3X2	T44.3X3	T44.3X4	T44.3X5	T44.3X6
Para-acetamidophenol	T39.1X1	T39.1X2	T39.1X3	T39.1X4	T39.1X5	T39.1X6
Para-aminobenzoic acid	T49.3X1	T49.3X2	T49.3X3	T49.3X4	T49.3X5	T49.3X6
Para-aminophenol derivatives	T39.1X1	T39.1X2	T39.1X3	T39.1X4	T39.1X5	T39.1X6
Para-aminosalicylic acid	T37.1X1	T37.1X2	T37.1X3	T37.1X4	T37.1X5	T37.1X6
Paracetaldehyde	T42.6X1	T42.6X2	T42.6X3	T42.6X4	T42.6X5	T42.6X6
Paracetamol	T39.1X1	T39.1X2	T39.1X3	T39.1X4	T39.1X5	T39.1X6
Parachlorophenol (camphorated)	T49.0X1	T49.0X2	T49.0X3	T49.0X4	T49.0X5	T49.0X6
Paracodin	T40.2X1	T40.2X2	T40.2X3	T40.2X4	T40.2X5	T40.2X6
Paradione	T42.2X1	T42.2X2	T42.2X3	T42.2X4	T42.2X5	T42.2X6
Paraffin(s) (wax)	T52.0X1	T52.0X2	T52.0X3	T52.0X4	—	—
liquid (medicinal)	T47.4X1	T47.4X2	T47.4X3	T47.4X4	T47.4X5	T47.4X6
nonmedicinal	T52.0X1	T52.0X2	T52.0X3	T52.0X4	—	—
Paraformaldehyde	T60.3X1	T60.3X2	T60.3X3	T60.3X4	—	—
Paraldehyde	T42.6X1	T42.6X2	T42.6X3	T42.6X4	T42.6X5	T42.6X6
Paramethadione	T42.2X1	T42.2X2	T42.2X3	T42.2X4	T42.2X5	T42.2X6
Paramethasone	T38.0X1	T38.0X2	T38.0X3	T38.0X4	T38.0X5	T38.0X6
acetate	T49.0X1	T49.0X2	T49.0X3	T49.0X4	T49.0X5	T49.0X6
Paraoxon	T60.0X1	T60.0X2	T60.0X3	T60.0X4	—	—
Paraquat	T60.3X1	T60.3X2	T60.3X3	T60.3X4	—	—
Parasympatholytic NEC	T44.3X1	T44.3X2	T44.3X3	T44.3X4	T44.3X5	T44.3X6
Parasympathomimetic drug NEC	T44.1X1	T44.1X2	T44.1X3	T44.1X4	T44.1X5	T44.1X6
Parathion	T60.0X1	T60.0X2	T60.0X3	T60.0X4	—	—
Parathormone	T50.991	T50.992	T50.993	T50.994	T50.995	T50.996
Parathyroid extract	T50.991	T50.992	T50.993	T50.994	T50.995	T50.996
Paratyphoid vaccine	T50.A91	T50.A92	T50.A93	T50.A94	T50.A95	T50.A96
Paredrine	T44.4X1	T44.4X2	T44.4X3	T44.4X4	T44.4X5	T44.4X6
Paregoric	T40.0X1	T40.0X2	T40.0X3	T40.0X4	T40.0X5	T40.0X6
Pargyline	T46.5X1	T46.5X2	T46.5X3	T46.5X4	T46.5X5	T46.5X6
Paris green	T57.0X1	T57.0X2	T57.0X3	T57.0X4	—	—
insecticide	T57.0X1	T57.0X2	T57.0X3	T57.0X4	—	—
Parnate	T43.1X1	T43.1X2	T43.1X3	T43.1X4	T43.1X5	T43.1X6
Paromomycin	T36.5X1	T36.5X2	T36.5X3	T36.5X4	T36.5X5	T36.5X6
Paroxypropione	T45.1X1	T45.1X2	T45.1X3	T45.1X4	T45.1X5	T45.1X6
Parzone	T40.2X1	T40.2X2	T40.2X3	T40.2X4	T40.2X5	T40.2X6
PAS	T37.1X1	T37.1X2	T37.1X3	T37.1X4	T37.1X5	T37.1X6
Pasiniazid	T37.1X1	T37.1X2	T37.1X3	T37.1X4	T37.1X5	T37.1X6
PBB (polybrominated biphenyls)	T65.891	T65.892	T65.893	T65.894	—	—
PCB	T65.891	T65.892	T65.893	T65.894	—	—
PCP						
meaning pentachlorophenol	T60.1X1	T60.1X2	T60.1X3	T60.1X4	—	—
fungicide	T60.3X1	T60.3X2	T60.3X3	T60.3X4	—	—
herbicide	T60.3X1	T60.3X2	T60.3X3	T60.3X4	—	—
insecticide	T60.1X1	T60.1X2	T60.1X3	T60.1X4	—	—
meaning phencyclidine	T40.991	T40.992	T40.993	T40.994	—	—

Substance	Poisoning, Accidental (unintentional)	Poisoning, Intentional self-harm	Poisoning, Assault	Poisoning, Undetermined	Adverse effect	Underdosing
Peach kernel oil (emulsion)	T47.4X1	T47.4X2	T47.4X3	T47.4X4	T47.4X5	T47.4X6
Peanut oil (emulsion) NEC	T47.4X1	T47.4X2	T47.4X3	T47.4X4	T47.4X5	T47.4X6
topical	T49.3X1	T49.3X2	T49.3X3	T49.3X4	T49.3X5	T49.3X6
Pearly Gates (morning glory seeds)	T40.991	T40.992	T40.993	T40.994	—	—
Pecazine	T43.3X1	T43.3X2	T43.3X3	T43.3X4	T43.3X5	T43.3X6
Pectin	T47.6X1	T47.6X2	T47.6X3	T47.6X4	T47.6X5	T47.6X6
Pefloxacin	T37.8X1	T37.8X2	T37.8X3	T37.8X4	T37.8X5	T37.8X6
Pegademase, bovine	T50.Z91	T50.Z92	T50.Z93	T50.Z94	T50.Z95	T50.Z96
Pelletierine tannate	T37.4X1	T37.4X2	T37.4X3	T37.4X4	T37.4X5	T37.4X6
Pemirolast (potassium)	T48.6X1	T48.6X2	T48.6X3	T48.6X4	T48.6X5	T48.6X6
Pemoline	T50.7X1	T50.7X2	T50.7X3	T50.7X4	T50.7X5	T50.7X6
Pempidine	T44.2X1	T44.2X2	T44.2X3	T44.2X4	T44.2X5	T44.2X6
Penamecillin	T36.0X1	T36.0X2	T36.0X3	T36.0X4	T36.0X5	T36.0X6
Penbutolol	T44.7X1	T44.7X2	T44.7X3	T44.7X4	T44.7X5	T44.7X6
Penethamate	T36.0X1	T36.0X2	T36.0X3	T36.0X4	T36.0X5	T36.0X6
Penfluridol	T43.591	T43.592	T43.593	T43.594	T43.595	T43.596
Penflutizide	T50.2X1	T50.2X2	T50.2X3	T50.2X4	T50.2X5	T50.2X6
Pengitoxin	T46.0X1	T46.0X2	T46.0X3	T46.0X4	T46.0X5	T46.0X6
Penicillamine	T50.6X1	T50.6X2	T50.6X3	T50.6X4	T50.6X5	T50.6X6
Penicillin (any)	T36.0X1	T36.0X2	T36.0X3	T36.0X4	T36.0X5	T36.0X6
Penicillinase	T45.3X1	T45.3X2	T45.3X3	T45.3X4	T45.3X5	T45.3X6
Penicilloyl polylysine	T50.8X1	T50.8X2	T50.8X3	T50.8X4	T50.8X5	T50.8X6
Penimepicycline	T36.4X1	T36.4X2	T36.4X3	T36.4X4	T36.4X5	T36.4X6
Pentachloroethane	T53.6X1	T53.6X2	T53.6X3	T53.6X4	—	—
Pentachloronaphthalene	T53.7X1	T53.7X2	T53.7X3	T53.7X4	—	—
Pentachlorophenol (pesticide)	T60.1X1	T60.1X2	T60.1X3	T60.1X4	—	—
fungicide	T60.3X1	T60.3X2	T60.3X3	T60.3X4	—	—
herbicide	T60.3X1	T60.3X2	T60.3X3	T60.3X4	—	—
insecticide	T60.1X1	T60.1X2	T60.1X3	T60.1X4	—	—
Pentaerythritol	T46.3X1	T46.3X2	T46.3X3	T46.3X4	T46.3X5	T46.3X6
chloral	T42.6X1	T42.6X2	T42.6X3	T42.6X4	T42.6X5	T42.6X6
tetranitrate NEC	T46.3X1	T46.3X2	T46.3X3	T46.3X4	T46.3X5	T46.3X6
Pentaerythrityl tetranitrate	T46.3X1	T46.3X2	T46.3X3	T46.3X4	T46.3X5	T46.3X6
Pentagastrin	T50.8X1	T50.8X2	T50.8X3	T50.8X4	T50.8X5	T50.8X6
Pentalin	T53.6X1	T53.6X2	T53.6X3	T53.6X4	—	—
Pentamethonium bromide	T44.2X1	T44.2X2	T44.2X3	T44.2X4	T44.2X5	T44.2X6
Pentamidine	T37.3X1	T37.3X2	T37.3X3	T37.3X4	T37.3X5	T37.3X6
Pentanol	T51.3X1	T51.3X2	T51.3X3	T51.3X4	—	—
Pentapyrrolinium (bitartrate)	T44.2X1	T44.2X2	T44.2X3	T44.2X4	T44.2X5	T44.2X6
Pentaquine	T37.2X1	T37.2X2	T37.2X3	T37.2X4	T37.2X5	T37.2X6
Pentazocine	T40.491	T40.492	T40.493	T40.494	T40.495	T40.496
Pentetrazole	T50.7X1	T50.7X2	T50.7X3	T50.7X4	T50.7X5	T50.7X6
Penthienate bromide	T44.3X1	T44.3X2	T44.3X3	T44.3X4	T44.3X5	T44.3X6
Pentifylline	T46.7X1	T46.7X2	T46.7X3	T46.7X4	T46.7X5	T46.7X6
Pentobarbital	T42.3X1	T42.3X2	T42.3X3	T42.3X4	T42.3X5	T42.3X6
sodium	T42.3X1	T42.3X2	T42.3X3	T42.3X4	T42.3X5	T42.3X6
Pentobarbitone	T42.3X1	T42.3X2	T42.3X3	T42.3X4	T42.3X5	T42.3X6
Pentolonium tartrate	T44.2X1	T44.2X2	T44.2X3	T44.2X4	T44.2X5	T44.2X6
Pentosan polysulfate (sodium)	T39.8X1	T39.8X2	T39.8X3	T39.8X4	T39.8X5	T39.8X6
Pentostatin	T45.1X1	T45.1X2	T45.1X3	T45.1X4	T45.1X5	T45.1X6
Pentothal	T41.1X1	T41.1X2	T41.1X3	T41.1X4	T41.1X5	T41.1X6
Pentoxifylline	T46.7X1	T46.7X2	T46.7X3	T46.7X4	T46.7X5	T46.7X6
Pentoxyverine	T48.3X1	T48.3X2	T48.3X3	T48.3X4	T48.3X5	T48.3X6
Pentrinat	T46.3X1	T46.3X2	T46.3X3	T46.3X4	T46.3X5	T46.3X6
Pentylenetetrazole	T50.7X1	T50.7X2	T50.7X3	T50.7X4	T50.7X5	T50.7X6
Pentylsalicylamide	T37.1X1	T37.1X2	T37.1X3	T37.1X4	T37.1X5	T37.1X6
Pentymal	T42.3X1	T42.3X2	T42.3X3	T42.3X4	T42.3X5	T42.3X6
Peplomycin	T45.1X1	T45.1X2	T45.1X3	T45.1X4	T45.1X5	T45.1X6
Peppermint (oil)	T47.5X1	T47.5X2	T47.5X3	T47.5X4	T47.5X5	T47.5X6
Pepsin	T47.5X1	T47.5X2	T47.5X3	T47.5X4	T47.5X5	T47.5X6
digestant	T47.5X1	T47.5X2	T47.5X3	T47.5X4	T47.5X5	T47.5X6
Pepstatin	T47.1X1	T47.1X2	T47.1X3	T47.1X4	T47.1X5	T47.1X6
Peptavlon	T50.8X1	T50.8X2	T50.8X3	T50.8X4	T50.8X5	T50.8X6
Perazine	T43.3X1	T43.3X2	T43.3X3	T43.3X4	T43.3X5	T43.3X6
Percaine (spinal)	T41.3X1	T41.3X2	T41.3X3	T41.3X4	T41.3X5	T41.3X6
topical (surface)	T41.3X1	T41.3X2	T41.3X3	T41.3X4	T41.3X5	T41.3X6
Perchloroethylene	T53.3X1	T53.3X2	T53.3X3	T53.3X4	—	—
medicinal	T37.4X1	T37.4X2	T37.4X3	T37.4X4	T37.4X5	T37.4X6
vapor	T53.3X1	T53.3X2	T53.3X3	T53.3X4	—	—
Percodan	T40.2X1	T40.2X2	T40.2X3	T40.2X4	T40.2X5	T40.2X6
Percogesic—see also acetaminophen	T45.0X1	T45.0X2	T45.0X3	T45.0X4	T45.0X5	T45.0X6
Percorten	T38.0X1	T38.0X2	T38.0X3	T38.0X4	T38.0X5	T38.0X6
Pergolide	T42.8X1	T42.8X2	T42.8X3	T42.8X4	T42.8X5	T42.8X6
Pergonal	T38.811	T38.812	T38.813	T38.814	T38.815	T38.816
Perhexilene	T46.3X1	T46.3X2	T46.3X3	T46.3X4	T46.3X5	T46.3X6
Perhexiline (maleate)	T46.3X1	T46.3X2	T46.3X3	T46.3X4	T46.3X5	T46.3X6
Periactin	T45.0X1	T45.0X2	T45.0X3	T45.0X4	T45.0X5	T45.0X6
Periciazine	T43.3X1	T43.3X2	T43.3X3	T43.3X4	T43.3X5	T43.3X6
Periclor	T42.6X1	T42.6X2	T42.6X3	T42.6X4	T42.6X5	T42.6X6
Perindopril	T46.4X1	T46.4X2	T46.4X3	T46.4X4	T46.4X5	T46.4X6
Perisoxal	T39.8X1	T39.8X2	T39.8X3	T39.8X4	T39.8X5	T39.8X6
Peritoneal dialysis solution	T50.3X1	T50.3X2	T50.3X3	T50.3X4	T50.3X5	T50.3X6
Peritrate	T46.3X1	T46.3X2	T46.3X3	T46.3X4	T46.3X5	T46.3X6
Perlapine	T42.4X1	T42.4X2	T42.4X3	T42.4X4	T42.4X5	T42.4X6
Permanganate	T65.891	T65.892	T65.893	T65.894	—	—
Permethrin	T60.1X1	T60.1X2	T60.1X3	T60.1X4	—	—
Pernocton	T42.3X1	T42.3X2	T42.3X3	T42.3X4	T42.3X5	T42.3X6
Pernoston	T42.3X1	T42.3X2	T42.3X3	T42.3X4	T42.3X5	T42.3X6
Peronine	T40.2X1	T40.2X2	T40.2X3	T40.2X4	—	—
Perphenazine	T43.3X1	T43.3X2	T43.3X3	T43.3X4	T43.3X5	T43.3X6
Pertofrane	T43.011	T43.012	T43.013	T43.014	T43.015	T43.016

Substance	Poisoning, Accidental (unintentional)	Poisoning, Intentional self-harm	Poisoning, Assault	Poisoning, Undetermined	Adverse effect	Underdosing
Pertussis						
immune serum (human)	T50.Z11	T50.Z12	T50.Z13	T50.Z14	T50.Z15	T50.Z16
vaccine (with diphtheria toxoid) (with tetanus toxoid)	T50.A11	T50.A12	T50.A13	T50.A14	T50.A15	T50.A16
Peruvian balsam	T49.0X1	T49.0X2	T49.0X3	T49.0X4	T49.0X5	T49.0X6
Peruvoside	T46.0X1	T46.0X2	T46.0X3	T46.0X4	T46.0X5	T46.0X6
Pesticide (dust) (fumes) (vapor) NEC	T60.91	T60.92	T60.93	T60.94	—	—
arsenic	T57.0X1	T57.0X2	T57.0X3	T57.0X4	—	—
chlorinated	T60.1X1	T60.1X2	T60.1X3	T60.1X4	—	—
cyanide	T65.0X1	T65.0X2	T65.0X3	T65.0X4	—	—
kerosene	T52.0X1	T52.0X2	T52.0X3	T52.0X4	—	—
mixture (of compounds)	T60.91	T60.92	T60.93	T60.94	—	—
naphthalene	T60.2X1	T60.2X2	T60.2X3	T60.2X4	—	—
organochlorine (compounds)	T60.1X1	T60.1X2	T60.1X3	T60.1X4	—	—
petroleum (distillate) (products) NEC	T60.8X1	T60.8X2	T60.8X3	T60.8X4	—	—
specified ingredient NEC	T60.8X1	T60.8X2	T60.8X3	T60.8X4	—	—
strychnine	T65.1X1	T65.1X2	T65.1X3	T65.1X4	—	—
thallium	T60.4X1	T60.4X2	T60.4X3	T60.4X4	—	—
Pethidine	T40.491	T40.492	T40.493	T40.494	T40.495	T40.496
Petrichloral	T42.6X1	T42.6X2	T42.6X3	T42.6X4	T42.6X5	T42.6X6
Petrol	T52.0X1	T52.0X2	T52.0X3	T52.0X4	—	—
vapor	T52.0X1	T52.0X2	T52.0X3	T52.0X4	—	—
Petrolatum	T49.3X1	T49.3X2	T49.3X3	T49.3X4	T49.3X5	T49.3X6
hydrophilic	T49.3X1	T49.3X2	T49.3X3	T49.3X4	T49.3X5	T49.3X6
liquid	T47.4X1	T47.4X2	T47.4X3	T47.4X4	T47.4X5	T47.4X6
topical	T49.3X1	T49.3X2	T49.3X3	T49.3X4	T49.3X5	T49.3X6
nonmedicinal	T52.0X1	T52.0X2	T52.0X3	T52.0X4	—	—
red veterinary	T49.3X1	T49.3X2	T49.3X3	T49.3X4	T49.3X5	T49.3X6
white	T49.3X1	T49.3X2	T49.3X3	T49.3X4	T49.3X5	T49.3X6
Petroleum (products) NEC	T52.0X1	T52.0X2	T52.0X3	T52.0X4	—	—
benzine(s)—see Ligroin						
ether—see Ligroin						
jelly—see Petrolatum						
naphtha—see Ligroin						
pesticide	T60.8X1	T60.8X2	T60.8X3	T60.8X4	—	—
solids	T52.0X1	T52.0X2	T52.0X3	T52.0X4	—	—
solvents	T52.0X1	T52.0X2	T52.0X3	T52.0X4	—	—
vapor	T52.0X1	T52.0X2	T52.0X3	T52.0X4	—	—
Peyote	T40.991	T40.992	T40.993	T40.994	—	—
Phanodorm, phanodorn	T42.3X1	T42.3X2	T42.3X3	T42.3X4	T42.3X5	T42.3X6
Phanquinone	T37.3X1	T37.3X2	T37.3X3	T37.3X4	T37.3X5	T37.3X6
Phanquone	T37.3X1	T37.3X2	T37.3X3	T37.3X4	T37.3X5	T37.3X6
Pharmaceutical						
adjunct NEC	T50.901	T50.902	T50.903	T50.904	T50.905	T50.906
excipient NEC	T50.901	T50.902	T50.903	T50.904	T50.905	T50.906
sweetener	T50.901	T50.902	T50.903	T50.904	T50.905	T50.906
viscous agent	T50.901	T50.902	T50.903	T50.904	T50.905	T50.906

Substance	Poisoning, Accidental (unintentional)	Poisoning, Intentional self-harm	Poisoning, Assault	Poisoning, Undetermined	Adverse effect	Underdosing
Phemitone	T42.3X1	T42.3X2	T42.3X3	T42.3X4	T42.3X5	T42.3X6
Phenacaine	T41.3X1	T41.3X2	T41.3X3	T41.3X4	T41.3X5	T41.3X6
Phenacemide	T42.6X1	T42.6X2	T42.6X3	T42.6X4	T42.6X5	T42.6X6
Phenacetin	T39.1X1	T39.1X2	T39.1X3	T39.1X4	T39.1X5	T39.1X6
Phenadoxone	T40.2X1	T40.2X2	T40.2X3	T40.2X4	—	—
Phenaglycodol	T43.591	T43.592	T43.593	T43.594	T43.595	T43.596
Phenantoin	T42.0X1	T42.0X2	T42.0X3	T42.0X4	T42.0X5	T42.0X6
Phenaphthazine reagent	T50.991	T50.992	T50.993	T50.994	T50.995	T50.996
Phenazocine	T40.491	T40.492	T40.493	T40.494	T40.495	T40.496
Phenazone	T39.2X1	T39.2X2	T39.2X3	T39.2X4	T39.2X5	T39.2X6
Phenazopyridine	T39.8X1	T39.8X2	T39.8X3	T39.8X4	T39.8X5	T39.8X6
Phenbenicillin	T36.0X1	T36.0X2	T36.0X3	T36.0X4	T36.0X5	T36.0X6
Phenbutrazate	T50.5X1	T50.5X2	T50.5X3	T50.5X4	T50.5X5	T50.5X6
Phencyclidine	T40.991	T40.992	T40.993	T40.994	T40.995	T40.996
Phendimetrazine	T50.5X1	T50.5X2	T50.5X3	T50.5X4	T50.5X5	T50.5X6
Phenelzine	T43.1X1	T43.1X2	T43.1X3	T43.1X4	T43.1X5	T43.1X6
Phenemal	T42.3X1	T42.3X2	T42.3X3	T42.3X4	T42.3X5	T42.3X6
Phenergan	T42.6X1	T42.6X2	T42.6X3	T42.6X4	T42.6X5	T42.6X6
Pheneticillin	T36.0X1	T36.0X2	T36.0X3	T36.0X4	T36.0X5	T36.0X6
Pheneturide	T42.6X1	T42.6X2	T42.6X3	T42.6X4	T42.6X5	T42.6X6
Phenformin	T38.3X1	T38.3X2	T38.3X3	T38.3X4	T38.3X5	T38.3X6
Phenglutarimide	T44.3X1	T44.3X2	T44.3X3	T44.3X4	T44.3X5	T44.3X6
Phenicarbazide	T39.8X1	T39.8X2	T39.8X3	T39.8X4	T39.8X5	T39.8X6
Phenindamine	T45.0X1	T45.0X2	T45.0X3	T45.0X4	T45.0X5	T45.0X6
Phenindione	T45.511	T45.512	T45.513	T45.514	T45.515	T45.516
Pheniprazine	T43.1X1	T43.1X2	T43.1X3	T43.1X4	T43.1X5	T43.1X6
Pheniramine	T45.0X1	T45.0X2	T45.0X3	T45.0X4	T45.0X5	T45.0X6
Phenisatin	T47.2X1	T47.2X2	T47.2X3	T47.2X4	T47.2X5	T47.2X6
Phenmetrazine	T50.5X1	T50.5X2	T50.5X3	T50.5X4	T50.5X5	T50.5X6
Phenobal	T42.3X1	T42.3X2	T42.3X3	T42.3X4	T42.3X5	T42.3X6
Phenobarbital	T42.3X1	T42.3X2	T42.3X3	T42.3X4	T42.3X5	T42.3X6
with						
mephenytoin	T42.3X1	T42.3X2	T42.3X3	T42.3X4	T42.3X5	T42.3X6
phenytoin	T42.3X1	T42.3X2	T42.3X3	T42.3X4	T42.3X5	T42.3X6
sodium	T42.3X1	T42.3X2	T42.3X3	T42.3X4	T42.3X5	T42.3X6
Phenobarbitone	T42.3X1	T42.3X2	T42.3X3	T42.3X4	T42.3X5	T42.3X6
Phenobutiodil	T50.8X1	T50.8X2	T50.8X3	T50.8X4	T50.8X5	T50.8X6
Phenoctide	T49.0X1	T49.0X2	T49.0X3	T49.0X4	T49.0X5	T49.0X6
Phenol	T49.0X1	T49.0X2	T49.0X3	T49.0X4	T49.0X5	T49.0X6
disinfectant	T54.0X1	T54.0X2	T54.0X3	T54.0X4	—	—
in oil injection	T46.8X1	T46.8X2	T46.8X3	T46.8X4	T46.8X5	T46.8X6
medicinal	T49.1X1	T49.1X2	T49.1X3	T49.1X4	T49.1X5	T49.1X6
nonmedicinal NEC	T54.0X1	T54.0X2	T54.0X3	T54.0X4	—	—
pesticide	T60.8X1	T60.8X2	T60.8X3	T60.8X4	—	—
red	T50.8X1	T50.8X2	T50.8X3	T50.8X4	T50.8X5	T50.8X6
Phenolic preparation	T49.1X1	T49.1X2	T49.1X3	T49.1X4	T49.1X5	T49.1X6
Phenolphthalein	T47.2X1	T47.2X2	T47.2X3	T47.2X4	T47.2X5	T47.2X6
Phenolsulfonphthalein	T50.8X1	T50.8X2	T50.8X3	T50.8X4	T50.8X5	T50.8X6
Phenomorphan	T40.2X1	T40.2X2	T40.2X3	T40.2X4	—	—
Phenonyl	T42.3X1	T42.3X2	T42.3X3	T42.3X4	T42.3X5	T42.3X6

Substance	Poisoning, Accidental (unintentional)	Poisoning, Intentional self-harm	Poisoning, Assault	Poisoning, Undetermined	Adverse effect	Underdosing
Phenoperidine	T40.491	T40.492	T40.493	T40.494	—	—
Phenopyrazone	T46.991	T46.992	T46.993	T46.994	T46.995	T46.996
Phenoquin	T50.4X1	T50.4X2	T50.4X3	T50.4X4	T50.4X5	T50.4X6
Phenothiazine (psychotropic) NEC	T43.3X1	T43.3X2	T43.3X3	T43.3X4	T43.3X5	T43.3X6
insecticide	T60.2X1	T60.2X2	T60.2X3	T60.2X4	—	—
Phenothrin	T49.0X1	T49.0X2	T49.0X3	T49.0X4	T49.0X5	T49.0X6
Phenoxybenzamine	T46.7X1	T46.7X2	T46.7X3	T46.7X4	T46.7X5	T46.7X6
Phenoxyethanol	T49.0X1	T49.0X2	T49.0X3	T49.0X4	T49.0X5	T49.0X6
Phenoxymethyl penicillin	T36.0X1	T36.0X2	T36.0X3	T36.0X4	T36.0X5	T36.0X6
Phenprobamate	T42.8X1	T42.8X2	T42.8X3	T42.8X4	T42.8X5	T42.8X6
Phenprocoumon	T45.511	T45.512	T45.513	T45.514	T45.515	T45.516
Phensuximide	T42.2X1	T42.2X2	T42.2X3	T42.2X4	T42.2X5	T42.2X6
Phentermine	T50.5X1	T50.5X2	T50.5X3	T50.5X4	T50.5X5	T50.5X6
Phenthicillin	T36.0X1	T36.0X2	T36.0X3	T36.0X4	T36.0X5	T36.0X6
Phentolamine	T46.7X1	T46.7X2	T46.7X3	T46.7X4	T46.7X5	T46.7X6
Phenyl						
butazone	T39.2X1	T39.2X2	T39.2X3	T39.2X4	T39.2X5	T39.2X6
enediamine	T65.3X1	T65.3X2	T65.3X3	T65.3X4	—	—
hydrazine	T65.3X1	T65.3X2	T65.3X3	T65.3X4	—	—
antineoplastic	T45.1X1	T45.1X2	T45.1X3	T45.1X4	T45.1X5	T45.1X6
mercuric compounds—see Mercury						
salicylate	T49.3X1	T49.3X2	T49.3X3	T49.3X4	T49.3X5	T49.3X6
Phenylalanine mustard	T45.1X1	T45.1X2	T45.1X3	T45.1X4	T45.1X5	T45.1X6
Phenylbutazone	T39.2X1	T39.2X2	T39.2X3	T39.2X4	T39.2X5	T39.2X6
Phenylenediamine	T65.3X1	T65.3X2	T65.3X3	T65.3X4	—	—
Phenylephrine	T44.4X1	T44.4X2	T44.4X3	T44.4X4	T44.4X5	T44.4X6
Phenylethylbiguanide	T38.3X1	T38.3X2	T38.3X3	T38.3X4	T38.3X5	T38.3X6
Phenylmercuric						
acetate	T49.0X1	T49.0X2	T49.0X3	T49.0X4	T49.0X5	T49.0X6
borate	T49.0X1	T49.0X2	T49.0X3	T49.0X4	T49.0X5	T49.0X6
nitrate	T49.0X1	T49.0X2	T49.0X3	T49.0X4	T49.0X5	T49.0X6
Phenylmethylbarbitone	T42.3X1	T42.3X2	T42.3X3	T42.3X4	T42.3X5	T42.3X6
Phenylpropanol	T47.5X1	T47.5X2	T47.5X3	T47.5X4	T47.5X5	T47.5X6
Phenylpropanolamine	T44.991	T44.992	T44.993	T44.994	T44.995	T44.996
Phenylsulfthion	T60.0X1	T60.0X2	T60.0X3	T60.0X4	—	—
Phenyltoloxamine	T45.0X1	T45.0X2	T45.0X3	T45.0X4	T45.0X5	T45.0X6
Phenyramidol, phenyramidon	T39.8X1	T39.8X2	T39.8X3	T39.8X4	T39.8X5	T39.8X6
Phenytoin	T42.0X1	T42.0X2	T42.0X3	T42.0X4	T42.0X5	T42.0X6
with Phenobarbital	T42.3X1	T42.3X2	T42.3X3	T42.3X4	T42.3X5	T42.3X6
pHisoHex	T49.2X1	T49.2X2	T49.2X3	T49.2X4	T49.2X5	T49.2X6
Pholcodine	T48.3X1	T48.3X2	T48.3X3	T48.3X4	T48.3X5	T48.3X6
Pholedrine	T46.991	T46.992	T46.993	T46.994	T46.995	T46.996
Phorate	T60.0X1	T60.0X2	T60.0X3	T60.0X4	—	—
Phosdrin	T60.0X1	T60.0X2	T60.0X3	T60.0X4	—	—
Phosfolan	T60.0X1	T60.0X2	T60.0X3	T60.0X4	—	—
Phosgene (gas)	T59.891	T59.892	T59.893	T59.894	—	—
Phosphamidon	T60.0X1	T60.0X2	T60.0X3	T60.0X4	—	—
Phosphate	T65.891	T65.892	T65.893	T65.894	—	—
laxative	T47.4X1	T47.4X2	T47.4X3	T47.4X4	T47.4X5	T47.4X6
organic	T60.0X1	T60.0X2	T60.0X3	T60.0X4	—	—
solvent	T52.91	T52.92	T52.93	T52.94	—	—
tricresyl	T65.891	T65.892	T65.893	T65.894	—	—
Phosphine	T57.1X1	T57.1X2	T57.1X3	T57.1X4	—	—
fumigant	T57.1X1	T57.1X2	T57.1X3	T57.1X4	—	—
Phospholine	T49.5X1	T49.5X2	T49.5X3	T49.5X4	T49.5X5	T49.5X6
Phosphoric acid	T54.2X1	T54.2X2	T54.2X3	T54.2X4	—	—
Phosphorus (compound) NEC	T57.1X1	T57.1X2	T57.1X3	T57.1X4	—	—
pesticide	T60.0X1	T60.0X2	T60.0X3	T60.0X4	—	—
Phthalates	T65.891	T65.892	T65.893	T65.894	—	—
Phthalic anhydride	T65.891	T65.892	T65.893	T65.894	—	—
Phthalimidoglutarimide	T42.6X1	T42.6X2	T42.6X3	T42.6X4	T42.6X5	T42.6X6
Phthalylsulfathiazole	T37.0X1	T37.0X2	T37.0X3	T37.0X4	T37.0X5	T37.0X6
Phylloquinone	T45.7X1	T45.7X2	T45.7X3	T45.7X4	T45.7X5	T45.7X6
Physeptone	T40.3X1	T40.3X2	T40.3X3	T40.3X4	T40.3X5	T40.3X6
Physostigma venenosum	T62.2X1	T62.2X2	T62.2X3	T62.2X4	—	—
Physostigmine	T49.5X1	T49.5X2	T49.5X3	T49.5X4	T49.5X5	T49.5X6
Phytolacca decandra	T62.2X1	T62.2X2	T62.2X3	T62.2X4	—	—
berries	T62.1X1	T62.1X2	T62.1X3	T62.1X4	—	—
Phytomenadione	T45.7X1	T45.7X2	T45.7X3	T45.7X4	T45.7X5	T45.7X6
Phytonadione	T45.7X1	T45.7X2	T45.7X3	T45.7X4	T45.7X5	T45.7X6
Picoperine	T48.3X1	T48.3X2	T48.3X3	T48.3X4	T48.3X5	T48.3X6
Picosulfate (sodium)	T47.2X1	T47.2X2	T47.2X3	T47.2X4	T47.2X5	T47.2X6
Picric (acid)	T54.2X1	T54.2X2	T54.2X3	T54.2X4	—	—
Picrotoxin	T50.7X1	T50.7X2	T50.7X3	T50.7X4	T50.7X5	T50.7X6
Piketoprofen	T49.0X1	T49.0X2	T49.0X3	T49.0X4	T49.0X5	T49.0X6
Pilocarpine	T44.1X1	T44.1X2	T44.1X3	T44.1X4	T44.1X5	T44.1X6
Pilocarpus (jaborandi) extract	T44.1X1	T44.1X2	T44.1X3	T44.1X4	T44.1X5	T44.1X6
Pilsicainide (hydrochloride)	T46.2X1	T46.2X2	T46.2X3	T46.2X4	T46.2X5	T46.2X6
Pimaricin	T36.7X1	T36.7X2	T36.7X3	T36.7X4	T36.7X5	T36.7X6
Pimeclone	T50.7X1	T50.7X2	T50.7X3	T50.7X4	T50.7X5	T50.7X6
Pimelic ketone	T52.8X1	T52.8X2	T52.8X3	T52.8X4	—	—
Pimethixene	T45.0X1	T45.0X2	T45.0X3	T45.0X4	T45.0X5	T45.0X6
Piminodine	T40.2X1	T40.2X2	T40.2X3	T40.2X4	T40.2X5	T40.2X6
Pimozide	T43.591	T43.592	T43.593	T43.594	T43.595	T43.596
Pinacidil	T46.5X1	T46.5X2	T46.5X3	T46.5X4	T46.5X5	T46.5X6
Pinaverium bromide	T44.3X1	T44.3X2	T44.3X3	T44.3X4	T44.3X5	T44.3X6
Pinazepam	T42.4X1	T42.4X2	T42.4X3	T42.4X4	T42.4X5	T42.4X6
Pindolol	T44.7X1	T44.7X2	T44.7X3	T44.7X4	T44.7X5	T44.7X6
Pindone	T60.4X1	T60.4X2	T60.4X3	T60.4X4	—	—
Pine oil (disinfectant)	T65.891	T65.892	T65.893	T65.894	—	—
Pinkroot	T37.4X1	T37.4X2	T37.4X3	T37.4X4	T37.4X5	T37.4X6
Pipadone	T40.2X1	T40.2X2	T40.2X3	T40.2X4	—	—
Pipamazine	T45.0X1	T45.0X2	T45.0X3	T45.0X4	T45.0X5	T45.0X6
Pipamperone	T43.4X1	T43.4X2	T43.4X3	T43.4X4	T43.4X5	T43.4X6
Pipazetate	T48.3X1	T48.3X2	T48.3X3	T48.3X4	T48.3X5	T48.3X6

Substance	Poisoning, Accidental (unintentional)	Poisoning, Intentional self-harm	Poisoning, Assault	Poisoning, Undetermined	Adverse effect	Underdosing
Pipemidic acid	T37.8X1	T37.8X2	T37.8X3	T37.8X4	T37.8X5	T37.8X6
Pipenzolate bromide	T44.3X1	T44.3X2	T44.3X3	T44.3X4	T44.3X5	T44.3X6
Piperacetazine	T43.3X1	T43.3X2	T43.3X3	T43.3X4	T43.3X5	T43.3X6
Piperacillin	T36.0X1	T36.0X2	T36.0X3	T36.0X4	T36.0X5	T36.0X6
Piperazine	T37.4X1	T37.4X2	T37.4X3	T37.4X4	T37.4X5	T37.4X6
estrone sulfate	T38.5X1	T38.5X2	T38.5X3	T38.5X4	T38.5X5	T38.5X6
Piper cubeba	T62.2X1	T62.2X2	T62.2X3	T62.2X4	—	—
Piperidione	T48.3X1	T48.3X2	T48.3X3	T48.3X4	T48.3X5	T48.3X6
Piperidolate	T44.3X1	T44.3X2	T44.3X3	T44.3X4	T44.3X5	T44.3X6
Piperocaine	T41.3X1	T41.3X2	T41.3X3	T41.3X4	T41.3X5	T41.3X6
infiltration (subcutaneous)	T41.3X1	T41.3X2	T41.3X3	T41.3X4	T41.3X5	T41.3X6
nerve block (peripheral) (plexus)	T41.3X1	T41.3X2	T41.3X3	T41.3X4	T41.3X5	T41.3X6
topical (surface)	T41.3X1	T41.3X2	T41.3X3	T41.3X4	T41.3X5	T41.3X6
Piperonyl butoxide	T60.8X1	T60.8X2	T60.8X3	T60.8X4	—	—
Pipethanate	T44.3X1	T44.3X2	T44.3X3	T44.3X4	T44.3X5	T44.3X6
Pipobroman	T45.1X1	T45.1X2	T45.1X3	T45.1X4	T45.1X5	T45.1X6
Pipotiazine	T43.3X1	T43.3X2	T43.3X3	T43.3X4	T43.3X5	T43.3X6
Pipoxizine	T45.0X1	T45.0X2	T45.0X3	T45.0X4	T45.0X5	T45.0X6
Pipradrol	T43.691	T43.692	T43.693	T43.694	T43.695	T43.696
Piprinhydrinate	T45.0X1	T45.0X2	T45.0X3	T45.0X4	T45.0X5	T45.0X6
Pirarubicin	T45.1X1	T45.1X2	T45.1X3	T45.1X4	T45.1X5	T45.1X6
Pirazinamide	T37.1X1	T37.1X2	T37.1X3	T37.1X4	T37.1X5	T37.1X6
Pirbuterol	T48.6X1	T48.6X2	T48.6X3	T48.6X4	T48.6X5	T48.6X6
Pirenzepine	T47.1X1	T47.1X2	T47.1X3	T47.1X4	T47.1X5	T47.1X6
Piretanide	T50.1X1	T50.1X2	T50.1X3	T50.1X4	T50.1X5	T50.1X6
Piribedil	T42.8X1	T42.8X2	T42.8X3	T42.8X4	T42.8X5	T42.8X6
Piridoxilate	T46.3X1	T46.3X2	T46.3X3	T46.3X4	T46.3X5	T46.3X6
Piritramide	T40.491	T40.492	T40.493	T40.494	—	—
Piromidic acid	T37.8X1	T37.8X2	T37.8X3	T37.8X4	T37.8X5	T37.8X6
Piroxicam	T39.391	T39.392	T39.393	T39.394	T39.395	T39.396
beta-cyclodextrin complex	T39.8X1	T39.8X2	T39.8X3	T39.8X4	T39.8X5	T39.8X6
Pirozadil	T46.6X1	T46.6X2	T46.6X3	T46.6X4	T46.6X5	T46.6X6
Piscidia (bark) (erythrina)	T39.8X1	T39.8X2	T39.8X3	T39.8X4	T39.8X5	T39.8X6
Pitch	T65.891	T65.892	T65.893	T65.894	—	—
Pitkin's solution	T41.3X1	T41.3X2	T41.3X3	T41.3X4	T41.3X5	T41.3X6
Pitocin	T48.0X1	T48.0X2	T48.0X3	T48.0X4	T48.0X5	T48.0X6
Pitressin (tannate)	T38.891	T38.892	T38.893	T38.894	T38.895	T38.896
Pituitary extracts (posterior)	T38.891	T38.892	T38.893	T38.894	T38.895	T38.896
anterior	T38.811	T38.812	T38.813	T38.814	T38.815	T38.816
Pituitrin	T38.891	T38.892	T38.893	T38.894	T38.895	T38.896
Pivampicillin	T36.0X1	T36.0X2	T36.0X3	T36.0X4	T36.0X5	T36.0X6
Pivmecillinam	T36.0X1	T36.0X2	T36.0X3	T36.0X4	T36.0X5	T36.0X6
Placental hormone	T38.891	T38.892	T38.893	T38.894	T38.895	T38.896
Placidyl	T42.6X1	T42.6X2	T42.6X3	T42.6X4	T42.6X5	T42.6X6
Plague vaccine	T50.A91	T50.A92	T50.A93	T50.A94	T50.A95	T50.A96

Substance	Poisoning, Accidental (unintentional)	Poisoning, Intentional self-harm	Poisoning, Assault	Poisoning, Undetermined	Adverse effect	Underdosing
Plant						
food or fertilizer NEC	T65.891	T65.892	T65.893	T65.894	—	—
containing herbicide	T60.3X1	T60.3X2	T60.3X3	T60.3X4	—	—
noxious, used as food	T62.2X1	T62.2X2	T62.2X3	T62.2X4	—	—
berries	T62.1X1	T62.1X2	T62.1X3	T62.1X4	—	—
seeds	T62.2X1	T62.2X2	T62.2X3	T62.2X4	—	—
specified type NEC	T62.2X1	T62.2X2	T62.2X3	T62.2X4	—	—
Plasma	T45.8X1	T45.8X2	T45.8X3	T45.8X4	T45.8X5	T45.8X6
expander NEC	T45.8X1	T45.8X2	T45.8X3	T45.8X4	T45.8X5	T45.8X6
protein fraction (human)	T45.8X1	T45.8X2	T45.8X3	T45.8X4	T45.8X5	T45.8X6
Plasmanate	T45.8X1	T45.8X2	T45.8X3	T45.8X4	T45.8X5	T45.8X6
Plasminogen (tissue) activator	T45.611	T45.612	T45.613	T45.614	T45.615	T45.616
Plaster dressing	T49.3X1	T49.3X2	T49.3X3	T49.3X4	T49.3X5	T49.3X6
Plastic dressing	T49.3X1	T49.3X2	T49.3X3	T49.3X4	T49.3X5	T49.3X6
Plegicil	T43.3X1	T43.3X2	T43.3X3	T43.3X4	T43.3X5	T43.3X6
Plicamycin	T45.1X1	T45.1X2	T45.1X3	T45.1X4	T45.1X5	T45.1X6
Podophyllotoxin	T49.8X1	T49.8X2	T49.8X3	T49.8X4	T49.8X5	T49.8X6
Podophyllum (resin)	T49.4X1	T49.4X2	T49.4X3	T49.4X4	T49.4X5	T49.4X6
Poison NEC	T65.91	T65.92	T65.93	T65.94	—	—
Poisonous berries	T62.1X1	T62.1X2	T62.1X3	T62.1X4	—	—
Pokeweed (any part)	T62.2X1	T62.2X2	T62.2X3	T62.2X4	—	—
Poldine metilsulfate	T44.3X1	T44.3X2	T44.3X3	T44.3X4	T44.3X5	T44.3X6
Polidexide (sulfate)	T46.6X1	T46.6X2	T46.6X3	T46.6X4	T46.6X5	T46.6X6
Polidocanol	T46.8X1	T46.8X2	T46.8X3	T46.8X4	T46.8X5	T46.8X6
Poliomyelitis vaccine	T50.B91	T50.B92	T50.B93	T50.B94	T50.B95	T50.B96
Polish (car) (floor) (furniture) (metal) (porcelain) (silver)	T65.891	T65.892	T65.893	T65.894	—	
abrasive	T65.891	T65.892	T65.893	T65.894	—	—
porcelain	T65.891	T65.892	T65.893	T65.894	—	—
Poloxalkol	T47.4X1	T47.4X2	T47.4X3	T47.4X4	T47.4X5	T47.4X6
Poloxamer	T47.4X1	T47.4X2	T47.4X3	T47.4X4	T47.4X5	T47.4X6
Polyaminostyrene resins	T50.3X1	T50.3X2	T50.3X3	T50.3X4	T50.3X5	T50.3X6
Polycarbophil	T47.4X1	T47.4X2	T47.4X3	T47.4X4	T47.4X5	T47.4X6
Polychlorinated biphenyl	T65.891	T65.892	T65.893	T65.894	—	—
Polycycline	T36.4X1	T36.4X2	T36.4X3	T36.4X4	T36.4X5	T36.4X6
Polyester fumes	T59.891	T59.892	T59.893	T59.894	—	—
Polyester resin hardener	T52.91	T52.92	T52.93	T52.94	—	—
fumes	T59.891	T59.892	T59.893	T59.894	—	—
Polyestradiol phosphate	T38.5X1	T38.5X2	T38.5X3	T38.5X4	T38.5X5	T38.5X6
Polyethanolamine alkyl sulfate	T49.2X1	T49.2X2	T49.2X3	T49.2X4	T49.2X5	T49.2X6
Polyethylene adhesive	T49.3X1	T49.3X2	T49.3X3	T49.3X4	T49.3X5	T49.3X6
Polyferose	T45.4X1	T45.4X2	T45.4X3	T45.4X4	T45.4X5	T45.4X6
Polygeline	T45.8X1	T45.8X2	T45.8X3	T45.8X4	T45.8X5	T45.8X6
Polymyxin	T36.8X1	T36.8X2	T36.8X3	T36.8X4	T36.8X5	T36.8X6
B	T36.8X1	T36.8X2	T36.8X3	T36.8X4	T36.8X5	T36.8X6
ENT agent	T49.6X1	T49.6X2	T49.6X3	T49.6X4	T49.6X5	T49.6X6

Substance	Poisoning, Accidental (unintentional)	Poisoning, Intentional self-harm	Poisoning, Assault	Poisoning, Undetermined	Adverse effect	Underdosing
Polymyxin — *Continued*						
ophthalmic preparation	T49.5X1	T49.5X2	T49.5X3	T49.5X4	T49.5X5	T49.5X6
topical NEC	T49.0X1	T49.0X2	T49.0X3	T49.0X4	T49.0X5	T49.0X6
E sulfate (eye preparation)	T49.5X1	T49.5X2	T49.5X3	T49.5X4	T49.5X5	T49.5X6
Polynoxylin	T49.0X1	T49.0X2	T49.0X3	T49.0X4	T49.0X5	T49.0X6
Polyoestradiol phosphate	T38.5X1	T38.5X2	T38.5X3	T38.5X4	T38.5X5	T38.5X6
Polyoxymethyleneurea	T49.0X1	T49.0X2	T49.0X3	T49.0X4	T49.0X5	T49.0X6
Polysilane	T47.8X1	T47.8X2	T47.8X3	T47.8X4	T47.8X5	T47.8X6
Polytetrafluoroethylene (inhaled)	T59.891	T59.892	T59.893	T59.894	—	—
Polythiazide	T50.2X1	T50.2X2	T50.2X3	T50.2X4	T50.2X5	T50.2X6
Polyvidone	T45.8X1	T45.8X2	T45.8X3	T45.8X4	T45.8X5	T45.8X6
Polyvinylpyrrolidone	T45.8X1	T45.8X2	T45.8X3	T45.8X4	T45.8X5	T45.8X6
Pontocaine (hydrochloride) (infiltration) (topical)	T41.3X1	T41.3X2	T41.3X3	T41.3X4	T41.3X5	T41.3X6
nerve block (peripheral) (plexus)	T41.3X1	T41.3X2	T41.3X3	T41.3X4	T41.3X5	T41.3X6
spinal	T41.3X1	T41.3X2	T41.3X3	T41.3X4	T41.3X5	T41.3X6
Porfiromycin	T45.1X1	T45.1X2	T45.1X3	T45.1X4	T45.1X5	T45.1X6
Posterior pituitary hormone NEC	T38.891	T38.892	T38.893	T38.894	T38.895	T38.896
Pot	T40.711	T40.712	T40.713	T40.714	T40.715	T40.716
Potash (caustic)	T54.3X1	T54.3X2	T54.3X3	T54.3X4	—	—
Potassic saline injection (lactated)	T50.3X1	T50.3X2	T50.3X3	T50.3X4	T50.3X5	T50.3X6
Potassium (salts) NEC	T50.3X1	T50.3X2	T50.3X3	T50.3X4	T50.3X5	T50.3X6
aminobenzoate	T45.8X1	T45.8X2	T45.8X3	T45.8X4	T45.8X5	T45.8X6
aminosalicylate	T37.1X1	T37.1X2	T37.1X3	T37.1X4	T37.1X5	T37.1X6
antimony 'tartrate'	T37.8X1	T37.8X2	T37.8X3	T37.8X4	T37.8X5	T37.8X6
arsenite (solution)	T57.0X1	T57.0X2	T57.0X3	T57.0X4	—	—
bichromate	T56.2X1	T56.2X2	T56.2X3	T56.2X4	—	—
bisulfate	T47.3X1	T47.3X2	T47.3X3	T47.3X4	T47.3X5	T47.3X6
bromide	T42.6X1	T42.6X2	T42.6X3	T42.6X4	T42.6X5	T42.6X6
canrenoate	T50.0X1	T50.0X2	T50.0X3	T50.0X4	T50.0X5	T50.0X6
carbonate	T54.3X1	T54.3X2	T54.3X3	T54.3X4	—	—
chlorate NEC	T65.891	T65.892	T65.893	T65.894	—	—
chloride	T50.3X1	T50.3X2	T50.3X3	T50.3X4	T50.3X5	T50.3X6
citrate	T50.991	T50.992	T50.993	T50.994	T50.995	T50.996
cyanide	T65.0X1	T65.0X2	T65.0X3	T65.0X4	—	—
ferric hexacyano-ferrate (medicinal)	T50.6X1	T50.6X2	T50.6X3	T50.6X4	T50.6X5	T50.6X6
nonmedicinal	T65.891	T65.892	T65.893	T65.894	—	—
Fluoride	T57.8X1	T57.8X2	T57.8X3	T57.8X4	—	—
glucaldrate	T47.1X1	T47.1X2	T47.1X3	T47.1X4	T47.1X5	T47.1X6
hydroxide	T54.3X1	T54.3X2	T54.3X3	T54.3X4	—	—
iodate	T49.0X1	T49.0X2	T49.0X3	T49.0X4	T49.0X5	T49.0X6
iodide	T48.4X1	T48.4X2	T48.4X3	T48.4X4	T48.4X5	T48.4X6
nitrate	T57.8X1	T57.8X2	T57.8X3	T57.8X4	—	—
oxalate	T65.891	T65.892	T65.893	T65.894	—	—
Potassium — *Continued*						
perchlorate (nonmedicinal) NEC	T65.891	T65.892	T65.893	T65.894	—	—
antithyroid	T38.2X1	T38.2X2	T38.2X3	T38.2X4	T38.2X5	T38.2X6
medicinal	T38.2X1	T38.2X2	T38.2X3	T38.2X4	T38.2X5	T38.2X6
Permanganate (nonmedicinal)	T65.891	T65.892	T65.893	T65.894	—	—
medicinal	T49.0X1	T49.0X2	T49.0X3	T49.0X4	T49.0X5	T49.0X6
sulfate	T47.2X1	T47.2X2	T47.2X3	T47.2X4	T47.2X5	T47.2X6
Potassium-removing resin	T50.3X1	T50.3X2	T50.3X3	T50.3X4	T50.3X5	T50.3X6
Potassium-retaining drug	T50.3X1	T50.3X2	T50.3X3	T50.3X4	T50.3X5	T50.3X6
Povidone	T45.8X1	T45.8X2	T45.8X3	T45.8X4	T45.8X5	T45.8X6
iodine	T49.0X1	T49.0X2	T49.0X3	T49.0X4	T49.0X5	T49.0X6
Practolol	T44.7X1	T44.7X2	T44.7X3	T44.7X4	T44.7X5	T44.7X6
Prajmalium bitartrate	T46.2X1	T46.2X2	T46.2X3	T46.2X4	T46.2X5	T46.2X6
Pralidoxime (iodide)	T50.6X1	T50.6X2	T50.6X3	T50.6X4	T50.6X5	T50.6X6
chloride	T50.6X1	T50.6X2	T50.6X3	T50.6X4	T50.6X5	T50.6X6
Pramiverine	T44.3X1	T44.3X2	T44.3X3	T44.3X4	T44.3X5	T44.3X6
Pramocaine	T49.1X1	T49.1X2	T49.1X3	T49.1X4	T49.1X5	T49.1X6
Pramoxine	T49.1X1	T49.1X2	T49.1X3	T49.1X4	T49.1X5	T49.1X6
Prasterone	T38.7X1	T38.7X2	T38.7X3	T38.7X4	T38.7X5	T38.7X6
Pravastatin	T46.6X1	T46.6X2	T46.6X3	T46.6X4	T46.6X5	T46.6X6
Prazepam	T42.4X1	T42.4X2	T42.4X3	T42.4X4	T42.4X5	T42.4X6
Praziquantel	T37.4X1	T37.4X2	T37.4X3	T37.4X4	T37.4X5	T37.4X6
Prazitone	T43.291	T43.292	T43.293	T43.294	T43.295	T43.296
Prazosin	T44.6X1	T44.6X2	T44.6X3	T44.6X4	T44.6X5	T44.6X6
Prednicarbate	T49.0X1	T49.0X2	T49.0X3	T49.0X4	T49.0X5	T49.0X6
Prednimustine	T45.1X1	T45.1X2	T45.1X3	T45.1X4	T45.1X5	T45.1X6
Prednisolone	T38.0X1	T38.0X2	T38.0X3	T38.0X4	T38.0X5	T38.0X6
ENT agent	T49.6X1	T49.6X2	T49.6X3	T49.6X4	T49.6X5	T49.6X6
ophthalmic preparation	T49.5X1	T49.5X2	T49.5X3	T49.5X4	T49.5X5	T49.5X6
steaglate	T49.0X1	T49.0X2	T49.0X3	T49.0X4	T49.0X5	T49.0X6
topical NEC	T49.0X1	T49.0X2	T49.0X3	T49.0X4	T49.0X5	T49.0X6
Prednisone	T38.0X1	T38.0X2	T38.0X3	T38.0X4	T38.0X5	T38.0X6
Prednylidene	T38.0X1	T38.0X2	T38.0X3	T38.0X4	T38.0X5	T38.0X6
Pregnandiol	T38.5X1	T38.5X2	T38.5X3	T38.5X4	T38.5X5	T38.5X6
Pregneninolone	T38.5X1	T38.5X2	T38.5X3	T38.5X4	T38.5X5	T38.5X6
Preludin	T43.691	T43.692	T43.693	T43.694	T43.695	T43.696
Premarin	T38.5X1	T38.5X2	T38.5X3	T38.5X4	T38.5X5	T38.5X6
Premedication anesthetic	T41.201	T41.202	T41.203	T41.204	T41.205	T41.206
Prenalterol	T44.5X1	T44.5X2	T44.5X3	T44.5X4	T44.5X5	T44.5X6
Prenoxdiazine	T48.3X1	T48.3X2	T48.3X3	T48.3X4	T48.3X5	T48.3X6
Prenylamine	T46.3X1	T46.3X2	T46.3X3	T46.3X4	T46.3X5	T46.3X6
Preparation H	T49.8X1	T49.8X2	T49.8X3	T49.8X4	T49.8X5	T49.8X6
Preparation, local	T49.4X1	T49.4X2	T49.4X3	T49.4X4	T49.4X5	T49.4X6
Preservative (nonmedicinal)	T65.891	T65.892	T65.893	T65.894	—	—
medicinal	T50.901	T50.902	T50.903	T50.904	T50.905	T50.906
wood	T60.91	T60.92	T60.93	T60.94	—	—

Substance	Poisoning, Accidental (unintentional)	Poisoning, Intentional self-harm	Poisoning, Assault	Poisoning, Undetermined	Adverse effect	Underdosing
Prethcamide	T50.7X1	T50.7X2	T50.7X3	T50.7X4	T50.7X5	T50.7X6
Pride of China	T62.2X1	T62.2X2	T62.2X3	T62.2X4	—	—
Pridinol	T44.3X1	T44.3X2	T44.3X3	T44.3X4	T44.3X5	T44.3X6
Prifinium bromide	T44.3X1	T44.3X2	T44.3X3	T44.3X4	T44.3X5	T44.3X6
Prilocaine	T41.3X1	T41.3X2	T41.3X3	T41.3X4	T41.3X5	T41.3X6
infiltration (subcutaneous)	T41.3X1	T41.3X2	T41.3X3	T41.3X4	T41.3X5	T41.3X6
nerve block (peripheral) (plexus)	T41.3X1	T41.3X2	T41.3X3	T41.3X4	T41.3X5	T41.3X6
regional	T41.3X1	T41.3X2	T41.3X3	T41.3X4	T41.3X5	T41.3X6
Primaquine	T37.2X1	T37.2X2	T37.2X3	T37.2X4	T37.2X5	T37.2X6
Primidone	T42.6X1	T42.6X2	T42.6X3	T42.6X4	T42.6X5	T42.6X6
Primula (veris)	T62.2X1	T62.2X2	T62.2X3	T62.2X4	—	—
Prinadol	T40.2X1	T40.2X2	T40.2X3	T40.2X4	T40.2X5	T40.2X6
Priscol, Priscoline	T44.6X1	T44.6X2	T44.6X3	T44.6X4	T44.6X5	T44.6X6
Pristinamycin	T36.3X1	T36.3X2	T36.3X3	T36.3X4	T36.3X5	T36.3X6
Privet	T62.2X1	T62.2X2	T62.2X3	T62.2X4	—	—
berries	T62.1X1	T62.1X2	T62.1X3	T62.1X4	—	—
Privine	T44.4X1	T44.4X2	T44.4X3	T44.4X4	T44.4X5	T44.4X6
Pro-Banthine	T44.3X1	T44.3X2	T44.3X3	T44.3X4	T44.3X5	T44.3X6
Probarbital	T42.3X1	T42.3X2	T42.3X3	T42.3X4	T42.3X5	T42.3X6
Probenecid	T50.4X1	T50.4X2	T50.4X3	T50.4X4	T50.4X5	T50.4X6
Probucol	T46.6X1	T46.6X2	T46.6X3	T46.6X4	T46.6X5	T46.6X6
Procainamide	T46.2X1	T46.2X2	T46.2X3	T46.2X4	T46.2X5	T46.2X6
Procaine	T41.3X1	T41.3X2	T41.3X3	T41.3X4	T41.3X5	T41.3X6
benzylpenicillin	T36.0X1	T36.0X2	T36.0X3	T36.0X4	T36.0X5	T36.0X6
nerve block (periphreal) (plexus)	T41.3X1	T41.3X2	T41.3X3	T41.3X4	T41.3X5	T41.3X6
penicillin G	T36.0X1	T36.0X2	T36.0X3	T36.0X4	T36.0X5	T36.0X6
regional	T41.3X1	T41.3X2	T41.3X3	T41.3X4	T41.3X5	T41.3X6
spinal	T41.3X1	T41.3X2	T41.3X3	T41.3X4	T41.3X5	T41.3X6
Procalmidol	T43.591	T43.592	T43.593	T43.594	T43.595	T43.596
Procarbazine	T45.1X1	T45.1X2	T45.1X3	T45.1X4	T45.1X5	T45.1X6
Procaterol	T44.5X1	T44.5X2	T44.5X3	T44.5X4	T44.5X5	T44.5X6
Prochlorperazine	T43.3X1	T43.3X2	T43.3X3	T43.3X4	T43.3X5	T43.3X6
Procyclidine	T44.3X1	T44.3X2	T44.3X3	T44.3X4	T44.3X5	T44.3X6
Producer gas	T58.8X1	T58.8X2	T58.8X3	T58.8X4	—	—
Profadol	T40.491	T40.492	T40.493	T40.494	T40.495	T40.496
Profenamine	T44.3X1	T44.3X2	T44.3X3	T44.3X4	T44.3X5	T44.3X6
Profenil	T44.3X1	T44.3X2	T44.3X3	T44.3X4	T44.3X5	T44.3X6
Proflavine	T49.0X1	T49.0X2	T49.0X3	T49.0X4	T49.0X5	T49.0X6
Progabide	T42.6X1	T42.6X2	T42.6X3	T42.6X4	T42.6X5	T42.6X6
Progesterone	T38.5X1	T38.5X2	T38.5X3	T38.5X4	T38.5X5	T38.5X6
Progestin	T38.5X1	T38.5X2	T38.5X3	T38.5X4	T38.5X5	T38.5X6
oral contraceptive	T38.4X1	T38.4X2	T38.4X3	T38.4X4	T38.4X5	T38.4X6
Progestogen NEC	T38.5X1	T38.5X2	T38.5X3	T38.5X4	T38.5X5	T38.5X6
Progestone	T38.5X1	T38.5X2	T38.5X3	T38.5X4	T38.5X5	T38.5X6
Proglumide	T47.1X1	T47.1X2	T47.1X3	T47.1X4	T47.1X5	T47.1X6
Proguanil	T37.2X1	T37.2X2	T37.2X3	T37.2X4	T37.2X5	T37.2X6
Prolactin	T38.811	T38.812	T38.813	T38.814	T38.815	T38.816
Prolintane	T43.691	T43.692	T43.693	T43.694	T43.695	T43.696
Proloid	T38.1X1	T38.1X2	T38.1X3	T38.1X4	T38.1X5	T38.1X6
Proluton	T38.5X1	T38.5X2	T38.5X3	T38.5X4	T38.5X5	T38.5X6
Promacetin	T37.1X1	T37.1X2	T37.1X3	T37.1X4	T37.1X5	T37.1X6
Promazine	T43.3X1	T43.3X2	T43.3X3	T43.3X4	T43.3X5	T43.3X6
Promedol	T40.2X1	T40.2X2	T40.2X3	T40.2X4	—	—
Promegestone	T38.5X1	T38.5X2	T38.5X3	T38.5X4	T38.5X5	T38.5X6
Promethazine (teoclate)	T43.3X1	T43.3X2	T43.3X3	T43.3X4	T43.3X5	T43.3X6
Promin	T37.1X1	T37.1X2	T37.1X3	T37.1X4	T37.1X5	T37.1X6
Pronase	T45.3X1	T45.3X2	T45.3X3	T45.3X4	T45.3X5	T45.3X6
Pronestyl (hydrochloride)	T46.2X1	T46.2X2	T46.2X3	T46.2X4	T46.2X5	T46.2X6
Pronetalol	T44.7X1	T44.7X2	T44.7X3	T44.7X4	T44.7X5	T44.7X6
Prontosil	T37.0X1	T37.0X2	T37.0X3	T37.0X4	T37.0X5	T37.0X6
Propachlor	T60.3X1	T60.3X2	T60.3X3	T60.3X4	—	—
Propafenone	T46.2X1	T46.2X2	T46.2X3	T46.2X4	T46.2X5	T46.2X6
Propallylonal	T42.3X1	T42.3X2	T42.3X3	T42.3X4	T42.3X5	T42.3X6
Propamidine	T49.0X1	T49.0X2	T49.0X3	T49.0X4	T49.0X5	T49.0X6
Propane (distributed in mobile container)	T59.891	T59.892	T59.893	T59.894	—	—
distributed through pipes	T59.891	T59.892	T59.893	T59.894	—	—
incomplete combustion	T58.11	T58.12	T58.13	T58.14	—	—
Propanidid	T41.291	T41.292	T41.293	T41.294	T41.295	T41.296
Propanil	T60.3X1	T60.3X2	T60.3X3	T60.3X4	—	—
1-Propanol	T51.3X1	T51.3X2	T51.3X3	T51.3X4	—	—
2-Propanol	T51.2X1	T51.2X2	T51.2X3	T51.2X4	—	—
Propantheline	T44.3X1	T44.3X2	T44.3X3	T44.3X4	T44.3X5	T44.3X6
bromide	T44.3X1	T44.3X2	T44.3X3	T44.3X4	T44.3X5	T44.3X6
Proparacaine	T41.3X1	T41.3X2	T41.3X3	T41.3X4	T41.3X5	T41.3X6
Propatylnitrate	T46.3X1	T46.3X2	T46.3X3	T46.3X4	T46.3X5	T46.3X6
Propicillin	T36.0X1	T36.0X2	T36.0X3	T36.0X4	T36.0X5	T36.0X6
Propiolactone	T49.0X1	T49.0X2	T49.0X3	T49.0X4	T49.0X5	T49.0X6
Propiomazine	T45.0X1	T45.0X2	T45.0X3	T45.0X4	T45.0X5	T45.0X6
Propionaldehyde (medicinal)	T42.6X1	T42.6X2	T42.6X3	T42.6X4	T42.6X5	T42.6X6
Propionate (calcium) (sodium)	T49.0X1	T49.0X2	T49.0X3	T49.0X4	T49.0X5	T49.0X6
Propion gel	T49.0X1	T49.0X2	T49.0X3	T49.0X4	T49.0X5	T49.0X6
Propitocaine	T41.3X1	T41.3X2	T41.3X3	T41.3X4	T41.3X5	T41.3X6
infiltration (subcutaneous)	T41.3X1	T41.3X2	T41.3X3	T41.3X4	T41.3X5	T41.3X6
nerve block (peripheral) (plexus)	T41.3X1	T41.3X2	T41.3X3	T41.3X4	T41.3X5	T41.3X6
Propofol	T41.291	T41.292	T41.293	T41.294	T41.295	T41.296
Propoxur	T60.0X1	T60.0X2	T60.0X3	T60.0X4	—	—
Propoxycaine	T41.3X1	T41.3X2	T41.3X3	T41.3X4	T41.3X5	T41.3X6
infiltration (subcutaneous)	T41.3X1	T41.3X2	T41.3X3	T41.3X4	T41.3X5	T41.3X6
nerve block (peripheral) (plexus)	T41.3X1	T41.3X2	T41.3X3	T41.3X4	T41.3X5	T41.3X6
topical (surface)	T41.3X1	T41.3X2	T41.3X3	T41.3X4	T41.3X5	T41.3X6

Substance	Poisoning, Accidental (unintentional)	Poisoning, Intentional self-harm	Poisoning, Assault	Poisoning, Undetermined	Adverse effect	Underdosing
Propoxyphene	T40.491	T40.492	T40.493	T40.494	T40.495	T40.496
Propranolol	T44.7X1	T44.7X2	T44.7X3	T44.7X4	T44.7X5	T44.7X6
Propyl						
alcohol	T51.3X1	T51.3X2	T51.3X3	T51.3X4	—	—
carbinol	T51.3X1	T51.3X2	T51.3X3	T51.3X4	—	—
hexadrine	T44.4X1	T44.4X2	T44.4X3	T44.4X4	T44.4X5	T44.4X6
iodone	T50.8X1	T50.8X2	T50.8X3	T50.8X4	T50.8X5	T50.8X6
thiouracil	T38.2X1	T38.2X2	T38.2X3	T38.2X4	T38.2X5	T38.2X6
Propylaminophenothiazine	T43.3X1	T43.3X2	T43.3X3	T43.3X4	T43.3X5	T43.3X6
Propylene	T59.891	T59.892	T59.893	T59.894	—	—
Propylhexedrine	T48.5X1	T48.5X2	T48.5X3	T48.5X4	T48.5X5	T48.5X6
Propyliodone	T50.8X1	T50.8X2	T50.8X3	T50.8X4	T50.8X5	T50.8X6
Propylparaben (ophthalmic)	T49.5X1	T49.5X2	T49.5X3	T49.5X4	T49.5X5	T49.5X6
Propylthiouracil	T38.2X1	T38.2X2	T38.2X3	T38.2X4	T38.2X5	T38.2X6
Propyphenazone	T39.2X1	T39.2X2	T39.2X3	T39.2X4	T39.2X5	T39.2X6
Proquazone	T39.391	T39.392	T39.393	T39.394	T39.395	T39.396
Proscillaridin	T46.0X1	T46.0X2	T46.0X3	T46.0X4	T46.0X5	T46.0X6
Prostacyclin	T45.521	T45.522	T45.523	T45.524	T45.525	T45.526
Prostaglandin (I2)	T45.521	T45.522	T45.523	T45.524	T45.525	T45.526
E1	T46.7X1	T46.7X2	T46.7X3	T46.7X4	T46.7X5	T46.7X6
E2	T48.0X1	T48.0X2	T48.0X3	T48.0X4	T48.0X5	T48.0X6
F2 alpha	T48.0X1	T48.0X2	T48.0X3	T48.0X4	T48.0X5	T48.0X6
Prostigmin	T44.0X1	T44.0X2	T44.0X3	T44.0X4	T44.0X5	T44.0X6
Prosultiamine	T45.2X1	T45.2X2	T45.2X3	T45.2X4	T45.2X5	T45.2X6
Protamine sulfate	T45.7X1	T45.7X2	T45.7X3	T45.7X4	T45.7X5	T45.7X6
zinc insulin	T38.3X1	T38.3X2	T38.3X3	T38.3X4	T38.3X5	T38.3X6
Protease	T47.5X1	T47.5X2	T47.5X3	T47.5X4	T47.5X5	T47.5X6
Protectant, skin NEC	T49.3X1	T49.3X2	T49.3X3	T49.3X4	T49.3X5	T49.3X6
Protein hydrolysate	T50.991	T50.992	T50.993	T50.994	T50.995	T50.996
Prothiaden—see Dothiepin hydrochloride						
Prothionamide	T37.1X1	T37.1X2	T37.1X3	T37.1X4	T37.1X5	T37.1X6
Prothipendyl	T43.591	T43.592	T43.593	T43.594	T43.595	T43.596
Prothoate	T60.0X1	T60.0X2	T60.0X3	T60.0X4	—	—
Prothrombin						
activator	T45.7X1	T45.7X2	T45.7X3	T45.7X4	T45.7X5	T45.7X6
synthesis inhibitor	T45.511	T45.512	T45.513	T45.514	T45.515	T45.516
Protionamide	T37.1X1	T37.1X2	T37.1X3	T37.1X4	T37.1X5	T37.1X6
Protirelin	T38.891	T38.892	T38.893	T38.894	T38.895	T38.896
Protokylol	T48.6X1	T48.6X2	T48.6X3	T48.6X4	T48.6X5	T48.6X6
Protopam	T50.6X1	T50.6X2	T50.6X3	T50.6X4	T50.6X5	T50.6X6
Protoveratrine (s) (A) (B)	T46.5X1	T46.5X2	T46.5X3	T46.5X4	T46.5X5	T46.5X6
Protriptyline	T43.011	T43.012	T43.013	T43.014	T43.015	T43.016
Provera	T38.5X1	T38.5X2	T38.5X3	T38.5X4	T38.5X5	T38.5X6
Provitamin A	T45.2X1	T45.2X2	T45.2X3	T45.2X4	T45.2X5	T45.2X6
Proxibarbal	T42.3X1	T42.3X2	T42.3X3	T42.3X4	T42.3X5	T42.3X6
Proxymetacaine	T41.3X1	T41.3X2	T41.3X3	T41.3X4	T41.3X5	T41.3X6
Proxyphylline	T48.6X1	T48.6X2	T48.6X3	T48.6X4	T48.6X5	T48.6X6

Substance	Poisoning, Accidental (unintentional)	Poisoning, Intentional self-harm	Poisoning, Assault	Poisoning, Undetermined	Adverse effect	Underdosing
Prozac—see Fluoxetine hydrochloride						
Prunus						
laurocerasus	T62.2X1	T62.2X2	T62.2X3	T62.2X4	—	—
virginiana	T62.2X1	T62.2X2	T62.2X3	T62.2X4	—	—
Prussian blue						
commercial	T65.891	T65.892	T65.893	T65.894	—	—
therapeutic	T50.6X1	T50.6X2	T50.6X3	T50.6X4	T50.6X5	T50.6X6
Prussic acid	T65.0X1	T65.0X2	T65.0X3	T65.0X4	—	—
vapor	T57.3X1	T57.3X2	T57.3X3	T57.3X4	—	—
Pseudoephedrine	T44.991	T44.992	T44.993	T44.994	T44.995	T44.996
Psilocin	T40.991	T40.992	T40.993	T40.994	—	—
Psilocybin	T40.991	T40.992	T40.993	T40.994	—	—
Psilocybine	T40.991	T40.992	T40.993	T40.994	—	—
Psoralene (nonmedicinal)	T65.891	T65.892	T65.893	T65.894	—	—
Psoralens (medicinal)	T50.991	T50.992	T50.993	T50.994	T50.995	T50.996
PSP (phenolsulfonphthalein)	T50.8X1	T50.8X2	T50.8X3	T50.8X4	T50.8X5	T50.8X6
Psychodysleptic drug NOS	T40.901	T40.902	T40.903	T40.904	T40.905	T40.906
specified NEC	T40.991	T40.992	T40.993	T40.994	T40.995	T40.996
Psychostimulant	T43.601	T43.602	T43.603	T43.604	T43.605	T43.606
amphetamine	T43.621	T43.622	T43.623	T43.624	T43.625	T43.626
caffeine	T43.611	T43.612	T43.613	T43.614	T43.615	T43.616
methylphenidate	T43.631	T43.632	T43.633	T43.634	T43.635	T43.636
specified NEC	T43.691	T43.692	T43.693	T43.694	T43.695	T43.696
Psychotherapeutic drug NEC	T43.91	T43.92	T43.93	T43.94	T43.95	T43.96
antidepressants—see also Antidepressant	T43.201	T43.202	T43.203	T43.204	T43.205	T43.206
specified NEC	T43.8X1	T43.8X2	T43.8X3	T43.8X4	T43.8X5	T43.8X6
tranquilizers NEC	T43.501	T43.502	T43.503	T43.504	T43.505	T43.506
Psychotomimetic agents	T40.901	T40.902	T40.903	T40.904	T40.905	T40.906
Psychotropic drug NEC	T43.91	T43.92	T43.93	T43.94	T43.95	T43.96
specified NEC	T43.8X1	T43.8X2	T43.8X3	T43.8X4	T43.8X5	T43.8X6
Psyllium hydrophilic mucilloid	T47.4X1	T47.4X2	T47.4X3	T47.4X4	T47.4X5	T47.4X6
Pteroylglutamic acid	T45.8X1	T45.8X2	T45.8X3	T45.8X4	T45.8X5	T45.8X6
Pteroyltriglutamate	T45.1X1	T45.1X2	T45.1X3	T45.1X4	T45.1X5	T45.1X6
PTFE—see Polytetrafluoroethylene						
Pulp						
devitalizing paste	T49.7X1	T49.7X2	T49.7X3	T49.7X4	T49.7X5	T49.7X6
dressing	T49.7X1	T49.7X2	T49.7X3	T49.7X4	T49.7X5	T49.7X6
Pulsatilla	T62.2X1	T62.2X2	T62.2X3	T62.2X4	—	—
Pumpkin seed extract	T37.4X1	T37.4X2	T37.4X3	T37.4X4	T37.4X5	T37.4X6
Purex (bleach)	T54.91	T54.92	T54.93	T54.94	—	—
Purgative NEC—see also Cathartic	T47.4X1	T47.4X2	T47.4X3	T47.4X4	T47.4X5	T47.4X6
Purine analogue (antineoplastic)	T45.1X1	T45.1X2	T45.1X3	T45.1X4	T45.1X5	T45.1X6

Substance	Poisoning, Accidental (unintentional)	Poisoning, Intentional self-harm	Poisoning, Assault	Poisoning, Undetermined	Adverse effect	Underdosing
Purine diuretics	T50.2X1	T50.2X2	T50.2X3	T50.2X4	T50.2X5	T50.2X6
Purinethol	T45.1X1	T45.1X2	T45.1X3	T45.1X4	T45.1X5	T45.1X6
PVP	T45.8X1	T45.8X2	T45.8X3	T45.8X4	T45.8X5	T45.8X6
Pyrabital	T39.8X1	T39.8X2	T39.8X3	T39.8X4	T39.8X5	T39.8X6
Pyramidon	T39.2X1	T39.2X2	T39.2X3	T39.2X4	T39.2X5	T39.2X6
Pyrantel	T37.4X1	T37.4X2	T37.4X3	T37.4X4	T37.4X5	T37.4X6
Pyrathiazine	T45.0X1	T45.0X2	T45.0X3	T45.0X4	T45.0X5	T45.0X6
Pyrazinamide	T37.1X1	T37.1X2	T37.1X3	T37.1X4	T37.1X5	T37.1X6
Pyrazinoic acid (amide)	T37.1X1	T37.1X2	T37.1X3	T37.1X4	T37.1X5	T37.1X6
Pyrazole (derivatives)	T39.2X1	T39.2X2	T39.2X3	T39.2X4	T39.2X5	T39.2X6
Pyrazolone analgesic NEC	T39.2X1	T39.2X2	T39.2X3	T39.2X4	T39.2X5	T39.2X6
Pyrethrin, pyrethrum (nonmedicinal)	T60.2X1	T60.2X2	T60.2X3	T60.2X4	—	—
Pyrethrum extract	T49.0X1	T49.0X2	T49.0X3	T49.0X4	T49.0X5	T49.0X6
Pyribenzamine	T45.0X1	T45.0X2	T45.0X3	T45.0X4	T45.0X5	T45.0X6
Pyridine	T52.8X1	T52.8X2	T52.8X3	T52.8X4	—	—
aldoxime methiodide	T50.6X1	T50.6X2	T50.6X3	T50.6X4	T50.6X5	T50.6X6
aldoxime methyl chloride	T50.6X1	T50.6X2	T50.6X3	T50.6X4	T50.6X5	T50.6X6
vapor	T59.891	T59.892	T59.893	T59.894	—	—
Pyridium	T39.8X1	T39.8X2	T39.8X3	T39.8X4	T39.8X5	T39.8X6
Pyridostigmine bromide	T44.0X1	T44.0X2	T44.0X3	T44.0X4	T44.0X5	T44.0X6
Pyridoxal phosphate	T45.2X1	T45.2X2	T45.2X3	T45.2X4	T45.2X5	T45.2X6
Pyridoxine	T45.2X1	T45.2X2	T45.2X3	T45.2X4	T45.2X5	T45.2X6
Pyrilamine	T45.0X1	T45.0X2	T45.0X3	T45.0X4	T45.0X5	T45.0X6
Pyrimethamine	T37.2X1	T37.2X2	T37.2X3	T37.2X4	T37.2X5	T37.2X6
with sulfadoxine	T37.2X1	T37.2X2	T37.2X3	T37.2X4	T37.2X5	T37.2X6
Pyrimidine antagonist	T45.1X1	T45.1X2	T45.1X3	T45.1X4	T45.1X5	T45.1X6
Pyriminil	T60.4X1	T60.4X2	T60.4X3	T60.4X4	—	—
Pyrithione zinc	T49.4X1	T49.4X2	T49.4X3	T49.4X4	T49.4X5	T49.4X6
Pyrithyldione	T42.6X1	T42.6X2	T42.6X3	T42.6X4	T42.6X5	T42.6X6
Pyrogallic acid	T49.0X1	T49.0X2	T49.0X3	T49.0X4	T49.0X5	T49.0X6
Pyrogallol	T49.0X1	T49.0X2	T49.0X3	T49.0X4	T49.0X5	T49.0X6
Pyroxylin	T49.3X1	T49.3X2	T49.3X3	T49.3X4	T49.3X5	T49.3X6
Pyrrobutamine	T45.0X1	T45.0X2	T45.0X3	T45.0X4	T45.0X5	T45.0X6
Pyrrolizidine alkaloids	T62.8X1	T62.8X2	T62.8X3	T62.8X4	—	—
Pyrvinium chloride	T37.4X1	T37.4X2	T37.4X3	T37.4X4	T37.4X5	T37.4X6
PZI	T38.3X1	T38.3X2	T38.3X3	T38.3X4	T38.3X5	T38.3X6
Q						
Quaalude	T42.6X1	T42.6X2	T42.6X3	T42.6X4	T42.6X5	T42.6X6
Quarternary ammonium						
anti-infective	T49.0X1	T49.0X2	T49.0X3	T49.0X4	T49.0X5	T49.0X6
ganglion blocking	T44.2X1	T44.2X2	T44.2X3	T44.2X4	T44.2X5	T44.2X6
parasympatholytic	T44.3X1	T44.3X2	T44.3X3	T44.3X4	T44.3X5	T44.3X6
Quazepam	T42.4X1	T42.4X2	T42.4X3	T42.4X4	T42.4X5	T42.4X6
Quicklime	T54.3X1	T54.3X2	T54.3X3	T54.3X4	—	—
Quillaja extract	T48.4X1	T48.4X2	T48.4X3	T48.4X4	T48.4X5	T48.4X6
Quinacrine	T37.2X1	T37.2X2	T37.2X3	T37.2X4	T37.2X5	T37.2X6
Quinaglute	T46.2X1	T46.2X2	T46.2X3	T46.2X4	T46.2X5	T46.2X6
Quinalbarbital	T42.3X1	T42.3X2	T42.3X3	T42.3X4	T42.3X5	T42.3X6
Quinalbarbitone sodium	T42.3X1	T42.3X2	T42.3X3	T42.3X4	T42.3X5	T42.3X6
Quinalphos	T60.0X1	T60.0X2	T60.0X3	T60.0X4	—	—
Quinapril	T46.4X1	T46.4X2	T46.4X3	T46.4X4	T46.4X5	T46.4X6
Quinestradiol	T38.5X1	T38.5X2	T38.5X3	T38.5X4	T38.5X5	T38.5X6
Quinestradol	T38.5X1	T38.5X2	T38.5X3	T38.5X4	T38.5X5	T38.5X6
Quinestrol	T38.5X1	T38.5X2	T38.5X3	T38.5X4	T38.5X5	T38.5X6
Quinethazone	T50.2X1	T50.2X2	T50.2X3	T50.2X4	T50.2X5	T50.2X6
Quingestanol	T38.4X1	T38.4X2	T38.4X3	T38.4X4	T38.4X5	T38.4X6
Quinidine	T46.2X1	T46.2X2	T46.2X3	T46.2X4	T46.2X5	T46.2X6
Quinine	T37.2X1	T37.2X2	T37.2X3	T37.2X4	T37.2X5	T37.2X6
Quiniobine	T37.8X1	T37.8X2	T37.8X3	T37.8X4	T37.8X5	T37.8X6
Quinisocaine	T49.1X1	T49.1X2	T49.1X3	T49.1X4	T49.1X5	T49.1X6
Quinocide	T37.2X1	T37.2X2	T37.2X3	T37.2X4	T37.2X5	T37.2X6
Quinoline (derivatives) NEC	T37.8X1	T37.8X2	T37.8X3	T37.8X4	T37.8X5	T37.8X6
Quinupramine	T43.011	T43.012	T43.013	T43.014	T43.015	T43.016
Quotane	T41.3X1	T41.3X2	T41.3X3	T41.3X4	T41.3X5	T41.3X6
R						
Rabies						
immune globulin (human)	T50.Z11	T50.Z12	T50.Z13	T50.Z14	T50.Z15	T50.Z16
vaccine	T50.B91	T50.B92	T50.B93	T50.B94	T50.B95	T50.B96
Racemoramide	T40.2X1	T40.2X2	T40.2X3	T40.2X4	—	—
Racemorphan	T40.2X1	T40.2X2	T40.2X3	T40.2X4	T40.2X5	T40.2X6
Racepinefrin	T44.5X1	T44.5X2	T44.5X3	T44.5X4	T44.5X5	T44.5X6
Raclopride	T43.591	T43.592	T43.593	T43.594	T43.595	T43.596
Radiator alcohol	T51.1X1	T51.1X2	T51.1X3	T51.1X4	—	—
Radioactive drug NEC	T50.8X1	T50.8X2	T50.8X3	T50.8X4	T50.8X5	T50.8X6
Radio-opaque (drugs) (materials)	T50.8X1	T50.8X2	T50.8X3	T50.8X4	T50.8X5	T50.8X6
Ramifenazone	T39.2X1	T39.2X2	T39.2X3	T39.2X4	T39.2X5	T39.2X6
Ramipril	T46.4X1	T46.4X2	T46.4X3	T46.4X4	T46.4X5	T46.4X6
Ranitidine	T47.0X1	T47.0X2	T47.0X3	T47.0X4	T47.0X5	T47.0X6
Ranunculus	T62.2X1	T62.2X2	T62.2X3	T62.2X4	—	—
Rat poison NEC	T60.4X1	T60.4X2	T60.4X3	T60.4X4	—	—
Rattlesnake (venom)	T63.011	T63.012	T63.013	T63.014	—	—
Raubasine	T46.7X1	T46.7X2	T46.7X3	T46.7X4	T46.7X5	T46.7X6
Raudixin	T46.5X1	T46.5X2	T46.5X3	T46.5X4	T46.5X5	T46.5X6
Rautensin	T46.5X1	T46.5X2	T46.5X3	T46.5X4	T46.5X5	T46.5X6
Rautina	T46.5X1	T46.5X2	T46.5X3	T46.5X4	T46.5X5	T46.5X6
Rautotal	T46.5X1	T46.5X2	T46.5X3	T46.5X4	T46.5X5	T46.5X6
Rauwiloid	T46.5X1	T46.5X2	T46.5X3	T46.5X4	T46.5X5	T46.5X6
Rauwoldin	T46.5X1	T46.5X2	T46.5X3	T46.5X4	T46.5X5	T46.5X6
Rauwolfia (alkaloids)	T46.5X1	T46.5X2	T46.5X3	T46.5X4	T46.5X5	T46.5X6
Razoxane	T45.1X1	T45.1X2	T45.1X3	T45.1X4	T45.1X5	T45.1X6
Realgar	T57.0X1	T57.0X2	T57.0X3	T57.0X4	—	—
Recombinant(R)—see specific protein						
Red blood cells, packed	T45.8X1	T45.8X2	T45.8X3	T45.8X4	T45.8X5	T45.8X6
Red squill (scilliroside)	T60.4X1	T60.4X2	T60.4X3	T60.4X4	—	—
Reducing agent, industrial NEC	T65.891	T65.892	T65.893	T65.894	—	—

Substance	Poisoning, Accidental (unintentional)	Poisoning, Intentional self-harm	Poisoning, Assault	Poisoning, Undetermined	Adverse effect	Underdosing
Refrigerant gas (chlorofluoro-carbon)	T53.5X1	T53.5X2	T53.5X3	T53.5X4	—	—
not chlorofluoro-carbon	T59.891	T59.892	T59.893	T59.894	—	—
Regroton	T50.2X1	T50.2X2	T50.2X3	T50.2X4	T50.2X5	T50.2X6
Rehydration salts (oral)	T50.3X1	T50.3X2	T50.3X3	T50.3X4	T50.3X5	T50.3X6
Rela	T42.8X1	T42.8X2	T42.8X3	T42.8X4	T42.8X5	T42.8X6
Relaxant, muscle						
anesthetic	T48.1X1	T48.1X2	T48.1X3	T48.1X4	T48.1X5	T48.1X6
central nervous system	T42.8X1	T42.8X2	T42.8X3	T42.8X4	T42.8X5	T42.8X6
skeletal NEC	T48.1X1	T48.1X2	T48.1X3	T48.1X4	T48.1X5	T48.1X6
smooth NEC	T44.3X1	T44.3X2	T44.3X3	T44.3X4	T44.3X5	T44.3X6
Remoxipride	T43.591	T43.592	T43.593	T43.594	T43.595	T43.596
Renese	T50.2X1	T50.2X2	T50.2X3	T50.2X4	T50.2X5	T50.2X6
Renografin	T50.8X1	T50.8X2	T50.8X3	T50.8X4	T50.8X5	T50.8X6
Replacement solution	T50.3X1	T50.3X2	T50.3X3	T50.3X4	T50.3X5	T50.3X6
Reproterol	T48.6X1	T48.6X2	T48.6X3	T48.6X4	T48.6X5	T48.6X6
Rescinnamine	T46.5X1	T46.5X2	T46.5X3	T46.5X4	T46.5X5	T46.5X6
Reserpin(e)	T46.5X1	T46.5X2	T46.5X3	T46.5X4	T46.5X5	T46.5X6
Resorcin, resorcinol (nonmedicinal)	T65.891	T65.892	T65.893	T65.894	—	—
medicinal	T49.4X1	T49.4X2	T49.4X3	T49.4X4	T49.4X5	T49.4X6
Respaire	T48.4X1	T48.4X2	T48.4X3	T48.4X4	T48.4X5	T48.4X6
Respiratory drug NEC	T48.901	T48.902	T48.903	T48.904	T48.905	T48.906
antiasthmatic NEC	T48.6X1	T48.6X2	T48.6X3	T48.6X4	T48.6X5	T48.6X6
anti-common-cold NEC	T48.5X1	T48.5X2	T48.5X3	T48.5X4	T48.5X5	T48.5X6
expectorant NEC	T48.4X1	T48.4X2	T48.4X3	T48.4X4	T48.4X5	T48.4X6
stimulant	T48.901	T48.902	T48.903	T48.904	T48.905	T48.906
Retinoic acid	T49.0X1	T49.0X2	T49.0X3	T49.0X4	T49.0X5	T49.0X6
Retinol	T45.2X1	T45.2X2	T45.2X3	T45.2X4	T45.2X5	T45.2X6
Rh(D) immune globulin (human)	T50.Z11	T50.Z12	T50.Z13	T50.Z14	T50.Z15	T50.Z16
Rhodine	T39.011	T39.012	T39.013	T39.014	T39.015	T39.016
RhoGAM	T50.Z11	T50.Z12	T50.Z13	T50.Z14	T50.Z15	T50.Z16
Rhubarb						
dry extract	T47.2X1	T47.2X2	T47.2X3	T47.2X4	T47.2X5	T47.2X6
tincture, compound	T47.2X1	T47.2X2	T47.2X3	T47.2X4	T47.2X5	T47.2X6
Ribavirin	T37.5X1	T37.5X2	T37.5X3	T37.5X4	T37.5X5	T37.5X6
Riboflavin	T45.2X1	T45.2X2	T45.2X3	T45.2X4	T45.2X5	T45.2X6
Ribostamycin	T36.5X1	T36.5X2	T36.5X3	T36.5X4	T36.5X5	T36.5X6
Ricin	T62.2X1	T62.2X2	T62.2X3	T62.2X4	—	—
Ricinus communis	T62.2X1	T62.2X2	T62.2X3	T62.2X4	—	—
Rickettsial vaccine NEC	T50.A91	T50.A92	T50.A93	T50.A94	T50.A95	T50.A96
Rifabutin	T36.6X1	T36.6X2	T36.6X3	T36.6X4	T36.6X5	T36.6X6
Rifamide	T36.6X1	T36.6X2	T36.6X3	T36.6X4	T36.6X5	T36.6X6
Rifampicin	T36.6X1	T36.6X2	T36.6X3	T36.6X4	T36.6X5	T36.6X6
with isoniazid	T37.1X1	T37.1X2	T37.1X3	T37.1X4	T37.1X5	T37.1X6
Rifampin	T36.6X1	T36.6X2	T36.6X3	T36.6X4	T36.6X5	T36.6X6
Rifamycin	T36.6X1	T36.6X2	T36.6X3	T36.6X4	T36.6X5	T36.6X6
Rifaximin	T36.6X1	T36.6X2	T36.6X3	T36.6X4	T36.6X5	T36.6X6

Substance	Poisoning, Accidental (unintentional)	Poisoning, Intentional self-harm	Poisoning, Assault	Poisoning, Undetermined	Adverse effect	Underdosing
Rimantadine	T37.5X1	T37.5X2	T37.5X3	T37.5X4	T37.5X5	T37.5X6
Rimazolium metilsulfate	T39.8X1	T39.8X2	T39.8X3	T39.8X4	T39.8X5	T39.8X6
Rimifon	T37.1X1	T37.1X2	T37.1X3	T37.1X4	T37.1X5	T37.1X6
Rimiterol	T48.6X1	T48.6X2	T48.6X3	T48.6X4	T48.6X5	T48.6X6
Ringer (lactate) solution	T50.3X1	T50.3X2	T50.3X3	T50.3X4	T50.3X5	T50.3X6
Ristocetin	T36.8X1	T36.8X2	T36.8X3	T36.8X4	T36.8X5	T36.8X6
Ritalin	T43.631	T43.632	T43.633	T43.634	T43.635	T43.636
Ritodrine	T44.5X1	T44.5X2	T44.5X3	T44.5X4	T44.5X5	T44.5X6
Roach killer—see Insecticide						
Rociverine	T44.3X1	T44.3X2	T44.3X3	T44.3X4	T44.3X5	T44.3X6
Rocky Mountain spotted fever vaccine	T50.A91	T50.A92	T50.A93	T50.A94	T50.A95	T50.A96
Rodenticide NEC	T60.4X1	T60.4X2	T60.4X3	T60.4X4	—	—
Rohypnol	T42.4X1	T42.4X2	T42.4X3	T42.4X4	T42.4X5	T42.4X6
Rokitamycin	T36.3X1	T36.3X2	T36.3X3	T36.3X4	T36.3X5	T36.3X6
Rolaids	T47.1X1	T47.1X2	T47.1X3	T47.1X4	T47.1X5	T47.1X6
Rolitetracycline	T36.4X1	T36.4X2	T36.4X3	T36.4X4	T36.4X5	T36.4X6
Romilar	T48.3X1	T48.3X2	T48.3X3	T48.3X4	T48.3X5	T48.3X6
Ronifibrate	T46.6X1	T46.6X2	T46.6X3	T46.6X4	T46.6X5	T46.6X6
Rosaprostol	T47.1X1	T47.1X2	T47.1X3	T47.1X4	T47.1X5	T47.1X6
Rose bengal sodium (131I)	T50.8X1	T50.8X2	T50.8X3	T50.8X4	T50.8X5	T50.8X6
Rose water ointment	T49.3X1	T49.3X2	T49.3X3	T49.3X4	T49.3X5	T49.3X6
Rosoxacin	T37.8X1	T37.8X2	T37.8X3	T37.8X4	T37.8X5	T37.8X6
Rotenone	T60.2X1	T60.2X2	T60.2X3	T60.2X4	—	—
Rotoxamine	T45.0X1	T45.0X2	T45.0X3	T45.0X4	T45.0X5	T45.0X6
Rough-on-rats	T60.4X1	T60.4X2	T60.4X3	T60.4X4	—	—
Roxatidine	T47.0X1	T47.0X2	T47.0X3	T47.0X4	T47.0X5	T47.0X6
Roxithromycin	T36.3X1	T36.3X2	T36.3X3	T36.3X4	T36.3X5	T36.3X6
Rt-PA	T45.611	T45.612	T45.613	T45.614	T45.615	T45.616
Rubbing alcohol	T51.2X1	T51.2X2	T51.2X3	T51.2X4	—	—
Rubefacient	T49.4X1	T49.4X2	T49.4X3	T49.4X4	T49.4X5	T49.4X6
Rubella vaccine	T50.B91	T50.B92	T50.B93	T50.B94	T50.B95	T50.B96
Rubeola vaccine	T50.B91	T50.B92	T50.B93	T50.B94	T50.B95	T50.B96
Rubidium chloride Rb82	T50.8X1	T50.8X2	T50.8X3	T50.8X4	T50.8X5	T50.8X6
Rubidomycin	T45.1X1	T45.1X2	T45.1X3	T45.1X4	T45.1X5	T45.1X6
Rue	T62.2X1	T62.2X2	T62.2X3	T62.2X4	—	—
Rufocromomycin	T45.1X1	T45.1X2	T45.1X3	T45.1X4	T45.1X5	T45.1X6
Russel's viper venin	T45.7X1	T45.7X2	T45.7X3	T45.7X4	T45.7X5	T45.7X6
Ruta (graveolens)	T62.2X1	T62.2X2	T62.2X3	T62.2X4	—	—
Rutinum	T46.991	T46.992	T46.993	T46.994	T46.995	T46.996
Rutoside	T46.991	T46.992	T46.993	T46.994	T46.995	T46.996
S						
Sabadilla (plant)	T62.2X1	T62.2X2	T62.2X3	T62.2X4	—	—
pesticide	T60.2X1	T60.2X2	T60.2X3	T60.2X4	—	—
Saccharated iron oxide	T45.8X1	T45.8X2	T45.8X3	T45.8X4	T45.8X5	T45.8X6
Saccharin	T50.901	T50.902	T50.903	T50.904	T50.905	T50.906
Saccharomyces boulardii	T47.6X1	T47.6X2	T47.6X3	T47.6X4	T47.6X5	T47.6X6
Safflower oil	T46.6X1	T46.6X2	T46.6X3	T46.6X4	T46.6X5	T46.6X6
Safrazine	T43.1X1	T43.1X2	T43.1X3	T43.1X4	T43.1X5	T43.1X6

Substance	Poisoning, Accidental (unintentional)	Poisoning, Intentional self-harm	Poisoning, Assault	Poisoning, Undetermined	Adverse effect	Underdosing
Salazosulfapyridine	T37.0X1	T37.0X2	T37.0X3	T37.0X4	T37.0X5	T37.0X6
Salbutamol	T48.6X1	T48.6X2	T48.6X3	T48.6X4	T48.6X5	T48.6X6
Salicylamide	T39.091	T39.092	T39.093	T39.094	T39.095	T39.096
Salicylate NEC	T39.091	T39.092	T39.093	T39.094	T39.095	T39.096
methyl	T49.3X1	T49.3X2	T49.3X3	T49.3X4	T49.3X5	T49.3X6
theobromine calcium	T50.2X1	T50.2X2	T50.2X3	T50.2X4	T50.2X5	T50.2X6
Salicylazosulfapyridine	T37.0X1	T37.0X2	T37.0X3	T37.0X4	T37.0X5	T37.0X6
Salicylhydroxamic acid	T49.0X1	T49.0X2	T49.0X3	T49.0X4	T49.0X5	T49.0X6
Salicylic acid	T49.4X1	T49.4X2	T49.4X3	T49.4X4	T49.4X5	T49.4X6
with benzoic acid	T49.4X1	T49.4X2	T49.4X3	T49.4X4	T49.4X5	T49.4X6
congeners	T39.091	T39.092	T39.093	T39.094	T39.095	T39.096
derivative	T39.091	T39.092	T39.093	T39.094	T39.095	T39.096
salts	T39.091	T39.092	T39.093	T39.094	T39.095	T39.096
Salinazid	T37.1X1	T37.1X2	T37.1X3	T37.1X4	T37.1X5	T37.1X6
Salmeterol	T48.6X1	T48.6X2	T48.6X3	T48.6X4	T48.6X5	T48.6X6
Salol	T49.3X1	T49.3X2	T49.3X3	T49.3X4	T49.3X5	T49.3X6
Salsalate	T39.091	T39.092	T39.093	T39.094	T39.095	T39.096
Salt substitute	T50.901	T50.902	T50.903	T50.904	T50.905	T50.906
Salt-replacing drug	T50.901	T50.902	T50.903	T50.904	T50.905	T50.906
Salt-retaining mineralocorticoid	T50.0X1	T50.0X2	T50.0X3	T50.0X4	T50.0X5	T50.0X6
Saluretic NEC	T50.2X1	T50.2X2	T50.2X3	T50.2X4	T50.2X5	T50.2X6
Saluron	T50.2X1	T50.2X2	T50.2X3	T50.2X4	T50.2X5	T50.2X6
Salvarsan 606 (neosilver) (silver)	T37.8X1	T37.8X2	T37.8X3	T37.8X4	T37.8X5	T37.8X6
Sambucus canadensis	T62.2X1	T62.2X2	T62.2X3	T62.2X4	—	—
berry	T62.1X1	T62.1X2	T62.1X3	T62.1X4	—	—
Sandril	T46.5X1	T46.5X2	T46.5X3	T46.5X4	T46.5X5	T46.5X6
Sanguinaria canadensis	T62.2X1	T62.2X2	T62.2X3	T62.2X4	—	—
Saniflush (cleaner)	T54.2X1	T54.2X2	T54.2X3	T54.2X4	—	—
Santonin	T37.4X1	T37.4X2	T37.4X3	T37.4X4	T37.4X5	T37.4X6
Santyl	T49.8X1	T49.8X2	T49.8X3	T49.8X4	T49.8X5	T49.8X6
Saralasin	T46.5X1	T46.5X2	T46.5X3	T46.5X4	T46.5X5	T46.5X6
Sarcolysin	T45.1X1	T45.1X2	T45.1X3	T45.1X4	T45.1X5	T45.1X6
Sarkomycin	T45.1X1	T45.1X2	T45.1X3	T45.1X4	T45.1X5	T45.1X6
Saroten	T43.011	T43.012	T43.013	T43.014	T43.015	T43.016
Saturnine—see Lead						
Savin (oil)	T49.4X1	T49.4X2	T49.4X3	T49.4X4	T49.4X5	T49.4X6
Scammony	T47.2X1	T47.2X2	T47.2X3	T47.2X4	T47.2X5	T47.2X6
Scarlet red	T49.8X1	T49.8X2	T49.8X3	T49.8X4	T49.8X5	T49.8X6
Scheele's green	T57.0X1	T57.0X2	T57.0X3	T57.0X4	—	—
insecticide	T57.0X1	T57.0X2	T57.0X3	T57.0X4	—	—
Schizontozide (blood) (tissue)	T37.2X1	T37.2X2	T37.2X3	T37.2X4	T37.2X5	T37.2X6
Schradan	T60.0X1	T60.0X2	T60.0X3	T60.0X4	—	—
Schweinfurth green	T57.0X1	T57.0X2	T57.0X3	T57.0X4	—	—
insecticide	T57.0X1	T57.0X2	T57.0X3	T57.0X4	—	—
Scilla, rat poison	T60.4X1	T60.4X2	T60.4X3	T60.4X4	—	—
Scillaren	T60.4X1	T60.4X2	T60.4X3	T60.4X4	—	—
Sclerosing agent	T46.8X1	T46.8X2	T46.8X3	T46.8X4	T46.8X5	T46.8X6
Scombrotoxin	T61.11	T61.12	T61.13	T61.14	—	—
Scopolamine	T44.3X1	T44.3X2	T44.3X3	T44.3X4	T44.3X5	T44.3X6
Scopolia extract	T44.3X1	T44.3X2	T44.3X3	T44.3X4	T44.3X5	T44.3X6
Scouring powder	T65.891	T65.892	T65.893	T65.894	—	—
Sea						
anemone (sting)	T63.631	T63.632	T63.633	T63.634	—	—
cucumber (sting)	T63.691	T63.692	T63.693	T63.694	—	—
snake (bite) (venom)	T63.091	T63.092	T63.093	T63.094	—	—
urchin spine (puncture)	T63.691	T63.692	T63.693	T63.694	—	—
Seafood	T61.91	T61.92	T61.93	T61.94	—	—
specified NEC	T61.8X1	T61.8X2	T61.8X3	T61.8X4	—	—
Secbutabarbital	T42.3X1	T42.3X2	T42.3X3	T42.3X4	T42.3X5	T42.3X6
Secbutabarbitone	T42.3X1	T42.3X2	T42.3X3	T42.3X4	T42.3X5	T42.3X6
Secnidazole	T37.3X1	T37.3X2	T37.3X3	T37.3X4	T37.3X5	T37.3X6
Secobarbital	T42.3X1	T42.3X2	T42.3X3	T42.3X4	T42.3X5	T42.3X6
Seconal	T42.3X1	T42.3X2	T42.3X3	T42.3X4	T42.3X5	T42.3X6
Secretin	T50.8X1	T50.8X2	T50.8X3	T50.8X4	T50.8X5	T50.8X6
Sedative NEC	T42.71	T42.72	T42.73	T42.74	T42.75	T42.76
mixed NEC	T42.6X1	T42.6X2	T42.6X3	T42.6X4	T42.6X5	T42.6X6
Sedormid	T42.6X1	T42.6X2	T42.6X3	T42.6X4	T42.6X5	T42.6X6
Seed disinfectant or dressing	T60.8X1	T60.8X2	T60.8X3	T60.8X4	—	—
Seeds (poisonous)	T62.2X1	T62.2X2	T62.2X3	T62.2X4	—	—
Selegiline	T42.8X1	T42.8X2	T42.8X3	T42.8X4	T42.8X5	T42.8X6
Selenium NEC	T56.891	T56.892	T56.893	T56.894	—	—
disulfide or sulfide	T49.4X1	T49.4X2	T49.4X3	T49.4X4	T49.4X5	T49.4X6
fumes	T59.891	T59.892	T59.893	T59.894	—	—
sulfide	T49.4X1	T49.4X2	T49.4X3	T49.4X4	T49.4X5	T49.4X6
Selenomethionine (75Se)	T50.8X1	T50.8X2	T50.8X3	T50.8X4	T50.8X5	T50.8X6
Selsun	T49.4X1	T49.4X2	T49.4X3	T49.4X4	T49.4X5	T49.4X6
Semustine	T45.1X1	T45.1X2	T45.1X3	T45.1X4	T45.1X5	T45.1X6
Senega syrup	T48.4X1	T48.4X2	T48.4X3	T48.4X4	T48.4X5	T48.4X6
Senna	T47.2X1	T47.2X2	T47.2X3	T47.2X4	T47.2X5	T47.2X6
Sennoside A+B	T47.2X1	T47.2X2	T47.2X3	T47.2X4	T47.2X5	T47.2X6
Septisol	T49.2X1	T49.2X2	T49.2X3	T49.2X4	T49.2X5	T49.2X6
Seractide	T38.811	T38.812	T38.813	T38.814	T38.815	T38.816
Serax	T42.4X1	T42.4X2	T42.4X3	T42.4X4	T42.4X5	T42.4X6
Serenesil	T42.6X1	T42.6X2	T42.6X3	T42.6X4	T42.6X5	T42.6X6
Serenium (hydrochloride)	T37.91	T37.92	T37.93	T37.94	T37.95	T37.96
Serepax—see Oxazepam						
Sermorelin	T38.891	T38.892	T38.893	T38.894	T38.895	T38.896
Sernyl	T41.1X1	T41.1X2	T41.1X3	T41.1X4	T41.1X5	T41.1X6
Serotonin	T50.991	T50.992	T50.993	T50.994	T50.995	T50.996
Serpasil	T46.5X1	T46.5X2	T46.5X3	T46.5X4	T46.5X5	T46.5X6
Serrapeptase	T45.3X1	T45.3X2	T45.3X3	T45.3X4	T45.3X5	T45.3X6
Serum						
antibotulinus	T50.Z11	T50.Z12	T50.Z13	T50.Z14	T50.Z15	T50.Z16
anticytotoxic	T50.Z11	T50.Z12	T50.Z13	T50.Z14	T50.Z15	T50.Z16
antidiphtheria	T50.Z11	T50.Z12	T50.Z13	T50.Z14	T50.Z15	T50.Z16
antimeningococcus	T50.Z11	T50.Z12	T50.Z13	T50.Z14	T50.Z15	T50.Z16
anti-Rh	T50.Z11	T50.Z12	T50.Z13	T50.Z14	T50.Z15	T50.Z16

Substance	Poisoning, Accidental (unintentional)	Poisoning, Intentional self-harm	Poisoning, Assault	Poisoning, Undetermined	Adverse effect	Underdosing
Serum — *Continued*						
anti-snake-bite	T50.Z11	T50.Z12	T50.Z13	T50.Z14	T50.Z15	T50.Z16
antitetanic	T50.Z11	T50.Z12	T50.Z13	T50.Z14	T50.Z15	T50.Z16
antitoxic	T50.Z11	T50.Z12	T50.Z13	T50.Z14	T50.Z15	T50.Z16
complement (inhibitor)	T45.8X1	T45.8X2	T45.8X3	T45.8X4	T45.8X5	T45.8X6
convalescent	T50.Z11	T50.Z12	T50.Z13	T50.Z14	T50.Z15	T50.Z16
hemolytic complement	T45.8X1	T45.8X2	T45.8X3	T45.8X4	T45.8X5	T45.8X6
immune (human)	T50.Z11	T50.Z12	T50.Z13	T50.Z14	T50.Z15	T50.Z16
protective NEC	T50.Z11	T50.Z12	T50.Z13	T50.Z14	T50.Z15	T50.Z16
Setastine	T45.0X1	T45.0X2	T45.0X3	T45.0X4	T45.0X5	T45.0X6
Setoperone	T43.591	T43.592	T43.593	T43.594	T43.595	T43.596
Sewer gas	T59.91	T59.92	T59.93	T59.94	—	—
Shampoo	T55.0X1	T55.0X2	T55.0X3	T55.0X4	—	—
Shellfish, noxious, nonbacterial	T61.781	T61.782	T61.783	T61.784	—	—
Sildenafil	T46.7X1	T46.7X2	T46.7X3	T46.7X4	T46.7X5	T46.7X6
Silibinin	T50.991	T50.992	T50.993	T50.994	T50.995	T50.996
Silicone NEC	T65.891	T65.892	T65.893	T65.894	—	—
medicinal	T49.3X1	T49.3X2	T49.3X3	T49.3X4	T49.3X5	T49.3X6
Silvadene	T49.0X1	T49.0X2	T49.0X3	T49.0X4	T49.0X5	T49.0X6
Silver	T49.0X1	T49.0X2	T49.0X3	T49.0X4	T49.0X5	T49.0X6
anti-infectives	T49.0X1	T49.0X2	T49.0X3	T49.0X4	T49.0X5	T49.0X6
arsphenamine	T37.8X1	T37.8X2	T37.8X3	T37.8X4	T37.8X5	T37.8X6
colloidal	T49.0X1	T49.0X2	T49.0X3	T49.0X4	T49.0X5	T49.0X6
nitrate	T49.0X1	T49.0X2	T49.0X3	T49.0X4	T49.0X5	T49.0X6
ophthalmic preparation	T49.5X1	T49.5X2	T49.5X3	T49.5X4	T49.5X5	T49.5X6
toughened (keratolytic)	T49.4X1	T49.4X2	T49.4X3	T49.4X4	T49.4X5	T49.4X6
nonmedicinal (dust)	T56.891	T56.892	T56.893	T56.894	—	—
protein	T49.5X1	T49.5X2	T49.5X3	T49.5X4	T49.5X5	T49.5X6
salvarsan	T37.8X1	T37.8X2	T37.8X3	T37.8X4	T37.8X5	T37.8X6
sulfadiazine	T49.4X1	T49.4X2	T49.4X3	T49.4X4	T49.4X5	T49.4X6
Silymarin	T50.991	T50.992	T50.993	T50.994	T50.995	T50.996
Simaldrate	T47.1X1	T47.1X2	T47.1X3	T47.1X4	T47.1X5	T47.1X6
Simazine	T60.3X1	T60.3X2	T60.3X3	T60.3X4	—	—
Simethicone	T47.1X1	T47.1X2	T47.1X3	T47.1X4	T47.1X5	T47.1X6
Simfibrate	T46.6X1	T46.6X2	T46.6X3	T46.6X4	T46.6X5	T46.6X6
Simvastatin	T46.6X1	T46.6X2	T46.6X3	T46.6X4	T46.6X5	T46.6X6
Sincalide	T50.8X1	T50.8X2	T50.8X3	T50.8X4	T50.8X5	T50.8X6
Sinequan	T43.011	T43.012	T43.013	T43.014	T43.015	T43.016
Singoserp	T46.5X1	T46.5X2	T46.5X3	T46.5X4	T46.5X5	T46.5X6
Sintrom	T45.511	T45.512	T45.513	T45.514	T45.515	T45.516
Sisomicin	T36.5X1	T36.5X2	T36.5X3	T36.5X4	T36.5X5	T36.5X6
Sitosterols	T46.6X1	T46.6X2	T46.6X3	T46.6X4	T46.6X5	T46.6X6
Skeletal muscle relaxants	T48.1X1	T48.1X2	T48.1X3	T48.1X4	T48.1X5	T48.1X6
Skin						
agents (external)	T49.91	T49.92	T49.93	T49.94	T49.95	T49.96
specified NEC	T49.8X1	T49.8X2	T49.8X3	T49.8X4	T49.8X5	T49.8X6
test antigen	T50.8X1	T50.8X2	T50.8X3	T50.8X4	T50.8X5	T50.8X6

Substance	Poisoning, Accidental (unintentional)	Poisoning, Intentional self-harm	Poisoning, Assault	Poisoning, Undetermined	Adverse effect	Underdosing
Sleep-eze	T45.0X1	T45.0X2	T45.0X3	T45.0X4	T45.0X5	T45.0X6
Sleeping draught, pill	T42.71	T42.72	T42.73	T42.74	T42.75	T42.76
Smallpox vaccine	T50.B11	T50.B12	T50.B13	T50.B14	T50.B15	T50.B16
Smelter fumes NEC	T56.91	T56.92	T56.93	T56.94	—	—
Smog	T59.1X1	T59.1X2	T59.1X3	T59.1X4	—	—
Smoke NEC	T59.811	T59.812	T59.813	T59.814	—	—
Smooth muscle relaxant	T44.3X1	T44.3X2	T44.3X3	T44.3X4	T44.3X5	T44.3X6
Snail killer NEC	T60.8X1	T60.8X2	T60.8X3	T60.8X4	—	—
Snake venom or bite	T63.001	T63.002	T63.003	T63.004	—	—
hemocoagulase	T45.7X1	T45.7X2	T45.7X3	T45.7X4	T45.7X5	T45.7X6
Snuff	T65.211	T65.212	T65.213	T65.214	—	—
Soap (powder) (product)	T55.0X1	T55.0X2	T55.0X3	T55.0X4	—	—
enema	T47.4X1	T47.4X2	T47.4X3	T47.4X4	T47.4X5	T47.4X6
medicinal, soft	T49.2X1	T49.2X2	T49.2X3	T49.2X4	T49.2X5	T49.2X6
superfatted	T49.2X1	T49.2X2	T49.2X3	T49.2X4	T49.2X5	T49.2X6
Sobrerol	T48.4X1	T48.4X2	T48.4X3	T48.4X4	T48.4X5	T48.4X6
Soda (caustic)	T54.3X1	T54.3X2	T54.3X3	T54.3X4	—	—
bicarb	T47.1X1	T47.1X2	T47.1X3	T47.1X4	T47.1X5	T47.1X6
chlorinated—see Sodium, hypochlorite						
Sodium						
acetosulfone	T37.1X1	T37.1X2	T37.1X3	T37.1X4	T37.1X5	T37.1X6
acetrizoate	T50.8X1	T50.8X2	T50.8X3	T50.8X4	T50.8X5	T50.8X6
acid phosphate	T50.3X1	T50.3X2	T50.3X3	T50.3X4	T50.3X5	T50.3X6
alginate	T47.8X1	T47.8X2	T47.8X3	T47.8X4	T47.8X5	T47.8X6
amidotrizoate	T50.8X1	T50.8X2	T50.8X3	T50.8X4	T50.8X5	T50.8X6
aminopterin	T45.1X1	T45.1X2	T45.1X3	T45.1X4	T45.1X5	T45.1X6
amylosulfate	T47.8X1	T47.8X2	T47.8X3	T47.8X4	T47.8X5	T47.8X6
amytal	T42.3X1	T42.3X2	T42.3X3	T42.3X4	T42.3X5	T42.3X6
antimony gluconate	T37.3X1	T37.3X2	T37.3X3	T37.3X4	T37.3X5	T37.3X6
arsenate	T57.0X1	T57.0X2	T57.0X3	T57.0X4	—	—
aurothiomalate	T39.4X1	T39.4X2	T39.4X3	T39.4X4	T39.4X5	T39.4X6
aurothiosulfate	T39.4X1	T39.4X2	T39.4X3	T39.4X4	T39.4X5	T39.4X6
barbiturate	T42.3X1	T42.3X2	T42.3X3	T42.3X4	T42.3X5	T42.3X6
basic phosphate	T47.4X1	T47.4X2	T47.4X3	T47.4X4	T47.4X5	T47.4X6
bicarbonate	T47.1X1	T47.1X2	T47.1X3	T47.1X4	T47.1X5	T47.1X6
bichromate	T57.8X1	T57.8X2	T57.8X3	T57.8X4	—	—
biphosphate	T50.3X1	T50.3X2	T50.3X3	T50.3X4	T50.3X5	T50.3X6
bisulfate	T65.891	T65.892	T65.893	T65.894	—	—
borate						
cleanser	T57.8X1	T57.8X2	T57.8X3	T57.8X4	—	—
eye	T49.5X1	T49.5X2	T49.5X3	T49.5X4	T49.5X5	T49.5X6
therapeutic	T49.8X1	T49.8X2	T49.8X3	T49.8X4	T49.8X5	T49.8X6
bromide	T42.6X1	T42.6X2	T42.6X3	T42.6X4	T42.6X5	T42.6X6
cacodylate (nonmedicinal) NEC	T50.8X1	T50.8X2	T50.8X3	T50.8X4	T50.8X5	T50.8X6
anti-infective	T37.8X1	T37.8X2	T37.8X3	T37.8X4	T37.8X5	T37.8X6
herbicide	T60.3X1	T60.3X2	T60.3X3	T60.3X4	—	—
calcium edetate	T45.8X1	T45.8X2	T45.8X3	T45.8X4	T45.8X5	T45.8X6
carbonate NEC	T54.3X1	T54.3X2	T54.3X3	T54.3X4	—	—
chlorate NEC	T65.891	T65.892	T65.893	T65.894	—	—

Substance	Poisoning, Accidental (unintentional)	Poisoning, Intentional self-harm	Poisoning, Assault	Poisoning, Undetermined	Adverse effect	Underdosing
Sodium — *Continued*						
herbicide	T54.91	T54.92	T54.93	T54.94	—	—
chloride	T50.3X1	T50.3X2	T50.3X3	T50.3X4	T50.3X5	T50.3X6
with glucose	T50.3X1	T50.3X2	T50.3X3	T50.3X4	T50.3X5	T50.3X6
chromate	T65.891	T65.892	T65.893	T65.894	—	—
citrate	T50.991	T50.992	T50.993	T50.994	T50.995	T50.996
cromoglicate	T48.6X1	T48.6X2	T48.6X3	T48.6X4	T48.6X5	T48.6X6
cyanide	T65.0X1	T65.0X2	T65.0X3	T65.0X4	—	—
cyclamate	T50.3X1	T50.3X2	T50.3X3	T50.3X4	T50.3X5	T50.3X6
dehydrocholate	T45.8X1	T45.8X2	T45.8X3	T45.8X4	T45.8X5	T45.8X6
diatrizoate	T50.8X1	T50.8X2	T50.8X3	T50.8X4	T50.8X5	T50.8X6
dibunate	T48.4X1	T48.4X2	T48.4X3	T48.4X4	T48.4X5	T48.4X6
dioctyl sulfosuccinate	T47.4X1	T47.4X2	T47.4X3	T47.4X4	T47.4X5	T47.4X6
dipantoyl ferrate	T45.8X1	T45.8X2	T45.8X3	T45.8X4	T45.8X5	T45.8X6
edetate	T45.8X1	T45.8X2	T45.8X3	T45.8X4	T45.8X5	T45.8X6
ethacrynate	T50.1X1	T50.1X2	T50.1X3	T50.1X4	T50.1X5	T50.1X6
feredetate	T45.8X1	T45.8X2	T45.8X3	T45.8X4	T45.8X5	T45.8X6
Fluoride—see Fluoride						
fluoroacetate (dust) (pesticide)	T60.4X1	T60.4X2	T60.4X3	T60.4X4	—	—
free salt	T50.3X1	T50.3X2	T50.3X3	T50.3X4	T50.3X5	T50.3X6
fusidate	T36.8X1	T36.8X2	T36.8X3	T36.8X4	T36.8X5	T36.8X6
glucaldrate	T47.1X1	T47.1X2	T47.1X3	T47.1X4	T47.1X5	T47.1X6
glucosulfone	T37.1X1	T37.1X2	T37.1X3	T37.1X4	T37.1X5	T37.1X6
glutamate	T45.8X1	T45.8X2	T45.8X3	T45.8X4	T45.8X5	T45.8X6
hydrogen carbonate	T50.3X1	T50.3X2	T50.3X3	T50.3X4	T50.3X5	T50.3X6
hydroxide	T54.3X1	T54.3X2	T54.3X3	T54.3X4	—	—
hypochlorite (bleach) NEC	T54.3X1	T54.3X2	T54.3X3	T54.3X4	—	—
disinfectant	T54.3X1	T54.3X2	T54.3X3	T54.3X4	—	—
medicinal (anti-infective) (external)	T49.0X1	T49.0X2	T49.0X3	T49.0X4	T49.0X5	T49.0X6
vapor	T54.3X1	T54.3X2	T54.3X3	T54.3X4	—	—
hyposulfite	T49.0X1	T49.0X2	T49.0X3	T49.0X4	T49.0X5	T49.0X6
indigotin disulfonate	T50.8X1	T50.8X2	T50.8X3	T50.8X4	T50.8X5	T50.8X6
iodide	T50.991	T50.992	T50.993	T50.994	T50.995	T50.996
I-131	T50.8X1	T50.8X2	T50.8X3	T50.8X4	T50.8X5	T50.8X6
therapeutic	T38.2X1	T38.2X2	T38.2X3	T38.2X4	T38.2X5	T38.2X6
iodohippurate (131I)	T50.8X1	T50.8X2	T50.8X3	T50.8X4	T50.8X5	T50.8X6
iopodate	T50.8X1	T50.8X2	T50.8X3	T50.8X4	T50.8X5	T50.8X6
iothalamate	T50.8X1	T50.8X2	T50.8X3	T50.8X4	T50.8X5	T50.8X6
iron edetate	T45.4X1	T45.4X2	T45.4X3	T45.4X4	T45.4X5	T45.4X6
lactate (compound solution)	T45.8X1	T45.8X2	T45.8X3	T45.8X4	T45.8X5	T45.8X6
lauryl (sulfate)	T49.2X1	T49.2X2	T49.2X3	T49.2X4	T49.2X5	T49.2X6
L-triiodothyronine	T38.1X1	T38.1X2	T38.1X3	T38.1X4	T38.1X5	T38.1X6
magnesium citrate	T50.991	T50.992	T50.993	T50.994	T50.995	T50.996
mersalate	T50.2X1	T50.2X2	T50.2X3	T50.2X4	T50.2X5	T50.2X6
metasilicate	T65.891	T65.892	T65.893	T65.894	—	—
metrizoate	T50.8X1	T50.8X2	T50.8X3	T50.8X4	T50.8X5	T50.8X6
monofluoroacetate (pesticide)	T60.1X1	T60.1X2	T60.1X3	T60.1X4	—	—
Sodium — *Continued*						
morrhuate	T46.8X1	T46.8X2	T46.8X3	T46.8X4	T46.8X5	T46.8X6
nafcillin	T36.0X1	T36.0X2	T36.0X3	T36.0X4	T36.0X5	T36.0X6
nitrate (oxidizing agent)	T65.891	T65.892	T65.893	T65.894	—	—
nitrite	T50.6X1	T50.6X2	T50.6X3	T50.6X4	T50.6X5	T50.6X6
nitroferricyanide	T46.5X1	T46.5X2	T46.5X3	T46.5X4	T46.5X5	T46.5X6
nitroprusside	T46.5X1	T46.5X2	T46.5X3	T46.5X4	T46.5X5	T46.5X6
oxalate	T65.891	T65.892	T65.893	T65.894	—	—
oxide/peroxide	T65.891	T65.892	T65.893	T65.894	—	—
oxybate	T41.291	T41.292	T41.293	T41.294	T41.295	T41.296
para-aminohippurate	T50.8X1	T50.8X2	T50.8X3	T50.8X4	T50.8X5	T50.8X6
perborate (nonmedicinal) NEC	T65.891	T65.892	T65.893	T65.894	—	—
medicinal	T49.0X1	T49.0X2	T49.0X3	T49.0X4	T49.0X5	T49.0X6
soap	T55.0X1	T55.0X2	T55.0X3	T55.0X4	—	—
percarbonate—see Sodium, perborate						
pertechnetate Tc99m	T50.8X1	T50.8X2	T50.8X3	T50.8X4	T50.8X5	T50.8X6
phosphate						
cellulose	T45.8X1	T45.8X2	T45.8X3	T45.8X4	T45.8X5	T45.8X6
dibasic	T47.2X1	T47.2X2	T47.2X3	T47.2X4	T47.2X5	T47.2X6
monobasic	T47.2X1	T47.2X2	T47.2X3	T47.2X4	T47.2X5	T47.2X6
phytate	T50.6X1	T50.6X2	T50.6X3	T50.6X4	T50.6X5	T50.6X6
picosulfate	T47.2X1	T47.2X2	T47.2X3	T47.2X4	T47.2X5	T47.2X6
polyhydroxyaluminium monocarbonate	T47.1X1	T47.1X2	T47.1X3	T47.1X4	T47.1X5	T47.1X6
polystyrene sulfonate	T50.3X1	T50.3X2	T50.3X3	T50.3X4	T50.3X5	T50.3X6
propionate	T49.0X1	T49.0X2	T49.0X3	T49.0X4	T49.0X5	T49.0X6
propyl hydroxybenzoate	T50.991	T50.992	T50.993	T50.994	T50.995	T50.996
psylliate	T46.8X1	T46.8X2	T46.8X3	T46.8X4	T46.8X5	T46.8X6
removing resins	T50.3X1	T50.3X2	T50.3X3	T50.3X4	T50.3X5	T50.3X6
salicylate	T39.091	T39.092	T39.093	T39.094	T39.095	T39.096
salt NEC	T50.3X1	T50.3X2	T50.3X3	T50.3X4	T50.3X5	T50.3X6
selenate	T60.2X1	T60.2X2	T60.2X3	T60.2X4	—	—
stibogluconate	T37.3X1	T37.3X2	T37.3X3	T37.3X4	T37.3X5	T37.3X6
sulfate	T47.4X1	T47.4X2	T47.4X3	T47.4X4	T47.4X5	T47.4X6
sulfoxone	T37.1X1	T37.1X2	T37.1X3	T37.1X4	T37.1X5	T37.1X6
tetradecyl sulfate	T46.8X1	T46.8X2	T46.8X3	T46.8X4	T46.8X5	T46.8X6
thiopental	T41.1X1	T41.1X2	T41.1X3	T41.1X4	T41.1X5	T41.1X6
thiosalicylate	T39.091	T39.092	T39.093	T39.094	T39.095	T39.096
thiosulfate	T50.6X1	T50.6X2	T50.6X3	T50.6X4	T50.6X5	T50.6X6
tolbutamide	T38.3X1	T38.3X2	T38.3X3	T38.3X4	T38.3X5	T38.3X6
(L)-triiodothyronine	T38.1X1	T38.1X2	T38.1X3	T38.1X4	T38.1X5	T38.1X6
tyropanoate	T50.8X1	T50.8X2	T50.8X3	T50.8X4	T50.8X5	T50.8X6
valproate	T42.6X1	T42.6X2	T42.6X3	T42.6X4	T42.6X5	T42.6X6
versenate	T50.6X1	T50.6X2	T50.6X3	T50.6X4	T50.6X5	T50.6X6
Sodium-free salt	T50.901	T50.902	T50.903	T50.904	T50.905	T50.906
Sodium-removing resin	T50.3X1	T50.3X2	T50.3X3	T50.3X4	T50.3X5	T50.3X6
Soft soap	T55.0X1	T55.0X2	T55.0X3	T55.0X4	—	—
Solanine	T62.2X1	T62.2X2	T62.2X3	T62.2X4	—	—
berries	T62.1X1	T62.1X2	T62.1X3	T62.1X4	—	—

Substance	Poisoning, Accidental (unintentional)	Poisoning, Intentional self-harm	Poisoning, Assault	Poisoning, Undetermined	Adverse effect	Underdosing
Solanum dulcamara	T62.2X1	T62.2X2	T62.2X3	T62.2X4	—	—
berries	T62.1X1	T62.1X2	T62.1X3	T62.1X4	—	—
Solapsone	T37.1X1	T37.1X2	T37.1X3	T37.1X4	T37.1X5	T37.1X6
Solar lotion	T49.3X1	T49.3X2	T49.3X3	T49.3X4	T49.3X5	T49.3X6
Solasulfone	T37.1X1	T37.1X2	T37.1X3	T37.1X4	T37.1X5	T37.1X6
Soldering fluid	T65.891	T65.892	T65.893	T65.894	—	—
Solid substance	T65.91	T65.92	T65.93	T65.94	—	—
specified NEC	T65.891	T65.892	T65.893	T65.894	—	—
Solvent, industrial NEC	T52.91	T52.92	T52.93	T52.94	—	—
naphtha	T52.0X1	T52.0X2	T52.0X3	T52.0X4	—	—
petroleum	T52.0X1	T52.0X2	T52.0X3	T52.0X4	—	—
specified NEC	T52.8X1	T52.8X2	T52.8X3	T52.8X4	—	—
Soma	T42.8X1	T42.8X2	T42.8X3	T42.8X4	T42.8X5	T42.8X6
Somatorelin	T38.891	T38.892	T38.893	T38.894	T38.895	T38.896
Somatostatin	T38.991	T38.992	T38.993	T38.994	T38.995	T38.996
Somatotropin	T38.811	T38.812	T38.813	T38.814	T38.815	T38.816
Somatrem	T38.811	T38.812	T38.813	T38.814	T38.815	T38.816
Somatropin	T38.811	T38.812	T38.813	T38.814	T38.815	T38.816
Sominex	T45.0X1	T45.0X2	T45.0X3	T45.0X4	T45.0X5	T45.0X6
Somnos	T42.6X1	T42.6X2	T42.6X3	T42.6X4	T42.6X5	T42.6X6
Somonal	T42.3X1	T42.3X2	T42.3X3	T42.3X4	T42.3X5	T42.3X6
Soneryl	T42.3X1	T42.3X2	T42.3X3	T42.3X4	T42.3X5	T42.3X6
Soothing syrup	T50.901	T50.902	T50.903	T50.904	T50.905	T50.906
Sopor	T42.6X1	T42.6X2	T42.6X3	T42.6X4	T42.6X5	T42.6X6
Soporific	T42.71	T42.72	T42.73	T42.74	T42.75	T42.76
Soporific drug	T42.71	T42.72	T42.73	T42.74	T42.75	T42.76
specified type NEC	T42.6X1	T42.6X2	T42.6X3	T42.6X4	T42.6X5	T42.6X6
Sorbide nitrate	T46.3X1	T46.3X2	T46.3X3	T46.3X4	T46.3X5	T46.3X6
Sorbitol	T47.4X1	T47.4X2	T47.4X3	T47.4X4	T47.4X5	T47.4X6
Sotalol	T44.7X1	T44.7X2	T44.7X3	T44.7X4	T44.7X5	T44.7X6
Sotradecol	T46.8X1	T46.8X2	T46.8X3	T46.8X4	T46.8X5	T46.8X6
Soysterol	T46.6X1	T46.6X2	T46.6X3	T46.6X4	T46.6X5	T46.6X6
Spacoline	T44.3X1	T44.3X2	T44.3X3	T44.3X4	T44.3X5	T44.3X6
Spanish fly	T49.8X1	T49.8X2	T49.8X3	T49.8X4	T49.8X5	T49.8X6
Sparine	T43.3X1	T43.3X2	T43.3X3	T43.3X4	T43.3X5	T43.3X6
Sparteine	T48.0X1	T48.0X2	T48.0X3	T48.0X4	T48.0X5	T48.0X6
Spasmolytic						
anticholinergics	T44.3X1	T44.3X2	T44.3X3	T44.3X4	T44.3X5	T44.3X6
autonomic	T44.3X1	T44.3X2	T44.3X3	T44.3X4	T44.3X5	T44.3X6
bronchial NEC	T48.6X1	T48.6X2	T48.6X3	T48.6X4	T48.6X5	T48.6X6
quaternary ammonium	T44.3X1	T44.3X2	T44.3X3	T44.3X4	T44.3X5	T44.3X6
skeletal muscle NEC	T48.1X1	T48.1X2	T48.1X3	T48.1X4	T48.1X5	T48.1X6
Spectinomycin	T36.5X1	T36.5X2	T36.5X3	T36.5X4	T36.5X5	T36.5X6
Speed	T43.621	T43.622	T43.623	T43.624	T43.625	T43.626
Spermicide	T49.8X1	T49.8X2	T49.8X3	T49.8X4	T49.8X5	T49.8X6
Spider (bite) (venom)	T63.391	T63.392	T63.393	T63.394	—	—
antivenin	T50.Z11	T50.Z12	T50.Z13	T50.Z14	T50.Z15	T50.Z16
Spigelia (root)	T37.4X1	T37.4X2	T37.4X3	T37.4X4	T37.4X5	T37.4X6
Spindle inactivator	T50.4X1	T50.4X2	T50.4X3	T50.4X4	T50.4X5	T50.4X6
Spiperone	T43.4X1	T43.4X2	T43.4X3	T43.4X4	T43.4X5	T43.4X6

Substance	Poisoning, Accidental (unintentional)	Poisoning, Intentional self-harm	Poisoning, Assault	Poisoning, Undetermined	Adverse effect	Underdosing
Spiramycin	T36.3X1	T36.3X2	T36.3X3	T36.3X4	T36.3X5	T36.3X6
Spirapril	T46.4X1	T46.4X2	T46.4X3	T46.4X4	T46.4X5	T46.4X6
Spirilene	T43.591	T43.592	T43.593	T43.594	T43.595	T43.596
Spirit(s) (neutral) NEC	T51.0X1	T51.0X2	T51.0X3	T51.0X4	—	—
beverage	T51.0X1	T51.0X2	T51.0X3	T51.0X4	—	—
industrial	T51.0X1	T51.0X2	T51.0X3	T51.0X4	—	—
mineral	T52.0X1	T52.0X2	T52.0X3	T52.0X4	—	—
of salt—see Hydrochloric acid						
surgical	T51.0X1	T51.0X2	T51.0X3	T51.0X4	—	—
Spironolactone	T50.0X1	T50.0X2	T50.0X3	T50.0X4	T50.0X5	T50.0X6
Spiroperidol	T43.4X1	T43.4X2	T43.4X3	T43.4X4	T43.4X5	T43.4X6
Sponge, absorbable (gelatin)	T45.7X1	T45.7X2	T45.7X3	T45.7X4	T45.7X5	T45.7X6
Sporostacin	T49.0X1	T49.0X2	T49.0X3	T49.0X4	T49.0X5	T49.0X6
Spray (aerosol)	T65.91	T65.92	T65.93	T65.94	—	—
cosmetic	T65.891	T65.892	T65.893	T65.894	—	—
medicinal NEC	T50.901	T50.902	T50.903	T50.904	T50.905	T50.906
pesticides—see Pesticides						
specified content—see specific substance						
Spurge flax	T62.2X1	T62.2X2	T62.2X3	T62.2X4	—	—
Spurges	T62.2X1	T62.2X2	T62.2X3	T62.2X4	—	—
Sputum viscosity-lowering drug	T48.4X1	T48.4X2	T48.4X3	T48.4X4	T48.4X5	T48.4X6
Squill	T46.0X1	T46.0X2	T46.0X3	T46.0X4	T46.0X5	T46.0X6
rat poison	T60.4X1	T60.4X2	T60.4X3	T60.4X4	—	—
Squirting cucumber (cathartic)	T47.2X1	T47.2X2	T47.2X3	T47.2X4	T47.2X5	T47.2X6
Stains	T65.6X1	T65.6X2	T65.6X3	T65.6X4	—	—
Stannous fluoride	T49.7X1	T49.7X2	T49.7X3	T49.7X4	T49.7X5	T49.7X6
Stanolone	T38.7X1	T38.7X2	T38.7X3	T38.7X4	T38.7X5	T38.7X6
Stanozolol	T38.7X1	T38.7X2	T38.7X3	T38.7X4	T38.7X5	T38.7X6
Staphisagria or stavesacre (pediculicide)	T49.0X1	T49.0X2	T49.0X3	T49.0X4	T49.0X5	T49.0X6
Starch	T50.901	T50.902	T50.903	T50.904	T50.905	T50.906
Stelazine	T43.3X1	T43.3X2	T43.3X3	T43.3X4	T43.3X5	T43.3X6
Stemetil	T43.3X1	T43.3X2	T43.3X3	T43.3X4	T43.3X5	T43.3X6
Stepronin	T48.4X1	T48.4X2	T48.4X3	T48.4X4	T48.4X5	T48.4X6
Sterculia	T47.4X1	T47.4X2	T47.4X3	T47.4X4	T47.4X5	T47.4X6
Sternutator gas	T59.891	T59.892	T59.893	T59.894	—	—
Steroid	T38.0X1	T38.0X2	T38.0X3	T38.0X4	T38.0X5	T38.0X6
anabolic	T38.7X1	T38.7X2	T38.7X3	T38.7X4	T38.7X5	T38.7X6
androgenic	T38.7X1	T38.7X2	T38.7X3	T38.7X4	T38.7X5	T38.7X6
antineoplastic, hormone	T38.7X1	T38.7X2	T38.7X3	T38.7X4	T38.7X5	T38.7X6
estrogen	T38.5X1	T38.5X2	T38.5X3	T38.5X4	T38.5X5	T38.5X6
ENT agent	T49.6X1	T49.6X2	T49.6X3	T49.6X4	T49.6X5	T49.6X6
ophthalmic preparation	T49.5X1	T49.5X2	T49.5X3	T49.5X4	T49.5X5	T49.5X6
topical NEC	T49.0X1	T49.0X2	T49.0X3	T49.0X4	T49.0X5	T49.0X6
Stibine	T56.891	T56.892	T56.893	T56.894	—	—
Stibogluconate	T37.3X1	T37.3X2	T37.3X3	T37.3X4	T37.3X5	T37.3X6

Substance	Poisoning, Accidental (unintentional)	Poisoning, Intentional self-harm	Poisoning, Assault	Poisoning, Undetermined	Adverse effect	Underdosing
Stibophen	T37.4X1	T37.4X2	T37.4X3	T37.4X4	T37.4X5	T37.4X6
Stilbamidine (isetionate)	T37.3X1	T37.3X2	T37.3X3	T37.3X4	T37.3X5	T37.3X6
Stilbestrol	T38.5X1	T38.5X2	T38.5X3	T38.5X4	T38.5X5	T38.5X6
Stilboestrol	T38.5X1	T38.5X2	T38.5X3	T38.5X4	T38.5X5	T38.5X6
Stimulant						
central nervous system—see also Psychostimulant	T43.601	T43.602	T43.603	T43.604	T43.605	T43.606
analeptics	T50.7X1	T50.7X2	T50.7X3	T50.7X4	T50.7X5	T50.7X6
opiate antagonist	T50.7X1	T50.7X2	T50.7X3	T50.7X4	T50.7X5	T50.7X6
psychotherapeutic NEC—see also Psychotherapeutic drug	T43.601	T43.602	T43.603	T43.604	T43.605	T43.606
specified NEC	T43.691	T43.692	T43.693	T43.694	T43.695	T43.696
respiratory	T48.901	T48.902	T48.903	T48.904	T48.905	T48.906
Stone-dissolving drug	T50.901	T50.902	T50.903	T50.904	T50.905	T50.906
Storage battery (cells) (acid)	T54.2X1	T54.2X2	T54.2X3	T54.2X4	—	—
Stovaine	T41.3X1	T41.3X2	T41.3X3	T41.3X4	T41.3X5	T41.3X6
infiltration (subcutaneous)	T41.3X1	T41.3X2	T41.3X3	T41.3X4	T41.3X5	T41.3X6
nerve block (peripheral) (plexus)	T41.3X1	T41.3X2	T41.3X3	T41.3X4	T41.3X5	T41.3X6
spinal	T41.3X1	T41.3X2	T41.3X3	T41.3X4	T41.3X5	T41.3X6
topical (surface)	T41.3X1	T41.3X2	T41.3X3	T41.3X4	T41.3X5	T41.3X6
Stovarsal	T37.8X1	T37.8X2	T37.8X3	T37.8X4	T37.8X5	T37.8X6
Stove gas—see Gas, stove						
Stoxil	T49.5X1	T49.5X2	T49.5X3	T49.5X4	T49.5X5	T49.5X6
Stramonium	T48.6X1	T48.6X2	T48.6X3	T48.6X4	T48.6X5	T48.6X6
natural state	T62.2X1	T62.2X2	T62.2X3	T62.2X4	—	—
Streptodornase	T45.3X1	T45.3X2	T45.3X3	T45.3X4	T45.3X5	T45.3X6
Streptoduocin	T36.5X1	T36.5X2	T36.5X3	T36.5X4	T36.5X5	T36.5X6
Streptokinase	T45.611	T45.612	T45.613	T45.614	T45.615	T45.616
Streptomycin (derivative)	T36.5X1	T36.5X2	T36.5X3	T36.5X4	T36.5X5	T36.5X6
Streptonivicin	T36.5X1	T36.5X2	T36.5X3	T36.5X4	T36.5X5	T36.5X6
Streptovarycin	T36.5X1	T36.5X2	T36.5X3	T36.5X4	T36.5X5	T36.5X6
Streptozocin	T45.1X1	T45.1X2	T45.1X3	T45.1X4	T45.1X5	T45.1X6
Streptozotocin	T45.1X1	T45.1X2	T45.1X3	T45.1X4	T45.1X5	T45.1X6
Stripper (paint) (solvent)	T52.8X1	T52.8X2	T52.8X3	T52.8X4	—	—
Strobane	T60.1X1	T60.1X2	T60.1X3	T60.1X4	—	—
Strofantina	T46.0X1	T46.0X2	T46.0X3	T46.0X4	T46.0X5	T46.0X6
Strophanthin (g) (k)	T46.0X1	T46.0X2	T46.0X3	T46.0X4	T46.0X5	T46.0X6
Strophanthus	T46.0X1	T46.0X2	T46.0X3	T46.0X4	T46.0X5	T46.0X6
Strophantin	T46.0X1	T46.0X2	T46.0X3	T46.0X4	T46.0X5	T46.0X6
Strophantin-g	T46.0X1	T46.0X2	T46.0X3	T46.0X4	T46.0X5	T46.0X6
Strychnine (nonmedicinal) (pesticide) (salts)	T65.1X1	T65.1X2	T65.1X3	T65.1X4	—	—
medicinal	T48.291	T48.292	T48.293	T48.294	T48.295	T48.296
Strychnos (ignatii)—see Strychnine						
Styramate	T42.8X1	T42.8X2	T42.8X3	T42.8X4	T42.8X5	T42.8X6
Styrene	T65.891	T65.892	T65.893	T65.894	—	—
Succinimide, antiepileptic or anticonvulsant	T42.2X1	T42.2X2	T42.2X3	T42.2X4	T42.2X5	T42.2X6
mercuric—see Mercury						
Succinylcholine	T48.1X1	T48.1X2	T48.1X3	T48.1X4	T48.1X5	T48.1X6
Succinylsulfathiazole	T37.0X1	T37.0X2	T37.0X3	T37.0X4	T37.0X5	T37.0X6
Sucralfate	T47.1X1	T47.1X2	T47.1X3	T47.1X4	T47.1X5	T47.1X6
Sucrose	T50.3X1	T50.3X2	T50.3X3	T50.3X4	T50.3X5	T50.3X6
Sufentanil	T40.411	T40.412	T40.413	T40.414	T40.415	T40.416
Sulbactam	T36.0X1	T36.0X2	T36.0X3	T36.0X4	T36.0X5	T36.0X6
Sulbenicillin	T36.0X1	T36.0X2	T36.0X3	T36.0X4	T36.0X5	T36.0X6
Sulbentine	T49.0X1	T49.0X2	T49.0X3	T49.0X4	T49.0X5	T49.0X6
Sulfacetamide	T49.0X1	T49.0X2	T49.0X3	T49.0X4	T49.0X5	T49.0X6
ophthalmic preparation	T49.5X1	T49.5X2	T49.5X3	T49.5X4	T49.5X5	T49.5X6
Sulfachlorpyridazine	T37.0X1	T37.0X2	T37.0X3	T37.0X4	T37.0X5	T37.0X6
Sulfacitine	T37.0X1	T37.0X2	T37.0X3	T37.0X4	T37.0X5	T37.0X6
Sulfadiasulfone sodium	T37.0X1	T37.0X2	T37.0X3	T37.0X4	T37.0X5	T37.0X6
Sulfadiazine	T37.0X1	T37.0X2	T37.0X3	T37.0X4	T37.0X5	T37.0X6
silver (topical)	T49.0X1	T49.0X2	T49.0X3	T49.0X4	T49.0X5	T49.0X6
Sulfadimethoxine	T37.0X1	T37.0X2	T37.0X3	T37.0X4	T37.0X5	T37.0X6
Sulfadimidine	T37.0X1	T37.0X2	T37.0X3	T37.0X4	T37.0X5	T37.0X6
Sulfadoxine	T37.0X1	T37.0X2	T37.0X3	T37.0X4	T37.0X5	T37.0X6
with pyrimethamine	T37.2X1	T37.2X2	T37.2X3	T37.2X4	T37.2X5	T37.2X6
Sulfaethidole	T37.0X1	T37.0X2	T37.0X3	T37.0X4	T37.0X5	T37.0X6
Sulfafurazole	T37.0X1	T37.0X2	T37.0X3	T37.0X4	T37.0X5	T37.0X6
Sulfaguanidine	T37.0X1	T37.0X2	T37.0X3	T37.0X4	T37.0X5	T37.0X6
Sulfalene	T37.0X1	T37.0X2	T37.0X3	T37.0X4	T37.0X5	T37.0X6
Sulfaloxate	T37.0X1	T37.0X2	T37.0X3	T37.0X4	T37.0X5	T37.0X6
Sulfaloxic acid	T37.0X1	T37.0X2	T37.0X3	T37.0X4	T37.0X5	T37.0X6
Sulfamazone	T39.2X1	T39.2X2	T39.2X3	T39.2X4	T39.2X5	T39.2X6
Sulfamerazine	T37.0X1	T37.0X2	T37.0X3	T37.0X4	T37.0X5	T37.0X6
Sulfameter	T37.0X1	T37.0X2	T37.0X3	T37.0X4	T37.0X5	T37.0X6
Sulfamethazine	T37.0X1	T37.0X2	T37.0X3	T37.0X4	T37.0X5	T37.0X6
Sulfamethizole	T37.0X1	T37.0X2	T37.0X3	T37.0X4	T37.0X5	T37.0X6
Sulfamethoxazole	T37.0X1	T37.0X2	T37.0X3	T37.0X4	T37.0X5	T37.0X6
with trimethoprim	T36.8X1	T36.8X2	T36.8X3	T36.8X4	T36.8X5	T36.8X6
Sulfamethoxydiazine	T37.0X1	T37.0X2	T37.0X3	T37.0X4	T37.0X5	T37.0X6
Sulfamethoxypyridazine	T37.0X1	T37.0X2	T37.0X3	T37.0X4	T37.0X5	T37.0X6
Sulfamethylthiazole	T37.0X1	T37.0X2	T37.0X3	T37.0X4	T37.0X5	T37.0X6
Sulfametoxydiazine	T37.0X1	T37.0X2	T37.0X3	T37.0X4	T37.0X5	T37.0X6
Sulfamidopyrine	T39.2X1	T39.2X2	T39.2X3	T39.2X4	T39.2X5	T39.2X6
Sulfamonomethoxine	T37.0X1	T37.0X2	T37.0X3	T37.0X4	T37.0X5	T37.0X6
Sulfamoxole	T37.0X1	T37.0X2	T37.0X3	T37.0X4	T37.0X5	T37.0X6
Sulfamylon	T49.0X1	T49.0X2	T49.0X3	T49.0X4	T49.0X5	T49.0X6
Sulfan blue (diagnostic dye)	T50.8X1	T50.8X2	T50.8X3	T50.8X4	T50.8X5	T50.8X6
Sulfanilamide	T37.0X1	T37.0X2	T37.0X3	T37.0X4	T37.0X5	T37.0X6
Sulfanilylguanidine	T37.0X1	T37.0X2	T37.0X3	T37.0X4	T37.0X5	T37.0X6
Sulfaperin	T37.0X1	T37.0X2	T37.0X3	T37.0X4	T37.0X5	T37.0X6

Substance	Poisoning, Accidental (unintentional)	Poisoning, Intentional self-harm	Poisoning, Assault	Poisoning, Undetermined	Adverse effect	Underdosing
Sulfaphenazole	T37.0X1	T37.0X2	T37.0X3	T37.0X4	T37.0X5	T37.0X6
Sulfaphenylthiazole	T37.0X1	T37.0X2	T37.0X3	T37.0X4	T37.0X5	T37.0X6
Sulfaproxyline	T37.0X1	T37.0X2	T37.0X3	T37.0X4	T37.0X5	T37.0X6
Sulfapyridine	T37.0X1	T37.0X2	T37.0X3	T37.0X4	T37.0X5	T37.0X6
Sulfapyrimidine	T37.0X1	T37.0X2	T37.0X3	T37.0X4	T37.0X5	T37.0X6
Sulfarsphenamine	T37.8X1	T37.8X2	T37.8X3	T37.8X4	T37.8X5	T37.8X6
Sulfasalazine	T37.0X1	T37.0X2	T37.0X3	T37.0X4	T37.0X5	T37.0X6
Sulfasuxidine	T37.0X1	T37.0X2	T37.0X3	T37.0X4	T37.0X5	T37.0X6
Sulfasymazine	T37.0X1	T37.0X2	T37.0X3	T37.0X4	T37.0X5	T37.0X6
Sulfated amylopectin	T47.8X1	T47.8X2	T47.8X3	T47.8X4	T47.8X5	T47.8X6
Sulfathiazole	T37.0X1	T37.0X2	T37.0X3	T37.0X4	T37.0X5	T37.0X6
Sulfatostearate	T49.2X1	T49.2X2	T49.2X3	T49.2X4	T49.2X5	T49.2X6
Sulfinpyrazone	T50.4X1	T50.4X2	T50.4X3	T50.4X4	T50.4X5	T50.4X6
Sulfiram	T49.0X1	T49.0X2	T49.0X3	T49.0X4	T49.0X5	T49.0X6
Sulfisomidine	T37.0X1	T37.0X2	T37.0X3	T37.0X4	T37.0X5	T37.0X6
Sulfisoxazole	T37.0X1	T37.0X2	T37.0X3	T37.0X4	T37.0X5	T37.0X6
ophthalmic preparation	T49.5X1	T49.5X2	T49.5X3	T49.5X4	T49.5X5	T49.5X6
Sulfobromophthalein (sodium)	T50.8X1	T50.8X2	T50.8X3	T50.8X4	T50.8X5	T50.8X6
Sulfobromphthalein	T50.8X1	T50.8X2	T50.8X3	T50.8X4	T50.8X5	T50.8X6
Sulfogaiacol	T48.4X1	T48.4X2	T48.4X3	T48.4X4	T48.4X5	T48.4X6
Sulfomyxin	T36.8X1	T36.8X2	T36.8X3	T36.8X4	T36.8X5	T36.8X6
Sulfonal	T42.6X1	T42.6X2	T42.6X3	T42.6X4	T42.6X5	T42.6X6
Sulfonamide NEC	T37.0X1	T37.0X2	T37.0X3	T37.0X4	T37.0X5	T37.0X6
eye	T49.5X1	T49.5X2	T49.5X3	T49.5X4	T49.5X5	T49.5X6
Sulfonazide	T37.1X1	T37.1X2	T37.1X3	T37.1X4	T37.1X5	T37.1X6
Sulfones	T37.1X1	T37.1X2	T37.1X3	T37.1X4	T37.1X5	T37.1X6
Sulfonethylmethane	T42.6X1	T42.6X2	T42.6X3	T42.6X4	T42.6X5	T42.6X6
Sulfonmethane	T42.6X1	T42.6X2	T42.6X3	T42.6X4	T42.6X5	T42.6X6
Sulfonphthal, sulfonphthol	T50.8X1	T50.8X2	T50.8X3	T50.8X4	T50.8X5	T50.8X6
Sulfonylurea derivatives, oral	T38.3X1	T38.3X2	T38.3X3	T38.3X4	T38.3X5	T38.3X6
Sulforidazine	T43.3X1	T43.3X2	T43.3X3	T43.3X4	T43.3X5	T43.3X6
Sulfoxone	T37.1X1	T37.1X2	T37.1X3	T37.1X4	T37.1X5	T37.1X6
Sulfur, sulfurated, sulfuric, sulfurous, sulfuryl (compounds NEC) (medicinal)	T49.4X1	T49.4X2	T49.4X3	T49.4X4	T49.4X5	T49.4X6
acid	T54.2X1	T54.2X2	T54.2X3	T54.2X4	—	—
dioxide (gas)	T59.1X1	T59.1X2	T59.1X3	T59.1X4	—	—
ether—see Ether(s)						
hydrogen	T59.6X1	T59.6X2	T59.6X3	T59.6X4	—	—
medicinal (keratolytic) (ointment) NEC	T49.4X1	T49.4X2	T49.4X3	T49.4X4	T49.4X5	T49.4X6
ointment	T49.0X1	T49.0X2	T49.0X3	T49.0X4	T49.0X5	T49.0X6
pesticide (vapor)	T60.91	T60.92	T60.93	T60.94	—	—
vapor NEC	T59.891	T59.892	T59.893	T59.894	—	—
Sulfuric acid	T54.2X1	T54.2X2	T54.2X3	T54.2X4	—	—
Sulglicotide	T47.1X1	T47.1X2	T47.1X3	T47.1X4	T47.1X5	T47.1X6
Sulindac	T39.391	T39.392	T39.393	T39.394	T39.395	T39.396
Sulisatin	T47.2X1	T47.2X2	T47.2X3	T47.2X4	T47.2X5	T47.2X6
Sulisobenzone	T49.3X1	T49.3X2	T49.3X3	T49.3X4	T49.3X5	T49.3X6
Sulkowitch's reagent	T50.8X1	T50.8X2	T50.8X3	T50.8X4	T50.8X5	T50.8X6
Sulmetozine	T44.3X1	T44.3X2	T44.3X3	T44.3X4	T44.3X5	T44.3X6
Suloctidil	T46.7X1	T46.7X2	T46.7X3	T46.7X4	T46.7X5	T46.7X6
Sulph-—see also Sulf-						
Sulphadiazine	T37.0X1	T37.0X2	T37.0X3	T37.0X4	T37.0X5	T37.0X6
Sulphadimethoxine	T37.0X1	T37.0X2	T37.0X3	T37.0X4	T37.0X5	T37.0X6
Sulphadimidine	T37.0X1	T37.0X2	T37.0X3	T37.0X4	T37.0X5	T37.0X6
Sulphadione	T37.1X1	T37.1X2	T37.1X3	T37.1X4	T37.1X5	T37.1X6
Sulphafurazole	T37.0X1	T37.0X2	T37.0X3	T37.0X4	T37.0X5	T37.0X6
Sulphamethizole	T37.0X1	T37.0X2	T37.0X3	T37.0X4	T37.0X5	T37.0X6
Sulphamethoxazole	T37.0X1	T37.0X2	T37.0X3	T37.0X4	T37.0X5	T37.0X6
Sulphan blue	T50.8X1	T50.8X2	T50.8X3	T50.8X4	T50.8X5	T50.8X6
Sulphaphenazole	T37.0X1	T37.0X2	T37.0X3	T37.0X4	T37.0X5	T37.0X6
Sulphapyridine	T37.0X1	T37.0X2	T37.0X3	T37.0X4	T37.0X5	T37.0X6
Sulphasalazine	T37.0X1	T37.0X2	T37.0X3	T37.0X4	T37.0X5	T37.0X6
Sulphinpyrazone	T50.4X1	T50.4X2	T50.4X3	T50.4X4	T50.4X5	T50.4X6
Sulpiride	T43.591	T43.592	T43.593	T43.594	T43.595	T43.596
Sulprostone	T48.0X1	T48.0X2	T48.0X3	T48.0X4	T48.0X5	T48.0X6
Sulpyrine	T39.2X1	T39.2X2	T39.2X3	T39.2X4	T39.2X5	T39.2X6
Sultamicillin	T36.0X1	T36.0X2	T36.0X3	T36.0X4	T36.0X5	T36.0X6
Sulthiame	T42.6X1	T42.6X2	T42.6X3	T42.6X4	T42.6X5	T42.6X6
Sultiame	T42.6X1	T42.6X2	T42.6X3	T42.6X4	T42.6X5	T42.6X6
Sultopride	T43.591	T43.592	T43.593	T43.594	T43.595	T43.596
Sumatriptan	T39.8X1	T39.8X2	T39.8X3	T39.8X4	T39.8X5	T39.8X6
Sunflower seed oil	T46.6X1	T46.6X2	T46.6X3	T46.6X4	T46.6X5	T46.6X6
Superinone	T48.4X1	T48.4X2	T48.4X3	T48.4X4	T48.4X5	T48.4X6
Suprofen	T39.311	T39.312	T39.313	T39.314	T39.315	T39.316
Suramin (sodium)	T37.4X1	T37.4X2	T37.4X3	T37.4X4	T37.4X5	T37.4X6
Surfacaine	T41.3X1	T41.3X2	T41.3X3	T41.3X4	T41.3X5	T41.3X6
Surital	T41.1X1	T41.1X2	T41.1X3	T41.1X4	T41.1X5	T41.1X6
Sutilains	T45.3X1	T45.3X2	T45.3X3	T45.3X4	T45.3X5	T45.3X6
Suxamethonium (chloride)	T48.1X1	T48.1X2	T48.1X3	T48.1X4	T48.1X5	T48.1X6
Suxethonium (chloride)	T48.1X1	T48.1X2	T48.1X3	T48.1X4	T48.1X5	T48.1X6
Suxibuzone	T39.2X1	T39.2X2	T39.2X3	T39.2X4	T39.2X5	T39.2X6
Sweet niter spirit	T46.3X1	T46.3X2	T46.3X3	T46.3X4	T46.3X5	T46.3X6
Sweet oil (birch)	T49.3X1	T49.3X2	T49.3X3	T49.3X4	T49.3X5	T49.3X6
Sweetener	T50.901	T50.902	T50.903	T50.904	T50.905	T50.906
Sym-dichloroethyl ether	T53.6X1	T53.6X2	T53.6X3	T53.6X4	—	—
Sympatholytic NEC	T44.8X1	T44.8X2	T44.8X3	T44.8X4	T44.8X5	T44.8X6
haloalkylamine	T44.8X1	T44.8X2	T44.8X3	T44.8X4	T44.8X5	T44.8X6
Sympathomimetic NEC	T44.901	T44.902	T44.903	T44.904	T44.905	T44.906
anti-common-cold	T48.5X1	T48.5X2	T48.5X3	T48.5X4	T48.5X5	T48.5X6
bronchodilator	T48.6X1	T48.6X2	T48.6X3	T48.6X4	T48.6X5	T48.6X6
specified NEC	T44.991	T44.992	T44.993	T44.994	T44.995	T44.996
Synagis	T50.B91	T50.B92	T50.B93	T50.B94	T50.B95	T50.B96
Synalar	T49.0X1	T49.0X2	T49.0X3	T49.0X4	T49.0X5	T49.0X6
Synthetic cannabinoids	T40.721	T40.722	T40.723	T40.724	T40.725	T40.726
Synthroid	T38.1X1	T38.1X2	T38.1X3	T38.1X4	T38.1X5	T38.1X6
Syntocinon	T48.0X1	T48.0X2	T48.0X3	T48.0X4	T48.0X5	T48.0X6

Substance	Poisoning, Accidental (unintentional)	Poisoning, Intentional self-harm	Poisoning, Assault	Poisoning, Undetermined	Adverse effect	Underdosing
Syrosingopine	T46.5X1	T46.5X2	T46.5X3	T46.5X4	T46.5X5	T46.5X6
Systemic drug	T45.91	T45.92	T45.93	T45.94	T45.95	T45.96
specified NEC	T45.8X1	T45.8X2	T45.8X3	T45.8X4	T45.8X5	T45.8X6
2,4,5-T	T60.3X1	T60.3X2	T60.3X3	T60.3X4	—	—
T						
Tablets—see also specified substance	T50.901	T50.902	T50.903	T50.904	T50.905	T50.906
Tace	T38.5X1	T38.5X2	T38.5X3	T38.5X4	T38.5X5	T38.5X6
Tacrine	T44.0X1	T44.0X2	T44.0X3	T44.0X4	T44.0X5	T44.0X6
Tadalafil	T46.7X1	T46.7X2	T46.7X3	T46.7X4	T46.7X5	T46.7X6
Talampicillin	T36.0X1	T36.0X2	T36.0X3	T36.0X4	T36.0X5	T36.0X6
Talbutal	T42.3X1	T42.3X2	T42.3X3	T42.3X4	T42.3X5	T42.3X6
Talc powder	T49.3X1	T49.3X2	T49.3X3	T49.3X4	T49.3X5	T49.3X6
Talcum	T49.3X1	T49.3X2	T49.3X3	T49.3X4	T49.3X5	T49.3X6
Taleranol	T38.6X1	T38.6X2	T38.6X3	T38.6X4	T38.6X5	T38.6X6
Tamoxifen	T38.6X1	T38.6X2	T38.6X3	T38.6X4	T38.6X5	T38.6X6
Tamsulosin	T44.6X1	T44.6X2	T44.6X3	T44.6X4	T44.6X5	T44.6X6
Tandearil, tanderil	T39.2X1	T39.2X2	T39.2X3	T39.2X4	T39.2X5	T39.2X6
Tannic acid	T49.2X1	T49.2X2	T49.2X3	T49.2X4	T49.2X5	T49.2X6
medicinal (astringent)	T49.2X1	T49.2X2	T49.2X3	T49.2X4	T49.2X5	T49.2X6
Tannin—see Tannic acid						
Tansy	T62.2X1	T62.2X2	T62.2X3	T62.2X4	—	—
TAO	T36.3X1	T36.3X2	T36.3X3	T36.3X4	T36.3X5	T36.3X6
Tapazole	T38.2X1	T38.2X2	T38.2X3	T38.2X4	T38.2X5	T38.2X6
Tar NEC	T52.0X1	T52.0X2	T52.0X3	T52.0X4	—	—
camphor	T60.1X1	T60.1X2	T60.1X3	T60.1X4	—	—
distillate	T49.1X1	T49.1X2	T49.1X3	T49.1X4	T49.1X5	T49.1X6
fumes	T59.891	T59.892	T59.893	T59.894	—	—
medicinal	T49.1X1	T49.1X2	T49.1X3	T49.1X4	T49.1X5	T49.1X6
ointment	T49.1X1	T49.1X2	T49.1X3	T49.1X4	T49.1X5	T49.1X6
Taractan	T43.591	T43.592	T43.593	T43.594	T43.595	T43.596
Tarantula (venomous)	T63.321	T63.322	T63.323	T63.324	—	—
Tartar emetic	T37.8X1	T37.8X2	T37.8X3	T37.8X4	T37.8X5	T37.8X6
Tartaric acid	T65.891	T65.892	T65.893	T65.894	—	—
Tartrate, laxative	T47.4X1	T47.4X2	T47.4X3	T47.4X4	T47.4X5	T47.4X6
Tartrated antimony (anti-infective)	T37.8X1	T37.8X2	T37.8X3	T37.8X4	T37.8X5	T37.8X6
Tauromustine	T45.1X1	T45.1X2	T45.1X3	T45.1X4	T45.1X5	T45.1X6
TCA—see Trichloroacetic acid						
TCDD	T53.7X1	T53.7X2	T53.7X3	T53.7X4	—	—
TDI (vapor)	T65.0X1	T65.0X2	T65.0X3	T65.0X4	—	—
Tear						
gas	T59.3X1	T59.3X2	T59.3X3	T59.3X4	—	—
solution	T49.5X1	T49.5X2	T49.5X3	T49.5X4	T49.5X5	T49.5X6
Teclothiazide	T50.2X1	T50.2X2	T50.2X3	T50.2X4	T50.2X5	T50.2X6
Teclozan	T37.3X1	T37.3X2	T37.3X3	T37.3X4	T37.3X5	T37.3X6
Tegafur	T45.1X1	T45.1X2	T45.1X3	T45.1X4	T45.1X5	T45.1X6
Tegretol	T42.1X1	T42.1X2	T42.1X3	T42.1X4	T42.1X5	T42.1X6
Teicoplanin	T36.8X1	T36.8X2	T36.8X3	T36.8X4	T36.8X5	T36.8X6
Telepaque	T50.8X1	T50.8X2	T50.8X3	T50.8X4	T50.8X5	T50.8X6

Substance	Poisoning, Accidental (unintentional)	Poisoning, Intentional self-harm	Poisoning, Assault	Poisoning, Undetermined	Adverse effect	Underdosing
Tellurium	T56.891	T56.892	T56.893	T56.894	—	—
fumes	T56.891	T56.892	T56.893	T56.894	—	—
TEM	T45.1X1	T45.1X2	T45.1X3	T45.1X4	T45.1X5	T45.1X6
Temazepam	T42.4X1	T42.4X2	T42.4X3	T42.4X4	T42.4X5	T42.4X6
Temocillin	T36.0X1	T36.0X2	T36.0X3	T36.0X4	T36.0X5	T36.0X6
Tenamfetamine	T43.621	T43.622	T43.623	T43.624	T43.625	T43.626
Teniposide	T45.1X1	T45.1X2	T45.1X3	T45.1X4	T45.1X5	T45.1X6
Tenitramine	T46.3X1	T46.3X2	T46.3X3	T46.3X4	T46.3X5	T46.3X6
Tenoglicin	T48.4X1	T48.4X2	T48.4X3	T48.4X4	T48.4X5	T48.4X6
Tenonitrozole	T37.3X1	T37.3X2	T37.3X3	T37.3X4	T37.3X5	T37.3X6
Tenoxicam	T39.391	T39.392	T39.393	T39.394	T39.395	T39.396
TEPA	T45.1X1	T45.1X2	T45.1X3	T45.1X4	T45.1X5	T45.1X6
TEPP	T60.0X1	T60.0X2	T60.0X3	T60.0X4	—	—
Teprotide	T46.5X1	T46.5X2	T46.5X3	T46.5X4	T46.5X5	T46.5X6
Terazosin	T44.6X1	T44.6X2	T44.6X3	T44.6X4	T44.6X5	T44.6X6
Terbufos	T60.0X1	T60.0X2	T60.0X3	T60.0X4	—	—
Terbutaline	T48.6X1	T48.6X2	T48.6X3	T48.6X4	T48.6X5	T48.6X6
Terconazole	T49.0X1	T49.0X2	T49.0X3	T49.0X4	T49.0X5	T49.0X6
Terfenadine	T45.0X1	T45.0X2	T45.0X3	T45.0X4	T45.0X5	T45.0X6
Teriparatide (acetate)	T50.991	T50.992	T50.993	T50.994	T50.995	T50.996
Terizidone	T37.1X1	T37.1X2	T37.1X3	T37.1X4	T37.1X5	T37.1X6
Terlipressin	T38.891	T38.892	T38.893	T38.894	T38.895	T38.896
Terodiline	T46.3X1	T46.3X2	T46.3X3	T46.3X4	T46.3X5	T46.3X6
Teroxalene	T37.4X1	T37.4X2	T37.4X3	T37.4X4	T37.4X5	T37.4X6
Terpin(cis) hydrate	T48.4X1	T48.4X2	T48.4X3	T48.4X4	T48.4X5	T48.4X6
Terramycin	T36.4X1	T36.4X2	T36.4X3	T36.4X4	T36.4X5	T36.4X6
Tertatolol	T44.7X1	T44.7X2	T44.7X3	T44.7X4	T44.7X5	T44.7X6
Tessalon	T48.3X1	T48.3X2	T48.3X3	T48.3X4	T48.3X5	T48.3X6
Testolactone	T38.7X1	T38.7X2	T38.7X3	T38.7X4	T38.7X5	T38.7X6
Testosterone	T38.7X1	T38.7X2	T38.7X3	T38.7X4	T38.7X5	T38.7X6
Tetanus toxoid or vaccine	T50.A91	T50.A92	T50.A93	T50.A94	T50.A95	T50.A96
antitoxin	T50.Z11	T50.Z12	T50.Z13	T50.Z14	T50.Z15	T50.Z16
immune globulin (human)	T50.Z11	T50.Z12	T50.Z13	T50.Z14	T50.Z15	T50.Z16
toxoid	T50.A91	T50.A92	T50.A93	T50.A94	T50.A95	T50.A96
with diphtheria toxoid	T50.A21	T50.A22	T50.A23	T50.A24	T50.A25	T50.A26
with pertussis	T50.A11	T50.A12	T50.A13	T50.A14	T50.A15	T50.A16
Tetrabenazine	T43.591	T43.592	T43.593	T43.594	T43.595	T43.596
Tetracaine	T41.3X1	T41.3X2	T41.3X3	T41.3X4	T41.3X5	T41.3X6
nerve block (peripheral) (plexus)	T41.3X1	T41.3X2	T41.3X3	T41.3X4	T41.3X5	T41.3X6
regional	T41.3X1	T41.3X2	T41.3X3	T41.3X4	T41.3X5	T41.3X6
spinal	T41.3X1	T41.3X2	T41.3X3	T41.3X4	T41.3X5	T41.3X6
Tetrachlorethylene—see Tetrachloroethylene						
Tetrachlormethiazide	T50.2X1	T50.2X2	T50.2X3	T50.2X4	T50.2X5	T50.2X6
2,3,7,8-Tetrachlorodi-benzo-p-dioxin	T53.7X1	T53.7X2	T53.7X3	T53.7X4	—	—
Tetrachloroethane	T53.6X1	T53.6X2	T53.6X3	T53.6X4	—	—
vapor	T53.6X1	T53.6X2	T53.6X3	T53.6X4	—	—

Substance	Poisoning, Accidental (unintentional)	Poisoning, Intentional self-harm	Poisoning, Assault	Poisoning, Undetermined	Adverse effect	Underdosing
Tetrachloroethane — *Continued*						
paint or varnish	T53.6X1	T53.6X2	T53.6X3	T53.6X4	—	—
Tetrachloroethylene (liquid)	T53.3X1	T53.3X2	T53.3X3	T53.3X4	—	—
medicinal	T37.4X1	T37.4X2	T37.4X3	T37.4X4	T37.4X5	T37.4X6
vapor	T53.3X1	T53.3X2	T53.3X3	T53.3X4	—	—
Tetrachloromethane—see Carbon tetrachloride						
Tetracosactide	T38.811	T38.812	T38.813	T38.814	T38.815	T38.816
Tetracosactrin	T38.811	T38.812	T38.813	T38.814	T38.815	T38.816
Tetracycline	T36.4X1	T36.4X2	T36.4X3	T36.4X4	T36.4X5	T36.4X6
ophthalmic preparation	T49.5X1	T49.5X2	T49.5X3	T49.5X4	T49.5X5	T49.5X6
topical NEC	T49.0X1	T49.0X2	T49.0X3	T49.0X4	T49.0X5	T49.0X6
Tetradifon	T60.8X1	T60.8X2	T60.8X3	T60.8X4	—	—
Tetradotoxin	T61.771	T61.772	T61.773	T61.774	—	—
Tetraethyl						
lead	T56.0X1	T56.0X2	T56.0X3	T56.0X4	—	—
pyrophosphate	T60.0X1	T60.0X2	T60.0X3	T60.0X4	—	—
Tetraethylammonium chloride	T44.2X1	T44.2X2	T44.2X3	T44.2X4	T44.2X5	T44.2X6
Tetraethylthiuram disulfide	T50.6X1	T50.6X2	T50.6X3	T50.6X4	T50.6X5	T50.6X6
Tetrahydroamino-acridine	T44.0X1	T44.0X2	T44.0X3	T44.0X4	T44.0X5	T44.0X6
Tetrahydrocannabinol	T40.711	T40.712	T40.713	T40.714	T40.715	T40.716
Tetrahydrofuran	T52.8X1	T52.8X2	T52.8X3	T52.8X4	—	—
Tetrahydronaphthalene	T52.8X1	T52.8X2	T52.8X3	T52.8X4	—	—
Tetrahydrozoline	T49.5X1	T49.5X2	T49.5X3	T49.5X4	T49.5X5	T49.5X6
Tetralin	T52.8X1	T52.8X2	T52.8X3	T52.8X4	—	—
Tetramethrin	T60.2X1	T60.2X2	T60.2X3	T60.2X4	—	—
Tetramethylthiuram (disulfide) NEC	T60.3X1	T60.3X2	T60.3X3	T60.3X4	—	—
medicinal	T49.0X1	T49.0X2	T49.0X3	T49.0X4	T49.0X5	T49.0X6
Tetramisole	T37.4X1	T37.4X2	T37.4X3	T37.4X4	T37.4X5	T37.4X6
Tetranicotinoyl fructose	T46.7X1	T46.7X2	T46.7X3	T46.7X4	T46.7X5	T46.7X6
Tetrazepam	T42.4X1	T42.4X2	T42.4X3	T42.4X4	T42.4X5	T42.4X6
Tetronal	T42.6X1	T42.6X2	T42.6X3	T42.6X4	T42.6X5	T42.6X6
Tetryl	T65.3X1	T65.3X2	T65.3X3	T65.3X4	—	—
Tetrylammonium chloride	T44.2X1	T44.2X2	T44.2X3	T44.2X4	T44.2X5	T44.2X6
Tetryzoline	T49.5X1	T49.5X2	T49.5X3	T49.5X4	T49.5X5	T49.5X6
Thalidomide	T45.1X1	T45.1X2	T45.1X3	T45.1X4	T45.1X5	T45.1X6
Thallium (compounds) (dust) NEC	T56.811	T56.812	T56.813	T56.814	—	—
pesticide	T60.4X1	T60.4X2	T60.4X3	T60.4X4	—	—
THC	T40.711	T40.712	T40.713	T40.714	T40.715	T40.716
Thebacon	T48.3X1	T48.3X2	T48.3X3	T48.3X4	T48.3X5	T48.3X6
Thebaine	T40.2X1	T40.2X2	T40.2X3	T40.2X4	T40.2X5	T40.2X6
Thenoic acid	T49.6X1	T49.6X2	T49.6X3	T49.6X4	T49.6X5	T49.6X6
Thenyldiamine	T45.0X1	T45.0X2	T45.0X3	T45.0X4	T45.0X5	T45.0X6
Theobromine (calcium salicylate)	T48.6X1	T48.6X2	T48.6X3	T48.6X4	T48.6X5	T48.6X6
sodium salicylate	T48.6X1	T48.6X2	T48.6X3	T48.6X4	T48.6X5	T48.6X6
Theophyllamine	T48.6X1	T48.6X2	T48.6X3	T48.6X4	T48.6X5	T48.6X6
Theophylline	T48.6X1	T48.6X2	T48.6X3	T48.6X4	T48.6X5	T48.6X6
aminobenzoic acid	T48.6X1	T48.6X2	T48.6X3	T48.6X4	T48.6X5	T48.6X6
ethylenediamine	T48.6X1	T48.6X2	T48.6X3	T48.6X4	T48.6X5	T48.6X6
piperazine p-amino-benzoate	T48.6X1	T48.6X2	T48.6X3	T48.6X4	T48.6X5	T48.6X6
Thiabendazole	T37.4X1	T37.4X2	T37.4X3	T37.4X4	T37.4X5	T37.4X6
Thialbarbital	T41.1X1	T41.1X2	T41.1X3	T41.1X4	T41.1X5	T41.1X6
Thiamazole	T38.2X1	T38.2X2	T38.2X3	T38.2X4	T38.2X5	T38.2X6
Thiambutosine	T37.1X1	T37.1X2	T37.1X3	T37.1X4	T37.1X5	T37.1X6
Thiamine	T45.2X1	T45.2X2	T45.2X3	T45.2X4	T45.2X5	T45.2X6
Thiamphenicol	T36.2X1	T36.2X2	T36.2X3	T36.2X4	T36.2X5	T36.2X6
Thiamylal	T41.1X1	T41.1X2	T41.1X3	T41.1X4	T41.1X5	T41.1X6
sodium	T41.1X1	T41.1X2	T41.1X3	T41.1X4	T41.1X5	T41.1X6
Thiazesim	T43.291	T43.292	T43.293	T43.294	T43.295	T43.296
Thiazides (diuretics)	T50.2X1	T50.2X2	T50.2X3	T50.2X4	T50.2X5	T50.2X6
Thiazinamium metilsulfate	T43.3X1	T43.3X2	T43.3X3	T43.3X4	T43.3X5	T43.3X6
Thiethylperazine	T43.3X1	T43.3X2	T43.3X3	T43.3X4	T43.3X5	T43.3X6
Thimerosal	T49.0X1	T49.0X2	T49.0X3	T49.0X4	T49.0X5	T49.0X6
ophthalmic preparation	T49.5X1	T49.5X2	T49.5X3	T49.5X4	T49.5X5	T49.5X6
Thioacetazone	T37.1X1	T37.1X2	T37.1X3	T37.1X4	T37.1X5	T37.1X6
with isoniazid	T37.1X1	T37.1X2	T37.1X3	T37.1X4	T37.1X5	T37.1X6
Thiobarbital sodium	T41.1X1	T41.1X2	T41.1X3	T41.1X4	T41.1X5	T41.1X6
Thiobarbiturate anesthetic	T41.1X1	T41.1X2	T41.1X3	T41.1X4	T41.1X5	T41.1X6
Thiobismol	T37.8X1	T37.8X2	T37.8X3	T37.8X4	T37.8X5	T37.8X6
Thiobutabarbital sodium	T41.1X1	T41.1X2	T41.1X3	T41.1X4	T41.1X5	T41.1X6
Thiocarbamate (insecticide)	T60.0X1	T60.0X2	T60.0X3	T60.0X4	—	—
Thiocarbamide	T38.2X1	T38.2X2	T38.2X3	T38.2X4	T38.2X5	T38.2X6
Thiocarbarsone	T37.8X1	T37.8X2	T37.8X3	T37.8X4	T37.8X5	T37.8X6
Thiocarlide	T37.1X1	T37.1X2	T37.1X3	T37.1X4	T37.1X5	T37.1X6
Thioctamide	T50.991	T50.992	T50.993	T50.994	T50.995	T50.996
Thioctic acid	T50.991	T50.992	T50.993	T50.994	T50.995	T50.996
Thiofos	T60.0X1	T60.0X2	T60.0X3	T60.0X4	—	—
Thioglycolate	T49.4X1	T49.4X2	T49.4X3	T49.4X4	T49.4X5	T49.4X6
Thioglycolic acid	T65.891	T65.892	T65.893	T65.894	—	—
Thioguanine	T45.1X1	T45.1X2	T45.1X3	T45.1X4	T45.1X5	T45.1X6
Thiomercaptomerin	T50.2X1	T50.2X2	T50.2X3	T50.2X4	T50.2X5	T50.2X6
Thiomerin	T50.2X1	T50.2X2	T50.2X3	T50.2X4	T50.2X5	T50.2X6
Thiomersal	T49.0X1	T49.0X2	T49.0X3	T49.0X4	T49.0X5	T49.0X6
Thionazin	T60.0X1	T60.0X2	T60.0X3	T60.0X4	—	—
Thiopental (sodium)	T41.1X1	T41.1X2	T41.1X3	T41.1X4	T41.1X5	T41.1X6
Thiopentone (sodium)	T41.1X1	T41.1X2	T41.1X3	T41.1X4	T41.1X5	T41.1X6
Thiopropazate	T43.3X1	T43.3X2	T43.3X3	T43.3X4	T43.3X5	T43.3X6
Thioproperazine	T43.3X1	T43.3X2	T43.3X3	T43.3X4	T43.3X5	T43.3X6

Substance	Poisoning, Accidental (unintentional)	Poisoning, Intentional self-harm	Poisoning, Assault	Poisoning, Undetermined	Adverse effect	Underdosing
Thioridazine	T43.3X1	T43.3X2	T43.3X3	T43.3X4	T43.3X5	T43.3X6
Thiosinamine	T49.3X1	T49.3X2	T49.3X3	T49.3X4	T49.3X5	T49.3X6
Thiotepa	T45.1X1	T45.1X2	T45.1X3	T45.1X4	T45.1X5	T45.1X6
Thiothixene	T43.4X1	T43.4X2	T43.4X3	T43.4X4	T43.4X5	T43.4X6
Thiouracil (benzyl) (methyl) (propyl)	T38.2X1	T38.2X2	T38.2X3	T38.2X4	T38.2X5	T38.2X6
Thiourea	T38.2X1	T38.2X2	T38.2X3	T38.2X4	T38.2X5	T38.2X6
Thiphenamil	T44.3X1	T44.3X2	T44.3X3	T44.3X4	T44.3X5	T44.3X6
Thiram	T60.3X1	T60.3X2	T60.3X3	T60.3X4	—	—
medicinal	T49.2X1	T49.2X2	T49.2X3	T49.2X4	T49.2X5	T49.2X6
Thonzylamine (systemic)	T45.0X1	T45.0X2	T45.0X3	T45.0X4	T45.0X5	T45.0X6
mucosal decongestant	T48.5X1	T48.5X2	T48.5X3	T48.5X4	T48.5X5	T48.5X6
Thorazine	T43.3X1	T43.3X2	T43.3X3	T43.3X4	T43.3X5	T43.3X6
Thorium dioxide suspension	T50.8X1	T50.8X2	T50.8X3	T50.8X4	T50.8X5	T50.8X6
Thornapple	T62.2X1	T62.2X2	T62.2X3	T62.2X4	—	—
Throat drug NEC	T49.6X1	T49.6X2	T49.6X3	T49.6X4	T49.6X5	T49.6X6
Thrombin	T45.7X1	T45.7X2	T45.7X3	T45.7X4	T45.7X5	T45.7X6
Thrombolysin	T45.611	T45.612	T45.613	T45.614	T45.615	T45.616
Thromboplastin	T45.7X1	T45.7X2	T45.7X3	T45.7X4	T45.7X5	T45.7X6
Thurfyl nicotinate	T46.7X1	T46.7X2	T46.7X3	T46.7X4	T46.7X5	T46.7X6
Thymol	T49.0X1	T49.0X2	T49.0X3	T49.0X4	T49.0X5	T49.0X6
Thymopentin	T37.5X1	T37.5X2	T37.5X3	T37.5X4	T37.5X5	T37.5X6
Thymoxamine	T46.7X1	T46.7X2	T46.7X3	T46.7X4	T46.7X5	T46.7X6
Thymus extract	T38.891	T38.892	T38.893	T38.894	T38.895	T38.896
Thyreotrophic hormone	T38.811	T38.812	T38.813	T38.814	T38.815	T38.816
Thyroglobulin	T38.1X1	T38.1X2	T38.1X3	T38.1X4	T38.1X5	T38.1X6
Thyroid (hormone)	T38.1X1	T38.1X2	T38.1X3	T38.1X4	T38.1X5	T38.1X6
Thyrolar	T38.1X1	T38.1X2	T38.1X3	T38.1X4	T38.1X5	T38.1X6
Thyrotrophin	T38.811	T38.812	T38.813	T38.814	T38.815	T38.816
Thyrotropic hormone	T38.811	T38.812	T38.813	T38.814	T38.815	T38.816
Thyroxine	T38.1X1	T38.1X2	T38.1X3	T38.1X4	T38.1X5	T38.1X6
Tiabendazole	T37.4X1	T37.4X2	T37.4X3	T37.4X4	T37.4X5	T37.4X6
Tiamizide	T50.2X1	T50.2X2	T50.2X3	T50.2X4	T50.2X5	T50.2X6
Tianeptine	T43.291	T43.292	T43.293	T43.294	T43.295	T43.296
Tiapamil	T46.1X1	T46.1X2	T46.1X3	T46.1X4	T46.1X5	T46.1X6
Tiapride	T43.591	T43.592	T43.593	T43.594	T43.595	T43.596
Tiaprofenic acid	T39.311	T39.312	T39.313	T39.314	T39.315	T39.316
Tiaramide	T39.8X1	T39.8X2	T39.8X3	T39.8X4	T39.8X5	T39.8X6
Ticarcillin	T36.0X1	T36.0X2	T36.0X3	T36.0X4	T36.0X5	T36.0X6
Ticlatone	T49.0X1	T49.0X2	T49.0X3	T49.0X4	T49.0X5	T49.0X6
Ticlopidine	T45.521	T45.522	T45.523	T45.524	T45.525	T45.526
Ticrynafen	T50.1X1	T50.1X2	T50.1X3	T50.1X4	T50.1X5	T50.1X6
Tidiacic	T50.991	T50.992	T50.993	T50.994	T50.995	T50.996
Tiemonium	T44.3X1	T44.3X2	T44.3X3	T44.3X4	T44.3X5	T44.3X6
iodide	T44.3X1	T44.3X2	T44.3X3	T44.3X4	T44.3X5	T44.3X6
Tienilic acid	T50.1X1	T50.1X2	T50.1X3	T50.1X4	T50.1X5	T50.1X6
Tifenamil	T44.3X1	T44.3X2	T44.3X3	T44.3X4	T44.3X5	T44.3X6
Tigan	T45.0X1	T45.0X2	T45.0X3	T45.0X4	T45.0X5	T45.0X6
Tigloidine	T44.3X1	T44.3X2	T44.3X3	T44.3X4	T44.3X5	T44.3X6
Tilactase	T47.5X1	T47.5X2	T47.5X3	T47.5X4	T47.5X5	T47.5X6
Tiletamine	T41.291	T41.292	T41.293	T41.294	T41.295	T41.296
Tilidine	T40.491	T40.492	T40.493	T40.494	—	—
Timepidium bromide	T44.3X1	T44.3X2	T44.3X3	T44.3X4	T44.3X5	T44.3X6
Timiperone	T43.4X1	T43.4X2	T43.4X3	T43.4X4	T43.4X5	T43.4X6
Timolol	T44.7X1	T44.7X2	T44.7X3	T44.7X4	T44.7X5	T44.7X6
Tin (chloride) (dust) (oxide) NEC	T56.6X1	T56.6X2	T56.6X3	T56.6X4	—	—
anti-infectives	T37.8X1	T37.8X2	T37.8X3	T37.8X4	T37.8X5	T37.8X6
Tincture, iodine—see Iodine						
Tindal	T43.3X1	T43.3X2	T43.3X3	T43.3X4	T43.3X5	T43.3X6
Tinidazole	T37.3X1	T37.3X2	T37.3X3	T37.3X4	T37.3X5	T37.3X6
Tinoridine	T39.8X1	T39.8X2	T39.8X3	T39.8X4	T39.8X5	T39.8X6
Tiocarlide	T37.1X1	T37.1X2	T37.1X3	T37.1X4	T37.1X5	T37.1X6
Tioclomarol	T45.511	T45.512	T45.513	T45.514	T45.515	T45.516
Tioconazole	T49.0X1	T49.0X2	T49.0X3	T49.0X4	T49.0X5	T49.0X6
Tioguanine	T45.1X1	T45.1X2	T45.1X3	T45.1X4	T45.1X5	T45.1X6
Tiopronin	T50.991	T50.992	T50.993	T50.994	T50.995	T50.996
Tiotixene	T43.4X1	T43.4X2	T43.4X3	T43.4X4	T43.4X5	T43.4X6
Tioxolone	T49.4X1	T49.4X2	T49.4X3	T49.4X4	T49.4X5	T49.4X6
Tipepidine	T48.3X1	T48.3X2	T48.3X3	T48.3X4	T48.3X5	T48.3X6
Tiquizium bromide	T44.3X1	T44.3X2	T44.3X3	T44.3X4	T44.3X5	T44.3X6
Tiratricol	T38.1X1	T38.1X2	T38.1X3	T38.1X4	T38.1X5	T38.1X6
Tisopurine	T50.4X1	T50.4X2	T50.4X3	T50.4X4	T50.4X5	T50.4X6
Titanium (compounds) (vapor)	T56.891	T56.892	T56.893	T56.894	—	—
dioxide	T49.3X1	T49.3X2	T49.3X3	T49.3X4	T49.3X5	T49.3X6
ointment	T49.3X1	T49.3X2	T49.3X3	T49.3X4	T49.3X5	T49.3X6
oxide	T49.3X1	T49.3X2	T49.3X3	T49.3X4	T49.3X5	T49.3X6
tetrachloride	T56.891	T56.892	T56.893	T56.894	—	—
Titanocene	T56.891	T56.892	T56.893	T56.894	—	—
Titroid	T38.1X1	T38.1X2	T38.1X3	T38.1X4	T38.1X5	T38.1X6
Tizanidine	T42.8X1	T42.8X2	T42.8X3	T42.8X4	T42.8X5	T42.8X6
TMTD	T60.3X1	T60.3X2	T60.3X3	T60.3X4	—	—
TNT (fumes)	T65.3X1	T65.3X2	T65.3X3	T65.3X4	—	—
Toadstool	T62.0X1	T62.0X2	T62.0X3	T62.0X4	—	—
Tobacco NEC	T65.291	T65.292	T65.293	T65.294	—	—
cigarettes	T65.221	T65.222	T65.223	T65.224	—	—
Indian	T62.2X1	T62.2X2	T62.2X3	T62.2X4	—	—
smoke, second-hand	T65.221	T65.222	T65.223	T65.224	—	—
Tobramycin	T36.5X1	T36.5X2	T36.5X3	T36.5X4	T36.5X5	T36.5X6
Tocainide	T46.2X1	T46.2X2	T46.2X3	T46.2X4	T46.2X5	T46.2X6
Tocoferol	T45.2X1	T45.2X2	T45.2X3	T45.2X4	T45.2X5	T45.2X6
Tocopherol	T45.2X1	T45.2X2	T45.2X3	T45.2X4	T45.2X5	T45.2X6
acetate	T45.2X1	T45.2X2	T45.2X3	T45.2X4	T45.2X5	T45.2X6
Tocosamine	T48.0X1	T48.0X2	T48.0X3	T48.0X4	T48.0X5	T48.0X6
Todralazine	T46.5X1	T46.5X2	T46.5X3	T46.5X4	T46.5X5	T46.5X6
Tofisopam	T42.4X1	T42.4X2	T42.4X3	T42.4X4	T42.4X5	T42.4X6
Tofranil	T43.011	T43.012	T43.013	T43.014	T43.015	T43.016
Toilet deodorizer	T65.891	T65.892	T65.893	T65.894	—	—

Substance	Poisoning, Accidental (unintentional)	Poisoning, Intentional self-harm	Poisoning, Assault	Poisoning, Undetermined	Adverse effect	Underdosing
Tolamolol	T44.7X1	T44.7X2	T44.7X3	T44.7X4	T44.7X5	T44.7X6
Tolazamide	T38.3X1	T38.3X2	T38.3X3	T38.3X4	T38.3X5	T38.3X6
Tolazoline	T46.7X1	T46.7X2	T46.7X3	T46.7X4	T46.7X5	T46.7X6
Tolbutamide (sodium)	T38.3X1	T38.3X2	T38.3X3	T38.3X4	T38.3X5	T38.3X6
Tolciclate	T49.0X1	T49.0X2	T49.0X3	T49.0X4	T49.0X5	T49.0X6
Tolmetin	T39.391	T39.392	T39.393	T39.394	T39.395	T39.396
Tolnaftate	T49.0X1	T49.0X2	T49.0X3	T49.0X4	T49.0X5	T49.0X6
Tolonidine	T46.5X1	T46.5X2	T46.5X3	T46.5X4	T46.5X5	T46.5X6
Toloxatone	T42.6X1	T42.6X2	T42.6X3	T42.6X4	T42.6X5	T42.6X6
Tolperisone	T44.3X1	T44.3X2	T44.3X3	T44.3X4	T44.3X5	T44.3X6
Tolserol	T42.8X1	T42.8X2	T42.8X3	T42.8X4	T42.8X5	T42.8X6
Toluene (liquid)	T52.2X1	T52.2X2	T52.2X3	T52.2X4	—	—
diisocyanate	T65.0X1	T65.0X2	T65.0X3	T65.0X4	—	—
Toluidine	T65.891	T65.892	T65.893	T65.894	—	—
vapor	T59.891	T59.892	T59.893	T59.894	—	—
Toluol (liquid)	T52.2X1	T52.2X2	T52.2X3	T52.2X4	—	—
vapor	T52.2X1	T52.2X2	T52.2X3	T52.2X4	—	—
Toluylenediamine	T65.3X1	T65.3X2	T65.3X3	T65.3X4	—	—
Tolylene-2,4-diisocyanate	T65.0X1	T65.0X2	T65.0X3	T65.0X4	—	—
Tonic NEC	T50.901	T50.902	T50.903	T50.904	T50.905	T50.906
Topical action drug NEC	T49.91	T49.92	T49.93	T49.94	T49.95	T49.96
ear, nose or throat	T49.6X1	T49.6X2	T49.6X3	T49.6X4	T49.6X5	T49.6X6
eye	T49.5X1	T49.5X2	T49.5X3	T49.5X4	T49.5X5	T49.5X6
skin	T49.91	T49.92	T49.93	T49.94	T49.95	T49.96
specified NEC	T49.8X1	T49.8X2	T49.8X3	T49.8X4	T49.8X5	T49.8X6
Toquizine	T44.3X1	T44.3X2	T44.3X3	T44.3X4	T44.3X5	T44.3X6
Toremifene	T38.6X1	T38.6X2	T38.6X3	T38.6X4	T38.6X5	T38.6X6
Tosylchloramide sodium	T49.8X1	T49.8X2	T49.8X3	T49.8X4	T49.8X5	T49.8X6
Toxaphene (dust) (spray)	T60.1X1	T60.1X2	T60.1X3	T60.1X4	—	—
Toxin, diphtheria (Schick Test)	T50.8X1	T50.8X2	T50.8X3	T50.8X4	T50.8X5	T50.8X6
Toxoid						
combined	T50.A21	T50.A22	T50.A23	T50.A24	T50.A25	T50.A26
diphtheria	T50.A91	T50.A92	T50.A93	T50.A94	T50.A95	T50.A96
tetanus	T50.A91	T50.A92	T50.A93	T50.A94	T50.A95	T50.A96
Trace element NEC	T45.8X1	T45.8X2	T45.8X3	T45.8X4	T45.8X5	T45.8X6
Tractor fuel NEC	T52.0X1	T52.0X2	T52.0X3	T52.0X4	—	—
Tragacanth	T50.991	T50.992	T50.993	T50.994	T50.995	T50.996
Tramadol	T40.421	T40.422	T40.423	T40.424	T40.425	T40.426
Tramazoline	T48.5X1	T48.5X2	T48.5X3	T48.5X4	T48.5X5	T48.5X6
Tranexamic acid	T45.621	T45.622	T45.623	T45.624	T45.625	T45.626
Tranilast	T45.0X1	T45.0X2	T45.0X3	T45.0X4	T45.0X5	T45.0X6
Tranquilizer NEC	T43.501	T43.502	T43.503	T43.504	T43.505	T43.506
with hypnotic or sedative	T42.6X1	T42.6X2	T42.6X3	T42.6X4	T42.6X5	T42.6X6
benzodiazepine NEC	T42.4X1	T42.4X2	T42.4X3	T42.4X4	T42.4X5	T42.4X6
butyrophenone NEC	T43.4X1	T43.4X2	T43.4X3	T43.4X4	T43.4X5	T43.4X6
carbamate	T43.591	T43.592	T43.593	T43.594	T43.595	T43.596
dimethylamine	T43.3X1	T43.3X2	T43.3X3	T43.3X4	T43.3X5	T43.3X6
ethylamine	T43.3X1	T43.3X2	T43.3X3	T43.3X4	T43.3X5	T43.3X6
Tranquilizer NEC — *Continued*						
hydroxyzine	T43.591	T43.592	T43.593	T43.594	T43.595	T43.596
major NEC	T43.501	T43.502	T43.503	T43.504	T43.505	T43.506
penothiazine NEC	T43.3X1	T43.3X2	T43.3X3	T43.3X4	T43.3X5	T43.3X6
phenothiazine-based	T43.3X1	T43.3X2	T43.3X3	T43.3X4	T43.3X5	T43.3X6
piperazine NEC	T43.3X1	T43.3X2	T43.3X3	T43.3X4	T43.3X5	T43.3X6
piperidine	T43.3X1	T43.3X2	T43.3X3	T43.3X4	T43.3X5	T43.3X6
propylamine	T43.3X1	T43.3X2	T43.3X3	T43.3X4	T43.3X5	T43.3X6
specified NEC	T43.591	T43.592	T43.593	T43.594	T43.595	T43.596
thioxanthene NEC	T43.591	T43.592	T43.593	T43.594	T43.595	T43.596
Tranxene	T42.4X1	T42.4X2	T42.4X3	T42.4X4	T42.4X5	T42.4X6
Tranylcypromine	T43.1X1	T43.1X2	T43.1X3	T43.1X4	T43.1X5	T43.1X6
Trapidil	T46.3X1	T46.3X2	T46.3X3	T46.3X4	T46.3X5	T46.3X6
Trasentine	T44.3X1	T44.3X2	T44.3X3	T44.3X4	T44.3X5	T44.3X6
Travert	T50.3X1	T50.3X2	T50.3X3	T50.3X4	T50.3X5	T50.3X6
Trazodone	T43.211	T43.212	T43.213	T43.214	T43.215	T43.216
Trecator	T37.1X1	T37.1X2	T37.1X3	T37.1X4	T37.1X5	T37.1X6
Treosulfan	T45.1X1	T45.1X2	T45.1X3	T45.1X4	T45.1X5	T45.1X6
Tretamine	T45.1X1	T45.1X2	T45.1X3	T45.1X4	T45.1X5	T45.1X6
Tretinoin	T49.0X1	T49.0X2	T49.0X3	T49.0X4	T49.0X5	T49.0X6
Tretoquinol	T48.6X1	T48.6X2	T48.6X3	T48.6X4	T48.6X5	T48.6X6
Triacetin	T49.0X1	T49.0X2	T49.0X3	T49.0X4	T49.0X5	T49.0X6
Triacetoxyanthracene	T49.4X1	T49.4X2	T49.4X3	T49.4X4	T49.4X5	T49.4X6
Triacetyloleandomycin	T36.3X1	T36.3X2	T36.3X3	T36.3X4	T36.3X5	T36.3X6
Triamcinolone	T38.0X1	T38.0X2	T38.0X3	T38.0X4	T38.0X5	T38.0X6
ENT agent	T49.6X1	T49.6X2	T49.6X3	T49.6X4	T49.6X5	T49.6X6
hexacetonide	T49.0X1	T49.0X2	T49.0X3	T49.0X4	T49.0X5	T49.0X6
ophthalmic preparation	T49.5X1	T49.5X2	T49.5X3	T49.5X4	T49.5X5	T49.5X6
topical NEC	T49.0X1	T49.0X2	T49.0X3	T49.0X4	T49.0X5	T49.0X6
Triampyzine	T44.3X1	T44.3X2	T44.3X3	T44.3X4	T44.3X5	T44.3X6
Triamterene	T50.2X1	T50.2X2	T50.2X3	T50.2X4	T50.2X5	T50.2X6
Triazine (herbicide)	T60.3X1	T60.3X2	T60.3X3	T60.3X4	—	—
Triaziquone	T45.1X1	T45.1X2	T45.1X3	T45.1X4	T45.1X5	T45.1X6
Triazolam	T42.4X1	T42.4X2	T42.4X3	T42.4X4	T42.4X5	T42.4X6
Triazole (herbicide)	T60.3X1	T60.3X2	T60.3X3	T60.3X4	—	—
Tribenoside	T46.991	T46.992	T46.993	T46.994	T46.995	T46.996
Tribromacetaldehyde	T42.6X1	T42.6X2	T42.6X3	T42.6X4	T42.6X5	T42.6X6
Tribromoethanol, rectal	T41.291	T41.292	T41.293	T41.294	T41.295	T41.296
Tribromomethane	T42.6X1	T42.6X2	T42.6X3	T42.6X4	T42.6X5	T42.6X6
Trichlorethane	T53.2X1	T53.2X2	T53.2X3	T53.2X4	—	—
Trichlorethylene	T53.2X1	T53.2X2	T53.2X3	T53.2X4	—	—
Trichlorfon	T60.0X1	T60.0X2	T60.0X3	T60.0X4	—	—
Trichlormethiazide	T50.2X1	T50.2X2	T50.2X3	T50.2X4	T50.2X5	T50.2X6
Trichlormethine	T45.1X1	T45.1X2	T45.1X3	T45.1X4	T45.1X5	T45.1X6
Trichloroacetic acid, Trichloracetic acid	T54.2X1	T54.2X2	T54.2X3	T54.2X4	—	—
medicinal	T49.4X1	T49.4X2	T49.4X3	T49.4X4	T49.4X5	T49.4X6
Trichloroethane	T53.2X1	T53.2X2	T53.2X3	T53.2X4	—	—
Trichloroethanol	T42.6X1	T42.6X2	T42.6X3	T42.6X4	T42.6X5	T42.6X6

Substance	Poisoning, Accidental (unintentional)	Poisoning, Intentional self-harm	Poisoning, Assault	Poisoning, Undetermined	Adverse effect	Underdosing
Trichloroethyl phosphate	T42.6X1	T42.6X2	T42.6X3	T42.6X4	T42.6X5	T42.6X6
Trichloroethylene (liquid) (vapor)	T53.2X1	T53.2X2	T53.2X3	T53.2X4	—	—
anesthetic (gas)	T41.0X1	T41.0X2	T41.0X3	T41.0X4	T41.0X5	T41.0X6
vapor NEC	T53.2X1	T53.2X2	T53.2X3	T53.2X4	—	—
Trichlorofluoromethane NEC	T53.5X1	T53.5X2	T53.5X3	T53.5X4	—	—
Trichloronate	T60.0X1	T60.0X2	T60.0X3	T60.0X4	—	—
2,4,5-Trichlorophen-oxyacetic acid	T60.3X1	T60.3X2	T60.3X3	T60.3X4	—	—
Trichloropropane	T53.6X1	T53.6X2	T53.6X3	T53.6X4	—	—
Trichlorotriethylamine	T45.1X1	T45.1X2	T45.1X3	T45.1X4	T45.1X5	T45.1X6
Trichomonacides NEC	T37.3X1	T37.3X2	T37.3X3	T37.3X4	T37.3X5	T37.3X6
Trichomycin	T36.7X1	T36.7X2	T36.7X3	T36.7X4	T36.7X5	T36.7X6
Triclobisonium chloride	T49.0X1	T49.0X2	T49.0X3	T49.0X4	T49.0X5	T49.0X6
Triclocarban	T49.0X1	T49.0X2	T49.0X3	T49.0X4	T49.0X5	T49.0X6
Triclofos	T42.6X1	T42.6X2	T42.6X3	T42.6X4	T42.6X5	T42.6X6
Triclosan	T49.0X1	T49.0X2	T49.0X3	T49.0X4	T49.0X5	T49.0X6
Tricresyl phosphate	T65.891	T65.892	T65.893	T65.894	—	—
solvent	T52.91	T52.92	T52.93	T52.94	—	—
Tricyclamol chloride	T44.3X1	T44.3X2	T44.3X3	T44.3X4	T44.3X5	T44.3X6
Tridesilon	T49.0X1	T49.0X2	T49.0X3	T49.0X4	T49.0X5	T49.0X6
Tridihexethyl iodide	T44.3X1	T44.3X2	T44.3X3	T44.3X4	T44.3X5	T44.3X6
Tridione	T42.2X1	T42.2X2	T42.2X3	T42.2X4	T42.2X5	T42.2X6
Trientine	T45.8X1	T45.8X2	T45.8X3	T45.8X4	T45.8X5	T45.8X6
Triethanolamine NEC	T54.3X1	T54.3X2	T54.3X3	T54.3X4	—	—
detergent	T54.3X1	T54.3X2	T54.3X3	T54.3X4	—	—
trinitrate (biphosphate)	T46.3X1	T46.3X2	T46.3X3	T46.3X4	T46.3X5	T46.3X6
Triethanomelamine	T45.1X1	T45.1X2	T45.1X3	T45.1X4	T45.1X5	T45.1X6
Triethylenemelamine	T45.1X1	T45.1X2	T45.1X3	T45.1X4	T45.1X5	T45.1X6
Triethylenephos-phoramide	T45.1X1	T45.1X2	T45.1X3	T45.1X4	T45.1X5	T45.1X6
Triethylenethiophos-phoramide	T45.1X1	T45.1X2	T45.1X3	T45.1X4	T45.1X5	T45.1X6
Trifluoperazine	T43.3X1	T43.3X2	T43.3X3	T43.3X4	T43.3X5	T43.3X6
Trifluoroethyl vinyl ether	T41.0X1	T41.0X2	T41.0X3	T41.0X4	T41.0X5	T41.0X6
Trifluperidol	T43.4X1	T43.4X2	T43.4X3	T43.4X4	T43.4X5	T43.4X6
Triflupromazine	T43.3X1	T43.3X2	T43.3X3	T43.3X4	T43.3X5	T43.3X6
Trifluridine	T37.5X1	T37.5X2	T37.5X3	T37.5X4	T37.5X5	T37.5X6
Triflusal	T45.521	T45.522	T45.523	T45.524	T45.525	T45.526
Trihexyphenidyl	T44.3X1	T44.3X2	T44.3X3	T44.3X4	T44.3X5	T44.3X6
Triiodothyronine	T38.1X1	T38.1X2	T38.1X3	T38.1X4	T38.1X5	T38.1X6
Trilene	T41.0X1	T41.0X2	T41.0X3	T41.0X4	T41.0X5	T41.0X6
Trilostane	T38.991	T38.992	T38.993	T38.994	T38.995	T38.996
Trimebutine	T44.3X1	T44.3X2	T44.3X3	T44.3X4	T44.3X5	T44.3X6
Trimecaine	T41.3X1	T41.3X2	T41.3X3	T41.3X4	T41.3X5	T41.3X6
Trimeprazine (tartrate)	T44.3X1	T44.3X2	T44.3X3	T44.3X4	T44.3X5	T44.3X6
Trimetaphan camsilate	T44.2X1	T44.2X2	T44.2X3	T44.2X4	T44.2X5	T44.2X6
Trimetazidine	T46.7X1	T46.7X2	T46.7X3	T46.7X4	T46.7X5	T46.7X6
Trimethadione	T42.2X1	T42.2X2	T42.2X3	T42.2X4	T42.2X5	T42.2X6
Trimethaphan	T44.2X1	T44.2X2	T44.2X3	T44.2X4	T44.2X5	T44.2X6
Trimethidinium	T44.2X1	T44.2X2	T44.2X3	T44.2X4	T44.2X5	T44.2X6
Trimethobenzamide	T45.0X1	T45.0X2	T45.0X3	T45.0X4	T45.0X5	T45.0X6
Trimethoprim	T37.8X1	T37.8X2	T37.8X3	T37.8X4	T37.8X5	T37.8X6
with sulfamethoxazole	T36.8X1	T36.8X2	T36.8X3	T36.8X4	T36.8X5	T36.8X6
Trimethylcarbinol	T51.3X1	T51.3X2	T51.3X3	T51.3X4	—	—
Trimethylpsoralen	T49.3X1	T49.3X2	T49.3X3	T49.3X4	T49.3X5	T49.3X6
Trimeton	T45.0X1	T45.0X2	T45.0X3	T45.0X4	T45.0X5	T45.0X6
Trimetrexate	T45.1X1	T45.1X2	T45.1X3	T45.1X4	T45.1X5	T45.1X6
Trimipramine	T43.011	T43.012	T43.013	T43.014	T43.015	T43.016
Trimustine	T45.1X1	T45.1X2	T45.1X3	T45.1X4	T45.1X5	T45.1X6
Trinitrine	T46.3X1	T46.3X2	T46.3X3	T46.3X4	T46.3X5	T46.3X6
Trinitrobenzol	T65.3X1	T65.3X2	T65.3X3	T65.3X4	—	—
Trinitrophenol	T65.3X1	T65.3X2	T65.3X3	T65.3X4	—	—
Trinitrotoluene (fumes)	T65.3X1	T65.3X2	T65.3X3	T65.3X4	—	—
Trional	T42.6X1	T42.6X2	T42.6X3	T42.6X4	T42.6X5	T42.6X6
Triorthocresyl phosphate	T65.891	T65.892	T65.893	T65.894	—	—
Trioxide of arsenic	T57.0X1	T57.0X2	T57.0X3	T57.0X4	—	—
Trioxysalen	T49.4X1	T49.4X2	T49.4X3	T49.4X4	T49.4X5	T49.4X6
Tripamide	T50.2X1	T50.2X2	T50.2X3	T50.2X4	T50.2X5	T50.2X6
Triparanol	T46.6X1	T46.6X2	T46.6X3	T46.6X4	T46.6X5	T46.6X6
Tripelennamine	T45.0X1	T45.0X2	T45.0X3	T45.0X4	T45.0X5	T45.0X6
Triperiden	T44.3X1	T44.3X2	T44.3X3	T44.3X4	T44.3X5	T44.3X6
Triperidol	T43.4X1	T43.4X2	T43.4X3	T43.4X4	T43.4X5	T43.4X6
Triphenylphosphate	T65.891	T65.892	T65.893	T65.894	—	—
Triple						
bromides	T42.6X1	T42.6X2	T42.6X3	T42.6X4	T42.6X5	T42.6X6
carbonate	T47.1X1	T47.1X2	T47.1X3	T47.1X4	T47.1X5	T47.1X6
vaccine						
DPT	T50.A11	T50.A12	T50.A13	T50.A14	T50.A15	T50.A16
including pertussis	T50.A11	T50.A12	T50.A13	T50.A14	T50.A15	T50.A16
MMR	T50.B91	T50.B92	T50.B93	T50.B94	T50.B95	T50.B96
Triprolidine	T45.0X1	T45.0X2	T45.0X3	T45.0X4	T45.0X5	T45.0X6
Trisodium hydrogen edetate	T50.6X1	T50.6X2	T50.6X3	T50.6X4	T50.6X5	T50.6X6
Trisoralen	T49.3X1	T49.3X2	T49.3X3	T49.3X4	T49.3X5	T49.3X6
Trisulfapyrimidines	T37.0X1	T37.0X2	T37.0X3	T37.0X4	T37.0X5	T37.0X6
Trithiozine	T44.3X1	T44.3X2	T44.3X3	T44.3X4	T44.3X5	T44.3X6
Tritiozine	T44.3X1	T44.3X2	T44.3X3	T44.3X4	T44.3X5	T44.3X6
Tritoqualine	T45.0X1	T45.0X2	T45.0X3	T45.0X4	T45.0X5	T45.0X6
Trofosfamide	T45.1X1	T45.1X2	T45.1X3	T45.1X4	T45.1X5	T45.1X6
Troleandomycin	T36.3X1	T36.3X2	T36.3X3	T36.3X4	T36.3X5	T36.3X6
Trolnitrate (phosphate)	T46.3X1	T46.3X2	T46.3X3	T46.3X4	T46.3X5	T46.3X6
Tromantadine	T37.5X1	T37.5X2	T37.5X3	T37.5X4	T37.5X5	T37.5X6
Trometamol	T50.2X1	T50.2X2	T50.2X3	T50.2X4	T50.2X5	T50.2X6
Tromethamine	T50.2X1	T50.2X2	T50.2X3	T50.2X4	T50.2X5	T50.2X6
Tronothane	T41.3X1	T41.3X2	T41.3X3	T41.3X4	T41.3X5	T41.3X6
Tropacine	T44.3X1	T44.3X2	T44.3X3	T44.3X4	T44.3X5	T44.3X6
Tropatepine	T44.3X1	T44.3X2	T44.3X3	T44.3X4	T44.3X5	T44.3X6

Substance	Poisoning, Accidental (unintentional)	Poisoning, Intentional self-harm	Poisoning, Assault	Poisoning, Undetermined	Adverse effect	Underdosing
Tropicamide	T44.3X1	T44.3X2	T44.3X3	T44.3X4	T44.3X5	T44.3X6
Trospium chloride	T44.3X1	T44.3X2	T44.3X3	T44.3X4	T44.3X5	T44.3X6
Troxerutin	T46.991	T46.992	T46.993	T46.994	T46.995	T46.996
Troxidone	T42.2X1	T42.2X2	T42.2X3	T42.2X4	T42.2X5	T42.2X6
Tryparsamide	T37.3X1	T37.3X2	T37.3X3	T37.3X4	T37.3X5	T37.3X6
Trypsin	T45.3X1	T45.3X2	T45.3X3	T45.3X4	T45.3X5	T45.3X6
Tryptizol	T43.011	T43.012	T43.013	T43.014	T43.015	T43.016
TSH	T38.811	T38.812	T38.813	T38.814	T38.815	T38.816
Tuaminoheptane	T48.5X1	T48.5X2	T48.5X3	T48.5X4	T48.5X5	T48.5X6
Tuberculin, purified protein derivative (PPD)	T50.8X1	T50.8X2	T50.8X3	T50.8X4	T50.8X5	T50.8X6
Tubocurare	T48.1X1	T48.1X2	T48.1X3	T48.1X4	T48.1X5	T48.1X6
Tubocurarine (chloride)	T48.1X1	T48.1X2	T48.1X3	T48.1X4	T48.1X5	T48.1X6
Tulobuterol	T48.6X1	T48.6X2	T48.6X3	T48.6X4	T48.6X5	T48.6X6
Turpentine (spirits of)	T52.8X1	T52.8X2	T52.8X3	T52.8X4	—	—
vapor	T52.8X1	T52.8X2	T52.8X3	T52.8X4	—	—
Tybamate	T43.591	T43.592	T43.593	T43.594	T43.595	T43.596
Tyloxapol	T48.4X1	T48.4X2	T48.4X3	T48.4X4	T48.4X5	T48.4X6
Tymazoline	T48.5X1	T48.5X2	T48.5X3	T48.5X4	T48.5X5	T48.5X6
Typhoid-paratyphoid vaccine	T50.A91	T50.A92	T50.A93	T50.A94	T50.A95	T50.A96
Typhus vaccine	T50.A91	T50.A92	T50.A93	T50.A94	T50.A95	T50.A96
Tyropanoate	T50.8X1	T50.8X2	T50.8X3	T50.8X4	T50.8X5	T50.8X6
Tyrothricin	T49.6X1	T49.6X2	T49.6X3	T49.6X4	T49.6X5	T49.6X6
ENT agent	T49.6X1	T49.6X2	T49.6X3	T49.6X4	T49.6X5	T49.6X6
ophthalmic preparation	T49.5X1	T49.5X2	T49.5X3	T49.5X4	T49.5X5	T49.5X6
U						
Ufenamate	T39.391	T39.392	T39.393	T39.394	T39.395	T39.396
Ultraviolet light protectant	T49.3X1	T49.3X2	T49.3X3	T49.3X4	T49.3X5	T49.3X6
Undecenoic acid	T49.0X1	T49.0X2	T49.0X3	T49.0X4	T49.0X5	T49.0X6
Undecoylium	T49.0X1	T49.0X2	T49.0X3	T49.0X4	T49.0X5	T49.0X6
Undecylenic acid (derivatives)	T49.0X1	T49.0X2	T49.0X3	T49.0X4	T49.0X5	T49.0X6
Unna's boot	T49.3X1	T49.3X2	T49.3X3	T49.3X4	T49.3X5	T49.3X6
Unsaturated fatty acid	T46.6X1	T46.6X2	T46.6X3	T46.6X4	T46.6X5	T46.6X6
Uracil mustard	T45.1X1	T45.1X2	T45.1X3	T45.1X4	T45.1X5	T45.1X6
Uramustine	T45.1X1	T45.1X2	T45.1X3	T45.1X4	T45.1X5	T45.1X6
Urapidil	T46.5X1	T46.5X2	T46.5X3	T46.5X4	T46.5X5	T46.5X6
Urari	T48.1X1	T48.1X2	T48.1X3	T48.1X4	T48.1X5	T48.1X6
Urate oxidase	T50.4X1	T50.4X2	T50.4X3	T50.4X4	T50.4X5	T50.4X6
Urea	T47.3X1	T47.3X2	T47.3X3	T47.3X4	T47.3X5	T47.3X6
peroxide	T49.0X1	T49.0X2	T49.0X3	T49.0X4	T49.0X5	T49.0X6
stibamine	T37.4X1	T37.4X2	T37.4X3	T37.4X4	T37.4X5	T37.4X6
topical	T49.8X1	T49.8X2	T49.8X3	T49.8X4	T49.8X5	T49.8X6
Urethane	T45.1X1	T45.1X2	T45.1X3	T45.1X4	T45.1X5	T45.1X6
Urginea (maritima) (scilla)—see Squill						
Uric acid metabolism drug NEC	T50.4X1	T50.4X2	T50.4X3	T50.4X4	T50.4X5	T50.4X6
Uricosuric agent	T50.4X1	T50.4X2	T50.4X3	T50.4X4	T50.4X5	T50.4X6
Urinary anti-infective	T37.8X1	T37.8X2	T37.8X3	T37.8X4	T37.8X5	T37.8X6
Urofollitropin	T38.811	T38.812	T38.813	T38.814	T38.815	T38.816
Urokinase	T45.611	T45.612	T45.613	T45.614	T45.615	T45.616
Urokon	T50.8X1	T50.8X2	T50.8X3	T50.8X4	T50.8X5	T50.8X6
Ursodeoxycholic acid	T50.991	T50.992	T50.993	T50.994	T50.995	T50.996
Ursodiol	T50.991	T50.992	T50.993	T50.994	T50.995	T50.996
Urtica	T62.2X1	T62.2X2	T62.2X3	T62.2X4	—	—
Utility gas—see Gas, utility						
V						
Vaccine NEC	T50.Z91	T50.Z92	T50.Z93	T50.Z94	T50.Z95	T50.Z96
antineoplastic	T50.Z91	T50.Z92	T50.Z93	T50.Z94	T50.Z95	T50.Z96
bacterial NEC	T50.A91	T50.A92	T50.A93	T50.A94	T50.A95	T50.A96
with						
other bacterial component	T50.A21	T50.A22	T50.A23	T50.A24	T50.A25	T50.A26
pertussis component	T50.A11	T50.A12	T50.A13	T50.A14	T50.A15	T50.A16
viral-rickettsial component	T50.A21	T50.A22	T50.A23	T50.A24	T50.A25	T50.A26
mixed NEC	T50.A21	T50.A22	T50.A23	T50.A24	T50.A25	T50.A26
BCG	T50.A91	T50.A92	T50.A93	T50.A94	T50.A95	T50.A96
cholera	T50.A91	T50.A92	T50.A93	T50.A94	T50.A95	T50.A96
diphtheria	T50.A91	T50.A92	T50.A93	T50.A94	T50.A95	T50.A96
with tetanus	T50.A21	T50.A22	T50.A23	T50.A24	T50.A25	T50.A26
and pertussis	T50.A11	T50.A12	T50.A13	T50.A14	T50.A15	T50.A16
influenza	T50.B91	T50.B92	T50.B93	T50.B94	T50.B95	T50.B96
measles	T50.B91	T50.B92	T50.B93	T50.B94	T50.B95	T50.B96
with mumps and rubella	T50.B91	T50.B92	T50.B93	T50.B94	T50.B95	T50.B96
meningococcal	T50.A91	T50.A92	T50.A93	T50.A94	T50.A95	T50.A96
mumps	T50.B91	T50.B92	T50.B93	T50.B94	T50.B95	T50.B96
paratyphoid	T50.A91	T50.A92	T50.A93	T50.A94	T50.A95	T50.A96
pertussis	T50.A11	T50.A12	T50.A13	T50.A14	T50.A15	T50.A16
with diphtheria	T50.A11	T50.A12	T50.A13	T50.A14	T50.A15	T50.A16
and tetanus	T50.A11	T50.A12	T50.A13	T50.A14	T50.A15	T50.A16
with other component	T50.A11	T50.A12	T50.A13	T50.A14	T50.A15	T50.A16
plague	T50.A91	T50.A92	T50.A93	T50.A94	T50.A95	T50.A96
poliomyelitis	T50.B91	T50.B92	T50.B93	T50.B94	T50.B95	T50.B96
poliovirus	T50.B91	T50.B92	T50.B93	T50.B94	T50.B95	T50.B96
rabies	T50.B91	T50.B92	T50.B93	T50.B94	T50.B95	T50.B96
respiratory syncytial virus	T50.B91	T50.B92	T50.B93	T50.B94	T50.B95	T50.B96
rickettsial NEC	T50.A91	T50.A92	T50.A93	T50.A94	T50.A95	T50.A96
with						
bacterial component	T50.A21	T50.A22	T50.A23	T50.A24	T50.A25	T50.A26
Rocky Mountain spotted fever	T50.A91	T50.A92	T50.A93	T50.A94	T50.A95	T50.A96
rubella	T50.B91	T50.B92	T50.B93	T50.B94	T50.B95	T50.B96
sabin oral	T50.B91	T50.B92	T50.B93	T50.B94	T50.B95	T50.B96
smallpox	T50.B11	T50.B12	T50.B13	T50.B14	T50.B15	T50.B16
TAB	T50.A91	T50.A92	T50.A93	T50.A94	T50.A95	T50.A96
tetanus	T50.A91	T50.A92	T50.A93	T50.A94	T50.A95	T50.A96

Substance	Poisoning, Accidental (unintentional)	Poisoning, Intentional self-harm	Poisoning, Assault	Poisoning, Undetermined	Adverse effect	Underdosing
Vaccine NEC — *Continued*						
typhoid	T50.A91	T50.A92	T50.A93	T50.A94	T50.A95	T50.A96
typhus	T50.A91	T50.A92	T50.A93	T50.A94	T50.A95	T50.A96
viral NEC	T50.B91	T50.B92	T50.B93	T50.B94	T50.B95	T50.B96
yellow fever	T50.B91	T50.B92	T50.B93	T50.B94	T50.B95	T50.B96
Vaccinia immune globulin	T50.Z11	T50.Z12	T50.Z13	T50.Z14	T50.Z15	T50.Z16
Vaginal contraceptives	T49.8X1	T49.8X2	T49.8X3	T49.8X4	T49.8X5	T49.8X6
Valerian						
root	T42.6X1	T42.6X2	T42.6X3	T42.6X4	T42.6X5	T42.6X6
tincture	T42.6X1	T42.6X2	T42.6X3	T42.6X4	T42.6X5	T42.6X6
Valethamate bromide	T44.3X1	T44.3X2	T44.3X3	T44.3X4	T44.3X5	T44.3X6
Valisone	T49.0X1	T49.0X2	T49.0X3	T49.0X4	T49.0X5	T49.0X6
Valium	T42.4X1	T42.4X2	T42.4X3	T42.4X4	T42.4X5	T42.4X6
Valmid	T42.6X1	T42.6X2	T42.6X3	T42.6X4	T42.6X5	T42.6X6
Valnoctamide	T42.6X1	T42.6X2	T42.6X3	T42.6X4	T42.6X5	T42.6X6
Valproate (sodium)	T42.6X1	T42.6X2	T42.6X3	T42.6X4	T42.6X5	T42.6X6
Valproic acid	T42.6X1	T42.6X2	T42.6X3	T42.6X4	T42.6X5	T42.6X6
Valpromide	T42.6X1	T42.6X2	T42.6X3	T42.6X4	T42.6X5	T42.6X6
Vanadium	T56.891	T56.892	T56.893	T56.894	—	—
Vancomycin	T36.8X1	T36.8X2	T36.8X3	T36.8X4	T36.8X5	T36.8X6
Vapor—see also Gas	T59.91	T59.92	T59.93	T59.94	—	—
kiln (carbon monoxide)	T58.8X1	T58.8X2	T58.8X3	T58.8X4	—	—
lead—see lead						
specified source NEC	T59.891	T59.892	T59.893	T59.894	—	—
Vardenafil	T46.7X1	T46.7X2	T46.7X3	T46.7X4	T46.7X5	T46.7X6
Varicose reduction drug	T46.8X1	T46.8X2	T46.8X3	T46.8X4	T46.8X5	T46.8X6
Varnish	T65.4X1	T65.4X2	T65.4X3	T65.4X4	—	—
cleaner	T52.91	T52.92	T52.93	T52.94	—	—
Vaseline	T49.3X1	T49.3X2	T49.3X3	T49.3X4	T49.3X5	T49.3X6
Vasodilan	T46.7X1	T46.7X2	T46.7X3	T46.7X4	T46.7X5	T46.7X6
Vasodilator						
coronary NEC	T46.3X1	T46.3X2	T46.3X3	T46.3X4	T46.3X5	T46.3X6
peripheral NEC	T46.7X1	T46.7X2	T46.7X3	T46.7X4	T46.7X5	T46.7X6
Vasopressin	T38.891	T38.892	T38.893	T38.894	T38.895	T38.896
Vasopressor drugs	T38.891	T38.892	T38.893	T38.894	T38.895	T38.896
Vecuronium bromide	T48.1X1	T48.1X2	T48.1X3	T48.1X4	T48.1X5	T48.1X6
Vegetable extract, astringent	T49.2X1	T49.2X2	T49.2X3	T49.2X4	T49.2X5	T49.2X6
Venlafaxine	T43.211	T43.212	T43.213	T43.214	T43.215	T43.216
Venom, venomous (bite) (sting)	T63.91	T63.92	T63.93	T63.94	—	—
amphibian NEC	T63.831	T63.832	T63.833	T63.834	—	—
animal NEC	T63.891	T63.892	T63.893	T63.894	—	—
ant	T63.421	T63.422	T63.423	T63.424	—	—
arthropod NEC	T63.481	T63.482	T63.483	T63.484	—	—
bee	T63.441	T63.442	T63.443	T63.444	—	—
centipede	T63.411	T63.412	T63.413	T63.414	—	—
fish	T63.591	T63.592	T63.593	T63.594	—	—
frog	T63.811	T63.812	T63.813	T63.814	—	—

Substance	Poisoning, Accidental (unintentional)	Poisoning, Intentional self-harm	Poisoning, Assault	Poisoning, Undetermined	Adverse effect	Underdosing
Venom, venomous — *Continued*						
hornet	T63.451	T63.452	T63.453	T63.454	—	—
insect NEC	T63.481	T63.482	T63.483	T63.484	—	—
lizard	T63.121	T63.122	T63.123	T63.124	—	—
marine						
animals	T63.691	T63.692	T63.693	T63.694	—	—
bluebottle	T63.611	T63.612	T63.613	T63.614	—	—
jellyfish NEC	T63.621	T63.622	T63.623	T63.624	—	—
Portuguese Man-o-war	T63.611	T63.612	T63.613	T63.614	—	—
sea anemone	T63.631	T63.632	T63.633	T63.634	—	—
specified NEC	T63.691	T63.692	T63.693	T63.694	—	—
fish	T63.591	T63.592	T63.593	T63.594	—	—
plants	T63.711	T63.712	T63.713	T63.714	—	—
sting ray	T63.511	T63.512	T63.513	T63.514	—	—
millipede (tropical)	T63.411	T63.412	T63.413	T63.414	—	—
plant NEC	T63.791	T63.792	T63.793	T63.794	—	—
marine	T63.711	T63.712	T63.713	T63.714	—	—
reptile	T63.191	T63.192	T63.193	T63.194	—	—
gila monster	T63.111	T63.112	T63.113	T63.114	—	—
lizard NEC	T63.121	T63.122	T63.123	T63.124	—	—
scorpion	T63.2X1	T63.2X2	T63.2X3	T63.2X4	—	—
snake	T63.001	T63.002	T63.003	T63.004	—	—
African NEC	T63.081	T63.082	T63.083	T63.084	—	—
American (North) (South) NEC	T63.061	T63.062	T63.063	T63.064	—	—
Asian	T63.081	T63.082	T63.083	T63.084	—	—
Australian	T63.071	T63.072	T63.073	T63.074	—	—
cobra	T63.041	T63.042	T63.043	T63.044	—	—
coral snake	T63.021	T63.022	T63.023	T63.024	—	—
rattlesnake	T63.011	T63.012	T63.013	T63.014	—	—
specified NEC	T63.091	T63.092	T63.093	T63.094	—	—
taipan	T63.031	T63.032	T63.033	T63.034	—	—
specified NEC	T63.891	T63.892	T63.893	T63.894	—	—
spider	T63.301	T63.302	T63.303	T63.304	—	—
black widow	T63.311	T63.312	T63.313	T63.314	—	—
brown recluse	T63.331	T63.332	T63.333	T63.334	—	—
specified NEC	T63.391	T63.392	T63.393	T63.394	—	—
tarantula	T63.321	T63.322	T63.323	T63.324	—	—
sting ray	T63.511	T63.512	T63.513	T63.514	—	—
toad	T63.821	T63.822	T63.823	T63.824	—	—
wasp	T63.461	T63.462	T63.463	T63.464	—	—
Venous sclerosing drug NEC	T46.8X1	T46.8X2	T46.8X3	T46.8X4	T46.8X5	T46.8X6
Ventolin—see Albuterol						
Veramon	T42.3X1	T42.3X2	T42.3X3	T42.3X4	T42.3X5	T42.3X6
Verapamil	T46.1X1	T46.1X2	T46.1X3	T46.1X4	T46.1X5	T46.1X6
Veratrine	T46.5X1	T46.5X2	T46.5X3	T46.5X4	T46.5X5	T46.5X6
Veratrum						
album	T62.2X1	T62.2X2	T62.2X3	T62.2X4	—	—
alkaloids	T46.5X1	T46.5X2	T46.5X3	T46.5X4	T46.5X5	T46.5X6

Substance	Poisoning, Accidental (unintentional)	Poisoning, Intentional self-harm	Poisoning, Assault	Poisoning, Undetermined	Adverse effect	Underdosing
Veratrum — *Continued*						
viride	T62.2X1	T62.2X2	T62.2X3	T62.2X4	—	—
Verdigris	T60.3X1	T60.3X2	T60.3X3	T60.3X4	—	—
Veronal	T42.3X1	T42.3X2	T42.3X3	T42.3X4	T42.3X5	T42.3X6
Veroxil	T37.4X1	T37.4X2	T37.4X3	T37.4X4	T37.4X5	T37.4X6
Versenate	T50.6X1	T50.6X2	T50.6X3	T50.6X4	T50.6X5	T50.6X6
Versidyne	T39.8X1	T39.8X2	T39.8X3	T39.8X4	T39.8X5	T39.8X6
Vetrabutine	T48.0X1	T48.0X2	T48.0X3	T48.0X4	T48.0X5	T48.0X6
Vidarabine	T37.5X1	T37.5X2	T37.5X3	T37.5X4	T37.5X5	T37.5X6
Vienna						
green	T57.0X1	T57.0X2	T57.0X3	T57.0X4	—	—
insecticide	T60.2X1	T60.2X2	T60.2X3	T60.2X4	—	—
red	T57.0X1	T57.0X2	T57.0X3	T57.0X4	—	—
pharmaceutical dye	T50.991	T50.992	T50.993	T50.994	T50.995	T50.996
Vigabatrin	T42.6X1	T42.6X2	T42.6X3	T42.6X4	T42.6X5	T42.6X6
Viloxazine	T43.291	T43.292	T43.293	T43.294	T43.295	T43.296
Viminol	T39.8X1	T39.8X2	T39.8X3	T39.8X4	T39.8X5	T39.8X6
Vinbarbital, vinbarbitone	T42.3X1	T42.3X2	T42.3X3	T42.3X4	T42.3X5	T42.3X6
Vinblastine	T45.1X1	T45.1X2	T45.1X3	T45.1X4	T45.1X5	T45.1X6
Vinburnine	T46.7X1	T46.7X2	T46.7X3	T46.7X4	T46.7X5	T46.7X6
Vincamine	T45.1X1	T45.1X2	T45.1X3	T45.1X4	T45.1X5	T45.1X6
Vincristine	T45.1X1	T45.1X2	T45.1X3	T45.1X4	T45.1X5	T45.1X6
Vindesine	T45.1X1	T45.1X2	T45.1X3	T45.1X4	T45.1X5	T45.1X6
Vinesthene, vinethene	T41.0X1	T41.0X2	T41.0X3	T41.0X4	T41.0X5	T41.0X6
Vinorelbine tartrate	T45.1X1	T45.1X2	T45.1X3	T45.1X4	T45.1X5	T45.1X6
Vinpocetine	T46.7X1	T46.7X2	T46.7X3	T46.7X4	T46.7X5	T46.7X6
Vinyl						
acetate	T65.891	T65.892	T65.893	T65.894	—	—
bital	T42.3X1	T42.3X2	T42.3X3	T42.3X4	T42.3X5	T42.3X6
bromide	T65.891	T65.892	T65.893	T65.894	—	—
chloride	T59.891	T59.892	T59.893	T59.894	—	—
ether	T41.0X1	T41.0X2	T41.0X3	T41.0X4	T41.0X5	T41.0X6
Vinylbital	T42.3X1	T42.3X2	T42.3X3	T42.3X4	T42.3X5	T42.3X6
Vinylidene chloride	T65.891	T65.892	T65.893	T65.894	—	—
Vioform	T37.8X1	T37.8X2	T37.8X3	T37.8X4	T37.8X5	T37.8X6
topical	T49.0X1	T49.0X2	T49.0X3	T49.0X4	T49.0X5	T49.0X6
Viomycin	T36.8X1	T36.8X2	T36.8X3	T36.8X4	T36.8X5	T36.8X6
Viosterol	T45.2X1	T45.2X2	T45.2X3	T45.2X4	T45.2X5	T45.2X6
Viper (venom)	T63.091	T63.092	T63.093	T63.094	—	—
Viprynium	T37.4X1	T37.4X2	T37.4X3	T37.4X4	T37.4X5	T37.4X6
Viquidil	T46.7X1	T46.7X2	T46.7X3	T46.7X4	T46.7X5	T46.7X6
Viral vaccine NEC	T50.B91	T50.B92	T50.B93	T50.B94	T50.B95	T50.B96
Virginiamycin	T36.8X1	T36.8X2	T36.8X3	T36.8X4	T36.8X5	T36.8X6
Virugon	T37.5X1	T37.5X2	T37.5X3	T37.5X4	T37.5X5	T37.5X6
Viscous agent	T50.901	T50.902	T50.903	T50.904	T50.905	T50.906
Visine	T49.5X1	T49.5X2	T49.5X3	T49.5X4	T49.5X5	T49.5X6
Visnadine	T46.3X1	T46.3X2	T46.3X3	T46.3X4	T46.3X5	T46.3X6
Vitamin NEC	T45.2X1	T45.2X2	T45.2X3	T45.2X4	T45.2X5	T45.2X6
A	T45.2X1	T45.2X2	T45.2X3	T45.2X4	T45.2X5	T45.2X6
B NEC	T45.2X1	T45.2X2	T45.2X3	T45.2X4	T45.2X5	T45.2X6

Substance	Poisoning, Accidental (unintentional)	Poisoning, Intentional self-harm	Poisoning, Assault	Poisoning, Undetermined	Adverse effect	Underdosing
Vitamin NEC — *Continued*						
nicotinic acid	T46.7X1	T46.7X2	T46.7X3	T46.7X4	T46.7X5	T46.7X6
B1	T45.2X1	T45.2X2	T45.2X3	T45.2X4	T45.2X5	T45.2X6
B2	T45.2X1	T45.2X2	T45.2X3	T45.2X4	T45.2X5	T45.2X6
B6	T45.2X1	T45.2X2	T45.2X3	T45.2X4	T45.2X5	T45.2X6
B12	T45.2X1	T45.2X2	T45.2X3	T45.2X4	T45.2X5	T45.2X6
B15	T45.2X1	T45.2X2	T45.2X3	T45.2X4	T45.2X5	T45.2X6
C	T45.2X1	T45.2X2	T45.2X3	T45.2X4	T45.2X5	T45.2X6
D	T45.2X1	T45.2X2	T45.2X3	T45.2X4	T45.2X5	T45.2X6
D2	T45.2X1	T45.2X2	T45.2X3	T45.2X4	T45.2X5	T45.2X6
D3	T45.2X1	T45.2X2	T45.2X3	T45.2X4	T45.2X5	T45.2X6
E	T45.2X1	T45.2X2	T45.2X3	T45.2X4	T45.2X5	T45.2X6
E acetate	T45.2X1	T45.2X2	T45.2X3	T45.2X4	T45.2X5	T45.2X6
hematopoietic	T45.8X1	T45.8X2	T45.8X3	T45.8X4	T45.8X5	T45.8X6
K NEC	T45.7X1	T45.7X2	T45.7X3	T45.7X4	T45.7X5	T45.7X6
K1	T45.7X1	T45.7X2	T45.7X3	T45.7X4	T45.7X5	T45.7X6
K2	T45.7X1	T45.7X2	T45.7X3	T45.7X4	T45.7X5	T45.7X6
PP	T45.2X1	T45.2X2	T45.2X3	T45.2X4	T45.2X5	T45.2X6
ulceroprotectant	T47.1X1	T47.1X2	T47.1X3	T47.1X4	T47.1X5	T47.1X6
Vleminckx's solution	T49.4X1	T49.4X2	T49.4X3	T49.4X4	T49.4X5	T49.4X6
Voltaren—see Diclofenac sodium						
W						
Warfarin	T45.511	T45.512	T45.513	T45.514	T45.515	T45.516
rodenticide	T60.4X1	T60.4X2	T60.4X3	T60.4X4	—	—
sodium	T45.511	T45.512	T45.513	T45.514	T45.515	T45.516
Wasp (sting)	T63.461	T63.462	T63.463	T63.464	—	—
Water						
balance drug	T50.3X1	T50.3X2	T50.3X3	T50.3X4	T50.3X5	T50.3X6
distilled	T50.3X1	T50.3X2	T50.3X3	T50.3X4	T50.3X5	T50.3X6
gas—see Gas, water						
incomplete combustion of—see Carbon, monoxide, fuel, utility						
hemlock	T62.2X1	T62.2X2	T62.2X3	T62.2X4	—	—
moccasin (venom)	T63.061	T63.062	T63.063	T63.064	—	—
purified	T50.3X1	T50.3X2	T50.3X3	T50.3X4	T50.3X5	T50.3X6
Wax (paraffin) (petroleum)	T52.0X1	T52.0X2	T52.0X3	T52.0X4	—	—
automobile	T65.891	T65.892	T65.893	T65.894	—	—
floor	T52.0X1	T52.0X2	T52.0X3	T52.0X4	—	—
Weed killers NEC	T60.3X1	T60.3X2	T60.3X3	T60.3X4	—	—
Welldorm	T42.6X1	T42.6X2	T42.6X3	T42.6X4	T42.6X5	T42.6X6
White						
arsenic	T57.0X1	T57.0X2	T57.0X3	T57.0X4	—	—
hellebore	T62.2X1	T62.2X2	T62.2X3	T62.2X4	—	—
lotion (keratolytic)	T49.4X1	T49.4X2	T49.4X3	T49.4X4	T49.4X5	T49.4X6
spirit	T52.0X1	T52.0X2	T52.0X3	T52.0X4	—	—
Whitewash	T65.891	T65.892	T65.893	T65.894	—	—
Whole blood (human)	T45.8X1	T45.8X2	T45.8X3	T45.8X4	T45.8X5	T45.8X6

Substance	Poisoning, Accidental (unintentional)	Poisoning, Intentional self-harm	Poisoning, Assault	Poisoning, Undetermined	Adverse effect	Underdosing
Wild						
black cherry	T62.2X1	T62.2X2	T62.2X3	T62.2X4	—	—
poisonous plants NEC	T62.2X1	T62.2X2	T62.2X3	T62.2X4	—	—
Window cleaning fluid	T65.891	T65.892	T65.893	T65.894	—	—
Wintergreen (oil)	T49.3X1	T49.3X2	T49.3X3	T49.3X4	T49.3X5	T49.3X6
Wisterine	T62.2X1	T62.2X2	T62.2X3	T62.2X4	—	—
Witch hazel	T49.2X1	T49.2X2	T49.2X3	T49.2X4	T49.2X5	T49.2X6
Wood alcohol or spirit	T51.1X1	T51.1X2	T51.1X3	T51.1X4	—	—
Wool fat (hydrous)	T49.3X1	T49.3X2	T49.3X3	T49.3X4	T49.3X5	T49.3X6
Woorali	T48.1X1	T48.1X2	T48.1X3	T48.1X4	T48.1X5	T48.1X6
Wormseed, American	T37.4X1	T37.4X2	T37.4X3	T37.4X4	T37.4X5	T37.4X6
X						
Xamoterol	T44.5X1	T44.5X2	T44.5X3	T44.5X4	T44.5X5	T44.5X6
Xanthine diuretics	T50.2X1	T50.2X2	T50.2X3	T50.2X4	T50.2X5	T50.2X6
Xanthinol nicotinate	T46.7X1	T46.7X2	T46.7X3	T46.7X4	T46.7X5	T46.7X6
Xanthotoxin	T49.3X1	T49.3X2	T49.3X3	T49.3X4	T49.3X5	T49.3X6
Xantinol nicotinate	T46.7X1	T46.7X2	T46.7X3	T46.7X4	T46.7X5	T46.7X6
Xantocillin	T36.0X1	T36.0X2	T36.0X3	T36.0X4	T36.0X5	T36.0X6
Xenon (127Xe) (133Xe)	T50.8X1	T50.8X2	T50.8X3	T50.8X4	T50.8X5	T50.8X6
Xenysalate	T49.4X1	T49.4X2	T49.4X3	T49.4X4	T49.4X5	T49.4X6
Xibornol	T37.8X1	T37.8X2	T37.8X3	T37.8X4	T37.8X5	T37.8X6
Xigris	T45.511	T45.512	T45.513	T45.514	T45.515	T45.516
Xipamide	T50.2X1	T50.2X2	T50.2X3	T50.2X4	T50.2X5	T50.2X6
Xylene (vapor)	T52.2X1	T52.2X2	T52.2X3	T52.2X4	—	—
Xylocaine (infiltration) (topical)	T41.3X1	T41.3X2	T41.3X3	T41.3X4	T41.3X5	T41.3X6
nerve block (peripheral) (plexus)	T41.3X1	T41.3X2	T41.3X3	T41.3X4	T41.3X5	T41.3X6
spinal	T41.3X1	T41.3X2	T41.3X3	T41.3X4	T41.3X5	T41.3X6
Xylol (vapor)	T52.2X1	T52.2X2	T52.2X3	T52.2X4	—	—
Xylometazoline	T48.5X1	T48.5X2	T48.5X3	T48.5X4	T48.5X5	T48.5X6
Y						
Yeast	T45.2X1	T45.2X2	T45.2X3	T45.2X4	T45.2X5	T45.2X6
dried	T45.2X1	T45.2X2	T45.2X3	T45.2X4	T45.2X5	T45.2X6
Yellow						
fever vaccine	T50.B91	T50.B92	T50.B93	T50.B94	T50.B95	T50.B96
jasmine	T62.2X1	T62.2X2	T62.2X3	T62.2X4	—	—
phenolphthalein	T47.2X1	T47.2X2	T47.2X3	T47.2X4	T47.2X5	T47.2X6
Yew	T62.2X1	T62.2X2	T62.2X3	T62.2X4	—	—
Yohimbic acid	T40.991	T40.992	T40.993	T40.994	T40.995	T40.996
Z						
Zactane	T39.8X1	T39.8X2	T39.8X3	T39.8X4	T39.8X5	T39.8X6

Substance	Poisoning, Accidental (unintentional)	Poisoning, Intentional self-harm	Poisoning, Assault	Poisoning, Undetermined	Adverse effect	Underdosing
Zalcitabine	T37.5X1	T37.5X2	T37.5X3	T37.5X4	T37.5X5	T37.5X6
Zaroxolyn	T50.2X1	T50.2X2	T50.2X3	T50.2X4	T50.2X5	T50.2X6
Zephiran (topical)	T49.0X1	T49.0X2	T49.0X3	T49.0X4	T49.0X5	T49.0X6
ophthalmic preparation	T49.5X1	T49.5X2	T49.5X3	T49.5X4	T49.5X5	T49.5X6
Zeranol	T38.7X1	T38.7X2	T38.7X3	T38.7X4	T38.7X5	T38.7X6
Zerone	T51.1X1	T51.1X2	T51.1X3	T51.1X4	—	—
Zidovudine	T37.5X1	T37.5X2	T37.5X3	T37.5X4	T37.5X5	T37.5X6
Zimeldine	T43.221	T43.222	T43.223	T43.224	T43.225	T43.226
Zinc (compounds) (fumes) (vapor) NEC	T56.5X1	T56.5X2	T56.5X3	T56.5X4	—	—
anti-infectives	T49.0X1	T49.0X2	T49.0X3	T49.0X4	T49.0X5	T49.0X6
antivaricose	T46.8X1	T46.8X2	T46.8X3	T46.8X4	T46.8X5	T46.8X6
bacitracin	T49.0X1	T49.0X2	T49.0X3	T49.0X4	T49.0X5	T49.0X6
chloride (mouthwash)	T49.6X1	T49.6X2	T49.6X3	T49.6X4	T49.6X5	T49.6X6
chromate	T56.5X1	T56.5X2	T56.5X3	T56.5X4	—	—
gelatin	T49.3X1	T49.3X2	T49.3X3	T49.3X4	T49.3X5	T49.3X6
oxide	T49.3X1	T49.3X2	T49.3X3	T49.3X4	T49.3X5	T49.3X6
plaster	T49.3X1	T49.3X2	T49.3X3	T49.3X4	T49.3X5	T49.3X6
peroxide	T49.0X1	T49.0X2	T49.0X3	T49.0X4	T49.0X5	T49.0X6
pesticides	T56.5X1	T56.5X2	T56.5X3	T56.5X4	—	—
phosphide	T60.4X1	T60.4X2	T60.4X3	T60.4X4	—	—
pyrithionate	T49.4X1	T49.4X2	T49.4X3	T49.4X4	T49.4X5	T49.4X6
stearate	T49.3X1	T49.3X2	T49.3X3	T49.3X4	T49.3X5	T49.3X6
sulfate	T49.5X1	T49.5X2	T49.5X3	T49.5X4	T49.5X5	T49.5X6
ENT agent	T49.6X1	T49.6X2	T49.6X3	T49.6X4	T49.6X5	T49.6X6
ophthalmic solution	T49.5X1	T49.5X2	T49.5X3	T49.5X4	T49.5X5	T49.5X6
topical NEC	T49.0X1	T49.0X2	T49.0X3	T49.0X4	T49.0X5	T49.0X6
undecylenate	T49.0X1	T49.0X2	T49.0X3	T49.0X4	T49.0X5	T49.0X6
Zineb	T60.0X1	T60.0X2	T60.0X3	T60.0X4	—	—
Zinostatin	T45.1X1	T45.1X2	T45.1X3	T45.1X4	T45.1X5	T45.1X6
Zipeprol	T48.3X1	T48.3X2	T48.3X3	T48.3X4	T48.3X5	T48.3X6
Zofenopril	T46.4X1	T46.4X2	T46.4X3	T46.4X4	T46.4X5	T46.4X6
Zolpidem	T42.6X1	T42.6X2	T42.6X3	T42.6X4	T42.6X5	T42.6X6
Zomepirac	T39.391	T39.392	T39.393	T39.394	T39.395	T39.396
Zopiclone	T42.6X1	T42.6X2	T42.6X3	T42.6X4	T42.6X5	T42.6X6
Zorubicin	T45.1X1	T45.1X2	T45.1X3	T45.1X4	T45.1X5	T45.1X6
Zotepine	T43.591	T43.592	T43.593	T43.594	T43.595	T43.596
Zovant	T45.511	T45.512	T45.513	T45.514	T45.515	T45.516
Zoxazolamine	T42.8X1	T42.8X2	T42.8X3	T42.8X4	T42.8X5	T42.8X6
Zuclopenthixol	T43.4X1	T43.4X2	T43.4X3	T43.4X4	T43.4X5	T43.4X6
Zygadenus (venenosus)	T62.2X1	T62.2X2	T62.2X3	T62.2X4	—	—
Zyprexa	T43.591	T43.592	T43.593	T43.594	T43.595	T43.596

External Cause of Injuries Index

A

Accident *(continued)*
- transport *(continued)*
  - aircraft NEC *(continued)*
    - occupant injured *(continued)*
      - nonpowered craft accident *(continued)*
        - balloon *(continued)*
          - fire V96.04
          - forced landing V96.02
          - specified type NEC V96.09
        - glider V96.20
          - collision V96.23
          - crash V96.21
          - explosion V96.25
          - fire V96.24
          - forced landing V96.22
          - specified type NEC V96.29
        - hang glider V96.10
          - collision V96.13
          - crash V96.11
          - explosion V96.15
          - fire V96.14
          - forced landing V96.12
          - specified type NEC V96.19
        - specified craft NEC V96.8
      - powered craft accident V95.9
        - fixed wing NEC
          - commercial V95.30
            - collision V95.33
            - crash V95.31
            - explosion V95.35
            - fire V95.34
            - forced landing V95.32
            - specified type NEC V95.39
          - private V95.20
            - collision V95.23
            - crash V95.21
            - explosion V95.25
            - fire V95.24
            - forced landing V95.22
            - specified type NEC V95.29
        - glider V95.10
          - collision V95.13
          - crash V95.11
          - explosion V95.15
          - fire V95.14
          - forced landing V95.12
          - specified type NEC V95.19
        - helicopter V95.00
          - collision V95.03
          - crash V95.01
          - explosion V95.05
          - fire V95.04
          - forced landing V95.02
          - specified type NEC V95.09
        - spacecraft V95.40
          - collision V95.43
          - crash V95.41
          - explosion V95.45
          - fire V95.44
          - forced landing V95.42
          - specified type NEC V95.49
        - specified craft NEC V95.8
        - ultralight V95.10
          - collision V95.13
          - crash V95.11
          - explosion V95.15
          - fire V95.14
          - forced landing V95.12
          - specified type NEC V95.19

Accident *(continued)*
- transport *(continued)*
  - aircraft NEC *(continued)*
    - occupant injured *(continued)*
      - specified accident NEC V97.0
      - while boarding or alighting V97.1
    - person (injured by)
      - falling from, in or on aircraft V97.0
      - machinery on aircraft V97.89
      - on ground with aircraft involvement V97.39
      - rotating propeller V97.32
      - struck by object falling from aircraft V97.31
      - sucked into aircraft jet V97.33
      - while boarding or alighting aircraft V97.1
  - airport (battery-powered) passenger vehicle *—see* Accident, transport, industrial vehicle occupant
  - all-terrain vehicle occupant (nontraffic) V86.95
    - driver V86.55
    - dune buggy *—see* Accident, transport, dune buggy occupant
    - hanger-on V86.75
    - passenger V86.65
    - snowmobile *—see* Accident, transport, snowmobile occupant
    - specified type NEC V86.99
      - driver V86.59
      - passenger V86.69
      - person on outside V86.79
    - traffic V86.35
      - driver V86.05
      - hanger-on V86.25
      - passenger V86.15
    - while boarding or alighting V86.45
  - ambulance occupant (traffic) V86.31
    - driver V86.01
    - hanger-on V86.21
    - nontraffic V86.91
      - driver V86.51
      - hanger-on V86.71
      - passenger V86.61
    - passenger V86.11
    - while boarding or alighting V86.41
  - animal-drawn vehicle occupant (in) V80.929
    - collision (with)
      - animal V80.12
        - being ridden V80.711
      - animal-drawn vehicle V80.721
      - bus V80.42
      - car V80.42
      - fixed or stationary object V80.82
      - military vehicle V80.920
      - nonmotor vehicle V80.791
      - pedal cycle V80.22
      - pedestrian V80.12
      - pickup V80.42
      - railway train or vehicle V80.62
      - specified motor vehicle NEC V80.52
      - streetcar V80.731
      - truck V80.42
      - two- or three-wheeled motor vehicle V80.32
      - van V80.42

Accident *(continued)*
- transport *(continued)*
  - animal-drawn vehicle occupant *(continued)*
    - noncollision V80.02
    - specified circumstance NEC V80.928
  - animal-rider V80.919
    - collision (with)
      - animal V80.11
        - being ridden V80.710
      - animal-drawn vehicle V80.720
      - bus V80.41
      - car V80.41
      - fixed or stationary object V80.81
      - military vehicle V80.910
      - nonmotor vehicle V80.790
      - pedal cycle V80.21
      - pedestrian V80.11
      - pickup V80.41
      - railway train or vehicle V80.61
      - specified motor vehicle NEC V80.51
      - streetcar V80.730
      - truck V80.41
      - two- or three-wheeled motor vehicle V80.31
      - van V80.41
    - noncollision V80.018
      - specified as horse rider V80.010
    - specified circumstance NEC V80.918
  - armored car *—see* Accident, transport, truck occupant
  - battery-powered truck (baggage) (mail) *—see* Accident, transport, industrial vehicle occupant
  - bus occupant V79.9
    - collision (with)
      - animal (traffic) V70.9
        - being ridden (traffic) V76.9
          - nontraffic V76.3
          - while boarding or alighting V76.4
        - nontraffic V70.3
        - while boarding or alighting V70.4
      - animal-drawn vehicle (traffic) V76.9
        - nontraffic V76.3
        - while boarding or alighting V76.4
      - bus (traffic) V74.9
        - nontraffic V74.3
        - while boarding or alighting V74.4
      - car (traffic) V73.9
        - nontraffic V73.3
        - while boarding or alighting V73.4
      - motor vehicle NOS (traffic) V79.60
        - nontraffic V79.20
        - specified type NEC (traffic) V79.69
          - nontraffic V79.29
      - pedal cycle (traffic) V71.9
        - nontraffic V71.3
        - while boarding or alighting V71.4
      - pickup truck (traffic) V73.9
        - nontraffic V73.3
        - while boarding or alighting V73.4
      - railway vehicle (traffic) V75.9
        - nontraffic V75.3
        - while boarding or alighting V75.4

Accident *(continued)*
- transport *(continued)*
  - bus occupant *(continued)*
    - collision *(continued)*
      - specified vehicle NEC (traffic) V76.9
        - nontraffic V76.3
        - while boarding or alighting V76.4
      - stationary object (traffic) V77.9
        - nontraffic V77.3
        - while boarding or alighting V77.4
      - streetcar (traffic) V76.9
        - nontraffic V76.3
        - while boarding or alighting V76.4
      - three wheeled motor vehicle (traffic) V72.9
        - nontraffic V72.3
        - while boarding or alighting V72.4
      - truck (traffic) V74.9
        - nontraffic V74.3
        - while boarding or alighting V74.4
      - two wheeled motor vehicle (traffic) V72.9
        - nontraffic V72.3
        - while boarding or alighting V72.4
      - van (traffic) V73.9
        - nontraffic V73.3
        - while boarding or alighting V73.4
    - driver
      - collision (with)
        - animal (traffic) V70.5
          - being ridden (traffic) V76.5
            - nontraffic V76.0
          - nontraffic V70.0
        - animal-drawn vehicle (traffic) V76.5
          - nontraffic V76.0
        - bus (traffic) V74.5
          - nontraffic V74.0
        - car (traffic) V73.5
          - nontraffic V73.0
        - motor vehicle NOS (traffic) V79.40
          - nontraffic V79.00
          - specified type NEC (traffic) V79.49
            - nontraffic V79.09
        - pedal cycle (traffic) V71.5
          - nontraffic V71.0
        - pickup truck (traffic) V73.5
          - nontraffic V73.0
        - railway vehicle (traffic) V75.5
          - nontraffic V75.0
        - specified vehicle NEC (traffic) V76.5
          - nontraffic V76.0
        - stationary object (traffic) V77.5
          - nontraffic V77.0
        - streetcar (traffic) V76.5
          - nontraffic V76.0
        - three wheeled motor vehicle (traffic) V72.5
          - nontraffic V72.0
        - truck (traffic) V74.5
          - nontraffic V74.0
        - two wheeled motor vehicle (traffic) V72.5
          - nontraffic V72.0

Accident *(continued)*
transport *(continued)*
car occupant *(continued)*
passenger
collision (with)
animal (traffic) V40.6
being ridden (traffic) V46.6
nontraffic V46.1
nontraffic V40.1
animal-drawn vehicle (traffic) V46.6
nontraffic V46.1
bus (traffic) V44.6
nontraffic V44.1
car (traffic) V43.62
nontraffic V43.12
motor vehicle NOS (traffic) V49.50
nontraffic V49.10
specified type NEC (traffic) V49.59
nontraffic V49.19
pedal cycle (traffic) V41.6
nontraffic V41.1
pickup truck (traffic) V43.63
nontraffic V43.13
railway vehicle (traffic) V45.6
nontraffic V45.1
specified vehicle NEC (traffic) V46.6
nontraffic V46.1
sport utility vehicle (traffic) V43.61
nontraffic V43.11
stationary object (traffic) V47.6
nontraffic V47.1
streetcar (traffic) V46.6
nontraffic V46.1
three wheeled motor vehicle (traffic) V42.6
nontraffic V42.1
truck (traffic) V44.6
nontraffic V44.1
two wheeled motor vehicle (traffic) V42.6
nontraffic V42.1
van (traffic) V43.64
nontraffic V43.14
noncollision accident (traffic) V48.6
nontraffic V48.1
specified type NEC V49.88
military vehicle V49.81
coal car —*see* Accident, transport, industrial vehicle occupant
construction vehicle occupant (nontraffic) V85.9
driver V85.5
hanger-on V85.7
passenger V85.6
traffic V85.3
driver V85.0
hanger-on V85.2
passenger V85.1
while boarding or alighting V85.4
dirt bike rider (nontraffic) V86.96
driver V86.56
hanger-on V86.76
passenger V86.66
traffic V86.36
driver V86.06
hanger-on V86.26
passenger V86.16

Accident *(continued)*
transport *(continued)*
dirt bike rider *(continued)*
while boarding or alighting V86.46
due to cataclysm —*see* Forces of nature, by type
dune buggy occupant (nontraffic) V86.93
driver V86.53
hanger-on V86.73
passenger V86.63
traffic V86.33
driver V86.03
hanger-on V86.23
passenger V86.13
while boarding or alighting V86.43
forklift —*see* Accident, transport, industrial vehicle occupant
go cart —*see* Accident, transport, all-terrain vehicle occupant
golf cart —*see* Accident, transport, all-terrain vehicle occupant
heavy transport vehicle occupant —*see* Accident, transport, truck occupant
hoverboard V00.848
ice yacht V98.2
industrial vehicle occupant (nontraffic) V83.9
driver V83.5
hanger-on V83.7
passenger V83.6
traffic V83.3
driver V83.0
hanger-on V83.2
passenger V83.1
while boarding or alighting V83.4
interurban electric car —*see* Accident, transport, streetcar
land yacht V98.1
logging car —*see* Accident, transport, industrial vehicle occupant
military vehicle occupant (traffic) V86.34
driver V86.04
hanger-on V86.24
nontraffic V86.94
driver V86.54
hanger-on V86.74
passenger V86.64
passenger V86.14
while boarding or alighting V86.44
mine tram —*see* Accident, transport, industrial vehicle occupant
motorcoach —*see* Accident, transport, bus occupant
motorcyclist V29.9
collision (with)
animal (traffic) V20.9
being ridden (traffic) V26.9
nontraffic V26.2
while boarding or alighting V26.3
nontraffic V20.2
while boarding or alighting V20.3
animal-drawn vehicle (traffic) V26.9
nontraffic V26.2

Accident *(continued)*
transport *(continued)*
motorcyclist *(continued)*
collision *(continued)*
animal-drawn vehicle *(continued)*
while boarding or alighting V26.3
bus (traffic) V24.9
nontraffic V24.2
while boarding or alighting V24.3
car (traffic) V23.9
nontraffic V23.2
while boarding or alighting V23.3
motor vehicle NOS (traffic) V29.60
nontraffic V29.20
specified type NEC (traffic) V29.69
nontraffic V29.29
pedal cycle (traffic) V21.9
nontraffic V21.2
while boarding or alighting V21.3
pickup truck (traffic) V23.9
nontraffic V23.2
while boarding or alighting V23.3
railway vehicle (traffic) V25.9
nontraffic V25.2
while boarding or alighting V25.3
specified vehicle NEC (traffic) V26.9
nontraffic V26.2
while boarding or alighting V26.3
stationary object (traffic) V27.9
nontraffic V27.2
while boarding or alighting V27.3
streetcar (traffic) V26.9
nontraffic V26.2
while boarding or alighting V26.3
three wheeled motor vehicle (traffic) V22.9
nontraffic V22.2
while boarding or alighting V22.3
truck (traffic) V24.9
nontraffic V24.2
while boarding or alighting V24.3
two wheeled motor vehicle (traffic) V22.9
nontraffic V22.2
while boarding or alighting V22.3
van (traffic) V23.9
nontraffic V23.2
while boarding or alighting V23.3
driver
collision (with)
animal (traffic) V20.4
being ridden (traffic) V26.4
nontraffic V26.0
nontraffic V20.0
animal-drawn vehicle (traffic) V26.4
nontraffic V26.0
bus (traffic) V24.4
nontraffic V24.0
car (traffic) V23.4
nontraffic V23.0

Accident *(continued)*
transport *(continued)*
motorcyclist *(continued)*
driver *(continued)*
collision *(continued)*
motor vehicle NOS (traffic) V29.40
nontraffic V29.00
specified type NEC (traffic) V29.49
nontraffic V29.09
pedal cycle (traffic) V21.4
nontraffic V21.0
pickup truck (traffic) V23.4
nontraffic V23.0
railway vehicle (traffic) V25.4
nontraffic V25.0
specified vehicle NEC (traffic) V26.4
nontraffic V26.0
stationary object (traffic) V27.4
nontraffic V27.0
streetcar (traffic) V26.4
nontraffic V26.0
three wheeled motor vehicle (traffic) V22.4
nontraffic V22.0
truck (traffic) V24.4
nontraffic V24.0
two wheeled motor vehicle (traffic) V22.4
nontraffic V22.0
van (traffic) V23.4
nontraffic V23.0
noncollision accident (traffic) V28.4
nontraffic V28.0
noncollision accident (traffic) V28.9
nontraffic V28.2
while boarding or alighting V28.3
nontraffic V29.3
passenger
collision (with)
animal (traffic) V20.5
being ridden (traffic) V26.5
nontraffic V26.1
nontraffic V20.1
animal-drawn vehicle (traffic) V26.5
nontraffic V26.1
bus (traffic) V24.5
nontraffic V24.1
car (traffic) V23.5
nontraffic V23.1
motor vehicle NOS (traffic) V29.50
nontraffic V29.10
specified type NEC (traffic) V29.59
nontraffic V29.19
pedal cycle (traffic) V21.5
nontraffic V21.1
pickup truck (traffic) V23.5
nontraffic V23.1
railway vehicle (traffic) V25.5
nontraffic V25.1
specified vehicle NEC (traffic) V26.5
nontraffic V26.1
stationary object (traffic) V27.5

Accident *(continued)*
transport *(continued)*
pedal cyclist *(continued)*
collision *(continued)*
truck (traffic) V14.9
nontraffic V14.2
while boarding or alighting V14.3
two wheeled motor vehicle (traffic) V12.9
nontraffic V12.2
while boarding or alighting V12.3
van (traffic) V13.9
nontraffic V13.2
while boarding or alighting V13.3
driver
collision (with)
animal (traffic) V10.4
being ridden (traffic) V16.4
nontraffic V16.0
nontraffic V10.0
animal-drawn vehicle (traffic) V16.4
nontraffic V16.0
bus (traffic) V14.4
nontraffic V14.0
car (traffic) V13.4
nontraffic V13.0
motor vehicle NOS (traffic) V19.40
nontraffic V19.00
specified type NEC (traffic) V19.49
nontraffic V19.09
pedal cycle (traffic) V11.4
nontraffic V11.0
pickup truck (traffic) tV13.4
nontraffic V13.0
railway vehicle (traffic) V15.4
nontraffic V15.0
specified vehicle NEC (traffic) V16.4
nontraffic V16.0
stationary object (traffic) V17.4
nontraffic V17.0
streetcar (traffic) V16.4
nontraffic V16.0
three wheeled motor vehicle (traffic) V12.4
nontraffic V12.0
truck (traffic) V14.4
nontraffic V14.0
two wheeled motor vehicle (traffic) V12.4
nontraffic V12.0
van (traffic) V13.4
nontraffic V13.0
noncollision accident (traffic) V18.4
nontraffic V18.0
noncollision accident (traffic) V18.9
nontraffic V18.2
while boarding or alighting V18.3
nontraffic V19.3
passenger
collision (with)
animal (traffic) V10.5
being ridden (traffic) V16.5
nontraffic V16.1
nontraffic V10.1
animal-drawn vehicle (traffic) V16.5

Accident *(continued)*
transport *(continued)*
pedal cyclist *(continued)*
passenger *(continued)*
collision *(continued)*
animal-drawn vehicle *(continued)*
nontraffic V16.1
bus (traffic) V14.5
nontraffic V14.1
car (traffic) V13.5
nontraffic V13.1
motor vehicle NOS (traffic) V19.50
nontraffic V19.10
specified type NEC (traffic) V19.59
nontraffic V19.19
pedal cycle (traffic) V11.5
nontraffic V11.1
pickup truck (traffic) V13.5
nontraffic V13.1
railway vehicle (traffic) V15.5
nontraffic V15.1
specified vehicle NEC (traffic) V16.5
nontraffic V16.1
stationary object (traffic) V17.5
nontraffic V17.1
streetcar (traffic) V16.5
nontraffic V16.1
three wheeled motor vehicle (traffic) V12.5
nontraffic V12.1
truck (traffic) V14.5
nontraffic V14.1
two wheeled motor vehicle (traffic) V12.5
nontraffic V12.1
van (traffic) V13.5
nontraffic V13.1
noncollision accident (traffic) V18.5
nontraffic V18.1
specified type NEC V19.88
military vehicle V19.81
pedestrian
conveyance (occupant) V09.9
baby stroller V00.828
collision (with) V09.9
animal being ridden or animal drawn vehicle V06.99
nontraffic V06.09
traffic V06.19
bus or heavy transport V04.99
nontraffic V04.09
traffic V04.19
car V03.99
nontraffic V03.09
traffic V03.19
pedal cycle V01.99
nontraffic V01.09
traffic V01.19
pick-up truck or van V03.99
nontraffic V03.09
traffic V03.19
railway (train) (vehicle) V05.99
nontraffic V05.09
traffic V05.19
streetcar V06.99
nontraffic V06.09
traffic V06.19
stationary object V00.822

Accident *(continued)*
transport *(continued)*
pedestrian *(continued)*
conveyance *(continued)*
baby stroller *(continued)*
collision *(continued)*
two- or three-wheeled motor vehicle V02.99
nontraffic V02.09
traffic V02.19
vehicle V09.9
animal-drawn V06.99
nontraffic V06.09
traffic V06.19
motor
nontraffic V09.00
traffic V09.20
fall V00.821
nontraffic V09.1
involving motor vehicle NEC V09.00
traffic V09.3
involving motor vehicle NEC V09.20
flat-bottomed NEC V00.388
collision (with) V09.9
animal being ridden or animal drawn vehicle V06.99
nontraffic V06.09
traffic V06.19
bus or heavy transport V04.99
nontraffic V04.09
traffic V04.19
car V03.99
nontraffic V03.09
traffic V03.19
pedal cycle V01.99
nontraffic V01.09
traffic V01.19
pick-up truck or van V03.99
nontraffic V03.09
traffic V03.19
railway (train) (vehicle) V05.99
nontraffic V05.09
traffic V05.19
stationary object V00.382
streetcar V06.99
nontraffic V06.09
traffic V06.19
two- or three-wheeled motor vehicle V02.99
nontraffic V02.09
traffic V02.19
vehicle V09.9
animal-drawn V06.99
nontraffic V06.09
traffic V06.19
motor
nontraffic V09.00
traffic V09.20
fall V00.381
nontraffic V09.1
involving motor vehicle NEC V09.00
snow
board —*see* Accident, transport, pedestrian, conveyance, snow board
ski —*see* Accident, transport, pedestrian, conveyance, skis (snow)
traffic V09.3

Accident *(continued)*
transport *(continued)*
pedestrian *(continued)*
conveyance *(continued)*
flat-bottomed NEC *(continued)*
traffic *(continued)*
involving motor vehicle NEC V09.20
gliding type NEC V00.288
collision (with) V09.9
animal being ridden or animal drawn vehicle V06.99
nontraffic V06.09
traffic V06.19
bus or heavy transport V04.99
nontraffic V04.09
traffic V04.19
car V03.99
nontraffic V03.09
traffic V03.19
pedal cycle V01.99
nontraffic V01.09
traffic V01.19
pick-up truck or van V03.99
nontraffic V03.09
traffic V03.19
railway (train) (vehicle) V05.99
nontraffic V05.09
traffic V05.19
stationary object V00.282
streetcar V06.99
nontraffic V06.09
traffic V06.19
two- or three-wheeled motor vehicle V02.99
nontraffic V02.09
traffic V02.19
vehicle V09.9
animal-drawn V06.99
nontraffic V06.09
traffic V06.19
motor
nontraffic V09.00
traffic V09.20
fall V00.281
heelies —*see* Accident, transport, pedestrian, conveyance, heelies
ice skate —*see* Accident, transport, pedestrian, conveyance, ice skate
nontraffic V09.1
involving motor vehicle NEC V09.00
sled —*see* Accident, transport, pedestrian, conveyance, sled
traffic V09.3
involving motor vehicle NEC V09.20
wheelies —*see* Accident, transport, pedestrian, conveyance, heelies
heelies V00.158
colliding with stationary object V00.152
fall V00.151
hoverboard
collision with
animal being ridden or animal drawn vehicle V06.938
nontraffic V06.038
traffic V06.138

- **Accident** *(continued)*
  - transport *(continued)*
    - pedestrian *(continued)*
      - conveyance *(continued)*
        - Segway *(continued)*
          - collision *(continued)*
            - pedal cycle V01.938
              - nontraffic V01.038
              - traffic V01.138
            - pick-up or van V03.938
              - nontraffic V03.038
              - traffic V03.138
            - railway (train) (vehicle) V05.938
              - nontraffic V05.038
              - traffic V05.138
            - streetcar V06.938
              - nontraffic V06.038
              - traffic V06.138
            - three-wheeled motor vehicle V02.938
              - nontraffic V02.038
              - traffic V02.138
            - two-wheeled motor vehicle V02.938
              - nontraffic V02.038
              - traffic V02.138
            - vehicle, nonmotor, specified NEC V06.938
              - nontraffic V06.038
              - traffic V06.138
          - fall V00.848
        - skate board V00.138
          - collision (with) V09.9
            - animal being ridden or animal drawn vehicle V06.92
              - nontraffic V06.02
              - traffic V06.12
            - bus or heavy transport V04.92
              - nontraffic V04.02
              - traffic V04.12
            - car V03.92
              - nontraffic V03.02
              - traffic V03.12
            - pedal cycle V01.92
              - nontraffic V01.02
              - traffic V01.12
            - pick-up truck or van V03.92
              - nontraffic V03.02
              - traffic V03.12
            - railway (train) (vehicle) V05.92
              - nontraffic V05.02
              - traffic V05.12
            - streetcar V06.92
              - nontraffic V06.02
              - traffic V06.12
            - stationary object V00.132
            - two- or three-wheeled motor vehicle V02.92
              - nontraffic V02.02
              - traffic V02.12
            - vehicle V09.9
              - animal-drawn V06.92
                - nontraffic V06.02
                - traffic V06.12
              - motor
                - nontraffic V09.00
                - traffic V09.20
          - fall V00.131

- **Accident** *(continued)*
  - transport *(continued)*
    - pedestrian *(continued)*
      - conveyance *(continued)*
        - skate board *(continued)*
          - nontraffic V09.1
            - involving motor vehicle NEC V09.00
          - traffic V09.3
            - involving motor vehicle NEC V09.20
        - sled V00.228
          - collision (with) V09.9
            - animal being ridden or animal drawn vehicle V06.99
              - nontraffic V06.09
              - traffic V06.19
            - bus or heavy transport V04.99
              - nontraffic V04.09
              - traffic V04.19
            - car V03.99
              - nontraffic V03.09
              - traffic V03.19
            - pedal cycle V01.99
              - nontraffic V01.09
              - traffic V01.19
            - pick-up truck or van V03.99
              - nontraffic V03.09
              - traffic V03.19
            - railway (train) (vehicle) V05.99
              - nontraffic V05.09
              - traffic V05.19
            - streetcar V06.99
              - nontraffic V06.09
              - traffic V06.19
            - stationary object V00.222
            - two- or three-wheeled motor vehicle V02.99
              - nontraffic V02.09
              - traffic V02.19
            - vehicle V09.9
              - animal-drawn V06.99
                - nontraffic V06.09
                - traffic V06.19
              - motor
                - nontraffic V09.00
                - traffic V09.20
          - fall V00.221
          - nontraffic V09.1
            - involving motor vehicle NEC V09.00
          - traffic V09.3
            - involving motor vehicle NEC V09.20
        - skis (snow) V00.328
          - collision (with) V09.9
            - animal being ridden or animal drawn vehicle V06.99
              - nontraffic V06.09
              - traffic V06.19
            - bus or heavy transport V04.99
              - nontraffic V04.09
              - traffic V04.19
            - car V03.99
              - nontraffic V03.09
              - traffic V03.19
            - pedal cycle V01.99
              - nontraffic V01.09
              - traffic V01.19

- **Accident** *(continued)*
  - transport *(continued)*
    - pedestrian *(continued)*
      - conveyance *(continued)*
        - skis *(continued)*
          - collision *(continued)*
            - pick-up truck or van V03.99
              - nontraffic V03.09
              - traffic V03.19
            - railway (train) (vehicle) V05.99
              - nontraffic V05.09
              - traffic V05.19
            - streetcar V06.99
              - nontraffic V06.09
              - traffic V06.19
            - stationary object V00.322
            - two- or three-wheeled motor vehicle V02.99
              - nontraffic V02.09
              - traffic V02.19
            - vehicle V09.9
              - animal-drawn V06.99
                - nontraffic V06.09
                - traffic V06.19
              - motor
                - nontraffic V09.00
                - traffic V09.20
          - fall V00.321
          - nontraffic V09.1
            - involving motor vehicle NEC V09.00
          - traffic V09.3
            - involving motor vehicle NEC V09.20
        - snow board V00.318
          - collision (with) V09.9
            - animal being ridden or animal drawn vehicle V06.99
              - nontraffic V06.09
              - traffic V06.19
            - bus or heavy transport V04.99
              - nontraffic V04.09
              - traffic V04.19
            - car V03.99
              - nontraffic V03.09
              - traffic V03.19
            - pedal cycle V01.99
              - nontraffic V01.09
              - traffic V01.19
            - pick-up truck or van V03.99
              - nontraffic V03.09
              - traffic V03.19
            - railway (train) (vehicle) V05.99
              - nontraffic V05.09
              - traffic V05.19
            - streetcar V06.99
              - nontraffic V06.09
              - traffic V06.19
            - stationary object V00.312
            - two- or three-wheeled motor vehicle V02.99
              - nontraffic V02.09
              - traffic V02.19
            - vehicle V09.9
              - animal-drawn V06.99
                - nontraffic V06.09
                - traffic V06.19

- **Accident** *(continued)*
  - transport *(continued)*
    - pedestrian *(continued)*
      - conveyance *(continued)*
        - snow board *(continued)*
          - collision *(continued)*
            - vehicle *(continued)*
              - motor
                - nontraffic V09.00
                - traffic V09.20
          - fall V00.311
          - nontraffic V09.1
            - involving motor vehicle NEC V09.00
          - traffic V09.3
            - involving motor vehicle NEC V09.20
        - specified type NEC V00.898
          - collision (with) V09.9
            - animal being ridden or animal drawn vehicle V06.99
              - nontraffic V06.09
              - traffic V06.19
            - bus or heavy transport V04.99
              - nontraffic V04.09
              - traffic V04.19
            - car V03.99
              - nontraffic V03.09
              - traffic V03.19
            - pedal cycle V01.99
              - nontraffic V01.09
              - traffic V01.19
            - pick-up truck or van V03.99
              - nontraffic V03.09
              - traffic V03.19
            - railway (train) (vehicle) V05.99
              - nontraffic V05.09
              - traffic V05.19
            - streetcar V06.99
              - nontraffic V06.09
              - traffic V06.19
            - stationary object V00.892
            - two- or three-wheeled motor vehicle V02.99
              - nontraffic V02.09
              - traffic V02.19
            - vehicle V09.9
              - animal-drawn V06.99
                - nontraffic V06.09
                - traffic V06.19
              - motor
                - nontraffic V09.00
                - traffic V09.20
          - fall V00.891
          - nontraffic V09.1
            - involving motor vehicle NEC V09.00
          - traffic V09.3
            - involving motor vehicle NEC V09.20
        - Standing
          - electric scooter
            - collision with
              - animal being ridden or animal drawn vehicle V06.931
                - nontraffic V06.031
                - traffic V06.131
              - bus or heavy transport V04.931
                - nontraffic V04.031
                - traffic V04.131

Accident *(continued)*
transport *(continued)*
three-wheeled motor vehicle occupant *(continued)*
collision *(continued)*
stationary object (traffic) V37.9
nontraffic V37.3
while boarding or alighting V37.4
streetcar (traffic) V36.9
nontraffic V36.3
while boarding or alighting V36.4
three wheeled motor vehicle (traffic) V32.9
nontraffic V32.3
while boarding or alighting V32.4
truck (traffic) V34.9
nontraffic V34.3
while boarding or alighting V34.4
two wheeled motor vehicle (traffic) V32.9
nontraffic V32.3
while boarding or alighting V32.4
van (traffic) V33.9
nontraffic V33.3
while boarding or alighting V33.4
driver
collision (with)
animal (traffic) V30.5
being ridden (traffic) V36.5
nontraffic V36.0
nontraffic V30.0
animal-drawn vehicle (traffic) V36.5
nontraffic V36.0
bus (traffic) V34.5
nontraffic V34.0
car (traffic) V33.5
nontraffic V33.0
motor vehicle NOS (traffic) V39.40
nontraffic V39.00
specified type NEC (traffic) V39.49
nontraffic V39.09
pedal cycle (traffic) V31.5
nontraffic V31.0
pickup truck (traffic) V33.5
nontraffic V33.0
railway vehicle (traffic) V35.5
nontraffic V35.0
specified vehicle NEC (traffic) V36.5
nontraffic V36.0
stationary object (traffic) V37.5
nontraffic V37.0
streetcar (traffic) V36.5
nontraffic V36.0
three wheeled motor vehicle (traffic) V32.5
nontraffic V32.0
truck (traffic) V34.5
nontraffic V34.0
two wheeled motor vehicle (traffic) V32.5
nontraffic V32.0
van (traffic) V33.5
nontraffic V33.0
noncollision accident (traffic) V38.5
nontraffic V38.0

Accident *(continued)*
transport *(continued)*
three-wheeled motor vehicle occupant *(continued)*
noncollision accident (traffic) V38.9
nontraffic V38.3
while boarding or alighting V38.4
nontraffic V39.3
hanger-on
collision (with)
animal (traffic) V30.7
being ridden (traffic) V36.7
nontraffic V36.2
nontraffic V30.2
animal-drawn vehicle (traffic) V36.7
nontraffic V36.2
bus (traffic) V34.7
nontraffic V34.2
car (traffic) V33.7
nontraffic V33.2
pedal cycle (traffic) V31.7
nontraffic V31.2
pickup truck (traffic) V33.7
nontraffic V33.2
railway vehicle (traffic) V35.7
nontraffic V35.2
specified vehicle NEC (traffic) V36.7
nontraffic V36.2
stationary object (traffic) V37.7
nontraffic V37.2
streetcar (traffic) V36.7
nontraffic V36.2
three wheeled motor vehicle (traffic) V32.7
nontraffic V32.2
truck (traffic) V34.7
nontraffic V34.2
two wheeled motor vehicle (traffic) V32.7
nontraffic V32.2
van (traffic) V33.7
nontraffic V33.2
noncollision accident (traffic) V38.7
nontraffic V38.2
passenger
collision (with)
animal (traffic) V30.6
being ridden (traffic) V36.6
nontraffic V36.1
nontraffic V30.1
animal-drawn vehicle (traffic) V36.6
nontraffic V36.1
bus (traffic) V34.6
nontraffic V34.1
car (traffic) V33.6
nontraffic V33.1
motor vehicle NOS (traffic) V39.50
nontraffic V39.10
specified type NEC (traffic) V39.59
nontraffic V39.19
pedal cycle (traffic) V31.6
nontraffic V31.1
pickup truck (traffic) V33.6
nontraffic V33.1
railway vehicle (traffic) V35.6
nontraffic V35.1

Accident *(continued)*
transport *(continued)*
three-wheeled motor vehicle occupant *(continued)*
passenger *(continued)*
collision *(continued)*
specified vehicle NEC (traffic) V36.6
nontraffic V36.1
stationary object (traffic) V37.6
nontraffic V37.1
streetcar (traffic) V36.6
nontraffic V36.1
three wheeled motor vehicle (traffic) V32.6
nontraffic V32.1
truck (traffic) V34.6
nontraffic V34.1
two wheeled motor vehicle (traffic) V32.6
nontraffic V32.1
van (traffic) V33.6
nontraffic V33.1
noncollision accident (traffic) V38.6
nontraffic V38.1
specified type NEC V39.89
military vehicle V39.81
tractor (farm) (and trailer) —*see* Accident, transport, agricultural vehicle occupant
tram —*see* Accident, transport, streetcar
in mine or quarry —*see* Accident, transport, industrial vehicle occupant
trolley —*see* Accident, transport, streetcar
in mine or quarry —*see* Accident, transport, industrial vehicle occupant
truck occupant V69.9
collision (with)
animal (traffic) V60.9
being ridden (traffic) V66.9
nontraffic V66.3
while boarding or alighting V66.4
nontraffic V60.3
while boarding or alighting V60.4
animal-drawn vehicle (traffic) V66.9
nontraffic V66.3
while boarding or alighting V66.4
bus (traffic) V64.9
nontraffic V64.3
while boarding or alighting V64.4
car (traffic) V63.9
nontraffic V63.3
while boarding or alighting V63.4
motor vehicle NOS (traffic) V69.60
nontraffic V69.20
specified type NEC (traffic) V69.69
nontraffic V69.29
pedal cycle (traffic) V61.9
nontraffic V61.3
while boarding or alighting V61.4
pickup truck (traffic) V63.9
nontraffic V63.3
while boarding or alighting V63.4

Accident *(continued)*
transport *(continued)*
truck occupant *(continued)*
collision *(continued)*
railway vehicle (traffic) V65.9
nontraffic V65.3
while boarding or alighting V65.4
specified vehicle NEC (traffic) V66.9
nontraffic V66.3
while boarding or alighting V66.4
stationary object (traffic) V67.9
nontraffic V67.3
while boarding or alighting V67.4
streetcar (traffic) V66.9
nontraffic V66.3
while boarding or alighting V66.4
three wheeled motor vehicle (traffic) V62.9
nontraffic V62.3
while boarding or alighting V62.4
truck (traffic) V64.9
nontraffic V64.3
while boarding or alighting V64.4
two wheeled motor vehicle (traffic) V62.9
nontraffic V62.3
while boarding or alighting V62.4
van (traffic) V63.9
nontraffic V63.3
while boarding or alighting V63.4
driver
collision (with)
animal (traffic) V60.5
being ridden (traffic) V66.5
nontraffic V66.0
nontraffic V60.0
animal-drawn vehicle (traffic) V66.5
nontraffic V66.0
bus (traffic) V64.5
nontraffic V64.0
car (traffic) V63.5
nontraffic V63.0
motor vehicle NOS (traffic) V69.40
nontraffic V69.00
specified type NEC (traffic) V69.49
nontraffic V69.09
pedal cycle (traffic) V61.5
nontraffic V61.0
pickup truck (traffic) V63.5
nontraffic V63.0
railway vehicle (traffic) V65.5
nontraffic V65.0
specified vehicle NEC (traffic) V66.5
nontraffic V66.0
stationary object (traffic) V67.5
nontraffic V67.0
streetcar (traffic) V66.5
nontraffic V66.0
three wheeled motor vehicle (traffic) V62.5
nontraffic V62.0
truck (traffic) V64.5
nontraffic V64.0

- **Accident** *(continued)*
  - transport *(continued)*
    - van occupant *(continued)*
      - passenger *(continued)*
        - collision (with)
          - motor vehicle NOS (traffic) V59.50
            - nontraffic V59.10
            - specified type NEC (traffic) V59.59
              - nontraffic V59.19
          - pedal cycle (traffic) V51.6
            - nontraffic V51.1
          - pickup truck (traffic) V53.6
            - nontraffic V53.1
          - railway vehicle (traffic) V55.6
            - nontraffic V55.1
          - specified vehicle NEC (traffic) V56.6
            - nontraffic V56.1
          - stationary object (traffic) V57.6
            - nontraffic V57.1
          - streetcar (traffic) V56.6
            - nontraffic V56.1
          - three wheeled motor vehicle (traffic) V52.6
            - nontraffic V52.1
          - truck (traffic) V54.6
            - nontraffic V54.1
          - two wheeled motor vehicle (traffic) V52.6
            - nontraffic V52.1
          - van (traffic) V53.6
            - nontraffic V53.1
        - noncollision accident (traffic) V58.6
          - nontraffic V58.1
      - specified type NEC V59.88
        - military vehicle V59.81
    - watercraft occupant —*see* Accident, watercraft
  - vehicle NEC V89.9
    - animal-drawn NEC —*see* Accident, transport, animal-drawn vehicle occupant
    - special
      - agricultural —*see* Accident, transport, agricultural vehicle occupant
      - construction —*see* Accident, transport, construction vehicle occupant
      - industrial —*see* Accident, transport, industrial vehicle occupant
    - three-wheeled NEC (motorized) —*see* Accident, transport, three-wheeled motor vehicle occupant
  - watercraft V94.9
    - causing
      - drowning —*see* Drowning, due to, accident to, watercraft
      - injury NEC V91.89
        - crushed between craft and object V91.19
          - powered craft V91.13
            - ferry boat V91.11
            - fishing boat V91.12
            - jetskis V91.13
            - liner V91.11
            - merchant ship V91.10
            - passenger ship V91.11
          - unpowered craft V91.18
            - canoe V91.15
            - inflatable V91.16
            - kayak V91.15

- **Accident** *(continued)*
  - watercraft *(continued)*
    - causing *(continued)*
      - injury NEC *(continued)*
        - crushed between craft and object *(continued)*
          - unpowered craft *(continued)*
            - sailboat V91.14
            - surf-board V91.18
            - windsurfer V91.18
        - fall on board V91.29
          - powered craft V91.23
            - ferry boat V91.21
            - fishing boat V91.22
            - jetskis V91.23
            - liner V91.21
            - merchant ship V91.20
            - passenger ship V91.21
          - unpowered craft
            - canoe V91.25
            - inflatable V91.26
            - kayak V91.25
            - sailboat V91.24
        - fire on board causing burn V91.09
          - powered craft V91.03
            - ferry boat V91.01
            - fishing boat V91.02
            - jetskis V91.03
            - liner V91.01
            - merchant ship V91.00
            - passenger ship V91.01
          - unpowered craft V91.08
            - canoe V91.05
            - inflatable V91.06
            - kayak V91.05
            - sailboat V91.04
            - surf-board V91.08
            - water skis V91.07
            - windsurfer V91.08
        - hit by falling object V91.39
          - powered craft V91.33
            - ferry boat V91.31
            - fishing boat V91.32
            - jetskis V91.33
            - liner V91.31
            - merchant ship V91.30
            - passenger ship V91.31
          - unpowered craft V91.38
            - canoe V91.35
            - inflatable V91.36
            - kayak V91.35
            - sailboat V91.34
            - surf-board V91.38
            - water skis V91.37
            - windsurfer V91.38
        - specified type NEC V91.89
          - powered craft V91.83
            - ferry boat V91.81
            - fishing boat V91.82
            - jetskis V91.83
            - liner V91.81
            - merchant ship V91.80
            - passenger ship V91.81
          - unpowered craft V91.88
            - canoe V91.85
            - inflatable V91.86
            - kayak V91.85
            - sailboat V91.84
            - surf-board V91.88
            - water skis V91.87
            - windsurfer V91.88
    - due to, caused by cataclysm —*see* Forces of nature, by type
    - military NEC V94.818
      - with civilian watercraft V94.810
      - civilian in water injured by V94.811

- **Accident** *(continued)*
  - watercraft *(continued)*
    - nonpowered, struck by
      - nonpowered vessel V94.22
      - powered vessel V94.21
    - specified type NEC V94.89
    - striking swimmer
      - powered V94.11
      - unpowered V94.12

- **Acid throwing (assault)** Y08.89

- **Activity** (involving) (of victim at time of event) Y93.9
  - aerobic and step exercise (class) Y93.A3
  - alpine skiing Y93.23
  - animal care NEC Y93.K9
  - arts and handcrafts NEC Y93.D9
  - athletics NEC Y93.79
  - athletics played as a team or group NEC Y93.69
  - athletics played individually NEC Y93.59
  - baking Y93.G3
  - ballet Y93.41
  - barbells Y93.B3
  - BASE (Building, Antenna, Span, Earth) jumping Y93.33
  - baseball Y93.64
  - basketball Y93.67
  - bathing (personal) Y93.E1
  - beach volleyball Y93.68
  - bike riding Y93.55
  - blackout game Y93.85
  - boogie boarding Y93.18
  - bowling Y93.54
  - boxing Y93.71
  - brass instrument playing Y93.J4
  - building construction Y93.H3
  - bungee jumping Y93.34
  - calisthenics Y93.A2
  - canoeing (in calm and turbulent water) Y93.16
  - capture the flag Y93.6A
  - cardiorespiratory exercise NEC Y93.A9
  - caregiving (providing) NEC Y93 F9
    - bathing Y93.F1
    - lifting Y93.F2
  - cellular
    - communication device Y93.C2
    - telephone Y93.C2
  - challenge course Y93.A5
  - cheerleading Y93.45
  - choking game Y93.85
  - circuit training Y93.A4
  - cleaning
    - floor Y93.E5
  - climbing NEC Y93.39
    - mountain Y93.31
    - rock Y93.31
    - wall Y93.31
  - clothing care and maintenance NEC Y93.E9
  - combatives Y93.75
  - computer
    - keyboarding Y93.C1
    - technology NEC Y93.C9
  - confidence course Y93.A5
  - construction (building) Y93.H3
  - cooking and baking Y93.G3
  - cool down exercises Y93.A2
  - cricket Y93.69
  - crocheting Y93.D1
  - cross country skiing Y93.24
  - dancing (all types) Y93.41
  - digging
    - dirt Y93.H1
  - dirt digging Y93.H1
  - dishwashing Y93.G1

- **Activity** *(continued)*
  - diving (platform) (springboard) Y93.12
    - underwater Y93.15
  - dodge ball Y93.6A
  - downhill skiing Y93.23
  - drum playing Y93.J2
  - dumbbells Y93.B3
  - electronic
    - devices NEC Y93.C9
      - hand held interactive Y93.C2
    - game playing (using) (with)
      - interactive device Y93.C2
      - keyboard or other stationary device Y93.C1
  - elliptical machine Y93.A1
  - exercise(s)
    - machines ((primarily) for)
      - cardiorespiratory conditioning Y93.A1
      - muscle strengthening Y93.B1
    - muscle strengthening (non-machine) NEC Y93.B9
  - external motion NEC Y93.I9
    - rollercoaster Y93.I1
  - fainting game Y93.85
  - field hockey Y93.65
  - figure skating (pairs) (singles) Y93.21
  - flag football Y93.62
  - floor mopping and cleaning Y93.E5
  - food preparation and clean up Y93.G1
  - football (American) NOS Y93.61
    - flag Y93.62
    - tackle Y93.61
    - touch Y93.62
  - four square Y93.6A
  - free weights Y93.B3
  - frisbee (ultimate) Y93.74
  - furniture
    - building Y93.D3
    - finishing Y93.D3
    - repair Y93.D3
  - game playing (electronic)
    - using keyboard or other stationary device Y93.C1
    - using interactive device Y93.C2
  - gardening Y93.H2
  - golf Y93.53
  - grass drills Y93.A6
  - grilling and smoking food Y93.G2
  - grooming and shearing an animal Y93.K3
  - guerilla drills Y93.A6
  - gymnastics (rhythmic) Y93.43
  - handball Y93.73
  - handcrafts NEC Y93.D9
  - hand held interactive electronic device Y93.C2
  - hang gliding Y93.35
  - hiking (on level or elevated terrain) Y93.01
  - hockey (ice) Y93.22
    - field Y93.65
  - horseback riding Y93.52
  - household (interior) maintenance NEC Y93.E9
  - ice NEC Y93.29
    - dancing Y93.21
    - hockey Y93.22
    - skating Y93.21
  - inline roller skating Y93.51
  - ironing Y93.E4
  - judo Y93.75
  - jumping (off) NEC Y93.39
    - BASE (Building, Antenna, Span, Earth) Y93.33
    - bungee Y93.34
    - jacks Y93.A2
    - rope Y93.56
  - jumping jacks Y93.A2

Assault *(continued)*
gunshot (wound) NEC —*see* Assault, firearm, by type
incendiary device X97
injury Y09
to child due to criminal abortion attempt NEC Y08.89
knife X99.1
late effect of —*see* X92-Y08 with 7th character S
placing before moving object NEC Y02.8
motor vehicle Y02.0
poisoning —*see* categories T36-T65 with 7th character S
puncture, any part of body —*see* Assault, cutting or piercing instrument
pushing
before moving object NEC Y02.8
motor vehicle Y02.0
subway train Y02.1
train Y02.1
from high place Y01
rape T74.2-
scalding —*see* Assault, burning
sequelae of —*see* X92-Y08 with 7th character S
sexual (by bodily force) T74.2-
shooting —*see* Assault, firearm
specified means NEC Y08.89
stab, any part of body —*see* Assault, cutting or piercing instrument
steam X98.0
striking against
other person Y04.2
sports equipment Y08.09
baseball bat Y08.02
hockey stick Y08.01
struck by
sports equipment Y08.09
baseball bat Y08.02
hockey stick Y08.01
submersion —*see* Assault, drowning
violence Y09
weapon Y09
blunt Y00
cutting or piercing —*see* Assault, cutting or piercing instrument
firearm —*see* Assault, firearm
wound Y09
cutting —*see* Assault, cutting or piercing instrument
gunshot —*see* Assault, firearm
knife X99.1
piercing —*see* Assault, cutting or piercing instrument
puncture —*see* Assault, cutting or piercing instrument
stab —*see* Assault, cutting or piercing instrument

Attack by mammals NEC W55.89

Avalanche —*see* Landslide

Aviator's disease —*see* Air, pressure

B

Barotitis, barodontalgia, barosinusitis, barotrauma (otitic) (sinus) —*see* Air, pressure

Battered (baby) (child) (person) (syndrome) X58

Bayonet wound W26.1
in
legal intervention —*see* Legal, intervention, sharp object, bayonet
war operations —*see* War operations, combat
stated as undetermined whether accidental or intentional Y28.8
suicide (attempt) X78.2

Bean in nose —*see* categories T17 and T18

Bed set on fire NEC —*see* Exposure, fire, uncontrolled, building, bed

Beheading (by guillotine)
homicide X99.9
legal execution —*see* Legal, intervention

Bending, injury in (prolonged) (static) X50.1

Bends —*see* Air, pressure, change

Bite, bitten by
alligator W58.01
arthropod (nonvenomous) NEC W57
bull W55.21
cat W55.01
cow W55.21
crocodile W58.11
dog W54.0
goat W55.31
hoof stock NEC W55.31
horse W55.11
human being (accidentally) W50.3
with intent to injure or kill Y04.1
as, or caused by, a crowd or human stampede (with fall) W52
assault Y04.1
homicide (attempt) Y04.1
in
fight Y04.1
insect (nonvenomous) W57
lizard (nonvenomous) W59.01
mammal NEC W55.81
marine W56.31
marine animal (nonvenomous) W56.81
millipede W57
moray eel W56.51
mouse W53.01
person(s) (accidentally) W50.3
with intent to injure or kill Y04.1
as, or caused by, a crowd or human stampede (with fall) W52
assault Y04.1
homicide (attempt) Y04.1
in
fight Y04.1
pig W55.41
raccoon W55.51
rat W53.11
reptile W59.81
lizard W59.01
snake W59.11
turtle W59.21
terrestrial W59.81
rodent W53.81
mouse W53.01
rat W53.11
specified NEC W53.81
squirrel W53.21
shark W56.41
sheep W55.31
snake (nonvenomous) W59.11
spider (nonvenomous) W57
squirrel W53.21

Blast (air) **in war operations** —*see* War operations, blast

Blizzard X37.2

Blood alcohol level Y90.9
less than 20mg/100ml Y90.0
presence in blood, level not specified Y90.9
20-39mg/100ml Y90.1
40-59mg/100ml Y90.2
60-79mg/100ml Y90.3
80-99mg/100ml Y90.4
100-119mg/100ml Y90.5
120-199mg/100ml Y90.6
200-239mg/100ml Y90.7

Blow X58
by law-enforcing agent, police (on duty) —*see* Legal, intervention, manhandling
blunt object —*see* Legal, intervention, blunt object

Blowing up —*see* Explosion

Brawl (hand) (fists) (foot) Y04.0

Breakage (accidental) (part of)
ladder (causing fall) W11
scaffolding (causing fall) W12

Broken
glass, contact with —*see* Contact, with, glass
power line (causing electric shock) W85

Bumping against, into (accidentally)
object NEC W22.8
with fall —*see* Fall, due to, bumping against, object
caused by crowd or human stampede (with fall) W52
sports equipment W21.9
person(s) W51
with fall W03
due to ice or snow W00.0
assault Y04.2
caused by, a crowd or human stampede (with fall) W52
homicide (attempt) Y04.2
sports equipment W21.9

Burn, burned, burning (accidental) (by) (from) (on)
acid NEC —*see* Table of Drugs and Chemicals
bed linen —*see* Exposure, fire, uncontrolled, in building, bed
blowtorch X08.8
with ignition of clothing NEC X06.2
nightwear X05
bonfire, campfire (controlled) —*see also* Exposure, fire, controlled, not in building
uncontrolled —*see* Exposure, fire, uncontrolled, not in building
candle X08.8
with ignition of clothing NEC X06.2
nightwear X05
caustic liquid, substance (external) (internal) NEC —*see* Table of Drugs and Chemicals
chemical (external) (internal) —*see also* Table of Drugs and Chemicals
in war operations —*see* War operations. fire
cigar(s) or cigarette(s) X08.8
with ignition of clothing NEC X06.2
nightwear X05
clothes, clothing NEC (from controlled fire) X06.2
with conflagration —*see* Exposure, fire, uncontrolled, building

Burn, burned, burning *(continued)*
clothes, clothing NEC *(continued)*
with conflagration *(continued)*
not in building or structure —*see* Exposure, fire, uncontrolled, not in building
cooker (hot) X15.8
stated as undetermined whether accidental or intentional Y27.3
suicide (attempt) X77.3
electric blanket X16
engine (hot) X17
fire, flames —*see* Exposure, fire
flare, Very pistol —*see* Discharge, firearm NEC
heat
from appliance (electrical) (household) X15.8
cooker X15.8
hotplate X15.2
kettle X15.8
light bulb X15.8
saucepan X15.3
skillet X15.3
stove X15.0
stated as undetermined whether accidental or intentional Y27.3
suicide (attempt) X77.3
toaster X15.1
in local application or packing during medical or surgical procedure Y63.5
heating
appliance, radiator or pipe X16
homicide (attempt) —*see* Assault, burning
hot
air X14.1
cooker X15.8
drink X10.0
engine X17
fat X10.2
fluid NEC X12
food X10.1
gases X14.1
heating appliance X16
household appliance NEC X15.8
kettle X15.8
liquid NEC X12
machinery X17
metal (molten) (liquid) NEC X18
object (not producing fire or flames) NEC X19
oil (cooking) X10.2
pipe(s) X16
radiator X16
saucepan (glass) (metal) X15.3
stove (kitchen) X15.0
substance NEC X19
caustic or corrosive NEC —*see* Table of Drugs and Chemicals
toaster X15.1
tool X17
vapor X13.1
water (tap) —*see* Contact, with, hot, tap water
hotplate X15.2
suicide (attempt) X77.3
ignition —*see* Ignition
in war operations —*see* War operations, fire
inflicted by other person X97
by hot objects, hot vapor, and steam —*see* Assault, burning, hot object

Burn, burned, burning *(continued)*
- internal, from swallowed caustic, corrosive liquid, substance —*see* Table of Drugs and Chemicals
- iron (hot) X15.8
  - stated as undetermined whether accidental or intentional Y27.3
  - suicide (attempt) X77.3
- kettle (hot) X15.8
  - stated as undetermined whether accidental or intentional Y27.3
  - suicide (attempt) X77.3
- lamp (flame) X08.8
  - with ignition of clothing NEC X06.2
    - nightwear X05
- lighter (cigar) (cigarette) X08.8
  - with ignition of clothing NEC X06.2
    - nightwear X05
- lightning —*see* subcategory T75.0
  - causing fire —*see* Exposure, fire
- liquid (boiling) (hot) NEC X12
  - stated as undetermined whether accidental or intentional Y27.2
  - suicide (attempt) X77.2
- local application of externally applied substance in medical or surgical care Y63.5
- machinery (hot) X17
- matches X08.8
  - with ignition of clothing NEC X06.2
    - nightwear X05
- mattress —*see* Exposure, fire, uncontrolled, building, bed
- medicament, externally applied Y63.5
- metal (hot) (liquid) (molten) NEC X18
- nightwear (nightclothes, nightdress, gown, pajamas, robe) X05
- object (hot) NEC X19
- on board watercraft
  - due to
    - accident to watercraft V91.09
      - powered craft V91.03
        - ferry boat V91.01
        - fishing boat V91.02
        - jetskis V91.03
        - liner V91.01
        - merchant ship V91.00
        - passenger ship V91.01
      - unpowered craft V91.08
        - canoe V91.05
        - inflatable V91.06
        - kayak V91.05
        - sailboat V91.04
        - surf-board V91.08
        - water skis V91.07
        - windsurfer V91.08
    - fire on board V93.09
      - ferry boat V93.01
      - fishing boat V93.02
      - jetskis V93.03
      - liner V93.01
      - merchant ship V93.00
      - passenger ship V93.01
      - powered craft NEC V93.03
      - sailboat V93.04
    - specified heat source NEC on board V93.19
      - ferry boat V93.11
      - fishing boat V93.12
      - jetskis V93.13
      - liner V93.11
      - merchant ship V93.10
      - passenger ship V93.11
      - powered craft NEC V93.13
      - sailboat V93.14

Burn, burned, burning *(continued)*
- pipe (hot) X16
  - smoking X08.8
    - with ignition of clothing NEC X06.2
      - nightwear X05
- powder —*see* Powder burn
- radiator (hot) X16
- saucepan (hot) (glass) (metal) X15.3
  - stated as undetermined whether accidental or intentional Y27.3
  - suicide (attempt) X77.3
- self-inflicted X76
  - stated as undetermined whether accidental or intentional Y26
- steam X13.1
  - pipe X16
    - stated as undetermined whether accidental or intentional Y27.8
  - stated as undetermined whether accidental or intentional Y27.0
  - suicide (attempt) X77.0
- stove (hot) (kitchen) X15.0
  - stated as undetermined whether accidental or intentional Y27.3
  - suicide (attempt) X77.3
- substance (hot) NEC X19
  - boiling X12
    - stated as undetermined whether accidental or intentional Y27.2
    - suicide (attempt) X77.2
  - molten (metal) X18
- suicide (attempt) NEC X76
  - hot
    - household appliance X77.3
    - object X77.9
- therapeutic misadventure
  - heat in local application or packing during medical or surgical procedure Y63.5
  - overdose of radiation Y63.2
- toaster (hot) X15.1
  - stated as undetermined whether accidental or intentional Y27.3
  - suicide (attempt) X77.3
- tool (hot) X17
- torch, welding X08.8
  - with ignition of clothing NEC X06.2
    - nightwear X05
- trash fire (controlled) —*see* Exposure, fire, controlled, not in building
  - uncontrolled —*see* Exposure, fire, uncontrolled, not in building
- vapor (hot) X13.1
  - stated as undetermined whether accidental or intentional Y27.0
  - suicide (attempt) X77.0
- Very pistol —*see* Discharge, firearm NEC

Butted by animal W55.82
- bull W55.22
- cow W55.22
- goat W55.32
- horse W55.12
- pig W55.42
- sheep W55.32

C

Caisson disease —*see* Air, pressure, change

Campfire (exposure to) (controlled) —*see also* Exposure, fire, controlled, not in building

Campfire *(continued)*
- uncontrolled —*see* Exposure, fire, uncontrolled, not in building

Capital punishment (any means) —*see* Legal, intervention

Car sickness T75.3

Casualty (not due to war) NEC X58
- war —*see* War operations

Cat
- bite W55.01
- scratch W55.03

Cataclysm, cataclysmic (any injury) NEC —*see* Forces of nature

Catching fire —*see* Exposure, fire

Caught
- between
  - folding object W23.0
  - objects (moving) (stationary and moving) W23.0
    - and machinery —*see* Contact, with, by type of machine
    - stationary W23.1
  - sliding door and door frame W23.0
- by, in
  - machinery (moving parts of) —*see* Contact, with, by type of machine
  - washing-machine wringer W23.0
- under packing crate (due to losing grip) W23.1

Cave-in caused by cataclysmic earth surface movement or eruption —*see* Landslide

Change(s) in air pressure —*see* Air, pressure, change

Choked, choking (on) (any object except food or vomitus)
- food (bone) (seed) —*see* categories T17 and T18
- vomitus T17.81-

Civil insurrection —*see* War operations

Cloudburst (any injury) X37.8

Cold, exposure to (accidental) (excessive) (extreme) (natural) (place) NEC —*see* Exposure, cold

Collapse
- building W20.1
  - burning (uncontrolled fire) X00.2
- dam or man-made structure (causing earth movement) X36.0
- machinery —*see* Contact, with, by type of machine
- structure W20.1
  - burning (uncontrolled fire) X00.2

Collision (accidental) NEC —*see also* Accident, transport V89.9
- pedestrian W51
  - with fall W03
  - due to ice or snow W00.0
    - involving pedestrian conveyance —*see* Accident, transport, pedestrian, conveyance
  - and
    - crowd or human stampede (with fall) W52
    - object W22.8
      - with fall —*see* Fall, due to, bumping against, object
- person(s) —*see* Collision, pedestrian
- transport vehicle NEC V89.9

Collision *(continued)*
- transport vehicle NEC *(continued)*
  - and
    - avalanche, fallen or not moving —*see* Accident, transport
      - falling or moving —*see* Landslide
    - landslide, fallen or not moving —*see* Accident, transport
      - falling or moving —*see* Landslide
  - due to cataclysm —*see* Forces of nature, by type
  - intentional, purposeful suicide (attempt) —*see* Suicide, collision

Combustion, spontaneous —*see* Ignition

Complication (delayed) of or following (medical or surgical procedure) Y84.9
- with misadventure —*see* Misadventure
- amputation of limb(s) Y83.5
- anastomosis (arteriovenous) (blood vessel) (gastrojejunal) (tendon) (natural or artificial material) Y83.2
- aspiration (of fluid) Y84.4
  - tissue Y84.8
- biopsy Y84.8
- blood
  - sampling Y84.7
  - transfusion
    - procedure Y84.8
- bypass Y83.2
- catheterization (urinary) Y84.6
  - cardiac Y84.0
- colostomy Y83.3
- cystostomy Y83.3
- dialysis (kidney) Y84.1
- drug —*see* Table of Drugs and Chemicals
- due to misadventure —*see* Misadventure
- duodenostomy Y83.3
- electroshock therapy Y84.3
- external stoma, creation of Y83.3
- formation of external stoma Y83.3
- gastrostomy Y83.3
- graft Y83.2
- hypothermia (medically-induced) Y84.8
- implant, implantation (of)
  - artificial
    - internal device (cardiac pacemaker) (electrodes in brain) (heart valve prosthesis) (orthopedic) Y83.1
    - material or tissue (for anastomosis or bypass) Y83.2
  - with creation of external stoma Y83.3
  - natural tissues (for anastomosis or bypass) Y83.2
    - with creation of external stoma Y83.3
- infusion
  - procedure Y84.8
- injection —*see* Table of Drugs and Chemicals
  - procedure Y84.8
- insertion of gastric or duodenal sound Y84.5
- insulin-shock therapy Y84.3
- paracentesis (abdominal) (thoracic) (aspirative) Y84.4

Complication *(continued)*
- procedures other than surgical operation *—see* Complication of or following, by type of procedure
- radiological procedure or therapy Y84.2
- removal of organ (partial) (total) NEC Y83.6
- sampling
  - blood Y84.7
  - fluid NEC Y84.4
  - tissue Y84.8
- shock therapy Y84.3
- surgical operation NEC *—see also* Complication of or following, by type of operation Y83.9
  - reconstructive NEC Y83.4
    - with
      - anastomosis, bypass or graft Y83.2
      - formation of external stoma Y83.3
  - specified NEC Y83.8
- transfusion *—see also* Table of Drugs and Chemicals
  - procedure Y84.8
- transplant, transplantation (heart) (kidney) (liver) (whole organ, any) Y83.0
  - partial organ Y83.4
- ureterostomy Y83.3
- vaccination *—see also* Table of Drugs and Chemicals
  - procedure Y84.8

Compression
- divers' squeeze *—see* Air, pressure, change
- trachea by
  - food (lodged in esophagus) *—see* categories T17 and T18
  - vomitus (lodged in esophagus) T17.81-

Conflagration *—see* Exposure, fire, uncontrolled

Constriction (external)
- hair W49.01
- jewelry W49.04
- ring W49.04
- rubber band W49.03
- specified item NEC W49.09
- string W49.02
- thread W49.02

Contact (accidental)
- with
  - abrasive wheel (metalworking) W31.1
  - alligator W58.09
    - bite W58.01
    - crushing W58.03
    - strike W58.02
  - amphibian W62.9
    - frog W62.0
    - toad W62.1
  - animal (nonvenomous) NEC W64
    - marine W56.89
      - bite W56.81
      - dolphin *—see* Contact, with, dolphin
      - fish NEC *—see* Contact, with, fish
      - mammal *—see* Contact, with, mammal, marine
      - orca *—see* Contact, with, orca
      - sea lion *—see* Contact, with, sea lion

Contact *(continued)*
- with *(continued)*
  - animal *(continued)*
    - marine *(continued)*
      - shark *—see* Contact, with, shark
      - strike W56.82
  - animate mechanical force NEC W64
  - arrow W21.89
    - not thrown, projected or falling W45.8
  - arthropods (nonvenomous) W57
  - axe W27.0
  - band-saw (industrial) W31.2
  - bayonet *—see* Bayonet wound
  - bee(s) X58
  - bench-saw (industrial) W31.2
  - bird W61.99
    - bite W61.91
    - chicken *—see* Contact, with, chicken
    - duck *—see* Contact, with, duck
    - goose *—see* Contact, with, goose
    - macaw *—see* Contact, with, macaw
    - parrot *—see* Contact, with, parrot
    - psittacine *—see* Contact, with, psittacine
    - strike W61.92
    - turkey *—see* Contact, with, turkey
  - blender W29.0
  - boiling water X12
    - stated as undetermined whether accidental or intentional Y27.2
    - suicide (attempt) X77.2
  - bore, earth-drilling or mining (land) (seabed) W31.0
  - buffalo *—see* Contact, with, hoof stock NEC
  - bull W55.29
    - bite W55.21
    - gored W55.22
    - strike W55.22
  - bumper cars W31.81
  - camel *—see* Contact, with, hoof stock NEC
  - can
    - lid W26.8
    - opener W27.4
      - powered W29.0
  - cat W55.09
    - bite W55.01
    - scratch W55.03
  - caterpillar (venomous) X58
  - centipede (venomous) X58
  - chain
    - hoist W24.0
      - agricultural operations W30.89
    - saw W29.3
  - chicken W61.39
    - peck W61.33
    - strike W61.32
  - chisel W27.0
  - circular saw W31.2
  - cobra X58
  - combine (harvester) W30.0
  - conveyer belt W24.1
  - cooker (hot) X15.8
    - stated as undetermined whether accidental or intentional Y27.3
    - suicide (attempt) X77.3
  - coral X58

Contact *(continued)*
- with *(continued)*
  - cotton gin W31.82
  - cow W55.29
    - bite W55.21
    - strike W55.22
  - crane W24.0
    - agricultural operations W30.89
  - crocodile W58.19
    - bite W58.11
    - crushing W58.13
    - strike W58.12
  - dagger W26.1
    - stated as undetermined whether accidental or intentional Y28.2
    - suicide (attempt) X78.2
  - dairy equipment W31.82
  - dart W21.89
    - not thrown, projected or falling W45.8
  - deer *—see* Contact, with, hoof stock NEC
  - derrick W24.0
    - agricultural operations W30.89
      - hay W30.2
  - dog W54.8
    - bite W54.0
    - strike W54.1
  - dolphin W56.09
    - bite W56.01
    - strike W56.02
  - donkey *—see* Contact, with, hoof stock NEC
  - drill (powered) W29.8
    - earth (land) (seabed) W31.0
    - nonpowered W27.8
  - drive belt W24.0
    - agricultural operations W30.89
  - dry ice *—see* Exposure, cold, man-made
  - dryer (clothes) (powered) (spin) W29.2
  - duck W61.69
    - bite W61.61
    - strike W61.62
  - earth (-)
    - drilling machine (industrial) W31.0
    - scraping machine in stationary use W31.83
  - edge of stiff paper W26.2
  - electric
    - beater W29.0
    - blanket X16
    - fan W29.2
      - commercial W31.82
    - knife W29.1
    - mixer W29.0
  - elevator (building) W24.0
    - agricultural operations W30.89
      - grain W30.3
  - engine(s), hot NEC X17
  - excavating machine W31.0
  - farm machine W30.9
  - feces *—see* Contact, with, by type of animal
  - fer de lance X58
  - fish W56.59
    - bite W56.51
    - shark *—see* Contact, with, shark
    - strike W56.52
  - flying horses W31.81
  - forging (metalworking) machine W31.1
  - fork W27.4
  - forklift (truck) W24.0

Contact *(continued)*
- with *(continued)*
  - forklift *(continued)*
    - agricultural operations W30.89
  - frog W62.0
  - garden
    - cultivator (powered) W29.3
      - riding W30.89
    - fork W27.1
  - gas turbine W31.3
  - Gila monster X58
  - giraffe *—see* Contact, with, hoof stock NEC
  - glass (sharp) (broken) W25
    - with subsequent fall W18.02
    - assault X99.0
    - due to fall *—see* Fall, by type
    - stated as undetermined whether accidental or intentional Y28.0
    - suicide (attempt) X78.0
  - goat W55.39
    - bite W55.31
    - strike W55.32
  - goose W61.59
    - bite W61.51
    - strike W61.52
  - hand
    - saw W27.0
    - tool (not powered) NEC W27.8
      - powered W29.8
  - harvester W30.0
  - hay-derrick W30.2
  - heat NEC X19
    - from appliance (electrical) (household) *—see* Contact, with, hot, household appliance
      - heating appliance X16
  - heating
    - appliance (hot) X16
    - pad (electric) X16
  - hedge-trimmer (powered) W29.3
  - hoe W27.1
  - hoist (chain) (shaft) NEC W24.0
    - agricultural W30.89
  - hoof stock NEC W55.39
    - bite W55.31
    - strike W55.32
  - hornet(s) X58
  - horse W55.19
    - bite W55.11
    - strike W55.12
  - hot
    - air X14.1
      - inhalation X14.0
    - cooker X15.8
    - drinks X10.0
    - engine X17
    - fats X10.2
    - fluids NEC X12
      - assault X98.2
      - suicide (attempt) X77.2
      - undetermined whether accidental or intentional Y27.2
    - food X10.1
    - gases X14.1
      - inhalation X14.0
    - heating appliance X16
    - household appliance X15.8
      - assault X98.3
      - cooker X15.8
      - hotplate X15.2
      - kettle X15.8
      - light bulb X15.8
      - object NEC X19
        - assault X98.8

D

Fight (hand) (fists) (foot) —*see* Assault, fight

Fire (accidental) —*see* Exposure, fire

Firearm discharge —*see* Discharge, firearm

Fireball effects from nuclear explosion in war operations —*see* War operations, nuclear weapons

Fireworks (explosion) W39

Flash burns from explosion —*see* Explosion

Flood (any injury) (caused by) X38
- collapse of man-made structure causing earth movement X36.0
- tidal wave —*see* Forces of nature, tidal wave

Food (any type) in
- air passages (with asphyxia, obstruction, or suffocation) —*see* categories T17 and T18
- alimentary tract causing asphyxia (due to compression of trachea) —*see* categories T17 and T18

Forces of nature X39.8
- avalanche X36.1
  - causing transport accident —*see* Accident, transport, by type of vehicle
- blizzard X37.2
- cataclysmic storm X37.9
  - with flood X38
  - blizzard X37.2
  - cloudburst X37.8
  - cyclone X37.1
  - dust storm X37.3
  - hurricane X37.0
  - specified storm NEC X37.8
  - storm surge X37.0
  - tornado X37.1
  - twister X37.1
  - typhoon X37.0
- cloudburst X37.8
- cold (natural) X31
- cyclone X37.1
- dam collapse causing earth movementX36.0
- dust storm X37.3
- earth movement X36.1
  - earthquake X34
  - caused by dam or structure collapse X36.0
- earthquake X34
- flood (caused by) X38
  - dam collapse X36.0
  - tidal wave —*see* Forces of nature, tidal wave
- heat (natural) X30
- hurricane X37.0
- landslide X36.1
  - causing transport accident —*see* Accident, transport, by type of vehicle
- lightning —*see subcategory* T75.0
  - causing fire —*see* Exposure, fire
- mudslide X36.1
  - causing transport accident —*see* Accident, transport, by type of vehicle
- radiation (natural) X39.08
  - radon X39.01
- radon X39.01
- specified force NEC X39.8
- storm surge X37.0

Forces of nature *(continued)*
- structure collapse causing earth movement X36.0
- sunlight X32
- tidal wave X37.41
  - due to
    - earthquake X37.41
    - landslide X37.43
    - storm X37.42
    - volcanic eruption X37.41
- tornado X37.1
- tsunami X37.41
- twister X37.1
- typhoon X37.0
- volcanic eruption X35

Foreign body
- aspiration —*see* Index to Diseases and Injuries, Foreign body, respiratory tract
- embedded in skin W45.-

entering through skin W45.8
- can lid W26.8
- nail W45.0
- paper W26.2
- specified NEC W45.8
- splinter W45.8

Forest fire (exposure to) —*see* Exposure, fire, uncontrolled, not in building

Found injured X58
- from exposure (to) —*see* Exposure
- on
  - highway, road (way), street V89.9
  - railway right of way V81.9

Fracture (circumstances unknown or unspecified) X58
- due to specified cause NEC X58

Freezing —*see* Exposure, cold

Frostbite X31
- due to man-made conditions —*see* Exposure, cold, man-made

Frozen —*see* Exposure, cold

G

Gored by bull W55.22

Gunshot wound W34.00

H

Hailstones, injured by X39.8

Hanged herself or himself —*see* Hanging, self-inflicted

Hanging (accidental) —*see also* category T71
- legal execution —*see* Legal, intervention, specified means NEC

Heat (effects of) (excessive) X30
- due to
  - man-made conditions W92
    - on board watercraft V93.29
      - fishing boat V93.22
      - merchant ship V93.20
      - passenger ship V93.21
      - sailboat V93.24
      - specified powered craft NEC V93.23
  - weather (conditions) X30
- from
  - electric heating apparatus causing burning X16
  - nuclear explosion in war operations —*see* War operations, nuclear weapons

Heat *(continued)*
- inappropriate in local application or packing in medical or surgical procedure Y63.5

Hemorrhage
- delayed following medical or surgical treatment without mention of misadventure —*see* Index to Diseases and Injuries, Complication(s)
- during medical or surgical treatment as misadventure —*see* Index to Diseases and Injuries, Complication(s)

High
- altitude (effects) —*see* Air, pressure, low
- level of radioactivity, effects —*see* Radiation
- pressure (effects) —*see* Air, pressure, high
- temperature, effects —*see* Heat

Hit, hitting (accidental) by —*see* Struck by

Hitting against —*see* Striking against

Homicide (attempt) (justifiable) —*see* Assault

Hot
- place, effects —*see also* Heat
- weather, effects X30

House fire (uncontrolled) —*see* Exposure, fire, uncontrolled, building

Humidity, causing problem X39.8

Hunger X58

Hurricane (any injury) X37.0

Hypobarism, hypobaropathy —*see* Air, pressure, low

I

Ictus
- caloris —*see also* Heat
- solaris X30

Ignition (accidental) —*see also* Exposure, fire X08.8
- anesthetic gas in operating room W40.1
- apparel X06.2
  - from highly flammable material X04
  - nightwear X05
- bed linen (sheets) (spreads) (pillows) (mattress) —*see* Exposure, fire, uncontrolled, building, bed
- benzine X04
- clothes, clothing NEC (from controlled fire) X06.2
  - from
    - highly flammable material X04
- ether X04
  - in operating room W40.1
- explosive material —*see* Explosion
- gasoline X04
- jewelry (plastic) (any) X06.0
- kerosene X04
- material
  - explosive —*see* Explosion
  - highly flammable with secondary explosion X04
- nightwear X05
- paraffin X04
- petrol X04

Immersion (accidental) —*see also* Drowning
- hand or foot due to cold (excessive) X31

Implantation of quills of porcupine W55.89

Inanition (from) (hunger) X58
- thirst X58

Inappropriate operation performed
- correct operation on wrong side or body part (wrong side) (wrong site) Y65.53
- operation intended for another patient done on wrong patient Y65.52
- wrong operation performed on correct patient Y65.51

Inattention after, at birth (homicidal intent) (infanticidal intent) X58

Incident, adverse
- device
  - anesthesiology Y70.8
    - accessory Y70.2
    - diagnostic Y70.0
    - miscellaneous Y70.8
    - monitoring Y70.0
    - prosthetic Y70.2
    - rehabilitative Y70.1
    - surgical Y70.3
    - therapeutic Y70.1
  - cardiovascular Y71.8
    - accessory Y71.2
    - diagnostic Y71.0
    - miscellaneous Y71.8
    - monitoring Y71.0
    - prosthetic Y71.2
    - rehabilitative Y71.1
    - surgical Y71.3
    - therapeutic Y71.1
  - gastroenterology Y73.8
    - accessory Y73.2
    - diagnostic Y73.0
    - miscellaneous Y73.8
    - monitoring Y73.0
    - prosthetic Y73.2
    - rehabilitative Y73.1
    - surgical Y73.3
    - therapeutic Y73.1
  - general
    - hospital Y74.8
      - accessory Y74.2
      - diagnostic Y74.0
      - miscellaneous Y74.8
      - monitoring Y74.0
      - prosthetic Y74.2
      - rehabilitative Y74.1
      - surgical Y74.3
      - therapeutic Y74.1
    - surgical Y81.8
      - accessory Y81.2
      - diagnostic Y81.0
      - miscellaneous Y81.8
      - monitoring Y81.0
      - prosthetic Y81.2
      - rehabilitative Y81.1
      - surgical Y81.3
      - therapeutic Y81.1
  - gynecological Y76.8
    - accessory Y76.2
    - diagnostic Y76.0
    - miscellaneous Y76.8
    - monitoring Y76.0
    - prosthetic Y76.2
    - rehabilitative Y76.1
    - surgical Y76.3
    - therapeutic Y76.1
  - medical Y82.9
    - specified type NEC Y82.8

Knocked down *(continued)*
- crowd or human stampede W52
- person W51
  - in brawl, fight Y04.0
- transport vehicle NEC —*see also* Accident, transport V09.9

L

Laceration NEC —*see* Injury

Lack of
- care (helpless person) (infant) (newborn) X58
- food except as result of abandonment or neglect X58
  - due to abandonment or neglect X58
- water except as result of transport accident X58
  - due to transport accident —*see* Accident, transport, by type
  - helpless person, infant, newborn X58

Landslide (falling on transport vehicle) X36.1
- caused by collapse of man-made structure X36.0

Late effect —*see* Sequelae

Legal
- execution (any method) —*see* Legal, intervention
- intervention (by)
  - baton —*see* Legal, intervention, blunt object, baton
  - bayonet —*see* Legal, intervention, sharp object, bayonet
  - blow —*see* Legal, intervention, manhandling
  - blunt object
    - baton
      - injuring
        - bystander Y35.312
        - law enforcement personnel Y35.311
        - suspect Y35.313
        - unspecified person Y35.319
    - injuring
      - bystander Y35.302
      - law enforcement personnel Y35.301
      - suspect Y35.303
      - unspecified person Y35.309
    - specified NEC
      - injuring
        - bystander Y35.392
        - law enforcement personnel Y35.391
        - suspect Y35.393
        - unspecified person Y35.399
    - stave
      - injuring
        - bystander Y35.392
        - law enforcement personnel Y35.391
        - suspect Y35.393
        - unspecified person Y35.399
  - bomb —*see* Legal, intervention, explosive
  - conducted energy device
    - injuring
      - bystander Y35.832
      - law enforcement personnel Y35.831
      - suspect Y35.833
      - unspecified person Y35.839
  - cutting or piercing instrument —*see* Legal, intervention, sharp object

Legal *(continued)*
- intervention *(continued)*
  - dynamite —*see* Legal, intervention, explosive, dynamite
  - electroshock device (taser)
    - injuring
      - bystander Y35.832
      - law enforcement personnel Y35.831
      - suspect Y35.833
      - unspecified person Y35.839
  - explosive(s)
    - dynamite
      - injuring
        - bystander Y35.112
        - law enforcement personnel Y35.111
        - suspect Y35.113
        - unspecified person Y35.119
    - grenade
      - injuring
        - bystander Y35.192
        - law enforcement personnel Y35.191
        - suspect Y35.193
        - unspecified person Y35.199
    - injuring
      - bystander Y35.102
      - law enforcement personnel Y35.101
      - suspect Y35.103
      - unspecified person Y35.109
    - mortar bomb
      - injuring
        - bystander Y35.192
        - law enforcement personnel Y35.191
        - suspect Y35.193
        - unspecified person Y35.199
    - shell
      - injuring
        - bystander Y35.122
        - law enforcement personnel Y35.121
        - suspect Y35.123
        - unspecified person Y35.129
    - specified NEC
      - injuring
        - bystander Y35.192
        - law enforcement personnel Y35.191
        - suspect Y35.193
        - unspecified person Y35.199
  - firearm(s) (discharge)
    - handgun
      - injuring
        - bystander Y35.022
        - law enforcement personnel Y35.021
        - suspect Y35.023
        - unspecified person Y35.029
    - injuring
      - bystander Y35.002
      - law enforcement personnel Y35.001
      - suspect Y35.003
      - unspecified person Y35.009
    - machine gun
      - injuring
        - bystander Y35.012
        - law enforcement personnel Y35.011
        - suspect Y35.013
        - unspecified person Y35.019

Legal *(continued)*
- intervention *(continued)*
  - firearm *(continued)*
    - rifle pellet
      - injuring
        - bystander Y35.032
        - law enforcement personnel Y35.031
        - suspect Y35.033
        - unspecified person Y35.039
    - rubber bullet
      - injuring
        - bystander Y35.042
        - law enforcement personnel Y35.041
        - suspect Y35.043
        - unspecified person Y35.049
    - shotgun —*see* Legal, intervention, firearm, specified NEC
    - specified NEC
      - injuring
        - bystander Y35.092
        - law enforcement personnel Y35.091
        - suspect Y35.093
        - unspecified person Y35.099
  - gas (asphyxiation) (poisoning)
    - injuring
      - bystander Y35.202
      - law enforcement personnel Y35.201
      - suspect Y35.203
      - unspecified person Y35.209
    - specified NEC
      - injuring
        - bystander Y35.292
        - law enforcement personnel Y35.291
        - suspect Y35.293
        - unspecified person Y35.299
    - tear gas
      - injuring
        - bystander Y35.212
        - law enforcement personnel Y35.211
        - suspect Y35.213
        - unspecified person Y35.219
  - grenade —*see* Legal, intervention, explosive, grenade
  - injuring
    - bystander Y35.92
    - law enforcement personnel Y35.91
    - suspect Y35.93
    - unspecified person Y35.99
  - late effect (of) —*see* with 7th character S Y35
  - manhandling
    - injuring
      - bystander Y35.812
      - law enforcement personnel Y35.811
      - suspect Y35.813
      - unspecified person Y35.819
  - sequelae (of) —*see* with 7th character S Y35
  - sharp objects
    - bayonet
      - injuring
        - bystander Y35.412
        - law enforcement personnel Y35.411
        - suspect Y35.413
        - unspecified person Y35.419

Legal *(continued)*
- intervention *(continued)*
  - sharp object *(continued)*
    - injuring
      - bystander Y35.402
      - law enforcement personnel Y35.401
      - suspect Y35.403
      - unspecified person Y35.409
    - specified NEC
      - injuring
        - bystander Y35.492
        - law enforcement personnel Y35.491
        - suspect Y35.493
        - unspecified person Y35.499
  - specified means NEC
    - injuring
      - bystander Y35.892
      - law enforcement personnel Y35.891
      - suspect Y35.893
      - unspecified person Y35.899
  - stabbing —*see* Legal, intervention, sharp object
  - stave —*see* Legal, intervention, blunt object, stave
  - stun gun
    - injuring
      - bystander Y35.832
      - law enforcement personnel Y35.831
      - suspect Y35.833
      - unspecified person Y35.839
  - taser
    - injuring
      - bystander Y35.832
      - law enforcement personnel Y35.831
      - suspect Y35.833
      - unspecified person Y35.839
  - tear gas —*see* Legal, intervention, gas, tear gas
  - truncheon —*see* Legal, intervention, blunt object, stave

Lifting - *see also* Overexertion
- heavy objects X50.0
- weights X50.0

Lightning (shock) (stroke) (struck by) —*see* subcategory T75.0
- causing fire —*see* Exposure, fire

Loss of control (transport vehicle) NEC —*see* Accident, transport

Lost at sea NOS —*see* Drowning, due to, fall overboard

Low
- pressure (effects) —*see* Air, pressure, low
- temperature (effects) —*see* Exposure, cold

Lying before train, vehicle or other moving object X81.8
- subway train X81.1
- train X81.1
- undetermined whether accidental or intentional Y31

Lynching —*see* Assault

M

Malfunction (mechanism or component) (of)
- firearm W34.10
  - airgun W34.110
  - BB gun W34.110
  - gas, air or spring-operated gun NEC W34.118
  - handgun W32.1

Misadventure(s) to patient(s) during surgical or medical care *(continued)*
- puncture *—see* Index to Diseases and Injuries, Complication(s)
- specified type NEC Y65.8
  - failure
    - suture or ligature during surgical operation Y65.2
    - to introduce or to remove tube or instrument *—see* Failure, to
  - infusion of wrong fluid Y65.1
  - performance of inappropriate operation *—see* Inappropriate operation performed
  - transfusion of mismatched blood Y65.0
  - wrong
    - drug given in error *—see* Table of Drugs and Chemicals
    - fluid in infusion Y65.1
    - placement of endotracheal tube during anesthetic procedure Y65.3
- transfusion *—see* Misadventure, by type, transfusion
  - excessive amount of blood Y63.0
  - mismatched blood Y65.0
- wrong
  - drug given in error *—see* Table of Drugs and Chemicals
  - fluid in infusion Y65.1
  - placement of endotracheal tube during anesthetic procedure Y65.3

Mismatched blood in transfusion Y65.0

Motion sickness T75.3

Mountain sickness W94.11

Mudslide (of cataclysmic nature) *—see* Landslide

Murder (attempt) *—see* Assault

N

Nail
- contact with W45.0
  - gun W29.4
- embedded in skin W45.0

Neglect (criminal) (homicidal intent) X58

Noise (causing injury) (pollution) W42.9
- supersonic W42.0

Nonadministration (of)
- drug or biological substance (necessary) Y63.6
- surgical and medical care Y66

Nosocomial condition Y95

O

Object
- falling
  - from, in, on, hitting
    - machinery *—see* Contact, with, by type of machine
- set in motion by
  - accidental explosion or rupture of pressure vessel W38
  - firearm *—see* Discharge, firearm, by type
  - machine (ry) *—see* Contact, with, by type of machine

Overdose (drug) *—see* Table of Drugs and Chemicals
- radiation Y63.2

Overexertion X50.9
- from
  - prolonged static or awkward postures X50.1
  - repetitive movements X50.3
  - specified strenuous movements or postures NEC X50.9
  - strenuous movement or load X50.0

Overexposure (accidental) (to)
- cold *—see also* Exposure, cold X31
  - due to man-made conditions *—see* Exposure, cold, man-made
- heat *—see also* Heat X30
- radiation *—see* Radiation
- radioactivity W88.0
- sun (sunburn) X32
- weather NEC *—see* Forces of nature
- wind NEC *—see* Forces of nature

Overheated *—see* Heat

Overturning (accidental)
- machinery *—see* Contact, with, by type of machine
- transport vehicle NEC *—see also* Accident, transport V89.9
- watercraft (causing drowning, submersion) *—see also* Drowning, due to, accident to, watercraft, overturning
  - causing injury except drowning or submersion *—see* Accident, watercraft, causing, injury NEC

P

Parachute descent (voluntary) (without accident to aircraft) V97.29
- due to accident to aircraft *—see* Accident, transport, aircraft

Pecked by bird W61.99

Perforation during medical or surgical treatment as misadventure *—see* Index to Diseases and Injuries, Complication(s)

Perpetrator, perpetration, of assault, maltreatment and neglect (by) Y07.9
- boyfriend Y07.03
- brother Y07.410
  - stepbrother Y07.435
- coach Y07.53
- cousin
  - female Y07.491
  - male Y07.490
- daycare provider Y07.519
  - at-home
    - adult care Y07.512
    - childcare Y07.510
  - care center
    - adult care Y07.513
    - childcare Y07.511
- family member NEC Y07.499
- father Y07.11
  - adoptive Y07.13
  - foster Y07.420
  - stepfather Y07.430
- foster father Y07.420
- foster mother Y07.421

Perpetrator, perpetration, of assault, maltreatment and neglect *(continued)*
- girl friend Y07.04
- healthcare provider Y07.529
  - mental health Y07.521
  - specified NEC Y07.528
- husband Y07.01
- instructor Y07.53
- mother Y07.12
  - adoptive Y07.14
  - foster Y07.421
  - stepmother Y07.433
- multiple perpetrators Y07.6
- nonfamily member Y07.50
  - specified NEC Y07.59
- nurse Y07.528
- occupational therapist Y07.528
- partner of parent
  - female Y07.434
  - male Y07.432
- physical therapist Y07.528
- sister Y07.411
- speech therapist Y07.528
- stepbrother Y07.435
- stepfather Y07.430
- stepmother Y07.433
- stepsister Y07.436
- teacher Y07.53
- wife Y07.02

Piercing *—see* Contact, with, by type of object or machine

Pinched
- between objects (moving) (stationary and moving) W23.0
  - stationary W23.1

Pinned under machine (ry) *—see* Contact, with, by type of machine

Place of occurrence Y92.9
- abandoned house Y92.89
- airplane Y92.813
- airport Y92.520
- ambulatory health services establishment NEC Y92.538
- ambulatory surgery center Y92.530
- amusement park Y92.831
- apartment (co-op) *—see* Place of occurrence, residence, apartment
- assembly hall Y92.29
- bank Y92.510
- barn Y92.71
- baseball field Y92.320
- basketball court Y92.310
- beach Y92.832
- boarding house *—see* Place of occurrence, residence, boarding house
- boat Y92.814
- bowling alley Y92.39
- bridge Y92.89
- building under construction Y92.61
- bus Y92.811
  - station Y92.521
- cafe Y92.511
- campsite Y92.833
- campus *—see* Place of occurrence, school
- canal Y92.89
- car Y92.810
- casino Y92.59
- children's home *—see* Place of occurrence, residence, institutional, orphanage
- church Y92.22
- cinema Y92.26
- clubhouse Y92.29
- coal pit Y92.64
- college (community) Y92.214

Place of occurrence *(continued)*
- condominium *—see* Place of occurrence, residence, apartment
- construction area *—see* Place of occurrence, industrial and construction area
- convalescent home *—see* Place of occurrence, residence, institutional, nursing home
- court-house Y92.240
- cricket ground Y92.328
- cultural building Y92.258
  - art gallery Y92.250
  - museum Y92.251
  - music hall Y92.252
  - opera house Y92.253
  - specified NEC Y92.258
  - theater Y92.254
- dancehall Y92.252
- day nursery Y92.210
- dentist office Y92.531
- derelict house Y92.89
- desert Y92.820
- dock NOS Y92.89
- dockyard Y92.62
- doctor's office Y92.531
- dormitory *—see* Place of occurrence, residence, institutional, school dormitory
- dry dock Y92.62
- factory (building) (premises) Y92.63
- farm (land under cultivation) (outbuildings) Y92.79
  - barn Y92.71
  - chicken coop Y92.72
  - field Y92.73
  - hen house Y92.72
  - house *—see* Place of occurrence, residence, house
  - orchard Y92.74
  - specified NEC Y92.79
- football field Y92.321
- forest Y92.821
- freeway Y92.411
- gallery Y92.250
- garage (commercial) Y92.59
  - boarding house Y92.044
  - military base Y92.135
  - mobile home Y92.025
  - nursing home Y92.124
  - orphanage Y92.114
  - private house Y92.015
  - reform school Y92.155
- gas station Y92.524
- gasworks Y92.69
- golf course Y92.39
- gravel pit Y92.64
- grocery Y92.512
- gymnasium Y92.39
- handball court Y92.318
- harbor Y92.89
- harness racing course Y92.39
- healthcare provider office Y92.531
- highway (interstate) Y92.411
- hill Y92.828
- hockey rink Y92.330
- home *—see* Place of occurrence, residence
- hospice *—see* Place of occurrence, residence, institutional, nursing home
- hospital Y92.239
  - cafeteria Y92.233
  - corridor Y92.232
  - operating room Y92.234
  - patient
    - bathroom Y92.231
    - room Y92.230
  - specified NEC Y92.238

Place of occurrence *(continued)*
- hotel Y92.59
- house *—see also* Place of occurrence, residence
  - abandoned Y92.89
  - under construction Y92.61
- industrial and construction area (yard) Y92.69
  - building under construction Y92.61
  - dock Y92.62
  - dry dock Y92.62
  - factory Y92.63
  - gasworks Y92.69
  - mine Y92.64
  - oil rig Y92.65
  - pit Y92.64
  - power station Y92.69
  - shipyard Y92.62
  - specified NEC Y92.69
  - tunnel under construction Y92.69
  - workshop Y92.69
- kindergarten Y92.211
- lacrosse field Y92.328
- lake Y92.828
- library Y92.241
- mall Y92.59
- market Y92.512
- marsh Y92.828
- military
  - base *—see* Place of occurrence, residence, institutional, military base
  - training ground Y92.84
- mine Y92.64
- mosque Y92.22
- motel Y92.59
- motorway (interstate) Y92.411
- mountain Y92.828
- movie-house Y92.26
- museum Y92.251
- music-hall Y92.252
- not applicable Y92.9
- nuclear power station Y92.69
- nursing home *—see* Place of occurrence, residence, institutional, nursing home
- office building Y92.59
- offshore installation Y92.65
- oil rig Y92.65
- old people's home *—see* Place of occurrence, residence, institutional, specified NEC
- opera-house Y92.253
- orphanage *—see* Place of occurrence, residence, institutional, orphanage
- outpatient surgery center Y92.530
- park (public) Y92.830
  - amusement Y92.831
- parking garage Y92.89
  - lot Y92.481
- pavement Y92.480
- physician office Y92.531
- polo field Y92.328
- pond Y92.828
- post office Y92.242
- power station Y92.69
- prairie Y92.828
- prison *—see* Place of occurrence, residence, institutional, prison
- public
  - administration building Y92.248
    - city hall Y92.243
    - courthouse Y92.240
    - library Y92.241
    - post office Y92.242
    - specified NEC Y92.248
  - building NEC Y92.29
  - hall Y92.29

Place of occurrence *(continued)*
- public *(continued)*
  - place NOS Y92.89
- race course Y92.39
- radio station Y92.59
- railway line (bridge) Y92.85
- ranch (outbuildings) *—see* Place of occurrence, farm
- recreation area Y92.838
  - amusement park Y92.831
  - beach Y92.832
  - campsite Y92.833
  - park (public) Y92.830
  - seashore Y92.832
  - specified NEC Y92.838
- religious institution Y92.22
- reform school *—see* Place of occurrence, residence, institutional, reform school
- residence (non-institutional) (private) Y92.009
  - apartment Y92.039
    - bathroom Y92.031
    - bedroom Y92.032
    - kitchen Y92.030
    - specified NEC Y92.038
  - bathroom Y92.002
  - bedroom Y92.003
  - boarding house Y92.049
    - bathroom Y92.041
    - bedroom Y92.042
    - driveway Y92.043
    - garage Y92.044
    - garden Y92.046
    - kitchen Y92.040
    - specified NEC Y92.048
    - swimming pool Y92.045
    - yard Y92.046
  - dining room Y92.001
  - garden Y92.007
  - home Y92.009
  - house, single family Y92.019
    - bathroom Y92.012
    - bedroom Y92.013
    - dining room Y92.011
    - driveway Y92.014
    - garage Y92.015
    - garden Y92.017
    - kitchen Y92.010
    - specified NEC Y92.018
    - swimming pool Y92.016
    - yard Y92.017
  - institutional Y92.10
    - children's home *—see* Place of occurrence, residence, institutional, orphanage
    - hospice *—see* Place of occurrence, residence, institutional, nursing home
    - military base Y92.139
      - barracks Y92.133
      - garage Y92.135
      - garden Y92.137
      - kitchen Y92.130
      - mess hall Y92.131
      - specified NEC Y92.138
      - swimming pool Y92.136
      - yard Y92.137
    - nursing home Y92.129
      - bathroom Y92.121
      - bedroom Y92.122
      - driveway Y92.123
      - garage Y92.124
      - garden Y92.126
      - kitchen Y92.120
      - specified NEC Y92.128
      - swimming pool Y92.125
      - yard Y92.126
    - orphanage Y92.119
      - bathroom Y92.111

Place of occurrence *(continued)*
- residence *(continued)*
  - institutional *(continued)*
    - orphanage *(continued)*
      - bedroom Y92.112
      - driveway Y92.113
      - garage Y92.114
      - garden Y92.116
      - kitchen Y92.110
      - specified NEC Y92.118
      - swimming pool Y92.115
      - yard Y92.116
    - prison Y92.149
      - bathroom Y92.142
      - cell Y92.143
      - courtyard Y92.147
      - dining room Y92.141
      - kitchen Y92.140
      - specified NEC Y92.148
      - swimming pool Y92.146
    - reform school Y92.159
      - bathroom Y92.152
      - bedroom Y92.153
      - dining room Y92.151
      - driveway Y92.154
      - garage Y92.155
      - garden Y92.157
      - kitchen Y92.150
      - specified NEC Y92.158
      - swimming pool Y92.156
      - yard Y92.157
    - school dormitory Y92.169
      - bathroom Y92.162
      - bedroom Y92.163
      - dining room Y92.161
      - kitchen Y92.160
      - specified NEC Y92.168
    - specified NEC Y92.199
      - bathroom Y92.192
      - bedroom Y92.193
      - dining room Y92.191
      - driveway Y92.194
      - garage Y92.195
      - garden Y92.197
      - kitchen Y92.190
      - specified NEC Y92.198
      - swimming pool Y92.196
      - yard Y92.197
  - kitchen Y92.000
  - mobile home Y92.029
    - bathroom Y92.022
    - bedroom Y92.023
    - dining room Y92.021
    - driveway Y92.024
    - garage Y92.025
    - garden Y92.027
    - kitchen Y92.020
    - specified NEC Y92.028
    - swimming pool Y92.026
    - yard Y92.027
  - specified place in residence NEC Y92.008
  - specified residence type NEC Y92.099
    - bathroom Y92.091
    - bedroom Y92.092
    - driveway Y92.093
    - garage Y92.094
    - garden Y92.096
    - kitchen Y92.090
    - specified NEC Y92.098
    - swimming pool Y92.095
    - yard Y92.096
- restaurant Y92.511
- riding school Y92.39
- river Y92.828
- road Y92.410
- rodeo ring Y92.39
- rugby field Y92.328
- same day surgery center Y92.530
- sand pit Y92.64

Place of occurrence *(continued)*
- school (private) (public) (state) Y92.219
  - college Y92.214
  - daycare center Y92.210
  - elementary school Y92.211
  - high school Y92.213
  - kindergarten Y92.211
  - middle school Y92.212
  - specified NEC Y92.218
  - trace school Y92.215
  - university Y92.214
  - vocational school Y92.215
- sea (shore) Y92.832
- senior citizen center Y92.29
- service area
  - airport Y92.520
  - bus station Y92.521
  - gas station Y92.524
  - highway rest stop Y92.523
  - railway station Y92.522
- shipyard Y92.62
- shop (commercial) Y92.513
- sidewalk Y92.480
- silo Y92.79
- skating rink (roller) Y92.331
  - ice Y92.330
- slaughter house Y92.86
- soccer field Y92.322
- specified place NEC Y92.89
- sports area Y92.39
  - athletic
    - court Y92.318
      - basketball Y92.310
      - specified NEC Y92.318
      - squash Y92.311
      - tennis Y92.312
    - field Y92.328
      - baseball Y92.320
      - cricket ground Y92.328
      - football Y92.321
      - hockey Y92.328
      - soccer Y92.322
      - specified NEC Y92.328
  - golf course Y92.39
  - gymnasium Y92.39
  - riding school Y92.39
  - skating rink (roller) Y92.331
    - ice Y92.330
  - stadium Y92.39
  - swimming pool Y92.34
- squash court Y92.311
- stadium Y92.39
- steeplechasing course Y92.39
- store Y92.512
- stream Y92.828
- street and highway Y92.410
  - bike path Y92.482
  - freeway Y92.411
  - highway ramp Y92.415
  - interstate highway Y92.411
  - local residential or business street Y92.414
  - motorway Y92.411
  - parkway Y92.412
  - parking lot Y92.481
  - sidewalk Y92.480
  - specified NEC Y92.488
  - state road Y92.413
- subway car Y92.816
- supermarket Y92.512
- swamp Y92.828
- swimming pool (public) Y92.34
  - private (at) Y92.095
    - boarding house Y92.045
    - military base Y92.136
    - mobile home Y92.026
    - nursing home Y92.125
    - orphanage Y92.115
    - prison Y92.146
    - reform school Y92.156

Place of occurrence *(continued)*
- swimming pool *(continued)*
  - private *(continued)*
    - single family residence Y92.016
- synagogue Y92.22
- television station Y92.59
- tennis court Y92.312
- theater Y92.254
- trade area Y92.59
  - bank Y92.510
  - cafe Y92.511
  - casino Y92.59
  - garage Y92.59
  - hotel Y92.59
  - market Y92.512
  - office building Y92.59
  - radio station Y92.59
  - restaurant Y92.511
  - shop Y92.513
  - shopping mall Y92.59
  - store Y92.512
  - supermarket Y92.512
  - television station Y92.59
  - warehouse Y92.59
- trailer park, residential —*see* Place of occurrence, residence, mobile home
- trailer site NOS Y92.89
- train Y92.815
  - station Y92.522
- truck Y92.812
- tunnel under construction Y92.69
- urgent (health) care center Y92.532
- university Y92.214
- vehicle (transport) Y92.818
  - airplane Y92.813
  - boat Y92.814
  - bus Y92.811
  - car Y92.810
  - specified NEC Y92.818
  - subway car Y92.816
  - train Y92.815
  - truck Y92.812
- warehouse Y92.59
- water reservoir Y92.89
- wilderness area Y92.828
  - desert Y92.820
  - forest Y92.821
  - marsh Y92.828
  - mountain Y92.828
  - prairie Y92.828
  - specified NEC Y92.828
  - swamp Y92.828
- workshop Y92.69
- yard, private Y92.096
  - boarding house Y92.046
  - single family house Y92.017
  - mobile home Y92.027
- youth center Y92.29
- zoo (zoological garden) Y92.834

Plumbism —*see* Table of Drugs and Chemicals, lead

Poisoning (accidental) (by) —*see also* Table of Drugs and Chemicals
- by plant, thorns, spines, sharp leaves or other mechanisms NEC X58
- carbon monoxide
  - generated by
    - motor vehicle —*see* Accident, transport
    - watercraft (in transit) (not in transit) V93.89
      - ferry boat V93.81
      - fishing boat V93.82
      - jet skis V93.83
      - liner V93.81

Poisoning *(continued)*
- carbon monoxide *(continued)*
  - generated by *(continued)*
    - watercraft *(continued)*
      - merchant ship V93.80
      - passenger ship V93.81
      - powered craft NEC V93.83
- caused by injection of poisons into skin by plant thorns, spines, sharp leaves X58
  - marine or sea plants (venomous) X58
- exhaust gas
  - generated by
    - motor vehicle —*see* Accident, transport
    - watercraft (in transit) (not in transit) V93.89
      - ferry boat V93.81
      - fishing boat V93.82
      - jet skis V93.83
      - liner V93.81
      - merchant ship V93.80
      - passenger ship V93.81
      - powered craft NEC V93.83
- fumes or smoke due to
  - explosion —*see also* Explosion W40.9
  - fire —*see* Exposure, fire
  - ignition —*see* Ignition gas
  - in legal intervention —*see* Legal, intervention, gas
  - legal execution —*see* Legal, intervention, gas
- in war operations —*see* War operations

Powder burn (by) (from)
- airgun W34.110
- BB gun W34.110
- firearn NEC W34.19
- gas, air or spring-operated gun NEC W34.118
- handgun W32.1
- hunting rifle W33.12
- larger firearm W33.10
  - specified NEC W33.19
- machine gun W33.13
- paintball gun W34.111
- pellet gun W34.110
- shotgun W33.11
- Very pistol [flare] W34.19

Premature cessation (of) surgical and medical care Y66

Privation (food) (water) X58

Procedure (operation)
- correct, on wrong side or body part (wrong side) (wrong site) Y65.53
- intended for another patient done on wrong patient Y65.52
- performed on patient not scheduled for surgery Y65.52
- performed on wrong patient Y65.52
- wrong, performed on correct patient Y65.51

Prolonged
- sitting in transport vehicle —*see* Travel, by type of vehicle
- stay in
  - high altitude as cause of anoxia, barodontalgia, barotitis or hypoxia W94.11
  - weightless environment X52

Pulling, excessive (*see also* Overexertion) X50.9

Puncture, puncturing —*see also* Contact, with, by type of object or machine
- by
  - plant thorns, spines, sharp leaves or other mechanisms NEC W60
- during medical or surgical treatment as misadventure —*see* Index to Diseases and Injuries, Complication(s)

Pushed, pushing (accidental) (injury in)
- by other person(s) (accidental) W51
  - with fall W03
    - due to ice or snow W00.0
  - as, or caused by, a crowd or human stampede (with fall) W52
  - before moving object NEC Y02.8
    - motor vehicle Y02.0
    - subway train Y02.1
    - train Y02.1
  - from
    - high place NEC
      - in accidental circumstances W17.89
      - stated as
        - intentional, homicide (attempt) Y01
        - undetermined whether accidental or intentional Y30
    - transport vehicle NEC —*see also* Accident, transport V89.9
      - stated as
        - intentional, homicide (attempt) Y08.89
- overexertion X50.9

R

Radiation (exposure to)
- arc lamps W89.0
- atomic power plant (malfunction) NEC W88.1
- complication of or abnormal reaction to medical radiotherapy Y84.2
- electromagnetic, ionizing W88.0
- gamma rays W88.1
- in
  - war operations (from or following nuclear explosion) —*see* War operations
- inadvertent exposure of patient (receiving test or therapy) Y63.3
- infrared (heaters and lamps) W90.1
  - excessive heat from W92
- ionized, ionizing (particles, artificially accelerated)
  - radioisotopes W88.1
  - specified NEC W88.8
  - x-rays W88.0
- isotopes, radioactive —*see* Radiation, radioactive isotopes
- laser(s) W90.2
  - in war operations —*see* War operations
  - misadventure in medical care Y63.2
- light sources (man-made visible and ultraviolet) W89.9
  - natural X32
  - specified NEC W89.8
  - tanning bed W89.1
  - welding light W89.0

Radiation *(continued)*
- man-made visible light W89.9
  - specified NEC W89.8
  - tanning bed W89.1
  - welding light W89.0
- microwave W90.8
- misadventure in medical or surgical procedure Y63.2
- natural NEC X39.08
  - radon X39.01
- overdose (in medical or surgical procedure) Y63.2
- radar W90.0
- radioactive isotopes (any) W88.1
  - atomic power plant malfunction W88.1
  - misadventure in medical or surgical treatment Y63.2
- radiofrequency W90.0
- radium NEC W88.1
- sun X32
- ultraviolet (light) (man-made) W89.9
  - natural X32
  - specified NEC W89.8
  - tanning bed W89.1
  - welding light W89.0
- welding arc, torch, or light W89.0
  - excessive heat from W92
- x-rays (hard) (soft) W88.0

Range disease W94.11

Rape (attempted) T74.2-

Rat bite W53.11

Reaching (prolonged) (static) X50.1

Reaction, abnormal to medical procedure —*see also* Complication of or following, by type of procedure Y84.9
- with misadventure —*see* Misadventure
- biologicals —*see* Table of Drugs and Chemicals
- drugs —*see* Table of Drugs and Chemicals
- vaccine —*see* Table of Drugs and Chemicals

Recoil
- airgun W34.110
- BB gun W34.110
- firearn NEC W34.19
- gas, air or spring-operated gun NEC W34.118
- handgun W32.1
- hunting rifle W33.12
- larger firearm W33.10
  - specified NEC W33.19
- machine gun W33.13
- paintball gun W34.111
- pellet W34.110
- shotgun W33.11
- Very pistol [flare] W34.19

Reduction in
- atmospheric pressure —*see* Air, pressure, change

Rock falling on or hitting (accidentally) (person) W20.8
- in cave-in W20.0

Run over (accidentally) (by)
- animal (not being ridden) NEC W55.89
- machinery —*see* Contact, with, by specified type of machine
- transport vehicle NEC —*see also* Accident, transport V09.9
  - intentional homicide (attempt) Y03.0
  - motor NEC V09.20
    - intentional homicide (attempt) Y03.0

Running
- before moving object X81.8
  - motor vehicle X81.0

Running off, away
- animal (being ridden) —*see also* Accident, transport V80.918
  - not being ridden W55.89
- animal-drawn vehicle NEC —*see also* Accident, transport V80.928
- highway, road (way), street
  - transport vehicle NEC —*see also* Accident, transport V89.9

Rupture pressurized devices —*see* Explosion, by type of device

S

Saturnism —*see* Table of Drugs and Chemicals, lead

Scald, scalding (accidental) (by) (from) (in) X19
- air (hot) X14.1
- gases (hot) X14.1
- homicide (attempt) —*see* Assault, burning, hot object
- inflicted by other person
  - stated as intentional, homicide (attempt) —*see* Assault, burning, hot object
- liquid (boiling) (hot) NEC X12
  - stated as undetermined whether accidental or intentional Y27.2
  - suicide (attempt) X77.2
- local application of externally applied substance in medical or surgical care Y63.5
- metal (molten) (liquid) (hot) NEC X18
- self-inflicted X77.9
- stated as undetermined whether accidental or intentional Y27.8
- steam X13.1
  - assault X98.0
  - stated as undetermined whether accidental or intentional Y27.0
  - suicide (attempt) X77.0
- suicide (attempt) X77.9
- vapor (hot) X13.1
  - assault X98.0
  - stated as undetermined whether accidental or intentional Y27.0
  - suicide (attempt) X77.0

Scratched by
- cat W55.03
- person(s) (accidentally) W50.4
  - with intent to injure or kill Y04.0
  - as, or caused by, a crowd or human stampede (with fall) W52
  - assault Y04.0
  - homicide (attempt) Y04.0
  - in
    - fight Y04.0
    - legal intervention
      - injuring
        - bystander Y35.892
        - law enforcement personnel Y35.891
        - suspect Y35.893
        - unspecified person Y35.899

Seasickness T75.3

Self-harm NEC —*see also* External cause by type, undetermined whether accidental or intentional
- intentional —*see* Suicide
- poisoning NEC —*see* Table of drugs and biologicals, accident

Self-inflicted (injury) NEC —*see also* External cause by type, undetermined whether accidental or intentional
- intentional —*see* Suicide
- poisoning NEC —*see* Table of drugs and biologicals, accident

Sequelae (of)
- accident NEC —*see* W00-X58 with 7th character S
- assault (homicidal) (any means) —*see* X92-Y08 with 7th character S
- homicide, attempt (any means) —*see* X92-Y08 with 7th character S
- injury undetermined whether accidentally or purposely inflicted —*see* Y21-Y33 with 7th character S
- intentional self-harm (classifiable to X71-X83) —*see* X71-X83 with 7th character S
- legal intervention —*see* with 7th character S Y35
- motor vehicle accident —*see* V00-V99 with 7th character S
- suicide, attempt (any means) —*see* X71-X83 with 7th character S
- transport accident —*see* V00-V99 with 7th character S
- war operations —*see* War operations

Shock
- electric —*see* Exposure, electric current
- from electric appliance (any) (faulty) W86.8
  - domestic W86.0
  - suicide (attempt) X83.1

Shooting, shot (accidental(ly)) —*see also* Discharge, firearm, by type
- herself or himself —*see* Discharge, firearm by type, self-inflicted
- homicide (attempt) —*see* Discharge, firearm by type, homicide
- in war operations —*see* War operations
- inflicted by other person —*see* Discharge, firearm by type, homicide
  - accidental —*see* Discharge, firearm, by type of firearm
- legal
  - execution —*see* Legal, intervention, firearm
  - intervention —*see* Legal, intervention, firearm
- self-inflicted —*see* Discharge, firearm by type, suicide
  - accidental —*see* Discharge, firearm, by type of firearm
- suicide (attempt) —*see* Discharge, firearm by type, suicide

Shoving (accidentally) by other person —*see* Pushed, by other person

Sickness
- alpine W94.11
- motion —*see* Motion
- mountain W94.11

Sinking (accidental)
- watercraft (causing drowning, submersion) —*see also* Drowning, due to, accident to, watercraft, sinking
  - causing injury except drowning or submersion —*see* Accident, watercraft, causing, injury NEC

Siriasis X32

Sitting (prolonged) (static) X50.1

Slashed wrists —*see* Cut, self-inflicted

Slipping (accidental) (on same level) (with fall) W01.0
- on
  - ice W00.0
    - with skates —*see* Accident, transport, pedestrian, conveyance
  - mud W01.0
  - oil W01.0
  - snow W00.0
    - with skis —*see* Accident, transport, pedestrian, conveyance
  - surface (slippery) (wet) NEC W01.0
- without fall W18.40
  - due to
    - specified NEC W18.49
    - stepping from one level to another W18.43
    - stepping into hole or opening W18.42
    - stepping on object W18.41

Sliver, wood, contact with W45.8

Smoldering (due to fire) —*see* Exposure, fire

Sodomy (attempted) by force T74.2-

Sound waves (causing injury) W42.9
- supersonic W42.0

Splinter, contact with W45.8

Stab, stabbing —*see* Cut

Standing (prolonged) (static) X50.1

Starvation X58

Status of external cause Y99.9
- child assisting in compensated work for family Y99.8
- civilian activity done for financial or other compensation Y99.0
- civilian activity done for income or pay Y99.0
- family member assisting in compensated work for other family member Y99.8
- hobby not done for income Y99.8
- leisure activity Y99.8
- military activity Y99.1
- off-duty activity of military personnel Y99.8
- recreation or sport not for income or while a student Y99.8
- specified NEC Y99.8
- student activity Y99.8
- volunteer activity Y99.2

Stepped on
- by
  - animal (not being ridden) NEC W55.89
  - crowd or human stampede W52
  - person W50.0

Stepping on
- object W22.8
  - with fall W18.31
  - sports equipment W21.9
  - stationary W22.09
    - sports equipment W21.89
- person W51
  - by crowd or human stampede W52
- sports equipment W21.9

Sting
- arthropod, nonvenomous W57
- insect, nonvenomous W57

Storm (cataclysmic) —see Forces of nature, cataclysmic storm

Straining, excessive —(*see also* Overexertion) X50.9

Strangling —*see* Strangulation

Strangulation (accidental) —*see* categories T71

Strenuous movements (*see also* Overexertion) X50.9

Striking against
- airbag (automobile) W22.10
  - driver side W22.11
  - front passenger side W22.12
  - specified NEC W22.19
- bottom when
  - diving or jumping into water (in) W16.822
    - causing drowning W16.821
    - from boat W16.722
      - causing drowning W16.721
    - natural body W16.622
      - causing drowning W16.821
    - swimming pool W16.522
      - causing drowning W16.521
  - falling into water (in) W16.322
    - causing drowning W16.321
    - fountain —*see* Striking against, bottom when, falling into water, specified NEC
    - natural body W16.122
      - causing drowning W16.121
    - reservoir —*see* Striking against, bottom when, falling into water, specified NEC
    - specified NEC W16.322
      - causing drowning W16.321
    - swimming pool W16.022
      - causing drowning W16.021
- diving board (swimming-pool) W21.4
- object W22.8
  - with
    - drowning or submersion —*see* Drowning
    - fall —*see* Fall, due to, bumping against, object
  - caused by crowd or human stampede (with fall) W52
  - furniture W22.03
  - lamppost W22.02
  - sports equipment W21.9
  - stationary W22.09
    - sports equipment W21.89
  - wall W22.01
- person(s) W51
  - with fall W03
    - due to ice or snow W00.0
  - as, or caused by, a crowd or human stampede (with fall) W52
  - assault Y04.2
  - homicide (attempt) Y04.2
- sports equipment W21.9
- wall (when) W22.01
  - diving or jumping into water (in) W16.832
    - causing drowning W16.831
    - swimming pool W16.532
      - causing drowning W16.531
  - falling into water (in) W16.332
    - causing drowning W16.331
    - fountain —*see* Striking against, wall when, falling into water, specified NEC
    - natural body W16.132
      - causing drowning W16.131

Tabular List of Diseases and Injuries

Table of Contents

Instructional Notations

Includes:

The word 'Includes' appears immediately under certain categories to further define, or give examples of, the content of the category.

Excludes Notes

The ICD-10-CM has two types of excludes notes. Each note has a different definition for use but they are both similar in that they indicate that codes excluded from each other are independent of each other.

Excludes1

A type 1 Excludes note is a pure excludes. It means 'NOT CODED HERE!' An Excludes1 note indicates that the code excluded should never be used at the same time as the code above the Excludes1 note. An Excludes1 is used when two conditions cannot occur together, such as a congenital form versus an acquired form of the same condition.

Excludes2

A type 2 excludes note represents 'Not included here'. An Excludes2 note indicates that the condition excluded is not part of the condition it is excluded from but a patient may have both conditions at the same time. When an Excludes2 note appears under a code it is acceptable to use both the code and the excluded code together.

Code First/Use Additional Code notes (etiology/manifestation paired codes)

Certain conditions have both an underlying etiology and multiple body system manifestations due to the underlying etiology. For such conditions the ICD-10-CM has a coding convention that requires the underlying condition be sequenced first followed by the manifestation. Wherever such a combination exists there is a 'use additional code' note at the etiology code, and a 'code first' note at the manifestation code. These instructional notes indicate the proper sequencing order of the codes, etiology followed by manifestation.

In most cases the manifestation codes will have in the code title, 'in diseases classified elsewhere.' Codes with this title are a component of the etiology/ manifestation convention. The code title indicates that it is a manifestation code. 'In diseases classified elsewhere' codes are never permitted to be used as first listed or principal diagnosis codes. They must be used in conjunction with an underlying condition code and they must be listed following the underlying condition.

Code Also

A "code also" note instructs that two codes may be required to fully describe a condition, but this note does not provide sequencing direction. **The sequencing depends on the circumstances of the encounter**.

7th characters and placeholder X

Certain ICD-10-CM categories have applicable 7th characters. The applicable 7th character is required for all codes within the category, or as the notes in the Tabular List instruct. The 7th character must always be the 7th character in the data field. If a code that requires a 7th character is not 6 characters, a placeholder X must be used to fill in the empty characters.

Chapter 1: Certain Infectious and Parasitic Diseases (A00-B99)

Includes: diseases generally recognized as communicable or transmissible

Use additional code to identify resistance to antimicrobial drugs (Z16-)

Excludes1: *certain localized infections - see body system-related chapters*

Excludes2: *carrier or suspected carrier of infectious disease (Z22.-)*
infectious and parasitic diseases specific to the perinatal period (P35-P39)
infectious and parasitic diseases complicating pregnancy, childbirth and the puerperium (O98.-)
influenza and other acute respiratory infections (J00-J22)

This chapter contains the following category blocks:

A00-A09	Intestinal infectious diseases
A15-A19	Tuberculosis
A20-A28	Certain zoonotic bacterial diseases
A30-A49	Other bacterial diseases
A50-A64	Infections with a predominantly sexual mode of transmission
A65-A69	Other spirochetal diseases
A70-A74	Other diseases caused by chlamydiae
A75-A79	Rickettsioses
A80-A89	Viral and prion infections of the central nervous system
A90-A99	Arthropod-borne viral fevers and viral hemorrhagic fevers
B00-B09	Viral infections characterized by skin and mucous membrane lesions
B10	Other human herpesviruses
B15-B19	Viral hepatitis
B20	Human immunodeficiency virus [HIV] disease
B25-B34	Other viral diseases
B35-B49	Mycoses
B50-B64	Protozoal diseases
B65-B83	Helminthiases
B85-B89	Pediculosis, acariasis and other infestations
B90-B94	Sequelae of infectious and parasitic diseases
B95-B97	Bacterial and viral infectious agents
B99	Other infectious diseases

C. Chapter-Specific Coding Guidelines

In addition to general coding guidelines, there are guidelines for specific diagnoses and/or conditions in the classification. Unless otherwise indicated, these guidelines apply to all health care settings. Please refer to Section II for guidelines on the selection of principal diagnosis.

1. Chapter 1: Certain Infectious and Parasitic Diseases (A00-B99), ***U07.1***

a. Human Immunodeficiency Virus (HIV) Infections

1) Code only confirmed cases

Code only confirmed cases of HIV infection/illness. This is an exception to the hospital inpatient guideline Section II, H.

In this context, "confirmation" does not require documentation of positive serology or culture for HIV; the provider's diagnostic statement that the patient is HIV positive, or has an HIV-related illness is sufficient.

2) Selection and sequencing of HIV codes

(a) Patient admitted for HIV-related condition

If a patient is admitted for an HIV-related condition, the principal diagnosis should be B20, Human immunodeficiency virus [HIV] disease followed by additional diagnosis codes for all reported HIV-related conditions.

(b) Patient with HIV disease admitted for unrelated condition

If a patient with HIV disease is admitted for an unrelated condition (such as a traumatic injury), the code for the unrelated condition (e.g., the nature of injury code) should be the principal diagnosis. Other diagnoses would be B20 followed by additional diagnosis codes for all reported HIV-related conditions.

(c) Whether the patient is newly diagnosed

Whether the patient is newly diagnosed or has had previous admissions/encounters for HIV conditions is irrelevant to the sequencing decision.

(d) Asymptomatic human immunodeficiency virus

Z21, Asymptomatic human immunodeficiency virus [HIV] infection status, is to be applied when the patient without any documentation of symptoms is listed as being "HIV positive," "known HIV," "HIV test positive," or similar terminology. Do not use this code if the term "AIDS" is used or if the patient is treated for any HIV-related illness or is described as having any condition(s) resulting from his/her HIV positive status; use B20 in these cases.

(e) Patients with inconclusive HIV serology

Patients with inconclusive HIV serology, but no definitive diagnosis or manifestations of the illness, may be assigned code R75, Inconclusive laboratory evidence of human immunodeficiency virus [HIV].

(f) Previously diagnosed HIV-related illness

Patients with any known prior diagnosis of an HIV-related illness should be coded to B20. Once a patient has developed an HIV-related illness, the patient should always be assigned code B20 on every subsequent admission/encounter. Patients previously diagnosed with any HIV illness (B20) should never be assigned to R75 or Z21, Asymptomatic human immunodeficiency virus [HIV] infection status.

(g) HIV Infection in Pregnancy, Childbirth and the Puerperium

During pregnancy, childbirth or the puerperium, a patient admitted (or presenting for a health care encounter) because of an HIV-related illness should receive a principal diagnosis code of O98.7-, Human immunodeficiency [HIV] disease complicating pregnancy, childbirth and the puerperium, followed by B20 and the code(s) for the HIV-related illness(es). Codes from Chapter 15 always take sequencing priority. Patients with asymptomatic HIV infection status admitted (or presenting for a health care encounter) during pregnancy, childbirth, or the puerperium should receive codes of O98.7- and Z21.

(h) Encounters for testing for HIV

If a patient is being seen to determine his/her HIV status, use code Z11.4, Encounter for screening for human immunodeficiency virus [HIV]. Use additional codes for any associated high risk behavior.

If a patient with signs or symptoms is being seen for HIV testing, code the signs and symptoms. An additional counseling code Z71.7, Human immunodeficiency virus [HIV] counseling, may be used if counseling is provided during the encounter for the test.

When a patient returns to be informed of his/her HIV test results and the test result is negative, use code Z71.7, Human immunodeficiency virus [HIV] counseling.

If the results are positive, see previous guidelines and assign codes as appropriate.

(i) History of HIV managed by medication

If a patient with documented history of HIV disease is currently managed on antiretroviral medications, assign code B20, Human immunodeficiency virus [HIV] disease. Code Z79.899, Other long term (current) drug therapy, may be assigned as an additional code to identify the long-term (current) use of antiretroviral medications.

b. Infectious agents as the cause of diseases classified to other chapters

Certain infections are classified in chapters other than Chapter 1 and no organism is identified as part of the infection code. In these instances, it is necessary to use an additional code from Chapter 1 to identify the organism. A code from category B95, Streptococcus, Staphylococcus, and Enterococcus as the cause of diseases classified to other chapters, B96, Other bacterial agents as the cause of diseases classified to other chapters, or B97, Viral agents as the cause of diseases classified to other chapters, is to be used as an additional code to identify the organism. An instructional note will be found at the infection code advising that an additional organism code is required.

c. Infections resistant to antibiotics

Many bacterial infections are resistant to current antibiotics. It is necessary to identify all infections documented as antibiotic resistant. Assign a code from category Z16, Resistance to antimicrobial drugs, following the infection code only if the infection code does not identify drug resistance.

d. Sepsis, Severe Sepsis, and Septic Shock

1) Coding of Sepsis and Severe Sepsis

(a) Sepsis

For a diagnosis of sepsis, assign the appropriate code for the underlying systemic infection. If the type of infection or causal organism is not further specified, assign code A41.9, Sepsis, unspecified organism.

A code from subcategory R65.2, Severe sepsis, should not be assigned unless severe sepsis or an associated acute organ dysfunction is documented.

(i) Negative or inconclusive blood cultures and sepsis

Negative or inconclusive blood cultures do not preclude a diagnosis of sepsis in patients with clinical evidence of the condition, however, the provider should be queried.

(ii) Urosepsis

The term urosepsis is a nonspecific term. It is not to be considered synonymous with sepsis. It has no default code in the Alphabetic Index. Should a provider use this term, he/she must be queried for clarification.

(iii) Sepsis with organ dysfunction

If a patient has sepsis and associated acute organ dysfunction or multiple organ dysfunction (MOD), follow the instructions for coding severe sepsis.

(iv) Acute organ dysfunction that is not clearly associated with the sepsis

If a patient has sepsis and an acute organ dysfunction, but the medical record documentation indicates that the acute organ dysfunction is related to a medical condition other than the sepsis, do not assign a code from subcategory R65.2, Severe sepsis. An acute organ dysfunction must be associated with the sepsis in order to assign the severe sepsis code. If the documentation is not clear as to whether an acute organ dysfunction is related to the sepsis or another medical condition, query the provider.

(b) Severe sepsis

The coding of severe sepsis requires a minimum of 2 codes: first a code for the underlying systemic infection, followed by a code from subcategory R65.2, Severe sepsis. If the causal organism is not documented, assign code A41.9, Sepsis, unspecified organism, for the infection. Additional code(s) for the associated acute organ dysfunction are also required.

Due to the complex nature of severe sepsis, some cases may require querying the provider prior to assignment of the codes.

2) Septic shock

(a) Septic shock generally refers to circulatory failure associated with severe sepsis, and therefore, it represents a type of acute organ dysfunction.

For cases of septic shock, the code for the systemic infection should be sequenced first, followed by code R65.21, Severe sepsis with septic shock or code T81.12, Postprocedural septic shock. Any additional codes for the other acute organ dysfunctions should also be assigned. As noted in the sequencing instructions in the Tabular List, the code for septic shock cannot be assigned as a principal diagnosis.

3) Sequencing of severe sepsis

If severe sepsis is present on admission, and meets the definition of principal diagnosis, the underlying systemic infection should be assigned as principal diagnosis followed by the appropriate code from subcategory R65.2 as required by the sequencing rules in the Tabular List. A code from subcategory R65.2 can never be assigned as a principal diagnosis.

When severe sepsis develops during an encounter (it was not present on admission) the underlying systemic infection and the appropriate code from subcategory R65.2 should be assigned as secondary diagnoses.

Severe sepsis may be present on admission but the diagnosis may not be confirmed until sometime after admission. If the documentation is not clear whether severe sepsis was present on admission, the provider should be queried.

4) Sepsis or severe sepsis with a localized infection

If the reason for admission is both sepsis or severe sepsis and a localized infection, such as pneumonia or cellulitis, a code(s) for the underlying systemic infection should be assigned first and the code for the localized infection should be assigned as a secondary diagnosis. If the patient has severe sepsis, a code from subcategory R65.2 should also be assigned as a secondary diagnosis. If the patient is admitted with a localized infection, such as pneumonia, and sepsis/severe sepsis doesn't develop until after admission, the localized infection should be assigned first, followed by the appropriate sepsis/severe sepsis codes.

5) Sepsis due to a postprocedural infection

(a) Documentation of causal relationship

As with all postprocedural complications, code assignment is based on the provider's documentation of the relationship between the infection and the procedure.

(b) Sepsis due to a postprocedural infection

For infections following a procedure, a code from T81.40, to T81.43, Infection following a procedure, or a code from O86.00 to O86.03, Infection of obstetric surgical wound, that identifies the site of the infection should be coded first, if known. Assign an additional code for sepsis following a procedure (T81.44) or sepsis following an obstetrical procedure (O86.04). Use an additional code to identify the infectious agent. If the patient has severe sepsis the appropriate code from subcategory R65.2 should also be assigned with the additional code(s) for any acute organ dysfunction.

For infections following infusion, transfusion, therapeutic injection, or immunization, a code from subcategory T80.2, Infections following infusion, transfusion, and therapeutic injection, or code T88.0-, Infection following immunization, should be coded first, followed by the code for the specific infection. If the patient has severe sepsis, the appropriate code from subcategory R65.2 should also be assigned, with the additional code(s) for any acute organ dysfunction.

(c) Postprocedural infection and postprocedural septic shock

If a postprocedural infection has resulted in postprocedural septic shock, assign the codes indicated above for sepsis due to a postprocedural infection, followed by code T81.12-, Postprocedural septic shock. Do not assign code R65.21, Severe sepsis with septic shock. Additional code(s) should be assigned for any acute organ dysfunction.

6) Sepsis and severe sepsis associated with a noninfectious process (condition)

In some cases a noninfectious process (condition), such as trauma, may lead to an infection which can result in sepsis or severe sepsis. If sepsis or severe sepsis is documented as associated with a noninfectious condition, such as a burn or serious injury, and this condition meets the definition for principal diagnosis, the code for the noninfectious condition should be sequenced first, followed by the code for the resulting infection. If severe sepsis, is present a code from subcategory R65.2 should also be assigned with any associated organ dysfunction(s) codes. It is not necessary to assign a code from subcategory R65.1, Systemic inflammatory response syndrome (SIRS) of non-infectious origin, for these cases.

If the infection meets the definition of principal diagnosis it should be sequenced before the non-infectious condition. When both the associated non-infectious condition and the infection meet the definition of principal diagnosis either may be assigned as principal diagnosis.

Only one code from category R65, Symptoms and signs specifically associated with systemic inflammation and infection, should be assigned. Therefore, when a non-infectious condition leads to an infection resulting in severe sepsis, assign the appropriate code from subcategory R65.2, Severe sepsis. Do not additionally assign a code from subcategory R65.1, Systemic inflammatory response syndrome (SIRS) of non-infectious origin.

See Section I.C.18. SIRS due to non-infectious process

7) Sepsis and septic shock complicating abortion, pregnancy, childbirth, and the puerperium

See Section I.C.15. Sepsis and septic shock complicating abortion, pregnancy, childbirth and the puerperium

8) Newborn sepsis

See Section I.C.16. f. Bacterial sepsis of Newborn

e. Methicillin Resistant *Staphylococcus aureus* (MRSA) Conditions

1) Selection and sequencing of MRSA codes

(a) Combination codes for MRSA infection

When a patient is diagnosed with an infection that is due to methicillin resistant Staphylococcus aureus (MRSA), and that infection has a combination code that includes the causal organism (e.g., sepsis, pneumonia) assign the appropriate combination code for the condition (e.g., code A41.02, Sepsis due to Methicillin resistant Staphylococcus aureus or code J15.212, Pneumonia due to Methicillin resistant Staphylococcus aureus). Do not assign code B95.62, Methicillin resistant Staphylococcus aureus infection as the cause of diseases classified elsewhere, as an additional code because the combination code includes the type of infection and the MRSA organism. Do not assign a code from subcategory Z16.11, Resistance to penicillins, as an additional diagnosis.

See Section C.1. for instructions on coding and sequencing of sepsis and severe sepsis.

(b) Other codes for MRSA infection

When there is documentation of a current infection (e.g., wound infection, stitch abscess, urinary tract infection) due to MRSA, and that infection does not have a combination code that includes the causal organism, assign the appropriate code to identify the condition along with code B95.62, Methicillin resistant Staphylococcus aureus infection as the cause of diseases classified elsewhere for the MRSA infection. Do not assign a code from subcategory Z16.11, Resistance to penicillins.

(c) Methicillin susceptible Staphylococcus aureus (MSSA) and MRSA colonization

The condition or state of being colonized or carrying MSSA or MRSA is called colonization or carriage, while an individual person is described as being colonized or being a carrier. Colonization means that MSSA or MSRA is present on or in the body without necessarily causing illness. A positive MRSA colonization test might be documented by the provider as "MRSA screen positive" or "MRSA nasal swab positive".

Assign code Z22.322, Carrier or suspected carrier of Methicillin resistant Staphylococcus aureus, for patients documented as having MRSA colonization. Assign code Z22.321, Carrier or suspected carrier of Methicillin susceptible Staphylococcus aureus, for patient documented as having MSSA colonization. Colonization is not necessarily indicative of a disease process or as the cause of a specific condition the patient may have unless documented as such by the provider.

(d) MRSA colonization and infection

If a patient is documented as having both MRSA colonization and infection during a hospital admission, code Z22.322, Carrier or suspected carrier of Methicillin resistant Staphylococcus aureus, and a code for the MRSA infection may both be assigned.

f. Zika virus infections

1) Code only confirmed cases

Code only a confirmed diagnosis of Zika virus (A92.5, Zika virus disease) as documented by the provider. This is an exception to the hospital inpatient guideline Section II, H. In this context, "confirmation" does not require documentation of the type of test performed; the provider's diagnostic statement that the condition is confirmed is sufficient. This code should be assigned regardless of the stated mode of transmission.

If the provider documents "suspected", "possible" or "provable" Zika, do not assign code A92.5. Assign a code(s) explaining the reason for encounter (such as fever, rash, or joint pain) or Z20.821, Contact with and (suspected) exposure to Zika virus.

g. Coronavirus infections

1) COVID-19 infection (infection due to SARS-CoV-2)

(a) Code only confirmed cases

Code only a confirmed diagnosis of the 2019 novel coronavirus disease (COVID-19) as documented by the provider or documentation of a positive COVID-19 test result. For a confirmed diagnosis, assign code U07.1, COVID-19. This is an exception to the hospital inpatient guideline Section II, H. In this context, "confirmation" does not require documentation of a positive test result for COVID-19; the provider's documentation that the individual has COVID-19 is sufficient.

If the provider documents "suspected," "possible," "probable," or "inconclusive" COVID-19, do not assign code U07.1. Instead, code the signs and symptoms reported.

See guideline I.C.1.g.1.g.

(b) Sequencing of codes

When COVID-19 meets the definition of principle diagnosis, code U07.1, COVID-19, should be sequenced first, followed by the appropriate codes for associated manifestations, except when another guideline requires that certain codes be sequenced first, such as obstetrics, sepsis, or transplant complications.

For a COVID-19 infection that progresses to sepsis, see Section I.C.1.d Sepsis, Severe Sepsis, and Septic Shock

See Section I.C.15.s. for COVID-19 infection in pregnancy, childbirth, and the puerperium

See Section I.C.16.h. for COVID-19 infection in newborn

For a COVID-19 infection in a lung transplant patient, see Section I.C.19.g.3.a. Transplant complications other than kidney

(c) Acute respiratory manifestations of COVID-19

When the reason for the encounter/admission is a respiratory manifestation of COVID-19, assign code U07.1, COVID-19, as the principal/first-listed diagnosis and assign code(s) for the respiratory manifestation(s) as additional diagnoses.

The following conditions are examples of common respiratory manifestations of COVID-19.

(i) Pneumonia

For a patient with pneumonia confirmed as due to COVID-19, assign codes U07.1, COVID-19, and J12.82, Pneumonia due to coronavirus disease 2019.

(ii) Acute bronchitis

For a patient with acute bronchitis confirmed as due to COVID-19, assign codes U07.1, and J20.8, Acute bronchitis due to other specified organisms.

Bronchitis not otherwise specified (NOS) due to COVID-19 should be coded using code U07.1 and J40, Bronchitis, not specified as acute or chronic.

(iii) Lower respiratory infection

If the COVID-19 is documented as being associated with lower respiratory infection, not otherwise specified (NOS), or an acute respiratory infection, NOS, codes U07.1 and J22, Unspecified acute lower respiratory infection, should be assigned.

If the COVID-19 is documented as being associated with a respiratory infection, NOS, codes U07.1 and J98.8, Other specified respiratory disorders, should be assigned.

(iv) Acute respiratory distress syndrome

For acute respiratory distress syndrome (ARDS) due to COVID-19, assign codes U07.1 and J80, Acute respiratory distress syndrome.

(v) Acute respiratory failure

For acute respiratory failure due to COVID-19, assign code U07.1 and code J96.0-, Acute respiratory failure.

(d) Non-respiratory manifestations of COVID-19

When the reason for the encounter/admission is a non-respiratory manifestation (e.g., viral enteritis) of COVID-19, assign code U07.1, COVID-19, as the principal/first-listed diagnosis and assign code(s) for the manifestation(s) as additional diagnoses.

(e) Exposure to COVID-19

For asymptomatic individuals with actual or suspected exposure to COVID-19, assign code Z20.822, Contact with and (suspected) exposure to COVID-19.

For symptomatic individuals with actual or suspected exposure to COVID-19 and the infection has been ruled out, or test results are inconclusive or unknown, assign code Z20.822, Contact with and (suspected) exposure to COVID-19.

See guidelines I.C.21.c.1, Contact/Exposure, for additional guidance regarding the use of category Z20 codes.

If COVID-19 is confirmed, see guidelines I.C.1.g.1.a.

(f) Screening for COVID-19

During the COVID-19 pandemic, a screening code is generally not appropriate. Do not assign code Z11.52, Encounter for screening for COVID-19. For encounters for COVID-19 testing, including preoperative testing, code as exposure to COVID-19 (guideline I.C.1.g.1.e).

Coding guidance will be updated as new information concerning any changes in the pandemic status becomes available.

(g) Signs and symptoms without definitive diagnosis of COVID-19

For patient presenting with any signs/symptoms associated with COVID-19 (such as fever, etc.) but a definitive diagnosis has not been established, assign the appropriate code(s) for each of the presenting signs and symptoms such as:

- R05.**1, Acute** cough, **or R05.9, Cough, unspecified**
- R06.02 Shortness of breath
- R50.9 Fever, unspecified

If a patient with signs/symptoms associated with COVID-19 also has an actual or suspected contact with or exposure to COVID-19, assign Z20.828, Contact with and (suspected) exposure to other viral communicable diseases, as an additional code.

(h) Asymptomatic individuals who test positive for COVID-19

For asymptomatic individuals who test positive for COVID-19, *see guideline I.C.1.g.1.a.* Although the individual is asymptomatic, the individual has tested positive and is considered to have a COVID-19 infection.

(i) Personal history of COVID-19

For patients with a history of COVID-19, assign code Z86.16, Personal history of COVID-19.

(j) Follow-up visits after COVID-19 infection has resolved

For individuals who previously had COVID-19, **without residual symptom(s) or condition(s)** and are being seen for follow-up evaluation, and COVID-19 test results are negative, assign codes Z09, Encounter for follow-up examination after completed treatment for conditions other than malignant neoplasm, and Z86.16, Personal history of COVID-19.

For follow-up visits for individuals with symptom(s) or condition(s) related to a previous COVID-19 infection, see guideline I.C.1.g.1.m.

See Section I.C.21.c.8, Factors influencing health states and contact with health services, Follow-up.

(k) **Encounter for antibody testing**

For an encounter for antibody testing that is not being performed to confirm a current COVID-19 infection, nor is a follow-up test after resolution of COVID-19, assign Z01.84, Encounter for antibody response examination.

Follow the applicable guidelines above if the individual is being tested to confirm a current COVID-19 infection.

For follow-up testing after a COVID-19 infection, see guideline I.C.1.g.1.j

(l) **Multisystem Inflammatory Syndrome**

For individuals with multisystem inflammatory syndrome (MIS) and COVID-19, assign code U07.1, COVID-19, as the principal/first-listed diagnosis and assign code M35.81, Multisystem inflammatory syndrome, as an additional diagnosis.

If an individual with a history of COVID-19 develops MIS, assign codes M35.81, Multisystem inflammatory syndrome, and **U09.9, Post COVID-19 condition, unspecified**.

If an individual with a known or suspected exposure to COVID-19, and no current COVID-19 infection or history of COVID-19, develops MIS, assign codes M35.81, Muyltisystem Inflammatory Syndrome, and Z20.822, Contact with and (suspected) exposure to COVID-19.

Additional codes should be assigned for any associated complications of MIS.

(m) **Post COVID-19 Condition**

For sequela of COVID-19, or associated symptoms or conditions that develop following a previous COVID-19 infection, assign a code(s) for the specific symptom(s) or condition(s) related to the previous COVID-19 infection, if known, and code U09.9, Post COVID-19 condition, unspecified.

Code U09.9 should not be assigned for manifestations of an active (current) COVID-19 infection.

If a patient has a condition(s) associated with a previous COVID-19 infection and develops a new active (current) COVID-19 infection, code U09.9 may be assigned in conjunction with code U07.1, COVID-19, to identify that the patient also has a condition(s) associated with a previous COVID-19 infection. Code(s) for the specific condition(s) associated with the previous COVID-19 infection and code(s) for manifestation(s) of the new active (current) COVID-19 infection should also be assigned.

Intestinal infectious diseases (A00-A09)

A00 Cholera

CC **A00.0 Cholera due to Vibrio cholerae 01, biovar cholerae**
Classical cholera

CC **A00.1 Cholera due to Vibrio cholerae 01, biovar eltor**
Cholera eltor

CC **A00.9 Cholera, unspecified**

A01 Typhoid and paratyphoid fevers

\+ **A01.0 Typhoid fever**
Infection due to Salmonella typhi

CC **A01.00 Typhoid fever, unspecified**
CC **A01.01 Typhoid meningitis**
CC **A01.02 Typhoid fever with heart involvement**
Typhoid endocarditis
Typhoid myocarditis

CC **A01.03 Typhoid pneumonia**
CC **A01.04 Typhoid arthritis**
CC **A01.05 Typhoid osteomyelitis**
CC **A01.09 Typhoid fever with other complications**

CC **A01.1 Paratyphoid fever A**
CC **A01.2 Paratyphoid fever B**
CC **A01.3 Paratyphoid fever C**
CC **A01.4 Paratyphoid fever, unspecified**
Infection due to Salmonella paratyphi NOS

A02 Other salmonella infections

Includes: infection or foodborne intoxication due to any Salmonella species other than S. typhi and S. paratyphi

CC **A02.0 Salmonella enteritis**
Salmonellosis

MCC **A02.1 Salmonella sepsis**
Review coding guideline C.1.d

\+ **A02.2 Localized salmonella infections**

A02.20 Localized salmonella infection, unspecified
MCC **A02.21 Salmonella meningitis**
MCC **A02.22 Salmonella pneumonia**
CC **A02.23 Salmonella arthritis**
CC **A02.24 Salmonella osteomyelitis**
CC **A02.25 Salmonella pyelonephritis**
Salmonella tubulo-interstitial nephropathy
CC **A02.29 Salmonella with other localized infection**

CC **A02.8 Other specified salmonella infections**
CC **A02.9 Salmonella infection, unspecified**

A03 Shigellosis

CC **A03.0 Shigellosis due to Shigella dysenteriae**
Group A shigellosis [Shiga-Kruse dysentery]

A03.1 Shigellosis due to Shigella flexneri
Group B shigellosis

A03.2 Shigellosis due to Shigella boydii
Group C shigellosis

A03.3 Shigellosis due to Shigella sonnei
Group D shigellosis

A03.8 Other shigellosis

A03.9 Shigellosis, unspecified
Bacillary dysentery NOS

A04 Other bacterial intestinal infections

Excludes1: *bacterial foodborne intoxications, NEC (A05.-)*
tuberculous enteritis (A18.32)

CC **A04.0 Enteropathogenic Escherichia coli infection**
CC **A04.1 Enterotoxigenic Escherichia coli infection**
CC **A04.2 Enteroinvasive Escherichia coli infection**
CC **A04.3 Enterohemorrhagic Escherichia coli infection**
CC **A04.4 Other intestinal Escherichia coli infections**
Escherichia coli enteritis NOS

CC **A04.5 Campylobacter enteritis**
CC **A04.6 Enteritis due to Yersinia enterocolitica**
Excludes1: *extraintestinal yersiniosis (A28.2)*

\+ **A04.7 Enterocolitis due to Clostridium difficile**
Foodborne intoxication by Clostridium difficile
Pseudomembraneous colitis
AHA CC: 4Q, 2017, 4

CC **A04.71 Enterocolitis due to clostridium difficile, recurrent**
AHA CC: 1Q, 2020, 18

CC **A04.72 Enterocolitis due to clostridium difficile, not specified as recurrent**

CC **A04.8 Other specified bacterial intestinal infections**
CC **A04.9 Bacterial intestinal infection, unspecified**
Bacterial enteritis NOS

A05 Other bacterial foodborne intoxications, not elsewhere classified

Excludes1: *Clostridium difficile foodborne intoxication and infection (A04.7-)*
Escherichia coli infection (A04.0-A04.4)
listeriosis (A32.-)
salmonella foodborne intoxication and infection (A02.-)
toxic effect of noxious foodstuffs (T61-T62)

CC **A05.0 Foodborne staphylococcal intoxication**
CC **A05.1 Botulism food poisoning**
Botulism NOS
Classical foodborne intoxication due to Clostridium botulinum
Excludes1: *infant botulism (A48.51)*
wound botulism (A48.52)

CC **A05.2 Foodborne Clostridium perfringens [Clostridium welchii] intoxication**
Enteritis necroticans
Pig-bel

CC **A05.3 Foodborne Vibrio parahaemolyticus intoxication**
CC **A05.4 Foodborne Bacillus cereus intoxication**
CC **A05.5 Foodborne Vibrio vulnificus intoxication**
CC **A05.8 Other specified bacterial foodborne intoxications**
A05.9 Bacterial foodborne intoxication, unspecified

A06 Amebiasis

Includes: infection due to Entamoeba histolytica
Excludes1: *other protozoal intestinal diseases (A07.-)*
Excludes2: *acanthamebiasis (B60.1-)*
Naegleriasis (B60.2)

CC **A06.0 Acute amebic dysentery**
Acute amebiasis
Intestinal amebiasis NOS
CC **A06.1 Chronic intestinal amebiasis**
CC **A06.2 Amebic nondysenteric colitis**
CC **A06.3 Ameboma of intestine**
Ameboma NOS
MCC **A06.4 Amebic liver abscess**
Hepatic amebiasis
MCC **A06.5 Amebic lung abscess**
Amebic abscess of lung (and liver)
MCC **A06.6 Amebic brain abscess**
Amebic abscess of brain (and liver) (and lung)
A06.7 Cutaneous amebiasis
\+ **A06.8 Amebic infection of other sites**
CC **A06.81 Amebic cystitis**
CC **A06.82 Other amebic genitourinary infections**
Amebic balanitis
Amebic vesiculitis
Amebic vulvovaginitis
CC **A06.89 Other amebic infections**
Amebic appendicitis
Amebic splenic abscess
A06.9 Amebiasis, unspecified

A07 Other protozoal intestinal diseases

A07.0 Balantidiasis
Balantidial dysentery
CC **A07.1 Giardiasis [lambliasis]**
CC **A07.2 Cryptosporidiosis**
CC **A07.3 Isosporiasis**
Infection due to Isospora belli and Isospora hominis
Intestinal coccidiosis
Isosporosis
CC **A07.4 Cyclosporiasis**
CC **A07.8 Other specified protozoal intestinal diseases**
Intestinal microsporidiosis
Intestinal trichomoniasis
Sarcocystosis
Sarcosporidiosis
CC **A07.9 Protozoal intestinal disease, unspecified**
Flagellate diarrhea
Protozoal colitis
Protozoal diarrhea
Protozoal dysentery

A08 Viral and other specified intestinal infections

Excludes1: *influenza with involvement of gastrointestinal tract (J09.X3, J10.2, J11.2)*

CC **A08.0 Rotaviral enteritis**
\+ **A08.1 Acute gastroenteropathy due to Norwalk agent and other small round viruses**
CC **A08.11 Acute gastroenteropathy due to Norwalk agent**
Acute gastroenteropathy due to Norovirus
Acute gastroenteropathy due to Norwalk-like agent
CC **A08.19 Acute gastroenteropathy due to other small round viruses**
Acute gastroenteropathy due to small round virus [SRV] NOS
CC **A08.2 Adenoviral enteritis**
\+ **A08.3 Other viral enteritis**
CC **A08.31 Calicivirus enteritis**
CC **A08.32 Astrovirus enteritis**
CC **A08.39 Other viral enteritis**
Coxsackie virus enteritis
Echovirus enteritis
Enterovirus enteritis NEC
Torovirus enteritis
A08.4 Viral intestinal infection, unspecified
Viral enteritis NOS
Viral gastroenteritis NOS
Viral gastroenteropathy NOS
AHA CC: 3Q, 2016, 12
A08.8 Other specified intestinal infections

CC **A09 Infectious gastroenteritis and colitis, unspecified**

Infectious colitis NOS
Infectious enteritis NOS
Infectious gastroenteritis NOS
Excludes1: *colitis NOS (K52.9)*
diarrhea NOS (R19.7)
enteritis NOS (K52.9)
gastroenteritis NOS (K52.9)
noninfective gastroenteritis and colitis, unspecified (K52.9)
Valid 3-character code, no further characters required

Tuberculosis (A15-A19)

Includes: infections due to Mycobacterium tuberculosis and Mycobacterium bovis
Excludes1: *congenital tuberculosis (P37.0)*
nonspecific reaction to test for tuberculosis without active tuberculosis (R76.1-)
pneumoconiosis associated with tuberculosis, any type in A15 (J65)
positive PPD (R76.11)
positive tuberculin skin test without active tuberculosis (R76.11)
sequelae of tuberculosis (B90.-)
silicotuberculosis (J65)

A15 Respiratory tuberculosis

CC **A15.0 Tuberculosis of lung**
Tuberculous bronchiectasis
Tuberculous fibrosis of lung
Tuberculous pneumonia
Tuberculous pneumothorax
CC **A15.4 Tuberculosis of intrathoracic lymph nodes**
Tuberculosis of hilar lymph nodes
Tuberculosis of mediastinal lymph nodes
Tuberculosis of tracheobronchial lymph nodes
Excludes1: *tuberculosis specified as primary (A15.7)*
CC **A15.5 Tuberculosis of larynx, trachea and bronchus**
Tuberculosis of bronchus
Tuberculosis of glottis
Tuberculosis of larynx
Tuberculosis of trachea
CC **A15.6 Tuberculous pleurisy**
Tuberculosis of pleura Tuberculous empyema
Excludes1: *primary respiratory tuberculosis (A15.7)*
CC **A15.7 Primary respiratory tuberculosis**
CC **A15.8 Other respiratory tuberculosis**
Mediastinal tuberculosis
Nasopharyngeal tuberculosis
Tuberculosis of nose
Tuberculosis of sinus [any nasal]
CC **A15.9 Respiratory tuberculosis unspecified**

A17 Tuberculosis of nervous system

MCC **A17.0 Tuberculous meningitis**
Tuberculosis of meninges (cerebral)(spinal)
Tuberculous leptomeningitis
Excludes1: *tuberculous meningoencephalitis (A17.82)*
MCC **A17.1 Meningeal tuberculoma**
Tuberculoma of meninges (cerebral) (spinal)
Excludes2: *tuberculoma of brain and spinal cord (A17.81)*
\+ **A17.8 Other tuberculosis of nervous system**
MCC **A17.81 Tuberculoma of brain and spinal cord**
Tuberculous abscess of brain and spinal cord
MCC **A17.82 Tuberculous meningoencephalitis**
Tuberculous myelitis
MCC **A17.83 Tuberculous neuritis**
Tuberculous mononeuropathy
MCC **A17.89 Other tuberculosis of nervous system**
Tuberculous polyneuropathy
CC **A17.9 Tuberculosis of nervous system, unspecified**

A18 Tuberculosis of other organs

\+ **A18.0 Tuberculosis of bones and joints**
CC **A18.01 Tuberculosis of spine**
Pott's disease or curvature of spine
Tuberculous arthritis
Tuberculous osteomyelitis of spine
Tuberculous spondylitis
CC **A18.02 Tuberculous arthritis of other joints**
Tuberculosis of hip (joint)
Tuberculosis of knee (joint)

CC **A18.03** **Tuberculosis of other bones**
Tuberculous mastoiditis
Tuberculous osteomyelitis
CC **A18.09** **Other musculoskeletal tuberculosis**
Tuberculous myositis
Tuberculous synovitis
Tuberculous tenosynovitis
+ **A18.1** **Tuberculosis of genitourinary system**
CC **A18.10** **Tuberculosis of genitourinary system, unspecified**
CC **A18.11** **Tuberculosis of kidney and ureter**
CC **A18.12** **Tuberculosis of bladder**
CC **A18.13** **Tuberculosis of other urinary organs**
Tuberculous urethritis
● ♂ CC **A18.14** **Tuberculosis of prostate**
♂ CC **A18.15** **Tuberculosis of other male genital organs**
♀ CC **A18.16** **Tuberculosis of cervix**
♀ CC **A18.17** **Tuberculous female pelvic inflammatory disease**
Tuberculous endometritis
Tuberculous oophoritis and salpingitis
♀ CC **A18.18** **Tuberculosis of other female genital organs**
Tuberculous ulceration of vulva
CC **A18.2** **Tuberculous peripheral lymphadenopathy**
Tuberculous adenitis
Excludes2: *tuberculosis of bronchial and mediastinal lymph nodes (A15.4)*
tuberculosis of mesenteric and retroperitoneal lymph nodes (A18.39)
tuberculous tracheobronchial adenopathy (A15.4)
+ **A18.3** **Tuberculosis of intestines, peritoneum and mesenteric glands**
MCC **A18.31** **Tuberculous peritonitis**
Tuberculous ascites
CC **A18.32** **Tuberculous enteritis**
Tuberculosis of anus and rectum
Tuberculosis of intestine (large) (small)
CC **A18.39** **Retroperitoneal tuberculosis**
Tuberculosis of mesenteric glands
Tuberculosis of retroperitoneal (lymph glands)
CC **A18.4** **Tuberculosis of skin and subcutaneous tissue**
Erythema induratum, tuberculous
Lupus excedens
Lupus vulgaris NOS
Lupus vulgaris of eyelid
Scrofuloderma
Tuberculosis of external ear
Excludes2: *lupus erythematosus (L93.-)*
systemic lupus erythematosus (M32.-)
+ **A18.5** **Tuberculosis of eye**
Excludes2: *lupus vulgaris of eyelid (A18.4)*
CC **A18.50** **Tuberculosis of eye, unspecified**
CC **A18.51** **Tuberculous episcleritis**
CC **A18.52** **Tuberculous keratitis**
Tuberculous interstitial keratitis
Tuberculous keratoconjunctivitis (interstitial) (phlyctenular)
CC **A18.53** **Tuberculous chorioretinitis**
CC **A18.54** **Tuberculous iridocyclitis**
CC **A18.59** **Other tuberculosis of eye**
Tuberculous conjunctivitis
CC **A18.6** **Tuberculosis of (inner) (middle) ear**
Tuberculous otitis media
Excludes2: *tuberculosis of external ear (A18.4)*
tuberculous mastoiditis (A18.03)
CC **A18.7** **Tuberculosis of adrenal glands**
Tuberculous Addison's disease
+ **A18.8** **Tuberculosis of other specified organs**
CC **A18.81** **Tuberculosis of thyroid gland**
CC **A18.82** **Tuberculosis of other endocrine glands**
Tuberculosis of pituitary gland
Tuberculosis of thymus gland
CC **A18.83** **Tuberculosis of digestive tract organs, not elsewhere classified**
Excludes1: *tuberculosis of intestine (A18.32)*
CC **A18.84** **Tuberculosis of heart**
Tuberculous cardiomyopathy
Tuberculous endocarditis
Tuberculous myocarditis
Tuberculous pericarditis
CC **A18.85** **Tuberculosis of spleen**
CC **A18.89** **Tuberculosis of other sites**
Tuberculosis of muscle
Tuberculous cerebral arteritis

A19 **Miliary tuberculosis**
Includes: disseminated tuberculosis
generalized tuberculosis
tuberculous polyserositis
MCC **A19.0** **Acute miliary tuberculosis of a single specified site**
MCC **A19.1** **Acute miliary tuberculosis of multiple sites**
MCC **A19.2** **Acute miliary tuberculosis, unspecified**
MCC **A19.8** **Other miliary tuberculosis**
MCC **A19.9** **Miliary tuberculosis, unspecified**

Certain zoonotic bacterial diseases (A20-A28)

A20 **Plague**
Includes: infection due to Yersinia pestis
MCC **A20.0** **Bubonic plague**
MCC **A20.1** **Cellulocutaneous plague**
MCC **A20.2** **Pneumonic plague**
MCC **A20.3** **Plague meningitis**
MCC **A20.7** **Septicemic plague**
Review coding guideline C.1.d
MCC **A20.8** **Other forms of plague**
Abortive plague
Asymptomatic plague
Pestis minor
MCC **A20.9** **Plague, unspecified**
A21 **Tularemia**
Includes: deer-fly fever
infection due to Francisella tularensis
rabbit fever
CC **A21.0** **Ulceroglandular tularemia**
CC **A21.1** **Oculoglandular tularemia**
Ophthalmic tularemia
CC **A21.2** **Pulmonary tularemia**
CC **A21.3** **Gastrointestinal tularemia**
Abdominal tularemia
CC **A21.7** **Generalized tularemia**
Review coding guideline C.1.d
CC **A21.8** **Other forms of tularemia**
CC **A21.9** **Tularemia, unspecified**
A22 **Anthrax**
Includes: infection due to Bacillus anthracis
CC **A22.0** **Cutaneous anthrax**
Malignant carbuncle
Malignant pustule
MCC **A22.1** **Pulmonary anthrax**
Inhalation anthrax
Ragpicker's disease
Woolsorter's disease
CC **A22.2** **Gastrointestinal anthrax**
MCC **A22.7** **Anthrax sepsis**
Review coding guideline C.1.d
CC **A22.8** **Other forms of anthrax**
Anthrax meningitis
CC **A22.9** **Anthrax, unspecified**
A23 **Brucellosis**
Includes: Malta fever
Mediterranean fever
undulant fever
A23.0 **Brucellosis due to Brucella melitensis**
A23.1 **Brucellosis due to Brucella abortus**
A23.2 **Brucellosis due to Brucella suis**
A23.3 **Brucellosis due to Brucella canis**
CC **A23.8** **Other brucellosis**
CC **A23.9** **Brucellosis, unspecified**
Review coding guideline C.1.d
A24 **Glanders and melioidosis**
CC **A24.0** **Glanders**
Infection due to Pseudomonas mallei
Malleus
Review coding guideline C.1.d
CC **A24.1** **Acute and fulminating melioidosis**
Melioidosis pneumonia
Melioidosis sepsis
Review coding guideline C.1.d

CC **A24.2 Subacute and chronic melioidosis**
CC **A24.3 Other melioidosis**
CC **A24.9 Melioidosis, unspecified**
Infection due to Pseudomonas pseudomallei NOS
Whitmore's disease

A25 Rat-bite fevers
CC **A25.0 Spirillosis**
Sodoku
CC **A25.1 Streptobacillosis**
Epidemic arthritic erythema
Haverhill fever
Streptobacillary rat-bite fever
CC **A25.9 Rat-bite fever, unspecified**

A26 Erysipeloid
A26.0 Cutaneous erysipeloid
Erythema migrans
MCC **A26.7 Erysipelothrix sepsis**
Review coding guideline C.1.d
A26.8 Other forms of erysipeloid
A26.9 Erysipeloid, unspecified

A27 Leptospirosis
CC **A27.0 Leptospirosis icterohemorrhagica**
Leptospiral or spirochetal jaundice (hemorrhagic)
Weil's disease
\+ **A27.8 Other forms of leptospirosis**
MCC **A27.81 Aseptic meningitis in leptospirosis**
CC **A27.89 Other forms of leptospirosis**
CC **A27.9 Leptospirosis, unspecified**

A28 Other zoonotic bacterial diseases, not elsewhere classified
CC **A28.0 Pasteurellosis**
Review coding guideline C.1.d
CC **A28.1 Cat-scratch disease**
Cat-scratch fever
CC **A28.2 Extraintestinal yersiniosis**
Excludes1: *enteritis due to Yersinia enterocolitica (A04.6)*
plague (A20.-)
Review coding guideline C.1.d
CC **A28.8 Other specified zoonotic bacterial diseases, not elsewhere classified**
CC **A28.9 Zoonotic bacterial disease, unspecified**

Other bacterial diseases (A30-A49)

A30 Leprosy [Hansen's disease]
Includes: infection due to Mycobacterium leprae
Excludes1: *sequelae of leprosy (B92)*
CC **A30.0 Indeterminate leprosy**
I leprosy
CC **A30.1 Tuberculoid leprosy**
TT leprosy
CC **A30.2 Borderline tuberculoid leprosy**
BT leprosy
CC **A30.3 Borderline leprosy**
BB leprosy
CC **A30.4 Borderline lepromatous leprosy**
BL leprosy
CC **A30.5 Lepromatous leprosy**
LL leprosy
CC **A30.8 Other forms of leprosy**
CC **A30.9 Leprosy, unspecified**

A31 Infection due to other mycobacteria
Excludes2: *leprosy (A30.-)*
tuberculosis (A15-A19)
CC **A31.0 Pulmonary mycobacterial infection**
Infection due to Mycobacterium avium
Infection due to Mycobacterium intracellulare [Battey bacillus]
Infection due to Mycobacterium kansasii
CC **A31.1 Cutaneous mycobacterial infection**
Buruli ulcer
Infection due to Mycobacterium marinum
Infection due to Mycobacterium ulcerans
CC **A31.2 Disseminated mycobacterium avium-intracellulare complex (DMAC)**
MAC sepsis
CC **A31.8 Other mycobacterial infections**
CC **A31.9 Mycobacterial infection, unspecified**
Atypical mycobacterial infection NOS
Mycobacteriosis NOS

A32 Listeriosis
Includes: listerial foodborne infection
Excludes1: *neonatal (disseminated) listeriosis (P37.2)*
CC **A32.0 Cutaneous listeriosis**
\+ **A32.1 Listerial meningitis and meningoencephalitis**
CC **A32.11 Listerial meningitis**
CC **A32.12 Listerial meningoencephalitis**
MCC **A32.7 Listerial sepsis**
Review coding guideline C.1.d
\+ **A32.8 Other forms of listeriosis**
CC **A32.81 Oculoglandular listeriosis**
CC **A32.82 Listerial endocarditis**
CC **A32.89 Other forms of listeriosis**
Listerial cerebral arteritis
CC **A32.9 Listeriosis, unspecified**

MCC ● **A33 Tetanus neonatorum**
Valid 3-character code, no further characters required

♀ CC ● **A34 Obstetrical tetanus**
Valid 3-character code, no further characters required

MCC **A35 Other tetanus**
Tetanus NOS
Excludes1: *obstetrical tetanus (A34)*
tetanus neonatorum (A33)
Valid 3-character code, no further characters required

A36 Diphtheria
CC **A36.0 Pharyngeal diphtheria**
Diphtheritic membranous angina
Tonsillar diphtheria
CC **A36.1 Nasopharyngeal diphtheria**
CC **A36.2 Laryngeal diphtheria**
Diphtheritic laryngotracheitis
CC **A36.3 Cutaneous diphtheria**
Excludes2: *erythrasma (L08.1)*
\+ **A36.8 Other diphtheria**
CC **A36.81 Diphtheritic cardiomyopathy**
Diphtheritic myocarditis
CC **A36.82 Diphtheritic radiculomyelitis**
CC **A36.83 Diphtheritic polyneuritis**
CC **A36.84 Diphtheritic tubulo-interstitial nephropathy**
CC **A36.85 Diphtheritic cystitis**
CC **A36.86 Diphtheritic conjunctivitis**
CC **A36.89 Other diphtheritic complications**
Diphtheritic peritonitis
CC **A36.9 Diphtheria, unspecified**

A37 Whooping cough
\+ **A37.0 Whooping cough due to Bordetella pertussis**
CC **A37.00 Whooping cough due to Bordetella pertussis without pneumonia**
Paroxysmal cough due to Bordetella pertussis without pneumonia
MCC **A37.01 Whooping cough due to Bordetella pertussis with pneumonia**
Paroxysmal cough due to Bordetella pertussis with pneumonia
\+ **A37.1 Whooping cough due to Bordetella parapertussis**
CC **A37.10 Whooping cough due to Bordetella parapertussis without pneumonia**
MCC **A37.11 Whooping cough due to Bordetella parapertussis with pneumonia**
\+ **A37.8 Whooping cough due to other Bordetella species**
CC **A37.80 Whooping cough due to other Bordetella species without pneumonia**
MCC **A37.81 Whooping cough due to other Bordetella species with pneumonia**
\+ **A37.9 Whooping cough, unspecified species**
CC **A37.90 Whooping cough, unspecified species without pneumonia**
MCC **A37.91 Whooping cough, unspecified species with pneumonia**

A38 Scarlet fever

Includes: scarlatina
Excludes2: *streptococcal sore throat (J02.0)*

CC **A38.0 Scarlet fever with otitis media**
CC **A38.1 Scarlet fever with myocarditis**
CC **A38.8 Scarlet fever with other complications**
CC **A38.9 Scarlet fever, uncomplicated**
Scarlet fever, NOS

A39 Meningococcal infection

MCC **A39.0 Meningococcal meningitis**
MCC **A39.1 Waterhouse-Friderichsen syndrome**
Meningococcal hemorrhagic adrenalitis
Meningococcic adrenal syndrome
Review coding guideline C.1.d
MCC **A39.2 Acute meningococcemia**
Review coding guideline C.1.d
MCC **A39.3 Chronic meningococcemia**
Review coding guideline C.1.d
MCC **A39.4 Meningococcemia, unspecified**
Review coding guideline C.1.d
\+ **A39.5 Meningococcal heart disease**
MCC **A39.50 Meningococcal carditis, unspecified**
MCC **A39.51 Meningococcal endocarditis**
MCC **A39.52 Meningococcal myocarditis**
MCC **A39.53 Meningococcal pericarditis**
\+ **A39.8 Other meningococcal infections**
MCC **A39.81 Meningococcal encephalitis**
CC **A39.82 Meningococcal retrobulbar neuritis**
CC **A39.83 Meningococcal arthritis**
CC **A39.84 Postmeningococcal arthritis**
CC **A39.89 Other meningococcal infections**
Meningococcal conjunctivitis
CC **A39.9 Meningococcal infection, unspecified**
Meningococcal disease NOS

A40 Streptococcal sepsis

Code first:
postprocedural streptococcal sepsis (T81.4-)
streptococcal sepsis during labor (O75.3)
streptococcal sepsis following abortion or ectopic or molar pregnancy (O03-O07, O08.0)
streptococcal sepsis following immunization (T88.0)
streptococcal sepsis following infusion, transfusion or therapeutic injection (T80.2-)
Excludes1: *neonatal (P36.0-P36.1)*
puerperal sepsis (O85)
sepsis due to Streptococcus, group D (A41.81)
Review coding guideline C.1.d

MCC **A40.0 Sepsis due to streptococcus, group A**
MCC **A40.1 Sepsis due to streptococcus, group B**
AHA CC: 4Q, 2018, 89; 1Q, 2019, 14
MCC **A40.3 Sepsis due to Streptococcus pneumoniae**
Pneumococcal sepsis
MCC **A40.8 Other streptococcal sepsis**
MCC **A40.9 Streptococcal sepsis, unspecified**

A41 Other sepsis

Code first:
postprocedural sepsis (T81.4-)
sepsis during labor (O75.3)
sepsis following abortion, ectopic or molar pregnancy (O03-O07, O08.0)
sepsis following immunization (T88.0)
sepsis following infusion, transfusion or therapeutic injection (T80.2-)
Excludes1: *bacteremia NOS (R78.81)*
neonatal (P36.-)
puerperal sepsis (O85)
streptococcal sepsis (A40.-)
Excludes2: *sepsis (due to) (in) actinomycotic (A42.7)*
sepsis (due to) (in) anthrax (A22.7)
sepsis (due to) (in) candidal (B37.7)
sepsis (due to) (in) Erysipelothrix (A26.7)
sepsis (due to) (in) extraintestinal yersiniosis (A28.2)
sepsis (due to) (in) gonococcal (A54.86)
sepsis (due to) (in) herpesviral (B00.7)
sepsis (due to) (in) listerial (A32.7)
sepsis (due to) (in) melioidosis (A24.1)
sepsis (due to) (in) meningococcal (A39.2-A39.4)
sepsis (due to) (in) plague (A20.7)
sepsis (due to) (in) tularemia (A21.7)
toxic shock syndrome (A48.3)
Review coding guideline C.1.d

\+ **A41.0 Sepsis due to Staphylococcus aureus**
MCC **A41.01 Sepsis due to Methicillin susceptible Staphylococcus aureus**
MSSA sepsis
Staphylococcus aureus sepsis NOS
AHA CC: 2Q, 2020, 17-18
MCC **A41.02 Sepsis due to Methicillin resistant Staphylococcus aureus**
Review coding guideline C.1.e.1.a
MCC **A41.1 Sepsis due to other specified staphylococcus**
Coagulase negative staphylococcus sepsis
MCC **A41.2 Sepsis due to unspecified staphylococcus**
MCC **A41.3 Sepsis due to Hemophilus influenzae**
MCC **A41.4 Sepsis due to anaerobes**
Excludes1: *gas gangrene (A48.0)*
\+ **A41.5 Sepsis due to other Gram-negative organisms**
MCC **A41.50 Gram-negative sepsis, unspecified**
Gram-negative sepsis NOS
AHA CC: 2Q, 2020, 29
MCC **A41.51 Sepsis due to Escherichia coli [E. coli]**
AHA CC: 1Q, 2018, 16; 2Q, 2020, 17-18
MCC **A41.52 Sepsis due to Pseudomonas**
Pseudomonas aeroginosa
MCC **A41.53 Sepsis due to Serratia**
MCC **A41.59 Other Gram-negative sepsis**
AHA CC: 1Q, 2019, 13
\+ **A41.8 Other specified sepsis**
MCC **A41.81 Sepsis due to Enterococcus**
MCC **A41.89 Other specified sepsis**
AHA CC: 3Q, 2016, 9-14; 2Q, 2020, 8; 1Q, 2021, 33
MCC **A41.9 Sepsis, unspecified organism**
Septicemia NOS
AHA CC: 4Q, 2018, 18; 2Q, 2020, 28

A42 Actinomycosis

Excludes1: *actinomycetoma (B47.1)*
CC **A42.0 Pulmonary actinomycosis**
CC **A42.1 Abdominal actinomycosis**
CC **A42.2 Cervicofacial actinomycosis**
MCC **A42.7 Actinomycotic sepsis**
Review coding guideline C.1.d
\+ **A42.8 Other forms of actinomycosis**
CC **A42.81 Actinomycotic meningitis**
CC **A42.82 Actinomycotic encephalitis**
CC **A42.89 Other forms of actinomycosis**
CC **A42.9 Actinomycosis, unspecified**

A43 Nocardiosis

CC **A43.0 Pulmonary nocardiosis**
CC **A43.1 Cutaneous nocardiosis**
CC **A43.8 Other forms of nocardiosis**
CC **A43.9 Nocardiosis, unspecified**

A44 Bartonellosis

CC **A44.0 Systemic bartonellosis**
Oroya fever
CC **A44.1 Cutaneous and mucocutaneous bartonellosis**
Verruga peruana
CC **A44.8 Other forms of bartonellosis**
CC **A44.9 Bartonellosis, unspecified**

A46 Erysipelas

Excludes1: *postpartum or puerperal erysipelas (O86.89)*
Valid 3-character code, no further characters required

A48 Other bacterial diseases, not elsewhere classified

Excludes1: *actinomycetoma (B47.1)*
MCC **A48.0 Gas gangrene**
Clostridial cellulitis
Clostridial myonecrosis
AHA CC: 4Q, 2017, 102
MCC **A48.1 Legionnaires' disease**
A48.2 Nonpneumonic Legionnaires' disease [Pontiac fever]
MCC **A48.3 Toxic shock syndrome**
Use additional code to identify the organism (B95, B96)
Excludes1: *endotoxic shock NOS (R57.8)*
sepsis NOS (A41.9)
A48.4 Brazilian purpuric fever
Systemic Hemophilus aegyptius infection

+ A48.5 **Other specified botulism**
Non-foodborne intoxication due to toxins of Clostridium botulinum [C. botulinum]
Excludes1: *food poisoning due to toxins of Clostridium botulinum (A05.1)*
• CC A48.51 **Infant botulism**
CC A48.52 **Wound botulism**
Non-foodborne botulism NOS
Use additional code for associated wound
A48.8 **Other specified bacterial diseases**

A49 **Bacterial infection of unspecified site**
Excludes1: *bacterial agents as the cause of diseases classified elsewhere (B95-B96)*
chlamydial infection NOS (A74.9)
meningococcal infection NOS (A39.9)
rickettsial infection NOS (A79.9)
spirochetal infection NOS (A69.9)
+ A49.0 **Staphylococcal infection, unspecified site**
A49.01 **Methicillin susceptible Staphylococcus aureus infection, unspecified site**
Methicillin susceptible Staphylococcus aureus (MSSA) infection
Staphylococcus aureus infection NOS
A49.02 **Methicillin resistant Staphylococcus aureus infection, unspecified site**
Methicillin resistant Staphylococcus aureus (MRSA) infection
A49.1 **Streptococcal infection, unspecified site**
A49.2 **Hemophilus influenzae infection, unspecified site**
A49.3 **Mycoplasma infection, unspecified site**
A49.8 **Other bacterial infections of unspecified site**
A49.9 **Bacterial infection, unspecified**
Excludes1: *bacteremia NOS (R78.81)*

Infections with a predominantly sexual mode of transmission (A50-A64)

Excludes1: *human immunodeficiency virus [HIV] disease (B20)*
nonspecific and nongonococcal urethritis (N34.1)
Reiter's disease (M02.3-)

A50 **Congenital syphilis**
+ A50.0 **Early congenital syphilis, symptomatic**
Any congenital syphilitic condition specified as early or manifest less than two years after birth.
CC A50.01 **Early congenital syphilitic oculopathy**
CC A50.02 **Early congenital syphilitic osteochondropathy**
CC A50.03 **Early congenital syphilitic pharyngitis**
Early congenital syphilitic laryngitis
CC A50.04 **Early congenital syphilitic pneumonia**
CC A50.05 **Early congenital syphilitic rhinitis**
CC A50.06 **Early cutaneous congenital syphilis**
CC A50.07 **Early mucocutaneous congenital syphilis**
CC A50.08 **Early visceral congenital syphilis**
CC A50.09 **Other early congenital syphilis, symptomatic**
A50.1 **Early congenital syphilis, latent**
Congenital syphilis without clinical manifestations, with positive serological reaction and negative spinal fluid test, less than two years after birth.
CC A50.2 **Early congenital syphilis, unspecified**
Congenital syphilis NOS less than two years after birth.
+ A50.3 **Late congenital syphilitic oculopathy**
Excludes1: *Hutchinson's triad (A50.53)*
CC A50.30 **Late congenital syphilitic oculopathy, unspecified**
CC A50.31 **Late congenital syphilitic interstitial keratitis**
CC A50.32 **Late congenital syphilitic chorioretinitis**
CC A50.39 **Other late congenital syphilitic oculopathy**
+ A50.4 **Late congenital neurosyphilis [juvenile neurosyphilis]**
Use additional code to identify any associated mental disorder
Excludes1: *Hutchinson's triad (A50.53)*
CC A50.40 **Late congenital neurosyphilis, unspecified**
Juvenile neurosyphilis NOS
MCC A50.41 **Late congenital syphilitic meningitis**
MCC A50.42 **Late congenital syphilitic encephalitis**
CC A50.43 **Late congenital syphilitic polyneuropathy**
CC A50.44 **Late congenital syphilitic optic nerve atrophy**
CC A50.45 **Juvenile general paresis**
Dementia paralytica juvenilis
Juvenile tabetoparetic neurosyphilis
CC A50.49 **Other late congenital neurosyphilis**
Juvenile tabes dorsalis
+ A50.5 **Other late congenital syphilis, symptomatic**
Any congenital syphilitic condition specified as late or manifest two years or more after birth.
CC A50.51 **Clutton's joints**
CC A50.52 **Hutchinson's teeth**
CC A50.53 **Hutchinson's triad**
CC A50.54 **Late congenital cardiovascular syphilis**
CC A50.55 **Late congenital syphilitic arthropathy**
CC A50.56 **Late congenital syphilitic osteochondropathy**
CC A50.57 **Syphilitic saddle nose**
CC A50.59 **Other late congenital syphilis, symptomatic**
A50.6 **Late congenital syphilis, latent**
Congenital syphilis without clinical manifestations, with positive serological reaction and negative spinal fluid test, two years or more after birth.
A50.7 **Late congenital syphilis, unspecified**
Congenital syphilis NOS two years or more after birth.
A50.9 **Congenital syphilis, unspecified**

A51 **Early syphilis**
A51.0 **Primary genital syphilis**
Syphilitic chancre NOS
A51.1 **Primary anal syphilis**
A51.2 **Primary syphilis of other sites**
+ A51.3 **Secondary syphilis of skin and mucous membranes**
CC A51.31 **Condyloma latum**
CC A51.32 **Syphilitic alopecia**
CC A51.39 **Other secondary syphilis of skin**
Syphilitic leukoderma
Syphilitic mucous patch
Excludes1: *late syphilitic leukoderma (A52.79)*
+ A51.4 **Other secondary syphilis**
MCC A51.41 **Secondary syphilitic meningitis**
♀ CC A51.42 **Secondary syphilitic female pelvic disease**
CC A51.43 **Secondary syphilitic oculopathy**
Secondary syphilitic chorioretinitis
Secondary syphilitic iridocyclitis, iritis
Secondary syphilitic uveitis
CC A51.44 **Secondary syphilitic nephritis**
CC A51.45 **Secondary syphilitic hepatitis**
CC A51.46 **Secondary syphilitic osteopathy**
CC A51.49 **Other secondary syphilitic conditions**
Secondary syphilitic lymphadenopathy
Secondary syphilitic myositis
A51.5 **Early syphilis, latent**
Syphilis (acquired) without clinical manifestations, with positive serological reaction and negative spinal fluid test, less than two years after infection.
A51.9 **Early syphilis, unspecified**

A52 **Late syphilis**
+ A52.0 **Cardiovascular and cerebrovascular syphilis**
CC A52.00 **Cardiovascular syphilis, unspecified**
CC A52.01 **Syphilitic aneurysm of aorta**
CC A52.02 **Syphilitic aortitis**
CC A52.03 **Syphilitic endocarditis**
Syphilitic aortic valve incompetence or stenosis
Syphilitic mitral valve stenosis
Syphilitic pulmonary valve regurgitation
CC A52.04 **Syphilitic cerebral arteritis**
CC A52.05 **Other cerebrovascular syphilis**
Syphilitic cerebral aneurysm (ruptured) (non-ruptured)
Syphilitic cerebral thrombosis
CC A52.06 **Other syphilitic heart involvement**
Syphilitic coronary artery disease
Syphilitic myocarditis
Syphilitic pericarditis
CC A52.09 **Other cardiovascular syphilis**
+ A52.1 **Symptomatic neurosyphilis**
CC A52.10 **Symptomatic neurosyphilis, unspecified**
CC A52.11 **Tabes dorsalis**
Locomotor ataxia (progressive)
Tabetic neurosyphilis
CC A52.12 **Other cerebrospinal syphilis**
MCC A52.13 **Late syphilitic meningitis**
MCC A52.14 **Late syphilitic encephalitis**
CC A52.15 **Late syphilitic neuropathy**
Late syphilitic acoustic neuritis
Late syphilitic optic (nerve) atrophy
Late syphilitic polyneuropathy
Late syphilitic retrobulbar neuritis

CC A52.16 **Charcôt's arthropathy (tabetic)**
CC A52.17 **General paresis**
Dementia paralytica
CC A52.19 **Other symptomatic neurosyphilis**
Syphilitic parkinsonism
CC A52.2 **Asymptomatic neurosyphilis**
CC A52.3 **Neurosyphilis, unspecified**
Gumma (syphilitic)
Syphilis (late)
Syphiloma
AHA CC: 2Q, 2021, 6
+ A52.7 **Other symptomatic late syphilis**
CC A52.71 **Late syphilitic oculopathy**
Late syphilitic chorioretinitis
Late syphilitic episcleritis
A52.72 **Syphilis of lung and bronchus**
CC A52.73 **Symptomatic late syphilis of other respiratory organs**
CC A52.74 **Syphilis of liver and other viscera**
Late syphilitic peritonitis
CC A52.75 **Syphilis of kidney and ureter**
Syphilitic glomerular disease
CC A52.76 **Other genitourinary symptomatic late syphilis**
Late syphilitic female pelvic inflammatory disease
CC A52.77 **Syphilis of bone and joint**
CC A52.78 **Syphilis of other musculoskeletal tissue**
Late syphilitic bursitis
Syphilis [stage unspecified] of bursa
Syphilis [stage unspecified] of muscle
Syphilis [stage unspecified] of synovium
Syphilis [stage unspecified] of tendon
CC A52.79 **Other symptomatic late syphilis**
Late syphilitic leukoderma
Syphilis of adrenal gland
Syphilis of pituitary gland
Syphilis of thyroid gland
Syphilitic splenomegaly
Excludes1: *syphilitic leukoderma (secondary) (A51.39)*
A52.8 **Late syphilis, latent**
Syphilis (acquired) without clinical manifestations, with positive serological reaction and negative spinal fluid test, two years or more after infection
A52.9 **Late syphilis, unspecified**

A53 **Other and unspecified syphilis**
A53.0 **Latent syphilis, unspecified as early or late**
Latent syphilis NOS
Positive serological reaction for syphilis
A53.9 **Syphilis, unspecified**
Infection due to Treponema pallidum NOS
Syphilis (acquired) NOS
Excludes1: *syphilis NOS under two years of age (A50.2)*

A54 **Gonococcal infection**
+ A54.0 **Gonococcal infection of lower genitourinary tract without periurethral or accessory gland abscess**
Excludes1: *gonococcal infection with genitourinary gland abscess (A54.1)*
gonococcal infection with periurethral abscess (A54.1)
CC A54.00 **Gonococcal infection of lower genitourinary tract, unspecified**
CC A54.01 **Gonococcal cystitis and urethritis, unspecified**
♀ CC A54.02 **Gonococcal vulvovaginitis, unspecified**
♀ CC A54.03 **Gonococcal cervicitis, unspecified**
CC A54.09 **Other gonococcal infection of lower genitourinary tract**
CC A54.1 **Gonococcal infection of lower genitourinary tract with periurethral and accessory gland abscess**
Gonococcal Bartholin's gland abscess
+ A54.2 **Gonococcal pelviperitonitis and other gonococcal genitourinary infection**
CC A54.21 **Gonococcal infection of kidney and ureter**
♂ CC A54.22 **Gonococcal prostatitis**
♂ CC A54.23 **Gonococcal infection of other male genital organs**
Gonococcal epididymitis
Gonococcal orchitis
♀ CC A54.24 **Gonococcal female pelvic inflammatory disease**
Gonococcal pelviperitonitis
Excludes1: *gonococcal peritonitis (A54.85)*
CC A54.29 **Other gonococcal genitourinary infections**
+ A54.3 **Gonococcal infection of eye**
CC A54.30 **Gonococcal infection of eye, unspecified**
CC A54.31 **Gonococcal conjunctivitis**
Ophthalmia neonatorum due to gonococcus
CC A54.32 **Gonococcal iridocyclitis**
CC A54.33 **Gonococcal keratitis**
CC A54.39 **Other gonococcal eye infection**
Gonococcal endophthalmia
+ A54.4 **Gonococcal infection of musculoskeletal system**
CC A54.40 **Gonococcal infection of musculoskeletal system, unspecified**
CC A54.41 **Gonococcal spondylopathy**
CC A54.42 **Gonococcal arthritis**
Excludes2: *gonococcal infection of spine (A54.41)*
CC A54.43 **Gonococcal osteomyelitis**
Excludes2: *gonococcal infection of spine (A54.41)*
CC A54.49 **Gonococcal infection of other musculoskeletal tissue**
Gonococcal bursitis
Gonococcal myositis
Gonococcal synovitis
Gonococcal tenosynovitis
A54.5 **Gonococcal pharyngitis**
A54.6 **Gonococcal infection of anus and rectum**
+ A54.8 **Other gonococcal infections**
MCC A54.81 **Gonococcal meningitis**
CC A54.82 **Gonococcal brain abscess**
CC A54.83 **Gonococcal heart infection**
Gonococcal endocarditis
Gonococcal myocarditis
Gonococcal pericarditis
CC A54.84 **Gonococcal pneumonia**
CC A54.85 **Gonococcal peritonitis**
Excludes1: *gonococcal pelviperitonitis (A54.24)*
MCC A54.86 **Gonococcal sepsis**
Review coding guideline C.1.d
CC A54.89 **Other gonococcal infections**
Gonococcal keratoderma
Gonococcal lymphadenitis
CC A54.9 **Gonococcal infection, unspecified**

A55 **Chlamydial lymphogranuloma (venereum)**
Climatic or tropical bubo
Durand-Nicolas-Favre disease
Esthiomene
Lymphogranuloma inguinale
Valid 3-character code, no further characters required

A56 **Other sexually transmitted chlamydial diseases**
Includes: sexually transmitted diseases due to Chlamydia trachomatis
Excludes1: *neonatal chlamydial conjunctivitis (P39.1)*
neonatal chlamydial pneumonia (P23.1)
Excludes2: *chlamydial lymphogranuloma (A55)*
conditions classified to A74.-
+ A56.0 **Chlamydial infection of lower genitourinary tract**
A56.00 **Chlamydial infection of lower genitourinary tract, unspecified**
A56.01 **Chlamydial cystitis and urethritis**
♀ A56.02 **Chlamydial vulvovaginitis**
A56.09 **Other chlamydial infection of lower genitourinary tract**
Chlamydial cervicitis
+ A56.1 **Chlamydial infection of pelviperitoneum and other genitourinary organs**
♀ A56.11 **Chlamydial female pelvic inflammatory disease**
A56.19 **Other chlamydial genitourinary infection**
Chlamydial epididymitis
Chlamydial orchitis
A56.2 **Chlamydial infection of genitourinary tract, unspecified**
A56.3 **Chlamydial infection of anus and rectum**
A56.4 **Chlamydial infection of pharynx**
A56.8 **Sexually transmitted chlamydial infection of other sites**

A57 **Chancroid**
Ulcus molle
Valid 3-character code, no further characters required

A58 **Granuloma inguinale**
Donovanosis
Valid 3-character code, no further characters required

A59 Trichomoniasis

Excludes2: *intestinal trichomoniasis (A07.8)*

+ **A59.0 Urogenital trichomoniasis**
  - **A59.00 Urogenital trichomoniasis, unspecified**
    - Fluor (vaginalis) due to Trichomonas
    - Leukorrhea (vaginalis) due to Trichomonas
  - ♀ **A59.01 Trichomonal vulvovaginitis**
  - ♂ **A59.02 Trichomonal prostatitis**
  - **A59.03 Trichomonal cystitis and urethritis**
  - **A59.09 Other urogenital trichomoniasis**
    - Trichomonas cervicitis

A59.8 Trichomoniasis of other sites

A59.9 Trichomoniasis, unspecified

A60 Anogenital herpesviral [herpes simplex] infections

+ **A60.0 Herpesviral infection of genitalia and urogenital tract**
  - **A60.00 Herpesviral infection of urogenital system, unspecified**
  - ♂ **A60.01 Herpesviral infection of penis**
  - ♂ **A60.02 Herpesviral infection of other male genital organs**
  - ♀ **A60.03 Herpesviral cervicitis**
  - ♀ **A60.04 Herpesviral vulvovaginitis**
    - Herpesviral [herpes simplex] ulceration
    - Herpesviral [herpes simplex] vaginitis
    - Herpesviral [herpes simplex] vulvitis
  - **A60.09 Herpesviral infection of other urogenital tract**

A60.1 Herpesviral infection of perianal skin and rectum

A60.9 Anogenital herpesviral infection, unspecified

AHA CC: 1Q, 2020, 20

A63 Other predominantly sexually transmitted diseases, not elsewhere classified

Excludes2: *molluscum contagiosum (B08.1)*
papilloma of cervix (D26.0)

A63.0 Anogenital (venereal) warts
- Anogenital warts due to (human) papillomavirus [HPV]
- Condyloma acuminatum

A63.8 Other specified predominantly sexually transmitted diseases

A64 Unspecified sexually transmitted disease

Valid 3-character code, no further characters required

Other spirochetal diseases (A65-A69)

Excludes2: *leptospirosis (A27.-)*
syphilis (A50-A53)

A65 Nonvenereal syphilis
- Bejel
- Endemic syphilis
- Njovera

Valid 3-character code, no further characters required

A66 Yaws

Includes: bouba
frambesia (tropica)
pian

A66.0 Initial lesions of yaws
- Chancre of yaws
- Frambesia, initial or primary
- Initial frambesial ulcer
- Mother yaw

A66.1 Multiple papillomata and wet crab yaws
- Frambesioma
- Pianoma
- Plantar or palmar papilloma of yaws

A66.2 Other early skin lesions of yaws
- Cutaneous yaws, less than five years after infection
- Early yaws (cutaneous)(macular)(maculopapular)(micropapular)(papular)
- Frambeside of early yaws

A66.3 Hyperkeratosis of yaws
- Ghoul hand
- Hyperkeratosis, palmar or plantar (early) (late) due to yaws
- Worm-eaten soles

A66.4 Gummata and ulcers of yaws
- Gummatous frambeside
- Nodular late yaws (ulcerated)

A66.5 Gangosa
- Rhinopharyngitis mutilans

A66.6 Bone and joint lesions of yaws
- Yaws ganglion
- Yaws goundou
- Yaws gumma, bone
- Yaws gummatous osteitis or periostitis
- Yaws hydrarthrosis
- Yaws osteitis
- Yaws periostitis (hypertrophic)

A66.7 Other manifestations of yaws
- Juxta-articular nodules of yaws
- Mucosal yaws

A66.8 Latent yaws
- Yaws without clinical manifestations, with positive serology

A66.9 Yaws, unspecified

A67 Pinta [carate]

A67.0 Primary lesions of pinta
- Chancre (primary) of pinta
- Papule (primary) of pinta

A67.1 Intermediate lesions of pinta
- Erythematous plaques of pinta
- Hyperchromic lesions of pinta
- Hyperkeratosis of pinta
- Pintids

A67.2 Late lesions of pinta
- Achromic skin lesions of pinta
- Cicatricial skin lesions of pinta
- Dyschromic skin lesions of pinta

A67.3 Mixed lesions of pinta
- Achromic with hyperchromic skin lesions of pinta [carate]

A67.9 Pinta, unspecified

A68 Relapsing fevers

Includes: recurrent fever
Excludes2: *Lyme disease (A69.2-)*

CC **A68.0 Louse-borne relapsing fever**
- Relapsing fever due to Borrelia recurrentis

CC **A68.1 Tick-borne relapsing fever**
- Relapsing fever due to any Borrelia species other than Borrelia recurrentis

CC **A68.9 Relapsing fever, unspecified**

A69 Other spirochetal infections

A69.0 Necrotizing ulcerative stomatitis
- Cancrum oris
- Fusospirochetal gangrene
- Noma
- Stomatitis gangrenosa

CC **A69.1 Other Vincent's infections**
- Fusospirochetal pharyngitis
- Necrotizing ulcerative (acute) gingivitis
- Necrotizing ulcerative (acute) gingivostomatitis
- Spirochetal stomatitis
- Trench mouth
- Vincent's angina
- Vincent's gingivitis

+ **A69.2 Lyme disease**
  - Erythema chronicum migrans due to Borrelia burgdorferi
  - CC **A69.20 Lyme disease, unspecified**
  - CC **A69.21 Meningitis due to Lyme disease**
  - CC **A69.22 Other neurologic disorders in Lyme disease**
    - Cranial neuritis
    - Meningoencephalitis
    - Polyneuropathy
  - CC **A69.23 Arthritis due to Lyme disease**
  - CC **A69.29 Other conditions associated with Lyme disease**
    - Myopericarditis due to Lyme disease
    - *AHA CC: 3Q, 2016, 12*

A69.8 Other specified spirochetal infections

A69.9 Spirochetal infection, unspecified

Other diseases caused by chlamydiae (A70-A74)

Excludes1: *sexually transmitted chlamydial diseases (A55-A56)*

CC **A70 Chlamydia psittaci infections**
Ornithosis
Parrot fever
Psittacosis
Valid 3-character code, no further characters required

A71 Trachoma
Excludes1: *sequelae of trachoma (B94.0)*
A71.0 Initial stage of trachoma
Trachoma dubium
A71.1 Active stage of trachoma
Granular conjunctivitis (trachomatous)
Trachomatous follicular conjunctivitis
Trachomatous pannus
A71.9 Trachoma, unspecified

A74 Other diseases caused by chlamydiae
Excludes1: *neonatal chlamydial conjunctivitis (P39.1)*
neonatal chlamydial pneumonia (P23.1)
Reiter's disease (M02.3-)
sexually transmitted chlamydial diseases (A55-A56)
Excludes2: *chlamydial pneumonia (J16.0)*
A74.0 Chlamydial conjunctivitis
Paratrachoma
\+ **A74.8 Other chlamydial diseases**
A74.81 Chlamydial peritonitis
A74.89 Other chlamydial diseases
A74.9 Chlamydial infection, unspecified
Chlamydiosis NOS

Rickettsioses (A75-A79)

A75 Typhus fever
Excludes1: *rickettsiosis due to Ehrlichia sennetsu (A79.81)*
CC **A75.0 Epidemic louse-borne typhus fever due to Rickettsia prowazekii**
Classical typhus (fever)
Epidemic (louse-borne) typhus
CC **A75.1 Recrudescent typhus [Brill's disease]**
Brill-Zinsser disease
CC **A75.2 Typhus fever due to Rickettsia typhi**
Murine (flea-borne) typhus
CC **A75.3 Typhus fever due to Rickettsia tsutsugamushi**
Scrub (mite-borne) typhus
Typhus fever due to Orientia Tsutsugamushi (scrub typhus)
Tsutsugamushi fever
CC **A75.9 Typhus fever, unspecified**
Typhus (fever) NOS

A77 Spotted fever [tick-borne rickettsioses]
CC **A77.0 Spotted fever due to Rickettsia rickettsii**
Rocky Mountain spotted fever
Sao Paulo fever
CC **A77.1 Spotted fever due to Rickettsia conorii**
African tick typhus
Boutonneuse fever
India tick typhus
Kenya tick typhus
Marseilles fever
Mediterranean tick fever
CC **A77.2 Spotted fever due to Rickettsia siberica**
North Asian tick fever
Siberian tick typhus
CC **A77.3 Spotted fever due to Rickettsia australis**
Queensland tick typhus
\+ **A77.4 Ehrlichiosis**
Excludes1: *anaplasmosis [A. phagocytophilum] (A79.82)*
rickettsiosis due to Ehrlichia sennetsu (A79.81)
CC **A77.40 Ehrlichiosis, unspecified**
CC **A77.41 Ehrlichiosis chafeensis [E. chafeensis]**
CC **A77.49 Other ehrlichiosis**
Ehrlichiosis due to E. ewingii
Ehrlichiosis due to E. muris euclairensis
CC **A77.8 Other spotted fevers**
Rickettsia 364D/R. philipii (Pacific Coast tick fever)
Spotted fever due to Rickettsia africae (African tick bite fever)
Spotted fever due to Rickettsia parkeri
CC **A77.9 Spotted fever, unspecified**
Tick-borne typhus NOS

CC **A78 Q fever**
Infection due to Coxiella burnetii
Nine Mile fever
Quadrilateral fever
Valid 3-character code, no further characters required

A79 Other rickettsioses
CC **A79.0 Trench fever**
Quintan fever
Wolhynian fever
CC **A79.1 Rickettsialpox due to Rickettsia akari**
Kew Garden fever
Vesicular rickettsiosis
\+ **A79.8 Other specified rickettsioses**
CC **A79.81 Rickettsiosis due to Ehrlichia sennetsu**
Rickettsiosis due to Neorickettsia sennetsu
Excludes1: *rickettsiosis due to Ehrlichia sennetsu (A79.81)*
CC **A79.82 Anaplasmosis [A. phagocytophilum]**
Transfusion transmitted A. phagocytophilum
CC **A79.89 Other specified rickettsioses**
CC **A79.9 Rickettsiosis, unspecified**
Rickettsial infection NOS

Viral and prion infections of the central nervous system (A80-A89)

Excludes1: *postpolio syndrome (G14)*
sequelae of poliomyelitis (B91)
sequelae of viral encephalitis (B94.1)

A80 Acute poliomyelitis
Excludes1: *acute flaccid myelitis (G04.82)*
MCC **A80.0 Acute paralytic poliomyelitis, vaccine-associated**
MCC **A80.1 Acute paralytic poliomyelitis, wild virus, imported**
MCC **A80.2 Acute paralytic poliomyelitis, wild virus, indigenous**
\+ **A80.3 Acute paralytic poliomyelitis, other and unspecified**
MCC **A80.30 Acute paralytic poliomyelitis, unspecified**
MCC **A80.39 Other acute paralytic poliomyelitis**
A80.4 Acute nonparalytic poliomyelitis
A80.9 Acute poliomyelitis, unspecified

A81 Atypical virus infections of central nervous system
Includes: diseases of the central nervous system caused by prions
Use additional code to identify:
dementia with behavioral disturbance (F02.81)
dementia without behavioral disturbance (F02.80)
\+ **A81.0 Creutzfeldt-Jakob disease**
CC **A81.00 Creutzfeldt-Jakob disease, unspecified**
Jakob-Creutzfeldt disease, unspecified
CC **A81.01 Variant Creutzfeldt-Jakob disease**
CJD
CC **A81.09 Other Creutzfeldt-Jakob disease**
CJD
Familial Creutzfeldt-Jakob disease
Iatrogenic Creutzfeldt-Jakob disease
Sporadic Creutzfeldt-Jakob disease
Subacute spongiform encephalopathy (with dementia)
CC **A81.1 Subacute sclerosing panencephalitis**
Dawson's inclusion body encephalitis
Van Bogaert's sclerosing leukoencephalopathy
CC **A81.2 Progressive multifocal leukoencephalopathy**
Multifocal leukoencephalopathy NOS
\+ **A81.8 Other atypical virus infections of central nervous system**
CC **A81.81 Kuru**
CC **A81.82 Gerstmann-Sträussler-Scheinker syndrome**
GSS syndrome
CC **A81.83 Fatal familial insomnia**
FFI
CC **A81.89 Other atypical virus infections of central nervous system**
CC **A81.9 Atypical virus infection of central nervous system, unspecified**
Prion diseases of the central nervous system NOS

A82 Rabies

CC **A82.0 Sylvatic rabies**
CC **A82.1 Urban rabies**
CC **A82.9 Rabies, unspecified**

A83 Mosquito-borne viral encephalitis

Includes: mosquito-borne viral meningoencephalitis
Excludes2: *Venezuelan equine encephalitis (A92.2)*
West Nile fever (A92.3-)
West Nile virus (A92.3-)

MCC **A83.0 Japanese encephalitis**
MCC **A83.1 Western equine encephalitis**
MCC **A83.2 Eastern equine encephalitis**
MCC **A83.3 St Louis encephalitis**
MCC **A83.4 Australian encephalitis**
Kunjin virus disease
MCC **A83.5 California encephalitis**
California meningoencephalitis
La Crosse encephalitis
MCC **A83.6 Rocio virus disease**
MCC **A83.8 Other mosquito-borne viral encephalitis**
MCC **A83.9 Mosquito-borne viral encephalitis, unspecified**

A84 Tick-borne viral encephalitis

Includes: tick-borne viral meningoencephalitis

MCC **A84.0 Far Eastern tick-borne encephalitis [Russian spring-summer encephalitis]**
MCC **A84.1 Central European tick-borne encephalitis**
\+ **A84.8 Other tick-borne viral encephalitis**
MCC **A84.81 Powassan virus disease**
AHA CC: 4Q, 2020, 4-5
MCC **A84.89 Other tick-borne viral encephalitis**
Louping ill
Code first, if applicable, transfusion related infection (T80.22-)
MCC **A84.9 Tick-borne viral encephalitis, unspecified**

A85 Other viral encephalitis, not elsewhere classified

Includes: specified viral encephalomyelitis NEC
specified viral meningoencephalitis NEC
Excludes1: *benign myalgic encephalomyelitis (G93.3)*
encephalitis due to cytomegalovirus (B25.8)
encephalitis due to herpesvirus NEC (B10.0-)
encephalitis due to herpesvirus [herpes simplex] (B00.4)
encephalitis due to measles virus (B05.0)
encephalitis due to mumps virus (B26.2)
encephalitis due to poliomyelitis virus (A80.-)
encephalitis due to zoster (B02.0)
lymphocytic choriomeningitis (A87.2)

CC **A85.0 Enteroviral encephalitis**
Enteroviral encephalomyelitis
CC **A85.1 Adenoviral encephalitis**
Adenoviral meningoencephalitis
MCC **A85.2 Arthropod-borne viral encephalitis, unspecified**
Excludes1: *West nile virus with encephalitis (A92.31)*
CC **A85.8 Other specified viral encephalitis**
Encephalitis lethargica
Von Economo-Cruchet disease

CC **A86 Unspecified viral encephalitis**

Viral encephalomyelitis NOS
Viral meningoencephalitis NOS
Valid 3-character code, no further characters required

A87 Viral meningitis

Excludes1: *meningitis due to herpesvirus [herpes simplex] (B00.3)*
meningitis due to herpesvirus [herpes simplex] (B00.3)
meningitis due to measles virus (B05.1)
meningitis due to mumps virus (B26.1)
meningitis due to poliomyelitis virus (A80.-)
meningitis due to zoster (B02.1)

CC **A87.0 Enteroviral meningitis**
Coxsackievirus meningitis
Echovirus meningitis
CC **A87.1 Adenoviral meningitis**
CC **A87.2 Lymphocytic choriomeningitis**
Lymphocytic meningoencephalitis
CC **A87.8 Other viral meningitis**
CC **A87.9 Viral meningitis, unspecified**

A88 Other viral infections of central nervous system, not elsewhere classified

Excludes1: *viral encephalitis NOS (A86)*
viral meningitis NOS (A87.9)

CC **A88.0 Enteroviral exanthematous fever [Boston exanthem]**
A88.1 Epidemic vertigo
CC **A88.8 Other specified viral infections of central nervous system**

CC **A89 Unspecified viral infection of central nervous system**

Valid 3-character code, no further characters required

Arthropod-borne viral fevers and viral hemorrhagic fevers (A90-A99)

CC **A90 Dengue fever [classical dengue]**

Excludes1: *dengue hemorrhagic fever (A91)*
AHA CC: 3Q, 2016, 13
Valid 3-character code, no further characters required

CC **A91 Dengue hemorrhagic fever**

Valid 3-character code, no further characters required

A92 Other mosquito-borne viral fevers

Excludes1: *Ross River disease (B33.1)*

CC **A92.0 Chikungunya virus disease**
Chikungunya (hemorrhagic) fever
CC **A92.1 O'nyong-nyong fever**
CC **A92.2 Venezuelan equine fever**
Venezuelan equine encephalitis
Venezuelan equine encephalomyelitis virus disease
\+ **A92.3 West Nile virus infection**
West Nile fever
MCC **A92.30 West Nile virus infection, unspecified**
West Nile fever NOS
West Nile fever without complications
West Nile virus NOS
MCC **A92.31 West Nile virus infection with encephalitis**
West Nile encephalitis
West Nile encephalomyelitis
AHA CC: 3Q, 2016, 12-13
MCC **A92.32 West Nile virus infection with other neurologic manifestation**
Use additional code to specify the neurologic manifestation
MCC **A92.39 West Nile virus infection with other complications**
Use additional code to specify the other conditions
CC **A92.4 Rift Valley fever**
CC **A92.5 Zika virus disease**
Zika virus fever
Zika virus infection
Zika NOS
Excludes1: *congenital Zika virus disease (P35.4)*
Review coding guideline C.1.f
AHA CC: 4Q, 2016, 4-7
CC **A92.8 Other specified mosquito-borne viral fevers**
CC **A92.9 Mosquito-borne viral fever, unspecified**

A93 Other arthropod-borne viral fevers, not elsewhere classified

CC **A93.0 Oropouche virus disease**
Oropouche fever
CC **A93.1 Sandfly fever**
Pappataci fever
Phlebotomus fever
CC **A93.2 Colorado tick fever**
CC **A93.8 Other specified arthropod-borne viral fevers**
Piry virus disease
Vesicular stomatitis virus disease [Indiana fever]

CC **A94 Unspecified arthropod-borne viral fever**

Arboviral fever NOS
Arbovirus infection NOS
Valid 3-character code, no further characters required

A95 Yellow fever

CC **A95.0 Sylvatic yellow fever**
Jungle yellow fever
CC **A95.1 Urban yellow fever**
CC **A95.9 Yellow fever, unspecified**

A96 Arenaviral hemorrhagic fever

CC **A96.0 Junin hemorrhagic fever**
Argentinian hemorrhagic fever

CC **A96.1 Machupo hemorrhagic fever**
Bolivian hemorrhagic fever

A96.2 Lassa fever

CC **A96.8 Other arenaviral hemorrhagic fevers**

CC **A96.9 Arenaviral hemorrhagic fever, unspecified**

A98 Other viral hemorrhagic fevers, not elsewhere classified

Excludes1: *chikungunya hemorrhagic fever (A92.0)*
dengue hemorrhagic fever (A91)

CC **A98.0 Crimean-Congo hemorrhagic fever**
Central Asian hemorrhagic fever

CC **A98.1 Omsk hemorrhagic fever**

CC **A98.2 Kyasanur Forest disease**

A98.3 Marburg virus disease

A98.4 Ebola virus disease

CC **A98.5 Hemorrhagic fever with renal syndrome**
Epidemic hemorrhagic fever
Korean hemorrhagic fever
Russian hemorrhagic fever
Hantaan virus disease
Hantavirus disease with renal manifestations
Nephropathia epidemica
Songo fever
Excludes1: *hantavirus (cardio)-pulmonary syndrome (B33.4)*

CC **A98.8 Other specified viral hemorrhagic fevers**

CC **A99 Unspecified viral hemorrhagic fever**
Valid 3-character code, no further characters

Viral infections characterized by skin and mucous membrane lesions (B00-B09)

B00 Herpesviral [herpes simplex] infections

Excludes1: *congenital herpesviral infections (P35.2)*
Excludes2: *anogenital herpesviral infection (A60.-)*
gammaherpesviral mononucleosis (B27.0-)
herpangina (B08.5)

B00.0 Eczema herpeticum
Kaposi's varicelliform eruption

B00.1 Herpesviral vesicular dermatitis
Herpes simplex facialis
Herpes simplex labialis
Herpes simplex otitis externa
Vesicular dermatitis of ear
Vesicular dermatitis of lip

CC **B00.2 Herpesviral gingivostomatitis and pharyngotonsillitis**
Herpesviral pharyngitis

MCC **B00.3 Herpesviral meningitis**

MCC **B00.4 Herpesviral encephalitis**
Herpesviral meningoencephalitis
Simian B disease
Excludes1: *herpesviral encephalitis due to herpesvirus 6 and 7 (B10.01, B10.09)*
non-simplex herpesviral encephalitis (B10.0-)

\+ **B00.5 Herpesviral ocular disease**

CC **B00.50 Herpesviral ocular disease, unspecified**

CC **B00.51 Herpesviral iridocyclitis**
Herpesviral iritis
Herpesviral uveitis, anterior

CC **B00.52 Herpesviral keratitis**
Herpesviral keratoconjunctivitis

CC **B00.53 Herpesviral conjunctivitis**

CC **B00.59 Other herpesviral disease of eye**
Herpesviral dermatitis of eyelid

MCC **B00.7 Disseminated herpesviral disease**
Herpesviral sepsis
Review coding guideline C.1.d

\+ **B00.8 Other forms of herpesviral infections**

CC **B00.81 Herpesviral hepatitis**

MCC **B00.82 Herpes simplex myelitis**

CC **B00.89 Other herpesviral infection**
Herpesviral whitlow

B00.9 Herpesviral infection, unspecified
Herpes simplex infection NOS

B01 Varicella [chickenpox]

CC **B01.0 Varicella meningitis**

\+ **B01.1 Varicella encephalitis, myelitis and encephalomyelitis**
Postchickenpox encephalitis, myelitis and encephalomyelitis

MCC **B01.11 Varicella encephalitis and encephalomyelitis**
Postchickenpox encephalitis and encephalomyelitis

MCC **B01.12 Varicella myelitis**
Postchickenpox myelitis

MCC **B01.2 Varicella pneumonia**

\+ **B01.8 Varicella with other complications**

CC **B01.81 Varicella keratitis**

CC **B01.89 Other varicella complications**

CC **B01.9 Varicella without complication**
Varicella NOS

B02 Zoster [herpes zoster]

Includes: shingles
zona

CC **B02.0 Zoster encephalitis**
Zoster meningoencephalitis

MCC **B02.1 Zoster meningitis**
AHA CC: 1Q, 2019, 18

\+ **B02.2 Zoster with other nervous system involvement**

CC **B02.21 Postherpetic geniculate ganglionitis**

CC **B02.22 Postherpetic trigeminal neuralgia**

CC **B02.23 Postherpetic polyneuropathy**

MCC **B02.24 Postherpetic myelitis**
Herpes zoster myelitis

CC **B02.29 Other postherpetic nervous system involvement**
Postherpetic radiculopathy

\+ **B02.3 Zoster ocular disease**

CC **B02.30 Zoster ocular disease, unspecified**

CC **B02.31 Zoster conjunctivitis**

CC **B02.32 Zoster iridocyclitis**

CC **B02.33 Zoster keratitis**
Herpes zoster keratoconjunctivitis

CC **B02.34 Zoster scleritis**

CC **B02.39 Other herpes zoster eye disease**
Zoster blepharitis

CC **B02.7 Disseminated zoster**

CC **B02.8 Zoster with other complications**
Herpes zoster otitis externa

B02.9 Zoster without complications
Zoster NOS

CC **B03 Smallpox**

NOTE In 1980 the 33rd World Health Assembly declared that smallpox had been eradicated.
The classification is maintained for surveillance purposes.

Valid 3-character code, no further characters required

CC **B04 Monkeypox**
Valid 3-character code, no further characters required

B05 Measles

Includes: morbilli
Excludes1: *subacute sclerosing panencephalitis (A81.1)*

MCC **B05.0 Measles complicated by encephalitis**
Postmeasles encephalitis

CC **B05.1 Measles complicated by meningitis**
Postmeasles meningitis

MCC **B05.2 Measles complicated by pneumonia**
Postmeasles pneumonia

B05.3 Measles complicated by otitis media
Postmeasles otitis media

CC **B05.4 Measles with intestinal complications**

\+ **B05.8 Measles with other complications**

CC **B05.81 Measles keratitis and keratoconjunctivitis**

CC **B05.89 Other measles complications**

B05.9 Measles without complication
Measles NOS

B06 Rubella [German measles]

Excludes1: *congenital rubella (P35.0)*

\+ **B06.0 Rubella with neurological complications**

CC **B06.00 Rubella with neurological complication, unspecified**

MCC **B06.01 Rubella encephalitis**

Rubella meningoencephalitis

CC **B06.02 Rubella meningitis**

CC **B06.09 Other neurological complications of rubella**

\+ **B06.8 Rubella with other complications**

CC **B06.81 Rubella pneumonia**

CC **B06.82 Rubella arthritis**

CC **B06.89 Other rubella complications**

B06.9 Rubella without complication

Rubella NOS

B07 Viral warts

Includes: verruca simplex
verruca vulgaris
viral warts due to human papillomavirus

Excludes2: *anogenital (venereal) warts (A63.0)*
papilloma of bladder (D41.4)
papilloma of cervix (D26.0)
papilloma larynx (D14.1)

B07.0 Plantar wart

Verruca plantaris

B07.8 Other viral warts

Common wart
Flat wart
Verruca plana

B07.9 Viral wart, unspecified

B08 Other viral infections characterized by skin and mucous membrane lesions, not elsewhere classified

Excludes1: *vesicular stomatitis virus disease (A93.8)*

B08.0 Other orthopoxvirus infections

Excludes2: *monkeypox (B04)*

\+ **B08.01 Cowpox and vaccinia not from vaccine**

B08.010 Cowpox

B08.011 Vaccinia not from vaccine

Excludes1: *vaccinia (from vaccination) (generalized) (T88.1)*

B08.02 Orf virus disease

Contagious pustular dermatitis
Ecthyma contagiosum

B08.03 Pseudocowpox [milker's node]

B08.04 Paravaccinia, unspecified

B08.09 Other orthopoxvirus infections

Orthopoxvirus infection NOS

B08.1 Molluscum contagiosum

\+ **B08.2 Exanthema subitum [sixth disease]**

Roseola infantum

• **B08.20 Exanthema subitum [sixth disease], unspecified**

Roseola infantum, unspecified

• **B08.21 Exanthema subitum [sixth disease] due to human herpesvirus 6**

Roseola infantum due to human herpesvirus 6

• **B08.22 Exanthema subitum [sixth disease] due to human herpesvirus 7**

Roseola infantum due to human herpesvirus 7

CC **B08.3 Erythema infectiosum [fifth disease]**

B08.4 Enteroviral vesicular stomatitis with exanthem

Hand, foot and mouth disease

B08.5 Enteroviral vesicular pharyngitis

Herpangina

\+ **B08.6 Parapoxvirus infections**

B08.60 Parapoxvirus infection, unspecified

B08.61 Bovine stomatitis

B08.62 Sealpox

B08.69 Other parapoxvirus infections

\+ **B08.7 Yatapoxvirus infections**

B08.70 Yatapoxvirus infection, unspecified

CC **B08.71 Tanapox virus disease**

B08.72 Yaba pox virus disease

Yaba monkey tumor disease

B08.79 Other yatapoxvirus infections

B08.8 Other specified viral infections characterized by skin and mucous membrane lesions

Enteroviral lymphonodular pharyngitis
Foot-and-mouth disease
Poxvirus NEC

B09 Unspecified viral infection characterized by skin and mucous membrane lesions

Viral enanthema NOS
Viral exanthema NOS
Valid 3-character code, no further characters required

Other human herpesviruses (B10)

B10 Other human herpesviruses

Excludes2: *cytomegalovirus (B25.9)*
Epstein-Barr virus (B27.0-)
herpes NOS (B00.9)
herpes simplex (B00.-)
herpes zoster (B02.-)
human herpesvirus NOS (B00.-)
human herpesvirus 1 and 2 (B00.-)
human herpesvirus 3 (B01.-, B02.-)
human herpesvirus 4 (B27.0-)
human herpesvirus 5 (B25.-)
varicella (B01.-)
zoster (B02.-)

\+ **B10.0 Other human herpesvirus encephalitis**

Excludes2: *herpes encephalitis NOS (B00.4)*
herpes simplex encephalitis (B00.4)
human herpesvirus encephalitis (B00.4)
simian B herpes virus encephalitis (B00.4)

MCC **B10.01 Human herpesvirus 6 encephalitis**

MCC **B10.09 Other human herpesvirus encephalitis**

Human herpesvirus 7 encephalitis

\+ **B10.8 Other human herpesvirus infection**

B10.81 Human herpesvirus 6 infection

B10.82 Human herpesvirus 7 infection

B10.89 Other human herpesvirus infection

Human herpesvirus 8 infection
Kaposi's sarcoma-associated herpesvirus infection

Viral hepatitis (B15-B19)

Excludes1: *sequelae of viral hepatitis (B94.2)*

Excludes2: *cytomegaloviral hepatitis (B25.1)*
herpesviral [herpes simplex] hepatitis (B00.81)

B15 Acute hepatitis A

MCC **B15.0 Hepatitis A with hepatic coma**

CC **B15.9 Hepatitis A without hepatic coma**

Hepatitis A (acute)(viral) NOS

B16 Acute hepatitis B

MCC **B16.0 Acute hepatitis B with delta-agent with hepatic coma**

CC **B16.1 Acute hepatitis B with delta-agent without hepatic coma**

MCC **B16.2 Acute hepatitis B without delta-agent with hepatic coma**

CC **B16.9 Acute hepatitis B without delta-agent and without hepatic coma**

Hepatitis B (acute) (viral) NOS
AHA CC: 3Q, 2016, 13

B17 Other acute viral hepatitis

CC **B17.0 Acute delta-(super) infection of hepatitis B carrier**

\+ **B17.1 Acute hepatitis C**

CC **B17.10 Acute hepatitis C without hepatic coma**

Acute hepatitis C NOS

MCC **B17.11 Acute hepatitis C with hepatic coma**

CC **B17.2 Acute hepatitis E**

CC **B17.8 Other specified acute viral hepatitis**

Hepatitis non-A non-B (acute) (viral) NEC

CC **B17.9 Acute viral hepatitis, unspecified**

Acute hepatitis NOS
Acute infectious hepatitis NOS

B18 Chronic viral hepatitis

Includes: Carrier of viral hepatitis

CC **B18.0 Chronic viral hepatitis B with delta-agent**

CC **B18.1 Chronic viral hepatitis B without delta-agent**

Carrier of viral hepatitis B
Chronic (viral) hepatitis B

B18.2 Chronic viral hepatitis C

Carrier of viral hepatitis C
AHA CC: 1Q, 2017, 41; 1Q, 2018, 4-5

CC **B18.8 Other chronic viral hepatitis**

Carrier of other viral hepatitis

CC **B18.9 Chronic viral hepatitis, unspecified**

Carrier of unspecified viral hepatitis

B19 Unspecified viral hepatitis

MCC **B19.0 Unspecified viral hepatitis with hepatic coma**
\+ **B19.1 Unspecified viral hepatitis B**
CC **B19.10 Unspecified viral hepatitis B without hepatic coma**
Unspecified viral hepatitis B NOS
MCC **B19.11 Unspecified viral hepatitis B with hepatic coma**
\+ **B19.2 Unspecified viral hepatitis C**
B19.20 Unspecified viral hepatitis C without hepatic coma
Viral hepatitis C NOS
MCC **B19.21 Unspecified viral hepatitis C with hepatic coma**
CC **B19.9 Unspecified viral hepatitis without hepatic coma**
Viral hepatitis NOS

Human immunodeficiency virus [HIV] disease (B20)

CC **B20 Human immunodeficiency virus [HIV] disease**

Includes: acquired immune deficiency syndrome [AIDS]
AIDS-related complex [ARC]
HIV infection, symptomatic

Code first Human immunodeficiency virus [HIV] disease complicating pregnancy, childbirth and the puerperium, if applicable (O98.7-)

Use additional code(s) to identify all manifestations of HIV infection

Excludes1: *asymptomatic human immunodeficiency virus [HIV] infection status (Z21)*
exposure to HIV virus (Z20.6)
inconclusive serologic evidence of HIV (R75)

Review coding guideline C.1.a
AHA CC: 1Q, 2019, 8-11; 4Q, 2020, 97-98; 1Q, 2021, 52; 2Q, 2021, 6
Valid 3-character code, no further characters required

Other viral diseases (B25-B34)

B25 Cytomegaloviral disease

Excludes1: *congenital cytomegalovirus infection (P35.1)*
cytomegaloviral mononucleosis (B27.1-)

MCC **B25.0 Cytomegaloviral pneumonitis**
CC **B25.1 Cytomegaloviral hepatitis**
MCC **B25.2 Cytomegaloviral pancreatitis**
CC **B25.8 Other cytomegaloviral diseases**
Cytomegaloviral encephalitis
CC **B25.9 Cytomegaloviral disease, unspecified**

B26 Mumps

Includes: epidemic parotitis
infectious parotitis

♂ CC **B26.0 Mumps orchitis**
MCC **B26.1 Mumps meningitis**
MCC **B26.2 Mumps encephalitis**
CC **B26.3 Mumps pancreatitis**
\+ **B26.8 Mumps with other complications**
CC **B26.81 Mumps hepatitis**
CC **B26.82 Mumps myocarditis**
CC **B26.83 Mumps nephritis**
CC **B26.84 Mumps polyneuropathy**
CC **B26.85 Mumps arthritis**
CC **B26.89 Other mumps complications**
B26.9 Mumps without complication
Mumps NOS
Mumps parotitis NOS

B27 Infectious mononucleosis

Includes: glandular fever
monocytic angina
Pfeiffer's disease

\+ **B27.0 Gammaherpesviral mononucleosis**
Mononucleosis due to Epstein-Barr virus
B27.00 Gammaherpesviral mononucleosis without complication
B27.01 Gammaherpesviral mononucleosis with polyneuropathy
B27.02 Gammaherpesviral mononucleosis with meningitis
B27.09 Gammaherpesviral mononucleosis with other complications
Hepatomegaly in gammaherpesviral mononucleosis

\+ **B27.1 Cytomegaloviral mononucleosis**
B27.10 Cytomegaloviral mononucleosis without complications
B27.11 Cytomegaloviral mononucleosis with polyneuropathy
B27.12 Cytomegaloviral mononucleosis with meningitis
B27.19 Cytomegaloviral mononucleosis with other complication
Hepatomegaly in cytomegaloviral mononucleosis
\+ **B27.8 Other infectious mononucleosis**
B27.80 Other infectious mononucleosis without complication
B27.81 Other infectious mononucleosis with polyneuropathy
B27.82 Other infectious mononucleosis with meningitis
B27.89 Other infectious mononucleosis with other complication
Hepatomegaly in other infectious mononucleosis
\+ **B27.9 Infectious mononucleosis, unspecified**
B27.90 Infectious mononucleosis, unspecified without complication
B27.91 Infectious mononucleosis, unspecified with polyneuropathy
B27.92 Infectious mononucleosis, unspecified with meningitis
B27.99 Infectious mononucleosis, unspecified with other complication
Hepatomegaly in unspecified infectious mononucleosis

B30 Viral conjunctivitis

Excludes1: *herpesviral [herpes simplex] ocular disease (B00.5)*
ocular zoster (B02.3)

B30.0 Keratoconjunctivitis due to adenovirus
Epidemic keratoconjunctivitis
Shipyard eye
B30.1 Conjunctivitis due to adenovirus
Acute adenoviral follicular conjunctivitis
Swimming-pool conjunctivitis
B30.2 Viral pharyngoconjunctivitis
B30.3 Acute epidemic hemorrhagic conjunctivitis (enteroviral)
Conjunctivitis due to coxsackievirus 24
Conjunctivitis due to enterovirus 70
Hemorrhagic conjunctivitis (acute)(epidemic)
B30.8 Other viral conjunctivitis
Newcastle conjunctivitis
B30.9 Viral conjunctivitis, unspecified

B33 Other viral diseases, not elsewhere classified

B33.0 Epidemic myalgia
Bornholm disease
CC **B33.1 Ross River disease**
Epidemic polyarthritis and exanthema
Ross River fever
\+ **B33.2 Viral carditis**
Coxsackie (virus) carditis
CC **B33.20 Viral carditis, unspecified**
CC **B33.21 Viral endocarditis**
CC **B33.22 Viral myocarditis**
CC **B33.23 Viral pericarditis**
B33.24 Viral cardiomyopathy
B33.3 Retrovirus infections, not elsewhere classified
Retrovirus infection NOS
CC **B33.4 Hantavirus (cardio)-pulmonary syndrome [HPS] [HCPS]**
Hantavirus disease with pulmonary manifestations
Sin nombre virus disease
Use additional code to identify any associated acute kidney failure (N17.9)

Excludes1: *hantavirus disease with renal manifestations (A98.5)*
hemorrhagic fever with renal manifestations (A98.5)

B33.8 Other specified viral diseases

Excludes1: *anogenital human papillomavirus infection (A63.0)*
viral warts due to human papillomavirus infection (B07)

B34 Viral infection of unspecified site

Excludes1: *anogenital human papillomavirus infection (A63.0)*
cytomegaloviral disease NOS (B25.9)
herpesvirus [herpes simplex] infection NOS (B00.9)
retrovirus infection NOS (B33.3)
viral agents as the cause of diseases classified elsewhere (B97.-)
viral warts due to human papillomavirus infection (B07)

B34.0 Adenovirus infection, unspecified
B34.1 Enterovirus infection, unspecified
Coxsackievirus infection NOS
Echovirus infection NOS
B34.2 Coronavirus infection, unspecified
Excludes1: *COVID-19 (U07.1)*
pneumonia due to SARS associated coronavirus (J12.81)
AHA CC: 1Q, 2020, 34-36
CC **B34.3 Parvovirus infection, unspecified**
B34.4 Papovavirus infection, unspecified
B34.8 Other viral infections of unspecified site
B34.9 Viral infection, unspecified
Viremia NOS
AHA CC: 3Q, 2016, 10

Mycoses (B35-B49)

Excludes2: *hypersensitivity pneumonitis due to organic dust (J67.-)*
mycosis fungoides (C84.0-)

B35 Dermatophytosis

Includes: favus
infections due to species of Epidermophyton, Micro-sporum and Trichophyton
tinea, any type except those in B36.-

B35.0 Tinea barbae and tinea capitis
Beard ringworm
Kerion
Scalp ringworm
Sycosis, mycotic
B35.1 Tinea unguium
Dermatophytic onychia
Dermatophytosis of nail
Onychomycosis
Ringworm of nails
B35.2 Tinea manuum
Dermatophytosis of hand
Hand ringworm
B35.3 Tinea pedis
Athlete's foot
Dermatophytosis of foot
Foot ringworm
B35.4 Tinea corporis
Ringworm of the body
B35.5 Tinea imbricata
Tokelau
B35.6 Tinea cruris
Dhobi itch
Groin ringworm
Jock itch
B35.8 Other dermatophytoses
Disseminated dermatophytosis
Granulomatous dermatophytosis
B35.9 Dermatophytosis, unspecified
Ringworm NOS

B36 Other superficial mycoses

B36.0 Pityriasis versicolor
Tinea flava
Tinea versicolor
B36.1 Tinea nigra
Keratomycosis nigricans palmaris
Microsporosis nigra
Pityriasis nigra
B36.2 White piedra
Tinea blanca
B36.3 Black piedra
B36.8 Other specified superficial mycoses
B36.9 Superficial mycosis, unspecified

B37 Candidiasis

Includes: candidosis
moniliasis
Excludes1: *neonatal candidiasis (P37.5)*

CC **B37.0 Candidal stomatitis**
Oral thrush
MCC **B37.1 Pulmonary candidiasis**
Candidal bronchitis
Candidal pneumonia
B37.2 Candidiasis of skin and nail
Candidal onychia
Candidal paronychia
Excludes2: *diaper dermatitis (L22)*
♀ **B37.3 Candidiasis of vulva and vagina**
Candidal vulvovaginitis
Monilial vulvovaginitis
Vaginal thrush
\+ **B37.4 Candidiasis of other urogenital sites**
CC **B37.41 Candidal cystitis and urethritis**
HAC see Appendix B for HAC conditional logic
♂ **B37.42 Candidal balanitis**
CC **B37.49 Other urogenital candidiasis**
Candidal pyelonephritis
HAC see Appendix B for HAC conditional logic
MCC **B37.5 Candidal meningitis**
MCC **B37.6 Candidal endocarditis**
MCC **B37.7 Candidal sepsis**
Disseminated candidiasis
Systemic candidiasis
Review coding guideline C.1.d
AHA CC: 4Q, 2014, 46
\+ **B37.8 Candidiasis of other sites**
CC **B37.81 Candidal esophagitis**
CC **B37.82 Candidal enteritis**
Candidal proctitis
CC **B37.83 Candidal cheilitis**
CC **B37.84 Candidal otitis externa**
CC **B37.89 Other sites of candidiasis**
Candidal osteomyelitis
B37.9 Candidiasis, unspecified
Thrush NOS

B38 Coccidioidomycosis

CC **B38.0 Acute pulmonary coccidioidomycosis**
CC **B38.1 Chronic pulmonary coccidioidomycosis**
CC **B38.2 Pulmonary coccidioidomycosis, unspecified**
CC **B38.3 Cutaneous coccidioidomycosis**
MCC **B38.4 Coccidioidomycosis meningitis**
CC **B38.7 Disseminated coccidioidomycosis**
Generalized coccidioidomycosis
\+ **B38.8 Other forms of coccidioidomycosis**
♂ CC **B38.81 Prostatic coccidioidomycosis**
CC **B38.89 Other forms of coccidioidomycosis**
CC **B38.9 Coccidioidomycosis, unspecified**

B39 Histoplasmosis

Code first associated AIDS (B20)

Use additional code for any associated manifestations, such as:
endocarditis (I39)
meningitis (G02)
pericarditis (I32)
retinitis (H32)

MCC **B39.0 Acute pulmonary histoplasmosis capsulati**
MCC **B39.1 Chronic pulmonary histoplasmosis capsulati**
MCC **B39.2 Pulmonary histoplasmosis capsulati, unspecified**
CC **B39.3 Disseminated histoplasmosis capsulati**
Generalized histoplasmosis capsulati
B39.4 Histoplasmosis capsulati, unspecified
American histoplasmosis
B39.5 Histoplasmosis duboisii
African histoplasmosis
B39.9 Histoplasmosis, unspecified

B40 Blastomycosis

Excludes1: *Brazilian blastomycosis (B41.-)*
keloidal blastomycosis (B48.0)

CC **B40.0 Acute pulmonary blastomycosis**
CC **B40.1 Chronic pulmonary blastomycosis**
CC **B40.2 Pulmonary blastomycosis, unspecified**
CC **B40.3 Cutaneous blastomycosis**
CC **B40.7 Disseminated blastomycosis**
Generalized blastomycosis
+ **B40.8 Other forms of blastomycosis**
CC **B40.81 Blastomycotic meningoencephalitis**
Meningomyelitis due to blastomycosis
CC **B40.89 Other forms of blastomycosis**
CC **B40.9 Blastomycosis, unspecified**

B41 Paracoccidioidomycosis

Includes: Brazilian blastomycosis
Lutz' disease

CC **B41.0 Pulmonary paracoccidioidomycosis**
CC **B41.7 Disseminated paracoccidioidomycosis**
Generalized paracoccidioidomycosis
CC **B41.8 Other forms of paracoccidioidomycosis**
CC **B41.9 Paracoccidioidomycosis, unspecified**

B42 Sporotrichosis

B42.0 Pulmonary sporotrichosis
B42.1 Lymphocutaneous sporotrichosis
B42.7 Disseminated sporotrichosis
Generalized sporotrichosis
+ **B42.8 Other forms of sporotrichosis**
B42.81 Cerebral sporotrichosis
Meningitis due to sporotrichosis
B42.82 Sporotrichosis arthritis
B42.89 Other forms of sporotrichosis
B42.9 Sporotrichosis, unspecified

B43 Chromomycosis and pheomycotic abscess

B43.0 Cutaneous chromomycosis
Dermatitis verrucosa
B43.1 Pheomycotic brain abscess
Cerebral chromomycosis
B43.2 Subcutaneous pheomycotic abscess and cyst
B43.8 Other forms of chromomycosis
B43.9 Chromomycosis, unspecified

B44 Aspergillosis

Includes: aspergilloma

MCC **B44.0 Invasive pulmonary aspergillosis**
CC **B44.1 Other pulmonary aspergillosis**
CC **B44.2 Tonsillar aspergillosis**
CC **B44.7 Disseminated aspergillosis**
Generalized aspergillosis
+ **B44.8 Other forms of aspergillosis**
CC **B44.81 Allergic bronchopulmonary aspergillosis**
CC **B44.89 Other forms of aspergillosis**
CC **B44.9 Aspergillosis, unspecified**

B45 Cryptococcosis

CC **B45.0 Pulmonary cryptococcosis**
MCC **B45.1 Cerebral cryptococcosis**
Cryptococcal meningitis
Cryptococcosis meningocerebralis
CC **B45.2 Cutaneous cryptococcosis**
CC **B45.3 Osseous cryptococcosis**
CC **B45.7 Disseminated cryptococcosis**
Generalized cryptococcosis
CC **B45.8 Other forms of cryptococcosis**
CC **B45.9 Cryptococcosis, unspecified**

B46 Zygomycosis

MCC **B46.0 Pulmonary mucormycosis**
MCC **B46.1 Rhinocerebral mucormycosis**
MCC **B46.2 Gastrointestinal mucormycosis**
MCC **B46.3 Cutaneous mucormycosis**
Subcutaneous mucormycosis
MCC **B46.4 Disseminated mucormycosis**
Generalized mucormycosis
MCC **B46.5 Mucormycosis, unspecified**
MCC **B46.8 Other zygomycoses**
Entomophthoromycosis
MCC **B46.9 Zygomycosis, unspecified**
Phycomycosis NOS

B47 Mycetoma

CC **B47.0 Eumycetoma**
Madura foot, mycotic
Maduromycosis
CC **B47.1 Actinomycetoma**
CC **B47.9 Mycetoma, unspecified**
Madura foot NOS

B48 Other mycoses, not elsewhere classified

B48.0 Lobomycosis
Keloidal blastomycosis
Lobo's disease
B48.1 Rhinosporidiosis
CC **B48.2 Allescheriasis**
Infection due to Pseudallescheria boydii
Excludes1: *eumycetoma (B47.0)*
CC **B48.3 Geotrichosis**
Geotrichum stomatitis
CC **B48.4 Penicillosis**
Talaromycosis
CC **B48.8 Other specified mycoses**
Adiaspiromycosis
Infection of tissue and organs by Alternaria
Infection of tissue and organs by Drechslera
Infection of tissue and organs by Fusarium
Infection of tissue and organs by saprophytic fungi NEC
AHA CC: 2Q, 2014, 13; 4Q, 2014, 46

CC **B49 Unspecified mycosis**

Fungemia NOS
Valid 3-character code, no further characters required

Protozoal diseases (B50-B64)

Excludes1: *amebiasis (A06.-)*
other protozoal intestinal diseases (A07.-)

B50 Plasmodium falciparum malaria

Includes: mixed infections of Plasmodium falciparum with any other Plasmodium species

CC **B50.0 Plasmodium falciparum malaria with cerebral complications**
Cerebral malaria NOS
CC **B50.8 Other severe and complicated Plasmodium falciparum malaria**
Severe or complicated Plasmodium falciparum malaria NOS
MCC **B50.9 Plasmodium falciparum malaria, unspecified**

B51 Plasmodium vivax malaria

Includes: mixed infections of Plasmodium vivax with other Plasmodium species, except Plasmodium falciparum
Excludes1: *plasmodium vivax with Plasmodium falciparum (B50.-)*

CC **B51.0 Plasmodium vivax malaria with rupture of spleen**
CC **B51.8 Plasmodium vivax malaria with other complications**
CC **B51.9 Plasmodium vivax malaria without complication**
Plasmodium vivax malaria NOS

B52 Plasmodium malariae malaria

Includes: mixed infections of Plasmodium malariae with other Plasmodium species, except Plasmodium falciparum and Plasmodium vivax
Excludes1: *Plasmodium falciparum (B50.-)*
Plasmodium vivax (B51.-)

CC **B52.0 Plasmodium malariae malaria with nephropathy**
CC **B52.8 Plasmodium malariae malaria with other complications**
CC **B52.9 Plasmodium malariae malaria without complication**
Plasmodium malariae malaria NOS

B53 Other specified malaria

CC **B53.0 Plasmodium ovale malaria**
Excludes1: *Plasmodium ovale with Plasmodium falciparum (B50.-)*
Plasmodium ovale with Plasmodium malariae (B52.-)
Plasmodium ovale with Plasmodium vivax (B51.-)
CC **B53.1 Malaria due to simian plasmodia**
Excludes1: *Malaria due to simian plasmodia with Plasmodium falciparum (B50.-)*
Malaria due to simian plasmodia with Plasmodium malariae (B52.-)
Malaria due to simian plasmodia with Plasmodium ovale (B53.0)
Malaria due to simian plasmodia with Plasmodium vivax (B51.-)
CC **B53.8 Other malaria, not elsewhere classified**

CC **B54 Unspecified malaria**

Valid 3-character code, no further characters required

B55 Leishmaniasis

CC **B55.0 Visceral leishmaniasis**
Kala-azar
Post-kala-azar dermal leishmaniasis

CC **B55.1 Cutaneous leishmaniasis**

CC **B55.2 Mucocutaneous leishmaniasis**

CC **B55.9 Leishmaniasis, unspecified**

B56 African trypanosomiasis

CC **B56.0 Gambiense trypanosomiasis**
Infection due to Trypanosoma brucei gambiense
West African sleeping sickness

CC **B56.1 Rhodesiense trypanosomiasis**
East African sleeping sickness
Infection due to Trypanosoma brucei rhodesiense

CC **B56.9 African trypanosomiasis, unspecified**
Sleeping sickness NOS

B57 Chagas' disease

Includes: American trypanosomiasis
infection due to Trypanosoma cruzi

CC **B57.0 Acute Chagas' disease with heart involvement**
Acute Chagas' disease with myocarditis

CC **B57.1 Acute Chagas' disease without heart involvement**
Acute Chagas' disease NOS

CC **B57.2 Chagas' disease (chronic) with heart involvement**
American trypanosomiasis NOS
Chagas' disease (chronic) NOS
Chagas' disease (chronic) with myocarditis
Trypanosomiasis NOS

\+ **B57.3 Chagas' disease (chronic) with digestive system involvement**

CC **B57.30 Chagas' disease with digestive system involvement, unspecified**

CC **B57.31 Megaesophagus in Chagas' disease**

CC **B57.32 Megacolon in Chagas' disease**

CC **B57.39 Other digestive system involvement in Chagas' disease**

\+ **B57.4 Chagas' disease (chronic) with nervous system involvement**

CC **B57.40 Chagas' disease with nervous system involvement, unspecified**

CC **B57.41 Meningitis in Chagas' disease**

CC **B57.42 Meningoencephalitis in Chagas' disease**

CC **B57.49 Other nervous system involvement in Chagas' disease**

CC **B57.5 Chagas' disease (chronic) with other organ involvement**

B58 Toxoplasmosis

Includes: infection due to Toxoplasma gondii
Excludes1: *congenital toxoplasmosis (P37.1)*

\+ **B58.0 Toxoplasma oculopathy**

CC **B58.00 Toxoplasma oculopathy, unspecified**

CC **B58.01 Toxoplasma chorioretinitis**

CC **B58.09 Other toxoplasma oculopathy**
Toxoplasma uveitis

CC **B58.1 Toxoplasma hepatitis**

MCC **B58.2 Toxoplasma meningoencephalitis**

MCC **B58.3 Pulmonary toxoplasmosis**

\+ **B58.8 Toxoplasmosis with other organ involvement**

MCC **B58.81 Toxoplasma myocarditis**

CC **B58.82 Toxoplasma myositis**

CC **B58.83 Toxoplasma tubulo-interstitial nephropathy**
Toxoplasma pyelonephritis

CC **B58.89 Toxoplasmosis with other organ involvement**

CC **B58.9 Toxoplasmosis, unspecified**

B59 Pneumocystosis

MCC
Pneumonia due to Pneumocystis carinii
Pneumonia due to Pneumocystis jiroveci
Valid 3-character code, no further characters required

B60 Other protozoal diseases, not elsewhere classified

Excludes1: *cryptosporidiosis (A07.2)*
intestinal microsporidiosis (A07.8)
isosporiasis (A07.3)

\+ **B60.0 Babesiosis**
AHA CC: 4Q, 2020, 5-6

CC **B60.00 Babesiosis, unspecified**
Babesiosis due to unspecified Babesia species
Piroplasmosis, unspecified

CC **B60.01 Babesiosis due to Babesia microti**
Infection due to B. microti

CC **B60.02 Babesiosis due to Babesia duncani**
Infection due to B. duncani and B. duncani-type species

CC **B60.03 Babesiosis due to Babesia divergens**
Babesiosis due to Babesia MO-1
Infection due to B. divergens and B. divergens-like strains

CC **B60.09 Other babesiosis**
Babesiosis due to Babesia KO-1
Babesiosis due to Babesia venatorum
Infection due to other Babesia species
Infection due to other protozoa of the order Piroplasmida
Other piroplasmosis

\+ **B60.1 Acanthamebiasis**

CC **B60.10 Acanthamebiasis, unspecified**

B60.11 Meningoencephalitis due to Acanthamoeba (culbertsoni)

B60.12 Conjunctivitis due to Acanthamoeba

B60.13 Keratoconjunctivitis due to Acanthamoeba

CC **B60.19 Other acanthamebic disease**

CC **B60.2 Naegleriasis**
Primary amebic meningoencephalitis

B60.8 Other specified protozoal diseases
Microsporidiosis

B64 Unspecified protozoal disease

Valid 3-character code, no further characters required

Helminthiases (B65-B83)

B65 Schistosomiasis [bilharziasis]

Includes: snail fever

CC **B65.0 Schistosomiasis due to Schistosoma haematobium [urinary schistosomiasis]**

CC **B65.1 Schistosomiasis due to Schistosoma mansoni [intestinal schistosomiasis]**

CC **B65.2 Schistosomiasis due to Schistosoma japonicum**
Asiatic schistosomiasis

CC **B65.3 Cercarial dermatitis**
Swimmer's itch

CC **B65.8 Other schistosomiasis**
Infection due to Schistosoma intercalatum
Infection due to Schistosoma mattheei
Infection due to Schistosoma mekongi

CC **B65.9 Schistosomiasis, unspecified**

B66 Other fluke infections

CC **B66.0 Opisthorchiasis**
Infection due to cat liver fluke
Infection due to Opisthorchis (felineus)(viverrini)

CC **B66.1 Clonorchiasis**
Chinese liver fluke disease
Infection due to Clonorchis sinensis
Oriental liver fluke disease

CC **B66.2 Dicroceliasis**
Infection due to Dicrocoelium dendriticum
Lancet fluke infection

CC **B66.3 Fascioliasis**
Infection due to Fasciola gigantica
Infection due to Fasciola hepatica
Infection due to Fasciola indica
Sheep liver fluke disease

CC **B66.4 Paragonimiasis**
Infection due to Paragonimus species
Lung fluke disease
Pulmonary distomiasis

CC **B66.5 Fasciolopsiasis**
Infection due to Fasciolopsis buski
Intestinal distomiasis
CC **B66.8 Other specified fluke infections**
Echinostomiasis
Heterophyiasis
Metagonimiasis
Nanophyetiasis
Watsoniasis
B66.9 Fluke infection, unspecified

B67 Echinococcosis

Includes: hydatidosis
CC **B67.0 Echinococcus granulosus infection of liver**
CC **B67.1 Echinococcus granulosus infection of lung**
CC **B67.2 Echinococcus granulosus infection of bone**
\+ **B67.3 Echinococcus granulosus infection, other and multiple sites**
CC **B67.31 Echinococcus granulosus infection, thyroid gland**
CC **B67.32 Echinococcus granulosus infection, multiple sites**
CC **B67.39 Echinococcus granulosus infection, other sites**
CC **B67.4 Echinococcus granulosus infection, unspecified**
Dog tapeworm (infection)
CC **B67.5 Echinococcus multilocularis infection of liver**
\+ **B67.6 Echinococcus multilocularis infection, other and multiple sites**
CC **B67.61 Echinococcus multilocularis infection, multiple sites**
CC **B67.69 Echinococcus multilocularis infection, other sites**
CC **B67.7 Echinococcus multilocularis infection, unspecified**
CC **B67.8 Echinococcosis, unspecified, of liver**
\+ **B67.9 Echinococcosis, other and unspecified**
CC **B67.90 Echinococcosis, unspecified**
Echinococcosis NOS
CC **B67.99 Other echinococcosis**

B68 Taeniasis

Excludes1: *cysticercosis (B69.-)*
CC **B68.0 Taenia solium taeniasis**
Pork tapeworm (infection)
CC **B68.1 Taenia saginata taeniasis**
Beef tapeworm (infection)
Infection due to adult tapeworm Taenia saginata
CC **B68.9 Taeniasis, unspecified**

B69 Cysticercosis

Includes: cysticerciasis infection due to larval form of Taenia solium
CC **B69.0 Cysticercosis of central nervous system**
CC **B69.1 Cysticercosis of eye**
\+ **B69.8 Cysticercosis of other sites**
CC **B69.81 Myositis in cysticercosis**
CC **B69.89 Cysticercosis of other sites**
CC **B69.9 Cysticercosis, unspecified**

B70 Diphyllobothriasis and sparganosis

CC **B70.0 Diphyllobothriasis**
Diphyllobothrium (adult) (latum) (pacificum) infection
Fish tapeworm (infection)
Excludes2: *larval diphyllobothriasis (B70.1)*
CC **B70.1 Sparganosis**
Infection due to Sparganum (mansoni) (proliferum)
Infection due to Spirometra larva
Larval diphyllobothriasis
Spirometrosis

B71 Other cestode infections

CC **B71.0 Hymenolepiasis**
Dwarf tapeworm infection
Rat tapeworm (infection)
CC **B71.1 Dipylidiasis**
CC **B71.8 Other specified cestode infections**
Coenurosis
B71.9 Cestode infection, unspecified
Tapeworm (infection) NOS

CC **B72 Dracunculiasis**

Includes: guinea worm infection
infection due to Dracunculus medinensis
Valid 3-character code, no further characters required

B73 Onchocerciasis

Includes: onchocerca volvulus infection
onchocercosis
river blindness
\+ **B73.0 Onchocerciasis with eye disease**
CC **B73.00 Onchocerciasis with eye involvement, unspecified**
CC **B73.01 Onchocerciasis with endophthalmitis**
CC **B73.02 Onchocerciasis with glaucoma**
CC **B73.09 Onchocerciasis with other eye involvement**
Infestation of eyelid due to onchocerciasis
CC **B73.1 Onchocerciasis without eye disease**

B74 Filariasis

Excludes2: *onchocerciasis (B73)*
tropical (pulmonary) eosinophilia NOS (J82.89)
CC **B74.0 Filariasis due to Wuchereria bancrofti**
Bancroftian elephantiasis
Bancroftian filariasis
CC **B74.1 Filariasis due to Brugia malayi**
CC **B74.2 Filariasis due to Brugia timori**
CC **B74.3 Loiasis**
Calabar swelling
Eyeworm disease of Africa
Loa loa infection
CC **B74.4 Mansonelliasis**
Infection due to Mansonella ozzardi
Infection due to Mansonella perstans
Infection due to Mansonella streptocerca
CC **B74.8 Other filariases**
Dirofilariasis
CC **B74.9 Filariasis, unspecified**

CC **B75 Trichinellosis**

Includes: infection due to Trichinella species
trichiniasis
Valid 3-character code, no further characters required

B76 Hookworm diseases

Includes: uncinariasis
CC **B76.0 Ancylostomiasis**
Infection due to Ancylostoma species
CC **B76.1 Necatoriasis**
Infection due to Necator americanus
CC **B76.8 Other hookworm diseases**
CC **B76.9 Hookworm disease, unspecified**
Cutaneous larva migrans NOS

B77 Ascariasis

Includes: ascaridiasis
roundworm infection
CC **B77.0 Ascariasis with intestinal complications**
\+ **B77.8 Ascariasis with other complications**
MCC **B77.81 Ascariasis pneumonia**
CC **B77.89 Ascariasis with other complications**
CC **B77.9 Ascariasis, unspecified**

B78 Strongyloidiasis

Excludes1: *trichostrongyliasis (B81.2)*
CC **B78.0 Intestinal strongyloidiasis**
B78.1 Cutaneous strongyloidiasis
CC **B78.7 Disseminated strongyloidiasis**
CC **B78.9 Strongyloidiasis, unspecified**

CC **B79 Trichuriasis**

Includes: trichocephaliasis
whipworm (disease)(infection)
Valid 3-character code, no further characters required

CC **B80 Enterobiasis**

Includes: oxyuriasis
pinworm infection
threadworm infection
Valid 3-character code, no further characters required

B81 Other intestinal helminthiases, not elsewhere classified

Excludes1: *angiostrongyliasis due to:*
Angiostrongylus cantonensis (B83.2)
Parastrongylus cantonensis (B83.2)

CC **B81.0 Anisakiasis**
Infection due to Anisakis larva

CC **B81.1 Intestinal capillariasis**
Capillariasis NOS
Infection due to Capillaria philippinensis
Excludes2: *hepatic capillariasis (B83.8)*

CC **B81.2 Trichostrongyliasis**

CC **B81.3 Intestinal angiostrongyliasis**
Angiostrongyliasis due to:
Angiostrongylus costaricensis
Parastrongylus cantonensis

CC **B81.4 Mixed intestinal helminthiases**
Infection due to intestinal helminths classified to more than one of the categories B65.0-B81.3 and B81.8
Mixed helminthiasis NOS

CC **B81.8 Other specified intestinal helminthiases**
Infection due to Oesophagostomum species [esophagostomiasis]
Infection due to Ternidens diminutus [ternidensiasis]

B82 Unspecified intestinal parasitism

CC **B82.0 Intestinal helminthiasis, unspecified**

B82.9 Intestinal parasitism, unspecified

B83 Other helminthiases

Excludes1: *capillariasis NOS (B81.1)*
Excludes2: *intestinal capillariasis (B81.1)*

B83.0 Visceral larva migrans
Toxocariasis

B83.1 Gnathostomiasis
Wandering swelling

B83.2 Angiostrongyliasis due to Parastrongylus cantonensis
Eosinophilic meningoencephalitis due to Parastrongylus cantonensis
Excludes2: *intestinal angiostrongyliasis (B81.3)*

B83.3 Syngamiasis
Syngamosis

B83.4 Internal hirudiniasis
Excludes2: *external hirudiniasis (B88.3)*

B83.8 Other specified helminthiases
Acanthocephaliasis
Gongylonemiasis
Hepatic capillariasis
Metastrongyliasis
Thelaziasis

B83.9 Helminthiasis, unspecified
Worms NOS
Excludes1: *intestinal helminthiasis NOS (B82.0)*

Pediculosis, acariasis and other infestations (B85-B89)

B85 Pediculosis and phthiriasis

B85.0 Pediculosis due to Pediculus humanus capitis
Head-louse infestation

B85.1 Pediculosis due to Pediculus humanus corporis
Body-louse infestation

B85.2 Pediculosis, unspecified

B85.3 Phthiriasis
Infestation by crab-louse
Infestation by Phthirus pubis

B85.4 Mixed pediculosis and phthiriasis
Infestation classifiable to more than one of the categories B85.0-B85.3

B86 Scabies

Sarcoptic itch
Valid 3-character code, no further characters required

B87 Myiasis

Includes: infestation by larva of flies

B87.0 Cutaneous myiasis
Creeping myiasis

B87.1 Wound myiasis
Traumatic myiasis

B87.2 Ocular myiasis

B87.3 Nasopharyngeal myiasis
Laryngeal myiasis

B87.4 Aural myiasis

\+ **B87.8 Myiasis of other sites**

B87.81 Genitourinary myiasis

B87.82 Intestinal myiasis

B87.89 Myiasis of other sites

B87.9 Myiasis, unspecified

B88 Other infestations

B88.0 Other acariasis
Acarine dermatitis
Dermatitis due to Demodex species
Dermatitis due to Dermanyssus gallinae
Dermatitis due to Liponyssoides sanguineus
Trombiculosis
Excludes2: *scabies (B86)*

B88.1 Tungiasis [sandflea infestation]

B88.2 Other arthropod infestations
Scarabiasis

B88.3 External hirudiniasis
Leech infestation NOS
Excludes2: *internal hirudiniasis (B83.4)*

B88.8 Other specified infestations
Ichthyoparasitism due to Vandellia cirrhosa
Linguatulosis
Porocephaliasis

B88.9 Infestation, unspecified
Infestation (skin) NOS
Infestation by mites NOS
Skin parasites NOS

B89 Unspecified parasitic disease

Valid 3-character code, no further characters required

Sequelae of infectious and parasitic diseases (B90-B94)

NOTE Categories B90-B94 are to be used to indicate conditions in categories A00-B89 as the cause of sequelae, which are themselves classified elsewhere. The 'sequelae' include conditions specified as such; they also include residuals of diseases classifiable to the above categories if there is evidence that the disease itself is no longer present. Codes from these categories are not to be used for chronic infections. Code chronic current infections to active infectious disease as appropriate.

Code first condition resulting from (sequela) the infectious or parasitic disease

B90 Sequelae of tuberculosis

B90.0 Sequelae of central nervous system tuberculosis

B90.1 Sequelae of genitourinary tuberculosis

B90.2 Sequelae of tuberculosis of bones and joints

B90.8 Sequelae of tuberculosis of other organs
Excludes2: *sequelae of respiratory tuberculosis (B90.9)*

B90.9 Sequelae of respiratory and unspecified tuberculosis
Sequelae of tuberculosis NOS

B91 Sequelae of poliomyelitis

Excludes1: *postpolio syndrome (G14)*
Valid 3-character code, no further characters required

B92 Sequelae of leprosy

Valid 3-character code, no further characters required

B94 Sequelae of other and unspecified infectious and parasitic diseases

B94.0 Sequelae of trachoma

B94.1 Sequelae of viral encephalitis

B94.2 Sequelae of viral hepatitis

B94.8 Sequelae of other specified infectious and parasitic diseases
AHA CC: 4Q, 2017, 109; 3Q, 2020, 10-14; 1Q, 2021, 35, 44-46, 48

B94.9 Sequelae of unspecified infectious and parasitic disease
Excludes2: *post COVID-19 condition (U09.9)*

Bacterial and viral infectious agents (B95-B97)

NOTE These categories are provided for use as supplementary or additional codes to identify the infectious agent(s) in diseases classified elsewhere.

B95 Streptococcus, Staphylococcus, and Enterococcus as the cause of diseases classified elsewhere

Review coding guideline C.1.b

B95.0 Streptococcus, group A, as the cause of diseases classified elsewhere

B95.1 Streptococcus, group B, as the cause of diseases classified elsewhere

AHA CC: 4Q, 2018, 23; 2Q, 2019, 9-10; 1Q, 2020, 10

B95.2 Enterococcus as the cause of diseases classified elsewhere

B95.3 Streptococcus pneumoniae as the cause of diseases classified elsewhere

B95.4 Other streptococcus as the cause of diseases classified elsewhere

B95.5 Unspecified streptococcus as the cause of diseases classified elsewhere

\+ **B95.6 Staphylococcus aureus as the cause of diseases classified elsewhere**

B95.61 Methicillin susceptible Staphylococcus aureus infection as the cause of diseases classified elsewhere

Methicillin susceptible Staphylococcus aureus (MSSA) infection as the cause of diseases classified elsewhere

Staphylococcus aureus infection NOS as the cause of diseases classified elsewhere

B95.62 Methicillin resistant Staphylococcus aureus infection as the cause of diseases classified elsewhere

Methicillin resistant staphylococcus aureus (MRSA) infection as the cause of diseases classified elsewhere

Review coding guidelines C.1.e.1.a and C.1.e.1.b

AHA CC: 1Q, 2016, 12-13

B95.7 Other staphylococcus as the cause of diseases classified elsewhere

B95.8 Unspecified staphylococcus as the cause of diseases classified elsewhere

B96 Other bacterial agents as the cause of diseases classified elsewhere

Review coding guideline C.1.b

B96.0 Mycoplasma pneumoniae [M. pneumoniae] as the cause of diseases classified elsewhere

Pleuro-pneumonia-like-organism [PPLO]

B96.1 Klebsiella pneumoniae [K. pneumoniae] as the cause of diseases classified elsewhere

\+ **B96.2 Escherichia coli [E. coli] as the cause of diseases classified elsewhere**

B96.20 Unspecified Escherichia coli [E. coli] as the cause of diseases classified elsewhere

Escherichia coli [E. coli] NOS

AHA CC: 1Q, 2018, 16; 4Q, 2018, 34

B96.21 Shiga toxin-producing Escherichia coli [E. coli] [STEC] O157 as the cause of diseases classified elsewhere

E. coli O157:H- (nonmotile) with confirmation of Shiga toxin

E. coli O157 with confirmation of Shiga toxin when H antigen is unknown, or is not H7

O157:H7 Escherichia coli [E.coli] with or without confirmation of Shiga toxin-production

Shiga toxin-producing Escherichia coli [E.coli] O157:H7 with or without confirmation of Shiga toxin-production

STEC O157:H7 with or without confirmation of Shiga toxin-production

B96.22 Other specified Shiga toxin-producing Escherichia coli [E. coli] [STEC] as the cause of diseases classified elsewhere

Non-O157 Shiga toxin-producing Escherichia coli [E.coli]

Non-O157 Shiga toxin-producing Escherichia coli [E.coli] with known O group

B96.23 Unspecified Shiga toxin-producing Escherichia coli [E. coli] [STEC] as the cause of diseases classified elsewhere

Shiga toxin-producing Escherichia coli [E. coli] with unspecified O group

STEC NOS

B96.29 Other Escherichia coli [E. coli] as the cause of diseases classified elsewhere

Non-Shiga toxin-producing E. coli

B96.3 Hemophilus influenzae [H. influenzae] as the cause of diseases classified elsewhere

B96.4 Proteus (mirabilis) (morganii) as the cause of diseases classified elsewhere

B96.5 Pseudomonas (aeruginosa) (mallei) (pseudomallei) as the cause of diseases classified elsewhere

AHA CC: 1Q, 2015, 18-19

B96.6 Bacteroides fragilis [B. fragilis] as the cause of diseases classified elsewhere

B96.7 Clostridium perfringens [C. perfringens] as the cause of diseases classified elsewhere

\+ **B96.8 Other specified bacterial agents as the cause of diseases classified elsewhere**

B96.81 Helicobacter pylori [H. pylori] as the cause of diseases classified elsewhere

B96.82 Vibrio vulnificus as the cause of diseases classified elsewhere

B96.89 Other specified bacterial agents as the cause of diseases classified elsewhere

B97 Viral agents as the cause of diseases classified elsewhere

Review coding guideline C.1.b

B97.0 Adenovirus as the cause of diseases classified elsewhere

\+ **B97.1 Enterovirus as the cause of diseases classified elsewhere**

B97.10 Unspecified enterovirus as the cause of diseases classified elsewhere

B97.11 Coxsackievirus as the cause of diseases classified elsewhere

B97.12 Echovirus as the cause of diseases classified elsewhere

B97.19 Other enterovirus as the cause of diseases classified elsewhere

\+ **B97.2 Coronavirus as the cause of diseases classified elsewhere**

CC **B97.21 SARS-associated coronavirus as the cause of diseases classified elsewhere**

Excludes1: *pneumonia due to SARS-associated coronavirus (J12.81)*

B97.29 Other coronavirus as the cause of diseases classified elsewhere

AHA CC: 1Q, 2020, 34-36

\+ **B97.3 Retrovirus as the cause of diseases classified elsewhere**

Excludes1: *Human immunodeficiency virus [HIV] disease (B20)*

B97.30 Unspecified retrovirus as the cause of diseases classified elsewhere

B97.31 Lentivirus as the cause of diseases classified elsewhere

B97.32 Oncovirus as the cause of diseases classified elsewhere

CC **B97.33 Human T-cell lymphotrophic virus, type I [HTLV-I] as the cause of diseases classified elsewhere**

CC **B97.34 Human T-cell lymphotrophic virus, type II [HTLV-II] as the cause of diseases classified elsewhere**

CC **B97.35 Human immunodeficiency virus, type 2 [HIV 2] as the cause of diseases classified elsewhere**

B97.39 Other retrovirus as the cause of diseases classified elsewhere

B97.4 Respiratory syncytial virus as the cause of diseases classified elsewhere

RSV as the cause of diseases classified elsewhere

Code first related disorders, such as:

otitis media (H65.-)

upper respiratory infection (J06.9)

Excludes1: *acute bronchiolitis due to respiratory syncytial virus (RSV) (J21.0)*

acute bronchitis due to respiratory syncytial virus (RSV) (J20.5)

respiratory syncytial virus (RSV) pneumonia (J12.1)

B97.5 **Reovirus as the cause of diseases classified elsewhere**
B97.6 **Parvovirus as the cause of diseases classified elsewhere**
B97.7 **Papillomavirus as the cause of diseases classified elsewhere**
+ **B97.8** **Other viral agents as the cause of diseases classified elsewhere**
B97.81 **Human metapneumovirus as the cause of diseases classified elsewhere**
B97.89 **Other viral agents as the cause of diseases classified elsewhere**
AHA CC: 3Q, 2016, 9-14

Other infectious diseases (B99)

B99 **Other and unspecified infectious diseases**
B99.8 **Other infectious disease**
B99.9 **Unspecified infectious disease**

Chapter 2: Neoplasms (C00-D49)

NOTE **Functional activity**

All neoplasms are classified in this chapter, whether they are functionally active or not. An additional code from Chapter 4 may be used, to identify functional activity associated with any neoplasm.

Morphology [Histology]

Chapter 2 classifies neoplasms primarily by site (topography), with broad groupings for behavior, malignant, in situ, benign, etc. The Table of Neoplasms should be used to identify the correct topography code. In a few cases, such as for malignant melanoma and certain neuroendocrine tumors, the morphology (histologic type) is included in the category and codes.

Primary malignant neoplasms overlapping site boundaries

A primary malignant neoplasm that overlaps two or more contiguous (next to each other) sites should be classified to the subcategory/ code .8 ('overlapping lesion'), unless the combination is specifically indexed elsewhere. For multiple neoplasms of the same site that are not contiguous, such as tumors in different quadrants of the same breast, codes for each site should be assigned.

Malignant neoplasm of ectopic tissue

Malignant neoplasms of ectopic tissue are to be coded to the site mentioned, e.g., ectopic pancreatic malignant neoplasms are coded to pancreas, unspecified (C25.9).

This chapter contains the following category blocks:

C00-C14	Malignant neoplasms of lip, oral cavity and pharynx
C15-C26	Malignant neoplasms of digestive organs
C30-C39	Malignant neoplasms of respiratory and intrathoracic organs
C40-C41	Malignant neoplasms of bone and articular cartilage
C43-C44	Melanoma and other malignant neoplasms of skin
C45-C49	Malignant neoplasms of mesothelial and soft tissue
C50	Malignant neoplasms of breast
C51-C58	Malignant neoplasms of female genital organs
C60-C63	Malignant neoplasms of male genital organs
C64-C68	Malignant neoplasms of urinary tract
C69-C72	Malignant neoplasms of eye, brain and other parts of central nervous system
C73-C75	Malignant neoplasms of thyroid and other endocrine glands
C7A	Malignant neuroendocrine tumors
C7B	Secondary neuroendocrine tumors
C76-C80	Malignant neoplasms of ill-defined, other secondary and unspecified sites
C81-C96	Malignant neoplasms of lymphoid, hematopoietic and related tissue
D00-D09	In situ neoplasms
D10-D36	Benign neoplasms, except benign neuroendocrine tumors
D3A	Benign neuroendocrine tumors
D37-D48	Neoplasms of uncertain behavior, polycythemia vera and myelodysplastic syndromes
D49	Neoplasms of unspecified behavior

C. Chapter-Specific Coding Guidelines

In addition to general coding guidelines, there are guidelines for specific diagnoses and/or conditions in the classification. Unless otherwise indicated, these guidelines apply to all health care settings. Please refer to Section II for guidelines on the selection of principal diagnosis.

2. Chapter 2: Neoplasms (C00-D49)

General guidelines

Chapter 2 of the ICD-10-CM contains the codes for most benign and all malignant neoplasms. Certain benign neoplasms, such as prostatic adenomas, may be found in the specific body system chapters. To properly code a neoplasm it is necessary to determine from the record if the neoplasm is benign, in-situ, malignant, or of uncertain histologic behavior. If malignant, any secondary (metastatic) sites should also be determined.

Primary malignant neoplasms overlapping site boundaries

A primary malignant neoplasm that overlaps two or more contiguous (next to each other) sites should be classified to the subcategory/code .8 ('overlapping lesion'), unless the combination is specifically indexed elsewhere. For multiple neoplasms of the same site that are not contiguous such as tumors in different quadrants of the same breast, codes for each site should be assigned.

Malignant neoplasm of ectopic tissue

Malignant neoplasms of ectopic tissue are to be coded to the site of origin mentioned, e.g., ectopic pancreatic malignant neoplasms involving the stomach are coded to malignant neoplasm of pancreas, unspecified (C25.9).

The neoplasm table in the Alphabetic Index should be referenced first. However, if the histological term is documented, that term should be referenced first, rather than going immediately to the Neoplasm Table, in order to determine which column in the Neoplasm Table is appropriate. For example, if the documentation indicates "adenoma," refer to the term in the Alphabetic Index to review the entries under this term and the instructional note to "see also neoplasm, by site, benign." The table provides the proper code based on the type of neoplasm and the site. It is important to select the proper column in the table that corresponds to the type of neoplasm. The Tabular List should then be referenced to verify that the correct code has been selected from the table and that a more specific site code does not exist.

See Section I.C.21. Factors influencing health status and contact with health services, Status, for information regarding Z15.0, codes for genetic susceptibility to cancer.

a. Treatment directed at the malignancy

If the treatment is directed at the malignancy, designate the malignancy as the principal diagnosis.

The only exception to this guideline is if a patient admission/encounter is solely for the administration of chemotherapy, immunotherapy or external beam radiation therapy, assign the appropriate Z51.-- code as the first-listed or principal diagnosis, and the diagnosis or problem for which the service is being performed as a secondary diagnosis.

b. Treatment of secondary site

When a patient is admitted because of a primary neoplasm with metastasis and treatment is directed toward the secondary site only, the secondary neoplasm is designated as the principal diagnosis even though the primary malignancy is still present.

c. Coding and sequencing of complications

Coding and sequencing of complications associated with the malignancies or with the therapy thereof are subject to the following guidelines:

1) Anemia associated with malignancy

When admission/encounter is for management of an anemia associated with the malignancy, and the treatment is only for anemia, the appropriate code for the malignancy is sequenced as the principal or first-listed diagnosis followed by the appropriate code for the anemia (such as code D63.0, Anemia in neoplastic disease).

2) Anemia associated with chemotherapy, immunotherapy and radiation therapy

When the admission/encounter is for management of an anemia associated with an adverse effect of the administration of chemotherapy or immunotherapy and the only treatment is for the anemia, the anemia code is sequenced first followed by the appropriate codes for the neoplasm and the adverse effect (T45.1X5-, Adverse effect of antineoplastic and immunosuppressive drugs).

When the admission/encounter is for management of an anemia associated with an adverse effect of radiotherapy, the anemia code should be sequenced first, followed by the appropriate neoplasm code and code Y84.2, Radiological procedure and radiotherapy as the cause of abnormal reaction of the patient, or of later complication, without mention of misadventure at the time of the procedure.

3) Management of dehydration due to the malignancy

When the admission/encounter is for management of dehydration due to the malignancy and only the dehydration is being treated (intravenous rehydration), the dehydration is sequenced first, followed by the code(s) for the malignancy.

4) Treatment of a complication resulting from a surgical procedure

When the admission/encounter is for treatment of a complication resulting from a surgical procedure, designate the complication as the principal or first-listed diagnosis if treatment is directed at resolving the complication.

d. Primary malignancy previously excised

When a primary malignancy has been previously excised or eradicated from its site and there is no further treatment directed to that site and there is no evidence of any existing primary malignancy at that site, a code from category Z85, Personal history of malignant neoplasm, should be used to indicate the former site of the malignancy. Any mention of extension, invasion, or metastasis to another site is coded as a secondary malignant neoplasm to that site. The secondary site may be the principal or first-listed diagnosis with the Z85 code used as a secondary code.

e. Admissions/Encounters involving chemotherapy, immunotherapy and radiation therapy

1) Episode of care involves surgical removal of neoplasm

When an episode of care involves the surgical removal of a neoplasm, primary or secondary site, followed by adjunct chemotherapy or radiation treatment during the same episode of care, the code for the neoplasm should be assigned as principal or first-listed diagnosis.

2) **Patient admission/encounter solely for administration of chemotherapy, immunotherapy and radiation therapy**

If a patient admission/encounter is solely for the administration of chemotherapy, immunotherapy or external beam radiation therapy assign code Z51.0, Encounter for antineoplastic radiation therapy, or Z51.11, Encounter for antineoplastic chemotherapy, or Z51.12, Encounter for antineoplastic immunotherapy as the first-listed or principal diagnosis. If a patient receives more than one of these therapies during the same admission more than one of these codes may be assigned, in any sequence.

The malignancy for which the therapy is being administered should be assigned as a secondary diagnosis.

If a patient admission/encounter is for the insertion or implantation of radioactive elements (e.g., brachytherapy) the appropriate code for the malignancy is sequenced as the principal or first-listed diagnosis. Code Z51.0 should not be assigned.

3) **Patient admitted for radiation therapy, chemotherapy or immunotherapy and develops complications**

When a patient is admitted for the purpose of external beam radiotherapy, immunotherapy or chemotherapy and develops complications such as uncontrolled nausea and vomiting or dehydration, the principal or first-listed diagnosis is Z51.0, Encounter for antineoplastic radiation therapy, or Z51.11, Encounter for antineoplastic chemotherapy, or Z51.12, Encounter for antineoplastic immunotherapy followed by any codes for the complications.

When a patient is admitted for the purpose of insertion or implantation of radioactive elements (e.g., brachytherapy) and develops complications such as uncontrolled nausea and vomiting or dehydration, the principal or first-listed diagnosis is the appropriate code for the malignancy followed by any codes for the complications.

f. **Admission/encounter to determine extent of malignancy**

When the reason for admission/encounter is to determine the extent of the malignancy, or for a procedure such as paracentesis or thoracentesis, the primary malignancy or appropriate metastatic site is designated as the principal or first-listed diagnosis, even though chemotherapy or radiotherapy is administered.

g. **Symptoms, signs, and abnormal findings listed in Chapter 18 associated with neoplasms**

Symptoms, signs, and ill-defined conditions listed in Chapter 18 characteristic of, or associated with, an existing primary or secondary site malignancy cannot be used to replace the malignancy as principal or first-listed diagnosis, regardless of the number of admissions or encounters for treatment and care of the neoplasm.

See section I.C.21. Factors influencing health status and contact with health services, Encounter for prophylactic organ removal.

h. **Admission/encounter for pain control/management**

See Section I.C.6. for information on coding admission/encounter for pain control/management.

i. **Malignancy in two or more noncontiguous sites**

A patient may have more than one malignant tumor in the same organ. These tumors may represent different primaries or metastatic disease, depending on the site. Should the documentation be unclear, the provider should be queried as to the status of each tumor so that the correct codes can be assigned.

j. **Disseminated malignant neoplasm, unspecified**

Code C80.0, Disseminated malignant neoplasm, unspecified, is for use only in those cases where the patient has advanced metastatic disease and no known primary or secondary sites are specified. It should not be used in place of assigning codes for the primary site and all known secondary sites.

k. **Malignant neoplasm without specification of site**

Code C80.1, Malignant (primary) neoplasm, unspecified, equates to Cancer, unspecified. This code should only be used when no determination can be made as to the primary site of a malignancy. This code should rarely be used in the inpatient setting.

l. **Sequencing of neoplasm codes**

1) **Encounter for treatment of primary malignancy**

If the reason for the encounter is for treatment of a primary malignancy, assign the malignancy as the principal/first-listed diagnosis. The primary site is to be sequenced first, followed by any metastatic sites.

2) **Encounter for treatment of secondary malignancy**

When an encounter is for a primary malignancy with metastasis and treatment is directed toward the metastatic (secondary) site(s) only, the metastatic site(s) is designated as the principal/first-listed diagnosis. The primary malignancy is coded as an additional code.

3) **Malignant neoplasm in a pregnant patient**

When a pregnant woman has a malignant neoplasm, a code from subcategory O9A.1-, Malignant neoplasm complicating pregnancy, childbirth, and the puerperium, should be sequenced first, followed by the appropriate code from Chapter 2 to indicate the type of neoplasm.

4) **Encounter for complication associated with a neoplasm**

When an encounter is for management of a complication associated with a neoplasm, such as dehydration, and the treatment is only for the complication, the complication is coded first, followed by the appropriate code(s) for the neoplasm.

The exception to this guideline is anemia. When the admission/encounter is for management of an anemia associated with the malignancy, and the treatment is only for anemia, the appropriate code for the malignancy is sequenced as the principal or first-listed diagnosis followed by code D63.0, Anemia in neoplastic disease.

5) **Complication from surgical procedure for treatment of a neoplasm**

When an encounter is for treatment of a complication resulting from a surgical procedure performed for the treatment of the neoplasm, designate the complication as the principal/first-listed diagnosis. See the guideline regarding the coding of a current malignancy versus personal history to determine if the code for the neoplasm should also be assigned.

6) **Pathologic fracture due to a neoplasm**

When an encounter is for a pathological fracture due to a neoplasm, and the focus of treatment is the fracture, a code from subcategory M84.5, Pathological fracture in neoplastic disease, should be sequenced first, followed by the code for the neoplasm.

If the focus of treatment is the neoplasm with an associated pathological fracture, the neoplasm code should be sequenced first, followed by a code from M84.5 for the pathological fracture.

m. **Current malignancy versus personal history of malignancy**

When a primary malignancy has been excised but further treatment, such as an additional surgery for the malignancy, radiation therapy or chemotherapy is directed to that site, the primary malignancy code should be used until treatment is completed.

When a primary malignancy has been previously excised or eradicated from its site, there is no further treatment (of the malignancy) directed to that site, and there is no evidence of any existing primary malignancy at that site, a code from category Z85, Personal history of malignant neoplasm, should be used to indicate the former site of the malignancy.

Subcategories Z85.0 - Z85.7 should only be assigned for the former site of a primary malignancy, not the site of a secondary malignancy. Codes from subcategory Z85.8-, may be assigned for the former site(s) of either a primary or secondary malignancy included in this subcategory.

See Section I.C.21. Factors influencing health status and contact with health services, History (of)

n. **Leukemia, Multiple Myeloma, and Malignant Plasma Cell Neoplasms in remission versus personal history**

The categories for leukemia, and category C90, Multiple myeloma and malignant plasma cell neoplasms, have codes indicating whether or not the leukemia has achieved remission. There are also codes Z85.6, Personal history of leukemia, and Z85.79, Personal history of other malignant neoplasms of lymphoid, hematopoietic and related tissues. If the documentation is unclear, as to whether the leukemia has achieved remission, the provider should be queried.

See Section I.C.21. Factors influencing health status and contact with health services, History (of)

o. **Aftercare following surgery for neoplasm**

See Section I.C.21. Factors influencing health status and contact with health services, Aftercare

p. **Follow-up care for completed treatment of a malignancy**

See Section I.C.21. Factors influencing health status and contact with health services, Follow-up

q. **Prophylactic organ removal for prevention of malignancy**

See Section I.C. 21, Factors influencing health status and contact with health services, Prophylactic organ removal

r. **Malignant neoplasm associated with transplanted organ**

A malignant neoplasm of a transplanted organ should be coded as a transplant complication. Assign first the appropriate code from category T86.-, Complications of transplanted organs and tissue, followed by code C80.2, Malignant neoplasm associated with transplanted organ. Use an additional code for the specific malignancy.

s. **Breast Implant Associated Anaplastic Large Cell Lymphoma**

Breast implant associated anaplastic large cell lymphoma (BIA-ALCL) is a type of lymphoma that can develop around breast implants. Assign code C84.7A, Anaplastic large cell lymphoma, ALK-negative, breast, for BIA-ALCL. Do not assign a complication code from chapter 19.

Malignant neoplasms (C00-C96)

Malignant neoplasms, stated or presumed to be primary (of specified sites), and certain specified histologies, except neuroendocrine, and of lymphoid, hematopoietic and related tissue (C00-C75)

Malignant neoplasms of lip, oral cavity and pharynx (C00-C14)

C00 Malignant neoplasm of lip

Use additional code to identify:
alcohol abuse and dependence (F10.-)
history of tobacco dependence (Z87.891)
tobacco dependence (F17.-)
tobacco use (Z72.0)

Excludes1: *malignant melanoma of lip (C43.0)*
Merkel cell carcinoma of lip (C4A.0)
other and unspecified malignant neoplasm of skin of lip (C44.0-)

C00.0 Malignant neoplasm of external upper lip
Malignant neoplasm of lipstick area of upper lip
Malignant neoplasm of upper lip NOS
Malignant neoplasm of vermilion border of upper lip

C00.1 Malignant neoplasm of external lower lip
Malignant neoplasm of lower lip NOS
Malignant neoplasm of lipstick area of lower lip
Malignant neoplasm of vermilion border of lower lip

C00.2 Malignant neoplasm of external lip, unspecified
Malignant neoplasm of vermilion border of lip NOS

C00.3 Malignant neoplasm of upper lip, inner aspect
Malignant neoplasm of buccal aspect of upper lip
Malignant neoplasm of frenulum of upper lip
Malignant neoplasm of mucosa of upper lip
Malignant neoplasm of oral aspect of upper lip

C00.4 Malignant neoplasm of lower lip, inner aspect
Malignant neoplasm of buccal aspect of lower lip
Malignant neoplasm of frenulum of lower lip
Malignant neoplasm of mucosa of lower lip
Malignant neoplasm of oral aspect of lower lip

C00.5 Malignant neoplasm of lip, unspecified, inner aspect
Malignant neoplasm of buccal aspect of lip, unspecified
Malignant neoplasm of frenulum of lip, unspecified
Malignant neoplasm of mucosa of lip, unspecified
Malignant neoplasm of oral aspect of lip, unspecified

C00.6 Malignant neoplasm of commissure of lip, unspecified

C00.8 Malignant neoplasm of overlapping sites of lip

C00.9 Malignant neoplasm of lip, unspecified

C01 Malignant neoplasm of base of tongue

Malignant neoplasm of dorsal surface of base of tongue
Malignant neoplasm of fixed part of tongue NOS
Malignant neoplasm of posterior third of tongue

Use additional code to identify:
alcohol abuse and dependence (F10.-)
history of tobacco dependence (Z87.891)
tobacco dependence (F17.-)
tobacco use (Z72.0)

Valid 3-character code, no further characters required

C02 Malignant neoplasm of other and unspecified parts of tongue

Use additional code to identify:
alcohol abuse and dependence (F10.-)
history of tobacco dependence (Z87.891)
tobacco dependence (F17.-)
tobacco use (Z72.0)

C02.0 Malignant neoplasm of dorsal surface of tongue
Malignant neoplasm of anterior two-thirds of tongue, dorsal surface

Excludes2: *malignant neoplasm of dorsal surface of base of tongue (C01)*

C02.1 Malignant neoplasm of border of tongue
Malignant neoplasm of tip of tongue

C02.2 Malignant neoplasm of ventral surface of tongue
Malignant neoplasm of anterior two-thirds of tongue, ventral surface
Malignant neoplasm of frenulum linguae

C02.3 Malignant neoplasm of anterior two-thirds of tongue, part unspecified
Malignant neoplasm of middle third of tongue NOS
Malignant neoplasm of mobile part of tongue NOS

C02.4 Malignant neoplasm of lingual tonsil

Excludes2: *malignant neoplasm of tonsil NOS (C09.9)*

C02.8 Malignant neoplasm of overlapping sites of tongue
Malignant neoplasm of two or more contiguous sites of tongue

C02.9 Malignant neoplasm of tongue, unspecified

C03 Malignant neoplasm of gum

Includes: malignant neoplasm of alveolar (ridge) mucosa
malignant neoplasm of gingiva

Use additional code to identify:
alcohol abuse and dependence (F10.-)
history of tobacco dependence (Z87.891)
tobacco dependence (F17.-)
tobacco use (Z72.0)

Excludes2: *malignant odontogenic neoplasms (C41.0-C41.1)*

C03.0 Malignant neoplasm of upper gum

C03.1 Malignant neoplasm of lower gum

C03.9 Malignant neoplasm of gum, unspecified

C04 Malignant neoplasm of floor of mouth

Use additional code to identify:
alcohol abuse and dependence (F10.-)
history of tobacco dependence (Z87.891)
tobacco dependence (F17.-)
tobacco use (Z72.0)

C04.0 Malignant neoplasm of anterior floor of mouth
Malignant neoplasm of anterior to the premolar-canine junction

C04.1 Malignant neoplasm of lateral floor of mouth

C04.8 Malignant neoplasm of overlapping sites of floor of mouth

C04.9 Malignant neoplasm of floor of mouth, unspecified

C05 Malignant neoplasm of palate

Use additional code to identify:
alcohol abuse and dependence (F10.-)
history of tobacco dependence (Z87.891)
tobacco dependence (F17.-)
tobacco use (Z72.0)

Excludes1: *Kaposi's sarcoma of palate (C46.2)*

C05.0 Malignant neoplasm of hard palate

C05.1 Malignant neoplasm of soft palate

Excludes2: *malignant neoplasm of nasopharyngeal surface of soft palate (C11.3)*

C05.2 Malignant neoplasm of uvula

C05.8 Malignant neoplasm of overlapping sites of palate

C05.9 Malignant neoplasm of palate, unspecified
Malignant neoplasm of roof of mouth

C06 Malignant neoplasm of other and unspecified parts of mouth

Use additional code to identify:
alcohol abuse and dependence (F10.-)
history of tobacco dependence (Z87.891)
tobacco dependence (F17.-)
tobacco use (Z72.0)

C06.0 Malignant neoplasm of cheek mucosa
Malignant neoplasm of buccal mucosa NOS
Malignant neoplasm of internal cheek

C06.1 Malignant neoplasm of vestibule of mouth
Malignant neoplasm of buccal sulcus (upper) (lower)
Malignant neoplasm of labial sulcus (upper) (lower)

C06.2 Malignant neoplasm of retromolar area

\+ **C06.8 Malignant neoplasm of overlapping sites of other and unspecified parts of mouth**

C06.80 Malignant neoplasm of overlapping sites of unspecified parts of mouth

C06.89 Malignant neoplasm of overlapping sites of other parts of mouth
'book leaf' neoplasm [ventral surface of tongue and floor of mouth]

C06.9 Malignant neoplasm of mouth, unspecified
Malignant neoplasm of minor salivary gland, unspecified site
Malignant neoplasm of oral cavity NOS

Tumor Biology and Chemotherapy

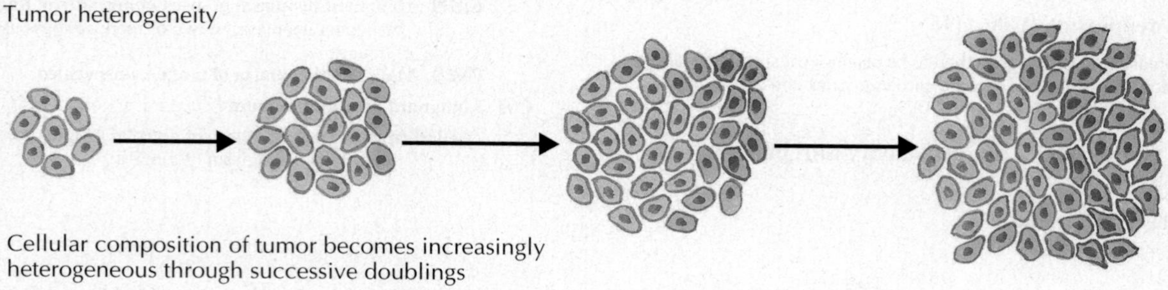

Cellular composition of tumor becomes increasingly heterogeneous through successive doublings

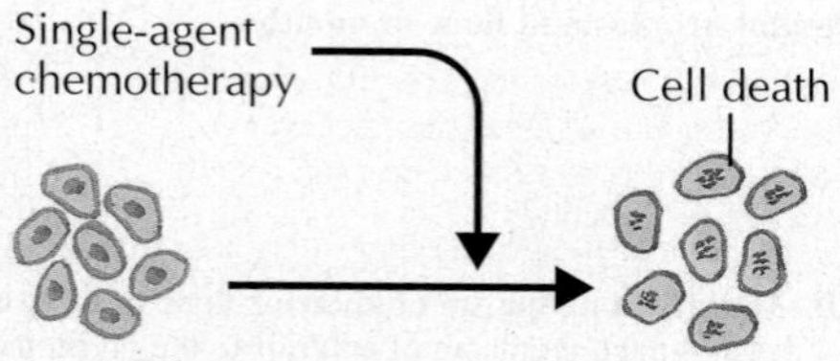

Single-agent chemotherapy *may* be successful in susceptible homogeneous tumors

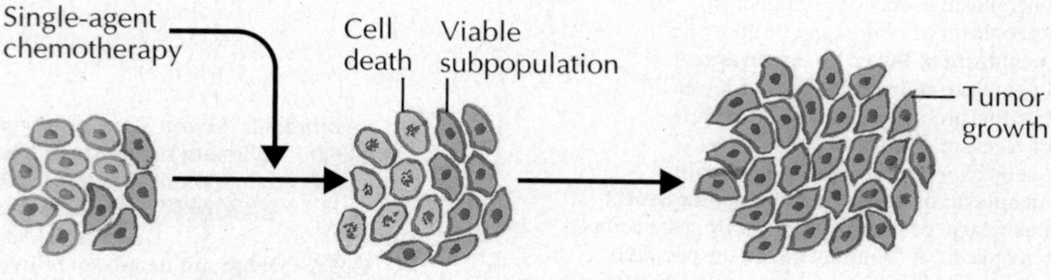

Single-agent chemotherapy for heterogeneous tumors may result only in death of susceptible cell line, selecting nonresponsive cells for growth and spread

JOHN A.CRAIG—AD

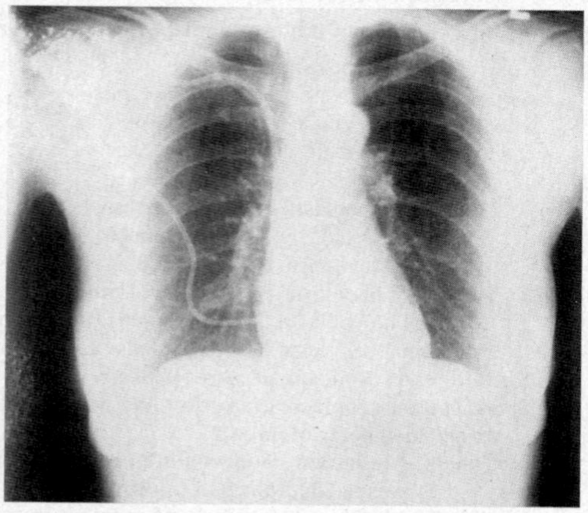

Radiograph of lungs after multiple-agent chemotherapy

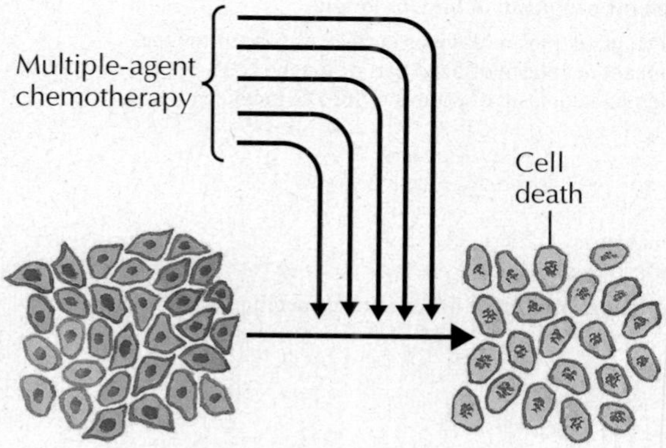

Multiple-agent chemotherapy affects subpopulations of heterogeneous tumors

C07 Malignant neoplasm of parotid gland

Use additional code to identify:
alcohol abuse and dependence (F10.-)
exposure to environmental tobacco smoke (Z77.22)
exposure to tobacco smoke in the perinatal period (P96.81)
history of tobacco dependence (Z87.891)
occupational exposure to environmental tobacco smoke (Z57.31)
tobacco dependence (F17.-)
tobacco use (Z72.0)

Valid 3-character code, no further characters required

C08 Malignant neoplasm of other and unspecified major salivary glands

Includes: malignant neoplasm of salivary ducts
Use additional code to identify:
alcohol abuse and dependence (F10.-)
exposure to environmental tobacco smoke (Z77.22)
exposure to tobacco smoke in the perinatal period (P96.81)
history of tobacco dependence (Z87.891)
occupational exposure to environmental tobacco smoke (Z57.31)
tobacco dependence (F17.-)
tobacco use (Z72.0)

Excludes1: *malignant neoplasms of specified minor salivary glands which are classified according to their anatomical location*

Excludes2: *malignant neoplasms of minor salivary glands NOS (C06.9)*
malignant neoplasm of parotid gland (C07)

C08.0 Malignant neoplasm of submandibular gland
Malignant neoplasm of submaxillary gland

C08.1 Malignant neoplasm of sublingual gland

C08.9 Malignant neoplasm of major salivary gland, unspecified
Malignant neoplasm of salivary gland (major) NOS

C09 Malignant neoplasm of tonsil

Use additional code to identify:
alcohol abuse and dependence (F10.-)
exposure to environmental tobacco smoke (Z77.22)
exposure to tobacco smoke in the perinatal period (P96.81)
history of tobacco dependence (Z87.891)
occupational exposure to environmental tobacco smoke (Z57.31)
tobacco dependence (F17.-)
tobacco use (Z72.0)

Excludes2: *malignant neoplasm of lingual tonsil (C02.4)*
malignant neoplasm of pharyngeal tonsil (C11.1)

C09.0 Malignant neoplasm of tonsillar fossa

C09.1 Malignant neoplasm of tonsillar pillar (anterior) (posterior)

C09.8 Malignant neoplasm of overlapping sites of tonsil

C09.9 Malignant neoplasm of tonsil, unspecified
Malignant neoplasm of tonsil NOS
Malignant neoplasm of faucial tonsils
Malignant neoplasm of palatine tonsils

C10 Malignant neoplasm of oropharynx

Use additional code to identify:
alcohol abuse and dependence (F10.-)
exposure to environmental tobacco smoke (Z77.22)
exposure to tobacco smoke in the perinatal period (P96.81)
history of tobacco dependence (Z87.891)
occupational exposure to environmental tobacco smoke (Z57.31)
tobacco dependence (F17.-)
tobacco use (Z72.0)

Excludes2: *malignant neoplasm of tonsil (C09.-)*

C10.0 Malignant neoplasm of vallecula

C10.1 Malignant neoplasm of anterior surface of epiglottis
Malignant neoplasm of epiglottis, free border [margin]
Malignant neoplasm of glossoepiglottic fold(s)

Excludes2: *malignant neoplasm of epiglottis (suprahyoid portion) NOS (C32.1)*

C10.2 Malignant neoplasm of lateral wall of oropharynx

C10.3 Malignant neoplasm of posterior wall of oropharynx

C10.4 Malignant neoplasm of branchial cleft
Malignant neoplasm of branchial cyst [site of neoplasm]

C10.8 Malignant neoplasm of overlapping sites of oropharynx
Malignant neoplasm of junctional region of oropharynx

C10.9 Malignant neoplasm of oropharynx, unspecified

C11 Malignant neoplasm of nasopharynx

Use additional code to identify:
exposure to environmental tobacco smoke (Z77.22)
exposure to tobacco smoke in the perinatal period (P96.81)
history of tobacco dependence (Z87.891)
occupational exposure to environmental tobacco smoke (Z57.31)
tobacco dependence (F17.-)
tobacco use (Z72.0)

C11.0 Malignant neoplasm of superior wall of nasopharynx
Malignant neoplasm of roof of nasopharynx

C11.1 Malignant neoplasm of posterior wall of nasopharynx
Malignant neoplasm of adenoid
Malignant neoplasm of pharyngeal tonsil

C11.2 Malignant neoplasm of lateral wall of nasopharynx
Malignant neoplasm of fossa of Rosenmüller
Malignant neoplasm of opening of auditory tube
Malignant neoplasm of pharyngeal recess

C11.3 Malignant neoplasm of anterior wall of nasopharynx
Malignant neoplasm of floor of nasopharynx
Malignant neoplasm of nasopharyngeal (anterior) (posterior) surface of soft palate
Malignant neoplasm of posterior margin of nasal choana
Malignant neoplasm of posterior margin of nasal septum

C11.8 Malignant neoplasm of overlapping sites of nasopharynx

C11.9 Malignant neoplasm of nasopharynx, unspecified
Malignant neoplasm of nasopharyngeal wall NOS

C12 Malignant neoplasm of pyriform sinus

Malignant neoplasm of pyriform fossa
Use additional code to identify:
exposure to environmental tobacco smoke (Z77.22)
exposure to tobacco smoke in the perinatal period (P96.81)
history of tobacco dependence (Z87.891)
occupational exposure to environmental tobacco smoke (Z57.31)
tobacco dependence (F17.-)
tobacco use (Z72.0)

Valid 3-character code, no further characters required

C13 Malignant neoplasm of hypopharynx

Use additional code to identify:
exposure to environmental tobacco smoke (Z77.22)
exposure to tobacco smoke in the perinatal period (P96.81)
history of tobacco dependence (Z87.891)
occupational exposure to environmental tobacco smoke (Z57.31)
tobacco dependence (F17.-)
tobacco use (Z72.0)

Excludes2: *malignant neoplasm of pyriform sinus (C12)*

C13.0 Malignant neoplasm of postcricoid region

C13.1 Malignant neoplasm of aryepiglottic fold, hypopharyngeal aspect
Malignant neoplasm of aryepiglottic fold NOS
Malignant neoplasm of interarytenoid fold NOS
Malignant neoplasm of aryepiglottic fold, marginal zone
Malignant neoplasm of interarytenoid fold, marginal zone

Excludes2: *malignant neoplasm of aryepiglottic fold or interarytenoid fold, laryngeal aspect (C32.1)*

C13.2 Malignant neoplasm of posterior wall of hypopharynx

C13.8 Malignant neoplasm of overlapping sites of hypopharynx

C13.9 Malignant neoplasm of hypopharynx, unspecified
Malignant neoplasm of hypopharyngeal wall NOS

C14 Malignant neoplasm of other and ill-defined sites in the lip, oral cavity and pharynx

Use additional code to identify:
alcohol abuse and dependence (F10.-)
exposure to environmental tobacco smoke (Z77.22)
exposure to tobacco smoke in the perinatal period (P96.81)
history of tobacco dependence (Z87.891)
occupational exposure to environmental tobacco smoke (Z57.31)
tobacco dependence (F17.-)
tobacco use (Z72.0)

Excludes1: *malignant neoplasm of oral cavity NOS (C06.9)*

C14.0 Malignant neoplasm of pharynx, unspecified

C14.2 Malignant neoplasm of Waldeyer's ring

C14.8 Malignant neoplasm of overlapping sites of lip, oral cavity and pharynx
Primary malignant neoplasm of two or more contiguous sites of lip, oral cavity and pharynx

Excludes1: *'book leaf' neoplasm [ventral surface of tongue and floor of mouth] (C06.89)*

Malignant neoplasms of digestive organs (C15-C26)

Excludes1: *Kaposi's sarcoma of gastrointestinal sites (C46.4)*

Excludes2: *gastrointestinal stromal tumors (C49.A-)*

C15 Malignant neoplasm of esophagus

Use additional code to identify:
alcohol abuse and dependence (F10.-)

CC **C15.3 Malignant neoplasm of upper third of esophagus**
CC **C15.4 Malignant neoplasm of middle third of esophagus**
CC **C15.5 Malignant neoplasm of lower third of esophagus**
Excludes1: *malignant neoplasm of cardio-esophageal junction (C16.0)*
CC **C15.8 Malignant neoplasm of overlapping sites of esophagus**
CC **C15.9 Malignant neoplasm of esophagus, unspecified**

C16 Malignant neoplasm of stomach

Use additional code to identify:
alcohol abuse and dependence (F10.-)

Excludes2: *malignant carcinoid tumor of the stomach (C7A.092)*

CC **C16.0 Malignant neoplasm of cardia**
Malignant neoplasm of cardiac orifice
Malignant neoplasm of cardio-esophageal junction
Malignant neoplasm of esophagus and stomach
Malignant neoplasm of gastro-esophageal junction
CC **C16.1 Malignant neoplasm of fundus of stomach**
CC **C16.2 Malignant neoplasm of body of stomach**
CC **C16.3 Malignant neoplasm of pyloric antrum**
Malignant neoplasm of gastric antrum
CC **C16.4 Malignant neoplasm of pylorus**
Malignant neoplasm of prepylorus
Malignant neoplasm of pyloric canal
CC **C16.5 Malignant neoplasm of lesser curvature of stomach, unspecified**
Malignant neoplasm of lesser curvature of stomach, not classifiable to C16.1-C16.4
CC **C16.6 Malignant neoplasm of greater curvature of stomach, unspecified**
Malignant neoplasm of greater curvature of stomach, not classifiable to C16.0-C16.4
CC **C16.8 Malignant neoplasm of overlapping sites of stomach**
CC **C16.9 Malignant neoplasm of stomach, unspecified**
Gastric cancer NOS

C17 Malignant neoplasm of small intestine

Excludes1: *malignant carcinoid tumors of the small intestine (C7A.01)*

CC **C17.0 Malignant neoplasm of duodenum**
CC **C17.1 Malignant neoplasm of jejunum**
CC **C17.2 Malignant neoplasm of ileum**
Excludes1: *malignant neoplasm of ileocecal valve (C18.0)*
CC **C17.3 Meckel's diverticulum, malignant**
Excludes1: *Meckel's diverticulum, congenital (Q43.0)*
CC **C17.8 Malignant neoplasm of overlapping sites of small intestine**
CC **C17.9 Malignant neoplasm of small intestine, unspecified**

C18 Malignant neoplasm of colon

Excludes1: *malignant carcinoid tumors of the colon (C7A.02-)*

CC **C18.0 Malignant neoplasm of cecum**
Malignant neoplasm of ileocecal valve
CC **C18.1 Malignant neoplasm of appendix**
CC **C18.2 Malignant neoplasm of ascending colon**
CC **C18.3 Malignant neoplasm of hepatic flexure**
CC **C18.4 Malignant neoplasm of transverse colon**
CC **C18.5 Malignant neoplasm of splenic flexure**
CC **C18.6 Malignant neoplasm of descending colon**
CC **C18.7 Malignant neoplasm of sigmoid colon**
Malignant neoplasm of sigmoid (flexure)
Excludes1: *malignant neoplasm of rectosigmoid junction (C19)*
CC **C18.8 Malignant neoplasm of overlapping sites of colon**
CC **C18.9 Malignant neoplasm of colon, unspecified**
Malignant neoplasm of large intestine NOS

CC C19 Malignant neoplasm of rectosigmoid junction

Malignant neoplasm of colon with rectum
Malignant neoplasm of rectosigmoid (colon)
Excludes1: *malignant carcinoid tumors of the colon (C7A.02-)*
Valid 3-character code, no further characters required

CC C20 Malignant neoplasm of rectum

Malignant neoplasm of rectal ampulla
Excludes1: *malignant carcinoid tumor of the rectum (C7A.026)*
Valid 3-character code, no further characters required

CC C21 Malignant neoplasm of anus and anal canal

Excludes2: *malignant carcinoid tumors of the colon (C7A.02-)*
malignant melanoma of anal margin (C43.51)
malignant melanoma of anal skin (C43.51)
malignant melanoma of perianal skin (C43.51)
other and unspecified malignant neoplasm of anal margin (C44.500, C44.510, C44.520, C44.590)
other and unspecified malignant neoplasm of anal skin (C44.500, C44.510, C44.520, C44.590)
other and unspecified malignant neoplasm of perianal skin (C44.500, C44.510, C44.520, C44.590)

CC **C21.0 Malignant neoplasm of anus, unspecified**
CC **C21.1 Malignant neoplasm of anal canal**
Malignant neoplasm of anal sphincter
CC **C21.2 Malignant neoplasm of cloacogenic zone**
CC **C21.8 Malignant neoplasm of overlapping sites of rectum, anus and anal canal**
Malignant neoplasm of anorectal junction
Malignant neoplasm of anorectum
Primary malignant neoplasm of two or more contiguous sites of rectum, anus and anal canal

C22 Malignant neoplasm of liver and intrahepatic bile ducts

Excludes1: *malignant neoplasm of biliary tract NOS (C24.9)*
secondary malignant neoplasm of liver and intrahepatic bile duct (C78.7)

Use additional code to identify:
alcohol abuse and dependence (F10.-)
hepatitis B (B16.-, B18.0-B18.1)
hepatitis C (B17.1-, B18.2)

CC **C22.0 Liver cell carcinoma**
Hepatocellular carcinoma
Hepatoma
AHA CC: 1Q, 2016, 18-19
CC **C22.1 Intrahepatic bile duct carcinoma**
Cholangiocarcinoma
Excludes1: *malignant neoplasm of hepatic duct (C24.0)*
CC **C22.2 Hepatoblastoma**
CC **C22.3 Angiosarcoma of liver**
Kupffer cell sarcoma
CC **C22.4 Other sarcomas of liver**
CC **C22.7 Other specified carcinomas of liver**
CC **C22.8 Malignant neoplasm of liver, primary, unspecified as to type**
CC **C22.9 Malignant neoplasm of liver, not specified as primary or secondary**

CC C23 Malignant neoplasm of gallbladder

Valid 3-character code, no further characters required

C24 Malignant neoplasm of other and unspecified parts of biliary tract

Excludes1: *malignant neoplasm of intrahepatic bile duct (C22.1)*

CC **C24.0 Malignant neoplasm of extrahepatic bile duct**
Malignant neoplasm of biliary duct or passage NOS
Malignant neoplasm of common bile duct
Malignant neoplasm of cystic duct
Malignant neoplasm of hepatic duct
CC **C24.1 Malignant neoplasm of ampulla of Vater**
CC **C24.8 Malignant neoplasm of overlapping sites of biliary tract**
Malignant neoplasm involving both intrahepatic and extrahepatic bile ducts
Primary malignant neoplasm of two or more contiguous sites of biliary tract
CC **C24.9 Malignant neoplasm of biliary tract, unspecified**

C25 Malignant neoplasm of pancreas

Code also, if applicable, exocrine pancreatic insufficiency (K86.81)

Use additional code to identify:
alcohol abuse and dependence (F10.-)

CC **C25.0 Malignant neoplasm of head of pancreas**
CC **C25.1 Malignant neoplasm of body of pancreas**
AHA CC: 4Q, 2018, 40
CC **C25.2 Malignant neoplasm of tail of pancreas**
CC **C25.3 Malignant neoplasm of pancreatic duct**
CC **C25.4 Malignant neoplasm of endocrine pancreas**
Malignant neoplasm of islets of Langerhans
Use additional code to identify any functional activity.

CC **C25.7 Malignant neoplasm of other parts of pancreas**
Malignant neoplasm of neck of pancreas

CC **C25.8 Malignant neoplasm of overlapping sites of pancreas**

CC **C25.9 Malignant neoplasm of pancreas, unspecified**

C26 Malignant neoplasm of other and ill-defined digestive organs

Excludes1: *malignant neoplasm of peritoneum and retroperitoneum (C48.-)*

C26.0 Malignant neoplasm of intestinal tract, part unspecified
Malignant neoplasm of intestine NOS

C26.1 Malignant neoplasm of spleen
Excludes1: *Hodgkin lymphoma (C81.-)*
non-Hodgkin lymphoma (C82-C85)

C26.9 Malignant neoplasm of ill-defined sites within the digestive system
Malignant neoplasm of alimentary canal or tract NOS
Malignant neoplasm of gastrointestinal tract NOS
Excludes1: *malignant neoplasm of abdominal NOS (C76.2)*
malignant neoplasm of intra-abdominal NOS (C76.2)

Malignant neoplasms of respiratory and intrathoracic organs (C30-C39)

Includes: malignant neoplasm of middle ear

Excludes1: *mesothelioma (C45.-)*

C30 Malignant neoplasm of nasal cavity and middle ear

C30.0 Malignant neoplasm of nasal cavity
Malignant neoplasm of cartilage of nose
Malignant neoplasm of nasal concha
Malignant neoplasm of internal nose
Malignant neoplasm of septum of nose
Malignant neoplasm of vestibule of nose
Excludes1: *malignant neoplasm of nasal bone (C41.0)*
malignant neoplasm of nose NOS (C76.0)
malignant neoplasm of olfactory bulb (C72.2-)
malignant neoplasm of posterior margin of nasal septum and choana (C11.3)
malignant melanoma of skin of nose (C43.31)
malignant neoplasm of turbinates (C41.0)
other and unspecified malignant neoplasm of skin of nose (C44.301, C44.311, C44.321, C44.391)

C30.1 Malignant neoplasm of middle ear
Malignant neoplasm of antrum tympanicum
Malignant neoplasm of auditory tube
Malignant neoplasm of eustachian tube
Malignant neoplasm of inner ear
Malignant neoplasm of mastoid air cells
Malignant neoplasm of tympanic cavity
Excludes1: *malignant neoplasm of auricular canal (external) (C43.2-,C44.2-)*
malignant neoplasm of bone of ear (meatus) (C41.0)
malignant neoplasm of cartilage of ear (C49.0)
malignant melanoma of skin of (external) ear (C43.2-)
other and unspecified malignant neoplasm of skin of (external) ear (C44.2-)

C31 Malignant neoplasm of accessory sinuses

C31.0 Malignant neoplasm of maxillary sinus
Malignant neoplasm of antrum (Highmore) (maxillary)

C31.1 Malignant neoplasm of ethmoidal sinus

C31.2 Malignant neoplasm of frontal sinus

C31.3 Malignant neoplasm of sphenoid sinus

C31.8 Malignant neoplasm of overlapping sites of accessory sinuses

C31.9 Malignant neoplasm of accessory sinus, unspecified

C32 Malignant neoplasm of larynx

Use additional code to identify:
alcohol abuse and dependence (F10.-)
exposure to environmental tobacco smoke (Z77.22)
exposure to tobacco smoke in the perinatal period (P96.81)
history of tobacco dependence (Z87.891)
occupational exposure to environmental tobacco smoke (Z57.31)
tobacco dependence (F17.-)
tobacco use (Z72.0)

C32.0 Malignant neoplasm of glottis
Malignant neoplasm of intrinsic larynx
Malignant neoplasm of laryngeal commissure (anterior) (posterior)
Malignant neoplasm of vocal cord (true) NOS

C32.1 Malignant neoplasm of supraglottis
Malignant neoplasm of aryepiglottic fold or interarytenoid fold, laryngeal aspect
Malignant neoplasm of epiglottis (suprahyoid portion) NOS
Malignant neoplasm of extrinsic larynx
Malignant neoplasm of false vocal cord
Malignant neoplasm of posterior (laryngeal) surface of epiglottis
Malignant neoplasm of ventricular bands
Excludes2: *malignant neoplasm of anterior surface of epiglottis (C10.1)*
malignant neoplasm of aryepiglottic fold or interarytenoid fold, hypopharyngeal aspect (C13.1)
malignant neoplasm of aryepiglottic fold or interarytenoid fold, marginal zone (C13.1)
malignant neoplasm of aryepiglottic fold or interarytenoid fold NOS (C13.1)

C32.2 Malignant neoplasm of subglottis

C32.3 Malignant neoplasm of laryngeal cartilage

C32.8 Malignant neoplasm of overlapping sites of larynx

C32.9 Malignant neoplasm of larynx, unspecified

CC **C33 Malignant neoplasm of trachea**

Use additional code to identify:
exposure to environmental tobacco smoke (Z77.22)
exposure to tobacco smoke in the perinatal period (P96.81)
history of tobacco dependence (Z87.891)
occupational exposure to environmental tobacco smoke (Z57.31)
tobacco dependence (F17.-)
tobacco use (Z72.0)

Valid 3-character code, no further characters required

Lungs

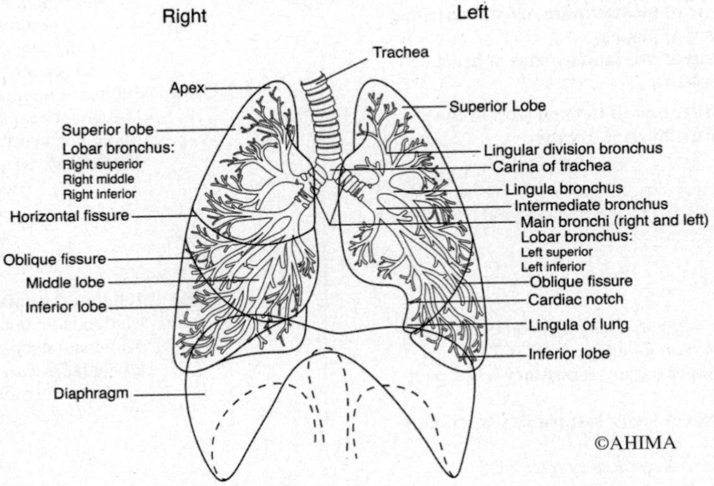

C34 Malignant neoplasm of bronchus and lung

Use additional code to identify:
exposure to environmental tobacco smoke (Z77.22)
exposure to tobacco smoke in the perinatal period (P96.81)
history of tobacco dependence (Z87.891)
occupational exposure to environmental tobacco smoke (Z57.31)
tobacco dependence (F17.-)
tobacco use (Z72.0)

Excludes1: *Kaposi's sarcoma of lung (C46.5-)*
malignant carcinoid tumor of the bronchus and lung (C7A.090)

+ **C34.0 Malignant neoplasm of main bronchus**
  Malignant neoplasm of carina
  Malignant neoplasm of hilus (of lung)
  CC **C34.00 Malignant neoplasm of unspecified main bronchus**
  CC **C34.01 Malignant neoplasm of right main bronchus**
  CC **C34.02 Malignant neoplasm of left main bronchus**
+ **C34.1 Malignant neoplasm of upper lobe, bronchus or lung**
  CC **C34.10 Malignant neoplasm of upper lobe, unspecified bronchus or lung**
  CC **C34.11 Malignant neoplasm of upper lobe, right bronchus or lung**
  CC **C34.12 Malignant neoplasm of upper lobe, left bronchus or lung**

CC **C34.2 Malignant neoplasm of middle lobe, bronchus or lung**

+ **C34.3 Malignant neoplasm of lower lobe, bronchus or lung**
  CC **C34.30 Malignant neoplasm of lower lobe, unspecified bronchus or lung**
  CC **C34.31 Malignant neoplasm of lower lobe, right bronchus or lung**
  CC **C34.32 Malignant neoplasm of lower lobe, left bronchus or lung**
+ **C34.8 Malignant neoplasm of overlapping sites of bronchus and lung**
  CC **C34.80 Malignant neoplasm of overlapping sites of unspecified bronchus and lung**
  CC **C34.81 Malignant neoplasm of overlapping sites of right bronchus and lung**
  CC **C34.82 Malignant neoplasm of overlapping sites of left bronchus and lung**
+ **C34.9 Malignant neoplasm of unspecified part of bronchus or lung**
  CC **C34.90 Malignant neoplasm of unspecified part of unspecified bronchus or lung**
  Lung cancer NOS
  AHA CC: 2Q, 2014, 10
  CC **C34.91 Malignant neoplasm of unspecified part of right bronchus or lung**
  CC **C34.92 Malignant neoplasm of unspecified part of left bronchus or lung**

CC **C37 Malignant neoplasm of thymus**

Excludes1: *malignant carcinoid tumor of the thymus (C7A.091)*
Valid 3-character code, no further characters required

C38 Malignant neoplasm of heart, mediastinum and pleura

Excludes1: *mesothelioma (C45.-)*

CC **C38.0 Malignant neoplasm of heart**
Malignant neoplasm of pericardium
Excludes1: *malignant neoplasm of great vessels (C49.3)*
CC **C38.1 Malignant neoplasm of anterior mediastinum**
CC **C38.2 Malignant neoplasm of posterior mediastinum**
CC **C38.3 Malignant neoplasm of mediastinum, part unspecified**
CC **C38.4 Malignant neoplasm of pleura**
CC **C38.8 Malignant neoplasm of overlapping sites of heart, mediastinum and pleura**

C39 Malignant neoplasm of other and ill-defined sites in the respiratory system and intrathoracic organs

Use additional code to identify:
exposure to environmental tobacco smoke (Z77.22)
exposure to tobacco smoke in the perinatal period (P96.81)
history of tobacco dependence (Z87.891)
occupational exposure to environmental tobacco smoke (Z57.31)
tobacco dependence (F17.-)
tobacco use (Z72.0)

Excludes1: *intrathoracic malignant neoplasm NOS (C76.1)*
thoracic malignant neoplasm NOS (C76.1)

C39.0 Malignant neoplasm of upper respiratory tract, part unspecified
C39.9 Malignant neoplasm of lower respiratory tract, part unspecified
Malignant neoplasm of respiratory tract NOS

Malignant neoplasms of bone and articular cartilage (C40-C41)

Includes: malignant neoplasm of cartilage (articular) (joint)
malignant neoplasm of periosteum

Excludes1: *malignant neoplasm of bone marrow NOS (C96.9)*
malignant neoplasm of synovia (C49.-)

C40 Malignant neoplasm of bone and articular cartilage of limbs

Use additional code to identify major osseous defect, if applicable (M89.7-)

+ **C40.0 Malignant neoplasm of scapula and long bones of upper limb**
  CC **C40.00 Malignant neoplasm of scapula and long bones of unspecified upper limb**
  CC **C40.01 Malignant neoplasm of scapula and long bones of right upper limb**
  CC **C40.02 Malignant neoplasm of scapula and long bones of left upper limb**
+ **C40.1 Malignant neoplasm of short bones of upper limb**
  CC **C40.10 Malignant neoplasm of short bones of unspecified upper limb**
  CC **C40.11 Malignant neoplasm of short bones of right upper limb**
  CC **C40.12 Malignant neoplasm of short bones of left upper limb**
+ **C40.2 Malignant neoplasm of long bones of lower limb**
  CC **C40.20 Malignant neoplasm of long bones of unspecified lower limb**
  CC **C40.21 Malignant neoplasm of long bones of right lower limb**
  CC **C40.22 Malignant neoplasm of long bones of left lower limb**
+ **C40.3 Malignant neoplasm of short bones of lower limb**
  CC **C40.30 Malignant neoplasm of short bones of unspecified lower limb**
  CC **C40.31 Malignant neoplasm of short bones of right lower limb**
  CC **C40.32 Malignant neoplasm of short bones of left lower limb**
+ **C40.8 Malignant neoplasm of overlapping sites of bone and articular cartilage of limb**
  CC **C40.80 Malignant neoplasm of overlapping sites of bone and articular cartilage of unspecified limb**
  CC **C40.81 Malignant neoplasm of overlapping sites of bone and articular cartilage of right limb**
  CC **C40.82 Malignant neoplasm of overlapping sites of bone and articular cartilage of left limb**
+ **C40.9 Malignant neoplasm of unspecified bones and articular cartilage of limb**
  CC **C40.90 Malignant neoplasm of unspecified bones and articular cartilage of unspecified limb**
  CC **C40.91 Malignant neoplasm of unspecified bones and articular cartilage of right limb**
  CC **C40.92 Malignant neoplasm of unspecified bones and articular cartilage of left limb**

C41 Malignant neoplasm of bone and articular cartilage of other and unspecified sites

Excludes1: *malignant neoplasm of bones of limbs (C40.-)*
malignant neoplasm of cartilage of ear (C49.0)
malignant neoplasm of cartilage of eyelid (C49.0)
malignant neoplasm of cartilage of larynx (C32.3)
malignant neoplasm of cartilage of limbs (C40.-)
malignant neoplasm of cartilage of nose (C30.0)

CC **C41.0 Malignant neoplasm of bones of skull and face**
Malignant neoplasm of maxilla (superior)
Malignant neoplasm of orbital bone
Excludes2: *carcinoma, any type except intraosseous or odontogenic of:*
maxillary sinus (C31.0)
upper jaw (C03.0)
malignant neoplasm of jaw bone (lower) (C41.1)

CC **C41.1 Malignant neoplasm of mandible**
Malignant neoplasm of inferior maxilla
Malignant neoplasm of lower jaw bone
Excludes2: *carcinoma, any type except intraosseous or odontogenic of:*
jaw NOS (C03.9)
lower (C03.1)
malignant neoplasm of upper jaw bone (C41.0)

CC **C41.2** **Malignant neoplasm of vertebral column**
Excludes1: *malignant neoplasm of sacrum and coccyx (C41.4)*
CC **C41.3** **Malignant neoplasm of ribs, sternum and clavicle**
CC **C41.4** **Malignant neoplasm of pelvic bones, sacrum and coccyx**
CC **C41.9** **Malignant neoplasm of bone and articular cartilage, unspecified**

Melanoma and other malignant neoplasms of skin (C43-C44)

C43 Malignant melanoma of skin

Excludes1: *melanoma in situ (D03.-)*
Excludes2: *malignant melanoma of skin of genital organs (C51-C52, C60.-, C63.-)*
Merkel cell carcinoma (C4A.-)
sites other than skin-code to malignant neoplasm of the site

C43.0 **Malignant melanoma of lip**
Excludes1: *malignant neoplasm of vermilion border of lip (C00.0-C00.2)*

\+ **C43.1** **Malignant melanoma of eyelid, including canthus**
C43.10 **Malignant melanoma of unspecified eyelid, including canthus**
\+ **C43.11** **Malignant melanoma of right eyelid, including canthus**
C43.111 **Malignant melanoma of right upper eyelid, including canthus**
C43.112 **Malignant melanoma of right lower eyelid, including canthus**
\+ **C43.12** **Malignant melanoma of left eyelid, including canthus**
C43.121 **Malignant melanoma of left upper eyelid, including canthus**
C43.122 **Malignant melanoma of left lower eyelid, including canthus**

\+ **C43.2** **Malignant melanoma of ear and external auricular canal**
C43.20 **Malignant melanoma of unspecified ear and external auricular canal**
C43.21 **Malignant melanoma of right ear and external auricular canal**
C43.22 **Malignant melanoma of left ear and external auricular canal**

\+ **C43.3** **Malignant melanoma of other and unspecified parts of face**
C43.30 **Malignant melanoma of unspecified part of face**
C43.31 **Malignant melanoma of nose**
C43.39 **Malignant melanoma of other parts of face**

C43.4 **Malignant melanoma of scalp and neck**

\+ **C43.5** **Malignant melanoma of trunk**
Excludes2: *malignant neoplasm of anus NOS (C21.0)*
malignant neoplasm of scrotum (C63.2)
C43.51 **Malignant melanoma of anal skin**
Malignant melanoma of anal margin
Malignant melanoma of perianal skin
C43.52 **Malignant melanoma of skin of breast**
C43.59 **Malignant melanoma of other part of trunk**

\+ **C43.6** **Malignant melanoma of upper limb, including shoulder**
C43.60 **Malignant melanoma of unspecified upper limb, including shoulder**
C43.61 **Malignant melanoma of right upper limb, including shoulder**
C43.62 **Malignant melanoma of left upper limb, including shoulder**

\+ **C43.7** **Malignant melanoma of lower limb, including hip**
C43.70 **Malignant melanoma of unspecified lower limb, including hip**
C43.71 **Malignant melanoma of right lower limb, including hip**
C43.72 **Malignant melanoma of left lower limb, including hip**

C43.8 **Malignant melanoma of overlapping sites of skin**
C43.9 **Malignant melanoma of skin, unspecified**
Malignant melanoma of unspecified site of skin
Melanoma (malignant) NOS

C4A Merkel cell carcinoma

C4A.0 **Merkel cell carcinoma of lip**
Excludes1: *malignant neoplasm of vermilion border of lip (C00.0-C00.2)*

\+ **C4A.1** **Merkel cell carcinoma of eyelid, including canthus**
C4A.10 **Merkel cell carcinoma of unspecified eyelid, including canthus**
\+ **C4A.11** **Merkel cell carcinoma of right eyelid, including canthus**
C4A.111 **Merkel cell carcinoma of right upper eyelid, including canthus**
C4A.112 **Merkel cell carcinoma of right lower eyelid, including canthus**
\+ **C4A.12** **Merkel cell carcinoma of left eyelid, including canthus**
C4A.121 **Merkel cell carcinoma of left upper eyelid, including canthus**
C4A.122 **Merkel cell carcinoma of left lower eyelid, including canthus**

\+ **C4A.2** **Merkel cell carcinoma of ear and external auricular canal**
C4A.20 **Merkel cell carcinoma of unspecified ear and external auricular canal**
C4A.21 **Merkel cell carcinoma of right ear and external auricular canal**
C4A.22 **Merkel cell carcinoma of left ear and external auricular canal**

\+ **C4A.3** **Merkel cell carcinoma of other and unspecified parts of face**
C4A.30 **Merkel cell carcinoma of unspecified part of face**
C4A.31 **Merkel cell carcinoma of nose**
C4A.39 **Merkel cell carcinoma of other parts of face**

C4A.4 **Merkel cell carcinoma of scalp and neck**

\+ **C4A.5** **Merkel cell carcinoma of trunk**
Excludes2: *malignant neoplasm of anus NOS (C21.0)*
malignant neoplasm of scrotum (C63.2)
C4A.51 **Merkel cell carcinoma of anal skin**
Merkel cell carcinoma of anal margin
Merkel cell carcinoma of perianal skin
C4A.52 **Merkel cell carcinoma of skin of breast**
C4A.59 **Merkel cell carcinoma of other part of trunk**

\+ **C4A.6** **Merkel cell carcinoma of upper limb, including shoulder**
C4A.60 **Merkel cell carcinoma of unspecified upper limb, including shoulder**
C4A.61 **Merkel cell carcinoma of right upper limb, including shoulder**
C4A.62 **Merkel cell carcinoma of left upper limb, including shoulder**

\+ **C4A.7** **Merkel cell carcinoma of lower limb, including hip**
C4A.70 **Merkel cell carcinoma of unspecified lower limb, including hip**
C4A.71 **Merkel cell carcinoma of right lower limb, including hip**
C4A.72 **Merkel cell carcinoma of left lower limb, including hip**

C4A.8 **Merkel cell carcinoma of overlapping sites**
C4A.9 **Merkel cell carcinoma, unspecified**
Merkel cell carcinoma of unspecified site
Merkel cell carcinoma NOS

C44 Other and unspecified malignant neoplasm of skin

Includes: malignant neoplasm of sebaceous glands
malignant neoplasm of sweat glands
Excludes1: *Kaposi's sarcoma of skin (C46.0)*
malignant melanoma of skin (C43.-)
malignant neoplasm of skin of genital organs (C51-C52, C60.-, C63.2)
Merkel cell carcinoma (C4A.-)

\+ **C44.0** **Other and unspecified malignant neoplasm of skin of lip**
Excludes1: *malignant neoplasm of lip (C00.-)*
C44.00 **Unspecified malignant neoplasm of skin of lip**
C44.01 **Basal cell carcinoma of skin of lip**
C44.02 **Squamous cell carcinoma of skin of lip**
C44.09 **Other specified malignant neoplasm of skin of lip**

+ C44.1 Other and unspecified malignant neoplasm of skin of eyelid, including canthus

Excludes1: *connective tissue of eyelid (C49.0)*

+ C44.10 Unspecified malignant neoplasm of skin of eyelid, including canthus

C44.101 Unspecified malignant neoplasm of skin of unspecified eyelid, including canthus

+ C44.102 Unspecified malignant neoplasm of skin of right eyelid, including canthus

C44.1021 Unspecified malignant neoplasm of skin of right upper eyelid, including canthus

C44.1022 Unspecified malignant neoplasm of skin of right lower eyelid, including canthus

+ C44.109 Unspecified malignant neoplasm of skin of left eyelid, including canthus

C44.1091 Unspecified malignant neoplasm of skin of left upper eyelid, including canthus

C44.1092 Unspecified malignant neoplasm of skin of left lower eyelid, including canthus

+ C44.11 Basal cell carcinoma of skin of eyelid, including canthus

C44.111 Basal cell carcinoma of skin of unspecified eyelid, including canthus

+ C44.112 Basal cell carcinoma of skin of right eyelid, including canthus

C44.1121 Basal cell carcinoma of skin of right upper eyelid, including canthus

C44.1122 Basal cell carcinoma of skin of right lower eyelid, including canthus

+ C44.119 Basal cell carcinoma of skin of left eyelid, including canthus

C44.1191 Basal cell carcinoma of skin of left upper eyelid, including canthus

C44.1192 Basal cell carcinoma of skin of left lower eyelid, including canthus

+ C44.12 Squamous cell carcinoma of skin of eyelid, including canthus

C44.121 Squamous cell carcinoma of skin of unspecified eyelid, including canthus

+ C44.122 Squamous cell carcinoma of skin of right eyelid, including canthus

C44.1221 Squamous cell carcinoma of skin of right upper eyelid, including canthus

C44.1222 Squamous cell carcinoma of skin of right lower eyelid, including canthus

+ C44.129 Squamous cell carcinoma of skin of left eyelid, including canthus

C44.1291 Squamous cell carcinoma of skin of left upper eyelid, including canthus

C44.1292 Squamous cell carcinoma of skin of left lower eyelid, including canthus

+ C44.13 Sebaceous cell carcinoma of skin of eyelid, including canthus

C44.131 Sebaceous cell carcinoma of skin of unspecified eyelid, including canthus

+ C44.132 Sebaceous cell carcinoma of skin of right eyelid, including canthus

C44.1321 Sebaceous cell carcinoma of skin of right upper eyelid, including canthus

C44.1322 Sebaceous cell carcinoma of skin of right lower eyelid, including canthus

+ C44.139 Sebaceous cell carcinoma of skin of left eyelid, including canthus

C44.1391 Sebaceous cell carcinoma of skin of left upper eyelid, including canthus

C44.1392 Sebaceous cell carcinoma of skin of left lower eyelid, including canthus

+ C44.19 Other specified malignant neoplasm of skin of eyelid, including canthus

C44.191 Other specified malignant neoplasm of skin of unspecified eyelid, including canthus

+ C44.192 Other specified malignant neoplasm of skin of right eyelid, including canthus

C44.1921 Other specified malignant neoplasm of skin of right upper eyelid, including canthus

C44.1922 Other specified malignant neoplasm of skin of right lower eyelid, including canthus

+ C44.199 Other specified malignant neoplasm of skin of left eyelid, including canthus

C44.1991 Other specified malignant neoplasm of skin of left upper eyelid, including canthus

C44.1992 Other specified malignant neoplasm of skin of left lower eyelid, including canthus

+ C44.2 Other and unspecified malignant neoplasm of skin of ear and external auricular canal

Excludes1: *connective tissue of ear (C49.0)*

+ C44.20 Unspecified malignant neoplasm of skin of ear and external auricular canal

C44.201 Unspecified malignant neoplasm of skin of unspecified ear and external auricular canal

C44.202 Unspecified malignant neoplasm of skin of right ear and external auricular canal

C44.209 Unspecified malignant neoplasm of skin of left ear and external auricular canal

+ C44.21 Basal cell carcinoma of skin of ear and external auricular canal

C44.211 Basal cell carcinoma of skin of unspecified ear and external auricular canal

C44.212 Basal cell carcinoma of skin of right ear and external auricular canal

C44.219 Basal cell carcinoma of skin of left ear and external auricular canal

+ C44.22 Squamous cell carcinoma of skin of ear and external auricular canal

C44.221 Squamous cell carcinoma of skin of unspecified ear and external auricular canal

C44.222 Squamous cell carcinoma of skin of right ear and external auricular canal

C44.229 Squamous cell carcinoma of skin of left ear and external auricular canal

+ C44.29 Other specified malignant neoplasm of skin of ear and external auricular canal
  - C44.291 Other specified malignant neoplasm of skin of unspecified ear and external auricular canal
  - C44.292 Other specified malignant neoplasm of skin of right ear and external auricular canal
  - C44.299 Other specified malignant neoplasm of skin of left ear and external auricular canal

+ C44.3 Other and unspecified malignant neoplasm of skin of other and unspecified parts of face

+ C44.30 Unspecified malignant neoplasm of skin of other and unspecified parts of face
  - C44.300 Unspecified malignant neoplasm of skin of unspecified part of face
  - C44.301 Unspecified malignant neoplasm of skin of nose
  - C44.309 Unspecified malignant neoplasm of skin of other parts of face

+ C44.31 Basal cell carcinoma of skin of other and unspecified parts of face
  - C44.310 Basal cell carcinoma of skin of unspecified parts of face
  - C44.311 Basal cell carcinoma of skin of nose
  - C44.319 Basal cell carcinoma of skin of other parts of face
    AHA CC: 1Q, 2017, 4

+ C44.32 Squamous cell carcinoma of skin of other and unspecified parts of face
  - C44.320 Squamous cell carcinoma of skin of unspecified parts of face
  - C44.321 Squamous cell carcinoma of skin of nose
  - C44.329 Squamous cell carcinoma of skin of other parts of face

+ C44.39 Other specified malignant neoplasm of skin of other and unspecified parts of face
  - C44.390 Other specified malignant neoplasm of skin of unspecified parts of face
  - C44.391 Other specified malignant neoplasm of skin of nose
  - C44.399 Other specified malignant neoplasm of skin of other parts of face

+ C44.4 Other and unspecified malignant neoplasm of skin of scalp and neck
  - C44.40 Unspecified malignant neoplasm of skin of scalp and neck
  - C44.41 Basal cell carcinoma of skin of scalp and neck
  - C44.42 Squamous cell carcinoma of skin of scalp and neck
  - C44.49 Other specified malignant neoplasm of skin of scalp and neck

+ C44.5 Other and unspecified malignant neoplasm of skin of trunk
  Excludes1: *anus NOS (C21.0)*
  scrotum (C63.2)

+ C44.50 Unspecified malignant neoplasm of skin of trunk
  - C44.500 Unspecified malignant neoplasm of anal skin
    Unspecified malignant neoplasm of anal margin
    Unspecified malignant neoplasm of perianal skin
  - C44.501 Unspecified malignant neoplasm of skin of breast
  - C44.509 Unspecified malignant neoplasm of skin of other part of trunk

+ C44.51 Basal cell carcinoma of skin of trunk
  - C44.510 Basal cell carcinoma of anal skin
    Basal cell carcinoma of anal margin
    Basal cell carcinoma of perianal skin
  - C44.511 Basal cell carcinoma of skin of breast
  - C44.519 Basal cell carcinoma of skin of other part of trunk

+ C44.52 Squamous cell carcinoma of skin of trunk
  - C44.520 Squamous cell carcinoma of anal skin
    Squamous cell carcinoma of anal margin
    Squamous cell carcinoma of perianal skin
  - C44.521 Squamous cell carcinoma of skin of breast
  - C44.529 Squamous cell carcinoma of skin of other part of trunk

+ C44.59 Other specified malignant neoplasm of skin of trunk
  - C44.590 Other specified malignant neoplasm of anal skin
    Other specified malignant neoplasm of anal margin
    Other specified malignant neoplasm of perianal skin
  - C44.591 Other specified malignant neoplasm of skin of breast
  - C44.599 Other specified malignant neoplasm of skin of other part of trunk

+ C44.6 Other and unspecified malignant neoplasm of skin of upper limb, including shoulder

+ C44.60 Unspecified malignant neoplasm of skin of upper limb, including shoulder
  - C44.601 Unspecified malignant neoplasm of skin of unspecified upper limb, including shoulder
  - C44.602 Unspecified malignant neoplasm of skin of right upper limb, including shoulder
  - C44.609 Unspecified malignant neoplasm of skin of left upper limb, including shoulder

+ C44.61 Basal cell carcinoma of skin of upper limb, including shoulder
  - C44.611 Basal cell carcinoma of skin of unspecified upper limb, including shoulder
  - C44.612 Basal cell carcinoma of skin of right upper limb, including shoulder
  - C44.619 Basal cell carcinoma of skin of left upper limb, including shoulder

+ C44.62 Squamous cell carcinoma of skin of upper limb, including shoulder
  - C44.621 Squamous cell carcinoma of skin of unspecified upper limb, including shoulder
  - C44.622 Squamous cell carcinoma of skin of right upper limb, including shoulder
  - C44.629 Squamous cell carcinoma of skin of left upper limb, including shoulder

+ C44.69 Other specified malignant neoplasm of skin of upper limb, including shoulder
  - C44.691 Other specified malignant neoplasm of skin of unspecified upper limb, including shoulder
  - C44.692 Other specified malignant neoplasm of skin of right upper limb, including shoulder
  - C44.699 Other specified malignant neoplasm of skin of left upper limb, including shoulder

+ C44.7 Other and unspecified malignant neoplasm of skin of lower limb, including hip

+ C44.70 Unspecified malignant neoplasm of skin of lower limb, including hip
  - C44.701 Unspecified malignant neoplasm of skin of unspecified lower limb, including hip
  - C44.702 Unspecified malignant neoplasm of skin of right lower limb, including hip
  - C44.709 Unspecified malignant neoplasm of skin of left lower limb, including hip

+ C44.71 Basal cell carcinoma of skin of lower limb, including hip
  - C44.711 Basal cell carcinoma of skin of unspecified lower limb, including hip
  - C44.712 Basal cell carcinoma of skin of right lower limb, including hip
  - C44.719 Basal cell carcinoma of skin of left lower limb, including hip

+ C44.72 **Squamous cell carcinoma of skin of lower limb, including hip**
  - C44.721 **Squamous cell carcinoma of skin of unspecified lower limb, including hip**
  - C44.722 **Squamous cell carcinoma of skin of right lower limb, including hip**
  - C44.729 **Squamous cell carcinoma of skin of left lower limb, including hip**

+ C44.79 **Other specified malignant neoplasm of skin of lower limb, including hip**
  - C44.791 **Other specified malignant neoplasm of skin of unspecified lower limb, including hip**
  - C44.792 **Other specified malignant neoplasm of skin of right lower limb, including hip**
  - C44.799 **Other specified malignant neoplasm of skin of left lower limb, including hip**

+ C44.8 **Other and unspecified malignant neoplasm of overlapping sites of skin**
  - C44.80 **Unspecified malignant neoplasm of overlapping sites of skin**
  - C44.81 **Basal cell carcinoma of overlapping sites of skin**
  - C44.82 **Squamous cell carcinoma of overlapping sites of skin**
  - C44.89 **Other specified malignant neoplasm of overlapping sites of skin**

+ C44.9 **Other and unspecified malignant neoplasm of skin, unspecified**
  - C44.90 **Unspecified malignant neoplasm of skin, unspecified**
    Malignant neoplasm of unspecified site of skin
  - C44.91 **Basal cell carcinoma of skin, unspecified**
  - C44.92 **Squamous cell carcinoma of skin, unspecified**
  - C44.99 **Other specified malignant neoplasm of skin, unspecified**

Malignant neoplasms of mesothelial and soft tissue (C45-C49)

C45 Mesothelioma

CC **C45.0 Mesothelioma of pleura**
Excludes1: *other malignant neoplasm of pleura (C38.4)*
AHA CC: 2Q, 2017, 11

CC **C45.1 Mesothelioma of peritoneum**
Mesothelioma of cul-de-sac
Mesothelioma of mesentery
Mesothelioma of mesocolon
Mesothelioma of omentum
Mesothelioma of peritoneum (parietal) (pelvic)
Excludes1: *other malignant neoplasm of soft tissue of peritoneum (C48.-)*

CC **C45.2 Mesothelioma of pericardium**
Excludes1: *other malignant neoplasm of pericardium (C38.0)*

C45.7 Mesothelioma of other sites
C45.9 Mesothelioma, unspecified

C46 Kaposi's sarcoma

Code first any human immunodeficiency virus [HIV] disease (B20)

CC **C46.0 Kaposi's sarcoma of skin**
CC **C46.1 Kaposi's sarcoma of soft tissue**
Kaposi's sarcoma of blood vessel
Kaposi's sarcoma of connective tissue
Kaposi's sarcoma of fascia
Kaposi's sarcoma of ligament
Kaposi's sarcoma of lymphatic(s) NEC
Kaposi's sarcoma of muscle
Excludes2: *Kaposi's sarcoma of lymph glands and nodes (C46.3)*

CC **C46.2 Kaposi's sarcoma of palate**
CC **C46.3 Kaposi's sarcoma of lymph nodes**
CC **C46.4 Kaposi's sarcoma of gastrointestinal sites**
+ **C46.5 Kaposi's sarcoma of lung**
  - CC **C46.50 Kaposi's sarcoma of unspecified lung**
  - CC **C46.51 Kaposi's sarcoma of right lung**
  - CC **C46.52 Kaposi's sarcoma of left lung**

CC **C46.7 Kaposi's sarcoma of other sites**
CC **C46.9 Kaposi's sarcoma, unspecified**
Kaposi's sarcoma of unspecified site

C47 Malignant neoplasm of peripheral nerves and autonomic nervous system

Includes: malignant neoplasm of sympathetic and parasympathetic nerves and ganglia
Excludes1: *Kaposi's sarcoma of soft tissue (C46.1)*

CC **C47.0 Malignant neoplasm of peripheral nerves of head, face and neck**
Excludes1: *malignant neoplasm of peripheral nerves of orbit (C69.6-)*

+ **C47.1 Malignant neoplasm of peripheral nerves of upper limb, including shoulder**
  - CC **C47.10 Malignant neoplasm of peripheral nerves of unspecified upper limb, including shoulder**
  - CC **C47.11 Malignant neoplasm of peripheral nerves of right upper limb, including shoulder**
  - CC **C47.12 Malignant neoplasm of peripheral nerves of left upper limb, including shoulder**

+ **C47.2 Malignant neoplasm of peripheral nerves of lower limb, including hip**
  - CC **C47.20 Malignant neoplasm of peripheral nerves of unspecified lower limb, including hip**
  - CC **C47.21 Malignant neoplasm of peripheral nerves of right lower limb, including hip**
  - CC **C47.22 Malignant neoplasm of peripheral nerves of left lower limb, including hip**

CC **C47.3 Malignant neoplasm of peripheral nerves of thorax**
CC **C47.4 Malignant neoplasm of peripheral nerves of abdomen**
CC **C47.5 Malignant neoplasm of peripheral nerves of pelvis**
CC **C47.6 Malignant neoplasm of peripheral nerves of trunk, unspecified**
Malignant neoplasm of peripheral nerves of unspecified part of trunk
CC **C47.8 Malignant neoplasm of overlapping sites of peripheral nerves and autonomic nervous system**
CC **C47.9 Malignant neoplasm of peripheral nerves and autonomic nervous system, unspecified**
Malignant neoplasm of unspecified site of peripheral nerves and autonomic nervous system

C48 Malignant neoplasm of retroperitoneum and peritoneum

Excludes1: *Kaposi's sarcoma of connective tissue (C46.1)*
mesothelioma (C45.-)

CC **C48.0 Malignant neoplasm of retroperitoneum**
CC **C48.1 Malignant neoplasm of specified parts of peritoneum**
Malignant neoplasm of cul-de-sac
Malignant neoplasm of mesentery
Malignant neoplasm of mesocolon
Malignant neoplasm of omentum
Malignant neoplasm of parietal peritoneum
Malignant neoplasm of pelvic peritoneum
CC **C48.2 Malignant neoplasm of peritoneum, unspecified**
CC **C48.8 Malignant neoplasm of overlapping sites of retroperitoneum and peritoneum**

C49 Malignant neoplasm of other connective and soft tissue

Includes: malignant neoplasm of blood vessel
malignant neoplasm of bursa
malignant neoplasm of cartilage
malignant neoplasm of fascia
malignant neoplasm of fat
malignant neoplasm of ligament, except uterine
malignant neoplasm of lymphatic vessel
malignant neoplasm of muscle
malignant neoplasm of synovia
malignant neoplasm of tendon (sheath)

Excludes1: *malignant neoplasm of cartilage (of):*
articular (C40-C41)
larynx (C32.3)
nose (C30.0)
malignant neoplasm of connective tissue of breast (C50.-)

Excludes2: *Kaposi's sarcoma of soft tissue (C46.1)*
malignant neoplasm of heart (C38.0)
malignant neoplasm of peripheral nerves and autonomic nervous system (C47.-)
malignant neoplasm of peritoneum (C48.2)
malignant neoplasm of retroperitoneum (C48.0)
malignant neoplasm of uterine ligament (C57.3)
mesothelioma (C45.-)

CC **C49.0 Malignant neoplasm of connective and soft tissue of head, face and neck**

Malignant neoplasm of connective tissue of ear

Malignant neoplasm of connective tissue of eyelid

Excludes1: *connective tissue of orbit (C69.6-)*

\+ **C49.1 Malignant neoplasm of connective and soft tissue of upper limb, including shoulder**

CC **C49.10 Malignant neoplasm of connective and soft tissue of unspecified upper limb, including shoulder**

CC **C49.11 Malignant neoplasm of connective and soft tissue of right upper limb, including shoulder**

CC **C49.12 Malignant neoplasm of connective and soft tissue of left upper limb, including shoulder**

\+ **C49.2 Malignant neoplasm of connective and soft tissue of lower limb, including hip**

CC **C49.20 Malignant neoplasm of connective and soft tissue of unspecified lower limb, including hip**

CC **C49.21 Malignant neoplasm of connective and soft tissue of right lower limb, including hip**

CC **C49.22 Malignant neoplasm of connective and soft tissue of left lower limb, including hip**

CC **C49.3 Malignant neoplasm of connective and soft tissue of thorax**

Malignant neoplasm of axilla

Malignant neoplasm of diaphragm

Malignant neoplasm of great vessels

Excludes1: *malignant neoplasm of breast (C50.-)*
malignant neoplasm of heart (C38.0)
malignant neoplasm of mediastinum (C38.1-C38.3)
malignant neoplasm of thymus (C37)

AHA CC: 3Q, 2015, 19-20

CC **C49.4 Malignant neoplasm of connective and soft tissue of abdomen**

Malignant neoplasm of abdominal wall

Malignant neoplasm of hypochondrium

CC **C49.5 Malignant neoplasm of connective and soft tissue of pelvis**

Malignant neoplasm of buttock

Malignant neoplasm of groin

Malignant neoplasm of perineum

CC **C49.6 Malignant neoplasm of connective and soft tissue of trunk, unspecified**

Malignant neoplasm of back NOS

CC **C49.8 Malignant neoplasm of overlapping sites of connective and soft tissue**

Primary malignant neoplasm of two or more contiguous sites of connective and soft tissue

CC **C49.9 Malignant neoplasm of connective and soft tissue, unspecified**

\+ **C49.A Gastrointestinal stromal tumor**

AHA CC: 4Q, 2016, 8

CC **C49.A0 Gastrointestinal stromal tumor, unspecified site**

CC **C49.A1 Gastrointestinal stromal tumor of esophagus**

CC **C49.A2 Gastrointestinal stromal tumor of stomach**

CC **C49.A3 Gastrointestinal stromal tumor of small intestine**

CC **C49.A4 Gastrointestinal stromal tumor of large intestine**

CC **C49.A5 Gastrointestinal stromal tumor of rectum**

CC **C49.A9 Gastrointestinal stromal tumor of other sites**

Malignant neoplasms of breast (C50)

C50 Malignant neoplasm of breast

Includes: connective tissue of breast
Paget's disease of breast
Paget's disease of nipple

Use additional code to identify estrogen receptor status (Z17.0, Z17.1)

Excludes1: *skin of breast (C44.501, C44.511, C44.521, C44.591)*

\+ **C50.0 Malignant neoplasm of nipple and areola**

\+ **C50.01 Malignant neoplasm of nipple and areola, female**

♀ **C50.011 Malignant neoplasm of nipple and areola, right female breast**

♀ **C50.012 Malignant neoplasm of nipple and areola, left female breast**

♀ **C50.019 Malignant neoplasm of nipple and areola, unspecified female breast**

\+ **C50.02 Malignant neoplasm of nipple and areola, male**

♂ **C50.021 Malignant neoplasm of nipple and areola, right male breast**

♂ **C50.022 Malignant neoplasm of nipple and areola, left male breast**

♂ **C50.029 Malignant neoplasm of nipple and areola, unspecified male breast**

\+ **C50.1 Malignant neoplasm of central portion of breast**

\+ **C50.11 Malignant neoplasm of central portion of breast, female**

♀ **C50.111 Malignant neoplasm of central portion of right female breast**

♀ **C50.112 Malignant neoplasm of central portion of left female breast**

♀ **C50.119 Malignant neoplasm of central portion of unspecified female breast**

\+ **C50.12 Malignant neoplasm of central portion of breast, male**

♂ **C50.121 Malignant neoplasm of central portion of right male breast**

♂ **C50.122 Malignant neoplasm of central portion of left male breast**

♂ **C50.129 Malignant neoplasm of central portion of unspecified male breast**

\+ **C50.2 Malignant neoplasm of upper-inner quadrant of breast**

\+ **C50.21 Malignant neoplasm of upper-inner quadrant of breast, female**

♀ **C50.211 Malignant neoplasm of upper-inner quadrant of right female breast**

♀ **C50.212 Malignant neoplasm of upper-inner quadrant of left female breast**

♀ **C50.219 Malignant neoplasm of upper-inner quadrant of unspecified female breast**

\+ **C50.22 Malignant neoplasm of upper-inner quadrant of breast, male**

♂ **C50.221 Malignant neoplasm of upper-inner quadrant of right male breast**

♂ **C50.222 Malignant neoplasm of upper-inner quadrant of left male breast**

♂ **C50.229 Malignant neoplasm of upper-inner quadrant of unspecified male breast**

\+ **C50.3 Malignant neoplasm of lower-inner quadrant of breast**

\+ **C50.31 Malignant neoplasm of lower-inner quadrant of breast, female**

♀ **C50.311 Malignant neoplasm of lower-inner quadrant of right female breast**

♀ **C50.312 Malignant neoplasm of lower-inner quadrant of left female breast**

♀ **C50.319 Malignant neoplasm of lower-inner quadrant of unspecified female breast**

\+ **C50.32 Malignant neoplasm of lower-inner quadrant of breast, male**

♂ **C50.321 Malignant neoplasm of lower-inner quadrant of right male breast**

♂ **C50.322 Malignant neoplasm of lower-inner quadrant of left male breast**

♂ **C50.329 Malignant neoplasm of lower-inner quadrant of unspecified male breast**

\+ **C50.4 Malignant neoplasm of upper-outer quadrant of breast**

\+ **C50.41 Malignant neoplasm of upper-outer quadrant of breast, female**

♀ **C50.411 Malignant neoplasm of upper-outer quadrant of right female breast**

♀ **C50.412 Malignant neoplasm of upper-outer quadrant of left female breast**

♀ **C50.419 Malignant neoplasm of upper-outer quadrant of unspecified female breast**

\+ **C50.42 Malignant neoplasm of upper-outer quadrant of breast, male**

♂ **C50.421 Malignant neoplasm of upper-outer quadrant of right male breast**

♂ **C50.422 Malignant neoplasm of upper-outer quadrant of left male breast**

♂ **C50.429 Malignant neoplasm of upper-outer quadrant of unspecified male breast**

+ C50.5 **Malignant neoplasm of lower-outer quadrant of breast**
+ C50.51 **Malignant neoplasm of lower-outer quadrant of breast, female**
♀ C50.511 **Malignant neoplasm of lower-outer quadrant of right female breast**
♀ C50.512 **Malignant neoplasm of lower-outer quadrant of left female breast**
♀ C50.519 **Malignant neoplasm of lower-outer quadrant of unspecified female breast**
+ C50.52 **Malignant neoplasm of lower-outer quadrant of breast, male**
♂ C50.521 **Malignant neoplasm of lower-outer quadrant of right male breast**
♂ C50.522 **Malignant neoplasm of lower-outer quadrant of left male breast**
♂ C50.529 **Malignant neoplasm of lower-outer quadrant of unspecified male breast**
+ C50.6 **Malignant neoplasm of axillary tail of breast**
+ C50.61 **Malignant neoplasm of axillary tail of breast, female**
♀ C50.611 **Malignant neoplasm of axillary tail of right female breast**
♀ C50.612 **Malignant neoplasm of axillary tail of left female breast**
♀ C50.619 **Malignant neoplasm of axillary tail of unspecified female breast**
+ C50.62 **Malignant neoplasm of axillary tail of breast, male**
♂ C50.621 **Malignant neoplasm of axillary tail of right male breast**
♂ C50.622 **Malignant neoplasm of axillary tail of left male breast**
♂ C50.629 **Malignant neoplasm of axillary tail of unspecified male breast**
+ C50.8 **Malignant neoplasm of overlapping sites of breast**
+ C50.81 **Malignant neoplasm of overlapping sites of breast, female**
♀ C50.811 **Malignant neoplasm of overlapping sites of right female breast**
♀ C50.812 **Malignant neoplasm of overlapping sites of left female breast**
♀ C50.819 **Malignant neoplasm of overlapping sites of unspecified female breast**
+ C50.82 **Malignant neoplasm of overlapping sites of breast, male**
♂ C50.821 **Malignant neoplasm of overlapping sites of right male breast**
♂ C50.822 **Malignant neoplasm of overlapping sites of left male breast**
♂ C50.829 **Malignant neoplasm of overlapping sites of unspecified male breast**
+ C50.9 **Malignant neoplasm of breast of unspecified site**
+ C50.91 **Malignant neoplasm of breast of unspecified site, female**
♀ C50.911 **Malignant neoplasm of unspecified site of right female breast**
♀ C50.912 **Malignant neoplasm of unspecified site of left female breast**
♀ C50.919 **Malignant neoplasm of unspecified site of unspecified female breast**
+ C50.92 **Malignant neoplasm of breast of unspecified site, male**
♂ C50.921 **Malignant neoplasm of unspecified site of right male breast**
♂ C50.922 **Malignant neoplasm of unspecified site of left male breast**
♂ C50.929 **Malignant neoplasm of unspecified site of unspecified male breast**

Malignant neoplasms of female genital organs (C51-C58)

Includes: malignant neoplasm of skin of female genital organs

C51 **Malignant neoplasm of vulva**

Excludes1: *carcinoma in situ of vulva (D07.1)*

♀ C51.0 **Malignant neoplasm of labium majus**
Malignant neoplasm of Bartholin's [greater vestibular] gland
♀ C51.1 **Malignant neoplasm of labium minus**
♀ C51.2 **Malignant neoplasm of clitoris**
♀ C51.8 **Malignant neoplasm of overlapping sites of vulva**
♀ C51.9 **Malignant neoplasm of vulva, unspecified**
Malignant neoplasm of external female genitalia NOS
Malignant neoplasm of pudendum

♀ C52 **Malignant neoplasm of vagina**

Excludes1: *carcinoma in situ of vagina (D07.2)*

Valid 3-character code, no further characters required

C53 **Malignant neoplasm of cervix uteri**

Excludes1: *carcinoma in situ of cervix uteri (D06.-)*

♀ C53.0 **Malignant neoplasm of endocervix**
♀ C53.1 **Malignant neoplasm of exocervix**
♀ C53.8 **Malignant neoplasm of overlapping sites of cervix uteri**
♀ C53.9 **Malignant neoplasm of cervix uteri, unspecified**
AHA CC: 4Q, 2017, 103-104

C54 **Malignant neoplasm of corpus uteri**

♀ C54.0 **Malignant neoplasm of isthmus uteri**
Malignant neoplasm of lower uterine segment
♀ C54.1 **Malignant neoplasm of endometrium**
♀ C54.2 **Malignant neoplasm of myometrium**
♀ C54.3 **Malignant neoplasm of fundus uteri**
♀ C54.8 **Malignant neoplasm of overlapping sites of corpus uteri**
♀ C54.9 **Malignant neoplasm of corpus uteri, unspecified**

♀ C55 **Malignant neoplasm of uterus, part unspecified**

Valid 3-character code, no further characters required

C56 **Malignant neoplasm of ovary**

Use additional code to identify any functional activity

♀ CC C56.1 **Malignant neoplasm of right ovary**
♀ CC C56.2 **Malignant neoplasm of left ovary**
♀ CC C56.3 **Malignant neoplasm of bilateral ovaries**
♀ CC C56.9 **Malignant neoplasm of unspecified ovary**

C57 **Malignant neoplasm of other and unspecified female genital organs**

+ C57.0 **Malignant neoplasm of fallopian tube**
Malignant neoplasm of oviduct
Malignant neoplasm of uterine tube
♀ C57.00 **Malignant neoplasm of unspecified fallopian tube**
♀ C57.01 **Malignant neoplasm of right fallopian tube**
♀ C57.02 **Malignant neoplasm of left fallopian tube**
+ C57.1 **Malignant neoplasm of broad ligament**
♀ C57.10 **Malignant neoplasm of unspecified broad ligament**
♀ C57.11 **Malignant neoplasm of right broad ligament**
♀ C57.12 **Malignant neoplasm of left broad ligament**
+ C57.2 **Malignant neoplasm of round ligament**
♀ C57.20 **Malignant neoplasm of unspecified round ligament**
♀ C57.21 **Malignant neoplasm of right round ligament**
♀ C57.22 **Malignant neoplasm of left round ligament**
♀ C57.3 **Malignant neoplasm of parametrium**
Malignant neoplasm of uterine ligament NOS
♀ C57.4 **Malignant neoplasm of uterine adnexa, unspecified**
♀ C57.7 **Malignant neoplasm of other specified female genital organs**
Malignant neoplasm of wolffian body or duct
♀ C57.8 **Malignant neoplasm of overlapping sites of female genital organs**
Primary malignant neoplasm of two or more contiguous sites of the female genital organs whose point of origin cannot be determined
Primary tubo-ovarian malignant neoplasm whose point of origin cannot be determined
Primary utero-ovarian malignant neoplasm whose point of origin cannot be determined
♀ C57.9 **Malignant neoplasm of female genital organ, unspecified**
Malignant neoplasm of female genitourinary tract NOS

♀ C58 **Malignant neoplasm of placenta**

Includes: choriocarcinoma NOS
chorionepithelioma NOS

Excludes1: *chorioadenoma (destruens) (D39.2)*
hydatidiform mole NOS (O01.9)
invasive hydatidiform mole (D39.2)
male choriocarcinoma NOS (C62.9-)
malignant hydatidiform mole (D39.2)

Valid 3-character code, no further characters required

Malignant neoplasms of male genital organs (C60-C63)

Includes: malignant neoplasm of skin of male genital organs

C60 Malignant neoplasm of penis

♂ **C60.0 Malignant neoplasm of prepuce**
Malignant neoplasm of foreskin

♂ **C60.1 Malignant neoplasm of glans penis**

♂ **C60.2 Malignant neoplasm of body of penis**
Malignant neoplasm of corpus cavernosum

♂ **C60.8 Malignant neoplasm of overlapping sites of penis**

♂ **C60.9 Malignant neoplasm of penis, unspecified**
Malignant neoplasm of skin of penis NOS

♂ **C61 Malignant neoplasm of prostate**

Use additional code to identify:
hormone sensitivity status (Z19.1-Z19.2)
rising PSA following treatment for malignant neoplasm of prostate (R97.21)

Excludes1: *malignant neoplasm of seminal vesicle (C63.7)*

AHA CC: 1Q, 2017, 17-18

Valid 3-character code, no further characters required

C62 Malignant neoplasm of testis

Use additional code to identify any functional activity

\+ **C62.0 Malignant neoplasm of undescended testis**
Malignant neoplasm of ectopic testis
Malignant neoplasm of retained testis

♂ **C62.00 Malignant neoplasm of unspecified undescended testis**

♂ **C62.01 Malignant neoplasm of undescended right testis**

♂ **C62.02 Malignant neoplasm of undescended left testis**

\+ **C62.1 Malignant neoplasm of descended testis**
Malignant neoplasm of scrotal testis

♂ **C62.10 Malignant neoplasm of unspecified descended testis**

♂ **C62.11 Malignant neoplasm of descended right testis**

♂ **C62.12 Malignant neoplasm of descended left testis**

\+ **C62.9 Malignant neoplasm of testis, unspecified whether descended or undescended**

♂ **C62.90 Malignant neoplasm of unspecified testis, unspecified whether descended or undescended**
Malignant neoplasm of testis NOS

♂ **C62.91 Malignant neoplasm of right testis, unspecified whether descended or undescended**

♂ **C62.92 Malignant neoplasm of left testis, unspecified whether descended or undescended**

C63 Malignant neoplasm of other and unspecified male genital organs

\+ **C63.0 Malignant neoplasm of epididymis**

♂ **C63.00 Malignant neoplasm of unspecified epididymis**

♂ **C63.01 Malignant neoplasm of right epididymis**

♂ **C63.02 Malignant neoplasm of left epididymis**

\+ **C63.1 Malignant neoplasm of spermatic cord**

♂ **C63.10 Malignant neoplasm of unspecified spermatic cord**

♂ **C63.11 Malignant neoplasm of right spermatic cord**

♂ **C63.12 Malignant neoplasm of left spermatic cord**

♂ **C63.2 Malignant neoplasm of scrotum**
Malignant neoplasm of skin of scrotum

♂ **C63.7 Malignant neoplasm of other specified male genital organs**
Malignant neoplasm of seminal vesicle
Malignant neoplasm of tunica vaginalis

♂ **C63.8 Malignant neoplasm of overlapping sites of male genital organs**
Primary malignant neoplasm of two or more contiguous sites of male genital organs whose point of origin cannot be determined

♂ **C63.9 Malignant neoplasm of male genital organ, unspecified**
Malignant neoplasm of male genitourinary tract NOS

Malignant neoplasms of urinary tract (C64-C68)

C64 Malignant neoplasm of kidney, except renal pelvis

Excludes1: *malignant carcinoid tumor of the kidney (C7A.093)*
malignant neoplasm of renal calyces (C65.-)
malignant neoplasm of renal pelvis (C65.-)

CC **C64.1 Malignant neoplasm of right kidney, except renal pelvis**

CC **C64.2 Malignant neoplasm of left kidney, except renal pelvis**

CC **C64.9 Malignant neoplasm of unspecified kidney, except renal pelvis**

C65 Malignant neoplasm of renal pelvis

Includes: malignant neoplasm of pelviureteric junction
malignant neoplasm of renal calyces

CC **C65.1 Malignant neoplasm of right renal pelvis**

CC **C65.2 Malignant neoplasm of left renal pelvis**

CC **C65.9 Malignant neoplasm of unspecified renal pelvis**

C66 Malignant neoplasm of ureter

Excludes1: *malignant neoplasm of ureteric orifice of bladder (C67.6)*

CC **C66.1 Malignant neoplasm of right ureter**

CC **C66.2 Malignant neoplasm of left ureter**

CC **C66.9 Malignant neoplasm of unspecified ureter**

C67 Malignant neoplasm of bladder

C67.0 Malignant neoplasm of trigone of bladder

C67.1 Malignant neoplasm of dome of bladder

C67.2 Malignant neoplasm of lateral wall of bladder

C67.3 Malignant neoplasm of anterior wall of bladder

C67.4 Malignant neoplasm of posterior wall of bladder

C67.5 Malignant neoplasm of bladder neck
Malignant neoplasm of internal urethral orifice

C67.6 Malignant neoplasm of ureteric orifice

C67.7 Malignant neoplasm of urachus

C67.8 Malignant neoplasm of overlapping sites of bladder

C67.9 Malignant neoplasm of bladder, unspecified

AHA CC: 1Q, 2016, 19; 1Q, 2017, 6

C68 Malignant neoplasm of other and unspecified urinary organs

Excludes1: *malignant neoplasm of female genitourinary tract NOS (C57.9)*
malignant neoplasm of male genitourinary tract NOS (C63.9)

CC **C68.0 Malignant neoplasm of urethra**

Excludes1: *malignant neoplasm of urethral orifice of bladder (C67.5)*

CC **C68.1 Malignant neoplasm of paraurethral glands**

CC **C68.8 Malignant neoplasm of overlapping sites of urinary organs**
Primary malignant neoplasm of two or more contiguous sites of urinary organs whose point of origin cannot be determined

CC **C68.9 Malignant neoplasm of urinary organ, unspecified**
Malignant neoplasm of urinary system NOS

Malignant neoplasms of eye, brain and other parts of central nervous system (C69-C72)

C69 Malignant neoplasm of eye and adnexa

Excludes1: *malignant neoplasm of connective tissue of eyelid (C49.0)*
malignant neoplasm of eyelid (skin) (C43.1-, C44.1-)
malignant neoplasm of optic nerve (C72.3-)

\+ **C69.0 Malignant neoplasm of conjunctiva**

C69.00 Malignant neoplasm of unspecified conjunctiva

C69.01 Malignant neoplasm of right conjunctiva

C69.02 Malignant neoplasm of left conjunctiva

\+ **C69.1 Malignant neoplasm of cornea**

C69.10 Malignant neoplasm of unspecified cornea

C69.11 Malignant neoplasm of right cornea

C69.12 Malignant neoplasm of left cornea

\+ **C69.2 Malignant neoplasm of retina**

Excludes1: *dark area on retina (D49.81)*
neoplasm of unspecified behavior of retina and choroid (D49.81)
retinal freckle (D49.81)

C69.20 Malignant neoplasm of unspecified retina

C69.21 Malignant neoplasm of right retina

C69.22 Malignant neoplasm of left retina

\+ **C69.3 Malignant neoplasm of choroid**

C69.30 Malignant neoplasm of unspecified choroid

C69.31 Malignant neoplasm of right choroid

C69.32 Malignant neoplasm of left choroid

\+ **C69.4 Malignant neoplasm of ciliary body**

C69.40 Malignant neoplasm of unspecified ciliary body

C69.41 Malignant neoplasm of right ciliary body

C69.42 Malignant neoplasm of left ciliary body

\+ **C69.5 Malignant neoplasm of lacrimal gland and duct**
Malignant neoplasm of lacrimal sac
Malignant neoplasm of nasolacrimal duct

C69.50 **Malignant neoplasm of unspecified lacrimal gland and duct**
C69.51 **Malignant neoplasm of right lacrimal gland and duct**
C69.52 **Malignant neoplasm of left lacrimal gland and duct**

+ C69.6 **Malignant neoplasm of orbit**
Malignant neoplasm of connective tissue of orbit
Malignant neoplasm of extraocular muscle
Malignant neoplasm of peripheral nerves of orbit
Malignant neoplasm of retrobulbar tissue
Malignant neoplasm of retro-ocular tissue
Excludes1: *malignant neoplasm of orbital bone (C41.0)*
C69.60 **Malignant neoplasm of unspecified orbit**
C69.61 **Malignant neoplasm of right orbit**
C69.62 **Malignant neoplasm of left orbit**

+ C69.8 **Malignant neoplasm of overlapping sites of eye and adnexa**
C69.80 **Malignant neoplasm of overlapping sites of unspecified eye and adnexa**
C69.81 **Malignant neoplasm of overlapping sites of right eye and adnexa**
C69.82 **Malignant neoplasm of overlapping sites of left eye and adnexa**

+ C69.9 **Malignant neoplasm of unspecified site of eye**
Malignant neoplasm of eyeball
C69.90 **Malignant neoplasm of unspecified site of unspecified eye**
C69.91 **Malignant neoplasm of unspecified site of right eye**
C69.92 **Malignant neoplasm of unspecified site of left eye**

C70 Malignant neoplasm of meninges
CC C70.0 **Malignant neoplasm of cerebral meninges**
CC C70.1 **Malignant neoplasm of spinal meninges**
CC C70.9 **Malignant neoplasm of meninges, unspecified**

C71 Malignant neoplasm of brain
Excludes1: *malignant neoplasm of cranial nerves (C72.2-C72.5)*
retrobulbar malignant neoplasm (C69.6-)
CC C71.0 **Malignant neoplasm of cerebrum, except lobes and ventricles**
Malignant neoplasm of supratentorial NOS
CC C71.1 **Malignant neoplasm of frontal lobe**
CC C71.2 **Malignant neoplasm of temporal lobe**
CC C71.3 **Malignant neoplasm of parietal lobe**
CC C71.4 **Malignant neoplasm of occipital lobe**
CC C71.5 **Malignant neoplasm of cerebral ventricle**
Excludes1: *malignant neoplasm of fourth cerebral ventricle (C71.7)*
CC C71.6 **Malignant neoplasm of cerebellum**
CC C71.7 **Malignant neoplasm of brain stem**
Malignant neoplasm of fourth cerebral ventricle
Infratentorial malignant neoplasm NOS
CC C71.8 **Malignant neoplasm of overlapping sites of brain**
CC C71.9 **Malignant neoplasm of brain, unspecified**
AHA CC: 3Q, 2014, 3-4

C72 Malignant neoplasm of spinal cord, cranial nerves and other parts of central nervous system
Excludes1: *malignant neoplasm of meninges (C70.-)*
malignant neoplasm of peripheral nerves and autonomic nervous system (C47.-)
CC C72.0 **Malignant neoplasm of spinal cord**
CC C72.1 **Malignant neoplasm of cauda equina**
+ C72.2 **Malignant neoplasm of olfactory nerve**
Malignant neoplasm of olfactory bulb
CC C72.20 **Malignant neoplasm of unspecified olfactory nerve**
CC C72.21 **Malignant neoplasm of right olfactory nerve**
CC C72.22 **Malignant neoplasm of left olfactory nerve**
+ C72.3 **Malignant neoplasm of optic nerve**
CC C72.30 **Malignant neoplasm of unspecified optic nerve**
CC C72.31 **Malignant neoplasm of right optic nerve**
CC C72.32 **Malignant neoplasm of left optic nerve**
+ C72.4 **Malignant neoplasm of acoustic nerve**
CC C72.40 **Malignant neoplasm of unspecified acoustic nerve**
CC C72.41 **Malignant neoplasm of right acoustic nerve**
CC C72.42 **Malignant neoplasm of left acoustic nerve**
+ C72.5 **Malignant neoplasm of other and unspecified cranial nerves**
CC C72.50 **Malignant neoplasm of unspecified cranial nerve**
Malignant neoplasm of cranial nerve NOS
CC C72.59 **Malignant neoplasm of other cranial nerves**
CC C72.9 **Malignant neoplasm of central nervous system, unspecified**
Malignant neoplasm of unspecified site of central nervous system
Malignant neoplasm of nervous system NOS

Malignant neoplasms of thyroid and other endocrine glands (C73-C75)

C73 **Malignant neoplasm of thyroid gland**
Use additional code to identify any functional activity
Valid 3-character code, no further characters required

C74 Malignant neoplasm of adrenal gland
+ C74.0 **Malignant neoplasm of cortex of adrenal gland**
CC C74.00 **Malignant neoplasm of cortex of unspecified adrenal gland**
CC C74.01 **Malignant neoplasm of cortex of right adrenal gland**
CC C74.02 **Malignant neoplasm of cortex of left adrenal gland**
+ C74.1 **Malignant neoplasm of medulla of adrenal gland**
CC C74.10 **Malignant neoplasm of medulla of unspecified adrenal gland**
CC C74.11 **Malignant neoplasm of medulla of right adrenal gland**
CC C74.12 **Malignant neoplasm of medulla of left adrenal gland**
+ C74.9 **Malignant neoplasm of unspecified part of adrenal gland**
CC C74.90 **Malignant neoplasm of unspecified part of unspecified adrenal gland**
CC C74.91 **Malignant neoplasm of unspecified part of right adrenal gland**
CC C74.92 **Malignant neoplasm of unspecified part of left adrenal gland**

C75 Malignant neoplasm of other endocrine glands and related structures
Excludes1: *malignant carcinoid tumors (C7A.0-)*
malignant neoplasm of adrenal gland (C74.-)
malignant neoplasm of endocrine pancreas (C25.4)
malignant neoplasm of islets of Langerhans (C25.4)
malignant neoplasm of ovary (C56.-)
malignant neoplasm of testis (C62.-)
malignant neoplasm of thymus (C37)
malignant neoplasm of thyroid gland (C73)
malignant neuroendocrine tumors (C7A.-)
CC C75.0 **Malignant neoplasm of parathyroid gland**
CC C75.1 **Malignant neoplasm of pituitary gland**
CC C75.2 **Malignant neoplasm of craniopharyngeal duct**
CC C75.3 **Malignant neoplasm of pineal gland**
CC C75.4 **Malignant neoplasm of carotid body**
CC C75.5 **Malignant neoplasm of aortic body and other paraganglia**
CC C75.8 **Malignant neoplasm with pluriglandular involvement, unspecified**
CC C75.9 **Malignant neoplasm of endocrine gland, unspecified**

Malignant neuroendocrine tumors (C7A)

C7A Malignant neuroendocrine tumors
Code also any associated multiple endocrine neoplasia [MEN] syndromes (E31.2-)
Use additional code to identify any associated endocrine syndrome, such as:
carcinoid syndrome (E34.0)
Excludes2: *malignant pancreatic islet cell tumors (C25.4)*
Merkel cell carcinoma (C4A.-)
+ C7A.0 **Malignant carcinoid tumors**
CC C7A.00 **Malignant carcinoid tumor of unspecified site**
+ C7A.01 **Malignant carcinoid tumors of the small intestine**
CC C7A.010 **Malignant carcinoid tumor of the duodenum**
CC C7A.011 **Malignant carcinoid tumor of the jejunum**
CC C7A.012 **Malignant carcinoid tumor of the ileum**
CC C7A.019 **Malignant carcinoid tumor of the small intestine, unspecified portion**
+ C7A.02 **Malignant carcinoid tumors of the appendix, large intestine, and rectum**
CC C7A.020 **Malignant carcinoid tumor of the appendix**
CC C7A.021 **Malignant carcinoid tumor of the cecum**
CC C7A.022 **Malignant carcinoid tumor of the ascending colon**
CC C7A.023 **Malignant carcinoid tumor of the transverse colon**
CC C7A.024 **Malignant carcinoid tumor of the descending colon**

CC **C7A.025 Malignant carcinoid tumor of the sigmoid colon**

CC **C7A.026 Malignant carcinoid tumor of the rectum**

CC **C7A.029 Malignant carcinoid tumor of the large intestine, unspecified portion**

Malignant carcinoid tumor of the colon NOS

\+ **C7A.09 Malignant carcinoid tumors of other sites**

CC **C7A.090 Malignant carcinoid tumor of the bronchus and lung**

CC **C7A.091 Malignant carcinoid tumor of the thymus**

CC **C7A.092 Malignant carcinoid tumor of the stomach**

CC **C7A.093 Malignant carcinoid tumor of the kidney**

CC **C7A.094 Malignant carcinoid tumor of the foregut, unspecified**

CC **C7A.095 Malignant carcinoid tumor of the midgut, unspecified**

CC **C7A.096 Malignant carcinoid tumor of the hindgut, unspecified**

CC **C7A.098 Malignant carcinoid tumors of other sites**

CC **C7A.1 Malignant poorly differentiated neuroendocrine tumors**

Malignant poorly differentiated neuroendocrine tumor NOS

Malignant poorly differentiated neuroendocrine carcinoma, any site

High grade neuroendocrine carcinoma, any site

CC **C7A.8 Other malignant neuroendocrine tumors**

AHA CC: 3Q, 2019, 7-8

Secondary neuroendocrine tumors (C7B)

C7B Secondary neuroendocrine tumors

Use additional code to identify any functional activity

\+ **C7B.0 Secondary carcinoid tumors**

C7B.00 Secondary carcinoid tumors, unspecified site

CC **C7B.01 Secondary carcinoid tumors of distant lymph nodes**

CC **C7B.02 Secondary carcinoid tumors of liver**

CC **C7B.03 Secondary carcinoid tumors of bone**

CC **C7B.04 Secondary carcinoid tumors of peritoneum**

Mesentary metastasis of carcinoid tumor

CC **C7B.09 Secondary carcinoid tumors of other sites**

C7B.1 Secondary Merkel cell carcinoma

Merkel cell carcinoma nodal presentation

Merkel cell carcinoma visceral metastatic presentation

CC **C7B.8 Other secondary neuroendocrine tumors**

AHA CC: 3Q, 2019, 7-8

Malignant neoplasms of ill-defined, other secondary and unspecified sites (C76-C80)

Review coding guidelines C.2.b and C.2.l.2

C76 Malignant neoplasm of other and ill-defined sites

Excludes1: *malignant neoplasm of female genitourinary tract NOS (C57.9)*
malignant neoplasm of male genitourinary tract NOS (C63.9)
malignant neoplasm of lymphoid, hematopoietic and related tissue (C81-C96)
malignant neoplasm of skin (C44.-)
malignant neoplasm of unspecified site NOS (C80.1)

C76.0 Malignant neoplasm of head, face and neck

Malignant neoplasm of cheek NOS

Malignant neoplasm of nose NOS

C76.1 Malignant neoplasm of thorax

Intrathoracic malignant neoplasm NOS

Malignant neoplasm of axilla NOS

Thoracic malignant neoplasm NOS

C76.2 Malignant neoplasm of abdomen

C76.3 Malignant neoplasm of pelvis

Malignant neoplasm of groin NOS

Malignant neoplasm of sites overlapping systems within the pelvis

Rectovaginal (septum) malignant neoplasm

Rectovesical (septum) malignant neoplasm

\+ **C76.4 Malignant neoplasm of upper limb**

C76.40 Malignant neoplasm of unspecified upper limb

C76.41 Malignant neoplasm of right upper limb

C76.42 Malignant neoplasm of left upper limb

\+ **C76.5 Malignant neoplasm of lower limb**

C76.50 Malignant neoplasm of unspecified lower limb

C76.51 Malignant neoplasm of right lower limb

C76.52 Malignant neoplasm of left lower limb

C76.8 Malignant neoplasm of other specified ill-defined sites

Malignant neoplasm of overlapping ill-defined sites

\+ **C77 Secondary and unspecified malignant neoplasm of lymph nodes**

Excludes1: *malignant neoplasm of lymph nodes, specified as primary (C81-C86, C88, C96.-)*
mesentary metastasis of carcinoid tumor (C7B.04)
secondary carcinoid tumors of distant lymph nodes (C7B.01)

CC **C77.0 Secondary and unspecified malignant neoplasm of lymph nodes of head, face and neck**

Secondary and unspecified malignant neoplasm of supraclavicular lymph nodes

CC **C77.1 Secondary and unspecified malignant neoplasm of intrathoracic lymph nodes**

CC **C77.2 Secondary and unspecified malignant neoplasm of intra-abdominal lymph nodes**

CC **C77.3 Secondary and unspecified malignant neoplasm of axilla and upper limb lymph nodes**

Secondary and unspecified malignant neoplasm of pectoral lymph nodes

CC **C77.4 Secondary and unspecified malignant neoplasm of inguinal and lower limb lymph nodes**

CC **C77.5 Secondary and unspecified malignant neoplasm of intrapelvic lymph nodes**

CC **C77.8 Secondary and unspecified malignant neoplasm of lymph nodes of multiple regions**

CC **C77.9 Secondary and unspecified malignant neoplasm of lymph node, unspecified**

C78 Secondary malignant neoplasm of respiratory and digestive organs

Excludes1: *secondary carcinoid tumors of liver (C7B.02)*
secondary carcinoid tumors of peritoneum (C7B.04)

Excludes2: *lymph node metastases (C77.0)*

\+ **C78.0 Secondary malignant neoplasm of lung**

CC **C78.00 Secondary malignant neoplasm of unspecified lung**

CC **C78.01 Secondary malignant neoplasm of right lung**

CC **C78.02 Secondary malignant neoplasm of left lung**

CC **C78.1 Secondary malignant neoplasm of mediastinum**

CC **C78.2 Secondary malignant neoplasm of pleura**

\+ **C78.3 Secondary malignant neoplasm of other and unspecified respiratory organs**

CC **C78.30 Secondary malignant neoplasm of unspecified respiratory organ**

CC **C78.39 Secondary malignant neoplasm of other respiratory organs**

CC **C78.4 Secondary malignant neoplasm of small intestine**

CC **C78.5 Secondary malignant neoplasm of large intestine and rectum**

CC **C78.6 Secondary malignant neoplasm of retroperitoneum and peritoneum**

AHA CC: 2Q, 2017, 12

CC **C78.7 Secondary malignant neoplasm of liver and intrahepatic bile duct**

\+ **C78.8 Secondary malignant neoplasm of other and unspecified digestive organs**

CC **C78.80 Secondary malignant neoplasm of unspecified digestive organ**

CC **C78.89 Secondary malignant neoplasm of other digestive organs**

Code also exocrine pancreatic insufficiency (K86.81)

C79 Secondary malignant neoplasm of other and unspecified sites

Excludes1: *secondary carcinoid tumors (C7B.-)*
secondary neuroendocrine tumors (C7B.-)

\+ **C79.0 Secondary malignant neoplasm of kidney and renal pelvis**

CC **C79.00 Secondary malignant neoplasm of unspecified kidney and renal pelvis**

CC **C79.01 Secondary malignant neoplasm of right kidney and renal pelvis**

CC **C79.02 Secondary malignant neoplasm of left kidney and renal pelvis**

+ **C79.1 Secondary malignant neoplasm of bladder and other and unspecified urinary organs**
  - CC **C79.10 Secondary malignant neoplasm of unspecified urinary organs**
  - CC **C79.11 Secondary malignant neoplasm of bladder**
    - ***Excludes2:*** *lymph node metastases (C77.0)*
  - CC **C79.19 Secondary malignant neoplasm of other urinary organs**

CC **C79.2 Secondary malignant neoplasm of skin**
- ***Excludes1:*** *secondary Merkel cell carcinoma (C7B.1)*

+ **C79.3 Secondary malignant neoplasm of brain and cerebral meninges**
  - CC **C79.31 Secondary malignant neoplasm of brain**
  - CC **C79.32 Secondary malignant neoplasm of cerebral meninges**
    - *AHA CC: 1Q, 2020, 13-14*

+ **C79.4 Secondary malignant neoplasm of other and unspecified parts of nervous system**
  - CC **C79.40 Secondary malignant neoplasm of unspecified part of nervous system**
  - CC **C79.49 Secondary malignant neoplasm of other parts of nervous system**

+ **C79.5 Secondary malignant neoplasm of bone and bone marrow**
  - ***Excludes1:*** *secondary carcinoid tumors of bone (C7B.03)*
  - CC **C79.51 Secondary malignant neoplasm of bone**
  - CC **C79.52 Secondary malignant neoplasm of bone marrow**

+ **C79.6 Secondary malignant neoplasm of ovary**
  - ♀ CC **C79.60 Secondary malignant neoplasm of unspecified ovary**
  - ♀ CC **C79.61 Secondary malignant neoplasm of right ovary**
  - ♀ CC **C79.62 Secondary malignant neoplasm of left ovary**
  - ♀ CC **C79.63 Secondary malignant neoplasm of bilateral ovaries**

+ **C79.7 Secondary malignant neoplasm of adrenal gland**
  - CC **C79.70 Secondary malignant neoplasm of unspecified adrenal gland**
  - CC **C79.71 Secondary malignant neoplasm of right adrenal gland**
  - CC **C79.72 Secondary malignant neoplasm of left adrenal gland**

+ **C79.8 Secondary malignant neoplasm of other specified sites**
  - CC **C79.81 Secondary malignant neoplasm of breast**
  - CC **C79.82 Secondary malignant neoplasm of genital organs**
  - CC **C79.89 Secondary malignant neoplasm of other specified sites**
    - *AHA CC: 2Q, 2017, 11*

CC **C79.9 Secondary malignant neoplasm of unspecified site**
- Metastatic cancer NOS
- Metastatic disease NOS
- ***Excludes1:*** *carcinomatosis NOS (C80.0)*
  generalized cancer NOS (C80.0)
  malignant (primary) neoplasm of unspecified site (C80.1)

C80 Malignant neoplasm without specification of site

Excludes1: *malignant carcinoid tumor of unspecified site (C7A.00)*
malignant neoplasm of specified multiple sites- code to each site

CC **C80.0 Disseminated malignant neoplasm, unspecified**
- Carcinomatosis NOS
- Generalized cancer, unspecified site (primary) (secondary)
- Generalized malignancy, unspecified site (primary) (secondary)
- **Review coding guideline C.2.j**

C80.1 Malignant (primary) neoplasm, unspecified
- Cancer NOS
- Cancer unspecified site (primary)
- Carcinoma unspecified site (primary)
- Malignancy unspecified site (primary)
- ***Excludes1:*** *secondary malignant neoplasm of unspecified site (C79.9)*
- **Review coding guideline C.2.k**

CC **C80.2 Malignant neoplasm associated with transplanted organ**
- Code first complication of transplanted organ (T86.-)
- Use additional code to identify the specific malignancy
- **Review coding guideline C.2.r**

Malignant neoplasms of lymphoid, hematopoietic and related tissue (C81-C96)

Excludes2: *Kaposi's sarcoma of lymph nodes (C46.3)*
secondary and unspecified neoplasm of lymph nodes (C77.-)
secondary neoplasm of bone marrow (C79.52)
secondary neoplasm of spleen (C78.89)

C81 Hodgkin lymphoma

Excludes1: *personal history of Hodgkin lymphoma (Z85.71)*

+ **C81.0 Nodular lymphocyte predominant Hodgkin lymphoma**
  - CC **C81.00 Nodular lymphocyte predominant Hodgkin lymphoma, unspecified site**
  - CC **C81.01 Nodular lymphocyte predominant Hodgkin lymphoma, lymph nodes of head, face, and neck**
  - CC **C81.02 Nodular lymphocyte predominant Hodgkin lymphoma, intrathoracic lymph nodes**
  - CC **C81.03 Nodular lymphocyte predominant Hodgkin lymphoma, intra-abdominal lymph nodes**
  - CC **C81.04 Nodular lymphocyte predominant Hodgkin lymphoma, lymph nodes of axilla and upper limb**
  - CC **C81.05 Nodular lymphocyte predominant Hodgkin lymphoma, lymph nodes of inguinal region and lower limb**
  - CC **C81.06 Nodular lymphocyte predominant Hodgkin lymphoma, intrapelvic lymph nodes**
  - CC **C81.07 Nodular lymphocyte predominant Hodgkin lymphoma, spleen**
  - CC **C81.08 Nodular lymphocyte predominant Hodgkin lymphoma, lymph nodes of multiple sites**
  - CC **C81.09 Nodular lymphocyte predominant Hodgkin lymphoma, extranodal and solid organ sites**

+ **C81.1 Nodular sclerosis Hodgkin lymphoma**
  - Nodular sclerosis classical Hodgkin lymphoma
  - CC **C81.10 Nodular sclerosis Hodgkin lymphoma, unspecified site**
  - CC **C81.11 Nodular sclerosis Hodgkin lymphoma, lymph nodes of head, face, and neck**
  - CC **C81.12 Nodular sclerosis Hodgkin lymphoma, intrathoracic lymph nodes**
  - CC **C81.13 Nodular sclerosis Hodgkin lymphoma, intra-abdominal lymph nodes**
  - CC **C81.14 Nodular sclerosis Hodgkin lymphoma, lymph nodes of axilla and upper limb**
  - CC **C81.15 Nodular sclerosis Hodgkin lymphoma, lymph nodes of inguinal region and lower limb**
  - CC **C81.16 Nodular sclerosis Hodgkin lymphoma, intrapelvic lymph nodes**
  - CC **C81.17 Nodular sclerosis Hodgkin lymphoma, spleen**
  - CC **C81.18 Nodular sclerosis Hodgkin lymphoma, lymph nodes of multiple sites**
  - CC **C81.19 Nodular sclerosis Hodgkin lymphoma, extranodal and solid organ sites**

+ **C81.2 Mixed cellularity Hodgkin lymphoma**
  - Mixed cellularity classical Hodgkin lymphoma
  - CC **C81.20 Mixed cellularity Hodgkin lymphoma, unspecified site**
  - CC **C81.21 Mixed cellularity Hodgkin lymphoma, lymph nodes of head, face, and neck**
  - CC **C81.22 Mixed cellularity Hodgkin lymphoma, intrathoracic lymph nodes**
  - CC **C81.23 Mixed cellularity Hodgkin lymphoma, intra-abdominal lymph nodes**
  - CC **C81.24 Mixed cellularity Hodgkin lymphoma, lymph nodes of axilla and upper limb**
  - CC **C81.25 Mixed cellularity Hodgkin lymphoma, lymph nodes of inguinal region and lower limb**
  - CC **C81.26 Mixed cellularity Hodgkin lymphoma, intrapelvic lymph nodes**
  - CC **C81.27 Mixed cellularity Hodgkin lymphoma, spleen**
  - CC **C81.28 Mixed cellularity Hodgkin lymphoma, lymph nodes of multiple sites**
  - CC **C81.29 Mixed cellularity Hodgkin lymphoma, extranodal and solid organ sites**

+ **C81.3 Lymphocyte depleted Hodgkin lymphoma**
  - Lymphocyte depleted classical Hodgkin lymphoma
  - CC **C81.30 Lymphocyte depleted Hodgkin lymphoma, unspecified site**
  - CC **C81.31 Lymphocyte depleted Hodgkin lymphoma, lymph nodes of head, face, and neck**
  - CC **C81.32 Lymphocyte depleted Hodgkin lymphoma, intrathoracic lymph nodes**
  - CC **C81.33 Lymphocyte depleted Hodgkin lymphoma, intra-abdominal lymph nodes**
  - CC **C81.34 Lymphocyte depleted Hodgkin lymphoma, lymph nodes of axilla and upper limb**

Lymphatic System

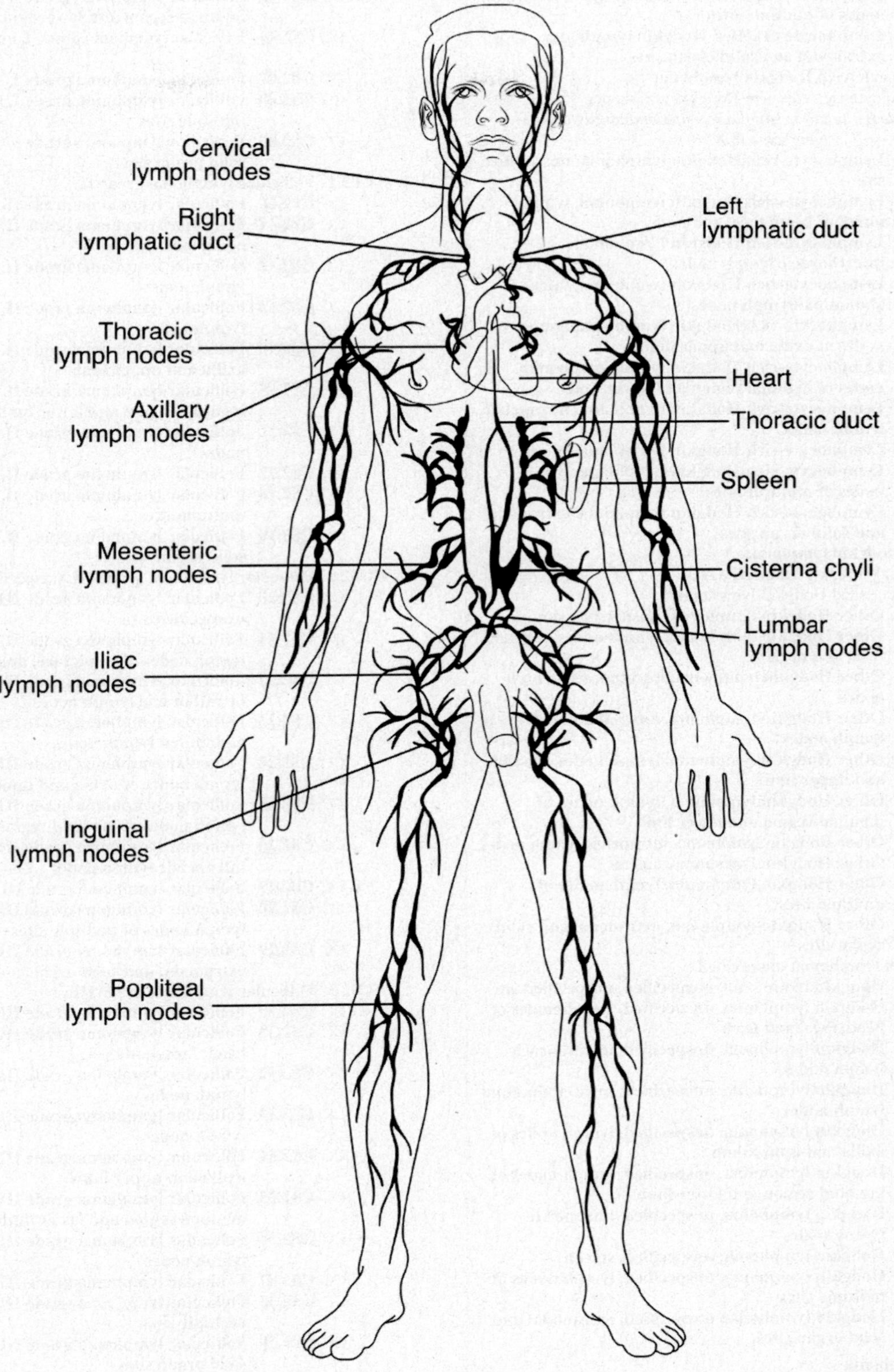

©AHIMA

CC **C81.35** **Lymphocyte depleted Hodgkin lymphoma, lymph nodes of inguinal region and lower limb**
CC **C81.36** **Lymphocyte depleted Hodgkin lymphoma, intrapelvic lymph nodes**
CC **C81.37** **Lymphocyte depleted Hodgkin lymphoma, spleen**
CC **C81.38** **Lymphocyte depleted Hodgkin lymphoma, lymph nodes of multiple sites**
CC **C81.39** **Lymphocyte depleted Hodgkin lymphoma, extranodal and solid organ sites**

+ **C81.4 Lymphocyte-rich Hodgkin lymphoma**
Lymphocyte-rich classical Hodgkin lymphoma
Excludes1: *nodular lymphocyte predominant Hodgkin lymphoma (C81.0-)*

CC **C81.40** **Lymphocyte-rich Hodgkin lymphoma, unspecified site**
CC **C81.41** **Lymphocyte-rich Hodgkin lymphoma, lymph nodes of head, face, and neck**
CC **C81.42** **Lymphocyte-rich Hodgkin lymphoma, intrathoracic lymph nodes**
CC **C81.43** **Lymphocyte-rich Hodgkin lymphoma, intra-abdominal lymph nodes**
CC **C81.44** **Lymphocyte-rich Hodgkin lymphoma, lymph nodes of axilla and upper limb**
CC **C81.45** **Lymphocyte-rich Hodgkin lymphoma, lymph nodes of inguinal region and lower limb**
CC **C81.46** **Lymphocyte-rich Hodgkin lymphoma, intrapelvic lymph nodes**
CC **C81.47** **Lymphocyte-rich Hodgkin lymphoma, spleen**
CC **C81.48** **Lymphocyte-rich Hodgkin lymphoma, lymph nodes of multiple sites**
CC **C81.49** **Lymphocyte-rich Hodgkin lymphoma, extranodal and solid organ sites**

+ **C81.7 Other Hodgkin lymphoma**
Classical Hodgkin lymphoma NOS
Other classical Hodgkin lymphoma

CC **C81.70** **Other Hodgkin lymphoma, unspecified site**
CC **C81.71** **Other Hodgkin lymphoma, lymph nodes of head, face, and neck**
CC **C81.72** **Other Hodgkin lymphoma, intrathoracic lymph nodes**
CC **C81.73** **Other Hodgkin lymphoma, intra-abdominal lymph nodes**
CC **C81.74** **Other Hodgkin lymphoma, lymph nodes of axilla and upper limb**
CC **C81.75** **Other Hodgkin lymphoma, lymph nodes of inguinal region and lower limb**
CC **C81.76** **Other Hodgkin lymphoma, intrapelvic lymph nodes**
CC **C81.77** **Other Hodgkin lymphoma, spleen**
CC **C81.78** **Other Hodgkin lymphoma, lymph nodes of multiple sites**
CC **C81.79** **Other Hodgkin lymphoma, extranodal and solid organ sites**

+ **C81.9 Hodgkin lymphoma, unspecified**

CC **C81.90** **Hodgkin lymphoma, unspecified, unspecified site**
CC **C81.91** **Hodgkin lymphoma, unspecified, lymph nodes of head, face, and neck**
CC **C81.92** **Hodgkin lymphoma, unspecified, intrathoracic lymph nodes**
CC **C81.93** **Hodgkin lymphoma, unspecified, intra-abdominal lymph nodes**
CC **C81.94** **Hodgkin lymphoma, unspecified, lymph nodes of axilla and upper limb**
CC **C81.95** **Hodgkin lymphoma, unspecified, lymph nodes of inguinal region and lower limb**
CC **C81.96** **Hodgkin lymphoma, unspecified, intrapelvic lymph nodes**
CC **C81.97** **Hodgkin lymphoma, unspecified, spleen**
CC **C81.98** **Hodgkin lymphoma, unspecified, lymph nodes of multiple sites**
CC **C81.99** **Hodgkin lymphoma, unspecified, extranodal and solid organ sites**

C82 Follicular lymphoma

Includes: follicular lymphoma with or without diffuse areas
Excludes1: *mature T/NK-cell lymphomas (C84.-)*
personal history of non-Hodgkin lymphoma (Z85.72)

+ **C82.0 Follicular lymphoma grade I**

CC **C82.00** **Follicular lymphoma grade I, unspecified site**
CC **C82.01** **Follicular lymphoma grade I, lymph nodes of head, face, and neck**
CC **C82.02** **Follicular lymphoma grade I, intrathoracic lymph nodes**
CC **C82.03** **Follicular lymphoma grade I, intra-abdominal lymph nodes**
CC **C82.04** **Follicular lymphoma grade I, lymph nodes of axilla and upper limb**
CC **C82.05** **Follicular lymphoma grade I, lymph nodes of inguinal region and lower limb**
CC **C82.06** **Follicular lymphoma grade I, intrapelvic lymph nodes**
CC **C82.07** **Follicular lymphoma grade I, spleen**
CC **C82.08** **Follicular lymphoma grade I, lymph nodes of multiple sites**
CC **C82.09** **Follicular lymphoma grade I, extranodal and solid organ sites**

+ **C82.1 Follicular lymphoma grade II**

CC **C82.10** **Follicular lymphoma grade II, unspecified site**
CC **C82.11** **Follicular lymphoma grade II, lymph nodes of head, face, and neck**
CC **C82.12** **Follicular lymphoma grade II, intrathoracic lymph nodes**
CC **C82.13** **Follicular lymphoma grade II, intra-abdominal lymph nodes**
CC **C82.14** **Follicular lymphoma grade II, lymph nodes of axilla and upper limb**
CC **C82.15** **Follicular lymphoma grade II, lymph nodes of inguinal region and lower limb**
CC **C82.16** **Follicular lymphoma grade II, intrapelvic lymph nodes**
CC **C82.17** **Follicular lymphoma grade II, spleen**
CC **C82.18** **Follicular lymphoma grade II, lymph nodes of multiple sites**
CC **C82.19** **Follicular lymphoma grade II, extranodal and solid organ sites**

+ **C82.2 Follicular lymphoma grade III, unspecified**

CC **C82.20** **Follicular lymphoma grade III, unspecified, unspecified site**
CC **C82.21** **Follicular lymphoma grade III, unspecified, lymph nodes of head, face, and neck**
CC **C82.22** **Follicular lymphoma grade III, unspecified, intrathoracic lymph nodes**
CC **C82.23** **Follicular lymphoma grade III, unspecified, intra-abdominal lymph nodes**
CC **C82.24** **Follicular lymphoma grade III, unspecified, lymph nodes of axilla and upper limb**
CC **C82.25** **Follicular lymphoma grade III, unspecified, lymph nodes of inguinal region and lower limb**
CC **C82.26** **Follicular lymphoma grade III, unspecified, intrapelvic lymph nodes**
CC **C82.27** **Follicular lymphoma grade III, unspecified, spleen**
CC **C82.28** **Follicular lymphoma grade III, unspecified, lymph nodes of multiple sites**
CC **C82.29** **Follicular lymphoma grade III, unspecified, extranodal and solid organ sites**

+ **C82.3 Follicular lymphoma grade IIIa**

CC **C82.30** **Follicular lymphoma grade IIIa, unspecified site**
CC **C82.31** **Follicular lymphoma grade IIIa, lymph nodes of head, face, and neck**
CC **C82.32** **Follicular lymphoma grade IIIa, intrathoracic lymph nodes**
CC **C82.33** **Follicular lymphoma grade IIIa, intra-abdominal lymph nodes**
CC **C82.34** **Follicular lymphoma grade IIIa, lymph nodes of axilla and upper limb**
CC **C82.35** **Follicular lymphoma grade IIIa, lymph nodes of inguinal region and lower limb**
CC **C82.36** **Follicular lymphoma grade IIIa, intrapelvic lymph nodes**
CC **C82.37** **Follicular lymphoma grade IIIa, spleen**
CC **C82.38** **Follicular lymphoma grade IIIa, lymph nodes of multiple sites**
CC **C82.39** **Follicular lymphoma grade IIIa, extranodal and solid organ sites**

+ **C82.4 Follicular lymphoma grade IIIb**

CC **C82.40** **Follicular lymphoma grade IIIb, unspecified site**
CC **C82.41** **Follicular lymphoma grade IIIb, lymph nodes of head, face, and neck**
CC **C82.42** **Follicular lymphoma grade IIIb, intrathoracic lymph nodes**
CC **C82.43** **Follicular lymphoma grade IIIb, intra-abdominal lymph nodes**

CC **C82.44** **Follicular lymphoma grade IIIb, lymph nodes of axilla and upper limb**
CC **C82.45** **Follicular lymphoma grade IIIb, lymph nodes of inguinal region and lower limb**
CC **C82.46** **Follicular lymphoma grade IIIb, intrapelvic lymph nodes**
CC **C82.47** **Follicular lymphoma grade IIIb, spleen**
CC **C82.48** **Follicular lymphoma grade IIIb, lymph nodes of multiple sites**
CC **C82.49** **Follicular lymphoma grade IIIb, extranodal and solid organ sites**

+ **C82.5 Diffuse follicle center lymphoma**
CC **C82.50** **Diffuse follicle center lymphoma, unspecified site**
CC **C82.51** **Diffuse follicle center lymphoma, lymph nodes of head, face, and neck**
CC **C82.52** **Diffuse follicle center lymphoma, intrathoracic lymph nodes**
CC **C82.53** **Diffuse follicle center lymphoma, intra-abdominal lymph nodes**
CC **C82.54** **Diffuse follicle center lymphoma, lymph nodes of axilla and upper limb**
CC **C82.55** **Diffuse follicle center lymphoma, lymph nodes of inguinal region and lower limb**
CC **C82.56** **Diffuse follicle center lymphoma, intrapelvic lymph nodes**
CC **C82.57** **Diffuse follicle center lymphoma, spleen**
CC **C82.58** **Diffuse follicle center lymphoma, lymph nodes of multiple sites**
CC **C82.59** **Diffuse follicle center lymphoma, extranodal and solid organ sites**

+ **C82.6** Cutaneous follicle center lymphoma
CC **C82.60** **Cutaneous follicle center lymphoma, unspecified site**
CC **C82.61** **Cutaneous follicle center lymphoma, lymph nodes of head, face, and neck**
CC **C82.62** **Cutaneous follicle center lymphoma, intrathoracic lymph nodes**
CC **C82.63** **Cutaneous follicle center lymphoma, intra-abdominal lymph nodes**
CC **C82.64** **Cutaneous follicle center lymphoma, lymph nodes of axilla and upper limb**
CC **C82.65** **Cutaneous follicle center lymphoma, lymph nodes of inguinal region and lower limb**
CC **C82.66** **Cutaneous follicle center lymphoma, intrapelvic lymph nodes**
CC **C82.67** **Cutaneous follicle center lymphoma, spleen**
CC **C82.68** **Cutaneous follicle center lymphoma, lymph nodes of multiple sites**
CC **C82.69** **Cutaneous follicle center lymphoma, extranodal and solid organ sites**

+ **C82.8** Other types of follicular lymphoma
CC **C82.80** **Other types of follicular lymphoma, unspecified site**
CC **C82.81** **Other types of follicular lymphoma, lymph nodes of head, face, and neck**
CC **C82.82** **Other types of follicular lymphoma, intrathoracic lymph nodes**
CC **C82.83** **Other types of follicular lymphoma, intra-abdominal lymph nodes**
CC **C82.84** **Other types of follicular lymphoma, lymph nodes of axilla and upper limb**
CC **C82.85** **Other types of follicular lymphoma, lymph nodes of inguinal region and lower limb**
CC **C82.86** **Other types of follicular lymphoma, intrapelvic lymph nodes**
CC **C82.87** **Other types of follicular lymphoma, spleen**
CC **C82.88** **Other types of follicular lymphoma, lymph nodes of multiple sites**
CC **C82.89** **Other types of follicular lymphoma, extranodal and solid organ sites**

+ **C82.9** Follicular lymphoma, unspecified
CC **C82.90** **Follicular lymphoma, unspecified, unspecified site**
CC **C82.91** **Follicular lymphoma, unspecified, lymph nodes of head, face, and neck**
CC **C82.92** **Follicular lymphoma, unspecified, intrathoracic lymph nodes**
CC **C82.93** **Follicular lymphoma, unspecified, intra-abdominal lymph nodes**
CC **C82.94** **Follicular lymphoma, unspecified, lymph nodes of axilla and upper limb**
CC **C82.95** **Follicular lymphoma, unspecified, lymph nodes of inguinal region and lower limb**
CC **C82.96** **Follicular lymphoma, unspecified, intrapelvic lymph nodes**
CC **C82.97** **Follicular lymphoma, unspecified, spleen**
CC **C82.98** **Follicular lymphoma, unspecified, lymph nodes of multiple sites**
CC **C82.99** **Follicular lymphoma, unspecified, extranodal and solid organ sites**

C83 Non-follicular lymphoma

Excludes1: *personal history of non-Hodgkin lymphoma (Z85.72)*

+ **C83.0 Small cell B-cell lymphoma**
Lymphoplasmacytic lymphoma
Nodal marginal zone lymphoma
Non-leukemic variant of B-CLL
Splenic marginal zone lymphoma
Excludes1: *chronic lymphocytic leukemia (C91.1)*
mature T/NK-cell lymphomas (C84.-)
Waldenström macroglobulinemia (C88.0)

CC **C83.00** **Small cell B-cell lymphoma, unspecified site**
CC **C83.01** **Small cell B-cell lymphoma, lymph nodes of head, face, and neck**
CC **C83.02** **Small cell B-cell lymphoma, intrathoracic lymph nodes**
CC **C83.03** **Small cell B-cell lymphoma, intra-abdominal lymph nodes**
CC **C83.04** **Small cell B-cell lymphoma, lymph nodes of axilla and upper limb**
CC **C83.05** **Small cell B-cell lymphoma, lymph nodes of inguinal region and lower limb**
CC **C83.06** **Small cell B-cell lymphoma, intrapelvic lymph nodes**
CC **C83.07** **Small cell B-cell lymphoma, spleen**
CC **C83.08** **Small cell B-cell lymphoma, lymph nodes of multiple sites**
CC **C83.09** **Small cell B-cell lymphoma, extranodal and solid organ sites**

+ **C83.1 Mantle cell lymphoma**
Centrocytic lymphoma
Malignant lymphomatous polyposis
CC **C83.10** **Mantle cell lymphoma, unspecified site**
CC **C83.11** **Mantle cell lymphoma, lymph nodes of head, face, and neck**
CC **C83.12** **Mantle cell lymphoma, intrathoracic lymph nodes**
CC **C83.13** **Mantle cell lymphoma, intra-abdominal lymph nodes**
CC **C83.14** **Mantle cell lymphoma, lymph nodes of axilla and upper limb**
CC **C83.15** **Mantle cell lymphoma, lymph nodes of inguinal region and lower limb**
CC **C83.16** **Mantle cell lymphoma, intrapelvic lymph nodes**
CC **C83.17** **Mantle cell lymphoma, spleen**
CC **C83.18** **Mantle cell lymphoma, lymph nodes of multiple sites**
CC **C83.19** **Mantle cell lymphoma, extranodal and solid organ sites**

+ **C83.3 Diffuse large B-cell lymphoma**
Anaplastic diffuse large B-cell lymphoma
CD30-positive diffuse large B-cell lymphoma
Centroblastic diffuse large B-cell lymphoma
Diffuse large B-cell lymphoma, subtype not specified
Immunoblastic diffuse large B-cell lymphoma
Plasmablastic diffuse large B-cell lymphoma
Diffuse large B-cell lymphoma, subtype not specified
T-cell rich diffuse large B-cell lymphoma
Excludes1: *mediastinal (thymic) large B-cell lymphoma (C85.2-)*
mature T/NK-cell lymphomas (C84.-)

CC **C83.30** **Diffuse large B-cell lymphoma, unspecified site**
CC **C83.31** **Diffuse large B-cell lymphoma, lymph nodes of head, face, and neck**
CC **C83.32** **Diffuse large B-cell lymphoma, intrathoracic lymph nodes**
CC **C83.33** **Diffuse large B-cell lymphoma, intra-abdominal lymph nodes**
CC **C83.34** **Diffuse large B-cell lymphoma, lymph nodes of axilla and upper limb**
CC **C83.35** **Diffuse large B-cell lymphoma, lymph nodes of inguinal region and lower limb**
CC **C83.36** **Diffuse large B-cell lymphoma, intrapelvic lymph nodes**
CC **C83.37** **Diffuse large B-cell lymphoma, spleen**

CC **C83.38 Diffuse large B-cell lymphoma, lymph nodes of multiple sites**
CC **C83.39 Diffuse large B-cell lymphoma, extranodal and solid organ sites**

\+ **C83.5 Lymphoblastic (diffuse) lymphoma**
B-precursor lymphoma
Lymphoblastic B-cell lymphoma
Lymphoblastic lymphoma NOS
Lymphoblastic T-cell lymphoma
T-precursor lymphoma

CC **C83.50 Lymphoblastic (diffuse) lymphoma, unspecified site**
CC **C83.51 Lymphoblastic (diffuse) lymphoma, lymph nodes of head, face, and neck**
CC **C83.52 Lymphoblastic (diffuse) lymphoma, intrathoracic lymph nodes**
CC **C83.53 Lymphoblastic (diffuse) lymphoma, intra-abdominal lymph nodes**
CC **C83.54 Lymphoblastic (diffuse) lymphoma, lymph nodes of axilla and upper limb**
CC **C83.55 Lymphoblastic (diffuse) lymphoma, lymph nodes of inguinal region and lower limb**
CC **C83.56 Lymphoblastic (diffuse) lymphoma, intrapelvic lymph nodes**
CC **C83.57 Lymphoblastic (diffuse) lymphoma, spleen**
CC **C83.58 Lymphoblastic (diffuse) lymphoma, lymph nodes of multiple sites**
CC **C83.59 Lymphoblastic (diffuse) lymphoma, extranodal and solid organ sites**

\+ **C83.7 Burkitt lymphoma**
Atypical Burkitt lymphoma
Burkitt-like lymphoma
Excludes1: *mature B-cell leukemia Burkitt type (C91.A-)*

CC **C83.70 Burkitt lymphoma, unspecified site**
CC **C83.71 Burkitt lymphoma, lymph nodes of head, face, and neck**
CC **C83.72 Burkitt lymphoma, intrathoracic lymph nodes**
CC **C83.73 Burkitt lymphoma, intra-abdominal lymph nodes**
CC **C83.74 Burkitt lymphoma, lymph nodes of axilla and upper limb**
CC **C83.75 Burkitt lymphoma, lymph nodes of inguinal region and lower limb**
CC **C83.76 Burkitt lymphoma, intrapelvic lymph nodes**
CC **C83.77 Burkitt lymphoma, spleen**
CC **C83.78 Burkitt lymphoma, lymph nodes of multiple sites**
CC **C83.79 Burkitt lymphoma, extranodal and solid organ sites**

\+ **C83.8 Other non-follicular lymphoma**
Intravascular large B-cell lymphoma
Lymphoid granulomatosis
Primary effusion B-cell lymphoma
Excludes1: *mediastinal (thymic) large B-cell lymphoma (C85.2-)*
T-cell rich B-cell lymphoma (C83.3-)

CC **C83.80 Other non-follicular lymphoma, unspecified site**
CC **C83.81 Other non-follicular lymphoma, lymph nodes of head, face, and neck**
CC **C83.82 Other non-follicular lymphoma, intrathoracic lymph nodes**
CC **C83.83 Other non-follicular lymphoma, intra-abdominal lymph nodes**
CC **C83.84 Other non-follicular lymphoma, lymph nodes of axilla and upper limb**
CC **C83.85 Other non-follicular lymphoma, lymph nodes of inguinal region and lower limb**
CC **C83.86 Other non-follicular lymphoma, intrapelvic lymph nodes**
CC **C83.87 Other non-follicular lymphoma, spleen**
CC **C83.88 Other non-follicular lymphoma, lymph nodes of multiple sites**
CC **C83.89 Other non-follicular lymphoma, extranodal and solid organ sites**

\+ **C83.9 Non-follicular (diffuse) lymphoma, unspecified**

CC **C83.90 Non-follicular (diffuse) lymphoma, unspecified, unspecified site**
CC **C83.91 Non-follicular (diffuse) lymphoma, unspecified, lymph nodes of head, face, and neck**
CC **C83.92 Non-follicular (diffuse) lymphoma, unspecified, intrathoracic lymph nodes**
CC **C83.93 Non-follicular (diffuse) lymphoma, unspecified, intra-abdominal lymph nodes**
CC **C83.94 Non-follicular (diffuse) lymphoma, unspecified, lymph nodes of axilla and upper limb**
CC **C83.95 Non-follicular (diffuse) lymphoma, unspecified, lymph nodes of inguinal region and lower limb**
CC **C83.96 Non-follicular (diffuse) lymphoma, unspecified, intrapelvic lymph nodes**
CC **C83.97 Non-follicular (diffuse) lymphoma, unspecified, spleen**
CC **C83.98 Non-follicular (diffuse) lymphoma, unspecified, lymph nodes of multiple sites**
CC **C83.99 Non-follicular (diffuse) lymphoma, unspecified, extranodal and solid organ sites**

C84 Mature T/NK-cell lymphomas

Excludes1: *personal history of non-Hodgkin lymphoma (Z85.72)*

\+ **C84.0 Mycosis fungoides**
Excludes1: *peripheral T-cell lymphoma, not classified (C84.4-)*

CC **C84.00 Mycosis fungoides, unspecified site**
CC **C84.01 Mycosis fungoides, lymph nodes of head, face, and neck**
CC **C84.02 Mycosis fungoides, intrathoracic lymph nodes**
CC **C84.03 Mycosis fungoides, intra-abdominal lymph nodes**
CC **C84.04 Mycosis fungoides, lymph nodes of axilla and upper limb**
CC **C84.05 Mycosis fungoides, lymph nodes of inguinal region and lower limb**
CC **C84.06 Mycosis fungoides, intrapelvic lymph nodes**
CC **C84.07 Mycosis fungoides, spleen**
CC **C84.08 Mycosis fungoides, lymph nodes of multiple sites**
CC **C84.09 Mycosis fungoides, extranodal and solid organ sites**

\+ **C84.1 Sézary disease**

CC **C84.10 Sézary disease, unspecified site**
CC **C84.11 Sézary disease, lymph nodes of head, face, and neck**
CC **C84.12 Sézary disease, intrathoracic lymph nodes**
CC **C84.13 Sézary disease, intra-abdominal lymph nodes**
CC **C84.14 Sézary disease, lymph nodes of axilla and upper limb**
CC **C84.15 Sézary disease, lymph nodes of inguinal region and lower limb**
CC **C84.16 Sézary disease, intrapelvic lymph nodes**
CC **C84.17 Sézary disease, spleen**
CC **C84.18 Sézary disease, lymph nodes of multiple sites**
CC **C84.19 Sézary disease, extranodal and solid organ sites**

\+ **C84.4 Peripheral T-cell lymphoma, not classified**
Lennert's lymphoma
Lymphoepithelioid lymphoma
Mature T-cell lymphoma, not elsewhere classified

CC **C84.40 Peripheral T-cell lymphoma, not classified, unspecified site**
CC **C84.41 Peripheral T-cell lymphoma, not classified, lymph nodes of head, face, and neck**
CC **C84.42 Peripheral T-cell lymphoma, not classified, intrathoracic lymph nodes**
CC **C84.43 Peripheral T-cell lymphoma, not classified, intra-abdominal lymph nodes**
CC **C84.44 Peripheral T-cell lymphoma, not classified, lymph nodes of axilla and upper limb**
CC **C84.45 Peripheral T-cell lymphoma, not classified, lymph nodes of inguinal region and lower limb**
CC **C84.46 Peripheral T-cell lymphoma, not classified, intrapelvic lymph nodes**
CC **C84.47 Peripheral T-cell lymphoma, not classified, spleen**
CC **C84.48 Peripheral T-cell lymphoma, not classified, lymph nodes of multiple sites**
CC **C84.49 Peripheral T-cell lymphoma, not classified, extranodal and solid organ sites**

\+ **C84.6 Anaplastic large cell lymphoma, ALK-positive**
Anaplastic large cell lymphoma, CD30-positive

CC **C84.60 Anaplastic large cell lymphoma, ALK-positive, unspecified site**
CC **C84.61 Anaplastic large cell lymphoma, ALK-positive, lymph nodes of head, face, and neck**
CC **C84.62 Anaplastic large cell lymphoma, ALK-positive, intrathoracic lymph nodes**
CC **C84.63 Anaplastic large cell lymphoma, ALK-positive, intra-abdominal lymph nodes**
CC **C84.64 Anaplastic large cell lymphoma, ALK-positive, lymph nodes of axilla and upper limb**
CC **C84.65 Anaplastic large cell lymphoma, ALK-positive, lymph nodes of inguinal region and lower limb**

CC **C84.66** **Anaplastic large cell lymphoma, ALK-positive, intrapelvic lymph nodes**
CC **C84.67** **Anaplastic large cell lymphoma, ALK-positive, spleen**
CC **C84.68** **Anaplastic large cell lymphoma, ALK-positive, lymph nodes of multiple sites**
CC **C84.69** **Anaplastic large cell lymphoma, ALK-positive, extranodal and solid organ sites**

\+ **C84.7 Anaplastic large cell lymphoma, ALK-negative**
Excludes1: *primary cutaneous CD30-positive T-cell proliferations (C86.6-)*

CC **C84.70** **Anaplastic large cell lymphoma, ALK-negative, unspecified site**
CC **C84.71** **Anaplastic large cell lymphoma, ALK-negative, lymph nodes of head, face, and neck**
CC **C84.72** **Anaplastic large cell lymphoma, ALK-negative, intrathoracic lymph nodes**
CC **C84.73** **Anaplastic large cell lymphoma, ALK-negative, intra-abdominal lymph nodes**
CC **C84.74** **Anaplastic large cell lymphoma, ALK-negative, lymph nodes of axilla and upper limb**
CC **C84.75** **Anaplastic large cell lymphoma, ALK-negative, lymph nodes of inguinal region and lower limb**
CC **C84.76** **Anaplastic large cell lymphoma, ALK-negative, intrapelvic lymph nodes**
CC **C84.77** **Anaplastic large cell lymphoma, ALK-negative, spleen**
CC **C84.78** **Anaplastic large cell lymphoma, ALK-negative, lymph nodes of multiple sites**
CC **C84.79** **Anaplastic large cell lymphoma, ALK-negative, extranodal and solid organ sites**
CC **C84.7A** **Anaplastic large cell lymphoma, ALK-negative, breast**
Breast implant associated anaplastic large cell lymphoma (BIA-ALCL)
Use additional code to identify:
breast implant status (Z98.82)
personal history of breast implant removal (Z98.86)

\+ **C84.A Cutaneous T-cell lymphoma, unspecified**

CC **C84.A0** **Cutaneous T-cell lymphoma, unspecified, unspecified site**
CC **C84.A1** **Cutaneous T-cell lymphoma, unspecified lymph nodes of head, face, and neck**
CC **C84.A2** **Cutaneous T-cell lymphoma, unspecified, intrathoracic lymph nodes**
CC **C84.A3** **Cutaneous T-cell lymphoma, unspecified, intra-abdominal lymph nodes**
CC **C84.A4** **Cutaneous T-cell lymphoma, unspecified, lymph nodes of axilla and upper limb**
CC **C84.A5** **Cutaneous T-cell lymphoma, unspecified, lymph nodes of inguinal region and lower limb**
CC **C84.A6** **Cutaneous T-cell lymphoma, unspecified, intrapelvic lymph nodes**
CC **C84.A7** **Cutaneous T-cell lymphoma, unspecified, spleen**
AHA CC: 2Q, 2021, 6-7
CC **C84.A8** **Cutaneous T-cell lymphoma, unspecified, lymph nodes of multiple sites**
AHA CC: 2Q, 2021, 6-7
CC **C84.A9** **Cutaneous T-cell lymphoma, unspecified, extranodal and solid organ sites**

\+ **C84.Z Other mature T/NK-cell lymphomas**
NOTE If T-cell lineage or involvement is mentioned in conjunction with a specific lymphoma, code to the more specific description.
Excludes1: *angioimmunoblastic T-cell lymphoma (C86.5)*
blastic NK-cell lymphoma (C86.4)
enteropathy-type T-cell lymphoma (C86.2)
extranodal NK-cell lymphoma, nasal type (C86.0)
hepatosplenic T-cell lymphoma (C86.1)
primary cutaneous CD30-positive T-cell proliferations (C86.6)
subcutaneous panniculitis-like T-cell lymphoma (C86.3)
T-cell leukemia (C91.1-)

CC **C84.Z0** **Other mature T/NK-cell lymphomas, unspecified site**
CC **C84.Z1** **Other mature T/NK-cell lymphomas, lymph nodes of head, face, and neck**
CC **C84.Z2** **Other mature T/NK-cell lymphomas, intrathoracic lymph nodes**
CC **C84.Z3** **Other mature T/NK-cell lymphomas, intra-abdominal lymph nodes**
CC **C84.Z4** **Other mature T/NK-cell lymphomas, lymph nodes of axilla and upper limb**
CC **C84.Z5** **Other mature T/NK-cell lymphomas, lymph nodes of inguinal region and lower limb**
CC **C84.Z6** **Other mature T/NK-cell lymphomas, intrapelvic lymph nodes**
CC **C84.Z7** **Other mature T/NK-cell lymphomas, spleen**
CC **C84.Z8** **Other mature T/NK-cell lymphomas, lymph nodes of multiple sites**
CC **C84.Z9** **Other mature T/NK-cell lymphomas, extranodal and solid organ sites**

\+ **C84.9 Mature T/NK-cell lymphomas, unspecified**
NK/T cell lymphoma NOS
Excludes1: *mature T-cell lymphoma, not elsewhere classified (C84.4-)*

CC **C84.90** **Mature T/NK-cell lymphomas, unspecified, unspecified site**
CC **C84.91** **Mature T/NK-cell lymphomas, unspecified, lymph nodes of head, face, and neck**
CC **C84.92** **Mature T/NK-cell lymphomas, unspecified, intrathoracic lymph nodes**
CC **C84.93** **Mature T/NK-cell lymphomas, unspecified, intra-abdominal lymph nodes**
CC **C84.94** **Mature T/NK-cell lymphomas, unspecified, lymph nodes of axilla and upper limb**
CC **C84.95** **Mature T/NK-cell lymphomas, unspecified, lymph nodes of inguinal region and lower limb**
CC **C84.96** **Mature T/NK-cell lymphomas, unspecified, intrapelvic lymph nodes**
CC **C84.97** **Mature T/NK-cell lymphomas, unspecified, spleen**
CC **C84.98** **Mature T/NK-cell lymphomas, unspecified, lymph nodes of multiple sites**
CC **C84.99** **Mature T/NK-cell lymphomas, unspecified, extranodal and solid organ sites**

C85 Other specified and unspecified types of non-Hodgkin lymphoma

Excludes1: *other specified types of T/NK-cell lymphoma (C86.-)*
personal history of non-Hodgkin lymphoma (Z85.72)

\+ **C85.1 Unspecified B-cell lymphoma**
NOTE If B-cell lineage or involvement is mentioned in conjunction with a specific lymphoma, code to the more specific description.

CC **C85.10** **Unspecified B-cell lymphoma, unspecified site**
CC **C85.11** **Unspecified B-cell lymphoma, lymph nodes of head, face, and neck**
CC **C85.12** **Unspecified B-cell lymphoma, intrathoracic lymph nodes**
CC **C85.13** **Unspecified B-cell lymphoma, intra-abdominal lymph nodes**
CC **C85.14** **Unspecified B-cell lymphoma, lymph nodes of axilla and upper limb**
CC **C85.15** **Unspecified B-cell lymphoma, lymph nodes of inguinal region and lower limb**
CC **C85.16** **Unspecified B-cell lymphoma, intrapelvic lymph nodes**
CC **C85.17** **Unspecified B-cell lymphoma, spleen**
CC **C85.18** **Unspecified B-cell lymphoma, lymph nodes of multiple sites**
CC **C85.19** **Unspecified B-cell lymphoma, extranodal and solid organ sites**

\+ **C85.2 Mediastinal (thymic) large B-cell lymphoma**

CC **C85.20** **Mediastinal (thymic) large B-cell lymphoma, unspecified site**
CC **C85.21** **Mediastinal (thymic) large B-cell lymphoma, lymph nodes of head, face, and neck**
CC **C85.22** **Mediastinal (thymic) large B-cell lymphoma, intrathoracic lymph nodes**
CC **C85.23** **Mediastinal (thymic) large B-cell lymphoma, intra-abdominal lymph nodes**
CC **C85.24** **Mediastinal (thymic) large B-cell lymphoma, lymph nodes of axilla and upper limb**
CC **C85.25** **Mediastinal (thymic) large B-cell lymphoma, lymph nodes of inguinal region and lower limb**
CC **C85.26** **Mediastinal (thymic) large B-cell lymphoma, intrapelvic lymph nodes**
CC **C85.27** **Mediastinal (thymic) large B-cell lymphoma, spleen**

CC **C85.28 Mediastinal (thymic) large B-cell lymphoma, lymph nodes of multiple sites**
CC **C85.29 Mediastinal (thymic) large B-cell lymphoma, extranodal and solid organ sites**

+ **C85.8 Other specified types of non-Hodgkin lymphoma**
CC **C85.80 Other specified types of non-Hodgkin lymphoma, unspecified site**
CC **C85.81 Other specified types of non-Hodgkin lymphoma, lymph nodes of head, face, and neck**
CC **C85.82 Other specified types of non-Hodgkin lymphoma, intrathoracic lymph nodes**
CC **C85.83 Other specified types of non-Hodgkin lymphoma, intra-abdominal lymph nodes**
CC **C85.84 Other specified types of non-Hodgkin lymphoma, lymph nodes of axilla and upper limb**
CC **C85.85 Other specified types of non-Hodgkin lymphoma, lymph nodes of inguinal region and lower limb**
CC **C85.86 Other specified types of non-Hodgkin lymphoma, intrapelvic lymph nodes**
CC **C85.87 Other specified types of non-Hodgkin lymphoma, spleen**
CC **C85.88 Other specified types of non-Hodgkin lymphoma, lymph nodes of multiple sites**
CC **C85.89 Other specified types of non-Hodgkin lymphoma, extranodal and solid organ sites**

+ **C85.9 Non-Hodgkin lymphoma, unspecified**
Lymphoma NOS
Malignant lymphoma NOS
Non-Hodgkin lymphoma NOS
CC **C85.90 Non-Hodgkin lymphoma, unspecified, unspecified site**
CC **C85.91 Non-Hodgkin lymphoma, unspecified, lymph nodes of head, face, and neck**
CC **C85.92 Non-Hodgkin lymphoma, unspecified, intrathoracic lymph nodes**
CC **C85.93 Non-Hodgkin lymphoma, unspecified, intra-abdominal lymph nodes**
CC **C85.94 Non-Hodgkin lymphoma, unspecified, lymph nodes of axilla and upper limb**
CC **C85.95 Non-Hodgkin lymphoma, unspecified, lymph nodes of inguinal region and lower limb**
CC **C85.96 Non-Hodgkin lymphoma, unspecified, intrapelvic lymph nodes**
CC **C85.97 Non-Hodgkin lymphoma, unspecified, spleen**
CC **C85.98 Non-Hodgkin lymphoma, unspecified, lymph nodes of multiple sites**
CC **C85.99 Non-Hodgkin lymphoma, unspecified, extranodal and solid organ sites**

C86 Other specified types of T/NK-cell lymphoma
Excludes1: *anaplastic large cell lymphoma, ALK negative (C84.7-)*
anaplastic large cell lymphoma, ALK positive (C84.6-)
mature T/NK-cell lymphomas (C84.-)
other specified types of non-Hodgkin lymphoma (C85.8-)
CC **C86.0 Extranodal NK/T-cell lymphoma, nasal type**
CC **C86.1 Hepatosplenic T-cell lymphoma**
Alpha-beta and gamma delta types
CC **C86.2 Enteropathy-type (intestinal) T-cell lymphoma**
Enteropathy associated T-cell lymphoma
CC **C86.3 Subcutaneous panniculitis-like T-cell lymphoma**
CC **C86.4 Blastic NK-cell lymphoma**
Blastic plasmacytoid dendritic cell neoplasm (BPDCN)
CC **C86.5 Angioimmunoblastic T-cell lymphoma**
Angioimmunoblastic lymphadenopathy with dysproteinemia (AILD)
CC **C86.6 Primary cutaneous CD30-positive T-cell proliferations**
Lymphomatoid papulosis
Primary cutaneous anaplastic large cell lymphoma
Primary cutaneous CD30-positive large T-cell lymphoma

C88 Malignant immunoproliferative diseases and certain other B-cell lymphomas
Excludes1: *B-cell lymphoma, unspecified (C85.1-)*
personal history of other malignant neoplasms of lymphoid, hematopoietic and related tissues (Z85.79)
C88.0 Waldenström macroglobulinemia
Lymphoplasmacytic lymphoma with IgM-production
Macroglobulinemia (idiopathic) (primary)
Excludes1: *small cell B-cell lymphoma (C83.0)*
CC **C88.2 Heavy chain disease**
Franklin disease
Gamma heavy chain disease
Mu heavy chain disease
CC **C88.3 Immunoproliferative small intestinal disease**
Alpha heavy chain disease
Mediterranean lymphoma
CC **C88.4 Extranodal marginal zone B-cell lymphoma of mucosa-associated lymphoid tissue [MALT-lymphoma]**
Lymphoma of skin-associated lymphoid tissue [SALT-lymphoma]
Lymphoma of bronchial-associated lymphoid tissue [BALT-lymphoma]
Excludes1: *high malignant (diffuse large B-cell) lymphoma (C83.3-)*
CC **C88.8 Other malignant immunoproliferative diseases**
CC **C88.9 Malignant immunoproliferative disease, unspecified**
Immunoproliferative disease NOS

C90 Multiple myeloma and malignant plasma cell neoplasms
Excludes1: *personal history of other malignant neoplasms of lymphoid, hematopoietic and related tissues (Z85.79)*

+ **C90.0 Multiple myeloma**
Kahler's disease
Medullary plasmacytoma
Myelomatosis
Plasma cell myeloma
Excludes1: *solitary myeloma (C90.3-)*
solitary plasmactyoma (C90.3-)
CC **C90.00 Multiple myeloma not having achieved remission**
Multiple myeloma with failed remission
Multiple myeloma NOS
AHA CC: 4Q, 2020, 11-12, 14
CC **C90.01 Multiple myeloma in remission**
CC **C90.02 Multiple myeloma in relapse**

+ **C90.1 Plasma cell leukemia**
Plasmacytic leukemia
CC **C90.10 Plasma cell leukemia not having achieved remission**
Plasma cell leukemia with failed remission
Plasma cell leukemia NOS
AHA CC: 2Q, 2019, 30
CC **C90.11 Plasma cell leukemia in remission**
CC **C90.12 Plasma cell leukemia in relapse**

+ **C90.2 Extramedullary plasmacytoma**
CC **C90.20 Extramedullary plasmacytoma not having achieved remission**
Extramedullary plasmacytoma with failed remission
Extramedullary plasmacytoma NOS
CC **C90.21 Extramedullary plasmacytoma in remission**
CC **C90.22 Extramedullary plasmacytoma in relapse**

+ **C90.3 Solitary plasmacytoma**
Localized malignant plasma cell tumor NOS
Plasmacytoma NOS
Solitary myeloma
CC **C90.30 Solitary plasmacytoma not having achieved remission**
Solitary plasmacytoma with failed remission
Solitary plasmacytoma NOS
CC **C90.31 Solitary plasmacytoma in remission**
CC **C90.32 Solitary plasmacytoma in relapse**

C91 Lymphoid leukemia

Excludes1: *personal history of leukemia (Z85.6)*

+ **C91.0 Acute lymphoblastic leukemia [ALL]**

  NOTE Codes in subcategory C91.0- should only be used for T-cell and B-cell precursor leukemia

  CC **C91.00 Acute lymphoblastic leukemia not having achieved remission**
  Acute lymphoblastic leukemia with failed remission
  Acute lymphoblastic leukemia NOS
  AHA CC: 4Q, 2020, 14-15

  CC **C91.01 Acute lymphoblastic leukemia, in remission**

  CC **C91.02 Acute lymphoblastic leukemia, in relapse**

+ **C91.1 Chronic lymphocytic leukemia of B-cell type**
  Lymphoplasmacytic leukemia
  Richter syndrome
  Excludes1: *lymphoplasmacytic lymphoma (C83.0-)*

  CC **C91.10 Chronic lymphocytic leukemia of B-cell type not having achieved remission**
  Chronic lymphocytic leukemia of B-cell type with failed remission
  Chronic lymphocytic leukemia of B-cell type NOS

  CC **C91.11 Chronic lymphocytic leukemia of B-cell type in remission**

  CC **C91.12 Chronic lymphocytic leukemia of B-cell type in relapse**

+ **C91.3 Prolymphocytic leukemia of B-cell type**

  CC **C91.30 Prolymphocytic leukemia of B-cell type not having achieved remission**
  Prolymphocytic leukemia of B-cell type with failed remission
  Prolymphocytic leukemia of B-cell type NOS

  CC **C91.31 Prolymphocytic leukemia of B-cell type, in remission**

  CC **C91.32 Prolymphocytic leukemia of B-cell type, in relapse**

+ **C91.4 Hairy cell leukemia**
  Leukemic reticuloendotheliosis

  CC **C91.40 Hairy cell leukemia not having achieved remission**
  Hairy cell leukemia with failed remission
  Hairy cell leukemia NOS

  CC **C91.41 Hairy cell leukemia, in remission**

  CC **C91.42 Hairy cell leukemia, in relapse**

+ **C91.5 Adult T-cell lymphoma/leukemia (HTLV-1-associated)**
  Acute variant of adult T-cell lymphoma/leukemia (HTLV-1-associated)
  Chronic variant of adult T-cell lymphoma/leukemia (HTLV-1-associated)
  Lymphomatoid variant of adult T-cell lymphoma/leukemia (HTLV-1-associated)
  Smouldering variant of adult T-cell lymphoma/leukemia (HTLV-1-associated)

  • CC **C91.50 Adult T-cell lymphoma/leukemia (HTLV-1-associated) not having achieved remission**
  Adult T-cell lymphoma/leukemia (HTLV-1-associated) with failed remission
  Adult T-cell lymphoma/leukemia (HTLV-1-associated) NOS

  • CC **C91.51 Adult T-cell lymphoma/leukemia (HTLV-1-associated), in remission**

  • CC **C91.52 Adult T-cell lymphoma/leukemia (HTLV-1-associated), in relapse**

+ **C91.6 Prolymphocytic leukemia of T-cell type**

  CC **C91.60 Prolymphocytic leukemia of T-cell type not having achieved remission**
  Prolymphocytic leukemia of T-cell type with failed remission
  Prolymphocytic leukemia of T-cell type NOS

  CC **C91.61 Prolymphocytic leukemia of T-cell type, in remission**

  CC **C91.62 Prolymphocytic leukemia of T-cell type, in relapse**

+ **C91.A Mature B-cell leukemia Burkitt-type**
  Excludes1: *Burkitt lymphoma (C83.7-)*

  CC **C91.A0 Mature B-cell leukemia Burkitt-type not having achieved remission**
  Mature B-cell leukemia Burkitt-type with failed remission
  Mature B-cell leukemia Burkitt-type NOS

  CC **C91.A1 Mature B-cell leukemia Burkitt-type, in remission**

  CC **C91.A2 Mature B-cell leukemia Burkitt-type, in relapse**

+ **C91.Z Other lymphoid leukemia**
  T-cell large granular lymphocytic leukemia (associated with rheumatoid arthritis)

  CC **C91.Z0 Other lymphoid leukemia not having achieved remission**
  Other lymphoid leukemia with failed remission
  Other lymphoid leukemia NOS
  AHA CC: 2Q, 2019, 24-26

  CC **C91.Z1 Other lymphoid leukemia, in remission**

  CC **C91.Z2 Other lymphoid leukemia, in relapse**

+ **C91.9 Lymphoid leukemia, unspecified**

  CC **C91.90 Lymphoid leukemia, unspecified not having achieved remission**
  Lymphoid leukemia with failed remission
  Lymphoid leukemia NOS

  CC **C91.91 Lymphoid leukemia, unspecified, in remission**

  CC **C91.92 Lymphoid leukemia, unspecified, in relapse**

C92 Myeloid leukemia

Includes: granulocytic leukemia
myelogenous leukemia
Excludes1: *personal history of leukemia (Z85.6)*
AHA CC: 1Q, 2019, 16-17

+ **C92.0 Acute myeloblastic leukemia**
  Acute myeloblastic leukemia, minimal differentiation
  Acute myeloblastic leukemia (with maturation)
  Acute myeloblastic leukemia 1/ETO
  Acute myeloblastic leukemia M0
  Acute myeloblastic leukemia M1
  Acute myeloblastic leukemia M2
  Acute myeloblastic leukemia with t(8;21)
  Acute myeloblastic leukemia (without a FAB classification) NOS
  Refractory anemia with excess blasts in transformation [RAEB T]
  Excludes1: *acute exacerbation of chronic myeloid leukemia (C92.10)*
  refractory anemia with excess of blasts not in transformation (D46.2-)
  AHA CC: 4Q, 2018, 87

  CC **C92.00 Acute myeloblastic leukemia, not having achieved remission**
  Acute myeloblastic leukemia with failed remission
  Acute myeloblastic leukemia NOS

  CC **C92.01 Acute myeloblastic leukemia, in remission**

  CC **C92.02 Acute myeloblastic leukemia, in relapse**

+ **C92.1 Chronic myeloid leukemia, BCR/ABL-positive**
  Chronic myelogenous leukemia, Philadelphia chromosome (Ph1) positive
  Chronic myelogenous leukemia, t(9;22) (q34;q11)
  Chronic myelogenous leukemia with crisis of blast cells
  Excludes1: *atypical chronic myeloid leukemia BCR/ABL-negative (C92.2-)*
  chronic myelomonocytic leukemia (C93.1-)
  chronic myeloproliferative disease (D47.1)

  CC **C92.10 Chronic myeloid leukemia, BCR/ABL-positive, not having achieved remission**
  Chronic myeloid leukemia, BCR/ABL-positive with failed remission
  Chronic myeloid leukemia, BCR/ABL-positive NOS
  AHA CC: 1Q, 2017, 7

  CC **C92.11 Chronic myeloid leukemia, BCR/ABL-positive, in remission**

  CC **C92.12 Chronic myeloid leukemia, BCR/ABL-positive, in relapse**

+ **C92.2 Atypical chronic myeloid leukemia, BCR/ABL-negative**

  CC **C92.20 Atypical chronic myeloid leukemia, BCR/ABL-negative, not having achieved remission**
  Atypical chronic myeloid leukemia, BCR/ABL-negative with failed remission
  Atypical chronic myeloid leukemia, BCR/ABL-negative NOS

  CC **C92.21 Atypical chronic myeloid leukemia, BCR/ABL-negative, in remission**

  CC **C92.22 Atypical chronic myeloid leukemia, BCR/ABL-negative, in relapse**

+ C92.3 **Myeloid sarcoma**
A malignant tumor of immature myeloid cells
Chloroma
Granulocytic sarcoma

CC **C92.30 Myeloid sarcoma, not having achieved remission**
Myeloid sarcoma with failed remission
Myeloid sarcoma NOS

CC **C92.31 Myeloid sarcoma, in remission**

CC **C92.32 Myeloid sarcoma, in relapse**

+ C92.4 **Acute promyelocytic leukemia**
AML M3
AML Me with t(15;17) and variants

CC **C92.40 Acute promyelocytic leukemia, not having achieved remission**
Acute promyelocytic leukemia with failed remission
Acute promyelocytic leukemia NOS

CC **C92.41 Acute promyelocytic leukemia, in remission**

CC **C92.42 Acute promyelocytic leukemia, in relapse**

+ C92.5 **Acute myelomonocytic leukemia**
AML M4
AML M4 Eo with inv(16) or t(16;16)

CC **C92.50 Acute myelomonocytic leukemia, not having achieved remission**
Acute myelomonocytic leukemia with failed remission
Acute myelomonocytic leukemia NOS

CC **C92.51 Acute myelomonocytic leukemia, in remission**

CC **C92.52 Acute myelomonocytic leukemia, in relapse**

+ C92.6 **Acute myeloid leukemia with 11q23-abnormality**
Acute myeloid leukemia with variation of MLL-gene

CC **C92.60 Acute myeloid leukemia with 11q23-abnormality not having achieved remission**
Acute myeloid leukemia with 11q23-abnormality with failed remission
Acute myeloid leukemia with 11q23-abnormality NOS

CC **C92.61 Acute myeloid leukemia with 11q23-abnormality in remission**

CC **C92.62 Acute myeloid leukemia with 11q23-abnormality in relapse**

+ C92.A **Acute myeloid leukemia with multilineage dysplasia**
Acute myeloid leukemia with dysplasia of remaining hematopoesis and/or myelodysplastic disease in its history

CC **C92.A0 Acute myeloid leukemia with multilineage dysplasia, not having achieved remission**
Acute myeloid leukemia with multilineage dysplasia with failed remission
Acute myeloid leukemia with multilineage dysplasia NOS

CC **C92.A1 Acute myeloid leukemia with multilineage dysplasia, in remission**

CC **C92.A2 Acute myeloid leukemia with multilineage dysplasia, in relapse**

+ C92.Z **Other myeloid leukemia**

CC **C92.Z0 Other myeloid leukemia not having achieved remission**
Myeloid leukemia NEC with failed remission
Myeloid leukemia NEC

CC **C92.Z1 Other myeloid leukemia, in remission**

CC **C92.Z2 Other myeloid leukemia, in relapse**

+ C92.9 **Myeloid leukemia, unspecified**

CC **C92.90 Myeloid leukemia, unspecified, not having achieved remission**
Myeloid leukemia, unspecified with failed remission
Myeloid leukemia, unspecified NOS

CC **C92.91 Myeloid leukemia, unspecified in remission**

CC **C92.92 Myeloid leukemia, unspecified in relapse**

C93 Monocytic leukemia

Includes: monocytoid leukemia
Excludes1: *personal history of leukemia (Z85.6)*

+ C93.0 **Acute monoblastic/monocytic leukemia**
AML M5
AML M5a
AML M5b

CC **C93.00 Acute monoblastic/monocytic leukemia, not having achieved remission**
Acute monoblastic/monocytic leukemia with failed remission
Acute monoblastic/monocytic leukemia NOS

CC **C93.01 Acute monoblastic/monocytic leukemia, in remission**

CC **C93.02 Acute monoblastic/monocytic leukemia, in relapse**

+ C93.1 **Chronic myelomonocytic leukemia**
Chronic monocytic leukemia
CMML-1
CMML-2
CMML with eosinophilia
Code also, if applicable, eosinophilia (D72.18)

CC **C93.10 Chronic myelomonocytic leukemia not having achieved remission**
Chronic myelomonocytic leukemia with failed remission
Chronic myelomonocytic leukemia NOS

CC **C93.11 Chronic myelomonocytic leukemia, in remission**

CC **C93.12 Chronic myelomonocytic leukemia, in relapse**

+ C93.3 **Juvenile myelomonocytic leukemia**

• CC **C93.30 Juvenile myelomonocytic leukemia, not having achieved remission**
Juvenile myelomonocytic leukemia with failed remission
Juvenile myelomonocytic leukemia NOS

• CC **C93.31 Juvenile myelomonocytic leukemia, in remission**

• CC **C93.32 Juvenile myelomonocytic leukemia, in relapse**

+ C93.Z **Other monocytic leukemia**

CC **C93.Z0 Other monocytic leukemia, not having achieved remission**
Other monocytic leukemia NOS

CC **C93.Z1 Other monocytic leukemia, in remission**

CC **C93.Z2 Other monocytic leukemia, in relapse**

+ C93.9 **Monocytic leukemia, unspecified**

CC **C93.90 Monocytic leukemia, unspecified, not having achieved remission**
Monocytic leukemia, unspecified with failed remission
Monocytic leukemia, unspecified NOS

CC **C93.91 Monocytic leukemia, unspecified in remission**

CC **C93.92 Monocytic leukemia, unspecified in relapse**

C94 Other leukemias of specified cell type

Excludes1: *leukemic reticuloendotheliosis (C91.4-)*
myelodysplastic syndromes (D46.-)
personal history of leukemia (Z85.6)
plasma cell leukemia (C90.1-)

+ C94.0 **Acute erythroid leukemia**
Acute myeloid leukemia M6(a)(b)
Erythroleukemia

CC **C94.00 Acute erythroid leukemia, not having achieved remission**
Acute erythroid leukemia with failed remission
Acute erythroid leukemia NOS

CC **C94.01 Acute erythroid leukemia, in remission**

CC **C94.02 Acute erythroid leukemia, in relapse**

+ C94.2 **Acute megakaryoblastic leukemia**
Acute myeloid leukemia M7
Acute megakaryocytic leukemia

CC **C94.20 Acute megakaryoblastic leukemia not having achieved remission**
Acute megakaryoblastic leukemia with failed remission
Acute megakaryoblastic leukemia NOS

CC **C94.21 Acute megakaryoblastic leukemia, in remission**

CC **C94.22 Acute megakaryoblastic leukemia, in relapse**

+ C94.3 **Mast cell leukemia**
AHA CC: 4Q, 2017, 5
CC **C94.30 Mast cell leukemia not having achieved remission**
Mast cell leukemia with failed remission
Mast cell leukemia NOS
CC **C94.31 Mast cell leukemia, in remission**
CC **C94.32 Mast cell leukemia, in relapse**
+ C94.4 **Acute panmyelosis with myelofibrosis**
Acute myelofibrosis
Excludes1: *myelofibrosis NOS (D75.81)*
secondary myelofibrosis NOS (D75.81)
CC **C94.40 Acute panmyelosis with myelofibrosis not having achieved remission**
Acute myelofibrosis NOS
Acute panmyelosis with myelofibrosis with failed remission
Acute panmyelosis NOS
CC **C94.41 Acute panmyelosis with myelofibrosis, in remission**
CC **C94.42 Acute panmyelosis with myelofibrosis, in relapse**
CC **C94.6 Myelodysplastic disease, not classified**
Myeloproliferative disease, not classified
+ C94.8 **Other specified leukemias**
Aggressive NK-cell leukemia
Acute basophilic leukemia
CC **C94.80 Other specified leukemias not having achieved remission**
Other specified leukemia with failed remission
Other specified leukemias NOS
CC **C94.81 Other specified leukemias, in remission**
CC **C94.82 Other specified leukemias, in relapse**

C95 Leukemia of unspecified cell type
Excludes1: *personal history of leukemia (Z85.6)*
+ C95.0 **Acute leukemia of unspecified cell type**
Acute bilineal leukemia
Acute mixed lineage leukemia
Biphenotypic acute leukemia
Stem cell leukemia of unclear lineage
Excludes1: *acute exacerbation of unspecified chronic leukemia (C95.10)*
CC **C95.00 Acute leukemia of unspecified cell type not having achieved remission**
Acute leukemia of unspecified cell type with failed remission
Acute leukemia NOS
CC **C95.01 Acute leukemia of unspecified cell type, in remission**
CC **C95.02 Acute leukemia of unspecified cell type, in relapse**
+ C95.1 **Chronic leukemia of unspecified cell type**
CC **C95.10 Chronic leukemia of unspecified cell type not having achieved remission**
Chronic leukemia of unspecified cell type with failed remission
Chronic leukemia NOS
CC **C95.11 Chronic leukemia of unspecified cell type, in remission**
CC **C95.12 Chronic leukemia of unspecified cell type, in relapse**
+ C95.9 **Leukemia, unspecified**
CC **C95.90 Leukemia, unspecified not having achieved remission**
Leukemia, unspecified with failed remission
Leukemia NOS
CC **C95.91 Leukemia, unspecified, in remission**
CC **C95.92 Leukemia, unspecified, in relapse**

C96 Other and unspecified malignant neoplasms of lymphoid, hematopoietic and related tissue
Excludes1: *personal history of other malignant neoplasms of lymphoid, hematopoietic and related tissues (Z85.79)*
CC **C96.0 Multifocal and multisystemic (disseminated) Langerhans-cell histiocytosis**
Histiocytosis X, multisystemic
Letterer-Siwe disease
Excludes1: *adult pulmonary Langerhans cell histiocytosis (J84.82)*
multifocal and unisystemic Langerhans-cell histiocytosis (C96.5)
unifocal Langerhans-cell histiocytosis (C96.6)
+ C96.2 **Malignant mast cell neoplasm**
Excludes1: *indolent mastocytosis (D47.02)*
mast cell leukemia (C94.30)
mastocytosis (congenital) (cutaneous) (Q82.2)
AHA CC: 4Q, 2017, 5
CC **C96.20 Malignant mast cell neoplasm, unspecified**
CC **C96.21 Aggressive systemic mastocytosis**
CC **C96.22 Mast cell sarcoma**
CC **C96.29 Other malignant mast cell neoplasm**
CC **C96.4 Sarcoma of dendritic cells (accessory cells)**
Follicular dendritic cell sarcoma
Interdigitating dendritic cell sarcoma
Langerhans cell sarcoma
CC **C96.5 Multifocal and unisystemic Langerhans-cell histiocytosis**
Hand-Schüller-Christian disease
Histiocytosis X, multifocal
Excludes1: *multifocal and multisystemic (disseminated) Langerhans-cell histiocytosis (C96.0)*
unifocal Langerhans-cell histiocytosis (C96.6)
CC **C96.6 Unifocal Langerhans-cell histiocytosis**
Eosinophilic granuloma
Histiocytosis X, unifocal
Histiocytosis X NOS
Langerhans-cell histiocytosis NOS
Excludes1: *multifocal and multisysemic (disseminated) Langerhans-cell histiocytosis (C96.0)*
multifocal and unisystemic Langerhans-cell histiocytosis (C96.5)
CC **C96.A Histiocytic sarcoma**
Malignant histiocytosis
CC **C96.Z Other specified malignant neoplasms of lymphoid, hematopoietic and related tissue**
CC **C96.9 Malignant neoplasm of lymphoid, hematopoietic and related tissue, unspecified**

In situ neoplasms (D00-D09)

Includes: Bowen's disease
erythroplasia
grade III intraepithelial neoplasia
Queyrat's erythroplasia

D00 Carcinoma in situ of oral cavity, esophagus and stomach
Excludes1: *melanoma in situ (D03.-)*
+ D00.0 **Carcinoma in situ of lip, oral cavity and pharynx**
Use additional code to identify:
exposure to environmental tobacco smoke (Z77.22)
exposure to tobacco smoke in the perinatal period (P96.81)
history of tobacco dependence (Z87.891)
occupational exposure to environmental tobacco smoke (Z57.31)
tobacco dependence (F17.-)
tobacco use (Z72.0)
Excludes1: *carcinoma in situ of aryepiglottic fold or interarytenoid fold, laryngeal aspect (D02.0)*
carcinoma in situ of epiglottis NOS (D02.0)
carcinoma in situ of epiglottis suprahyoid portion (D02.0)
carcinoma in situ of skin of lip (D03.0, D04.0)
D00.00 Carcinoma in situ of oral cavity, unspecified site
D00.01 Carcinoma in situ of labial mucosa and vermilion border
D00.02 Carcinoma in situ of buccal mucosa
D00.03 Carcinoma in situ of gingiva and edentulous alveolar ridge
D00.04 Carcinoma in situ of soft palate
D00.05 Carcinoma in situ of hard palate
D00.06 Carcinoma in situ of floor of mouth
D00.07 Carcinoma in situ of tongue
D00.08 Carcinoma in situ of pharynx
Carcinoma in situ of aryepiglottic fold NOS
Carcinoma in situ of hypopharyngeal aspect of aryepiglottic fold
Carcinoma in situ of marginal zone of aryepiglottic fold
D00.1 Carcinoma in situ of esophagus
D00.2 Carcinoma in situ of stomach

D01 Carcinoma in situ of other and unspecified digestive organs

Excludes1: *melanoma in situ (D03.-)*

D01.0 Carcinoma in situ of colon

Excludes1: *carcinoma in situ of rectosigmoid junction (D01.1)*

D01.1 Carcinoma in situ of rectosigmoid junction

D01.2 Carcinoma in situ of rectum

D01.3 Carcinoma in situ of anus and anal canal

Anal intraepithelial neoplasia III [AIN III]

Severe dysplasia of anus

Excludes1: *anal intraepithelial neoplasia I and II [AIN I and AIN II] (K62.82)*
carcinoma in situ of anal margin (D04.5)
carcinoma in situ of anal skin (D04.5)
carcinoma in situ of perianal skin (D04.5)

\+ **D01.4 Carcinoma in situ of other and unspecified parts of intestine**

Excludes1: *carcinoma in situ of ampulla of Vater (D01.5)*

D01.40 Carcinoma in situ of unspecified part of intestine

D01.49 Carcinoma in situ of other parts of intestine

D01.5 Carcinoma in situ of liver, gallbladder and bile ducts

Carcinoma in situ of ampulla of Vater

D01.7 Carcinoma in situ of other specified digestive organs

Carcinoma in situ of pancreas

D01.9 Carcinoma in situ of digestive organ, unspecified

D02 Carcinoma in situ of middle ear and respiratory system

Use additional code to identify:
exposure to environmental tobacco smoke (Z77.22)
exposure to tobacco smoke in the perinatal period (P96.81)
history of tobacco dependence (Z87.891)
occupational exposure to environmental tobacco smoke (Z57.31)
tobacco dependence (F17.-)
tobacco use (Z72.0)

Excludes1: *melanoma in situ (D03.-)*

D02.0 Carcinoma in situ of larynx

Carcinoma in situ of aryepiglottic fold or interarytenoid fold, laryngeal aspect

Carcinoma in situ of epiglottis (suprahyoid portion)

Excludes1: *carcinoma in situ of aryepiglottic fold or interarytenoid fold NOS (D00.08)*
carcinoma in situ of hypopharyngeal aspect (D00.08)
carcinoma in situ of marginal zone (D00.08)

D02.1 Carcinoma in situ of trachea

\+ **D02.2 Carcinoma in situ of bronchus and lung**

D02.20 Carcinoma in situ of unspecified bronchus and lung

D02.21 Carcinoma in situ of right bronchus and lung

D02.22 Carcinoma in situ of left bronchus and lung

D02.3 Carcinoma in situ of other parts of respiratory system

Carcinoma in situ of accessory sinuses
Carcinoma in situ of middle ear
Carcinoma in situ of nasal cavities

Excludes1: *carcinoma in situ of ear (external) (skin) (D04.2-)*
carcinoma in situ of nose NOS (D09.8)
carcinoma in situ of skin of nose (D04.3)

D02.4 Carcinoma in situ of respiratory system, unspecified

D03 Melanoma in situ

D03.0 Melanoma in situ of lip

\+ **D03.1 Melanoma in situ of eyelid, including canthus**

D03.10 Melanoma in situ of unspecified eyelid, including canthus

\+ **D03.11 Melanoma in situ of right eyelid, including canthus**

D03.111 Melanoma in situ of right upper eyelid, including canthus

D03.112 Melanoma in situ of right lower eyelid, including canthus

\+ **D03.12 Melanoma in situ of left eyelid, including canthus**

D03.121 Melanoma in situ of left upper eyelid, including canthus

D03.122 Melanoma in situ of left lower eyelid, including canthus

\+ **D03.2 Melanoma in situ of ear and external auricular canal**

D03.20 Melanoma in situ of unspecified ear and external auricular canal

D03.21 Melanoma in situ of right ear and external auricular canal

D03.22 Melanoma in situ of left ear and external auricular canal

\+ **D03.3 Melanoma in situ of other and unspecified parts of face**

D03.30 Melanoma in situ of unspecified part of face

D03.39 Melanoma in situ of other parts of face

D03.4 Melanoma in situ of scalp and neck

\+ **D03.5 Melanoma in situ of trunk**

D03.51 Melanoma in situ of anal skin

Melanoma in situ of anal margin
Melanoma in situ of perianal skin

D03.52 Melanoma in situ of breast (skin) (soft tissue)

D03.59 Melanoma in situ of other part of trunk

\+ **D03.6 Melanoma in situ of upper limb, including shoulder**

D03.60 Melanoma in situ of unspecified upper limb, including shoulder

D03.61 Melanoma in situ of right upper limb, including shoulder

D03.62 Melanoma in situ of left upper limb, including shoulder

\+ **D03.7 Melanoma in situ of lower limb, including hip**

D03.70 Melanoma in situ of unspecified lower limb, including hip

D03.71 Melanoma in situ of right lower limb, including hip

D03.72 Melanoma in situ of left lower limb, including hip

D03.8 Melanoma in situ of other sites

Melanoma in situ of scrotum

Excludes1: *carcinoma in situ of scrotum (D07.61)*

D03.9 Melanoma in situ, unspecified

D04 Carcinoma in situ of skin

Excludes1: *erythroplasia of Queyrat (penis) NOS (D07.4)*
melanoma in situ (D03.-)

D04.0 Carcinoma in situ of skin of lip

Excludes2: *carcinoma in situ of vermilion border of lip (D00.01)*

\+ **D04.1 Carcinoma in situ of skin of eyelid, including canthus**

D04.10 Carcinoma in situ of skin of unspecified eyelid, including canthus

\+ **D04.11 Carcinoma in situ of skin of right eyelid, including canthus**

D04.111 Carcinoma in situ of skin of right upper eyelid, including canthus

D04.112 Carcinoma in situ of skin of right lower eyelid, including canthus

\+ **D04.12 Carcinoma in situ of skin of left eyelid, including canthus**

D04.121 Carcinoma in situ of skin of left upper eyelid, including canthus

D04.122 Carcinoma in situ of skin of left lower eyelid, including canthus

\+ **D04.2 Carcinoma in situ of skin of ear and external auricular canal**

D04.20 Carcinoma in situ of skin of unspecified ear and external auricular canal

D04.21 Carcinoma in situ of skin of right ear and external auricular canal

D04.22 Carcinoma in situ of skin of left ear and external auricular canal

\+ **D04.3 Carcinoma in situ of skin of other and unspecified parts of face**

D04.30 Carcinoma in situ of skin of unspecified part of face

D04.39 Carcinoma in situ of skin of other parts of face

D04.4 Carcinoma in situ of skin of scalp and neck

D04.5 Carcinoma in situ of skin of trunk

Carcinoma in situ of anal margin
Carcinoma in situ of anal skin
Carcinoma in situ of perianal skin
Carcinoma in situ of skin of breast

Excludes1: *carcinoma in situ of anus NOS (D01.3)*
carcinoma in situ of scrotum (D07.61)
carcinoma in situ of skin of genital organs (D07.-)

+ D04.6 **Carcinoma in situ of skin of upper limb, including shoulder**
D04.60 **Carcinoma in situ of skin of unspecified upper limb, including shoulder**
D04.61 **Carcinoma in situ of skin of right upper limb, including shoulder**
D04.62 **Carcinoma in situ of skin of left upper limb, including shoulder**
+ D04.7 **Carcinoma in situ of skin of lower limb, including hip**
D04.70 **Carcinoma in situ of skin of unspecified lower limb, including hip**
D04.71 **Carcinoma in situ of skin of right lower limb, including hip**
D04.72 **Carcinoma in situ of skin of left lower limb, including hip**
D04.8 **Carcinoma in situ of skin of other sites**
D04.9 **Carcinoma in situ of skin, unspecified**

D05 Carcinoma in situ of breast

Excludes1: *carcinoma in situ of skin of breast (D04.5)*
melanoma in situ of breast (skin) (D03.5)
Paget's disease of breast or nipple (C50.-)

+ D05.0 **Lobular carcinoma in situ of breast**
D05.00 **Lobular carcinoma in situ of unspecified breast**
D05.01 **Lobular carcinoma in situ of right breast**
D05.02 **Lobular carcinoma in situ of left breast**
+ D05.1 **Intraductal carcinoma in situ of breast**
D05.10 **Intraductal carcinoma in situ of unspecified breast**
D05.11 **Intraductal carcinoma in situ of right breast**
D05.12 **Intraductal carcinoma in situ of left breast**
+ D05.8 **Other specified type of carcinoma in situ of breast**
D05.80 **Other specified type of carcinoma in situ of unspecified breast**
D05.81 **Other specified type of carcinoma in situ of right breast**
D05.82 **Other specified type of carcinoma in situ of left breast**
+ D05.9 **Unspecified type of carcinoma in situ of breast**
D05.90 **Unspecified type of carcinoma in situ of unspecified breast**
D05.91 **Unspecified type of carcinoma in situ of right breast**
D05.92 **Unspecified type of carcinoma in situ of left breast**

D06 Carcinoma in situ of cervix uteri

Includes: cervical adenocarcinoma in situ
cervical intraepithelial glandular neoplasia
cervical intraepithelial neoplasia III [CIN III]
severe dysplasia of cervix uteri

Excludes1: *cervical intraepithelial neoplasia II [CIN II] (N87.1)*
cytologic evidence of malignancy of cervix without histologic confirmation (R87.614)
high grade squamous intraepithelial lesion (HGSIL) of cervix (R87.613)
melanoma in situ of cervix (D03.5)
moderate cervical dysplasia (N87.1)

♀ D06.0 **Carcinoma in situ of endocervix**
♀ D06.1 **Carcinoma in situ of exocervix**
♀ D06.7 **Carcinoma in situ of other parts of cervix**
♀ D06.9 **Carcinoma in situ of cervix, unspecified**

D07 Carcinoma in situ of other and unspecified genital organs

Excludes1: *melanoma in situ of trunk (D03.5)*

♀ D07.0 **Carcinoma in situ of endometrium**
♀ D07.1 **Carcinoma in situ of vulva**
Severe dysplasia of vulva
Vulvar intraepithelial neoplasia III [VIN III]
Excludes1: *moderate dysplasia of vulva (N90.1)*
vulvar intraepithelial neoplasia II [VIN II] (N90.1)
♀ D07.2 **Carcinoma in situ of vagina**
Severe dysplasia of vagina
Vaginal intraepithelial neoplasia III [VAIN III]
Excludes1: *moderate dysplasia of vagina (N89.1)*
vaginal intraepithelial neoplasia II [VIN II] (N89.1)
+ D07.3 **Carcinoma in situ of other and unspecified female genital organs**
♀ D07.30 **Carcinoma in situ of unspecified female genital organs**
♀ D07.39 **Carcinoma in situ of other female genital organs**
♂ D07.4 **Carcinoma in situ of penis**
Erythroplasia of Queyrat NOS
♂ D07.5 **Carcinoma in situ of prostate**
Prostatic intraepithelial neoplasia III (PIN III)
Severe dysplasia of prostate
Excludes1: *dysplasia (mild) (moderate) of prostate (N42.3-)*
prostatic intraepithelial neoplasia II [PIN II] (N42.3-)
+ D07.6 **Carcinoma in situ of other and unspecified male genital organs**
♂ D07.60 **Carcinoma in situ of unspecified male genital organs**
♂ D07.61 **Carcinoma in situ of scrotum**
♂ D07.69 **Carcinoma in situ of other male genital organs**

D09 Carcinoma in situ of other and unspecified sites

Excludes1: *melanoma in situ (D03.-)*

D09.0 **Carcinoma in situ of bladder**
+ D09.1 **Carcinoma in situ of other and unspecified urinary organs**
D09.10 **Carcinoma in situ of unspecified urinary organ**
D09.19 **Carcinoma in situ of other urinary organs**
+ D09.2 **Carcinoma in situ of eye**
Excludes1: *carcinoma in situ of skin of eyelid (D04.1-)*
D09.20 **Carcinoma in situ of unspecified eye**
D09.21 **Carcinoma in situ of right eye**
D09.22 **Carcinoma in situ of left eye**
D09.3 **Carcinoma in situ of thyroid and other endocrine glands**
Excludes1: *carcinoma in situ of endocrine pancreas (D01.7)*
carcinoma in situ of ovary (D07.39)
carcinoma in situ of testis (D07.69)
D09.8 **Carcinoma in situ of other specified sites**
D09.9 **Carcinoma in situ, unspecified**

Benign neoplasms, except benign neuroendocrine tumors (D10-D36)

D10 Benign neoplasm of mouth and pharynx

D10.0 **Benign neoplasm of lip**
Benign neoplasm of lip (frenulum) (inner aspect) (mucosa) (vermilion border)
Excludes1: *benign neoplasm of skin of lip (D22.0, D23.0)*
D10.1 **Benign neoplasm of tongue**
Benign neoplasm of lingual tonsil
D10.2 **Benign neoplasm of floor of mouth**
+ D10.3 **Benign neoplasm of other and unspecified parts of mouth**
D10.30 **Benign neoplasm of unspecified part of mouth**
D10.39 **Benign neoplasm of other parts of mouth**
Benign neoplasm of minor salivary gland NOS
Excludes1: *benign odontogenic neoplasms (D16.4-D16.5)*
benign neoplasm of mucosa of lip (D10.0)
benign neoplasm of nasopharyngeal surface of soft palate (D10.6)
D10.4 **Benign neoplasm of tonsil**
Benign neoplasm of tonsil (faucial) (palatine)
Excludes1: *benign neoplasm of lingual tonsil (D10.1)*
benign neoplasm of pharyngeal tonsil (D10.6)
benign neoplasm of tonsillar fossa (D10.5)
benign neoplasm of tonsillar pillars (D10.5)
D10.5 **Benign neoplasm of other parts of oropharynx**
Benign neoplasm of epiglottis, anterior aspect
Benign neoplasm of tonsillar fossa
Benign neoplasm of tonsillar pillars
Benign neoplasm of vallecula
Excludes1: *benign neoplasm of epiglottis NOS (D14.1)*
benign neoplasm of epiglottis, suprahyoid portion (D14.1)
D10.6 **Benign neoplasm of nasopharynx**
Benign neoplasm of pharyngeal tonsil
Benign neoplasm of posterior margin of septum and choanae
D10.7 **Benign neoplasm of hypopharynx**
D10.9 **Benign neoplasm of pharynx, unspecified**

D11 Benign neoplasm of major salivary glands

Excludes1: *benign neoplasms of specified minor salivary glands which are classified according to their anatomical location*
benign neoplasms of minor salivary glands NOS (D10.39)

D11.0 Benign neoplasm of parotid gland

D11.7 Benign neoplasm of other major salivary glands
Benign neoplasm of sublingual salivary gland
Benign neoplasm of submandibular salivary gland

D11.9 Benign neoplasm of major salivary gland, unspecified

D12 Benign neoplasm of colon, rectum, anus and anal canal

Excludes1: *benign carcinoid tumors of the large intestine, and rectum (D3A.02-)*
polyp of colon NOS (K63.5)

D12.0 Benign neoplasm of cecum
Benign neoplasm of ileocecal valve
AHA CC: 3Q, 2018, 22

D12.1 Benign neoplasm of appendix
Excludes1: *benign carcinoid tumor of the appendix (D3A.020)*

D12.2 Benign neoplasm of ascending colon
AHA CC: 2Q, 2018, 14

D12.3 Benign neoplasm of transverse colon
Benign neoplasm of hepatic flexure
Benign neoplasm of splenic flexure

D12.4 Benign neoplasm of descending colon

D12.5 Benign neoplasm of sigmoid colon

D12.6 Benign neoplasm of colon, unspecified
Adenomatosis of colon
Benign neoplasm of large intestine NOS
Polyposis (hereditary) of colon
Excludes1: *inflammatory polyp of colon (K51.4-)*
AHA CC: 1Q, 2017, 8-9

D12.7 Benign neoplasm of rectosigmoid junction

D12.8 Benign neoplasm of rectum
Excludes1: *benign carcinoid tumor of the rectum (D3A.026)*
AHA CC: 1Q, 2018, 6-7

D12.9 Benign neoplasm of anus and anal canal
Benign neoplasm of anus NOS
Excludes1: *benign neoplasm of anal margin (D22.5, D23.5)*
benign neoplasm of anal skin (D22.5, D23.5)
benign neoplasm of perianal skin (D22.5, D23.5)

D13 Benign neoplasm of other and ill-defined parts of digestive system

Excludes1: *benign stromal tumors of digestive system (D21.4)*

D13.0 Benign neoplasm of esophagus

D13.1 Benign neoplasm of stomach
Excludes1: *benign carcinoid tumor of the stomach (D3A.092)*

D13.2 Benign neoplasm of duodenum
Excludes1: *benign carcinoid tumor of the duodenum (D3A.010)*

\+ **D13.3 Benign neoplasm of other and unspecified parts of small intestine**
Excludes1: *benign carcinoid tumors of the small intestine (D3A.01-)*
benign neoplasm of ileocecal valve (D12.0)

D13.30 Benign neoplasm of unspecified part of small intestine

D13.39 Benign neoplasm of other parts of small intestine

D13.4 Benign neoplasm of liver
Benign neoplasm of intrahepatic bile ducts

D13.5 Benign neoplasm of extrahepatic bile ducts

D13.6 Benign neoplasm of pancreas
Excludes1: *benign neoplasm of endocrine pancreas (D13.7)*

D13.7 Benign neoplasm of endocrine pancreas
Islet cell tumor
Benign neoplasm of islets of Langerhans
Use additional code to identify any functional activity.

D13.9 Benign neoplasm of ill-defined sites within the digestive system
Benign neoplasm of digestive system NOS
Benign neoplasm of intestine NOS
Benign neoplasm of spleen

D14 Benign neoplasm of middle ear and respiratory system

D14.0 Benign neoplasm of middle ear, nasal cavity and accessory sinuses
Benign neoplasm of cartilage of nose
Excludes1: *benign neoplasm of auricular canal (external) (D22.2-, D23.2-)*
benign neoplasm of bone of ear (D16.4)
benign neoplasm of bone of nose (D16.4)
benign neoplasm of cartilage of ear (D21.0)
benign neoplasm of ear (external)(skin) (D22.2-, D23.2-)
benign neoplasm of nose NOS (D36.7)
benign neoplasm of skin of nose (D22.39, D23.39)
benign neoplasm of olfactory bulb (D33.3)
benign neoplasm of posterior margin of septum and choanae (D10.6)
polyp of accessory sinus (J33.8)
polyp of ear (middle) (H74.4)
polyp of nasal (cavity) (J33.-)

D14.1 Benign neoplasm of larynx
Adenomatous polyp of larynx
Benign neoplasm of epiglottis (suprahyoid portion)
Excludes1: *benign neoplasm of epiglottis, anterior aspect (D10.5)*
polyp (nonadenomatous) of vocal cord or larynx (J38.1)

D14.2 Benign neoplasm of trachea

\+ **D14.3 Benign neoplasm of bronchus and lung**
Excludes1: *benign carcinoid tumor of the bronchus and lung (D3A.090)*

D14.30 Benign neoplasm of unspecified bronchus and lung

D14.31 Benign neoplasm of right bronchus and lung

D14.32 Benign neoplasm of left bronchus and lung

D14.4 Benign neoplasm of respiratory system, unspecified

D15 Benign neoplasm of other and unspecified intrathoracic organs

Excludes1: *benign neoplasm of mesothelial tissue (D19.-)*

D15.0 Benign neoplasm of thymus
Excludes1: *benign carcinoid tumor of the thymus (D3A.091)*

D15.1 Benign neoplasm of heart
Excludes1: *benign neoplasm of great vessels (D21.3)*

D15.2 Benign neoplasm of mediastinum

D15.7 Benign neoplasm of other specified intrathoracic organs

D15.9 Benign neoplasm of intrathoracic organ, unspecified

D16 Benign neoplasm of bone and articular cartilage

Excludes1: *benign neoplasm of connective tissue of ear (D21.0)*
benign neoplasm of connective tissue of eyelid (D21.0)
benign neoplasm of connective tissue of larynx (D14.1)
benign neoplasm of connective tissue of nose (D14.0)
benign neoplasm of synovia (D21.-)

\+ **D16.0 Benign neoplasm of scapula and long bones of upper limb**

D16.00 Benign neoplasm of scapula and long bones of unspecified upper limb

D16.01 Benign neoplasm of scapula and long bones of right upper limb

D16.02 Benign neoplasm of scapula and long bones of left upper limb

\+ **D16.1 Benign neoplasm of short bones of upper limb**

D16.10 Benign neoplasm of short bones of unspecified upper limb

D16.11 Benign neoplasm of short bones of right upper limb

D16.12 Benign neoplasm of short bones of left upper limb

\+ **D16.2 Benign neoplasm of long bones of lower limb**

D16.20 Benign neoplasm of long bones of unspecified lower limb

D16.21 Benign neoplasm of long bones of right lower limb

D16.22 Benign neoplasm of long bones of left lower limb

\+ **D16.3 Benign neoplasm of short bones of lower limb**

D16.30 Benign neoplasm of short bones of unspecified lower limb

D16.31 Benign neoplasm of short bones of right lower limb

D16.32 Benign neoplasm of short bones of left lower limb

D16.4 Benign neoplasm of bones of skull and face
Benign neoplasm of maxilla (superior)
Benign neoplasm of orbital bone
Keratocyst of maxilla
Keratocystic odontogenic tumor of maxilla
Excludes2: *benign neoplasm of lower jaw bone (D16.5)*

D16.5 Benign neoplasm of lower jaw bone
Keratocyst of mandible
Keratocystic odontogenic tumor of mandible

D16.6 Benign neoplasm of vertebral column
Excludes1: *benign neoplasm of sacrum and coccyx (D16.8)*

D16.7 Benign neoplasm of ribs, sternum and clavicle
D16.8 Benign neoplasm of pelvic bones, sacrum and coccyx
D16.9 Benign neoplasm of bone and articular cartilage, unspecified

D17 Benign lipomatous neoplasm

D17.0 Benign lipomatous neoplasm of skin and subcutaneous tissue of head, face and neck
D17.1 Benign lipomatous neoplasm of skin and subcutaneous tissue of trunk
+ **D17.2 Benign lipomatous neoplasm of skin and subcutaneous tissue of limb**
  - **D17.20 Benign lipomatous neoplasm of skin and subcutaneous tissue of unspecified limb**
  - **D17.21 Benign lipomatous neoplasm of skin and subcutaneous tissue of right arm**
  - **D17.22 Benign lipomatous neoplasm of skin and subcutaneous tissue of left arm**
  - **D17.23 Benign lipomatous neoplasm of skin and subcutaneous tissue of right leg**
  - **D17.24 Benign lipomatous neoplasm of skin and subcutaneous tissue of left leg**

+ **D17.3 Benign lipomatous neoplasm of skin and subcutaneous tissue of other and unspecified sites**
  - **D17.30 Benign lipomatous neoplasm of skin and subcutaneous tissue of unspecified sites**
  - **D17.39 Benign lipomatous neoplasm of skin and subcutaneous tissue of other sites**

D17.4 Benign lipomatous neoplasm of intrathoracic organs
D17.5 Benign lipomatous neoplasm of intra-abdominal organs
Excludes1: *benign lipomatous neoplasm of peritoneum and retroperitoneum (D17.79)*

♂ **D17.6 Benign lipomatous neoplasm of spermatic cord**
+ **D17.7 Benign lipomatous neoplasm of other sites**
  - **D17.71 Benign lipomatous neoplasm of kidney**
  - **D17.72 Benign lipomatous neoplasm of other genitourinary organ**
  - **D17.79 Benign lipomatous neoplasm of other sites**
    Benign lipomatous neoplasm of peritoneum
    Benign lipomatous neoplasm of retroperitoneum

D17.9 Benign lipomatous neoplasm, unspecified
Lipoma NOS

D18 Hemangioma and lymphangioma, any site

Excludes1: *benign neoplasm of glomus jugulare (D35.6)*
blue or pigmented nevus (D22.-)
nevus NOS (D22.-)
vascular nevus (Q82.5)

+ **D18.0 Hemangioma**
  Angioma NOS
  Cavernous nevus
  - **D18.00 Hemangioma unspecified site**
  - **D18.01 Hemangioma of skin and subcutaneous tissue**
  - **D18.02 Hemangioma of intracranial structures**
  - **D18.03 Hemangioma of intra-abdominal structures**
  - **D18.09 Hemangioma of other sites**

D18.1 Lymphangioma, any site
AHA CC: 2Q, 2018, 13; 3Q, 2018, 31

D19 Benign neoplasm of mesothelial tissue

D19.0 Benign neoplasm of mesothelial tissue of pleura
D19.1 Benign neoplasm of mesothelial tissue of peritoneum
D19.7 Benign neoplasm of mesothelial tissue of other sites
D19.9 Benign neoplasm of mesothelial tissue, unspecified
Benign mesothelioma NOS

D20 Benign neoplasm of soft tissue of retroperitoneum and peritoneum

Excludes1: *benign lipomatous neoplasm of peritoneum and retroperitoneum (D17.79)*
benign neoplasm of mesothelial tissue (D19.-)

D20.0 Benign neoplasm of soft tissue of retroperitoneum
D20.1 Benign neoplasm of soft tissue of peritoneum

D21 Other benign neoplasms of connective and other soft tissue

Includes: benign neoplasm of blood vessel
benign neoplasm of bursa
benign neoplasm of cartilage
benign neoplasm of fascia
benign neoplasm of fat
benign neoplasm of ligament, except uterine
benign neoplasm of lymphatic channel
benign neoplasm of muscle
benign neoplasm of synovia
benign neoplasm of tendon (sheath)
benign stromal tumors

Excludes1: *benign neoplasm of articular cartilage (D16.-)*
benign neoplasm of cartilage of larynx (D14.1)
benign neoplasm of cartilage of nose (D14.0)
benign neoplasm of connective tissue of breast (D24.-)
benign neoplasm of peripheral nerves and autonomic nervous system (D36.1-)
benign neoplasm of peritoneum (D20.1)
benign neoplasm of retroperitoneum (D20.0)
benign neoplasm of uterine ligament, any (D28.2)
benign neoplasm of vascular tissue (D18.-)
hemangioma (D18.0-)
lipomatous neoplasm (D17.-)
lymphangioma (D18.1)
uterine leiomyoma (D25.-)

D21.0 Benign neoplasm of connective and other soft tissue of head, face and neck
Benign neoplasm of connective tissue of ear
Benign neoplasm of connective tissue of eyelid
Excludes1: *benign neoplasm of connective tissue of orbit (D31.6-)*

+ **D21.1 Benign neoplasm of connective and other soft tissue of upper limb, including shoulder**
  - **D21.10 Benign neoplasm of connective and other soft tissue of unspecified upper limb, including shoulder**
  - **D21.11 Benign neoplasm of connective and other soft tissue of right upper limb, including shoulder**
  - **D21.12 Benign neoplasm of connective and other soft tissue of left upper limb, including shoulder**

+ **D21.2 Benign neoplasm of connective and other soft tissue of lower limb, including hip**
  - **D21.20 Benign neoplasm of connective and other soft tissue of unspecified lower limb, including hip**
  - **D21.21 Benign neoplasm of connective and other soft tissue of right lower limb, including hip**
  - **D21.22 Benign neoplasm of connective and other soft tissue of left lower limb, including hip**

D21.3 Benign neoplasm of connective and other soft tissue of thorax
Benign neoplasm of axilla
Benign neoplasm of diaphragm
Benign neoplasm of great vessels
Excludes1: *benign neoplasm of heart (D15.1)*
benign neoplasm of mediastinum (D15.2)
benign neoplasm of thymus (D15.0)

D21.4 Benign neoplasm of connective and other soft tissue of abdomen
Benign stromal tumors of abdomen

D21.5 Benign neoplasm of connective and other soft tissue of pelvis
Excludes1: *benign neoplasm of any uterine ligament (D28.2)*
uterine leiomyoma (D25.-)

D21.6 Benign neoplasm of connective and other soft tissue of trunk, unspecified
Benign neoplasm of connective and other soft tissue of back NOS

D21.9 Benign neoplasm of connective and other soft tissue, unspecified

D22 Melanocytic nevi

Includes: atypical nevus
blue hairy pigmented nevus
nevus NOS

D22.0 Melanocytic nevi of lip
+ **D22.1 Melanocytic nevi of eyelid, including canthus**
D22.10 Melanocytic nevi of unspecified eyelid, including canthus
+ **D22.11 Melanocytic nevi of right eyelid, including canthus**
D22.111 Melanocytic nevi of right upper eyelid, including canthus
D22.112 Melanocytic nevi of right lower eyelid, including canthus
+ **D22.12 Melanocytic nevi of left eyelid, including canthus**
D22.121 Melanocytic nevi of left upper eyelid, including canthus
D22.122 Melanocytic nevi of left lower eyelid, including canthus
+ **D22.2 Melanocytic nevi of ear and external auricular canal**
D22.20 Melanocytic nevi of unspecified ear and external auricular canal
D22.21 Melanocytic nevi of right ear and external auricular canal
D22.22 Melanocytic nevi of left ear and external auricular canal
+ **D22.3 Melanocytic nevi of other and unspecified parts of face**
D22.30 Melanocytic nevi of unspecified part of face
D22.39 Melanocytic nevi of other parts of face
D22.4 Melanocytic nevi of scalp and neck
D22.5 Melanocytic nevi of trunk
Melanocytic nevi of anal margin
Melanocytic nevi of anal skin
Melanocytic nevi of perianal skin
Melanocytic nevi of skin of breast
+ **D22.6 Melanocytic nevi of upper limb, including shoulder**
D22.60 Melanocytic nevi of unspecified upper limb, including shoulder
D22.61 Melanocytic nevi of right upper limb, including shoulder
D22.62 Melanocytic nevi of left upper limb, including shoulder
+ **D22.7 Melanocytic nevi of lower limb, including hip**
D22.70 Melanocytic nevi of unspecified lower limb, including hip
D22.71 Melanocytic nevi of right lower limb, including hip
D22.72 Melanocytic nevi of left lower limb, including hip
D22.9 Melanocytic nevi, unspecified

D23 Other benign neoplasms of skin

Includes: benign neoplasm of hair follicles
benign neoplasm of sebaceous glands
benign neoplasm of sweat glands

Excludes1: *benign lipomatous neoplasms of skin (D17.0-D17.3)*
Excludes2: *melanocytic nevi (D22.-)*

D23.0 Other benign neoplasm of skin of lip
Excludes1: *benign neoplasm of vermilion border of lip (D10.0)*
+ **D23.1 Other benign neoplasm of skin of eyelid, including canthus**
D23.10 Other benign neoplasm of skin of unspecified eyelid, including canthus
+ **D23.11 Other benign neoplasm of skin of right eyelid, including canthus**
D23.111 Other benign neoplasm of skin of right upper eyelid, including canthus
D23.112 Other benign neoplasm of skin of right lower eyelid, including canthus
+ **D23.12 Other benign neoplasm of skin of left eyelid, including canthus**
D23.121 Other benign neoplasm of skin of left upper eyelid, including canthus
D23.122 Other benign neoplasm of skin of left lower eyelid, including canthus
+ **D23.2 Other benign neoplasm of skin of ear and external auricular canal**
D23.20 Other benign neoplasm of skin of unspecified ear and external auricular canal
D23.21 Other benign neoplasm of skin of right ear and external auricular canal
D23.22 Other benign neoplasm of skin of left ear and external auricular canal
+ **D23.3 Other benign neoplasm of skin of other and unspecified parts of face**
D23.30 Other benign neoplasm of skin of unspecified part of face
D23.39 Other benign neoplasm of skin of other parts of face
D23.4 Other benign neoplasm of skin of scalp and neck
D23.5 Other benign neoplasm of skin of trunk
Other benign neoplasm of anal margin
Other benign neoplasm of anal skin
Other benign neoplasm of perianal skin
Other benign neoplasm of skin of breast
Excludes1: *benign neoplasm of anus NOS (D12.9)*
+ **D23.6 Other benign neoplasm of skin of upper limb, including shoulder**
D23.60 Other benign neoplasm of skin of unspecified upper limb, including shoulder
D23.61 Other benign neoplasm of skin of right upper limb, including shoulder
D23.62 Other benign neoplasm of skin of left upper limb, including shoulder
+ **D23.7 Other benign neoplasm of skin of lower limb, including hip**
D23.70 Other benign neoplasm of skin of unspecified lower limb, including hip
D23.71 Other benign neoplasm of skin of right lower limb, including hip
D23.72 Other benign neoplasm of skin of left lower limb, including hip
D23.9 Other benign neoplasm of skin, unspecified

D24 Benign neoplasm of breast

Includes: benign neoplasm of connective tissue of breast
benign neoplasm of soft parts of breast
fibroadenoma of breast

Excludes2: *adenofibrosis of breast (N60.2)*
benign cyst of breast (N60.-)
benign mammary dysplasia (N60.-)
benign neoplasm of skin of breast (D22.5, D23.5)
fibrocystic disease of breast (N60.-)

D24.1 Benign neoplasm of right breast
AHA CC: 1Q, 2017, 5-6
D24.2 Benign neoplasm of left breast
D24.9 Benign neoplasm of unspecified breast

D25 Leiomyoma of uterus

Includes: uterine fibroid
uterine fibromyoma
uterine myoma

♀ **D25.0 Submucous leiomyoma of uterus**
♀ **D25.1 Intramural leiomyoma of uterus**
Interstitial leiomyoma of uterus
♀ **D25.2 Subserosal leiomyoma of uterus**
Subperitoneal leiomyoma of uterus
♀ **D25.9 Leiomyoma of uterus, unspecified**

D26 Other benign neoplasms of uterus

♀ **D26.0 Other benign neoplasm of cervix uteri**
♀ **D26.1 Other benign neoplasm of corpus uteri**
♀ **D26.7 Other benign neoplasm of other parts of uterus**
♀ **D26.9 Other benign neoplasm of uterus, unspecified**

D27 Benign neoplasm of ovary

Use additional code to identify any functional activity.

Excludes2: *corpus albicans cyst (N83.2-)*
corpus luteum cyst (N83.1-)
endometrial cyst (N80.1)
follicular (atretic) cyst (N83.0-)
graafian follicle cyst (N83.0-)
ovarian cyst NEC (N83.2-)
ovarian retention cyst (N83.2-)

♀ **D27.0 Benign neoplasm of right ovary**
♀ **D27.1 Benign neoplasm of left ovary**
♀ **D27.9 Benign neoplasm of unspecified ovary**

D28 Benign neoplasm of other and unspecified female genital organs

Includes: adenomatous polyp
benign neoplasm of skin of female genital organs
benign teratoma

Excludes1: *epoophoron cyst (Q50.5)*
fimbrial cyst (Q50.4)
Gartner's duct cyst (Q52.4)
parovarian cyst (Q50.5)

♀ **D28.0 Benign neoplasm of vulva**
♀ **D28.1 Benign neoplasm of vagina**
♀ **D28.2 Benign neoplasm of uterine tubes and ligaments**
Benign neoplasm of fallopian tube
Benign neoplasm of uterine ligament (broad) (round)
♀ **D28.7 Benign neoplasm of other specified female genital organs**
♀ **D28.9 Benign neoplasm of female genital organ, unspecified**

D29 Benign neoplasm of male genital organs

Includes: benign neoplasm of skin of male genital organs

♂ **D29.0 Benign neoplasm of penis**
♂ **D29.1 Benign neoplasm of prostate**
Excludes1: *enlarged prostate (N40.-)*
\+ **D29.2 Benign neoplasm of testis**
Use additional code to identify any functional activity.
♂ **D29.20 Benign neoplasm of unspecified testis**
♂ **D29.21 Benign neoplasm of right testis**
♂ **D29.22 Benign neoplasm of left testis**
\+ **D29.3 Benign neoplasm of epididymis**
♂ **D29.30 Benign neoplasm of unspecified epididymis**
♂ **D29.31 Benign neoplasm of right epididymis**
♂ **D29.32 Benign neoplasm of left epididymis**
♂ **D29.4 Benign neoplasm of scrotum**
Benign neoplasm of skin of scrotum
♂ **D29.8 Benign neoplasm of other specified male genital organs**
Benign neoplasm of seminal vesicle
Benign neoplasm of spermatic cord
Benign neoplasm of tunica vaginalis
♂ **D29.9 Benign neoplasm of male genital organ, unspecified**

D30 Benign neoplasm of urinary organs

\+ **D30.0 Benign neoplasm of kidney**
Excludes1: *benign carcinoid tumor of the kidney (D3A.093)*
benign neoplasm of renal calyces (D30.1-)
benign neoplasm of renal pelvis (D30.1-)
D30.00 Benign neoplasm of unspecified kidney
D30.01 Benign neoplasm of right kidney
D30.02 Benign neoplasm of left kidney
\+ **D30.1 Benign neoplasm of renal pelvis**
D30.10 Benign neoplasm of unspecified renal pelvis
D30.11 Benign neoplasm of right renal pelvis
D30.12 Benign neoplasm of left renal pelvis
\+ **D30.2 Benign neoplasm of ureter**
Excludes1: *benign neoplasm of ureteric orifice of bladder (D30.3)*
D30.20 Benign neoplasm of unspecified ureter
D30.21 Benign neoplasm of right ureter
D30.22 Benign neoplasm of left ureter
D30.3 Benign neoplasm of bladder
Benign neoplasm of ureteric orifice of bladder
Benign neoplasm of urethral orifice of bladder
D30.4 Benign neoplasm of urethra
Excludes1: *benign neoplasm of urethral orifice of bladder (D30.3)*
D30.8 Benign neoplasm of other specified urinary organs
Benign neoplasm of paraurethral glands
D30.9 Benign neoplasm of urinary organ, unspecified
Benign neoplasm of urinary system NOS

D31 Benign neoplasm of eye and adnexa

Excludes1: *benign neoplasm of connective tissue of eyelid (D21.0)*
benign neoplasm of optic nerve (D33.3)
benign neoplasm of skin of eyelid (D22.1-, D23.1-)

\+ **D31.0 Benign neoplasm of conjunctiva**
D31.00 Benign neoplasm of unspecified conjunctiva
D31.01 Benign neoplasm of right conjunctiva
D31.02 Benign neoplasm of left conjunctiva
\+ **D31.1 Benign neoplasm of cornea**
D31.10 Benign neoplasm of unspecified cornea
D31.11 Benign neoplasm of right cornea
D31.12 Benign neoplasm of left cornea
\+ **D31.2 Benign neoplasm of retina**
Excludes1: *dark area on retina (D49.81)*
hemangioma of retina (D49.81)
neoplasm of unspecified behavior of retina and choroid (D49.81)
retinal freckle (D49.81)
D31.20 Benign neoplasm of unspecified retina
D31.21 Benign neoplasm of right retina
D31.22 Benign neoplasm of left retina
\+ **D31.3 Benign neoplasm of choroid**
D31.30 Benign neoplasm of unspecified choroid
D31.31 Benign neoplasm of right choroid
D31.32 Benign neoplasm of left choroid
\+ **D31.4 Benign neoplasm of ciliary body**
D31.40 Benign neoplasm of unspecified ciliary body
D31.41 Benign neoplasm of right ciliary body
D31.42 Benign neoplasm of left ciliary body
\+ **D31.5 Benign neoplasm of lacrimal gland and duct**
Benign neoplasm of lacrimal sac
Benign neoplasm of nasolacrimal duct
D31.50 Benign neoplasm of unspecified lacrimal gland and duct
D31.51 Benign neoplasm of right lacrimal gland and duct
D31.52 Benign neoplasm of left lacrimal gland and duct
\+ **D31.6 Benign neoplasm of unspecified site of orbit**
Benign neoplasm of connective tissue of orbit
Benign neoplasm of extraocular muscle
Benign neoplasm of peripheral nerves of orbit
Benign neoplasm of retrobulbar tissue
Benign neoplasm of retro-ocular tissue
Excludes1: *benign neoplasm of orbital bone (D16.4)*
D31.60 Benign neoplasm of unspecified site of unspecified orbit
D31.61 Benign neoplasm of unspecified site of right orbit
D31.62 Benign neoplasm of unspecified site of left orbit
\+ **D31.9 Benign neoplasm of unspecified part of eye**
Benign neoplasm of eyeball
D31.90 Benign neoplasm of unspecified part of unspecified eye
D31.91 Benign neoplasm of unspecified part of right eye
D31.92 Benign neoplasm of unspecified part of left eye

D32 Benign neoplasm of meninges

D32.0 Benign neoplasm of cerebral meninges
D32.1 Benign neoplasm of spinal meninges
D32.9 Benign neoplasm of meninges, unspecified
Meningioma NOS

D33 Benign neoplasm of brain and other parts of central nervous system

Excludes1: *angioma (D18.0-)*
benign neoplasm of meninges (D32.-)
benign neoplasm of peripheral nerves and autonomic nervous system (D36.1-)
hemangioma (D18.0-)
neurofibromatosis (Q85.0-)
retro-ocular benign neoplasm (D31.6-)

D33.0 Benign neoplasm of brain, supratentorial
Benign neoplasm of cerebral ventricle
Benign neoplasm of cerebrum
Benign neoplasm of frontal lobe
Benign neoplasm of occipital lobe
Benign neoplasm of parietal lobe
Benign neoplasm of temporal lobe
Excludes1: *benign neoplasm of fourth ventricle (D33.1)*
D33.1 Benign neoplasm of brain, infratentorial
Benign neoplasm of brain stem
Benign neoplasm of cerebellum
Benign neoplasm of fourth ventricle
D33.2 Benign neoplasm of brain, unspecified
D33.3 Benign neoplasm of cranial nerves
Benign neoplasm of olfactory bulb
D33.4 Benign neoplasm of spinal cord
D33.7 Benign neoplasm of other specified parts of central nervous system
D33.9 Benign neoplasm of central nervous system, unspecified
Benign neoplasm of nervous system (central) NOS

D34 Benign neoplasm of thyroid gland

Use additional code to identify any functional activity
Valid 3-character code, no further characters required

D35 Benign neoplasm of other and unspecified endocrine glands

Use additional code to identify any functional activity
Excludes1: *benign neoplasm of endocrine pancreas (D13.7)*
benign neoplasm of ovary (D27.-)
benign neoplasm of testis (D29.2.-)
benign neoplasm of thymus (D15.0)

+ **D35.0 Benign neoplasm of adrenal gland**
  - **D35.00 Benign neoplasm of unspecified adrenal gland**
  - **D35.01 Benign neoplasm of right adrenal gland**
  - **D35.02 Benign neoplasm of left adrenal gland**

D35.1 Benign neoplasm of parathyroid gland
D35.2 Benign neoplasm of pituitary gland
AHA CC: 3Q, 2014, 22-23
D35.3 Benign neoplasm of craniopharyngeal duct
D35.4 Benign neoplasm of pineal gland
D35.5 Benign neoplasm of carotid body
D35.6 Benign neoplasm of aortic body and other paraganglia
Benign tumor of glomus jugulare
D35.7 Benign neoplasm of other specified endocrine glands
D35.9 Benign neoplasm of endocrine gland, unspecified
Benign neoplasm of unspecified endocrine gland

D36 Benign neoplasm of other and unspecified sites

D36.0 Benign neoplasm of lymph nodes
Excludes1: *lymphangioma (D18.1)*

+ **D36.1 Benign neoplasm of peripheral nerves and autonomic nervous system**
Excludes1: *benign neoplasm of peripheral nerves of orbit (D31.6-)*
neurofibromatosis (Q85.0-)
  - **D36.10 Benign neoplasm of peripheral nerves and autonomic nervous system, unspecified**
  - **D36.11 Benign neoplasm of peripheral nerves and autonomic nervous system of face, head, and neck**
  - **D36.12 Benign neoplasm of peripheral nerves and autonomic nervous system, upper limb, including shoulder**
  - **D36.13 Benign neoplasm of peripheral nerves and autonomic nervous system of lower limb, including hip**
  - **D36.14 Benign neoplasm of peripheral nerves and autonomic nervous system of thorax**
  - **D36.15 Benign neoplasm of peripheral nerves and autonomic nervous system of abdomen**
  - **D36.16 Benign neoplasm of peripheral nerves and autonomic nervous system of pelvis**
  - **D36.17 Benign neoplasm of peripheral nerves and autonomic nervous system of trunk, unspecified**

D36.7 Benign neoplasm of other specified sites
Benign neoplasm of nose NOS
Benign neoplasm of back NOS
D36.9 Benign neoplasm, unspecified site

Benign neuroendocrine tumors (D3A)

D3A Benign neuroendocrine tumors

Code also any associated multiple endocrine neoplasia [MEN] syndromes (E31.2-)

Use additional code to identify any associated endocrine syndrome, such as:
carcinoid syndrome (E34.0)
Excludes2: *benign pancreatic islet cell tumors (D13.7)*

+ **D3A.0 Benign carcinoid tumors**
  - **D3A.00 Benign carcinoid tumor of unspecified site**
    Carcinoid tumor NOS
  - + **D3A.01 Benign carcinoid tumors of the small intestine**
    - **D3A.010 Benign carcinoid tumor of the duodenum**
    - **D3A.011 Benign carcinoid tumor of the jejunum**
    - **D3A.012 Benign carcinoid tumor of the ileum**
    - **D3A.019 Benign carcinoid tumor of the small intestine, unspecified portion**
  - + **D3A.02 Benign carcinoid tumors of the appendix, large intestine, and rectum**
    - **D3A.020 Benign carcinoid tumor of the appendix**
    - **D3A.021 Benign carcinoid tumor of the cecum**
    - **D3A.022 Benign carcinoid tumor of the ascending colon**
    - **D3A.023 Benign carcinoid tumor of the transverse colon**
    - **D3A.024 Benign carcinoid tumor of the descending colon**
    - **D3A.025 Benign carcinoid tumor of the sigmoid colon**
    - **D3A.026 Benign carcinoid tumor of the rectum**
    - **D3A.029 Benign carcinoid tumor of the large intestine, unspecified portion**
      Benign carcinoid tumor of the colon NOS
  - + **D3A.09 Benign carcinoid tumors of other sites**
    - **D3A.090 Benign carcinoid tumor of the bronchus and lung**
    - **D3A.091 Benign carcinoid tumor of the thymus**
    - **D3A.092 Benign carcinoid tumor of the stomach**
    - **D3A.093 Benign carcinoid tumor of the kidney**
    - **D3A.094 Benign carcinoid tumor of the foregut, unspecified**
    - **D3A.095 Benign carcinoid tumor of the midgut, unspecified**
    - **D3A.096 Benign carcinoid tumor of the hindgut, unspecified**
    - **D3A.098 Benign carcinoid tumors of other sites**

D3A.8 Other benign neuroendocrine tumors
Neuroendocrine tumor NOS

Neoplasms of uncertain behavior, polycythemia vera and myelodysplastic syndromes (D37-D48)

NOTE Categories D37-D44, and D48 classify by site neoplasms of uncertain behavior, i.e., histologic confirmation whether the neoplasm is malignant or benign cannot be made.

Excludes1: *neoplasms of unspecified behavior (D49.-)*

D37 Neoplasm of uncertain behavior of oral cavity and digestive organs

Excludes1: *stromal tumors of uncertain behavior of digestive system (D48.1)*

+ **D37.0 Neoplasm of uncertain behavior of lip, oral cavity and pharynx**
Excludes1: *neoplasm of uncertain behavior of aryepiglottic fold or interarytenoid fold, laryngeal aspect (D38.0)*
neoplasm of uncertain behavior of epiglottis NOS (D38.0)
neoplasm of uncertain behavior of skin of lip (D48.5)
neoplasm of uncertain behavior of suprahyoid portion of epiglottis (D38.0)
  - **D37.01 Neoplasm of uncertain behavior of lip**
    Neoplasm of uncertain behavior of vermilion border of lip
  - **D37.02 Neoplasm of uncertain behavior of tongue**
  - + **D37.03 Neoplasm of uncertain behavior of the major salivary glands**
    - **D37.030 Neoplasm of uncertain behavior of the parotid salivary glands**
    - **D37.031 Neoplasm of uncertain behavior of the sublingual salivary glands**
    - **D37.032 Neoplasm of uncertain behavior of the submandibular salivary glands**
    - **D37.039 Neoplasm of uncertain behavior of the major salivary glands, unspecified**

D37.04 Neoplasm of uncertain behavior of the minor salivary glands
Neoplasm of uncertain behavior of submucosal salivary glands of lip
Neoplasm of uncertain behavior of submucosal salivary glands of cheek
Neoplasm of uncertain behavior of submucosal salivary glands of hard palate
Neoplasm of uncertain behavior of submucosal salivary glands of soft palate

D37.05 Neoplasm of uncertain behavior of pharynx
Neoplasm of uncertain behavior of aryepiglottic fold of pharynx NOS
Neoplasm of uncertain behavior of hypopharyngeal aspect of aryepiglottic fold of pharynx
Neoplasm of uncertain behavior of marginal zone of aryepiglottic fold of pharynx

D37.09 Neoplasm of uncertain behavior of other specified sites of the oral cavity

D37.1 Neoplasm of uncertain behavior of stomach
D37.2 Neoplasm of uncertain behavior of small intestine
D37.3 Neoplasm of uncertain behavior of appendix
D37.4 Neoplasm of uncertain behavior of colon
D37.5 Neoplasm of uncertain behavior of rectum
Neoplasm of uncertain behavior of rectosigmoid junction

D37.6 Neoplasm of uncertain behavior of liver, gallbladder and bile ducts
Neoplasm of uncertain behavior of ampulla of Vater

D37.8 Neoplasm of uncertain behavior of other specified digestive organs
Neoplasm of uncertain behavior of anal canal
Neoplasm of uncertain behavior of anal sphincter
Neoplasm of uncertain behavior of anus NOS
Neoplasm of uncertain behavior of esophagus
Neoplasm of uncertain behavior of intestine NOS
Neoplasm of uncertain behavior of pancreas
Excludes1: *neoplasm of uncertain behavior of anal margin (D48.5)*
neoplasm of uncertain behavior of anal skin (D48.5)
neoplasm of uncertain behavior of perianal skin (D48.5)

D37.9 Neoplasm of uncertain behavior of digestive organ, unspecified

D38 Neoplasm of uncertain behavior of middle ear and respiratory and intrathoracic organs

Excludes1: *neoplasm of uncertain behavior of heart (D48.7)*

D38.0 Neoplasm of uncertain behavior of larynx
Neoplasm of uncertain behavior of aryepiglottic fold or interarytenoid fold, laryngeal aspect
Neoplasm of uncertain behavior of epiglottis (suprahyoid portion)
Excludes1: *neoplasm of uncertain behavior of aryepiglottic fold or interarytenoid fold NOS (D37.05)*
neoplasm of uncertain behavior of hypopharyngeal aspect of aryepiglottic fold (D37.05)
neoplasm of uncertain behavior of marginal zone of aryepiglottic fold (D37.05)

D38.1 Neoplasm of uncertain behavior of trachea, bronchus and lung
D38.2 Neoplasm of uncertain behavior of pleura
D38.3 Neoplasm of uncertain behavior of mediastinum
D38.4 Neoplasm of uncertain behavior of thymus
D38.5 Neoplasm of uncertain behavior of other respiratory organs
Neoplasm of uncertain behavior of accessory sinuses
Neoplasm of uncertain behavior of cartilage of nose
Neoplasm of uncertain behavior of middle ear
Neoplasm of uncertain behavior of nasal cavities
Excludes1: *neoplasm of uncertain behavior of ear (external) (skin) (D48.5)*
neoplasm of uncertain behavior of nose NOS (D48.7)
neoplasm of uncertain behavior of skin of nose (D48.5)

D38.6 Neoplasm of uncertain behavior of respiratory organ, unspecified

D39 Neoplasm of uncertain behavior of female genital organs

♀ **D39.0 Neoplasm of uncertain behavior of uterus**
\+ **D39.1 Neoplasm of uncertain behavior of ovary**
Use additional code to identify any functional activity.
♀ **D39.10 Neoplasm of uncertain behavior of unspecified ovary**
♀ **D39.11 Neoplasm of uncertain behavior of right ovary**
♀ **D39.12 Neoplasm of uncertain behavior of left ovary**
• ♀ **D39.2 Neoplasm of uncertain behavior of placenta**
Chorioadenoma destruens
Invasive hydatidiform mole
Malignant hydatidiform mole
Excludes1: *hydatidiform mole NOS (O01.9)*
♀ **D39.8 Neoplasm of uncertain behavior of other specified female genital organs**
Neoplasm of uncertain behavior of skin of female genital organs
♀ **D39.9 Neoplasm of uncertain behavior of female genital organ, unspecified**

D40 Neoplasm of uncertain behavior of male genital organs

♂ **D40.0 Neoplasm of uncertain behavior of prostate**
\+ **D40.1 Neoplasm of uncertain behavior of testis**
♂ **D40.10 Neoplasm of uncertain behavior of unspecified testis**
♂ **D40.11 Neoplasm of uncertain behavior of right testis**
♂ **D40.12 Neoplasm of uncertain behavior of left testis**
♂ **D40.8 Neoplasm of uncertain behavior of other specified male genital organs**
Neoplasm of uncertain behavior of skin of male genital organs
♂ **D40.9 Neoplasm of uncertain behavior of male genital organ, unspecified**

D41 Neoplasm of uncertain behavior of urinary organs

\+ **D41.0 Neoplasm of uncertain behavior of kidney**
Excludes1: *neoplasm of uncertain behavior of renal pelvis (D41.1-)*
D41.00 Neoplasm of uncertain behavior of unspecified kidney
D41.01 Neoplasm of uncertain behavior of right kidney
D41.02 Neoplasm of uncertain behavior of left kidney
\+ **D41.1 Neoplasm of uncertain behavior of renal pelvis**
D41.10 Neoplasm of uncertain behavior of unspecified renal pelvis
D41.11 Neoplasm of uncertain behavior of right renal pelvis
D41.12 Neoplasm of uncertain behavior of left renal pelvis
\+ **D41.2 Neoplasm of uncertain behavior of ureter**
D41.20 Neoplasm of uncertain behavior of unspecified ureter
D41.21 Neoplasm of uncertain behavior of right ureter
D41.22 Neoplasm of uncertain behavior of left ureter
D41.3 Neoplasm of uncertain behavior of urethra
D41.4 Neoplasm of uncertain behavior of bladder
D41.8 Neoplasm of uncertain behavior of other specified urinary organs
D41.9 Neoplasm of uncertain behavior of unspecified urinary organ

D42 Neoplasm of uncertain behavior of meninges

D42.0 Neoplasm of uncertain behavior of cerebral meninges
D42.1 Neoplasm of uncertain behavior of spinal meninges
D42.9 Neoplasm of uncertain behavior of meninges, unspecified

D43 Neoplasm of uncertain behavior of brain and central nervous system

Excludes1: *neoplasm of uncertain behavior of peripheral nerves and autonomic nervous system (D48.2)*

D43.0 Neoplasm of uncertain behavior of brain, supratentorial
Neoplasm of uncertain behavior of cerebral ventricle
Neoplasm of uncertain behavior of cerebrum
Neoplasm of uncertain behavior of frontal lobe
Neoplasm of uncertain behavior of occipital lobe
Neoplasm of uncertain behavior of parietal lobe
Neoplasm of uncertain behavior of temporal lobe
Excludes1: *neoplasm of uncertain behavior of fourth ventricle (D43.1)*

D43.1 Neoplasm of uncertain behavior of brain, infratentorial
Neoplasm of uncertain behavior of brain stem
Neoplasm of uncertain behavior of cerebellum
Neoplasm of uncertain behavior of fourth ventricle

D43.2 Neoplasm of uncertain behavior of brain, unspecified
D43.3 Neoplasm of uncertain behavior of cranial nerves
D43.4 Neoplasm of uncertain behavior of spinal cord
D43.8 Neoplasm of uncertain behavior of other specified parts of central nervous system
D43.9 Neoplasm of uncertain behavior of central nervous system, unspecified
Neoplasm of uncertain behavior of nervous system (central) NOS

D44 Neoplasm of uncertain behavior of endocrine glands
Excludes1: *multiple endocrine adenomatosis (E31.2-)*
multiple endocrine neoplasia (E31.2-)
neoplasm of uncertain behavior of endocrine pancreas (D37.8)
neoplasm of uncertain behavior of ovary (D39.1-)
neoplasm of uncertain behavior of testis (D40.1-)
neoplasm of uncertain behavior of thymus (D38.4)
D44.0 Neoplasm of uncertain behavior of thyroid gland
+ **D44.1 Neoplasm of uncertain behavior of adrenal gland**
Use additional code to identify any functional activity.
D44.10 Neoplasm of uncertain behavior of unspecified adrenal gland
D44.11 Neoplasm of uncertain behavior of right adrenal gland
D44.12 Neoplasm of uncertain behavior of left adrenal gland
D44.2 Neoplasm of uncertain behavior of parathyroid gland
D44.3 Neoplasm of uncertain behavior of pituitary gland
Use additional code to identify any functional activity.
D44.4 Neoplasm of uncertain behavior of craniopharyngeal duct
D44.5 Neoplasm of uncertain behavior of pineal gland
D44.6 Neoplasm of uncertain behavior of carotid body
D44.7 Neoplasm of uncertain behavior of aortic body and other paraganglia
AHA CC: 4Q, 2016, 26; 2Q, 2021, 7
D44.9 Neoplasm of uncertain behavior of unspecified endocrine gland

D45 Polycythemia vera
Excludes1: *familial polycythemia (D75.0)*
secondary polycythemia (D75.1)
Valid 3-character code, no further characters required

D46 Myelodysplastic syndromes
Use additional code for adverse effect, if applicable, to identify drug (T36-T50 with fifth or sixth character 5)
Excludes2: *drug-induced aplastic anemia (D61.1)*
D46.0 Refractory anemia without ring sideroblasts, so stated
Refractory anemia without sideroblasts, without excess of blasts
D46.1 Refractory anemia with ring sideroblasts
RARS
+ **D46.2 Refractory anemia with excess of blasts [RAEB]**
D46.20 Refractory anemia with excess of blasts, unspecified
RAEB NOS
D46.21 Refractory anemia with excess of blasts 1
RAEB 1
CC **D46.22 Refractory anemia with excess of blasts 2**
RAEB 2
D46.A Refractory cytopenia with multilineage dysplasia
D46.B Refractory cytopenia with multilineage dysplasia and ring sideroblasts
RCMD RS
CC **D46.C Myelodysplastic syndrome with isolated del(5q) chromosomal abnormality**
Myelodysplastic syndrome with 5q deletion
5q minus syndrome NOS
D46.4 Refractory anemia, unspecified
D46.Z Other myelodysplastic syndromes
Excludes1: *chronic myelomonocytic leukemia (C93.1-)*
D46.9 Myelodysplastic syndrome, unspecified
Myelodysplasia NOS

D47 Other neoplasms of uncertain behavior of lymphoid, hematopoietic and related tissue
D47.0 Mast cell neoplasms of uncertain behavior
Excludes1: *congenital cutaneous mastocytosis (Q82.2)*
histiocytic neoplasms of uncertain behavior (D47.Z9)
malignant mast cell neoplasm (C96.2-)
AHA CC: 4Q, 2017, 5
CC **D47.01 Cutaneous mastocytosis**
Diffuse cutaneous mastocytosis
Maculopapular cutaneous mastocytosis
Solitary mastocytoma
Telangiectasia macularis eruptiva perstans
Urticaria pigmentosa
Excludes1: *congenital (diffuse) (maculopapular) cutaneous mastocytosis (Q82.2)*
congenital urticaria pigmentosa (Q82.2)
extracutaneous mastocytoma (D47.09)
CC **D47.02 Systemic mastocytosis**
Indolent systemic mastocytosis
Isolated bone marrow mastocytosis
Smoldering systemic mastocytosis
Systemic mastocytosis, with an associated hematological non-mast cell lineage disease (SM-AHNMD)
Code also, if applicable, any associated hematological non-mast cell lineage disease, such as:
acute myeloid leukemia (C92.6-, C92.A-)
chronic myelomonocytic leukemia (C93.1-)
essential thrombocytosis (D47.3)
hypereosinophilic syndrome (D72.1)
myelodysplastic syndrome (D46.9)
myeloproliferative syndrome (D47.1)
non-Hodgkin lymphoma (C82-C85)
plasma cell myeloma (C90.0-)
polycythemia vera (D45)
Excludes1: *aggressive systemic mastocytosis (C96.21)*
mast cell leukemia (C94.3-)
CC **D47.09 Other mast cell neoplasms of uncertain behavior**
Extracutaneous mastocytoma
Mast cell tumor NOS
Mastocytoma NOS
Mastocytosis NOS
Excludes1: *malignant mast cell tumor (C96.2)*
mastocytosis (congenital) (cutaneous) (Q82.2)
CC **D47.1 Chronic myeloproliferative disease**
Chronic neutrophilic leukemia
Myeloproliferative disease, unspecified
Excludes1: *atypical chronic myeloid leukemia BCR/ABL-negative (C92.2-)*
chronic myeloid leukemia BCR/ABL-positive (C92.1-)
myelofibrosis NOS (D75.81)
myelophthisic anemia (D61.82)
myelophthisis (D61.82)
secondary myelofibrosis NOS (D75.81)
D47.2 Monoclonal gammopathy
Monoclonal gammopathy of undetermined significance [MGUS]
D47.3 Essential (hemorrhagic) thrombocythemia
Essential thrombocytosis
Idiopathic hemorrhagic thrombocythemia
Primary thrombocytosis
Excludes2: *reactive thrombocytosis (D75.838)*
secondary thrombocytosis (D75.838)
thrombocythemia NOS (D75.839)
thrombocytosis NOS (D75.839)
D47.4 Osteomyelofibrosis
Chronic idiopathic myelofibrosis
Myelofibrosis (idiopathic) (with myeloid metaplasia)
Myelosclerosis (megakaryocytic) with myeloid metaplasia
Secondary myelofibrosis in myeloproliferative disease
Excludes1: *acute myelofibrosis (C94.4-)*

+ **D47.Z Other specified neoplasms of uncertain behavior of lymphoid, hematopoietic and related tissue**

CC **D47.Z1 Post-transplant lymphoproliferative disorder (PTLD)**

Code first complications of transplanted organs and tissue (T86.-)

CC **D47.Z2 Castleman disease**

Code also, if applicable, human herpesvirus 8 infection (B10.89)

Excludes2: *Kaposi's sarcoma (C46.-)*

AHA CC: 4Q, 2016, 8

CC **D47.Z9 Other specified neoplasms of uncertain behavior of lymphoid, hematopoietic and related tissue**

Histiocytic tumors of uncertain behavior

CC **D47.9 Neoplasm of uncertain behavior of lymphoid, hematopoietic and related tissue, unspecified**

Lymphoproliferative disease NOS

D48 Neoplasm of uncertain behavior of other and unspecified sites

Excludes1: *neurofibromatosis (nonmalignant) (Q85.0-)*

D48.0 Neoplasm of uncertain behavior of bone and articular cartilage

Excludes1: *neoplasm of uncertain behavior of cartilage of ear (D48.1)*
neoplasm of uncertain behavior of cartilage of larynx (D38.0)
neoplasm of uncertain behavior of cartilage of nose (D38.5)
neoplasm of uncertain behavior of connective tissue of eyelid (D48.1)
neoplasm of uncertain behavior of synovia (D48.1)

D48.1 Neoplasm of uncertain behavior of connective and other soft tissue

Neoplasm of uncertain behavior of connective tissue of ear
Neoplasm of uncertain behavior of connective tissue of eyelid
Stromal tumors of uncertain behavior of digestive system

Excludes1: *neoplasm of uncertain behavior of articular cartilage (D48.0)*
neoplasm of uncertain behavior of cartilage of larynx (D38.0)
neoplasm of uncertain behavior of cartilage of nose (D38.5)
neoplasm of uncertain behavior of connective tissue of breast (D48.6-)

D48.2 Neoplasm of uncertain behavior of peripheral nerves and autonomic nervous system

Excludes1: *neoplasm of uncertain behavior of peripheral nerves of orbit (D48.7)*

D48.3 Neoplasm of uncertain behavior of retroperitoneum

D48.4 Neoplasm of uncertain behavior of peritoneum

D48.5 Neoplasm of uncertain behavior of skin

Neoplasm of uncertain behavior of anal margin
Neoplasm of uncertain behavior of anal skin
Neoplasm of uncertain behavior of perianal skin
Neoplasm of uncertain behavior of skin of breast

Excludes1: *neoplasm of uncertain behavior of anus NOS (D37.8)*
neoplasm of uncertain behavior of skin of genital organs (D39.8, D40.8)
neoplasm of uncertain behavior of vermilion border of lip (D37.0)

+ **D48.6 Neoplasm of uncertain behavior of breast**

Neoplasm of uncertain behavior of connective tissue of breast
Cystosarcoma phyllodes

Excludes1: *neoplasm of uncertain behavior of skin of breast (D48.5)*

D48.60 Neoplasm of uncertain behavior of unspecified breast

D48.61 Neoplasm of uncertain behavior of right breast

D48.62 Neoplasm of uncertain behavior of left breast

D48.7 Neoplasm of uncertain behavior of other specified sites

Neoplasm of uncertain behavior of eye
Neoplasm of uncertain behavior of heart
Neoplasm of uncertain behavior of peripheral nerves of orbit

Excludes1: *neoplasm of uncertain behavior of connective tissue (D48.1)*
neoplasm of uncertain behavior of skin of eyelid (D48.5)

D48.9 Neoplasm of uncertain behavior, unspecified

Neoplasms of unspecified behavior (D49)

D49 Neoplasms of unspecified behavior

NOTE Category D49 classifies by site neoplasms ofunspecified morphology and behavior. The term'mass', unless otherwise stated, is not to be regarded as a neoplastic growth.

Includes: 'growth' NOS
neoplasm NOS
new growth NOS
tumor NOS

Excludes1: *neoplasms of uncertain behavior (D37-D44, D48)*

D49.0 Neoplasm of unspecified behavior of digestive system

Excludes1: *neoplasm of unspecified behavior of margin of anus (D49.2)*
neoplasm of unspecified behavior of perianal skin (D49.2)
neoplasm of unspecified behavior of skin of anus (D49.2)

D49.1 Neoplasm of unspecified behavior of respiratory system

D49.2 Neoplasm of unspecified behavior of bone, soft tissue, and skin

Excludes1: *neoplasm of unspecified behavior of anal canal (D49.0)*
neoplasm of unspecified behavior of anus NOS (D49.0)
neoplasm of unspecified behavior of bone marrow (D49.89)
neoplasm of unspecified behavior of cartilage of larynx (D49.1)
neoplasm of unspecified behavior of cartilage of nose (D49.1)
neoplasm of unspecified behavior of connective tissue of breast (D49.3)
neoplasm of unspecified behavior of skin of genital organs (D49.59)
neoplasm of unspecified behavior of vermilion border of lip (D49.0)

D49.3 Neoplasm of unspecified behavior of breast

Excludes1: *neoplasm of unspecified behavior of skin of breast (D49.2)*

D49.4 Neoplasm of unspecified behavior of bladder

+ **D49.5 Neoplasm of unspecified behavior of other genitourinary organs**

AHA CC: 4Q, 2016, 9

+ **D49.51 Neoplasm of unspecified behavior of kidney**

D49.511 Neoplasm of unspecified behavior of right kidney

D49.512 Neoplasm of unspecified behavior of left kidney

D49.519 Neoplasm of unspecified behavior of unspecified kidney

D49.59 Neoplasm unspecified behavior of other genitourinary organ

D49.6 Neoplasm of unspecified behavior of brain

Excludes1: *neoplasm of unspecified behavior of cerebral meninges (D49.7)*
neoplasm of unspecified behavior of cranial nerves (D49.7)

D49.7 Neoplasm of unspecified behavior of endocrine glands and other parts of nervous system

Excludes1: *neoplasm of unspecified behavior of peripheral, sympathetic,andparasympatheticnerves and ganglia (D49.2)*

+ **D49.8 Neoplasm of unspecified behavior of other specified sites**

Excludes1: *neoplasm of unspecified behavior of eyelid (skin) (D49.2)*
neoplasm of unspecified behavior of eyelid cartilage (D49.2)
neoplasm of unspecified behavior of great vessels (D49.2)
neoplasm of unspecified behavior of optic nerve (D49.7)

D49.81 Neoplasm of unspecified behavior of retina and choroid

Dark area on retina
Retinal freckle

D49.89 Neoplasm of unspecified behavior of other specified sites

D49.9 Neoplasm of unspecified behavior of unspecified site

Chapter 3: Diseases of the Blood and Blood-Forming Organs and Certain Disorders Involving the Immune Mechanism (D50-D89)

Excludes2: *autoimmune disease (systemic) NOS (M35.9)*
certain conditions originating in the perinatal period (P00-P96)
complications of pregnancy, childbirth and the puerperium (O00-O9A)
congenital malformations, deformations and chromosomal abnormalities (Q00-Q99)
endocrine, nutritional and metabolic diseases (E00-E88)
human immunodeficiency virus [HIV] disease (B20)
injury, poisoning and certain other consequences of external causes (S00-T88)
neoplasms (C00-D49)
symptoms, signs and abnormal clinical and laboratory findings, not elsewhere classified (R00-R94)

This chapter contains the following category blocks:

D50-D53	Nutritional anemias
D55-D59	Hemolytic anemias
D60-D64	Aplastic and other anemias and other bone marrow failure syndromes
D65-D69	Coagulation defects, purpura and other hemorrhagic conditions
D70-D77	Other disorders of blood and blood-forming organs
D78	Intraoperative and postprocedural complications of the spleen
D80-D89	Certain disorders involving the immune mechanism

C. Chapter-Specific Coding Guidelines

In addition to general coding guidelines, there are guidelines for specific diagnoses and/or conditions in the classification. Unless otherwise indicated, these guidelines apply to all health care settings. Please refer to Section II for guidelines on the selection of principal diagnosis.

3. Chapter 3: Diseases of the Blood and Blood-Forming Organs and Certain Disorders Involving the Immune Mechanism (D50-D89)

Reserved for future guideline expansion

Nutritional anemias (D50-D53)

D50 Iron deficiency anemia

Includes: asiderotic anemia
hypochromic anemia

D50.0 Iron deficiency anemia secondary to blood loss (chronic)
Posthemorrhagic anemia (chronic)
Excludes1: *acute posthemorrhagic anemia (D62)*
congenital anemia from fetal blood loss (P61.3)

D50.1 Sideropenic dysphagia
Kelly-Paterson syndrome
Plummer-Vinson syndrome

D50.8 Other iron deficiency anemias
Iron deficiency anemia due to inadequate dietary iron intake

D50.9 Iron deficiency anemia, unspecified

D51 Vitamin B12 deficiency anemia

Excludes1: *vitamin B12 deficiency (E53.8)*

D51.0 Vitamin B12 deficiency anemia due to intrinsic factor deficiency
Addison anemia
Biermer anemia
Pernicious (congenital) anemia
Congenital intrinsic factor deficiency

D51.1 Vitamin B12 deficiency anemia due to selective vitamin B12 malabsorption with proteinuria
Imerslund (Gräsbeck) syndrome
Megaloblastic hereditary anemia

D51.2 Transcobalamin II deficiency

D51.3 Other dietary vitamin B12 deficiency anemia
Vegan anemia

D51.8 Other vitamin B12 deficiency anemias

D51.9 Vitamin B12 deficiency anemia, unspecified

D52 Folate deficiency anemia

Excludes1: *folate deficiency without anemia (E53.8)*

D52.0 Dietary folate deficiency anemia
Nutritional megaloblastic anemia

D52.1 Drug-induced folate deficiency anemia
Use additional code for adverse effect, if applicable, to identify drug (T36-T50 with fifth or sixth character 5)

D52.8 Other folate deficiency anemias

D52.9 Folate deficiency anemia, unspecified
Folic acid deficiency anemia NOS

D53 Other nutritional anemias

Includes: megaloblastic anemia unresponsive to vitamin B12 or folate therapy

D53.0 Protein deficiency anemia
Amino-acid deficiency anemia
Orotaciduric anemia
Excludes1: *Lesch-Nyhan syndrome (E79.1)*

D53.1 Other megaloblastic anemias, not elsewhere classified
Megaloblastic anemia NOS
Excludes1: *Di Guglielmo's disease (C94.0)*

D53.2 Scorbutic anemia
Excludes1: *scurvy (E54)*

D53.8 Other specified nutritional anemias
Anemia associated with deficiency of copper
Anemia associated with deficiency of molybdenum
Anemia associated with deficiency of zinc
Excludes1: *nutritional deficiencies without anemia, such as:*
copper deficiency NOS (E61.0)
molybdenum deficiency NOS (E61.5)
zinc deficiency NOS (E60)

D53.9 Nutritional anemia, unspecified
Simple chronic anemia
Excludes1: *anemia NOS (D64.9)*
AHA CC: 4Q, 2018, 88

Hemolytic anemias (D55-D59)

D55 Anemia due to enzyme disorders

Excludes1: *drug-induced enzyme deficiency anemia (D59.2)*

D55.0 Anemia due to glucose-6-phosphate dehydrogenase [G6PD] deficiency
Favism
G6PD deficiency anemia
Excludes1: *glucose-6-phosphate dehydrogenase (G6PD) deficiency without anemia (D75.A)*

D55.1 Anemia due to other disorders of glutathione metabolism
Anemia (due to) enzyme deficiencies, except G6PD, related to the hexose monophosphate [HMP] shunt pathway
Anemia (due to) hemolytic nonspherocytic (hereditary), type I

\+ **D55.2 Anemia due to disorders of glycolytic enzymes**
Excludes1: *disorders of glycolysis not associated with anemia (E74.81-)*

D55.21 Anemia due to pyruvate kinase deficiency
PK deficiency anemia
Pyruvate kinase deficiency anemia

D55.29 Anemia due to other disorders of glycolytic enzymes
Hexokinase deficiency anemia
Triose-phosphate isomerase deficiency anemia

D55.3 Anemia due to disorders of nucleotide metabolism

D55.8 Other anemias due to enzyme disorders

D55.9 Anemia due to enzyme disorder, unspecified

D56 Thalassemia

Excludes1: *sickle-cell thalassemia (D57.4-)*

D56.0 Alpha thalassemia
Alpha thalassemia major
Hemoglobin H Constant Spring
Hemoglobin H disease
Hydrops fetalis due to alpha thalassemia
Severe alpha thalassemia
Triple gene defect alpha thalassemia
Use additional code, if applicable, for hydrops fetalis due to alpha thalassemia (P56.99)
Excludes1: *alpha thalassemia trait or minor (D56.3)*
asymptomatic alpha thalassemia (D56.3)
hydrops fetalis due to isoimmunization (P56.0)
hydrops fetalis not due to immune hemolysis (P83.2)

D56.1 Beta thalassemia
Beta thalassemia major
Cooley's anemia
Homozygous beta thalassemia
Severe beta thalassemia
Thalassemia intermedia
Thalassemia major
Excludes1: *beta thalassemia minor (D56.3)*
beta thalassemia trait (D56.3)
delta-beta thalassemia (D56.2)
hemoglobin E-beta thalassemia (D56.5)
sickle-cell beta thalassemia (D57.4-)

D56.2 Delta-beta thalassemia
Homozygous delta-beta thalassemia
Excludes1: *delta-beta thalassemia minor (D56.3)*
delta-beta thalassemia trait (D56.3)

D56.3 Thalassemia minor
Alpha thalassemia minor
Alpha thalassemia silent carrier
Alpha thalassemia trait
Beta thalassemia minor
Beta thalassemia trait
Delta-beta thalassemia minor
Delta-beta thalassemia trait
Thalassemia trait NOS
Excludes1: *alpha thalassemia (D56.0)*
beta thalassemia (D56.1)
delta-beta thalassemia (D56.2)
hemoglobin E-beta thalassemia (D56.5)
sickle-cell trait (D57.3)

D56.4 Hereditary persistence of fetal hemoglobin [HPFH]

D56.5 Hemoglobin E-beta thalassemia
Excludes1: *beta thalassemia (D56.1)*
beta thalassemia minor (D56.3)
beta thalassemia trait (D56.3)
delta-beta thalassemia (D56.2)
delta-beta thalassemia trait (D56.3)
hemoglobin E disease (D58.2)
other hemoglobinopathies (D58.2)
sickle-cell beta thalassemia (D57.4-)

D56.8 Other thalassemias
Dominant thalassemia
Hemoglobin C thalassemia
Mixed thalassemia
Thalassemia with other hemoglobinopathy
Excludes1: *hemoglobin C disease (D58.2)*
hemoglobin E disease (D58.2)
other hemoglobinopathies (D58.2)
sickle-cell anemia (D57.-)
sickle-cell thalassemia (D57.4)

D56.9 Thalassemia, unspecified
Mediterranean anemia (with other hemoglobinopathy)

D57 Sickle-cell disorders
Use additional code for any associated fever (R50.81)
Excludes1: *other hemoglobinopathies (D58.-)*
AHA CC: 4Q, 2020, 6-7

\+ **D57.0 Hb-SS disease with crisis**
Sickle-cell disease with crisis
Hb-SS disease with vasoocclusive pain

MCC **D57.00 Hb-SS disease with crisis, unspecified**
Hb-SS disease with (painful) crisis NOS
Hb-SS disease with vasoocclusive pain NOS

MCC **D57.01 Hb-SS disease with acute chest syndrome**

MCC **D57.02 Hb-SS disease with splenic sequestration**

MCC **D57.03 Hb-SS disease with cerebral vascular involvement**
Code also, if applicable, cerebral infarction (I63.-)

MCC **D57.09 Hb-SS disease with crisis with other specified complication**
Use additional code to identify complications, such as:
cholelithiasis (K80.-)
priapism (N48.32)

D57.1 Sickle-cell disease without crisis
Hb-SS disease without crisis
Sickle-cell anemia NOS
Sickle-cell disease NOS
Sickle-cell disorder NOS

\+ **D57.2 Sickle-cell/Hb-C disease**
Hb-SC disease
Hb-S/Hb-C disease

D57.20 Sickle-cell/Hb-C disease without crisis

\+ **D57.21 Sickle-cell/Hb-C disease with crisis**

MCC **D57.211 Sickle-cell/Hb-C disease with acute chest syndrome**

MCC **D57.212 Sickle-cell/Hb-C disease with splenic sequestration**

MCC **D57.213 Sickle-cell/Hb-C disease with cerebral vascular involvement**
Code also, if applicable, cerebral infarction (I63.-)

MCC **D57.218 Sickle-cell/Hb-C disease with crisis with other specified complication**
Use additional code to identify complications, such as:
cholelithiasis (K80.-)
priapism (N48.32)

MCC **D57.219 Sickle-cell/Hb-C disease with crisis, unspecified**
Sickle-cell/Hb-C disease with crisis NOS
Sickle-cell/Hb-C disease with vasoocclusive pain NOS

D57.3 Sickle-cell trait
Hb-S trait
Heterozygous hemoglobin S

\+ **D57.4 Sickle-cell thalassemia**
Sickle-cell beta thalassemia
Thalassemia Hb-S disease

D57.40 Sickle-cell thalassemia without crisis
Microdrepanocytosis
Sickle-cell thalassemia NOS

\+ **D57.41 Sickle-cell thalassemia, unspecified, with crisis**
Sickle-cell thalassemia with (painful) crisis NOS
Sickle-cell thalassemia with vasoocclusive pain NOS

MCC **D57.411 Sickle-cell thalassemia, unspecified, with acute chest syndrome**

MCC **D57.412 Sickle-cell thalassemia, unspecified, with splenic sequestration**

MCC **D57.413 Sickle-cell thalassemia, unspecified, with cerebral vascular involvement**
Code also, if applicable, cerebral infarction (I63.-)

MCC **D57.418 Sickle-cell thalassemia, unspecified, with crisis with other specified complication**
Use additional code to identify complications, such as:
cholelithiasis (K80.-)
priapism (N48.32)

MCC **D57.419 Sickle-cell thalassemia, unspecified, with crisis**
Sickle-cell thalassemia with (painful) crisis NOS
Sickle-cell thalassemia with vasoocclusive pain NOS

D57.42 Sickle-cell thalassemia beta zero without crisis
HbS-beta zero without crisis
Sickle-cell beta zero without crisis

\+ **D57.43 Sickle-cell thalassemia beta zero with crisis**
HbS-beta zero with crisis
Sickle-cell beta zero with crisis

MCC **D57.431 Sickle-cell thalassemia beta zero with acute chest syndrome**
HbS-beta zero with acute chest syndrome
Sickle-cell beta zero with acute chest syndrome

MCC **D57.432 Sickle-cell thalassemia beta zero with splenic sequestration**
HbS-beta zero with splenic sequestration
Sickle-cell beta zero with splenic sequestration

MCC **D57.433 Sickle-cell thalassemia beta zero with cerebral vascular involvement**
HbS-beta zero with cerebral vascular involvement
Sickle-cell beta zero with cerebral vascular involvement
Code also, if applicable, cerebral infarction (I63.-)

MCC **D57.438 Sickle-cell thalassemia beta zero with crisis with other specified complication**
HbS-beta zero with other specified complication
Sickle-cell beta zero with other specified complication
Use additional code to identify complications, such as:
cholelithiasis (K80.-)
priapism (N48.32)

MCC **D57.439 Sickle-cell thalassemia beta zero with crisis, unspecified**
HbS-beta zero with other specified complication
Sickle-cell beta zero with crisis unspecified
Sickle-cell thalassemia beta zero with (painful) crisis NOS
Sickle-cell thalassemia beta zero with vasoocclusive pain NOS

D57.44 Sickle-cell thalassemia beta plus without crisis
HbS-beta plus without crisis
Sickle-cell beta plus without crisis

+ **D57.45 Sickle-cell thalassemia beta plus with crisis**
HbS-beta plus with crisis
Sickle-cell beta plus with crisis

MCC **D57.451 Sickle-cell thalassemia beta plus with acute chest syndrome**
HbS-beta plus with acute chest syndrome
Sickle-cell beta plus with acute chest syndrome

MCC **D57.452 Sickle-cell thalassemia beta plus with splenic sequestration**
HbS-beta plus with splenic sequestration
Sickle-cell beta plus with splenic sequestration

MCC **D57.453 Sickle-cell thalassemia beta plus with cerebral vascular involvement**
HbS-beta plus with cerebral vascular involvement
Sickle-cell beta plus with cerebral vascular involvement
Code also, if applicable, cerebral infarction (I63.-)

MCC **D57.458 Sickle-cell thalassemia beta plus with crisis with other specified complication**
HbS-beta plus with crisis with other specified complication
Sickle-cell beta plus with crisis with other specified complication
Use additional code to identify complications, such as:
cholelithiasis (K80.-)
priapism (N48.32)

MCC **D57.459 Sickle-cell thalassemia beta plus with crisis, unspecified**
HbS-beta plus with crisis with unspecified complication
Sickle-cell beta plus with crisis with unspecified complication
Sickle-cell thalassemia beta plus with (painful) crisis NOS
Sickle-cell thalassemia beta plus with vasoocclusive pain NOS

+ **D57.8 Other sickle-cell disorders**
Hb-SD disease
Hb-SE disease

D57.80 Other sickle-cell disorders without crisis

+ **D57.81 Other sickle-cell disorders with crisis**

MCC **D57.811 Other sickle-cell disorders with acute chest syndrome**

MCC **D57.812 Other sickle-cell disorders with splenic sequestration**

MCC **D57.813 Other sickle-cell disorders with cerebral vascular involvement**
Code also, if applicable, cerebral infarction (I63.-)

MCC **D57.818 Other sickle-cell disorders with crisis with other specified complication**
Use additional code to identify complications, such as:
cholelithiasis (K80.-)
priapism (N48.32)

MCC **D57.819 Other sickle-cell disorders with crisis, unspecified**
Other sickle-cell disorders with crisis NOS
Other sickle-cell disorders with vasoocclusive pain NOS

D58 Other hereditary hemolytic anemias

Excludes1: *hemolytic anemia of the newborn (P55.-)*

D58.0 Hereditary spherocytosis
Acholuric (familial) jaundice
Congenital (spherocytic) hemolytic icterus
Minkowski-Chauffard syndrome

D58.1 Hereditary elliptocytosis
Elliptocytosis (congenital)
Ovalocytosis (congenital) (hereditary)

D58.2 Other hemoglobinopathies
Abnormal hemoglobin NOS
Congenital Heinz body anemia
Hb-C disease
Hb-D disease
Hb-E disease
Hemoglobinopathy NOS
Unstable hemoglobin hemolytic disease
Excludes1: *familial polycythemia (D75.0)*
Hb-M disease (D74.0)
hemoglobin E-beta thalassemia (D56.5)
hereditary persistence of fetal hemoglobin [HPFH] (D56.4)
high-altitude polycythemia (D75.1)
methemoglobinemia (D74.-)
other hemoglobinopathies with thalassemia (D56.8)

CC **D58.8 Other specified hereditary hemolytic anemias**
Stomatocytosis

CC **D58.9 Hereditary hemolytic anemia, unspecified**

D59 Acquired hemolytic anemia

CC **D59.0 Drug-induced autoimmune hemolytic anemia**
Use additional code for adverse effect, if applicable, to identify drug (T36-T50 with fifth or sixth character 5)

+ **D59.1 Other autoimmune hemolytic anemias**
Excludes2: *Evans syndrome (D69.41)*
hemolytic disease of newborn (P55.-)
paroxysmal cold hemoglobinuria (D59.6)
AHA CC: 4Q, 2020, 7-8

CC **D59.10 Autoimmune hemolytic anemia, unspecified**

CC **D59.11 Warm autoimmune hemolytic anemia**
Warm type (primary) (secondary) (symptomatic) autoimmune hemolytic anemia
Warm type autoimmune hemolytic disease

CC **D59.12 Cold autoimmune hemolytic anemia**
Chronic cold hemagglutinin disease
Cold agglutinin disease
Cold agglutinin hemoglobinuria
Cold type (primary) (secondary) (symptomatic) autoimmune hemolytic anemia
Cold type autoimmune hemolytic disease

CC **D59.13 Mixed type autoimmune hemolytic anemia**
Mixed type autoimmune hemolytic disease
Mixed type, cold and warm, (primary) (secondary) (symptomatic) autoimmune hemolytic anemia

CC **D59.19 Other autoimmune hemolytic anemia**

CC **D59.2 Drug-induced nonautoimmune hemolytic anemia**
Drug-induced enzyme deficiency anemia
Use additional code for adverse effect, if applicable, to identify drug (T36-T50 with fifth or sixth character 5)

MCC **D59.3 Hemolytic-uremic syndrome**
Use additional code to identify associated:
E. coli infection (B96.2-)
Pneumococcal pneumonia (J13)
Shigella dysenteriae (A03.9)

CC **D59.4 Other nonautoimmune hemolytic anemias**
Mechanical hemolytic anemia
Microangiopathic hemolytic anemia
Toxic hemolytic anemia

D59.5 Paroxysmal nocturnal hemoglobinuria [Marchiafava-Micheli]
Excludes1: *hemoglobinuria NOS (R82.3)*

D59.6 Hemoglobinuria due to hemolysis from other external causes
Hemoglobinuria from exertion
March hemoglobinuria
Paroxysmal cold hemoglobinuria
Use additional code (Chapter 20) to identify external cause
Excludes1: *hemoglobinuria NOS (R82.3)*

D59.8 Other acquired hemolytic anemias

CC **D59.9 Acquired hemolytic anemia, unspecified**
Idiopathic hemolytic anemia, chronic

Aplastic and other anemias and other bone marrow failure syndromes (D60-D64)

D60 Acquired pure red cell aplasia [erythroblastopenia]
Includes: red cell aplasia (acquired) (adult) (with thymoma)
Excludes1: *congenital red cell aplasia (D61.01)*

MCC **D60.0 Chronic acquired pure red cell aplasia**
MCC **D60.1 Transient acquired pure red cell aplasia**
MCC **D60.8 Other acquired pure red cell aplasias**
MCC **D60.9 Acquired pure red cell aplasia, unspecified**

D61 Other aplastic anemias and other bone marrow failure syndromes
Excludes2: neutropenia (D70.-)

\+ **D61.0 Constitutional aplastic anemia**

CC **D61.01 Constitutional (pure) red blood cell aplasia**
Blackfan-Diamond syndrome
Congenital (pure) red cell aplasia
Familial hypoplastic anemia
Primary (pure) red cell aplasia
Red cell (pure) aplasia of infants
Excludes1: *acquired red cell aplasia (D60.9)*

CC **D61.09 Other constitutional aplastic anemia**
Fanconi's anemia
Pancytopenia with malformations

MCC **D61.1 Drug-induced aplastic anemia**
Use additional code for adverse effect, if applicable, to identify drug (T36-T50 with fifth or sixth character 5)

MCC **D61.2 Aplastic anemia due to other external agents**
Code first, if applicable, toxic effects of substances chiefly nonmedicinal as to source (T51-T65)

MCC **D61.3 Idiopathic aplastic anemia**

\+ **D61.8 Other specified aplastic anemias and other bone marrow failure syndromes**

\+ **D61.81 Pancytopenia**
Excludes1: *pancytopenia (due to) (with) aplastic anemia (D61.9)*
pancytopenia (due to) (with) bone marrow infiltration (D61.82)
pancytopenia (due to) (with) congenital (pure) red cell aplasia (D61.01)
pancytopenia (due to) (with) hairy cell leukemia (C91.4-)
pancytopenia (due to) (with) human immunodeficiency virus disease (B20.-)
pancytopenia (due to) (with) leukoerythroblastic anemia (D61.82)
pancytopenia (due to) (with) myeloproliferative disease (D47.1)
Excludes2: *pancytopenia (due to) (with) myelodysplastic syndromes (D46.-)*

MCC **D61.810 Antineoplastic chemotherapy induced pancytopenia**
Excludes2: *aplastic anemia due to antineoplastic chemotherapy (D61.1)*
AHA CC: 3Q, 2020, 22-23

MCC **D61.811 Other drug-induced pancytopenia**
Excludes2: *aplastic anemia due to drugs (D61.1)*

CC **D61.818 Other pancytopenia**
AHA CC: 1Q, 2019, 16-17

CC **D61.82 Myelophthisis**
Leukoerythroblastic anemia
Myelophthisic anemia
Panmyelophthisis
Code also the underlying disorder, such as:
malignant neoplasm of breast (C50.-)
tuberculosis (A15.-)
Excludes1: *idiopathic myelofibrosis (D47.1)*
myelofibrosis NOS (D75.81)
myelofibrosis with myeloid metaplasia (D47.4)
primary myelofibrosis (D47.1)
secondary myelofibrosis (D75.81)

MCC **D61.89 Other specified aplastic anemias and other bone marrow failure syndromes**

CC **D61.9 Aplastic anemia, unspecified**
Hypoplastic anemia NOS
Medullary hypoplasia

CC **D62 Acute posthemorrhagic anemia**
Excludes1: *anemia due to chronic blood loss (D50.0)*
blood loss anemia NOS (D50.0)
congenital anemia from fetal blood loss (P61.3)
AHA CC: 3Q, 2019, 11-12, 17
Valid 3-character code, no further characters required

D63 Anemia in chronic diseases classified elsewhere

D63.0 Anemia in neoplastic disease
Code first neoplasm (C00-D49)
Excludes1: *aplastic anemia due to antineoplastic chemotherapy (D61.1)*
Excludes2: *anemia due to antineoplastic chemotherapy (D64.81)*
Review coding guidelines C.2.c.1, C.2.c.2 and C.2.l.4

D63.1 Anemia in chronic kidney disease
Erythropoietin resistant anemia (EPO resistant anemia)
Code first underlying chronic kidney disease (CKD) (N18.-)

D63.8 Anemia in other chronic diseases classified elsewhere
Code first underlying disease, such as:
diphyllobothriasis (B70.0)
hookworm disease (B76.0-B76.9)
hypothyroidism (E00.0-E03.9)
malaria (B50.0-B54)
symptomatic late syphilis (A52.79)
tuberculosis (A18.89)

D64 Other anemias
Excludes1: *refractory anemia (D46.-)*
refractory anemia with excess blasts in transformation [RAEB T] (C92.0-)

D64.0 Hereditary sideroblastic anemia
Sex-linked hypochromic sideroblastic anemia

D64.1 Secondary sideroblastic anemia due to disease
Code first underlying disease

D64.2 Secondary sideroblastic anemia due to drugs and toxins
Code first poisoning due to drug or toxin, if applicable (T36-T65 with fifth or sixth character 1-4 or 6)

Use additional code for adverse effect, if applicable, to identify drug (T36-T50 with fifth or sixth character 5)

D64.3 Other sideroblastic anemias
Sideroblastic anemia NOS
Pyridoxine-responsive sideroblastic anemia NEC

D64.4 Congenital dyserythropoietic anemia
Dyshematopoietic anemia (congenital)
Excludes1: *Blackfan-Diamond syndrome (D61.01)*
Di Guglielmo's disease (C94.0)

+ **D64.8 Other specified anemias**

D64.81 Anemia due to antineoplastic chemotherapy
Antineoplastic chemotherapy induced anemia
Excludes2: *anemia in neoplastic disease (D63.0)*
aplastic anemia due to antineoplastic chemotherapy (D61.1)
AHA CC: 4Q, 2014, 22-23

D64.89 Other specified anemias
Infantile pseudoleukemia

D64.9 Anemia, unspecified
AHA CC: 4Q, 2018, 88

Coagulation defects, purpura and other hemorrhagic conditions (D65-D69)

MCC **D65 Disseminated intravascular coagulation [defibrination syndrome]**
Afibrinogenemia, acquired
Consumption coagulopathy
Diffuse or disseminated intravascular coagulation [DIC]
Fibrinolytic hemorrhage, acquired
Fibrinolytic purpura
Purpura fulminans
Excludes1: *disseminated intravascular coagulation (complicating):*
abortion or ectopic or molar pregnancy (O00-O07, O08.1)
in newborn (P60)
pregnancy, childbirth and the puerperium (O45.0, O46.0, O67.0, O72.3)
AHA CC: 1Q, 2021, 39
Valid 3-character code, no further characters required

MCC **D66 Hereditary factor VIII deficiency**
Classical hemophilia
Deficiency factor VIII (with functional defect)
Hemophilia NOS
Hemophilia A
Excludes1: *factor VIII deficiency with vascular defect (D68.0)*
Valid 3-character code, no further characters required

MCC **D67 Hereditary factor IX deficiency**
Christmas disease
Factor IX deficiency (with functional defect)
Hemophilia B
Plasma thromboplastin component [PTC] deficiency
Valid 3-character code, no further characters required

D68 Other coagulation defects
Excludes1: *abnormal coagulation profile (R79.1)*
coagulation defects complicating abortion or ectopic or molar pregnancy (O00-O07, O08.1)
coagulation defects complicating pregnancy, childbirth and the puerperium (O45.0, O46.0, O67.0, O72.3)

CC **D68.0 Von Willebrand's disease**
Angiohemophilia
Factor VIII deficiency with vascular defect
Vascular hemophilia
Excludes1: *capillary fragility (hereditary) (D69.8)*
factor VIII deficiency NOS (D66)
factor VIII deficiency with functional defect (D66)

CC **D68.1 Hereditary factor XI deficiency**
Hemophilia C
Plasma thromboplastin antecedent [PTA] deficiency
Rosenthal's disease

CC **D68.2 Hereditary deficiency of other clotting factors**
AC globulin deficiency
Congenital afibrinogenemia
Deficiency of factor I [fibrinogen]
Deficiency of factor II [prothrombin]
Deficiency of factor V [labile]
Deficiency of factor VII [stable]
Deficiency of factor X [Stuart-Prower]
Deficiency of factor XII [Hageman]
Deficiency of factor XIII [fibrin stabilizing]
Dysfibrinogenemia (congenital)
Hypoproconvertinemia
Owren's disease
Proaccelerin deficiency

+ **D68.3 Hemorrhagic disorder due to circulating anticoagulants**

+ **D68.31 Hemorrhagic disorder due to intrinsic circulating anticoagulants, antibodies, or inhibitors**

CC **D68.311 Acquired hemophilia**
Autoimmune hemophilia
Autoimmune inhibitors to clotting factors
Secondary hemophilia

CC **D68.312 Antiphospholipid antibody with hemorrhagic disorder**
Lupus anticoagulant (LAC) with hemorrhagic disorder
Systemic lupus erythematosus [SLE] inhibitor with hemorrhagic disorder
Excludes1: *antiphospholipid antibody, finding without diagnosis (R76.0)*
antiphospholipid antibody syndrome (D68.61)
antiphospholipid antibody with hypercoagulable state (D68.61)
lupus anticoagulant (LAC) finding without diagnosis (R76.0)
lupus anticoagulant (LAC) with hypercoagulable state (D68.62)
systemic lupus erythematosus [SLE] inhibitor finding without diagnosis (R76.0)
systemic lupus erythematosus [SLE] inhibitor with hypercoagulable state (D68.62)

CC **D68.318 Other hemorrhagic disorder due to intrinsic circulating anticoagulants, antibodies, or inhibitors**
Antithromboplastinemia
Antithromboplastinogenemia
Hemorrhagic disorder due to intrinsic increase in antithrombin
Hemorrhagic disorder due to intrinsic increase in anti-VIIIa
Hemorrhagic disorder due to intrinsic increase in anti-IXa
Hemorrhagic disorder due to intrinsic increase in anti-XIa

CC **D68.32 Hemorrhagic disorder due to extrinsic circulating anticoagulants**
Drug-induced hemorrhagic disorder
Hemorrhagic disorder due to increase in anti-IIa
Hemorrhagic disorder due to increase in anti-Xa
Hyperheparinemia
Use additional code for adverse effect, if applicable, to identify drug (T45.515, T45.525)
AHA CC: 1Q, 2016, 14-15; 1Q, 2021, 4-5

CC **D68.4 Acquired coagulation factor deficiency**
Deficiency of coagulation factor due to liver disease
Deficiency of coagulation factor due to vitamin K deficiency
Excludes1: *vitamin K deficiency of newborn (P53)*

+ **D68.5 Primary thrombophilia**
Primary hypercoagulable states
Excludes1: *antiphospholipid syndrome (D68.61)*
lupus anticoagulant (D68.62)
secondary activated protein C resistance (D68.69)
secondary antiphospholipid antibody syndrome (D68.69)
secondary lupus anticoagulant with hypercoagulable state (D68.69)
secondary systemic lupus erythematosus [SLE] inhibitor with hypercoagulable state (D68.69)
systemic lupus erythematosus [SLE] inhibitor finding without diagnosis (R76.0)
systemic lupus erythematosus [SLE] inhibitor with hemorrhagic disorder (D68.312)
thrombotic thrombocytopenic purpura (M31.19)

CC **D68.51 Activated protein C resistance**
Factor V Leiden mutation

CC **D68.52 Prothrombin gene mutation**

CC **D68.59 Other primary thrombophilia**
Antithrombin III deficiency
Hypercoagulable state NOS
Primary hypercoagulable state NEC
Primary thrombophilia NEC
Protein C deficiency
Protein S deficiency
Thrombophilia NOS
AHA CC: 2Q, 2021, 8-9

+ **D68.6 Other thrombophilia**
Other hypercoagulable states
Excludes1: *diffuse or disseminated intravascular coagulation [DIC] (D65)*
heparin induced thrombocytopenia (HIT) (D75.82)
hyperhomocysteinemia (E72.11)

CC **D68.61 Antiphospholipid syndrome**
Anticardiolipin syndrome
Antiphospholipid antibody syndrome
Excludes1: *anti-phospholipid antibody, finding without diagnosis (R76.0)*
anti-phospholipid antibody with hemorrhagic disorder (D68.312)
lupus anticoagulant syndrome (D68.62)

CC **D68.62 Lupus anticoagulant syndrome**
Lupus anticoagulant
Presence of systemic lupus erythematosus [SLE] inhibitor
Excludes1: *anticardiolipin syndrome (D68.61)*
antiphospholipid syndrome (D68.61)
lupus anticoagulant (LAC) finding without diagnosis (R76.0)
lupus anticoagulant (LAC) with hemorrhagic disorder (D68.312)

CC **D68.69 Other thrombophilia**
Hypercoagulable states NEC
Secondary hypercoagulable state NOS
AHA CC: 2Q, 2021, 8

CC **D68.8 Other specified coagulation defects**
Excludes1: *hemorrhagic disease of newborn (P53)*
AHA CC: 1Q, 2021, 39-40

CC **D68.9 Coagulation defect, unspecified**

D69 Purpura and other hemorrhagic conditions
Excludes1: *benign hypergammaglobulinemic purpura (D89.0)*
cryoglobulinemic purpura (D89.1)
essential (hemorrhagic) thrombocythemia (D47.3)
hemorrhagic thrombocythemia (D47.3)
purpura fulminans (D65)
thrombotic thrombocytopenic purpura (M31.19)
Waldenström hypergammaglobulinemic purpura (D89.0)

CC **D69.0 Allergic purpura**
Allergic vasculitis
Nonthrombocytopenic hemorrhagic purpura
Nonthrombocytopenic idiopathic purpura
Purpura anaphylactoid
Purpura Henoch(-Schönlein)
Purpura rheumatica
Vascular purpura
Excludes1: *thrombocytopenic hemorrhagic purpura (D69.3)*
AHA CC: 3Q, 2020, 26-27

CC **D69.1 Qualitative platelet defects**
Bernard-Soulier [giant platelet] syndrome
Glanzmann's disease
Grey platelet syndrome
Thromboasthenia (hemorrhagic) (hereditary)
Thrombocytopathy
Excludes1: *von Willebrand's disease (D68.0)*

D69.2 Other nonthrombocytopenic purpura
Purpura NOS
Purpura simplex
Senile purpura

CC **D69.3 Immune thrombocytopenic purpura**
Hemorrhagic (thrombocytopenic) purpura
Idiopathic thrombocytopenic purpura
Tidal platelet dysgenesis

+ **D69.4 Other primary thrombocytopenia**
Excludes1: *transient neonatal thrombocytopenia (P61.0)*
Wiskott-Aldrich syndrome (D82.0)

CC **D69.41 Evans syndrome**

CC **D69.42 Congenital and hereditary thrombocytopenia purpura**
Congenital thrombocytopenia
Hereditary thrombocytopenia
Code first congential or hereditary disorder, such as:
thrombocytopenia with absent radius (TAR syndrome) (Q87.2)

D69.49 Other primary thrombocytopenia
Megakaryocytic hypoplasia
Primary thrombocytopenia NOS

+ **D69.5 Secondary thrombocytopenia**
Excludes1: *heparin induced thrombocytopenia (HIT) (D75.82)*
transient thrombocytopenia of newborn (P61.0)

D69.51 Posttransfusion purpura
Posttransfusion purpura from whole blood (fresh) or blood products PTP

D69.59 Other secondary thrombocytopenia
AHA CC: 4Q, 2014, 22-23

D69.6 Thrombocytopenia, unspecified

D69.8 Other specified hemorrhagic conditions
Capillary fragility (hereditary)
Vascular pseudohemophilia

D69.9 Hemorrhagic condition, unspecified

Other disorders of blood and blood-forming organs (D70-D77)

D70 Neutropenia
Includes: agranulocytosis
decreased absolute neurophile count (ANC)
Use additional code for any associated:
fever (R50.81)
mucositis (J34.81, K12.3-, K92.81, N76.81)
Excludes1: *neutropenic splenomegaly (D73.81)*
transient neonatal neutropenia (P61.5)

D70.0 Congenital agranulocytosis
Congenital neutropenia
Infantile genetic agranulocytosis
Kostmann's disease

D70.1 Agranulocytosis secondary to cancer chemotherapy
Use additional code for adverse effect, if applicable, to identify drug (T45.1X5)

Code also underlying neoplasm
AHA CC: 4Q, 2014, 22-23

D70.2 Other drug-induced agranulocytosis
Use additional code for adverse effect, if applicable, to identify drug (T36-T50 with fifth or sixth character 5)

D70.3 Neutropenia due to infection

D70.4 Cyclic neutropenia
Cyclic hematopoiesis
Periodic neutropenia

D70.8 Other neutropenia

D70.9 Neutropenia, unspecified
AHA CC: 2Q, 2019, 24-26

D71 Functional disorders of polymorphonuclear neutrophils
Cell membrane receptor complex [CR3] defect
Chronic (childhood) granulomatous disease
Congenital dysphagocytosis
Progressive septic granulomatosis
Valid 3-character code, no further characters required

D72 Other disorders of white blood cells

Excludes1: *basophilia (D72.824)*
immunity disorders (D80-D89)
neutropenia (D70)
preleukemia (syndrome) (D46.9)

D72.0 Genetic anomalies of leukocytes
Alder (granulation) (granulocyte) anomaly
Alder syndrome
Hereditary leukocytic hypersegmentation
Hereditary leukocytic hyposegmentation
Hereditary leukomelanopathy
May-Hegglin (granulation) (granulocyte) anomaly
May-Hegglin syndrome
Pelger-Huët (granulation) (granulocyte) anomaly
Pelger-Huët syndrome
Excludes1: *Chédiak (-Steinbrinck)-Higashi syndrome (E70.330)*

+ **D72.1 Eosinophilia**
Excludes2: *Löffler's syndrome (J82.89)*
pulmonary eosinophilia (J82.-)
AHA CC: 4Q, 2020, 8-10

D72.10 Eosinophilia, unspecified
+ **D72.11 Hypereosinophilic syndrome [HES]**
D72.110 Idiopathic hypereosinophilic syndrome [IHES]
D72.111 Lymphocytic Variant Hypereosinophilic Syndrome [LHES]
Lymphocyte variant hypereosinophilia
Code also, if applicable, any associated lymphocytic neoplastic disorder
AHA CC: 4Q, 2020, 10
D72.118 Other hypereosinophilic syndrome
Episodic angioendema with eosinophilia
Gleich's syndrome
D72.119 Hypereosinophilic syndrome [HES], unspecified
D72.12 Drug rash with eosinophilia and systemic symptoms syndrome
DRESS syndrome
Use additional code for adverse effect, if applicable, to identify drug (T36-T50 with fifth or sixth character 5)
D72.18 Eosinophilia in diseases classified elsewhere
Code first underlying disease, such as:
chronic myelomonocytic leukemia (C93.1-)
D72.19 Other eosinophilia
Familial eosinophilia
Hereditary eosinophilia

+ **D72.8 Other specified disorders of white blood cells**
Excludes1: *leukemia (C91-C95)*

+ **D72.81 Decreased white blood cell count**
Excludes1: *neutropenia (D70.-)*
D72.810 Lymphocytopenia
Decreased lymphocytes
D72.818 Other decreased white blood cell count
Basophilic leukopenia
Eosinophilic leukopenia
Monocytopenia
Other decreased leukocytes
Plasmacytopenia
D72.819 Decreased white blood cell count, unspecified
Decreased leukocytes, unspecified
Leukocytopenia, unspecified
Leukopenia
Excludes1: *malignant leukopenia (D70.9)*

+ **D72.82 Elevated white blood cell count**
Excludes1: *eosinophilia (D72.1)*
D72.820 Lymphocytosis (symptomatic)
Elevated lymphocytes
D72.821 Monocytosis (symptomatic)
Excludes1: *infectious mononucleosis (B27.-)*
D72.822 Plasmacytosis
D72.823 Leukemoid reaction
Basophilic leukemoid reaction
Leukemoid reaction NOS
Lymphocytic leukemoid reaction
Monocytic leukemoid reaction
Myelocytic leukemoid reaction
Neutrophilic leukemoid reaction
D72.824 Basophilia
D72.825 Bandemia
Bandemia without diagnosis of specific infection
Excludes1: *confirmed infection - code to infection*
leukemia (C91.-, C92.-, C93.-, C94.-, C95.-)
D72.828 Other elevated white blood cell count
D72.829 Elevated white blood cell count, unspecified
Elevated leukocytes, unspecified
Leukocytosis, unspecified

D72.89 Other specified disorders of white blood cells
Abnormality of white blood cells NEC

D72.9 Disorder of white blood cells, unspecified
Abnormal leukocyte differential NOS

D73 Diseases of spleen

D73.0 Hyposplenism
Atrophy of spleen
Excludes1: *asplenia (congenital) (Q89.01)*
postsurgical absence of spleen (Z90.81)

D73.1 Hypersplenism
Excludes1: *neutropenic splenomegaly (D73.81)*
primary splenic neutropenia (D73.81)
splenitis, splenomegaly in late syphilis (A52.79)
splenitis, splenomegaly in tuberculosis (A18.85)
splenomegaly NOS (R16.1)
splenomegaly congenital (Q89.0)

D73.2 Chronic congestive splenomegaly
D73.3 Abscess of spleen
D73.4 Cyst of spleen
D73.5 Infarction of spleen
Splenic rupture, nontraumatic
Torsion of spleen
Excludes1: *rupture of spleen due to Plasmodium vivax malaria (B51.0)*
traumatic rupture of spleen (S36.03-)

+ **D73.8 Other diseases of spleen**
D73.81 Neutropenic splenomegaly
Werner-Schultz disease
D73.89 Other diseases of spleen
Fibrosis of spleen NOS
Perisplenitis
Splenitis NOS

D73.9 Disease of spleen, unspecified

D74 Methemoglobinemia

CC **D74.0 Congenital methemoglobinemia**
Congenital NADH-methemoglobin reductase deficiency
Hemoglobin-M [Hb-M] disease
Methemoglobinemia, hereditary

CC **D74.8 Other methemoglobinemias**
Acquired methemoglobinemia (with sulfhemoglobinemia)
Toxic methemoglobinemia

CC **D74.9 Methemoglobinemia, unspecified**

D75 Other and unspecified diseases of blood and blood-forming organs

Excludes2: *acute lymphadenitis (L04.-)*
chronic lymphadenitis (I88.1)
enlarged lymph nodes (R59.-)
hypergammaglobulinemia NOS (D89.2)
lymphadenitis NOS (I88.9)
mesenteric lymphadenitis (acute) (chronic) (I88.0)

D75.0 Familial erythrocytosis
Benign polycythemia
Familial polycythemia
Excludes1: *hereditary ovalocytosis (D58.1)*

D75.1 Secondary polycythemia
Acquired polycythemia
Emotional polycythemia
Erythrocytosis NOS
Hypoxemic polycythemia
Nephrogenous polycythemia
Polycythemia due to erythropoietin
Polycythemia due to fall in plasma volume
Polycythemia due to high altitude
Polycythemia due to stress
Polycythemia NOS
Relative polycythemia
Excludes1: *polycythemia neonatorum (P61.1)*
polycythemia vera (D45)

+ **D75.8 Other specified diseases of blood and blood-forming organs**
CC **D75.81 Myelofibrosis**
Myelofibrosis NOS
Secondary myelofibrosis NOS
Code first the underlying disorder, such as:
malignant neoplasm of breast (C50.-)
Use additional code, if applicable, for associated therapy-related myelodysplastic syndrome (D46.-)
Use additional code for adverse effect, if applicable, to identify drug (T45.1X5)
Excludes1: *acute myelofibrosis (C94.4-)*
idiopathic myelofibrosis (D47.1)
leukoerythroblastic anemia (D61.82)
myelofibrosis with myeloid metaplasia (D47.4)
myelophthisic anemia (D61.82)
myelophthisis (D61.82)
primary myelofibrosis (D47.1)
D75.82 Heparin induced thrombocytopenia (HIT)
+ **D75.83 Thrombocytosis**
Excludes2: *essential thrombocythemia (D47.3)*
D75.838 Other thrombocytosis
Reactive thrombocytosis
Secondary thrombocytosis
Code also underlying condition, if known and applicable
D75.839 Thrombocytosis, unspecified
Thrombocythemia NOS
Thrombocytosis NOS
D75.89 Other specified diseases of blood and blood-forming organs
D75.9 Disease of blood and blood-forming organs, unspecified
D75.A Glucose-6-phosphate dehydrogenase (G6PD) deficiency without anemia
Excludes1: *glucose-6-phosphate dehydrogenase (G6PD) deficiency with anemia (D55.0)*
AHA CC: 4Q, 2019, 4-5

D76 Other specified diseases with participation of lymphoreticular and reticulohistiocytic tissue
Excludes1: *(Abt-) Letterer-Siwe disease (C96.0)*
eosinophilic granuloma (C96.6)
Hand-Schüller-Christian disease (C96.5)
histiocytic medullary reticulosis (C96.9)
histiocytic sarcoma (C96.A)
histiocytosis X, multifocal (C96.5)
histiocytosis X, unifocal (C96.6)
Langerhans-cell histiocytosis, multifocal (C96.5)
Langerhans-cell histiocytosis NOS (C96.6)
Langerhans-cell histiocytosis, unifocal (C96.6)
leukemic reticuloendotheliosis (C91.4-)
lipomelanotic reticulosis (I89.8)
malignant histiocytosis (C96.A)
malignant reticulosis (C86.0)
nonlipid reticuloendotheliosis (C96.0)
CC **D76.1 Hemophagocytic lymphohistiocytosis**
Familial hemophagocytic reticulosis
Histiocytoses of mononuclear phagocytes
CC **D76.2 Hemophagocytic syndrome, infection-associated**
Use additional code to identify infectious agent or disease.
CC **D76.3 Other histiocytosis syndromes**
Reticulohistiocytoma (giant-cell)
Sinus histiocytosis with massive lymphadenopathy
Xanthogranuloma

D77 Other disorders of blood and blood-forming organs in diseases classified elsewhere
Code first underlying disease, such as:
amyloidosis (E85.-)
congenital early syphilis (A50.0)
echinococcosis (B67.0-B67.9)
malaria (B50.0-B54)
schistosomiasis [bilharziasis] (B65.0-B65.9)
vitamin C deficiency (E54)
Excludes1: *rupture of spleen due to Plasmodium vivax malaria (B51.0)*
splenitis, splenomegaly in late syphilis (A52.79)
splenitis, splenomegaly in tuberculosis (A18.85)
Valid 3-character code, no further characters required

Intraoperative and postprocedural complications of the spleen (D78)

D78 Intraoperative and postprocedural complications of the spleen
AHA CC: 4Q, 2016, 9-10
+ **D78.0 Intraoperative hemorrhage and hematoma of the spleen complicating a procedure**
Excludes1: *intraoperative hemorrhage and hematoma of the spleen due to accidental puncture or laceration during a procedure (D78.1-)*
CC **D78.01 Intraoperative hemorrhage and hematoma of the spleen complicating a procedure on the spleen**
CC **D78.02 Intraoperative hemorrhage and hematoma of the spleen complicating other procedure**
+ **D78.1 Accidental puncture and laceration of the spleen during a procedure**
CC **D78.11 Accidental puncture and laceration of the spleen during a procedure on the spleen**
CC **D78.12 Accidental puncture and laceration of the spleen during other procedure**
+ **D78.2 Postprocedural hemorrhage of the spleen following a procedure**
CC **D78.21 Postprocedural hemorrhage of the spleen following a procedure on the spleen**
CC **D78.22 Postprocedural hemorrhage of the spleen following other procedure**
+ **D78.3 Postprocedural hematoma and seroma of the spleen following a procedure**
CC **D78.31 Postprocedural hematoma of the spleen following a procedure on the spleen**
CC **D78.32 Postprocedural hematoma of the spleen following other procedure**
CC **D78.33 Postprocedural seroma of the spleen following a procedure on the spleen**
CC **D78.34 Postprocedural seroma of the spleen following other procedure**
+ **D78.8 Other intraoperative and postprocedural complications of the spleen**
Use additional code, if applicable, to further specify disorder
CC **D78.81 Other intraoperative complications of the spleen**
CC **D78.89 Other postprocedural complications of the spleen**

Certain disorders involving the immune mechanism (D80-D89)

Includes: defects in the complement system
immunodeficiency disorders, except human immunodeficiency virus [HIV] disease sarcoidosis
Excludes1: *autoimmune disease (systemic) NOS (M35.9)*
functional disorders of polymorphonuclear neutrophils (D71)
human immunodeficiency virus [HIV] disease (B20)

D80 Immunodeficiency with predominantly antibody defects
CC **D80.0 Hereditary hypogammaglobulinemia**
Autosomal recessive agammaglobulinemia (Swiss type)
X-linked agammaglobulinemia [Bruton] (with growth hormone deficiency)

CC **D80.1 Nonfamilial hypogammaglobulinemia**
Agammaglobulinemia with immunoglobulin-bearing B-lymphocytes
Common variable agammaglobulinemia [CVAgamma]
Hypogammaglobulinemia NOS
CC **D80.2 Selective deficiency of immunoglobulin A [IgA]**
CC **D80.3 Selective deficiency of immunoglobulin G [IgG] subclasses**
CC **D80.4 Selective deficiency of immunoglobulin M [IgM]**
CC **D80.5 Immunodeficiency with increased immunoglobulin M [IgM]**
CC **D80.6 Antibody deficiency with near-normal immunoglobulins or with hyperimmunoglobulinemia**
CC **D80.7 Transient hypogammaglobulinemia of infancy**
CC **D80.8 Other immunodeficiencies with predominantly antibody defects**
Kappa light chain deficiency
CC **D80.9 Immunodeficiency with predominantly antibody defects, unspecified**

D81 Combined immunodeficiencies
Excludes1: *autosomal recessive agammaglobulinemia (Swiss type) (D80.0)*
CC **D81.0 Severe combined immunodeficiency [SCID] with reticular dysgenesis**
CC **D81.1 Severe combined immunodeficiency [SCID] with low T- and B-cell numbers**
CC **D81.2 Severe combined immunodeficiency [SCID] with low or normal B-cell numbers**
+D81.3 Adenosine deaminase [ADA] deficiency
AHA CC: 4Q, 2019, 5-6
CC **D81.30 Adenosine deaminase deficiency, unspecified**
ADA deficiency NOS
CC **D81.31 Severe combined immunodeficiency due to adenosine deaminase deficiency**
ADA deficiency with SCID
Adenosine deaminase [ADA] deficiency with severe combined immunodeficiency
CC **D81.32 Adenosine deaminase 2 deficiency**
ADA2 deficiency
Adenosine deaminase deficiency type 2
Code also, if applicable, any associated manifestations, such as:
polyarteritis nodosa (M30.0)
stroke (I63.-)
CC **D81.39 Other adenosine deaminase deficiency**
Adenosine deaminase [ADA] deficiency type 1, NOS
Adenosine deaminase [ADA] deficiency type 1, without SCID
Adenosine deaminase [ADA] deficiency type 1, without severe combined immunodeficiency
Partial ADA deficiency (type 1)
Partial adenosine deaminase deficiency (type 1)
CC **D81.4 Nezelof's syndrome**
CC **D81.5 Purine nucleoside phosphorylase [PNP] deficiency**
CC **D81.6 Major histocompatibility complex class I deficiency**
Bare lymphocyte syndrome
CC **D81.7 Major histocompatibility complex class II deficiency**
+ D81.8 Other combined immunodeficiencies
+ D81.81 Biotin-dependent carboxylase deficiency
Multiple carboxylase deficiency
Excludes1: *biotin-dependent carboxylase deficiency due to dietary deficiency of biotin (E53.8)*
D81.810 Biotinidase deficiency
D81.818 Other biotin-dependent carboxylase deficiency
Holocarboxylase synthetase deficiency
Other multiple carboxylase deficiency
D81.819 Biotin-dependent carboxylase deficiency, unspecified
Multiple carboxylase deficiency, unspecified
CC **D81.89 Other combined immunodeficiencies**
CC **D81.9 Combined immunodeficiency, unspecified**
Severe combined immunodeficiency disorder [SCID] NOS

D82 Immunodeficiency associated with other major defects
Excludes1: *ataxia telangiectasia [Louis-Bar] (G11.3)*
CC **D82.0 Wiskott-Aldrich syndrome**
Immunodeficiency with thrombocytopenia and eczema
CC **D82.1 Di George's syndrome**
Pharyngeal pouch syndrome
Thymic alymphoplasia
Thymic aplasia or hypoplasia with immunodeficiency
AHA CC: 3Q, 2019, 14-15
D82.2 Immunodeficiency with short-limbed stature
D82.3 Immunodeficiency following hereditary defective response to Epstein-Barr virus
X-linked lymphoproliferative disease
D82.4 Hyperimmunoglobulin E [IgE] syndrome
D82.8 Immunodeficiency associated with other specified major defects
D82.9 Immunodeficiency associated with major defect, unspecified

D83 Common variable immunodeficiency
CC **D83.0 Common variable immunodeficiency with predominant abnormalities of B-cell numbers and function**
CC **D83.1 Common variable immunodeficiency with predominant immunoregulatory T-cell disorders**
CC **D83.2 Common variable immunodeficiency with autoantibodies to B- or T-cells**
CC **D83.8 Other common variable immunodeficiencies**
CC **D83.9 Common variable immunodeficiency, unspecified**

D84 Other immunodeficiencies
D84.0 Lymphocyte function antigen-1 [LFA-1] defect
D84.1 Defects in the complement system
C1 esterase inhibitor [C1-INH] deficiency
+ D84.8 Other specified immunodeficiencies
AHA CC: 4Q, 2020, 10-11
CC **D84.81 Immunodeficiency due to conditions classified elsewhere**
Code first underlying condition, such as:
chromosomal abnormalities (Q90-Q99)
diabetes mellitus (E08-E13)
malignant neoplasms (C00-C96)
Excludes1: *certain disorders involving the immune mechanism (D80-D83, D84.0, D84.1, D84.9)*
human immunodeficiency virus [HIV] disease (B20)
AHA CC: 1Q, 2021, 52
+ D84.82 Immunodeficiency due to drugs and external causes
CC **D84.821 Immunodeficiency due to drugs**
Immunodeficiency due to (current or past) medication
Use additional code for adverse effect if applicable, to identify adverse effect of drug (T36-T50 with fifth or sixth character 5)
Use additional code, if applicable, for associated long term (current) drug therapy drug or medication such as:
long term (current) drug therapy systemic steroids (Z79.52)
other long term (current) drug therapy (Z79.899)
AHA CC: 4Q, 2020, 11-12
CC **D84.822 Immunodeficiency due to external causes**
Code also, if applicable, radiological procedure and radiotherapy (Y84.2)
Use additional code for external cause such as:
exposure to ionizing radiation (W88)
CC **D84.89 Other immunodeficiencies**
CC **D84.9 Immunodeficiency, unspecified**
Immunocompromised NOS
Immunodeficient NOS
Immunosuppressed NOS

D86 Sarcoidosis

D86.0 Sarcoidosis of lung

D86.1 Sarcoidosis of lymph nodes

D86.2 Sarcoidosis of lung with sarcoidosis of lymph nodes

D86.3 Sarcoidosis of skin

+ **D86.8 Sarcoidosis of other sites**

D86.81 Sarcoid meningitis

D86.82 Multiple cranial nerve palsies in sarcoidosis

D86.83 Sarcoid iridocyclitis

D86.84 Sarcoid pyelonephritis

Tubulo-interstitial nephropathy in sarcoidosis

D86.85 Sarcoid myocarditis

D86.86 Sarcoid arthropathy

Polyarthritis in sarcoidosis

D86.87 Sarcoid myositis

D86.89 Sarcoidosis of other sites

Hepatic granuloma

Uveoparotid fever [Heerfordt]

D86.9 Sarcoidosis, unspecified

D89 Other disorders involving the immune mechanism, not elsewhere classified

Excludes1: *hyperglobulinemia NOS (R77.1)*
monoclonal gammopathy (of undetermined significance) (D47.2)

Excludes2: *transplant failure and rejection (T86.-)*

D89.0 Polyclonal hypergammaglobulinemia

Benign hypergammaglobulinemic purpura

Polyclonal gammopathy NOS

D89.1 Cryoglobulinemia

Cryoglobulinemic purpura
Cryoglobulinemic vasculitis
Essential cryoglobulinemia
Idiopathic cryoglobulinemia
Mixed cryoglobulinemia
Primary cryoglobulinemia
Secondary cryoglobulinemia

D89.2 Hypergammaglobulinemia, unspecified

D89.3 Immune reconstitution syndrome

Immune reconstitution inflammatory syndrome [IRIS]

Use additional code for adverse effect, if applicable, to identify drug (T36-T50 with fifth or sixth character 5)

Add the following new codes after D89.3.

+ **D89.4 Mast cell activation syndrome and related disorders**

Excludes1: *aggressive systemic mastocytosis (C96.21)*
congenital cutaneous mastocytosis (Q82.2)
(indolent) systemic mastocytosis (D47.02)
malignant mast cell neoplasm (C96.2-)
malignant mastocytoma (C96.29)
mast cell sarcoma (C96.22)
mastocytoma NOS *(D47.09)*
(non-congenital) cutaneous mastocytosis (D47.01)
other mast cell neoplasms of uncertain behavior (D47.09)
systemic mastocytosis associated with a clonal hematologic non-mast cell lineage disease (SM-AHNMD) (D47.02)

AHA CC: 4Q, 2016, 11

D89.40 Mast cell activation, unspecified

Mast cell activation disorder, unspecified
Mast cell activation syndrome, NOS

D89.41 Monoclonal mast cell activation syndrome

D89.42 Idiopathic mast cell activation syndrome

D89.43 Secondary mast cell activation

Secondary mast cell activation syndrome

Code also underlying etiology, if known

D89.44 Hereditary alpha tryptasemia

Use additional code, if applicable, for:
allergy status, other than to drugs and biological substances (Z91.0-)
personal history of anaphylaxis (Z87.892)

D89.49 Other mast cell activation disorder

Other mast cell activation syndrome

+ **D89.8 Other specified disorders involving the immune mechanism, not elsewhere classified**

+ **D89.81 Graft-versus-host disease**

Code first underlying cause, such as:
complications of transplanted organs and tissues (T86.-)
complications of blood transfusion (T80.89)

Use additional code to identify associated manifestations, such as:
desquamative dermatitis (L30.8)
diarrhea (R19.7)
elevated bilirubin (R17)
hair loss (L65.9)

CC **D89.810 Acute graft-versus-host disease**

CC **D89.811 Chronic graft-versus-host disease**

CC **D89.812 Acute on chronic graft-versus-host disease**

CC **D89.813 Graft-versus-host disease, unspecified**

D89.82 Autoimmune lymphoproliferative syndrome [ALPS]

+ **D89.83 Cytokine release syndrome**

Code first underlying cause, such as:
complications following infusion, transfusion and therapeutic injection (T80.89-)
complications of transplanted organs and tissues (T86.-)

Use additional code to identify associated manifestations

AHA CC: 4Q, 2020, 12-13

D89.831 Cytokine release syndrome, grade 1

D89.832 Cytokine release syndrome, grade 2

AHA CC: 4Q, 2020, 14-15

CC **D89.833 Cytokine release syndrome, grade 3**

AHA CC: 4Q, 2020, 14

CC **D89.834 Cytokine release syndrome, grade 4**

CC **D89.835 Cytokine release syndrome, grade 5**

D89.839 Cytokine release syndrome, grade unspecified

D89.89 Other specified disorders involving the immune mechanism, not elsewhere classified

Excludes1: *human immunodeficiency virus disease (B20)*

AHA CC: 4Q, 2017, 109

D89.9 Disorder involving the immune mechanism, unspecified

Immune disease NOS

AHA CC: 3Q, 2015, 22

Chapter 4: Endocrine, Nutritional and Metabolic Disease (E00-E89)

NOTE All neoplasms, whether functionally active or not, are classified in Chapter 2. Appropriate codes in this chapter (i.e. E05.8, E07.0, E16-E31, E34.-) may be used as additional codes to indicate either functional activity by neoplasms and ectopic endocrine tissue or hyperfunction and hypofunction of endocrine glands associated with neoplasms and other conditions classified elsewhere.

Excludes1: *transitory endocrine and metabolic disorders specific to newborn (P70-P74)*

This chapter contains the following category blocks:

E00-E07	Disorders of thyroid gland
E08-E13	Diabetes mellitus
E15-E16	Other disorders of glucose regulation and pancreatic internal secretion
E20-E35	Disorders of other endocrine glands
E36	Intraoperative complications of endocrine system
E40-E46	Malnutrition
E50-E64	Other nutritional deficiencies
E65-E68	Overweight, obesity and other hyperalimentation
E70-E88	Metabolic disorders
E89	Postprocedural endocrine and metabolic complications and disorders, not elsewhere classified

C. Chapter-Specific Coding Guidelines

In addition to general coding guidelines, there are guidelines for specific diagnoses and/or conditions in the classification. Unless otherwise indicated, these guidelines apply to all health care settings. Please refer to Section II for guidelines on the selection of principal diagnosis.

4. Chapter 4: Endocrine, Nutritional and Metabolic Diseases (E00-E89)

a. Diabetes mellitus

The diabetes mellitus codes are combination codes that include the type of diabetes mellitus, the body system affected, and the complications affecting that body system. As many codes within a particular category as are necessary to describe all of the complications of the disease may be used. They should be sequenced based on the reason for a particular encounter. Assign as many codes from categories E08 – E13 as needed to identify all of the associated conditions that the patient has.

1) Type of diabetes

The age of a patient is not the sole determining factor, though most type 1 diabetics develop the condition before reaching puberty. For this reason type 1 diabetes mellitus is also referred to as juvenile diabetes.

2) Type of diabetes mellitus not documented

If the type of diabetes mellitus is not documented in the medical record the default is E11.-, Type 2 diabetes mellitus.

3) Diabetes mellitus and the use of insulin and oral hypoglycemics

If the documentation in a medical record does not indicate the type of diabetes but does indicate that the patient uses insulin, code E11-, Type 2 diabetes mellitus, should be assigned. **Additional** code**(s)** should be assigned from category Z79 to identify the long-term (current) use of insulin, oral hypoglycemic drugs, **or injectable non-insulin antidiabetic, as follows:**

If the patient is treated with both oral medications and insulin, **both code Z79.4, Long term (current) use of insulin, and code Z79.84, Long term (current) use of oral hypoglycemic drugs,** should be assigned. If the patient is treated with both insulin and an injectable non-insulin antidiabetic drug, assign codes Z79.4, Long-term (current) use of insulin, and Z79.899, Other long term (current) drug therapy. If the patient is treated with both oral hypoglycemic drugs and an injectable non-insulin antidiabetic drug, assign codes Z79.84, Long-term (current) use of oral hypoglycemic drugs, and Z79.899, Other long-term (current) drug therapy. Code Z79.4 should not be assigned if insulin is given temporarily to bring a type 2 patient's blood sugar under control during an encounter.

4) Diabetes mellitus in pregnancy and gestational diabetes

See Section I.C.15. Diabetes mellitus in pregnancy.

See Section I.C.15. Gestational (pregnancy induced) diabetes

5) Complications due to insulin pump malfunction

(a) Underdose of insulin due to insulin pump failure

An underdose of insulin due to an insulin pump failure should be assigned to a code from subcategory T85.6, Mechanical complication of other specified internal and external prosthetic devices, implants and grafts, that specifies the type of pump malfunction, as the principal or first-listed code, followed by code T38.3x6-, Underdosing of insulin and oral hypoglycemic [antidiabetic] drugs. Additional codes for the type of diabetes mellitus and any associated complications due to the underdosing should also be assigned.

(b) Overdose of insulin due to insulin pump failure

The principal or first-listed code for an encounter due to an insulin pump malfunction resulting in an overdose of insulin, should also be T85.6-, Mechanical complication of other specified internal and external prosthetic devices, implants and grafts, followed by code T38.3x1-, Poisoning by insulin and oral hypoglycemic [antidiabetic] drugs, accidental (unintentional).

6) Secondary diabetes mellitus

Codes under categories E08, Diabetes mellitus due to underlying condition, E09, Drug or chemical induced diabetes mellitus, and E13, Other specified diabetes mellitus, identify complications/manifestations associated with secondary diabetes mellitus. Secondary diabetes is always caused by another condition or event (e.g., cystic fibrosis, malignant neoplasm of pancreas, pancreatectomy, adverse effect of drug, or poisoning).

(a) Secondary diabetes mellitus and the use of insulin or *oral* hypoglycemic drugs

For patients with secondary diabetes mellitus who routinely use insulin or oral hypoglycemic drugs, **or injectable non-insulin drugs,** an additional code(s) from category Z79 should be assigned to identify the long-term (current) use of insulin, oral hypoglycemic drugs **or non-injectable non-insulin drugs as follows:** If the patient is treated with both oral medications and insulin, **both code Z79.4, Long term (current) use of insulin, and code Z79.84, Long term (current) use of oral hypoglycemic drugs,** should be assigned. If the patient is treated with both insulin and an injectable non-insulin antidiabetic drug, assign codes Z79.4, Long-term (current) use of insulin, and Z79.899, Other long term (current) drug therapy. If the patient is treated with both oral hypoglycemic drugs and an injectable non-insulin antidiabetic drug, assign codes Z79.84, Long-term (current) use of oral hypoglycemic drugs, and Z79.899, Other long-term (current) drug therapy. Code Z79.4 should not be assigned if insulin is given temporarily to bring a secondary diabetic patient's blood sugar under control during an encounter.

(b) Assigning and sequencing secondary diabetes codes and its causes

The sequencing of the secondary diabetes codes in relationship to codes for the cause of the diabetes is based on the Tabular List instructions for categories E08, E09 and E13.

(i) Secondary diabetes mellitus due to pancreatectomy

For postpancreatectomy diabetes mellitus (lack of insulin due to the surgical removal of all or part of the pancreas), assign code E89.1, Postprocedural hypoinsulinemia. Assign a code from category E13 and a code from subcategory Z90.41-, Acquired absence of pancreas, as additional codes.

(ii) Secondary diabetes due to drugs

Secondary diabetes may be caused by an adverse effect of correctly administered medications, poisoning or sequela of poisoning.

See section I.C.19.e for coding of adverse effects and poisoning, and section I.C.20 for external cause code reporting.

Disorders of thyroid gland (E00-E07)

E00 Congenital iodine-deficiency syndrome

Use additional code (F70-F79) to identify associated intellectual disabilities.

Excludes1: *subclinical iodine-deficiency hypothyroidism (E02)*

E00.0 Congenital iodine-deficiency syndrome, neurological type
Endemic cretinism, neurological type

E00.1 Congenital iodine-deficiency syndrome, myxedematous type
Endemic hypothyroid cretinism
Endemic cretinism, myxedematous type

E00.2 Congenital iodine-deficiency syndrome, mixed type
Endemic cretinism, mixed type

E00.9 Congenital iodine-deficiency syndrome, unspecified
Congenital iodine-deficiency hypothyroidism NOS
Endemic cretinism NOS

E01 Iodine-deficiency related thyroid disorders and allied conditions

Excludes1: *congenital iodine-deficiency syndrome (E00.-)*
subclinical iodine-deficiency hypothyroidism (E02)

E01.0 Iodine-deficiency related diffuse (endemic) goiter

E01.1 Iodine-deficiency related multinodular (endemic) goiter
Iodine-deficiency related nodular goiter

E01.2 Iodine-deficiency related (endemic) goiter, unspecified
Endemic goiter NOS

E01.8 Other iodine-deficiency related thyroid disorders and allied conditions
Acquired iodine-deficiency hypothyroidism NOS

Endocrine System

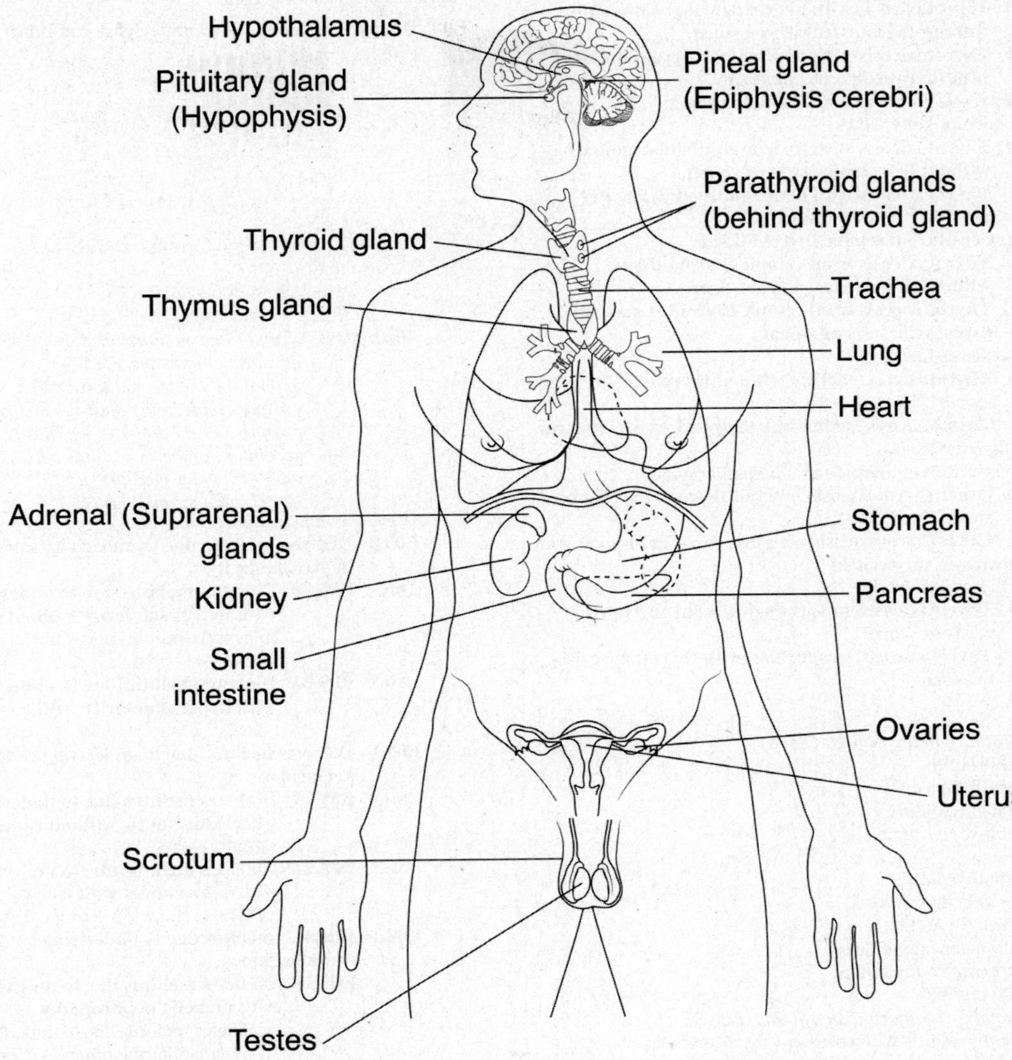

E02 Subclinical iodine-deficiency hypothyroidism

AHA CC: 1Q, 2021, 8-9

Valid 3-character code, no further characters required

E03 Other hypothyroidism

Excludes1: *iodine-deficiency related hypothyroidism (E00-E02)*
postprocedural hypothyroidism (E89.0)

E03.0 Congenital hypothyroidism with diffuse goiter
Congenital parenchymatous goiter (nontoxic)
Congenital goiter (nontoxic) NOS
Excludes1: *transitory congenital goiter with normal function (P72.0)*

E03.1 Congenital hypothyroidism without goiter
Aplasia of thyroid (with myxedema)
Congenital atrophy of thyroid
Congenital hypothyroidism NOS

E03.2 Hypothyroidism due to medicaments and other exogenous substances
Code first poisoning due to drug or toxin, if applicable (T36-T65 with fifth or sixth character 1-4 or 6)

Use additional code for adverse effect, if applicable, to identify drug (T36-T50 with fifth or sixth character 5)

E03.3 Postinfectious hypothyroidism

E03.4 Atrophy of thyroid (acquired)
Excludes1: *congenital atrophy of thyroid (E03.1)*

MCC **E03.5 Myxedema coma**

E03.8 Other specified hypothyroidism
AHA CC: 1Q, 2021, 8-9

E03.9 Hypothyroidism, unspecified
Myxedema NOS

E04 Other nontoxic goiter

Excludes1: *congenital goiter (NOS) (diffuse) (parenchymatous) (E03.0)*
iodine-deficiency related goiter (E00-E02)

E04.0 Nontoxic diffuse goiter
Diffuse (colloid) nontoxic goiter
Simple nontoxic goiter

E04.1 Nontoxic single thyroid nodule
Colloid nodule (cystic) (thyroid)
Nontoxic uninodular goiter
Thyroid (cystic) nodule NOS

E04.2 Nontoxic multinodular goiter
Cystic goiter NOS
Multinodular (cystic) goiter NOS

E04.8 Other specified nontoxic goiter

E04.9 Nontoxic goiter, unspecified
Goiter NOS
Nodular goiter (nontoxic) NOS

E05 Thyrotoxicosis [hyperthyroidism]

Excludes1: *chronic thyroiditis with transient thyrotoxicosis (E06.2)*
neonatal thyrotoxicosis (P72.1)

\+ **E05.0 Thyrotoxicosis with diffuse goiter**
Exophthalmic or toxic goiter NOS
Graves' disease
Toxic diffuse goiter

E05.00 Thyrotoxicosis with diffuse goiter without thyrotoxic crisis or storm

MCC **E05.01 Thyrotoxicosis with diffuse goiter with thyrotoxic crisis or storm**

+ **E05.1 Thyrotoxicosis with toxic single thyroid nodule**
  Thyrotoxicosis with toxic uninodular goiter
  E05.10 Thyrotoxicosis with toxic single thyroid nodule without thyrotoxic crisis or storm
  MCC **E05.11 Thyrotoxicosis with toxic single thyroid nodule with thyrotoxic crisis or storm**
+ **E05.2 Thyrotoxicosis with toxic multinodular goiter**
  Toxic nodular goiter NOS
  E05.20 Thyrotoxicosis with toxic multinodular goiter without thyrotoxic crisis or storm
  MCC **E05.21 Thyrotoxicosis with toxic multinodular goiter with thyrotoxic crisis or storm**
+ **E05.3 Thyrotoxicosis from ectopic thyroid tissue**
  E05.30 Thyrotoxicosis from ectopic thyroid tissue without thyrotoxic crisis or storm
  MCC **E05.31 Thyrotoxicosis from ectopic thyroid tissue with thyrotoxic crisis or storm**
+ **E05.4 Thyrotoxicosis factitia**
  E05.40 Thyrotoxicosis factitia without thyrotoxic crisis or storm
  MCC **E05.41 Thyrotoxicosis factitia with thyrotoxic crisis or storm**
+ **E05.8 Other thyrotoxicosis**
  Overproduction of thyroid-stimulating hormone
  E05.80 Other thyrotoxicosis without thyrotoxic crisis or storm
  MCC **E05.81 Other thyrotoxicosis with thyrotoxic crisis or storm**
+ **E05.9 Thyrotoxicosis, unspecified**
  Hyperthyroidism NOS
  E05.90 Thyrotoxicosis, unspecified without thyrotoxic crisis or storm
  MCC **E05.91 Thyrotoxicosis, unspecified with thyrotoxic crisis or storm**

E06 Thyroiditis

Excludes1: *postpartum thyroiditis (O90.5)*

CC **E06.0 Acute thyroiditis**
  Abscess of thyroid
  Pyogenic thyroiditis
  Suppurative thyroiditis
  Use additional code (B95-B97) to identify infectious agent.

E06.1 Subacute thyroiditis
  de Quervain thyroiditis
  Giant-cell thyroiditis
  Granulomatous thyroiditis
  Nonsuppurative thyroiditis
  Viral thyroiditis
  Excludes1: *autoimmune thyroiditis (E06.3)*

E06.2 Chronic thyroiditis with transient thyrotoxicosis
  Excludes1: *autoimmune thyroiditis (E06.3)*

E06.3 Autoimmune thyroiditis
  Hashimoto's thyroiditis
  Hashitoxicosis (transient)
  Lymphadenoid goiter
  Lymphocytic thyroiditis
  Struma lymphomatosa

E06.4 Drug-induced thyroiditis
  Use additional code for adverse effect, if applicable, to identify drug (T36-T50 with fifth or sixth character 5)

E06.5 Other chronic thyroiditis
  Chronic fibrous thyroiditis
  Chronic thyroiditis NOS
  Ligneous thyroiditis
  Riedel thyroiditis

E06.9 Thyroiditis, unspecified

E07 Other disorders of thyroid

E07.0 Hypersecretion of calcitonin
  C-cell hyperplasia of thyroid
  Hypersecretion of thyrocalcitonin

E07.1 Dyshormogenetic goiter
  Familial dyshormogenetic goiter
  Pendred's syndrome
  Excludes1: *transitory congenital goiter with normal function (P72.0)*

+ **E07.8 Other specified disorders of thyroid**
  E07.81 Sick-euthyroid syndrome
  Euthyroid sick-syndrome
  E07.89 Other specified disorders of thyroid
  Abnormality of thyroid-binding globulin
  Hemorrhage of thyroid
  Infarction of thyroid

E07.9 Disorder of thyroid, unspecified

Diabetes mellitus (E08-E13)

Review coding guideline C.4.a

E08 Diabetes mellitus due to underlying condition

Code first the underlying condition, such as:
  congenital rubella (P35.0)
  Cushing's syndrome (E24.-)
  cystic fibrosis (E84.-)
  malignant neoplasm (C00-C96)
  malnutrition (E40-E46)
  pancreatitis and other diseases of the pancreas (K85-K86.-)

Use additional code to identify control using:
  insulin (Z79.4)
  oral antidiabetic drugs (Z79.84)
  oral hypoglycemic drugs (Z79.84)

Excludes1: *drug or chemical induced diabetes mellitus (E09.-)*
gestational diabetes (O24.4-)
neonatal diabetes mellitus (P70.2)
postpancreatectomy diabetes mellitus (E13.-)
postprocedural diabetes mellitus (E13.-)
secondary diabetes mellitus NEC (E13.-)
type 1 diabetes mellitus (E10.-)
type 2 diabetes mellitus (E11.-)

Review coding guideline C.4.a.6.a

+ **E08.0 Diabetes mellitus due to underlying condition with hyperosmolarity**
  MCC **E08.00 Diabetes mellitus due to underlying condition with hyperosmolarity without nonketotic hyperglycemic-hyperosmolar coma (NKHHC)**
  HAC see Appendix B for HAC conditional logic
  MCC **E08.01 Diabetes mellitus due to underlying condition with hyperosmolarity with coma**
  HAC see Appendix B for HAC conditional logic
+ **E08.1 Diabetes mellitus due to underlying condition with ketoacidosis**
  MCC **E08.10 Diabetes mellitus due to underlying condition with ketoacidosis without coma**
  HAC see Appendix B for HAC conditional logic
  MCC **E08.11 Diabetes mellitus due to underlying condition with ketoacidosis with coma**
  HAC see Appendix B for HAC conditional logic
+ **E08.2 Diabetes mellitus due to underlying condition with kidney complications**
  E08.21 Diabetes mellitus due to underlying condition with diabetic nephropathy
  Diabetes mellitus due to underlying condition with intercapillary glomerulosclerosis
  Diabetes mellitus due to underlying condition with intracapillary glomerulonephrosis
  Diabetes mellitus due to underlying condition with Kimmelstiel-Wilson disease
  E08.22 Diabetes mellitus due to underlying condition with diabetic chronic kidney disease
  Use additional code to identify stage of chronic kidney disease (N18.1-N18.6)
  E08.29 Diabetes mellitus due to underlying condition with other diabetic kidney complication
  Renal tubular degeneration in diabetes mellitus due to underlying condition
+ **E08.3 Diabetes mellitus due to underlying condition with ophthalmic complications**
  AHA CC: 4Q, 2016, 11-13
  + **E08.31 Diabetes mellitus due to underlying condition with unspecified diabetic retinopathy**
  E08.311 Diabetes mellitus due to underlying condition with unspecified diabetic retinopathy with macular edema
  E08.319 Diabetes mellitus due to underlying condition with unspecified diabetic retinopathy without macular edema

\+ E08.32 **Diabetes mellitus due to underlying condition with mild nonproliferative diabetic retinopathy**

Diabetes mellitus due to underlying condition with nonproliferative diabetic retinopathy NOS

One of the following 7th characters is to be assigned to codes in subcategory **E08.32** to designate laterality of the disease:
1 right eye
2 left eye
3 bilateral
9 unspecified eye

+7th **E08.321** **Diabetes mellitus due to underlying condition with mild nonproliferative diabetic retinopathy with macular edema**

+7th **E08.329** **Diabetes mellitus due to underlying condition with mild nonproliferative diabetic retinopathy without macular edema**

\+ E08.33 **Diabetes mellitus due to underlying condition with moderate nonproliferative diabetic retinopathy**

One of the following 7th characters is to be assigned to codes in subcategory **E08.33** to designate laterality of the disease:
1 right eye
2 left eye
3 bilateral
9 unspecified eye

+7th **E08.331** **Diabetes mellitus due to underlying condition with moderate nonproliferative diabetic retinopathy with macular edema**

+7th **E08.339** **Diabetes mellitus due to underlying condition with moderate nonproliferative diabetic retinopathy without macular edema**

\+ E08.34 **Diabetes mellitus due to underlying condition with severe nonproliferative diabetic retinopathy**

One of the following 7th characters is to be assigned to codes in subcategory **E08.34** to designate laterality of the disease:
1 right eye
2 left eye
3 bilateral
9 unspecified eye

+7th **E08.341** **Diabetes mellitus due to underlying condition with severe nonproliferative diabetic retinopathy with macular edema**

+7th **E08.349** **Diabetes mellitus due to underlying condition with severe nonproliferative diabetic retinopathy without macular edema**

\+ E08.35 **Diabetes mellitus due to underlying condition with proliferative diabetic retinopathy**

One of the following 7th characters is to be assigned to codes in subcategory **E08.35** to designate laterality of the disease:
1 right eye
2 left eye
3 bilateral
9 unspecified eye

+7th **E08.351** **Diabetes mellitus due to underlying condition with proliferative diabetic retinopathy with macular edema**

+7th **E08.352** **Diabetes mellitus due to underlying condition with proliferative diabetic retinopathy with traction retinal detachment involving the macula**

+7th **E08.353** **Diabetes mellitus due to underlying condition with proliferative diabetic retinopathy with traction retinal detachment not involving the macula**

+7th **E08.354** **Diabetes mellitus due to underlying condition with proliferative diabetic retinopathy with combined traction retinal detachment and rhegmatogenous retinal detachment**

+7th **E08.355** **Diabetes mellitus due to underlying condition with stable proliferative diabetic retinopathy**

+7th **E08.359** **Diabetes mellitus due to underlying condition with proliferative diabetic retinopathy without macular edema**

E08.36 **Diabetes mellitus due to underlying condition with diabetic cataract**

X+7th **E08.37** **Diabetes mellitus due to underlying condition with diabetic macular edema, resolved following treatment**

One of the following 7th characters is to be assigned to codes in subcategory **E08.37** to designate laterality of the disease:
1 right eye
2 left eye
3 bilateral
9 unspecified eye

E08.39 **Diabetes mellitus due to underlying condition with other diabetic ophthalmic complication**

Use additional code to identify manifestation, such as:
diabetic glaucoma (H40-H42)

\+ E08.4 **Diabetes mellitus due to underlying condition with neurological complications**

E08.40 **Diabetes mellitus due to underlying condition with diabetic neuropathy, unspecified**

E08.41 **Diabetes mellitus due to underlying condition with diabetic mononeuropathy**

E08.42 **Diabetes mellitus due to underlying condition with diabetic polyneuropathy**

Diabetes mellitus due to underlying condition with diabetic neuralgia

E08.43 **Diabetes mellitus due to underlying condition with diabetic autonomic (poly)neuropathy**

Diabetes mellitus due to underlying condition with diabetic gastroparesis

AHA CC: 3Q, 2013, 114-115

E08.44 **Diabetes mellitus due to underlying condition with diabetic amyotrophy**

E08.49 **Diabetes mellitus due to underlying condition with other diabetic neurological complication**

\+ E08.5 **Diabetes mellitus due to underlying condition with circulatory complications**

E08.51 **Diabetes mellitus due to underlying condition with diabetic peripheral angiopathy without gangrene**

CC **E08.52** **Diabetes mellitus due to underlying condition with diabetic peripheral angiopathy with gangrene**

Diabetes mellitus due to underlying condition with diabetic gangrene

E08.59 **Diabetes mellitus due to underlying condition with other circulatory complications**

\+ E08.6 **Diabetes mellitus due to underlying condition with other specified complications**

\+ E08.61 **Diabetes mellitus due to underlying condition with diabetic arthropathy**

E08.610 **Diabetes mellitus due to underlying condition with diabetic neuropathic arthropathy**

Diabetes mellitus due to underlying condition with Charcôt's joints

E08.618 **Diabetes mellitus due to underlying condition with other diabetic arthropathy**

+ **E08.62 Diabetes mellitus due to underlying condition with skin complications**
  - **E08.620 Diabetes mellitus due to underlying condition with diabetic dermatitis**
    Diabetes mellitus due to underlying condition with diabetic necrobiosis lipoidica
  - **E08.621 Diabetes mellitus due to underlying condition with foot ulcer**
    Use additional code to identify site of ulcer (L97.4-, L97.5-)
  - **E08.622 Diabetes mellitus due to underlying condition with other skin ulcer**
    Use additional code to identify site of ulcer (L97.1-L97.9, L98.41-L98.49)
  - **E08.628 Diabetes mellitus due to underlying condition with other skin complications**

+ **E08.63 Diabetes mellitus due to underlying condition with oral complications**
  - **E08.630 Diabetes mellitus due to underlying condition with periodontal disease**
  - **E08.638 Diabetes mellitus due to underlying condition with other oral complications**

+ **E08.64 Diabetes mellitus due to underlying condition with hypoglycemia**
  - MCC **E08.641 Diabetes mellitus due to underlying condition with hypoglycemia with coma**
  - **E08.649 Diabetes mellitus due to underlying condition with hypoglycemia without coma**

E08.65 Diabetes mellitus due to underlying condition with hyperglycemia

E08.69 Diabetes mellitus due to underlying condition with other specified complication
Use additional code to identify complication

E08.8 Diabetes mellitus due to underlying condition with unspecified complications

E08.9 Diabetes mellitus due to underlying condition without complications

E09 Drug or chemical induced diabetes mellitus

Code first poisoning due to drug or toxin, if applicable (T36-T65 with fifth or sixth character 1-4 or 6)

Use additional code for adverse effect, if applicable, to identify drug (T36-T50 with fifth or sixth character 5)

Use additional code to identify control using:
insulin (Z79.4)
oral antidiabetic drugs (Z79.84)
oral hypoglycemic drugs (Z79.84)

Excludes1: *diabetes mellitus due to underlying condition (E08.-)*
gestational diabetes (O24.4-)
neonatal diabetes mellitus (P70.2)
postpancreatectomy diabetes mellitus (E13.-)
postprocedural diabetes mellitus (E13.-)
secondary diabetes mellitus NEC (E13.-)
type 1 diabetes mellitus (E10.-)
type 2 diabetes mellitus (E11.-)

Review coding guideline C.4.a.6.a

+ **E09.0 Drug or chemical induced diabetes mellitus with hyperosmolarity**
  - MCC **E09.00 Drug or chemical induced diabetes mellitus with hyperosmolarity without nonketotic hyperglycemic-hyperosmolar coma (NKHHC)**
    HAC see Appendix B for HAC conditional logic
  - MCC **E09.01 Drug or chemical induced diabetes mellitus with hyperosmolarity with coma**
    HAC see Appendix B for HAC conditional logic

+ **E09.1 Drug or chemical induced diabetes mellitus with ketoacidosis**
  - MCC **E09.10 Drug or chemical induced diabetes mellitus with ketoacidosis without coma**
    HAC see Appendix B for HAC conditional logic
  - MCC **E09.11 Drug or chemical induced diabetes mellitus with ketoacidosis with coma**
    HAC see Appendix B for HAC conditional logic

+ **E09.2 Drug or chemical induced diabetes mellitus with kidney complications**
  - **E09.21 Drug or chemical induced diabetes mellitus with diabetic nephropathy**
    Drug or chemical induced diabetes mellitus with intercapillary glomerulosclerosis
    Drug or chemical induced diabetes mellitus with intracapillary glomerulonephrosis
    Drug or chemical induced diabetes mellitus with Kimmelstiel-Wilson disease
  - **E09.22 Drug or chemical induced diabetes mellitus with diabetic chronic kidney disease**
    Use additional code to identify stage of chronic kidney disease (N18.1-N18.6)
  - **E09.29 Drug or chemical induced diabetes mellitus with other diabetic kidney complication**
    Drug or chemical induced diabetes mellitus with renal tubular degeneration

+ **E09.3 Drug or chemical induced diabetes mellitus with ophthalmic complications**
  AHA CC: 4Q, 2016, 11-13
  + **E09.31 Drug or chemical induced diabetes mellitus with unspecified diabetic retinopathy**
    - **E09.311 Drug or chemical induced diabetes mellitus with unspecified diabetic retinopathy with macular edema**
    - **E09.319 Drug or chemical induced diabetes mellitus with unspecified diabetic retinopathy without macular edema**
  + **E09.32 Drug or chemical induced diabetes mellitus with mild nonproliferative diabetic retinopathy**
    Drug or chemical induced diabetes mellitus with nonproliferative diabetic retinopathy NOS

    One of the following 7th characters is to be assigned to codes in subcategory **E09.32** to designate laterality of the disease:
    1 right eye
    2 left eye
    3 bilateral
    9 unspecified eye

    - +7th **E09.321 Drug or chemical induced diabetes mellitus with mild nonproliferative diabetic retinopathy with macular edema**
    - +7th **E09.329 Drug or chemical induced diabetes mellitus with mild nonproliferative diabetic retinopathy without macular edema**
  +7th **E09.33 Drug or chemical induced diabetes mellitus with moderate nonproliferative diabetic retinopathy**

    One of the following 7th characters is to be assigned to codes in subcategory **E09.33** to designate laterality of the disease:
    1 right eye
    2 left eye
    3 bilateral
    9 unspecified eye

    - +7th **E09.331 Drug or chemical induced diabetes mellitus with moderate nonproliferative diabetic retinopathy with macular edema**
    - +7th **E09.339 Drug or chemical induced diabetes mellitus with moderate nonproliferative diabetic retinopathy without macular edema**
  + **E09.34 Drug or chemical induced diabetes mellitus with severe nonproliferative diabetic retinopathy**

    One of the following 7th characters is to be assigned to codes in subcategory **E09.34** to designate laterality of the disease:
    1 right eye
    2 left eye
    3 bilateral
    9 unspecified eye

+7th **E09.341** **Drug or chemical induced diabetes mellitus with severe nonproliferative diabetic retinopathy with macular edema**

+7th **E09.349** **Drug or chemical induced diabetes mellitus with severe nonproliferative diabetic retinopathy without macular edema**

\+ **E09.35** **Drug or chemical induced diabetes mellitus with proliferative diabetic retinopathy**

One of the following 7th characters is to be assigned to codes in subcategory **E09.35** to designate laterality of the disease:
1 right eye
2 left eye
3 bilateral
9 unspecified eye

+7th **E09.351** **Drug or chemical induced diabetes mellitus with proliferative diabetic retinopathy with macular edema**

+7th **E09.352** **Drug or chemical induced diabetes mellitus with proliferative diabetic retinopathy with traction retinal detachment involving the macula**

+7th **E09.353** **Drug or chemical induced diabetes mellitus with proliferative diabetic retinopathy with traction retinal detachment not involving the macula**

+7th **E09.354** **Drug or chemical induced diabetes mellitus with proliferative diabetic retinopathy with combined traction retinal detachment and rhegmatogenous retinal detachment**

+7th **E09.355** **Drug or chemical induced diabetes mellitus with stable proliferative diabetic retinopathy**

+7th **E09.359** **Drug or chemical induced diabetes mellitus with proliferative diabetic retinopathy without macular edema**

E09.36 **Drug or chemical induced diabetes mellitus with diabetic cataract**

X+7th **E09.37** **Drug or chemical induced diabetes mellitus with diabetic macular edema, resolved following treatment**

One of the following 7th characters is to be assigned to codes in subcategory **E09.37** to designate laterality of the disease:
1 right eye
2 left eye
3 bilateral
9 unspecified eye

E09.39 **Drug or chemical induced diabetes mellitus with other diabetic ophthalmic complication**
Use additional code to identify manifestation, such as:
diabetic glaucoma (H40-H42)

\+ **E09.4** **Drug or chemical induced diabetes mellitus with neurological complications**

E09.40 **Drug or chemical induced diabetes mellitus with neurological complications with diabetic neuropathy, unspecified**

E09.41 **Drug or chemical induced diabetes mellitus with neurological complications with diabetic mononeuropathy**

E09.42 **Drug or chemical induced diabetes mellitus with neurological complications with diabetic polyneuropathy**
Drug or chemical induced diabetes mellitus with diabetic neuralgia

E09.43 **Drug or chemical induced diabetes mellitus with neurological complications with diabetic autonomic (poly)neuropathy**
Drug or chemical induced diabetes mellitus with diabetic gastroparesis
AHA CC: 3Q, 2013, 114-115

E09.44 **Drug or chemical induced diabetes mellitus with neurological complications with diabetic amyotrophy**

E09.49 **Drug or chemical induced diabetes mellitus with neurological complications with other diabetic neurological complication**

\+ **E09.5** **Drug or chemical induced diabetes mellitus with circulatory complications**

E09.51 **Drug or chemical induced diabetes mellitus with diabetic peripheral angiopathy without gangrene**

CC **E09.52** **Drug or chemical induced diabetes mellitus with diabetic peripheral angiopathy with gangrene**
Drug or chemical induced diabetes mellitus with diabetic gangrene

E09.59 **Drug or chemical induced diabetes mellitus with other circulatory complications**

\+ **E09.6** **Drug or chemical induced diabetes mellitus with other specified complications**

\+ **E09.61** **Drug or chemical induced diabetes mellitus with diabetic arthropathy**

E09.610 **Drug or chemical induced diabetes mellitus with diabetic neuropathic arthropathy**
Drug or chemical induced diabetes mellitus with Charcôt's joints

E09.618 **Drug or chemical induced diabetes mellitus with other diabetic arthropathy**

\+ **E09.62** **Drug or chemical induced diabetes mellitus with skin complications**

E09.620 **Drug or chemical induced diabetes mellitus with diabetic dermatitis**
Drug or chemical induced diabetes mellitus with diabetic necrobiosis lipoidica

E09.621 **Drug or chemical induced diabetes mellitus with foot ulcer**
Use additional code to identify site of ulcer (L97.4-, L97.5-)

E09.622 **Drug or chemical induced diabetes mellitus with other skin ulcer**
Use additional code to identify site of ulcer (L97.1-L97.9, L98.41-L98.49)

E09.628 **Drug or chemical induced diabetes mellitus with other skin complications**

\+ **E09.63** **Drug or chemical induced diabetes mellitus with oral complications**

E09.630 **Drug or chemical induced diabetes mellitus with periodontal disease**

E09.638 **Drug or chemical induced diabetes mellitus with other oral complications**

\+ **E09.64** **Drug or chemical induced diabetes mellitus with hypoglycemia**

MCC **E09.641** **Drug or chemical induced diabetes mellitus with hypoglycemia with coma**

E09.649 **Drug or chemical induced diabetes mellitus with hypoglycemia without coma**

CC **E09.65** **Drug or chemical induced diabetes mellitus with hyperglycemia**

CC **E09.69** **Drug or chemical induced diabetes mellitus with other specified complication**
Use additional code to identify complication

CC **E09.8** **Drug or chemical induced diabetes mellitus with unspecified complications**

CC **E09.9** **Drug or chemical induced diabetes mellitus without complications**

E10 Type 1 diabetes mellitus

Includes: brittle diabetes (mellitus)
diabetes (mellitus) due to autoimmune process
diabetes (mellitus) due to immune mediated pancreatic islet beta-cell destruction
idiopathic diabetes (mellitus)
juvenile onset diabetes (mellitus)
ketosis-prone diabetes (mellitus)

Excludes1: *diabetes mellitus due to underlying condition (E08.-)*
drug or chemical induced diabetes mellitus (E09.-)
gestational diabetes (O24.4-)
hyperglycemia NOS (R73.9)
neonatal diabetes mellitus (P70.2)
postpancreatectomy diabetes mellitus (E13.-)
postprocedural diabetes mellitus (E13.-)
secondary diabetes mellitus NEC (E13.-)
type 2 diabetes mellitus (E11.-)

Diabetes Mellitus and Its Complications: Micro and Macrovascular Complications

Diabetic retinopathy

Diabetic retinopathy can be easily detected during a dilated eye exam and is the leading cause of blindness among adults in theUnited States. Visual loss can be prevented with early recognition and treatment of retinopathy.

Cerebrovascular disease

The high incidence of vascular complications among patients with diabetes is related not only to blood glucose elevations, but also to the frequent association of dyslipidemia, hypertension, a procoagulant state and the tendency to form unstable plaques in the arterial wall.

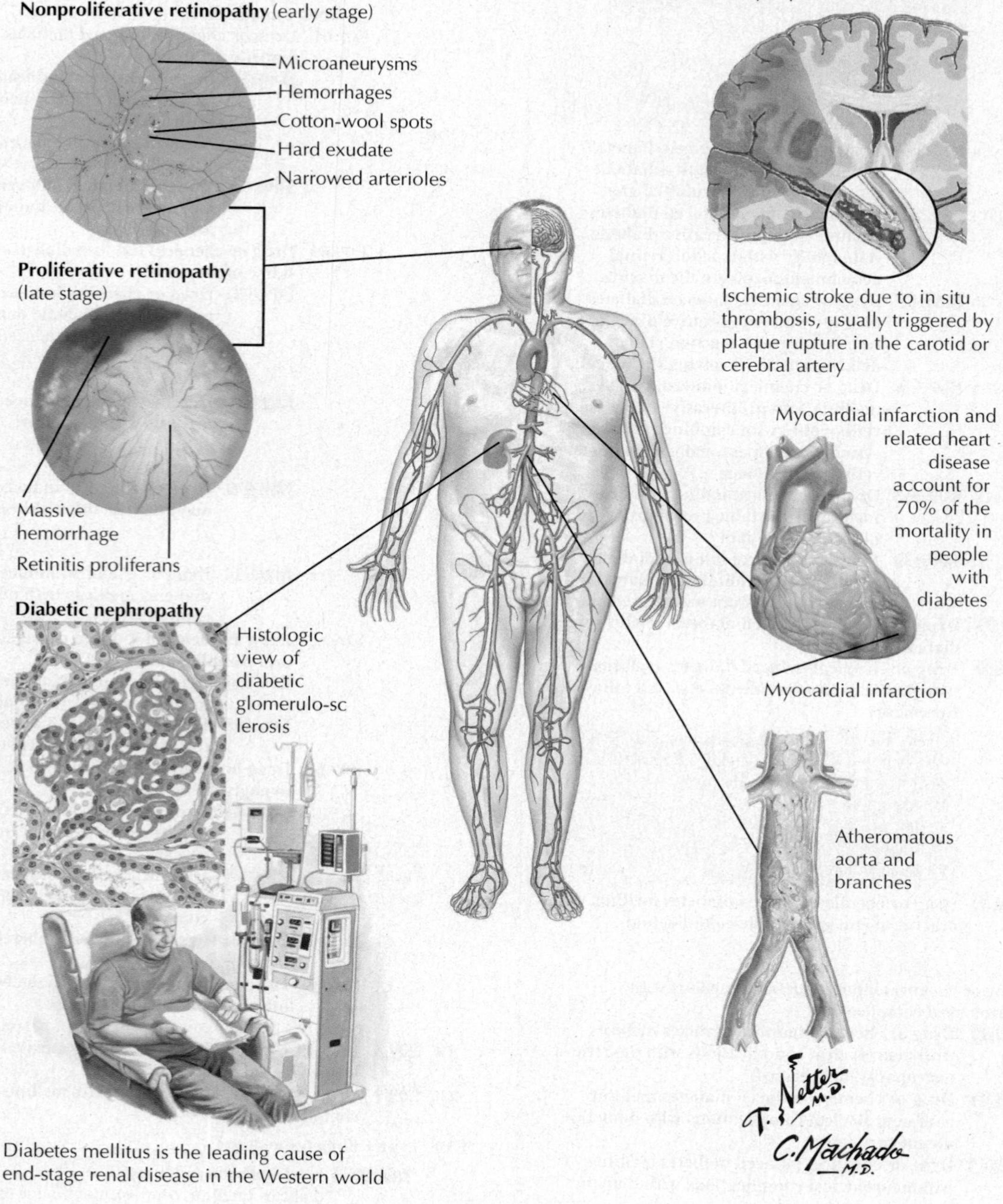

Diabetes mellitus is the leading cause of end-stage renal disease in the Western world

+ E10.1 **Type 1 diabetes mellitus with ketoacidosis**

MCC **E10.10** **Type 1 diabetes mellitus with ketoacidosis without coma**

HAC see Appendix B for HAC conditional logic

AHA CC: 3Q, 2013, 20

MCC **E10.11** **Type 1 diabetes mellitus with ketoacidosis with coma**

HAC see Appendix B for HAC conditional logic

+ E10.2 **Type 1 diabetes mellitus with kidney complications**

E10.21 **Type 1 diabetes mellitus with diabetic nephropathy**

Type 1 diabetes mellitus with intercapillary glomerulosclerosis

Type 1 diabetes mellitus with intracapillary glomerulonephrosis

Type 1 diabetes mellitus with Kimmelstiel-Wilson disease

E10.22 **Type 1 diabetes mellitus with diabetic chronic kidney disease**

Use additional code to identify stage of chronic kidney disease (N18.1-N18.6)

E10.29 **Type 1 diabetes mellitus with other diabetic kidney complication**

Type 1 diabetes mellitus with renal tubular degeneration

+ E10.3 **Type 1 diabetes mellitus with ophthalmic complications**

AHA CC: 4Q, 2016, 11-13

+ E10.31 **Type 1 diabetes mellitus with unspecified diabetic retinopathy**

E10.311 **Type 1 diabetes mellitus with unspecified diabetic retinopathy with macular edema**

E10.319 **Type 1 diabetes mellitus with unspecified diabetic retinopathy without macular edema**

+ E10.32 **Type 1 diabetes mellitus with mild nonproliferative diabetic retinopathy**

Type 1 diabetes mellitus with nonproliferative diabetic retinopathy NOS

One of the following 7th characters is to be assigned to codes in subcategory **E10.32** to designate laterality of the disease:
1 right eye
2 left eye
3 bilateral
9 unspecified eye

+7th **E10.321** **Type 1 diabetes mellitus with mild nonproliferative diabetic retinopathy with macular edema**

+7th **E10.329** **Type 1 diabetes mellitus with mild nonproliferative diabetic retinopathy without macular edema**

+ E10.33 **Type 1 diabetes mellitus with moderate nonproliferative diabetic retinopathy**

One of the following 7th characters is to be assigned to codes in subcategory **E10.33** to designate laterality of the disease:
1 right eye
2 left eye
3 bilateral
9 unspecified eye

+7th **E10.331** **Type 1 diabetes mellitus with moderate nonproliferative diabetic retinopathy with macular edema**

+7th **E10.339** **Type 1 diabetes mellitus with moderate nonproliferative diabetic retinopathy without macular edema**

+ E10.34 **Type 1 diabetes mellitus with severe nonproliferative diabetic retinopathy**

One of the following 7th characters is to be assigned to codes in subcategory **E10.34** to designate laterality of the disease:
1 right eye
2 left eye
3 bilateral
9 unspecified eye

+7th **E10.341** **Type 1 diabetes mellitus with severe nonproliferative diabetic retinopathy with macular edema**

+7th **E10.349** **Type 1 diabetes mellitus with severe nonproliferative diabetic retinopathy without macular edema**

+ E10.35 **Type 1 diabetes mellitus with proliferative diabetic retinopathy**

One of the following 7th characters is to be assigned to codes in subcategory **E10.35** to designate laterality of the disease:
1 right eye
2 left eye
3 bilateral
9 unspecified eye

+7th **E10.351** **Type 1 diabetes mellitus with proliferative diabetic retinopathy with macular edema**

+7th **E10.352** **Type 1 diabetes mellitus with proliferative diabetic retinopathy with traction retinal detachment involving the macula**

+7th **E10.353** **Type 1 diabetes mellitus with proliferative diabetic retinopathy with traction retinal detachment not involving the macula**

+7th **E10.354** **Type 1 diabetes mellitus with proliferative diabetic retinopathy with combined traction retinal detachment and rhegmatogenous retinal detachment**

+7th **E10.355** **Type 1 diabetes mellitus with stable proliferative diabetic retinopathy**

+7th **E10.359** **Type 1 diabetes mellitus with proliferative diabetic retinopathy without macular edema**

E10.36 **Type 1 diabetes mellitus with diabetic cataract**

X+7th **E10.37** **Type 1 diabetes mellitus with diabetic macular edema, resolved following treatment**

One of the following 7th characters is to be assigned to codes in subcategory **E10.37** to designate laterality of the disease:
1 right eye
2 left eye
3 bilateral
9 unspecified eye

E10.39 **Type 1 diabetes mellitus with other diabetic ophthalmic complication**

Use additional code to identify manifestation, such as: diabetic glaucoma (H40-H42)

+ E10.4 **Type 1 diabetes mellitus with neurological complications**

E10.40 **Type 1 diabetes mellitus with diabetic neuropathy, unspecified**

E10.41 **Type 1 diabetes mellitus with diabetic mononeuropathy**

E10.42 **Type 1 diabetes mellitus with diabetic polyneuropathy**

Type 1 diabetes mellitus with diabetic neuralgia

E10.43 **Type 1 diabetes mellitus with diabetic autonomic (poly)neuropathy**

Type 1 diabetes mellitus with diabetic gastroparesis

AHA CC: 3Q, 2013, 114-115

E10.44 **Type 1 diabetes mellitus with diabetic amyotrophy**

E10.49 **Type 1 diabetes mellitus with other diabetic neurological complication**

+ E10.5 **Type 1 diabetes mellitus with circulatory complications**

E10.51 **Type 1 diabetes mellitus with diabetic peripheral angiopathy without gangrene**

CC **E10.52** **Type 1 diabetes mellitus with diabetic peripheral angiopathy with gangrene**

Type 1 diabetes mellitus with diabetic gangrene

E10.59 **Type 1 diabetes mellitus with other circulatory complications**

+ E10.6 **Type 1 diabetes mellitus with other specified complications**

+ E10.61 **Type 1 diabetes mellitus with diabetic arthropathy**

E10.610 **Type 1 diabetes mellitus with diabetic neuropathic arthropathy**
Type 1 diabetes mellitus with Charcôt's joints

E10.618 **Type 1 diabetes mellitus with other diabetic arthropathy**

+ E10.62 **Type 1 diabetes mellitus with skin complications**

E10.620 **Type 1 diabetes mellitus with diabetic dermatitis**
Type 1 diabetes mellitus with diabetic necrobiosis lipoidica

E10.621 **Type 1 diabetes mellitus with foot ulcer**
Use additional code to identify site of ulcer (L97.4-, L97.5-)

E10.622 **Type 1 diabetes mellitus with other skin ulcer**
Use additional code to identify site of ulcer (L97.1-L97.9, L98.41-L98.49)

E10.628 **Type 1 diabetes mellitus with other skin complications**

+ E10.63 **Type 1 diabetes mellitus with oral complications**

E10.630 **Type 1 diabetes mellitus with periodontal disease**

E10.638 **Type 1 diabetes mellitus with other oral complications**

+ E10.64 **Type 1 diabetes mellitus with hypoglycemia**

MCC E10.641 **Type 1 diabetes mellitus with hypoglycemia with coma**

E10.649 **Type 1 diabetes mellitus with hypoglycemia without coma**
AHA CC: 1Q, 2016, 13

E10.65 **Type 1 diabetes mellitus with hyperglycemia**

E10.69 **Type 1 diabetes mellitus with other specified complication**
Use additional code to identify complication

E10.8 **Type 1 diabetes mellitus with unspecified complications**

E10.9 **Type 1 diabetes mellitus without complications**

E11 **Type 2 diabetes mellitus**

Includes: diabetes (mellitus) due to insulin secretory defect
diabetes NOS
insulin resistant diabetes (mellitus)

Use additional code to identify control using:
insulin (Z79.4)
oral antidiabetic drugs (Z79.84)
oral hypoglycemic drugs (Z79.84)

Excludes1: *diabetes mellitus due to underlying condition (E08.-)*
drug or chemical induced diabetes mellitus (E09.-)
gestational diabetes (O24.4-)
neonatal diabetes mellitus (P70.2)
postpancreatectomy diabetes mellitus (E13.-)
postprocedural diabetes mellitus (E13.-)
secondary diabetes mellitus NEC (E13.-)
type 1 diabetes mellitus (E10.-)

Review coding guidelines C.4.a.2 and C.4.a.3

+ E11.0 **Type 2 diabetes mellitus with hyperosmolarity**
AHA CC: 4Q, 2017, 6

MCC E11.00 **Type 2 diabetes mellitus with hyperosmolarity without nonketotic hyperglycemic-hyperosmolar coma (NKHHC)**
HAC see Appendix B for HAC conditional logic

MCC E11.01 **Type 2 diabetes mellitus with hyperosmolarity with coma**
HAC see Appendix B for HAC conditional logic

+ E11.1 **Type 2 diabetes mellitus with ketoacidosis**

MCC E11.10 **Type 2 diabetes mellitus with ketoacidosis without coma**
HAC see Appendix B for HAC conditional logic

MCC E11.11 **Type 2 diabetes mellitus with ketoacidosis with coma**
AHA CC: 4Q, 2017, 6
HAC see Appendix B for HAC conditional logic

+ E11.2 **Type 2 diabetes mellitus with kidney complications**

E11.21 **Type 2 diabetes mellitus with diabetic nephropathy**
Type 2 diabetes mellitus with intercapillary glomerulosclerosis
Type 2 diabetes mellitus with intracapillary glomerulonephrosis
Type 2 diabetes mellitus with Kimmelstiel-Wilson disease

E11.22 **Type 2 diabetes mellitus with diabetic chronic kidney disease**
Use additional code to identify stage of chronic kidney disease (N18.1-N18.6)
AHA CC: 4Q, 2018, 88-89; 3Q, 2019, 3

E11.29 **Type 2 diabetes mellitus with other diabetic kidney complication**
Type 2 diabetes mellitus with renal tubular degeneration

+ E11.3 **Type 2 diabetes mellitus with ophthalmic complications**
AHA CC: 4Q, 2016, 11-13

+ E11.31 **Type 2 diabetes mellitus with unspecified diabetic retinopathy**

E11.311 **Type 2 diabetes mellitus with unspecified diabetic retinopathy with macular edema**

E11.319 **Type 2 diabetes mellitus with unspecified diabetic retinopathy without macular edema**
AHA CC: 3Q, 2013, 20

+ E11.32 **Type 2 diabetes mellitus with mild nonproliferative diabetic retinopathy**
Type 2 diabetes mellitus with nonproliferative diabetic retinopathy NOS

One of the following 7th characters is to be assigned to codes in subcategory **E11.32** to designate laterality of the disease:
1 right eye
2 left eye
3 bilateral
9 unspecified eye

+7th E11.321 **Type 2 diabetes mellitus with mild nonproliferative diabetic retinopathy with macular edema**

+7th E11.329 **Type 2 diabetes mellitus with mild nonproliferative diabetic retinopathy without macular edema**

+ E11.33 **Type 2 diabetes mellitus with moderate nonproliferative diabetic retinopathy**

One of the following 7th characters is to be assigned to codes in subcategory **E11.33** to designate laterality of the disease:
1 right eye
2 left eye
3 bilateral
9 unspecified eye

+7th E11.331 **Type 2 diabetes mellitus with moderate nonproliferative diabetic retinopathy with macular edema**

+7th E11.339 **Type 2 diabetes mellitus with moderate nonproliferative diabetic retinopathy without macular edema**

+ E11.34 **Type 2 diabetes mellitus with severe nonproliferative diabetic retinopathy**

One of the following 7th characters is to be assigned to codes in subcategory **E11.34** to designate laterality of the disease:
1 right eye
2 left eye
3 bilateral
9 unspecified eye

+7th E11.341 **Type 2 diabetes mellitus with severe nonproliferative diabetic retinopathy with macular edema**

+7th E11.349 **Type 2 diabetes mellitus with severe nonproliferative diabetic retinopathy without macular edema**

+ E11.35 **Type 2 diabetes mellitus with proliferative diabetic retinopathy**

One of the following 7th characters is to be assigned to codes in subcategory **E11.35** to designate laterality of the disease:
1 right eye
2 left eye
3 bilateral
9 unspecified eye

+7th **E11.351 Type 2 diabetes mellitus with proliferative diabetic retinopathy with macular edema**

+7th **E11.352 Type 2 diabetes mellitus with proliferative diabetic retinopathy with traction retinal detachment involving the macula**

+7th **E11.353 Type 2 diabetes mellitus with proliferative diabetic retinopathy with traction retinal detachment not involving the macula**

+7th **E11.354 Type 2 diabetes mellitus with proliferative diabetic retinopathy with combined traction retinal detachment and rhegmatogenous retinal detachment**

+7th **E11.355 Type 2 diabetes mellitus with stable proliferative diabetic retinopathy**

+7th **E11.359 Type 2 diabetes mellitus with proliferative diabetic retinopathy without macular edema**

E11.36 Type 2 diabetes mellitus with diabetic cataract
AHA CC: 2Q, 2019, 30-31

X+7th **E11.37 Type 2 diabetes mellitus with diabetic macular edema, resolved following treatment**

One of the following 7th characters is to be assigned to codes in subcategory **E11.37** to designate laterality of the disease:
1 right eye
2 left eye
3 bilateral
9 unspecified eye

E11.39 Type 2 diabetes mellitus with other diabetic ophthalmic complication
Use additional code to identify manifestation, such as:
diabetic glaucoma (H40-H42)

+ E11.4 **Type 2 diabetes mellitus with neurological complications**

E11.40 Type 2 diabetes mellitus with diabetic neuropathy, unspecified
AHA CC: 4Q, 2013, 129; 3Q, 2018, 3-4

E11.41 Type 2 diabetes mellitus with diabetic mononeuropathy

E11.42 Type 2 diabetes mellitus with diabetic polyneuropathy
Type 2 diabetes mellitus with diabetic neuralgia
AHA CC: 1Q, 2020, 12

E11.43 Type 2 diabetes mellitus with diabetic autonomic (poly)neuropathy
Type 2 diabetes mellitus with diabetic gastroparesis
AHA CC: 4Q, 2013, 114-115

E11.44 Type 2 diabetes mellitus with diabetic amyotrophy

E11.49 Type 2 diabetes mellitus with other diabetic neurological complication

+ E11.5 **Type 2 diabetes mellitus with circulatory complications**

E11.51 Type 2 diabetes mellitus with diabetic peripheral angiopathy without gangrene
AHA CC: 3Q, 2018, 3-4

CC **E11.52 Type 2 diabetes mellitus with diabetic peripheral angiopathy with gangrene**
Type 2 diabetes mellitus with diabetic gangrene
AHA CC: 4Q, 2017, 102

E11.59 Type 2 diabetes mellitus with other circulatory complications

+ E11.6 **Type 2 diabetes mellitus with other specified complications**

+ E11.61 **Type 2 diabetes mellitus with diabetic arthropathy**

E11.610 Type 2 diabetes mellitus with diabetic neuropathic arthropathy
Type 2 diabetes mellitus with Charcôt's joints

E11.618 Type 2 diabetes mellitus with other diabetic arthropathy

+ E11.62 **Type 2 diabetes mellitus with skin complications**

E11.620 Type 2 diabetes mellitus with diabetic dermatitis
Type 2 diabetes mellitus with diabetic necrobiosis lipoidica

E11.621 Type 2 diabetes mellitus with foot ulcer
Use additional code to identify site of ulcer (L97.4-, L97.5-)
AHA CC: 1Q, 2016, 12-13; 1Q, 2020, 12; 2Q, 2020, 19

E11.622 Type 2 diabetes mellitus with other skin ulcer
Use additional code to identify site of ulcer (L97.1-L97.9, L98.41-L98.49)
AHA CC: 4Q, 2017, 17; 1Q, 2021, 7-8

E11.628 Type 2 diabetes mellitus with other skin complications

+ E11.63 **Type 2 diabetes mellitus with oral complications**

E11.630 Type 2 diabetes mellitus with periodontal disease

E11.638 Type 2 diabetes mellitus with other oral complications

+ E11.64 **Type 2 diabetes mellitus with hypoglycemia**

MCC **E11.641 Type 2 diabetes mellitus with hypoglycemia with coma**

E11.649 Type 2 diabetes mellitus with hypoglycemia without coma
AHA CC: 3Q, 2015, 21; 3Q, 2016, 42

E11.65 Type 2 diabetes mellitus with hyperglycemia
AHA CC: 3Q, 2013, 20

E11.69 Type 2 diabetes mellitus with other specified complication
Use additional code to identify complication
AHA CC: 4Q, 2016, 141-142; 1Q, 2020, 12

E11.8 Type 2 diabetes mellitus with unspecified complications

E11.9 Type 2 diabetes mellitus without complications
AHA CC: 4Q, 2013, 128; 2Q, 2020, 18

E13 Other specified diabetes mellitus

Includes: diabetes mellitus due to genetic defects of beta-cell function diabetes mellitus due to genetic defects in insulin action postpancreatectomy diabetes mellitus postprocedural diabetes mellitus secondary diabetes mellitus NEC

Use additional code to identify control using:
insulin (Z79.4)
oral antidiabetic drugs (Z79.84)
oral hypoglycemic drugs (Z79.84)

Excludes1: *diabetes (mellitus) due to autoimmune process (E10.-)*
diabetes (mellitus) due to immune mediated pancreatic islet beta-cell destruction (E10.-)
diabetes mellitus due to underlying condition (E08.-)
drug or chemical induced diabetes mellitus (E09.-)
gestational diabetes (O24.4-)
neonatal diabetes mellitus (P70.2)
type 1 diabetes mellitus (E10.-)

AHA CC: 3Q, 2018, 4-5

Review coding guidelines C.4.a.6.a and C.4.a.6.b.i

+ E13.0 **Other specified diabetes mellitus with hyperosmolarity**

MCC **E13.00 Other specified diabetes mellitus with hyperosmolarity without nonketotic hyperglycemic-hyperosmolar coma (NKHHC)**
Excludes2: *type 2 diabetes mellitus (E11.-)*
HAC see Appendix B for HAC conditional logic

MCC **E13.01 Other specified diabetes mellitus with hyperosmolarity with coma**
HAC see Appendix B for HAC conditional logic

+ E13.1 **Other specified diabetes mellitus with ketoacidosis**

MCC **E13.10 Other specified diabetes mellitus with ketoacidosis without coma**
HAC see Appendix B for HAC conditional logic
AHA CC: 1Q, 2013, 26-27; 2Q, 2016,10

MCC **E13.11 Other specified diabetes mellitus with ketoacidosis with coma**
HAC see Appendix B for HAC conditional logic

+ **E13.2 Other specified diabetes mellitus with kidney complications**

E13.21 Other specified diabetes mellitus with diabetic nephropathy
Other specified diabetes mellitus with intercapillary glomerulosclerosis
Other specified diabetes mellitus with intracapillary glomerulonephrosis
Other specified diabetes mellitus with Kimmelstiel-Wilson disease

E13.22 Other specified diabetes mellitus with diabetic chronic kidney disease
Use additional code to identify stage of chronic kidney disease (N18.1-N18.6)

E13.29 Other specified diabetes mellitus with other diabetic kidney complication
Other specified diabetes mellitus with renal tubular degeneration

+ **E13.3 Other specified diabetes mellitus with ophthalmic complications**
AHA CC: 4Q, 2016, 11-13

+ **E13.31 Other specified diabetes mellitus with unspecified diabetic retinopathy**

E13.311 Other specified diabetes mellitus with unspecified diabetic retinopathy with macular edema

E13.319 Other specified diabetes mellitus with unspecified diabetic retinopathy without macular edema

+ **E13.32 Other specified diabetes mellitus with mild nonproliferative diabetic retinopathy**
Other specified diabetes mellitus with nonproliferative diabetic retinopathy NOS

One of the following 7th characters is to be assigned to codes in subcategory **E13.32** to designate laterality of the disease:
1 right eye
2 left eye
3 bilateral
9 unspecified eye

+7th **E13.321 Other specified diabetes mellitus with mild nonproliferative diabetic retinopathy with macular edema**

+7th **E13.329 Other specified diabetes mellitus with mild nonproliferative diabetic retinopathy without macular edema**

+ **E13.33 Other specified diabetes mellitus with moderate nonproliferative diabetic retinopathy**

One of the following 7th characters is to be assigned to codes in subcategory **E13.33** to designate laterality of the disease:
1 right eye
2 left eye
3 bilateral
9 unspecified eye

+7th **E13.331 Other specified diabetes mellitus with moderate nonproliferative diabetic retinopathy with macular edema**

+7th **E13.339 Other specified diabetes mellitus with moderate nonproliferative diabetic retinopathy without macular edema**

+ **E13.34 Other specified diabetes mellitus with severe nonproliferative diabetic retinopathy**

One of the following 7th characters is to be assigned to codes in subcategory **E13.34** to designate laterality of the disease:
1 right eye
2 left eye
3 bilateral
9 unspecified eye

+7th **E13.341 Other specified diabetes mellitus with severe nonproliferative diabetic retinopathy with macular edema**

+7th **E13.349 Other specified diabetes mellitus with severe nonproliferative diabetic retinopathy without macular edema**

+ **E13.35 Other specified diabetes mellitus with proliferative diabetic retinopathy**

One of the following 7th characters is to be assigned to codes in subcategory **E13.35** to designate laterality of the disease:
1 right eye
2 left eye
3 bilateral
9 unspecified eye

+7th **E13.351 Other specified diabetes mellitus with proliferative diabetic retinopathy with macular edema**

+7th **E13.352 Other specified diabetes mellitus with proliferative diabetic retinopathy with traction retinal detachment involving the macula**

+7th **E13.353 Other specified diabetes mellitus with proliferative diabetic retinopathy with traction retinal detachment not involving the macula**

+7th **E13.354 Other specified diabetes mellitus with proliferative diabetic retinopathy with combined traction retinal detachment and rhegmatogenous retinal detachment**

+7th **E13.355 Other specified diabetes mellitus with stable proliferative diabetic retinopathy**

+7th **E13.359 Other specified diabetes mellitus with proliferative diabetic retinopathy without macular edema**

E13.36 Other specified diabetes mellitus with diabetic cataract

X+7th **E13.37 Other specified diabetes mellitus with diabetic macular edema, resolved following treatment**

One of the following 7th characters is to be assigned to codes in subcategory **E13.37** to designate laterality of the disease:
1 right eye
2 left eye
3 bilateral
9 unspecified eye

E13.39 Other specified diabetes mellitus with other diabetic ophthalmic complication
Use additional code to identify manifestation, such as: diabetic glaucoma (H40-H42)

+ **E13.4 Other specified diabetes mellitus with neurological complications**

E13.40 Other specified diabetes mellitus with diabetic neuropathy, unspecified
AHA CC: 4Q, 2013, 129

E13.41 Other specified diabetes mellitus with diabetic mononeuropathy

E13.42 Other specified diabetes mellitus with diabetic polyneuropathy
Other specified diabetes mellitus with diabetic neuralgia

E13.43 Other specified diabetes mellitus with diabetic autonomic (poly)neuropathy
Other specified diabetes mellitus with diabetic gastroparesis
AHA CC: 4Q, 2013, 114-115

E13.44 Other specified diabetes mellitus with diabetic amyotrophy

E13.49 Other specified diabetes mellitus with other diabetic neurological complication

+ **E13.5 Other specified diabetes mellitus with circulatory complications**

E13.51 Other specified diabetes mellitus with diabetic peripheral angiopathy without gangrene

CC **E13.52 Other specified diabetes mellitus with diabetic peripheral angiopathy with gangrene**
Other specified diabetes mellitus with diabetic gangrene

E13.59 Other specified diabetes mellitus with other circulatory complications

+ E13.6 **Other specified diabetes mellitus with other specified complications**
+ E13.61 **Other specified diabetes mellitus with diabetic arthropathy**
E13.610 **Other specified diabetes mellitus with diabetic neuropathic arthropathy**
Other specified diabetes mellitus with Charcôt's joints
E13.618 **Other specified diabetes mellitus with other diabetic arthropathy**
+ E13.62 **Other specified diabetes mellitus with skin complications**
E13.620 **Other specified diabetes mellitus with diabetic dermatitis**
Other specified diabetes mellitus with diabetic necrobiosis lipoidica
E13.621 **Other specified diabetes mellitus with foot ulcer**
Use additional code to identify site of ulcer (L97.4-, L97.5-)
E13.622 **Other specified diabetes mellitus with other skin ulcer**
Use additional code to identify site of ulcer (L97.1-L97.9, L98.41-L98.49)
E13.628 **Other specified diabetes mellitus with other skin complications**
+ E13.63 **Other specified diabetes mellitus with oral complications**
E13.630 **Other specified diabetes mellitus with periodontal disease**
E13.638 **Other specified diabetes mellitus with other oral complications**
+ E13.64 **Other specified diabetes mellitus with hypoglycemia**
MCC E13.641 **Other specified diabetes mellitus with hypoglycemia with coma**
E13.649 **Other specified diabetes mellitus with hypoglycemia without coma**
E13.65 **Other specified diabetes mellitus with hyperglycemia**
AHA CC: 3Q, 2018, 4-5
E13.69 **Other specified diabetes mellitus with other specified complication**
Use additional code to identify complication
E13.8 **Other specified diabetes mellitus with unspecified complications**
E13.9 **Other specified diabetes mellitus without complications**

Other disorders of glucose regulation and pancreatic internal secretion (E15-E16)

CC E15 **Nondiabetic hypoglycemic coma**
Includes: drug-induced insulin coma in nondiabetic
hyperinsulinism with hypoglycemic coma
hypoglycemic coma NOS
HAC see Appendix B for HAC conditional logic
Valid 3-character code, no further characters required

E16 **Other disorders of pancreatic internal secretion**
E16.0 **Drug-induced hypoglycemia without coma**
Use additional code for adverse effect, if applicable, to identify drug (T36-T50 with fifth or sixth character 5)
Excludes1: *diabetes with hypoglycemia without coma (E09.649)*
E16.1 **Other hypoglycemia**
Functional hyperinsulinism
Functional nonhyperinsulinemic hypoglycemia
Hyperinsulinism NOS
Hyperplasia of pancreatic islet beta cells NOS
Excludes1: *diabetes with hypoglycemia (E08.649, E10.649, E11.649, E13.649)*
hypoglycemia in infant of diabetic mother (P70.1)
neonatal hypoglycemia (P70.4)
E16.2 **Hypoglycemia, unspecified**
Excludes1: *diabetes with hypoglycemia (E08.649, E10.649, E11.649, E13.649)*
E16.3 **Increased secretion of glucagon**
Hyperplasia of pancreatic endocrine cells with glucagon excess
E16.4 **Increased secretion of gastrin**
Hypergastrinemia
Hyperplasia of pancreatic endocrine cells with gastrin excess
Zollinger-Ellison syndrome
E16.8 **Other specified disorders of pancreatic internal secretion**
Increased secretion from endocrine pancreas of growth hormone-releasing hormone
Increased secretion from endocrine pancreas of pancreatic polypeptide
Increased secretion from endocrine pancreas of somatostatin
Increased secretion from endocrine pancreas of vasoactive-intestinal polypeptide
E16.9 **Disorder of pancreatic internal secretion, unspecified**
Islet-cell hyperplasia NOS
Pancreatic endocrine cell hyperplasia NOS

Disorders of other endocrine glands (E20-E35)

Excludes1: *galactorrhea (N64.3)*
gynecomastia (N62)

E20 **Hypoparathyroidism**
Excludes1: *Di George's syndrome (D82.1)*
postprocedural hypoparathyroidism (E89.2)
tetany NOS (R29.0)
transitory neonatal hypoparathyroidism (P71.4)
E20.0 **Idiopathic hypoparathyroidism**
E20.1 **Pseudohypoparathyroidism**
E20.8 **Other hypoparathyroidism**
E20.9 **Hypoparathyroidism, unspecified**
Parathyroid tetany

E21 **Hyperparathyroidism and other disorders of parathyroid gland**
Excludes1: *adult osteomalacia (M83.-)*
ectopic hyperparathyroidism (E34.2)
hungry bone syndrome (E83.81)
infantile and juvenile osteomalacia (E55.0)
Excludes2: *familial hypocalciuric hypercalcemia (E83.52)*
E21.0 **Primary hyperparathyroidism**
Hyperplasia of parathyroid
Osteitis fibrosa cystica generalisata [von Recklinghausen's disease of bone]
E21.1 **Secondary hyperparathyroidism, not elsewhere classified**
Excludes1: *secondary hyperparathyroidism of renal origin (N25.81)*
E21.2 **Other hyperparathyroidism**
Tertiary hyperparathyroidism
Excludes1: *familial hypocalciuric hypercalcemia (E83.52)*
E21.3 **Hyperparathyroidism, unspecified**
E21.4 **Other specified disorders of parathyroid gland**
E21.5 **Disorder of parathyroid gland, unspecified**

E22 **Hyperfunction of pituitary gland**
Excludes1: *Cushing's syndrome (E24.-)*
Nelson's syndrome (E24.1)
overproduction of ACTH not associated with Cushing's disease (E27.0)
overproduction of pituitary ACTH (E24.0)
overproduction of thyroid-stimulating hormone (E05.8-)
E22.0 **Acromegaly and pituitary gigantism**
Overproduction of growth hormone
Excludes1: *constitutional gigantism (E34.4)*
constitutional tall stature (E34.4)
increased secretion from endocrine pancreas of growth hormone-releasing hormone (E16.8)
CC E22.1 **Hyperprolactinemia**
Use additional code for adverse effect, if applicable, to identify drug (T36-T50 with fifth or sixth character 5)
CC E22.2 **Syndrome of inappropriate secretion of antidiuretic hormone**
CC E22.8 **Other hyperfunction of pituitary gland**
Central precocious puberty
CC E22.9 **Hyperfunction of pituitary gland, unspecified**

E23 Hypofunction and other disorders of the pituitary gland

Includes: the listed conditions whether the disorder is in the pituitary or the hypothalamus

Excludes1: *postprocedural hypopituitarism (E89.3)*

CC **E23.0 Hypopituitarism**
Fertile eunuch syndrome
Hypogonadotropic hypogonadism
Idiopathic growth hormone deficiency
Isolated deficiency of gonadotropin
Isolated deficiency of growth hormone
Isolated deficiency of pituitary hormone
Kallmann's syndrome
Lorain-Levi short stature
Necrosis of pituitary gland (postpartum)
Panhypopituitarism
Pituitary cachexia
Pituitary insufficiency NOS
Pituitary short stature
Sheehan's syndrome
Simmonds' disease

E23.1 Drug-induced hypopituitarism
Use additional code for adverse effect, if applicable, to identify drug (T36-T50 with fifth or sixth character 5)

CC **E23.2 Diabetes insipidus**
Excludes1: *nephrogenic diabetes insipidus (N25.1)*

E23.3 Hypothalamic dysfunction, not elsewhere classified
Excludes1: *Prader-Willi syndrome (Q87.11)*
Russell-Silver syndrome (Q87.19)

E23.6 Other disorders of pituitary gland
Abscess of pituitary
Adiposogenital dystrophy

E23.7 Disorder of pituitary gland, unspecified

E24 Cushing's syndrome

Excludes1: *congenital adrenal hyperplasia (E25.0)*

CC **E24.0 Pituitary-dependent Cushing's disease**
Overproduction of pituitary ACTH
Pituitary-dependent hypercorticalism

E24.1 Nelson's syndrome

CC **E24.2 Drug-induced Cushing's syndrome**
Use additional code for adverse effect, if applicable, to identify drug (T36-T50 with fifth or sixth character 5)

CC **E24.3 Ectopic ACTH syndrome**

CC **E24.4 Alcohol-induced pseudo-Cushing's syndrome**

CC **E24.8 Other Cushing's syndrome**

CC **E24.9 Cushing's syndrome, unspecified**

E25 Adrenogenital disorders

Includes: adrenogenital syndromes, virilizing or feminizing, whether acquired or due to adrenal hyperplasia consequent on inborn enzyme defects in hormone synthesis
Female adrenal pseudohermaphroditism
Female heterosexual precocious pseudopuberty
Male isosexual precocious pseudopuberty
Male macrogenitosomia praecox
Male sexual precocity with adrenal hyperplasia
Male virilization (female)

Excludes1: *indeterminate sex and pseudohermaphroditism (Q56)*
chromosomal abnormalities (Q90-Q99)

E25.0 Congenital adrenogenital disorders associated with enzyme deficiency
Congenital adrenal hyperplasia
21-Hydroxylase deficiency
Salt-losing congenital adrenal hyperplasia

E25.8 Other adrenogenital disorders
Idiopathic adrenogenital disorder
Use additional code for adverse effect, if applicable, to identify drug (T36-T50 with fifth or sixth character 5)

E25.9 Adrenogenital disorder, unspecified
Adrenogenital syndrome NOS

E26 Hyperaldosteronism

+ **E26.0 Primary hyperaldosteronism**

E26.01 Conn's syndrome
Code also adrenal adenoma (D35.0-)

E26.02 Glucocorticoid-remediable aldosteronism
Familial aldosteronism type I

E26.09 Other primary hyperaldosteronism
Primary aldosteronism due to adrenal hyperplasia (bilateral)

E26.1 Secondary hyperaldosteronism

+ **E26.8 Other hyperaldosteronism**

E26.81 Bartter's syndrome

E26.89 Other hyperaldosteronism

E26.9 Hyperaldosteronism, unspecified
Aldosteronism NOS
Hyperaldosteronism NOS

E27 Other disorders of adrenal gland

CC **E27.0 Other adrenocortical overactivity**
Overproduction of ACTH, not associated with Cushing's disease
Premature adrenarche
Excludes1: *Cushing's syndrome (E24.-)*

CC **E27.1 Primary adrenocortical insufficiency**
Addison's disease
Autoimmune adrenalitis
Excludes1: *Addison only phenotype adrenoleukodystrophy (E71.528)*
amyloidosis (E85.-)
tuberculous Addison's disease (A18.7)
Waterhouse-Friderichsen syndrome (A39.1)

CC **E27.2 Addisonian crisis**
Adrenal crisis
Adrenocortical crisis

CC **E27.3 Drug-induced adrenocortical insufficiency**
Use additional code for adverse effect, if applicable, to identify drug (T36-T50 with fifth or sixth character 5)

+ **E27.4 Other and unspecified adrenocortical insufficiency**
Excludes1: *adrenoleukodystrophy [Addison-Schilder] (E71.528)*
Waterhouse-Friderichsen syndrome (A39.1)

CC **E27.40 Unspecified adrenocortical insufficiency**
Adrenocortical insufficiency NOS
Hypoaldosteronism

CC **E27.49 Other adrenocortical insufficiency**
Adrenal hemorrhage
Adrenal infarction

CC **E27.5 Adrenomedullary hyperfunction**
Adrenomedullary hyperplasia
Catecholamine hypersecretion

E27.8 Other specified disorders of adrenal gland
Abnormality of cortisol-binding globulin

E27.9 Disorder of adrenal gland, unspecified

E28 Ovarian dysfunction

Excludes1: *isolated gonadotropin deficiency (E23.0)*
postprocedural ovarian failure (E89.4-)

♀ **E28.0 Estrogen excess**
Use additional code for adverse effect, if applicable, to identify drug (T36-T50 with fifth or sixth character 5)

♀ **E28.1 Androgen excess**
Hypersecretion of ovarian androgens
Use additional code for adverse effect, if applicable, to identify drug (T36-T50 with fifth or sixth character 5)

♀ **E28.2 Polycystic ovarian syndrome**
Sclerocystic ovary syndrome
Stein-Leventhal syndrome

+ **E28.3 Primary ovarian failure**
Excludes1: *pure gonadal dysgenesis (Q99.1)*
Turner's syndrome (Q96.-)

+ **E28.31 Premature menopause**

● ♀ **E28.310 Symptomatic premature menopause**
Symptoms such as flushing, sleeplessness, headache, lack of concentration, associated with premature menopause

● ♀ **E28.319 Asymptomatic premature menopause**
Premature menopause NOS

♀ **E28.39 Other primary ovarian failure**
Decreased estrogen
Resistant ovary syndrome

♀ **E28.8 Other ovarian dysfunction**
Ovarian hyperfunction NOS
Excludes1: *postprocedural ovarian failure (E89.4-)*

♀ **E28.9 Ovarian dysfunction, unspecified**

E29 Testicular dysfunction

Excludes1: *androgen insensitivity syndrome (E34.5-)*
azoospermia or oligospermia NOS (N46.0-N46.1)
isolated gonadotropin deficiency (E23.0)
Klinefelter's syndrome (Q98.0-Q98.1, Q98.4)

♂ **E29.0 Testicular hyperfunction**
Hypersecretion of testicular hormones

♂ **E29.1 Testicular hypofunction**
Defective biosynthesis of testicular androgen NOS
5-delta-Reductase deficiency (with male pseudohermaphroditism)
Testicular hypogonadism NOS
Use additional code for adverse effect, if applicable, to identify drug (T36-T50 with fifth or sixth character 5)
Excludes1: *postprocedural testicular hypofunction (E89.5)*

♂ **E29.8 Other testicular dysfunction**

♂ **E29.9 Testicular dysfunction, unspecified**

E30 Disorders of puberty, not elsewhere classified

E30.0 Delayed puberty
Constitutional delay of puberty
Delayed sexual development

• **E30.1 Precocious puberty**
Precocious menstruation
Excludes1: *Albright (-McCune) (-Sternberg) syndrome (Q78.1)*
central precocious puberty (E22.8)
congenital adrenal hyperplasia (E25.0)
female heterosexual precocious pseudopuberty (E25.-)
male isosexual precocious pseudopuberty (E25.-)

• **E30.8 Other disorders of puberty**
Premature thelarche

E30.9 Disorder of puberty, unspecified

E31 Polyglandular dysfunction

Excludes1: *ataxia telangiectasia [Louis-Bar] (G11.3)*
dystrophia myotonica [Steinert] (G71.11)
pseudohypoparathyroidism (E20.1)

E31.0 Autoimmune polyglandular failure
Schmidt's syndrome

E31.1 Polyglandular hyperfunction
Excludes1: *multiple endocrine adenomatosis (E31.2-)*
multiple endocrine neoplasia (E31.2-)

\+ **E31.2 Multiple endocrine neoplasia [MEN] syndromes**
Multiple endocrine adenomatosis
Code also any associated malignancies and other conditions associated with the syndromes

E31.20 Multiple endocrine neoplasia [MEN] syndrome, unspecified
Multiple endocrine adenomatosis NOS
Multiple endocrine neoplasia [MEN] syndrome NOS

E31.21 Multiple endocrine neoplasia [MEN] type I
Wermer's syndrome

E31.22 Multiple endocrine neoplasia [MEN] type IIA
Sipple's syndrome

E31.23 Multiple endocrine neoplasia [MEN] type IIB

E31.8 Other polyglandular dysfunction

E31.9 Polyglandular dysfunction, unspecified

E32 Diseases of thymus

Excludes1: *aplasia or hypoplasia of thymus with immunodeficiency (D82.1)*
myasthenia gravis (G70.0)

E32.0 Persistent hyperplasia of thymus
Hypertrophy of thymus

CC **E32.1 Abscess of thymus**

E32.8 Other diseases of thymus
Excludes1: *aplasia or hypoplasia with immunodeficiency (D82.1)*
thymoma (D15.0)

E32.9 Disease of thymus, unspecified

E34 Other endocrine disorders

Excludes1: *pseudohypoparathyroidism (E20.1)*

CC **E34.0 Carcinoid syndrome**
NOTE May be used as an additional code to identify functional activity associated with a carcinoid tumor.

E34.1 Other hypersecretion of intestinal hormones

E34.2 Ectopic hormone secretion, not elsewhere classified
Excludes1: *ectopic ACTH syndrome (E24.3)*

E34.3 Short stature due to endocrine disorder
Constitutional short stature
Laron-type short stature
Excludes1: *achondroplastic short stature (Q77.4)*
hypochondroplastic short stature (Q77.4)
nutritional short stature (E45)
pituitary short stature (E23.0)
progeria (E34.8)
renal short stature (N25.0)
Russell-Silver syndrome (Q87.19)
short-limbed stature with immunodeficiency (D82.2)
short stature in specific dysmorphic syndromes - code to syndrome - see Alphabetical Index
short stature NOS (R62.52)

E34.4 Constitutional tall stature
Constitutional gigantism

\+ **E34.5 Androgen insensitivity syndrome**

E34.50 Androgen insensitivity syndrome, unspecified
Androgen insensitivity NOS

E34.51 Complete androgen insensitivity syndrome
Complete androgen insensitivity
de Quervain syndrome
Goldberg-Maxwell syndrome

E34.52 Partial androgen insensitivity syndrome
Partial androgen insensitivity
Reifenstein syndrome

E34.8 Other specified endocrine disorders
Pineal gland dysfunction
Progeria
Excludes2: *pseudohypoparathyroidism (E20.1)*

E34.9 Endocrine disorder, unspecified
Endocrine disturbance NOS
Hormone disturbance NOS

E35 Disorders of endocrine glands in diseases classified elsewhere

Code first underlying disease, such as:
late congenital syphilis of thymus gland [Dubois disease] (A50.5)

Use additional code, if applicable, to identify:
sequelae of tuberculosis of other organs (B90.8)

Excludes1: *Echinococcus granulosus infection of thyroid gland (B67.3)*
meningococcal hemorrhagic adrenalitis (A39.1)
syphilis of endocrine gland (A52.79)
tuberculosis of adrenal gland, except calcification (A18.7)
tuberculosis of endocrine gland NEC (A18.82)
tuberculosis of thyroid gland (A18.81)
Waterhouse-Friderichsen syndrome (A39.1)

Valid 3-character code, no further characters required

Intraoperative complications of endocrine system (E36)

E36 Intraoperative complications of endocrine system

Excludes2: *postprocedural endocrine and metabolic complications and disorders, not elsewhere classified (E89.-)*

\+ **E36.0 Intraoperative hemorrhage and hematoma of an endocrine system organ or structure complicating a procedure**
Excludes1: *intraoperative hemorrhage and hematoma of an endocrine system organ or structure due to accidental puncture or laceration during a procedure (E36.1-)*

CC **E36.01 Intraoperative hemorrhage and hematoma of an endocrine system organ or structure complicating an endocrine system procedure**
AHA CC: 1Q, 2020, 19

CC **E36.02 Intraoperative hemorrhage and hematoma of an endocrine system organ or structure complicating other procedure**

+ **E36.1 Accidental puncture and laceration of an endocrine system organ or structure during a procedure**
  - CC **E36.11 Accidental puncture and laceration of an endocrine system organ or structure during an endocrine system procedure**
  - CC **E36.12 Accidental puncture and laceration of an endocrine system organ or structure during other procedure**

E36.8 Other intraoperative complications of endocrine system
Use additional code, if applicable, to further specify disorder

Malnutrition (E40-E46)

Excludes1: *intestinal malabsorption (K90.-)*
sequelae of protein-calorie malnutrition (E64.0)
Excludes2: *nutritional anemias (D50-D53)*
starvation (T73.0)

MCC **E40 Kwashiorkor**
Severe malnutrition with nutritional edema with dyspigmentation of skin and hair
Excludes1: *marasmic kwashiorkor (E42)*
AHA CC: 3Q, 2017, 25-26
Valid 3-character code, no further characters required

MCC **E41 Nutritional marasmus**
Severe malnutrition with marasmus
Excludes1: *marasmic kwashiorkor (E42)*
AHA CC: 3Q, 2017, 24-25
Valid 3-character code, no further characters required

MCC **E42 Marasmic kwashiorkor**
Intermediate form severe protein-calorie malnutrition
Severe protein-calorie malnutrition with signs of both kwashiorkor and marasmus
AHA CC: 3Q, 2017, 25-26
Valid 3-character code, no further characters required

MCC **E43 Unspecified severe protein-calorie malnutrition**
Starvation edema
AHA CC: 3Q, 2017, 25-26; 4Q, 2017, 108-109; 1Q, 2020, 4-7
Valid 3-character code, no further characters required

E44 Protein-calorie malnutrition of moderate and mild degree
- CC **E44.0 Moderate protein-calorie malnutrition**
- CC **E44.1 Mild protein-calorie malnutrition**

CC **E45 Retarded development following protein-calorie malnutrition**
Nutritional short stature
Nutritional stunting
Physical retardation due to malnutrition
Valid 3-character code, no further characters required

CC **E46 Unspecified protein-calorie malnutrition**
Malnutrition NOS
Protein-calorie imbalance NOS
Excludes1: *nutritional deficiency NOS (E63.9)*
Valid 3-character code, no further characters required

Other nutritional deficiencies (E50-E64)

Excludes2: *nutritional anemias (D50-D53)*

E50 Vitamin A deficiency
Excludes1: *sequelae of vitamin A deficiency (E64.1)*
- **E50.0 Vitamin A deficiency with conjunctival xerosis**
- **E50.1 Vitamin A deficiency with Bitot's spot and conjunctival xerosis**
  Bitot's spot in the young child
- **E50.2 Vitamin A deficiency with corneal xerosis**
- **E50.3 Vitamin A deficiency with corneal ulceration and xerosis**
- **E50.4 Vitamin A deficiency with keratomalacia**
- **E50.5 Vitamin A deficiency with night blindness**
- **E50.6 Vitamin A deficiency with xerophthalmic scars of cornea**
- **E50.7 Other ocular manifestations of vitamin A deficiency**
  Xerophthalmia NOS
- **E50.8 Other manifestations of vitamin A deficiency**
  Follicular keratosis
  Xeroderma
- **E50.9 Vitamin A deficiency, unspecified**
  Hypovitaminosis A NOS

E51 Thiamine deficiency
Excludes1: *sequelae of thiamine deficiency (E64.8)*
+ **E51.1 Beriberi**
  - CC **E51.11 Dry beriberi**
    Beriberi NOS
    Beriberi with polyneuropathy
  - CC **E51.12 Wet beriberi**
    Beriberi with cardiovascular manifestations
    Cardiovascular beriberi
    Shoshin disease
- CC **E51.2 Wernicke's encephalopathy**
- CC **E51.8 Other manifestations of thiamine deficiency**
- CC **E51.9 Thiamine deficiency, unspecified**

E52 Niacin deficiency [pellagra]
Niacin (-tryptophan) deficiency
Nicotinamide deficiency
Pellagra (alcoholic)
Excludes1: *sequelae of niacin deficiency (E64.8)*
Valid 3-character code, no further characters required

E53 Deficiency of other B group vitamins
Excludes1: *sequelae of vitamin B deficiency (E64.8)*
- CC **E53.0 Riboflavin deficiency**
  Ariboflavinosis
  Vitamin B2 deficiency
- **E53.1 Pyridoxine deficiency**
  Vitamin B6 deficiency
  Excludes1: *pyridoxine-responsive sideroblastic anemia (D64.3)*
- **E53.8 Deficiency of other specified B group vitamins**
  Biotin deficiency
  Cyanocobalamin deficiency
  Folate deficiency
  Folic acid deficiency
  Pantothenic acid deficiency
  Vitamin B12 deficiency
  Excludes1: *folate deficiency anemia (D52.-)*
  vitamin B12 deficiency anemia (D51.-)
- **E53.9 Vitamin B deficiency, unspecified**

E54 Ascorbic acid deficiency
Deficiency of vitamin C
Scurvy
Excludes1: *scorbutic anemia (D53.2)*
sequelae of vitamin C deficiency (E64.2)
Valid 3-character code, no further characters required

E55 Vitamin D deficiency
Excludes1: *adult osteomalacia (M83.-)*
osteoporosis (M80.-)
sequelae of rickets (E64.3)
- CC **E55.0 Rickets, active**
  Infantile osteomalacia
  Juvenile osteomalacia
  Excludes1: *celiac rickets (K90.0)*
  Crohn's rickets (K50.-)
  hereditary vitamin D-dependent rickets (E83.32)
  inactive rickets (E64.3)
  renal rickets (N25.0)
  sequelae of rickets (E64.3)
  vitamin D-resistant rickets (E83.31)
- **E55.9 Vitamin D deficiency, unspecified**
  Avitaminosis D

E56 Other vitamin deficiencies
Excludes1: *sequelae of other vitamin deficiencies (E64.8)*
- **E56.0 Deficiency of vitamin E**
- **E56.1 Deficiency of vitamin K**
  Excludes1: *deficiency of coagulation factor due to vitamin K deficiency (D68.4)*
  vitamin K deficiency of newborn (P53)
- **E56.8 Deficiency of other vitamins**
- **E56.9 Vitamin deficiency, unspecified**

E58 Dietary calcium deficiency
Excludes1: *disorders of calcium metabolism (E83.5-)*
sequelae of calcium deficiency (E64.8)
Valid 3-character code, no further characters required

E59 Dietary selenium deficiency
Keshan disease
Excludes1: *sequelae of selenium deficiency (E64.8)*
Valid 3-character code, no further characters required

E60 Dietary zinc deficiency
Valid 3-character code, no further characters required

E61 Deficiency of other nutrient elements

Use additional code for adverse effect, if applicable, to identify drug (T36-T50 with fifth or sixth character 5)

Excludes1: *disorders of mineral metabolism (E83.-)*
iodine deficiency related thyroid disorders (E00-E02)
sequelae of malnutrition and other nutritional deficiencies (E64.-)

E61.0 Copper deficiency
E61.1 Iron deficiency
Excludes1: *iron deficiency anemia (D50.-)*
E61.2 Magnesium deficiency
E61.3 Manganese deficiency
E61.4 Chromium deficiency
E61.5 Molybdenum deficiency
E61.6 Vanadium deficiency
E61.7 Deficiency of multiple nutrient elements
E61.8 Deficiency of other specified nutrient elements
E61.9 Deficiency of nutrient element, unspecified

E63 Other nutritional deficiencies

Excludes2: *dehydration (E86.0)*
failure to thrive, adult (R62.7)
failure to thrive, child (R62.51)
feeding problems in newborn (P92.-)
sequelae of malnutrition and other nutritional deficiencies (E64.-)

E63.0 Essential fatty acid [EFA] deficiency
E63.1 Imbalance of constituents of food intake
E63.8 Other specified nutritional deficiencies
E63.9 Nutritional deficiency, unspecified

E64 Sequelae of malnutrition and other nutritional deficiencies

NOTE This category is to be used to indicate conditions in categories E43, E44, E46, E50-E63 as the cause of sequelae, which are themselves classified elsewhere. The 'sequelae' include conditions specified as such; they also include the late effects of diseases classifiable to the above categories if the disease itself is no longer present

Code first condition resulting from (sequela) of malnutrition and other nutritional deficiencies

CC **E64.0 Sequelae of protein-calorie malnutrition**
Excludes2: *retarded development following protein-calorie malnutrition (E45)*
E64.1 Sequelae of vitamin A deficiency
E64.2 Sequelae of vitamin C deficiency
E64.3 Sequelae of rickets
E64.8 Sequelae of other nutritional deficiencies
E64.9 Sequelae of unspecified nutritional deficiency

Overweight, obesity and other hyperalimentation (E65-E68)

E65 Localized adiposity

Fat pad
Valid 3-character code, no further characters required

E66 Overweight and obesity

Code first obesity complicating pregnancy, childbirth and the puerperium, if applicable (O99.21-)

Use additional code to identify body mass index (BMI), if known (Z68.-)

Excludes1: *adiposogenital dystrophy (E23.6)*
lipomatosis NOS (E88.2)
lipomatosis dolorosa [Dercum] (E88.2)
Prader-Willi syndrome (Q87.11)

AHA CC: 4Q, 2018, 80

\+ **E66.0 Obesity due to excess calories**
E66.01 Morbid (severe) obesity due to excess calories
Excludes1: *morbid (severe) obesity with alveolar hypoventilation (E66.2)*
AHA CC: 4Q, 2018, 79
HAC see Appendix B for HAC conditional logic
E66.09 Other obesity due to excess calories
E66.1 Drug-induced obesity
Use additional code for adverse effect, if applicable, to identify drug (T36-T50 with fifth or sixth character 5)
CC **E66.2 Morbid (severe) obesity with alveolar hypoventilation**
Obesity hypoventilation syndrome (OHS)
Pickwickian syndrome
E66.3 Overweight
E66.8 Other obesity
E66.9 Obesity, unspecified
Obesity NOS
AHA CC: 4Q, 2013, 129; 2Q, 2021, 10-11

E67 Other hyperalimentation

Excludes1: *hyperalimentation NOS (R63.2)*
sequelae of hyperalimentation (E68)

E67.0 Hypervitaminosis A
E67.1 Hypercarotenemia
E67.2 Megavitamin-B6 syndrome
E67.3 Hypervitaminosis D
E67.8 Other specified hyperalimentation

E68 Sequelae of hyperalimentation

Code first condition resulting from (sequela) of hyperalimentation
Valid 3-character code, no further characters required

Metabolic disorders (E70-E88)

Excludes1: *androgen insensitivity syndrome (E34.5-)*
congenital adrenal hyperplasia (E25.0)
hemolytic anemias attributable to enzyme disorders (D55.-)
Marfan's syndrome (Q87.4)
5-alpha-reductase deficiency (E29.1)

Excludes2: *Ehlers-Danlos syndromes (Q79.6-)*

E70 Disorders of aromatic amino-acid metabolism

CC **E70.0 Classical phenylketonuria**
CC **E70.1 Other hyperphenylalaninemias**
\+ **E70.2 Disorders of tyrosine metabolism**
Excludes1: *transitory tyrosinemia of newborn (P74.5)*
CC **E70.20 Disorder of tyrosine metabolism, unspecified**
CC **E70.21 Tyrosinemia**
Hypertyrosinemia
CC **E70.29 Other disorders of tyrosine metabolism**
Alkaptonuria
Ochronosis
\+ **E70.3 Albinism**
CC **E70.30 Albinism, unspecified**
\+ **E70.31 Ocular albinism**
CC **E70.310 X-linked ocular albinism**
CC **E70.311 Autosomal recessive ocular albinism**
CC **E70.318 Other ocular albinism**
CC **E70.319 Ocular albinism, unspecified**
\+ **E70.32 Oculocutaneous albinism**
Excludes1: *Chediak-Higashi syndrome (E70.330)*
Hermansky-Pudlak syndrome (E70.331)
CC **E70.320 Tyrosinase negative oculocutaneous albinism**
Albinism I
Oculocutaneous albinism ty-neg
CC **E70.321 Tyrosinase positive oculocutaneous albinism**
Albinism II
Oculocutaneous albinism ty-pos
CC **E70.328 Other oculocutaneous albinism**
Cross syndrome
CC **E70.329 Oculocutaneous albinism, unspecified**
\+ **E70.33 Albinism with hematologic abnormality**
CC **E70.330 Chediak-Higashi syndrome**
CC **E70.331 Hermansky-Pudlak syndrome**
CC **E70.338 Other albinism with hematologic abnormality**
CC **E70.339 Albinism with hematologic abnormality, unspecified**
CC **E70.39 Other specified albinism**
Piebaldism
\+ **E70.4 Disorders of histidine metabolism**
CC **E70.40 Disorders of histidine metabolism, unspecified**
CC **E70.41 Histidinemia**
CC **E70.49 Other disorders of histidine metabolism**
CC **E70.5 Disorders of tryptophan metabolism**
\+ **E70.8 Other disorders of aromatic amino-acid metabolism**
CC **E70.81 Aromatic L-amino acid decarboxylase deficiency**
AADC deficiency
AHA CC: 4Q, 2020, 15-16
CC **E70.89 Other disorders of aromatic amino-acid metabolism**
\+ **E70.9 Disorder of aromatic amino-acid metabolism, unspecified**

E71 **Disorders of branched-chain amino-acid metabolism and fatty-acid metabolism**

CC **E71.0 Maple-syrup-urine disease**
+ E71.1 **Other disorders of branched-chain amino-acid metabolism**
+ E71.11 **Branched-chain organic acidurias**
CC **E71.110 Isovaleric acidemia**
CC **E71.111 3-methylglutaconic aciduria**
CC **E71.118 Other branched-chain organic acidurias**
+ E71.12 **Disorders of propionate metabolism**
CC **E71.120 Methylmalonic acidemia**
CC **E71.121 Propionic acidemia**
CC **E71.128 Other disorders of propionate metabolism**
CC **E71.19 Other disorders of branched-chain amino-acid metabolism**
Hyperleucine-isoleucinemia
Hypervalinemia
CC **E71.2 Disorder of branched-chain amino-acid metabolism, unspecified**
+ E71.3 **Disorders of fatty-acid metabolism**
Excludes1: *peroxisomal disorders (E71.5)*
Refsum's disease (G60.1)
Schilder's disease (G37.0)
Excludes2: *carnitine deficiency due to inborn error of metabolism (E71.42)*
E71.30 **Disorder of fatty-acid metabolism, unspecified**
+ E71.31 **Disorders of fatty-acid oxidation**
CC **E71.310 Long chain/very long chain acyl CoA dehydrogenase deficiency**
LCAD
VLCAD
CC **E71.311 Medium chain acyl CoA dehydrogenase deficiency**
MCAD
CC **E71.312 Short chain acyl CoA dehydrogenase deficiency**
SCAD
CC **E71.313 Glutaric aciduria type II**
Glutaric aciduria type II A
Glutaric aciduria type II B
Glutaric aciduria type II C
Excludes1: *glutaric aciduria (type 1) NOS (E72.3)*
CC **E71.314 Muscle carnitine palmitoyltransferase deficiency**
CC **E71.318 Other disorders of fatty-acid oxidation**
CC **E71.32 Disorders of ketone metabolism**
CC **E71.39 Other disorders of fatty-acid metabolism**
+ E71.4 **Disorders of carnitine metabolism**
Excludes1: *Muscle carnitine palmitoyltransferase deficiency (E71.314)*
E71.40 Disorder of carnitine metabolism, unspecified
E71.41 Primary carnitine deficiency
E71.42 Carnitine deficiency due to inborn errors of metabolism
Code also associated inborn error or metabolism
E71.43 Iatrogenic carnitine deficiency
Carnitine deficiency due to hemodialysis
Carnitine deficiency due to Valproic acid therapy
+ E71.44 **Other secondary carnitine deficiency**
E71.440 Ruvalcaba-Myhre-Smith syndrome
E71.448 Other secondary carnitine deficiency
+ E71.5 **Peroxisomal disorders**
Excludes1: *Schilder's disease (G37.0)*
CC **E71.50 Peroxisomal disorder, unspecified**
+ E71.51 **Disorders of peroxisome biogenesis**
Group 1 peroxisomal disorders
Excludes1: *Refsum's disease (G60.1)*
CC **E71.510 Zellweger syndrome**
CC **E71.511 Neonatal adrenoleukodystrophy**
Excludes1: *X-linked adrenoleukodystrophy (E71.42-)*
CC **E71.518 Other disorders of peroxisome biogenesis**
+ E71.52 **X-linked adrenoleukodystrophy**
CC **E71.520 Childhood cerebral X-linked adrenoleukodystrophy**
CC **E71.521 Adolescent X-linked adrenoleukodystrophy**
CC **E71.522 Adrenomyeloneuropathy**
CC **E71.528 Other X-linked adrenoleukodystrophy**
Addison only phenotype adrenoleukodystrophy
Addison-Schilder adrenoleukodystrophy
CC **E71.529 X-linked adrenoleukodystrophy, unspecified type**
CC **E71.53 Other group 2 peroxisomal disorders**
+ E71.54 **Other peroxisomal disorders**
CC **E71.540 Rhizomelic chondrodysplasia punctata**
Excludes1: *chondrodysplasia punctata NOS (Q77.3)*
CC **E71.541 Zellweger-like syndrome**
CC **E71.542 Other group 3 peroxisomal disorders**
CC **E71.548 Other peroxisomal disorders**

E72 **Other disorders of amino-acid metabolism**
Excludes1: *disorders of:*
aromatic amino-acid metabolism (E70.-)
branched-chain amino-acid metabolism (E71.0-E71.2)
fatty-acid metabolism (E71.3)
purine and pyrimidine metabolism (E79.-)
gout (M1A.-, M10.-)
+ E72.0 **Disorders of amino-acid transport**
Excludes1: *disorders of tryptophan metabolism (E70.5)*
CC **E72.00 Disorders of amino-acid transport, unspecified**
CC **E72.01 Cystinuria**
CC **E72.02 Hartnup's disease**
CC **E72.03 Lowe's syndrome**
Use additional code for associated glaucoma (H42)
CC **E72.04 Cystinosis**
Fanconi (-de Toni) (-Debré) syndrome with cystinosis
Excludes1: *Fanconi (-de Toni) (-Debré) syndrome without cystinosis (E72.09)*
CC **E72.09 Other disorders of amino-acid transport**
Fanconi (-de Toni) (-Debré) syndrome, unspecified
+ E72.1 **Disorders of sulfur-bearing amino-acid metabolism**
Excludes1: *cystinosis (E72.04)*
cystinuria (E72.01)
transcobalamin II deficiency (D51.2)
CC **E72.10 Disorders of sulfur-bearing amino-acid metabolism, unspecified**
CC **E72.11 Homocystinuria**
Cystathionine synthase deficiency
CC **E72.12 Methylenetetrahydrofolate reductase deficiency**
CC **E72.19 Other disorders of sulfur-bearing amino-acid metabolism**
Cystathioninuria
Methioninemia
Sulfite oxidase deficiency
+ E72.2 **Disorders of urea cycle metabolism**
Excludes1: *disorders of ornithine metabolism (E72.4)*
CC **E72.20 Disorder of urea cycle metabolism, unspecified**
Hyperammonemia
Excludes1: *hyperammonemia-hyperornithinemia-homocitrullinemia syndrome E72.4*
transient hyperammonemia of newborn (P74.6)
CC **E72.21 Argininemia**
CC **E72.22 Arginosuccinic aciduria**
CC **E72.23 Citrullinemia**
CC **E72.29 Other disorders of urea cycle metabolism**
CC **E72.3 Disorders of lysine and hydroxylysine metabolism**
Glutaric aciduria NOS
Glutaric aciduria (type I)
Hydroxylysinemia
Hyperlysinemia
Excludes1: *glutaric aciduria type II (E71.313)*
Refsum's disease (G60.1)
Zellweger syndrome (E71.510)

CC E72.4 **Disorders of ornithine metabolism**
Hyperammonemia-Hyperornithinemia-Homocitrullinemia syndrome
Ornithinemia (types I, II)
Ornithine transcarbamylase deficiency
Excludes1: *hereditary choroidal dystrophy (H31.2-)*

+ E72.5 **Disorders of glycine metabolism**
CC E72.50 **Disorder of glycine metabolism, unspecified**
CC E72.51 **Non-ketotic hyperglycinemia**
CC E72.52 **Trimethylaminuria**
CC E72.53 **Primary hyperoxaluria**
Oxalosis
Oxaluria
AHA CC: 4Q, 2018, 29
CC E72.59 **Other disorders of glycine metabolism**
D-glycericacidemia
Hyperhydroxyprolinemia
Hyperprolinemia (types I, II)
Sarcosinemia

+ E72.8 **Other specified disorders of amino-acid metabolism**
CC E72.81 **Disorders of gamma aminobutyric acid metabolism**
4-hydroxybutyric aciduria
Disorders of GABA metabolism
GABA metabolic defect
GABA transaminase deficiency
GABA-T deficiency
Gamma-hydroxybutyric aciduria
SSADHA
Succinic semialdehyde dehydrogenase deficiency
AHA CC: 4Q, 2018, 5
CC E72.89 **Other specified disorders of amino-acid metabolism**
Disorders of beta-amino-acid metabolism
Disorders of gamma-glutamyl cycle

CC E72.9 **Disorder of amino-acid metabolism, unspecified**

E73 Lactose intolerance

E73.0 **Congenital lactase deficiency**
E73.1 **Secondary lactase deficiency**
E73.8 **Other lactose intolerance**
E73.9 **Lactose intolerance, unspecified**

E74 Other disorders of carbohydrate metabolism

Excludes1: *diabetes mellitus (E08-E13)*
NOS (E16.2)
increased secretion of glucagon (E16.3)
mucopolysaccharidosis (E76.0-E76.3)

+ E74.0 **Glycogen storage disease**
CC E74.00 **Glycogen storage disease, unspecified**
CC E74.01 **von Gierke disease**
Type I glycogen storage disease
CC E74.02 **Pompe disease**
Cardiac glycogenosis
Type II glycogen storage disease
CC E74.03 **Cori disease**
Forbes disease
Type III glycogen storage disease
CC E74.04 **McArdle disease**
Type V glycogen storage disease
CC E74.09 **Other glycogen storage disease**
Andersen disease
Hers disease
Tauri disease
Glycogen storage disease, types 0, IV, VI-XI
Liver phosphorylase deficiency
Muscle phosphofructokinase deficiency

+ E74.1 **Disorders of fructose metabolism**
Excludes1: *muscle phosphofructokinase deficiency (E74.09)*
E74.10 **Disorder of fructose metabolism, unspecified**
E74.11 **Essential fructosuria**
Fructokinase deficiency
E74.12 **Hereditary fructose intolerance**
Fructosemia
E74.19 **Other disorders of fructose metabolism**
Fructose-1, 6-diphosphatase deficiency

+ E74.2 **Disorders of galactose metabolism**
CC E74.20 **Disorders of galactose metabolism, unspecified**
CC E74.21 **Galactosemia**
CC E74.29 **Other disorders of galactose metabolism**
Galactokinase deficiency

+ E74.3 **Other disorders of intestinal carbohydrate absorption**
Excludes2: *lactose intolerance (E73.-)*
E74.31 **Sucrase-isomaltase deficiency**
E74.39 **Other disorders of intestinal carbohydrate absorption**
Disorder of intestinal carbohydrate absorption NOS
Glucose-galactose malabsorption
Sucrase deficiency

CC E74.4 **Disorders of pyruvate metabolism and gluconeogenesis**
Deficiency of phosphoenolpyruvate carboxykinase
Deficiency of pyruvate carboxylase
Deficiency of pyruvate dehydrogenase
Excludes1: *disorders of pyruvate metabolism and gluconeogenesis with anemia (D55.-)*
Leigh's syndrome (G31.82)

+ E74.8 **Other specified disorders of carbohydrate metabolism**
+ E74.81 **Disorders of glucose transport, not elsewhere classified**
AHA CC: 4Q, 2020, 16
CC E74.810 **Glucose transporter protein type 1 deficiency**
De Vivo syndrome
Glucose transport defect, blood-brain barrier
Glut1 deficiency
GLUT1 deficiency syndrome 1, infantile onset
GLUT1 deficiency syndrome 2, childhood onset
CC E74.818 **Other disorders of glucose transport**
(Familial) renal glycosuria
CC E74.819 **Disorders of glucose transport, unspecified**
CC E74.89 **Other specified disorders of carbohydrate metabolism**
Essential pentosuria

E74.9 **Disorder of carbohydrate metabolism, unspecified**

E75 Disorders of sphingolipid metabolism and other lipid storage disorders

Excludes1: *mucolipidosis, types I-III (E77.0-E77.1)*
Refsum's disease (G60.1)

+ E75.0 **GM2 gangliosidosis**
CC E75.00 **GM2 gangliosidosis, unspecified**
CC E75.01 **Sandhoff disease**
CC E75.02 **Tay-Sachs disease**
CC E75.09 **Other GM2 gangliosidosis**
Adult GM2 gangliosidosis
Juvenile GM2 gangliosidosis

+ E75.1 **Other and unspecified gangliosidosis**
CC E75.10 **Unspecified gangliosidosis**
Gangliosidosis NOS
CC E75.11 **Mucolipidosis IV**
CC E75.19 **Other gangliosidosis**
GM1 gangliosidosis
GM3 gangliosidosis

+ E75.2 **Other sphingolipidosis**
Excludes1: *adrenoleukodystrophy [Addison-Schilder] (E71.528)*
E75.21 **Fabry (-Anderson) disease**
E75.22 **Gaucher disease**
CC E75.23 **Krabbe disease**
+ E75.24 **Niemann-Pick disease**
Acid sphingomyelinase deficiency (ASMD)
E75.240 **Niemann-Pick disease type A**
Acid sphingomyelinase deficiency type A (ASMD type A)
Infantile neurovisceral acid sphingomyelinase deficiency
E75.241 **Niemann-Pick disease type B**
Acid sphingomyelinase deficiency type B (ASMD type B)
Chronic visceral acid sphingomyelinase deficiency
E75.242 **Niemann-Pick disease type C**
E75.243 **Niemann-Pick disease type D**
E75.244 **Niemann-Pick disease type A/B**
Acid sphingomyelinase deficiency type A/B (ASMD type A/B)
Chronic neurovisceral acid sphingomyelinase deficiency
E75.248 **Other Niemann-Pick disease**
E75.249 **Niemann-Pick disease, unspecified**
Acid sphingomyelinase deficiency (ASMD) NOS

CC **E75.25 Metachromatic leukodystrophy**
CC **E75.26 Sulfatase deficiency**
Multiple sulfatase deficiency (MSD)
AHA CC: 4Q, 2018, 5-6
CC **E75.29 Other sphingolipidosis**
Farber's syndrome
Sulfatide lipidosis
E75.3 Sphingolipidosis, unspecified
CC **E75.4 Neuronal ceroid lipofuscinosis**
Batten disease
Bielschowsky-Jansky disease
Kufs disease
Spielmeyer-Vogt disease
E75.5 Other lipid storage disorders
Cerebrotendinous cholesterosis [van Bogaert-Scherer-Epstein]
Wolman's disease
E75.6 Lipid storage disorder, unspecified

E76 Disorders of glycosaminoglycan metabolism

+ **E76.0 Mucopolysaccharidosis, type I**
CC **E76.01 Hurler's syndrome**
CC **E76.02 Hurler-Scheie syndrome**
CC **E76.03 Scheie's syndrome**
CC **E76.1 Mucopolysaccharidosis, type II**
Hunter's syndrome
+ **E76.2 Other mucopolysaccharidoses**
+ **E76.21 Morquio mucopolysaccharidoses**
CC **E76.210 Morquio A mucopolysaccharidoses**
Classic Morquio syndrome
Morquio syndrome A
Mucopolysaccharidosis, type IVA
CC **E76.211 Morquio B mucopolysaccharidoses**
Morquio-like mucopolysaccharidoses
Morquio-like syndrome
Morquio syndrome B
Mucopolysaccharidosis, type IVB
CC **E76.219 Morquio mucopolysaccharidoses, unspecified**
Morquio syndrome
Mucopolysaccharidosis, type IV
CC **E76.22 Sanfilippo mucopolysaccharidoses**
Mucopolysaccharidosis, type III (A) (B) (C) (D)
Sanfilippo A syndrome
Sanfilippo B syndrome
Sanfilippo C syndrome
Sanfilippo D syndrome
CC **E76.29 Other mucopolysaccharidoses**
beta-Glucuronidase deficiency
Maroteaux-Lamy (mild) (severe) syndrome
Mucopolysaccharidosis, types VI, VII
CC **E76.3 Mucopolysaccharidosis, unspecified**
CC **E76.8 Other disorders of glucosaminoglycan metabolism**
CC **E76.9 Glucosaminoglycan metabolism disorder, unspecified**

E77 Disorders of glycoprotein metabolism

E77.0 Defects in post-translational modification of lysosomal enzymes
Mucolipidosis II [I-cell disease]
Mucolipidosis III [pseudo-Hurler polydystrophy]
E77.1 Defects in glycoprotein degradation
Aspartylglucosaminuria
Fucosidosis
Mannosidosis
Sialidosis [mucolipidosis I]
E77.8 Other disorders of glycoprotein metabolism
E77.9 Disorder of glycoprotein metabolism, unspecified

E78 Disorders of lipoprotein metabolism and other lipidemias

Excludes1: *sphingolipidosis (E75.0-E75.3)*
+ **E78.0 Pure hypercholesterolemia**
E78.00 Pure hypercholesterolemia, unspecified
Fedrickson's hyperlipoproteinemia, type IIa
Hyperbetalipoproteinemia
Low-density-lipoprotein-type [LDL] hyperlipoproteinemia
(Pure) hypercholesterolemia, NOS
AHA CC: 4Q, 2016, 13-14
E78.01 Familial hypercholesterolemia
E78.1 Pure hyperglyceridemia
Elevated fasting triglycerides
Endogenous hyperglyceridemia
Fredrickson's hyperlipoproteinemia, type IV
Hyperlipidemia, group B
Hyperprebetalipoproteinemia
Very-low-density-lipoprotein-type [VLDL] hyperlipoproteinemia
E78.2 Mixed hyperlipidemia
Broad- or floating-betalipoproteinemia
Combined hyperlipidemia NOS
Elevated cholesterol with elevated triglycerides NEC
Fredrickson's hyperlipoproteinemia, type IIb or III
Hyperbetalipoproteinemia with prebetalipoproteinemia
Hypercholesteremia with endogenous hyperglyceridemia
Hyperlipidemia, group C
Tubo-eruptive xanthoma
Xanthoma tuberosum
Excludes1: *cerebrotendinous cholesterosis [van Bogaert-Scherer-Epstein] (E75.5)*
familial combined hyperlipidemia (E78.49)
E78.3 Hyperchylomicronemia
Chylomicron retention disease
Fredrickson's hyperlipoproteinemia, type I or V
Hyperlipidemia, group D
Mixed hyperglyceridemia
+ **E78.4 Other hyperlipidemia**
AHA CC: 4Q, 2018, 6
E78.41 Elevated Lipoprotein(a)
Elevated Lp(a)
E78.49 Other hyperlipidemia
Familial combined hyperlipidemia
E78.5 Hyperlipidemia, unspecified
E78.6 Lipoprotein deficiency
Abetalipoproteinemia
Depressed HDL cholesterol
High-density lipoprotein deficiency
Hypoalphalipoproteinemia
Hypobetalipoproteinemia (familial)
Lecithin cholesterol acyltransferase deficiency
Tangier disease
+ **E78.7 Disorders of bile acid and cholesterol metabolism**
Excludes1: *Niemann-Pick disease type C (E75.242)*
E78.70 Disorder of bile acid and cholesterol metabolism, unspecified
CC **E78.71 Barth syndrome**
CC **E78.72 Smith-Lemli-Opitz syndrome**
E78.79 Other disorders of bile acid and cholesterol metabolism
+ **E78.8 Other disorders of lipoprotein metabolism**
E78.81 Lipoid dermatoarthritis
E78.89 Other lipoprotein metabolism disorders
E78.9 Disorder of lipoprotein metabolism, unspecified

E79 Disorders of purine and pyrimidine metabolism

Excludes1: *Ataxia-telangiectasia (Q87.19)*
Bloom's syndrome (Q82.8)
Cockayne's syndrome (Q87.19)
calculus of kidney (N20.0)
combined immunodeficiency disorders (D81.-)
Fanconi's anemia (D61.09)
gout (M1A.-, M10.-)
orotaciduric anemia (D53.0)
progeria (E34.8)
Werner's syndrome (E34.8)
xeroderma pigmentosum (Q82.1)
E79.0 Hyperuricemia without signs of inflammatory arthritis and tophaceous disease
Asymptomatic hyperuricemia
CC **E79.1 Lesch-Nyhan syndrome**
HGPRT deficiency
CC **E79.2 Myoadenylate deaminase deficiency**
CC **E79.8 Other disorders of purine and pyrimidine metabolism**
Hereditary xanthinuria
CC **E79.9 Disorder of purine and pyrimidine metabolism, unspecified**

E80 Disorders of porphyrin and bilirubin metabolism

Includes: defects of catalase and peroxidase
CC **E80.0 Hereditary erythropoietic porphyria**
Congenital erythropoietic porphyria
Erythropoietic protoporphyria
CC **E80.1 Porphyria cutanea tarda**
+ **E80.2 Other and unspecified porphyria**
CC **E80.20 Unspecified porphyria**
Porphyria NOS

CC **E80.21 Acute intermittent (hepatic) porphyria**
CC **E80.29 Other porphyria**
Hereditary coproporphyria
CC **E80.3 Defects of catalase and peroxidase**
Acatalasia [Takahara]
E80.4 Gilbert syndrome
E80.5 Crigler-Najjar syndrome
E80.6 Other disorders of bilirubin metabolism
Dubin-Johnson syndrome
Rotor's syndrome
E80.7 Disorder of bilirubin metabolism, unspecified

E83 Disorders of mineral metabolism
Excludes1: *dietary mineral deficiency (E58-E61)*
parathyroid disorders (E20-E21)
vitamin D deficiency (E55.-)
\+ **E83.0 Disorders of copper metabolism**
E83.00 Disorder of copper metabolism, unspecified
E83.01 Wilson's disease
Code also associated Kayser Fleischer ring (H18.04-)
E83.09 Other disorders of copper metabolism
Menkes' (kinky hair) (steely hair) disease
\+ **E83.1 Disorders of iron metabolism**
Excludes1: *iron deficiency anemia (D50.-)*
sideroblastic anemia (D64.0-D64.3)
E83.10 Disorder of iron metabolism, unspecified
\+ **E83.11 Hemochromatosis**
Excludes1: *GALD (P78.84)*
Gestational alloimmune liver disease (P78.84)
Neonatal hemochromatosis (P78.84)
E83.110 Hereditary hemochromatosis
Bronzed diabetes
Pigmentary cirrhosis (of liver)
Primary (hereditary) hemochromatosis
E83.111 Hemochromatosis due to repeated red blood cell transfusions
Iron overload due to repeated red blood cell transfusions
Transfusion (red blood cell) associated hemochromatosis
E83.118 Other hemochromatosis
E83.119 Hemochromatosis, unspecified
E83.19 Other disorders of iron metabolism
Use additional code, if applicable, for idiopathic pulmonary hemosiderosis (J84.03)
E83.2 Disorders of zinc metabolism
Acrodermatitis enteropathica
\+ **E83.3 Disorders of phosphorus metabolism and phosphatases**
Excludes1: *adult osteomalacia (M83.-)*
osteoporosis (M80.-)
E83.30 Disorder of phosphorus metabolism, unspecified
E83.31 Familial hypophosphatemia
Vitamin D-resistant osteomalacia
Vitamin D-resistant rickets
Excludes1: *vitamin D-deficiency rickets (E55.0)*
E83.32 Hereditary vitamin D-dependent rickets (type 1) (type 2)
25-hydroxyvitamin D 1-alpha-hydroxylase deficiency
Pseudovitamin D deficiency
Vitamin D receptor defect
E83.39 Other disorders of phosphorus metabolism
Acid phosphatase deficiency
Hypophosphatasia
\+ **E83.4 Disorders of magnesium metabolism**
E83.40 Disorders of magnesium metabolism, unspecified
E83.41 Hypermagnesemia
AHA CC: 4Q, 2016, 54-55
E83.42 Hypomagnesemia
E83.49 Other disorders of magnesium metabolism
\+ **E83.5 Disorders of calcium metabolism**
Excludes1: *chondrocalcinosis (M11.1-M11.2)*
hungry bone syndrome (E83.81)
hyperparathyroidism (E21.0-E21.3)
E83.50 Unspecified disorder of calcium metabolism
E83.51 Hypocalcemia
E83.52 Hypercalcemia
Familial hypocalciuric hypercalcemia
E83.59 Other disorders of calcium metabolism
\+ **E83.8 Other disorders of mineral metabolism**
E83.81 Hungry bone syndrome
E83.89 Other disorders of mineral metabolism
E83.9 Disorder of mineral metabolism, unspecified

E84 Cystic fibrosis
Code also exocrine pancreatic insufficiency (K86.81)
Includes: mucoviscidosis
MCC **E84.0 Cystic fibrosis with pulmonary manifestations**
Use additional code to identify any infectious organism present, such as:
Pseudomonas (B96.5)
AHA CC: 1Q, 2021, 23-24
\+ **E84.1 Cystic fibrosis with intestinal manifestations**
• MCC **E84.11 Meconium ileus in cystic fibrosis**
Excludes1: *meconium ileus not due to cystic fibrosis (P76.0)*
CC **E84.19 Cystic fibrosis with other intestinal manifestations**
Distal intestinal obstruction syndrome
CC **E84.8 Cystic fibrosis with other manifestations**
CC **E84.9 Cystic fibrosis, unspecified**

E85 Amyloidosis
Excludes2: *Alzheimer's disease (G30.0-)*
CC **E85.0 Non-neuropathic heredofamilial amyloidosis**
Hereditary amyloid nephropathy
Code also associated disorders, such as:
autoinflammatory syndromes (M04.-)
Excludes2: *Transthyretin-related (ATTR) familial amyloid cardiomyopathy (E85.4)*
CC **E85.1 Neuropathic heredofamilial amyloidosis**
Amyloid polyneuropathy (Portuguese)
Transthyretin-related (ATTR) familial amyloid polyneuropathy
AHA CC: 4Q, 2012, 99-101
CC **E85.2 Heredofamilial amyloidosis, unspecified**
CC **E85.3 Secondary systemic amyloidosis**
Hemodialysis-associated amyloidosis
CC **E85.4 Organ-limited amyloidosis**
Localized amyloidosis
Transthyretin-related (ATTR) familial amyloid cardiomyopathy
\+ **E85.8 Other amyloidosis**
AHA CC: 4Q, 2017, 7
CC **E85.81 Light chain (AL) amyloidosis**
CC **E85.82 Wild-type transthyretin-related (ATTR) amyloidosis**
Senile systemic amyloidosis (SSA)
CC **E85.89 Other amyloidosis**
CC **E85.9 Amyloidosis, unspecified**

E86 Volume depletion
Use Additional code(s) for any associated disorders of electrolyte and acid-base balance (E87.-)
Excludes1: *dehydration of newborn (P74.1)*
postprocedural hypovolemic shock (T81.19)
traumatic hypovolemic shock (T79.4)
Excludes2: *hypovolemic shock NOS (R57.1)*
E86.0 Dehydration
Review coding guidelines C.2.c.3
AHA CC: 1Q, 2014, 7; 2Q, 2019, 7-8
E86.1 Hypovolemia
Depletion of volume of plasma
E86.9 Volume depletion, unspecified
AHA CC: 2Q, 2019, 7-8

E87 Other disorders of fluid, electrolyte and acid-base balance
Excludes1: *diabetes insipidus (E23.2)*
electrolyte imbalance associated with hyperemesis gravidarum (O21.1)
electrolyte imbalance following ectopic or molar pregnancy (O08.5)
familial periodic paralysis (G72.3)
CC **E87.0 Hyperosmolality and hypernatremia**
Sodium [Na] excess
Sodium [Na] overload
AHA CC: 1Q, 2014, 7
CC **E87.1 Hypo-osmolality and hyponatremia**
Sodium [Na] deficiency
Excludes1: *syndrome of inappropriate secretion of antidiuretic hormone (E22.2)*
AHA CC: 1Q, 2014, 7

CC **E87.2 Acidosis**
Acidosis NOS
Lactic acidosis
Metabolic acidosis
Respiratory acidosis
Excludes1: *diabetic acidosis - see categories E08-E10, E11, E13 with ketoacidosis*
AHA CC: 3Q, 2020, 30-31

CC **E87.3 Alkalosis**
Alkalosis NOS
Metabolic alkalosis
Respiratory alkalosis

CC **E87.4 Mixed disorder of acid-base balance**

E87.5 Hyperkalemia
Potassium [K] excess
Potassium [K] overload

E87.6 Hypokalemia
Potassium [K] deficiency

\+ **E87.7 Fluid overload**
Excludes1: *edema NOS (R60.9)*
fluid retention (R60.9)

E87.70 Fluid overload, unspecified

E87.71 Transfusion associated circulatory overload
Fluid overload due to transfusion (blood) (blood components)
TACO

E87.79 Other fluid overload

E87.8 Other disorders of electrolyte and fluid balance, not elsewhere classified
Electrolyte imbalance NOS
Hyperchloremia
Hypochloremia

E88 Other and unspecified metabolic disorders
Use additional codes for associated conditions
Excludes1: *histiocytosis X (chronic) (C96.6)*

\+ **E88.0 Disorders of plasma-protein metabolism, not elsewhere classified**
Excludes1: *monoclonal gammopathy (of undetermined significance) (D47.2)*
polyclonal hypergammaglobulinemia (D89.0)
Waldenström macroglobulinemia (C88.0)
Excludes2: *disorder of lipoprotein metabolism (E78.-)*

E88.01 Alpha-1-antitrypsin deficiency
AAT deficiency

CC **E88.02 Plasminogen deficiency**
Dysplasminogenemia
Hypoplasminogenemia
Type 1 plasminogen deficiency
Type 2 plasminogen deficiency
Code also, if applicable, ligneous conjunctivitis (H10.51)

Use additional code for associated findings, such as:
hydrocephalus (G91.4)
otitis media (H67.-)
respiratory disorder related to plasminogen deficiency (J99)
AHA CC: 4Q, 2018, 6-7

E88.09 Other disorders of plasma-protein metabolism, not elsewhere classified
Bisalbuminemia

E88.1 Lipodystrophy, not elsewhere classified
Lipodystrophy NOS
Excludes1: *Whipple's disease (K90.81)*

E88.2 Lipomatosis, not elsewhere classified
Lipomatosis NOS
Lipomatosis (Check) dolorosa [Dercum]

MCC **E88.3 Tumor lysis syndrome**
Tumor lysis syndrome (spontaneous)
Tumor lysis syndrome following antineoplastic drug chemotherapy
Use additional code for adverse effect, if applicable, to identify drug (T45.1X5)
AHA CC: 2Q, 2019, 24-26

\+ **E88.4 Mitochondrial metabolism disorders**
Excludes1: disorders of pyruvate metabolism (E74.4)
Kearns-Sayre syndrome (H49.81)
Leber's disease (H47.22)
Leigh's encephalopathy (G31.82)
Mitochondrial myopathy, NEC (G71.3)
Reye's syndrome (G93.7)

CC **E88.40 Mitochondrial metabolism disorder, unspecified**

CC **E88.41 MELAS syndrome**
Mitochondrial myopathy, encephalopathy, lactic acidosis and stroke-like episodes

CC **E88.42 MERRF syndrome**
Myoclonic epilepsy associated with ragged-red fibers
Code also progressive myoclonic epilepsy (G40.3-)

CC **E88.49 Other mitochondrial metabolism disorders**

\+ **E88.8 Other specified metabolic disorders**

E88.81 Metabolic syndrome
Dysmetabolic syndrome X
Use additional codes for associated manifestations, such as:
obesity (E66.-)

E88.89 Other specified metabolic disorders
Launois-Bensaude adenolipomatosis
Excludes1: *adult pulmonary Langerhans cell histiocytosis (J84.82)*

E88.9 Metabolic disorder, unspecified

Postprocedural endocrine and metabolic complications and disorders, not elsewhere classified (E89)

E89 Postprocedural endocrine and metabolic complications and disorders, not elsewhere classified
Excludes2: *intraoperative complications of endocrine system organ or structure (E36.0-, E36.1-, E36.8)*

E89.0 Postprocedural hypothyroidism
Postirradiation hypothyroidism
Postsurgical hypothyroidism

CC **E89.1 Postprocedural hypoinsulinemia**
Postpancreatectomy hyperglycemia
Postsurgical hypoinsulinemia
Use additional code, if applicable, to identify:
acquired absence of pancreas (Z90.41-)
diabetes mellitus (postpancreatectomy) (postprocedural) (E13.-)
insulin use (Z79.4)
Excludes1: *transient postprocedural hyperglycemia (R73.9)*
transient postprocedural hypoglycemia (E16.2)
Review coding guideline C.4.a.6.b.i

E89.2 Postprocedural hypoparathyroidism
Parathyroprival tetany

E89.3 Postprocedural hypopituitarism
Postirradiation hypopituitarism

\+ **E89.4 Postprocedural ovarian failure**

♀ **E89.40 Asymptomatic postprocedural ovarian failure**
Postprocedural ovarian failure NOS

♀ **E89.41 Symptomatic postprocedural ovarian failure**
Symptoms such as flushing, sleeplessness, headache, lack of concentration, associated with postprocedural menopause

♂ **E89.5 Postprocedural testicular hypofunction**

CC **E89.6 Postprocedural adrenocortical (-medullary) hypofunction**

\+ **E89.8 Other postprocedural endocrine and metabolic complications and disorders**
AHA CC: 4Q, 2016, 9-10

\+ **E89.81 Postprocedural hemorrhage of an endocrine system organ or structure following a procedure**

CC **E89.810 Postprocedural hemorrhage of an endocrine system organ or structure following an endocrine system procedure**

CC **E89.811 Postprocedural hemorrhage of an endocrine system organ or structure following other procedure**

\+ **E89.82 Postprocedural hematoma and seroma of an endocrine system organ or structre**

CC **E89.820 Postprocedural hematoma of an endocrine system organ or structure following an endocrine system procedure**

CC **E89.821 Postprocedural hematoma of an endocrine system organ or structure following other procedure**

CC **E89.822 Postprocedural seroma of an endocrine system organ or structure following an endocrine system procedure**

CC **E89.823 Postprocedural seroma of an endocrine system organ or structure following other procedure**

CC **E89.89 Other postprocedural endocrine and metabolic complications and disorders**
Use additional code, if applicable, to further specify disorder

Chapter 5: Mental, Behavioral and Neurodevelopmental Disorders (F01-F99)

Includes: disorders of psychological development

Excludes2: *symptoms, signs and abnormal clinical laboratory findings, not elsewhere classified (R00-R99)*

This chapter contains the following category blocks:

F01-F09 Mental disorders due to known physiological conditions
F10-F19 Mental and behavioral disorders due to psychoactive substance use
F20-F29 Schizophrenia, schizotypal, delusional, and other non-mood psychotic disorders
F30-F39 Mood [affective] disorders
F40-F48 Anxiety, dissociative, stress-related, somatoform and other nonpsychotic mental disorders
F50-F59 Behavioral syndromes associated with physiological disturbances and physical factors
F60-F69 Disorders of adult personality and behavior
F70-F79 Intellectual disabilities
F80-F89 Pervasive and specific developmental disorders
F90-F98 Behavioral and emotional disorders with onset usually occurring in childhood and adolescence
F99 Unspecified mental disorder

C. Chapter-Specific Coding Guidelines

In addition to general coding guidelines, there are guidelines for specific diagnoses and/or conditions in the classification. Unless otherwise indicated, these guidelines apply to all health care settings. Please refer to Section II for guidelines on the selection of principal diagnosis.

5. Chapter 5: Mental, Behavioral and Neurodevelopmental Disorders (F01-F99)

a. Pain disorders related to psychological factors

Assign code F45.41, for pain that is exclusively related to psychological disorders. As indicated by the Excludes 1 note under category G89, a code from category G89 should not be assigned with code F45.41

Code F45.42, Pain disorders with related psychological factors, should be used with a code from category G89, Pain, not elsewhere classified, if there is documentation of a psychological component for a patient with acute or chronic pain.

See Section I.C.6. Pain

b. Mental and behavioral disorders due to psychoactive substance use

1) In Remission

Selection of codes for "in remission" for categories F10-F19, Mental and behavioral disorders due to psychoactive substance use (categories F10-F19 with -.11, -.21) requires the provider's clinical judgment. The appropriate codes for "in remission" are assigned only on the basis of provider documentation (as defined in the Official Guidelines for Coding and Reporting), unless otherwise instructed by the classification.

Mild substance use disorders in early or sustained remission are classified to the appropriate codes for substance abuse in remission, and moderate or severe substance use disorders in early or sustained remission are classified to the appropriate codes for substance dependence in remission.

2) Psychoactive Substance Use, Abuse And Dependence

When the provider documentation refers to use, abuse and dependence of the same substance (e.g. alcohol, opioid, cannabis, etc.), only one code should be assigned to identify the pattern of use based on the following hierarchy:

- If both use and abuse are documented, assign only the code for abuse
- If both abuse and dependence are documented, assign only the code for dependence
- If use, abuse and dependence are all documented, assign only the code for dependence
- If both use and dependence are documented, assign only the code for dependence.

3) Psychoactive Substance Use Unspecified

As with all other unspecified diagnoses, the codes for unspecified psychoactive substance use disorders (F10.9-, F11.9-, F12.9-, F13.9-, F14.9-, F15.9-, F16.9-, F18.9-, F19.9-) should only be assigned based on provider documentation and when they meet the definition of a reportable diagnosis (see Section III, Reporting Additional Diagnoses). These codes are to be used only when the psychoactive substance use is associated with a **substance related** disorder (chapter 5 **disorders** such as sexual dysfunction, sleep disorder, or a mental or behavioral disorder) **or medical condition**, and such a relationship is documented by the provider.

4) Medical Conditions Due to Psychoactive Substance Use, Abuse and Dependence

Medical conditions due to substance use, abuse, and dependence are not classified as substance-induced disorders. Assign the diagnosis code for the medical condition as directed by the Alphabetical Index along with the appropriate psychoactive substance use, abuse or dependence code. For example, for alcoholic pancreatitis due to alcohol dependence, assign the appropriate code from subcategory K85.2, Alcohol induced acute pancreatitis, and the appropriate code from subcategory F10.2, such as code F10.20, Alcohol dependence, uncomplicated. It would not be appropriate to assign code F10.288, Alcohol dependence with other alcohol-induced disorder.

5) Blood Alcohol Level

A code from category Y90, Evidence of alcohol involvement determined by blood alcohol level, may be assigned when this information is documented and the patient's provider has documented a condition classifiable to category F10, Alcohol related disorders. The blood alcohol level does not need to be documented by the patient's provider in order for it to be coded.

c. Factitious Disorder

Factitious disorder imposed on self or Munchausen's syndrome is a disorder in which a person falsely reports or causes his or her own physical or psychological signs or symptoms. For patients with documented factitious disorder on self or Munchausen's syndrome, assign the appropriate code from subcategory F68.1-, Factitious disorder imposed on self.

Munchausen's syndrome by proxy (MSBP) is a disorder in which a caregiver (perpetrator) falsely reports or causes an illness or injury in another person (victim) under his or her care, such as a child, an elderly adult, or a person who has a disability. The conditions is also referred to as "factitious disorder imposed on another" or "factitious disorder by proxy." The perpetrator, not the victim, receives this diagnosis. Assign code F68.A, Factitious disorder imposed on another, to the perpetrator's record. For the victim of a patient suffering from MSBP, assign the appropriate code from categories T74, Adult and child abuse, neglect and other maltreatment, confirmed, or T76, Adult and child abuse, neglect and other maltreatment, suspected.

See Section I.C.19.f. Adult and child abuse, neglect and other maltreatment

Mental disorders due to known physiological conditions (F01-F09)

NOTE This block comprises a range of mental disorders grouped together on the basis of their having in common a demonstrable etiology in cerebral disease, brain injury, or other insult leading to cerebral dysfunction. The dysfunction may be primary, as in diseases, injuries, and insults that affect the brain directly and selectively; or secondary, as in systemic diseases and disorders that attack the brain only as one of the multiple organs or systems of the body that are involved.

F01 Vascular dementia

Vascular dementia as a result of infarction of the brain due to vascular disease, including hypertensive cerebrovascular disease.

Includes: arteriosclerotic dementia

Code first the underlying physiological condition or sequelae of cerebrovascular disease.

+ **F01.5 Vascular dementia**

• **F01.50 Vascular dementia without behavioral disturbance**

Major neurocognitive disorder without behavioral disturbance

AHA CC: 2Q, 2021, 4

• CC **F01.51 Vascular dementia with behavioral disturbance**

Major neurocognitive disorder due to vascular disease, with behavioral disturbance
Major neurocognitive disorder with aggressive behavior
Major neurocognitive disorder with combative behavior
Major neurocognitive disorder with violent behavior
Vascular dementia with aggressive behavior
Vascular dementia with combative behavior
Vascular dementia with violent behavior

Use additional code, if applicable, to identify wandering in vascular dementia (Z91.83)

F02 Dementia in other diseases classified elsewhere

Includes: Major neurocognitive disorder in other diseases classified elsewhere

Code first the underlying physiological condition, such as:
Alzheimer's (G30.-)
cerebral lipidosis (E75.4)
Creutzfeldt-Jakob disease (A81.0-)
dementia with Lewy bodies (G31.83)
dementia with Parkinsonism (G31.83)
epilepsy and recurrent seizures (G40.-)
frontotemporal dementia (G31.09)
hepatolenticular degeneration (E83.0)
human immunodeficiency virus [HIV] disease (B20)
Huntington's disease (G10)
hypercalcemia (E83.52)
hypothyroidism, acquired (E00-E03.-)
intoxications (T36-T65)
Jakob-Creutzfeldt disease (A81.0-)
multiple sclerosis (G35)
neurosyphilis (A52.17)
niacin deficiency [pellagra] (E52)
Parkinson's disease (G20)
Pick's disease (G31.01)
polyarteritis nodosa (M30.0)
prion disease (A81.9)
systemic lupus erythematosus (M32.-)
traumatic brain injury (S06.-)
trypanosomiasis (B56.-, B57.-)
vitamin B deficiency (E53.8)

Excludes2: *dementia in alcohol and psychoactive substance disorders (F10-F19, with .17, .27, .97)*
vascular dementia (F01.5-)

\+ **F02.8 Dementia in other diseases classified elsewhere**

F02.80 Dementia in other diseases classified elsewhere without behavioral disturbance
Dementia in other diseases classified elsewhere NOS
Major neurocognitive disorder in other diseases classified elsewhere
AHA CC: 2Q, 2016, 6; 4Q, 2016, 141; 1Q, 2017, 43-44

CC **F02.81 Dementia in other diseases classified elsewhere with behavioral disturbance**
Dementia in other diseases classified elsewhere with aggressive behavior
Dementia in other diseases classified elsewhere with combative behavior
Dementia in other diseases classified elsewhere with violent behavior
Major neurocognitive disorder in other diseases classified elsewhere with aggressive behavior
Major neurocognitive disorder in other diseases classified elsewhere with combative behavior
Major neurocognitive disorder in other diseases classified elsewhere with violent behavior
Use additional code, if applicable, to identify wandering in dementia in conditions classified elsewhere (Z91.83)
AHA CC: 2Q, 2017, 7-8

F03 Unspecified dementia

Presenile dementia NOS
Presenile psychosis NOS
Primary degenerative dementia NOS
Senile dementia NOS
Senile dementia depressed or paranoid type
Senile psychosis NOS

Excludes1: *senility NOS (R41.81)*

Excludes2: *mild memory disturbance due to known physiological condition (F06.8)*
senile dementia with delirium or acute confusional state (F05)

\+ **F03.9 Unspecified dementia**

• **F03.90 Unspecified dementia without behavioral disturbance**
Dementia NOS
AHA CC: 4Q, 2012, 92-93; 2Q, 2021, 4

• CC **F03.91 Unspecified dementia with behavioral disturbance**
Unspecified dementia with aggressive behavior
Unspecified dementia with combative behavior
Unspecified dementia with violent behavior
Use additional code, if applicable, to identify wandering in unspecified dementia (Z91.83)

F04 Amnestic disorder due to known physiological condition

Korsakov's psychosis or syndrome, nonalcoholic
Code first the underlying physiological condition

Excludes1: *amnesia NOS (R41.3)*
anterograde amnesia (R41.1)
dissociative amnesia (F44.0)
retrograde amnesia (R41.2)

Excludes2: *alcohol-induced or unspecified Korsakov's syndrome (F10.26, F10.96)*
Korsakov's syndrome induced by other psychoactive substances (F13.26, F13.96, F19.16, F19.26, F19.96)

Valid 3-character code, no further characters required

CC **F05 Delirium due to known physiological condition**

Acute or subacute brain syndrome
Acute or subacute confusional state (nonalcoholic)
Acute or subacute infective psychosis
Acute or subacute organic reaction
Acute or subacute psycho-organic syndrome
Delirium of mixed etiology
Delirium superimposed on dementia
Sundowning
Code first the underlying physiological condition

Excludes1: *delirium NOS (R41.0)*

Excludes2: *delirium tremens alcohol-induced or unspecified (F10.231, F10.921)*

AHA CC: 2Q, 2019, 34

Valid 3-character code, no further characters required

F06 Other mental disorders due to known physiological condition

Includes: mental disorders due to endocrine disorder
mental disorders due to exogenous hormone
mental disorders due to exogenous toxic substance
mental disorders due to primary cerebral disease
mental disorders due to somatic illness
mental disorders due to systemic disease affecting the brain

Code first the underlying physiological condition

Excludes1: *unspecified dementia (F03)*

Excludes2: *delirium due to known physiological condition (F05)*
dementia as classified in F01-F02
other mental disorders associated with alcohol and other psychoactive substances (F10-F19)

CC **F06.0 Psychotic disorder with hallucinations due to known physiological condition**
Organic hallucinatory state (nonalcoholic)
Excludes2: *hallucinations and perceptual disturbance induced by alcohol and other psychoactive substances (F10-F19 with .151, .251, .951)*
schizophrenia (F20.-)

F06.1 Catatonic disorder due to known physiological condition
Catatonia associated with another mental disorder
Catatonia NOS
Excludes1: *catatonic stupor (R40.1)*
stupor NOS (R40.1)
Excludes2: *catatonic schizophrenia (F20.2)*
dissociative stupor (F44.2)

CC **F06.2 Psychotic disorder with delusions due to known physiological condition**
Paranoid and paranoid-hallucinatory organic states
Schizophrenia-like psychosis in epilepsy
Excludes2: *alcohol and drug-induced psychotic disorder (F10-F19 with .150, .250, .950)*
brief psychotic disorder (F23)
delusional disorder (F22)
schizophrenia (F20.-)

\+ **F06.3 Mood disorder due to known physiological condition**
Excludes2: *mood disorders due to alcohol and other psychoactive substances (F10-F19 with .14, .24, .94)*
mood disorders, not due to known physiological condition or unspecified (F30-F39)

F06.30 Mood disorder due to known physiological condition, unspecified

F06.31 Mood disorder due to known physiological condition with depressive features
Depressive disorder due to known physiological condition, with depressive features

F06.32 Mood disorder due to known physiological condition with major depressive-like episode
Depressive disorder due to known physiological condition, with major depressive-like episode

F06.33 Mood disorder due to known physiological condition with manic features
Bipolar and related disorder due to a known physiological condition, with manic features
Bipolar and related disorder due to known physiological condition, with manic- or hypomanic-like episodes

F06.34 Mood disorder due to known physiological condition with mixed features
Bipolar and related disorder due to known physiological condition, with mixed features
Depressive disorder due to known physiological condition, with mixed features

F06.4 Anxiety disorder due to known physiological condition
Excludes2: *anxiety disorders due to alcohol and other psychoactive substances (F10-F19 with .180, .280, .980)*
anxiety disorders, not due to known physiological condition or unspecified (F40.-, F41.-)

F06.8 Other specified mental disorders due to known physiological condition
Epileptic psychosis NOS
Obsessive-compulsive and related disorder due to a known physiological condition
Organic dissociative disorder
Organic emotionally labile [asthenic] disorder

F07 Personality and behavioral disorders due to known physiological condition
Code first the underlying physiological condition

F07.0 Personality change due to known physiological condition
Frontal lobe syndrome
Limbic epilepsy personality syndrome
Lobotomy syndrome
Organic personality disorder
Organic pseudopsychopathic personality
Organic pseudoretarded personality
Postleucotomy syndrome
Code first underlying physiological condition
Excludes1: *mild cognitive impairment (G31.84)*
postconcussional syndrome (F07.81)
postencephalitic syndrome (F07.89)
signs and symptoms involving emotional state (R45.-)
Excludes2: *specific personality disorder (F60.-)*

+ **F07.8 Other personality and behavioral disorders due to known physiological condition**

F07.81 Postconcussional syndrome
Postcontusional syndrome (encephalopathy)
Post-traumatic brain syndrome, nonpsychotic
Use additional code to identify associated post-traumatic headache, if applicable (G44.3-)
Excludes1: *current concussion (brain) (S06.0-)*
postencephalitic syndrome (F07.89)

F07.89 Other personality and behavioral disorders due to known physiological condition
Postencephalitic syndrome
Right hemispheric organic affective disorder

F07.9 Unspecified personality and behavioral disorder due to known physiological condition
Organic psychosyndrome

F09 Unspecified mental disorder due to known physiological condition
Mental disorder NOS due to known physiological condition
Organic brain syndrome NOS
Organic mental disorder NOS
Organic psychosis NOS
Symptomatic psychosis NOS
Code first the underlying physiological condition
Excludes1: *psychosis NOS (F29)*
Valid 3-character code, no further characters required

Mental and behavioral disorders due to psychoactive substance use (F10-F19)

Review coding guideline C.5.b
AHA CC: 4Q, 2017, 8; 1Q, 2020, 9

F10 Alcohol related disorders
Use additional code for blood alcohol level, if applicable (Y90.-)

+ **F10.1 Alcohol abuse**
Excludes1: *alcohol dependence (F10.2-)*
alcohol use, unspecified (F10.9-)

F10.10 Alcohol abuse, uncomplicated
Alcohol use disorder, mild

F10.11 Alcohol abuse, in remission
Alcohol use disorder, mild, in early remission
Alcohol use disorder, mild, in sustained remission

+ **F10.12 Alcohol abuse with intoxication**
F10.120 Alcohol abuse with intoxication, uncomplicated
CC **F10.121 Alcohol abuse with intoxication delirium**
F10.129 Alcohol abuse with intoxication, unspecified

+ **F10.13 Alcohol abuse, with withdrawal**
AHA CC: 4Q, 2020, 16-17
CC **F10.130 Alcohol abuse with withdrawal, uncomplicated**
CC **F10.131 Alcohol abuse with withdrawal delirium**
CC **F10.132 Alcohol abuse with withdrawal with perceptual disturbance**
CC **F10.139 Alcohol abuse with withdrawal, unspecified**

CC **F10.14 Alcohol abuse with alcohol-induced mood disorder**
Alcohol use disorder, mild, with alcohol-induced bipolar or related disorder
Alcohol use disorder, mild, with alcohol-induced depressive disorder

+ **F10.15 Alcohol abuse with alcohol-induced psychotic disorder**
F10.150 Alcohol abuse with alcohol-induced psychotic disorder with delusions
CC **F10.151 Alcohol abuse with alcohol-induced psychotic disorder with hallucinations**
CC **F10.159 Alcohol abuse with alcohol-induced psychotic disorder, unspecified**

+ **F10.18 Alcohol abuse with other alcohol-induced disorders**
CC **F10.180 Alcohol abuse with alcohol-induced anxiety disorder**
CC **F10.181 Alcohol abuse with alcohol-induced sexual dysfunction**
F10.182 Alcohol abuse with alcohol-induced sleep disorder
CC **F10.188 Alcohol abuse with other alcohol-induced disorder**

CC **F10.19 Alcohol abuse with unspecified alcohol-induced disorder**

+ **F10.2 Alcohol dependence**
Excludes1: *alcohol abuse (F10.1-)*
alcohol use, unspecified (F10.9-)
Excludes2: *toxic effect of alcohol (T51.0-)*

F10.20 Alcohol dependence, uncomplicated
Alcohol use disorder, moderate
Alcohol use disorder, severe
AHA CC: 1Q, 2020, 9

F10.21 Alcohol dependence, in remission
Alcohol use disorder, moderate, in early remission
Alcohol use disorder, moderate, in sustained remission
Alcohol use disorder, severe, in early remission
Alcohol use disorder, severe, in sustained remission

+ **F10.22 Alcohol dependence with intoxication**
Acute drunkenness (in alcoholism)
Excludes2: *alcohol dependence with withdrawal (F10.23-)*
F10.220 Alcohol dependence with intoxication, uncomplicated
CC **F10.221 Alcohol dependence with intoxication delirium**
F10.229 Alcohol dependence with intoxication, unspecified

+ **F10.23 Alcohol dependence with withdrawal**
  Excludes2: *Alcohol dependence with intoxication (F10.22-)*
  - CC **F10.230 Alcohol dependence with withdrawal, uncomplicated**
  - CC **F10.231 Alcohol dependence with withdrawal delirium**
  - CC **F10.232 Alcohol dependence with withdrawal with perceptual disturbance**
  - CC **F10.239 Alcohol dependence with withdrawal, unspecified**

CC **F10.24 Alcohol dependence with alcohol-induced mood disorder**
Alcohol use disorder, moderate, with alcohol-induced bipolar or related disorder
Alcohol use disorder, moderate, with alcohol-induced depressive disorder
Alcohol use disorder, severe, with alcohol-induced bipolar or related disorder
Alcohol use disorder, severe, with alcohol-induced depressive disorder

+ **F10.25 Alcohol dependence with alcohol-induced psychotic disorder**
  - **F10.250 Alcohol dependence with alcohol-induced psychotic disorder with delusions**
  - CC **F10.251 Alcohol dependence with alcohol-induced psychotic disorder with hallucinations**
  - CC **F10.259 Alcohol dependence with alcohol-induced psychotic disorder, unspecified**

F10.26 Alcohol dependence with alcohol-induced persisting amnestic disorder
Alcohol use disorder, moderate, with alcohol-induced major neurocognitive disorder, amnestic-confabulatory type
Alcohol use disorder, severe, with alcohol-induced major neurocognitive disorder, amnestic-confabulatory type

CC **F10.27 Alcohol dependence with alcohol-induced persisting dementia**
Alcohol use disorder, moderate, with alcohol-induced major neurocognitive disorder, nonamnestic-confabulatory type
Alcohol use disorder, severe, with alcohol-induced major neurocognitive disorder, nonamnestic-confabulatory type

+ **F10.28 Alcohol dependence with other alcohol-induced disorders**
  - CC **F10.280 Alcohol dependence with alcohol-induced anxiety disorder**
  - CC **F10.281 Alcohol dependence with alcohol-induced sexual dysfunction**
  - **F10.282 Alcohol dependence with alcohol-induced sleep disorder**
  - CC **F10.288 Alcohol dependence with other alcohol-induced disorder**
    Alcohol use disorder, moderate, with alcohol-induced mild neurocognitive disorder
    Alcohol use disorder, severe, with alcohol-induced mild neurocognitive disorder

CC **F10.29 Alcohol dependence with unspecified alcohol-induced disorder**

+ **F10.9 Alcohol use, unspecified**
  Excludes1: *alcohol abuse (F10.1-)*
  alcohol dependence (F10.2-)

+ **F10.92 Alcohol use, unspecified with intoxication**
  - **F10.920 Alcohol use, unspecified with intoxication, uncomplicated**
  - CC **F10.921 Alcohol use, unspecified with intoxication delirium**
  - **F10.929 Alcohol use, unspecified with intoxication, unspecified**

+ **F10.93 Alcohol use, unspecified with withdrawal**
  AHA CC: 4Q, 2020, 16-17
  - CC **F10.930 Alcohol use, unspecified with withdrawal, uncomplicated**
  - CC **F10.931 Alcohol use, unspecified with withdrawal delirium**
  - CC **F10.932 Alcohol use, unspecified with withdrawal with perceptual disturbance**
  - CC **F10.939 Alcohol use, unspecified with withdrawal, unspecified**

CC **F10.94 Alcohol use, unspecified with alcohol-induced mood disorder**
Alcohol-induced bipolar or related disorder, without use disorder
Alcohol-induced depressive disorder, without use disorder

+ **F10.95 Alcohol use, unspecified with alcohol-induced psychotic disorder**
  - **F10.950 Alcohol use, unspecified with alcohol-induced psychotic disorder with delusions**
  - CC **F10.951 Alcohol use, unspecified with alcohol-induced psychotic disorder with hallucinations**
  - CC **F10.959 Alcohol use, unspecified with alcohol-induced psychotic disorder, unspecified**
    Alcohol-induced psychotic disorder without use disorder

F10.96 Alcohol use, unspecified with alcohol-induced persisting amnestic disorder
Alcohol-induced major neurocognitive disorder, amnestic-confabulatory type, without use disorder

F10.97 Alcohol use, unspecified with alcohol-induced persisting dementia
Alcohol-induced major neurocognitive disorder, nonamnestic-confabulatory type, without use disorder

+ **F10.98 Alcohol use, unspecified with other alcohol-induced disorders**
  - CC **F10.980 Alcohol use, unspecified with alcohol-induced anxiety disorder**
    Alcohol-induced anxiety disorder, without use disorder
  - CC **F10.981 Alcohol use, unspecified with alcohol-induced sexual dysfunction**
    Alcohol-induced sexual dysfunction, without use disorder
  - **F10.982 Alcohol use, unspecified with alcohol-induced sleep disorder**
    Alcohol-induced sleep disorder, without use disorder
  - CC **F10.988 Alcohol use, unspecified with other alcohol-induced disorder**
    Alcohol-induced mild neurocognitive disorder, without use disorder
    AHA CC: 3Q, 2019, 8

CC **F10.99 Alcohol use, unspecified with unspecified alcohol-induced disorder**

F11 Opioid related disorders

+ **F11.1 Opioid abuse**
  Excludes1: *opioid dependence (F11.2-)*
  opioid use, unspecified (F11.9-)

F11.10 Opioid abuse, uncomplicated
Opioid use disorder, mild

F11.11 Opioid abuse, in remission
Opioid use disorder, mild, in early remission
Opioid use disorder, mild, in sustained remission

+ **F11.12 Opioid abuse with intoxication**
  - **F11.120 Opioid abuse with intoxication, uncomplicated**
  - CC **F11.121 Opioid abuse with intoxication delirium**
  - **F11.122 Opioid abuse with intoxication with perceptual disturbance**
  - **F11.129 Opioid abuse with intoxication, unspecified**

CC **F11.13 Opioid abuse with withdrawal**
AHA CC: 4Q, 2020, 16-17

F11.14 Opioid abuse with opioid-induced mood disorder
Opioid use disorder, mild, with opioid-induced depressive disorder

+ F11.15 **Opioid abuse with opioid-induced psychotic disorder**
CC **F11.150** **Opioid abuse with opioid-induced psychotic disorder with delusions**
CC **F11.151** **Opioid abuse with opioid-induced psychotic disorder with hallucinations**
F11.159 **Opioid abuse with opioid-induced psychotic disorder, unspecified**
+ **F11.18** **Opioid abuse with other opioid-induced disorder**
F11.181 **Opioid abuse with opioid-induced sexual dysfunction**
F11.182 **Opioid abuse with opioid-induced sleep disorder**
F11.188 **Opioid abuse with other opioid-induced disorder**
F11.19 **Opioid abuse with unspecified opioid-induced disorder**
+ **F11.2** **Opioid dependence**
Excludes1: *opioid abuse (F11.1-)*
opioid use, unspecified (F11.9-)
Excludes2: *opioid poisoning (T40.0-T40.2-)*
CC **F11.20** **Opioid dependence, uncomplicated**
Opioid use disorder, moderate
Opioid use disorder, severe
F11.21 **Opioid dependence, in remission**
Opioid use disorder, moderate, in early remission
Opioid use disorder, moderate, in sustained remission
Opioid use disorder, severe, in early remission
Opioid use disorder, severe, in sustained remission
+ **F11.22** **Opioid dependence with intoxication**
Excludes1: *opioid dependence with withdrawal (F11.23)*
F11.220 **Opioid dependence with intoxication, uncomplicated**
CC **F11.221** **Opioid dependence with intoxication delirium**
CC **F11.222** **Opioid dependence with intoxication with perceptual disturbance**
F11.229 **Opioid dependence with intoxication, unspecified**
CC **F11.23** **Opioid dependence with withdrawal**
Excludes1: *opioid dependence with intoxication (F11.22-)*
F11.24 **Opioid dependence with opioid-induced mood disorder**
Opioid use disorder, moderate, with opioid-induced depressive disorder
+ **F11.25** **Opioid dependence with opioid-induced psychotic disorder**
CC **F11.250** **Opioid dependence with opioid-induced psychotic disorder with delusions**
CC **F11.251** **Opioid dependence with opioid-induced psychotic disorder with hallucinations**
CC **F11.259** **Opioid dependence with opioid-induced psychotic disorder, unspecified**
+ **F11.28** **Opioid dependence with other opioid-induced disorder**
CC **F11.281** **Opioid dependence with opioid-induced sexual dysfunction**
CC **F11.282** **Opioid dependence with opioid-induced sleep disorder**
CC **F11.288** **Opioid dependence with other opioid-induced disorder**
F11.29 **Opioid dependence with unspecified opioid-induced disorder**
+ **F11.9** **Opioid use, unspecified**
Excludes1: *opioid abuse (F11.1-)*
opioid dependence (F11.2-)
F11.90 **Opioid use, unspecified, uncomplicated**
+ **F11.92** **Opioid use, unspecified with intoxication**
Excludes1: *opioid use, unspecified with withdrawal (F11.93)*
F11.920 **Opioid use, unspecified with intoxication, uncomplicated**
CC **F11.921** **Opioid use, unspecified with intoxication delirium**
Opioid use delirium
F11.922 **Opioid use, unspecified with intoxication with perceptual disturbance**
F11.929 **Opioid use, unspecified with intoxication, unspecified**
CC **F11.93** **Opioid use, unspecified with withdrawal**
Excludes1: *opioid use, unspecified with intoxication (F11.92-)*
F11.94 **Opioid use, unspecified with opioid-induced mood disorder**
Opioid-induced depressive disorder, without use disorder
+ **F11.95** **Opioid use, unspecified with opioid-induced psychotic disorder**
CC **F11.950** **Opioid use, unspecified with opioid-induced psychotic disorder with delusions**
CC **F11.951** **Opioid use, unspecified with opioid-induced psychotic disorder with hallucinations**
F11.959 **Opioid use, unspecified with opioid-induced psychotic disorder, unspecified**
+ **F11.98** **Opioid use, unspecified with other specified opioid-induced disorder**
F11.981 **Opioid use, unspecified with opioid-induced sexual dysfunction**
Opioid-induced sexual dysfunction, without use disorder
F11.982 **Opioid use, unspecified with opioid-induced sleep disorder**
Opioid-induced sleep disorder, without use disorder
F11.988 **Opioid use, unspecified with other opioid-induced disorder**
Opioid-induced anxiety disorder, without use disorder
F11.99 **Opioid use, unspecified with unspecified opioid-induced disorder**

F12 Cannabis related disorders
Includes: marijuana
AHA CC: 1Q, 2020, 8
+ **F12.1** **Cannabis abuse**
Excludes1: *cannabis dependence (F12.2-)*
cannabis use, unspecified (F12.9-)
F12.10 **Cannabis abuse, uncomplicated**
Cannabis use disorder, mild
F12.11 **Cannabis abuse, in remission**
Cannabis use disorder, mild, in early remission
Cannabis use disorder, mild, in sustained remission
+ **F12.12** **Cannabis abuse with intoxication**
F12.120 **Cannabis abuse with intoxication, uncomplicated**
CC **F12.121** **Cannabis abuse with intoxication delirium**
F12.122 **Cannabis abuse with intoxication with perceptual disturbance**
F12.129 **Cannabis abuse with intoxication, unspecified**
CC **F12.13** **Cannabis abuse with withdrawal**
AHA CC: 4Q, 2020, 16-17
+ **F12.15** **Cannabis abuse with psychotic disorder**
CC **F12.150** **Cannabis abuse with psychotic disorder with delusions**
CC **F12.151** **Cannabis abuse with psychotic disorder with hallucinations**
F12.159 **Cannabis abuse with psychotic disorder, unspecified**
+ **F12.18** **Cannabis abuse with other cannabis-induced disorder**
F12.180 **Cannabis abuse with cannabis-induced anxiety disorder**
F12.188 **Cannabis abuse with other cannabis-induced disorder**
Cannabis use disorder, mild, with cannabis-induced sleep disorder
F12.19 **Cannabis abuse with unspecified cannabis-induced disorder**

+ F12.2 **Cannabis dependence**
Excludes1: *cannabis abuse (F12.1-)*
cannabis use, unspecified (F12.9-)
Excludes2: *cannabis poisoning (T40.7-)*
F12.20 **Cannabis dependence, uncomplicated**
Cannabis use disorder, moderate
Cannabis use disorder, severe
F12.21 **Cannabis dependence, in remission**
Cannabis use disorder, moderate, in early remission
Cannabis use disorder, moderate, in sustained remission
Cannabis use disorder, severe, in early remission
Cannabis use disorder, severe, in sustained remission
+ F12.22 **Cannabis dependence with intoxication**
F12.220 **Cannabis dependence with intoxication, uncomplicated**
CC F12.221 **Cannabis dependence with intoxication delirium**
F12.222 **Cannabis dependence with intoxication with perceptual disturbance**
F12.229 **Cannabis dependence with intoxication, unspecified**
F12.23 **Cannabis dependence with withdrawal**
AHA CC: 4Q, 2018, 7
+ F12.25 **Cannabis dependence with psychotic disorder**
CC F12.250 **Cannabis dependence with psychotic disorder with delusions**
CC F12.251 **Cannabis dependence with psychotic disorder with hallucinations**
F12.259 **Cannabis dependence with psychotic disorder, unspecified**
+ F12.28 **Cannabis dependence with other cannabis-induced disorder**
F12.280 **Cannabis dependence with cannabis-induced anxiety disorder**
F12.288 **Cannabis dependence with other cannabis-induced disorder**
Cannabis use disorder, moderate, with cannabis-induced sleep disorder
Cannabis use disorder, severe, with cannabis-induced sleep disorder
F12.29 **Cannabis dependence with unspecified cannabis-induced disorder**
+ F12.9 **Cannabis use, unspecified**
Excludes1: *cannabis abuse (F12.1-)*
cannabis dependence (F12.2-)
F12.90 **Cannabis use, unspecified, uncomplicated**
+ F12.92 **Cannabis use, unspecified with intoxication**
F12.920 **Cannabis use, unspecified with intoxication, uncomplicated**
CC F12.921 **Cannabis use, unspecified with intoxication delirium**
F12.922 **Cannabis use, unspecified with intoxication with perceptual disturbance**
F12.929 **Cannabis use, unspecified with intoxication, unspecified**
F12.93 **Cannabis use, unspecified with withdrawal**
AHA CC: 4Q, 2018, 7
+ F12.95 **Cannabis use, unspecified with psychotic disorder**
CC F12.950 **Cannabis use, unspecified with psychotic disorder with delusions**
CC F12.951 **Cannabis use, unspecified with psychotic disorder with hallucinations**
F12.959 **Cannabis use, unspecified with psychotic disorder, unspecified**
Cannabis-induced psychotic disorder, without use disorder
+ F12.98 **Cannabis use, unspecified with other cannabis-induced disorder**
F12.980 **Cannabis use, unspecified with anxiety disorder**
Cannabis-induced anxiety disorder, without use disorder
F12.988 **Cannabis use, unspecified with other cannabis-induced disorder**
Cannabis-induced sleep disorder, without use disorder
F12.99 **Cannabis use, unspecified with unspecified cannabis-induced disorder**

F13 **Sedative, hypnotic, or anxiolytic related disorders**
+ F13.1 **Sedative, hypnotic or anxiolytic-related abuse**
Excludes1: *sedative, hypnotic or anxiolytic-related dependence (F13.2-)*
sedative, hypnotic, or anxiolytic use, unspecified (F13.9-)
F13.10 **Sedative, hypnotic or anxiolytic abuse, uncomplicated**
Sedative, hypnotic, or anxiolytic use disorder, mild
F13.11 **Sedative, hypnotic or anxiolytic abuse, in remission**
Sedative, hypnotic or anxiolytic use disorder, mild, in early remission
Sedative, hypnotic or anxiolytic use disorder, mild, in sustained remission
+ F13.12 **Sedative, hypnotic or anxiolytic abuse with intoxication**
F13.120 **Sedative, hypnotic or anxiolytic abuse with intoxication, uncomplicated**
CC F13.121 **Sedative, hypnotic or anxiolytic abuse with intoxication delirium**
F13.129 **Sedative, hypnotic or anxiolytic abuse with intoxication, unspecified**
+ F13.13 **Sedative, hypnotic or anxiolytic abuse with withdrawal**
AHA CC: 4Q, 2020, 16-17
CC F13.130 **Sedative, hypnotic or anxiolytic abuse with withdrawal, uncomplicated**
CC F13.131 **Sedative, hypnotic or anxiolytic abuse with withdrawal delirium**
CC F13.132 **Sedative, hypnotic or anxiolytic abuse with withdrawal with perceptual disturbance**
CC F13.139 **Sedative, hypnotic or anxiolytic abuse with withdrawal, unspecified**
F13.14 **Sedative, hypnotic or anxiolytic abuse with sedative, hypnotic or anxiolytic-induced mood disorder**
Sedative, hypnotic, or anxiolytic use disorder, mild, with sedative, hypnotic, or anxiolytic-induced bipolar or related disorder
Sedative, hypnotic, or anxiolytic use disorder, mild, with sedative, hypnotic, or anxiolytic-induced depressive disorder
+ F13.15 **Sedative, hypnotic or anxiolytic abuse with sedative, hypnotic or anxiolytic-induced psychotic disorder**
CC F13.150 **Sedative, hypnotic or anxiolytic abuse with sedative, hypnotic or anxiolytic-induced psychotic disorder with delusions**
CC F13.151 **Sedative, hypnotic or anxiolytic abuse with sedative, hypnotic or anxiolytic-induced psychotic disorder with hallucinations**
F13.159 **Sedative, hypnotic or anxiolytic abuse with sedative, hypnotic or anxiolytic-induced psychotic disorder, unspecified**
+ F13.18 **Sedative, hypnotic or anxiolytic abuse with other sedative, hypnotic or anxiolytic-induced disorders**
F13.180 **Sedative, hypnotic or anxiolytic abuse with sedative, hypnotic or anxiolytic-induced anxiety disorder**
F13.181 **Sedative, hypnotic or anxiolytic abuse with sedative, hypnotic or anxiolytic-induced sexual dysfunction**
F13.182 **Sedative, hypnotic or anxiolytic abuse with sedative, hypnotic or anxiolytic-induced sleep disorder**
F13.188 **Sedative, hypnotic or anxiolytic abuse with other sedative, hypnotic or anxiolytic-induced disorder**
F13.19 **Sedative, hypnotic or anxiolytic abuse with unspecified sedative, hypnotic or anxiolytic-induced disorder**

+ F13.2 Sedative, hypnotic or anxiolytic-related dependence

Excludes1: *sedative, hypnotic or anxiolytic-related abuse (F13.1-)*
sedative, hypnotic, or anxiolytic use, unspecified (F13.9-)

Excludes2: *sedative, hypnotic, or anxiolytic poisoning (T42.-)*

CC **F13.20 Sedative, hypnotic or anxiolytic dependence, uncomplicated**

F13.21 Sedative, hypnotic or anxiolytic dependence, in remission

Sedative, hypnotic or anxiolytic use disorder, moderate, in early remission
Sedative, hypnotic or anxiolytic use disorder, moderate, in sustained remission
Sedative, hypnotic or anxiolytic use disorder, severe, in early remission
Sedative, hypnotic or anxiolytic use disorder, severe, in sustained remission

+ F13.22 Sedative, hypnotic or anxiolytic dependence with intoxication

Excludes1: *sedative, hypnotic or anxiolytic dependence with withdrawal (F13.23-)*

F13.220 Sedative, hypnotic or anxiolytic dependence with intoxication, uncomplicated

CC **F13.221 Sedative, hypnotic or anxiolytic dependence with intoxication delirium**

F13.229 Sedative, hypnotic or anxiolytic dependence with intoxication, unspecified

+ F13.23 Sedative, hypnotic or anxiolytic dependence with withdrawal

Sedative, hypnotic, or anxiolytic use disorder, moderate
Sedative, hypnotic, or anxiolytic use disorder, severe

Excludes1: *sedative, hypnotic or anxiolytic dependence with intoxication (F13.22-)*

CC **F13.230 Sedative, hypnotic or anxiolytic dependence with withdrawal, uncomplicated**

CC **F13.231 Sedative, hypnotic or anxiolytic dependence with withdrawal delirium**

CC **F13.232 Sedative, hypnotic or anxiolytic dependence with withdrawal with perceptual disturbance**

Sedative, hypnotic, or anxiolytic withdrawal with perceptual disturbances

CC **F13.239 Sedative, hypnotic or anxiolytic dependence with withdrawal, unspecified**

Sedative, hypnotic, or anxiolytic withdrawal without perceptual disturbances

F13.24 Sedative, hypnotic or anxiolytic dependence with sedative, hypnotic or anxiolytic-induced mood disorder

Sedative, hypnotic, or anxiolytic use disorder, moderate, with sedative, hypnotic, or anxiolytic-induced bipolar or related disorder
Sedative, hypnotic, or anxiolytic use disorder, moderate, with sedative, hypnotic, or anxiolytic-induced depressive disorder
Sedative, hypnotic, or anxiolytic use disorder, severe, with sedative, hypnotic, or anxiolytic-induced bipolar or related disorder
Sedative, hypnotic, or anxiolytic use disorder, severe, with sedative, hypnotic, or anxiolytic-induced depressive disorder

+ F13.25 Sedative, hypnotic or anxiolytic dependence with sedative, hypnotic or anxiolytic-induced psychotic disorder

CC **F13.250 Sedative, hypnotic or anxiolytic dependence with sedative, hypnotic or anxiolytic-induced psychotic disorder with delusions**

CC **F13.251 Sedative, hypnotic or anxiolytic dependence with sedative, hypnotic or anxiolytic-induced psychotic disorder with hallucinations**

CC **F13.259 Sedative, hypnotic or anxiolytic dependence with sedative, hypnotic or anxiolytic-induced psychotic disorder, unspecified**

CC **F13.26 Sedative, hypnotic or anxiolytic dependence with sedative, hypnotic or anxiolytic-induced persisting amnestic disorder**

CC **F13.27 Sedative, hypnotic or anxiolytic dependence with sedative, hypnotic or anxiolytic-induced persisting dementia**

Sedative, hypnotic, or anxiolytic use disorder, moderate, with sedative, hypnotic, or anxiolytic-induced major neurocognitive disorder
Sedative, hypnotic, or anxiolytic use disorder, severe, with sedative, hypnotic, or anxiolytic-induced major neurocognitive disorder

+ F13.28 Sedative, hypnotic or anxiolytic dependence with other sedative, hypnotic or anxiolytic-induced disorders

CC **F13.280 Sedative, hypnotic or anxiolytic dependence with sedative, hypnotic or anxiolytic-induced anxiety disorder**

CC **F13.281 Sedative, hypnotic or anxiolytic dependence with sedative, hypnotic or anxiolytic-induced sexual dysfunction**

CC **F13.282 Sedative, hypnotic or anxiolytic dependence with sedative, hypnotic or anxiolytic-induced sleep disorder**

CC **F13.288 Sedative, hypnotic or anxiolytic dependence with other sedative, hypnotic or anxiolytic-induced disorder**

Sedative, hypnotic, or anxiolytic use disorder, moderate, with sedative, hypnotic, or anxiolytic-induced mild neurocognitive disorder
Sedative, hypnotic, or anxiolytic use disorder, severe, with sedative, hypnotic, or anxiolytic-induced mild neurocognitive disorder

F13.29 Sedative, hypnotic or anxiolytic dependence with unspecified sedative, hypnotic or anxiolytic-induced disorder

+ F13.9 Sedative, hypnotic or anxiolytic-related use, unspecified

Excludes1: *sedative, hypnotic or anxiolytic-related abuse (F13.1-)*
sedative, hypnotic or anxiolytic-related dependence (F13.2-)

Review coding guideline C.5.b.3

F13.90 Sedative, hypnotic, or anxiolytic use, unspecified, uncomplicated

+ F13.92 Sedative, hypnotic or anxiolytic use, unspecified with intoxication

Excludes1: *sedative, hypnotic or anxiolytic use, unspecified with withdrawal (F13.93-)*

F13.920 Sedative, hypnotic or anxiolytic use, unspecified with intoxication, uncomplicated

CC **F13.921 Sedative, hypnotic or anxiolytic use, unspecified with intoxication delirium**

Sedative, hypnotic, or anxiolytic-induced delirium

F13.929 Sedative, hypnotic or anxiolytic use, unspecified with intoxication, unspecified

+ **F13.93 Sedative, hypnotic or anxiolytic use, unspecified with withdrawal**
  Excludes1: *sedative, hypnotic or anxiolytic use, unspecified with intoxication (F13.92-)*
  CC **F13.930 Sedative, hypnotic or anxiolytic use, unspecified with withdrawal, uncomplicated**
  CC **F13.931 Sedative, hypnotic or anxiolytic use, unspecified with withdrawal delirium**
  CC **F13.932 Sedative, hypnotic or anxiolytic use, unspecified with withdrawal with perceptual disturbances**
  CC **F13.939 Sedative, hypnotic or anxiolytic use, unspecified with withdrawal, unspecified**

F13.94 Sedative, hypnotic or anxiolytic use, unspecified with sedative, hypnotic or anxiolytic-induced mood disorder
Sedative, hypnotic, or anxiolytic-induced bipolar or related disorder, without use disorder
Sedative, hypnotic, or anxiolytic-induced depressive disorder, without use disorder

+ **F13.95 Sedative, hypnotic or anxiolytic use, unspecified with sedative, hypnotic or anxiolytic-induced psychotic disorder**
  CC **F13.950 Sedative, hypnotic or anxiolytic use, unspecified with sedative, hypnotic or anxiolytic-induced psychotic disorder with delusions**
  CC **F13.951 Sedative, hypnotic or anxiolytic use, unspecified with sedative, hypnotic or anxiolytic-induced psychotic disorder with hallucinations**
  F13.959 Sedative, hypnotic or anxiolytic use, unspecified with sedative, hypnotic or anxiolytic-induced psychotic disorder, unspecified
  Sedative, hypnotic, or anxiolytic-induced psychotic disorder, without use disorder

F13.96 Sedative, hypnotic or anxiolytic use, unspecified with sedative, hypnotic or anxiolytic-induced persisting amnestic disorder

CC **F13.97 Sedative, hypnotic or anxiolytic use, unspecified with sedative, hypnotic or anxiolytic-induced persisting dementia**
Sedative, hypnotic, or anxiolytic-induced major neurocognitive disorder, without use disorder

+ **F13.98 Sedative, hypnotic or anxiolytic use, unspecified with other sedative, hypnotic or anxiolytic-induced disorders**
  F13.980 Sedative, hypnotic or anxiolytic use, unspecified with sedative, hypnotic or anxiolytic-induced anxiety disorder
  Sedative, hypnotic, or anxiolytic-induced anxiety disorder, without use disorder
  F13.981 Sedative, hypnotic or anxiolytic use, unspecified with sedative, hypnotic or anxiolytic-induced sexual dysfunction
  Sedative, hypnotic, or anxiolytic-induced sexual dysfunction, without use disorder
  F13.982 Sedative, hypnotic or anxiolytic use, unspecified with sedative, hypnotic or anxiolytic-induced sleep disorder
  Sedative, hypnotic, or anxiolytic-induced sleep, without use disorder
  F13.988 Sedative, hypnotic or anxiolytic use, unspecified with other sedative, hypnotic or anxiolytic-induced disorder
  Sedative, hypnotic, or anxiolytic-induced mild neurocognitive disorder

F13.99 Sedative, hypnotic or anxiolytic use, unspecified with unspecified sedative, hypnotic or anxiolytic-induced disorder

F14 Cocaine related disorders

Excludes2: *other stimulant-related disorders (F15.-)*

+ **F14.1 Cocaine abuse**
  Excludes1: *cocaine dependence (F14.2-)*
  cocaine use, unspecified (F14.9-)
  F14.10 Cocaine abuse, uncomplicated
  Cocaine use disorder, mild
  F14.11 Cocaine abuse, in remission
  Cocaine use disorder, mild, in early remission
  Cocaine use disorder, mild, in sustained remission
  + **F14.12 Cocaine abuse with intoxication**
    F14.120 Cocaine abuse with intoxication, uncomplicated
    CC **F14.121 Cocaine abuse with intoxication with delirium**
    F14.122 Cocaine abuse with intoxication with perceptual disturbance
    F14.129 Cocaine abuse with intoxication, unspecified
  CC **F14.13 Cocaine abuse, unspecified with withdrawal**
  AHA CC: 4Q, 2020, 16-17
  F14.14 Cocaine abuse with cocaine-induced mood disorder
  Cocaine use disorder, mild, with cocaine-induced bipolar or related disorder
  Cocaine use disorder, mild, with cocaine-induced depressive disorder
  + **F14.15 Cocaine abuse with cocaine-induced psychotic disorder**
    CC **F14.150 Cocaine abuse with cocaine-induced psychotic disorder with delusions**
    CC **F14.151 Cocaine abuse with cocaine-induced psychotic disorder with hallucinations**
    F14.159 Cocaine abuse with cocaine-induced psychotic disorder, unspecified
  + **F14.18 Cocaine abuse with other cocaine-induced disorder**
    F14.180 Cocaine abuse with cocaine-induced anxiety disorder
    F14.181 Cocaine abuse with cocaine-induced sexual dysfunction
    F14.182 Cocaine abuse with cocaine-induced sleep disorder
    F14.188 Cocaine abuse with other cocaine-induced disorder
    Cocaine use disorder, mild, with cocaine-induced obsessive compulsive or related disorder
  F14.19 Cocaine abuse with unspecified cocaine-induced disorder

+ **F14.2 Cocaine dependence**
  Excludes1: *cocaine abuse (F14.1-)*
  cocaine use, unspecified (F14.9-)
  Excludes2: *cocaine poisoning (T40.5-)*
  CC **F14.20 Cocaine dependence, uncomplicated**
  Cocaine use disorder, moderate
  Cocaine use disorder, severe
  F14.21 Cocaine dependence, in remission
  Cocaine use disorder, moderate, in early remission
  Cocaine use disorder, moderate, in sustained remission
  Cocaine use disorder, severe, in early remission
  Cocaine use disorder, severe, in sustained remission
  AHA CC: 2Q, 2017, 26-28
  + **F14.22 Cocaine dependence with intoxication**
    Excludes1: *cocaine dependence with withdrawal (F14.23)*
    F14.220 Cocaine dependence with intoxication, uncomplicated
    CC **F14.221 Cocaine dependence with intoxication delirium**
    CC **F14.222 Cocaine dependence with intoxication with perceptual disturbance**
    CC **F14.229 Cocaine dependence with intoxication, unspecified**

CC **F14.23** **Cocaine dependence with withdrawal**
Excludes1: *cocaine dependence with intoxication (F14.22-)*

F14.24 **Cocaine dependence with cocaine-induced mood disorder**
Cocaine use disorder, moderate, with cocaine-induced bipolar or related disorder
Cocaine use disorder, moderate, with cocaine-induced depressive disorder
Cocaine use disorder, severe, with cocaine-induced bipolar or related disorder
Cocaine use disorder, severe, with cocaine-induced depressive disorder

\+ **F14.25** **Cocaine dependence with cocaine-induced psychotic disorder**
CC **F14.250** **Cocaine dependence with cocaine-induced psychotic disorder with delusions**
CC **F14.251** **Cocaine dependence with cocaine-induced psychotic disorder with hallucinations**
CC **F14.259** **Cocaine dependence with cocaine-induced psychotic disorder, unspecified**

\+ **F14.28** **Cocaine dependence with other cocaine-induced disorder**
CC **F14.280** **Cocaine dependence with cocaine-induced anxiety disorder**
CC **F14.281** **Cocaine dependence with cocaine-induced sexual dysfunction**
CC **F14.282** **Cocaine dependence with cocaine-induced sleep disorder**
CC **F14.288** **Cocaine dependence with other cocaine-induced disorder**
Cocaine use disorder, moderate, with cocaine-induced obsessive compulsive or related disorder
Cocaine use disorder, severe, with cocaine-induced obsessive compulsive or related disorder

F14.29 **Cocaine dependence with unspecified cocaine-induced disorder**

\+ **F14.9** **Cocaine use, unspecified**
Excludes1: *cocaine abuse (F14.1-)*
cocaine dependence (F14.2-)
Review coding guideline C.5.b.3

F14.90 **Cocaine use, unspecified, uncomplicated**
AHA CC: 2Q, 2018, 10-11

\+ **F14.92** **Cocaine use, unspecified with intoxication**
F14.920 **Cocaine use, unspecified with intoxication, uncomplicated**
CC **F14.921** **Cocaine use, unspecified with intoxication delirium**
F14.922 **Cocaine use, unspecified with intoxication with perceptual disturbance**
F14.929 **Cocaine use, unspecified with intoxication, unspecified**

CC **F14.93** **Cocaine use, unspecified with withdrawal**
AHA CC: 4Q, 2020, 16-17

F14.94 **Cocaine use, unspecified with cocaine-induced mood disorder**
Cocaine-induced bipolar or related disorder, without use disorder
Cocaine-induced depressive disorder, without use disorder

\+ **F14.95** **Cocaine use, unspecified with cocaine-induced psychotic disorder**
CC **F14.950** **Cocaine use, unspecified with cocaine-induced psychotic disorder with delusions**
CC **F14.951** **Cocaine use, unspecified with cocaine-induced psychotic disorder with hallucinations**
F14.959 **Cocaine use, unspecified with cocaine-induced psychotic disorder, unspecified**
Cocaine-induced psychotic disorder, without use disorder

\+ **F14.98** **Cocaine use, unspecified with other specified cocaine-induced disorder**
F14.980 **Cocaine use, unspecified with cocaine-induced anxiety disorder**
Cocaine-induced anxiety disorder, without use disorder
F14.981 **Cocaine use, unspecified with cocaine-induced sexual dysfunction**
Cocaine-induced sexual dysfunction, without use disorder
F14.982 **Cocaine use, unspecified with cocaine-induced sleep disorder**
Cocaine-induced sleep disorder, without use disorder
F14.988 **Cocaine use, unspecified with other cocaine-induced disorder**
Cocaine-induced obsessive compulsive or related disorder

F14.99 **Cocaine use, unspecified with unspecified cocaine-induced disorder**

F15 Other stimulant related disorders

Includes: amphetamine-related disorders
caffeine
Excludes2: *cocaine-related disorders (F14.-)*

\+ **F15.1** **Other stimulant abuse**
Excludes1: *other stimulant dependence (F15.2-)*
other stimulant use, unspecified (F15.9-)

F15.10 **Other stimulant abuse, uncomplicated**
Amphetamine type substance use disorder, mild
Other or unspecified stimulant use disorder, mild

F15.11 **Other stimulant abuse, in remission**
Amphetamine type substance use disorder, mild, in early remission
Amphetamine type substance use disorder, mild, in sustained remission
Other or unspecified stimulant use disorder, mild, in early remission
Other or unspecified stimulant use disorder, mild, in sustained remission

\+ **F15.12** **Other stimulant abuse with intoxication**
F15.120 **Other stimulant abuse with intoxication, uncomplicated**
CC **F15.121** **Other stimulant abuse with intoxication delirium**
F15.122 **Other stimulant abuse with intoxication with perceptual disturbance**
Amphetamine or other stimulant use disorder, mild, with amphetamine or other stimulant intoxication, with perceptual disturbances
F15.129 **Other stimulant abuse with intoxication, unspecified**
Amphetamine or other stimulant use disorder, mild, with amphetamine or other stimulant intoxication, without perceptual disturbances

CC **F15.13** **Other stimulant abuse with withdrawal**
AHA CC: 4Q, 2020, 16-17

F15.14 **Other stimulant abuse with stimulant-induced mood disorder**
Amphetamine or other stimulant use disorder, mild, with amphetamine or other stimulant-induced bipolar or related disorder
Amphetamine or other stimulant use disorder, mild, with amphetamine or other stimulant-induced depressive disorder

\+ **F15.15** **Other stimulant abuse with stimulant-induced psychotic disorder**
CC **F15.150** **Other stimulant abuse with stimulant-induced psychotic disorder with delusions**
CC **F15.151** **Other stimulant abuse with stimulant-induced psychotic disorder with hallucinations**
F15.159 **Other stimulant abuse with stimulant-induced psychotic disorder, unspecified**

+ **F15.18 Other stimulant abuse with other stimulant-induced disorder**
  - **F15.180 Other stimulant abuse with stimulant-induced anxiety disorder**
  - **F15.181 Other stimulant abuse with stimulant-induced sexual dysfunction**
  - **F15.182 Other stimulant abuse with stimulant-induced sleep disorder**
  - **F15.188 Other stimulant abuse with other stimulant-induced disorder**
    Amphetamine or other stimulant use disorder, mild, with amphetamine or other stimulant-induced obsessive-compulsive or related disorder

F15.19 Other stimulant abuse with unspecified stimulant-induced disorder

+ **F15.2 Other stimulant dependence**
  Excludes1: *other stimulant abuse (F15.1-)*
  other stimulant use, unspecified (F15.9-)

CC **F15.20 Other stimulant dependence, uncomplicated**
Amphetamine type substance use disorder, moderate
Amphetamine type substance use disorder, severe
Other or unspecified stimulant use disorder, moderate
Other or unspecified stimulant use disorder, severe

F15.21 Other stimulant dependence, in remission
Amphetamine type substance use disorder, moderate, in early remission
Amphetamine type substance use disorder, moderate, in sustained remission
Amphetamine type substance use disorder, severe, in early remission
Amphetamine type substance use disorder, severe, in sustained remission
Other or unspecified stimulant use disorder, moderate, in early remission
Other or unspecified stimulant use disorder, moderate, in sustained remission
Other or unspecified stimulant use disorder, severe, in early remission
Other or unspecified stimulant use disorder, severe, in sustained remission

+ **F15.22 Other stimulant dependence with intoxication**
  Excludes1: *other stimulant dependence with withdrawal (F15.23)*
  - **F15.220 Other stimulant dependence with intoxication, uncomplicated**
  - CC **F15.221 Other stimulant dependence with intoxication delirium**
  - CC **F15.222 Other stimulant dependence with intoxication with perceptual disturbance**
    Amphetamine or other stimulant use disorder, moderate, with amphetamine or other stimulant intoxication, with perceptual disturbances
    Amphetamine or other stimulant use disorder, severe, with amphetamine or other stimulant intoxication, with perceptual disturbances
  - **F15.229 Other stimulant dependence with intoxication, unspecified**
    Amphetamine or other stimulant use disorder, moderate, with amphetamine or other stimulant intoxication, without perceptual disturbances
    Amphetamine or other stimulant use disorder, severe, with amphetamine or other stimulant intoxication, without perceptual disturbances

CC **F15.23 Other stimulant dependence with withdrawal**
Amphetamine or other stimulant withdrawal
Excludes1: *other stimulant dependence with intoxication (F15.22-)*

F15.24 Other stimulant dependence with stimulant-induced mood disorder
Amphetamine or other stimulant use disorder, moderate, with amphetamine or other stimulant-induced bipolar or related disorder
Amphetamine or other stimulant use disorder, moderate, with amphetamine or other stimulant-induced depressive disorder
Amphetamine or other stimulant use disorder, severe, with amphetamine or other stimulant-induced bipolar or related disorder
Amphetamine or other stimulant use disorder, severe, with amphetamine or other stimulant-induced depressive disorder

+ **F15.25 Other stimulant dependence with stimulant-induced psychotic disorder**
  - CC **F15.250 Other stimulant dependence with stimulant-induced psychotic disorder with delusions**
  - CC **F15.251 Other stimulant dependence with stimulant-induced psychotic disorder with hallucinations**
  - CC **F15.259 Other stimulant dependence with stimulant-induced psychotic disorder, unspecified**

+ **F15.28 Other stimulant dependence with other stimulant-induced disorder**
  - CC **F15.280 Other stimulant dependence with stimulant-induced anxiety disorder**
  - CC **F15.281 Other stimulant dependence with stimulant-induced sexual dysfunction**
  - CC **F15.282 Other stimulant dependence with stimulant-induced sleep disorder**
  - CC **F15.288 Other stimulant dependence with other stimulant-induced disorder**
    Amphetamine or other stimulant use disorder, moderate, with amphetamine or other stimulant-induced obsessive-compulsive or related disorder
    Amphetamine or other stimulant use disorder, severe, with amphetamine or other stimulant-induced obsessive-compulsive or related disorder

F15.29 Other stimulant dependence with unspecified stimulant-induced disorder

+ **F15.9 Other stimulant use, unspecified**
  Excludes1: *other stimulant abuse (F15.1-)*
  other stimulant dependence (F15.2-)
  Review coding guideline C.5.b.3

F15.90 Other stimulant use, unspecified, uncomplicated

+ **F15.92 Other stimulant use, unspecified with intoxication**
  Excludes1: *other stimulant use, unspecified with withdrawal (F15.93)*
  - **F15.920 Other stimulant use, unspecified with intoxication, uncomplicated**
  - CC **F15.921 Other stimulant use, unspecified with intoxication delirium**
    Amphetamine or other stimulant-induced delirium
  - **F15.922 Other stimulant use, unspecified with intoxication with perceptual disturbance**
  - **F15.929 Other stimulant use, unspecified with intoxication, unspecified**
    Caffeine intoxication

CC **F15.93 Other stimulant use, unspecified with withdrawal**
Caffeine withdrawal
Excludes1: *other stimulant use, unspecified with intoxication (F15.92-)*

F15.94 Other stimulant use, unspecified with stimulant-induced mood disorder
Amphetamine or other stimulant-induced bipolar or related disorder, without use disorder
Amphetamine or other stimulant-induced depressive disorder, without use disorder

+ F15.95 **Other stimulant use, unspecified with stimulant-induced psychotic disorder**

CC **F15.950 Other stimulant use, unspecified with stimulant-induced psychotic disorder with delusions**

CC **F15.951 Other stimulant use, unspecified with stimulant-induced psychotic disorder with hallucinations**

F15.959 Other stimulant use, unspecified with stimulant-induced psychotic disorder, unspecified

Amphetamine or other stimulant-induced psychotic disorder, without use disorder

+ F15.98 **Other stimulant use, unspecified with other stimulant-induced disorder**

F15.980 Other stimulant use, unspecified with stimulant-induced anxiety disorder

Amphetamine or other stimulant-induced anxiety disorder, without use disorder

Caffeine induced anxiety disorder, without use disorder

F15.981 Other stimulant use, unspecified with stimulant-induced sexual dysfunction

Amphetamine or other stimulant-induced sexual dysfunction, without use disorder

F15.982 Other stimulant use, unspecified with stimulant-induced sleep disorder

Amphetamine or other stimulant-induced sleep disorder, without use disorder

Caffeine induced sleep disorder, without use disorder

F15.988 Other stimulant use, unspecified with other stimulant-induced disorder

Amphetamine or other stimulant-induced obsessive-compulsive or related disorder, without use disorder

F15.99 Other stimulant use, unspecified with unspecified stimulant-induced disorder

F16 Hallucinogen related disorders

Includes: ecstasy
PCP
phencyclidine

+ F16.1 **Hallucinogen abuse**

Excludes1: *hallucinogen dependence (F16.2-)*
hallucinogen use, unspecified (F16.9-)

F16.10 Hallucinogen abuse, uncomplicated

Other hallucinogen use disorder, mild
Phencyclidine use disorder, mild

AHA CC: 4Q, 2018, 31

F16.11 Hallucinogen abuse, in remission

Other hallucinogen use disorder, mild, in early remission
Other hallucinogen use disorder, mild, in sustained remission
Phencyclidine use disorder, mild, in early remission
Phencyclidine use disorder, mild, in sustained remission

+ F16.12 **Hallucinogen abuse with intoxication**

F16.120 Hallucinogen abuse with intoxication, uncomplicated

CC **F16.121 Hallucinogen abuse with intoxication with delirium**

F16.122 Hallucinogen abuse with intoxication with perceptual disturbance

F16.129 Hallucinogen abuse with intoxication, unspecified

F16.14 Hallucinogen abuse with hallucinogen-induced mood disorder

Other hallucinogen use disorder, mild, with other hallucinogen-induced bipolar or related disorder
Other hallucinogen use disorder, mild, with other hallucinogen-induced depressive disorder
Phencyclidine use disorder, mild, with other hallucinogen-induced bipolar or related disorder
Phencyclidine use disorder, mild, with other hallucinogen-induced depressive disorder

+ F16.15 **Hallucinogen abuse with hallucinogen-induced psychotic disorder**

CC **F16.150 Hallucinogen abuse with hallucinogen-induced psychotic disorder with delusions**

CC **F16.151 Hallucinogen abuse with hallucinogen-induced psychotic disorder with hallucinations**

F16.159 Hallucinogen abuse with hallucinogen-induced psychotic disorder, unspecified

+ F16.18 **Hallucinogen abuse with other hallucinogen-induced disorder**

F16.180 Hallucinogen abuse with hallucinogen-induced anxiety disorder

F16.183 Hallucinogen abuse with hallucinogen persisting perception disorder (flashbacks)

F16.188 Hallucinogen abuse with other hallucinogen-induced disorder

F16.19 Hallucinogen abuse with unspecified hallucinogen-induced disorder

+ F16.2 **Hallucinogen dependence**

Excludes1: *hallucinogen abuse (F16.1-)*
hallucinogen use, unspecified (F16.9-)

CC **F16.20 Hallucinogen dependence, uncomplicated**

Other hallucinogen use disorder, moderate
Other hallucinogen use disorder, severe
Phencyclidine use disorder, moderate
Phencyclidine use disorder, severe

F16.21 Hallucinogen dependence, in remission

Other hallucinogen use disorder, moderate, in early remission
Other hallucinogen use disorder, moderate, in sustained remission
Other hallucinogen use disorder, severe, in early remission
Other hallucinogen use disorder, severe, in sustained remission
Phencyclidine use disorder, moderate, in early remission
Phencyclidine use disorder, moderate, in sustained remission
Phencyclidine use disorder, severe, in early remission
Phencyclidine use disorder, severe, in sustained remission

+ F16.22 **Hallucinogen dependence with intoxication**

F16.220 Hallucinogen dependence with intoxication, uncomplicated

CC **F16.221 Hallucinogen dependence with intoxication with delirium**

F16.229 Hallucinogen dependence with intoxication, unspecified

F16.24 Hallucinogen dependence with hallucinogen-induced mood disorder

Other hallucinogen use disorder, moderate, with other hallucinogen-induced bipolar or related disorder
Other hallucinogen use disorder, moderate, with other hallucinogen-induced depressive disorder
Other hallucinogen use disorder, severe, with other hallucinogen-induced bipolar or related disorder
Other hallucinogen use disorder, severe, with other hallucinogen-induced depressive disorder
Phencyclidine use disorder, moderate, with other phencyclidine-induced bipolar or related disorder
Phencyclidine use disorder, moderate, with other phencyclidine-induced depressive disorder
Phencyclidine use disorder, severe, with other phencyclidine-induced bipolar or related disorder
Phencyclidine use disorder, severe, with other phencyclidine-induced depressive disorder

+ **F16.25 Hallucinogen dependence with hallucinogen-induced psychotic disorder**
  - CC **F16.250 Hallucinogen dependence with hallucinogen-induced psychotic disorder with delusions**
  - CC **F16.251 Hallucinogen dependence with hallucinogen-induced psychotic disorder with hallucinations**
  - CC **F16.259 Hallucinogen dependence with hallucinogen-induced psychotic disorder, unspecified**
+ **F16.28 Hallucinogen dependence with other hallucinogen-induced disorder**
  - CC **F16.280 Hallucinogen dependence with hallucinogen-induced anxiety disorder**
  - CC **F16.283 Hallucinogen dependence with hallucinogen persisting perception disorder (flashbacks)**
  - CC **F16.288 Hallucinogen dependence with other hallucinogen-induced disorder**

F16.29 Hallucinogen dependence with unspecified hallucinogen-induced disorder

+ **F16.9 Hallucinogen use, unspecified**

Excludes1: *hallucinogen abuse (F16.1-)*
hallucinogen dependence (F16.2-)

Review coding guideline C.5.b.3

F16.90 Hallucinogen use, unspecified, uncomplicated

+ **F16.92 Hallucinogen use, unspecified with intoxication**
  - **F16.920 Hallucinogen use, unspecified with intoxication, uncomplicated**
  - CC **F16.921 Hallucinogen use, unspecified with intoxication with delirium**
    Other hallucinogen intoxication delirium
  - **F16.929 Hallucinogen use, unspecified with intoxication, unspecified**

F16.94 Hallucinogen use, unspecified with hallucinogen-induced mood disorder
Other hallucinogen-induced bipolar or related disorder, without use disorder
Other hallucinogen-induced depressive disorder, without use disorder
Phencyclidine-induced bipolar or related disorder, without use disorder
Phencyclidine-induced depressive disorder, without use disorder

+ **F16.95 Hallucinogen use, unspecified with hallucinogen-induced psychotic disorder**
  - CC **F16.950 Hallucinogen use, unspecified with hallucinogen-induced psychotic disorder with delusions**
  - CC **F16.951 Hallucinogen use, unspecified with hallucinogen-induced psychotic disorder with hallucinations**
  - **F16.959 Hallucinogen use, unspecified with hallucinogen-induced psychotic disorder, unspecified**
    Other hallucinogen-induced psychotic disorder, without use disorder
    Phencyclidine-induced psychotic disorder, without use disorder
+ **F16.98 Hallucinogen use, unspecified with other specified hallucinogen-induced disorder**
  - **F16.980 Hallucinogen use, unspecified with hallucinogen-induced anxiety disorder**
    Other hallucinogen-induced anxiety disorder, without use disorder
    Phencyclidine-induced anxiety disorder, without use disorder
  - **F16.983 Hallucinogen use, unspecified with hallucinogen persisting perception disorder (flashbacks)**
  - **F16.988 Hallucinogen use, unspecified with other hallucinogen-induced disorder**

F16.99 Hallucinogen use, unspecified with unspecified hallucinogen-induced disorder

F17 Nicotine dependence

Excludes1: *history of tobacco dependence (Z87.891)*
tobacco use NOS (Z72.0)

Excludes2: *tobacco use (smoking) during pregnancy, childbirth and the puerperium (O99.33-)*
toxic effect of nicotine (T65.2-)

Review coding guideline C.15.1.2

+ **F17.2 Nicotine dependence**
+ **F17.20 Nicotine dependence, unspecified**
  - **F17.200 Nicotine dependence, unspecified, uncomplicated**
    Tobacco use disorder, mild
    Tobacco use disorder, moderate
    Tobacco use disorder, severe
    AHA CC: 4Q, 2013, 108; 1Q, 2016, 36-37
  - **F17.201 Nicotine dependence, unspecified, in remission**
    Tobacco use disorder, mild, in early remission
    Tobacco use disorder, mild, in sustained remission
    Tobacco use disorder, moderate, in early remission
    Tobacco use disorder, moderate, in sustained remission
    Tobacco use disorder, severe, in early remission
    Tobacco use disorder, severe, in sustained remission
  - CC **F17.203 Nicotine dependence unspecified, with withdrawal**
    Tobacco withdrawal
  - **F17.208 Nicotine dependence, unspecified, with other nicotine-induced disorders**
  - **F17.209 Nicotine dependence, unspecified, with unspecified nicotine-induced disorders**
+ **F17.21 Nicotine dependence, cigarettes**
  - **F17.210 Nicotine dependence, cigarettes, uncomplicated**
    AHA CC: 4Q, 2013, 109; 2Q, 2017, 28-29
  - **F17.211 Nicotine dependence, cigarettes, in remission**
    Tobacco use disorder, cigarettes, mild, in early remission
    Tobacco use disorder, cigarettes, mild, in sustained remission
    Tobacco use disorder, cigarettes, moderate, in early remission
    Tobacco use disorder, cigarettes, moderate, in sustained remission
    Tobacco use disorder, cigarettes, severe, in early remission
    Tobacco use disorder, cigarettes, severe, in sustained remission
  - CC **F17.213 Nicotine dependence, cigarettes, with withdrawal**
  - **F17.218 Nicotine dependence, cigarettes, with other nicotine-induced disorders**
  - **F17.219 Nicotine dependence, cigarettes, with unspecified nicotine-induced disorders**
+ **F17.22 Nicotine dependence, chewing tobacco**
  - **F17.220 Nicotine dependence, chewing tobacco, uncomplicated**
  - **F17.221 Nicotine dependence, chewing tobacco, in remission**
    Tobacco use disorder, chewing tobacco, mild, in early remission
    Tobacco use disorder, chewing tobacco, mild, in sustained remission
    Tobacco use disorder, chewing tobacco, moderate, in early remission
    Tobacco use disorder, chewing tobacco, moderate, in sustained remission
    Tobacco use disorder, chewing tobacco, severe, in early remission
    Tobacco use disorder, chewing tobacco, severe, in sustained remission

CC **F17.223 Nicotine dependence, chewing tobacco, with withdrawal**

F17.228 Nicotine dependence, chewing tobacco, with other nicotine-induced disorders

F17.229 Nicotine dependence, chewing tobacco, with unspecified nicotine-induced disorders

+ **F17.29 Nicotine dependence, other tobacco product**

F17.290 Nicotine dependence, other tobacco product, uncomplicated

AHA CC: 2Q, 2017, 28-29

F17.291 Nicotine dependence, other tobacco product, in remission

Tobacco use disorder, other tobacco product, mild, in early remission

Tobacco use disorder, other tobacco product, mild, in sustained remission

Tobacco use disorder, other tobacco product, moderate, in early remission

Tobacco use disorder, other tobacco product, moderate, in sustained remission

Tobacco use disorder, other tobacco product, severe, in early remission

Tobacco use disorder, other tobacco product, severe, in sustained remission

CC **F17.293 Nicotine dependence, other tobacco product, with withdrawal**

F17.298 Nicotine dependence, other tobacco product, with other nicotine-induced disorders

F17.299 Nicotine dependence, other tobacco product, with unspecified nicotine-induced disorders

F18 Inhalant related disorders

Includes: volatile solvents

+ **F18.1 Inhalant abuse**

Excludes1: *inhalant dependence (F18.2-)*
inhalant use, unspecified (F18.9-)

F18.10 Inhalant abuse, uncomplicated

Inhalant use disorder, mild

F18.11 Inhalant abuse, in remission

Inhalant use disorder, mild, in early remission

Inhalant use disorder, mild, in sustained remission

+ **F18.12 Inhalant abuse with intoxication**

F18.120 Inhalant abuse with intoxication, uncomplicated

CC **F18.121 Inhalant abuse with intoxication delirium**

F18.129 Inhalant abuse with intoxication, unspecified

F18.14 Inhalant abuse with inhalant-induced mood disorder

Inhalant use disorder, mild, with inhalant-induced depressive disorder

+ **F18.15 Inhalant abuse with inhalant-induced psychotic disorder**

CC **F18.150 Inhalant abuse with inhalant-induced psychotic disorder with delusions**

CC **F18.151 Inhalant abuse with inhalant-induced psychotic disorder with hallucinations**

F18.159 Inhalant abuse with inhalant-induced psychotic disorder, unspecified

CC **F18.17 Inhalant abuse with inhalant-induced dementia**

Inhalant use disorder, mild, with inhalant-induced major neurocognitive disorder

+ **F18.18 Inhalant abuse with other inhalant-induced disorders**

F18.180 Inhalant abuse with inhalant-induced anxiety disorder

F18.188 Inhalant abuse with other inhalant-induced disorder

Inhalant use disorder, mild, with inhalant-induced mild neurocognitive disorder

F18.19 Inhalant abuse with unspecified inhalant-induced disorder

+ **F18.2 Inhalant dependence**

Excludes1: *inhalant abuse (F18.1-)*
inhalant use, unspecified (F18.9-)

CC **F18.20 Inhalant dependence, uncomplicated**

Inhalant use disorder, moderate

Inhalant use disorder, severe

F18.21 Inhalant dependence, in remission

Inhalant use disorder, moderate, in early remission

Inhalant use disorder, moderate, in sustained remission

Inhalant use disorder, severe, in early remission

Inhalant use disorder, severe, in sustained remission

+ **F18.22 Inhalant dependence with intoxication**

F18.220 Inhalant dependence with intoxication, uncomplicated

CC **F18.221 Inhalant dependence with intoxication delirium**

F18.229 Inhalant dependence with intoxication, unspecified

F18.24 Inhalant dependence with inhalant-induced mood disorder

Inhalant use disorder, moderate, with inhalant-induced depressive disorder

Inhalant use disorder, severe, with inhalant-induced depressive disorder

+ **F18.25 Inhalant dependence with inhalant-induced psychotic disorder**

CC **F18.250 Inhalant dependence with inhalant-induced psychotic disorder with delusions**

CC **F18.251 Inhalant dependence with inhalant-induced psychotic disorder with hallucinations**

CC **F18.259 Inhalant dependence with inhalant-induced psychotic disorder, unspecified**

CC **F18.27 Inhalant dependence with inhalant-induced dementia**

Inhalant use disorder, moderate, with inhalant-induced major neurocognitive disorder

Inhalant use disorder, severe, with inhalant-induced major neurocognitive disorder

+ **F18.28 Inhalant dependence with other inhalant-induced disorders**

CC **F18.280 Inhalant dependence with inhalant-induced anxiety disorder**

CC **F18.288 Inhalant dependence with other inhalant-induced disorder**

Inhalant use disorder, moderate, with inhalant-induced mild neurocognitive disorder

Inhalant use disorder, severe, with inhalant-induced mild neurocognitive disorder

F18.29 Inhalant dependence with unspecified inhalant-induced disorder

+ **F18.9 Inhalant use, unspecified**

Excludes1: *inhalant abuse (F18.1-)*
inhalant dependence (F18.2-)

Review coding guideline C.5.b.3

F18.90 Inhalant use, unspecified, uncomplicated

+ **F18.92 Inhalant use, unspecified with intoxication**

F18.920 Inhalant use, unspecified with intoxication, uncomplicated

CC **F18.921 Inhalant use, unspecified with intoxication with delirium**

F18.929 Inhalant use, unspecified with intoxication, unspecified

F18.94 Inhalant use, unspecified with inhalant-induced mood disorder

Inhalant-induced depressive disorder

+ F18.95 Inhalant use, unspecified with inhalant-induced psychotic disorder

CC F18.950 Inhalant use, unspecified with inhalant-induced psychotic disorder with delusions

CC F18.951 Inhalant use, unspecified with inhalant-induced psychoticdisorder with hallucinations

F18.959 Inhalant use, unspecified with inhalant-induced psychotic disorder, unspecified

CC F18.97 Inhalant use, unspecified with inhalant-induced persisting dementia

Inhalant-induced major neurocognitive disorder

+ F18.98 Inhalant use, unspecified with other inhalant-induced disorders

F18.980 Inhalant use, unspecified with inhalant-induced anxiety disorder

F18.988 Inhalant use, unspecified with other inhalant-induced disorder

Inhalant-induced mild neurocognitive disorder

F18.99 Inhalant use, unspecified with unspecified inhalant-induced disorder

F19 Other psychoactive substance related disorders

Includes: polysubstance drug use (indiscriminate drug use)

+ F19.1 Other psychoactive substance abuse

Excludes1: *other psychoactive substance dependence (F19.2-)*

other psychoactive substance use, unspecified (F19.9-)

F19.10 Other psychoactive substance abuse, uncomplicated

Other (or unknown) substance use disorder, mild

F19.11 Other psychoactive substance abuse, in remission

Other (or unknown) substance use disorder, mild, in early remission

Other (or unknown) substance use disorder, mild, in sustained remission

+ F19.12 Other psychoactive substance abuse with intoxication

F19.120 Other psychoactive substance abuse with intoxication, uncomplicated

CC F19.121 Other psychoactive substance abuse with intoxication delirium

F19.122 Other psychoactive substance abuse with intoxication with perceptual disturbances

F19.129 Other psychoactive substance abuse with intoxication, unspecified

+ F19.13 Other psychoactive substance abuse with withdrawal

AHA CC: 4Q, 2020, 16-17

CC F19.130 Other psychoactive substance abuse with withdrawal, uncomplicated

CC F19.131 Other psychoactive substance abuse with withdrawal delirium

CC F19.132 Other psychoactive substance abuse with withdrawal with perceptual disturbance

CC F19.139 Other psychoactive substance abuse with withdrawal, unspecified

F19.14 Other psychoactive substance abuse with psychoactive substance-induced mood disorder

Other (or unknown) substance use disorder, mild, with other (or known) substance-induced bipolar or related disorder

Other (or unknown) substance use disorder, mild, with other (or known) substance-induced depressive disorder

+ F19.15 Other psychoactive substance abuse with psychoactive substance-induced psychotic disorder

CC F19.150 Other psychoactive substance abuse with psychoactive substance-induced psychotic disorder with delusions

CC F19.151 Other psychoactive substance abuse with psychoactive substance-induced psychotic disorder with hallucinations

F19.159 Other psychoactive substance abuse with psychoactive substance-induced psychotic disorder, unspecified

F19.16 Other psychoactive substance abuse with psychoactive substance-induced persisting amnestic disorder

CC F19.17 Other psychoactive substance abuse with psychoactive substance-induced persisting dementia

Other (or unknown) substance use disorder, mild, with other (or known) substance-induced major neurocognitive disorder

+ F19.18 Other psychoactive substance abuse with other psychoactive substance-induced disorders

F19.180 Other psychoactive substance abuse with psychoactive substance-induced anxiety disorder

F19.181 Other psychoactive substance abuse with psychoactive substance-induced sexual dysfunction

F19.182 Other psychoactive substance abuse with psychoactive substance-induced sleep disorder

F19.188 Other psychoactive substance abuse with other psychoactive substance-induced disorder

Other (or unknown) substance use disorder, mild, with other (or known) substance-induced mild neurocognitive disorder

Other (or unknown) substance use disorder, mild, with other (or known) substance-induced obsessive-compulsive disorder

F19.19 Other psychoactive substance abuse with unspecified psychoactive substance-induced disorder

+ F19.2 Other psychoactive substance dependence

Excludes1: *other psychoactive substance abuse (F19.1-)*

other psychoactive substance use, unspecified (F19.9-)

CC F19.20 Other psychoactive substance dependence, uncomplicated

Other (or unknown) substance use disorder, moderate

Other (or unknown) substance use disorder, severe

F19.21 Other psychoactive substance dependence, in remission

Other (or unknown) substance use disorder, moderate, in early remission

Other (or unknown) substance use disorder, moderate, in sustained remission

Other (or unknown) substance use disorder, severe, in early remission

Other (or unknown) substance use disorder, severe, in sustained remission

+ F19.22 Other psychoactive substance dependence with intoxication

Excludes1: *other psychoactive substance dependence with withdrawal (F19.23-)*

F19.220 Other psychoactive substance dependence with intoxication, uncomplicated

CC F19.221 Other psychoactive substance dependence with intoxication delirium

CC F19.222 Other psychoactive substance dependence with intoxication with perceptual disturbance

F19.229 Other psychoactive substance dependence with intoxication, unspecified

+ F19.23 **Other psychoactive substance dependence with withdrawal**

Excludes1: *other psychoactive substance dependence with intoxication (F19.22-)*

CC **F19.230** **Other psychoactive substance dependence with withdrawal, uncomplicated**

CC **F19.231** **Other psychoactive substance dependence with withdrawal delirium**

CC **F19.232** **Other psychoactive substance dependence with withdrawal with perceptual disturbance**

CC **F19.239** **Other psychoactive substance dependence with withdrawal, unspecified**

F19.24 **Other psychoactive substance dependence with psychoactive substance-induced mood disorder**

Other (or known) substance use disorder, moderate, with other (or unknown) substance-induced bipolar or related disorder

Other (or known) substance use disorder, moderate, with other (or unknown) substance-induced depressive disorder

Other (or known) substance use disorder, severe, with other (or unknown) substance-induced bipolar or related disorder

Other (or known) substance use disorder, severe, with other (or unknown) substance-induced depressive disorder

+ F19.25 **Other psychoactive substance dependence with psychoactive substance-induced psychotic disorder**

CC **F19.250** **Other psychoactive substance dependence with psychoactive substance-induced psychotic disorder with delusions**

CC **F19.251** **Other psychoactive substance dependence with psychoactive substance-induced psychotic disorder with hallucinations**

CC **F19.259** **Other psychoactive substance dependence with psychoactive substance-induced psychotic disorder, unspecified**

CC **F19.26** **Other psychoactive substance dependence with psychoactive substance-induced persisting amnestic disorder**

CC **F19.27** **Other psychoactive substance dependence with psychoactive substance-induced persisting dementia**

Other (or unknown) substance use disorder, moderate, with other (or known) substance-induced major neurocognitive disorder

Other (or unknown) substance use disorder, severe, with other (or known) substance-induced major neurocognitive disorder

+ F19.28 **Other psychoactive substance dependence with other psychoactive substance-induced disorders**

CC **F19.280** **Other psychoactive substance dependence with psychoactive substance-induced anxiety disorder**

CC **F19.281** **Other psychoactive substance dependence with psychoactive substance-induced sexual dysfunction**

CC **F19.282** **Other psychoactive substance dependence with psychoactive substance-induced sleep disorder**

CC **F19.288** **Other psychoactive substance dependence with other psychoactive substance-induced disorder**

Other (or unknown) substance use disorder, moderate, with other (or known) substance-induced mild neurocognitive disorder

Other (or unknown) substance use disorder, moderate, with other (or known) substance-induced obsessive-compulsive disorder

Other (or unknown) substance use disorder, severe, with other (or known) substance-induced mild neurocognitive disorder

Other (or unknown) substance use disorder, severe, with other (or known) substance-induced obsessive-compulsive disorder

F19.29 **Other psychoactive substance dependence with unspecified psychoactive substance-induced disorder**

+ F19.9 **Other psychoactive substance use, unspecified**

Excludes1: *other psychoactive substance abuse (F19.1-)*
other psychoactive substance dependence (F19.2-)

Review coding guideline C.5.b.3

F19.90 **Other psychoactive substance use, unspecified, uncomplicated**

+ F19.92 **Other psychoactive substance use, unspecified with intoxication**

Excludes1: *other psychoactive substance use, unspecified with withdrawal (F19.93)*

F19.920 **Other psychoactive substance use, unspecified with intoxication, uncomplicated**

CC **F19.921** **Other psychoactive substance use, unspecified with intoxication with delirium**

Other (or unknown) substance-induced delirium

F19.922 **Other psychoactive substance use, unspecified with intoxication with perceptual disturbance**

F19.929 **Other psychoactive substance use, unspecified with intoxication, unspecified**

+ F19.93 **Other psychoactive substance use, unspecified with withdrawal**

Excludes1: *other psychoactive substance use, unspecified with intoxication (F19.92-)*

CC **F19.930** **Other psychoactive substance use, unspecified with withdrawal, uncomplicated**

CC **F19.931** **Other psychoactive substance use, unspecified with withdrawal delirium**

CC **F19.932** **Other psychoactive substance use, unspecified with withdrawal with perceptual disturbance**

CC **F19.939** **Other psychoactive substance use, unspecified with withdrawal, unspecified**

F19.94 **Other psychoactive substance use, unspecified with psychoactive substance-induced mood disorder**

Other (or unknown) substance-induced bipolar or related disorder, without use disorder

Other (or unknown) substance-induced depressive disorder, without use disorder

\+ **F19.95 Other psychoactive substance use, unspecified with psychoactive substance-induced psychotic disorder**

CC **F19.950 Other psychoactive substance use, unspecified with psychoactive substance-induced psychotic disorder with delusions**

CC **F19.951 Other psychoactive substance use, unspecified with psychoactive substance-induced psychotic disorder with hallucinations**

F19.959 Other psychoactive substance use, unspecified with psychoactive substance-induced psychotic disorder, unspecified

Other (or unknown) substance-induced psychotic disorder, without use disorder

F19.96 Other psychoactive substance use, unspecified with psychoactive substance-induced persisting amnestic disorder

CC **F19.97 Other psychoactive substance use, unspecified with psychoactive substance-induced persisting dementia**

Other (or unknown) substance-induced major neurocognitive disorder, without use disorder

\+ **F19.98 Other psychoactive substance use, unspecified with other psychoactive substance-induced disorders**

F19.980 Other psychoactive substance use, unspecified with psychoactive substance-induced anxiety disorder

Other (or unknown) substance-induced anxiety disorder, without use disorder

F19.981 Other psychoactive substance use, unspecified with psychoactive substance-induced sexual dysfunction

Other (or unknown) substance-induced sexual dysfunction, without use disorder

F19.982 Other psychoactive substance use, unspecified with psychoactive substance-induced sleep disorder

Other (or unknown) substance-induced sleep disorder, without use disorder

F19.988 Other psychoactive substance use, unspecified with other psychoactive substance-induced disorder

Other (or unknown) substance-induced mild neurocognitive disorder, without use disorder

Other (or unknown) substance-induced obsessive-compulsive or related disorder, without use disorder

F19.99 Other psychoactive substance use, unspecified with unspecified psychoactive substance-induced disorder

Schizophrenia, schizotypal, delusional, and other non-mood psychotic disorders (F20-F29)

F20 Schizophrenia

Excludes1: *brief psychotic disorder (F23)*
cyclic schizophrenia (F25.0)
mood [affective] disorders with psychotic symptoms (F30.2, F31.2, F31.5, F31.64, F32.3, F33.3)
schizoaffective disorder (F25.-)
schizophrenic reaction NOS (F23)

Excludes2: *schizophrenic reaction in:*
alcoholism (F10.15-, F10.25-, F10.95-)
brain disease (F06.2)
epilepsy (F06.2)
psychoactive drug use (F11-F19 with .15. .25, .95)
schizotypal disorder (F21)

CC **F20.0 Paranoid schizophrenia**

Paraphrenic schizophrenia

Excludes1: *involutional paranoid state (F22)*
paranoia (F22)

CC **F20.1 Disorganized schizophrenia**

Hebephrenic schizophrenia
Hebephrenia

CC **F20.2 Catatonic schizophrenia**

Schizophrenic catalepsy
Schizophrenic catatonia
Schizophrenic flexibilitas cerea

Excludes1: *catatonic stupor (R40.1)*

F20.3 Undifferentiated schizophrenia

Atypical schizophrenia

Excludes1: *acute schizophrenia-like psychotic disorder (F23)*

Excludes2: *post-schizophrenic depression (F32.89)*

CC **F20.5 Residual schizophrenia**

Restzustand (schizophrenic)
Schizophrenic residual state

\+ **F20.8 Other schizophrenia**

CC **F20.81 Schizophreniform disorder**

Schizophreniform psychosis NOS

CC **F20.89 Other schizophrenia**

Cenesthopathic schizophrenia
Simple schizophrenia

F20.9 Schizophrenia, unspecified

AHA CC: 2Q, 2019, 32

F21 Schizotypal disorder

Borderline schizophrenia
Latent schizophrenia
Latent schizophrenic reaction
Prepsychotic schizophrenia
Prodromal schizophrenia
Pseudoneurotic schizophrenia
Pseudopsychopathic schizophrenia
Schizotypal personality disorder

Excludes2: *Asperger's syndrome (F84.5)*
schizoid personality disorder (F60.1)

Valid 3-character code, no further characters required

F22 Delusional disorders

Delusional dysmorphophobia
Involutional paranoid state
Paranoia
Paranoia querulans
Paranoid psychosis
Paranoid state
Paraphrenia (late)
Sensitiver Beziehungswahn

Excludes1: *mood [affective] disorders with psychotic symptoms (F30.2, F31.2, F31.5, F31.64, F32.3, F33.3)*
paranoid schizophrenia (F20.0)

Excludes2: *paranoid personality disorder (F60.0)*
paranoid psychosis, psychogenic (F23)
paranoid reaction (F23)

Valid 3-character code, no further characters required

CC **F23 Brief psychotic disorder**

Paranoid reaction
Psychogenic paranoid psychosis

Excludes2: *mood [affective] disorders with psychotic symptoms (F30.2, F31.2, F31.5, F31.64, F32.3, F33.3)*

Valid 3-character code, no further characters required

F24 Shared psychotic disorder

Folie à deux
Induced paranoid disorder
Induced psychotic disorder

Valid 3-character code, no further characters required

F25 Schizoaffective disorders

Excludes1: *mood [affective] disorders with psychotic symptoms (F30.2, F31.2, F31.5, F31.64, F32.3, F33.3)*
schizophrenia (F20.-)

F25.0 Schizoaffective disorder, bipolar type

Cyclic schizophrenia
Schizoaffective disorder, manic type
Schizoaffective disorder, mixed type
Schizoaffective psychosis, bipolar type

F25.1 Schizoaffective disorder, depressive type

Schizoaffective psychosis, depressive type

F25.8 Other schizoaffective disorders

F25.9 Schizoaffective disorder, unspecified

Schizoaffective psychosis NOS

F28 Other psychotic disorder not due to a substance or known physiological condition

Chronic hallucinatory psychosis
Other specified schizophrenia spectrum and other psychotic disorder

Valid 3-character code, no further characters required

F29 Unspecified psychosis not due to a substance or known physiological condition

Psychosis NOS
Unspecified schizophrenia spectrum and other psychotic disorder
Excludes1: *mental disorder NOS (F99)*
unspecified mental disorder due to known physiological condition (F09)
Valid 3-character code, no further characters required

Mood [affective] disorders (F30-F39)

F30 Manic episode

Includes: bipolar disorder, single manic episode
mixed affective episode
Excludes1: *bipolar disorder (F31.-)*
major depressive disorder, single episode (F32.-)
major depressive disorder, recurrent (F33.-)

\+ **F30.1 Manic episode without psychotic symptoms**
CC **F30.10 Manic episode without psychotic symptoms, unspecified**
CC **F30.11 Manic episode without psychotic symptoms, mild**
CC **F30.12 Manic episode without psychotic symptoms, moderate**
CC **F30.13 Manic episode, severe, without psychotic symptoms**

CC **F30.2 Manic episode, severe with psychotic symptoms**
Manic stupor
Mania with mood-congruent psychotic symptoms
Mania with mood-incongruent psychotic symptoms

F30.3 Manic episode in partial remission
F30.4 Manic episode in full remission
F30.8 Other manic episodes
Hypomania
CC **F30.9 Manic episode, unspecified**
Mania NOS

F31 Bipolar disorder

Includes: bipolar I disorder
bipolar type I disorder
manic-depressive illness
manic-depressive psychosis
manic-depressive reaction
Excludes1: *bipolar disorder, single manic episode (F30.-)*
major depressive disorder, single episode (F32.-)
major depressive disorder, recurrent (F33.-)
Excludes2: *cyclothymia (F34.0)*

CC **F31.0 Bipolar disorder, current episode hypomanic**
\+ **F31.1 Bipolar disorder, current episode manic without psychotic features**
CC **F31.10 Bipolar disorder, current episode manic without psychotic features, unspecified**
CC **F31.11 Bipolar disorder, current episode manic without psychotic features, mild**
CC **F31.12 Bipolar disorder, current episode manic without psychotic features, moderate**
CC **F31.13 Bipolar disorder, current episode manic without psychotic features, severe**

CC **F31.2 Bipolar disorder, current episode manic severe with psychotic features**
Bipolar disorder, current episode manic with mood-congruent psychotic symptoms
Bipolar disorder, current episode manic with mood-incongruent psychotic symptoms
Bipolar I disorder, current or most recent episode manic, with psychotic features

\+ **F31.3 Bipolar disorder, current episode depressed, mild or moderate severity**
CC **F31.30 Bipolar disorder, current episode depressed, mild or moderate severity, unspecified**
CC **F31.31 Bipolar disorder, current episode depressed, mild**
CC **F31.32 Bipolar disorder, current episode depressed, moderate**

CC **F31.4 Bipolar disorder, current episode depressed, severe, without psychotic features**

CC **F31.5 Bipolar disorder, current episode depressed, severe, with psychotic features**
Bipolar disorder, current episode depressed with mood-incongruent psychotic symptoms
Bipolar disorder, current episode depressed with mood-congruent psychotic symptoms
Bipolar I disorder, current or most recent episode depressed, with psychotic features

\+ **F31.6 Bipolar disorder, current episode mixed**
CC **F31.60 Bipolar disorder, current episode mixed, unspecified**
CC **F31.61 Bipolar disorder, current episode mixed, mild**
CC **F31.62 Bipolar disorder, current episode mixed, moderate**
CC **F31.63 Bipolar disorder, current episode mixed, severe, without psychotic features**
CC **F31.64 Bipolar disorder, current episode mixed, severe, with psychotic features**
Bipolar disorder, current episode mixed with mood-congruent psychotic symptoms
Bipolar disorder, current episode mixed with mood-incongruent psychotic symptoms

\+ **F31.7 Bipolar disorder, currently in remission**
F31.70 Bipolar disorder, currently in remission, most recent episode unspecified
F31.71 Bipolar disorder, in partial remission, most recent episode hypomanic
F31.72 Bipolar disorder, in full remission, most recent episode hypomanic
F31.73 Bipolar disorder, in partial remission, most recent episode manic
F31.74 Bipolar disorder, in full remission, most recent episode manic
F31.75 Bipolar disorder, in partial remission, most recent episode depressed
F31.76 Bipolar disorder, in full remission, most recent episode depressed
F31.77 Bipolar disorder, in partial remission, most recent episode mixed
F31.78 Bipolar disorder, in full remission, most recent episode mixed

\+ **F31.8 Other bipolar disorders**
CC **F31.81 Bipolar II disorder**
Bipolar disorder, type 2
CC **F31.89 Other bipolar disorder**
Recurrent manic episodes NOS

F31.9 Bipolar disorder, unspecified
Manic depression
AHA CC: 1Q, 2020, 23

F32 Depressive episode

Includes: single episode of agitated depression
single episode of depressive reaction
single episode of major depression
single episode of psychogenic depression
single episode of reactive depression
single episode of vital depression
Excludes1: *bipolar disorder (F31.-)*
manic episode (F30.-)
recurrent depressive disorder (F33.-)
Excludes2: *adjustment disorder (F43.2)*

CC **F32.0 Major depressive disorder, single episode, mild**
CC **F32.1 Major depressive disorder, single episode, moderate**
CC **F32.2 Major depressive disorder, single episode, severe without psychotic features**
CC **F32.3 Major depressive disorder, single episode, severe with psychotic features**
Single episode of major depression with mood-congruent psychotic symptoms
Single episode of major depression with mood-incongruent psychotic symptoms
Single episode of major depression with psychotic symptoms
Single episode of psychogenic depressive psychosis
Single episode of psychotic depression
Single episode of reactive depressive psychosis
F32.4 Major depressive disorder, single episode, in partial remission
F32.5 Major depressive disorder, single episode, in full remission

+ F32.8 **Other depressive episodes**
AHA CC: 4Q, 2016, 14

♀ F32.81 **Premenstrual dysphoric disorder**
Excludes1: *premenstrual tension syndrome (N94.3)*

F32.89 **Other specified depressive episodes**
Atypical depression
Post-schizophrenic depression
Single episode of 'masked' depression NOS

F32.9 **Major depressive disorder, single episode, unspecified**
Major depression NOS
AHA CC: 4Q, 2013, 107-108; 1Q, 2021, 10-11

F32.A **Depression, unspecified**
Depression NOS
Depressive disorder NOS

F33 **Major depressive disorder, recurrent**

Includes: recurrent episodes of depressive reaction
recurrent episodes of endogenous depression
recurrent episodes of major depression
recurrent episodes of psychogenic depression
recurrent episodes of reactive depression
recurrent episodes of seasonal depressive disorder
recurrent episodes of vital depression

Excludes1: *bipolar disorder (F31.-)*
manic episode (F30.-)

CC F33.0 **Major depressive disorder, recurrent, mild**
CC F33.1 **Major depressive disorder, recurrent, moderate**
CC F33.2 **Major depressive disorder, recurrent severe without psychotic features**
CC F33.3 **Major depressive disorder, recurrent, severe with psychotic symptoms**
Endogenous depression with psychotic symptoms
Major depressive disorder, recurrent, with psychotic features
Recurrent severe episodes of major depression with mood-congruent psychotic symptoms
Recurrent severe episodes of major depression with mood-incongruent psychotic symptoms
Recurrent severe episodes of major depression with psychotic symptoms
Recurrent severe episodes of psychogenic depressive psychosis
Recurrent severe episodes of psychotic depression
Recurrent severe episodes of reactive depressive psychosis

+ F33.4 **Major depressive disorder, recurrent, in remission**
CC F33.40 **Major depressive disorder, recurrent, in remission, unspecified**
F33.41 **Major depressive disorder, recurrent, in partial remission**
F33.42 **Major depressive disorder, recurrent, in full remission**

CC F33.8 **Other recurrent depressive disorders**
Recurrent brief depressive episodes

CC F33.9 **Major depressive disorder, recurrent, unspecified**
Monopolar depression NOS

F34 **Persistent mood [affective] disorders**

F34.0 **Cyclothymic disorder**
Affective personality disorder
Cycloid personality
Cyclothymia
Cyclothymic personality

F34.1 **Dysthymic disorder**
Depressive neurosis
Depressive personality disorder
Dysthymia
Neurotic depression
Persistent depressive disorder
Persistent anxiety depression
Excludes2: *anxiety depression (mild or not persistent) (F41.8)*

+ F34.8 **Other persistent mood [affective] disorders**
AHA CC: 4Q, 2016, 14

CC F34.81 **Disruptive mood dysregulation disorder**
CC F34.89 **Other specified persistent mood disorders**

CC F34.9 **Persistent mood [affective] disorder, unspecified**

F39 **Unspecified mood [affective] disorder**

Affective psychosis NOS
Valid 3-character code, no further characters required

Anxiety, dissociative, stress-related, somatoform and other nonpsychotic mental disorders (F40-F48)

F40 **Phobic anxiety disorders**

+ F40.0 **Agoraphobia**
F40.00 **Agoraphobia, unspecified**
F40.01 **Agoraphobia with panic disorder**
Panic disorder with agoraphobia
Excludes1: *panic disorder without agoraphobia (F41.0)*
F40.02 **Agoraphobia without panic disorder**

+ F40.1 **Social phobias**
Anthropophobia
Social anxiety disorder
Social anxiety disorder of childhood
Social neurosis
F40.10 **Social phobia, unspecified**
F40.11 **Social phobia, generalized**

+ F40.2 **Specific (isolated) phobias**
Excludes2: *dysmorphophobia (nondelusional) (F45.22)*
nosophobia (F45.22)

+ F40.21 **Animal type phobia**
F40.210 **Arachnophobia**
Fear of spiders
F40.218 **Other animal type phobia**

+ F40.22 **Natural environment type phobia**
F40.220 **Fear of thunderstorms**
F40.228 **Other natural environment type phobia**

+ F40.23 **Blood, injection, injury type phobia**
F40.230 **Fear of blood**
F40.231 **Fear of injections and transfusions**
F40.232 **Fear of other medical care**
F40.233 **Fear of injury**

+ F40.24 **Situational type phobia**
F40.240 **Claustrophobia**
F40.241 **Acrophobia**
F40.242 **Fear of bridges**
F40.243 **Fear of flying**
F40.248 **Other situational type phobia**

+ F40.29 **Other specified phobia**
F40.290 **Androphobia**
Fear of men
F40.291 **Gynephobia**
Fear of women
F40.298 **Other specified phobia**

F40.8 **Other phobic anxiety disorders**
Phobic anxiety disorder of childhood

F40.9 **Phobic anxiety disorder, unspecified**
Phobia NOS
Phobic state NOS

F41 **Other anxiety disorders**

Excludes2: *anxiety in:*
acute stress reaction (F43.0)
transient adjustment reaction (F43.2)
neurasthenia (F48.8)
psychophysiologic disorders (F45.-)
separation anxiety (F93.0)

F41.0 **Panic disorder [episodic paroxysmal anxiety]**
Panic attack
Panic state
Excludes1: *panic disorder with agoraphobia (F40.01)*

F41.1 **Generalized anxiety disorder**
Anxiety neurosis
Anxiety reaction
Anxiety state
Overanxious disorder
Excludes2: *neurasthenia (F48.8)*

F41.3 **Other mixed anxiety disorders**

F41.8 **Other specified anxiety disorders**
Anxiety depression (mild or not persistent)
Anxiety hysteria
Mixed anxiety and depressive disorder

F41.9 **Anxiety disorder, unspecified**
Anxiety NOS
AHA CC: 1Q, 2021, 10-11

F42 Obsessive-compulsive disorder

Excludes2: *obsessive-compulsive personality (disorder) (F60.5)*
obsessive-compulsive symptoms occurring in depression (F32-F33)
obsessive-compulsive symptoms occurring in schizophrenia (F20.-)

AHA CC: 4Q, 2016, 14-15

F42.2 Mixed obsessional thoughts and acts

F42.3 Hoarding disorder

F42.4 Excoriation (skin-picking) disorder

Excludes1: *factitial dermatitis (L98.1)*
other specified behavioral and emotional disorders with onset usually occurring in early childhood and adolescence (F98.8)

F42.8 Other obsessive compulsive disorder

Anancastic neurosis
Obsessive-compulsive neurosis

F42.9 Obsessive-compulsive disorder, unspecified

F43 Reaction to severe stress, and adjustment disorders

F43.0 Acute stress reaction

Acute crisis reaction
Acute reaction to stress
Combat and operational stress reaction
Combat fatigue
Crisis state
Psychic shock

+ **F43.1 Post-traumatic stress disorder (PTSD)**

Traumatic neurosis

F43.10 Post-traumatic stress disorder, unspecified

F43.11 Post-traumatic stress disorder, acute

F43.12 Post-traumatic stress disorder, chronic

+ **F43.2 Adjustment disorders**

Culture shock
Grief reaction
Hospitalism in children

Excludes2: *separation anxiety disorder of childhood (F93.0)*

F43.20 Adjustment disorder, unspecified

F43.21 Adjustment disorder with depressed mood

AHA CC: 1Q, 2014, 25

F43.22 Adjustment disorder with anxiety

F43.23 Adjustment disorder with mixed anxiety and depressed mood

F43.24 Adjustment disorder with disturbance of conduct

F43.25 Adjustment disorder with mixed disturbance of emotions and conduct

F43.29 Adjustment disorder with other symptoms

F43.8 Other reactions to severe stress

Other specified trauma and stressor-related disorder

F43.9 Reaction to severe stress, unspecified

Trauma and stressor-related disorder, NOS

F44 Dissociative and conversion disorders

Includes: conversion hysteria
conversion reaction
hysteria
hysterical psychosis

Excludes2: *malingering [conscious simulation] (Z76.5)*

F44.0 Dissociative amnesia

Excludes1: *amnesia NOS (R41.3)*
anterograde amnesia (R41.1)
dissociative amnesia with dissociative fugue (F44.1)
retrograde amnesia (R41.2)

Excludes2: *alcohol-or other psychoactive substance-induced amnestic disorder (F10, F13, F19 with .26, .96)*
amnestic disorder due to known physiological condition (F04)
postictal amnesia in epilepsy (G40.-)

F44.1 Dissociative fugue

Dissociative amnesia with dissociative fugue

Excludes2: *postictal fugue in epilepsy (G40.-)*

F44.2 Dissociative stupor

Excludes1: *catatonic stupor (R40.1)*
stupor NOS (R40.1)

Excludes2: *catatonic disorder due to known physiological condition (F06.1)*
depressive stupor (F32, F33)
manic stupor (F30, F31)

F44.4 Conversion disorder with motor symptom or deficit

Conversion disorder with abnormal movement
Conversion disorder with speech symptoms
Conversion disorder with swallowing symptoms
Conversion disorder with weakness/paralysis
Dissociative motor disorders
Psychogenic aphonia
Psychogenic dysphonia

F44.5 Conversion disorder with seizures or convulsions

Conversion disorder with attacks or seizures
Dissociative convulsions

AHA CC: 1Q, 2019, 19

F44.6 Conversion disorder with sensory symptom or deficit

Conversion disorder with anesthesia or sensory loss
Conversion disorder with special sensory symptoms
Dissociative anesthesia and sensory loss
Psychogenic deafness

F44.7 Conversion disorder with mixed symptom presentation

+ **F44.8 Other dissociative and conversion disorders**

F44.81 Dissociative identity disorder

Multiple personality disorder

F44.89 Other dissociative and conversion disorders

Ganser's syndrome
Psychogenic confusion
Psychogenic twilight state
Trance and possession disorders

F44.9 Dissociative and conversion disorder, unspecified

Dissociative disorder NOS

F45 Somatoform disorders

Excludes2: *dissociative and conversion disorders (F44.-)*
factitious disorders (F68.1-, F68.A)
hair-plucking (F63.3)
lalling (F80.0)
lisping (F80.0)
malingering [conscious simulation] (Z76.5)
nail-biting (F98.8)
psychological or behavioral factors associated with disorders or diseases classified elsewhere (F54)
sexual dysfunction, not due to a substance or known physiological condition (F52.-)
thumb-sucking (F98.8)
tic disorders (in childhood and adolescence) (F95.-)
Tourette's syndrome (F95.2)
trichotillomania (F63.3)

F45.0 Somatization disorder

Briquet's disorder
Multiple psychosomatic disorder

F45.1 Undifferentiated somatoform disorder

Somatic symptom disorder
Undifferentiated psychosomatic disorder

+ **F45.2 Hypochondriacal disorders**

Excludes2: *delusional dysmorphophobia (F22)*
fixed delusions about bodily functions or shape (F22)

F45.20 Hypochondriacal disorder, unspecified

F45.21 Hypochondriasis

Hypochondriacal neurosis
Illness anxiety disorder

F45.22 Body dysmorphic disorder

Dysmorphophobia (nondelusional)
Nosophobia

F45.29 Other hypochondriacal disorders

+ **F45.4 Pain disorders related to psychological factors**

Excludes1: *pain NOS (R52)*

F45.41 Pain disorder exclusively related to psychological factors

Somatoform pain disorder (persistent)
Review coding guideline C.5.a

F45.42 Pain disorder with related psychological factors

Code also associated acute or chronic pain (G89.-)
Review coding guideline C.5.a

F45.8 Other somatoform disorders
Psychogenic dysmenorrhea
Psychogenic dysphagia, including 'globus hystericus'
Psychogenic pruritus
Psychogenic torticollis
Somatoform autonomic dysfunction
Teeth grinding
Excludes1: *sleep related teeth grinding (G47.63)*

F45.9 Somatoform disorder, unspecified
Psychosomatic disorder NOS

F48 Other nonpsychotic mental disorders

F48.1 Depersonalization-derealization syndrome

F48.2 Pseudobulbar affect
Involuntary emotional expression disorder
Code first underlying cause, if known, such as:
amyotrophic lateral sclerosis (G12.21)
multiple sclerosis (G35)
sequelae of cerebrovascular disease (I69.-)
sequelae of traumatic intracranial injury (S06.-)

F48.8 Other specified nonpsychotic mental disorders
Dhat syndrome
Neurasthenia
Occupational neurosis, including writer's cramp
Psychasthenia
Psychasthenic neurosis
Psychogenic syncope

F48.9 Nonpsychotic mental disorder, unspecified
Neurosis NOS

Behavioral syndromes associated with physiological disturbances and physical factors (F50-F59)

F50 Eating disorders
Excludes1: *anorexia NOS (R63.0)*
feeding problems of newborn (P92.-)
polyphagia (R63.2)
Excludes2: *feeding difficulties (R63.3)*
feeding disorder in infancy or childhood (F98.2-)

\+ **F50.0 Anorexia nervosa**
Excludes1: *loss of appetite (R63.0)*
psychogenic loss of appetite (F50.89)

CC **F50.00 Anorexia nervosa, unspecified**

CC **F50.01 Anorexia nervosa, restricting type**

CC **F50.02 Anorexia nervosa, binge eating/purging type**
Excludes1: *bulimia nervosa (F50.2)*

CC **F50.2 Bulimia nervosa**
Bulimia NOS
Hyperorexia nervosa
Excludes1: *anorexia nervosa, binge eating/purging type (F50.02)*

\+ **F50.8 Other eating disorders**
Excludes2: *pica of infancy and childhood (F98.3)*
AHA CC: 4Q, 2016, 15-16

F50.81 Binge eating disorder

F50.82 Avoidant/restrictive food intake disorder
AHA CC: 4Q, 2017, 9

F50.89 Other specified eating disorder
Pica in adults
Psychogenic loss of appetite

F50.9 Eating disorder, unspecified
Atypical anorexia nervosa
Atypical bulimia nervosa
Feeding or eating disorder, unspecified
Other specified feeding disorder

F51 Sleep disorders not due to a substance or known physiological condition
Excludes2: *organic sleep disorders (G47.-)*

\+ **F51.0 Insomnia not due to a substance or known physiological condition**
Excludes2: *alcohol related insomnia (F10.182, F10.282, F10.982)*
drug-related insomnia (F11.182, F11.282, F11.982, F13.182, F13.282, F13.982, F14.182, F14.282, F14.982, F15.182, F15.282, F15.982, F19.182, F19.282, F19.982)
insomnia NOS (G47.0-)
insomnia due to known physiological condition (G47.0-)
organic insomnia (G47.0-)
sleep deprivation (Z72.820)

F51.01 Primary insomnia
Idiopathic insomnia

F51.02 Adjustment insomnia

F51.03 Paradoxical insomnia

F51.04 Psychophysiologic insomnia

F51.05 Insomnia due to other mental disorder
Code also associated mental disorder

F51.09 Other insomnia not due to a substance or known physiological condition

\+ **F51.1 Hypersomnia not due to a substance or known physiological condition**
Excludes2: *alcohol related hypersomnia (F10.182, F10.282, F10.982)*
drug-related hypersomnia (F11.182, F11.282, F11.982, F13.182, F13.282, F13.982, F14.182, F14.282, F14.982, F15.182, F15.282, F15.982, F19.182, F19.282, F19.982)
hypersomnia NOS (G47.10)
hypersomnia due to known physiological condition (G47.10)
idiopathic hypersomnia (G47.11, G47.12)
narcolepsy (G47.4-)

F51.11 Primary hypersomnia

F51.12 Insufficient sleep syndrome
Excludes1: *sleep deprivation (Z72.820)*

F51.13 Hypersomnia due to other mental disorder
Code also associated mental disorder

F51.19 Other hypersomnia not due to a substance or known physiological condition

F51.3 Sleepwalking [somnambulism]
Non-rapid eye movement sleep arousal disorders, sleepwalking type

F51.4 Sleep terrors [night terrors]
Non-rapid eye movement sleep arousal disorders, sleep terror type

F51.5 Nightmare disorder
Dream anxiety disorder

F51.8 Other sleep disorders not due to a substance or known physiological condition

F51.9 Sleep disorder not due to a substance or known physiological condition, unspecified
Emotional sleep disorder NOS

F52 Sexual dysfunction not due to a substance or known physiological condition
Excludes2: *Dhat syndrome (F48.8)*

F52.0 Hypoactive sexual desire disorder
Lack or loss of sexual desire
Male hypoactive sexual desire disorder
Sexual anhedonia
Excludes1: *decreased libido (R68.82)*

F52.1 Sexual aversion disorder
Sexual aversion and lack of sexual enjoyment

\+ **F52.2 Sexual arousal disorders**
Failure of genital response

♂ **F52.21 Male erectile disorder**
Erectile disorder
Psychogenic impotence
Excludes1: *impotence of organic origin (N52.-)*
impotence NOS (N52.-)

♀ **F52.22 Female sexual arousal disorder**
Female sexual interest/arousal disorder

+ **F52.3 Orgasmic disorder**
Inhibited orgasm
Psychogenic anorgasmy
♀ **F52.31 Female orgasmic disorder**
♂ **F52.32 Male orgasmic disorder**
Delayed ejaculation

♂ **F52.4 Premature ejaculation**

♀ **F52.5 Vaginismus not due to a substance or known physiological condition**
Psychogenic vaginismus
Excludes2: *vaginismus (due to a known physiological condition) (N94.2)*

F52.6 Dyspareunia not due to a substance or known physiological condition
Genito-pelvic pain penetration disorder
Psychogenic dyspareunia
Excludes2: *dyspareunia (due to a known physiological condition) (N94.1-)*

F52.8 Other sexual dysfunction not due to a substance or known physiological condition
Excessive sexual drive
Nymphomania
Satyriasis

F52.9 Unspecified sexual dysfunction not due to a substance or known physiological condition
Sexual dysfunction NOS

F53 Mental and behavioral disorders associated with the puerperium, not elsewhere classified
Excludes1: *mood disorders with psychotic features (F30.2, F31.2, F31.5, F31.64, F32.3, F33.3)*
postpartum dysphoria (O90.6)
psychosis in schizophrenia, schizotypal, delusional, and other psychotic disorders (F20-F29)
AHA CC: 4Q, 2018, 8-9

•♀ **F53.0 Postpartum depression**
Postnatal depression, NOS
Postpartum depression, NOS

•♀ **F53.1 Puerperal psychosis**
Postpartum psychosis
Puerperal psychosis, NOS

F54 Psychological and behavioral factors associated with disorders or diseases classified elsewhere
Psychological factors affecting physical conditions
Code first the associated physical disorder, such as:
asthma (J45.-)
dermatitis (L23-L25)
gastric ulcer (K25.-)
mucous colitis (K58.-)
ulcerative colitis (K51.-)
urticaria (L50.-)
Excludes2: *tension-type headache (G44.2)*
Valid 3-character code, no further characters required

F55 Abuse of non-psychoactive substances
Excludes2: *abuse of psychoactive substances (F10-F19)*
F55.0 Abuse of antacids
F55.1 Abuse of herbal or folk remedies
F55.2 Abuse of laxatives
F55.3 Abuse of steroids or hormones
F55.4 Abuse of vitamins
F55.8 Abuse of other non-psychoactive substances

F59 Unspecified behavioral syndromes associated with physiological disturbances and physical factors
Psychogenic physiological dysfunction NOS
Valid 3-character code, no further characters required

Disorders of adult personality and behavior (F60-F69)

F60 Specific personality disorders

F60.0 Paranoid personality disorder
Expansive paranoid personality (disorder)
Fanatic personality (disorder)
Querulant personality (disorder)
Paranoid personality (disorder)
Sensitive paranoid personality (disorder)
Excludes2: *paranoia (F22)*
paranoia querulans (F22)
paranoid psychosis (F22)
paranoid schizophrenia (F20.0)
paranoid state (F22)

F60.1 Schizoid personality disorder
Excludes2: *Asperger's syndrome (F84.5)*
delusional disorder (F22)
schizoid disorder of childhood (F84.5)
schizophrenia (F20.-)
schizotypal disorder (F21)

F60.2 Antisocial personality disorder
Amoral personality (disorder)
Asocial personality (disorder)
Dissocial personality disorder
Psychopathic personality (disorder)
Sociopathic personality (disorder)
Excludes1: *conduct disorders (F91.-)*
Excludes2: *borderline personality disorder (F60.3)*

F60.3 Borderline personality disorder
Aggressive personality (disorder)
Emotionally unstable personality disorder
Explosive personality (disorder)
Excludes2: *antisocial personality disorder (F60.2)*

F60.4 Histrionic personality disorder
Hysterical personality (disorder)
Psychoinfantile personality (disorder)

F60.5 Obsessive-compulsive personality disorder
Anankastic personality (disorder)
Compulsive personality (disorder)
Obsessional personality (disorder)
Excludes2: *obsessive-compulsive disorder (F42.-)*

F60.6 Avoidant personality disorder
Anxious personality disorder

F60.7 Dependent personality disorder
Asthenic personality (disorder)
Inadequate personality (disorder)
Passive personality (disorder)

+ **F60.8 Other specific personality disorders**
F60.81 Narcissistic personality disorder
F60.89 Other specific personality disorders
Eccentric personality disorder
'Haltlose' type personality disorder
Immature personality disorder
Passive-aggressive personality disorder
Psychoneurotic personality disorder
Self-defeating personality disorder

F60.9 Personality disorder, unspecified
Character disorder NOS
Character neurosis NOS
Pathological personality NOS

F63 Impulse disorders
Excludes2: *habitual excessive use of alcohol or psychoactive substances (F10-F19)*
impulse disorders involving sexual behavior (F65.-)

F63.0 Pathological gambling
Compulsive gambling
Gambling disorder
Excludes1: *gambling and betting NOS (Z72.6)*
Excludes2: *excessive gambling by manic patients (F30, F31)*
gambling in antisocial personality disorder (F60.2)

F63.1 Pyromania
Pathological fire-setting
Excludes2: *fire-setting (by) (in):*
adult with antisocial personality disorder (F60.2)
alcohol or psychoactive substance intoxication (F10-F19)
conduct disorders (F91.-)
mental disorders due to known physiological condition (F01-F09)
schizophrenia (F20.-)

F63.2 Kleptomania
Pathological stealing
Excludes1: *shoplifting as the reason for observation for suspected mental disorder (Z03.8)*
Excludes2: *depressive disorder with stealing (F31-F33)*
stealing due to underlying mental condition-code to mental condition
stealing in mental disorders due to known physiological condition (F01-F09)

F63.3 Trichotillomania
Hair plucking
Excludes2: *other stereotyped movement disorder (F98.4)*

+ **F63.8 Other impulse disorders**
  - **F63.81 Intermittent explosive disorder**
  - **F63.89 Other impulse disorders**

F63.9 Impulse disorder, unspecified
Impulse control disorder NOS

F64 Gender identity disorders
AHA CC: 4Q, 2016, 16

F64.0 Transsexualism
Gender identify disorder in adolescence and adulthood
Gender dysphoria in adolescents and adults

F64.1 Dual role transvestism
Use additional code to identify sex reassignment status (Z87.890)
Excludes1: *gender identity disorder in childhood (F64.2)*
Excludes2: *fetishistic transvestism (F65.1)*

• **F64.2 Gender identity disorder of childhood**
Gender dysphoria in children
Excludes1: *gender identity disorder in adolescence and adulthood (F64.0)*
Excludes2: *sexual maturation disorder (F66)*

F64.8 Other gender identity disorders
Other specified gender dysphoria

F64.9 Gender identity disorder, unspecified
Gender dysphoria, unspecified
Gender-role disorder NOS

F65 Paraphilias

F65.0 Fetishism
Fetishistic disorder

F65.1 Transvestic fetishism
Fetishistic transvestism
Transvestic disorder

F65.2 Exhibitionism
Exhibitionistic disorder

F65.3 Voyeurism
Voyeuristic disorder

F65.4 Pedophilia
Pedophilic disorder

+ **F65.5 Sadomasochism**

F65.50 Sadomasochism, unspecified

F65.51 Sexual masochism
Sexual masochism disorder

F65.52 Sexual sadism
Sexual sadism disorder

+ **F65.8 Other paraphilias**

F65.81 Frotteurism
Frotteuristic disorder

F65.89 Other paraphilias
Necrophilia
Other specified paraphilic disorder

F65.9 Paraphilia, unspecified
Paraphillic disorder, unspecified
Sexual deviation NOS

F66 Other sexual disorders
Sexual maturation disorder
Sexual relationship disorder
Valid 3-character code, no further characters required

F68 Other disorders of adult personality and behavior

+ **F68.1 Factitious disorder imposed on self**
Compensation neurosis
Elaboration of physical symptoms for psychological reasons
Hospital hopper syndrome
Münchausen's syndrome
Peregrinating patient
Excludes2: *factitial dermatitis (L98.1)*
person feigning illness (with obvious motivation) (Z76.5)
AHA CC: 4Q, 2018, 9
Review coding guideline C.5.c

CC **F68.10 Factitious disorder imposed on self, unspecified**

F68.11 Factitious disorder imposed on self with predominantly psychological signs and symptoms

CC **F68.12 Factitious disorder imposed on self with predominantly physical signs and symptoms**

F68.13 Factitious disorder imposed on self with combined psychological and physical signs and symptoms

CC **F68.A Factitious disorder imposed on another**
Factitious disorder by proxy
Münchaüsen's by proxy
AHA CC: 4Q, 2018, 9
Review coding guideline C.5.c

F68.8 Other specified disorders of adult personality and behavior

• **F69 Unspecified disorder of adult personality and behavior**
Valid 3-character code, no further characters required

Intellectual Disabilities (F70-F79)

Code first any associated physical or developmental disorders
Excludes1: *borderline intellectual functioning, IQ above 70 to 84 (R41.83)*

F70 Mild intellectual disabilities
IQ level 50-55 to approximately 70
Mild mental subnormality
Valid 3-character code, no further characters required

F71 Moderate intellectual disabilities
IQ level 35-40 to 50-55
Moderate mental subnormality
Valid 3-character code, no further characters required

CC **F72 Severe intellectual disabilities**
IQ 20-25 to 35-40
Severe mental subnormality
Valid 3-character code, no further characters required

CC **F73 Profound intellectual disabilities**
IQ level below 20-25
Profound mental subnormality
Valid 3-character code, no further characters required

F78 Other intellectual disabilities

+ **F78.A Other genetic related intellectual disability**

F78.A1 SYNGAP1-related intellectual disability
Code also, if applicable, any associated:
autism spectrum disorder (F84.0)
autistic disorder (F84.0)
encephalopathy (G93.4-)
epilepsy and recurrent seizures (G40.-)
other pervasive developmental disorders (F84.8)
pervasive developmental disorder, NOS (F84.9)

F78.A9 Other genetic related intellectual disability
Code also, if applicable, any associated disorders

F79 Unspecified intellectual disabilities
Mental deficiency NOS
Mental subnormality NOS
Valid 3-character code, no further characters required

Pervasive and specific developmental disorders (F80-F89)

F80 Specific developmental disorders of speech and language

F80.0 Phonological disorder
Dyslalia
Functional speech articulation disorder
Lalling
Lisping
Phonological developmental disorder
Speech articulation developmental disorder
Speech-sound disorder
Excludes1: *speech articulation impairment due to aphasia NOS (R47.01)*
speech articulation impairment due to apraxia (R48.2)
Excludes2: *speech articulation impairment due to hearing loss (F80.4)*
speech articulation impairment due to intellectual disabilities (F70-F79)
speech articulation impairment with expressive language developmental disorder (F80.1)
speech articulation impairment with mixed receptive expressive language developmental disorder (F80.2)

F80.1 Expressive language disorder
Developmental dysphasia or aphasia, expressive type
Excludes1: *mixed receptive-expressive language disorder (F80.2)*
dysphasia and aphasia NOS (R47.-)
Excludes2: *acquired aphasia with epilepsy [Landau-Kleffner] (G40.80-)*
selective mutism (F94.0)
intellectual disabilities (F70-F79)
pervasive developmental disorders (F84.-)

F80.2 Mixed receptive-expressive language disorder
Developmental dysphasia or aphasia, receptive type
Developmental Wernicke's aphasia
Excludes1: *central auditory processing disorder (H93.25)*
dysphasia or aphasia NOS (R47.-)
expressive language disorder (F80.1)
expressive type dysphasia or aphasia (F80.1)
word deafness (H93.25)
Excludes2: *acquired aphasia with epilepsy [Landau-Kleffner] (G40.80-)*
pervasive developmental disorders (F84.-)
selective mutism (F94.0)
intellectual disabilities (F70-F79)

F80.4 Speech and language development delay due to hearing loss
Code also type of hearing loss (H90.-, H91.-)

+ **F80.8 Other developmental disorders of speech and language**

F80.81 Childhood onset fluency disorder
Cluttering NOS
Stuttering NOS
Excludes1: *adult onset fluency disorder (F98.5)*
fluency disorder in conditions classified elsewhere (R47.82)
fluency disorder (stuttering) following cerebrovascular disease (I69. with final characters -23)

F80.82 Social pragmatic communication disorder
Excludes1: *Asperger's syndrome (F84.5)*
autistic disorder (F84.0)
AHA CC: 4Q, 2016, 16

F80.89 Other developmental disorders of speech and language
AHA CC: 1Q, 2017, 27-28

F80.9 Developmental disorder of speech and language, unspecified
Communication disorder NOS
Language disorder NOS

F81 Specific developmental disorders of scholastic skills

F81.0 Specific reading disorder
'Backward reading'
Developmental dyslexia
Specific learning disorder, with impairment in reading
Specific reading retardation
Excludes1: *alexia NOS (R48.0)*
dyslexia NOS (R48.0)

F81.2 Mathematics disorder
Developmental acalculia
Developmental arithmetical disorder
Developmental Gerstmann's syndrome
Specific learning disorder, with impairment in mathematics
Excludes1: *acalculia NOS (R48.8)*
Excludes2: *arithmetical difficulties associated with a reading disorder (F81.0)*
arithmetical difficulties associated with a spelling disorder (F81.81)
arithmetical difficulties due to inadequate teaching (Z55.8)

+ **F81.8 Other developmental disorders of scholastic skills**

F81.81 Disorder of written expression
Specific learning disorder, with impairment in written expression
Specific spelling disorder

F81.89 Other developmental disorders of scholastic skills

F81.9 Developmental disorder of scholastic skills, unspecified
Knowledge acquisition disability NOS
Learning disability NOS
Learning disorder NOS

F82 Specific developmental disorder of motor function
Clumsy child syndrome
Developmental coordination disorder
Developmental dyspraxia
Excludes1: *abnormalities of gait and mobility (R26.-)*
lack of coordination (R27.-)
Excludes2: *lack of coordination secondary to intellectual disabilities (F70-F79)*
Valid 3-character code, no further characters required

F84 Pervasive developmental disorders
Code also any associated medical condition and intellectual disabilities.

CC **F84.0 Autistic disorder**
Autism spectrum disorder
Infantile autism
Infantile psychosis
Kanner's syndrome
Excludes1: *Asperger's syndrome (F84.5)*
AHA CC: 1Q, 2017, 27-28

CC **F84.2 Rett's syndrome**
Excludes1: *Asperger's syndrome (F84.5)*
Autistic disorder (F84.0)
Other childhood disintegrative disorder (F84.3)

• CC **F84.3 Other childhood disintegrative disorder**
Dementia infantilis
Disintegrative psychosis
Heller's syndrome
Symbiotic psychosis
Use additional code to identify any associated neurological condition.
Excludes1: *Asperger's syndrome (F84.5)*
Autistic disorder (F84.0)
Rett's syndrome (F84.2)

CC **F84.5 Asperger's syndrome**
Asperger's disorder
Autistic psychopathy
Schizoid disorder of childhood

CC **F84.8 Other pervasive developmental disorders**
Overactive disorder associated with intellectual disabilities and stereotyped movements

CC **F84.9 Pervasive developmental disorder, unspecified**
Atypical autism

F88 Other disorders of psychological development
Developmental agnosia
Global developmental delay
Other specified neurodevelopmental disorder
Valid 3-character code, no further characters required

F89 Unspecified disorder of psychological development
Developmental disorder NOS
Neurodevelopmental disorder NOS
Valid 3-character code, no further characters required

Behavioral and emotional disorders with onset usually occurring in childhood and adolescence (F90-F98)

NOTE Codes within categories F90-F98 may be used regardless of the age of a patient. These disorders generally have onset within the childhood or adolescent years, but may continue throughout life or not be diagnosed until adulthood

F90 Attention-deficit hyperactivity disorders
Includes: attention deficit disorder with hyperactivity
attention deficit syndrome with hyperactivity
Excludes2: *anxiety disorders (F40.-, F41.-)*
mood [affective] disorders (F30-F39)
pervasive developmental disorders (F84.-)
schizophrenia (F20.-)

F90.0 Attention-deficit hyperactivity disorder, predominantly inattentive type
Attention-deficit/hyperactivity disorder, predominantly inattentive presentation

F90.1 Attention-deficit hyperactivity disorder, predominantly hyperactive type
Attention-deficit/hyperactivity disorder, predominantly hyperactive impulsive presentation

F90.2 Attention-deficit hyperactivity disorder, combined type
Attention-deficit/hyperactivity disorder, combined presentation

F90.8 Attention-deficit hyperactivity disorder, other type

F90.9 Attention-deficit hyperactivity disorder, unspecified type

Attention-deficit hyperactivity disorder of childhood or adolescence NOS

Attention-deficit hyperactivity disorder NOS

F91 Conduct disorders

Excludes1: *antisocial behavior (Z72.81-)*
antisocial personality disorder (F60.2)

Excludes2: *conduct problems associated with attention-deficit hyperactivity disorder (F90.-)*
mood [affective] disorders (F30-F39)
pervasive developmental disorders (F84.-)
schizophrenia (F20.-)

F91.0 Conduct disorder confined to family context

F91.1 Conduct disorder, childhood-onset type

Unsocialized conduct disorder

Conduct disorder, solitary aggressive type

Unsocialized aggressive disorder

F91.2 Conduct disorder, adolescent-onset type

Socialized conduct disorder

Conduct disorder, group type

F91.3 Oppositional defiant disorder

F91.8 Other conduct disorders

Other specified conduct disorder

Other specified disruptive disorder

F91.9 Conduct disorder, unspecified

Behavioral disorder NOS

Conduct disorder NOS

Disruptive behavior disorder NOS

Disruptive disorder NOS

F93 Emotional disorders with onset specific to childhood

F93.0 Separation anxiety disorder of childhood

Excludes2: *mood [affective] disorders (F30-F39)*
nonpsychotic mental disorders (F40-F48)
phobic anxiety disorder of childhood (F40.8)
social phobia (F40.1)

F93.8 Other childhood emotional disorders

Identity disorder

Excludes2: *gender identity disorder of childhood (F64.2)*

F93.9 Childhood emotional disorder, unspecified

F94 Disorders of social functioning with onset specific to childhood and adolescence

F94.0 Selective mutism

Elective mutism

Excludes2: *pervasive developmental disorders (F84.-)*
schizophrenia (F20.-)
specific developmental disorders of speech and language (F80.-)
transient mutism as part of separation anxiety in young children (F93.0)

F94.1 Reactive attachment disorder of childhood

Use additional code to identify any associated failure to thrive or growth retardation

Excludes1: *disinhibited attachment disorder of childhood (F94.2)*
normal variation in pattern of selective attachment

Excludes2: *Asperger's syndrome (F84.5)*
maltreatment syndromes (T74.-)
sexual or physical abuse in childhood, resulting in psychosocial problems (Z62.81-)

F94.2 Disinhibited attachment disorder of childhood

Affectionless psychopathy

Institutional syndrome

Excludes1: *reactive attachment disorder of childhood (F94.1)*

Excludes2: *Asperger's syndrome (F84.5)*
attention-deficit hyperactivity disorders (F90.-)
hospitalism in children (F43.2-)

F94.8 Other childhood disorders of social functioning

F94.9 Childhood disorder of social functioning, unspecified

F95 Tic disorder

F95.0 Transient tic disorder

Provisional tic disorder

F95.1 Chronic motor or vocal tic disorder

F95.2 Tourette's disorder

Combined vocal and multiple motor tic disorder [de la Tourette]

Tourette's syndrome

F95.8 Other tic disorders

F95.9 Tic disorder, unspecified

Tic NOS

F98 Other behavioral and emotional disorders with onset usually occurring in childhood and adolescence

Excludes2: *breath-holding spells (R06.89)*
gender identity disorder of childhood (F64.2)
Kleine-Levin syndrome (G47.13)
obsessive-compulsive disorder (F42.-)
sleep disorders not due to a substance or known physiological condition (F51.-)

F98.0 Enuresis not due to a substance or known physiological condition

Enuresis (primary) (secondary) of nonorganic origin

Functional enuresis

Psychogenic enuresis

Urinary incontinence of nonorganic origin

Excludes1: *enuresis NOS (R32)*

F98.1 Encopresis not due to a substance or known physiological condition

Functional encopresis

Incontinence of feces of nonorganic origin

Psychogenic encopresis

Use additional code to identify the cause of any coexisting constipation.

Excludes1: *encopresis NOS (R15.-)*

+ F98.2 Other feeding disorders of infancy and childhood

Excludes2: *anorexia nervosa and other eating disorders (F50.-)*
feeding difficulties (R63.3)
feeding problems of newborn (P92.-)
pica of infancy or childhood (F98.3)

F98.21 Rumination disorder of infancy

F98.29 Other feeding disorders of infancy and early childhood

F98.3 Pica of infancy and childhood

F98.4 Stereotyped movement disorders

Stereotype/habit disorder

Excludes1: *abnormal involuntary movements (R25.-)*

Excludes2: *compulsions in obsessive-compulsive disorder (F42.-)*
hair plucking (F63.3)
movement disorders of organic origin (G20-G25)
nail-biting (F98.8)
nose-picking (F98.8)
stereotypies that are part of a broader psychiatric condition (F01-F95)
thumb-sucking (F98.8)
tic disorders (F95.-)
trichotillomania (F63.3)

F98.5 Adult onset fluency disorder

Excludes1: *childhood onset fluency disorder (F80.81)*
dysphasia (R47.02)
fluency disorder in conditions classified elsewhere (R47.82)
fluency disorder (stuttering) following cerebrovascular disease (I69. with final characters -23)
tic disorders (F95.-)

F98.8 Other specified behavioral and emotional disorders with onset usually occurring in childhood and adolescence

Excessive masturbation

Nail-biting

Nose-picking

Thumb-sucking

F98.9 Unspecified behavioral and emotional disorders with onset usually occurring in childhood and adolescence

Unspecified mental disorder (F99)

F99 Mental disorder, not otherwise specified

Mental illness NOS

Excludes1: *unspecified mental disorder due to known physiological condition (F09)*

Valid 3-character code, no further characters required

Chapter 6: Diseases of the Nervous System (G00-G99)

Excludes2: *certain conditions originating in the perinatal period (P04-P96)*
certain infectious and parasitic diseases (A00-B99)
complications of pregnancy, childbirth and the puerperium (O00-O9A)
congenital malformations, deformations, and chromosomal abnormalities (Q00-Q99)
endocrine, nutritional and metabolic diseases (E00-E88)
injury, poisoning and certain other consequences of external causes (S00-T88)
neoplasms (C00-D49)
symptoms, signs and abnormal clinical and laboratory findings, not elsewhere classified (R00-R94)

This chapter contains the following category blocks:

G00-G09	Inflammatory diseases of the central nervous system
G10-G14	Systemic atrophies primarily affecting the central nervous system
G20-G26	Extrapyramidal and movement disorders
G30-G32	Other degenerative diseases of the nervous system
G35-G37	Demyelinating diseases of the central nervous system
G40-G47	Episodic and paroxysmal disorders
G50-G59	Nerve, nerve root and plexus disorders
G60-G65	Polyneuropathies and other disorders of the peripheral nervous system
G70-G73	Diseases of myoneural junction and muscle
G80-G83	Cerebral palsy and other paralytic syndromes
G89-G99	Other disorders of the nervous system

C. Chapter-Specific Coding Guidelines

In addition to general coding guidelines, there are guidelines for specific diagnoses and/or conditions in the classification. Unless otherwise indicated, these guidelines apply to all health care settings. Please refer to Section II for guidelines on the selection of principal diagnosis.

6. Chapter 6: Diseases of the Nervous System (G00-G99)

a. Dominant/nondominant side

Codes from category G81, Hemiplegia and hemiparesis, and subcategories, G83.1, Monoplegia of lower limb, G83.2, Monoplegia of upper limb, and G83.3, Monoplegia, unspecified, identify whether the dominant or nondominant side is affected. Should the affected side be documented, but not specified as dominant or nondominant, and the classification system does not indicate a default, code selection is as follows:

- For ambidextrous patients, the default should be dominant.
- If the left side is affected, the default is non-dominant.
- If the right side is affected, the default is dominant.

b. Pain-Category G89

1) General coding information

Codes in category G89, Pain, not elsewhere classified, may be used in conjunction with codes from other categories and chapters to provide more detail about acute or chronic pain and neoplasm-related pain, unless otherwise indicated below.

If the pain is not specified as acute or chronic, post- thoracotomy, post procedural, or neoplasm-related, do not assign codes from category G89.

A code from category G89 should not be assigned if the underlying (definitive) diagnosis is known, unless the reason for the encounter is pain control/management and not management of the underlying condition.

When an admission or encounter is for a procedure aimed at treating the underlying condition (e.g., spinal fusion, kyphoplasty), a code for the underlying condition (e.g., vertebral fracture, spinal stenosis) should be assigned as the principal diagnosis. No code from category G89 should be assigned.

(a) Category G89 Codes as Principal or First-Listed Diagnosis

Category G89 codes are acceptable as principal diagnosis or the first-listed code:

- When pain control or pain management is the reason for the admission/encounter (e.g., a patient with displaced intervertebral disc, nerve impingement and severe back pain presents for injection of steroid into the spinal canal). The underlying cause of the pain should be reported as an additional diagnosis, if known.
- When a patient is admitted for the insertion of a neurostimulator for pain control, assign the appropriate pain code as the principal or first-listed diagnosis. When an admission or encounter is for a procedure aimed at treating the underlying condition and a neurostimulator is inserted for pain control during the same admission/encounter, a code for the underlying condition should be assigned as the principal diagnosis and the appropriate pain code should be assigned as a secondary diagnosis.

(b) Use of Category G89 Codes in Conjunction with Site Specific Pain Codes

(i) Assigning Category G89 and Site-Specific Pain Codes

Codes from category G89 may be used in conjunction with codes that identify the site of pain (including codes from chapter 18) if the category G89 code provides additional information. For example, if the code describes the site of the pain, but does not fully describe whether the pain is acute or chronic, then both codes should be assigned.

(ii) Sequencing of Category G89 Codes with Site- Specific Pain Codes

The sequencing of category G89 codes with site-specific pain codes (including chapter 18 codes), is dependent on the circumstances of the encounter/admission as follows:

- If the encounter is for pain control or pain management, assign the code from category G89 followed by the code identifying the specific site of pain (e.g., encounter for pain management for acute neck pain from trauma is assigned code G89.11, Acute pain due to trauma, followed by code M54.2, Cervicalgia, to identify the site of pain).
- If the encounter is for any other reason except pain control or pain management, and a related definitive diagnosis has not been established (confirmed) by the provider, assign the code for the specific site of pain first, followed by the appropriate code from category G89.

2) Pain due to devices, implants and grafts

See Section I.C.19. Pain due to medical devices

3) Postoperative Pain

The provider's documentation should be used to guide the coding of postoperative pain, as well as *Section III. Reporting Additional Diagnoses and Section IV. Diagnostic Coding* and *Reporting in the Outpatient Setting.*

The default for post-thoracotomy and other postoperative pain not specified as acute or chronic is the code for the acute form.

Routine or expected postoperative pain immediately after surgery should not be coded.

(a) Postoperative pain not associated with specific postoperative complication

Postoperative pain not associated with a specific postoperative complication is assigned to the appropriate postoperative pain code in category G89.

(b) Postoperative pain associated with specific postoperative complication

Postoperative pain associated with a specific postoperative complication (such as painful wire sutures) is assigned to the appropriate code(s) found in Chapter 19, Injury, poisoning, and certain other consequences of external causes. If appropriate, use additional code(s) from category G89 to identify acute or chronic pain (G89.18 or G89.28).

4) Chronic pain

Chronic pain is classified to subcategory G89.2. There is no time frame defining when pain becomes chronic pain. The provider's documentation should be used to guide use of these codes.

5) Neoplasm Related Pain

Code G89.3 is assigned to pain documented as being related, associated or due to cancer, primary or secondary malignancy, or tumor. This code is assigned regardless of whether the pain is acute or chronic.

This code may be assigned as the principal or first- listed code when the stated reason for the admission/encounter is documented as pain control/pain management. The underlying neoplasm should be reported as an additional diagnosis.

When the reason for the admission/encounter is management of the neoplasm and the pain associated with the neoplasm is also documented, code G89.3 may be assigned as an additional diagnosis. It is not necessary to assign an additional code for the site of the pain.

See Section I.C.2 for instructions on the sequencing of neoplasms for all other stated reasons for the admission/encounter (except for pain control/pain management).

6) Chronic pain syndrome

Central pain syndrome (G89.0) and chronic pain syndrome (G89.4) are different than the term "chronic pain," and therefore codes should only be used when the provider has specifically documented this condition.

See Section I.C.5. Pain disorders related to psychological factors

Inflammatory diseases of the central nervous system (G00-G09)

G00 Bacterial meningitis, not elsewhere classified

Includes: bacterial arachnoiditis
bacterial leptomeningitis
bacterial meningitis
bacterial pachymeningitis

Excludes1: *bacterial meningoencephalitis (G04.2)*
bacterial meningomyelitis (G04.2)

MCC **G00.0 Hemophilus meningitis**
Meningitis due to Hemophilus influenzae

MCC **G00.1 Pneumococcal meningitis**
Meningitis due to Streptococcal pneumoniae

MCC **G00.2 Streptococcal meningitis**
Use additional code to further identify organism (B95.0-B95.5)

MCC **G00.3 Staphylococcal meningitis**
Use additional code to further identify organism (B95.61-B95.8)

MCC **G00.8 Other bacterial meningitis**
Meningitis due to Escherichia coli
Meningitis due to Friedländer's bacillus
Meningitis due to Klebsiella
Use additional code to further identify organism (B96.-)

MCC **G00.9 Bacterial meningitis, unspecified**
Meningitis due to gram-negative bacteria, unspecified
Purulent meningitis NOS
Pyogenic meningitis NOS
Suppurative meningitis NOS

MCC **G01 Meningitis in bacterial diseases classified elsewhere**

Code first underlying disease

Excludes1: *meningitis (in):*
gonococcal (A54.81)
leptospirosis (A27.81)
listeriosis (A32.11)
Lyme disease (A69.21)
meningococcal (A39.0)
neurosyphilis (A52.13)
tuberculosis (A17.0)
meningoencephalitis and meningomyelitis in bacterial diseases classified elsewhere (G05)

Valid 3-character code, no further characters required

MCC **G02 Meningitis in other infectious and parasitic diseases classified elsewhere**

Code first underlying disease, such as:
African trypanosomiasis (B56.-)
poliovirus infection (A80.-)

Excludes1: *candidal meningitis (B37.5)*
coccidioidomycosis meningitis (B38.4)
cryptococcal meningitis (B45.1)
herpesviral [herpes simplex] meningitis (B00.3)
infectious mononucleosis complicated by meningitis (B27.- with fifth character 2)
measles complicated by meningitis (B05.1)
meningoencephalitis and meningomyelitis in other infectious and parasitic diseases classified elsewhere (G05)
mumps meningitis (B26.1)
rubella meningitis (B06.02)
varicella [chickenpox] meningitis (B01.0)
zoster meningitis (B02.1)

Valid 3-character code, no further characters required

G03 Meningitis due to other and unspecified causes

Includes: arachnoiditis NOS
leptomeningitis NOS
meningitis NOS
pachymeningitis NOS

Excludes1: *meningoencephalitis (G04.-)*
meningomyelitis (G04.-)

MCC **G03.0 Nonpyogenic meningitis**
Aseptic meningitis
Nonbacterial meningitis

CC **G03.1 Chronic meningitis**

CC **G03.2 Benign recurrent meningitis [Mollaret]**

MCC **G03.8 Meningitis due to other specified causes**

MCC **G03.9 Meningitis, unspecified**
Arachnoiditis (spinal) NOS

G04 Encephalitis, myelitis and encephalomyelitis

Includes: acute ascending myelitis
meningoencephalitis
meningomyelitis

Excludes1: *encephalopathy NOS (G93.40)*

Excludes2: *acute transverse myelitis (G37.3-)*
alcoholic encephalopathy (G31.2)
benign myalgic encephalomyelitis (G93.3)
multiple sclerosis (G35)
subacute necrotizing myelitis (G37.4)
toxic encephalitis (G92.8)
toxic encephalopathy (G92.8)

\+ **G04.0 Acute disseminated encephalitis and encephalomyelitis (ADEM)**

Excludes1: *acute necrotizing hemorrhagic encephalopathy (G04.3-)*
other noninfectious acute disseminated encephalomyelitis (noninfectious ADEM) (G04.81)

MCC **G04.00 Acute disseminated encephalitis and encephalomyelitis, unspecified**

MCC **G04.01 Postinfectious acute disseminated encephalitis and encephalomyelitis (postinfectious ADEM)**

Excludes1: *post chickenpox encephalitis (B01.1)*
post measles encephalitis (B05.0)
post measles myelitis (B05.1)

MCC **G04.02 Postimmunization acute disseminated encephalitis, myelitis and encephalomyelitis**
Encephalitis, post immunization
Encephalomyelitis, post immunization
Use additional code to identify the vaccine (T50.A-, T50.B-, T50.Z-)

CC **G04.1 Tropical spastic paraplegia**

MCC **G04.2 Bacterial meningoencephalitis and meningomyelitis, not elsewhere classified**

\+ **G04.3 Acute necrotizing hemorrhagic encephalopathy**

Excludes1: *acute disseminated encephalitis and encephalomyelitis (G04.0-)*

MCC **G04.30 Acute necrotizing hemorrhagic encephalopathy, unspecified**

MCC **G04.31 Postinfectious acute necrotizing hemorrhagic encephalopathy**

MCC **G04.32 Postimmunization acute necrotizing hemorrhagic encephalopathy**
Use additional code to identify the vaccine (T50.A-, T50.B-, T50.Z-)

MCC **G04.39 Other acute necrotizing hemorrhagic encephalopathy**
Code also underlying etiology, if applicable

\+ **G04.8 Other encephalitis, myelitis and encephalomyelitis**
Code also any associated seizure (G40.-, R56.9)

MCC **G04.81 Other encephalitis and encephalomyelitis**
Noninfectious acute disseminated encephalomyelitis (noninfectious ADEM)

MCC **G04.82 Acute flaccid myelitis**

Excludes1: *transverse myelitis (G37.3)*

MCC **G04.89 Other myelitis**
AHA CC: 1Q, 2020, 14

\+ **G04.9 Encephalitis, myelitis and encephalomyelitis, unspecified**

MCC **G04.90 Encephalitis and encephalomyelitis, unspecified**
Ventriculitis (cerebral) NOS

MCC **G04.91 Myelitis, unspecified**

G05 Encephalitis, myelitis and encephalomyelitis in diseases classified elsewhere

Code first underlying disease, such as:
congenital toxoplasmosis encephalitis, myelitis and encephalomyelitis (P37.1)
cytomegaloviral encephalitis, myelitis and encephalomyelitis (B25.8)
encephalitis, myelitis and encephalomyelitis (in) systemic lupus erythematosus (M32.19)
eosinophilic meningoencephalitis (B83.2)
human immunodeficiency virus [HIV] disease (B20)
poliovirus (A80.-)
suppurative otitis media (H66.01-H66.4)
trichinellosis (B75)

Excludes1: *adenoviral encephalitis, myelitis and encephalomyelitis (A85.1)*
encephalitis, myelitis and encephalomyelitis (in) measles (B05.0)
enteroviral encephalitis, myelitis and encephalomyelitis (A85.0)
herpesviral [herpes simplex] encephalitis, myelitis and encephalomyelitis (B00.4)
listerial encephalitis, myelitis and encephalomyelitis (A32.12)
meningococcal encephalitis, myelitis and encephalomyelitis (A39.81)
mumps encephalitis, myelitis and encephalomyelitis (B26.2)
postchickenpox encephalitis, myelitis and encephalomyelitis (B01.1-)
rubella encephalitis, myelitis and encephalomyelitis (B06.01)
toxoplasmosis encephalitis, myelitis and encephalomyelitis (B58.2)
zoster encephalitis, myelitis and encephalomyelitis (B02.0)

MCC **G05.3 Encephalitis and encephalomyelitis in diseases classified elsewhere**
Meningoencephalitis in diseases classified elsewhere

MCC **G05.4 Myelitis in diseases classified elsewhere**
Meningomyelitis in diseases classified elsewhere

G06 Intracranial and intraspinal abscess and granuloma

Use additional code (B95-B97) to identify infectious agent.

MCC **G06.0 Intracranial abscess and granuloma**
Brain [any part] abscess (embolic)
Cerebellar abscess (embolic)
Cerebral abscess (embolic)
Intracranial epidural abscess or granuloma
Intracranial extradural abscess or granuloma
Intracranial subdural abscess or granuloma
Otogenic abscess (embolic)
Excludes1: *tuberculous intracranial abscess and granuloma (A17.81)*

MCC **G06.1 Intraspinal abscess and granuloma**
Abscess (embolic) of spinal cord [any part]
Intraspinal epidural abscess or granuloma
Intraspinal extradural abscess or granuloma
Intraspinal subdural abscess or granuloma
Excludes1: *tuberculous intraspinal abscess and granuloma (A17.81)*

MCC **G06.2 Extradural and subdural abscess, unspecified**

G07 Intracranial and intraspinal abscess and granuloma in diseases classified elsewhere MCC

Code first underlying disease such as:
schistosomiasis granuloma of brain (B65.-)

Excludes1: *abscess of brain:*
amebic (A06.6)
chromomycotic (B43.1)
gonococcal (A54.82)
tuberculous (A17.81)
tuberculoma of meninges (A17.1)

Valid 3-character code, no further characters required

MCC **G08 Intracranial and intraspinal phlebitis and thrombophlebitis**

Septic embolism of intracranial or intraspinal venous sinuses and veins
Septic endophlebitis of intracranial or intraspinal venous sinuses and veins
Septic phlebitis of intracranial or intraspinal venous sinuses and veins
Septic thrombophlebitis of intracranial or intraspinal venous sinuses and veins
Septic thrombosis of intracranial or intraspinal venous sinuses and veins

Excludes1: *intracranial phlebitis and thrombophlebitis complicating:*
abortion, ectopic or molar pregnancy (O00-O07, O08.7)
pregnancy, childbirth and the puerperium (O22.5, O87.3)
nonpyogenic intracranial phlebitis and thrombophlebitis (I67.6)

Excludes2: *intracranial phlebitis and thrombophlebitis complicating nonpyogenic intraspinal phlebitis and thrombophlebitis (G95.1)*

Valid 3-character code, no further characters required

G09 Sequelae of inflammatory diseases of central nervous system

NOTE Category G09 is to be used to indicate conditions whose primary classification is to G00-G08 as the cause of sequelae, themselves classifiable elsewhere. The 'sequelae' include conditions specified as residuals.

Code first condition resulting from (sequela) of inflammatory diseases of central nervous system

Valid 3-character code, no further characters required

Systemic atrophies primarily affecting the central nervous system (G10-G14)

CC **G10 Huntington's disease**

Huntington's chorea
Huntington's dementia
Code also dementia in other diseases classified elsewhere without behavioral disturbance (F02.80)

Valid 3-character code, no further characters required

G11 Hereditary ataxia

Excludes2: *cerebral palsy (G80.-)*
hereditary and idiopathic neuropathy (G60.-)
metabolic disorders (E70-E88)

CC **G11.0 Congenital nonprogressive ataxia**

\+ **G11.1 Early-onset cerebellar ataxia**
AHA CC: 4Q, 2020, 17-18

CC **G11.10 Early-onset cerebellar ataxia, unspecified**

CC **G11.11 Friedreich ataxia**
Autosomal recessive Friedreich ataxia
Friedreich ataxia with retained reflexes

CC **G11.19 Other early-onset cerebellar ataxia**
Early-onset cerebellar ataxia with essential tremor
Early-onset cerebellar ataxia with myoclonus [Hunt's ataxia]
Early-onset cerebellar ataxia with retained tendon reflexes
X-linked recessive spinocerebellar ataxia

• CC **G11.2 Late-onset cerebellar ataxia**

CC **G11.3 Cerebellar ataxia with defective DNA repair**
Ataxia telangiectasia [Louis-Bar]
Excludes2: *Cockayne's syndrome (Q87.19)*
other disorders of purine and pyrimidine metabolism (E79.-)
xeroderma pigmentosum (Q82.19)

CC **G11.4 Hereditary spastic paraplegia**

CC **G11.8 Other hereditary ataxias**

CC **G11.9 Hereditary ataxia, unspecified**
Hereditary cerebellar ataxia NOS
Hereditary cerebellar degeneration
Hereditary cerebellar disease
Hereditary cerebellar syndrome

G12 Spinal muscular atrophy and related syndromes

CC **G12.0 Infantile spinal muscular atrophy, type I [Werdnig-Hoffman]**

CC **G12.1 Other inherited spinal muscular atrophy**
Adult form spinal muscular atrophy
Childhood form, type II spinal muscular atrophy
Distal spinal muscular atrophy
Juvenile form, type III spinal muscular atrophy [Kugelberg-Welander]
Progressive bulbar palsy of childhood [Fazio-Londe]
Scapuloperoneal form spinal muscular atrophy

+ **G12.2 Motor neuron disease**

CC **G12.20 Motor neuron disease, unspecified**

• CC **G12.21 Amyotrophic lateral sclerosis**

CC **G12.22 Progressive bulbar palsy**

CC **G12.23 Primary lateral sclerosis**
AHA CC: 4Q, 2017, 9-10

CC **G12.24 Familial motor neuron disease**
AHA CC: 4Q, 2017, 9-10

CC **G12.25 Progressive spinal muscle atrophy**
AHA CC: 4Q, 2017, 9-10

CC **G12.29 Other motor neuron disease**

CC **G12.8 Other spinal muscular atrophies and related syndromes**

CC **G12.9 Spinal muscular atrophy, unspecified**

G13 Systemic atrophies primarily affecting central nervous system in diseases classified elsewhere

G13.0 Paraneoplastic neuromyopathy and neuropathy
Carcinomatous neuromyopathy
Sensorial paraneoplastic neuropathy [Denny Brown]
Code first underlying neoplasm (C00-D49)

G13.1 Other systemic atrophy primarily affecting central nervous system in neoplastic disease
Paraneoplastic limbic encephalopathy
Code first underlying neoplasm (C00-D49)

G13.2 Systemic atrophy primarily affecting the central nervous system in myxedema
Code first underlying disease, such as:
hypothyroidism (E03.-)
myxedematous congenital iodine deficiency (E00.1)

G13.8 Systemic atrophy primarily affecting central nervous system in other diseases classified elsewhere
Code first underlying disease

G14 Postpolio syndrome

Includes: postpolio myelitic syndrome
Excludes1: *sequelae of poliomyelitis (B91)*
Valid 3-character code, no further characters required

Extrapyramidal and movement disorders (G20-G26)

G20 Parkinson's disease

Hemiparkinsonism
Idiopathic Parkinsonism or Parkinson's disease
Paralysis agitans
Parkinsonism or Parkinson's disease NOS
Primary Parkinsonism or Parkinson's disease
Excludes1: *dementia with Parkinsonism (G31.83)*
Use additional code to identify:
dementia with behavioral disturbance (F02.81)
dementia without behavioral disturbance (F02.80)
AHA CC: 2Q, 2016, 6-7; 2Q, 2017, 7-8
Valid 3-character code, no further characters required

G21 Secondary parkinsonism

Excludes1: *dementia with Parkinsonism (G31.83)*
Huntington's disease (G10)
Shy-Drager syndrome (G90.3)
syphilitic Parkinsonism (A52.19)

MCC **G21.0 Malignant neuroleptic syndrome**
Use additional code for adverse effect, if applicable, to identify drug (T43.3X5, T43.4X5, T43.505, T43.595)
Excludes1: *neuroleptic induced parkinsonism (G21.11)*

+ **G21.1 Other drug-induced secondary parkinsonism**

CC **G21.11 Neuroleptic induced parkinsonism**
Use additional code for adverse effect, if applicable, to identify drug (T43.3X5, T43.4X5, T43.505, T43.595)
Excludes1: *malignant neuroleptic syndrome (G21.0)*

CC **G21.19 Other drug induced secondary parkinsonism**
Other medication-induced parkinsonism
Use additional code for adverse effect, if applicable, to identify drug (T36-T50 with fifth or sixth character 5)

CC **G21.2 Secondary parkinsonism due to other external agents**
Code first (T51-T65) to identify external agent

CC **G21.3 Postencephalitic parkinsonism**

G21.4 Vascular parkinsonism

CC **G21.8 Other secondary parkinsonism**

CC **G21.9 Secondary parkinsonism, unspecified**

G23 Other degenerative diseases of basal ganglia

Excludes2: *multi-system degeneration of the autonomic nervous system (G90.3)*

CC **G23.0 Hallervorden-Spatz disease**
Pigmentary pallidal degeneration

CC **G23.1 Progressive supranuclear ophthalmoplegia [Steele-Richardson-Olszewski]**
Progressive supranuclear palsy

CC **G23.2 Striatonigral degeneration**

CC **G23.8 Other specified degenerative diseases of basal ganglia**
Calcification of basal ganglia

CC **G23.9 Degenerative disease of basal ganglia, unspecified**

G24 Dystonia

Includes: dyskinesia
Excludes2: *athetoid cerebral palsy (G80.3)*

+ **G24.0 Drug induced dystonia**
Use additional code for adverse effect, if applicable, to identify drug (T36-T50 with fifth or sixth character 5)

G24.01 Drug induced subacute dyskinesia
Drug induced blepharospasm
Drug induced orofacial dyskinesia
Neuroleptic induced tardive dyskinesia
Tardive dyskinesia

CC **G24.02 Drug induced acute dystonia**
Acute dystonic reaction to drugs
Neuroleptic induced acute dystonia

CC **G24.09 Other drug induced dystonia**

G24.1 Genetic torsion dystonia
Dystonia deformans progressiva
Dystonia musculorum deformans
Familial torsion dystonia
Idiopathic familial dystonia
Idiopathic (torsion) dystonia NOS
(Schwalbe-) Ziehen-Oppenheim disease

CC **G24.2 Idiopathic nonfamilial dystonia**

G24.3 Spasmodic torticollis
Excludes1: *congenital torticollis (Q68.0)*
hysterical torticollis (F44.4)
ocular torticollis (R29.891)
psychogenic torticollis (F45.8)
torticollis NOS (M43.6)
traumatic recurrent torticollis (S13.4)

G24.4 Idiopathic orofacial dystonia
Orofacial dyskinesia
Excludes1: *drug induced orofacial dyskinesia (G24.01)*

G24.5 Blepharospasm
Excludes1: *drug induced blepharospasm (G24.01)*

CC **G24.8 Other dystonia**
Acquired torsion dystonia NOS

G24.9 Dystonia, unspecified
Dyskinesia NOS

G25 Other extrapyramidal and movement disorders

Excludes2: *sleep related movement disorders (G47.6-)*

G25.0 Essential tremor

Familial tremor

Excludes1: *tremor NOS (R25.1)*

G25.1 Drug-induced tremor

Use additional code for adverse effect, if applicable, to identify drug (T36-T50 with fifth or sixth character 5)

G25.2 Other specified forms of tremor

Intention tremor

G25.3 Myoclonus

Drug-induced myoclonus

Palatal myoclonus

Use additional code for adverse effect, if applicable, to identify drug (T36-T50 with fifth or sixth character 5)

Excludes1: *facial myokymia (G51.4)*
myoclonic epilepsy (G40.-)

G25.4 Drug-induced chorea

Use additional code for adverse effect, if applicable, to identify drug (T36-T50 with fifth or sixth character 5)

G25.5 Other chorea

Chorea NOS

Excludes1: *chorea NOS with heart involvement (I02.0)*
Huntington's chorea (G10)
rheumatic chorea (I02.-)
Sydenham's chorea (I02.-)

+ **G25.6 Drug induced tics and other tics of organic origin**

G25.61 Drug induced tics

Use additional code for adverse effect, if applicable, to identify drug (T36-T50 with fifth or sixth character 5)

G25.69 Other tics of organic origin

Excludes1: *habit spasm (F95.9)*
tic NOS (F95.9)
Tourette's syndrome (F95.2)

+ **G25.7 Other and unspecified drug induced movement disorders**

Use additional code for adverse effect, if applicable, to identify drug (T36-T50 with fifth or sixth character 5)

G25.70 Drug induced movement disorder, unspecified

G25.71 Drug induced akathisia

Drug induced acathisia

Neuroleptic induced acute akathisia

Tardive akathisia

G25.79 Other drug induced movement disorders

+ **G25.8 Other specified extrapyramidal and movement disorders**

G25.81 Restless legs syndrome

CC **G25.82 Stiff-man syndrome**

G25.83 Benign shuddering attacks

G25.89 Other specified extrapyramidal and movement disorders

CC **G25.9 Extrapyramidal and movement disorder, unspecified**

G26 Extrapyramidal and movement disorders in diseases classified elsewhere

Code first underlying disease

Valid 3-character code, no further characters required

Other degenerative diseases of the nervous system (G30-G32)

G30 Alzheimer's disease

Includes: Alzheimer's dementia senile and presenile forms

Use additional code to identify:
delirium, if applicable (F05)
dementia with behavioral disturbance (F02.81)
dementia without behavioral disturbance (F02.80)

Excludes1: *senile degeneration of brain NEC (G31.1)*
senile dementia NOS (F03)
senility NOS (R41.81)

G30.0 Alzheimer's disease with early onset

• **G30.1 Alzheimer's disease with late onset**

G30.8 Other Alzheimer's disease

G30.9 Alzheimer's disease, unspecified

AHA CC: 4Q, 2012, 95-96; 2Q, 2016, 6; 1Q, 2017, 43-44

G31 Other degenerative diseases of nervous system, not elsewhere classified

For codes G31.0-G31.83, G31.85-G31.9, use additional code to identify::
dementia with behavioral disturbance (F02.81)
dementia without behavioral disturbance (F02.80)

Excludes2: *Reye's syndrome (G93.7)*

+ **G31.0 Frontotemporal dementia**

G31.01 Pick's disease

Primary progressive aphasia

Progressive isolated aphasia

G31.09 Other frontotemporal dementia

Frontal dementia

G31.1 Senile degeneration of brain, not elsewhere classified

Excludes1: *Alzheimer's disease (G30.-)*
senility NOS (R41.81)

G31.2 Degeneration of nervous system due to alcohol

Alcoholic cerebellar ataxia

Alcoholic cerebellar degeneration

Alcoholic cerebral degeneration

Alcoholic encephalopathy

Dysfunction of the autonomic nervous system due to alcohol

Code also associated alcoholism (F10.-)

+ **G31.8 Other specified degenerative diseases of nervous system**

CC **G31.81 Alpers disease**

Grey-matter degeneration

CC **G31.82 Leigh's disease**

Subacute necrotizing encephalopathy

G31.83 Dementia with Lewy bodies

Dementia with Parkinsonism

Lewy body dementia

Lewy body disease

AHA CC: 4Q, 2016, 141

G31.84 Mild cognitive impairment, so stated

Mild neurocognitive disorder

Excludes1: *age related cognitive decline (R41.81)*
altered mental status (R41.82)
cerebral degeneration (G31.9)
change in mental status (R41.82)
cognitive deficits following (sequelae of) cerebral hemorrhage or infarction (I69.01-, I69.11-, I69.21-, I69.31-, I69.81-, I69.91-)
cognitive impairment due to intracranial or head injury (S06.-)
dementia (F01.-, F02.-, F03)
mild memory disturbance (F06.8)
neurologic neglect syndrome (R41.4)
personality change, nonpsychotic (F68.8)

G31.85 Corticobasal degeneration

G31.89 Other specified degenerative diseases of nervous system

G31.9 Degenerative disease of nervous system, unspecified

G32 Other degenerative disorders of nervous system in diseases classified elsewhere

CC **G32.0 Subacute combined degeneration of spinal cord in diseases classified elsewhere**

Dana-Putnam syndrome

Sclerosis of spinal cord (combined) (dorsolateral) (posterolateral)

Code first underlying disease, such as:
anemia (D51.9)
dietary (D51.3)
pernicious (D51.0)
vitamin B12 deficiency (E53.8)

Excludes1: *syphilitic combined degeneration of spinal cord (A52.11)*

+ **G32.8 Other specified degenerative disorders of nervous system in diseases classified elsewhere**

Code first underlying disease, such as:
amyloidosis cerebral degeneration (E85.-)
cerebral degeneration (due to) hypothyroidism (E00.0-E03.9)
cerebral degeneration (due to) neoplasm (C00-D49)
cerebral degeneration (due to) vitamin B deficiency, except thiamine (E52-E53.-)
non-celiac gluten ataxia (M35.9)

Excludes1: *superior hemorrhagic polioencephalitis [Wernicke's encephalopathy] (E51.2)*

CC **G32.81 Cerebellar ataxia in diseases classified elsewhere**
Code first underlying disease, such as:
celiac disease (with gluten ataxia) (K90.0)
cerebellar ataxia (in) neoplastic disease (paraneoplastic cerebellar degeneration) (C00-D49)
non-celiac gluten ataxia (M35.9)
Excludes1: *systemic atrophy primarily affecting the central nervous system in alcoholic cerebellar ataxia (G31.2)*
systemic atrophy primarily affecting the central nervous system in myxedema (G13.2)

G32.89 Other specified degenerative disorders of nervous system in diseases classified elsewhere
Degenerative encephalopathy in diseases classified elsewhere

Demyelinating diseases of the central nervous system (G35-G37)

G35 Multiple sclerosis
Disseminated multiple sclerosis
Generalized multiple sclerosis
Multiple sclerosis NOS
Multiple sclerosis of brain stem
Multiple sclerosis of cord
AHA CC: 1Q, 2021, 7
Valid 3-character code, no further characters required

G36 Other acute disseminated demyelination
Excludes1: *postinfectious encephalitis and encephalomyelitis NOS (G04.01)*

CC **G36.0 Neuromyelitis optica [Devic]**
Demyelination in optic neuritis
Excludes1: *optic neuritis NOS (H46)*

CC **G36.1 Acute and subacute hemorrhagic leukoencephalitis [Hurst]**
CC **G36.8 Other specified acute disseminated demyelination**
CC **G36.9 Acute disseminated demyelination, unspecified**

G37 Other demyelinating diseases of central nervous system

CC **G37.0 Diffuse sclerosis of central nervous system**
Periaxial encephalitis
Schilder's disease
Excludes1: *X linked adrenoleukodystrophy (E71.52-)*

CC **G37.1 Central demyelination of corpus callosum**
CC **G37.2 Central pontine myelinolysis**
CC **G37.3 Acute transverse myelitis in demyelinating disease of central nervous system**
Acute transverse myelitis NOS
Acute transverse myelopathy
Excludes1: *acute flaccid myelitis (G04.82)*
multiple sclerosis (G35)
neuromyelitis optica [Devic] (G36.0)

MCC **G37.4 Subacute necrotizing myelitis of central nervous system**
CC **G37.5 Concentric sclerosis [Balo] of central nervous system**
CC **G37.8 Other specified demyelinating diseases of central nervous system**
CC **G37.9 Demyelinating disease of central nervous system, unspecified**

Episodic and paroxysmal disorders (G40-G47)

G40 Epilepsy and recurrent seizures
NOTE the following terms are to be considered equivalent to intractable: pharmacoresistant (pharmacologically resistant), treatment resistant, refractory (medically) and poorly controlled
Excludes1: *conversion disorder with seizures (F44.5)*
convulsions NOS (R56.9)
post traumatic seizures (R56.1)
seizure (convulsive) NOS (R56.9)
seizure of newborn (P90)
Excludes2: *hippocampal sclerosis (G93.81)*
mesial temporal sclerosis (G93.81)
temporal sclerosis (G93.81)
Todd's paralysis (G83.84)

\+ **G40.0 Localization-related (focal) (partial) idiopathic epilepsy and epileptic syndromes with seizures of localized onset**
Benign childhood epilepsy with centrotemporal EEG spikes
Childhood epilepsy with occipital EEG paroxysms
Excludes1: *adult onset localization-related epilepsy (G40.1-, G40.2-)*

\+ **G40.00 Localization-related (focal) (partial) idiopathic epilepsy and epileptic syndromes with seizures of localized onset, not intractable**
Localization-related (focal) (partial) idiopathic epilepsy and epileptic syndromes with seizures of localized onset without intractability

CC **G40.001 Localization-related (focal) (partial) idiopathic epilepsy and epileptic syndromes with seizures of localized onset, not intractable, with status epilepticus**

CC **G40.009 Localization-related (focal) (partial) idiopathic epilepsy and epileptic syndromes with seizures of localized onset, not intractable, without status epilepticus**
Localization-related (focal) (partial) idiopathic epilepsy and epileptic syndromes with seizures of localized onset NOS

\+ **G40.01 Localization-related (focal) (partial) idiopathic epilepsy and epileptic syndromes with seizures of localized onset, intractable**

CC **G40.011 Localization-related (focal) (partial) idiopathic epilepsy and epileptic syndromes with seizures of localized onset, intractable, with status epilepticus**

CC **G40.019 Localization-related (focal) (partial) idiopathic epilepsy and epileptic syndromes with seizures of localized onset, intractable, without status epilepticus**

\+ **G40.1 Localization-related (focal) (partial) symptomatic epilepsy and epileptic syndromes with simple partial seizures**
Attacks without alteration of consciousness
Epilepsia partialis continua [Kozhevnikof]
Simple partial seizures developing into secondarily generalized seizures

\+ **G40.10 Localization-related (focal) (partial) symptomatic epilepsy and epileptic syndromes with simple partial seizures, not intractable**
Localization-related (focal) (partial) symptomatic epilepsy and epileptic syndromes with simple partial seizures without intractability

CC **G40.101 Localization-related (focal) (partial) symptomatic epilepsy and epileptic syndromes with simple partial seizures, not intractable, with status epilepticus**

CC **G40.109 Localization-related (focal) (partial) symptomatic epilepsy and epileptic syndromes with simple partial seizures, not intractable, without status epilepticus**
Localization-related (focal) (partial) symptomatic epilepsy and epileptic syndromes with simple partial seizures NOS

\+ **G40.11 Localization-related (focal) (partial) symptomatic epilepsy and epileptic syndromes with simple partial seizures, intractable**

CC **G40.111 Localization-related (focal) (partial) symptomatic epilepsy and epileptic syndromes with simple partial seizures, intractable, with status epilepticus**

CC **G40.119 Localization-related (focal) (partial) symptomatic epilepsy and epileptic syndromes with simple partial seizures, intractable, without status epilepticus**

\+ **G40.2 Localization-related (focal) (partial) symptomatic epilepsy and epileptic syndromes with complex partial seizures**
Attacks with alteration of consciousness, often with automatisms
Complex partial seizures developing into secondarily generalized seizures

\+ **G40.20 Localization-related (focal) (partial) symptomatic epilepsy and epileptic syndromes with complex partial seizures, not intractable**
Localization-related (focal) (partial) symptomatic epilepsy and epileptic syndromes with complex partial seizures without intractability

CC **G40.201 Localization-related (focal) (partial) symptomatic epilepsy and epileptic syndromes with complex partial seizures, not intractable, with status epilepticus**

CC **G40.209 Localization-related (focal) (partial) symptomatic epilepsy and epileptic syndromes with complex partial seizures, not intractable, without status epilepticus**
Localization-related (focal) (partial) symptomatic epilepsy and epileptic syndromes with complex partial seizures NOS

+ **G40.21 Localization-related (focal) (partial) symptomatic epilepsy and epileptic syndromes with complex partial seizures, intractable**

CC **G40.211 Localization-related (focal) (partial) symptomatic epilepsy and epileptic syndromes with complex partial seizures, intractable, with status epilepticus**

CC **G40.219 Localization-related (focal) (partial) symptomatic epilepsy and epileptic syndromes with complex partial seizures, intractable, without status epilepticus**

+ **G40.3 Generalized idiopathic epilepsy and epileptic syndromes**
Code also MERRF syndrome, if applicable (E88.42)

+ **G40.30 Generalized idiopathic epilepsy and epileptic syndromes, not intractable**
Generalized idiopathic epilepsy and epileptic syndromes without intractability

MCC **G40.301 Generalized idiopathic epilepsy and epileptic syndromes, not intractable, with status epilepticus**

G40.309 Generalized idiopathic epilepsy and epileptic syndromes, not intractable, without status epilepticus
Generalized idiopathic epilepsy and epileptic syndromes NOS

+ **G40.31 Generalized idiopathic epilepsy and epileptic syndromes, intractable**

MCC **G40.311 Generalized idiopathic epilepsy and epileptic syndromes, intractable, with status epilepticus**

MCC **G40.319 Generalized idiopathic epilepsy and epileptic syndromes, intractable, without status epilepticus**

+ **G40.A Absence epileptic syndrome**
Childhood absence epilepsy [pyknolepsy]
Juvenile absence epilepsy
Absence epileptic syndrome, NOS

+ **G40.A0 Absence epileptic syndrome, not intractable**

G40.A01 Absence epileptic syndrome, not intractable, with status epilepticus

G40.A09 Absence epileptic syndrome, not intractable, without status epilepticus

+ **G40.A1 Absence epileptic syndrome, intractable**

CC **G40.A11 Absence epileptic syndrome, intractable, with status epilepticus**

CC **G40.A19 Absence epileptic syndrome, intractable, without status epilepticus**

+ **G40.B Juvenile myoclonic epilepsy [impulsive petit mal]**

+ **G40.B0 Juvenile myoclonic epilepsy, not intractable**

CC **G40.B01 Juvenile myoclonic epilepsy, not intractable, with status epilepticus**

CC **G40.B09 Juvenile myoclonic epilepsy, not intractable, without status epilepticus**

+ **G40.B1 Juvenile myoclonic epilepsy, intractable**

CC **G40.B11 Juvenile myoclonic epilepsy, intractable, with status epilepticus**

CC **G40.B19 Juvenile myoclonic epilepsy, intractable, without status epilepticus**

+ **G40.4 Other generalized epilepsy and epileptic syndromes**
Epilepsy with grand mal seizures on awakening
Epilepsy with myoclonic absences
Epilepsy with myoclonic-astatic seizures
Grand mal seizure NOS
Nonspecific atonic epileptic seizures
Nonspecific clonic epileptic seizures
Nonspecific myoclonic epileptic seizures
Nonspecific tonic epileptic seizures
Nonspecific tonic-clonic epileptic seizures
Symptomatic early myoclonic encephalopathy

+ **G40.40 Other generalized epilepsy and epileptic syndromes, not intractable**
Other generalized epilepsy and epileptic syndromes without intractability
Other generalized epilepsy and epileptic syndromes NOS

G40.401 Other generalized epilepsy and epileptic syndromes, not intractable, with status epilepticus

G40.409 Other generalized epilepsy and epileptic syndromes, not intractable, without status epilepticus

+ **G40.41 Other generalized epilepsy and epileptic syndromes, intractable**

CC **G40.411 Other generalized epilepsy and epileptic syndromes, intractable, with status epilepticus**

CC **G40.419 Other generalized epilepsy and epileptic syndromes, intractable, without status epilepticus**

G40.42 Cyclin-Dependent Kinase-Like 5 Deficiency Disorder
CDKL5
Use additional code, if known, to identify associated manifestations, such as:
cortical blindness (H47.61-)
global developmental delay (F88)
AHA CC: 4Q, 2020, 18-19

+ **G40.5 Epileptic seizures related to external causes**
Epileptic seizures related to alcohol
Epileptic seizures related to drugs
Epileptic seizures related to hormonal changes
Epileptic seizures related to sleep deprivation
Epileptic seizures related to stress
Use additional code for adverse effect, if applicable, to identify drug (T36-T50 with fifth or sixth character 5)
Code also if applicable, associated epilepsy and recurrent seizures (G40.-)

+ **G40.50 Epileptic seizures related to external causes, not intractable**

CC **G40.501 Epileptic seizures related to external causes, not intractable, with status epilepticus**

CC **G40.509 Epileptic seizures related to external causes, not intractable, without status epilepticus**
Epileptic seizures related to external causes, NOS

+ **G40.8 Other epilepsy and recurrent seizures**
Epilepsies and epileptic syndromes undetermined as to whether they are focal or generalized
Landau-Kleffner syndrome

+ **G40.80 Other epilepsy**

CC **G40.801 Other epilepsy, not intractable, with status epilepticus**
Other epilepsy without intractability with status epilepticus

CC **G40.802 Other epilepsy, not intractable, without status epilepticus**
Other epilepsy NOS
Other epilepsy without intractability without status epilepticus

CC **G40.803 Other epilepsy, intractable, with status epilepticus**

CC **G40.804 Other epilepsy, intractable, without status epilepticus**

+ **G40.81 Lennox-Gastaut syndrome**

CC **G40.811 Lennox-Gastaut syndrome, not intractable, with status epilepticus**

CC **G40.812 Lennox-Gastaut syndrome, not intractable, without status epilepticus**

CC **G40.813 Lennox-Gastaut syndrome, intractable, with status epilepticus**

CC **G40.814 Lennox-Gastaut syndrome, intractable, without status epilepticus**

+ **G40.82 Epileptic spasms**
Infantile spasms
Salaam attacks
West's syndrome

CC **G40.821 Epileptic spasms, not intractable, with status epilepticus**

CC **G40.822 Epileptic spasms, not intractable, without status epilepticus**

CC **G40.823 Epileptic spasms, intractable, with status epilepticus**

CC **G40.824 Epileptic spasms, intractable, without status epilepticus**

\+ **G40.83 Dravet syndrome**
Polymorphic epilepsy in infancy (PMEI)
Severe myoclonic epilepsy in infancy (SMEI)
AHA CC: 4Q, 2020, 19

CC **G40.833 Dravet syndrome, intractable, with status epilepticus**

CC **G40.834 Dravet syndrome, intractable, without status epilepticus**
Dravet syndrome NOS

CC **G40.89 Other seizures**
Excludes1: *post traumatic seizures (R56.1)*
recurrent seizures NOS (G40.909)
seizure NOS (R56.9)

\+ **G40.9 Epilepsy, unspecified**

\+ **G40.90 Epilepsy, unspecified, not intractable**
Epilepsy, unspecified, without intractability

G40.901 Epilepsy, unspecified, not intractable, with status epilepticus

G40.909 Epilepsy, unspecified, not intractable, without status epilepticus
Epilepsy NOS
Epileptic convulsions NOS
Epileptic fits NOS
Epileptic seizures NOS
Recurrent seizures NOS
Seizure disorder NOS
AHA CC: 2Q, 2021, 3-4

\+ **G40.91 Epilepsy, unspecified, intractable**
Intractable seizure disorder NOS

CC **G40.911 Epilepsy, unspecified, intractable, with status epilepticus**

CC **G40.919 Epilepsy, unspecified, intractable, without status epilepticus**

G43 Migraine

NOTE The following terms are to be considered equivalent to intractable: pharmacoresistant (pharmacologically resistant), treatment resistant, refractory (medically) and poorly controlled

Use additional code for adverse effect, if applicable, to identify drug (T36-T50 with fifth or sixth character 5)
Excludes1: *headache NOS (R51.9)*
lower half migraine (G44.00)
Excludes2: *headache syndromes (G44.-)*

\+ **G43.0 Migraine without aura**
Common migraine
Excludes1: *chronic migraine without aura (G43.7-)*

\+ **G43.00 Migraine without aura, not intractable**
Migraine without aura without mention of refractory migraine

G43.001 Migraine without aura, not intractable, with status migrainosus

G43.009 Migraine without aura, not intractable, without status migrainosus
Migraine without aura NOS

\+ **G43.01 Migraine without aura, intractable**
Migraine without aura with refractory migraine

G43.011 Migraine without aura, intractable, with status migrainosus

G43.019 Migraine without aura, intractable, without status migrainosus

\+ **G43.1 Migraine with aura**
Basilar migraine
Classical migraine
Migraine equivalents
Migraine preceded or accompanied by transient focal neurological phenomena
Migraine triggered seizures
Migraine with acute-onset aura
Migraine with aura without headache (migraine equivalents)
Migraine with prolonged aura
Migraine with typical aura
Retinal migraine
Code also any associated seizure (G40.-, R56.9)
Excludes1: *persistent migraine aura (G43.5-, G43.6-)*

\+ **G43.10 Migraine with aura, not intractable**
Migraine with aura without mention of refractory migraine

G43.101 Migraine with aura, not intractable, with status migrainosus

G43.109 Migraine with aura, not intractable, without status migrainosus
Migraine with aura NOS

\+ **G43.11 Migraine with aura, intractable**
Migraine with aura with refractory migraine

G43.111 Migraine with aura, intractable, with status migrainosus

G43.119 Migraine with aura, intractable, without status migrainosus

\+ **G43.4 Hemiplegic migraine**
Familial migraine
Sporadic migraine

\+ **G43.40 Hemiplegic migraine, not intractable**
Hemiplegic migraine without refractory migraine

G43.401 Hemiplegic migraine, not intractable, with status migrainosus

G43.409 Hemiplegic migraine, not intractable, without status migrainosus
Hemiplegic migraine NOS

\+ **G43.41 Hemiplegic migraine, intractable**
Hemiplegic migraine with refractory migraine

G43.411 Hemiplegic migraine, intractable, with status migrainosus

G43.419 Hemiplegic migraine, intractable, without status migrainosus

\+ **G43.5 Persistent migraine aura without cerebral infarction**

\+ **G43.50 Persistent migraine aura without cerebral infarction, not intractable**
Persistent migraine aura without cerebral infarction, without refractory migraine

G43.501 Persistent migraine aura without cerebral infarction, not intractable, with status migrainosus

G43.509 Persistent migraine aura without cerebral infarction, not intractable, without status migrainosus
Persistent migraine aura NOS

\+ **G43.51 Persistent migraine aura without cerebral infarction, intractable**
Persistent migraine aura without cerebral infarction, with refractory migraine

G43.511 Persistent migraine aura without cerebral infarction, intractable, with status migrainosus

G43.519 Persistent migraine aura without cerebral infarction, intractable, without status migrainosus

\+ **G43.6 Persistent migraine aura with cerebral infarction**
Code also the type of cerebral infarction (I63.-)

\+ **G43.60 Persistent migraine aura with cerebral infarction, not intractable**
Persistent migraine aura with cerebral infarction, without refractory migraine

CC **G43.601 Persistent migraine aura with cerebral infarction, not intractable, with status migrainosus**

CC **G43.609 Persistent migraine aura with cerebral infarction, not intractable, without status migrainosus**

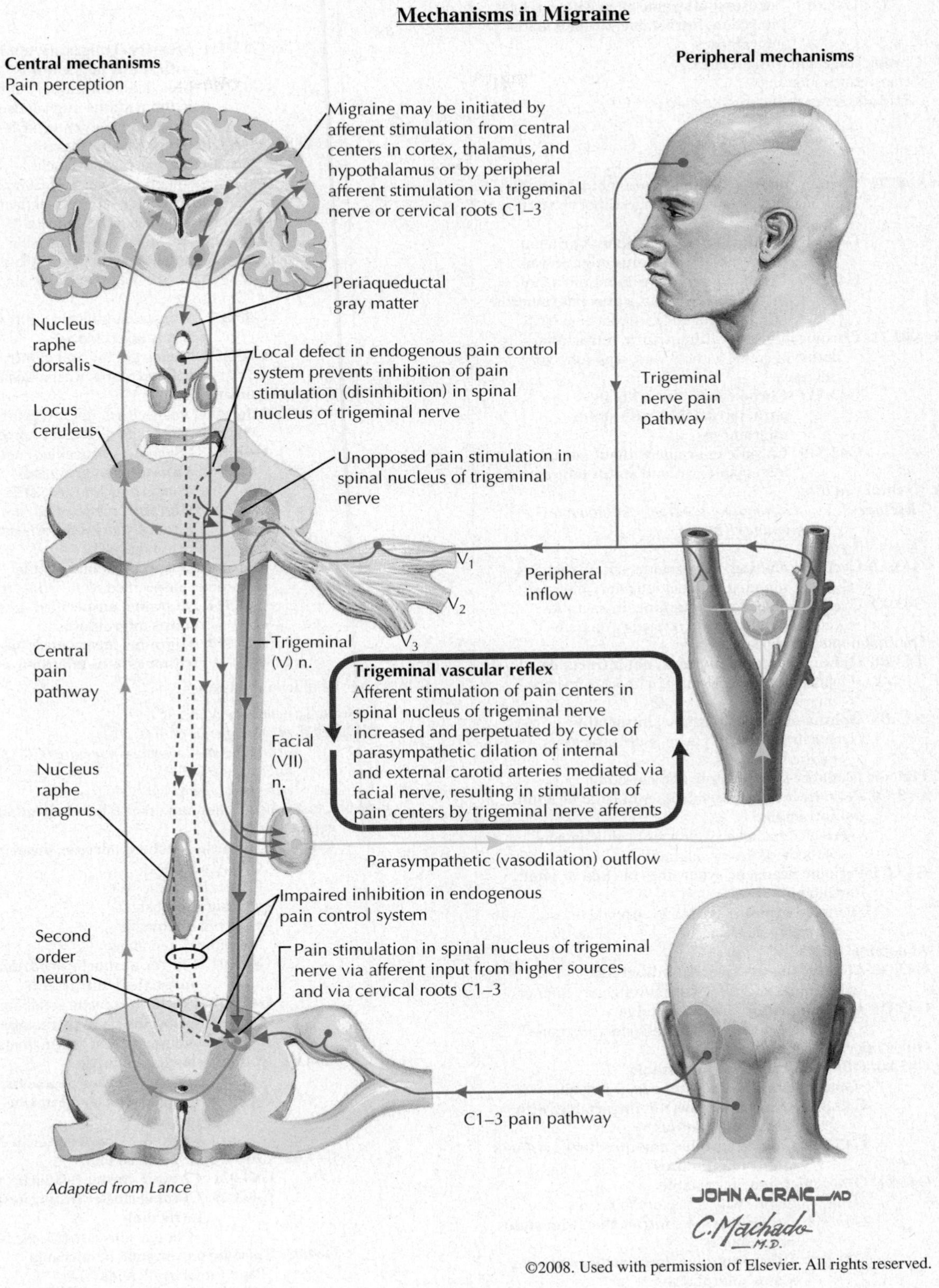
Mechanisms in Migraine
Central mechanisms
Pain perception
Peripheral mechanisms
Migraine may be initiated by afferent stimulation from central centers in cortex, thalamus, and hypothalamus or by peripheral afferent stimulation via trigeminal nerve or cervical roots C1–3
Periaqueductal gray matter
Nucleus raphe dorsalis
Local defect in endogenous pain control system prevents inhibition of pain stimulation (disinhibition) in spinal nucleus of trigeminal nerve
Locus ceruleus
Trigeminal nerve pain pathway
Unopposed pain stimulation in spinal nucleus of trigeminal nerve
V_1
Peripheral inflow
V_2
V_3
Trigeminal (V) n.
Central pain pathway
Trigeminal vascular reflex
Afferent stimulation of pain centers in spinal nucleus of trigeminal nerve increased and perpetuated by cycle of parasympathetic dilation of internal and external carotid arteries mediated via facial nerve, resulting in stimulation of pain centers by trigeminal nerve afferents
Facial (VII) n.
Nucleus raphe magnus
Parasympathetic (vasodilation) outflow
Impaired inhibition in endogenous pain control system
Second order neuron
Pain stimulation in spinal nucleus of trigeminal nerve via afferent input from higher sources and via cervical roots C1–3
C1–3 pain pathway
Adapted from Lance
JOHN A.CRAIG—AD
C.Machado—M.D.

+ **G43.61 Persistent migraine aura with cerebral infarction, intractable**
  Persistent migraine aura with cerebral infarction, with refractory migraine
  - CC **G43.611 Persistent migraine aura with cerebral infarction, intractable, with status migrainosus**
  - CC **G43.619 Persistent migraine aura with cerebral infarction, intractable, without status migrainosus**

+ **G43.7 Chronic migraine without aura**
  Transformed migraine
  Excludes1: *migraine without aura (G43.0-)*

+ **G43.70 Chronic migraine without aura, not intractable**
  Chronic migraine without aura, without refractory migraine
  - **G43.701 Chronic migraine without aura, not intractable, with status migrainosus**
  - **G43.709 Chronic migraine without aura, not intractable, without status migrainosus**
    Chronic migraine without aura NOS

+ **G43.71 Chronic migraine without aura, intractable**
  Chronic migraine without aura, with refractory migraine
  - **G43.711 Chronic migraine without aura, intractable, with status migrainosus**
  - **G43.719 Chronic migraine without aura, intractable, without status migrainosus**

+ **G43.A Cyclical vomiting**
  Excludes1: *cyclical vomiting syndrome unrelated to migraine (R11.15)*
  AHA CC: 4Q, 2019, 15
  - **G43.A0 Cyclical vomiting, in migraine, not intractable**
    Cyclical vomiting, without refractory migraine
  - **G43.A1 Cyclical vomiting, in migraine, intractable**
    Cyclical vomiting, with refractory migraine

+ **G43.B Ophthalmoplegic migraine**
  - **G43.B0 Ophthalmoplegic migraine, not intractable**
    Ophthalmoplegic migraine, without refractory migraine
  - **G43.B1 Ophthalmoplegic migraine, intractable**
    Ophthalmoplegic migraine, with refractory migraine

+ **G43.C Periodic headache syndromes in child or adult**
  - **G43.C0 Periodic headache syndromes in child or adult, not intractable**
    Periodic headache syndromes in child or adult, without refractory migraine
  - **G43.C1 Periodic headache syndromes in child or adult, intractable**
    Periodic headache syndromes in child or adult, with refractory migraine

+ **G43.D Abdominal migraine**
  - **G43.D0 Abdominal migraine, not intractable**
    Abdominal migraine, without refractory migraine
  - **G43.D1 Abdominal migraine, intractable**
    Abdominal migraine, with refractory migraine

+ **G43.8 Other migraine**

+ **G43.80 Other migraine, not intractable**
  Other migraine, without refractory migraine
  - **G43.801 Other migraine, not intractable, with status migrainosus**
  - **G43.809 Other migraine, not intractable, without status migrainosus**

+ **G43.81 Other migraine, intractable**
  Other migraine, with refractory migraine
  - **G43.811 Other migraine, intractable, with status migrainosus**
  - **G43.819 Other migraine, intractable, without status migrainosus**

+ **G43.82 Menstrual migraine, not intractable**
  Menstrual headache, not intractable
  Menstrual migraine, without refractory migraine
  Menstrually related migraine, not intractable
  Pre-menstrual headache, not intractable
  Pre-menstrual migraine, not intractable
  Pure menstrual migraine, not intractable
  Code also associated premenstrual tension syndrome (N94.3)
  - ♀ **G43.821 Menstrual migraine, not intractable, with status migrainosus**
  - ♀ **G43.829 Menstrual migraine, not intractable, without status migrainosus**
    Menstrual migraine NOS

+ **G43.83 Menstrual migraine, intractable**
  Menstrual headache, intractable
  Menstrual migraine, with refractory migraine
  Menstrually related migraine, intractable
  Pre-menstrual headache, intractable
  Pre-menstrual migraine, intractable
  Pure menstrual migraine, intractable
  Code also associated premenstrual tension syndrome (N94.3)
  - ♀ **G43.831 Menstrual migraine, intractable, with status migrainosus**
  - ♀ **G43.839 Menstrual migraine, intractable, without status migrainosus**

+ **G43.9 Migraine, unspecified**

+ **G43.90 Migraine, unspecified, not intractable**
  Migraine, unspecified, without refractory migraine
  - **G43.901 Migraine, unspecified, not intractable, with status migrainosus**
    Status migrainosus NOS
  - **G43.909 Migraine, unspecified, not intractable, without status migrainosus**
    Migraine NOS

+ **G43.91 Migraine, unspecified, intractable**
  Migraine, unspecified, with refractory migraine
  - **G43.911 Migraine, unspecified, intractable, with status migrainosus**
  - **G43.919 Migraine, unspecified, intractable, without status migrainosus**

G44 Other headache syndromes

Excludes1: *headache NOS (R51.9)*
Excludes2: *atypical facial pain (G50.1)*
headache due to lumbar puncture (G97.1)
migraines (G43.-)
trigeminal neuralgia (G50.0)

+ **G44.0 Cluster headaches and other trigeminal autonomic cephalgias (TAC)**

+ **G44.00 Cluster headache syndrome, unspecified**
  Ciliary neuralgia
  Cluster headache NOS
  Histamine cephalgia
  Lower half migraine
  Migrainous neuralgia
  - **G44.001 Cluster headache syndrome, unspecified, intractable**
  - **G44.009 Cluster headache syndrome, unspecified, not intractable**
    Cluster headache syndrome NOS

+ **G44.01 Episodic cluster headache**
  - **G44.011 Episodic cluster headache, intractable**
  - **G44.019 Episodic cluster headache, not intractable**
    Episodic cluster headache NOS

+ **G44.02 Chronic cluster headache**
  - **G44.021 Chronic cluster headache, intractable**
  - **G44.029 Chronic cluster headache, not intractable**
    Chronic cluster headache NOS

+ **G44.03 Episodic paroxysmal hemicrania**
  Paroxysmal hemicrania NOS
  - **G44.031 Episodic paroxysmal hemicrania, intractable**
  - **G44.039 Episodic paroxysmal hemicrania, not intractable**
    Episodic paroxysmal hemicrania NOS

+ **G44.04 Chronic paroxysmal hemicrania**
  - **G44.041 Chronic paroxysmal hemicrania, intractable**
  - **G44.049 Chronic paroxysmal hemicrania, not intractable**
    Chronic paroxysmal hemicrania NOS
+ **G44.05 Short lasting unilateral neuralgiform headache with conjunctival injection and tearing (SUNCT)**
  - **G44.051 Short lasting unilateral neuralgiform headache with conjunctival injection and tearing (SUNCT), intractable**
  - **G44.059 Short lasting unilateral neuralgiform headache with conjunctival injection and tearing (SUNCT), not intractable**
    Short lasting unilateral neuralgiform headache with conjunctival injection and tearing (SUNCT) NOS
+ **G44.09 Other trigeminal autonomic cephalgias (TAC)**
  - **G44.091 Other trigeminal autonomic cephalgias (TAC), intractable**
  - **G44.099 Other trigeminal autonomic cephalgias (TAC), not intractable**

G44.1 Vascular headache, not elsewhere classified
Excludes2: *cluster headache (G44.0)*
complicated headache syndromes (G44.5-)
drug-induced headache (G44.4-)
migraine (G43.-)
other specified headache syndromes (G44.8-)
post-traumatic headache (G44.3-)
tension-type headache (G44.2-)

+ **G44.2 Tension-type headache**
+ **G44.20 Tension-type headache, unspecified**
  - **G44.201 Tension-type headache, unspecified, intractable**
  - **G44.209 Tension-type headache, unspecified, not intractable**
    Tension headache NOS
+ **G44.21 Episodic tension-type headache**
  - **G44.211 Episodic tension-type headache, intractable**
  - **G44.219 Episodic tension-type headache, not intractable**
    Episodic tension-type headache NOS
+ **G44.22 Chronic tension-type headache**
  - **G44.221 Chronic tension-type headache, intractable**
  - **G44.229 Chronic tension-type headache, not intractable**
    Chronic tension-type headache NOS

+ **G44.3 Post-traumatic headache**
+ **G44.30 Post-traumatic headache, unspecified**
  - **G44.301 Post-traumatic headache, unspecified, intractable**
  - **G44.309 Post-traumatic headache, unspecified, not intractable**
    Post-traumatic headache NOS
+ **G44.31 Acute post-traumatic headache**
  - **G44.311 Acute post-traumatic headache, intractable**
  - **G44.319 Acute post-traumatic headache, not intractable**
    Acute post-traumatic headache NOS
+ **G44.32 Chronic post-traumatic headache**
  - **G44.321 Chronic post-traumatic headache, intractable**
  - **G44.329 Chronic post-traumatic headache, not intractable**
    Chronic post-traumatic headache NOS

+ **G44.4 Drug-induced headache, not elsewhere classified**
Medication overuse headache
Use additional code for adverse effect, if applicable, to identify drug (T36-T50 with fifth or sixth character 5)
  - **G44.40 Drug-induced headache, not elsewhere classified, not intractable**
  - **G44.41 Drug-induced headache, not elsewhere classified, intractable**

+ **G44.5 Complicated headache syndromes**
  - **G44.51 Hemicrania continua**
  - **G44.52 New daily persistent headache (NDPH)**
  - **G44.53 Primary thunderclap headache**
  - **G44.59 Other complicated headache syndrome**

+ **G44.8 Other specified headache syndromes**
Excludes2: *headache with orthostatic or positional component, not elsewhere classified (R51.0)*
  - **G44.81 Hypnic headache**
  - **G44.82 Headache associated with sexual activity**
    Orgasmic headache
    Preorgasmic headache
  - **G44.83 Primary cough headache**
  - **G44.84 Primary exertional headache**
  - **G44.85 Primary stabbing headache**
  - **G44.86 Cervicogenic headache**
    Code also associated cervical spinal condition, if known
  - **G44.89 Other headache syndrome**

G45 Transient cerebral ischemic attacks and related syndromes

Excludes1: *neonatal cerebral ischemia (P91.0)*
transient retinal artery occlusion (H34.0-)

CC **G45.0 Vertebro-basilar artery syndrome**
CC **G45.1 Carotid artery syndrome (hemispheric)**
CC **G45.2 Multiple and bilateral precerebral artery syndromes**
CC **G45.3 Amaurosis fugax**
G45.4 Transient global amnesia
Excludes1: *amnesia NOS (R41.3)*
CC **G45.8 Other transient cerebral ischemic attacks and related syndromes**
CC **G45.9 Transient cerebral ischemic attack, unspecified**
Spasm of cerebral artery
TIA
Transient cerebral ischemia NOS

G46 Vascular syndromes of brain in cerebrovascular diseases

Code first underlying cerebrovascular disease (I60-I69)

CC **G46.0 Middle cerebral artery syndrome**
CC **G46.1 Anterior cerebral artery syndrome**
CC **G46.2 Posterior cerebral artery syndrome**
G46.3 Brain stem stroke syndrome
Benedikt syndrome
Claude syndrome
Foville syndrome
Millard-Gubler syndrome
Wallenberg syndrome
Weber syndrome
G46.4 Cerebellar stroke syndrome
G46.5 Pure motor lacunar syndrome
G46.6 Pure sensory lacunar syndrome
G46.7 Other lacunar syndromes
G46.8 Other vascular syndromes of brain in cerebrovascular diseases

G47 Sleep disorders

Excludes2: *nightmares (F51.5)*
nonorganic sleep disorders (F51.-)
sleep terrors (F51.4)
sleepwalking (F51.3)

+ **G47.0 Insomnia**
Excludes2: *alcohol related insomnia (F10.182, F10.282, F10.982)*
drug-related insomnia (F11.182, F11.282, F11.982, F13.182, F13.282, F13.982, F14.182, F14.282, F14.982, F15.182, F15.282, F15.982, F19.182, F19.282, F19.982)
idiopathic insomnia (F51.01)
insomnia due to a mental disorder (F51.05)
insomnia not due to a substance or known physiological condition (F51.0-)
nonorganic insomnia (F51.0-)
primary insomnia (F51.01)
sleep apnea (G47.3-)
  - **G47.00 Insomnia, unspecified**
    Insomnia NOS
  - **G47.01 Insomnia due to medical condition**
    Code also associated medical condition
  - **G47.09 Other insomnia**

Medial Views of Cerebrum

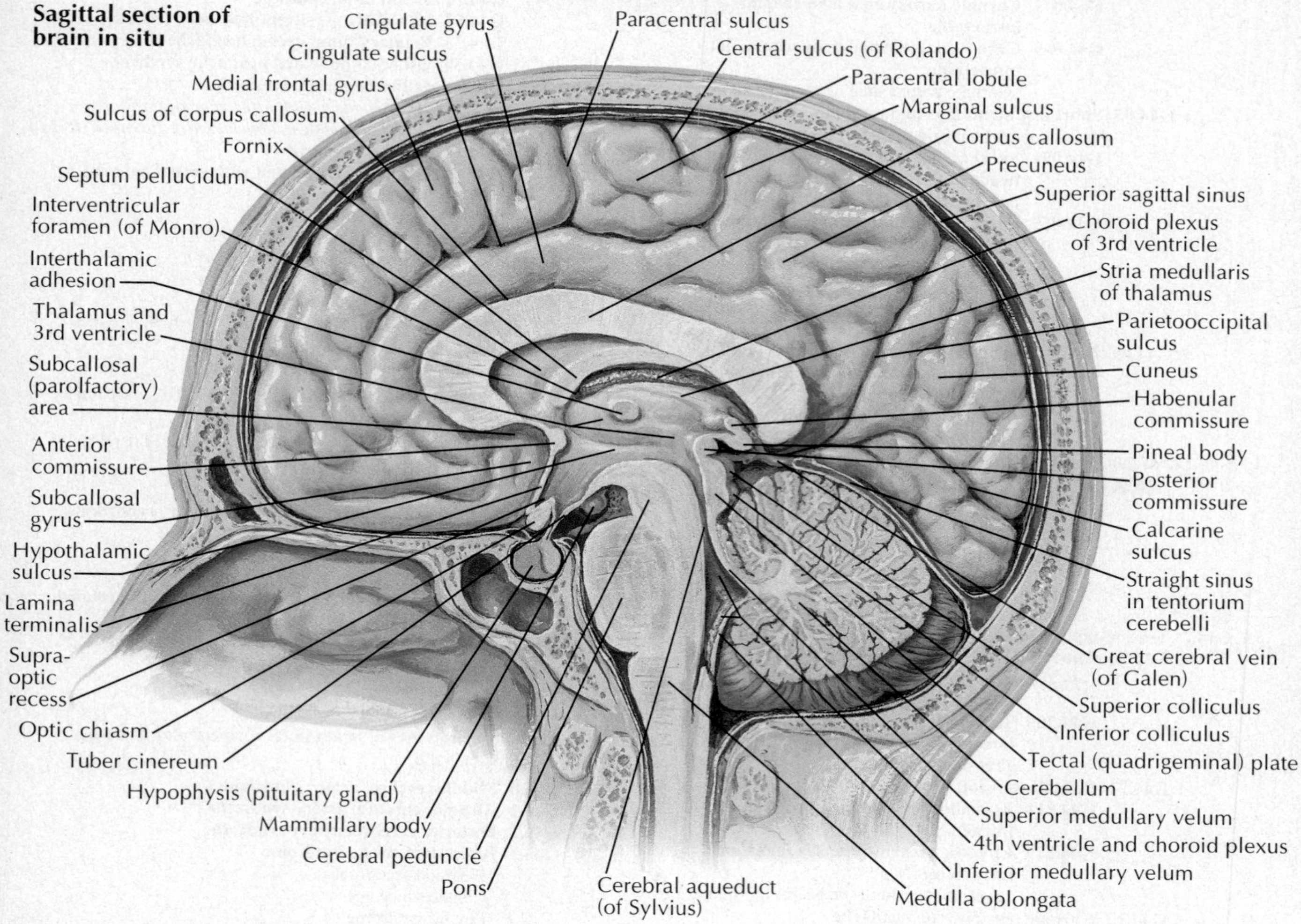

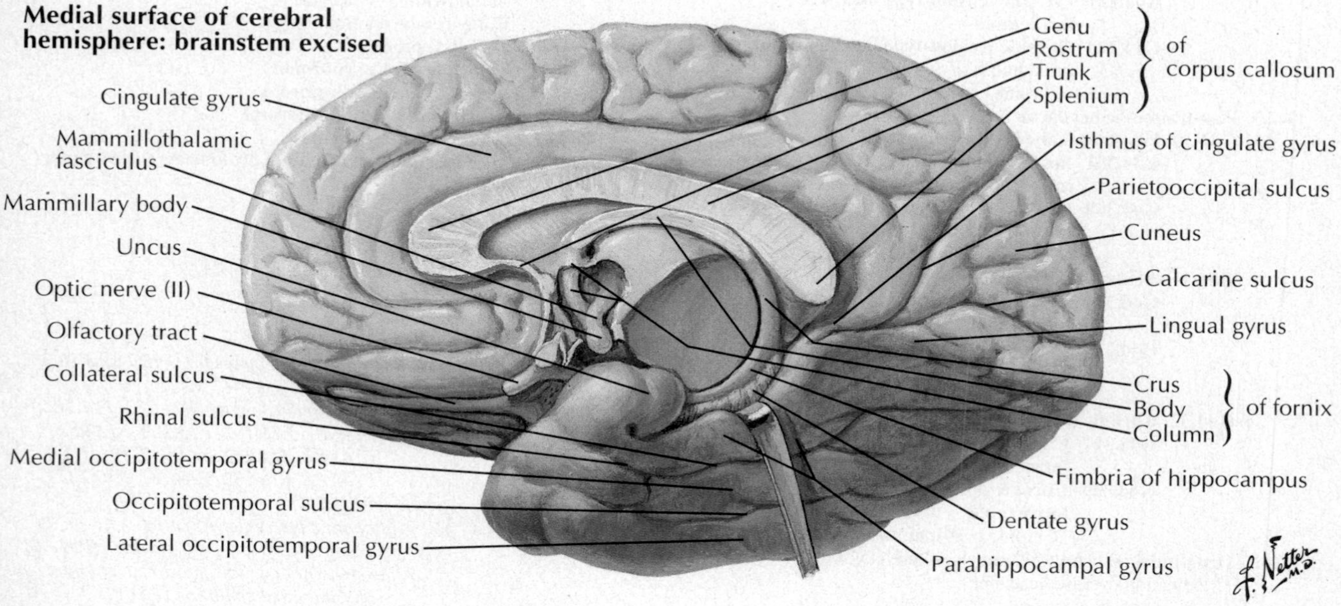

Cranial Nerves: Schema

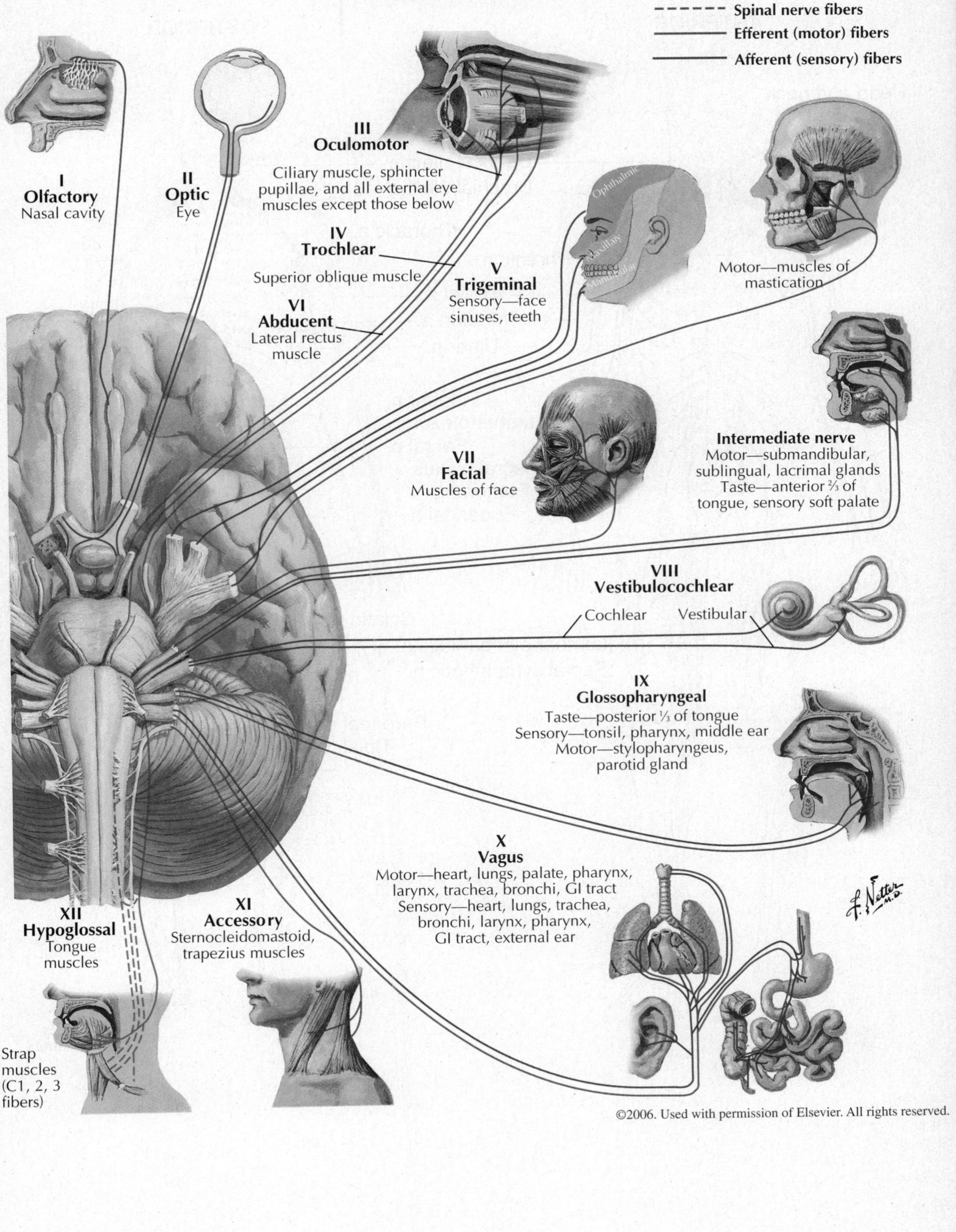

Peripheral Nervous System

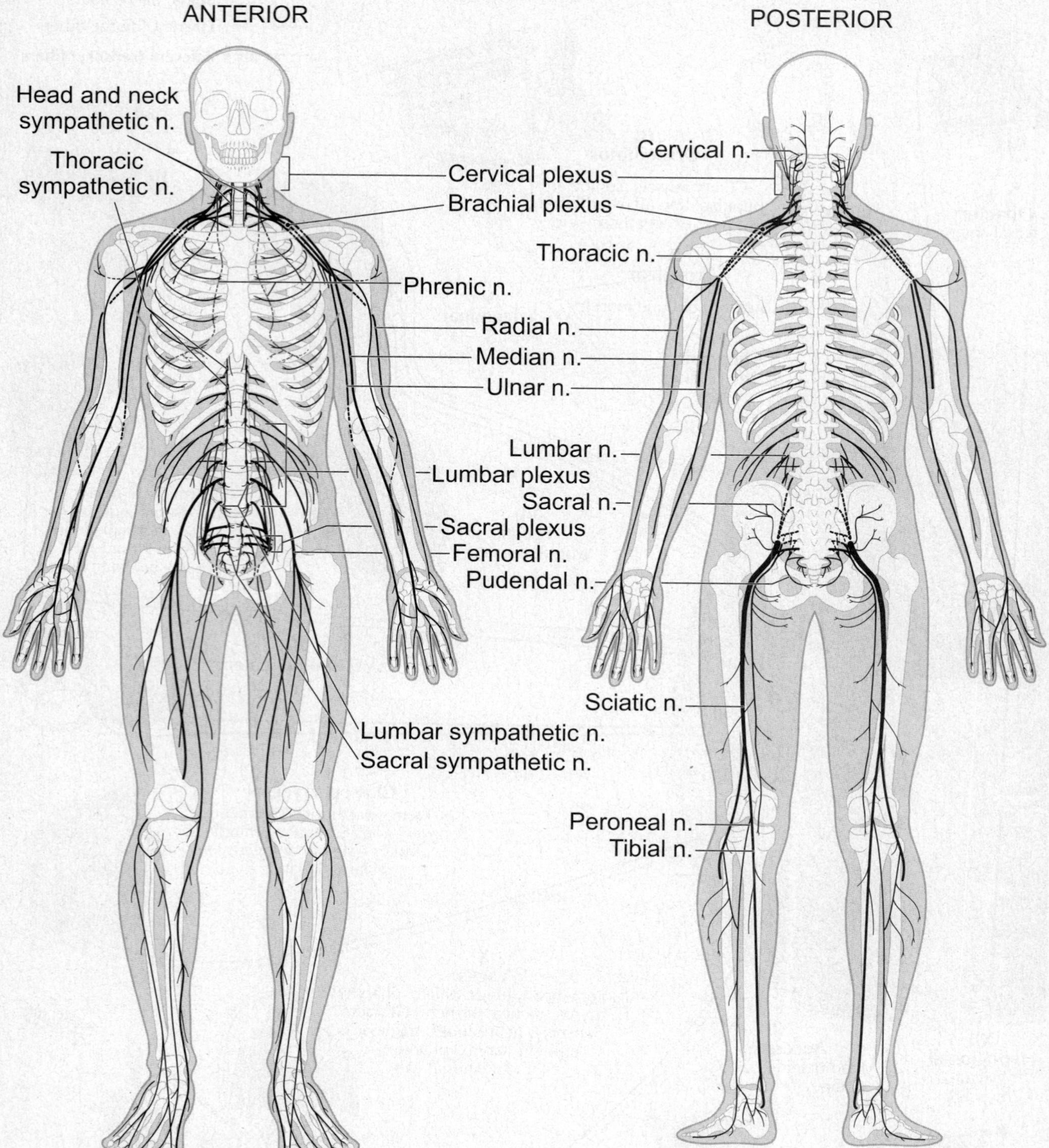

+ **G47.1 Hypersomnia**

Excludes2: *alcohol-related hypersomnia (F10.182, F10.282, F10.982)*
drug-related hypersomnia (F11.182, F11.282, F11.982, F13.182, F13.282, F13.982, F14.182, F14.282, F14.982, F15.182, F15.282, F15.982, F19.182, F19.282, F19.982)
hypersomnia due to a mental disorder (F51.13)
hypersomnia not due to a substance or known physiological condition (F51.1-)
primary hypersomnia (F51.11)
sleep apnea (G47.3-)

G47.10 Hypersomnia, unspecified
Hypersomnia NOS
G47.11 Idiopathic hypersomnia with long sleep time
Idiopathic hypersomnia NOS
G47.12 Idiopathic hypersomnia without long sleep time
G47.13 Recurrent hypersomnia
Kleine-Levin syndrome
Menstrual related hypersomnia
G47.14 Hypersomnia due to medical condition
Code also associated medical condition
G47.19 Other hypersomnia

+ **G47.2 Circadian rhythm sleep disorders**
Disorders of the sleep wake schedule
Inversion of nyctohemeral rhythm
Inversion of sleep rhythm
G47.20 Circadian rhythm sleep disorder, unspecified type
Sleep wake schedule disorder NOS
G47.21 Circadian rhythm sleep disorder, delayed sleep phase type
Delayed sleep phase syndrome
G47.22 Circadian rhythm sleep disorder, advanced sleep phase type
G47.23 Circadian rhythm sleep disorder, irregular sleep wake type
Irregular sleep-wake pattern
G47.24 Circadian rhythm sleep disorder, free running type
Circadian rhythm sleep disorder, non-24-hour sleep-wake type
G47.25 Circadian rhythm sleep disorder, jet lag type
G47.26 Circadian rhythm sleep disorder, shift work type
G47.27 Circadian rhythm sleep disorder in conditions classified elsewhere
Code first underlying condition
G47.29 Other circadian rhythm sleep disorder

+ **G47.3 Sleep apnea**
Code also any associated underlying condition
Excludes1: *apnea NOS (R06.81)*
Cheyne-Stokes breathing (R06.3)
pickwickian syndrome (E66.2)
sleep apnea of newborn (P28.3)
G47.30 Sleep apnea, unspecified
Sleep apnea NOS
G47.31 Primary central sleep apnea
Idiopathic central sleep apnea
G47.32 High altitude periodic breathing
G47.33 Obstructive sleep apnea (adult) (pediatric)
Obstructive sleep apnea hypopnea
Excludes1: *obstructive sleep apnea of newborn (P28.3)*
G47.34 Idiopathic sleep related nonobstructive alveolar hypoventilation
Sleep related hypoxia
G47.35 Congenital central alveolar hypoventilation syndrome
G47.36 Sleep related hypoventilation in conditions classified elsewhere
Sleep related hypoxemia in conditions classified elsewhere
Code first underlying condition
G47.37 Central sleep apnea in conditions classified elsewhere
Code first underlying condition
G47.39 Other sleep apnea

+ **G47.4 Narcolepsy and cataplexy**
+ **G47.41 Narcolepsy**
G47.411 Narcolepsy with cataplexy
G47.419 Narcolepsy without cataplexy
Narcolepsy NOS
+ **G47.42 Narcolepsy in conditions classified elsewhere**
Code first underlying condition
G47.421 Narcolepsy in conditions classified elsewhere with cataplexy
G47.429 Narcolepsy in conditions classified elsewhere without cataplexy

+ **G47.5 Parasomnia**
Excludes1: *alcohol induced parasomnia (F10.182, F10.282, F10.982)*
drug induced parasomnia (F11.182, F11.282, F11.982, F13.182, F13.282, F13.982, F14.182, F14.282, F14.982, F15.182, F15.282, F15.982, F19.182, F19.282, F19.982)
parasomnia not due to a substance or known physiological condition (F51.8)
G47.50 Parasomnia, unspecified
Parasomnia NOS
G47.51 Confusional arousals
G47.52 REM sleep behavior disorder
G47.53 Recurrent isolated sleep paralysis
G47.54 Parasomnia in conditions classified elsewhere
Code first underlying condition
G47.59 Other parasomnia

+ **G47.6 Sleep related movement disorders**
Excludes2: *restless legs syndrome (G25.81)*
G47.61 Periodic limb movement disorder
G47.62 Sleep related leg cramps
G47.63 Sleep related bruxism
Excludes1: *psychogenic bruxism (F45.8)*
G47.69 Other sleep related movement disorders

G47.8 Other sleep disorders
Other specified sleep-wake disorder
G47.9 Sleep disorder, unspecified
Sleep disorder NOS
Unspecified sleep-wake disorder

Nerve, nerve root and plexus disorders (G50-G59)

Excludes1: *current traumatic nerve, nerve root and plexus disorders - see Injury, nerve by body region*
neuralgia NOS (M79.2)
neuritis NOS (M79.2)
peripheral neuritis in pregnancy (O26.82-)
radiculitis NOS (M54.1-)

G50 Disorders of trigeminal nerve
Includes: disorders of 5th cranial nerve
G50.0 Trigeminal neuralgia
Syndrome of paroxysmal facial pain
Tic douloureux
G50.1 Atypical facial pain
G50.8 Other disorders of trigeminal nerve
G50.9 Disorder of trigeminal nerve, unspecified

G51 Facial nerve disorders
Includes: disorders of 7th cranial nerve
G51.0 Bell's palsy
Facial palsy
G51.1 Geniculate ganglionitis
Excludes1: *postherpetic geniculate ganglionitis (B02.21)*
G51.2 Melkersson's syndrome
Melkersson-Rosenthal syndrome
+ **G51.3 Clonic hemifacial spasm**
AHA CC: 4Q, 2018, 10
G51.31 Clonic hemifacial spasm, right
G51.32 Clonic hemifacial spasm, left
AHA CC: 4Q, 2018, 10
G51.33 Clonic hemifacial spasm, bilateral
G51.39 Clonic hemifacial spasm, unspecified
G51.4 Facial myokymia
G51.8 Other disorders of facial nerve
G51.9 Disorder of facial nerve, unspecified

G52 Disorders of other cranial nerves

Excludes2: *disorders of acoustic [8th] nerve (H93.3)*
disorders of optic [2nd] nerve (H46, H47.0)
paralytic strabismus due to nerve palsy (H49.0-H49.2)

G52.0 Disorders of olfactory nerve
Disorders of 1st cranial nerve

G52.1 Disorders of glossopharyngeal nerve
Disorder of 9th cranial nerve
Glossopharyngeal neuralgia

G52.2 Disorders of vagus nerve
Disorders of pneumogastric [10th] nerve

G52.3 Disorders of hypoglossal nerve
Disorders of 12th cranial nerve

G52.7 Disorders of multiple cranial nerves
Polyneuritis cranialis

G52.8 Disorders of other specified cranial nerves

G52.9 Cranial nerve disorder, unspecified

G53 Cranial nerve disorders in diseases classified elsewhere

Code first underlying disease, such as:
neoplasm (C00-D49)

Excludes1: *multiple cranial nerve palsy in sarcoidosis (D86.82)*
multiple cranial nerve palsy in syphilis (A52.15)
postherpetic geniculate ganglionitis (B02.21)
postherpetic trigeminal neuralgia (B02.22)

Valid 3-character code, no further characters required

G54 Nerve root and plexus disorders

Excludes1: *current traumatic nerve root and plexus disorders - see nerve injury by body region*
intervertebral disc disorders (M50-M51)
neuralgia or neuritis NOS (M79.2)
neuritis or radiculitis brachial NOS (M54.13)
neuritis or radiculitis lumbar NOS (M54.16)
neuritis or radiculitis lumbosacral NOS (M54.17)
neuritis or radiculitis thoracic NOS (M54.14)
radiculitis NOS (M54.10)
radiculopathy NOS (M54.10)
spondylosis (M47.-)

G54.0 Brachial plexus disorders
Thoracic outlet syndrome

G54.1 Lumbosacral plexus disorders

G54.2 Cervical root disorders, not elsewhere classified

G54.3 Thoracic root disorders, not elsewhere classified

G54.4 Lumbosacral root disorders, not elsewhere classified

G54.5 Neuralgic amyotrophy
Parsonage-Aldren-Turner syndrome
Shoulder-girdle neuritis
Excludes1: *neuralgic amyotrophy in diabetes mellitus (E08-E13 with .44)*

G54.6 Phantom limb syndrome with pain

G54.7 Phantom limb syndrome without pain
Phantom limb syndrome NOS

G54.8 Other nerve root and plexus disorders

G54.9 Nerve root and plexus disorder, unspecified

G55 Nerve root and plexus compressions in diseases classified elsewhere

Code first underlying disease, such as:
neoplasm (C00-D49)

Excludes1: *nerve root compression (due to) (in) ankylosing spondylitis (M45.-)*
nerve root compression (due to) (in) dorsopathies (M53.-, M54.-)
nerve root compression (due to) (in) intervertebral disc disorders (M50.1.-, M51.1.-)
nerve root compression (due to) (in) spondylopathies (M46.-, M48.-)
nerve root compression (due to) (in) spondylosis (M47.0-, M47.2-)

Valid 3-character code, no further characters required

G56 Mononeuropathies of upper limb

Excludes1: *current traumatic nerve disorder - see nerve injury by body region*

AHA CC: 4Q, 2016, 17-18

\+ **G56.0 Carpal tunnel syndrome**
G56.00 Carpal tunnel syndrome, unspecified upper limb
G56.01 Carpal tunnel syndrome, right upper limb
G56.02 Carpal tunnel syndrome, left upper limb
G56.03 Carpal tunnel syndrome, bilateral upper limbs

\+ **G56.1 Other lesions of median nerve**
G56.10 Other lesions of median nerve, unspecified upper limb
G56.11 Other lesions of median nerve, right upper limb
G56.12 Other lesions of median nerve, left upper limb
G56.13 Other lesions of median nerve, bilateral upper limbs

\+ **G56.2 Lesion of ulnar nerve**
Tardy ulnar nerve palsy
G56.20 Lesion of ulnar nerve, unspecified upper limb
G56.21 Lesion of ulnar nerve, right upper limb
G56.22 Lesion of ulnar nerve, left upper limb
G56.23 Lesion of ulnar nerve, bilateral upper limbs

\+ **G56.3 Lesion of radial nerve**
G56.30 Lesion of radial nerve, unspecified upper limb
G56.31 Lesion of radial nerve, right upper limb
G56.32 Lesion of radial nerve, left upper limb
G56.33 Lesion of radial nerve, bilateral upper limbs

\+ **G56.4 Causalgia of upper limb**
Complex regional pain syndrome II of upper limb
Excludes1: *complex regional pain syndrome I of lower limb (G90.52-)*
complex regional pain syndrome I of upper limb (G90.51-)
complex regional pain syndrome II of lower limb (G57.7-)
reflex sympathetic dystrophy of lower limb (G90.52-)
reflex sympathetic dystrophy of upper limb (G90.51-)
G56.40 Causalgia of unspecified upper limb
G56.41 Causalgia of right upper limb
G56.42 Causalgia of left upper limb
G56.43 Causalgia of bilateral upper limbs

\+ **G56.8 Other specified mononeuropathies of upper limb**
Interdigital neuroma of upper limb
G56.80 Other specified mononeuropathies of unspecified upper limb
G56.81 Other specified mononeuropathies of right upper limb
G56.82 Other specified mononeuropathies of left upper limb
G56.83 Other specified mononeuropathies of bilateral upper limbs

\+ **G56.9 Unspecified mononeuropathy of upper limb**
G56.90 Unspecified mononeuropathy of unspecified upper limb
G56.91 Unspecified mononeuropathy of right upper limb
G56.92 Unspecified mononeuropathy of left upper limb
G56.93 Unspecified mononeuropathy of bilateral upper limbs

G57 Mononeuropathies of lower limb

Excludes1: *current traumatic nerve disorder - see nerve injury by body region*

AHA CC: 4Q, 2016, 17-18

\+ **G57.0 Lesion of sciatic nerve**
Excludes1: *sciatica NOS (M54.3-)*
Excludes2: *sciatica attributed to intervertebral disc disorder (M51.1.-)*
G57.00 Lesion of sciatic nerve, unspecified lower limb
G57.01 Lesion of sciatic nerve, right lower limb
G57.02 Lesion of sciatic nerve, left lower limb
G57.03 Lesion of sciatic nerve, bilateral lower limbs

+ G57.1 **Meralgia paresthetica**
Lateral cutaneous nerve of thigh syndrome
G57.10 **Meralgia paresthetica, unspecified lower limb**
G57.11 **Meralgia paresthetica, right lower limb**
G57.12 **Meralgia paresthetica, left lower limb**
G57.13 **Meralgia paresthetica, bilateral lower limbs**

+ G57.2 **Lesion of femoral nerve**
G57.20 **Lesion of femoral nerve, unspecified lower limb**
G57.21 **Lesion of femoral nerve, right lower limb**
G57.22 **Lesion of femoral nerve, left lower limb**
G57.23 **Lesion of femoral nerve, bilateral lower limbs**

+ G57.3 **Lesion of lateral popliteal nerve**
Peroneal nerve palsy
G57.30 **Lesion of lateral popliteal nerve, unspecified lower limb**
G57.31 **Lesion of lateral popliteal nerve, right lower limb**
AHA CC: 3Q, 2020, 12
G57.32 **Lesion of lateral popliteal nerve, left lower limb**
G57.33 **Lesion of lateral popliteal nerve, bilateral lower limbs**

+ G57.4 **Lesion of medial popliteal nerve**
G57.40 **Lesion of medial popliteal nerve, unspecified lower limb**
G57.41 **Lesion of medial popliteal nerve, right lower limb**
G57.42 **Lesion of medial popliteal nerve, left lower limb**
G57.43 **Lesion of medial popliteal nerve, bilateral lower limbs**

+ G57.5 **Tarsal tunnel syndrome**
G57.50 **Tarsal tunnel syndrome, unspecified lower limb**
G57.51 **Tarsal tunnel syndrome, right lower limb**
G57.52 **Tarsal tunnel syndrome, left lower limb**
G57.53 **Tarsal tunnel syndrome, bilateral lower limbs**

+ G57.6 **Lesion of plantar nerve**
Morton's metatarsalgia
G57.60 **Lesion of plantar nerve, unspecified lower limb**
G57.61 **Lesion of plantar nerve, right lower limb**
G57.62 **Lesion of plantar nerve, left lower limb**
G57.63 **Lesion of plantar nerve, bilateral lower limbs**

+ G57.7 **Causalgia of lower limb**
Complex regional pain syndrome II of lower limb
Excludes1: *complex regional pain syndrome I of lower limb (G90.52-)*
complex regional pain syndrome I of upper limb (G90.51-)
complex regional pain syndrome II of upper limb (G56.4-)
reflex sympathetic dystrophy of lower limb (G90.52-)
reflex sympathetic dystrophy of upper limb (G90.51-)
G57.70 **Causalgia of unspecified lower limb**
G57.71 **Causalgia of right lower limb**
G57.72 **Causalgia of left lower limb**
G57.73 **Causalgia of bilateral lower limbs**

+ G57.8 **Other specified mononeuropathies of lower limb**
Interdigital neuroma of lower limb
G57.80 **Other specified mononeuropathies of unspecified lower limb**
G57.81 **Other specified mononeuropathies of right lower limb**
G57.82 **Other specified mononeuropathies of left lower limb**
G57.83 **Other specified mononeuropathies of bilateral lower limbs**

+ G57.9 **Unspecified mononeuropathy of lower limb**
G57.90 **Unspecified mononeuropathy of unspecified lower limb**
G57.91 **Unspecified mononeuropathy of right lower limb**
G57.92 **Unspecified mononeuropathy of left lower limb**
G57.93 **Unspecified mononeuropathy of bilateral lower limbs**

G58 Other mononeuropathies
G58.0 **Intercostal neuropathy**
G58.7 **Mononeuritis multiplex**
G58.8 **Other specified mononeuropathies**
G58.9 **Mononeuropathy, unspecified**

G59 Mononeuropathy in diseases classified elsewhere
Code first underlying disease
Excludes1: *diabetic mononeuropathy (E08-E13 with .41)*
syphilitic nerve paralysis (A52.19)
syphilitic neuritis (A52.15)
tuberculous mononeuropathy (A17.83)
Valid 3-character code, no further characters required

Polyneuropathies and other disorders of the peripheral nervous system (G60-G65)

Excludes1: *neuralgia NOS (M79.2)*
neuritis NOS (M79.2)
peripheral neuritis in pregnancy (O26.82-)
radiculitis NOS (M54.10)

G60 Hereditary and idiopathic neuropathy
G60.0 **Hereditary motor and sensory neuropathy**
Charcot-Marie-Tooth disease
Déjérine-Sottas disease
Hereditary motor and sensory neuropathy, types I-IV
Hypertrophic neuropathy of infancy
Peroneal muscular atrophy (axonal type) (hypertrophic type)
Roussy-Levy syndrome
CC G60.1 **Refsum's disease**
Infantile Refsum disease
G60.2 **Neuropathy in association with hereditary ataxia**
G60.3 **Idiopathic progressive neuropathy**
G60.8 **Other hereditary and idiopathic neuropathies**
Dominantly inherited sensory neuropathy
Morvan's disease
Nelaton's syndrome
Recessively inherited sensory neuropathy
G60.9 **Hereditary and idiopathic neuropathy, unspecified**

G61 Inflammatory polyneuropathy
CC G61.0 **Guillain-Barre syndrome**
Acute (post-)infective polyneuritis
Miller Fisher Syndrome
AHA CC: 2Q, 2014, 4; 3Q, 2020, 12
G61.1 **Serum neuropathy**
Use additional code for adverse effect, if applicable, to identify serum (T50.-)
G61.8 **Other inflammatory polyneuropathies**
CC G61.81 **Chronic inflammatory demyelinating polyneuritis**
G61.82 **Multifocal motor neuropathy**
MMN
AHA CC: 4Q, 2016, 18
G61.89 **Other inflammatory polyneuropathies**
G61.9 **Inflammatory polyneuropathy, unspecified**

G62 Other and unspecified polyneuropathies
G62.0 **Drug-induced polyneuropathy**
Use additional code for adverse effect, if applicable, to identify drug (T36-T50 with fifth or sixth character 5)
G62.1 **Alcoholic polyneuropathy**
AHA CC: 3Q, 2019, 8
G62.2 **Polyneuropathy due to other toxic agents**
Code first (T51-T65) to identify toxic agent
+ G62.8 **Other specified polyneuropathies**
CC G62.81 **Critical illness polyneuropathy**
Acute motor neuropathy
G62.82 **Radiation-induced polyneuropathy**
Use additional external cause code (W88-W90, X39.0-) to identify cause
G62.89 **Other specified polyneuropathies**
AHA CC: 2Q, 2016, 11
G62.9 **Polyneuropathy, unspecified**
Neuropathy NOS

G63 Polyneuropathy in diseases classified elsewhere

Code first underlying disease, such as:
amyloidosis (E85.-)
endocrine disease, except diabetes (E00-E07, E15-E16, E20-E34)
metabolic diseases (E70-E88)
neoplasm (C00-D49)
nutritional deficiency (E40-E64)

Excludes1: *polyneuropathy (in):*
diabetes mellitus (E08-E13 with .42)
diphtheria (A36.83)
infectious mononucleosis complicated by polyneuropathy (B27.0-B27.9 with fifth character 1)
Lyme disease (A69.22)
mumps (B26.84)
postherpetic (B02.23)
rheumatoid arthritis (M05.5-)
scleroderma (M34.83)
systemic lupus erythematosus (M32.19)

AHA CC: 4Q, 2012, 99-101; 1Q, 2021, 7
Valid 3-character code, no further characters required

G64 Other disorders of peripheral nervous system

Disorder of peripheral nervous system NOS
Valid 3-character code, no further characters required

G65 Sequelae of inflammatory and toxic polyneuropathies

Code first condition resulting from (sequela) of inflammatory and toxic polyneuropathies

G65.0 Sequelae of Guillain-Barré syndrome
G65.1 Sequelae of other inflammatory polyneuropathy
G65.2 Sequelae of toxic polyneuropathy

Diseases of myoneural junction and muscle (G70-G73)

G70 Myasthenia gravis and other myoneural disorders

Excludes1: *botulism (A05.1, A48.51-A48.52)*
transient neonatal myasthenia gravis (P94.0)

\+ **G70.0 Myasthenia gravis**
G70.00 Myasthenia gravis without (acute) exacerbation
Myasthenia gravis NOS
MCC **G70.01 Myasthenia gravis with (acute) exacerbation**
Myasthenia gravis in crisis
G70.1 Toxic myoneural disorders
Code first (T51-T65) to identify toxic agent
G70.2 Congenital and developmental myasthenia
\+ **G70.8 Other specified myoneural disorders**
CC **G70.80 Lambert-Eaton syndrome, unspecified**
Lambert-Eaton syndrome NOS
CC **G70.81 Lambert-Eaton syndrome in disease classified elsewhere**
Code first underlying disease
Excludes1: *Lambert-Eaton syndrome in neoplastic disease (G73.1)*
G70.89 Other specified myoneural disorders
G70.9 Myoneural disorder, unspecified

G71 Primary disorders of muscles

Excludes2: *arthrogryposis multiplex congenita (Q74.3)*
metabolic disorders (E70-E88)
myositis (M60.-)

\+ **G71.0 Muscular dystrophy**
AHA CC: 4Q, 2018, 11
G71.00 Muscular dystrophy, unspecified
G71.01 Duchenne or Becker muscular dystrophy
Autosomal recessive, childhood type, muscular dystrophy resembling Duchenne or Becker muscular dystrophy
Benign [Becker] muscular dystrophy
Severe [Duchenne] muscular dystrophy
G71.02 Facioscapulohumeral muscular dystrophy
Scapulohumeral muscular dystrophy
AHA CC: 4Q, 2018, 12-13
G71.09 Other specified muscular dystrophies
Benign scapuloperoneal muscular dystrophy with early contractures [Emery-Dreifuss]
Congenital muscular dystrophy NOS
Congenital muscular dystrophy with specific morphological abnormalities of the muscle fiber
Distal muscular dystrophy
Limb-girdle muscular dystrophy
Ocular muscular dystrophy
Oculopharyngeal muscular dystrophy
Scapuloperoneal muscular dystrophy

\+ **G71.1 Myotonic disorders**
G71.11 Myotonic muscular dystrophy
Dystrophia myotonica [Steinert]
Myotonia atrophica
Myotonic dystrophy
Proximal myotonic myopathy (PROMM)
Steinert disease
G71.12 Myotonia congenita
Acetazolamide responsive myotonia congenita
Dominant myotonia congenita [Thomsen disease]
Myotonia levior
Recessive myotonia congenita [Becker disease]
G71.13 Myotonic chondrodystrophy
Chondrodystrophic myotonia
Congenital myotonic chondrodystrophy
Schwartz-Jampel disease
G71.14 Drug induced myotonia
Use additional code for adverse effect, if applicable, to identify drug (T36-T50 with fifth or sixth character 5)
G71.19 Other specified myotonic disorders
Myotonia fluctuans
Myotonia permanens
Neuromyotonia [Isaacs]
Paramyotonia congenita (of von Eulenburg)
Pseudomyotonia
Symptomatic myotonia

\+ **G71.2 Congenital myopathies**
Excludes2: *arthrogryposis multiplex congenita (Q74.3)*
AHA CC: 4Q, 2020, 19-21
CC **G71.20 Congenital myopathy, unspecified**
CC **G71.21 Nemaline myopathy**
\+ **G71.22 Centronuclear myopathy**
CC **G71.220 X-linked myotubular myopathy**
Myotubular (centronuclear) myopathy
CC **G71.228 Other centronuclear myopathy**
Autosomal centronuclear myopathy
Autosomal dominant centronuclear myopathy
Autosomal recessive centronuclear myopathy
Centronuclear myopathy, NOS
CC **G71.29 Other congenital myopathy**
Central core disease
Minicore disease
Multicore disease
Multiminicore disease

G71.3 Mitochondrial myopathy, not elsewhere classified
Excludes1: *Kearns-Sayre syndrome (H49.81)*
Leber's disease (H47.21)
Leigh's encephalopathy (G31.82)
mitochondrial metabolism disorders (E88.4.-)
Reye's syndrome (G93.7)

G71.8 Other primary disorders of muscles

G71.9 Primary disorder of muscle, unspecified
Hereditary myopathy NOS

G72 Other and unspecified myopathies
Excludes1: *arthrogryposis multiplex congenita (Q74.3)*
dermatopolymyositis (M33.-)
ischemic infarction of muscle (M62.2-)
myositis (M60.-)
polymyositis (M33.2.-)

CC **G72.0 Drug-induced myopathy**
Use additional code for adverse effect, if applicable, to identify drug (T36-T50 with fifth or sixth character 5)

CC **G72.1 Alcoholic myopathy**
Use additional code to identify alcoholism (F10.-)

CC **G72.2 Myopathy due to other toxic agents**
Code first (T51-T65) to identify toxic agent

G72.3 Periodic paralysis
Familial periodic paralysis
Hyperkalemic periodic paralysis (familial)
Hypokalemic periodic paralysis (familial)
Myotonic periodic paralysis (familial)
Normokalemic paralysis (familial)
Potassium sensitive periodic paralysis
Excludes1: *paramyotonia congenita (of von Eulenburg) (G71.19)*

\+ **G72.4 Inflammatory and immune myopathies, not elsewhere classified**
G72.41 Inclusion body myositis [IBM]
G72.49 Other inflammatory and immune myopathies, not elsewhere classified
Inflammatory myopathy NOS

\+ **G72.8 Other specified myopathies**
CC **G72.81 Critical illness myopathy**
Acute necrotizing myopathy
Acute quadriplegic myopathy
Intensive care (ICU) myopathy
Myopathy of critical illness
AHA CC: 3Q, 2020, 12
G72.89 Other specified myopathies

G72.9 Myopathy, unspecified

G73 Disorders of myoneural junction and muscle in diseases classified elsewhere

CC **G73.1 Lambert-Eaton syndrome in neoplastic disease**
Code first underlying neoplasm (C00-D49)
Excludes1: *Lambert-Eaton syndrome not associated with neoplasm (G70.80-G70.81)*

CC **G73.3 Myasthenic syndromes in other diseases classified elsewhere**
Code first underlying disease, such as:
neoplasm (C00-D49)
thyrotoxicosis (E05.-)

G73.7 Myopathy in diseases classified elsewhere
Code first underlying disease, such as:
hyperparathyroidism (E21.0, E21.3)
hypoparathyroidism (E20.-)
glycogen storage disease (E74.0)
lipid storage disorders (E75.-)
Excludes1: *myopathy in:*
rheumatoid arthritis (M05.32)
sarcoidosis (D86.87)
scleroderma (M34.82)
Sjögren syndrome (M35.03)
systemic lupus erythematosus (M32.19)

Cerebral palsy and other paralytic syndromes (G80-G83)

G80 Cerebral palsy
Excludes1: *hereditary spastic paraplegia (G11.4)*

MCC **G80.0 Spastic quadriplegic cerebral palsy**
Congenital spastic paralysis (cerebral)

CC **G80.1 Spastic diplegic cerebral palsy**
Spastic cerebral palsy NOS

CC **G80.2 Spastic hemiplegic cerebral palsy**

CC **G80.3 Athetoid cerebral palsy**
Double athetosis (syndrome)
Dyskinetic cerebral palsy
Dystonic cerebral palsy
Vogt disease

G80.4 Ataxic cerebral palsy

G80.8 Other cerebral palsy
Mixed cerebral palsy syndromes

G80.9 Cerebral palsy, unspecified
Cerebral palsy NOS

G81 Hemiplegia and hemiparesis
NOTE This category is to be used only when hemiplegia (complete) (incomplete) is reported without further specification, or is stated to be old or longstanding but of unspecified cause. The category is also for use in multiple coding to identify these types of hemiplegia resulting from any cause.
Excludes1: *congenital cerebral palsy (G80.-)*
hemiplegia and hemiparesis due to sequela of cerebrovascular disease (I69.05-, I69.15-, I69.25-, I69.35-, I69.85-, I69.95-)
Review coding guideline C.6.a

\+ **G81.0 Flaccid hemiplegia**
CC **G81.00 Flaccid hemiplegia affecting unspecified side**
CC **G81.01 Flaccid hemiplegia affecting right dominant side**
CC **G81.02 Flaccid hemiplegia affecting left dominant side**
CC **G81.03 Flaccid hemiplegia affecting right nondominant side**
CC **G81.04 Flaccid hemiplegia affecting left nondominant side**

\+ **G81.1 Spastic hemiplegia**
CC **G81.10 Spastic hemiplegia affecting unspecified side**
CC **G81.11 Spastic hemiplegia affecting right dominant side**
CC **G81.12 Spastic hemiplegia affecting left dominant side**
CC **G81.13 Spastic hemiplegia affecting right nondominant side**
CC **G81.14 Spastic hemiplegia affecting left nondominant side**

\+ **G81.9 Hemiplegia, unspecified**
CC **G81.90 Hemiplegia, unspecified affecting unspecified side**
CC **G81.91 Hemiplegia, unspecified affecting right dominant side**
CC **G81.92 Hemiplegia, unspecified affecting left dominant side**
CC **G81.93 Hemiplegia, unspecified affecting right nondominant side**
CC **G81.94 Hemiplegia, unspecified affecting left nondominant side**
AHA CC: 1Q, 2015, 26

G82 Paraplegia (paraparesis) and quadriplegia (quadriparesis)

NOTE This category is to be used only when the listed conditions are reported without further specification, or are stated to be old or longstanding but of unspecified cause. The category is also for use in multiple coding to identify these conditions resulting from any cause

Excludes1: *congenital cerebral palsy (G80.-)*
functional quadriplegia (R53.2)
hysterical paralysis (F44.4)

\+ **G82.2 Paraplegia**
Paralysis of both lower limbs NOS
Paraparesis (lower) NOS
Paraplegia (lower) NOS

CC **G82.20 Paraplegia, unspecified**
AHA CC: 3Q, 2017, 3

CC **G82.21 Paraplegia, complete**
CC **G82.22 Paraplegia, incomplete**

\+ **G82.5 Quadriplegia**
MCC **G82.50 Quadriplegia, unspecified**
MCC **G82.51 Quadriplegia, C1-C4 complete**
MCC **G82.52 Quadriplegia, C1-C4 incomplete**
MCC **G82.53 Quadriplegia, C5-C7 complete**
MCC **G82.54 Quadriplegia, C5-C7 incomplete**

G83 Other paralytic syndromes

NOTE This category is to be used only when the listed conditions are reported without further specification, or are stated to be old or longstanding but of unspecified cause. The category is also for use in multiple coding to identify these conditions resulting from any cause.

Includes: paralysis (complete) (incomplete), except as in G80-G82

CC **G83.0 Diplegia of upper limbs**
Diplegia (upper)
Paralysis of both upper limbs

\+ **G83.1 Monoplegia of lower limb**
Paralysis of lower limb
Excludes1: *monoplegia of lower limbs due to sequela of cerebrovascular disease (I69.04-, I69.14-, I69.24-, I69.34-, I69.84-, I69.94-)*
Review coding guideline C.6.a

G83.10 Monoplegia of lower limb affecting unspecified side
G83.11 Monoplegia of lower limb affecting right dominant side
G83.12 Monoplegia of lower limb affecting left dominant side
G83.13 Monoplegia of lower limb affecting right nondominant side
G83.14 Monoplegia of lower limb affecting left nondominant side

\+ **G83.2 Monoplegia of upper limb**
Paralysis of upper limb
Excludes1: *monoplegia of upper limbs due to sequela of cerebrovascular disease (I69.03-, I69.13-, I69.23-, I69.33-, I69.83-, I69.93-)*
Review coding guideline C.6.a

G83.20 Monoplegia of upper limb affecting unspecified side
G83.21 Monoplegia of upper limb affecting right dominant side
G83.22 Monoplegia of upper limb affecting left dominant side
G83.23 Monoplegia of upper limb affecting right nondominant side
G83.24 Monoplegia of upper limb affecting left nondominant side

\+ **G83.3 Monoplegia, unspecified**
Review coding guideline C.6.a

G83.30 Monoplegia, unspecified affecting unspecified side
G83.31 Monoplegia, unspecified affecting right dominant side
G83.32 Monoplegia, unspecified affecting left dominant side
G83.33 Monoplegia, unspecified affecting right nondominant side
G83.34 Monoplegia, unspecified affecting left nondominant side

CC **G83.4 Cauda equina syndrome**
Neurogenic bladder due to cauda equina syndrome
Excludes1: *cord bladder NOS (G95.89)*
neurogenic bladder NOS (N31.9)
AHA CC: 3Q, 2020, 24

MCC **G83.5 Locked-in state**

\+ **G83.8 Other specified paralytic syndromes**
Excludes1: *paralytic syndromes due to current spinal cord injury-code to spinal cord injury (S14, S24, S34)*

G83.81 Brown-Séquard syndrome
G83.82 Anterior cord syndrome
G83.83 Posterior cord syndrome
G83.84 Todd's paralysis (postepileptic)
G83.89 Other specified paralytic syndromes

G83.9 Paralytic syndrome, unspecified

Other disorders of the nervous system (G89-G99)

G89 Pain, not elsewhere classified

Code also related psychological factors associated with pain (F45.42)

Excludes1: *generalized pain NOS (R52)*
pain disorders exclusively related to psychological factors (F45.41)
pain NOS (R52)

Excludes2: *atypical face pain (G50.1)*
headache syndromes (G44.-)
localized pain, unspecified type - code to pain by site, such as:
abdomen pain (R10.-)
back pain (M54.9)
breast pain (N64.4)
chest pain (R07.1-R07.9)
ear pain (H92.0-)
eye pain (H57.1)
headache (R51.9)
joint pain (M25.5-)
limb pain (M79.6-)
lumbar region pain (M54.5-)
painful urination (R30.9)
pelvic and perineal pain (R10.2)
shoulder pain (M25.51-)
spine pain (M54.-)
throat pain (R07.0)
tongue pain (K14.6)
tooth pain (K08.8)
renal colic (N23)
migraines (G43.-)
myalgia (M79.1-)
pain from prosthetic devices, implants, and grafts (T82.84, T83.84, T84.84, T85.84-)
phantom limb syndrome with pain (G54.6)
vulvar vestibulitis (N94.810)
vulvodynia (N94.81-)

Review coding guideline C.5.a
Review coding guidelines C.6.b.1 and C.6.b.3
Review coding guideline C.19.g.2

G89.0 Central pain syndrome
Déjérine-Roussy syndrome
Myelopathic pain syndrome
Thalamic pain syndrome (hyperesthetic)
Review coding guideline C.6.b.6

\+ **G89.1 Acute pain, not elsewhere classified**
G89.11 Acute pain due to trauma
G89.12 Acute post-thoracotomy pain
Post-thoracotomy pain NOS
G89.18 Other acute postprocedural pain
Postoperative pain NOS
Postprocedural pain NOS

+ **G89.2 Chronic pain, not elsewhere classified**
Excludes1: *causalgia, lower limb (G57.7-)*
causalgia, upper limb (G56.4-)
central pain syndrome (G89.0)
chronic pain syndrome (G89.4)
complex regional pain syndrome II, lower limb (G57.7-)
complex regional pain syndrome II, upper limb (G56.4-)
neoplasm related chronic pain (G89.3)
reflex sympathetic dystrophy (G90.5-)
Review coding guideline C.6.b.4
G89.21 Chronic pain due to trauma
G89.22 Chronic post-thoracotomy pain
G89.28 Other chronic postprocedural pain
Other chronic postoperative pain
G89.29 Other chronic pain
G89.3 Neoplasm related pain (acute) (chronic)
Cancer associated pain
Pain due to malignancy (primary) (secondary)
Tumor associated pain
Review coding guideline C.6.b.5
G89.4 Chronic pain syndrome
Chronic pain associated with significant psychosocial dysfunction
Review coding guideline C.6.b.6

G90 Disorders of autonomic nervous system
Excludes1: *dysfunction of the autonomic nervous system due to alcohol (G31.2)*
+ **G90.0 Idiopathic peripheral autonomic neuropathy**
G90.01 Carotid sinus syncope
Carotid sinus syndrome
G90.09 Other idiopathic peripheral autonomic neuropathy
Idiopathic peripheral autonomic neuropathy NOS
G90.1 Familial dysautonomia [Riley-Day]
G90.2 Horner's syndrome
Bernard(-Horner) syndrome
Cervical sympathetic dystrophy or paralysis
CC **G90.3 Multi-system degeneration of the autonomic nervous system**
Neurogenic orthostatic hypotension [Shy-Drager]
Excludes1: *orthostatic hypotension NOS (I95.1)*
G90.4 Autonomic dysreflexia
Use additional code to identify the cause, such as:
fecal impaction (K56.41)
pressure ulcer (pressure area) (L89.-)
urinary tract infection (N39.0)
+ **G90.5 Complex regional pain syndrome I (CRPS I)**
Reflex sympathetic dystrophy
Excludes1: *causalgia of lower limb (G57.7-)*
causalgia of upper limb (G56.4-)
complex regional pain syndrome II of lower limb (G57.7-)
complex regional pain syndrome II of upper limb (G56.4-)
CC **G90.50 Complex regional pain syndrome I, unspecified**
+ **G90.51 Complex regional pain syndrome I of upper limb**
CC **G90.511 Complex regional pain syndrome I of right upper limb**
CC **G90.512 Complex regional pain syndrome I of left upper limb**
CC **G90.513 Complex regional pain syndrome I of upper limb, bilateral**
CC **G90.519 Complex regional pain syndrome I of unspecified upper limb**
+ **G90.52 Complex regional pain syndrome I of lower limb**
CC **G90.521 Complex regional pain syndrome I of right lower limb**
CC **G90.522 Complex regional pain syndrome I of left lower limb**
CC **G90.523 Complex regional pain syndrome I of lower limb, bilateral**
CC **G90.529 Complex regional pain syndrome I of unspecified lower limb**
CC **G90.59 Complex regional pain syndrome I of other specified site**
G90.8 Other disorders of autonomic nervous system
G90.9 Disorder of the autonomic nervous system, unspecified

G91 Hydrocephalus
Includes: acquired hydrocephalus
Excludes1: *Arnold-Chiari syndrome with hydrocephalus (Q07.-)*
congenital hydrocephalus (Q03.-)
spina bifida with hydrocephalus (Q05.-)
CC **G91.0 Communicating hydrocephalus**
Secondary normal pressure hydrocephalus
CC **G91.1 Obstructive hydrocephalus**
CC **G91.2 (Idiopathic) normal pressure hydrocephalus**
Normal pressure hydrocephalus NOS
CC **G91.3 Post-traumatic hydrocephalus, unspecified**
G91.4 Hydrocephalus in diseases classified elsewhere
Code first underlying condition, such as:
congenital syphilis (A50.4-)
neoplasm (C00-D49)
plasminogen deficiency (E88.02)
Excludes1: *hydrocephalus due to congenital toxoplasmosis (P37.1)*
AHA CC: 3Q, 2014, 3-4
CC **G91.8 Other hydrocephalus**
CC **G91.9 Hydrocephalus, unspecified**

G92 Toxic encephalopathy
AHA CC: 1Q, 2017, 39-40; 4Q, 2020, 14; 1Q, 2021, 13
+ **G92.0 Immune effector cell-associated neurotoxicity syndrome**
Code first underlying cause such as:
complications of immune effector cellular therapy (T80.82)
Code also associated signs and symptoms, such as seizures and cerebral edema
Code also, if applicable,
cerebral edema (G93.6)
unspecified convulsions (R56.9)
G92.00 Immune effector cell-associated neurotoxicity syndrome, grade unspecified
ICANS, grade unspecified
G92.01 Immune effector cell-associated neurotoxicity syndrome, grade 1
ICANS, grade 1
G92.02 Immune effector cell-associated neurotoxicity syndrome, grade 2
ICANS, grade 2
CC **G92.03 Immune effector cell-associated neurotoxicity syndrome, grade 3**
ICANS, grade 3
CC **G92.04 Immune effector cell-associated neurotoxicity syndrome, grade 4**
ICANS, grade 4
CC **G92.05 Immune effector cell-associated neurotoxicity syndrome, grade 5**
ICANS, grade 5
MCC **G92.8 Other toxic encephalopathy**
Toxic encephalitis
Toxic metabolic encephalopathy
Code first poisoning due to drug or toxin, if applicable, (T36-T65 with fifth or sixth character 1-4 or 6)
Use additional code for adverse effect, if applicable, to identify drug (T36-T50 with fifth or sixth character 5)
MCC **G92.9 Unspecified toxic encephalopathy**
Code first poisoning due to drug or toxin, if applicable, (T36-T65 with fifth or sixth character 1-4 or 6)
Use additional code for adverse effect, if applicable, to identify drug (T36-T50 with fifth or sixth character 5)

G93 Other disorders of brain

G93.0 Cerebral cysts
Arachnoid cyst
Porencephalic cyst, acquired
Excludes1: *acquired periventricular cysts of newborn (P91.1)*
congenital cerebral cysts (Q04.6)

CC **G93.1 Anoxic brain damage, not elsewhere classified**
Excludes1: *cerebral anoxia due to anesthesia during labor and delivery (O74.3)*
cerebral anoxia due to anesthesia during the puerperium (O89.2)
neonatal anoxia (P84)

G93.2 Benign intracranial hypertension
Pseudotumor
Excludes1: *hypertensive encephalopathy (I67.4)*
obstructive hydrocephalus (G91.1)

G93.3 Postviral fatigue syndrome
Benign myalgic encephalomyelitis
Excludes1: *chronic fatigue syndrome NOS (R53.82)*

+ **G93.4 Other and unspecified encephalopathy**
Excludes1: *alcoholic encephalopathy (G31.2)*
encephalopathy in diseases classified elsewhere (G94)
hypertensive encephalopathy (I67.4)
Excludes2: *toxic (metabolic) encephalopathy (G92.8)*
AHA CC: 2Q, 2017, 8-9

CC **G93.40 Encephalopathy, unspecified**

MCC **G93.41 Metabolic encephalopathy**
Septic encephalopathy
AHA CC: 3Q, 2015, 21; 3Q, 2016, 42

CC **G93.49 Other encephalopathy**
Encephalopathy NEC
AHA CC: 2Q, 2017, 9; 2Q, 2018, 22, 25; 4Q, 2018, 16; 2Q, 2021, 3-4

MCC **G93.5 Compression of brain**
Arnold-Chiari type 1 compression of brain
Compression of brain (stem)
Herniation of brain (stem)
Excludes1: *traumatic compression of brain (S06.A-)*
AHA CC: 2Q, 2020, 31

MCC **G93.6 Cerebral edema**
Excludes1: *cerebral edema due to birth injury (P11.0)*
traumatic cerebral edema (S06.1-)

• MCC **G93.7 Reye's syndrome**
Code first poisoning due to salicylates, if applicable (T39.0-, with sixth character 1-4)
Use additional code for adverse effect due to salicylates, if applicable (T39.0-, with sixth character 5)

+ **G93.8 Other specified disorders of brain**

G93.81 Temporal sclerosis
Hippocampal sclerosis
Mesial temporal sclerosis

MCC **G93.82 Brain death**

G93.89 Other specified disorders of brain
Postradiation encephalopathy
AHA CC: 4Q, 2016, 4-7; 3Q, 2019, 8-9; 2Q, 2020, 24

G93.9 Disorder of brain, unspecified

G94 Other disorders of brain in diseases classified elsewhere
Code first underlying disease
Excludes1: *encephalopathy in congenital syphilis (A50.49)*
encephalopathy in influenza (J09.X9, J10.81, J11.81)
encephalopathy in syphilis (A52.19)
hydrocephalus in diseases classified elsewhere (G91.4)
AHA CC: 2Q, 2017, 8-9
Valid 3-character code, no further characters required

G95 Other and unspecified diseases of spinal cord
Excludes2: *myelitis (G04.-)*

CC **G95.0 Syringomyelia and syringobulbia**

+ **G95.1 Vascular myelopathies**
Excludes2: *intraspinal phlebitis and thrombophlebitis, except non-pyogenic (G08)*

MCC **G95.11 Acute infarction of spinal cord (embolic) (nonembolic)**
Anoxia of spinal cord
Arterial thrombosis of spinal cord

MCC **G95.19 Other vascular myelopathies**
Edema of spinal cord
Hematomyelia
Nonpyogenic intraspinal phlebitis and thrombophlebitis
Subacute necrotic myelopathy

+ **G95.2 Other and unspecified cord compression**

CC **G95.20 Unspecified cord compression**

CC **G95.29 Other cord compression**

+ **G95.8 Other specified diseases of spinal cord**
Excludes1: *neurogenic bladder NOS (N31.9)*
neurogenic bladder due to cauda equina syndrome (G83.4)
neuromuscular dysfunction of bladder without spinal cord lesion (N31.-)

CC **G95.81 Conus medullaris syndrome**

CC **G95.89 Other specified diseases of spinal cord**
Cord bladder NOS
Drug-induced myelopathy
Radiation-induced myelopathy
Excludes1: *myelopathy NOS (G95.9)*

CC **G95.9 Disease of spinal cord, unspecified**
Myelopathy NOS

G96 Other disorders of central nervous system

+ **G96.0 Cerebrospinal fluid leak**
Excludes1: *cerebrospinal fluid leak from spinal puncture (G97.0)*
Code also if applicable:
intracranial hypotension (G96.81-)
AHA CC: 2Q, 2018, 13; 4Q, 2020, 21-22

CC **G96.00 Cerebrospinal fluid leak, unspecified**
Code also if applicable:
head injury (S00.- to S09.-)

CC **G96.01 Cranial cerebrospinal fluid leak, spontaneous**
Otorrhea due to spontaneous cerebrospinal fluid CSF leak
Rhinorrhea due to spontaneous cerebrospinal fluid CSF leak
Spontaneous cerebrospinal fluid leak from skull base

CC **G96.02 Spinal cerebrospinal fluid leak, spontaneous**
Spontaneous cerebrospinal fluid leak from spine

CC **G96.08 Other cranial cerebrospinal fluid leak**
Postoperative cranial cerebrospinal fluid leak
Traumatic cranial cerebrospinal fluid leak
Code also if applicable:
head injury (S00.- to S09.-)

CC **G96.09 Other spinal cerebrospinal fluid leak**
Other spinal CSF leak
Postoperative spinal cerebrospinal fluid leak
Traumatic spinal cerebrospinal fluid leak
Code also if applicable:
head injury (S00.- to S09.-)

+ **G96.1 Disorders of meninges, not elsewhere classified**

CC **G96.11 Dural tear**
Excludes1: *accidental puncture or laceration of dura during a procedure (G97.41)*
Code also intracranial hypotension, if applicable (G96.81-)
AHA CC: 4Q, 2014, 24

G96.12 Meningeal adhesions (cerebral) (spinal)

+ **G96.19 Other disorders of meninges, not elsewhere classified**
AHA CC: 4Q, 2020, 22
G96.191 Perineural cyst
Cervical nerve root cyst
Lumbar nerve root cyst
Sacral nerve root cyst
Tarlov cyst
Thoracic nerve root cyst
G96.198 Other disorders of meninges, not elsewhere classified

+ **G96.8 Other specified disorders of central nervous system**
+ **G96.81 Intracranial hypotension**
Code also any associated diagnoses, such as:
Brachial amyotrophy (G54.5)
Cerebrospinal fluid leak from spine (G96.02)
Cranial nerve disorders in diseases classified elsewhere (G53)
Nerve root and compressions in diseases classified elsewhere (G55)
Nonpyogenic thrombosis of intracranial venous system (I67.6)
Nontraumatic intracerebral hemorrhage (I61.-)
Nontraumatic subdural hemorrhage (I62.0-)
Other and unspecified cord compression (G95.2-)
Other secondary parkinsonism (G21.8)
Reversible cerebrovascular vasoconstriction syndrome (I67.841)
Spinal cord herniation (G95.89)
Stroke (I63.-)
Syringomyelia (G95.0)
AHA CC: 4Q, 2020, 23
G96.810 Intracranial hypotension, unspecified
G96.811 Intracranial hypotension, spontaneous
AHA CC: 4Q, 2020, 24
G96.819 Other intracranial hypotension
G96.89 Other specified disorders of central nervous system
G96.9 Disorder of central nervous system, unspecified

G97 Intraoperative and postprocedural complications and disorders of nervous system, not elsewhere classified

Excludes2: *intraoperative and postprocedural cerebrovascular infarction (I97.81-, I97.82-)*
AHA CC: 4Q, 2016, 9-10

CC **G97.0 Cerebrospinal fluid leak from spinal puncture**
Code also any associated diagnoses or complications, such as:
intracranial hypotension following a procedure (G97.83-G97.84)
G97.1 Other reaction to spinal and lumbar puncture
Headache due to lumbar puncture
Other reaction to spinal dural puncture
Code also, if applicable, any associated headache with orthostatic component (R51.0)
CC **G97.2 Intracranial hypotension following ventricular shunting**
Code also any associated diagnoses or complications
+ **G97.3 Intraoperative hemorrhage and hematoma of a nervous system organ or structure complicating a procedure**
Excludes1: *intraoperative hemorrhage and hematoma of a nervous system organ or structure due to accidental puncture and laceration during a procedure (G97.4-)*
CC **G97.31 Intraoperative hemorrhage and hematoma of a nervous system organ or structure complicating a nervous system procedure**
CC **G97.32 Intraoperative hemorrhage and hematoma of a nervous system organ or structure complicating other procedure**

+ **G97.4 Accidental puncture and laceration of a nervous system organ or structure during a procedure**
CC **G97.41 Accidental puncture or laceration of dura during a procedure**
Incidental (inadvertent) durotomy
Code also any associated diagnoses or complications
CC **G97.48 Accidental puncture and laceration of other nervous system organ or structure during a nervous system procedure**
CC **G97.49 Accidental puncture and laceration of other nervous system organ or structure during other procedure**
+ **G97.5 Postprocedural hemorrhage of a nervous system organ or structure following a procedure**
CC **G97.51 Postprocedural hemorrhage of a nervous system organ or structure following a nervous system procedure**
CC **G97.52 Postprocedural hemorrhage of a nervous system organ or structure following other procedure**
+ **G97.6 Postprocedural hematoma and seroma of a nervous system organ or structure following a procedure**
CC **G97.61 Postprocedural hematoma of a nervous system organ or structure following a nervous system procedure**
AHA CC: 3Q, 2020, 24
CC **G97.62 Postprocedural hematoma of a nervous system organ or structure following other procedure**
CC **G97.63 Postprocedural seroma of a nervous system organ or structure following a nervous system procedure**
CC **G97.64 Postprocedural seroma of a nervous system organ or structure following other procedure**
+ **G97.8 Other intraoperative and postprocedural complications and disorders of nervous system**
Use additional code to further specify disorder
AHA CC: 4Q, 2020, 23-24
CC **G97.81 Other intraoperative complications of nervous system**
CC **G97.82 Other postprocedural complications and disorders of nervous system**
CC **G97.83 Intracranial hypotension following lumbar cerebrospinal fluid shunting**
Code also any associated diagnoses or complications
CC **G97.84 Intracranial hypotension following other procedure**
Code also, if applicable:
accidental puncture or laceration of dura during a procedure (G97.41)
cerebrospinal fluid leak from spinal puncture (G97.0)

G98 Other disorders of nervous system not elsewhere classified

Includes: nervous system disorder NOS
G98.0 Neurogenic arthritis, not elsewhere classified
Nonsyphilitic neurogenic arthropathy NEC
Nonsyphilitic neurogenic spondylopathy NEC
Excludes1: *spondylopathy (in):*
syringomyelia and syringobulbia (G95.0)
tabes dorsalis (A52.11)
G98.8 Other disorders of nervous system
Nervous system disorder NOS

G99 Other disorders of nervous system in diseases classified elsewhere

CC **G99.0 Autonomic neuropathy in diseases classified elsewhere**

Code first underlying disease, such as:
- amyloidosis (E85.-)
- gout (M1A.-, M10.-)
- hyperthyroidism (E05.-)

Excludes1: *diabetic autonomic neuropathy (E08-E13 with .43)*

CC **G99.2 Myelopathy in diseases classified elsewhere**

Code first underlying disease, such as:
- neoplasm (C00-D49)

Excludes1: *myelopathy in:*
- *intervertebral disease (M50.0-, M51.0-)*
- *spondylosis (M47.0-, M47.1-)*

AHA CC: 3Q, 2018, 18-19

G99.8 Other specified disorders of nervous system in diseases classified elsewhere

Code first underlying disorder, such as:
- amyloidosis (E85.-)
- avitaminosis (E56.9)

Excludes1: *nervous system involvement in:*
- *cysticercosis (B69.0)*
- *rubella (B06.0-)*
- *syphilis (A52.1-)*

Chapter 7: Diseases of the Eye and Adnexa (H00-H59)

NOTE Use an external cause code following the code for the eye condition, if applicable, to identify the cause of the eye condition

Excludes2: *certain conditions originating in the perinatal period (P04-P96)*
certain infectious and parasitic diseases (A00-B99)
complications of pregnancy, childbirth and the puerperium (O00-O9A)
congenital malformations, deformations, and chromosomal abnormalities (Q00-Q99)
diabetes mellitus related eye conditions (E09.3-, E10.3-, E11.3-, E13.3-)
endocrine, nutritional and metabolic diseases (E00-E88)
injury (trauma) of eye and orbit (S05.-)
injury, poisoning and certain other consequences of external causes (S00-T88)
neoplasms (C00-D49)
symptoms, signs and abnormal clinical and laboratory findings, not elsewhere classified (R00-R94)
syphilis related eye disorders (A50.01, A50.3-, A51.43, A52.71)

This chapter contains the following category blocks:

H00-H05	Disorders of eyelid, lacrimal system and orbit
H10-H11	Disorders of conjunctiva
H15-H22	Disorders of sclera, cornea, iris and ciliary body
H25-H28	Disorders of lens
H30-H36	Disorders of choroid and retina
H40-H42	Glaucoma
H43-H44	Disorders of vitreous body and globe
H46-H47	Disorders of optic nerve and visual pathways
H49-H52	Disorders of ocular muscles, binocular movement, accommodation and refraction
H53-H54	Visual disturbances and blindness
H55-H57	Other disorders of eye and adnexa
H59	Intraoperative and postprocedural complications and disorders of eye and adnexa, not elsewhere classified

C. Chapter-Specific Coding Guidelines

In addition to general coding guidelines, there are guidelines for specific diagnoses and/or conditions in the classification. Unless otherwise indicated, these guidelines apply to all health care settings. Please refer to Section II for guidelines on the selection of principal diagnosis.

7. Chapter 7: Diseases of the Eye and Adnexa (H00-H59)

a. Glaucoma

1) Assigning Glaucoma Codes

Assign as many codes from category H40, Glaucoma, as needed to identify the type of glaucoma, the affected eye, and the glaucoma stage.

2) Bilateral glaucoma with same type and stage

When a patient has bilateral glaucoma and both eyes are documented as being the same type and stage, and there is a code for bilateral glaucoma, report only the code for the type of glaucoma, bilateral, with the seventh character for the stage.

When a patient has bilateral glaucoma and both eyes are documented as being the same type and stage, and the classification does not provide a code for bilateral glaucoma (i.e. subcategories H40.10, H40.11 and H40.20) report only one code for the type of glaucoma with the appropriate seventh character for the stage.

3) Bilateral glaucoma stage with different types or stages

When a patient has bilateral glaucoma and each eye is documented as having a different type or stage, and the classification distinguishes laterality, assign the appropriate code for each eye rather than the code for bilateral glaucoma.

When a patient has bilateral glaucoma and each eye is documented as having a different type, and the classification does not distinguish laterality (i.e. subcategories H40.10, H40.11 and H40.20), assign one code for each type of glaucoma with the appropriate seventh character for the stage.

When a patient has bilateral glaucoma and each eye is documented as having the same type, but different stage, and the classification does not distinguish laterality (i.e. subcategories H40.10, H40.11 and H40.20), assign a code for the type of glaucoma for each eye with the seventh character for the specific glaucoma stage documented for each eye.

4) Patient admitted with glaucoma and stage evolves during the admission

If a patient is admitted with glaucoma and the stage progresses during the admission, assign the code for highest stage documented.

5) Indeterminate stage glaucoma

Assignment of the seventh character "4" for "indeterminate stage" should be based on the clinical documentation. The seventh character "4" is used for glaucomas whose stage cannot be clinically determined. This seventh character should not be confused with the seventh character "0", unspecified, which should be assigned when there is no documentation regarding the stage of the glaucoma.

b. Blindness

If "blindness" or "low vision" of both eyes is documented but the visual impairment category is not documented, assign code H54.3, Unqualified visual loss, both eyes. If "blindness" or "low vision" in one eye is documented but the visual impairment category is not documented, assign a code from H54.6-, Unqualified visual loss, one eye. If "blindness" or "visual loss" is documented without any information about whether one or both eyes are affected, assign code H54.7, Unspecified visual loss.

Disorders of eyelid, lacrimal system and orbit (H00-H05)

Excludes2: *open wound of eyelid (S01.1-)*
superficial injury of eyelid (S00.1-, S00.2-)

H00 Hordeolum and chalazion

+ **H00.0 Hordeolum (externum) (internum) of eyelid**
  + **H00.01 Hordeolum externum**
    Hordeolum NOS
    Stye
    H00.011 Hordeolum externum right upper eyelid
    H00.012 Hordeolum externum right lower eyelid
    H00.013 Hordeolum externum right eye, unspecified eyelid
    H00.014 Hordeolum externum left upper eyelid
    H00.015 Hordeolum externum left lower eyelid
    H00.016 Hordeolum externum left eye, unspecified eyelid
    H00.019 Hordeolum externum unspecified eye, unspecified eyelid
  + **H00.02 Hordeolum internum**
    Infection of meibomian gland
    H00.021 Hordeolum internum right upper eyelid
    H00.022 Hordeolum internum right lower eyelid
    H00.023 Hordeolum internum right eye, unspecified eyelid
    H00.024 Hordeolum internum left upper eyelid
    H00.025 Hordeolum internum left lower eyelid
    H00.026 Hordeolum internum left eye, unspecified eyelid
    H00.029 Hordeolum internum unspecified eye, unspecified eyelid
  + **H00.03 Abscess of eyelid**
    Furuncle of eyelid
    H00.031 Abscess of right upper eyelid
    H00.032 Abscess of right lower eyelid
    H00.033 Abscess of eyelid right eye, unspecified eyelid
    H00.034 Abscess of left upper eyelid
    H00.035 Abscess of left lower eyelid
    H00.036 Abscess of eyelid left eye, unspecified eyelid
    H00.039 Abscess of eyelid unspecified eye, unspecified eyelid
+ **H00.1 Chalazion**
  Meibomian (gland) cyst
  Excludes2: *infected meibomian gland (H00.02-)*
  H00.11 Chalazion right upper eyelid
  H00.12 Chalazion right lower eyelid
  H00.13 Chalazion right eye, unspecified eyelid
  H00.14 Chalazion left upper eyelid
  H00.15 Chalazion left lower eyelid
  H00.16 Chalazion left eye, unspecified eyelid
  H00.19 Chalazion unspecified eye, unspecified eyelid

H01 Other inflammation of eyelid

+ **H01.0 Blepharitis**
  Excludes1: *blepharoconjunctivitis (H10.5-)*
  AHA CC: 4Q, 2018, 13
  + **H01.00 Unspecified blepharitis**
    H01.001 Unspecified blepharitis right upper eyelid
    H01.002 Unspecified blepharitis right lower eyelid
    H01.003 Unspecified blepharitis right eye, unspecified eyelid
    H01.004 Unspecified blepharitis left upper eyelid
    H01.005 Unspecified blepharitis left lower eyelid

Eye

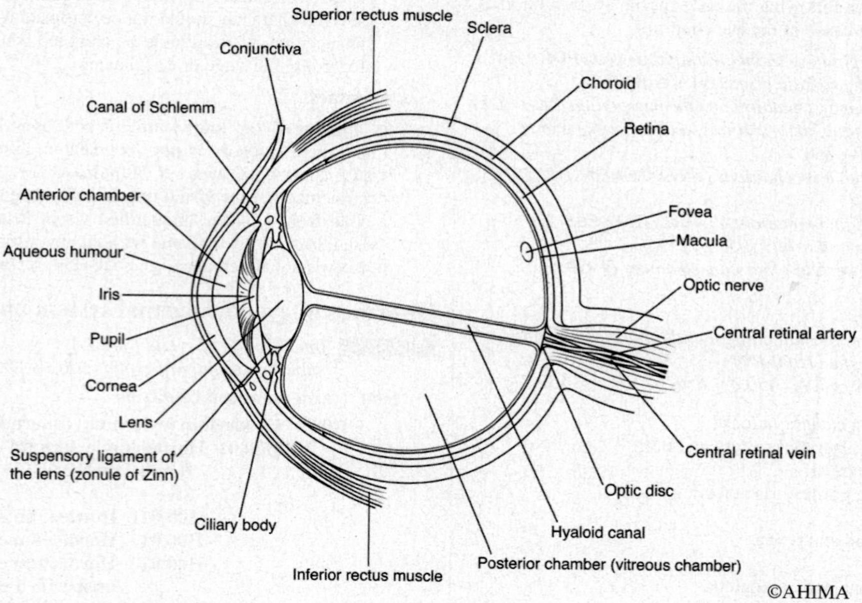

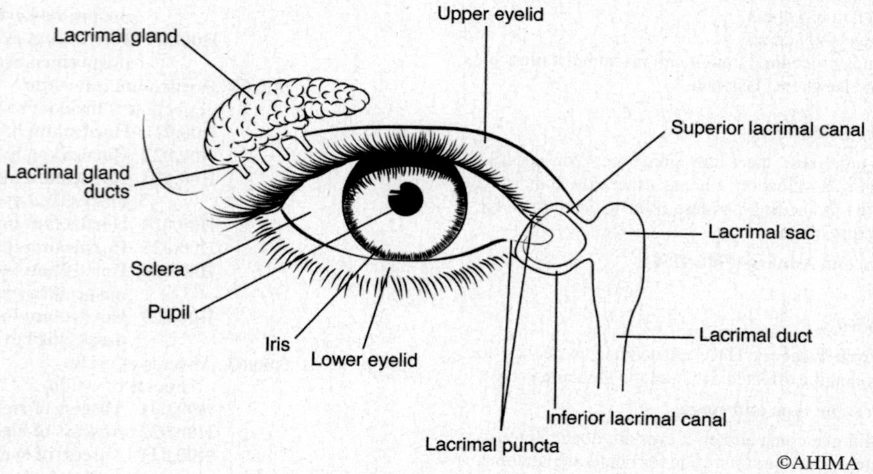

Muscles of the Eye

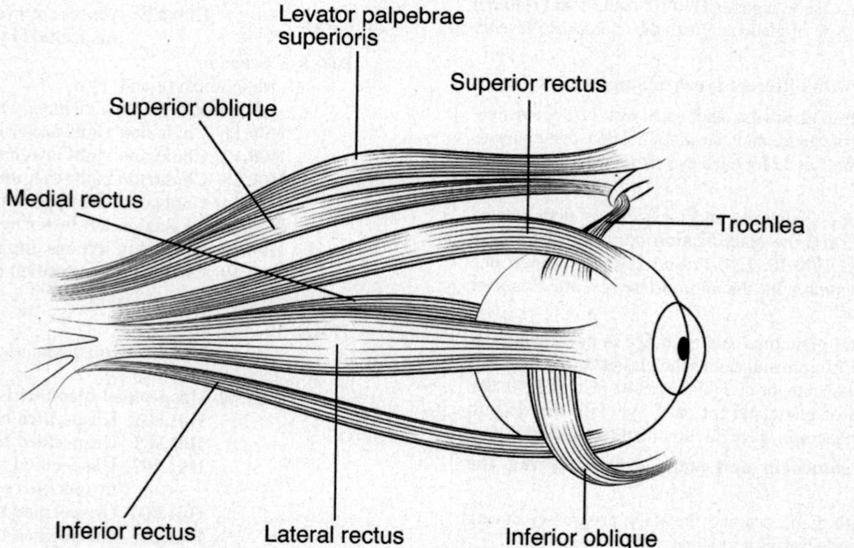

H01.006 Unspecified blepharitis left eye, unspecified eyelid
H01.009 Unspecified blepharitis unspecified eye, unspecified eyelid
H01.00A Unspecified blepharitis right eye, upper and lower eyelids
H01.00B Unspecified blepharitis left eye, upper and lower eyelids
+ H01.01 Ulcerative blepharitis
H01.011 Ulcerative blepharitis right upper eyelid
H01.012 Ulcerative blepharitis right lower eyelid
H01.013 Ulcerative blepharitis right eye, unspecified eyelid
H01.014 Ulcerative blepharitis left upper eyelid
H01.015 Ulcerative blepharitis left lower eyelid
H01.016 Ulcerative blepharitis left eye, unspecified eyelid
H01.019 Ulcerative blepharitis unspecified eye, unspecified eyelid
H01.01A Ulcerative blepharitis right eye, upper and lower eyelids
H01.01B Ulcerative blepharitis left eye, upper and lower eyelids
+ H01.02 Squamous blepharitis
H01.021 Squamous blepharitis right upper eyelid
H01.022 Squamous blepharitis right lower eyelid
H01.023 Squamous blepharitis right eye, unspecified eyelid
H01.024 Squamous blepharitis left upper eyelid
H01.025 Squamous blepharitis left lower eyelid
H01.026 Squamous blepharitis left eye, unspecified eyelid
H01.029 Squamous blepharitis unspecified eye, unspecified eyelid
H01.02A Squamous blepharitis right eye, upper and lower eyelids
H01.02B Squamous blepharitis left eye, upper and lower eyelids
+ H01.1 Noninfectious dermatoses of eyelid
+ H01.11 Allergic dermatitis of eyelid
Contact dermatitis of eyelid
H01.111 Allergic dermatitis of right upper eyelid
H01.112 Allergic dermatitis of right lower eyelid
H01.113 Allergic dermatitis of right eye, unspecified eyelid
H01.114 Allergic dermatitis of left upper eyelid
H01.115 Allergic dermatitis of left lower eyelid
H01.116 Allergic dermatitis of left eye, unspecified eyelid
H01.119 Allergic dermatitis of unspecified eye, unspecified eyelid
+ H01.12 Discoid lupus erythematosus of eyelid
H01.121 Discoid lupus erythematosus of right upper eyelid
H01.122 Discoid lupus erythematosus of right lower eyelid
H01.123 Discoid lupus erythematosus of right eye, unspecified eyelid
H01.124 Discoid lupus erythematosus of left upper eyelid
H01.125 Discoid lupus erythematosus of left lower eyelid
H01.126 Discoid lupus erythematosus of left eye, unspecified eyelid
H01.129 Discoid lupus erythematosus of unspecified eye, unspecified eyelid
+ H01.13 Eczematous dermatitis of eyelid
H01.131 Eczematous dermatitis of right upper eyelid
H01.132 Eczematous dermatitis of right lower eyelid
H01.133 Eczematous dermatitis of right eye, unspecified eyelid
H01.134 Eczematous dermatitis of left upper eyelid
H01.135 Eczematous dermatitis of left lower eyelid
H01.136 Eczematous dermatitis of left eye, unspecified eyelid
H01.139 Eczematous dermatitis of unspecified eye, unspecified eyelid
+ H01.14 Xeroderma of eyelid
H01.141 Xeroderma of right upper eyelid
H01.142 Xeroderma of right lower eyelid
H01.143 Xeroderma of right eye, unspecified eyelid
H01.144 Xeroderma of left upper eyelid
H01.145 Xeroderma of left lower eyelid
H01.146 Xeroderma of left eye, unspecified eyelid
H01.149 Xeroderma of unspecified eye, unspecified eyelid
H01.8 Other specified inflammations of eyelid
H01.9 Unspecified inflammation of eyelid
Inflammation of eyelid NOS

H02 Other disorders of eyelid

Excludes1: *congenital malformations of eyelid (Q10.0-Q10.3)*

+ H02.0 Entropion and trichiasis of eyelid
+ H02.00 Unspecified entropion of eyelid
H02.001 Unspecified entropion of right upper eyelid
H02.002 Unspecified entropion of right lower eyelid
H02.003 Unspecified entropion of right eye, unspecified eyelid
H02.004 Unspecified entropion of left upper eyelid
H02.005 Unspecified entropion of left lower eyelid
H02.006 Unspecified entropion of left eye, unspecified eyelid
H02.009 Unspecified entropion of unspecified eye, unspecified eyelid
+ H02.01 Cicatricial entropion of eyelid
H02.011 Cicatricial entropion of right upper eyelid
H02.012 Cicatricial entropion of right lower eyelid
H02.013 Cicatricial entropion of right eye, unspecified eyelid
H02.014 Cicatricial entropion of left upper eyelid
H02.015 Cicatricial entropion of left lower eyelid
H02.016 Cicatricial entropion of left eye, unspecified eyelid
H02.019 Cicatricial entropion of unspecified eye, unspecified eyelid
+ H02.02 Mechanical entropion of eyelid
H02.021 Mechanical entropion of right upper eyelid
H02.022 Mechanical entropion of right lower eyelid
H02.023 Mechanical entropion of right eye, unspecified eyelid
H02.024 Mechanical entropion of left upper eyelid
H02.025 Mechanical entropion of left lower eyelid
H02.026 Mechanical entropion of left eye, unspecified eyelid
H02.029 Mechanical entropion of unspecified eye, unspecified eyelid
+ H02.03 Senile entropion of eyelid
• H02.031 Senile entropion of right upper eyelid
• H02.032 Senile entropion of right lower eyelid
• H02.033 Senile entropion of right eye, unspecified eyelid
• H02.034 Senile entropion of left upper eyelid
• H02.035 Senile entropion of left lower eyelid
• H02.036 Senile entropion of left eye, unspecified eyelid
• H02.039 Senile entropion of unspecified eye, unspecified eyelid
+ H02.04 Spastic entropion of eyelid
H02.041 Spastic entropion of right upper eyelid
H02.042 Spastic entropion of right lower eyelid
H02.043 Spastic entropion of right eye, unspecified eyelid
H02.044 Spastic entropion of left upper eyelid
H02.045 Spastic entropion of left lower eyelid
H02.046 Spastic entropion of left eye, unspecified eyelid
H02.049 Spastic entropion of unspecified eye, unspecified eyelid

+ **H02.05** Trichiasis without entropion
  - **H02.051** Trichiasis without entropion right upper eyelid
  - **H02.052** Trichiasis without entropion right lower eyelid
  - **H02.053** Trichiasis without entropion right eye, unspecified eyelid
  - **H02.054** Trichiasis without entropion left upper eyelid
  - **H02.055** Trichiasis without entropion left lower eyelid
  - **H02.056** Trichiasis without entropion left eye, unspecified eyelid
  - **H02.059** Trichiasis without entropion unspecified eye, unspecified eyelid

+ **H02.1** Ectropion of eyelid

+ **H02.10** Unspecified ectropion of eyelid
  - **H02.101** Unspecified ectropion of right upper eyelid
  - **H02.102** Unspecified ectropion of right lower eyelid
  - **H02.103** Unspecified ectropion of right eye, unspecified eyelid
  - **H02.104** Unspecified ectropion of left upper eyelid
  - **H02.105** Unspecified ectropion of left lower eyelid
  - **H02.106** Unspecified ectropion of left eye, unspecified eyelid
  - **H02.109** Unspecified ectropion of unspecified eye, unspecified eyelid

+ **H02.11** Cicatricial ectropion of eyelid
  - **H02.111** Cicatricial ectropion of right upper eyelid
  - **H02.112** Cicatricial ectropion of right lower eyelid
  - **H02.113** Cicatricial ectropion of right eye, unspecified eyelid
  - **H02.114** Cicatricial ectropion of left upper eyelid
  - **H02.115** Cicatricial ectropion of left lower eyelid
  - **H02.116** Cicatricial ectropion of left eye, unspecified eyelid
  - **H02.119** Cicatricial ectropion of unspecified eye, unspecified eyelid

+ **H02.12** Mechanical ectropion of eyelid
  - **H02.121** Mechanical ectropion of right upper eyelid
  - **H02.122** Mechanical ectropion of right lower eyelid
  - **H02.123** Mechanical ectropion of right eye, unspecified eyelid
  - **H02.124** Mechanical ectropion of left upper eyelid
  - **H02.125** Mechanical ectropion of left lower eyelid
  - **H02.126** Mechanical ectropion of left eye, unspecified eyelid
  - **H02.129** Mechanical ectropion of unspecified eye, unspecified eyelid

+ **H02.13** Senile ectropion of eyelid
  - ● **H02.131** Senile ectropion of right upper eyelid
  - ● **H02.132** Senile ectropion of right lower eyelid
  - ● **H02.133** Senile ectropion of right eye, unspecified eyelid
  - ● **H02.134** Senile ectropion of left upper eyelid
  - ● **H02.135** Senile ectropion of left lower eyelid
  - ● **H02.136** Senile ectropion of left eye, unspecified eyelid
  - ● **H02.139** Senile ectropion of unspecified eye, unspecified eyelid

+ **H02.14** Spastic ectropion of eyelid
  - **H02.141** Spastic ectropion of right upper eyelid
  - **H02.142** Spastic ectropion of right lower eyelid
  - **H02.143** Spastic ectropion of right eye, unspecified eyelid
  - **H02.144** Spastic ectropion of left upper eyelid
  - **H02.145** Spastic ectropion of left lower eyelid
  - **H02.146** Spastic ectropion of left eye, unspecified eyelid
  - **H02.149** Spastic ectropion of unspecified eye, unspecified eyelid

+ **H02.15** Paralytic ectropion of eyelid

  AHA CC: 4Q, 2018, 13
  - **H02.151** Paralytic ectropion of right upper eyelid
  - **H02.152** Paralytic ectropion of right lower eyelid
  - **H02.153** Paralytic ectropion of right eye, unspecified eyelid
  - **H02.154** Paralytic ectropion of left upper eyelid
  - **H02.155** Paralytic ectropion of left lower eyelid
  - **H02.156** Paralytic ectropion of left eye, unspecified eyelid
  - **H02.159** Paralytic ectropion of unspecified eye, unspecified eyelid

+ **H02.2** Lagophthalmos

  AHA CC: 4Q, 2018, 14

+ **H02.20** Unspecified lagophthalmos
  - **H02.201** Unspecified lagophthalmos right upper eyelid
  - **H02.202** Unspecified lagophthalmos right lower eyelid
  - **H02.203** Unspecified lagophthalmos right eye, unspecified eyelid
  - **H02.204** Unspecified lagophthalmos left upper eyelid
  - **H02.205** Unspecified lagophthalmos left lower eyelid
  - **H02.206** Unspecified lagophthalmos left eye, unspecified eyelid
  - **H02.209** Unspecified lagophthalmos unspecified eye, unspecified eyelid
  - **H02.20A** Unspecified lagophthalmos right eye, upper and lower eyelids
  - **H02.20B** Unspecified lagophthalmos left eye, upper and lower eyelids
  - **H02.20C** Unspecified lagophthalmos, bilateral, upper and lower eyelids

+ **H02.21** Cicatricial lagophthalmos
  - **H02.211** Cicatricial lagophthalmos right upper eyelid
  - **H02.212** Cicatricial lagophthalmos right lower eyelid
  - **H02.213** Cicatricial lagophthalmos right eye, unspecified eyelid
  - **H02.214** Cicatricial lagophthalmos left upper eyelid
  - **H02.215** Cicatricial lagophthalmos left lower eyelid
  - **H02.216** Cicatricial lagophthalmos left eye, unspecified eyelid
  - **H02.219** Cicatricial lagophthalmos unspecified eye, unspecified eyelid
  - **H02.21A** Cicatricial lagophthalmos right eye, upper and lower eyelids
  - **H02.21B** Cicatricial lagophthalmos left eye, upper and lower eyelids
  - **H02.21C** Cicatricial lagophthalmos, bilateral, upper and lower eyelids

+ **H02.22** Mechanical lagophthalmos
  - **H02.221** Mechanical lagophthalmos right upper eyelid
  - **H02.222** Mechanical lagophthalmos right lower eyelid
  - **H02.223** Mechanical lagophthalmos right eye, unspecified eyelid
  - **H02.224** Mechanical lagophthalmos left upper eyelid
  - **H02.225** Mechanical lagophthalmos left lower eyelid
  - **H02.226** Mechanical lagophthalmos left eye, unspecified eyelid
  - **H02.229** Mechanical lagophthalmos unspecified eye, unspecified eyelid
  - **H02.22A** Mechanical lagophthalmos right eye, upper and lower eyelids
  - **H02.22B** Mechanical lagophthalmos left eye, upper and lower eyelids
  - **H02.22C** Mechanical lagophthalmos, bilateral, upper and lower eyelids

+ **H02.23 Paralytic lagophthalmos**
  - **H02.231 Paralytic lagophthalmos right upper eyelid**
  - **H02.232 Paralytic lagophthalmos right lower eyelid**
  - **H02.233 Paralytic lagophthalmos right eye, unspecified eyelid**
  - **H02.234 Paralytic lagophthalmos left upper eyelid**
  - **H02.235 Paralytic lagophthalmos left lower eyelid**
  - **H02.236 Paralytic lagophthalmos left eye, unspecified eyelid**
  - **H02.239 Paralytic lagophthalmos unspecified eye, unspecified eyelid**
  - **H02.23A Paralytic lagophthalmos right eye, upper and lower eyelids**
  - **H02.23B Paralytic lagophthalmos left eye, upper and lower eyelids**
  - **H02.23C Paralytic lagophthalmos, bilateral, upper and lower eyelids**

+ **H02.3 Blepharochalasis**
  Pseudoptosis
  - **H02.30 Blepharochalasis unspecified eye, unspecified eyelid**
  - **H02.31 Blepharochalasis right upper eyelid**
  - **H02.32 Blepharochalasis right lower eyelid**
  - **H02.33 Blepharochalasis right eye, unspecified eyelid**
  - **H02.34 Blepharochalasis left upper eyelid**
  - **H02.35 Blepharochalasis left lower eyelid**
  - **H02.36 Blepharochalasis left eye, unspecified eyelid**

+ **H02.4 Ptosis of eyelid**

+ **H02.40 Unspecified ptosis of eyelid**
  - **H02.401 Unspecified ptosis of right eyelid**
  - **H02.402 Unspecified ptosis of left eyelid**
  - **H02.403 Unspecified ptosis of bilateral eyelids**
  - **H02.409 Unspecified ptosis of unspecified eyelid**

+ **H02.41 Mechanical ptosis of eyelid**
  - **H02.411 Mechanical ptosis of right eyelid**
  - **H02.412 Mechanical ptosis of left eyelid**
  - **H02.413 Mechanical ptosis of bilateral eyelids**
  - **H02.419 Mechanical ptosis of unspecified eyelid**

+ **H02.42 Myogenic ptosis of eyelid**
  - **H02.421 Myogenic ptosis of right eyelid**
  - **H02.422 Myogenic ptosis of left eyelid**
  - **H02.423 Myogenic ptosis of bilateral eyelids**
  - **H02.429 Myogenic ptosis of unspecified eyelid**

+ **H02.43 Paralytic ptosis of eyelid**
  Neurogenic ptosis of eyelid
  - **H02.431 Paralytic ptosis of right eyelid**
  - **H02.432 Paralytic ptosis of left eyelid**
  - **H02.433 Paralytic ptosis of bilateral eyelids**
  - **H02.439 Paralytic ptosis unspecified eyelid**

+ **H02.5 Other disorders affecting eyelid function**
  Excludes2: *blepharospasm (G24.5)*
  organic tic (G25.69)
  psychogenic tic (F95.-)

+ **H02.51 Abnormal innervation syndrome**
  - **H02.511 Abnormal innervation syndrome right upper eyelid**
  - **H02.512 Abnormal innervation syndrome right lower eyelid**
  - **H02.513 Abnormal innervation syndrome right eye, unspecified eyelid**
  - **H02.514 Abnormal innervation syndrome left upper eyelid**
  - **H02.515 Abnormal innervation syndrome left lower eyelid**
  - **H02.516 Abnormal innervation syndrome left eye, unspecified eyelid**
  - **H02.519 Abnormal innervation syndrome unspecified eye, unspecified eyelid**

+ **H02.52 Blepharophimosis**
  Ankyloblepharon
  - **H02.521 Blepharophimosis right upper eyelid**
  - **H02.522 Blepharophimosis right lower eyelid**
  - **H02.523 Blepharophimosis right eye, unspecified eyelid**
  - **H02.524 Blepharophimosis left upper eyelid**
  - **H02.525 Blepharophimosis left lower eyelid**
  - **H02.526 Blepharophimosis left eye, unspecified eyelid**
  - **H02.529 Blepharophimosis unspecified eye, unspecified lid**

+ **H02.53 Eyelid retraction**
  Eyelid lag
  - **H02.531 Eyelid retraction right upper eyelid**
  - **H02.532 Eyelid retraction right lower eyelid**
  - **H02.533 Eyelid retraction right eye, unspecified eyelid**
  - **H02.534 Eyelid retraction left upper eyelid**
  - **H02.535 Eyelid retraction left lower eyelid**
  - **H02.536 Eyelid retraction left eye, unspecified eyelid**
  - **H02.539 Eyelid retraction unspecified eye, unspecified lid**

H02.59 Other disorders affecting eyelid function
  Deficient blink reflex
  Sensory disorders

+ **H02.6 Xanthelasma of eyelid**
  - **H02.60 Xanthelasma of unspecified eye, unspecified eyelid**
  - **H02.61 Xanthelasma of right upper eyelid**
  - **H02.62 Xanthelasma of right lower eyelid**
  - **H02.63 Xanthelasma of right eye, unspecified eyelid**
  - **H02.64 Xanthelasma of left upper eyelid**
  - **H02.65 Xanthelasma of left lower eyelid**
  - **H02.66 Xanthelasma of left eye, unspecified eyelid**

+ **H02.7 Other and unspecified degenerative disorders of eyelid and periocular area**
  - **H02.70 Unspecified degenerative disorders of eyelid and periocular area**

+ **H02.71 Chloasma of eyelid and periocular area**
  Dyspigmentation of eyelid
  Hyperpigmentation of eyelid
  - **H02.711 Chloasma of right upper eyelid and periocular area**
  - **H02.712 Chloasma of right lower eyelid and periocular area**
  - **H02.713 Chloasma of right eye, unspecified eyelid and periocular area**
  - **H02.714 Chloasma of left upper eyelid and periocular area**
  - **H02.715 Chloasma of left lower eyelid and periocular area**
  - **H02.716 Chloasma of left eye, unspecified eyelid and periocular area**
  - **H02.719 Chloasma of unspecified eye, unspecified eyelid and periocular area**

+ **H02.72 Madarosis of eyelid and periocular area**
  Hypotrichosis of eyelid
  - **H02.721 Madarosis of right upper eyelid and periocular area**
  - **H02.722 Madarosis of right lower eyelid and periocular area**
  - **H02.723 Madarosis of right eye, unspecified eyelid and periocular area**
  - **H02.724 Madarosis of left upper eyelid and periocular area**
  - **H02.725 Madarosis of left lower eyelid and periocular area**
  - **H02.726 Madarosis of left eye, unspecified eyelid and periocular area**
  - **H02.729 Madarosis of unspecified eye, unspecified eyelid and periocular area**

+ **H02.73 Vitiligo of eyelid and periocular area**
  Hypopigmentation of eyelid
  - **H02.731 Vitiligo of right upper eyelid and periocular area**
  - **H02.732 Vitiligo of right lower eyelid and periocular area**
  - **H02.733 Vitiligo of right eye, unspecified eyelid and periocular area**
  - **H02.734 Vitiligo of left upper eyelid and periocular area**
  - **H02.735 Vitiligo of left lower eyelid and periocular area**
  - **H02.736 Vitiligo of left eye, unspecified eyelid and periocular area**
  - **H02.739 Vitiligo of unspecified eye, unspecified eyelid and periocular area**

H02.79 Other degenerative disorders of eyelid and periocular area

+ H02.8 Other specified disorders of eyelid
+ H02.81 Retained foreign body in eyelid
Use additional code to identify the type of retained foreign body (Z18.-)
Excludes1: *laceration of eyelid with foreign body (S01.12-)*
retained intraocular foreign body (H44.6-, H44.7-)
superficial foreign body of eyelid and periocular area (S00.25-)
H02.811 Retained foreign body in right upper eyelid
H02.812 Retained foreign body in right lower eyelid
H02.813 Retained foreign body in right eye, unspecified eyelid
H02.814 Retained foreign body in left upper eyelid
H02.815 Retained foreign body in left lower eyelid
H02.816 Retained foreign body in left eye, unspecified eyelid
H02.819 Retained foreign body in unspecified eye, unspecified eyelid
+ H02.82 Cysts of eyelid
Sebaceous cyst of eyelid
H02.821 Cysts of right upper eyelid
H02.822 Cysts of right lower eyelid
H02.823 Cysts of right eye, unspecified eyelid
H02.824 Cysts of left upper eyelid
H02.825 Cysts of left lower eyelid
H02.826 Cysts of left eye, unspecified eyelid
H02.829 Cysts of unspecified eye, unspecified eyelid
+ H02.83 Dermatochalasis of eyelid
H02.831 Dermatochalasis of right upper eyelid
H02.832 Dermatochalasis of right lower eyelid
H02.833 Dermatochalasis of right eye, unspecified eyelid
H02.834 Dermatochalasis of left upper eyelid
H02.835 Dermatochalasis of left lower eyelid
H02.836 Dermatochalasis of left eye, unspecified eyelid
H02.839 Dermatochalasis of unspecified eye, unspecified eyelid
+ H02.84 Edema of eyelid
Hyperemia of eyelid
H02.841 Edema of right upper eyelid
H02.842 Edema of right lower eyelid
H02.843 Edema of right eye, unspecified eyelid
H02.844 Edema of left upper eyelid
H02.845 Edema of left lower eyelid
H02.846 Edema of left eye, unspecified eyelid
H02.849 Edema of unspecified eye, unspecified eyelid
+ H02.85 Elephantiasis of eyelid
H02.851 Elephantiasis of right upper eyelid
H02.852 Elephantiasis of right lower eyelid
H02.853 Elephantiasis of right eye, unspecified eyelid
H02.854 Elephantiasis of left upper eyelid
H02.855 Elephantiasis of left lower eyelid
H02.856 Elephantiasis of left eye, unspecified eyelid
H02.859 Elephantiasis of unspecified eye, unspecified eyelid
+ H02.86 Hypertrichosis of eyelid
H02.861 Hypertrichosis of right upper eyelid
H02.862 Hypertrichosis of right lower eyelid
H02.863 Hypertrichosis of right eye, unspecified eyelid
H02.864 Hypertrichosis of left upper eyelid
H02.865 Hypertrichosis of left lower eyelid
H02.866 Hypertrichosis of left eye, unspecified eyelid
H02.869 Hypertrichosis of unspecified eye, unspecified eyelid
+ H02.87 Vascular anomalies of eyelid
H02.871 Vascular anomalies of right upper eyelid
H02.872 Vascular anomalies of right lower eyelid
H02.873 Vascular anomalies of right eye, unspecified eyelid
H02.874 Vascular anomalies of left upper eyelid
H02.875 Vascular anomalies of left lower eyelid
H02.876 Vascular anomalies of left eye, unspecified eyelid
H02.879 Vascular anomalies of unspecified eye, unspecified eyelid
+ H02.88 Meibomian gland dysfunction of eyelid
AHA CC: 4Q, 2018, 14-15
H02.881 Meibomian gland dysfunction right upper eyelid
H02.882 Meibomian gland dysfunction right lower eyelid
H02.883 Meibomian gland dysfunction of right eye, unspecified eyelid
H02.884 Meibomian gland dysfunction left upper eyelid
H02.885 Meibomian gland dysfunction left lower eyelid
H02.886 Meibomian gland dysfunction of left eye, unspecified eyelid
H02.889 Meibomian gland dysfunction of unspecified eye, unspecified eyelid
H02.88A Meibomian gland dysfunction right eye, upper and lower eyelids
H02.88B Meibomian gland dysfunction left eye, upper and lower eyelids
H02.89 Other specified disorders of eyelid
Hemorrhage of eyelid
H02.9 Unspecified disorder of eyelid
Disorder of eyelid NOS

H04 Disorders of lacrimal system
Excludes1: *congenital malformations of lacrimal system (Q10.4-Q10.6)*
+ H04.0 Dacryoadenitis
+ H04.00 Unspecified dacryoadenitis
H04.001 Unspecified dacryoadenitis, right lacrimal gland
H04.002 Unspecified dacryoadenitis, left lacrimal gland
H04.003 Unspecified dacryoadenitis, bilateral lacrimal glands
H04.009 Unspecified dacryoadenitis, unspecified lacrimal gland
+ H04.01 Acute dacryoadenitis
H04.011 Acute dacryoadenitis, right lacrimal gland
H04.012 Acute dacryoadenitis, left lacrimal gland
H04.013 Acute dacryoadenitis, bilateral lacrimal glands
H04.019 Acute dacryoadenitis, unspecified lacrimal gland
+ H04.02 Chronic dacryoadenitis
H04.021 Chronic dacryoadenitis, right lacrimal gland
H04.022 Chronic dacryoadenitis, left lacrimal gland
H04.023 Chronic dacryoadenitis, bilateral lacrimal gland
H04.029 Chronic dacryoadenitis, unspecified lacrimal gland
+ H04.03 Chronic enlargement of lacrimal gland
H04.031 Chronic enlargement of right lacrimal gland
H04.032 Chronic enlargement of left lacrimal gland
H04.033 Chronic enlargement of bilateral lacrimal glands
H04.039 Chronic enlargement of unspecified lacrimal gland
+ H04.1 Other disorders of lacrimal gland
+ H04.11 Dacryops
H04.111 Dacryops of right lacrimal gland
H04.112 Dacryops of left lacrimal gland
H04.113 Dacryops of bilateral lacrimal glands
H04.119 Dacryops of unspecified lacrimal gland

+ **H04.12 Dry eye syndrome**
Tear film insufficiency, NOS
H04.121 Dry eye syndrome of right lacrimal gland
H04.122 Dry eye syndrome of left lacrimal gland
H04.123 Dry eye syndrome of bilateral lacrimal glands
H04.129 Dry eye syndrome of unspecified lacrimal gland

+ **H04.13 Lacrimal cyst**
Lacrimal cystic degeneration
H04.131 Lacrimal cyst, right lacrimal gland
H04.132 Lacrimal cyst, left lacrimal gland
H04.133 Lacrimal cyst, bilateral lacrimal glands
H04.139 Lacrimal cyst, unspecified lacrimal gland

+ **H04.14 Primary lacrimal gland atrophy**
H04.141 Primary lacrimal gland atrophy, right lacrimal gland
H04.142 Primary lacrimal gland atrophy, left lacrimal gland
H04.143 Primary lacrimal gland atrophy, bilateral lacrimal glands
H04.149 Primary lacrimal gland atrophy, unspecified lacrimal gland

+ **H04.15 Secondary lacrimal gland atrophy**
H04.151 Secondary lacrimal gland atrophy, right lacrimal gland
H04.152 Secondary lacrimal gland atrophy, left lacrimal gland
H04.153 Secondary lacrimal gland atrophy, bilateral lacrimal glands
H04.159 Secondary lacrimal gland atrophy, unspecified lacrimal gland

+ **H04.16 Lacrimal gland dislocation**
H04.161 Lacrimal gland dislocation, right lacrimal gland
H04.162 Lacrimal gland dislocation, left lacrimal gland
H04.163 Lacrimal gland dislocation, bilateral lacrimal glands
H04.169 Lacrimal gland dislocation, unspecified lacrimal gland

H04.19 Other specified disorders of lacrimal gland

+ **H04.2 Epiphora**

+ **H04.20 Unspecified epiphora**
H04.201 Unspecified epiphora, right side
H04.202 Unspecified epiphora, left side
H04.203 Unspecified epiphora, bilateral
H04.209 Unspecified epiphora, unspecified side

+ **H04.21 Epiphora due to excess lacrimation**
H04.211 Epiphora due to excess lacrimation, right lacrimal gland
H04.212 Epiphora due to excess lacrimation, left lacrimal gland
H04.213 Epiphora due to excess lacrimation, bilateral lacrimal glands
H04.219 Epiphora due to excess lacrimation, unspecified lacrimal gland

+ **H04.22 Epiphora due to insufficient drainage**
H04.221 Epiphora due to insufficient drainage, right side
H04.222 Epiphora due to insufficient drainage, left side
H04.223 Epiphora due to insufficient drainage, bilateral
H04.229 Epiphora due to insufficient drainage, unspecified side

+ **H04.3 Acute and unspecified inflammation of lacrimal passages**
Excludes1: *neonatal dacryocystitis (P39.1)*

+ **H04.30 Unspecified dacryocystitis**
H04.301 Unspecified dacryocystitis of right lacrimal passage
H04.302 Unspecified dacryocystitis of left lacrimal passage
H04.303 Unspecified dacryocystitis of bilateral lacrimal passages
H04.309 Unspecified dacryocystitis of unspecified lacrimal passage

+ **H04.31 Phlegmonous dacryocystitis**
H04.311 Phlegmonous dacryocystitis of right lacrimal passage
H04.312 Phlegmonous dacryocystitis of left lacrimal passage
H04.313 Phlegmonous dacryocystitis of bilateral lacrimal passages
H04.319 Phlegmonous dacryocystitis of unspecified lacrimal passage

+ **H04.32 Acute dacryocystitis**
Acute dacryopericystitis
H04.321 Acute dacryocystitis of right lacrimal passage
H04.322 Acute dacryocystitis of left lacrimal passage
H04.323 Acute dacryocystitis of bilateral lacrimal passages
H04.329 Acute dacryocystitis of unspecified lacrimal passage

+ **H04.33 Acute lacrimal canaliculitis**
H04.331 Acute lacrimal canaliculitis of right lacrimal passage
H04.332 Acute lacrimal canaliculitis of left lacrimal passage
H04.333 Acute lacrimal canaliculitis of bilateral lacrimal passages
H04.339 Acute lacrimal canaliculitis of unspecified lacrimal passage

+ **H04.4 Chronic inflammation of lacrimal passages**

+ **H04.41 Chronic dacryocystitis**
H04.411 Chronic dacryocystitis of right lacrimal passage
H04.412 Chronic dacryocystitis of left lacrimal passage
H04.413 Chronic dacryocystitis of bilateral lacrimal passages
H04.419 Chronic dacryocystitis of unspecified lacrimal passage

+ **H04.42 Chronic lacrimal canaliculitis**
H04.421 Chronic lacrimal canaliculitis of right lacrimal passage
H04.422 Chronic lacrimal canaliculitis of left lacrimal passage
H04.423 Chronic lacrimal canaliculitis of bilateral lacrimal passages
H04.429 Chronic lacrimal canaliculitis of unspecified lacrimal passage

+ **H04.43 Chronic lacrimal mucocele**
H04.431 Chronic lacrimal mucocele of right lacrimal passage
H04.432 Chronic lacrimal mucocele of left lacrimal passage
H04.433 Chronic lacrimal mucocele of bilateral lacrimal passages
H04.439 Chronic lacrimal mucocele of unspecified lacrimal passage

+ **H04.5 Stenosis and insufficiency of lacrimal passages**

+ **H04.51 Dacryolith**
H04.511 Dacryolith of right lacrimal passage
H04.512 Dacryolith of left lacrimal passage
H04.513 Dacryolith of bilateral lacrimal passages
H04.519 Dacryolith of unspecified lacrimal passage

+ **H04.52 Eversion of lacrimal punctum**
H04.521 Eversion of right lacrimal punctum
H04.522 Eversion of left lacrimal punctum
H04.523 Eversion of bilateral lacrimal punctum
H04.529 Eversion of unspecified lacrimal punctum

+ **H04.53 Neonatal obstruction of nasolacrimal duct**
Excludes1: *congenital stenosis and stricture of lacrimal duct (Q10.5)*
• **H04.531 Neonatal obstruction of right nasolacrimal duct**
• **H04.532 Neonatal obstruction of left nasolacrimal duct**
• **H04.533 Neonatal obstruction of bilateral nasolacrimal duct**
• **H04.539 Neonatal obstruction of unspecified nasolacrimal duct**

+ **H04.54 Stenosis of lacrimal canaliculi**
  - **H04.541 Stenosis of right lacrimal canaliculi**
  - **H04.542 Stenosis of left lacrimal canaliculi**
  - **H04.543 Stenosis of bilateral lacrimal canaliculi**
  - **H04.549 Stenosis of unspecified lacrimal canaliculi**

+ **H04.55 Acquired stenosis of nasolacrimal duct**
  - **H04.551 Acquired stenosis of right nasolacrimal duct**
  - **H04.552 Acquired stenosis of left nasolacrimal duct**
  - **H04.553 Acquired stenosis of bilateral nasolacrimal duct**
  - **H04.559 Acquired stenosis of unspecified nasolacrimal duct**

+ **H04.56 Stenosis of lacrimal punctum**
  - **H04.561 Stenosis of right lacrimal punctum**
  - **H04.562 Stenosis of left lacrimal punctum**
  - **H04.563 Stenosis of bilateral lacrimal punctum**
  - **H04.569 Stenosis of unspecified lacrimal punctum**

+ **H04.57 Stenosis of lacrimal sac**
  - **H04.571 Stenosis of right lacrimal sac**
  - **H04.572 Stenosis of left lacrimal sac**
  - **H04.573 Stenosis of bilateral lacrimal sac**
  - **H04.579 Stenosis of unspecified lacrimal sac**

+ **H04.6 Other changes of lacrimal passages**

+ **H04.61 Lacrimal fistula**
  - **H04.611 Lacrimal fistula right lacrimal passage**
  - **H04.612 Lacrimal fistula left lacrimal passage**
  - **H04.613 Lacrimal fistula bilateral lacrimal passages**
  - **H04.619 Lacrimal fistula unspecified lacrimal passage**

H04.69 Other changes of lacrimal passages

+ **H04.8 Other disorders of lacrimal system**

+ **H04.81 Granuloma of lacrimal passages**
  - **H04.811 Granuloma of right lacrimal passage**
  - **H04.812 Granuloma of left lacrimal passage**
  - **H04.813 Granuloma of bilateral lacrimal passages**
  - **H04.819 Granuloma of unspecified lacrimal passage**

H04.89 Other disorders of lacrimal system

H04.9 Disorder of lacrimal system, unspecified

H05 Disorders of orbit

Excludes1: *congenital malformation of orbit (Q10.7)*

+ **H05.0 Acute inflammation of orbit**

H05.00 Unspecified acute inflammation of orbit

+ **H05.01 Cellulitis of orbit**

Abscess of orbit

  - CC **H05.011 Cellulitis of right orbit**
  - CC **H05.012 Cellulitis of left orbit**
  - CC **H05.013 Cellulitis of bilateral orbits**
  - CC **H05.019 Cellulitis of unspecified orbit**

+ **H05.02 Osteomyelitis of orbit**
  - CC **H05.021 Osteomyelitis of right orbit**
  - CC **H05.022 Osteomyelitis of left orbit**
  - CC **H05.023 Osteomyelitis of bilateral orbits**
  - CC **H05.029 Osteomyelitis of unspecified orbit**

+ **H05.03 Periostitis of orbit**
  - CC **H05.031 Periostitis of right orbit**
  - CC **H05.032 Periostitis of left orbit**
  - CC **H05.033 Periostitis of bilateral orbits**
  - CC **H05.039 Periostitis of unspecified orbit**

+ **H05.04 Tenonitis of orbit**
  - **H05.041 Tenonitis of right orbit**
  - **H05.042 Tenonitis of left orbit**
  - **H05.043 Tenonitis of bilateral orbits**
  - **H05.049 Tenonitis of unspecified orbit**

+ **H05.1 Chronic inflammatory disorders of orbit**

H05.10 Unspecified chronic inflammatory disorders of orbit

+ **H05.11 Granuloma of orbit**

Pseudotumor (inflammatory) of orbit

  - **H05.111 Granuloma of right orbit**
  - **H05.112 Granuloma of left orbit**
  - **H05.113 Granuloma of bilateral orbits**
  - **H05.119 Granuloma of unspecified orbit**

+ **H05.12 Orbital myositis**
  - **H05.121 Orbital myositis, right orbit**
  - **H05.122 Orbital myositis, left orbit**
  - **H05.123 Orbital myositis, bilateral**
  - **H05.129 Orbital myositis, unspecified orbit**

+ **H05.2 Exophthalmic conditions**

H05.20 Unspecified exophthalmos

+ **H05.21 Displacement (lateral) of globe**
  - **H05.211 Displacement (lateral) of globe, right eye**
  - **H05.212 Displacement (lateral) of globe, left eye**
  - **H05.213 Displacement (lateral) of globe, bilateral**
  - **H05.219 Displacement (lateral) of globe, unspecified eye**

+ **H05.22 Edema of orbit**

Orbital congestion

  - **H05.221 Edema of right orbit**
  - **H05.222 Edema of left orbit**
  - **H05.223 Edema of bilateral orbit**
  - **H05.229 Edema of unspecified orbit**

+ **H05.23 Hemorrhage of orbit**
  - **H05.231 Hemorrhage of right orbit**
  - **H05.232 Hemorrhage of left orbit**
  - **H05.233 Hemorrhage of bilateral orbit**
  - **H05.239 Hemorrhage of unspecified orbit**

+ **H05.24 Constant exophthalmos**
  - **H05.241 Constant exophthalmos, right eye**
  - **H05.242 Constant exophthalmos, left eye**
  - **H05.243 Constant exophthalmos, bilateral**
  - **H05.249 Constant exophthalmos, unspecified eye**

+ **H05.25 Intermittent exophthalmos**
  - **H05.251 Intermittent exophthalmos, right eye**
  - **H05.252 Intermittent exophthalmos, left eye**
  - **H05.253 Intermittent exophthalmos, bilateral**
  - **H05.259 Intermittent exophthalmos, unspecified eye**

+ **H05.26 Pulsating exophthalmos**
  - **H05.261 Pulsating exophthalmos, right eye**
  - **H05.262 Pulsating exophthalmos, left eye**
  - **H05.263 Pulsating exophthalmos, bilateral**
  - **H05.269 Pulsating exophthalmos, unspecified eye**

+ **H05.3 Deformity of orbit**

Excludes1: *congenital deformity of orbit (Q10.7)*
hypertelorism (Q75.2)

H05.30 Unspecified deformity of orbit

+ **H05.31 Atrophy of orbit**
  - **H05.311 Atrophy of right orbit**
  - **H05.312 Atrophy of left orbit**
  - **H05.313 Atrophy of bilateral orbit**
  - **H05.319 Atrophy of unspecified orbit**

+ **H05.32 Deformity of orbit due to bone disease**

Code also associated bone disease

  - **H05.321 Deformity of right orbit due to bone disease**
  - **H05.322 Deformity of left orbit due to bone disease**
  - **H05.323 Deformity of bilateral orbits due to bone disease**
  - **H05.329 Deformity of unspecified orbit due to bone disease**

+ **H05.33 Deformity of orbit due to trauma or surgery**
  - **H05.331 Deformity of right orbit due to trauma or surgery**
  - **H05.332 Deformity of left orbit due to trauma or surgery**
  - **H05.333 Deformity of bilateral orbits due to trauma or surgery**
  - **H05.339 Deformity of unspecified orbit due to trauma or surgery**

+ **H05.34 Enlargement of orbit**
  - **H05.341 Enlargement of right orbit**
  - **H05.342 Enlargement of left orbit**
  - **H05.343 Enlargement of bilateral orbits**
  - **H05.349 Enlargement of unspecified orbit**

+ **H05.35 Exostosis of orbit**
  - **H05.351 Exostosis of right orbit**
  - **H05.352 Exostosis of left orbit**
  - **H05.353 Exostosis of bilateral orbits**
  - **H05.359 Exostosis of unspecified orbit**

+ **H05.4 Enophthalmos**
  + **H05.40 Unspecified enophthalmos**
    - **H05.401 Unspecified enophthalmos, right eye**
    - **H05.402 Unspecified enophthalmos, left eye**
    - **H05.403 Unspecified enophthalmos, bilateral**
    - **H05.409 Unspecified enophthalmos, unspecified eye**
  + **H05.41 Enophthalmos due to atrophy of orbital tissue**
    - **H05.411 Enophthalmos due to atrophy of orbital tissue, right eye**
    - **H05.412 Enophthalmos due to atrophy of orbital tissue, left eye**
    - **H05.413 Enophthalmos due to atrophy of orbital tissue, bilateral**
    - **H05.419 Enophthalmos due to atrophy of orbital tissue, unspecified eye**
  + **H05.42 Enophthalmos due to trauma or surgery**
    - **H05.421 Enophthalmos due to trauma or surgery, right eye**
    - **H05.422 Enophthalmos due to trauma or surgery, left eye**
    - **H05.423 Enophthalmos due to trauma or surgery, bilateral**
    - **H05.429 Enophthalmos due to trauma or surgery, unspecified eye**

+ **H05.5 Retained (old) foreign body following penetrating wound of orbit**

  Retrobulbar foreign body

  Use additional code to identify the type of retained foreign body (Z18.-)

  Excludes1: *current penetrating wound of orbit (S05.4-)*

  Excludes2: *retained foreign body of eyelid (H02.81-)*
  retained intraocular foreign body (H44.6-, H44.7-)

  - **H05.50 Retained (old) foreign body following penetrating wound of unspecified orbit**
  - **H05.51 Retained (old) foreign body following penetrating wound of right orbit**
  - **H05.52 Retained (old) foreign body following penetrating wound of left orbit**
  - **H05.53 Retained (old) foreign body following penetrating wound of bilateral orbits**

+ **H05.8 Other disorders of orbit**
  + **H05.81 Cyst of orbit**

    Encephalocele of orbit

    - **H05.811 Cyst of right orbit**
    - **H05.812 Cyst of left orbit**
    - **H05.813 Cyst of bilateral orbits**
    - **H05.819 Cyst of unspecified orbit**
  + **H05.82 Myopathy of extraocular muscles**
    - **H05.821 Myopathy of extraocular muscles, right orbit**
    - **H05.822 Myopathy of extraocular muscles, left orbit**
    - **H05.823 Myopathy of extraocular muscles, bilateral**
    - **H05.829 Myopathy of extraocular muscles, unspecified orbit**
  - **H05.89 Other disorders of orbit**
- **H05.9 Unspecified disorder of orbit**

Disorders of conjunctiva (H10-H11)

H10 Conjunctivitis

Excludes1: *keratoconjunctivitis (H16.2-)*

+ **H10.0 Mucopurulent conjunctivitis**
  + **H10.01 Acute follicular conjunctivitis**
    - **H10.011 Acute follicular conjunctivitis, right eye**
    - **H10.012 Acute follicular conjunctivitis, left eye**
    - **H10.013 Acute follicular conjunctivitis, bilateral**
    - **H10.019 Acute follicular conjunctivitis, unspecified eye**
  + **H10.02 Other mucopurulent conjunctivitis**
    - **H10.021 Other mucopurulent conjunctivitis, right eye**
    - **H10.022 Other mucopurulent conjunctivitis, left eye**
    - **H10.023 Other mucopurulent conjunctivitis, bilateral**
    - **H10.029 Other mucopurulent conjunctivitis, unspecified eye**

+ **H10.1 Acute atopic conjunctivitis**

  Acute papillary conjunctivitis

  - **H10.10 Acute atopic conjunctivitis, unspecified eye**
  - **H10.11 Acute atopic conjunctivitis, right eye**
  - **H10.12 Acute atopic conjunctivitis, left eye**
  - **H10.13 Acute atopic conjunctivitis, bilateral**

+ **H10.2 Other acute conjunctivitis**
  + **H10.21 Acute toxic conjunctivitis**

    Acute chemical conjunctivitis

    Code first (T51-T65) to identify chemical and intent

    Excludes1: *burn and corrosion of eye and adnexa (T26.-)*

    - **H10.211 Acute toxic conjunctivitis, right eye**
    - **H10.212 Acute toxic conjunctivitis, left eye**
    - **H10.213 Acute toxic conjunctivitis, bilateral**
    - **H10.219 Acute toxic conjunctivitis, unspecified eye**
  + **H10.22 Pseudomembranous conjunctivitis**
    - **H10.221 Pseudomembranous conjunctivitis, right eye**
    - **H10.222 Pseudomembranous conjunctivitis, left eye**
    - **H10.223 Pseudomembranous conjunctivitis, bilateral**
    - **H10.229 Pseudomembranous conjunctivitis, unspecified eye**
  + **H10.23 Serous conjunctivitis, except viral**

    Excludes1: *viral conjunctivitis (B30.-)*

    - **H10.231 Serous conjunctivitis, except viral, right eye**
    - **H10.232 Serous conjunctivitis, except viral, left eye**
    - **H10.233 Serous conjunctivitis, except viral, bilateral**
    - **H10.239 Serous conjunctivitis, except viral, unspecified eye**

+ **H10.3 Unspecified acute conjunctivitis**

  Excludes1: *ophthalmia neonatorum NOS (P39.1)*

  - **H10.30 Unspecified acute conjunctivitis, unspecified eye**
  - **H10.31 Unspecified acute conjunctivitis, right eye**
  - **H10.32 Unspecified acute conjunctivitis, left eye**
  - **H10.33 Unspecified acute conjunctivitis, bilateral**

+ **H10.4 Chronic conjunctivitis**
  + **H10.40 Unspecified chronic conjunctivitis**
    - **H10.401 Unspecified chronic conjunctivitis, right eye**
    - **H10.402 Unspecified chronic conjunctivitis, left eye**
    - **H10.403 Unspecified chronic conjunctivitis, bilateral**
    - **H10.409 Unspecified chronic conjunctivitis, unspecified eye**
  + **H10.41 Chronic giant papillary conjunctivitis**
    - **H10.411 Chronic giant papillary conjunctivitis, right eye**
    - **H10.412 Chronic giant papillary conjunctivitis, left eye**
    - **H10.413 Chronic giant papillary conjunctivitis, bilateral**
    - **H10.419 Chronic giant papillary conjunctivitis, unspecified eye**
  + **H10.42 Simple chronic conjunctivitis**
    - **H10.421 Simple chronic conjunctivitis, right eye**
    - **H10.422 Simple chronic conjunctivitis, left eye**
    - **H10.423 Simple chronic conjunctivitis, bilateral**
    - **H10.429 Simple chronic conjunctivitis, unspecified eye**
  + **H10.43 Chronic follicular conjunctivitis**
    - **H10.431 Chronic follicular conjunctivitis, right eye**
    - **H10.432 Chronic follicular conjunctivitis, left eye**
    - **H10.433 Chronic follicular conjunctivitis, bilateral**
    - **H10.439 Chronic follicular conjunctivitis, unspecified eye**
  - **H10.44 Vernal conjunctivitis**

    Excludes1: *vernal keratoconjunctivitis with limbar and corneal involvement (H16.26-)*
  - **H10.45 Other chronic allergic conjunctivitis**

+ **H10.5 Blepharoconjunctivitis**
  + **H10.50 Unspecified blepharoconjunctivitis**
    - **H10.501 Unspecified blepharoconjunctivitis, right eye**
    - **H10.502 Unspecified blepharoconjunctivitis, left eye**
    - **H10.503 Unspecified blepharoconjunctivitis, bilateral**
    - **H10.509 Unspecified blepharoconjunctivitis, unspecified eye**
  + **H10.51 Ligneous conjunctivitis**
    Code also underlying condition if known, such as: plasminogen deficiency (E88.02)
    - **H10.511 Ligneous conjunctivitis, right eye**
    - **H10.512 Ligneous conjunctivitis, left eye**
    - **H10.513 Ligneous conjunctivitis, bilateral**
    - **H10.519 Ligneous conjunctivitis, unspecified eye**
  + **H10.52 Angular blepharoconjunctivitis**
    - **H10.521 Angular blepharoconjunctivitis, right eye**
    - **H10.522 Angular blepharoconjunctivitis, left eye**
    - **H10.523 Angular blepharoconjunctivitis, bilateral**
    - **H10.529 Angular blepharoconjunctivitis, unspecified eye**
  + **H10.53 Contact blepharoconjunctivitis**
    - **H10.531 Contact blepharoconjunctivitis, right eye**
    - **H10.532 Contact blepharoconjunctivitis, left eye**
    - **H10.533 Contact blepharoconjunctivitis, bilateral**
    - **H10.539 Contact blepharoconjunctivitis, unspecified eye**

+ **H10.8 Other conjunctivitis**
  AHA CC: 4Q, 2018, 15
  + **H10.81 Pingueculitis**
    Excludes1: *pinguecula (H11.15-)*
    - **H10.811 Pingueculitis, right eye**
    - **H10.812 Pingueculitis, left eye**
    - **H10.813 Pingueculitis, bilateral**
    - **H10.819 Pingueculitis, unspecified eye**
  + **H10.82 Rosacea conjunctivitis**
    Code first underlying rosacea dermatitis (L71.-)
    - **H10.821 Rosacea conjunctivitis, right eye**
    - **H10.822 Rosacea conjunctivitis, left eye**
    - **H10.823 Rosacea conjunctivitis, bilateral**
      AHA CC: 4Q, 2018, 15
    - **H10.829 Rosacea conjunctivitis, unspecified eye**
  - **H10.89 Other conjunctivitis**

H10.9 Unspecified conjunctivitis

H11 Other disorders of conjunctiva

Excludes1: *keratoconjunctivitis (H16.2-)*

+ **H11.0 Pterygium of eye**
  Excludes1: *pseudopterygium (H11.81-)*
  + **H11.00 Unspecified pterygium of eye**
    - **H11.001 Unspecified pterygium of right eye**
    - **H11.002 Unspecified pterygium of left eye**
    - **H11.003 Unspecified pterygium of eye, bilateral**
    - **H11.009 Unspecified pterygium of unspecified eye**
  + **H11.01 Amyloid pterygium**
    - **H11.011 Amyloid pterygium of right eye**
    - **H11.012 Amyloid pterygium of left eye**
    - **H11.013 Amyloid pterygium of eye, bilateral**
    - **H11.019 Amyloid pterygium of unspecified eye**
  + **H11.02 Central pterygium of eye**
    - **H11.021 Central pterygium of right eye**
    - **H11.022 Central pterygium of left eye**
    - **H11.023 Central pterygium of eye, bilateral**
    - **H11.029 Central pterygium of unspecified eye**
  + **H11.03 Double pterygium of eye**
    - **H11.031 Double pterygium of right eye**
    - **H11.032 Double pterygium of left eye**
    - **H11.033 Double pterygium of eye, bilateral**
    - **H11.039 Double pterygium of unspecified eye**
  + **H11.04 Peripheral pterygium of eye, stationary**
    - **H11.041 Peripheral pterygium, stationary, right eye**
    - **H11.042 Peripheral pterygium, stationary, left eye**
    - **H11.043 Peripheral pterygium, stationary, bilateral**
    - **H11.049 Peripheral pterygium, stationary, unspecified eye**
  + **H11.05 Peripheral pterygium of eye, progressive**
    - **H11.051 Peripheral pterygium, progressive, right eye**
    - **H11.052 Peripheral pterygium, progressive, left eye**
    - **H11.053 Peripheral pterygium, progressive, bilateral**
    - **H11.059 Peripheral pterygium, progressive, unspecified eye**
  + **H11.06 Recurrent pterygium of eye**
    - **H11.061 Recurrent pterygium of right eye**
    - **H11.062 Recurrent pterygium of left eye**
    - **H11.063 Recurrent pterygium of eye, bilateral**
    - **H11.069 Recurrent pterygium of unspecified eye**

+ **H11.1 Conjunctival degenerations and deposits**
  Excludes2: *pseudopterygium (H11.81)*
  - **H11.10 Unspecified conjunctival degenerations**
  + **H11.11 Conjunctival deposits**
    - **H11.111 Conjunctival deposits, right eye**
    - **H11.112 Conjunctival deposits, left eye**
    - **H11.113 Conjunctival deposits, bilateral**
    - **H11.119 Conjunctival deposits, unspecified eye**
  + **H11.12 Conjunctival concretions**
    - **H11.121 Conjunctival concretions, right eye**
    - **H11.122 Conjunctival concretions, left eye**
    - **H11.123 Conjunctival concretions, bilateral**
    - **H11.129 Conjunctival concretions, unspecified eye**
  + **H11.13 Conjunctival pigmentations**
    Conjunctival argyrosis [argyria]
    - **H11.131 Conjunctival pigmentations, right eye**
    - **H11.132 Conjunctival pigmentations, left eye**
    - **H11.133 Conjunctival pigmentations, bilateral**
    - **H11.139 Conjunctival pigmentations, unspecified eye**
  + **H11.14 Conjunctival xerosis, unspecified**
    Excludes1: *xerosis of conjunctiva due to vitamin A deficiency (E50.0, E50.1)*
    - **H11.141 Conjunctival xerosis, unspecified, right eye**
    - **H11.142 Conjunctival xerosis, unspecified, left eye**
    - **H11.143 Conjunctival xerosis, unspecified, bilateral**
    - **H11.149 Conjunctival xerosis, unspecified, unspecified eye**
  + **H11.15 Pinguecula**
    Excludes1: *pingueculitis (H10.81-)*
    - **H11.151 Pinguecula, right eye**
    - **H11.152 Pinguecula, left eye**
    - **H11.153 Pinguecula, bilateral**
    - **H11.159 Pinguecula, unspecified eye**

+ **H11.2 Conjunctival scars**
  + **H11.21 Conjunctival adhesions and strands (localized)**
    - **H11.211 Conjunctival adhesions and strands (localized), right eye**
    - **H11.212 Conjunctival adhesions and strands (localized), left eye**
    - **H11.213 Conjunctival adhesions and strands (localized), bilateral**
    - **H11.219 Conjunctival adhesions and strands (localized), unspecified eye**
  + **H11.22 Conjunctival granuloma**
    - **H11.221 Conjunctival granuloma, right eye**
    - **H11.222 Conjunctival granuloma, left eye**
    - **H11.223 Conjunctival granuloma, bilateral**
    - **H11.229 Conjunctival granuloma, unspecified**
  + **H11.23 Symblepharon**
    - **H11.231 Symblepharon, right eye**
    - **H11.232 Symblepharon, left eye**
    - **H11.233 Symblepharon, bilateral**
    - **H11.239 Symblepharon, unspecified eye**
  + **H11.24 Scarring of conjunctiva**
    - **H11.241 Scarring of conjunctiva, right eye**
    - **H11.242 Scarring of conjunctiva, left eye**
    - **H11.243 Scarring of conjunctiva, bilateral**
    - **H11.249 Scarring of conjunctiva, unspecified eye**

+ **H11.3 Conjunctival hemorrhage**
  Subconjunctival hemorrhage
  - **H11.30 Conjunctival hemorrhage, unspecified eye**
  - **H11.31 Conjunctival hemorrhage, right eye**
  - **H11.32 Conjunctival hemorrhage, left eye**
  - **H11.33 Conjunctival hemorrhage, bilateral**

+ **H11.4 Other conjunctival vascular disorders and cysts**
+ **H11.41 Vascular abnormalities of conjunctiva**
Conjunctival aneurysm
H11.411 Vascular abnormalities of conjunctiva, right eye
H11.412 Vascular abnormalities of conjunctiva, left eye
H11.413 Vascular abnormalities of conjunctiva, bilateral
H11.419 Vascular abnormalities of conjunctiva, unspecified eye
+ **H11.42 Conjunctival edema**
H11.421 Conjunctival edema, right eye
H11.422 Conjunctival edema, left eye
H11.423 Conjunctival edema, bilateral
H11.429 Conjunctival edema, unspecified eye
+ **H11.43 Conjunctival hyperemia**
H11.431 Conjunctival hyperemia, right eye
H11.432 Conjunctival hyperemia, left eye
H11.433 Conjunctival hyperemia, bilateral
H11.439 Conjunctival hyperemia, unspecified eye
+ **H11.44 Conjunctival cysts**
H11.441 Conjunctival cysts, right eye
H11.442 Conjunctival cysts, left eye
H11.443 Conjunctival cysts, bilateral
H11.449 Conjunctival cysts, unspecified eye
+ **H11.8 Other specified disorders of conjunctiva**
+ **H11.81 Pseudopterygium of conjunctiva**
H11.811 Pseudopterygium of conjunctiva, right eye
H11.812 Pseudopterygium of conjunctiva, left eye
H11.813 Pseudopterygium of conjunctiva, bilateral
H11.819 Pseudopterygium of conjunctiva, unspecified eye
+ **H11.82 Conjunctivochalasis**
H11.821 Conjunctivochalasis, right eye
H11.822 Conjunctivochalasis, left eye
H11.823 Conjunctivochalasis, bilateral
H11.829 Conjunctivochalasis, unspecified eye
H11.89 Other specified disorders of conjunctiva
H11.9 Unspecified disorder of conjunctiva

Disorders of sclera, cornea, iris and ciliary body (H15-H22)

+ **H15 Disorders of sclera**
+ **H15.0 Scleritis**
+ **H15.00 Unspecified scleritis**
H15.001 Unspecified scleritis, right eye
H15.002 Unspecified scleritis, left eye
H15.003 Unspecified scleritis, bilateral
H15.009 Unspecified scleritis, unspecified eye
+ **H15.01 Anterior scleritis**
H15.011 Anterior scleritis, right eye
H15.012 Anterior scleritis, left eye
H15.013 Anterior scleritis, bilateral
H15.019 Anterior scleritis, unspecified eye
+ **H15.02 Brawny scleritis**
H15.021 Brawny scleritis, right eye
H15.022 Brawny scleritis, left eye
H15.023 Brawny scleritis, bilateral
H15.029 Brawny scleritis, unspecified eye
+ **H15.03 Posterior scleritis**
Sclerotenonitis
H15.031 Posterior scleritis, right eye
H15.032 Posterior scleritis, left eye
H15.033 Posterior scleritis, bilateral
H15.039 Posterior scleritis, unspecified eye
+ **H15.04 Scleritis with corneal involvement**
H15.041 Scleritis with corneal involvement, right eye
H15.042 Scleritis with corneal involvement, left eye
H15.043 Scleritis with corneal involvement, bilateral
H15.049 Scleritis with corneal involvement, unspecified eye
+ **H15.05 Scleromalacia perforans**
H15.051 Scleromalacia perforans, right eye
H15.052 Scleromalacia perforans, left eye
H15.053 Scleromalacia perforans, bilateral
H15.059 Scleromalacia perforans, unspecified eye
+ **H15.09 Other scleritis**
Scleral abscess
H15.091 Other scleritis, right eye
H15.092 Other scleritis, left eye
H15.093 Other scleritis, bilateral
H15.099 Other scleritis, unspecified eye
+ **H15.1 Episcleritis**
+ **H15.10 Unspecified episcleritis**
H15.101 Unspecified episcleritis, right eye
H15.102 Unspecified episcleritis, left eye
H15.103 Unspecified episcleritis, bilateral
H15.109 Unspecified episcleritis, unspecified eye
+ **H15.11 Episcleritis periodica fugax**
H15.111 Episcleritis periodica fugax, right eye
H15.112 Episcleritis periodica fugax, left eye
H15.113 Episcleritis periodica fugax, bilateral
H15.119 Episcleritis periodica fugax, unspecified eye
+ **H15.12 Nodular episcleritis**
H15.121 Nodular episcleritis, right eye
H15.122 Nodular episcleritis, left eye
H15.123 Nodular episcleritis, bilateral
H15.129 Nodular episcleritis, unspecified eye
+ **H15.8 Other disorders of sclera**
Excludes2: *blue sclera (Q13.5)*
degenerative myopia (H44.2-)
+ **H15.81 Equatorial staphyloma**
H15.811 Equatorial staphyloma, right eye
H15.812 Equatorial staphyloma, left eye
H15.813 Equatorial staphyloma, bilateral
H15.819 Equatorial staphyloma, unspecified eye
+ **H15.82 Localized anterior staphyloma**
H15.821 Localized anterior staphyloma, right eye
H15.822 Localized anterior staphyloma, left eye
H15.823 Localized anterior staphyloma, bilateral
H15.829 Localized anterior staphyloma, unspecified eye
+ **H15.83 Staphyloma posticum**
H15.831 Staphyloma posticum, right eye
H15.832 Staphyloma posticum, left eye
H15.833 Staphyloma posticum, bilateral
H15.839 Staphyloma posticum, unspecified eye
+ **H15.84 Scleral ectasia**
H15.841 Scleral ectasia, right eye
H15.842 Scleral ectasia, left eye
H15.843 Scleral ectasia, bilateral
H15.849 Scleral ectasia, unspecified eye
+ **H15.85 Ring staphyloma**
H15.851 Ring staphyloma, right eye
H15.852 Ring staphyloma, left eye
H15.853 Ring staphyloma, bilateral
H15.859 Ring staphyloma, unspecified eye
H15.89 Other disorders of sclera
H15.9 Unspecified disorder of sclera

H16 Keratitis
+ **H16.0 Corneal ulcer**
+ **H16.00 Unspecified corneal ulcer**
H16.001 Unspecified corneal ulcer, right eye
H16.002 Unspecified corneal ulcer, left eye
H16.003 Unspecified corneal ulcer, bilateral
H16.009 Unspecified corneal ulcer, unspecified eye
+ **H16.01 Central corneal ulcer**
H16.011 Central corneal ulcer, right eye
H16.012 Central corneal ulcer, left eye
H16.013 Central corneal ulcer, bilateral
H16.019 Central corneal ulcer, unspecified eye
+ **H16.02 Ring corneal ulcer**
H16.021 Ring corneal ulcer, right eye
H16.022 Ring corneal ulcer, left eye
H16.023 Ring corneal ulcer, bilateral
H16.029 Ring corneal ulcer, unspecified eye

+ **H16.03 Corneal ulcer with hypopyon**
  - **H16.031 Corneal ulcer with hypopyon, right eye**
  - **H16.032 Corneal ulcer with hypopyon, left eye**
  - **H16.033 Corneal ulcer with hypopyon, bilateral**
  - **H16.039 Corneal ulcer with hypopyon, unspecified eye**

+ **H16.04 Marginal corneal ulcer**
  - **H16.041 Marginal corneal ulcer, right eye**
  - **H16.042 Marginal corneal ulcer, left eye**
  - **H16.043 Marginal corneal ulcer, bilateral**
  - **H16.049 Marginal corneal ulcer, unspecified eye**

+ **H16.05 Mooren's corneal ulcer**
  - **H16.051 Mooren's corneal ulcer, right eye**
  - **H16.052 Mooren's corneal ulcer, left eye**
  - **H16.053 Mooren's corneal ulcer, bilateral**
  - **H16.059 Mooren's corneal ulcer, unspecified eye**

+ **H16.06 Mycotic corneal ulcer**
  - **H16.061 Mycotic corneal ulcer, right eye**
  - **H16.062 Mycotic corneal ulcer, left eye**
  - **H16.063 Mycotic corneal ulcer, bilateral**
  - **H16.069 Mycotic corneal ulcer, unspecified eye**

+ **H16.07 Perforated corneal ulcer**
  - **H16.071 Perforated corneal ulcer, right eye**
  - **H16.072 Perforated corneal ulcer, left eye**
  - **H16.073 Perforated corneal ulcer, bilateral**
  - **H16.079 Perforated corneal ulcer, unspecified eye**

+ **H16.1 Other and unspecified superficial keratitis without conjunctivitis**

+ **H16.10 Unspecified superficial keratitis**
  - **H16.101 Unspecified superficial keratitis, right eye**
  - **H16.102 Unspecified superficial keratitis, left eye**
  - **H16.103 Unspecified superficial keratitis, bilateral**
  - **H16.109 Unspecified superficial keratitis, unspecified eye**

+ **H16.11 Macular keratitis**

  Areolar keratitis
  Nummular keratitis
  Stellate keratitis
  Striate keratitis
  - **H16.111 Macular keratitis, right eye**
  - **H16.112 Macular keratitis, left eye**
  - **H16.113 Macular keratitis, bilateral**
  - **H16.119 Macular keratitis, unspecified eye**

+ **H16.12 Filamentary keratitis**
  - **H16.121 Filamentary keratitis, right eye**
  - **H16.122 Filamentary keratitis, left eye**
  - **H16.123 Filamentary keratitis, bilateral**
  - **H16.129 Filamentary keratitis, unspecified eye**

+ **H16.13 Photokeratitis**

  Snow blindness
  Welders keratitis
  - **H16.131 Photokeratitis, right eye**
  - **H16.132 Photokeratitis, left eye**
  - **H16.133 Photokeratitis, bilateral**
  - **H16.139 Photokeratitis, unspecified eye**

+ **H16.14 Punctate keratitis**
  - **H16.141 Punctate keratitis, right eye**
  - **H16.142 Punctate keratitis, left eye**
  - **H16.143 Punctate keratitis, bilateral**
  - **H16.149 Punctate keratitis, unspecified eye**

+ **H16.2 Keratoconjunctivitis**

+ **H16.20 Unspecified keratoconjunctivitis**

  Superficial keratitis with conjunctivitis NOS
  - **H16.201 Unspecified keratoconjunctivitis, right eye**
  - **H16.202 Unspecified keratoconjunctivitis, left eye**
  - **H16.203 Unspecified keratoconjunctivitis, bilateral**
  - **H16.209 Unspecified keratoconjunctivitis, unspecified eye**

+ **H16.21 Exposure keratoconjunctivitis**
  - **H16.211 Exposure keratoconjunctivitis, right eye**
  - **H16.212 Exposure keratoconjunctivitis, left eye**
  - **H16.213 Exposure keratoconjunctivitis, bilateral**
  - **H16.219 Exposure keratoconjunctivitis, unspecified eye**

+ **H16.22 Keratoconjunctivitis sicca, not specified as Sjögren's**

  Excludes1: *Sjögren's syndrome (M35.01)*
  - **H16.221 Keratoconjunctivitis sicca, not specified as Sjögren's, right eye**
  - **H16.222 Keratoconjunctivitis sicca, not specified as Sjögren's, left eye**
  - **H16.223 Keratoconjunctivitis sicca, not specified as Sjögren's, bilateral**
  - **H16.229 Keratoconjunctivitis sicca, not specified as Sjögren's, unspecified eye**

+ **H16.23 Neurotrophic keratoconjunctivitis**
  - **H16.231 Neurotrophic keratoconjunctivitis, right eye**
  - **H16.232 Neurotrophic keratoconjunctivitis, left eye**
  - **H16.233 Neurotrophic keratoconjunctivitis, bilateral**
  - **H16.239 Neurotrophic keratoconjunctivitis, unspecified eye**

+ **H16.24 Ophthalmia nodosa**
  - **H16.241 Ophthalmia nodosa, right eye**
  - **H16.242 Ophthalmia nodosa, left eye**
  - **H16.243 Ophthalmia nodosa, bilateral**
  - **H16.249 Ophthalmia nodosa, unspecified eye**

+ **H16.25 Phlyctenular keratoconjunctivitis**
  - **H16.251 Phlyctenular keratoconjunctivitis, right eye**
  - **H16.252 Phlyctenular keratoconjunctivitis, left eye**
  - **H16.253 Phlyctenular keratoconjunctivitis, bilateral**
  - **H16.259 Phlyctenular keratoconjunctivitis, unspecified eye**

+ **H16.26 Vernal keratoconjunctivitis, with limbar and corneal involvement**

  Excludes1: *vernal conjunctivitis without limbar and corneal involvement (H10.44)*
  - **H16.261 Vernal keratoconjunctivitis, with limbar and corneal involvement, right eye**
  - **H16.262 Vernal keratoconjunctivitis, with limbar and corneal involvement, left eye**
  - **H16.263 Vernal keratoconjunctivitis, with limbar and corneal involvement, bilateral**
  - **H16.269 Vernal keratoconjunctivitis, with limbar and corneal involvement, unspecified eye**

+ **H16.29 Other keratoconjunctivitis**
  - **H16.291 Other keratoconjunctivitis, right eye**
  - **H16.292 Other keratoconjunctivitis, left eye**
  - **H16.293 Other keratoconjunctivitis, bilateral**
  - **H16.299 Other keratoconjunctivitis, unspecified eye**

+ **H16.3 Interstitial and deep keratitis**

+ **H16.30 Unspecified interstitial keratitis**
  - **H16.301 Unspecified interstitial keratitis, right eye**
  - **H16.302 Unspecified interstitial keratitis, left eye**
  - **H16.303 Unspecified interstitial keratitis, bilateral**
  - **H16.309 Unspecified interstitial keratitis, unspecified eye**

+ **H16.31 Corneal abscess**
  - **H16.311 Corneal abscess, right eye**
  - **H16.312 Corneal abscess, left eye**
  - **H16.313 Corneal abscess, bilateral**
  - **H16.319 Corneal abscess, unspecified eye**

+ **H16.32 Diffuse interstitial keratitis**

  Cogan's syndrome
  - **H16.321 Diffuse interstitial keratitis, right eye**
  - **H16.322 Diffuse interstitial keratitis, left eye**
  - **H16.323 Diffuse interstitial keratitis, bilateral**
  - **H16.329 Diffuse interstitial keratitis, unspecified eye**

+ **H16.33 Sclerosing keratitis**
  - **H16.331 Sclerosing keratitis, right eye**
  - **H16.332 Sclerosing keratitis, left eye**
  - **H16.333 Sclerosing keratitis, bilateral**
  - **H16.339 Sclerosing keratitis, unspecified eye**

+ H16.39 Other interstitial and deep keratitis
H16.391 Other interstitial and deep keratitis, right eye
H16.392 Other interstitial and deep keratitis, left eye
H16.393 Other interstitial and deep keratitis, bilateral
H16.399 Other interstitial and deep keratitis, unspecified eye
+ H16.4 Corneal neovascularization
+ H16.40 Unspecified corneal neovascularization
H16.401 Unspecified corneal neovascularization, right eye
H16.402 Unspecified corneal neovascularization, left eye
H16.403 Unspecified corneal neovascularization, bilateral
H16.409 Unspecified corneal neovascularization, unspecified eye
+ H16.41 Ghost vessels (corneal)
H16.411 Ghost vessels (corneal), right eye
H16.412 Ghost vessels (corneal), left eye
H16.413 Ghost vessels (corneal), bilateral
H16.419 Ghost vessels (corneal), unspecified eye
+ H16.42 Pannus (corneal)
H16.421 Pannus (corneal), right eye
H16.422 Pannus (corneal), left eye
H16.423 Pannus (corneal), bilateral
H16.429 Pannus (corneal), unspecified eye
+ H16.43 Localized vascularization of cornea
H16.431 Localized vascularization of cornea, right eye
H16.432 Localized vascularization of cornea, left eye
H16.433 Localized vascularization of cornea, bilateral
H16.439 Localized vascularization of cornea, unspecified eye
+ H16.44 Deep vascularization of cornea
H16.441 Deep vascularization of cornea, right eye
H16.442 Deep vascularization of cornea, left eye
H16.443 Deep vascularization of cornea, bilateral
H16.449 Deep vascularization of cornea, unspecified eye
H16.8 Other keratitis
H16.9 Unspecified keratitis

H17 Corneal scars and opacities

+ H17.0 Adherent leukoma
H17.00 Adherent leukoma, unspecified eye
H17.01 Adherent leukoma, right eye
H17.02 Adherent leukoma, left eye
H17.03 Adherent leukoma, bilateral
+ H17.1 Central corneal opacity
H17.10 Central corneal opacity, unspecified eye
H17.11 Central corneal opacity, right eye
H17.12 Central corneal opacity, left eye
H17.13 Central corneal opacity, bilateral
+ H17.8 Other corneal scars and opacities
+ H17.81 Minor opacity of cornea
Corneal nebula
H17.811 Minor opacity of cornea, right eye
H17.812 Minor opacity of cornea, left eye
H17.813 Minor opacity of cornea, bilateral
H17.819 Minor opacity of cornea, unspecified eye
+ H17.82 Peripheral opacity of cornea
H17.821 Peripheral opacity of cornea, right eye
H17.822 Peripheral opacity of cornea, left eye
H17.823 Peripheral opacity of cornea, bilateral
H17.829 Peripheral opacity of cornea, unspecified eye
H17.89 Other corneal scars and opacities
H17.9 Unspecified corneal scar and opacity

H18 Other disorders of cornea

+ H18.0 Corneal pigmentations and deposits
+ H18.00 Unspecified corneal deposit
H18.001 Unspecified corneal deposit, right eye
H18.002 Unspecified corneal deposit, left eye
H18.003 Unspecified corneal deposit, bilateral
H18.009 Unspecified corneal deposit, unspecified eye
+ H18.01 Anterior corneal pigmentations
Staehli's line
H18.011 Anterior corneal pigmentations, right eye
H18.012 Anterior corneal pigmentations, left eye
H18.013 Anterior corneal pigmentations, bilateral
H18.019 Anterior corneal pigmentations, unspecified eye
+ H18.02 Argentous corneal deposits
H18.021 Argentous corneal deposits, right eye
H18.022 Argentous corneal deposits, left eye
H18.023 Argentous corneal deposits, bilateral
H18.029 Argentous corneal deposits, unspecified eye
+ H18.03 Corneal deposits in metabolic disorders
Code also associated metabolic disorder
H18.031 Corneal deposits in metabolic disorders, right eye
H18.032 Corneal deposits in metabolic disorders, left eye
H18.033 Corneal deposits in metabolic disorders, bilateral
H18.039 Corneal deposits in metabolic disorders, unspecified eye
+ H18.04 Kayser-Fleischer ring
Code also associated Wilson's disease (E83.01)
H18.041 Kayser-Fleischer ring, right eye
H18.042 Kayser-Fleischer ring, left eye
H18.043 Kayser-Fleischer ring, bilateral
H18.049 Kayser-Fleischer ring, unspecified eye
+ H18.05 Posterior corneal pigmentations
Krukenberg's spindle
H18.051 Posterior corneal pigmentations, right eye
H18.052 Posterior corneal pigmentations, left eye
H18.053 Posterior corneal pigmentations, bilateral
H18.059 Posterior corneal pigmentations, unspecified eye
+ H18.06 Stromal corneal pigmentations
Hematocornea
H18.061 Stromal corneal pigmentations, right eye
H18.062 Stromal corneal pigmentations, left eye
H18.063 Stromal corneal pigmentations, bilateral
H18.069 Stromal corneal pigmentations, unspecified eye
+ H18.1 Bullous keratopathy
H18.10 Bullous keratopathy, unspecified eye
H18.11 Bullous keratopathy, right eye
H18.12 Bullous keratopathy, left eye
H18.13 Bullous keratopathy, bilateral
+ H18.2 Other and unspecified corneal edema
H18.20 Unspecified corneal edema
+ H18.21 Corneal edema secondary to contact lens
Excludes2: *other corneal disorders due to contact lens (H18.82-)*
H18.211 Corneal edema secondary to contact lens, right eye
H18.212 Corneal edema secondary to contact lens, left eye
H18.213 Corneal edema secondary to contact lens, bilateral
H18.219 Corneal edema secondary to contact lens, unspecified eye

+ **H18.22 Idiopathic corneal edema**
  - **H18.221 Idiopathic corneal edema, right eye**
  - **H18.222 Idiopathic corneal edema, left eye**
  - **H18.223 Idiopathic corneal edema, bilateral**
  - **H18.229 Idiopathic corneal edema, unspecified eye**

+ **H18.23 Secondary corneal edema**
  - **H18.231 Secondary corneal edema, right eye**
  - **H18.232 Secondary corneal edema, left eye**
  - **H18.233 Secondary corneal edema, bilateral**
  - **H18.239 Secondary corneal edema, unspecified eye**

+ **H18.3 Changes of corneal membranes**
  - **H18.30 Unspecified corneal membrane change**

+ **H18.31 Folds and rupture in Bowman's membrane**
  - **H18.311 Folds and rupture in Bowman's membrane, right eye**
  - **H18.312 Folds and rupture in Bowman's membrane, left eye**
  - **H18.313 Folds and rupture in Bowman's membrane, bilateral**
  - **H18.319 Folds and rupture in Bowman's membrane, unspecified eye**

+ **H18.32 Folds in Descemet's membrane**
  - **H18.321 Folds in Descemet's membrane, right eye**
  - **H18.322 Folds in Descemet's membrane, left eye**
  - **H18.323 Folds in Descemet's membrane, bilateral**
  - **H18.329 Folds in Descemet's membrane, unspecified eye**

+ **H18.33 Rupture in Descemet's membrane**
  - **H18.331 Rupture in Descemet's membrane, right eye**
  - **H18.332 Rupture in Descemet's membrane, left eye**
  - **H18.333 Rupture in Descemet's membrane, bilateral**
  - **H18.339 Rupture in Descemet's membrane, unspecified eye**

+ **H18.4 Corneal degeneration**

Excludes1: *Mooren's ulcer (H16.0-)*
recurrent erosion of cornea (H18.83-)

- **H18.40 Unspecified corneal degeneration**

+ **H18.41 Arcus senilis**

  Senile corneal changes
  - **H18.411 Arcus senilis, right eye**
  - **H18.412 Arcus senilis, left eye**
  - **H18.413 Arcus senilis, bilateral**
  - **H18.419 Arcus senilis, unspecified eye**

+ **H18.42 Band keratopathy**
  - **H18.421 Band keratopathy, right eye**
  - **H18.422 Band keratopathy, left eye**
  - **H18.423 Band keratopathy, bilateral**
  - **H18.429 Band keratopathy, unspecified eye**

- **H18.43 Other calcerous corneal degeneration**

+ **H18.44 Keratomalacia**

  Excludes1: *keratomalacia due to vitamin A deficiency (E50.4)*
  - **H18.441 Keratomalacia, right eye**
  - **H18.442 Keratomalacia, left eye**
  - **H18.443 Keratomalacia, bilateral**
  - **H18.449 Keratomalacia, unspecified eye**

+ **H18.45 Nodular corneal degeneration**
  - **H18.451 Nodular corneal degeneration, right eye**
  - **H18.452 Nodular corneal degeneration, left eye**
  - **H18.453 Nodular corneal degeneration, bilateral**
  - **H18.459 Nodular corneal degeneration, unspecified eye**

+ **H18.46 Peripheral corneal degeneration**
  - **H18.461 Peripheral corneal degeneration, right eye**
  - **H18.462 Peripheral corneal degeneration, left eye**
  - **H18.463 Peripheral corneal degeneration, bilateral**
  - **H18.469 Peripheral corneal degeneration, unspecified eye**

- **H18.49 Other corneal degeneration**

+ **H18.5 Hereditary corneal dystrophies**

  AHA CC: 4Q, 2020, 24

+ **H18.50 Unspecified hereditary corneal dystrophies**
  - **H18.501 Unspecified hereditary corneal dystrophies, right eye**
  - **H18.502 Unspecified hereditary corneal dystrophies, left eye**
  - **H18.503 Unspecified hereditary corneal dystrophies, bilateral**
  - **H18.509 Unspecified hereditary corneal dystrophies, unspecified eye**

+ **H18.51 Endothelial corneal dystrophy**

  Fuchs' dystrophy
  - **H18.511 Endothelial corneal dystrophy, right eye**
  - **H18.512 Endothelial corneal dystrophy, left eye**
  - **H18.513 Endothelial corneal dystrophy, bilateral**
  - **H18.519 Endothelial corneal dystrophy, unspecified eye**

+ **H18.52 Epithelial (juvenile) corneal dystrophy**
  - **H18.521 Epithelial (juvenile) corneal dystrophy, right eye**
  - **H18.522 Epithelial (juvenile) corneal dystrophy, left eye**
  - **H18.523 Epithelial (juvenile) corneal dystrophy, bilateral**
  - **H18.529 Epithelial (juvenile) corneal dystrophy, unspecified eye**

+ **H18.53 Granular corneal dystrophy**
  - **H18.531 Granular corneal dystrophy, right eye**
  - **H18.532 Granular corneal dystrophy, left eye**
  - **H18.533 Granular corneal dystrophy, bilateral**
  - **H18.539 Granular corneal dystrophy, unspecified eye**

+ **H18.54 Lattice corneal dystrophy**
  - **H18.541 Lattice corneal dystrophy, right eye**
  - **H18.542 Lattice corneal dystrophy, left eye**
  - **H18.543 Lattice corneal dystrophy, bilateral**
  - **H18.549 Lattice corneal dystrophy, unspecified eye**

+ **H18.55 Macular corneal dystrophy**
  - **H18.551 Macular corneal dystrophy, right eye**
  - **H18.552 Macular corneal dystrophy, left eye**
  - **H18.553 Macular corneal dystrophy, bilateral**
  - **H18.559 Macular corneal dystrophy, unspecified eye**

+ **H18.59 Other hereditary corneal dystrophies**
  - **H18.591 Other hereditary corneal dystrophies, right eye**
  - **H18.592 Other hereditary corneal dystrophies, left eye**
  - **H18.593 Other hereditary corneal dystrophies, bilateral**
  - **H18.599 Other hereditary corneal dystrophies, unspecified eye**

+ **H18.6 Keratoconus**

+ **H18.60 Keratoconus, unspecified**
  - **H18.601 Keratoconus, unspecified, right eye**
  - **H18.602 Keratoconus, unspecified, left eye**
  - **H18.603 Keratoconus, unspecified, bilateral**
  - **H18.609 Keratoconus, unspecified, unspecified eye**

+ **H18.61 Keratoconus, stable**
  - **H18.611 Keratoconus, stable, right eye**
  - **H18.612 Keratoconus, stable, left eye**
  - **H18.613 Keratoconus, stable, bilateral**
  - **H18.619 Keratoconus, stable, unspecified eye**

+ **H18.62 Keratoconus, unstable**

  Acute hydrops
  - **H18.621 Keratoconus, unstable, right eye**
  - **H18.622 Keratoconus, unstable, left eye**
  - **H18.623 Keratoconus, unstable, bilateral**
  - **H18.629 Keratoconus, unstable, unspecified eye**

+ **H18.7 Other and unspecified corneal deformities**

  Excludes1: *congenital malformations of cornea (Q13.3-Q13.4)*

- **H18.70 Unspecified corneal deformity**

+ **H18.71 Corneal ectasia**
  - **H18.711 Corneal ectasia, right eye**
  - **H18.712 Corneal ectasia, left eye**
  - **H18.713 Corneal ectasia, bilateral**
  - **H18.719 Corneal ectasia, unspecified eye**

+ **H18.72 Corneal staphyloma**
  - **H18.721 Corneal staphyloma, right eye**
  - **H18.722 Corneal staphyloma, left eye**

H18.723 Corneal staphyloma, bilateral
H18.729 Corneal staphyloma, unspecified eye
+ H18.73 Descemetocele
H18.731 Descemetocele, right eye
H18.732 Descemetocele, left eye
H18.733 Descemetocele, bilateral
H18.739 Descemetocele, unspecified eye
+ H18.79 Other corneal deformities
H18.791 Other corneal deformities, right eye
H18.792 Other corneal deformities, left eye
H18.793 Other corneal deformities, bilateral
H18.799 Other corneal deformities, unspecified eye
+ H18.8 Other specified disorders of cornea
+ H18.81 Anesthesia and hypoesthesia of cornea
H18.811 Anesthesia and hypoesthesia of cornea, right eye
H18.812 Anesthesia and hypoesthesia of cornea, left eye
H18.813 Anesthesia and hypoesthesia of cornea, bilateral
H18.819 Anesthesia and hypoesthesia of cornea, unspecified eye
+ H18.82 Corneal disorder due to contact lens
Excludes2: *corneal edema due to contact lens (H18.21-)*
H18.821 Corneal disorder due to contact lens, right eye
H18.822 Corneal disorder due to contact lens, left eye
H18.823 Corneal disorder due to contact lens, bilateral
H18.829 Corneal disorder due to contact lens, unspecified eye
+ H18.83 Recurrent erosion of cornea
H18.831 Recurrent erosion of cornea, right eye
H18.832 Recurrent erosion of cornea, left eye
H18.833 Recurrent erosion of cornea, bilateral
H18.839 Recurrent erosion of cornea, unspecified eye
+ H18.89 Other specified disorders of cornea
H18.891 Other specified disorders of cornea, right eye
H18.892 Other specified disorders of cornea, left eye
H18.893 Other specified disorders of cornea, bilateral
H18.899 Other specified disorders of cornea, unspecified eye
H18.9 Unspecified disorder of cornea

H20 Iridocyclitis

+ H20.0 Acute and subacute iridocyclitis
Acute anterior uveitis
Acute cyclitis
Acute iritis
Subacute anterior uveitis
Subacute cyclitis
Subacute iritis
Excludes1: *iridocyclitis, iritis, uveitis (due to) (in) diabetes mellitus (E08-E13 with .39)*
iridocyclitis, iritis, uveitis (due to) (in) diphtheria (A36.89)
iridocyclitis, iritis, uveitis (due to) (in) gonococcal (A54.32)
iridocyclitis, iritis, uveitis (due to) (in) herpes (simplex) (B00.51)
iridocyclitis, iritis, uveitis (due to) (in) herpes zoster (B02.32)
iridocyclitis, iritis, uveitis (due to) (in) late congenital syphilis (A50.39)
iridocyclitis, iritis, uveitis (due to) (in) late syphilis (A52.71)
iridocyclitis, iritis, uveitis (due to) (in) sarcoidosis (D86.83)
iridocyclitis, iritis, uveitis (due to) (in) syphilis (A51.43)
iridocyclitis, iritis, uveitis (due to) (in) toxoplasmosis (B58.09)
iridocyclitis, iritis, uveitis (due to) (in) tuberculosis (A18.54)
CC H20.00 Unspecified acute and subacute iridocyclitis
+ H20.01 Primary iridocyclitis
CC H20.011 Primary iridocyclitis, right eye
CC H20.012 Primary iridocyclitis, left eye
CC H20.013 Primary iridocyclitis, bilateral
CC H20.019 Primary iridocyclitis, unspecified eye
+ H20.02 Recurrent acute iridocyclitis
CC H20.021 Recurrent acute iridocyclitis, right eye
CC H20.022 Recurrent acute iridocyclitis, left eye
CC H20.023 Recurrent acute iridocyclitis, bilateral
CC H20.029 Recurrent acute iridocyclitis, unspecified eye
+ H20.03 Secondary infectious iridocyclitis
CC H20.031 Secondary infectious iridocyclitis, right eye
CC H20.032 Secondary infectious iridocyclitis, left eye
CC H20.033 Secondary infectious iridocyclitis, bilateral
CC H20.039 Secondary infectious iridocyclitis, unspecified eye
+ H20.04 Secondary noninfectious iridocyclitis
H20.041 Secondary noninfectious iridocyclitis, right eye
H20.042 Secondary noninfectious iridocyclitis, left eye
H20.043 Secondary noninfectious iridocyclitis, bilateral
H20.049 Secondary noninfectious iridocyclitis, unspecified eye
+ H20.05 Hypopyon
H20.051 Hypopyon, right eye
H20.052 Hypopyon, left eye
H20.053 Hypopyon, bilateral
H20.059 Hypopyon, unspecified eye
+ H20.1 Chronic iridocyclitis
Use additional code for any associated cataract (H26.21-)
Excludes2: *posterior cyclitis (H30.2-)*
H20.10 Chronic iridocyclitis, unspecified eye
H20.11 Chronic iridocyclitis, right eye
H20.12 Chronic iridocyclitis, left eye
H20.13 Chronic iridocyclitis, bilateral
+ H20.2 Lens-induced iridocyclitis
H20.20 Lens-induced iridocyclitis, unspecified eye
H20.21 Lens-induced iridocyclitis, right eye
H20.22 Lens-induced iridocyclitis, left eye
H20.23 Lens-induced iridocyclitis, bilateral
+ H20.8 Other iridocyclitis
Excludes2: *glaucomatocyclitis crises (H40.4-)*
posterior cyclitis (H30.2-)
sympathetic uveitis (H44.13-)
+ H20.81 Fuchs' heterochromic cyclitis
H20.811 Fuchs' heterochromic cyclitis, right eye
H20.812 Fuchs' heterochromic cyclitis, left eye
H20.813 Fuchs' heterochromic cyclitis, bilateral
H20.819 Fuchs' heterochromic cyclitis, unspecified eye
+ H20.82 Vogt-Koyanagi syndrome
H20.821 Vogt-Koyanagi syndrome, right eye
H20.822 Vogt-Koyanagi syndrome, left eye
H20.823 Vogt-Koyanagi syndrome, bilateral
H20.829 Vogt-Koyanagi syndrome, unspecified eye
CC H20.9 Unspecified iridocyclitis
Uveitis NOS

H21 Other disorders of iris and ciliary body

Excludes2: *sympathetic uveitis (H44.1-)*
+ H21.0 Hyphema
Excludes1: *traumatic hyphema (S05.1-)*
H21.00 Hyphema, unspecified eye
H21.01 Hyphema, right eye
H21.02 Hyphema, left eye
H21.03 Hyphema, bilateral

+ **H21.1 Other vascular disorders of iris and ciliary body**
  Neovascularization of iris or ciliary body
  Rubeosis iridis
  Rubeosis of iris
  + **H21.1X Other vascular disorders of iris and ciliary body**
    H21.1X1 Other vascular disorders of iris and ciliary body, right eye
    H21.1X2 Other vascular disorders of iris and ciliary body, left eye
    H21.1X3 Other vascular disorders of iris and ciliary body, bilateral
    H21.1X9 Other vascular disorders of iris and ciliary body, unspecified eye
+ **H21.2 Degeneration of iris and ciliary body**
  + **H21.21 Degeneration of chamber angle**
    H21.211 Degeneration of chamber angle, right eye
    H21.212 Degeneration of chamber angle, left eye
    H21.213 Degeneration of chamber angle, bilateral
    H21.219 Degeneration of chamber angle, unspecified eye
  + **H21.22 Degeneration of ciliary body**
    H21.221 Degeneration of ciliary body, right eye
    H21.222 Degeneration of ciliary body, left eye
    H21.223 Degeneration of ciliary body, bilateral
    H21.229 Degeneration of ciliary body, unspecified eye
  + **H21.23 Degeneration of iris (pigmentary)**
    Translucency of iris
    H21.231 Degeneration of iris (pigmentary), right eye
    H21.232 Degeneration of iris (pigmentary), left eye
    H21.233 Degeneration of iris (pigmentary), bilateral
    H21.239 Degeneration of iris (pigmentary), unspecified eye
  + **H21.24 Degeneration of pupillary margin**
    H21.241 Degeneration of pupillary margin, right eye
    H21.242 Degeneration of pupillary margin, left eye
    H21.243 Degeneration of pupillary margin, bilateral
    H21.249 Degeneration of pupillary margin, unspecified eye
  + **H21.25 Iridoschisis**
    H21.251 Iridoschisis, right eye
    H21.252 Iridoschisis, left eye
    H21.253 Iridoschisis, bilateral
    H21.259 Iridoschisis, unspecified eye
  + **H21.26 Iris atrophy (essential) (progressive)**
    H21.261 Iris atrophy (essential) (progressive), right eye
    H21.262 Iris atrophy (essential) (progressive), left eye
    H21.263 Iris atrophy (essential) (progressive), bilateral
    H21.269 Iris atrophy (essential) (progressive), unspecified eye
  + **H21.27 Miotic pupillary cyst**
    H21.271 Miotic pupillary cyst, right eye
    H21.272 Miotic pupillary cyst, left eye
    H21.273 Miotic pupillary cyst, bilateral
    H21.279 Miotic pupillary cyst, unspecified eye
  H21.29 Other iris atrophy
+ **H21.3 Cyst of iris, ciliary body and anterior chamber**
  Excludes2: *miotic pupillary cyst (H21.27-)*
  + **H21.30 Idiopathic cysts of iris, ciliary body or anterior chamber**
    Cyst of iris, ciliary body or anterior chamber NOS
    H21.301 Idiopathic cysts of iris, ciliary body or anterior chamber, right eye
    H21.302 Idiopathic cysts of iris, ciliary body or anterior chamber, left eye
    H21.303 Idiopathic cysts of iris, ciliary body or anterior chamber, bilateral
    H21.309 Idiopathic cysts of iris, ciliary body or anterior chamber, unspecified eye
  + **H21.31 Exudative cysts of iris or anterior chamber**
    H21.311 Exudative cysts of iris or anterior chamber, right eye
    H21.312 Exudative cysts of iris or anterior chamber, left eye
    H21.313 Exudative cysts of iris or anterior chamber, bilateral
    H21.319 Exudative cysts of iris or anterior chamber, unspecified eye
  + **H21.32 Implantation cysts of iris, ciliary body or anterior chamber**
    H21.321 Implantation cysts of iris, ciliary body or anterior chamber, right eye
    H21.322 Implantation cysts of iris, ciliary body or anterior chamber, left eye
    H21.323 Implantation cysts of iris, ciliary body or anterior chamber, bilateral
    H21.329 Implantation cysts of iris, ciliary body or anterior chamber, unspecified eye
  + **H21.33 Parasitic cyst of iris, ciliary body or anterior chamber**
    CC **H21.331 Parasitic cyst of iris, ciliary body or anterior chamber, right eye**
    CC **H21.332 Parasitic cyst of iris, ciliary body or anterior chamber, left eye**
    CC **H21.333 Parasitic cyst of iris, ciliary body or anterior chamber, bilateral**
    CC **H21.339 Parasitic cyst of iris, ciliary body or anterior chamber, unspecified eye**
  + **H21.34 Primary cyst of pars plana**
    H21.341 Primary cyst of pars plana, right eye
    H21.342 Primary cyst of pars plana, left eye
    H21.343 Primary cyst of pars plana, bilateral
    H21.349 Primary cyst of pars plana, unspecified eye
  + **H21.35 Exudative cyst of pars plana**
    H21.351 Exudative cyst of pars plana, right eye
    H21.352 Exudative cyst of pars plana, left eye
    H21.353 Exudative cyst of pars plana, bilateral
    H21.359 Exudative cyst of pars plana, unspecified eye
+ **H21.4 Pupillary membranes**
  Iris bombé
  Pupillary occlusion
  Pupillary seclusion
  Excludes1: *congenital pupillary membranes (Q13.8)*
  H21.40 Pupillary membranes, unspecified eye
  H21.41 Pupillary membranes, right eye
  H21.42 Pupillary membranes, left eye
  H21.43 Pupillary membranes, bilateral
+ **H21.5 Other and unspecified adhesions and disruptions of iris and ciliary body**
  Excludes1: *corectopia (Q13.2)*
  + **H21.50 Unspecified adhesions of iris**
    Synechia (iris) NOS
    H21.501 Unspecified adhesions of iris, right eye
    H21.502 Unspecified adhesions of iris, left eye
    H21.503 Unspecified adhesions of iris, bilateral
    H21.509 Unspecified adhesions of iris and ciliary body, unspecified eye
  + **H21.51 Anterior synechiae (iris)**
    H21.511 Anterior synechiae (iris), right eye
    H21.512 Anterior synechiae (iris), left eye
    H21.513 Anterior synechiae (iris), bilateral
    H21.519 Anterior synechiae (iris), unspecified eye
  + **H21.52 Goniosynechiae**
    H21.521 Goniosynechiae, right eye
    H21.522 Goniosynechiae, left eye
    H21.523 Goniosynechiae, bilateral
    H21.529 Goniosynechiae, unspecified eye

+ **H21.53 Iridodialysis**
H21.531 Iridodialysis, right eye
H21.532 Iridodialysis, left eye
H21.533 Iridodialysis, bilateral
H21.539 Iridodialysis, unspecified eye

+ **H21.54 Posterior synechiae (iris)**
H21.541 Posterior synechiae (iris), right eye
H21.542 Posterior synechiae (iris), left eye
H21.543 Posterior synechiae (iris), bilateral
H21.549 Posterior synechiae (iris), unspecified eye

+ **H21.55 Recession of chamber angle**
H21.551 Recession of chamber angle, right eye
H21.552 Recession of chamber angle, left eye
H21.553 Recession of chamber angle, bilateral
H21.559 Recession of chamber angle, unspecified eye

+ **H21.56 Pupillary abnormalities**
Deformed pupil
Ectopic pupil
Rupture of sphincter, pupil
Excludes1: *congenital deformity of pupil (Q13.2-)*
H21.561 Pupillary abnormality, right eye
H21.562 Pupillary abnormality, left eye
H21.563 Pupillary abnormality, bilateral
H21.569 Pupillary abnormality, unspecified eye

+ **H21.8 Other specified disorders of iris and ciliary body**
H21.81 Floppy iris syndrome
Intraoperative floppy iris syndrome (IFIS)
Use additional code for adverse effect, if applicable, to identify drug (T36-T50 with fifth or sixth character 5)
H21.82 Plateau iris syndrome (post-iridectomy) (postprocedural)
H21.89 Other specified disorders of iris and ciliary body
H21.9 Unspecified disorder of iris and ciliary body

H22 Disorders of iris and ciliary body in diseases classified elsewhere
Code first underlying disease, such as:
gout (M1A.-, M10.-)
leprosy (A30.-)
parasitic disease (B89)
Valid 3-character code, no further characters required

Disorders of lens (H25-H28)

H25 Age-related cataract
Senile cataract
Excludes2: *capsular glaucoma with pseudoexfoliation of lens (H40.1-)*

+ **H25.0 Age-related incipient cataract**
+ **H25.01 Cortical age-related cataract**
• **H25.011 Cortical age-related cataract, right eye**
• **H25.012 Cortical age-related cataract, left eye**
• **H25.013 Cortical age-related cataract, bilateral**
• **H25.019 Cortical age-related cataract, unspecified eye**
+ **H25.03 Anterior subcapsular polar age-related cataract**
• **H25.031 Anterior subcapsular polar age-related cataract, right eye**
• **H25.032 Anterior subcapsular polar age-related cataract, left eye**
• **H25.033 Anterior subcapsular polar age-related cataract, bilateral**
• **H25.039 Anterior subcapsular polar age-related cataract, unspecified eye**
+ **H25.04 Posterior subcapsular polar age-related cataract**
• **H25.041 Posterior subcapsular polar age-related cataract, right eye**
• **H25.042 Posterior subcapsular polar age-related cataract, left eye**
• **H25.043 Posterior subcapsular polar age-related cataract, bilateral**
• **H25.049 Posterior subcapsular polar age-related cataract, unspecified eye**
+ **H25.09 Other age-related incipient cataract**
Coronary age-related cataract
Punctate age-related cataract
Water clefts
• **H25.091 Other age-related incipient cataract, right eye**
• **H25.092 Other age-related incipient cataract, left eye**
• **H25.093 Other age-related incipient cataract, bilateral**
• **H25.099 Other age-related incipient cataract, unspecified eye**

+ **H25.1 Age-related nuclear cataract**
Cataracta brunescens
Nuclear sclerosis cataract
• **H25.10 Age-related nuclear cataract, unspecified eye**
• **H25.11 Age-related nuclear cataract, right eye**
AHA CC: 2Q, 2019, 31
• **H25.12 Age-related nuclear cataract, left eye**
AHA CC: 1Q, 2016, 32-33
• **H25.13 Age-related nuclear cataract, bilateral**
AHA CC: 1Q, 2016, 32-33

+ **H25.2 Age-related cataract, morgagnian type**
Age-related hypermature cataract
• **H25.20 Age-related cataract, morgagnian type, unspecified eye**
• **H25.21 Age-related cataract, morgagnian type, right eye**
• **H25.22 Age-related cataract, morgagnian type, left eye**
• **H25.23 Age-related cataract, morgagnian type, bilateral**

+ **H25.8 Other age-related cataract**
+ **H25.81 Combined forms of age-related cataract**
• **H25.811 Combined forms of age-related cataract, right eye**
• **H25.812 Combined forms of age-related cataract, left eye**
• **H25.813 Combined forms of age-related cataract, bilateral**
AHA CC: 2Q, 2019, 30
• **H25.819 Combined forms of age-related cataract, unspecified eye**
• **H25.89 Other age-related cataract**
• **H25.9 Unspecified age-related cataract**

H26 Other cataract
Excludes1: *congenital cataract (Q12.0)*
+ **H26.0 Infantile and juvenile cataract**
+ **H26.00 Unspecified infantile and juvenile cataract**
• **H26.001 Unspecified infantile and juvenile cataract, right eye**
• **H26.002 Unspecified infantile and juvenile cataract, left eye**
• **H26.003 Unspecified infantile and juvenile cataract, bilateral**
• **H26.009 Unspecified infantile and juvenile cataract, unspecified eye**
+ **H26.01 Infantile and juvenile cortical, lamellar, or zonular cataract**
• **H26.011 Infantile and juvenile cortical, lamellar, or zonular cataract, right eye**
• **H26.012 Infantile and juvenile cortical, lamellar, or zonular cataract, left eye**
• **H26.013 Infantile and juvenile cortical, lamellar, or zonular cataract, bilateral**
• **H26.019 Infantile and juvenile cortical, lamellar, or zonular cataract, unspecified eye**
+ **H26.03 Infantile and juvenile nuclear cataract**
• **H26.031 Infantile and juvenile nuclear cataract, right eye**
• **H26.032 Infantile and juvenile nuclear cataract, left eye**
• **H26.033 Infantile and juvenile nuclear cataract, bilateral**
• **H26.039 Infantile and juvenile nuclear cataract, unspecified eye**

+ H26.04 Anterior subcapsular polar infantile and juvenile cataract
- **H26.041 Anterior subcapsular polar infantile and juvenile cataract, right eye**
- **H26.042 Anterior subcapsular polar infantile and juvenile cataract, left eye**
- **H26.043 Anterior subcapsular polar infantile and juvenile cataract, bilateral**
- **H26.049 Anterior subcapsular polar infantile and juvenile cataract, unspecified eye**

+ H26.05 Posterior subcapsular polar infantile and juvenile cataract
- **H26.051 Posterior subcapsular polar infantile and juvenile cataract, right eye**
- **H26.052 Posterior subcapsular polar infantile and juvenile cataract, left eye**
- **H26.053 Posterior subcapsular polar infantile and juvenile cataract, bilateral**
- **H26.059 Posterior subcapsular polar infantile and juvenile cataract, unspecified eye**

+ H26.06 Combined forms of infantile and juvenile cataract
- **H26.061 Combined forms of infantile and juvenile cataract, right eye**
- **H26.062 Combined forms of infantile and juvenile cataract, left eye**
- **H26.063 Combined forms of infantile and juvenile cataract, bilateral**
- **H26.069 Combined forms of infantile and juvenile cataract, unspecified eye**

• **H26.09 Other infantile and juvenile cataract**

+ H26.1 Traumatic cataract

Use additional code (Chapter 20) to identify external cause

+ H26.10 Unspecified traumatic cataract
H26.101 Unspecified traumatic cataract, right eye
H26.102 Unspecified traumatic cataract, left eye
H26.103 Unspecified traumatic cataract, bilateral
H26.109 Unspecified traumatic cataract, unspecified eye

+ H26.11 Localized traumatic opacities
H26.111 Localized traumatic opacities, right eye
H26.112 Localized traumatic opacities, left eye
H26.113 Localized traumatic opacities, bilateral
H26.119 Localized traumatic opacities, unspecified eye

+ H26.12 Partially resolved traumatic cataract
H26.121 Partially resolved traumatic cataract, right eye
H26.122 Partially resolved traumatic cataract, left eye
H26.123 Partially resolved traumatic cataract, bilateral
H26.129 Partially resolved traumatic cataract, unspecified eye

+ H26.13 Total traumatic cataract
H26.131 Total traumatic cataract, right eye
H26.132 Total traumatic cataract, left eye
H26.133 Total traumatic cataract, bilateral
H26.139 Total traumatic cataract, unspecified eye

+ H26.2 Complicated cataract

H26.20 Unspecified complicated cataract
Cataracta complicata NOS

+ H26.21 Cataract with neovascularization
Code also associated condition, such as:
chronic iridocyclitis (H20.1-)
H26.211 Cataract with neovascularization, right eye
H26.212 Cataract with neovascularization, left eye
H26.213 Cataract with neovascularization, bilateral
H26.219 Cataract with neovascularization, unspecified eye

+ H26.22 Cataract secondary to ocular disorders (degenerative) (inflammatory)
Code also associated ocular disorder
H26.221 Cataract secondary to ocular disorders (degenerative) (inflammatory), right eye
H26.222 Cataract secondary to ocular disorders (degenerative) (inflammatory), left eye
H26.223 Cataract secondary to ocular disorders (degenerative) (inflammatory), bilateral
H26.229 Cataract secondary to ocular disorders (degenerative) (inflammatory), unspecified eye

+ H26.23 Glaucomatous flecks (subcapsular)
Code first underlying glaucoma (H40-H42)
H26.231 Glaucomatous flecks (subcapsular), right eye
H26.232 Glaucomatous flecks (subcapsular), left eye
H26.233 Glaucomatous flecks (subcapsular), bilateral
H26.239 Glaucomatous flecks (subcapsular), unspecified eye

+ H26.3 Drug-induced cataract

Toxic cataract

Use additional code for adverse effect, if applicable, to identify drug (T36-T50 with fifth or sixth character 5)

H26.30 Drug-induced cataract, unspecified eye
H26.31 Drug-induced cataract, right eye
H26.32 Drug-induced cataract, left eye
H26.33 Drug-induced cataract, bilateral

+ H26.4 Secondary cataract

H26.40 Unspecified secondary cataract

+ H26.41 Soemmering's ring
H26.411 Soemmering's ring, right eye
H26.412 Soemmering's ring, left eye
H26.413 Soemmering's ring, bilateral
H26.419 Soemmering's ring, unspecified eye

+ H26.49 Other secondary cataract
H26.491 Other secondary cataract, right eye
H26.492 Other secondary cataract, left eye
AHA CC: 2Q, 2018, 14
H26.493 Other secondary cataract, bilateral
H26.499 Other secondary cataract, unspecified eye

H26.8 Other specified cataract

H26.9 Unspecified cataract

H27 Other disorders of lens

Excludes1: *congenital lens malformations (Q12.-)*
mechanical complications of intraocular lens implant (T85.2)
pseudophakia (Z96.1)

+ H27.0 Aphakia

Acquired absence of lens
Acquired aphakia
Aphakia due to trauma

Excludes1: *cataract extraction status (Z98.4-)*
congenital absence of lens (Q12.3)
congenital aphakia (Q12.3)

H27.00 Aphakia, unspecified eye
H27.01 Aphakia, right eye
H27.02 Aphakia, left eye
H27.03 Aphakia, bilateral

+ H27.1 Dislocation of lens

H27.10 Unspecified dislocation of lens

+ H27.11 Subluxation of lens
H27.111 Subluxation of lens, right eye
H27.112 Subluxation of lens, left eye
H27.113 Subluxation of lens, bilateral
H27.119 Subluxation of lens, unspecified eye

+ H27.12 Anterior dislocation of lens
H27.121 Anterior dislocation of lens, right eye
H27.122 Anterior dislocation of lens, left eye
H27.123 Anterior dislocation of lens, bilateral
H27.129 Anterior dislocation of lens, unspecified eye

+ H27.13 Posterior dislocation of lens
H27.131 Posterior dislocation of lens, right eye
H27.132 Posterior dislocation of lens, left eye
H27.133 Posterior dislocation of lens, bilateral
H27.139 Posterior dislocation of lens, unspecified eye

H27.8 Other specified disorders of lens

H27.9 Unspecified disorder of lens

H28 Cataract in diseases classified elsewhere

Code first underlying disease, such as:
hypoparathyroidism (E20.-)
myotonia (G71.1-)
myxedema (E03.-)
protein-calorie malnutrition (E40-E46)

Excludes1: *cataract in diabetes mellitus (E08.36, E09.36, E10.36, E11.36, E13.36)*

Valid 3-character code, no further characters required

Disorders of choroid and retina (H30-H36)

H30 Chorioretinal inflammation

+ H30.0 Focal chorioretinal inflammation
Focal chorioretinitis
Focal choroiditis
Focal retinitis
Focal retinochoroiditis

+ H30.00 Unspecified focal chorioretinal inflammation
Focal chorioretinitis NOS
Focal choroiditis NOS
Focal retinitis NOS
Focal retinochoroiditis NOS

H30.001 Unspecified focal chorioretinal inflammation, right eye
H30.002 Unspecified focal chorioretinal inflammation, left eye
H30.003 Unspecified focal chorioretinal inflammation, bilateral
H30.009 Unspecified focal chorioretinal inflammation, unspecified eye

+ H30.01 Focal chorioretinal inflammation, juxtapapillary
H30.011 Focal chorioretinal inflammation, juxtapapillary, right eye
H30.012 Focal chorioretinal inflammation, juxtapapillary, left eye
H30.013 Focal chorioretinal inflammation, juxtapapillary, bilateral
H30.019 Focal chorioretinal inflammation, juxtapapillary, unspecified eye

+ H30.02 Focal chorioretinal inflammation of posterior pole
H30.021 Focal chorioretinal inflammation of posterior pole, right eye
H30.022 Focal chorioretinal inflammation of posterior pole, left eye
H30.023 Focal chorioretinal inflammation of posterior pole, bilateral
H30.029 Focal chorioretinal inflammation of posterior pole, unspecified eye

+ H30.03 Focal chorioretinal inflammation, peripheral
H30.031 Focal chorioretinal inflammation, peripheral, right eye
H30.032 Focal chorioretinal inflammation, peripheral, left eye
H30.033 Focal chorioretinal inflammation, peripheral, bilateral
H30.039 Focal chorioretinal inflammation, peripheral, unspecified eye

+ H30.04 Focal chorioretinal inflammation, macular or paramacular
H30.041 Focal chorioretinal inflammation, macular or paramacular, right eye
H30.042 Focal chorioretinal inflammation, macular or paramacular, left eye
H30.043 Focal chorioretinal inflammation, macular or paramacular, bilateral
H30.049 Focal chorioretinal inflammation, macular or paramacular, unspecified eye

+ H30.1 Disseminated chorioretinal inflammation
Disseminated chorioretinitis
Disseminated choroiditis
Disseminated retinitis
Disseminated retinochoroiditis
Excludes2: *exudative retinopathy (H35.02-)*

+ H30.10 Unspecified disseminated chorioretinal inflammation
Disseminated chorioretinitis NOS
Disseminated choroiditis NOS
Disseminated retinitis NOS
Disseminated retinochoroiditis NOS

CC **H30.101 Unspecified disseminated chorioretinal inflammation, right eye**
CC **H30.102 Unspecified disseminated chorioretinal inflammation, left eye**
CC **H30.103 Unspecified disseminated chorioretinal inflammation, bilateral**
CC **H30.109 Unspecified disseminated chorioretinal inflammation, unspecified eye**

+ H30.11 Disseminated chorioretinal inflammation of posterior pole
CC **H30.111 Disseminated chorioretinal inflammation of posterior pole, right eye**
CC **H30.112 Disseminated chorioretinal inflammation of posterior pole, left eye**
CC **H30.113 Disseminated chorioretinal inflammation of posterior pole, bilateral**
CC **H30.119 Disseminated chorioretinal inflammation of posterior pole, unspecified eye**

+ H30.12 Disseminated chorioretinal inflammation, peripheral
CC **H30.121 Disseminated chorioretinal inflammation, peripheral right eye**
CC **H30.122 Disseminated chorioretinal inflammation, peripheral, left eye**
CC **H30.123 Disseminated chorioretinal inflammation, peripheral, bilateral**
CC **H30.129 Disseminated chorioretinal inflammation, peripheral, unspecified eye**

+ H30.13 Disseminated chorioretinal inflammation, generalized
CC **H30.131 Disseminated chorioretinal inflammation, generalized, right eye**
CC **H30.132 Disseminated chorioretinal inflammation, generalized, left eye**
CC **H30.133 Disseminated chorioretinal inflammation, generalized, bilateral**
CC **H30.139 Disseminated chorioretinal inflammation, generalized, unspecified eye**

+ H30.14 Acute posterior multifocal placoid pigment epitheliopathy
CC **H30.141 Acute posterior multifocal placoid pigment epitheliopathy, right eye**
CC **H30.142 Acute posterior multifocal placoid pigment epitheliopathy, left eye**
CC **H30.143 Acute posterior multifocal placoid pigment epitheliopathy, bilateral**
CC **H30.149 Acute posterior multifocal placoid pigment epitheliopathy, unspecified eye**

+ H30.2 Posterior cyclitis
Pars planitis
H30.20 Posterior cyclitis, unspecified eye
H30.21 Posterior cyclitis, right eye
H30.22 Posterior cyclitis, left eye
H30.23 Posterior cyclitis, bilateral

+ H30.8 Other chorioretinal inflammations
+ H30.81 Harada's disease
H30.811 Harada's disease, right eye
H30.812 Harada's disease, left eye
H30.813 Harada's disease, bilateral
H30.819 Harada's disease, unspecified eye

+ H30.89 Other chorioretinal inflammations
CC **H30.891 Other chorioretinal inflammations, right eye**
CC **H30.892 Other chorioretinal inflammations, left eye**
CC **H30.893 Other chorioretinal inflammations, bilateral**
CC **H30.899 Other chorioretinal inflammations, unspecified eye**

+ H30.9 Unspecified chorioretinal inflammation
Chorioretinitis NOS
Choroiditis NOS
Neuroretinitis NOS
Retinitis NOS
Retinochoroiditis NOS
CC **H30.90 Unspecified chorioretinal inflammation, unspecified eye**
CC **H30.91 Unspecified chorioretinal inflammation, right eye**
CC **H30.92 Unspecified chorioretinal inflammation, left eye**
CC **H30.93 Unspecified chorioretinal inflammation, bilateral**

H31 Other disorders of choroid

+ **H31.0 Chorioretinal scars**
  Excludes2: *postsurgical chorioretinal scars (H59.81-)*
  + **H31.00 Unspecified chorioretinal scars**
    - **H31.001 Unspecified chorioretinal scars, righ eye**
    - **H31.002 Unspecified chorioretinal scars, left eye**
    - **H31.003 Unspecified chorioretinal scars, bilateral**
    - **H31.009 Unspecified chorioretinal scars, unspecified eye**
  + **H31.01 Macula scars of posterior pole (postinflammatory) (post-traumatic)**
    Excludes1: *postprocedural chorioretinal scar (H59.81-)*
    - **H31.011 Macula scars of posterior pole (postinflammatory) (post-traumatic), right eye**
    - **H31.012 Macula scars of posterior pole (postinflammatory) (post-traumatic), left eye**
    - **H31.013 Macula scars of posterior pole (postinflammatory) (post-traumatic), bilateral**
    - **H31.019 Macula scars of posterior pole (postinflammatory) (post-traumatic), unspecified eye**
  + **H31.02 Solar retinopathy**
    - **H31.021 Solar retinopathy, right eye**
    - **H31.022 Solar retinopathy, left eye**
    - **H31.023 Solar retinopathy, bilateral**
    - **H31.029 Solar retinopathy, unspecified eye**
  + **H31.09 Other chorioretinal scars**
    - **H31.091 Other chorioretinal scars, right eye**
    - **H31.092 Other chorioretinal scars, left eye**
    - **H31.093 Other chorioretinal scars, bilateral**
    - **H31.099 Other chorioretinal scars, unspecified eye**

+ **H31.1 Choroidal degeneration**
  Excludes2: *angioid streaks of macula (H35.33)*
  + **H31.10 Unspecified choroidal degeneration**
    Choroidal sclerosis NOS
    - **H31.101 Choroidal degeneration, unspecified, right eye**
    - **H31.102 Choroidal degeneration, unspecified, left eye**
    - **H31.103 Choroidal degeneration, unspecified, bilateral**
    - **H31.109 Choroidal degeneration, unspecified, unspecified eye**
  + **H31.11 Age-related choroidal atrophy**
    - ● **H31.111 Age-related choroidal atrophy, right eye**
    - ● **H31.112 Age-related choroidal atrophy, left eye**
    - ● **H31.113 Age-related choroidal atrophy, bilateral**
    - ● **H31.119 Age-related choroidal atrophy, unspecified eye**
  + **H31.12 Diffuse secondary atrophy of choroid**
    - **H31.121 Diffuse secondary atrophy of choroid, right eye**
    - **H31.122 Diffuse secondary atrophy of choroid, left eye**
    - **H31.123 Diffuse secondary atrophy of choroid, bilateral**
    - **H31.129 Diffuse secondary atrophy of choroid, unspecified eye**

+ **H31.2 Hereditary choroidal dystrophy**
  Excludes2: *hyperornithinemia (E72.4)*
  ornithinemia (E72.4)
  - **H31.20 Hereditary choroidal dystrophy, unspecified**
  - **H31.21 Choroideremia**
  - **H31.22 Choroidal dystrophy (central areolar) (generalized) (peripapillary)**
  - **H31.23 Gyrate atrophy, choroid**
  - **H31.29 Other hereditary choroidal dystrophy**

+ **H31.3 Choroidal hemorrhage and rupture**
  + **H31.30 Unspecified choroidal hemorrhage**
    - **H31.301 Unspecified choroidal hemorrhage, right eye**
    - **H31.302 Unspecified choroidal hemorrhage, left eye**
    - **H31.303 Unspecified choroidal hemorrhage, bilateral**
    - **H31.309 Unspecified choroidal hemorrhage, unspecified eye**
  + **H31.31 Expulsive choroidal hemorrhage**
    - **H31.311 Expulsive choroidal hemorrhage, right eye**
    - **H31.312 Expulsive choroidal hemorrhage, left eye**
    - **H31.313 Expulsive choroidal hemorrhage, bilateral**
    - **H31.319 Expulsive choroidal hemorrhage, unspecified eye**
  + **H31.32 Choroidal rupture**
    - CC **H31.321 Choroidal rupture, right eye**
    - CC **H31.322 Choroidal rupture, left eye**
    - CC **H31.323 Choroidal rupture, bilateral**
    - CC **H31.329 Choroidal rupture, unspecified eye**

+ **H31.4 Choroidal detachment**
  + **H31.40 Unspecified choroidal detachment**
    - CC **H31.401 Unspecified choroidal detachment, right eye**
    - CC **H31.402 Unspecified choroidal detachment, left eye**
    - CC **H31.403 Unspecified choroidal detachment, bilateral**
    - CC **H31.409 Unspecified choroidal detachment, unspecified eye**
  + **H31.41 Hemorrhagic choroidal detachment**
    - CC **H31.411 Hemorrhagic choroidal detachment, right eye**
    - CC **H31.412 Hemorrhagic choroidal detachment, left eye**
    - CC **H31.413 Hemorrhagic choroidal detachment, bilateral**
    - CC **H31.419 Hemorrhagic choroidal detachment, unspecified eye**
  + **H31.42 Serous choroidal detachment**
    - CC **H31.421 Serous choroidal detachment, right eye**
    - CC **H31.422 Serous choroidal detachment, left eye**
    - CC **H31.423 Serous choroidal detachment, bilateral**
    - CC **H31.429 Serous choroidal detachment, unspecified eye**

H31.8 Other specified disorders of choroid
H31.9 Unspecified disorder of choroid

H32 Chorioretinal disorders in diseases classified elsewhere

Code first underlying disease, such as:
congenital toxoplasmosis (P37.1)
histoplasmosis (B39.-)
leprosy (A30.-)

Excludes1: *chorioretinitis (in):*
toxoplasmosis (acquired) (B58.01)
tuberculosis (A18.53)

Valid 3-character code, no further characters required

H33 Retinal detachments and breaks

Excludes1: *detachment of retinal pigment epithelium (H35.72-, H35.73-)*

\+ **H33.0 Retinal detachment with retinal break**

Rhegmatogenous retinal detachment

Excludes1: *serous retinal detachment (without retinal break) (H33.2-)*

\+ **H33.00 Unspecified retinal detachment with retinal break**

H33.001 Unspecified retinal detachment with retinal break, right eye

H33.002 Unspecified retinal detachment with retinal break, left eye

H33.003 Unspecified retinal detachment with retinal break, bilateral

H33.009 Unspecified retinal detachment with retinal break, unspecified eye

\+ **H33.01 Retinal detachment with single break**

H33.011 Retinal detachment with single break, right eye

H33.012 Retinal detachment with single break, left eye

H33.013 Retinal detachment with single break, bilateral

H33.019 Retinal detachment with single break, unspecified eye

\+ **H33.02 Retinal detachment with multiple breaks**

H33.021 Retinal detachment with multiple breaks, right eye

H33.022 Retinal detachment with multiple breaks, left eye

H33.023 Retinal detachment with multiple breaks, bilateral

H33.029 Retinal detachment with multiple breaks, unspecified eye

\+ **H33.03 Retinal detachment with giant retinal tear**

H33.031 Retinal detachment with giant retinal tear, right eye

H33.032 Retinal detachment with giant retinal tear, left eye

H33.033 Retinal detachment with giant retinal tear, bilateral

H33.039 Retinal detachment with giant retinal tear, unspecified eye

\+ **H33.04 Retinal detachment with retinal dialysis**

H33.041 Retinal detachment with retinal dialysis, right eye

H33.042 Retinal detachment with retinal dialysis, left eye

H33.043 Retinal detachment with retinal dialysis, bilateral

H33.049 Retinal detachment with retinal dialysis, unspecified eye

\+ **H33.05 Total retinal detachment**

H33.051 Total retinal detachment, right eye

H33.052 Total retinal detachment, left eye

H33.053 Total retinal detachment, bilateral

H33.059 Total retinal detachment, unspecified eye

\+ **H33.1 Retinoschisis and retinal cysts**

Excludes1: *congenital retinoschisis (Q14.1)*
microcystoid degeneration of retina (H35.42-)

\+ **H33.10 Unspecified retinoschisis**

H33.101 Unspecified retinoschisis, right eye

H33.102 Unspecified retinoschisis, left eye

H33.103 Unspecified retinoschisis, bilateral

H33.109 Unspecified retinoschisis, unspecified eye

\+ **H33.11 Cyst of ora serrata**

H33.111 Cyst of ora serrata, right eye

H33.112 Cyst of ora serrata, left eye

H33.113 Cyst of ora serrata, bilateral

H33.119 Cyst of ora serrata, unspecified eye

\+ **H33.12 Parasitic cyst of retina**

CC **H33.121 Parasitic cyst of retina, right eye**

CC **H33.122 Parasitic cyst of retina, left eye**

CC **H33.123 Parasitic cyst of retina, bilateral**

CC **H33.129 Parasitic cyst of retina, unspecified eye**

\+ **H33.19 Other retinoschisis and retinal cysts**

Pseudocyst of retina

H33.191 Other retinoschisis and retinal cysts, right eye

H33.192 Other retinoschisis and retinal cysts, left eye

H33.193 Other retinoschisis and retinal cysts, bilateral

H33.199 Other retinoschisis and retinal cysts, unspecified eye

\+ **H33.2 Serous retinal detachment**

Retinal detachment NOS

Retinal detachment without retinal break

Excludes1: *central serous chorioretinopathy (H35.71-)*

CC **H33.20 Serous retinal detachment, unspecified eye**

CC **H33.21 Serous retinal detachment, right eye**

CC **H33.22 Serous retinal detachment, left eye**

CC **H33.23 Serous retinal detachment, bilateral**

\+ **H33.3 Retinal breaks without detachment**

Excludes1: *chorioretinal scars after surgery for detachment (H59.81-)*
peripheral retinal degeneration without break (H35.4-)

\+ **H33.30 Unspecified retinal break**

H33.301 Unspecified retinal break, right eye

H33.302 Unspecified retinal break, left eye

H33.303 Unspecified retinal break, bilateral

H33.309 Unspecified retinal break, unspecified eye

\+ **H33.31 Horseshoe tear of retina without detachment**

Operculum of retina without detachment

H33.311 Horseshoe tear of retina without detachment, right eye

H33.312 Horseshoe tear of retina without detachment, left eye

H33.313 Horseshoe tear of retina without detachment, bilateral

H33.319 Horseshoe tear of retina without detachment, unspecified eye

\+ **H33.32 Round hole of retina without detachment**

H33.321 Round hole, right eye

H33.322 Round hole, left eye

H33.323 Round hole, bilateral

H33.329 Round hole, unspecified eye

\+ **H33.33 Multiple defects of retina without detachment**

H33.331 Multiple defects of retina without detachment, right eye

H33.332 Multiple defects of retina without detachment, left eye

H33.333 Multiple defects of retina without detachment, bilateral

H33.339 Multiple defects of retina without detachment, unspecified eye

\+ **H33.4 Traction detachment of retina**

Proliferative vitreo-retinopathy with retinal detachment

CC **H33.40 Traction detachment of retina, unspecified eye**

CC **H33.41 Traction detachment of retina, right eye**

CC **H33.42 Traction detachment of retina, left eye**

CC **H33.43 Traction detachment of retina, bilateral**

CC **H33.8 Other retinal detachments**

H34 Retinal vascular occlusions

Excludes1: *amaurosis fugax (G45.3)*

+ **H34.0 Transient retinal artery occlusion**
  - CC **H34.00 Transient retinal artery occlusion, unspecified eye**
  - CC **H34.01 Transient retinal artery occlusion, right eye**
  - CC **H34.02 Transient retinal artery occlusion, left eye**
  - CC **H34.03 Transient retinal artery occlusion, bilateral**
+ **H34.1 Central retinal artery occlusion**
  - CC **H34.10 Central retinal artery occlusion, unspecified eye**
  - CC **H34.11 Central retinal artery occlusion, right eye**
  - CC **H34.12 Central retinal artery occlusion, left eye**
  - CC **H34.13 Central retinal artery occlusion, bilateral**
+ **H34.2 Other retinal artery occlusions**
  + **H34.21 Partial retinal artery occlusion**
    Hollenhorst's plaque
    Retinal microembolism
    - CC **H34.211 Partial retinal artery occlusion, right eye**
    - CC **H34.212 Partial retinal artery occlusion, left eye**
    - CC **H34.213 Partial retinal artery occlusion, bilateral**
    - CC **H34.219 Partial retinal artery occlusion, unspecified eye**
  + **H34.23 Retinal artery branch occlusion**
    - CC **H34.231 Retinal artery branch occlusion, right eye**
    - CC **H34.232 Retinal artery branch occlusion, left eye**
    - CC **H34.233 Retinal artery branch occlusion, bilateral**
    - CC **H34.239 Retinal artery branch occlusion, unspecified eye**
+ **H34.8 Other retinal vascular occlusions**
  AHA CC: 4Q, 2016, 19
  + **H34.81 Central retinal vein occlusion**

    One of the following 7th characters is to be assigned to codes in subcategory **H34.81** to designate the severity of the occlusion:
    0 with macular edema
    1 with retinal neovascularization
    2 stable
    Old central retinal vein occlusion

    - +7th CC **H34.811 Central retinal vein occlusion, right eye**
    - +7th CC **H34.812 Central retinal vein occlusion, left eye**
    - +7th CC **H34.813 Central retinal vein occlusion, bilateral**
    - +7th CC **H34.819 Central retinal vein occlusion, unspecified eye**
  + **H34.82 Venous engorgement**
    Incipient retinal vein occlusion
    Partial retinal vein occlusion
    - **H34.821 Venous engorgement, right eye**
    - **H34.822 Venous engorgement, left eye**
    - **H34.823 Venous engorgement, bilateral**
    - **H34.829 Venous engorgement, unspecified eye**
  + **H34.83 Tributary (branch) retinal vein occlusion**

    One of the following 7th characters is to be assigned to codes in subcategory **H34.83** to designate the severity of the occlusion:
    0 with macular edema
    1 with retinal neovascularization
    2 stable
    Old central retinal vein occlusion

    - +7th **H34.831 Tributary (branch) retinal vein occlusion, right eye**
    - +7th **H34.832 Tributary (branch) retinal vein occlusion, left eye**
    - +7th **H34.833 Tributary (branch) retinal vein occlusion, bilateral**
    - +7th **H34.839 Tributary (branch) retinal vein occlusion, unspecified eye**
- CC **H34.9 Unspecified retinal vascular occlusion**

H35 Other retinal disorders

Excludes2: *diabetic retinal disorders (E08.311-E08.359, E09.311-E09.359, E10.311-E10.359, E11.311-E11.359, E13.311-E13.359)*

+ **H35.0 Background retinopathy and retinal vascular changes**
  Review coding guideline C.9.a.5
  Code also any associated hypertension (I10)
  - **H35.00 Unspecified background retinopathy**
  + **H35.01 Changes in retinal vascular appearance**
    Retinal vascular sheathing
    - **H35.011 Changes in retinal vascular appearance, right eye**
    - **H35.012 Changes in retinal vascular appearance, left eye**
    - **H35.013 Changes in retinal vascular appearance, bilateral**
    - **H35.019 Changes in retinal vascular appearance, unspecified eye**
  + **H35.02 Exudative retinopathy**
    Coats retinopathy
    - **H35.021 Exudative retinopathy, right eye**
    - **H35.022 Exudative retinopathy, left eye**
    - **H35.023 Exudative retinopathy, bilateral**
    - **H35.029 Exudative retinopathy, unspecified eye**
  + **H35.03 Hypertensive retinopathy**
    - **H35.031 Hypertensive retinopathy, right eye**
    - **H35.032 Hypertensive retinopathy, left eye**
    - **H35.033 Hypertensive retinopathy, bilateral**
    - **H35.039 Hypertensive retinopathy, unspecified eye**
  + **H35.04 Retinal micro-aneurysms, unspecified**
    - **H35.041 Retinal micro-aneurysms, unspecified, right eye**
    - **H35.042 Retinal micro-aneurysms, unspecified, left eye**
    - **H35.043 Retinal micro-aneurysms, unspecified, bilateral**
    - **H35.049 Retinal micro-aneurysms, unspecified, unspecified eye**
  + **H35.05 Retinal neovascularization, unspecified**
    - **H35.051 Retinal neovascularization, unspecified, right eye**
    - **H35.052 Retinal neovascularization, unspecified, left eye**
    - **H35.053 Retinal neovascularization, unspecified, bilateral**
    - **H35.059 Retinal neovascularization, unspecified, unspecified eye**
  + **H35.06 Retinal vasculitis**
    Eales disease
    Retinal perivasculitis
    - **H35.061 Retinal vasculitis, right eye**
    - **H35.062 Retinal vasculitis, left eye**
    - **H35.063 Retinal vasculitis, bilateral**
    - **H35.069 Retinal vasculitis, unspecified eye**
  + **H35.07 Retinal telangiectasis**
    - **H35.071 Retinal telangiectasis, right eye**
    - **H35.072 Retinal telangiectasis, left eye**
    - **H35.073 Retinal telangiectasis, bilateral**
    - **H35.079 Retinal telangiectasis, unspecified eye**
  - **H35.09 Other intraretinal microvascular abnormalities**
    Retinal varices
+ **H35.1 Retinopathy of prematurity**
  + **H35.10 Retinopathy of prematurity, unspecified**
    Retinopathy of prematurity NOS

H35.101 **Retinopathy of prematurity, unspecified, right eye**
H35.102 **Retinopathy of prematurity, unspecified, left eye**
H35.103 **Retinopathy of prematurity, unspecified, bilateral**
H35.109 **Retinopathy of prematurity, unspecified, unspecified eye**

\+ H35.11 **Retinopathy of prematurity, stage 0**
H35.111 **Retinopathy of prematurity, stage 0, right eye**
H35.112 **Retinopathy of prematurity, stage 0, left eye**
H35.113 **Retinopathy of prematurity, stage 0, bilateral**
H35.119 **Retinopathy of prematurity, stage 0, unspecified eye**

\+ H35.12 **Retinopathy of prematurity, stage 1**
H35.121 **Retinopathy of prematurity, stage 1, right eye**
H35.122 **Retinopathy of prematurity, stage 1, left eye**
H35.123 **Retinopathy of prematurity, stage 1, bilateral**
H35.129 **Retinopathy of prematurity, stage 1, unspecified eye**

\+ H35.13 **Retinopathy of prematurity, stage 2**
H35.131 **Retinopathy of prematurity, stage 2, right eye**
H35.132 **Retinopathy of prematurity, stage 2, left eye**
H35.133 **Retinopathy of prematurity, stage 2, bilateral**
H35.139 **Retinopathy of prematurity, stage 2, unspecified eye**

\+ H35.14 **Retinopathy of prematurity, stage 3**
H35.141 **Retinopathy of prematurity, stage 3, right eye**
H35.142 **Retinopathy of prematurity, stage 3, left eye**
H35.143 **Retinopathy of prematurity, stage 3, bilateral**
H35.149 **Retinopathy of prematurity, stage 3, unspecified eye**

\+ H35.15 **Retinopathy of prematurity, stage 4**
H35.151 **Retinopathy of prematurity, stage 4, right eye**
H35.152 **Retinopathy of prematurity, stage 4, left eye**
H35.153 **Retinopathy of prematurity, stage 4, bilateral**
H35.159 **Retinopathy of prematurity, stage 4, unspecified eye**

\+ H35.16 **Retinopathy of prematurity, stage 5**
H35.161 **Retinopathy of prematurity, stage 5, right eye**
H35.162 **Retinopathy of prematurity, stage 5, left eye**
H35.163 **Retinopathy of prematurity, stage 5, bilateral**
H35.169 **Retinopathy of prematurity, stage 5, unspecified eye**

\+ H35.17 **Retrolental fibroplasia**
H35.171 **Retrolental fibroplasia, right eye**
H35.172 **Retrolental fibroplasia, left eye**
H35.173 **Retrolental fibroplasia, bilateral**
H35.179 **Retrolental fibroplasia, unspecified eye**

\+ H35.2 **Other non-diabetic proliferative retinopathy**
Proliferative vitreo-retinopathy
Excludes1: *proliferative vitreo-retinopathy with retinal detachment (H33.4-)*
H35.20 **Other non-diabetic proliferative retinopathy, unspecified eye**
H35.21 **Other non-diabetic proliferative retinopathy, right eye**
H35.22 **Other non-diabetic proliferative retinopathy, left eye**
H35.23 **Other non-diabetic proliferative retinopathy, bilateral**

\+ H35.3 **Degeneration of macula and posterior pole**
AHA CC: 4Q, 2016, 20-21
• H35.30 **Unspecified macular degeneration**
Age-related macular degeneration

\+ H35.31 **Nonexudative age-related macular degeneration**
Atrophic age-related macular degeneration
Dry age-related macular degeneration

One of the following 7th characters is to be assigned to codes in subcategory **H35.31** to designate the stage of the disease:
0 stage unspecified
1 early dry stage
2 intermediate dry stage
3 advanced atrophic without subfoveal involvement advanced dry stage
4 advanced atrophic with sobfoveal involvement

• +7th H35.311 **Nonexudative age-related macular degeneration, right eye**
AHA CC: 4Q, 2016, 21
• +7th H35.312 **Nonexudative age-related macular degeneration, left eye**
AHA CC: 4Q, 2016, 21
• +7th H35.313 **Nonexudative age-related macular degeneration, bilateral**
• +7th H35.319 **Nonexudative age-related macular degeneration, unspecified eye**

\+ H35.32 **Exudative age-related macular degeneration**
Wet age-related macular degeneration

One of the following 7th characters is to be assigned to codes in subcategory **H35.32** to designate the stage of the disease:
0 stage unspecified
1 with active choroidal neovascularization
2 with inactive choroidal neovascularization with involuted or regressed neovascularization
3 with inactive scar

• +7th H35.321 **Exudative age-related macular degeneration, right eye**
• +7th H35.322 **Exudative age-related macular degeneration, left eye**
• +7th H35.323 **Exudative age-related macular degeneration, bilateral**
• +7th H35.329 **Exudative age-related macular degeneration, unspecified eye**

H35.33 **Angioid streaks of macula**

\+ H35.34 **Macular cyst, hole, or pseudohole**
H35.341 **Macular cyst, hole, or pseudohole, right eye**
H35.342 **Macular cyst, hole, or pseudohole, left eye**
H35.343 **Macular cyst, hole, or pseudohole, bilateral**
H35.349 **Macular cyst, hole, or pseudohole, unspecified eye**

\+ H35.35 **Cystoid macular degeneration**
Excludes1: *cystoid macular edema following cataract surgery (H59.03-)*
H35.351 **Cystoid macular degeneration, right eye**
H35.352 **Cystoid macular degeneration, left eye**
H35.353 **Cystoid macular degeneration, bilateral**
H35.359 **Cystoid macular degeneration, unspecified eye**

+ **H35.36 Drusen (degenerative) of macula**
  - **H35.361 Drusen (degenerative) of macula, right eye**
  - **H35.362 Drusen (degenerative) of macula, left eye**
    AHA CC: 4Q, 2016, 21
  - **H35.363 Drusen (degenerative) of macula, bilateral**
    AHA CC: 4Q, 2016, 21; 1Q, 2017, 51
  - **H35.369 Drusen (degenerative) of macula, unspecified eye**

+ **H35.37 Puckering of macula**
  - **H35.371 Puckering of macula, right eye**
  - **H35.372 Puckering of macula, left eye**
  - **H35.373 Puckering of macula, bilateral**
  - **H35.379 Puckering of macula, unspecified eye**

+ **H35.38 Toxic maculopathy**
  Code first poisoning due to drug or toxin, if applicable (T36-T65 with fifth or sixth character 1-4 or 6)
  Use additional code for adverse effect, if applicable, to identify drug (T36-T50 with fifth or sixth character 5)
  - **H35.381 Toxic maculopathy, right eye**
  - **H35.382 Toxic maculopathy, left eye**
  - **H35.383 Toxic maculopathy, bilateral**
  - **H35.389 Toxic maculopathy, unspecified eye**

+ **H35.4 Peripheral retinal degeneration**
  Excludes1: *hereditary retinal degeneration (dystrophy) (H35.5-)*
  peripheral retinal degeneration with retinal break (H33.3-)
  - **H35.40 Unspecified peripheral retinal degeneration**
  - + **H35.41 Lattice degeneration of retina**
    Palisade degeneration of retina
    - **H35.411 Lattice degeneration of retina, right eye**
    - **H35.412 Lattice degeneration of retina, left eye**
    - **H35.413 Lattice degeneration of retina, bilateral**
    - **H35.419 Lattice degeneration of retina, unspecified eye**
  - + **H35.42 Microcystoid degeneration of retina**
    - **H35.421 Microcystoid degeneration of retina, right eye**
    - **H35.422 Microcystoid degeneration of retina, left eye**
    - **H35.423 Microcystoid degeneration of retina, bilateral**
    - **H35.429 Microcystoid degeneration of retina, unspecified eye**
  - + **H35.43 Paving stone degeneration of retina**
    - **H35.431 Paving stone degeneration of retina, right eye**
    - **H35.432 Paving stone degeneration of retina, left eye**
    - **H35.433 Paving stone degeneration of retina, bilateral**
    - **H35.439 Paving stone degeneration of retina, unspecified eye**
  - + **H35.44 Age-related reticular degeneration of retina**
    - ● **H35.441 Age-related reticular degeneration of retina, right eye**
    - ● **H35.442 Age-related reticular degeneration of retina, left eye**
    - ● **H35.443 Age-related reticular degeneration of retina, bilateral**
    - ● **H35.449 Age-related reticular degeneration of retina, unspecified eye**
  - + **H35.45 Secondary pigmentary degeneration**
    - **H35.451 Secondary pigmentary degeneration, right eye**
    - **H35.452 Secondary pigmentary degeneration, left eye**
    - **H35.453 Secondary pigmentary degeneration, bilateral**
    - **H35.459 Secondary pigmentary degeneration, unspecified eye**
  - + **H35.46 Secondary vitreoretinal degeneration**
    - **H35.461 Secondary vitreoretinal degeneration, right eye**
    - **H35.462 Secondary vitreoretinal degeneration, left eye**
    - **H35.463 Secondary vitreoretinal degeneration, bilateral**
    - **H35.469 Secondary vitreoretinal degeneration, unspecified eye**

+ **H35.5 Hereditary retinal dystrophy**
  Excludes1: *dystrophies primarily involving Bruch's membrane (H31.1-)*
  - **H35.50 Unspecified hereditary retinal dystrophy**
  - **H35.51 Vitreoretinal dystrophy**
  - **H35.52 Pigmentary retinal dystrophy**
    Albipunctate retinal dystrophy
    Retinitis pigmentosa
    Tapetoretinal dystrophy
  - **H35.53 Other dystrophies primarily involving the sensory retina**
    Stargardt's disease
  - **H35.54 Dystrophies primarily involving the retinal pigment epithelium**
    Vitelliform retinal dystrophy

+ **H35.6 Retinal hemorrhage**
  - **H35.60 Retinal hemorrhage, unspecified eye**
  - **H35.61 Retinal hemorrhage, right eye**
  - **H35.62 Retinal hemorrhage, left eye**
  - **H35.63 Retinal hemorrhage, bilateral**

+ **H35.7 Separation of retinal layers**
  Excludes1: *retinal detachment (serous) (H33.2-)*
  rhegmatogenous retinal detachment (H33.0-)
  - CC **H35.70 Unspecified separation of retinal layers**
  - + **H35.71 Central serous chorioretinopathy**
    - **H35.711 Central serous chorioretinopathy, right eye**
    - **H35.712 Central serous chorioretinopathy, left eye**
    - **H35.713 Central serous chorioretinopathy, bilateral**
    - **H35.719 Central serous chorioretinopathy, unspecified eye**
  - + **H35.72 Serous detachment of retinal pigment epithelium**
    - CC **H35.721 Serous detachment of retinal pigment epithelium, right eye**
    - CC **H35.722 Serous detachment of retinal pigment epithelium, left eye**
    - CC **H35.723 Serous detachment of retinal pigment epithelium, bilateral**
    - CC **H35.729 Serous detachment of retinal pigment epithelium, unspecified eye**
  - + **H35.73 Hemorrhagic detachment of retinal pigment epithelium**
    - CC **H35.731 Hemorrhagic detachment of retinal pigment epithelium, right eye**
    - CC **H35.732 Hemorrhagic detachment of retinal pigment epithelium, left eye**
    - CC **H35.733 Hemorrhagic detachment of retinal pigment epithelium, bilateral**
    - CC **H35.739 Hemorrhagic detachment of retinal pigment epithelium, unspecified eye**

+ **H35.8 Other specified retinal disorders**
  Excludes2: *retinal hemorrhage (H35.6-)*
  - **H35.81 Retinal edema**
    Retinal cotton wool spots
  - CC **H35.82 Retinal ischemia**
  - **H35.89 Other specified retinal disorders**

H35.9 Unspecified retinal disorder

H36 **Retinal disorders in diseases classified elsewhere**

Code first underlying disease, such as:
lipid storage disorders (E75.-)
sickle-cell disorders (D57.-)

Excludes1: *arteriosclerotic retinopathy (H35.0-)*
diabetic retinopathy (E08.3-, E09.3-, E10.3-, E11.3-, E13.3-)

Valid 3-character code, no further characters required

Glaucoma (H40-H42)

H40 Glaucoma

Excludes1: *absolute glaucoma (H44.51-)*
congenital glaucoma (Q15.0)
traumatic glaucoma due to birth injury (P15.3)

Review coding guideline C.7.a

+ **H40.0 Glaucoma suspect**
+ **H40.00 Preglaucoma, unspecified**
H40.001 Preglaucoma, unspecified, right eye
H40.002 Preglaucoma, unspecified, left eye
H40.003 Preglaucoma, unspecified, bilateral
H40.009 Preglaucoma, unspecified, unspecified eye
+ **H40.01 Open angle with borderline findings, low risk**
Open angle, low risk
H40.011 Open angle with borderline findings, low risk, right eye
H40.012 Open angle with borderline findings, low risk, left eye
H40.013 Open angle with borderline findings, low risk, bilateral
H40.019 Open angle with borderline findings, low risk, unspecified eye
+ **H40.02 Open angle with borderline findings, high risk**
Open angle, high risk
H40.021 Open angle with borderline findings, high risk, right eye
H40.022 Open angle with borderline findings, high risk, left eye
H40.023 Open angle with borderline findings, high risk, bilateral
H40.029 Open angle with borderline findings, high risk, unspecified eye
+ **H40.03 Anatomical narrow angle**
Primary angle closure suspect
H40.031 Anatomical narrow angle, right eye
H40.032 Anatomical narrow angle, left eye
H40.033 Anatomical narrow angle, bilateral
H40.039 Anatomical narrow angle, unspecified eye
+ **H40.04 Steroid responder**
H40.041 Steroid responder, right eye
H40.042 Steroid responder, left eye
H40.043 Steroid responder, bilateral
H40.049 Steroid responder, unspecified eye
+ **H40.05 Ocular hypertension**
H40.051 Ocular hypertension, right eye
H40.052 Ocular hypertension, left eye
H40.053 Ocular hypertension, bilateral
H40.059 Ocular hypertension, unspecified eye
+ **H40.06 Primary angle closure without glaucoma damage**
H40.061 Primary angle closure without glaucoma damage, right eye
H40.062 Primary angle closure without glaucoma damage, left eye
H40.063 Primary angle closure without glaucoma damage, bilateral
H40.069 Primary angle closure without glaucoma damage, unspecified eye

+ **H40.1 Open-angle glaucoma**
AHA CC: 4Q, 2016, 22

X+7th **H40.10 Unspecified open-angle glaucoma**

One of the following 7th characters is to be assigned to code **H40.10** to designate the stage of glaucoma
0 stage unspecified
1 mild stage
2 moderate stage
3 severe stage
4 indeterminate stage

+ **H40.11 Primary open-angle glaucoma**
Chronic simple glaucoma

One of the following 7th characters is to be assigned to each code in subcategory **H40.11** to designate the stage of glaucoma
0 stage unspecified
1 mild stage
2 moderate stage
3 severe stage
4 indeterminate stage

+7th **H40.111 Primary open-angle glaucoma, right eye**
AHA CC: 2Q, 2019, 31
+7th **H40.112 Primary open-angle glaucoma, left eye**
+7th **H40.113 Primary open-angle glaucoma, bilateral**
+7th **H40.119 Primary open-angle glaucoma, unspecified eye**

+ **H40.12 Low-tension glaucoma**

One of the following 7th characters is to be assigned to each code in subcategory **H40.12** to designate the stage of glaucoma
0 stage unspecified
1 mild stage
2 moderate stage
3 severe stage
4 indeterminate stage

+7th **H40.121 Low-tension glaucoma, right eye**
+7th **H40.122 Low-tension glaucoma, left eye**
+7th **H40.123 Low-tension glaucoma, bilateral**
+7th **H40.129 Low-tension glaucoma, unspecified eye**

+ **H40.13 Pigmentary glaucoma**

One of the following 7th characters is to be assigned to each code in subcategory **H40.13** to designate the stage of glaucoma
0 stage unspecified
1 mild stage
2 moderate stage
3 severe stage
4 indeterminate stage

+7th **H40.131 Pigmentary glaucoma, right eye**
+7th **H40.132 Pigmentary glaucoma, left eye**
+7th **H40.133 Pigmentary glaucoma, bilateral**
+7th **H40.139 Pigmentary glaucoma, unspecified eye**

+ **H40.14 Capsular glaucoma with pseudoexfoliation of lens**

One of the following 7th characters is to be assigned to each code in subcategory **H40.14** to designate the stage of glaucoma
0 stage unspecified
1 mild stage
2 moderate stage
3 severe stage
4 indeterminate stage

+7th **H40.141 Capsular glaucoma with pseudoexfoliation of lens, right eye**
+7th **H40.142 Capsular glaucoma with pseudoexfoliation of lens, left eye**
+7th **H40.143 Capsular glaucoma with pseudoexfoliation of lens, bilateral**
+7th **H40.149 Capsular glaucoma with pseudoexfoliation of lens, unspecified eye**

+ H40.15 **Residual stage of open-angle glaucoma**
 - H40.151 **Residual stage of open-angle glaucoma, right eye**
 - H40.152 **Residual stage of open-angle glaucoma, left eye**
 - H40.153 **Residual stage of open-angle glaucoma, bilateral**
 - H40.159 **Residual stage of open-angle glaucoma, unspecified eye**

+ H40.2 **Primary angle-closure glaucoma**

Excludes1: *aqueous misdirection (H40.83-)*
malignant glaucoma (H40.83-)

X+7th **H40.20 Unspecified primary angle-closure glaucoma**

One of the following 7th characters is to be assigned to code **H40.20** to designate the stage of glaucoma
0 stage unspecified
1 mild stage
2 moderate stage
3 severe stage
4 indeterminate stage

+ **H40.21 Acute angle-closure glaucoma**
Acute angle-closure glaucoma attack
Acute angle-closure glaucoma crisis
 - CC **H40.211 Acute angle-closure glaucoma, right eye**
 - CC **H40.212 Acute angle-closure glaucoma, left eye**
 - CC **H40.213 Acute angle-closure glaucoma, bilateral**
 - CC **H40.219 Acute angle-closure glaucoma, unspecified eye**

+ **H40.22 Chronic angle-closure glaucoma**
Chronic primary angle closure glaucoma

One of the following 7th characters is to be assigned to each code in subcategory **H40.22** to designate the stage of glaucoma
0 stage unspecified
1 mild stage
2 moderate stage
3 severe stage
4 indeterminate stage

 - +7th **H40.221 Chronic angle-closure glaucoma, right eye**
 - +7th **H40.222 Chronic angle-closure glaucoma, left eye**
 - +7th **H40.223 Chronic angle-closure glaucoma, bilateral**
 - +7th **H40.229 Chronic angle-closure glaucoma, unspecified eye**

+ **H40.23 Intermittent angle-closure glaucoma**
 - **H40.231 Intermittent angle-closure glaucoma, right eye**
 - **H40.232 Intermittent angle-closure glaucoma, left eye**
 - **H40.233 Intermittent angle-closure glaucoma, bilateral**
 - **H40.239 Intermittent angle-closure glaucoma, unspecified eye**

+ **H40.24 Residual stage of angle-closure glaucoma**
 - **H40.241 Residual stage of angle-closure glaucoma, right eye**
 - **H40.242 Residual stage of angle-closure glaucoma, left eye**
 - **H40.243 Residual stage of angle-closure glaucoma, bilateral**
 - **H40.249 Residual stage of angle-closure glaucoma, unspecified eye**

+ **H40.3 Glaucoma secondary to eye trauma**
Code also underlying condition

One of the following 7th characters is to be assigned to each code in subcategory **H40.3** to designate the stage of glaucoma
0 stage unspecified
1 mild stage
2 moderate stage
3 severe stage
4 indeterminate stage

 - X+7th **H40.30 Glaucoma secondary to eye trauma, unspecified eye**
 - X+7th **H40.31 Glaucoma secondary to eye trauma, right eye**
 - X+7th **H40.32 Glaucoma secondary to eye trauma, left eye**
 - X+7th **H40.33 Glaucoma secondary to eye trauma, bilateral**

+ **H40.4 Glaucoma secondary to eye inflammation**
Code also underlying condition

One of the following 7th characters is to be assigned to each code in subcategory **H40.4** to designate the stage of glaucoma
0 stage unspecified
1 mild stage
2 moderate stage
3 severe stage
4 indeterminate stage

 - X+7th **H40.40 Glaucoma secondary to eye inflammation, unspecified eye**
 - X+7th **H40.41 Glaucoma secondary to eye inflammation, right eye**
 - X+7th **H40.42 Glaucoma secondary to eye inflammation, left eye**
 - X+7th **H40.43 Glaucoma secondary to eye inflammation, bilateral**

+ **H40.5 Glaucoma secondary to other eye disorders**
Code also underlying eye disorder

One of the following 7th characters is to be assigned to each code in subcategory **H40.5** to designate the stage of glaucoma
0 stage unspecified
1 mild stage
2 moderate stage
3 severe stage
4 indeterminate stage

 - X+7th **H40.50 Glaucoma secondary to other eye disorders, unspecified eye**
 - X+7th **H40.51 Glaucoma secondary to other eye disorders, right eye**
 - X+7th **H40.52 Glaucoma secondary to other eye disorders, left eye**
 - X+7th **H40.53 Glaucoma secondary to other eye disorders, bilateral**

+ **H40.6 Glaucoma secondary to drugs**
Use additional code for adverse effect, if applicable, to identify drug (T36-T50 with fifth or sixth character 5)

One of the following 7th characters is to be assigned to each code in subcategory **H40.6** to designate the stage of glaucoma
0 stage unspecified
1 mild stage
2 moderate stage
3 severe stage
4 indeterminate stage

 - X+7th **H40.60 Glaucoma secondary to drugs, unspecified eye**
 - X+7th **H40.61 Glaucoma secondary to drugs, right eye**
 - X+7th **H40.62 Glaucoma secondary to drugs, left eye**
 - X+7th **H40.63 Glaucoma secondary to drugs, bilateral**

+ **H40.8 Other glaucoma**

+ **H40.81 Glaucoma with increased episcleral venous pressure**
 - **H40.811 Glaucoma with increased episcleral venous pressure, right eye**
 - **H40.812 Glaucoma with increased episcleral venous pressure, left eye**
 - **H40.813 Glaucoma with increased episcleral venous pressure, bilateral**
 - **H40.819 Glaucoma with increased episcleral venous pressure, unspecified eye**

+ **H40.82 Hypersecretion glaucoma**
 - **H40.821 Hypersecretion glaucoma, right eye**
 - **H40.822 Hypersecretion glaucoma, left eye**
 - **H40.823 Hypersecretion glaucoma, bilateral**
 - **H40.829 Hypersecretion glaucoma, unspecified eye**

+ **H40.83 Aqueous misdirection**
Malignant glaucoma
 - **H40.831 Aqueous misdirection, right eye**
 - **H40.832 Aqueous misdirection, left eye**
 - **H40.833 Aqueous misdirection, bilateral**
 - **H40.839 Aqueous misdirection, unspecified eye**

H40.89 Other specified glaucoma

H40.9 Unspecified glaucoma

H42 Glaucoma in diseases classified elsewhere

Code first underlying condition, such as:
amyloidosis (E85.-)
aniridia (Q13.1)
glaucoma (in) diabetes mellitus (E08.39, E09.39, E10.39, E11.39, E13.39)
Lowe's syndrome (E72.03)
Reiger's anomaly (Q13.81)
specified metabolic disorder (E70-E88)

Excludes1: *glaucoma (in) onchocerciasis (B73.02)*
glaucoma (in) syphilis (A52.71)
glaucoma (in) tuberculous (A18.59)

Valid 3-character code, no further characters required

Disorders of vitreous body and globe (H43-H44)

H43 Disorders of vitreous body

+ **H43.0 Vitreous prolapse**
  Excludes1: *vitreous syndrome following cataract surgery (H59.0-)*
  traumatic vitreous prolapse (S05.2-)
  H43.00 Vitreous prolapse, unspecified eye
  H43.01 Vitreous prolapse, right eye
  H43.02 Vitreous prolapse, left eye
  H43.03 Vitreous prolapse, bilateral
+ **H43.1 Vitreous hemorrhage**
  H43.10 Vitreous hemorrhage, unspecified eye
  H43.11 Vitreous hemorrhage, right eye
  H43.12 Vitreous hemorrhage, left eye
  H43.13 Vitreous hemorrhage, bilateral
+ **H43.2 Crystalline deposits in vitreous body**
  H43.20 Crystalline deposits in vitreous body, unspecified eye
  H43.21 Crystalline deposits in vitreous body, right eye
  H43.22 Crystalline deposits in vitreous body, left eye
  H43.23 Crystalline deposits in vitreous body, bilateral
+ **H43.3 Other vitreous opacities**
  + **H43.31 Vitreous membranes and strands**
    H43.311 Vitreous membranes and strands, right eye
    H43.312 Vitreous membranes and strands, left eye
    H43.313 Vitreous membranes and strands, bilateral
    H43.319 Vitreous membranes and strands, unspecified eye
  + **H43.39 Other vitreous opacities**
    Vitreous floaters
    H43.391 Other vitreous opacities, right eye
    H43.392 Other vitreous opacities, left eye
    H43.393 Other vitreous opacities, bilateral
    H43.399 Other vitreous opacities, unspecified eye
+ **H43.8 Other disorders of vitreous body**
  Excludes1: *proliferative vitreo-retinopathy with retinal detachment (H33.4-)*
  Excludes2: *vitreous abscess (H44.02-)*
  + **H43.81 Vitreous degeneration**
    Vitreous detachment
    H43.811 Vitreous degeneration, right eye
    H43.812 Vitreous degeneration, left eye
    H43.813 Vitreous degeneration, bilateral
    H43.819 Vitreous degeneration, unspecified eye
  + **H43.82 Vitreomacular adhesion**
    Vitreomacular traction
    ● **H43.821 Vitreomacular adhesion, right eye**
    ● **H43.822 Vitreomacular adhesion, left eye**
    ● **H43.823 Vitreomacular adhesion, bilateral**
    ● **H43.829 Vitreomacular adhesion, unspecified eye**
  H43.89 Other disorders of vitreous body
H43.9 Unspecified disorder of vitreous body

H44 Disorders of globe

Includes: disorders affecting multiple structures of eye

+ **H44.0 Purulent endophthalmitis**
  Use additional code to identify organism
  Excludes1: *bleb associated endophthalmitis (H59.4-)*
  + **H44.00 Unspecified purulent endophthalmitis**
    CC **H44.001 Unspecified purulent endophthalmitis, right eye**
    CC **H44.002 Unspecified purulent endophthalmitis, left eye**
    CC **H44.003 Unspecified purulent endophthalmitis, bilateral**
    CC **H44.009 Unspecified purulent endophthalmitis, unspecified eye**
  + **H44.01 Panophthalmitis (acute)**
    CC **H44.011 Panophthalmitis (acute), right eye**
    CC **H44.012 Panophthalmitis (acute), left eye**
    CC **H44.013 Panophthalmitis (acute), bilateral**
    CC **H44.019 Panophthalmitis (acute), unspecified eye**
  + **H44.02 Vitreous abscess (chronic)**
    CC **H44.021 Vitreous abscess (chronic), right eye**
    CC **H44.022 Vitreous abscess (chronic), left eye**
    CC **H44.023 Vitreous abscess (chronic), bilateral**
    CC **H44.029 Vitreous abscess (chronic), unspecified eye**
+ **H44.1 Other endophthalmitis**
  Excludes1: *bleb associated endophthalmitis (H59.4-)*
  Excludes2: *ophthalmia nodosa (H16.2-)*
  + **H44.11 Panuveitis**
    CC **H44.111 Panuveitis, right eye**
    CC **H44.112 Panuveitis, left eye**
    CC **H44.113 Panuveitis, bilateral**
    CC **H44.119 Panuveitis, unspecified eye**
  + **H44.12 Parasitic endophthalmitis, unspecified**
    CC **H44.121 Parasitic endophthalmitis, unspecified, right eye**
    CC **H44.122 Parasitic endophthalmitis, unspecified, left eye**
    CC **H44.123 Parasitic endophthalmitis, unspecified, bilateral**
    CC **H44.129 Parasitic endophthalmitis, unspecified, unspecified eye**
  + **H44.13 Sympathetic uveitis**
    CC **H44.131 Sympathetic uveitis, right eye**
    CC **H44.132 Sympathetic uveitis, left eye**
    CC **H44.133 Sympathetic uveitis, bilateral**
    CC **H44.139 Sympathetic uveitis, unspecified eye**
  CC **H44.19 Other endophthalmitis**
+ **H44.2 Degenerative myopia**
  Malignant myopia
  AHA CC: 4Q, 2017, 10-11
  H44.20 Degenerative myopia, unspecified eye
  H44.21 Degenerative myopia, right eye
  H44.22 Degenerative myopia, left eye
  H44.23 Degenerative myopia, bilateral
  + **H44.2A Degenerative myopia with choroidal neovascularization**
    Use additional code for any associated choroid disorders (H31.-)
    H44.2A1 Degenerative myopia with choroidal neovascularization, right eye
    H44.2A2 Degenerative myopia with choroidal neovascularization, left eye
    H44.2A3 Degenerative myopia with choroidal neovascularization, bilateral eye
    H44.2A9 Degenerative myopia with choroidal neovascularization, unspecified eye

+ H44.2B Degenerative myopia with macular hole
  - H44.2B1 Degenerative myopia with macular hole, right eye
  - H44.2B2 Degenerative myopia with macular hole, left eye
  - H44.2B3 Degenerative myopia with macular hole, bilateral eye
  - H44.2B9 Degenerative myopia with macular hole, unspecified eye

+ H44.2C Degenerative myopia with retinal detachment

  Use additional code to identify the retinal detachment (H33.-)
  - H44.2C1 Degenerative myopia with retinal detachment, right eye
  - H44.2C2 Degenerative myopia with retinal detachment, left eye
  - H44.2C3 Degenerative myopia with retinal detachment, bilateral eye
  - H44.2C9 Degenerative myopia with retinal detachment, unspecified eye

+ H44.2D Degenerative myopia with foveoschisis
  - H44.2D1 Degenerative myopia with foveoschisis, right eye
  - H44.2D2 Degenerative myopia with foveoschisis, left eye
  - H44.2D3 Degenerative myopia with foveoschisis, bilateral eye
  - H44.2D9 Degenerative myopia with foveoschisis, unspecified eye

+ H44.2E Degenerative myopia with other maculopathy
  - H44.2E1 Degenerative myopia with other maculopathy, right eye
  - H44.2E2 Degenerative myopia with other maculopathy, left eye
  - H44.2E3 Degenerative myopia with other maculopathy, bilateral eye
  - H44.2E9 Degenerative myopia with other maculopathy, unspecified eye

+ H44.3 Other and unspecified degenerative disorders of globe
  - H44.30 Unspecified degenerative disorder of globe
  - + H44.31 Chalcosis
    - H44.311 Chalcosis, right eye
    - H44.312 Chalcosis, left eye
    - H44.313 Chalcosis, bilateral
    - H44.319 Chalcosis, unspecified eye
  - + H44.32 Siderosis of eye
    - H44.321 Siderosis of eye, right eye
    - H44.322 Siderosis of eye, left eye
    - H44.323 Siderosis of eye, bilateral
    - H44.329 Siderosis of eye, unspecified eye
  - + H44.39 Other degenerative disorders of globe
    - H44.391 Other degenerative disorders of globe, right eye
    - H44.392 Other degenerative disorders of globe, left eye
    - H44.393 Other degenerative disorders of globe, bilateral
    - H44.399 Other degenerative disorders of globe, unspecified eye

+ H44.4 Hypotony of eye
  - H44.40 Unspecified hypotony of eye
  - + H44.41 Flat anterior chamber hypotony of eye
    - H44.411 Flat anterior chamber hypotony of right eye
    - H44.412 Flat anterior chamber hypotony of left eye
    - H44.413 Flat anterior chamber hypotony of eye, bilateral
    - H44.419 Flat anterior chamber hypotony of unspecified eye
  - + H44.42 Hypotony of eye due to ocular fistula
    - H44.421 Hypotony of right eye due to ocular fistula
    - H44.422 Hypotony of left eye due to ocular fistula
    - H44.423 Hypotony of eye due to ocular fistula, bilateral
    - H44.429 Hypotony of unspecified eye due to ocular fistula
  - + H44.43 Hypotony of eye due to other ocular disorders
    - H44.431 Hypotony of eye due to other ocular disorders, right eye
    - H44.432 Hypotony of eye due to other ocular disorders, left eye
    - H44.433 Hypotony of eye due to other ocular disorders, bilateral
    - H44.439 Hypotony of eye due to other ocular disorders, unspecified eye
  - + H44.44 Primary hypotony of eye
    - H44.441 Primary hypotony of right eye
    - H44.442 Primary hypotony of left eye
    - H44.443 Primary hypotony of eye, bilateral
    - H44.449 Primary hypotony of unspecified eye

+ H44.5 Degenerated conditions of globe
  - H44.50 Unspecified degenerated conditions of globe
  - + H44.51 Absolute glaucoma
    - H44.511 Absolute glaucoma, right eye
    - H44.512 Absolute glaucoma, left eye
    - H44.513 Absolute glaucoma, bilateral
    - H44.519 Absolute glaucoma, unspecified eye
  - + H44.52 Atrophy of globe

    Phthisis bulbi
    - H44.521 Atrophy of globe, right eye
    - H44.522 Atrophy of globe, left eye
    - H44.523 Atrophy of globe, bilateral
    - H44.529 Atrophy of globe, unspecified eye
  - + H44.53 Leucocoria
    - H44.531 Leucocoria, right eye
    - H44.532 Leucocoria, left eye
    - H44.533 Leucocoria, bilateral
    - H44.539 Leucocoria, unspecified eye

+ H44.6 Retained (old) intraocular foreign body, magnetic

  Use additional code to identify magnetic foreign body (Z18.11)

  Excludes1: *current intraocular foreign body (S05.-)*

  Excludes2: *retained foreign body in eyelid (H02.81-)*
  retained (old) foreign body following penetrating wound of orbit (H05.5-)
  retained (old) intraocular foreign body, nonmagnetic (H44.7-)
  - + H44.60 Unspecified retained (old) intraocular foreign body, magnetic
    - H44.601 Unspecified retained (old) intraocular foreign body, magnetic, right eye
    - H44.602 Unspecified retained (old) intraocular foreign body, magnetic, left eye
    - H44.603 Unspecified retained (old) intraocular foreign body, magnetic, bilateral
    - H44.609 Unspecified retained (old) intraocular foreign body, magnetic, unspecified eye

+ **H44.61 Retained (old) magnetic foreign body in anterior chamber**
  - **H44.611 Retained (old) magnetic foreign body in anterior chamber, right eye**
  - **H44.612 Retained (old) magnetic foreign body in anterior chamber, left eye**
  - **H44.613 Retained (old) magnetic foreign body in anterior chamber, bilateral**
  - **H44.619 Retained (old) magnetic foreign body in anterior chamber, unspecified eye**

+ **H44.62 Retained (old) magnetic foreign body in iris or ciliary body**
  - **H44.621 Retained (old) magnetic foreign body in iris or ciliary body, right eye**
  - **H44.622 Retained (old) magnetic foreign body in iris or ciliary body, left eye**
  - **H44.623 Retained (old) magnetic foreign body in iris or ciliary body, bilateral**
  - **H44.629 Retained (old) magnetic foreign body in iris or ciliary body, unspecified eye**

+ **H44.63 Retained (old) magnetic foreign body in lens**
  - **H44.631 Retained (old) magnetic foreign body in lens, right eye**
  - **H44.632 Retained (old) magnetic foreign body in lens, left eye**
  - **H44.633 Retained (old) magnetic foreign body in lens, bilateral**
  - **H44.639 Retained (old) magnetic foreign body in lens, unspecified eye**

+ **H44.64 Retained (old) magnetic foreign body in posterior wall of globe**
  - **H44.641 Retained (old) magnetic foreign body in posterior wall of globe, right eye**
  - **H44.642 Retained (old) magnetic foreign body in posterior wall of globe, left eye**
  - **H44.643 Retained (old) magnetic foreign body in posterior wall of globe, bilateral**
  - **H44.649 Retained (old) magnetic foreign body in posterior wall of globe, unspecified eye**

+ **H44.65 Retained (old) magnetic foreign body in vitreous body**
  - **H44.651 Retained (old) magnetic foreign body in vitreous body, right eye**
  - **H44.652 Retained (old) magnetic foreign body in vitreous body, left eye**
  - **H44.653 Retained (old) magnetic foreign body in vitreous body, bilateral**
  - **H44.659 Retained (old) magnetic foreign body in vitreous body, unspecified eye**

+ **H44.69 Retained (old) intraocular foreign body, magnetic, in other or multiple sites**
  - **H44.691 Retained (old) intraocular foreign body, magnetic, in other or multiple sites, right eye**
  - **H44.692 Retained (old) intraocular foreign body, magnetic, in other or multiple sites, left eye**
  - **H44.693 Retained (old) intraocular foreign body, magnetic, in other or multiple sites, bilateral**
  - **H44.699 Retained (old) intraocular foreign body, magnetic, in other or multiple sites, unspecified eye**

+ **H44.7 Retained (old) intraocular foreign body, nonmagnetic**

Use additional code to identify nonmagnetic foreign body (Z18.01-Z18.10, Z18.12, Z18.2-Z18.9)

Excludes1: *current intraocular foreign body (S05.-)*

Excludes2: *retained foreign body in eyelid (H02.81-)*
retained (old) foreign body following penetrating wound of orbit (H05.5-)
retained (old) intraocular foreign body, magnetic (H44.6-)

+ **H44.70 Unspecified retained (old) intraocular foreign body, nonmagnetic**
  - **H44.701 Unspecified retained (old) intraocular foreign body, nonmagnetic, right eye**
  - **H44.702 Unspecified retained (old) intraocular foreign body, nonmagnetic, left eye**
  - **H44.703 Unspecified retained (old) intraocular foreign body, nonmagnetic, bilateral**
  - **H44.709 Unspecified retained (old) intraocular foreign body, nonmagnetic, unspecified eye**
    Retained (old) intraocular foreign body NOS

+ **H44.71 Retained (nonmagnetic) (old) foreign body in anterior chamber**
  - **H44.711 Retained (nonmagnetic) (old) foreign body in anterior chamber, right eye**
  - **H44.712 Retained (nonmagnetic) (old) foreign body in anterior chamber, left eye**
  - **H44.713 Retained (nonmagnetic) (old) foreign body in anterior chamber, bilateral**
  - **H44.719 Retained (nonmagnetic) (old) foreign body in anterior chamber, unspecified eye**

+ **H44.72 Retained (nonmagnetic) (old) foreign body in iris or ciliary body**
  - **H44.721 Retained (nonmagnetic) (old) foreign body in iris or ciliary body, right eye**
  - **H44.722 Retained (nonmagnetic) (old) foreign body in iris or ciliary body, left eye**
  - **H44.723 Retained (nonmagnetic) (old) foreign body in iris or ciliary body, bilateral**
  - **H44.729 Retained (nonmagnetic) (old) foreign body in iris or ciliary body, unspecified eye**

+ **H44.73 Retained (nonmagnetic) (old) foreign body in lens**
  - **H44.731 Retained (nonmagnetic) (old) foreign body in lens, right eye**
  - **H44.732 Retained (nonmagnetic) (old) foreign body in lens, left eye**
  - **H44.733 Retained (nonmagnetic) (old) foreign body in lens, bilateral**
  - **H44.739 Retained (nonmagnetic) (old) foreign body in lens, unspecified eye**

+ **H44.74 Retained (nonmagnetic) (old) foreign body in posterior wall of globe**
  - **H44.741 Retained (nonmagnetic) (old) foreign body in posterior wall of globe, right eye**
  - **H44.742 Retained (nonmagnetic) (old) foreign body in posterior wall of globe, left eye**
  - **H44.743 Retained (nonmagnetic) (old) foreign body in posterior wall of globe, bilateral**
  - **H44.749 Retained (nonmagnetic) (old) foreign body in posterior wall of globe, unspecified eye**

+ **H44.75 Retained (nonmagnetic) (old) foreign body in vitreous body**
  - **H44.751 Retained (nonmagnetic) (old) foreign body in vitreous body, right eye**
  - **H44.752 Retained (nonmagnetic) (old) foreign body in vitreous body, left eye**
  - **H44.753 Retained (nonmagnetic) (old) foreign body in vitreous body, bilateral**
  - **H44.759 Retained (nonmagnetic) (old) foreign body in vitreous body, unspecified eye**

+ **H44.79 Retained (old) intraocular foreign body, nonmagnetic, in other or multiple sites**
  - **H44.791 Retained (old) intraocular foreign body, nonmagnetic, in other or multiple sites, right eye**

H44.792 Retained (old) intraocular foreign body, nonmagnetic, in other or multiple sites, left eye
H44.793 Retained (old) intraocular foreign body, nonmagnetic, in other or multiple sites, bilateral
H44.799 Retained (old) intraocular foreign body, nonmagnetic, in other or multiple sites, unspecified eye
+ H44.8 Other disorders of globe
+ H44.81 Hemophthalmos
H44.811 Hemophthalmos, right eye
H44.812 Hemophthalmos, left eye
H44.813 Hemophthalmos, bilateral
H44.819 Hemophthalmos, unspecified eye
+ H44.82 Luxation of globe
H44.821 Luxation of globe, right eye
H44.822 Luxation of globe, left eye
H44.823 Luxation of globe, bilateral
H44.829 Luxation of globe, unspecified eye
H44.89 Other disorders of globe
H44.9 Unspecified disorder of globe

Disorders of optic nerve and visual pathways (H46-H47)

H46 Optic neuritis

Excludes2: *ischemic optic neuropathy (H47.01-)*
neuromyelitis optica [Devic] (G36.0)

+ H46.0 Optic papillitis
CC H46.00 Optic papillitis, unspecified eye
CC H46.01 Optic papillitis, right eye
CC H46.02 Optic papillitis, left eye
CC H46.03 Optic papillitis, bilateral
+ H46.1 Retrobulbar neuritis
Retrobulbar neuritis NOS
Excludes1: *syphilitic retrobulbar neuritis (A52.15)*
CC H46.10 Retrobulbar neuritis, unspecified eye
CC H46.11 Retrobulbar neuritis, right eye
CC H46.12 Retrobulbar neuritis, left eye
CC H46.13 Retrobulbar neuritis, bilateral
H46.2 Nutritional optic neuropathy
H46.3 Toxic optic neuropathy
Code first (T51-T65) to identify cause
CC H46.8 Other optic neuritis
CC H46.9 Unspecified optic neuritis

H47 Other disorders of optic [2nd] nerve and visual pathways

+ H47.0 Disorders of optic nerve, not elsewhere classified
+ H47.01 Ischemic optic neuropathy
H47.011 Ischemic optic neuropathy, right eye
H47.012 Ischemic optic neuropathy, left eye
H47.013 Ischemic optic neuropathy, bilateral
H47.019 Ischemic optic neuropathy, unspecified eye
+ H47.02 Hemorrhage in optic nerve sheath
H47.021 Hemorrhage in optic nerve sheath, right eye
H47.022 Hemorrhage in optic nerve sheath, left eye
H47.023 Hemorrhage in optic nerve sheath, bilateral
H47.029 Hemorrhage in optic nerve sheath, unspecified eye
+ H47.03 Optic nerve hypoplasia
H47.031 Optic nerve hypoplasia, right eye
H47.032 Optic nerve hypoplasia, left eye
H47.033 Optic nerve hypoplasia, bilateral
H47.039 Optic nerve hypoplasia, unspecified eye
+ H47.09 Other disorders of optic nerve, not elsewhere classified
Compression of optic nerve
H47.091 Other disorders of optic nerve, not elsewhere classified, right eye
H47.092 Other disorders of optic nerve, not elsewhere classified, left eye
H47.093 Other disorders of optic nerve, not elsewhere classified, bilateral
H47.099 Other disorders of optic nerve, not elsewhere classified, unspecified eye
+ H47.1 Papilledema
CC H47.10 Unspecified papilledema
CC H47.11 Papilledema associated with increased intracranial pressure
H47.12 Papilledema associated with decreased ocular pressure
H47.13 Papilledema associated with retinal disorder
+ H47.14 Foster-Kennedy syndrome
H47.141 Foster-Kennedy syndrome, right eye
H47.142 Foster-Kennedy syndrome, left eye
H47.143 Foster-Kennedy syndrome, bilateral
H47.149 Foster-Kennedy syndrome, unspecified eye
+ H47.2 Optic atrophy
H47.20 Unspecified optic atrophy
+ H47.21 Primary optic atrophy
H47.211 Primary optic atrophy, right eye
H47.212 Primary optic atrophy, left eye
H47.213 Primary optic atrophy, bilateral
H47.219 Primary optic atrophy, unspecified eye
H47.22 Hereditary optic atrophy
Leber's optic atrophy
+ H47.23 Glaucomatous optic atrophy
H47.231 Glaucomatous optic atrophy, right eye
H47.232 Glaucomatous optic atrophy, left eye
H47.233 Glaucomatous optic atrophy, bilateral
H47.239 Glaucomatous optic atrophy, unspecified eye
+ H47.29 Other optic atrophy
Temporal pallor of optic disc
H47.291 Other optic atrophy, right eye
H47.292 Other optic atrophy, left eye
H47.293 Other optic atrophy, bilateral
H47.299 Other optic atrophy, unspecified eye
+ H47.3 Other disorders of optic disc
+ H47.31 Coloboma of optic disc
H47.311 Coloboma of optic disc, right eye
H47.312 Coloboma of optic disc, left eye
H47.313 Coloboma of optic disc, bilateral
H47.319 Coloboma of optic disc, unspecified eye
+ H47.32 Drusen of optic disc
H47.321 Drusen of optic disc, right eye
H47.322 Drusen of optic disc, left eye
H47.323 Drusen of optic disc, bilateral
H47.329 Drusen of optic disc, unspecified eye
+ H47.33 Pseudopapilledema of optic disc
H47.331 Pseudopapilledema of optic disc, right eye
H47.332 Pseudopapilledema of optic disc, left eye
H47.333 Pseudopapilledema of optic disc, bilateral
H47.339 Pseudopapilledema of optic disc, unspecified eye
+ H47.39 Other disorders of optic disc
H47.391 Other disorders of optic disc, right eye
H47.392 Other disorders of optic disc, left eye
H47.393 Other disorders of optic disc, bilateral
H47.399 Other disorders of optic disc, unspecified eye
+ H47.4 Disorders of optic chiasm
Code also underlying condition
CC H47.41 Disorders of optic chiasm in (due to) inflammatory disorders
CC H47.42 Disorders of optic chiasm in (due to) neoplasm
CC H47.43 Disorders of optic chiasm in (due to) vascular disorders
CC H47.49 Disorders of optic chiasm in (due to) other disorders
+ H47.5 Disorders of other visual pathways
Disorders of optic tracts, geniculate nuclei and optic radiations
Code also underlying condition
+ H47.51 Disorders of visual pathways in (due to) inflammatory disorders
CC H47.511 Disorders of visual pathways in (due to) inflammatory disorders, right side
CC H47.512 Disorders of visual pathways in (due to) inflammatory disorders, left side
CC H47.519 Disorders of visual pathways in (due to) inflammatory disorders, unspecified side

+ H47.52 Disorders of visual pathways in (due to) neoplasm
CC H47.521 Disorders of visual pathways in (due to) neoplasm, right side
CC H47.522 Disorders of visual pathways in (due to) neoplasm, left side
CC H47.529 Disorders of visual pathways in (due to) neoplasm, unspecified side
+ H47.53 Disorders of visual pathways in (due to) vascular disorders
CC H47.531 Disorders of visual pathways in (due to) vascular disorders, right side
CC H47.532 Disorders of visual pathways in (due to) vascular disorders, left side
CC H47.539 Disorders of visual pathways in (due to) vascular disorders, unspecified side
+ H47.6 Disorders of visual cortex
Code also underlying condition
Excludes1: *injury to visual cortex S04.04-*
+ H47.61 Cortical blindness
H47.611 Cortical blindness, right side of brain
H47.612 Cortical blindness, left side of brain
H47.619 Cortical blindness, unspecified side of brain
+ H47.62 Disorders of visual cortex in (due to) inflammatory disorders
CC H47.621 Disorders of visual cortex in (due to) inflammatory disorders, right side of brain
CC H47.622 Disorders of visual cortex in (due to) inflammatory disorders, left side of brain
CC H47.629 Disorders of visual cortex in (due to) inflammatory disorders, unspecified side of brain
+ H47.63 Disorders of visual cortex in (due to) neoplasm
CC H47.631 Disorders of visual cortex in (due to) neoplasm, right side of brain
CC H47.632 Disorders of visual cortex in (due to) neoplasm, left side of brain
CC H47.639 Disorders of visual cortex in (due to) neoplasm, unspecified side of brain
+ H47.64 Disorders of visual cortex in (due to) vascular disorders
CC H47.641 Disorders of visual cortex in (due to) vascular disorders, right side of brain
CC H47.642 Disorders of visual cortex in (due to) vascular disorders, left side of brain
CC H47.649 Disorders of visual cortex in (due to) vascular disorders, unspecified side of brain
H47.9 Unspecified disorder of visual pathways

Disorders of ocular muscles, binocular movement, accommodation and refraction (H49-H52)

Excludes2: *nystagmus and other irregular eye movements (H55)*

H49 Paralytic strabismus

Excludes2: *internal ophthalmoplegia (H52.51-)*
internuclear ophthalmoplegia (H51.2-)
progressive supranuclear ophthalmoplegia (G23.1)

+ H49.0 Third [oculomotor] nerve palsy
H49.00 Third [oculomotor] nerve palsy, unspecified eye
H49.01 Third [oculomotor] nerve palsy, right eye
H49.02 Third [oculomotor] nerve palsy, left eye
H49.03 Third [oculomotor] nerve palsy, bilateral
+ H49.1 Fourth [trochlear] nerve palsy
H49.10 Fourth [trochlear] nerve palsy, unspecified eye
H49.11 Fourth [trochlear] nerve palsy, right eye
H49.12 Fourth [trochlear] nerve palsy, left eye
H49.13 Fourth [trochlear] nerve palsy, bilateral
+ H49.2 Sixth [abducent] nerve palsy
H49.20 Sixth [abducent] nerve palsy, unspecified eye
H49.21 Sixth [abducent] nerve palsy, right eye
H49.22 Sixth [abducent] nerve palsy, left eye
H49.23 Sixth [abducent] nerve palsy, bilateral
+ H49.3 Total (external) ophthalmoplegia
H49.30 Total (external) ophthalmoplegia, unspecified eye
H49.31 Total (external) ophthalmoplegia, right eye
H49.32 Total (external) ophthalmoplegia, left eye
H49.33 Total (external) ophthalmoplegia, bilateral
+ H49.4 Progressive external ophthalmoplegia
Excludes1: *Kearns-Sayre syndrome (H49.81-)*
H49.40 Progressive external ophthalmoplegia, unspecified eye
H49.41 Progressive external ophthalmoplegia, right eye
H49.42 Progressive external ophthalmoplegia, left eye
H49.43 Progressive external ophthalmoplegia, bilateral
+ H49.8 Other paralytic strabismus
+ H49.81 Kearns-Sayre syndrome
Progressive external ophthalmoplegia with pigmentary retinopathy
Use additional code for other manifestation, such as: heart block (I45.9)
CC H49.811 Kearns-Sayre syndrome, right eye
CC H49.812 Kearns-Sayre syndrome, left eye
CC H49.813 Kearns-Sayre syndrome, bilateral
CC H49.819 Kearns-Sayre syndrome, unspecified eye
+ H49.88 Other paralytic strabismus
External ophthalmoplegia NOS
H49.881 Other paralytic strabismus, right eye
H49.882 Other paralytic strabismus, left eye
H49.883 Other paralytic strabismus, bilateral
H49.889 Other paralytic strabismus, unspecified eye
H49.9 Unspecified paralytic strabismus

H50 Other strabismus

+ H50.0 Esotropia
Convergent concomitant strabismus
Excludes1: *intermittent esotropia (H50.31-, H50.32)*
H50.00 Unspecified esotropia
+ H50.01 Monocular esotropia
H50.011 Monocular esotropia, right eye
H50.012 Monocular esotropia, left eye
+ H50.02 Monocular esotropia with A pattern
H50.021 Monocular esotropia with A pattern, right eye
H50.022 Monocular esotropia with A pattern, left eye
+ H50.03 Monocular esotropia with V pattern
H50.031 Monocular esotropia with V pattern, right eye
H50.032 Monocular esotropia with V pattern, left eye
+ H50.04 Monocular esotropia with other noncomitancies
H50.041 Monocular esotropia with other noncomitancies, right eye
H50.042 Monocular esotropia with other noncomitancies, left eye
H50.05 Alternating esotropia
H50.06 Alternating esotropia with A pattern
H50.07 Alternating esotropia with V pattern
H50.08 Alternating esotropia with other noncomitancies
+ H50.1 Exotropia
Divergent concomitant strabismus
Excludes1: *intermittent exotropia (H50.33-, H50.34)*
H50.10 Unspecified exotropia
+ H50.11 Monocular exotropia
H50.111 Monocular exotropia, right eye
H50.112 Monocular exotropia, left eye
+ H50.12 Monocular exotropia with A pattern
H50.121 Monocular exotropia with A pattern, right eye
H50.122 Monocular exotropia with A pattern, left eye
+ H50.13 Monocular exotropia with V pattern
H50.131 Monocular exotropia with V pattern, right eye
H50.132 Monocular exotropia with V pattern, left eye
+ H50.14 Monocular exotropia with other noncomitancies
H50.141 Monocular exotropia with other noncomitancies, right eye
H50.142 Monocular exotropia with other noncomitancies, left eye
H50.15 Alternating exotropia
H50.16 Alternating exotropia with A pattern
H50.17 Alternating exotropia with V pattern
H50.18 Alternating exotropia with other noncomitancies

+ **H50.2 Vertical strabismus**
  Hypertropia
  H50.21 Vertical strabismus, right eye
  H50.22 Vertical strabismus, left eye
+ **H50.3 Intermittent heterotropia**
  H50.30 Unspecified intermittent heterotropia
  + **H50.31 Intermittent monocular esotropia**
    H50.311 Intermittent monocular esotropia, right eye
    H50.312 Intermittent monocular esotropia, left eye
  H50.32 Intermittent alternating esotropia
  + **H50.33 Intermittent monocular exotropia**
    H50.331 Intermittent monocular exotropia, right eye
    H50.332 Intermittent monocular exotropia, left eye
  H50.34 Intermittent alternating exotropia
+ **H50.4 Other and unspecified heterotropia**
  H50.40 Unspecified heterotropia
  + **H50.41 Cyclotropia**
    H50.411 Cyclotropia, right eye
    H50.412 Cyclotropia, left eye
  H50.42 Monofixation syndrome
  H50.43 Accommodative component in esotropia
+ **H50.5 Heterophoria**
  H50.50 Unspecified heterophoria
  H50.51 Esophoria
  H50.52 Exophoria
  H50.53 Vertical heterophoria
  H50.54 Cyclophoria
  H50.55 Alternating heterophoria
+ **H50.6 Mechanical strabismus**
  H50.60 Mechanical strabismus, unspecified
  + **H50.61 Brown's sheath syndrome**
    H50.611 Brown's sheath syndrome, right eye
    H50.612 Brown's sheath syndrome, left eye
  H50.69 Other mechanical strabismus
  Strabismus due to adhesions
  Traumatic limitation of duction of eye muscle
+ **H50.8 Other specified strabismus**
  + **H50.81 Duane's syndrome**
    H50.811 Duane's syndrome, right eye
    H50.812 Duane's syndrome, left eye
  H50.89 Other specified strabismus
H50.9 Unspecified strabismus

H51 Other disorders of binocular movement
H51.0 Palsy (spasm) of conjugate gaze
+ **H51.1 Convergence insufficiency and excess**
  H51.11 Convergence insufficiency
  H51.12 Convergence excess
+ **H51.2 Internuclear ophthalmoplegia**
  H51.20 Internuclear ophthalmoplegia, unspecified eye
  H51.21 Internuclear ophthalmoplegia, right eye
  H51.22 Internuclear ophthalmoplegia, left eye
  H51.23 Internuclear ophthalmoplegia, bilateral
H51.8 Other specified disorders of binocular movement
H51.9 Unspecified disorder of binocular movement

H52 Disorders of refraction and accommodation
+ **H52.0 Hypermetropia**
  H52.00 Hypermetropia, unspecified eye
  H52.01 Hypermetropia, right eye
  H52.02 Hypermetropia, left eye
  H52.03 Hypermetropia, bilateral
+ **H52.1 Myopia**
  Excludes1: *degenerative myopia (H44.2-)*
  H52.10 Myopia, unspecified eye
  H52.11 Myopia, right eye
  H52.12 Myopia, left eye
  H52.13 Myopia, bilateral
+ **H52.2 Astigmatism**
  + **H52.20 Unspecified astigmatism**
    H52.201 Unspecified astigmatism, right eye
    H52.202 Unspecified astigmatism, left eye
    H52.203 Unspecified astigmatism, bilateral
    H52.209 Unspecified astigmatism, unspecified eye
  + **H52.21 Irregular astigmatism**
    H52.211 Irregular astigmatism, right eye
    H52.212 Irregular astigmatism, left eye
    H52.213 Irregular astigmatism, bilateral
    H52.219 Irregular astigmatism, unspecified eye
  + **H52.22 Regular astigmatism**
    H52.221 Regular astigmatism, right eye
    H52.222 Regular astigmatism, left eye
    H52.223 Regular astigmatism, bilateral
    H52.229 Regular astigmatism, unspecified eye
+ **H52.3 Anisometropia and aniseikonia**
  H52.31 Anisometropia
  H52.32 Aniseikonia
H52.4 Presbyopia
+ **H52.5 Disorders of accommodation**
  + **H52.51 Internal ophthalmoplegia (complete) (total)**
    H52.511 Internal ophthalmoplegia (complete) (total), right eye
    H52.512 Internal ophthalmoplegia (complete) (total), left eye
    H52.513 Internal ophthalmoplegia (complete) (total), bilateral
    H52.519 Internal ophthalmoplegia (complete) (total), unspecified eye
  + **H52.52 Paresis of accommodation**
    H52.521 Paresis of accommodation, right eye
    H52.522 Paresis of accommodation, left eye
    H52.523 Paresis of accommodation, bilateral
    H52.529 Paresis of accommodation, unspecified eye
  + **H52.53 Spasm of accommodation**
    H52.531 Spasm of accommodation, right eye
    H52.532 Spasm of accommodation, left eye
    H52.533 Spasm of accommodation, bilateral
    H52.539 Spasm of accommodation, unspecified eye
H52.6 Other disorders of refraction
H52.7 Unspecified disorder of refraction

Visual disturbances and blindness (H53-H54)

H53 Visual disturbances
+ **H53.0 Amblyopia ex anopsia**
  Excludes1: *amblyopia due to vitamin A deficiency (E50.5)*
  + **H53.00 Unspecified amblyopia**
    H53.001 Unspecified amblyopia, right eye
    H53.002 Unspecified amblyopia, left eye
    H53.003 Unspecified amblyopia, bilateral
    H53.009 Unspecified amblyopia, unspecified eye
  + **H53.01 Deprivation amblyopia**
    H53.011 Deprivation amblyopia, right eye
    H53.012 Deprivation amblyopia, left eye
    H53.013 Deprivation amblyopia, bilateral
    H53.019 Deprivation amblyopia, unspecified eye
  + **H53.02 Refractive amblyopia**
    H53.021 Refractive amblyopia, right eye
    H53.022 Refractive amblyopia, left eye
    H53.023 Refractive amblyopia, bilateral
    H53.029 Refractive amblyopia, unspecified eye
  + **H53.03 Strabismic amblyopia**
    Excludes1: *strabismus (H50.-)*
    H53.031 Strabismic amblyopia, right eye
    H53.032 Strabismic amblyopia, left eye
    H53.033 Strabismic amblyopia, bilateral
    H53.039 Strabismic amblyopia, unspecified eye
  + **H53.04 Amblyopia suspect**
    AHA CC: 4Q, 2016, 22-23
    H53.041 Amblyopia suspect, right eye
    H53.042 Amblyopia suspect, left eye
    H53.043 Amblyopia suspect, bilateral
    H53.049 Amblyopia suspect, unspecified eye
+ **H53.1 Subjective visual disturbances**
  Excludes1: *subjective visual disturbances due to vitamin A deficiency (E50.5)*
  visual hallucinations (R44.1)
  H53.10 Unspecified subjective visual disturbances
  H53.11 Day blindness
  Hemeralopia
  + **H53.12 Transient visual loss**
    Scintillating scotoma
    Excludes1: *amaurosis fugax (G45.3-)*
    transient retinal artery occlusion (H34.0-)
    CC **H53.121 Transient visual loss, right eye**
    CC **H53.122 Transient visual loss, left eye**
    CC **H53.123 Transient visual loss, bilateral**
    CC **H53.129 Transient visual loss, unspecified eye**

+ **H53.13 Sudden visual loss**
CC **H53.131 Sudden visual loss, right eye**
CC **H53.132 Sudden visual loss, left eye**
CC **H53.133 Sudden visual loss, bilateral**
CC **H53.139 Sudden visual loss, unspecified eye**
+ **H53.14 Visual discomfort**
Asthenopia
Photophobia
H53.141 Visual discomfort, right eye
H53.142 Visual discomfort, left eye
H53.143 Visual discomfort, bilateral
H53.149 Visual discomfort, unspecified
H53.15 Visual distortions of shape and size
Metamorphopsia
H53.16 Psychophysical visual disturbances
H53.19 Other subjective visual disturbances
Visual halos
H53.2 Diplopia
Double vision
+ **H53.3 Other and unspecified disorders of binocular vision**
H53.30 Unspecified disorder of binocular vision
H53.31 Abnormal retinal correspondence
H53.32 Fusion with defective stereopsis
H53.33 Simultaneous visual perception without fusion
H53.34 Suppression of binocular vision
+ **H53.4 Visual field defects**
H53.40 Unspecified visual field defects
+ **H53.41 Scotoma involving central area**
Central scotoma
H53.411 Scotoma involving central area, right eye
H53.412 Scotoma involving central area, left eye
H53.413 Scotoma involving central area, bilateral
H53.419 Scotoma involving central area, unspecified eye
+ **H53.42 Scotoma of blind spot area**
Enlarged blind spot
H53.421 Scotoma of blind spot area, right eye
H53.422 Scotoma of blind spot area, left eye
H53.423 Scotoma of blind spot area, bilateral
H53.429 Scotoma of blind spot area, unspecified eye
+ **H53.43 Sector or arcuate defects**
Arcuate scotoma
Bjerrum scotoma
H53.431 Sector or arcuate defects, right eye
H53.432 Sector or arcuate defects, left eye
H53.433 Sector or arcuate defects, bilateral
H53.439 Sector or arcuate defects, unspecified eye
+ **H53.45 Other localized visual field defect**
Peripheral visual field defect
Ring scotoma NOS
Scotoma NOS
H53.451 Other localized visual field defect, right eye
H53.452 Other localized visual field defect, left eye
H53.453 Other localized visual field defect, bilateral
H53.459 Other localized visual field defect, unspecified eye
+ **H53.46 Homonymous bilateral field defects**
Homonymous hemianopsia
Quadrant anopia
Quadrant anopsia
H53.461 Homonymous bilateral field defects, right side
H53.462 Homonymous bilateral field defects, left side
H53.469 Homonymous bilateral field defects, unspecified side
Homonymous bilateral field defects NOS
H53.47 Heteronymous bilateral field defects
Heteronymous hemianop(s)ia
+ **H53.48 Generalized contraction of visual field**
H53.481 Generalized contraction of visual field, right eye
H53.482 Generalized contraction of visual field, left eye
H53.483 Generalized contraction of visual field, bilateral
H53.489 Generalized contraction of visual field, unspecified eye
+ **H53.5 Color vision deficiencies**
Color blindness
Excludes2: *day blindness (H53.11)*
H53.50 Unspecified color vision deficiencies
Color blindness NOS
H53.51 Achromatopsia
H53.52 Acquired color vision deficiency
H53.53 Deuteranomaly
Deuteranopia
H53.54 Protanomaly
Protanopia
H53.55 Tritanomaly
Tritanopia
H53.59 Other color vision deficiencies
+ **H53.6 Night blindness**
Excludes1: *night blindness due to vitamin A deficiency (E50.5)*
H53.60 Unspecified night blindness
H53.61 Abnormal dark adaptation curve
H53.62 Acquired night blindness
H53.63 Congenital night blindness
H53.69 Other night blindness
+ **H53.7 Vision sensitivity deficiencies**
H53.71 Glare sensitivity
H53.72 Impaired contrast sensitivity
H53.8 Other visual disturbances
H53.9 Unspecified visual disturbance

H54 Blindness and low vision
NOTE For definition of visual impairment categories see table below
Code first any associated underlying cause of the blindness
Excludes1: *amaurosis fugax (G45.3)*
AHA CC: 4Q, 2017, 11-12
+ **H54.0 Blindness, both eyes**
Visual impairment categories 3, 4, 5 in both eyes.
H54.0X Blindness, both eyes, different category levels
+ **H54.0X3 Blindness right eye, category 3**
H54.0X33 Blindness right eye category 3, blindness left eye category 3
H54.0X34 Blindness right eye category 3, blindness left eye category 4
H54.0X35 Blindness right eye category 3, blindness left eye category 5
+ **H54.0X4 Blindness right eye, category 4**
H54.0X43 Blindness right eye category 4, blindness left eye category 3
H54.0X44 Blindness right eye category 4, blindness left eye category 4
H54.0X45 Blindness right eye category 4, blindness left eye category 5
+ **H54.0X5 Blindness right eye, category 5**
H54.0X53 Blindness right eye category 5, blindness left eye category 3
H54.0X54 Blindness right eye category 5, blindness left eye category 4
H54.0X55 Blindness right eye category 5, blindness left eye category 5
+ **H54.1 Blindness, one eye, low vision other eye**
Visual impairment categories 3, 4, 5 in one eye, with categories 1 or 2 in the other eye.
H54.10 Blindness, one eye, low vision other eye, unspecified eyes
+ **H54.11 Blindness, right eye, low vision left eye**
+ **H54.113 Blindness right eye category 3, low vision left eye**
H54.1131 Blindness right eye category 3, low vision left eye category 1
H54.1132 Blindness right eye category 3, low vision left eye category 2
+ **H54.114 Blindness right eye category 4, low vision left eye**
H54.1141 Blindness right eye category 4, low vision left eye category 1
H54.1142 Blindness right eye category 4, low vision left eye category 2

+ **H54.115 Blindness right eye category 5, low vision left eye**
  - **H54.1151 Blindness right eye category 5, low vision left eye category 1**
  - **H54.1152 Blindness right eye category 5, low vision left eye category 2**

+ **H54.12 Blindness, left eye, low vision right eye**
  + **H54.121 Low vision right eye category 1, blindness left eye**
    - **H54.1213 Low vision right eye category 1, blindness left eye category 3**
    - **H54.1214 Low vision right eye category 1, blindness left eye category 4**
    - **H54.1215 Low vision right eye category 1, blindness left eye category 5**
  + **H54.122 Low vision right eye category 2, blindness left eye**
    - **H54.1223 Low vision right eye category 2, blindness left eye category 3**
    - **H54.1224 Low vision right eye category 2, blindness left eye category 4**
    - **H54.1225 Low vision right eye category 2, blindness left eye category 5**

+ **H54.2 Low vision, both eyes**

Visual impairment categories 1 or 2 in both eyes.

+ **H54.2X Low vision, both eyes, different category levels**
  + **H54.2X1 Low vision, right eye, category 1**
    - **H54.2X11 Low vision, right eye, category 1, low vision left eye category 1**
    - **H54.2X12 Low vision, right eye, category 1, low vision left eye category 2**
  + **H54.2X2 Low vision, right eye, category 2**
    - **H54.2X21 Low vision, right eye, category 2, low vision left eye category 1**
    - **H54.2X22 Low vision, right eye, category 2, low vision left eye category 2**

H54.3 Unqualified visual loss, both eyes

Visual impairment category 9 in both eyes.

Review coding guideline C.7.b

+ **H54.4 Blindness, one eye**

Visual impairment categories 3, 4, 5 in one eye [normal vision in other eye]

H54.40 Blindness, one eye, unspecified eye

+ **H54.41 Blindness, right eye, normal vision left eye**
  + **H54.413 Blindness, right eye, category 3**
    - **H54.413A Blindness right eye category 3, normal vision left eye**
  + **H54.414 Blindness, right eye, category 4**
    - **H54.414A Blindness right eye category 4, normal vision left eye**
  + **H54.415 Blindness, right eye, category 5**
    - **H54.415A Blindness right eye category 5, normal vision left eye**
+ **H54.42 Blindness, left eye, normal vision right eye**
  + **H54.42A Blindness, left eye, category 3-5**
    - **H54.42A3 Blindness left eye category 3, normal vision right eye**
    - **H54.42A4 Blindness left eye category 4, normal vision right eye**
    - **H54.42A5 Blindness left eye category 5, normal vision right eye**

+ **H54.5 Low vision, one eye**

Visual impairment categories 1 or 2 in one eye [normal vision in other eye].

H54.50 Low vision, one eye, unspecified eye

+ **H54.51 Low vision, right eye, normal vision left eye**
  + **H54.511 Low vision, right eye, category 1-2**
    - **H54.511A Low vision right eye category 1, normal vision left eye**
    - **H54.512A Low vision right eye category 2, normal vision left eye**
+ **H54.52 Low vision, left eye, normal vision right eye**
  + **H54.52A Low vision, left eye, category 1-2**
    - **H54.52A1 Low vision left eye category 1, normal vision right eye**
    - **H54.52A2 Low vision left eye category 2, normal vision right eye**

+ **H54.6 Unqualified visual loss, one eye**

Visual impairment category 9 in one eye [normal vision in other eye].

Review coding guideline C.7.b

H54.60 Unqualified visual loss, one eye, unspecified

H54.61 Unqualified visual loss, right eye, normal vision left eye

H54.62 Unqualified visual loss, left eye, normal vision right eye

H54.7 Unspecified visual loss

Visual impairment category 9 NOS

Review coding guideline C.7.b

H54.8 Legal blindness, as defined in USA

Blindness NOS according to USA definition

Excludes1: *legal blindness with specification of impairment level (H54.0-H54.7)*

NOTE The table below gives a classification of severity of visual impairment recommended by a WHO Study Group on the Prevention of Blindness, Geneva, 6-10 November 1972.

The term 'low vision' in category H54 comprises categories 1 and 2 of the table, the term 'blindness' categories 3, 4 and 5, and the term 'unqualified visual loss' category 9.

If the extent of the visual field is taken into account, patients with a field no greater than 10 but greater than 5 around central fixation should be placed in category 3 and patients with a field no greater than 5 around central fixation should be placed in category 4, even if the central acuity is not impaired.

Category of visual impairment	Visual acuity with best possible correction	
	Maximum less than:	Minimum equal to or better than:
	6/18	6/60
3/10(0.3)	1/10(0.1)	
20/70	20/200	
	6/60	3/60
1/10(0.1)	1/20(0.05)	
20/200	20/400	
	3/60	1/60(finger counting at one meter)
1/20(0.05)	1/50(0.02)	
20/400	5/300(20/1200)	
	1/60(finger counting at one meter)	Light perception
1/50(0.02)		
5/300		
	No light perception	
	Undetermined or unspecified	

Note: Document 508 compliance requires all cells in the above table to be filled.

Other disorders of eye and adnexa (H55-H57)

H55 Nystagmus and other irregular eye movements

+ **H55.0 Nystagmus**
  - **H55.00 Unspecified nystagmus**
  - **H55.01 Congenital nystagmus**
  - **H55.02 Latent nystagmus**
  - **H55.03 Visual deprivation nystagmus**
  - **H55.04 Dissociated nystagmus**
  - **H55.09 Other forms of nystagmus**
+ **H55.8 Other irregular eye movements**
  AHA CC: 4Q, 2020, 25
  - **H55.81 Deficient saccadic eye movements**
  - **H55.82 Deficient smooth pursuit eye movements**
  - **H55.89 Other irregular eye movements**

H57 Other disorders of eye and adnexa

+ **H57.0 Anomalies of pupillary function**
  - **H57.00 Unspecified anomaly of pupillary function**
  - **H57.01 Argyll Robertson pupil, atypical**
    Excludes1: *syphilitic Argyll Robertson pupil (A52.19)*
  - **H57.02 Anisocoria**
  - **H57.03 Miosis**
  - **H57.04 Mydriasis**
  - + **H57.05 Tonic pupil**
    - **H57.051 Tonic pupil, right eye**
    - **H57.052 Tonic pupil, left eye**
    - **H57.053 Tonic pupil, bilateral**
    - **H57.059 Tonic pupil, unspecified eye**
  - **H57.09 Other anomalies of pupillary function**
+ **H57.1 Ocular pain**
  - **H57.10 Ocular pain, unspecified eye**
  - **H57.11 Ocular pain, right eyew**
  - **H57.12 Ocular pain, left eye**
  - **H57.13 Ocular pain, bilateral**
+ **H57.8 Other specified disorders of eye and adnexa**
  AHA CC: 4Q, 2018, 15-16
  - + **H57.81 Brow ptosis**
    - **H57.811 Brow ptosis, right**
    - **H57.812 Brow ptosis, left**
    - **H57.813 Brow ptosis, bilateral**
    - **H57.819 Brow ptosis, unspecified**
  - **H57.89 Other specified disorders of eye and adnexa**
- **H57.9 Unspecified disorder of eye and adnexa**

Intraoperative and postprocedural complications and disorders of eye and adnexa, not elsewhere classified (H59)

H59 Intraoperative and postprocedural complications and disorders of eye and adnexa, not elsewhere classified

Excludes1: *mechanical complication of intraocular lens (T85.2)*
mechanical complication of other ocular prosthetic devices, implants and grafts (T85.3)
pseudophakia (Z96.1)
secondary cataracts (H26.4-)

+ **H59.0 Disorders of the eye following cataract surgery**
  - + **H59.01 Keratopathy (bullous aphakic) following cataract surgery**
    Vitreal corneal syndrome
    Vitreous (touch) syndrome
    - CC **H59.011 Keratopathy (bullous aphakic) following cataract surgery, right eye**
    - CC **H59.012 Keratopathy (bullous aphakic) following cataract surgery, left eye**
    - CC **H59.013 Keratopathy (bullous aphakic) following cataract surgery, bilateral**
    - CC **H59.019 Keratopathy (bullous aphakic) following cataract surgery, unspecified eye**
  - + **H59.02 Cataract (lens) fragments in eye following cataract surgery**
    - **H59.021 Cataract (lens) fragments in eye following cataract surgery, right eye**
    - **H59.022 Cataract (lens) fragments in eye following cataract surgery, left eye**
    - **H59.023 Cataract (lens) fragments in eye following cataract surgery, bilateral**
    - **H59.029 Cataract (lens) fragments in eye following cataract surgery, unspecified eye**
  - + **H59.03 Cystoid macular edema following cataract surgery**
    - CC **H59.031 Cystoid macular edema following cataract surgery, right eye**
    - CC **H59.032 Cystoid macular edema following cataract surgery, left eye**
    - CC **H59.033 Cystoid macular edema following cataract surgery, bilateral**
    - CC **H59.039 Cystoid macular edema following cataract surgery, unspecified eye**
  - + **H59.09 Other disorders of the eye following cataract surgery**
    - CC **H59.091 Other disorders of the right eye following cataract surgery**
    - CC **H59.092 Other disorders of the left eye following cataract surgery**
    - CC **H59.093 Other disorders of the eye following cataract surgery, bilateral**
    - CC **H59.099 Other disorders of unspecified eye following cataract surgery**
+ **H59.1 Intraoperative hemorrhage and hematoma of eye and adnexa complicating a procedure**
  Excludes1: *intraoperative hemorrhage and hematoma of eye and adnexa due to accidental puncture or laceration during a procedure (H59.2-)*
  - + **H59.11 Intraoperative hemorrhage and hematoma of eye and adnexa complicating an ophthalmic procedure**
    - CC **H59.111 Intraoperative hemorrhage and hematoma of right eye and adnexa complicating an ophthalmic procedure**
    - CC **H59.112 Intraoperative hemorrhage and hematoma of left eye and adnexa complicating an ophthalmic procedure**
    - CC **H59.113 Intraoperative hemorrhage and hematoma of eye and adnexa complicating an ophthalmic procedure, bilateral**
    - CC **H59.119 Intraoperative hemorrhage and hematoma of unspecified eye and adnexa complicating an ophthalmic procedure**
  - + **H59.12 Intraoperative hemorrhage and hematoma of eye and adnexa complicating other procedure**
    - CC **H59.121 Intraoperative hemorrhage and hematoma of right eye and adnexa complicating other procedure**
    - CC **H59.122 Intraoperative hemorrhage and hematoma of left eye and adnexa complicating other procedure**
    - CC **H59.123 Intraoperative hemorrhage and hematoma of eye and adnexa complicating other procedure, bilateral**
    - CC **H59.129 Intraoperative hemorrhage and hematoma of unspecified eye and adnexa complicating other procedure**
+ **H59.2 Accidental puncture and laceration of eye and adnexa during a procedure**
  - + **H59.21 Accidental puncture and laceration of eye and adnexa during an ophthalmic procedure**
    - CC **H59.211 Accidental puncture and laceration of right eye and adnexa during an ophthalmic procedure**
    - CC **H59.212 Accidental puncture and laceration of left eye and adnexa during an ophthalmic procedure**
    - CC **H59.213 Accidental puncture and laceration of eye and adnexa during an ophthalmic procedure, bilateral**
    - CC **H59.219 Accidental puncture and laceration of unspecified eye and adnexa during an ophthalmic procedure**

+ **H59.22 Accidental puncture and laceration of eye and adnexa during other procedure**
  - CC **H59.221 Accidental puncture and laceration of right eye and adnexa during other procedure**
  - CC **H59.222 Accidental puncture and laceration of left eye and adnexa during other procedure**
  - CC **H59.223 Accidental puncture and laceration of eye and adnexa during other procedure, bilateral**
  - CC **H59.229 Accidental puncture and laceration of unspecified eye and adnexa during other procedure**

+ **H59.3 Postprocedural hemorrhage, hematoma and seroma of eye and adnexa following a procedure**
  AHA CC: 4Q, 2016, 9-10
  + **H59.31 Postprocedural hemorrhage of eye and adnexa following an ophthalmic procedure**
    - CC **H59.311 Postprocedural hemorrhage of right eye and adnexa following an ophthalmic procedure**
    - CC **H59.312 Postprocedural hemorrhage of left eye and adnexa following an ophthalmic procedure**
    - CC **H59.313 Postprocedural hemorrhage of eye and adnexa following an ophthalmic procedure, bilateral**
    - CC **H59.319 Postprocedural hemorrhage of unspecified eye and adnexa following an ophthalmic procedure**
  + **H59.32 Postprocedural hemorrhage of eye and adnexa following other procedure**
    - CC **H59.321 Postprocedural hemorrhage of right eye and adnexa following other procedure**
    - CC **H59.322 Postprocedural hemorrhage of left eye and adnexa following other procedure**
    - CC **H59.323 Postprocedural hemorrhage of eye and adnexa following other procedure, bilateral**
    - CC **H59.329 Postprocedural hemorrhage of unspecified eye and adnexa following other procedure**
  + **H59.33 Postprocedural hematoma of eye and adnexa following an ophthalmic procedure**
    - CC **H59.331 Postprocedural hematoma of right eye and adnexa following an ophthalmic procedure**
    - CC **H59.332 Postprocedural hematoma of left eye and adnexa following an ophthalmic procedure**
    - CC **H59.333 Postprocedural hematoma of eye and adnexa following an ophthalmic procedure, bilateral**
    - CC **H59.339 Postprocedural hematoma of unspecified eye and adnexa following an ophthalmic procedure**
  + **H59.34 Postprocedural hematoma of eye and adnexa following other procedure**
    - CC **H59.341 Postprocedural hematoma of right eye and adnexa following other procedure**
    - CC **H59.342 Postprocedural hematoma of left eye and adnexa following other procedure**
    - CC **H59.343 Postprocedural hematoma of eye and adnexa following other procedure, bilateral**
    - CC **H59.349 Postprocedural hematoma of unspecified eye and adnexa following other procedure**
  + **H59.35 Postprocedural seroma of eye and adnexa following an ophthalmic procedure**
    - CC **H59.351 Postprocedural seroma of right eye and adnexa following an ophthalmic procedure**
    - CC **H59.352 Postprocedural seroma of left eye and adnexa following an ophthalmic procedure**
    - CC **H59.353 Postprocedural seroma of eye and adnexa following an ophthalmic procedure, bilateral**
    - CC **H59.359 Postprocedural seroma of unspecified eye and adnexa following an ophthalmic procedure**
  + **H59.36 Postprocedural seroma of eye and adnexa following other procedure**
    - CC **H59.361 Postprocedural seroma of right eye and adnexa following other procedure**
    - CC **H59.362 Postprocedural seroma of left eye and adnexa following other procedure**
    - CC **H59.363 Postprocedural seroma of eye and adnexa following other procedure, bilateral**
    - CC **H59.369 Postprocedural seroma of unspecified eye and adnexa following other procedure**

+ **H59.4 Inflammation (infection) of postprocedural bleb**
  Postprocedural blebitis
  Excludes1: *filtering (vitreous) bleb after glaucoma surgery status (Z98.83)*
  - **H59.40 Inflammation (infection) of postprocedural bleb, unspecified**
  - **H59.41 Inflammation (infection) of postprocedural bleb, stage 1**
  - **H59.42 Inflammation (infection) of postprocedural bleb, stage 2**
  - **H59.43 Inflammation (infection) of postprocedural bleb, stage 3**
    Bleb endophthalmitis

+ **H59.8 Other intraoperative and postprocedural complications and disorders of eye and adnexa, not elsewhere classified**
  + **H59.81 Chorioretinal scars after surgery for detachment**
    - CC **H59.811 Chorioretinal scars after surgery for detachment, right eye**
    - CC **H59.812 Chorioretinal scars after surgery for detachment, left eye**
    - CC **H59.813 Chorioretinal scars after surgery for detachment, bilateral**
    - CC **H59.819 Chorioretinal scars after surgery for detachment, unspecified eye**
  - CC **H59.88 Other intraoperative complications of eye and adnexa, not elsewhere classified**
  - CC **H59.89 Other postprocedural complications and disorders of eye and adnexa, not elsewhere classified**
    AHA CC: 3Q, 2020, 29

Chapter 8: Diseases of the Ear and Mastoid Process (H60-H95)

NOTE Use an external cause code following the code for the ear condition, if applicable, to identify the cause of the ear condition

Excludes2: *certain conditions originating in the perinatal period (P04-P96)*
certain infectious and parasitic diseases (A00-B99)
complications of pregnancy, childbirth and the puerperium (O00-O9A)
congenital malformations, deformations and chromosomal abnormalities (Q00-Q99)
endocrine, nutritional and metabolic diseases (E00-E88)
injury, poisoning and certain other consequences of external causes (S00-T88)
neoplasms (C00-D49)
symptoms, signs and abnormal clinical and laboratory findings, not elsewhere classified (R00-R94)

This chapter contains the following category blocks:

- H60-H62 Diseases of external ear
- H65-H75 Diseases of middle ear and mastoid
- H80-H83 Diseases of inner ear
- H90-H94 Other disorders of ear
- H95 Intraoperative and postprocedural complications and disorders of ear and mastoid process, not elsewhere classified

C. Chapter-Specific Coding Guidelines

In addition to general coding guidelines, there are guidelines for specific diagnoses and/or conditions in the classification. Unless otherwise indicated, these guidelines apply to all health care settings. Please refer to Section II for guidelines on the selection of principal diagnosis.

8. Chapter 8: Diseases of the Ear and Mastoid Process (H60-H95)

Reserved for future guideline expansion

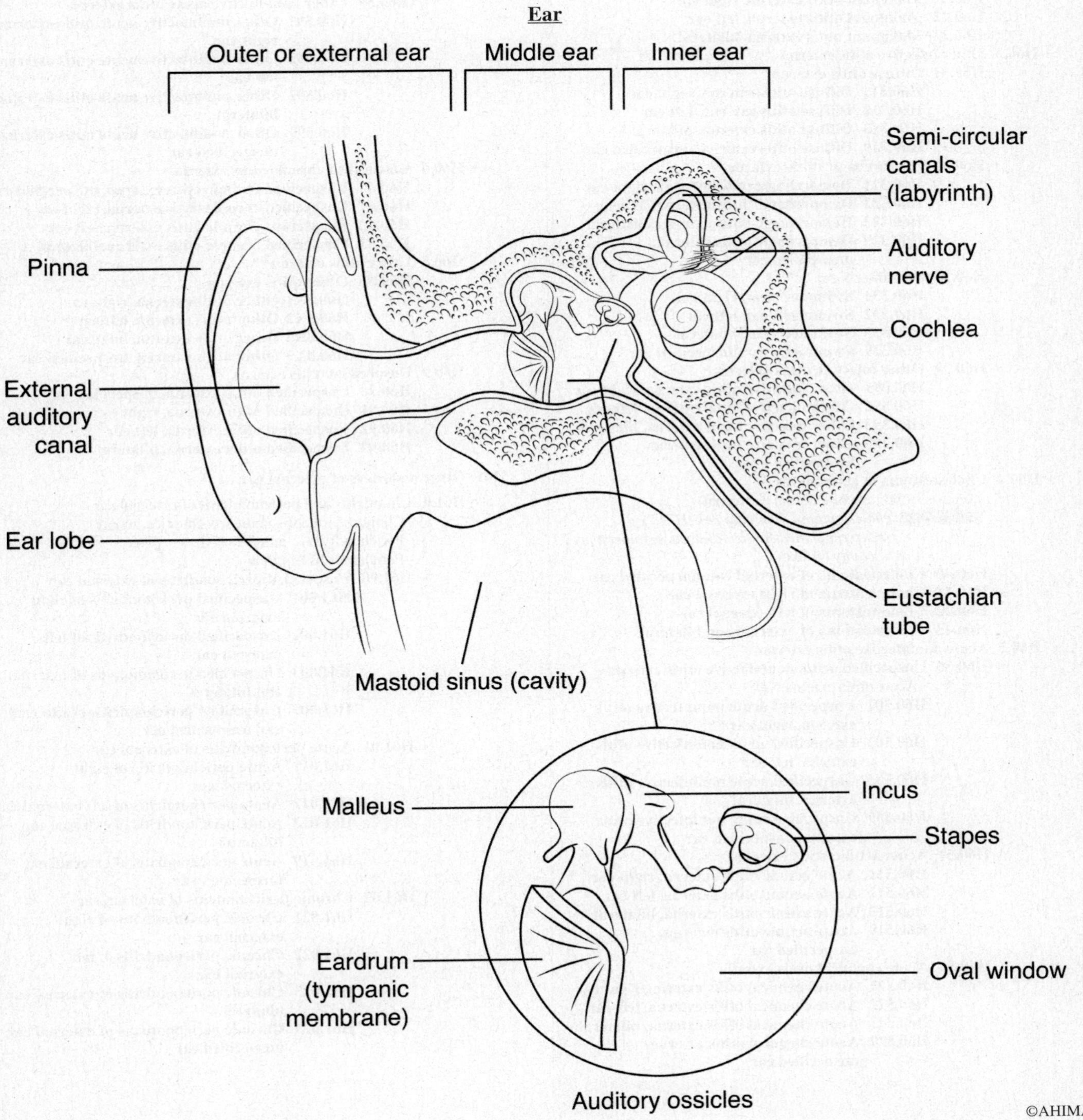

Diseases of external ear (H60-H62)

H60 Otitis externa

+ **H60.0 Abscess of external ear**
  Boil of external ear
  Carbuncle of auricle or external auditory canal
  Furuncle of external ear
  H60.00 Abscess of external ear, unspecified ear
  H60.01 Abscess of right external ear
  H60.02 Abscess of left external ear
  H60.03 Abscess of external ear, bilateral

+ **H60.1 Cellulitis of external ear**
  Cellulitis of auricle
  Cellulitis of external auditory canal
  H60.10 Cellulitis of external ear, unspecified ear
  H60.11 Cellulitis of right external ear
  H60.12 Cellulitis of left external ear
  H60.13 Cellulitis of external ear, bilateral

+ **H60.2 Malignant otitis externa**
  CC **H60.20 Malignant otitis externa, unspecified ear**
  CC **H60.21 Malignant otitis externa, right ear**
  CC **H60.22 Malignant otitis externa, left ear**
  CC **H60.23 Malignant otitis externa, bilateral**

+ **H60.3 Other infective otitis externa**
  + **H60.31 Diffuse otitis externa**
    H60.311 Diffuse otitis externa, right ear
    H60.312 Diffuse otitis externa, left ear
    H60.313 Diffuse otitis externa, bilateral
    H60.319 Diffuse otitis externa, unspecified ear
  + **H60.32 Hemorrhagic otitis externa**
    H60.321 Hemorrhagic otitis externa, right ear
    H60.322 Hemorrhagic otitis externa, left ear
    H60.323 Hemorrhagic otitis externa, bilateral
    H60.329 Hemorrhagic otitis externa, unspecified ear
  + **H60.33 Swimmer's ear**
    H60.331 Swimmer's ear, right ear
    H60.332 Swimmer's ear, left ear
    H60.333 Swimmer's ear, bilateral
    H60.339 Swimmer's ear, unspecified ear
  + **H60.39 Other infective otitis externa**
    H60.391 Other infective otitis externa, right ear
    H60.392 Other infective otitis externa, left ear
    H60.393 Other infective otitis externa, bilateral
    H60.399 Other infective otitis externa, unspecified ear

+ **H60.4 Cholesteatoma of external ear**
  Keratosis obturans of external ear (canal)
  Excludes2: *cholesteatoma of middle ear (H71.-)*
  recurrent cholesteatoma of postmastoidectomy cavity (H95.0-)
  H60.40 Cholesteatoma of external ear, unspecified ear
  H60.41 Cholesteatoma of right external ear
  H60.42 Cholesteatoma of left external ear
  H60.43 Cholesteatoma of external ear, bilateral

+ **H60.5 Acute noninfective otitis externa**
  + **H60.50 Unspecified acute noninfective otitis externa**
    Acute otitis externa NOS
    H60.501 Unspecified acute noninfective otitis externa, right ear
    H60.502 Unspecified acute noninfective otitis externa, left ear
    H60.503 Unspecified acute noninfective otitis externa, bilateral
    H60.509 Unspecified acute noninfective otitis externa, unspecified ear
  + **H60.51 Acute actinic otitis externa**
    H60.511 Acute actinic otitis externa, right ear
    H60.512 Acute actinic otitis externa, left ear
    H60.513 Acute actinic otitis externa, bilateral
    H60.519 Acute actinic otitis externa, unspecified ear
  + **H60.52 Acute chemical otitis externa**
    H60.521 Acute chemical otitis externa, right ear
    H60.522 Acute chemical otitis externa, left ear
    H60.523 Acute chemical otitis externa, bilateral
    H60.529 Acute chemical otitis externa, unspecified ear
  + **H60.53 Acute contact otitis externa**
    H60.531 Acute contact otitis externa, right ear
    H60.532 Acute contact otitis externa, left ear
    H60.533 Acute contact otitis externa, bilateral
    H60.539 Acute contact otitis externa, unspecified ear
  + **H60.54 Acute eczematoid otitis externa**
    H60.541 Acute eczematoid otitis externa, right ear
    H60.542 Acute eczematoid otitis externa, left ear
    H60.543 Acute eczematoid otitis externa, bilateral
    H60.549 Acute eczematoid otitis externa, unspecified ear
  + **H60.55 Acute reactive otitis externa**
    H60.551 Acute reactive otitis externa, right ear
    H60.552 Acute reactive otitis externa, left ear
    H60.553 Acute reactive otitis externa, bilateral
    H60.559 Acute reactive otitis externa, unspecified ear
  + **H60.59 Other noninfective acute otitis externa**
    H60.591 Other noninfective acute otitis externa, right ear
    H60.592 Other noninfective acute otitis externa, left ear
    H60.593 Other noninfective acute otitis externa, bilateral
    H60.599 Other noninfective acute otitis externa, unspecified ear

+ **H60.6 Unspecified chronic otitis externa**
  H60.60 Unspecified chronic otitis externa, unspecified ear
  H60.61 Unspecified chronic otitis externa, right ear
  H60.62 Unspecified chronic otitis externa, left ear
  H60.63 Unspecified chronic otitis externa, bilateral

+ **H60.8 Other otitis externa**
  + **H60.8X Other otitis externa**
    H60.8X1 Other otitis externa, right ear
    H60.8X2 Other otitis externa, left ear
    H60.8X3 Other otitis externa, bilateral
    H60.8X9 Other otitis externa, unspecified ear

+ **H60.9 Unspecified otitis externa**
  H60.90 Unspecified otitis externa, unspecified ear
  H60.91 Unspecified otitis externa, right ear
  H60.92 Unspecified otitis externa, left ear
  H60.93 Unspecified otitis externa, bilateral

H61 Other disorders of external ear

+ **H61.0 Chondritis and perichondritis of external ear**
  Chondrodermatitis nodularis chronica helicis
  Perichondritis of auricle
  Perichondritis of pinna
  + **H61.00 Unspecified perichondritis of external ear**
    H61.001 Unspecified perichondritis of right external ear
    H61.002 Unspecified perichondritis of left external ear
    H61.003 Unspecified perichondritis of external ear, bilateral
    H61.009 Unspecified perichondritis of external ear, unspecified ear
  + **H61.01 Acute perichondritis of external ear**
    H61.011 Acute perichondritis of right external ear
    H61.012 Acute perichondritis of left external ear
    H61.013 Acute perichondritis of external ear, bilateral
    H61.019 Acute perichondritis of external ear, unspecified ear
  + **H61.02 Chronic perichondritis of external ear**
    H61.021 Chronic perichondritis of right external ear
    H61.022 Chronic perichondritis of left external ear
    H61.023 Chronic perichondritis of external ear, bilateral
    H61.029 Chronic perichondritis of external ear, unspecified ear

+ **H61.03 Chondritis of external ear**
  Chondritis of auricle
  Chondritis of pinna
  H61.031 Chondritis of right external ear
  H61.032 Chondritis of left external ear
  AHA CC: 1Q, 2015, 18-19
  H61.033 Chondritis of external ear, bilateral
  H61.039 Chondritis of external ear, unspecified ear

+ **H61.1 Noninfective disorders of pinna**
  Excludes2: *cauliflower ear (M95.1-)*
  gouty tophi of ear (M1A.-)

+ **H61.10 Unspecified noninfective disorders of pinna**
  Disorder of pinna NOS
  H61.101 Unspecified noninfective disorders of pinna, right ear
  H61.102 Unspecified noninfective disorders of pinna, left ear
  H61.103 Unspecified noninfective disorders of pinna, bilateral
  H61.109 Unspecified noninfective disorders of pinna, unspecified ear

+ **H61.11 Acquired deformity of pinna**
  Acquired deformity of auricle
  Excludes2: *cauliflower ear (M95.1-)*
  H61.111 Acquired deformity of pinna, right ear
  H61.112 Acquired deformity of pinna, left ear
  H61.113 Acquired deformity of pinna, bilateral
  H61.119 Acquired deformity of pinna, unspecified ear

+ **H61.12 Hematoma of pinna**
  Hematoma of auricle
  H61.121 Hematoma of pinna, right ear
  H61.122 Hematoma of pinna, left ear
  H61.123 Hematoma of pinna, bilateral
  H61.129 Hematoma of pinna, unspecified ear

+ **H61.19 Other noninfective disorders of pinna**
  H61.191 Noninfective disorders of pinna, right ear
  H61.192 Noninfective disorders of pinna, left ear
  H61.193 Noninfective disorders of pinna, bilateral
  H61.199 Noninfective disorders of pinna, unspecified ear

+ **H61.2 Impacted cerumen**
  Wax in ear
  H61.20 Impacted cerumen, unspecified ear
  H61.21 Impacted cerumen, right ear
  H61.22 Impacted cerumen, left ear
  H61.23 Impacted cerumen, bilateral

+ **H61.3 Acquired stenosis of external ear canal**
  Collapse of external ear canal
  Excludes1: *postprocedural stenosis of external ear canal (H95.81-)*

+ **H61.30 Acquired stenosis of external ear canal, unspecified**
  H61.301 Acquired stenosis of right external ear canal, unspecified
  H61.302 Acquired stenosis of left external ear canal, unspecified
  H61.303 Acquired stenosis of external ear canal, unspecified, bilateral
  H61.309 Acquired stenosis of external ear canal, unspecified, unspecified ear

+ **H61.31 Acquired stenosis of external ear canal secondary to trauma**
  H61.311 Acquired stenosis of right external ear canal secondary to trauma
  H61.312 Acquired stenosis of left external ear canal secondary to trauma
  H61.313 Acquired stenosis of external ear canal secondary to trauma, bilateral
  H61.319 Acquired stenosis of external ear canal secondary to trauma, unspecified ear

+ **H61.32 Acquired stenosis of external ear canal secondary to inflammation and infection**
  H61.321 Acquired stenosis of right external ear canal secondary to inflammation and infection
  H61.322 Acquired stenosis of left external ear canal secondary to inflammation and infection
  H61.323 Acquired stenosis of external ear canal secondary to inflammation and infection, bilateral
  H61.329 Acquired stenosis of external ear canal secondary to inflammation and infection, unspecified ear

+ **H61.39 Other acquired stenosis of external ear canal**
  H61.391 Other acquired stenosis of right external ear canal
  H61.392 Other acquired stenosis of left external ear canal
  H61.393 Other acquired stenosis of external ear canal, bilateral
  H61.399 Other acquired stenosis of external ear canal, unspecified ear

+ **H61.8 Other specified disorders of external ear**

+ **H61.81 Exostosis of external canal**
  H61.811 Exostosis of right external canal
  H61.812 Exostosis of left external canal
  H61.813 Exostosis of external canal, bilateral
  H61.819 Exostosis of external canal, unspecified ear

+ **H61.89 Other specified disorders of external ear**
  H61.891 Other specified disorders of right external ear
  H61.892 Other specified disorders of left external ear
  H61.893 Other specified disorders of external ear, bilateral
  H61.899 Other specified disorders of external ear, unspecified ear

+ **H61.9 Disorder of external ear, unspecified**
  H61.90 Disorder of external ear, unspecified, unspecified ear
  H61.91 Disorder of right external ear, unspecified
  H61.92 Disorder of left external ear, unspecified
  H61.93 Disorder of external ear, unspecified, bilateral

H62 Disorders of external ear in diseases classified elsewhere

+ **H62.4 Otitis externa in other diseases classified elsewhere**
  Code first underlying disease, such as:
  erysipelas (A46)
  impetigo (L01.0)
  Excludes1: *otitis externa (in):*
  candidiasis (B37.84)
  herpes viral [herpes simplex] (B00.1)
  herpes zoster (B02.8)
  H62.40 Otitis externa in other diseases classified elsewhere, unspecified ear
  H62.41 Otitis externa in other diseases classified elsewhere, right ear
  H62.42 Otitis externa in other diseases classified elsewhere, left ear
  H62.43 Otitis externa in other diseases classified elsewhere, bilateral

+ **H62.8 Other disorders of external ear in diseases classified elsewhere**
  Code first underlying disease, such as:
  gout (M1A.-, M10.-)

+ **H62.8X Other disorders of external ear in diseases classified elsewhere**
  H62.8X1 Other disorders of right external ear in diseases classified elsewhere
  H62.8X2 Other disorders of left external ear in diseases classified elsewhere
  H62.8X3 Other disorders of external ear in diseases classified elsewhere, bilateral
  H62.8X9 Other disorders of external ear in diseases classified elsewhere, unspecified ear

Diseases of middle ear and mastoid (H65-H75)

H65 Nonsuppurative otitis media

Includes: nonsuppurative otitis media with myringitis

Use additional code for any associated perforated tympanic membrane (H72.-)

Use additional code, if applicable, to identify:
- exposure to environmental tobacco smoke (Z77.22)
- exposure to tobacco smoke in the perinatal period (P96.81)
- history of tobacco dependence (Z87.891)
- infectious agent (B95-B97)
- occupational exposure to environmental tobacco smoke (Z57.31)
- tobacco dependence (F17.-)
- tobacco use (Z72.0)

+ **H65.0 Acute serous otitis media**

Acute and subacute secretory otitis

H65.00 Acute serous otitis media, unspecified ear
H65.01 Acute serous otitis media, right ear
H65.02 Acute serous otitis media, left ear
H65.03 Acute serous otitis media, bilateral
H65.04 Acute serous otitis media, recurrent, right ear
H65.05 Acute serous otitis media, recurrent, left ear
H65.06 Acute serous otitis media, recurrent, bilateral
H65.07 Acute serous otitis media, recurrent, unspecified ear

+ **H65.1 Other acute nonsuppurative otitis media**

Excludes1: *otitic barotrauma (T70.0)*
otitis media (acute) NOS (H66.9)

+ **H65.11 Acute and subacute allergic otitis media (mucoid) (sanguinous) (serous)**

H65.111 Acute and subacute allergic otitis media (mucoid) (sanguinous) (serous), right ear
H65.112 Acute and subacute allergic otitis media (mucoid) (sanguinous) (serous), left ear
H65.113 Acute and subacute allergic otitis media (mucoid) (sanguinous) (serous), bilateral
H65.114 Acute and subacute allergic otitis media (mucoid) (sanguinous) (serous), recurrent, right ear
H65.115 Acute and subacute allergic otitis media (mucoid) (sanguinous) (serous), recurrent, left ear
H65.116 Acute and subacute allergic otitis media (mucoid) (sanguinous) (serous), recurrent, bilateral
H65.117 Acute and subacute allergic otitis media (mucoid) (sanguinous) (serous), recurrent, unspecified ear
H65.119 Acute and subacute allergic otitis media (mucoid) (sanguinous) (serous), unspecified ear

+ **H65.19 Other acute nonsuppurative otitis media**

Acute and subacute mucoid otitis media
Acute and subacute nonsuppurative otitis media NOS
Acute and subacute sanguinous otitis media
Acute and subacute seromucinous otitis media

H65.191 Other acute nonsuppurative otitis media, right ear
H65.192 Other acute nonsuppurative otitis media, left ear
H65.193 Other acute nonsuppurative otitis media, bilateral
H65.194 Other acute nonsuppurative otitis media, recurrent, right ear
H65.195 Other acute nonsuppurative otitis media, recurrent, left ear
H65.196 Other acute nonsuppurative otitis media, recurrent, bilateral
H65.197 Other acute nonsuppurative otitis media recurrent, unspecified ear
H65.199 Other acute nonsuppurative otitis media, unspecified ear

+ **H65.2 Chronic serous otitis media**

Chronic tubotympanal catarrh

H65.20 Chronic serous otitis media, unspecified ear
H65.21 Chronic serous otitis media, right ear
H65.22 Chronic serous otitis media, left ear
H65.23 Chronic serous otitis media, bilateral

+ **H65.3 Chronic mucoid otitis media**

Chronic mucinous otitis media
Chronic secretory otitis media
Chronic transudative otitis media
Glue ear

Excludes1: *adhesive middle ear disease (H74.1)*

H65.30 Chronic mucoid otitis media, unspecified ear
H65.31 Chronic mucoid otitis media, right ear
H65.32 Chronic mucoid otitis media, left ear
H65.33 Chronic mucoid otitis media, bilateral

+ **H65.4 Other chronic nonsuppurative otitis media**

+ **H65.41 Chronic allergic otitis media**

H65.411 Chronic allergic otitis media, right ear
H65.412 Chronic allergic otitis media, left ear
H65.413 Chronic allergic otitis media, bilateral
H65.419 Chronic allergic otitis media, unspecified ear

+ **H65.49 Other chronic nonsuppurative otitis media**

Chronic exudative otitis media
Chronic nonsuppurative otitis media NOS
Chronic otitis media with effusion (nonpurulent)
Chronic seromucinous otitis media

H65.491 Other chronic nonsuppurative otitis media, right ear
H65.492 Other chronic nonsuppurative otitis media, left ear
H65.493 Other chronic nonsuppurative otitis media, bilateral
H65.499 Other chronic nonsuppurative otitis media, unspecified ear

+ **H65.9 Unspecified nonsuppurative otitis media**

Allergic otitis media NOS
Catarrhal otitis media NOS
Exudative otitis media NOS
Mucoid otitis media NOS
Otitis media with effusion (nonpurulent) NOS
Secretory otitis media NOS
Seromucinous otitis media NOS
Serous otitis media NOS
Transudative otitis media NOS

H65.90 Unspecified nonsuppurative otitis media, unspecified ear
H65.91 Unspecified nonsuppurative otitis media, right ear
H65.92 Unspecified nonsuppurative otitis media, left ear
H65.93 Unspecified nonsuppurative otitis media, bilateral

H66 Suppurative and unspecified otitis media

Includes: suppurative and unspecified otitis media with myringitis

Use additional code to identify:
- exposure to environmental tobacco smoke (Z77.22)
- exposure to tobacco smoke in the perinatal period (P96.81)
- history of tobacco dependence (Z87.891)
- occupational exposure to environmental tobacco smoke (Z57.31)
- tobacco dependence (F17.-)
- tobacco use (Z72.0)

+ **H66.0 Acute suppurative otitis media**

+ **H66.00 Acute suppurative otitis media without spontaneous rupture of ear drum**

H66.001 Acute suppurative otitis media without spontaneous rupture of ear drum, right ear
H66.002 Acute suppurative otitis media without spontaneous rupture of ear drum, left ear
H66.003 Acute suppurative otitis media without spontaneous rupture of ear drum, bilateral
H66.004 Acute suppurative otitis media without spontaneous rupture of ear drum, recurrent, right ear
H66.005 Acute suppurative otitis media without spontaneous rupture of ear drum, recurrent, left ear
H66.006 Acute suppurative otitis media without spontaneous rupture of ear drum, recurrent, bilateral
H66.007 Acute suppurative otitis media without spontaneous rupture of ear drum, recurrent, unspecified ear
H66.009 Acute suppurative otitis media without spontaneous rupture of ear drum, unspecified ear

+ **H66.01 Acute suppurative otitis media with spontaneous rupture of ear drum**
H66.011 Acute suppurative otitis media with spontaneous rupture of ear drum, right ear
H66.012 Acute suppurative otitis media with spontaneous rupture of ear drum, left ear
H66.013 Acute suppurative otitis media with spontaneous rupture of ear drum, bilateral
H66.014 Acute suppurative otitis media with spontaneous rupture of ear drum, recurrent, right ear
H66.015 Acute suppurative otitis media with spontaneous rupture of ear drum, recurrent, left ear
H66.016 Acute suppurative otitis media with spontaneous rupture of ear drum, recurrent, bilateral
H66.017 Acute suppurative otitis media with spontaneous rupture of ear drum, recurrent, unspecified ear
H66.019 Acute suppurative otitis media with spontaneous rupture of ear drum, unspecified ear

+ **H66.1 Chronic tubotympanic suppurative otitis media**
Benign chronic suppurative otitis media
Chronic tubotympanic disease
Use additional code for any associated perforated tympanic membrane (H72.-)
H66.10 Chronic tubotympanic suppurative otitis media, unspecified
H66.11 Chronic tubotympanic suppurative otitis media, right ear
H66.12 Chronic tubotympanic suppurative otitis media, left ear
H66.13 Chronic tubotympanic suppurative otitis media, bilateral

+ **H66.2 Chronic atticoantral suppurative otitis media**
Chronic atticoantral disease
Use additional code for any associated perforated tympanic membrane (H72.-)
H66.20 Chronic atticoantral suppurative otitis media, unspecified ear
H66.21 Chronic atticoantral suppurative otitis media, right ear
H66.22 Chronic atticoantral suppurative otitis media, left ear
H66.23 Chronic atticoantral suppurative otitis media, bilateral

+ **H66.3 Other chronic suppurative otitis media**
Chronic suppurative otitis media NOS
Use additional code for any associated perforated tympanic membrane (H72.-)
Excludes1: *tuberculous otitis media (A18.6)*
+ **H66.3X Other chronic suppurative otitis media**
H66.3X1 Other chronic suppurative otitis media, right ear
H66.3X2 Other chronic suppurative otitis media, left ear
H66.3X3 Other chronic suppurative otitis media, bilateral
H66.3X9 Other chronic suppurative otitis media, unspecified ear

+ **H66.4 Suppurative otitis media, unspecified**
Purulent otitis media NOS
Use additional code for any associated perforated tympanic membrane (H72.-)
H66.40 Suppurative otitis media, unspecified, unspecified ear
H66.41 Suppurative otitis media, unspecified, right ear
H66.42 Suppurative otitis media, unspecified, left ear
H66.43 Suppurative otitis media, unspecified, bilateral

+ **H66.9 Otitis media, unspecified**
Otitis media NOS
Acute otitis media NOS
Chronic otitis media NOS
Use additional code for any associated perforated tympanic membrane (H72.-)
H66.90 Otitis media, unspecified, unspecified ear
H66.91 Otitis media, unspecified, right ear
H66.92 Otitis media, unspecified, left ear
AHA CC: 4Q, 2020, 11-12
H66.93 Otitis media, unspecified, bilateral

H67 Otitis media in diseases classified elsewhere
Code first underlying disease, such as:
plasminogen deficiency (E88.02)
viral disease NEC (B00-B34)

Use additional code for any associated perforated tympanic membrane (H72.-)
Excludes1: *otitis media in:*
influenza (J09.X9, J10.83, J11.83)
measles (B05.3)
scarlet fever (A38.0)
tuberculosis (A18.6)
H67.1 Otitis media in diseases classified elsewhere, right ear
H67.2 Otitis media in diseases classified elsewhere, left ear
H67.3 Otitis media in diseases classified elsewhere, bilateral
H67.9 Otitis media in diseases classified elsewhere, unspecified ear

H68 Eustachian salpingitis and obstruction
+ **H68.0 Eustachian salpingitis**
+ **H68.00 Unspecified Eustachian salpingitis**
H68.001 Unspecified Eustachian salpingitis, right ear
H68.002 Unspecified Eustachian salpingitis, left ear
H68.003 Unspecified Eustachian salpingitis, bilateral
H68.009 Unspecified Eustachian salpingitis, unspecified ear
+ **H68.01 Acute Eustachian salpingitis**
H68.011 Acute Eustachian salpingitis, right ear
H68.012 Acute Eustachian salpingitis, left ear
H68.013 Acute Eustachian salpingitis, bilateral
H68.019 Acute Eustachian salpingitis, unspecified ear
+ **H68.02 Chronic Eustachian salpingitis**
H68.021 Chronic Eustachian salpingitis, right ear
H68.022 Chronic Eustachian salpingitis, left ear
H68.023 Chronic Eustachian salpingitis, bilateral
H68.029 Chronic Eustachian salpingitis, unspecified ear

+ **H68.1 Obstruction of Eustachian tube**
Stenosis of Eustachian tube
Stricture of Eustachian tube
+ **H68.10 Unspecified obstruction of Eustachian tube**
H68.101 Unspecified obstruction of Eustachian tube, right ear
H68.102 Unspecified obstruction of Eustachian tube, left ear
H68.103 Unspecified obstruction of Eustachian tube, bilateral
H68.109 Unspecified obstruction of Eustachian tube, unspecified ear
+ **H68.11 Osseous obstruction of Eustachian tube**
H68.111 Osseous obstruction of Eustachian tube, right ear
H68.112 Osseous obstruction of Eustachian tube, left ear
H68.113 Osseous obstruction of Eustachian tube, bilateral
H68.119 Osseous obstruction of Eustachian tube, unspecified ear
+ **H68.12 Intrinsic cartilagenous obstruction of Eustachian tube**
H68.121 Intrinsic cartilagenous obstruction of Eustachian tube, right ear
H68.122 Intrinsic cartilagenous obstruction of Eustachian tube, left ear
H68.123 Intrinsic cartilagenous obstruction of Eustachian tube, bilateral
H68.129 Intrinsic cartilagenous obstruction of Eustachian tube, unspecified ear

+ **H68.13 Extrinsic cartilagenous obstruction of Eustachian tube**
Compression of Eustachian tube
H68.131 Extrinsic cartilagenous obstruction of Eustachian tube, right ear
H68.132 Extrinsic cartilagenous obstruction of Eustachian tube, left ear
H68.133 Extrinsic cartilagenous obstruction of Eustachian tube, bilateral
H68.139 Extrinsic cartilagenous obstruction of Eustachian tube, unspecified ear

H69 Other and unspecified disorders of Eustachian tube

+ **H69.0 Patulous Eustachian tube**
H69.00 Patulous Eustachian tube, unspecified ear
H69.01 Patulous Eustachian tube, right ear
H69.02 Patulous Eustachian tube, left ear
H69.03 Patulous Eustachian tube, bilateral
+ **H69.8 Other specified disorders of Eustachian tube**
H69.80 Other specified disorders of Eustachian tube, unspecified ear
H69.81 Other specified disorders of Eustachian tube, right ear
H69.82 Other specified disorders of Eustachian tube, left ear
H69.83 Other specified disorders of Eustachian tube, bilateral
+ **H69.9 Unspecified Eustachian tube disorder**
H69.90 Unspecified Eustachian tube disorder, unspecified ear
H69.91 Unspecified Eustachian tube disorder, right ear
H69.92 Unspecified Eustachian tube disorder, left ear
H69.93 Unspecified Eustachian tube disorder, bilateral

H70 Mastoiditis and related conditions

+ **H70.0 Acute mastoiditis**
Abscess of mastoid
Empyema of mastoid
+ **H70.00 Acute mastoiditis without complications**
CC **H70.001 Acute mastoiditis without complications, right ear**
CC **H70.002 Acute mastoiditis without complications, left ear**
CC **H70.003 Acute mastoiditis without complications, bilateral**
CC **H70.009 Acute mastoiditis without complications, unspecified ear**
+ **H70.01 Subperiosteal abscess of mastoid**
CC **H70.011 Subperiosteal abscess of mastoid, right ear**
CC **H70.012 Subperiosteal abscess of mastoid, left ear**
CC **H70.013 Subperiosteal abscess of mastoid, bilateral**
CC **H70.019 Subperiosteal abscess of mastoid, unspecified ear**
+ **H70.09 Acute mastoiditis with other complications**
CC **H70.091 Acute mastoiditis with other complications, right ear**
CC **H70.092 Acute mastoiditis with other complications, left ear**
CC **H70.093 Acute mastoiditis with other complications, bilateral**
CC **H70.099 Acute mastoiditis with other complications, unspecified ear**
+ **H70.1 Chronic mastoiditis**
Caries of mastoid
Fistula of mastoid
Excludes1: *tuberculous mastoiditis (A18.03)*
H70.10 Chronic mastoiditis, unspecified ear
H70.11 Chronic mastoiditis, right ear
H70.12 Chronic mastoiditis, left ear
H70.13 Chronic mastoiditis, bilateral
+ **H70.2 Petrositis**
Inflammation of petrous bone
+ **H70.20 Unspecified petrositis**
H70.201 Unspecified petrositis, right ear
H70.202 Unspecified petrositis, left ear
H70.203 Unspecified petrositis, bilateral
H70.209 Unspecified petrositis, unspecified ear
+ **H70.21 Acute petrositis**
H70.211 Acute petrositis, right ear
H70.212 Acute petrositis, left ear
H70.213 Acute petrositis, bilateral
H70.219 Acute petrositis, unspecified ear
+ **H70.22 Chronic petrositis**
H70.221 Chronic petrositis, right ear
H70.222 Chronic petrositis, left ear
H70.223 Chronic petrositis, bilateral
H70.229 Chronic petrositis, unspecified ear
+ **H70.8 Other mastoiditis and related conditions**
Excludes1: *preauricular sinus and cyst (Q18.1)*
sinus, fistula, and cyst of branchial cleft (Q18.0)
+ **H70.81 Postauricular fistula**
H70.811 Postauricular fistula, right ear
H70.812 Postauricular fistula, left ear
H70.813 Postauricular fistula, bilateral
H70.819 Postauricular fistula, unspecified ear
+ **H70.89 Other mastoiditis and related conditions**
H70.891 Other mastoiditis and related conditions, right ear
H70.892 Other mastoiditis and related conditions, left ear
H70.893 Other mastoiditis and related conditions, bilateral
H70.899 Other mastoiditis and related conditions, unspecified ear
+ **H70.9 Unspecified mastoiditis**
H70.90 Unspecified mastoiditis, unspecified ear
H70.91 Unspecified mastoiditis, right ear
H70.92 Unspecified mastoiditis, left ear
H70.93 Unspecified mastoiditis, bilateral

H71 Cholesteatoma of middle ear

Excludes2: *cholesteatoma of external ear (H60.4-)*
recurrent cholesteatoma of postmastoidectomy cavity (H95.0-)
+ **H71.0 Cholesteatoma of attic**
H71.00 Cholesteatoma of attic, unspecified ear
H71.01 Cholesteatoma of attic, right ear
H71.02 Cholesteatoma of attic, left ear
H71.03 Cholesteatoma of attic, bilateral
+ **H71.1 Cholesteatoma of tympanum**
H71.10 Cholesteatoma of tympanum, unspecified ear
H71.11 Cholesteatoma of tympanum, right ear
H71.12 Cholesteatoma of tympanum, left ear
H71.13 Cholesteatoma of tympanum, bilateral
+ **H71.2 Cholesteatoma of mastoid**
H71.20 Cholesteatoma of mastoid, unspecified ear
H71.21 Cholesteatoma of mastoid, right ear
H71.22 Cholesteatoma of mastoid, left ear
H71.23 Cholesteatoma of mastoid, bilateral
+ **H71.3 Diffuse cholesteatosis**
H71.30 Diffuse cholesteatosis, unspecified ear
H71.31 Diffuse cholesteatosis, right ear
H71.32 Diffuse cholesteatosis, left ear
H71.33 Diffuse cholesteatosis, bilateral
+ **H71.9 Unspecified cholesteatoma**
H71.90 Unspecified cholesteatoma, unspecified ear
H71.91 Unspecified cholesteatoma, right ear
H71.92 Unspecified cholesteatoma, left ear
H71.93 Unspecified cholesteatoma, bilateral

H72 Perforation of tympanic membrane

Includes: persistent post-traumatic perforation of ear drum
postinflammatory perforation of ear drum
Code first any associated otitis media (H65.-, H66.1-, H66.2-, H66.3-, H66.4-, H66.9-, H67.-)
Excludes1: *acute suppurative otitis media with rupture of the tympanic membrane (H66.01-)*
traumatic rupture of ear drum (S09.2-)
+ **H72.0 Central perforation of tympanic membrane**
H72.00 Central perforation of tympanic membrane, unspecified ear
H72.01 Central perforation of tympanic membrane, right ear
H72.02 Central perforation of tympanic membrane, left ear
H72.03 Central perforation of tympanic membrane, bilateral

+ **H72.1 Attic perforation of tympanic membrane**
Perforation of pars flaccida
H72.10 Attic perforation of tympanic membrane, unspecified ear
H72.11 Attic perforation of tympanic membrane, right ear
H72.12 Attic perforation of tympanic membrane, left ear
H72.13 Attic perforation of tympanic membrane, bilateral

+ **H72.2 Other marginal perforations of tympanic membrane**
+ **H72.2X Other marginal perforations of tympanic membrane**
H72.2X1 Other marginal perforations of tympanic membrane, right ear
H72.2X2 Other marginal perforations of tympanic membrane, left ear
H72.2X3 Other marginal perforations of tympanic membrane, bilateral
H72.2X9 Other marginal perforations of tympanic membrane, unspecified ear

+ **H72.8 Other perforations of tympanic membrane**
+ **H72.81 Multiple perforations of tympanic membrane**
H72.811 Multiple perforations of tympanic membrane, right ear
H72.812 Multiple perforations of tympanic membrane, left ear
H72.813 Multiple perforations of tympanic membrane, bilateral
H72.819 Multiple perforations of tympanic membrane, unspecified ear
+ **H72.82 Total perforations of tympanic membrane**
H72.821 Total perforations of tympanic membrane, right ear
H72.822 Total perforations of tympanic membrane, left ear
H72.823 Total perforations of tympanic membrane, bilateral
H72.829 Total perforations of tympanic membrane, unspecified ear

+ **H72.9 Unspecified perforation of tympanic membrane**
H72.90 Unspecified perforation of tympanic membrane, unspecified ear
H72.91 Unspecified perforation of tympanic membrane, right ear
H72.92 Unspecified perforation of tympanic membrane, left ear
H72.93 Unspecified perforation of tympanic membrane, bilateral

H73 Other disorders of tympanic membrane

+ **H73.0 Acute myringitis**
Excludes1: *acute myringitis with otitis media (H65, H66)*
+ **H73.00 Unspecified acute myringitis**
Acute tympanitis NOS
H73.001 Acute myringitis, right ear
H73.002 Acute myringitis, left ear
H73.003 Acute myringitis, bilateral
H73.009 Acute myringitis, unspecified ear
+ **H73.01 Bullous myringitis**
H73.011 Bullous myringitis, right ear
H73.012 Bullous myringitis, left ear
H73.013 Bullous myringitis, bilateral
H73.019 Bullous myringitis, unspecified ear
+ **H73.09 Other acute myringitis**
H73.091 Other acute myringitis, right ear
H73.092 Other acute myringitis, left ear
H73.093 Other acute myringitis, bilateral
H73.099 Other acute myringitis, unspecified ear

+ **H73.1 Chronic myringitis**
Chronic tympanitis
Excludes1: *chronic myringitis with otitis media (H65, H66)*
H73.10 Chronic myringitis, unspecified ear
H73.11 Chronic myringitis, right ear
H73.12 Chronic myringitis, left ear
H73.13 Chronic myringitis, bilateral

+ **H73.2 Unspecified myringitis**
H73.20 Unspecified myringitis, unspecified ear
H73.21 Unspecified myringitis, right ear
H73.22 Unspecified myringitis, left ear
H73.23 Unspecified myringitis, bilateral

+ **H73.8 Other specified disorders of tympanic membrane**
+ **H73.81 Atrophic flaccid tympanic membrane**
H73.811 Atrophic flaccid tympanic membrane, right ear
H73.812 Atrophic flaccid tympanic membrane, left ear
H73.813 Atrophic flaccid tympanic membrane, bilateral
H73.819 Atrophic flaccid tympanic membrane, unspecified ear
+ **H73.82 Atrophic nonflaccid tympanic membrane**
H73.821 Atrophic nonflaccid tympanic membrane, right ear
H73.822 Atrophic nonflaccid tympanic membrane, left ear
H73.823 Atrophic nonflaccid tympanic membrane, bilateral
H73.829 Atrophic nonflaccid tympanic membrane, unspecified ear
+ **H73.89 Other specified disorders of tympanic membrane**
H73.891 Other specified disorders of tympanic membrane, right ear
H73.892 Other specified disorders of tympanic membrane, left ear
H73.893 Other specified disorders of tympanic membrane, bilateral
H73.899 Other specified disorders of tympanic membrane, unspecified ear

+ **H73.9 Unspecified disorder of tympanic membrane**
H73.90 Unspecified disorder of tympanic membrane, unspecified ear
H73.91 Unspecified disorder of tympanic membrane, right ear
H73.92 Unspecified disorder of tympanic membrane, left ear
H73.93 Unspecified disorder of tympanic membrane, bilateral

H74 Other disorders of middle ear mastoid

Excludes2: *mastoiditis (H70.-)*

+ **H74.0 Tympanosclerosis**
H74.01 Tympanosclerosis, right ear
H74.02 Tympanosclerosis, left ear
H74.03 Tympanosclerosis, bilateral
H74.09 Tympanosclerosis, unspecified ear

+ **H74.1 Adhesive middle ear disease**
Adhesive otitis
Excludes1: *glue ear (H65.3-)*
H74.11 Adhesive right middle ear disease
H74.12 Adhesive left middle ear disease
H74.13 Adhesive middle ear disease, bilateral
H74.19 Adhesive middle ear disease, unspecified ear

+ **H74.2 Discontinuity and dislocation of ear ossicles**
H74.20 Discontinuity and dislocation of ear ossicles, unspecified ear
H74.21 Discontinuity and dislocation of right ear ossicles
H74.22 Discontinuity and dislocation of left ear ossicles
H74.23 Discontinuity and dislocation of ear ossicles, bilateral

+ **H74.3 Other acquired abnormalities of ear ossicles**
+ **H74.31 Ankylosis of ear ossicles**
H74.311 Ankylosis of ear ossicles, right ear
H74.312 Ankylosis of ear ossicles, left ear
H74.313 Ankylosis of ear ossicles, bilateral
H74.319 Ankylosis of ear ossicles, unspecified ear
+ **H74.32 Partial loss of ear ossicles**
H74.321 Partial loss of ear ossicles, right ear
H74.322 Partial loss of ear ossicles, left ear
H74.323 Partial loss of ear ossicles, bilateral
H74.329 Partial loss of ear ossicles, unspecified ear
+ **H74.39 Other acquired abnormalities of ear ossicles**
H74.391 Other acquired abnormalities of right ear ossicles
H74.392 Other acquired abnormalities of left ear ossicles
H74.393 Other acquired abnormalities of ear ossicles, bilateral
H74.399 Other acquired abnormalities of ear ossicles, unspecified ear

+ **H74.4 Polyp of middle ear**
  - **H74.40 Polyp of middle ear, unspecified ear**
  - **H74.41 Polyp of right middle ear**
  - **H74.42 Polyp of left middle ear**
  - **H74.43 Polyp of middle ear, bilateral**

+ **H74.8 Other specified disorders of middle ear and mastoid**
  + **H74.8X Other specified disorders of middle ear and mastoid**
    - **H74.8X1 Other specified disorders of right middle ear and mastoid**
    - **H74.8X2 Other specified disorders of left middle ear and mastoid**
    - **H74.8X3 Other specified disorders of middle ear and mastoid, bilateral**
    - **H74.8X9 Other specified disorders of middle ear and mastoid, unspecified ear**

+ **H74.9 Unspecified disorder of middle ear and mastoid**
  - **H74.90 Unspecified disorder of middle ear and mastoid, unspecified ear**
  - **H74.91 Unspecified disorder of right middle ear and mastoid**
  - **H74.92 Unspecified disorder of left middle ear and mastoid**
  - **H74.93 Unspecified disorder of middle ear and mastoid, bilateral**

H75 Other disorders of middle ear and mastoid in diseases classified elsewhere

Code first underlying disease

+ **H75.0 Mastoiditis in infectious and parasitic diseases classified elsewhere**

  Excludes1: *mastoiditis (in):*
  syphilis (A52.77)
  tuberculosis (A18.03)

  - **H75.00 Mastoiditis in infectious and parasitic diseases classified elsewhere, unspecified ear**
  - **H75.01 Mastoiditis in infectious and parasitic diseases classified elsewhere, right ear**
  - **H75.02 Mastoiditis in infectious and parasitic diseases classified elsewhere, left ear**
  - **H75.03 Mastoiditis in infectious and parasitic diseases classified elsewhere, bilateral**

+ **H75.8 Other specified disorders of middle ear and mastoid in diseases classified elsewhere**
  - **H75.80 Other specified disorders of middle ear and mastoid in diseases classified elsewhere, unspecified ear**
  - **H75.81 Other specified disorders of right middle ear and mastoid in diseases classified elsewhere**
  - **H75.82 Other specified disorders of left middle ear and mastoid in diseases classified elsewhere**
  - **H75.83 Other specified disorders of middle ear and mastoid in diseases classified elsewhere, bilateral**

Diseases of inner ear (H80-H83)

H80 Otosclerosis

Includes: Otospongiosis

+ **H80.0 Otosclerosis involving oval window, nonobliterative**
  - **H80.00 Otosclerosis involving oval window, nonobliterative, unspecified ear**
  - **H80.01 Otosclerosis involving oval window, nonobliterative, right ear**
  - **H80.02 Otosclerosis involving oval window, nonobliterative, left ear**
  - **H80.03 Otosclerosis involving oval window, nonobliterative, bilateral**

+ **H80.1 Otosclerosis involving oval window, obliterative**
  - **H80.10 Otosclerosis involving oval window, obliterative, unspecified ear**
  - **H80.11 Otosclerosis involving oval window, obliterative, right ear**
  - **H80.12 Otosclerosis involving oval window, obliterative, left ear**
  - **H80.13 Otosclerosis involving oval window, obliterative, bilateral**

+ **H80.2 Cochlear otosclerosis**

  Otosclerosis involving otic capsule
  Otosclerosis involving round window

  - **H80.20 Cochlear otosclerosis, unspecified ear**
  - **H80.21 Cochlear otosclerosis, right ear**
  - **H80.22 Cochlear otosclerosis, left ear**
  - **H80.23 Cochlear otosclerosis, bilateral**

+ **H80.8 Other otosclerosis**
  - **H80.80 Other otosclerosis, unspecified ear**
  - **H80.81 Other otosclerosis, right ear**
  - **H80.82 Other otosclerosis, left ear**
  - **H80.83 Other otosclerosis, bilateral**

+ **H80.9 Unspecified otosclerosis**
  - **H80.90 Unspecified otosclerosis, unspecified ear**
  - **H80.91 Unspecified otosclerosis, right ear**
  - **H80.92 Unspecified otosclerosis, left ear**
  - **H80.93 Unspecified otosclerosis, bilateral**

H81 Disorders of vestibular function

Excludes1: *epidemic vertigo (A88.1)*
vertigo NOS (R42)

+ **H81.0 Ménière's disease**

  Labyrinthine hydrops
  Ménière's syndrome or vertigo

  - **H81.01 Ménière's disease, right ear**
  - **H81.02 Ménière's disease, left ear**
  - **H81.03 Ménière's disease, bilateral**
  - **H81.09 Ménière's disease, unspecified ear**

+ **H81.1 Benign paroxysmal vertigo**
  - **H81.10 Benign paroxysmal vertigo, unspecified ear**
  - **H81.11 Benign paroxysmal vertigo, right ear**
  - **H81.12 Benign paroxysmal vertigo, left ear**
  - **H81.13 Benign paroxysmal vertigo, bilateral**

+ **H81.2 Vestibular neuronitis**
  - **H81.20 Vestibular neuronitis, unspecified ear**
  - **H81.21 Vestibular neuronitis, right ear**
  - **H81.22 Vestibular neuronitis, left ear**
  - **H81.23 Vestibular neuronitis, bilateral**

+ **H81.3 Other peripheral vertigo**
  + **H81.31 Aural vertigo**
    - **H81.311 Aural vertigo, right ear**
    - **H81.312 Aural vertigo, left ear**
    - **H81.313 Aural vertigo, bilateral**
    - **H81.319 Aural vertigo, unspecified ear**
  + **H81.39 Other peripheral vertigo**

    Lermoyez' syndrome
    Otogenic vertigo
    Peripheral vertigo NOS

    - **H81.391 Other peripheral vertigo, right ear**
    - **H81.392 Other peripheral vertigo, left ear**
    - **H81.393 Other peripheral vertigo, bilateral**
    - **H81.399 Other peripheral vertigo, unspecified ear**

H81.4 Vertigo of central origin

Central positional nystagmus
AHA CC: 4Q, 2019, 4

+ **H81.8 Other disorders of vestibular function**
  + **H81.8X Other disorders of vestibular function**
    - **H81.8X1 Other disorders of vestibular function, right ear**
    - **H81.8X2 Other disorders of vestibular function, left ear**
    - **H81.8X3 Other disorders of vestibular function, bilateral**
    - **H81.8X9 Other disorders of vestibular function, unspecified ear**

+ **H81.9 Unspecified disorder of vestibular function**

  Vertiginous syndrome NOS

  - **H81.90 Unspecified disorder of vestibular function, unspecified ear**
  - **H81.91 Unspecified disorder of vestibular function, right ear**
  - **H81.92 Unspecified disorder of vestibular function, left ear**
  - **H81.93 Unspecified disorder of vestibular function, bilateral**

H82 Vertiginous syndromes in diseases classified elsewhere
Code first underlying disease
Excludes1: *epidemic vertigo (A88.1)*
H82.1 Vertiginous syndromes in diseases classified elsewhere, right ear
H82.2 Vertiginous syndromes in diseases classified elsewhere, left ear
H82.3 Vertiginous syndromes in diseases classified elsewhere, bilateral
H82.9 Vertiginous syndromes in diseases classified elsewhere, unspecified ear

H83 Other diseases of inner ear
+ H83.0 Labyrinthitis
H83.01 Labyrinthitis, right ear
H83.02 Labyrinthitis, left ear
H83.03 Labyrinthitis, bilateral
H83.09 Labyrinthitis, unspecified ear
+ H83.1 Labyrinthine fistula
H83.11 Labyrinthine fistula, right ear
H83.12 Labyrinthine fistula, left ear
H83.13 Labyrinthine fistula, bilateral
H83.19 Labyrinthine fistula, unspecified ear
+ H83.2 Labyrinthine dysfunction
Labyrinthine hypersensitivity
Labyrinthine hypofunction
Labyrinthine loss of function
+ H83.2X Labyrinthine dysfunction
H83.2X1 Labyrinthine dysfunction, right ear
H83.2X2 Labyrinthine dysfunction, left ear
H83.2X3 Labyrinthine dysfunction, bilateral
H83.2X9 Labyrinthine dysfunction, unspecified ear
+ H83.3 Noise effects on inner ear
Acoustic trauma of inner ear
Noise-induced hearing loss of inner ear
+ H83.3X Noise effects on inner ear
H83.3X1 Noise effects on right inner ear
H83.3X2 Noise effects on left inner ear
H83.3X3 Noise effects on inner ear, bilateral
H83.3X9 Noise effects on inner ear, unspecified ear
+ H83.8 Other specified diseases of inner ear
+ H83.8X Other specified diseases of inner ear
H83.8X1 Other specified diseases of right inner ear
H83.8X2 Other specified diseases of left inner ear
H83.8X3 Other specified diseases of inner ear, bilateral
H83.8X9 Other specified diseases of inner ear, unspecified ear
+ H83.9 Unspecified disease of inner ear
H83.90 Unspecified disease of inner ear, unspecified ear
H83.91 Unspecified disease of right inner ear
H83.92 Unspecified disease of left inner ear
H83.93 Unspecified disease of inner ear, bilateral

Other disorders of ear (H90-H94)

H90 Conductive and sensorineural hearing loss
Excludes1: *deaf nonspeaking NEC (H91.3)*
deafness NOS (H91.9-)
hearing loss NOS (H91.9-)
noise-induced hearing loss (H83.3-)
ototoxic hearing loss (H91.0-)
sudden (idiopathic) hearing loss (H91.2-)
H90.0 Conductive hearing loss, bilateral
+ H90.1 Conductive hearing loss, unilateral with unrestricted hearing on the contralateral side
H90.11 Conductive hearing loss, unilateral, right ear, with unrestricted hearing on the contralateral side
H90.12 Conductive hearing loss, unilateral, left ear, with unrestricted hearing on the contralateral side
H90.2 Conductive hearing loss, unspecified
Conductive deafness NOS
H90.3 Sensorineural hearing loss, bilateral
+ H90.4 Sensorineural hearing loss, unilateral with unrestricted hearing on the contralateral side
H90.41 Sensorineural hearing loss, unilateral, right ear, with unrestricted hearing on the contralateral side
H90.42 Sensorineural hearing loss, unilateral, left ear, with unrestricted hearing on the contralateral side
H90.5 Unspecified sensorineural hearing loss
Central hearing loss NOS
Congenital deafness NOS
Neural hearing loss NOS
Perceptive hearing loss NOS
Sensorineural deafness NOS
Sensory hearing loss NOS
Excludes1: *abnormal auditory perception (H93.2-)*
psychogenic deafness (F44.6)
H90.6 Mixed conductive and sensorineural hearing loss, bilateral
AHA CC: 2Q, 2015, 7
+ H90.7 Mixed conductive and sensorineural hearing loss, unilateral with unrestricted hearing on the contralateral side
H90.71 Mixed conductive and sensorineural hearing loss, unilateral, right ear, with unrestricted hearing on the contralateral side
H90.72 Mixed conductive and sensorineural hearing loss, unilateral, left ear, with unrestricted hearing on the contralateral side
H90.8 Mixed conductive and sensorineural hearing loss, unspecified
+ H90.A Conductive and sensorineural hearing loss with restricted hearing on the contralateral side
AHA CC: 4Q, 2016, 23-24
+ H90.A1 Conductive hearing loss, unilateral, with restricted hearing on the contralateral side
H90.A11 Conductive hearing loss, unilateral, right ear with restricted hearing on the contralateral side
H90.A12 Conductive hearing loss, unilateral, left ear with restricted hearing on the contralateral side
AHA CC: 4Q, 2016, 24-25
+ H90.A2 Sensorineural hearing loss, unilateral, with restricted hearing on the contralateral side
H90.A21 Sensorineural hearing loss, unilateral, right ear, with restricted hearing on the contralateral side
AHA CC: 4Q, 2016, 24-25
H90.A22 Sensorineural hearing loss, unilateral, left ear, with restricted hearing on the contralateral side
+ H90.A3 Mixed conductive and sensorineural hearing loss, unilateral with restricted hearing on the contralateral side
H90.A31 Mixed conductive and sensorineural hearing loss, unilateral, right ear with restricted hearing on the contralateral side
H90.A32 Mixed conductive and sensorineural hearing, unilateral, left ear with restricted hearing on the contralateral side

H91 Other and unspecified hearing loss
Excludes1: *abnormal auditory perception (H93.2-)*
hearing loss as classified in H90.-
impacted cerumen (H61.2-)
noise-induced hearing loss (H83.3-)
psychogenic deafness (F44.6)
transient ischemic deafness (H93.01-)

\+ **H91.0 Ototoxic hearing loss**
Code first poisoning due to drug or toxin, if applicable (T36-T65 with fifth or sixth character 1-4 or 6)
Use additional code for adverse effect, if applicable, to identify drug (T36-T50 with fifth or sixth character 5)
H91.01 Ototoxic hearing loss, right ear
H91.02 Ototoxic hearing loss, left ear
H91.03 Ototoxic hearing loss, bilateral
H91.09 Ototoxic hearing loss, unspecified ear

\+ **H91.1 Presbycusis**
Presbyacusia
H91.10 Presbycusis, unspecified ear
H91.11 Presbycusis, right ear
H91.12 Presbycusis, left ear
H91.13 Presbycusis, bilateral

\+ **H91.2 Sudden idiopathic hearing loss**
Sudden hearing loss NOS
H91.20 Sudden idiopathic hearing loss, unspecified ear
H91.21 Sudden idiopathic hearing loss, right ear
H91.22 Sudden idiopathic hearing loss, left ear
H91.23 Sudden idiopathic hearing loss, bilateral

H91.3 Deaf nonspeaking, not elsewhere classified

\+ **H91.8 Other specified hearing loss**
\+ **H91.8X Other specified hearing loss**
H91.8X1 Other specified hearing loss, right ear
H91.8X2 Other specified hearing loss, left ear
H91.8X3 Other specified hearing loss, bilateral
H91.8X9 Other specified hearing loss, unspecified ear

\+ **H91.9 Unspecified hearing loss**
Deafness NOS
High frequency deafness
Low frequency deafness
H91.90 Unspecified hearing loss, unspecified ear
H91.91 Unspecified hearing loss, right ear
H91.92 Unspecified hearing loss, left ear
H91.93 Unspecified hearing loss, bilateral

H92 Otalgia and effusion of ear

\+ **H92.0 Otalgia**
H92.01 Otalgia, right ear
H92.02 Otalgia, left ear
H92.03 Otalgia, bilateral
H92.09 Otalgia, unspecified ear

\+ **H92.1 Otorrhea**
Excludes1: *leakage of cerebrospinal fluid through ear (G96.0)*
H92.10 Otorrhea, unspecified ear
H92.11 Otorrhea, right ear
H92.12 Otorrhea, left ear
H92.13 Otorrhea, bilateral

\+ **H92.2 Otorrhagia**
Excludes1: *traumatic otorrhagia - code to injury*
H92.20 Otorrhagia, unspecified ear
H92.21 Otorrhagia, right ear
H92.22 Otorrhagia, left ear
H92.23 Otorrhagia, bilateral

H93 Other disorders of ear, not elsewhere classified

\+ **H93.0 Degenerative and vascular disorders of ear**
Excludes1: *presbycusis (H91.1)*
\+ **H93.01 Transient ischemic deafness**
H93.011 Transient ischemic deafness, right ear
H93.012 Transient ischemic deafness, left ear
H93.013 Transient ischemic deafness, bilateral
H93.019 Transient ischemic deafness, unspecified ear
\+ **H93.09 Unspecified degenerative and vascular disorders of ear**
H93.091 Unspecified degenerative and vascular disorders of right ear
H93.092 Unspecified degenerative and vascular disorders of left ear
H93.093 Unspecified degenerative and vascular disorders of ear, bilateral
H93.099 Unspecified degenerative and vascular disorders of unspecified ear

\+ **H93.1 Tinnitus**
H93.11 Tinnitus, right ear
H93.12 Tinnitus, left ear
H93.13 Tinnitus, bilateral
H93.19 Tinnitus, unspecified ear

\+ **H93.A Pulsatile tinnitus**
AHA CC: 4Q, 2016, 25-26
H93.A1 Pulsatile tinnitus, right ear
AHA CC: 4Q, 2016, 26
H93.A2 Pulsatile tinnitus, left ear
H93.A3 Pulsatile tinnitus, bilateral
H93.A9 Pulsatile tinnitus, unspecified ear

\+ **H93.2 Other abnormal auditory perceptions**
Excludes2: *auditory hallucinations (R44.0)*
\+ **H93.21 Auditory recruitment**
H93.211 Auditory recruitment, right ear
H93.212 Auditory recruitment, left ear
H93.213 Auditory recruitment, bilateral
H93.219 Auditory recruitment, unspecified ear
\+ **H93.22 Diplacusis**
H93.221 Diplacusis, right ear
H93.222 Diplacusis, left ear
H93.223 Diplacusis, bilateral
H93.229 Diplacusis, unspecified ear
\+ **H93.23 Hyperacusis**
H93.231 Hyperacusis, right ear
H93.232 Hyperacusis, left ear
H93.233 Hyperacusis, bilateral
H93.239 Hyperacusis, unspecified ear
\+ **H93.24 Temporary auditory threshold shift**
H93.241 Temporary auditory threshold shift, right ear
H93.242 Temporary auditory threshold shift, left ear
H93.243 Temporary auditory threshold shift, bilateral
H93.249 Temporary auditory threshold shift, unspecified ear
H93.25 Central auditory processing disorder
Congenital auditory imperception
Word deafness
Excludes1: *mixed receptive-expressive language disorder (F80.2)*
\+ **H93.29 Other abnormal auditory perceptions**
H93.291 Other abnormal auditory perceptions, right ear
H93.292 Other abnormal auditory perceptions, left ear
H93.293 Other abnormal auditory perceptions, bilateral
H93.299 Other abnormal auditory perceptions, unspecified ear

\+ **H93.3 Disorders of acoustic nerve**
Disorder of 8th cranial nerve
Excludes1: *acoustic neuroma (D33.3)*
syphilitic acoustic neuritis (A52.15)
\+ **H93.3X Disorders of acoustic nerve**
H93.3X1 Disorders of right acoustic nerve
H93.3X2 Disorders of left acoustic nerve
H93.3X3 Disorders of bilateral acoustic nerves
H93.3X9 Disorders of unspecified acoustic nerve

\+ **H93.8 Other specified disorders of ear**
\+ **H93.8X Other specified disorders of ear**
H93.8X1 Other specified disorders of right ear
H93.8X2 Other specified disorders of left ear
H93.8X3 Other specified disorders of ear, bilateral
H93.8X9 Other specified disorders of ear, unspecified ear

\+ **H93.9 Unspecified disorder of ear**
H93.90 Unspecified disorder of ear, unspecified ear
H93.91 Unspecified disorder of right ear
H93.92 Unspecified disorder of left ear
H93.93 Unspecified disorder of ear, bilateral

H94 Other disorders of ear in diseases classified elsewhere

+ **H94.0 Acoustic neuritis in infectious and parasitic diseases classified elsewhere**
  Code first underlying disease, such as:
  parasitic disease (B65-B89)
  Excludes1: *acoustic neuritis (in):*
  herpes zoster (B02.29)
  syphilis (A52.15)
  H94.00 Acoustic neuritis in infectious and parasitic diseases classified elsewhere, unspecified ear
  H94.01 Acoustic neuritis in infectious and parasitic diseases classified elsewhere, right ear
  H94.02 Acoustic neuritis in infectious and parasitic diseases classified elsewhere, left ear
  H94.03 Acoustic neuritis in infectious and parasitic diseases classified elsewhere, bilateral
+ **H94.8 Other specified disorders of ear in diseases classified elsewhere**
  Code first underlying disease, such as:
  congenital syphilis (A50.0)
  Excludes1: *aural myiasis (B87.4)*
  syphilitic labyrinthitis (A52.79)
  H94.80 Other specified disorders of ear in diseases classified elsewhere, unspecified ear
  H94.81 Other specified disorders of right ear in diseases classified elsewhere
  H94.82 Other specified disorders of left ear in diseases classified elsewhere
  H94.83 Other specified disorders of ear in diseases classified elsewhere, bilateral

Intraoperative and postprocedural complications and disorders of ear and mastoid process, not elsewhere classified (H95)

H95 Intraoperative and postprocedural complications and disorders of ear and mastoid process, not elsewhere classified
AHA CC: 4Q, 2016, 9-10

+ **H95.0 Recurrent cholesteatoma of postmastoidectomy cavity**
  H95.00 Recurrent cholesteatoma of postmastoidectomy cavity, unspecified ear
  H95.01 Recurrent cholesteatoma of postmastoidectomy cavity, right ear
  H95.02 Recurrent cholesteatoma of postmastoidectomy cavity, left ear
  H95.03 Recurrent cholesteatoma of postmastoidectomy cavity, bilateral ears
+ **H95.1 Other disorders of ear and mastoid process following mastoidectomy**
  + **H95.11 Chronic inflammation of postmastoidectomy cavity**
    H95.111 Chronic inflammation of postmastoidectomy cavity, right ear
    H95.112 Chronic inflammation of postmastoidectomy cavity, left ear
    H95.113 Chronic inflammation of postmastoidectomy cavity, bilateral ears
    H95.119 Chronic inflammation of postmastoidectomy cavity, unspecified ear
  + **H95.12 Granulation of postmastoidectomy cavity**
    H95.121 Granulation of postmastoidectomy cavity, right ear
    H95.122 Granulation of postmastoidectomy cavity, left ear
    H95.123 Granulation of postmastoidectomy cavity, bilateral ears
    H95.129 Granulation of postmastoidectomy cavity, unspecified ear
  + **H95.13 Mucosal cyst of postmastoidectomy cavity**
    H95.131 Mucosal cyst of postmastoidectomy cavity, right ear
    H95.132 Mucosal cyst of postmastoidectomy cavity, left ear
    H95.133 Mucosal cyst of postmastoidectomy cavity, bilateral ears
    H95.139 Mucosal cyst of postmastoidectomy cavity, unspecified ear
  + **H95.19 Other disorders following mastoidectomy**
    H95.191 Other disorders following mastoidectomy, right ear
    H95.192 Other disorders following mastoidectomy, left ear
    H95.193 Other disorders following mastoidectomy, bilateral ears
    H95.199 Other disorders following mastoidectomy, unspecified ear
+ **H95.2 Intraoperative hemorrhage and hematoma of ear and mastoid process complicating a procedure**
  Excludes1: *intraoperative hemorrhage and hematoma of ear and mastoid process due to accidental puncture or laceration during a procedure (H95.3-)*
  CC **H95.21 Intraoperative hemorrhage and hematoma of ear and mastoid process complicating a procedure on the ear and mastoid process**
  CC **H95.22 Intraoperative hemorrhage and hematoma of ear and mastoid process complicating other procedure**
+ **H95.3 Accidental puncture and laceration of ear and mastoid process during a procedure**
  CC **H95.31 Accidental puncture and laceration of the ear and mastoid process during a procedure on the ear and mastoid process**
  CC **H95.32 Accidental puncture and laceration of the ear and mastoid process during other procedure**
+ **H95.4 Postprocedural hemorrhage of ear and mastoid process following a procedure**
  CC **H95.41 Postprocedural hemorrhage of ear and mastoid process following a procedure on the ear and mastoid process**
  CC **H95.42 Postprocedural hemorrhage of ear and mastoid process following other procedure**
+ **H95.5 Postprocedural hematoma and seroma of ear and mastoid process following a procedure**
  CC **H95.51 Postprocedural hematoma of ear and mastoid process following a procedure on the ear and mastoid process**
  CC **H95.52 Postprocedural hematoma of ear and mastoid process following other procedure**
  CC **H95.53 Postprocedureal seroma of ear and mastoid process following a procedure on the ear and mastoid process**
  CC **H95.54 Postprocedureal seroma of ear and mastoid process following other procedure**
+ **H95.8 Other intraoperative and postprocedural complications and disorders of the ear and mastoid process, not elsewhere classified**
  Excludes2: *postprocedural complications and disorders following mastoidectomy (H95.0-, H95.1-)*
  + **H95.81 Postprocedural stenosis of external ear canal**
    CC **H95.811 Postprocedural stenosis of right external ear canal**
    CC **H95.812 Postprocedural stenosis of left external ear canal**
    CC **H95.813 Postprocedural stenosis of external ear canal, bilateral**
    CC **H95.819 Postprocedural stenosis of unspecified external ear canal**
  CC **H95.88 Other intraoperative complications and disorders of the ear and mastoid process, not elsewhere classified**
  Use additional code, if applicable, to further specify disorder
  CC **H95.89 Other postprocedural complications and disorders of the ear and mastoid process, not elsewhere classified**
  Use additional code, if applicable, to further specify disorder

Chapter 9: Diseases of the Circulatory System (I00-I99)

Excludes2: *certain conditions originating in the perinatal period (P04-P96)*
certain infectious and parasitic diseases (A00-B99)
complications of pregnancy, childbirth and the puerperium (O00-O9A)
congenital malformations, deformations, and chromosomal abnormalities (Q00-Q99)
endocrine, nutritional and metabolic diseases (E00-E88)
injury, poisoning and certain other consequences of external causes (S00-T88)
neoplasms (C00-D49)
symptoms, signs and abnormal clinical and laboratory findings, not elsewhere classified (R00-R94)
systemic connective tissue disorders (M30-M36)
transient cerebral ischemic attacks and related syndromes (G45.-)

This chapter contains the following category blocks:

I00-I02 Acute rheumatic fever
I05-I09 Chronic rheumatic heart diseases
I10-I16 Hypertensive diseases
I20-I25 Ischemic heart diseases
I26-I28 Pulmonary heart disease and diseases of pulmonary circulation
I30-I5A Other forms of heart disease
I60-I69 Cerebrovascular diseases
I70-I79 Diseases of arteries, arterioles and capillaries
I80-I89 Diseases of veins, lymphatic vessels and lymph nodes, not elsewhere classified
I95-I99 Other and unspecified disorders of the circulatory system

C. Chapter-Specific Coding Guidelines

In addition to general coding guidelines, there are guidelines for specific diagnoses and/or conditions in the classification. Unless otherwise indicated, these guidelines apply to all health care settings. Please refer to Section II for guidelines on the selection of principal diagnosis.

9. Chapter 9: Diseases of the Circulatory System (I00-I99)

a. Hypertension

The classification presumes a causal relationship between hypertension and heart involvement and between hypertension and kidney involvement, as the two conditions are linked by the term "with" in the Alphabetic Index. These conditions should be coded as related even in the absence of provider documentation explicitly linking them, unless the documentation clearly states the conditions are unrelated.

For hypertension and conditions not specifically linked by relational terms such as "with," "associated with" or "due to" in the classification, provider documentation must link the conditions in order to code them as related.

1) Hypertension with Heart Disease

Hypertension with heart conditions classified to I50.- or I51.4-I51.7, I51.89, I51.9, are assigned to, a code from category I11, Hypertensive heart disease. Use an additional code(s) from category I50, Heart failure, to identify the type(s) of heart failure in those patients with heart failure.

The same heart conditions (I50.-, I51.4-I51.7, I51.89, I51.9) with hypertension are coded separately if the provider has documented they are unrelated to the hypertension. Sequence according to the circumstances of the admission/encounter.

2) Hypertensive Chronic Kidney Disease

Assign codes from category I12, Hypertensive chronic kidney disease, when both hypertension and a condition classifiable to category N18, Chronic kidney disease (CKD), are present. CKD should not be coded as hypertensive if the provider indicates the CKD is not related to the hypertension.

The appropriate code from category N18 should be used as a secondary code with a code from category I12 to identify the stage of chronic kidney disease.

See Section I.C.14. Chronic kidney disease.

If a patient has hypertensive chronic kidney disease and acute renal failure, the acute renal failure should also be coded. Sequence according to the circumstances of the admission/encounter.

3) Hypertensive Heart and Chronic Kidney Disease

Assign codes from combination category I13, Hypertensive heart and chronic kidney disease, when there is hypertension with both heart and kidney involvement. If heart failure is present, assign an additional code from category I50 to identify the type of heart failure.

The appropriate code from category N18, Chronic kidney disease, should be used as a secondary code with a code from category I13 to identify the stage of chronic kidney disease.

See Section I.C.14. Chronic kidney disease.

The codes in category I13, Hypertensive heart and chronic kidney disease, are combination codes that include hypertension, heart disease and chronic kidney disease. The Includes note at I13 specifies that the conditions included at I11 and I12 are included together in I13. If a patient has hypertension, heart disease and chronic kidney disease then a code from I13 should be used, not individual codes for hypertension, heart disease and chronic kidney disease, or codes from I11 or I12.

For patients with both acute renal failure and chronic kidney disease the acute renal failure should also be coded. Sequence according to the circumstances of the admission/encounter.

4) Hypertensive Cerebrovascular Disease

For hypertensive cerebrovascular disease, first assign the appropriate code from categories I60-I69, followed by the appropriate hypertension code.

5) Hypertensive Retinopathy

Subcategory H35.0, Background retinopathy and retinal vascular changes, should be used with a code from category I10 – I15, Hypertensive disease to include the systemic hypertension. The sequencing is based on the reason for the encounter.

6) Hypertension, Secondary

Secondary hypertension is due to an underlying condition. Two codes are required: one to identify the underlying etiology and one from category I15 to identify the hypertension. Sequencing of codes is determined by the reason for admission/encounter.

7) Hypertension, Transient

Assign code R03.0, Elevated blood pressure reading without diagnosis of hypertension, unless patient has an established diagnosis of hypertension. Assign code O13.-, Gestational [pregnancy-induced] hypertension without significant proteinuria, or O14.-, Pre-eclampsia, for transient hypertension of pregnancy.

8) Hypertension, Controlled

This diagnostic statement usually refers to an existing state of hypertension under control by therapy. Assign the appropriate code from categories I10-I15, Hypertensive diseases.

9) Hypertension, Uncontrolled

Uncontrolled hypertension may refer to untreated hypertension or hypertension not responding to current therapeutic regimen. In either case, assign the appropriate code from categories I10-I15, Hypertensive diseases.

10) Hypertensive Crisis

Assign a code from category I16, Hypertensive crisis, for documented hypertensive urgency, hypertensive emergency or unspecified hypertensive crisis. Code also any identified hypertensive disease (I10-I15). The sequencing is based on the reason for the encounter.

11) Pulmonary Hypertension

Pulmonary hypertension is classified to category I27, Other pulmonary heart diseases. For secondary pulmonary hypertension (I27.1, I27.2-), code also any associated conditions or adverse effects of drugs or toxins. The sequencing is based on the reason for the encounter, except for adverse effects of drugs (See Section I.C.19.e).

b. Atherosclerotic Coronary Artery Disease and Angina

ICD-10-CM has combination codes for atherosclerotic heart disease with angina pectoris. The subcategories for these codes are I25.11, Atherosclerotic heart disease of native coronary artery with angina pectoris and I25.7, Atherosclerosis of coronary artery bypass graft(s) and coronary artery of transplanted heart with angina pectoris.

When using one of these combination codes it is not necessary to use an additional code for angina pectoris. A causal relationship can be assumed in a patient with both atherosclerosis and angina pectoris, unless the documentation indicates the angina is due to something other than the atherosclerosis.

If a patient with coronary artery disease is admitted due to an acute myocardial infarction (AMI), the AMI should be sequenced before the coronary artery disease.

See Section I.C.9. Acute myocardial infarction (AMI)

c. Intraoperative and Postprocedural Cerebrovascular Accident

Medical record documentation should clearly specify the cause- and-effect relationship between the medical intervention and the cerebrovascular accident in order to assign a code for intraoperative or postprocedural cerebrovascular accident.

Proper code assignment depends on whether it was an infarction or hemorrhage and whether it occurred intraoperatively or postoperatively. If it was a cerebral hemorrhage, code assignment depends on the type of procedure performed.

d. Sequelae of Cerebrovascular Disease

1) Category I69, Sequelae of Cerebrovascular disease

Category I69 is used to indicate conditions classifiable to categories I60-I67 as the causes of sequela (neurologic deficits), themselves classified elsewhere. These "late effects" include neurologic deficits that persist after initial onset of conditions classifiable to categories I60-I67. The neurologic deficits caused by cerebrovascular disease may be present from the onset or may arise at any time after the onset of the condition classifiable to categories I60-I67.

Codes from category I69, Sequelae of cerebrovascular disease, that specify hemiplegia, hemiparesis and monoplegia identify whether the dominant or nondominant side is affected. Should the affected side be documented, but not specified as dominant or nondominant, and the classification system does not indicate a default, code selection is as follows:

- For ambidextrous patients, the default should be dominant.
- If the left side is affected, the default is non-dominant.
- If the right side is affected, the default is dominant.

2) Codes from category I69 with codes from I60-I67

Codes from category I69 may be assigned on a health care record with codes from I60-I67, if the patient has a current cerebrovascular disease and deficits from an old cerebrovascular disease.

3) Codes from category I69 and Personal history of transient ischemic attack (TIA) and cerebral infarction (Z86.73)

Codes from category I69 should not be assigned if the patient does not have neurologic deficits.

See Section I.C.21. 4. History (of) for use of personal history codes

e. Acute myocardial infarction (AMI)

1) ST elevation myocardial infarction (STEMI) and non ST elevation myocardial infarction (NSTEMI)

The ICD-10-CM codes for type 1 acute myocardial infarction (AMI) identify the site, such as anterolateral wall or true posterior wall. Subcategories I21.0-I21.2 and code I21.3 are used for type 1 ST elevation myocardial infarction (STEMI). Code I21.4, Non-ST elevation (NSTEMI) myocardial infarction, is used for type 1 non ST elevation myocardial infarction (NSTEMI) and nontransmural MIs.

If a type 1 NSTEMI evolves to STEMI, assign the STEMI code. If a type 1 STEMI converts to NSTEMI due to thrombolytic therapy, it is still coded as STEMI.

For encounters occurring while the myocardial infarction is equal to, or less than, four weeks old, including transfers to another acute setting or a postacute setting, and the myocardial infarction meets the definition for "other diagnoses" (see Section III, Reporting Additional Diagnoses), codes from category I21 may continue to be reported. For encounters after the 4 week time frame and the patient is still receiving care related to the myocardial infarction, the appropriate aftercare code should be assigned, rather than a code from category I21. For old or healed myocardial infarctions not requiring further care, code I25.2, Old myocardial infarction, may be assigned.

2) Acute myocardial infarction, unspecified

Code I21.9, Acute myocardial infarction, unspecified, is the default for unspecified acute myocardial infarction or unspecified type. If only type 1 STEMI or transmural MI without the site is documented, assign code I21.3, ST elevation (STEMI) myocardial infarction of unspecified site.

3) AMI documented as nontransmural or subendocardial but site provided

If an AMI is documented as nontransmural or subendocardial, but the site is provided, it is still coded as a subendocardial AMI.

See Section I.C.21.3 for information on coding status post administration of tPA in a different facility within the last 24 hours.

4) Subsequent acute myocardial infarction

A code from category I22, Subsequent ST elevation (STEMI) and non-ST elevation (NSTEMI) myocardial infarction, is to be used when a patient who has suffered a type 1 or unspecified AMI has a new AMI within the 4 week time frame of the initial AMI. A code from category I22 must be used in conjunction with a code from category I21. The sequencing of the I22 and I21 codes depends on the circumstances of the encounter.

Do not assign code I22 for subsequent myocardial infarctions other than type 1 or unspecified. For subsequent type 2 AMI assign only code I21.A1. For subsequent type 4 or type 5 AMI, assign only code I21.A9.

If a subsequent myocardial infarction of one type occurs within 4 weeks of a myocardial infarction of a different type, assign the appropriate codes from category I21 to identify each type. Do not assign a code from I22. Codes from category I22 should only be assigned if both the initial and subsequent myocardial infarctions are type 1 or unspecified.

5) Other Types of Myocardial Infarction

The ICD-10-CM provides codes for different types of myocardial infarction. Type 1 myocardial infarctions are assigned to codes I21.0-I21.4.

Type 2 myocardial infarction (myocardial infarction due to demand ischemia or secondary to ischemic imbalance) is assigned to code I21.A1, Myocardial infarction type 2 with the underlying cause coded first. Do not assign code I24.8, Other forms of acute ischemic heart disease, for the demand ischemia. If a type 2 AMI is described as NSTEMI or STEMI, only assign code I21.A1. Codes I21.0-I21.4 should only be assigned for type 1 AMIs.

Acute myocardial infarctions type 3, 4a, 4b, 4c and 5 are assigned to code I21.A9, Other myocardial infarction type.

The "Code also" and "Code first" notes should be followed related to complications, and for coding of postprocedural myocardial infarctions during or following cardiac surgery.

Acute rheumatic fever (I00-I02)

I00 Rheumatic fever without heart involvement

Includes: arthritis, rheumatic, acute or subacute
Excludes1: *rheumatic fever with heart involvement (I01.0-I01.9)*
Valid 3-character code, no further characters required

I01 Rheumatic fever with heart involvement

Excludes1: *chronic diseases of rheumatic origin (I05-I09) unless rheumatic fever is also present or there is evidence of reactivation or activity of the rheumatic process.*

CC **I01.0 Acute rheumatic pericarditis**
Any condition in I00 with pericarditis
Rheumatic pericarditis (acute)
Excludes1: *acute pericarditis not specified as rheumatic (I30.-)*

CC **I01.1 Acute rheumatic endocarditis**
Any condition in I00 with endocarditis or valvulitis
Acute rheumatic valvulitis

CC **I01.2 Acute rheumatic myocarditis**
Any condition in I00 with myocarditis

CC **I01.8 Other acute rheumatic heart disease**
Any condition in I00 with other or multiple types of heart involvement
Acute rheumatic pancarditis

CC **I01.9 Acute rheumatic heart disease, unspecified**
Any condition in I00 with unspecified type of heart involvement
Rheumatic carditis, acute
Rheumatic heart disease, active or acute

I02 Rheumatic chorea

Includes: Sydenham's chorea
Excludes1: *chorea NOS (G25.5)*
Huntington's chorea (G10)

CC **I02.0 Rheumatic chorea with heart involvement**
Chorea NOS with heart involvement
Rheumatic chorea with heart involvement of any type classifiable under I01.-

CC **I02.9 Rheumatic chorea without heart involvement**
Rheumatic chorea NOS

Atria, Ventricles, and Interventricular Septum

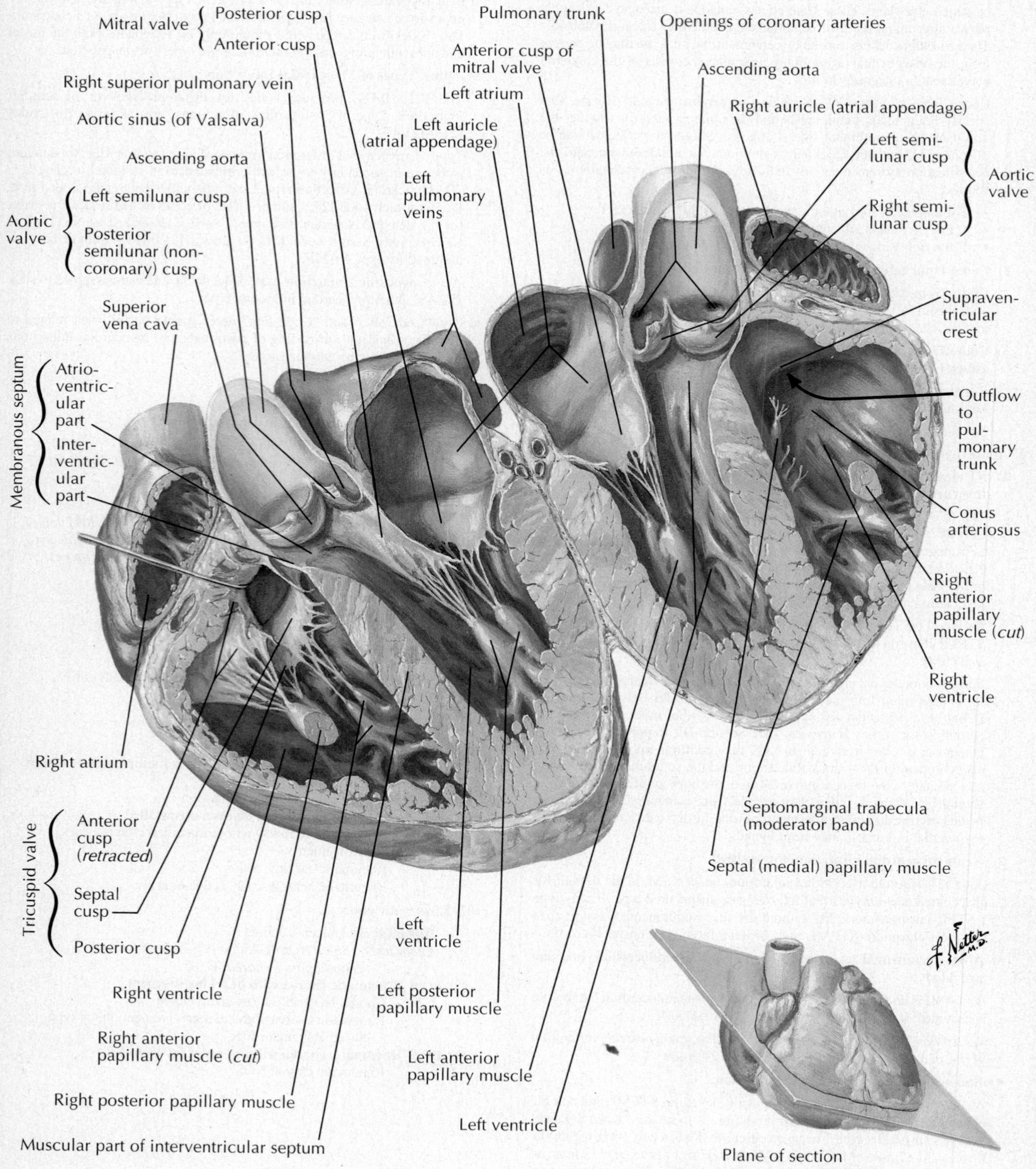

Veins

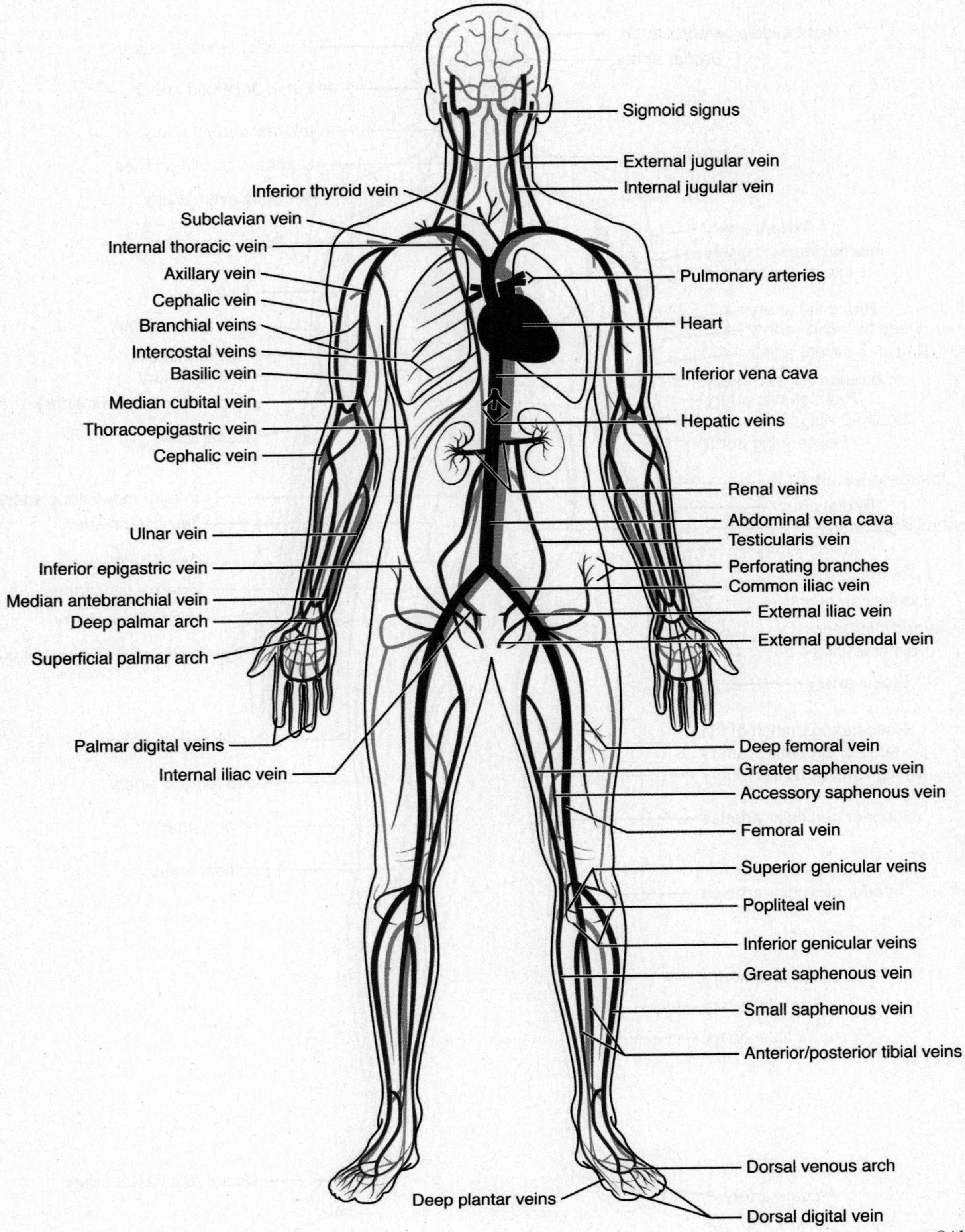
Sigmoid signus
External jugular vein
Internal jugular vein
Inferior thyroid vein
Subclavian vein
Internal thoracic vein
Axillary vein
Cephalic vein
Branchial veins
Intercostal veins
Basilic vein
Median cubital vein
Thoracoepigastric vein
Cephalic vein
Pulmonary arteries
Heart
Inferior vena cava
Hepatic veins
Renal veins
Abdominal vena cava
Testicularis vein
Perforating branches
Common iliac vein
External iliac vein
External pudendal vein
Ulnar vein
Inferior epigastric vein
Median antebranchial vein
Deep palmar arch
Superficial palmar arch
Palmar digital veins
Internal iliac vein
Deep femoral vein
Greater saphenous vein
Accessory saphenous vein
Femoral vein
Superior genicular veins
Popliteal vein
Inferior genicular veins
Great saphenous vein
Small saphenous vein
Anterior/posterior tibial veins
Dorsal venous arch
Deep plantar veins
Dorsal digital vein

Arteries

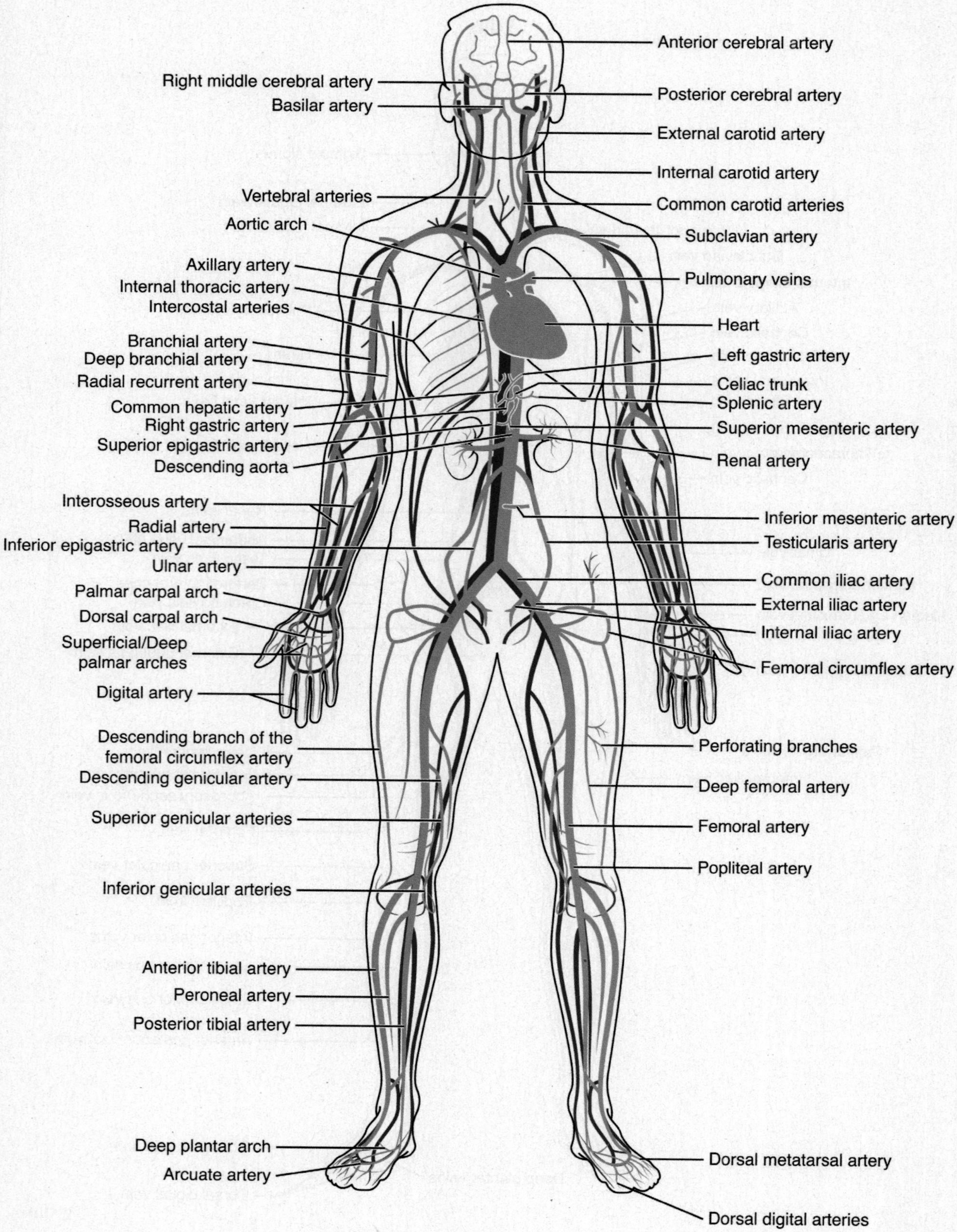
Anterior cerebral artery
Right middle cerebral artery
Posterior cerebral artery
Basilar artery
External carotid artery
Internal carotid artery
Vertebral arteries
Common carotid arteries
Aortic arch
Subclavian artery
Axillary artery
Pulmonary veins
Internal thoracic artery
Intercostal arteries
Heart
Branchial artery
Deep branchial artery
Left gastric artery
Radial recurrent artery
Celiac trunk
Common hepatic artery
Splenic artery
Right gastric artery
Superior mesenteric artery
Superior epigastric artery
Descending aorta
Renal artery
Interosseous artery
Inferior mesenteric artery
Radial artery
Inferior epigastric artery
Testicularis artery
Ulnar artery
Common iliac artery
Palmar carpal arch
External iliac artery
Dorsal carpal arch
Internal iliac artery
Superficial/Deep palmar arches
Femoral circumflex artery
Digital artery
Descending branch of the femoral circumflex artery
Perforating branches
Descending genicular artery
Deep femoral artery
Superior genicular arteries
Femoral artery
Popliteal artery
Inferior genicular arteries
Anterior tibial artery
Peroneal artery
Posterior tibial artery
Deep plantar arch
Dorsal metatarsal artery
Arcuate artery
Dorsal digital arteries

Chronic rheumatic heart diseases (I05-I09)

I05 Rheumatic mitral valve diseases

Includes: conditions classifiable to both I05.0 and I05.2-I05.9, whether specified as rheumatic or not

Excludes1: *mitral valve disease specified as nonrheumatic (I34.-)*
mitral valve disease with aortic and/or tricuspid valve involvement (I08.-)

I05.0 Rheumatic mitral stenosis
Mitral (valve) obstruction (rheumatic)

I05.1 Rheumatic mitral insufficiency
Rheumatic mitral incompetence
Rheumatic mitral regurgitation
Excludes1: *mitral insufficiency not specified as rheumatic (I34.0)*

I05.2 Rheumatic mitral stenosis with insufficiency
Rheumatic mitral stenosis with incompetence or regurgitation

I05.8 Other rheumatic mitral valve diseases
Rheumatic mitral (valve) failure

I05.9 Rheumatic mitral valve disease, unspecified
Rheumatic mitral (valve) disorder (chronic) NOS

I06 Rheumatic aortic valve diseases

Excludes1: *aortic valve disease not specified as rheumatic (I35.-)*
aortic valve disease with mitral and/or tricuspid valve involvement (I08.-)

I06.0 Rheumatic aortic stenosis
Rheumatic aortic (valve) obstruction

I06.1 Rheumatic aortic insufficiency
Rheumatic aortic incompetence
Rheumatic aortic regurgitation

I06.2 Rheumatic aortic stenosis with insufficiency
Rheumatic aortic stenosis with incompetence or regurgitation

I06.8 Other rheumatic aortic valve diseases

I06.9 Rheumatic aortic valve disease, unspecified
Rheumatic aortic (valve) disease NOS

I07 Rheumatic tricuspid valve diseases

Includes: rheumatic tricuspid valve diseases specified as rheumatic or unspecified

Excludes1: *tricuspid valve disease specified as nonrheumatic (I36.-)*
tricuspid valve disease with aortic and/or mitral valve involvement (I08.-)

I07.0 Rheumatic tricuspid stenosis
Tricuspid (valve) stenosis (rheumatic)

I07.1 Rheumatic tricuspid insufficiency
Tricuspid (valve) insufficiency (rheumatic)

I07.2 Rheumatic tricuspid stenosis and insufficiency

I07.8 Other rheumatic tricuspid valve diseases

I07.9 Rheumatic tricuspid valve disease, unspecified
Rheumatic tricuspid valve disorder NOS

I08 Multiple valve diseases

Includes: multiple valve diseases specified as rheumatic or unspecified

Excludes1: *endocarditis, valve unspecified (I38)*
multiple valve disease specified a nonrheumatic (I34.-, I35.-, I36.-, I37.-, I38.-, Q22.-, Q23.-, Q24.8-)
rheumatic valve disease NOS (I09.1)

I08.0 Rheumatic disorders of both mitral and aortic valves
Involvement of both mitral and aortic valves specified as rheumatic or unspecified
AHA CC: 2Q, 2019, 5

I08.1 Rheumatic disorders of both mitral and tricuspid valves

I08.2 Rheumatic disorders of both aortic and tricuspid valves

I08.3 Combined rheumatic disorders of mitral, aortic and tricuspid valves

I08.8 Other rheumatic multiple valve diseases

I08.9 Rheumatic multiple valve disease, unspecified

I09 Other rheumatic heart diseases

CC **I09.0 Rheumatic myocarditis**
Excludes1: *myocarditis not specified as rheumatic (I51.4)*

I09.1 Rheumatic diseases of endocardium, valve unspecified
Rheumatic endocarditis (chronic)
Rheumatic valvulitis (chronic)
Excludes1: *endocarditis, valve unspecified (I38)*

CC **I09.2 Chronic rheumatic pericarditis**
Adherent pericardium, rheumatic
Chronic rheumatic mediastinopericarditis
Chronic rheumatic myopericarditis
Excludes1: *chronic pericarditis not specified as rheumatic (I31.-)*

+ **I09.8 Other specified rheumatic heart diseases**

CC **I09.81 Rheumatic heart failure**
Use additional code to identify type of heart failure (I50.-)

I09.89 Other specified rheumatic heart diseases
Rheumatic disease of pulmonary valve

I09.9 Rheumatic heart disease, unspecified
Rheumatic carditis
Excludes1: *rheumatoid carditis (M05.31)*

Hypertensive diseases (I10-I16)

Use additional code to identify:
exposure to environmental tobacco smoke (Z77.22)
history of tobacco dependence (Z87.891)
occupational exposure to environmental tobacco smoke (Z57.31)
tobacco dependence (F17.-)
tobacco use (Z72.0)

Excludes1: *neonatal hypertension (P29.2)*
primary pulmonary hypertension (I27.0)

Excludes2: *hypertensive disease complicating pregnancy, childbirth and the puerperium (O10-O11, O13-O16)*

Review coding guidelines C.9, C.9.a.5, C.9.a.8 and C.9.a.9

I10 Essential (primary) hypertension

Includes: high blood pressure
hypertension (arterial) (benign) (essential) (malignant) (primary) (systemic)

Excludes1: *hypertensive disease complicating pregnancy, childbirth and the puerperium (O10-O11, O13-O16)*

Excludes2: *essential (primary) hypertension involving vessels of brain (I60-I69)*
essential (primary) hypertension involving vessels of eye (H35.0-)

AHA CC: 4Q, 2013, 128; 4Q, 2016, 27-28; 2Q, 2018, 9-10
Valid 3-character code, no further characters required

I11 Hypertensive heart disease

Includes: any condition in I50.-or I51.4-I51.7, I51.89, I51.9 due to hypertension

Review coding guidelines C.9.a.1 and C.9.a.3

I11.0 Hypertensive heart disease with heart failure
Hypertensive heart failure
Use additional code to identify type of heart failure (I50.-)
AHA CC: 1Q, 2017, 47

I11.9 Hypertensive heart disease without heart failure
Hypertensive heart disease NOS

I12 Hypertensive chronic kidney disease

Includes: any condition in N18 and N26 - due to hypertension
arteriosclerosis of kidney
arteriosclerotic nephritis (chronic) (interstitial)
hypertensive nephropathy
nephrosclerosis

Excludes1: *hypertension due to kidney disease (I15.0, I15.1)*
renovascular hypertension (I15.0)
secondary hypertension (I15.-)

Excludes2: *acute kidney failure (N17.-)*

Review coding guidelines C.9.a.2 and C.9.a.3

CC **I12.0 Hypertensive chronic kidney disease with stage 5 chronic kidney disease or end stage renal disease**
Use additional code to identify the stage of chronic kidney disease (N18.5, N18.6)

Hypertension and CHF

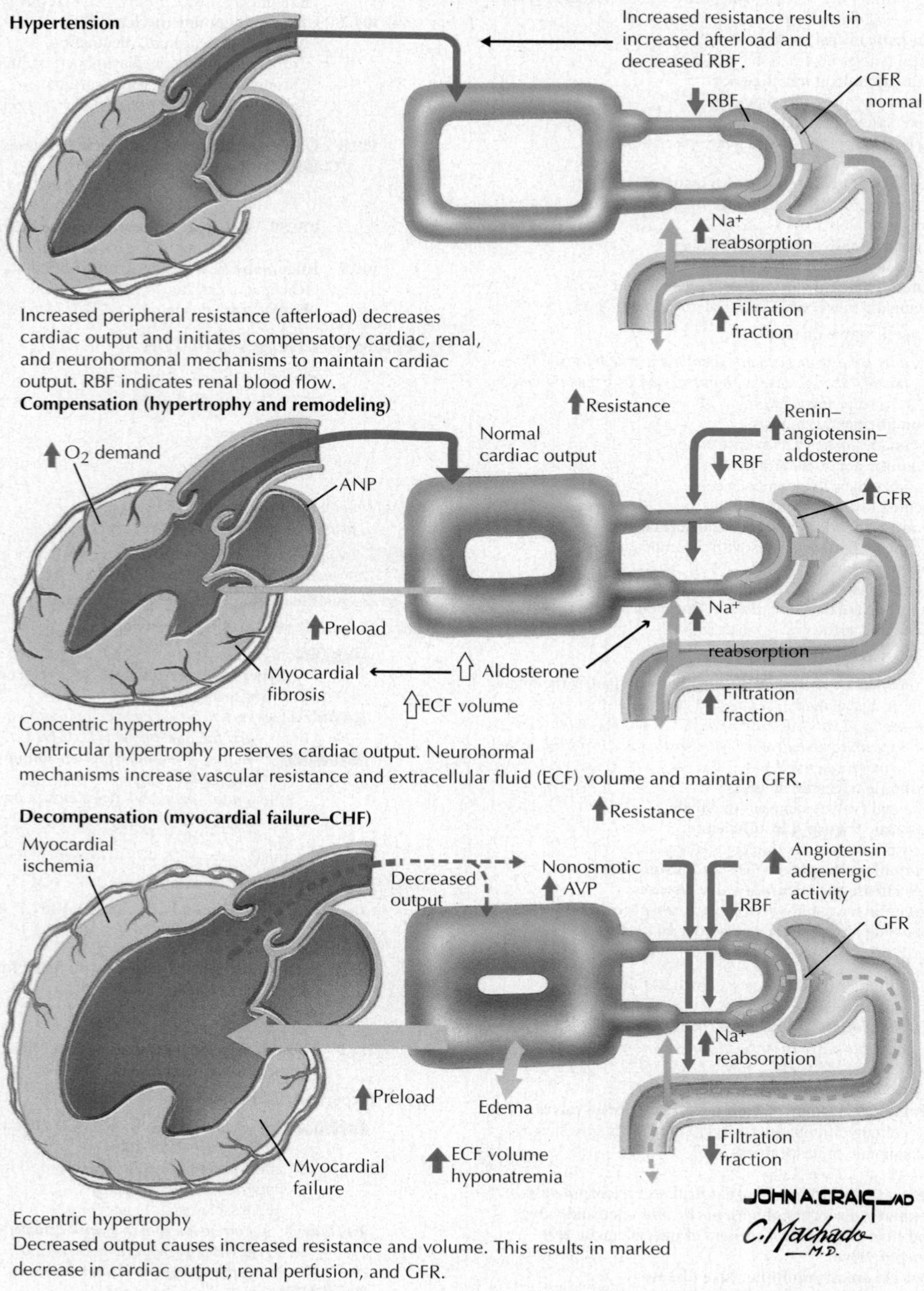

The Kidneys in Congestive Heart Failure (CHF)

Effects of Left Heart Failure on Renal Blood Flow and Tubular Function

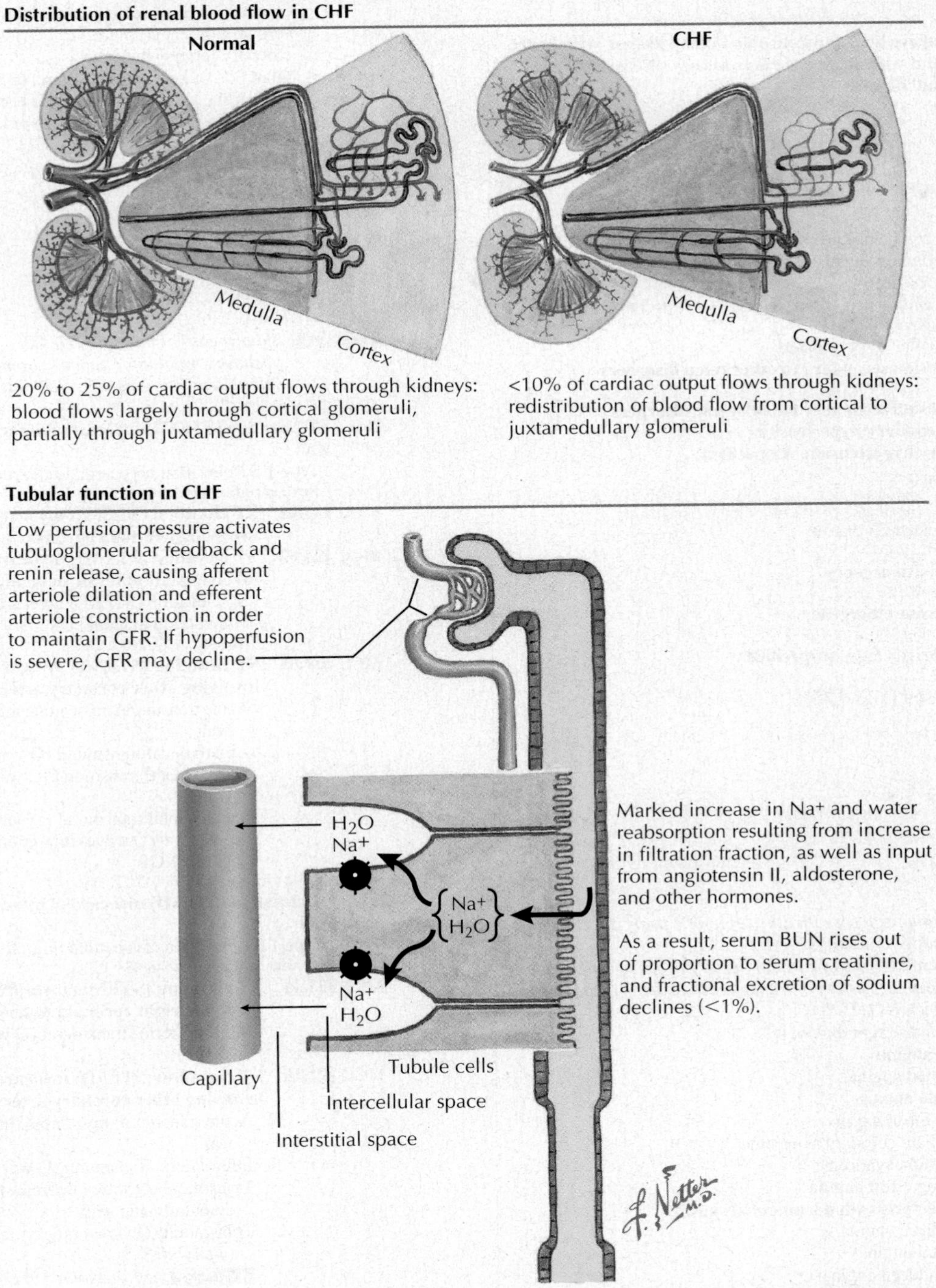

I12.9 Hypertensive chronic kidney disease with stage 1 through stage 4 chronic kidney disease, or unspecified chronic kidney disease

Hypertensive chronic kidney disease NOS

Hypertensive renal disease NOS

Use additional code to identify the stage of chronic kidney disease (N18.1-N18.4, N18.9)

AHA CC: 4Q, 2018, 88-89

I13 Hypertensive heart and chronic kidney disease

Includes: any condition in I11.- with any condition in I12.-
cardiorenal disease
cardiovascular renal disease

Review coding guideline C.9.a.3

CC **I13.0 Hypertensive heart and chronic kidney disease with heart failure and stage 1 through stage 4 chronic kidney disease, or unspecified chronic kidney disease**

Use additional code to identify type of heart failure (I50.-)

Use additional code to identify stage of chronic kidney disease (N18.1-N18.4, N18.9)

\+ **I13.1 Hypertensive heart and chronic kidney disease without heart failure**

I13.10 Hypertensive heart and chronic kidney disease without heart failure, with stage 1 through stage 4 chronic kidney disease, or unspecified chronic kidney disease

Hypertensive heart disease and hypertensive chronic kidney disease NOS

Use additional code to identify the stage of chronic kidney disease (N18.1-N18.4, N18.9)

CC **I13.11 Hypertensive heart and chronic kidney disease without heart failure, with stage 5 chronic kidney disease, or end stage renal disease**

Use additional code to identify the stage of chronic kidney disease (N18.5, N18.6)

CC **I13.2 Hypertensive heart and chronic kidney disease with heart failure and with stage 5 chronic kidney disease, or end stage renal disease**

Use additional code to identify type of heart failure (I50.-)

Use additional code to identify the stage of chronic kidney disease (N18.5, N18.6)

I15 Secondary hypertension

Code also underlying condition

Excludes1: *postprocedural hypertension (I97.3)*

Excludes2: *secondary hypertension involving vessels of brain (I60-I69)*

secondary hypertension involving vessels of eye (H35.0-)

Review coding guideline C.9.a.6

I15.0 Renovascular hypertension

I15.1 Hypertension secondary to other renal disorders

AHA CC: 3Q, 2016, 22-23

I15.2 Hypertension secondary to endocrine disorders

I15.8 Other secondary hypertension

I15.9 Secondary hypertension, unspecified

I16 Hypertensive crisis

Code also any identified hypertensive disease (I10-I15)

Review coding guideline C.9.a.10

AHA CC: 4Q, 2016, 26-28

I16.0 Hypertensive urgency

AHA CC: 4Q, 2016, 27-28

CC **I16.1 Hypertensive emergency**

AHA CC: 4Q, 2016, 27-28

CC **I16.9 Hypertensive crisis, unspecified**

Ischemic heart diseases (I20-I25)

Code also the presence of hypertension (I10-I16)

I20 Angina pectoris

Use additional code to identify:
exposure to environmental tobacco smoke (Z77.22)
history of tobacco dependence (Z87.891)
occupational exposure to environmental tobacco smoke (Z57.31)
tobacco dependence (F17.-)
tobacco use (Z72.0)

Excludes1: *angina pectoris with atherosclerotic heart disease of native coronary arteries (I25.1-)*

atherosclerosis of coronary artery bypass graft(s) and coronary artery of transplanted heart with angina pectoris (I25.7-)

postinfarction angina (I23.7)

CC **I20.0 Unstable angina**

Accelerated angina
Crescendo angina
De novo effort angina
Intermediate coronary syndrome
Preinfarction syndrome
Worsening effort angina

CC **I20.1 Angina pectoris with documented spasm**

Angiospastic angina
Prinzmetal angina
Spasm-induced angina
Variant angina

I20.8 Other forms of angina pectoris

Angina equivalent
Angina of effort
Coronary slow flow syndrome
Stable angina
Stenocardia
Use additional code(s) for symptoms associated with angina equivalent

I20.9 Angina pectoris, unspecified

Angina NOS
Anginal syndrome
Cardiac angina
Ischemic chest pain

I21 Acute myocardial infarction

Includes: cardiac infarction
coronary (artery) embolism
coronary (artery) occlusion
coronary (artery) rupture
coronary (artery) thrombosis
infarction of heart, myocardium, or ventricle
myocardial infarction specified as acute or with a stated duration of 4 weeks (28 days) or less from onset

Use additional code, if applicable, to identify:
exposure to environmental tobacco smoke (Z77.22)
history of tobacco dependence (Z87.891)
occupational exposure to environmental tobacco smoke (Z57.31)
status post administration of tPA (rtPA) in a different facility within the last 24 hours prior to admission to current facility (Z92.82)
tobacco dependence (F17.-)
tobacco use (Z72.0)

Excludes2: *old myocardial infarction (I25.2)*

postmyocardial infarction syndrome (I24.1)

subsequent type 1 myocardial infarction (I22.-)

AHA CC: 1Q, 2013, 25; 4Q, 2016, 140

\+ **I21.0 ST elevation (STEMI) myocardial infarction of anterior wall**

Type 1 ST elevation myocardial infarction of anterior wall

Review coding guideline C.9.e.1

MCC **I21.01 ST elevation (STEMI) myocardial infarction involving left main coronary artery**

MCC **I21.02 ST elevation (STEMI) myocardial infarction involving left anterior descending coronary artery**

ST elevation (STEMI) myocardial infarction involving diagonal coronary artery

AHA CC: 1Q, 2013, 25-26

MCC **I21.09 ST elevation (STEMI) myocardial infarction involving other coronary artery of anterior wall**

Acute transmural myocardial infarction of anterior wall
Anteroapical transmural (Q wave) infarction (acute)
Anterolateral transmural (Q wave) infarction (acute)
Anteroseptal transmural (Q wave) infarction (acute)
Transmural (Q wave) infarction (acute) (of) anterior (wall) NOS

AHA CC: 4Q, 2012, 102-104

\+ **I21.1 ST elevation (STEMI) myocardial infarction of inferior wall**

Type 1 ST elevation myocardial infarction of inferior wall

Review coding guideline C.9.e.1

MCC **I21.11 ST elevation (STEMI) myocardial infarction involving right coronary artery**

Inferoposterior transmural (Q wave) infarction (acute)

MCC **I21.19 ST elevation (STEMI) myocardial infarction involving other coronary artery of inferior wall**

Acute transmural myocardial infarction of inferior wall
Inferolateral transmural (Q wave) infarction (acute)
Transmural (Q wave) infarction (acute) (of) diaphragmatic wall
Transmural (Q wave) infarction (acute) (of) inferior (wall) NOS

Excludes2: *ST elevation (STEMI) myocardial infarction involving left circumflex coronary artery (I21.21)*

AHA CC: 4Q, 2012, 97

\+ **I21.2 ST elevation (STEMI) myocardial infarction of other sites**

Type 1 ST elevation myocardial infarction of other sites

Review coding guideline C.9.e.1

MCC **I21.21 ST elevation (STEMI) myocardial infarction involving left circumflex coronary artery**

ST elevation (STEMI) myocardial infarction involving oblique marginal coronary artery

Localization of Anterior and Posterior Infarcts

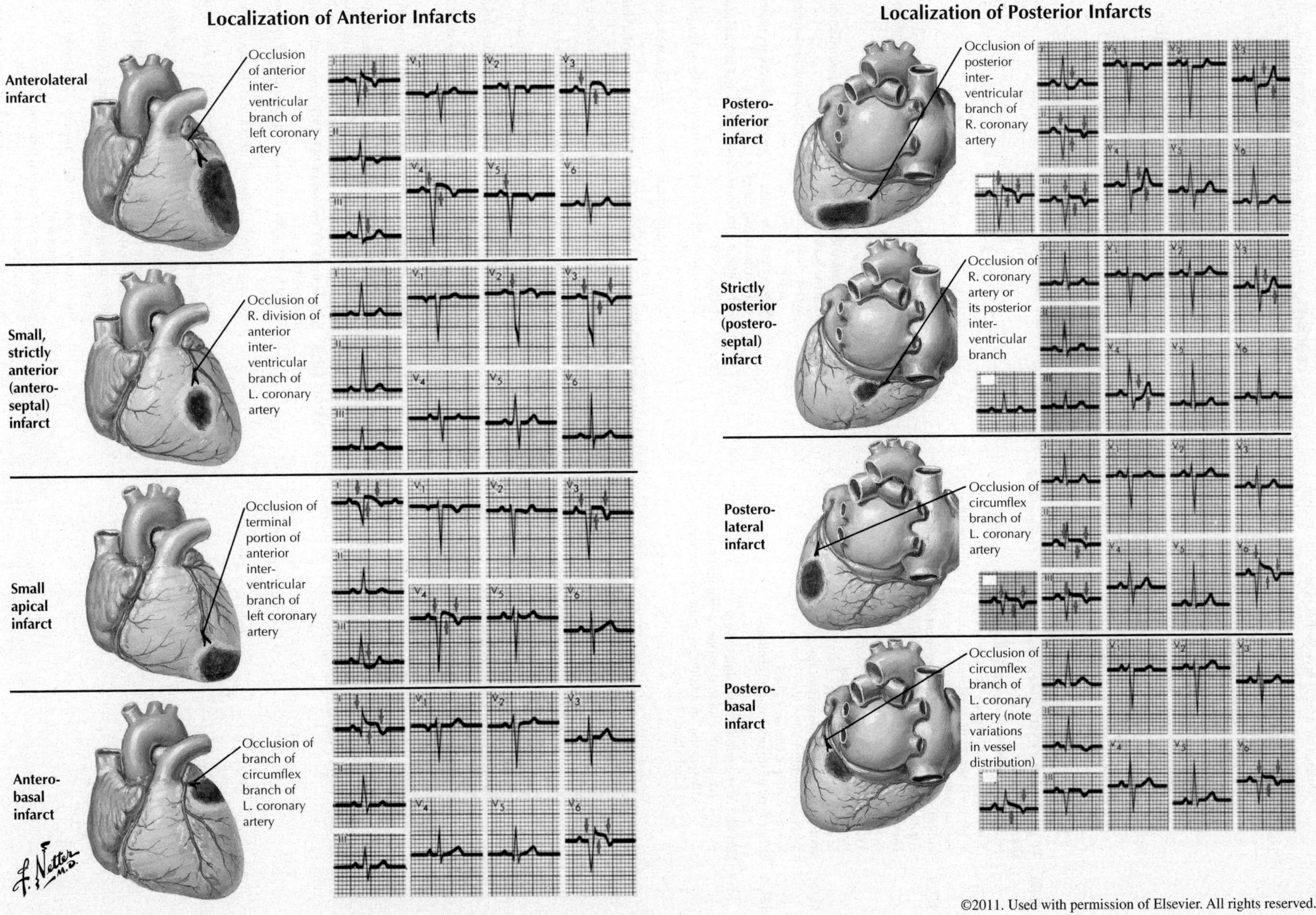

MCC **I21.29 ST elevation (STEMI) myocardial infarction involving other sites**
Acute transmural myocardial infarction of other sites
Apical-lateral transmural (Q wave) infarction (acute)
Basal-lateral transmural (Q wave) infarction (acute)
High lateral transmural (Q wave) infarction (acute)
Lateral (wall) NOS transmural (Q wave) infarction (acute)
Posterior (true) transmural (Q wave) infarction (acute)
Posterobasal transmural (Q wave) infarction (acute)
Posterolateral transmural (Q wave) infarction (acute)
Posteroseptal transmural (Q wave) infarction (acute)
Septal transmural (Q wave) infarction (acute) NOS

MCC **I21.3 ST elevation (STEMI) myocardial infarction of unspecified site**
Acute transmural myocardial infarction of unspecified site
Transmural (Q wave) myocardial infarction NOS
Type 1 ST elevation myocardial infarction of unspecified site
Review coding guidelines C.9.e.1 and C.9.e.2

MCC **I21.4 Non-ST elevation (NSTEMI) myocardial infarction**
Acute subendocardial myocardial infarction
Non-Q wave myocardial infarction NOS
Nontransmural myocardial infarction NOS
Type 1 non-ST elevation myocardial infarction
Review coding guideline C.9.e.1
AHA CC: 2Q, 2015, 16-17; 1Q, 2017, 44-45

MCC **I21.9 Acute myocardial infarction, unspecified**
Myocardial infarction (acute) NOS
Review coding guideline C.9.e.5

\+ **I21.A Other type of myocardial infarction**
AHA CC: 4Q, 2017, 12-14

MCC **I21.A1 Myocardial infarction type 2**
Myocardial infarction due to demand ischemia
Myocardial infarction secondary to ischemic imbalance
Code first the underlying cause, such as:
anemia (D50.0-D64.9)
chronic obstructive pulmonary disease (J44.-)
paroxysmal tachycardia (I47.0-I47.9)
shock (R57.0-R57.9)

MCC **I21.A9 Other myocardial infarction type**
Myocardial infarction associated with revascularization procedure
Myocardial infarction type 3
Myocardial infarction type 4a
Myocardial infarction type 4b
Myocardial infarction type 4c
Myocardial infarction type 5
Code first, if applicable, postprocedural myocardial infarction following cardiac surgery (I97.190), or postprocedural myocardial infarction during cardiac surgery (I97.790)
Code also complication, if known and applicable, such as:
(acute) stent occlusion (T82.897-)
(acute) stent stenosis (T82.855-)
(acute) stent thrombosis (T82.867-)
cardiac arrest due to underlying cardiac condition (I46.2)
complication of percutaneous coronary intervention (PCI) (I97.89)
occlusion of coronary artery bypass graft (T82.218-)
AHA CC: 2Q, 2019, 32-33

I22 Subsequent ST elevation (STEMI) and non-ST elevation (NSTEMI) myocardial infarction

Includes: acute myocardial infarction occurring within four weeks (28 days) of a previous acute myocardial infarction, regardless of site
cardiac infarction
coronary (artery) embolism
coronary (artery) occlusion
coronary (artery) rupture
coronary (artery) thrombosis
infarction of heart, myocardium, or ventricle
recurrent myocardial infarction
reinfarction of myocardium
rupture of heart, myocardium, or ventricle
subsequent type 1 myocardial infarction

Use additional code, if applicable, to identify:
exposure to environmental tobacco smoke (Z77.22)
history of tobacco dependence (Z87.891)
occupational exposure to environmental tobacco smoke (Z57.31)
status post administration of tPA (rtPA) in a different facility within the last 24 hours prior to admission to current facility (Z92.82)
tobacco dependence (F17.-)
tobacco use (Z72.0)

Excludes1: *subsequent myocardial infarction, type 2 (I21.A1)*
subsequent myocardial infarction of other type (type 3) (type 4) (type 5) (I21.A9)

Review coding guideline C.9.e.4
AHA CC: 1Q, 2013, 25

MCC **I22.0 Subsequent ST elevation (STEMI) myocardial infarction of anterior wall**
Subsequent acute transmural myocardial infarction of anterior wall
Subsequent transmural (Q wave) infarction (acute)(of) anterior (wall) NOS
Subsequent anteroapical transmural (Q wave) infarction (acute)
Subsequent anterolateral transmural (Q wave) infarction (acute)
Subsequent anteroseptal transmural (Q wave) infarction (acute)

MCC **I22.1 Subsequent ST elevation (STEMI) myocardial infarction of inferior wall**
Subsequent acute transmural myocardial infarction of inferior wall
Subsequent transmural (Q wave) infarction (acute)(of) diaphragmatic wall
Subsequent transmural (Q wave) infarction (acute)(of) inferior (wall) NOS
Subsequent inferolateral transmural (Q wave) infarction (acute)
Subsequent inferoposterior transmural (Q wave) infarction (acute)
AHA CC: 4Q, 2012, 102-104

MCC **I22.2 Subsequent non-ST elevation (NSTEMI) myocardial infarction**
Subsequent acute subendocardial myocardial infarction
Subsequent non-Q wave myocardial infarction NOS
Subsequent nontransmural myocardial infarction NOS

MCC **I22.8 Subsequent ST elevation (STEMI) myocardial infarction of other sites**
Subsequent acute transmural myocardial infarction of other sites
Subsequent apical-lateral transmural (Q wave) myocardial infarction (acute)
Subsequent basal-lateral transmural (Q wave) myocardial infarction (acute)
Subsequent high lateral transmural (Q wave) myocardial infarction (acute)
Subsequent transmural (Q wave) myocardial infarction (acute)(of) lateral (wall) NOS
Subsequent posterior (true) transmural (Q wave) myocardial infarction (acute)
Subsequent posterobasal transmural (Q wave) myocardial infarction (acute)
Subsequent posterolateral transmural (Q wave) myocardial infarction (acute)
Subsequent posteroseptal transmural (Q wave) myocardial infarction (acute)
Subsequent septal NOS transmural (Q wave) myocardial infarction (acute)

MCC **I22.9** **Subsequent ST elevation (STEMI) myocardial infarction of unspecified site**
Subsequent acute myocardial infarction of unspecified site
Subsequent myocardial infarction (acute) NOS

I23 **Certain current complications following ST elevation (STEMI) and non-ST elevation (NSTEMI) myocardial infarction (within the 28 day period)**

• CC **I23.0** **Hemopericardium as current complication following acute myocardial infarction**
Excludes1: *hemopericardium not specified as current complication following acute myocardial infarction (I31.2)*

• CC **I23.1** **Atrial septal defect as current complication following acute myocardial infarction**
Excludes1: *acquired atrial septal defect not specified as current complication following acute myocardial infarction (I51.0)*

• CC **I23.2** **Ventricular septal defect as current complication following acute myocardial infarction**
Excludes1: *acquired ventricular septal defect not specified as current complication following acute myocardial infarction (I51.0)*

• CC **I23.3** **Rupture of cardiac wall without hemopericardium as current complication following acute myocardial infarction**
AHA CC: 2Q, 2017, 11-12

MCC **I23.4** **Rupture of chordae tendineae as current complication following acute myocardial infarction**
Excludes1: *rupture of chordae tendineae not specified as current complication following acute myocardial infarction (I51.1)*

MCC **I23.5** **Rupture of papillary muscle as current complication following acute myocardial infarction**
Excludes1: *rupture of papillary muscle not specified as current complication following acute myocardial infarction (I51.2)*

• CC **I23.6** **Thrombosis of atrium, auricular appendage, and ventricle as current complications following acute myocardial infarction**
Excludes1: *thrombosis of atrium, auricular appendage, and ventricle not specified as current complication following acute myocardial infarction (I51.3)*

• CC **I23.7** **Postinfarction angina**
AHA CC: 2Q, 2015, 16-17

• CC **I23.8** **Other current complications following acute myocardial infarction**

I24 **Other acute ischemic heart diseases**
Excludes1: *angina pectoris (I20.-)*
transient myocardial ischemia in newborn (P29.4)
Excludes2: *non-ischemic myocardial injury (I5A)*

CC **I24.0** **Acute coronary thrombosis not resulting in myocardial infarction**
Acute coronary (artery) (vein) embolism not resulting in myocardial infarction
Acute coronary (artery) (vein) occlusion not resulting in myocardial infarction
Acute coronary (artery) (vein) thromboembolism not resulting in myocardial infarction
Excludes1: *atherosclerotic heart disease (I25.1-)*

CC **I24.1** **Dressler's syndrome**
Postmyocardial infarction syndrome
Excludes1: *postinfarction angina (I23.7)*

CC **I24.8** **Other forms of acute ischemic heart disease**
Excludes1: *myocardial infarction due to demand ischemia (I21.A1)*

CC **I24.9** **Acute ischemic heart disease, unspecified**
Excludes1: *ischemic heart disease (chronic) NOS (I25.9)*

I25 **Chronic ischemic heart disease**
Use additional code to identify:
chronic total occlusion of coronary artery (I25.82)
exposure to environmental tobacco smoke (Z77.22)
history of tobacco dependence (Z87.891)
occupational exposure to environmental tobacco smoke (Z57.31)
tobacco dependence (F17.-)
tobacco use (Z72.0)
Excludes2: *non-ischemic myocardial injury (I5A)*

\+ **I25.1** **Atherosclerotic heart disease of native coronary artery**
Atherosclerotic cardiovascular disease
Coronary (artery) atheroma
Coronary (artery) atherosclerosis
Coronary (artery) disease
Coronary (artery) sclerosis
Use additional code, if applicable, to identify:
coronary atherosclerosis due to calcified coronary lesion (I25.84)
coronary atherosclerosis due to lipid rich plaque (I25.83)
Excludes2: *atheroembolism (I75.-)*
atherosclerosis of coronary artery bypass graft(s) and transplanted heart (I25.7-)

• **I25.10** **Atherosclerotic heart disease of native coronary artery without angina pectoris**
Atherosclerotic heart disease NOS
AHA CC: 4Q, 2012, 92-92; 4Q, 2013, 128

\+ **I25.11** **Atherosclerotic heart disease of native coronary artery with angina pectoris**
Review coding guideline C.9.b

Great Vessels of the Heart

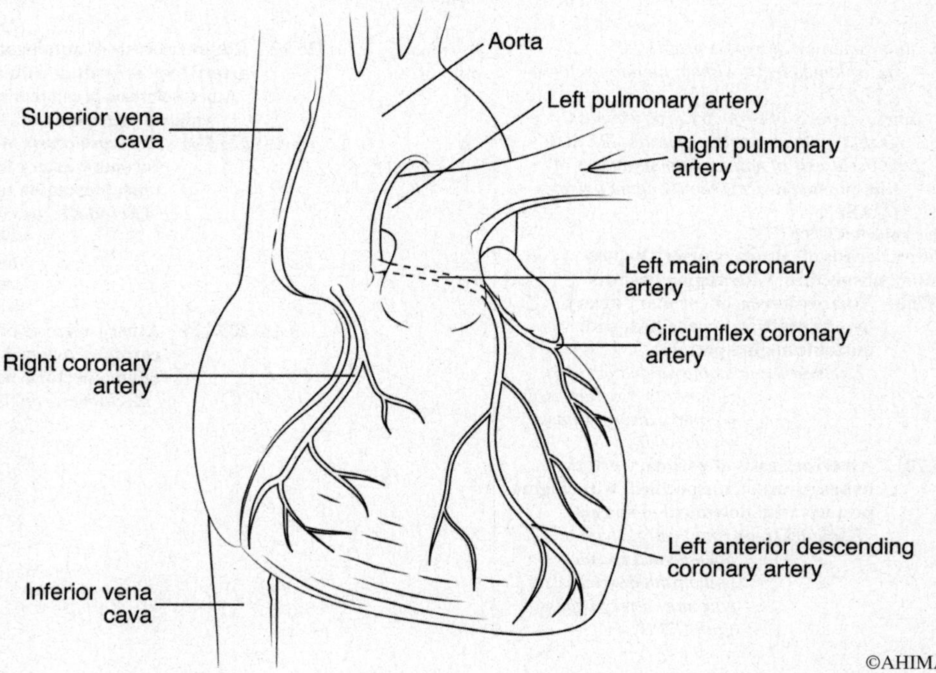

• CC **I25.110** **Atherosclerotic heart disease of native coronary artery with unstable angina pectoris**
Excludes1: *unstable angina without atherosclerotic heart disease (I20.0)*

• **I25.111** **Atherosclerotic heart disease of native coronary artery with angina pectoris with documented spasm**
Excludes1: *angina pectoris with documented spasm without atherosclerotic heart disease (I20.1)*

• **I25.118** **Atherosclerotic heart disease of native coronary artery with other forms of angina pectoris**
Excludes1: *other forms of angina pectoris without atherosclerotic heart disease (I20.8)*
AHA CC: 2Q, 2015, 16-17

• **I25.119** **Atherosclerotic heart disease of native coronary artery with unspecified angina pectoris**
Atherosclerotic heart disease with angina NOS
Atherosclerotic heart disease with ischemic chest pain
Excludes1: *unspecified angina pectoris without atherosclerotic heart disease (I20.9)*

I25.2 **Old myocardial infarction**
Healed myocardial infarction
Past myocardial infarction diagnosed by ECG or other investigation, but currently presenting no symptoms

CC **I25.3** **Aneurysm of heart**
Mural aneurysm
Ventricular aneurysm

\+ **I25.4** **Coronary artery aneurysm and dissection**

I25.41 **Coronary artery aneurysm**
Coronary arteriovenous fistula, acquired
Excludes1: *congenital coronary (artery) aneurysm (Q24.5)*

MCC **I25.42** **Coronary artery dissection**

I25.5 **Ischemic cardiomyopathy**
Excludes2: *coronary atherosclerosis (I25.1-, I25.7-)*

I25.6 **Silent myocardial ischemia**

\+ **I25.7** **Atherosclerosis of coronary artery bypass graft(s) and coronary artery of transplanted heart with angina pectoris**
Use additional code, if applicable, to identify:
coronary atherosclerosis due to calcified coronary lesion (I25.84)
coronary atherosclerosis due to lipid rich plaque (I25.83)
Excludes1: *atherosclerosis of bypass graft(s) of transplanted heart without angina pectoris (I25.812)*
atherosclerosis of coronary artery bypass graft(s) without angina pectoris (I25.810)
atherosclerosis of native coronary artery of transplanted heart without angina pectoris (I25.811)
Review coding guideline C.9.b

\+ **I25.70** **Atherosclerosis of coronary artery bypass graft(s), unspecified, with angina pectoris**

• CC **I25.700** **Atherosclerosis of coronary artery bypass graft(s), unspecified, with unstable angina pectoris**
Excludes1: *unstable angina pectoris without atherosclerosis of coronary artery bypass graft (I20.0)*

• **I25.701** **Atherosclerosis of coronary artery bypass graft(s), unspecified, with angina pectoris with documented spasm**
Excludes1: *angina pectoris with documented spasm without atherosclerosis of coronary artery bypass graft (I20.1)*

• **I25.708** **Atherosclerosis of coronary artery bypass graft(s), unspecified, with other forms of angina pectoris**
Excludes1: *other forms of angina pectoris without atherosclerosis of coronary artery bypass graft (I20.8)*

• **I25.709** **Atherosclerosis of coronary artery bypass graft(s), unspecified, with unspecified angina pectoris**
Excludes1: *unspecified angina pectoris without atherosclerosis of coronary artery bypass graft (I20.9)*

\+ **I25.71** **Atherosclerosis of autologous vein coronary artery bypass graft(s) with angina pectoris**

• CC **I25.710** **Atherosclerosis of autologous vein coronary artery bypass graft(s) with unstable angina pectoris**
Excludes1: *unstable angina without atherosclerosis of autologous vein coronary artery bypass graft(s) (I20.0)*
Excludes2: *embolism or thrombus of coronary artery bypass graft(s) (T82.8-)*

• CC **I25.711** **Atherosclerosis of autologous vein coronary artery bypass graft(s) with angina pectoris with documented spasm**
Excludes1: *angina pectoris with documented spasm without atherosclerosis of autologous vein coronary artery bypass graft(s) (I20.1)*

• CC **I25.718** **Atherosclerosis of autologous vein coronary artery bypass graft(s) with other forms of angina pectoris**
Excludes1: *other forms of angina pectoris without atherosclerosis of autologous vein coronary artery bypass graft(s) (I20.8)*

• CC **I25.719** **Atherosclerosis of autologous vein coronary artery bypass graft(s) with unspecified angina pectoris**
Excludes1: *unspecified angina pectoris without atherosclerosis of autologous vein coronary artery bypass graft(s) (I20.9)*

\+ **I25.72** **Atherosclerosis of autologous artery coronary artery bypass graft(s) with angina pectoris**
Atherosclerosis of internal mammary artery graft with angina pectoris

• CC **I25.720** **Atherosclerosis of autologous artery coronary artery bypass graft(s) with unstable angina pectoris**
Excludes1: *unstable angina without atherosclerosis of autologous artery coronary artery bypass graft(s) (I20.0)*

• CC **I25.721** **Atherosclerosis of autologous artery coronary artery bypass graft(s) with angina pectoris with documented spasm**
Excludes1: *angina pectoris with documented spasm without atherosclerosis of autologous artery coronary artery bypass graft(s) (I20.1)*

Pathologic Changes in CAD; Types and Degrees of Coronary Atherosclerotic Narrowing or Occlusion

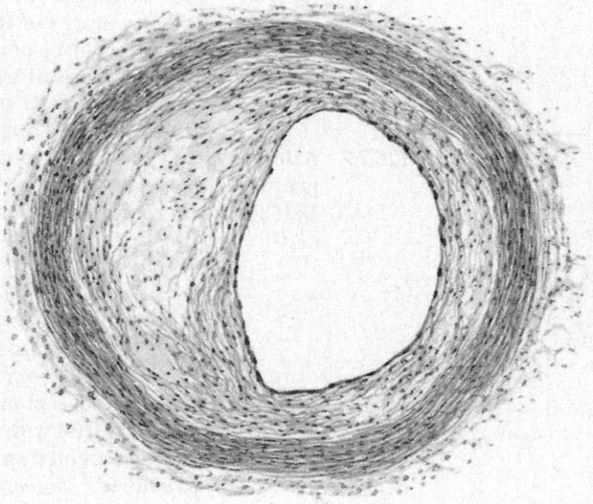

Moderate atherosclerotic narrowing of lumen

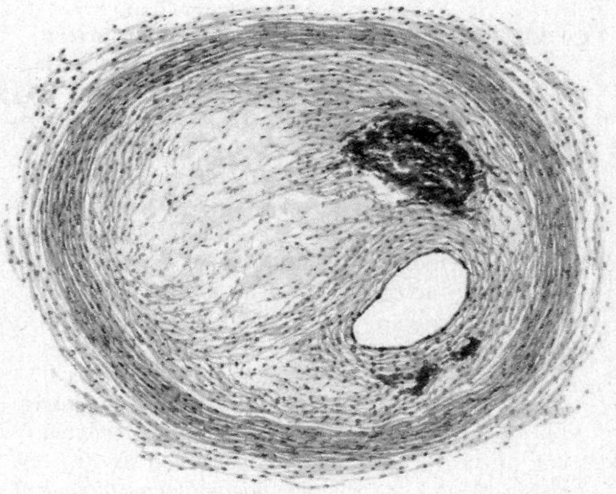

Almost complete occlusion by intimal atherosclerosis with calcium deposition

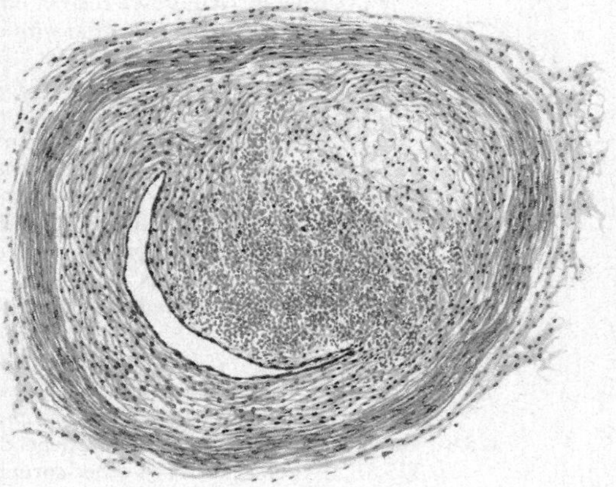

Hemorrhage into atheroma, leaving only a slit-like lumen

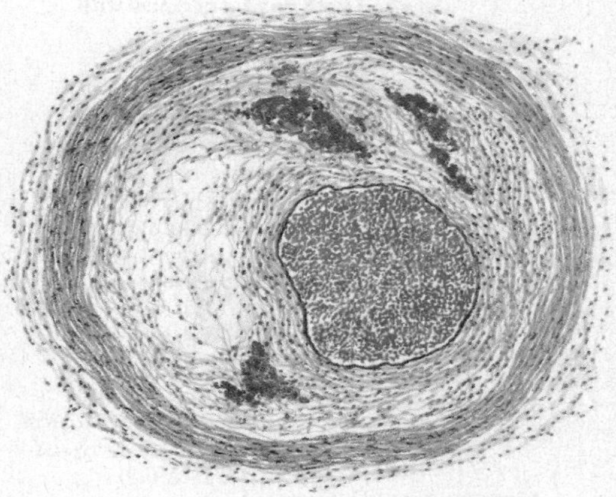

Complete occlusion by thrombus in lumen greatly narrowed by atheroma

F. Netter M.D.

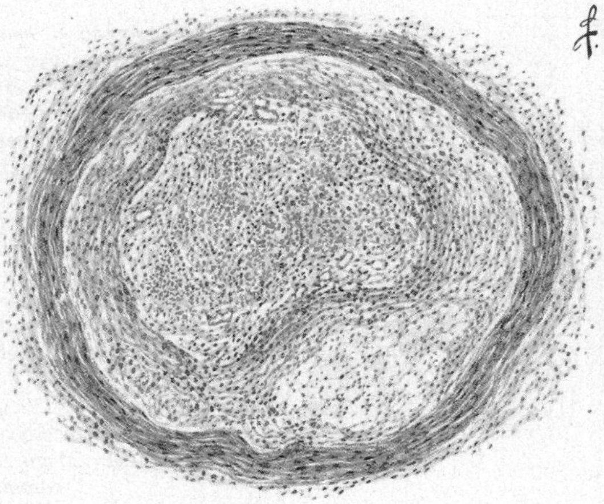

Organization of thrombus

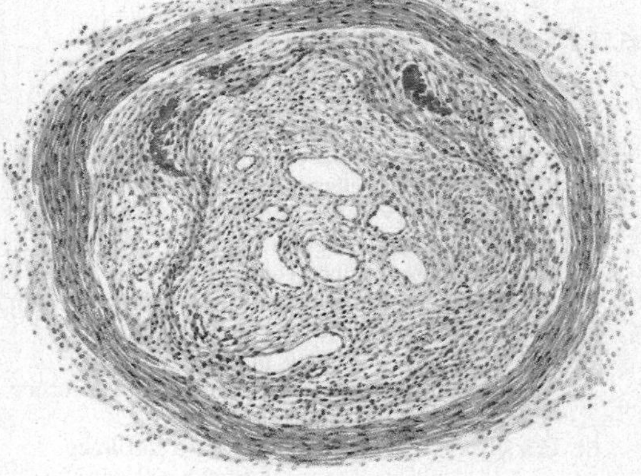

Organization with recanalization may occur

• CC **I25.728** **Atherosclerosis of autologous artery coronary artery bypass graft(s) with other forms of angina pectoris**
Excludes1: *other forms of angina pectoris without atherosclerosis of autologous artery coronary artery bypass graft(s) (I20.8)*

• CC **I25.729** **Atherosclerosis of autologous artery coronary artery bypass graft(s) with unspecified angina pectoris**
Excludes1: *unspecified angina pectoris without atherosclerosis of autologous artery coronary artery bypass graft(s) (I20.9)*

+ **I25.73** **Atherosclerosis of nonautologous biological coronary artery bypass graft(s) with angina pectoris**

• CC **I25.730** **Atherosclerosis of nonautologous biological coronary artery bypass graft(s) with unstable angina pectoris**
Excludes1: *unstable angina without atherosclerosis of nonautologousbiological coronary artery bypass graft(s) (I20.0)*

• CC **I25.731** **Atherosclerosis of nonautologous biological coronary artery bypass graft(s) with angina pectoris with documented spasm**
Excludes1: *angina pectoris with documented spasm withoutatherosclerosisof nonautologousbiological coronary artery bypass graft(s) (I20.1)*

• CC **I25.738** **Atherosclerosis of nonautologous biological coronary artery bypass graft(s) with other forms of angina pectoris**
Excludes1: *other forms of angina pectoris without atherosclerosis of nonautologousbiological coronary artery bypass graft(s) (I20.8)*

• CC **I25.739** **Atherosclerosis of nonautologous biological coronary artery bypass graft(s) with unspecified angina pectoris**
Excludes1: *unspecified angina pectoris withoutatherosclerosisof nonautologousbiological coronary artery bypass graft(s) (I20.9)*

+ **I25.75** **Atherosclerosis of native coronary artery of transplanted heart with angina pectoris**
Excludes1: *atherosclerosis of native coronary arteryoftransplantedheartwithout angina pectoris (I25.811)*

CC **I25.750** **Atherosclerosis of native coronary artery of transplanted heart with unstable angina**

CC **I25.751** **Atherosclerosis of native coronary artery of transplanted heart with angina pectoris with documented spasm**

CC **I25.758** **Atherosclerosis of native coronary artery of transplanted heart with other forms of angina pectoris**

CC **I25.759** **Atherosclerosis of native coronary artery of transplanted heart with unspecified angina pectoris**

+ **I25.76** **Atherosclerosis of bypass graft of coronary artery of transplanted heart with angina pectoris**
Excludes1: *atherosclerosis of bypass graft of coronary artery of transplanted heart without angina pectoris (I25.812)*

• CC **I25.760** **Atherosclerosis of bypass graft of coronary artery of transplanted heart with unstable angina**

• CC **I25.761** **Atherosclerosis of bypass graft of coronary artery of transplanted heart with angina pectoris with documented spasm**

• CC **I25.768** **Atherosclerosis of bypass graft of coronary artery of transplanted heart with other forms of angina pectoris**

• CC **I25.769** **Atherosclerosis of bypass graft of coronary artery of transplanted heart with unspecified angina pectoris**

+ **I25.79** **Atherosclerosis of other coronary artery bypass graft(s) with angina pectoris**

• CC **I25.790** **Atherosclerosis of other coronary artery bypass graft(s) with unstable angina pectoris**
Excludes1: *unstable angina without atherosclerosis of other coronary artery bypass graft(s) (I20.0)*

• CC **I25.791** **Atherosclerosis of other coronary artery bypass graft(s) with angina pectoris with documented spasm**
Excludes1: *angina pectoris with documented spasm without atherosclerosis of other coronary artery bypass graft(s) (I20.1)*

• CC **I25.798** **Atherosclerosis of other coronary artery bypass graft(s) with other forms of angina pectoris**
Excludes1: *other forms of angina pectoris without atherosclerosis of other coronary artery bypass graft(s) (I20.8)*

• CC **I25.799** **Atherosclerosis of other coronary artery bypass graft(s) with unspecified angina pectoris**
Excludes1: *unspecified angina pectoris without atherosclerosis of other coronary artery bypass graft(s) (I20.9)*

+ **I25.8** **Other forms of chronic ischemic heart disease**

+ **I25.81** **Atherosclerosis of other coronary vessels without angina pectoris**
Use additional code, if applicable, to identify:
coronary atherosclerosis due to calcified coronary lesion (I25.84)
coronary atherosclerosis due to lipid rich plaque (I25.83)
Excludes2: *atherosclerotic heart disease of native coronary artery without angina pectoris (I25.10)*

• CC **I25.810** **Atherosclerosis of coronary artery bypass graft(s) without angina pectoris**
Atherosclerosis of coronary artery bypass graft NOS
Excludes1: *atherosclerosis of coronary bypassgraft(s)withangina pectoris (I25.70-I25.73-, I25.79-)*

CC **I25.811** **Atherosclerosis of native coronary artery of transplanted heart without angina pectoris**
Atherosclerosis of native coronary artery of transplanted heart NOS
Excludes1: *atherosclerosis of native coronary artery of transplanted heart with anginapectoris(I25.75-)*

• CC **I25.812** **Atherosclerosis of bypass graft of coronary artery of transplanted heart without angina pectoris**
Atherosclerosis of bypass graft of transplanted heart NOS
Excludes1: *atherosclerosis of bypass graft of transplanted heartwithanginapectoris (I25.76)*

I25.82 **Chronic total occlusion of coronary artery**
Complete occlusion of coronary artery
Total occlusion of coronary artery
Code first coronary atherosclerosis (I25.1-, I25.7-, I25.81-)
Excludes1: *acute coronary occlusion with myocardial infarction (I21.0-I21.9, I22.-)*
acute coronary occlusion without myocardial infarction (I24.0)
AHA CC: 3Q, 2018, 5-6

• **I25.83** **Coronary atherosclerosis due to lipid rich plaque**
Code first coronary atherosclerosis (I25.1-, I25.7-, I25.81-)

I25.84 **Coronary atherosclerosis due to calcified coronary lesion**
Coronary atherosclerosis due to severely calcified coronary lesion
Code first coronary atherosclerosis (I25.1-, I25.7-, I25.81-)

I25.89 **Other forms of chronic ischemic heart disease**

I25.9 **Chronic ischemic heart disease, unspecified**
Ischemic heart disease (chronic) NOS

Pulmonary heart disease and diseases of pulmonary circulation (I26-I28)

I26 **Pulmonary embolism**

Includes: pulmonary (acute) (artery)(vein) infarction
pulmonary (acute) (artery)(vein) thromboembolism
pulmonary (acute) (artery)(vein) thrombosis
Excludes2: *chronic pulmonary embolism (I27.82)*
personal history of pulmonary embolism (Z86.711)
pulmonary embolism due to trauma (T79.0, T79.1)
pulmonary embolism due to complications of surgical and medical care (T80.0, T81.7-, T82.8-)
pulmonary embolism complicating abortion, ectopic or molar pregnancy (O00-O07, O08.2)
pulmonary embolism complicating pregnancy, childbirth and the puerperium (O88.-)
septic (non-pulmonary) arterial embolism (I76)

\+ **I26.0** **Pulmonary embolism with acute cor pulmonale**

MCC **I26.01** **Septic pulmonary embolism with acute cor pulmonale**
Code first underlying infection

MCC **I26.02** **Saddle embolus of pulmonary artery with acute cor pulmonale**
HAC *see Appendix B for HAC conditional logic*

MCC **I26.09** **Other pulmonary embolism with acute cor pulmonale**
HAC *see Appendix B for HAC conditional logic*

\+ **I26.9** **Pulmonary embolism without acute cor pulmonale**

MCC **I26.90** **Septic pulmonary embolism without acute cor pulmonale**
Code first underlying infection

MCC **I26.92** **Saddle embolus of pulmonary artery without acute cor pulmonale**
HAC *see Appendix B for HAC conditional logic*

MCC **I26.93** **Single subsegmental pulmonary embolism without acute cor pulmonale**
Subsegmental pulmonary embolism NOS
AHA CC: 4Q, 2019, 6-7
HAC *see Appendix B for HAC conditional logic*

MCC **I26.94** **Multiple subsegmental pulmonary emboli without acute cor pulmonale**
AHA CC: 4Q, 2019, 6-7; 2Q, 2021, 9-10
HAC *see Appendix B for HAC conditional logic*

MCC **I26.99** **Other pulmonary embolism without acute cor pulmonale**
Acute pulmonary embolism NOS
Pulmonary embolism NOS
AHA CC: 2Q, 2019, 22-23; 3Q, 2020, 10-11
HAC *see Appendix B for HAC conditional logic*

I27 **Other pulmonary heart diseases**
Review coding guideline C.9.a.11

CC **I27.0** **Primary pulmonary hypertension**
Heritable pulmonary arterial hypertension
Idiopathic pulmonary arterial hypertension
Primary group 1 pulmonary hypertension
Primary pulmonary arterial hypertension
Excludes1: *persistent pulmonary hypertension of newborn (P29.30)*
pulmonary hypertension NOS (I27.20)
secondary pulmonary arterial hypertension (I27.21)
secondary pulmonary hypertension (I27.29)
AHA CC: 4Q, 2017, 14-15

CC **I27.1** **Kyphoscoliotic heart disease**

\+ **I27.2** **Other secondary pulmonary hypertension**
Code also associated underlying condition
Excludes1: *Eisenmenger's syndrome (I27.83)*
AHA CC: 4Q, 2014, 21-22; 2Q, 2016, 8; 4Q, 2017, 14-15

I27.20 **Pulmonary hypertension, unspecified**
Pulmonary hypertension NOS

I27.21 **Secondary pulmonary arterial hypertension**
(Associated) (drug-induced) (toxin-induced) pulmonary arterial hypertension NOS
(Associated) (drug-induced) (toxin-induced) (secondary) group 1 pulmonary hypertension
Code also associated conditions if applicable, or adverse effects of drugs or toxins, such as:
adverse effect of appetite depressants (T50.5X5)
congenital heart disease (Q20-Q28)
human immunodeficiency virus [HIV] disease (B20)
polymyositis (M33.2-)
portal hypertension (K76.6)
rheumatoid arthritis (M05.-)
schistosomiasis (B65.-)
Sjögren syndrome (M35.0-)
systemic sclerosis (M34.-)

I27.22 **Pulmonary hypertension due to left heart disease**
Group 2 pulmonary hypertension
Code also associated left heart disease, if known, such as:
multiple valve disease (I08.-)
rheumatic mitral valve diseases (I05.-)
rheumatic aortic valve diseases (I06.-)

I27.23 **Pulmonary hypertension due to lung diseases and hypoxia**
Group 3 pulmonary hypertension
Code also associated lung disease, if known, such as:
bronchiectasis (J47.-)
cystic fibrosis with pulmonary manifestations (E84.0)
interstitial lung disease (J84.-)
pleural effusion (J90)
sleep apnea (G47.3-)

I27.24 **Chronic thromboembolic pulmonary hypertension**
Group 4 pulmonary hypertension
Code also associated pulmonary embolism, if applicable (I26.-, I27.82)

I27.29 **Other secondary pulmonary hypertension**
Group 5 pulmonary hypertension
Pulmonary hypertension with unclear multifactorial mechanisms
Pulmonary hypertension due to hematologic disorders
Pulmonary hypertension due to metabolic disorders
Pulmonary hypertension due to other systemic disorders
Code also other associated disorders, if known, such as:
chronic myeloid leukemia (C92.10-C92.22)
essential thrombocythemia (D47.3)
Gaucher disease (E75.22)
hypertensive chronic kidney disease with end stage renal disease (I12.0, I13.11, I13.2)
hyperthyroidism (E05.-)
hypothyroidism (E00-E03)
polycythemia vera (D45)
sarcoidosis (D86.-)

+ **I27.8 Other specified pulmonary heart diseases**

I27.81 Cor pulmonale (chronic)

Cor pulmonale NOS

Excludes1: *acute cor pulmonale (I26.0-)*

AHA CC: 4Q, 2014, 21-22

CC **I27.82 Chronic pulmonary embolism**

Use additional code, if applicable, for associated long-term (current) use of anticoagulants (Z79.01)

Excludes1: *personal history of pulmonary embolism (Z86.711)*

AHA CC: 2Q, 2021, 9-10

I27.83 Eisenmenger's syndrome

Eisenmenger's complex

(Irreversible) Eisenmenger's disease

Pulmonary hypertension with right to left shunt related to congential heart disease

Code also underlying heart defect, if known, such as:

atrial septal defect (Q21.1)

Eisenmenger's defect (Q21.8)

patent ductus arteriosus (Q25.0)

ventricular septal defect (Q21.0)

I27.89 Other specified pulmonary heart diseases

I27.9 Pulmonary heart disease, unspecified

Chronic cardiopulmonary disease

I28 Other diseases of pulmonary vessels

CC **I28.0 Arteriovenous fistula of pulmonary vessels**

Excludes1: *congenital arteriovenous fistula (Q25.72)*

CC **I28.1 Aneurysm of pulmonary artery**

Excludes1: *congenital aneurysm (Q25.79)*
congenital arteriovenous aneurysm (Q25.72)

I28.8 Other diseases of pulmonary vessels

Pulmonary arteritis

Pulmonary endarteritis

Rupture of pulmonary vessels

Stenosis of pulmonary vessels

Stricture of pulmonary vessels

I28.9 Disease of pulmonary vessels, unspecified

Other forms of heart disease (I30-I5A)

I30 Acute pericarditis

Includes: acute mediastinopericarditis
acute myopericarditis
acute pericardial effusion
acute pleuropericarditis
acute pneumopericarditis

Excludes1: *Dressler's syndrome (I24.1)*
rheumatic pericarditis (acute) (I01.0)
viral pericarditis due to Coxsakie virus (B33.23)

CC **I30.0 Acute nonspecific idiopathic pericarditis**

CC **I30.1 Infective pericarditis**

Pneumococcal pericarditis

Pneumopyopericardium

Purulent pericarditis

Pyopericarditis

Pyopericardium

Pyopneumopericardium

Staphylococcal pericarditis

Streptococcal pericarditis

Suppurative pericarditis

Viral pericarditis

Use additional code (B95-B97) to identify infectious agent

CC **I30.8 Other forms of acute pericarditis**

CC **I30.9 Acute pericarditis, unspecified**

I31 Other diseases of pericardium

Excludes1: *diseases of pericardium specified as rheumatic (I09.2)*
postcardiotomy syndrome (I97.0)
traumatic injury to pericardium (S26.-)

CC **I31.0 Chronic adhesive pericarditis**

Accretio cordis

Adherent pericardium

Adhesive mediastinopericarditis

CC **I31.1 Chronic constrictive pericarditis**

Concretio cordis

Pericardial calcification

CC **I31.2 Hemopericardium, not elsewhere classified**

Excludes1: *hemopericardium as current complication following acute myocardial infarction (I23.0)*

CC **I31.3 Pericardial effusion (noninflammatory)**

Chylopericardium

Excludes1: *acute pericardial effusion (I30.9)*

AHA CC: 1Q, 2019, 16

CC **I31.4 Cardiac tamponade**

Code first underlying cause

CC **I31.8 Other specified diseases of pericardium**

Epicardial plaques

Focal pericardial adhesions

CC **I31.9 Disease of pericardium, unspecified**

Pericarditis (chronic) NOS

CC **I32 Pericarditis in diseases classified elsewhere**

Code first underlying disease

Excludes1: *pericarditis (in):*
coxsackie (virus) (B33.23)
gonococcal (A54.83)
meningococcal (A39.53)
rheumatoid (arthritis) (M05.31)
syphilitic (A52.06)
systemic lupus erythematosus (M32.12)
tuberculosis (A18.84)

Valid 3-character code, no further characters required

I33 Acute and subacute endocarditis

Excludes1: *acute rheumatic endocarditis (I01.1)*
endocarditis NOS (I38)

MCC **I33.0 Acute and subacute infective endocarditis**

Bacterial endocarditis (acute) (subacute)

Infective endocarditis (acute) (subacute) NOS

Endocarditis lenta (acute) (subacute)

Malignant endocarditis (acute) (subacute)

Purulent endocarditis (acute) (subacute)

Septic endocarditis (acute) (subacute)

Ulcerative endocarditis (acute) (subacute)

Vegetative endocarditis (acute) (subacute)

Use additional code (B95-B97) to identify infectious agent

MCC **I33.9 Acute and subacute endocarditis, unspecified**

Acute endocarditis NOS

Acute myoendocarditis NOS

Acute periendocarditis NOS

Subacute endocarditis NOS

Subacute myoendocarditis NOS

Subacute periendocarditis NOS

I34 Nonrheumatic mitral valve disorders

Excludes1: *mitral valve disease (I05.9)*
mitral valve failure (I05.8)
mitral valve stenosis (I05.0)
mitral valve disorder of unspecified cause with diseases of aortic and/or tricuspid valve(s) (I08.-)
mitral valve disorder of unspecified cause with mitral stenosis or obstruction (I05.0)
mitral valve disorder specified as congenital (Q23.2, Q23.9)
mitral valve disorder specified as rheumatic (I05.-)

I34.0 Nonrheumatic mitral (valve) insufficiency

Nonrheumatic mitral (valve) incompetence NOS

Nonrheumatic mitral (valve) regurgitation NOS

I34.1 Nonrheumatic mitral (valve) prolapse

Floppy nonrheumatic mitral valve syndrome

Excludes1: *Marfan's syndrome (Q87.4-)*

I34.2 Nonrheumatic mitral (valve) stenosis

I34.8 Other nonrheumatic mitral valve disorders

I34.9 Nonrheumatic mitral valve disorder, unspecified

I35 Nonrheumatic aortic valve disorders

Excludes1: *aortic valve disorder of unspecified cause but with diseases of mitral and/or tricuspid valve(s) (I08.-)*
aortic valve disorder specified as congenital (Q23.0, Q23.1)
aortic valve disorder specified as rheumatic (I06.-)
hypertrophic subaortic stenosis (I42.1)

I35.0 Nonrheumatic aortic (valve) stenosis
I35.1 Nonrheumatic aortic (valve) insufficiency
Nonrheumatic aortic (valve) incompetence NOS
Nonrheumatic aortic (valve) regurgitation NOS
I35.2 Nonrheumatic aortic (valve) stenosis with insufficiency
I35.8 Other nonrheumatic aortic valve disorders
I35.9 Nonrheumatic aortic valve disorder, unspecified

I36 Nonrheumatic tricuspid valve disorders

Excludes1: *tricuspid valve disorders of unspecified cause (I07.-)*
tricuspid valve disorders specified as congenital (Q22.4, Q22.8, Q22.9)
tricuspid valve disorders specified as rheumatic (I07.-)
tricuspid valve disorders with aortic and/or mitral valve involvement (I08.-)

I36.0 Nonrheumatic tricuspid (valve) stenosis
I36.1 Nonrheumatic tricuspid (valve) insufficiency
Nonrheumatic tricuspid (valve) incompetence
Nonrheumatic tricuspid (valve) regurgitation
I36.2 Nonrheumatic tricuspid (valve) stenosis with insufficiency
I36.8 Other nonrheumatic tricuspid valve disorders
I36.9 Nonrheumatic tricuspid valve disorder, unspecified

I37 Nonrheumatic pulmonary valve disorders

Excludes1: *pulmonary valve disorder specified as congenital (Q22.1, Q22.2, Q22.3)*
pulmonary valve disorder specified as rheumatic (I09.89)

I37.0 Nonrheumatic pulmonary valve stenosis
I37.1 Nonrheumatic pulmonary valve insufficiency
Nonrheumatic pulmonary valve incompetence
Nonrheumatic pulmonary valve regurgitation
I37.2 Nonrheumatic pulmonary valve stenosis with insufficiency
I37.8 Other nonrheumatic pulmonary valve disorders
I37.9 Nonrheumatic pulmonary valve disorder, unspecified

CC **I38 Endocarditis, valve unspecified**

Includes: endocarditis (chronic) NOS
valvular incompetence NOS
valvular insufficiency NOS
valvular regurgitation NOS
valvular stenosis NOS
valvulitis (chronic) NOS

Excludes1: *congenital insufficiency of cardiac valve NOS (Q24.8)*
congenital stenosis of cardiac valve NOS (Q24.8)
endocardial fibroelastosis (I42.4)
endocarditis specified as rheumatic (I09.1)

Valid 3-character code, no further characters required

CC **I39 Endocarditis and heart valve disorders in diseases classified elsewhere**

Code first underlying disease, such as:
Q fever (A78)

Excludes1: *endocardial involvement in:*
candidiasis (B37.6)
gonococcal infection (A54.83)
Libman-Sacks disease (M32.11)
listerosis (A32.82)
meningococcal infection (A39.51)
rheumatoid arthritis (M05.31)
syphilis (A52.03)
tuberculosis (A18.84)
typhoid fever (A01.02)

Valid 3-character code, no further characters required

I40 Acute myocarditis

Includes: subacute myocarditis
Excludes1: *acute rheumatic myocarditis (I01.2)*

MCC **I40.0 Infective myocarditis**
Septic myocarditis
Use additional code (B95-B97) to identify infectious agent
MCC **I40.1 Isolated myocarditis**
Fiedler's myocarditis
Giant cell myocarditis
Idiopathic myocarditis
MCC **I40.8 Other acute myocarditis**
MCC **I40.9 Acute myocarditis, unspecified**

MCC **I41 Myocarditis in diseases classified elsewhere**

Code first underlying disease, such as:
typhus (A75.0-A75.9)

Excludes1: *myocarditis (in):*
Chagas' disease (chronic) (B57.2)
acute (B57.0)
coxsackie (virus) infection (B33.22)
diphtheritic (A36.81)
gonococcal (A54.83)
influenzal (J09.X9, J10.82, J11.82)
meningococcal (A39.52)
mumps (B26.82)
rheumatoid arthritis (M05.31)
sarcoid (D86.85)
syphilis (A52.06)
toxoplasmosis (B58.81)
tuberculous (A18.84)

Valid 3-character code, no further characters required

I42 Cardiomyopathy

Includes: myocardiopathy
Code first pre-existing cardiomyopathy complicating pregnancy and puerperium (O99.4)

Excludes2: *ischemic cardiomyopathy (I25.5)*
peripartum cardiomyopathy (O90.3)
ventricular hypertrophy (I51.7)

CC **I42.0 Dilated cardiomyopathy**
Congestive cardiomyopathy
CC **I42.1 Obstructive hypertrophic cardiomyopathy**
Hypertrophic subaortic stenosis (idiopathic)
CC **I42.2 Other hypertrophic cardiomyopathy**
Nonobstructive hypertrophic cardiomyopathy
CC **I42.3 Endomyocardial (eosinophilic) disease**
Endomyocardial (tropical) fibrosis
Löffler's endocarditis
CC **I42.4 Endocardial fibroelastosis**
Congenital cardiomyopathy
Elastomyofibrosis
CC **I42.5 Other restrictive cardiomyopathy**
Constrictive cardiomyopathy NOS
CC **I42.6 Alcoholic cardiomyopathy**
Code also presence of alcoholism (F10.-)
CC **I42.7 Cardiomyopathy due to drug and external agent**
Code first poisoning due to drug or toxin, if applicable (T36-T65 with fifth or sixth character 1-4 or 6)
Use additional code for adverse effect, if applicable, to identify drug (T36-T50 with fifth or sixth character 5)
CC **I42.8 Other cardiomyopathies**
CC **I42.9 Cardiomyopathy, unspecified**
Cardiomyopathy (primary) (secondary) NOS

CC **I43 Cardiomyopathy in diseases classified elsewhere**

Code first underlying disease, such as:
amyloidosis (E85.-)
glycogen storage disease (E74.0)
gout (M10.0-)
thyrotoxicosis (E05.0-E05.9-)

Excludes1: *cardiomyopathy (in):*
coxsackie (virus) (B33.24)
diphtheria (A36.81)
sarcoidosis (D86.85)
tuberculosis (A18.84)

Valid 3-character code, no further characters required

I44 Atrioventricular and left bundle-branch block

I44.0 Atrioventricular block, first degree

I44.1 Atrioventricular block, second degree
Atrioventricular block, type I and II
Möbitz block, type I and II
Second degree block, type I and II
Wenckebach's block

CC **I44.2 Atrioventricular block, complete**
Complete heart block NOS
Third degree block
AHA CC: 2Q, 2019, 4

\+ **I44.3 Other and unspecified atrioventricular block**
Atrioventricular block NOS

I44.30 Unspecified atrioventricular block

I44.39 Other atrioventricular block

I44.4 Left anterior fascicular block

I44.5 Left posterior fascicular block

\+ **I44.6 Other and unspecified fascicular block**

I44.60 Unspecified fascicular block
Left bundle-branch hemiblock NOS

I44.69 Other fascicular block

I44.7 Left bundle-branch block, unspecified

I45 Other conduction disorders

I45.0 Right fascicular block

\+ **I45.1 Other and unspecified right bundle-branch block**

I45.10 Unspecified right bundle-branch block
Right bundle-branch block NOS

I45.19 Other right bundle-branch block

CC **I45.2 Bifascicular block**

CC **I45.3 Trifascicular block**

I45.4 Nonspecific intraventricular block
Bundle-branch block NOS

I45.5 Other specified heart block
Sinoatrial block
Sinoauricular block
Excludes1: *heart block NOS (I45.9)*

I45.6 Pre-excitation syndrome
Accelerated atrioventricular conduction
Accessory atrioventricular conduction
Anomalous atrioventricular excitation
Lown-Ganong-Levine syndrome
Pre-excitation atrioventricular conduction
Wolff-Parkinson-White syndrome

\+ **I45.8 Other specified conduction disorders**

I45.81 Long QT syndrome

CC **I45.89 Other specified conduction disorders**
Atrioventricular [AV] dissociation
Interference dissociation
Isorhythmic dissociation
Nonparoxysmal AV nodal tachycardia
AHA CC: 2Q, 2013, 31-32

I45.9 Conduction disorder, unspecified
Heart block NOS
Stokes-Adams syndrome

I46 Cardiac arrest

Excludes2: *cardiogenic shock (R57.0)*

MCC **I46.2 Cardiac arrest due to underlying cardiac condition**
Code first underlying cardiac condition

MCC **I46.8 Cardiac arrest due to other underlying condition**
Code first underlying condition

MCC **I46.9 Cardiac arrest, cause unspecified**
AHA CC: 3Q, 2020, 26

I47 Paroxysmal tachycardia

Code first tachycardia complicating:
abortion or ectopic or molar pregnancy (O00-O07, O08.8)
obstetric surgery and procedures (O75.4)
Excludes1: *tachycardia NOS (R00.0)*
sinoauricular tachycardia NOS (R00.0)
sinus [sinusal] tachycardia NOS (R00.0)

CC **I47.0 Re-entry ventricular arrhythmia**

CC **I47.1 Supraventricular tachycardia**
Atrial (paroxysmal) tachycardia
Atrioventricular [AV] (paroxysmal) tachycardia
Atrioventricular re-entrant (nodal) tachycardia [AVNRT] [AVRT]
Junctional (paroxysmal) tachycardia
Nodal (paroxysmal) tachycardia

CC **I47.2 Ventricular tachycardia**
AHA CC: 3Q, 2013, 23-24

I47.9 Paroxysmal tachycardia, unspecified
Bouveret (-Hoffman) syndrome

I48 Atrial fibrillation and flutter
AHA CC: 4Q, 2019, 7

I48.0 Paroxysmal atrial fibrillation

\+ **I48.1 Persistent atrial fibrillation**
Excludes1: *Permanent atrial fibrillation (I48.21)*
AHA CC: 2Q, 2019, 3-4

CC **I48.11 Longstanding persistent atrial fibrillation**

CC **I48.19 Other persistent atrial fibrillation**
Chronic persistent atrial fibrillation
Persistent atrial fibrillation, NOS

\+ **I48.2 Chronic atrial fibrillation**
AHA CC: 4Q, 2013, 128; 3Q, 2018, 6

CC **I48.20 Chronic atrial fibrillation, unspecified**
Excludes1: *Chronic persistent atrial fibrillation (I48.19)*

CC **I48.21 Permanent atrial fibrillation**

I48.3 Typical atrial flutter
Type I atrial flutter

CC **I48.4 Atypical atrial flutter**
Type II atrial flutter

\+ **I48.9 Unspecified atrial fibrillation and atrial flutter**

I48.91 Unspecified atrial fibrillation

CC **I48.92 Unspecified atrial flutter**

I49 Other cardiac arrhythmias

Code first cardiac arrhythmia complicating:
abortion or ectopic or molar pregnancy (O00-O07, O08.8)
obstetric surgery and procedures (O75.4)
Excludes1: *neonatal dysrhythmia (P29.1-)*
sinoatrial bradycardia (R00.1)
sinus bradycardia (R00.1)
vagal bradycardia (R00.1)
Excludes2: *bradycardia NOS (R00.1)*

\+ **I49.0 Ventricular fibrillation and flutter**

MCC **I49.01 Ventricular fibrillation**

MCC **I49.02 Ventricular flutter**

I49.1 Atrial premature depolarization
Atrial premature beats

CC **I49.2 Junctional premature depolarization**

I49.3 Ventricular premature depolarization
AHA CC: 2Q, 2020, 23-24

\+ **I49.4 Other and unspecified premature depolarization**

I49.40 Unspecified premature depolarization
Premature beats NOS

I49.49 Other premature depolarization
Ectopic beats
Extrasystoles
Extrasystolic arrhythmias
Premature contractions

I49.5 Sick sinus syndrome
Tachycardia-bradycardia syndrome
AHA CC: 1Q, 2019, 33-34

I49.8 Other specified cardiac arrhythmias
Brugada syndrome
Coronary sinus rhythm disorder
Ectopic rhythm disorder
Nodal rhythm disorder

I49.9 Cardiac arrhythmia, unspecified
Arrhythmia (cardiac) NOS

I50 Heart failure

Code first:
heart failure complicating abortion or ectopic or molar pregnancy O00-O07, O08.8)
heart failure due to hypertension (I11.0)
heart failure due to hypertension with chronic kidney disease (I13.-)
heart failure following surgery (I97.13-)
obstetrics surgery and procedures (O75.4)
rheumatic heart failure (I09.81)

Excludes2: *cardiac arrest (I46.-)*
neonatal cardiac failure (P29.0)

Review coding guidelines C.9.a.1 and C.9.a.3

AHA CC: 1Q, 2017, 47

CC **I50.1 Left ventricular failure, unspecified**
Cardiac asthma
Edema of lung with heart disease NOS
Edema of lung with heart failure
Left heart failure
Pulmonary edema with heart disease NOS
Pulmonary edema with heart failure
Excludes1: *edema of lung without heart disease or heart failure (J81.-)*
pulmonary edema without heart disease or failure (J81.-)

\+ **I50.2 Systolic (congestive) heart failure**
Heart failure with reduced ejection fraction [HFrEF]
Systolic left ventricular heart failure
Code also end stage heart failure, if applicable (I50.84)
Excludes1: *combined systolic (congestive) and diastolic (congestive) heart failure (I50.4-)*

CC **I50.20 Unspecified systolic (congestive) heart failure**
MCC **I50.21 Acute systolic (congestive) heart failure**
CC **I50.22 Chronic systolic (congestive) heart failure**
MCC **I50.23 Acute on chronic systolic (congestive) heart failure**
AHA CC: 2Q, 2013, 33

\+ **I50.3 Diastolic (congestive) heart failure**
Diastolic left ventricular heart failure
Heart failure with normal ejection fraction
Heart failure with preserved ejection fraction [HFpEF]
Code also end stage heart failure, if applicable (I50.84)
Excludes1: *combined systolic (congestive) and diastolic (congestive) heart failure (I50.4-)*

CC **I50.30 Unspecified diastolic (congestive) heart failure**
MCC **I50.31 Acute diastolic (congestive) heart failure**
AHA CC: 1Q, 2017, 46
CC **I50.32 Chronic diastolic (congestive) heart failure**
AHA CC: 3Q, 2020, 32
MCC **I50.33 Acute on chronic diastolic (congestive) heart failure**

\+ **I50.4 Combined systolic (congestive) and diastolic (congestive) heart failure**
Combined systolic and diastolic left ventricular heart failure
Heart failure with reduced ejection fraction and diastolic dysfunction
Code also end stage heart failure, if applicable (I50.84)

CC **I50.40 Unspecified combined systolic (congestive) and diastolic (congestive) heart failure**
MCC **I50.41 Acute combined systolic (congestive) and diastolic (congestive) heart failure**
CC **I50.42 Chronic combined systolic (congestive) and diastolic (congestive) heart failure**
MCC **I50.43 Acute on chronic combined systolic (congestive) and diastolic (congestive) heart failure**

\+ **I50.8 Other heart failure**
AHA CC: 4Q, 2017, 15-16

\+ **I50.81 Right heart failure**
Right ventricular failure

I50.810 Right heart failure, unspecified
Right heart failure without mention of left heart failure
Right ventricular failure NOS

I50.811 Acute right heart failure
Acute isolated right heart failure
Acute (isolated) right ventricular failure

I50.812 Chronic right heart failure
Chronic isolated right heart failure
Chronic (isolated) right ventricular failure

I50.813 Acute on chronic right heart failure
Acute on chronic isolated right heart failure
Acute on chronic (isolated) right ventricular failure
Acute decompensation of chronic (isolated) right ventricular failure
Acute exacerbation of chronic (isolated) right ventricular failure

I50.814 Right heart failure, unspecified
Right ventricular failure secondary to left ventricular failure
Code also the type of left ventricular failure, if known (I50.2-I50.43)
Excludes1: *right heart failure with but not due to left heart failure (I50.82)*

I50.82 Biventricular heart failure
Code also the type of left ventricular failure as systolic, diastolic, or combined, if known (I50.2-I50.43)

I50.83 High output heart failure

I50.84 End stage heart failure
Stage D heart failure
Code also the type of heart failure as systolic, diastolic, or combined, if known (I50.2-I50.43)

I50.89 Heart failure, unspecified

I50.9 Heart failure, unspecified
Cardiac, heart or myocardial failure NOS
Congestive heart disease
Congestive heart failure NOS
Excludes2: *fluid overload unrelated to congestive heart failure (E87.70)*
AHA CC: 4Q, 2012, 92-93; 4Q, 2014, 21-22; 1Q, 2017, 46

I51 Complications and ill-defined descriptions of heart disease

Excludes1: *any condition in I51.4-I51.9 due to hypertension (I11.-)*
any condition in I51.4-I51.9 due to hypertension and chronic kidney disease (I13.-)
heart disease specified as rheumatic (I00-I09)

• CC **I51.0 Cardiac septal defect, acquired**
Acquired septal atrial defect (old)
Acquired septal auricular defect (old)
Acquired septal ventricular defect (old)
Excludes1: *cardiac septal defect as current complication following acute myocardial infarction (I23.1, I23.2)*

MCC **I51.1 Rupture of chordae tendineae, not elsewhere classified**
Excludes1: *rupture of chordae tendineae as current complication following acute myocardial infarction (I23.4)*

MCC **I51.2 Rupture of papillary muscle, not elsewhere classified**
Excludes1: *rupture of papillary muscle as current complication following acute myocardial infarction (I23.5)*

I51.3 Intracardiac thrombosis, not elsewhere classified
Apical thrombosis (old)
Atrial thrombosis (old)
Auricular thrombosis (old)
Mural thrombosis (old)
Ventricular thrombosis (old)
Excludes1: *intracardiac thrombosis as current complication following acute myocardial infarction (I23.6)*
AHA CC: 1Q, 2013, 24

I51.4 Myocarditis, unspecified
Chronic (interstitial) myocarditis
Myocardial fibrosis
Myocarditis NOS
Excludes1: *acute or subacute myocarditis (I40.-)*
Review coding guideline C.9.a.1

I51.5 Myocardial degeneration
Fatty degeneration of heart or myocardium
Myocardial disease
Senile degeneration of heart or myocardium
Review coding guideline C.9.a.1

I51.7 Cardiomegaly
Cardiac dilatation
Cardiac hypertrophy
Ventricular dilatation
Review coding guideline C.9.a.1

+ **I51.8 Other ill-defined heart diseases**
Review coding guideline C.9.a.1

CC **I51.81 Takotsubo syndrome**
Reversible left ventricular dysfunction following sudden emotional stress
Stress induced cardiomyopathy
Takotsubo cardiomyopathy
Transient left ventricular apical ballooning syndrome
AHA CC: 2Q, 2018, 9-10

I51.89 Other ill-defined heart diseases
Carditis (acute)(chronic)
Pancarditis (acute)(chronic)
AHA CC: 2Q, 2019, 5-6

I51.9 Heart disease, unspecified
Review coding guideline C.9.a.1

I52 Other heart disorders in diseases classified elsewhere
Code first underlying disease, such as:
congenital syphilis (A50.5)
mucopolysaccharidosis (E76.3)
schistosomiasis (B65.0-B65.9)
Excludes1: *heart disease (in):*
gonococcal infection (A54.83)
meningococcal infection (A39.50)
rheumatoid arthritis (M05.31)
syphilis (A52.06)
Valid 3-character code, no further characters required

CC **I5A Non-ischemic myocardial injury (non-traumatic)**
Acute (non-ischemic) myocardial injury
Chronic (non-ischemic) myocardial injury
Unspecified (non-ischemic) myocardial injury
Code first the underlying cause, if known and applicable, such as:
acute kidney failure (N17.-)
acute myocarditis (I40.-)
cardiomyopathy (I42.-)
chronic kidney disease (CKD) (N18.-)
heart failure (I50.-)
hypertensive urgency (I16.0)
nonrheumatic aortic valve disorders (I35.-)
paroxysmal tachycardia (I47.-)
pulmonary embolism (I26.-)
pulmonary hypertension (I27.0, I27.2-)
sepsis (A41.-)
takotsubo syndrome (I51.81)
Excludes1: *acute myocardial infarction (I21.-)*
injury of heart (S26.-)
Excludes2: *other acute ischemic heart diseases (I24.-)*
Valid 3-character code, no further characters required

Cerebrovascular diseases (I60-I69)

Use additional code to identify presence of:
alcohol abuse and dependence (F10.-)
exposure to environmental tobacco smoke (Z77.22)
history of tobacco dependence (Z87.891)
hypertension (I10-I16)
occupational exposure to environmental tobacco smoke (Z57.31)
tobacco dependence (F17.-)
tobacco use (Z72.0)

Excludes1: *traumatic intracranial hemorrhage (S06.-)*
Review coding guidelines C.9.a.4 and C.9.d

I60 Nontraumatic subarachnoid hemorrhage
Excludes1: *syphilitic ruptured cerebral aneurysm (A52.05)*
Excludes2: *sequelae of subarachnoid hemorrhage (I69.0-)*

+ **I60.0 Nontraumatic subarachnoid hemorrhage from carotid siphon and bifurcation**
MCC **I60.00 Nontraumatic subarachnoid hemorrhage from unspecified carotid siphon and bifurcation**
MCC **I60.01 Nontraumatic subarachnoid hemorrhage from right carotid siphon and bifurcation**
MCC **I60.02 Nontraumatic subarachnoid hemorrhage from left carotid siphon and bifurcation**

+ **I60.1 Nontraumatic subarachnoid hemorrhage from middle cerebral artery**
MCC **I60.10 Nontraumatic subarachnoid hemorrhage from unspecified middle cerebral artery**
MCC **I60.11 Nontraumatic subarachnoid hemorrhage from right middle cerebral artery**
MCC **I60.12 Nontraumatic subarachnoid hemorrhage from left middle cerebral artery**

MCC **I60.2 Nontraumatic subarachnoid hemorrhage from anterior communicating artery**

+ **I60.3 Nontraumatic subarachnoid hemorrhage from posterior communicating artery**
MCC **I60.30 Nontraumatic subarachnoid hemorrhage from unspecified posterior communicating artery**
MCC **I60.31 Nontraumatic subarachnoid hemorrhage from right posterior communicating artery**
MCC **I60.32 Nontraumatic subarachnoid hemorrhage from left posterior communicating artery**

MCC **I60.4 Nontraumatic subarachnoid hemorrhage from basilar artery**

+ **I60.5 Nontraumatic subarachnoid hemorrhage from vertebral artery**
MCC **I60.50 Nontraumatic subarachnoid hemorrhage from unspecified vertebral artery**
MCC **I60.51 Nontraumatic subarachnoid hemorrhage from right vertebral artery**
MCC **I60.52 Nontraumatic subarachnoid hemorrhage from left vertebral artery**

MCC **I60.6 Nontraumatic subarachnoid hemorrhage from other intracranial arteries**

MCC **I60.7 Nontraumatic subarachnoid hemorrhage from unspecified intracranial artery**
Ruptured (congenital) berry aneurysm
Ruptured (congenital) cerebral aneurysm
Subarachnoid hemorrhage (nontraumatic) from cerebral artery NOS
Subarachnoid hemorrhage (nontraumatic) from communicating artery NOS
Excludes1: *berry aneurysm, nonruptured (I67.1)*

MCC **I60.8 Other nontraumatic subarachnoid hemorrhage**
Meningeal hemorrhage
Rupture of cerebral arteriovenous malformation

MCC **I60.9 Nontraumatic subarachnoid hemorrhage, unspecified**

I61 Nontraumatic intracerebral hemorrhage
Excludes2: *sequelae of intracerebral hemorrhage (I69.1-)*
AHA CC: 2Q, 2017, 10

MCC **I61.0 Nontraumatic intracerebral hemorrhage in hemisphere, subcortical**
Deep intracerebral hemorrhage (nontraumatic)
MCC **I61.1 Nontraumatic intracerebral hemorrhage in hemisphere, cortical**
Cerebral lobe hemorrhage (nontraumatic)
Superficial intracerebral hemorrhage (nontraumatic)
MCC **I61.2 Nontraumatic intracerebral hemorrhage in hemisphere, unspecified**
MCC **I61.3 Nontraumatic intracerebral hemorrhage in brain stem**
MCC **I61.4 Nontraumatic intracerebral hemorrhage in cerebellum**
MCC **I61.5 Nontraumatic intracerebral hemorrhage, intraventricular**
MCC **I61.6 Nontraumatic intracerebral hemorrhage, multiple localized**
MCC **I61.8 Other nontraumatic intracerebral hemorrhage**
MCC **I61.9 Nontraumatic intracerebral hemorrhage, unspecified**

I62 Other and unspecified nontraumatic intracranial hemorrhage
Excludes2: *sequelae of intracranial hemorrhage (I69.2)*

+ **I62.0 Nontraumatic subdural hemorrhage**
MCC **I62.00 Nontraumatic subdural hemorrhage, unspecified**
MCC **I62.01 Nontraumatic acute subdural hemorrhage**
MCC **I62.02 Nontraumatic subacute subdural hemorrhage**
MCC **I62.03 Nontraumatic chronic subdural hemorrhage**

MCC **I62.1 Nontraumatic extradural hemorrhage**
Nontraumatic epidural hemorrhage

CC **I62.9 Nontraumatic intracranial hemorrhage, unspecified**

I63 Cerebral infarction

Includes: occlusion and stenosis of cerebral and precerebral arteries, resulting in cerebral infarction

Use additional code, if applicable, to identify status post administration of tPA (rtPA) in a different facility within the last 24 hours prior to admission to current facility (Z92.82)

Use additional code, if known, to indicate National Institutes of Health Stroke Scale (NIHSS) score (R29.7-)

Excludes1: *neonatal cerebral infarction (P91.82-)*

Excludes2: *sequelae of cerebral infarction (I69.3-)*

AHA CC: 4Q, 2016, 28

+ **I63.0 Cerebral infarction due to thrombosis of precerebral arteries**
  - MCC **I63.00 Cerebral infarction due to thrombosis of unspecified precerebral artery**
  - + **I63.01 Cerebral infarction due to thrombosis of vertebral artery**
    - MCC **I63.011 Cerebral infarction due to thrombosis of right vertebral artery**
    - MCC **I63.012 Cerebral infarction due to thrombosis of left vertebral artery**
    - MCC **I63.013 Cerebral infarction due to thrombosis of bilateral vertebral arteries**
    - MCC **I63.019 Cerebral infarction due to thrombosis of unspecified vertebral artery**
  - MCC **I63.02 Cerebral infarction due to thrombosis of basilar artery**
  - + **I63.03 Cerebral infarction due to thrombosis of carotid artery**
    - MCC **I63.031 Cerebral infarction due to thrombosis of right carotid artery**
    - MCC **I63.032 Cerebral infarction due to thrombosis of left carotid artery**
    - MCC **I63.033 Cerebral infarction due to thrombosis of bilateral carotid arteries**
    - MCC **I63.039 Cerebral infarction due to thrombosis of unspecified carotid artery**
  - MCC **I63.09 Cerebral infarction due to thrombosis of other precerebral artery**

+ **I63.1 Cerebral infarction due to embolism of precerebral arteries**
  - MCC **I63.10 Cerebral infarction due to embolism of unspecified precerebral artery**
  - + **I63.11 Cerebral infarction due to embolism of vertebral artery**
    - MCC **I63.111 Cerebral infarction due to embolism of right vertebral artery**
    - MCC **I63.112 Cerebral infarction due to embolism of left vertebral artery**
    - MCC **I63.113 Cerebral infarction due to embolism of bilateral vertebral arteries**
    - MCC **I63.119 Cerebral infarction due to embolism of unspecified vertebral artery**
  - MCC **I63.12 Cerebral infarction due to embolism of basilar artery**
  - + **I63.13 Cerebral infarction due to embolism of carotid artery**
    - MCC **I63.131 Cerebral infarction due to embolism of right carotid artery**
    - MCC **I63.132 Cerebral infarction due to embolism of left carotid artery**
    - MCC **I63.133 Cerebral infarction due to embolism of bilateral carotid arteries**
    - MCC **I63.139 Cerebral infarction due to embolism of unspecified carotid artery**
  - MCC **I63.19 Cerebral infarction due to embolism of other precerebral artery**

+ **I63.2 Cerebral infarction due to unspecified occlusion or stenosis of precerebral arteries**
  - MCC **I63.20 Cerebral infarction due to unspecified occlusion or stenosis of unspecified precerebral arteries**
  - + **I63.21 Cerebral infarction due to unspecified occlusion or stenosis of vertebral arteries**
    - MCC **I63.211 Cerebral infarction due to unspecified occlusion or stenosis of right vertebral artery**
    - MCC **I63.212 Cerebral infarction due to unspecified occlusion or stenosis of left vertebral artery**
    - MCC **I63.213 Cerebral infarction due to unspecified occlusion or stenosis of bilateral vertebral arteries**
    - MCC **I63.219 Cerebral infarction due to unspecified occlusion or stenosis of unspecified vertebral artery**
  - MCC **I63.22 Cerebral infarction due to unspecified occlusion or stenosis of basilar artery**
  - + **I63.23 Cerebral infarction due to unspecified occlusion or stenosis of carotid arteries**
    - MCC **I63.231 Cerebral infarction due to unspecified occlusion or stenosis of right carotid arteries**

      AHA CC: 3Q, 2020, 28-29
    - MCC **I63.232 Cerebral infarction due to unspecified occlusion or stenosis of left carotid arteries**
    - MCC **I63.233 Cerebral infarction due to unspecified occlusion or stenosis of bilateral carotid arteries**
    - MCC **I63.239 Cerebral infarction due to unspecified occlusion or stenosis of unspecified carotid artery**
  - MCC **I63.29 Cerebral infarction due to unspecified occlusion or stenosis of other precerebral arteries**

+ **I63.3 Cerebral infarction due to thrombosis of cerebral arteries**
  - MCC **I63.30 Cerebral infarction due to thrombosis of unspecified cerebral artery**
  - + **I63.31 Cerebral infarction due to thrombosis of middle cerebral artery**
    - MCC **I63.311 Cerebral infarction due to thrombosis of right middle cerebral artery**
    - MCC **I63.312 Cerebral infarction due to thrombosis of left middle cerebral artery**
    - MCC **I63.313 Cerebral infarction due to thrombosis of bilateral middle cerebral arteries**
    - MCC **I63.319 Cerebral infarction due to thrombosis of unspecified middle cerebral artery**
  - + **I63.32 Cerebral infarction due to thrombosis of anterior cerebral artery**
    - MCC **I63.321 Cerebral infarction due to thrombosis of right anterior cerebral artery**
    - MCC **I63.322 Cerebral infarction due to thrombosis of left anterior cerebral artery**
    - MCC **I63.323 Cerebral infarction due to thrombosis of bilateral anterior cerebral arteries**
    - MCC **I63.329 Cerebral infarction due to thrombosis of unspecified anterior cerebral artery**
  - + **I63.33 Cerebral infarction due to thrombosis of posterior cerebral artery**
    - MCC **I63.331 Cerebral infarction due to thrombosis of right posterior cerebral artery**
    - MCC **I63.332 Cerebral infarction due to thrombosis of left posterior cerebral artery**
    - MCC **I63.333 Cerebral infarction due to thrombosis of bilateral posterior cerebral arteries**
    - MCC **I63.339 Cerebral infarction due to thrombosis of unspecified posterior cerebral artery**
  - + **I63.34 Cerebral infarction due to thrombosis of cerebellar artery**
    - MCC **I63.341 Cerebral infarction due to thrombosis of right cerebellar artery**
    - MCC **I63.342 Cerebral infarction due to thrombosis of left cerebellar artery**
    - MCC **I63.343 Cerebral infarction due to thrombosis of bilateral cerebellar arteries**
    - MCC **I63.349 Cerebral infarction due to thrombosis of unspecified cerebellar artery**
  - MCC **I63.39 Cerebral infarction due to thrombosis of other cerebral artery**

+ **I63.4 Cerebral infarction due to embolism of cerebral arteries**
  - MCC **I63.40** **Cerebral infarction due to embolism of unspecified cerebral artery**
  - + **I63.41** **Cerebral infarction due to embolism of middle cerebral artery**
    - MCC **I63.411** **Cerebral infarction due to embolism of right middle cerebral artery**
    - MCC **I63.412** **Cerebral infarction due to embolism of left middle cerebral artery**
    - MCC **I63.413** **Cerebral infarction due to embolism of bilateral middle cerebral arteries**
    - MCC **I63.419** **Cerebral infarction due to embolism of unspecified middle cerebral artery**
  - + **I63.42** **Cerebral infarction due to embolism of anterior cerebral artery**
    - MCC **I63.421** **Cerebral infarction due to embolism of right anterior cerebral artery**
    - MCC **I63.422** **Cerebral infarction due to embolism of left anterior cerebral artery**
    - MCC **I63.423** **Cerebral infarction due to embolism of bilateral anterior cerebral arteries**
    - MCC **I63.429** **Cerebral infarction due to embolism of unspecified anterior cerebral artery**
  - + **I63.43** **Cerebral infarction due to embolism of posterior cerebral artery**
    - MCC **I63.431** **Cerebral infarction due to embolism of right posterior cerebral artery**
    - MCC **I63.432** **Cerebral infarction due to embolism of left posterior cerebral artery**
    - MCC **I63.433** **Cerebral infarction due to embolism of bilateral posterior cerebral arteries**
    - MCC **I63.439** **Cerebral infarction due to embolism of unspecified posterior cerebral artery**
  - + **I63.44** **Cerebral infarction due to embolism of cerebellar artery**
    - MCC **I63.441** **Cerebral infarction due to embolism of right cerebellar artery**
    - MCC **I63.442** **Cerebral infarction due to embolism of left cerebellar artery**
    - MCC **I64.443** **Cerebral infarction due to embolism of bilateral cerebellar arteries**
    - MCC **I63.449** **Cerebral infarction due to embolism of unspecified cerebellar artery**
  - MCC **I63.49** **Cerebral infarction due to embolism of other cerebral artery**

+ **I63.5 Cerebral infarction due to unspecified occlusion or stenosis of cerebral arteries**
  - MCC **I63.50** **Cerebral infarction due to unspecified occlusion or stenosis of unspecified cerebral artery**
  - + **I63.51** **Cerebral infarction due to unspecified occlusion or stenosis of middle cerebral artery**
    - MCC **I63.511** **Cerebral infarction due to unspecified occlusion or stenosis of right middle cerebral artery**
    - MCC **I63.512** **Cerebral infarction due to unspecified occlusion or stenosis of left middle cerebral artery**
    - MCC **I63.513** **Cerebral infarction due to unspecified occlusion or stenosis of bilateral middle cerebral arteries**
    - MCC **I63.519** **Cerebral infarction due to unspecified occlusion or stenosis of unspecified middle cerebral artery**
  - + **I63.52** **Cerebral infarction due to unspecified occlusion or stenosis of anterior cerebral artery**
    - MCC **I63.521** **Cerebral infarction due to unspecified occlusion or stenosis of right anterior cerebral artery**
    - MCC **I63.522** **Cerebral infarction due to unspecified occlusion or stenosis of left anterior cerebral artery**
    - MCC **I63.523** **Cerebral infarction due to unspecified occlusion or stenosis of bilateral anterior cerebral arteries**
    - MCC **I63.529** **Cerebral infarction due to unspecified occlusion or stenosis of unspecified anterior cerebral artery**
  - + **I63.53** **Cerebral infarction due to unspecified occlusion or stenosis of posterior cerebral artery**
    - MCC **I63.531** **Cerebral infarction due to unspecified occlusion or stenosis of right posterior cerebral artery**
    - MCC **I63.532** **Cerebral infarction due to unspecified occlusion or stenosis of left posterior cerebral artery**
      AHA CC: 2Q, 2017, 10
    - MCC **I63.533** **Cerebral infarction due to unspecified occlusion or stenosis of bilateral posterior cerebral arteries**
    - MCC **I63.539** **Cerebral infarction due to unspecified occlusion or stenosis of unspecified posterior cerebral artery**
  - + **I63.54** **Cerebral infarction due to unspecified occlusion or stenosis of cerebellar artery**
    - MCC **I63.541** **Cerebral infarction due to unspecified occlusion or stenosis of right cerebellar artery**
    - MCC **I63.542** **Cerebral infarction due to unspecified occlusion or stenosis of left cerebellar artery**
    - MCC **I63.543** **Cerebral infarction due to unspecified occlusion or stenosis of bilateral cerebellar arteries**
    - MCC **I63.549** **Cerebral infarction due to unspecified occlusion or stenosis of unspecified cerebellar artery**
  - MCC **I63.59** **Cerebral infarction due to unspecified occlusion or stenosis of other cerebral artery**

MCC **I63.6** **Cerebral infarction due to cerebral venous thrombosis, nonpyogenic**

+ **I63.8** **Other cerebral infarction**
  AHA CC: 2Q, 2017, 9-10; 4Q, 2018, 16
  - MCC **I63.81** **Other cerebral infarction due to occlusion or stenosis of small artery**
    Lacunar infarction
    AHA CC: 4Q, 2018, 16; 3Q, 2020, 27-28
  - MCC **I63.89** **Other cerebral infarction**

MCC **I63.9** **Cerebral infarction, unspecified**
Stroke NOS
Excludes2: *transient cerebral ischemic attacks and related syndromes (G45.-)*
AHA CC: 1Q, 2015, 26; 4Q, 2016, 61-62

I65 Occlusion and stenosis of precerebral arteries, not resulting in cerebral infarction

Includes: embolism of precerebral artery
narrowing of precerebral artery
obstruction (complete) (partial) of precerebral artery
thrombosis of precerebral artery

Excludes1: *insufficiency, NOS, of precerebral artery (G45.-)*
insufficiency of precerebral arteries causing cerebral infarction (I63.0-I63.2)

+ **I65.0** **Occlusion and stenosis of vertebral artery**
  - **I65.01** **Occlusion and stenosis of right vertebral artery**
  - **I65.02** **Occlusion and stenosis of left vertebral artery**
  - **I65.03** **Occlusion and stenosis of bilateral vertebral arteries**
  - **I65.09** **Occlusion and stenosis of unspecified vertebral artery**

I65.1 **Occlusion and stenosis of basilar artery**

+ **I65.2** **Occlusion and stenosis of carotid artery**
  - **I65.21** **Occlusion and stenosis of right carotid artery**
  - **I65.22** **Occlusion and stenosis of left carotid artery**
    AHA CC: 3Q, 2020, 28-29
  - **I65.23** **Occlusion and stenosis of bilateral carotid arteries**
    AHA CC: 2Q, 2018, 9; 1Q, 2021, 4
  - **I65.29** **Occlusion and stenosis of unspecified carotid artery**

I65.8 **Occlusion and stenosis of other precerebral arteries**

I65.9 **Occlusion and stenosis of unspecified precerebral artery**
Occlusion and stenosis of precerebral artery NOS

I66 Occlusion and stenosis of cerebral arteries, not resulting in cerebral infarction

Includes: embolism of cerebral artery
narrowing of cerebral artery
obstruction (complete) (partial) of cerebral artery
thrombosis of cerebral artery

Excludes1: *Occlusion and stenosis of cerebral artery causing cerebral infarction (I63.3-I63.5)*

\+ **I66.0 Occlusion and stenosis of middle cerebral artery**
I66.01 Occlusion and stenosis of right middle cerebral artery
I66.02 Occlusion and stenosis of left middle cerebral artery
I66.03 Occlusion and stenosis of bilateral middle cerebral arteries
I66.09 Occlusion and stenosis of unspecified middle cerebral artery

\+ **I66.1 Occlusion and stenosis of anterior cerebral artery**
I66.11 Occlusion and stenosis of right anterior cerebral artery
I66.12 Occlusion and stenosis of left anterior cerebral artery
I66.13 Occlusion and stenosis of bilateral anterior cerebral arteries
I66.19 Occlusion and stenosis of unspecified anterior cerebral artery

\+ **I66.2 Occlusion and stenosis of posterior cerebral artery**
I66.21 Occlusion and stenosis of right posterior cerebral artery
I66.22 Occlusion and stenosis of left posterior cerebral artery
I66.23 Occlusion and stenosis of bilateral posterior cerebral arteries
I66.29 Occlusion and stenosis of unspecified posterior cerebral artery

I66.3 Occlusion and stenosis of cerebellar arteries
I66.8 Occlusion and stenosis of other cerebral arteries
Occlusion and stenosis of perforating arteries
I66.9 Occlusion and stenosis of unspecified cerebral artery

I67 Other cerebrovascular diseases

Excludes2: *sequelae of the listed conditions (I69.8)*

MCC **I67.0 Dissection of cerebral arteries, nonruptured**
Excludes1: *ruptured cerebral arteries (I60.7)*

I67.1 Cerebral aneurysm, nonruptured
Cerebral aneurysm NOS
Cerebral arteriovenous fistula, acquired
Internal carotid artery aneurysm, intracranial portion
Internal carotid artery aneurysm, NOS
Excludes1: *congenital cerebral aneurysm, nonruptured (Q28.-)*
ruptured cerebral aneurysm (I60.7)

• **I67.2 Cerebral atherosclerosis**
Atheroma of cerebral and precerebral arteries

CC **I67.3 Progressive vascular leukoencephalopathy**
Binswanger's disease

CC **I67.4 Hypertensive encephalopathy**
Excludes2: *insufficiency, NOS, of precerebral arteries (G45.2)*

CC **I67.5 Moyamoya disease**

CC **I67.6 Nonpyogenic thrombosis of intracranial venous system**
Nonpyogenic thrombosis of cerebral vein
Nonpyogenic thrombosis of intracranial venous sinus
Excludes1: *nonpyogenic thrombosis of intracranial venous system causing infarction (I63.6)*

CC **I67.7 Cerebral arteritis, not elsewhere classified**
Granulomatous angiitis of the nervous system
Excludes1: *allergic granulomatous angiitis (M30.1)*

\+ **I67.8 Other specified cerebrovascular diseases**
AHA CC: 4Q, 2018, 17

CC **I67.81 Acute cerebrovascular insufficiency**
Acute cerebrovascular insufficiency unspecified as to location or reversibility

CC **I67.82 Cerebral ischemia**
Chronic cerebral ischemia

MCC **I67.83 Posterior reversible encephalopathy syndrome**
PRES

\+ **I67.84 Cerebral vasospasm and vasoconstriction**

CC **I67.841 Reversible cerebrovascular vasoconstriction syndrome**
Call-Fleming syndrome
Code first underlying condition, if applicable, such as eclampsia (O15.00-O15.9)

CC **I67.848 Other cerebrovascular vasospasm and vasoconstriction**

\+ **I67.85 Hereditary cerebrovascular diseases**

CC **I67.850 Cerebral autosomal dominant arteriopathy with subcortical infarcts and leukoencephalopathy**
CADASIL
Code also any associated diagnoses, such as:
epilepsy (G40.-)
stroke (I63.-)
vascular dementia (F01.-)

CC **I67.858 Other hereditary cerebrovascular disease**

CC **I67.89 Other cerebrovascular disease**

I67.9 Cerebrovascular disease, unspecified

I68 Cerebrovascular disorders in diseases classified elsewhere

I68.0 Cerebral amyloid angiopathy
Code first underlying amyloidosis (E85.-)

CC **I68.2 Cerebral arteritis in other diseases classified elsewhere**
Code first underlying disease
Excludes1: *cerebral arteritis (in):*
listerosis (A32.89)
systemic lupus erythematosus (M32.19)
syphilis (A52.04)
tuberculosis (A18.89)

I68.8 Other cerebrovascular disorders in diseases classified elsewhere
Code first underlying disease
Excludes1: *syphilitic cerebral aneurysm (A52.05)*

I69 Sequelae of cerebrovascular disease

NOTE Category I69 is to be used to indicate conditions in I60-I67 as the cause of sequelae. The 'sequelae' include conditions specified as such or as residuals which may occur at any time after the onset of the causal condition

Excludes1: *personal history of cerebral infarction without residual deficit (Z86.73)*
personal history of prolonged reversible ischemic neurologic deficit (PRIND) (Z86.73)
personal history of reversible ischemic neurologcial deficit (RIND) (Z86.73)
sequelae of traumatic intracranial injury (S06.-)

Review coding guideline C.9.d
AHA CC: 4Q, 2016, 28

\+ **I69.0 Sequelae of nontraumatic subarachnoid hemorrhage**
I69.00 Unspecified sequelae of nontraumatic subarachnoid hemorrhage
\+ **I69.01 Cognitive deficits following nontraumatic subarachnoid hemorrhage**
I69.010 Attention and concentration deficit following nontraumatic subarachnoid hemorrhage
I69.011 Memory deficit following nontraumatic subarachnoid hemorrhage
I69.012 Visuospatial deficit and spatial neglect following nontraumatic subarachnoid hemorrhage
I69.013 Psychomotor deficit following nontraumatic subarachnoid hemorrhage
I69.014 Frontal lobe and executive function deficit following nontraumatic subarachnoid hemorrhage
I69.015 Cognitive social or emotional deficit following nontraumatic subarachnoid hemorrhage
I69.018 Other symptoms and signs involving cognitive functions following nontraumatic subarachnoid hemorrhage
I69.019 Unspecified symptoms and signs involving cognitive functions following nontraumatic subarachnoid hemorrhage

+ **I69.02 Speech and language deficits following nontraumatic subarachnoid hemorrhage**
  - **I69.020 Aphasia following nontraumatic subarachnoid hemorrhage**
  - **I69.021 Dysphasia following nontraumatic subarachnoid hemorrhage**
  - **I69.022 Dysarthria following nontraumatic subarachnoid hemorrhage**
  - **I69.023 Fluency disorder following nontraumatic subarachnoid hemorrhage**
    Stuttering following nontraumatic subarachnoid hemorrhage
  - **I69.028 Other speech and language deficits following nontraumatic subarachnoid hemorrhage**

+ **I69.03 Monoplegia of upper limb following nontraumatic subarachnoid hemorrhage**
  - **I69.031 Monoplegia of upper limb following nontraumatic subarachnoid hemorrhage affecting right dominant side**
  - **I69.032 Monoplegia of upper limb following nontraumatic subarachnoid hemorrhage affecting left dominant side**
  - **I69.033 Monoplegia of upper limb following nontraumatic subarachnoid hemorrhage affecting right non-dominant side**
  - **I69.034 Monoplegia of upper limb following nontraumatic subarachnoid hemorrhage affecting left non-dominant side**
  - **I69.039 Monoplegia of upper limb following nontraumatic subarachnoid hemorrhage affecting unspecified side**

+ **I69.04 Monoplegia of lower limb following nontraumatic subarachnoid hemorrhage**
  - **I69.041 Monoplegia of lower limb following nontraumatic subarachnoid hemorrhage affecting right dominant side**
  - **I69.042 Monoplegia of lower limb following nontraumatic subarachnoid hemorrhage affecting left dominant side**
  - **I69.043 Monoplegia of lower limb following nontraumatic subarachnoid hemorrhage affecting right non-dominant side**
  - **I69.044 Monoplegia of lower limb following nontraumatic subarachnoid hemorrhage affecting left non-dominant side**
  - **I69.049 Monoplegia of lower limb following nontraumatic subarachnoid hemorrhage affecting unspecified side**

+ **I69.05 Hemiplegia and hemiparesis following nontraumatic subarachnoid hemorrhage**
  - CC **I69.051 Hemiplegia and hemiparesis following nontraumatic subarachnoid hemorrhage affecting right dominant side**
  - CC **I69.052 Hemiplegia and hemiparesis following nontraumatic subarachnoid hemorrhage affecting left dominant side**
  - CC **I69.053 Hemiplegia and hemiparesis following nontraumatic subarachnoid hemorrhage affecting right non-dominant side**
  - CC **I69.054 Hemiplegia and hemiparesis following nontraumatic subarachnoid hemorrhage affecting left non-dominant side**
  - CC **I69.059 Hemiplegia and hemiparesis following nontraumatic subarachnoid hemorrhage affecting unspecified side**

+ **I69.06 Other paralytic syndrome following nontraumatic subarachnoid hemorrhage**
  Use additional code to identify type of paralytic syndrome, such as:
  locked-in state (G83.5)
  quadriplegia (G82.5-)
  Excludes1: *hemiplegia/hemiparesis following nontraumatic subarachnoid hemorrhage (I69.05-)*
  monoplegia of lower limb following nontraumatic subarachnoid hemorrhage (I69.04-)
  monoplegia of upper limb following nontraumatic subarachnoid hemorrhage (I69.03-)
  - **I69.061 Other paralytic syndrome following nontraumatic subarachnoid hemorrhage affecting right dominant side**
  - **I69.062 Other paralytic syndrome following nontraumatic subarachnoid hemorrhage affecting left dominant side**
  - **I69.063 Other paralytic syndrome following nontraumatic subarachnoid hemorrhage affecting right non-dominant side**
  - **I69.064 Other paralytic syndrome following nontraumatic subarachnoid hemorrhage affecting left non-dominant side**
  - **I69.065 Other paralytic syndrome following nontraumatic subarachnoid hemorrhage, bilateral**
  - **I69.069 Other paralytic syndrome following nontraumatic subarachnoid hemorrhage affecting unspecified side**

+ **I69.09 Other sequelae of nontraumatic subarachnoid hemorrhage**
  - **I69.090 Apraxia following nontraumatic subarachnoid hemorrhage**
  - **I69.091 Dysphagia following nontraumatic subarachnoid hemorrhage**
    Use additional code to identify the type of dysphagia, if known (R13.1-)
  - **I69.092 Facial weakness following nontraumatic subarachnoid hemorrhage**
    Facial droop following nontraumatic subarachnoid hemorrhage
  - **I69.093 Ataxia following nontraumatic subarachnoid hemorrhage**
  - **I69.098 Other sequelae following nontraumatic subarachnoid hemorrhage**
    Alterations of sensation following nontraumatic subarachnoid hemorrhage
    Disturbance of vision following nontraumatic subarachnoid hemorrhage
    Use additional code to identify the sequelae

+ **I69.1 Sequelae of nontraumatic intracerebral hemorrhage**
  - **I69.10 Unspecified sequelae of nontraumatic intracerebral hemorrhage**

+ **I69.11 Cognitive deficits following nontraumatic intracerebral hemorrhage**
  - **I69.110 Attention and concentration deficit following nontraumatic intracerebral hemorrhage**
  - **I69.111 Memory deficit following nontraumatic intracerebral hemorrhage**
  - **I69.112 Visuospatial deficit and spatial neglect following nontraumatic intracerebral hemorrhage**
  - **I69.113 Psychomotor deficit following nontraumatic intracerebral hemorrhage**
  - **I69.114 Frontal lobe and executive function deficit following nontraumatic intracerebral hemorrhage**

I69.115 **Cognitive social or emotional deficit following nontraumatic intracerebral hemorrhage**

I69.118 **Other symptoms and signs involving cognitive functions following nontraumatic intracerebral hemorrhage**

I69.119 **Unspecified symptoms and signs involving cognitive functions following nontraumatic intracerebral hemorrhage**

\+ **I69.12 Speech and language deficits following nontraumatic intracerebral hemorrhage**

I69.120 **Aphasia following nontraumatic intracerebral hemorrhage**

I69.121 **Dysphasia following nontraumatic intracerebral hemorrhage**

I69.122 **Dysarthria following nontraumatic intracerebral hemorrhage**

I69.123 **Fluency disorder following nontraumatic intracerebral hemorrhage**

Stuttering following nontraumatic intracerebral hemorrhage

I69.128 **Other speech and language deficits following nontraumatic intracerebral hemorrhage**

\+ **I69.13 Monoplegia of upper limb following nontraumatic intracerebral hemorrhage**

I69.131 **Monoplegia of upper limb following nontraumatic intracerebral hemorrhage affecting right dominant side**

I69.132 **Monoplegia of upper limb following nontraumatic intracerebral hemorrhage affecting left dominant side**

I69.133 **Monoplegia of upper limb following nontraumatic intracerebral hemorrhage affecting right non-dominant side**

I69.134 **Monoplegia of upper limb following nontraumatic intracerebral hemorrhage affecting left non-dominant side**

I69.139 **Monoplegia of upper limb following nontraumatic intracerebral hemorrhage affecting unspecified side**

\+ **I69.14 Monoplegia of lower limb following nontraumatic intracerebral hemorrhage**

I69.141 **Monoplegia of lower limb following nontraumatic intracerebral hemorrhage affecting right dominant side**

I69.142 **Monoplegia of lower limb following nontraumatic intracerebral hemorrhage affecting left dominant side**

I69.143 **Monoplegia of lower limb following nontraumatic intracerebral hemorrhage affecting right non-dominant side**

I69.144 **Monoplegia of lower limb following nontraumatic intracerebral hemorrhage affecting left non-dominant side**

I69.149 **Monoplegia of lower limb following nontraumatic intracerebral hemorrhage affecting unspecified side**

\+ **I69.15 Hemiplegia and hemiparesis following nontraumatic intracerebral hemorrhage**

CC I69.151 **Hemiplegia and hemiparesis following nontraumatic intracerebral hemorrhage affecting right dominant side**

CC I69.152 **Hemiplegia and hemiparesis following nontraumatic intracerebral hemorrhage affecting left dominant side**

CC I69.153 **Hemiplegia and hemiparesis following nontraumatic intracerebral hemorrhage affecting right non-dominant side**

CC I69.154 **Hemiplegia and hemiparesis following nontraumatic intracerebral hemorrhage affecting left non-dominant side**

CC I69.159 **Hemiplegia and hemiparesis following nontraumatic intracerebral hemorrhage affecting unspecified side**

\+ **I69.16 Other paralytic syndrome following nontraumatic intracerebral hemorrhage**

Use additional code to identify type of paralytic syndrome, such as:
locked-in state (G83.5)
quadriplegia (G82.5-)

Excludes1: *hemiplegia/hemiparesis following nontraumatic intracerebral hemorrhage (I69.15-)*
monoplegia of lower limb following nontraumatic intracerebral hemorrhage (I69.14-)
monoplegia of upper limb following nontraumatic intracerebral hemorrhage (I69.13-)

I69.161 **Other paralytic syndrome following nontraumatic intracerebral hemorrhage affecting right dominant side**

I69.162 **Other paralytic syndrome following nontraumatic intracerebral hemorrhage affecting left dominant side**

I69.163 **Other paralytic syndrome following nontraumatic intracerebral hemorrhage affecting right non-dominant side**

I69.164 **Other paralytic syndrome following nontraumatic intracerebral hemorrhage affecting left non-dominant side**

I69.165 **Other paralytic syndrome following nontraumatic intracerebral hemorrhage, bilateral**

I69.169 **Other paralytic syndrome following nontraumatic intracerebral hemorrhage affecting unspecified side**

\+ **I69.19 Other sequelae of nontraumatic intracerebral hemorrhage**

I69.190 **Apraxia following nontraumatic intracerebral hemorrhage**

I69.191 **Dysphagia following nontraumatic intracerebral hemorrhage**

Use additional code to identify the type of dysphagia, if known (R13.1-)

I69.192 **Facial weakness following nontraumatic intracerebral hemorrhage**

Facial droop following nontraumatic intracerebral hemorrhage

I69.193 **Ataxia following nontraumatic intracerebral hemorrhage**

I69.198 **Other sequelae of nontraumatic intracerebral hemorrhage**

Alteration of sensations following nontraumatic intracerebral hemorrhage
Disturbance of vision following nontraumatic intracerebral hemorrhage
Use additional code to identify the sequelae

\+ **I69.2 Sequelae of other nontraumatic intracranial hemorrhage**

I69.20 **Unspecified sequelae of other nontraumatic intracranial hemorrhage**

\+ **I69.21 Cognitive deficits following other nontraumatic intracranial hemorrhage**

I69.210 **Attention and concentration deficit following other nontraumatic intracranial hemorrhage**

I69.211 **Memory deficit following other nontraumatic intracranial hemorrhage**

I69.212 **Visuospatial deficit and spatial neglect following other nontraumatic intracranial hemorrhage**

I69.213 **Psychomotor deficit following other nontraumatic intracranial hemorrhage**

I69.214 **Frontal lobe and executive function deficit following other nontraumatic intracranial hemorrhage**

I69.215 **Cognitive social or emotional deficit following other nontraumatic intracranial hemorrhage**

I69.218 Other symptoms and signs involving cognitive functions following other nontraumatic intracranial hemorrhage

I69.219 Unspecified symptoms and signs involving cognitive functions following other nontraumatic intracranial hemorrhage

+ I69.22 Speech and language deficits following other nontraumatic intracranial hemorrhage

I69.220 Aphasia following other nontraumatic intracranial hemorrhage

I69.221 Dysphasia following other nontraumatic intracranial hemorrhage

I69.222 Dysarthria following other nontraumatic intracranial hemorrhage

I69.223 Fluency disorder following other nontraumatic intracranial hemorrhage

Stuttering following other nontraumatic intracranial hemorrhage

I69.228 Other speech and language deficits following other nontraumatic intracranial hemorrhage

+ I69.23 Monoplegia of upper limb following other nontraumatic intracranial hemorrhage

I69.231 Monoplegia of upper limb following other nontraumatic intracranial hemorrhage affecting right dominant side

I69.232 Monoplegia of upper limb following other nontraumatic intracranial hemorrhage affecting left dominant side

I69.233 Monoplegia of upper limb following other nontraumatic intracranial hemorrhage affecting right non-dominant side

I69.234 Monoplegia of upper limb following other nontraumatic intracranial hemorrhage affecting left non-dominant side

I69.239 Monoplegia of upper limb following other nontraumatic intracranial hemorrhage affecting unspecified side

+ I69.24 Monoplegia of lower limb following other nontraumatic intracranial hemorrhage

I69.241 Monoplegia of lower limb following other nontraumatic intracranial hemorrhage affecting right dominant side

I69.242 Monoplegia of lower limb following other nontraumatic intracranial hemorrhage affecting left dominant side

I69.243 Monoplegia of lower limb following other nontraumatic intracranial hemorrhage affecting right non-dominant side

I69.244 Monoplegia of lower limb following other nontraumatic intracranial hemorrhage affecting left non-dominant side

I69.249 Monoplegia of lower limb following other nontraumatic intracranial hemorrhage affecting unspecified side

+ I69.25 Hemiplegia and hemiparesis following other nontraumatic intracranial hemorrhage

CC **I69.251 Hemiplegia and hemiparesis following other nontraumatic intracranial hemorrhage affecting right dominant side**

CC **I69.252 Hemiplegia and hemiparesis following other nontraumatic intracranial hemorrhage affecting left dominant side**

CC **I69.253 Hemiplegia and hemiparesis following other nontraumatic intracranial hemorrhage affecting right non-dominant side**

CC **I69.254 Hemiplegia and hemiparesis following other nontraumatic intracranial hemorrhage affecting left non-dominant side**

CC **I69.259 Hemiplegia and hemiparesis following other nontraumatic intracranial hemorrhage affecting unspecified side**

+ I69.26 Other paralytic syndrome following other nontraumatic intracranial hemorrhage

Use additional code to identify type of paralytic syndrome, such as:
locked-in state (G83.5)
quadriplegia (G82.5-)

Excludes1: *hemiplegia/hemiparesis following other nontraumatic intracranial hemorrhage (I69.25-)*
monoplegia of lower limb following other nontraumatic intracranial hemorrhage (I69.24-)
monoplegia of upper limb following other nontraumatic intracranial hemorrhage (I69.23-)

I69.261 Other paralytic syndrome following other nontraumatic intracranial hemorrhage affecting right dominant side

I69.262 Other paralytic syndrome following other nontraumatic intracranial hemorrhage affecting left dominant side

I69.263 Other paralytic syndrome following other nontraumatic intracranial hemorrhage affecting right non-dominant side

I69.264 Other paralytic syndrome following other nontraumatic intracranial hemorrhage affecting left non-dominant side

I69.265 Other paralytic syndrome following other nontraumatic intracranial hemorrhage, bilateral

I69.269 Other paralytic syndrome following other nontraumatic intracranial hemorrhage affecting unspecified side

+ I69.29 Other sequelae of other nontraumatic intracranial hemorrhage

I69.290 Apraxia following other nontraumatic intracranial hemorrhage

I69.291 Dysphagia following other nontraumatic intracranial hemorrhage

Use additional code to identify the type of dysphagia, if known (R13.1-)

I69.292 Facial weakness following other nontraumatic intracranial hemorrhage

Facial droop following other nontraumatic intracranial hemorrhage

I69.293 Ataxia following other nontraumatic intracranial hemorrhage

I69.298 Other sequelae of other nontraumatic intracranial hemorrhage

Alteration of sensation following other nontraumatic intracranial hemorrhage
Disturbance of vision following other nontraumatic intracranial hemorrhage
Use additional code to identify the sequelae

+ I69.3 Sequelae of cerebral infarction

Sequelae of stroke NOS
AHA CC: 4Q, 2012, 95; 4Q, 2013, 127-128

I69.30 Unspecified sequelae of cerebral infarction

+ I69.31 Cognitive deficits following cerebral infarction

I69.310 Attention and concentration deficit following cerebral infarction

I69.311 Memory deficit following cerebral infarction

I69.312 Visuospatial deficit and spatial neglect following cerebral infarction

I69.313 Psychomotor deficit following cerebral infarction

I69.314 **Frontal lobe and executive function deficit following cerebral infarction**

I69.315 **Cognitive social or emotional deficit following cerebral infarction**

I69.318 **Other symptoms and signs involving cognitive functions following cerebral infarction**

I69.319 **Unspecified symptoms and signs involving cognitive functions following cerebral infarction**

\+ **I69.32** **Speech and language deficits following cerebral infarction**

I69.320 **Aphasia following cerebral infarction**
AHA CC: 4Q, 2013, 128

I69.321 **Dysphasia following cerebral infarction**
AHA CC: 4Q, 2012, 91

I69.322 **Dysarthria following cerebral infarction**
Excludes2: *transient ischemic attach (TIA) (G45.9)*

I69.323 **Fluency disorder following cerebral infarction**
Stuttering following cerebral hemorrhage

I69.328 **Other speech and language deficits following cerebral infarction**

\+ **I69.33** **Monoplegia of upper limb following cerebral infarction**
AHA CC: 1Q, 2017, 47-48

I69.331 **Monoplegia of upper limb following cerebral infarction affecting right dominant side**

I69.332 **Monoplegia of upper limb following cerebral infarction affecting left dominant side**

I69.333 **Monoplegia of upper limb following cerebral infarction affecting right non-dominant side**

I69.334 **Monoplegia of upper limb following cerebral infarction affecting left non-dominant side**

I69.339 **Monoplegia of upper limb following cerebral infarction affecting unspecified side**

\+ **I69.34** **Monoplegia of lower limb following cerebral infarction**
AHA CC: 1Q, 2017, 47-48

I69.341 **Monoplegia of lower limb following cerebral infarction affecting right dominant side**

I69.342 **Monoplegia of lower limb following cerebral infarction affecting left dominant side**

I69.343 **Monoplegia of lower limb following cerebral infarction affecting right non-dominant side**

I69.344 **Monoplegia of lower limb following cerebral infarction affecting left non-dominant side**

I69.349 **Monoplegia of lower limb following cerebral infarction affecting unspecified side**

\+ **I69.35** **Hemiplegia and hemiparesis following cerebral infarction**

CC **I69.351** **Hemiplegia and hemiparesis following cerebral infarction affecting right dominant side**
Excludes2: *transient ischemic attach (TIA) (G45.9)*
AHA CC: 4Q, 2013, 128; 1Q, 2015, 25

CC **I69.352** **Hemiplegia and hemiparesis following cerebral infarction affecting left dominant side**

CC **I69.353** **Hemiplegia and hemiparesis following cerebral infarction affecting right non-dominant side**

CC **I69.354** **Hemiplegia and hemiparesis following cerebral infarction affecting left non-dominant side**
AHA CC: 4Q, 2012, 91

CC **I69.359** **Hemiplegia and hemiparesis following cerebral infarction affecting unspecified side**

\+ **I69.36** **Other paralytic syndrome following cerebral infarction**
Use additional code to identify type of paralytic syndrome, such as:
locked-in state (G83.5)
quadriplegia (G82.5-)
Excludes1: *hemiplegia/hemiparesis following cerebral infarction (I69.35-)*
monoplegia of lower limb following cerebral infarction (I69.34-)
monoplegia of upper limb following cerebral infarction (I69.33-)

I69.361 **Other paralytic syndrome following cerebral infarction affecting right dominant side**

I69.362 **Other paralytic syndrome following cerebral infarction affecting left dominant side**

I69.363 **Other paralytic syndrome following cerebral infarction affecting right non-dominant side**

I69.364 **Other paralytic syndrome following cerebral infarction affecting left non-dominant side**

I69.365 **Other paralytic syndrome following cerebral infarction, bilateral**

I69.369 **Other paralytic syndrome following cerebral infarction affecting unspecified side**

\+ **I69.39** **Other sequelae of cerebral infarction**

I69.390 **Apraxia following cerebral infarction**

I69.391 **Dysphagia following cerebral infarction**
Use additional code to identify the type of dysphagia, if known (R13.1-)

I69.392 **Facial weakness following cerebral infarction**
Facial droop following cerebral infarction

I69.393 **Ataxia following cerebral infarction**

I69.398 **Other sequelae of cerebral infarction**
Alteration of sensation following cerebral infarction
Disturbance of vision following cerebral infarction
Use additional code to identify the sequelae
AHA CC: 2Q, 2020, 29

\+ **I69.8** **Sequelae of other cerebrovascular diseases**
Excludes1: *sequelae of traumatic intracranial injury (S06.-)*

I69.80 **Unspecified sequelae of other cerebrovascular disease**

\+ **I69.81** **Cognitive deficits following other cerebrovascular disease**

I69.810 **Attention and concentration deficit following other cerebrovascular disease**

I69.811 **Memory deficit following other cerebrovascular disease**

I69.812 **Visuospatial deficit and spatial neglect following other cerebrovascular disease**

I69.813 **Psychomotor deficit following other cerebrovascular disease**

I69.814 **Frontal lobe and executive function deficit following other cerebrovascular disease**

I69.815 **Cognitive social or emotional deficit following other cerebrovascular disease**

I69.818 **Other symptoms and signs involving cognitive functions following other cerebrovascular disease**

I69.819 **Unspecified symptoms and signs involving cognitive functions following other cerebrovascular disease**

\+ **I69.82** **Speech and language deficits following other cerebrovascular disease**

I69.820 **Aphasia following other cerebrovascular disease**

I69.821 **Dysphasia following other cerebrovascular disease**

I69.822 **Dysarthria following other cerebrovascular disease**

I69.823 **Fluency disorder following other cerebrovascular disease**
Stuttering following other cerebrovascular disease hemorrhage

I69.828 **Other speech and language deficits following other cerebrovascular disease**
AHA CC: 3Q, 2019, 8-9

+ I69.83 **Monoplegia of upper limb following other cerebrovascular disease**

I69.831 **Monoplegia of upper limb following other cerebrovascular disease affecting right dominant side**

I69.832 **Monoplegia of upper limb following other cerebrovascular disease affecting left dominant side**

I69.833 **Monoplegia of upper limb following other cerebrovascular disease affecting right non-dominant side**

I69.834 **Monoplegia of upper limb following other cerebrovascular disease affecting left non-dominant side**

I69.839 **Monoplegia of upper limb following other cerebrovascular disease affecting unspecified side**

+ I69.84 **Monoplegia of lower limb following other cerebrovascular disease**

I69.841 **Monoplegia of lower limb following other cerebrovascular disease affecting right dominant side**

I69.842 **Monoplegia of lower limb following other cerebrovascular disease affecting left dominant side**

I69.843 **Monoplegia of lower limb following other cerebrovascular disease affecting right non-dominant side**

I69.844 **Monoplegia of lower limb following other cerebrovascular disease affecting left non-dominant side**

I69.849 **Monoplegia of lower limb following other cerebrovascular disease affecting unspecified side**

+ I69.85 **Hemiplegia and hemiparesis following other cerebrovascular disease**

CC I69.851 **Hemiplegia and hemiparesis following other cerebrovascular disease affecting right dominant side**

CC I69.852 **Hemiplegia and hemiparesis following other cerebrovascular disease affecting left dominant side**

CC I69.853 **Hemiplegia and hemiparesis following other cerebrovascular disease affecting right non-dominant side**

CC I69.854 **Hemiplegia and hemiparesis following other cerebrovascular disease affecting left non-dominant side**

CC I69.859 **Hemiplegia and hemiparesis following other cerebrovascular disease affecting unspecified side**

+ I69.86 **Other paralytic syndrome following other cerebrovascular disease**
Use additional code to identify type of paralytic syndrome, such as:
locked-in state (G83.5)
quadriplegia (G82.5-)
Excludes1: *hemiplegia/hemiparesis following other cerebrovascular disease (I69.85-)*
monoplegia of lower limb following other cerebrovascular disease (I69.84-)
monoplegia of upper limb following other cerebrovascular disease (I69.83-)

I69.861 **Other paralytic syndrome following other cerebrovascular disease affecting right dominant side**

I69.862 **Other paralytic syndrome following other cerebrovascular disease affecting left dominant side**

I69.863 **Other paralytic syndrome following other cerebrovascular disease affecting right non-dominant side**

I69.864 **Other paralytic syndrome following other cerebrovascular disease affecting left non-dominant side**

I69.865 **Other paralytic syndrome following other cerebrovascular disease, bilateral**

I69.869 **Other paralytic syndrome following other cerebrovascular disease affecting unspecified side**

+ I69.89 **Other sequelae of other cerebrovascular disease**

I69.890 **Apraxia following other cerebrovascular disease**

I69.891 **Dysphagia following other cerebrovascular disease**
Use additional code to identify the type of dysphagia, if known (R13.1-)

I69.892 **Facial weakness following other cerebrovascular disease**
Facial droop following other cerebrovascular disease

I69.893 **Ataxia following other cerebrovascular disease**

I69.898 **Other sequelae of other cerebrovascular disease**
Alteration of sensation following other cerebrovascular disease
Disturbance of vision following other cerebrovascular disease
Use additional code to identify the sequelae

+ I69.9 **Sequelae of unspecified cerebrovascular diseases**
Excludes1: *sequelae of stroke (I69.3)*
sequelae of traumatic intracranial injury (S06.-)

I69.90 **Unspecified sequelae of unspecified cerebrovascular disease**

+ I69.91 **Cognitive deficits following unspecified cerebrovascular disease**

I69.910 **Attention and concentration deficit following unspecified cerebrovascular disease**

I69.911 **Memory deficit following unspecified cerebrovascular disease**

I69.912 **Visuospatial deficit and spatial neglect following unspecified cerebrovascular disease**

I69.913 **Psychomotor deficit following unspecified cerebrovascular disease**

I69.914 **Frontal lobe and executive function deficit following unspecified cerebrovascular disease**

I69.915 **Cognitive social or emotional deficit following unspecified cerebrovascular disease**

I69.918 **Other symptoms and signs involving cognitive functions following unspecified cerebrovascular disease**

I69.919 **Unspecified symptoms and signs involving cognitive functions following unspecified cerebrovascular disease**

+ I69.92 **Speech and language deficits following unspecified cerebrovascular disease**

I69.920 **Aphasia following unspecified cerebrovascular disease**

I69.921 **Dysphasia following unspecified cerebrovascular disease**

I69.922 **Dysarthria following unspecified cerebrovascular disease**

I69.923 **Fluency disorder following unspecified cerebrovascular disease**
Stuttering following unspecified cerebrovascular disease

I69.928 **Other speech and language deficits following unspecified cerebrovascular disease**

+ I69.93 **Monoplegia of upper limb following unspecified cerebrovascular disease**

I69.931 **Monoplegia of upper limb following unspecified cerebrovascular disease affecting right dominant side**

I69.932 **Monoplegia of upper limb following unspecified cerebrovascular disease affecting left dominant side**

I69.933 **Monoplegia of upper limb following unspecified cerebrovascular disease affecting right non-dominant side**

I69.934 **Monoplegia of upper limb following unspecified cerebrovascular disease affecting left non-dominant side**

I69.939 **Monoplegia of upper limb following unspecified cerebrovascular disease affecting unspecified side**

+ I69.94 **Monoplegia of lower limb following unspecified cerebrovascular disease**

I69.941 **Monoplegia of lower limb following unspecified cerebrovascular disease affecting right dominant side**

I69.942 **Monoplegia of lower limb following unspecified cerebrovascular disease affecting left dominant side**

I69.943 **Monoplegia of lower limb following unspecified cerebrovascular disease affecting right non-dominant side**

I69.944 **Monoplegia of lower limb following unspecified cerebrovascular disease affecting left non-dominant side**

I69.949 **Monoplegia of lower limb following unspecified cerebrovascular disease affecting unspecified side**

+ I69.95 **Hemiplegia and hemiparesis following unspecified cerebrovascular disease**

CC **I69.951** **Hemiplegia and hemiparesis following unspecified cerebrovascular disease affecting right dominant side**

CC **I69.952** **Hemiplegia and hemiparesis following unspecified cerebrovascular disease affecting left dominant side**

CC **I69.953** **Hemiplegia and hemiparesis following unspecified cerebrovascular disease affecting right non-dominant side**

CC **I69.954** **Hemiplegia and hemiparesis following unspecified cerebrovascular disease affecting left non-dominant side**

CC **I69.959** **Hemiplegia and hemiparesis following unspecified cerebrovascular disease affecting unspecified side**

+ I69.96 **Other paralytic syndrome following unspecified cerebrovascular disease**

Use additional code to identify type of paralytic syndrome, such as:
locked-in state (G83.5)
quadriplegia (G82.5-)

Excludes1: *hemiplegia/hemiparesis following unspecifiedcerebrovasculardisease (I69.95-)*
monoplegia of lower limb following unspecified cerebrovascular disease (I69.94-)
monoplegia of upper limb following unspecified cerebrovascular disease (I69.93-)

I69.961 **Other paralytic syndrome following unspecified cerebrovascular disease affecting right dominant side**

I69.962 **Other paralytic syndrome following unspecified cerebrovascular disease affecting left dominant side**

I69.963 **Other paralytic syndrome following unspecified cerebrovascular disease affecting right non-dominant side**

I69.964 **Other paralytic syndrome following unspecified cerebrovascular disease affecting left non-dominant side**

I69.965 **Other paralytic syndrome following unspecified cerebrovascular disease, bilateral**

I69.969 **Other paralytic syndrome following unspecified cerebrovascular disease affecting unspecified side**

+ I69.99 **Other sequelae of unspecified cerebrovascular disease**

I69.990 **Apraxia following unspecified cerebrovascular disease**

I69.991 **Dysphagia following unspecified cerebrovascular disease**

Use additional code to identify the type of dysphagia, if known (R13.1-)

I69.992 **Facial weakness following unspecified cerebrovascular disease**

Facial droop following unspecified cerebrovascular disease

I69.993 **Ataxia following unspecified cerebrovascular disease**

I69.998 **Other sequelae following unspecified cerebrovascular disease**

Alteration in sensation following unspecified cerebrovascular disease
Disturbance of vision following unspecified cerebrovascular disease
Use additional code to identify the sequelae

Diseases of arteries, arterioles and capillaries (I70-I79)

I70 Atherosclerosis

Includes: arteriolosclerosis
arterial degeneration
arteriosclerosis
arteriosclerotic vascular disease
arteriovascular degeneration
atheroma
endarteritis deformans or obliterans
senile arteritis
senile endarteritis
vascular degeneration

Use additional code to identify:
exposure to environmental tobacco smoke (Z77.22)
history of tobacco dependence (Z87.891)
occupational exposure to environmental tobacco smoke (Z57.31)
tobacco dependence (F17.-)
tobacco use (Z72.0)

Excludes2: *arteriosclerotic cardiovascular disease (I25.1-)*
arteriosclerotic heart disease (I25.1-)
atheroembolism (I75.-)
cerebral atherosclerosis (I67.2)
coronary atherosclerosis (I25.1-)
mesenteric atherosclerosis (K55.1)
precerebral atherosclerosis (I67.2)
primary pulmonary atherosclerosis (I27.0)

AHA CC: 4Q, 2020, 98-99

• **I70.0** **Atherosclerosis of aorta**

• **I70.1** **Atherosclerosis of renal artery**

Goldblatt's kidney

Excludes2: *atherosclerosis of renal arterioles (I12.-)*

+ I70.2 **Atherosclerosis of native arteries of the extremities**

Mönckeberg's (medial) sclerosis

Use additional code, if applicable, to identify chronic total occlusion of artery of extremity (I70.92)

Excludes2: *atherosclerosis of bypass graft of extremities (I70.30-I70.79)*

AHA CC: 3Q, 2018, 4

+ I70.20 **Unspecified atherosclerosis of native arteries of extremities**

• **I70.201** **Unspecified atherosclerosis of native arteries of extremities, right leg**

• **I70.202** **Unspecified atherosclerosis of native arteries of extremities, left leg**

• **I70.203** **Unspecified atherosclerosis of native arteries of extremities, bilateral legs**

• **I70.208** **Unspecified atherosclerosis of native arteries of extremities, other extremity**

• **I70.209** **Unspecified atherosclerosis of native arteries of extremities, unspecified extremity**

+ **I70.21 Atherosclerosis of native arteries of extremities with intermittent claudication**
- **I70.211 Atherosclerosis of native arteries of extremities with intermittent claudication, right leg**
- **I70.212 Atherosclerosis of native arteries of extremities with intermittent claudication, left leg**
- **I70.213 Atherosclerosis of native arteries of extremities with intermittent claudication, bilateral legs**
- **I70.218 Atherosclerosis of native arteries of extremities with intermittent claudication, other extremity**
- **I70.219 Atherosclerosis of native arteries of extremities with intermittent claudication, unspecified extremity**

+ **I70.22 Atherosclerosis of native arteries of extremities with rest pain**

Includes: any condition classifiable to I70.21-
chronic limb-threatening ischemia NOS of native arteries of the extremities
chronic limb-threatening ischemia of native arteries of the extremities with rest pain
critical limb ischemia NOS of native arteries of the extremities
critical limb ischemia of native arteries of the extremities with rest pain

- **I70.221 Atherosclerosis of native arteries of extremities with rest pain, right leg**
- **I70.222 Atherosclerosis of native arteries of extremities with rest pain, left leg**
- **I70.223 Atherosclerosis of native arteries of extremities with rest pain, bilateral legs**
- **I70.228 Atherosclerosis of native arteries of extremities with rest pain, other extremity**
- **I70.229 Atherosclerosis of native arteries of extremities with rest pain, unspecified extremity**

+ **I70.23 Atherosclerosis of native arteries of right leg with ulceration**

Includes: any condition classifiable to I70.211 and I70.221
chronic limb-threatening ischemia of native arteries of right leg with ulceration
critical limb ischemia of native arteries of right leg with ulceration

Use additional code to identify severity of ulcer (L97.-)

- **I70.231 Atherosclerosis of native arteries of right leg with ulceration of thigh**
- **I70.232 Atherosclerosis of native arteries of right leg with ulceration of calf**
- **I70.233 Atherosclerosis of native arteries of right leg with ulceration of ankle**
- **I70.234 Atherosclerosis of native arteries of right leg with ulceration of heel and midfoot**
  Atherosclerosis of native arteries of right leg with ulceration of plantar surface of midfoot
- **I70.235 Atherosclerosis of native arteries of right leg with ulceration of other part of foot**
  Atherosclerosis of native arteries of right leg extremities with ulceration of toe
- **I70.238 Atherosclerosis of native arteries of right leg with ulceration of other part of lower leg**
- **I70.239 Atherosclerosis of native arteries of right leg with ulceration of unspecified site**

+ **I70.24 Atherosclerosis of native arteries of left leg with ulceration**

Includes: any condition classifiable to I70.212 and I70.222
chronic limb-threatening ischemia of native arteries of left leg with ulceration
critical limb ischemia of native arteries of left leg with ulceration

Use additional code to identify severity of ulcer (L97.-)

- **I70.241 Atherosclerosis of native arteries of left leg with ulceration of thigh**
- **I70.242 Atherosclerosis of native arteries of left leg with ulceration of calf**
- **I70.243 Atherosclerosis of native arteries of left leg with ulceration of ankle**
- **I70.244 Atherosclerosis of native arteries of left leg with ulceration of heel and midfoot**
  Atherosclerosis of native arteries of left leg with ulceration of plantar surface of midfoot
- **I70.245 Atherosclerosis of native arteries of left leg with ulceration of other part of foot**
  Atherosclerosis of native arteries of left leg extremities with ulceration of toe
- **I70.248 Atherosclerosis of native arteries of left leg with ulceration of other part of lower leg**
- **I70.249 Atherosclerosis of native arteries of left leg with ulceration of unspecified site**

• **I70.25 Atherosclerosis of native arteries of other extremities with ulceration**

Includes: any condition classifiable to I70.218 and I70.228

Use additional code to identify the severity of the ulcer (L98.49-)

+ **I70.26 Atherosclerosis of native arteries of extremities with gangrene**

Includes: any condition classifiable to I70.21-, I70.22-, I70.23-, I70.24-, and I70.25-
chronic limb-threatening ischemia of native arteries of extremities with gangrene
critical limb ischemia of native arteries of extremities with gangrene

Use additional code to identify the severity of any ulcer (L97.-, L98.49-), if applicable

- CC **I70.261 Atherosclerosis of native arteries of extremities with gangrene, right leg**
- CC **I70.262 Atherosclerosis of native arteries of extremities with gangrene, left leg**
- CC **I70.263 Atherosclerosis of native arteries of extremities with gangrene, bilateral legs**
- CC **I70.268 Atherosclerosis of native arteries of extremities with gangrene, other extremity**
- CC **I70.269 Atherosclerosis of native arteries of extremities with gangrene, unspecified extremity**

+ **I70.29 Other atherosclerosis of native arteries of extremities**
- **I70.291 Other atherosclerosis of native arteries of extremities, right leg**
- **I70.292 Other atherosclerosis of native arteries of extremities, left leg**
- **I70.293 Other atherosclerosis of native arteries of extremities, bilateral legs**
- **I70.298 Other atherosclerosis of native arteries of extremities, other extremity**
- **I70.299 Other atherosclerosis of native arteries of extremities, unspecified extremity**

+ I70.3 Atherosclerosis of unspecified type of bypass graft(s) of the extremities

Use additional code, if applicable, to identify chronic total occlusion of artery of extremity (I70.92)

Excludes1: *embolism or thrombus of bypass graft(s) of extremities (T82.8-)*

+ I70.30 Unspecified atherosclerosis of unspecified type of bypass graft(s) of the extremities

- **I70.301 Unspecified atherosclerosis of unspecified type of bypass graft(s) of the extremities, right leg**
- **I70.302 Unspecified atherosclerosis of unspecified type of bypass graft(s) of the extremities, left leg**
- **I70.303 Unspecified atherosclerosis of unspecified type of bypass graft(s) of the extremities, bilateral legs**
- **I70.308 Unspecified atherosclerosis of unspecified type of bypass graft(s) of the extremities, other extremity**
- **I70.309 Unspecified atherosclerosis of unspecified type of bypass graft(s) of the extremities, unspecified extremity**

+ I70.31 Atherosclerosis of unspecified type of bypass graft(s) of the extremities with intermittent claudication

- **I70.311 Atherosclerosis of unspecified type of bypass graft(s) of the extremities with intermittent claudication, right leg**
- **I70.312 Atherosclerosis of unspecified type of bypass graft(s) of the extremities with intermittent claudication, left leg**
- **I70.313 Atherosclerosis of unspecified type of bypass graft(s) of the extremities with intermittent claudication, bilateral legs**
- **I70.318 Atherosclerosis of unspecified type of bypass graft(s) of the extremities with intermittent claudication, other extremity**
- **I70.319 Atherosclerosis of unspecified type of bypass graft(s) of the extremities with intermittent claudication, unspecified extremity**

+ I70.32 Atherosclerosis of unspecified type of bypass graft(s) of the extremities with rest pain

Includes: any condition classifiable to I70.31-
chronic limb-threatening ischemia NOS of unspecified type of bypass graft(s) of the extremities
chronic limb-threatening ischemia of unspecified type of bypass graft(s) of the extremities with rest pain
critical limb ischemia NOS of unspecified type of bypass graft(s) of the extremities
critical limb ischemia of unspecified type of bypass graft(s) of the extremities with rest pain

- **I70.321 Atherosclerosis of unspecified type of bypass graft(s) of the extremities with rest pain, right leg**
- **I70.322 Atherosclerosis of unspecified type of bypass graft(s) of the extremities with rest pain, left leg**
- **I70.323 Atherosclerosis of unspecified type of bypass graft(s) of the extremities with rest pain, bilateral legs**
- **I70.328 Atherosclerosis of unspecified type of bypass graft(s) of the extremities with rest pain, other extremity**
- **I70.329 Atherosclerosis of unspecified type of bypass graft(s) of the extremities with rest pain, unspecified extremity**

+ I70.33 Atherosclerosis of unspecified type of bypass graft(s) of the right leg with ulceration

Includes: any condition classifiable to I70.311 and I70.321
chronic limb-threatening ischemia of unspecified type of bypass graft(s) of right leg with ulceration
critical limb ischemia of unspecified type of bypass graft(s) of right leg with ulceration

Use additional code to identify severity of ulcer (L97.-)

- CC **I70.331 Atherosclerosis of unspecified type of bypass graft(s) of the right leg with ulceration of thigh**
- CC **I70.332 Atherosclerosis of unspecified type of bypass graft(s) of the right leg with ulceration of calf**
- CC **I70.333 Atherosclerosis of unspecified type of bypass graft(s) of the right leg with ulceration of ankle**
- CC **I70.334 Atherosclerosis of unspecified type of bypass graft(s) of the right leg with ulceration of heel and midfoot**
  Atherosclerosis of unspecified type of bypass graft(s) of right leg with ulceration of plantar surface of midfoot
- **I70.335 Atherosclerosis of unspecified type of bypass graft(s) of the right leg with ulceration of other part of foot**
  Atherosclerosis of unspecified type of bypass graft(s) of the right leg with ulceration of toe
- CC **I70.338 Atherosclerosis of unspecified type of bypass graft(s) of the right leg with ulceration of other part of lower leg**
- CC **I70.339 Atherosclerosis of unspecified type of bypass graft(s) of the right leg with ulceration of unspecified site**

+ I70.34 Atherosclerosis of unspecified type of bypass graft(s) of the left leg with ulceration

Includes: any condition classifiable to I70.312 and I70.322
chronic limb-threatening ischemia of unspecified type of bypass graft(s) of left leg with ulceration
critical limb ischemia of unspecified type of bypass graft(s) of left leg with ulceration

Use additional code to identify severity of ulcer (L97.-)

- CC **I70.341 Atherosclerosis of unspecified type of bypass graft(s) of the left leg with ulceration of thigh**
- CC **I70.342 Atherosclerosis of unspecified type of bypass graft(s) of the left leg with ulceration of calf**
- CC **I70.343 Atherosclerosis of unspecified type of bypass graft(s) of the left leg with ulceration of ankle**
- CC **I70.344 Atherosclerosis of unspecified type of bypass graft(s) of the left leg with ulceration of heel and midfoot**
  Atherosclerosis of unspecified type of bypass graft(s) of left leg with ulceration of plantar surface of midfoot
- **I70.345 Atherosclerosis of unspecified type of bypass graft(s) of the left leg with ulceration of other part of foot**
  Atherosclerosis of unspecified type of bypass graft(s) of the left leg with ulceration of toe
- CC **I70.348 Atherosclerosis of unspecified type of bypass graft(s) of the left leg with ulceration of other part of lower leg**
- CC **I70.349 Atherosclerosis of unspecified type of bypass graft(s) of the left leg with ulceration of unspecified site**

• **I70.35 Atherosclerosis of unspecified type of bypass graft(s) of other extremity with ulceration**
Includes: any condition classifiable to I70.318 and I70.328
Use additional code to identify severity of ulcer (L98.49-)

+ **I70.36 Atherosclerosis of unspecified type of bypass graft(s) of the extremities with gangrene**
Includes: any condition classifiable to I70.31-, I70.32-, I70.33-, I70.34-, I70.35
chronic limb-threatening ischemia of unspecified type of bypass graft(s) of the extremities with gangrene
critical limb ischemia of unspecified type of bypass graft(s) of the extremities with gangrene
Use additional code to identify the severity of any ulcer (L97.-, L98.49-), if applicable

• CC **I70.361 Atherosclerosis of unspecified type of bypass graft(s) of the extremities with gangrene, right leg**
• CC **I70.362 Atherosclerosis of unspecified type of bypass graft(s) of the extremities with gangrene, left leg**
• CC **I70.363 Atherosclerosis of unspecified type of bypass graft(s) of the extremities with gangrene, bilateral legs**
• CC **I70.368 Atherosclerosis of unspecified type of bypass graft(s) of the extremities with gangrene, other extremity**
• CC **I70.369 Atherosclerosis of unspecified type of bypass graft(s) of the extremities with gangrene, unspecified extremity**

+ **I70.39 Other atherosclerosis of unspecified type of bypass graft(s) of the extremities**
• **I70.391 Other atherosclerosis of unspecified type of bypass graft(s) of the extremities, right leg**
• **I70.392 Other atherosclerosis of unspecified type of bypass graft(s) of the extremities, left leg**
• **I70.393 Other atherosclerosis of unspecified type of bypass graft(s) of the extremities, bilateral legs**
• **I70.398 Other atherosclerosis of unspecified type of bypass graft(s) of the extremities, other extremity**
• **I70.399 Other atherosclerosis of unspecified type of bypass graft(s) of the extremities, unspecified extremity**

+ **I70.4 Atherosclerosis of autologous vein bypass graft(s) of the extremities**
Use additional code, if applicable, to identify chronic total occlusion of artery of extremity (I70.92)

+ **I70.40 Unspecified atherosclerosis of autologous vein bypass graft(s) of the extremities**
• **I70.401 Unspecified atherosclerosis of autologous vein bypass graft(s) of the extremities, right leg**
• **I70.402 Unspecified atherosclerosis of autologous vein bypass graft(s) of the extremities, left leg**
• **I70.403 Unspecified atherosclerosis of autologous vein bypass graft(s) of the extremities, bilateral legs**
• **I70.408 Unspecified atherosclerosis of autologous vein bypass graft(s) of the extremities, other extremity**
• **I70.409 Unspecified atherosclerosis of autologous vein bypass graft(s) of the extremities, unspecified extremity**

+ **I70.41 Atherosclerosis of autologous vein bypass graft(s) of the extremities with intermittent claudication**
• **I70.411 Atherosclerosis of autologous vein bypass graft(s) of the extremities with intermittent claudication, right leg**
• **I70.412 Atherosclerosis of autologous vein bypass graft(s) of the extremities with intermittent claudication, left leg**
• **I70.413 Atherosclerosis of autologous vein bypass graft(s) of the extremities with intermittent claudication, bilateral legs**
• **I70.418 Atherosclerosis of autologous vein bypass graft(s) of the extremities with intermittent claudication, other extremity**
• **I70.419 Atherosclerosis of autologous vein bypass graft(s) of the extremities with intermittent claudication, unspecified extremity**

+ **I70.42 Atherosclerosis of autologous vein bypass graft(s) of the extremities with rest pain**
Includes: any condition classifiable to I70.41-
chronic limb-threatening ischemia NOS of autologous vein bypass graft(s) of the extremities
chronic limb-threatening ischemia of autologous vein bypass graft(s) of the extremities with rest pain
critical limb ischemia NOS of autologous vein bypass graft(s) of the extremities
critical limb ischemia of autologous vein bypass graft(s) of the extremities with rest pain

• **I70.421 Atherosclerosis of autologous vein bypass graft(s) of the extremities with rest pain, right leg**
• **I70.422 Atherosclerosis of autologous vein bypass graft(s) of the extremities with rest pain, left leg**
• **I70.423 Atherosclerosis of autologous vein bypass graft(s) of the extremities with rest pain, bilateral legs**
• **I70.428 Atherosclerosis of autologous vein bypass graft(s) of the extremities with rest pain, other extremity**
• **I70.429 Atherosclerosis of autologous vein bypass graft(s) of the extremities with rest pain, unspecified extremity**

+ **I70.43 Atherosclerosis of autologous vein bypass graft(s) of the right leg with ulceration**
Includes: any condition classifiable to I70.411 and I70.421
chronic limb-threatening ischemia of autologous vein bypass graft(s) of right leg with ulceration
critical limb ischemia of autologous vein bypass graft(s) of right leg with ulceration
Use additional code to identify severity of ulcer (L97.-)

• CC **I70.431 Atherosclerosis of autologous vein bypass graft(s) of the right leg with ulceration of thigh**
• CC **I70.432 Atherosclerosis of autologous vein bypass graft(s) of the right leg with ulceration of calf**
• CC **I70.433 Atherosclerosis of autologous vein bypass graft(s) of the right leg with ulceration of ankle**
• CC **I70.434 Atherosclerosis of autologous vein bypass graft(s) of the right leg with ulceration of heel and midfoot**
Atherosclerosis of autologous vein bypass graft(s) of right leg with ulceration of plantar surface of midfoot
• **I70.435 Atherosclerosis of autologous vein bypass graft(s) of the right leg with ulceration of other part of foot**
Atherosclerosis of autologous vein bypass graft(s) of right leg with ulceration of toe
• CC **I70.438 Atherosclerosis of autologous vein bypass graft(s) of the right leg with ulceration of other part of lower leg**
• CC **I70.439 Atherosclerosis of autologous vein bypass graft(s) of the right leg with ulceration of unspecified site**

+ **I70.44 Atherosclerosis of autologous vein bypass graft(s) of the left leg with ulceration**
  Includes: any condition classifiable to I70.412 and I70.422
  chronic limb-threatening ischemia of autologous vein bypass graft(s) of left leg with ulceration
  critical limb ischemia of autologous vein bypass graft(s) of left leg with ulceration
  Use additional code to identify severity of ulcer (L97.-)
• CC **I70.441 Atherosclerosis of autologous vein bypass graft(s) of the left leg with ulceration of thigh**
• CC **I70.442 Atherosclerosis of autologous vein bypass graft(s) of the left leg with ulceration of calf**
• CC **I70.443 Atherosclerosis of autologous vein bypass graft(s) of the left leg with ulceration of ankle**
• CC **I70.444 Atherosclerosis of autologous vein bypass graft(s) of the left leg with ulceration of heel and midfoot**
  Atherosclerosis of autologous vein bypass graft(s) of left leg with ulceration of plantar surface of midfoot
• **I70.445 Atherosclerosis of autologous vein bypass graft(s) of the left leg with ulceration of other part of foot**
  Atherosclerosis of autologous vein bypass graft(s) of left leg with ulceration of toe
• CC **I70.448 Atherosclerosis of autologous vein bypass graft(s) of the left leg with ulceration of other part of lower leg**
• CC **I70.449 Atherosclerosis of autologous vein bypass graft(s) of the left leg with ulceration of unspecified site**
• **I70.45 Atherosclerosis of autologous vein bypass graft(s) of other extremity with ulceration**
  Includes: any condition classifiable to I70.418, I70.428, and I70.438
  Use additional code to identify severity of ulcer (L98.49)
+ **I70.46 Atherosclerosis of autologous vein bypass graft(s) of the extremities with gangrene**
  Includes: any condition classifiable to I70.41-, I70.42-, and I70.43-, I70.44-, I70.45
  chronic limb-threatening ischemia of autologous vein bypass graft(s) of the extremities with gangrene
  critical limb ischemia of autologous vein bypass graft(s) of the extremities with gangrene
  Use additional code to identify the severity of any ulcer (L97.-, L98.49-), if applicable
• CC **I70.461 Atherosclerosis of autologous vein bypass graft(s) of the extremities with gangrene, right leg**
• CC **I70.462 Atherosclerosis of autologous vein bypass graft(s) of the extremities with gangrene, left leg**
• CC **I70.463 Atherosclerosis of autologous vein bypass graft(s) of the extremities with gangrene, bilateral legs**
• CC **I70.468 Atherosclerosis of autologous vein bypass graft(s) of the extremities with gangrene, other extremity**
• CC **I70.469 Atherosclerosis of autologous vein bypass graft(s) of the extremities with gangrene, unspecified extremity**
+ **I70.49 Other atherosclerosis of autologous vein bypass graft(s) of the extremities**
• **I70.491 Other atherosclerosis of autologous vein bypass graft(s) of the extremities, right leg**
• **I70.492 Other atherosclerosis of autologous vein bypass graft(s) of the extremities, left leg**
• **I70.493 Other atherosclerosis of autologous vein bypass graft(s) of the extremities, bilateral legs**
• **I70.498 Other atherosclerosis of autologous vein bypass graft(s) of the extremities, other extremity**
• **I70.499 Other atherosclerosis of autologous vein bypass graft(s) of the extremities, unspecified extremity**
+ **I70.5 Atherosclerosis of nonautologous biological bypass graft(s) of the extremities**
  Use additional code, if applicable, to identify chronic total occlusion of artery of extremity (I70.92)
+ **I70.50 Unspecified atherosclerosis of nonautologous biological bypass graft(s) of the extremities**
• **I70.501 Unspecified atherosclerosis of nonautologous biological bypass graft(s) of the extremities, right leg**
• **I70.502 Unspecified atherosclerosis of nonautologous biological bypass graft(s) of the extremities, left leg**
• **I70.503 Unspecified atherosclerosis of nonautologous biological bypass graft(s) of the extremities, bilateral legs**
• **I70.508 Unspecified atherosclerosis of nonautologous biological bypass graft(s) of the extremities, other extremity**
• **I70.509 Unspecified atherosclerosis of nonautologous biological bypass graft(s) of the extremities, unspecified extremity**
+ **I70.51 Atherosclerosis of nonautologous biological bypass graft(s) of the extremities intermittent claudication**
• **I70.511 Atherosclerosis of nonautologous biological bypass graft(s) of the extremities with intermittent claudication, right leg**
• **I70.512 Atherosclerosis of nonautologous biological bypass graft(s) of the extremities with intermittent claudication, left leg**
• **I70.513 Atherosclerosis of nonautologous biological bypass graft(s) of the extremities with intermittent claudication, bilateral legs**
• **I70.518 Atherosclerosis of nonautologous biological bypass graft(s) of the extremities with intermittent claudication, other extremity**
• **I70.519 Atherosclerosis of nonautologous biological bypass graft(s) of the extremities with intermittent claudication, unspecified extremity**
+ **I70.52 Atherosclerosis of nonautologous biological bypass graft(s) of the extremities with rest pain**
  Includes: any condition classifiable to I70.51-
  chronic limb-threatening ischemia NOS of nonautologous vein bypass graft(s) of the extremities
  chronic limb-threatening ischemia of nonautologous vein bypass graft(s) of the extremities with rest pain
  critical limb ischemia NOS of nonautologous vein bypass graft(s) of the extremities
  critical limb ischemia of nonautologous vein bypass graft(s) of the extremities with rest pain
• **I70.521 Atherosclerosis of nonautologous biological bypass graft(s) of the extremities with rest pain, right leg**
• **I70.522 Atherosclerosis of nonautologous biological bypass graft(s) of the extremities with rest pain, left leg**
• **I70.523 Atherosclerosis of nonautologous biological bypass graft(s) of the extremities with rest pain, bilateral legs**

• **I70.528** **Atherosclerosis of nonautologous biological bypass graft(s) of the extremities with rest pain, other extremity**

• **I70.529** **Atherosclerosis of nonautologous biological bypass graft(s) of the extremities with rest pain, unspecified extremity**

+ **I70.53** **Atherosclerosis of nonautologous biological bypass graft(s) of the right leg with ulceration**

Includes: any condition classifiable to I70.511 and I70.521
chronic limb-threatening ischemia of nonautologous vein bypass graft(s) of right leg with ulceration
critical limb ischemia of nonautologous vein bypass graft(s) of right leg with ulceration

Use additional code to identify severity of ulcer (L97.-)

• CC **I70.531** **Atherosclerosis of nonautologous biological bypass graft(s) of the right leg with ulceration of thigh**

• CC **I70.532** **Atherosclerosis of nonautologous biological bypass graft(s) of the right leg with ulceration of calf**

• CC **I70.533** **Atherosclerosis of nonautologous biological bypass graft(s) of the right leg with ulceration of ankle**

• CC **I70.534** **Atherosclerosis of nonautologous biological bypass graft(s) of the right leg with ulceration of heel and midfoot**

Atherosclerosis of nonautologous biological bypass graft(s) of right leg with ulceration of plantar surface of midfoot

• **I70.535** **Atherosclerosis of nonautologous biological bypass graft(s) of the right leg with ulceration of other part of foot**

Atherosclerosis of nonautologous biological bypass graft(s) of the right leg with ulceration of toe

• CC **I70.538** **Atherosclerosis of nonautologous biological bypass graft(s) of the right leg with ulceration of other part of lower leg**

• CC **I70.539** **Atherosclerosis of nonautologous biological bypass graft(s) of the right leg with ulceration of unspecified site**

+ **I70.54** **Atherosclerosis of nonautologous biological bypass graft(s) of the left leg with ulceration**

Includes: any condition classifiable to I70.512 and I70.522
chronic limb-threatening ischemia of nonautologous vein bypass graft(s) of left leg with ulceration
critical limb ischemia of nonautologous vein bypass graft(s) of left leg with ulceration

Use additional code to identify severity of ulcer (L97.-)

• CC **I70.541** **Atherosclerosis of nonautologous biological bypass graft(s) of the left leg with ulceration of thigh**

• CC **I70.542** **Atherosclerosis of nonautologous biological bypass graft(s) of the left leg with ulceration of calf**

• CC **I70.543** **Atherosclerosis of nonautologous biological bypass graft(s) of the left leg with ulceration of ankle**

• CC **I70.544** **Atherosclerosis of nonautologous biological bypass graft(s) of the left leg with ulceration of heel and midfoot**

Atherosclerosis of nonautologous biological bypass graft(s) of left leg with ulceration of plantar surface of midfoot

• **I70.545** **Atherosclerosis of nonautologous biological bypass graft(s) of the left leg with ulceration of other part of foot**

Atherosclerosis of nonautologous biological bypass graft(s) of the left leg with ulceration of toe

• CC **I70.548** **Atherosclerosis of nonautologous biological bypass graft(s) of the left leg with ulceration of other part of lower leg**

• CC **I70.549** **Atherosclerosis of nonautologous biological bypass graft(s) of the left leg with ulceration of unspecified site**

• **I70.55** **Atherosclerosis of nonautologous biological bypass graft(s) of other extremity with ulceration**

Includes: any condition classifiable to I70.518, I70.528, and I70.538

Use additional code to identify severity of ulcer (L98.49)

+ **I70.56** **Atherosclerosis of nonautologous biological bypass graft(s) of the extremities with gangrene**

Includes: any condition classifiable to I70.51-, I70.52-, and I70.53-, I70.54-, I70.55
chronic limb-threatening ischemia of nonautologous vein bypass graft(s) of the extremities with gangrene
critical limb ischemia of nonautologous vein bypass graft(s) of the extremities with gangrene

Use additional code to identify the severity of any ulcer (L97.-, L98.49-), if applicable

• CC **I70.561** **Atherosclerosis of nonautologous biological bypass graft(s) of the extremities with gangrene, right leg**

• CC **I70.562** **Atherosclerosis of nonautologous biological bypass graft(s) of the extremities with gangrene, left leg**

• CC **I70.563** **Atherosclerosis of nonautologous biological bypass graft(s) of the extremities with gangrene, bilateral legs**

• CC **I70.568** **Atherosclerosis of nonautologous biological bypass graft(s) of the extremities with gangrene, other extremity**

• CC **I70.569** **Atherosclerosis of nonautologous biological bypass graft(s) of the extremities with gangrene, unspecified extremity**

+ **I70.59** **Other atherosclerosis of nonautologous biological bypass graft(s) of the extremities**

• **I70.591** **Other atherosclerosis of nonautologous biological bypass graft(s) of the extremities, right leg**

• **I70.592** **Other atherosclerosis of nonautologous biological bypass graft(s) of the extremities, left leg**

• **I70.593** **Other atherosclerosis of nonautologous biological bypass graft(s) of the extremities, bilateral legs**

• **I70.598** **Other atherosclerosis of nonautologous biological bypass graft(s) of the extremities, other extremity**

• **I70.599** **Other atherosclerosis of nonautologous biological bypass graft(s) of the extremities, unspecified extremity**

+ **I70.6** **Atherosclerosis of nonbiological bypass graft(s) of the extremities**

Use additional code, if applicable, to identify chronic total occlusion of artery of extremity (I70.92)

+ **I70.60** **Unspecified atherosclerosis of nonbiological bypass graft(s) of the extremities**

• **I70.601** **Unspecified atherosclerosis of nonbiological bypass graft(s) of the extremities, right leg**

• **I70.602** **Unspecified atherosclerosis of nonbiological bypass graft(s) of the extremities, left leg**

• **I70.603** **Unspecified atherosclerosis of nonbiological bypass graft(s) of the extremities, bilateral legs**

- I70.608 **Unspecified atherosclerosis of nonbiological bypass graft(s) of the extremities, other extremity**
- I70.609 **Unspecified atherosclerosis of nonbiological bypass graft(s) of the extremities, unspecified extremity**

+ **I70.61 Atherosclerosis of nonbiological bypass graft(s) of the extremities with intermittent claudication**
- I70.611 **Atherosclerosis of nonbiological bypass graft(s) of the extremities with intermittent claudication, right leg**
- I70.612 **Atherosclerosis of nonbiological bypass graft(s) of the extremities with intermittent claudication, left leg**
- I70.613 **Atherosclerosis of nonbiological bypass graft(s) of the extremities with intermittent claudication, bilateral legs**
- I70.618 **Atherosclerosis of nonbiological bypass graft(s) of the extremities with intermittent claudication, other extremity**
- I70.619 **Atherosclerosis of nonbiological bypass graft(s) of the extremities with intermittent claudication, unspecified extremity**

+ **I70.62 Atherosclerosis of nonbiological bypass graft(s) of the extremities with rest pain**

Includes: any condition classifiable to I70.61-
chronic limb-threatening ischemia NOS of nonbiological bypass graft(s) of the extremities
chronic limb-threatening ischemia of nonbiological bypass graft(s) of the extremities with rest pain
critical limb ischemia NOS of nonbiological bypass graft(s) of the extremities
critical limb ischemia of nonbiological bypass graft(s) of the extremities with rest pain

- I70.621 **Atherosclerosis of nonbiological bypass graft(s) of the extremities with rest pain, right leg**
- I70.622 **Atherosclerosis of nonbiological bypass graft(s) of the extremities with rest pain, left leg**
- I70.623 **Atherosclerosis of nonbiological bypass graft(s) of the extremities with rest pain, bilateral legs**
- I70.628 **Atherosclerosis of nonbiological bypass graft(s) of the extremities with rest pain, other extremity**
- I70.629 **Atherosclerosis of nonbiological bypass graft(s) of the extremities with rest pain, unspecified extremity**

+ **I70.63 Atherosclerosis of nonbiological bypass graft(s) of the right leg with ulceration**

Includes: any condition classifiable to I70.611 and I70.621
chronic limb-threatening ischemia of nonbiological bypass graft(s) of the right leg with ulceration
critical limb ischemia of nonbiological bypass graft(s) of the right leg with ulceration

Use additional code to identify severity of ulcer (L97.-)

- CC I70.631 **Atherosclerosis of nonbiological bypass graft(s) of the right leg with ulceration of thigh**
- CC I70.632 **Atherosclerosis of nonbiological bypass graft(s) of the right leg with ulceration of calf**
- CC I70.633 **Atherosclerosis of nonbiological bypass graft(s) of the right leg with ulceration of ankle**
- CC I70.634 **Atherosclerosis of nonbiological bypass graft(s) of the right leg with ulceration of heel and midfoot**
  Atherosclerosis of nonbiological bypass graft(s) of right leg with ulceration of plantar surface of midfoot
- I70.635 **Atherosclerosis of nonbiological bypass graft(s) of the right leg with ulceration of other part of foot**
  Atherosclerosis of nonbiological bypass graft(s) of the right leg with ulceration of toe
- CC I70.638 **Atherosclerosis of nonbiological bypass graft(s) of the right leg with ulceration of other part of lower leg**
- CC I70.639 **Atherosclerosis of nonbiological bypass graft(s) of the right leg with ulceration of unspecified site**

+ **I70.64 Atherosclerosis of nonbiological bypass graft(s) of the left leg with ulceration**

Includes: any condition classifiable to I70.612 and I70.622
chronic limb-threatening ischemia of nonbiological bypass graft(s) of the left leg with ulceration
critical limb ischemia of nonbiological bypass graft(s) of the left leg with ulceration

Use additional code to identify severity of ulcer (L97.-)

- CC I70.641 **Atherosclerosis of nonbiological bypass graft(s) of the left leg with ulceration of thigh**
- CC I70.642 **Atherosclerosis of nonbiological bypass graft(s) of the left leg with ulceration of calf**
- CC I70.643 **Atherosclerosis of nonbiological bypass graft(s) of the left leg with ulceration of ankle**
- CC I70.644 **Atherosclerosis of nonbiological bypass graft(s) of the left leg with ulceration of heel and midfoot**
  Atherosclerosis of nonbiological bypass graft(s) of left leg with ulceration of plantar surface of midfoot
- I70.645 **Atherosclerosis of nonbiological bypass graft(s) of the left leg with ulceration of other part of foot**
  Atherosclerosis of nonbiological bypass graft(s) of the left leg with ulceration of toe
- CC I70.648 **Atherosclerosis of nonbiological bypass graft(s) of the left leg with ulceration of other part of lower leg**
- CC I70.649 **Atherosclerosis of nonbiological bypass graft(s) of the left leg with ulceration of unspecified site**

- **I70.65 Atherosclerosis of nonbiological bypass graft(s) of other extremity with ulceration**

Includes: any condition classifiable to I70.618 and I70.628

Use additional code to identify severity of ulcer (L98.49)

+ **I70.66 Atherosclerosis of nonbiological bypass graft(s) of the extremities with gangrene**

Includes: any condition classifiable to I70.61-, I70.62-, I70.63-, I70.64-, I70.65
chronic limb-threatening ischemia of nonbiological bypass graft(s) of the extremities with gangrene
critical limb ischemia of nonbiological bypass graft(s) of the extremities with gangrene

Use additional code to identify the severity of any ulcer (L97.-, L98.49-), if applicable

- CC I70.661 **Atherosclerosis of nonbiological bypass graft(s) of the extremities with gangrene, right leg**
- CC I70.662 **Atherosclerosis of nonbiological bypass graft(s) of the extremities with gangrene, left leg**
- CC I70.663 **Atherosclerosis of nonbiological bypass graft(s) of the extremities with gangrene, bilateral legs**

• CC **I70.668** **Atherosclerosis of nonbiological bypass graft(s) of the extremities with gangrene, other extremity**

• CC **I70.669** **Atherosclerosis of nonbiological bypass graft(s) of the extremities with gangrene, unspecified extremity**

+ **I70.69** **Other atherosclerosis of nonbiological bypass graft(s) of the extremities**

• **I70.691** **Other atherosclerosis of nonbiological bypass graft(s) of the extremities, right leg**

• **I70.692** **Other atherosclerosis of nonbiological bypass graft(s) of the extremities, left leg**

• **I70.693** **Other atherosclerosis of nonbiological bypass graft(s) of the extremities, bilateral legs**

• **I70.698** **Other atherosclerosis of nonbiological bypass graft(s) of the extremities, other extremity**

• **I70.699** **Other atherosclerosis of nonbiological bypass graft(s) of the extremities, unspecified extremity**

+ **I70.7** **Atherosclerosis of other type of bypass graft(s) of the extremities**

Use additional code, if applicable, to identify chronic total occlusion of artery of extremity (I70.92)

+ **I70.70** **Unspecified atherosclerosis of other type of bypass graft(s) of the extremities**

• **I70.701** **Unspecified atherosclerosis of other type of bypass graft(s) of the extremities, right leg**

• **I70.702** **Unspecified atherosclerosis of other type of bypass graft(s) of the extremities, left leg**

• **I70.703** **Unspecified atherosclerosis of other type of bypass graft(s) of the extremities, bilateral legs**

• **I70.708** **Unspecified atherosclerosis of other type of bypass graft(s) of the extremities, other extremity**

• **I70.709** **Unspecified atherosclerosis of other type of bypass graft(s) of the extremities, unspecified extremity**

+ **I70.71** **Atherosclerosis of other type of bypass graft(s) of the extremities with intermittent claudication**

• **I70.711** **Atherosclerosis of other type of bypass graft(s) of the extremities with intermittent claudication, right leg**

• **I70.712** **Atherosclerosis of other type of bypass graft(s) of the extremities with intermittent claudication, left leg**

• **I70.713** **Atherosclerosis of other type of bypass graft(s) of the extremities with intermittent claudication, bilateral legs**

• **I70.718** **Atherosclerosis of other type of bypass graft(s) of the extremities with intermittent claudication, other extremity**

• **I70.719** **Atherosclerosis of other type of bypass graft(s) of the extremities with intermittent claudication, unspecified extremity**

+ **I70.72** **Atherosclerosis of other type of bypass graft(s) of the extremities with rest pain**

Includes: any condition classifiable to I70.71-
chronic limb-threatening ischemia NOS of other type of bypass graft(s) of the extremities
chronic limb-threatening ischemia of other type of bypass graft(s) of the extremities with rest pain
critical limb ischemia NOS of other type of bypass graft(s) of the extremities
critical limb ischemia of other type of bypass graft(s) of the extremities with rest pain

• **I70.721** **Atherosclerosis of other type of bypass graft(s) of the extremities with rest pain, right leg**

• **I70.722** **Atherosclerosis of other type of bypass graft(s) of the extremities with rest pain, left leg**

• **I70.723** **Atherosclerosis of other type of bypass graft(s) of the extremities with rest pain, bilateral legs**

• **I70.728** **Atherosclerosis of other type of bypass graft(s) of the extremities with rest pain, other extremity**

• **I70.729** **Atherosclerosis of other type of bypass graft(s) of the extremities with rest pain, unspecified extremity**

+ **I70.73** **Atherosclerosis of other type of bypass graft(s) of the right leg with ulceration**

Includes: any condition classifiable to I70.711 and I70.721
chronic limb-threatening ischemia of other type of bypass graft(s) of the right leg with ulceration
critical limb ischemia of other type of bypass graft(s) of the right leg with ulceration

Use additional code to identify severity of ulcer (L97.-)

• CC **I70.731** **Atherosclerosis of other type of bypass graft(s) of the right leg with ulceration of thigh**

• CC **I70.732** **Atherosclerosis of other type of bypass graft(s) of the right leg with ulceration of calf**

• CC **I70.733** **Atherosclerosis of other type of bypass graft(s) of the right leg with ulceration of ankle**

• CC **I70.734** **Atherosclerosis of other type of bypass graft(s) of the right leg with ulceration of heel and midfoot**

Atherosclerosis of other type of bypass graft(s) of right leg with ulceration of plantar surface of midfoot

• **I70.735** **Atherosclerosis of other type of bypass graft(s) of the right leg with ulceration of other part of foot**

Atherosclerosis of other type of bypass graft(s) of right leg with ulceration of toe

• CC **I70.738** **Atherosclerosis of other type of bypass graft(s) of the right leg with ulceration of other part of lower leg**

• CC **I70.739** **Atherosclerosis of other type of bypass graft(s) of the right leg with ulceration of unspecified site**

+ **I70.74** **Atherosclerosis of other type of bypass graft(s) of the left leg with ulceration**

Includes: any condition classifiable to I70.712 and I70.722
chronic limb-threatening ischemia of other type of bypass graft(s) of the left leg with ulceration
critical limb ischemia of other type of bypass graft(s) of the left leg with ulceration

Use additional code to identify severity of ulcer (L97.-)

• CC **I70.741** **Atherosclerosis of other type of bypass graft(s) of the left leg with ulceration of thigh**

• CC **I70.742** **Atherosclerosis of other type of bypass graft(s) of the left leg with ulceration of calf**

• CC **I70.743** **Atherosclerosis of other type of bypass graft(s) of the left leg with ulceration of ankle**

• CC **I70.744** **Atherosclerosis of other type of bypass graft(s) of the left leg with ulceration of heel and midfoot**

Atherosclerosis of other type of bypass graft(s) of left leg with ulceration of plantar surface of midfoot

• **I70.745** **Atherosclerosis of other type of bypass graft(s) of the left leg with ulceration of other part of foot**

Atherosclerosis of other type of bypass graft(s) of left leg with ulceration of toe

• CC **I70.748** **Atherosclerosis of other type of bypass graft(s) of the left leg with ulceration of other part of lower leg**

• CC **I70.749** **Atherosclerosis of other type of bypass graft(s) of the left leg with ulceration of unspecified site**

• **I70.75** **Atherosclerosis of other type of bypass graft(s) of other extremity with ulceration**
Includes: any condition classifiable to I70.718 and I70.728
Use additional code to identify severity of ulcer (L98.49)

+ **I70.76** **Atherosclerosis of other type of bypass graft(s) of the extremities with gangrene**
Includes: any condition classifiable to I70.71-, I70.72-, I70.73-, I70.74-, I70.75
chronic limb-threatening ischemia of other type of bypass graft(s) of the extremities with gangrene
critical limb ischemia of other type of bypass graft(s) of the extremities with gangrene
Use additional code to identify the severity of any ulcer (L97.-, L98.49-), if applicable

• CC **I70.761** **Atherosclerosis of other type of bypass graft(s) of the extremities with gangrene, right leg**

• CC **I70.762** **Atherosclerosis of other type of bypass graft(s) of the extremities with gangrene, left leg**

• CC **I70.763** **Atherosclerosis of other type of bypass graft(s) of the extremities with gangrene, bilateral legs**

• CC **I70.768** **Atherosclerosis of other type of bypass graft(s) of the extremities with gangrene, other extremity**

• CC **I70.769** **Atherosclerosis of other type of bypass graft(s) of the extremities with gangrene, unspecified extremity**

+ **I70.79** **Other atherosclerosis of other type of bypass graft(s) of the extremities**

• **I70.791** **Other atherosclerosis of other type of bypass graft(s) of the extremities, right leg**

• **I70.792** **Other atherosclerosis of other type of bypass graft(s) of the extremities, left leg**

• **I70.793** **Other atherosclerosis of other type of bypass graft(s) of the extremities, bilateral legs**

• **I70.798** **Other atherosclerosis of other type of bypass graft(s) of the extremities, other extremity**

• **I70.799** **Other atherosclerosis of other type of bypass graft(s) of the extremities, unspecified extremity**

• **I70.8** **Atherosclerosis of other arteries**

+ **I70.9** **Other and unspecified atherosclerosis**

• **I70.90** **Unspecified atherosclerosis**

• **I70.91** **Generalized atherosclerosis**

• CC **I70.92** **Chronic total occlusion of artery of the extremities**
Complete occlusion of artery of the extremities
Total occlusion of artery of the extremities
Code first atherosclerosis of arteries of the extremities (I70.2-, I70.3-, I70.4-, I70.5-, I70.6-, I70.7-)

I71 Aortic aneurysm and dissection

Excludes1: *aortic ectasia (I77.81-)*
syphilitic aortic aneurysm (A52.01)
traumatic aortic aneurysm (S25.09, S35.09)

+ **I71.0** **Dissection of aorta**

MCC **I71.00** **Dissection of unspecified site of aorta**

MCC **I71.01** **Dissection of thoracic aorta**

MCC **I71.02** **Dissection of abdominal aorta**

MCC **I71.03** **Dissection of thoracoabdominal aorta**

MCC **I71.1** **Thoracic aortic aneurysm, ruptured**

I71.2 **Thoracic aortic aneurysm, without rupture**

MCC **I71.3** **Abdominal aortic aneurysm, ruptured**

I71.4 **Abdominal aortic aneurysm, without rupture**

MCC **I71.5** **Thoracoabdominal aortic aneurysm, ruptured**

I71.6 **Thoracoabdominal aortic aneurysm, without rupture**

MCC **I71.8** **Aortic aneurysm of unspecified site, ruptured**
Rupture of aorta NOS

I71.9 **Aortic aneurysm of unspecified site, without rupture**
Aneurysm of aorta
Dilatation of aorta
Hyaline necrosis of aorta

I72 Other aneurysm

Includes: aneurysm (cirsoid) (false) (ruptured)
Excludes2: *acquired aneurysm (I77.0)*
aneurysm (of) aorta (I71.-)
aneurysm (of) arteriovenous NOS (Q27.3-)
carotid artery dissection (I77.71)
cerebral (nonruptured) aneurysm (I67.1)
coronary aneurysm (I25.4)
coronary artery dissection (I25.42)
dissection of artery NEC (I77.79)
dissection of precerebral artery, congenital (nonruptured) (Q28.1)
heart aneurysm (I25.3)
iliac artery dissection (I77.72)
precerebral artery, congenital (nonruptured) (Q28.1)
pulmonary artery aneurysm (I28.1)
renal artery dissection (I77.73)
retinal aneurysm (H35.0)
ruptured cerebral aneurysm (I60.7)
varicose aneurysm (I77.0)
vertebral artery dissection (I77.74)

I72.0 **Aneurysm of carotid artery**
Aneurysm of common carotid artery
Aneurysm of external carotid artery
Aneurysm of internal carotid artery, extracranial portion
Excludes1: *aneurysm of internal carotid artery, intracranial portion (I67.1)*
aneurysm of internal carotid artery NOS (I67.1)

I72.1 **Aneurysm of artery of upper extremity**

I72.2 **Aneurysm of renal artery**

I72.3 **Aneurysm of iliac artery**

I72.4 **Aneurysm of artery of lower extremity**
AHA CC: 2Q, 2019, 21-22

I72.5 **Aneurysm of other precerebral arteries**
Aneurysm of basilar artery (trunk)
Excludes2: *aneurysm of carotid artery (I72.0)*
aneurysm of vertebral artery (I72.6)
dissection of carotid artery (I77.71)
dissection of other precerebral arteries (I77.75)
dissection of vertebral artery (I77.74)
AHA CC: 4Q, 2016, 28-29

I72.6 **Aneurysm of vertebral artery**
Excludes2: *dissection of vertebral artery (I77.74)*
AHA CC: 4Q, 2016, 28-29

I72.8 **Aneurysm of other specified arteries**

I72.9 **Aneurysm of unspecified site**

I73 Other peripheral vascular diseases

Excludes2: *chilblains (T69.1)*
frostbite (T33-T34)
immersion hand or foot (T69.0-)
spasm of cerebral artery (G45.9)

+ **I73.0** **Raynaud's syndrome**
Raynaud's disease
Raynaud's phenomenon (secondary)

I73.00 **Raynaud's syndrome without gangrene**

CC **I73.01** **Raynaud's syndrome with gangrene**

I73.1 **Thromboangiitis obliterans [Buerger's disease]**

+ **I73.8** **Other specified peripheral vascular diseases**
Excludes1: *diabetic (peripheral) angiopathy (E08-E13 with .51-.52)*

I73.81 **Erythromelalgia**

I73.89 **Other specified peripheral vascular diseases**
Acrocyanosis
Erythrocyanosis
Simple acroparesthesia [Schultze's type]
Vasomotor acroparesthesia [Nothnagel's type]

I73.9 **Peripheral vascular disease, unspecified**
Intermittent claudication
Peripheral angiopathy NOS
Spasm of artery
Excludes1: *atherosclerosis of the extremities (I70.2--I70.7-)*

I74 Arterial embolism and thrombosis

Includes: embolic infarction
embolic occlusion
thrombotic infarction
thrombotic occlusion

Code first embolism and thrombosis complicating abortion or ectopic or molar pregnancy (O00-O07, O08.2)
embolism and thrombosis complicating pregnancy, childbirth and the puerperium (O88.-)

Excludes2: *atheroembolism (I75.-)*
basilar embolism and thrombosis (I63.0-I63.2, I65.1)
carotid embolism and thrombosis (I63.0-I63.2, I65.2)
cerebral embolism and thrombosis (I63.3-I63.5, I66.-)
coronary embolism and thrombosis (I21-I25)
mesenteric embolism and thrombosis (K55.0-)
ophthalmic embolism and thrombosis (H34.-)
precerebral embolism and thrombosis NOS (I63.0-I63.2, I65.9)
pulmonary embolism and thrombosis (I26.-)
renal embolism and thrombosis (N28.0)
retinal embolism and thrombosis (H34.-)
septic embolism and thrombosis (I76)
vertebral embolism and thrombosis (I63.0-I63.2, I65.0)

\+ **I74.0 Embolism and thrombosis of abdominal aorta**

MCC **I74.01 Saddle embolus of abdominal aorta**

CC **I74.09 Other arterial embolism and thrombosis of abdominal aorta**
Aortic bifurcation syndrome
Aortoiliac obstruction
Leriche's syndrome

\+ **I74.1 Embolism and thrombosis of other and unspecified parts of aorta**

CC **I74.10 Embolism and thrombosis of unspecified parts of aorta**

CC **I74.11 Embolism and thrombosis of thoracic aorta**

CC **I74.19 Embolism and thrombosis of other parts of aorta**

CC **I74.2 Embolism and thrombosis of arteries of the upper extremities**

CC **I74.3 Embolism and thrombosis of arteries of the lower extremities**

CC **I74.4 Embolism and thrombosis of arteries of extremities, unspecified**
Peripheral arterial embolism NOS

CC **I74.5 Embolism and thrombosis of iliac artery**

CC **I74.8 Embolism and thrombosis of other arteries**

CC **I74.9 Embolism and thrombosis of unspecified artery**

I75 Atheroembolism

Includes: atherothrombotic microembolism
cholesterol embolism

\+ **I75.0 Atheroembolism of extremities**

\+ **I75.01 Atheroembolism of upper extremity**

CC **I75.011 Atheroembolism of right upper extremity**

CC **I75.012 Atheroembolism of left upper extremity**

CC **I75.013 Atheroembolism of bilateral upper extremities**

CC **I75.019 Atheroembolism of unspecified upper extremity**

\+ **I75.02 Atheroembolism of lower extremity**

CC **I75.021 Atheroembolism of right lower extremity**

CC **I75.022 Atheroembolism of left lower extremity**

CC **I75.023 Atheroembolism of bilateral lower extremities**

CC **I75.029 Atheroembolism of unspecified lower extremity**

\+ **I75.8 Atheroembolism of other sites**

CC **I75.81 Atheroembolism of kidney**
Use additional code for any associated acute kidney failure and chronic kidney disease (N17.-, N18.-)

CC **I75.89 Atheroembolism of other site**

CC **I76 Septic arterial embolism**

Code first underlying infection, such as:
infective endocarditis (I33.0)
lung abscess (J85.-)

Use additional code to identify the site of the embolism (I74.-)

Excludes2: *septic pulmonary embolism (I26.01, I26.90)*

Valid 3-character code, no further characters required

I77 Other disorders of arteries and arterioles

Excludes2: *collagen (vascular) diseases (M30-M36)*
hypersensitivity angiitis (M31.0)
pulmonary artery (I28.-)

I77.0 Arteriovenous fistula, acquired
Aneurysmal varix
Arteriovenous aneurysm, acquired

Excludes1: *arteriovenous aneurysm NOS (Q27.3-)*
presence of arteriovenous shunt (fistula) for dialysis (Z99.2)
traumatic - see injury of blood vessel by body region

Excludes2: *cerebral (I67.1)*
coronary (I25.4)

I77.1 Stricture of artery
Narrowing of artery

CC **I77.2 Rupture of artery**
Erosion of artery
Fistula of artery
Ulcer of artery

Excludes1: *traumatic rupture of artery - see injury of blood vessel by body region*

I77.3 Arterial fibromuscular dysplasia
Fibromuscular hyperplasia (of) carotid artery
Fibromuscular hyperplasia (of) renal artery

CC **I77.4 Celiac artery compression syndrome**

CC **I77.5 Necrosis of artery**

I77.6 Arteritis, unspecified
Aortitis NOS
Endarteritis NOS

Excludes1: *arteritis or endarteritis:*
aortic arch (M31.4)
cerebral NEC (I67.7)
coronary (I25.89)
deformans (I70.-)
giant cell (M31.5, M31.6)
obliterans (I70.-)
senile (I70.-)

\+ **I77.7 Other arterial dissection**

Excludes2: *dissection of aorta (I71.0-)*
dissection of coronary artery (I25.42)

MCC **I77.70 Dissection of unspecified artery**
AHA CC: 4Q, 2016, 28-29

MCC **I77.71 Dissection of carotid artery**

MCC **I77.72 Dissection of iliac artery**

MCC **I77.73 Dissection of renal artery**

MCC **I77.74 Dissection of vertebral artery**

Excludes2: *aneurysm of vertebral artery (I72.6)*

MCC **I77.75 Dissection of other precerebral arteries**
Dissection of basilar artery (trunk)

Excludes2: *aneurysm of carotid artery (I72.0)*
aneurysm of other precerebral arteries (I72.5)
aneurysm of vertebral artery (I72.6)
dissection of carotid artery (I77.71)
dissection of vertebral artery (I77.74)

AHA CC: 4Q, 2016, 28-29

MCC **I77.76 Dissection of artery of upper extremity**
AHA CC: 4Q, 2016, 28-29

MCC **I77.77 Dissection of artery of lower extremity**
AHA CC: 4Q, 2016, 28-29

MCC **I77.79 Dissection of other specified artery**

\+ **I77.8 Other specified disorders of arteries and arterioles**

\+ **I77.81 Aortic ectasia**
Ectasis aorta

Excludes1: *aortic aneurysm and dissection (I71.0-)*

I77.810 Thoracic aortic ectasia

I77.811 Abdominal aortic ectasia

I77.812 Thoracoabdominal aortic ectasia

I77.819 Aortic ectasia, unspecified site

I77.89 Other specified disorders of arteries and arterioles
AHA CC: 1Q, 2021, 23

I77.9 Disorder of arteries and arterioles, unspecified
AHA CC: 1Q, 2021, 4

I78 Diseases of capillaries

I78.0 Hereditary hemorrhagic telangiectasia
Rendu-Osler-Weber disease

I78.1 Nevus, non-neoplastic
Araneus nevus
Senile nevus
Spider nevus
Stellar nevus
Excludes1: *nevus NOS (D22.-)*
vascular NOS (Q82.5)
Excludes2: *blue nevus (D22.-)*
flammeus nevus (Q82.5)
hairy nevus (D22.-)
melanocytic nevus (D22.-)
pigmented nevus (D22.-)
portwine nevus (Q82.5)
sanguineous nevus (Q82.5)
strawberry nevus (Q82.5)
verrucous nevus (Q82.5)

I78.8 Other diseases of capillaries

I78.9 Disease of capillaries, unspecified

I79 Disorders of arteries, arterioles and capillaries in diseases classified elsewhere

I79.0 Aneurysm of aorta in diseases classified elsewhere
Code first underlying disease
Excludes1: *syphilitic aneurysm (A52.01)*

I79.1 Aortitis in diseases classified elsewhere
Code first underlying disease
Excludes1: *syphilitic aortitis (A52.02)*

I79.8 Other disorders of arteries, arterioles and capillaries in diseases classified elsewhere
Code first underlying disease, such as:
amyloidosis (E85.-)
Excludes1: *diabetic (peripheral) angiopathy (E08-E13 with .51-.52)*
syphilitic endarteritis (A52.09)
tuberculous endarteritis (A18.89)

Diseases of veins, lymphatic vessels and lymph nodes, not elsewhere classified (I80-I89)

I80 Phlebitis and thrombophlebitis

Includes: endophlebitis
inflammation, vein
periphlebitis
suppurative phlebitis

Code first phlebitis and thrombophlebitis complicating abortion, ectopic or molar pregnancy (O00-O07, O08.7)
phlebitis and thrombophlebitis complicating pregnancy, childbirth and the puerperium (O22.-, O87.-)

Excludes1: *venous embolism and thrombosis of lower extremities (I82.4-, I82.5-, I82.81-)*

+ I80.0 Phlebitis and thrombophlebitis of superficial vessels of lower extremities
Phlebitis and thrombophlebitis of femoropopliteal vein

I80.00 Phlebitis and thrombophlebitis of superficial vessels of unspecified lower extremity

I80.01 Phlebitis and thrombophlebitis of superficial vessels of right lower extremity

I80.02 Phlebitis and thrombophlebitis of superficial vessels of left lower extremity

I80.03 Phlebitis and thrombophlebitis of superficial vessels of lower extremities, bilateral

+ I80.1 Phlebitis and thrombophlebitis of femoral vein
Phlebitis and thrombophlebitis of common femoral vein
Phlebitis and thrombophlebitis of deep femoral vein

CC **I80.10 Phlebitis and thrombophlebitis of unspecified femoral vein**

CC **I80.11 Phlebitis and thrombophlebitis of right femoral vein**

CC **I80.12 Phlebitis and thrombophlebitis of left femoral vein**

CC **I80.13 Phlebitis and thrombophlebitis of femoral vein, bilateral**

+ I80.2 Phlebitis and thrombophlebitis of other and unspecified deep vessels of lower extremities

+ I80.20 Phlebitis and thrombophlebitis of unspecified deep vessels of lower extremities

CC **I80.201 Phlebitis and thrombophlebitis of unspecified deep vessels of right lower extremity**

CC **I80.202 Phlebitis and thrombophlebitis of unspecified deep vessels of left lower extremity**

CC **I80.203 Phlebitis and thrombophlebitis of unspecified deep vessels of lower extremities, bilateral**

CC **I80.209 Phlebitis and thrombophlebitis of unspecified deep vessels of unspecified lower extremity**

+ I80.21 Phlebitis and thrombophlebitis of iliac vein
Phlebitis and thrombophlebitis of common iliac vein
Phlebitis and thrombophlebitis of external iliac vein
Phlebitis and thrombophlebitis of internal iliac vein

CC **I80.211 Phlebitis and thrombophlebitis of right iliac vein**

CC **I80.212 Phlebitis and thrombophlebitis of left iliac vein**

CC **I80.213 Phlebitis and thrombophlebitis of iliac vein, bilateral**

CC **I80.219 Phlebitis and thrombophlebitis of unspecified iliac vein**

+ I80.22 Phlebitis and thrombophlebitis of popliteal vein

CC **I80.221 Phlebitis and thrombophlebitis of right popliteal vein**

CC **I80.222 Phlebitis and thrombophlebitis of left popliteal vein**

CC **I80.223 Phlebitis and thrombophlebitis of popliteal vein, bilateral**

CC **I80.229 Phlebitis and thrombophlebitis of unspecified popliteal vein**

+ I80.23 Phlebitis and thrombophlebitis of tibial vein
Phlebitis and thrombophlebitis of anterior tibial vein
Phlebitis and thrombophlebitis of posterior tibial vein

CC **I80.231 Phlebitis and thrombophlebitis of right tibial vein**

CC **I80.232 Phlebitis and thrombophlebitis of left tibial vein**

CC **I80.233 Phlebitis and thrombophlebitis of tibial vein, bilateral**

CC **I80.239 Phlebitis and thrombophlebitis of unspecified tibial vein**

+ I80.24 Phlebitis and thrombophlebitis of peroneal vein
AHA CC: 4Q, 2019, 8

CC **I80.241 Phlebitis and thrombophlebitis of right peroneal vein**

CC **I80.242 Phlebitis and thrombophlebitis of left peroneal vein**

CC **I80.243 Phlebitis and thrombophlebitis of peroneal vein, bilateral**

CC **I80.249 Phlebitis and thrombophlebitis of unspecified peroneal vein**

+ I80.25 Phlebitis and thrombophlebitis of calf muscular vein
Phlebitis and thrombophlebitis of calf muscular vein, NOS
Phlebitis and thrombophlebitis of gastocnemial vein
Phlebitis and thrombophlebitis of soleal vein
AHA CC: 4Q, 2019, 8

I80.251 Phlebitis and thrombophlebitis of right calf muscular vein

I80.252 Phlebitis and thrombophlebitis of left calf muscular vein

I80.253 Phlebitis and thrombophlebitis of calf muscular vein, bilateral

I80.259 Phlebitis and thrombophlebitis of unspecified calf muscular vein

+ I80.29 Phlebitis and thrombophlebitis of other deep vessels of lower extremities

CC **I80.291 Phlebitis and thrombophlebitis of other deep vessels of right lower extremity**

CC **I80.292 Phlebitis and thrombophlebitis of other deep vessels of left lower extremity**

CC **I80.293** **Phlebitis and thrombophlebitis of other deep vessels of lower extremity, bilateral**
CC **I80.299** **Phlebitis and thrombophlebitis of other deep vessels of unspecified lower extremity**
I80.3 **Phlebitis and thrombophlebitis of lower extremities, unspecified**
I80.8 **Phlebitis and thrombophlebitis of other sites**
I80.9 **Phlebitis and thrombophlebitis of unspecified site**

MCC **I81** **Portal vein thrombosis**
Portal (vein) obstruction
Excludes2: *hepatic vein thrombosis (I82.0)*
phlebitis of portal vein (K75.1)
Valid 3-character code, no further characters required

I82 **Other venous embolism and thrombosis**
Code first venous embolism and thrombosis complicating:
abortion, ectopic or molar pregnancy (O00-O07, O08.7)
pregnancy, childbirth and the puerperium (O22.-, O87.-)
Excludes2: *venous embolism and thrombosis (of):*
cerebral (I63.6, I67.6)
coronary (I21-I25)
intracranial and intraspinal, septic or NOS (G08)
intracranial, nonpyogenic (I67.6)
intraspinal, nonpyogenic (G95.1)
mesenteric (K55.0-)
portal (I81)
pulmonary (I26.-)

MCC **I82.0** **Budd-Chiari syndrome**
Hepatic vein thrombosis
CC **I82.1** **Thrombophlebitis migrans**
+ **I82.2** **Embolism and thrombosis of vena cava and other thoracic veins**
+ **I82.21** **Embolism and thrombosis of superior vena cava**
CC **I82.210** **Acute embolism and thrombosis of superior vena cava**
Embolism and thrombosis of superior vena cava NOS
CC **I82.211** **Chronic embolism and thrombosis of superior vena cava**
+ **I82.22** **Embolism and thrombosis of inferior vena cava**
MCC **I82.220** **Acute embolism and thrombosis of inferior vena cava**
Embolism and thrombosis of inferior vena cava NOS
MCC **I82.221** **Chronic embolism and thrombosis of inferior vena cava**
+ **I82.29** **Embolism and thrombosis of other thoracic veins**
Embolism and thrombosis of brachiocephalic (innominate) vein
CC **I82.290** **Acute embolism and thrombosis of other thoracic veins**
CC **I82.291** **Chronic embolism and thrombosis of other thoracic veins**
CC **I82.3** **Embolism and thrombosis of renal vein**
+ **I82.4** **Acute embolism and thrombosis of deep veins of lower extremity**
AHA CC: 4Q, 2019, 8-10
+ **I82.40** **Acute embolism and thrombosis of unspecified deep veins of lower extremity**
Deep vein thrombosis NOS
DVT NOS
Excludes1: *acute embolism and thrombosis of unspecified deep veins of distal lower extremity (I82.4Z-)*
acute embolism and thrombosis of unspecified deep veins of proximal lower extremity (I82.4Y-)
CC **I82.401** **Acute embolism and thrombosis of unspecified deep veins of right lower extremity**
HAC see Appendix B for HAC conditional logic
CC **I82.402** **Acute embolism and thrombosis of unspecified deep veins of left lower extremity**
HAC see Appendix B for HAC conditional logic
CC **I82.403** **Acute embolism and thrombosis of unspecified deep veins of lower extremity, bilateral**
HAC see Appendix B for HAC conditional logic
CC **I82.409** **Acute embolism and thrombosis of unspecified deep veins of unspecified lower extremity**
HAC see Appendix B for HAC conditional logic
+ **I82.41** **Acute embolism and thrombosis of femoral vein**
Acute embolism and thrombosis of common femoral vein
Acute embolism and thrombosis of deep femoral vein
CC **I82.411** **Acute embolism and thrombosis of right femoral vein**
HAC see Appendix B for HAC conditional logic
CC **I82.412** **Acute embolism and thrombosis of left femoral vein**
HAC see Appendix B for HAC conditional logic
CC **I82.413** **Acute embolism and thrombosis of femoral vein, bilateral**
HAC see Appendix B for HAC conditional logic
CC **I82.419** **Acute embolism and thrombosis of unspecified femoral vein**
HAC see Appendix B for HAC conditional logic
+ **I82.42** **Acute embolism and thrombosis of iliac vein**
Acute embolism and thrombosis of common iliac vein
Acute embolism and thrombosis of external iliac vein
Acute embolism and thrombosis of internal iliac vein
CC **I82.421** **Acute embolism and thrombosis of right iliac vein**
HAC see Appendix B for HAC conditional logic
CC **I82.422** **Acute embolism and thrombosis of left iliac vein**
HAC see Appendix B for HAC conditional logic
CC **I82.423** **Acute embolism and thrombosis of iliac vein, bilateral**
HAC see Appendix B for HAC conditional logic
CC **I82.429** **Acute embolism and thrombosis of unspecified iliac vein**
HAC see Appendix B for HAC conditional logic
+ **I82.43** **Acute embolism and thrombosis of popliteal vein**
CC **I82.431** **Acute embolism and thrombosis of right popliteal vein**
HAC see Appendix B for HAC conditional logic
CC **I82.432** **Acute embolism and thrombosis of left popliteal vein**
HAC see Appendix B for HAC conditional logic
CC **I82.433** **Acute embolism and thrombosis of popliteal vein, bilateral**
HAC see Appendix B for HAC conditional logic
CC **I82.439** **Acute embolism and thrombosis of unspecified popliteal vein**
HAC see Appendix B for HAC conditional logic
+ **I82.44** **Acute embolism and thrombosis of tibial vein**
Acute embolism and thrombosis of anterior tibial vein
Acute embolism and thrombosis of posterior tibial vein
CC **I82.441** **Acute embolism and thrombosis of right tibial vein**
HAC see Appendix B for HAC conditional logic
CC **I82.442** **Acute embolism and thrombosis of left tibial vein**
HAC see Appendix B for HAC conditional logic

CC **I82.443 Acute embolism and thrombosis of tibial vein, bilateral**
HAC see Appendix B for HAC conditional logic

CC **I82.449 Acute embolism and thrombosis of unspecified tibial vein**
HAC see Appendix B for HAC conditional logic

+ **I82.45 Acute embolism and thrombosis of peroneal vein**

CC **I82.451 Acute embolism and thrombosis of right peroneal vein**
HAC see Appendix B for HAC conditional logic

CC **I82.452 Acute embolism and thrombosis of left peroneal vein**
HAC see Appendix B for HAC conditional logic

CC **I82.453 Acute embolism and thrombosis of peroneal vein, bilateral**
HAC see Appendix B for HAC conditional logic

CC **I82.459 Acute embolism and thrombosis of unspecified peroneal vein**
HAC see Appendix B for HAC conditional logic

+ **I82.46 Acute embolism and thrombosis of calf muscular vein**
Acute embolism and thrombosis of calf muscular vein, NOS
Acute embolism and thrombosis of gastocnemial vein
Acute embolism and thrombosis of soleal vein

I82.461 Acute embolism and thrombosis of right calf muscular vein

I82.462 Acute embolism and thrombosis of left calf muscular vein

I82.463 Acute embolism and thrombosis of calf muscular vein, bilateral

I82.469 Acute embolism and thrombosis of unspecified calf muscular vein

+ **I82.49 Acute embolism and thrombosis of other specified deep vein of lower extremity**

CC **I82.491 Acute embolism and thrombosis of other specified deep vein of right lower extremity**
HAC see Appendix B for HAC conditional logic

CC **I82.492 Acute embolism and thrombosis of other specified deep vein of left lower extremity**
HAC see Appendix B for HAC conditional logic

CC **I82.493 Acute embolism and thrombosis of other specified deep vein of lower extremity, bilateral**
HAC see Appendix B for HAC conditional logic

CC **I82.499 Acute embolism and thrombosis of other specified deep vein of unspecified lower extremity**
HAC see Appendix B for HAC conditional logic

+ **I82.4Y Acute embolism and thrombosis of unspecified deep veins of proximal lower extremity**
Acute embolism and thrombosis of deep vein of thigh NOS
Acute embolism and thrombosis of deep vein of upper leg NOS

CC **I82.4Y1 Acute embolism and thrombosis of unspecified deep veins of right proximal lower extremity**
HAC see Appendix B for HAC conditional logic

CC **I82.4Y2 Acute embolism and thrombosis of unspecified deep veins of left proximal lower extremity**
HAC see Appendix B for HAC conditional logic

CC **I82.4Y3 Acute embolism and thrombosis of unspecified deep veins of proximal lower extremity, bilateral**
HAC see Appendix B for HAC conditional logic

CC **I82.4Y9 Acute embolism and thrombosis of unspecified deep veins of unspecified proximal lower extremity**
HAC see Appendix B for HAC conditional logic

+ **I82.4Z Acute embolism and thrombosis of unspecified deep veins of distal lower extremity**
Acute embolism and thrombosis of deep vein of calf NOS
Acute embolism and thrombosis of deep vein of lower leg NOS

CC **I82.4Z1 Acute embolism and thrombosis of unspecified deep veins of right distal lower extremity**
HAC see Appendix B for HAC conditional logic

CC **I82.4Z2 Acute embolism and thrombosis of unspecified deep veins of left distal lower extremity**
HAC see Appendix B for HAC conditional logic

CC **I82.4Z3 Acute embolism and thrombosis of unspecified deep veins of distal lower extremity, bilateral**
HAC see Appendix B for HAC conditional logic

CC **I82.4Z9 Acute embolism and thrombosis of unspecified deep veins of unspecified distal lower extremity**
HAC see Appendix B for HAC conditional logic

+ **I82.5 Chronic embolism and thrombosis of deep veins of lower extremity**
Use additional code, if applicable, for associated long-term (current) use of anticoagulants (Z79.01)
Excludes1: *personal history of venous embolism and thrombosis (Z86.718)*
AHA CC: 4Q, 2019, 8-10

+ **I82.50 Chronic embolism and thrombosis of unspecified deep veins of lower extremity**
Excludes1: *chronic embolism and thrombosis of unspecified deep veins of distal lower extremity (I82.5Z-)*
chronic embolism and thrombosis of unspecified deep veins of proximal lower extremity (I82.5Y-)

CC **I82.501 Chronic embolism and thrombosis of unspecified deep veins of right lower extremity**

CC **I82.502 Chronic embolism and thrombosis of unspecified deep veins of left lower extremity**

CC **I82.503 Chronic embolism and thrombosis of unspecified deep veins of lower extremity, bilateral**

CC **I82.509 Chronic embolism and thrombosis of unspecified deep veins of unspecified lower extremity**

+ **I82.51 Chronic embolism and thrombosis of femoral vein**
Chronic embolism and thrombosis of common femoral vein
Chronic embolism and thrombosis of deep femoral vein

CC **I82.511 Chronic embolism and thrombosis of right femoral vein**

CC **I82.512 Chronic embolism and thrombosis of left femoral vein**

CC **I82.513 Chronic embolism and thrombosis of femoral vein, bilateral**

CC **I82.519 Chronic embolism and thrombosis of unspecified femoral vein**

+ **I82.52 Chronic embolism and thrombosis of iliac vein**
Chronic embolism and thrombosis of common iliac vein
Chronic embolism and thrombosis of external iliac vein
Chronic embolism and thrombosis of internal iliac vein
CC **I82.521 Chronic embolism and thrombosis of right iliac vein**
CC **I82.522 Chronic embolism and thrombosis of left iliac vein**
CC **I82.523 Chronic embolism and thrombosis of iliac vein, bilateral**
CC **I82.529 Chronic embolism and thrombosis of unspecified iliac vein**

+ **I82.53 Chronic embolism and thrombosis of popliteal vein**
CC **I82.531 Chronic embolism and thrombosis of right popliteal vein**
CC **I82.532 Chronic embolism and thrombosis of left popliteal vein**
CC **I82.533 Chronic embolism and thrombosis of popliteal vein, bilateral**
CC **I82.539 Chronic embolism and thrombosis of unspecified popliteal vein**

+ **I82.54 Chronic embolism and thrombosis of tibial vein**
Chronic embolism and thrombosis of anterior tibial vein
Chronic embolism and thrombosis of posterior tibial vein
CC **I82.541 Chronic embolism and thrombosis of right tibial vein**
CC **I82.542 Chronic embolism and thrombosis of left tibial vein**
CC **I82.543 Chronic embolism and thrombosis of tibial vein, bilateral**
CC **I82.549 Chronic embolism and thrombosis of unspecified tibial vein**

+ **I82.55 Acute embolism and thrombosis of peroneal vein**
CC **I82.551 Chronic embolism and thrombosis of right peroneal vein**
CC **I82.552 Chronic embolism and thrombosis of left peroneal vein**
CC **I82.553 Chronic embolism and thrombosis of peroneal vein, bilateral**
CC **I82.559 Chronic embolism and thrombosis of unspecified peroneal vein**

+ **I82.56 Acute embolism and thrombosis of calf muscular vein**
Acute embolism and thrombosis of calf muscular vein, NOS
Acute embolism and thrombosis of gastocnemial vein
Acute embolism and thrombosis of soleal vein
I82.561 Chronic embolism and thrombosis of right calf muscular vein
I82.562 Chronic embolism and thrombosis of left calf muscular vein
I82.563 Chronic embolism and thrombosis of calf muscular vein, bilateral
I82.569 Chronic embolism and thrombosis of unspecified calf muscular vein

+ **I82.59 Chronic embolism and thrombosis of other specified deep vein of lower extremity**
CC **I82.591 Chronic embolism and thrombosis of other specified deep vein of right lower extremity**
CC **I82.592 Chronic embolism and thrombosis of other specified deep vein of left lower extremity**
CC **I82.593 Chronic embolism and thrombosis of other specified deep vein of lower extremity, bilateral**
CC **I82.599 Chronic embolism and thrombosis of other specified deep vein of unspecified lower extremity**

+ **I82.5Y Chronic embolism and thrombosis of unspecified deep veins of proximal lower extremity**
Chronic embolism and thrombosis of deep veins of thigh NOS
Chronic embolism and thrombosis of deep veins of upper leg NOS
CC **I82.5Y1 Chronic embolism and thrombosis of unspecified deep veins of right proximal lower extremity**
CC **I82.5Y2 Chronic embolism and thrombosis of unspecified deep veins of left proximal lower extremity**
CC **I82.5Y3 Chronic embolism and thrombosis of unspecified deep veins of proximal lower extremity, bilateral**
CC **I82.5Y9 Chronic embolism and thrombosis of unspecified deep veins of unspecified proximal lower extremity**

+ **I82.5Z Chronic embolism and thrombosis of unspecified deep veins of distal lower extremity**
Chronic embolism and thrombosis of deep veins of calf NOS
Chronic embolism and thrombosis of deep veins of lower leg NOS
CC **I82.5Z1 Chronic embolism and thrombosis of unspecified deep veins of right distal lower extremity**
CC **I82.5Z2 Chronic embolism and thrombosis of unspecified deep veins of left distal lower extremity**
CC **I82.5Z3 Chronic embolism and thrombosis of unspecified deep veins of distal lower extremity, bilateral**
CC **I82.5Z9 Chronic embolism and thrombosis of unspecified deep veins of unspecified distal lower extremity**

+ **I82.6 Acute embolism and thrombosis of veins of upper extremity**

+ **I82.60 Acute embolism and thrombosis of unspecified veins of upper extremity**
CC **I82.601 Acute embolism and thrombosis of unspecified veins of right upper extremity**
CC **I82.602 Acute embolism and thrombosis of unspecified veins of left upper extremity**
CC **I82.603 Acute embolism and thrombosis of unspecified veins of upper extremity, bilateral**
CC **I82.609 Acute embolism and thrombosis of unspecified veins of unspecified upper extremity**

+ **I82.61 Acute embolism and thrombosis of superficial veins of upper extremity**
Acute embolism and thrombosis of antecubital vein
Acute embolism and thrombosis of basilic vein
Acute embolism and thrombosis of cephalic vein
CC **I82.611 Acute embolism and thrombosis of superficial veins of right upper extremity**
CC **I82.612 Acute embolism and thrombosis of superficial veins of left upper extremity**
CC **I82.613 Acute embolism and thrombosis of superficial veins of upper extremity, bilateral**
CC **I82.619 Acute embolism and thrombosis of superficial veins of unspecified upper extremity**

+ **I82.62 Acute embolism and thrombosis of deep veins of upper extremity**
Acute embolism and thrombosis of brachial vein
Acute embolism and thrombosis of radial vein
Acute embolism and thrombosis of ulnar vein
CC **I82.621 Acute embolism and thrombosis of deep veins of right upper extremity**
CC **I82.622 Acute embolism and thrombosis of deep veins of left upper extremity**
CC **I82.623 Acute embolism and thrombosis of deep veins of upper extremity, bilateral**
CC **I82.629 Acute embolism and thrombosis of deep veins of unspecified upper extremity**

+ I82.7 **Chronic embolism and thrombosis of veins of upper extremity**
Use additional code, if applicable, for associated long-term (current) use of anticoagulants (Z79.01)
Excludes1: *personal history of venous embolism and thrombosis (Z86.718)*

+ I82.70 **Chronic embolism and thrombosis of unspecified veins of upper extremity**
CC I82.701 **Chronic embolism and thrombosis of unspecified veins of right upper extremity**
CC I82.702 **Chronic embolism and thrombosis of unspecified veins of left upper extremity**
CC I82.703 **Chronic embolism and thrombosis of unspecified veins of upper extremity, bilateral**
CC I82.709 **Chronic embolism and thrombosis of unspecified veins of unspecified upper extremity**

+ I82.71 **Chronic embolism and thrombosis of superficial veins of upper extremity**
Chronic embolism and thrombosis of antecubital vein
Chronic embolism and thrombosis of basilic vein
Chronic embolism and thrombosis of cephalic vein
CC I82.711 **Chronic embolism and thrombosis of superficial veins of right upper extremity**
CC I82.712 **Chronic embolism and thrombosis of superficial veins of left upper extremity**
CC I82.713 **Chronic embolism and thrombosis of superficial veins of upper extremity, bilateral**
CC I82.719 **Chronic embolism and thrombosis of superficial veins of unspecified upper extremity**

+ I82.72 **Chronic embolism and thrombosis of deep veins of upper extremity**
Chronic embolism and thrombosis of brachial vein
Chronic embolism and thrombosis of radial vein
Chronic embolism and thrombosis of ulnar vein
CC I82.721 **Chronic embolism and thrombosis of deep veins of right upper extremity**
CC I82.722 **Chronic embolism and thrombosis of deep veins of left upper extremity**
CC I82.723 **Chronic embolism and thrombosis of deep veins of upper extremity, bilateral**
CC I82.729 **Chronic embolism and thrombosis of deep veins of unspecified upper extremity**

+ I82.A **Embolism and thrombosis of axillary vein**

+ I82.A1 **Acute embolism and thrombosis of axillary vein**
CC I82.A11 **Acute embolism and thrombosis of right axillary vein**
CC I82.A12 **Acute embolism and thrombosis of left axillary vein**
CC I82.A13 **Acute embolism and thrombosis of axillary vein, bilateral**
CC I82.A19 **Acute embolism and thrombosis of unspecified axillary vein**

+ I82.A2 **Chronic embolism and thrombosis of axillary vein**
CC I82.A21 **Chronic embolism and thrombosis of right axillary vein**
CC I82.A22 **Chronic embolism and thrombosis of left axillary vein**
CC I82.A23 **Chronic embolism and thrombosis of axillary vein, bilateral**
CC I82.A29 **Chronic embolism and thrombosis of unspecified axillary vein**

+ I82.B **Embolism and thrombosis of subclavian vein**

+ I82.B1 **Acute embolism and thrombosis of subclavian≈vein**
CC I82.B11 **Acute embolism and thrombosis of right subclavian vein**
CC I82.B12 **Acute embolism and thrombosis of left subclavian vein**
CC I82.B13 **Acute embolism and thrombosis of subclavian vein, bilateral**
CC I82.B19 **Acute embolism and thrombosis of unspecified subclavian vein**

+ I82.B2 **Chronic embolism and thrombosis of subclavian vein**
CC I82.B21 **Chronic embolism and thrombosis of right subclavian vein**
CC I82.B22 **Chronic embolism and thrombosis of left subclavian vein**
CC I82.B23 **Chronic embolism and thrombosis of subclavian vein, bilateral**
CC I82.B29 **Chronic embolism and thrombosis of unspecified subclavian vein**

+ I82.C **Embolism and thrombosis of internal jugular vein**

+ I82.C1 **Acute embolism and thrombosis of internal jugular vein**
CC I82.C11 **Acute embolism and thrombosis of right internal jugular vein**
CC I82.C12 **Acute embolism and thrombosis of left internal jugular vein**
CC I82.C13 **Acute embolism and thrombosis of internal jugular vein, bilateral**
CC I82.C19 **Acute embolism and thrombosis of unspecified internal jugular vein**

+ I82.C2 **Chronic embolism and thrombosis of internal jugular vein**
CC I82.C21 **Chronic embolism and thrombosis of right internal jugular vein**
CC I82.C22 **Chronic embolism and thrombosis of left internal jugular vein**
CC I82.C23 **Chronic embolism and thrombosis of internal jugular vein, bilateral**
CC I82.C29 **Chronic embolism and thrombosis of unspecified internal jugular vein**

+ I82.8 **Embolism and thrombosis of other specified veins**
Use additional code, if applicable, for associated long-term (current) use of anticoagulants (Z79.01)

+ I82.81 **Embolism and thrombosis of superficial veins of lower extremities**
Embolism and thrombosis of saphenous vein (greater) (lesser)
CC I82.811 **Embolism and thrombosis of superficial veins of right lower extremity**
CC I82.812 **Embolism and thrombosis of superficial veins of left lower extremity**
CC I82.813 **Embolism and thrombosis of superficial veins of lower extremities, bilateral**
CC I82.819 **Embolism and thrombosis of superficial veins of unspecified lower extremity**

+ I82.89 **Embolism and thrombosis of other specified veins**
CC I82.890 **Acute embolism and thrombosis of other specified veins**
CC I82.891 **Chronic embolism and thrombosis of other specified veins**

+ I82.9 **Embolism and thrombosis of unspecified vein**
CC I82.90 **Acute embolism and thrombosis of unspecified vein**
Embolism of vein NOS
Thrombosis (vein) NOS
CC I82.91 **Chronic embolism and thrombosis of unspecified vein**

I83 **Varicose veins of lower extremities**
Excludes2: *varicose veins complicating pregnancy (O22.0-)*
varicose veins complicating the puerperium (O87.4)

+ I83.0 **Varicose veins of lower extremities with ulcer**
Use additional code to identify severity of ulcer (L97.-)

+ I83.00 **Varicose veins of unspecified lower extremity with ulcer**
• I83.001 **Varicose veins of unspecified lower extremity with ulcer of thigh**
• I83.002 **Varicose veins of unspecified lower extremity with ulcer of calf**
• I83.003 **Varicose veins of unspecified lower extremity with ulcer of ankle**
• I83.004 **Varicose veins of unspecified lower extremity with ulcer of heel and midfoot**
Varicose veins of unspecified lower extremity with ulcer of plantar surface of midfoot
• I83.005 **Varicose veins of unspecified lower extremity with ulcer other part of foot**
Varicose veins of unspecified lower extremity with ulcer of toe

- I83.008 **Varicose veins of unspecified lower extremity with ulcer other part of lower leg**
- I83.009 **Varicose veins of unspecified lower extremity with ulcer of unspecified site**

\+ I83.01 **Varicose veins of right lower extremity with ulcer**
- I83.011 **Varicose veins of right lower extremity with ulcer of thigh**
- I83.012 **Varicose veins of right lower extremity with ulcer of calf**
- I83.013 **Varicose veins of right lower extremity with ulcer of ankle**
- I83.014 **Varicose veins of right lower extremity with ulcer of heel and midfoot**
  Varicose veins of right lower extremity with ulcer of plantar surface of midfoot
- I83.015 **Varicose veins of right lower extremity with ulcer other part of foot**
  Varicose veins of right lower extremity with ulcer of toe
- I83.018 **Varicose veins of right lower extremity with ulcer other part of lower leg**
- I83.019 **Varicose veins of right lower extremity with ulcer of unspecified site**

\+ I83.02 **Varicose veins of left lower extremity with ulcer**
- I83.021 **Varicose veins of left lower extremity with ulcer of thigh**
- I83.022 **Varicose veins of left lower extremity with ulcer of calf**
- I83.023 **Varicose veins of left lower extremity with ulcer of ankle**
- I83.024 **Varicose veins of left lower extremity with ulcer of heel and midfoot**
  Varicose veins of left lower extremity with ulcer of plantar surface of midfoot
- I83.025 **Varicose veins of left lower extremity with ulcer other part of foot**
  Varicose veins of left lower extremity with ulcer of toe
- I83.028 **Varicose veins of left lower extremity with ulcer other part of lower leg**
- I83.029 **Varicose veins of left lower extremity with ulcer of unspecified site**

\+ I83.1 **Varicose veins of lower extremities with inflammation**
- I83.10 **Varicose veins of unspecified lower extremity with inflammation**
- I83.11 **Varicose veins of right lower extremity with inflammation**
- I83.12 **Varicose veins of left lower extremity with inflammation**

\+ I83.2 **Varicose veins of lower extremities with both ulcer and inflammation**
Use additional code to identify severity of ulcer (L97.-)

\+ I83.20 **Varicose veins of unspecified lower extremity with both ulcer and inflammation**
- CC I83.201 **Varicose veins of unspecified lower extremity with both ulcer of thigh and inflammation**
- CC I83.202 **Varicose veins of unspecified lower extremity with both ulcer of calf and inflammation**
- CC I83.203 **Varicose veins of unspecified lower extremity with both ulcer of ankle and inflammation**
- CC I83.204 **Varicose veins of unspecified lower extremity with both ulcer of heel and midfoot and inflammation**
  Varicose veins of unspecified lower extremity with both ulcer of plantar surface of midfoot and inflammation
- CC I83.205 **Varicose veins of unspecified lower extremity with both ulcer other part of foot and inflammation**
  Varicose veins of unspecified lower extremity with both ulcer of toe and inflammation
- CC I83.208 **Varicose veins of unspecified lower extremity with both ulcer of other part of lower extremity and inflammation**
- CC I83.209 **Varicose veins of unspecified lower extremity with both ulcer of unspecified site and inflammation**

\+ I83.21 **Varicose veins of right lower extremity with both ulcer and inflammation**
- CC I83.211 **Varicose veins of right lower extremity with both ulcer of thigh and inflammation**
- CC I83.212 **Varicose veins of right lower extremity with both ulcer of calf and inflammation**
- CC I83.213 **Varicose veins of right lower extremity with both ulcer of ankle and inflammation**
- CC I83.214 **Varicose veins of right lower extremity with both ulcer of heel and midfoot and inflammation**
  Varicose veins of right lower extremity with both ulcer of plantar surface of midfoot and inflammation
- CC I83.215 **Varicose veins of right lower extremity with both ulcer other part of foot and inflammation**
  Varicose veins of right lower extremity with both ulcer of toe and inflammation
- CC I83.218 **Varicose veins of right lower extremity with both ulcer of other part of lower extremity and inflammation**
- CC I83.219 **Varicose veins of right lower extremity with both ulcer of unspecified site and inflammation**

\+ I83.22 **Varicose veins of left lower extremity with both ulcer and inflammation**
- CC I83.221 **Varicose veins of left lower extremity with both ulcer of thigh and inflammation**
- CC I83.222 **Varicose veins of left lower extremity with both ulcer of calf and inflammation**
- CC I83.223 **Varicose veins of left lower extremity with both ulcer of ankle and inflammation**
- CC I83.224 **Varicose veins of left lower extremity with both ulcer of heel and midfoot and inflammation**
  Varicose veins of left lower extremity with both ulcer of plantar surface of midfoot and inflammation
- CC I83.225 **Varicose veins of left lower extremity with both ulcer other part of foot and inflammation**
  Varicose veins of left lower extremity with both ulcer of toe and inflammation
- CC I83.228 **Varicose veins of left lower extremity with both ulcer of other part of lower extremity and inflammation**
- CC I83.229 **Varicose veins of left lower extremity with both ulcer of unspecified site and inflammation**

\+ I83.8 **Varicose veins of lower extremities with other complications**

\+ I83.81 **Varicose veins of lower extremities with pain**
- I83.811 **Varicose veins of right lower extremity with pain**
- I83.812 **Varicose veins of left lower extremity with pain**
- I83.813 **Varicose veins of bilateral lower extremities with pain**
- I83.819 **Varicose veins of unspecified lower extremity with pain**

+ **I83.89 Varicose veins of lower extremities with other complications**
Varicose veins of lower extremities with edema
Varicose veins of lower extremities with swelling
• **I83.891 Varicose veins of right lower extremity with other complications**
• **I83.892 Varicose veins of left lower extremity with other complications**
• **I83.893 Varicose veins of bilateral lower extremities with other complications**
• **I83.899 Varicose veins of unspecified lower extremity with other complications**

+ **I83.9 Asymptomatic varicose veins of lower extremities**
Phlebectasia of lower extremities
Varicose veins of lower extremities
Varix of lower extremities
• **I83.90 Asymptomatic varicose veins of unspecified lower extremity**
Varicose veins NOS
• **I83.91 Asymptomatic varicose veins of right lower extremity**
• **I83.92 Asymptomatic varicose veins of left lower extremity**
• **I83.93 Asymptomatic varicose veins of bilateral lower extremities**

I85 Esophageal varices
Use additional code to identify:
alcohol abuse and dependence (F10.-)
+ **I85.0 Esophageal varices**
Idiopathic esophageal varices
Primary esophageal varices
CC **I85.00 Esophageal varices without bleeding**
Esophageal varices NOS
MCC **I85.01 Esophageal varices with bleeding**
+ **I85.1 Secondary esophageal varices**
Esophageal varices secondary to alcoholic liver disease
Esophageal varices secondary to cirrhosis of liver
Esophageal varices secondary to schistosomiasis
Esophageal varices secondary to toxic liver disease
Code first underlying disease
CC **I85.10 Secondary esophageal varices without bleeding**
MCC **I85.11 Secondary esophageal varices with bleeding**

I86 Varicose veins of other sites
Excludes1: *varicose veins of unspecified site (I83.9-)*
Excludes2: *retinal varices (H35.0-)*
I86.0 Sublingual varices
♂ **I86.1 Scrotal varices**
Varicocele
I86.2 Pelvic varices
♀ **I86.3 Vulval varices**
Excludes1: *vulval varices complicating childbirth and the puerperium (O87.8)*
vulval varices complicating pregnancy (O22.1-)
I86.4 Gastric varices
• **I86.8 Varicose veins of other specified sites**
Varicose ulcer of nasal septum

I87 Other disorders of veins
+ **I87.0 Postthrombotic syndrome**
Chronic venous hypertension due to deep vein thrombosis
Postphlebitic syndrome
Excludes1: *chronic venous hypertension without deep vein thrombosis (I87.3-)*
+ **I87.00 Postthrombotic syndrome without complications**
Asymptomatic Postthrombotic syndrome
I87.001 Postthrombotic syndrome without complications of right lower extremity
I87.002 Postthrombotic syndrome without complications of left lower extremity
I87.003 Postthrombotic syndrome without complications of bilateral lower extremity
I87.009 Postthrombotic syndrome without complications of unspecified extremity
Postthrombotic syndrome NOS
+ **I87.01 Postthrombotic syndrome with ulcer**
Use additional code to specify site and severity of ulcer (L97.-)
CC **I87.011 Postthrombotic syndrome with ulcer of right lower extremity**
CC **I87.012 Postthrombotic syndrome with ulcer of left lower extremity**
CC **I87.013 Postthrombotic syndrome with ulcer of bilateral lower extremity**
CC **I87.019 Postthrombotic syndrome with ulcer of unspecified lower extremity**
+ **I87.02 Postthrombotic syndrome with inflammation**
I87.021 Postthrombotic syndrome with inflammation of right lower extremity
I87.022 Postthrombotic syndrome with inflammation of left lower extremity
I87.023 Postthrombotic syndrome with inflammation of bilateral lower extremity
I87.029 Postthrombotic syndrome with inflammation of unspecified lower extremity
+ **I87.03 Postthrombotic syndrome with ulcer and inflammation**
Use additional code to specify site and severity of ulcer (L97.-)
CC **I87.031 Postthrombotic syndrome with ulcer and inflammation of right lower extremity**
CC **I87.032 Postthrombotic syndrome with ulcer and inflammation of left lower extremity**
CC **I87.033 Postthrombotic syndrome with ulcer and inflammation of bilateral lower extremity**
CC **I87.039 Postthrombotic syndrome with ulcer and inflammation of unspecified lower extremity**
+ **I87.09 Postthrombotic syndrome with other complications**
I87.091 Postthrombotic syndrome with other complications of right lower extremity
I87.092 Postthrombotic syndrome with other complications of left lower extremity
I87.093 Postthrombotic syndrome with other complications of bilateral lower extremity
I87.099 Postthrombotic syndrome with other complications of unspecified lower extremity
CC **I87.1 Compression of vein**
Stricture of vein
Vena cava syndrome (inferior) (superior)
Excludes2: *compression of pulmonary vein (I28.8)*
I87.2 Venous insufficiency (chronic) (peripheral)
Stasis dermatitis
Excludes1: *stasis dermatitis with varicose veins of lower extremities (I83.1-, I83.2-)*
+ **I87.3 Chronic venous hypertension (idiopathic)**
Stasis edema
Excludes1: *chronic venous hypertension due to deep vein thrombosis (I87.0-)*
varicose veins of lower extremities (I83.-)
+ **I87.30 Chronic venous hypertension (idiopathic) without complications**
Asymptomatic chronic venous hypertension (idiopathic)
I87.301 Chronic venous hypertension (idiopathic) without complications of right lower extremity
I87.302 Chronic venous hypertension (idiopathic) without complications of left lower extremity
I87.303 Chronic venous hypertension (idiopathic) without complications of bilateral lower extremity
I87.309 Chronic venous hypertension (idiopathic) without complications of unspecified lower extremity
Chronic venous hypertension NOS

+ **I87.31 Chronic venous hypertension (idiopathic) with ulcer**
Use additional code to specify site and severity of ulcer (L97.-)
CC **I87.311 Chronic venous hypertension (idiopathic) with ulcer of right lower extremity**
CC **I87.312 Chronic venous hypertension (idiopathic) with ulcer of left lower extremity**
CC **I87.313 Chronic venous hypertension (idiopathic) with ulcer of bilateral lower extremity**
CC **I87.319 Chronic venous hypertension (idiopathic) with ulcer of unspecified lower extremity**
+ **I87.32 Chronic venous hypertension (idiopathic) with inflammation**
I87.321 Chronic venous hypertension (idiopathic) with inflammation of right lower extremity
I87.322 Chronic venous hypertension (idiopathic) with inflammation of left lower extremity
I87.323 Chronic venous hypertension (idiopathic) with inflammation of bilateral lower extremity
I87.329 Chronic venous hypertension (idiopathic) with inflammation of unspecified lower extremity
+ **I87.33 Chronic venous hypertension (idiopathic) with ulcer and inflammation**
Use additional code to specify site and severity of ulcer (L97.-)
CC **I87.331 Chronic venous hypertension (idiopathic) with ulcer and inflammation of right lower extremity**
CC **I87.332 Chronic venous hypertension (idiopathic) with ulcer and inflammation of left lower extremity**
CC **I87.333 Chronic venous hypertension (idiopathic) with ulcer and inflammation of bilateral lower extremity**
CC **I87.339 Chronic venous hypertension (idiopathic) with ulcer and inflammation of unspecified lower extremity**
+ **I87.39 Chronic venous hypertension (idiopathic) with other complications**
I87.391 Chronic venous hypertension (idiopathic) with other complications of right lower extremity
I87.392 Chronic venous hypertension (idiopathic) with other complications of left lower extremity
I87.393 Chronic venous hypertension (idiopathic) with other complications of bilateral lower extremity
I87.399 Chronic venous hypertension (idiopathic) with other complications of unspecified lower extremity

I87.8 Other specified disorders of veins
Phlebosclerosis
Venofibrosis
I87.9 Disorder of vein, unspecified

I88 Nonspecific lymphadenitis
Excludes1: *acute lymphadenitis, except mesenteric (L04.-)*
enlarged lymph nodes NOS (R59.-)
human immunodeficiency virus [HIV] disease resulting in generalized lymphadenopathy (B20)
I88.0 Nonspecific mesenteric lymphadenitis
Mesenteric lymphadenitis (acute)(chronic)
I88.1 Chronic lymphadenitis, except mesenteric
Adenitis
Lymphadenitis
I88.8 Other nonspecific lymphadenitis
I88.9 Nonspecific lymphadenitis, unspecified
Lymphadenitis NOS

I89 Other noninfective disorders of lymphatic vessels and lymph nodes
Excludes1: *chylocele, tunica vaginalis (nonfilarial) NOS (N50.89)*
enlarged lymph nodes NOS (R59.-)
filarial chylocele (B74.-)
hereditary lymphedema (Q82.0)
I89.0 Lymphedema, not elsewhere classified
Elephantiasis (nonfilarial) NOS
Lymphangiectasis
Obliteration, lymphatic vessel
Praecox lymphedema
Secondary lymphedema
Excludes1: *postmastectomy lymphedema (I97.2)*
I89.1 Lymphangitis
Chronic lymphangitis
Lymphangitis NOS
Subacute lymphangitis
Excludes1: *acute lymphangitis (L03.-)*
I89.8 Other specified noninfective disorders of lymphatic vessels and lymph nodes
Chylocele (nonfilarial)
Chylous ascites
Chylous cyst
Lipomelanotic reticulosis
Lymph node or vessel fistula
Lymph node or vessel infarction
Lymph node or vessel rupture
I89.9 Noninfective disorder of lymphatic vessels and lymph nodes, unspecified
Disease of lymphatic vessels NOS

Other and unspecified disorders of the circulatory system (I95-I99)

I95 Hypotension
Excludes1: *cardiovascular collapse (R57.9)*
maternal hypotension syndrome (O26.5-)
nonspecific low blood pressure reading NOS (R03.1)
I95.0 Idiopathic hypotension
I95.1 Orthostatic hypotension
Hypotension, postural
Excludes1: *neurogenic orthostatic hypotension [Shy-Drager] (G90.3)*
orthostatic hypotension due to drugs (I95.2)
I95.2 Hypotension due to drugs
Orthostatic hypotension due to drugs
Use additional code for adverse effect, if applicable, to identify drug (T36-T50 with fifth or sixth character 5)
I95.3 Hypotension of hemodialysis
Intra-dialytic hypotension
I95.8 Other hypotension
I95.81 Postprocedural hypotension
I95.89 Other hypotension
Chronic hypotension
I95.9 Hypotension, unspecified

CC **I96 Gangrene, not elsewhere classified**
Gangrenous cellulitis
Excludes1: *gangrene in atherosclerosis of native arteries of the extremities (I70.26)*
gangrene in hernia (K40.1, K40.4, K41.1, K41.4, K42.1, K43.1-, K44.1, K45.1, K46.1)
gangrene in other peripheral vascular diseases (I73.-)
gangrene of certain specified sites - see Alphabetical Index
gas gangrene (A48.0)
pyoderma gangrenosum (L88)
Excludes2: *gangrene in diabetes mellitus (E08-E13 with .52)*
AHA CC: Q2, 2013, 34-35; 3Q, 2017, 6; 3Q, 2018, 3-4
Valid 3-character code, no further characters required

I97 Intraoperative and postprocedural complications and disorders of circulatory system, not elsewhere classified

Excludes2: *postprocedural shock (T81.1-)*

AHA CC: 1Q, 2021, 13-14

I97.0 Postcardiotomy syndrome

+ **I97.1 Other postprocedural cardiac functional disturbances**

Excludes2: *acute pulmonary insufficiency following thoracic surgery (J95.1)*

intraoperative cardiac functional disturbances (I97.7-)

+ **I97.11 Postprocedural cardiac insufficiency**

CC **I97.110 Postprocedural cardiac insufficiency following cardiac surgery**

CC **I97.111 Postprocedural cardiac insufficiency following other surgery**

+ **I97.12 Postprocedural cardiac arrest**

CC **I97.120 Postprocedural cardiac arrest following cardiac surgery**

CC **I97.121 Postprocedural cardiac arrest following other surgery**

+ **I97.13 Postprocedural heart failure**

Use additional code to identify the heart failure (I50.-)

CC **I97.130 Postprocedural heart failure following cardiac surgery**

CC **I97.131 Postprocedural heart failure following other surgery**

+ **I97.19 Other postprocedural cardiac functional disturbances**

Use additional code, if applicable, to further specify disorder

CC **I97.190 Other postprocedural cardiac functional disturbances following cardiac surgery**

Use additional code, if applicable, for type 4 or type 5 myocardial infarction, to further specify disorder

AHA CC: 2Q, 2019, 32-33

CC **I97.191 Other postprocedural cardiac functional disturbances following other surgery**

• **I97.2 Postmastectomy lymphedema syndrome**

Elephantiasis due to mastectomy

Obliteration of lymphatic vessels

I97.3 Postprocedural hypertension

+ **I97.4 Intraoperative hemorrhage and hematoma of a circulatory system organ or structure complicating a procedure**

Excludes1: *intraoperative hemorrhage and hematoma of a circulatory system organ or structure due to accidental puncture and laceration during a procedure (I97.5-)*

Excludes2: *intraoperative cerebrovascular hemorrhage complicating a procedure (G97.3-)*

+ **I97.41 Intraoperative hemorrhage and hematoma of a circulatory system organ or structure complicating a circulatory system procedure**

CC **I97.410 Intraoperative hemorrhage and hematoma of a circulatory system organ or structure complicating a cardiac catheterization**

CC **I97.411 Intraoperative hemorrhage and hematoma of a circulatory system organ or structure complicating a cardiac bypass**

CC **I97.418 Intraoperative hemorrhage and hematoma of a circulatory system organ or structure complicating other circulatory system procedure**

CC **I97.42 Intraoperative hemorrhage and hematoma of a circulatory system organ or structure complicating other procedure**

AHA CC: 4Q, 2016, 100-101

+ **I97.5 Accidental puncture and laceration of a circulatory system organ or structure during a procedure**

Excludes2: *accidental puncture and laceration of brain during a procedure (G97.4-)*

CC **I97.51 Accidental puncture and laceration of a circulatory system organ or structure during a circulatory system procedure**

AHA CC: 2Q, 2019, 24

CC **I97.52 Accidental puncture and laceration of a circulatory system organ or structure during other procedure**

+ **I97.6 Postprocedural hemorrhage, hematoma and seroma of a circulatory system organ or structure following a procedure**

Excludes2: *postprocedural cerebrovascular hemorrhage complicating a procedure (G97.5-)*

AHA CC: 4Q, 2016, 9-10

+ **I97.61 Postprocedural hemorrhage of a circulatory system organ or structure following a circulatory system procedure**

CC **I97.610 Postprocedural hemorrhage of a circulatory system organ or structure following a cardiac catheterization**

CC **I97.611 Postprocedural hemorrhage of a circulatory system organ or structure following cardiac bypass**

CC **I97.618 Postprocedural hemorrhage of a circulatory system organ or structure following other circulatory system procedure**

+ **I97.62 Postprocedural hemorrhage, hematoma and seroma of a circulatory system organ or structure following other procedure**

CC **I97.620 Postprocedural hemorrhage of a circulatory system organ or structure following other procedure**

CC **I97.621 Postprocedural hematoma of a circulatory system organ or structure following other procedure**

CC **I97.622 Postprocedural seroma of a circulatory system organ or structure following other procedure**

+ **I97.63 Postprocedural hematoma of a circulatory system organ or structure following a circulatory system procedure**

CC **I97.630 Postprocedural hematoma of a circulatory system organ or structure following a cardiac catheterization**

CC **I97.631 Postprocedural hematoma of a circulatory system organ or structure following cardiac bypass**

CC **I97.638 Postprocedural hematoma of a circulatory system organ or structure following other circulatory system procedure**

I97.64 Postprocedural seroma of a circulatory system organ or structure following a circulatory system procedure

CC **I97.640 Postprocedural seroma of a circulatory system organ or structure following a cardiac catheterization**

CC **I97.641 Postprocedural seroma of a circulatory system organ or structure following cardiac bypass**

CC **I97.648 Postprocedural seroma of a circulatory system organ or structure following other circulatory system procedure**

+ **I97.7 Intraoperative cardiac functional disturbances**

Excludes2: *acute pulmonary insufficiency following thoracic surgery (J95.1)*

postprocedural cardiac functional disturbances (I97.1-)

+ **I97.71 Intraoperative cardiac arrest**

CC **I97.710 Intraoperative cardiac arrest during cardiac surgery**

CC **I97.711 Intraoperative cardiac arrest during other surgery**

+ I97.79 **Other intraoperative cardiac functional disturbances**
Use additional code, if applicable, to further specify disorder
CC I97.790 **Other intraoperative cardiac functional disturbances during cardiac surgery**
CC I97.791 **Other intraoperative cardiac functional disturbances during other surgery**

+ I97.8 **Other intraoperative and postprocedural complications and disorders of the circulatory system, not elsewhere classified**
Use additional code, if applicable, to further specify disorder

+ I97.81 **Intraoperative cerebrovascular infarction**
CC I97.810 **Intraoperative cerebrovascular infarction cardiac surgery**
CC I97.811 **Intraoperative cerebrovascular infarction during other surgery**

+ I97.82 **Postprocedural cerebrovascular infarction**
CC I97.820 **Postprocedural cerebrovascular infarction following cardiac surgery**
CC I97.821 **Postprocedural cerebrovascular infarction following other surgery**

CC I97.88 **Other intraoperative complications of the circulatory system, not elsewhere classified**
CC I97.89 **Other postprocedural complications and disorders of the circulatory system, not elsewhere classified**
AHA CC: 3Q, 2020, 4, 7-8

I99 Other and unspecified disorders of circulatory system
I99.8 Other disorder of circulatory system
I99.9 Unspecified disorder of circulatory system

Chapter 10: Diseases of the Respiratory System (J00-J99)

NOTE When a respiratory condition is described as occurring in more than one site and is not specifically indexed, it should be classified to the lower anatomic site (e.g. tracheobronchitis to bronchitis in J40).

Use additional code, where applicable, to identify:
exposure to environmental tobacco smoke (Z77.22)
exposure to tobacco smoke in the perinatal period (P96.81)
history of tobacco dependence (Z87.891)
occupational exposure to environmental tobacco smoke (Z57.31)
tobacco dependence (F17.-)
tobacco use (Z72.0)

Excludes2: *certain conditions originating in the perinatal period (P04-P96)*
certain infectious and parasitic diseases (A00-B99)
complications of pregnancy, childbirth and the puerperium (O00-O9A)
congenital malformations, deformations and chromosomal abnormalities (Q00-Q99)
endocrine, nutritional and metabolic diseases (E00-E88)
injury, poisoning and certain other consequences of external causes (S00-T88)
neoplasms (C00-D49)
smoke inhalation (T59.81-)
symptoms, signs and abnormal clinical and laboratory findings, not elsewhere classified (R00-R94)

This chapter contains the following category blocks:

J00-J06	Acute upper respiratory infections
J09-J18	Influenza and pneumonia
J20-J22	Other acute lower respiratory infections
J30-J39	Other diseases of upper respiratory tract
J40-J47	Chronic lower respiratory diseases
J60-J70	Lung diseases due to external agents
J80-J84	Other respiratory diseases principally affecting the interstitium
J85-J86	Suppurative and necrotic conditions of the lower respiratory tract
J90-J94	Other diseases of the pleura
J95	Intraoperative and postprocedural complications and disorders of respiratory system, not elsewhere classified
J96-J99	Other diseases of the respiratory system

C. Chapter-Specific Coding Guidelines

In addition to general coding guidelines, there are guidelines for specific diagnoses and/or conditions in the classification. Unless otherwise indicated, these guidelines apply to all health care settings. Please refer to Section II for guidelines on the selection of principal diagnosis.

10. Chapter 10: Diseases of the Respiratory System (J00-J99), U07.0

a. Chronic Obstructive Pulmonary Disease [COPD] and Asthma

1) Acute exacerbation of chronic obstructive bronchitis and asthma

The codes in categories J44 and J45 distinguish between uncomplicated cases and those in acute exacerbation. An acute exacerbation is a worsening or a decompensation of a chronic condition. An acute exacerbation is not equivalent to an infection superimposed on a chronic condition, though an exacerbation may be triggered by an infection.

b. Acute Respiratory Failure

1) Acute respiratory failure as principal diagnosis

A code from subcategory J96.0, Acute respiratory failure, or subcategory J96.2, Acute and chronic respiratory failure, may be assigned as a principal diagnosis when it is the condition established after study to be chiefly responsible for occasioning the admission to the hospital, and the selection is supported by the Alphabetic Index and Tabular List. However, chapter- specific coding guidelines (such as obstetrics, poisoning, HIV, newborn) that provide sequencing direction take precedence.

2) Acute respiratory failure as secondary diagnosis

Respiratory failure may be listed as a secondary diagnosis if it occurs after admission, or if it is present on admission, but does not meet the definition of principal diagnosis.

3) Sequencing of acute respiratory failure and another acute condition

When a patient is admitted with respiratory failure and another acute condition, (e.g., myocardial infarction, cerebrovascular accident, aspiration pneumonia), the principal diagnosis will not be the same in every situation. This applies whether the other acute condition is a respiratory or nonrespiratory condition. Selection of the principal diagnosis will be dependent on the circumstances of admission. If both the respiratory failure and the other acute condition are equally responsible for occasioning the admission to the hospital, and there are no chapter-specific sequencing rules, the guideline regarding two or more diagnoses that equally meet the definition for principal diagnosis *(Section II, C.)* may be applied in these situations.

If the documentation is not clear as to whether acute respiratory failure and another condition are equally responsible for occasioning the admission, query the provider for clarification.

c. Influenza due to certain identified influenza viruses

Code only confirmed cases of influenza due to certain identified influenza viruses (category J09), and due to other identified influenza virus (category J10). This is an exception to the hospital inpatient guideline Section II, H. (Uncertain Diagnosis).

In this context, "confirmation" does not require documentation of positive laboratory testing specific for avian or other novel influenza A or other identified influenza virus. However, coding should be based on the provider's diagnostic statement that the patient has avian influenza, or other novel influenza A, for category J09, or has another particular identified strain of influenza, such as H1N1 or H3N2, but not identified as novel or variant, for category J10.

If the provider records "suspected" or "possible" or "probable" avian influenza, or novel influenza, or other identified influenza, then the appropriate influenza code from category J11, Influenza due to unidentified influenza virus, should be assigned. A code from category J09, Influenza due to certain identified influenza viruses, should not be assigned nor should a code from category J10, Influenza due to other identified influenza virus.

d. Ventilator associated Pneumonia

1) Documentation of Ventilator associated Pneumonia

As with all procedural or postprocedural complications, code assignment is based on the provider's documentation of the relationship between the condition and the procedure.

Code J95.851, Ventilator associated pneumonia, should be assigned only when the provider has documented ventilator associated pneumonia (VAP). An additional code to identify the organism (e.g., Pseudomonas aeruginosa, code B96.5) should also be assigned. Do not assign an additional code from categories J12-J18 to identify the type of pneumonia.

Code J95.851 should not be assigned for cases where the patient has pneumonia and is on a mechanical ventilator and the provider has not specifically stated that the pneumonia is ventilator-associated pneumonia. If the documentation is unclear as to whether the patient has a pneumonia that is a complication attributable to the mechanical ventilator, query the provider.

2) Ventilator associated Pneumonia Develops after Admission

A patient may be admitted with one type of pneumonia (e.g., code J13, Pneumonia due to Streptococcus pneumonia) and subsequently develop VAP. In this instance, the principal diagnosis would be the appropriate code from categories J12- J18 for the pneumonia diagnosed at the time of admission. Code J95.851, Ventilator associated pneumonia, would be assigned as an additional diagnosis when the provider has also documented the presence of ventilator associated pneumonia.

e. Vaping-related disorders

For patients presenting with condition(s) related to vaping, assign code U07.0, Vaping-related disorder, as the principal diagnosis. For lung injury due to vaping, assign only code U07.0. Assign additional codes for other manifestations, such as acute respiratory failure (subcategory J96.0-) or pneumonitis (code J68.0)

Associated respiratory signs and symptoms due to vaping, such as cough, shortness of breath, etc., are not coded separately, when a definitive diagnosis has been established. However, it would be appropriate to code separately any gastrointestinal symptoms, such as diarrhea and abdominal pain.

See Section I.C.1.g.1.c.i. for Pneumonia confirmed as due to COVID-19

Acute upper respiratory infections (J00-J06)

Excludes1: *chronic obstructive pulmonary disease with acute lower respiratory infection (J44.0)*

J00 Acute nasopharyngitis [common cold]

Acute rhinitis
Coryza (acute)
Infective nasopharyngitis NOS
Infective rhinitis
Nasal catarrh, acute
Nasopharyngitis NOS

Excludes1: *acute pharyngitis (J02.-)*
acute sore throat NOS (J02.9)
influenza virus with other respiratory manifestations (J09.X2, J10.1, J11.1)
pharyngitis NOS (J02.9)
rhinitis NOS (J31.0)
sore throat NOS (J02.9)

Nose and Sinuses

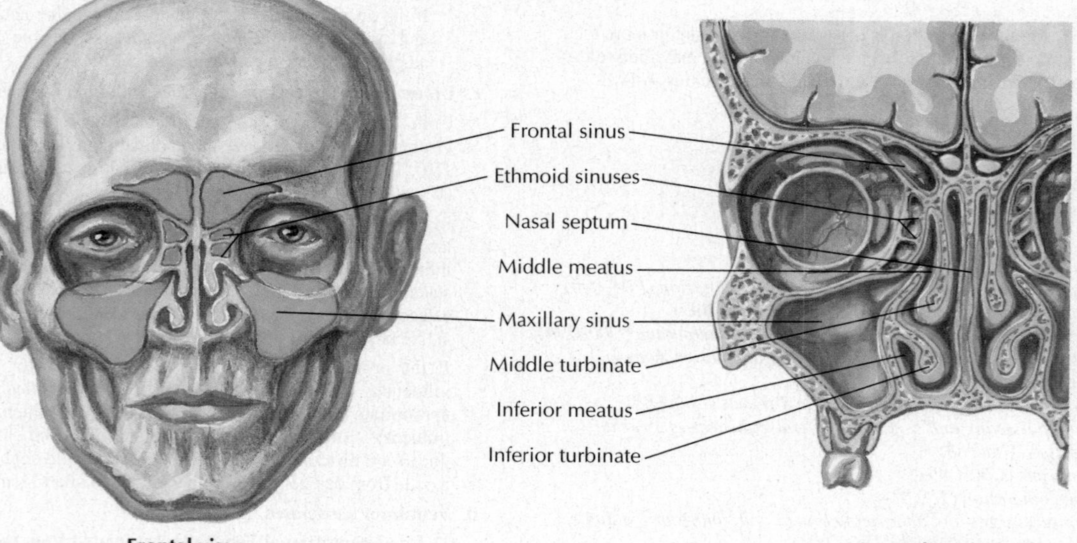

Frontal view **Coronal section**

Anatomy of nasal cavity and sinuses

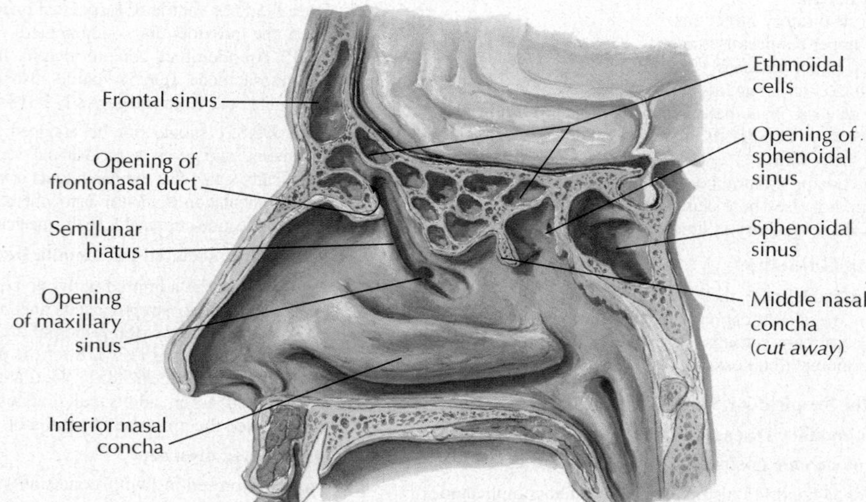

Sagittal section

Paranasal sinuses

F. Netter M.D.
JOHN A.CRAIG—AD

Excludes2: *allergic rhinitis (J30.1-J30.9)*
chronic pharyngitis (J31.2)
chronic rhinitis (J31.0)
chronic sore throat (J31.2)
nasopharyngitis, chronic (J31.1)
vasomotor rhinitis (J30.0)

Valid 3-character code, no further characters required

J01 Acute sinusitis

Includes: acute abscess of sinus
acute empyema of sinus
acute infection of sinus
acute inflammation of sinus
acute suppuration of sinus

Use additional code (B95-B97) to identify infectious agent

Excludes1: *sinusitis NOS (J32.9)*
Excludes2: *chronic sinusitis (J32.0-J32.8)*

+ **J01.0 Acute maxillary sinusitis**
  Acute antritis
  J01.00 Acute maxillary sinusitis, unspecified
  J01.01 Acute recurrent maxillary sinusitis
+ **J01.1 Acute frontal sinusitis**
  J01.10 Acute frontal sinusitis, unspecified
  J01.11 Acute recurrent frontal sinusitis
+ **J01.2 Acute ethmoidal sinusitis**
  J01.20 Acute ethmoidal sinusitis, unspecified
  J01.21 Acute recurrent ethmoidal sinusitis
+ **J01.3 Acute sphenoidal sinusitis**
  J01.30 Acute sphenoidal sinusitis, unspecified
  J01.31 Acute recurrent sphenoidal sinusitis
+ **J01.4 Acute pansinusitis**
  J01.40 Acute pansinusitis, unspecified
  J01.41 Acute recurrent pansinusitis

+ J01.8 **Other acute sinusitis**
  - J01.80 **Other acute sinusitis**
    Acute sinusitis involving more than one sinus but not pansinusitis
  - J01.81 **Other acute recurrent sinusitis**
    Acute recurrent sinusitis involving more than one sinus but not pansinusitis

+ J01.9 **Acute sinusitis, unspecified**
  - J01.90 **Acute sinusitis, unspecified**
  - J01.91 **Acute recurrent sinusitis, unspecified**

J02 Acute pharyngitis

Includes: acute sore throat
Excludes1: *acute laryngopharyngitis (J06.0)*
peritonsillar abscess (J36)
pharyngeal abscess (J39.1)
retropharyngeal abscess (J39.0)
Excludes2: *chronic pharyngitis (J31.2)*

J02.0 Streptococcal pharyngitis
Septic pharyngitis
Streptococcal sore throat
Excludes2: *scarlet fever (A38.-)*

J02.8 Acute pharyngitis due to other specified organisms
Use additional code (B95-B97) to identify infectious agent
Excludes1: *acute pharyngitis due to coxsackie virus (B08.5)*
acute pharyngitis due to gonococcus (A54.5)
acute pharyngitis due to herpes [simplex] virus (B00.2)
acute pharyngitis due to infectious mononucleosis (B27.-)
enteroviral vesicular pharyngitis (B08.5)

J02.9 Acute pharyngitis, unspecified
Gangrenous pharyngitis (acute)
Infective pharyngitis (acute) NOS
Pharyngitis (acute) NOS
Sore throat (acute) NOS
Suppurative pharyngitis (acute)
Ulcerative pharyngitis (acute)
Excludes1: *influenza virus with other respiratory manifestations (J09.X2, J10.1, J11.1)*

J03 Acute tonsillitis

Excludes1: *acute sore throat (J02.-)*
hypertrophy of tonsils (J35.1)
peritonsillar abscess (J36)
sore throat NOS (J02.9)
streptococcal sore throat (J02.0)
Excludes2: *chronic tonsillitis (J35.0)*

+ J03.0 **Streptococcal tonsillitis**
  - J03.00 **Acute streptococcal tonsillitis, unspecified**
  - J03.01 **Acute recurrent streptococcal tonsillitis**

+ J03.8 **Acute tonsillitis due to other specified organisms**
Use additional code (B95-B97) to identify infectious agent
Excludes1: *diphtheritic tonsillitis (A36.0)*
herpesviral pharyngotonsillitis (B00.2)
streptococcal tonsillitis (J03.0)
tuberculous tonsillitis (A15.8)
Vincent's tonsillitis (A69.1)
  - J03.80 **Acute tonsillitis due to other specified organisms**
  - J03.81 **Acute recurrent tonsillitis due to other specified organisms**

+ J03.9 **Acute tonsillitis, unspecified**
Follicular tonsillitis (acute)
Gangrenous tonsillitis (acute)
Infective tonsillitis (acute)
Tonsillitis (acute) NOS
Ulcerative tonsillitis (acute)
Excludes1: *influenza virus with other respiratory manifestations (J09.X2, J10.1, J11.1)*
  - J03.90 **Acute tonsillitis, unspecified**
  - J03.91 **Acute recurrent tonsillitis, unspecified**

J04 Acute laryngitis and tracheitis

Code also influenza, if present, such as:
influenza due to identified novel influenza A virus with other respiratory manifestations (J09.X2)
influenza due to other identified influenza virus with other respiratory manifestations (J10.1)
influenza due to unidentified influenza virus with other respiratory manifestations (J11.1)

Use additional code (B95-B97) to identify infectious agent
Excludes1: *acute obstructive laryngitis [croup] and epiglottitis (J05.-)*
Excludes2: *laryngismus (stridulus) (J38.5)*

J04.0 Acute laryngitis
Edematous laryngitis (acute)
Laryngitis (acute) NOS
Subglottic laryngitis (acute)
Suppurative laryngitis (acute)
Ulcerative laryngitis (acute)
Excludes1: *acute obstructive laryngitis (J05.0)*
Excludes2: *chronic laryngitis (J37.0)*

+ J04.1 **Acute tracheitis**
Acute viral tracheitis
Catarrhal tracheitis (acute)
Tracheitis (acute) NOS
Excludes2: *chronic tracheitis (J42)*
  - J04.10 **Acute tracheitis without obstruction**
  - MCC J04.11 **Acute tracheitis with obstruction**

J04.2 Acute laryngotracheitis
Laryngotracheitis NOS
Tracheitis (acute) with laryngitis (acute)
Excludes1: *acute obstructive laryngotracheitis (J05.0)*
Excludes2: *chronic laryngotracheitis (J37.1)*

+ J04.3 **Supraglottitis, unspecified**
  - J04.30 **Supraglottitis, unspecified, without obstruction**
  - MCC J04.31 **Supraglottitis, unspecified, with obstruction**

J05 Acute obstructive laryngitis [croup] and epiglottitis

Code also, influenza, if present, such as:
influenza due to identified novel influenza A virus with other respiratory manifestations (J09.X2)
influenza due to other identified influenza virus with other respiratory manifestations (J10.1)
influenza due to unidentified influenza virus with other respiratory manifestations (J11.1)

Use additional code (B95-B97) to identify infectious agent

J05.0 Acute obstructive laryngitis [croup]
Obstructive laryngitis (acute) NOS
Obstructive laryngotracheitis NOS

+ J05.1 **Acute epiglottitis**
Excludes2: *epiglottitis, chronic (J37.0)*
  - CC J05.10 **Acute epiglottitis without obstruction**
    Epiglottitis NOS
  - MCC J05.11 **Acute epiglottitis with obstruction**

J06 Acute upper respiratory infections of multiple and unspecified sites

Excludes1: *acute respiratory infection NOS (J22)*
influenza virus with other respiratory manifestations (J09.X2, J10.1, J11.1)
streptococcal pharyngitis (J02.0)

J06.0 Acute laryngopharyngitis

J06.9 Acute upper respiratory infection, unspecified
Upper respiratory disease, acute
Upper respiratory infection NOS
Use additional code (B95-B97) to identify infectious agent, if known, such as:
respiratory syncytial virus (RSV) (B97.4)

Influenza and pneumonia (J09-J18)

Excludes2: *allergic or eosinophilic pneumonia (J82)*
aspiration pneumonia NOS (J69.0)
meconium pneumonia (P24.01)
neonatal aspiration pneumonia (P24.-)
pneumonia due to solids and liquids (J69-)
congenital pneumonia (P23.9)
lipid pneumonia (J69.1)
rheumatic pneumonia (I00)
ventilator associated pneumonia (J95.851)

J09 Influenza due to certain identified influenza viruses

Excludes1: *influenza A/H1N1 (J10.-)*
influenza due to other identified influenza virus (J10.-)
influenza due to unidentified influenza virus (J11.-)
seasonal influenza due to other identified influenza virus (J10.-)
seasonal influenza due to unidentified influenza virus (J11.-)

Review coding guideline C.10.c

+ J09.X **Influenza due to identified novel influenza A virus**
Avian influenza
Bird influenza

Lungs

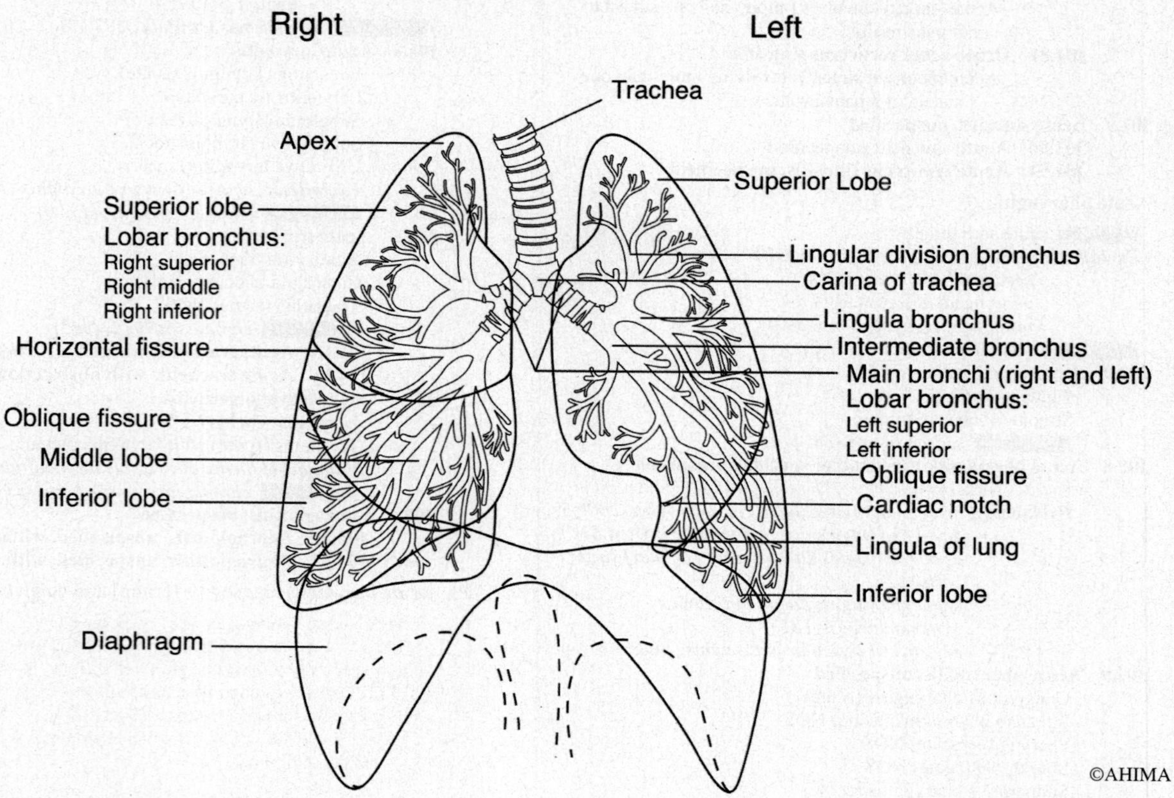

©AHIMA

Influenza A/H5N1
Influenza of other animal origin, not bird or swine
Swine influenza virus (viruses that normally cause infections in pigs)

MCC **J09.X1 Influenza due to identified novel influenza A virus with pneumonia**
Code also if applicable, associated:
lung abscess (J85.1)
other specified type of pneumonia

J09.X2 Influenza due to identified novel influenza A virus with other respiratory manifestations
Influenza due to identified novel influenza A virus NOS
Influenza due to identified novel influenza A virus with laryngitis
Influenza due to identified novel influenza A virus with pharyngitis
Influenza due to identified novel influenza A virus with upper respiratory symptoms
Use additional code, if applicable, for associated:
pleural effusion (J91.8)
sinusitis (J01.-)

J09.X3 Influenza due to identified novel influenza A virus with gastrointestinal manifestations
Influenza due to identified novel influenza A virus gastroenteritis
Excludes1: *'intestinal flu' [viral gastroenteritis] (A08.-)*

J09.X9 Influenza due to identified novel influenza A virus with other manifestations
Influenza due to identified novel influenza A virus with encephalopathy
Influenza due to identified novel influenza A virus with myocarditis
Influenza due to identified novel influenza A virus with otitis media
Use additional code to identify manifestation

J10 Influenza due to other identified influenza virus
Includes: *influenza A (non-novel)*
influenza B
influenza C
Excludes1: *influenza due to avian influenza virus (J09.X-)*
influenza due to swine flu (J09.X-)
influenza due to unidentifed influenza virus (J11.-)
Review coding guideline C.10.c

\+ **J10.0 Influenza due to other identified influenza virus with pneumonia**
Code also associated lung abscess, if applicable (J85.1)

MCC **J10.00 Influenza due to other identified influenza virus with unspecified type of pneumonia**

MCC **J10.01 Influenza due to other identified influenza virus with the same other identified influenza virus pneumonia**

MCC **J10.08 Influenza due to other identified influenza virus with other specified pneumonia**
Code also other specified type of pneumonia
AHA CC: 4Q, 2017, 96

J10.1 Influenza due to other identified influenza virus with other respiratory manifestations
Influenza due to other identified influenza virus NOS
Influenza due to other identified influenza virus with laryngitis
Influenza due to other identified influenza virus with pharyngitis
Influenza due to other identified influenza virus with upper respiratory symptoms
Use additional code for associated pleural effusion, if applicable (J91.8)
Use additional code for associated sinusitis, if applicable (J01.-)
AHA CC: 3Q, 2016, 10-11

J10.2 Influenza due to other identified influenza virus with gastrointestinal manifestations
Influenza due to other identified influenza virus gastroenteritis
Excludes1: *'intestinal flu' [viral gastroenteritis] (A08.-)*

\+ **J10.8 Influenza due to other identified influenza virus with other manifestations**

J10.81 Influenza due to other identified influenza virus with encephalopathy

J10.82 Influenza due to other identified influenza virus with myocarditis

J10.83 **Influenza due to other identified influenza virus with otitis media**
Use additional code for any associated perforated tympanic membrane (H72.-)

J10.89 **Influenza due to other identified influenza virus with other manifestations**
Use additional codes to identify the manifestations

J11 Influenza due to unidentified influenza virus

+ **J11.0 Influenza due to unidentified influenza virus with pneumonia**
Code also associated lung abscess, if applicable (J85.1)

MCC **J11.00 Influenza due to unidentified influenza virus with unspecified type of pneumonia**
Influenza with pneumonia NOS
AHA CC: 3Q, 2016, 11-12

MCC **J11.08 Influenza due to unidentified influenza virus with specified pneumonia**
Code also other specified type of pneumonia

J11.1 Influenza due to unidentified influenza virus with other respiratory manifestations
Influenza NOS
Influenzal laryngitis NOS
Influenzal pharyngitis NOS
Influenza with upper respiratory symptoms NOS
Use additional code for associated pleural effusion, if applicable (J91.8)

Use additional code for associated sinusitis, if applicable (J01.-)

J11.2 Influenza due to unidentified influenza virus with gastrointestinal manifestations
Influenza gastroenteritis NOS
Excludes1: *'intestinal flu' [viral gastroenteritis] (A08.-)*

+ **J11.8 Influenza due to unidentified influenza virus with other manifestations**

J11.81 Influenza due to unidentified influenza virus with encephalopathy
Influenzal encephalopathy NOS

J11.82 Influenza due to unidentified influenza virus with myocarditis
Influenzal myocarditis NOS

J11.83 Influenza due to unidentified influenza virus with otitis media
Influenzal otitis media NOS
Use additional code for any associated perforated tympanic membrane (H72.-)

J11.89 Influenza due to unidentified influenza virus with other manifestations
Use additional codes to identify the manifestations

J12 Viral pneumonia, not elsewhere classified

Includes: bronchopneumonia due to viruses other than influenza viruses
Code first associated influenza, if applicable (J09.X1, J10.0-, J11.0-)

Code also associated abscess, if applicable (J85.1)
Excludes1: *aspiration pneumonia due to anesthesia during labor and delivery (O74.0)*
aspiration pneumonia due to anesthesia during pregnancy (O29)
aspiration pneumonia due to anesthesia during puerperium (O89.0)
aspiration pneumonia due to solids and liquids (J69.-)
aspiration pneumonia NOS (J69.0)
congenital pneumonia (P23.0)
congenital rubella pneumonitis (P35.0)
interstitial pneumonia NOS (J84.9)
lipid pneumonia (J69.1)
neonatal aspiration pneumonia (P24.-)

MCC **J12.0 Adenoviral pneumonia**
MCC **J12.1 Respiratory syncytial virus pneumonia**
RSV pneumonia
MCC **J12.2 Parainfluenza virus pneumonia**
MCC **J12.3 Human metapneumovirus pneumonia**
+ **J12.8 Other viral pneumonia**

MCC **J12.81 Pneumonia due to SARS-associated coronavirus**
Severe acute respiratory syndrome NOS

MCC **J12.82 Pneumonia due to coronavirus disease 2019**
Pneumonia due to 2019 novel coronavirus (SARS-CoV-2)
Pneumonia due to COVID-19
Code first COVID-19 (U07.1)
AHA CC: 1Q, 2021, 33-34, 41-42, 46-49

MCC **J12.89 Other viral pneumonia**
AHA CC: 1Q, 2020, 34-36; 2Q, 2020, 8,11; 1Q, 2021, 33-34
Review coding guideline C.1.g.1.c.i

MCC **J12.9 Viral pneumonia, unspecified**

MCC **J13 Pneumonia due to Streptococcus pneumoniae**

Bronchopneumonia due to S. pneumoniae
Code first associated influenza, if applicable (J09.X1, J10.0-, J11.0-)

Code also associated abscess, if applicable (J85.1)
Excludes1: *congenital pneumonia due to S. pneumoniae (P23.6)*
lobar pneumonia, unspecified organism (J18.1)
pneumonia due to other streptococci (J15.3-J15.4)
Valid 3-character code, no further characters required

MCC **J14 Pneumonia due to Hemophilus influenzae**

Bronchopneumonia due to H. influenzae
Code first associated influenza, if applicable (J09.X1, J10.0-, J11.0-)

Code also associated abscess, if applicable (J85.1)
Excludes1: *congenital pneumonia due to H. influenzae (P23.6)*
Valid 3-character code, no further characters required

J15 Bacterial pneumonia, not elsewhere classified

Includes: bronchopneumonia due to bacteria other than S. pneumoniae and H. influenzae
Code first associated influenza, if applicable (J09.X1, J10.0-, J11.0-)

Code also associated abscess, if applicable (J85.1)
Excludes1: *chlamydial pneumonia (J16.0)*
congenital pneumonia (P23.-)
Legionnaires' disease (A48.1)
spirochetal pneumonia (A69.8)

MCC **J15.0 Pneumonia due to Klebsiella pneumoniae**
MCC **J15.1 Pneumonia due to Pseudomonas**
+ **J15.2 Pneumonia due to staphylococcus**

MCC **J15.20 Pneumonia due to staphylococcus, unspecified**
+ **J15.21 Pneumonia due to staphylococcus aureus**

MCC **J15.211 Pneumonia due to Methicillin susceptible Staphylococcus aureus**
MSSA pneumonia
Pneumonia due to Staphylococcus aureus NOS

MCC **J15.212 Pneumonia due to Methicillin resistant Staphylococcus aureus**
Review coding guideline C.1.e.1.a

MCC **J15.29 Pneumonia due to other staphylococcus**
MCC **J15.3 Pneumonia due to streptococcus, group B**
MCC **J15.4 Pneumonia due to other streptococci**
Excludes1: *pneumonia due to streptococcus, group B (J15.3)*
pneumonia due to Streptococcus pneumoniae (J13)

MCC **J15.5 Pneumonia due to Escherichia coli**
MCC **J15.6 Pneumonia due to other Gram-negative bacteria**
Pneumonia due to other aerobic Gram-negative bacteria
Pneumonia due to Serratia marcescens
AHA CC: 2Q, 2020, 29

MCC **J15.7 Pneumonia due to Mycoplasma pneumoniae**
MCC **J15.8 Pneumonia due to other specified bacteria**
MCC **J15.9 Unspecified bacterial pneumonia**
Pneumonia due to gram-positive bacteria
AHA CC: 4Q, 2017, 96

J16 Pneumonia due to other infectious organisms, not elsewhere classified

Code first associated influenza, if applicable (J09.X1, J10.0-, J11.0-)

Code also associated abscess, if applicable (J85.1)
Excludes1: *congenital pneumonia (P23.-)*
ornithosis (A70)
pneumocystosis (B59)
pneumonia NOS (J18.9)

MCC **J16.0 Chlamydial pneumonia**
MCC **J16.8 Pneumonia due to other specified infectious organisms**

MCC **J17 Pneumonia in diseases classified elsewhere**

Code first underlying disease, such as:
Q fever (A78)
rheumatic fever (I00)
schistosomiasis (B65.0-B65.9)

Excludes1: *candidial pneumonia (B37.1)*
chlamydial pneumonia (J16.0)
gonorrheal pneumonia (A54.84)
histoplasmosis pneumonia (B39.0-B39.2)
measles pneumonia (B05.2)
nocardiosis pneumonia (A43.0)
pneumocystosis (B59)
pneumonia due to Pneumocystis carinii (B59)
pneumonia due to Pneumocystis jiroveci (B59)
pneumonia in actinomycosis (A42.0)
pneumonia in anthrax (A22.1)
pneumonia in ascariasis (B77.81)
pneumonia in aspergillosis (B44.0-B44.1)
pneumonia in coccidioidomycosis (B38.0-B38.2)
pneumonia in cytomegalovirus disease(B25.0)
pneumonia in toxoplasmosis (B58.3)
rubella pneumonia (B06.81)
salmonella pneumonia (A02.22)
spirochetal infection NEC with pneumonia (A69.8)
tularemia pneumonia (A21.2)
typhoid fever with pneumonia (A01.03)
varicella pneumonia (B01.2)
whooping cough with pneumonia (A37 with fifth-character 1)

Valid 3-character code, no further characters required

J18 Pneumonia, unspecified organism

Code first associated influenza, if applicable (J09.X1, J10.0-, J11.0-)

Excludes1: *abscess of lung with pneumonia (J85.1)*
aspiration pneumonia due to anesthesia during labor and delivery (O74.0)
aspiration pneumonia due to anesthesia during pregnancy (O29)
aspiration pneumonia due to anesthesia during puerperium (O89.0)
aspiration pneumonia due to solids and liquids (J69.-)
aspiration pneumonia NOS (J69.0)
congenital pneumonia (P23.0)
drug-induced interstitial lung disorder (J70.2-J70.4)
interstitial pneumonia NOS (J84.9)
lipid pneumonia (J69.1)
neonatal aspiration pneumonia (P24.-)
pneumonitis due to external agents (J67-J70)
pneumonitis due to fumes and vapors (J68.0)
usual interstitial pneumonia (J84.178)

MCC **J18.0 Bronchopneumonia, unspecified organism**
Excludes1: *hypostatic bronchopneumonia (J18.2)*
lipid pneumonia (J69.1)
Excludes2: *acute bronchiolitis (J21.-)*
chronic bronchiolitis (J44.9)

MCC **J18.1 Lobar pneumonia, unspecified organism**
AHA CC: 3Q, 2016, 15

CC **J18.2 Hypostatic pneumonia, unspecified organism**
Hypostatic bronchopneumonia
Passive pneumonia

MCC **J18.8 Other pneumonia, unspecified organism**

MCC **J18.9 Pneumonia, unspecified organism**
AHA CC: 4Q, 2012, 94; 3Q, 2014, 4; 3Q, 2016, 15-16; 1Q, 2019, 35-36; 3Q, 2019, 15; 2Q, 2020, 28

Other acute lower respiratory infections (J20-J22)

Excludes2: *chronic obstructive pulmonary disease with acute lower respiratory infection (J44.0)*

J20 Acute bronchitis

Includes: acute and subacute bronchitis (with) bronchospasm
acute and subacute bronchitis (with) tracheitis
acute and subacute bronchitis (with) tracheobronchitis, acute
acute and subacute fibrinous bronchitis
acute and subacute membranous bronchitis
acute and subacute purulent bronchitis
acute and subacute septic bronchitis

Excludes1: *bronchitis NOS (J40)*
tracheobronchitis NOS (J40)
Excludes2: *acute bronchitis with bronchiectasis (J47.0)*
acute bronchitis with chronic obstructive asthma (J44.0)
acute bronchitis with chronic obstructive pulmonary disease (J44.0)
allergic bronchitis NOS (J45.909-)
bronchitis due to chemicals, fumes and vapors (J68.0)
chronic bronchitis NOS (J42)
chronic mucopurulent bronchitis (J41.1)
chronic obstructive bronchitis (J44.-)
chronic obstructive tracheobronchitis (J44.-)
chronic simple bronchitis (J41.0)
chronic tracheobronchitis (J42)

J20.0 Acute bronchitis due to Mycoplasma pneumoniae
J20.1 Acute bronchitis due to Hemophilus influenzae
J20.2 Acute bronchitis due to streptococcus
J20.3 Acute bronchitis due to coxsackievirus
J20.4 Acute bronchitis due to parainfluenza virus
J20.5 Acute bronchitis due to respiratory syncytial virus
Acute bronchitis due to RSV
J20.6 Acute bronchitis due to rhinovirus
AHA CC: 3Q, 2016, 10
J20.7 Acute bronchitis due to echovirus
J20.8 Acute bronchitis due to other specified organisms
AHA CC: 3Q, 2016, 10-11; 1Q, 2020, 34-36; 4Q, 2020, 11-12
Review coding guideline C.1.g.1.c.ii
J20.9 Acute bronchitis, unspecified
AHA CC: 3Q, 2016, 16; 1Q, 2019, 35

J21 Acute bronchiolitis

Includes: *acute bronchiolitis with bronchospasm*
Excludes2: *respiratory bronchiolitis interstitial lung disease (J84.115)*

CC **J21.0 Acute bronchiolitis due to respiratory syncytial virus**
Acute bronchiolitis due to RSV
CC **J21.1 Acute bronchiolitis due to human metapneumovirus**
CC **J21.8 Acute bronchiolitis due to other specified organisms**
CC **J21.9 Acute bronchiolitis, unspecified**
Bronchiolitis (acute)
Excludes1: *chronic bronchiolitis (J44.-)*

J22 Unspecified acute lower respiratory infection

Acute (lower) respiratory (tract) infection NOS
Excludes1: *upper respiratory infection (acute) (J06.9)*
AHA CC: 1Q, 2020, 22-23, 34-36
Review coding guideline C.1.g.1.c.iii
Valid 3-character code, no further characters required

Other diseases of upper respiratory tract (J30-J39)

J30 Vasomotor and allergic rhinitis

Includes: spasmodic rhinorrhea
Excludes1: *allergic rhinitis with asthma (bronchial) (J45.909)*
rhinitis NOS (J31.0)

J30.0 Vasomotor rhinitis
J30.1 Allergic rhinitis due to pollen
Allergy NOS due to pollen
Hay fever
Pollinosis
J30.2 Other seasonal allergic rhinitis
J30.5 Allergic rhinitis due to food
\+ **J30.8 Other allergic rhinitis**
J30.81 Allergic rhinitis due to animal (cat) (dog) hair and dander
J30.89 Other allergic rhinitis
Perennial allergic rhinitis
J30.9 Allergic rhinitis, unspecified

J31 Chronic rhinitis, nasopharyngitis and pharyngitis

Use additional code to identify:
exposure to environmental tobacco smoke (Z77.22)
exposure to tobacco smoke in the perinatal period (P96.81)
history of tobacco dependence (Z87.891)
occupational exposure to environmental tobacco smoke (Z57.31)
tobacco dependence (F17.-)
tobacco use (Z72.0)

J31.0 Chronic rhinitis
Atrophic rhinitis (chronic)
Granulomatous rhinitis (chronic)
Hypertrophic rhinitis (chronic)
Obstructive rhinitis (chronic)
Ozena
Purulent rhinitis (chronic)
Rhinitis (chronic) NOS
Ulcerative rhinitis (chronic)
Excludes1: *allergic rhinitis (J30.1-J30.9)*
vasomotor rhinitis (J30.0)

J31.1 Chronic nasopharyngitis
Excludes2: *acute nasopharyngitis (J00)*

J31.2 Chronic pharyngitis
Chronic sore throat
Atrophic pharyngitis (chronic)
Granular pharyngitis (chronic)
Hypertrophic pharyngitis (chronic)
Excludes2: *acute pharyngitis (J02.9)*

J32 Chronic sinusitis

Includes: sinus abscess
sinus empyema
sinus infection
sinus suppuration

Use additional code to identify:
exposure to environmental tobacco smoke (Z77.22)
exposure to tobacco smoke in the perinatal period (P96.81)
history of tobacco dependence (Z87.891)
infectious agent (B95-B97)
occupational exposure to environmental tobacco smoke (Z57.31)
tobacco dependence (F17.-)
tobacco use (Z72.0)

Excludes2: *acute sinusitis (J01.-)*

J32.0 Chronic maxillary sinusitis
Antritis (chronic)
Maxillary sinusitis NOS

J32.1 Chronic frontal sinusitis
Frontal sinusitis NOS

J32.2 Chronic ethmoidal sinusitis
Ethmoidal sinusitis NOS
Excludes1: *Woakes' ethmoiditis (J33.1)*

J32.3 Chronic sphenoidal sinusitis
Sphenoidal sinusitis NOS

J32.4 Chronic pansinusitis
Pansinusitis NOS

J32.8 Other chronic sinusitis
Sinusitis (chronic) involving more than one sinus but not pansinusitis

J32.9 Chronic sinusitis, unspecified
Sinusitis (chronic) NOS

J33 Nasal polyp

Use additional code to identify:
exposure to environmental tobacco smoke (Z77.22)
exposure to tobacco smoke in the perinatal period (P96.81)
history of tobacco dependence (Z87.891)
occupational exposure to environmental tobacco smoke (Z57.31)
tobacco dependence (F17.-)
tobacco use (Z72.0)

Excludes1: *adenomatous polyps (D14.0)*

J33.0 Polyp of nasal cavity
Choanal polyp
Nasopharyngeal polyp

J33.1 Polypoid sinus degeneration
Woakes' syndrome or ethmoiditis

J33.8 Other polyp of sinus
Accessory polyp of sinus
Ethmoidal polyp of sinus
Maxillary polyp of sinus
Sphenoidal polyp of sinus

J33.9 Nasal polyp, unspecified

J34 Other and unspecified disorders of nose and nasal sinuses

Excludes2: *varicose ulcer of nasal septum (I86.8)*

J34.0 Abscess, furuncle and carbuncle of nose
Cellulitis of nose
Necrosis of nose
Ulceration of nose

J34.1 Cyst and mucocele of nose and nasal sinus

J34.2 Deviated nasal septum
Deflection or deviation of septum (nasal) (acquired)
Excludes1: *congenital deviated nasal septum (Q67.4)*

J34.3 Hypertrophy of nasal turbinates

\+ **J34.8 Other specified disorders of nose and nasal sinuses**

J34.81 Nasal mucositis (ulcerative)
Code also type of associated therapy, such as:
antineoplastic and immunosuppressive drugs (T45.1X-)
radiological procedure and radiotherapy (Y84.2)
Excludes2: *gastrointestinal mucositis (ulcerative) (K92.81)*
mucositis (ulcerative) of vagina and vulva (N76.81)
oral mucositis (ulcerative) (K12.3-)

J34.89 Other specified disorders of nose and nasal sinuses
Perforation of nasal septum NOS
Rhinolith

J34.9 Unspecified disorder of nose and nasal sinuses

J35 Chronic diseases of tonsils and adenoids

Use additional code to identify:
exposure to environmental tobacco smoke (Z77.22)
exposure to tobacco smoke in the perinatal period (P96.81)
history of tobacco dependence (Z87.891)
occupational exposure to environmental tobacco smoke (Z57.31)
tobacco dependence (F17.-)
tobacco use (Z72.0)

\+ **J35.0 Chronic tonsillitis and adenoiditis**
Excludes2: *acute tonsillitis (J03.-)*

J35.01 Chronic tonsillitis

J35.02 Chronic adenoiditis

J35.03 Chronic tonsillitis and adenoiditis

J35.1 Hypertrophy of tonsils
Enlargement of tonsils
Excludes1: *hypertrophy of tonsils with tonsillitis (J35.0-)*

J35.2 Hypertrophy of adenoids
Enlargement of adenoids
Excludes1: *hypertrophy of adenoids with adenoiditis (J35.0-)*

J35.3 Hypertrophy of tonsils with hypertrophy of adenoids
Excludes1: *hypertrophy of tonsils and adenoids with tonsillitis and adenoiditis (J35.03)*

J35.8 Other chronic diseases of tonsils and adenoids
Adenoid vegetations
Amygdalolith
Calculus, tonsil
Cicatrix of tonsil (and adenoid)
Tonsillar tag
Ulcer of tonsil

J35.9 Chronic disease of tonsils and adenoids, unspecified
Disease (chronic) of tonsils and adenoids NOS

CC J36 Peritonsillar abscess

Includes: abscess of tonsil
peritonsillar cellulitis
quinsy

Use additional code (B95-B97) to identify infectious agent

Excludes1: *acute tonsillitis (J03.-)*
chronic tonsillitis (J35.0)
retropharyngeal abscess (J39.0)
tonsillitis NOS (J03.9-)

Valid 3-character code, no further characters required

J37 Chronic laryngitis and laryngotracheitis

Use additional code to identify:
exposure to environmental tobacco smoke (Z77.22)
exposure to tobacco smoke in the perinatal period (P96.81)
history of tobacco dependence (Z87.891)
infectious agent (B95-B97)
occupational exposure to environmental tobacco smoke (Z57.31)
tobacco dependence (F17.-)
tobacco use (Z72.0)

J37.0 Chronic laryngitis
Catarrhal laryngitis
Hypertrophic laryngitis
Sicca laryngitis
Excludes2: *acute laryngitis (J04.0)*
obstructive (acute) laryngitis (J05.0)

J37.1 **Chronic laryngotracheitis**
Laryngitis, chronic, with tracheitis (chronic)
Tracheitis, chronic, with laryngitis
Excludes1: *chronic tracheitis (J42)*
Excludes2: *acute laryngotracheitis (J04.2)*
acute tracheitis (J04.1)

J38 Diseases of vocal cords and larynx, not elsewhere classified
Use additional code to identify:
exposure to environmental tobacco smoke (Z77.22)
exposure to tobacco smoke in the perinatal period (P96.81)
history of tobacco dependence (Z87.891)
occupational exposure to environmental tobacco smoke (Z57.31)
tobacco dependence (F17.-)
tobacco use (Z72.0)
Excludes1: *congenital laryngeal stridor (P28.89)*
obstructive laryngitis (acute) (J05.0)
postprocedural subglottic stenosis (J95.5)
stridor (R06.1)
ulcerative laryngitis (J04.0)

\+ **J38.0 Paralysis of vocal cords and larynx**
Laryngoplegia
Paralysis of glottis
J38.00 Paralysis of vocal cords and larynx, unspecified
J38.01 Paralysis of vocal cords and larynx, unilateral
J38.02 Paralysis of vocal cords and larynx, bilateral

J38.1 Polyp of vocal cord and larynx
Excludes1: *adenomatous polyps (D14.1)*

J38.2 Nodules of vocal cords
Chorditis (fibrinous)(nodosa)(tuberosa)
Singer's nodes
Teacher's nodes

J38.3 Other diseases of vocal cords
Abscess of vocal cords
Cellulitis of vocal cords
Granuloma of vocal cords
Leukokeratosis of vocal cords
Leukoplakia of vocal cords

J38.4 Edema of larynx
Edema (of) glottis
Subglottic edema
Supraglottic edema
Excludes1: *acute obstructive laryngitis [croup] (J05.0)*
edematous laryngitis (J04.0)

J38.5 Laryngeal spasm
Laryngismus (stridulus)

J38.6 Stenosis of larynx

J38.7 Other diseases of larynx
Abscess of larynx
Cellulitis of larynx
Disease of larynx NOS
Necrosis of larynx
Pachyderma of larynx
Perichondritis of larynx
Ulcer of larynx

J39 Other diseases of upper respiratory tract
Excludes1: *acute respiratory infection NOS (J22)*
acute upper respiratory infection (J06.9)
upper respiratory inflammation due to chemicals, gases, fumes or vapors (J68.2)

CC **J39.0 Retropharyngeal and parapharyngeal abscess**
Peripharyngeal abscess
Excludes1: *peritonsillar abscess (J36)*

CC **J39.1 Other abscess of pharynx**
Cellulitis of pharynx
Nasopharyngeal abscess

J39.2 Other diseases of pharynx
Cyst of pharynx
Edema of pharynx
Excludes2: *chronic pharyngitis (J31.2)*
ulcerative pharyngitis (J02.9)

J39.3 Upper respiratory tract hypersensitivity reaction, site unspecified
Excludes1: *hypersensitivity reaction of upper respiratory tract, such as:*
extrinsic allergic alveolitis (J67.9)
pneumoconiosis (J60-J67.9)

J39.8 Other specified diseases of upper respiratory tract

J39.9 Disease of upper respiratory tract, unspecified

Chronic lower respiratory diseases (J40-J47)

Excludes1: *bronchitis due to chemicals, gases, fumes and vapors (J68.0)*
Excludes2: *cystic fibrosis (E84.-)*

J40 Bronchitis, not specified as acute or chronic
Bronchitis NOS
Bronchitis with tracheitis NOS
Catarrhal bronchitis
Tracheobronchitis NOS
Use additional code to identify:
exposure to environmental tobacco smoke (Z77.22)
exposure to tobacco smoke in the perinatal period (P96.81)
history of tobacco dependence (Z87.891)
occupational exposure to environmental tobacco smoke (Z57.31)
tobacco dependence (F17.-)
tobacco use (Z72.0)
Excludes1: *allergic bronchitis NOS (J45.909-)*
asthmatic bronchitis NOS (J45.9-)
acute bronchitis (J20.-)
bronchitis due to chemicals, gases, fumes and vapors (J68.0)
AHA CC: 1Q, 2020 34-36
Review coding guideline C.1.g.1.c.ii
Valid 3-character code, no further characters required

J41 Simple and mucopurulent chronic bronchitis
Use additional code to identify:
exposure to environmental tobacco smoke (Z77.22)
exposure to tobacco smoke in the perinatal period (P96.81)
history of tobacco dependence (Z87.891)
occupational exposure to environmental tobacco smoke (Z57.31)
tobacco dependence (F17.-)
tobacco use (Z72.0)
Excludes1: *chronic bronchitis NOS (J42)*
chronic obstructive bronchitis (J44.-)
J41.0 Simple chronic bronchitis
J41.1 Mucopurulent chronic bronchitis
J41.8 Mixed simple and mucopurulent chronic bronchitis

J42 Unspecified chronic bronchitis
Chronic bronchitis NOS
Chronic tracheitis
Chronic tracheobronchitis
Use additional code to identify:
exposure to environmental tobacco smoke (Z77.22)
exposure to tobacco smoke in the perinatal period (P96.81)
history of tobacco dependence (Z87.891)
occupational exposure to environmental tobacco smoke (Z57.31)
tobacco dependence (F17.-)
tobacco use (Z72.0)
Excludes1: *chronic asthmatic bronchitis (J44.-)*
chronic bronchitis with airways obstruction (J44.-)
chronic emphysematous bronchitis (J44.-)
chronic obstructive pulmonary disease NOS (J44.9)
simple and mucopurulent chronic bronchitis (J41.-)
Valid 3-character code, no further characters required

J43 Emphysema
Use additional code to identify:
exposure to environmental tobacco smoke (Z77.22)
history of tobacco dependence (Z87.891)
occupational exposure to environmental tobacco smoke (Z57.31)
tobacco dependence (F17.-)
tobacco use (Z72.0)
Excludes1: *compensatory emphysema (J98.3)*
emphysema due to inhalation of chemicals, gases, fumes or vapors (J68.4)
emphysema with chronic (obstructive) bronchitis (J44.-)
emphysematous (obstructive) bronchitis (J44.-)
interstitial emphysema (J98.2)
mediastinal emphysema (J98.2)
neonatal interstitial emphysema (P25.0)
surgical (subcutaneous) emphysema (T81.82)
Excludes2: *traumatic subcutaneous emphysema (T79.7)*

J43.0 Unilateral pulmonary emphysema [MacLeod's syndrome]
Swyer-James syndrome
Unilateral emphysema
Unilateral hyperlucent lung
Unilateral pulmonary artery functional hypoplasia
Unilateral transparency of lung

J43.1 Panlobular emphysema
Panacinar emphysema

Chronic Obstructive Pulmonary Disease

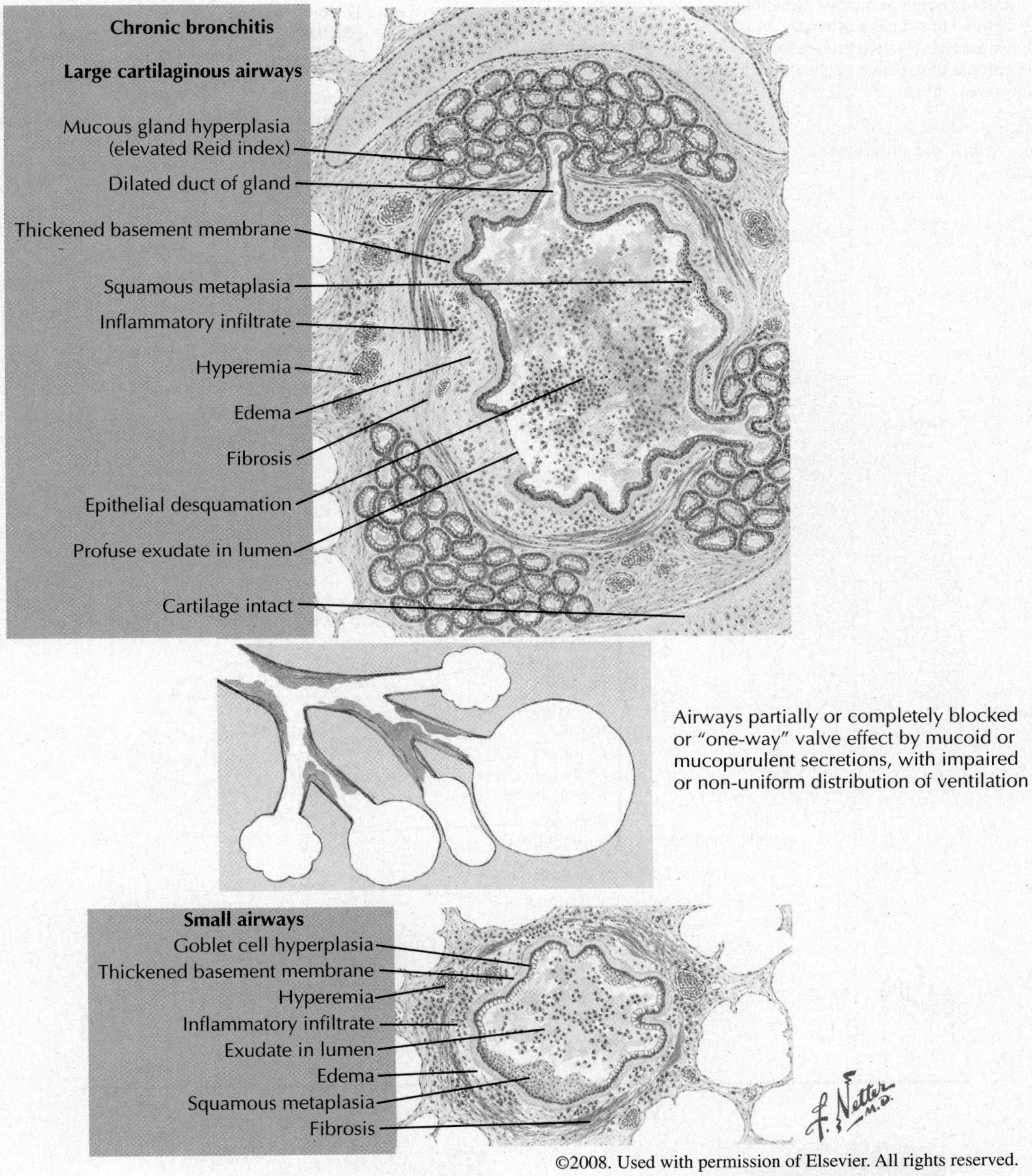

J43.2 **Centrilobular emphysema**
J43.8 **Other emphysema**
J43.9 **Emphysema, unspecified**
Bullous emphysema (lung)(pulmonary)
Emphysema (lung)(pulmonary) NOS
Emphysematous bleb
Vesicular emphysema (lung)(pulmonary)
AHA CC: 4Q, 2017, 97-98; 1Q, 2019, 34-37

J44 **Other chronic obstructive pulmonary disease**

Includes: asthma with chronic obstructive pulmonary disease
chronic asthmatic (obstructive) bronchitis
chronic bronchitis with airway obstruction
chronic bronchitis with emphysema
chronic emphysematous bronchitis
chronic obstructive asthma
chronic obstructive bronchitis
chronic obstructive tracheobronchitis

Code also type of asthma, if applicable (J45.-)

Use additional code to identify:
exposure to environmental tobacco smoke (Z77.22)
history of tobacco dependence (Z87.891)
occupational exposure to environmental tobacco smoke (Z57.31)
tobacco dependence (F17.-)
tobacco use (Z72.0)

Excludes1: *bronchiectasis (J47.-)*
chronic bronchitis NOS (J42)
chronic simple and mucopurulent bronchitis (J41.-)
chronic tracheitis (J42)
chronic tracheobronchitis (J42)
emphysema without chronic bronchitis (J43.-)

Review coding guideline C.10.a.1

CC **J44.0** **Chronic obstructive pulmonary disease with (acute) lower respiratory infection**
Code also to identify the infection
AHA CC: 3Q, 2016, 15-16; 4Q, 2017, 96

CC **J44.1** **Chronic obstructive pulmonary disease with (acute) exacerbation**
Decompensated COPD
Decompensated COPD with (acute) exacerbation
Excludes2: *chronic obstructive pulmonary disease [COPD] with acute bronchitis (J44.0)*
lung diseases due to external agents (J60-J70)
AHA CC: 1Q, 2016, 36; 3Q, 2016, 15-16; 1Q, 2017, 26; 4Q, 2017, 96

J44.9 **Chronic obstructive pulmonary disease, unspecified**
Chronic obstructive airway disease NOS
Chronic obstructive lung disease NOS
Excludes2: *lung diseases due to external agents (J60-J70)*
AHA CC: 4Q, 2013, 109, 129; 4Q, 2014, 21-22; 1Q, 2016, 36-37; 1Q, 2017, 24-25; 4Q, 2017, 96-97

Pathology of Asthma

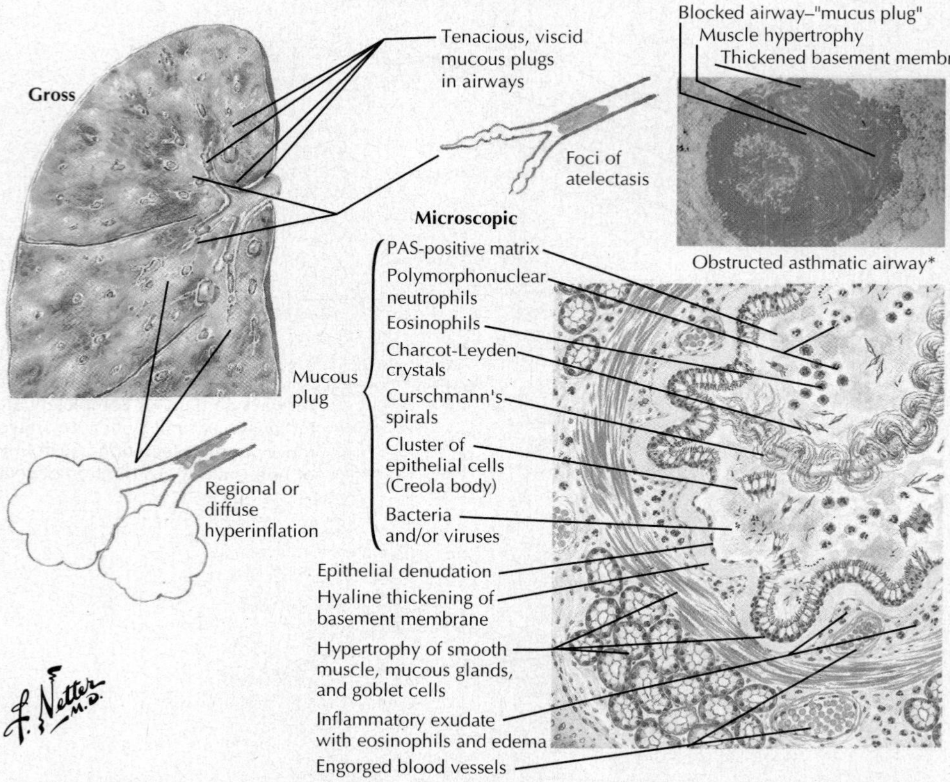

Microscopy of Airway

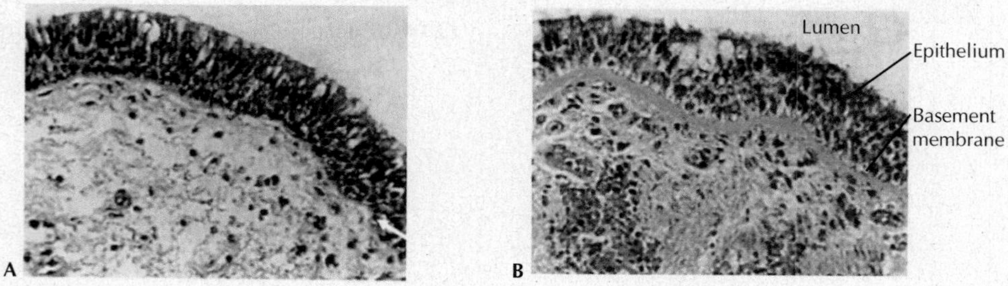

(**A**) Normal airway. (**B**) Asthmatic airway before therapy with high-dose inhaled steroids demonstrating remodeling.

J45 Asthma

Includes: allergic (predominantly) asthma
allergic bronchitis NOS
allergic rhinitis with asthma
atopic asthma
extrinsic allergic asthma
hay fever with asthma
idiosyncratic asthma
intrinsic nonallergic asthma
nonallergic asthma

Use additional code to identify:
eosinophilic asthma (J82.83)
exposure to environmental tobacco smoke (Z77.22)
exposure to tobacco smoke in the perinatal period (P96.81)
history of tobacco dependence (Z87.891)
occupational exposure to environmental tobacco smoke (Z57.31)
tobacco dependence (F17.-)
tobacco use (Z72.0)

Excludes1: *detergent asthma (J69.8)*
eosinophilic asthma (J82)
miner's asthma (J60)
wheezing NOS (R06.2)
wood asthma (J67.8)

Excludes2: *asthma with chronic obstructive pulmonary disease (J44.9)*
chronic asthmatic (obstructive) bronchitis (J44.9)
chronic obstructive asthma (J44.9)

AHA CC: 1Q, 2019, 36-37

Review coding guideline C.10.a.1

\+ **J45.2 Mild intermittent asthma**
J45.20 Mild intermittent asthma, uncomplicated
Mild intermittent asthma NOS
CC **J45.21 Mild intermittent asthma with (acute) exacerbation**
CC **J45.22 Mild intermittent asthma with status asthmaticus**

\+ **J45.3 Mild persistent asthma**
J45.30 Mild persistent asthma, uncomplicated
Mild persistent asthma NOS
CC **J45.31 Mild persistent asthma with (acute) exacerbation**
AHA CC: 1Q, 2016, 35
CC **J45.32 Mild persistent asthma with status asthmaticus**

\+ **J45.4 Moderate persistent asthma**
J45.40 Moderate persistent asthma, uncomplicated
Moderate persistent asthma NOS
CC **J45.41 Moderate persistent asthma with (acute) exacerbation**
AHA CC: 1Q, 2017, 26
CC **J45.42 Moderate persistent asthma with status asthmaticus**

\+ **J45.5 Severe persistent asthma**
J45.50 Severe persistent asthma, uncomplicated
Severe persistent asthma NOS
CC **J45.51 Severe persistent asthma with (acute) exacerbation**
AHA CC: 4Q, 2020, 27
CC **J45.52 Severe persistent asthma with status asthmaticus**

\+ **J45.9 Other and unspecified asthma**
\+ **J45.90 Unspecified asthma**
Asthmatic bronchitis NOS
Childhood asthma NOS
Late onset asthma
CC **J45.901 Unspecified asthma with (acute) exacerbation**
AHA CC: 4Q, 2017, 96-97
CC **J45.902 Unspecified asthma with status asthmaticus**
J45.909 Unspecified asthma, uncomplicated
Asthma NOS
Excludes2: *lung diseases due to external agents (J60-J70)*
\+ **J45.99 Other asthma**
J45.990 Exercise induced bronchospasm
J45.991 Cough variant asthma
J45.998 Other asthma

J47 Bronchiectasis

Includes: bronchiolectasis

Use additional code to identify:
exposure to environmental tobacco smoke (Z77.22)
exposure to tobacco smoke in the perinatal period (P96.81)
history of tobacco dependence (Z87.891)
occupational exposure to environmental tobacco smoke (Z57.31)
tobacco dependence (F17.-)
tobacco use (Z72.0)

Excludes1: *congenital bronchiectasis (Q33.4)*
tuberculous bronchiectasis (current disease) (A15.0)

CC **J47.0 Bronchiectasis with acute lower respiratory infection**
Bronchiectasis with acute bronchitis
Code also to identify infection, if applicable
CC **J47.1 Bronchiectasis with (acute) exacerbation**
AHA CC: 1Q, 2021, 23-24
J47.9 Bronchiectasis, uncomplicated
Bronchiectasis NOS

Lung diseases due to external agents (J60-J70)

Excludes2: *asthma (J45.-)*
malignant neoplasm of bronchus and lung (C34.-)

● **J60 Coalworker's pneumoconiosis**
Anthracosilicosis
Anthracosis
Black lung disease
Coalworker's lung
Excludes1: *coalworker pneumoconiosis with tuberculosis, any type in A15 (J65)*
Valid 3-character code, no further characters required

● **J61 Pneumoconiosis due to asbestos and other mineral fibers**
Asbestosis
Excludes1: *pleural plaque with asbestosis (J92.0)*
pneumoconiosis with tuberculosis, any type in A15 (J65)
Valid 3-character code, no further characters required

J62 Pneumoconiosis due to dust containing silica
Includes: silicotic fibrosis (massive) of lung
Excludes1: *pneumoconiosis with tuberculosis, any type in A15 (J65)*
J62.0 Pneumoconiosis due to talc dust
J62.8 Pneumoconiosis due to other dust containing silica
Silicosis NOS

J63 Pneumoconiosis due to other inorganic dusts
Excludes1: *pneumoconiosis with tuberculosis, any type in A15 (J65)*
J63.0 Aluminosis (of lung)
J63.1 Bauxite fibrosis (of lung)
J63.2 Berylliosis
J63.3 Graphite fibrosis (of lung)
J63.4 Siderosis
J63.5 Stannosis
J63.6 Pneumoconiosis due to other specified inorganic dusts

J64 Unspecified pneumoconiosis
Excludes1: *pneumonoconiosis with tuberculosis, any type in A15 (J65)*
Valid 3-character code, no further characters required

J65 Pneumoconiosis associated with tuberculosis
Any condition in J60-J64 with tuberculosis, any type in A15
Silicotuberculosis
Valid 3-character code, no further characters required

J66 Airway disease due to specific organic dust
Excludes2: *allergic alveolitis (J67.-)*
asbestosis (J61)
bagassosis (J67.1)
farmer's lung (J67.0)
hypersensitivity pneumonitis due to organic dust (J67.-)
reactive airways dysfunction syndrome (J68.3)
J66.0 Byssinosis
Airway disease due to cotton dust
J66.1 Flax-dressers' disease
J66.2 Cannabinosis
J66.8 Airway disease due to other specific organic dusts

J67 Hypersensitivity pneumonitis due to organic dust

Includes: allergic alveolitis and pneumonitis due to inhaled organic dust and particles of fungal, actinomycetic or other origin

Excludes1: *pneumonitis due to inhalation of chemicals, gases, fumes or vapors (J68.0)*

J67.0 Farmer's lung
Harvester's lung
Haymaker's lung
Moldy hay disease

J67.1 Bagassosis
Bagasse disease
Bagasse pneumonitis

J67.2 Bird fancier's lung
Budgerigar fancier's disease or lung
Pigeon fancier's disease or lung

J67.3 Suberosis
Corkhandler's disease or lung
Corkworker's disease or lung

J67.4 Maltworker's lung
Alveolitis due to Aspergillus clavatus

J67.5 Mushroom-worker's lung

J67.6 Maple-bark-stripper's lung
Alveolitis due to Cryptostroma corticale
Cryptostromosis

CC **J67.7 Air conditioner and humidifier lung**
Allergic alveolitis due to fungal, thermophilic actinomycetes and other organisms growing in ventilation [air conditioning] systems

CC **J67.8 Hypersensitivity pneumonitis due to other organic dusts**
Cheese-washer's lung
Coffee-worker's lung
Fish-meal worker's lung
Furrier's lung
Sequoiosis

CC **J67.9 Hypersensitivity pneumonitis due to unspecified organic dust**
Allergic alveolitis (extrinsic) NOS
Hypersensitivity pneumonitis NOS

J68 Respiratory conditions due to inhalation of chemicals, gases, fumes and vapors

Code first (T51-T65) to identify cause

Use additional code to identify associated respiratory conditions, such as: acute respiratory failure (J96.0-)

CC **J68.0 Bronchitis and pneumonitis due to chemicals, gases, fumes and vapors**
Chemical bronchitis (acute)
AHA CC: 2Q, 2019, 31-32
Review coding guideline C.11.e

MCC **J68.1 Pulmonary edema due to chemicals, gases, fumes and vapors**
Chemical pulmonary edema (acute) (chronic)
Excludes1: *pulmonary edema (acute) (chronic) NOS (J81.-)*

J68.2 Upper respiratory inflammation due to chemicals, gases, fumes and vapors, not elsewhere classified

J68.3 Other acute and subacute respiratory conditions due to chemicals, gases, fumes and vapors
Reactive airways dysfunction syndrome

J68.4 Chronic respiratory conditions due to chemicals, gases, fumes and vapors
Emphysema (diffuse) (chronic) due to inhalation of chemicals, gases, fumes and vapors
Obliterative bronchiolitis (chronic) (subacute) due to inhalation of chemicals, gases, fumes and vapors
Pulmonary fibrosis (chronic) due to inhalation of chemicals, gases, fumes and vapors
Excludes1: *chronic pulmonary edema due to chemicals, gases, fumes and vapors (J68.1)*

J68.8 Other respiratory conditions due to chemicals, gases, fumes and vapors

J68.9 Unspecified respiratory condition due to chemicals, gases, fumes and vapors

J69 Pneumonitis due to solids and liquids

Excludes1: *neonatal aspiration syndromes (P24.-)*
postprocedural pneumonitis (J95.4)

AHA CC: 2Q, 2020, 11, 28-29

MCC **J69.0 Pneumonitis due to inhalation of food and vomit**
Aspiration pneumonia NOS
Aspiration pneumonia (due to) food (regurgitated)
Aspiration pneumonia (due to) gastric secretions
Aspiration pneumonia (due to) milk
Aspiration pneumonia (due to) vomit
Code also any associated foreign body in respiratory tract (T17.-)
Excludes1: *chemical pneumonitis due to anesthesia (J95.4)*
obstetric aspiration pneumonitis (O74.0)
AHA CC: 1Q, 2017, 24; 2Q, 2019, 6-7, 31-32

MCC **J69.1 Pneumonitis due to inhalation of oils and essences**
Exogenous lipoid pneumonia
Lipid pneumonia NOS
Code first (T51-T65) to identify substance
Excludes1: *endogenous lipoid pneumonia (J84.89)*

MCC **J69.8 Pneumonitis due to inhalation of other solids and liquids**
Pneumonitis due to aspiration of blood
Pneumonitis due to aspiration of detergent
Code first (T51-T65) to identify substance

J70 Respiratory conditions due to other external agents

CC **J70.0 Acute pulmonary manifestations due to radiation**
Radiation pneumonitis
Use additional code (W88-W90, X39.0-) to identify the external cause

CC **J70.1 Chronic and other pulmonary manifestations due to radiation**
Fibrosis of lung following radiation
Use additional code (W88-W90, X39.0-) to identify the external cause

J70.2 Acute drug-induced interstitial lung disorders
Use additional code for adverse effect, if applicable, to identify drug (T36-T50 with fifth or sixth character 5)
AHA CC: 2Q, 2019, 28
Excludes1: *interstitial pneumonia NOS (J84.9)*
lymphoid interstitial pneumonia (J84.2)

J70.3 Chronic drug-induced interstitial lung disorders
Use additional code for adverse effect, if applicable, to identify drug (T36-T50 with fifth or sixth character 5)
Excludes1: *interstitial pneumonia NOS (J84.9)*
lymphoid interstitial pneumonia (J84.2)

J70.4 Drug-induced interstitial lung disorders, unspecified
Use additional code for adverse effect, if applicable, to identify drug (T36-T50 with fifth or sixth character 5)
AHA CC: 2Q, 2019, 28
Excludes1: *interstitial pneumonia NOS (J84.9)*
lymphoid interstitial pneumonia (J84.2)

J70.5 Respiratory conditions due to smoke inhalation
Code first smoke inhalation (T59.81-)
Excludes2: *smoke inhalation due to chemicals, gases, fumes and vapors (J68.9)*

J70.8 Respiratory conditions due to other specified external agents
Code first (T51-T65) to identify the external agent

J70.9 Respiratory conditions due to unspecified external agent
Code first (T51-T65) to identify the external agent

Other respiratory diseases principally affecting the interstitium (J80-J84)

MCC **J80 Acute respiratory distress syndrome**

Acute respiratory distress syndrome in adult or child
Adult hyaline membrane disease
Excludes1: *respiratory distress syndrome in newborn (perinatal) (P22.0)*
AHA CC: 1Q, 2017, 26-27; 1Q, 2020, 34-36; 4Q, 2020, 96-97; 2Q, 2021, 23
Review coding guideline C.1.g.1.c.iv
Valid 3-character code, no further characters required

J81 Pulmonary edema

Use additional code to identify:
exposure to environmental tobacco smoke (Z77.22)
history of tobacco dependence (Z87.891)
occupational exposure to environmental tobacco smoke (Z57.31)
tobacco dependence (F17.-)
tobacco use (Z72.0)

Excludes1: *chemical (acute) pulmonary edema (J68.1)*
hypostatic pneumonia (J18.2)
passive pneumonia (J18.2)
pulmonary edema due to external agents (J60-J70)
pulmonary edema with heart disease NOS (I50.1)
pulmonary edema with heart failure (I50.1)

MCC **J81.0 Acute pulmonary edema**
Acute edema of lung
AHA CC: 3Q, 2020, 27

CC **J81.1 Chronic pulmonary edema**
Pulmonary congestion (chronic) (passive)
Pulmonary edema NOS

J82 Pulmonary eosinophilia, not elsewhere classified

Excludes2: *pulmonary eosinophilia due to aspergillosis (B44.-)*
pulmonary eosinophilia due to drugs (J70.2-J70.4)
pulmonary eosinophilia due to specified parasitic infection (B50-B83)
pulmonary eosinophilia due to systemic connective tissue disorders (M30-M36)
pulmonary infiltrate NOS (R91.8)

\+ **J82.8 Pulmonary eosinophilia, not elsewhere classified**
AHA CC: 4Q, 2020, 25-27

CC **J82.81 Chronic eosinophilic pneumonia**
Eosinophilic pneumonia, NOS

CC **J82.82 Acute eosinophilic pneumonia**

CC **J82.83 Eosinophilic asthma**
Code first asthma, by type, such as:
mild intermittent asthma (J45.2-)
mild persistent asthma (J45.3-)
moderate persistent asthma (J45.4-)
severe persistent asthma (J45.5-)
AHA CC: 4Q, 2020, 27

CC **J82.89 Other pulmonary eosinophilia, not elsewhere classified**
Allergic pneumonia
Löffler's pneumonia
Tropical (pulmonary) eosinophilia NOS

J84 Other interstitial pulmonary diseases

Excludes1: *drug-induced interstitial lung disorders (J70.2-J70.4)*
interstitial emphysema (J98.2)
Excludes2: *lung diseases due to external agents (J60-J70)*

\+ **J84.0 Alveolar and parieto-alveolar conditions**

CC **J84.01 Alveolar proteinosis**

CC **J84.02 Pulmonary alveolar microlithiasis**

CC **J84.03 Idiopathic pulmonary hemosiderosis**
Essential brown induration of lung
Code first underlying disease, such as:
disorders of iron metabolism (E83.1-)
Excludes1: *acute idiopathic pulmonary hemorrhage in infants [AIPHI] (R04.81)*

CC **J84.09 Other alveolar and parieto-alveolar conditions**

\+ **J84.1 Other interstitial pulmonary diseases with fibrosis**
Excludes1: *pulmonary fibrosis (chronic) due to inhalation of chemicals, gases, fumes or vapors (J68.4)*
pulmonary fibrosis (chronic) following radiation (J70.1)

J84.10 Pulmonary fibrosis, unspecified
Capillary fibrosis of lung
Cirrhosis of lung (chronic) NOS
Fibrosis of lung (atrophic) (chronic) (confluent) (massive) (perialveolar) (peribronchial) NOS
Induration of lung (chronic) NOS
Postinflammatory pulmonary fibrosis

\+ **J84.11 Idiopathic interstitial pneumonia**
Excludes1: *lymphoid interstitial pneumonia (J84.2)*
pneumocystis pneumonia (B59)

J84.111 Idiopathic interstitial pneumonia, not otherwise specified

J84.112 Idiopathic pulmonary fibrosis
Cryptogenic fibrosing alveolitis
Idiopathic fibrosing alveolitis

J84.113 Idiopathic non-specific interstitial pneumonitis
Excludes1: *non-specific interstitial pneumoniaNOS,ordueto known underlying cause (J84.89)*

CC **J84.114 Acute interstitial pneumonitis**
Hamman-Rich syndrome
Excludes1: *pneumocystis pneumonia (B59)*

J84.115 Respiratory bronchiolitis interstitial lung disease

CC **J84.116 Cryptogenic organizing pneumonia**
Excludes1: *organizing pneumonia NOS, or due to known underlyingcause(J84.89)*

CC **J84.117 Desquamative interstitial pneumonia**

J84.17 Other interstitial pulmonary diseases with fibrosis in diseases classified elsewhere
AHA CC: 4Q, 2020, 27-28

J84.170 Interstitial lung disease with progressive fibrotic phenotype in diseases classified elsewhere
Progressive fibrotic interstitial lung disease
Code first underlying disease, such as:
lung diseases due to external agents (J60-J70)
rheumatoid arthritis (M05.00-M06.9)
sarcoidosis (D86)
systemic connective tissue disorders (M30-M36)

J84.178 Other interstitial pulmonary diseases with fibrosis in diseases classified elsewhere
Interstitial pneumonia (nonspecific) (usual) due to collagen vascular disease
Interstitial pneumonia (nonspecific) (usual) in diseases classified elsewhere
Organizing pneumonia due to collagen vascular disease
Organizing pneumonia in diseases classified elsewhere
Code first underlying diseases, such as:
progressive systemic sclerosis (M34.0)
rheumatoid arthritis (M05.00-M06.9)
systemic lupus erythematosis (M32.0-M32.9)

CC **J84.2 Lymphoid interstitial pneumonia**
Lymphoid interstitial pneumonitis

\+ **J84.8 Other specified interstitial pulmonary diseases**
Excludes1: *exogenous lipoid pneumonia (J69.1)*
unspecified lipoid pneumonia (J69.1)

MCC **J84.81 Lymphangioleiomyomatosis**
Lymphangiomyomatosis

• CC **J84.82 Adult pulmonary Langerhans cell histiocytosis**
Adult PLCH

MCC **J84.83 Surfactant mutations of the lung**

\+ **J84.84 Other interstitial lung diseases of childhood**

MCC **J84.841 Neuroendocrine cell hyperplasia of infancy**

MCC **J84.842 Pulmonary interstitial glycogenosis**

MCC **J84.843 Alveolar capillary dysplasia with vein misalignment**

MCC **J84.848 Other interstitial lung diseases of childhood**

J84.89 Other specified interstitial pulmonary diseases
Endogenous lipoid pneumonia
Interstitial pneumonitis
Non-specific interstitial pneumonitis NOS
Organizing pneumonia NOS
Code first if applicable:
poisoning due to drug or toxin (T51-T65 with fifth or sixth character to indicate intent), for toxic pneumonopathy
underlying cause of pneumonopathy, if known

Use additional code, for adverse effect, to identify drug (T36-T50 with fifth or sixth character 5), if drug-induced
Excludes1: *cryptogenic organizing pneumonia (J84.116)*
idiopathic non-specific interstitial pneumonitis (J84.113)
lipoid pneumonia, exogenous or unspecified (J69.1)
lymphoid interstitial pneumonia (J84.2)
AHA CC: 2Q, 2019, 28; 1Q, 2021, 48

CC **J84.9 Interstitial pulmonary disease, unspecified**
Interstitial pneumonia NOS

Suppurative and necrotic conditions of the lower respiratory tract (J85-J86)

J85 Abscess of lung and mediastinum

Use additional code (B95-B97) to identify infectious agent

MCC **J85.0 Gangrene and necrosis of lung**

MCC **J85.1 Abscess of lung with pneumonia**

Code also the type of pneumonia

MCC **J85.2 Abscess of lung without pneumonia**

Abscess of lung NOS

MCC **J85.3 Abscess of mediastinum**

J86 Pyothorax

Use additional code (B95-B97) to identify infectious agent

Excludes1: *abscess of lung (J85.-)*
pyothorax due to tuberculosis (A15.6)

MCC **J86.0 Pyothorax with fistula**

Bronchocutaneous fistula
Bronchopleural fistula
Hepatopleural fistula
Mediastinal fistula
Pleural fistula
Thoracic fistula
Any condition classifiable to J86.9 with fistula

MCC **J86.9 Pyothorax without fistula**

Abscess of pleura
Abscess of thorax
Empyema (chest) (lung) (pleura)
Fibrinopurulent pleurisy
Purulent pleurisy
Pyopneumothorax
Septic pleurisy
Seropurulent pleurisy
Suppurative pleurisy

Other diseases of the pleura (J90-J94)

CC **J90 Pleural effusion, not elsewhere classified**

Encysted pleurisy
Pleural effusion NOS
Pleurisy with effusion (exudative) (serous)

Excludes1: *chylous (pleural) effusion (J94.0)*
malignant pleural effusion (J91.0)
pleurisy NOS (R09.1)
tuberculous pleural effusion (A15.6)

Valid 3-character code, no further characters required

J91 Pleural effusion in conditions classified elsewhere

Excludes2: *pleural effusion in heart failure (I50.-)*
pleural effusion in systemic lupus erythematosus (M32.13)

CC **J91.0 Malignant pleural effusion**

Code first underlying neoplasm

CC **J91.8 Pleural effusion in other conditions classified elsewhere**

Code first underlying disease, such as:
filariasis (B74.0-B74.9)
influenza (J09.X2, J10.1, J11.1)

AHA CC: 2Q, 2015, 15-16

J92 Pleural plaque

Includes: pleural thickening

J92.0 Pleural plaque with presence of asbestos

J92.9 Pleural plaque without asbestos

Pleural plaque NOS

J93 Pneumothorax and air leak

Excludes1: *congenital or perinatal pneumothorax (P25.1)*
postprocedural air leak (J95.812)
postprocedural pneumothorax (J95.811)
traumatic pneumothorax (S27.0)
tuberculous (current disease) pneumothorax (A15.-)
pyopneumothorax (J86.-)

MCC **J93.0 Spontaneous tension pneumothorax**

\+ **J93.1 Other spontaneous pneumothorax**

CC **J93.11 Primary spontaneous pneumothorax**

CC **J93.12 Secondary spontaneous pneumothorax**

Code first underlying condition, such as:
catamenial pneumothorax due to endometriosis (N80.8)
cystic fibrosis (E84.-)
eosinophilic pneumonia (J82)
lymphangioleiomyomatosis (J84.81)
malignant neoplasm of bronchus and lung (C34.-)
Marfan's syndrome (Q87.4)
pneumonia due to Pneumocystis carinii (B59)
secondary malignant neoplasm of lung (C78.0-)
spontaneous rupture of the esophagus (K22.3)

\+ **J93.8 Other pneumothorax and air leak**

CC **J93.81 Chronic pneumothorax**

CC **J93.82 Other air leak**

Persistent air leak

CC **J93.83 Other pneumothorax**

Acute pneumothorax
Spontaneous pneumothorax NOS

AHA CC: 3Q, 2020, 9-10

CC **J93.9 Pneumothorax, unspecified**

Pneumothorax NOS

J94 Other pleural conditions

Excludes1: *pleurisy NOS (R09.1)*
traumatic hemopneumothorax (S27.2)
traumatic hemothorax (S27.1)
tuberculous pleural conditions (current disease) (A15.-)

CC **J94.0 Chylous effusion**

Chyliform effusion

J94.1 Fibrothorax

CC **J94.2 Hemothorax**

Hemopneumothorax

CC **J94.8 Other specified pleural conditions**

Hydropneumothorax
Hydrothorax

AHA CC: 1Q, 2021, 48-49

J94.9 Pleural condition, unspecified

Intraoperative and postprocedural complications and disorders of respiratory system, not elsewhere classified (J95)

J95 Intraoperative and postprocedural complications and disorders of respiratory system, not elsewhere classified

Excludes2: *aspiration pneumonia (J69.-)*
emphysema (subcutaneous) resulting from a procedure (T81.82)
hypostatic pneumonia (J18.2)
pulmonary manifestations due to radiation (J70.0-J70.1)

\+ **J95.0 Tracheostomy complications**

CC **J95.00 Unspecified tracheostomy complication**

CC **J95.01 Hemorrhage from tracheostomy stoma**

CC **J95.02 Infection of tracheostomy stoma**

Use additional code to identify type of infection, such as:
cellulitis of neck (L03.221)
sepsis (A40, A41.-)

CC **J95.03 Malfunction of tracheostomy stoma**

Mechanical complication of tracheostomy stoma
Obstruction of tracheostomy airway
Tracheal stenosis due to tracheostomy

CC **J95.04 Tracheo-esophageal fistula following tracheostomy**

CC **J95.09 Other tracheostomy complication**

MCC **J95.1 Acute pulmonary insufficiency following thoracic surgery**

Excludes2: *Functional disturbances following cardiac surgery (I97.0, I97.1-)*

MCC **J95.2 Acute pulmonary insufficiency following nonthoracic surgery**
Excludes2: *Functional disturbances following cardiac surgery (I97.0, I97.1-)*

MCC **J95.3 Chronic pulmonary insufficiency following surgery**
Excludes2: *Functional disturbances following cardiac surgery (I97.0, I97.1-)*

CC **J95.4 Chemical pneumonitis due to anesthesia**
Mendelson's syndrome
Postprocedural aspiration pneumonia
Use additional code for adverse effect, if applicable, to identify drug (T41.- with fifth or sixth character 5)
Excludes1: *aspiration pneumonitis due to anesthesia complicating labor and delivery (O74.0)*
aspiration pneumonitis due to anesthesia complicating pregnancy (O29)
aspiration pneumonitis due to anesthesia complicating the puerperium (O89.01)

CC **J95.5 Postprocedural subglottic stenosis**

\+ **J95.6 Intraoperative hemorrhage and hematoma of a respiratory system organ or structure complicating a procedure**
Excludes1: *intraoperative hemorrhage and hematoma of a respiratory system organ or structure due to accidental puncture and laceration during procedure (J95.7-)*

CC **J95.61 Intraoperative hemorrhage and hematoma of a respiratory system organ or structure complicating a respiratory system procedure**

CC **J95.62 Intraoperative hemorrhage and hematoma of a respiratory system organ or structure complicating other procedure**

\+ **J95.7 Accidental puncture and laceration of a respiratory system organ or structure during a procedure**
Excludes2: *postprocedural pneumothorax (J95.811)*

CC **J95.71 Accidental puncture and laceration of a respiratory system organ or structure during a respiratory system procedure**

CC **J95.72 Accidental puncture and laceration of a respiratory system organ or structure during other procedure**

\+ **J95.8 Other intraoperative and postprocedural complications and disorders of respiratory system, not elsewhere classified**
AHA CC: 4Q, 2016, 9-10

\+ **J95.81 Postprocedural pneumothorax and air leak**

CC **J95.811 Postprocedural pneumothorax**
AHA CC: 1Q, 2021, 48-49
HAC see Appendix B for HAC conditional logic

CC **J95.812 Postprocedural air leak**

\+ **J95.82 Postprocedural respiratory failure**
Excludes1: *Respiratory failure in other conditions (J96.-)*

MCC **J95.821 Acute postprocedural respiratory failure**
Postprocedural respiratory failure NOS

MCC **J95.822 Acute and chronic postprocedural respiratory failure**

\+ **J95.83 Postprocedural hemorrhage of a respiratory system organ or structure following a procedure**

CC **J95.830 Postprocedural hemorrhage of a respiratory system organ or structure following a respiratory system procedure**

CC **J95.831 Postprocedural hemorrhage of a respiratory system organ or structure following other procedure**

CC **J95.84 Transfusion-related acute lung injury (TRALI)**

\+ **J95.85 Complication of respirator [ventilator]**

CC **J95.850 Mechanical complication of respirator**
Excludes1: *encounter for respirator [ventilator] dependence during power failure (Z99.12)*

CC **J95.851 Ventilator associated pneumonia**
Ventilator associated pneumonitis
Use additional code to identify the organism, if known (B95.-, B96.-, B97.-)
Excludes1: *ventilator lung in newborn (P27.8)*
Review coding guideline C.10.d.1
AHA CC: 1Q, 2017, 25; 2Q, 2020, 17-18

CC **J95.859 Other complication of respirator [ventilator]**
AHA CC: 1Q, 2021, 48-49

\+ **J95.86 Postprocedural hematoma and seroma of a respiratory system organ or structure following a procedure**

CC **J95.860 Postprocedural hematoma of a respiratory system organ or structure following a respiratory system procedure**

CC **J95.861 Postprocedural hematoma of a respiratory system organ or structure following other procedure**

CC **J95.862 Postprocedural seroma of a respiratory system organ or structure following a respiratory system procedure**

CC **J95.863 Postprocedural seroma of a respiratory system organ or structure following other procedure**

CC **J95.88 Other intraoperative complications of respiratory system, not elsewhere classified**

CC **J95.89 Other postprocedural complications and disorders of respiratory system, not elsewhere classified**
Use additional code to identify disorder, such as:
aspiration pneumonia (J69.-)
bacterial or viral pneumonia (J12-J18)
Excludes2: *acute pulmonary insufficiency following thoracic surgery (J95.1)*
postprocedural subglottic stenosis (J95.5)

Other diseases of the respiratory system (J96-J99)

J96 Respiratory failure, not elsewhere classified
Excludes1: *acute respiratory distress syndrome (J80)*
cardiorespiratory failure (R09.2)
newborn respiratory distress syndrome (P22.0)
postprocedural respiratory failure (J95.82-)
respiratory arrest (R09.2)
respiratory arrest of newborn (P28.81)
respiratory failure of newborn (P28.5)

\+ **J96.0 Acute respiratory failure**
AHA CC: 1Q, 2021, 34
Review coding guideline C.10.b and C.11.e

MCC **J96.00 Acute respiratory failure, unspecified whether with hypoxia or hypercapnia**
AHA CC: 4Q, 2013, 121; 3Q, 2016, 14

MCC **J96.01 Acute respiratory failure with hypoxia**
AHA CC: 3Q, 2020, 12

MCC **J96.02 Acute respiratory failure with hypercapnia**

\+ **J96.1 Chronic respiratory failure**

CC **J96.10 Chronic respiratory failure, unspecified whether with hypoxia or hypercapnia**
AHA CC: 1Q, 2015, 21; 1Q, 2021, 45-46

CC **J96.11 Chronic respiratory failure with hypoxia**
AHA CC: 4Q, 2013, 129

CC **J96.12 Chronic respiratory failure with hypercapnia**

\+ **J96.2 Acute and chronic respiratory failure**
Acute on chronic respiratory failure
Review coding guideline C.10.b

MCC **J96.20 Acute and chronic respiratory failure, unspecified whether with hypoxia or hypercapnia**

MCC **J96.21 Acute and chronic respiratory failure with hypoxia**

MCC **J96.22 Acute and chronic respiratory failure with hypercapnia**

\+ **J96.9 Respiratory failure, unspecified**

MCC **J96.90 Respiratory failure, unspecified, unspecified whether with hypoxia or hypercapnia**

MCC **J96.91 Respiratory failure, unspecified with hypoxia**

MCC **J96.92 Respiratory failure, unspecified with hypercapnia**

J98 Other respiratory disorders

Use additional code to identify:
exposure to environmental tobacco smoke (Z77.22)
exposure to tobacco smoke in the perinatal period (P96.81)
history of tobacco dependence (Z87.891)
occupational exposure to environmental tobacco smoke (Z57.31)
tobacco dependence (F17.-)
tobacco use (Z72.0)

Excludes1: *newborn apnea (P28.4)*
newborn sleep apnea (P28.3)

Excludes2: *apnea NOS (R06.81)*
sleep apnea (G47.3-)

+ **J98.0 Diseases of bronchus, not elsewhere classified**

J98.01 Acute bronchospasm

Excludes1: *acute bronchiolitis with bronchospasm (J21.-)*
acute bronchitis with bronchospasm (J20.-)
asthma (J45.-)
exercise induced bronchospasm (J45.990)

J98.09 Other diseases of bronchus, not elsewhere classified

Broncholithiasis
Calcification of bronchus
Stenosis of bronchus
Tracheobronchial collapse
Tracheobronchial dyskinesia
Ulcer of bronchus

+ **J98.1 Pulmonary collapse**

Excludes1: *therapeutic collapse of lung status (Z98.3)*

CC **J98.11 Atelectasis**

Excludes1: *newborn atelectasis tuberculous atelectasis (current disease) (A15)*

CC **J98.19 Other pulmonary collapse**

J98.2 Interstitial emphysema

Mediastinal emphysema

Excludes1: *emphysema NOS (J43.9)*
emphysema in newborn (P25.0)
surgical emphysema (subcutaneous) (T81.82)
traumatic subcutaneous emphysema (T79.7)

J98.3 Compensatory emphysema

J98.4 Other disorders of lung

Calcification of lung
Cystic lung disease (acquired)
Lung disease NOS
Pulmolithiasis

Excludes1: *acute interstitial pneumonitis (J84.114)*
pulmonary insufficiency following surgery (J95.1-J95.2)

+ **J98.5 Diseases of mediastinum, not elsewhere classified**

Excludes2: *abscess of mediastinum (J85.3)*

AHA CC: 4Q, 2016, 29

MCC **J98.51 Mediastinitis**

Code first underlying condition, if applicable, such as postoperative mediastinitis (T81.-)

MCC **J98.59 Other diseases of mediastinum, not elsewhere classified**

Fibrosis of mediastinum
Hernia of mediastinum
Retraction of mediastinum

J98.6 Disorders of diaphragm

Diaphragmatitis
Paralysis of diaphragm
Relaxation of diaphragm

Excludes1: *congenital malformation of diaphragm NEC (Q79.1)*
congenital diaphragmatic hernia (Q79.0)

Excludes2: *diaphragmatic hernia (K44.-)*

J98.8 Other specified respiratory disorders

AHA CC: 1Q, 2020, 34-36

Review coding guideline C.1.g.1.c.iii

J98.9 Respiratory disorder, unspecified

Respiratory disease (chronic) NOS

J99 Respiratory disorders in diseases classified elsewhere

Code first underlying disease, such as:
amyloidosis (E85.-)
ankylosing spondylitis (M45)
congenital syphilis (A50.5)
cryoglobulinemia (D89.1)
early congenital syphilis (A50.0)
plasminogen deficiency (E88.02)
schistosomiasis (B65.0-B65.9)

Excludes1: *respiratory disorders in:*
amebiasis (A06.5)
blastomycosis (B40.0-B40.2)
candidiasis (B37.1)
coccidioidomycosis (B38.0-B38.2)
cystic fibrosis with pulmonary manifestations (E84.0)
dermatomyositis (M33.01, M33.11)
histoplasmosis (B39.0-B39.2)
late syphilis (A52.72, A52.73)
polymyositis (M33.21)
Sjögren syndrome (M35.02)
systemic lupus erythematosus (M32.13)
systemic sclerosis (M34.81)
Wegener's granulomatosis (M31.30-M31.31)

Valid 3-character code, no further characters required

Chapter 11: Diseases of the Digestive System (K00-K95)

Excludes2: *certain conditions originating in the perinatal period (P04-P96)*
certain infectious and parasitic diseases (A00-B99)
complications of pregnancy, childbirth and the puerperium (O00-O9A)
congenital malformations, deformations and chromosomal abnormalities (Q00-Q99)
endocrine, nutritional and metabolic diseases (E00-E88)
injury, poisoning and certain other consequences of external causes (S00-T88)
neoplasms (C00-D49)
symptoms, signs and abnormal clinical and laboratory findings, not elsewhere classified (R00-R94)

This chapter contains the following category blocks:
K00-K14 Diseases of oral cavity and salivary glands
K20-K31 Diseases of esophagus, stomach and duodenum
K35-K38 Diseases of appendix
K40-K46 Hernia
K50-K52 Noninfective enteritis and colitis
K55-K64 Other diseases of intestines
K65-K68 Diseases of peritoneum and retroperitoneum
K70-K77 Diseases of liver
K80-K87 Disorders of gallbladder, biliary tract and pancreas
K90-K95 Other diseases of the digestive system

C. Chapter-Specific Coding Guidelines

In addition to general coding guidelines, there are guidelines for specific diagnoses and/or conditions in the classification. Unless otherwise indicated, these guidelines apply to all health care settings. Please refer to Section II for guidelines on the selection of principal diagnosis.

11. Chapter 11: Diseases of the Digestive System (K00-K95)

Reserved for future guideline expansion

Diseases of oral cavity and salivary glands (K00-K14)

K00 Disorders of tooth development and eruption

Excludes2: *embedded and impacted teeth (K01.-)*

K00.0 Anodontia
Hypodontia
Oligodontia
Excludes1: *acquired absence of teeth (K08.1-)*

K00.1 Supernumerary teeth
Distomolar
Fourth molar
Mesiodens
Paramolar
Supplementary teeth
Excludes2: *supernumerary roots (K00.2)*

K00.2 Abnormalities of size and form of teeth
Concrescence of teeth
Fusion of teeth
Gemination of teeth
Dens evaginatus
Dens in dente
Dens invaginatus
Enamel pearls
Macrodontia
Microdontia
Peg-shaped [conical] teeth
Supernumerary roots
Taurodontism
Tuberculum paramolare
Excludes1: *abnormalities of teeth due to congenital syphilis (A50.5)*
tuberculum Carabelli, which is regarded as a normal variation and should not be coded

K00.3 Mottled teeth
Dental fluorosis
Mottling of enamel
Nonfluoride enamel opacities
Excludes2: *deposits [accretions] on teeth (K03.6)*

K00.4 Disturbances in tooth formation
Aplasia and hypoplasia of cementum
Dilaceration of tooth
Enamel hypoplasia (neonatal) (postnatal) (prenatal)
Regional odontodysplasia
Turner's tooth
Excludes1: *Hutchinson's teeth and mulberry molars in congenital syphilis (A50.5)*
Excludes2: *mottled teeth (K00.3)*

K00.5 Hereditary disturbances in tooth structure, not elsewhere classified
Amelogenesis imperfecta
Dentinogenesis imperfecta
Odontogenesis imperfecta
Dentinal dysplasia
Shell teeth

Oral Cavity

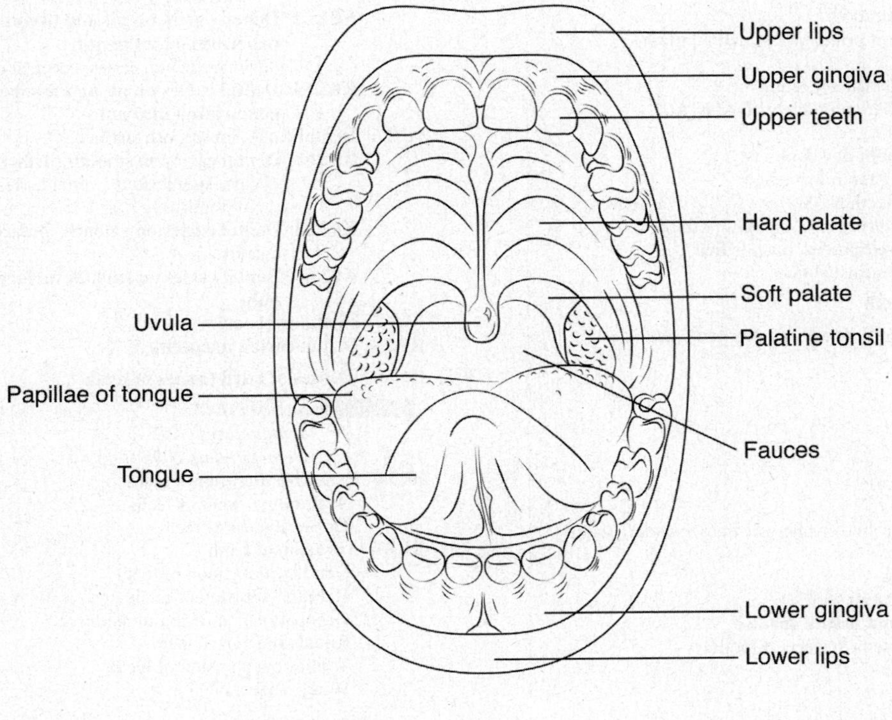

Glands of the Oral Cavity

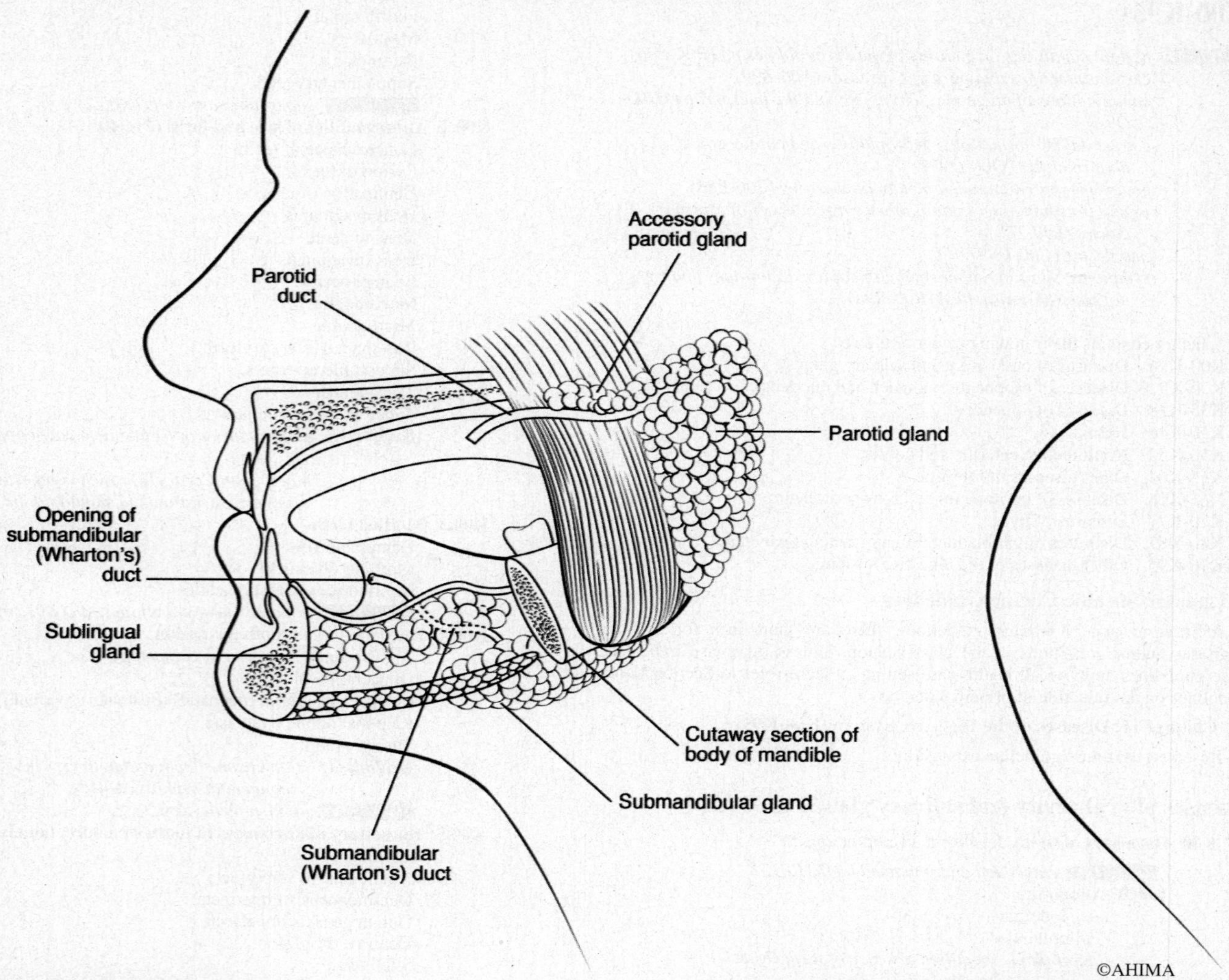

K00.6 Disturbances in tooth eruption
Dentia praecox
Natal tooth
Neonatal tooth
Premature eruption of tooth
Premature shedding of primary [deciduous] tooth
Prenatal teeth
Retained [persistent] primary tooth
Excludes2: *embedded and impacted teeth (K01.-)*

K00.7 Teething syndrome

K00.8 Other disorders of tooth development
Color changes during tooth formation
Intrinsic staining of teeth NOS
Excludes2: *posteruptive color changes (K03.7)*

K00.9 Disorder of tooth development, unspecified
Disorder of odontogenesis NOS

K01 Embedded and impacted teeth

Excludes1: *abnormal position of fully erupted teeth (M26.3-)*

K01.0 Embedded teeth

K01.1 Impacted teeth

K02 Dental caries

Includes: caries of dentine
dental cavities
early childhood caries
pre-eruptive caries
recurrent caries (dentino enamel junction) (enamel) (to the pulp) tooth decay

K02.3 Arrested dental caries
Arrested coronal and root caries

+ K02.5 Dental caries on pit and fissure surface
Dental caries on chewing surface of tooth

K02.51 Dental caries on pit and fissure surface limited to enamel
White spot lesions [initial caries] on pit and fissure surface of tooth

K02.52 Dental caries on pit and fissure surface penetrating into dentin
Primary dental caries, cervical origin

K02.53 Dental caries on pit and fissure surface penetrating into pulp

+ K02.6 Dental caries on smooth surface

K02.61 Dental caries on smooth surface limited to enamel
White spot lesions [initial caries] on smooth surface of tooth

K02.62 Dental caries on smooth surface penetrating into dentin

K02.63 Dental caries on smooth surface penetrating into pulp

K02.7 Dental root caries

K02.9 Dental caries, unspecified

K03 Other diseases of hard tissues of teeth

Excludes2: *bruxism (F45.8)*
dental caries (K02.-)
teeth-grinding NOS (F45.8)

K03.0 Excessive attrition of teeth
Approximal wear of teeth
Occlusal wear of teeth

K03.1 Abrasion of teeth
Dentifrice abrasion of teeth
Habitual abrasion of teeth
Occupational abrasion of teeth
Ritual abrasion of teeth
Traditional abrasion of teeth
Wedge defect NOS

K03.2 Erosion of teeth
Erosion of teeth due to diet
Erosion of teeth due to drugs and medicaments
Erosion of teeth due to persistent vomiting
Erosion of teeth NOS
Idiopathic erosion of teeth
Occupational erosion of teeth
K03.3 Pathological resorption of teeth
Internal granuloma of pulp
Resorption of teeth (external)
K03.4 Hypercementosis
Cementation hyperplasia
K03.5 Ankylosis of teeth
K03.6 Deposits [accretions] on teeth
Betel deposits [accretions] on teeth
Black deposits [accretions] on teeth
Extrinsic staining of teeth NOS
Green deposits [accretions] on teeth
Materia alba deposits [accretions] on teeth
Orange deposits [accretions] on teeth
Staining of teeth NOS
Subgingival dental calculus
Supragingival dental calculus
Tobacco deposits [accretions] on teeth
K03.7 Posteruptive color changes of dental hard tissues
Excludes2: *deposits [accretions] on teeth (K03.6)*
\+ **K03.8 Other specified diseases of hard tissues of teeth**
K03.81 Cracked tooth
Excludes1: *asymptomatic craze lines in enamel - omit code*
broken or fractured tooth due to trauma (S02.5)
K03.89 Other specified diseases of hard tissues of teeth
K03.9 Disease of hard tissues of teeth, unspecified

K04 Diseases of pulp and periapical tissues
AHA CC: 4Q, 2016, 29-30

\+ **K04.0 Pulpitis**
Acute pulpitis
Chronic (hyperplastic) (ulcerative) pulpitis
CC **K04.01 Reversible pulpitis**
CC **K04.02 Irreversible pulpitis**
K04.1 Necrosis of pulp
Pulpal gangrene
K04.2 Pulp degeneration
Denticles
Pulpal calcifications
Pulpal stones
K04.3 Abnormal hard tissue formation in pulp
Secondary or irregular dentine
CC **K04.4 Acute apical periodontitis of pulpal origin**
Acute apical periodontitis NOS
Excludes1: *acute periodontitis (K05.2-)*
K04.5 Chronic apical periodontitis
Apical or periapical granuloma
Apical periodontitis NOS
Excludes1: *chronic periodontitis (K05.3-)*
K04.6 Periapical abscess with sinus
Dental abscess with sinus
Dentoalveolar abscess with sinus
K04.7 Periapical abscess without sinus
Dental abscess without sinus
Dentoalveolar abscess without sinus
K04.8 Radicular cyst
Apical (periodontal) cyst
Periapical cyst
Residual radicular cyst
Excludes2: *lateral periodontal cyst (K09.0)*
\+ **K04.9 Other and unspecified diseases of pulp and periapical tissues**
K04.90 Unspecified diseases of pulp and periapical tissues
K04.99 Other diseases of pulp and periapical tissues

K05 Gingivitis and periodontal diseases
Use additional code to identify:
alcohol abuse and dependence (F10.-)
exposure to environmental tobacco smoke (Z77.22)
exposure to tobacco smoke in the perinatal period (P96.81)
history of tobacco dependence (Z87.891)
occupational exposure to environmental tobacco smoke (Z57.31)
tobacco dependence (F17.-)
tobacco use (Z72.0)
AHA CC: 4Q, 2016, 29-30

\+ **K05.0 Acute gingivitis**
Excludes1: *acute necrotizing ulcerative gingivitis (A69.1)*
herpesviral [herpes simplex] gingivostomatitis (B00.2)
K05.00 Acute gingivitis, plaque induced
Acute gingivitis NOS
Plaque induced gingival disease
K05.01 Acute gingivitis, non-plaque induced
\+ **K05.1 Chronic gingivitis**
Desquamative gingivitis (chronic)
Gingivitis (chronic) NOS
Hyperplastic gingivitis (chronic)
Pregnancy associated gingivitis
Simple marginal gingivitis (chronic)
Ulcerative gingivitis (chronic)
Code first, if applicable, diseases of the digestive system complicating pregnancy (O99.61-)
K05.10 Chronic gingivitis, plaque induced
Chronic gingivitis NOS
Gingivitis NOS
K05.11 Chronic gingivitis, non-plaque induced
\+ **K05.2 Aggressive periodontitis**
Acute pericoronitis
Excludes1: *acute apical periodontitis (K04.4)*
periapical abscess (K04.7)
periapical abscess with sinus (K04.6)
K05.20 Aggressive periodontitis, unspecified
\+ **K05.21 Aggressive periodontitis, localized**
Periodontal abscess
K05.211 Aggressive periodontitis, localized, slight
K05.212 Aggressive periodontitis, localized, moderate
K05.213 Aggressive periodontitis, localized, severe
K05.219 Aggressive periodontitis, localized, unspecified severity
\+ **K05.22 Aggressive periodontitis, generalized**
K05.221 Aggressive periodontitis, generalized, slight
K05.222 Aggressive periodontitis, generalized, moderate
K05.223 Aggressive periodontitis, generalized, severe
K05.229 Aggressive periodontitis, generalized, unspecified severity
\+ **K05.3 Chronic periodontitis**
Chronic pericoronitis
Complex periodontitis
Periodontitis NOS
Simplex periodontitis
Excludes1: *chronic apical periodontitis (K04.5)*
K05.30 Chronic periodontitis, unspecified
\+ **K05.31 Chronic periodontitis, localized**
K05.311 Chronic periodontitis, localized, slight
K05.312 Chronic periodontitis, localized, moderate
K05.313 Chronic periodontitis, localized, severe
K05.319 Chronic periodontitis, localized, unspecified severity
\+ **K05.32 Chronic periodontitis, generalized**
K05.321 Chronic periodontitis, generalized, slight
K05.322 Chronic periodontitis, generalized, moderate
K05.323 Chronic periodontitis, generalized, severe
K05.329 Chronic periodontitis, generalized, unspecified severity
K05.4 Periodontosis
Juvenile periodontosis
K05.5 Other periodontal diseases
Combined periodontic-endodontic lesion
Narrow gingival width (of periodontal soft tissue)
Excludes2: *leukoplakia of gingiva (K13.21)*
K05.6 Periodontal disease, unspecified

K06 Other disorders of gingiva and edentulous alveolar ridge

Excludes2: *acute gingivitis (K05.0)*
atrophy of edentulous alveolar ridge (K08.2)
chronic gingivitis (K05.1)
gingivitis NOS (K05.1)

AHA CC: 4Q, 2016, 29-30

K06.0 Gingival recession
Gingival recession (postinfective) (postprocedural)
AHA CC: 4Q, 2017, 16

+ **K06.01 Gingival recession, localized**
K06.010 Localized gingival recession, unspecified
Localized gingival recession, NOS
K06.011 Localized gingival recession, minimal
K06.012 Localized gingival recession, moderate
K06.013 Localized gingival recession, severe

+ **K06.02 Gingival recession, generalized**
K06.020 Generalized gingival recession, unspecified
Generalized gingival recession, NOS
K06.021 Generalized gingival recession, minimal
K06.022 Generalized gingival recession, moderate
K06.023 Generalized gingival recession, severe

K06.1 Gingival enlargement
Gingival fibromatosis

K06.2 Gingival and edentulous alveolar ridge lesions associated with trauma
Irritative hyperplasia of edentulous ridge [denture hyperplasia]
Use additional code (Chapter 20) to identify external cause or denture status (Z97.2)

K06.3 Horizontal alveolar bone loss

K06.8 Other specified disorders of gingiva and edentulous alveolar ridge
Fibrous epulis
Flabby alveolar ridge
Giant cell epulis
Peripheral giant cell granuloma of gingiva
Pyogenic granuloma of gingiva
Vertical ridge deficiency
Excludes2: *gingival cyst (K09.0)*

K06.9 Disorder of gingiva and edentulous alveolar ridge, unspecified

K08 Other disorders of teeth and supporting structures

Excludes2: *dentofacial anomalies [including malocclusion] (M26.-)*
disorders of jaw (M27.-)

AHA CC: 4Q, 2016, 29-30

K08.0 Exfoliation of teeth due to systemic causes
Code also underlying systemic condition

+ **K08.1 Complete loss of teeth**
Acquired loss of teeth, complete
Excludes1: *congenital absence of teeth (K00.0)*
exfoliation of teeth due to systemic causes (K08.0)
partial loss of teeth (K08.4-)

+ **K08.10 Complete loss of teeth, unspecified cause**
K08.101 Complete loss of teeth, unspecified cause, class I
K08.102 Complete loss of teeth, unspecified cause, class II
K08.103 Complete loss of teeth, unspecified cause, class III
K08.104 Complete loss of teeth, unspecified cause, class IV
K08.109 Complete loss of teeth, unspecified cause, unspecified class
Edentulism NOS

+ **K08.11 Complete loss of teeth due to trauma**
K08.111 Complete loss of teeth due to trauma, class I
K08.112 Complete loss of teeth due to trauma, class II
K08.113 Complete loss of teeth due to trauma, class III
K08.114 Complete loss of teeth due to trauma, class IV
K08.119 Complete loss of teeth due to trauma, unspecified class

+ **K08.12 Complete loss of teeth due to periodontal diseases**
K08.121 Complete loss of teeth due to periodontal diseases, class I
K08.122 Complete loss of teeth due to periodontal diseases, class II
K08.123 Complete loss of teeth due to periodontal diseases, class III
K08.124 Complete loss of teeth due to periodontal diseases, class IV
K08.129 Complete loss of teeth due to periodontal diseases, unspecified class

+ **K08.13 Complete loss of teeth due to caries**
K08.131 Complete loss of teeth due to caries, class I
K08.132 Complete loss of teeth due to caries, class II
K08.133 Complete loss of teeth due to caries, class III
K08.134 Complete loss of teeth due to caries, class IV
K08.139 Complete loss of teeth due to caries, unspecified class

+ **K08.19 Complete loss of teeth due to other specified cause**
K08.191 Complete loss of teeth due to other specified cause, class I
K08.192 Complete loss of teeth due to other specified cause, class II
K08.193 Complete loss of teeth due to other specified cause, class III
K08.194 Complete loss of teeth due to other specified cause, class IV
K08.199 Complete loss of teeth due to other specified cause, unspecified class

+ **K08.2 Atrophy of edentulous alveolar ridge**
K08.20 Unspecified atrophy of edentulous alveolar ridge
Atrophy of the mandible NOS
Atrophy of the maxilla NOS
K08.21 Minimal atrophy of the mandible
Minimal atrophy of the edentulous mandible
K08.22 Moderate atrophy of the mandible
Moderate atrophy of the edentulous mandible
K08.23 Severe atrophy of the mandible
Severe atrophy of the edentulous mandible
K08.24 Minimal atrophy of maxilla
Minimal atrophy of the edentulous maxilla
K08.25 Moderate atrophy of the maxilla
Moderate atrophy of the edentulous maxilla
K08.26 Severe atrophy of the maxilla
Severe atrophy of the edentulous maxilla

K08.3 Retained dental root

+ **K08.4 Partial loss of teeth**
Acquired loss of teeth, partial
Excludes1: *complete loss of teeth (K08.1-)*
congenital absence of teeth (K00.0)
Excludes2: *exfoliation of teeth due to systemic causes (K08.0)*

+ **K08.40 Partial loss of teeth, unspecified cause**
K08.401 Partial loss of teeth, unspecified cause, class I
K08.402 Partial loss of teeth, unspecified cause, class II
K08.403 Partial loss of teeth, unspecified cause, class III
K08.404 Partial loss of teeth, unspecified cause, class IV
K08.409 Partial loss of teeth, unspecified cause, unspecified class
Tooth extraction status NOS

+ **K08.41 Partial loss of teeth due to trauma**
K08.411 Partial loss of teeth due to trauma, class I
K08.412 Partial loss of teeth due to trauma, class II
K08.413 Partial loss of teeth due to trauma, class III
K08.414 Partial loss of teeth due to trauma, class IV
K08.419 Partial loss of teeth due to trauma, unspecified class

+ **K08.42 Partial loss of teeth due to periodontal diseases**
  - **K08.421 Partial loss of teeth due to periodontal diseases, class I**
  - **K08.422 Partial loss of teeth due to periodontal diseases, class II**
  - **K08.423 Partial loss of teeth due to periodontal diseases, class III**
  - **K08.424 Partial loss of teeth due to periodontal diseases, class IV**
  - **K08.429 Partial loss of teeth due to periodontal diseases, unspecified class**

+ **K08.43 Partial loss of teeth due to caries**
  - **K08.431 Partial loss of teeth due to caries, class I**
  - **K08.432 Partial loss of teeth due to caries, class II**
  - **K08.433 Partial loss of teeth due to caries, class III**
  - **K08.434 Partial loss of teeth due to caries, class IV**
  - **K08.439 Partial loss of teeth due to caries, unspecified class**

+ **K08.49 Partial loss of teeth due to other specified cause**
  - **K08.491 Partial loss of teeth due to other specified cause, class I**
  - **K08.492 Partial loss of teeth due to other specified cause, class II**
  - **K08.493 Partial loss of teeth due to other specified cause, class III**
  - **K08.494 Partial loss of teeth due to other specified cause, class IV**
  - **K08.499 Partial loss of teeth due to other specified cause, unspecified class**

+ **K08.5 Unsatisfactory restoration of tooth**

Defective bridge, crown, filling
Defective dental restoration

Excludes1: *dental restoration status (Z98.811)*

Excludes2: *endosseous dental implant failure (M27.6-)*
unsatisfactory endodontic treatment (M27.5-)

K08.50 Unsatisfactory restoration of tooth, unspecified
Defective dental restoration NOS

K08.51 Open restoration margins of tooth
Dental restoration failure of marginal integrity
Open margin on tooth restoration
Poor gingival margin to tooth restoration

K08.52 Unrepairable overhanging of dental restorative materials
Overhanging of tooth restoration

+ **K08.53 Fractured dental restorative material**

Excludes1: *cracked tooth (K03.81)*
traumatic fracture of tooth (S02.5)

- **K08.530 Fractured dental restorative material without loss of material**
- **K08.531 Fractured dental restorative material with loss of material**
- **K08.539 Fractured dental restorative material, unspecified**

K08.54 Contour of existing restoration of tooth biologically incompatible with oral health
Dental restoration failure of periodontal anatomical integrity
Unacceptable contours of existing restoration of tooth
Unacceptable morphology of existing restoration of tooth

K08.55 Allergy to existing dental restorative material
Use additional code to identify the specific type of allergy

K08.56 Poor aesthetic of existing restoration of tooth
Dental restoration aesthetically inadequate or displeasing

K08.59 Other unsatisfactory restoration of tooth
Other defective dental restoration

+ **K08.8 Other specified disorders of teeth and supporting structures**

K08.81 Primary occlusal trauma

K08.82 Secondary occlusal trauma

K08.89 Other specified disorders of teeth and supporting structures
Enlargement of alveolar ridge NOS
Insufficient anatomic crown height
Insufficient clinical crown length
Irregular alveolar process
Toothache NOS

K08.9 Disorder of teeth and supporting structures, unspecified

K09 Cysts of oral region, not elsewhere classified

Includes: lesions showing histological features both of aneurysmal cyst and of another fibro-osseous lesion

Excludes2: *cysts of jaw (M27.0-, M27.4-)*
radicular cyst (K04.8)

K09.0 Developmental odontogenic cysts
Dentigerous cyst
Eruption cyst
Follicular cyst
Gingival cyst
Lateral periodontal cyst
Primordial cyst

Excludes2: *keratocysts (D16.4, D16.5)*
odontogenic keratocystic tumors (D16.4, D16.5)

K09.1 Developmental (nonodontogenic) cysts of oral region
Cyst (of) incisive canal
Cyst (of) palatine of papilla
Globulomaxillary cyst
Median palatal cyst
Nasoalveolar cyst
Nasolabial cyst
Nasopalatine duct cyst

K09.8 Other cysts of oral region, not elsewhere classified
Dermoid cyst
Epidermoid cyst
Lymphoepithelial cyst
Epstein's pearl

K09.9 Cyst of oral region, unspecified

K11 Diseases of salivary glands

Use additional code to identify:
alcohol abuse and dependence (F10.-)
exposure to environmental tobacco smoke (Z77.22)
exposure to tobacco smoke in the perinatal period (P96.81)
history of tobacco dependence (Z87.891)
occupational exposure to environmental tobacco smoke (Z57.31)
tobacco dependence (F17.-)
tobacco use (Z72.0)

K11.0 Atrophy of salivary gland

K11.1 Hypertrophy of salivary gland

+ **K11.2 Sialoadenitis**

Parotitis

Excludes1: *epidemic parotitis (B26.-)*
mumps (B26.-)
uveoparotid fever [Heerfordt] (D86.89)

- **K11.20 Sialoadenitis, unspecified**
- **K11.21 Acute sialoadenitis**
  Excludes1: *acute recurrent sialoadenitis (K11.22)*
- **K11.22 Acute recurrent sialoadenitis**
- **K11.23 Chronic sialoadenitis**

CC **K11.3 Abscess of salivary gland**

CC **K11.4 Fistula of salivary gland**

Excludes1: *congenital fistula of salivary gland (Q38.4)*

K11.5 Sialolithiasis
Calculus of salivary gland or duct
Stone of salivary gland or duct

K11.6 Mucocele of salivary gland
Mucous extravasation cyst of salivary gland
Mucous retention cyst of salivary gland
Ranula

K11.7 Disturbances of salivary secretion
Hypoptyalism
Ptyalism
Xerostomia

Excludes2: *dry mouth NOS (R68.2)*

K11.8 Other diseases of salivary glands
Benign lymphoepithelial lesion of salivary gland
Mikulicz' disease
Necrotizing sialometaplasia
Sialectasia
Stenosis of salivary duct
Stricture of salivary duct

Excludes1: *Sjögren syndrome (M35.0-)*

K11.9 Disease of salivary gland, unspecified
Sialoadenopathy NOS

K12 Stomatitis and related lesions

Use additional code to identify:
alcohol abuse and dependence (F10.-)
exposure to environmental tobacco smoke (Z77.22)
exposure to tobacco smoke in the perinatal period (P96.81)
history of tobacco dependence (Z87.891)
occupational exposure to environmental tobacco smoke (Z57.31)
tobacco dependence (F17.-)
tobacco use (Z72.0)

Excludes1: *cancrum oris (A69.0)*
cheilitis (K13.0)
gangrenous stomatitis (A69.0)
herpesviral [herpes simplex] gingivostomatitis (B00.2)
noma (A69.0)

K12.0 Recurrent oral aphthae
Aphthous stomatitis (major) (minor)
Bednar's aphthae
Periadenitis mucosa necrotica recurrens
Recurrent aphthous ulcer
Stomatitis herpetiformis

K12.1 Other forms of stomatitis
Stomatitis NOS
Denture stomatitis
Ulcerative stomatitis
Vesicular stomatitis
Excludes1: *acute necrotizing ulcerative stomatitis (A69.1)*
Vincent's stomatitis (A69.1)

CC **K12.2 Cellulitis and abscess of mouth**
Cellulitis of mouth (floor)
Submandibular abscess
Excludes2: *abscess of salivary gland (K11.3)*
abscess of tongue (K14.0)
periapical abscess (K04.6-K04.7)
periodontal abscess (K05.21)
peritonsillar abscess (J36)

\+ **K12.3 Oral mucositis (ulcerative)**
Mucositis (oral) (oropharyneal)
Excludes2: *gastrointestinal mucositis (ulcerative) (K92.81)*
mucositis (ulcerative) of vagina and vulva (N76.81)
nasal mucositis (ulcerative) (J34.81)

K12.30 Oral mucositis (ulcerative), unspecified

K12.31 Oral mucositis (ulcerative) due to antineoplastic therapy
Use additional code for adverse effect, if applicable, to identify antineoplastic and immunosuppressive drugs (T45.1X5)
Use additional code for other antineoplastic therapy, such as: radiological procedure and radiotherapy (Y84.2)

K12.32 Oral mucositis (ulcerative) due to other drugs
Use additional code for adverse effect, if applicable, to identify drug (T36-T50 with fifth or sixth character 5)

K12.33 Oral mucositis (ulcerative) due to radiation
Use additional external cause code (W88-W90, X39.0-) to identify cause

K12.39 Other oral mucositis (ulcerative)
Viral oral mucositis (ulcerative)

K13 Other diseases of lip and oral mucosa

Includes: epithelial disturbances of tongue
Use additional code to identify:
alcohol abuse and dependence (F10.-)
exposure to environmental tobacco smoke (Z77.22)
exposure to tobacco smoke in the perinatal period (P96.81)
history of tobacco dependence (Z87.891)
occupational exposure to environmental tobacco smoke (Z57.31)
tobacco dependence (F17.-)
tobacco use (Z72.0)
Excludes2: *certain disorders of gingiva and edentulous alveolar ridge (K05-K06)*
cysts of oral region (K09.-)
diseases of tongue (K14.-)
stomatitis and related lesions (K12.-)

K13.0 Diseases of lips
Abscess of lips
Angular cheilitis
Cellulitis of lips
Cheilitis NOS
Cheilodynia
Cheilosis
Exfoliative cheilitis
Fistula of lips
Glandular cheilitis
Hypertrophy of lips
Perlèche NEC
Excludes1: *ariboflavinosis (E53.0)*
cheilitis due to radiation-related disorders (L55-L59)
congenital fistula of lips (Q38.0)
congenital hypertrophy of lips (Q18.6)
Perlèche due to candidiasis (B37.83)
Perlèche due to riboflavin deficiency (E53.0)

K13.1 Cheek and lip biting

\+ **K13.2 Leukoplakia and other disturbances of oral epithelium, including tongue**
Excludes1: *carcinoma in situ of oral epithelium (D00.0-)*
hairy leukoplakia (K13.3)

K13.21 Leukoplakia of oral mucosa, including tongue
Leukokeratosis of oral mucosa
Leukoplakia of gingiva, lips, tongue
Excludes1: *hairy leukoplakia (K13.3)*
leukokeratosis nicotina palati (K13.24)

K13.22 Minimal keratinized residual ridge mucosa
Minimal keratinization of alveolar ridge mucosa

K13.23 Excessive keratinized residual ridge mucosa
Excessive keratinization of alveolar ridge mucosa

K13.24 Leukokeratosis nicotina palati
Smoker's palate

K13.29 Other disturbances of oral epithelium, including tongue
Erythroplakia of mouth or tongue
Focal epithelial hyperplasia of mouth or tongue
Leukoedema of mouth or tongue
Other oral epithelium disturbances

K13.3 Hairy leukoplakia

K13.4 Granuloma and granuloma-like lesions of oral mucosa
Eosinophilic granuloma
Granuloma pyogenicum
Verrucous xanthoma

K13.5 Oral submucous fibrosis
Submucous fibrosis of tongue

K13.6 Irritative hyperplasia of oral mucosa
Excludes2: *irritative hyperplasia of edentulous ridge [denture hyperplasia] (K06.2)*

\+ **K13.7 Other and unspecified lesions of oral mucosa**

K13.70 Unspecified lesions of oral mucosa

K13.79 Other lesions of oral mucosa
Focal oral mucinosis

K14 Diseases of tongue

Use additional code to identify:
alcohol abuse and dependence (F10.-)
exposure to environmental tobacco smoke (Z77.22)
history of tobacco dependence (Z87.891)
occupational exposure to environmental tobacco smoke (Z57.31)
tobacco dependence (F17.-)
tobacco use (Z72.0)
Excludes2: *erythroplakia (K13.29)*
focal epithelial hyperplasia (K13.29)
leukedema of tongue (K13.29)
leukoplakia of tongue (K13.21)
hairy leukoplakia (K13.3)
macroglossia (congenital) (Q38.2)
submucous fibrosis of tongue (K13.5)

K14.0 Glossitis
Abscess of tongue
Ulceration (traumatic) of tongue
Excludes1: *atrophic glossitis (K14.4)*

K14.1 Geographic tongue
Benign migratory glossitis
Glossitis areata exfoliativa
K14.2 Median rhomboid glossitis
K14.3 Hypertrophy of tongue papillae
Black hairy tongue
Coated tongue
Hypertrophy of foliate papillae
Lingua villosa nigra
K14.4 Atrophy of tongue papillae
Atrophic glossitis
K14.5 Plicated tongue
Fissured tongue
Furrowed tongue
Scrotal tongue
Excludes1: *fissured tongue, congenital (Q38.3)*
K14.6 Glossodynia
Glossopyrosis
Painful tongue
K14.8 Other diseases of tongue
Atrophy of tongue
Crenated tongue
Enlargement of tongue
Glossocele
Glossoptosis
Hypertrophy of tongue
K14.9 Disease of tongue, unspecified
Glossopathy NOS

Diseases of esophagus, stomach and duodenum (K20-K31)

Excludes2: *hiatus hernia (K44.-)*

K20 Esophagitis
Use additional code to identify:
alcohol abuse and dependence (F10.-)
Excludes1: *erosion of esophagus (K22.1-)*
esophagitis with gastro-esophageal reflux disease (K21.0-)
reflux esophagitis (K21.0-)
ulcerative esophagitis (K22.1-)
Excludes2: *eosinophilic gastritis or gastroenteritis (K52.81)*
K20.0 Eosinophilic esophagitis
AHA CC: 4Q, 2020, 9-10
+ **K20.8 Other esophagitis**
AHA CC: 4Q, 2020, 28-29
K20.80 Other esophagitis without bleeding
Abscess of esophagus
Other esophagitis NOS
MCC **K20.81 Other esophagitis with bleeding**
+ **K20.9 Esophagitis, unspecified**
AHA CC: 4Q, 2020, 28-29
K20.90 Esophagitis, unspecified without bleeding
Esophagitis NOS
MCC **K20.91 Esophagitis, unspecified with bleeding**

K21 Gastro-esophageal reflux disease
Excludes1: *newborn esophageal reflux (P78.83)*
+ **K21.0 Gastro-esophageal reflux disease with esophagitis**
AHA CC: 4Q, 2020, 28-29
K21.00 Gastro-esophageal reflux disease with esophagitis, without bleeding
Reflux esophagitis
MCC **K21.01 Gastro-esophageal reflux disease with esophagitis, with bleeding**
K21.9 Gastro-esophageal reflux disease without esophagitis
Esophageal reflux NOS
CC AHA: 1Q, 2016, 18

Gastroesophageal Reflux Disease

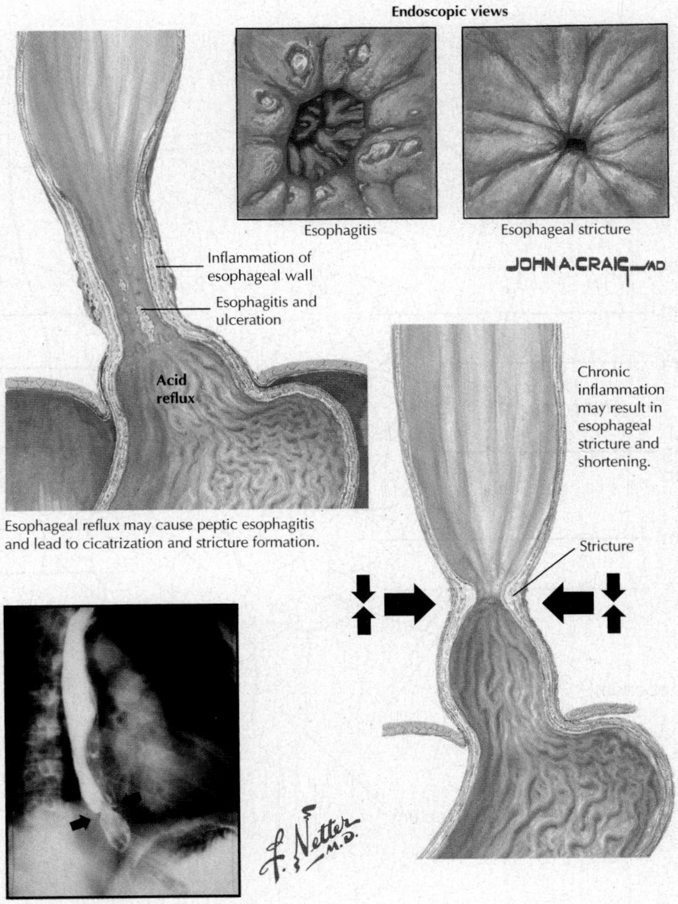

Esophageal reflux may cause peptic esophagitis and lead to cicatrization and stricture formation.

Barium study shows esophageal stricture.

Gastrointestinal System Side View

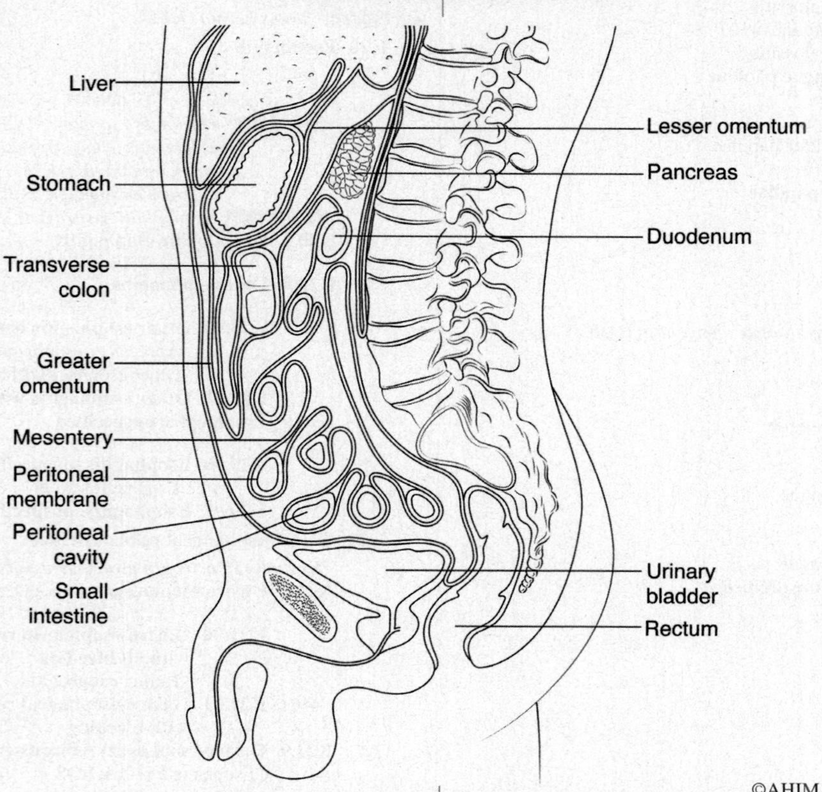

©AHIMA

Gastrointestinal System Front View

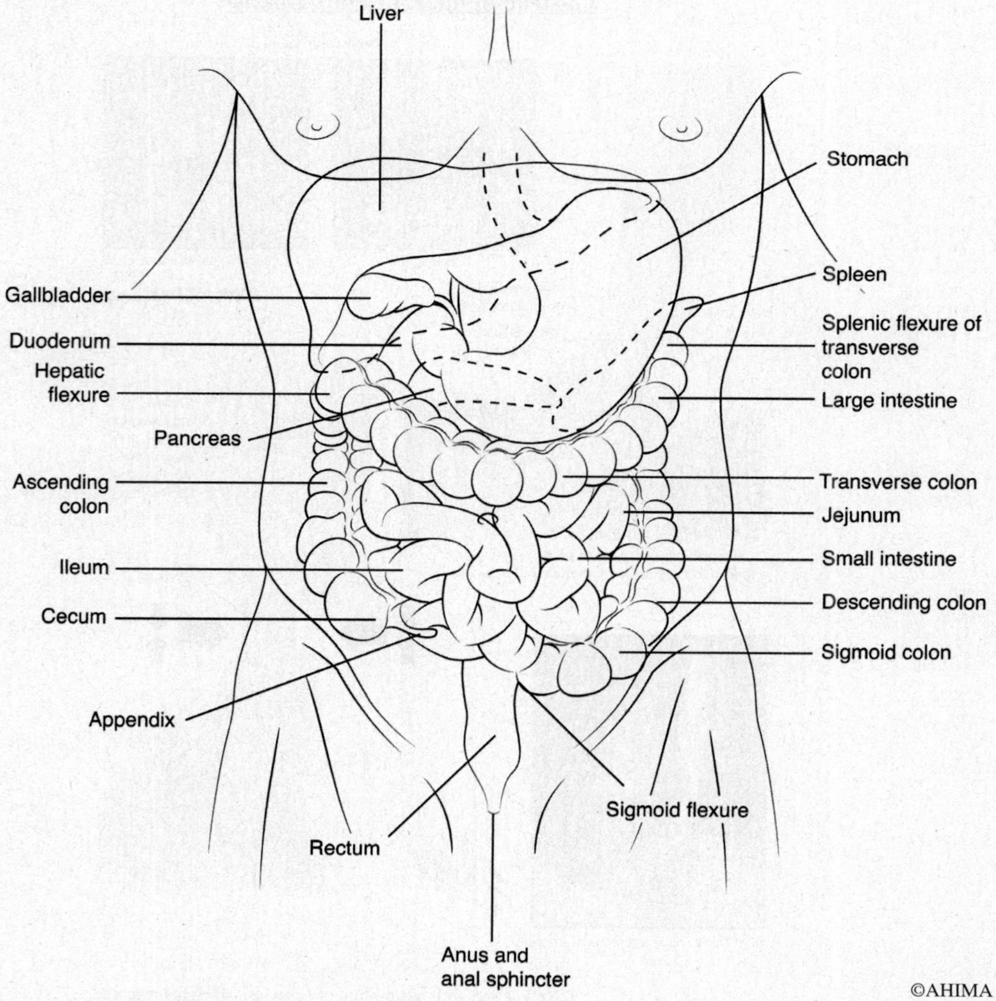

©AHIMA

Upper Gastrointestinal System

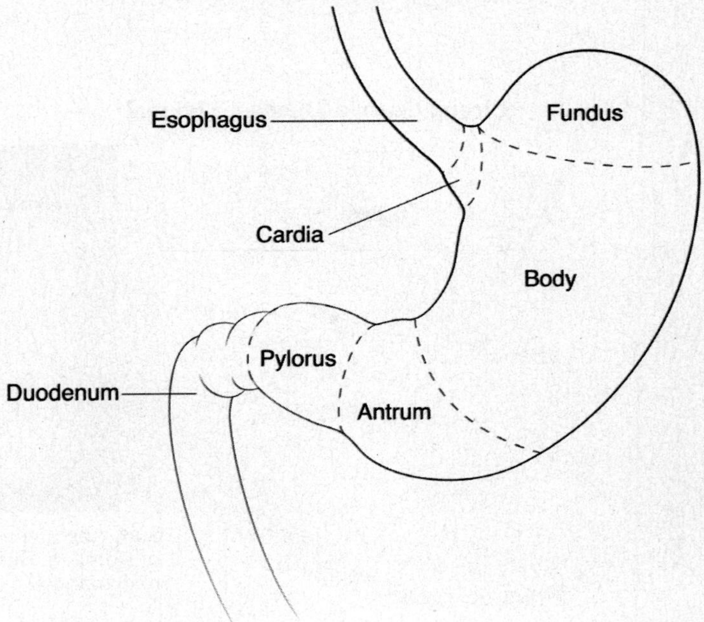

©AHIMA

K22 Other diseases of esophagus

Excludes2: *esophageal varices (I85.-)*

K22.0 Achalasia of cardia
Achalasia NOS
Cardiospasm
Excludes1: *congenital cardiospasm (Q39.5)*

+ **K22.1 Ulcer of esophagus**
Barrett's ulcer
Erosion of esophagus
Fungal ulcer of esophagus
Peptic ulcer of esophagus
Ulcer of esophagus due to ingestion of chemicals
Ulcer of esophagus due to ingestion of drugs and medicaments
Ulcerative esophagitis
Code first poisoning due to drug or toxin, if applicable (T36-T65 with fifth or sixth character 1-4 or 6)

Use additional code for adverse effect, if applicable, to identify drug (T36-T50 with fifth or sixth character 5)
Excludes1: *Barrett's esophagus (K22.7-)*

CC **K22.10 Ulcer of esophagus without bleeding**
Ulcer of esophagus NOS

MCC **K22.11 Ulcer of esophagus with bleeding**
Excludes2: *bleeding esophageal varices (I85.01, I85.11)*
AHA CC: 3Q, 2018, 22-23

K22.2 Esophageal obstruction
Compression of esophagus
Constriction of esophagus
Stenosis of esophagus
Stricture of esophagus
Excludes1: *congenital stenosis or stricture of esophagus (Q39.3)*

MCC **K22.3 Perforation of esophagus**
Rupture of esophagus
Excludes1: *traumatic perforation of (thoracic) esophagus (S27.8-)*

K22.4 Dyskinesia of esophagus
Corkscrew esophagus
Diffuse esophageal spasm
Spasm of esophagus
Excludes1: *cardiospasm (K22.0)*

K22.5 Diverticulum of esophagus, acquired
Esophageal pouch, acquired
Excludes1: *diverticulum of esophagus (congenital) (Q39.6)*

MCC **K22.6 Gastro-esophageal laceration-hemorrhage syndrome**
Mallory-Weiss syndrome

+ **K22.7 Barrett's esophagus**
Barrett's disease
Barrett's syndrome
Excludes1: *Barrett's ulcer (K22.1)*
malignant neoplasm of esophagus (C15.-)

K22.70 Barrett's esophagus without dysplasia
Barrett's esophagus NOS

+ **K22.71 Barrett's esophagus with dysplasia**

K22.710 Barrett's esophagus with low grade dysplasia

K22.711 Barrett's esophagus with high grade dysplasia

K22.719 Barrett's esophagus with dysplasia, unspecified

+ **K22.8 Other specified diseases of esophagus**
Excludes2: *esophageal varices (I85.-)*
Paterson-Kelly syndrome (D50.1)
AHA CC: 1Q, 2020, 16

K22.81 Esophageal polyp
Excludes1: *benign neoplasm of esophagus (D13.0)*

K22.82 Esophagogastric junction polyp
Excludes1: *benign neoplasm of stomach (D13.1)*

K22.89 Other specified disease of esophagus
Hemorrhage of esophagus NOS

K22.9 Disease of esophagus, unspecified

K23 Disorders of esophagus in diseases classified elsewhere

Code first underlying disease, such as:
congenital syphilis (A50.5)
Excludes1: *late syphilis (A52.79)*
megaesophagus due to Chagas' disease (B57.31)
tuberculosis (A18.83)

Valid 3-character code, no further characters required

K25 Gastric ulcer

Includes: erosion (acute) of stomach
pylorus ulcer (peptic)
stomach ulcer (peptic)
Use additional code to identify:
alcohol abuse and dependence (F10.-)
Excludes1: *acute gastritis (K29.0-)*
peptic ulcer NOS (K27.-)

MCC **K25.0 Acute gastric ulcer with hemorrhage**
MCC **K25.1 Acute gastric ulcer with perforation**
MCC **K25.2 Acute gastric ulcer with both hemorrhage and perforation**
CC **K25.3 Acute gastric ulcer without hemorrhage or perforation**
MCC **K25.4 Chronic or unspecified gastric ulcer with hemorrhage**
AHA CC: 3Q, 2017, 27
MCC **K25.5 Chronic or unspecified gastric ulcer with perforation**
MCC **K25.6 Chronic or unspecified gastric ulcer with both hemorrhage and perforation**

Ulcers: Gastric, Duodena, Jejunal

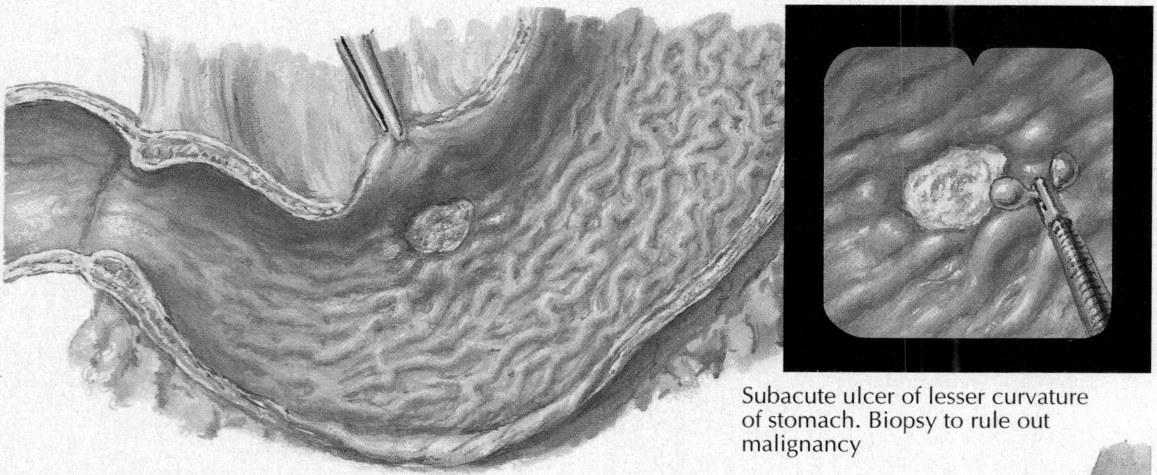

Subacute ulcer of lesser curvature of stomach. Biopsy to rule out malignancy

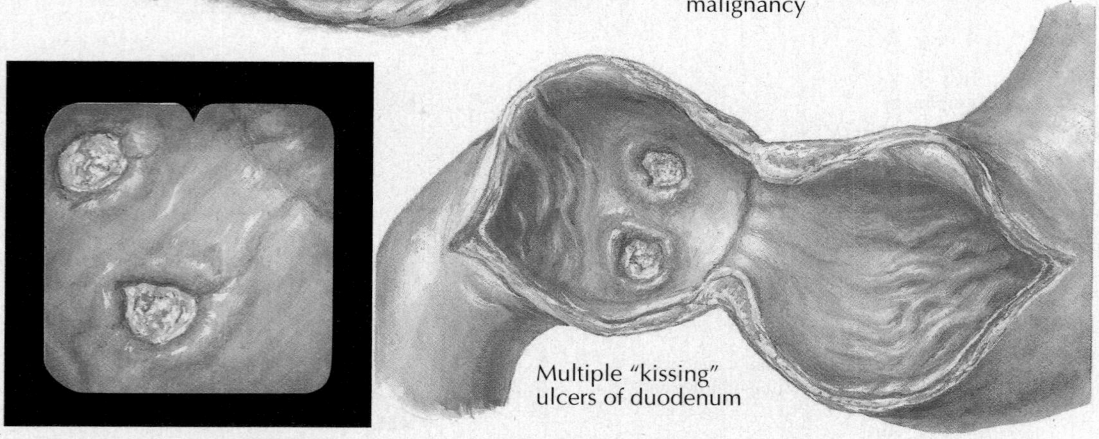

Multiple “kissing” ulcers of duodenum

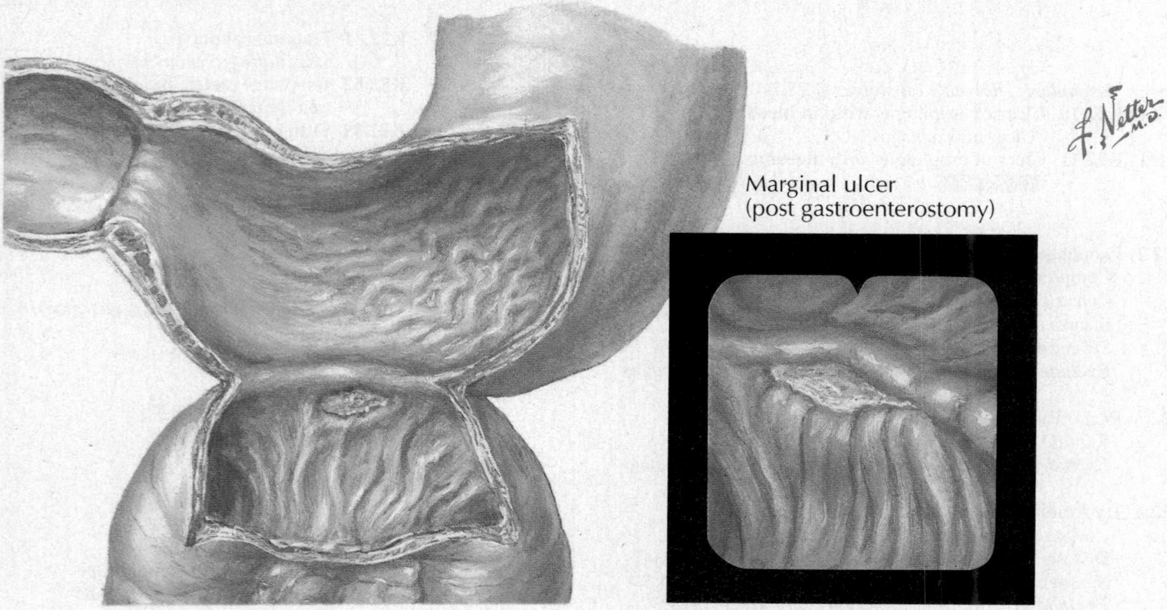

Marginal ulcer (post gastroenterostomy)

K25.7 Chronic gastric ulcer without hemorrhage or perforation
K25.9 Gastric ulcer, unspecified as acute or chronic, without hemorrhage or perforation
AHA CC: 1Q, 2021, 11-12

K26 Duodenal ulcer

Includes: erosion (acute) of duodenum
duodenum ulcer (peptic)
postpyloric ulcer (peptic)
Use additional code to identify:
alcohol abuse and dependence (F10.-)
Excludes1: *peptic ulcer NOS (K27.-)*

MCC **K26.0 Acute duodenal ulcer with hemorrhage**
K26.1 Acute duodenal ulcer with perforation
K26.2 Acute duodenal ulcer with both hemorrhage and perforation
CC **K26.3 Acute duodenal ulcer without hemorrhage or perforation**
MCC **K26.4 Chronic or unspecified duodenal ulcer with hemorrhage**
CC AHA: 1Q, 2016, 14
MCC **K26.5 Chronic or unspecified duodenal ulcer with perforation**
MCC **K26.6 Chronic or unspecified duodenal ulcer with both hemorrhage and perforation**
K26.7 Chronic duodenal ulcer without hemorrhage or perforation
K26.9 Duodenal ulcer, unspecified as acute or chronic, without hemorrhage or perforation

K27 Peptic ulcer, site unspecified

Includes: gastroduodenal ulcer NOS
peptic ulcer NOS
Use additional code to identify:
alcohol abuse and dependence (F10.-)
Excludes1: *peptic ulcer of newborn (P78.82)*

MCC **K27.0 Acute peptic ulcer, site unspecified, with hemorrhage**
MCC **K27.1 Acute peptic ulcer, site unspecified, with perforation**
K27.2 Acute peptic ulcer, site unspecified, with both hemorrhage and perforation
CC **K27.3 Acute peptic ulcer, site unspecified, without hemorrhage or perforation**
MCC **K27.4 Chronic or unspecified peptic ulcer, site unspecified, with hemorrhage**
MCC **K27.5 Chronic or unspecified peptic ulcer, site unspecified, with perforation**
MCC **K27.6 Chronic or unspecified peptic ulcer, site unspecified, with both hemorrhage and perforation**
K27.7 Chronic peptic ulcer, site unspecified, without hemorrhage or perforation
K27.9 Peptic ulcer, site unspecified, unspecified as acute or chronic, without hemorrhage or perforation

K28 Gastrojejunal ulcer

Includes: anastomotic ulcer (peptic) or erosion
gastrocolic ulcer (peptic) or erosion
gastrointestinal ulcer (peptic) or erosion
gastrojejunal ulcer (peptic) or erosion
jejunal ulcer (peptic) or erosion
marginal ulcer (peptic) or erosion
stomal ulcer (peptic) or erosion
Use additional code to identify:
alcohol abuse and dependence (F10.-)
Excludes1: *primary ulcer of small intestine (K63.3)*

MCC **K28.0 Acute gastrojejunal ulcer with hemorrhage**
MCC **K28.1 Acute gastrojejunal ulcer with perforation**
MCC **K28.2 Acute gastrojejunal ulcer with both hemorrhage and perforation**
CC **K28.3 Acute gastrojejunal ulcer without hemorrhage or perforation**
MCC **K28.4 Chronic or unspecified gastrojejunal ulcer with hemorrhage**
MCC **K28.5 Chronic or unspecified gastrojejunal ulcer with perforation**
MCC **K28.6 Chronic or unspecified gastrojejunal ulcer with both hemorrhage and perforation**
K28.7 Chronic gastrojejunal ulcer without hemorrhage or perforation
K28.9 Gastrojejunal ulcer, unspecified as acute or chronic, without hemorrhage or perforation

K29 Gastritis and duodenitis

Excludes1: *eosinophilic gastritis or gastroenteritis (K52.81)*
Zollinger-Ellison syndrome (E16.4)

\+ **K29.0 Acute gastritis**
Use additional code to identify:
alcohol abuse and dependence (F10.-)
Excludes1: *erosion (acute) of stomach (K25.-)*
K29.00 Acute gastritis without bleeding
MCC **K29.01 Acute gastritis with bleeding**

\+ **K29.2 Alcoholic gastritis**
Use additional code to identify:
alcohol abuse and dependence (F10.-)
K29.20 Alcoholic gastritis without bleeding
MCC **K29.21 Alcoholic gastritis with bleeding**
\+ **K29.3 Chronic superficial gastritis**
K29.30 Chronic superficial gastritis without bleeding
MCC **K29.31 Chronic superficial gastritis with bleeding**
\+ **K29.4 Chronic atrophic gastritis**
Gastric atrophy
K29.40 Chronic atrophic gastritis without bleeding
MCC **K29.41 Chronic atrophic gastritis with bleeding**
\+ **K29.5 Unspecified chronic gastritis**
Chronic antral gastritis
Chronic fundal gastritis
K29.50 Unspecified chronic gastritis without bleeding
MCC **K29.51 Unspecified chronic gastritis with bleeding**
\+ **K29.6 Other gastritis**
Giant hypertrophic gastritis
Granulomatous gastritis
Ménétrier's disease
K29.60 Other gastritis without bleeding
MCC **K29.61 Other gastritis with bleeding**
\+ **K29.7 Gastritis, unspecified**
K29.70 Gastritis, unspecified, without bleeding
MCC **K29.71 Gastritis, unspecified, with bleeding**
\+ **K29.8 Duodenitis**
K29.80 Duodenitis without bleeding
MCC **K29.81 Duodenitis with bleeding**
AHA CC: 3Q, 2018, 22-23
\+ **K29.9 Gastroduodenitis, unspecified**
K29.90 Gastroduodenitis, unspecified, without bleeding
MCC **K29.91 Gastroduodenitis, unspecified, with bleeding**

K30 Functional dyspepsia

Indigestion
Excludes1: *dyspepsia NOS (R10.13)*
heartburn (R12)
nervous dyspepsia (F45.8)
neurotic dyspepsia (F45.8)
psychogenic dyspepsia (F45.8)
Valid 3-character code, no further characters required

K31 Other diseases of stomach and duodenum

Includes: functional disorders of stomach
Excludes2: *diabetic gastroparesis (E08.43, E09.43, E10.43, E11.43, E13.43)*
diverticulum of duodenum (K57.00-K57.13)

K31.0 Acute dilatation of stomach
Acute distention of stomach
• **K31.1 Adult hypertrophic pyloric stenosis**
Pyloric stenosis NOS
Excludes1: *congenital or infantile pyloric stenosis (Q40.0)*
K31.2 Hourglass stricture and stenosis of stomach
Excludes1: *congenital hourglass stomach (Q40.2)*
hourglass contraction of stomach (K31.89)
K31.3 Pylorospasm, not elsewhere classified
Excludes1: *congenital or infantile pylorospasm (Q40.0)*
neurotic pylorospasm (F45.8)
psychogenic pylorospasm (F45.8)v
K31.4 Gastric diverticulum
Excludes1: *congenital diverticulum of stomach (Q40.2)*
CC **K31.5 Obstruction of duodenum**
Constriction of duodenum
Duodenal ileus (chronic)
Stenosis of duodenum
Stricture of duodenum
Volvulus of duodenum
Excludes1: *congenital stenosis of duodenum (Q41.0)*
CC **K31.6 Fistula of stomach and duodenum**
Gastrocolic fistula
Gastrojejunocolic fistula
K31.7 Polyp of stomach and duodenum
Excludes1: *adenomatous polyp of stomach (D13.1)*
AHA CC: 1Q, 2020, 16
\+ **K31.8 Other specified diseases of stomach and duodenum**
\+ **K31.81 Angiodysplasia of stomach and duodenum**
MCC **K31.811 Angiodysplasia of stomach and duodenum with bleeding**

K31.819 Angiodysplasia of stomach and duodenum without bleeding
Angiodysplasia of stomach and duodenum NOS
MCC **K31.82 Dieulafoy lesion (hemorrhagic) of stomach and duodenum**
Excludes2: *Dieulafoy lesion of intestine (K63.81)*
K31.83 Achlorhydria
K31.84 Gastroparesis
Gastroparalysis
Code first underlying disease, if known, such as:
anorexia nervosa (F50.0-)
diabetes mellitus (E08.43, E09.43, E10.43, E11.43, E13.43)
scleroderma (M34.-)
AHA CC: 4Q, 2013, 114-115
K31.89 Other diseases of stomach and duodenum
AHA CC: 1Q, 2017, 28; 1Q, 2020, 15
K31.9 Disease of stomach and duodenum, unspecified
+ **K31.A Gastric intestinal metaplasia**
K31.A0 Gastric intestinal metaplasia, unspecified
Gastric intestinal metaplasia definite for dysplasia
Gastric intestinal metaplasia NOS
+ **K31.A1 Gastric intestinal metaplasia without dysplasia**
K31.A11 Gastric intestinal metaplasia without dysplasia, involving the antrum
K31.A12 Gastric intestinal metaplasia without dysplasia, involving the body (corpus)
K31.A13 Gastric intestinal metaplasia without dysplasia, involving the fundus
K31.A14 Gastric intestinal metaplasia without dysplasia, involving the cardia
K31.A15 Gastric intestinal metaplasia without dysplasia, involving the multiple sites
K31.A19 Gastric intestinal metaplasia without dysplasia, unspecified site
+ **K31.A2 Gastric intestinal metaplasia with dysplasia**
K31.A21 Gastric intestinal metaplasia with low grade dysplasia
K31.A22 Gastric intestinal metaplasia with high grade dysplasia
K31.A29 Gastric intestinal metaplasia with dysplasia, unspecified

Diseases of appendix (K35-K38)

K35 Acute appendicitis
+ **K35.2 Acute appendicitis with generalized peritonitis**
Appendicitis (acute) with generalized (diffuse) peritonitis following rupture or perforation of appendix
AHA CC: 4Q, 2018, 17-18
CC **K35.20 Acute appendicitis with generalized peritonitis, without abscess**
(Acute) appendicitis with generalized peritonitis NOS
AHA CC: 4Q, 2018, 18
MCC **K35.21 Acute appendicitis with generalized peritonitis, with abscess**
+ **K35.3 Acute appendicitis with localized peritonitis**
AHA CC: 4Q, 2018, 17-18
CC **K35.30 Acute appendicitis with localized peritonitis, without perforation or gangrene**
Acute appendicitis with localized peritonitis NOS
CC **K35.31 Acute appendicitis with localized peritonitis and gangrene, without perforation**
MCC **K35.32 Acute appendicitis with perforation and localized peritonitis, without abscess**
(Acute) appendicitis with perforation NOS
Perforated appendix NOS
Ruptured appendix (with localized peritonitis) NOS
AHA CC: 4Q, 2018, 18; 1Q, 2020, 16
MCC **K35.33 Acute appendicitis with perforation and localized peritonitis, with abscess**
(Acute) appendicitis with (peritoneal) abscess NOS
Ruptured appendix with localized peritonitis and abscess
+ **K35.8 Other and unspecified acute appendicitis**
CC **K35.80 Unspecified acute appendicitis**
Acute appendicitis NOS
Acute appendicitis without (localized) (generalized) peritonitis
+ **K35.89 Other acute appendicitis**
AHA CC: 4Q, 2018, 17-18
CC **K35.890 Other acute appendicitis without perforation or gangrene**
CC **K35.891 Other acute appendicitis without perforation, with gangrene**
(Acute) appendicitis with gangrene NOS

K36 Other appendicitis
Chronic appendicitis
Recurrent appendicitis
Valid 3-character code, no further characters required

K37 Unspecified appendicitis
Excludes1: *unspecified appendicitis with peritonitis (K35.2-, K35.3-)*
Valid 3-character code, no further characters required

K38 Other diseases of appendix
K38.0 Hyperplasia of appendix
K38.1 Appendicular concretions
Fecalith of appendix
Stercolith of appendix
K38.2 Diverticulum of appendix
K38.3 Fistula of appendix
K38.8 Other specified diseases of appendix
Intussusception of appendix
K38.9 Disease of appendix, unspecified

Abdominal Wall: Inguinal Hernia

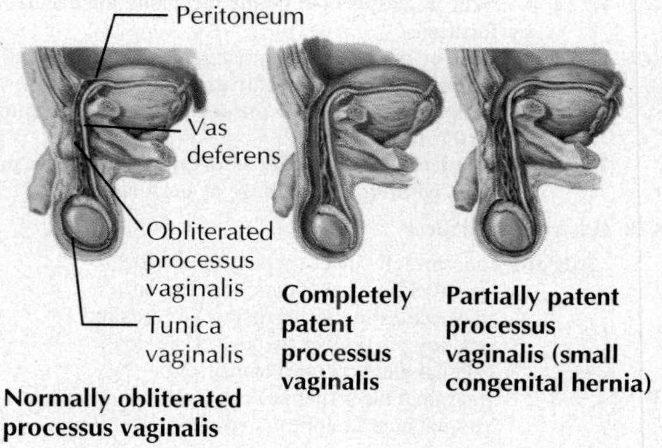

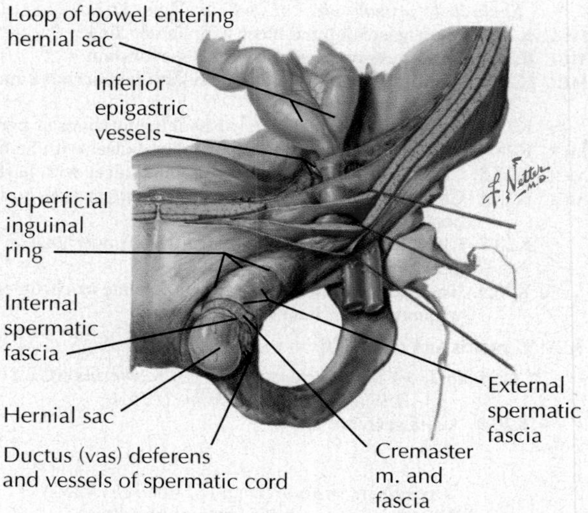

Hernia (K40-K46)

NOTE Hernia with both gangrene and obstruction is classified to hernia with gangrene.

Includes: acquired hernia
congenital [except diaphragmatic or hiatus] hernia
recurrent hernia

K40 Inguinal hernia

Includes: bubonocele
direct inguinal hernia
double inguinal hernia
indirect inguinal hernia
inguinal hernia NOS
oblique inguinal hernia
scrotal hernia

+ **K40.0 Bilateral inguinal hernia, with obstruction, without gangrene**
Inguinal hernia (bilateral) causing obstruction without gangrene
Incarcerated inguinal hernia (bilateral) without gangrene
Irreducible inguinal hernia (bilateral) without gangrene
Strangulated inguinal hernia (bilateral) without gangrene

CC **K40.00 Bilateral inguinal hernia, with obstruction, without gangrene, not specified as recurrent**
Bilateral inguinal hernia, with obstruction, without gangrene NOS

CC **K40.01 Bilateral inguinal hernia, with obstruction, without gangrene, recurrent**

+ **K40.1 Bilateral inguinal hernia, with gangrene**

MCC **K40.10 Bilateral inguinal hernia, with gangrene, not specified as recurrent**
Bilateral inguinal hernia, with gangrene NOS

MCC **K40.11 Bilateral inguinal hernia, with gangrene, recurrent**

+ **K40.2 Bilateral inguinal hernia, without obstruction or gangrene**

K40.20 Bilateral inguinal hernia, without obstruction or gangrene, not specified as recurrent
Bilateral inguinal hernia NOS

K40.21 Bilateral inguinal hernia, without obstruction or gangrene, recurrent

+ **K40.3 Unilateral inguinal hernia, with obstruction, without gangrene**
Inguinal hernia (unilateral) causing obstruction without gangrene
Incarcerated inguinal hernia (unilateral) without gangrene
Irreducible inguinal hernia (unilateral) without gangrene
Strangulated inguinal hernia (unilateral) without gangrene

CC **K40.30 Unilateral inguinal hernia, with obstruction, without gangrene, not specified as recurrent**
Inguinal hernia, with obstruction NOS
Unilateral inguinal hernia, with obstruction, without gangrene NOS

CC **K40.31 Unilateral inguinal hernia, with obstruction, without gangrene, recurrent**

+ **K40.4 Unilateral inguinal hernia, with gangrene**

MCC **K40.40 Unilateral inguinal hernia, with gangrene, not specified as recurrent**
Inguinal hernia with gangrene NOS
Unilateral inguinal hernia with gangrene NOS

MCC **K40.41 Unilateral inguinal hernia, with gangrene, recurrent**

+ **K40.9 Unilateral inguinal hernia, without obstruction or gangrene**

K40.90 Unilateral inguinal hernia, without obstruction or gangrene, not specified as recurrent
Inguinal hernia NOS
Unilateral inguinal hernia NOS

K40.91 Unilateral inguinal hernia, without obstruction or gangrene, recurrent

K41 Femoral hernia

+ **K41.0 Bilateral femoral hernia, with obstruction, without gangrene**
Femoral hernia (bilateral) causing obstruction, without gangrene
Incarcerated femoral hernia (bilateral), without gangrene
Irreducible femoral hernia (bilateral), without gangrene
Strangulated femoral hernia (bilateral), without gangrene

CC **K41.00 Bilateral femoral hernia, with obstruction, without gangrene, not specified as recurrent**
Bilateral femoral hernia, with obstruction, without gangrene NOS

CC **K41.01 Bilateral femoral hernia, with obstruction, without gangrene, recurrent**

+ **K41.1 Bilateral femoral hernia, with gangrene**

MCC **K41.10 Bilateral femoral hernia, with gangrene, not specified as recurrent**
Bilateral femoral hernia, with gangrene NOS

MCC **K41.11 Bilateral femoral hernia, with gangrene, recurrent**

+ **K41.2 Bilateral femoral hernia, without obstruction or gangrene**

K41.20 Bilateral femoral hernia, without obstruction or gangrene, not specified as recurrent
Bilateral femoral hernia NOS

K41.21 Bilateral femoral hernia, without obstruction or gangrene, recurrent

+ **K41.3 Unilateral femoral hernia, with obstruction, without gangrene**
Femoral hernia (unilateral) causing obstruction, without gangrene
Incarcerated femoral hernia (unilateral), without gangrene
Irreducible femoral hernia (unilateral), without gangrene
Strangulated femoral hernia (unilateral), without gangrene

CC **K41.30 Unilateral femoral hernia, with obstruction, without gangrene, not specified as recurrent**
Femoral hernia, with obstruction NOS
Unilateral femoral hernia, with obstruction NOS

CC **K41.31 Unilateral femoral hernia, with obstruction, without gangrene, recurrent**

+ **K41.4 Unilateral femoral hernia, with gangrene**

CC **K41.40 Unilateral femoral hernia, with gangrene, not specified as recurrent**
Femoral hernia, with gangrene NOS
Unilateral femoral hernia, with gangrene NOS

CC **K41.41 Unilateral femoral hernia, with gangrene, recurrent**

+ **K41.9 Unilateral femoral hernia, without obstruction or gangrene**

K41.90 Unilateral femoral hernia, without obstruction or gangrene, not specified as recurrent
Femoral hernia NOS
Unilateral femoral hernia NOS

K41.91 Unilateral femoral hernia, without obstruction or gangrene, recurrent

K42 Umbilical hernia

Includes: paraumbilical hernia
Excludes1: *omphalocele (Q79.2)*

K42.0 Umbilical hernia with obstruction, without gangrene
Umbilical hernia causing obstruction, without gangrene
Incarcerated umbilical hernia, without gangrene
Irreducible umbilical hernia, without gangrene
Strangulated umbilical hernia, without gangrene

K42.1 Umbilical hernia with gangrene
Gangrenous umbilical hernia

K42.9 Umbilical hernia without obstruction or gangrene
Umbilical hernia NOS

K43 Ventral hernia

K43.0 Incisional hernia with obstruction, without gangrene
Incisional hernia causing obstruction, without gangrene
Incarcerated incisional hernia, without gangrene
Irreducible incisional hernia, without gangrene
Strangulated incisional hernia, without gangrene

K43.1 Incisional hernia with gangrene
Gangrenous incisional hernia
AHA CC: 2Q, 2020, 22

K43.2 Incisional hernia without obstruction or gangrene
Incisional hernia NOS

K43.3 Parastomal hernia with obstruction, without gangrene
Incarcerated parastomal hernia, without gangrene
Irreducible parastomal hernia, without gangrene
Parastomal hernia causing obstruction, without gangrene
Strangulated parastomal hernia, without gangrene

K43.4 Parastomal hernia with gangrene
Gangrenous parastomal hernia

K43.5 Parastomal hernia without obstruction or gangrene
Parastomal hernia NOS

K43.6 Other and unspecified ventral hernia with obstruction, without gangrene
Epigastric hernia causing obstruction, without gangrene
Hypogastric hernia causing obstruction, without gangrene
Incarcerated epigastric hernia without gangrene
Incarcerated hypogastric hernia without gangrene
Incarcerated midline hernia without gangrene
Incarcerated spigelian hernia without gangrene
Incarcerated subxiphoid hernia without gangrene
Irreducible epigastric hernia without gangrene
Irreducible hypogastric hernia without gangrene
Irreducible midline hernia without gangrene
Irreducible spigelian hernia without gangrene
Irreducible subxiphoid hernia without gangrene
Midline hernia causing obstruction, without gangrene
Spigelian hernia causing obstruction, without gangrene
Strangulated epigastric hernia without gangrene
Strangulated hypogastric hernia without gangrene
Strangulated midline hernia without gangrene
Strangulated spigelian hernia without gangrene
Strangulated subxiphoid hernia without gangrene
Subxiphoid hernia causing obstruction, without gangrene

K43.7 Other and unspecified ventral hernia with gangrene
Any condition listed under K43.6 specified as gangrenous

K43.9 Ventral hernia without obstruction or gangrene
Epigastric hernia
Ventral hernia NOS

K44 Diaphragmatic hernia

Includes: hiatus hernia (esophageal) (sliding)
paraesophageal hernia

Excludes1: *congenital diaphragmatic hernia (Q79.0)*
congenital hiatus hernia (Q40.1)

K44.0 Diaphragmatic hernia with obstruction, without gangrene
Diaphragmatic hernia causing obstruction
Incarcerated diaphragmatic hernia
Irreducible diaphragmatic hernia
Strangulated diaphragmatic hernia

K44.1 Diaphragmatic hernia with gangrene
Gangrenous diaphragmatic hernia

K44.9 Diaphragmatic hernia without obstruction or gangrene
Diaphragmatic hernia NOS

K45 Other abdominal hernia

Includes: abdominal hernia, specified site NEC
lumbar hernia
obturator hernia
pudendal hernia
retroperitoneal hernia
sciatic hernia

K45.0 Other specified abdominal hernia with obstruction, without gangrene
Other specified abdominal hernia causing obstruction
Other specified incarcerated abdominal hernia
Other specified irreducible abdominal hernia
Other specified strangulated abdominal hernia

K45.1 Other specified abdominal hernia with gangrene
Any condition listed under K45 specified as gangrenous

K45.8 Other specified abdominal hernia without obstruction or gangrene

K46 Unspecified abdominal hernia

Includes: enterocele
epiplocele
hernia NOS
interstitial hernia
intestinal hernia
intra-abdominal hernia

Excludes1: *vaginal enterocele (N81.5)*

K46.0 Unspecified abdominal hernia with obstruction, without gangrene
Unspecified abdominal hernia causing obstruction
Unspecified incarcerated abdominal hernia
Unspecified irreducible abdominal hernia
Unspecified strangulated abdominal hernia

K46.1 Unspecified abdominal hernia with gangrene
Any condition listed under K46 specified as gangrenous

K46.9 Unspecified abdominal hernia without obstruction or gangrene
Abdominal hernia NOS

Noninfective enteritis and colitis (K50-K52)

Includes: noninfective inflammatory bowel disease

Excludes1: *irritable bowel syndrome (K58.-)*
megacolon (K59.3-)

K50 Crohn's disease [regional enteritis]

Includes: granulomatous enteritis
Use additional code to identify manifestations, such as:
pyoderma gangrenosum (L88)

Excludes1: *ulcerative colitis (K51.-)*

\+ **K50.0 Crohn's disease of small intestine**
Crohn's disease [regional enteritis] of duodenum
Crohn's disease [regional enteritis] of ileum
Crohn's disease [regional enteritis] of jejunum
Regional ileitis
Terminal ileitis

Excludes1: *Crohn's disease of both small and large intestine (K50.8-)*

CC **K50.00 Crohn's disease of small intestine without complications**

\+ **K50.01 Crohn's disease of small intestine with complications**

CC **K50.011 Crohn's disease of small intestine with rectal bleeding**

CC **K50.012 Crohn's disease of small intestine with intestinal obstruction**

CC **K50.013 Crohn's disease of small intestine with fistula**

CC **K50.014 Crohn's disease of small intestine with abscess**
AHA CC: 4Q, 2012, 104

CC **K50.018 Crohn's disease of small intestine with other complication**

CC **K50.019 Crohn's disease of small intestine with unspecified complications**

\+ **K50.1 Crohn's disease of large intestine**
Crohn's disease [regional enteritis] of colon
Crohn's disease [regional enteritis] of large bowel
Crohn's disease [regional enteritis] of rectum
Granulomatous colitis
Regional colitis

Excludes1: *Crohn's disease of both small and large intestine (K50.8)*

CC **K50.10 Crohn's disease of large intestine without complications**

\+ **K50.11 Crohn's disease of large intestine with complications**

CC **K50.111 Crohn's disease of large intestine with rectal bleeding**

CC **K50.112 Crohn's disease of large intestine with intestinal obstruction**

CC **K50.113 Crohn's disease of large intestine with fistula**

CC **K50.114 Crohn's disease of large intestine with abscess**
AHA CC: 4Q, 2012, 104

CC **K50.118 Crohn's disease of large intestine with other complication**

CC **K50.119 Crohn's disease of large intestine with unspecified complications**

Inflammatory Bowel Disease: Progression of Inflammatory Process in Chron's Disease

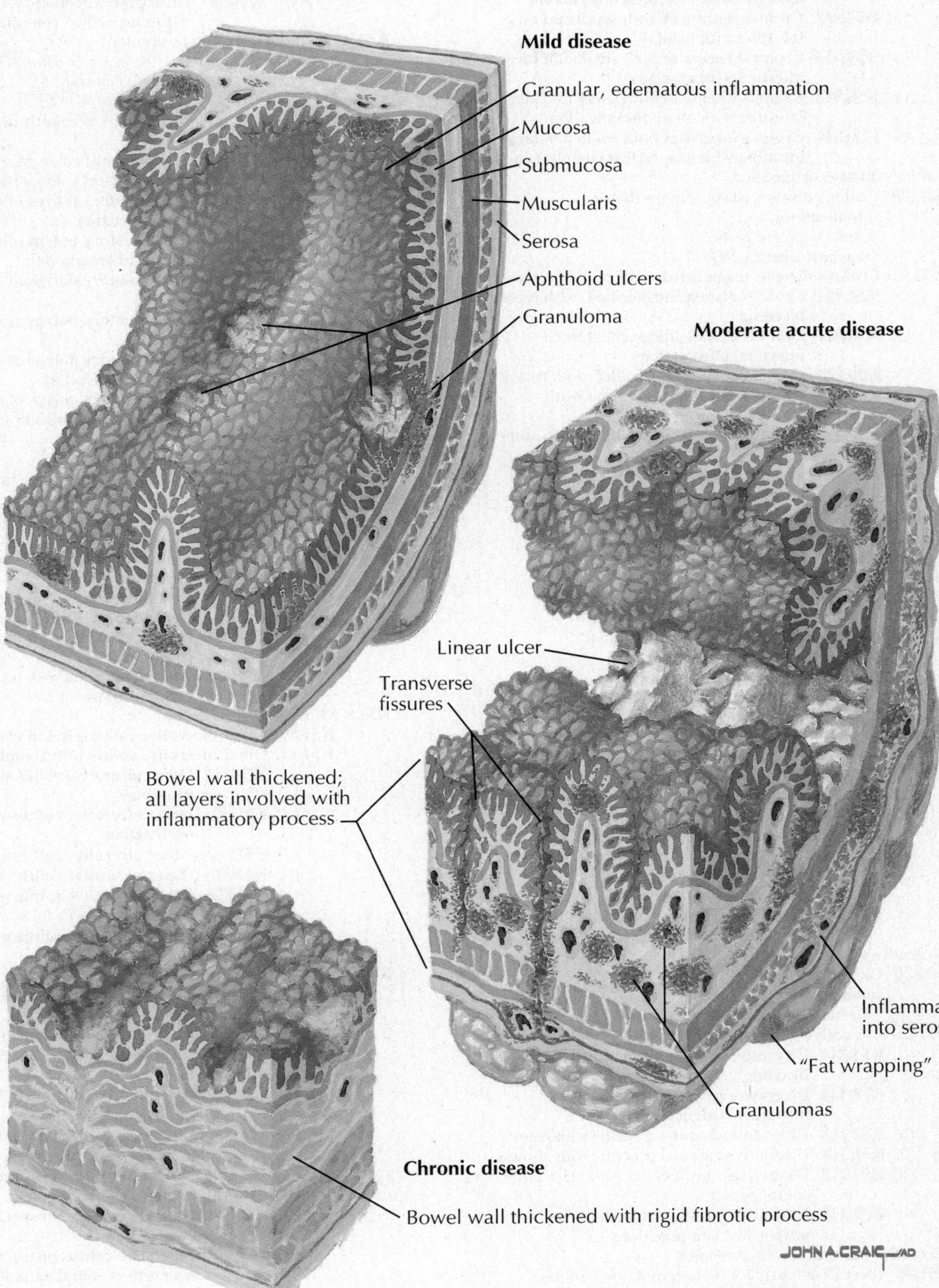

+ **K50.8 Crohn's disease of both small and large intestine**
  - CC **K50.80 Crohn's disease of both small and large intestine without complications**
  - + **K50.81 Crohn's disease of both small and large intestine with complications**
    - CC **K50.811 Crohn's disease of both small and large intestine with rectal bleeding**
    - CC **K50.812 Crohn's disease of both small and large intestine with intestinal obstruction**
    - CC **K50.813 Crohn's disease of both small and large intestine with fistula**
    - CC **K50.814 Crohn's disease of both small and large intestine with abscess**
    - CC **K50.818 Crohn's disease of both small and large intestine with other complication**
    - CC **K50.819 Crohn's disease of both small and large intestine with unspecified complications**

+ **K50.9 Crohn's disease, unspecified**
  - CC **K50.90 Crohn's disease, unspecified, without complications**
    - Crohn's disease NOS
    - Regional enteritis NOS
  - + **K50.91 Crohn's disease, unspecified, with complications**
    - CC **K50.911 Crohn's disease, unspecified, with rectal bleeding**
    - CC **K50.912 Crohn's disease, unspecified, with intestinal obstruction**
    - CC **K50.913 Crohn's disease, unspecified, with fistula**
    - CC **K50.914 Crohn's disease, unspecified, with abscess**
    - CC **K50.918 Crohn's disease, unspecified, with other complication**
    - CC **K50.919 Crohn's disease, unspecified, with unspecified complications**

K51 Ulcerative colitis

Use additional code to identify manifestations, such as:
pyoderma gangrenosum (L88)

Excludes1: *Crohn's disease [regional enteritis] (K50.-)*

+ **K51.0 Ulcerative (chronic) pancolitis**
  - Backwash ileitis
  - CC **K51.00 Ulcerative (chronic) pancolitis without complications**
    - Ulcerative (chronic) pancolitis NOS
  - + **K51.01 Ulcerative (chronic) pancolitis with complications**
    - CC CC **K51.011 Ulcerative (chronic) pancolitis with rectal bleeding**
    - CC **K51.012 Ulcerative (chronic) pancolitis with intestinal obstruction**
    - CC **K51.013 Ulcerative (chronic) pancolitis with fistula**
    - CC **K51.014 Ulcerative (chronic) pancolitis with abscess**
    - CC **K51.018 Ulcerative (chronic) pancolitis with other complication**
    - CC **K51.019 Ulcerative (chronic) pancolitis with unspecified complications**

+ **K51.2 Ulcerative (chronic) proctitis**
  - CC **K51.20 Ulcerative (chronic) proctitis without complications**
    - Ulcerative (chronic) proctitis NOS
  - + **K51.21 Ulcerative (chronic) proctitis with complications**
    - CC **K51.211 Ulcerative (chronic) proctitis with rectal bleeding**
    - **K51.212 Ulcerative (chronic) proctitis with intestinal obstruction**
    - CC **K51.213 Ulcerative (chronic) proctitis with fistula**
    - CC **K51.214 Ulcerative (chronic) proctitis with abscess**
    - CC **K51.218 Ulcerative (chronic) proctitis with other complication**
    - CC **K51.219 Ulcerative (chronic) proctitis with unspecified complications**

+ **K51.3 Ulcerative (chronic) rectosigmoiditis**
  - CC **K51.30 Ulcerative (chronic) rectosigmoiditis without complications**
    - Ulcerative (chronic) rectosigmoiditis NOS
  - + **K51.31 Ulcerative (chronic) rectosigmoiditis with complications**
    - CC **K51.311 Ulcerative (chronic) rectosigmoiditis with rectal bleeding**
    - CC **K51.312 Ulcerative (chronic) rectosigmoiditis with intestinal obstruction**
    - CC **K51.313 Ulcerative (chronic) rectosigmoiditis with fistula**
    - CC **K51.314 Ulcerative (chronic) rectosigmoiditis with abscess**
    - CC **K51.318 Ulcerative (chronic) rectosigmoiditis with other complication**
    - CC **K51.319 Ulcerative (chronic) rectosigmoiditis with unspecified complications**

+ **K51.4 Inflammatory polyps of colon**
  - ***Excludes1:*** *adenomatous polyp of colon (D12.6)*
    polyposis of colon (D12.6)
    polyps of colon NOS (K63.5)
  - CC **K51.40 Inflammatory polyps of colon without complications**
    - Inflammatory polyps of colon NOS
  - + **K51.41 Inflammatory polyps of colon with complications**
    - CC **K51.411 Inflammatory polyps of colon with rectal bleeding**
    - CC **K51.412 Inflammatory polyps of colon with intestinal obstruction**
    - CC **K51.413 Inflammatory polyps of colon with fistula**
    - CC **K51.414 Inflammatory polyps of colon with abscess**
    - CC **K51.418 Inflammatory polyps of colon with other complication**
    - CC **K51.419 Inflammatory polyps of colon with unspecified complications**

+ **K51.5 Left sided colitis**
  - Left hemicolitis
  - CC **K51.50 Left sided colitis without complications**
    - Left sided colitis NOS
  - + **K51.51 Left sided colitis with complications**
    - CC **K51.511 Left sided colitis with rectal bleeding**
    - CC **K51.512 Left sided colitis with intestinal obstruction**
    - CC **K51.513 Left sided colitis with fistula**
    - CC **K51.514 Left sided colitis with abscess**
    - CC **K51.518 Left sided colitis with other complication**
    - CC **K51.519 Left sided colitis with unspecified complications**

+ **K51.8 Other ulcerative colitis**
  - CC **K51.80 Other ulcerative colitis without complications**
  - + **K51.81 Other ulcerative colitis with complications**
    - CC **K51.811 Other ulcerative colitis with rectal bleeding**
    - CC **K51.812 Other ulcerative colitis with intestinal obstruction**
    - CC **K51.813 Other ulcerative colitis with fistula**
    - CC **K51.814 Other ulcerative colitis with abscess**
    - CC **K51.818 Other ulcerative colitis with other complication**
    - CC **K51.819 Other ulcerative colitis with unspecified complications**

+ **K51.9 Ulcerative colitis, unspecified**
  - CC **K51.90 Ulcerative colitis, unspecified, without complications**
  - + **K51.91 Ulcerative colitis, unspecified, with complications**
    - CC **K51.911 Ulcerative colitis, unspecified with rectal bleeding**
    - CC **K51.912 Ulcerative colitis, unspecified with intestinal obstruction**
    - CC **K51.913 Ulcerative colitis, unspecified with fistula**
    - CC **K51.914 Ulcerative colitis, unspecified with abscess**
    - CC **K51.918 Ulcerative colitis, unspecified with other complication**
    - CC **K51.919 Ulcerative colitis, unspecified with unspecified complications**

K52 Other and unspecified noninfective gastroenteritis and colitis
AHA CC: 4Q, 2016, 30-31

CC **K52.0 Gastroenteritis and colitis due to radiation**

CC **K52.1 Toxic gastroenteritis and colitis**
Drug-induced gastroenteritis and colitis
Code first (T51-T65) to identify toxic agent
Use additional code for adverse effect, if applicable, to identify drug (T36-T50 with fifth or sixth character 5)
AHA CC: 1Q, 2019, 17

\+ **K52.2 Allergic and dietetic gastroenteritis and colitis**
Food hypersensitivity gastroenteritis or colitis
Use additional code to identify type of food allergy (Z91.01-, Z91.02-)
Excludes2: *allergic eosinophilic colitis (K52.82)*
allergic eosinophilic esophagitis (K20.0)
allergic eosinophilic gastritis (K52.81)
allergic eosinophilic gastroenteritis (K52.81)

K52.21 Food protein-induced enterocolitis syndrome
FPIES
Use additional code for hypovolemic shock, if present (R57.1)

K52.22 Food protein-induced enteropathy

K52.29 Other allergic and dietetic gastroenteritis and colitis
Allergic proctocolitis
Food hypersensitivity gastroenteritis or colitis
Food-induced eosinophilic proctocolitis
Food protein-induced proctocolitis
Immediate gastrointestinal hypersensitivity
Milk protein-induced proctocolitis

K52.3 Indeterminate colitis
Colonic inflammatory bowel disease unclassified (IBDU)
Excludes1: *unspecified colitis (K52.9)*

\+ **K52.8 Other specified noninfective gastroenteritis and colitis**

K52.81 Eosinophilic gastritis or gastroenteritis
Eosinophilic enteritis
Excludes2: *eosinophilic esophagitis (K20.0)*

K52.82 Eosinophilic colitis
Excludes2: *allergic protocolitis (K52.29)*
food-induced eosinophilic proctocolitis (K52.29)
food protein-induced enterocolitis syndrome (FPIES) (K52.21)
food protein-induced proctocolitis (K52.29)
milk protein induced proctocolitis (K52.29)

\+ **K52.83 Microscopic colitis**
K52.831 Collagenous colitis
K52.832 Lymphocytic colitis
K52.838 Other microscopic colitis
K52.839 Microscopic colitis, unspecified

K52.89 Other specified noninfective gastroenteritis and colitis
AHA CC: 1Q, 2019, 20-21

K52.9 Noninfective gastroenteritis and colitis, unspecified
Colitis NOS
Enteritis NOS
Gastroenteritis NOS
Ileitis NOS
Jejunitis NOS
Sigmoiditis NOS
Excludes1: *diarrhea NOS (R19.7)*
functional diarrhea (K59.1)
infectious gastroenteritis and colitis NOS (A09)
neonatal diarrhea (noninfective) (P78.3)
psychogenic diarrhea (F45.8)

Other diseases of intestines (K55-K64)

K55 Vascular disorders of intestine
Excludes1: *necrotizing enterocolitis of newborn (P77.-)*
AHA CC: 4Q, 2016, 32-33

\+ **K55.0 Acute vascular disorders of intestine**
Infarction of appendices epiploicae
Mesenteric (artery) (vein) embolism
Mesenteric (artery) (vein) infarction
Mesenteric (artery) (vein) thrombosis

\+ **K55.01 Acute (reversible) ischemia of small intestine**
MCC **K55.011 Focal (segmental) acute (reversible) ischemia of small intestine**
MCC **K55.012 Diffuse acute (reversible) ischemia of small intestine**
MCC **K55.019 Acute (reversible) ischemia of small intestine, extent unspecified**

\+ **K55.02 Acute infarction of small intestine**
Gangrene of small intestine
Necrosis of small intestine
MCC **K55.021 Focal (segmental) acute infarction of small intestine**
MCC **K55.022 Diffuse acute infarction of small intestine**
MCC **K55.029 Acute infarction of small intestine, extent unspecified**

\+ **K55.03 Acute (reversible) ischemia of large intestine**
Acute fulminant ischemic colitis
Subacute ischemic colitis
MCC **K55.031 Focal (segmental) acute (reversible) ischemia of large intestine**
MCC **K55.032 Diffuse acute (reversible) ischemia of large intestine**
MCC **K55.039 Acute (reversible) ischemia of large intestine, extent unspecified**
AHA CC: 4Q, 2019, 68

\+ **K55.04 Acute infarction of large intestine**
Gangrene of large intestine
Necrosis of large intestine
MCC **K55.041 Focal (segmental) acute infarction of large intestine**
MCC **K55.042 Diffuse acute infarction of large intestine**
MCC **K55.049 Acute infarction of large intestine, extent unspecified**

\+ **K55.05 Acute (reversible) ischemia of intestine, part unspecified**
MCC **K55.051 Focal (segmental) acute (reversible) ischemia of intestine, part unspecified**
MCC **K55.052 Diffuse acute (reversible) ischemia of intestine, part unspecified**
MCC **K55.059 Acute (reversible) ischemia of intestine, part and extent unspecified**

\+ **K55.06 Acute infarction of intestine, part unspecified**
Acute intestinal infarction
Gangrene of intestine
Necrosis of intestine
MCC **K55.061 Focal (segmental) acute infarction of intestine, part unspecified**
MCC **K55.062 Diffuse acute infarction of intestine, part unspecified**
MCC **K55.069 Acute infarction of intestine, part and extent unspecified**

CC **K55.1 Chronic vascular disorders of intestine**
Chronic ischemic colitis
Chronic ischemic enteritis
Chronic ischemic enterocolitis
Ischemic stricture of intestine
Mesenteric atherosclerosis
Mesenteric vascular insufficiency

\+ **K55.2 Angiodysplasia of colon**
K55.20 Angiodysplasia of colon without hemorrhage
MCC **K55.21 Angiodysplasia of colon with hemorrhage**
AHA CC: 3Q, 2018, 21

\+ **K55.3 Necrotizing enterocolitis**
Excludes1: *necrotizing enterocolitis of newborn (P77.-)*
Excludes2: *necrotizing enterocolitis due to Clostridium difficile (A04.7-)*
MCC **K55.30 Necrotizing enterocolitis, unspecified**
Necrotizing enterocolitis, NOS
MCC **K55.31 Stage 1 necrotizing enterocolitis**
Necrotizing enterocolitis without pneumatosis, without perforation
MCC **K55.32 Stage 2 necrotizing enterocolitis**
Necrotizing enterocolitis with pneumatosis, without perforation
MCC **K55.33 Stage 3 necrotizing enterocolitis**
Necrotizing enterocolitis with perforation
Necrotizing enterocolitis with pneumatosis and perforation

CC **K55.8 Other vascular disorders of intestine**

CC **K55.9 Vascular disorder of intestine, unspecified**
Ischemic colitis
Ischemic enteritis
Ischemic enterocolitis

K56 Paralytic ileus and intestinal obstruction without hernia

Excludes1: *congenital stricture or stenosis of intestine (Q41-Q42)*
cystic fibrosis with meconium ileus (E84.11)
ischemic stricture of intestine (K55.1)
meconium ileus NOS (P76.0)
neonatal intestinal obstructions classifiable to P76.-
obstruction of duodenum (K31.5)
postprocedural intestinal obstruction (K91.3-)

Excludes2: *stenosis of anus or rectum (K62.4)*

CC **K56.0 Paralytic ileus**
Paralysis of bowel
Paralysis of colon
Paralysis of intestine
Excludes1: *gallstone ileus (K56.3)*
ileus NOS (K56.7)
obstructive ileus NOS (K56.69-)

CC **K56.1 Intussusception**
Intussusception or invagination of bowel
Intussusception or invagination of colon
Intussusception or invagination of intestine
Intussusception or invagination of rectum
Excludes2: *intussusception of appendix (K38.8)*

MCC **K56.2 Volvulus**
Strangulation of colon or intestine
Torsion of colon or intestine
Twist of colon or intestine
Excludes2: *volvulus of duodenum (K31.5)*

K56.3 Gallstone ileus
Obstruction of intestine by gallstone

\+ **K56.4 Other impaction of intestine**

K56.41 Fecal impaction
Excludes1: *constipation (K59.0-)*
incomplete defecation (R15.0)

CC **K56.49 Other impaction of intestine**

\+ **K56.5 Intestinal adhesions [bands] with obstruction (postinfection)**
Abdominal hernia due to adhesions with obstruction
Peritoneal adhesions [bands] with intestinal obstruction (postinfection)
AHA CC: 4Q, 2017, 16-17

CC **K56.50 Intestinal adhesions [bands], unspecified as to partial versus complete obstruction**
Intestinal adhesions with obstruction NOS

CC **K56.51 Intestinal adhesions [bands], with partial obstruction**
Intestinal adhesions with incomplete obstruction

CC **K56.52 Intestinal adhesions [bands] with complete obstruction**

\+ **K56.6 Other and unspecified intestinal obstruction**
AHA CC: 4Q, 2017, 16-17

\+ **K56.60 Unspecified intestinal obstruction**

CC **K56.600 Partial intestinal obstruction, unspecified as to cause**
Incomplete intestinal obstruction, NOS

CC **K56.601 Complete intestinal obstruction, unspecified as to cause**

CC **K56.609 Unspecified intestinal obstruction, unspecified as to partial versus complete obstruction**
Intestinal obstruction NOS

\+ **K56.69 Other intestinal obstruction**
Enterostenosis NOS
Obstructive ileus NOS
Occlusion of colon or intestine NOS
Stenosis of colon or intestine NOS
Stricture of colon or intestine NOS
Excludes1: *intestinal obstruction due to specified condition-code to condition*

CC **K56.690 Other partial intestinal obstruction**
Other incomplete intestinal obstruction

CC **K56.691 Other complete intestinal obstruction**

CC **K56.699 Other intestinal obstruction unspecified as to partial versus complete obstruction**
Other intestinal obstruction, NEC

CC **K56.7 Ileus, unspecified**
Excludes1: *obstructive ileus (K56.69-)*
Excludes2: *intestinal obstruction with hernia (K40-K46)*
AHA CC: 1Q, 2017, 40-41

K57 Diverticular disease of intestine

Excludes1: *congenital diverticulum of intestine (Q43.8)*
Meckel's diverticulum (Q43.0)

Excludes2: *diverticulum of appendix (K38.2)*

Code also if applicable peritonitis K65.-

\+ **K57.0 Diverticulitis of small intestine with perforation and abscess**
Excludes1: *diverticulitis of both small and large intestine with perforation and abscess (K57.4-)*

CC **K57.00 Diverticulitis of small intestine with perforation and abscess without bleeding**

MCC **K57.01 Diverticulitis of small intestine with perforation and abscess with bleeding**

\+ **K57.1 Diverticular disease of small intestine without perforation or abscess**
Excludes1: *diverticular disease of both small and large intestine without perforation or abscess (K57.5-)*

K57.10 Diverticulosis of small intestine without perforation or abscess without bleeding
Diverticular disease of small intestine NOS

MCC **K57.11 Diverticulosis of small intestine without perforation or abscess with bleeding**

CC **K57.12 Diverticulitis of small intestine without perforation or abscess without bleeding**

MCC **K57.13 Diverticulitis of small intestine without perforation or abscess with bleeding**

\+ **K57.2 Diverticulitis of large intestine with perforation and abscess**
Excludes1: *diverticulitis of both small and large intestine with perforation and abscess (K57.4-)*

CC **K57.20 Diverticulitis of large intestine with perforation and abscess without bleeding**

MCC **K57.21 Diverticulitis of large intestine with perforation and abscess with bleeding**

\+ **K57.3 Diverticular disease of large intestine without perforation or abscess**
Excludes1: *diverticular disease of both small and large intestine without perforation or abscess (K57.5-)*

K57.30 Diverticulosis of large intestine without perforation or abscess without bleeding
Diverticular disease of colon NOS

MCC **K57.31 Diverticulosis of large intestine without perforation or abscess with bleeding**
AHA CC: 3Q, 2018, 21-22

CC **K57.32 Diverticulitis of large intestine without perforation or abscess without bleeding**

MCC **K57.33 Diverticulitis of large intestine without perforation or abscess with bleeding**

\+ **K57.4 Diverticulitis of both small and large intestine with perforation and abscess**

CC **K57.40 Diverticulitis of both small and large intestine with perforation and abscess without bleeding**

MCC **K57.41 Diverticulitis of both small and large intestine with perforation and abscess with bleeding**

\+ **K57.5 Diverticular disease of both small and large intestine without perforation or abscess**

K57.50 Diverticulosis of both small and large intestine without perforation or abscess without bleeding
Diverticular disease of both small and large intestine NOS

MCC **K57.51 Diverticulosis of both small and large intestine without perforation or abscess with bleeding**

CC **K57.52 Diverticulitis of both small and large intestine without perforation or abscess without bleeding**

MCC **K57.53 Diverticulitis of both small and large intestine without perforation or abscess with bleeding**

\+ **K57.8 Diverticulitis of intestine, part unspecified, with perforation and abscess**

CC **K57.80 Diverticulitis of intestine, part unspecified, with perforation and abscess without bleeding**

MCC **K57.81 Diverticulitis of intestine, part unspecified, with perforation and abscess with bleeding**

\+ **K57.9 Diverticular disease of intestine, part unspecified, without perforation or abscess**

K57.90 Diverticulosis of intestine, part unspecified, without perforation or abscess without bleeding
Diverticular disease of intestine NOS
AHA CC: 1Q, 2021, 11-12

MCC **K57.91 Diverticulosis of intestine, part unspecified, without perforation or abscess with bleeding**

CC **K57.92 Diverticulitis of intestine, part unspecified, without perforation or abscess without bleeding**

MCC **K57.93 Diverticulitis of intestine, part unspecified, without perforation or abscess with bleeding**

K58 Irritable bowel syndrome

Includes: irritable colon
spastic colon

K58.0 Irritable bowel syndrome with diarrhea

K58.1 Irritable bowel syndrome with constipation
AHA CC: 4Q, 2016, 32-33

K58.2 Mixed irritable bowel syndrome
AHA CC: 4Q, 2016, 32-33

K58.8 Other irritable bowel syndrome
AHA CC: 4Q, 2016, 32-33

K58.9 Irritable bowel syndrome without diarrhea
Irritable bowel syndrome NOS

K59 Other functional intestinal disorders

Excludes1: *change in bowel habit NOS (R19.4)*
intestinal malabsorption (K90.-)
psychogenic intestinal disorders (F45.8)

Excludes2: *functional disorders of stomach (K31.-)*

\+ **K59.0 Constipation**

Excludes1: *fecal impaction (K56.41)*
incomplete defecation (R15.0)

K59.00 Constipation, unspecified

K59.01 Slow transit constipation

K59.02 Outlet dysfunction constipation

K59.03 Drug induced constipation
Use additional code for adverse effect, if applicable, to identify drug (T36-T50 with fifth or sixth character 5)
AHA CC: 4Q, 2016, 33

K59.04 Chronic idiopathic constipation
Functional constipation
AHA CC: 4Q, 2016, 33

K59.09 Other constipation
Chronic constipation

K59.1 Functional diarrhea

Excludes1: *diarrhea NOS (R19.7)*
irritable bowel syndrome with diarrhea (K58.0)

CC **K59.2 Neurogenic bowel, not elsewhere classified**

\+ **K59.3 Megacolon, not elsewhere classified**
Dilatation of colon
Code first, if applicable (T51-T65) to identify toxic agent

Excludes1: *congenital megacolon (aganglionic) (Q43.1)*
megacolon (due to) (in) Chagas' disease (B57.32)
megacolon (due to) (in) Clostridium difficile (A04.7-)
megacolon (due to) (in) Hirschsprung's disease (Q43.1)

AHA CC: 4Q, 2016, 33-34

CC **K59.31 Toxic megacolon**

CC **K59.39 Other megacolon**
Megacolon NOS

K59.4 Anal spasm
Proctalgia fugax

\+ **K59.8 Other specified functional intestinal disorders**
AHA CC: 4Q, 2020, 29-30

K59.81 Ogilvie syndrome
Acute colonic pseudo-obstruction (ACPO)

K59.89 Other specified functional intestinal disorders
Atony of colon
Pseudo-obstruction (acute) (chronic) of intestine

K59.9 Functional intestinal disorder, unspecified

K60 Fissure and fistula of anal and rectal regions

Excludes1: *fissure and fistula of anal and rectal regions with abscess or cellulitis (K61.-)*

Excludes2: *anal sphincter tear (healed) (nontraumatic) (old) (K62.81)*

K60.0 Acute anal fissure

K60.1 Chronic anal fissure

K60.2 Anal fissure, unspecified

K60.3 Anal fistula

K60.4 Rectal fistula
Fistula of rectum to skin

Excludes1: *rectovaginal fistula (N82.3)*
vesicorectal fistual (N32.1)

K60.5 Anorectal fistula

K61 Abscess of anal and rectal regions

Includes: abscess of anal and rectal regions
cellulitis of anal and rectal regions

CC **K61.0 Anal abscess**
Perianal abscess

Excludes2: *intrasphincteric abscess (K61.4)*

CC **K61.1 Rectal abscess**
Perirectal abscess

Excludes1: *ischiorectal abscess (K61.39)*

CC **K61.2 Anorectal abscess**

\+ **K61.3 Ischiorectal abscess**
AHA CC: 4Q, 2018, 19

CC **K61.31 Horseshoe abscess**

CC **K61.32 Ischiorectal abscess, NOS**

K61.39 Other ischiorectal abscess
Abscess of ischiorectal fossa
Ischiorectal abscess, NOS

CC **K61.4 Intrasphincteric abscess**
Intersphincteric abscess
AHA CC: 4Q, 2018, 19

CC **K61.5 Supralevator abscess**
AHA CC: 4Q, 2018, 19

K62 Other diseases of anus and rectum

Includes: anal canal

Excludes2: *colostomy and enterostomy malfunction (K94.0-, K94.1-)*
fecal incontinence (R15.-)
hemorrhoids (K64.-)

K62.0 Anal polyp

K62.1 Rectal polyp

Excludes1: *adenomatous polyp (D12.8)*

K62.2 Anal prolapse
Prolapse of anal canal

K62.3 Rectal prolapse
Prolapse of rectal mucosa

K62.4 Stenosis of anus and rectum
Stricture of anus (sphincter)
AHA CC: 2Q, 2019, 13

CC **K62.5 Hemorrhage of anus and rectum**

Excludes1: *gastrointestinal bleeding NOS (K92.2)*
melena (K92.1)
neonatal rectal hemorrhage (P54.2)

AHA CC: 1Q, 2019, 21

CC **K62.6 Ulcer of anus and rectum**
Solitary ulcer of anus and rectum
Stercoral ulcer of anus and rectum

Excludes1: *fissure and fistula of anus and rectum (K60.-)*
ulcerative colitis (K51.-)

K62.7 Radiation proctitis
Use additional code to identify the type of radiation (W88.-) or radiation therapy (Y84.2)
AHA CC: 1Q, 2019, 21

\+ **K62.8 Other specified diseases of anus and rectum**

Excludes2: *ulcerative proctitis (K51.2)*

K62.81 Anal sphincter tear (healed) (nontraumatic) (old)
Tear of anus, nontraumatic
Use additional code for any associated fecal incontinence (R15.-)

Excludes2: *anal fissure (K60.-)*
anal sphincter tear (healed) (old) complicating delivery (O34.7-)
traumatic tear of anal sphincter (S31.831)

K62.82 Dysplasia of anus
Anal intraepithelial neoplasia I and II (AIN I and II) (histologically confirmed)
Dysplasia of anus NOS
Mild and moderate dysplasia of anus (histologically confirmed)
Excludes1: *abnormal results from anal cytologic examination without histologic confirmation (R85.61-)*
anal intraepithelial neoplasia III (D01.3)
carcinoma in situ of anus (D01.3)
HGSIL of anus (R85.613)
severe dysplasia of anus (D01.3)

K62.89 Other specified diseases of anus and rectum
Proctitis NOS
Use additional code for any associated fecal incontinence (R15.-)

K62.9 Disease of anus and rectum, unspecified

K63 Other diseases of intestine

CC **K63.0 Abscess of intestine**
Excludes1: *abscess of intestine with Crohn's disease (K50.014, K50.114, K50.814, K50.914,)*
abscess of intestine with diverticular disease (K57.0, K57.2, K57.4, K57.8)
abscess of intestine with ulcerative colitis (K51.014, K51.214, K51.314, K51.414, K51.514, K51.814, K51.914)
Excludes2: *abscess of anal and rectal regions (K61.-)*
abscess of appendix (K35.3-)

MCC **K63.1 Perforation of intestine (nontraumatic)**
Perforation (nontraumatic) of rectum
Excludes1: *perforation (nontraumatic) of duodenum (K26.-)*
perforation (nontraumatic) of intestine with diverticular disease (K57.0, K57.2, K57.4, K57.8)
Excludes2: *perforation (nontraumatic) of appendix (K35.2-, K35.3-)*
AHA CC: 2Q, 2020, 22

CC **K63.2 Fistula of intestine**
Excludes1: *fistula of duodenum (K31.6)*
fistula of intestine with Crohn's disease (K50.013, K50.113, K50.813, K50.913,)
fistula of intestine with ulcerative colitis (K51.013, K51.213, K51.313, K51.413, K51.513, K51.813, K51.913)
Excludes2: *fistula of anal and rectal regions (K60.-)*
fistula of appendix (K38.3)
intestinal-genital fistula, female (N82.2-N82.4)
vesicointestinal fistula (N32.1)
AHA CC: 3Q, 2017, 4-5

CC **K63.3 Ulcer of intestine**
Primary ulcer of small intestine
Excludes1: *duodenal ulcer (K26.-)*
gastrointestinal ulcer (K28.-)
gastrojejunal ulcer (K28.-)
jejunal ulcer (K28.-)
peptic ulcer, site unspecified (K27.-)
ulcer of intestine with perforation (K63.1)
ulcer of anus or rectum (K62.6)
ulcerative colitis (K51.-)

CC **K63.4 Enteroptosis**

K63.5 Polyp of colon
Excludes1: *adenomatous polyp of colon (D12.-)*
inflammatory polyp of colon (K51.4-)
polyposis of colon (D12.6)
AHA CC: 2Q, 2015, 14; 1Q, 2017, 15-16; 1Q, 2019, 33

\+ **K63.8 Other specified diseases of intestine**

MCC **K63.81 Dieulafoy lesion of intestine**
Excludes2: *Dieulafoy lesion of stomach and duodenum (K31.82)*

K63.89 Other specified diseases of intestine

K63.9 Disease of intestine, unspecified

K64 Hemorrhoids and perianal venous thrombosis
Includes: piles
Excludes1: *hemorrhoids complicating childbirth and the puerperium (O87.2)*
hemorrhoids complicating pregnancy (O22.4)

K64.0 First degree hemorrhoids
Grade/stage I hemorrhoids
Hemorrhoids (bleeding) without prolapse outside of anal canal

K64.1 Second degree hemorrhoids
Grade/stage II hemorrhoids
Hemorrhoids (bleeding) that prolapse with straining, but retract spontaneously

K64.2 Third degree hemorrhoids
Grade/stage III hemorrhoids
Hemorrhoids (bleeding) that prolapse with straining and require manual replacement back inside anal canal

K64.3 Fourth degree hemorrhoids
Grade/stage IV hemorrhoids
Hemorrhoids (bleeding) with prolapsed tissue that cannot be manually replaced

K64.4 Residual hemorrhoidal skin tags
External hemorrhoids, NOS
Skin tags of anus

K64.5 Perianal venous thrombosis
External hemorrhoids with thrombosis
Perianal hematoma
Thrombosed hemorrhoids NOS

K64.8 Other hemorrhoids
Internal hemorrhoids, without mention of degree
Prolapsed hemorrhoids, degree not specified
AHA CC: 3Q, 2018, 22

K64.9 Unspecified hemorrhoids
Hemorrhoids (bleeding) NOS
Hemorrhoids (bleeding) without mention of degree

Diseases of peritoneum and retroperitoneum (K65-K68)

K65 Peritonitis
Use additional code (B95-B97), to identify infectious agent, if known
Code also if applicable diverticular disease of intestine (K57.-)
Excludes1: *acute appendicitis with generalized peritonitis (K35.2-)*
aseptic peritonitis (T81.6)
benign paroxysmal peritonitis (E85.0)
chemical peritonitis (T81.6)
gonococcal peritonitis (A54.85)
neonatal peritonitis (P78.0-P78.1)
pelvic peritonitis, female (N73.3-N73.5)
periodic familial peritonitis (E85.0)
peritonitis due to talc or other foreign substance (T81.6)
peritonitis in chlamydia (A74.81)
peritonitis in diphtheria (A36.89)
peritonitis in syphilis (late) (A52.74)
peritonitis in tuberculosis (A18.31)
peritonitis with or following abortion or ectopic or molar pregnancy (O00-O07, O08.0)
peritonitis with or following appendicitis (K35.-)
puerperal peritonitis (O85)
retroperitoneal infections (K68.-)

MCC **K65.0 Generalized (acute) peritonitis**
Pelvic peritonitis (acute), male
Subphrenic peritonitis (acute)
Suppurative peritonitis (acute)

MCC **K65.1 Peritoneal abscess**
Abdominopelvic abscess
Abscess (of) omentum
Abscess (of) peritoneum
Mesenteric abscess
Retrocecal abscess
Subdiaphragmatic abscess
Subhepatic abscess
Subphrenic abscess
AHA CC: 1Q, 2019, 15-16

MCC **K65.2 Spontaneous bacterial peritonitis**
Excludes1: *bacterial peritonitis NOS (K65.9)*

MCC **K65.3 Choleperitonitis**
Peritonitis due to bile

CC **K65.4 Sclerosing mesenteritis**
Fat necrosis of peritoneum
(Idiopathic) sclerosing mesenteric fibrosis
Mesenteric lipodystrophy
Mesenteric panniculitis
Retractile mesenteritis

MCC **K65.8 Other peritonitis**
Chronic proliferative peritonitis
Peritonitis due to urine

MCC **K65.9 Peritonitis, unspecified**
Bacterial peritonitis NOS
AHA CC: 2Q, 2013, 31

K66 Other disorders of peritoneum

Excludes2: *ascites (R18.-)*
peritoneal effusion (chronic) (R18.8)

K66.0 Peritoneal adhesions (postprocedural) (postinfection)
Adhesions (of) abdominal (wall)
Adhesions (of) diaphragm
Adhesions (of) intestine
Adhesions (of) male pelvis
Adhesions (of) omentum
Adhesions (of) stomach
Adhesive bands
Mesenteric adhesions
Excludes1: *female pelvic adhesions [bands] (N73.6)*
peritoneal adhesions with intestinal obstruction (K56.5-)

MCC **K66.1 Hemoperitoneum**
Excludes1: *traumatic hemoperitoneum (S36.8-)*

K66.8 Other specified disorders of peritoneum

K66.9 Disorder of peritoneum, unspecified

MCC **K67 Disorders of peritoneum in infectious diseases classified elsewhere**

Code first underlying disease, such as:
congenital syphilis (A50.0)
helminthiasis (B65.0-B83.9)

Excludes1: *peritonitis in chlamydia (A74.81)*
peritonitis in diphtheria (A36.89)
peritonitis in gonococcal (A54.85)
peritonitis in syphilis (late) (A52.74)
peritonitis in tuberculosis (A18.31)

Valid 3-character code, no further characters required

K68 Disorders of retroperitoneum

\+ **K68.1 Retroperitoneal abscess**

CC **K68.11 Postprocedural retroperitoneal abscess**
Excludes2: *infection following procedure (T81.4-)*
HAC see Appendix B for HAC conditional logic

MCC **K68.12 Psoas muscle abscess**

MCC **K68.19 Other retroperitoneal abscess**
AHA CC: 1Q, 2019, 15-16

MCC **K68.9 Other disorders of retroperitoneum**

Diseases of liver (K70-K77)

Excludes1: *jaundice NOS (R17)*

Excludes2: *hemochromatosis (E83.11-)*
Reye's syndrome (G93.7)
viral hepatitis (B15-B19)
Wilson's disease (E83.0)

K70 Alcoholic liver disease

Use additional code to identify:
alcohol abuse and dependence (F10.-)

• **K70.0 Alcoholic fatty liver**

\+ **K70.1 Alcoholic hepatitis**

• **K70.10 Alcoholic hepatitis without ascites**

• **K70.11 Alcoholic hepatitis with ascites**

• **K70.2 Alcoholic fibrosis and sclerosis of liver**

\+ **K70.3 Alcoholic cirrhosis of liver**
Alcoholic cirrhosis NOS

• **K70.30 Alcoholic cirrhosis of liver without ascites**

• **K70.31 Alcoholic cirrhosis of liver with ascites**

\+ **K70.4 Alcoholic hepatic failure**
Acute alcoholic hepatic failure
Alcoholic hepatic failure NOS
Chronic alcoholic hepatic failure
Subacute alcoholic hepatic failure

• **K70.40 Alcoholic hepatic failure without coma**

• MCC **K70.41 Alcoholic hepatic failure with coma**

• **K70.9 Alcoholic liver disease, unspecified**

K71 Toxic liver disease

Includes: drug-induced idiosyncratic (unpredictable) liver disease
drug-induced toxic (predictable) liver disease

Code first poisoning due to drug or toxin, if applicable (T36-T65 with fifth or sixth character 1-4 or 6)

Use additional code for adverse effect, if applicable, to identify drug (T36-T50 with fifth or sixth character 5)

Excludes2: *alcoholic liver disease (K70.-)*
Budd-Chiari syndrome (I82.0)

K71.0 Toxic liver disease with cholestasis
Cholestasis with hepatocyte injury
'Pure' cholestasis

\+ **K71.1 Toxic liver disease with hepatic necrosis**
Hepatic failure (acute) (chronic) due to drugs

K71.10 Toxic liver disease with hepatic necrosis, without coma

MCC **K71.11 Toxic liver disease with hepatic necrosis, with coma**

K71.2 Toxic liver disease with acute hepatitis

K71.3 Toxic liver disease with chronic persistent hepatitis

K71.4 Toxic liver disease with chronic lobular hepatitis

\+ **K71.5 Toxic liver disease with chronic active hepatitis**
Toxic liver disease with lupoid hepatitis

K71.50 Toxic liver disease with chronic active hepatitis without ascites

K71.51 Toxic liver disease with chronic active hepatitis with ascites

K71.6 Toxic liver disease with hepatitis, not elsewhere classified

K71.7 Toxic liver disease with fibrosis and cirrhosis of liver

K71.8 Toxic liver disease with other disorders of liver
Toxic liver disease with focal nodular hyperplasia
Toxic liver disease with hepatic granulomas
Toxic liver disease with peliosis hepatis
Toxic liver disease with veno-occlusive disease of liver

K71.9 Toxic liver disease, unspecified

K72 Hepatic failure, not elsewhere classified

Includes: fulminant hepatitis NEC, with hepatic failure
hepatic encephalopathy NOS
liver (cell) necrosis with hepatic failure
malignant hepatitis NEC, with hepatic failure
yellow liver atrophy or dystrophy

Excludes1: *alcoholic hepatic failure (K70.4)*
hepatic failure with toxic liver disease (K71.1-)
icterus of newborn (P55-P59)
postprocedural hepatic failure (K91.82)

Excludes2: *hepatic failure complicating abortion or ectopic or molar pregnancy (O00-O07, O08.8)*
hepatic failure complicating pregnancy, childbirth and the puerperium (O26.6-)
viral hepatitis with hepatic coma (B15-B19)

\+ **K72.0 Acute and subacute hepatic failure**
Acute non-viral hepatitis NOS
AHA CC: 2Q, 2014, 13

MCC **K72.00 Acute and subacute hepatic failure without coma**
AHA CC: 1Q, 2021, 13

MCC **K72.01 Acute and subacute hepatic failure with coma**

\+ **K72.1 Chronic hepatic failure**
End stage liver disease

K72.10 Chronic hepatic failure without coma
AHA CC: 1Q, 2017, 41; 1Q, 2021, 13

MCC **K72.11 Chronic hepatic failure with coma**

\+ **K72.9 Hepatic failure, unspecified**

K72.90 Hepatic failure, unspecified without coma
AHA CC: 2Q, 2016, 35; 4Q, 2018, 21

MCC **K72.91 Hepatic failure, unspecified with coma**
Hepatic coma NOS

K73 Chronic hepatitis, not elsewhere classified

Excludes1: *alcoholic hepatitis (chronic) (K70.1-)*
drug-induced hepatitis (chronic) (K71.-)
granulomatous hepatitis (chronic) NEC (K75.3)
reactive, nonspecific hepatitis (chronic) (K75.2)
viral hepatitis (chronic) (B15-B19)

K73.0 Chronic persistent hepatitis, not elsewhere classified

K73.1 Chronic lobular hepatitis, not elsewhere classified

K73.2 Chronic active hepatitis, not elsewhere classified

K73.8 Other chronic hepatitis, not elsewhere classified

K73.9 Chronic hepatitis, unspecified

Surfaces and Bed of Liver

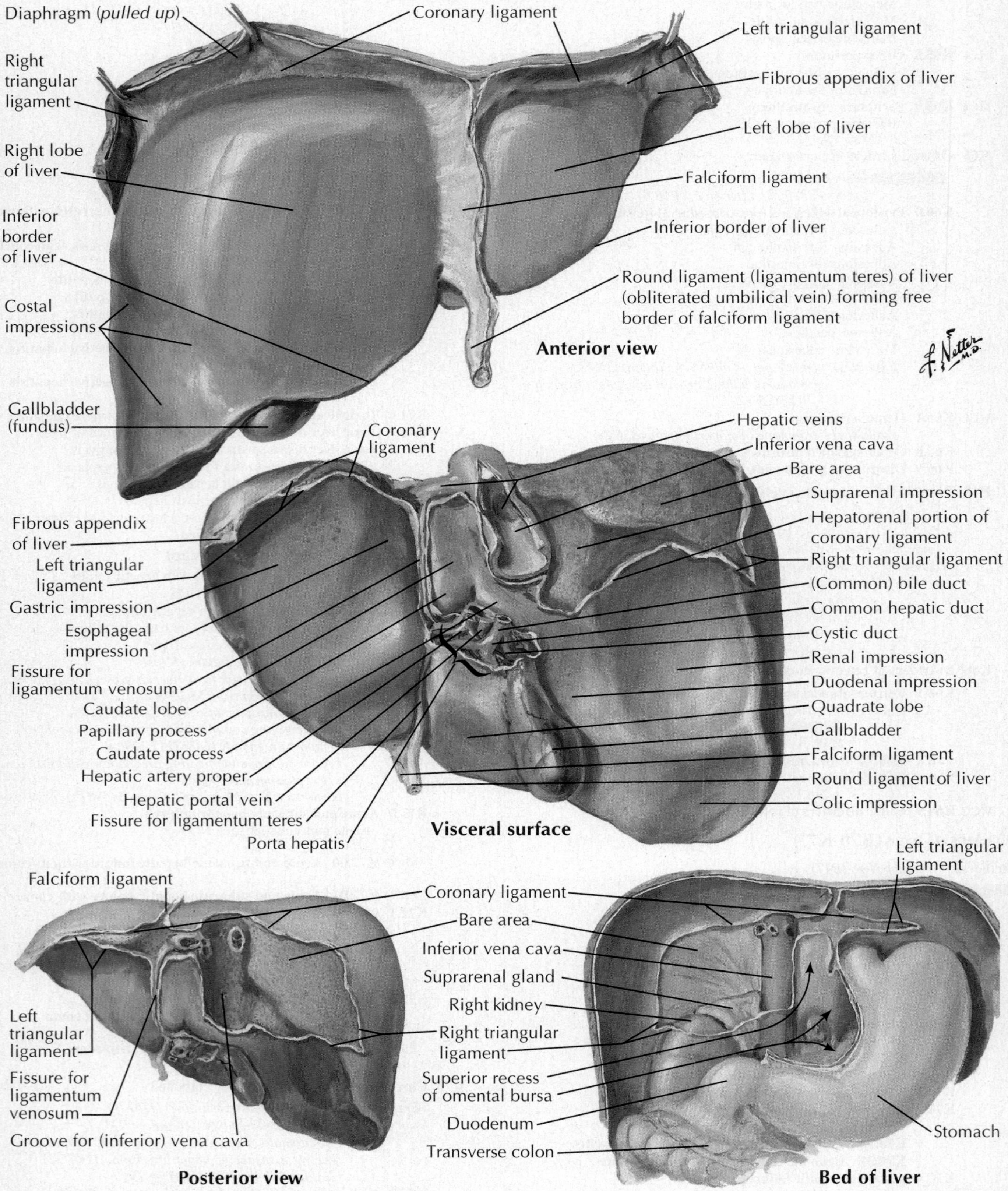

K74 Fibrosis and cirrhosis of liver

Code also, if applicable, viral hepatitis (acute) (chronic) (B15-B19)

Excludes1: *alcoholic cirrhosis (of liver) (K70.3)*
alcoholic fibrosis of liver (K70.2)
cardiac sclerosis of liver (K76.1)
cirrhosis (of liver) with toxic liver disease (K71.7)
congenital cirrhosis (of liver) (P78.81)
pigmentary cirrhosis (of liver) (E83.110)

\+ **K74.0 Hepatic fibrosis**
Code first underlying liver disease such as:
nonalcoholic steatohepatitis (NASH) (K57.81)
AHA CC: 4Q, 2020, 30-31

K74.00 Hepatic fibrosis, unspecified
K74.01 Hepatic fibrosis, early fibrosis
Hepatic fibrosis, stage F1 or stage F2
K74.02 Hepatic fibrosis, advanced fibrosis
Hepatic fibrosis, stage 3
Excludes1: *cirrhosis of liver (K74.6-)*
hepatic fibrosis, stage F4 (K74.6-)

K74.1 Hepatic sclerosis
K74.2 Hepatic fibrosis with hepatic sclerosis
K74.3 Primary biliary cirrhosis
Chronic nonsuppurative destructive cholangitis
Primary biliary cholangitis
Excludes2: *primary sclerosing cholangitis (K83.01)*
K74.4 Secondary biliary cirrhosis
K74.5 Biliary cirrhosis, unspecified
\+ **K74.6 Other and unspecified cirrhosis of liver**
K74.60 Unspecified cirrhosis of liver
Cirrhosis (of liver) NOS
AHA CC: 1Q, 2018, 4-5
K74.69 Other cirrhosis of liver
Cryptogenic cirrhosis (of liver)
Macronodular cirrhosis (of liver)
Micronodular cirrhosis (of liver)
Mixed type cirrhosis (of liver)
Portal cirrhosis (of liver)
Postnecrotic cirrhosis (of liver)

K75 Other inflammatory liver diseases

Excludes2: *toxic liver disease (K71.-)*

MCC **K75.0 Abscess of liver**
Cholangitic hepatic abscess
Hematogenic hepatic abscess
Hepatic abscess NOS
Lymphogenic hepatic abscess
Pylephlebitic hepatic abscess
Excludes1: *amebic liver abscess (A06.4)*
cholangitis without liver abscess (K83.09)
pylephlebitis without liver abscess (K75.1)
Excludes2: *acute or subacute hepatitis NOS (B17.9)*
acute or subacute non-viral hepatitis (K72.0)
chronic hepatitis NEC (K73.8)
MCC **K75.1 Phlebitis of portal vein**
Pylephlebitis
Excludes1: *pylephlebitic liver abscess (K75.0)*
K75.2 Nonspecific reactive hepatitis
Excludes1: *acute or subacute hepatitis (K72.0-)*
chronic hepatitis NEC (K73.-)
viral hepatitis (B15-B19)
K75.3 Granulomatous hepatitis, not elsewhere classified
Excludes1: *acute or subacute hepatitis (K72.0-)*
chronic hepatitis NEC (K73.-)
viral hepatitis (B15-B19)
K75.4 Autoimmune hepatitis
Lupoid hepatitis NEC
\+ **K75.8 Other specified inflammatory liver diseases**
K75.81 Nonalcoholic steatohepatitis (NASH)
Use additional code, if applicable, hepatic fibrosis (K74.0-)
K75.89 Other specified inflammatory liver diseases
K75.9 Inflammatory liver disease, unspecified
Hepatitis NOS
Excludes1: *acute or subacute hepatitis (K72.0-)*
chronic hepatitis NEC (K73.-)
viral hepatitis (B15-B19)

K76 Other diseases of liver

Excludes2: *alcoholic liver disease (K70.-)*
amyloid degeneration of liver (E85.-)
cystic disease of liver (congenital) (Q44.6)
hepatic vein thrombosis (I82.0)
hepatomegaly NOS (R16.0)
pigmentary cirrhosis (of liver) (E83.110)
portal vein thrombosis (I81)
toxic liver disease (K71.-)

K76.0 Fatty (change of) liver, not elsewhere classified
Nonalcoholic fatty liver disease (NAFLD)
Excludes1: *nonalcoholic steatohepatitis (NASH) (K75.81)*
K76.1 Chronic passive congestion of liver
Cardiac cirrhosis
Cardiac sclerosis
MCC **K76.2 Central hemorrhagic necrosis of liver**
Excludes1: *liver necrosis with hepatic failure (K72.-)*
MCC **K76.3 Infarction of liver**
K76.4 Peliosis hepatis
Hepatic angiomatosis
K76.5 Hepatic veno-occlusive disease
Excludes1: *Budd-Chiari syndrome (I82.0)*
CC **K76.6 Portal hypertension**
Use additional code for any associated complications, such as:
portal hypertensive gastropathy (K31.89)
AHA CC: 1Q, 2020, 15
MCC **K76.7 Hepatorenal syndrome**
Excludes1: *hepatorenal syndrome following labor and delivery (O90.4)*
postprocedural hepatorenal syndrome (K91.83)
\+ **K76.8 Other specified diseases of liver**
K76.81 Hepatopulmonary syndrome
Code first underlying liver disease, such as:
alcoholic cirrhosis of liver (K70.3-)
cirrhosis of liver without mention of alcohol (K74.6-)
K76.89 Other specified diseases of liver
Cyst (simple) of liver
Focal nodular hyperplasia of liver
Hepatoptosis
K76.9 Liver disease, unspecified

CC **K77 Liver disorders in diseases classified elsewhere**

Code first underlying disease, such as:
amyloidosis (E85.-)
congenital syphilis (A50.0, A50.5)
congenital toxoplasmosis (P37.1)
infectious mononucleosis with liver disease (B27.0-B27.9 with .9)
schistosomiasis (B65.0-B65.9)
Excludes1: *alcoholic hepatitis (K70.1-)*
alcoholic liver disease (K70.-)
cytomegaloviral hepatitis (B25.1)
herpesviral [herpes simplex] hepatitis (B00.81)
mumps hepatitis (B26.81)
sarcoidosis with liver disease (D86.89)
secondary syphilis with liver disease (A51.45)
syphilis (late) with liver disease (A52.74)
toxoplasmosis (acquired) hepatitis (B58.1)
tuberculosis with liver disease (A18.83)
Valid 3-character code, no further characters required

Disorders of gallbladder, biliary tract and pancreas (K80-K87)

K80 Cholelithiasis

Excludes1: *retained cholelithiasis following cholecystectomy (K91.86)*

\+ **K80.0 Calculus of gallbladder with acute cholecystitis**
Any condition listed in K80.2 with acute cholecystitis
Use additional code if applicable for associated gangrene of gallbladder (K82.A1), or perforation of gallbladder (K82.A2)
CC **K80.00 Calculus of gallbladder with acute cholecystitis without obstruction**
AHA CC: 4Q, 2018, 20
CC **K80.01 Calculus of gallbladder with acute cholecystitis with obstruction**

Cholelithiasis (Gallstones)

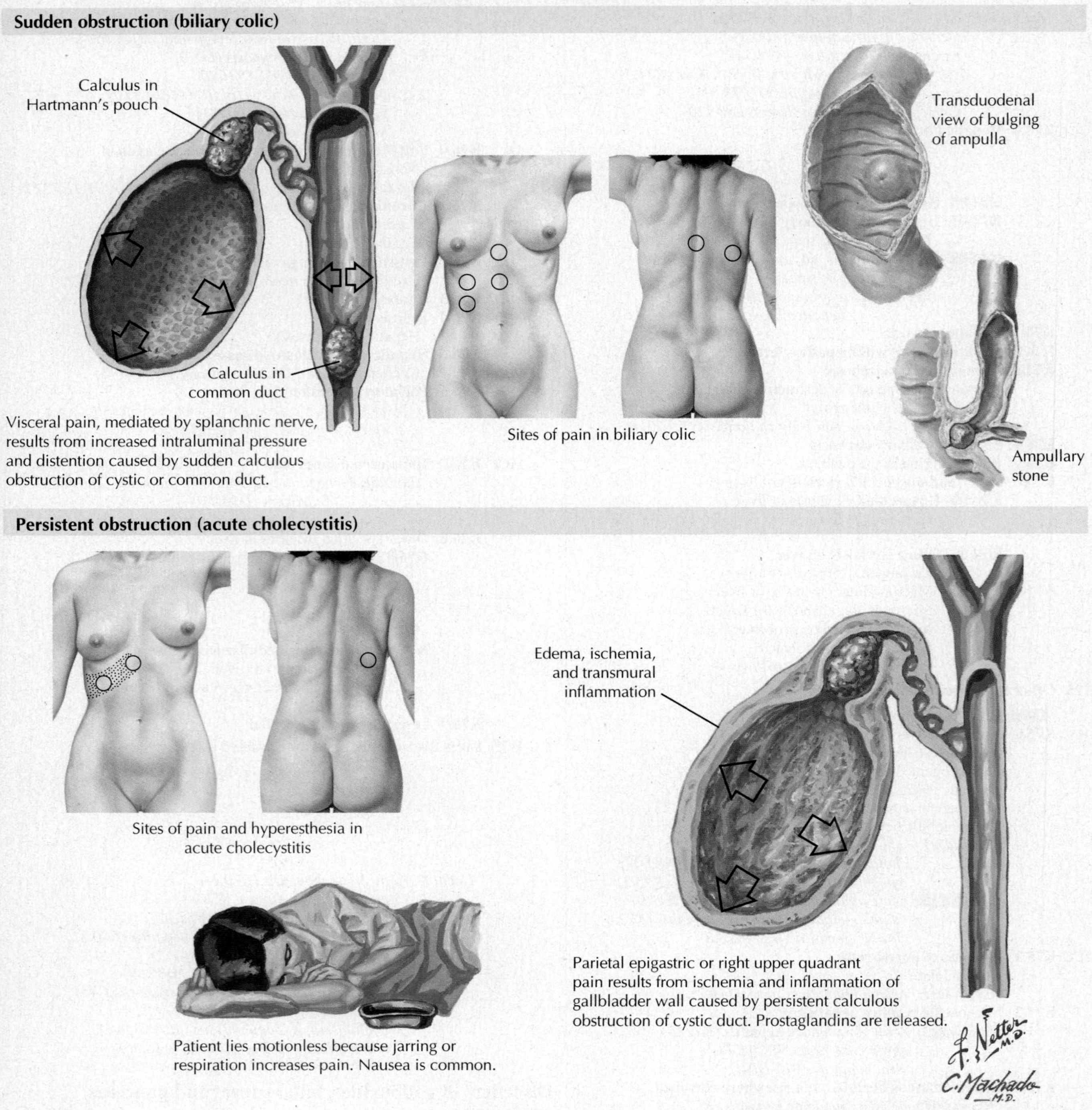

+ **K80.1 Calculus of gallbladder with other cholecystitis**
  Use additional code if applicable for associated gangrene of gallbladder (K82.A1), or perforation of gallbladder (K82.A2)
  - CC **K80.10 Calculus of gallbladder with chronic cholecystitis without obstruction**
    Cholelithiasis with cholecystitis NOS
  - CC **K80.11 Calculus of gallbladder with chronic cholecystitis with obstruction**
  - CC **K80.12 Calculus of gallbladder with acute and chronic cholecystitis without obstruction**
  - CC **K80.13 Calculus of gallbladder with acute and chronic cholecystitis with obstruction**
  - CC **K80.18 Calculus of gallbladder with other cholecystitis without obstruction**
  - CC **K80.19 Calculus of gallbladder with other cholecystitis with obstruction**

+ **K80.2 Calculus of gallbladder without cholecystitis**
  Cholecystolithiasis without cholecystitis
  Cholelithiasis (without cholecystitis)
  Colic (recurrent) of gallbladder (without cholecystitis)
  Gallstone (impacted) of cystic duct (without cholecystitis)
  Gallstone (impacted) of gallbladder (without cholecystitis)
  - **K80.20 Calculus of gallbladder without cholecystitis without obstruction**
  - CC **K80.21 Calculus of gallbladder without cholecystitis with obstruction**

+ **K80.3 Calculus of bile duct with cholangitis**
  Any condition listed in K80.5 with cholangitis
  - CC **K80.30 Calculus of bile duct with cholangitis, unspecified, without obstruction**
  - CC **K80.31 Calculus of bile duct with cholangitis, unspecified, with obstruction**
  - CC **K80.32 Calculus of bile duct with acute cholangitis without obstruction**

CC **K80.33 Calculus of bile duct with acute cholangitis with obstruction**

CC **K80.34 Calculus of bile duct with chronic cholangitis without obstruction**

CC **K80.35 Calculus of bile duct with chronic cholangitis with obstruction**

CC **K80.36 Calculus of bile duct with acute and chronic cholangitis without obstruction**

CC **K80.37 Calculus of bile duct with acute and chronic cholangitis with obstruction**

+ **K80.4 Calculus of bile duct with cholecystitis**

Any condition listed in K80.5 with cholecystitis (with cholangitis)

Code also fistula of bile duct (K83.3)

Use additional code if applicable for associated gangrene of gallbladder (K82.A1), or perforation of gallbladder (K82.A2)

CC **K80.40 Calculus of bile duct with cholecystitis, unspecified, without obstruction**

CC **K80.41 Calculus of bile duct with cholecystitis, unspecified, with obstruction**

AHA CC: 1Q, 2019, 17-18

CC **K80.42 Calculus of bile duct with acute cholecystitis without obstruction**

CC **K80.43 Calculus of bile duct with acute cholecystitis with obstruction**

CC **K80.44 Calculus of bile duct with chronic cholecystitis without obstruction**

CC **K80.45 Calculus of bile duct with chronic cholecystitis with obstruction**

CC **K80.46 Calculus of bile duct with acute and chronic cholecystitis without obstruction**

CC **K80.47 Calculus of bile duct with acute and chronic cholecystitis with obstruction**

+ **K80.5 Calculus of bile duct without cholangitis or cholecystitis**

Choledocholithiasis (without cholangitis or cholecystitis)

Gallstone (impacted) of bile duct NOS (without cholangitis or cholecystitis)

Gallstone (impacted) of common duct (without cholangitis or cholecystitis)

Gallstone (impacted) of hepatic duct (without cholangitis or cholecystitis)

Hepatic cholelithiasis (without cholangitis or cholecystitis)

Hepatic colic (recurrent) (without cholangitis or cholecystitis)

K80.50 Calculus of bile duct without cholangitis or cholecystitis without obstruction

CC **K80.51 Calculus of bile duct without cholangitis or cholecystitis with obstruction**

+ **K80.6 Calculus of gallbladder and bile duct with cholecystitis**

Use additional code if applicable for associated gangrene of gallbladder (K82.A1), or perforation of gallbladder (K82.A2)

CC **K80.60 Calculus of gallbladder and bile duct with cholecystitis, unspecified, without obstruction**

CC **K80.61 Calculus of gallbladder and bile duct with cholecystitis, unspecified, with obstruction**

CC **K80.62 Calculus of gallbladder and bile duct with acute cholecystitis without obstruction**

CC **K80.63 Calculus of gallbladder and bile duct with acute cholecystitis with obstruction**

CC **K80.64 Calculus of gallbladder and bile duct with chronic cholecystitis without obstruction**

CC **K80.65 Calculus of gallbladder and bile duct with chronic cholecystitis with obstruction**

CC **K80.66 Calculus of gallbladder and bile duct with acute and chronic cholecystitis without obstruction**

MCC **K80.67 Calculus of gallbladder and bile duct with acute and chronic cholecystitis with obstruction**

+ **K80.7 Calculus of gallbladder and bile duct without cholecystitis**

K80.70 Calculus of gallbladder and bile duct without cholecystitis without obstruction

CC **K80.71 Calculus of gallbladder and bile duct without cholecystitis with obstruction**

+ **K80.8 Other cholelithiasis**

K80.80 Other cholelithiasis without obstruction

CC **K80.81 Other cholelithiasis with obstruction**

K81 Cholecystitis

Excludes1: *cholecystitis with cholelithiasis (K80.-)*

Use additional code if applicable for associated gangrene of gallbladder (K82.A1), or perforation of gallbladder (K82.A2)

K81.0 Acute cholecystitis

Abscess of gallbladder

Angiocholecystitis

Emphysematous (acute) cholecystitis

Empyema of gallbladder

Gangrene of gallbladder

Gangrenous cholecystitis

Suppurative cholecystitis

K81.1 Chronic cholecystitis

CC **K81.2 Acute cholecystitis with chronic cholecystitis**

K81.9 Cholecystitis, unspecified

K82 Other diseases of gallbladder

Excludes1: *nonvisualization of gallbladder (R93.2)*
postcholecystectomy syndrome (K91.5)

CC **K82.0 Obstruction of gallbladder**

Occlusion of cystic duct or gallbladder without cholelithiasis

Stenosis of cystic duct or gallbladder without cholelithiasis

Stricture of cystic duct or gallbladder without cholelithiasis

Excludes1: *obstruction of gallbladder with cholelithiasis (K80.-)*

CC **K82.1 Hydrops of gallbladder**

Mucocele of gallbladder

MCC **K82.2 Perforation of gallbladder**

Rupture of cystic duct or gallbladder

Exlcudes1: *Perforation of gallbladder in cholecystitis (K82.A2)*

CC **K82.3 Fistula of gallbladder**

Cholecystocolic fistula

Cholecystoduodenal fistula

K82.4 Cholesterolosis of gallbladder

Strawberry gallbladder

Excludes1: *cholesterolosis of gallbladder with cholecystitis (K81.-)*
cholesterolosis of gallbladder with cholelithiasis (K80.-)

K82.8 Other specified diseases of gallbladder

Adhesions of cystic duct or gallbladder

Atrophy of cystic duct or gallbladder

Cyst of cystic duct or gallbladder

Dyskinesia of cystic duct or gallbladder

Hypertrophy of cystic duct or gallbladder

Nonfunctioning of cystic duct or gallbladder

Ulcer of cystic duct or gallbladder

K82.9 Disease of gallbladder, unspecified

+ **K82.A Disorders of gallbladder in diseases classified elsewhere**

Code first the type of cholecystitis (K81.-), or cholelithiasis with cholecystitis (K80.00-K80.19, K80.40-K80.47, K80.60-K80.67)

K82.A1 Gangrene of gallbladder in cholecystitis

AHA CC: 4Q, 2018, 19-20

CC **K82.A2 Perforation of gallbladder in cholecystitis**

AHA CC: 4Q, 2018, 19-20

K83 Other diseases of biliary tract

Excludes1: *postcholecystectomy syndrome (K91.5)*

Excludes2: *conditions involving the gallbladder (K81-K82)*
conditions involving the cystic duct (K81-K82)

+ **K83.0 Cholangitis**

Excludes1: *cholangitic liver abscess (K75.0)*
cholangitis with choledocholithiasis (K80.3-, K80.4-)

Excludes2: *chronic nonsuppurative destructive cholangitis (K74.3)*
primary biliary cholangitis (K74.3)
primary biliary cirrhosis (K74.3)

AHA CC: 4Q, 2018, 20

CC **K83.01 Primary sclerosing cholangitis**

AHA CC: 4Q, 2018, 21

CC **K83.09 Other cholangitis**

Ascending cholangitis

Cholangitis NOS

Primary cholangitis

Recurrent cholangitis

Sclerosing cholangitis

Secondary cholangitis

Stenosing cholangitis

Suppurative cholangitis

Acute Pancreatitis

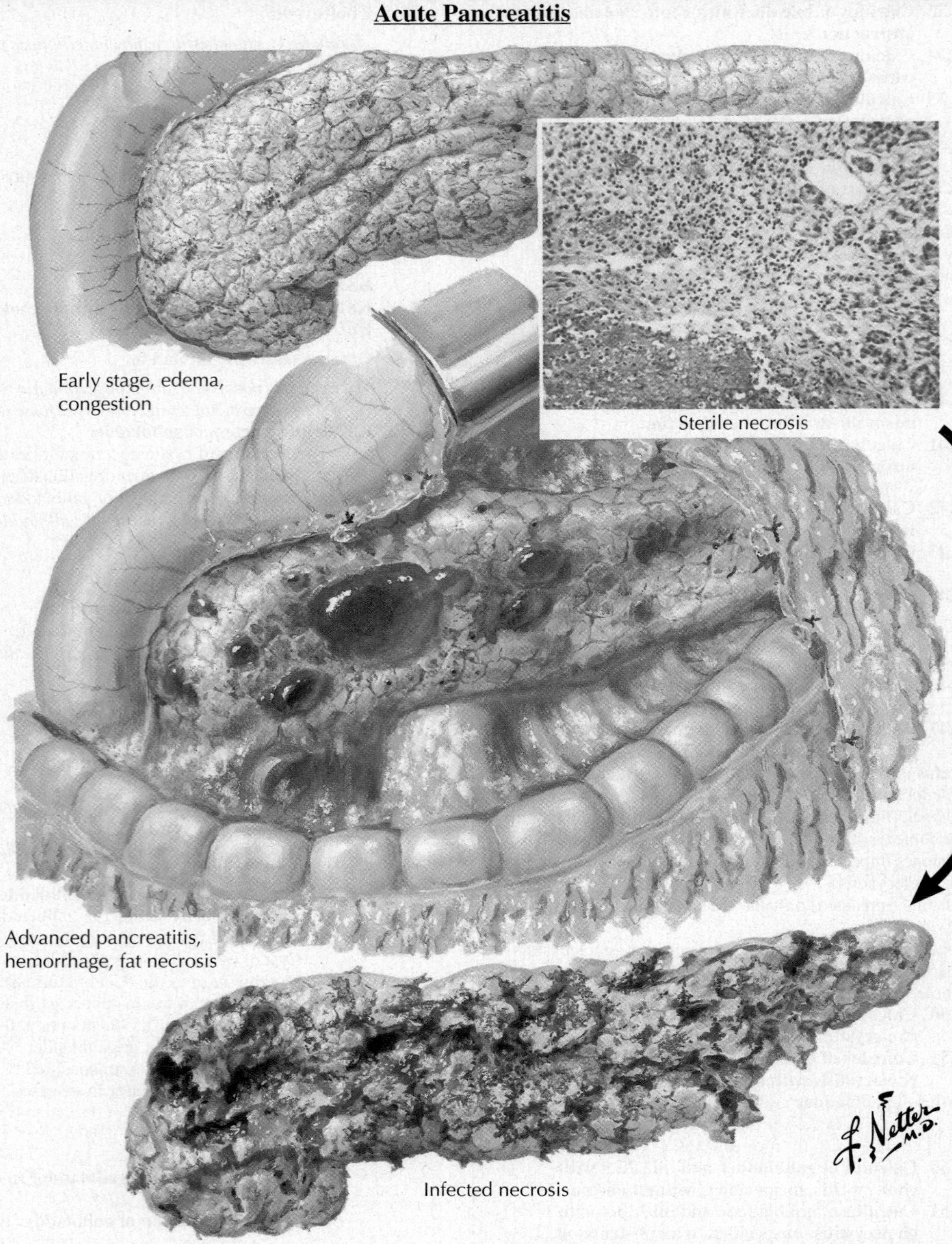

MCC **K83.1 Obstruction of bile duct**
Occlusion of bile duct without cholelithiasis
Stenosis of bile duct without cholelithiasis
Stricture of bile duct without cholelithiasis
Excludes1: *congenital obstruction of bile duct (Q44.3)*
obstruction of bile duct with cholelithiasis (K80.-)
CC AHA: 1Q, 2016, 18-19

MCC **K83.2 Perforation of bile duct**
Rupture of bile duct

CC **K83.3 Fistula of bile duct**
Choledochoduodenal fistula
AHA CC: 1Q, 2019, 17-18

K83.4 Spasm of sphincter of Oddi

K83.5 Biliary cyst

K83.8 Other specified diseases of biliary tract
Adhesions of biliary tract
Atrophy of biliary tract
Hypertrophy of biliary tract
Ulcer of biliary tract

K83.9 Disease of biliary tract, unspecified

K85 Acute pancreatitis
Includes: acute (recurrent) pancreatitis
subacute pancreatitis
AHA CC: 4Q, 2016, 34

\+ **K85.0 Idiopathic acute pancreatitis**
MCC **K85.00 Idiopathic acute pancreatitis without necrosis or infection**
MCC **K85.01 Idiopathic acute pancreatitis with uninfected necrosis**
MCC **K85.02 Idiopathic acute pancreatitis with infected necrosis**

\+ **K85.1 Biliary acute pancreatitis**
Gallstone pancreatitis
MCC **K85.10 Biliary acute pancreatitis without necrosis or infection**
MCC **K85.11 Biliary acute pancreatitis with uninfected necrosis**
MCC **K85.12 Biliary acute pancreatitis with infected necrosis**

+ **K85.2 Alcohol induced acute pancreatitis**
Excludes2: alcohol induced chronic pancreatitis (K86.0)
MCC **K85.20 Alcohol induced acute pancreatitis without necrosis or infection**
AHA CC: 1Q, 2020, 9
MCC **K85.21 Alcohol induced acute pancreatitis with uninfected necrosis**
MCC **K85.22 Alcohol induced acute pancreatitis with infected necrosis**
+ **K85.3 Drug induced acute pancreatitis**
Use additional code for adverse effect, if applicable, to identify drug (T36-T50 with fifth or sixth character 5)

Use additional code to identify drug abuse and dependence (F11.-F17.-)
MCC **K85.30 Drug induced acute pancreatitis without necrosis or infection**
MCC **K85.31 Drug induced acute pancreatitis with uninfected necrosis**
MCC **K85.32 Drug induced acute pancreatitis with infected necrosis**
+ **K85.8 Other acute pancreatitis**
MCC **K85.80 Other acute pancreatitis without necrosis or infection**
MCC **K85.81 Other acute pancreatitis with uninfected necrosis**
MCC **K85.82 Other acute pancreatitis with infected necrosis**
+ **K85.9 Acute pancreatitis, unspecified**
Pancreatitis NOS
MCC **K85.90 Acute pancreatitis without necrosis or infection, unspecified**
MCC **K85.91 Acute pancreatitis with uninfected necrosis, unspecified**
MCC **K85.92 Acute pancreatitis with infected necrosis, unspecified**

K86 Other diseases of pancreas
Excludes2: fibrocystic disease of pancreas (E84.-)
islet cell tumor (of pancreas) (D13.7)
pancreatic steatorrhea (K90.3)
CC **K86.0 Alcohol-induced chronic pancreatitis**
Use additional code to identify:
alcohol abuse and dependence (F10.-)

Code also exocrine pancreatic insufficiency (K86.81)
Excludes2: alcohol induced acute pancreatitis (K85.2-)
CC **K86.1 Other chronic pancreatitis**
Chronic pancreatitis NOS
Infectious chronic pancreatitis
Recurrent chronic pancreatitis
Relapsing chronic pancreatitis
Code also exocrine pancreatic insufficiency (K86.81)
CC **K86.2 Cyst of pancreas**
CC **K86.3 Pseudocyst of pancreas**
+ **K86.8 Other specified diseases of pancreas**
AHA CC: 4Q, 2016, 33
K86.81 Exocrine pancreatic insufficiency
K86.89 Other specified diseases of pancreas
Aseptic pancreatic necrosis, unrelated to acute pancreatitis
Atrophy of pancreas
Calculus of pancreas
Cirrhosis of pancreas
Fibrosis of pancreas
Pancreatic fat necrosis, unrelated to acute pancreatitis
Pancreatic infantilism
Pancreatic necrosis NOS, unrelated to acute pancreatitis
K86.9 Disease of pancreas, unspecified

K87 Disorders of gallbladder, biliary tract and pancreas in diseases classified elsewhere
Code first underlying disease
Excludes1: cytomegaloviral pancreatitis (B25.2)
mumps pancreatitis (B26.3)
syphilitic gallbladder (A52.74)
syphilitic pancreas (A52.74)
tuberculosis of gallbladder (A18.83)
tuberculosis of pancreas (A18.83)
Valid 3-character code, no further characters required

Other diseases of the digestive system (K90-K95)

K90 Intestinal malabsorption
Excludes1: intestinal malabsorption following gastrointestinal surgery (K91.2)
K90.0 Celiac disease
Celiac disease with steatorrhea
Celiac gluten-sensitive enteropathy
Nontropical sprue
Code also exocrine pancreatic insufficiency (K86.81)

Use additional code for associated disorders including:
dermatitis herpetiformis (L13.0)
gluten ataxia (G32.81)
CC **K90.1 Tropical sprue**
Sprue NOS
Tropical steatorrhea
CC **K90.2 Blind loop syndrome, not elsewhere classified**
Blind loop syndrome NOS
Excludes1: congenital blind loop syndrome (Q43.8)
postsurgical blind loop syndrome (K91.2)
CC **K90.3 Pancreatic steatorrhea**
+ **K90.4 Other malabsorption due to intolerance**
Excludes2: celiac gluten-sensitive enteropathy (K90.0)
lactose intolerance (E73.-)
CC **K90.41 Non-celiac gluten sensitivity**
Gluten sensitivity NOS
Non-celiac gluten sensitive enteropathy
AHA CC: 4Q, 2016, 35-36
CC **K90.49 Malabsorption due to intolerance, not elsewhere classified**
Malabsorption due to intolerance to carbohydrate
Malabsorption due to intolerance to fat
Malabsorption due to intolerance to protein
Malabsorption due to intolerance to starch
+ **K90.8 Other intestinal malabsorption**
CC **K90.81 Whipple's disease**
CC **K90.89 Other intestinal malabsorption**
CC **K90.9 Intestinal malabsorption, unspecified**
AHA CC: 4Q, 2017, 108-109

K91 Intraoperative and postprocedural complications and disorders of digestive system, not elsewhere classified
Excludes2: complications of artificial opening of digestive system (K94.-)
complications of bariatric procedures (K95.-)
gastrojejunal ulcer (K28.-)
postprocedural (radiation) retroperitoneal abscess (K68.11)
radiation colitis (K52.0)
radiation gastroenteritis (K52.0)
radiation proctitis (K62.7)
AHA CC: 4Q, 2016, 9-10
K91.0 Vomiting following gastrointestinal surgery
K91.1 Postgastric surgery syndromes
Dumping syndrome
Postgastrectomy syndrome
Postvagotomy syndrome
CC **K91.2 Postsurgical malabsorption, not elsewhere classified**
Postsurgical blind loop syndrome
Excludes1: malabsorption osteomalacia in adults (M83.2)
malabsorption osteoporosis, postsurgical (M80.8-, M81.8)
+ **K91.3 Postprocedural intestinal obstruction**
AHA CC: 4Q, 2017, 16-17
CC **K91.30 Postprocedural intestinal obstruction, unspecified as to partial versus complete**
Postprocedural intestinal obstruction NOS
CC **K91.31 Postprocedural partial intestinal obstruction**
Postprocedural incomplete intestinal obstruction
CC **K91.32 Postprocedural complete intestinal obstruction**
K91.5 Postcholecystectomy syndrome

+ **K91.6 Intraoperative hemorrhage and hematoma of a digestive system organ or structure complicating a procedure**
  Excludes1: *intraoperative hemorrhage and hematoma of a digestive system organ or structure due to accidental puncture and laceration during a procedure (K91.7-)*
  - CC **K91.61 Intraoperative hemorrhage and hematoma of a digestive system organ or structure complicating a digestive sytem procedure**
    AHA CC: 1Q, 2020, 19-20
  - CC **K91.62 Intraoperative hemorrhage and hematoma of a digestive system organ or structure complicating other procedure**

+ **K91.7 Accidental puncture and laceration of a digestive system organ or structure during a procedure**
  - CC **K91.71 Accidental puncture and laceration of a digestive system organ or structure during a digestive system procedure**
    AHA CC: 2Q, 2021, 11-12
  - CC **K91.72 Accidental puncture and laceration of a digestive system organ or structure during other procedure**
    AHA CC: 2Q, 2019, 23-24

+ **K91.8 Other intraoperative and postprocedural complications and disorders of digestive system**
  - CC **K91.81 Other intraoperative complications of digestive system**
  - CC **K91.82 Postprocedural hepatic failure**
  - CC **K91.83 Postprocedural hepatorenal syndrome**
  - + **K91.84 Postprocedural hemorrhage of a digestive system organ or structure following a procedure**
    - CC **K91.840 Postprocedural hemorrhage of a digestive system organ or structure following a digestive system procedure**
      AHA CC: 1Q, 2016, 15
    - CC **K91.841 Postprocedural hemorrhage of a digestive system organ or structure following other procedure**
  - + **K91.85 Complications of intestinal pouch**
    - CC **K91.850 Pouchitis**
      Inflammation of internal ileoanal pouch
    - CC **K91.858 Other complications of intestinal pouch**
      AHA CC: 2Q, 2019, 13
  - CC **K91.86 Retained cholelithiasis following cholecystectomy**
  - + **K91.87 Postprocedural hematoma and seroma of a digestive system organ or structure following a procedure**
    - CC **K91.870 Postprocedural hematoma of a digestive system organ or structure following a digestive system procedure**
    - CC **K91.871 Postprocedural hematoma of a digestive system organ or structure following other procedure**
    - CC **K91.872 Postprocedural seroma of a digestive system organ or structure following a digestive system procedure**
    - CC **K91.873 Postprocedural seroma of a digestive system organ or structure following other procedure**
  - CC **K91.89 Other postprocedural complications and disorders of digestive system**
    Use additional code, if applicable, to further specify disorder
    Excludes2: *postprocedural retroperitoneal abscess (K68.11)*
    AHA CC: 1Q, 2017, 40-41; 2Q, 2020, 22-23

K92 Other diseases of digestive system

Excludes1: *neonatal gastrointestinal hemorrhage (P54.0-P54.3)*

- CC **K92.0 Hematemesis**
- CC **K92.1 Melena**
  Excludes1: *occult blood in feces (R19.5)*
- CC **K92.2 Gastrointestinal hemorrhage, unspecified**
  Gastric hemorrhage NOS
  Intestinal hemorrhage NOS
  Excludes1: *acute hemorrhagic gastritis (K29.01)*
  hemorrhage of anus and rectum (K62.5)
  angiodysplasia of stomach with hemorrhage (K31.811)
  diverticular disease with hemorrhage (K57.-)
  gastritis and duodenitis with hemorrhage (K29.-)
  peptic ulcer with hemorrhage (K25-K28)
  AHA CC: 1Q, 2021, 11-12
- + **K92.8 Other specified diseases of the digestive system**
  - CC **K92.81 Gastrointestinal mucositis (ulcerative)**
    Code also type of associated therapy, such as:
    antineoplastic and immunosuppressive drugs (T45.1X-)
    radiological procedure and radiotherapy (Y84.2)
    Excludes2: *mucositis (ulcerative) of vagina and vulva (N76.81)*
    nasal mucositis (ulcerative) (J34.81)
    oral mucositis (ulcerative) (K12.3-)
  - **K92.89 Other specified diseases of the digestive system**
- **K92.9 Disease of digestive system, unspecified**

K94 Complications of artificial openings of the digestive system

+ **K94.0 Colostomy complications**
  - **K94.00 Colostomy complication, unspecified**
  - CC **K94.01 Colostomy hemorrhage**
  - CC **K94.02 Colostomy infection**
    Use additional code to specify type of infection, such as:
    cellulitis of abdominal wall (L03.311)
    sepsis (A40.-, A41.-)
  - CC **K94.03 Colostomy malfunction**
    Mechanical complication of colostomy
  - **K94.09 Other complications of colostomy**
+ **K94.1 Enterostomy complications**
  - **K94.10 Enterostomy complication, unspecified**
  - CC **K94.11 Enterostomy hemorrhage**
  - CC **K94.12 Enterostomy infection**
    Use additional code to specify type of infection, such as:
    cellulitis of abdominal wall (L03.311)
    sepsis (A40.-, A41.-)
  - CC **K94.13 Enterostomy malfunction**
    Mechanical complication of enterostomy
  - CC **K94.19 Other complications of enterostomy**
+ **K94.2 Gastrostomy complications**
  - **K94.20 Gastrostomy complication, unspecified**
  - **K94.21 Gastrostomy hemorrhage**
  - CC **K94.22 Gastrostomy infection**
    Use additional code to specify type of infection, such as:
    cellulitis of abdominal wall (L03.311)
    sepsis (A40.-, A41.-)
  - CC **K94.23 Gastrostomy malfunction**
    Mechanical complication of gastrostomy
    AHA CC: 1Q, 2019, 26
  - **K94.29 Other complications of gastrostomy**
+ **K94.3 Esophagostomy complications**
  - CC **K94.30 Esophagostomy complications, unspecified**
  - CC **K94.31 Esophagostomy hemorrhage**
  - CC **K94.32 Esophagostomy infection**
    Use additional code to identify the infection
  - CC **K94.33 Esophagostomy malfunction**
    Mechanical complication of esophagostomy
  - CC **K94.39 Other complications of esophagostomy**

+ K95 Complications of bariatric procedures

+ **K95.0 Complications of gastric band procedure**
  - CC **K95.01 Infection due to gastric band procedure**
    Use additional code to specify type of infection or organism, such as:
    bacterial and viral infectious agents (B95.-, B96.-)
    cellulitis of abdominal wall (L03.311)
    sepsis (A40.-, A41.-)
    HAC see Appendix B for HAC conditional logic
  - CC **K95.09 Other complications of gastric band procedure**
    Use additional code, if applicable, to further specify complication
+ **K95.8 Complications of other bariatric procedure**
  Excludes1: *complications of gastric band surgery (K95.0-)*
  - CC **K95.81 Infection due to other bariatric procedure**
    Use additional code to specify type of infection or organism, such as:
    bacterial and viral infectious agents (B95.-, B96.-)
    cellulitis of abdominal wall (L03.311)
    sepsis (A40.-, A41.-)
    HAC see Appendix B for HAC conditional logic
  - CC **K95.89 Other complications of other bariatric procedure**
    Use additional code, if applicable, to further specify complication

Chapter 12: Diseases of the Skin and Subcutaneous Tissue (L00-L99)

Excludes2: certain conditions originating in the perinatal period (P04-P96)
certain infectious and parasitic diseases (A00-B99)
complications of pregnancy, childbirth and the puerperium (O00-O9A)
congenital malformations, deformations, and chromosomal abnormalities (Q00-Q99)
endocrine, nutritional and metabolic diseases (E00-E88)
lipomelanotic reticulosis (I89.8)
neoplasms (C00-D49)
symptoms, signs and abnormal clinical and laboratory findings, not elsewhere classified (R00-R94)
systemic connective tissue disorders (M30-M36)
viral warts (B07.-)

This chapter contains the following category blocks:

L00-L08	Infections of the skin and subcutaneous tissue
L10-L14	Bullous disorders
L20-L30	Dermatitis and eczema
L40-L45	Papulosquamous disorders
L49-L54	Urticaria and erythema
L55-L59	Radiation-related disorders of the skin and subcutaneous tissue
L60-L75	Disorders of skin appendages
L76	Intraoperative and postprocedural complications of skin and subcutaneous tissue
L80-L99	Other disorders of the skin and subcutaneous tissue

C. Chapter-Specific Coding Guidelines

In addition to general coding guidelines, there are guidelines for specific diagnoses and/or conditions in the classification. Unless otherwise indicated, these guidelines apply to all health care settings. Please refer to Section II for guidelines on the selection of principal diagnosis.

12. Chapter 12: Diseases of the Skin and Subcutaneous Tissue (L00-L99)

a. Pressure ulcer stage codes

1) Pressure ulcer stages

Codes in category L89, Pressure ulcer, identify the site and stage of the pressure ulcer.

The ICD-10-CM classifies pressure ulcer stages based on severity, which is designated by stages 1-4 deep tissue pressure injury, unspecified stage and unstageable.

Assign as many codes from category L89 as needed to identify all the pressure ulcers the patient has, if applicable.

See Section I.B.14 for pressure ulcer stage documentation by clinicians other than patient's provider.

2) Unstageable pressure ulcers

Assignment of the code for unstageable pressure ulcer (L89.--0) should be based on the clinical documentation. These codes are used for pressure ulcers whose stage cannot be clinically determined (e.g., the ulcer is covered by eschar or has been treated with a skin or muscle graft) and pressure ulcers that are documented as deep tissue injury but not documented as due to trauma. This code should not be confused with the codes for unspecified stage (L89.--9). When there is no documentation regarding the stage of the pressure ulcer, assign the appropriate code for unspecified stage (L89.--9).

If during an encounter, the stage of an unstageable pressure ulcer is revealed after debridement, assign only the code for the stage revealed following debridement.

3) Documented pressure ulcer stage

Assignment of the pressure ulcer stage code should be guided by clinical documentation of the stage or documentation of the terms found in the Alphabetic Index. For clinical terms describing the stage that are not found in the Alphabetic Index, and there is no documentation of the stage, the provider should be queried.

4) Patients admitted with pressure ulcers documented as healed

No code is assigned if the documentation states that the pressure ulcer is completely healed at the time of admission.

5) Patients admitted with pressure ulcers documented as healing

Pressure ulcers described as healing should be assigned the appropriate pressure ulcer stage code based on the documentation in the medical record. If the documentation does not provide information about the stage of the healing pressure ulcer, assign the appropriate code for unspecified stage.

If the documentation is unclear as to whether the patient has a current (new) pressure ulcer or if the patient is being treated for a healing pressure ulcer, query the provider.

For ulcers that were present on admission but healed at the time of discharge, assign the code for the site and stage of the pressure ulcer at the time of admission.

6) Patient admitted with pressure ulcer evolving into another stage during the admission

If a patient is admitted to an inpatient hospital with a pressure ulcer at one stage and it progresses to a higher stage, two separate codes should be assigned: one code for the site and stage of the ulcer on admission and a second code for the same ulcer site and the highest stage reported during the stay.

7) Pressure-induced deep tissue damage

For pressure-induced deep tissue damage or deep tissue pressure injury, assign only the appropriate code for pressure-induced deep tissue damage (L89.--6).

b. Non-Pressure Chronic Ulcers

1) Patients admitted with non-pressure ulcers documented as healed

No code is assigned if the documentation states that the non-pressure ulcer is completely healed at the time of admission.

2) Patients admitted with non-pressure ulcers documented as healing

Non-pressure ulcers described as healing should be assigned the appropriate non-pressure ulcer code based on the documentation in the medical record. If the documentation does not provide information about the severity of the healing non-pressure ulcer, assign the appropriate code unspecified severity.

If the documentation is unclear as to whether the patient has a current (new) non-pressure ulcer or if the patient is being treated for a healing non-pressure ulcer, query the provider.

For ulcers that were present on admission but healed at the time of discharge, assign the code for the site and severity of the non-pressure ulcer at the time of admission.

3) Patient admitted with non-pressure ulcer that progresses to another severity level during the admission

If a patient is admitted to an inpatient hospital with a non-pressure ulcer at one severity level and it progresses to a higher severity level, two separate codes should be assigned; one code for the site and severity level of the ulcer on admission and a second code for the same ulcer site and the highest severity level reported during the stay.

See Section I.B.14 for pressure ulcer stage documentation by clinicians other than patient's provider.

Infections of the skin and subcutaneous tissue (L00-L08)

Use additional code (B95-B97) to identify infectious agent

Excludes2: *hordeolum (H00.0)*
infective dermatitis (L30.3)
local infections of skin classified in Chapter 1
lupus panniculitis (L93.2)
panniculitis NOS (M79.3)
panniculitis of neck and back (M54.0-)
Perlèche NOS (K13.0)
Perlèche due to candidiasis (B37.0)
Perlèche due to riboflavin deficiency (E53.0)
pyogenic granuloma (L98.0)
relapsing panniculitis [Weber-Christian] (M35.6)
viral warts (B07.-)
zoster (B02.-)

L00 Staphylococcal scalded skin syndrome
Ritter's disease
Use additional code to identify percentage of skin exfoliation (L49.-)
Excludes1: *bullous impetigo (L01.03)*
pemphigus neonatorum (L01.03)
toxic epidermal necrolysis [Lyell] (L51.2)
Valid 3-character code, no further characters required

L01 Impetigo
Excludes1: *impetigo herpetiformis (L40.1)*

+ **L01.0 Impetigo**
Impetigo contagiosa
Impetigo vulgaris
L01.00 Impetigo, unspecified
Impetigo NOS
L01.01 Non-bullous impetigo
L01.02 Bockhart's impetigo
Impetigo follicularis
Perifolliculitis NOS
Superficial pustular perifolliculitis

Cross-Section of the Skin Showing Layers and Types of Infection

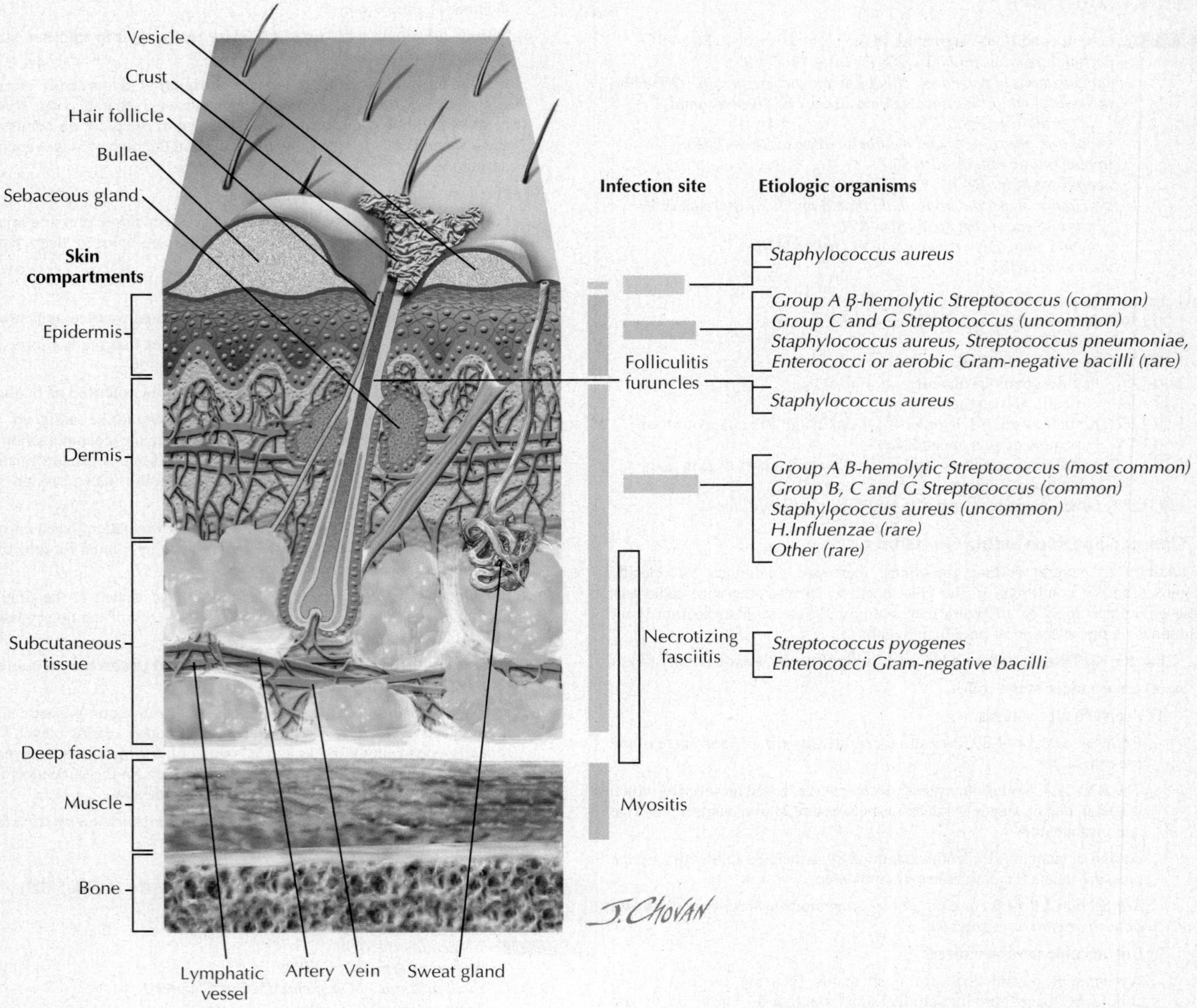

L01.03 Bullous impetigo
Impetigo neonatorum
Pemphigus neonatorum

L01.09 Other impetigo
Ulcerative impetigo

L01.1 Impetiginization of other dermatoses

L02 Cutaneous abscess, furuncle and carbuncle
Use additional code to identify organism (B95-B96)
Excludes2: *abscess of anus and rectal regions (K61.-)*
abscess of female genital organs (external) (N76.4)
abscess of male genital organs (external) (N48.2, N49.-)

\+ **L02.0 Cutaneous abscess, furuncle and carbuncle of face**
Excludes2: *abscess of ear, external (H60.0)*
abscess of eyelid (H00.0)
abscess of head [any part, except face] (L02.8)
abscess of lacrimal gland (H04.0)
abscess of lacrimal passages (H04.3)
abscess of mouth (K12.2)
abscess of nose (J34.0)
abscess of orbit (H05.0)
submandibular abscess (K12.2)

CC **L02.01 Cutaneous abscess of face**

L02.02 Furuncle of face
Boil of face
Folliculitis of face

L02.03 Carbuncle of face

\+ **L02.1 Cutaneous abscess, furuncle and carbuncle of neck**

CC **L02.11 Cutaneous abscess of neck**

L02.12 Furuncle of neck
Boil of neck
Folliculitis of neck

L02.13 Carbuncle of neck

\+ **L02.2 Cutaneous abscess, furuncle and carbuncle of trunk**
Excludes1: *non-newborn omphalitis (L08.82)*
omphalitis of newborn (P38.-)
Excludes2: *abscess of breast (N61.1)*
abscess of buttocks (L02.3)
abscess of female external genital organs (N76.4)
abscess of male external genital organs (N48.2, N49.-)
abscess of hip (L02.4)

CC **L02.21 Cutaneous abscess of trunk**

CC **L02.211 Cutaneous abscess of abdominal wall**

CC **L02.212 Cutaneous abscess of back [any part, except buttock]**

CC **L02.213 Cutaneous abscess of chest wall**

CC **L02.214 Cutaneous abscess of groin**

CC **L02.215 Cutaneous abscess of perineum**

CC **L02.216 Cutaneous abscess of umbilicus**

CC **L02.219 Cutaneous abscess of trunk, unspecified**

+ **L02.22 Furuncle of trunk**
Boil of trunk
Folliculitis of trunk
L02.221 Furuncle of abdominal wall
L02.222 Furuncle of back [any part, except buttock]
L02.223 Furuncle of chest wall
L02.224 Furuncle of groin
L02.225 Furuncle of perineum
L02.226 Furuncle of umbilicus
L02.229 Furuncle of trunk, unspecified
+ **L02.23 Carbuncle of trunk**
L02.231 Carbuncle of abdominal wall
L02.232 Carbuncle of back [any part, except buttock]
L02.233 Carbuncle of chest wall
L02.234 Carbuncle of groin
L02.235 Carbuncle of perineum
L02.236 Carbuncle of umbilicus
L02.239 Carbuncle of trunk, unspecified
+ **L02.3 Cutaneous abscess, furuncle and carbuncle of buttock**
Excludes1: *pilonidal cyst with abscess (L05.01)*
CC **L02.31 Cutaneous abscess of buttock**
Cutaneous abscess of gluteal region
L02.32 Furuncle of buttock
Boil of buttock
Folliculitis of buttock
Furuncle of gluteal region
L02.33 Carbuncle of buttock
Carbuncle of gluteal region
+ **L02.4 Cutaneous abscess, furuncle and carbuncle of limb**
Excludes2: *Cutaneous abscess, furuncle and carbuncle of groin (L02.214, L02.224, L02.234)*
Cutaneous abscess, furuncle and carbuncle of hand (L02.5-)
Cutaneous abscess, furuncle and carbuncle of foot (L02.6-)
+ **L02.41 Cutaneous abscess of limb**
CC **L02.411 Cutaneous abscess of right axilla**
CC **L02.412 Cutaneous abscess of left axilla**
CC **L02.413 Cutaneous abscess of right upper limb**
CC **L02.414 Cutaneous abscess of left upper limb**
CC **L02.415 Cutaneous abscess of right lower limb**
CC **L02.416 Cutaneous abscess of left lower limb**
CC **L02.419 Cutaneous abscess of limb, unspecified**
+ **L02.42 Furuncle of limb**
Boil of limb
Folliculitis of limb
L02.421 Furuncle of right axilla
L02.422 Furuncle of left axilla
L02.423 Furuncle of right upper limb
L02.424 Furuncle of left upper limb
L02.425 Furuncle of right lower limb
L02.426 Furuncle of left lower limb
L02.429 Furuncle of limb, unspecified
+ **L02.43 Carbuncle of limb**
L02.431 Carbuncle of right axilla
L02.432 Carbuncle of left axilla
L02.433 Carbuncle of right upper limb
L02.434 Carbuncle of left upper limb
L02.435 Carbuncle of right lower limb
L02.436 Carbuncle of left lower limb
L02.439 Carbuncle of limb, unspecified
+ **L02.5 Cutaneous abscess, furuncle and carbuncle of hand**
+ **L02.51 Cutaneous abscess of hand**
CC **L02.511 Cutaneous abscess of right hand**
CC **L02.512 Cutaneous abscess of left hand**
CC **L02.519 Cutaneous abscess of unspecified hand**
+ **L02.52 Furuncle hand**
Boil of hand
Folliculitis of hand
L02.521 Furuncle right hand
L02.522 Furuncle left hand
L02.529 Furuncle unspecified hand
+ **L02.53 Carbuncle of hand**
L02.531 Carbuncle of right hand
L02.532 Carbuncle of left hand
L02.539 Carbuncle of unspecified hand
+ **L02.6 Cutaneous abscess, furuncle and carbuncle of foot**
+ **L02.61 Cutaneous abscess of foot**
CC **L02.611 Cutaneous abscess of right foot**
CC **L02.612 Cutaneous abscess of left foot**
CC **L02.619 Cutaneous abscess of unspecified foot**
+ **L02.62 Furuncle of foot**
Boil of foot
Folliculitis of foot
L02.621 Furuncle of right foot
L02.622 Furuncle of left foot
L02.629 Furuncle of unspecified foot
+ **L02.63 Carbuncle of foot**
L02.631 Carbuncle of right foot
L02.632 Carbuncle of left foot
L02.639 Carbuncle of unspecified foot
+ **L02.8 Cutaneous abscess, furuncle and carbuncle of other sites**
+ **L02.81 Cutaneous abscess of other sites**
CC **L02.811 Cutaneous abscess of head [any part, except face]**
CC **L02.818 Cutaneous abscess of other sites**
+ **L02.82 Furuncle of other sites**
Boil of other sites
Folliculitis of other sites
L02.821 Furuncle of head [any part, except face]
L02.828 Furuncle of other sites
+ **L02.83 Carbuncle of other sites**
L02.831 Carbuncle of head [any part, except face]
L02.838 Carbuncle of other sites
+ **L02.9 Cutaneous abscess, furuncle and carbuncle, unspecified**
CC **L02.91 Cutaneous abscess, unspecified**
L02.92 Furuncle, unspecified
Boil NOS
Furunculosis NOS
L02.93 Carbuncle, unspecified

L03 Cellulitis and acute lymphangitis

Excludes2: *cellulitis of anal and rectal region (K61.-)*
cellulitis of external auditory canal (H60.1)
cellulitis of eyelid (H00.0)
cellulitis of female external genital organs (N76.4)
cellulitis of lacrimal apparatus (H04.3)
cellulitis of male external genital organs (N48.2, N49.-)
cellulitis of mouth (K12.2)
cellulitis of nose (J34.0)
eosinophilic cellulitis [Wells] (L98.3)
febrile neutrophilic dermatosis [Sweet] (L98.2)
lymphangitis (chronic) (subacute) (I89.1)
+ **L03.0 Cellulitis and acute lymphangitis of finger and toe**
Infection of nail
Onychia
Paronychia
Perionychia
+ **L03.01 Cellulitis of finger**
Felon
Whitlow
Excludes1: herpetic whitlow (B00.89)
L03.011 Cellulitis of right finger
AHA CC: 4Q, 2020, 11
L03.012 Cellulitis of left finger
L03.019 Cellulitis of unspecified finger
+ **L03.02 Acute lymphangitis of finger**
Hangnail with lymphangitis of finger
L03.021 Acute lymphangitis of right finger
L03.022 Acute lymphangitis of left finger
L03.029 Acute lymphangitis of unspecified finger
+ **L03.03 Cellulitis of toe**
L03.031 Cellulitis of right toe
L03.032 Cellulitis of left toe
L03.039 Cellulitis of unspecified toe
+ **L03.04 Acute lymphangitis of toe**
Hangnail with lymphangitis of toe
L03.041 Acute lymphangitis of right toe
L03.042 Acute lymphangitis of left toe
L03.049 Acute lymphangitis of unspecified toe

+ **L03.1 Cellulitis and acute lymphangitis of other parts of limb**
  + **L03.11 Cellulitis of other parts of limb**
    Excludes2: *cellulitis of fingers (L03.01-)*
    cellulitis of toes (L03.03-)
    groin (L03.314)
    CC **L03.111 Cellulitis of right axilla**
    CC **L03.112 Cellulitis of left axilla**
    CC **L03.113 Cellulitis of right upper limb**
    CC **L03.114 Cellulitis of left upper limb**
    AHA CC: 1Q, 2019, 13
    CC **L03.115 Cellulitis of right lower limb**
    CC **L03.116 Cellulitis of left lower limb**
    CC **L03.119 Cellulitis of unspecified part of limb**
  + **L03.12 Acute lymphangitis of other parts of limb**
    Excludes2: *acute lymphangitis of fingers (L03.2-)*
    acute lymphangitis of toes (L03.04-)
    acute lymphangitis of groin (L03.324)
    CC **L03.121 Acute lymphangitis of right axilla**
    CC **L03.122 Acute lymphangitis of left axilla**
    CC **L03.123 Acute lymphangitis of right upper limb**
    CC **L03.124 Acute lymphangitis of left upper limb**
    CC **L03.125 Acute lymphangitis of right lower limb**
    CC **L03.126 Acute lymphangitis of left lower limb**
    CC **L03.129 Acute lymphangitis of unspecified part of limb**
+ **L03.2 Cellulitis and acute lymphangitis of face and neck**
  + **L03.21 Cellulitis and acute lymphangitis of face**
    CC **L03.211 Cellulitis of face**
    Excludes2: *abscess of orbit (H05.01-)*
    cellulitis of ear (H60.1-)
    cellulitis of eyelid (H00.0-)
    cellulitis of head (L03.81)
    cellulitis of lacrimal apparatus (H04.3)
    cellulitis of lip (K13.0)
    cellulitis of mouth (K12.2)
    cellulitis of nose (internal) (J34.0)
    cellulitis of orbit (H05.01-)
    cellulitis of scalp (L03.81)
    AHA CC: 4Q, 2013, 123
    CC **L03.212 Acute lymphangitis of face**
    CC **L03.213 Periorbital cellulitis**
    Preseptal cellulitis
    AHA CC: 4Q, 2016, 36
  + **L03.22 Cellulitis and acute lymphangitis of neck**
    CC **L03.221 Cellulitis of neck**
    CC **L03.222 Acute lymphangitis of neck**
+ **L03.3 Cellulitis and acute lymphangitis of trunk**
  + **L03.31 Cellulitis of trunk**
    Excludes2: *cellulitis of anal and rectal regions (K61.-)*
    cellulitis of breast NOS (N61.0)
    cellulitis of female external genital organs (N76.4)
    cellulitis of male external genital organs (N48.2, N49.-)
    omphalitis of newborn (P38.-)
    puerperal cellulitis of breast (O91.2)
    CC **L03.311 Cellulitis of abdominal wall**
    Excludes2: *cellulitis of umbilicus (L03.316)*
    cellulitis of groin (L03.314)
    CC **L03.312 Cellulitis of back [any part except buttock]**
    CC **L03.313 Cellulitis of chest wall**
    CC **L03.314 Cellulitis of groin**
    CC **L03.315 Cellulitis of perineum**
    CC **L03.316 Cellulitis of umbilicus**
    CC **L03.317 Cellulitis of buttock**
    CC **L03.319 Cellulitis of trunk, unspecified**
  + **L03.32 Acute lymphangitis of trunk**
    CC **L03.321 Acute lymphangitis of abdominal wall**
    CC **L03.322 Acute lymphangitis of back [any part except buttock]**
    CC **L03.323 Acute lymphangitis of chest wall**
    CC **L03.324 Acute lymphangitis of groin**
    CC **L03.325 Acute lymphangitis of perineum**
    CC **L03.326 Acute lymphangitis of umbilicus**
    CC **L03.327 Acute lymphangitis of buttock**
    CC **L03.329 Acute lymphangitis of trunk, unspecified**
+ **L03.8 Cellulitis and acute lymphangitis of other sites**
  + **L03.81 Cellulitis of other sites**
    CC **L03.811 Cellulitis of head [any part, except face]**
    Cellulitis of scalp
    Excludes2: *cellulitis of face (L03.211)*
    CC **L03.818 Cellulitis of other sites**
  + **L03.89 Acute lymphangitis of other sites**
    CC **L03.891 Acute lymphangitis of head [any part, except face]**
    CC **L03.898 Acute lymphangitis of other sites**
+ **L03.9 Cellulitis and acute lymphangitis, unspecified**
  CC **L03.90 Cellulitis, unspecified**
  CC **L03.91 Acute lymphangitis, unspecified**
  Excludes1: *lymphangitis NOS (I89.1)*

L04 Acute lymphadenitis

Includes: abscess (acute) of lymph nodes, except mesenteric
acute lymphadenitis, except mesenteric
Excludes1: *chronic or subacute lymphadenitis, except mesenteric (I88.1)*
enlarged lymph nodes (R59.-)
human immunodeficiency virus [HIV] disease resulting in generalized lymphadenopathy (B20)
lymphadenitis NOS (I88.9)
nonspecific mesenteric lymphadenitis (I88.0)

L04.0 Acute lymphadenitis of face, head and neck
L04.1 Acute lymphadenitis of trunk
L04.2 Acute lymphadenitis of upper limb
Acute lymphadenitis of axilla
Acute lymphadenitis of shoulder
L04.3 Acute lymphadenitis of lower limb
Acute lymphadenitis of hip
Excludes2: *acute lymphadenitis of groin (L04.1)*
L04.8 Acute lymphadenitis of other sites
L04.9 Acute lymphadenitis, unspecified

L05 Pilonidal cyst and sinus

+ **L05.0 Pilonidal cyst and sinus with abscess**
  CC **L05.01 Pilonidal cyst with abscess**
  Pilonidal abscess
  Pilonidal dimple with abscess
  Postanal dimple with abscess
  Excludes2: *congenital sacral dimple (Q82.6)*
  parasacral dimple (Q82.6)
  CC **L05.02 Pilonidal sinus with abscess**
  Coccygeal fistula with abscess
  Coccygeal sinus with abscess
  Pilonidal fistula with abscess
+ **L05.9 Pilonidal cyst and sinus without abscess**
  L05.91 Pilonidal cyst without abscess
  Pilonidal dimple
  Postanal dimple
  Pilonidal cyst NOS
  Excludes2: *congenital sacral dimple (Q82.6)*
  parasacral dimple (Q82.6)
  L05.92 Pilonidal sinus without abscess
  Coccygeal fistula
  Coccygeal sinus without abscess
  Pilonidal fistula

L08 Other local infections of skin and subcutaneous tissue

L08.0 Pyoderma
Dermatitis gangrenosa
Purulent dermatitis
Septic dermatitis
Suppurative dermatitis
Excludes1: *pyoderma gangrenosum (L88)*
pyoderma vegetans (L08.81)
CC **L08.1 Erythrasma**
+ **L08.8 Other specified local infections of the skin and subcutaneous tissue**
  L08.81 Pyoderma vegetans
  Excludes1: *pyoderma gangrenosum (L88)*
  pyoderma NOS (L08.0)
  L08.82 Omphalitis not of newborn
  Excludes1: *omphalitis of newborn (P38.-)*
  L08.89 Other specified local infections of the skin and subcutaneous tissue
L08.9 Local infection of the skin and subcutaneous tissue, unspecified

Bullous disorders (L10-L14)

Excludes1: *benign familial pemphigus [Hailey-Hailey] (Q82.8)*
staphylococcal scalded skin syndrome (L00)
toxic epidermal necrolysis [Lyell] (L51.2)

L10 Pemphigus

Excludes1: *pemphigus neonatorum (L01.03)*

CC **L10.0 Pemphigus vulgaris**
CC **L10.1 Pemphigus vegetans**
CC **L10.2 Pemphigus foliaceous**
CC **L10.3 Brazilian pemphigus [fogo selvagem]**
CC **L10.4 Pemphigus erythematosus**
Senear-Usher syndrome
CC **L10.5 Drug-induced pemphigus**
Use additional code for adverse effect, if applicable, to identify drug (T36-T50 with fifth or sixth character 5)
+ **L10.8 Other pemphigus**
CC **L10.81 Paraneoplastic pemphigus**
CC **L10.89 Other pemphigus**
CC **L10.9 Pemphigus, unspecified**

L11 Other acantholytic disorders

L11.0 Acquired keratosis follicularis
Excludes1: *keratosis follicularis (congenital) [Darier-White] (Q82.8)*
L11.1 Transient acantholytic dermatosis [Grover]
L11.8 Other specified acantholytic disorders
L11.9 Acantholytic disorder, unspecified

L12 Pemphigoid

Excludes1: *herpes gestationis (O26.4-)*
impetigo herpetiformis (L40.1)

CC **L12.0 Bullous pemphigoid**
L12.1 Cicatricial pemphigoid
Benign mucous membrane pemphigoid
• **L12.2 Chronic bullous disease of childhood**
Juvenile dermatitis herpetiformis
+ **L12.3 Acquired epidermolysis bullosa**
Excludes1: *epidermolysis bullosa (congenital) (Q81.-)*
CC **L12.30 Acquired epidermolysis bullosa, unspecified**
CC **L12.31 Epidermolysis bullosa due to drug**
Use additional code for adverse effect, if applicable, to identify drug (T36-T50 with fifth or sixth character 5)
CC **L12.35 Other acquired epidermolysis bullosa**
CC **L12.8 Other pemphigoid**
CC **L12.9 Pemphigoid, unspecified**

L13 Other bullous disorders

L13.0 Dermatitis herpetiformis
Duhring's disease
Hydroa herpetiformis
Excludes1: *juvenile dermatitis herpetiformis (L12.2)*
senile dermatitis herpetiformis (L12.0)
L13.1 Subcorneal pustular dermatitis
Sneddon-Wilkinson disease
L13.8 Other specified bullous disorders
L13.9 Bullous disorder, unspecified

L14 Bullous disorders in diseases classified elsewhere

Code first underlying disease
Valid 3-character code, no further characters required

Dermatitis and eczema (L20-L30)

NOTE In this block the terms dermatitis and eczema are used synonymously and interchangeably.

Excludes2: *chronic (childhood) granulomatous disease (D71)*
dermatitis gangrenosa (L08.0)
dermatitis herpetiformis (L13.0)
dry skin dermatitis (L85.3)
factitial dermatitis (L98.1)
perioral dermatitis (L71.0)
radiation-related disorders of the skin and subcutaneous tissue (L55-L59)
stasis dermatitis (I87.2)

L20 Atopic dermatitis

L20.0 Besnier's prurigo
+ **L20.8 Other atopic dermatitis**
Excludes2: *circumscribed neurodermatitis (L28.0)*
L20.81 Atopic neurodermatitis
Diffuse neurodermatitis
L20.82 Flexural eczema
• **L20.83 Infantile (acute) (chronic) eczema**
L20.84 Intrinsic (allergic) eczema
L20.89 Other atopic dermatitis
L20.9 Atopic dermatitis, unspecified

L21 Seborrheic dermatitis

Excludes2: *infective dermatitis (L30.3)*
seborrheic keratosis (L82.-)

L21.0 Seborrhea capitis
Cradle cap
AHA CC: 1Q, 2018, 6
• **L21.1 Seborrheic infantile dermatitis**
L21.8 Other seborrheic dermatitis
L21.9 Seborrheic dermatitis, unspecified
Seborrhea NOS

L22 Diaper dermatitis

Diaper erythema
Diaper rash
Psoriasiform diaper rash
Valid 3-character code, no further characters required

L23 Allergic contact dermatitis

Excludes1: *allergy NOS (T78.40)*
contact dermatitis NOS (L25.9)
dermatitis NOS (L30.9)
Excludes2: *dermatitis due to substances taken internally (L27.-)*
dermatitis of eyelid (H01.1-)
diaper dermatitis (L22)
eczema of external ear (H60.5-)
irritant contact dermatitis (L24.-)
perioral dermatitis (L71.0)
radiation-related disorders of the skin and subcutaneous tissue (L55-L59)

L23.0 Allergic contact dermatitis due to metals
Allergic contact dermatitis due to chromium
Allergic contact dermatitis due to nickel
L23.1 Allergic contact dermatitis due to adhesives
L23.2 Allergic contact dermatitis due to cosmetics
L23.3 Allergic contact dermatitis due to drugs in contact with skin
Use additional code for adverse effect, if applicable, to identify drug (T36-T50 with fifth or sixth character 5)
Excludes2: *dermatitis due to ingested drugs and medicaments (L27.0-L27.1)*
L23.4 Allergic contact dermatitis due to dyes
L23.5 Allergic contact dermatitis due to other chemical products
Allergic contact dermatitis due to cement
Allergic contact dermatitis due to insecticide
Allergic contact dermatitis due to plastic
Allergic contact dermatitis due to rubber
L23.6 Allergic contact dermatitis due to food in contact with the skin
Excludes2: *dermatitis due to ingested food (L27.2)*
L23.7 Allergic contact dermatitis due to plants, except food
Excludes2: *allergy NOS due to pollen (J30.1)*
+ **L23.8 Allergic contact dermatitis due to other agents**
L23.81 Allergic contact dermatitis due to animal (cat) (dog) dander
Allergic contact dermatitis due to animal (cat) (dog) hair
L23.89 Allergic contact dermatitis due to other agents
L23.9 Allergic contact dermatitis, unspecified cause
Allergic contact eczema NOS

L24 Irritant contact dermatitis

Excludes1: *allergy NOS (T78.40)*
contact dermatitis NOS (L25.9)
dermatitis NOS (L30.9)

Excludes2: *allergic contact dermatitis (L23.-)*
dermatitis due to substances taken internally (L27.-)
dermatitis of eyelid (H01.1-)
diaper dermatitis (L22)
eczema of external ear (H60.5-)
perioral dermatitis (L71.0)
radiation-related disorders of the skin and subcutaneous tissue (L55-L59)

L24.0 Irritant contact dermatitis due to detergents

L24.1 Irritant contact dermatitis due to oils and greases

L24.2 Irritant contact dermatitis due to solvents
Irritant contact dermatitis due to chlorocompound
Irritant contact dermatitis due to cyclohexane
Irritant contact dermatitis due to ester
Irritant contact dermatitis due to glycol
Irritant contact dermatitis due to hydrocarbon
Irritant contact dermatitis due to ketone

L24.3 Irritant contact dermatitis due to cosmetics

L24.4 Irritant contact dermatitis due to drugs in contact with skin
Use additional code for adverse effect, if applicable, to identify drug (T36-T50 with fifth or sixth character 5)

L24.5 Irritant contact dermatitis due to other chemical products
Irritant contact dermatitis due to cement
Irritant contact dermatitis due to insecticide
Irritant contact dermatitis due to plastic
Irritant contact dermatitis due to rubber

L24.6 Irritant contact dermatitis due to food in contact with skin
Excludes2: *dermatitis due to ingested food (L27.2)*

L24.7 Irritant contact dermatitis due to plants, except food
Excludes2: *allergy NOS to pollen (J30.1)*

\+ **L24.8 Irritant contact dermatitis due to other agents**

L24.81 Irritant contact dermatitis due to metals
Irritant contact dermatitis due to chromium
Irritant contact dermatitis due to nickel

L24.89 Irritant contact dermatitis due to other agents
Irritant contact dermatitis due to dyes

L24.9 Irritant contact dermatitis, unspecified cause
Irritant contact eczema NOS

\+ **L24.A Irritant contact dermatitis due to friction or contact with body fluids**
Excludes1: *irritant contact dermatitis related to stoma or fistula (L24.B-)*
Excludes2: *erythema intertrigo (L30.4)*

L24.A0 Irritant contact dermatitis due to friction or contact with body fluids, unspecified

L24.A1 Irritant contact dermatitis due to saliva

L24.A2 Irritant contact dermatitis due to fecal, urinary or dual incontinence
Excludes1: *diaper dermatitis (L22)*

L24.A9 Irritant contact dermatitis due to friction or contact with other specified body fluids
Irritant contact dermatitis related to endotracheal tube
Wound fluids, exudate

\+ **L24.B Irritant contact dermatitis related to stoma or fistula**
Use additional code to identify any artificial opening status (Z93.-), if applicable, for contact dermatitis related to stoma secretions

L24.B0 Irritant contact dermatitis related to unspecified stoma or fistula
Irritant contact dermatitis related to fistula NOS
Irritant contact dermatitis related to stoma NOS

L24.B1 Irritant contact dermatitis related to digestive stoma or fistula
Irritant contact dermatitis related to gastrostomy
Irritant contact dermatitis related to jejunostomy
Irritant contact dermatitis related to saliva or spit fistula

L24.B2 Irritant contact dermatitis related to respiratory stoma or fistula
Irritant contact dermatitis related tracheostomy

L24.B3 Irritant contact dermatitis related to fecal or urinary stoma or fistula
Irritant contact dermatitis related to colostomy
Irritant contact dermatitis related to enterocutaneous fistua
Irritant contact dermatitis related to ileostomy

L25 Unspecified contact dermatitis

Excludes1: *allergic contact dermatitis (L23.-)*
allergy NOS (T78.40)
dermatitis NOS (L30.9)
irritant contact dermatitis (L24.-)

Excludes2: *dermatitis due to ingested substances (L27.-)*
dermatitis of eyelid (H01.1-)
eczema of external ear (H60.5-)
perioral dermatitis (L71.0)
radiation-related disorders of the skin and subcutaneous tissue (L55-L59)

L25.0 Unspecified contact dermatitis due to cosmetics

L25.1 Unspecified contact dermatitis due to drugs in contact with skin
Use additional code for adverse effect, if applicable, to identify drug (T36-T50 with fifth or sixth character 5)
Excludes2: *dermatitis due to ingested drugs and medicaments (L27.0-L27.1)*

L25.2 Unspecified contact dermatitis due to dyes

L25.3 Unspecified contact dermatitis due to other chemical products
Unspecified contact dermatitis due to cement
Unspecified contact dermatitis due to insecticide

L25.4 Unspecified contact dermatitis due to food in contact with skin
Excludes2: *dermatitis due to ingested food (L27.2)*

L25.5 Unspecified contact dermatitis due to plants, except food
Excludes1: *nettle rash (L50.9)*
Excludes2: *allergy NOS due to pollen (J30.1)*

L25.8 Unspecified contact dermatitis due to other agents

L25.9 Unspecified contact dermatitis, unspecified cause
Contact dermatitis (occupational) NOS
Contact eczema (occupational) NOS

L26 Exfoliative dermatitis

Hebra's pityriasis
Excludes1: *Ritter's disease (L00)*
Valid 3-character code, no further characters required

L27 Dermatitis due to substances taken internally

Excludes1: *allergy NOS (T78.40)*

Excludes2: *adverse food reaction, except dermatitis (T78.0-T78.1)*
contact dermatitis (L23-L25)
drug photoallergic response (L56.1)
drug phototoxic response (L56.0)
urticaria (L50.-)

L27.0 Generalized skin eruption due to drugs and medicaments taken internally
Use additional code for adverse effect, if applicable, to identify drug (T36-T50 with fifth or sixth character 5)

L27.1 Localized skin eruption due to drugs and medicaments taken internally
Use additional code for adverse effect, if applicable, to identify drug (T36-T50 with fifth or sixth character 5)

L27.2 Dermatitis due to ingested food
Excludes2: *dermatitis due to food in contact with skin (L23.6, L24.6, L25.4)*

L27.8 Dermatitis due to other substances taken internally

L27.9 Dermatitis due to unspecified substance taken internally

L28 Lichen simplex chronicus and prurigo

L28.0 Lichen simplex chronicus
Circumscribed neurodermatitis
Lichen NOS

L28.1 Prurigo nodularis

L28.2 Other prurigo
Prurigo NOS
Prurigo Hebra
Prurigo mitis
Urticaria papulosa

L29 Pruritus

Excludes1: *neurotic excoriation (L98.1)*
psychogenic pruritus (F45.8)

L29.0 Pruritus ani
♂ **L29.1 Pruritus scroti**
♀ **L29.2 Pruritus vulvae**
L29.3 Anogenital pruritus, unspecified
L29.8 Other pruritus
L29.9 Pruritus, unspecified
Itch NOS

L30 Other and unspecified dermatitis

Excludes2: *contact dermatitis (L23-L25)*
dry skin dermatitis (L85.3)
small plaque parapsoriasis (L41.3)
stasis dermatitis (I87.2)

L30.0 Nummular dermatitis
L30.1 Dyshidrosis [pompholyx]
L30.2 Cutaneous autosensitization
Candidid [levurid]
Dermatophytid
Eczematid
L30.3 Infective dermatitis
Infectious eczematoid dermatitis
L30.4 Erythema intertrigo
L30.5 Pityriasis alba
L30.8 Other specified dermatitis
L30.9 Dermatitis, unspecified
Eczema NOS

Papulosquamous disorders (L40-L45)

L40 Psoriasis

L40.0 Psoriasis vulgaris
Nummular psoriasis
Plaque psoriasis
L40.1 Generalized pustular psoriasis
Impetigo herpetiformis
Von Zumbusch's disease
L40.2 Acrodermatitis continua
L40.3 Pustulosis palmaris et plantaris
L40.4 Guttate psoriasis
+ **L40.5 Arthropathic psoriasis**
L40.50 Arthropathic psoriasis, unspecified
L40.51 Distal interphalangeal psoriatic arthropathy
L40.52 Psoriatic arthritis mutilans
L40.53 Psoriatic spondylitis
L40.54 Psoriatic juvenile arthropathy
L40.59 Other psoriatic arthropathy
L40.8 Other psoriasis
Flexural psoriasis
L40.9 Psoriasis, unspecified

L41 Parapsoriasis

Excludes1: *poikiloderma vasculare atrophicans (L94.5)*

L41.0 Pityriasis lichenoides et varioliformis acuta
Mucha-Habermann disease
L41.1 Pityriasis lichenoides chronica
L41.3 Small plaque parapsoriasis
L41.4 Large plaque parapsoriasis
L41.5 Retiform parapsoriasis
L41.8 Other parapsoriasis
L41.9 Parapsoriasis, unspecified

L42 Pityriasis rosea

Valid 3-character code, no further characters required

L43 Lichen planus

Excludes1: *lichen planopilaris (L66.1)*

L43.0 Hypertrophic lichen planus
L43.1 Bullous lichen planus
L43.2 Lichenoid drug reaction
Use additional code for adverse effect, if applicable, to identify drug (T36-T50 with fifth or sixth character 5)
L43.3 Subacute (active) lichen planus
Lichen planus tropicus
L43.8 Other lichen planus
L43.9 Lichen planus, unspecified

L44 Other papulosquamous disorders

L44.0 Pityriasis rubra pilaris
L44.1 Lichen nitidus
L44.2 Lichen striatus
L44.3 Lichen ruber moniliformis
• **L44.4 Infantile papular acrodermatitis [Gianotti-Crosti]**
L44.8 Other specified papulosquamous disorders
L44.9 Papulosquamous disorder, unspecified

L45 Papulosquamous disorders in diseases classified elsewhere

Code first underlying disease.
Valid 3-character code, no further characters required

Urticaria and erythema (L49-L54)

Excludes1: *Lyme disease (A69.2-)*
rosacea (L71.-)

L49 Exfoliation due to erythematous conditions according to extent of body surface involved

Code first erythematous condition causing exfoliation, such as:
Ritter's disease (L00)
(Staphylococcal) scalded skin syndrome (L00)
Stevens-Johnson syndrome (L51.1)
Stevens-Johnson syndrome-toxic epidermal necrolysis overlap syndrome (L51.3)
Toxic epidermal necrolysis (L51.2)

L49.0 Exfoliation due to erythematous condition involving less than 10 percent of body surface
Exfoliation due to erythematous condition NOS
L49.1 Exfoliation due to erythematous condition involving 10-19 percent of body surface
L49.2 Exfoliation due to erythematous condition involving 20-29 percent of body surface
CC **L49.3 Exfoliation due to erythematous condition involving 30-39 percent of body surface**
CC **L49.4 Exfoliation due to erythematous condition involving 40-49 percent of body surface**
CC **L49.5 Exfoliation due to erythematous condition involving 50-59 percent of body surface**
CC **L49.6 Exfoliation due to erythematous condition involving 60-69 percent of body surface**
CC **L49.7 Exfoliation due to erythematous condition involving 70-79 percent of body surface**
CC **L49.8 Exfoliation due to erythematous condition involving 80-89 percent of body surface**
CC **L49.9 Exfoliation due to erythematous condition involving 90 or more percent of body surface**

L50 Urticaria

Excludes1: *allergic contact dermatitis (L23.-)*
angioneurotic edema (T78.3)
giant urticaria (T78.3)
hereditary angio-edema (D84.1)
Quincke's edema (T78.3)
serum urticaria (T80.6-)
solar urticaria (L56.3)
urticaria neonatorum (P83.8)
urticaria papulosa (L28.2)
urticaria pigmentosa (D47.01)

L50.0 Allergic urticaria
L50.1 Idiopathic urticaria
L50.2 Urticaria due to cold and heat
Excludes2: *familial cold urticaria (M04.2)*
L50.3 Dermatographic urticaria
L50.4 Vibratory urticaria
L50.5 Cholinergic urticaria
L50.6 Contact urticaria
L50.8 Other urticaria
Chronic urticaria
Recurrent periodic urticaria
L50.9 Urticaria, unspecified

L51 Erythema multiforme

Use additional code for adverse effect, if applicable, to identify drug (T36-T50 with fifth or sixth character 5)

Use additional code to identify associated manifestations, such as:
- arthropathy associated with dermatological disorders (M14.8-)
- conjunctival edema (H11.42)
- conjunctivitis (H10.22-)
- corneal scars and opacities (H17.-)
- corneal ulcer (H16.0-)
- edema of eyelid (H02.84-)
- inflammation of eyelid (H01.8)
- keratoconjunctivitis sicca (H16.22-)
- mechanical lagophthalmos (H02.22-)
- stomatitis (K12.-)
- symblepharon (H11.23-)

Use additional code to identify percentage of skin exfoliation (L49.-)

Excludes1: *staphylococcal scalded skin syndrome (L00)*
Ritter's disease (L00)

L51.0 Nonbullous erythema multiforme
CC **L51.1 Stevens-Johnson syndrome**
CC **L51.2 Toxic epidermal necrolysis [Lyell]**
CC **L51.3 Stevens-Johnson syndrome-toxic epidermal necrolysis overlap syndrome**
SJS-TEN overlap syndrome
L51.8 Other erythema multiforme
L51.9 Erythema multiforme, unspecified
Erythema iris
Erythema multiforme major NOS
Erythema multiforme minor NOS
Herpes iris

L52 Erythema nodosum

Excludes1: *tuberculous erythema nodosum (A18.4)*

Valid 3-character code, no further characters required

L53 Other erythematous conditions

Excludes1: *erythema ab igne (L59.0)*
erythema due to external agents in contact with skin (L23-L25)
erythema intertrigo (L30.4)

CC **L53.0 Toxic erythema**
Code first poisoning due to drug or toxin, if applicable (T36-T65 with fifth or sixth character 1-4 or 6)

Use additional code for adverse effect, if applicable, to identify drug (T36-T50 with fifth or sixth character 5)

Excludes1: *neonatal erythema toxicum (P83.1)*

CC **L53.1 Erythema annulare centrifugum**
CC **L53.2 Erythema marginatum**
CC **L53.3 Other chronic figurate erythema**
L53.8 Other specified erythematous conditions
L53.9 Erythematous condition, unspecified
Erythema NOS
Erythroderma NOS

L54 Erythema in diseases classified elsewhere

Code first underlying disease

Valid 3-character code, no further characters required

Radiation-related disorders of the skin and subcutaneous tissue (L55-L59)

L55 Sunburn

L55.0 Sunburn of first degree
L55.1 Sunburn of second degree
L55.2 Sunburn of third degree
L55.9 Sunburn, unspecified

L56 Other acute skin changes due to ultraviolet radiation

Use additional code to identify the source of the ultraviolet radiation (W89, X32)

L56.0 Drug phototoxic response
Use additional code for adverse effect, if applicable, to identify drug (T36-T50 with fifth or sixth character 5)
L56.1 Drug photoallergic response
Use additional code for adverse effect, if applicable, to identify drug (T36-T50 with fifth or sixth character 5)
L56.2 Photocontact dermatitis [berloque dermatitis]
L56.3 Solar urticaria
L56.4 Polymorphous light eruption
L56.5 Disseminated superficial actinic porokeratosis (DSAP)
L56.8 Other specified acute skin changes due to ultraviolet radiation
L56.9 Acute skin change due to ultraviolet radiation, unspecified

L57 Skin changes due to chronic exposure to nonionizing radiation

Use additional code to identify the source of the ultraviolet radiation (W89), or other nonionizing radiation (W90)

L57.0 Actinic keratosis
Keratosis NOS
Senile keratosis
Solar keratosis
L57.1 Actinic reticuloid
L57.2 Cutis rhomboidalis nuchae
L57.3 Poikiloderma of Civatte
L57.4 Cutis laxa senilis
Elastosis senilis
L57.5 Actinic granuloma
L57.8 Other skin changes due to chronic exposure to nonionizing radiation
Farmer's skin
Sailor's skin
Solar dermatitis
L57.9 Skin changes due to chronic exposure to nonionizing radiation, unspecified

L58 Radiodermatitis

Use additional code to identify the source of the radiation (W88, W90)

L58.0 Acute radiodermatitis
L58.1 Chronic radiodermatitis
L58.9 Radiodermatitis, unspecified

L59 Other disorders of skin and subcutaneous tissue related to radiation

L59.0 Erythema ab igne [dermatitis ab igne]
L59.8 Other specified disorders of the skin and subcutaneous tissue related to radiation
AHA CC: 1Q, 2017, 33-34
L59.9 Disorder of the skin and subcutaneous tissue related to radiation, unspecified

Disorders of skin appendages (L60-L75)

Excludes1: *congenital malformations of integument (Q84.-)*

L60 Nail disorders

Excludes2: *clubbing of nails (R68.3)*
onychia and paronychia (L03.0-)

L60.0 Ingrowing nail
L60.1 Onycholysis
L60.2 Onychogryphosis
L60.3 Nail dystrophy
L60.4 Beau's lines
L60.5 Yellow nail syndrome
L60.8 Other nail disorders
L60.9 Nail disorder, unspecified

L62 Nail disorders in diseases classified elsewhere

Code first underlying disease, such as:
pachydermoperiostosis (M89.4-)

Valid 3-character code, no further characters required

L63 Alopecia areata

L63.0 Alopecia (capitis) totalis
L63.1 Alopecia universalis
L63.2 Ophiasis
L63.8 Other alopecia areata
L63.9 Alopecia areata, unspecified

L64 Androgenic alopecia

Includes: male-pattern baldness

L64.0 Drug-induced androgenic alopecia
Use additional code for adverse effect, if applicable, to identify drug (T36-T50 with fifth or sixth character 5)
L64.8 Other androgenic alopecia
L64.9 Androgenic alopecia, unspecified

L65 Other nonscarring hair loss

Use additional code for adverse effect, if applicable, to identify drug (T36-T50 with fifth or sixth character 5)

Excludes1: *trichotillomania (F63.3)*

L65.0 Telogen effluvium
L65.1 Anagen effluvium
L65.2 Alopecia mucinosa
L65.8 Other specified nonscarring hair loss
L65.9 Nonscarring hair loss, unspecified
Alopecia NOS

L66 Cicatricial alopecia [scarring hair loss]

L66.0 Pseudopelade
L66.1 Lichen planopilaris
Follicular lichen planus
L66.2 Folliculitis decalvans
L66.3 Perifolliculitis capitis abscedens
L66.4 Folliculitis ulerythematosa reticulata
L66.8 Other cicatricial alopecia
AHA CC: 1Q, 2015, 19
L66.9 Cicatricial alopecia, unspecified

L67 Hair color and hair shaft abnormalities

Excludes1: *monilethrix (Q84.1)*
pili annulati (Q84.1)
telogen effluvium (L65.0)

L67.0 Trichorrhexis nodosa
L67.1 Variations in hair color
Canities
Greyness, hair (premature)
Heterochromia of hair
Poliosis circumscripta, acquired
Poliosis NOS
L67.8 Other hair color and hair shaft abnormalities
Fragilitas crinium
L67.9 Hair color and hair shaft abnormality, unspecified

L68 Hypertrichosis

Includes: excess hair
Excludes1: *congenital hypertrichosis (Q84.2)*
persistent lanugo (Q84.2)

L68.0 Hirsutism
L68.1 Acquired hypertrichosis lanuginosa
L68.2 Localized hypertrichosis
L68.3 Polytrichia
L68.8 Other hypertrichosis
L68.9 Hypertrichosis, unspecified

L70 Acne

Excludes2: *acne keloid (L73.0)*

L70.0 Acne vulgaris
L70.1 Acne conglobata
L70.2 Acne varioliformis
Acne necrotica miliaris
L70.3 Acne tropica
• **L70.4 Infantile acne**
L70.5 Acné excoriée
Acné exocoriée des jeunes filles
Picker's acne
L70.8 Other acne
L70.9 Acne, unspecified

L71 Rosacea

Use additional code for adverse effect, if applicable, to identify drug (T36-T50 with fifth or sixth character 5)

L71.0 Perioral dermatitis
L71.1 Rhinophyma
L71.8 Other rosacea
AHA CC: 4Q, 2018, 15
L71.9 Rosacea, unspecified

L72 Follicular cysts of skin and subcutaneous tissue

L72.0 Epidermal cyst
\+ **L72.1 Pilar and trichodermal cyst**
L72.11 Pilar cyst
L72.12 Trichodermal cyst
Trichilemmal (proliferating) cyst
L72.2 Steatocystoma multiplex
L72.3 Sebaceous cyst
Excludes2: *pilar cyst (L72.11)*
trichilemmal (proliferating) cyst (L72.12)
L72.8 Other follicular cysts of the skin and subcutaneous tissue
L72.9 Follicular cyst of the skin and subcutaneous tissue, unspecified

L73 Other follicular disorders

L73.0 Acne keloid
L73.1 Pseudofolliculitis barbae
L73.2 Hidradenitis suppurativa
L73.8 Other specified follicular disorders
Sycosis barbae
L73.9 Follicular disorder, unspecified

L74 Eccrine sweat disorders

Excludes2: *generalized hyperhidrosis (R61)*

L74.0 Miliaria rubra
L74.1 Miliaria crystallina
L74.2 Miliaria profunda
Miliaria tropicalis
L74.3 Miliaria, unspecified
L74.4 Anhidrosis
Hypohidrosis
\+ **L74.5 Focal hyperhidrosis**
\+ **L74.51 Primary focal hyperhidrosis**
L74.510 Primary focal hyperhidrosis, axilla
L74.511 Primary focal hyperhidrosis, face
L74.512 Primary focal hyperhidrosis, palms
L74.513 Primary focal hyperhidrosis, soles
L74.519 Primary focal hyperhidrosis, unspecified
L74.52 Secondary focal hyperhidrosis
Frey's syndrome
L74.8 Other eccrine sweat disorders
L74.9 Eccrine sweat disorder, unspecified
Sweat gland disorder NOS

L75 Apocrine sweat disorders

Excludes1: *dyshidrosis (L30.1)*
hidradenitis suppurativa (L73.2)

L75.0 Bromhidrosis
L75.1 Chromhidrosis
L75.2 Apocrine miliaria
Fox-Fordyce disease
L75.8 Other apocrine sweat disorders
L75.9 Apocrine sweat disorder, unspecified

Intraoperative and postprocedural complications of skin and subcutaneous tissue (L76)

L76 Intraoperative and postprocedural complications of skin and subcutaneous tissue

AHA CC: 4Q, 2016, 9-10

\+ **L76.0 Intraoperative hemorrhage and hematoma of skin and subcutaneous tissue complicating a procedure**
Excludes1: *intraoperative hemorrhage and hematoma of skin and subcutaneous tissue due to accidental puncture and laceration during a procedure (L76.1-)*
CC **L76.01 Intraoperative hemorrhage and hematoma of skin and subcutaneous tissue complicating a dermatologic procedure**
CC **L76.02 Intraoperative hemorrhage and hematoma of skin and subcutaneous tissue complicating other procedure**
\+ **L76.1 Accidental puncture and laceration of skin and subcutaneous tissue during a procedure**
CC **L76.11 Accidental puncture and laceration of skin and subcutaneous tissue during a dermatologic procedure**
CC **L76.12 Accidental puncture and laceration of skin and subcutaneous tissue during other procedure**
\+ **L76.2 Postprocedural hemorrhage of skin and subcutaneous tissue following a procedure**
CC **L76.21 Postprocedural hemorrhage of skin and subcutaneous tissue following a dermatologic procedure**
CC **L76.22 Postprocedural hemorrhage of skin and subcutaneous tissue following other procedure**

+ **L76.3 Postprocedural hematoma and seroma of skin and subcutaneous issue following a procedure**
  - CC **L76.31 Postprocedural hematoma of skin and subcutaneous tissue following a dermatologic procedure**
  - CC **L76.32 Postprocedural hematoma of skin and subcutaneous tissue following other procedure**
  - CC **L76.33 Postprocedural seroma of skin and subcutaneous tissue following a dermatologic procedure**
  - CC **L76.34 Postprocedural seroma of skin and subcutaneous tissue following other procedure**

+ **L76.8 Other intraoperative and postprocedural complications of skin and subcutaneous tissue**
  Use additional code, if applicable, to further specify disorder
  - **L76.81 Other intraoperative complications of skin and subcutaneous tissue**
  - **L76.82 Other postprocedural complications of skin and subcutaneous tissue**
    AHA CC: 3Q, 2017, 6

Other disorders of the skin and subcutaneous tissue (L80-L99)

L80 Vitiligo
Excludes2: *vitiligo of eyelids (H02.73-)*
vitiligo of vulva (N90.89)
Valid 3-character code, no further characters required

L81 Other disorders of pigmentation
Excludes1: *birthmark NOS (Q82.5)*
Peutz-Jeghers syndrome (Q85.8)
Excludes2: *nevus - see Alphabetical Index*
- **L81.0 Postinflammatory hyperpigmentation**
- **L81.1 Chloasma**
- **L81.2 Freckles**
- **L81.3 Café au lait spots**
- **L81.4 Other melanin hyperpigmentation**
  Lentigo
- **L81.5 Leukoderma, not elsewhere classified**
- **L81.6 Other disorders of diminished melanin formation**
- **L81.7 Pigmented purpuric dermatosis**
  Angioma serpiginosum
- **L81.8 Other specified disorders of pigmentation**
  Iron pigmentation
  Tattoo pigmentation
- **L81.9 Disorder of pigmentation, unspecified**

L82 Seborrheic keratosis
Includes: basal cell papilloma
dermatosis papulosa nigra
Leser-Trélat disease
Excludes2: *seborrheic dermatitis (L21.-)*
- **L82.0 Inflamed seborrheic keratosis**
- **L82.1 Other seborrheic keratosis**
  Seborrheic keratosis NOS

L83 Acanthosis nigricans
Confluent and reticulated papillomatosis
Valid 3-character code, no further characters required

L84 Corns and callosities
Callus
Clavus
Valid 3-character code, no further characters required

L85 Other epidermal thickening
Excludes2: *hypertrophic disorders of the skin (L91.-)*
- **L85.0 Acquired ichthyosis**
  Excludes1: *congenital ichthyosis (Q80.-)*
- **L85.1 Acquired keratosis [keratoderma] palmaris et plantaris**
  Excludes1: *inherited keratosis palmaris et plantaris (Q82.8)*
- **L85.2 Keratosis punctata (palmaris et plantaris)**
- **L85.3 Xerosis cutis**
  Dry skin dermatitis
- **L85.8 Other specified epidermal thickening**
  Cutaneous horn
- **L85.9 Epidermal thickening, unspecified**

L86 Keratoderma in diseases classified elsewhere
Code first underlying disease, such as:
Reiter's disease (M02.3-)
Excludes1: *gonococcal keratoderma (A54.89)*
gonococcal keratosis (A54.89)
keratoderma due to vitamin A deficiency (E50.8)
keratosis due to vitamin A deficiency (E50.8)
xeroderma due to vitamin A deficiency (E50.8)
Valid 3-character code, no further characters required

L87 Transepidermal elimination disorders
Excludes1: *granuloma annulare (perforating) (L92.0)*
- **L87.0 Keratosis follicularis et parafollicularis in cutem penetrans**
  Kyrle disease
  Hyperkeratosis follicularis penetrans
- **L87.1 Reactive perforating collagenosis**
- **L87.2 Elastosis perforans serpiginosa**
- **L87.8 Other transepidermal elimination disorders**
- **L87.9 Transepidermal elimination disorder, unspecified**

CC **L88 Pyoderma gangrenosum**
Phagedenic pyoderma
Excludes1: *dermatitis gangrenosa (L08.0)*
Valid 3-character code, no further characters required

L89 Pressure ulcer
Includes: bed sore
decubitus ulcer
plaster ulcer
pressure area
pressure sore
Code first any associated gangrene (I96)
Excludes2: *decubitus (trophic) ulcer of cervix (uteri) (N86)*
diabetic ulcers (E08.621, E08.622, E09.621, E09.622, E10.621, E10.622, E11.621, E11.622, E13.621, E13.622)
non-pressure chronic ulcer of skin (L97.-)
skin infections (L00-L08)
varicose ulcer (I83.0, I83.2)
AHA CC: 2Q, 2018, 21-22; 4Q, 2019, 10-11
Review coding guidelines B.14 and C.12.a

+ **L89.0 Pressure ulcer of elbow**
  + **L89.00 Pressure ulcer of unspecified elbow**
    - **L89.000 Pressure ulcer of unspecified elbow, unstageable**
    - **L89.001 Pressure ulcer of unspecified elbow, stage 1**
      Healing pressure ulcer of unspecified elbow, stage 1
      Pressure pre-ulcer skin changes limited to persistent focal edema, unspecified elbow
    - **L89.002 Pressure ulcer of unspecified elbow, stage 2**
      Healing pressure ulcer of unspecified elbow, stage 2
      Pressure ulcer with abrasion, blister, partial thickness skin loss involving epidermis and/or dermis, unspecified elbow
    - MCC **L89.003 Pressure ulcer of unspecified elbow, stage 3**
      Healing pressure ulcer of unspecified elbow, stage 3
      Pressure ulcer with full thickness skin loss involving damage or necrosis of subcutaneous tissue, unspecified elbow
      HAC see Appendix B for HAC conditional logic
    - MCC **L89.004 Pressure ulcer of unspecified elbow, stage 4**
      Healing pressure ulcer of unspecified elbow, stage 4
      Pressure ulcer with necrosis of soft tissues through to underlying muscle, tendon, or bone, unspecified elbow
      HAC see Appendix B for HAC conditional logic

Pressure Ulcer

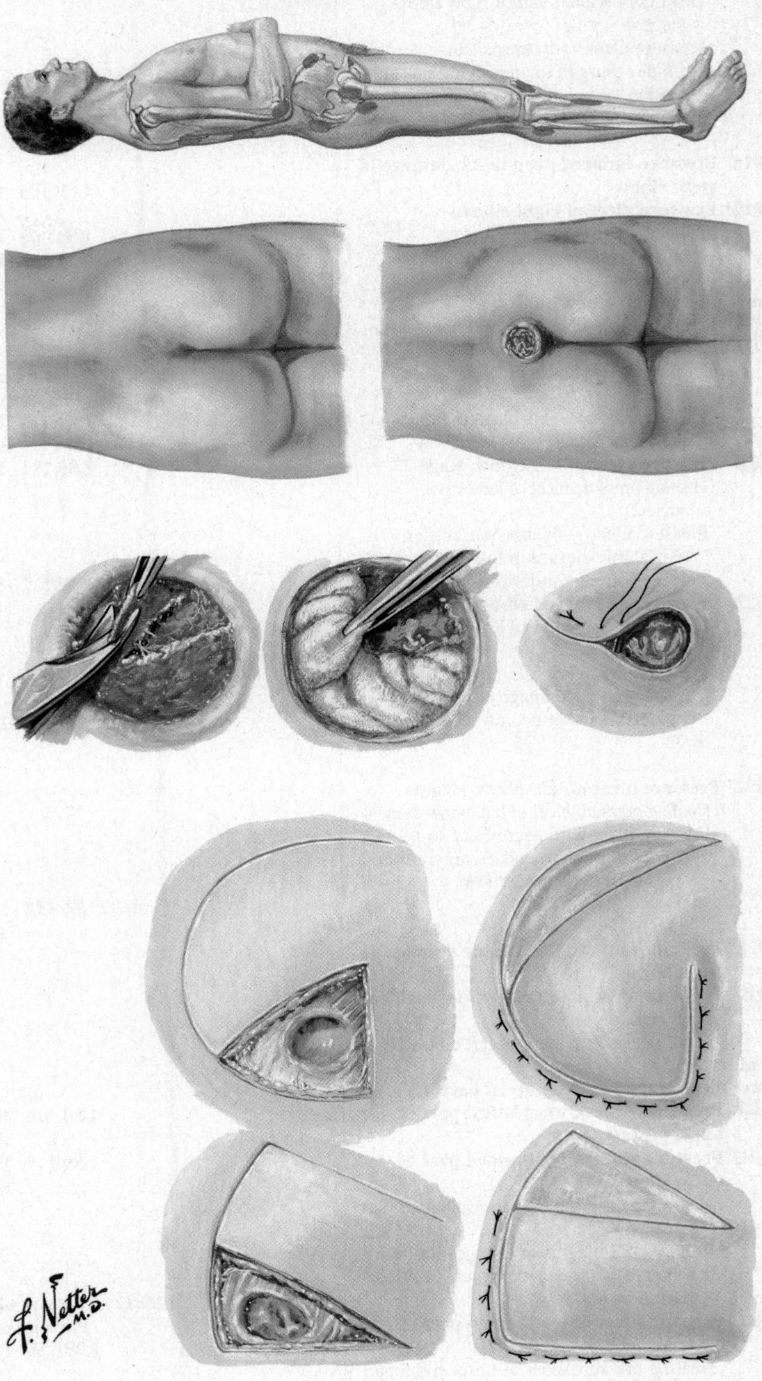

L89.006 Pressure-induced deep tissue damage of unspecified elbow

L89.009 Pressure ulcer of unspecified elbow, unspecified stage
- Healing pressure ulcer of elbow NOS
- Healing pressure ulcer of unspecified elbow, unspecified stage

+ L89.01 Pressure ulcer of right elbow

L89.010 Pressure ulcer of right elbow, unstageable

L89.011 Pressure ulcer of right elbow, stage 1
- Healing pressure ulcer of right elbow, stage 1
- Pressure pre-ulcer skin changes limited to persistent focal edema, right elbow

L89.012 Pressure ulcer of right elbow, stage 2
- Healing pressure ulcer of right elbow, stage 2
- Pressure ulcer with abrasion, blister, partial thickness skin loss involving epidermis and/or dermis, right elbow

MCC **L89.013 Pressure ulcer of right elbow, stage 3**
- Healing pressure ulcer of right elbow, stage 3
- Pressure ulcer with full thickness skin loss involving damage or necrosis of subcutaneous tissue, right elbow

HAC see Appendix B for HAC conditional logic

MCC **L89.014 Pressure ulcer of right elbow, stage 4**
Healing pressure ulcer of right elbow, stage 4
Pressure ulcer with necrosis of soft tissues through to underlying muscle, tendon, or bone, right elbow
HAC see Appendix B for HAC conditional logic

L89.016 Pressure-induced deep tissue damage of right elbow

L89.019 Pressure ulcer of right elbow, unspecified stage
Healing pressure ulcer of right elbow NOS

+ **L89.02 Pressure ulcer of left elbow**

L89.020 Pressure ulcer of left elbow, unstageable

L89.021 Pressure ulcer of left elbow, stage 1
Healing pressure ulcer of left elbow, stage 1
Pressure pre-ulcer skin changes limited to persistent focal edema, left elbow

L89.022 Pressure ulcer of left elbow, stage 2
Healing pressure ulcer of left elbow, stage 2
Pressure ulcer with abrasion, blister, partial thickness skin loss involving epidermis and/or dermis, left elbow

MCC **L89.023 Pressure ulcer of left elbow, stage 3**
Healing pressure ulcer of left elbow, stage 3
Pressure ulcer with full thickness skin loss involving damage or necrosis of subcutaneous tissue, left elbow
HAC see Appendix B for HAC conditional logic

MCC **L89.024 Pressure ulcer of left elbow, stage 4**
Healing pressure ulcer of left elbow, stage 4
Pressure ulcer with necrosis of soft tissues through to underlying muscle, tendon, or bone, left elbow
HAC see Appendix B for HAC conditional logic

L89.026 Pressure-induced deep tissue damage of left elbow

L89.029 Pressure ulcer of left elbow, unspecified stage
Healing pressure ulcer of left elbow NOS

+ **L89.1 Pressure ulcer of back**

+ **L89.10 Pressure ulcer of unspecified part of back**

L89.100 Pressure ulcer of unspecified part of back, unstageable

L89.101 Pressure ulcer of unspecified part of back, stage 1
Healing pressure ulcer of unspecified part of back, stage 1
Pressure pre-ulcer skin changes limited to persistent focal edema, unspecified part of back

L89.102 Pressure ulcer of unspecified part of back, stage 2
Healing pressure ulcer of unspecified part of back, stage 2
Pressure ulcer with abrasion, blister, partial thickness skin loss involving epidermis and/or dermis, unspecified part of back

MCC **L89.103 Pressure ulcer of unspecified part of back, stage 3**
Healing pressure ulcer of unspecified part of back, stage 3
Pressure ulcer with full thickness skin loss involving damage or necrosis of subcutaneous tissue, unspecified part of back
HAC see Appendix B for HAC conditional logic

MCC **L89.104 Pressure ulcer of unspecified part of back, stage 4**
Healing pressure ulcer of unspecified part of back, stage 4
Pressure ulcer with necrosis of soft tissues through to underlying muscle, tendon, or bone, unspecified part of back
HAC see Appendix B for HAC conditional logic

L89.106 Pressure-induced deep tissue damage of unspecified part of back

L89.109 Pressure ulcer of unspecified part of back, unspecified stage
Healing pressure ulcer of unspecified part of back NOS
Healing pressure ulcer of unspecified part of back, unspecified stage

+ **L89.11 Pressure ulcer of right upper back**
Pressure ulcer of right shoulder blade

L89.110 Pressure ulcer of right upper back, unstageable

L89.111 Pressure ulcer of right upper back, stage 1
Healing pressure ulcer of right upper back, stage 1
Pressure pre-ulcer skin changes limited to persistent focal edema, right upper back

L89.112 Pressure ulcer of right upper back, stage 2
Healing pressure ulcer of right upper back, stage 2
Pressure ulcer with abrasion, blister, partial thickness skin loss involving epidermis and/or dermis, right upper back

MCC **L89.113 Pressure ulcer of right upper back, stage 3**
Healing pressure ulcer of right upper back, stage 3
Pressure ulcer with full thickness skin loss involving damage or necrosis of subcutaneous tissue, right upper back
HAC see Appendix B for HAC conditional logic

MCC **L89.114 Pressure ulcer of right upper back, stage 4**
Healing pressure ulcer of right upper back, stage 4
Pressure ulcer with necrosis of soft tissues through to underlying muscle, tendon, or bone, right upper back
HAC see Appendix B for HAC conditional logic

L89.116 Pressure-induced deep tissue damage of right upper back

L89.119 Pressure ulcer of right upper back, unspecified stage
Healing pressure ulcer of right upper back NOS
Healing pressure ulcer of right upper back, unspecified stage

+ **L89.12 Pressure ulcer of left upper back**
Pressure ulcer of left shoulder blade

L89.120 Pressure ulcer of left upper back, unstageable

L89.121 Pressure ulcer of left upper back, stage 1
Healing pressure ulcer of left upper back, stage 1
Pressure pre-ulcer skin changes limited to persistent focal edema, left upper back

L89.122 Pressure ulcer of left upper back, stage 2
Healing pressure ulcer of left upper back, stage 2
Pressure ulcer with abrasion, blister, partial thickness skin loss involving epidermis and/or dermis, left upper back

MCC **L89.123 Pressure ulcer of left upper back, stage 3**
Healing pressure ulcer of left upper back, stage 3
Pressure ulcer with full thickness skin loss involving damage or necrosis of subcutaneous tissue, left upper back
HAC see Appendix B for HAC conditional logic

MCC **L89.124 Pressure ulcer of left upper back, stage 4**
Healing pressure ulcer of left upper back, stage 4
Pressure ulcer with necrosis of soft tissues through to underlying muscle, tendon, or bone, left upper back
HAC see Appendix B for HAC conditional logic

L89.126 Pressure-induced deep tissue damage of left upper back

L89.129 Pressure ulcer of left upper back, unspecified stage
Healing pressure ulcer of left upper back NOS
Healing pressure ulcer of left upper back, unspecified stage

+ L89.13 Pressure ulcer of right lower back

L89.130 Pressure ulcer of right lower back, unstageable

L89.131 Pressure ulcer of right lower back, stage 1
Healing pressure ulcer of right lower back, stage 1
Pressure pre-ulcer skin changes limited to persistent focal edema, right lower back

L89.132 Pressure ulcer of right lower back, stage 2
Healing pressure ulcer of right lower back, stage 2
Pressure ulcer with abrasion, blister, partial thickness skin loss involving epidermis and/or dermis, right lower back

MCC **L89.133 Pressure ulcer of right lower back, stage 3**
Healing pressure ulcer of right lower back, stage 3
Pressure ulcer with full thickness skin loss involving damage or necrosis of subcutaneous tissue, right lower back
HAC see Appendix B for HAC conditional logic

MCC **L89.134 Pressure ulcer of right lower back, stage 4**
Healing pressure ulcer of right lower back, stage 4
Pressure ulcer with necrosis of soft tissues through to underlying muscle, tendon, or bone, right lower back
HAC see Appendix B for HAC conditional logic

L89.136 Pressure-induced deep tissue damage of right lower back

L89.139 Pressure ulcer of right lower back, unspecified stage
Healing pressure ulcer of right lower back NOS
Healing pressure ulcer of right lower back, unspecified stage

+ L89.14 Pressure ulcer of left lower back

L89.140 Pressure ulcer of left lower back, unstageable

L89.141 Pressure ulcer of left lower back, stage 1
Healing pressure ulcer of left lower back, stage 1
Pressure pre-ulcer skin changes limited to persistent focal edema, left lower back

L89.142 Pressure ulcer of left lower back, stage 2
Healing pressure ulcer of left lower back, stage 2
Pressure ulcer with abrasion, blister, partial thickness skin loss involving epidermis and/or dermis, left lower back

MCC **L89.143 Pressure ulcer of left lower back, stage 3**
Healing pressure ulcer of left lower back, stage 3
Pressure ulcer with full thickness skin loss involving damage or necrosis of subcutaneous tissue, left lower back
HAC see Appendix B for HAC conditional logic

MCC **L89.144 Pressure ulcer of left lower back, stage 4**
Healing pressure ulcer of left lower back, stage 4
Pressure ulcer with necrosis of soft tissues through to underlying muscle, tendon, or bone, left lower back
HAC see Appendix B for HAC conditional logic

L89.146 Pressure-induced deep tissue damage of left lower back

L89.149 Pressure ulcer of left lower back, unspecified stage
Healing pressure ulcer of left lower back NOS
Healing pressure ulcer of left lower back, unspecified stage

+ L89.15 Pressure ulcer of sacral region
Pressure ulcer of coccyx
Pressure ulcer of tailbone

L89.150 Pressure ulcer of sacral region, unstageable

L89.151 Pressure ulcer of sacral region, stage 1
Healing pressure ulcer of sacral region, stage 1
Pressure pre-ulcer skin changes limited to persistent focal edema, sacral region

L89.152 Pressure ulcer of sacral region, stage 2
Healing pressure ulcer of sacral region, stage 2
Pressure ulcer with abrasion, blister, partial thickness skin loss involving epidermis and/or dermis, sacral region

MCC **L89.153 Pressure ulcer of sacral region, stage 3**
Healing pressure ulcer of sacral region, stage 3
Pressure ulcer with full thickness skin loss involving damage or necrosis of subcutaneous tissue, sacral region
HAC see Appendix B for HAC conditional logic

MCC **L89.154 Pressure ulcer of sacral region, stage 4**
Healing pressure ulcer of sacral region, stage 4
Pressure ulcer with necrosis of soft tissues through to underlying muscle, tendon, or bone, sacral region
AHA CC: 1Q, 2021, 24
HAC see Appendix B for HAC conditional logic

L89.156 Pressure-induced deep tissue damage of sacral region

L89.159 Pressure ulcer of sacral region, unspecified stage
Healing pressure ulcer of sacral region NOS
Healing pressure ulcer of sacral region, unspecified stage

+ L89.2 **Pressure ulcer of hip**

+ L89.20 **Pressure ulcer of unspecified hip**

L89.200 **Pressure ulcer of unspecified hip, unstageable**

L89.201 **Pressure ulcer of unspecified hip, stage 1**
Healing pressure ulcer of unspecified hip back, stage 1
Pressure pre-ulcer skin changes limited to persistent focal edema, unspecified hip

L89.202 **Pressure ulcer of unspecified hip, stage 2**
Healing pressure ulcer of unspecified hip, stage 2
Pressure ulcer with abrasion, blister, partial thickness skin loss involving epidermis and/or dermis, unspecified hip

MCC L89.203 **Pressure ulcer of unspecified hip, stage 3**
Healing pressure ulcer of unspecified hip, stage 3
Pressure ulcer with full thickness skin loss involving damage or necrosis of subcutaneous tissue, unspecified hip
HAC see Appendix B for HAC conditional logic

MCC L89.204 **Pressure ulcer of unspecified hip, stage 4**
Healing pressure ulcer of unspecified hip, stage 4
Pressure ulcer with necrosis of soft tissues through to underlying muscle, tendon, or bone, unspecified hip
HAC see Appendix B for HAC conditional logic

L89.206 **Pressure-induced deep tissue damage of unspecified hip**

L89.209 **Pressure ulcer of unspecified hip, unspecified stage**
Healing pressure ulcer of unspecified hip NOS
Healing pressure ulcer of unspecified hip, unspecified stage

+ L89.21 **Pressure ulcer of right hip**

L89.210 **Pressure ulcer of right hip, unstageable**

L89.211 **Pressure ulcer of right hip, stage 1**
Healing pressure ulcer of right hip back, stage 1
Pressure pre-ulcer skin changes limited to persistent focal edema, right hip

L89.212 **Pressure ulcer of right hip, stage 2**
Healing pressure ulcer of right hip, stage 2
Pressure ulcer with abrasion, blister, partial thickness skin loss involving epidermis and/or dermis, right hip

MCC L89.213 **Pressure ulcer of right hip, stage 3**
Healing pressure ulcer of right hip, stage 3
Pressure ulcer with full thickness skin loss involving damage or necrosis of subcutaneous tissue, right hip
HAC see Appendix B for HAC conditional logic

MCC L89.214 **Pressure ulcer of right hip, stage 4**
Healing pressure ulcer of right hip, stage 4
Pressure ulcer with necrosis of soft tissues through to underlying muscle, tendon, or bone, right hip
HAC see Appendix B for HAC conditional logic

L89.216 **Pressure-induced deep tissue damage of right hip**

L89.219 **Pressure ulcer of right hip, unspecified stage**
Healing pressure ulcer of right hip NOS
Healing pressure ulcer of right hip, unspecified stage

+ L89.22 **Pressure ulcer of left hip**

L89.220 **Pressure ulcer of left hip, unstageable**

L89.221 **Pressure ulcer of left hip, stage 1**
Healing pressure ulcer of left hip back, stage 1
Pressure pre-ulcer skin changes limited to persistent focal edema, left hip

L89.222 **Pressure ulcer of left hip, stage 2**
Healing pressure ulcer of left hip, stage 2
Pressure ulcer with abrasion, blister, partial thickness skin loss involving epidermis and/or dermis, left hip

MCC L89.223 **Pressure ulcer of left hip, stage 3**
Healing pressure ulcer of left hip, stage 3
Pressure ulcer with full thickness skin loss involving damage or necrosis of subcutaneous tissue, left hip
HAC see Appendix B for HAC conditional logic

MCC L89.224 **Pressure ulcer of left hip, stage 4**
Healing pressure ulcer of left hip, stage 4
Pressure ulcer with necrosis of soft tissues through to underlying muscle, tendon, or bone, left hip
HAC see Appendix B for HAC conditional logic

L89.226 **Pressure-induced deep tissue damage of left hip**

L89.229 **Pressure ulcer of left hip, unspecified stage**
Healing pressure ulcer of left hip NOS
Healing pressure ulcer of left hip, unspecified stage

+ L89.3 **Pressure ulcer of buttock**

+ L89.30 **Pressure ulcer of unspecified buttock**

L89.300 **Pressure ulcer of unspecified buttock, unstageable**

L89.301 **Pressure ulcer of unspecified buttock, stage 1**
Healing pressure ulcer of unspecified buttock, stage 1
Pressure pre-ulcer skin changes limited to persistent focal edema, unspecified buttock

L89.302 **Pressure ulcer of unspecified buttock, stage 2**
Healing pressure ulcer of unspecified buttock, stage 2
Pressure ulcer with abrasion, blister, partial thickness skin loss involving epidermis and/or dermis, unspecified buttock

MCC L89.303 **Pressure ulcer of unspecified buttock, stage 3**
Healing pressure ulcer of unspecified buttock, stage 3
Pressure ulcer with full thickness skin loss involving damage or necrosis of subcutaneous tissue, unspecified buttock
HAC see Appendix B for HAC conditional logic

MCC L89.304 **Pressure ulcer of unspecified buttock, stage 4**
Healing pressure ulcer of unspecified buttock, stage 4
Pressure ulcer with necrosis of soft tissues through to underlying muscle, tendon, or bone, unspecified buttock
HAC see Appendix B for HAC conditional logic

L89.306 **Pressure-induced deep tissue damage of unspecified buttock**

L89.309 **Pressure ulcer of unspecified buttock, unspecified stage**
Healing pressure ulcer of unspecified buttock NOS
Healing pressure ulcer of unspecified buttock, unspecified stage

+ L89.31 **Pressure ulcer of right buttock**

L89.310 **Pressure ulcer of right buttock, unstageable**

L89.311 **Pressure ulcer of right buttock, stage 1**
Healing pressure ulcer of right buttock, stage 1
Pressure pre-ulcer skin changes limited to persistent focal edema, right buttock

L89.312 **Pressure ulcer of right buttock, stage 2**
Healing pressure ulcer of right buttock, stage 2
Pressure ulcer with abrasion, blister, partial thickness skin loss involving epidermis and/or dermis, right buttock

MCC **L89.313** **Pressure ulcer of right buttock, stage 3**
Healing pressure ulcer of right buttock, stage 3
Pressure ulcer with full thickness skin loss involving damage or necrosis of subcutaneous tissue, right buttock
HAC see Appendix B for HAC conditional logic

MCC **L89.314** **Pressure ulcer of right buttock, stage 4**
Healing pressure ulcer of right buttock, stage 4
Pressure ulcer with necrosis of soft tissues through to underlying muscle, tendon, or bone, right buttock
HAC see Appendix B for HAC conditional logic

L89.316 **Pressure-induced deep tissue damage of right buttock**

L89.319 **Pressure ulcer of right buttock, unspecified stage**
Healing pressure ulcer of right buttock NOS
Healing pressure ulcer of right buttock, unspecified stage

+ L89.32 **Pressure ulcer of left buttock**

L89.320 **Pressure ulcer of left buttock, unstageable**

L89.321 **Pressure ulcer of left buttock, stage 1**
Healing pressure ulcer of left buttock, stage 1
Pressure pre-ulcer skin changes limited to persistent focal edema, left buttock

L89.322 **Pressure ulcer of left buttock, stage 2**
Healing pressure ulcer of left buttock, stage 2
Pressure ulcer with abrasion, blister, partial thickness skin loss involving epidermis and/or dermis, left buttock

MCC **L89.323** **Pressure ulcer of left buttock, stage 3**
Healing pressure ulcer of left buttock, stage 3
Pressure ulcer with full thickness skin loss involving damage or necrosis of subcutaneous tissue, left buttock
HAC see Appendix B for HAC conditional logic

MCC **L89.324** **Pressure ulcer of left buttock, stage 4**
Healing pressure ulcer of left buttock, stage 4
Pressure ulcer with necrosis of soft tissues through to underlying muscle, tendon, or bone, left buttock
HAC see Appendix B for HAC conditional logic

L89.326 **Pressure-induced deep tissue damage of left buttock**

L89.329 **Pressure ulcer of left buttock, unspecified stage**
Healing pressure ulcer of left buttock NOS
Healing pressure ulcer of left buttock, unspecified stage

+ L89.4 **Pressure ulcer of contiguous site of back, buttock and hip**

L89.40 **Pressure ulcer of contiguous site of back, buttock and hip, unspecified stage**
Healing pressure ulcer of contiguous site of back, buttock and hip NOS
Healing pressure ulcer of contiguous site of back, buttock and hip, unspecified stage

L89.41 **Pressure ulcer of contiguous site of back, buttock and hip, stage 1**
Healing pressure ulcer of contiguous site of back, buttock and hip, stage 1
Pressure pre-ulcer skin changes limited to persistent focal edema, contiguous site of back, buttock and hip

L89.42 **Pressure ulcer of contiguous site of back, buttock and hip, stage 2**
Healing pressure ulcer of contiguous site of back, buttock and hip, stage 2
Pressure ulcer with abrasion, blister, partial thickness skin loss involving epidermis and/or dermis, contiguous site of back, buttock and hip

MCC **L89.43** **Pressure ulcer of contiguous site of back, buttock and hip, stage 3**
Healing pressure ulcer of contiguous site of back, buttock and hip, stage 3
Pressure ulcer with full thickness skin loss involving damage or necrosis of subcutaneous tissue, contiguous site of back, buttock and hip
HAC see Appendix B for HAC conditional logic

MCC **L89.44** **Pressure ulcer of contiguous site of back, buttock and hip, stage 4**
Healing pressure ulcer of contiguous site of back, buttock and hip, stage 4
Pressure ulcer with necrosis of soft tissues through to underlying muscle, tendon, or bone, contiguous site of back, buttock and hip
HAC see Appendix B for HAC conditional logic

L89.45 **Pressure ulcer of contiguous site of back, buttock and hip, unstageable**

L89.46 **Pressure-induced deep tissue damage of contiguous site of back, buttock and hip**

+ L89.5 **Pressure ulcer of ankle**

+ L89.50 **Pressure ulcer of unspecified ankle**

L89.500 **Pressure ulcer of unspecified ankle, unstageable**

L89.501 **Pressure ulcer of unspecified ankle, stage 1**
Healing pressure ulcer of unspecified ankle, stage 1
Pressure pre-ulcer skin changes limited to persistent focal edema, unspecified ankle

L89.502 **Pressure ulcer of unspecified ankle, stage 2**
Healing pressure ulcer of unspecified ankle, stage 2
Pressure ulcer with abrasion, blister, partial thickness skin loss involving epidermis and/or dermis, unspecified ankle

MCC **L89.503** **Pressure ulcer of unspecified ankle, stage 3**
Healing pressure ulcer of unspecified ankle, stage 3
Pressure ulcer with full thickness skin loss involving damage or necrosis of subcutaneous tissue, unspecified ankle
HAC see Appendix B for HAC conditional logic

MCC **L89.504** **Pressure ulcer of unspecified ankle, stage 4**
Healing pressure ulcer of unspecified ankle, stage 4
Pressure ulcer with necrosis of soft tissues through to underlying muscle, tendon, or bone, unspecified ankle
HAC see Appendix B for HAC conditional logic

L89.506 Pressure-induced deep tissue damage of unspecified ankle

L89.509 Pressure ulcer of unspecified ankle, unspecified stage
Healing pressure ulcer of unspecified ankle NOS
Healing pressure ulcer of unspecified ankle, unspecified stage

+ L89.51 Pressure ulcer of right ankle

L89.510 Pressure ulcer of right ankle, unstageable

L89.511 Pressure ulcer of right ankle, stage 1
Healing pressure ulcer of right ankle, stage 1
Pressure pre-ulcer skin changes limited to persistent focal edema, right ankle

L89.512 Pressure ulcer of right ankle, stage 2
Healing pressure ulcer of right ankle, stage 2
Pressure ulcer with abrasion, blister, partial thickness skin loss involving epidermis and/or dermis, right ankle

MCC **L89.513 Pressure ulcer of right ankle, stage 3**
Healing pressure ulcer of right ankle, stage 3
Pressure ulcer with full thickness skin loss involving damage or necrosis of subcutaneous tissue, right ankle
HAC see Appendix B for HAC conditional logic

MCC **L89.514 Pressure ulcer of right ankle, stage 4**
Healing pressure ulcer of right ankle, stage 4
Pressure ulcer with necrosis of soft tissues through to underlying muscle, tendon, or bone, right ankle
HAC see Appendix B for HAC conditional logic

L89.516 Pressure-induced deep tissue damage of right ankle

L89.519 Pressure ulcer of right ankle, unspecified stage
Healing pressure ulcer of right ankle NOS
Healing pressure ulcer of right ankle, unspecified stage

+ L89.52 Pressure ulcer of left ankle

L89.520 Pressure ulcer of left ankle, unstageable

L89.521 Pressure ulcer of left ankle, stage 1
Healing pressure ulcer of left ankle, stage 1
Pressure pre-ulcer skin changes limited to persistent focal edema, left ankle

L89.522 Pressure ulcer of left ankle, stage 2
Healing pressure ulcer of left ankle, stage 2
Pressure ulcer with abrasion, blister, partial thickness skin loss involving epidermis and/or dermis, left ankle

MCC **L89.523 Pressure ulcer of left ankle, stage 3**
Healing pressure ulcer of left ankle, stage 3
Pressure ulcer with full thickness skin loss involving damage or necrosis of subcutaneous tissue, left ankle
HAC see Appendix B for HAC conditional logic

MCC **L89.524 Pressure ulcer of left ankle, stage 4**
Healing pressure ulcer of left ankle, stage 4
Pressure ulcer with necrosis of soft tissues through to underlying muscle, tendon, or bone, left ankle
HAC see Appendix B for HAC conditional logic

L89.526 Pressure-induced deep tissue damage of left ankle

L89.529 Pressure ulcer of left ankle, unspecified stage
Healing pressure ulcer of left ankle NOS
Healing pressure ulcer of left ankle, unspecified stage

+ L89.6 Pressure ulcer of heel

+ L89.60 Pressure ulcer of unspecified heel

L89.600 Pressure ulcer of unspecified heel, unstageable

L89.601 Pressure ulcer of unspecified heel, stage 1
Healing pressure ulcer of unspecified heel, stage 1
Pressure pre-ulcer skin changes limited to persistent focal edema, unspecified heel

L89.602 Pressure ulcer of unspecified heel, stage 2
Healing pressure ulcer of unspecified heel, stage 2
Pressure ulcer with abrasion, blister, partial thickness skin loss involving epidermis and/or dermis, unspecified heel

MCC **L89.603 Pressure ulcer of unspecified heel, stage 3**
Healing pressure ulcer of unspecified heel, stage 3
Pressure ulcer with full thickness skin loss involving damage or necrosis of subcutaneous tissue, unspecified heel
HAC see Appendix B for HAC conditional logic

MCC **L89.604 Pressure ulcer of unspecified heel, stage 4**
Healing pressure ulcer of unspecified heel, stage 4
Pressure ulcer with necrosis of soft tissues through to underlying muscle, tendon, or bone, unspecified heel
HAC see Appendix B for HAC conditional logic

L89.606 Pressure-induced deep tissue damage of unspecified heel

L89.609 Pressure ulcer of unspecified heel, unspecified stage
Healing pressure ulcer of unspecified heel NOS
Healing pressure ulcer of unspecified heel, unspecified stage

+ L89.61 Pressure ulcer of right heel

L89.610 Pressure ulcer of right heel, unstageable

L89.611 Pressure ulcer of right heel, stage 1
Healing pressure ulcer of right heel, stage 1
Pressure pre-ulcer skin changes limited to persistent focal edema, right heel

L89.612 Pressure ulcer of right heel, stage 2
Healing pressure ulcer of right heel, stage 2
Pressure ulcer with abrasion, blister, partial thickness skin loss involving epidermis and/or dermis, right heel

MCC **L89.613 Pressure ulcer of right heel, stage 3**
Healing pressure ulcer of right heel, stage 3
Pressure ulcer with full thickness skin loss involving damage or necrosis of subcutaneous tissue, right heel
HAC see Appendix B for HAC conditional logic

MCC **L89.614 Pressure ulcer of right heel, stage 4**
Healing pressure ulcer of right heel, stage 4
Pressure ulcer with necrosis of soft tissues through to underlying muscle, tendon, or bone, right heel
HAC see Appendix B for HAC conditional logic

L89.616 **Pressure-induced deep tissue damage of right heel**
L89.619 **Pressure ulcer of right heel, unspecified stage**
Healing pressure ulcer of right heel NOS
Healing pressure ulcer of right heel, unspecified stage

+ L89.62 **Pressure ulcer of left heel**
L89.620 **Pressure ulcer of left heel, unstageable**
L89.621 **Pressure ulcer of left heel, stage 1**
Healing pressure ulcer of left heel, stage 1
Pressure pre-ulcer skin changes limited to persistent focal edema, left heel
L89.622 **Pressure ulcer of left heel, stage 2**
Healing pressure ulcer of left heel, stage 2
Pressure ulcer with abrasion, blister, partial thickness skin loss involving epidermis and/or dermis, left heel
AHA CC: 4Q, 2016, 144
MCC L89.623 **Pressure ulcer of left heel, stage 3**
Healing pressure ulcer of left heel, stage 3
Pressure ulcer with full thickness skin loss involving damage or necrosis of subcutaneous tissue, left heel
AHA CC: 4Q, 2016, 144; 3Q, 2018, 3-4
HAC see Appendix B for HAC conditional logic
MCC L89.624 **Pressure ulcer of left heel, stage 4**
Healing pressure ulcer of left heel, stage 4
Pressure ulcer with necrosis of soft tissues through to underlying muscle, tendon, or bone, left heel
HAC see Appendix B for HAC conditional logic
L89.626 **Pressure-induced deep tissue damage of left heel**
L89.629 **Pressure ulcer of left heel, unspecified stage**
Healing pressure ulcer of left heel NOS
Healing pressure ulcer of left heel, unspecified stage

+ L89.8 **Pressure ulcer of other site**
+ L89.81 **Pressure ulcer of head**
Pressure ulcer of face
L89.810 **Pressure ulcer of head, unstageable**
L89.811 **Pressure ulcer of head, stage 1**
Healing pressure ulcer of head, stage 1
Pressure pre-ulcer skin changes limited to persistent focal edema, head
L89.812 **Pressure ulcer of head, stage 2**
Healing pressure ulcer of head, stage 2
Pressure ulcer with abrasion, blister, partial thickness skin loss involving epidermis and/or dermis, head
MCC L89.813 **Pressure ulcer of head, stage 3**
Healing pressure ulcer of head, stage 3
Pressure ulcer with full thickness skin loss involving damage or necrosis of subcutaneous tissue, head
HAC see Appendix B for HAC conditional logic
MCC L89.814 **Pressure ulcer of head, stage 4**
Healing pressure ulcer of head, stage 4
Pressure ulcer with necrosis of soft tissues through to underlying muscle, tendon, or bone, head
HAC see Appendix B for HAC conditional logic
L89.816 **Pressure-induced deep tissue damage of head**
L89.819 **Pressure ulcer of head, unspecified stage**
Healing pressure ulcer of head NOS
Healing pressure ulcer of head, unspecified stage

+ L89.89 **Pressure ulcer of other site**
L89.890 **Pressure ulcer of other site, unstageable**
L89.891 **Pressure ulcer of other site, stage 1**
Healing pressure ulcer of other site, stage 1
Pressure pre-ulcer skin changes limited to persistent focal edema, other site
L89.892 **Pressure ulcer of other site, stage 2**
Healing pressure ulcer of other site, stage 2
Pressure ulcer with abrasion, blister, partial thickness skin loss involving epidermis and/or dermis, other site
MCC L89.893 **Pressure ulcer of other site, stage 3**
Healing pressure ulcer of other site, stage 3
Pressure ulcer with full thickness skin loss involving damage or necrosis of subcutaneous tissue, other site
HAC see Appendix B for HAC conditional logic
MCC L89.894 **Pressure ulcer of other site, stage 4**
Healing pressure ulcer of other site, stage 4
Pressure ulcer with necrosis of soft tissues through to underlying muscle, tendon, or bone, other site
HAC see Appendix B for HAC conditional logic
L89.896 **Pressure-induced deep tissue damage of other site**
L89.899 **Pressure ulcer of other site, unspecified stage**
Healing pressure ulcer of other site NOS
Healing pressure ulcer of other site, unspecified stage

+ L89.9 **Pressure ulcer of unspecified site**
L89.90 **Pressure ulcer of unspecified site, unspecified stage**
Healing pressure ulcer of unspecified site NOS
Healing pressure ulcer of unspecified site, unspecified stage
L89.91 **Pressure ulcer of unspecified site, stage 1**
Healing pressure ulcer of unspecified site, stage 1
Pressure pre-ulcer skin changes limited to persistent focal edema, unspecified site
L89.92 **Pressure ulcer of unspecified site, stage 2**
Healing pressure ulcer of unspecified site, stage 2
Pressure ulcer with abrasion, blister, partial thickness skin loss involving epidermis and/or dermis, unspecified site
MCC L89.93 **Pressure ulcer of unspecified site, stage 3**
Healing pressure ulcer of unspecified site, stage 3
Pressure ulcer with full thickness skin loss involving damage or necrosis of subcutaneous tissue, unspecified site
HAC see Appendix B for HAC conditional logic
MCC L89.94 **Pressure ulcer of unspecified site, stage 4**
Healing pressure ulcer of unspecified site, stage 4
Pressure ulcer with necrosis of soft tissues through to underlying muscle, tendon, or bone, unspecified site
HAC see Appendix B for HAC conditional logic
L89.95 **Pressure ulcer of unspecified site, unstageable**
L89.96 **Pressure-induced deep tissue damage of unspecified site**

L90 Atrophic disorders of skin

L90.0 **Lichen sclerosus et atrophicus**
Excludes2: *lichen sclerosus of external female genital organs (N90.4)*
lichen sclerosus of external male genital organs (N48.0)
L90.1 **Anetoderma of Schweninger-Buzzi**
L90.2 **Anetoderma of Jadassohn-Pellizzari**
L90.3 **Atrophoderma of Pasini and Pierini**
L90.4 **Acrodermatitis chronica atrophicans**

L90.5 Scar conditions and fibrosis of skin
Adherent scar (skin)
Cicatrix
Disfigurement of skin due to scar
Fibrosis of skin NOS
Scar NOS
Excludes2: *hypertrophic scar (L91.0)*
keloid scar (L91.0)
AHA CC: 1Q, 2015, 19; 2Q, 2016, 5

L90.6 Striae atrophicae
L90.8 Other atrophic disorders of skin
L90.9 Atrophic disorder of skin, unspecified

L91 Hypertrophic disorders of skin

L91.0 Hypertrophic scar
Keloid
Keloid scar
Excludes2: *acne keloid (L73.0)*
scar NOS (L90.5)

L91.8 Other hypertrophic disorders of the skin
L91.9 Hypertrophic disorder of the skin, unspecified

L92 Granulomatous disorders of skin and subcutaneous tissue

Excludes2: *actinic granuloma (L57.5)*

L92.0 Granuloma annulare
Perforating granuloma annulare

L92.1 Necrobiosis lipoidica, not elsewhere classified
Excludes1: *necrobiosis lipoidica associated with diabetes mellitus (E08-E13 with .620)*

L92.2 Granuloma faciale [eosinophilic granuloma of skin]
L92.3 Foreign body granuloma of the skin and subcutaneous tissue
Use additional code to identify the type of retained foreign body (Z18.-)

L92.8 Other granulomatous disorders of the skin and subcutaneous tissue
L92.9 Granulomatous disorder of the skin and subcutaneous tissue, unspecified
Excludes2: *umbilical granuloma (P83.81)*

L93 Lupus erythematosus

Use additional code for adverse effect, if applicable, to identify drug (T36-T50 with fifth or sixth character 5)

Excludes1: *lupus exedens (A18.4)*
lupus vulgaris (A18.4)
scleroderma (M34.-)
systemic lupus erythematosus (M32.-)

L93.0 Discoid lupus erythematosus
Lupus erythematosus NOS

L93.1 Subacute cutaneous lupus erythematosus
L93.2 Other local lupus erythematosus
Lupus erythematosus profundus
Lupus panniculitis

L94 Other localized connective tissue disorders

Excludes1: *systemic connective tissue disorders (M30-M36)*

L94.0 Localized scleroderma [morphea]
Circumscribed scleroderma

L94.1 Linear scleroderma
En coup de sabre lesion

L94.2 Calcinosis cutis
L94.3 Sclerodactyly
L94.4 Gottron's papules
L94.5 Poikiloderma vasculare atrophicans
L94.6 Ainhum
L94.8 Other specified localized connective tissue disorders
L94.9 Localized connective tissue disorder, unspecified

L95 Vasculitis limited to skin, not elsewhere classified

Excludes1: *angioma serpiginosum (L81.7)*
Henoch(-Schönlein) purpura (D69.0)
hypersensitivity angiitis (M31.0)
lupus panniculitis (L93.2)
panniculitis NOS (M79.3)
panniculitis of neck and back (M54.0-)
polyarteritis nodosa (M30.0)
relapsing panniculitis (M35.6)
rheumatoid vasculitis (M05.2)
serum sickness (T80.6-)
urticaria (L50.-)
Wegener's granulomatosis (M31.3-)

L95.0 Livedoid vasculitis
Atrophie blanche (en plaque)

L95.1 Erythema elevatum diutinum
L95.8 Other vasculitis limited to the skin
L95.9 Vasculitis limited to the skin, unspecified

L97 Non-pressure chronic ulcer of lower limb, not elsewhere classified

Includes: chronic ulcer of skin of lower limb NOS
non-healing ulcer of skin
non-infected sinus of skin
trophic ulcer NOS
tropical ulcer NOS
ulcer of skin of lower limb NOS

Code first any associated underlying condition, such as:
any associated gangrene (I96)
atherosclerosis of the lower extremities (I70.23-, I70.24-, I70.33-, I70.34-, I70.43-, I70.44-, I70.53-, I70.54-, I70.63-, I70.64-, I70.73-, I70.74-)
chronic venous hypertension (I87.31-, I87.33-)
diabetic ulcers (E08.621, E08.622, E09.621, E09.622, E10.621, E10.622, E11.621, E11.622, E13.621, E13.622)
postphlebitic syndrome (I87.01-, I87.03-)
postthrombotic syndrome (I87.01-, I87.03-)
varicose ulcer (I83.0-, I83.2-)

Excludes2: *pressure ulcer (pressure area) (L89.-)*
skin infections (L00-L08)
specific infections classified to A00-B99

AHA CC: 4Q, 2017, 17
Review coding guidelines B.14 and C.12.b

+ **L97.1 Non-pressure chronic ulcer of thigh**
  + **L97.10 Non-pressure chronic ulcer of unspecified thigh**
    - CC **L97.101 Non-pressure chronic ulcer of unspecified thigh limited to breakdown of skin**
    - CC **L97.102 Non-pressure chronic ulcer of unspecified thigh with fat layer exposed**
    - CC **L97.103 Non-pressure chronic ulcer of unspecified thigh with necrosis of muscle**
    - CC **L97.104 Non-pressure chronic ulcer of unspecified thigh with necrosis of bone**
    - CC **L97.105 Non-pressure chronic ulcer of unspecified thigh with muscle involvement without evidence of necrosis**
    - CC **L97.106 Non-pressure chronic ulcer of unspecified thigh with bone involvement without evidence of necrosis**
    - CC **L97.108 Non-pressure chronic ulcer of unspecified thigh with other specified severity**
    - CC **L97.109 Non-pressure chronic ulcer of unspecified thigh with unspecified severity**

+ L97.11 Non-pressure chronic ulcer of right thigh
  - CC L97.111 Non-pressure chronic ulcer of right thigh limited to breakdown of skin
  - CC L97.112 Non-pressure chronic ulcer of right thigh with fat layer exposed
  - CC L97.113 Non-pressure chronic ulcer of right thigh with necrosis of muscle
  - CC L97.114 Non-pressure chronic ulcer of right thigh with necrosis of bone
  - CC L97.115 Non-pressure chronic ulcer of right thigh with muscle involvement without evidence of necrosis
  - CC L97.116 Non-pressure chronic ulcer of right thigh with bone involvement without evidence of necrosis
  - CC L97.118 Non-pressure chronic ulcer of right thigh with other specified severity
  - CC L97.119 Non-pressure chronic ulcer of right thigh with unspecified severity

+ L97.12 Non-pressure chronic ulcer of left thigh
  - CC L97.121 Non-pressure chronic ulcer of left thigh limited to breakdown of skin
  - CC L97.122 Non-pressure chronic ulcer of left thigh with fat layer exposed
  - CC L97.123 Non-pressure chronic ulcer of left thigh with necrosis of muscle
  - CC L97.124 Non-pressure chronic ulcer of left thigh with necrosis of bone
  - CC L97.125 Non-pressure chronic ulcer of left thigh with muscle involvement without evidence of necrosis
  - CC L97.126 Non-pressure chronic ulcer of left thigh with bone involvement without evidence of necrosis
  - CC L97.128 Non-pressure chronic ulcer of left thigh with other specified severity
  - CC L97.129 Non-pressure chronic ulcer of left thigh with unspecified severity

+ L97.2 Non-pressure chronic ulcer of calf

+ L97.20 Non-pressure chronic ulcer of unspecified calf
  - CC L97.201 Non-pressure chronic ulcer of unspecified calf limited to breakdown of skin
  - CC L97.202 Non-pressure chronic ulcer of unspecified calf with fat layer exposed
  - CC L97.203 Non-pressure chronic ulcer of unspecified calf with necrosis of muscle
  - CC L97.204 Non-pressure chronic ulcer of unspecified calf with necrosis of bone
  - CC L97.205 Non-pressure chronic ulcer of unspecified calf with muscle involvement without evidence of necrosis
  - CC L97.206 Non-pressure chronic ulcer of unspecified calf with bone involvement without evidence of necrosis
  - CC L97.208 Non-pressure chronic ulcer of unspecified calf with other specified severity
  - CC L97.209 Non-pressure chronic ulcer of unspecified calf with unspecified severity

+ L97.21 Non-pressure chronic ulcer of right calf
  - CC L97.211 Non-pressure chronic ulcer of right calf limited to breakdown of skin
  - CC L97.212 Non-pressure chronic ulcer of right calf with fat layer exposed
  - CC L97.213 Non-pressure chronic ulcer of right calf with necrosis of muscle
  - CC L97.214 Non-pressure chronic ulcer of right calf with necrosis of bone
  - CC L97.215 Non-pressure chronic ulcer of right calf with muscle involvement without evidence of necrosis
  - CC L97.216 Non-pressure chronic ulcer of right calf with bone involvement without evidence of necrosis
  - CC L97.218 Non-pressure chronic ulcer of right calf with other specified severity
  - CC L97.219 Non-pressure chronic ulcer of right calf with unspecified severity

+ L97.22 Non-pressure chronic ulcer of left calf
  - CC L97.221 Non-pressure chronic ulcer of left calf limited to breakdown of skin
  - CC L97.222 Non-pressure chronic ulcer of left calf with fat layer exposed
    AHA CC: 1Q, 2016, 12-13
  - CC L97.223 Non-pressure chronic ulcer of left calf with necrosis of muscle
  - CC L97.224 Non-pressure chronic ulcer of left calf with necrosis of bone
  - CC L97.225 Non-pressure chronic ulcer of left calf with muscle involvement without evidence of necrosis
  - CC L97.226 Non-pressure chronic ulcer of left calf with bone involvement without evidence of necrosis
  - CC L97.228 Non-pressure chronic ulcer of left calf with other specified severity
  - CC L97.229 Non-pressure chronic ulcer of left calf with unspecified severity

+ L97.3 Non-pressure chronic ulcer of ankle

+ L97.30 Non-pressure chronic ulcer of unspecified ankle
  - CC L97.301 Non-pressure chronic ulcer of unspecified ankle limited to breakdown of skin
  - CC L97.302 Non-pressure chronic ulcer of unspecified ankle with fat layer exposed
  - CC L97.303 Non-pressure chronic ulcer of unspecified ankle with necrosis of muscle
  - CC L97.304 Non-pressure chronic ulcer of unspecified ankle with necrosis of bone
  - CC L97.305 Non-pressure chronic ulcer of unspecified ankle with muscle involvement without evidence of necrosis
  - CC L97.306 Non-pressure chronic ulcer of unspecified ankle with bone involvement without evidence of necrosis
  - CC L97.308 Non-pressure chronic ulcer of unspecified ankle with other specified severity
  - CC L97.309 Non-pressure chronic ulcer of unspecified ankle with unspecified severity

+ L97.31 Non-pressure chronic ulcer of right ankle
  - CC L97.311 Non-pressure chronic ulcer of right ankle limited to breakdown of skin
  - CC L97.312 Non-pressure chronic ulcer of right ankle with fat layer exposed
  - CC L97.313 Non-pressure chronic ulcer of right ankle with necrosis of muscle
  - CC L97.314 Non-pressure chronic ulcer of right ankle with necrosis of bone
  - CC L97.315 Non-pressure chronic ulcer of right ankle with muscle involvement without evidence of necrosis
    AHA CC: 4Q, 2017, 17
  - CC L97.316 Non-pressure chronic ulcer of right ankle with bone involvement without evidence of necrosis
  - CC L97.318 Non-pressure chronic ulcer of right ankle with other specified severity
  - CC L97.319 Non-pressure chronic ulcer of right ankle with unspecified severity

+ **L97.32 Non-pressure chronic ulcer of left ankle**
  - CC **L97.321** **Non-pressure chronic ulcer of left ankle limited to breakdown of skin**
  - CC **L97.322** **Non-pressure chronic ulcer of left ankle with fat layer exposed**
    AHA CC: 1Q, 2021, 7-8
  - CC **L97.323** **Non-pressure chronic ulcer of left ankle with necrosis of muscle**
  - CC **L97.324** **Non-pressure chronic ulcer of left ankle with necrosis of bone**
  - CC **L97.325** **Non-pressure chronic ulcer of left ankle with muscle involvement without evidence of necrosis**
  - CC **L97.326** **Non-pressure chronic ulcer of left ankle with bone involvement without evidence of necrosis**
  - CC **L97.328** **Non-pressure chronic ulcer of left ankle with other specified severity**
  - CC **L97.329** **Non-pressure chronic ulcer of left ankle with unspecified severity**

+ **L97.4 Non-pressure chronic ulcer of heel and midfoot**
  Non-pressure chronic ulcer of plantar surface of midfoot

+ **L97.40 Non-pressure chronic ulcer of unspecified heel and midfoot**
  - CC **L97.401** **Non-pressure chronic ulcer of unspecified heel and midfoot limited to breakdown of skin**
  - CC **L97.402** **Non-pressure chronic ulcer of unspecified heel and midfoot with fat layer exposed**
  - CC **L97.403** **Non-pressure chronic ulcer of unspecified heel and midfoot with necrosis of muscle**
  - CC **L97.404** **Non-pressure chronic ulcer of unspecified heel and midfoot with necrosis of bone**
  - CC **L97.405** **Non-pressure chronic ulcer of unspecified heel and midfoot with muscle involvement without evidence of necrosis**
  - CC **L97.406** **Non-pressure chronic ulcer of unspecified heel and midfoot with bone involvement without evidence of necrosis**
  - CC **L97.408** **Non-pressure chronic ulcer of unspecified heel and midfoot with other specified severity**
  - CC **L97.409** **Non-pressure chronic ulcer of unspecified heel and midfoot with unspecified severity**

+ **L97.41 Non-pressure chronic ulcer of right heel and midfoot**
  - CC **L97.411** **Non-pressure chronic ulcer of right heel and midfoot limited to breakdown of skin**
  - CC **L97.412** **Non-pressure chronic ulcer of right heel and midfoot with fat layer exposed**
    AHA CC: 2Q, 2020, 19
  - CC **L97.413** **Non-pressure chronic ulcer of right heel and midfoot with necrosis of muscle**
  - CC **L97.414** **Non-pressure chronic ulcer of right heel and midfoot with necrosis of bone**
  - CC **L97.415** **Non-pressure chronic ulcer of right heel and midfoot with muscle involvement without evidence of necrosis**
  - CC **L97.416** **Non-pressure chronic ulcer of right heel and midfoot with bone involvement without evidence of necrosis**
  - CC **L97.418** **Non-pressure chronic ulcer of right heel and midfoot with other specified severity**
  - CC **L97.419** **Non-pressure chronic ulcer of right heel and midfoot with unspecified severity**

+ **L97.42 Non-pressure chronic ulcer of left heel and midfoot**
  - CC **L97.421** **Non-pressure chronic ulcer of left heel and midfoot limited to breakdown of skin**
  - CC **L97.422** **Non-pressure chronic ulcer of left heel and midfoot with fat layer exposed**
  - CC **L97.423** **Non-pressure chronic ulcer of left heel and midfoot with necrosis of muscle**
  - CC **L97.424** **Non-pressure chronic ulcer of left heel and midfoot with necrosis of bone**
  - CC **L97.425** **Non-pressure chronic ulcer of left heel and midfoot with muscle involvement without evidence of necrosis**
  - CC **L97.426** **Non-pressure chronic ulcer of left heel and midfoot with bone involvement without evidence of necrosis**
  - CC **L97.428** **Non-pressure chronic ulcer of left heel and midfoot with other specified severity**
  - CC **L97.429** **Non-pressure chronic ulcer of left heel and midfoot with unspecified severity**

+ **L97.5 Non-pressure chronic ulcer of other part of foot**
  Non-pressure chronic ulcer of toe

+ **L97.50 Non-pressure chronic ulcer of other part of unspecified foot**
  - **L97.501** **Non-pressure chronic ulcer of other part of unspecified foot limited to breakdown of skin**
  - **L97.502** **Non-pressure chronic ulcer of other part of unspecified foot with fat layer exposed**
  - **L97.503** **Non-pressure chronic ulcer of other part of unspecified foot with necrosis of muscle**
  - **L97.504** **Non-pressure chronic ulcer of other part of unspecified foot with necrosis of bone**
  - CC **L97.505** **Non-pressure chronic ulcer of other part of unspecified foot with muscle involvement without evidence of necrosis**
  - CC **L97.506** **Non-pressure chronic ulcer of other part of unspecified foot with bone involvement without evidence of necrosis**
  - CC **L97.508** **Non-pressure chronic ulcer of other part of unspecified foot with other specified severity**
  - **L97.509** **Non-pressure chronic ulcer of other part of unspecified foot with unspecified severity**

+ **L97.51 Non-pressure chronic ulcer of other part of right foot**
  - **L97.511** **Non-pressure chronic ulcer of other part of right foot limited to breakdown of skin**
    AHA CC: 1Q, 2020, 12
  - **L97.512** **Non-pressure chronic ulcer of other part of right foot with fat layer exposed**
    AHA CC: 2Q, 2020, 19-20
  - **L97.513** **Non-pressure chronic ulcer of other part of right foot with necrosis of muscle**
  - **L97.514** **Non-pressure chronic ulcer of other part of right foot with necrosis of bone**
  - CC **L97.515** **Non-pressure chronic ulcer of other part of right foot with muscle involvement without evidence of necrosis**
  - CC **L97.516** **Non-pressure chronic ulcer of other part of right foot with bone involvement without evidence of necrosis**
  - CC **L97.518** **Non-pressure chronic ulcer of other part of right foot with other specified severity**
  - **L97.519** **Non-pressure chronic ulcer of other part of right foot with unspecified severity**

+ L97.52 Non-pressure chronic ulcer of other part of left foot
L97.521 Non-pressure chronic ulcer of other part of left foot limited to breakdown of skin
L97.522 Non-pressure chronic ulcer of other part of left foot with fat layer exposed
L97.523 Non-pressure chronic ulcer of other part of left foot with necrosis of muscle
L97.524 Non-pressure chronic ulcer of other part of left foot with necrosis of bone
CC L97.525 Non-pressure chronic ulcer of other part of left foot with muscle involvement without evidence of necrosis
CC L97.526 Non-pressure chronic ulcer of other part of left foot with bone involvement without evidence of necrosis
CC L97.528 Non-pressure chronic ulcer of other part of left foot with other specified severity
L97.529 Non-pressure chronic ulcer of other part of left foot with unspecified severity
+ L97.8 Non-pressure chronic ulcer of other part of lower leg
+ L97.80 Non-pressure chronic ulcer of other part of unspecified lower leg
CC L97.801 Non-pressure chronic ulcer of other part of unspecified lower leg limited to breakdown of skin
CC L97.802 Non-pressure chronic ulcer of other part of unspecified lower leg with fat layer exposed
CC L97.803 Non-pressure chronic ulcer of other part of unspecified lower leg with necrosis of muscle
CC L97.804 Non-pressure chronic ulcer of other part of unspecified lower leg with necrosis of bone
CC L97.805 Non-pressure chronic ulcer of other part of unspecified lower leg with muscle involvement without evidence of necrosis
CC L97.806 Non-pressure chronic ulcer of other part of unspecified lower leg with bone involvement without evidence of necrosis
CC L97.808 Non-pressure chronic ulcer of other part of unspecified lower leg with other specified severity
CC L97.809 Non-pressure chronic ulcer of other part of unspecified lower leg with unspecified severity
+ L97.81 Non-pressure chronic ulcer of other part of right lower leg
CC L97.811 Non-pressure chronic ulcer of other part of right lower leg limited to breakdown of skin
CC L97.812 Non-pressure chronic ulcer of other part of right lower leg with fat layer exposed
CC L97.813 Non-pressure chronic ulcer of other part of right lower leg with necrosis of muscle
CC L97.814 Non-pressure chronic ulcer of other part of right lower leg with necrosis of bone
CC L97.815 Non-pressure chronic ulcer of other part of right lower leg with muscle involvement without evidence of necrosis
CC L97.816 Non-pressure chronic ulcer of other part of right lower leg with bone involvement without evidence of necrosis
CC L97.818 Non-pressure chronic ulcer of other part of right lower leg with other specified severity
CC L97.819 Non-pressure chronic ulcer of other part of right lower leg with unspecified severity
+ L97.82 Non-pressure chronic ulcer of other part of left lower leg
CC L97.821 Non-pressure chronic ulcer of other part of left lower leg limited to breakdown of skin
CC L97.822 Non-pressure chronic ulcer of other part of left lower leg with fat layer exposed
CC L97.823 Non-pressure chronic ulcer of other part of left lower leg with necrosis of muscle
CC L97.824 Non-pressure chronic ulcer of other part of left lower leg with necrosis of bone
CC L97.825 Non-pressure chronic ulcer of other part of left lower leg with muscle involvement without evidence of necrosis
CC L97.826 Non-pressure chronic ulcer of other part of left lower leg with bone involvement without evidence of necrosis
CC L97.828 Non-pressure chronic ulcer of other part of left lower leg with other specified severity
CC L97.829 Non-pressure chronic ulcer of other part of left lower leg with unspecified severity
+ L97.9 Non-pressure chronic ulcer of unspecified part of lower leg
+ L97.90 Non-pressure chronic ulcer of unspecified part of unspecified lower leg
CC L97.901 Non-pressure chronic ulcer of unspecified part of unspecified lower leg limited to breakdown of skin
CC L97.902 Non-pressure chronic ulcer of unspecified part of unspecified lower leg with fat layer exposed
CC L97.903 Non-pressure chronic ulcer of unspecified part of unspecified lower leg with necrosis of muscle
CC L97.904 Non-pressure chronic ulcer of unspecified part of unspecified lower leg with necrosis of bone
CC L97.905 Non-pressure chronic ulcer of unspecified part of unspecified lower leg with muscle involvement without evidence of necrosis
CC L97.906 Non-pressure chronic ulcer of unspecified part of unspecified lower leg with bone involvement without evidence of necrosis
CC L97.908 Non-pressure chronic ulcer of unspecified part of unspecified lower leg with other specified severity
CC L97.909 Non-pressure chronic ulcer of unspecified part of unspecified lower leg with unspecified severity
+ L97.91 Non-pressure chronic ulcer of unspecified part of right lower leg
CC L97.911 Non-pressure chronic ulcer of unspecified part of right lower leg limited to breakdown of skin
CC L97.912 Non-pressure chronic ulcer of unspecified part of right lower leg with fat layer exposed
CC L97.913 Non-pressure chronic ulcer of unspecified part of right lower leg with necrosis of muscle

CC **L97.914 Non-pressure chronic ulcer of unspecified part of right lower leg with necrosis of bone**

CC **L97.915 Non-pressure chronic ulcer of unspecified part of right lower leg with muscle involvement without evidence of necrosis**

CC **L97.916 Non-pressure chronic ulcer of unspecified part of right lower leg with bone involvement without evidence of necrosis**

CC **L97.918 Non-pressure chronic ulcer of unspecified part of right lower leg with other specified severity**

CC **L97.919 Non-pressure chronic ulcer of unspecified part of right lower leg with unspecified severity**

+ **L97.92 Non-pressure chronic ulcer of unspecified part of left lower leg**

CC **L97.921 Non-pressure chronic ulcer of unspecified part of left lower leg limited to breakdown of skin**

CC **L97.922 Non-pressure chronic ulcer of unspecified part of left lower leg with fat layer exposed**

CC **L97.923 Non-pressure chronic ulcer of unspecified part of left lower leg with necrosis of muscle**

CC **L97.924 Non-pressure chronic ulcer of unspecified part of left lower leg with necrosis of bone**

CC **L97.925 Non-pressure chronic ulcer of unspecified part of left lower leg with muscle involvement without evidence of necrosis**

CC **L97.926 Non-pressure chronic ulcer of unspecified part of left lower leg with bone involvement without evidence of necrosis**

CC **L97.928 Non-pressure chronic ulcer of unspecified part of left lower leg with other specified severity**

CC **L97.929 Non-pressure chronic ulcer of unspecified part of left lower leg with unspecified severity**

L98 Other disorders of skin and subcutaneous tissue, not elsewhere classified

L98.0 Pyogenic granuloma

Excludes2: *pyogenic granuloma of gingiva (K06.8)*
pyogenic granuloma of maxillary alveolar ridge (K04.5)
pyogenic granuloma of oral mucosa (K13.4)

L98.1 Factitial dermatitis

Neurotic excoriation

Excludes1: *Excoriation (skin-picking) disorder (F42.4)*

L98.2 Febrile neutrophilic dermatosis [Sweet]

CC **L98.3 Eosinophilic cellulitis [Wells]**

+ **L98.4 Non-pressure chronic ulcer of skin, not elsewhere classified**

Chronic ulcer of skin NOS
Tropical ulcer NOS
Ulcer of skin NOS

Excludes2: *pressure ulcer (pressure area) (L89.-)*
gangrene (I96)
skin infections (L00-L08)
specific infections classified to A00-B99
ulcer of lower limb NEC (L97.-)
varicose ulcer (I83.0-I83.93)

AHA CC: 4Q, 2017, 17

+ **L98.41 Non-pressure chronic ulcer of buttock**

L98.411 Non-pressure chronic ulcer of buttock limited to breakdown of skin

L98.412 Non-pressure chronic ulcer of buttock with fat layer exposed

L98.413 Non-pressure chronic ulcer of buttock with necrosis of muscle

L98.414 Non-pressure chronic ulcer of buttock with necrosis of bone

CC **L98.415 Non-pressure chronic ulcer of buttock with muscle involvement without evidence of necrosis**

CC **L98.416 Non-pressure chronic ulcer of buttock with bone involvement without evidence of necrosis**

CC **L98.418 Non-pressure chronic ulcer of buttock with other specified severity**

L98.419 Non-pressure chronic ulcer of buttock with unspecified severity

+ **L98.42 Non-pressure chronic ulcer of back**

L98.421 Non-pressure chronic ulcer of back limited to breakdown of skin

L98.422 Non-pressure chronic ulcer of back with fat layer exposed

L98.423 Non-pressure chronic ulcer of back with necrosis of muscle

L98.424 Non-pressure chronic ulcer of back with necrosis of bone

CC **L98.425 Non-pressure chronic ulcer of back with muscle involvement without evidence of necrosis**

CC **L98.426 Non-pressure chronic ulcer of back with bone involvement without evidence of necrosis**

CC **L98.428 Non-pressure chronic ulcer of back with other specified severity**

L98.429 Non-pressure chronic ulcer of back with unspecified severity

+ **L98.49 Non-pressure chronic ulcer of skin of other sites**

Non-pressure chronic ulcer of skin NOS

L98.491 Non-pressure chronic ulcer of skin of other sites limited to breakdown of skin

L98.492 Non-pressure chronic ulcer of skin of other sites with fat layer exposed

L98.493 Non-pressure chronic ulcer of skin of other sites with necrosis of muscle

L98.494 Non-pressure chronic ulcer of skin of other sites with necrosis of bone

CC **L98.495 Non-pressure chronic ulcer of skin of other sites with muscle involvement without evidence of necrosis**

CC **L98.496 Non-pressure chronic ulcer of skin of other sites with bone involvement without evidence of necrosis**

CC **L98.498 Non-pressure chronic ulcer of skin of other sites with other specified severity**

L98.499 Non-pressure chronic ulcer of skin of other sites with unspecified severity

L98.5 Mucinosis of the skin

Focal mucinosis
Lichen myxedematosus
Reticular erythematous mucinosis

Excludes1: *focal oral mucinosis (K13.79)*
myxedema (E03.9)

L98.6 Other infiltrative disorders of the skin and subcutaneous tissue

Excludes1: *hyalinosis cutis et mucosae (E78.89)*

L98.7 Excessive and redundant skin and subcutaneous tissue

Loose or sagging skin following bariatric surgery weight loss

Loose or sagging skin following dietary weight loss

Loose or sagging skin, NOS

Excludes2: *acquired excess or redundant skin of eyelid (H02.3-)*
congenital excess or redundant skin or eyelid (Q10.3)
skin changes due to chronic exposure to nonionizing radiation (L57.-)

AHA CC: 4Q, 2016, 36

L98.8 Other specified disorders of the skin and subcutaneous tissue

AHA CC: 2Q, 2013, 32-33

L98,9 Disorder of the skin and subcutaneous tissue, unspecified

L99 Other disorders of skin and subcutaneous tissue in diseases classified elsewhere

Code first underlying disease, such as:
amyloidosis (E85.-)

Excludes1: *skin disorders in diabetes (E08-E13 with .62-)*
skin disorders in gonorrhea (A54.89)
skin disorders in syphilis (A51.31, A52.79)

AHA CC: 1Q, 2021, 39-40

Valid 3-character code, no further characters required

Intervertebral Joint

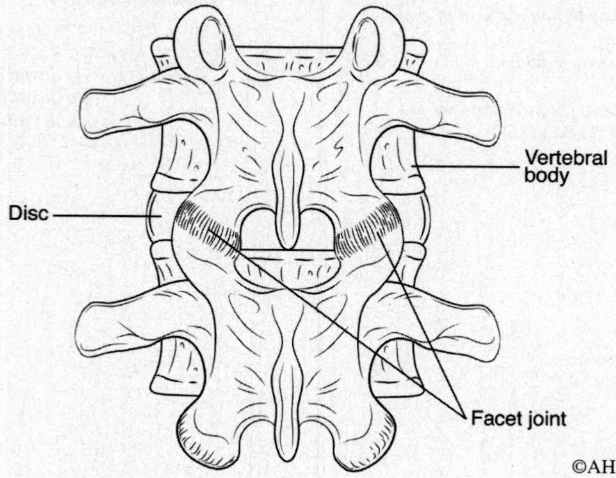

Shoulder Joint

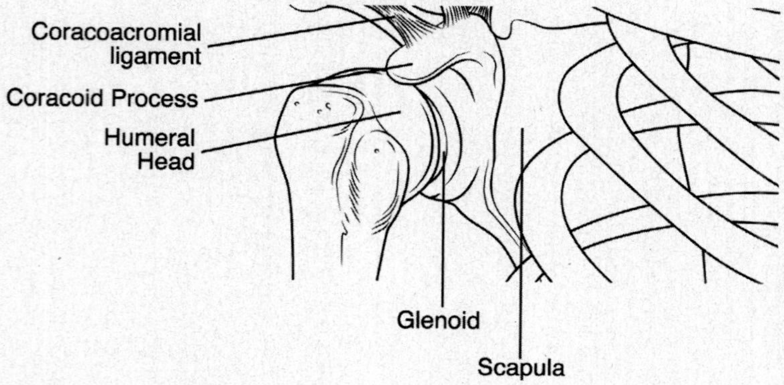

Elbow

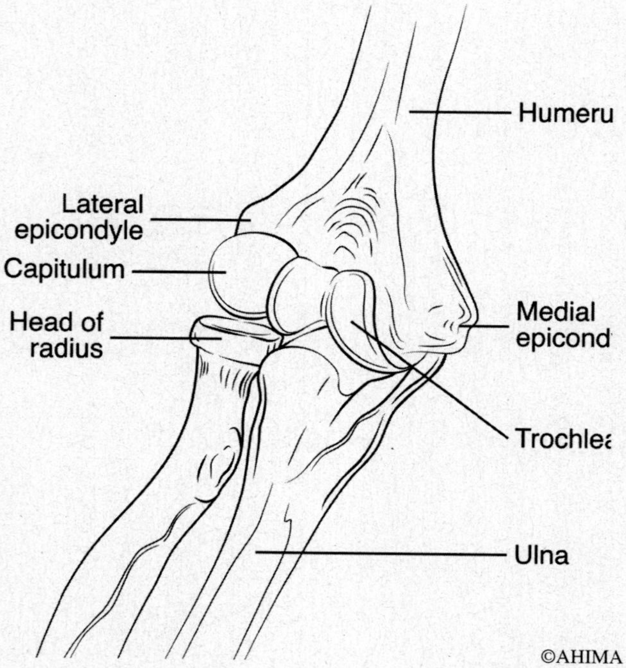

Wrist

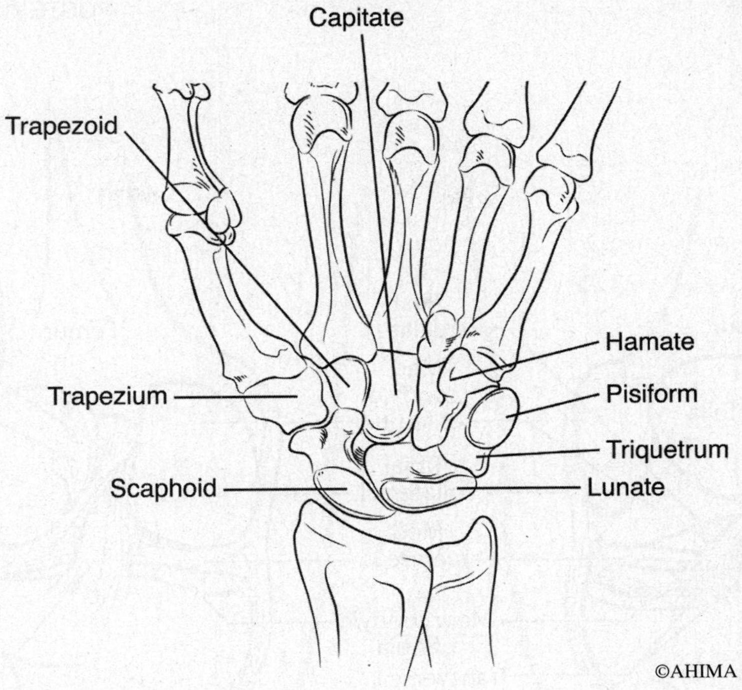

Hip Joint

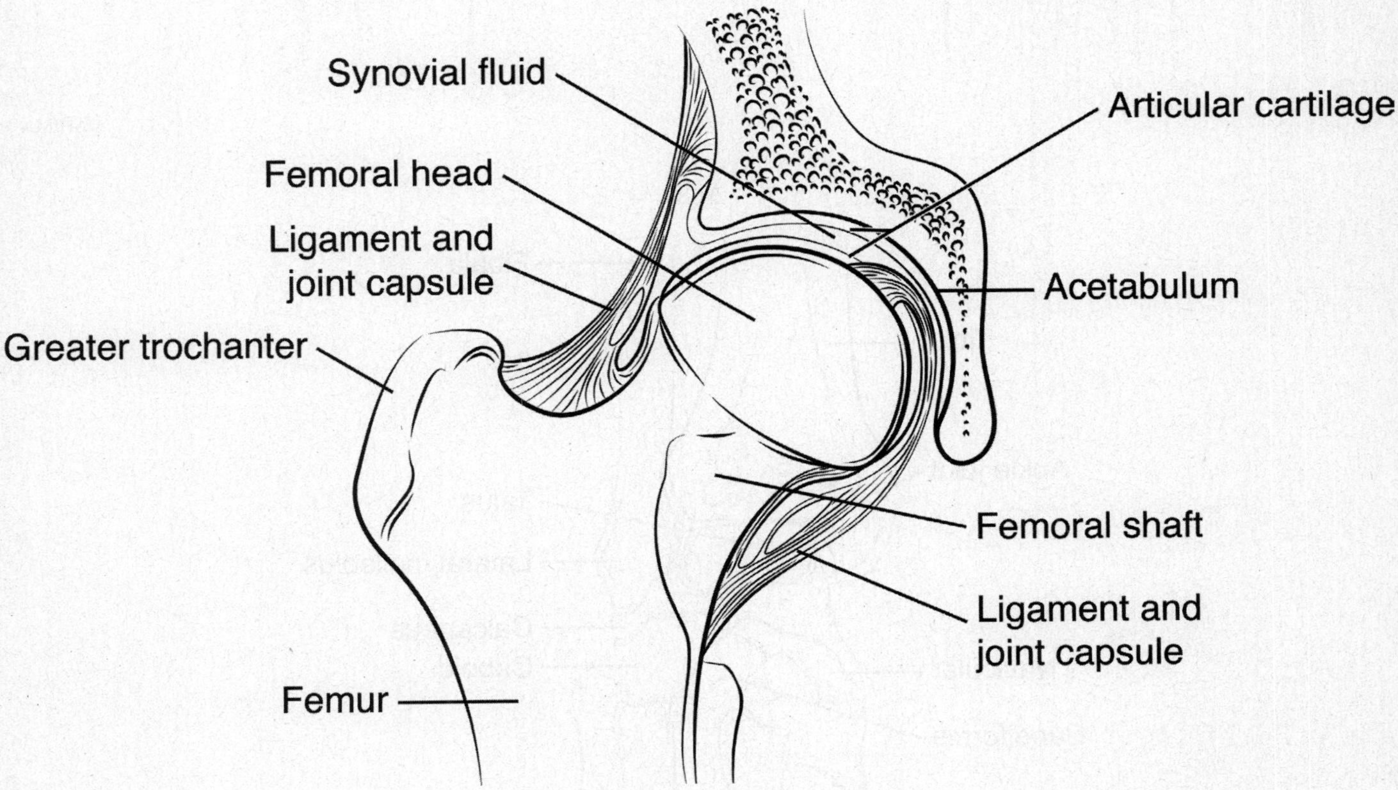

Knee Joint

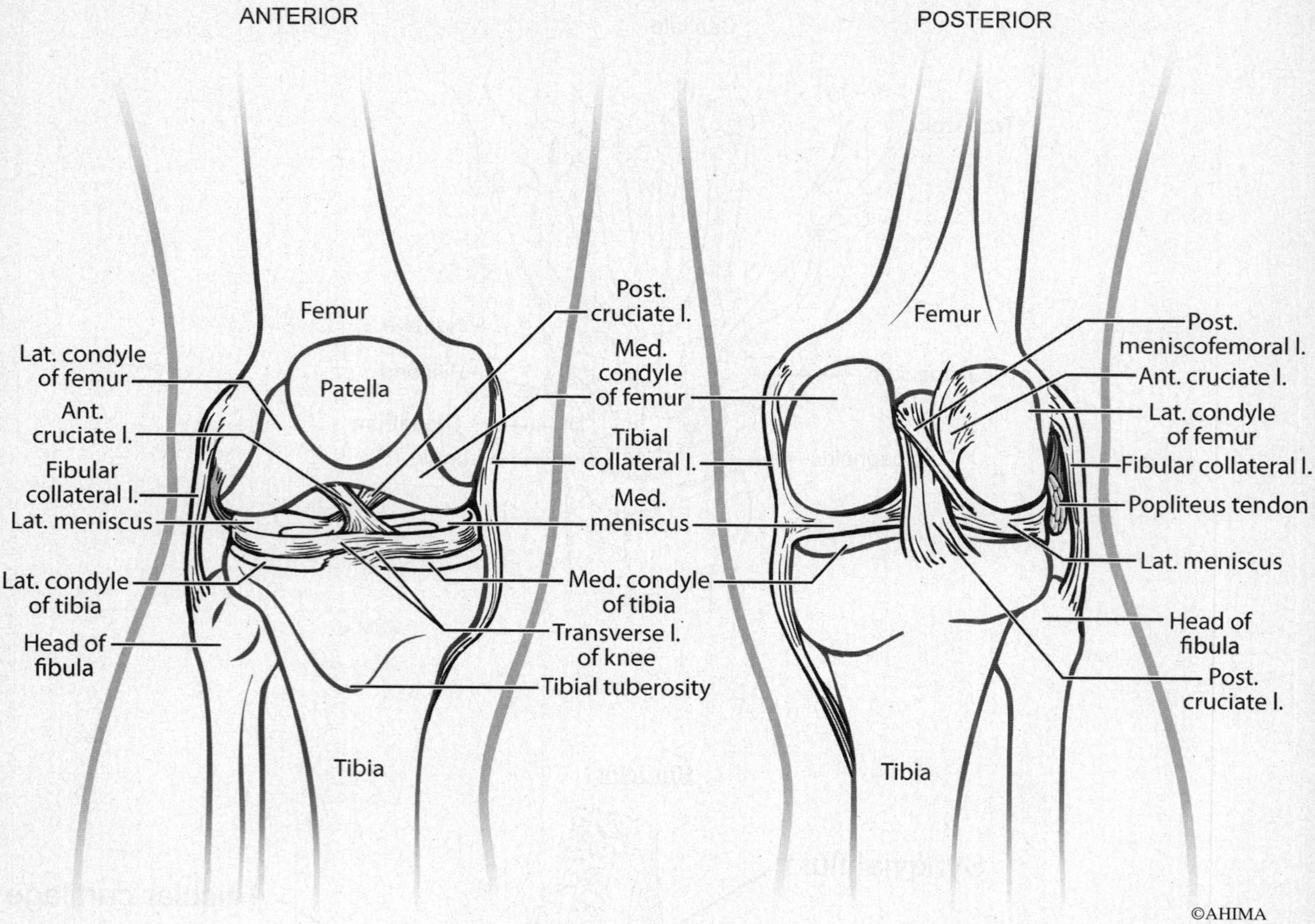

Ankle

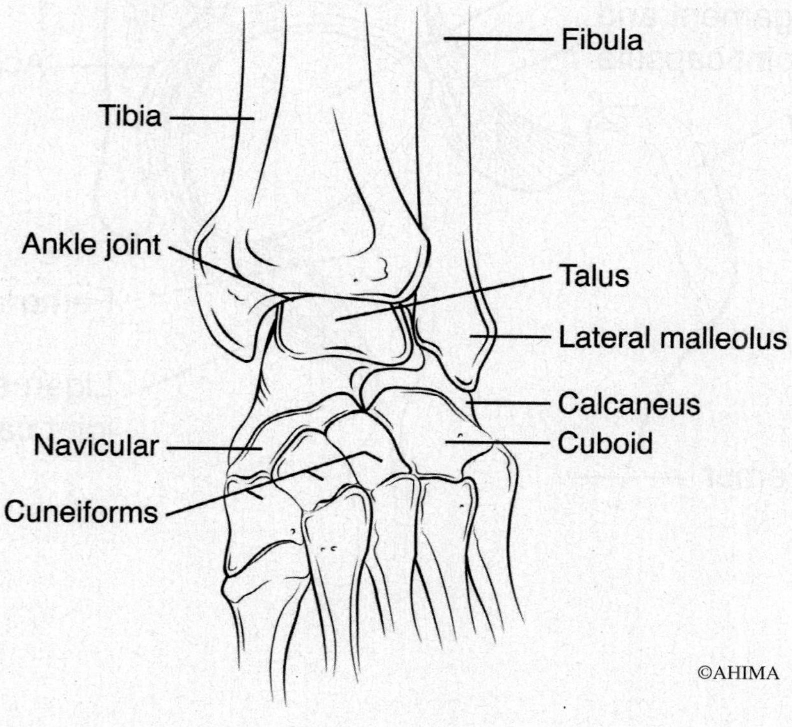

Chapter 13: Diseases of the Musculoskeletal System and Connective Tissue (M00-M99)

NOTE Use an external cause code following the code for the musculoskeletal condition, if applicable, to identify the cause of the musculoskeletal condition

Excludes2: *arthropathic psoriasis (L40.5-)*
certain conditions originating in the perinatal period (P04-P96)
certain infectious and parasitic diseases (A00-B99)
compartment syndrome (traumatic) (T79.A-)
complications of pregnancy, childbirth and the puerperium (O00-O9A)
congenital malformations, deformations, and chromosomal abnormalities (Q00-Q99)
endocrine, nutritional and metabolic diseases (E00-E88)
injury, poisoning and certain other consequences of external causes (S00-T88)
neoplasms (C00-D49)
symptoms, signs and abnormal clinical and laboratory findings, not elsewhere classified (R00-R94)

This chapter contains the following category blocks:

M00-M02	Infectious arthropathies
M04	Autoinflammatory syndromes
M05-M14	Inflammatory polyarthropathies
M15-M19	Osteoarthritis
M20-M25	Other joint disorders
M26-M27	Dentofacial anomalies [including malocclusion] and other disorders of jaw
M30-M36	Systemic connective tissue disorders
M40-M43	Deforming dorsopathies
M45-M49	Spondylopathies
M50-M54	Other dorsopathies
M60-M63	Disorders of muscles
M65-M67	Disorders of synovium and tendon
M70-M79	Other soft tissue disorders
M80-M85	Disorders of bone density and structure
M86-M90	Other osteopathies
M91-M94	Chondropathies
M95	Other disorders of the musculoskeletal system and connective tissue
M96	Intraoperative and postprocedural complications and disorders of musculoskeletal system, not elsewhere classified
M97	Periprosthetic fracture around internal prosthetic joint
M99	Biomechanical lesions, not elsewhere classified

C. Chapter-Specific Coding Guidelines

In addition to general coding guidelines, there are guidelines for specific diagnoses and/or conditions in the classification. Unless otherwise indicated, these guidelines apply to all health care settings. Please refer to Section II for guidelines on the selection of principal diagnosis.

13. Chapter 13: Diseases of the Musculoskeletal System and Connective Tissue (M00-M99)

a. Site and laterality

Most of the codes within Chapter 13 have site and laterality designations. The site represents the bone, joint or the muscle involved. For some conditions where more than one bone, joint or muscle is usually involved, such as osteoarthritis, there is a "multiple sites" code available. For categories where no multiple site code is provided and more than one bone, joint or muscle is involved, multiple codes should be used to indicate the different sites involved.

1) Bone versus joint

For certain conditions, the bone may be affected at the upper or lower end, (e.g., avascular necrosis of bone, M87, Osteoporosis, M80, M81). Though the portion of the bone affected may be at the joint, the site designation will be the bone, not the joint.

b. Acute traumatic versus chronic or recurrent musculoskeletal conditions

Many musculoskeletal conditions are a result of previous injury or trauma to a site, or are recurrent conditions. Bone, joint or muscle conditions that are the result of a healed injury are usually found in chapter 13. Recurrent bone, joint or muscle conditions are also usually found in chapter 13. Any current, acute injury should be coded to the appropriate injury code from chapter 19. Chronic or recurrent conditions should generally be coded with a code from chapter 13. If it is difficult to determine from the documentation in the record which code is best to describe a condition, query the provider.

c. Coding of Pathologic Fractures

7th character A is for use as long as the patient is receiving active treatment for the fracture. While the patient may be seen by a new or different provider over the course of treatment for a pathological fracture, assignment of the 7th character is based on whether the patient is undergoing active treatment and not whether the provider is seeing the patient for the first time.

7th character, D is to be used for encounters after the patient has completed active treatment for the fracture and is receiving routine care for the fracture during the healing or recovery phase. The other 7th characters, listed under each subcategory in the Tabular List, are to be used for subsequent encounters for routine care of fractures during the healing and recovery phase as well as treatment of problems associated with the healing, such as malunions, nonunions, and sequelae.

Care for complications of surgical treatment for fracture repairs during the healing or recovery phase should be coded with the appropriate complication codes.

See Section I.C.19. Coding of traumatic fractures.

d. Osteoporosis

Osteoporosis is a systemic condition, meaning that all bones of the musculoskeletal system are affected. Therefore, site is not a component of the codes under category M81, Osteoporosis without current pathological fracture. The site codes under category M80, Osteoporosis with current pathological fracture, identify the site of the fracture, not the osteoporosis.

1) Osteoporosis without pathological fracture

Category M81, Osteoporosis without current pathological fracture, is for use for patients with osteoporosis who do not currently have a pathologic fracture due to the osteoporosis, even if they have had a fracture in the past. For patients with a history of osteoporosis fractures, status code Z87.310, Personal history of (healed) osteoporosis fracture, should follow the code from M81.

2) Osteoporosis with current pathological fracture

Category M80, Osteoporosis with current pathological fracture, is for patients who have a current pathologic fracture at the time of an encounter. The codes under M80 identify the site of the fracture. A code from category M80, not a traumatic fracture code, should be used for any patient with known osteoporosis who suffers a fracture, even if the patient had a minor fall or trauma, if that fall or trauma would not usually break a normal, healthy bone.

e. Multisystem Inflammatory Syndrome

See Section I.C.1.g.1.l for Multisystem Inflammatory Syndrome

ARTHROPATHIES (M00-M25)

Includes: Disorders affecting predominantly peripheral (limb) joints

Infectious arthropathies (M00-M02)

NOTE This block comprises arthropathies due to microbiological agents. Distinction is made between the following types of etiological relationship:
a) direct infection of joint, where organisms invade synovial tissue and microbial antigen is present in the joint;
b) indirect infection, which may be of two types: a reactive arthropathy, where microbial infection of the body is established but neither organisms nor antigens can be identified in the joint, and a postinfective arthropathy, where microbial antigen is present but recovery of an organism is inconstant and evidence of local multiplication is lacking.

M00 Pyogenic arthritis

Excludes2: *infection and inflammatory reaction due to internal joint prosthesis (T84.5-)*

\+ **M00.0 Staphylococcal arthritis and polyarthritis**
Use additional code (B95.61-B95.8) to identify bacterial agent

CC **M00.00 Staphylococcal arthritis, unspecified joint**
\+ **M00.01 Staphylococcal arthritis, shoulder**
M00.011 Staphylococcal arthritis, right shoulder
M00.012 Staphylococcal arthritis, left shoulder
CC **M00.019 Staphylococcal arthritis, unspecified shoulder**
\+ **M00.02 Staphylococcal arthritis, elbow**
M00.021 Staphylococcal arthritis, right elbow
M00.022 Staphylococcal arthritis, left elbow
CC **M00.029 Staphylococcal arthritis, unspecified elbow**

+ **M00.03 Staphylococcal arthritis, wrist**
  Staphylococcal arthritis of carpal bones
  M00.031 Staphylococcal arthritis, right wrist
  M00.032 Staphylococcal arthritis, left wrist
  CC **M00.039 Staphylococcal arthritis, unspecified wrist**
+ **M00.04 Staphylococcal arthritis, hand**
  Staphylococcal arthritis of metacarpus and phalanges
  M00.041 Staphylococcal arthritis, right hand
  M00.042 Staphylococcal arthritis, left hand
  CC **M00.049 Staphylococcal arthritis, unspecified hand**
+ **M00.05 Staphylococcal arthritis, hip**
  M00.051 Staphylococcal arthritis, right hip
  M00.052 Staphylococcal arthritis, left hip
  CC **M00.059 Staphylococcal arthritis, unspecified hip**
+ **M00.06 Staphylococcal arthritis, knee**
  M00.061 Staphylococcal arthritis, right knee
  M00.062 Staphylococcal arthritis, left knee
  CC **M00.069 Staphylococcal arthritis, unspecified knee**
+ **M00.07 Staphylococcal arthritis, ankle and foot**
  Staphylococcal arthritis, tarsus, metatarsus and phalanges
  M00.071 Staphylococcal arthritis, right ankle and foot
  M00.072 Staphylococcal arthritis, left ankle and foot
  CC **M00.079 Staphylococcal arthritis, unspecified ankle and foot**
CC **M00.08 Staphylococcal arthritis, vertebrae**
CC **M00.09 Staphylococcal polyarthritis**
+ **M00.1 Pneumococcal arthritis and polyarthritis**
CC **M00.10 Pneumococcal arthritis, unspecified joint**
+ **M00.11 Pneumococcal arthritis, shoulder**
  CC **M00.111 Pneumococcal arthritis, right shoulder**
  CC **M00.112 Pneumococcal arthritis, left shoulder**
  CC **M00.119 Pneumococcal arthritis, unspecified shoulder**
+ **M00.12 Pneumococcal arthritis, elbow**
  CC **M00.121 Pneumococcal arthritis, right elbow**
  CC **M00.122 Pneumococcal arthritis, left elbow**
  CC **M00.129 Pneumococcal arthritis, unspecified elbow**
+ **M00.13 Pneumococcal arthritis, wrist**
  Pneumococcal arthritis of carpal bones
  CC **M00.131 Pneumococcal arthritis, right wrist**
  CC **M00.132 Pneumococcal arthritis, left wrist**
  CC **M00.139 Pneumococcal arthritis, unspecified wrist**
+ **M00.14 Pneumococcal arthritis, hand**
  Pneumococcal arthritis of metacarpus and phalanges
  CC **M00.141 Pneumococcal arthritis, right hand**
  CC **M00.142 Pneumococcal arthritis, left hand**
  CC **M00.149 Pneumococcal arthritis, unspecified hand**
+ **M00.15 Pneumococcal arthritis, hip**
  CC **M00.151 Pneumococcal arthritis, right hip**
  CC **M00.152 Pneumococcal arthritis, left hip**
  CC **M00.159 Pneumococcal arthritis, unspecified hip**
+ **M00.16 Pneumococcal arthritis, knee**
  CC **M00.161 Pneumococcal arthritis, right knee**
  CC **M00.162 Pneumococcal arthritis, left knee**
  CC **M00.169 Pneumococcal arthritis, unspecified knee**
+ **M00.17 Pneumococcal arthritis, ankle and foot**
  Pneumococcal arthritis, tarsus, metatarsus and phalanges
  CC **M00.171 Pneumococcal arthritis, right ankle and foot**
  CC **M00.172 Pneumococcal arthritis, left ankle and foot**
  CC **M00.179 Pneumococcal arthritis, unspecified ankle and foot**
CC **M00.18 Pneumococcal arthritis, vertebrae**
CC **M00.19 Pneumococcal polyarthritis**
+ **M00.2 Other streptococcal arthritis and polyarthritis**
  Use additional code (B95.0-B95.2, B95.4-B95.5) to identify bacterial agent
CC **M00.20 Other streptococcal arthritis, unspecified joint**
+ **M00.21 Other streptococcal arthritis, shoulder**
  CC **M00.211 Other streptococcal arthritis, right shoulder**
  CC **M00.212 Other streptococcal arthritis, left shoulder**
  CC **M00.219 Other streptococcal arthritis, unspecified shoulder**
+ **M00.22 Other streptococcal arthritis, elbow**
  CC **M00.221 Other streptococcal arthritis, right elbow**
  CC **M00.222 Other streptococcal arthritis, left elbow**
  CC **M00.229 Other streptococcal arthritis, unspecified elbow**
+ **M00.23 Other streptococcal arthritis, wrist**
  Other streptococcal arthritis of carpal bones
  CC **M00.231 Other streptococcal arthritis, right wrist**
  CC **M00.232 Other streptococcal arthritis, left wrist**
  CC **M00.239 Other streptococcal arthritis, unspecified wrist**
+ **M00.24 Other streptococcal arthritis, hand**
  Other streptococcal arthritis metacarpus and phalanges
  CC **M00.241 Other streptococcal arthritis, right hand**
  CC **M00.242 Other streptococcal arthritis, left hand**
  CC **M00.249 Other streptococcal arthritis, unspecified hand**
+ **M00.25 Other streptococcal arthritis, hip**
  CC **M00.251 Other streptococcal arthritis, right hip**
  CC **M00.252 Other streptococcal arthritis, left hip**
  CC **M00.259 Other streptococcal arthritis, unspecified hip**
+ **M00.26 Other streptococcal arthritis, knee**
  CC **M00.261 Other streptococcal arthritis, right knee**
  CC **M00.262 Other streptococcal arthritis, left knee**
  CC **M00.269 Other streptococcal arthritis, unspecified knee**
+ **M00.27 Other streptococcal arthritis, ankle and foot**
  Other streptococcal arthritis, tarsus, metatarsus and phalanges
  CC **M00.271 Other streptococcal arthritis, right ankle and foot**
  CC **M00.272 Other streptococcal arthritis, left ankle and foot**
  CC **M00.279 Other streptococcal arthritis, unspecified ankle and foot**
CC **M00.28 Other streptococcal arthritis, vertebrae**
CC **M00.29 Other streptococcal polyarthritis**
+ **M00.8 Arthritis and polyarthritis due to other bacteria**
  Use additional code (B96) to identify bacteria
CC **M00.80 Arthritis due to other bacteria, unspecified joint**
+ **M00.81 Arthritis due to other bacteria, shoulder**
  CC **M00.811 Arthritis due to other bacteria, right shoulder**
  CC **M00.812 Arthritis due to other bacteria, left shoulder**
  CC **M00.819 Arthritis due to other bacteria, unspecified shoulder**
+ **M00.82 Arthritis due to other bacteria, elbow**
  CC **M00.821 Arthritis due to other bacteria, right elbow**
  CC **M00.822 Arthritis due to other bacteria, left elbow**
  CC **M00.829 Arthritis due to other bacteria, unspecified elbow**
+ **M00.83 Arthritis due to other bacteria, wrist**
  Arthritis due to other bacteria, carpal bones
  CC **M00.831 Arthritis due to other bacteria, right wrist**
  CC **M00.832 Arthritis due to other bacteria, left wrist**
  CC **M00.839 Arthritis due to other bacteria, unspecified wrist**

+ M00.84 **Arthritis due to other bacteria, hand**
Arthritis due to other bacteria, metacarpus and phalanges
CC **M00.841 Arthritis due to other bacteria, right hand**
CC **M00.842 Arthritis due to other bacteria, left hand**
CC **M00.849 Arthritis due to other bacteria, unspecified hand**
+ M00.85 **Arthritis due to other bacteria, hip**
CC **M00.851 Arthritis due to other bacteria, right hip**
CC **M00.852 Arthritis due to other bacteria, left hip**
CC **M00.859 Arthritis due to other bacteria, unspecified hip**
+ M00.86 **Arthritis due to other bacteria, knee**
CC **M00.861 Arthritis due to other bacteria, right knee**
CC **M00.862 Arthritis due to other bacteria, left knee**
AHA CC: 3Q, 2019, 16-17
CC **M00.869 Arthritis due to other bacteria, unspecified knee**
+ M00.87 **Arthritis due to other bacteria, ankle and foot**
Arthritis due to other bacteria, tarsus, metatarsus, and phalanges
CC **M00.871 Arthritis due to other bacteria, right ankle and foot**
CC **M00.872 Arthritis due to other bacteria, left ankle and foot**
CC **M00.879 Arthritis due to other bacteria, unspecified ankle and foot**
CC **M00.88 Arthritis due to other bacteria, vertebrae**
CC **M00.89 Polyarthritis due to other bacteria**
CC **M00.9 Pyogenic arthritis, unspecified**
Infective arthritis NOS

M01 Direct infections of joint in infectious and parasitic diseases classified elsewhere
Code first underlying disease, such as:
leprosy [Hansen's disease] (A30.-)
mycoses (B35-B49)
O'nyong-nyong fever (A92.1)
paratyphoid fever (A01.1-A01.4)
Excludes1: *arthropathy in Lyme disease (A69.23)*
gonococcal arthritis (A54.42)
meningococcal arthritis (A39.83)
mumps arthritis (B26.85)
postinfective arthropathy (M02.-)
postmeningococcal arthritis (39.84)
reactive arthritis (M02.3)
rubella arthritis (B06.82)
sarcoidosis arthritis (D86.86)
tuberculosis arthritis (A18.01-A18.02)
typhoid fever arthritis (A01.04)

+ **M01.X Direct infection of joint in infectious and parasitic diseases classified elsewhere**
CC **M01.X0 Direct infection of unspecified joint in infectious and parasitic diseases classified elsewhere**
+ **M01.X1 Direct infection of shoulder joint in infectious and parasitic diseases classified elsewhere**
CC **M01.X11 Direct infection of right shoulder in infectious and parasitic diseases classified elsewhere**
CC **M01.X12 Direct infection of left shoulder in infectious and parasitic diseases classified elsewhere**
CC **M01.X19 Direct infection of unspecified shoulder in infectious and parasitic diseases classified elsewhere**
+ **M01.X2 Direct infection of elbow in infectious and parasitic diseases classified elsewhere**
CC **M01.X21 Direct infection of right elbow in infectious and parasitic diseases classified elsewhere**
CC **M01.X22 Direct infection of left elbow in infectious and parasitic diseases classified elsewhere**
CC **M01.X29 Direct infection of unspecified elbow in infectious and parasitic diseases classified elsewhere**
+ **M01.X3 Direct infection of wrist in infectious and parasitic diseases classified elsewhere**
Direct infection of carpal bones in infectious and parasitic diseases classified elsewhere
CC **M01.X31 Direct infection of right wrist in infectious and parasitic diseases classified elsewhere**
CC **M01.X32 Direct infection of left wrist in infectious and parasitic diseases classified elsewhere**
CC **M01.X39 Direct infection of unspecified wrist in infectious and parasitic diseases classified elsewhere**
+ **M01.X4 Direct infection of hand in infectious and parasitic diseases classified elsewhere**
Direct infection of metacarpus and phalanges in infectious and parasitic diseases classified elsewhere
CC **M01.X41 Direct infection of right hand in infectious and parasitic diseases classified elsewhere**
CC **M01.X42 Direct infection of left hand in infectious and parasitic diseases classified elsewhere**
CC **M01.X49 Direct infection of unspecified hand in infectious and parasitic diseases classified elsewhere**
+ **M01.X5 Direct infection of hip in infectious and parasitic diseases classified elsewhere**
CC **M01.X51 Direct infection of right hip in infectious and parasitic diseases classified elsewhere**
CC **M01.X52 Direct infection of left hip in infectious and parasitic diseases classified elsewhere**
CC **M01.X59 Direct infection of unspecified hip in infectious and parasitic diseases classified elsewhere**
+ **M01.X6 Direct infection of knee in infectious and parasitic diseases classified elsewhere**
CC **M01.X61 Direct infection of right knee in infectious and parasitic diseases classified elsewhere**
CC **M01.X62 Direct infection of left knee in infectious and parasitic diseases classified elsewhere**
CC **M01.X69 Direct infection of unspecified knee in infectious and parasitic diseases classified elsewhere**
+ **M01.X7 Direct infection of ankle and foot in infectious and parasitic diseases classified elsewhere**
Direct infection of tarsus, metatarsus and phalanges in infectious and parasitic diseases classified elsewhere
CC **M01.X71 Direct infection of right ankle and foot in infectious and parasitic diseases classified elsewhere**
CC **M01.X72 Direct infection of left ankle and foot in infectious and parasitic diseases classified elsewhere**
CC **M01.X79 Direct infection of unspecified ankle and foot in infectious and parasitic diseases classified elsewhere**
CC **M01.X8 Direct infection of vertebrae in infectious and parasitic diseases classified elsewhere**
CC **M01.X9 Direct infection of multiple joints in infectious and parasitic diseases classified elsewhere**

M02 Postinfective and reactive arthropathies

Code first underlying disease, such as:
- congenital syphilis [Clutton's joints] (A50.5)
- enteritis due to Yersinia enterocolitica (A04.6)
- infective endocarditis (I33.0)
- viral hepatitis (B15-B19)

Excludes1: *Behçet's disease (M35.2)*
direct infections of joint in infectious and parasitic diseases classified elsewhere (M01.-)
postmeningcoccal arthritis (A39.84)
mumps arthritis (B26.85)
rubella arthritis (B06.82)
syphilis arthritis (late) (A52.77)
rheumatic fever (I00)
tabetic arthropathy [Charcôt's] (A52.16)

+ **M02.0 Arthropathy following intestinal bypass**
M02.00 Arthropathy following intestinal bypass, unspecified site
+ **M02.01 Arthropathy following intestinal bypass, shoulder**
M02.011 Arthropathy following intestinal bypass, right shoulder
M02.012 Arthropathy following intestinal bypass, left shoulder
M02.019 Arthropathy following intestinal bypass, unspecified shoulder
+ **M02.02 Arthropathy following intestinal bypass, elbow**
M02.021 Arthropathy following intestinal bypass, right elbow
M02.022 Arthropathy following intestinal bypass, left elbow
M02.029 Arthropathy following intestinal bypass, unspecified elbow
+ **M02.03 Arthropathy following intestinal bypass, wrist**
Arthropathy following intestinal bypass, carpal bones
M02.031 Arthropathy following intestinal bypass, right wrist
M02.032 Arthropathy following intestinal bypass, left wrist
M02.039 Arthropathy following intestinal bypass, unspecified wrist
+ **M02.04 Arthropathy following intestinal bypass, hand**
Arthropathy following intestinal bypass, metacarpals and phalanges
M02.041 Arthropathy following intestinal bypass, right hand
M02.042 Arthropathy following intestinal bypass, left hand
M02.049 Arthropathy following intestinal bypass, unspecified hand
+ **M02.05 Arthropathy following intestinal bypass, hip**
M02.051 Arthropathy following intestinal bypass, right hip
M02.052 Arthropathy following intestinal bypass, left hip
M02.059 Arthropathy following intestinal bypass, unspecified hip
+ **M02.06 Arthropathy following intestinal bypass, knee**
M02.061 Arthropathy following intestinal bypass, right knee
M02.062 Arthropathy following intestinal bypass, left knee
M02.069 Arthropathy following intestinal bypass, unspecified knee
+ **M02.07 Arthropathy following intestinal bypass, ankle and foot**
Arthropathy following intestinal bypass, tarsus, metatarsus and phalanges
M02.071 Arthropathy following intestinal bypass, right ankle and foot
M02.072 Arthropathy following intestinal bypass, left ankle and foot
M02.079 Arthropathy following intestinal bypass, unspecified ankle and foot
M02.08 Arthropathy following intestinal bypass, vertebrae
M02.09 Arthropathy following intestinal bypass, multiple sites

+ **M02.1 Postdysenteric arthropathy**
CC **M02.10 Postdysenteric arthropathy, unspecified site**
+ **M02.11 Postdysenteric arthropathy, shoulder**
CC **M02.111 Postdysenteric arthropathy, right shoulder**
CC **M02.112 Postdysenteric arthropathy, left shoulder**
CC **M02.119 Postdysenteric arthropathy, unspecified shoulder**
+ **M02.12 Postdysenteric arthropathy, elbow**
CC **M02.121 Postdysenteric arthropathy, right elbow**
CC **M02.122 Postdysenteric arthropathy, left elbow**
CC **M02.129 Postdysenteric arthropathy, unspecified elbow**
+ **M02.13 Postdysenteric arthropathy, wrist**
Postdysenteric arthropathy, carpal bones
CC **M02.131 Postdysenteric arthropathy, right wrist**
CC **M02.132 Postdysenteric arthropathy, left wrist**
CC **M02.139 Postdysenteric arthropathy, unspecified wrist**
+ **M02.14 Postdysenteric arthropathy, hand**
Postdysenteric arthropathy, metacarpus and phalanges
CC **M02.141 Postdysenteric arthropathy, right hand**
CC **M02.142 Postdysenteric arthropathy, left hand**
CC **M02.149 Postdysenteric arthropathy, unspecified hand**
+ **M02.15 Postdysenteric arthropathy, hip**
CC **M02.151 Postdysenteric arthropathy, right hip**
CC **M02.152 Postdysenteric arthropathy, left hip**
CC **M02.159 Postdysenteric arthropathy, unspecified hip**
+ **M02.16 Postdysenteric arthropathy, knee**
CC **M02.161 Postdysenteric arthropathy, right knee**
CC **M02.162 Postdysenteric arthropathy, left knee**
CC **M02.169 Postdysenteric arthropathy, unspecified knee**
+ **M02.17 Postdysenteric arthropathy, ankle and foot**
Postdysenteric arthropathy, tarsus, metatarsus and phalanges
CC **M02.171 Postdysenteric arthropathy, right ankle and foot**
CC **M02.172 Postdysenteric arthropathy, left ankle and foot**
CC **M02.179 Postdysenteric arthropathy, unspecified ankle and foot**
CC **M02.18 Postdysenteric arthropathy, vertebrae**
CC **M02.19 Postdysenteric arthropathy, multiple sites**
+ **M02.2 Postimmunization arthropathy**
M02.20 Postimmunization arthropathy, unspecified site
+ **M02.21 Postimmunization arthropathy, shoulder**
M02.211 Postimmunization arthropathy, right shoulder
M02.212 Postimmunization arthropathy, left shoulder
M02.219 Postimmunization arthropathy, unspecified shoulder
+ **M02.22 Postimmunization arthropathy, elbow**
M02.221 Postimmunization arthropathy, right elbow
M02.222 Postimmunization arthropathy, left elbow
M02.229 Postimmunization arthropathy, unspecified elbow
+ **M02.23 Postimmunization arthropathy, wrist**
Postimmunization arthropathy, carpal bones
M02.231 Postimmunization arthropathy, right wrist
M02.232 Postimmunization arthropathy, left wrist
M02.239 Postimmunization arthropathy, unspecified wrist
+ **M02.24 Postimmunization arthropathy, hand**
Postimmunization arthropathy, metacarpus and phalanges
M02.241 Postimmunization arthropathy, right hand

M02.242 Postimmunization arthropathy, left hand
M02.249 Postimmunization arthropathy, unspecified hand
+ M02.25 Postimmunization arthropathy, hip
M02.251 Postimmunization arthropathy, right hip
M02.252 Postimmunization arthropathy, left hip
M02.259 Postimmunization arthropathy, unspecified hip
+ M02.26 Postimmunization arthropathy, knee
M02.261 Postimmunization arthropathy, right knee
M02.262 Postimmunization arthropathy, left knee
M02.269 Postimmunization arthropathy, unspecified knee
+ M02.27 Postimmunization arthropathy, ankle and foot
Postimmunization arthropathy, tarsus, metatarsus and phalanges
M02.271 Postimmunization arthropathy, right ankle and foot
M02.272 Postimmunization arthropathy, left ankle and foot
M02.279 Postimmunization arthropathy, unspecified ankle and foot
M02.28 Postimmunization arthropathy, vertebrae
M02.29 Postimmunization arthropathy, multiple sites
+ M02.3 Reiter's disease
Reactive arthritis
CC **M02.30 Reiter's disease, unspecified site**
+ M02.31 Reiter's disease, shoulder
CC **M02.311 Reiter's disease, right shoulder**
CC **M02.312 Reiter's disease, left shoulder**
CC **M02.319 Reiter's disease, unspecified shoulder**
+ M02.32 Reiter's disease, elbow
CC **M02.321 Reiter's disease, right elbow**
CC **M02.322 Reiter's disease, left elbow**
CC **M02.329 Reiter's disease, unspecified elbow**
+ M02.33 Reiter's disease, wrist
Reiter's disease, carpal bones
CC **M02.331 Reiter's disease, right wrist**
CC **M02.332 Reiter's disease, left wrist**
CC **M02.339 Reiter's disease, unspecified wrist**
+ M02.34 Reiter's disease, hand
Reiter's disease, metacarpus and phalanges
CC **M02.341 Reiter's disease, right hand**
CC **M02.342 Reiter's disease, left hand**
CC **M02.349 Reiter's disease, unspecified hand**
+ M02.35 Reiter's disease, hip
CC **M02.351 Reiter's disease, right hip**
CC **M02.352 Reiter's disease, left hip**
CC **M02.359 Reiter's disease, unspecified hip**
+ M02.36 Reiter's disease, knee
CC **M02.361 Reiter's disease, right knee**
CC **M02.362 Reiter's disease, left knee**
CC **M02.369 Reiter's disease, unspecified knee**
+ M02.37 Reiter's disease, ankle and foot
Reiter's disease, tarsus, metatarsus and phalanges
CC **M02.371 Reiter's disease, right ankle and foot**
CC **M02.372 Reiter's disease, left ankle and foot**
CC **M02.379 Reiter's disease, unspecified ankle and foot**
CC **M02.38 Reiter's disease, vertebrae**
CC **M02.39 Reiter's disease, multiple sites**
+ M02.8 Other reactive arthropathies
CC **M02.80 Other reactive arthropathies, unspecified site**
+ M02.81 Other reactive arthropathies, shoulder
CC **M02.811 Other reactive arthropathies, right shoulder**
CC **M02.812 Other reactive arthropathies, left shoulder**
CC **M02.819 Other reactive arthropathies, unspecified shoulder**
+ M02.82 Other reactive arthropathies, elbow
CC **M02.821 Other reactive arthropathies, right elbow**
CC **M02.822 Other reactive arthropathies, left elbow**
CC **M02.829 Other reactive arthropathies, unspecified elbow**
+ M02.83 Other reactive arthropathies, wrist
Other reactive arthropathies, carpal bones
CC **M02.831 Other reactive arthropathies, right wrist**
CC **M02.832 Other reactive arthropathies, left wrist**
CC **M02.839 Other reactive arthropathies, unspecified wrist**
+ M02.84 Other reactive arthropathies, hand
Other reactive arthropathies, metacarpus and phalanges
CC **M02.841 Other reactive arthropathies, right hand**
CC **M02.842 Other reactive arthropathies, left hand**
CC **M02.849 Other reactive arthropathies, unspecified hand**
+ M02.85 Other reactive arthropathies, hip
CC **M02.851 Other reactive arthropathies, right hip**
CC **M02.852 Other reactive arthropathies, left hip**
CC **M02.859 Other reactive arthropathies, unspecified hip**
+ M02.86 Other reactive arthropathies, knee
CC **M02.861 Other reactive arthropathies, right knee**
CC **M02.862 Other reactive arthropathies, left knee**
CC **M02.869 Other reactive arthropathies, unspecified knee**
+ M02.87 Other reactive arthropathies, ankle and foot
Other reactive arthropathies, tarsus, metatarsus and phalanges
CC **M02.871 Other reactive arthropathies, right ankle and foot**
CC **M02.872 Other reactive arthropathies, left ankle and foot**
CC **M02.879 Other reactive arthropathies, unspecified ankle and foot**
CC **M02.88 Other reactive arthropathies, vertebrae**
CC **M02.89 Other reactive arthropathies, multiple sites**
M02.9 Reactive arthropathy, unspecified

Autoinflammatory syndromes (M04)

M04 Autoinflammatory syndromes
Excludes2: *Crohn's disease (K50.-)*
AHA CC: 4Q, 2016, 37
M04.1 Periodic fever syndromes
Familial Mediterranean fever
Hyperimmunoglobin D syndrome
Mevalonate kinase deficiency
Tumor necrosis factor receptor associated periodic syndrome [TRAPS]
M04.2 Cryopyrin-associated periodic syndromes
Chronic infantile neurological, cutaneous and articular syndrome [CINCA]
Familial cold autoinflammatory syndrome
Familial cold urticaria
Muckle-Wells syndrome
Neonatal onset multisystemic inflammatory disorder [NOMID]
M04.8 Other autoinflammatory syndromes
Blau syndrome
Deficiency of interleukin 1 receptor antagonist [DIRA]
Majeed syndrome
Periodic fever, aphthous stomatitis, pharyngitis, and adenopathy syndrome [PFAPA]
Pyogenic arthritis, pyoderma gangrenosum, and acne syndrome [PAPA]
M04.9 Autoinflammatory syndrome, unspecified

Inflammatory polyarthropathies (M05-M14)

M05 Rheumatoid arthritis with rheumatoid factor
Excludes1: *rheumatic fever (I00)*
juvenile rheumatoid arthritis (M08.-)
rheumatoid arthritis of spine (M45.-)
AHA CC: 4Q, 2020, 31-32
+ M05.0 Felty's syndrome
Rheumatoid arthritis with splenoadenomegaly and leukopenia
M05.00 Felty's syndrome, unspecified site

+ **M05.01 Felty's syndrome, shoulder**
  - **M05.011 Felty's syndrome, right shoulder**
  - **M05.012 Felty's syndrome, left shoulder**
  - **M05.019 Felty's syndrome, unspecified shoulder**
+ **M05.02 Felty's syndrome, elbow**
  - **M05.021 Felty's syndrome, right elbow**
  - **M05.022 Felty's syndrome, left elbow**
  - **M05.029 Felty's syndrome, unspecified elbow**
+ **M05.03 Felty's syndrome, wrist**
  Felty's syndrome, carpal bones
  - **M05.031 Felty's syndrome, right wrist**
  - **M05.032 Felty's syndrome, left wrist**
  - **M05.039 Felty's syndrome, unspecified wrist**
+ **M05.04 Felty's syndrome, hand**
  Felty's syndrome, metacarpus and phalanges
  - **M05.041 Felty's syndrome, right hand**
  - **M05.042 Felty's syndrome, left hand**
  - **M05.049 Felty's syndrome, unspecified hand**
+ **M05.05 Felty's syndrome, hip**
  - **M05.051 Felty's syndrome, right hip**
  - **M05.052 Felty's syndrome, left hip**
  - **M05.059 Felty's syndrome, unspecified hip**
+ **M05.06 Felty's syndrome, knee**
  - **M05.061 Felty's syndrome, right knee**
  - **M05.062 Felty's syndrome, left knee**
  - **M05.069 Felty's syndrome, unspecified knee**
+ **M05.07 Felty's syndrome, ankle and foot**
  Felty's syndrome, tarsus, metatarsus and phalanges
  - **M05.071 Felty's syndrome, right ankle and foot**
  - **M05.072 Felty's syndrome, left ankle and foot**
  - **M05.079 Felty's syndrome, unspecified ankle and foot**
- **M05.09 Felty's syndrome, multiple sites**

+ **M05.1 Rheumatoid lung disease with rheumatoid arthritis**
  - **M05.10 Rheumatoid lung disease with rheumatoid arthritis of unspecified site**
+ **M05.11 Rheumatoid lung disease with rheumatoid arthritis of shoulder**
  - **M05.111 Rheumatoid lung disease with rheumatoid arthritis of right shoulder**
  - **M05.112 Rheumatoid lung disease with rheumatoid arthritis of left shoulder**
  - **M05.119 Rheumatoid lung disease with rheumatoid arthritis of unspecified shoulder**
+ **M05.12 Rheumatoid lung disease with rheumatoid arthritis of elbow**
  - **M05.121 Rheumatoid lung disease with rheumatoid arthritis of right elbow**
  - **M05.122 Rheumatoid lung disease with rheumatoid arthritis of left elbow**
  - **M05.129 Rheumatoid lung disease with rheumatoid arthritis of unspecified elbow**
+ **M05.13 Rheumatoid lung disease with rheumatoid arthritis of wrist**
  Rheumatoid lung disease with rheumatoid arthritis, carpal bones
  - **M05.131 Rheumatoid lung disease with rheumatoid arthritis of right wrist**
  - **M05.132 Rheumatoid lung disease with rheumatoid arthritis of left wrist**
  - **M05.139 Rheumatoid lung disease with rheumatoid arthritis of unspecified wrist**
+ **M05.14 Rheumatoid lung disease with rheumatoid arthritis of hand**
  Rheumatoid lung disease with rheumatoid arthritis, metacarpus and phalanges
  - **M05.141 Rheumatoid lung disease with rheumatoid arthritis of right hand**
  - **M05.142 Rheumatoid lung disease with rheumatoid arthritis of left hand**
  - **M05.149 Rheumatoid lung disease with rheumatoid arthritis of unspecified hand**
+ **M05.15 Rheumatoid lung disease with rheumatoid arthritis of hip**
  - **M05.151 Rheumatoid lung disease with rheumatoid arthritis of right hip**
  - **M05.152 Rheumatoid lung disease with rheumatoid arthritis of left hip**
  - **M05.159 Rheumatoid lung disease with rheumatoid arthritis of unspecified hip**
+ **M05.16 Rheumatoid lung disease with rheumatoid arthritis of knee**
  - **M05.161 Rheumatoid lung disease with rheumatoid arthritis of right knee**
  - **M05.162 Rheumatoid lung disease with rheumatoid arthritis of left knee**
  - **M05.169 Rheumatoid lung disease with rheumatoid arthritis of unspecified knee**
+ **M05.17 Rheumatoid lung disease with rheumatoid arthritis of ankle and foot**
  Rheumatoid lung disease with rheumatoid arthritis, tarsus, metatarsus and phalanges
  - **M05.171 Rheumatoid lung disease with rheumatoid arthritis of right ankle and foot**
  - **M05.172 Rheumatoid lung disease with rheumatoid arthritis of left ankle and foot**
  - **M05.179 Rheumatoid lung disease with rheumatoid arthritis of unspecified ankle and foot**
- **M05.19 Rheumatoid lung disease with rheumatoid arthritis of multiple sites**

+ **M05.2 Rheumatoid vasculitis with rheumatoid arthritis**
  - **M05.20 Rheumatoid vasculitis with rheumatoid arthritis of unspecified site**
+ **M05.21 Rheumatoid vasculitis with rheumatoid arthritis of shoulder**
  - **M05.211 Rheumatoid vasculitis with rheumatoid arthritis of right shoulder**
  - **M05.212 Rheumatoid vasculitis with rheumatoid arthritis of left shoulder**
  - **M05.219 Rheumatoid vasculitis with rheumatoid arthritis of unspecified shoulder**
+ **M05.22 Rheumatoid vasculitis with rheumatoid arthritis of elbow**
  - **M05.221 Rheumatoid vasculitis with rheumatoid arthritis of right elbow**
  - **M05.222 Rheumatoid vasculitis with rheumatoid arthritis of left elbow**
  - **M05.229 Rheumatoid vasculitis with rheumatoid arthritis of unspecified elbow**
+ **M05.23 Rheumatoid vasculitis with rheumatoid arthritis of wrist**
  Rheumatoid vasculitis with rheumatoid arthritis, carpal bones
  - **M05.231 Rheumatoid vasculitis with rheumatoid arthritis of right wrist**
  - **M05.232 Rheumatoid vasculitis with rheumatoid arthritis of left wrist**
  - **M05.239 Rheumatoid vasculitis with rheumatoid arthritis of unspecified wrist**
+ **M05.24 Rheumatoid vasculitis with rheumatoid arthritis of hand**
  Rheumatoid vasculitis with rheumatoid arthritis, metacarpus and phalanges
  - **M05.241 Rheumatoid vasculitis with rheumatoid arthritis of right hand**
  - **M05.242 Rheumatoid vasculitis with rheumatoid arthritis of left hand**
  - **M05.249 Rheumatoid vasculitis with rheumatoid arthritis of unspecified hand**
+ **M05.25 Rheumatoid vasculitis with rheumatoid arthritis of hip**
  - **M05.251 Rheumatoid vasculitis with rheumatoid arthritis of right hip**
  - **M05.252 Rheumatoid vasculitis with rheumatoid arthritis of left hip**
  - **M05.259 Rheumatoid vasculitis with rheumatoid arthritis of unspecified hip**

+ **M05.26 Rheumatoid vasculitis with rheumatoid arthritis of knee**
  - **M05.261 Rheumatoid vasculitis with rheumatoid arthritis of right knee**
  - **M05.262 Rheumatoid vasculitis with rheumatoid arthritis of left knee**
  - **M05.269 Rheumatoid vasculitis with rheumatoid arthritis of unspecified knee**

+ **M05.27 Rheumatoid vasculitis with rheumatoid arthritis of ankle and foot**
  Rheumatoid vasculitis with rheumatoid arthritis, tarsus, metatarsus and phalanges
  - **M05.271 Rheumatoid vasculitis with rheumatoid arthritis of right ankle and foot**
  - **M05.272 Rheumatoid vasculitis with rheumatoid arthritis of left ankle and foot**
  - **M05.279 Rheumatoid vasculitis with rheumatoid arthritis of unspecified ankle and foot**

M05.29 Rheumatoid vasculitis with rheumatoid arthritis of multiple sites

+ **M05.3 Rheumatoid heart disease with rheumatoid arthritis**
  Rheumatoid carditis
  Rheumatoid endocarditis
  Rheumatoid myocarditis
  Rheumatoid pericarditis

M05.30 Rheumatoid heart disease with rheumatoid arthritis of unspecified site

+ **M05.31 Rheumatoid heart disease with rheumatoid arthritis of shoulder**
  - **M05.311 Rheumatoid heart disease with rheumatoid arthritis of right shoulder**
  - **M05.312 Rheumatoid heart disease with rheumatoid arthritis of left shoulder**
  - **M05.319 Rheumatoid heart disease with rheumatoid arthritis of unspecified shoulder**

+ **M05.32 Rheumatoid heart disease with rheumatoid arthritis of elbow**
  - **M05.321 Rheumatoid heart disease with rheumatoid arthritis of right elbow**
  - **M05.322 Rheumatoid heart disease with rheumatoid arthritis of left elbow**
  - **M05.329 Rheumatoid heart disease with rheumatoid arthritis of unspecified elbow**

+ **M05.33 Rheumatoid heart disease with rheumatoid arthritis of wrist**
  Rheumatoid heart disease with rheumatoid arthritis, carpal bones
  - **M05.331 Rheumatoid heart disease with rheumatoid arthritis of right wrist**
  - **M05.332 Rheumatoid heart disease with rheumatoid arthritis of left wrist**
  - **M05.339 Rheumatoid heart disease with rheumatoid arthritis of unspecified wrist**

+ **M05.34 Rheumatoid heart disease with rheumatoid arthritis of hand**
  Rheumatoid heart disease with rheumatoid arthritis, metacarpus and phalanges
  - **M05.341 Rheumatoid heart disease with rheumatoid arthritis of right hand**
  - **M05.342 Rheumatoid heart disease with rheumatoid arthritis of left hand**
  - **M05.349 Rheumatoid heart disease with rheumatoid arthritis of unspecified hand**

+ **M05.35 Rheumatoid heart disease with rheumatoid arthritis of hip**
  - **M05.351 Rheumatoid heart disease with rheumatoid arthritis of right hip**
  - **M05.352 Rheumatoid heart disease with rheumatoid arthritis of left hip**
  - **M05.359 Rheumatoid heart disease with rheumatoid arthritis of unspecified hip**

+ **M05.36 Rheumatoid heart disease with rheumatoid arthritis of knee**
  - **M05.361 Rheumatoid heart disease with rheumatoid arthritis of right knee**
  - **M05.362 Rheumatoid heart disease with rheumatoid arthritis of left knee**
  - **M05.369 Rheumatoid heart disease with rheumatoid arthritis of unspecified knee**

+ **M05.37 Rheumatoid heart disease with rheumatoid arthritis of ankle and foot**
  Rheumatoid heart disease with rheumatoid arthritis, tarsus, metatarsus and phalanges
  - **M05.371 Rheumatoid heart disease with rheumatoid arthritis of right ankle and foot**
  - **M05.372 Rheumatoid heart disease with rheumatoid arthritis of left ankle and foot**
  - **M05.379 Rheumatoid heart disease with rheumatoid arthritis of unspecified ankle and foot**

M05.39 Rheumatoid heart disease with rheumatoid arthritis of multiple sites

+ **M05.4 Rheumatoid myopathy with rheumatoid arthritis**

CC **M05.40 Rheumatoid myopathy with rheumatoid arthritis of unspecified site**

+ **M05.41 Rheumatoid myopathy with rheumatoid arthritis of shoulder**
  - CC **M05.411 Rheumatoid myopathy with rheumatoid arthritis of right shoulder**
  - CC **M05.412 Rheumatoid myopathy with rheumatoid arthritis of left shoulder**
  - CC **M05.419 Rheumatoid myopathy with rheumatoid arthritis of unspecified shoulder**

+ **M05.42 Rheumatoid myopathy with rheumatoid arthritis of elbow**
  - CC **M05.421 Rheumatoid myopathy with rheumatoid arthritis of right elbow**
  - CC **M05.422 Rheumatoid myopathy with rheumatoid arthritis of left elbow**
  - CC **M05.429 Rheumatoid myopathy with rheumatoid arthritis of unspecified elbow**

+ **M05.43 Rheumatoid myopathy with rheumatoid arthritis of wrist**
  Rheumatoid myopathy with rheumatoid arthritis, carpal bones
  - CC **M05.431 Rheumatoid myopathy with rheumatoid arthritis of right wrist**
  - CC **M05.432 Rheumatoid myopathy with rheumatoid arthritis of left wrist**
  - CC **M05.439 Rheumatoid myopathy with rheumatoid arthritis of unspecified wrist**

+ **M05.44 Rheumatoid myopathy with rheumatoid arthritis of hand**
  Rheumatoid myopathy with rheumatoid arthritis, metacarpus and phalanges
  - CC **M05.441 Rheumatoid myopathy with rheumatoid arthritis of right hand**
  - CC **M05.442 Rheumatoid myopathy with rheumatoid arthritis of left hand**
  - CC **M05.449 Rheumatoid myopathy with rheumatoid arthritis of unspecified hand**

+ **M05.45 Rheumatoid myopathy with rheumatoid arthritis of hip**
  - CC **M05.451 Rheumatoid myopathy with rheumatoid arthritis of right hip**
  - CC **M05.452 Rheumatoid myopathy with rheumatoid arthritis of left hip**
  - CC **M05.459 Rheumatoid myopathy with rheumatoid arthritis of unspecified hip**

+ **M05.46 Rheumatoid myopathy with rheumatoid arthritis of knee**
  - CC **M05.461 Rheumatoid myopathy with rheumatoid arthritis of right knee**
  - CC **M05.462 Rheumatoid myopathy with rheumatoid arthritis of left knee**
  - CC **M05.469 Rheumatoid myopathy with rheumatoid arthritis of unspecified knee**

+ **M05.47 Rheumatoid myopathy with rheumatoid arthritis of ankle and foot**
  Rheumatoid myopathy with rheumatoid arthritis, tarsus, metatarsus and phalanges
  - CC **M05.471 Rheumatoid myopathy with rheumatoid arthritis of right ankle and foot**

CC **M05.472 Rheumatoid myopathy with rheumatoid arthritis of left ankle and foot**

CC **M05.479 Rheumatoid myopathy with rheumatoid arthritis of unspecified ankle and foot**

CC **M05.49 Rheumatoid myopathy with rheumatoid arthritis of multiple sites**

\+ **M05.5 Rheumatoid polyneuropathy with rheumatoid arthritis**

M05.50 Rheumatoid polyneuropathy with rheumatoid arthritis of unspecified site

\+ **M05.51 Rheumatoid polyneuropathy with rheumatoid arthritis of shoulder**

M05.511 Rheumatoid polyneuropathy with rheumatoid arthritis of right shoulder

M05.512 Rheumatoid polyneuropathy with rheumatoid arthritis of left shoulder

M05.519 Rheumatoid polyneuropathy with rheumatoid arthritis of unspecified shoulder

\+ **M05.52 Rheumatoid polyneuropathy with rheumatoid arthritis of elbow**

M05.521 Rheumatoid polyneuropathy with rheumatoid arthritis of right elbow

M05.522 Rheumatoid polyneuropathy with rheumatoid arthritis of left elbow

M05.529 Rheumatoid polyneuropathy with rheumatoid arthritis of unspecified elbow

\+ **M05.53 Rheumatoid polyneuropathy with rheumatoid arthritis of wrist**

Rheumatoid polyneuropathy with rheumatoid arthritis, carpal bones

M05.531 Rheumatoid polyneuropathy with rheumatoid arthritis of right wrist

M05.532 Rheumatoid polyneuropathy with rheumatoid arthritis of left wrist

M05.539 Rheumatoid polyneuropathy with rheumatoid arthritis of unspecified wrist

\+ **M05.54 Rheumatoid polyneuropathy with rheumatoid arthritis of hand**

Rheumatoid polyneuropathy with rheumatoid arthritis, metacarpus and phalanges

M05.541 Rheumatoid polyneuropathy with rheumatoid arthritis of right hand

M05.542 Rheumatoid polyneuropathy with rheumatoid arthritis of left hand

M05.549 Rheumatoid polyneuropathy with rheumatoid arthritis of unspecified hand

\+ **M05.55 Rheumatoid polyneuropathy with rheumatoid arthritis of hip**

M05.551 Rheumatoid polyneuropathy with rheumatoid arthritis of right hip

M05.552 Rheumatoid polyneuropathy with rheumatoid arthritis of left hip

M05.559 Rheumatoid polyneuropathy with rheumatoid arthritis of unspecified hip

\+ **M05.56 Rheumatoid polyneuropathy with rheumatoid arthritis of knee**

M05.561 Rheumatoid polyneuropathy with rheumatoid arthritis of right knee

M05.562 Rheumatoid polyneuropathy with rheumatoid arthritis of left knee

M05.569 Rheumatoid polyneuropathy with rheumatoid arthritis of unspecified knee

\+ **M05.57 Rheumatoid polyneuropathy with rheumatoid arthritis of ankle and foot**

Rheumatoid polyneuropathy with rheumatoid arthritis, tarsus, metatarsus and phalanges

M05.571 Rheumatoid polyneuropathy with rheumatoid arthritis of right ankle and foot

M05.572 Rheumatoid polyneuropathy with rheumatoid arthritis of left ankle and foot

M05.579 Rheumatoid polyneuropathy with rheumatoid arthritis of unspecified ankle and foot

M05.59 Rheumatoid polyneuropathy with rheumatoid arthritis of multiple sites

\+ **M05.6 Rheumatoid arthritis with involvement of other organs and systems**

M05.60 Rheumatoid arthritis of unspecified site with involvement of other organs and systems

\+ **M05.61 Rheumatoid arthritis of shoulder with involvement of other organs and systems**

M05.611 Rheumatoid arthritis of right shoulder with involvement of other organs and systems

M05.612 Rheumatoid arthritis of left shoulder with involvement of other organs and systems

M05.619 Rheumatoid arthritis of unspecified shoulder with involvement of other organs and systems

\+ **M05.62 Rheumatoid arthritis of elbow with involvement of other organs and systems**

M05.621 Rheumatoid arthritis of right elbow with involvement of other organs and systems

M05.622 Rheumatoid arthritis of left elbow with involvement of other organs and systems

M05.629 Rheumatoid arthritis of unspecified elbow with involvement of other organs and systems

\+ **M05.63 Rheumatoid arthritis of wrist with involvement of other organs and systems**

Rheumatoid arthritis of carpal bones with involvement of other organs and systems

M05.631 Rheumatoid arthritis of right wrist with involvement of other organs and systems

M05.632 Rheumatoid arthritis of left wrist with involvement of other organs and systems

M05.639 Rheumatoid arthritis of unspecified wrist with involvement of other organs and systems

\+ **M05.64 Rheumatoid arthritis of hand with involvement of other organs and systems**

Rheumatoid arthritis of metacarpus and phalanges with involvement of other organs and systems

M05.641 Rheumatoid arthritis of right hand with involvement of other organs and systems

M05.642 Rheumatoid arthritis of left hand with involvement of other organs and systems

M05.649 Rheumatoid arthritis of unspecified hand with involvement of other organs and systems

\+ **M05.65 Rheumatoid arthritis of hip with involvement of other organs and systems**

M05.651 Rheumatoid arthritis of right hip with involvement of other organs and systems

M05.652 Rheumatoid arthritis of left hip with involvement of other organs and systems

M05.659 Rheumatoid arthritis of unspecified hip with involvement of other organs and systems

\+ **M05.66 Rheumatoid arthritis of knee with involvement of other organs and systems**

M05.661 Rheumatoid arthritis of right knee with involvement of other organs and systems

M05.662 Rheumatoid arthritis of left knee with involvement of other organs and systems

M05.669 Rheumatoid arthritis of unspecified knee with involvement of other organs and systems

+ M05.67 Rheumatoid arthritis of ankle and foot with involvement of other organs and systems
Rheumatoid arthritis of tarsus, metatarsus and phalanges with involvement of other organs and systems
M05.671 Rheumatoid arthritis of right ankle and foot with involvement of other organs and systems
M05.672 Rheumatoid arthritis of left ankle and foot with involvement of other organs and systems
M05.679 Rheumatoid arthritis of unspecified ankle and foot with involvement of other organs and systems
M05.69 Rheumatoid arthritis of multiple sites with involvement of other organs and systems
+ M05.7 Rheumatoid arthritis with rheumatoid factor without organ or systems involvement
M05.70 Rheumatoid arthritis with rheumatoid factor of unspecified site without organ or systems involvement
+ M05.71 Rheumatoid arthritis with rheumatoid factor of shoulder without organ or systems involvement
M05.711 Rheumatoid arthritis with rheumatoid factor of right shoulder without organ or systems involvement
M05.712 Rheumatoid arthritis with rheumatoid factor of left shoulder without organ or systems involvement
M05.719 Rheumatoid arthritis with rheumatoid factor of unspecified shoulder without organ or systems involvement
+ M05.72 Rheumatoid arthritis with rheumatoid factor of elbow without organ or systems involvement
M05.721 Rheumatoid arthritis with rheumatoid factor of right elbow without organ or systems involvement
M05.722 Rheumatoid arthritis with rheumatoid factor of left elbow without organ or systems involvement
M05.729 Rheumatoid arthritis with rheumatoid factor of unspecified elbow without organ or systems involvement
+ M05.73 Rheumatoid arthritis with rheumatoid factor of wrist without organ or systems involvement
M05.731 Rheumatoid arthritis with rheumatoid factor of right wrist without organ or systems involvement
M05.732 Rheumatoid arthritis with rheumatoid factor of left wrist without organ or systems involvement
M05.739 Rheumatoid arthritis with rheumatoid factor of unspecified wrist without organ or systems involvement
+ M05.74 Rheumatoid arthritis with rheumatoid factor of hand without organ or systems involvement
M05.741 Rheumatoid arthritis with rheumatoid factor of right hand without organ or systems involvement
M05.742 Rheumatoid arthritis with rheumatoid factor of left hand without organ or systems involvement
M05.749 Rheumatoid arthritis with rheumatoid factor of unspecified hand without organ or systems involvement
+ M05.75 Rheumatoid arthritis with rheumatoid factor of hip without organ or systems involvement
M05.751 Rheumatoid arthritis with rheumatoid factor of right hip without organ or systems involvement
M05.752 Rheumatoid arthritis with rheumatoid factor of left hip without organ or systems involvement
M05.759 Rheumatoid arthritis with rheumatoid factor of unspecified hip without organ or systems involvement
+ M05.76 Rheumatoid arthritis with rheumatoid factor of knee without organ or systems involvement
M05.761 Rheumatoid arthritis with rheumatoid factor of right knee without organ or systems involvement
M05.762 Rheumatoid arthritis with rheumatoid factor of left knee without organ or systems involvement
M05.769 Rheumatoid arthritis with rheumatoid factor of unspecified knee without organ or systems involvement
+ M05.77 Rheumatoid arthritis with rheumatoid factor of ankle and foot without organ or systems involvement
M05.771 Rheumatoid arthritis with rheumatoid factor of right ankle and foot without organ or systems involvement
M05.772 Rheumatoid arthritis with rheumatoid factor of left ankle and foot without organ or systems involvement
M05.779 Rheumatoid arthritis with rheumatoid factor of unspecified ankle and foot without organ or systems involvement
M05.79 Rheumatoid arthritis with rheumatoid factor of multiple sites without organ or systems involvement
M05.7A Rheumatoid arthritis with rheumatoid factor of other specified site without organ or systems involvement
+ M05.8 Other rheumatoid arthritis with rheumatoid factor
M05.80 Other rheumatoid arthritis with rheumatoid factor of unspecified site
+ M05.81 Other rheumatoid arthritis with rheumatoid factor of shoulder
M05.811 Other rheumatoid arthritis with rheumatoid factor of right shoulder
M05.812 Other rheumatoid arthritis with rheumatoid factor of left shoulder
M05.819 Other rheumatoid arthritis with rheumatoid factor of unspecified shoulder
+ M05.82 Other rheumatoid arthritis with rheumatoid factor of elbow
M05.821 Other rheumatoid arthritis with rheumatoid factor of right elbow
M05.822 Other rheumatoid arthritis with rheumatoid factor of left elbow
M05.829 Other rheumatoid arthritis with rheumatoid factor of unspecified elbow
+ M05.83 Other rheumatoid arthritis with rheumatoid factor of wrist
M05.831 Other rheumatoid arthritis with rheumatoid factor of right wrist
M05.832 Other rheumatoid arthritis with rheumatoid factor of left wrist
M05.839 Other rheumatoid arthritis with rheumatoid factor of unspecified wrist
+ M05.84 Other rheumatoid arthritis with rheumatoid factor of hand
M05.841 Other rheumatoid arthritis with rheumatoid factor of right hand
M05.842 Other rheumatoid arthritis with rheumatoid factor of left hand
M05.849 Other rheumatoid arthritis with rheumatoid factor of unspecified hand
+ M05.85 Other rheumatoid arthritis with rheumatoid factor of hip
M05.851 Other rheumatoid arthritis with rheumatoid factor of right hip
M05.852 Other rheumatoid arthritis with rheumatoid factor of left hip
M05.859 Other rheumatoid arthritis with rheumatoid factor of unspecified hip

+ M05.86 Other rheumatoid arthritis with rheumatoid factor of knee
  - M05.861 Other rheumatoid arthritis with rheumatoid factor of right knee
  - M05.862 Other rheumatoid arthritis with rheumatoid factor of left knee
  - M05.869 Other rheumatoid arthritis with rheumatoid factor of unspecified knee

+ M05.87 Other rheumatoid arthritis with rheumatoid factor of ankle and foot
  - M05.871 Other rheumatoid arthritis with rheumatoid factor of right ankle and foot
  - M05.872 Other rheumatoid arthritis with rheumatoid factor of left ankle and foot
  - M05.879 Other rheumatoid arthritis with rheumatoid factor of unspecified ankle and foot

M05.89 Other rheumatoid arthritis with rheumatoid factor of multiple sites

M05.8A Other rheumatoid arthritis with rheumatoid factor of other specified site

M05.9 Rheumatoid arthritis with rheumatoid factor, unspecified

M06 Other rheumatoid arthritis

AHA CC: 4Q, 2020, 31-32

+ M06.0 Rheumatoid arthritis without rheumatoid factor
  - M06.00 Rheumatoid arthritis without rheumatoid factor, unspecified site
  - + M06.01 Rheumatoid arthritis without rheumatoid factor, shoulder
    - M06.011 Rheumatoid arthritis without rheumatoid factor, right shoulder
    - M06.012 Rheumatoid arthritis without rheumatoid factor, left shoulder
    - M06.019 Rheumatoid arthritis without rheumatoid factor, unspecified shoulder
  - + M06.02 Rheumatoid arthritis without rheumatoid factor, elbow
    - M06.021 Rheumatoid arthritis without rheumatoid factor, right elbow
    - M06.022 Rheumatoid arthritis without rheumatoid factor, left elbow
    - M06.029 Rheumatoid arthritis without rheumatoid factor, unspecified elbow
  - + M06.03 Rheumatoid arthritis without rheumatoid factor, wrist
    - M06.031 Rheumatoid arthritis without rheumatoid factor, right wrist
    - M06.032 Rheumatoid arthritis without rheumatoid factor, left wrist
    - M06.039 Rheumatoid arthritis without rheumatoid factor, unspecified wrist
  - + M06.04 Rheumatoid arthritis without rheumatoid factor, hand
    - M06.041 Rheumatoid arthritis without rheumatoid factor, right hand
    - M06.042 Rheumatoid arthritis without rheumatoid factor, left hand
    - M06.049 Rheumatoid arthritis without rheumatoid factor, unspecified hand
  - + M06.05 Rheumatoid arthritis without rheumatoid factor, hip
    - M06.051 Rheumatoid arthritis without rheumatoid factor, right hip
    - M06.052 Rheumatoid arthritis without rheumatoid factor, left hip
    - M06.059 Rheumatoid arthritis without rheumatoid factor, unspecified hip
  - + M06.06 Rheumatoid arthritis without rheumatoid factor, knee
    - M06.061 Rheumatoid arthritis without rheumatoid factor, right knee
    - M06.062 Rheumatoid arthritis without rheumatoid factor, left knee
    - M06.069 Rheumatoid arthritis without rheumatoid factor, unspecified knee
  - + M06.07 Rheumatoid arthritis without rheumatoid factor, ankle and foot
    - M06.071 Rheumatoid arthritis without rheumatoid factor, right ankle and foot
    - M06.072 Rheumatoid arthritis without rheumatoid factor, left ankle and foot
    - M06.079 Rheumatoid arthritis without rheumatoid factor, unspecified ankle and foot
  - M06.08 Rheumatoid arthritis without rheumatoid factor, vertebrae
  - M06.09 Rheumatoid arthritis without rheumatoid factor, multiple sites
  - M06.0A Rheumatoid arthritis without rheumatoid factor, other specified site

• M06.1 Adult-onset Still's disease

Excludes1: Still's disease NOS (M08.2-)

+ M06.2 Rheumatoid bursitis
  - M06.20 Rheumatoid bursitis, unspecified site
  - + M06.21 Rheumatoid bursitis, shoulder
    - M06.211 Rheumatoid bursitis, right shoulder
    - M06.212 Rheumatoid bursitis, left shoulder
    - M06.219 Rheumatoid bursitis, unspecified shoulder
  - + M06.22 Rheumatoid bursitis, elbow
    - M06.221 Rheumatoid bursitis, right elbow
    - M06.222 Rheumatoid bursitis, left elbow
    - M06.229 Rheumatoid bursitis, unspecified elbow
  - + M06.23 Rheumatoid bursitis, wrist
    - M06.231 Rheumatoid bursitis, right wrist
    - M06.232 Rheumatoid bursitis, left wrist
    - M06.239 Rheumatoid bursitis, unspecified wrist
  - + M06.24 Rheumatoid bursitis, hand
    - M06.241 Rheumatoid bursitis, right hand
    - M06.242 Rheumatoid bursitis, left hand
    - M06.249 Rheumatoid bursitis, unspecified hand
  - + M06.25 Rheumatoid bursitis, hip
    - M06.251 Rheumatoid bursitis, right hip
    - M06.252 Rheumatoid bursitis, left hip
    - M06.259 Rheumatoid bursitis, unspecified hip
  - + M06.26 Rheumatoid bursitis, knee
    - M06.261 Rheumatoid bursitis, right knee
    - M06.262 Rheumatoid bursitis, left knee
    - M06.269 Rheumatoid bursitis, unspecified knee
  - + M06.27 Rheumatoid bursitis, ankle and foot
    - M06.271 Rheumatoid bursitis, right ankle and foot
    - M06.272 Rheumatoid bursitis, left ankle and foot
    - M06.279 Rheumatoid bursitis, unspecified ankle and foot
  - M06.28 Rheumatoid bursitis, vertebrae
  - M06.29 Rheumatoid bursitis, multiple sites

+ M06.3 Rheumatoid nodule
  - M06.30 Rheumatoid nodule, unspecified site
  - + M06.31 Rheumatoid nodule, shoulder
    - M06.311 Rheumatoid nodule, right shoulder
    - M06.312 Rheumatoid nodule, left shoulder
    - M06.319 Rheumatoid nodule, unspecified shoulder
  - + M06.32 Rheumatoid nodule, elbow
    - M06.321 Rheumatoid nodule, right elbow
    - M06.322 Rheumatoid nodule, left elbow
    - M06.329 Rheumatoid nodule, unspecified elbow
  - + M06.33 Rheumatoid nodule, wrist
    - M06.331 Rheumatoid nodule, right wrist
    - M06.332 Rheumatoid nodule, left wrist
    - M06.339 Rheumatoid nodule, unspecified wrist
  - + M06.34 Rheumatoid nodule, hand
    - M06.341 Rheumatoid nodule, right hand
    - M06.342 Rheumatoid nodule, left hand
    - M06.349 Rheumatoid nodule, unspecified hand
  - + M06.35 Rheumatoid nodule, hip
    - M06.351 Rheumatoid nodule, right hip
    - M06.352 Rheumatoid nodule, left hip
    - M06.359 Rheumatoid nodule, unspecified hip
  - + M06.36 Rheumatoid nodule, knee
    - M06.361 Rheumatoid nodule, right knee
    - M06.362 Rheumatoid nodule, left knee
    - M06.369 Rheumatoid nodule, unspecified knee
  - + M06.37 Rheumatoid nodule, ankle and foot
    - M06.371 Rheumatoid nodule, right ankle and foot
    - M06.372 Rheumatoid nodule, left ankle and foot
    - M06.379 Rheumatoid nodule, unspecified ankle and foot

M06.38 Rheumatoid nodule, vertebrae
M06.39 Rheumatoid nodule, multiple sites
M06.4 Inflammatory polyarthropathy
Excludes1: *polyarthritis NOS (M13.0)*
+ M06.8 Other specified rheumatoid arthritis
M06.80 Other specified rheumatoid arthritis, unspecified site
+ M06.81 Other specified rheumatoid arthritis, shoulder
M06.811 Other specified rheumatoid arthritis, right shoulder
M06.812 Other specified rheumatoid arthritis, left shoulder
M06.819 Other specified rheumatoid arthritis, unspecified shoulder
+ M06.82 Other specified rheumatoid arthritis, elbow
M06.821 Other specified rheumatoid arthritis, right elbow
M06.822 Other specified rheumatoid arthritis, left elbow
M06.829 Other specified rheumatoid arthritis, unspecified elbow
+ M06.83 Other specified rheumatoid arthritis, wrist
M06.831 Other specified rheumatoid arthritis, right wrist
M06.832 Other specified rheumatoid arthritis, left wrist
M06.839 Other specified rheumatoid arthritis, unspecified wrist
+ M06.84 Other specified rheumatoid arthritis, hand
M06.841 Other specified rheumatoid arthritis, right hand
M06.842 Other specified rheumatoid arthritis, left hand
M06.849 Other specified rheumatoid arthritis, unspecified hand
+ M06.85 Other specified rheumatoid arthritis, hip
M06.851 Other specified rheumatoid arthritis, right hip
M06.852 Other specified rheumatoid arthritis, left hip
M06.859 Other specified rheumatoid arthritis, unspecified hip
+ M06.86 Other specified rheumatoid arthritis, knee
M06.861 Other specified rheumatoid arthritis, right knee
M06.862 Other specified rheumatoid arthritis, left knee
M06.869 Other specified rheumatoid arthritis, unspecified knee
+ M06.87 Other specified rheumatoid arthritis, ankle and foot
M06.871 Other specified rheumatoid arthritis, right ankle and foot
M06.872 Other specified rheumatoid arthritis, left ankle and foot
M06.879 Other specified rheumatoid arthritis, unspecified ankle and foot
M06.88 Other specified rheumatoid arthritis, vertebrae
M06.89 Other specified rheumatoid arthritis, multiple sites
M06.8A Other specified rheumatoid arthritis, other specified site
M06.9 Rheumatoid arthritis, unspecified

M07 Enteropathic arthropathies

Code also associated enteropathy, such as:
regional enteritis [Crohn's disease] (K50.-)
ulcerative colitis (K51.-)
Excludes1: *psoriatic arthropathies (L40.5-)*
+ M07.6 Enteropathic arthropathies
M07.60 Enteropathic arthropathies, unspecified site
+ M07.61 Enteropathic arthropathies, shoulder
M07.611 Enteropathic arthropathies, right shoulder
M07.612 Enteropathic arthropathies, left shoulder
M07.619 Enteropathic arthropathies, unspecified shoulder
+ M07.62 Enteropathic arthropathies, elbow
M07.621 Enteropathic arthropathies, right elbow
M07.622 Enteropathic arthropathies, left elbow
M07.629 Enteropathic arthropathies, unspecified elbow
+ M07.63 Enteropathic arthropathies, wrist
M07.631 Enteropathic arthropathies, right wrist
M07.632 Enteropathic arthropathies, left wrist
M07.639 Enteropathic arthropathies, unspecified wrist
+ M07.64 Enteropathic arthropathies, hand
M07.641 Enteropathic arthropathies, right hand
M07.642 Enteropathic arthropathies, lefthand
M07.649 Enteropathic arthropathies, unspecified hand
+ M07.65 Enteropathic arthropathies, hip
M07.651 Enteropathic arthropathies, right hip
M07.652 Enteropathic arthropathies, left hip
M07.659 Enteropathic arthropathies, unspecified hip
+ M07.66 Enteropathic arthropathies, knee
M07.661 Enteropathic arthropathies, right knee
M07.662 Enteropathic arthropathies, left knee
M07.669 Enteropathic arthropathies, unspecified knee
+ M07.67 Enteropathic arthropathies, ankle and foot
M07.671 Enteropathic arthropathies, right ankle and foot
M07.672 Enteropathic arthropathies, left ankle and foot
M07.679 Enteropathic arthropathies, unspecified ankle and foot
M07.68 Enteropathic arthropathies, vertebrae
M07.69 Enteropathic arthropathies, multiple sites

M08 Juvenile arthritis

Code also any associated underlying condition, such as:
regional enteritis [Crohn's disease] (K50.-)
ulcerative colitis (K51.-)
Excludes1: *arthropathy in Whipple's disease (M14.8)*
Felty's syndrome (M05.0)
juvenile dermatomyositis (M33.0-)
psoriatic juvenile arthropathy (L40.54)
AHA CC: 4Q, 2020, 31-32
+ M08.0 Unspecified juvenile rheumatoid arthritis
Juvenile rheumatoid arthritis with or without rheumatoid factor
M08.00 Unspecified juvenile rheumatoid arthritis of unspecified site
+ M08.01 Unspecified juvenile rheumatoid arthritis, shoulder
M08.011 Unspecified juvenile rheumatoid arthritis, right shoulder
M08.012 Unspecified juvenile rheumatoid arthritis, left shoulder
M08.019 Unspecified juvenile rheumatoid arthritis, unspecified shoulder
+ M08.02 Unspecified juvenile rheumatoid arthritis of elbow
M08.021 Unspecified juvenile rheumatoid arthritis, right elbow
M08.022 Unspecified juvenile rheumatoid arthritis, left elbow
M08.029 Unspecified juvenile rheumatoid arthritis, unspecified elbow
+ M08.03 Unspecified juvenile rheumatoid arthritis, wrist
M08.031 Unspecified juvenile rheumatoid arthritis, right wrist
M08.032 Unspecified juvenile rheumatoid arthritis, left wrist
M08.039 Unspecified juvenile rheumatoid arthritis, unspecified wrist
+ M08.04 Unspecified juvenile rheumatoid arthritis, hand
M08.041 Unspecified juvenile rheumatoid arthritis, right hand
M08.042 Unspecified juvenile rheumatoid arthritis, left hand
M08.049 Unspecified juvenile rheumatoid arthritis, unspecified hand
+ M08.05 Unspecified juvenile rheumatoid arthritis, hip
M08.051 Unspecified juvenile rheumatoid arthritis, right hip

M08.052 Unspecified juvenile rheumatoid arthritis, left hip
M08.059 Unspecified juvenile rheumatoid arthritis, unspecified hip
+ M08.06 Unspecified juvenile rheumatoid arthritis, knee
M08.061 Unspecified juvenile rheumatoid arthritis, right knee
M08.062 Unspecified juvenile rheumatoid arthritis, left knee
M08.069 Unspecified juvenile rheumatoid arthritis, unspecified knee
+ M08.07 Unspecified juvenile rheumatoid arthritis, ankle and foot
M08.071 Unspecified juvenile rheumatoid arthritis, right ankle and foot
M08.072 Unspecified juvenile rheumatoid arthritis, left ankle and foot
M08.079 Unspecified juvenile rheumatoid arthritis, unspecified ankle and foot
M08.08 Unspecified juvenile rheumatoid arthritis, vertebrae
M08.09 Unspecified juvenile rheumatoid arthritis, multiple sites
M08.0A Unspecified juvenile rheumatoid arthritis, other specified site
M08.1 Juvenile ankylosing spondylitis
Excludes1: ankylosing spondylitis in adults (M45.0-)
+ M08.2 Juvenile rheumatoid arthritis with systemic onset
Still's disease NOS
Excludes1: adult-onset Still's disease (M06.1-)
M08.20 Juvenile rheumatoid arthritis with systemic onset, unspecified site
+ M08.21 Juvenile rheumatoid arthritis with systemic onset, shoulder
M08.211 Juvenile rheumatoid arthritis with systemic onset, right shoulder
M08.212 Juvenile rheumatoid arthritis with systemic onset, left shoulder
M08.219 Juvenile rheumatoid arthritis with systemic onset, unspecified shoulder
+ M08.22 Juvenile rheumatoid arthritis with systemic onset, elbow
M08.221 Juvenile rheumatoid arthritis with systemic onset, right elbow
M08.222 Juvenile rheumatoid arthritis with systemic onset, left elbow
M08.229 Juvenile rheumatoid arthritis with systemic onset, unspecified elbow
+ M08.23 Juvenile rheumatoid arthritis with systemic onset, wrist
M08.231 Juvenile rheumatoid arthritis with systemic onset, right wrist
M08.232 Juvenile rheumatoid arthritis with systemic onset, left wrist
M08.239 Juvenile rheumatoid arthritis with systemic onset, unspecified wrist
+ M08.24 Juvenile rheumatoid arthritis with systemic onset, hand
M08.241 Juvenile rheumatoid arthritis with systemic onset, right hand
M08.242 Juvenile rheumatoid arthritis with systemic onset, left hand
M08.249 Juvenile rheumatoid arthritis with systemic onset, unspecified hand
+ M08.25 Juvenile rheumatoid arthritis with systemic onset, hip
M08.251 Juvenile rheumatoid arthritis with systemic onset, right hip
M08.252 Juvenile rheumatoid arthritis with systemic onset, left hip
M08.259 Juvenile rheumatoid arthritis with systemic onset, unspecified hip
+ M08.26 Juvenile rheumatoid arthritis with systemic onset, knee
M08.261 Juvenile rheumatoid arthritis with systemic onset, right knee
M08.262 Juvenile rheumatoid arthritis with systemic onset, left knee
M08.269 Juvenile rheumatoid arthritis with systemic onset, unspecified knee
+ M08.27 Juvenile rheumatoid arthritis with systemic onset, ankle and foot
M08.271 Juvenile rheumatoid arthritis with systemic onset, right ankle and foot
M08.272 Juvenile rheumatoid arthritis with systemic onset, left ankle and foot
M08.279 Juvenile rheumatoid arthritis with systemic onset, unspecified ankle and foot
M08.28 Juvenile rheumatoid arthritis with systemic onset, vertebrae
M08.29 Juvenile rheumatoid arthritis with systemic onset, multiple sites
M08.2A Juvenile rheumatoid arthritis with systemic onset, other specified site
M08.3 Juvenile rheumatoid polyarthritis (seronegative)
+ M08.4 Pauciarticular juvenile rheumatoid arthritis
M08.40 Pauciarticular juvenile rheumatoid arthritis, unspecified site
+ M08.41 Pauciarticular juvenile rheumatoid arthritis, shoulder
M08.411 Pauciarticular juvenile rheumatoid arthritis, right shoulder
M08.412 Pauciarticular juvenile rheumatoid arthritis, left shoulder
M08.419 Pauciarticular juvenile rheumatoid arthritis, unspecified shoulder
+ M08.42 Pauciarticular juvenile rheumatoid arthritis, elbow
M08.421 Pauciarticular juvenile rheumatoid arthritis, right elbow
M08.422 Pauciarticular juvenile rheumatoid arthritis, left elbow
M08.429 Pauciarticular juvenile rheumatoid arthritis, unspecified elbow
+ M08.43 Pauciarticular juvenile rheumatoid arthritis, wrist
M08.431 Pauciarticular juvenile rheumatoid arthritis, right wrist
M08.432 Pauciarticular juvenile rheumatoid arthritis, left wrist
M08.439 Pauciarticular juvenile rheumatoid arthritis, unspecified wrist
+ M08.44 Pauciarticular juvenile rheumatoid arthritis, hand
M08.441 Pauciarticular juvenile rheumatoid arthritis, right hand
M08.442 Pauciarticular juvenile rheumatoid arthritis, left hand
M08.449 Pauciarticular juvenile rheumatoid arthritis, unspecified hand
+ M08.45 Pauciarticular juvenile rheumatoid arthritis, hip
M08.451 Pauciarticular juvenile rheumatoid arthritis, right hip
M08.452 Pauciarticular juvenile rheumatoid arthritis, left hip
M08.459 Pauciarticular juvenile rheumatoid arthritis, unspecified hip
+ M08.46 Pauciarticular juvenile rheumatoid arthritis, knee
M08.461 Pauciarticular juvenile rheumatoid arthritis, right knee
M08.462 Pauciarticular juvenile rheumatoid arthritis, left knee
M08.469 Pauciarticular juvenile rheumatoid arthritis, unspecified knee
+ M08.47 Pauciarticular juvenile rheumatoid arthritis, ankle and foot
M08.471 Pauciarticular juvenile rheumatoid arthritis, right ankle and foot
M08.472 Pauciarticular juvenile rheumatoid arthritis, left ankle and foot
M08.479 Pauciarticular juvenile rheumatoid arthritis, unspecified ankle and foot
M08.48 Pauciarticular juvenile rheumatoid arthritis, vertebrae
M08.4A Pauciarticular juvenile rheumatoid arthritis, other specified site

+ M08.8 Other juvenile arthritis
M08.80 Other juvenile arthritis, unspecified site
+ M08.81 Other juvenile arthritis, shoulder
M08.811 Other juvenile arthritis, right shoulder
M08.812 Other juvenile arthritis, left shoulder
M08.819 Other juvenile arthritis, unspecified shoulder
+ M08.82 Other juvenile arthritis, elbow
M08.821 Other juvenile arthritis, right elbow
M08.822 Other juvenile arthritis, left elbow
M08.829 Other juvenile arthritis, unspecified elbow
+ M08.83 Other juvenile arthritis, wrist
M08.831 Other juvenile arthritis, right wrist
M08.832 Other juvenile arthritis, left wrist
M08.839 Other juvenile arthritis, unspecified wrist
+ M08.84 Other juvenile arthritis, hand
M08.841 Other juvenile arthritis, right hand
M08.842 Other juvenile arthritis, left hand
M08.849 Other juvenile arthritis, unspecified hand
+ M08.85 Other juvenile arthritis, hip
M08.851 Other juvenile arthritis, right hip
M08.852 Other juvenile arthritis, left hip
M08.859 Other juvenile arthritis, unspecified hip
+ M08.86 Other juvenile arthritis, knee
M08.861 Other juvenile arthritis, right knee
M08.862 Other juvenile arthritis, left knee
M08.869 Other juvenile arthritis, unspecified knee
+ M08.87 Other juvenile arthritis, ankle and foot
M08.871 Other juvenile arthritis, right ankle and foot
M08.872 Other juvenile arthritis, left ankle and foot
M08.879 Other juvenile arthritis, unspecified ankle and foot
M08.88 Other juvenile arthritis, other specified site
Other juvenile arthritis, vertebrae
M08.89 Other juvenile arthritis, multiple sites
+ M08.9 Juvenile arthritis, unspecified
Excludes1: *juvenile rheumatoid arthritis, unspecified (M08.0-)*
M08.90 Juvenile arthritis, unspecified, unspecified site
+ M08.91 Juvenile arthritis, unspecified, shoulder
M08.911 Juvenile arthritis, unspecified, right shoulder
M08.912 Juvenile arthritis, unspecified, left shoulder
M08.919 Juvenile arthritis, unspecified, unspecified shoulder
+ M08.92 Juvenile arthritis, unspecified, elbow
M08.921 Juvenile arthritis, unspecified, right elbow
M08.922 Juvenile arthritis, unspecified, left elbow
M08.929 Juvenile arthritis, unspecified, unspecified elbow
+ M08.93 Juvenile arthritis, unspecified, wrist
M08.931 Juvenile arthritis, unspecified, right wrist
M08.932 Juvenile arthritis, unspecified, left wrist
M08.939 Juvenile arthritis, unspecified, unspecified wrist
+ M08.94 Juvenile arthritis, unspecified, hand
M08.941 Juvenile arthritis, unspecified, right hand
M08.942 Juvenile arthritis, unspecified, left hand
M08.949 Juvenile arthritis, unspecified, unspecified hand
+ M08.95 Juvenile arthritis, unspecified, hip
M08.951 Juvenile arthritis, unspecified, right hip
M08.952 Juvenile arthritis, unspecified, left hip
M08.959 Juvenile arthritis, unspecified, unspecified hip
+ M08.96 Juvenile arthritis, unspecified, knee
M08.961 Juvenile arthritis, unspecified, right knee
M08.962 Juvenile arthritis, unspecified, left knee
M08.969 Juvenile arthritis, unspecified, unspecified knee
+ M08.97 Juvenile arthritis, unspecified, ankle and foot
M08.971 Juvenile arthritis, unspecified, right ankle and foot
M08.972 Juvenile arthritis, unspecified, left ankle and foot
M08.979 Juvenile arthritis, unspecified, unspecified ankle and foot
M08.98 Juvenile arthritis, unspecified, vertebrae
M08.99 Juvenile arthritis, unspecified, multiple sites
M08.9A Juvenile arthritis, unspecified, other specified site

M1A Chronic gout

Use additional code to identify:
Autonomic neuropathy in diseases classified elsewhere (G99.0)
Calculus of urinary tract in diseases classified elsewhere (N22)
Cardiomyopathy in diseases classified elsewhere (I43)
Disorders of external ear in diseases classified elsewhere (H61.1-, H62.8-)
Disorders of iris and ciliary body in diseases classified elsewhere (H22)
Glomerular disorders in diseases classified elsewhere (N08)
Excludes1: *gout NOS (M10.-)*
Excludes2: *acute gout (M10.-)*

The appropriate 7th character is to be added to each code from category M1A
0 without tophus (tophi)
1 with tophus (tophi)

+ M1A.0 Idiopathic chronic gout
Chronic gouty bursitis
Primary chronic gout
X+7th M1A.00 Idiopathic chronic gout, unspecified site
+ M1A.01 Idiopathic chronic gout, shoulder
+7th M1A.011 Idiopathic chronic gout, right shoulder
+7th M1A.012 Idiopathic chronic gout, left shoulder
+7th M1A.019 Idiopathic chronic gout, unspecified shoulder
+ M1A.02 Idiopathic chronic gout, elbow
+7th M1A.021 Idiopathic chronic gout, right elbow
+7th M1A.022 Idiopathic chronic gout, left elbow
+7th M1A.029 Idiopathic chronic gout, unspecified elbow
+ M1A.03 Idiopathic chronic gout, wrist
+7th M1A.031 Idiopathic chronic gout, right wrist
+7th M1A.032 Idiopathic chronic gout, left wrist
+7th M1A.039 Idiopathic chronic gout, unspecified wrist
+ M1A.04 Idiopathic chronic gout, hand
+7th M1A.041 Idiopathic chronic gout, right hand
+7th M1A.042 Idiopathic chronic gout, left hand
+7th M1A.049 Idiopathic chronic gout, unspecified hand
+ M1A.05 Idiopathic chronic gout, hip
+7th M1A.051 Idiopathic chronic gout, right hip
+7th M1A.052 Idiopathic chronic gout, left hip
+7th M1A.059 Idiopathic chronic gout, unspecified hip
+ M1A.06 Idiopathic chronic gout, knee
+7th M1A.061 Idiopathic chronic gout, right knee
+7th M1A.062 Idiopathic chronic gout, left knee
+7th M1A.069 Idiopathic chronic gout, unspecified knee
+ M1A.07 Idiopathic chronic gout, ankle and foot
+7th M1A.071 Idiopathic chronic gout, right ankle and foot
+7th M1A.072 Idiopathic chronic gout, left ankle and foot
+7th M1A.079 Idiopathic chronic gout, unspecified ankle and foot
X+7th M1A.08 Idiopathic chronic gout, vertebrae
M1A.09 Idiopathic chronic gout, multiple sites
+ M1A.1 Lead-induced chronic gout
Code first toxic effects of lead and its compounds (T56.0-)
X+7th M1A.10 Lead-induced chronic gout, unspecified site
+ M1A.11 Lead-induced chronic gout, shoulder
+7th M1A.111 Lead-induced chronic gout, right shoulder
+7th M1A.112 Lead-induced chronic gout, left shoulder
+7th M1A.119 Lead-induced chronic gout, unspecified shoulder

+ **M1A.12 Lead-induced chronic gout, elbow**
  - +7th **M1A.121 Lead-induced chronic gout, right elbow**
  - +7th **M1A.122 Lead-induced chronic gout, left elbow**
  - +7th **M1A.129 Lead-induced chronic gout, unspecified elbow**
+ **M1A.13 Lead-induced chronic gout, wrist**
  - +7th **M1A.131 Lead-induced chronic gout, right wrist**
  - +7th **M1A.132 Lead-induced chronic gout, left wrist**
  - +7th **M1A.139 Lead-induced chronic gout, unspecified wrist**
+ **M1A.14 Lead-induced chronic gout, hand**
  - +7th **M1A.141 Lead-induced chronic gout, right hand**
  - +7th **M1A.142 Lead-induced chronic gout, left hand**
  - +7th **M1A.149 Lead-induced chronic gout, unspecified hand**
+ **M1A.15 Lead-induced chronic gout, hip**
  - +7th **M1A.151 Lead-induced chronic gout, right hip**
  - +7th **M1A.152 Lead-induced chronic gout, left hip**
  - +7th **M1A.159 Lead-induced chronic gout, unspecified hip**
+ **M1A.16 Lead-induced chronic gout, knee**
  - +7th **M1A.161 Lead-induced chronic gout, right knee**
  - +7th **M1A.162 Lead-induced chronic gout, left knee**
  - +7th **M1A.169 Lead-induced chronic gout, unspecified knee**
+ **M1A.17 Lead-induced chronic gout, ankle and foot**
  - +7th **M1A.171 Lead-induced chronic gout, right ankle and foot**
  - +7th **M1A.172 Lead-induced chronic gout, left ankle and foot**
  - +7th **M1A.179 Lead-induced chronic gout, unspecified ankle and foot**

X+7th **M1A.18 Lead-induced chronic gout, vertebrae**

X+7th **M1A.19 Lead-induced chronic gout, multiple sites**

+ **M1A.2 Drug-induced chronic gout**

  Use additional code for adverse effect, if applicable, to identify drug (T36-T50 with fifth or sixth character 5)

X+7th **M1A.20 Drug-induced chronic gout, unspecified site**

+ **M1A.21 Drug-induced chronic gout, shoulder**
  - +7th **M1A.211 Drug-induced chronic gout, right shoulder**
  - +7th **M1A.212 Drug-induced chronic gout, left shoulder**
  - +7th **M1A.219 Drug-induced chronic gout, unspecified shoulder**
+ **M1A.22 Drug-induced chronic gout, elbow**
  - +7th **M1A.221 Drug-induced chronic gout, right elbow**
  - +7th **M1A.222 Drug-induced chronic gout, left elbow**
  - +7th **M1A.229 Drug-induced chronic gout, unspecified elbow**
+ **M1A.23 Drug-induced chronic gout, wrist**
  - +7th **M1A.231 Drug-induced chronic gout, right wrist**
  - +7th **M1A.232 Drug-induced chronic gout, left wrist**
  - +7th **M1A.239 Drug-induced chronic gout, unspecified wrist**
+ **M1A.24 Drug-induced chronic gout, hand**
  - +7th **M1A.241 Drug-induced chronic gout, right hand**
  - +7th **M1A.242 Drug-induced chronic gout, left hand**
  - +7th **M1A.249 Drug-induced chronic gout, unspecified hand**
+ **M1A.25 Drug-induced chronic gout, hip**
  - +7th **M1A.251 Drug-induced chronic gout, right hip**
  - +7th **M1A.252 Drug-induced chronic gout, left hip**
  - +7th **M1A.259 Drug-induced chronic gout, unspecified hip**
+ **M1A.26 Drug-induced chronic gout, knee**
  - +7th **M1A.261 Drug-induced chronic gout, right knee**
  - +7th **M1A.262 Drug-induced chronic gout, left knee**
  - +7th **M1A.269 Drug-induced chronic gout, unspecified knee**
+ **M1A.27 Drug-induced chronic gout, ankle and foot**
  - +7th **M1A.271 Drug-induced chronic gout, right ankle and foot**
  - +7th **M1A.272 Drug-induced chronic gout, left ankle and foot**
  - +7th **M1A.279 Drug-induced chronic gout, unspecified ankle and foot**

X+7th **M1A.28 Drug-induced chronic gout, vertebrae**

X+7th **M1A.29 Drug-induced chronic gout, multiple sites**

+ **M1A.3 Chronic gout due to renal impairment**

  Code first associated renal disease

X+7th **M1A.30 Chronic gout due to renal impairment, unspecified site**

+ **M1A.31 Chronic gout due to renal impairment, shoulder**
  - +7th **M1A.311 Chronic gout due to renal impairment, right shoulder**
  - +7th **M1A.312 Chronic gout due to renal impairment, left shoulder**
  - +7th **M1A.319 Chronic gout due to renal impairment, unspecified shoulder**
+ **M1A.32 Chronic gout due to renal impairment, elbow**
  - +7th **M1A.321 Chronic gout due to renal impairment, right elbow**
  - +7th **M1A.322 Chronic gout due to renal impairment, left elbow**
  - +7th **M1A.329 Chronic gout due to renal impairment, unspecified elbow**
+ **M1A.33 Chronic gout due to renal impairment, wrist**
  - +7th **M1A.331 Chronic gout due to renal impairment, right wrist**
  - +7th **M1A.332 Chronic gout due to renal impairment, left wrist**
  - +7th **M1A.339 Chronic gout due to renal impairment, unspecified wrist**
+ **M1A.34 Chronic gout due to renal impairment, hand**
  - +7th **M1A.341 Chronic gout due to renal impairment, right hand**
  - +7th **M1A.342 Chronic gout due to renal impairment, left hand**
  - +7th **M1A.349 Chronic gout due to renal impairment, unspecified hand**
+ **M1A.35 Chronic gout due to renal impairment, hip**
  - +7th **M1A.351 Chronic gout due to renal impairment, right hip**
  - +7th **M1A.352 Chronic gout due to renal impairment, left hip**
  - +7th **M1A.359 Chronic gout due to renal impairment, unspecified hip**
+ **M1A.36 Chronic gout due to renal impairment, knee**
  - +7th **M1A.361 Chronic gout due to renal impairment, right knee**
  - +7th **M1A.362 Chronic gout due to renal impairment, left knee**
  - +7th **M1A.369 Chronic gout due to renal impairment, unspecified knee**
+ **M1A.37 Chronic gout due to renal impairment, ankle and foot**
  - +7th **M1A.371 Chronic gout due to renal impairment, right ankle and foot**
  - +7th **M1A.372 Chronic gout due to renal impairment, left ankle and foot**
  - +7th **M1A.379 Chronic gout due to renal impairment, unspecified ankle and foot**

X+7th **M1A.38 Chronic gout due to renal impairment, vertebrae**

X+7th **M1A.39 Chronic gout due to renal impairment, multiple sites**

+ **M1A.4 Other secondary chronic gout**

  Code first associated condition

X+7th **M1A.40 Other secondary chronic gout, unspecified site**

+ **M1A.41 Other secondary chronic gout, shoulder**
  - +7th **M1A.411 Other secondary chronic gout, right shoulder**
  - +7th **M1A.412 Other secondary chronic gout, left shoulder**
  - +7th **M1A.419 Other secondary chronic gout, unspecified shoulder**
+ **M1A.42 Other secondary chronic gout, elbow**
  - +7th **M1A.421 Other secondary chronic gout, right elbow**
  - +7th **M1A.422 Other secondary chronic gout, left elbow**
  - +7th **M1A.429 Other secondary chronic gout, unspecified elbow**

+ M1A.43 Other secondary chronic gout, wrist
+7th M1A.431 Other secondary chronic gout, right wrist
+7th M1A.432 Other secondary chronic gout, left wrist
+7th M1A.439 Other secondary chronic gout, unspecified wrist
+ M1A.44 Other secondary chronic gout, hand
+7th M1A.441 Other secondary chronic gout, right hand
+7th M1A.442 Other secondary chronic gout, left hand
+7th M1A.449 Other secondary chronic gout, unspecified hand
+ M1A.45 Other secondary chronic gout, hip
+7th M1A.451 Other secondary chronic gout, right hip
+7th M1A.452 Other secondary chronic gout, left hip
+7th M1A.459 Other secondary chronic gout, unspecified hip
+ M1A.46 Other secondary chronic gout, knee
+7th M1A.461 Other secondary chronic gout, right knee
+7th M1A.462 Other secondary chronic gout, left knee
+7th M1A.469 Other secondary chronic gout, unspecified knee
+ M1A.47 Other secondary chronic gout, ankle and foot
+7th M1A.471 Other secondary chronic gout, right ankle and foot
+7th M1A.472 Other secondary chronic gout, left ankle and foot
+7th M1A.479 Other secondary chronic gout, unspecified ankle and foot
X+7th M1A.48 Other secondary chronic gout, vertebrae
X+7th M1A.49 Other secondary chronic gout, multiple sites
X+7th M1A.9 Chronic gout, unspecified

M10 Gout

Acute gout
Gout attack
Gout flare
Podagra
Use additional code to identify:
Autonomic neuropathy in diseases classified elsewhere (G99.0)
Calculus of urinary tract in diseases classified elsewhere (N22)
Cardiomyopathy in diseases classified elsewhere (I43)
Disorders of external ear in diseases classified elsewhere (H61.1-, H62.8-)
Disorders of iris and ciliary body in diseases classified elsewhere (H22)
Glomerular disorders in diseases classified elsewhere (N08)

Excludes2: *chronic gout (M1A.-)*

+ M10.0 Idiopathic gout
Gouty bursitis
Primary gout
M10.00 Idiopathic gout, unspecified site
+ M10.01 Idiopathic gout, shoulder
M10.011 Idiopathic gout, right shoulder
M10.012 Idiopathic gout, left shoulder
M10.019 Idiopathic gout, unspecified shoulder
+ M10.02 Idiopathic gout, elbow
M10.021 Idiopathic gout, right elbow
M10.022 Idiopathic gout, left elbow
M10.029 Idiopathic gout, unspecified elbow
+ M10.03 Idiopathic gout, wrist
M10.031 Idiopathic gout, right wrist
M10.032 Idiopathic gout, left wrist
M10.039 Idiopathic gout, unspecified wrist
+ M10.04 Idiopathic gout, hand
M10.041 Idiopathic gout, right hand
M10.042 Idiopathic gout, left hand
M10.049 Idiopathic gout, unspecified hand
+ M10.05 Idiopathic gout, hip
M10.051 Idiopathic gout, right hip
M10.052 Idiopathic gout, left hip
M10.059 Idiopathic gout, unspecified hip
+ M10.06 Idiopathic gout, knee
M10.061 Idiopathic gout, right knee
M10.062 Idiopathic gout, left knee
M10.069 Idiopathic gout, unspecified knee
+ M10.07 Idiopathic gout, ankle and foot
M10.071 Idiopathic gout, right ankle and foot
M10.072 Idiopathic gout, left ankle and foot
M10.079 Idiopathic gout, unspecified ankle and foot
M10.08 Idiopathic gout, vertebrae
M10.09 Idiopathic gout, multiple sites
+ M10.1 Lead-induced gout
Code first toxic effects of lead and its compounds (T56.0-)
M10.10 Lead-induced gout, unspecified site
+ M10.11 Lead-induced gout, shoulder
M10.111 Lead-induced gout, right shoulder
M10.112 Lead-induced gout, left shoulder
M10.119 Lead-induced gout, unspecified shoulder
+ M10.12 Lead-induced gout, elbow
M10.121 Lead-induced gout, right elbow
M10.122 Lead-induced gout, left elbow
M10.129 Lead-induced gout, unspecified elbow
+ M10.13 Lead-induced gout, wrist
M10.131 Lead-induced gout, right wrist
M10.132 Lead-induced gout, left wrist
M10.139 Lead-induced gout, unspecified wrist
+ M10.14 Lead-induced gout, hand
M10.141 Lead-induced gout, right hand
M10.142 Lead-induced gout, left hand
M10.149 Lead-induced gout, unspecified hand
+ M10.15 Lead-induced gout, hip
M10.151 Lead-induced gout, right hip
M10.152 Lead-induced gout, left hip
M10.159 Lead-induced gout, unspecified hip
+ M10.16 Lead-induced gout, knee
M10.161 Lead-induced gout, right knee
M10.162 Lead-induced gout, left knee
M10.169 Lead-induced gout, unspecified knee
+ M10.17 Lead-induced gout, ankle and foot
M10.171 Lead-induced gout, right ankle and foot
M10.172 Lead-induced gout, left ankle and foot
M10.179 Lead-induced gout, unspecified ankle and foot
M10.18 Lead-induced gout, vertebrae
M10.19 Lead-induced gout, multiple sites
+ M10.2 Drug-induced gout
Use additional code for adverse effect, if applicable, to identify drug (T36-T50 with fifth or sixth character 5)
M10.20 Drug-induced gout, unspecified site
+ M10.21 Drug-induced gout, shoulder
M10.211 Drug-induced gout, right shoulder
M10.212 Drug-induced gout, left shoulder
M10.219 Drug-induced gout, unspecified shoulder
+ M10.22 Drug-induced gout, elbow
M10.221 Drug-induced gout, right elbow
M10.222 Drug-induced gout, left elbow
M10.229 Drug-induced gout, unspecified elbow
+ M10.23 Drug-induced gout, wrist
M10.231 Drug-induced gout, right wrist
M10.232 Drug-induced gout, left wrist
M10.239 Drug-induced gout, unspecified wrist
+ M10.24 Drug-induced gout, hand
M10.241 Drug-induced gout, right hand
M10.242 Drug-induced gout, left hand
M10.249 Drug-induced gout, unspecified hand
+ M10.25 Drug-induced gout, hip
M10.251 Drug-induced gout, right hip
M10.252 Drug-induced gout, left hip
M10.259 Drug-induced gout, unspecified hip
+ M10.26 Drug-induced gout, knee
M10.261 Drug-induced gout, right knee
M10.262 Drug-induced gout, left knee
M10.269 Drug-induced gout, unspecified knee
+ M10.27 Drug-induced gout, ankle and foot
M10.271 Drug-induced gout, right ankle and foot
M10.272 Drug-induced gout, left ankle and foot
M10.279 Drug-induced gout, unspecified ankle and foot
M10.28 Drug-induced gout, vertebrae
M10.29 Drug-induced gout, multiple sites

+ **M10.3 Gout due to renal impairment**
  Code first associated renal disease
  M10.30 Gout due to renal impairment, unspecified site
  + **M10.31 Gout due to renal impairment, shoulder**
    M10.311 Gout due to renal impairment, right shoulder
    M10.312 Gout due to renal impairment, left shoulder
    M10.319 Gout due to renal impairment, unspecified shoulder
  + **M10.32 Gout due to renal impairment, elbow**
    M10.321 Gout due to renal impairment, right elbow
    M10.322 Gout due to renal impairment, left elbow
    M10.329 Gout due to renal impairment, unspecified elbow
  + **M10.33 Gout due to renal impairment, wrist**
    M10.331 Gout due to renal impairment, right wrist
    M10.332 Gout due to renal impairment, left wrist
    M10.339 Gout due to renal impairment, unspecified wrist
  + **M10.34 Gout due to renal impairment, hand**
    M10.341 Gout due to renal impairment, right hand
    M10.342 Gout due to renal impairment, left hand
    M10.349 Gout due to renal impairment, unspecified hand
  + **M10.35 Gout due to renal impairment, hip**
    M10.351 Gout due to renal impairment, right hip
    M10.352 Gout due to renal impairment, left hip
    M10.359 Gout due to renal impairment, unspecified hip
  + **M10.36 Gout due to renal impairment, knee**
    M10.361 Gout due to renal impairment, right knee
    M10.362 Gout due to renal impairment, left knee
    M10.369 Gout due to renal impairment, unspecified knee
  + **M10.37 Gout due to renal impairment, ankle and foot**
    M10.371 Gout due to renal impairment, right ankle and foot
    M10.372 Gout due to renal impairment, left ankle and foot
    M10.379 Gout due to renal impairment, unspecified ankle and foot
  M10.38 Gout due to renal impairment, vertebrae
  M10.39 Gout due to renal impairment, multiple sites

+ **M10.4 Other secondary gout**
  Code first associated condition
  M10.40 Other secondary gout, unspecified site
  + **M10.41 Other secondary gout, shoulder**
    M10.411 Other secondary gout, right shoulder
    M10.412 Other secondary gout, left shoulder
    M10.419 Other secondary gout, unspecified shoulder
  + **M10.42 Other secondary gout, elbow**
    M10.421 Other secondary gout, right elbow
    M10.422 Other secondary gout, left elbow
    M10.429 Other secondary gout, unspecified elbow
  + **M10.43 Other secondary gout, wrist**
    M10.431 Other secondary gout, right wrist
    M10.432 Other secondary gout, left wrist
    M10.439 Other secondary gout, unspecified wrist
  + **M10.44 Other secondary gout, hand**
    M10.441 Other secondary gout, right hand
    M10.442 Other secondary gout, left hand
    M10.449 Other secondary gout, unspecified hand
  + **M10.45 Other secondary gout, hip**
    M10.451 Other secondary gout, right hip
    M10.452 Other secondary gout, left hip
    M10.459 Other secondary gout, unspecified hip
  + **M10.46 Other secondary gout, knee**
    M10.461 Other secondary gout, right knee
    M10.462 Other secondary gout, left knee
    M10.469 Other secondary gout, unspecified knee
  + **M10.47 Other secondary gout, ankle and foot**
    M10.471 Other secondary gout, right ankle and foot
    M10.472 Other secondary gout, left ankle and foot
    M10.479 Other secondary gout, unspecified ankle and foot
  M10.48 Other secondary gout, vertebrae
  M10.49 Other secondary gout, multiple sites

M10.9 Gout, unspecified
  Gout NOS

M11 Other crystal arthropathies

+ **M11.0 Hydroxyapatite deposition disease**
  M11.00 Hydroxyapatite deposition disease, unspecified site
  + **M11.01 Hydroxyapatite deposition disease, shoulder**
    M11.011 Hydroxyapatite deposition disease, right shoulder
    M11.012 Hydroxyapatite deposition disease, left shoulder
    M11.019 Hydroxyapatite deposition disease, unspecified shoulder
  + **M11.02 Hydroxyapatite deposition disease, elbow**
    M11.021 Hydroxyapatite deposition disease, right elbow
    M11.022 Hydroxyapatite deposition disease, left elbow
    M11.029 Hydroxyapatite deposition disease, unspecified elbow
  + **M11.03 Hydroxyapatite deposition disease, wrist**
    M11.031 Hydroxyapatite deposition disease, right wrist
    M11.032 Hydroxyapatite deposition disease, left wrist
    M11.039 Hydroxyapatite deposition disease, unspecified wrist
  + **M11.04 Hydroxyapatite deposition disease, hand**
    M11.041 Hydroxyapatite deposition disease, right hand
    M11.042 Hydroxyapatite deposition disease, left hand
    M11.049 Hydroxyapatite deposition disease, unspecified hand
  + **M11.05 Hydroxyapatite deposition disease, hip**
    M11.051 Hydroxyapatite deposition disease, right hip
    M11.052 Hydroxyapatite deposition disease, left hip
    M11.059 Hydroxyapatite deposition disease, unspecified hip
  + **M11.06 Hydroxyapatite deposition disease, knee**
    M11.061 Hydroxyapatite deposition disease, right knee
    M11.062 Hydroxyapatite deposition disease, left knee
    M11.069 Hydroxyapatite deposition disease, unspecified knee
  + **M11.07 Hydroxyapatite deposition disease, ankle and foot**
    M11.071 Hydroxyapatite deposition disease, right ankle and foot
    M11.072 Hydroxyapatite deposition disease, left ankle and foot
    M11.079 Hydroxyapatite deposition disease, unspecified ankle and foot
  M11.08 Hydroxyapatite deposition disease, vertebrae
  M11.09 Hydroxyapatite deposition disease, multiple sites

+ **M11.1 Familial chondrocalcinosis**
  M11.10 Familial chondrocalcinosis, unspecified site
  + **M11.11 Familial chondrocalcinosis, shoulder**
    M11.111 Familial chondrocalcinosis, right shoulder
    M11.112 Familial chondrocalcinosis, left shoulder
    M11.119 Familial chondrocalcinosis, unspecified shoulder
  + **M11.12 Familial chondrocalcinosis, elbow**
    M11.121 Familial chondrocalcinosis, right elbow
    M11.122 Familial chondrocalcinosis, left elbow
    M11.129 Familial chondrocalcinosis, unspecified elbow

+ M11.13 Familial chondrocalcinosis, wrist
  - M11.131 Familial chondrocalcinosis, right wrist
  - M11.132 Familial chondrocalcinosis, left wrist
  - M11.139 Familial chondrocalcinosis, unspecified wrist

+ M11.14 Familial chondrocalcinosis, hand
  - M11.141 Familial chondrocalcinosis, right hand
  - M11.142 Familial chondrocalcinosis, left hand
  - M11.149 Familial chondrocalcinosis, unspecified hand

+ M11.15 Familial chondrocalcinosis, hip
  - M11.151 Familial chondrocalcinosis, right hip
  - M11.152 Familial chondrocalcinosis, left hip
  - M11.159 Familial chondrocalcinosis, unspecified hip

+ M11.16 Familial chondrocalcinosis, knee
  - M11.161 Familial chondrocalcinosis, right knee
  - M11.162 Familial chondrocalcinosis, left knee
  - M11.169 Familial chondrocalcinosis, unspecified knee

+ M11.17 Familial chondrocalcinosis, ankle and foot
  - M11.171 Familial chondrocalcinosis, right ankle and foot
  - M11.172 Familial chondrocalcinosis, left ankle and foot
  - M11.179 Familial chondrocalcinosis, unspecified ankle and foot

M11.18 Familial chondrocalcinosis, vertebrae

M11.19 Familial chondrocalcinosis, multiple sites

+ M11.2 Other chondrocalcinosis

Chondrocalcinosis NOS

M11.20 Other chondrocalcinosis, unspecified site

+ M11.21 Other chondrocalcinosis, shoulder
  - M11.211 Other chondrocalcinosis, right shoulder
  - M11.212 Other chondrocalcinosis, left shoulder
  - M11.219 Other chondrocalcinosis, unspecified shoulder

+ M11.22 Other chondrocalcinosis, elbow
  - M11.221 Other chondrocalcinosis, right elbow
  - M11.222 Other chondrocalcinosis, left elbow
  - M11.229 Other chondrocalcinosis, unspecified elbow

+ M11.23 Other chondrocalcinosis, wrist
  - M11.231 Other chondrocalcinosis, right wrist
  - M11.232 Other chondrocalcinosis, left wrist
  - M11.239 Other chondrocalcinosis, unspecified wrist

+ M11.24 Other chondrocalcinosis, hand
  - M11.241 Other chondrocalcinosis, right hand
  - M11.242 Other chondrocalcinosis, left hand
  - M11.249 Other chondrocalcinosis, unspecified hand

+ M11.25 Other chondrocalcinosis, hip
  - M11.251 Other chondrocalcinosis, right hip
  - M11.252 Other chondrocalcinosis, left hip
  - M11.259 Other chondrocalcinosis, unspecified hip

+ M11.26 Other chondrocalcinosis, knee
  - M11.261 Other chondrocalcinosis, right knee
  - M11.262 Other chondrocalcinosis, left knee

    AHA CC: 3Q, 2018, 20
  - M11.269 Other chondrocalcinosis, unspecified knee

+ M11.27 Other chondrocalcinosis, ankle and foot
  - M11.271 Other chondrocalcinosis, right ankle and foot
  - M11.272 Other chondrocalcinosis, left ankle and foot
  - M11.279 Other chondrocalcinosis, unspecified ankle and foot

M11.28 Other chondrocalcinosis, vertebrae

M11.29 Other chondrocalcinosis, multiple sites

+ M11.8 Other specified crystal arthropathies

M11.80 Other specified crystal arthropathies, unspecified site

+ M11.81 Other specified crystal arthropathies, shoulder
  - M11.811 Other specified crystal arthropathies, right shoulder
  - M11.812 Other specified crystal arthropathies, left shoulder
  - M11.819 Other specified crystal arthropathies, unspecified shoulder

+ M11.82 Other specified crystal arthropathies, elbow
  - M11.821 Other specified crystal arthropathies, right elbow
  - M11.822 Other specified crystal arthropathies, left elbow
  - M11.829 Other specified crystal arthropathies, unspecified elbow

+ M11.83 Other specified crystal arthropathies, wrist
  - M11.831 Other specified crystal arthropathies, right wrist
  - M11.832 Other specified crystal arthropathies, left wrist
  - M11.839 Other specified crystal arthropathies, unspecified wrist

+ M11.84 Other specified crystal arthropathies, hand
  - M11.841 Other specified crystal arthropathies, right hand
  - M11.842 Other specified crystal arthropathies, left hand
  - M11.849 Other specified crystal arthropathies, unspecified hand

+ M11.85 Other specified crystal arthropathies, hip
  - M11.851 Other specified crystal arthropathies, right hip
  - M11.852 Other specified crystal arthropathies, left hip
  - M11.859 Other specified crystal arthropathies, unspecified hip

+ M11.86 Other specified crystal arthropathies, knee
  - M11.861 Other specified crystal arthropathies, right knee
  - M11.862 Other specified crystal arthropathies, left knee
  - M11.869 Other specified crystal arthropathies, unspecified knee

+ M11.87 Other specified crystal arthropathies, ankle and foot
  - M11.871 Other specified crystal arthropathies, right ankle and foot
  - M11.872 Other specified crystal arthropathies, left ankle and foot
  - M11.879 Other specified crystal arthropathies, unspecified ankle and foot

M11.88 Other specified crystal arthropathies, vertebrae

M11.89 Other specified crystal arthropathies, multiple sites

M11.9 Crystal arthropathy, unspecified

M12 Other and unspecified arthropathy

Excludes1: *arthrosis (M15-M19)*
cricoarytenoid arthropathy (J38.7)

+ M12.0 Chronic postrheumatic arthropathy [Jaccoud]

M12.00 Chronic postrheumatic arthropathy [Jaccoud], unspecified site

+ M12.01 Chronic postrheumatic arthropathy [Jaccoud], shoulder
  - M12.011 Chronic postrheumatic arthropathy [Jaccoud], right shoulder
  - M12.012 Chronic postrheumatic arthropathy [Jaccoud], left shoulder
  - M12.019 Chronic postrheumatic arthropathy [Jaccoud], unspecified shoulder

+ M12.02 Chronic postrheumatic arthropathy [Jaccoud], elbow
  - M12.021 Chronic postrheumatic arthropathy [Jaccoud], right elbow
  - M12.022 Chronic postrheumatic arthropathy [Jaccoud], left elbow
  - M12.029 Chronic postrheumatic arthropathy [Jaccoud], unspecified elbow

+ M12.03 Chronic postrheumatic arthropathy [Jaccoud], wrist
  - M12.031 Chronic postrheumatic arthropathy [Jaccoud], right wrist
  - M12.032 Chronic postrheumatic arthropathy [Jaccoud], left wrist
  - M12.039 Chronic postrheumatic arthropathy [Jaccoud], unspecified wrist

+ **M12.04 Chronic postrheumatic arthropathy [Jaccoud], hand**
  - **M12.041 Chronic postrheumatic arthropathy [Jaccoud], right hand**
  - **M12.042 Chronic postrheumatic arthropathy [Jaccoud], left hand**
  - **M12.049 Chronic postrheumatic arthropathy [Jaccoud], unspecified hand**

+ **M12.05 Chronic postrheumatic arthropathy [Jaccoud], hip**
  - **M12.051 Chronic postrheumatic arthropathy [Jaccoud], right hip**
  - **M12.052 Chronic postrheumatic arthropathy [Jaccoud], left hip**
  - **M12.059 Chronic postrheumatic arthropathy [Jaccoud], unspecified hip**

+ **M12.06 Chronic postrheumatic arthropathy [Jaccoud], knee**
  - **M12.061 Chronic postrheumatic arthropathy [Jaccoud], right knee**
  - **M12.062 Chronic postrheumatic arthropathy [Jaccoud], left knee**
  - **M12.069 Chronic postrheumatic arthropathy [Jaccoud], unspecified knee**

+ **M12.07 Chronic postrheumatic arthropathy [Jaccoud], ankle and foot**
  - **M12.071 Chronic postrheumatic arthropathy [Jaccoud], right ankle and foot**
  - **M12.072 Chronic postrheumatic arthropathy [Jaccoud], left ankle and foot**
  - **M12.079 Chronic postrheumatic arthropathy [Jaccoud], unspecified ankle and foot**

M12.08 Chronic postrheumatic arthropathy [Jaccoud], other specified site
Chronic postrheumatic arthropathy [Jaccoud], vertebrae

M12.09 Chronic postrheumatic arthropathy [Jaccoud], multiple sites

+ **M12.1 Kaschin-Beck disease**
Osteochondroarthrosis deformans endemica

M12.10 Kaschin-Beck disease, unspecified site

+ **M12.11 Kaschin-Beck disease, shoulder**
  - **M12.111 Kaschin-Beck disease, right shoulder**
  - **M12.112 Kaschin-Beck disease, left shoulder**
  - **M12.119 Kaschin-Beck disease, unspecified shoulder**

+ **M12.12 Kaschin-Beck disease, elbow**
  - **M12.121 Kaschin-Beck disease, right elbow**
  - **M12.122 Kaschin-Beck disease, left elbow**
  - **M12.129 Kaschin-Beck disease, unspecified elbow**

+ **M12.13 Kaschin-Beck disease, wrist**
  - **M12.131 Kaschin-Beck disease, right wrist**
  - **M12.132 Kaschin-Beck disease, left wrist**
  - **M12.139 Kaschin-Beck disease, unspecified wrist**

+ **M12.14 Kaschin-Beck disease, hand**
  - **M12.141 Kaschin-Beck disease, right hand**
  - **M12.142 Kaschin-Beck disease, left hand**
  - **M12.149 Kaschin-Beck disease, unspecified hand**

+ **M12.15 Kaschin-Beck disease, hip**
  - **M12.151 Kaschin-Beck disease, right hip**
  - **M12.152 Kaschin-Beck disease, left hip**
  - **M12.159 Kaschin-Beck disease, unspecified hip**

+ **M12.16 Kaschin-Beck disease, knee**
  - **M12.161 Kaschin-Beck disease, right knee**
  - **M12.162 Kaschin-Beck disease, left knee**
  - **M12.169 Kaschin-Beck disease, unspecified knee**

+ **M12.17 Kaschin-Beck disease, ankle and foot**
  - **M12.171 Kaschin-Beck disease, right ankle and foot**
  - **M12.172 Kaschin-Beck disease, left ankle and foot**
  - **M12.179 Kaschin-Beck disease, unspecified ankle and foot**

M12.18 Kaschin-Beck disease, vertebrae

M12.19 Kaschin-Beck disease, multiple sites

+ **M12.2 Villonodular synovitis (pigmented)**

M12.20 Villonodular synovitis (pigmented), unspecified site

+ **M12.21 Villonodular synovitis (pigmented), shoulder**
  - **M12.211 Villonodular synovitis (pigmented), right shoulder**
  - **M12.212 Villonodular synovitis (pigmented), left shoulder**
  - **M12.219 Villonodular synovitis (pigmented), unspecified shoulder**

+ **M12.22 Villonodular synovitis (pigmented), elbow**
  - **M12.221 Villonodular synovitis (pigmented), right elbow**
  - **M12.222 Villonodular synovitis (pigmented), left elbow**
  - **M12.229 Villonodular synovitis (pigmented), unspecified elbow**

+ **M12.23 Villonodular synovitis (pigmented), wrist**
  - **M12.231 Villonodular synovitis (pigmented), right wrist**
  - **M12.232 Villonodular synovitis (pigmented), left wrist**
  - **M12.239 Villonodular synovitis (pigmented), unspecified wrist**

+ **M12.24 Villonodular synovitis (pigmented), hand**
  - **M12.241 Villonodular synovitis (pigmented), right hand**
  - **M12.242 Villonodular synovitis (pigmented), left hand**
  - **M12.249 Villonodular synovitis (pigmented), unspecified hand**

+ **M12.25 Villonodular synovitis (pigmented), hip**
  - **M12.251 Villonodular synovitis (pigmented), right hip**
  - **M12.252 Villonodular synovitis (pigmented), left hip**
  - **M12.259 Villonodular synovitis (pigmented), unspecified hip**

+ **M12.26 Villonodular synovitis (pigmented), knee**
  - **M12.261 Villonodular synovitis (pigmented), right knee**
  - **M12.262 Villonodular synovitis (pigmented), left knee**
  - **M12.269 Villonodular synovitis (pigmented), unspecified knee**

+ **M12.27 Villonodular synovitis (pigmented), ankle and foot**
  - **M12.271 Villonodular synovitis (pigmented), right ankle and foot**
  - **M12.272 Villonodular synovitis (pigmented), left ankle and foot**
  - **M12.279 Villonodular synovitis (pigmented), unspecified ankle and foot**

M12.28 Villonodular synovitis (pigmented), other specified site
Villonodular synovitis (pigmented), vertebrae

M12.29 Villonodular synovitis (pigmented), multiple sites

+ **M12.3 Palindromic rheumatism**

M12.30 Palindromic rheumatism, unspecified site

+ **M12.31 Palindromic rheumatism, shoulder**
  - **M12.311 Palindromic rheumatism, right shoulder**
  - **M12.312 Palindromic rheumatism, left shoulder**
  - **M12.319 Palindromic rheumatism, unspecified shoulder**

+ **M12.32 Palindromic rheumatism, elbow**
  - **M12.321 Palindromic rheumatism, right elbow**
  - **M12.322 Palindromic rheumatism, left elbow**
  - **M12.329 Palindromic rheumatism, unspecified elbow**

+ **M12.33 Palindromic rheumatism, wrist**
  - **M12.331 Palindromic rheumatism, right wrist**
  - **M12.332 Palindromic rheumatism, left wrist**
  - **M12.339 Palindromic rheumatism, unspecified wrist**

+ **M12.34 Palindromic rheumatism, hand**
  - **M12.341 Palindromic rheumatism, right hand**
  - **M12.342 Palindromic rheumatism, left hand**
  - **M12.349 Palindromic rheumatism, unspecified hand**

+ **M12.35 Palindromic rheumatism, hip**
M12.351 Palindromic rheumatism, right hip
M12.352 Palindromic rheumatism, left hip
M12.359 Palindromic rheumatism, unspecified hip
+ **M12.36 Palindromic rheumatism, knee**
M12.361 Palindromic rheumatism, right knee
M12.362 Palindromic rheumatism, left knee
M12.369 Palindromic rheumatism, unspecified knee
+ **M12.37 Palindromic rheumatism, ankle and foot**
M12.371 Palindromic rheumatism, right ankle and foot
M12.372 Palindromic rheumatism, left ankle and foot
M12.379 Palindromic rheumatism, unspecified ankle and foot
M12.38 Palindromic rheumatism, other specified site
Palindromic rheumatism, vertebrae
M12.39 Palindromic rheumatism, multiple sites
+ **M12.4 Intermittent hydrarthrosis**
M12.40 Intermittent hydrarthrosis, unspecified site
+ **M12.41 Intermittent hydrarthrosis, shoulder**
M12.411 Intermittent hydrarthrosis, right shoulder
M12.412 Intermittent hydrarthrosis, left shoulder
M12.419 Intermittent hydrarthrosis, unspecified shoulder
+ **M12.42 Intermittent hydrarthrosis, elbow**
M12.421 Intermittent hydrarthrosis, right elbow
M12.422 Intermittent hydrarthrosis, left elbow
M12.429 Intermittent hydrarthrosis, unspecified elbow
+ **M12.43 Intermittent hydrarthrosis, wrist**
M12.431 Intermittent hydrarthrosis, right wrist
M12.432 Intermittent hydrarthrosis, left wrist
M12.439 Intermittent hydrarthrosis, unspecified wrist
+ **M12.44 Intermittent hydrarthrosis, hand**
M12.441 Intermittent hydrarthrosis, right hand
M12.442 Intermittent hydrarthrosis, left hand
M12.449 Intermittent hydrarthrosis, unspecified hand
+ **M12.45 Intermittent hydrarthrosis, hip**
M12.451 Intermittent hydrarthrosis, right hip
M12.452 Intermittent hydrarthrosis, left hip
M12.459 Intermittent hydrarthrosis, unspecified hip
+ **M12.46 Intermittent hydrarthrosis, knee**
M12.461 Intermittent hydrarthrosis, right knee
M12.462 Intermittent hydrarthrosis, left knee
M12.469 Intermittent hydrarthrosis, unspecified knee
+ **M12.47 Intermittent hydrarthrosis, ankle and foot**
M12.471 Intermittent hydrarthrosis, right ankle and foot
M12.472 Intermittent hydrarthrosis, left ankle and foot
M12.479 Intermittent hydrarthrosis, unspecified ankle and foot
M12.48 Intermittent hydrarthrosis, other site
M12.49 Intermittent hydrarthrosis, multiple sites
+ **M12.5 Traumatic arthropathy**
Excludes1: *current injury-see Alphabetic Index*
post-traumatic osteoarthritis of first carpometacarpal joint (M18.2-M18.3)
post-traumatic osteoarthritis of hip (M16.4-M16.5)
post-traumatic osteoarthritis of knee (M17.2-M17.3)
post-traumatic osteoarthritis NOS (M19.1-)
post-traumatic osteoarthritis of other single joints (M19.1-)
M12.50 Traumatic arthropathy, unspecified site
+ **M12.51 Traumatic arthropathy, shoulder**
M12.511 Traumatic arthropathy, right shoulder
M12.512 Traumatic arthropathy, left shoulder
M12.519 Traumatic arthropathy, unspecified shoulder
+ **M12.52 Traumatic arthropathy, elbow**
M12.521 Traumatic arthropathy, right elbow
M12.522 Traumatic arthropathy, left elbow
M12.529 Traumatic arthropathy, unspecified elbow
+ **M12.53 Traumatic arthropathy, wrist**
M12.531 Traumatic arthropathy, right wrist
M12.532 Traumatic arthropathy, left wrist
M12.539 Traumatic arthropathy, unspecified wrist
+ **M12.54 Traumatic arthropathy, hand**
M12.541 Traumatic arthropathy, right hand
M12.542 Traumatic arthropathy, left hand
M12.549 Traumatic arthropathy, unspecified hand
+ **M12.55 Traumatic arthropathy, hip**
M12.551 Traumatic arthropathy, right hip
M12.552 Traumatic arthropathy, left hip
AHA CC: 1Q, 2015, 17-18
M12.559 Traumatic arthropathy, unspecified hip
+ **M12.56 Traumatic arthropathy, knee**
M12.561 Traumatic arthropathy, right knee
M12.562 Traumatic arthropathy, left knee
M12.569 Traumatic arthropathy, unspecified knee
+ **M12.57 Traumatic arthropathy, ankle and foot**
M12.571 Traumatic arthropathy, right ankle and foot
M12.572 Traumatic arthropathy, left ankle and foot
M12.579 Traumatic arthropathy, unspecified ankle and foot
M12.58 Traumatic arthropathy, other specified site
Traumatic arthropathy, vertebrae
M12.59 Traumatic arthropathy, multiple sites
+ **M12.8 Other specific arthropathies, not elsewhere classified**
Transient arthropathy
M12.80 Other specific arthropathies, not elsewhere classified, unspecified site
+ **M12.81 Other specific arthropathies, not elsewhere classified, shoulder**
M12.811 Other specific arthropathies, not elsewhere classified, right shoulder
M12.812 Other specific arthropathies, not elsewhere classified, left shoulder
M12.819 Other specific arthropathies, not elsewhere classified, unspecified shoulder
+ **M12.82 Other specific arthropathies, not elsewhere classified, elbow**
M12.821 Other specific arthropathies, not elsewhere classified, right elbow
M12.822 Other specific arthropathies, not elsewhere classified, left elbow
M12.829 Other specific arthropathies, not elsewhere classified, unspecified elbow
+ **M12.83 Other specific arthropathies, not elsewhere classified, wrist**
M12.831 Other specific arthropathies, not elsewhere classified, right wrist
M12.832 Other specific arthropathies, not elsewhere classified, left wrist
M12.839 Other specific arthropathies, not elsewhere classified, unspecified wrist
+ **M12.84 Other specific arthropathies, not elsewhere classified, hand**
M12.841 Other specific arthropathies, not elsewhere classified, right hand
M12.842 Other specific arthropathies, not elsewhere classified, left hand
M12.849 Other specific arthropathies, not elsewhere classified, unspecified hand
+ **M12.85 Other specific arthropathies, not elsewhere classified, hip**
M12.851 Other specific arthropathies, not elsewhere classified, right hip
M12.852 Other specific arthropathies, not elsewhere classified, left hip
M12.859 Other specific arthropathies, not elsewhere classified, unspecified hip

+ **M12.86 Other specific arthropathies, not elsewhere classified, knee**
  - **M12.861 Other specific arthropathies, not elsewhere classified, right knee**
  - **M12.862 Other specific arthropathies, not elsewhere classified, left knee**
  - **M12.869 Other specific arthropathies, not elsewhere classified, unspecified knee**

+ **M12.87 Other specific arthropathies, not elsewhere classified, ankle and foot**
  - **M12.871 Other specific arthropathies, not elsewhere classified, right ankle and foot**
  - **M12.872 Other specific arthropathies, not elsewhere classified, left ankle and foot**
  - **M12.879 Other specific arthropathies, not elsewhere classified, unspecified ankle and foot**

M12.88 Other specific arthropathies, not elsewhere classified, other specified site

Other specific arthropathies, not elsewhere classified, vertebrae

M12.89 Other specific arthropathies, not elsewhere classified, multiple sites

M12.9 Arthropathy, unspecified

M13 Other arthritis

Excludes1: *arthrosis (M15-M19)*
osteoarthritis (M15-M19)

M13.0 Polyarthritis, unspecified

+ **M13.1 Monoarthritis, not elsewhere classified**
  - **M13.10 Monoarthritis, not elsewhere classified, unspecified site**

+ **M13.11 Monoarthritis, not elsewhere classified, shoulder**
  - **M13.111 Monoarthritis, not elsewhere classified, right shoulder**
  - **M13.112 Monoarthritis, not elsewhere classified, left shoulder**
  - **M13.119 Monoarthritis, not elsewhere classified, unspecified shoulder**

+ **M13.12 Monoarthritis, not elsewhere classified, elbow**
  - **M13.121 Monoarthritis, not elsewhere classified, right elbow**
  - **M13.122 Monoarthritis, not elsewhere classified, left elbow**
  - **M13.129 Monoarthritis, not elsewhere classified, unspecified elbow**

+ **M13.13 Monoarthritis, not elsewhere classified, wrist**
  - **M13.131 Monoarthritis, not elsewhere classified, right wrist**
  - **M13.132 Monoarthritis, not elsewhere classified, left wrist**
  - **M13.139 Monoarthritis, not elsewhere classified, unspecified wrist**

+ **M13.14 Monoarthritis, not elsewhere classified, hand**
  - **M13.141 Monoarthritis, not elsewhere classified, right hand**
  - **M13.142 Monoarthritis, not elsewhere classified, left hand**
  - **M13.149 Monoarthritis, not elsewhere classified, unspecified hand**

+ **M13.15 Monoarthritis, not elsewhere classified, hip**
  - **M13.151 Monoarthritis, not elsewhere classified, right hip**
  - **M13.152 Monoarthritis, not elsewhere classified, left hip**
  - **M13.159 Monoarthritis, not elsewhere classified, unspecified hip**

+ **M13.16 Monoarthritis, not elsewhere classified, knee**
  - **M13.161 Monoarthritis, not elsewhere classified, right knee**
  - **M13.162 Monoarthritis, not elsewhere classified, left knee**
  - **M13.169 Monoarthritis, not elsewhere classified, unspecified knee**

+ **M13.17 Monoarthritis, not elsewhere classified, ankle and foot**
  - **M13.171 Monoarthritis, not elsewhere classified, right ankle and foot**
  - **M13.172 Monoarthritis, not elsewhere classified, left ankle and foot**
  - **M13.179 Monoarthritis, not elsewhere classified, unspecified ankle and foot**

+ **M13.8 Other specified arthritis**

Allergic arthritis

Excludes1: *osteoarthritis (M15-M19)*

M13.80 Other specified arthritis, unspecified site

+ **M13.81 Other specified arthritis, shoulder**
  - **M13.811 Other specified arthritis, right shoulder**
  - **M13.812 Other specified arthritis, left shoulder**
  - **M13.819 Other specified arthritis, unspecified shoulder**

+ **M13.82 Other specified arthritis, elbow**
  - **M13.821 Other specified arthritis, right elbow**
  - **M13.822 Other specified arthritis, left elbow**
  - **M13.829 Other specified arthritis, unspecified elbow**

+ **M13.83 Other specified arthritis, wrist**
  - **M13.831 Other specified arthritis, right wrist**
  - **M13.832 Other specified arthritis, left wrist**
  - **M13.839 Other specified arthritis, unspecified wrist**

+ **M13.84 Other specified arthritis, hand**
  - **M13.841 Other specified arthritis, right hand**
  - **M13.842 Other specified arthritis, left hand**
  - **M13.849 Other specified arthritis, unspecified hand**

+ **M13.85 Other specified arthritis, hip**
  - **M13.851 Other specified arthritis, right hip**
  - **M13.852 Other specified arthritis, left hip**
  - **M13.859 Other specified arthritis, unspecified hip**

+ **M13.86 Other specified arthritis, knee**
  - **M13.861 Other specified arthritis, right knee**
  - **M13.862 Other specified arthritis, left knee**
  - **M13.869 Other specified arthritis, unspecified knee**

+ **M13.87 Other specified arthritis, ankle and foot**
  - **M13.871 Other specified arthritis, right ankle and foot**
  - **M13.872 Other specified arthritis, left ankle and foot**
  - **M13.879 Other specified arthritis, unspecified ankle and foot**

M13.88 Other specified arthritis, other site

M13.89 Other specified arthritis, multiple sites

M14 Arthropathies in other diseases classified elsewhere

Excludes1: *arthropathy in:*
diabetes mellitus (E08-E13 with .61-)
hematological disorders (M36.2-M36.3)
hypersensitivity reactions (M36.4)
neoplastic disease (M36.1)
neurosyphillis (A52.16)
sarcoidosis (D86.86)
enteropathic arthropathies (M07.-)
juvenile psoriatic arthropathy (L40.54)
lipoid dermatoarthritis (E78.81)

+ **M14.6 Charcôt's joint**

Neuropathic arthropathy

Excludes1: *Charcôt's joint in diabetes mellitus (E08-E13 with .610)*
Charcôt's joint in tabes dorsalis (A52.16)

M14.60 Charcôt's joint, unspecified site

+ **M14.61 Charcôt's joint, shoulder**
  - **M14.611 Charcôt's joint, right shoulder**
  - **M14.612 Charcôt's joint, left shoulder**
  - **M14.619 Charcôt's joint, unspecified shoulder**

+ **M14.62 Charcôt's joint, elbow**
  - **M14.621 Charcôt's joint, right elbow**
  - **M14.622 Charcôt's joint, left elbow**
  - **M14.629 Charcôt's joint, unspecified elbow**

+ **M14.63 Charcôt's joint, wrist**
  - **M14.631 Charcôt's joint, right wrist**
  - **M14.632 Charcôt's joint, left wrist**
  - **M14.639 Charcôt's joint, unspecified wrist**

+ **M14.64 Charcôt's joint, hand**
  - **M14.641 Charcôt's joint, right hand**
  - **M14.642 Charcôt's joint, left hand**
  - **M14.649 Charcôt's joint, unspecified hand**

+ **M14.65 Charcôt's joint, hip**
  - **M14.651 Charcôt's joint, right hip**
  - **M14.652 Charcôt's joint, left hip**
  - **M14.659 Charcôt's joint, unspecified hip**

+ M14.66 Charcôt's joint, knee
M14.661 Charcôt's joint, right knee
M14.662 Charcôt's joint, left knee
M14.669 Charcôt's joint, unspecified knee
+ M14.67 Charcôt's joint, ankle and foot
M14.671 Charcôt's joint, right ankle and foot
M14.672 Charcôt's joint, left ankle and foot
M14.679 Charcôt's joint, unspecified ankle and foot
M14.68 Charcôt's joint, vertebrae
M14.69 Charcôt's joint, multiple sites
+ M14.8 Arthropathies in other specified diseases classified elsewhere
Code first underlying disease, such as:
amyloidosis (E85.-)
erythema multiforme (L51.-)
erythema nodosum (L52)
hemochromatosis (E83.11-)
hyperparathyroidism (E21.-)
hypothyroidism (E00-E03)
sickle-cell disorders (D57.-)
thyrotoxicosis [hyperthyroidism] (E05.-)
Whipple's disease (K90.81)
M14.80 Arthropathies in other specified diseases classified elsewhere, unspecified site
+ M14.81 Arthropathies in other specified diseases classified elsewhere, shoulder
M14.811 Arthropathies in other specified diseases classified elsewhere, right shoulder
M14.812 Arthropathies in other specified diseases classified elsewhere, left shoulder
M14.819 Arthropathies in other specified diseases classified elsewhere, unspecified shoulder
+ M14.82 Arthropathies in other specified diseases classified elsewhere, elbow
M14.821 Arthropathies in other specified diseases classified elsewhere, right elbow
M14.822 Arthropathies in other specified diseases classified elsewhere, left elbow
M14.829 Arthropathies in other specified diseases classified elsewhere, unspecified elbow
+ M14.83 Arthropathies in other specified diseases classified elsewhere, wrist
M14.831 Arthropathies in other specified diseases classified elsewhere, right wrist
M14.832 Arthropathies in other specified diseases classified elsewhere, left wrist
M14.839 Arthropathies in other specified diseases classified elsewhere, unspecified wrist
+ M14.84 Arthropathies in other specified diseases classified elsewhere, hand
M14.841 Arthropathies in other specified diseases classified elsewhere, right hand
M14.842 Arthropathies in other specified diseases classified elsewhere, left hand
M14.849 Arthropathies in other specified diseases classified elsewhere, unspecified hand
+ M14.85 Arthropathies in other specified diseases classified elsewhere, hip
M14.851 Arthropathies in other specified diseases classified elsewhere, right hip
M14.852 Arthropathies in other specified diseases classified elsewhere, left hip
M14.859 Arthropathies in other specified diseases classified elsewhere, unspecified hip
+ M14.86 Arthropathies in other specified diseases classified elsewhere, knee
M14.861 Arthropathies in other specified diseases classified elsewhere, right knee
M14.862 Arthropathies in other specified diseases classified elsewhere, left knee
M14.869 Arthropathies in other specified diseases classified elsewhere, unspecified knee
+ M14.87 Arthropathies in other specified diseases classified elsewhere, ankle and foot
M14.871 Arthropathies in other specified diseases classified elsewhere, right ankle and foot
M14.872 Arthropathies in other specified diseases classified elsewhere, left ankle and foot
M14.879 Arthropathies in other specified diseases classified elsewhere, unspecified ankle and foot
M14.88 Arthropathies in other specified diseases classified elsewhere, vertebrae
M14.89 Arthropathies in other specified diseases classified elsewhere, multiple sites

Osteoarthritis (M15-M19)

Excludes2: *osteoarthritis of spine (M47.-)*

M15 Polyosteoarthritis

Includes: arthritis of multiple sites
Excludes1: *bilateral involvement of single joint (M16-M19)*

M15.0 Primary generalized (osteo)arthritis
M15.1 Heberden's nodes (with arthropathy)
Interphalangeal distal osteoarthritis
M15.2 Bouchard's nodes (with arthropathy)
Juxtaphalangeal distal osteoarthritis
M15.3 Secondary multiple arthritis
Post-traumatic polyosteoarthritis
M15.4 Erosive (osteo)arthritis
M15.8 Other polyosteoarthritis
M15.9 Polyosteoarthritis, unspecified
Generalized osteoarthritis NOS

M16 Osteoarthritis of hip

M16.0 Bilateral primary osteoarthritis of hip
AHA CC: 4Q, 2016, 146; 2Q, 2018, 15
+ M16.1 Unilateral primary osteoarthritis of hip
Primary osteoarthritis of hip NOS
M16.10 Unilateral primary osteoarthritis, unspecified hip
M16.11 Unilateral primary osteoarthritis, right hip
M16.12 Unilateral primary osteoarthritis, left hip
M16.2 Bilateral osteoarthritis resulting from hip dysplasia
+ M16.3 Unilateral osteoarthritis resulting from hip dysplasia
Dysplastic osteoarthritis of hip NOS
M16.30 Unilateral osteoarthritis resulting from hip dysplasia, unspecified hip
M16.31 Unilateral osteoarthritis resulting from hip dysplasia, right hip
M16.32 Unilateral osteoarthritis resulting from hip dysplasia, left hip
M16.4 Bilateral post-traumatic osteoarthritis of hip
+ M16.5 Unilateral post-traumatic osteoarthritis of hip
Post-traumatic osteoarthritis of hip NOS
M16.50 Unilateral post-traumatic osteoarthritis, unspecified hip
M16.51 Unilateral post-traumatic osteoarthritis, right hip
M16.52 Unilateral post-traumatic osteoarthritis, left hip
M16.6 Other bilateral secondary osteoarthritis of hip
M16.7 Other unilateral secondary osteoarthritis of hip
Secondary osteoarthritis of hip NOS
M16.9 Osteoarthritis of hip, unspecified

M17 Osteoarthritis of knee

M17.0 Bilateral primary osteoarthritis of knee
+ M17.1 Unilateral primary osteoarthritis of knee
Primary osteoarthritis of knee NOS
M17.10 Unilateral primary osteoarthritis, unspecified knee
AHA CC: 4Q, 2016, 147
M17.11 Unilateral primary osteoarthritis, right knee
M17.12 Unilateral primary osteoarthritis, left knee
AHA CC: 4Q, 2016, 146
M17.2 Bilateral post-traumatic osteoarthritis of knee
+ M17.3 Unilateral post-traumatic osteoarthritis of knee
Post-traumatic osteoarthritis of knee NOS
M17.30 Unilateral post-traumatic osteoarthritis, unspecified knee
M17.31 Unilateral post-traumatic osteoarthritis, right knee
M17.32 Unilateral post-traumatic osteoarthritis, left knee
M17.4 Other bilateral secondary osteoarthritis of knee
M17.5 Other unilateral secondary osteoarthritis of knee
Secondary osteoarthritis of knee NOS
M17.9 Osteoarthritis of knee, unspecified

Pathology in Osteoarthritis

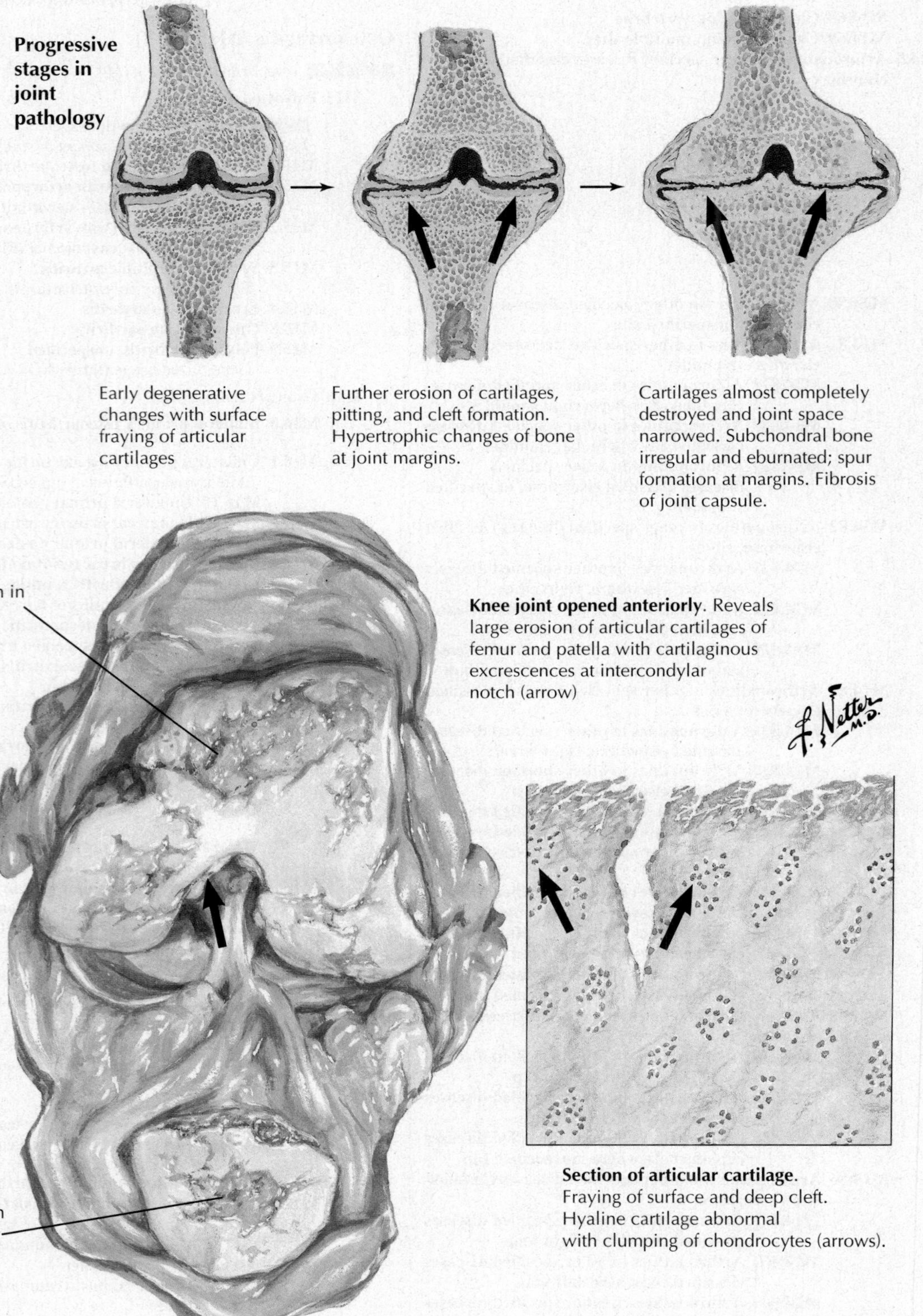

M18 Osteoarthritis of first carpometacarpal joint

M18.0 Bilateral primary osteoarthritis of first carpometacarpal joints

+ M18.1 Unilateravl primary osteoarthritis of first carpometacarpal joint

Primary osteoarthritis of first carpometacarpal joint NOS

M18.10 Unilateral primary osteoarthritis of first carpometacarpal joint, unspecified hand

M18.11 Unilateral primary osteoarthritis of first carpometacarpal joint, right hand

M18.12 Unilateral primary osteoarthritis of first carpometacarpal joint, left hand

M18.2 Bilateral post-traumatic osteoarthritis of first carpometacarpal joints

+ M18.3 Unilateral post-traumatic osteoarthritis of first carpometacarpal joint

Post-traumatic osteoarthritis of first carpometacarpal joint NOS

M18.30 Unilateral post-traumatic osteoarthritis of first carpometacarpal joint, unspecified hand

M18.31 Unilateral post-traumatic osteoarthritis of first carpometacarpal joint, right hand

M18.32 Unilateral post-traumatic osteoarthritis of first carpometacarpal joint, left hand

M18.4 Other bilateral secondary osteoarthritis of first carpometacarpal joints

+ M18.5 Other unilateral secondary osteoarthritis of first carpometacarpal joint

Secondary osteoarthritis of first carpometacarpal joint NOS

M18.50 Other unilateral secondary osteoarthritis of first carpometacarpal joint, unspecified hand

M18.51 Other unilateral secondary osteoarthritis of first carpometacarpal joint, right hand

M18.52 Other unilateral secondary osteoarthritis of first carpometacarpal joint, left hand

M18.9 Osteoarthritis of first carpometacarpal joint, unspecified

M19 Other and unspecified osteoarthritis

Excludes1: *polyarthritis (M15.-)*

Excludes2: *arthrosis of spine (M47.-)*
hallux rigidus (M20.2)
osteoarthritis of spine (M47.-)

AHA CC: 4Q, 2020, 31-32

+ M19.0 Primary osteoarthritis of other joints

+ M19.01 Primary osteoarthritis, shoulder

M19.011 Primary osteoarthritis, right shoulder

AHA CC: 4Q, 2016, 145

M19.012 Primary osteoarthritis, left shoulder

M19.019 Primary osteoarthritis, unspecified shoulder

+ M19.02 Primary osteoarthritis, elbow

M19.021 Primary osteoarthritis, right elbow

M19.022 Primary osteoarthritis, left elbow

M19.029 Primary osteoarthritis, unspecified elbow

+ M19.03 Primary osteoarthritis, wrist

M19.031 Primary osteoarthritis, right wrist

M19.032 Primary osteoarthritis, left wrist

M19.039 Primary osteoarthritis, unspecified wrist

+ M19.04 Primary osteoarthritis, hand

Excludes2: *primary osteoarthritis of first carpometacarpal joint (M18.0-, M18.1-)*

M19.041 Primary osteoarthritis, right hand

M19.042 Primary osteoarthritis, left hand

M19.049 Primary osteoarthritis, unspecified hand

+ M19.07 Primary osteoarthritis ankle and foot

M19.071 Primary osteoarthritis, right ankle and foot

M19.072 Primary osteoarthritis, left ankle and foot

M19.079 Primary osteoarthritis, unspecified ankle and foot

M19.09 Primary osteoarthritis, other specified site

+ M19.1 Post-traumatic osteoarthritis of other joints

+ M19.11 Post-traumatic osteoarthritis, shoulder

M19.111 Post-traumatic osteoarthritis, right shoulder

M19.112 Post-traumatic osteoarthritis, left shoulder

M19.119 Post-traumatic osteoarthritis, unspecified shoulder

+ M19.12 Post-traumatic osteoarthritis, elbow

M19.121 Post-traumatic osteoarthritis, right elbow

M19.122 Post-traumatic osteoarthritis, left elbow

M19.129 Post-traumatic osteoarthritis, unspecified elbow

+ M19.13 Post-traumatic osteoarthritis, wrist

M19.131 Post-traumatic osteoarthritis, right wrist

M19.132 Post-traumatic osteoarthritis, left wrist

M19.139 Post-traumatic osteoarthritis, unspecified wrist

+ M19.14 Post-traumatic osteoarthritis, hand

Excludes2: *post-traumatic osteoarthritis of first carpometacarpal joint (M18.2-, M18.3-)*

M19.141 Post-traumatic osteoarthritis, right hand

M19.142 Post-traumatic osteoarthritis, left hand

M19.149 Post-traumatic osteoarthritis, unspecified hand

+ M19.17 Post-traumatic osteoarthritis, ankle and foot

M19.171 Post-traumatic osteoarthritis, right ankle and foot

M19.172 Post-traumatic osteoarthritis, left ankle and foot

M19.179 Post-traumatic osteoarthritis, unspecified ankle and foot

M19.19 Post-traumatic osteoarthritis, other specified site

+ M19.2 Secondary osteoarthritis of other joints

+ M19.21 Secondary osteoarthritis, shoulder

M19.211 Secondary osteoarthritis, right shoulder

M19.212 Secondary osteoarthritis, left shoulder

M19.219 Secondary osteoarthritis, unspecified shoulder

+ M19.22 Secondary osteoarthritis, elbow

M19.221 Secondary osteoarthritis, right elbow

M19.222 Secondary osteoarthritis, left elbow

M19.229 Secondary osteoarthritis, unspecified elbow

+ M19.23 Secondary osteoarthritis, wrist

M19.231 Secondary osteoarthritis, right wrist

M19.232 Secondary osteoarthritis, left wrist

M19.239 Secondary osteoarthritis, unspecified wrist

+ M19.24 Secondary osteoarthritis, hand

M19.241 Secondary osteoarthritis, right hand

M19.242 Secondary osteoarthritis, left hand

M19.249 Secondary osteoarthritis, unspecified hand

+ M19.27 Secondary osteoarthritis, ankle and foot

M19.271 Secondary osteoarthritis, right ankle and foot

M19.272 Secondary osteoarthritis, left ankle and foot

M19.279 Secondary osteoarthritis, unspecified ankle and foot

M19.29 Secondary osteoarthritis, other specified site

+ M19.9 Osteoarthritis, unspecified site

M19.90 Unspecified osteoarthritis, unspecified site

Arthrosis NOS
Arthritis NOS
Osteoarthritis NOS

AHA CC: 4Q, 2016, 147

M19.91 Primary osteoarthritis, unspecified site

Primary osteoarthritis NOS

M19.92 Post-traumatic osteoarthritis, unspecified site

Post-traumatic osteoarthritis NOS

M19.93 Secondary osteoarthritis, unspecified site

Secondary osteoarthritis NOS

Other joint disorders (M20-M25)

Excludes2: *joints of the spine (M40-M54)*

M20 Acquired deformities of fingers and toes

Excludes1: *acquired absence of fingers and toes (Z89.-)*
congenital absence of fingers and toes (Q71.3-, Q72.3-)
congenital deformities and malformations of fingers and toes (Q66.-, Q68-Q70, Q74.-)

+ **M20.0 Deformity of finger(s)**
  Excludes1: *clubbing of fingers (R68.3)*
  palmar fascial fibromatosis [Dupuytren] (M72.0)
  trigger finger (M65.3)
  + **M20.00 Unspecified deformity of finger(s)**
    M20.001 Unspecified deformity of right finger(s)
    M20.002 Unspecified deformity of left finger(s)
    M20.009 Unspecified deformity of unspecified finger(s)
  + **M20.01 Mallet finger**
    M20.011 Mallet finger of right finger(s)
    M20.012 Mallet finger of left finger(s)
    M20.019 Mallet finger of unspecified finger(s)
  + **M20.02 Boutonnière deformity**
    M20.021 Boutonnière deformity of right finger(s)
    M20.022 Boutonnière deformity of left finger(s)
    M20.029 Boutonnière deformity of unspecified finger(s)
  + **M20.03 Swan-neck deformity**
    M20.031 Swan-neck deformity of right finger(s)
    M20.032 Swan-neck deformity of left finger(s)
    M20.039 Swan-neck deformity of unspecified finger(s)
  + **M20.09 Other deformity of finger(s)**
    M20.091 Other deformity of right finger(s)
    M20.092 Other deformity of left finger(s)
    M20.099 Other deformity of finger(s), unspecified finger(s)
+ **M20.1 Hallux valgus (acquired)**
  Excludes2: *bunion (M21.6-)*
  M20.10 Hallux valgus (acquired), unspecified foot
  M20.11 Hallux valgus (acquired), right foot
  M20.12 Hallux valgus (acquired), left foot
+ **M20.2 Hallux rigidus**
  M20.20 Hallux rigidus, unspecified foot
  M20.21 Hallux rigidus, right foot
  M20.22 Hallux rigidus, left foot
+ **M20.3 Hallux varus (acquired)**
  M20.30 Hallux varus (acquired), unspecified foot
  M20.31 Hallux varus (acquired), right foot
  M20.32 Hallux varus (acquired), left foot
+ **M20.4 Other hammer toe(s) (acquired)**
  M20.40 Other hammer toe(s) (acquired), unspecified foot
  M20.41 Other hammer toe(s) (acquired), right foot
  M20.42 Other hammer toe(s) (acquired), left foot
+ **M20.5 Other deformities of toe(s) (acquired)**
  + **M20.5X Other deformities of toe(s) (acquired)**
    M20.5X1 Other deformities of toe(s) (acquired), right foot
    M20.5X2 Other deformities of toe(s) (acquired), left foot
    M20.5X9 Other deformities of toe(s) (acquired), unspecified foot
+ **M20.6 Acquired deformities of toe(s), unspecified**
  M20.60 Acquired deformities of toe(s), unspecified, unspecified foot
  M20.61 Acquired deformities of toe(s), unspecified, right foot
  M20.62 Acquired deformities of toe(s), unspecified, left foot

M21 Other acquired deformities of limbs

Excludes1: *acquired absence of limb (Z89.-)*
congenital absence of limbs (Q71-Q73)
congenital deformities and malformations of limbs (Q65-Q66, Q68-Q74)

Excludes2: *acquired deformities of fingers or toes (M20.-)*
coxa plana (M91.2)

+ **M21.0 Valgus deformity, not elsewhere classified**
  Excludes1: *metatarsus valgus (Q66.6)*
  talipes calcaneovalgus (Q66.4-)
  M21.00 Valgus deformity, not elsewhere classified, unspecified site
  + **M21.02 Valgus deformity, not elsewhere classified, elbow**
    Cubitus valgus
    M21.021 Valgus deformity, not elsewhere classified, right elbow
    M21.022 Valgus deformity, not elsewhere classified, left elbow
    M21.029 Valgus deformity, not elsewhere classified, unspecified elbow
  + **M21.05 Valgus deformity, not elsewhere classified, hip**
    M21.051 Valgus deformity, not elsewhere classified, right hip
    M21.052 Valgus deformity, not elsewhere classified, left hip
    M21.059 Valgus deformity, not elsewhere classified, unspecified hip
  + **M21.06 Valgus deformity, not elsewhere classified, knee**
    Genu valgum
    Knock knee
    M21.061 Valgus deformity, not elsewhere classified, right knee
    M21.062 Valgus deformity, not elsewhere classified, left knee
    M21.069 Valgus deformity, not elsewhere classified, unspecified knee
  + **M21.07 Valgus deformity, not elsewhere classified, ankle**
    M21.071 Valgus deformity, not elsewhere classified, right ankle
    M21.072 Valgus deformity, not elsewhere classified, left ankle
    M21.079 Valgus deformity, not elsewhere classified, unspecified ankle
+ **M21.1 Varus deformity, not elsewhere classified**
  Excludes1: *metatarsus varus (Q66.22-)*
  tibia vara (M92.51-)
  M21.10 Varus deformity, not elsewhere classified, unspecified site
  + **M21.12 Varus deformity, not elsewhere classified, elbow**
    Cubitus varus, elbow
    M21.121 Varus deformity, not elsewhere classified, right elbow
    M21.122 Varus deformity, not elsewhere classified, left elbow
    M21.129 Varus deformity, not elsewhere classified, unspecified elbow
  + **M21.15 Varus deformity, not elsewhere classified, hip**
    M21.151 Varus deformity, not elsewhere classified, right hip
    M21.152 Varus deformity, not elsewhere classified, left hip
    M21.159 Varus deformity, not elsewhere classified, unspecified
  + **M21.16 Varus deformity, not elsewhere classified, knee**
    Bow leg
    Genu varum
    M21.161 Varus deformity, not elsewhere classified, right knee
    M21.162 Varus deformity, not elsewhere classified, left knee
    M21.169 Varus deformity, not elsewhere classified, unspecified knee
  + **M21.17 Varus deformity, not elsewhere classified, ankle**
    M21.171 Varus deformity, not elsewhere classified, right ankle
    M21.172 Varus deformity, not elsewhere classified, left ankle
    M21.179 Varus deformity, not elsewhere classified, unspecified ankle
+ **M21.2 Flexion deformity**
  M21.20 Flexion deformity, unspecified site
  + **M21.21 Flexion deformity, shoulder**
    M21.211 Flexion deformity, right shoulder
    M21.212 Flexion deformity, left shoulder
    M21.219 Flexion deformity, unspecified shoulder

+ M21.22 Flexion deformity, elbow
M21.221 Flexion deformity, right elbow
M21.222 Flexion deformity, left elbow
M21.229 Flexion deformity, unspecified elbow
+ M21.23 Flexion deformity, wrist
M21.231 Flexion deformity, right wrist
M21.232 Flexion deformity, left wrist
M21.239 Flexion deformity, unspecified wrist
+ M21.24 Flexion deformity, finger joints
M21.241 Flexion deformity, right finger joints
M21.242 Flexion deformity, left finger joints
M21.249 Flexion deformity, unspecified finger joints
+ M21.25 Flexion deformity, hip
M21.251 Flexion deformity, right hip
M21.252 Flexion deformity, left hip
M21.259 Flexion deformity, unspecified hip
+ M21.26 Flexion deformity, knee
M21.261 Flexion deformity, right knee
M21.262 Flexion deformity, left knee
M21.269 Flexion deformity, unspecified knee
+ M21.27 Flexion deformity, ankle and toes
M21.271 Flexion deformity, right ankle and toes
M21.272 Flexion deformity, left ankle and toes
M21.279 Flexion deformity, unspecified ankle and toes
+ M21.3 Wrist or foot drop (acquired)
+ M21.33 Wrist drop (acquired)
M21.331 Wrist drop, right wrist
M21.332 Wrist drop, left wrist
M21.339 Wrist drop, unspecified wrist
+ M21.37 Foot drop (acquired)
M21.371 Foot drop, right foot
M21.372 Foot drop, left foot
M21.379 Foot drop, unspecified foot
+ M21.4 Flat foot [pes planus] (acquired)
Excludes1: *congenital pes planus (Q66.5-)*
M21.40 Flat foot [pes planus] (acquired), unspecified foot
M21.41 Flat foot [pes planus] (acquired), right foot
M21.42 Flat foot [pes planus] (acquired), left foot
+ M21.5 Acquired clawhand, clubhand, clawfoot and clubfoot
Excludes1: *clubfoot, not specified as acquired (Q66.89)*
+ M21.51 Acquired clawhand
M21.511 Acquired clawhand, right hand
M21.512 Acquired clawhand, left hand
M21.519 Acquired clawhand, unspecified hand
+ M21.52 Acquired clubhand
M21.521 Acquired clubhand, right hand
M21.522 Acquired clubhand, left hand
M21.529 Acquired clubhand, unspecified hand
+ M21.53 Acquired clawfoot
M21.531 Acquired clawfoot, right foot
M21.532 Acquired clawfoot, left foot
M21.539 Acquired clawfoot, unspecified foot
+ M21.54 Acquired clubfoot
M21.541 Acquired clubfoot, right foot
M21.542 Acquired clubfoot, left foot
M21.549 Acquired clubfoot, unspecified foot
+ M21.6 Other acquired deformities of foot
Excludes2: *deformities of toe (acquired) (M20.1-M20.6-)*
AHA CC: 4Q, 2016, 38
+ M21.61 Bunion
M21.611 Bunion of right foot
M21.612 Bunion of left foot
M21.619 Bunion of unspecified foot
+ M21.62 Bunionette
M21.621 Bunionette of right foot
M21.622 Bunionette of left foot
M21.629 Bunionette of unspecified foot
+ M21.6X Other acquired deformities of foot
M21.6X1 Other acquired deformities of right foot
M21.6X2 Other acquired deformities of left foot
M21.6X9 Other acquired deformities of unspecified foot
+ M21.7 Unequal limb length (acquired)
NOTE The site used should correspond to the shorter limb
M21.70 Unequal limb length (acquired), unspecified site
+ M21.72 Unequal limb length (acquired), humerus
M21.721 Unequal limb length (acquired), right humerus
M21.722 Unequal limb length (acquired), left humerus
M21.729 Unequal limb length (acquired), unspecified humerus
+ M21.73 Unequal limb length (acquired), ulna and radius
M21.731 Unequal limb length (acquired), right ulna
M21.732 Unequal limb length (acquired), left ulna
M21.733 Unequal limb length (acquired), right radius
M21.734 Unequal limb length (acquired), left radius
M21.739 Unequal limb length (acquired), unspecified ulna and radius
+ M21.75 Unequal limb length (acquired), femur
M21.751 Unequal limb length (acquired), right femur
M21.752 Unequal limb length (acquired), left femur
M21.759 Unequal limb length (acquired), unspecified femur
+ M21.76 Unequal limb length (acquired), tibia and fibula
M21.761 Unequal limb length (acquired), right tibia
M21.762 Unequal limb length (acquired), left tibia
M21.763 Unequal limb length (acquired), right fibula
M21.764 Unequal limb length (acquired), left fibula
M21.769 Unequal limb length (acquired), unspecified tibia and fibula
+ M21.8 Other specified acquired deformities of limbs
Excludes2: *coxa plana (M91.2)*
M21.80 Other specified acquired deformities of unspecified limb
+ M21.82 Other specified acquired deformities of upper arm
M21.821 Other specified acquired deformities of right upper arm
M21.822 Other specified acquired deformities of left upper arm
M21.829 Other specified acquired deformities of unspecified upper arm
+ M21.83 Other specified acquired deformities of forearm
M21.831 Other specified acquired deformities of right forearm
M21.832 Other specified acquired deformities of left forearm
M21.839 Other specified acquired deformities of unspecified forearm
+ M21.85 Other specified acquired deformities of thigh
M21.851 Other specified acquired deformities of right thigh
M21.852 Other specified acquired deformities of left thigh
M21.859 Other specified acquired deformities of unspecified thigh
+ M21.86 Other specified acquired deformities of lower leg
M21.861 Other specified acquired deformities of right lower leg
M21.862 Other specified acquired deformities of left lower leg
M21.869 Other specified acquired deformities of unspecified lower leg
+ M21.9 Unspecified acquired deformity of limb and hand
M21.90 Unspecified acquired deformity of unspecified limb
+ M21.92 Unspecified acquired deformity of upper arm
M21.921 Unspecified acquired deformity of right upper arm
M21.922 Unspecified acquired deformity of left upper arm
M21.929 Unspecified acquired deformity of unspecified upper arm
+ M21.93 Unspecified acquired deformity of forearm
M21.931 Unspecified acquired deformity of right forearm
M21.932 Unspecified acquired deformity of left forearm
M21.939 Unspecified acquired deformity of unspecified forearm

+ **M21.94 Unspecified acquired deformity of hand**
  - **M21.941 Unspecified acquired deformity of hand, right hand**
  - **M21.942 Unspecified acquired deformity of hand, left hand**
  - **M21.949 Unspecified acquired deformity of hand, unspecified hand**

+ **M21.95 Unspecified acquired deformity of thigh**
  - **M21.951 Unspecified acquired deformity of right thigh**
  - **M21.952 Unspecified acquired deformity of left thigh**
  - **M21.959 Unspecified acquired deformity of unspecified thigh**

+ **M21.96 Unspecified acquired deformity of lower leg**
  - **M21.961 Unspecified acquired deformity of right lower leg**
  - **M21.962 Unspecified acquired deformity of left lower leg**
  - **M21.969 Unspecified acquired deformity of unspecified lower leg**

M22 Disorder of patella

Excludes2: *traumatic dislocation of patella (S83.0-)*

+ **M22.0 Recurrent dislocation of patella**
  - **M22.00 Recurrent dislocation of patella, unspecified knee**
  - **M22.01 Recurrent dislocation of patella, right knee**
  - **M22.02 Recurrent dislocation of patella, left knee**

+ **M22.1 Recurrent subluxation of patella**
  Incomplete dislocation of patella
  - **M22.10 Recurrent subluxation of patella, unspecified knee**
  - **M22.11 Recurrent subluxation of patella, right knee**
  - **M22.12 Recurrent subluxation of patella, left knee**

+ **M22.2 Patellofemoral disorders**
  + **M22.2X Patellofemoral disorders**
    - **M22.2X1 Patellofemoral disorders, right knee**
    - **M22.2X2 Patellofemoral disorders, left knee**
    - **M22.2X9 Patellofemoral disorders, unspecified knee**

+ **M22.3 Other derangements of patella**
  + **M22.3X Other derangements of patella**
    - **M22.3X1 Other derangements of patella, right knee**
    - **M22.3X2 Other derangements of patella, left knee**
    - **M22.3X9 Other derangements of patella, unspecified knee**

+ **M22.4 Chondromalacia patellae**
  - **M22.40 Chondromalacia patellae, unspecified knee**
  - **M22.41 Chondromalacia patellae, right knee**
  - **M22.42 Chondromalacia patellae, left knee**

+ **M22.8 Other disorders of patella**
  + **M22.8X Other disorders of patella**
    - **M22.8X1 Other disorders of patella, right knee**
    - **M22.8X2 Other disorders of patella, left knee**
    - **M22.8X9 Other disorders of patella, unspecified knee**

+ **M22.9 Unspecified disorder of patella**
  - **M22.90 Unspecified disorder of patella, unspecified knee**
  - **M22.91 Unspecified disorder of patella, right knee**
  - **M22.92 Unspecified disorder of patella, left knee**

M23 Internal derangement of knee

Excludes1: *ankylosis (M24.66)*
deformity of knee (M21.-)
osteochondritis dissecans (M93.2)

Excludes2: *current injury - see injury of knee and lower leg (S80-S89)*
recurrent dislocation or subluxation of joints (M24.4)
recurrent dislocation or subluxation of patella (M22.0-M22.1)

+ **M23.0 Cystic meniscus**
  + **M23.00 Cystic meniscus, unspecified meniscus**
    Cystic meniscus, unspecified lateral meniscus
    Cystic meniscus, unspecified medial meniscus
    - **M23.000 Cystic meniscus, unspecified lateral meniscus, right knee**
    - **M23.001 Cystic meniscus, unspecified lateral meniscus, left knee**
    - **M23.002 Cystic meniscus, unspecified lateral meniscus, unspecified knee**
    - **M23.003 Cystic meniscus, unspecified medial meniscus, right knee**
    - **M23.004 Cystic meniscus, unspecified medial meniscus, left knee**
    - **M23.005 Cystic meniscus, unspecified medial meniscus, unspecified knee**
    - **M23.006 Cystic meniscus, unspecified meniscus, right knee**
    - **M23.007 Cystic meniscus, unspecified meniscus, left knee**
    - **M23.009 Cystic meniscus, unspecified meniscus, unspecified knee**
  + **M23.01 Cystic meniscus, anterior horn of medial meniscus**
    - **M23.011 Cystic meniscus, anterior horn of medial meniscus, right knee**
    - **M23.012 Cystic meniscus, anterior horn of medial meniscus, left knee**
    - **M23.019 Cystic meniscus, anterior horn of medial meniscus, unspecified knee**
  + **M23.02 Cystic meniscus, posterior horn of medial meniscus**
    - **M23.021 Cystic meniscus, posterior horn of medial meniscus, right knee**
    - **M23.022 Cystic meniscus, posterior horn of medial meniscus, left knee**
    - **M23.029 Cystic meniscus, posterior horn of medial meniscus, unspecified knee**
  + **M23.03 Cystic meniscus, other medial meniscus**
    - **M23.031 Cystic meniscus, other medial meniscus, right knee**
    - **M23.032 Cystic meniscus, other medial meniscus, left knee**
    - **M23.039 Cystic meniscus, other medial meniscus, unspecified knee**
  + **M23.04 Cystic meniscus, anterior horn of lateral meniscus**
    - **M23.041 Cystic meniscus, anterior horn of lateral meniscus, right knee**
    - **M23.042 Cystic meniscus, anterior horn of lateral meniscus, left knee**
    - **M23.049 Cystic meniscus, anterior horn of lateral meniscus, unspecified knee**
  + **M23.05 Cystic meniscus, posterior horn of lateral meniscus**
    - **M23.051 Cystic meniscus, posterior horn of lateral meniscus, right knee**
    - **M23.052 Cystic meniscus, posterior horn of lateral meniscus, left knee**
    - **M23.059 Cystic meniscus, posterior horn of lateral meniscus, unspecified knee**
  + **M23.06 Cystic meniscus, other lateral meniscus**
    - **M23.061 Cystic meniscus, other lateral meniscus, right knee**
    - **M23.062 Cystic meniscus, other lateral meniscus, left knee**
    - **M23.069 Cystic meniscus, other lateral meniscus, unspecified knee**

+ **M23.2 Derangement of meniscus due to old tear or injury**
  Old bucket-handle tear
  + **M23.20 Derangement of unspecified meniscus due to old tear or injury**
    Derangement of unspecified lateral meniscus due to old tear or injury
    Derangement of unspecified medial meniscus due to old tear or injury
    - **M23.200 Derangement of unspecified lateral meniscus due to old tear or injury, right knee**
    - **M23.201 Derangement of unspecified lateral meniscus due to old tear or injury, left knee**
    - **M23.202 Derangement of unspecified lateral meniscus due to old tear or injury, unspecified knee**
    - **M23.203 Derangement of unspecified medial meniscus due to old tear or injury, right knee**
    - **M23.204 Derangement of unspecified medial meniscus due to old tear or injury, left knee**

M23.205 Derangement of unspecified medial meniscus due to old tear or injury, unspecified knee
M23.206 Derangement of unspecified meniscus due to old tear or injury, right knee
M23.207 Derangement of unspecified meniscus due to old tear or injury, left knee
M23.209 Derangement of unspecified meniscus due to old tear or injury, unspecified knee

+ M23.21 Derangement of anterior horn of medial meniscus due to old tear or injury
M23.211 Derangement of anterior horn of medial meniscus due to old tear or injury, right knee
M23.212 Derangement of anterior horn of medial meniscus due to old tear or injury, left knee
M23.219 Derangement of anterior horn of medial meniscus due to old tear or injury, unspecified knee

+ M23.22 Derangement of posterior horn of medial meniscus due to old tear or injury
M23.221 Derangement of posterior horn of medial meniscus due to old tear or injury, right knee
M23.222 Derangement of posterior horn of medial meniscus due to old tear or injury, left knee
M23.229 Derangement of posterior horn of medial meniscus due to old tear or injury, unspecified knee

+ M23.23 Derangement of other medial meniscus due to old tear or injury
M23.231 Derangement of other medial meniscus due to old tear or injury, right knee
M23.232 Derangement of other medial meniscus due to old tear or injury, left knee
M23.239 Derangement of other medial meniscus due to old tear or injury, unspecified knee

+ M23.24 Derangement of anterior horn of lateral meniscus due to old tear or injury
M23.241 Derangement of anterior horn of lateral meniscus due to old tear or injury, right knee
M23.242 Derangement of anterior horn of lateral meniscus due to old tear or injury, left knee
M23.249 Derangement of anterior horn of lateral meniscus due to old tear or injury, unspecified knee

+ M23.25 Derangement of posterior horn of lateral meniscus due to old tear or injury
M23.251 Derangement of posterior horn of lateral meniscus due to old tear or injury, right knee
M23.252 Derangement of posterior horn of lateral meniscus due to old tear or injury, left knee
M23.259 Derangement of posterior horn of lateral meniscus due to old tear or injury, unspecified knee

+ M23.26 Derangement of other lateral meniscus due to old tear or injury
M23.261 Derangement of other lateral meniscus due to old tear or injury, right knee
M23.262 Derangement of other lateral meniscus due to old tear or injury, left knee
M23.269 Derangement of other lateral meniscus due to old tear or injury, unspecified knee

+ M23.3 Other meniscus derangements
Degenerate meniscus
Detached meniscus
Retained meniscus

+ M23.30 Other meniscus derangements, unspecified meniscus
Other meniscus derangements, unspecified lateral meniscus
Other meniscus derangements, unspecified medial meniscus
M23.300 Other meniscus derangements, unspecified lateral meniscus, right knee
M23.301 Other meniscus derangements, unspecified lateral meniscus, left knee
M23.302 Other meniscus derangements, unspecified lateral meniscus, unspecified knee
M23.303 Other meniscus derangements, unspecified medial meniscus, right knee
M23.304 Other meniscus derangements, unspecified medial meniscus, left knee
M23.305 Other meniscus derangements, unspecified medial meniscus, unspecified knee
M23.306 Other meniscus derangements, unspecified meniscus, right knee
M23.307 Other meniscus derangements, unspecified meniscus, left knee
M23.309 Other meniscus derangements, unspecified meniscus, unspecified knee

+ M23.31 Other meniscus derangements, anterior horn of medial meniscus
M23.311 Other meniscus derangements, anterior horn of medial meniscus, right knee
M23.312 Other meniscus derangements, anterior horn of medial meniscus, left knee
M23.319 Other meniscus derangements, anterior horn of medial meniscus, unspecified knee

+ M23.32 Other meniscus derangements, posterior horn of medial meniscus
M23.321 Other meniscus derangements, posterior horn of medial meniscus, right knee
M23.322 Other meniscus derangements, posterior horn of medial meniscus, left knee
M23.329 Other meniscus derangements, posterior horn of medial meniscus, unspecified knee

+ M23.33 Other meniscus derangements, other medial meniscus
M23.331 Other meniscus derangements, other medial meniscus, right knee
M23.332 Other meniscus derangements, other medial meniscus, left knee
M23.339 Other meniscus derangements, other medial meniscus, unspecified knee

+ M23.34 Other meniscus derangements, anterior horn of lateral meniscus
M23.341 Other meniscus derangements, anterior horn of lateral meniscus, right knee
M23.342 Other meniscus derangements, anterior horn of lateral meniscus, left knee
M23.349 Other meniscus derangements, anterior horn of lateral meniscus, unspecified knee

+ M23.35 Other meniscus derangements, posterior horn of lateral meniscus
M23.351 Other meniscus derangements, posterior horn of lateral meniscus, right knee
M23.352 Other meniscus derangements, posterior horn of lateral meniscus, left knee
M23.359 Other meniscus derangements, posterior horn of lateral meniscus, unspecified knee

+ M23.36 Other meniscus derangements, other lateral meniscus
M23.361 Other meniscus derangements, other lateral meniscus, right knee
M23.362 Other meniscus derangements, other lateral meniscus, left knee
M23.369 Other meniscus derangements, other lateral meniscus, unspecified knee

+ M23.4 Loose body in knee
M23.40 Loose body in knee, unspecified knee
M23.41 Loose body in knee, right knee
M23.42 Loose body in knee, left knee

+ M23.5 Chronic instability of knee
M23.50 Chronic instability of knee, unspecified knee
M23.51 Chronic instability of knee, right knee
M23.52 Chronic instability of knee, left knee

+ **M23.6 Other spontaneous disruption of ligament(s) of knee**
  + **M23.60 Other spontaneous disruption of unspecified ligament of knee**
    - **M23.601 Other spontaneous disruption of unspecified ligament of right knee**
    - **M23.602 Other spontaneous disruption of unspecified ligament of left knee**
    - **M23.609 Other spontaneous disruption of unspecified ligament of unspecified knee**
  + **M23.61 Other spontaneous disruption of anterior cruciate ligament of knee**
    - **M23.611 Other spontaneous disruption of anterior cruciate ligament of right knee**
    - **M23.612 Other spontaneous disruption of anterior cruciate ligament of left knee**
    - **M23.619 Other spontaneous disruption of anterior cruciate ligament of unspecified knee**
  + **M23.62 Other spontaneous disruption of posterior cruciate ligament of knee**
    - **M23.621 Other spontaneous disruption of posterior cruciate ligament of right knee**
    - **M23.622 Other spontaneous disruption of posterior cruciate ligament of left knee**
    - **M23.629 Other spontaneous disruption of posterior cruciate ligament of unspecified knee**
  + **M23.63 Other spontaneous disruption of medial collateral ligament of knee**
    - **M23.631 Other spontaneous disruption of medial collateral ligament of right knee**
    - **M23.632 Other spontaneous disruption of medial collateral ligament of left knee**
    - **M23.639 Other spontaneous disruption of medial collateral ligament of unspecified knee**
  + **M23.64 Other spontaneous disruption of lateral collateral ligament of knee**
    - **M23.641 Other spontaneous disruption of lateral collateral ligament of right knee**
    - **M23.642 Other spontaneous disruption of lateral collateral ligament of left knee**
    - **M23.649 Other spontaneous disruption of lateral collateral ligament of unspecified knee**
  + **M23.67 Other spontaneous disruption of capsular ligament of knee**
    - **M23.671 Other spontaneous disruption of capsular ligament of right knee**
    - **M23.672 Other spontaneous disruption of capsular ligament of left knee**
    - **M23.679 Other spontaneous disruption of capsular ligament of unspecified knee**

+ **M23.8 Other internal derangements of knee**
  Laxity of ligament of knee
  Snapping knee
  + **M23.8X Other internal derangements of knee**
    - **M23.8X1 Other internal derangements of right knee**
    - **M23.8X2 Other internal derangements of left knee**
    - **M23.8X9 Other internal derangements of unspecified knee**

+ **M23.9 Unspecified internal derangement of knee**
  - **M23.90 Unspecified internal derangement of unspecified knee**
  - **M23.91 Unspecified internal derangement of right knee**
  - **M23.92 Unspecified internal derangement of left knee**

M24 Other specific joint derangements

Excludes1: *current injury - see injury of joint by body region*
Excludes2: *ganglion (M67.4)*
snapping knee (M23.8-)
temporomandibular joint disorders (M26.6-)

AHA CC: 4Q, 2020, 31-32.

+ **M24.0 Loose body in joint**
  Excludes2: *loose body in knee (M23.4)*
  - **M24.00 Loose body in unspecified joint**
  + **M24.01 Loose body in shoulder**
    - **M24.011 Loose body in right shoulder**
    - **M24.012 Loose body in left shoulder**
    - **M24.019 Loose body in unspecified shoulder**
  + **M24.02 Loose body in elbow**
    - **M24.021 Loose body in right elbow**
    - **M24.022 Loose body in left elbow**
    - **M24.029 Loose body in unspecified elbow**
  + **M24.03 Loose body in wrist**
    - **M24.031 Loose body in right wrist**
    - **M24.032 Loose body in left wrist**
    - **M24.039 Loose body in unspecified wrist**
  + **M24.04 Loose body in finger joints**
    - **M24.041 Loose body in right finger joint(s)**
    - **M24.042 Loose body in left finger joint(s)**
    - **M24.049 Loose body in unspecified finger joint(s)**
  + **M24.05 Loose body in hip**
    - **M24.051 Loose body in right hip**
    - **M24.052 Loose body in left hip**
    - **M24.059 Loose body in unspecified hip**
  + **M24.07 Loose body in ankle and toe joints**
    - **M24.071 Loose body in right ankle**
    - **M24.072 Loose body in left ankle**
    - **M24.073 Loose body in unspecified ankle**
    - **M24.074 Loose body in right toe joint(s)**
    - **M24.075 Loose body in left toe joint(s)**
    - **M24.076 Loose body in unspecified toe joints**
  - **M24.08 Loose body, other site**

+ **M24.1 Other articular cartilage disorders**
  Excludes2: *chondrocalcinosis (M11.1, M11.2-)*
  internal derangement of knee (M23.-)
  metastatic calcification (E83.5)
  ochronosis (E70.2)
  - **M24.10 Other articular cartilage disorders, unspecified site**
  + **M24.11 Other articular cartilage disorders, shoulder**
    - **M24.111 Other articular cartilage disorders, right shoulder**
    - **M24.112 Other articular cartilage disorders, left shoulder**
    - **M24.119 Other articular cartilage disorders, unspecified shoulder**
  + **M24.12 Other articular cartilage disorders, elbow**
    - **M24.121 Other articular cartilage disorders, right elbow**
    - **M24.122 Other articular cartilage disorders, left elbow**
    - **M24.129 Other articular cartilage disorders, unspecified elbow**
  + **M24.13 Other articular cartilage disorders, wrist**
    - **M24.131 Other articular cartilage disorders, right wrist**
    - **M24.132 Other articular cartilage disorders, left wrist**
    - **M24.139 Other articular cartilage disorders, unspecified wrist**
  + **M24.14 Other articular cartilage disorders, hand**
    - **M24.141 Other articular cartilage disorders, right hand**
    - **M24.142 Other articular cartilage disorders, left hand**
    - **M24.149 Other articular cartilage disorders, unspecified hand**
  + **M24.15 Other articular cartilage disorders, hip**
    - **M24.151 Other articular cartilage disorders, right hip**
    - **M24.152 Other articular cartilage disorders, left hip**
    - **M24.159 Other articular cartilage disorders, unspecified hip**
  + **M24.17 Other articular cartilage disorders, ankle and foot**
    - **M24.171 Other articular cartilage disorders, right ankle**
    - **M24.172 Other articular cartilage disorders, left ankle**
    - **M24.173 Other articular cartilage disorders, unspecified ankle**
    - **M24.174 Other articular cartilage disorders, right foot**
    - **M24.175 Other articular cartilage disorders, left foot**
    - **M24.176 Other articular cartilage disorders, unspecified foot**
  - **M24.19 Other articular cartilage disorders, other specified site**

+ **M24.2 Disorder of ligament**
Instability secondary to old ligament injury
Ligamentous laxity NOS
Excludes1: *familial ligamentous laxity (M35.7)*
Excludes2: *internal derangement of knee (M23.5-M23.8X9)*
M24.20 Disorder of ligament, unspecified site
+ **M24.21 Disorder of ligament, shoulder**
M24.211 Disorder of ligament, right shoulder
M24.212 Disorder of ligament, left shoulder
M24.219 Disorder of ligament, unspecified shoulder
+ **M24.22 Disorder of ligament, elbow**
M24.221 Disorder of ligament, right elbow
M24.222 Disorder of ligament, left elbow
M24.229 Disorder of ligament, unspecified elbow
+ **M24.23 Disorder of ligament, wrist**
M24.231 Disorder of ligament, right wrist
M24.232 Disorder of ligament, left wrist
M24.239 Disorder of ligament, unspecified wrist
+ **M24.24 Disorder of ligament, hand**
M24.241 Disorder of ligament, right hand
M24.242 Disorder of ligament, left hand
M24.249 Disorder of ligament, unspecified hand
+ **M24.25 Disorder of ligament, hip**
M24.251 Disorder of ligament, right hip
M24.252 Disorder of ligament, left hip
M24.259 Disorder of ligament, unspecified hip
+ **M24.27 Disorder of ligament, ankle and foot**
M24.271 Disorder of ligament, right ankle
M24.272 Disorder of ligament, left ankle
M24.273 Disorder of ligament, unspecified ankle
M24.274 Disorder of ligament, right foot
M24.275 Disorder of ligament, left foot
M24.276 Disorder of ligament, unspecifiedfoot
M24.28 Disorder of ligament, vertebrae
M24.29 Disorder of ligament, other specified site
+ **M24.3 Pathological dislocation of joint, not elsewhere classified**
Excludes1: *congenital dislocation or displacement of joint- see congenital malformations and deformations of the musculoskeletal system (Q65-Q79)*
current injury - see injury of joints and ligaments by body region
recurrent dislocation of joint (M24.4-)
M24.30 Pathological dislocation of unspecified joint, not elsewhere classified
+ **M24.31 Pathological dislocation of shoulder, not elsewhere classified**
M24.311 Pathological dislocation of right shoulder, not elsewhere classified
M24.312 Pathological dislocation of left shoulder, not elsewhere classified
M24.319 Pathological dislocation of unspecified shoulder, not elsewhere classified
+ **M24.32 Pathological dislocation of elbow, not elsewhere classified**
M24.321 Pathological dislocation of right elbow, not elsewhere classified
M24.322 Pathological dislocation of left elbow, not elsewhere classified
M24.329 Pathological dislocation of unspecified elbow, not elsewhere classified
+ **M24.33 Pathological dislocation of wrist, not elsewhere classified**
M24.331 Pathological dislocation of right wrist, not elsewhere classified
M24.332 Pathological dislocation of left wrist, not elsewhere classified
M24.339 Pathological dislocation of unspecified wrist, not elsewhere classified
+ **M24.34 Pathological dislocation of hand, not elsewhere classified**
M24.341 Pathological dislocation of right hand, not elsewhere classified
M24.342 Pathological dislocation of left hand, not elsewhere classified
M24.349 Pathological dislocation of unspecified hand, not elsewhere classified
+ **M24.35 Pathological dislocation of hip, not elsewhere classified**
M24.351 Pathological dislocation of right hip, not elsewhere classified
M24.352 Pathological dislocation of left hip, not elsewhere classified
M24.359 Pathological dislocation of unspecified hip, not elsewhere classified
+ **M24.36 Pathological dislocation of knee, not elsewhere classified**
M24.361 Pathological dislocation of right knee, not elsewhere classified
M24.362 Pathological dislocation of left knee, not elsewhere classified
M24.369 Pathological dislocation of unspecified knee, not elsewhere classified
+ **M24.37 Pathological dislocation of ankle and foot, not elsewhere classified**
M24.371 Pathological dislocation of right ankle, not elsewhere classified
M24.372 Pathological dislocation of left ankle, not elsewhere classified
M24.373 Pathological dislocation of unspecified ankle, not elsewhere classified
M24.374 Pathological dislocation of right foot, not elsewhere classified
M24.375 Pathological dislocation of left foot, not elsewhere classified
M24.376 Pathological dislocation of unspecified foot, not elsewhere classified
M24.39 Pathological dislocation of other specified joint, not elsewhere classified
+ **M24.4 Recurrent dislocation of joint**
Recurrent subluxation of joint
Excludes2: *recurrent dislocation of patella (M22.0-M22.1)*
recurrent vertebral dislocation (M43.3-, M43.4, M43.5-)
M24.40 Recurrent dislocation, unspecified joint
+ **M24.41 Recurrent dislocation, shoulder**
M24.411 Recurrent dislocation, right shoulder
M24.412 Recurrent dislocation, left shoulder
M24.419 Recurrent dislocation, unspecified shoulder
+ **M24.42 Recurrent dislocation, elbow**
M24.421 Recurrent dislocation, right elbow
M24.422 Recurrent dislocation, left elbow
M24.429 Recurrent dislocation, unspecified elbow
+ **M24.43 Recurrent dislocation, wrist**
M24.431 Recurrent dislocation, right wrist
M24.432 Recurrent dislocation, left wrist
M24.439 Recurrent dislocation, unspecified wrist
+ **M24.44 Recurrent dislocation, hand and finger(s)**
M24.441 Recurrent dislocation, right hand
M24.442 Recurrent dislocation, left hand
M24.443 Recurrent dislocation, unspecified hand
M24.444 Recurrent dislocation, right finger
M24.445 Recurrent dislocation, left finger
M24.446 Recurrent dislocation, unspecified finger
+ **M24.45 Recurrent dislocation, hip**
M24.451 Recurrent dislocation, right hip
M24.452 Recurrent dislocation, left hip
M24.459 Recurrent dislocation, unspecified hip
+ **M24.46 Recurrent dislocation, knee**
M24.461 Recurrent dislocation, right knee
M24.462 Recurrent dislocation, left knee
M24.469 Recurrent dislocation, unspecified knee
+ **M24.47 Recurrent dislocation, ankle, foot and toes**
M24.471 Recurrent dislocation, right ankle
M24.472 Recurrent dislocation, left ankle
M24.473 Recurrent dislocation, unspecified ankle
M24.474 Recurrent dislocation, right foot
M24.475 Recurrent dislocation, left foot
M24.476 Recurrent dislocation, unspecified foot
M24.477 Recurrent dislocation, right toe(s)
M24.478 Recurrent dislocation, left toe(s)
M24.479 Recurrent dislocation, unspecified toe(s)
M24.49 Recurrent dislocation, other specified joint

+ **M24.5 Contracture of joint**

Excludes1: *contracture of muscle without contracture of joint (M62.4-)*
contracture of tendon (sheath) without contracture of joint (M62.4-)
Dupuytren's contracture (M72.0)

Excludes2: *acquired deformities of limbs (M20-M21)*

AHA CC: 2Q, 2016, 6

M24.50 Contracture, unspecified joint
+ **M24.51 Contracture, shoulder**
M24.511 Contracture, right shoulder
M24.512 Contracture, left shoulder
M24.519 Contracture, unspecified shoulder
+ **M24.52 Contracture, elbow**
M24.521 Contracture, right elbow
M24.522 Contracture, left elbow
M24.529 Contracture, unspecified elbow
+ **M24.53 Contracture, wrist**
M24.531 Contracture, right wrist
M24.532 Contracture, left wrist
M24.539 Contracture, unspecified wrist
+ **M24.54 Contracture, hand**
M24.541 Contracture, right hand
M24.542 Contracture, left hand
M24.549 Contracture, unspecified hand
+ **M24.55 Contracture, hip**
M24.551 Contracture, right hip
M24.552 Contracture, left hip
M24.559 Contracture, unspecified hip
+ **M24.56 Contracture, knee**
M24.561 Contracture, right knee
M24.562 Contracture, left knee
M24.569 Contracture, unspecified knee
+ **M24.57 Contracture, ankle and foot**
M24.571 Contracture, right ankle
M24.572 Contracture, left ankle
M24.573 Contracture, unspecified ankle
M24.574 Contracture, right foot
M24.575 Contracture, left foot
M24.576 Contracture, unspecified foot
M24.59 Contracture, other specified joint

+ **M24.6 Ankylosis of joint**

Excludes1: *stiffness of joint without ankylosis (M25.6-)*

Excludes2: *spine (M43.2-)*

M24.60 Ankylosis, unspecified joint
+ **M24.61 Ankylosis, shoulder**
M24.611 Ankylosis, right shoulder
M24.612 Ankylosis, left shoulder
M24.619 Ankylosis, unspecified shoulder
+ **M24.62 Ankylosis, elbow**
M24.621 Ankylosis, right elbow
M24.622 Ankylosis, left elbow
M24.629 Ankylosis, unspecified elbow
+ **M24.63 Ankylosis, wrist**
M24.631 Ankylosis, right wrist
M24.632 Ankylosis, left wrist
M24.639 Ankylosis, unspecified wrist
+ **M24.64 Ankylosis, hand**
M24.641 Ankylosis, right hand
M24.642 Ankylosis, left hand
M24.649 Ankylosis, unspecified hand
+ **M24.65 Ankylosis, hip**
M24.651 Ankylosis, right hip
M24.652 Ankylosis, left hip
M24.659 Ankylosis, unspecified hip
+ **M24.66 Ankylosis, knee**
M24.661 Ankylosis, right knee
M24.662 Ankylosis, left knee
M24.669 Ankylosis, unspecified knee
+ **M24.67 Ankylosis, ankle and foot**
M24.671 Ankylosis, right ankle
M24.672 Ankylosis, left ankle
M24.673 Ankylosis, unspecified ankle
M24.674 Ankylosis, right foot
M24.675 Ankylosis, left foot
M24.676 Ankylosis, unspecified foot
M24.69 Ankylosis, other specified joint

M24.7 Protrusio acetabuli

+ **M24.8 Other specific joint derangements, not elsewhere classified**

Excludes2: *iliotibial band syndrome (M76.3)*

M24.80 Other specific joint derangements of unspecified joint, not elsewhere classified
+ **M24.81 Other specific joint derangements of shoulder, not elsewhere classified**
M24.811 Other specific joint derangements of right shoulder, not elsewhere classified
M24.812 Other specific joint derangements of left shoulder, not elsewhere classified
M24.819 Other specific joint derangements of unspecified shoulder, not elsewhere classified
+ **M24.82 Other specific joint derangements of elbow, not elsewhere classified**
M24.821 Other specific joint derangements of right elbow, not elsewhere classified
M24.822 Other specific joint derangements of left elbow, not elsewhere classified
M24.829 Other specific joint derangements of unspecified elbow, not elsewhere classified
+ **M24.83 Other specific joint derangements of wrist, not elsewhere classified**
M24.831 Other specific joint derangements of right wrist, not elsewhere classified
M24.832 Other specific joint derangements of left wrist, not elsewhere classified
M24.839 Other specific joint derangements of unspecified wrist, not elsewhere classified
+ **M24.84 Other specific joint derangements of hand, not elsewhere classified**
M24.841 Other specific joint derangements of right hand, not elsewhere classified
M24.842 Other specific joint derangements of left hand, not elsewhere classified
M24.849 Other specific joint derangements of unspecified hand, not elsewhere classified
+ **M24.85 Other specific joint derangements of hip, not elsewhere classified**
Irritable hip
M24.851 Other specific joint derangements of right hip, not elsewhere classified
M24.852 Other specific joint derangements of left hip, not elsewhere classified
M24.859 Other specific joint derangements of unspecified hip, not elsewhere classified
+ **M24.87 Other specific joint derangements of ankle and foot, not elsewhere classified**
M24.871 Other specific joint derangements of right ankle, not elsewhere classified
M24.872 Other specific joint derangements of left ankle, not elsewhere classified
M24.873 Other specific joint derangements of unspecified ankle, not elsewhere classified
M24.874 Other specific joint derangements of right foot, not elsewhere classified
M24.875 Other specific joint derangements left foot, not elsewhere classified
M24.876 Other specific joint derangements of unspecified foot, not elsewhere classified
M24.89 Other specific joint derangement of other specified joint, not elsewhere classified

M24.9 Joint derangement, unspecified

M25 Other joint disorder, not elsewhere classified

Excludes2: *abnormality of gait and mobility (R26.-)*
acquired deformities of limb (M20-M21)
calcification of bursa (M71.4-)
calcification of shoulder (joint) (M75.3)
calcification of tendon (M65.2-)
difficulty in walking (R26.2)
temporomandibular joint disorder (M26.6-)

AHA CC: 4Q, 2020, 31-32

+ **M25.0 Hemarthrosis**

Excludes1: *current injury - see injury of joint by body region*
hemophilic arthropathy (M36.2)

CC **M25.00 Hemarthrosis, unspecified joint**

+ **M25.01 Hemarthrosis, shoulder**
CC **M25.011 Hemarthrosis, right shoulder**
CC **M25.012 Hemarthrosis, left shoulder**
CC **M25.019 Hemarthrosis, unspecified shoulder**
+ **M25.02 Hemarthrosis, elbow**
CC **M25.021 Hemarthrosis, right elbow**
CC **M25.022 Hemarthrosis, left elbow**
CC **M25.029 Hemarthrosis, unspecified elbow**
+ **M25.03 Hemarthrosis, wrist**
CC **M25.031 Hemarthrosis, right wrist**
CC **M25.032 Hemarthrosis, left wrist**
CC **M25.039 Hemarthrosis, unspecified wrist**
+ **M25.04 Hemarthrosis, hand**
CC **M25.041 Hemarthrosis, right hand**
CC **M25.042 Hemarthrosis, left hand**
CC **M25.049 Hemarthrosis, unspecified hand**
+ **M25.05 Hemarthrosis, hip**
CC **M25.051 Hemarthrosis, right hip**
CC **M25.052 Hemarthrosis, left hip**
CC **M25.059 Hemarthrosis, unspecified hip**
+ **M25.06 Hemarthrosis, knee**
CC **M25.061 Hemarthrosis, right knee**
CC **M25.062 Hemarthrosis, left knee**
CC **M25.069 Hemarthrosis, unspecified knee**
+ **M25.07 Hemarthrosis, ankle and foot**
CC **M25.071 Hemarthrosis, right ankle**
CC **M25.072 Hemarthrosis, left ankle**
CC **M25.073 Hemarthrosis, unspecified ankle**
CC **M25.074 Hemarthrosis, right foot**
CC **M25.075 Hemarthrosis, left foot**
CC **M25.076 Hemarthrosis, unspecified foot**
CC **M25.08 Hemarthrosis, other specified site**
Hemarthrosis, vertebrae
+ **M25.1 Fistula of joint**
M25.10 Fistula, unspecified joint
+ **M25.11 Fistula, shoulder**
M25.111 Fistula, right shoulder
M25.112 Fistula, left shoulder
M25.119 Fistula, unspecified shoulder
+ **M25.12 Fistula, elbow**
M25.121 Fistula, right elbow
M25.122 Fistula, left elbow
M25.129 Fistula, unspecified elbow
+ **M25.13 Fistula, wrist**
M25.131 Fistula, right wrist
M25.132 Fistula, left wrist
M25.139 Fistula, unspecified wrist
+ **M25.14 Fistula, hand**
M25.141 Fistula, right hand
M25.142 Fistula, left hand
M25.149 Fistula, unspecified hand
+ **M25.15 Fistula, hip**
M25.151 Fistula, right hip
M25.152 Fistula, left hip
M25.159 Fistula, unspecified hip
+ **M25.16 Fistula, knee**
M25.161 Fistula, right knee
M25.162 Fistula, left knee
M25.169 Fistula, unspecified knee
+ **M25.17 Fistula, ankle and foot**
M25.171 Fistula, right ankle
M25.172 Fistula, left ankle
M25.173 Fistula, unspecified ankle
M25.174 Fistula, right foot
M25.175 Fistula, left foot
M25.176 Fistula, unspecified foot
M25.18 Fistula, other specified site
Fistula, vertebrae
+ **M25.2 Flail joint**
M25.20 Flail joint, unspecified joint
+ **M25.21 Flail joint, shoulder**
M25.211 Flail joint, right shoulder
M25.212 Flail joint, left shoulder
M25.219 Flail joint, unspecified shoulder
+ **M25.22 Flail joint, elbow**
M25.221 Flail joint, right elbow
M25.222 Flail joint, left elbow
M25.229 Flail joint, unspecified elbow
+ **M25.23 Flail joint, wrist**
M25.231 Flail joint, right wrist
M25.232 Flail joint, left wrist
M25.239 Flail joint, unspecified wrist
+ **M25.24 Flail joint, hand**
M25.241 Flail joint, right hand
M25.242 Flail joint, left hand
M25.249 Flail joint, unspecified hand
+ **M25.25 Flail joint, hip**
M25.251 Flail joint, right hip
M25.252 Flail joint, left hip
M25.259 Flail joint, unspecified hip
+ **M25.26 Flail joint, knee**
M25.261 Flail joint, right knee
M25.262 Flail joint, left knee
M25.269 Flail joint, unspecified knee
+ **M25.27 Flail joint, ankle and foot**
M25.271 Flail joint, right ankle and foot
M25.272 Flail joint, left ankle and foot
M25.279 Flail joint, unspecified ankle and foot
M25.28 Flail joint, other site
+ **M25.3 Other instability of joint**
Excludes1: *instability of joint secondary to old ligament injury (M24.2-)*
instability of joint secondary to removal of joint prosthesis (M96.8-)
Excludes2: *spinal instabilities (M53.2-)*
M25.30 Other instability, unspecified joint
+ **M25.31 Other instability, shoulder**
M25.311 Other instability, right shoulder
M25.312 Other instability, left shoulder
M25.319 Other instability, unspecified shoulder
+ **M25.32 Other instability, elbow**
M25.321 Other instability, right elbow
M25.322 Other instability, left elbow
M25.329 Other instability, unspecified elbow
+ **M25.33 Other instability, wrist**
M25.331 Other instability, right wrist
M25.332 Other instability, left wrist
M25.339 Other instability, unspecified wrist
+ **M25.34 Other instability, hand**
M25.341 Other instability, right hand
M25.342 Other instability, left hand
M25.349 Other instability, unspecified hand
+ **M25.35 Other instability, hip**
M25.351 Other instability, right hip
M25.352 Other instability, left hip
M25.359 Other instability, unspecified hip
+ **M25.36 Other instability, knee**
M25.361 Other instability, right knee
M25.362 Other instability, left knee
M25.369 Other instability, unspecified knee
+ **M25.37 Other instability, ankle and foot**
M25.371 Other instability, right ankle
M25.372 Other instability, left ankle
M25.373 Other instability, unspecified ankle
M25.374 Other instability, right foot
M25.375 Other instability, left foot
M25.376 Other instability, unspecified foot
M25.39 Other instability, other specified joint
+ **M25.4 Effusion of joint**
Excludes1: *hydrarthrosis in yaws (A66.6)*
intermittent hydrarthrosis (M12.4-)
other infective (teno)synovitis (M65.1-)
M25.40 Effusion, unspecified joint
+ **M25.41 Effusion, shoulder**
M25.411 Effusion, right shoulder
M25.412 Effusion, left shoulder
M25.419 Effusion, unspecified shoulder
+ **M25.42 Effusion, elbow**
M25.421 Effusion, right elbow
M25.422 Effusion, left elbow
M25.429 Effusion, unspecified elbow
+ **M25.43 Effusion, wrist**
M25.431 Effusion, right wrist
M25.432 Effusion, left wrist
M25.439 Effusion, unspecified wrist

+ **M25.44 Effusion, hand**
  - **M25.441 Effusion, right hand**
  - **M25.442 Effusion, left hand**
  - **M25.449 Effusion, unspecified hand**
+ **M25.45 Effusion, hip**
  - **M25.451 Effusion, right hip**
  - **M25.452 Effusion, left hip**
  - **M25.459 Effusion, unspecified hip**
+ **M25.46 Effusion, knee**
  - **M25.461 Effusion, right knee**
  - **M25.462 Effusion, left knee**
  - **M25.469 Effusion, unspecified knee**
+ **M25.47 Effusion, ankle and foot**
  - **M25.471 Effusion, right ankle**
  - **M25.472 Effusion, left ankle**
  - **M25.473 Effusion, unspecified ankle**
  - **M25.474 Effusion, right foot**
  - **M25.475 Effusion, left foot**
  - **M25.476 Effusion, unspecified foot**

M25.48 Effusion, other site

+ **M25.5 Pain in joint**

Excludes2: *pain in hand (M79.64-)*
pain in fingers (M79.64-)
pain in foot (M79.67-)
pain in limb (M79.6-)
pain in toes (M79.67-)

AHA CC: 4Q, 2016, 38

M25.50 Pain in unspecified joint

+ **M25.51 Pain in shoulder**
  - **M25.511 Pain in right shoulder**
  - **M25.512 Pain in left shoulder**
  - **M25.519 Pain in unspecified shoulder**
+ **M25.52 Pain in elbow**
  - **M25.521 Pain in right elbow**
  - **M25.522 Pain in left elbow**
  - **M25.529 Pain in unspecified elbow**
+ **M25.53 Pain in wrist**
  - **M25.531 Pain in right wrist**
  - **M25.532 Pain in left wrist**
  - **M25.539 Pain in unspecified wrist**
+ **M25.54 Pain in joints of hand**
  - **M25.541 Pain in joints of right hand**
  - **M25.542 Pain in joints of left hand**
  - **M25.549 Pain in joints of unspecified hand**
    Pain in joints of hand NOS
+ **M25.55 Pain in hip**
  - **M25.551 Pain in right hip**
  - **M25.552 Pain in left hip**
  - **M25.559 Pain in unspecified hip**
+ **M25.56 Pain in knee**
  - **M25.561 Pain in right knee**
  - **M25.562 Pain in left knee**
  - **M25.569 Pain in unspecified knee**
+ **M25.57 Pain in ankle and joints of foot**
  - **M25.571 Pain in right ankle and joints of right foot**
  - **M25.572 Pain in left ankle and joints of left foot**
  - **M25.579 Pain in unspecified ankle and joints of unspecified foot**

M25.59 Pain in other specified joint

+ **M25.6 Stiffness of joint, not elsewhere classified**

Excludes1: *ankylosis of joint (M24.6-)*
contracture of joint (M24.5-)

M25.60 Stiffness of unspecified joint, not elsewhere classified

+ **M25.61 Stiffness of shoulder, not elsewhere classified**
  - **M25.611 Stiffness of right shoulder, not elsewhere classified**
  - **M25.612 Stiffness of left shoulder, not elsewhere classified**
  - **M25.619 Stiffness of unspecified shoulder, not elsewhere classified**
+ **M25.62 Stiffness of elbow, not elsewhere classified**
  - **M25.621 Stiffness of right elbow, not elsewhere classified**
  - **M25.622 Stiffness of left elbow, not elsewhere classified**
  - **M25.629 Stiffness of unspecified elbow, not elsewhere classified**
+ **M25.63 Stiffness of wrist, not elsewhere classified**
  - **M25.631 Stiffness of right wrist, not elsewhere classified**
  - **M25.632 Stiffness of left wrist, not elsewhere classified**
  - **M25.639 Stiffness of unspecified wrist, not elsewhere classified**
+ **M25.64 Stiffness of hand, not elsewhere classified**
  - **M25.641 Stiffness of right hand, not elsewhere classified**
  - **M25.642 Stiffness of left hand, not elsewhere classified**
  - **M25.649 Stiffness of unspecified hand, not elsewhere classified**
+ **M25.65 Stiffness of hip, not elsewhere classified**
  - **M25.651 Stiffness of right hip, not elsewhere classified**
  - **M25.652 Stiffness of left hip, not elsewhere classified**
  - **M25.659 Stiffness of unspecified hip, not elsewhere classified**
+ **M25.66 Stiffness of knee, not elsewhere classified**
  - **M25.661 Stiffness of right knee, not elsewhere classified**
  - **M25.662 Stiffness of left knee, not elsewhere classified**
  - **M25.669 Stiffness of unspecified knee, not elsewhere classified**
+ **M25.67 Stiffness of ankle and foot, not elsewhere classified**
  - **M25.671 Stiffness of right ankle, not elsewhere classified**
  - **M25.672 Stiffness of left ankle, not elsewhere classified**
  - **M25.673 Stiffness of unspecified ankle, not elsewhere classified**
  - **M25.674 Stiffness of right foot, not elsewhere classified**
  - **M25.675 Stiffness of left foot, not elsewhere classified**
  - **M25.676 Stiffness of unspecified foot, not elsewhere classified**

M25.69 Stiffness of other specified joint, not elsewhere classified

+ **M25.7 Osteophyte**

M25.70 Osteophyte, unspecified joint

+ **M25.71 Osteophyte, shoulder**
  - **M25.711 Osteophyte, right shoulder**
  - **M25.712 Osteophyte, left shoulder**
  - **M25.719 Osteophyte, unspecified shoulder**
+ **M25.72 Osteophyte, elbow**
  - **M25.721 Osteophyte, right elbow**
  - **M25.722 Osteophyte, left elbow**
  - **M25.729 Osteophyte, unspecified elbow**
+ **M25.73 Osteophyte, wrist**
  - **M25.731 Osteophyte, right wrist**
  - **M25.732 Osteophyte, left wrist**
  - **M25.739 Osteophyte, unspecified wrist**
+ **M25.74 Osteophyte, hand**
  - **M25.741 Osteophyte, right hand**
  - **M25.742 Osteophyte, left hand**
  - **M25.749 Osteophyte, unspecified hand**
+ **M25.75 Osteophyte, hip**
  - **M25.751 Osteophyte, right hip**
  - **M25.752 Osteophyte, left hip**
  - **M25.759 Osteophyte, unspecified hip**
+ **M25.76 Osteophyte, knee**
  - **M25.761 Osteophyte, right knee**
  - **M25.762 Osteophyte, left knee**
  - **M25.769 Osteophyte, unspecified knee**
+ **M25.77 Osteophyte, ankle and foot**
  - **M25.771 Osteophyte, right ankle**
  - **M25.772 Osteophyte, left ankle**
  - **M25.773 Osteophyte, unspecified ankle**
  - **M25.774 Osteophyte, right foot**
  - **M25.775 Osteophyte, left foot**
  - **M25.776 Osteophyte, unspecified foot**

M25.78 Osteophyte, vertebrae

\+ M25.8 Other specified joint disorders
M25.80 Other specified joint disorders, unspecified joint
\+ M25.81 Other specified joint disorders, shoulder
M25.811 Other specified joint disorders, right shoulder
M25.812 Other specified joint disorders, left shoulder
M25.819 Other specified joint disorders, unspecified shoulder
\+ M25.82 Other specified joint disorders, elbow
M25.821 Other specified joint disorders, right elbow
M25.822 Other specified joint disorders, left elbow
M25.829 Other specified joint disorders, unspecified elbow
\+ M25.83 Other specified joint disorders, wrist
M25.831 Other specified joint disorders, right wrist
M25.832 Other specified joint disorders, left wrist
M25.839 Other specified joint disorders, unspecified wrist
\+ M25.84 Other specified joint disorders, hand
M25.841 Other specified joint disorders, right hand
M25.842 Other specified joint disorders, left hand
M25.849 Other specified joint disorders, unspecified hand
\+ M25.85 Other specified joint disorders, hip
M25.851 Other specified joint disorders, right hip
M25.852 Other specified joint disorders, left hip
AHA CC: 4Q, 2014, 25
M25.859 Other specified joint disorders, unspecified hip
\+ M25.86 Other specified joint disorders, knee
M25.861 Other specified joint disorders, right knee
M25.862 Other specified joint disorders, left knee
M25.869 Other specified joint disorders, unspecified knee
\+ M25.87 Other specified joint disorders, ankle and foot
M25.871 Other specified joint disorders, right ankle and foot
M25.872 Other specified joint disorders, left ankle and foot
M25.879 Other specified joint disorders, unspecified ankle and foot
M25.9 Joint disorder, unspecified

Dentofacial anomalies [including malocclusion] and other disorders of jaw (M26-M27)

Excludes1: *hemifacial atrophy or hypertrophy (Q67.4)*
unilateral condylar hyperplasia or hypoplasia (M27.8)

M26 Dentofacial anomalies [including malocclusion]
\+ M26.0 Major anomalies of jaw size
Excludes1: *acromegaly (E22.0)*
Robin's syndrome (Q87.0)
M26.00 Unspecified anomaly of jaw size
M26.01 Maxillary hyperplasia
M26.02 Maxillary hypoplasia
AHA CC: 3Q, 2014, 23-24
M26.03 Mandibular hyperplasia
M26.04 Mandibular hypoplasia
M26.05 Macrogenia
M26.06 Microgenia
M26.07 Excessive tuberosity of jaw
Entire maxillary tuberosity
M26.09 Other specified anomalies of jaw size
\+ M26.1 Anomalies of jaw-cranial base relationship
M26.10 Unspecified anomaly of jaw-cranial base relationship
M26.11 Maxillary asymmetry
M26.12 Other jaw asymmetry
M26.19 Other specified anomalies of jaw-cranial base relationship
AHA CC: 1Q, 2020, 21
\+ M26.2 Anomalies of dental arch relationship
M26.20 Unspecified anomaly of dental arch relationship
\+ M26.21 Malocclusion, Angle's class
M26.211 Malocclusion, Angle's class I
Neutro-occlusion
M26.212 Malocclusion, Angle's class II
Disto-occlusion Division I
Disto-occlusion Division II
M26.213 Malocclusion, Angle's class III
Mesio-occlusion
M26.219 Malocclusion, Angle's class, unspecified
\+ M26.22 Open occlusal relationship
M26.220 Open anterior occlusal relationship
Anterior open bite
M26.221 Open posterior occlusal relationship
Posterior open bite
M26.23 Excessive horizontal overlap
Excessive horizontal overjet
M26.24 Reverse articulation
Crossbite (anterior) (posterior)
M26.25 Anomalies of interarch distance
M26.29 Other anomalies of dental arch relationship
Midline deviation of dental arch
Overbite (excessive) deep
Overbite (excessive) horizontal
Overbite (excessive) vertical
Posterior lingual occlusion of mandibular teeth
\+ M26.3 Anomalies of tooth position of fully erupted tooth or teeth
Excludes2: *embedded and impacted teeth (K01.-)*
M26.30 Unspecified anomaly of tooth position of fully erupted tooth or teeth
Abnormal spacing of fully erupted tooth or teeth NOS
Displacement of fully erupted tooth or teeth NOS
Transposition of fully erupted tooth or teeth NOS
M26.31 Crowding of fully erupted teeth
M26.32 Excessive spacing of fully erupted teeth
Diastema of fully erupted tooth or teeth NOS
M26.33 Horizontal displacement of fully erupted tooth or teeth
Tipped tooth or teeth
Tipping of fully erupted tooth
M26.34 Vertical displacement of fully erupted tooth or teeth
Extruded tooth
Infraeruption of tooth or teeth
Supraeruption of tooth or teeth
M26.35 Rotation of fully erupted tooth or teeth
M26.36 Insufficient interocclusal distance of fully erupted teeth (ridge)
Lack of adequate intermaxillary vertical dimension of fully erupted teeth
M26.37 Excessive interocclusal distance of fully erupted teeth
Excessive intermaxillary vertical dimension of fully erupted teeth
Loss of occlusal vertical dimension of fully erupted teeth
M26.39 Other anomalies of tooth position of fully erupted tooth or teeth
M26.4 Malocclusion, unspecified
\+ M26.5 Dentofacial functional abnormalities
Excludes1: *bruxism (F45.8)*
teeth-grinding NOS (F45.8)
M26.50 Dentofacial functional abnormalities, unspecified
M26.51 Abnormal jaw closure
M26.52 Limited mandibular range of motion
M26.53 Deviation in opening and closing of the mandible
M26.54 Insufficient anterior guidance
Insufficient anterior occlusal guidance
M26.55 Centric occlusion maximum intercuspation discrepancy
Excludes1: *centric occlusion NOS (M26.59)*
M26.56 Non-working side interference
Balancing side interference
M26.57 Lack of posterior occlusal support
M26.59 Other dentofacial functional abnormalities
Centric occlusion (of teeth) NOS
Malocclusion due to abnormal swallowing
Malocclusion due to mouth breathing
Malocclusion due to tongue, lip or finger habits

+ **M26.6 Temporomandibular joint disorders**
  Excludes2: *current temporomandibular joint dislocation (S03.0)*
  current temporomandibular joint sprain (S03.4)
  AHA CC: 4Q, 2016, 38-39
  + **M26.60 Temporomandibular joint disorder, unspecified**
    M26.601 Right temporomandibular joint disorder, unspecified
    M26.602 Left temporomandibular joint disorder, unspecified
    M26.603 Bilateral temporomandibular joint disorder, unspecified
    M26.609 Unspecified temporomandibular joint disorder, unspecified side
    Temporomandibular joint disorder NOS
  + **M26.61 Adhesions and ankylosis of temporomandibular joint**
    M26.611 Adhesions and ankylosis of right temporomandibular joint
    M26.612 Adhesions and ankylosis of left temporomandibular joint
    M26.613 Adhesions and ankylosis of bilateral temporomandibular joint
    M26.619 Adhesions and ankylosis of temporomandibular joint, unspecified side
  + **M26.62 Arthralgia of temporomandibular joint**
    M26.621 Arthralgia of right temporomandibular joint
    M26.622 Arthralgia of left temporomandibular joint
    M26.623 Arthralgia of bilateral temporomandibular joint
    M26.629 Arthralgia of temporomandibular joint, unspecified side
  + **M26.63 Articular disc disorder of temporomandibular joint**
    M26.631 Articular disc disorder of right temporomandibular joint
    M26.632 Articular disc disorder of left temporomandibular joint
    M26.633 Articular disc disorder of bilateral temporomandibular joint
    M26.639 Articular disc disorder of temporomandibular joint, unspecified side
  + **M26.64 Arthritis of temporomandibular joint**
    AHA CC: 4Q, 2020, 32
    M26.641 Arthritis of right temporomandibular joint
    M26.642 Arthritis of left temporomandibular joint
    M26.643 Arthritis of bilateral temporomandibular joint
    M26.649 Arthritis of unspecified temporomandibular joint
  + **M26.65 Arthropathy of temporomandibular joing**
    AHA CC: 4Q, 2020, 32
    M26.651 Arthropathy of right temporomandibular joint
    M26.652 Arthropathy of left temporomandibular joint
    M26.653 Arthropathy of bilateral temporomandibular joint
    M26.659 Arthropathy of unspecified temporomandibular joint
  M26.69 Other specified disorders of temporomandibular joint

+ **M26.7 Dental alveolar anomalies**
  M26.70 Unspecified alveolar anomaly
  M26.71 Alveolar maxillary hyperplasia
  M26.72 Alveolar mandibular hyperplasia
  M26.73 Alveolar maxillary hypoplasia
  M26.74 Alveolar mandibular hypoplasia
  M26.79 Other specified alveolar anomalies

+ **M26.8 Other dentofacial anomalies**
  M26.81 Anterior soft tissue impingement
  Anterior soft tissue impingement on teeth
  M26.82 Posterior soft tissue impingement
  Posterior soft tissue impingement on teeth
  M26.89 Other dentofacial anomalies

M26.9 Dentofacial anomaly, unspecified

M27 Other diseases of jaws

M27.0 Developmental disorders of jaws
Latent bone cyst of jaw
Stafne's cyst
Torus mandibularis
Torus palatinus

M27.1 Giant cell granuloma, central
Giant cell granuloma NOS
Excludes1: *peripheral giant cell granuloma (K06.8)*

M27.2 Inflammatory conditions of jaws
Osteitis of jaw(s)
Osteomyelitis (neonatal) jaw(s)
Osteoradionecrosis jaw(s)
Periostitis jaw(s)
Sequestrum of jaw bone
Use additional code (W88-W90, X39.0) to identify radiation, if radiation-induced
Excludes2: *osteonecrosis of jaw due to drug (M87.180)*

M27.3 Alveolitis of jaws
Alveolar osteitis
Dry socket

+ **M27.4 Other and unspecified cysts of jaw**
  Excludes1: *cysts of oral region (K09.-)*
  latent bone cyst of jaw (M27.0)
  Stafne's cyst (M27.0)
  M27.40 Unspecified cyst of jaw
  Cyst of jaw NOS
  M27.49 Other cysts of jaw
  Aneurysmal cyst of jaw
  Hemorrhagic cyst of jaw
  Traumatic cyst of jaw

+ **M27.5 Periradicular pathology associated with previous endodontic treatment**
  M27.51 Perforation of root canal space due to endodontic treatment
  M27.52 Endodontic overfill
  M27.53 Endodontic underfill
  M27.59 Other periradicular pathology associated with previous endodontic treatment

+ **M27.6 Endosseous dental implant failure**
  M27.61 Osseointegration failure of dental implant
  Hemorrhagic complications of dental implant placement
  Iatrogenic osseointegration failure of dental implant
  Osseointegration failure of dental implant due to complications of systemic disease
  Osseointegration failure of dental implant due to poor bone quality
  Pre-integration failure of dental implant NOS
  Pre-osseointegration failure of dental implant
  M27.62 Post-osseointegration biological failure of dental implant
  Failure of dental implant due to lack of attached gingiva
  Failure of dental implant due to occlusal trauma (caused by poor prosthetic design)
  Failure of dental implant due to parafunctional habits
  Failure of dental implant due to periodontal infection (peri-implantitis)
  Failure of dental implant due to poor oral hygiene
  Iatrogenic post-osseointegration failure of dental implant
  Post-osseointegration failure of dental implant due to complications of systemic disease
  M27.63 Post-osseointegration mechanical failure of dental implant
  Failure of dental prosthesis causing loss of dental implant
  Fracture of dental implant
  Excludes2: *cracked tooth (K03.81)*
  fractured dental restorative material with loss of material (K08.531)
  fractured dental restorative material without loss of material (K08.530)
  fractured tooth (S02.5)
  M27.69 Other endosseous dental implant failure
  Dental implant failure NOS

M27.8 **Other specified diseases of jaws**
Cherubism
Exostosis
Fibrous dysplasia
Unilateral condylar hyperplasia
Unilateral condylar hypoplasia
Excludes1: *jaw pain (R68.84)*

M27.9 **Disease of jaws, unspecified**

Systemic connective tissue disorders (M30-M36)

Includes: autoimmune disease NOS
collagen (vascular) disease NOS
systemic autoimmune disease
systemic collagen (vascular) disease

Excludes1: *autoimmune disease, single organ or single cell-type -code to relevant condition category*

M30 **Polyarteritis nodosa and related conditions**

Excludes1: *microscopic polyarteritis (M31.7)*

CC M30.0 **Polyarteritis nodosa**

CC M30.1 **Polyarteritis with lung involvement [Churg-Strauss]**
Allergic granulomatous angiitis
Eosinophilic granulomatosis with polyangiitis [EGPA]
AHA CC: 1Q, 2021, 23

CC M30.2 **Juvenile polyarteritis**

CC M30.3 **Mucocutaneous lymph node syndrome [Kawasaki]**

CC M30.8 **Other conditions related to polyarteritis nodosa**
Polyangiitis overlap syndrome

M31 **Other necrotizing vasculopathies**

CC M31.0 **Hypersensitivity angiitis**
Goodpasture's syndrome

+ M31.1 **Thrombotic microangiopathy**

MCC M31.10 **Thrombotic microangiopathy, unspecified**

MCC M31.11 **Hematopoietic stem cell transplantation-associated thrombotic microangiopathy [HSCT-TMA]**
Transplant-associated thrombotic microangiopathy [TA-TMA]
Code first if applicable:
complications of bone marrow transplant (T86.0-)
complications of stem cell transplant (T86.5)

Use additional code to identify specific organ dysfunction, such as:
acute kidney failure (N17.-)
acute respiratory distress syndrome (J80)
capillary leak syndrome (I78.8)
diffuse alveolar hemorrhage (R04.89)
encephalopathy (metabolic) (septic) G93.41
fluid overload, unspecified (E87.70)
graft versus host disease (D89.81-)
hemolytic uremic syndrome (D59.3)
hepatic failure (K72.-)
hepatic veno-occlusive disease (K76.5)
idiopathic interstitial pneumonia (J84.11-)
sinusoidal obstruction syndrome (K76.5)

MCC M31.19 **Other thrombotic microangiopathy**
Thrombotic thrombocytopenic purpura

CC M31.2 **Lethal midline granuloma**

+ M31.3 **Wegener's granulomatosis**
Granulomatosis with polyangiitis
Necrotizing respiratory granulomatosis
AHA CC: 1Q, 2021, 23

CC M31.30 **Wegener's granulomatosis without renal involvement**
Wegener's granulomatosis NOS
AHA CC: 2Q, 2021, 10

CC M31.31 **Wegener's granulomatosis with renal involvement**

CC M31.4 **Aortic arch syndrome [Takayasu]**

M31.5 **Giant cell arteritis with polymyalgia rheumatica**

M31.6 **Other giant cell arteritis**

CC M31.7 **Microscopic polyangiitis**
Microscopic polyarteritis
Excludes1: *polyarteritis nodosa (M30.0)*
AHA CC: 1Q, 2021, 23

CC M31.8 **Other specified necrotizing vasculopathies**
Hypocomplementemic vasculitis
Septic vasculitis

CC M31.9 **Necrotizing vasculopathy, unspecified**

M32 **Systemic lupus erythematosus (SLE)**

Excludes1: *lupus erythematosus (discoid) (NOS) (L93.0)*
AHA CC: 3Q, 2018, 14-15

M32.0 **Drug-induced systemic lupus erythematosus**
Use additional code for adverse effect, if applicable, to identify drug (T36-T50 with fifth or sixth character 5)

+ M32.1 **Systemic lupus erythematosus with organ or system involvement**

M32.10 **Systemic lupus erythematosus, organ or system involvement unspecified**

CC M32.11 **Endocarditis in systemic lupus erythematosus**
Libman-Sacks disease

CC M32.12 **Pericarditis in systemic lupus erythematosus**
Lupus pericarditis

M32.13 **Lung involvement in systemic lupus erythematosus**
Pleural effusion due to systemic lupus erythematosus

M32.14 **Glomerular disease in systemic lupus erythematosus**
Lupus renal disease NOS
AHA CC: 4Q, 2013, 125

M32.15 **Tubulo-interstitial nephropathy in systemic lupus erythematosus**

M32.19 **Other organ or system involvement in systemic lupus erythematosus**

M32.8 **Other forms of systemic lupus erythematosus**

M32.9 **Systemic lupus erythematosus, unspecified**
SLE NOS
Systemic lupus erythematosus NOS
Systemic lupus erythematosus without organ involvement
AHA CC: 3Q, 2018, 14-15; 4Q, 2020, 11

M33 **Dermatopolymyositis**

+ M33.0 **Juvenile dermatomyositis**

CC M33.00 **Juvenile dermatomyositis, organ involvement unspecified**

CC M33.01 **Juvenile dermatomyositis with respiratory involvement**

CC M33.02 **Juvenile dermatomyositis with myopathy**

CC M33.03 **Juvenile dermatomyositis without myopathy**
AHA CC: 4Q, 2017, 18

CC M33.09 **Juvenile dermatomyositis with other organ involvement**

+ M33.1 **Other dermatomyositis**
Adult dematomyositis

CC M33.10 **Other dermatomyositis, organ involvement unspecified**

CC M33.11 **Other dermatomyositis with respiratory involvement**

CC M33.12 **Other dermatomyositis with myopathy**

CC M33.13 **Other dermatomyositis without myopathy**
Dermatomyositis NOS
AHA CC: 4Q, 2017, 18

CC M33.19 **Other dermatomyositis with other organ involvement**

+ M33.2 **Polymyositis**

CC M33.20 **Polymyositis, organ involvement unspecified**

CC M33.21 **Polymyositis with respiratory involvement**

CC M33.22 **Polymyositis with myopathy**

CC M33.29 **Polymyositis with other organ involvement**

+ M33.9 **Dermatopolymyositis, unspecified**

CC M33.90 **Dermatopolymyositis, unspecified, organ involvement unspecified**

CC M33.91 **Dermatopolymyositis, unspecified with respiratory involvement**

CC M33.92 **Dermatopolymyositis, unspecified with myopathy**

CC M33.93 **Dermatopolymyositis, unspecified without myopathy**
AHA CC: 4Q, 2017, 18

CC M33.99 **Dermatopolymyositis, unspecified with other organ involvement**

M34 **Systemic sclerosis [scleroderma]**

Excludes1: *circumscribed scleroderma (L94.0)*
neonatal scleroderma (P83.88)

M34.0 **Progressive systemic sclerosis**

M34.1 **CR(E)ST syndrome**
Combination of calcinosis, Raynaud's phenomenon, esophageal dysfunction, sclerodactyly, telangiectasia

M34.2 Systemic sclerosis induced by drug and chemical
Code first poisoning due to drug or toxin, if applicable (T36-T65 with fifth or sixth character 1-4 or 6)
Use additional code for adverse effect, if applicable, to identify drug (T36-T50 with fifth or sixth character 5)

+ **M34.8 Other forms of systemic sclerosis**
CC **M34.81 Systemic sclerosis with lung involvement**
Code also if applicable:
other interstitial pulmonary diseases (J84.89)
secondary pulmonary arterial hypertension (I27.21)
CC **M34.82 Systemic sclerosis with myopathy**
M34.83 Systemic sclerosis with polyneuropathy
M34.89 Other systemic sclerosis
M34.9 Systemic sclerosis, unspecified

M35 Other systemic involvement of connective tissue
Excludes1: *reactive perforating collagenosis (L87.1)*

+ **M35.0 Sjögren syndrome**
Sicca syndrome
Use additional code to identify associated manifestations
Excludes1: *dry mouth, unspecified (R68.2)*
M35.00 Sjögren syndrome, unspecified
M35.01 Sjögren syndrome with keratoconjunctivitis
M35.02 Sjögren syndrome with lung involvement
CC **M35.03 Sjögren syndrome with myopathy**
M35.04 Sjögren syndrome with tubulo-interstitial nephropathy
Renal tubular acidosis in sicca syndrome
M35.05 Sjögren syndrome with inflammatory arthritis
M35.06 Sjögren syndrome with peripheral nervous system involvement
CC **M35.07 Sjögren syndrome with central nervous system involvement**
M35.08 Sjögren syndrome with gastrointestinal involvement
M35.0A Sjögren syndrome with glomerular disease
M35.0B Sjögren syndrome with vasculitis
M35.0C Sjögren syndrome with dental involvement
M35.09 Sjögren syndrome with other organ involvement

CC **M35.1 Other overlap syndromes**
Mixed connective tissue disease
Excludes1: *polyangiitis overlap syndrome (M30.8)*
CC **M35.2 Behçet's disease**
M35.3 Polymyalgia rheumatica
Excludes1: *polymyalgia rheumatica with giant cell arteritis (M31.5)*
M35.4 Diffuse (eosinophilic) fasciitis
CC **M35.5 Multifocal fibrosclerosis**
M35.6 Relapsing panniculitis [Weber-Christian]
Excludes1: *lupus panniculitis (L93.2)*
panniculitis NOS (M79.3-)
M35.7 Hypermobility syndrome
Familial ligamentous laxity
Excludes1: *ligamentous laxity, NOS (M24.2-)*
Excludes2: *Ehlers-Danlos syndromes (Q79.6-)*
M35.8 Other specified systemic involvement of connective tissue
AHA CC: 3Q, 2020, 13-14; 1Q, 2021, 36-37
CC **M35.81 Multisystem inflammatory syndrome**
MIS-A
MIS-C
Multisystem inflammatory syndrome in adults
Multisystem inflammatory syndrome in children
Pediatric inflammatory multisystem syndrome
PIMS
Code first, if applicable, COVID-19 (U07.1)

Code also any associated complications such as:
acute hepatic failure (K72.0-)
acute kidney failure (N17.-)
acute myocarditis (I40.-)
acute respiratory distress syndrome (J80)
cardiac arrhythmia (I47-I49.-)
pneumonia due to COVID-19 (J12.82)
severe sepsis (R65.2-)
viral cardiomyopathy (B33.24)
viral pericarditis (B33.23)

Use additional code, if applicable, for:
exposure to COVID-19 or SARS-CoV-2 infection (Z20.822)
personal history of COVID-19 (Z86.16)
post COVID-19 condition (U09.9)
AHA CC: 1Q, 2021, 36-37, 41-42
CC **M35.89 Other specified systemic involvement of connective tissue**
M35.9 Systemic involvement of connective tissue, unspecified
Autoimmune disease (systemic) NOS
Collagen (vascular) disease NOS

M36 Systemic disorders of connective tissue in diseases classified elsewhere
Excludes2: *arthropathies in diseases classified elsewhere (M14.-)*
CC **M36.0 Dermato(poly)myositis in neoplastic disease**
Code first underlying neoplasm (C00-D49)
M36.1 Arthropathy in neoplastic disease
Code first underlying neoplasm, such as:
leukemia (C91-C95)
malignant histiocytosis (C96.A)
multiple myeloma (C90.0)
M36.2 Hemophilic arthropathy
Hemarthrosis in hemophilic arthropathy
Code first underlying disease, such as:
factor VIII deficiency (D66)
with vascular defect (D68.0)
factor IX deficiency (D67)
hemophilia (classical) (D66)
hemophilia B (D67)
hemophilia C (D68.1)
M36.3 Arthropathy in other blood disorders
M36.4 Arthropathy in hypersensitivity reactions classified elsewhere
Code first underlying disease, such as:
Henoch (-Schönlein) purpura (D69.0)
serum sickness (T80.6-)
M36.8 Systemic disorders of connective tissue in other diseases classified elsewhere
Code first underlying disease, such as:
alkaptonuria (E70.2)
hypogammaglobulinemia (D80.-)
ochronosis (E70.2)

DORSOPATHIES (M40-M54)

Deforming dorsopathies (M40-M43)

M40 Kyphosis and lordosis
Code first underlying disease
Excludes1: *congenital kyphosis and lordosis (Q76.4)*
kyphoscoliosis (M41.-)
postprocedural kyphosis and lordosis (M96.-)

+ **M40.0 Postural kyphosis**
Excludes1: *osteochondrosis of spine (M42.-)*
M40.00 Postural kyphosis, site unspecified
M40.03 Postural kyphosis, cervicothoracic region
M40.04 Postural kyphosis, thoracic region
M40.05 Postural kyphosis, thoracolumbar region

+ **M40.1 Other secondary kyphosis**
M40.10 Other secondary kyphosis, site unspecified
M40.12 Other secondary kyphosis, cervical region
M40.13 Other secondary kyphosis, cervicothoracic region
M40.14 Other secondary kyphosis, thoracic region
M40.15 Other secondary kyphosis, thoracolumbar region

+ **M40.2 Other and unspecified kyphosis**
+ **M40.20 Unspecified kyphosis**
M40.202 Unspecified kyphosis, cervical region
M40.203 Unspecified kyphosis, cervicothoracic region
M40.204 Unspecified kyphosis, thoracic region
M40.205 Unspecified kyphosis, thoracolumbar region
M40.209 Unspecified kyphosis, site unspecified
+ **M40.29 Other kyphosis**
M40.292 Other kyphosis, cervical region
M40.293 Other kyphosis, cervicothoracic region
M40.294 Other kyphosis, thoracic region
M40.295 Other kyphosis, thoracolumbar region
M40.299 Other kyphosis, site unspecified

+ M40.3 Flatback syndrome
M40.30 Flatback syndrome, site unspecified
M40.35 Flatback syndrome, thoracolumbar region
M40.36 Flatback syndrome, lumbar region
M40.37 Flatback syndrome, lumbosacral region
+ M40.4 Postural lordosis
Acquired lordosis
M40.40 Postural lordosis, site unspecified
M40.45 Postural lordosis, thoracolumbar region
M40.46 Postural lordosis, lumbar region
M40.47 Postural lordosis, lumbosacral region
+ M40.5 Lordosis, unspecified
M40.50 Lordosis, unspecified, site unspecified
M40.55 Lordosis, unspecified, thoracolumbar region
M40.56 Lordosis, unspecified, lumbar region
M40.57 Lordosis, unspecified, lumbosacral region

M41 Scoliosis

Includes: kyphoscoliosis
Excludes1: *congenital scoliosis NOS (Q67.5)*
congenital scoliosis due to bony malformation (Q76.3)
postural congenital scoliosis (Q67.5)
kyphoscoliotic heart disease (I27.1)
Excludes2: *postprocedural scoliosis (M96.-)*

+ M41.0 Infantile idiopathic scoliosis
M41.00 Infantile idiopathic scoliosis, site unspecified
M41.02 Infantile idiopathic scoliosis, cervical region
M41.03 Infantile idiopathic scoliosis, cervicothoracic region
M41.04 Infantile idiopathic scoliosis, thoracic region
AHA CC: 4Q, 2014, 26-27
M41.05 Infantile idiopathic scoliosis, thoracolumbar region
M41.06 Infantile idiopathic scoliosis, lumbar region
M41.07 Infantile idiopathic scoliosis, lumbosacral region
M41.08 Infantile idiopathic scoliosis, sacral and sacrococcygeal region
+ M41.1 Juvenile and adolescent idiopathic scoliosis
+ M41.11 Juvenile idiopathic scoliosis
M41.112 Juvenile idiopathic scoliosis, cervical region
M41.113 Juvenile idiopathic scoliosis, cervicothoracic region
M41.114 Juvenile idiopathic scoliosis, thoracic region
M41.115 Juvenile idiopathic scoliosis, thoracolumbar region
M41.116 Juvenile idiopathic scoliosis, lumbar region
M41.117 Juvenile idiopathic scoliosis, lumbosacral region
M41.119 Juvenile idiopathic scoliosis, site unspecified
AHA CC: 4Q, 2014, 28-29
+ M41.12 Adolescent scoliosis
M41.122 Adolescent idiopathic scoliosis, cervical region
M41.123 Adolescent idiopathic scoliosis, cervicothoracic region
M41.124 Adolescent idiopathic scoliosis, thoracic region
M41.125 Adolescent idiopathic scoliosis, thoracolumbar region
M41.126 Adolescent idiopathic scoliosis, lumbar region
M41.127 Adolescent idiopathic scoliosis, lumbosacral region
M41.129 Adolescent idiopathic scoliosis, site unspecified
+ M41.2 Other idiopathic scoliosis
M41.20 Other idiopathic scoliosis, site unspecified
M41.22 Other idiopathic scoliosis, cervical region
M41.23 Other idiopathic scoliosis, cervicothoracic region
M41.24 Other idiopathic scoliosis, thoracic region
M41.25 Other idiopathic scoliosis, thoracolumbar region
M41.26 Other idiopathic scoliosis, lumbar region
M41.27 Other idiopathic scoliosis, lumbosacral region
+ M41.3 Thoracogenic scoliosis
M41.30 Thoracogenic scoliosis, site unspecified
M41.34 Thoracogenic scoliosis, thoracic region
M41.35 Thoracogenic scoliosis, thoracolumbar region
+ M41.4 Neuromuscular scoliosis
Scoliosis secondary to cerebral palsy, Friedreich's ataxia, poliomyelitis and other neuromuscular disorders
Code also underlying condition
M41.40 Neuromuscular scoliosis, site unspecified
M41.41 Neuromuscular scoliosis, occipito-atlanto-axial region
M41.42 Neuromuscular scoliosis, cervical region
M41.43 Neuromuscular scoliosis, cervicothoracic region
M41.44 Neuromuscular scoliosis, thoracic region
M41.45 Neuromuscular scoliosis, thoracolumbar region
AHA CC: 4Q, 2014, 27-28
M41.46 Neuromuscular scoliosis, lumbar region
M41.47 Neuromuscular scoliosis, lumbosacral region
+ M41.5 Other secondary scoliosis
Code first underlying disease
AHA CC: 1Q, 2019, 19
M41.50 Other secondary scoliosis, site unspecified
M41.52 Other secondary scoliosis, cervical region
M41.53 Other secondary scoliosis, cervicothoracic region
M41.54 Other secondary scoliosis, thoracic region
M41.55 Other secondary scoliosis, thoracolumbar region
M41.56 Other secondary scoliosis, lumbar region
M41.57 Other secondary scoliosis, lumbosacral region
+ M41.8 Other forms of scoliosis
M41.80 Other forms of scoliosis, site unspecified
M41.82 Other forms of scoliosis, cervical region
M41.83 Other forms of scoliosis, cervicothoracic region
M41.84 Other forms of scoliosis, thoracic region
M41.85 Other forms of scoliosis, thoracolumbar region
M41.86 Other forms of scoliosis, lumbar region
M41.87 Other forms of scoliosis, lumbosacral region
M41.9 Scoliosis, unspecified

M42 Spinal osteochondrosis

+ M42.0 Juvenile osteochondrosis of spine
Calvé's disease
Scheuermann's disease
Excludes1: *postural kyphosis (M40.0)*
M42.00 Juvenile osteochondrosis of spine, site unspecified
M42.01 Juvenile osteochondrosis of spine, occipito-atlanto-axial region
M42.02 Juvenile osteochondrosis of spine, cervical region
M42.03 Juvenile osteochondrosis of spine, cervicothoracic region
M42.04 Juvenile osteochondrosis of spine, thoracic region
M42.05 Juvenile osteochondrosis of spine, thoracolumbar region
M42.06 Juvenile osteochondrosis of spine, lumbar region
M42.07 Juvenile osteochondrosis of spine, lumbosacral region
M42.08 Juvenile osteochondrosis of spine, sacral and sacrococcygeal region
M42.09 Juvenile osteochondrosis of spine, multiple sites in spine
+ M42.1 Adult osteochondrosis of spine
M42.10 Adult osteochondrosis of spine, site unspecified
• M42.11 Adult osteochondrosis of spine, occipito-atlanto-axial region
• M42.12 Adult osteochondrosis of spine, cervical region
• M42.13 Adult osteochondrosis of spine, cervicothoracic region
• M42.14 Adult osteochondrosis of spine, thoracic region
• M42.15 Adult osteochondrosis of spine, thoracolumbar region
• M42.16 Adult osteochondrosis of spine, lumbar region
• M42.17 Adult osteochondrosis of spine, lumbosacral region
• M42.18 Adult osteochondrosis of spine, sacral and sacrococcygeal region
• M42.19 Adult osteochondrosis of spine, multiple sites in spine
M42.9 Spinal osteochondrosis, unspecified

M43 Other deforming dorsopathies

Excludes1: *congenital spondylolysis and spondylolisthesis (Q76.2)*
hemivertebra (Q76.3-Q76.4)
Klippel-Feil syndrome (Q76.1)
lumbarization and sacralization (Q76.4)
platyspondylisis (Q76.4)
spina bifida occulta (Q76.0)
spinal curvature in osteoporosis (M80.-)
spinal curvature in Paget's disease of bone [osteitis deformans] (M88.-)

+ **M43.0 Spondylolysis**

Excludes1: *congenital spondylolysis (Q76.2)*
spondylolisthesis (M43.1)

M43.00 Spondylolysis, site unspecified
M43.01 Spondylolysis, occipito-atlanto-axial region
M43.02 Spondylolysis, cervical region
M43.03 Spondylolysis, cervicothoracic region
M43.04 Spondylolysis, thoracic region
M43.05 Spondylolysis, thoracolumbar region
M43.06 Spondylolysis, lumbar region
M43.07 Spondylolysis, lumbosacral region
M43.08 Spondylolysis, sacral and sacrococcygeal region
M43.09 Spondylolysis, multiple sites in spine

+ **M43.1 Spondylolisthesis**

Excludes1: *acute traumatic of lumbosacral region (S33.1)*
acute traumatic of sites other than lumbosacral- code to Fracture, vertebra, by region
congenital spondylolisthesis (Q76.2)

AHA CC: 2Q, 2020, 21

M43.10 Spondylolisthesis, site unspecified
M43.11 Spondylolisthesis, occipito-atlanto-axial region
M43.12 Spondylolisthesis, cervical region
M43.13 Spondylolisthesis, cervicothoracic region
M43.14 Spondylolisthesis, thoracic region
M43.15 Spondylolisthesis, thoracolumbar region
M43.16 Spondylolisthesis, lumbar region

AHA CC: 3Q, 2018, 18

M43.17 Spondylolisthesis, lumbosacral region
M43.18 Spondylolisthesis, sacral and sacrococcygeal region
M43.19 Spondylolisthesis, multiple sites in spine

+ **M43.2 Fusion of spine**

Ankylosis of spinal joint

Excludes1: *ankylosing spondylitis (M45.0-)*
congenital fusion of spine (Q76.4)

Excludes2: *arthrodesis status (Z98.1)*
pseudoarthrosis after fusion or arthrodesis (M96.0)

M43.20 Fusion of spine, site unspecified
M43.21 Fusion of spine, occipito-atlanto-axial region
M43.22 Fusion of spine, cervical region
M43.23 Fusion of spine, cervicothoracic region
M43.24 Fusion of spine, thoracic region
M43.25 Fusion of spine, thoracolumbar region
M43.26 Fusion of spine, lumbar region
M43.27 Fusion of spine, lumbosacral region
M43.28 Fusion of spine, sacral and sacrococcygeal region

M43.3 Recurrent atlantoaxial dislocation with myelopathy
M43.4 Other recurrent atlantoaxial dislocation

+ **M43.5 Other recurrent vertebral dislocation**

Excludes1: *biomechanical lesions NEC (M99.-)*

+ **M43.5X Other recurrent vertebral dislocation**

M43.5X2 Other recurrent vertebral dislocation, cervical region
M43.5X3 Other recurrent vertebral dislocation, cervicothoracic region
M43.5X4 Other recurrent vertebral dislocation, thoracic region
M43.5X5 Other recurrent vertebral dislocation, thoracolumbar region
M43.5X6 Other recurrent vertebral dislocation, lumbar region
M43.5X7 Other recurrent vertebral dislocation, lumbosacral region
M43.5X8 Other recurrent vertebral dislocation, sacral and sacrococcygeal region
M43.5X9 Other recurrent vertebral dislocation, site unspecified

M43.6 Torticollis

Excludes1: *congenital (sternomastoid) torticollis (Q68.0)*
current injury - see Injury, of spine, by body region
ocular torticollis (R29.891)
psychogenic torticollis (F45.8)
spasmodic torticollis (G24.3)
torticollis due to birth injury (P15.2)

+ **M43.8 Other specified deforming dorsopathies**

Excludes2: *kyphosis and lordosis (M40.-)*
scoliosis (M41.-)

+ **M43.8X Other specified deforming dorsopathies**

M43.8X1 Other specified deforming dorsopathies, occipito-atlanto-axial region
M43.8X2 Other specified deforming dorsopathies, cervical region
M43.8X3 Other specified deforming dorsopathies, cervicothoracic region
M43.8X4 Other specified deforming dorsopathies, thoracic region
M43.8X5 Other specified deforming dorsopathies, thoracolumbar region
M43.8X6 Other specified deforming dorsopathies, lumbar region
M43.8X7 Other specified deforming dorsopathies, lumbosacral region
M43.8X8 Other specified deforming dorsopathies, sacral and sacrococcygeal region
M43.8X9 Other specified deforming dorsopathies, site unspecified

M43.9 Deforming dorsopathy, unspecified

Curvature of spine NOS

Spondylopathies (M45-M49)

M45 Ankylosing spondylitis

Rheumatoid arthritis of spine

Excludes1: *arthropathy in Reiter's disease (M02.3-)*
juvenile (ankylosing) spondylitis (M08.1)

Excludes2: *Behçet's disease (M35.2)*

M45.0 Ankylosing spondylitis of multiple sites in spine
M45.1 Ankylosing spondylitis of occipito-atlanto-axial region
M45.2 Ankylosing spondylitis of cervical region
M45.3 Ankylosing spondylitis of cervicothoracic region
M45.4 Ankylosing spondylitis of thoracic region
M45.5 Ankylosing spondylitis of thoracolumbar region
M45.6 Ankylosing spondylitis lumbar region
M45.7 Ankylosing spondylitis of lumbosacral region
M45.8 Ankylosing spondylitis sacral and sacrococcygeal region
M45.9 Ankylosing spondylitis of unspecified sites in spine

+ **M45.A Non-radiographic axial spondyloarthritis**

M45.A0 Non-radiographic axial spondyloarthritis of unspecified sites in spine
M45.A1 Non-radiographic axial spondyloarthritis of occipito-atlanto-axial region
M45.A2 Non-radiographic axial spondyloarthritis of cervical region
M45.A3 Non-radiographic axial spondyloarthritis of cerviothoracic region
M45.A4 Non-radiographic axial spondyloarthritis of throacic region
M45.A5 Non-radiographic axial spondyloarthritis of thoracolumbar region
M45.A6 Non-radiographic axial spondyloarthritis of lumbar region
M45.A7 Non-radiographic axial spondyloarthritis of lumbosacral region
M45.A8 Non-radiographic axial spondyloarthritis of sacral and sacrococcygeal region
M45.AB Non-radiographic axial spondyloarthritis of multiple sites in spine

M46 Other inflammatory spondylopathies

+ **M46.0 Spinal enthesopathy**

Disorder of ligamentous or muscular attachments of spine

M46.00 Spinal enthesopathy, site unspecified
M46.01 Spinal enthesopathy, occipito-atlanto-axial region
M46.02 Spinal enthesopathy, cervical region
M46.03 Spinal enthesopathy, cervicothoracic region
M46.04 Spinal enthesopathy, thoracic region
M46.05 Spinal enthesopathy, thoracolumbar region

M46.06 Spinal enthesopathy, lumbar region
M46.07 Spinal enthesopathy, lumbosacral region
M46.08 Spinal enthesopathy, sacral and sacrococcygeal region
M46.09 Spinal enthesopathy, multiple sites in spine

M46.1 Sacroiliitis, not elsewhere classified
AHA CC: 2Q, 2020, 14

+ M46.2 Osteomyelitis of vertebra
CC M46.20 Osteomyelitis of vertebra, site unspecified
CC M46.21 Osteomyelitis of vertebra, occipito-atlanto-axial region
CC M46.22 Osteomyelitis of vertebra, cervical region
CC M46.23 Osteomyelitis of vertebra, cervicothoracic region
CC M46.24 Osteomyelitis of vertebra, thoracic region
CC M46.25 Osteomyelitis of vertebra, thoracolumbar region
CC M46.26 Osteomyelitis of vertebra, lumbar region
CC M46.27 Osteomyelitis of vertebra, lumbosacral region
CC M46.28 Osteomyelitis of vertebra, sacral and sacrococcygeal region

+ M46.3 Infection of intervertebral disc (pyogenic)
Use additional code (B95-B97) to identify infectious agent
CC M46.30 Infection of intervertebral disc (pyogenic), site unspecified
CC M46.31 Infection of intervertebral disc (pyogenic), occipito-atlanto-axial region
CC M46.32 Infection of intervertebral disc (pyogenic), cervical region
CC M46.33 Infection of intervertebral disc (pyogenic), cervicothoracic region
CC M46.34 Infection of intervertebral disc (pyogenic), thoracic region
CC M46.35 Infection of intervertebral disc (pyogenic), thoracolumbar region
CC M46.36 Infection of intervertebral disc (pyogenic), lumbar region
CC M46.37 Infection of intervertebral disc (pyogenic), lumbosacral region
CC M46.38 Infection of intervertebral disc (pyogenic), sacral and sacrococcygeal region
CC M46.39 Infection of intervertebral disc (pyogenic), multiple sites in spine

+ M46.4 Discitis, unspecified
M46.40 Discitis, unspecified, site unspecified
M46.41 Discitis, unspecified, occipito-atlanto-axial region
M46.42 Discitis, unspecified, cervical region
M46.43 Discitis, unspecified, cervicothoracic region
M46.44 Discitis, unspecified, thoracic region
M46.45 Discitis, unspecified, thoracolumbar region
M46.46 Discitis, unspecified, lumbar region
M46.47 Discitis, unspecified, lumbosacral region
M46.48 Discitis, unspecified, sacral and sacrococcygeal region
M46.49 Discitis, unspecified, multiple sites in spine

+ M46.5 Other infective spondylopathies
M46.50 Other infective spondylopathies, site unspecified
M46.51 Other infective spondylopathies, occipito-atlanto-axial region
M46.52 Other infective spondylopathies, cervical region
M46.53 Other infective spondylopathies, cervicothoracic region
M46.54 Other infective spondylopathies, thoracic region
M46.55 Other infective spondylopathies, thoracolumbar region
M46.56 Other infective spondylopathies, lumbar region
M46.57 Other infective spondylopathies, lumbosacral region
M46.58 Other infective spondylopathies, sacral and sacrococcygeal region
M46.59 Other infective spondylopathies, multiple sites in spine

+ M46.8 Other specified inflammatory spondylopathies
M46.80 Other specified inflammatory spondylopathies, site unspecified
M46.81 Other specified inflammatory spondylopathies, occipito-atlanto-axial region
M46.82 Other specified inflammatory spondylopathies, cervical region
M46.83 Other specified inflammatory spondylopathies, cervicothoracic region
M46.84 Other specified inflammatory spondylopathies, thoracic region
M46.85 Other specified inflammatory spondylopathies, thoracolumbar region
M46.86 Other specified inflammatory spondylopathies, lumbar region
M46.87 Other specified inflammatory spondylopathies, lumbosacral region
M46.88 Other specified inflammatory spondylopathies, sacral and sacrococcygeal region
M46.89 Other specified inflammatory spondylopathies, multiple sites in spine

+ M46.9 Unspecified inflammatory spondylopathy
M46.90 Unspecified inflammatory spondylopathy, site unspecified
M46.91 Unspecified inflammatory spondylopathy, occipito-atlanto-axial region
M46.92 Unspecified inflammatory spondylopathy, cervical region
M46.93 Unspecified inflammatory spondylopathy, cervicothoracic region
M46.94 Unspecified inflammatory spondylopathy, thoracic region
M46.95 Unspecified inflammatory spondylopathy, thoracolumbar region
M46.96 Unspecified inflammatory spondylopathy, lumbar region
M46.97 Unspecified inflammatory spondylopathy, lumbosacral region
M46.98 Unspecified inflammatory spondylopathy, sacral and sacrococcygeal region
M46.99 Unspecified inflammatory spondylopathy, multiple sites in spine

M47 Spondylosis

Includes: arthrosis or osteoarthritis of spine
degeneration of facet joints

+ M47.0 Anterior spinal and vertebral artery compression syndromes
+ M47.01 Anterior spinal artery compression syndromes
CC M47.011 Anterior spinal artery compression syndromes, occipito-atlanto-axial region
CC M47.012 Anterior spinal artery compression syndromes, cervical region
CC M47.013 Anterior spinal artery compression syndromes, cervicothoracic region
CC M47.014 Anterior spinal artery compression syndromes, thoracic region
CC M47.015 Anterior spinal artery compression syndromes, thoracolumbar region
CC M47.016 Anterior spinal artery compression syndromes, lumbar region
CC M47.019 Anterior spinal artery compression syndromes, site unspecified
+ M47.02 Vertebral artery compression syndromes
CC M47.021 Vertebral artery compression syndromes, occipito-atlanto-axial region
CC M47.022 Vertebral artery compression syndromes, cervical region
CC M47.029 Vertebral artery compression syndromes, site unspecified

+ M47.1 Other spondylosis with myelopathy
Spondylogenic compression of spinal cord
Excludes1: *vertebral subluxation (M43.3-M43.5X9)*
CC M47.10 Other spondylosis with myelopathy, site unspecified
CC M47.11 Other spondylosis with myelopathy, occipito-atlanto-axial region
CC M47.12 Other spondylosis with myelopathy, cervical region
AHA CC: 1Q, 2020, 17
CC M47.13 Other spondylosis with myelopathy, cervicothoracic region
CC M47.14 Other spondylosis with myelopathy, thoracic region
CC M47.15 Other spondylosis with myelopathy, thoracolumbar region
CC M47.16 Other spondylosis with myelopathy, lumbar region

+ M47.2 Other spondylosis with radiculopathy
M47.20 Other spondylosis with radiculopathy, site unspecified

M47.21 Other spondylosis with radiculopathy, occipito-atlanto-axial region
M47.22 Other spondylosis with radiculopathy, cervical region
AHA CC: 1Q, 2020, 17
M47.23 Other spondylosis with radiculopathy, cervicothoracic region
M47.24 Other spondylosis with radiculopathy, thoracic region
M47.25 Other spondylosis with radiculopathy, thoracolumbar region
M47.26 Other spondylosis with radiculopathy, lumbar region
M47.27 Other spondylosis with radiculopathy, lumbosacral region
M47.28 Other spondylosis with radiculopathy, sacral and sacrococcygeal region

\+ M47.8 Other spondylosis
\+ M47.81 Spondylosis without myelopathy or radiculopathy
M47.811 Spondylosis without myelopathy or radiculopathy, occipito-atlanto-axial region
M47.812 Spondylosis without myelopathy or radiculopathy, cervical region
AHA CC: 2Q, 2018, 14-15; 3Q, 2019, 10-11
M47.813 Spondylosis without myelopathy or radiculopathy, cervicothoracic region
M47.814 Spondylosis without myelopathy or radiculopathy, thoracic region
M47.815 Spondylosis without myelopathy or radiculopathy, thoracolumbar region
M47.816 Spondylosis without myelopathy or radiculopathy, lumbar region
M47.817 Spondylosis without myelopathy or radiculopathy, lumbosacral region
M47.818 Spondylosis without myelopathy or radiculopathy, sacral and sacrococcygeal region
M47.819 Spondylosis without myelopathy or radiculopathy, site unspecified
\+ M47.89 Other spondylosis
M47.891 Other spondylosis, occipito-atlanto-axial region
M47.892 Other spondylosis, cervical region
M47.893 Other spondylosis, cervicothoracic region
M47.894 Other spondylosis, thoracic region
M47.895 Other spondylosis, thoracolumbar region
M47.896 Other spondylosis, lumbar region
M47.897 Other spondylosis, lumbosacral region
M47.898 Other spondylosis, sacral and sacrococcygeal region
M47.899 Other spondylosis, site unspecified
M47.9 Spondylosis, unspecified

M48 Other spondylopathies

\+ M48.0 Spinal stenosis
Caudal stenosis
M48.00 Spinal stenosis, site unspecified
M48.01 Spinal stenosis, occipito-atlanto-axial region
M48.02 Spinal stenosis, cervical region
AHA CC: 3Q, 2018, 18-19; 1Q, 2020, 17
M48.03 Spinal stenosis, cervicothoracic region
M48.04 Spinal stenosis, thoracic region
M48.05 Spinal stenosis, thoracolumbar region
\+ M48.06 Spinal stenosis, lumbar region
AHA CC: 3Q, 2017, 24
M48.061 Spinal stenosis, lumbar region without neurogenic claudication
Spinal stenosis. lumbar region NOS
AHA CC: 4Q, 2017, 18-19; 3Q, 2018, 19-20
M48.062 Spinal stenosis, lumbar region with neurogenic claudication
AHA CC: 4Q, 2017, 18-19
M48.07 Spinal stenosis, lumbosacral region
AHA CC: 3Q, 2018, 19-20
M48.08 Spinal stenosis, sacral and sacrococcygeal region
\+ M48.1 Ankylosing hyperostosis [Forestier]
Diffuse idiopathic skeletal hyperostosis [DISH]
M48.10 Ankylosing hyperostosis [Forestier], site unspecified
M48.11 Ankylosing hyperostosis [Forestier], occipito-atlanto-axial region
M48.12 Ankylosing hyperostosis [Forestier], cervical region
M48.13 Ankylosing hyperostosis [Forestier], cervicothoracic region
M48.14 Ankylosing hyperostosis [Forestier], thoracic region
M48.15 Ankylosing hyperostosis [Forestier], thoracolumbar region
M48.16 Ankylosing hyperostosis [Forestier], lumbar region
M48.17 Ankylosing hyperostosis [Forestier], lumbosacral region
M48.18 Ankylosing hyperostosis [Forestier], sacral and sacrococcygeal region
M48.19 Ankylosing hyperostosis [Forestier], multiple sites in spine
\+ M48.2 Kissing spine
M48.20 Kissing spine, site unspecified
M48.21 Kissing spine, occipito-atlanto-axial region
M48.22 Kissing spine, cervical region
M48.23 Kissing spine, cervicothoracic region
M48.24 Kissing spine, thoracic region
M48.25 Kissing spine, thoracolumbar region
M48.26 Kissing spine, lumbar region
M48.27 Kissing spine, lumbosacral region
\+ M48.3 Traumatic spondylopathy
CC M48.30 Traumatic spondylopathy, site unspecified
CC M48.31 Traumatic spondylopathy, occipito-atlanto-axial region
CC M48.32 Traumatic spondylopathy, cervical region
CC M48.33 Traumatic spondylopathy, cervicothoracic region
CC M48.34 Traumatic spondylopathy, thoracic region
CC M48.35 Traumatic spondylopathy, thoracolumbar region
CC M48.36 Traumatic spondylopathy, lumbar region
CC M48.37 Traumatic spondylopathy, lumbosacral region
CC M48.38 Traumatic spondylopathy, sacral and sacrococcygeal region
\+ M48.4 Fatigue fracture of vertebra
Stress fracture of vertebra
Excludes1: *pathological fracture NOS (M84.4-)*
pathological fracture of vertebra due to neoplasm (M84.58)
pathological fracture of vertebra due to other diagnosis (M84.68)
pathological fracture of vertebra due to osteoporosis (M80.-)
traumatic fracture of vertebrae (S12.0-S12.3-, S22.0-, S32.0-)

The appropriate 7th character is to be added to each code from subcategory **M48.4**:
A initial encounter for fracture
D subsequent encounter for fracture with routine healing
G subsequent encounter for fracture with delayed healing
S sequela of fracture

X+7th M48.40 Fatigue fracture of vertebra, site unspecified
X+7th M48.41 Fatigue fracture of vertebra, occipito-atlanto-axial region
X+7th M48.42 Fatigue fracture of vertebra, cervical region
X+7th M48.43 Fatigue fracture of vertebra, cervicothoracic region
X+7th M48.44 Fatigue fracture of vertebra, thoracic region
X+7th M48.45 Fatigue fracture of vertebra, thoracolumbar region
X+7th M48.46 Fatigue fracture of vertebra, lumbar region
X+7th M48.47 Fatigue fracture of vertebra, lumbosacral region
X+7th M48.48 Fatigue fracture of vertebra, sacral and sacrococcygeal region

+ **M48.5 Collapsed vertebra, not elsewhere classified**
Collapsed vertebra NOS
Compression fracture of vertebra NOS
Wedging of vertebra NOS
Excludes1: *current injury - see Injury of spine, by body region*
fatigue fracture of vertebra (M48.4)
pathological fracture of vertebra due to neoplasm (M84.58)
pathological fracture of vertebra due to other diagnosis (M84.68)
pathological fracture of vertebra due to osteoporosis (M80.-)
pathological fracture NOS (M84.4-)
stress fracture of vertebra (M48.4-)
traumatic fracture of vertebra (S12.-, S22.-, S32.-)

The appropriate 7th character is to be added to each code from subcategory **M48.5**:
A initial encounter for fracture
D subsequent encounter for fracture with routine healing
G subsequent encounter for fracture with delayed healing
S sequela of fracture

CC X+7th **M48.50 Collapsed vertebra, not elsewhere classified, site unspecified**
CC X+7th **M48.51 Collapsed vertebra, not elsewhere classified, occipito-atlanto-axial region**
CC X+7th **M48.52 Collapsed vertebra, not elsewhere classified, cervical region**
CC X+7th **M48.53 Collapsed vertebra, not elsewhere classified, cervicothoracic region**
CC X+7th **M48.54 Collapsed vertebra, not elsewhere classified, thoracic region**
CC X+7th **M48.55 Collapsed vertebra, not elsewhere classified, thoracolumbar region**
CC X+7th **M48.56 Collapsed vertebra, not elsewhere classified, lumbar region**
CC X+7th **M48.57 Collapsed vertebra, not elsewhere classified, lumbosacral region**
CC X+7th **M48.58 Collapsed vertebra, not elsewhere classified, sacral and sacrococcygeal region**

+ **M48.8 Other specified spondylopathies**
Ossification of posterior longitudinal ligament
+ **M48.8X Other specified spondylopathies**
M48.8X1 Other specified spondylopathies, occipito-atlanto-axial region
M48.8X2 Other specified spondylopathies, cervical region
M48.8X3 Other specified spondylopathies, cervicothoracic region
M48.8X4 Other specified spondylopathies, thoracic region
M48.8X5 Other specified spondylopathies, thoracolumbar region
M48.8X6 Other specified spondylopathies, lumbar region
M48.8X7 Other specified spondylopathies, lumbosacral region
M48.8X8 Other specified spondylopathies, sacral and sacrococcygeal region
M48.8X9 Other specified spondylopathies, site unspecified

M48.9 Spondylopathy, unspecified

M49 Spondylopathies in diseases classified elsewhere
Includes: curvature of spine in diseases classified elsewhere
deformity of spine in diseases classified elsewhere
kyphosis in diseases classified elsewhere
scoliosis in diseases classified elsewhere
spondylopathy in diseases classified elsewhere
Code first *underlying disease, such as:*
brucellosis (A23.-)
Charcot-Marie-Tooth disease (G60.0)
enterobacterial infections (A01-A04)
osteitis fibrosa cystica (E21.0)
Excludes1: *curvature of spine in tuberculosis [Pott's] (A18.01)*
enteropathic arthropathies (M07.-)
gonococcal spondylitis (A54.41)
neuropathic [tabes dorsalis] spondylitis (A52.11)
neuropathic spondylopathy in syringomyelia (G95.0)
neuropathic spondylopathy in tabes dorsalis (A52.11)
nonsyphilitic neuropathic spondylopathy NEC (G98.0)
spondylitis in syphilis (acquired) (A52.77)
tuberculous spondylitis (A18.01)
typhoid fever spondylitis (A01.05)

+ **M49.8 Spondylopathy in diseases classified elsewhere**
M49.80 Spondylopathy in diseases classified elsewhere, site unspecified
M49.81 Spondylopathy in diseases classified elsewhere, occipito-atlanto-axial region
M49.82 Spondylopathy in diseases classified elsewhere, cervical region
M49.83 Spondylopathy in diseases classified elsewhere, cervicothoracic region
M49.84 Spondylopathy in diseases classified elsewhere, thoracic region
M49.85 Spondylopathy in diseases classified elsewhere, thoracolumbar region
M49.86 Spondylopathy in diseases classified elsewhere, lumbar region
M49.87 Spondylopathy in diseases classified elsewhere, lumbosacral region
M49.88 Spondylopathy in diseases classified elsewhere, sacral and sacrococcygeal region
M49.89 Spondylopathy in diseases classified elsewhere, multiple sites in spine

Other dorsopathies (M50-M54)

Excludes1: *current injury - see injury of spine by body region*
discitis NOS (M46.4-)

M50 Cervical disc disorders
NOTE code to the most superior level of disorder
Includes: cervicothoracic disc disorders with cervicalgia
cervicothoracic disc disorders

+ **M50.0 Cervical disc disorder with myelopathy**
CC **M50.00 Cervical disc disorder with myelopathy, unspecified cervical region**
CC **M50.01 Cervical disc disorder with myelopathy, high cervical region**
C2-C3 disc disorder with myelopathy
C3-C4 disc disorder with myelopathy
AHA CC: 1Q, 2016, 17
+ **M50.02 Cervical disc disorder with myelopathy, mid-cervical region**
AHA CC: 4Q, 2016, 39-40
CC **M50.020 Cervical disc disorder with myelopathy, mid-cervical region, unspecified level**
CC **M50.021 Cervical disc disorder at C4-C5 level with myelopathy**
C4-C5 disc disorder with myelopathy
CC **M50.022 Cervical disc disorder at C5-C6 level with myelopathy**
C5-C6 disc disorder with myelopathy
AHA CC: 3Q, 2018, 19
CC **M50.023 Cervical disc disorder at C6-C7 level with myelopathy**
C6-C7 disc disorder with myelopathy
CC **M50.03 Cervical disc disorder with myelopathy, cervicothoracic region**
C7-T1 disc disorder with myelopathy

Lumbar Disk Herniation: Clinical Manifestation

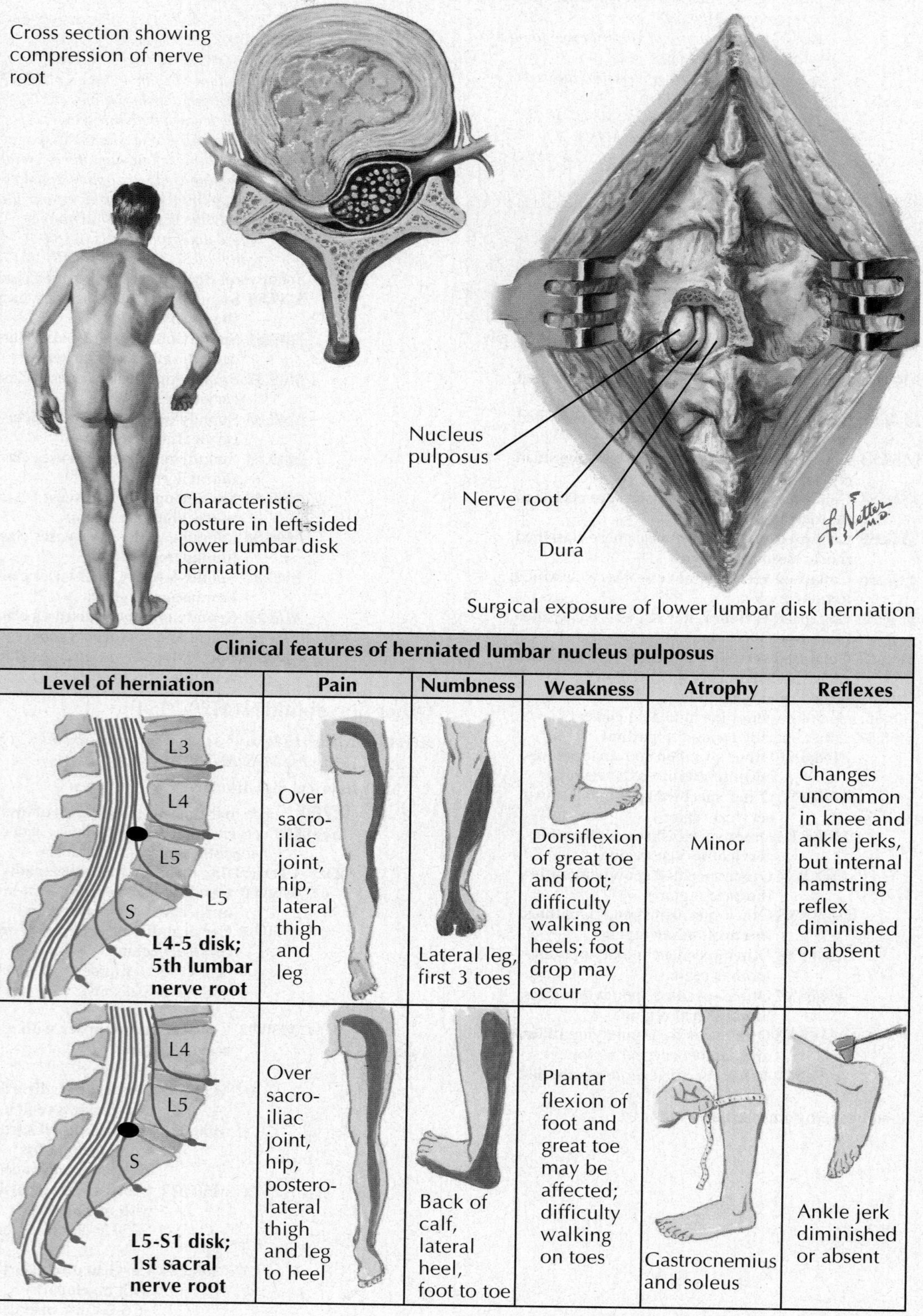

Clinical features of herniated lumbar nucleus pulposus					
Level of herniation	**Pain**	**Numbness**	**Weakness**	**Atrophy**	**Reflexes**
L3, L4, L5, L5, S **L4-5 disk; 5th lumbar nerve root**	Over sacro-iliac joint, hip, lateral thigh and leg	Lateral leg, first 3 toes	Dorsiflexion of great toe and foot; difficulty walking on heels; foot drop may occur	Minor	Changes uncommon in knee and ankle jerks, but internal hamstring reflex diminished or absent
L4, L5, S **L5-S1 disk; 1st sacral nerve root**	Over sacro-iliac joint, hip, postero-lateral thigh and leg to heel	Back of calf, lateral heel, foot to toe	Plantar flexion of foot and great toe may be affected; difficulty walking on toes	Gastrocnemius and soleus	Ankle jerk diminished or absent

+ **M50.1 Cervical disc disorder with radiculopathy**
Excludes2: *brachial radiculitis NOS (M54.13)*
M50.10 Cervical disc disorder with radiculopathy, unspecified cervical region
M50.11 Cervical disc disorder with radiculopathy, high cervical region
C2-C3 disc disorder with radiculopathy
C3 radiculopathy due to disc disorder
C3-C4 disc disorder with radiculopathy
C4 radiculopathy due to disc disorder
+ **M50.12 Cervical disc disorder with radiculopathy, mid-cervical region**
AHA CC: 4Q, 2016, 39-40
M50.120 Mid-cervical disc disorder, unspecified level
M50.121 Cervical disc disorder at C4-C5 level with radiculopathy
C4-C5 disc disorder with radiculopathy
C5 radiculopathy due to disc disorder
M50.122 Cervical disc disorder at C5-C6 level with radiculopathy
C5-C6 disc disorder with radiculopathy
C6 radiculopathy due to disc disorder
AHA CC: 3Q, 2018, 19
M50.123 Cervical disc disorder at C6-C7 level with radiculopathy
C6-C7 disc disorder with radiculopathy
C7 radiculopathy due to disc disorder
M50.13 Cervical disc disorder with radiculopathy, cervicothoracic region
C7-T1 disc disorder with radiculopathy
C8 radiculopathy due to disc disorder
+ **M50.2 Other cervical disc displacement**
M50.20 Other cervical disc displacement, unspecified cervical region
M50.21 Other cervical disc displacement, high cervical region
Other C2-C3 cervical disc displacement
Other C3-C4 cervical disc displacement
+ **M50.22 Other cervical disc displacement, mid-cervical region**
M50.220 Other cervical disc displacement, mid-cervical region, unspecified level
M50.221 Other cervical disc displacement at C4-C5 level
Other C4-C5 cervical disc displacement
M50.222 Other cervical disc displacement at C5-C6 level
Other C5-C6 cervical disc displacement
M50.223 Other cervical disc displacement at C6-C7 level
Other C6-C7 cervical disc displacement
M50.23 Other cervical disc displacement, cervicothoracic region
Other C7-T1 cervical disc displacement
+ **M50.3 Other cervical disc degeneration**
M50.30 Other cervical disc degeneration, unspecified cervical region
M50.31 Other cervical disc degeneration, high cervical region
Other C2-C3 cervical disc degeneration
Other C3-C4 cervical disc degeneration
+ **M50.32 Other cervical disc degeneration, mid-cervical region**
M50.320 Other cervical disc degeneration, mid-cervical region, unspecified level
M50.321 Other cervical disc degeneration at C4-C5 level
Other C4-C5 cervical disc degeneration
M50.322 Other cervical disc degeneration at C5-C6 level
Other C5-C6 cervical disc degeneration
M50.323 Other cervical disc degeneration at C6-C7 level
Other C6-C7 cervical disc degeneration
M50.33 Other cervical disc degeneration, cervicothoracic region
Other C7-T1 cervical disc degeneration

+ **M50.8 Other cervical disc disorders**
M50.80 Other cervical disc disorders, unspecified cervical region
M50.81 Other cervical disc disorders, high cervical region
Other C2-C3 cervical disc disorders
Other C3-C4 cervical disc disorders
+ **M50.82 Other cervical disc disorders, mid-cervical region**
M50.820 Other cervical disc disorders, mid-cervical region, unspecified level
M50.821 Other cervical disc disorders at C4-C5 level
Other C4-C5 cervical disc disorders
M50.822 Other cervical disc disorders at C5-C6 level
Other C5-C6 cervical disc disorders
M50.823 Other cervical disc disorders at C6-C7 level
Other C6-C7 cervical disc disorders
M50.83 Other cervical disc disorders, cervicothoracic region
Other C7-T1 cervical disc disorders
+ **M50.9 Cervical disc disorder, unspecified**
M50.90 Cervical disc disorder, unspecified, unspecified cervical region
M50.91 Cervical disc disorder, unspecified, high cervical region
Other C2-C3 cervical disc disorder, unspecified
Other C3-C4 cervical disc disorder, unspecified
+ **M50.92 Cervical disc disorder, unspecified, mid-cervical region**
M50.920 Unspecified cervical disc disorder, mid-cervical region, unspecified level
M50.921 Unspecified cervical disc disorder at C4-C5 level
Unspecified C4-C5 cervical disc disorder
M50.922 Unspecified cervical disc disorder at C5-C6 level
Unspecified C5-C6 cervical disc disorder
M50.923 Unspecified cervical disc disorder at C6-C7 level
Unspecified C6-C7 cervical disc disorder
M50.93 Cervical disc disorder, unspecified, cervicothoracic region
Other C7-T1 cervical disc disorder, unspecified

M51 Thoracic, thoracolumbar, and lumbosacral intervertebral disc disorders
Excludes2: *cervical and cervicothoracic disc disorders (M50.-)*
sacral and sacrococcygeal disorders (M53.3)
+ **M51.0 Thoracic, thoracolumbar and lumbosacral intervertebral disc disorders with myelopathy**
CC **M51.04 Intervertebral disc disorders with myelopathy, thoracic region**
CC **M51.05 Intervertebral disc disorders with myelopathy, thoracolumbar region**
CC **M51.06 Intervertebral disc disorders with myelopathy, lumbar region**
+ **M51.1 Thoracic, thoracolumbar and lumbosacral intervertebral disc disorders with radiculopathy**
Sciatica due to intervertebral disc disorder
Excludes1: *lumbar radiculitis NOS (M54.16)*
sciatica NOS (M54.3)
M51.14 Intervertebral disc disorders with radiculopathy, thoracic region
M51.15 Intervertebral disc disorders with radiculopathy, thoracolumbar region
M51.16 Intervertebral disc disorders with radiculopathy, lumbar region
M51.17 Intervertebral disc disorders with radiculopathy, lumbosacral region
+ **M51.2 Other thoracic, thoracolumbar and lumbosacral intervertebral disc displacement**
Lumbago due to displacement of intervertebral disc
M51.24 Other intervertebral disc displacement, thoracic region
M51.25 Other intervertebral disc displacement, thoracolumbar region

M51.26 Other intervertebral disc displacement, lumbar region
M51.27 Other intervertebral disc displacement, lumbosacral region
+ M51.3 Other thoracic, thoracolumbar and lumbosacral intervertebral disc degeneration
M51.34 Other intervertebral disc degeneration, thoracic region
M51.35 Other intervertebral disc degeneration, thoracolumbar region
M51.36 Other intervertebral disc degeneration, lumbar region
AHA CC: 2Q, 2018, 15
M51.37 Other intervertebral disc degeneration, lumbosacral region
+ M51.4 Schmorl's nodes
M51.44 Schmorl's nodes, thoracic region
M51.45 Schmorl's nodes, thoracolumbar region
M51.46 Schmorl's nodes, lumbar region
M51.47 Schmorl's nodes, lumbosacral region
+ M51.8 Other thoracic, thoracolumbar and lumbosacral intervertebral disc disorders
M51.84 Other intervertebral disc disorders, thoracic region
M51.85 Other intervertebral disc disorders, thoracolumbar region
M51.86 Other intervertebral disc disorders, lumbar region
M51.87 Other intervertebral disc disorders, lumbosacral region
M51.9 Unspecified thoracic, thoracolumbar and lumbosacral intervertebral disc disorder

M53 Other and unspecified dorsopathies, not elsewhere classified
M53.0 Cervicocranial syndrome
Posterior cervical sympathetic syndrome
M53.1 Cervicobrachial syndrome
Excludes2: *cervical disc disorder (M50.-)*
thoracic outlet syndrome (G54.0)
+ M53.2 Spinal instabilities
+ M53.2X Spinal instabilities
M53.2X1 Spinal instabilities, occipito-atlanto-axial region
M53.2X2 Spinal instabilities, cervical region
M53.2X3 Spinal instabilities, cervicothoracic region
M53.2X4 Spinal instabilities, thoracic region
M53.2X5 Spinal instabilities, thoracolumbar region
M53.2X6 Spinal instabilities, lumbar region
M53.2X7 Spinal instabilities, lumbosacral region
M53.2X8 Spinal instabilities, sacral and sacrococcygeal region
M53.2X9 Spinal instabilities, site unspecified
M53.3 Sacrococcygeal disorders, not elsewhere classified
Coccygodynia
+ M53.8 Other specified dorsopathies
M53.80 Other specified dorsopathies, site unspecified
M53.81 Other specified dorsopathies, occipito-atlanto-axial region
M53.82 Other specified dorsopathies, cervical region
M53.83 Other specified dorsopathies, cervicothoracic region
M53.84 Other specified dorsopathies, thoracic region
M53.85 Other specified dorsopathies, thoracolumbar region
M53.86 Other specified dorsopathies, lumbar region
M53.87 Other specified dorsopathies, lumbosacral region
M53.88 Other specified dorsopathies, sacral and sacrococcygeal region
M53.9 Dorsopathy, unspecified

M54 Dorsalgia
Excludes1: *psychogenic dorsalgia (F45.41)*
+ M54.0 Panniculitis affecting regions of neck and back
Excludes1: *lupus panniculitis (L93.2)*
panniculitis NOS (M79.3)
relapsing [Weber-Christian] panniculitis (M35.6)
M54.00 Panniculitis affecting regions of neck and back, site unspecified
M54.01 Panniculitis affecting regions of neck and back, occipito-atlanto-axial region
M54.02 Panniculitis affecting regions of neck and back, cervical region
M54.03 Panniculitis affecting regions of neck and back, cervicothoracic region
M54.04 Panniculitis affecting regions of neck and back, thoracic region
M54.05 Panniculitis affecting regions of neck and back, thoracolumbar region
M54.06 Panniculitis affecting regions of neck and back, lumbar region
M54.07 Panniculitis affecting regions of neck and back, lumbosacral region
M54.08 Panniculitis affecting regions of neck and back, sacral and sacrococcygeal region
M54.09 Panniculitis affecting regions, neck and back, multiple sites in spine
+ M54.1 Radiculopathy
Brachial neuritis or radiculitis NOS
Lumbar neuritis or radiculitis NOS
Lumbosacral neuritis or radiculitis NOS
Thoracic neuritis or radiculitis NOS
Radiculitis NOS
Excludes1: *neuralgia and neuritis NOS (M79.2)*
radiculopathy with cervical disc disorder (M50.1)
radiculopathy with lumbar and other intervertebral disc disorder (M51.1-)
radiculopathy with spondylosis (M47.2-)
M54.10 Radiculopathy, site unspecified
M54.11 Radiculopathy, occipito-atlanto-axial region
M54.12 Radiculopathy, cervical region
AHA CC: 3Q, 2018, 18-19
M54.13 Radiculopathy, cervicothoracic region
M54.14 Radiculopathy, thoracic region
M54.15 Radiculopathy, thoracolumbar region
M54.16 Radiculopathy, lumbar region
AHA CC: 3Q, 2018, 18
M54.17 Radiculopathy, lumbosacral region
M54.18 Radiculopathy, sacral and sacrococcygeal region
M54.2 Cervicalgia
Excludes1: *cervicalgia due to intervertebral cervical disc disorder (M50.-)*
+ M54.3 Sciatica
Excludes1: *lesion of sciatic nerve (G57.0)*
sciatica due to intervertebral disc disorder (M51.1-)
sciatica with lumbago (M54.4-)
M54.30 Sciatica, unspecified side
M54.31 Sciatica, right side
M54.32 Sciatica, left side
+ M54.4 Lumbago with sciatica
Excludes1: *lumbago with sciatica due to intervertebral disc disorder (M51.1-)*
M54.40 Lumbago with sciatica, unspecified side
M54.41 Lumbago with sciatica, right side
M54.42 Lumbago with sciatica, left side
AHA CC: 2Q, 2016, 7
+ M54.5 Low back pain
Excludes1: *low back strain (S39.012)*
lumbago due to intervertebral disc displacement (M51.2-)
lumbago with sciatica (M54.4-)
M54.50 Low pack pain, unspecified
Loin pain
Lumbago NOS
M54.51 Vertebrogenic low back pain
Low back vertebral endplate pain
M54.59 Other low back pain
M54.6 Pain in thoracic spine
Excludes1: *pain in thoracic spine due to intervertebral disc disorder (M51.-)*
+ M54.8 Other dorsalgia
Excludes1: *dorsalgia in thoracic region (M54.6)*
low back pain (M54.5-)
M54.81 Occipital neuralgia
M54.89 Other dorsalgia
M54.9 Dorsalgia, unspecified
Backache NOS
Back pain NOS

SOFT TISSUE DISORDERS (M60-M79)

Disorders of muscles (M60-M63)

Excludes1: *dermatopolymyositis (M33.-)*
muscular dystrophies and myopathies (G71-G72)
myopathy in amyloidosis (E85.-)
myopathy in polyarteritis nodosa (M30.0)
myopathy in rheumatoid arthritis (M05.32)
myopathy in scleroderma (M34.-)
myopathy in Sjögren's syndrome (M35.03)
myopathy in systemic lupus erythematosus (M32.-)

M60 Myositis

Excludes2: *inclusion body myositis [IBM] (G72.41)*

+ **M60.0 Infective myositis**
Tropical pyomyositis
Use additional code (B95-B97) to identify infectious agent
+ **M60.00 Infective myositis, unspecified site**
CC **M60.000 Infective myositis, unspecified right arm**
Infective myositis, right upper limb NOS
CC **M60.001 Infective myositis, unspecified left arm**
Infective myositis, left upper limb NOS
CC **M60.002 Infective myositis, unspecified arm**
Infective myositis, upper limb NOS
CC **M60.003 Infective myositis, unspecified right leg**
Infective myositis, right lower limb NOS
CC **M60.004 Infective myositis, unspecified left leg**
Infective myositis, left lower limb NOS
CC **M60.005 Infective myositis, unspecified leg**
Infective myositis, lower limb NOS
CC **M60.009 Infective myositis, unspecified site**
+ **M60.01 Infective myositis, shoulder**
CC **M60.011 Infective myositis, right shoulder**
CC **M60.012 Infective myositis, left shoulder**
CC **M60.019 Infective myositis, unspecified shoulder**
+ **M60.02 Infective myositis, upper arm**
CC **M60.021 Infective myositis, right upper arm**
CC **M60.022 Infective myositis, left upper arm**
CC **M60.029 Infective myositis, unspecified upper arm**
+ **M60.03 Infective myositis, forearm**
CC **M60.031 Infective myositis, right forearm**
CC **M60.032 Infective myositis, left forearm**
CC **M60.039 Infective myositis, unspecified forearm**
+ **M60.04 Infective myositis, hand and fingers**
CC **M60.041 Infective myositis, right hand**
CC **M60.042 Infective myositis, left hand**
CC **M60.043 Infective myositis, unspecified hand**
CC **M60.044 Infective myositis, right finger(s)**
CC **M60.045 Infective myositis, left finger(s)**
CC **M60.046 Infective myositis, unspecified finger(s)**
+ **M60.05 Infective myositis, thigh**
CC **M60.051 Infective myositis, right thigh**
CC **M60.052 Infective myositis, left thigh**
CC **M60.059 Infective myositis, unspecified thigh**
+ **M60.06 Infective myositis, lower leg**
CC **M60.061 Infective myositis, right lower leg**
CC **M60.062 Infective myositis, left lower leg**
CC **M60.069 Infective myositis, unspecified lower leg**
+ **M60.07 Infective myositis, ankle, foot and toes**
CC **M60.070 Infective myositis, right ankle**
CC **M60.071 Infective myositis, left ankle**
CC **M60.072 Infective myositis, unspecified ankle**
CC **M60.073 Infective myositis, right foot**
CC **M60.074 Infective myositis, left foot**
CC **M60.075 Infective myositis, unspecified foot**
CC **M60.076 Infective myositis, right toe(s)**
CC **M60.077 Infective myositis, left toe(s)**
CC **M60.078 Infective myositis, unspecified toe(s)**
CC **M60.08 Infective myositis, other site**
CC **M60.09 Infective myositis, multiple sites**
+ **M60.1 Interstitial myositis**
M60.10 Interstitial myositis of unspecified site
+ **M60.11 Interstitial myositis, shoulder**
M60.111 Interstitial myositis, right shoulder
M60.112 Interstitial myositis, left shoulder
M60.119 Interstitial myositis, unspecified shoulder
+ **M60.12 Interstitial myositis, upper arm**
M60.121 Interstitial myositis, right upper arm
M60.122 Interstitial myositis, left upper arm
M60.129 Interstitial myositis, unspecified upper arm
+ **M60.13 Interstitial myositis, forearm**
M60.131 Interstitial myositis, right forearm
M60.132 Interstitial myositis, left forearm
M60.139 Interstitial myositis, unspecified forearm
+ **M60.14 Interstitial myositis, hand**
M60.141 Interstitial myositis, right hand
M60.142 Interstitial myositis, left hand
M60.149 Interstitial myositis, unspecifiedhand
+ **M60.15 Interstitial myositis, thigh**
M60.151 Interstitial myositis, right thigh
M60.152 Interstitial myositis, left thigh
M60.159 Interstitial myositis, unspecifiedthigh
+ **M60.16 Interstitial myositis, lower leg**
M60.161 Interstitial myositis, right lower leg
M60.162 Interstitial myositis, left lower leg
M60.169 Interstitial myositis, unspecified lower leg
+ **M60.17 Interstitial myositis, ankle and foot**
M60.171 Interstitial myositis, right ankle and foot
M60.172 Interstitial myositis, left ankle and foot
M60.179 Interstitial myositis, unspecified ankle and foot
M60.18 Interstitial myositis, other site
M60.19 Interstitial myositis, multiple sites
+ **M60.2 Foreign body granuloma of soft tissue, not elsewhere classified**
Use additional code to identify the type of retained foreign body (Z18.-)
Excludes1: *foreign body granuloma of skin and subcutaneous tissue (L92.3)*
M60.20 Foreign body granuloma of soft tissue, not elsewhere classified, unspecified site
+ **M60.21 Foreign body granuloma of soft tissue, not elsewhere classified, shoulder**
M60.211 Foreign body granuloma of soft tissue, not elsewhere classified, right shoulder
M60.212 Foreign body granuloma of soft tissue, not elsewhere classified, left shoulder
M60.219 Foreign body granuloma of soft tissue, not elsewhere classified, unspecified shoulder
+ **M60.22 Foreign body granuloma of soft tissue, not elsewhere classified, upper arm**
M60.221 Foreign body granuloma of soft tissue, not elsewhere classified, right upper arm
M60.222 Foreign body granuloma of soft tissue, not elsewhere classified, left upper arm
M60.229 Foreign body granuloma of soft tissue, not elsewhere classified, unspecified upper arm
+ **M60.23 Foreign body granuloma of soft tissue, not elsewhere classified, forearm**
M60.231 Foreign body granuloma of soft tissue, not elsewhere classified, right forearm
M60.232 Foreign body granuloma of soft tissue, not elsewhere classified, left forearm
M60.239 Foreign body granuloma of soft tissue, not elsewhere classified, unspecified forearm
+ **M60.24 Foreign body granuloma of soft tissue, not elsewhere classified, hand**
M60.241 Foreign body granuloma of soft tissue, not elsewhere classified, right hand
M60.242 Foreign body granuloma of soft tissue, not elsewhere classified, left hand
M60.249 Foreign body granuloma of soft tissue, not elsewhere classified, unspecified hand

+ M60.25 Foreign body granuloma of soft tissue, not elsewhere classified, thigh
M60.251 Foreign body granuloma of soft tissue, not elsewhere classified, right thigh
M60.252 Foreign body granuloma of soft tissue, not elsewhere classified, left thigh
M60.259 Foreign body granuloma of soft tissue, not elsewhere classified, unspecified thigh
+ M60.26 Foreign body granuloma of soft tissue, not elsewhere classified, lower leg
M60.261 Foreign body granuloma of soft tissue, not elsewhere classified, right lower leg
M60.262 Foreign body granuloma of soft tissue, not elsewhere classified, left lower leg
M60.269 Foreign body granuloma of soft tissue, not elsewhere classified, unspecified lower leg
+ M60.27 Foreign body granuloma of soft tissue, not elsewhere classified, ankle and foot
M60.271 Foreign body granuloma of soft tissue, not elsewhere classified, right ankle and foot
M60.272 Foreign body granuloma of soft tissue, not elsewhere classified, left ankle and foot
M60.279 Foreign body granuloma of soft tissue, not elsewhere classified, unspecified ankle and foot
M60.28 Foreign body granuloma of soft tissue, not elsewhere classified, other site
+ M60.8 Other myositis
M60.80 Other myositis, unspecified site
+ M60.81 Other myositis shoulder
M60.811 Other myositis, right shoulder
M60.812 Other myositis, left shoulder
M60.819 Other myositis, unspecified shoulder
+ M60.82 Other myositis, upper arm
M60.821 Other myositis, right upper arm
M60.822 Other myositis, left upper arm
M60.829 Other myositis, unspecified upper arm
+ M60.83 Other myositis, forearm
M60.831 Other myositis, right forearm
M60.832 Other myositis, left forearm
M60.839 Other myositis, unspecified forearm
+ M60.84 Other myositis, hand
M60.841 Other myositis, right hand
M60.842 Other myositis, left hand
M60.849 Other myositis, unspecified hand
+ M60.85 Other myositis, thigh
M60.851 Other myositis, right thigh
M60.852 Other myositis, left thigh
M60.859 Other myositis, unspecified thigh
+ M60.86 Other myositis, lower leg
M60.861 Other myositis, right lower leg
M60.862 Other myositis, left lower leg
M60.869 Other myositis, unspecified lower leg
+ M60.87 Other myositis, ankle and foot
M60.871 Other myositis, right ankle and foot
M60.872 Other myositis, left ankle and foot
M60.879 Other myositis, unspecified ankle and foot
M60.88 Other myositis, other site
M60.89 Other myositis, multiple sites
M60.9 Myositis, unspecified

M61 Calcification and ossification of muscle
+ M61.0 Myositis ossificans traumatica
M61.00 Myositis ossificans traumatica, unspecified site
+ M61.01 Myositis ossificans traumatica, shoulder
M61.011 Myositis ossificans traumatica, right shoulder
M61.012 Myositis ossificans traumatica, left shoulder
M61.019 Myositis ossificans traumatica, unspecified shoulder
+ M61.02 Myositis ossificans traumatica, upper arm
M61.021 Myositis ossificans traumatica, right upper arm
M61.022 Myositis ossificans traumatica, left upper arm
M61.029 Myositis ossificans traumatica, unspecified upper arm
+ M61.03 Myositis ossificans traumatica, forearm
M61.031 Myositis ossificans traumatica, right forearm
M61.032 Myositis ossificans traumatica, left forearm
M61.039 Myositis ossificans traumatica, unspecified forearm
+ M61.04 Myositis ossificans traumatica, hand
M61.041 Myositis ossificans traumatica, right hand
M61.042 Myositis ossificans traumatica, left hand
M61.049 Myositis ossificans traumatica, unspecified hand
+ M61.05 Myositis ossificans traumatica, thigh
M61.051 Myositis ossificans traumatica, right thigh
M61.052 Myositis ossificans traumatica, left thigh
M61.059 Myositis ossificans traumatica, unspecified thigh
+ M61.06 Myositis ossificans traumatica, lower leg
M61.061 Myositis ossificans traumatica, right lower leg
M61.062 Myositis ossificans traumatica, left lower leg
M61.069 Myositis ossificans traumatica, unspecified lower leg
+ M61.07 Myositis ossificans traumatica, ankle and foot
M61.071 Myositis ossificans traumatica, right ankle and foot
M61.072 Myositis ossificans traumatica, left ankle and foot
M61.079 Myositis ossificans traumatica, unspecified ankle and foot
M61.08 Myositis ossificans traumatica, other site
M61.09 Myositis ossificans traumatica, multiple sites
+ M61.1 Myositis ossificans progressiva
Fibrodysplasia ossificans progressiva
M61.10 Myositis ossificans progressiva, unspecified site
+ M61.11 Myositis ossificans progressiva, shoulder
M61.111 Myositis ossificans progressiva, right shoulder
M61.112 Myositis ossificans progressiva, left shoulder
M61.119 Myositis ossificans progressiva, unspecified shoulder
+ M61.12 Myositis ossificans progressiva, upper arm
M61.121 Myositis ossificans progressiva, right upper arm
M61.122 Myositis ossificans progressiva, left upper arm
M61.129 Myositis ossificans progressiva, unspecified arm
+ M61.13 Myositis ossificans progressiva, forearm
M61.131 Myositis ossificans progressiva, right forearm
M61.132 Myositis ossificans progressiva, left forearm
M61.139 Myositis ossificans progressiva, unspecified forearm
+ M61.14 Myositis ossificans progressiva, hand and finger(s)
M61.141 Myositis ossificans progressiva, right hand
M61.142 Myositis ossificans progressiva, left hand
M61.143 Myositis ossificans progressiva, unspecified hand
M61.144 Myositis ossificans progressiva, right finger(s)
M61.145 Myositis ossificans progressiva, left finger(s)
M61.146 Myositis ossificans progressiva, unspecified finger(s)

+ M61.15 Myositis ossificans progressiva, thigh
M61.151 Myositis ossificans progressiva, right thigh
M61.152 Myositis ossificans progressiva, left thigh
M61.159 Myositis ossificans progressiva, unspecified thigh
+ M61.16 Myositis ossificans progressiva, lower leg
M61.161 Myositis ossificans progressiva, right lower leg
M61.162 Myositis ossificans progressiva, left lower leg
M61.169 Myositis ossificans progressiva, unspecified lower leg
+ M61.17 Myositis ossificans progressiva, ankle, foot and toe(s)
M61.171 Myositis ossificans progressiva, right ankle
M61.172 Myositis ossificans progressiva, left ankle
M61.173 Myositis ossificans progressiva, unspecified ankle
M61.174 Myositis ossificans progressiva, right foot
M61.175 Myositis ossificans progressiva, left foot
M61.176 Myositis ossificans progressiva, unspecified foot
M61.177 Myositis ossificans progressiva, right toe(s)
M61.178 Myositis ossificans progressiva, left toe(s)
M61.179 Myositis ossificans progressiva, unspecified toe(s)
M61.18 Myositis ossificans progressiva, other site
M61.19 Myositis ossificans progressiva, multiple sites
+ M61.2 Paralytic calcification and ossification of muscle
Myositis ossificans associated with quadriplegia or paraplegia
M61.20 Paralytic calcification and ossification of muscle, unspecified site
+ M61.21 Paralytic calcification and ossification of muscle, shoulder
M61.211 Paralytic calcification and ossification of muscle, right shoulder
M61.212 Paralytic calcification and ossification of muscle, left shoulder
M61.219 Paralytic calcification and ossification of muscle, unspecified shoulder
+ M61.22 Paralytic calcification and ossification of muscle, upper arm
M61.221 Paralytic calcification and ossification of muscle, right upper arm
M61.222 Paralytic calcification and ossification of muscle, left upper arm
M61.229 Paralytic calcification and ossification of muscle, unspecified upper arm
+ M61.23 Paralytic calcification and ossification of muscle, forearm
M61.231 Paralytic calcification and ossification of muscle, right forearm
M61.232 Paralytic calcification and ossification of muscle, left forearm
M61.239 Paralytic calcification and ossification of muscle, unspecified forearm
+ M61.24 Paralytic calcification and ossification of muscle, hand
M61.241 Paralytic calcification and ossification of muscle, right hand
M61.242 Paralytic calcification and ossification of muscle, left hand
M61.249 Paralytic calcification and ossification of muscle, unspecified hand
+ M61.25 Paralytic calcification and ossification of muscle, thigh
M61.251 Paralytic calcification and ossification of muscle, right thigh
M61.252 Paralytic calcification and ossification of muscle, left thigh
M61.259 Paralytic calcification and ossification of muscle, unspecified thigh
+ M61.26 Paralytic calcification and ossification of muscle, lower leg
M61.261 Paralytic calcification and ossification of muscle, right lower leg
M61.262 Paralytic calcification and ossification of muscle, left lower leg
M61.269 Paralytic calcification and ossification of muscle, unspecified lower leg
+ M61.27 Paralytic calcification and ossification of muscle, ankle and foot
M61.271 Paralytic calcification and ossification of muscle, right ankle and foot
M61.272 Paralytic calcification and ossification of muscle, left ankle and foot
M61.279 Paralytic calcification and ossification of muscle, unspecified ankle and foot
M61.28 Paralytic calcification and ossification of muscle, other site
M61.29 Paralytic calcification and ossification of muscle, multiple sites
+ M61.3 Calcification and ossification of muscles associated with burns
Myositis ossificans associated with burns
M61.30 Calcification and ossification of muscles associated with burns, unspecified site
+ M61.31 Calcification and ossification of muscles associated with burns, shoulder
M61.311 Calcification and ossification of muscles associated with burns, right shoulder
M61.312 Calcification and ossification of muscles associated with burns, left shoulder
M61.319 Calcification and ossification of muscles associated with burns, unspecified shoulder
+ M61.32 Calcification and ossification of muscles associated with burns, upper arm
M61.321 Calcification and ossification of muscles associated with burns, right upper arm
M61.322 Calcification and ossification of muscles associated with burns, left upper arm
M61.329 Calcification and ossification of muscles associated with burns, unspecified upper arm
+ M61.33 Calcification and ossification of muscles associated with burns, forearm
M61.331 Calcification and ossification of muscles associated with burns, right forearm
M61.332 Calcification and ossification of muscles associated with burns, left forearm
M61.339 Calcification and ossification of muscles associated with burns, unspecified forearm
+ M61.34 Calcification and ossification of muscles associated with burns, hand
M61.341 Calcification and ossification of muscles associated with burns, right hand
M61.342 Calcification and ossification of muscles associated with burns, left hand
M61.349 Calcification and ossification of muscles associated with burns, unspecified hand
+ M61.35 Calcification and ossification of muscles associated with burns, thigh
M61.351 Calcification and ossification of muscles associated with burns, right thigh
M61.352 Calcification and ossification of muscles associated with burns, left thigh
M61.359 Calcification and ossification of muscles associated with burns, unspecified thigh
+ M61.36 Calcification and ossification of muscles associated with burns, lower leg
M61.361 Calcification and ossification of muscles associated with burns, right lower leg
M61.362 Calcification and ossification of muscles associated with burns, left lower leg
M61.369 Calcification and ossification of muscles associated with burns, unspecified lower leg

+ M61.37 Calcification and ossification of muscles associated with burns, ankle and foot
M61.371 Calcification and ossification of muscles associated with burns, right ankle and foot
M61.372 Calcification and ossification of muscles associated with burns, left ankle and foot
M61.379 Calcification and ossification of muscles associated with burns, unspecified ankle and foot
M61.38 Calcification and ossification of muscles associated with burns, other site
M61.39 Calcification and ossification of muscles associated with burns, multiple sites
+ M61.4 Other calcification of muscle
Excludes1: *calcific tendinitis NOS (M65.2-)*
calcific tendinitis of shoulder (M75.3)
M61.40 Other calcification of muscle, unspecified site
+ M61.41 Other calcification of muscle, shoulder
M61.411 Other calcification of muscle, right shoulder
M61.412 Other calcification of muscle, left shoulder
M61.419 Other calcification of muscle, unspecified shoulder
+ M61.42 Other calcification of muscle, upper arm
M61.421 Other calcification of muscle, right upper arm
M61.422 Other calcification of muscle, left upper arm
M61.429 Other calcification of muscle, unspecified upper arm
+ M61.43 Other calcification of muscle, forearm
M61.431 Other calcification of muscle, right forearm
M61.432 Other calcification of muscle, left forearm
M61.439 Other calcification of muscle, unspecified forearm
+ M61.44 Other calcification of muscle, hand
M61.441 Other calcification of muscle, right hand
M61.442 Other calcification of muscle, left hand
M61.449 Other calcification of muscle, unspecified hand
+ M61.45 Other calcification of muscle, thigh
M61.451 Other calcification of muscle, right thigh
M61.452 Other calcification of muscle, left thigh
M61.459 Other calcification of muscle, unspecified thigh
+ M61.46 Other calcification of muscle, lower leg
M61.461 Other calcification of muscle, right lower leg
M61.462 Other calcification of muscle, left lower leg
M61.469 Other calcification of muscle, unspecified lower leg
+ M61.47 Other calcification of muscle, ankle and foot
M61.471 Other calcification of muscle, right ankle and foot
M61.472 Other calcification of muscle, left ankle and foot
M61.479 Other calcification of muscle, unspecified ankle and foot
M61.48 Other calcification of muscle, other site
M61.49 Other calcification of muscle, multiple sites
+ M61.5 Other ossification of muscle
M61.50 Other ossification of muscle, unspecified site
+ M61.51 Other ossification of muscle, shoulder
M61.511 Other ossification of muscle, right shoulder
M61.512 Other ossification of muscle, left shoulder
M61.519 Other ossification of muscle, unspecified shoulder
+ M61.52 Other ossification of muscle, upper arm
M61.521 Other ossification of muscle, right upper arm
M61.522 Other ossification of muscle, left upper arm
M61.529 Other ossification of muscle, unspecified upper arm
+ M61.53 Other ossification of muscle, forearm
M61.531 Other ossification of muscle, right forearm
M61.532 Other ossification of muscle, left forearm
M61.539 Other ossification of muscle, unspecified forearm
+ M61.54 Other ossification of muscle, hand
M61.541 Other ossification of muscle, right hand
M61.542 Other ossification of muscle, left hand
M61.549 Other ossification of muscle, unspecified hand
+ M61.55 Other ossification of muscle, thigh
M61.551 Other ossification of muscle, right thigh
M61.552 Other ossification of muscle, left thigh
M61.559 Other ossification of muscle, unspecified thigh
+ M61.56 Other ossification of muscle, lower leg
M61.561 Other ossification of muscle, right lower leg
M61.562 Other ossification of muscle, left lower leg
M61.569 Other ossification of muscle, unspecified lower leg
+ M61.57 Other ossification of muscle, ankle and foot
M61.571 Other ossification of muscle, right ankle and foot
M61.572 Other ossification of muscle, left ankle and foot
M61.579 Other ossification of muscle, unspecified ankle and foot
M61.58 Other ossification of muscle, other site
M61.59 Other ossification of muscle, multiple sites
M61.9 Calcification and ossification of muscle, unspecified

M62 Other disorders of muscle
Excludes1: *alcoholic myopathy (G72.1)*
cramp and spasm (R25.2)
drug-induced myopathy (G72.0)
myalgia (M79.1-)
stiff-man syndrome (G25.82)
Excludes2: *nontraumatic hematoma of muscle (M79.81)*
+ M62.0 Separation of muscle (nontraumatic)
Diastasis of muscle
Excludes1: *diastasis recti complicating pregnancy, labor and delivery (O71.8)*
traumatic separation of muscle- see strain of muscle by body region
M62.00 Separation of muscle (nontraumatic), unspecified site
+ M62.01 Separation of muscle (nontraumatic), shoulder
M62.011 Separation of muscle (nontraumatic), right shoulder
M62.012 Separation of muscle (nontraumatic), left shoulder
M62.019 Separation of muscle (nontraumatic), unspecified shoulder
+ M62.02 Separation of muscle (nontraumatic), upper arm
M62.021 Separation of muscle (nontraumatic), right upper arm
M62.022 Separation of muscle (nontraumatic), left upper arm
M62.029 Separation of muscle (nontraumatic), unspecified upper arm
+ M62.03 Separation of muscle (nontraumatic), forearm
M62.031 Separation of muscle (nontraumatic), right forearm
M62.032 Separation of muscle (nontraumatic), left forearm
M62.039 Separation of muscle (nontraumatic), unspecified forearm

+ M62.04 Separation of muscle (nontraumatic), hand
- **M62.041 Separation of muscle (nontraumatic), right hand**
- **M62.042 Separation of muscle (nontraumatic), left hand**
- **M62.049 Separation of muscle (nontraumatic), unspecified hand**

+ M62.05 Separation of muscle (nontraumatic), thigh
- **M62.051 Separation of muscle (nontraumatic), right thigh**
- **M62.052 Separation of muscle (nontraumatic), left thigh**
- **M62.059 Separation of muscle (nontraumatic), unspecified thigh**

+ M62.06 Separation of muscle (nontraumatic), lower leg
- **M62.061 Separation of muscle (nontraumatic), right lower leg**
- **M62.062 Separation of muscle (nontraumatic), left lower leg**
- **M62.069 Separation of muscle (nontraumatic), unspecified lower leg**

+ M62.07 Separation of muscle (nontraumatic), ankle and foot
- **M62.071 Separation of muscle (nontraumatic), right ankle and foot**
- **M62.072 Separation of muscle (nontraumatic), left ankle and foot**
- **M62.079 Separation of muscle (nontraumatic), unspecified ankle and foot**

M62.08 Separation of muscle (nontraumatic), other site

+ M62.1 Other rupture of muscle (nontraumatic)

Excludes1: *traumatic rupture of muscle - see strain of muscle by body region*

Excludes2: *rupture of tendon (M66.-)*

M62.10 Other rupture of muscle (nontraumatic), unspecified site

+ M62.11 Other rupture of muscle (nontraumatic), shoulder
- **M62.111 Other rupture of muscle (nontraumatic), right shoulder**
- **M62.112 Other rupture of muscle (nontraumatic), left shoulder**
- **M62.119 Other rupture of muscle (nontraumatic), unspecified shoulder**

+ M62.12 Other rupture of muscle (nontraumatic), upper arm
- **M62.121 Other rupture of muscle (nontraumatic), right upper arm**
- **M62.122 Other rupture of muscle (nontraumatic), left upper arm**
- **M62.129 Other rupture of muscle (nontraumatic), unspecified upper arm**

+ M62.13 Other rupture of muscle (nontraumatic), forearm
- **M62.131 Other rupture of muscle (nontraumatic), right forearm**
- **M62.132 Other rupture of muscle (nontraumatic), left forearm**
- **M62.139 Other rupture of muscle (nontraumatic), unspecified forearm**

+ M62.14 Other rupture of muscle (nontraumatic), hand
- **M62.141 Other rupture of muscle (nontraumatic), right hand**
- **M62.142 Other rupture of muscle (nontraumatic), left hand**
- **M62.149 Other rupture of muscle (nontraumatic), unspecified hand**

+ M62.15 Other rupture of muscle (nontraumatic), thigh
- **M62.151 Other rupture of muscle (nontraumatic), right thigh**
- **M62.152 Other rupture of muscle (nontraumatic), left thigh**
- **M62.159 Other rupture of muscle (nontraumatic), unspecified thigh**

+ M62.16 Other rupture of muscle (nontraumatic), lower leg
- **M62.161 Other rupture of muscle (nontraumatic), right lower leg**
- **M62.162 Other rupture of muscle (nontraumatic), left lower leg**
- **M62.169 Other rupture of muscle (nontraumatic), unspecified lower leg**

+ M62.17 Other rupture of muscle (nontraumatic), ankle and foot
- **M62.171 Other rupture of muscle (nontraumatic), right ankle and foot**
- **M62.172 Other rupture of muscle (nontraumatic), left ankle and foot**
- **M62.179 Other rupture of muscle (nontraumatic), unspecified ankle and foot**

M62.18 Other rupture of muscle (nontraumatic), other site

+ M62.2 Nontraumatic ischemic infarction of muscle

Excludes1: *compartment syndrome (traumatic) (T79.A-)*
nontraumatic compartment syndrome (M79.A-)
traumatic ischemia of muscle (T79.6)
rhabdomyolysis (M62.82)
Volkmann's ischemic contracture (T79.6)

M62.20 Nontraumatic ischemic infarction of muscle, unspecified site

+ M62.21 Nontraumatic ischemic infarction of muscle, shoulder
- **M62.211 Nontraumatic ischemic infarction of muscle, right shoulder**
- **M62.212 Nontraumatic ischemic infarction of muscle, left shoulder**
- **M62.219 Nontraumatic ischemic infarction of muscle, unspecified shoulder**

+ M62.22 Nontraumatic ischemic infarction of muscle, upper arm
- **M62.221 Nontraumatic ischemic infarction of muscle, right upper arm**
- **M62.222 Nontraumatic ischemic infarction of muscle, left upper arm**
- **M62.229 Nontraumatic ischemic infarction of muscle, unspecified upper arm**

+ M62.23 Nontraumatic ischemic infarction of muscle, forearm
- **M62.231 Nontraumatic ischemic infarction of muscle, right forearm**
- **M62.232 Nontraumatic ischemic infarction of muscle, left forearm**
- **M62.239 Nontraumatic ischemic infarction of muscle, unspecified forearm**

+ M62.24 Nontraumatic ischemic infarction of muscle, hand
- **M62.241 Nontraumatic ischemic infarction of muscle, right hand**
- **M62.242 Nontraumatic ischemic infarction of muscle, left hand**
- **M62.249 Nontraumatic ischemic infarction of muscle, unspecified hand**

+ M62.25 Nontraumatic ischemic infarction of muscle, thigh
- **M62.251 Nontraumatic ischemic infarction of muscle, right thigh**
- **M62.252 Nontraumatic ischemic infarction of muscle, left thigh**
- **M62.259 Nontraumatic ischemic infarction of muscle, unspecified thigh**

+ M62.26 Nontraumatic ischemic infarction of muscle, lower leg
- **M62.261 Nontraumatic ischemic infarction of muscle, right lower leg**
- **M62.262 Nontraumatic ischemic infarction of muscle, left lower leg**
- **M62.269 Nontraumatic ischemic infarction of muscle, unspecified lower leg**

+ M62.27 Nontraumatic ischemic infarction of muscle, ankle and foot
- **M62.271 Nontraumatic ischemic infarction of muscle, right ankle and foot**
- **M62.272 Nontraumatic ischemic infarction of muscle, left ankle and foot**
- **M62.279 Nontraumatic ischemic infarction of muscle, unspecified ankle and foot**

M62.28 Nontraumatic ischemic infarction of muscle, other site

M62.3 Immobility syndrome (paraplegic)

+ **M62.4 Contracture of muscle**
  Contracture of tendon (sheath)
  Excludes1: *contracture of joint (M24.5-)*
  M62.40 Contracture of muscle, unspecified site
  + **M62.41 Contracture of muscle, shoulder**
    M62.411 Contracture of muscle, right shoulder
    M62.412 Contracture of muscle, left shoulder
    M62.419 Contracture of muscle, unspecified shoulder
  + **M62.42 Contracture of muscle, upper arm**
    M62.421 Contracture of muscle, right upper arm
    M62.422 Contracture of muscle, left upper arm
    M62.429 Contracture of muscle, unspecified upper arm
  + **M62.43 Contracture of muscle, forearm**
    M62.431 Contracture of muscle, right forearm
    M62.432 Contracture of muscle, left forearm
    M62.439 Contracture of muscle, unspecified forearm
  + **M62.44 Contracture of muscle, hand**
    M62.441 Contracture of muscle, right hand
    M62.442 Contracture of muscle, left hand
    M62.449 Contracture of muscle, unspecified hand
  + **M62.45 Contracture of muscle, thigh**
    M62.451 Contracture of muscle, right thigh
    M62.452 Contracture of muscle, left thigh
    M62.459 Contracture of muscle, unspecified thigh
  + **M62.46 Contracture of muscle, lower leg**
    M62.461 Contracture of muscle, right lower leg
    M62.462 Contracture of muscle, left lower leg
    M62.469 Contracture of muscle, unspecified lower leg
  + **M62.47 Contracture of muscle, ankle and foot**
    M62.471 Contracture of muscle, right ankle and foot
    M62.472 Contracture of muscle, left ankle and foot
    M62.479 Contracture of muscle, unspecified ankle and foot
  M62.48 Contracture of muscle, other site
  M62.49 Contracture of muscle, multiple sites

+ **M62.5 Muscle wasting and atrophy, not elsewhere classified**
  Disuse atrophy NEC
  Excludes1: *neuralgic amyotrophy (G54.5)*
  progressive muscular atrophy (G12.21)
  sarcopenia (M62.84)
  Excludes2: *pelvic muscle wasting (N81.84)*
  M62.50 Muscle wasting and atrophy, not elsewhere classified, unspecified site
  + **M62.51 Muscle wasting and atrophy, not elsewhere classified, shoulder**
    M62.511 Muscle wasting and atrophy, not elsewhere classified, right shoulder
    M62.512 Muscle wasting and atrophy, not elsewhere classified, left shoulder
    M62.519 Muscle wasting and atrophy, not elsewhere classified, unspecified shoulder
  + **M62.52 Muscle wasting and atrophy, not elsewhere classified, upper arm**
    M62.521 Muscle wasting and atrophy, not elsewhere classified, right upper arm
    M62.522 Muscle wasting and atrophy, not elsewhere classified, left upper arm
    M62.529 Muscle wasting and atrophy, not elsewhere classified, unspecified upper arm
  + **M62.53 Muscle wasting and atrophy, not elsewhere classified, forearm**
    M62.531 Muscle wasting and atrophy, not elsewhere classified, right forearm
    M62.532 Muscle wasting and atrophy, not elsewhere classified, left forearm
    M62.539 Muscle wasting and atrophy, not elsewhere classified, unspecified forearm
  + **M62.54 Muscle wasting and atrophy, not elsewhere classified, hand**
    M62.541 Muscle wasting and atrophy, not elsewhere classified, right hand
    M62.542 Muscle wasting and atrophy, not elsewhere classified, left hand
    M62.549 Muscle wasting and atrophy, not elsewhere classified, unspecified hand
  + **M62.55 Muscle wasting and atrophy, not elsewhere classified, thigh**
    M62.551 Muscle wasting and atrophy, not elsewhere classified, right thigh
    M62.552 Muscle wasting and atrophy, not elsewhere classified, left thigh
    M62.559 Muscle wasting and atrophy, not elsewhere classified, unspecified thigh
  + **M62.56 Muscle wasting and atrophy, not elsewhere classified, lower leg**
    M62.561 Muscle wasting and atrophy, not elsewhere classified, right lower leg
    M62.562 Muscle wasting and atrophy, not elsewhere classified, left lower leg
    M62.569 Muscle wasting and atrophy, not elsewhere classified, unspecified lower leg
  + **M62.57 Muscle wasting and atrophy, not elsewhere classified, ankle and foot**
    M62.571 Muscle wasting and atrophy, not elsewhere classified, right ankle and foot
    M62.572 Muscle wasting and atrophy, not elsewhere classified, left ankle and foot
    M62.579 Muscle wasting and atrophy, not elsewhere classified, unspecified ankle and foot
  M62.58 Muscle wasting and atrophy, not elsewhere classified, other site
  M62.59 Muscle wasting and atrophy, not elsewhere classified, multiple sites

+ **M62.8 Other specified disorders of muscle**
  Excludes2: *nontraumatic hematoma of muscle (M79.81)*
  M62.81 Muscle weakness (generalized)
  Excludes1: *muscle weakness in sarcopenia (M62.84)*
  CC **M62.82 Rhabdomyolysis**
  Excludes1: *traumatic rhabdomyolysis (T79.6)*
  AHA CC: 2Q, 2019, 12-13
  + **M62.83 Muscle spasm**
    M62.830 Muscle spasm of back
    M62.831 Muscle spasm of calf
    Charley-horse
    M62.838 Other muscle spasm
  M62.84 Sarcopenia
  Age-related sarcopenia
  Code first underlying disease, if applicable, such as:
  disorders of myoneural junction and muscle disease
  in diseases classified elsewhere (G73.-)
  other and unspecified myopathies (G72.-)
  primary disorders of muscles (G71.-)
  AHA CC: 4Q, 2016, 41
  M62.89 Other specified disorders of muscle
  Muscle (sheath) hernia

M62.9 Disorder of muscle, unspecified

M63 Disorders of muscle in diseases classified elsewhere
Code first underlying disease, such as:
leprosy (A30.-)
neoplasm (C49.-, C79.89, D21.-, D48.1)
schistosomiasis (B65.-)
trichinellosis (B75)
Excludes1: *myopathy in cysticercosis (B69.81)*
myopathy in endocrine diseases (G73.7)
myopathy in metabolic diseases (G73.7)
myopathy in sarcoidosis (D86.87)
myopathy in secondary syphilis (A51.49)
myopathy in syphilis (late) (A52.78)
myopathy in toxoplasmosis (B58.82)
myopathy in tuberculosis (A18.09)

+ **M63.8 Disorders of muscle in diseases classified elsewhere**
  M63.80 Disorders of muscle in diseases classified elsewhere, unspecified site

+ M63.81 Disorders of muscle in diseases classified elsewhere, shoulder
  - M63.811 Disorders of muscle in diseases classified elsewhere, right shoulder
  - M63.812 Disorders of muscle in diseases classified elsewhere, left shoulder
  - M63.819 Disorders of muscle in diseases classified elsewhere, unspecified shoulder

+ M63.82 Disorders of muscle in diseases classified elsewhere, upper arm
  - M63.821 Disorders of muscle in diseases classified elsewhere, right upper arm
  - M63.822 Disorders of muscle in diseases classified elsewhere, left upper arm
  - M63.829 Disorders of muscle in diseases classified elsewhere, unspecified upper arm

+ M63.83 Disorders of muscle in diseases classified elsewhere, forearm
  - M63.831 Disorders of muscle in diseases classified elsewhere, right forearm
  - M63.832 Disorders of muscle in diseases classified elsewhere, left forearm
  - M63.839 Disorders of muscle in diseases classified elsewhere, unspecified forearm

+ M63.84 Disorders of muscle in diseases classified elsewhere, hand
  - M63.841 Disorders of muscle in diseases classified elsewhere, right hand
  - M63.842 Disorders of muscle in diseases classified elsewhere, left hand
  - M63.849 Disorders of muscle in diseases classified elsewhere, unspecified hand

+ M63.85 Disorders of muscle in diseases classified elsewhere, thigh
  - M63.851 Disorders of muscle in diseases classified elsewhere, right thigh
  - M63.852 Disorders of muscle in diseases classified elsewhere, left thigh
  - M63.859 Disorders of muscle in diseases classified elsewhere, unspecified thigh

+ M63.86 Disorders of muscle in diseases classified elsewhere, lower leg
  - M63.861 Disorders of muscle in diseases classified elsewhere, right lower leg
  - M63.862 Disorders of muscle in diseases classified elsewhere, left lower leg
  - M63.869 Disorders of muscle in diseases classified elsewhere, unspecified lower leg

+ M63.87 Disorders of muscle in diseases classified elsewhere, ankle and foot
  - M63.871 Disorders of muscle in diseases classified elsewhere, right ankle and foot
  - M63.872 Disorders of muscle in diseases classified elsewhere, left ankle and foot
  - M63.879 Disorders of muscle in diseases classified elsewhere, unspecified ankle and foot

M63.88 Disorders of muscle in diseases classified elsewhere, other site

M63.89 Disorders of muscle in diseases classified elsewhere, multiple sites

Disorders of synovium and tendon (M65-M67)

M65 Synovitis and tenosynovitis

Excludes1: *chronic crepitant synovitis of hand and wrist (M70.0-)*
current injury - see injury of ligament or tendon by body region
soft tissue disorders related to use, overuse and pressure (M70.-)

+ M65.0 Abscess of tendon sheath
  Use additional code (B95-B96) to identify bacterial agent
  - M65.00 Abscess of tendon sheath, unspecified site
  - + M65.01 Abscess of tendon sheath, shoulder
    - M65.011 Abscess of tendon sheath, right shoulder
    - M65.012 Abscess of tendon sheath, left shoulder
    - M65.019 Abscess of tendon sheath, unspecified shoulder
  - + M65.02 Abscess of tendon sheath, upper arm
    - M65.021 Abscess of tendon sheath, right upper arm
    - M65.022 Abscess of tendon sheath, left upper arm
    - M65.029 Abscess of tendon sheath, unspecified upper arm
  - + M65.03 Abscess of tendon sheath, forearm
    - M65.031 Abscess of tendon sheath, right forearm
    - M65.032 Abscess of tendon sheath, left forearm
    - M65.039 Abscess of tendon sheath, unspecified forearm
  - + M65.04 Abscess of tendon sheath, hand
    - M65.041 Abscess of tendon sheath, right hand
    - M65.042 Abscess of tendon sheath, left hand
    - M65.049 Abscess of tendon sheath, unspecified hand
  - + M65.05 Abscess of tendon sheath, thigh
    - M65.051 Abscess of tendon sheath, right thigh
    - M65.052 Abscess of tendon sheath, left thigh
    - M65.059 Abscess of tendon sheath, unspecified thigh
  - + M65.06 Abscess of tendon sheath, lower leg
    - M65.061 Abscess of tendon sheath, right lower leg
    - M65.062 Abscess of tendon sheath, left lower leg
    - M65.069 Abscess of tendon sheath, unspecified lower leg
  - + M65.07 Abscess of tendon sheath, ankle and foot
    - M65.071 Abscess of tendon sheath, right ankle and foot
    - M65.072 Abscess of tendon sheath, left ankle and foot
    - M65.079 Abscess of tendon sheath, unspecified ankle and foot
  - M65.08 Abscess of tendon sheath, other site

+ M65.1 Other infective (teno)synovitis
  - M65.10 Other infective (teno)synovitis, unspecified site
  - + M65.11 Other infective (teno)synovitis, shoulder
    - M65.111 Other infective (teno)synovitis, right shoulder
    - M65.112 Other infective (teno)synovitis, left shoulder
    - M65.119 Other infective (teno)synovitis, unspecified shoulder
  - + M65.12 Other infective (teno)synovitis, elbow
    - M65.121 Other infective (teno)synovitis, right elbow
    - M65.122 Other infective (teno)synovitis, left elbow
    - M65.129 Other infective (teno)synovitis, unspecified elbow
  - + M65.13 Other infective (teno)synovitis, wrist
    - M65.131 Other infective (teno)synovitis, right wrist
    - M65.132 Other infective (teno)synovitis, left wrist
    - M65.139 Other infective (teno)synovitis, unspecified wrist
  - + M65.14 Other infective (teno)synovitis, hand
    - M65.141 Other infective (teno)synovitis, right hand
    - M65.142 Other infective (teno)synovitis, left hand
    - M65.149 Other infective (teno)synovitis, unspecified hand
  - + M65.15 Other infective (teno)synovitis, hip
    - M65.151 Other infective (teno)synovitis, right hip
    - M65.152 Other infective (teno)synovitis, left hip
    - M65.159 Other infective (teno)synovitis, unspecified hip
  - + M65.16 Other infective (teno)synovitis, knee
    - M65.161 Other infective (teno)synovitis, right knee
    - M65.162 Other infective (teno)synovitis, left knee
    - M65.169 Other infective (teno)synovitis, unspecified knee

+ M65.17 Other infective (teno)synovitis, ankle and foot
M65.171 Other infective (teno)synovitis, right ankle and foot
M65.172 Other infective (teno)synovitis, left ankle and foot
M65.179 Other infective (teno)synovitis, unspecified ankle and foot
M65.18 Other infective (teno)synovitis, other site
M65.19 Other infective (teno)synovitis, multiple sites
+ M65.2 Calcific tendinitis
Excludes1: *tendinitis as classified in M75-M77*
calcified tendinitis of shoulder (M75.3)
M65.20 Calcific tendinitis, unspecified site
+ M65.22 Calcific tendinitis, upper arm
M65.221 Calcific tendinitis, right upper arm
M65.222 Calcific tendinitis, left upper arm
M65.229 Calcific tendinitis, unspecified upper arm
+ M65.23 Calcific tendinitis, forearm
M65.231 Calcific tendinitis, right forearm
M65.232 Calcific tendinitis, left forearm
M65.239 Calcific tendinitis, unspecified forearm
+ M65.24 Calcific tendinitis, hand
M65.241 Calcific tendinitis, right hand
M65.242 Calcific tendinitis, left hand
M65.249 Calcific tendinitis, unspecified hand
+ M65.25 Calcific tendinitis, thigh
M65.251 Calcific tendinitis, right thigh
M65.252 Calcific tendinitis, left thigh
M65.259 Calcific tendinitis, unspecified thigh
+ M65.26 Calcific tendinitis, lower leg
M65.261 Calcific tendinitis, right lower leg
M65.262 Calcific tendinitis, left lower leg
M65.269 Calcific tendinitis, unspecified lower leg
+ M65.27 Calcific tendinitis, ankle and foot
M65.271 Calcific tendinitis, right ankle and foot
M65.272 Calcific tendinitis, left ankle and foot
M65.279 Calcific tendinitis, unspecified ankle and foot
M65.28 Calcific tendinitis, other site
M65.29 Calcific tendinitis, multiple sites
+ M65.3 Trigger finger
Nodular tendinous disease
M65.30 Trigger finger, unspecified finger
+ M65.31 Trigger thumb
M65.311 Trigger thumb, right thumb
M65.312 Trigger thumb, left thumb
M65.319 Trigger thumb, unspecified thumb
+ M65.32 Trigger finger, index finger
M65.321 Trigger finger, right index finger
M65.322 Trigger finger, left index finger
M65.329 Trigger finger, unspecified index finger
+ M65.33 Trigger finger, middle finger
M65.331 Trigger finger, right middle finger
M65.332 Trigger finger, left middle finger
M65.339 Trigger finger, unspecified middle finger
+ M65.34 Trigger finger, ring finger
M65.341 Trigger finger, right ring finger
M65.342 Trigger finger, left ring finger
M65.349 Trigger finger, unspecified ring finger
+ M65.35 Trigger finger, little finger
M65.351 Trigger finger, right little finger
M65.352 Trigger finger, left little finger
M65.359 Trigger finger, unspecified little finger
M65.4 Radial styloid tenosynovitis [de Quervain]
+ M65.8 Other synovitis and tenosynovitis
M65.80 Other synovitis and tenosynovitis, unspecified site
+ M65.81 Other synovitis and tenosynovitis, shoulder
M65.811 Other synovitis and tenosynovitis, right shoulder
M65.812 Other synovitis and tenosynovitis, left shoulder
M65.819 Other synovitis and tenosynovitis, unspecified shoulder
+ M65.82 Other synovitis and tenosynovitis, upper arm
M65.821 Other synovitis and tenosynovitis, right upper arm
M65.822 Other synovitis and tenosynovitis, left upper arm
M65.829 Other synovitis and tenosynovitis, unspecified upper arm
+ M65.83 Other synovitis and tenosynovitis, forearm
M65.831 Other synovitis and tenosynovitis, right forearm
M65.832 Other synovitis and tenosynovitis, left forearm
M65.839 Other synovitis and tenosynovitis, unspecified forearm
+ M65.84 Other synovitis and tenosynovitis, hand
M65.841 Other synovitis and tenosynovitis, right hand
M65.842 Other synovitis and tenosynovitis, left hand
M65.849 Other synovitis and tenosynovitis, unspecified hand
+ M65.85 Other synovitis and tenosynovitis, thigh
M65.851 Other synovitis and tenosynovitis, right thigh
M65.852 Other synovitis and tenosynovitis, left thigh
M65.859 Other synovitis and tenosynovitis, unspecified thigh
+ M65.86 Other synovitis and tenosynovitis, lower leg
M65.861 Other synovitis and tenosynovitis, right lower leg
M65.862 Other synovitis and tenosynovitis, left lower leg
M65.869 Other synovitis and tenosynovitis, unspecified lower leg
+ M65.87 Other synovitis and tenosynovitis, ankle and foot
M65.871 Other synovitis and tenosynovitis, right ankle and foot
M65.872 Other synovitis and tenosynovitis, left ankle and foot
M65.879 Other synovitis and tenosynovitis, unspecified ankle and foot
M65.88 Other synovitis and tenosynovitis, other site
M65.89 Other synovitis and tenosynovitis, multiple sites
M65.9 Synovitis and tenosynovitis, unspecified

M66 Spontaneous rupture of synovium and tendon
Includes: rupture that occurs when a normal force is applied to tissues that are inferred to have less than normal strength
Excludes2: *rotator cuff syndrome (M75.1-)*
rupture where an abnormal force is applied to normal tissue - see injury of tendon by body region
M66.0 Rupture of popliteal cyst
+ M66.1 Rupture of synovium
Rupture of synovial cyst
Excludes2: *rupture of popliteal cyst (M66.0)*
M66.10 Rupture of synovium, unspecified joint
+ M66.11 Rupture of synovium, shoulder
M66.111 Rupture of synovium, right shoulder
M66.112 Rupture of synovium, left shoulder
M66.119 Rupture of synovium, unspecified shoulder
+ M66.12 Rupture of synovium, elbow
M66.121 Rupture of synovium, right elbow
M66.122 Rupture of synovium, left elbow
M66.129 Rupture of synovium, unspecified elbow
+ M66.13 Rupture of synovium, wrist
M66.131 Rupture of synovium, right wrist
M66.132 Rupture of synovium, left wrist
M66.139 Rupture of synovium, unspecified wrist
+ M66.14 Rupture of synovium, hand and fingers
M66.141 Rupture of synovium, right hand
M66.142 Rupture of synovium, left hand
M66.143 Rupture of synovium, unspecified hand
M66.144 Rupture of synovium, right finger(s)
M66.145 Rupture of synovium, left finger(s)
M66.146 Rupture of synovium, unspecified finger(s)
+ M66.15 Rupture of synovium, hip
M66.151 Rupture of synovium, right hip
M66.152 Rupture of synovium, left hip
M66.159 Rupture of synovium, unspecified hip
+ M66.17 Rupture of synovium, ankle, foot and toes
M66.171 Rupture of synovium, right ankle
M66.172 Rupture of synovium, left ankle
M66.173 Rupture of synovium, unspecified ankle
M66.174 Rupture of synovium, right foot

M66.175 Rupture of synovium, left foot
M66.176 Rupture of synovium, unspecified foot
M66.177 Rupture of synovium, right toe(s)
M66.178 Rupture of synovium, left toe(s)
M66.179 Rupture of synovium, unspecified toe(s)
M66.18 Rupture of synovium, other site
+ M66.2 Spontaneous rupture of extensor tendons
M66.20 Spontaneous rupture of extensor tendons, unspecified site
+ M66.21 Spontaneous rupture of extensor tendons, shoulder
M66.211 Spontaneous rupture of extensor tendons, right shoulder
M66.212 Spontaneous rupture of extensor tendons, left shoulder
M66.219 Spontaneous rupture of extensor tendons, unspecified shoulder
+ M66.22 Spontaneous rupture of extensor tendons, upper arm
M66.221 Spontaneous rupture of extensor tendons, right upper arm
M66.222 Spontaneous rupture of extensor tendons, left upper arm
M66.229 Spontaneous rupture of extensor tendons, unspecified upper arm
+ M66.23 Spontaneous rupture of extensor tendons, forearm
M66.231 Spontaneous rupture of extensor tendons, right forearm
M66.232 Spontaneous rupture of extensor tendons, left forearm
M66.239 Spontaneous rupture of extensor tendons, unspecified forearm
+ M66.24 Spontaneous rupture of extensor tendons, hand
M66.241 Spontaneous rupture of extensor tendons, right hand
M66.242 Spontaneous rupture of extensor tendons, left hand
M66.249 Spontaneous rupture of extensor tendons, unspecified hand
+ M66.25 Spontaneous rupture of extensor tendons, thigh
M66.251 Spontaneous rupture of extensor tendons, right thigh
M66.252 Spontaneous rupture of extensor tendons, left thigh
M66.259 Spontaneous rupture of extensor tendons, unspecified thigh
+ M66.26 Spontaneous rupture of extensor tendons, lower leg
M66.261 Spontaneous rupture of extensor tendons, right lower leg
M66.262 Spontaneous rupture of extensor tendons, left lower leg
M66.269 Spontaneous rupture of extensor tendons, unspecified lower leg
+ M66.27 Spontaneous rupture of extensor tendons, ankle and foot
M66.271 Spontaneous rupture of extensor tendons, right ankle and foot
M66.272 Spontaneous rupture of extensor tendons, left ankle and foot
M66.279 Spontaneous rupture of extensor tendons, unspecified ankle and foot
M66.28 Spontaneous rupture of extensor tendons, other site
M66.29 Spontaneous rupture of extensor tendons, multiple sites
+ M66.3 Spontaneous rupture of flexor tendons
M66.30 Spontaneous rupture of flexor tendons, unspecified site
+ M66.31 Spontaneous rupture of flexor tendons, shoulder
M66.311 Spontaneous rupture of flexor tendons, right shoulder
M66.312 Spontaneous rupture of flexor tendons, left shoulder
M66.319 Spontaneous rupture of flexor tendons, unspecified shoulder
+ M66.32 Spontaneous rupture of flexor tendons, upper arm
M66.321 Spontaneous rupture of flexor tendons, right upper arm
M66.322 Spontaneous rupture of flexor tendons, left upper arm
M66.329 Spontaneous rupture of flexor tendons, unspecified upper arm
+ M66.33 Spontaneous rupture of flexor tendons, forearm
M66.331 Spontaneous rupture of flexor tendons, right forearm
M66.332 Spontaneous rupture of flexor tendons, left forearm
M66.339 Spontaneous rupture of flexor tendons, unspecified forearm
+ M66.34 Spontaneous rupture of flexor tendons, hand
M66.341 Spontaneous rupture of flexor tendons, right hand
M66.342 Spontaneous rupture of flexor tendons, left hand
M66.349 Spontaneous rupture of flexor tendons, unspecified hand
+ M66.35 Spontaneous rupture of flexor tendons, thigh
M66.351 Spontaneous rupture of flexor tendons, right thigh
M66.352 Spontaneous rupture of flexor tendons, left thigh
M66.359 Spontaneous rupture of flexor tendons, unspecified thigh
+ M66.36 Spontaneous rupture of flexor tendons, lower leg
M66.361 Spontaneous rupture of flexor tendons, right lower leg
M66.362 Spontaneous rupture of flexor tendons, left lower leg
M66.369 Spontaneous rupture of flexor tendons, unspecified lower leg
+ M66.37 Spontaneous rupture of flexor tendons, ankle and foot
M66.371 Spontaneous rupture of flexor tendons, right ankle and foot
M66.372 Spontaneous rupture of flexor tendons, left ankle and foot
M66.379 Spontaneous rupture of flexor tendons, unspecified ankle and foot
M66.38 Spontaneous rupture of flexor tendons, other site
M66.39 Spontaneous rupture of flexor tendons, multiple sites
+ M66.8 Spontaneous rupture of other tendons
M66.80 Spontaneous rupture of other tendons, unspecified site
+ M66.81 Spontaneous rupture of other tendons, shoulder
M66.811 Spontaneous rupture of other tendons, right shoulder
M66.812 Spontaneous rupture of other tendons, left shoulder
M66.819 Spontaneous rupture of other tendons, unspecified shoulder
+ M66.82 Spontaneous rupture of other tendons, upper arm
M66.821 Spontaneous rupture of other tendons, right upper arm
M66.822 Spontaneous rupture of other tendons, left upper arm
M66.829 Spontaneous rupture of other tendons, unspecified upper arm
+ M66.83 Spontaneous rupture of other tendons, forearm
M66.831 Spontaneous rupture of other tendons, right forearm
M66.832 Spontaneous rupture of other tendons, left forearm
M66.839 Spontaneous rupture of other tendons, unspecified forearm
+ M66.84 Spontaneous rupture of other tendons, hand
M66.841 Spontaneous rupture of other tendons, right hand
M66.842 Spontaneous rupture of other tendons, left hand
M66.849 Spontaneous rupture of other tendons, unspecified hand

+ **M66.85 Spontaneous rupture of other tendons, thigh**
  - **M66.851 Spontaneous rupture of other tendons, right thigh**
  - **M66.852 Spontaneous rupture of other tendons, left thigh**
  - **M66.859 Spontaneous rupture of other tendons, unspecified thigh**

+ **M66.86 Spontaneous rupture of other tendons, lower leg**
  - **M66.861 Spontaneous rupture of other tendons, right lower leg**
  - **M66.862 Spontaneous rupture of other tendons, left lower leg**
  - **M66.869 Spontaneous rupture of other tendons, unspecified lower leg**

+ **M66.87 Spontaneous rupture of other tendons, ankle and foot**
  - **M66.871 Spontaneous rupture of other tendons, right ankle and foot**
  - **M66.872 Spontaneous rupture of other tendons, left ankle and foot**
  - **M66.879 Spontaneous rupture of other tendons, unspecified ankle and foot**

M66.88 Spontaneous rupture of other tendons, other sites

M66.89 Spontaneous rupture of other tendons, multiple sites

M66.9 Spontaneous rupture of unspecified tendon

Rupture at musculotendinous junction, nontraumatic

M67 Other disorders of synovium and tendon

Excludes1: *palmar fascial fibromatosis [Dupuytren] (M72.0)*
tendinitis NOS (M77.9-)
xanthomatosis localized to tendons (E78.2)

+ **M67.0 Short Achilles tendon (acquired)**
  - **M67.00 Short Achilles tendon (acquired), unspecified ankle**
  - **M67.01 Short Achilles tendon (acquired), right ankle**
  - **M67.02 Short Achilles tendon (acquired), left ankle**

+ **M67.2 Synovial hypertrophy, not elsewhere classified**

Excludes1: *villonodular synovitis (pigmented) (M12.2-)*

M67.20 Synovial hypertrophy, not elsewhere classified, unspecified site

+ **M67.21 Synovial hypertrophy, not elsewhere classified, shoulder**
  - **M67.211 Synovial hypertrophy, not elsewhere classified, right shoulder**
  - **M67.212 Synovial hypertrophy, not elsewhere classified, left shoulder**
  - **M67.219 Synovial hypertrophy, not elsewhere classified, unspecified shoulder**

+ **M67.22 Synovial hypertrophy, not elsewhere classified, upper arm**
  - **M67.221 Synovial hypertrophy, not elsewhere classified, right upper arm**
  - **M67.222 Synovial hypertrophy, not elsewhere classified, left upper arm**
  - **M67.229 Synovial hypertrophy, not elsewhere classified, unspecified upper arm**

+ **M67.23 Synovial hypertrophy, not elsewhere classified, forearm**
  - **M67.231 Synovial hypertrophy, not elsewhere classified, right forearm**
  - **M67.232 Synovial hypertrophy, not elsewhere classified, left forearm**
  - **M67.239 Synovial hypertrophy, not elsewhere classified, unspecified forearm**

+ **M67.24 Synovial hypertrophy, not elsewhere classified, hand**
  - **M67.241 Synovial hypertrophy, not elsewhere classified, right hand**
  - **M67.242 Synovial hypertrophy, not elsewhere classified, left hand**
  - **M67.249 Synovial hypertrophy, not elsewhere classified, unspecified hand**

+ **M67.25 Synovial hypertrophy, not elsewhere classified, thigh**
  - **M67.251 Synovial hypertrophy, not elsewhere classified, right thigh**
  - **M67.252 Synovial hypertrophy, not elsewhere classified, left thigh**
  - **M67.259 Synovial hypertrophy, not elsewhere classified, unspecified thigh**

+ **M67.26 Synovial hypertrophy, not elsewhere classified, lower leg**
  - **M67.261 Synovial hypertrophy, not elsewhere classified, right lower leg**
  - **M67.262 Synovial hypertrophy, not elsewhere classified, left lower leg**
  - **M67.269 Synovial hypertrophy, not elsewhere classified, unspecified lower leg**

+ **M67.27 Synovial hypertrophy, not elsewhere classified, ankle and foot**
  - **M67.271 Synovial hypertrophy, not elsewhere classified, right ankle and foot**
  - **M67.272 Synovial hypertrophy, not elsewhere classified, left ankle and foot**
  - **M67.279 Synovial hypertrophy, not elsewhere classified, unspecified ankle and foot**

M67.28 Synovial hypertrophy, not elsewhere classified, other site

M67.29 Synovial hypertrophy, not elsewhere classified, multiple sites

+ **M67.3 Transient synovitis**

Toxic synovitis

Excludes1: *palindromic rheumatism (M12.3-)*

M67.30 Transient synovitis, unspecified site

+ **M67.31 Transient synovitis, shoulder**
  - **M67.311 Transient synovitis, right shoulder**
  - **M67.312 Transient synovitis, left shoulder**
  - **M67.319 Transient synovitis, unspecified shoulder**

+ **M67.32 Transient synovitis, elbow**
  - **M67.321 Transient synovitis, right elbow**
  - **M67.322 Transient synovitis, left elbow**
  - **M67.329 Transient synovitis, unspecified elbow**

+ **M67.33 Transient synovitis, wrist**
  - **M67.331 Transient synovitis, right wrist**
  - **M67.332 Transient synovitis, left wrist**
  - **M67.339 Transient synovitis, unspecified wrist**

+ **M67.34 Transient synovitis, hand**
  - **M67.341 Transient synovitis, right hand**
  - **M67.342 Transient synovitis, left hand**
  - **M67.349 Transient synovitis, unspecified hand**

+ **M67.35 Transient synovitis, hip**
  - **M67.351 Transient synovitis, right hip**
  - **M67.352 Transient synovitis, left hip**
  - **M67.359 Transient synovitis, unspecified hip**

+ **M67.36 Transient synovitis, knee**
  - **M67.361 Transient synovitis, right knee**
  - **M67.362 Transient synovitis, left knee**
  - **M67.369 Transient synovitis, unspecified knee**

+ **M67.37 Transient synovitis, ankle and foot**
  - **M67.371 Transient synovitis, right ankle and foot**
  - **M67.372 Transient synovitis, left ankle and foot**
  - **M67.379 Transient synovitis, unspecified ankle and foot**

M67.38 Transient synovitis, other site

M67.39 Transient synovitis, multiple sites

+ **M67.4 Ganglion**

Ganglion of joint or tendon (sheath)

Excludes1: *ganglion in yaws (A66.6)*

Excludes2: *cyst of bursa (M71.2-M71.3)*
cyst of synovium (M71.2-M71.3)

M67.40 Ganglion, unspecified site

+ **M67.41 Ganglion, shoulder**
  - **M67.411 Ganglion, right shoulder**
  - **M67.412 Ganglion, left shoulder**
  - **M67.419 Ganglion, unspecified shoulder**

+ **M67.42 Ganglion, elbow**
  - **M67.421 Ganglion, right elbow**
  - **M67.422 Ganglion, left elbow**
  - **M67.429 Ganglion, unspecified elbow**

+ **M67.43 Ganglion, wrist**
  - **M67.431 Ganglion, right wrist**
  - **M67.432 Ganglion, left wrist**
  - **M67.439 Ganglion, unspecified wrist**

+ **M67.44 Ganglion, hand**
  - **M67.441 Ganglion, right hand**
  - **M67.442 Ganglion, left hand**
  - **M67.449 Ganglion, unspecified hand**

+ **M67.45 Ganglion, hip**
  - **M67.451 Ganglion, right hip**
  - **M67.452 Ganglion, left hip**
  - **M67.459 Ganglion, unspecified hip**

+ **M67.46 Ganglion, knee**
  - **M67.461 Ganglion, right knee**
  - **M67.462 Ganglion, left knee**
  - **M67.469 Ganglion, unspecified knee**

+ **M67.47 Ganglion, ankle and foot**
  - **M67.471 Ganglion, right ankle and foot**
  - **M67.472 Ganglion, left ankle and foot**
  - **M67.479 Ganglion, unspecified ankle and foot**

M67.48 Ganglion, other site

M67.49 Ganglion, multiple sites

+ **M67.5 Plica syndrome**
  Plica knee
  - **M67.50 Plica syndrome, unspecified knee**
  - **M67.51 Plica syndrome, right knee**
  - **M67.52 Plica syndrome, left knee**

+ **M67.8 Other specified disorders of synovium and tendon**
  - **M67.80 Other specified disorders of synovium and tendon, unspecified site**

+ **M67.81 Other specified disorders of synovium and tendon, shoulder**
  - **M67.811 Other specified disorders of synovium, right shoulder**
  - **M67.812 Other specified disorders of synovium, left shoulder**
  - **M67.813 Other specified disorders of tendon, right shoulder**
  - **M67.814 Other specified disorders of tendon, left shoulder**
  - **M67.819 Other specified disorders of synovium and tendon, unspecified shoulder**

+ **M67.82 Other specified disorders of synovium and tendon, elbow**
  - **M67.821 Other specified disorders of synovium, right elbow**
  - **M67.822 Other specified disorders of synovium, left elbow**
  - **M67.823 Other specified disorders of tendon, right elbow**
  - **M67.824 Other specified disorders of tendon, left elbow**
  - **M67.829 Other specified disorders of synovium and tendon, unspecified elbow**

+ **M67.83 Other specified disorders of synovium and tendon, wrist**
  - **M67.831 Other specified disorders of synovium, right wrist**
  - **M67.832 Other specified disorders of synovium, left wrist**
  - **M67.833 Other specified disorders of tendon, right wrist**
  - **M67.834 Other specified disorders of tendon, left wrist**
  - **M67.839 Other specified disorders of synovium and tendon, unspecified wrist**

+ **M67.84 Other specified disorders of synovium and tendon, hand**
  - **M67.841 Other specified disorders of synovium, right hand**
  - **M67.842 Other specified disorders of synovium, left hand**
  - **M67.843 Other specified disorders of tendon, right hand**
  - **M67.844 Other specified disorders of tendon, left hand**
  - **M67.849 Other specified disorders of synovium and tendon, unspecified hand**

+ **M67.85 Other specified disorders of synovium and tendon, hip**
  - **M67.851 Other specified disorders of synovium, right hip**
  - **M67.852 Other specified disorders of synovium, left hip**
  - **M67.853 Other specified disorders of tendon, right hip**
  - **M67.854 Other specified disorders of tendon, left hip**
  - **M67.859 Other specified disorders of synovium and tendon, unspecified hip**

+ **M67.86 Other specified disorders of synovium and tendon, knee**
  - **M67.861 Other specified disorders of synovium, right knee**
  - **M67.862 Other specified disorders of synovium, left knee**
  - **M67.863 Other specified disorders of tendon, right knee**
  - **M67.864 Other specified disorders of tendon, left knee**
  - **M67.869 Other specified disorders of synovium and tendon, unspecified knee**

+ **M67.87 Other specified disorders of synovium and tendon, ankle and foot**
  - **M67.871 Other specified disorders of synovium, right ankle and foot**
  - **M67.872 Other specified disorders of synovium, left ankle and foot**
  - **M67.873 Other specified disorders of tendon, right ankle and foot**
  - **M67.874 Other specified disorders of tendon, left ankle and foot**
  - **M67.879 Other specified disorders of synovium and tendon, unspecified ankle and foot**

M67.88 Other specified disorders of synovium and tendon, other site

M67.89 Other specified disorders of synovium and tendon, multiple sites

+ **M67.9 Unspecified disorder of synovium and tendon**
  - **M67.90 Unspecified disorder of synovium and tendon, unspecified site**

+ **M67.91 Unspecified disorder of synovium and tendon, shoulder**
  - **M67.911 Unspecified disorder of synovium and tendon, right shoulder**
  - **M67.912 Unspecified disorder of synovium and tendon, left shoulder**
  - **M67.919 Unspecified disorder of synovium and tendon, unspecified shoulder**

+ **M67.92 Unspecified disorder of synovium and tendon, upper arm**
  - **M67.921 Unspecified disorder of synovium and tendon, right upper arm**
  - **M67.922 Unspecified disorder of synovium and tendon, left upper arm**
  - **M67.929 Unspecified disorder of synovium and tendon, unspecified upper arm**

+ **M67.93 Unspecified disorder of synovium and tendon, forearm**
  - **M67.931 Unspecified disorder of synovium and tendon, right forearm**
  - **M67.932 Unspecified disorder of synovium and tendon, left forearm**
  - **M67.939 Unspecified disorder of synovium and tendon, unspecified forearm**

+ **M67.94 Unspecified disorder of synovium and tendon, hand**
  - **M67.941 Unspecified disorder of synovium and tendon, right hand**
  - **M67.942 Unspecified disorder of synovium and tendon, left hand**
  - **M67.949 Unspecified disorder of synovium and tendon, unspecified hand**

+ **M67.95 Unspecified disorder of synovium and tendon, thigh**
  - **M67.951 Unspecified disorder of synovium and tendon, right thigh**
  - **M67.952 Unspecified disorder of synovium and tendon, left thigh**
  - **M67.959 Unspecified disorder of synovium and tendon, unspecified thigh**

+ **M67.96 Unspecified disorder of synovium and tendon, lower leg**
  - **M67.961 Unspecified disorder of synovium and tendon, right lower leg**
  - **M67.962 Unspecified disorder of synovium and tendon, left lower leg**
  - **M67.969 Unspecified disorder of synovium and tendon, unspecified lower leg**

+ **M67.97 Unspecified disorder of synovium and tendon, ankle and foot**
  - **M67.971 Unspecified disorder of synovium and tendon, right ankle and foot**
  - **M67.972 Unspecified disorder of synovium and tendon, left ankle and foot**
  - **M67.979 Unspecified disorder of synovium and tendon, unspecified ankle and foot**

M67.98 Unspecified disorder of synovium and tendon, other site

M67.99 Unspecified disorder of synovium and tendon, multiple sites

Other soft tissue disorders (M70-M79)

M70 Soft tissue disorders related to use, overuse and pressure

Includes: soft tissue disorders of occupational origin

Use additional external cause code to identify activity causing disorder (Y93.-)

Excludes1: *bursitis NOS (M71.9-)*

Excludes2: *bursitis of shoulder (M75.5)*
enthesopathies (M76-M77)
pressure ulcer (pressure area) (L89.-)

+ **M70.0 Crepitant synovitis (acute) (chronic) of hand and wrist**

+ **M70.03 Crepitant synovitis (acute) (chronic), wrist**
  - **M70.031 Crepitant synovitis (acute) (chronic), right wrist**
  - **M70.032 Crepitant synovitis (acute) (chronic), left wrist**
  - **M70.039 Crepitant synovitis (acute) (chronic), unspecified wrist**

+ **M70.04 Crepitant synovitis (acute) (chronic), hand**
  - **M70.041 Crepitant synovitis (acute) (chronic), right hand**
  - **M70.042 Crepitant synovitis (acute) (chronic), left hand**
  - **M70.049 Crepitant synovitis (acute) (chronic), unspecified hand**

+ **M70.1 Bursitis of hand**
  - **M70.10 Bursitis, unspecified hand**
  - **M70.11 Bursitis, right hand**
  - **M70.12 Bursitis, left hand**

+ **M70.2 Olecranon bursitis**
  - **M70.20 Olecranon bursitis, unspecified elbow**
  - **M70.21 Olecranon bursitis, right elbow**
  - **M70.22 Olecranon bursitis, left elbow**

+ **M70.3 Other bursitis of elbow**
  - **M70.30 Other bursitis of elbow, unspecified elbow**
  - **M70.31 Other bursitis of elbow, right elbow**
  - **M70.32 Other bursitis of elbow, left elbow**

+ **M70.4 Prepatellar bursitis**
  - **M70.40 Prepatellar bursitis, unspecified knee**
  - **M70.41 Prepatellar bursitis, right knee**
  - **M70.42 Prepatellar bursitis, left knee**

+ **M70.5 Other bursitis of knee**
  - **M70.50 Other bursitis of knee, unspecified knee**
  - **M70.51 Other bursitis of knee, right knee**
  - **M70.52 Other bursitis of knee, left knee**

+ **M70.6 Trochanteric bursitis**
  Trochanteric tendinitis
  - **M70.60 Trochanteric bursitis, unspecified hip**
  - **M70.61 Trochanteric bursitis, right hip**
  - **M70.62 Trochanteric bursitis, left hip**

+ **M70.7 Other bursitis of hip**
  Ischial bursitis
  - **M70.70 Other bursitis of hip, unspecified hip**
  - **M70.71 Other bursitis of hip, right hip**
  - **M70.72 Other bursitis of hip, left hip**

+ **M70.8 Other soft tissue disorders related to use, overuse and pressure**

M70.80 Other soft tissue disorders related to use, overuse and pressure of unspecified site

+ **M70.81 Other soft tissue disorders related to use, overuse and pressure of shoulder**
  - **M70.811 Other soft tissue disorders related to use, overuse and pressure, right shoulder**
  - **M70.812 Other soft tissue disorders related to use, overuse and pressure, left shoulder**
  - **M70.819 Other soft tissue disorders related to use, overuse and pressure, unspecified shoulder**

+ **M70.82 Other soft tissue disorders related to use, overuse and pressure of upper arm**
  - **M70.821 Other soft tissue disorders related to use, overuse and pressure, right upper arm**
  - **M70.822 Other soft tissue disorders related to use, overuse and pressure, left upper arm**
  - **M70.829 Other soft tissue disorders related to use, overuse and pressure, unspecified upper arms**

+ **M70.83 Other soft tissue disorders related to use, overuse and pressure of forearm**
  - **M70.831 Other soft tissue disorders related to use, overuse and pressure, right forearm**
  - **M70.832 Other soft tissue disorders related to use, overuse and pressure, left forearm**
  - **M70.839 Other soft tissue disorders related to use, overuse and pressure, unspecified forearm**

+ **M70.84 Other soft tissue disorders related to use, overuse and pressure of hand**
  - **M70.841 Other soft tissue disorders related to use, overuse and pressure, right hand**
  - **M70.842 Other soft tissue disorders related to use, overuse and pressure, left hand**
  - **M70.849 Other soft tissue disorders related to use, overuse and pressure, unspecified hand**

+ **M70.85 Other soft tissue disorders related to use, overuse and pressure of thigh**
  - **M70.851 Other soft tissue disorders related to use, overuse and pressure, right thigh**
  - **M70.852 Other soft tissue disorders related to use, overuse and pressure, left thigh**
  - **M70.859 Other soft tissue disorders related to use, overuse and pressure, unspecified thigh**

+ **M70.86 Other soft tissue disorders related to use, overuse and pressure lower leg**
  - **M70.861 Other soft tissue disorders related to use, overuse and pressure, right lower leg**
  - **M70.862 Other soft tissue disorders related to use, overuse and pressure, left lower leg**
  - **M70.869 Other soft tissue disorders related to use, overuse and pressure, unspecified leg**

+ **M70.87 Other soft tissue disorders related to use, overuse and pressure of ankle and foot**
  - **M70.871 Other soft tissue disorders related to use, overuse and pressure, right ankle and foot**
  - **M70.872 Other soft tissue disorders related to use, overuse and pressure, left ankle and foot**
  - **M70.879 Other soft tissue disorders related to use, overuse and pressure, unspecified ankle and foot**

M70.88 Other soft tissue disorders related to use, overuse and pressure other site

M70.89 Other soft tissue disorders related to use, overuse and pressure multiple sites

+ **M70.9 Unspecified soft tissue disorder related to use, overuse and pressure**
M70.90 Unspecified soft tissue disorder related to use, overuse and pressure of unspecified site
+ **M70.91 Unspecified soft tissue disorder related to use, overuse and pressure of shoulder**
M70.911 Unspecified soft tissue disorder related to use, overuse and pressure, right shoulder
M70.912 Unspecified soft tissue disorder related to use, overuse and pressure, left shoulder
M70.919 Unspecified soft tissue disorder related to use, overuse and pressure, unspecified shoulder
+ **M70.92 Unspecified soft tissue disorder related to use, overuse and pressure of upper arm**
M70.921 Unspecified soft tissue disorder related to use, overuse and pressure, right upper arm
M70.922 Unspecified soft tissue disorder related to use, overuse and pressure, left upper arm
M70.929 Unspecified soft tissue disorder related to use, overuse and pressure, unspecified upper arm
+ **M70.93 Unspecified soft tissue disorder related to use, overuse and pressure of forearm**
M70.931 Unspecified soft tissue disorder related to use, overuse and pressure, right forearm
M70.932 Unspecified soft tissue disorder related to use, overuse and pressure, left forearm
M70.939 Unspecified soft tissue disorder related to use, overuse and pressure, unspecified forearm
+ **M70.94 Unspecified soft tissue disorder related to use, overuse and pressure of hand**
M70.941 Unspecified soft tissue disorder related to use, overuse and pressure, right hand
M70.942 Unspecified soft tissue disorder related to use, overuse and pressure, left hand
M70.949 Unspecified soft tissue disorder related to use, overuse and pressure, unspecified hand
+ **M70.95 Unspecified soft tissue disorder related to use, overuse and pressure of thigh**
M70.951 Unspecified soft tissue disorder related to use, overuse and pressure, right thigh
M70.952 Unspecified soft tissue disorder related to use, overuse and pressure, left thigh
M70.959 Unspecified soft tissue disorder related to use, overuse and pressure, unspecified thigh
+ **M70.96 Unspecified soft tissue disorder related to use, overuse and pressure lower leg**
M70.961 Unspecified soft tissue disorder related to use, overuse and pressure, right lower leg
M70.962 Unspecified soft tissue disorder related to use, overuse and pressure, left lower leg
M70.969 Unspecified soft tissue disorder related to use, overuse and pressure, unspecified lower leg
+ **M70.97 Unspecified soft tissue disorder related to use, overuse and pressure of ankle and foot**
M70.971 Unspecified soft tissue disorder related to use, overuse and pressure, right ankle and foot
M70.972 Unspecified soft tissue disorder related to use, overuse and pressure, left ankle and foot
M70.979 Unspecified soft tissue disorder related to use, overuse and pressure, unspecified ankle and foot
M70.98 Unspecified soft tissue disorder related to use, overuse and pressure other
M70.99 Unspecified soft tissue disorder related to use, overuse and pressure multiple sites

M71 Other bursopathies
Excludes1: *bunion (M20.1)*
bursitis related to use, overuse or pressure (M70.-)
enthesopathies (M76-M77)
+ **M71.0 Abscess of bursa**
Use additional code (B95.-, B96.-) to identify causative organism
M71.00 Abscess of bursa, unspecified site
+ **M71.01 Abscess of bursa, shoulder**
M71.011 Abscess of bursa, right shoulder
M71.012 Abscess of bursa, left shoulder
M71.019 Abscess of bursa, unspecified shoulder
+ **M71.02 Abscess of bursa, elbow**
M71.021 Abscess of bursa, right elbow
M71.022 Abscess of bursa, left elbow
M71.029 Abscess of bursa, unspecified elbow
+ **M71.03 Abscess of bursa, wrist**
M71.031 Abscess of bursa, right wrist
M71.032 Abscess of bursa, left wrist
M71.039 Abscess of bursa, unspecified wrist
+ **M71.04 Abscess of bursa, hand**
M71.041 Abscess of bursa, right hand
M71.042 Abscess of bursa, left hand
M71.049 Abscess of bursa, unspecified hand
+ **M71.05 Abscess of bursa, hip**
M71.051 Abscess of bursa, right hip
M71.052 Abscess of bursa, left hip
M71.059 Abscess of bursa, unspecified hip
+ **M71.06 Abscess of bursa, knee**
M71.061 Abscess of bursa, right knee
M71.062 Abscess of bursa, left knee
M71.069 Abscess of bursa, unspecified knee
+ **M71.07 Abscess of bursa, ankle and foot**
M71.071 Abscess of bursa, right ankle and foot
M71.072 Abscess of bursa, left ankle and foot
M71.079 Abscess of bursa, unspecified ankle and foot
M71.08 Abscess of bursa, other site
M71.09 Abscess of bursa, multiple sites
+ **M71.1 Other infective bursitis**
Use additional code (B95.-, B96.-) to identify causative organism
M71.10 Other infective bursitis, unspecified site
+ **M71.11 Other infective bursitis, shoulder**
M71.111 Other infective bursitis, right shoulder
M71.112 Other infective bursitis, left shoulder
M71.119 Other infective bursitis, unspecified shoulder
+ **M71.12 Other infective bursitis, elbow**
M71.121 Other infective bursitis, right elbow
M71.122 Other infective bursitis, left elbow
M71.129 Other infective bursitis, unspecified elbow
+ **M71.13 Other infective bursitis, wrist**
M71.131 Other infective bursitis, right wrist
M71.132 Other infective bursitis, left wrist
M71.139 Other infective bursitis, unspecified wrist
+ **M71.14 Other infective bursitis, hand**
M71.141 Other infective bursitis, right hand
M71.142 Other infective bursitis, left hand
M71.149 Other infective bursitis, unspecified hand
+ **M71.15 Other infective bursitis, hip**
M71.151 Other infective bursitis, right hip
M71.152 Other infective bursitis, left hip
M71.159 Other infective bursitis, unspecified hip
+ **M71.16 Other infective bursitis, knee**
M71.161 Other infective bursitis, right knee
M71.162 Other infective bursitis, left knee
M71.169 Other infective bursitis, unspecified knee
+ **M71.17 Other infective bursitis, ankle and foot**
M71.171 Other infective bursitis, right ankle and foot
M71.172 Other infective bursitis, left ankle and foot
M71.179 Other infective bursitis, unspecified ankle and foot
M71.18 Other infective bursitis, other site
M71.19 Other infective bursitis, multiple sites

+ **M71.2 Synovial cyst of popliteal space [Baker]**
  Excludes1: *synovial cyst of popliteal space with rupture (M66.0)*
  M71.20 Synovial cyst of popliteal space [Baker], unspecified knee
  M71.21 Synovial cyst of popliteal space [Baker], right knee
  M71.22 Synovial cyst of popliteal space [Baker], left knee
+ **M71.3 Other bursal cyst**
  Synovial cyst NOS
  Excludes1: *synovial cyst with rupture (M66.1-)*
  M71.30 Other bursal cyst, unspecified site
  + **M71.31 Other bursal cyst, shoulder**
    M71.311 Other bursal cyst, right shoulder
    M71.312 Other bursal cyst, left shoulder
    M71.319 Other bursal cyst, unspecified shoulder
  + **M71.32 Other bursal cyst, elbow**
    M71.321 Other bursal cyst, right elbow
    M71.322 Other bursal cyst, left elbow
    M71.329 Other bursal cyst, unspecified elbow
  + **M71.33 Other bursal cyst, wrist**
    M71.331 Other bursal cyst, right wrist
    M71.332 Other bursal cyst, left wrist
    M71.339 Other bursal cyst, unspecified wrist
  + **M71.34 Other bursal cyst, hand**
    M71.341 Other bursal cyst, right hand
    M71.342 Other bursal cyst, left hand
    M71.349 Other bursal cyst, unspecified hand
  + **M71.35 Other bursal cyst, hip**
    M71.351 Other bursal cyst, right hip
    M71.352 Other bursal cyst, left hip
    M71.359 Other bursal cyst, unspecified hip
  + **M71.37 Other bursal cyst, ankle and foot**
    M71.371 Other bursal cyst, right ankle and foot
    M71.372 Other bursal cyst, left ankle and foot
    M71.379 Other bursal cyst, unspecified ankle and foot
  M71.38 Other bursal cyst, other site
  M71.39 Other bursal cyst, multiple sites
+ **M71.4 Calcium deposit in bursa**
  Excludes2: *calcium deposit in bursa of shoulder (M75.3)*
  M71.40 Calcium deposit in bursa, unspecified site
  + **M71.42 Calcium deposit in bursa, elbow**
    M71.421 Calcium deposit in bursa, right elbow
    M71.422 Calcium deposit in bursa, left elbow
    M71.429 Calcium deposit in bursa, unspecified elbow
  + **M71.43 Calcium deposit in bursa, wrist**
    M71.431 Calcium deposit in bursa, right wrist
    M71.432 Calcium deposit in bursa, left wrist
    M71.439 Calcium deposit in bursa, unspecified wrist
  + **M71.44 Calcium deposit in bursa, hand**
    M71.441 Calcium deposit in bursa, right hand
    M71.442 Calcium deposit in bursa, left hand
    M71.449 Calcium deposit in bursa, unspecified hand
  + **M71.45 Calcium deposit in bursa, hip**
    M71.451 Calcium deposit in bursa, right hip
    M71.452 Calcium deposit in bursa, left hip
    M71.459 Calcium deposit in bursa, unspecified hip
  + **M71.46 Calcium deposit in bursa, knee**
    M71.461 Calcium deposit in bursa, right knee
    M71.462 Calcium deposit in bursa, left knee
    M71.469 Calcium deposit in bursa, unspecified knee
  + **M71.47 Calcium deposit in bursa, ankle and foot**
    M71.471 Calcium deposit in bursa, right ankle and foot
    M71.472 Calcium deposit in bursa, left ankle and foot
    M71.479 Calcium deposit in bursa, unspecified ankle and foot
  M71.48 Calcium deposit in bursa, other site
  M71.49 Calcium deposit in bursa, multiple sites
+ **M71.5 Other bursitis, not elsewhere classified**
  Excludes1: *bursitis NOS (M71.9-)*
  Excludes2: *bursitis of shoulder (M75.5)*
  bursitis of tibial collateral [Pellegrini-Stieda] (M76.4-)
  M71.50 Other bursitis, not elsewhere classified, unspecified site
  + **M71.52 Other bursitis, not elsewhere classified, elbow**
    M71.521 Other bursitis, not elsewhere classified, right elbow
    M71.522 Other bursitis, not elsewhere classified, left elbow
    M71.529 Other bursitis, not elsewhere classified, unspecified elbow
  + **M71.53 Other bursitis, not elsewhere classified, wrist**
    M71.531 Other bursitis, not elsewhere classified, right wrist
    M71.532 Other bursitis, not elsewhere classified, left wrist
    M71.539 Other bursitis, not elsewhere classified, unspecified wrist
  + **M71.54 Other bursitis, not elsewhere classified, hand**
    M71.541 Other bursitis, not elsewhere classified, right hand
    M71.542 Other bursitis, not elsewhere classified, left hand
    M71.549 Other bursitis, not elsewhere classified, unspecified hand
  + **M71.55 Other bursitis, not elsewhere classified, hip**
    M71.551 Other bursitis, not elsewhere classified, right hip
    M71.552 Other bursitis, not elsewhere classified, left hip
    M71.559 Other bursitis, not elsewhere classified, unspecified hip
  + **M71.56 Other bursitis, not elsewhere classified, knee**
    M71.561 Other bursitis, not elsewhere classified, right knee
    M71.562 Other bursitis, not elsewhere classified, left knee
    M71.569 Other bursitis, not elsewhere classified, unspecified knee
  + **M71.57 Other bursitis, not elsewhere classified, ankle and foot**
    M71.571 Other bursitis, not elsewhere classified, right ankle and foot
    M71.572 Other bursitis, not elsewhere classified, left ankle and foot
    M71.579 Other bursitis, not elsewhere classified, unspecified ankle and foot
  M71.58 Other bursitis, not elsewhere classified, other site
+ **M71.8 Other specified bursopathies**
  M71.80 Other specified bursopathies, unspecified site
  + **M71.81 Other specified bursopathies, shoulder**
    M71.811 Other specified bursopathies, right shoulder
    M71.812 Other specified bursopathies, left shoulder
    M71.819 Other specified bursopathies, unspecified shoulder
  + **M71.82 Other specified bursopathies, elbow**
    M71.821 Other specified bursopathies, right elbow
    M71.822 Other specified bursopathies, left elbow
    M71.829 Other specified bursopathies, unspecified elbow
  + **M71.83 Other specified bursopathies, wrist**
    M71.831 Other specified bursopathies, right wrist
    M71.832 Other specified bursopathies, left wrist
    M71.839 Other specified bursopathies, unspecified wrist
  + **M71.84 Other specified bursopathies, hand**
    M71.841 Other specified bursopathies, right hand
    M71.842 Other specified bursopathies, left hand
    M71.849 Other specified bursopathies, unspecified hand

+ **M71.85 Other specified bursopathies, hip**
  - **M71.851 Other specified bursopathies, right hip**
  - **M71.852 Other specified bursopathies, left hip**
  - **M71.859 Other specified bursopathies, unspecified hip**
+ **M71.86 Other specified bursopathies, knee**
  - **M71.861 Other specified bursopathies, right knee**
  - **M71.862 Other specified bursopathies, left knee**
  - **M71.869 Other specified bursopathies, unspecified knee**
+ **M71.87 Other specified bursopathies, ankle and foot**
  - **M71.871 Other specified bursopathies, right ankle and foot**
  - **M71.872 Other specified bursopathies, left ankle and foot**
  - **M71.879 Other specified bursopathies, unspecified ankle and foot**

M71.88 Other specified bursopathies, other site

M71.89 Other specified bursopathies, multiple sites

M71.9 Bursopathy, unspecified
Bursitis NOS

M72 Fibroblastic disorders

Excludes2: *retroperitoneal fibromatosis (D48.3)*

• **M72.0 Palmar fascial fibromatosis [Dupuytren]**

M72.1 Knuckle pads

M72.2 Plantar fascial fibromatosis
Plantar fasciitis

M72.4 Pseudosarcomatous fibromatosis
Nodular fasciitis

MCC **M72.6 Necrotizing fasciitis**
Use additional code (B95.-, B96.-) to identify causative organism

M72.8 Other fibroblastic disorders
Abscess of fascia
Fasciitis NEC
Other infective fasciitis
Use additional code to (B95.-, B96.-) identify causative organism
Excludes1: *diffuse (eosinophilic) fasciitis (M35.4)*
necrotizing fasciitis (M72.6)
nodular fasciitis (M72.4)
perirenal fasciitis NOS (N13.5)
perirenal fasciitis with infection (N13.6)
plantar fasciitis (M72.2)

M72.9 Fibroblastic disorder, unspecified
Fasciitis NOS
Fibromatosis NOS

M75 Shoulder lesions

Excludes2: *shoulder-hand syndrome (M89.0-)*

+ **M75.0 Adhesive capsulitis of shoulder**
  Frozen shoulder
  Periarthritis of shoulder
  - **M75.00 Adhesive capsulitis of unspecified shoulder**
  - **M75.01 Adhesive capsulitis of right shoulder**
  - **M75.02 Adhesive capsulitis of left shoulder**
+ **M75.1 Rotator cuff tear or rupture, not specified as traumatic**
  Rotator cuff syndrome
  Supraspinatus tear or rupture, not specified as traumatic
  Supraspinatus syndrome
  Excludes1: *tear of rotator cuff, traumatic (S46.01-)*
+ **M75.10 Unspecified rotator cuff tear or rupture, not specified as traumatic**
  - **M75.100 Unspecified rotator cuff tear or rupture of unspecified shoulder, not specified as traumatic**
  - **M75.101 Unspecified rotator cuff tear or rupture of right shoulder, not specified as traumatic**
  - **M75.102 Unspecified rotator cuff tear or rupture of left shoulder, not specified as traumatic**
+ **M75.11 Incomplete rotator cuff tear or rupture not specified as traumatic**
  - **M75.110 Incomplete rotator cuff tear or rupture of unspecified shoulder, not specified as traumatic**
  - **M75.111 Incomplete rotator cuff tear or rupture of right shoulder, not specified as traumatic**
  - **M75.112 Incomplete rotator cuff tear or rupture of left shoulder, not specified as traumatic**
+ **M75.12 Complete rotator cuff tear or rupture not specified as traumatic**
  - **M75.120 Complete rotator cuff tear or rupture of unspecified shoulder, not specified as traumatic**
  - **M75.121 Complete rotator cuff tear or rupture of right shoulder, not specified as traumatic**
  - **M75.122 Complete rotator cuff tear or rupture of left shoulder, not specified as traumatic**
+ **M75.2 Bicipital tendinitis**
  - **M75.20 Bicipital tendinitis, unspecified shoulder**
  - **M75.21 Bicipital tendinitis, right shoulder**
  - **M75.22 Bicipital tendinitis, left shoulder**
+ **M75.3 Calcific tendinitis of shoulder**
  Calcified bursa of shoulder
  - **M75.30 Calcific tendinitis of unspecified shoulder**
  - **M75.31 Calcific tendinitis of right shoulder**
  - **M75.32 Calcific tendinitis of left shoulder**
+ **M75.4 Impingement syndrome of shoulder**
  - **M75.40 Impingement syndrome of unspecified shoulder**
  - **M75.41 Impingement syndrome of right shoulder**
  - **M75.42 Impingement syndrome of left shoulder**
+ **M75.5 Bursitis of shoulder**
  - **M75.50 Bursitis of unspecified shoulder**
  - **M75.51 Bursitis of right shoulder**
  - **M75.52 Bursitis of left shoulder**
+ **M75.8 Other shoulder lesions**
  - **M75.80 Other shoulder lesions, unspecified shoulder**
  - **M75.81 Other shoulder lesions, right shoulder**
  - **M75.82 Other shoulder lesions, left shoulder**
+ **M75.9 Shoulder lesion, unspecified**
  - **M75.90 Shoulder lesion, unspecified, unspecified shoulder**
  - **M75.91 Shoulder lesion, unspecified, right shoulder**
  - **M75.92 Shoulder lesion, unspecified, left shoulder**

M76 Enthesopathies, lower limb, excluding foot

Excludes2: *bursitis due to use, overuse and pressure (M70.-)*
enthesopathies of ankle and foot (M77.5-)

+ **M76.0 Gluteal tendinitis**
  - **M76.00 Gluteal tendinitis, unspecified hip**
  - **M76.01 Gluteal tendinitis, right hip**
  - **M76.02 Gluteal tendinitis, left hip**
+ **M76.1 Psoas tendinitis**
  - **M76.10 Psoas tendinitis, unspecified hip**
  - **M76.11 Psoas tendinitis, right hip**
  - **M76.12 Psoas tendinitis, left hip**
+ **M76.2 Iliac crest spur**
  - **M76.20 Iliac crest spur, unspecified hip**
  - **M76.21 Iliac crest spur, right hip**
  - **M76.22 Iliac crest spur, left hip**
+ **M76.3 Iliotibial band syndrome**
  - **M76.30 Iliotibial band syndrome, unspecified leg**
  - **M76.31 Iliotibial band syndrome, right leg**
  - **M76.32 Iliotibial band syndrome, left leg**
+ **M76.4 Tibial collateral bursitis [Pellegrini-Stieda]**
  - **M76.40 Tibial collateral bursitis [Pellegrini-Stieda], unspecified leg**
  - **M76.41 Tibial collateral bursitis [Pellegrini-Stieda], right leg**
  - **M76.42 Tibial collateral bursitis [Pellegrini-Stieda], left leg**
+ **M76.5 Patellar tendinitis**
  - **M76.50 Patellar tendinitis, unspecified knee**
  - **M76.51 Patellar tendinitis, right knee**
  - **M76.52 Patellar tendinitis, left knee**

+ **M76.6 Achilles tendinitis**
  Achilles bursitis
  M76.60 Achilles tendinitis, unspecified leg
  M76.61 Achilles tendinitis, right leg
  M76.62 Achilles tendinitis, left leg
+ **M76.7 Peroneal tendinitis**
  M76.70 Peroneal tendinitis, unspecified leg
  M76.71 Peroneal tendinitis, right leg
  M76.72 Peroneal tendinitis, left leg
+ **M76.8 Other specified enthesopathies of lower limb, excluding foot**
  + **M76.81 Anterior tibial syndrome**
    M76.811 Anterior tibial syndrome, right leg
    M76.812 Anterior tibial syndrome, left leg
    M76.819 Anterior tibial syndrome, unspecified leg
  + **M76.82 Posterior tibial tendinitis**
    M76.821 Posterior tibial tendinitis, right leg
    M76.822 Posterior tibial tendinitis, left leg
    M76.829 Posterior tibial tendinitis, unspecified leg
  + **M76.89 Other specified enthesopathies of lower limb, excluding foot**
    M76.891 Other specified enthesopathies of right lower limb, excluding foot
    M76.892 Other specified enthesopathies of left lower limb, excluding foot
    M76.899 Other specified enthesopathies of unspecified lower limb, excluding foot
M76.9 Unspecified enthesopathy, lower limb, excluding foot

M77 Other enthesopathies
Excludes1: *bursitis NOS (M71.9-)*
Excludes2: *bursitis due to use, overuse and pressure (M70.-)*
osteophyte (M25.7)
spinal enthesopathy (M46.0-)
+ **M77.0 Medial epicondylitis**
  M77.00 Medial epicondylitis, unspecified elbow
  M77.01 Medial epicondylitis, right elbow
  M77.02 Medial epicondylitis, left elbow
+ **M77.1 Lateral epicondylitis**
  Tennis elbow
  M77.10 Lateral epicondylitis, unspecified elbow
  M77.11 Lateral epicondylitis, right elbow
  M77.12 Lateral epicondylitis, left elbow
+ **M77.2 Periarthritis of wrist**
  M77.20 Periarthritis, unspecified wrist
  M77.21 Periarthritis, right wrist
  M77.22 Periarthritis, left wrist
+ **M77.3 Calcaneal spur**
  M77.30 Calcaneal spur, unspecified foot
  M77.31 Calcaneal spur, right foot
  M77.32 Calcaneal spur, left foot
+ **M77.4 Metatarsalgia**
  Excludes1: *Morton's metatarsalgia (G57.6)*
  M77.40 Metatarsalgia, unspecified foot
  M77.41 Metatarsalgia, right foot
  M77.42 Metatarsalgia, left foot
+ **M77.5 Other enthesopathy of foot and ankle**
  M77.50 Other enthesopathy of unspecified foot and ankle
  M77.51 Other enthesopathy of right foot and ankle
  M77.52 Other enthesopathy of left foot and ankle
M77.8 Other enthesopathies, not elsewhere classified
M77.9 Enthesopathy, unspecified
  Bone spur NOS
  Capsulitis NOS
  Periarthritis NOS
  Tendinitis NOS

M79 Other and unspecified soft tissue disorders, not elsewhere classified
Excludes1: *psychogenic rheumatism (F45.8)*
soft tissue pain, psychogenic (F45.41)
M79.0 Rheumatism, unspecified
  Excludes1: *fibromyalgia (M79.7)*
  palindromic rheumatism (M12.3-)
+ **M79.1 Myalgia**
  Myofascial pain syndrome
  Excludes1: *fibromyalgia (M79.7)*
  myositis (M60.-)
  AHA CC: 4Q, 2018, 21
  M79.10 Myalgia, unspecified site
  M79.11 Myalgia of mastication muscle
  M79.12 Myalgia of auxiliary muscles, head and neck
  M79.18 Myalgia, other site
M79.2 Neuralgia and neuritis, unspecified
  Excludes1: *brachial radiculitis NOS (M54.1)*
  lumbosacral radiculitis NOS (M54.1)
  mononeuropathies (G56-G58)
  radiculitis NOS (M54.1)
  sciatica (M54.3-M54.4)
M79.3 Panniculitis, unspecified
  Excludes1: *lupus panniculitis (L93.2)*
  neck and back panniculitis (M54.0-)
  relapsing [Weber-Christian] panniculitis (M35.6)
M79.4 Hypertrophy of (infrapatellar) fat pad
M79.5 Residual foreign body in soft tissue
  Excludes1: *foreign body granuloma of skin and subcutaneous tissue (L92.3)*
  foreign body granuloma of soft tissue (M60.2-)
+ **M79.6 Pain in limb, hand, foot, fingers and toes**
  Excludes2: *pain in joint (M25.5-)*
  + **M79.60 Pain in limb, unspecified**
    M79.601 Pain in right arm
    Pain in right upper limb NOS
    M79.602 Pain in left arm
    Pain in left upper limb NOS
    M79.603 Pain in arm, unspecified
    Pain in upper limb NOS
    M79.604 Pain in right leg
    Pain in right lower limb NOS
    M79.605 Pain in left leg
    Pain in left lower limb NOS
    M79.606 Pain in leg, unspecified
    Pain in lower limb NOS
    M79.609 Pain in unspecified limb
    Pain in limb NOS
  + **M79.62 Pain in upper arm**
    Pain in axillary region
    M79.621 Pain in right upper arm
    M79.622 Pain in left upper arm
    M79.629 Pain in unspecified upper arm
  + **M79.63 Pain in forearm**
    M79.631 Pain in right forearm
    M79.632 Pain in left forearm
    M79.639 Pain in unspecified forearm
  + **M79.64 Pain in hand and fingers**
    M79.641 Pain in right hand
    M79.642 Pain in left hand
    M79.643 Pain in unspecified hand
    M79.644 Pain in right finger(s)
    M79.645 Pain in left finger(s)
    M79.646 Pain in unspecified finger(s)
  + **M79.65 Pain in thigh**
    M79.651 Pain in right thigh
    M79.652 Pain in left thigh
    M79.659 Pain in unspecified thigh
  + **M79.66 Pain in lower leg**
    M79.661 Pain in right lower leg
    M79.662 Pain in left lower leg
    M79.669 Pain in unspecified lower leg
  + **M79.67 Pain in foot and toes**
    M79.671 Pain in right foot
    M79.672 Pain in left foot
    M79.673 Pain in unspecified foot
    M79.674 Pain in right toe(s)
    M79.675 Pain in left toe(s)
    M79.676 Pain in unspecified toe(s)
M79.7 Fibromyalgia
  Fibromyositis
  Fibrositis
  Myofibrositis

Osteoporosis

Axial

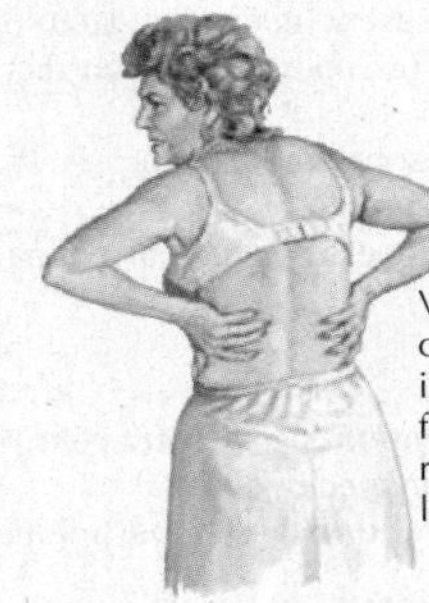

Vertebral compression fractures cause continuous (acute) or intermittent (chronic) back pain from midthoracic to midlumbar region, occasionally to lower lumbar region.

A change in backbone strength over time

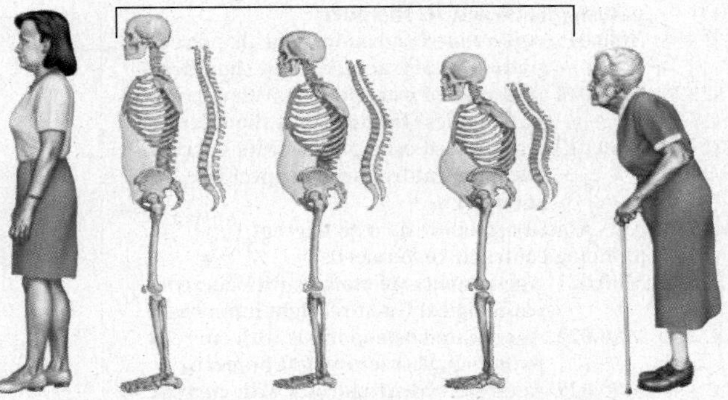

Osteoporosis is the thinning of the bones. Bones become fragile and loss of height is common as the back bones begin to collapse.

Characteristics of Osteoporosis	
Characteristic	**Description**
Etiology	Postmenopausal women, genetics, vitamin D synthesis deficiency, idiopathic
Prevalence	Approximately 10 million Americans (8 million of them women), white
Risk factors	Family history, white female, increasing age, estrogen deficiency, vitamin D deficiency, low calcium intake, smoking, excessive alcohol use, inactive lifestyle
Complications	Vertebral compression fractures, fracture of proximal femur or humerus, ribs, and distal radius (Colles' fracture)

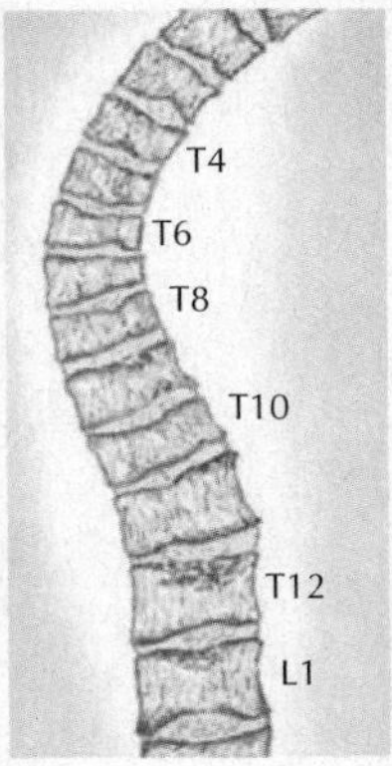

F. Netter M.D.
C. Machado M.D.

Multiple compression fractures of lower thoracic and upper lumbar vertebrae in patient with severe osteoporosis

Appendicular
Fractures caused by minimal trauma

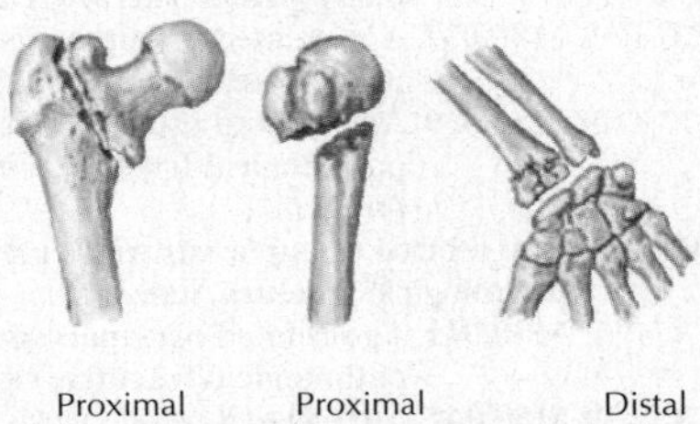

\+ **M79.A Nontraumatic compartment syndrome**
Code first if applicable, associated postprocedural complication
Excludes1: *compartment syndrome NOS (T79.A-)*
fibromyalgia (M79.7)
nontraumatic ischemic infarction of muscle (M62.2-)
traumatic compartment syndrome (T79.A-)

\+ **M79.A1 Nontraumatic compartment syndrome of upper extremity**
Nontraumatic compartment syndrome of shoulder, arm, forearm, wrist, hand, and fingers

CC **M79.A11 Nontraumatic compartment syndrome of right upper extremity**
CC **M79.A12 Nontraumatic compartment syndrome of left upper extremity**
CC **M79.A19 Nontraumatic compartment syndrome of unspecified upper extremity**

\+ **M79.A2 Nontraumatic compartment syndrome of lower extremity**
Nontraumatic compartment syndrome of hip, buttock, thigh, leg, foot, and toes

CC **M79.A21 Nontraumatic compartment syndrome of right lower extremity**
CC **M79.A22 Nontraumatic compartment syndrome of left lower extremity**
CC **M79.A29 Nontraumatic compartment syndrome of unspecified lower extremity**

CC **M79.A3 Nontraumatic compartment syndrome of abdomen**
CC **M79.A9 Nontraumatic compartment syndrome of other sites**

\+ **M79.8 Other specified soft tissue disorders**
M79.81 Nontraumatic hematoma of soft tissue
Nontraumatic hematoma of muscle
Nontraumatic seroma of muscle and soft tissue
M79.89 Other specified soft tissue disorders
Polyalgia

M79.9 Soft tissue disorder, unspecified

OSTEOPATHIES AND CHONDROPATHIES (M80-M94)

Disorders of bone density and structure (M80-M85)

M80 Osteoporosis with current pathological fracture
Includes: osteoporosis with current fragility fracture
Use additional code to identify major osseous defect, if applicable (M89.7-)
Excludes1: *collapsed vertebra NOS (M48.5)*
pathological fracture NOS (M84.4)
wedging of vertebra NOS (M48.5)
Excludes2: *personal history of (healed) osteoporosis fracture (Z87.310)*

The appropriate 7th character is to be added to each code from category M80:
A initial encounter for fracture
D subsequent encounter for fracture with routine healing
G subsequent encounter for fracture with delayed healing
K subsequent encounter for fracture with nonunion
P subsequent encounter for fracture with malunion
S sequela

Review coding guideline C.13.c
Review coding guideline C.19.c.1

\+ **M80.0 Age-related osteoporosis with current pathological fracture**
Involutional osteoporosis with current pathological fracture
Osteoporosis NOS with current pathological fracture
Postmenopausal osteoporosis with current pathological fracture
Senile osteoporosis with current pathological fracture

• CC X+7th **M80.00 Age-related osteoporosis with current pathological fracture, unspecified site**

+ **M80.01 Age-related osteoporosis with current pathological fracture, shoulder**

• CC +7th **M80.011 Age-related osteoporosis with current pathological fracture, right shoulder**

• CC +7th **M80.012 Age-related osteoporosis with current pathological fracture, left shoulder**

• CC +7th **M80.019 Age-related osteoporosis with current pathological fracture, unspecified shoulder**

+ **M80.02 Age-related osteoporosis with current pathological fracture, humerus**

• CC +7th **M80.021 Age-related osteoporosis with current pathological fracture, right humerus**

• CC +7th **M80.022 Age-related osteoporosis with current pathological fracture, left humerus**

• CC +7th **M80.029 Age-related osteoporosis with current pathological fracture, unspecified humerus**

+ **M80.03 Age-related osteoporosis with current pathological fracture, forearm**

Age-related osteoporosis with current pathological fracture of wrist

• CC +7th **M80.031 Age-related osteoporosis with current pathological fracture, right forearm**

• CC +7th **M80.032 Age-related osteoporosis with current pathological fracture, left forearm**

• CC +7th **M80.039 Age-related osteoporosis with current pathological fracture, unspecified forearm**

+ **M80.04 Age-related osteoporosis with current pathological fracture, hand**

• CC +7th **M80.041 Age-related osteoporosis with current pathological fracture, right hand**

• CC +7th **M80.042 Age-related osteoporosis with current pathological fracture, left hand**

• CC +7th **M80.049 Age-related osteoporosis with current pathological fracture, unspecified hand**

+ **M80.05 Age-related osteoporosis with current pathological fracture, femur**

Age-related osteoporosis with current pathological fracture of hip

• CC +7th **M80.051 Age-related osteoporosis with current pathological fracture, right femur**

AHA CC: 2Q, 2018, 12

• CC +7th **M80.052 Age-related osteoporosis with current pathological fracture, left femur**

• CC +7th **M80.059 Age-related osteoporosis with current pathological fracture, unspecified femur**

+ **M80.06 Age-related osteoporosis with current pathological fracture, lower leg**

• CC +7th **M80.061 Age-related osteoporosis with current pathological fracture, right lower leg**

• CC +7th **M80.062 Age-related osteoporosis with current pathological fracture, left lower leg**

• CC +7th **M80.069 Age-related osteoporosis with current pathological fracture, unspecified lower leg**

+ **M80.07 Age-related osteoporosis with current pathological fracture, ankle and foot**

• CC +7th **M80.071 Age-related osteoporosis with current pathological fracture, right ankle and foot**

• CC +7th **M80.072 Age-related osteoporosis with current pathological fracture, left ankle and foot**

• CC +7th **M80.079 Age-related osteoporosis with current pathological fracture, unspecified ankle and foot**

• CC X+7th **M80.08 Age-related osteoporosis with current pathological fracture, vertebra(e)**

• CC X+7th **M80.0A Age-related osteoporosis with current pathological fracture, other site**

AHA CC: 4Q, 2020, 32-33

+ **M80.8 Other osteoporosis with current pathological fracture**

Drug-induced osteoporosis with current pathological fracture
Idiopathic osteoporosis with current pathological fracture
Osteoporosis of disuse with current pathological fracture
Postoophorectomy osteoporosis with current pathological fracture
Postsurgical malabsorption osteoporosis with current pathological fracture
Post-traumatic osteoporosis with current pathological fracture

Use additional code for adverse effect, if applicable, to identify drug (T36-T50 with fifth or sixth character 5)

CC X+7th **M80.80 Other osteoporosis with current pathological fracture, unspecified site**

+ **M80.81 Other osteoporosis with pathological fracture, shoulder**

CC +7th **M80.811 Other osteoporosis with current pathological fracture, right shoulder**

CC +7th **M80.812 Other osteoporosis with current pathological fracture, left shoulder**

CC +7th **M80.819 Other osteoporosis with current pathological fracture, unspecified shoulder**

+ **M80.82 Other osteoporosis with current pathological fracture, humerus**

CC +7th **M80.821 Other osteoporosis with current pathological fracture, right humerus**

CC +7th **M80.822 Other osteoporosis with current pathological fracture, left humerus**

CC +7th **M80.829 Other osteoporosis with current pathological fracture, unspecified humerus**

+ **M80.83 Other osteoporosis with current pathological fracture, forearm**

Other osteoporosis with current pathological fracture of wrist

CC +7th **M80.831 Other osteoporosis with current pathological fracture, right forearm**

CC +7th **M80.832 Other osteoporosis with current pathological fracture, left forearm**

CC +7th **M80.839 Other osteoporosis with current pathological fracture, unspecified forearm**

+ **M80.84 Other osteoporosis with current pathological fracture, hand**

CC +7th **M80.841 Other osteoporosis with current pathological fracture, right hand**

CC +7th **M80.842 Other osteoporosis with current pathological fracture, left hand**

CC +7th **M80.849 Other osteoporosis with current pathological fracture, unspecified hand**

+ **M80.85 Other osteoporosis with current pathological fracture, femur**

Other osteoporosis with current pathological fracture of hip

CC +7th **M80.851 Other osteoporosis with current pathological fracture, right femur**

CC +7th **M80.852 Other osteoporosis with current pathological fracture, left femur**

CC +7th **M80.859 Other osteoporosis with current pathological fracture, unspecified femur**

+ **M80.86 Other osteoporosis with current pathological fracture, lower leg**

CC +7th **M80.861 Other osteoporosis with current pathological fracture, right lower leg**

CC +7th **M80.862 Other osteoporosis with current pathological fracture, left lower leg**

CC +7th **M80.869 Other osteoporosis with current pathological fracture, unspecified lower leg**

+ **M80.87 Other osteoporosis with current pathological fracture, ankle and foot**

CC +7th **M80.871 Other osteoporosis with current pathological fracture, right ankle and foot**

CC +7th **M80.872 Other osteoporosis with current pathological fracture, left ankle and foot**

CC +7th **M80.879 Other osteoporosis with current pathological fracture, unspecified ankle and foot**

CC X+7th **M80.88 Other osteoporosis with current pathological fracture, vertebra(e)**
CC X+7th **M80.8A Other osteoporosis with current pathological fracture, other site**
AHA CC: 4Q, 2020, 32

M81 Osteoporosis without current pathological fracture
Use additional code to identify:
major osseous defect, if applicable (M89.7-)
personal history of (healed) osteoporosis fracture, if applicable (Z87.310)
Excludes1: *osteoporosis with current pathological fracture (M80.-)*
Sudeck's atrophy (M89.0)
Review coding guideline C.13.d
• **M81.0 Age-related osteoporosis without current pathological fracture**
Involutional osteoporosis without current pathological fracture
Osteoporosis NOS
Postmenopausal osteoporosis without current pathological fracture
Senile osteoporosis without current pathological fracture
M81.6 Localized osteoporosis [Lequesne]
Excludes1: *Sudeck's atrophy (M89.0)*
M81.8 Other osteoporosis without current pathological fracture
Drug-induced osteoporosis without current pathological fracture
Idiopathic osteoporosis without current pathological fracture
Osteoporosis of disuse without current pathological fracture
Postoophorectomy osteoporosis without current pathological fracture
Postsurgical malabsorption osteoporosis without current pathological fracture
Post-traumatic osteoporosis without current pathological fracture
Use additional code for adverse effect, if applicable, to identify drug (T36-T50 with fifth or sixth character 5)

M83 Adult osteomalacia
Excludes1: *infantile and juvenile osteomalacia (E55.0)*
renal osteodystrophy (N25.0)
rickets (active) (E55.0)
rickets (active) sequelae (E64.3)
vitamin D-resistant osteomalacia (E83.3)
vitamin D-resistant rickets (active) (E83.3)
• ♀ **M83.0 Puerperal osteomalacia**
• **M83.1 Senile osteomalacia**
• **M83.2 Adult osteomalacia due to malabsorption**
Postsurgical malabsorption osteomalacia in adults
• **M83.3 Adult osteomalacia due to malnutrition**
M83.4 Aluminum bone disease
• **M83.5 Other drug-induced osteomalacia in adults**
Use additional code for adverse effect, if applicable, to identify drug (T36-T50 with fifth or sixth character 5)
• **M83.8 Other adult osteomalacia**
• **M83.9 Adult osteomalacia, unspecified**

M84 Disorder of continuity of bone
Excludes2: *traumatic fracture of bone-see fracture, by site*
+ **M84.3 Stress fracture**
Fatigue fracture
March fracture
Stress fracture NOS
Stress reaction
external cause code(s) to identify the cause of the stress fracture
Excludes1: *pathological fracture NOS (M84.4.-)*
pathological fracture due to osteoporosis (M80.-)
traumatic fracture (S12.-, S22.-, S32.-, S42.-, S52.-, S62.-, S72.-, S82.-, S92.-)
Excludes2: *personal history of (healed) stress (fatigue) fracture (Z87.312)*
stress fracture of vertebra (M48.4-)

The appropriate 7th character is to be added to each code from subcategory **M84.3**:
A initial encounter for fracture
D subsequent encounter for fracture with routine healing
G subsequent encounter for fracture with delayed healing
K subsequent encounter for fracture with nonunion
P subsequent encounter for fracture with malunion
S sequela

CC X+7th **M84.30 Stress fracture, unspecified site**
+ **M84.31 Stress fracture, shoulder**
CC +7th **M84.311 Stress fracture, right shoulder**
CC +7th **M84.312 Stress fracture, left shoulder**
CC +7th **M84.319 Stress fracture, unspecified shoulder**
+ **M84.32 Stress fracture, humerus**
CC +7th **M84.321 Stress fracture, right humerus**
CC +7th **M84.322 Stress fracture, left humerus**
CC +7th **M84.329 Stress fracture, unspecified humerus**
+ **M84.33 Stress fracture, ulna and radius**
CC +7th **M84.331 Stress fracture, right ulna**
CC +7th **M84.332 Stress fracture, left ulna**
CC +7th **M84.333 Stress fracture, right radius**
CC +7th **M84.334 Stress fracture, left radius**
CC +7th **M84.339 Stress fracture, unspecified ulna and radius**
+ **M84.34 Stress fracture, hand and fingers**
CC +7th **M84.341 Stress fracture, right hand**
CC +7th **M84.342 Stress fracture, left hand**
CC +7th **M84.343 Stress fracture, unspecified hand**
CC +7th **M84.344 Stress fracture, right finger(s)**
CC +7th **M84.345 Stress fracture, left finger(s)**
CC +7th **M84.346 Stress fracture, unspecified finger(s)**
+ **M84.35 Stress fracture, pelvis and femur**
Stress fracture, hip
CC +7th **M84.350 Stress fracture, pelvis**
CC +7th **M84.351 Stress fracture, right femur**
CC +7th **M84.352 Stress fracture, left femur**
CC +7th **M84.353 Stress fracture, unspecified femur**
CC +7th **M84.359 Stress fracture, hip, unspecified**
+ **M84.36 Stress fracture, tibia and fibula**
CC +7th **M84.361 Stress fracture, right tibia**
CC +7th **M84.362 Stress fracture, left tibia**
CC +7th **M84.363 Stress fracture, right fibula**
CC +7th **M84.364 Stress fracture, left fibula**
CC +7th **M84.369 Stress fracture, unspecified tibia and fibula**
+ **M84.37 Stress fracture, ankle, foot and toes**
CC +7th **M84.371 Stress fracture, right ankle**
CC +7th **M84.372 Stress fracture, left ankle**
CC +7th **M84.373 Stress fracture, unspecified ankle**
CC +7th **M84.374 Stress fracture, right foot**
CC +7th **M84.375 Stress fracture, left foot**
CC +7th **M84.376 Stress fracture, unspecified foot**
CC +7th **M84.377 Stress fracture, right toe(s)**
CC +7th **M84.378 Stress fracture, left toe(s)**
CC +7th **M84.379 Stress fracture, unspecified toe(s)**
CC X+7th **M84.38 Stress fracture, other site**
Excludes2: *stress fracture of vertebra (M48.4-)*

+ **M84.4 Pathological fracture, not elsewhere classified**
Chronic fracture
Pathological fracture NOS
Excludes1: *collapsed vertebra NEC (M48.5)*
pathological fracture in neoplastic disease (M84.5-)
pathological fracture in osteoporosis (M80.-)
pathological fracture in other disease (M84.6-)
stress fracture (M84.3-)
traumatic fracture (S12.-, S22.-, S32.-, S42.-, S52.-, S62.-, S72.-, S82.-, S92.-)
Excludes2: *personal history of (healed) pathological fracture (Z87.311)*

The appropriate 7th character is to be added to each code from subcategory **M84.4**:
A initial encounter for fracture
D subsequent encounter for fracture with routine healing
G subsequent encounter for fracture with delayed healing
K subsequent encounter for fracture with nonunion
P subsequent encounter for fracture with malunion
S sequela

CC X+7th **M84.40 Pathological fracture, unspecified site**
+ **M84.41 Pathological fracture, shoulder**
CC +7th **M84.411 Pathological fracture, right shoulder**
CC +7th **M84.412 Pathological fracture, left shoulder**
CC +7th **M84.419 Pathological fracture, unspecified shoulder**
+ **M84.42 Pathological fracture, humerus**
CC +7th **M84.421 Pathological fracture, right humerus**
CC +7th **M84.422 Pathological fracture, left humerus**
CC +7th **M84.429 Pathological fracture, unspecified humerus**
+ **M84.43 Pathological fracture, ulna and radius**
CC +7th **M84.431 Pathological fracture, right ulna**
CC +7th **M84.432 Pathological fracture, left ulna**
CC +7th **M84.433 Pathological fracture, right radius**
CC +7th **M84.434 Pathological fracture, left radius**
CC +7th **M84.439 Pathological fracture, unspecified ulna and radius**
+ **M84.44 Pathological fracture, hand and fingers**
CC +7th **M84.441 Pathological fracture, right hand**
CC +7th **M84.442 Pathological fracture, left hand**
CC +7th **M84.443 Pathological fracture, unspecified hand**
CC +7th **M84.444 Pathological fracture, right finger(s)**
CC +7th **M84.445 Pathological fracture, left finger(s)**
CC +7th **M84.446 Pathological fracture, unspecified finger(s)**
+ **M84.45 Pathological fracture, femur and pelvis**
CC +7th **M84.451 Pathological fracture, right femur**
CC +7th **M84.452 Pathological fracture, left femur**
CC +7th **M84.453 Pathological fracture, unspecified femur**
CC +7th **M84.454 Pathological fracture, pelvis**
AHA CC: 4Q, 2016, 42-43
CC +7th **M84.459 Pathological fracture, hip, unspecified**
+ **M84.46 Pathological fracture, tibia and fibula**
CC +7th **M84.461 Pathological fracture, right tibia**
CC +7th **M84.462 Pathological fracture, left tibia**
CC +7th **M84.463 Pathological fracture, right fibula**
CC +7th **M84.464 Pathological fracture, left fibula**
CC +7th **M84.469 Pathological fracture, unspecified tibia and fibula**
+ **M84.47 Pathological fracture, ankle, foot and toes**
CC +7th **M84.471 Pathological fracture, right ankle**
CC +7th **M84.472 Pathological fracture, left ankle**
CC +7th **M84.473 Pathological fracture, unspecified ankle**
CC +7th **M84.474 Pathological fracture, right foot**
CC +7th **M84.475 Pathological fracture, left foot**
CC +7th **M84.476 Pathological fracture, unspecified foot**
CC +7th **M84.477 Pathological fracture, right toe(s)**
CC +7th **M84.478 Pathological fracture, left toe(s)**
CC +7th **M84.479 Pathological fracture, unspecified toe(s)**
CC X+7th **M84.48 Pathological fracture, other site**

+ **M84.5 Pathological fracture in neoplastic disease**
Code also underlying neoplasm

The appropriate 7th character is to be added to each code from subcategory **M84.5**:
A initial encounter for fracture
D subsequent encounter for fracture with routine healing
G subsequent encounter for fracture with delayed healing
K subsequent encounter for fracture with nonunion
P subsequent encounter for fracture with malunion
S sequela

Review coding guideline C.2.l.6
CC X+7th **M84.50 Pathological fracture in neoplastic disease, unspecified site**
+ **M84.51 Pathological fracture in neoplastic disease, shoulder**
CC +7th **M84.511 Pathological fracture in neoplastic disease, right shoulder**
CC +7th **M84.512 Pathological fracture in neoplastic disease, left shoulder**
CC +7th **M84.519 Pathological fracture in neoplastic disease, unspecified shoulder**
+ **M84.52 Pathological fracture in neoplastic disease, humerus**
CC +7th **M84.521 Pathological fracture in neoplastic disease, right humerus**
CC +7th **M84.522 Pathological fracture in neoplastic disease, left humerus**
CC +7th **M84.529 Pathological fracture in neoplastic disease, unspecified humerus**
+ **M84.53 Pathological fracture in neoplastic disease, ulna and radius**
CC +7th **M84.531 Pathological fracture in neoplastic disease, right ulna**
CC +7th **M84.532 Pathological fracture in neoplastic disease, left ulna**
CC +7th **M84.533 Pathological fracture in neoplastic disease, right radius**
CC +7th **M84.534 Pathological fracture in neoplastic disease, left radius**
CC +7th **M84.539 Pathological fracture in neoplastic disease, unspecified ulna and radius**
+ **M84.54 Pathological fracture in neoplastic disease, hand**
CC +7th **M84.541 Pathological fracture in neoplastic disease, right hand**
CC +7th **M84.542 Pathological fracture in neoplastic disease, left hand**
CC +7th **M84.549 Pathological fracture in neoplastic disease, unspecified hand**
+ **M84.55 Pathological fracture in neoplastic disease, pelvis and femur**
CC +7th **M84.550 Pathological fracture in neoplastic disease, pelvis**
CC +7th **M84.551 Pathological fracture in neoplastic disease, right femur**
CC +7th **M84.552 Pathological fracture in neoplastic disease, left femur**
CC +7th **M84.553 Pathological fracture in neoplastic disease, unspecified femur**
CC +7th **M84.559 Pathological fracture in neoplastic disease, hip, unspecified**
+ **M84.56 Pathological fracture in neoplastic disease, tibia and fibula**
CC +7th **M84.561 Pathological fracture in neoplastic disease, right tibia**
CC +7th **M84.562 Pathological fracture in neoplastic disease, left tibia**
CC +7th **M84.563 Pathological fracture in neoplastic disease, right fibula**
CC +7th **M84.564 Pathological fracture in neoplastic disease, left fibula**
CC +7th **M84.569 Pathological fracture in neoplastic disease, unspecified tibia and fibula**
+ **M84.57 Pathological fracture in neoplastic disease, ankle and foot**
CC +7th **M84.571 Pathological fracture in neoplastic disease, right ankle**
CC +7th **M84.572 Pathological fracture in neoplastic disease, left ankle**

CC +7th **M84.573 Pathological fracture in neoplastic disease, unspecified ankle**
CC +7th **M84.574 Pathological fracture in neoplastic disease, right foot**
CC +7th **M84.575 Pathological fracture in neoplastic disease, left foot**
CC +7th **M84.576 Pathological fracture in neoplastic disease, unspecified foot**
CC X+7th **M84.58 Pathological fracture in neoplastic disease, other specified site**
Pathological fracture in neoplastic disease, vertebrae
\+ **M84.6 Pathological fracture in other disease**
Code also underlying condition
Excludes1: *pathological fracture in osteoporosis (M80.-)*

The appropriate 7th character is to be added to each code from subcategory **M84.6**:
A initial encounter for fracture
D subsequent encounter for fracture with routine healing
G subsequent encounter for fracture with delayed healing
K subsequent encounter for fracture with nonunion
P subsequent encounter for fracture with malunion
S sequela

CC X+7th **M84.60 Pathological fracture in other disease, unspecified site**
\+ **M84.61 Pathological fracture in other disease, shoulder**
CC +7th **M84.611 Pathological fracture in other disease, right shoulder**
CC +7th **M84.612 Pathological fracture in other disease, left shoulder**
CC +7th **M84.619 Pathological fracture in other disease, unspecified shoulder**
\+ **M84.62 Pathological fracture in other disease, humerus**
CC +7th **M84.621 Pathological fracture in other disease, right humerus**
CC +7th **M84.622 Pathological fracture in other disease, left humerus**
CC +7th **M84.629 Pathological fracture in other disease, unspecified humerus**
\+ **M84.63 Pathological fracture in other disease, ulna and radius**
CC +7th **M84.631 Pathological fracture in other disease, right ulna**
CC +7th **M84.632 Pathological fracture in other disease, left ulna**
CC +7th **M84.633 Pathological fracture in other disease, right radius**
CC +7th **M84.634 Pathological fracture in other disease, left radius**
CC +7th **M84.639 Pathological fracture in other disease, unspecified ulna and radius**
\+ **M84.64 Pathological fracture in other disease, hand**
CC +7th **M84.641 Pathological fracture in other disease, right hand**
CC +7th **M84.642 Pathological fracture in other disease, left hand**
CC +7th **M84.649 Pathological fracture in other disease, unspecified hand**
\+ **M84.65 Pathological fracture in other disease, pelvis and femur**
M84.650 Pathological fracture in other disease, pelvis
CC +7th **M84.651 Pathological fracture in other disease, right femur**
CC +7th **M84.652 Pathological fracture in other disease, left femur**
CC +7th **M84.653 Pathological fracture in other disease, unspecified femur**
CC +7th **M84.659 Pathological fracture in other disease, hip, unspecified**
\+ **M84.66 Pathological fracture in other disease, tibia and fibula**
CC +7th **M84.661 Pathological fracture in other disease, right tibia**
CC +7th **M84.662 Pathological fracture in other disease, left tibia**
CC +7th **M84.663 Pathological fracture in other disease, right fibula**
CC +7th **M84.664 Pathological fracture in other disease, left fibula**
CC +7th **M84.669 Pathological fracture in other disease, unspecified tibia and fibula**
\+ **M84.67 Pathological fracture in other disease, ankle and foot**
CC +7th **M84.671 Pathological fracture in other disease, right ankle**
CC +7th **M84.672 Pathological fracture in other disease, left ankle**
CC +7th **M84.673 Pathological fracture in other disease, unspecified ankle**
CC +7th **M84.674 Pathological fracture in other disease, right foot**
CC +7th **M84.675 Pathological fracture in other disease, left foot**
CC +7th **M84.676 Pathological fracture in other disease, unspecified foot**
CC X+7th **M84.68 Pathological fracture in other disease, other site**
\+ **M84.7 Nontraumatic fracture, not elsewhere classified**
\+ **M84.75 Atypical femoral fracture**
AHA CC: 4Q, 2016, 41-42

The appropriate 7th character is to be added to each code from subcategory **M84.75**:
A initial encounter for fracture
D subsequent encounter for fracture with routine healing
G subsequent encounter for fracture with delayed healing
K subsequent encounter for fracture with nonunion
P subsequent encounter for fracture with malunion
S sequela

CC +7th **M84.750 Atypical femoral fracture, unspecified**
CC +7th **M84.751 Incomplete atypical femoral fracture, right leg**
CC +7th **M84.752 Incomplete atypical femoral fracture, left leg**
CC +7th **M84.753 Incomplete atypical femoral fracture, unspecified leg**
CC +7th **M84.754 Complete transverse atypical femoral fracture, right leg**
CC +7th **M84.755 Complete transverse atypical femoral fracture, left leg**
CC +7th **M84.756 Complete transverse atypical femoral fracture, unspecified leg**
CC +7th **M84.757 Complete oblique atypical femoral fracture, right leg**
CC +7th **M84.758 Complete oblique atypical femoral fracture, left leg**
CC +7th **M84.759 Complete oblique atypical femoral fracture, unspecified leg**
\+ **M84.8 Other disorders of continuity of bone**
M84.80 Other disorders of continuity of bone, unspecified site
\+ **M84.81 Other disorders of continuity of bone, shoulder**
M84.811 Other disorders of continuity of bone, right shoulder
M84.812 Other disorders of continuity of bone, left shoulder
M84.819 Other disorders of continuity of bone, unspecified shoulder
\+ **M84.82 Other disorders of continuity of bone, humerus**
M84.821 Other disorders of continuity of bone, right humerus
M84.822 Other disorders of continuity of bone, left humerus
M84.829 Other disorders of continuity of bone, unspecified humerus
\+ **M84.83 Other disorders of continuity of bone, ulna and radius**
M84.831 Other disorders of continuity of bone, right ulna
M84.832 Other disorders of continuity of bone, left ulna
M84.833 Other disorders of continuity of bone, right radius
M84.834 Other disorders of continuity of bone, left radius
M84.839 Other disorders of continuity of bone, unspecified ulna and radius

+ M84.84 Other disorders of continuity of bone, hand
M84.841 Other disorders of continuity of bone, right hand
M84.842 Other disorders of continuity of bone, left hand
M84.849 Other disorders of continuity of bone, unspecified hand
+ M84.85 Other disorders of continuity of bone, pelvic region and thigh
M84.851 Other disorders of continuity of bone, right pelvic region and thigh
M84.852 Other disorders of continuity of bone, left pelvic region and thigh
M84.859 Other disorders of continuity of bone, unspecified pelvic region and thigh
+ M84.86 Other disorders of continuity of bone, tibia and fibula
M84.861 Other disorders of continuity of bone, right tibia
M84.862 Other disorders of continuity of bone, left tibia
M84.863 Other disorders of continuity of bone, right fibula
M84.864 Other disorders of continuity of bone, left fibula
M84.869 Other disorders of continuity of bone, unspecified tibia and fibula
+ M84.87 Other disorders of continuity of bone, ankle and foot
M84.871 Other disorders of continuity of bone, right ankle and foot
M84.872 Other disorders of continuity of bone, left ankle and foot
M84.879 Other disorders of continuity of bone, unspecified ankle and foot
M84.88 Other disorders of continuity of bone, other site
M84.9 Disorder of continuity of bone, unspecified

M85 Other disorders of bone density and structure

Excludes1: *osteogenesis imperfecta (Q78.0)*
osteopetrosis (Q78.2)
osteopoikilosis (Q78.8)
polyostotic fibrous dysplasia (Q78.1)

+ M85.0 Fibrous dysplasia (monostotic)
Excludes2: *fibrous dysplasia of jaw (M27.8)*
M85.00 Fibrous dysplasia (monostotic), unspecified site
+ M85.01 Fibrous dysplasia (monostotic), shoulder
M85.011 Fibrous dysplasia (monostotic), right shoulder
M85.012 Fibrous dysplasia (monostotic), left shoulder
M85.019 Fibrous dysplasia (monostotic), unspecified shoulder
+ M85.02 Fibrous dysplasia (monostotic), upper arm
M85.021 Fibrous dysplasia (monostotic), right upper arm
M85.022 Fibrous dysplasia (monostotic), left upper arm
M85.029 Fibrous dysplasia (monostotic), unspecified upper arm
+ M85.03 Fibrous dysplasia (monostotic), forearm
M85.031 Fibrous dysplasia (monostotic), right forearm
M85.032 Fibrous dysplasia (monostotic), left forearm
M85.039 Fibrous dysplasia (monostotic), unspecified forearm
+ M85.04 Fibrous dysplasia (monostotic), hand
M85.041 Fibrous dysplasia (monostotic), right hand
M85.042 Fibrous dysplasia (monostotic), left hand
M85.049 Fibrous dysplasia (monostotic), unspecified hand
+ M85.05 Fibrous dysplasia (monostotic), thigh
M85.051 Fibrous dysplasia (monostotic), right thigh
M85.052 Fibrous dysplasia (monostotic), left thigh
M85.059 Fibrous dysplasia (monostotic), unspecified thigh
+ M85.06 Fibrous dysplasia (monostotic), lower leg
M85.061 Fibrous dysplasia (monostotic), right lower leg
M85.062 Fibrous dysplasia (monostotic), left lower leg
M85.069 Fibrous dysplasia (monostotic), unspecified lower leg
+ M85.07 Fibrous dysplasia (monostotic), ankle and foot
M85.071 Fibrous dysplasia (monostotic), right ankle and foot
M85.072 Fibrous dysplasia (monostotic), left ankle and foot
M85.079 Fibrous dysplasia (monostotic), unspecified ankle and foot
M85.08 Fibrous dysplasia (monostotic), other site
M85.09 Fibrous dysplasia (monostotic), multiple sites
+ M85.1 Skeletal fluorosis
M85.10 Skeletal fluorosis, unspecified site
+ M85.11 Skeletal fluorosis, shoulder
M85.111 Skeletal fluorosis, right shoulder
M85.112 Skeletal fluorosis, left shoulder
M85.119 Skeletal fluorosis, unspecified shoulder
+ M85.12 Skeletal fluorosis, upper arm
M85.121 Skeletal fluorosis, right upper arm
M85.122 Skeletal fluorosis, left upper arm
M85.129 Skeletal fluorosis, unspecified upper arm
+ M85.13 Skeletal fluorosis, forearm
M85.131 Skeletal fluorosis, right forearm
M85.132 Skeletal fluorosis, left forearm
M85.139 Skeletal fluorosis, unspecified forearm
+ M85.14 Skeletal fluorosis, hand
M85.141 Skeletal fluorosis, right hand
M85.142 Skeletal fluorosis, left hand
M85.149 Skeletal fluorosis, unspecified hand
+ M85.15 Skeletal fluorosis, thigh
M85.151 Skeletal fluorosis, right thigh
M85.152 Skeletal fluorosis, left thigh
M85.159 Skeletal fluorosis, unspecified thigh
+ M85.16 Skeletal fluorosis, lower leg
M85.161 Skeletal fluorosis, right lower leg
M85.162 Skeletal fluorosis, left lower leg
M85.169 Skeletal fluorosis, unspecified lower leg
+ M85.17 Skeletal fluorosis, ankle and foot
M85.171 Skeletal fluorosis, right ankle and foot
M85.172 Skeletal fluorosis, left ankle and foot
M85.179 Skeletal fluorosis, unspecified ankle and foot
M85.18 Skeletal fluorosis, other site
M85.19 Skeletal fluorosis, multiple sites
M85.2 Hyperostosis of skull
+ M85.3 Osteitis condensans
M85.30 Osteitis condensans, unspecified site
+ M85.31 Osteitis condensans, shoulder
M85.311 Osteitis condensans, right shoulder
M85.312 Osteitis condensans, left shoulder
M85.319 Osteitis condensans, unspecified shoulder
+ M85.32 Osteitis condensans, upper arm
M85.321 Osteitis condensans, right upper arm
M85.322 Osteitis condensans, left upper arm
M85.329 Osteitis condensans, unspecified upper arm
+ M85.33 Osteitis condensans, forearm
M85.331 Osteitis condensans, right forearm
M85.332 Osteitis condensans, left forearm
M85.339 Osteitis condensans, unspecified forearm
+ M85.34 Osteitis condensans, hand
M85.341 Osteitis condensans, right hand
M85.342 Osteitis condensans, left hand
M85.349 Osteitis condensans, unspecified hand
+ M85.35 Osteitis condensans, thigh
M85.351 Osteitis condensans, right thigh
M85.352 Osteitis condensans, left thigh
M85.359 Osteitis condensans, unspecified thigh
+ M85.36 Osteitis condensans, lower leg
M85.361 Osteitis condensans, right lower leg
M85.362 Osteitis condensans, left lower leg
M85.369 Osteitis condensans, unspecified lower leg

+ **M85.37 Osteitis condensans, ankle and foot**
  - **M85.371 Osteitis condensans, right ankle and foot**
  - **M85.372 Osteitis condensans, left ankle and foot**
  - **M85.379 Osteitis condensans, unspecified ankle and foot**
- **M85.38 Osteitis condensans, other site**
- **M85.39 Osteitis condensans, multiple sites**

+ **M85.4 Solitary bone cyst**
  Excludes2: *solitary cyst of jaw (M27.4)*
  - **M85.40 Solitary bone cyst, unspecified site**
  + **M85.41 Solitary bone cyst, shoulder**
    - **M85.411 Solitary bone cyst, right shoulder**
    - **M85.412 Solitary bone cyst, left shoulder**
    - **M85.419 Solitary bone cyst, unspecified shoulder**
  + **M85.42 Solitary bone cyst, humerus**
    - **M85.421 Solitary bone cyst, right humerus**
    - **M85.422 Solitary bone cyst, left humerus**
    - **M85.429 Solitary bone cyst, unspecified humerus**
  + **M85.43 Solitary bone cyst, ulna and radius**
    - **M85.431 Solitary bone cyst, right ulna and radius**
    - **M85.432 Solitary bone cyst, left ulna and radius**
    - **M85.439 Solitary bone cyst, unspecified ulna and radius**
  + **M85.44 Solitary bone cyst, hand**
    - **M85.441 Solitary bone cyst, right hand**
    - **M85.442 Solitary bone cyst, left hand**
    - **M85.449 Solitary bone cyst, unspecified hand**
  + **M85.45 Solitary bone cyst, pelvis**
    - **M85.451 Solitary bone cyst, right pelvis**
    - **M85.452 Solitary bone cyst, left pelvis**
    - **M85.459 Solitary bone cyst, unspecified pelvis**
  + **M85.46 Solitary bone cyst, tibia and fibula**
    - **M85.461 Solitary bone cyst, right tibia and fibula**
    - **M85.462 Solitary bone cyst, left tibia and fibula**
    - **M85.469 Solitary bone cyst, unspecified tibia and fibula**
  + **M85.47 Solitary bone cyst, ankle and foot**
    - **M85.471 Solitary bone cyst, right ankle and foot**
    - **M85.472 Solitary bone cyst, left ankle and foot**
    - **M85.479 Solitary bone cyst, unspecified ankle and foot**
  - **M85.48 Solitary bone cyst, other site**

+ **M85.5 Aneurysmal bone cyst**
  Excludes2: *aneurysmal cyst of jaw (M27.4)*
  - **M85.50 Aneurysmal bone cyst, unspecified site**
  + **M85.51 Aneurysmal bone cyst, shoulder**
    - **M85.511 Aneurysmal bone cyst, right shoulder**
    - **M85.512 Aneurysmal bone cyst, left shoulder**
    - **M85.519 Aneurysmal bone cyst, unspecified shoulder**
  + **M85.52 Aneurysmal bone cyst, upper arm**
    - **M85.521 Aneurysmal bone cyst, right upper arm**
    - **M85.522 Aneurysmal bone cyst, left upper arm**
    - **M85.529 Aneurysmal bone cyst, unspecified upper arm**
  + **M85.53 Aneurysmal bone cyst, forearm**
    - **M85.531 Aneurysmal bone cyst, right forearm**
    - **M85.532 Aneurysmal bone cyst, left forearm**
    - **M85.539 Aneurysmal bone cyst, unspecified forearm**
  + **M85.54 Aneurysmal bone cyst, hand**
    - **M85.541 Aneurysmal bone cyst, right hand**
    - **M85.542 Aneurysmal bone cyst, left hand**
    - **M85.549 Aneurysmal bone cyst, unspecified hand**
  + **M85.55 Aneurysmal bone cyst, thigh**
    - **M85.551 Aneurysmal bone cyst, right thigh**
    - **M85.552 Aneurysmal bone cyst, left thigh**
    - **M85.559 Aneurysmal bone cyst, unspecified thigh**
  + **M85.56 Aneurysmal bone cyst, lower leg**
    - **M85.561 Aneurysmal bone cyst, right lower leg**
    - **M85.562 Aneurysmal bone cyst, left lower leg**
    - **M85.569 Aneurysmal bone cyst, unspecified lower leg**
  + **M85.57 Aneurysmal bone cyst, ankle and foot**
    - **M85.571 Aneurysmal bone cyst, right ankle and foot**
    - **M85.572 Aneurysmal bone cyst, left ankle and foot**
    - **M85.579 Aneurysmal bone cyst, unspecified ankle and foot**
  - **M85.58 Aneurysmal bone cyst, other site**
  - **M85.59 Aneurysmal bone cyst, multiple sites**

+ **M85.6 Other cyst of bone**
  Excludes1: *cyst of jaw NEC (M27.4)*
  osteitis fibrosa cystica generalisata [von Recklinghausen's disease of bone] (E21.0)
  - **M85.60 Other cyst of bone, unspecified site**
  + **M85.61 Other cyst of bone, shoulder**
    - **M85.611 Other cyst of bone, right shoulder**
    - **M85.612 Other cyst of bone, left shoulder**
    - **M85.619 Other cyst of bone, unspecified shoulder**
  + **M85.62 Other cyst of bone, upper arm**
    - **M85.621 Other cyst of bone, right upper arm**
    - **M85.622 Other cyst of bone, left upper arm**
    - **M85.629 Other cyst of bone, unspecified upper arm**
  + **M85.63 Other cyst of bone, forearm**
    - **M85.631 Other cyst of bone, right forearm**
    - **M85.632 Other cyst of bone, left forearm**
    - **M85.639 Other cyst of bone, unspecified forearm**
  + **M85.64 Other cyst of bone, hand**
    - **M85.641 Other cyst of bone, right hand**
    - **M85.642 Other cyst of bone, left hand**
    - **M85.649 Other cyst of bone, unspecified hand**
  + **M85.65 Other cyst of bone, thigh**
    - **M85.651 Other cyst of bone, right thigh**
    - **M85.652 Other cyst of bone, left thigh**
    - **M85.659 Other cyst of bone, unspecified thigh**
  + **M85.66 Other cyst of bone, lower leg**
    - **M85.661 Other cyst of bone, right lower leg**
    - **M85.662 Other cyst of bone, left lower leg**
    - **M85.669 Other cyst of bone, unspecified lower leg**
  + **M85.67 Other cyst of bone, ankle and foot**
    - **M85.671 Other cyst of bone, right ankle and foot**
    - **M85.672 Other cyst of bone, left ankle and foot**
    - **M85.679 Other cyst of bone, unspecified ankle and foot**
  - **M85.68 Other cyst of bone, other site**
  - **M85.69 Other cyst of bone, multiple sites**

+ **M85.8 Other specified disorders of bone density and structure**
  Hyperostosis of bones, except skull
  Osteosclerosis, acquired
  Excludes1: *diffuse idiopathic skeletal hyperostosis [DISH] (M48.1)*
  osteosclerosis congenita (Q77.4)
  osteosclerosis fragilitas (generalista) (Q78.2)
  osteosclerosis myelofibrosis (D75.81)
  - **M85.80 Other specified disorders of bone density and structure, unspecified site**
  + **M85.81 Other specified disorders of bone density and structure, shoulder**
    - **M85.811 Other specified disorders of bone density and structure, right shoulder**
    - **M85.812 Other specified disorders of bone density and structure, left shoulder**
    - **M85.819 Other specified disorders of bone density and structure, unspecified shoulder**
  + **M85.82 Other specified disorders of bone density and structure, upper arm**
    - **M85.821 Other specified disorders of bone density and structure, right upper arm**
    - **M85.822 Other specified disorders of bone density and structure, left upper arm**
    - **M85.829 Other specified disorders of bone density and structure, unspecified upper arm**

+ M85.83 Other specified disorders of bone density and structure, forearm
  - M85.831 Other specified disorders of bone density and structure, right forearm
  - M85.832 Other specified disorders of bone density and structure, left forearm
  - M85.839 Other specified disorders of bone density and structure, unspecified forearm

+ M85.84 Other specified disorders of bone density and structure, hand
  - M85.841 Other specified disorders of bone density and structure, right hand
  - M85.842 Other specified disorders of bone density and structure, left hand
  - M85.849 Other specified disorders of bone density and structure, unspecified hand

+ M85.85 Other specified disorders of bone density and structure, thigh
  - M85.851 Other specified disorders of bone density and structure, right thigh
  - M85.852 Other specified disorders of bone density and structure, left thigh
  - M85.859 Other specified disorders of bone density and structure, unspecified thigh

+ M85.86 Other specified disorders of bone density and structure, lower leg
  - M85.861 Other specified disorders of bone density and structure, right lower leg
  - M85.862 Other specified disorders of bone density and structure, left lower leg
  - M85.869 Other specified disorders of bone density and structure, unspecified lower leg

+ M85.87 Other specified disorders of bone density and structure, ankle and foot
  - M85.871 Other specified disorders of bone density and structure, right ankle and foot
  - M85.872 Other specified disorders of bone density and structure, left ankle and foot
  - M85.879 Other specified disorders of bone density and structure, unspecified ankle and foot

M85.88 Other specified disorders of bone density and structure, other site

M85.89 Other specified disorders of bone density and structure, multiple sites

M85.9 Disorder of bone density and structure, unspecified

Other osteopathies (M86-M90)

Excludes1: *postprocedural osteopathies (M96.-)*

M86 Osteomyelitis

Use additional code (B95-B97) to identify infectious agent

Use additional code to identify major osseous defect, if applicable (M89.7-)

Excludes1: *osteomyelitis due to:*
echinococcus (B67.2)
gonococcus (A54.43)
salmonella (A02.24)

Excludes2: *ostemyelitis of:*
orbit (H05.0-)
petrous bone (H70.2-)
vertebra (M46.2-)

+ M86.0 Acute hematogenous osteomyelitis
  - CC M86.00 Acute hematogenous osteomyelitis, unspecifiedsite
  - + M86.01 Acute hematogenous osteomyelitis, shoulder
    - CC M86.011 Acute hematogenous osteomyelitis, right shoulder
    - CC M86.012 Acute hematogenous osteomyelitis, left shoulder
    - CC M86.019 Acute hematogenous osteomyelitis, unspecified shoulder
  - + M86.02 Acute hematogenous osteomyelitis, humerus
    - CC M86.021 Acute hematogenous osteomyelitis, right humerus
    - CC M86.022 Acute hematogenous osteomyelitis, left humerus
    - CC M86.029 Acute hematogenous osteomyelitis, unspecified humerus
  - + M86.03 Acute hematogenous osteomyelitis, radius and ulna
    - CC M86.031 Acute hematogenous osteomyelitis, right radius and ulna
    - CC M86.032 Acute hematogenous osteomyelitis, left radius and ulna
    - CC M86.039 Acute hematogenous osteomyelitis, unspecified radius and ulna
  - + M86.04 Acute hematogenous osteomyelitis, hand
    - CC M86.041 Acute hematogenous osteomyelitis, right hand
    - CC M86.042 Acute hematogenous osteomyelitis, left hand
    - CC M86.049 Acute hematogenous osteomyelitis, unspecified hand
  - + M86.05 Acute hematogenous osteomyelitis, femur
    - CC M86.051 Acute hematogenous osteomyelitis, right femur
    - CC M86.052 Acute hematogenous osteomyelitis, left femur
    - CC M86.059 Acute hematogenous osteomyelitis, unspecified femur
  - + M86.06 Acute hematogenous osteomyelitis, tibia and fibula
    - CC M86.061 Acute hematogenous osteomyelitis, right tibia and fibula
    - CC M86.062 Acute hematogenous osteomyelitis, left tibia and fibula
    - CC M86.069 Acute hematogenous osteomyelitis, unspecified tibia and fibula
  - + M86.07 Acute hematogenous osteomyelitis, ankle and foot
    - CC M86.071 Acute hematogenous osteomyelitis, right ankle and foot
    - CC M86.072 Acute hematogenous osteomyelitis, left ankle and foot
    - CC M86.079 Acute hematogenous osteomyelitis, unspecified ankle and foot
  - CC M86.08 Acute hematogenous osteomyelitis, other sites
  - CC M86.09 Acute hematogenous osteomyelitis, multiple sites

+ M86.1 Other acute osteomyelitis
  - CC M86.10 Other acute osteomyelitis, unspecified site
  - + M86.11 Other acute osteomyelitis, shoulder
    - CC M86.111 Other acute osteomyelitis, right shoulder
    - CC M86.112 Other acute osteomyelitis, left shoulder
    - CC M86.119 Other acute osteomyelitis, unspecified shoulder
  - + M86.12 Other acute osteomyelitis, humerus
    - CC M86.121 Other acute osteomyelitis, right humerus
    - CC M86.122 Other acute osteomyelitis, left humerus
    - CC M86.129 Other acute osteomyelitis, unspecified humerus
  - + M86.13 Other acute osteomyelitis, radius and ulna
    - CC M86.131 Other acute osteomyelitis, right radius and ulna
    - CC M86.132 Other acute osteomyelitis, left radius and ulna
    - CC M86.139 Other acute osteomyelitis, unspecified radius and ulna
  - + M86.14 Other acute osteomyelitis, hand
    - CC M86.141 Other acute osteomyelitis, righthand
    - CC M86.142 Other acute osteomyelitis, left hand
    - CC M86.149 Other acute osteomyelitis, unspecified hand
  - + M86.15 Other acute osteomyelitis, femur
    - CC M86.151 Other acute osteomyelitis, right femur
    - CC M86.152 Other acute osteomyelitis, left femur
    - CC M86.159 Other acute osteomyelitis, unspecified femur

+ M86.16 Other acute osteomyelitis, tibia and fibula
  - CC M86.161 Other acute osteomyelitis, right tibia and fibula
  - CC M86.162 Other acute osteomyelitis, left tibia and fibula
  - CC M86.169 Other acute osteomyelitis, unspecified tibia and fibula

+ M86.17 Other acute osteomyelitis, ankle and foot
  - CC M86.171 Other acute osteomyelitis, right ankle and foot
    AHA CC: 1Q, 2020, 12
  - CC M86.172 Other acute osteomyelitis, left ankle and foot
  - CC M86.179 Other acute osteomyelitis, unspecified ankle and foot

CC M86.18 Other acute osteomyelitis, other site
CC M86.19 Other acute osteomyelitis, multiple sites

+ M86.2 Subacute osteomyelitis
  - CC M86.20 Subacute osteomyelitis, unspecified site
  - + M86.21 Subacute osteomyelitis, shoulder
    - CC M86.211 Subacute osteomyelitis, right shoulder
    - CC M86.212 Subacute osteomyelitis, left shoulder
    - CC M86.219 Subacute osteomyelitis, unspecified shoulder
  - + M86.22 Subacute osteomyelitis, humerus
    - CC M86.221 Subacute osteomyelitis, right humerus
    - CC M86.222 Subacute osteomyelitis, left humerus
    - CC M86.229 Subacute osteomyelitis, unspecified humerus
  - + M86.23 Subacute osteomyelitis, radius and ulna
    - CC M86.231 Subacute osteomyelitis, right radius and ulna
    - CC M86.232 Subacute osteomyelitis, left radius and ulna
    - CC M86.239 Subacute osteomyelitis, unspecified radius and ulna
  - + M86.24 Subacute osteomyelitis, hand
    - CC M86.241 Subacute osteomyelitis, right hand
    - CC M86.242 Subacute osteomyelitis, left hand
    - CC M86.249 Subacute osteomyelitis, unspecified hand
  - + M86.25 Subacute osteomyelitis, femur
    - CC M86.251 Subacute osteomyelitis, right femur
    - CC M86.252 Subacute osteomyelitis, left femur
    - CC M86.259 Subacute osteomyelitis, unspecified femur
  - + M86.26 Subacute osteomyelitis, tibia and fibula
    - CC M86.261 Subacute osteomyelitis, right tibia and fibula
    - CC M86.262 Subacute osteomyelitis, left tibia and fibula
    - CC M86.269 Subacute osteomyelitis, unspecified tibia and fibula
  - + M86.27 Subacute osteomyelitis, ankle and foot
    - CC M86.271 Subacute osteomyelitis, right ankle and foot
    - CC M86.272 Subacute osteomyelitis, left ankle and foot
    - CC M86.279 Subacute osteomyelitis, unspecified ankle and foot
  - CC M86.28 Subacute osteomyelitis, other site
  - CC M86.29 Subacute osteomyelitis, multiple sites

+ M86.3 Chronic multifocal osteomyelitis
  - CC M86.30 Chronic multifocal osteomyelitis, unspecified site
  - + M86.31 Chronic multifocal osteomyelitis, shoulder
    - CC M86.311 Chronic multifocal osteomyelitis, right shoulder
    - CC M86.312 Chronic multifocal osteomyelitis, left shoulder
    - CC M86.319 Chronic multifocal osteomyelitis, unspecified shoulder
  - + M86.32 Chronic multifocal osteomyelitis, humerus
    - CC M86.321 Chronic multifocal osteomyelitis, right humerus
    - CC M86.322 Chronic multifocal osteomyelitis, left humerus
    - CC M86.329 Chronic multifocal osteomyelitis, unspecified humerus
  - + M86.33 Chronic multifocal osteomyelitis, radius and ulna
    - CC M86.331 Chronic multifocal osteomyelitis, right radius and ulna
    - CC M86.332 Chronic multifocal osteomyelitis, left radius and ulna
    - CC M86.339 Chronic multifocal osteomyelitis, unspecified radius and ulna
  - + M86.34 Chronic multifocal osteomyelitis, hand
    - CC M86.341 Chronic multifocal osteomyelitis, right hand
    - CC M86.342 Chronic multifocal osteomyelitis, left hand
    - CC M86.349 Chronic multifocal osteomyelitis, unspecified hand
  - + M86.35 Chronic multifocal osteomyelitis, femur
    - CC M86.351 Chronic multifocal osteomyelitis, right femur
    - CC M86.352 Chronic multifocal osteomyelitis, left femur
    - CC M86.359 Chronic multifocal osteomyelitis, unspecified femur
  - + M86.36 Chronic multifocal osteomyelitis, tibia and fibula
    - CC M86.361 Chronic multifocal osteomyelitis, right tibia and fibula
    - CC M86.362 Chronic multifocal osteomyelitis, left tibia and fibula
    - CC M86.369 Chronic multifocal osteomyelitis, unspecified tibia and fibula
  - + M86.37 Chronic multifocal osteomyelitis, ankle and foot
    - CC M86.371 Chronic multifocal osteomyelitis, right ankle and foot
    - CC M86.372 Chronic multifocal osteomyelitis, left ankle and foot
    - CC M86.379 Chronic multifocal osteomyelitis, unspecified ankle and foot
  - CC M86.38 Chronic multifocal osteomyelitis, other site
  - CC M86.39 Chronic multifocal osteomyelitis, multiple sites

+ M86.4 Chronic osteomyelitis with draining sinus
  - CC M86.40 Chronic osteomyelitis with draining sinus, unspecified site
  - + M86.41 Chronic osteomyelitis with draining sinus, shoulder
    - CC M86.411 Chronic osteomyelitis with draining sinus, right shoulder
    - CC M86.412 Chronic osteomyelitis with draining sinus, left shoulder
    - CC M86.419 Chronic osteomyelitis with draining sinus, unspecified shoulder
  - + M86.42 Chronic osteomyelitis with draining sinus, humerus
    - CC M86.421 Chronic osteomyelitis with draining sinus, right humerus
    - CC M86.422 Chronic osteomyelitis with draining sinus, left humerus
    - CC M86.429 Chronic osteomyelitis with draining sinus, unspecified humerus
  - + M86.43 Chronic osteomyelitis with draining sinus, radius and ulna
    - CC M86.431 Chronic osteomyelitis with draining sinus, right radius and ulna
    - CC M86.432 Chronic osteomyelitis with draining sinus, left radius and ulna
    - CC M86.439 Chronic osteomyelitis with draining sinus, unspecified radius and ulna
  - + M86.44 Chronic osteomyelitis with draining sinus, hand
    - CC M86.441 Chronic osteomyelitis with draining sinus, right hand
    - CC M86.442 Chronic osteomyelitis with draining sinus, left hand
    - CC M86.449 Chronic osteomyelitis with draining sinus, unspecified hand
  - + M86.45 Chronic osteomyelitis with draining sinus, femur
    - CC M86.451 Chronic osteomyelitis with draining sinus, right femur
    - CC M86.452 Chronic osteomyelitis with draining sinus, left femur
    - CC M86.459 Chronic osteomyelitis with draining sinus, unspecified femur

+ M86.46 Chronic osteomyelitis with draining sinus, tibia and fibula
  - CC M86.461 Chronic osteomyelitis with draining sinus, right tibia and fibula
  - CC M86.462 Chronic osteomyelitis with draining sinus, left tibia and fibula
  - CC M86.469 Chronic osteomyelitis with draining sinus, unspecified tibia and fibula

+ M86.47 Chronic osteomyelitis with draining sinus, ankle and foot
  - CC M86.471 Chronic osteomyelitis with draining sinus, right ankle and foot
  - CC M86.472 Chronic osteomyelitis with draining sinus, left ankle and foot
  - CC M86.479 Chronic osteomyelitis with draining sinus, unspecified ankle and foot

CC M86.48 Chronic osteomyelitis with draining sinus, other site

CC M86.49 Chronic osteomyelitis with draining sinus, multiple sites

+ M86.5 Other chronic hematogenous osteomyelitis

CC M86.50 Other chronic hematogenous osteomyelitis, unspecified site

+ M86.51 Other chronic hematogenous osteomyelitis, shoulder
  - CC M86.511 Other chronic hematogenous osteomyelitis, right shoulder
  - CC M86.512 Other chronic hematogenous osteomyelitis, left shoulder
  - CC M86.519 Other chronic hematogenous osteomyelitis, unspecified shoulder

+ M86.52 Other chronic hematogenous osteomyelitis, humerus
  - CC M86.521 Other chronic hematogenous osteomyelitis, right humerus
  - CC M86.522 Other chronic hematogenous osteomyelitis, left humerus
  - CC M86.529 Other chronic hematogenous osteomyelitis, unspecified humerus

+ M86.53 Other chronic hematogenous osteomyelitis, radius and ulna
  - CC M86.531 Other chronic hematogenous osteomyelitis, right radius and ulna
  - CC M86.532 Other chronic hematogenous osteomyelitis, left radius and ulna
  - CC M86.539 Other chronic hematogenous osteomyelitis, unspecified radius and ulna

+ M86.54 Other chronic hematogenous osteomyelitis, hand
  - CC M86.541 Other chronic hematogenous osteomyelitis, right hand
  - CC M86.542 Other chronic hematogenous osteomyelitis, left hand
  - CC M86.549 Other chronic hematogenous osteomyelitis, unspecified hand

+ M86.55 Other chronic hematogenous osteomyelitis, femur
  - CC M86.551 Other chronic hematogenous osteomyelitis, right femur
  - CC M86.552 Other chronic hematogenous osteomyelitis, left femur
  - CC M86.559 Other chronic hematogenous osteomyelitis, unspecified femur

+ M86.56 Other chronic hematogenous osteomyelitis, tibia and fibula
  - CC M86.561 Other chronic hematogenous osteomyelitis, right tibia and fibula
  - CC M86.562 Other chronic hematogenous osteomyelitis, left tibia and fibula
  - CC M86.569 Other chronic hematogenous osteomyelitis, unspecified tibia and fibula

+ M86.57 Other chronic hematogenous osteomyelitis, ankle and foot
  - CC M86.571 Other chronic hematogenous osteomyelitis, right ankle and foot
  - CC M86.572 Other chronic hematogenous osteomyelitis, left ankle and foot
  - CC M86.579 Other chronic hematogenous osteomyelitis, unspecified ankle and foot

CC M86.58 Other chronic hematogenous osteomyelitis, other site

CC M86.59 Other chronic hematogenous osteomyelitis, multiple sites

+ M86.6 Other chronic osteomyelitis

CC M86.60 Other chronic osteomyelitis, unspecified site

+ M86.61 Other chronic osteomyelitis, shoulder
  - CC M86.611 Other chronic osteomyelitis, right shoulder
  - CC M86.612 Other chronic osteomyelitis, left shoulder
  - CC M86.619 Other chronic osteomyelitis, unspecified shoulder

+ M86.62 Other chronic osteomyelitis, humerus
  - CC M86.621 Other chronic osteomyelitis, right humerus
  - CC M86.622 Other chronic osteomyelitis, left humerus
  - CC M86.629 Other chronic osteomyelitis, unspecified humerus

+ M86.63 Other chronic osteomyelitis, radius and ulna
  - CC M86.631 Other chronic osteomyelitis, right radius and ulna
  - CC M86.632 Other chronic osteomyelitis, left radius and ulna
  - CC M86.639 Other chronic osteomyelitis, unspecified radius and ulna

+ M86.64 Other chronic osteomyelitis, hand
  - CC M86.641 Other chronic osteomyelitis, right hand
  - CC M86.642 Other chronic osteomyelitis, left hand
  - CC M86.649 Other chronic osteomyelitis, unspecified hand

+ M86.65 Other chronic osteomyelitis, thigh
  - CC M86.651 Other chronic osteomyelitis, right thigh
  - CC M86.652 Other chronic osteomyelitis, left thigh
  - CC M86.659 Other chronic osteomyelitis, unspecified thigh

+ M86.66 Other chronic osteomyelitis, tibia and fibula
  - CC M86.661 Other chronic osteomyelitis, right tibia and fibula
  - CC M86.662 Other chronic osteomyelitis, left tibia and fibula
  - CC M86.669 Other chronic osteomyelitis, unspecified tibia and fibula

+ M86.67 Other chronic osteomyelitis, ankle and foot
  - CC M86.671 Other chronic osteomyelitis, right ankle and foot

    AHA CC: 1Q, 2016, 13
  - CC M86.672 Other chronic osteomyelitis, left ankle and foot
  - CC M86.679 Other chronic osteomyelitis, unspecified ankle and foot

CC M86.68 Other chronic osteomyelitis, other site

CC M86.69 Other chronic osteomyelitis, multiple sites

+ M86.8 Other osteomyelitis

Brodie's abscess

+ M86.8X Other osteomyelitis
  - CC M86.8X0 Other osteomyelitis, multiple sites
  - CC M86.8X1 Other osteomyelitis, shoulder
  - CC M86.8X2 Other osteomyelitis, upper arm
  - CC M86.8X3 Other osteomyelitis, forearm
  - CC M86.8X4 Other osteomyelitis, hand
  - CC M86.8X5 Other osteomyelitis, thigh
  - CC M86.8X6 Other osteomyelitis, lower leg
  - CC M86.8X7 Other osteomyelitis, ankle and foot
  - CC M86.8X8 Other osteomyelitis, other site
  - CC M86.8X9 Other osteomyelitis, unspecified sites

CC M86.9 Osteomyelitis, unspecified

Infection of bone NOS

Periostitis without osteomyelitis

M87 Osteonecrosis

Includes: avascular necrosis of bone

Use additional code to identify major osseous defect, if applicable (M89.7-)

Excludes1: *juvenile osteonecrosis (M91-M92)*
osteochondropathies (M90-M93)

+ **M87.0 Idiopathic aseptic necrosis of bone**
  - CC **M87.00 Idiopathic aseptic necrosis of unspecifiedbone**
  - + **M87.01 Idiopathic aseptic necrosis of shoulder**
    Idiopathic aseptic necrosis of clavicle and scapula
    - CC **M87.011 Idiopathic aseptic necrosis of right shoulder**
    - CC **M87.012 Idiopathic aseptic necrosis of left shoulder**
    - CC **M87.019 Idiopathic aseptic necrosis of unspecified shoulder**
  - + **M87.02 Idiopathic aseptic necrosis of humerus**
    - CC **M87.021 Idiopathic aseptic necrosis of right humerus**
    - CC **M87.022 Idiopathic aseptic necrosis of left humerus**
    - CC **M87.029 Idiopathic aseptic necrosis of unspecified humerus**
  - + **M87.03 Idiopathic aseptic necrosis of radius, ulna and carpus**
    - CC **M87.031 Idiopathic aseptic necrosis of right radius**
    - CC **M87.032 Idiopathic aseptic necrosis of left radius**
    - CC **M87.033 Idiopathic aseptic necrosis of unspecified radius**
    - CC **M87.034 Idiopathic aseptic necrosis of right ulna**
    - CC **M87.035 Idiopathic aseptic necrosis of left ulna**
    - CC **M87.036 Idiopathic aseptic necrosis of unspecified ulna**
    - CC **M87.037 Idiopathic aseptic necrosis of right carpus**
    - CC **M87.038 Idiopathic aseptic necrosis of left carpus**
    - CC **M87.039 Idiopathic aseptic necrosis of unspecified carpus**
  - + **M87.04 Idiopathic aseptic necrosis of hand and fingers**
    Idiopathic aseptic necrosis of metacarpals and phalanges of hands
    - CC **M87.041 Idiopathic aseptic necrosis of right hand**
    - CC **M87.042 Idiopathic aseptic necrosis of left hand**
    - CC **M87.043 Idiopathic aseptic necrosis of unspecified hand**
    - CC **M87.044 Idiopathic aseptic necrosis of right finger(s)**
    - CC **M87.045 Idiopathic aseptic necrosis of left finger(s)**
    - CC **M87.046 Idiopathic aseptic necrosis of unspecified finger(s)**
  - + **M87.05 Idiopathic aseptic necrosis of pelvis and femur**
    - CC **M87.050 Idiopathic aseptic necrosis of pelvis**
    - CC **M87.051 Idiopathic aseptic necrosis of right femur**
    - CC **M87.052 Idiopathic aseptic necrosis of left femur**
    - CC **M87.059 Idiopathic aseptic necrosis of unspecified femur**
      Idiopathic aseptic necrosis of hip NOS
  - + **M87.06 Idiopathic aseptic necrosis of tibia and fibula**
    - CC **M87.061 Idiopathic aseptic necrosis of right tibia**
    - CC **M87.062 Idiopathic aseptic necrosis of left tibia**
    - CC **M87.063 Idiopathic aseptic necrosis of unspecified tibia**
    - CC **M87.064 Idiopathic aseptic necrosis of right fibula**
    - CC **M87.065 Idiopathic aseptic necrosis of left fibula**
    - CC **M87.066 Idiopathic aseptic necrosis of unspecified fibula**
  - + **M87.07 Idiopathic aseptic necrosis of ankle, foot and toes**
    Idiopathic aseptic necrosis of metatarsus, tarsus, and phalanges of toes
    - CC **M87.071 Idiopathic aseptic necrosis of right ankle**
    - CC **M87.072 Idiopathic aseptic necrosis of left ankle**
    - CC **M87.073 Idiopathic aseptic necrosis of unspecified ankle**
    - CC **M87.074 Idiopathic aseptic necrosis of right foot**
    - CC **M87.075 Idiopathic aseptic necrosis of left foot**
    - CC **M87.076 Idiopathic aseptic necrosis of unspecified foot**
    - CC **M87.077 Idiopathic aseptic necrosis of right toe(s)**
    - CC **M87.078 Idiopathic aseptic necrosis of left toe(s)**
    - CC **M87.079 Idiopathic aseptic necrosis of unspecified toe(s)**
  - CC **M87.08 Idiopathic aseptic necrosis of bone, other site**
  - CC **M87.09 Idiopathic aseptic necrosis of bone, multiple sites**

+ **M87.1 Osteonecrosis due to drugs**
  Use additional code for adverse effect, if applicable, to identify drug (T36-T50 with fifth or sixth character 5)
  - CC **M87.10 Osteonecrosis due to drugs, unspecified bone**
  - + **M87.11 Osteonecrosis due to drugs, shoulder**
    - CC **M87.111 Osteonecrosis due to drugs, right shoulder**
    - CC **M87.112 Osteonecrosis due to drugs, left shoulder**
    - CC **M87.119 Osteonecrosis due to drugs, unspecified shoulder**
  - + **M87.12 Osteonecrosis due to drugs, humerus**
    - CC **M87.121 Osteonecrosis due to drugs, right humerus**
    - CC **M87.122 Osteonecrosis due to drugs, left humerus**
    - CC **M87.129 Osteonecrosis due to drugs, unspecified humerus**
  - + **M87.13 Osteonecrosis due to drugs of radius, ulna and carpus**
    - CC **M87.131 Osteonecrosis due to drugs of right radius**
    - CC **M87.132 Osteonecrosis due to drugs of left radius**
    - CC **M87.133 Osteonecrosis due to drugs of unspecified radius**
    - CC **M87.134 Osteonecrosis due to drugs of right ulna**
    - CC **M87.135 Osteonecrosis due to drugs of left ulna**
    - CC **M87.136 Osteonecrosis due to drugs of unspecified ulna**
    - CC **M87.137 Osteonecrosis due to drugs of right carpus**
    - CC **M87.138 Osteonecrosis due to drugs of left carpus**
    - CC **M87.139 Osteonecrosis due to drugs of unspecified carpus**
  - + **M87.14 Osteonecrosis due to drugs, hand and fingers**
    - CC **M87.141 Osteonecrosis due to drugs, right hand**
    - CC **M87.142 Osteonecrosis due to drugs, left hand**
    - CC **M87.143 Osteonecrosis due to drugs, unspecified hand**
    - CC **M87.144 Osteonecrosis due to drugs, right finger(s)**
    - CC **M87.145 Osteonecrosis due to drugs, left finger(s)**
    - CC **M87.146 Osteonecrosis due to drugs, unspecified finger(s)**
  - + **M87.15 Osteonecrosis due to drugs, pelvis and femur**
    - CC **M87.150 Osteonecrosis due to drugs, pelvis**
    - CC **M87.151 Osteonecrosis due to drugs, right femur**
    - CC **M87.152 Osteonecrosis due to drugs, left femur**
    - CC **M87.159 Osteonecrosis due to drugs, unspecified femur**
  - + **M87.16 Osteonecrosis due to drugs, tibia and fibula**
    - CC **M87.161 Osteonecrosis due to drugs, right tibia**
    - CC **M87.162 Osteonecrosis due to drugs, left tibia**
    - CC **M87.163 Osteonecrosis due to drugs, unspecified tibia**
    - CC **M87.164 Osteonecrosis due to drugs, right fibula**
    - CC **M87.165 Osteonecrosis due to drugs, left fibula**
    - CC **M87.166 Osteonecrosis due to drugs, unspecified fibula**
  - + **M87.17 Osteonecrosis due to drugs, ankle, foot and toes**
    - CC **M87.171 Osteonecrosis due to drugs, right ankle**
    - CC **M87.172 Osteonecrosis due to drugs, left ankle**
    - CC **M87.173 Osteonecrosis due to drugs, unspecified ankle**
    - CC **M87.174 Osteonecrosis due to drugs, right foot**
    - CC **M87.175 Osteonecrosis due to drugs, left foot**
    - CC **M87.176 Osteonecrosis due to drugs, unspecified foot**

CC **M87.177** **Osteonecrosis due to drugs, right toe(s)**
CC **M87.178** **Osteonecrosis due to drugs, left toe(s)**
CC **M87.179** **Osteonecrosis due to drugs, unspecified toe(s)**
+ **M87.18** **Osteonecrosis due to drugs, other site**
CC **M87.180** **Osteonecrosis due to drugs, jaw**
CC **M87.188** **Osteonecrosis due to drugs, other site**
CC **M87.19** **Osteonecrosis due to drugs, multiple sites**
+ **M87.2** **Osteonecrosis due to previous trauma**
CC **M87.20** **Osteonecrosis due to previous trauma, unspecified bone**
+ **M87.21** **Osteonecrosis due to previous trauma, shoulder**
CC **M87.211** **Osteonecrosis due to previous trauma, right shoulder**
CC **M87.212** **Osteonecrosis due to previous trauma, left shoulder**
CC **M87.219** **Osteonecrosis due to previous trauma, unspecified shoulder**
+ **M87.22** **Osteonecrosis due to previous trauma, humerus**
CC **M87.221** **Osteonecrosis due to previous trauma, right humerus**
CC **M87.222** **Osteonecrosis due to previous trauma, left humerus**
CC **M87.229** **Osteonecrosis due to previous trauma, unspecified humerus**
+ **M87.23** **Osteonecrosis due to previous trauma of radius, ulna and carpus**
CC **M87.231** **Osteonecrosis due to previous trauma of right radius**
CC **M87.232** **Osteonecrosis due to previous trauma of left radius**
CC **M87.233** **Osteonecrosis due to previous trauma of unspecified radius**
CC **M87.234** **Osteonecrosis due to previous trauma of right ulna**
CC **M87.235** **Osteonecrosis due to previous trauma of left ulna**
CC **M87.236** **Osteonecrosis due to previous trauma of unspecified ulna**
CC **M87.237** **Osteonecrosis due to previous trauma of right carpus**
CC **M87.238** **Osteonecrosis due to previous trauma of left carpus**
CC **M87.239** **Osteonecrosis due to previous trauma of unspecified carpus**
+ **M87.24** **Osteonecrosis due to previous trauma, hand and fingers**
CC **M87.241** **Osteonecrosis due to previous trauma, right hand**
CC **M87.242** **Osteonecrosis due to previous trauma, left hand**
CC **M87.243** **Osteonecrosis due to previous trauma, unspecified hand**
CC **M87.244** **Osteonecrosis due to previous trauma, right finger(s)**
CC **M87.245** **Osteonecrosis due to previous trauma, left finger(s)**
CC **M87.246** **Osteonecrosis due to previous trauma, unspecified finger(s)**
+ **M87.25** **Osteonecrosis due to previous trauma, pelvis and femur**
CC **M87.250** **Osteonecrosis due to previous trauma, pelvis**
CC **M87.251** **Osteonecrosis due to previous trauma, right femur**
CC **M87.252** **Osteonecrosis due to previous trauma, left femur**
CC **M87.256** **Osteonecrosis due to previous trauma, unspecified femur**
+ **M87.26** **Osteonecrosis due to previous trauma, tibia and fibula**
CC **M87.261** **Osteonecrosis due to previous trauma, right tibia**
CC **M87.262** **Osteonecrosis due to previous trauma, left tibia**
CC **M87.263** **Osteonecrosis due to previous trauma, unspecified tibia**
CC **M87.264** **Osteonecrosis due to previous trauma, right fibula**
CC **M87.265** **Osteonecrosis due to previous trauma, left fibula**
CC **M87.266** **Osteonecrosis due to previous trauma, unspecified fibula**
+ **M87.27** **Osteonecrosis due to previous trauma, ankle, foot and toes**
CC **M87.271** **Osteonecrosis due to previous trauma, right ankle**
CC **M87.272** **Osteonecrosis due to previous trauma, left ankle**
CC **M87.273** **Osteonecrosis due to previous trauma, unspecified ankle**
CC **M87.274** **Osteonecrosis due to previous trauma, right foot**
CC **M87.275** **Osteonecrosis due to previous trauma, left foot**
CC **M87.276** **Osteonecrosis due to previous trauma, unspecified foot**
CC **M87.277** **Osteonecrosis due to previous trauma, right toe(s)**
CC **M87.278** **Osteonecrosis due to previous trauma, left toe(s)**
CC **M87.279** **Osteonecrosis due to previous trauma, unspecified toe(s)**
CC **M87.28** **Osteonecrosis due to previous trauma, other site**
CC **M87.29** **Osteonecrosis due to previous trauma, multiple sites**
+ **M87.3** **Other secondary osteonecrosis**
CC **M87.30** **Other secondary osteonecrosis, unspecified bone**
+ **M87.31** **Other secondary osteonecrosis, shoulder**
CC **M87.311** **Other secondary osteonecrosis, right shoulder**
CC **M87.312** **Other secondary osteonecrosis, left shoulder**
CC **M87.319** **Other secondary osteonecrosis, unspecified shoulder**
+ **M87.32** **Other secondary osteonecrosis, humerus**
CC **M87.321** **Other secondary osteonecrosis, right humerus**
CC **M87.322** **Other secondary osteonecrosis, left humerus**
CC **M87.329** **Other secondary osteonecrosis, unspecified humerus**
+ **M87.33** **Other secondary osteonecrosis of radius, ulna and carpus**
CC **M87.331** **Other secondary osteonecrosis of right radius**
CC **M87.332** **Other secondary osteonecrosis of left radius**
CC **M87.333** **Other secondary osteonecrosis of unspecified radius**
CC **M87.334** **Other secondary osteonecrosis of right ulna**
CC **M87.335** **Other secondary osteonecrosis of left ulna**
CC **M87.336** **Other secondary osteonecrosis of unspecified ulna**
CC **M87.337** **Other secondary osteonecrosis of right carpus**
CC **M87.338** **Other secondary osteonecrosis of left carpus**
CC **M87.339** **Other secondary osteonecrosis of unspecified carpus**
+ **M87.34** **Other secondary osteonecrosis, hand and fingers**
CC **M87.341** **Other secondary osteonecrosis, right hand**
CC **M87.342** **Other secondary osteonecrosis, left hand**
CC **M87.343** **Other secondary osteonecrosis, unspecified hand**
CC **M87.344** **Other secondary osteonecrosis, right finger(s)**
CC **M87.345** **Other secondary osteonecrosis, left finger(s)**
CC **M87.346** **Other secondary osteonecrosis, unspecified finger(s)**

+ **M87.35** Other secondary osteonecrosis, pelvis and femur
  - CC **M87.350** Other secondary osteonecrosis, pelvis
  - CC **M87.351** Other secondary osteonecrosis, right femur
  - CC **M87.352** Other secondary osteonecrosis, left femur
  - CC **M87.353** Other secondary osteonecrosis, unspecified femur

+ **M87.36** Other secondary osteonecrosis, tibia and fibula
  - CC **M87.361** Other secondary osteonecrosis, right tibia
  - CC **M87.362** Other secondary osteonecrosis, left tibia
  - CC **M87.363** Other secondary osteonecrosis, unspecified tibia
  - CC **M87.364** Other secondary osteonecrosis, right fibula
  - CC **M87.365** Other secondary osteonecrosis, left fibula
  - CC **M87.366** Other secondary osteonecrosis, unspecified fibula

+ **M87.37** Other secondary osteonecrosis, ankle and foot
  - CC **M87.371** Other secondary osteonecrosis, right ankle
  - CC **M87.372** Other secondary osteonecrosis, left ankle
  - CC **M87.373** Other secondary osteonecrosis, unspecified ankle
  - CC **M87.374** Other secondary osteonecrosis, right foot
  - CC **M87.375** Other secondary osteonecrosis, left foot
  - CC **M87.376** Other secondary osteonecrosis, unspecified foot
  - CC **M87.377** Other secondary osteonecrosis, right toe(s)
  - CC **M87.378** Other secondary osteonecrosis, left toe(s)
  - CC **M87.379** Other secondary osteonecrosis, unspecified toe(s)

CC **M87.38** Other secondary osteonecrosis, other site

CC **M87.39** Other secondary osteonecrosis, multiple sites

+ **M87.8** Other osteonecrosis

CC **M87.80** Other osteonecrosis, unspecified bone

+ **M87.81** Other osteonecrosis, shoulder
  - CC **M87.811** Other osteonecrosis, right shoulder
  - CC **M87.812** Other osteonecrosis, left shoulder
  - CC **M87.819** Other osteonecrosis, unspecified shoulder

+ **M87.82** Other osteonecrosis, humerus
  - CC **M87.821** Other osteonecrosis, right humerus
  - CC **M87.822** Other osteonecrosis, left humerus
  - CC **M87.829** Other osteonecrosis, unspecified humerus

+ **M87.83** Other osteonecrosis of radius, ulna and carpus
  - CC **M87.831** Other osteonecrosis of right radius
  - CC **M87.832** Other osteonecrosis of left radius
  - CC **M87.833** Other osteonecrosis of unspecified radius
  - CC **M87.834** Other osteonecrosis of right ulna
  - CC **M87.835** Other osteonecrosis of left ulna
  - CC **M87.836** Other osteonecrosis of unspecified ulna
  - CC **M87.837** Other osteonecrosis of right carpus
  - CC **M87.838** Other osteonecrosis of left carpus
  - CC **M87.839** Other osteonecrosis of unspecified carpus

+ **M87.84** Other osteonecrosis, hand and fingers
  - CC **M87.841** Other osteonecrosis, right hand
  - CC **M87.842** Other osteonecrosis, left hand
  - CC **M87.843** Other osteonecrosis, unspecified hand
  - CC **M87.844** Other osteonecrosis, right finger(s)
  - CC **M87.845** Other osteonecrosis, left finger(s)
  - CC **M87.849** Other osteonecrosis, unspecified finger(s)

+ **M87.85** Other osteonecrosis, pelvis and femur
  - CC **M87.850** Other osteonecrosis, pelvis
  - CC **M87.851** Other osteonecrosis, right femur
  - CC **M87.852** Other osteonecrosis, left femur
  - CC **M87.859** Other osteonecrosis, unspecified femur

+ **M87.86** Other osteonecrosis, tibia and fibula
  - CC **M87.861** Other osteonecrosis, right tibia
  - CC **M87.862** Other osteonecrosis, left tibia
  - CC **M87.863** Other osteonecrosis, unspecified tibia
  - CC **M87.864** Other osteonecrosis, right fibula
  - CC **M87.865** Other osteonecrosis, left fibula
  - CC **M87.869** Other osteonecrosis, unspecified fibula

+ **M87.87** Other osteonecrosis, ankle, foot and toes
  - CC **M87.871** Other osteonecrosis, right ankle
  - CC **M87.872** Other osteonecrosis, left ankle
  - CC **M87.873** Other osteonecrosis, unspecified ankle
  - CC **M87.874** Other osteonecrosis, right foot
  - CC **M87.875** Other osteonecrosis, left foot
  - CC **M87.876** Other osteonecrosis, unspecified foot
  - CC **M87.877** Other osteonecrosis, right toe(s)
  - CC **M87.878** Other osteonecrosis, left toe(s)
  - CC **M87.879** Other osteonecrosis, unspecified toe(s)

CC **M87.88** Other osteonecrosis, other site

CC **M87.89** Other osteonecrosis, multiple sites

CC **M87.9** Osteonecrosis, unspecified
Necrosis of bone NOS

M88 Osteitis deformans [Paget's disease of bone]

Excludes1: *osteitis deformans in neoplastic disease (M90.6)*

M88.0 Osteitis deformans of skull

M88.1 Osteitis deformans of vertebrae

+ **M88.8** Osteitis deformans of other bones

+ **M88.81** Osteitis deformans of shoulder
  - **M88.811** Osteitis deformans of right shoulder
  - **M88.812** Osteitis deformans of left shoulder
  - **M88.819** Osteitis deformans of unspecified shoulder

+ **M88.82** Osteitis deformans of upper arm
  - **M88.821** Osteitis deformans of right upper arm
  - **M88.822** Osteitis deformans of left upper arm
  - **M88.829** Osteitis deformans of unspecified upper arm

+ **M88.83** Osteitis deformans of forearm
  - **M88.831** Osteitis deformans of right forearm
  - **M88.832** Osteitis deformans of left forearm
  - **M88.839** Osteitis deformans of unspecified forearm

+ **M88.84** Osteitis deformans of hand
  - **M88.841** Osteitis deformans of right hand
  - **M88.842** Osteitis deformans of left hand
  - **M88.849** Osteitis deformans of unspecified hand

+ **M88.85** Osteitis deformans of thigh
  - **M88.851** Osteitis deformans of right thigh
  - **M88.852** Osteitis deformans of left thigh
  - **M88.859** Osteitis deformans of unspecified thigh

+ **M88.86** Osteitis deformans of lower leg
  - **M88.861** Osteitis deformans of right lower leg
  - **M88.862** Osteitis deformans of left lower leg
  - **M88.869** Osteitis deformans of unspecified lower leg

+ **M88.87** Osteitis deformans of ankle and foot
  - **M88.871** Osteitis deformans of right ankle and foot
  - **M88.872** Osteitis deformans of left ankle and foot
  - **M88.879** Osteitis deformans of unspecified ankle and foot

M88.88 Osteitis deformans of other bones

Excludes2: *osteitis deformans of skull (M88.0)*
osteitis deformans of vertebrae (M88.1)

M88.89 Osteitis deformans of multiple sites

M88.9 Osteitis deformans of unspecified bone

M89 Other disorders of bone

+ **M89.0** Algoneurodystrophy
Shoulder-hand syndrome
Sudeck's atrophy

Excludes1: *causalgia, lower limb (G57.7-)*
causalgia, upper limb (G56.4-)
complex regional pain syndrome II, lower limb (G57.7-)
complex regional pain syndrome II, upper limb (G56.4-)
reflex sympathetic dystrophy (G90.5-)

M89.00 Algoneurodystrophy, unspecified site

+ **M89.01** Algoneurodystrophy, shoulder
  - **M89.011** Algoneurodystrophy, right shoulder
  - **M89.012** Algoneurodystrophy, left shoulder
  - **M89.019** Algoneurodystrophy, unspecified shoulder

+ M89.02 Algoneurodystrophy, upper arm
  - M89.021 Algoneurodystrophy, right upper arm
  - M89.022 Algoneurodystrophy, left upper arm
  - M89.029 Algoneurodystrophy, unspecified upper arm
+ M89.03 Algoneurodystrophy, forearm
  - M89.031 Algoneurodystrophy, right forearm
  - M89.032 Algoneurodystrophy, left forearm
  - M89.039 Algoneurodystrophy, unspecified forearm
+ M89.04 Algoneurodystrophy, hand
  - M89.041 Algoneurodystrophy, right≈hand
  - M89.042 Algoneurodystrophy, left hand
  - M89.049 Algoneurodystrophy, unspecified hand
+ M89.05 Algoneurodystrophy, thigh
  - M89.051 Algoneurodystrophy, right thigh
  - M89.052 Algoneurodystrophy, left thigh
  - M89.059 Algoneurodystrophy, unspecified thigh
+ M89.06 Algoneurodystrophy, lower leg
  - M89.061 Algoneurodystrophy, right lower leg
  - M89.062 Algoneurodystrophy, left lower leg
  - M89.069 Algoneurodystrophy, unspecified lower leg
+ M89.07 Algoneurodystrophy, ankle and foot
  - M89.071 Algoneurodystrophy, right ankle and foot
  - M89.072 Algoneurodystrophy, left ankle and foot
  - M89.079 Algoneurodystrophy, unspecified ankle and foot

M89.08 Algoneurodystrophy, other site

M89.09 Algoneurodystrophy, multiple sites

+ M89.1 Physeal arrest
  Arrest of growth plate
  Epiphyseal arrest
  Growth plate arrest
+ M89.12 Physeal arrest, humerus
  - M89.121 Complete physeal arrest, right proximal humerus
  - M89.122 Complete physeal arrest, left proximal humerus
  - M89.123 Partial physeal arrest, right proximal humerus
  - M89.124 Partial physeal arrest, left proximal humerus
  - M89.125 Complete physeal arrest, right distal humerus
  - M89.126 Complete physeal arrest, left distal humerus
  - M89.127 Partial physeal arrest, right distal humerus
  - M89.128 Partial physeal arrest, left distal humerus
  - M89.129 Physeal arrest, humerus, unspecified
+ M89.13 Physeal arrest, forearm
  - M89.131 Complete physeal arrest, right distal radius
  - M89.132 Complete physeal arrest, left distal radius
  - M89.133 Partial physeal arrest, right distal radius
  - M89.134 Partial physeal arrest, left distal radius
  - M89.138 Other physeal arrest of forearm
  - M89.139 Physeal arrest, forearm, unspecified
+ M89.15 Physeal arrest, femur
  - M89.151 Complete physeal arrest, right proximal femur
  - M89.152 Complete physeal arrest, left proximal femur
  - M89.153 Partial physeal arrest, right proximal femur
  - M89.154 Partial physeal arrest, left proximal femur
  - M89.155 Complete physeal arrest, right distal femur
  - M89.156 Complete physeal arrest, left distal femur
  - M89.157 Partial physeal arrest, right distal femur
  - M89.158 Partial physeal arrest, left distal femur
  - M89.159 Physeal arrest, femur, unspecified
+ M89.16 Physeal arrest, lower leg
  - M89.160 Complete physeal arrest, right proximal tibia
  - M89.161 Complete physeal arrest, left proximal tibia
  - M89.162 Partial physeal arrest, right proximal tibia
  - M89.163 Partial physeal arrest, left proximal tibia
  - M89.164 Complete physeal arrest, right distal tibia
  - M89.165 Complete physeal arrest, left distal tibia
  - M89.166 Partial physeal arrest, right distal tibia
  - M89.167 Partial physeal arrest, left distal tibia
  - M89.168 Other physeal arrest of lower leg
  - M89.169 Physeal arrest, lower leg, unspecified

M89.18 Physeal arrest, other site

+ M89.2 Other disorders of bone development and growth

M89.20 Other disorders of bone development and growth, unspecified site

+ M89.21 Other disorders of bone development and growth, shoulder
  - M89.211 Other disorders of bone development and growth, right shoulder
  - M89.212 Other disorders of bone development and growth, left shoulder
  - M89.219 Other disorders of bone development and growth, unspecified shoulder
+ M89.22 Other disorders of bone development and growth, humerus
  - M89.221 Other disorders of bone development and growth, right humerus
  - M89.222 Other disorders of bone development and growth, left humerus
  - M89.229 Other disorders of bone development and growth, unspecified humerus
+ M89.23 Other disorders of bone development and growth, ulna and radius
  - M89.231 Other disorders of bone development and growth, right ulna
  - M89.232 Other disorders of bone development and growth, left ulna
  - M89.233 Other disorders of bone development and growth, right radius
  - M89.234 Other disorders of bone development and growth, left radius
  - M89.239 Other disorders of bone development and growth, unspecified ulna and radius
+ M89.24 Other disorders of bone development and growth, hand
  - M89.241 Other disorders of bone development and growth, right hand
  - M89.242 Other disorders of bone development and growth, left hand
  - M89.249 Other disorders of bone development and growth, unspecified hand
+ M89.25 Other disorders of bone development and growth, femur
  - M89.251 Other disorders of bone development and growth, right femur
  - M89.252 Other disorders of bone development and growth, left femur
  - M89.259 Other disorders of bone development and growth, unspecified femur
+ M89.26 Other disorders of bone development and growth, tibia and fibula
  - M89.261 Other disorders of bone development and growth, right tibia
  - M89.262 Other disorders of bone development and growth, left tibia
  - M89.263 Other disorders of bone development and growth, right fibula
  - M89.264 Other disorders of bone development and growth, left fibula
  - M89.269 Other disorders of bone development and growth, unspecified lower leg

+ **M89.27 Other disorders of bone development and growth, ankle and foot**
  - **M89.271 Other disorders of bone development and growth, right ankle and foot**
  - **M89.272 Other disorders of bone development and growth, left ankle and foot**
  - **M89.279 Other disorders of bone development and growth, unspecified ankle and foot**

M89.28 Other disorders of bone development and growth, other site

M89.29 Other disorders of bone development and growth, multiple sites

+ **M89.3 Hypertrophy of bone**

M89.30 Hypertrophy of bone, unspecified site

+ **M89.31 Hypertrophy of bone, shoulder**
  - **M89.311 Hypertrophy of bone, right shoulder**
  - **M89.312 Hypertrophy of bone, left shoulder**
  - **M89.319 Hypertrophy of bone, unspecified shoulder**

+ **M89.32 Hypertrophy of bone, humerus**
  - **M89.321 Hypertrophy of bone, right humerus**
  - **M89.322 Hypertrophy of bone, left humerus**
  - **M89.329 Hypertrophy of bone, unspecified humerus**

+ **M89.33 Hypertrophy of bone, ulna and radius**
  - **M89.331 Hypertrophy of bone, right ulna**
  - **M89.332 Hypertrophy of bone, left ulna**
  - **M89.333 Hypertrophy of bone, right radius**
  - **M89.334 Hypertrophy of bone, left radius**
  - **M89.339 Hypertrophy of bone, unspecified ulna and radius**

+ **M89.34 Hypertrophy of bone, hand**
  - **M89.341 Hypertrophy of bone, right hand**
  - **M89.342 Hypertrophy of bone, left hand**
  - **M89.349 Hypertrophy of bone, unspecified hand**

+ **M89.35 Hypertrophy of bone, femur**
  - **M89.351 Hypertrophy of bone, right femur**
  - **M89.352 Hypertrophy of bone, left femur**
  - **M89.359 Hypertrophy of bone, unspecified femur**

+ **M89.36 Hypertrophy of bone, tibia and fibula**
  - **M89.361 Hypertrophy of bone, right tibia**
  - **M89.362 Hypertrophy of bone, left tibia**
  - **M89.363 Hypertrophy of bone, right fibula**
  - **M89.364 Hypertrophy of bone, left fibula**
  - **M89.369 Hypertrophy of bone, unspecified tibia and fibula**

+ **M89.37 Hypertrophy of bone, ankle and foot**
  - **M89.371 Hypertrophy of bone, right ankle and foot**
  - **M89.372 Hypertrophy of bone, left ankle and foot**
  - **M89.379 Hypertrophy of bone, unspecified ankle and foot**

M89.38 Hypertrophy of bone, other site

M89.39 Hypertrophy of bone, multiple sites

+ **M89.4 Other hypertrophic osteoarthropathy**

Marie-Bamberger disease
Pachydermoperiostosis

M89.40 Other hypertrophic osteoarthropathy, unspecified site

+ **M89.41 Other hypertrophic osteoarthropathy, shoulder**
  - **M89.411 Other hypertrophic osteoarthropathy, right shoulder**
  - **M89.412 Other hypertrophic osteoarthropathy, left shoulder**
  - **M89.419 Other hypertrophic osteoarthropathy, unspecified shoulder**

+ **M89.42 Other hypertrophic osteoarthropathy, upper arm**
  - **M89.421 Other hypertrophic osteoarthropathy, right upper arm**
  - **M89.422 Other hypertrophic osteoarthropathy, left upper arm**
  - **M89.429 Other hypertrophic osteoarthropathy, unspecified upper arm**

+ **M89.43 Other hypertrophic osteoarthropathy, forearm**
  - **M89.431 Other hypertrophic osteoarthropathy, right forearm**
  - **M89.432 Other hypertrophic osteoarthropathy, left forearm**
  - **M89.439 Other hypertrophic osteoarthropathy, unspecified forearm**

+ **M89.44 Other hypertrophic osteoarthropathy, hand**
  - **M89.441 Other hypertrophic osteoarthropathy, right hand**
  - **M89.442 Other hypertrophic osteoarthropathy, left hand**
  - **M89.449 Other hypertrophic osteoarthropathy, unspecified hand**

+ **M89.45 Other hypertrophic osteoarthropathy, thigh**
  - **M89.451 Other hypertrophic osteoarthropathy, right thigh**
  - **M89.452 Other hypertrophic osteoarthropathy, left thigh**
  - **M89.459 Other hypertrophic osteoarthropathy, unspecified thigh**

+ **M89.46 Other hypertrophic osteoarthropathy, lower leg**
  - **M89.461 Other hypertrophic osteoarthropathy, right lower leg**
  - **M89.462 Other hypertrophic osteoarthropathy, left lower leg**
  - **M89.469 Other hypertrophic osteoarthropathy, unspecified lower leg**

+ **M89.47 Other hypertrophic osteoarthropathy, ankle and foot**
  - **M89.471 Other hypertrophic osteoarthropathy, right ankle and foot**
  - **M89.472 Other hypertrophic osteoarthropathy, left ankle and foot**
  - **M89.479 Other hypertrophic osteoarthropathy, unspecified ankle and foot**

M89.48 Other hypertrophic osteoarthropathy, other site

M89.49 Other hypertrophic osteoarthropathy, multiple sites

+ **M89.5 Osteolysis**

Use additional code to identify major osseous defect, if applicable (M89.7-)

Excludes2: *periprosthetic osteolysis of internal prosthetic joint (T84.05-)*

M89.50 Osteolysis, unspecified site

+ **M89.51 Osteolysis, shoulder**
  - **M89.511 Osteolysis, right shoulder**
  - **M89.512 Osteolysis, left shoulder**
  - **M89.519 Osteolysis, unspecified shoulder**

+ **M89.52 Osteolysis, upper arm**
  - **M89.521 Osteolysis, right upper arm**
  - **M89.522 Osteolysis, left upper arm**
  - **M89.529 Osteolysis, unspecified upper arm**

+ **M89.53 Osteolysis, forearm**
  - **M89.531 Osteolysis, right forearm**
  - **M89.532 Osteolysis, left forearm**
  - **M89.539 Osteolysis, unspecified forearm**

+ **M89.54 Osteolysis, hand**
  - **M89.541 Osteolysis, right hand**
  - **M89.542 Osteolysis, left hand**
  - **M89.549 Osteolysis, unspecified hand**

+ **M89.55 Osteolysis, thigh**
  - **M89.551 Osteolysis, right thigh**
  - **M89.552 Osteolysis, left thigh**
  - **M89.559 Osteolysis, unspecified thigh**

+ **M89.56 Osteolysis, lower leg**
  - **M89.561 Osteolysis, right lower leg**
  - **M89.562 Osteolysis, left lower leg**
  - **M89.569 Osteolysis, unspecified lower leg**

+ **M89.57 Osteolysis, ankle and foot**
  - **M89.571 Osteolysis, right ankle and foot**
  - **M89.572 Osteolysis, left ankle and foot**
  - **M89.579 Osteolysis, unspecified ankle and foot**

M89.58 Osteolysis, other site

M89.59 Osteolysis, multiple sites

+ **M89.6 Osteopathy after poliomyelitis**

Use additional code (B91) to identify previous poliomyelitis

Excludes1: *postpolio syndrome (G14)*

M89.60 Osteopathy after poliomyelitis, unspecified site

+ **M89.61 Osteopathy after poliomyelitis, shoulder**
  - **M89.611 Osteopathy after poliomyelitis, right shoulder**
  - **M89.612 Osteopathy after poliomyelitis, left shoulder**
  - **M89.619 Osteopathy after poliomyelitis, unspecified shoulder**

+ **M89.62 Osteopathy after poliomyelitis, upper arm**
  - **M89.621 Osteopathy after poliomyelitis, right upper arm**
  - **M89.622 Osteopathy after poliomyelitis, left upper arm**
  - **M89.629 Osteopathy after poliomyelitis, unspecified upper arm**

+ **M89.63 Osteopathy after poliomyelitis, forearm**
  - **M89.631 Osteopathy after poliomyelitis, right forearm**
  - **M89.632 Osteopathy after poliomyelitis, left forearm**
  - **M89.639 Osteopathy after poliomyelitis, unspecified forearm**

+ **M89.64 Osteopathy after poliomyelitis, hand**
  - **M89.641 Osteopathy after poliomyelitis, right hand**
  - **M89.642 Osteopathy after poliomyelitis, left hand**
  - **M89.649 Osteopathy after poliomyelitis, unspecified hand**

+ **M89.65 Osteopathy after poliomyelitis, thigh**
  - **M89.651 Osteopathy after poliomyelitis, right thigh**
  - **M89.652 Osteopathy after poliomyelitis, left thigh**
  - **M89.659 Osteopathy after poliomyelitis, unspecified thigh**

+ **M89.66 Osteopathy after poliomyelitis, lower leg**
  - **M89.661 Osteopathy after poliomyelitis, right lower leg**
  - **M89.662 Osteopathy after poliomyelitis, left lower leg**
  - **M89.669 Osteopathy after poliomyelitis, unspecified lower leg**

+ **M89.67 Osteopathy after poliomyelitis, ankle and foot**
  - **M89.671 Osteopathy after poliomyelitis, right ankle and foot**
  - **M89.672 Osteopathy after poliomyelitis, left ankle and foot**
  - **M89.679 Osteopathy after poliomyelitis, unspecified ankle and foot**

M89.68 Osteopathy after poliomyelitis, other site

M89.69 Osteopathy after poliomyelitis, multiple sites

+ **M89.7 Major osseous defect**

Code first underlying disease, if known, such as:
- aseptic necrosis of bone (M87.-)
- malignant neoplasm of bone (C40.-)
- osteolysis (M89.5)
- osteomyelitis (M86.-)
- osteonecrosis (M87.-)
- osteoporosis (M80.-, M81.-)
- periprosthetic osteolysis (T84.05-)

M89.70 Major osseous defect, unspecified site

+ **M89.71 Major osseous defect, shoulder region**

Major osseous defect clavicle or scapula
  - **M89.711 Major osseous defect, right shoulder region**
  - **M89.712 Major osseous defect, left shoulder region**
  - **M89.719 Major osseous defect, unspecified shoulder region**

+ **M89.72 Major osseous defect, humerus**
  - **M89.721 Major osseous defect, right humerus**
  - **M89.722 Major osseous defect, left humerus**
  - **M89.729 Major osseous defect, unspecified humerus**

+ **M89.73 Major osseous defect, forearm**

Major osseous defect of radius and ulna
  - **M89.731 Major osseous defect, right forearm**
  - **M89.732 Major osseous defect, left forearm**
  - **M89.739 Major osseous defect, unspecified forearm**

+ **M89.74 Major osseous defect, hand**

Major osseous defect of carpus, fingers, metacarpus
  - **M89.741 Major osseous defect, right hand**
  - **M89.742 Major osseous defect, left hand**
  - **M89.749 Major osseous defect, unspecified hand**

+ **M89.75 Major osseous defect, pelvic region and thigh**

Major osseous defect of femur and pelvis
  - **M89.751 Major osseous defect, right pelvic region and thigh**
  - **M89.752 Major osseous defect, left pelvic region and thigh**
  - **M89.759 Major osseous defect, unspecified pelvic region and thigh**

+ **M89.76 Major osseous defect, lower leg**

Major osseous defect of fibula and tibia
  - **M89.761 Major osseous defect, right lower leg**
  - **M89.762 Major osseous defect, left lower leg**
  - **M89.769 Major osseous defect, unspecified lower leg**

+ **M89.77 Major osseous defect, ankle and foot**

Major osseous defect of metatarsus, tarsus, toes
  - **M89.771 Major osseous defect, right ankle and foot**
  - **M89.772 Major osseous defect, left ankle and foot**
  - **M89.779 Major osseous defect, unspecified ankle and foot**

M89.78 Major osseous defect, other site

M89.79 Major osseous defect, multiple sites

+ **M89.8 Other specified disorders of bone**

Infantile cortical hyperostoses
Post-traumatic subperiosteal ossification

+ **M89.8X Other specified disorders of bone**
  - **M89.8X0 Other specified disorders of bone, multiple sites**
  - **M89.8X1 Other specified disorders of bone, shoulder**
  - **M89.8X2 Other specified disorders of bone, upper arm**
  - **M89.8X3 Other specified disorders of bone, forearm**
    AHA CC: 3Q, 2019, 9-10
  - **M89.8X4 Other specified disorders of bone, hand**
  - **M89.8X5 Other specified disorders of bone, thigh**
  - **M89.8X6 Other specified disorders of bone, lower leg**
  - **M89.8X7 Other specified disorders of bone, ankle and foot**
  - **M89.8X8 Other specified disorders of bone, other site**
  - **M89.8X9 Other specified disorders of bone, unspecified site**

M89.9 Disorder of bone, unspecified

M90 Osteopathies in diseases classified elsewhere

Excludes1: *osteochondritis, osteomyelitis, and osteopathy (in):*
cryptococcosis (B45.3)
diabetes mellitus (E08-E13 with .69-)
gonococcal (A54.43)
neurogenic syphilis (A52.11)
renal osteodystrophy (N25.0)
salmonellosis (A02.24)
secondary syphilis (A51.46)
syphilis (late) (A52.77)

+ **M90.5 Osteonecrosis in diseases classified elsewhere**

Code first underlying disease, such as:
- caisson disease (T70.3)
- hemoglobinopathy (D50-D64)

CC **M90.50 Osteonecrosis in diseases classified elsewhere, unspecified site**

+ **M90.51 Osteonecrosis in diseases classified elsewhere, shoulder**
  - CC **M90.511 Osteonecrosis in diseasesclassified elsewhere, rightshoulder**
  - CC **M90.512 Osteonecrosis in diseases classified elsewhere, left shoulder**
  - CC **M90.519 Osteonecrosis in diseases classified elsewhere, unspecified shoulder**

+ **M90.52 Osteonecrosis in diseases classified elsewhere, upper arm**
  - CC **M90.521 Osteonecrosis in diseases classified elsewhere, right upper arm**
  - CC **M90.522 Osteonecrosis in diseases classified elsewhere, left upper arm**
  - CC **M90.529 Osteonecrosis in diseases classified elsewhere, unspecified upper arm**

Knee Injuries and Problems

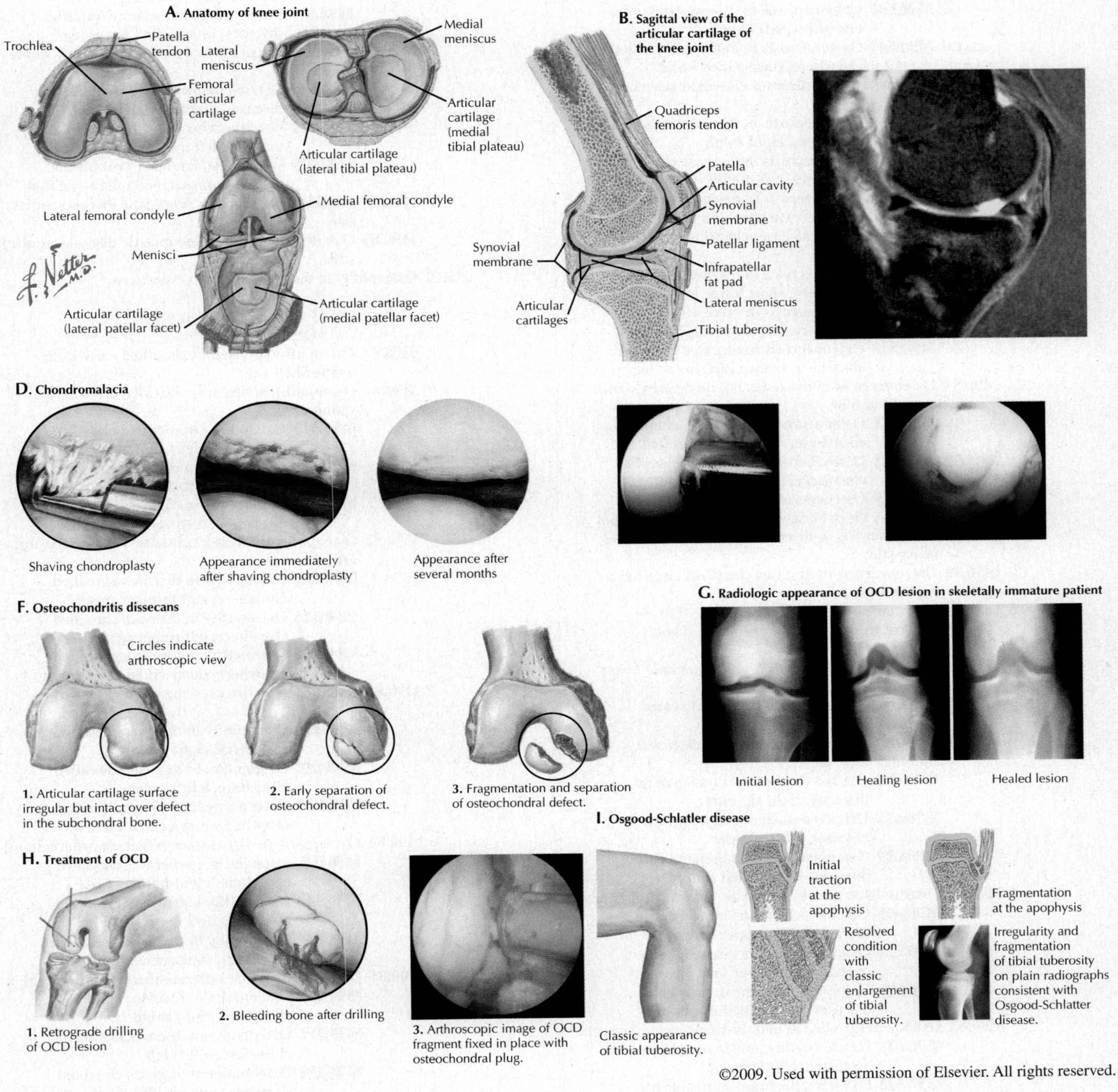

+ **M90.53** **Osteonecrosis in diseases classified elsewhere, forearm**
  - CC **M90.531** **Osteonecrosis in diseases classified elsewhere, right forearm**
  - CC **M90.532** **Osteonecrosis in diseases classified elsewhere, left forearm**
  - CC **M90.539** **Osteonecrosis in diseases classified elsewhere, unspecified forearm**

+ **M90.54** **Osteonecrosis in diseases classified elsewhere, hand**
  - CC **M90.541** **Osteonecrosis in diseases classified elsewhere, right hand**
  - CC **M90.542** **Osteonecrosis in diseases classified elsewhere, left hand**
  - CC **M90.549** **Osteonecrosis in diseases classified elsewhere, unspecified hand**

+ **M90.55** **Osteonecrosis in diseases classified elsewhere, thigh**
  - CC **M90.551** **Osteonecrosis in diseases classified elsewhere, right thigh**
  - CC **M90.552** **Osteonecrosis in diseases classified elsewhere, left thigh**
  - CC **M90.559** **Osteonecrosis in diseases classified elsewhere, unspecified thigh**

+ **M90.56** **Osteonecrosis in diseases classified elsewhere, lower leg**
  - CC **M90.561** **Osteonecrosis in diseases classified elsewhere, right lower leg**
  - CC **M90.562** **Osteonecrosis in diseases classified elsewhere, left lower leg**
  - CC **M90.569** **Osteonecrosis in diseases classified elsewhere, unspecified lower leg**

+ **M90.57** **Osteonecrosis in diseases classified elsewhere, ankle and foot**
  - CC **M90.571** **Osteonecrosis in diseases classified elsewhere, right ankle and foot**
  - CC **M90.572** **Osteonecrosis in diseases classified elsewhere, left ankle and foot**
  - CC **M90.579** **Osteonecrosis in diseases classified elsewhere, unspecified ankle and foot**

CC **M90.58** **Osteonecrosis in diseases classified elsewhere, other site**

CC **M90.59** **Osteonecrosis in diseases classified elsewhere, multiple sites**

+ **M90.6** **Osteitis deformans in neoplastic diseases**

Osteitis deformans in malignant neoplasm of bone

Code first the neoplasm (C40.-, C41.-)

Excludes1: *osteitis deformans [Paget's disease of bone] (M88.-)*

M90.60 **Osteitis deformans in neoplastic diseases, unspecified site**

+ **M90.61** **Osteitis deformans in neoplastic diseases, shoulder**
  - **M90.611** **Osteitis deformans in neoplastic diseases, right shoulder**
  - **M90.612** **Osteitis deformans in neoplastic diseases, left shoulder**
  - **M90.619** **Osteitis deformans in neoplastic diseases, unspecified shoulder**

+ **M90.62** **Osteitis deformans in neoplastic diseases, upper arm**
  - **M90.621** **Osteitis deformans in neoplastic diseases, right upper arm**
  - **M90.622** **Osteitis deformans in neoplastic diseases, left upper arm**
  - **M90.629** **Osteitis deformans in neoplastic diseases, unspecified upper arm**

+ **M90.63** **Osteitis deformans in neoplastic diseases, forearm**
  - **M90.631** **Osteitis deformans in neoplastic diseases, right forearm**
  - **M90.632** **Osteitis deformans in neoplastic diseases, left forearm**
  - **M90.639** **Osteitis deformans in neoplastic diseases, unspecified forearm**

+ **M90.64** **Osteitis deformans in neoplastic diseases, hand**
  - **M90.641** **Osteitis deformans in neoplastic diseases, right hand**
  - **M90.642** **Osteitis deformans in neoplastic diseases, left hand**
  - **M90.649** **Osteitis deformans in neoplastic diseases, unspecified hand**

+ **M90.65** **Osteitis deformans in neoplastic diseases, thigh**
  - **M90.651** **Osteitis deformans in neoplastic diseases, right thigh**
  - **M90.652** **Osteitis deformans in neoplastic diseases, left thigh**
  - **M90.659** **Osteitis deformans in neoplastic diseases, unspecified thigh**

+ **M90.66** **Osteitis deformans in neoplastic diseases, lower leg**
  - **M90.661** **Osteitis deformans in neoplastic diseases, right lower leg**
  - **M90.662** **Osteitis deformans in neoplastic diseases, left lower leg**
  - **M90.669** **Osteitis deformans in neoplastic diseases, unspecified lower leg**

+ **M90.67** **Osteitis deformans in neoplastic diseases, ankle and foot**
  - **M90.671** **Osteitis deformans in neoplastic diseases, right ankle and foot**
  - **M90.672** **Osteitis deformans in neoplastic diseases, left ankle and foot**
  - **M90.679** **Osteitis deformans in neoplastic diseases, unspecified ankle and foot**

M90.68 **Osteitis deformans in neoplastic diseases, other site**

M90.69 **Osteitis deformans in neoplastic diseases, multiple sites**

+ **M90.8** **Osteopathy in diseases classified elsewhere**

Code first underlying disease, such as:
- rickets (E55.0)
- vitamin-D-resistant rickets (E83.3)

M90.80 **Osteopathy in diseases classified elsewhere, unspecified site**

+ **M90.81** **Osteopathy in diseases classified elsewhere, shoulder**
  - **M90.811** **Osteopathy in diseases classified elsewhere, right shoulder**
  - **M90.812** **Osteopathy in diseases classified elsewhere, left shoulder**
  - **M90.819** **Osteopathy in diseases classified elsewhere, unspecified shoulder**

+ **M90.82** **Osteopathy in diseases classified elsewhere, upper arm**
  - **M90.821** **Osteopathy in diseases classified elsewhere, right upper arm**
  - **M90.822** **Osteopathy in diseases classified elsewhere, left upper arm**
  - **M90.829** **Osteopathy in diseases classified elsewhere, unspecified upper arm**

+ **M90.83** **Osteopathy in diseases classified elsewhere, forearm**
  - **M90.831** **Osteopathy in diseases classified elsewhere, right forearm**
  - **M90.832** **Osteopathy in diseases classified elsewhere, left forearm**
  - **M90.839** **Osteopathy in diseases classified elsewhere, unspecified forearm**

+ **M90.84** **Osteopathy in diseases classified elsewhere, hand**
  - **M90.841** **Osteopathy in diseases classified elsewhere, right hand**
  - **M90.842** **Osteopathy in diseases classified elsewhere, left hand**
  - **M90.849** **Osteopathy in diseases classified elsewhere, unspecified hand**

+ **M90.85** **Osteopathy in diseases classified elsewhere, thigh**
  - **M90.851** **Osteopathy in diseases classified elsewhere, right thigh**
  - **M90.852** **Osteopathy in diseases classified elsewhere, left thigh**
  - **M90.859** **Osteopathy in diseases classified elsewhere, unspecified thigh**

+ **M90.86** **Osteopathy in diseases classified elsewhere, lower leg**
  - **M90.861** **Osteopathy in diseases classified elsewhere, right lower leg**
  - **M90.862** **Osteopathy in diseases classified elsewhere, left lower leg**
  - **M90.869** **Osteopathy in diseases classified elsewhere, unspecified lower leg**

+ **M90.87 Osteopathy in diseases classified elsewhere, ankle and foot**
M90.871 Osteopathy in diseases classified elsewhere, right ankle and foot
M90.872 Osteopathy in diseases classified elsewhere, left ankle and foot
M90.879 Osteopathy in diseases classified elsewhere, unspecified ankle and foot
M90.88 Osteopathy in diseases classified elsewhere, other site
M90.89 Osteopathy in diseases classified elsewhere, multiple sites

Chondropathies (M91-M94)

Excludes1: *postprocedural chondropathies (M96.-)*

M91 Juvenile osteochondrosis of hip and pelvis
Excludes1: *slipped upper femoral epiphysis (nontraumatic) (M93.0)*
M91.0 Juvenile osteochondrosis of pelvis
Osteochondrosis (juvenile) of acetabulum
Osteochondrosis (juvenile) of iliac crest [Buchanan]
Osteochondrosis (juvenile) of ischiopubic synchondrosis [van Neck]
Osteochondrosis (juvenile) of symphysis pubis [Pierson]
+ **M91.1 Juvenile osteochondrosis of head of femur [Legg-Calvé-Perthes]**
M91.10 Juvenile osteochondrosis of head of femur [Legg-Calvé-Perthes], unspecified leg
M91.11 Juvenile osteochondrosis of head of femur [Legg-Calvé-Perthes], right leg
M91.12 Juvenile osteochondrosis of head of femur [Legg-Calvé-Perthes], left leg
+ **M91.2 Coxa plana**
Hip deformity due to previous juvenile osteochondrosis
M91.20 Coxa plana, unspecified hip
M91.21 Coxa plana, right hip
M91.22 Coxa plana, left hip
+ **M91.3 Pseudocoxalgia**
M91.30 Pseudocoxalgia, unspecified hip
M91.31 Pseudocoxalgia, right hip
M91.32 Pseudocoxalgia, left hip
+ **M91.4 Coxa magna**
M91.40 Coxa magna, unspecified hip
M91.41 Coxa magna, right hip
M91.42 Coxa magna, left hip
+ **M91.8 Other juvenile osteochondrosis of hip and pelvis**
Juvenile osteochondrosis after reduction of congenital dislocation of hip
M91.80 Other juvenile osteochondrosis of hip and pelvis, unspecified leg
M91.81 Other juvenile osteochondrosis of hip and pelvis, right leg
M91.82 Other juvenile osteochondrosis of hip and pelvis, left leg
+ **M91.9 Juvenile osteochondrosis of hip and pelvis, unspecified**
M91.90 Juvenile osteochondrosis of hip and pelvis, unspecified, unspecified leg
M91.91 Juvenile osteochondrosis of hip and pelvis, unspecified, right leg
M91.92 Juvenile osteochondrosis of hip and pelvis, unspecified, left leg

M92 Other juvenile osteochondrosis
+ **M92.0 Juvenile osteochondrosis of humerus**
Osteochondrosis (juvenile) of capitulum of humerus [Panner]
Osteochondrosis (juvenile) of head of humerus [Haas]
M92.00 Juvenile osteochondrosis of humerus, unspecified arm
M92.01 Juvenile osteochondrosis of humerus, right arm
M92.02 Juvenile osteochondrosis of humerus, left arm
+ **M92.1 Juvenile osteochondrosis of radius and ulna**
Osteochondrosis (juvenile) of lower ulna [Burns]
Osteochondrosis (juvenile) of radial head [Brailsford]
M92.10 Juvenile osteochondrosis of radius and ulna, unspecified arm
M92.11 Juvenile osteochondrosis of radius and ulna, right arm
M92.12 Juvenile osteochondrosis of radius and ulna, left arm
+ **M92.2 Juvenile osteochondrosis, hand**
+ **M92.20 Unspecified juvenile osteochondrosis, hand**
M92.201 Unspecified juvenile osteochondrosis, right hand
M92.202 Unspecified juvenile osteochondrosis, left hand
M92.209 Unspecified juvenile osteochondrosis, unspecified hand
+ **M92.21 Osteochondrosis (juvenile) of carpal lunate [Kienböck]**
M92.211 Osteochondrosis (juvenile) of carpal lunate [Kienböck], right hand
M92.212 Osteochondrosis (juvenile) of carpal lunate [Kienböck], left hand
M92.219 Osteochondrosis (juvenile) of carpal lunate [Kienböck], unspecified hand
+ **M92.22 Osteochondrosis (juvenile) of metacarpal heads [Mauclaire]**
M92.221 Osteochondrosis (juvenile) of metacarpal heads [Mauclaire], right hand
M92.222 Osteochondrosis (juvenile) of metacarpal heads [Mauclaire], left hand
M92.229 Osteochondrosis (juvenile) of metacarpal heads [Mauclaire], unspecified hand
+ **M92.29 Other juvenile osteochondrosis, hand**
M92.291 Other juvenile osteochondrosis, right hand
M92.292 Other juvenile osteochondrosis, left hand
M92.299 Other juvenile osteochondrosis, unspecified hand
+ **M92.3 Other juvenile osteochondrosis, upper limb**
M92.30 Other juvenile osteochondrosis, unspecified upper limb
M92.31 Other juvenile osteochondrosis, right upper limb
M92.32 Other juvenile osteochondrosis, left upper limb
+ **M92.4 Juvenile osteochondrosis of patella**
Osteochondrosis (juvenile) of primary patellar center [Köhler]
Osteochondrosis (juvenile) of secondary patellar centre [Sinding Larsen]
M92.40 Juvenile osteochondrosis of patella, unspecified knee
M92.41 Juvenile osteochondrosis of patella, right knee
M92.42 Juvenile osteochondrosis of patella, left knee
+ **M92.5 Juvenile osteochondrosis of tibia and fibula tubercle**
AHA CC: 4Q, 2020, 33-34
+ **M92.50 Unspecified juvenile osteochondrosis of tibia and fibula**
M92.501 Unspecified juvenile osteochondrosis, right leg
M92.502 Unspecified juvenile osteochondrosis, left leg
M92.503 Unspecified juvenile osteochondrosis, bilateral leg
M92.509 Unspecified juvenile osteochondrosis, unspecified leg
+ **M92.51 Juvenile osteochondrosis of proximal tibia**
Blount disease
Tibia vara
M92.511 Juvenile osteochondrosis of proximal tibia, right leg
M92.512 Juvenile osteochondrosis of proximal tibia, left leg
M92.513 Juvenile osteochondrosis of proximal tibia, bilateral
M92.519 Juvenile osteochondrosis of proximal tibia, unspecified leg
+ **M92.52 Juvenile osteochondrosis of tibia tubercle**
Osgood-Schlatter disease
M92.521 Juvenile osteochondrosis of tibia tubercle, right leg
M92.522 Juvenile osteochondrosis of tibia tubercle, left leg
M92.523 Juvenile osteochondrosis of tibia tubercle, bilateral
M92.529 Juvenile osteochondrosis of tibia tubercle, unspecified leg

+ M92.59 Other juvenile osteochondrosis of tibia and fibula
M92.591 Other juvenile osteochondrosis of tibia and fibula, right leg
M92.592 Other juvenile osteochondrosis of tibia and fibula, left leg
M92.593 Other juvenile osteochondrosis of tibia and fibula, bilateral
M92.599 Other juvenile osteochondrosis of tibia and fibula, unspecified leg
+ M92.6 Juvenile osteochondrosis of tarsus
Osteochondrosis (juvenile) of calcaneum [Sever]
Osteochondrosis (juvenile) of os tibiale externum [Haglund]
Osteochondrosis (juvenile) of talus [Diaz]
Osteochondrosis (juvenile) of tarsal navicular [Köhler]
M92.60 Juvenile osteochondrosis of tarsus, unspecified ankle
M92.61 Juvenile osteochondrosis of tarsus, right ankle
M92.62 Juvenile osteochondrosis of tarsus, left ankle
+ M92.7 Juvenile osteochondrosis of metatarsus
Osteochondrosis (juvenile) of fifth metatarsus [Iselin]
Osteochondrosis (juvenile) of second metatarsus [Freiberg]
M92.70 Juvenile osteochondrosis of metatarsus, unspecified foot
M92.71 Juvenile osteochondrosis of metatarsus, right foot
M92.72 Juvenile osteochondrosis of metatarsus, left foot
M92.8 Other specified juvenile osteochondrosis
Calcaneal apophysitis
M92.9 Juvenile osteochondrosis, unspecified
Juvenile apophysitis NOS
Juvenile epiphysitis NOS
Juvenile osteochondritis NOS
Juvenile osteochondrosis NOS

M93 Other osteochondropathies

Excludes2: *osteochondrosis of spine (M42.-)*

+ M93.0 Slipped upper femoral epiphysis (nontraumatic)
Use additional code for associated chondrolysis (M94.3)
+ M93.00 Unspecified slipped upper femoral epiphysis (nontraumatic)
M93.001 Unspecified slipped upper femoral epiphysis (nontraumatic), right hip
M93.002 Unspecified slipped upper femoral epiphysis (nontraumatic), left hip
M93.003 Unspecified slipped upper femoral epiphysis (nontraumatic), unspecified hip
+ M93.01 Acute slipped upper femoral epiphysis (nontraumatic)
M93.011 Acute slipped upper femoral epiphysis (nontraumatic), right hip
M93.012 Acute slipped upper femoral epiphysis (nontraumatic), left hip
M93.013 Acute slipped upper femoral epiphysis (nontraumatic), unspecified hip
+ M93.02 Chronic slipped upper femoral epiphysis (nontraumatic)
M93.021 Chronic slipped upper femoral epiphysis (nontraumatic), right hip
M93.022 Chronic slipped upper femoral epiphysis (nontraumatic), left hip
M93.023 Chronic slipped upper femoral epiphysis (nontraumatic), unspecified hip
+ M93.03 Acute on chronic slipped upper femoral epiphysis (nontraumatic)
M93.031 Acute on chronic slipped upper femoral epiphysis (nontraumatic), right hip
M93.032 Acute on chronic slipped upper femoral epiphysis (nontraumatic), left hip
M93.033 Acute on chronic slipped upper femoral epiphysis (nontraumatic), unspecified hip
● M93.1 Kienböck's disease of adults
Adult osteochondrosis of carpal lunates
+ M93.2 Osteochondritis dissecans
M93.20 Osteochondritis dissecans of unspecified site
+ M93.21 Osteochondritis dissecans of shoulder
M93.211 Osteochondritis dissecans, right shoulder
M93.212 Osteochondritis dissecans, left shoulder
M93.219 Osteochondritis dissecans, unspecified shoulder
+ M93.22 Osteochondritis dissecans of elbow
M93.221 Osteochondritis dissecans, right elbow
M93.222 Osteochondritis dissecans, left elbow
M93.229 Osteochondritis dissecans, unspecified elbow
+ M93.23 Osteochondritis dissecans of wrist
M93.231 Osteochondritis dissecans, right wrist
M93.232 Osteochondritis dissecans, left wrist
M93.239 Osteochondritis dissecans, unspecified wrist
+ M93.24 Osteochondritis dissecans of joints of hand
M93.241 Osteochondritis dissecans, joints of right hand
M93.242 Osteochondritis dissecans, joints of left hand
M93.249 Osteochondritis dissecans, joints of unspecified hand
+ M93.25 Osteochondritis dissecans of hip
M93.251 Osteochondritis dissecans, right hip
M93.252 Osteochondritis dissecans, left hip
M93.259 Osteochondritis dissecans, unspecified hip
+ M93.26 Osteochondritis dissecans knee
M93.261 Osteochondritis dissecans, right knee
M93.262 Osteochondritis dissecans, left knee
M93.269 Osteochondritis dissecans, unspecified knee
+ M93.27 Osteochondritis dissecans of ankle and joints of foot
M93.271 Osteochondritis dissecans, right ankle and joints of right foot
M93.272 Osteochondritis dissecans, left ankle and joints of left foot
M93.279 Osteochondritis dissecans, unspecified ankle and joints of foot
M93.28 Osteochondritis dissecans other site
M93.29 Osteochondritis dissecans multiple sites
+ M93.8 Other specified osteochondropathies
M93.80 Other specified osteochondropathies of unspecified site
+ M93.81 Other specified osteochondropathies of shoulder
M93.811 Other specified osteochondropathies, right shoulder
M93.812 Other specified osteochondropathies, left shoulder
M93.819 Other specified osteochondropathies, unspecified shoulder
+ M93.82 Other specified osteochondropathies of upper arm
M93.821 Other specified osteochondropathies, right upper arm
M93.822 Other specified osteochondropathies, left upper arm
M93.829 Other specified osteochondropathies, unspecified upper arm
+ M93.83 Other specified osteochondropathies of forearm
M93.831 Other specified osteochondropathies, right forearm
M93.832 Other specified osteochondropathies, left forearm
M93.839 Other specified osteochondropathies, unspecified forearm
+ M93.84 Other specified osteochondropathies of hand
M93.841 Other specified osteochondropathies, right hand
M93.842 Other specified osteochondropathies, left hand
M93.849 Other specified osteochondropathies, unspecified hand
+ M93.85 Other specified osteochondropathies of thigh
M93.851 Other specified osteochondropathies, right thigh
M93.852 Other specified osteochondropathies, left thigh
M93.859 Other specified osteochondropathies, unspecified thigh

+ M93.86 Other specified osteochondropathies lower leg
M93.861 Other specified osteochondropathies, right lower leg
M93.862 Other specified osteochondropathies, left lower leg
M93.869 Other specified osteochondropathies, unspecified lower leg
+ M93.87 Other specified osteochondropathies of ankle and foot
M93.871 Other specified osteochondropathies, right ankle and foot
M93.872 Other specified osteochondropathies, left ankle and foot
M93.879 Other specified osteochondropathies, unspecified ankle and foot
M93.88 Other specified osteochondropathies other
M93.89 Other specified osteochondropathies multiple sites
+ M93.9 Osteochondropathy, unspecified
Apophysitis NOS
Epiphysitis NOS
Osteochondritis NOS
Osteochondrosis NOS
M93.90 Osteochondropathy, unspecified of unspecified site
+ M93.91 Osteochondropathy, unspecified of shoulder
M93.911 Osteochondropathy, unspecified, right shoulder
M93.912 Osteochondropathy, unspecified, left shoulder
M93.919 Osteochondropathy, unspecified, unspecified shoulder
+ M93.92 Osteochondropathy, unspecified of upper arm
M93.921 Osteochondropathy, unspecified, right upper arm
M93.922 Osteochondropathy, unspecified, left upper arm
M93.929 Osteochondropathy, unspecified, unspecified upper arm
+ M93.93 Osteochondropathy, unspecified of forearm
M93.931 Osteochondropathy, unspecified, right forearm
M93.932 Osteochondropathy, unspecified, left forearm
M93.939 Osteochondropathy, unspecified, unspecified forearm
+ M93.94 Osteochondropathy, unspecified of hand
M93.941 Osteochondropathy, unspecified, right hand
M93.942 Osteochondropathy, unspecified, left hand
M93.949 Osteochondropathy, unspecified, unspecified hand
+ M93.95 Osteochondropathy, unspecified of thigh
M93.951 Osteochondropathy, unspecified, right thigh
M93.952 Osteochondropathy, unspecified, left thigh
M93.959 Osteochondropathy, unspecified, unspecified thigh
+ M93.96 Osteochondropathy, unspecified lower leg
M93.961 Osteochondropathy, unspecified, right lower leg
M93.962 Osteochondropathy, unspecified, left lower leg
M93.969 Osteochondropathy, unspecified, unspecified lower leg
+ M93.97 Osteochondropathy, unspecified of ankle and foot
M93.971 Osteochondropathy, unspecified, right ankle and foot
M93.972 Osteochondropathy, unspecified, left ankle and foot
M93.979 Osteochondropathy, unspecified, unspecified ankle and foot
M93.98 Osteochondropathy, unspecified other
M93.99 Osteochondropathy, unspecified multiple sites

M94 Other disorders of cartilage
M94.0 Chondrocostal junction syndrome [Tietze]
Costochondritis
M94.1 Relapsing polychondritis
+ M94.2 Chondromalacia
Excludes1: *chondromalacia patellae (M22.4)*
M94.20 Chondromalacia, unspecified site
+ M94.21 Chondromalacia, shoulder
M94.211 Chondromalacia, right shoulder
M94.212 Chondromalacia, left shoulder
M94.219 Chondromalacia, unspecified shoulder
+ M94.22 Chondromalacia, elbow
M94.221 Chondromalacia, right elbow
M94.222 Chondromalacia, left elbow
M94.229 Chondromalacia, unspecified elbow
+ M94.23 Chondromalacia, wrist
M94.231 Chondromalacia, right wrist
M94.232 Chondromalacia, left wrist
M94.239 Chondromalacia, unspecified wrist
+ M94.24 Chondromalacia, joints of hand
M94.241 Chondromalacia, joints of right hand
M94.242 Chondromalacia, joints of left hand
M94.249 Chondromalacia, joints of unspecified hand
+ M94.25 Chondromalacia, hip
M94.251 Chondromalacia, right hip
M94.252 Chondromalacia, left hip
M94.259 Chondromalacia, unspecified hip
+ M94.26 Chondromalacia, knee
M94.261 Chondromalacia, right knee
M94.262 Chondromalacia, left knee
M94.269 Chondromalacia, unspecified knee
+ M94.27 Chondromalacia, ankle and joints of foot
M94.271 Chondromalacia, right ankle and joints of right foot
M94.272 Chondromalacia, left ankle and joints of left foot
M94.279 Chondromalacia, unspecified ankle and joints of foot
M94.28 Chondromalacia, other site
M94.29 Chondromalacia, multiple sites
+ M94.3 Chondrolysis
Code first any associated slipped upper femoral epiphysis (nontraumatic) (M93.0-)
+ M94.35 Chondrolysis, hip
M94.351 Chondrolysis, right hip
M94.352 Chondrolysis, left hip
M94.359 Chondrolysis, unspecified hip
+ M94.8 Other specified disorders of cartilage
+ M94.8X Other specified disorders of cartilage
M94.8X0 Other specified disorders of cartilage, multiple sites
M94.8X1 Other specified disorders of cartilage, shoulder
M94.8X2 Other specified disorders of cartilage, upper arm
M94.8X3 Other specified disorders of cartilage, forearm
M94.8X4 Other specified disorders of cartilage, hand
M94.8X5 Other specified disorders of cartilage, thigh
M94.8X6 Other specified disorders of cartilage, lower leg
M94.8X7 Other specified disorders of cartilage, ankle and foot
M94.8X8 Other specified disorders of cartilage, other site
M94.8X9 Other specified disorders of cartilage, unspecified sites
M94.9 Disorder of cartilage, unspecified

Other disorders of the musculoskeletal system and connective tissue (M95)

M95 Other acquired deformities of musculoskeletal system and connective tissue

Excludes2: *acquired absence of limbs and organs (Z89-Z90)*
acquired deformities of limbs (M20-M21)
congenital malformations and deformations of the musculoskeletal system (Q65-Q79)
deforming dorsopathies (M40-M43)
dentofacial anomalies [including malocclusion] (M26.-)
postprocedural musculoskeletal disorders (M96.-)

M95.0 Acquired deformity of nose
Excludes2: *deviated nasal septum (J34.2)*

+ **M95.1 Cauliflower ear**
Excludes2: *other acquired deformities of ear (H61.1)*
M95.10 Cauliflower ear, unspecified ear
M95.11 Cauliflower ear, right ear
M95.12 Cauliflower ear, left ear

M95.2 Other acquired deformity of head
M95.3 Acquired deformity of neck
M95.4 Acquired deformity of chest and rib
AHA CC: 4Q, 2014, 26-27
M95.5 Acquired deformity of pelvis
Excludes1: *maternal care for known or suspected disproportion (O33.-)*
M95.8 Other specified acquired deformities of musculoskeletal system
M95.9 Acquired deformity of musculoskeletal system, unspecified

Intraoperative and postprocedural complications and disorders of musculoskeletal system, not elsewhere classified (M96)

M96 Intraoperative and postprocedural complications and disorders of musculoskeletal system, not elsewhere classified

Excludes2: *arthropathy following intestinal bypass (M02.0-)*
complications of internal orthopedic prosthetic devices, implants and grafts (T84.-)
disorders associated with osteoporosis (M80)
periprosthetic fracture around internal prosthetic joint (M97.-)
presence of functional implants and other devices (Z96-Z97)

CC **M96.0 Pseudarthrosis after fusion or arthrodesis**
M96.1 Postlaminectomy syndrome, not elsewhere classified
M96.2 Postradiation kyphosis
M96.3 Postlaminectomy kyphosis
M96.4 Postsurgical lordosis
M96.5 Postradiation scoliosis

+ **M96.6 Fracture of bone following insertion of orthopedic implant, joint prosthesis, or bone plate**
Intraoperative fracture of bone during insertion of orthopedic implant, joint prosthesis, or bone plate
Excludes2: *complication of internal orthopedic devices, implants or grafts (T84.-)*

+ **M96.62 Fracture of humerus following insertion of orthopedic implant, joint prosthesis, or bone plate**
CC **M96.621 Fracture of humerus following insertion of orthopedic implant, joint prosthesis, or bone plate, right arm**
CC **M96.622 Fracture of humerus following insertion of orthopedic implant, joint prosthesis, or bone plate, left arm**
CC **M96.629 Fracture of humerus following insertion of orthopedic implant, joint prosthesis, or bone plate, unspecified arm**

+ **M96.63 Fracture of radius or ulna following insertion of orthopedic implant, joint prosthesis, or bone plate**
CC **M96.631 Fracture of radius or ulna following insertion of orthopedic implant, joint prosthesis, or bone plate, right arm**
CC **M96.632 Fracture of radius or ulna following insertion of orthopedic implant, joint prosthesis, or bone plate, left arm**
CC **M96.639 Fracture of radius or ulna following insertion of orthopedic implant, joint prosthesis, or bone plate, unspecified arm**

CC **M96.65 Fracture of pelvis following insertion of orthopedic implant, joint prosthesis, or bone plate**

+ **M96.66 Fracture of femur following insertion of orthopedic implant, joint prosthesis, or bone plate**
CC **M96.661 Fracture of femur following insertion of orthopedic implant, joint prosthesis, or bone plate, right leg**
CC **M96.662 Fracture of femur following insertion of orthopedic implant, joint prosthesis, or bone plate, left leg**
CC **M96.669 Fracture of femur following insertion of orthopedic implant, joint prosthesis, or bone plate, unspecified leg**

+ **M96.67 Fracture of tibia or fibula following insertion of orthopedic implant, joint prosthesis, or bone plate**
CC **M96.671 Fracture of tibia or fibula following insertion of orthopedic implant, joint prosthesis, or bone plate, right leg**
CC **M96.672 Fracture of tibia or fibula following insertion of orthopedic implant, joint prosthesis, or bone plate, left leg**
CC **M96.679 Fracture of tibia or fibula following insertion of orthopedic implant, joint prosthesis, or bone plate, unspecified leg**

CC **M96.69 Fracture of other bone following insertion of orthopedic implant, joint prosthesis, or bone plate**

+ **M96.8 Other intraoperative and postprocedural complications and disorders of musculoskeletal system, not elsewhere classified**
AHA CC: 4Q, 2016, 9-10

+ **M96.81 Intraoperative hemorrhage and hematoma of a musculoskeletal structure complicating a procedure**
Excludes1: *intraoperative hemorrhage and hematoma of a musculoskeletal structure due to accidental puncture and laceration during a procedure (M96.82)*
CC **M96.810 Intraoperative hemorrhage and hematoma of a musculoskeletal structure complicating a musculoskeletal system procedure**
CC **M96.811 Intraoperative hemorrhage and hematoma of a musculoskeletal structure complicating other procedure**

+ **M96.82 Accidental puncture and laceration of a musculoskeletal structure during a procedure**
CC **M96.820 Accidental puncture and laceration of a musculoskeletal structure during a musculoskeletal system procedure**
CC **M96.821 Accidental puncture and laceration of a musculoskeletal structure during other procedure**

+ **M96.83 Postprocedural hemorrhage of a musculoskeletal structure following a procedure**
CC **M96.830 Postprocedural hemorrhage of a musculoskeletal structure following a musculoskeletal system procedure**
CC **M96.831 Postprocedural hemorrhage of a musculoskeletal structure following other procedure**

+ **M96.84 Postprocedural hematoma and seroma of a musculoskeletal structure following a procedure**
CC **M96.840 Postprocedural hematoma of a musculoskeletal structure following a musculoskeletal system procedure**
CC **M96.841 Postprocedural hematoma of a musculoskeletal structure following other procedure**
AHA CC: 4Q, 2016, 9-10
CC **M96.842 Postprocedural seroma of a musculoskeletal structure following a musculoskeletal system procedure**
CC **M96.843 Postprocedural seroma of a musculoskeletal structure following other procedure**
AHA CC: 3Q, 2018, 6

+ CC **M96.89 Other intraoperative and postprocedural complications and disorders of the musculoskeletal system**
Instability of joint secondary to removal of joint prosthesis
Use additional code, if applicable, to further specify disorder
AHA CC: 1Q, 2021, 5-6

Periprosthetic fracture around internal prosthetic joint (M97)

M97 Periprosthetic fracture around internal prosthetic joint
Excludes2: *fracture of bone following insertion of orthopedic implant, joint prosthesis or bone plate (M96.6-)*
breakage (fracture) of prosthetic joint (T84.01-)
AHA CC: 4Q, 2016, 42-43

The appropriate 7th character is to be added to each code from category M97:
A initial encounter
D subsequent encounter
S sequela

+ **M97.0 Periprosthetic fracture around internal prosthetic hip joint**
CC X+7th **M97.01 Periprosthetic fracture around internal prosthetic right hip joint**
AHA CC: 4Q, 2016, 42-43
CC X+7th **M97.02 Periprosthetic fracture around internal prosthetic left hip joint**
+ **M97.1 Periprosthetic fracture around internal prosthetic knee joint**
CC X+7th **M97.11 Periprosthetic fracture around internal prosthetic right knee joint**
CC X+7th **M97.12 Periprosthetic fracture around internal prosthetic left knee joint**
+ **M97.2 Periprosthetic fracture around internal prosthetic ankle joint**
CC X+7th **M97.21 Periprosthetic fracture around internal prosthetic right ankle joint**
CC X+7th **M97.22 Periprosthetic fracture around internal prosthetic left ankle joint**
+ **M97.3 Periprosthetic fracture around internal prosthetic shoulder joint**
CC X+7th **M97.31 Periprosthetic fracture around internal prosthetic right shoulder joint**
CC X+7th **M97.32 Periprosthetic fracture around internal prosthetic left shoulder joint**
+ **M97.4 Periprosthetic fracture around internal prosthetic elbow joint**
CC X+7th **M97.41 Periprosthetic fracture around internal prosthetic right elbow joint**
CC X+7th **M97.42 Periprosthetic fracture around internal prosthetic left elbow joint**
CC X+7th **M97.8 Periprosthetic fracture around other internal prosthetic joint**
Periprosthetic fracture around internal prosthetic finger joint
Periprosthetic fracture around internal prosthetic spinal joint
Periprosthetic fracture around internal prosthetic toe joint
Periprosthetic fracture around internal prosthetic wrist joint
Use additional code to identify the joint (Z96.6-)
CC X+7th **M97.9 Periprosthetic fracture around unspecified internal prosthetic joint**

Biomechanical lesions, not elsewhere classified (M99)

M99 Biomechanical lesions, not elsewhere classified
NOTE This category should not be used if the condition can be classified elsewhere.
+ **M99.0 Segmental and somatic dysfunction**
M99.00 Segmental and somatic dysfunction of head region
M99.01 Segmental and somatic dysfunction of cervical region
M99.02 Segmental and somatic dysfunction of thoracic region
M99.03 Segmental and somatic dysfunction of lumbar region
M99.04 Segmental and somatic dysfunction of sacral region
M99.05 Segmental and somatic dysfunction of pelvic region
M99.06 Segmental and somatic dysfunction of lower extremity
M99.07 Segmental and somatic dysfunction of upper extremity
M99.08 Segmental and somatic dysfunction of rib cage
M99.09 Segmental and somatic dysfunction of abdomen and other regions
+ **M99.1 Subluxation complex (vertebral)**
CC **M99.10 Subluxation complex (vertebral) of head region**
HAC see Appendix B for HAC conditional logic
CC **M99.11 Subluxation complex (vertebral) of cervical region**
HAC see Appendix B for HAC conditional logic
M99.12 Subluxation complex (vertebral) of thoracic region
M99.13 Subluxation complex (vertebral) of lumbar region
M99.14 Subluxation complex (vertebral) of sacral region
M99.15 Subluxation complex (vertebral) of pelvic region
M99.16 Subluxation complex (vertebral) of lower extremity
M99.17 Subluxation complex (vertebral) of upper extremity
CC **M99.18 Subluxation complex (vertebral) of rib cage**
HAC see Appendix B for HAC conditional logic
M99.19 Subluxation complex (vertebral) of abdomen and other regions
+ **M99.2 Subluxation stenosis of neural canal**
M99.20 Subluxation stenosis of neural canal of head region
M99.21 Subluxation stenosis of neural canal of cervical region
M99.22 Subluxation stenosis of neural canal of thoracic region
M99.23 Subluxation stenosis of neural canal of lumbar region
M99.24 Subluxation stenosis of neural canal of sacral region
M99.25 Subluxation stenosis of neural canal of pelvic region
M99.26 Subluxation stenosis of neural canal of lower extremity
M99.27 Subluxation stenosis of neural canal of upper extremity
M99.28 Subluxation stenosis of neural canal of rib cage
M99.29 Subluxation stenosis of neural canal of abdomen and other regions
+ **M99.3 Osseous stenosis of neural canal**
M99.30 Osseous stenosis of neural canal of head region
M99.31 Osseous stenosis of neural canal of cervical region
M99.32 Osseous stenosis of neural canal of thoracic region
M99.33 Osseous stenosis of neural canal of lumbar region
M99.34 Osseous stenosis of neural canal of sacral region
M99.35 Osseous stenosis of neural canal of pelvic region
M99.36 Osseous stenosis of neural canal of lower extremity
M99.37 Osseous stenosis of neural canal of upper extremity
M99.38 Osseous stenosis of neural canal of rib cage
M99.39 Osseous stenosis of neural canal of abdomen and other regions
+ **M99.4 Connective tissue stenosis of neural canal**
M99.40 Connective tissue stenosis of neural canal of head region
M99.41 Connective tissue stenosis of neural canal of cervical region
M99.42 Connective tissue stenosis of neural canal of thoracic region
M99.43 Connective tissue stenosis of neural canal of lumbar region
M99.44 Connective tissue stenosis of neural canal of sacral region
M99.45 Connective tissue stenosis of neural canal of pelvic region
M99.46 Connective tissue stenosis of neural canal of lower extremity
M99.47 Connective tissue stenosis of neural canal of upper extremity

M99.48 Connective tissue stenosis of neural canal of rib cage
M99.49 Connective tissue stenosis of neural canal of abdomen and other regions

+ M99.5 Intervertebral disc stenosis of neural canal
M99.50 Intervertebral disc stenosis of neural canal of head region
M99.51 Intervertebral disc stenosis of neural canal of cervical region
M99.52 Intervertebral disc stenosis of neural canal of thoracic region
M99.53 Intervertebral disc stenosis of neural canal of lumbar region
M99.54 Intervertebral disc stenosis of neural canal of sacral region
M99.55 Intervertebral disc stenosis of neural canal of pelvic region
M99.56 Intervertebral disc stenosis of neural canal of lower extremity
M99.57 Intervertebral disc stenosis of neural canal of upper extremity
M99.58 Intervertebral disc stenosis of neural canal of rib cage
M99.59 Intervertebral disc stenosis of neural canal of abdomen and other regions

+ M99.6 Osseous and subluxation stenosis of intervertebral foramina
M99.60 Osseous and subluxation stenosis of intervertebral foramina of head region
M99.61 Osseous and subluxation stenosis of intervertebral foramina of cervical region
M99.62 Osseous and subluxation stenosis of intervertebral foramina of thoracic region
M99.63 Osseous and subluxation stenosis of intervertebral foramina of lumbar region
M99.64 Osseous and subluxation stenosis of intervertebral foramina of sacral region
M99.65 Osseous and subluxation stenosis of intervertebral foramina of pelvic region
M99.66 Osseous and subluxation stenosis of intervertebral foramina of lower extremity
M99.67 Osseous and subluxation stenosis of intervertebral foramina of upper extremity
M99.68 Osseous and subluxation stenosis of intervertebral foramina of rib cage
M99.69 Osseous and subluxation stenosis of intervertebral foramina of abdomen and other regions

+ M99.7 Connective tissue and disc stenosis of intervertebral foramina
M99.70 Connective tissue and disc stenosis of intervertebral foramina of head region
M99.71 Connective tissue and disc stenosis of intervertebral foramina of cervical region
M99.72 Connective tissue and disc stenosis of intervertebral foramina of thoracic region
M99.73 Connective tissue and disc stenosis of intervertebral foramina of lumbar region
M99.74 Connective tissue and disc stenosis of intervertebral foramina of sacral region
M99.75 Connective tissue and disc stenosis of intervertebral foramina of pelvic region
M99.76 Connective tissue and disc stenosis of intervertebral foramina of lower extremity
M99.77 Connective tissue and disc stenosis of intervertebral foramina of upper extremity
M99.78 Connective tissue and disc stenosis of intervertebral foramina of rib cage
M99.79 Connective tissue and disc stenosis of intervertebral foramina of abdomen and other regions

+ M99.8 Other biomechanical lesions
M99.80 Other biomechanical lesions of head region
M99.81 Other biomechanical lesions of cervical region
M99.82 Other biomechanical lesions of thoracic region
M99.83 Other biomechanical lesions of lumbar region
M99.84 Other biomechanical lesions of sacral region
M99.85 Other biomechanical lesions of pelvic region
M99.86 Other biomechanical lesions of lower extremity
M99.87 Other biomechanical lesions of upper extremity
M99.88 Other biomechanical lesions of rib cage
M99.89 Other biomechanical lesions of abdomen and other regions

M99.9 Biomechanical lesion, unspecified

Chapter 14: Diseases of the Genitourinary System (N00-N99)

Excludes2: *certain conditions originating in the perinatal period (P04-P96)*
certain infectious and parasitic diseases (A00-B99)
complications of pregnancy, childbirth and the puerperium (O00-O9A)
congenital malformations, deformations and chromosomal abnormalities (Q00-Q99)
endocrine, nutritional and metabolic diseases (E00-E88)
injury, poisoning and certain other consequences of external causes (S00-T88)
neoplasms (C00-D49)
symptoms, signs and abnormal clinical and laboratory findings, not elsewhere classified (R00-R94)

This chapter contains the following category blocks:

- N00-N08 Glomerular diseases
- N10-N16 Renal tubulo-interstitial diseases
- N17-N19 Acute kidney failure and chronic kidney disease
- N20-N23 Urolithiasis
- N25-N29 Other disorders of kidney and ureter
- N30-N39 Other diseases of the urinary system
- N40-N53 Diseases of male genital organs
- N60-N65 Disorders of breast
- N70-N77 Inflammatory diseases of female pelvic organs
- N80-N98 Noninflammatory disorders of female genital tract
- N99 Intraoperative and postprocedural complications and disorders of genitourinary system, not elsewhere classified

C. Chapter-Specific Coding Guidelines

In addition to general coding guidelines, there are guidelines for specific diagnoses and/or conditions in the classification. Unless otherwise indicated, these guidelines apply to all health care settings. Please refer to Section II for guidelines on the selection of principal diagnosis.

14. Chapter 14: Diseases of the Genitourinary System (N00-N99)

a. Chronic kidney disease

1) Stages of chronic kidney disease (CKD)

The ICD-10-CM classifies CKD based on severity. The severity of CKD is designated by stages 1-5. Stage 2, code N18.2, equates to mild CKD; stage 3, code N18.3, equates to moderate CKD; and stage 4, code N18.4, equates to severe CKD. Code N18.6, End stage renal disease (ESRD), is assigned when the provider has documented end-stage-renal disease (ESRD).

If both a stage of CKD and ESRD are documented, assign code N18.6 only.

2) Chronic kidney disease and kidney transplant status

Patients who have undergone kidney transplant may still have some form of chronic kidney disease (CKD) because the kidney transplant may not fully restore kidney function. Therefore, the presence of CKD alone does not constitute a transplant complication. Assign the appropriate N18 code for the patient's stage of CKD and code Z94.0, Kidney transplant status. If a transplant complication such as failure or rejection or other transplant complication is documented, see section I.C.19.g for information on coding complications of a kidney transplant. If the documentation is unclear as to whether the patient has a complication of the transplant, query the provider.

3) Chronic kidney disease with other conditions

Patients with CKD may also suffer from other serious conditions, most commonly diabetes mellitus and hypertension. The sequencing of the CKD code in relationship to codes for other contributing conditions is based on the conventions in the Tabular List.

See I.C.9. Hypertensive chronic kidney disease.

See I.C.19. Chronic kidney disease and kidney transplant complications.

Urinary System

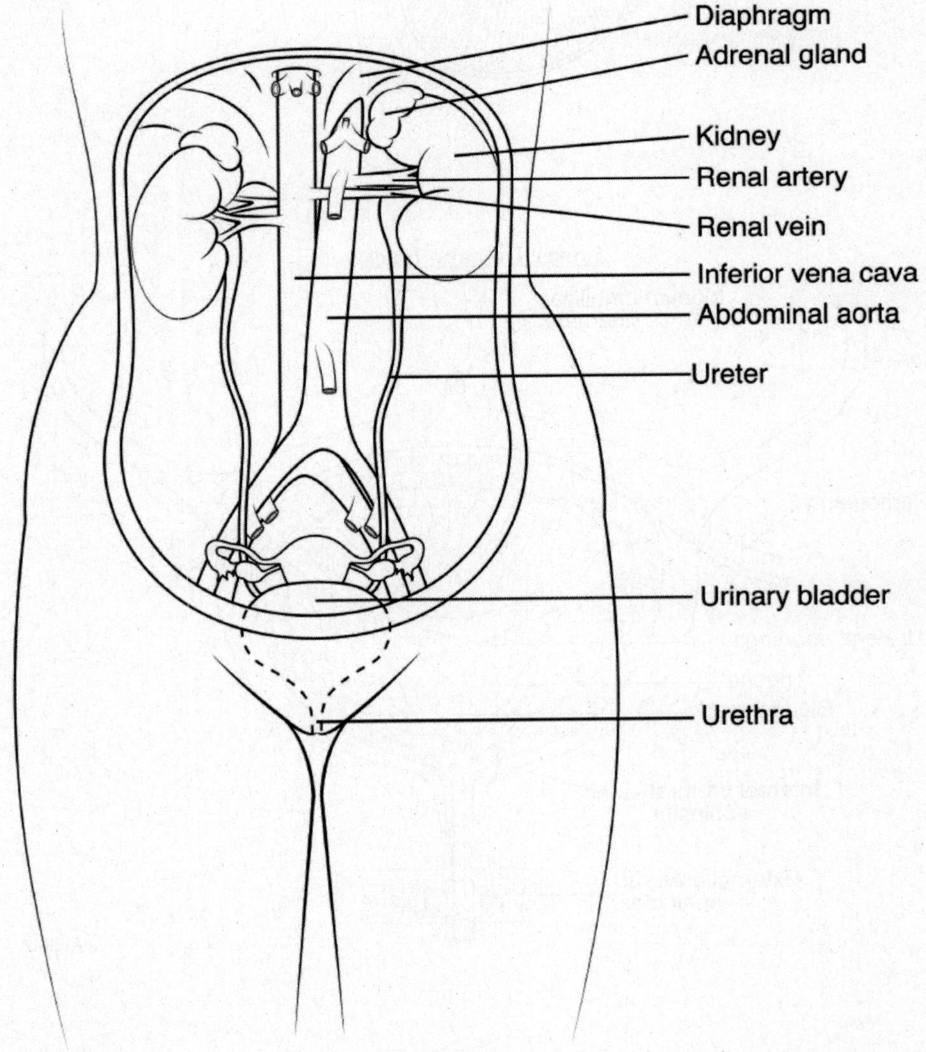

Kidney

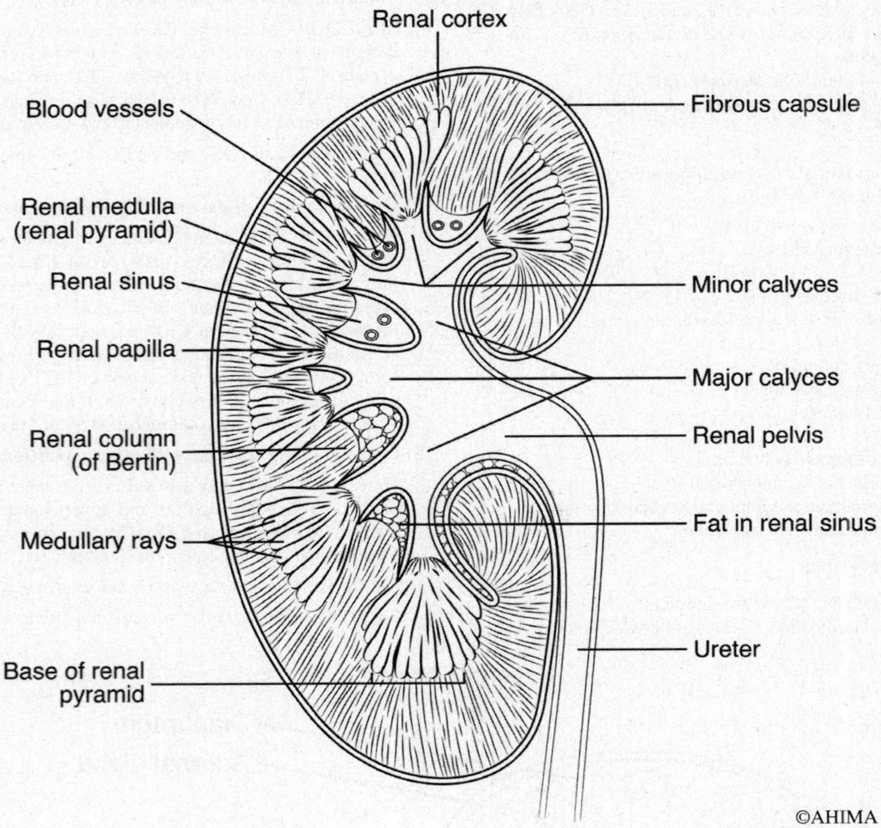

Lower Urinary Tract

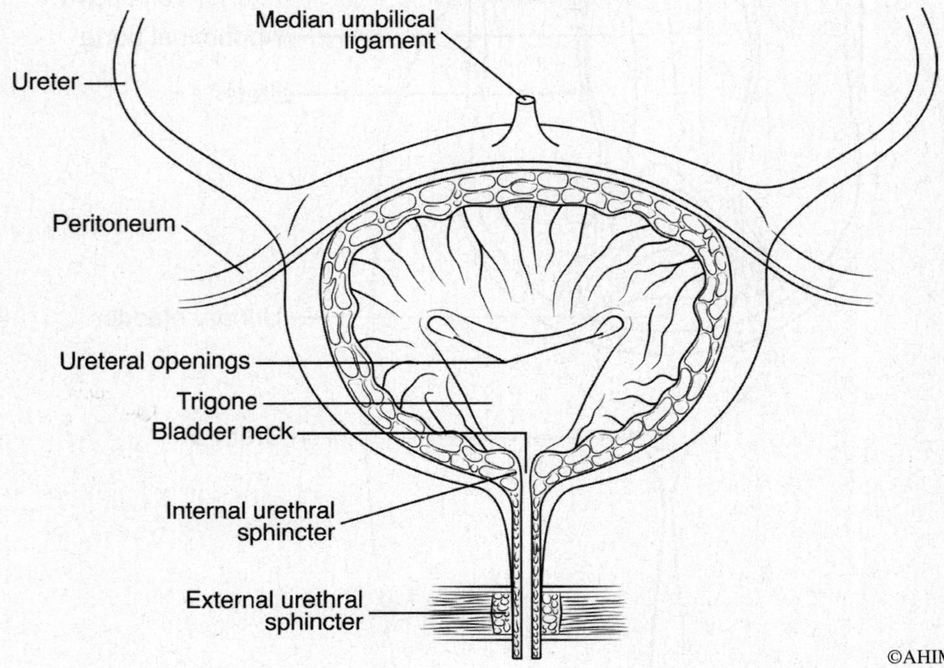

Glomerular diseases (N00-N08)

Code also any associated kidney failure (N17-N19)

Excludes1: *hypertensive chronic kidney disease (I12.-)*

AHA CC: 4Q, 2020, 34-35

N00 Acute nephritic syndrome

Includes: acute glomerular disease
acute glomerulonephritis
acute nephritis

Excludes1: *acute tubulo-interstitial nephritis (N10)*
nephritic syndrome NOS (N05.-)

MCC **N00.0 Acute nephritic syndrome with minor glomerular abnormality**
Acute nephritic syndrome with minimal change lesion

MCC **N00.1 Acute nephritic syndrome with focal and segmental glomerular lesions**
Acute nephritic syndrome with focal and segmental hyalinosis
Acute nephritic syndrome with focal and segmental sclerosis
Acute nephritic syndrome with focal glomerulonephritis

MCC **N00.2 Acute nephritic syndrome with diffuse membranous glomerulonephritis**

MCC **N00.3 Acute nephritic syndrome with diffuse mesangial proliferative glomerulonephritis**

MCC **N00.4 Acute nephritic syndrome with diffuse endocapillary proliferative glomerulonephritis**

MCC **N00.5 Acute nephritic syndrome with diffuse mesangiocapillary glomerulonephritis**
Acute nephritic syndrome with membranoproliferative glomerulonephritis, types 1 and 3, or NOS

Excludes1: *Acute nephritic syndrome with C3 glomerulonephritis (N00.A)*
Acute nephritic syndrome with C3 glomerulopathy (N00.A)

MCC **N00.6 Acute nephritic syndrome with dense deposit disease**
Acute nephritic syndrome with membranoproliferative glomerulonephritis, type 2
Acute nephritic syndrome with C3 glomerulopathy with dense deposit disease

MCC **N00.7 Acute nephritic syndrome with diffuse crescentic glomerulonephritis**
Acute nephritic syndrome with extracapillary glomerulonephritis

MCC **N00.8 Acute nephritic syndrome with other morphologic changes**
Acute nephritic syndrome with proliferative glomerulonephritis NOS

MCC **N00.9 Acute nephritic syndrome with unspecified morphologic changes**

MCC **N00.A Acute nephritic syndrome with C3 glomerulonephritis**
Acute nephritic syndrome with C3 glomerulopathy, NOS

Excludes1: *Acute nephritic syndrome (with C3 glomerulopathy) with dense deposit disease (N00.6)*

N01 Rapidly progressive nephritic syndrome

Includes: rapidly progressive glomerular disease
rapidly progressive glomerulonephritis
rapidly progressive nephritis

Excludes1: *nephritic syndrome NOS (N05.-)*

MCC **N01.0 Rapidly progressive nephritic syndrome with minor glomerular abnormality**
Rapidly progressive nephritic syndrome with minimal change lesion

MCC **N01.1 Rapidly progressive nephritic syndrome with focal and segmental glomerular lesions**
Rapidly progressive nephritic syndrome with focal and segmental hyalinosis
Rapidly progressive nephritic syndrome with focal and segmental sclerosis
Rapidly progressive nephritic syndrome with focal glomerulonephritis

MCC **N01.2 Rapidly progressive nephritic syndrome with diffuse membranous glomerulonephritis**

MCC **N01.3 Rapidly progressive nephritic syndrome with diffuse mesangial proliferative glomerulonephritis**

MCC **N01.4 Rapidly progressive nephritic syndrome with diffuse endocapillary proliferative glomerulonephritis**

MCC **N01.5 Rapidly progressive nephritic syndrome with diffuse mesangiocapillary glomerulonephritis**
Rapidly progressive nephritic syndrome with membranoproliferative glomerulonephritis, types 1 and 3, or NOS

Excludes1: *Rapidly progressive nephritic syndrome with C3 glomerulonephritis (N01.A)*
Rapidly progressive nephritic syndrome with C3 glomerulopathy (N01.A)

MCC **N01.6 Rapidly progressive nephritic syndrome with dense deposit disease**
Rapidly progressive nephritic syndrome with membranoproliferative glomerulonephritis, type 2
Rapidly progressive nephritic syndrome with C3 glomerulopathy with dense deposit disease

MCC **N01.7 Rapidly progressive nephritic syndrome with diffuse crescentic glomerulonephritis**
Rapidly progressive nephritic syndrome with extracapillary glomerulonephritis

MCC **N01.8 Rapidly progressive nephritic syndrome with other morphologic changes**
Rapidly progressive nephritic syndrome with proliferative glomerulonephritis NOS

MCC **N01.9 Rapidly progressive nephritic syndrome with unspecified morphologic changes**

MCC **N01.A Rapidly progressive nephritic syndrome with C3 glomerulonephritis**
Rapidly progressive nephritic syndrome with C3 glomerulopathy, NOS

Excludes1: *Rapidly progressive nephritic syndrome (with C3 glomerulopathy) with dense deposit disease (N01.6)*

N02 Recurrent and persistent hematuria

Excludes1: *acute cystitis with hematuria (N30.01)*
hematuria NOS (R31.9)
hematuria not associated with specified morphologic lesions (R31.-)

CC **N02.0 Recurrent and persistent hematuria with minor glomerular abnormality**
Recurrent and persistent hematuria with minimal change lesion

CC **N02.1 Recurrent and persistent hematuria with focal and segmental glomerular lesions**
Recurrent and persistent hematuria with focal and segmental hyalinosis
Recurrent and persistent hematuria with focal and segmental sclerosis
Recurrent and persistent hematuria with focal glomerulonephritis

CC **N02.2 Recurrent and persistent hematuria with diffuse membranous glomerulonephritis**

CC **N02.3 Recurrent and persistent hematuria with diffuse mesangial proliferative glomerulonephritis**

CC **N02.4 Recurrent and persistent hematuria with diffuse endocapillary proliferative glomerulonephritis**

CC **N02.5 Recurrent and persistent hematuria with diffuse mesangiocapillary glomerulonephritis**
Recurrent and persistent hematuria with membranoproliferative glomerulonephritis, types 1 and 3, or NOS

Excludes1: *Recurrent and persistent hematuria with C3 glomerulonephritis (N02.A)*
Recurrent and persistent hematuria with C3 glomerulopathy (N02.A)

CC **N02.6 Recurrent and persistent hematuria with dense deposit disease**
Recurrent and persistent hematuria with membranoproliferative glomerulonephritis, type 2
Recurrent and persistent hematuria with C3 glomerulopathy with dense deposit disease

CC **N02.7 Recurrent and persistent hematuria with diffuse crescentic glomerulonephritis**
Recurrent and persistent hematuria with extracapillary glomerulonephritis

CC **N02.8 Recurrent and persistent hematuria with other morphologic changes**
Recurrent and persistent hematuria with proliferative glomerulonephritis NOS

CC **N02.9 Recurrent and persistent hematuria with unspecified morphologic changes**
AHA CC: 2Q, 2017, 5

CC **N02.A Recurrent and persistent hematuria with C3 glomerulonephritis**
Recurrent and persistent hematuria with C3 glomerulopathy
Excludes1: *Recurrent and persistent hematuria (with C3 glomerulopathy) with dense deposit disease (N02.6)*

N03 Chronic nephritic syndrome

Includes: chronic glomerular disease
chronic glomerulonephritis
chronic nephritis

Excludes1: *chronic tubulo-interstitial nephritis (N11.-)*
diffuse sclerosing glomerulonephritis (N05.8-)
nephritic syndrome NOS (N05.-)

CC **N03.0 Chronic nephritic syndrome with minor glomerular abnormality**
Chronic nephritic syndrome with minimal change lesion

CC **N03.1 Chronic nephritic syndrome with focal and segmental glomerular lesions**
Chronic nephritic syndrome with focal and segmental hyalinosis
Chronic nephritic syndrome with focal and segmental sclerosis
Chronic nephritic syndrome with focal glomerulonephritis

CC **N03.2 Chronic nephritic syndrome with diffuse membranous glomerulonephritis**

CC **N03.3 Chronic nephritic syndrome with diffuse mesangial proliferative glomerulonephritis**

CC **N03.4 Chronic nephritic syndrome with diffuse endocapillary proliferative glomerulonephritis**

CC **N03.5 Chronic nephritic syndrome with diffuse mesangiocapillary glomerulonephritis**
Chronic nephritic syndrome with membranoproliferative glomerulonephritis, types 1 and 3, or NOS
Excludes1: *Chronic nephritic syndrome with C3 glomerulonephritis (N03.A)*
Chronic nephritic syndrome with C3 glomerulopathy (N03.A)

CC **N03.6 Chronic nephritic syndrome with dense deposit disease**
Chronic nephritic syndrome with membranoproliferative glomerulonephritis, type 2
Chronic nephritic syndrome with C3 glomerulopathy with dense deposit disease

CC **N03.7 Chronic nephritic syndrome with diffuse crescentic glomerulonephritis**
Chronic nephritic syndrome with extracapillary glomerulonephritis

CC **N03.8 Chronic nephritic syndrome with other morphologic changes**
Chronic nephritic syndrome with proliferative glomerulonephritis NOS

CC **N03.9 Chronic nephritic syndrome with unspecified morphologic changes**

CC **N03.A Chronic nephritic syndrome with C3 glomerulonephritis**
Chronic nephritic syndrome with C3 glomerulopathy
Excludes1: *Chronic nephritic syndrome (with C3 glomerulopathy) with dense deposit disease (N03.6)*

N04 Nephrotic syndrome

Includes: congenital nephrotic syndrome
lipoid nephrosis

CC **N04.0 Nephrotic syndrome with minor glomerular abnormality**
Nephrotic syndrome with minimal change lesion

CC **N04.1 Nephrotic syndrome with focal and segmental glomerular lesions**
Nephrotic syndrome with focal and segmental hyalinosis
Nephrotic syndrome with focal and segmental sclerosis
Nephrotic syndrome with focal glomerulonephritis

CC **N04.2 Nephrotic syndrome with diffuse membranous glomerulonephritis**

CC **N04.3 Nephrotic syndrome with diffuse mesangial proliferative glomerulonephritis**

CC **N04.4 Nephrotic syndrome with diffuse endocapillary proliferative glomerulonephritis**

CC **N04.5 Nephrotic syndrome with diffuse mesangiocapillary glomerulonephritis**
Nephrotic syndrome with membranoproliferative glomerulonephritis, types 1 and 3, or NOS
Excludes1: *Nephrotic syndrome with C3 glomerulonephritis (N04.A)*
Nephrotic syndrome with C3 glomerulopathy (N04.A)

CC **N04.6 Nephrotic syndrome with dense deposit disease**
Nephrotic syndrome with membranoproliferative glomerulonephritis, type 2
Nephrotic syndrome with C3 glomerulopathy with dense deposit disease

CC **N04.7 Nephrotic syndrome with diffuse crescentic glomerulonephritis**
Nephrotic syndrome with extracapillary glomerulonephritis

CC **N04.8 Nephrotic syndrome with other morphologic changes**
Nephrotic syndrome with proliferative glomerulonephritis NOS

CC **N04.9 Nephrotic syndrome with unspecified morphologic changes**

CC **N04.A Nephrotic syndrome with C3 glomerulonephritis**
Nephrotic syndrome with C3 glomerulopathy
Excludes1: *Nephrotic syndrome (with C3 glomerulopathy) with dense deposit disease (N04.6)*

N05 Unspecified nephritic syndrome

Includes: glomerular disease NOS
glomerulonephritis NOS
nephritis NOS
nephropathy NOS and renal disease NOS with morphological lesion specified in .0-.8

Excludes1: *nephropathy NOS with no stated morphological lesion (N28.9)*
renal disease NOS with no stated morphological lesion (N28.9)
tubulo-interstitial nephritis NOS (N12)

N05.0 Unspecified nephritic syndrome with minor glomerular abnormality
Unspecified nephritic syndrome with minimal change lesion

N05.1 Unspecified nephritic syndrome with focal and segmental glomerular lesions
Unspecified nephritic syndrome with focal and segmental hyalinosis
Unspecified nephritic syndrome with focal and segmental sclerosis
Unspecified nephritic syndrome with focal glomerulonephritis

CC **N05.2 Unspecified nephritic syndrome with diffuse membranous glomerulonephritis**

CC **N05.3 Unspecified nephritic syndrome with diffuse mesangial proliferative glomerulonephritis**

CC **N05.4 Unspecified nephritic syndrome with diffuse endocapillary proliferative glomerulonephritis**

CC **N05.5 Unspecified nephritic syndrome with diffuse mesangiocapillary glomerulonephritis**
Unspecified nephritic syndrome with membranoproliferative glomerulonephritis, types 1 and 3, or NOS
Excludes1: *Unspecified nephritic syndrome with C3 glomerulonephritis (N05.A)*
Unspecified nephritic syndrome with C3 glomerulopathy (N05.A)

N05.6 Unspecified nephritic syndrome with dense deposit disease
Unspecified nephritic syndrome with membranoproliferative glomerulonephritis, type 2
Unspecified nephritic syndrome with C3 glomerulopathy with dense deposit disease

N05.7 Unspecified nephritic syndrome with diffuse crescentic glomerulonephritis
Unspecified nephritic syndrome with extracapillary glomerulonephritis

N05.8 Unspecified nephritic syndrome with other morphologic changes
Unspecified nephritic syndrome with proliferative glomerulonephritis NOS

N05.9 Unspecified nephritic syndrome with unspecified morphologic changes

CC **N05.A Unspecified nephritic syndrome with C3 glomerulonephritis**
Unspecified nephritic syndrome with C3 glomerulopathy
Excludes1: *Unspecified nephritic syndrome (with C3 glomerulopathy) with dense deposit disease (N05.6)*

N06 Isolated proteinuria with specified morphological lesion

Excludes1: *Proteinuria not associated with specific morphologic lesions (R80.0)*

N06.0 Isolated proteinuria with minor glomerular abnormality
Isolated proteinuria with minimal change lesion

N06.1 Isolated proteinuria with focal and segmental glomerular lesions
Isolated proteinuria with focal and segmental hyalinosis
Isolated proteinuria with focal and segmental sclerosis
Isolated proteinuria with focal glomerulonephritis

CC **N06.2 Isolated proteinuria with diffuse membranous glomerulonephritis**

CC **N06.3 Isolated proteinuria with diffuse mesangial proliferative glomerulonephritis**

CC **N06.4 Isolated proteinuria with diffuse endocapillary proliferative glomerulonephritis**

CC **N06.5 Isolated proteinuria with diffuse mesangiocapillary glomerulonephritis**
Isolated proteinuria with membranoproliferative glomerulonephritis, types 1 and 3, or NOS
Excludes1: *Isolated proteinuria with C3 glomerulonephritis (N06.A)*
Isolated proteinuria with C3 glomerulopathy (N06.A)

N06.6 Isolated proteinuria with dense deposit disease
Isolated proteinuria with membranoproliferative glomerulonephritis, type 2
Isolated proteinuria with C3 glomerulopathy with dense deposit disease

N06.7 Isolated proteinuria with diffuse crescentic glomerulonephritis
Isolated proteinuria with extracapillary glomerulonephritis

N06.8 Isolated proteinuria with other morphologic lesion
Isolated proteinuria with proliferative glomerulonephritis NOS

N06.9 Isolated proteinuria with unspecified morphologic lesion

CC **N06.A Isolated proteinuria with C3 glomerulonephritis**
Isolated proteinuria with C3 glomerulopathy
Excludes1: *Isolated proteinuria (with C3 glomerulopathy) with dense deposit disease (N06.6)*

N07 Hereditary nephropathy, not elsewhere classified

Excludes2: *Alport's syndrome (Q87.81-)*
hereditary amyloid nephropathy (E85.-)
nail patella syndrome (Q87.2)
non-neuropathic heredofamilial amyloidosis (E85.-)

N07.0 Hereditary nephropathy, not elsewhere classified with minor glomerular abnormality
Hereditary nephropathy, not elsewhere classified with minimal change lesion

N07.1 Hereditary nephropathy, not elsewhere classified with focal and segmental glomerular lesions
Hereditary nephropathy, not elsewhere classified with focal and segmental hyalinosis
Hereditary nephropathy, not elsewhere classified with focal and segmental sclerosis
Hereditary nephropathy, not elsewhere classified with focal glomerulonephritis

CC **N07.2 Hereditary nephropathy, not elsewhere classified with diffuse membranous glomerulonephritis**

CC **N07.3 Hereditary nephropathy, not elsewhere classified with diffuse mesangial proliferative glomerulonephritis**

CC **N07.4 Hereditary nephropathy, not elsewhere classified with diffuse endocapillary proliferative glomerulonephritis**

CC **N07.5 Hereditary nephropathy, not elsewhere classified with diffuse mesangiocapillary glomerulonephritis**
Hereditary nephropathy, not elsewhere classified with membranoproliferative glomerulonephritis, types 1 and 3, or NOS
Excludes1: *Hereditary nephropathy, not elsewhere classified with C3 glomerulonephritis (N07.A)*
Hereditary nephropathy, not elsewhere classified with C3 glomerulopathy (N07.A)

N07.6 Hereditary nephropathy, not elsewhere classified with dense deposit disease
Hereditary nephropathy, not elsewhere classified with membranoproliferative glomerulonephritis, type 2
Hereditary nephropathy, not elsewhere classified with C3 glomerulopathy with dense deposit disease

N07.7 Hereditary nephropathy, not elsewhere classified with diffuse crescentic glomerulonephritis
Hereditary nephropathy, not elsewhere classified with extracapillary glomerulonephritis

N07.8 Hereditary nephropathy, not elsewhere classified with other morphologic lesions
Hereditary nephropathy, not elsewhere classified with proliferative glomerulonephritis NOS

N07.9 Hereditary nephropathy, not elsewhere classified with unspecified morphologic lesions

CC **N07.A Hereditary nephropathy, not elsewhere classified with C3 glomerulonephritis**
Hereditary nephropathy, not elsewhere classified with C3 glomerulopathy
Excludes1: *Hereditary nephropathy, not elsewhere classified (with C3 glomerulopathy) with dense deposit disease (N07.6)*

N08 Glomerular disorders in diseases classified elsewhere

Glomerulonephritis
Nephritis
Nephropathy
Code first underlying disease, such as:
amyloidosis (E85.-)
congenital syphilis (A50.5)
cryoglobulinemia (D89.1)
disseminated intravascular coagulation (D65)
gout (M1A.-, M10.-)
microscopic polyangiitis (M31.7)
multiple myeloma (C90.0-)
sepsis (A40.0-A41.9)
sickle-cell disease (D57.0-D57.8)
Excludes1: *glomerulonephritis, nephritis and nephropathy (in):*
antiglomerular basement membrane disease (M31.0)
diabetes (E08-E13 with .21)
gonococcal (A54.21)
Goodpasture's syndrome (M31.0)
hemolytic-uremic syndrome (D59.3)
lupus (M32.14)
mumps (B26.83)
syphilis (A52.75)
systemic lupus erythematosus (M32.14)
Wegener's granulomatosis (M31.31)
pyelonephritis in diseases classified elsewhere (N16)
renal tubulo-interstitial disorders classified elsewhere (N16)

Valid 3-character code, no further characters required

Renal tubulo-interstitial diseases (N10-N16)

Includes: pyelonephritis

Excludes1: *pyeloureteritis cystica (N28.85)*

CC **N10 Acute pyelonephritis**
Acute infectious interstitial nephritis
Acute pyelitis
Acute tubulo-interstitial nephritis
Hemoglobin nephrosis
Myoglobin nephrosis
Use additional code (B95-B97), to identify infectious agent
AHA CC: 3Q, 2019, 13-14; 3Q, 2020, 25-26
HAC see Appendix B for HAC conditional logic
Valid 3-character code, no further characters required

N11 Chronic tubulo-interstitial nephritis
Includes: chronic infectious interstitial nephritis
chronic pyelitis
chronic pyelonephritis
Use additional code (B95-B97), to identify infectious agent

N11.0 Nonobstructive reflux-associated chronic pyelonephritis
Pyelonephritis (chronic) associated with (vesicoureteral) reflux
Excludes1: *vesicoureteral reflux NOS (N13.70)*

CC **N11.1 Chronic obstructive pyelonephritis**
Pyelonephritis (chronic) associated with anomaly of pelviureteric junction
Pyelonephritis (chronic) associated with anomaly of pyeloureteric junction
Pyelonephritis (chronic) associated with crossing of vessel
Pyelonephritis (chronic) associated with kinking of ureter
Pyelonephritis (chronic) associated with obstruction of ureter
Pyelonephritis (chronic) associated with stricture of pelviureteric junction
Pyelonephritis (chronic) associated with stricture of ureter
Excludes1: *calculous pyelonephritis (N20.9)*
obstructive uropathy (N13.-)

CC **N11.8 Other chronic tubulo-interstitial nephritis**
Nonobstructive chronic pyelonephritis NOS

CC **N11.9 Chronic tubulo-interstitial nephritis, unspecified**
Chronic interstitial nephritis NOS
Chronic pyelitis NOS
Chronic pyelonephritis NOS
HAC see Appendix B for HAC conditional logic

CC **N12 Tubulo-interstitial nephritis, not specified as acute or chronic**
Interstitial nephritis NOS
Pyelitis NOS
Pyelonephritis NOS
Excludes1: *calculous pyelonephritis (N20.9)*
HAC see Appendix B for HAC conditional logic
Valid 3-character code, no further characters required

N13 Obstructive and reflux uropathy
Excludes2: *calculus of kidney and ureter without hydronephrosis (N20.-)*
congenital obstructive defects of renal pelvis and ureter (Q62.0-Q62.3)
hydronephrosis with ureteropelvic junction obstruction (Q62.11)
obstructive pyelonephritis (N11.1)

CC **N13.0 Hydronephrosis with ureteropelvic junction obstruction**
Hydronephrosis due to acquired occlusion of ureteropelvic junction
Excludes2: *Hydronephrosis with ureteropelvic junction obstruction due to calculus (N13.2)*
AHA CC: 4Q, 2016, 43

CC **N13.1 Hydronephrosis with ureteral stricture, not elsewhere classified**
Excludes1: *hydronephrosis with ureteral stricture with infection (N13.6)*

N13.2 Hydronephrosis with renal and ureteral calculous obstruction
Excludes1: *hydronephrosis with renal and ureteral calculous obstruction with infection (N13.6)*

+ **N13.3 Other and unspecified hydronephrosis**
Excludes1: *hydronephrosis with infection (N13.6)*
CC **N13.30 Unspecified hydronephrosis**
CC **N13.39 Other hydronephrosis**

CC **N13.4 Hydroureter**
Excludes1: *congenital hydroureter (Q62.3-)*
hydroureter with infection (N13.6)
vesicoureteral-reflux with hydroureter (N13.73-)

N13.5 Crossing vessel and stricture of ureter without hydronephrosis
Kinking and stricture of ureter without hydronephrosis
Excludes1: *Crossing vessel and stricture of ureter without hydronephrosis with infection (N13.6)*

CC **N13.6 Pyonephrosis**
Conditions in N13.0-N13.5 with infection
Obstructive uropathy with infection
Use additional code (B95-B97), to identify infectious agent
AHA CC: 2Q, 2018, 21
HAC see Appendix B for HAC conditional logic

+ **N13.7 Vesicoureteral-reflux**
Excludes1: *reflux-associated pyelonephritis (N11.0)*
N13.70 Vesicoureteral-reflux, unspecified
Vesicoureteral-reflux NOS
N13.71 Vesicoureteral-reflux without reflux nephropathy
+ **N13.72 Vesicoureteral-reflux with reflux nephropathy without hydroureter**
N13.721 Vesicoureteral-reflux with reflux nephropathy without hydroureter, unilateral
N13.722 Vesicoureteral-reflux with reflux nephropathy without hydroureter, bilateral
N13.729 Vesicoureteral-reflux with reflux nephropathy without hydroureter, unspecified
+ **N13.73 Vesicoureteral-reflux with reflux nephropathy with hydroureter**
N13.731 Vesicoureteral-reflux with reflux nephropathy with hydroureter, unilateral
N13.732 Vesicoureteral-reflux with reflux nephropathy with hydroureter, bilateral
N13.739 Vesicoureteral-reflux with reflux nephropathy with hydroureter, unspecified

CC **N13.8 Other obstructive and reflux uropathy**
Urinary tract obstruction due to specified cause
Code first, if applicable, any causal condition, such as:
enlarged prostate (N40.1)

N13.9 Obstructive and reflux uropathy, unspecified
Urinary tract obstruction NOS

N14 Drug- and heavy-metal-induced tubulo-interstitial and tubular conditions
Code first poisoning due to drug or toxin, if applicable (T36-T65 with fifth or sixth character 1-4 or 6)

Use additional code for adverse effect, if applicable, to identify drug (T36-T50 with fifth or sixth character 5)
N14.0 Analgesic nephropathy
N14.1 Nephropathy induced by other drugs, medicaments and biological substances
N14.2 Nephropathy induced by unspecified drug, medicament or biological substance
N14.3 Nephropathy induced by heavy metals
N14.4 Toxic nephropathy, not elsewhere classified

N15 Other renal tubulo-interstitial diseases
N15.0 Balkan nephropathy
Balkan endemic nephropathy
MCC **N15.1 Renal and perinephric abscess**
HAC see Appendix B for HAC conditional logic
N15.8 Other specified renal tubulo-interstitial diseases
N15.9 Renal tubulo-interstitial disease, unspecified
Infection of kidney NOS
Excludes1: *urinary tract infection NOS (N39.0)*

N16 Renal tubulo-interstitial disorders in diseases classified elsewhere
Pyelonephritis
Tubulo-interstitial nephritis
Code first underlying disease, such as:
brucellosis (A23.0-A23.9)
cryoglobulinemia (D89.1)
glycogen storage disease (E74.0)
leukemia (C91-C95)
lymphoma (C81.0-C85.9, C96.0-C96.9)
multiple myeloma (C90.0-)
sepsis (A40.0-A41.9)
Wilson's disease (E83.0)

Excludes1: *diphtheritic pyelonephritis and tubulo-interstitial nephritis (A36.84)*
pyelonephritis and tubulo-interstitial nephritis in candidiasis (B37.49)
pyelonephritis and tubulo-interstitial nephritis in cystinosis (E72.04)
pyelonephritis and tubulo-interstitial nephritis in salmonella infection (A02.25)
pyelonephritis and tubulo-interstitial nephritis in sarcoidosis (D86.84)
pyelonephritis and tubulo-interstitial nephritis in Sjögren's syndrome (M35.04)
pyelonephritis and tubulo-interstitial nephritis in systemic lupus erythematosus (M32.15)
pyelonephritis and tubulo-interstitial nephritis in toxoplasmosis (B58.83)
renal tubular degeneration in diabetes (E08-E13 with .29)
syphilitic pyelonephritis and tubulo-interstitial nephritis (A52.75)

Valid 3-character code, no further characters required

Acute kidney failure and chronic kidney disease (N17-N19)

Excludes2: *congenital renal failure (P96.0)*
drug- and heavy-metal-induced tubulo-interstitial and tubular conditions (N14.-)
extrarenal uremia (R39.2)
hemolytic-uremic syndrome (D59.3)
hepatorenal syndrome (K76.7)
postpartum hepatorenal syndrome (O90.4)
posttraumatic renal failure (T79.5)
prerenal uremia (R39.2)
renal failure complicating abortion or ectopic or molar pregnancy (O00-O07, O08.4)
renal failure following labor and delivery (O90.4)
renal failure postprocedural (N99.0)

N17 Acute kidney failure

Code also associated underlying condition

Excludes1: *posttraumatic renal failure (T79.5)*

MCC **N17.0 Acute kidney failure with tubular necrosis**

Acute tubular necrosis
Renal tubular necrosis
Tubular necrosis NOS

AHA CC: 3Q, 2020, 22

MCC **N17.1 Acute kidney failure with acute cortical necrosis**

Acute cortical necrosis
Cortical necrosis NOS
Renal cortical necrosis

N17.2 Acute kidney failure with medullary necrosis

Medullary [papillary] necrosis NOS
Acute medullary [papillary] necrosis
Renal medullary [papillary] necrosis

CC **N17.8 Other acute kidney failure**

CC **N17.9 Acute kidney failure, unspecified**

Acute kidney injury (nontraumatic)

Excludes2: *traumatic kidney injury (S37.0-)*

AHA CC: 2Q, 2019, 7, 24-26

N18 Chronic kidney disease (CKD)

Code first any associated:
diabetic chronic kidney disease (E08.22, E09.22, E10.22, E11.22, E13.22)
hypertensive chronic kidney disease (I12.-, I13.-)

Use additional code to identify kidney transplant status, if applicable, (Z94.0)

Review coding guidelines C.9.a.2 and C.9.a.3
Review coding guidelines C.14.a.1 and C.14.a.2

N18.1 Chronic kidney disease, stage 1

N18.2 Chronic kidney disease, stage 2 (mild)

\+ **N18.3 Chronic kidney disease, stage 3 (moderate)**

AHA CC: 4Q, 2020, 35

N18.30 Chronic kidney disease, stage 3 unspecified

N18.31 Chronic kidney disease, stage 3a

N18.32 Chronic kidney disease, stage 3b

CC **N18.4 Chronic kidney disease, stage 4 (severe)**

CC **N18.5 Chronic kidney disease, stage 5**

Excludes1: *chronic kidney disease, stage 5 requiring chronic dialysis (N18.6)*

MCC **N18.6 End stage renal disease**

Chronic kidney disease requiring chronic dialysis
Use additional code to identify dialysis status (Z99.2)

AHA CC: 4Q, 2013, 125; 3Q, 2016, 22-23

N18.9 Chronic kidney disease, unspecified

Chronic renal disease
Chronic renal failure NOS
Chronic renal insufficiency
Chronic uremia NOS
Diffuse sclerosing glomerulonephritis NOS

AHA CC: 4Q, 2018, 88-89

N19 Unspecified kidney failure

Uremia NOS

Excludes1: *acute kidney failure (N17.-)*
chronic kidney disease (N18.-)
chronic uremia (N18.9)
extrarenal uremia (R39.2)
prerenal uremia (R39.2)
renal insufficiency (acute) (N28.9)
uremia of newborn (P96.0)

Valid 3-character code, no further characters required

Urolithiasis (N20-N23)

N20 Calculus of kidney and ureter

Calculous pyelonephritis

Excludes1: *nephrocalcinosis (E83.5)*
that with hydronephrosis (N13.2)

N20.0 Calculus of kidney

Nephrolithiasis NOS
Renal calculus
Renal stone
Staghorn calculus
Stone in kidney

AHA CC: 1Q, 2017, 5; 3Q, 2019, 13-14

CC **N20.1 Calculus of ureter**

Calculus of the ureteropelvic junction
Ureteric stone

AHA CC: 3Q, 2016, 23-24

CC **N20.2 Calculus of kidney with calculus of ureter**

AHA CC: 2Q, 2015, 8-9

N20.9 Urinary calculus, unspecified

N21 Calculus of lower urinary tract

Includes: calculus of lower urinary tract with cystitis and urethritis

N21.0 Calculus in bladder

Calculus in diverticulum of bladder
Urinary bladder stone

Excludes2: *staghorn calculus (N20.0)*

N21.1 Calculus in urethra

Excludes2: *calculus of prostate (N42.0)*

N21.8 Other lower urinary tract calculus

N21.9 Calculus of lower urinary tract, unspecified

Excludes1: *calculus of urinary tract NOS (N20.9)*

N22 Calculus of urinary tract in diseases classified elsewhere

Code first underlying disease, such as:
gout (M1A.-, M10.-)
schistosomiasis (B65.0-B65.9)

Valid 3-character code, no further characters required

N23 Unspecified renal colic

Valid 3-character code, no further characters required

Other disorders of kidney and ureter (N25-N29)

Excludes2: *disorders of kidney and ureter with urolithiasis (N20-N23)*

N25 Disorders resulting from impaired renal tubular function

N25.0 Renal osteodystrophy
Azotemic osteodystrophy
Phosphate-losing tubular disorders
Renal rickets
Renal short stature
Excludes2: metabolic disorders classifiable to E70-E88

CC **N25.1 Nephrogenic diabetes insipidus**
Excludes1: *diabetes insipidus NOS (E23.2)*

+ **N25.8 Other disorders resulting from impaired renal tubular function**

CC **N25.81 Secondary hyperparathyroidism of renal origin**
Excludes1: *secondary hyperparathyroidism, non-renal (E21.1)*
Excludes2: *metabolic disorders classifiable to E70-E88*

N25.89 Other disorders resulting from impaired renal tubular function
Hypokalemic nephropathy
Lightwood-Albright syndrome
Renal tubular acidosis NOS

N25.9 Disorder resulting from impaired renal tubular function, unspecified

N26 Unspecified contracted kidney
Excludes1: *contracted kidney due to hypertension (I12.-)*
diffuse sclerosing glomerulonephritis (N05.8.-)
hypertensive nephrosclerosis (arteriolar) (arteriosclerotic) (I12.-)
small kidney of unknown cause (N27.-)

N26.1 Atrophy of kidney (terminal)
N26.2 Page kidney
N26.9 Renal sclerosis, unspecified

N27 Small kidney of unknown cause
Includes: oligonephronia
N27.0 Small kidney, unilateral
N27.1 Small kidney, bilateral
N27.9 Small kidney, unspecified

N28 Other disorders of kidney and ureter, not elsewhere classified

CC **N28.0 Ischemia and infarction of kidney**
Renal artery embolism
Renal artery obstruction
Renal artery occlusion
Renal artery thrombosis
Renal infarct
Excludes1: *atherosclerosis of renal artery (extrarenal part) (I70.1)*
congenital stenosis of renal artery (Q27.1)
Goldblatt's kidney (I70.1)

N28.1 Cyst of kidney, acquired
Cyst (multiple) (solitary) of kidney (acquired)
Excludes1: *cystic kidney disease (congenital) (Q61.-)*

+ **N28.8 Other specified disorders of kidney and ureter**
Excludes1: *hydroureter (N13.4)*
ureteric stricture with hydronephrosis (N13.1)
ureteric stricture without hydronephrosis (N13.5)

N28.81 Hypertrophy of kidney
N28.82 Megaloureter
N28.83 Nephroptosis
CC **N28.84 Pyelitis cystica**
HAC see Appendix B for HAC conditional logic
CC **N28.85 Pyeloureteritis cystica**
HAC see Appendix B for HAC conditional logic
CC **N28.86 Ureteritis cystica**
HAC see Appendix B for HAC conditional logic
N28.89 Other specified disorders of kidney and ureter

N28.9 Disorder of kidney and ureter, unspecified
Nephropathy NOS
Renal disease (acute) NOS
Renal insufficiency (acute)
Excludes1: *chronic renal insufficiency (N18.9)*
unspecified nephritic syndrome (N05.-)
AHA CC: 1Q, 2016, 13

N29 Other disorders of kidney and ureter in diseases classified elsewhere
Code first underlying disease, such as:
amyloidosis (E85.-)
nephrocalcinosis (E83.5)
schistosomiasis (B65.0-B65.9)
Excludes1: *disorders of kidney and ureter in:*
cystinosis (E72.0)
gonorrhea (A54.21)
syphilis (A52.75)
tuberculosis (A18.11)
Valid 3-character code, no further characters required

Other diseases of the urinary system (N30-N39)

Excludes2: *urinary infection (complicating):*
abortion or ectopic or molar pregnancy (O00-O07, O08.8)
pregnancy, childbirth and the puerperium (O23.-, O75.3, O86.2-)

N30 Cystitis
Use additional code to identify infectious agent (B95-B97)
Excludes1: *prostatocystitis (N41.3)*

+ **N30.0 Acute cystitis**
Excludes1: *irradiation cystitis (N30.4-)*
trigonitis (N30.3-)
CC **N30.00 Acute cystitis without hematuria**
HAC see Appendix B for HAC conditional logic
CC **N30.01 Acute cystitis with hematuria**
HAC see Appendix B for HAC conditional logic

+ **N30.1 Interstitial cystitis (chronic)**
N30.10 Interstitial cystitis (chronic) without hematuria
N30.11 Interstitial cystitis (chronic) with hematuria

+ **N30.2 Other chronic cystitis**
N30.20 Other chronic cystitis without hematuria
N30.21 Other chronic cystitis with hematuria

+ **N30.3 Trigonitis**
Urethrotrigonitis
N30.30 Trigonitis without hematuria
N30.31 Trigonitis with hematuria

+ **N30.4 Irradiation cystitis**
CC **N30.40 Irradiation cystitis without hematuria**
CC **N30.41 Irradiation cystitis with hematuria**

+ **N30.8 Other cystitis**
Abscess of bladder
N30.80 Other cystitis without hematuria
N30.81 Other cystitis with hematuria

+ **N30.9 Cystitis, unspecified**
N30.90 Cystitis, unspecified without hematuria
N30.91 Cystitis, unspecified with hematuria

N31 Neuromuscular dysfunction of bladder, not elsewhere classified
Use additional code to identify any associated urinary incontinence (N39.3-N39.4-)
Excludes1: *cord bladder NOS (G95.89)*
neurogenic bladder due to cauda equina syndrome (G83.4)
neuromuscular dysfunction due to spinal cord lesion (G95.89)

N31.0 Uninhibited neuropathic bladder, not elsewhere classified

Obstructive Uropathy: Etiology

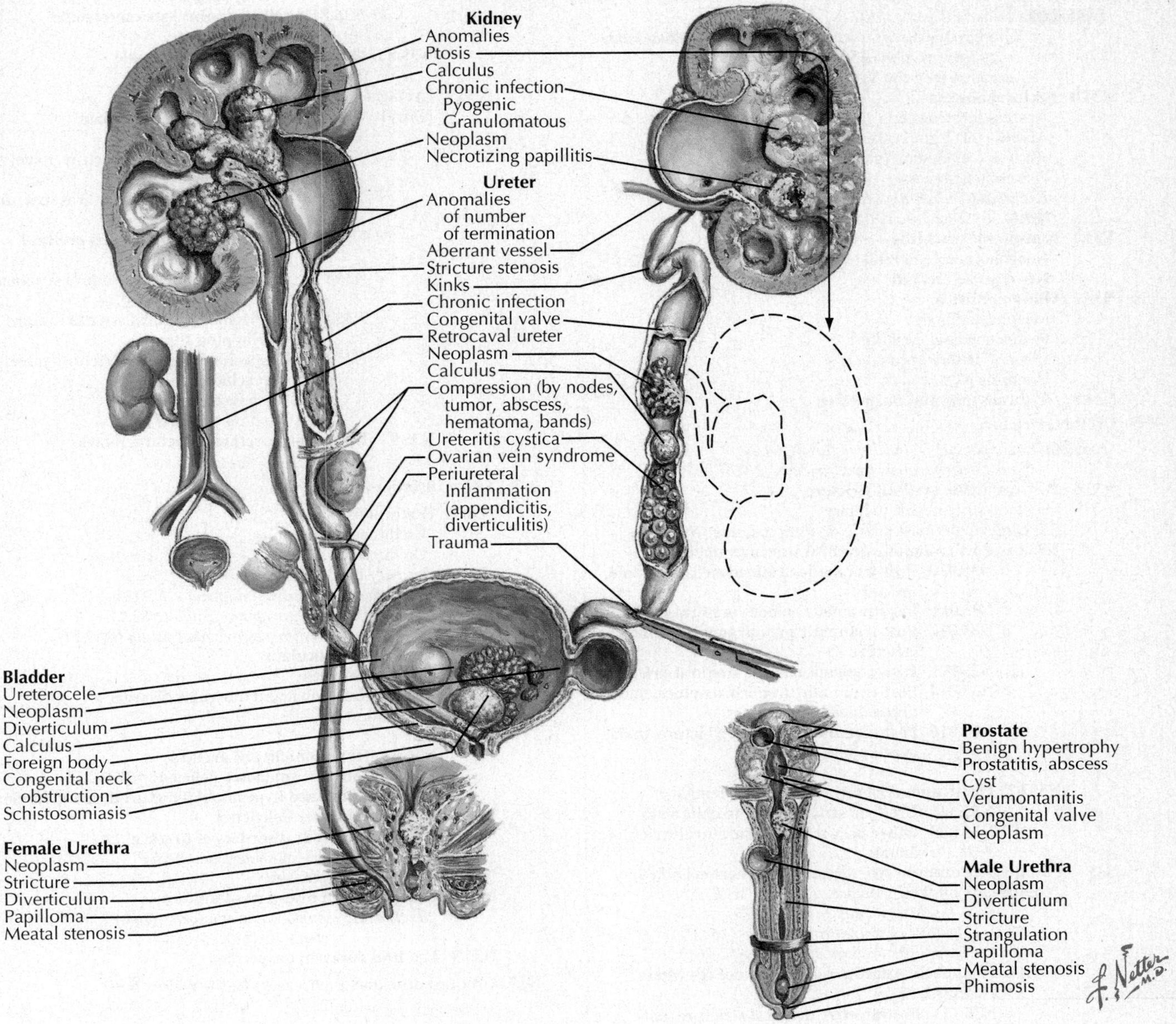

N31.1 Reflex neuropathic bladder, not elsewhere classified

N31.2 Flaccid neuropathic bladder, not elsewhere classified
- Atonic (motor) (sensory) neuropathic bladder
- Autonomous neuropathic bladder
- Nonreflex neuropathic bladder

N31.8 Other neuromuscular dysfunction of bladder

N31.9 Neuromuscular dysfunction of bladder, unspecified
- Neurogenic bladder dysfunction NOS

N32 Other disorders of bladder

Excludes2: *calculus of bladder (N21.0)*
cystocele (N81.1-)
hernia or prolapse of bladder, female (N81.1-)

N32.0 Bladder-neck obstruction
- Bladder-neck stenosis (acquired)

Excludes1: *congenital bladder-neck obstruction (Q64.3-)*

CC **N32.1 Vesicointestinal fistula**
- Vesicorectal fistula

CC **N32.2 Vesical fistula, not elsewhere classified**

Excludes1: *fistula between bladder and female genital tract (N82.0-N82.1)*

N32.3 Diverticulum of bladder

Excludes1: *congenital diverticulum of bladder (Q64.6)*
diverticulitis of bladder (N30.8-)

\+ **N32.8 Other specified disorders of bladder**

N32.81 Overactive bladder
- Detrusor muscle hyperactivity

Excludes1: *frequent urination due to specified bladdercondition-codetocondition*

N32.89 Other specified disorders of bladder
- Bladder hemorrhage
- Bladder hypertrophy
- Calcified bladder
- Contracted bladder

N32.9 Bladder disorder, unspecified

N33 Bladder disorders in diseases classified elsewhere

Code first underlying disease, such as:
schistosomiasis (B65.0-B65.9)

Excludes1: *bladder disorder in syphilis (A52.76)*
bladder disorder in tuberculosis (A18.12)
candidal cystitis (B37.41)
chlamydial cystitis (A56.01)
cystitis in gonorrhea (A54.01)
cystitis in neurogenic bladder (N31.-)
diphtheritic cystitis (A36.85)
syphilitic cystitis (A52.76)
trichomonal cystitis (A59.03)

Valid 3-character code, no further characters required

N34 Urethritis and urethral syndrome
Use additional code (B95-B97), to identify infectious agent.
Excludes2: *Reiter's disease (M02.3-)*
urethritis in diseases with a predominantly sexual mode of transmission (A50-A64)
urethrotrigonitis (N30.3-)

CC **N34.0 Urethral abscess**
Abscess (of) Cowper's gland
Abscess (of) Littré's gland
Abscess (of) urethral (gland)
Periurethral abscess
Excludes1: *urethral caruncle (N36.2)*
HAC see Appendix B for HAC conditional logic

N34.1 Nonspecific urethritis
Nongonococcal urethritis
Nonvenereal urethritis

N34.2 Other urethritis
Meatitis, urethral
Postmenopausal urethritis
Ulcer of urethra (meatus)
Urethritis NOS

N34.3 Urethral syndrome, unspecified

N35 Urethral stricture
Excludes1: *congenital urethral stricture (Q64.3-)*
postprocedural urethral stricture (N99.1-)

\+ **N35.0 Post-traumatic urethral stricture**
Urethral stricture due to injury
Excludes1: *postprocedural urethral stricture (N99.1-)*

\+ **N35.01 Post-traumatic urethral stricture, male**
♂ **N35.010 Post-traumatic urethral stricture, male, meatal**
♂ **N35.011 Post-traumatic bulbous urethral stricture**
♂ **N35.012 Post-traumatic membranous urethral stricture**
♂ **N35.013 Post-traumatic anterior urethral stricture**
♂ **N35.014 Post-traumatic urethral stricture, male, unspecified**
♂ **N35.016 Post-traumatic urethral stricture, male, overlapping sites**
AHA CC: 4Q, 2018, 21-22

\+ **N35.02 Post-traumatic urethral stricture, female**
♀ **N35.021 Urethral stricture due to childbirth**
♀ **N35.028 Other post-traumatic urethral stricture, female**

\+ **N35.1 Postinfective urethral stricture, not elsewhere classified**
Excludes1: *urethral stricture associated with schistosomiasis (B65.-, N29)*
gonococcal urethral stricture (A54.01)
syphilitic urethral stricture (A52.76)

\+ **N35.11 Postinfective urethral stricture, not elsewhere classified, male**
♂ **N35.111 Postinfective urethral stricture, not elsewhere classified, male, meatal**
♂ **N35.112 Postinfective bulbous urethral stricture, not elsewhere classified, male**
♂ **N35.113 Postinfective membranous urethral stricture, not elsewhere classified, male**
♂ **N35.114 Postinfective anterior urethral stricture, not elsewhere classified, male**
♂ **N35.116 Postinfective urethral stricture, not elsewhere classified, male, overlapping sites**
AHA CC: 4Q, 2018, 21-22
♂ **N35.119 Postinfective urethral stricture, not elsewhere classified, male, unspecified**

♀ **N35.12 Postinfective urethral stricture, not elsewhere classified, female**

\+ **N35.8 Other urethral stricture**
Excludes1: *postprocedural urethral stricture (N99.1-)*

\+ **N35.81 Other urethral stricture, male**
AHA CC: 4Q, 2018, 21-22
♂ **N35.811 Other urethral stricture, male, meatal**
♂ **N35.812 Other urethral bulbous stricture, male**
♂ **N35.813 Other membranous urethral stricture, male**
♂ **N35.814 Other anterior urethral stricture, male**
♂ **N35.816 Other urethral stricture, male, overlapping sites**
♂ **N35.819 Other urethral stricture, male, unspecified site**

♀ **N35.82 Other urethral stricture, female**
AHA CC: 4Q, 2018, 21-22

\+ **N35.9 Urethral stricture, unspecified**

\+ **N35.91 Urethral stricture, unspecified, male**
AHA CC: 4Q, 2018, 21-22
♂ **N35.911 Unspecified urethral stricture, male, meatal**
♂ **N35.912 Unspecified bulbous urethral stricture, male**
♂ **N35.913 Unspecified membranous urethral stricture, male**
♂ **N35.914 Unspecified anterior urethral stricture, male**
♂ **N35.916 Unspecified urethral stricture, male, overlapping sites**
♂ **N35.919 Unspecified urethral stricture, male, unspecified site**
Pinhole meatus NOS
Urethral stricture NOS

♀ **N35.92 Unspecified urethral stricture, female**
AHA CC: 4Q, 2018, 21-22

N36 Other disorders of urethra

CC **N36.0 Urethral fistula**
Urethroperineal fistula
Urethrorectal fistula
Urinary fistula NOS
Excludes1: *urethroscrotal fistula (N50.89)*
urethrovaginal fistula (N82.1)
urethrovesicovaginal fistula (N82.1)

N36.1 Urethral diverticulum

N36.2 Urethral caruncle

\+ **N36.4 Urethral functional and muscular disorders**
Use additional code to identify associated urinary stress incontinence (N39.3)
N36.41 Hypermobility of urethra
N36.42 Intrinsic sphincter deficiency (ISD)
N36.43 Combined hypermobility of urethra and intrinsic sphincter deficiency
N36.44 Muscular disorders of urethra
Bladder sphincter dyssynergy

N36.5 Urethral false passage

N36.8 Other specified disorders of urethra
Excludes1: *congenital urethrocele (Q64.7)*
female urethrocele (N81.0)

N36.9 Urethral disorder, unspecified

N37 Urethral disorders in diseases classified elsewhere
Code first underlying disease
Excludes1: *urethritis (in):*
candidal infection (B37.41)
chlamydial (A56.01)
gonorrhea (A54.01)
syphilis (A52.76)
trichomonal infection (A59.03)
tuberculosis (A18.13)
Valid 3-character code, no further characters required

N39 Other disorders of urinary system
Excludes2: *hematuria NOS (R31.-)*
recurrent or persistent hematuria (N02.-)
recurrent or persistent hematuria with specified morphological lesion (N02.-)
proteinuria NOS (R80.-)

CC **N39.0 Urinary tract infection, site not specified**
Use additional code (B95-B97), to identify infectious agent
Excludes1: *candidiasis of urinary tract (B37.4-)*
neonatal urinary tract infection (P39.3)
pyuria (R82.81)
urinary tract infection of specified site, such as:
cystitis (N30.-)
urethritis (N34.-)
HAC see Appendix B for HAC conditional logic
AHA CC: 4Q, 2012, 94; 1Q, 2018, 16; 2Q, 2018, 22

N39.3 Stress incontinence (female) (male)
Code also any associated overactive bladder (N32.81)
Excludes1: *mixed incontinence (N39.46)*

+ **N39.4 Other specified urinary incontinence**
Code also any associated overactive bladder (N32.81)
Excludes1: *enuresis NOS (R32)*
functional urinary incontinence (R39.81)
urinary incontinence associated with cognitive impairment (R39.81)
urinary incontinence NOS (R32)
urinary incontinence of nonorganic origin (F98.0)

N39.41 Urge incontinence
Excludes1: *mixed incontinence (N39.46)*

N39.42 Incontinence without sensory awareness
Insensible (urinary) incontinence

N39.43 Post-void dribbling

N39.44 Nocturnal enuresis
Excludes2: *nocturnal polyuria (R35.81)*

N39.45 Continuous leakage

N39.46 Mixed incontinence
Urge and stress incontinence

+ **N39.49 Other specified urinary incontinence**
AHA CC: 4Q, 2016, 44

N39.490 Overflow incontinence

N39.491 Coital incontinence

N39.492 Postural (urinary) incontinence

N39.498 Other specified urinary incontinence
Reflex incontinence
Total incontinence

N39.8 Other specified disorders of urinary system

N39.9 Disorder of urinary system, unspecified

Diseases of male genital organs (N40-N53)

N40 Benign prostatic hyperplasia

Includes: adenofibromatous hypertrophy of prostate
benign hypertrophy of the prostate
benign prostatic hypertrophy
BPH
enlarged prostate
nodular prostate
polyp of prostate

Excludes1: *benign neoplasms of prostate (adenoma, benign) (fibroadenoma) (fibroma) (myoma) (D29.1)*

Excludes2: *malignant neoplasm of prostate (C61)*

● ♂ **N40.0 Benign prostatic hyperplasia without lower urinary tract symptoms**
Enlarged prostate without LUTS
Enlarged prostate NOS

● ♂ **N40.1 Benign prostatic hyperplasia with lower urinary tract symptoms**
Enlarged prostate with LUTS
Use additional code for associated symptoms, when specified:
incomplete bladder emptying (R39.14)
nocturia (R35.1)
straining on urination (R39.16)
urinary frequency (R35.0)
urinary hesitancy (R39.11)
urinary incontinence (N39.4-)
urinary obstruction (N13.8)
urinary retention (R33.8)
urinary urgency (R39.15)
weak urinary stream (R39.12)

● ♂ **N40.2 Nodular prostate without lower urinary tract symptoms**
Nodular prostate without LUTS

● ♂ **N40.3 Nodular prostate with lower urinary tract symptoms**
Use additional code for associated symptoms, when specified:
incomplete bladder emptying (R39.14)
nocturia (R35.1)
straining on urination (R39.16)
urinary frequency (R35.0)
urinary hesitancy (R39.11)
urinary incontinence (N39.4-)
urinary obstruction (N13.8)
urinary retention (R33.8)
urinary urgency (R39.15)
weak urinary stream (R39.12)

N41 Inflammatory diseases of prostate
Use additional code (B95-B97), to identify infectious agent

● ♂ CC **N41.0 Acute prostatitis**

● ♂ **N41.1 Chronic prostatitis**

● ♂ CC **N41.2 Abscess of prostate**

● ♂ **N41.3 Prostatocystitis**

● ♂ **N41.4 Granulomatous prostatitis**

● ♂ **N41.8 Other inflammatory diseases of prostate**

● ♂ **N41.9 Inflammatory disease of prostate, unspecified**
Prostatitis NOS

N42 Other and unspecified disorders of prostate

● ♂ **N42.0 Calculus of prostate**
Prostatic stone

● ♂ **N42.1 Congestion and hemorrhage of prostate**
Excludes1: *enlarged prostate (N40.-)*
hematuria (R31.-)
hyperplasia of prostate (N40.-)
inflammatory diseases of prostate (N41.-)

+ **N42.3 Dysplasia of prostate**
AHA CC: 4Q, 2016, 44

♂ **N42.30 Unspecified dysplasia of prostate**

♂ **N42.31 Prostatic intraepithelial neoplasia**
PIN
Prostatic intraepithelial neoplasia I (PIN I)
Prostatic intraepithelial neoplasia II (PIN II)
Exlcudes1: *prostatic intraepithelial neoplasia III (PIN III) (D07.5)*

♂ **N42.32 Atypical small acinar proliferation of prostate**

♂ **N42.39 Other dysplasia of prostate**

+ **N42.8 Other specified disorders of prostate**

● ♂ **N42.81 Prostatodynia syndrome**
Painful prostate syndrome

● ♂ **N42.82 Prostatosis syndrome**

● ♂ **N42.83 Cyst of prostate**

● ♂ **N42.89 Other specified disorders of prostate**

● ♂ **N42.9 Disorder of prostate, unspecified**

N43 Hydrocele and spermatocele

Includes: hydrocele of spermatic cord, testis or tunica vaginalis
Excludes1: *congenital hydrocele (P83.5)*

♂ **N43.0 Encysted hydrocele**

CC ♂ **N43.1 Infected hydrocele**
Use additional code (B95-B97), to identify infectious agent

♂ **N43.2 Other hydrocele**

♂ **N43.3 Hydrocele, unspecified**

+ **N43.4 Spermatocele of epididymis**
Spermatic cyst

♂ **N43.40 Spermatocele of epididymis, unspecified**

♂ **N43.41 Spermatocele of epididymis, single**

♂ **N43.42 Spermatocele of epididymis, multiple**

N44 Noninflammatory disorders of testis

+ **N44.0 Torsion of testis**

CC ♂ **N44.00 Torsion of testis, unspecified**

CC ♂ **N44.01 Extravaginal torsion of spermatic cord**

CC ♂ **N44.02 Intravaginal torsion of spermatic cord**
Torsion of spermatic cord NOS

CC ♂ **N44.03 Torsion of appendix testis**

CC ♂ **N44.04 Torsion of appendix epididymis**

♂ **N44.1 Cyst of tunica albuginea testis**

♂ **N44.2 Benign cyst of testis**

♂ **N44.8 Other noninflammatory disorders of the testis**

N45 Orchitis and epididymitis
Use additional code (B95-B97), to identify infectious agent

♂ **N45.1 Epididymitis**

♂ **N45.2 Orchitis**

♂ **N45.3 Epididymo-orchitis**

CC ♂ **N45.4 Abscess of epididymis or testis**

N46 Male infertility

Excludes1: *vasectomy status (Z98.52)*

+ **N46.0 Azoospermia**
Absolute male infertility
Male infertility due to germinal (cell) aplasia
Male infertility due to spermatogenic arrest (complete)

● ♂ **N46.01 Organic azoospermia**
Azoospermia NOS

Male Reproductive System

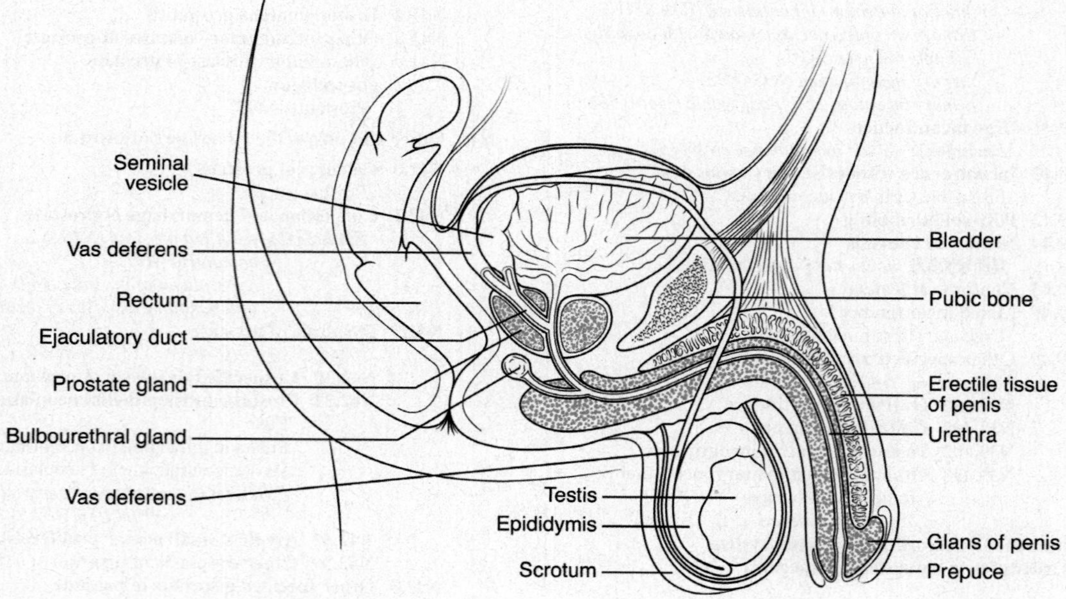

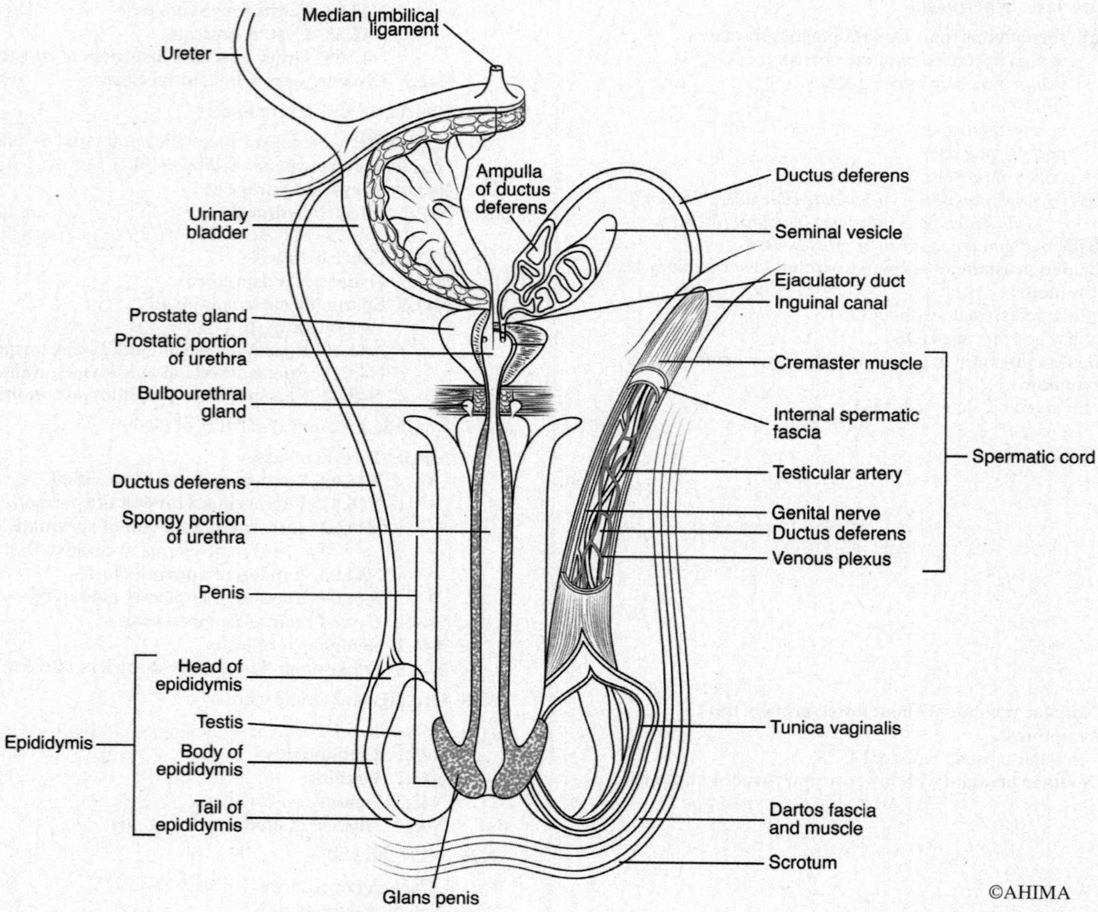

+ **N46.02 Azoospermia due to extratesticular causes**
Code also associated cause
- ● ♂ **N46.021 Azoospermia due to drug therapy**
- ● ♂ **N46.022 Azoospermia due to infection**
- ● ♂ **N46.023 Azoospermia due to obstruction of efferent ducts**
- ● ♂ **N46.024 Azoospermia due to radiation**
- ● ♂ **N46.025 Azoospermia due to systemic disease**
- ● ♂ **N46.029 Azoospermia due to other extratesticular causes**

+ **N46.1 Oligospermia**
Male infertility due to germinal cell desquamation
Male infertility due to hypospermatogenesis
Male infertility due to incomplete spermatogenic arrest
- ● ♂ **N46.11 Organic oligospermia**
Oligospermia NOS
- + **N46.12 Oligospermia due to extratesticular causes**
Code also associated cause
  - ● ♂ **N46.121 Oligospermia due to drug therapy**
  - ● ♂ **N46.122 Oligospermia due to infection**
  - ● ♂ **N46.123 Oligospermia due to obstruction of efferent ducts**
  - ● ♂ **N46.124 Oligospermia due to radiation**
  - ● ♂ **N46.125 Oligospermia due to systemic disease**
  - ● ♂ **N46.129 Oligospermia due to other extratesticular causes**

● ♂ **N46.8 Other male infertility**
● ♂ **N46.9 Male infertility, unspecified**

N47 Disorders of prepuce

● ♂ **N47.0 Adherent prepuce, newborn**
♂ **N47.1 Phimosis**
♂ **N47.2 Paraphimosis**
♂ **N47.3 Deficient foreskin**
♂ **N47.4 Benign cyst of prepuce**
♂ **N47.5 Adhesions of prepuce and glans penis**
♂ **N47.6 Balanoposthitis**
Use additional code (B95-B97), to identify infectious agent
Excludes1: *balanitis (N48.1)*
♂ **N47.7 Other inflammatory diseases of prepuce**
Use additional code (B95-B97), to identify infectious agent
♂ **N47.8 Other disorders of prepuce**

N48 Other disorders of penis

♂ **N48.0 Leukoplakia of penis**
Balanitis xerotica obliterans
Kraurosis of penis
Lichen sclerosus of external male genital organs
Excludes1: *carcinoma in situ of penis (D07.4)*

♂ **N48.1 Balanitis**
Use additional code (B95-B97), to identify infectious agent
Excludes1: *amebic balanitis (A06.8)*
balanitis xerotica obliterans (N48.0)
candidal balanitis (B37.42)
gonococcal balanitis (A54.23)
herpesviral [herpes simplex] balanitis (A60.01)

+ **N48.2 Other inflammatory disorders of penis**
Use additional code (B95-B97), to identify infectious agent
Excludes1: *balanitis (N48.1)*
balanitis xerotica obliterans (N48.0)
balanoposthitis (N47.6)
- ♂ **N48.21 Abscess of corpus cavernosum and penis**
- ♂ **N48.22 Cellulitis of corpus cavernosum and penis**
- ♂ **N48.29 Other inflammatory disorders of penis**

+ **N48.3 Priapism**
Painful erection
Code first underlying cause
- CC ♂ **N48.30 Priapism, unspecified**
- CC ♂ **N48.31 Priapism due to trauma**
- CC ♂ **N48.32 Priapism due to disease classified elsewhere**
- CC ♂ **N48.33 Priapism, drug-induced**
- CC ♂ **N48.39 Other priapism**

♂ **N48.5 Ulcer of penis**
♂ **N48.6 Induration penis plastica**
Peyronie's disease
Plastic induration of penis

+ **N48.8 Other specified disorders of penis**
- ♂ **N48.81 Thrombosis of superficial vein of penis**
- ♂ **N48.82 Acquired torsion of penis**
Acquired torsion of penis NOS
Excludes1: *congenital torsion of penis (Q55.63)*
- ♂ **N48.83 Acquired buried penis**
Excludes1: *congenital hidden penis (Q55.64)*
- ♂ **N48.89 Other specified disorders of penis**

♂ **N48.9 Disorder of penis, unspecified**

N49 Inflammatory disorders of male genital organs, not elsewhere classified

Use additional code (B95-B97), to identify infectious agent
Excludes1: *inflammation of penis (N48.1, N48.2-)*
orchitis and epididymitis (N45.-)

♂ **N49.0 Inflammatory disorders of seminal vesicle**
Vesiculitis NOS
♂ **N49.1 Inflammatory disorders of spermatic cord, tunica vaginalis and vas deferens**
Vasitis
♂ **N49.2 Inflammatory disorders of scrotum**
♂ **N49.3 Fournier gangrene**
AHA CC: 2Q, 2020, 18
♂ **N49.8 Inflammatory disorders of other specified male genital organs**
Inflammation of multiple sites in male genital organs
♂ **N49.9 Inflammatory disorder of unspecified male genital organ**
Abscess of unspecified male genital organ
Boil of unspecified male genital organ
Carbuncle of unspecified male genital organ
Cellulitis of unspecified male genital organ

N50 Other and unspecified disorders of male genital organs

Excludes2: *torsion of testis (N44.0-)*

♂ **N50.0 Atrophy of testis**
♂ **N50.1 Vascular disorders of male genital organs**
Hematocele, NOS, of male genital organs
Hemorrhage of male genital organs
Thrombosis of male genital organs
♂ **N50.3 Cyst of epididymis**
+ **N50.8 Other specified disorders of male genital organs**
AHA CC: 4Q, 2016, 45
- + **N50.81 Testicular pain**
  - ♂ **N50.811 Right testicular pain**
  - ♂ **N50.812 Left testicular pain**
  - ♂ **N50.819 Testicular pain, unspecified**
- ♂ **N50.82 Scrotal pain**
- ♂ **N50.89 Other specified disorders of the male genital organs**
Atrophy of scrotum, seminal vesicle, spermatic cord, tunica vaginalis and vas deferens
Chylocele, tunica vaginalis (nonfilarial) NOS
Edema of scrotum, seminal vesicle, spermatic cord, tunica vaginalis and vas deferens
Hypertrophy of scrotum, seminal vesicle, spermatic cord, tunica vaginalis and vas deferens
Stricture of spermatic cord, tunical vaginalis, and vas deferens
Ulcer of scrotum, seminal vesicle, spermatic cord, testis, tunica vaginalis and vas deferens
Urethroscrotal fistula

♂ **N50.9 Disorder of male genital organs, unspecified**

♂ N51 Disorders of male genital organs in diseases classified elsewhere

Code first underlying disease, such as:
filariasis (B74.0-B74.9)
Excludes1: *amebic balanitis (A06.8)*
candidal balanitis (B37.42)
gonococcal balanitis (A54.23)
gonococcal prostatitis (A54.22)
herpesviral [herpes simplex] balanitis (A60.01)
trichomonal prostatitis (A59.02)
tuberculous prostatitis (A18.14)
Valid 3-character code, no further characters required

N52 Male erectile dysfunction

Excludes1: *psychogenic impotence (F52.21)*

+ **N52.0 Vasculogenic erectile dysfunction**
- ● ♂ **N52.01 Erectile dysfunction due to arterial insufficiency**
- ● ♂ **N52.02 Corporo-venous occlusive erectile dysfunction**
- ● ♂ **N52.03 Combined arterial insufficiency and corporo-venous occlusive erectile dysfunction**

● ♂ CC **N52.1 Erectile dysfunction due to diseases classified elsewhere**
Code first underlying disease
● ♂ CC **N52.2 Drug-induced erectile dysfunction**

\+ **N52.3 Postprocedural erectile dysfunction**
AHA CC: 4Q, 2016, 45
• ♂ **N52.31 Erectile dysfunction following radical prostatectomy**
• ♂ **N52.32 Erectile dysfunction following radical cystectomy**
• ♂ **N52.33 Erectile dysfunction following urethral surgery**
• ♂ **N52.34 Erectile dysfunction following simple prostatectomy**
• ♂ **N52.35 Erectile dysfunction following radiation therapy**
• ♂ **N52.36 Erectile dysfunction following interstitial seed therapy**
• ♂ **N52.37 Erectile dysfunction following prostate ablative therapy**
Erectile dysfunction following cryotherapy
Erectile dysfunction following other prostate ablative therapies
Erectile dysfunction following ultrasound ablative therapies
• ♂ **N52.39 Other and unspecified postprocedural erectile dysfunction**
• ♂ **N52.8 Other male erectile dysfunction**
• ♂ **N52.9 Male erectile dysfunction, unspecified**
Impotence NOS

N53 Other male sexual dysfunction

Excludes1: *psychogenic sexual dysfunction (F52.-)*
\+ **N53.1 Ejaculatory dysfunction**
Excludes1: *premature ejaculation (F52.4)*
♂ **N53.11 Retarded ejaculation**
♂ **N53.12 Painful ejaculation**
♂ **N53.13 Anejaculatory orgasm**
♂ **N53.14 Retrograde ejaculation**
♂ **N53.19 Other ejaculatory dysfunction**
Ejaculatory dysfunction NOS
♂ **N53.8 Other male sexual dysfunction**
♂ **N53.9 Unspecified male sexual dysfunction**

Disorders of breast (N60-N65)

Excludes1: *disorders of breast associated with childbirth (O91-O92)*

N60 Benign mammary dysplasia

Includes: fibrocystic mastopathy
\+ **N60.0 Solitary cyst of breast**
Cyst of breast
N60.01 Solitary cyst of right breast
N60.02 Solitary cyst of left breast
N60.09 Solitary cyst of unspecified breast
\+ **N60.1 Diffuse cystic mastopathy**
Cystic breast
Fibrocystic disease of breast
Excludes1: *diffuse cystic mastopathy with epithelial proliferation (N60.3-)*
• **N60.11 Diffuse cystic mastopathy of right breast**
• **N60.12 Diffuse cystic mastopathy of left breast**
• **N60.19 Diffuse cystic mastopathy of unspecified breast**
\+ **N60.2 Fibroadenosis of breast**
Adenofibrosis of breast
Excludes2: *fibroadenoma of breast (D24.-)*
N60.21 Fibroadenosis of right breast
N60.22 Fibroadenosis of left breast
N60.29 Fibroadenosis of unspecified breast
\+ **N60.3 Fibrosclerosis of breast**
Cystic mastopathy with epithelial proliferation
N60.31 Fibrosclerosis of right breast
N60.32 Fibrosclerosis of left breast
N60.39 Fibrosclerosis of unspecified breast
\+ **N60.4 Mammary duct ectasia**
N60.41 Mammary duct ectasia of right breast
N60.42 Mammary duct ectasia of left breast
N60.49 Mammary duct ectasia of unspecified breast
\+ **N60.8 Other benign mammary dysplasias**
N60.81 Other benign mammary dysplasias of right breast
N60.82 Other benign mammary dysplasias of left breast
N60.89 Other benign mammary dysplasias of unspecified breast
\+ **N60.9 Unspecified benign mammary dysplasia**
N60.91 Unspecified benign mammary dysplasia of right breast
N60.92 Unspecified benign mammary dysplasia of left breast
N60.99 Unspecified benign mammary dysplasia of unspecified breast

N61 Inflammatory disorders of breast

Excludes1: *inflammatory carcinoma of breast (C50.9)*
inflammatory disorder of breast associated with childbirth (O91.-)
neonatal infective mastitis (P39.0)
thrombophlebitis of breast [Mondor's disease] (I80.8)
N61.0 Mastitis without abscess
Infective mastitis (acute) (nonpuerperal) (subacute)
Mastitis (acute) (nonpuerperal) (subacute) NOS
Cellulitis (acute) (nonpuerperal) (subacute) of breast NOS
Cellulitis (acute) (nonpuerperal) (subacute) of nipple NOS
N61.1 Abscess of the breast and nipple
Abscess (acute) (chronic) (nonpuerperal) of areola
Abscess (acute) (chronic) (nonpuerperal) of breast
Carbuncle of breast
Mastitis with abscess
\+ **N61.2 Granulomatous mastitis**
AHA CC: 4Q, 2020, 35
N61.20 Granulomatous mastitis, unspecified breast
N61.21 Granulomatous mastitis, right breast
N61.22 Granulomatous mastitis, left breast
N61.23 Granulomatous mastitis, bilateral breast

N62 Hypertrophy of breast

Gynecomastia
Hypertrophy of breast NOS
Massive pubertal hypertrophy of breast
Excludes1: *breast engorgement of newborn (P83.4)*
disproportion of reconstructed breast (N65.1)
Valid 3-character code, no further characters required

N63 Unspecified lump in breast

Nodule(s) NOS in breast
AHA CC: 4Q, 2017, 19
N63.0 Unspecified lump in unspecified breast
\+ **N63.1 Unspecified lump in the right breast**
N63.10 Unspecified lump in the right breast, unspecified quadrant
N63.11 Unspecified lump in the right breast, upper outer quadrant
N63.12 Unspecified lump in the right breast, upper inner quadrant
N63.13 Unspecified lump in the right breast, lower outer quadrant
N63.14 Unspecified lump in the right breast, lower inner quadrant
N63.15 Unspecified lump in the right breast, overlapping quadrants
AHA CC: 4Q, 2019, 12
\+ **N63.2 Unspecified lump in the left breast**
N63.20 Unspecified lump in the left breast, unspecified quadrant
N63.21 Unspecified lump in the left breast, upper outer quadrant
N63.22 Unspecified lump in the left breast, upper inner quadrant
N63.23 Unspecified lump in the left breast, lower outer quadrant
N63.24 Unspecified lump in the left breast, lower inner quadrant
N63.25 Unspecified lump in the left breast, overlapping quadrants
AHA CC: 4Q, 2019, 12
\+ **N63.3 Unspecified lump in axillary tail**
N63.31 Unspecified lump in axillary tail of the right breast
N63.32 Unspecified lump in axillary tail of the left breast
\+ **N63.4 Unspecified lump in breast, subareolar**
N63.41 Unspecified lump in right breast, subareolar
N63.42 Unspecified lump in left breast, subareolar

N64 Other disorders of breast

Excludes2: *mechanical complication of breast prosthesis and implant (T85.4-)*
N64.0 Fissure and fistula of nipple
N64.1 Fat necrosis of breast
Fat necrosis (segmental) of breast
Code first breast necrosis due to breast graft (T85.898)

Breast

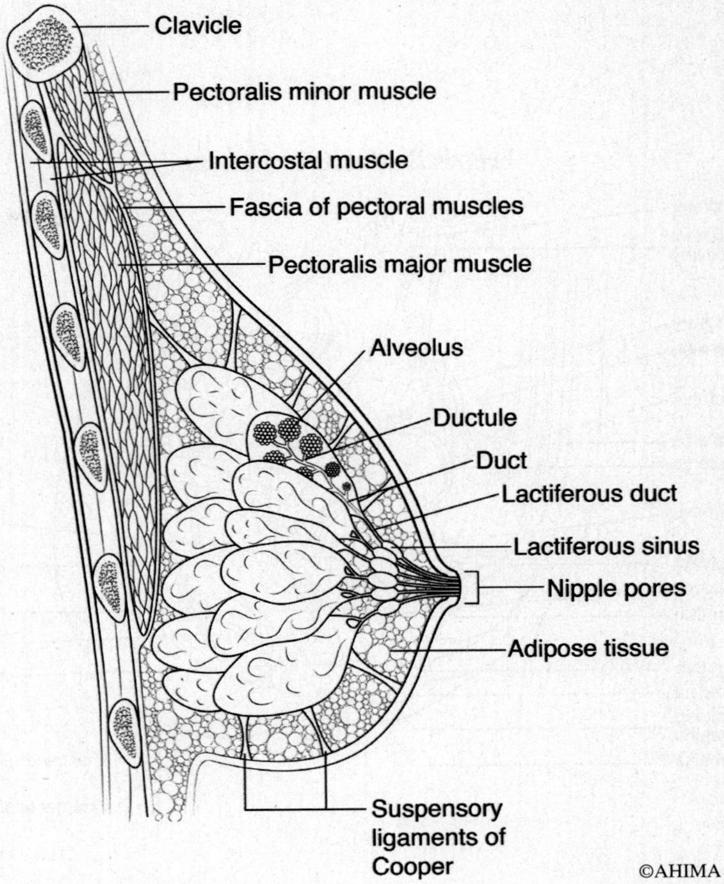

N64.2 Atrophy of breast
N64.3 Galactorrhea not associated with childbirth
N64.4 Mastodynia
\+ **N64.5 Other signs and symptoms in breast**
Excludes2: *abnormal findings on diagnostic imaging of breast (R92.-)*
N64.51 Induration of breast
N64.52 Nipple discharge
Excludes1: *abnormal findings in nipple discharge (R89.-)*
N64.53 Retraction of nipple
N64.59 Other signs and symptoms in breast
\+ **N64.8 Other specified disorders of breast**
● **N64.81 Ptosis of breast**
Excludes1: *ptosis of native breast in relation to reconstructed breast (N65.1)*
● **N64.82 Hypoplasia of breast**
Micromastia
Excludes1: *congenital absence of breast (Q83.0)*
hypoplasia of native breast in relation to reconstructed breast (N65.1)
N64.89 Other specified disorders of breast
Galactocele
Subinvolution of breast (postlactational)
AHA CC: 1Q, 2018, 3-4; 1Q, 2019, 32
N64.9 Disorder of breast, unspecified

N65 Deformity and disproportion of reconstructed breast
● **N65.0 Deformity of reconstructed breast**
Contour irregularity in reconstructed breast
Excess tissue in reconstructed breast
Misshapen reconstructed breast
● **N65.1 Disproportion of reconstructed breast**
Breast asymmetry between native breast and reconstructed breast
Disproportion between native breast and reconstructed breast

Inflammatory diseases of female pelvic organs (N70-N77)

Excludes1: *inflammatory diseases of female pelvic organs complicating:*
abortion or ectopic or molar pregnancy (O00-O07, O08.0)
pregnancy, childbirth and the puerperium (O23.-, O75.3, O85, O86.-)

N70 Salpingitis and oophoritis
Includes: abscess (of) fallopian tube
abscess (of) ovary
pyosalpinx
salpingo-oophoritis
tubo-ovarian abscess
tubo-ovarian inflammatory disease
Use additional code (B95-B97), to identify infectious agent
Excludes1: *gonococcal infection (A54.24)*
tuberculous infection (A18.17)
\+ **N70.0 Acute salpingitis and oophoritis**
♀ CC **N70.01 Acute salpingitis**
♀ CC **N70.02 Acute oophoritis**
♀ CC **N70.03 Acute salpingitis and oophoritis**
\+ **N70.1 Chronic salpingitis and oophoritis**
Hydrosalpinx
♀ **N70.11 Chronic salpingitis**
♀ **N70.12 Chronic oophoritis**
♀ **N70.13 Chronic salpingitis and oophoritis**
\+ **N70.9 Salpingitis and oophoritis, unspecified**
♀ **N70.91 Salpingitis, unspecified**
♀ **N70.92 Oophoritis, unspecified**
♀ **N70.93 Salpingitis and oophoritis, unspecified**

Female Reproductive System

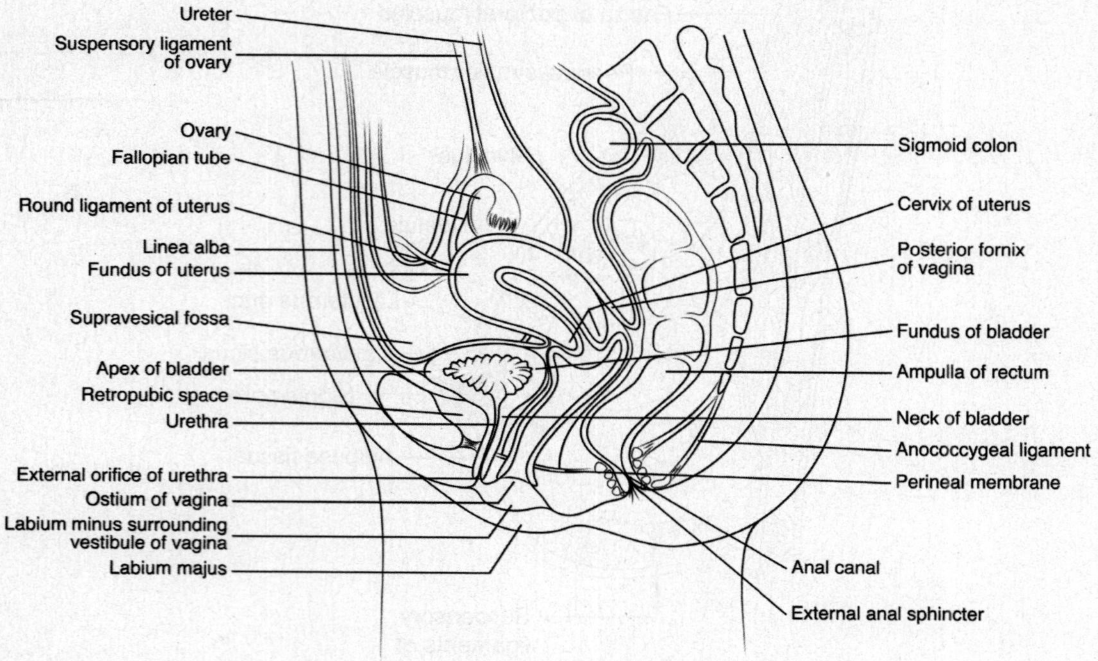

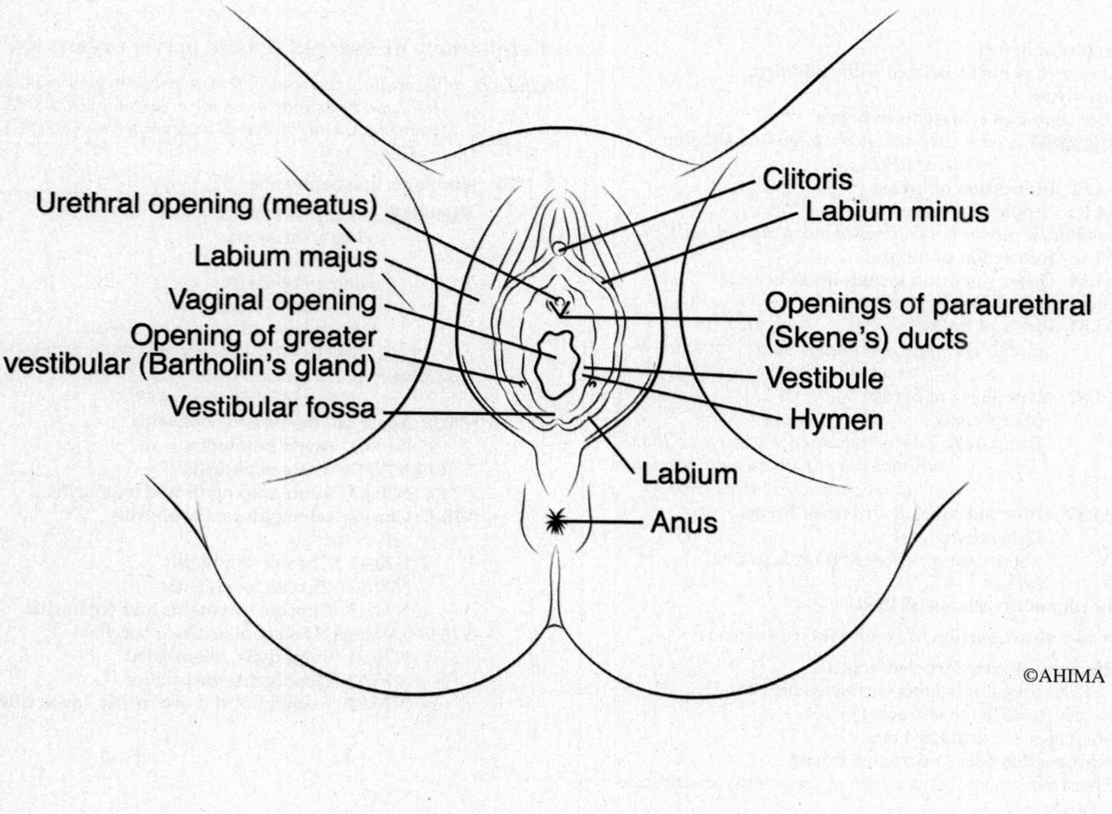

N71 Inflammatory disease of uterus, except cervix

Includes: endo (myo) metritis
metritis
myometritis
pyometra
uterine abscess

Use additional code (B95-B97), to identify infectious agent

Excludes1: *hyperplastic endometritis (N85.0-)*
infection of uterus following delivery (O85, O86.-)

♀ CC **N71.0 Acute inflammatory disease of uterus**
♀ **N71.1 Chronic inflammatory disease of uterus**
♀ **N71.9 Inflammatory disease of uterus, unspecified**

♀ **N72 Inflammatory disease of cervix uteri**

Includes: cervicitis (with or without erosion or ectropion)
endocervicitis (with or without erosion or ectropion)
exocervicitis (with or without erosion or ectropion)

Use additional code (B95-B97), to identify infectious agent

Excludes1: *erosion and ectropion of cervix without cervicitis (N86)*

Valid 3-character code, no further characters required

N73 Other female pelvic inflammatory diseases

Use additional code (B95-B97), to identify infectious agent

♀ CC **N73.0 Acute parametritis and pelvic cellulitis**
Abscess of broad ligament
Abscess of parametrium
Pelvic cellulitis, female

♀ **N73.1 Chronic parametritis and pelvic cellulitis**
Any condition in N73.0 specified as chronic
Excludes1: *tuberculous parametritis and pelvic cellultis (A18.17)*

♀ **N73.2 Unspecified parametritis and pelvic cellulitis**
Any condition in N73.0 unspecified whether acute or chronic

♀ MCC **N73.3 Female acute pelvic peritonitis**
♀ CC **N73.4 Female chronic pelvic peritonitis**
Excludes1: *tuberculous pelvic (female) peritonitis (A18.17)*

♀ **N73.5 Female pelvic peritonitis, unspecified**
♀ **N73.6 Female pelvic peritoneal adhesions (postinfective)**
Excludes2: *postprocedural pelvic peritoneal adhesions (N99.4)*
AHA CC: 1Q, 2014, 6

♀ **N73.8 Other specified female pelvic inflammatory diseases**
♀ **N73.9 Female pelvic inflammatory disease, unspecified**
Female pelvic infection or inflammation NOS

♀ **N74 Female pelvic inflammatory disorders in diseases classified elsewhere**

Code first underlying disease

Excludes1: *chlamydial cervicitis (A56.02)*
chlamydial pelvic inflammatory disease (A56.11)
gonococcal cervicitis (A54.03)
gonococcal pelvic inflammatory disease (A54.24)
herpesviral [herpes simplex] cervicitis (A60.03)
herpesviral [herpes simplex] pelvic inflammatory disease (A60.09)
syphilitic cervicitis (A52.76)
syphilitic pelvic inflammatory disease (A52.76)
trichomonal cervicitis (A59.09)
tuberculous cervicitis (A18.16)
tuberculous pelvic inflammatory disease (A18.17)

Valid 3-character code, no further characters required

N75 Diseases of Bartholin's gland

♀ **N75.0 Cyst of Bartholin's gland**
♀ CC **N75.1 Abscess of Bartholin's gland**
♀ **N75.8 Other diseases of Bartholin's gland**
Bartholinitis
♀ **N75.9 Disease of Bartholin's gland, unspecified**

N76 Other inflammation of vagina and vulva

Use additional code (B95-B97), to identify infectious agent

Excludes2: *senile (atrophic) vaginitis (N95.2)*
vulvar vestibulitis (N94.810)

♀ **N76.0 Acute vaginitis**
Acute vulvovaginitis
Vaginitis NOS
Vulvovaginitis NOS

♀ **N76.1 Subacute and chronic vaginitis**
Chronic vulvovaginitis
Subacute vulvovaginitis

♀ **N76.2 Acute vulvitis**
Vulvitis NOS

♀ **N76.3 Subacute and chronic vulvitis**
♀ CC **N76.4 Abscess of vulva**
Furuncle of vulva
♀ **N76.5 Ulceration of vagina**
♀ **N76.6 Ulceration of vulva**
\+ **N76.8 Other specified inflammation of vagina and vulva**

♀ CC **N76.81 Mucositis (ulcerative) of vagina and vulva**
Code also type of associated therapy, such as:
antineoplastic and immunosuppressive drugs (T45.1X-)
radiological procedure and radiotherapy (Y84.2)
Excludes2: *gastrointestinal mucositis (ulcerative) (K92.81)*
nasal mucositis (ulcerative) (J34.81)
oral mucositis (ulcerative) (K12.3-)

♀ **N76.89 Other specified inflammation of vagina and vulva**

N77 Vulvovaginal ulceration and inflammation in diseases classified elsewhere

♀ **N77.0 Ulceration of vulva in diseases classified elsewhere**
Code first underlying disease, such as:
Behçet's disease (M35.2)
Excludes1: *ulceration of vulva in gonococcal infection (A54.02)*
ulceration of vulva in herpesviral [herpes simplex] infection (A60.04)
ulceration of vulva in syphilis (A51.0)
ulceration of vulva in tuberculosis (A18.18)

♀ **N77.1 Vaginitis, vulvitis and vulvovaginitis in diseases classified elsewhere**
Code first underlying disease, such as:
pinworm (B80)
Excludes1: *candidal vulvovaginitis (B37.3)*
chlamydial vulvovaginitis (A56.02)
gonococcal vulvovaginitis (A54.02)
herpesviral [herpes simplex] vulvovaginitis (A60.04)
trichomonal vulvovaginitis (A59.01)
tuberculous vulvovaginitis (A18.18)
vulvovaginitis in early syphilis (A51.0)
vulvovaginitis in late syphilis (A52.76)

Noninflammatory disorders of female genital tract (N80-N98)

N80 Endometriosis

♀ **N80.0 Endometriosis of uterus**
Adenomyosis
Excludes1: *stromal endometriosis (D39.0)*

♀ **N80.1 Endometriosis of ovary**
♀ **N80.2 Endometriosis of fallopian tube**
♀ **N80.3 Endometriosis of pelvic peritoneum**
♀ **N80.4 Endometriosis of rectovaginal septum and vagina**
♀ **N80.5 Endometriosis of intestine**
♀ **N80.6 Endometriosis in cutaneous scar**
♀ **N80.8 Other endometriosis**
Endometriosis of thorax
♀ **N80.9 Endometriosis, unspecified**

N81 Female genital prolapse

See page 887 for Vaginal Prolapse illustration.

Excludes1: *genital prolapse complicating pregnancy, labor or delivery (O34.5-)*
prolapse and hernia of ovary and fallopian tube (N83.4-)
prolapse of vaginal vault after hysterectomy (N99.3)

♀ **N81.0 Urethrocele**
Excludes1: *urethrocele with cystocele (N81.1-)*
urethrocele with prolapse of uterus (N81.2-N81.4)

Vaginal Prolapse

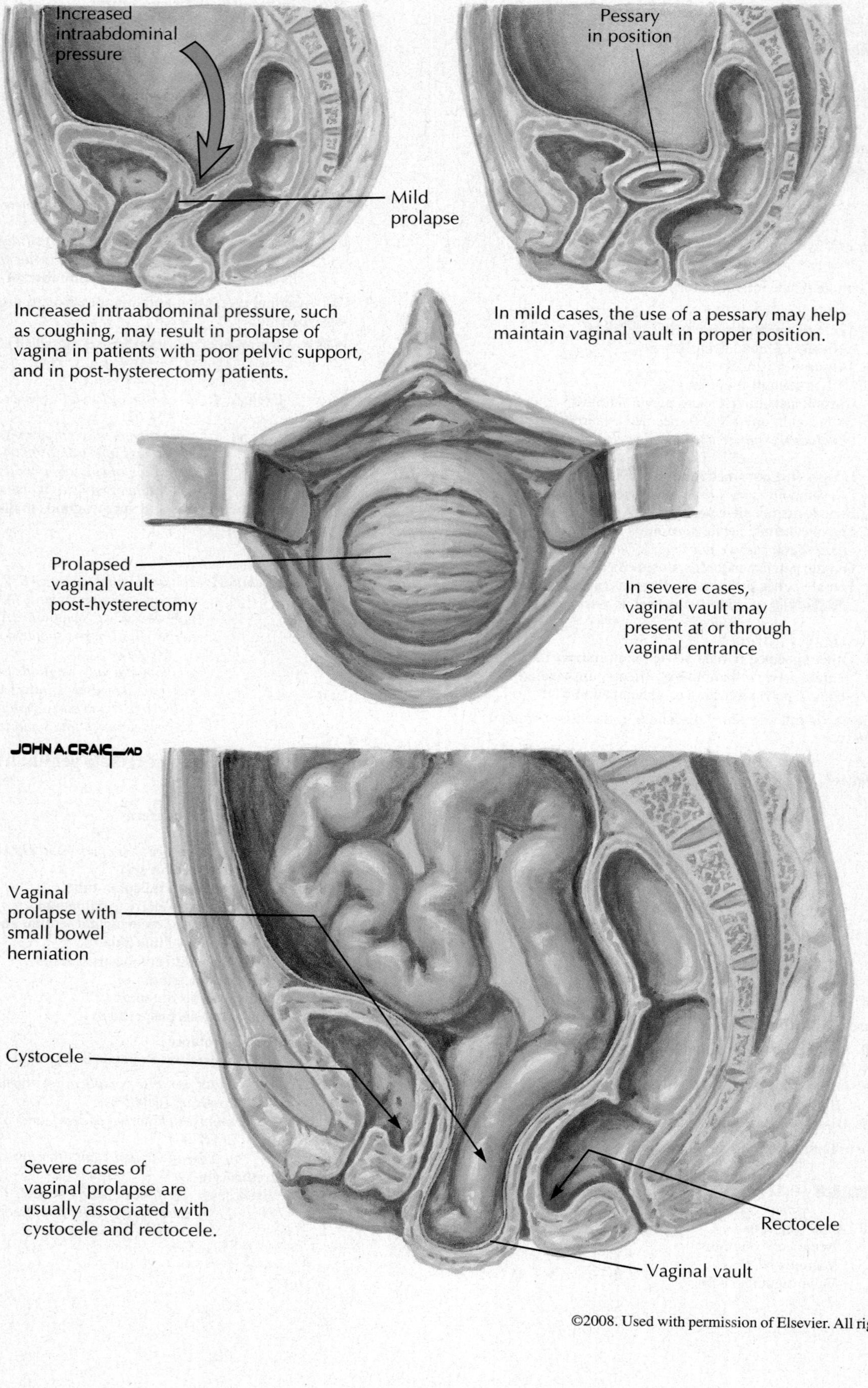

+ **N81.1 Cystocele**
Cystocele with urethrocele
Cystourethrocele
Excludes1: *cystocele with prolapse of uterus (N81.2-N81.4)*
♀ **N81.10 Cystocele, unspecified**
Prolapse of (anterior) vaginal wall NOS
♀ **N81.11 Cystocele, midline**
♀ **N81.12 Cystocele, lateral**
Paravaginal cystocele
♀ **N81.2 Incomplete uterovaginal prolapse**
First degree uterine prolapse
Prolapse of cervix NOS
Second degree uterine prolapse
Excludes1: *cervical stump prolapse (N81.85)*
♀ **N81.3 Complete uterovaginal prolapse**
Procidentia (uteri) NOS
Third degree uterine prolapse
♀ **N81.4 Uterovaginal prolapse, unspecified**
Prolapse of uterus NOS
♀ **N81.5 Vaginal enterocele**
Excludes1: *enterocele with prolapse of uterus (N81.2-N81.4)*
♀ **N81.6 Rectocele**
Prolapse of posterior vaginal wall
Use additional code for any associated fecal incontinence, if applicable (R15.-)
Excludes2: *perineocele (N81.81)*
rectal prolapse (K62.3)
rectocele with prolapse of uterus (N81.2-N81.4)
+ **N81.8 Other female genital prolapse**
♀ **N81.81 Perineocele**
♀ **N81.82 Incompetence or weakening of pubocervical tissue**
♀ **N81.83 Incompetence or weakening of rectovaginal tissue**
♀ **N81.84 Pelvic muscle wasting**
Disuse atrophy of pelvic muscles and anal sphincter
♀ **N81.85 Cervical stump prolapse**
♀ **N81.89 Other female genital prolapse**
Deficient perineum
Old laceration of muscles of pelvic floor
♀ **N81.9 Female genital prolapse, unspecified**

N82 Fistulae involving female genital tract

Excludes1: *vesicointestinal fistulae (N32.1)*
♀ CC **N82.0 Vesicovaginal fistula**
♀ CC **N82.1 Other female urinary-genital tract fistulae**
Cervicovesical fistula
Ureterovaginal fistula
Urethrovaginal fistula
Uteroureteric fistula
Uterovesical fistula
AHA CC: 3Q, 2017, 3-4
♀ CC **N82.2 Fistula of vagina to small intestine**
♀ CC **N82.3 Fistula of vagina to large intestine**
Rectovaginal fistula
♀ CC **N82.4 Other female intestinal-genital tract fistulae**
Intestinouterine fistula
♀ CC **N82.5 Female genital tract-skin fistulae**
Uterus to abdominal wall fistula
Vaginoperineal fistula
♀ CC **N82.8 Other female genital tract fistulae**
♀ CC **N82.9 Female genital tract fistula, unspecified**

N83 Noninflammatory disorders of ovary, fallopian tube and broad ligament

Excludes2: *hydrosalpinx (N70.1-)*
AHA CC: 4Q, 2016, 46
+ **N83.0 Follicular cyst of ovary**
Cyst of graafian follicle
Hemorrhagic follicular cyst (of ovary)
♀ **N83.00 Follicular cyst of ovary, unspecified side**
♀ **N83.01 Follicular cyst of right ovary**
♀ **N83.02 Follicular cyst of left ovary**
+ **N83.1 Corpus luteum cyst**
Hemorrhagic corpus luteum cyst
♀ **N83.10 Corpus luteum cyst of ovary, unspecified side**
♀ **N83.11 Corpus luteum cyst of right ovary**
♀ **N83.12 Corpus luteum cyst of left ovary**
+ **N83.2 Other and unspecified ovarian cysts**
Excludes1: *developmental ovarian cyst (Q50.1)*
neoplastic ovarian cyst (D27.-)
polycystic ovarian syndrome (E28.2)
Stein-Leventhal syndrome (E28.2)
+ **N83.20 Unspecified ovarian cysts**
♀ **N83.201 Unspecified ovarian cyst, right side**
♀ **N83.202 Unspecified ovarian cyst, left side**
♀ **N83.209 Unspecified ovarian cyst, unspecified side**
Ovarian cyst, NOS
+ **N83.29 Other ovarian cysts**
Retention cyst of ovary
Simple cyst of ovary
♀ **N83.291 Other ovarian cyst, right side**
♀ **N83.292 Other ovarian cyst, left side**
♀ **N83.299 Other ovarian cyst, unspecified side**
+ **N83.3 Acquired atrophy of ovary and fallopian tube**
+ **N83.31 Acquired atrophy of ovary**
♀ **N83.311 Acquired atrophy of right ovary**
♀ **N83.312 Acquired atrophy of left ovary**
♀ **N83.319 Acquired atrophy of ovary, unspecified side**
Acquired atrophy of ovary, NOS
+ **N83.32 Acquired atrophy of fallopian tube**
♀ **N83.321 Acquired atrophy of right fallopian tube**
♀ **N83.322 Acquired atrophy of left fallopian tube**
♀ **N83.329 Acquired atrophy of fallopian tube, unspecified side**
Acquired atrophy of fallopian tube, NOS
+ **N83.33 Acquired atrophy of ovary and fallopian tube**
♀ **N83.331 Acquired atrophy of right ovary and fallopian tube**
♀ **N83.332 Acquired atrophy of left ovary and fallopian tube**
♀ **N83.339 Acquired atrophy of ovary and fallopian tube, unspecified side**
Acquired atrophy of ovary and fallopian tube, NOS
+ **N83.4 Prolapse and hernia of ovary and fallopian tube**
♀ **N83.40 Prolapse and hernia of ovary and fallopian tube, unspecified side**
Prolapse and hernia of ovary and fallopian tube, NOS
♀ **N83.41 Prolapse and hernia of right ovary and fallopian tube**
♀ **N83.42 Prolapse and hernia of left ovary and fallopian tube**
+ **N83.5 Torsion of ovary, ovarian pedicle and fallopian tube**
Torsion of accessory tube
+ **N83.51 Torsion of ovary and ovarian pedicle**
♀ CC **N83.511 Torsion of right ovary and ovarian pedicle**
♀ CC **N83.512 Torsion of left ovary and ovarian pedicle**
♀ CC **N83.519 Torsion of ovary and ovarian pedicle, unspecified side**
Torsion of ovary and ovarian pedicle, NOS
+ **N83.52 Torsion of fallopian tube**
Torsion of hydatid of Morgagni
♀ CC **N83.521 Torsion of right fallopian tube**
♀ CC **N83.522 Torsion of left fallopian tube**
♀ CC **N83.529 Torsion of fallopian tube, unspecified side**
Torsion of fallopian tube, NOS
♀ CC **N83.53 Torsion of ovary, ovarian pedicle and fallopian tube**
♀ **N83.6 Hematosalpinx**
Excludes1: *hematosalpinx (with) (in):*
hematocolpos (N89.7)
hematometra (N85.7)
tubal pregnancy (O00.1-)
♀ **N83.7 Hematoma of broad ligament**
♀ **N83.8 Other noninflammatory disorders of ovary, fallopian tube and broad ligament**
Broad ligament laceration syndrome [Allen-Masters]
♀ **N83.9 Noninflammatory disorder of ovary, fallopian tube and broad ligament, unspecified**

N84 Polyp of female genital tract

Excludes1: *adenomatous polyp (D28.-)*
placental polyp (O90.89)

♀ **N84.0 Polyp of corpus uteri**
Polyp of endometrium
Polyp of uterus NOS
Excludes1: *polypoid endometrial hyperplasia (N85.0-)*

♀ **N84.1 Polyp of cervix uteri**
Mucous polyp of cervix

♀ **N84.2 Polyp of vagina**

♀ **N84.3 Polyp of vulva**
Polyp of labia

♀ **N84.8 Polyp of other parts of female genital tract**

♀ **N84.9 Polyp of female genital tract, unspecified**

N85 Other noninflammatory disorders of uterus, except cervix

Excludes1: *endometriosis (N80.-)*
inflammatory diseases of uterus (N71.-)
noninflammatory disorders of cervix, except malposition (N86-N88)
polyp of corpus uteri (N84.0)
uterine prolapse (N81.-)

\+ **N85.0 Endometrial hyperplasia**

♀ **N85.00 Endometrial hyperplasia, unspecified**
Hyperplasia (adenomatous) (cystic) (glandular) of endometrium
Hyperplastic endometritis

♀ **N85.01 Benign endometrial hyperplasia**
Endometrial hyperplasia (complex) (simple) without atypia

♀ **N85.02 Endometrial intraepithelial neoplasia [EIN]**
Endometrial hyperplasia with atypia
Excludes1: *malignant neoplasm of endometrium (with endometrial intraepithelial neoplasia [EIN]) (C54.1)*

♀ **N85.2 Hypertrophy of uterus**
Bulky or enlarged uterus
Excludes1: *puerperal hypertrophy of uterus (O90.89)*

♀ **N85.3 Subinvolution of uterus**
Excludes1: *puerperal subinvolution of uterus (O90.89)*

♀ **N85.4 Malposition of uterus**
Anteversion of uterus
Retroflexion of uterus
Retroversion of uterus
Excludes1: *malposition of uterus complicating pregnancy, labor or delivery (O34.5-, O65.5)*

♀ **N85.5 Inversion of uterus**
Excludes1: *current obstetric trauma (O71.2)*
postpartum inversion of uterus (O71.2)

♀ **N85.6 Intrauterine synechiae**

♀ **N85.7 Hematometra**
Hematosalpinx with hematometra
Excludes1: *hematometra with hematocolpos (N89.7)*

♀ **N85.8 Other specified noninflammatory disorders of uterus**
Atrophy of uterus, acquired
Fibrosis of uterus NOS

♀ **N85.9 Noninflammatory disorder of uterus, unspecified**
Disorder of uterus NOS

♀ **N86 Erosion and ectropion of cervix uteri**
Decubitus (trophic) ulcer of cervix
Eversion of cervix
Excludes1: *erosion and ectropion of cervix with cervicitis (N72)*
Valid 3-character code, no further characters required

N87 Dysplasia of cervix uteri

Excludes1: *abnormal results from cervical cytologic examination without histologic confirmation (R87.61-)*
carcinoma in situ of cervix uteri (D06.-)
cervical intraepithelial neoplasia III [CIN III] (D06.-)
HGSIL of cervix (R87.613)
severe dysplasia of cervix uteri (D06.-)

♀ **N87.0 Mild cervical dysplasia**
Cervical intraepithelial neoplasia I [CIN I]

♀ **N87.1 Moderate cervical dysplasia**
Cervical intraepithelial neoplasia II [CIN II]

♀ **N87.9 Dysplasia of cervix uteri, unspecified**
Anaplasia of cervix
Cervical atypism
Cervical dysplasia NOS

N88 Other noninflammatory disorders of cervix uteri

Excludes2: *inflammatory disease of cervix (N72)*
polyp of cervix (N84.1)

♀ **N88.0 Leukoplakia of cervix uteri**

♀ **N88.1 Old laceration of cervix uteri**
Adhesions of cervix
Excludes1: *current obstetric trauma (O71.3)*

♀ **N88.2 Stricture and stenosis of cervix uteri**
Excludes1: *stricture and stenosis of cervix uteri complicating labor (O65.5)*

♀ **N88.3 Incompetence of cervix uteri**
Investigation and management of (suspected) cervical incompetence in a nonpregnant woman
Excludes1: *cervical incompetence complicating pregnancy (O34.3-)*

♀ **N88.4 Hypertrophic elongation of cervix uteri**

♀ **N88.8 Other specified noninflammatory disorders of cervix uteri**
Excludes1: *current obstetric trauma (O71.3)*

♀ **N88.9 Noninflammatory disorder of cervix uteri, unspecified**

N89 Other noninflammatory disorders of vagina

Excludes1: *abnormal results from vaginal cytologic examination without histologic confirmation (R87.62-)*
carcinoma in situ of vagina (D07.2)
HGSIL of vagina (R87.623)
inflammation of vagina (N76.-)
senile (atrophic) vaginitis (N95.2)
severe dysplasia of vagina (D07.2)
trichomonal leukorrhea (A59.00)
vaginal intraepithelial neoplasia [VAIN], grade III (D07.2)

♀ **N89.0 Mild vaginal dysplasia**
Vaginal intraepithelial neoplasia [VAIN], grade I

♀ **N89.1 Moderate vaginal dysplasia**
Vaginal intraepithelial neoplasia [VAIN], grade II

♀ **N89.3 Dysplasia of vagina, unspecified**

♀ **N89.4 Leukoplakia of vagina**

♀ **N89.5 Stricture and atresia of vagina**
Vaginal adhesions
Vaginal stenosis
Excludes1: *congenital atresia or stricture (Q52.4)*
postprocedural adhesions of vagina (N99.2)

♀ **N89.6 Tight hymenal ring**
Rigid hymen
Tight introitus
Excludes1: *imperforate hymen (Q52.3)*

♀ **N89.7 Hematocolpos**
Hematocolpos with hematometra or hematosalpinx
AHA CC: 4Q, 2016, 58-59

♀ **N89.8 Other specified noninflammatory disorders of vagina**
Leukorrhea NOS
Old vaginal laceration
Pessary ulcer of vagina
Excludes1: *current obstetric trauma (O70.-, O71.4, O71.7-O71.8)*
old laceration involving muscles of pelvic floor (N81.8)

♀ **N89.9 Noninflammatory disorder of vagina, unspecified**

N90 Other noninflammatory disorders of vulva and perineum

Excludes1: *anogenital (venereal) warts (A63.0)*
carcinoma in situ of vulva (D07.1)
condyloma acuminatum (A63.0)
current obstetric trauma (O70.-, O71.7-O71.8)
inflammation of vulva (N76.-)
severe dysplasia of vulva (D07.1)
vulvar intraepithelial neoplasm III [VIN III] (D07.1)

♀ **N90.0 Mild vulvar dysplasia**
Vulvar intraepithelial neoplasia [VIN], grade I

♀ **N90.1 Moderate vulvar dysplasia**
Vulvar intraepithelial neoplasia [VIN], grade II

♀ **N90.3 Dysplasia of vulva, unspecified**

♀ **N90.4 Leukoplakia of vulva**
Dystrophy of vulva
Kraurosis of vulva
Lichen sclerosus of external female genital organs

♀ **N90.5 Atrophy of vulva**
Stenosis of vulva

+ N90.6 **Hypertrophy of vulva**
AHA CC: 4Q, 2016, 46
♀ N90.60 **Unspecified hypertrophy of vulva**
Unspecified hypertrophy of labia
♀ N90.61 **Childhood asymmetric labium majus enlargement**
CALME
♀ N90.69 **Other specified hypertrophy of vulva**
Other specified hypertrophy of labia
♀ N90.7 **Vulvar cyst**
+ N90.8 **Other specified noninflammatory disorders of vulva and perineum**
+ N90.81 **Female genital mutilation status**
Female genital cutting status
♀ N90.810 **Female genital mutilation status, unspecified**
Female genital cutting status, unspecified
Female genital mutilation status NOS
♀ N90.811 **Female genital mutilation Type I status**
Clitorectomy status
Female genital cutting Type I status
♀ N90.812 **Female genital mutilation Type II status**
Clitorectomy with excision of labia minora status
Female genital cutting Type II status
♀ N90.813 **Female genital mutilation Type III status**
Female genital cutting Type III status
Infibulation status
♀ N90.818 **Other female genital mutilation status**
Female genital cutting Type IV status
Female genital mutilation Type IV status
Other female genital cutting status
♀ N90.89 **Other specified noninflammatory disorders of vulva and perineum**
Adhesions of vulva
Hypertrophy of clitoris
♀ N90.9 **Noninflammatory disorder of vulva and perineum, unspecified**

N91 **Absent, scanty and rare menstruation**
Excludes1: *ovarian dysfunction (E28.-)*
♀ N91.0 **Primary amenorrhea**
♀ N91.1 **Secondary amenorrhea**
♀ N91.2 **Amenorrhea, unspecified**
♀ N91.3 **Primary oligomenorrhea**
♀ N91.4 **Secondary oligomenorrhea**
♀ N91.5 **Oligomenorrhea, unspecified**
Hypomenorrhea NOS

N92 **Excessive, frequent and irregular menstruation**
Excludes1: *postmenopausal bleeding (N95.0)*
precocious puberty (menstruation) (E30.1)
♀ N92.0 **Excessive and frequent menstruation with regular cycle**
Heavy periods NOS
Menorrhagia NOS
Polymenorrhea
♀ N92.1 **Excessive and frequent menstruation with irregular cycle**
Irregular intermenstrual bleeding
Irregular, shortened intervals between menstrual bleeding
Menometrorrhagia
Metrorrhagia
● ♀ N92.2 **Excessive menstruation at puberty**
Excessive bleeding associated with onset of menstrual periods
Pubertal menorrhagia
Puberty bleeding
♀ N92.3 **Ovulation bleeding**
Regular intermenstrual bleeding
♀ N92.4 **Excessive bleeding in the premenopausal period**
Climacteric menorrhagia or metrorrhagia
Menopausal menorrhagia or metrorrhagia
Perimenopausal bleeding
Perimenopausal menorrhagia or metrorrhagia
Preclimacteric menorrhagia or metrorrhagia
Premenopausal menorrhagia or metrorrhagia
♀ N92.5 **Other specified irregular menstruation**
♀ N92.6 **Irregular menstruation, unspecified**
Irregular bleeding NOS
Irregular periods NOS
Excludes1: *irregular menstruation with:*
lengthened intervals or scanty bleeding (N91.3-N91.5)
shortened intervals or excessive bleeding (N92.1)

N93 **Other abnormal uterine and vaginal bleeding**
Excludes1: *neonatal vaginal hemorrhage (P54.6)*
precocious puberty (menstruation) (E30.1)
pseudomenses (P54.6)
♀ N93.0 **Postcoital and contact bleeding**
♀ N93.1 **Pre-pubertal vaginal bleeding**
AHA CC: 4Q, 2016, 47
♀ N93.8 **Other specified abnormal uterine and vaginal bleeding**
Dysfunctional or functional uterine or vaginal bleeding NOS
♀ N93.9 **Abnormal uterine and vaginal bleeding,unspecified**

N94 **Pain and other conditions associated with female genital organs and menstrual cycle**
♀ N94.0 **Mittelschmerz**
+ N94.1 **Dyspareunia**
Excludes1: *psychogenic dyspareunia (F52.6)*
AHA CC: 4Q, 2016, 47
♀ N94.10 **Unspecified dyspareunia**
♀ N94.11 **Superficial (introital) dyspareunia**
♀ N94.12 **Deep dyspareunia**
♀ N94.19 **Other specified dyspareunia**
♀ N94.2 **Vaginismus**
Excludes1: *psychogenic vaginismus (F52.5)*
♀ N94.3 **Premenstrual tension syndrome**
Code also associated menstrual migraine (G43.82-, G43.83-)
Excludes1: *Premenstrual dysphoric disorder (F32.81)*
♀ N94.4 **Primary dysmenorrhea**
♀ N94.5 **Secondary dysmenorrhea**
♀ N94.6 **Dysmenorrhea, unspecified**
Excludes1: *psychogenic dysmenorrhea (F45.8)*
+ N94.8 **Other specified conditions associated with female genital organs and menstrual cycle**
+ N94.81 **Vulvodynia**
♀ N94.810 **Vulvar vestibulitis**
♀ N94.818 **Other vulvodynia**
♀ N94.819 **Vulvodynia, unspecified**
Vulvodynia NOS
♀ N94.89 **Other specified conditions associated with female genital organs and menstrual cycle**
♀ N94.9 **Unspecified condition associated with female genital organs and menstrual cycle**

N95 **Menopausal and other perimenopausal disorders**
Menopausal and other perimenopausal disorders due to naturally occurring (age-related) menopause and perimenopause
Excludes1: *excessive bleeding in the premenopausal period (N92.4)*
menopausal and perimenopausal disorders due to artificial or premature menopause (E89.4-, E28.31-)
premature menopause (E28.31-)
Excludes2: *postmenopausal osteoporosis (M81.0-)*
postmenopausal osteoporosis with current pathological fracture (M80.0-)
postmenopausal urethritis (N34.2)
♀ N95.0 **Postmenopausal bleeding**
♀ N95.1 **Menopausal and female climacteric states**
Symptoms such as flushing, sleeplessness, headache, lack of concentration, associated with natural (age-related) menopause
Use additional code for associated symptoms
Excludes1: *asymptomatic menopausal state (Z78.0)*
symptoms associated with artificial menopause (E89.41)
symptoms associated with premature menopause (E28.310)
♀ N95.2 **Postmenopausal atrophic vaginitis**
Senile (atrophic) vaginitis
♀ N95.8 **Other specified menopausal and perimenopausal disorders**
♀ N95.9 **Unspecified menopausal and perimenopausal disorder**

♀ **N96 Recurrent pregnancy loss**

Investigation or care in a nonpregnant woman with history of recurrent pregnancy loss

Excludes1: *recurrent pregancy loss with current pregnancy (O26.2-)*

Valid 3-character code, no further characters required

N97 Female infertility

Includes: inability to achieve a pregnancy
sterility, female NOS

Excludes2: *female infertility associated with:*
hypopituitarism (E23.0)
incompetence of cervix uteri (N88.3)
Stein-Leventhal syndrome (E28.2)

♀ **N97.0 Female infertility associated with anovulation**

♀ **N97.1 Female infertility of tubal origin**

Female infertility associated with congenital anomaly of tube
Female infertility due to tubal block
Female infertility due to tubal occlusion
Female infertility due to tubal stenosis

♀ **N97.2 Female infertility of uterine origin**

Female infertility associated with congenital anomaly of uterus
Female infertility due to nonimplantation of ovum

♀ **N97.8 Female infertility of other origin**

♀ **N97.9 Female infertility, unspecified**

N98 Complications associated with artificial fertilization

♀ CC **N98.0 Infection associated with artificial insemination**

♀ CC **N98.1 Hyperstimulation of ovaries**

Hyperstimulation of ovaries NOS
Hyperstimulation of ovaries associated with induced ovulation

♀ CC **N98.2 Complications of attempted introduction of fertilized ovum following in vitro fertilization**

♀ CC **N98.3 Complications of attempted introduction of embryo in embryo transfer**

♀ CC **N98.8 Other complications associated with artificial fertilization**

♀ **N98.9 Complication associated with artificial fertilization, unspecified**

Intraoperative and postprocedural complications and disorders of genitourinary system, not elsewhere classified (N99)

N99 Intraoperative and postprocedural complications and disorders of genitourinary system, not elsewhere classified

Excludes2: *irradiation cystitis (N30.4-)*
postoophorectomy osteoporosis with current pathological fracture (M80.8-)
postoophorectomy osteoporosis without current pathological fracture (M81.8)

N99.0 Postprocedural (acute) (chronic) kidney failure

Use additional code to type of kidney disease

\+ **N99.1 Postprocedural urethral stricture**

Postcatheterization urethral stricture

\+ **N99.11 Postprocedural urethral stricture, male**

♂ **N99.110 Postprocedural urethral stricture, male, meatal**

♂ **N99.111 Postprocedural bulbous urethral stricture, male**

♂ **N99.112 Postprocedural membranous urethral stricture, male**

♂ **N99.113 Postprocedural anterior bulbous urethral stricture, male**

AHA CC: 4Q, 2016, 47-48

♂ **N99.114 Postprocedural urethral stricture, male, unspecified**

♂ **N99.115 Postprocedural fossa navicularis urethral stricture**

AHA CC: 4Q, 2016, 47-48

♂ **N99.116 Postprocedural urethral stricture, male, overlapping sites**

AHA CC: 4Q, 2018, 21-22

♀ **N99.12 Postprocedural urethral stricture, female**

♀ **N99.2 Postprocedural adhesions of vagina**

♀ **N99.3 Prolapse of vaginal vault after hysterectomy**

N99.4 Postprocedural pelvic peritoneal adhesions

Excludes2: *pelvic peritoneal adhesions NOS (N73.6)*
postinfective pelvic peritoneal adhesions (N73.6)

\+ **N99.5 Complications of stoma of urinary tract**

Excludes2: *mechanical complication of urinary catheter (T83.0-)*

AHA CC: 4Q, 2016, 48

\+ **N99.51 Complication of cystostomy**

CC **N99.510 Cystostomy hemorrhage**

CC **N99.511 Cystostomy infection**

CC **N99.512 Cystostomy malfunction**

CC **N99.518 Other cystostomy complication**

\+ **N99.52 Complication of incontinent external stoma of urinary tract**

N99.520 Hemorrhage of incontinent external stoma of urinary tract

N99.521 Infection of incontinent external stoma of urinary tract

AHA CC: 4Q, 2016, 48

N99.522 Malfunction of incontinent external stoma of urinary tract

N99.523 Herniation of incontinent stoma of urinary tract

N99.524 Stenosis of incontinent stoma of urinary tract

N99.528 Other complication of incontinent external stoma of urinary tract

\+ **N99.53 Complication of continent stoma of urinary tract**

N99.530 Hemorrhage of continent stoma of urinary tract

N99.531 Infection of continent stoma of urinary tract

N99.532 Malfunction of continent stoma of urinary tract

N99.533 Herniation of continent stoma of urinary tract

N99.534 Stenosis of continent stoma of urinary tract

N99.538 Other complication of continent stoma of urinary tract

\+ **N99.6 Intraoperative hemorrhage and hematoma of a genitourinary system organ or structure complicating a procedure**

Excludes1: *intraoperative hemorrhage and hematoma of a genitourinary system organ or structure due to accidental puncture or laceration during a procedure (N99.7-)*

N99.61 Intraoperative hemorrhage and hematoma of a genitourinary system organ or structure complicating a genitourinary system procedure

CC **N99.62 Intraoperative hemorrhage and hematoma of a genitourinary system organ or structure complicating other procedure**

\+ **N99.7 Accidental puncture and laceration of a genitourinary system organ or structure during a procedure**

CC **N99.71 Accidental puncture and laceration of a genitourinary system organ or structure during a genitourinary system procedure**

CC **N99.72 Accidental puncture and laceration of a genitourinary system organ or structure during other procedure**

\+ **N99.8 Other intraoperative and postprocedural complications and disorders of genitourinary system**

AHA CC: 4Q, 2016, 9-10

N99.81 Other intraoperative complications of genitourinary system

\+ **N99.82 Postprocedural hemorrhage of a genitourinary system organ or structure following a procedure**

CC **N99.820 Postprocedural hemorrhage of a genitourinary system organ or structure following a genitourinary system procedure**

CC **N99.821 Postprocedural hemorrhage of a genitourinary system organ or structure following other procedure**

♀ **N99.83 Residual ovary syndrome**

\+ **N99.84 Postprocedural hematoma and seroma of a genitourinary system organ or structure following a procedure**

CC **N99.840 Postprocedural hematoma of a genitourinary system organ or structure following a genitourinary system procedure**

CC **N99.841 Postprocedural hematoma of a genitourinary system organ or structure following other procedure**

CC **N99.842 Postprocedural seroma of a genitourinary system organ or structure following a genitourinary system procedure**

CC **N99.843 Postprocedural seroma of a genitourinary system organ or structure following other procedure**

♀ **N99.85 Post endometrial ablation syndrome**

AHA CC: 4Q, 2019, 12

N99.89 Other postprocedural complications and disorders of genitourinary system

Chapter 15: Pregnancy, Childbirth and the Puerperium (O00-O9A)

NOTE Codes from this chapter are for use only on maternal records, never on newborn records
Codes from this chapter are for use for conditions related to or aggravated by the pregnancy, childbirth, or by the puerperium (maternal causes or obstetric causes)

NOTE Trimesters are counted from the first day of the last menstrual period. They are defined as follows:
1st trimester- less than 14 weeks 0 days
2nd trimester- 14 weeks 0 days to less than 28 weeks 0 days
3rd trimester- 28 weeks 0 days until delivery

Use additional code from category Z3A, Weeks of gestation, to identify the specific week of the pregnancy, if known

Excludes1: *supervision of normal pregnancy (Z34.-)*

Excludes2: *mental and behavioral disorders associated with the puerperium (F53.-)*
obstetrical tetanus (A34)
postpartum necrosis of pituitary gland (E23.0)
puerperal osteomalacia (M83.0)

This chapter contains the following category blocks:

O00-O08	Pregnancy with abortive outcome
O09	Supervision of high risk pregnancy
O10-O16	Edema, proteinuria and hypertensive disorders in pregnancy, childbirth and the puerperium
O20-O29	Other maternal disorders predominantly related to pregnancy
O30-O48	Maternal care related to the fetus and amniotic cavity and possible delivery problems
O60-O77	Complications of labor and delivery
O80-O82	Encounter for delivery
O85-O92	Complications predominantly related to the puerperium
O94-O9A	Other obstetric conditions, not elsewhere classified

C. Chapter-Specific Coding Guidelines

In addition to general coding guidelines, there are guidelines for specific diagnoses and/or conditions in the classification. Unless otherwise indicated, these guidelines apply to all health care settings. Please refer to Section II for guidelines on the selection of principal diagnosis.

15. Chapter 15: Pregnancy, Childbirth and the Puerperium (O00-O9A)

a. General Rules for Obstetric Cases

1) Codes from chapter 15 and sequencing priority

Obstetric cases require codes from chapter 15, codes in the range O00-O9A, Pregnancy, Childbirth, and the Puerperium. Chapter 15 codes have sequencing priority over codes from other chapters. Additional codes from other chapters may be used in conjunction with chapter 15 codes to further specify conditions. Should the provider document that the pregnancy is incidental to the encounter, then code Z33.1, Pregnant state, incidental, should be used in place of any chapter 15 codes. It is the provider's responsibility to state that the condition being treated is not affecting the pregnancy.

2) Chapter 15 codes used only on the maternal record

Chapter 15 codes are to be used only on the maternal record, never on the record of the newborn.

3) Final character for trimester

The majority of codes in Chapter 15 have a final character indicating the trimester of pregnancy. The timeframes for the trimesters are indicated at the beginning of the chapter. If trimester is not a component of a code it is because the condition always occurs in a specific trimester, or the concept of trimester of pregnancy is not applicable. Certain codes have characters for only certain trimesters because the condition does not occur in all trimesters, but it may occur in more than just one.

Assignment of the final character for trimester should be based on the provider's documentation of the trimester (or number of weeks) for the current admission/encounter. This applies to the assignment of trimester for pre-existing conditions as well as those that develop during or are due to the pregnancy. The provider's documentation of the number of weeks may be used to assign the appropriate code identifying the trimester.

Whenever delivery occurs during the current admission, and there is an "in childbirth" option for the obstetric complication being coded, the "in childbirth" code should be assigned. **When the classification does not provide an obstetric code with an "in childbirth" option, it is appropriate to assign a code describing the current trimester.**

4) Selection of trimester for inpatient admissions that encompass more than one trimester

In instances when a patient is admitted to a hospital for complications of pregnancy during one trimester and remains in the hospital into a subsequent trimester, the trimester character for the antepartum complication code should be assigned on the basis of the trimester when the complication developed, not the trimester of the discharge. If the condition developed prior to the current admission/encounter or represents a pre-existing condition, the trimester character for the trimester at the time of the admission/encounter should be assigned.

5) Unspecified trimester

Each category that includes codes for trimester has a code for "unspecified trimester." The "unspecified trimester" code should rarely be used, such as when the documentation in the record is insufficient to determine the trimester and it is not possible to obtain clarification.

6) 7th character for Fetus Identification

Where applicable, a 7th character is to be assigned for certain categories (O31, O32, O33.3 - O33.6, O35, O36, O40, O41, O60.1, O60.2, O64, and O69) to identify the fetus for which the complication code applies.

Assign 7th character "0":

- For single gestations
- When the documentation in the record is insufficient to determine the fetus affected and it is not possible to obtain clarification.
- When it is not possible to clinically determine which fetus is affected.

b. Selection of OB Principal or First-listed Diagnosis

1) Routine outpatient prenatal visits

For routine outpatient prenatal visits when no complications are present, a code from category Z34, Encounter for supervision of normal pregnancy, should be used as the first-listed diagnosis. These codes should not be used in conjunction with chapter 15 codes.

2) Supervision of High-Risk Pregnancy

Codes from category O09, Supervision of high-risk pregnancy, are intended for use only during the prenatal period. For complications during the labor or delivery episode as a result of a high-risk pregnancy, assign the applicable complication codes from Chapter 15. If there are no complications during the labor or delivery episode, assign code O80, Encounter for full-term uncomplicated delivery.

For routine prenatal outpatient visits for patients with high-risk pregnancies, a code from category O09, Supervision of high-risk pregnancy, should be used as the first-listed diagnosis. Secondary chapter 15 codes may be used in conjunction with these codes if appropriate.

3) Episodes when no delivery occurs

In episodes when no delivery occurs, the principal diagnosis should correspond to the principal complication of the pregnancy which necessitated the encounter. Should more than one complication exist, all of which are treated or monitored, any of the complications codes may be sequenced first.

4) When a delivery occurs

When an obstetric patient is admitted and delivers during that admission, the condition that prompted the admission should be sequenced as the principal diagnosis. If multiple conditions prompted the admission, sequence the one most related to the delivery as the principal diagnosis. A code for any complication of the delivery should be assigned as an additional diagnosis. In cases of cesarean delivery, if the patient was admitted with a condition that resulted in the performance of a cesarean procedure, that condition should be selected as the principal diagnosis. If the reason for the admission was unrelated to the condition resulting in the cesarean delivery, the condition related to the reason for the admission should be selected as the principal diagnosis.

5) Outcome of delivery

A code from category Z37, Outcome of delivery, should be included on every maternal record when a delivery has occurred. These codes are not to be used on subsequent records or on the newborn record.

c. Pre-existing conditions versus conditions due to the pregnancy

Certain categories in Chapter 15 distinguish between conditions of the mother that existed prior to pregnancy (pre-existing) and those that are a direct result of pregnancy. When assigning codes from Chapter 15, it is important to assess if a condition was pre-existing prior to pregnancy or developed during or due to the pregnancy in order to assign the correct code.

Categories that do not distinguish between pre-existing and pregnancy-related conditions may be used for either. It is acceptable to use codes specifically for the puerperium with codes complicating pregnancy and childbirth if a condition arises postpartum during the delivery encounter.

d. Pre-existing hypertension in pregnancy

Category O10, Pre-existing hypertension complicating pregnancy, childbirth and the puerperium, includes codes for hypertensive heart and hypertensive chronic kidney disease. When assigning one of the O10 codes that includes hypertensive heart disease or hypertensive chronic kidney disease, it is necessary to add a secondary code from the appropriate hypertension category to specify the type of heart failure or chronic kidney disease.

See Section I.C.9. Hypertension.

e. Fetal Conditions Affecting the Management of the Mother

1) Codes from categories O35 and O36

Codes from categories O35, Maternal care for known or suspected fetal abnormality and damage, and O36, Maternal care for other fetal problems, are assigned only when the fetal condition is actually responsible for modifying the management of the mother, i.e., by requiring diagnostic studies, additional observation, special care, or termination of pregnancy. The fact that the fetal condition exists does not justify assigning a code from this series to the mother's record.

2) In utero surgery

In cases when surgery is performed on the fetus, a diagnosis code from category O35, Maternal care for known or suspected fetal abnormality and damage, should be assigned identifying the fetal condition. Assign the appropriate procedure code for the procedure performed.

No code from Chapter 16, the perinatal codes, should be used on the mother's record to identify fetal conditions. Surgery performed in utero on a fetus is still to be coded as an obstetric encounter.

f. HIV Infection in Pregnancy, Childbirth and the Puerperium

During pregnancy, childbirth or the puerperium, a patient admitted because of an HIV-related illness should receive a principal diagnosis from subcategory O98.7-, Human immunodeficiency [HIV] disease complicating pregnancy, childbirth and the puerperium, followed by the code(s) for the HIV-related illness(es).

Patients with asymptomatic HIV infection status admitted during pregnancy, childbirth, or the puerperium should receive codes of O98.7- and Z21, Asymptomatic human immunodeficiency virus [HIV] infection status.

g. Diabetes mellitus in pregnancy

Diabetes mellitus is a significant complicating factor in pregnancy. Pregnant women who are diabetic should be assigned a code from category O24, Diabetes mellitus in pregnancy, childbirth, and the puerperium, first, followed by the appropriate diabetes code(s) (E08-E13) from Chapter 4.

h. Long term use of insulin and oral hypoglycemics

See section I.C.4.a.3 for information on the long term use of insulin and oral hypoglycemic.

i. Gestational (pregnancy induced) diabetes

Gestational (pregnancy induced) diabetes can occur during the second and third trimester of pregnancy in **patients** who were not diabetic prior to pregnancy. Gestational diabetes can cause complications in the pregnancy similar to those of pre-existing diabetes mellitus. It also puts the **patient** at greater risk of developing diabetes after the pregnancy. Codes for gestational diabetes are in subcategory O24.4, Gestational diabetes mellitus. No other code from category O24, Diabetes mellitus in pregnancy, childbirth, and the puerperium, should be used with a code from O24.4

The codes under subcategory O24.4 include diet controlled, insulin controlled, and controlled by oral hypoglycemic drugs. If a patient with gestational diabetes is treated with both diet and insulin, only the code for insulin-controlled is required. If a patient with gestational diabetes is treated with both diet and oral hypoglycemic medications, only the code for "controlled by oral hypoglycemic drugs" is required. Code Z79.4, Long-term (current) use of insulin or code Z79.84, Long-term (current) use of oral hypoglycemic drugs, should not be assigned with codes from subcategory O24.4.

An abnormal glucose tolerance in pregnancy is assigned a code from subcategory O99.81, Abnormal glucose complicating pregnancy, childbirth, and the puerperium.

j. Sepsis and septic shock complicating abortion, pregnancy, childbirth and the puerperium

When assigning a chapter 15 code for sepsis complicating abortion, pregnancy, childbirth, and the puerperium, a code for the specific type of infection should be assigned as an additional diagnosis. If severe sepsis is present, a code from subcategory R65.2, Severe sepsis, and code(s) for associated organ dysfunction(s) should also be assigned as additional diagnoses.

k. Puerperal sepsis

Code O85, Puerperal sepsis, should be assigned with a secondary code to identify the causal organism (e.g., for a bacterial infection, assign a code from category B95-B96, Bacterial infections in conditions classified elsewhere). A code from category A40, Streptococcal sepsis, or A41, Other sepsis, should not be used for puerperal sepsis. If applicable, use additional codes to identify severe sepsis (R65.2-) and any associated acute organ dysfunction.

Code O85 should not be assigned for sepsis following an obstetrical procedure (*See Section I.C.1.d.5b., Sepsis due to a postprocedural infection*).

l. Alcohol, tobacco and drug use during pregnancy, childbirth and the puerperium

1) Alcohol use during pregnancy, childbirth and the puerperium

Codes under subcategory O99.31, Alcohol use complicating pregnancy, childbirth, and the puerperium, should be assigned for any pregnancy case when a **patient** uses alcohol during the pregnancy or postpartum. A secondary code from category F10, Alcohol related disorders, should also be assigned to identify manifestations of the alcohol use.

2) Tobacco use during pregnancy, childbirth and the puerperium

Codes under subcategory O99.33, Smoking (tobacco) complicating pregnancy, childbirth, and the puerperium, should be assigned for any pregnancy case when a mother uses any type of tobacco product during the pregnancy or postpartum. A secondary code from category F17, Nicotine dependence, should also be assigned to identify the type of nicotine dependence.

3) Drug use during pregnancy, childbirth and the puerperium

Codes under subcategory O99.32, Drug use complicating pregnancy, childbirth, and the puerperium, should be assigned for any pregnancy case when a **patient** uses drugs during the pregnancy or postpartum. This can involve illegal drugs, or inappropriate use or abuse of prescription drugs. Secondary code(s) from categories F11-F16 and F18-F19 should also be assigned to identify manifestations of the drug use.

m. Poisoning, toxic effects, adverse effects and underdosing in a pregnant patient

A code from subcategory O9A.2, Injury, poisoning and certain other consequences of external causes complicating pregnancy, childbirth, and the puerperium, should be sequenced first, followed by the appropriate injury, poisoning, toxic effect, adverse effect or underdosing code, and then the additional code(s) that specifies the condition caused by the poisoning, toxic effect, adverse effect or underdosing.

See Section I.C.19. Adverse effects, poisoning, underdosing and toxic effects.

n. Normal Delivery, Code O80

1) Encounter for full term uncomplicated delivery

Code O80 should be assigned when a patient is admitted for a full-term normal delivery and delivers a single, healthy infant without any complications antepartum, during the delivery, or postpartum during the delivery episode. Code O80 is always a principal diagnosis. It is not to be used if any other code from chapter 15 is needed to describe a current complication of the antenatal, delivery, or postnatal period. Additional codes from other chapters may be used with code O80 if they are not related to or are in any way complicating the pregnancy.

2) Uncomplicated delivery with resolved antepartum complication

Code O80 may be used if the patient had a complication at some point during the pregnancy, but the complication is not present at the time of the admission for delivery.

3) Outcome of delivery for O80

Z37.0, Single live birth, is the only outcome of delivery code appropriate for use with O80.

o. The Peripartum and Postpartum Periods

1) Peripartum and Postpartum periods

The postpartum period begins immediately after delivery and continues for six weeks following delivery. The peripartum period is defined as the last month of pregnancy to five months postpartum.

2) Peripartum and postpartum complication

A postpartum complication is any complication occurring within the six-week period.

3) Pregnancy-related complications after 6 week period

Chapter 15 codes may also be used to describe pregnancy-related complications after the peripartum or postpartum period if the provider documents that a condition is pregnancy related.

4) Admission for routine postpartum care following delivery outside hospital

When the mother delivers outside the hospital prior to admission and is admitted for routine postpartum care and no complications are noted, code Z39.0, Encounter for care and examination of mother immediately after delivery, should be assigned as the principal diagnosis.

5) Pregnancy associated cardiomyopathy

Pregnancy associated cardiomyopathy, code O90.3, is unique in that it may be diagnosed in the third trimester of pregnancy but may continue to progress months after delivery. For this reason, it is referred to as peripartum cardiomyopathy. Code O90.3 is only for use when the cardiomyopathy develops as a result of pregnancy in a woman who did not have pre-existing heart disease.

p. Code O94, Sequelae of complication of pregnancy, childbirth, and the puerperium

1) Code O94

Code O94, Sequelae of complication of pregnancy, childbirth, and the puerperium, is for use in those cases when an initial complication of a pregnancy develops a sequelae requiring care or treatment at a future date.

2) After the initial postpartum period

This code may be used at any time after the initial postpartum period.

3) Sequencing of Code O94

This code, like all sequela codes, is to be sequenced following the code describing the sequelae of the complication.

q. Termination of Pregnancy and Spontaneous abortions

1) Abortion with Liveborn Fetus

When an attempted termination of pregnancy results in a liveborn fetus, assign code Z33.2, Encounter for elective termination of pregnancy and a code from category Z37, Outcome of Delivery.

2) Retained Products of Conception following an abortion

Subsequent encounters for retained products of conception following a spontaneous abortion or elective termination of pregnancy, without complications are assigned O03.4, Incomplete spontaneous, abortion without complication, or codes O07.4, Failed attempted termination of pregnancy without complication. This advice is appropriate even when the patient was discharged previously with a discharge diagnosis of complete abortion. If the patient has a specific complication associated with the spontaneous abortion or elective termination of pregnancy in addition to retained products of conception, assign the appropriate complication code (e.g., O03.-, O04.-, O07.-) instead of code O03.4 or O07.4.

3) Complications leading to abortion

Codes from Chapter 15 may be used as additional codes to identify any documented complications of the pregnancy in conjunction with codes in categories in O04, O07 and O08.

r. Abuse in a pregnant patient

For suspected or confirmed cases of abuse of a pregnant patient, a code(s) from subcategories O9A.3, Physical abuse complicating pregnancy, childbirth, and the puerperium, O9A.4, Sexual abuse complicating pregnancy, childbirth, and the puerperium, and O9A.5, Psychological abuse complicating pregnancy, childbirth, and the puerperium, should be sequenced first, followed by the appropriate codes (if applicable) to identify any associated current injury due to physical abuse, sexual abuse, and the perpetrator of abuse.

See Section I.C.19. Adult and child abuse, neglect and other maltreatment.

s. COVID-19 infection in pregnancy, childbirth, and the puerperium

During pregnancy, childbirth or the puerperium, when COVID-19 is the reason for admission/encounter, code O98.5-, Other viral diseases complicating pregnancy, childbirth and the puerperium, should be sequenced as the principal/first-listed diagnosis, and code U07.1, COVID-19, and the appropriate codes for associated manifestation(s) should be assigned as additional diagnoses. Codes from Chapter 15 always take sequencing priority.

If the reason for admission/encounter is unrelated to COVID-19 but the patient tests positive for COVID-19 during the admission/encounter, the appropriate code for the reason for admission/encounter should be sequenced as the principal/first-listed diagnosis, and code O98.5- and U07.1, as well as the appropriate codes for associated COVID-19 manifestations, should be assigned as additional diagnoses.

Pregnancy with abortive outcome (O00-O08)

Excludes1: *continuing pregnancy in multiple gestation after abortion of one fetus or more (O31.1-, O31.3-)*

O00 Ectopic pregnancy

Includes: ruptured ectopic pregnancy

Use additional code from category O08 to identify any associated complication

AHA CC: 4Q, 2016, 48-50

\+ **O00.0 Abdominal pregnancy**

Excludes1: *maternal care for viable fetus in abdominal pregnancy (O36.7-)*

• ♀ CC **O00.00 Abdominal pregnancy without intrauterine pregnancy**

Abdominal pregnancy NOS

• ♀ CC **O00.01 Abdominal pregnancy with intrauterine pregnancy**

\+ **O00.1 Tubal pregnancy**

Fallopian pregnancy

Rupture of (fallopian) tube due to pregnancy

Tubal abortion

AHA CC: 4Q, 2017, 20

\+ **O00.10 Tubal pregnancy without intrauterine pregnancy**

Tubal pregnancy NOS

• ♀ CC **O00.101 Right tubal pregnancy without intrauterine pregnancy**

• ♀ CC **O00.102 Left tubal pregnancy without intrauterine pregnancy**

• ♀ CC **O00.109 Unspecified tubal pregnancy without intrauterine pregnancy**

\+ **O00.11 Tubal pregnancy with intrauterine pregnancy**

• ♀ CC **O00.111 Right tubal pregnancy with intrauterine pregnancy**

• ♀ CC **O00.112 Left tubal pregnancy with intrauterine pregnancy**

• ♀ CC **O00.119 Unspecified tubal pregnancy with intrauterine pregnancy**

\+ **O00.2 Ovarian pregnancy**

AHA CC: 4Q, 2017, 20

\+ **O00.20 Ovarian pregnancy without intrauterine pregnancy**

Ovarian pregnancy NOS

• ♀ CC **O00.201 Right ovarian pregnancy without intrauterine pregnancy**

• ♀ CC **O00.202 Left ovarian pregnancy without intrauterine pregnancy**

• ♀ CC **O00.209 Unspecified ovarian pregnancy without intrauterine pregnancy**

\+ **O00.21 Ovarian pregnancy with intrauterine pregnancy**

• ♀ CC **O00.211 Right ovarian pregnancy with intrauterine pregnancy**

• ♀ CC **O00.212 Left ovarian pregnancy with intrauterine pregnancy**

• ♀ CC **O00.219 Unspecified ovarian pregnancy with intrauterine pregnancy**

\+ **O00.8 Other ectopic pregnancy**

Cervical pregnancy

Cornual pregnancy

Intraligamentous pregnancy

Mural pregnancy

• ♀ CC **O00.80 Other ectopic pregnancy without intrauterine pregnancy**

Other ectopic pregnancy NOS

• ♀ CC **O00.81 Other ectopic pregnancy with intrauterine pregnancy**

\+ **O00.9 Ectopic pregnancy, unspecified**

• ♀ CC **O00.90 Unspecified ectopic pregnancy without intrauterine pregnancy**

Ectopic pregnancy NOS

• ♀ CC **O00.91 Unspecified ectopic pregnancy with intrauterine pregnancy**

O01 Hydatidiform mole

Use additional code from category O08 to identify any associated complication

Excludes1: *chorioadenoma (destruens) (D39.2)*
malignant hydatidiform mole (D39.2)

• ♀ **O01.0 Classical hydatidiform mole**

Complete hydatidiform mole

• ♀ **O01.1 Incomplete and partial hydatidiform mole**

• ♀ **O01.9 Hydatidiform mole, unspecified**

Trophoblastic disease NOS

Vesicular mole NOS

O02 Other abnormal products of conception

Use additional code from category O08 to identify any associated complication

Excludes1: *papyraceous fetus (O31.0-)*

• ♀ **O02.0 Blighted ovum and nonhydatidiform mole**

Carneous mole

Fleshy mole

Intrauterine mole NOS

Molar pregnancy NEC

Pathological ovum

Ectopic Pregnancy I - Tubal Pregnancy

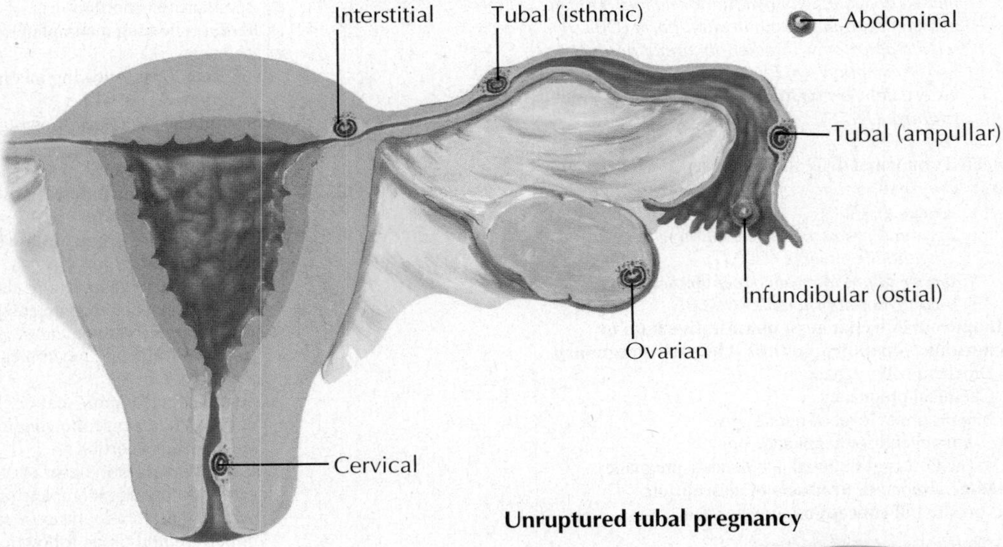

Unruptured tubal pregnancy

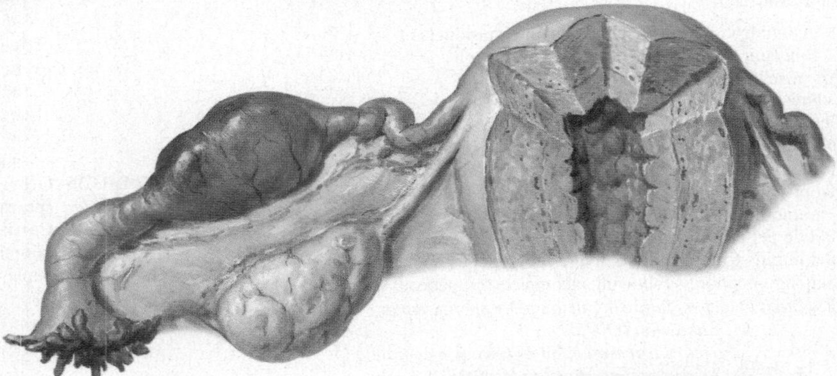

Section through tubal pregnancy

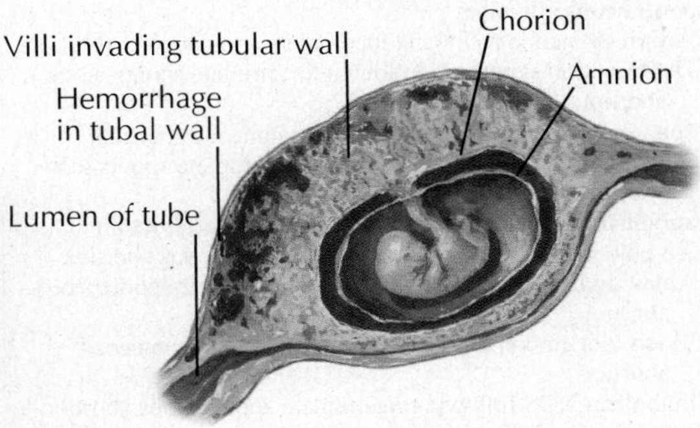

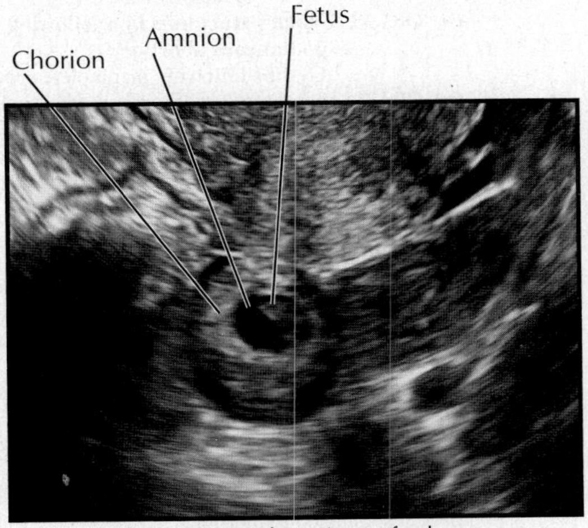

Ultrasonographic view of adnexa

● ♀ **O02.1 Missed abortion**
Early fetal death, before completion of 20 weeks of gestation, with retention of dead fetus
Excludes1: *failed induced abortion (O07.-)*
fetal death (intrauterine) (late) (O36.4)
missed abortion with blighted ovum (O02.0)
missed abortion with hydatidiform mole (O01.-)
missed abortion with nonhydatidiform (O02.0)
missed abortion with other abnormal products of conception (O02.8-)
missed delivery (O36.4)
stillbirth (P95)
AHA CC: 3Q, 2019, 11-12

\+ **O02.8 Other specified abnormal products of conception**
Excludes1: *abnormal products of conception with blighted ovum (O02.0)*
abnormal products of conception with hydatidiform mole (O01.-)
abnormal products of conception with nonhydatidiform mole (O02.0)

● ♀ **O02.81 Inappropriate change in quantitative human chorionic gonadotropin (hCG) in early pregnancy**
Biochemical pregnancy
Chemical pregnancy
Inappropriate level of quantitative human chorionic gonadotropin (hCG) for gestational age in early pregnancy

● ♀ **O02.89 Other abnormal products of conception**

● ♀ **O02.9 Abnormal product of conception, unspecified**

O03 Spontaneous abortion
NOTE Incomplete abortion includes retained products of conception following spontaneous abortion
Includes: miscarriage
Review coding guideline C.15.q.2

● ♀ CC **O03.0 Genital tract and pelvic infection following incomplete spontaneous abortion**
Endometritis following incomplete spontaneous abortion
Oophoritis following incomplete spontaneous abortion
Parametritis following incomplete spontaneous abortion
Pelvic peritonitis following incomplete spontaneous abortion
Salpingitis following incomplete spontaneous abortion
Salpingo-oophoritis following incomplete spontaneous abortion
Excludes1: *sepsis following incomplete spontaneous abortion (O03.37)*
urinary tract infection following incomplete spontaneous abortion (O03.38)

● ♀ **O03.1 Delayed or excessive hemorrhage following incomplete spontaneous abortion**
Afibrinogenemia following incomplete spontaneous abortion
Defibrination syndrome following incomplete spontaneous abortion
Hemolysis following incomplete spontaneous abortion
Intravascular coagulation following incomplete spontaneous abortion

● ♀ MCC **O03.2 Embolism following incomplete spontaneous abortion**
Air embolism following incomplete spontaneous abortion
Amniotic fluid embolism following incomplete spontaneous abortion
Blood-clot embolism following incomplete spontaneous abortion
Embolism NOS following incomplete spontaneous abortion
Fat embolism following incomplete spontaneous abortion
Pulmonary embolism following incomplete spontaneous abortion
Pyemic embolism following incomplete spontaneous abortion
Septic or septicopyemic embolism following incomplete spontaneous abortion
Soap embolism following incomplete spontaneous abortion
Review coding guideline C.15.j

\+ **O03.3 Other and unspecified complications following incomplete spontaneous abortion**

● ♀ CC **O03.30 Unspecified complication following incomplete spontaneous abortion**

● ♀ MCC **O03.31 Shock following incomplete spontaneous abortion**
Circulatory collapse following incomplete spontaneous abortion
Shock (postprocedural) following incomplete spontaneous abortion
Excludes1: *shock due to infection following incomplete spontaneous abortion (O03.37)*

● ♀ MCC **O03.32 Renal failure following incomplete spontaneous abortion**
Kidney failure (acute) following incomplete spontaneous abortion
Oliguria following incomplete spontaneous abortion
Renal shutdown following incomplete spontaneous abortion
Renal tubular necrosis following incomplete spontaneous abortion
Uremia following incomplete spontaneous abortion

● ♀ CC **O03.33 Metabolic disorder following incomplete spontaneous abortion**

● ♀ CC **O03.34 Damage to pelvic organs following incomplete spontaneous abortion**
Laceration, perforation, tear or chemical damage of bladder following incomplete spontaneous abortion
Laceration, perforation, tear or chemical damage of bowel following incomplete spontaneous abortion
Laceration, perforation, tear or chemical damage of broad ligament following incomplete spontaneous abortion
Laceration, perforation, tear or chemical damage of cervix following incomplete spontaneous abortion
Laceration, perforation, tear or chemical damage of periurethral tissue following incomplete spontaneous abortion
Laceration, perforation, tear or chemical damage of uterus following incomplete spontaneous abortion
Laceration, perforation, tear or chemical damage of vagina following incomplete spontaneous abortion

● ♀ CC **O03.35 Other venous complications following incomplete spontaneous abortion**

● ♀ CC **O03.36 Cardiac arrest following incomplete spontaneous abortion**

● ♀ CC **O03.37 Sepsis following incomplete spontaneous abortion**
Use additional code to identify infectious agent (B95-B97)
Use additional code to identify severe sepsis, if applicable (R65.2-)
Excludes1: *septic or septicopyemic embolism following incomplete spontaneous abortion (O03.2)*
Review coding guideline C.15.j

● ♀ CC **O03.38 Urinary tract infection following incomplete spontaneous abortion**
Cystitis following incomplete spontaneous abortion

● ♀ CC **O03.39 Incomplete spontaneous abortion with other complications**

● ♀ **O03.4 Incomplete spontaneous abortion without complication**

● ♀ CC **O03.5 Genital tract and pelvic infection following complete or unspecified spontaneous abortion**
Endometritis following complete or unspecified spontaneous abortion
Oophoritis following complete or unspecified spontaneous abortion
Parametritis following complete or unspecified spontaneous abortion
Pelvic peritonitis following complete or unspecified spontaneous abortion
Salpingitis following complete or unspecified spontaneous abortion
Salpingo-oophoritis following complete or unspecified spontaneous abortion
Excludes1: *sepsis following complete or unspecified spontaneous abortion (O03.87)*
urinary tract infection following complete or unspecified spontaneous abortion (O03.88)

• ♀ **O03.6 Delayed or excessive hemorrhage following complete or unspecified spontaneous abortion**
Afibrinogenemia following complete or unspecified spontaneous abortion
Defibrination syndrome following complete or unspecified spontaneous abortion
Hemolysis following complete or unspecified spontaneous abortion
Intravascular coagulation following complete or unspecified spontaneous abortion

• ♀ CC **O03.7 Embolism following complete or unspecified spontaneous abortion**
Air embolism following complete or unspecified spontaneous abortion
Amniotic fluid embolism following complete or unspecified spontaneous abortion
Blood-clot embolism following complete or unspecified spontaneous abortion
Embolism NOS following complete or unspecified spontaneous abortion
Fat embolism following complete or unspecified spontaneous abortion
Pulmonary embolism following complete or unspecified spontaneous abortion
Pyemic embolism following complete or unspecified spontaneous abortion
Septic or septicopyemic embolism following complete or unspecified spontaneous abortion
Soap embolism following complete or unspecified spontaneous abortion

+ **O03.8 Other and unspecified complications following complete or unspecified spontaneous abortion**

• ♀ CC **O03.80 Unspecified complication following complete or unspecified spontaneous abortion**

• ♀ MCC **O03.81 Shock following complete or unspecified spontaneous abortion**
Circulatory collapse following complete or unspecified spontaneous abortion
Shock (postprocedural) following complete or unspecified spontaneous abortion
Excludes1: *shock due to infection following complete or unspecified spontaneous abortion (O03.87)*

• ♀ MCC **O03.82 Renal failure following complete or unspecified spontaneous abortion**
Kidney failure (acute) following complete or unspecified spontaneous abortion
Oliguria following complete or unspecified spontaneous abortion
Renal shutdown following complete or unspecified spontaneous abortion
Renal tubular necrosis following complete or unspecified spontaneous abortion
Uremia following complete or unspecified spontaneous abortion

• ♀ CC **O03.83 Metabolic disorder following complete or unspecified spontaneous abortion**

• ♀ CC **O03.84 Damage to pelvic organs following complete or unspecified spontaneous abortion**
Laceration, perforation, tear or chemical damage of bladder following complete or unspecified spontaneous abortion
Laceration, perforation, tear or chemical damage of bowel following complete or unspecified spontaneous abortion
Laceration, perforation, tear or chemical damage of broad ligament following complete or unspecified spontaneous abortion
Laceration, perforation, tear or chemical damage of cervix following complete or unspecified spontaneous abortion
Laceration, perforation, tear or chemical damage of periurethral tissue following complete or unspecified spontaneous abortion
Laceration, perforation, tear or chemical damage of uterus following complete or unspecified spontaneous abortion
Laceration, perforation, tear or chemical damage of vagina following complete or unspecified spontaneous abortion

• ♀ CC **O03.85 Other venous complications following complete or unspecified spontaneous abortion**

• ♀ CC **O03.86 Cardiac arrest following complete or unspecified spontaneous abortion**

• ♀ CC **O03.87 Sepsis following complete or unspecified spontaneous abortion**
Use additional code to identify infectious agent (B95-B97)
Use additional code to identify severe sepsis, if applicable (R65.2-)
Excludes1: *septic or septicopyemic embolism following complete or unspecified spontaneous abortion (O03.7)*
Review coding guideline C.15.j

• ♀ CC **O03.88 Urinary tract infection following complete or unspecified spontaneous abortion**
Cystitis following complete or unspecified spontaneous abortion

• ♀ CC **O03.89 Complete or unspecified spontaneous abortion with other complications**

• ♀ **O03.9 Complete or unspecified spontaneous abortion without complication**
Miscarriage NOS
Spontaneous abortion NOS

O04 Complications following (induced) termination of pregnancy
Includes: complications following (induced) termination of pregnancy
Excludes1: *encounter for elective termination of pregnancy, uncomplicated (Z33.2)*
failed attempted termination of pregnancy (O07.-)

• ♀ CC **O04.5 Genital tract and pelvic infection following (induced) termination of pregnancy**
Endometritis following (induced) termination of pregnancy
Oophoritis following (induced) termination of pregnancy
Parametritis following (induced) termination of pregnancy
Pelvic peritonitis following (induced) termination of pregnancy
Salpingitis following (induced) termination of pregnancy
Salpingo-oophoritis following (induced) termination of pregnancy
Excludes1: *sepsis following (induced) termination of pregnancy (O04.87)*
urinary tract infection following (induced) termination of pregnancy (O04.88)

• ♀ **O04.6 Delayed or excessive hemorrhage following (induced) termination of pregnancy**
Afibrinogenemia following (induced) termination of pregnancy
Defibrination syndrome following (induced) termination of pregnancy
Hemolysis following (induced) termination of pregnancy
Intravascular coagulation following (induced) termination of pregnancy
AHA CC: 3Q, 2019, 11-12

• ♀ MCC **O04.7 Embolism following (induced) termination of pregnancy**
Air embolism following (induced) termination of pregnancy
Amniotic fluid embolism following (induced) termination of pregnancy
Blood-clot embolism following (induced) termination of pregnancy
Embolism NOS following (induced) termination of pregnancy
Fat embolism following (induced) termination of pregnancy
Pulmonary embolism following (induced) termination of pregnancy
Pyemic embolism following (induced) termination of pregnancy
Septic or septicopyemic embolism following (induced) termination of pregnancy
Soap embolism following (induced) termination of pregnancy

+ **O04.8 (Induced) termination of pregnancy with other and unspecified complications**

• ♀ CC **O04.80 (Induced) termination of pregnancy with unspecified complications**

• ♀ MCC **O04.81 Shock following (induced) termination of pregnancy**
Circulatory collapse following (induced) termination of pregnancy
Shock (postprocedural) following (induced) termination of pregnancy
Excludes1: *shock due to infection following (induced) termination of pregnancy (O04.87)*

● ♀ MCC **O04.82 Renal failure following (induced) termination of pregnancy**
Kidney failure (acute) following (induced) termination of pregnancy
Oliguria following (induced) termination of pregnancy
Renal shutdown following (induced) termination of pregnancy
Renal tubular necrosis following (induced) termination of pregnancy
Uremia following (induced) termination of pregnancy

● ♀ CC **O04.83 Metabolic disorder following (induced) termination of pregnancy**

● ♀ CC **O04.84 Damage to pelvic organs following (induced) termination of pregnancy**
Laceration, perforation, tear or chemical damage of bladder following (induced) termination of pregnancy
Laceration, perforation, tear or chemical damage of bowel following (induced) termination of pregnancy
Laceration, perforation, tear or chemical damage of broad ligament following (induced) termination of pregnancy
Laceration, perforation, tear or chemical damage of cervix following (induced) termination of pregnancy
Laceration, perforation, tear or chemical damage of periurethral tissue following (induced) termination of pregnancy
Laceration, perforation, tear or chemical damage of uterus following (induced) termination of pregnancy
Laceration, perforation, tear or chemical damage of vagina following (induced) termination of pregnancy

● ♀ CC **O04.85 Other venous complications following (induced) termination of pregnancy**

● ♀ CC **O04.86 Cardiac arrest following (induced) termination of pregnancy**

● ♀ CC **O04.87 Sepsis following (induced) termination of pregnancy**
Use additional code to identify infectious agent (B95-B97)
Use additional code to identify severe sepsis, if applicable (R65.2-)
Excludes1: *septic or septicopyemic embolism following (induced) termination of pregnancy (O04.7)*
Review coding guideline C.15.j

● ♀ CC **O04.88 Urinary tract infection following (induced) termination of pregnancy**
Cystitis following (induced) termination of pregnancy

● ♀ CC **O04.89 (Induced) termination of pregnancy with other complications**

O07 Failed attempted termination of pregnancy
Includes: failure of attempted induction of termination of pregnancy
incomplete elective abortion
Excludes1: *incomplete spontaneous abortion (O03.0-)*

● ♀ CC **O07.0 Genital tract and pelvic infection following failed attempted termination of pregnancy**
Endometritis following failed attempted termination of pregnancy
Oophoritis following failed attempted termination of pregnancy
Parametritis following failed attempted termination of pregnancy
Pelvic peritonitis following failed attempted termination of pregnancy
Salpingitis following failed attempted termination of pregnancy
Salpingo-oophoritis following failed attempted termination of pregnancy
Excludes1: *sepsis following failed attempted termination of pregnancy (O07.37)*
urinary tract infection following failed attempted termination of pregnancy (O07.38)

● ♀ CC **O07.1 Delayed or excessive hemorrhage following failed attempted termination of pregnancy**
Afibrinogenemia following failed attempted termination of pregnancy
Defibrination syndrome following failed attempted termination of pregnancy
Hemolysis following failed attempted termination of pregnancy
Intravascular coagulation following failed attempted termination of pregnancy

● ♀ MCC **O07.2 Embolism following failed attempted termination of pregnancy**
Air embolism following failed attempted termination of pregnancy
Amniotic fluid embolism following failed attempted termination of pregnancy
Blood-clot embolism following failed attempted termination of pregnancy
Embolism NOS following failed attempted termination of pregnancy
Fat embolism following failed attempted termination of pregnancy
Pulmonary embolism following failed attempted termination of pregnancy
Pyemic embolism following failed attempted termination of pregnancy
Septic or septicopyemic embolism following failed attempted termination of pregnancy
Soap embolism following failed attempted termination of pregnancy

\+ **O07.3 Failed attempted termination of pregnancy with other and unspecified complications**

● ♀ CC **O07.30 Failed attempted termination of pregnancy with unspecified complications**

● ♀ MCC **O07.31 Shock following failed attempted termination of pregnancy**
Circulatory collapse following failed attempted termination of pregnancy
Shock (postprocedural) following failed attempted termination of pregnancy
Excludes1: *shock due to infection following failed attempted termination of pregnancy (O07.37)*

● ♀ MCC **O07.32 Renal failure following failed attempted termination of pregnancy**
Kidney failure (acute) following failed attempted termination of pregnancy
Oliguria following failed attempted termination of pregnancy
Renal shutdown following failed attempted termination of pregnancy
Renal tubular necrosis following failed attempted termination of pregnancy
Uremia following failed attempted termination of pregnancy

● ♀ CC **O07.33 Metabolic disorder following failed attempted termination of pregnancy**

● ♀ CC **O07.34 Damage to pelvic organs following failed attempted termination of pregnancy**
Laceration, perforation, tear or chemical damage of bladder following failed attempted termination of pregnancy
Laceration, perforation, tear or chemical damage of bowel following failed attempted termination of pregnancy
Laceration, perforation, tear or chemical damage of broad ligament following failed attempted termination of pregnancy
Laceration, perforation, tear or chemical damage of cervix following failed attempted termination of pregnancy
Laceration, perforation, tear or chemical damage of periurethral tissue following failed attempted termination of pregnancy
Laceration, perforation, tear or chemical damage of uterus following failed attempted termination of pregnancy
Laceration, perforation, tear or chemical damage of vagina following failed attempted termination of pregnancy

• ♀ CC **O07.35 Other venous complications following failed attempted termination of pregnancy**

• ♀ CC **O07.36 Cardiac arrest following failed attempted termination of pregnancy**

• ♀ CC **O07.37 Sepsis following failed attempted termination of pregnancy**

Use additional code (B95-B97), to identify infectious agent

Use additional code (R65.2-) to identify severe sepsis, if applicable

Excludes1: *septic or septicopyemic embolism following failed attempted termination of pregnancy (O07.2)*

Review coding guideline C.15.j

• ♀ CC **O07.38 Urinary tract infection following failed attempted termination of pregnancy**

Cystitis following failed attempted termination of pregnancy

• ♀ CC **O07.39 Failed attempted termination of pregnancy with other complications**

• ♀ CC **O07.4 Failed attempted termination of pregnancy without complication**

Review coding guideline C.15.q.2

O08 Complications following ectopic and molar pregnancy

This category is for use with categories O00-O02 to identify any associated complications

• ♀ CC **O08.0 Genital tract and pelvic infection following ectopic and molar pregnancy**

Endometritis following ectopic and molar pregnancy
Oophoritis following ectopic and molar pregnancy
Parametritis following ectopic and molar pregnancy
Pelvic peritonitis following ectopic and molar pregnancy
Salpingitis following ectopic and molar pregnancy
Salpingo-oophoritis following ectopic and molar pregnancy

Excludes1: *sepsis following ectopic and molar pregnancy (O08.82)*
urinary tract infection (O08.83)

• ♀ CC **O08.1 Delayed or excessive hemorrhage following ectopic and molar pregnancy**

Afibrinogenemia following ectopic and molar pregnancy
Defibrination syndrome following ectopic and molar pregnancy
Hemolysis following ectopic and molar pregnancy
Intravascular coagulation following ectopic and molar pregnancy

Excludes1: *delayed or excessive hemorrhage due to incomplete abortion (O03.1)*

• ♀ MCC **O08.2 Embolism following ectopic and molar pregnancy**

Air embolism following ectopic and molar pregnancy
Amniotic fluid embolism following ectopic and molar pregnancy
Blood-clot embolism following ectopic and molar pregnancy
Embolism NOS following ectopic and molar pregnancy
Fat embolism following ectopic and molar pregnancy
Pulmonary embolism following ectopic and molar pregnancy
Pyemic embolism following ectopic and molar pregnancy
Septic or septicopyemic embolism following ectopic and molar pregnancy
Soap embolism following ectopic and molar pregnancy

• ♀ MCC **O08.3 Shock following ectopic and molar pregnancy**

Circulatory collapse following ectopic and molar pregnancy
Shock (postprocedural) following ectopic and molar pregnancy

Excludes1: *shock due to infection following ectopic and molar pregnancy (O08.82)*

• ♀ MCC **O08.4 Renal failure following ectopic and molar pregnancy**

Kidney failure (acute) following ectopic and molar pregnancy
Oliguria following ectopic and molar pregnancy
Renal shutdown following ectopic and molar pregnancy
Renal tubular necrosis following ectopic and molar pregnancy
Uremia following ectopic and molar pregnancy

• ♀ CC **O08.5 Metabolic disorders following an ectopic and molar pregnancy**

• ♀ CC **O08.6 Damage to pelvic organs and tissues following an ectopic and molar pregnancy**

Laceration, perforation, tear or chemical damage of bladder following an ectopic and molar pregnancy
Laceration, perforation, tear or chemical damage of bowel following an ectopic and molar pregnancy
Laceration, perforation, tear or chemical damage of broad ligament following an ectopic and molar pregnancy
Laceration, perforation, tear or chemical damage of cervix following an ectopic and molar pregnancy
Laceration, perforation, tear or chemical damage of periurethral tissue following an ectopic and molar pregnancy
Laceration, perforation, tear or chemical damage of uterus following an ectopic and molar pregnancy
Laceration, perforation, tear or chemical damage of vagina following an ectopic and molar pregnancy

• ♀ CC **O08.7 Other venous complications following an ectopic and molar pregnancy**

\+ **O08.8 Other complications following an ectopic and molar pregnancy**

• ♀ CC **O08.81 Cardiac arrest following an ectopic and molar pregnancy**

• ♀ CC **O08.82 Sepsis following ectopic and molar pregnancy**

Use additional code (B95-B97), to identify infectious agent

Use additional code (R65.2-) to identify severe sepsis, if applicable

Excludes1: *septic or septicopyemic embolism following ectopic and molar pregnancy (O08.2)*

Review coding guideline C.15.j

• ♀ CC **O08.83 Urinary tract infection following an ectopic and molar pregnancy**

Cystitis following an ectopic and molar pregnancy

• ♀ CC **O08.89 Other complications following an ectopic and molar pregnancy**

• ♀ CC **O08.9 Unspecified complication following an ectopic and molar pregnancy**

Supervision of high risk pregnancy (O09)

O09 Supervision of high risk pregnancy

Review coding guideline C.15.b.2
AHA CC: 4Q, 2016, 48-50

\+ **O09.0 Supervision of pregnancy with history of infertility**

• ♀ **O09.00 Supervision of pregnancy with history of infertility, unspecified trimester**

• ♀ **O09.01 Supervision of pregnancy with history of infertility, first trimester**

• ♀ **O09.02 Supervision of pregnancy with history of infertility, second trimester**

• ♀ **O09.03 Supervision of pregnancy with history of infertility, third trimester**

\+ **O09.1 Supervision of pregnancy with history of ectopic pregnancy**

• ♀ **O09.10 Supervision of pregnancy with history of ectopic pregnancy, unspecified trimester**

• ♀ **O09.11 Supervision of pregnancy with history of ectopic pregnancy, first trimester**

• ♀ **O09.12 Supervision of pregnancy with history of ectopic pregnancy, second trimester**

• ♀ **O09.13 Supervision of pregnancy with history of ectopic pregnancy, third trimester**

\+ **O09.A Supervision of pregnancy with history of molar pregnancy**

• ♀ **O09.A0 Supervision of pregnancy with history of molar pregnancy, unspecified trimester**

• ♀ **O09.A1 Supervision of pregnancy with history of molar pregnancy, first trimester**

• ♀ **O09.A2 Supervision of pregnancy with history of molar pregnancy, second trimester**

• ♀ **O09.A3 Supervision of pregnancy with history of molar pregnancy, third trimester**

+ **O09.2 Supervision of pregnancy with other poor reproductive or obstetric history**
  Excludes2: *pregnancy care for patient with history of recurrent pregnancy loss (O26.2-)*
  + **O09.21 Supervision of pregnancy with history of pre-term labor**
    • ♀ **O09.211 Supervision of pregnancy with history of pre-term labor, first trimester**
    • ♀ **O09.212 Supervision of pregnancy with history of pre-term labor, second trimester**
    • ♀ **O09.213 Supervision of pregnancy with history of pre-term labor, third trimester**
    • ♀ **O09.219 Supervision of pregnancy with history of pre-term labor, unspecified trimester**
  + **O09.29 Supervision of pregnancy with other poor reproductive or obstetric history**
    Supervision of pregnancy with history of neonatal death
    Supervision of pregnancy with history of stillbirth
    • ♀ **O09.291 Supervision of pregnancy with other poor reproductive or obstetric history, first trimester**
    • ♀ **O09.292 Supervision of pregnancy with other poor reproductive or obstetric history, second trimester**
    • ♀ **O09.293 Supervision of pregnancy with other poor reproductive or obstetric history, third trimester**
    • ♀ **O09.299 Supervision of pregnancy with other poor reproductive or obstetric history, unspecified trimester**

+ **O09.3 Supervision of pregnancy with insufficient antenatal care**
  Supervision of concealed pregnancy
  Supervision of hidden pregnancy
  • ♀ **O09.30 Supervision of pregnancy with insufficient antenatal care, unspecified trimester**
  • ♀ **O09.31 Supervision of pregnancy with insufficient antenatal care, first trimester**
  • ♀ **O09.32 Supervision of pregnancy with insufficient antenatal care, second trimester**
  • ♀ **O09.33 Supervision of pregnancy with insufficient antenatal care, third trimester**

+ **O09.4 Supervision of pregnancy with grand multiparity**
  • ♀ **O09.40 Supervision of pregnancy with grand multiparity, unspecified trimester**
  • ♀ **O09.41 Supervision of pregnancy with grand multiparity, first trimester**
  • ♀ **O09.42 Supervision of pregnancy with grand multiparity, second trimester**
  • ♀ **O09.43 Supervision of pregnancy with grand multiparity, third trimester**

+ **O09.5 Supervision of elderly primigravida and multigravida**
  Pregnancy for a female 35 years and older at expected date of delivery
  + **O09.51 Supervision of elderly primigravida**
    • ♀ **O09.511 Supervision of elderly primigravida, first trimester**
    • ♀ **O09.512 Supervision of elderly primigravida, second trimester**
    • ♀ **O09.513 Supervision of elderly primigravida, third trimester**
    • ♀ **O09.519 Supervision of elderly primigravida, unspecified trimester**
  + **O09.52 Supervision of elderly multigravida**
    • ♀ **O09.521 Supervision of elderly multigravida, first trimester**
    • ♀ **O09.522 Supervision of elderly multigravida, second trimester**
    • ♀ **O09.523 Supervision of elderly multigravida, third trimester**
    • ♀ **O09.529 Supervision of elderly multigravida, unspecified trimester**

+ **O09.6 Supervision of young primigravida and multigravida**
  Supervision of pregnancy for a female less than 16 years old at expected date of delivery
  + **O09.61 Supervision of young primigravida**
    • ♀ **O09.611 Supervision of young primigravida, first trimester**
    • ♀ **O09.612 Supervision of young primigravida, second trimester**
    • ♀ **O09.613 Supervision of young primigravida, third trimester**
    • ♀ **O09.619 Supervision of young primigravida, unspecified trimester**
  + **O09.62 Supervision of young multigravida**
    • ♀ **O09.621 Supervision of young multigravida, first trimester**
    • ♀ **O09.622 Supervision of young multigravida, second trimester**
    • ♀ **O09.623 Supervision of young multigravida, third trimester**
    • ♀ **O09.629 Supervision of young multigravida, unspecified trimester**

+ **O09.7 Supervision of high risk pregnancy due to social problems**
  • ♀ **O09.70 Supervision of high risk pregnancy due to social problems, unspecified trimester**
  • ♀ **O09.71 Supervision of high risk pregnancy due to social problems, first trimester**
  • ♀ **O09.72 Supervision of high risk pregnancy due to social problems, second trimester**
  • ♀ **O09.73 Supervision of high risk pregnancy due to social problems, third trimester**

+ **O09.8 Supervision of other high risk pregnancies**
  + **O09.81 Supervision of pregnancy resulting from assisted reproductive technology**
    Supervision of pregnancy resulting from in-vitro fertilization
    Excludes2: *gestational carrier status (Z33.3)*
    • ♀ **O09.811 Supervision of pregnancy resulting from assisted reproductive technology, first trimester**
    • ♀ **O09.812 Supervision of pregnancy resulting from assisted reproductive technology, second trimester**
    • ♀ **O09.813 Supervision of pregnancy resulting from assisted reproductive technology, third trimester**
    • ♀ **O09.819 Supervision of pregnancy resulting from assisted reproductive technology, unspecified trimester**
  + **O09.82 Supervision of pregnancy with history of in utero procedure during previous pregnancy**
    • ♀ **O09.821 Supervision of pregnancy with history of in utero procedure during previous pregnancy, first trimester**
    • ♀ **O09.822 Supervision of pregnancy with history of in utero procedure during previous pregnancy, second trimester**
    • ♀ **O09.823 Supervision of pregnancy with history of in utero procedure during previous pregnancy, third trimester**
    • ♀ **O09.829 Supervision of pregnancy with history of in utero procedure during previous pregnancy, unspecified trimester**
      Excludes1: *supervision of pregnancy affected by in utero procedure during current pregnancy (O35.7)*
  + **O09.89 Supervision of other high risk pregnancies**
    • ♀ **O09.891 Supervision of other high risk pregnancies, first trimester**
    • ♀ **O09.892 Supervision of other high risk pregnancies, second trimester**
    • ♀ **O09.893 Supervision of other high risk pregnancies, third trimester**
    • ♀ **O09.899 Supervision of other high risk pregnancies, unspecified trimester**

+ **O09.9 Supervision of high risk pregnancy, unspecified**
  • ♀ **O09.90 Supervision of high risk pregnancy, unspecified, unspecified trimester**
  • ♀ **O09.91 Supervision of high risk pregnancy, unspecified, first trimester**
  • ♀ **O09.92 Supervision of high risk pregnancy, unspecified, second trimester**
  • ♀ **O09.93 Supervision of high risk pregnancy, unspecified, third trimester**

Edema, proteinuria and hypertensive disorders in pregnancy, childbirth and the puerperium (O10-O16)

O10 Pre-existing hypertension complicating pregnancy, childbirth and the puerperium

Includes: pre-existing hypertension with pre-existing proteinuria complicating pregnancy, childbirth and the puerperium

Excludes2: *pre-existing hypertension with superimposed pre-eclampsia complicating pregnancy, childbirth and the puerperium (O11.-)*

Review coding guideline C.15.d

+ **O10.0 Pre-existing essential hypertension complicating pregnancy, childbirth and the puerperium**
  Any condition in I10 specified as a reason for obstetric care during pregnancy, childbirth or the puerperium
  + **O10.01 Pre-existing essential hypertension complicating pregnancy,**
    - ● ♀ CC **O10.011 Pre-existing essential hypertension complicating pregnancy, first trimester**
    - ● ♀ CC **O10.012 Pre-existing essential hypertension complicating pregnancy, second trimester**
    - ● ♀ CC **O10.013 Pre-existing essential hypertension complicating pregnancy, third trimester**
    - ● ♀ **O10.019 Pre-existing essential hypertension complicating pregnancy, unspecified trimester**
  - ● ♀ CC **O10.02 Pre-existing essential hypertension complicating childbirth**
  - ● ♀ **O10.03 Pre-existing essential hypertension complicating the puerperium**

+ **O10.1 Pre-existing hypertensive heart disease complicating pregnancy, childbirth and the puerperium**
  Any condition in I11 specified as a reason for obstetric care during pregnancy, childbirth or the puerperium
  Use additional code from I11 to identify the type of hypertensive heart disease
  + **O10.11 Pre-existing hypertensive heart disease complicating pregnancy**
    - ● ♀ **O10.111 Pre-existing hypertensive heart disease complicating pregnancy, first trimester**
    - ● ♀ **O10.112 Pre-existing hypertensive heart disease complicating pregnancy, second trimester**
    - ● ♀ **O10.113 Pre-existing hypertensive heart disease complicating pregnancy, third trimester**
    - ● ♀ **O10.119 Pre-existing hypertensive heart disease complicating pregnancy, unspecified trimester**
  - ● ♀ **O10.12 Pre-existing hypertensive heart disease complicating childbirth**
  - ● ♀ **O10.13 Pre-existing hypertensive heart disease complicating the puerperium**

+ **O10.2 Pre-existing hypertensive chronic kidney disease complicating pregnancy, childbirth and the puerperium**
  Any condition in I12 specified as a reason for obstetric care during pregnancy, childbirth or the puerperium
  Use additional code from I12 to identify the type of hypertensive chronic kidney disease
  + **O10.21 Pre-existing hypertensive chronic kidney disease complicating pregnancy**
    - ● ♀ **O10.211 Pre-existing hypertensive chronic kidney disease complicating pregnancy, first trimester**
    - ● ♀ **O10.212 Pre-existing hypertensive chronic kidney disease complicating pregnancy, second trimester**
    - ● ♀ **O10.213 Pre-existing hypertensive chronic kidney disease complicating pregnancy, third trimester**
    - ● ♀ **O10.219 Pre-existing hypertensive chronic kidney disease complicating pregnancy, unspecified trimester**
  - ● ♀ **O10.22 Pre-existing hypertensive chronic kidney disease complicating childbirth**
  - ● ♀ **O10.23 Pre-existing hypertensive chronic kidney disease complicating the puerperium**

+ **O10.3 Pre-existing hypertensive heart and chronic kidney disease complicating pregnancy, childbirth and the puerperium**
  Any condition in I13 specified as a reason for obstetric care during pregnancy, childbirth or the puerperium
  Use additional code from I13 to identify the type of hypertensive heart and chronic kidney disease
  + **O10.31 Pre-existing hypertensive heart and chronic kidney disease complicating pregnancy**
    - ● ♀ **O10.311 Pre-existing hypertensive heart and chronic kidney disease complicating pregnancy, first trimester**
    - ● ♀ **O10.312 Pre-existing hypertensive heart and chronic kidney disease complicating pregnancy, second trimester**
    - ● ♀ **O10.313 Pre-existing hypertensive heart and chronic kidney disease complicating pregnancy, third trimester**
    - ● ♀ **O10.319 Pre-existing hypertensive heart and chronic kidney disease complicating pregnancy, unspecified trimester**
  - ● ♀ **O10.32 Pre-existing hypertensive heart and chronic kidney disease complicating childbirth**
  - ● ♀ **O10.33 Pre-existing hypertensive heart and chronic kidney disease complicating the puerperium**

+ **O10.4 Pre-existing secondary hypertension complicating pregnancy, childbirth and the puerperium**
  Any condition in I15 specified as a reason for obstetric care during pregnancy, childbirth or the puerperium
  Use additional code from I15 to identify the type of secondary hypertension
  + **O10.41 Pre-existing secondary hypertension complicating pregnancy**
    - ● ♀ CC **O10.411 Pre-existing secondary hypertension complicating pregnancy, first trimester**
    - ● ♀ CC **O10.412 Pre-existing secondary hypertension complicating pregnancy, second trimester**
    - ● ♀ CC **O10.413 Pre-existing secondary hypertension complicating pregnancy, third trimester**
    - ● ♀ **O10.419 Pre-existing secondary hypertension complicating pregnancy, unspecified trimester**
  - ● ♀ MCC **O10.42 Pre-existing secondary hypertension complicating childbirth**
  - ● ♀ CC **O10.43 Pre-existing secondary hypertension complicating the puerperium**

+ **O10.9 Unspecified pre-existing hypertension complicating pregnancy, childbirth and the puerperium**
  + **O10.91 Unspecified pre-existing hypertension complicating pregnancy**
    - ● ♀ CC **O10.911 Unspecified pre-existing hypertension complicating pregnancy, first trimester**
    - ● ♀ CC **O10.912 Unspecified pre-existing hypertension complicating pregnancy, second trimester**
    - ● ♀ CC **O10.913 Unspecified pre-existing hypertension complicating pregnancy, third trimester**
    - ● ♀ **O10.919 Unspecified pre-existing hypertension complicating pregnancy, unspecified trimester**
  - ● ♀ CC **O10.92 Unspecified pre-existing hypertension complicating childbirth**
  - ● ♀ **O10.93 Unspecified pre-existing hypertension complicating the puerperium**

O11 Pre-existing hypertension with pre-eclampsia

Includes: conditions in O10 complicated by pre-eclampsia
pre-eclampsia superimposed pre-existing hypertension

Use additional code from O10 to identify the type of hypertension

AHA CC: 4Q, 2016, 50

- ● ♀ MCC **O11.1 Pre-existing hypertension with pre-eclampsia, first trimester**
- ● ♀ MCC **O11.2 Pre-existing hypertension with pre-eclampsia, second trimester**
- ● ♀ MCC **O11.3 Pre-existing hypertension with pre-eclampsia, third trimester**

- ♀ **O11.4 Pre-existing hypertension with pre-eclampsia, complicating childbirth**
- ♀ **O11.5 Pre-existing hypertension with pre-eclampsia, complicating the puerperium**
- ♀ **O11.9 Pre-existing hypertension with pre-eclampsia, unspecified trimester**

O12 Gestational [pregnancy-induced] edema and proteinuria without hypertension

AHA CC: 4Q, 2016, 50

+ **O12.0 Gestational edema**
  - ♀ **O12.00 Gestational edema, unspecified trimester**
  - ♀ **O12.01 Gestational edema, first trimester**
  - ♀ **O12.02 Gestational edema, second trimester**
  - ♀ **O12.03 Gestational edema, third trimester**
  - ♀ **O12.04 Gestational edema, complicating childbirth**
  - ♀ **O12.05 Gestational edema, complicating the puerperium**
+ **O12.1 Gestational proteinuria**
  - ♀ **O12.10 Gestational proteinuria, unspecified trimester**
  - ♀ CC **O12.11 Gestational proteinuria, first trimester**
  - ♀ CC **O12.12 Gestational proteinuria, second trimester**
  - ♀ CC **O12.13 Gestational proteinuria, third trimester**
  - ♀ **O12.14 Gestational proteinuria, complicating childbirth**
  - ♀ **O12.15 Gestational proteinuria, complicating the puerperium**
+ **O12.2 Gestational edema with proteinuria**
  - ♀ **O12.20 Gestational edema with proteinuria, unspecified trimester**
  - ♀ CC **O12.21 Gestational edema with proteinuria, first trimester**
  - ♀ CC **O12.22 Gestational edema with proteinuria, second trimester**
  - ♀ CC **O12.23 Gestational edema with proteinuria, third trimester**
  - ♀ **O12.24 Gestational edema with proteinuria, complicating childbirth**
  - ♀ **O12.25 Gestational edema with proteinuria, complicating the puerperium**

O13 Gestational [pregnancy-induced] hypertension without significant proteinuria

Includes: gestational hypertension NOS
transient hypertension of pregnancy

Review coding guideline C.9.a.7

AHA CC: 4Q, 2016, 50

- ♀ **O13.1 Gestational [pregnancy-induced] hypertension without significant proteinuria, first trimester**
- ♀ **O13.2 Gestational [pregnancy-induced] hypertension without significant proteinuria, second trimester**
- ♀ **O13.3 Gestational [pregnancy-induced] hypertension without significant proteinuria, third trimester**
- ♀ **O13.4 Gestational [pregnancy-induced] hypertension without significant proteinuria, complicating childbirth**
- ♀ **O13.5 Gestational [pregnancy-induced] hypertension without significant proteinuria, complicating the puerperium**
- ♀ **O13.9 Gestational [pregnancy-induced] hypertension without significant proteinuria, unspecified trimester**

O14 Pre-eclampsia

Excludes1: *pre-existing hypertension with pre-eclampsia (O11)*

Review coding guideline C.9.a.7

AHA CC: 4Q, 2016, 50

+ **O14.0 Mild to moderate pre-eclampsia**
  - ♀ **O14.00 Mild to moderate pre-eclampsia, unspecified trimester**
  - ♀ CC **O14.02 Mild to moderate pre-eclampsia, second trimester**
  - ♀ CC **O14.03 Mild to moderate pre-eclampsia, third trimester**
  - ♀ **O14.04 Mild to moderate pre-eclampsia, complicating childbirth**

    AHA CC: 2Q, 2019, 8
  - ♀ **O14.05 Mild to moderate pre-eclampsia, complicating the puerperium**
+ **O14.1 Severe pre-eclampsia**

  Excludes1: *HELLP syndrome (O14.2-)*

  AHA CC: 3Q, 2019, 12
  - ♀ **O14.10 Severe pre-eclampsia, unspecified trimester**
  - ♀ MCC **O14.12 Severe pre-eclampsia, second trimester**
  - ♀ MCC **O14.13 Severe pre-eclampsia, third trimester**
  - ♀ **O14.14 Severe pre-eclampsia complicating childbirth**
  - ♀ **O14.15 Severe pre-eclampsia, complicating the puerperium**
+ **O14.2 HELLP syndrome**

  Severe pre-eclampsia with hemolysis, elevated liver enzymes and low platelet count (HELLP)
  - ♀ **O14.20 HELLP syndrome (HELLP), unspecified trimester**
  - ♀ MCC **O14.22 HELLP syndrome (HELLP), second trimester**
  - ♀ MCC **O14.23 HELLP syndrome (HELLP), third trimester**
  - ♀ **O14.24 HELLP syndrome, complicating childbirth**
  - ♀ **O14.25 HELLP syndrome, complicating the puerperium**
+ **O14.9 Unspecified pre-eclampsia**
  - ♀ **O14.90 Unspecified pre-eclampsia, unspecified trimester**
  - ♀ CC **O14.92 Unspecified pre-eclampsia, second trimester**
  - ♀ CC **O14.93 Unspecified pre-eclampsia, third trimester**
  - ♀ **O14.94 Unspecified pre-eclampsia, complicating childbirth**
  - ♀ **O14.95 Unspecified pre-eclampsia, complicating the puerperium**

O15 Eclampsia

Includes: convulsions following conditions in O10-O14 and O16

+ **O15.0 Eclampsia complicating pregnancy**

  AHA CC: 4Q, 2016, 50
  - ♀ **O15.00 Eclampsia complicating pregnancy, unspecified trimester**
  - ♀ MCC **O15.02 Eclampsia complicating pregnancy, second trimester**
  - ♀ MCC **O15.03 Eclampsia complicating pregnancy, third trimester**
- ♀ MCC **O15.1 Eclampsia complicating labor**
- ♀ MCC **O15.2 Eclampsia complicating the puerperium**
- ♀ **O15.9 Eclampsia, unspecified as to time period**

  Eclampsia NOS

O16 Unspecified maternal hypertension

AHA CC: 4Q, 2016, 50

- ♀ CC **O16.1 Unspecified maternal hypertension, first trimester**
- ♀ CC **O16.2 Unspecified maternal hypertension, second trimester**
- ♀ CC **O16.3 Unspecified maternal hypertension, third trimester**
- ♀ **O16.4 Unspecified maternal hypertension, complicating childbirth**
- ♀ **O16.5 Unspecified maternal hypertension, complicating the puerperium**
- ♀ **O16.9 Unspecified maternal hypertension, unspecified trimester**

Other maternal disorders predominantly related to pregnancy (O20-O29)

Excludes2: *maternal care related to the fetus and amniotic cavity and possible delivery problems (O30-O48)*
maternal diseases classifiable elsewhere but complicating pregnancy, labor and delivery, and the puerperium (O98-O99)

O20 Hemorrhage in early pregnancy

Includes: hemorrhage before completion of 20 weeks gestation

Excludes1: *pregnancy with abortive outcome (O00-O08)*

- ♀ CC **O20.0 Threatened abortion**

  Hemorrhage specified as due to threatened abortion
- ♀ **O20.8 Other hemorrhage in early pregnancy**
- ♀ CC **O20.9 Hemorrhage in early pregnancy, unspecified**

O21 Excessive vomiting in pregnancy

- ♀ **O21.0 Mild hyperemesis gravidarum**

  Hyperemesis gravidarum, mild or unspecified, starting before the end of the 20th week of gestation
- ♀ **O21.1 Hyperemesis gravidarum with metabolic disturbance**

  Hyperemesis gravidarum, starting before the end of the 20th week of gestation, with metabolic disturbance such as carbohydrate depletion

  Hyperemesis gravidarum, starting before the end of the 20th week of gestation, with metabolic disturbance such as dehydration

  Hyperemesis gravidarum, starting before the end of the 20th week of gestation, with metabolic disturbance such as electrolyte imbalance
- ♀ **O21.2 Late vomiting of pregnancy**

  Excessive vomiting starting after 20 completed weeks of gestation
- ♀ **O21.8 Other vomiting complicating pregnancy**

  Vomiting due to diseases classified elsewhere, complicating pregnancy

  Use additional code, to identify cause.
- ♀ **O21.9 Vomiting of pregnancy, unspecified**

O22 Venous complications and hemorrhoids in pregnancy

Excludes1: *venous complications of:*
abortion NOS (O03.9)
ectopic or molar pregnancy (O08.7)
failed attempted abortion (O07.35)
induced abortion (O04.85)
spontaneous abortion (O03.89)

Excludes2: *obstetric pulmonary embolism (O88.-)*
venous complications and hemorrhoids of childbirth and the puerperium (O87.-)

\+ **O22.0 Varicose veins of lower extremity in pregnancy**
Varicose veins NOS in pregnancy
● ♀ **O22.00 Varicose veins of lower extremity in pregnancy, unspecified trimester**
● ♀ **O22.01 Varicose veins of lower extremity in pregnancy, first trimester**
● ♀ **O22.02 Varicose veins of lower extremity in pregnancy, second trimester**
● ♀ **O22.03 Varicose veins of lower extremity in pregnancy, third trimester**

\+ **O22.1 Genital varices in pregnancy**
Perineal varices in pregnancy
Vaginal varices in pregnancy
Vulval varices in pregnancy
● ♀ **O22.10 Genital varices in pregnancy, unspecified trimester**
● ♀ **O22.11 Genital varices in pregnancy, first trimester**
● ♀ **O22.12 Genital varices in pregnancy, second trimester**
● ♀ **O22.13 Genital varices in pregnancy, third trimester**

\+ **O22.2 Superficial thrombophlebitis in pregnancy**
Phlebitis in pregnancy NOS
Thrombophlebitis of legs in pregnancy
Thrombosis in pregnancy NOS
Use additional code to identify the superficial thrombophlebitis (I80.0-)
● ♀ CC **O22.20 Superficial thrombophlebitis in pregnancy, unspecified trimester**
● ♀ CC **O22.21 Superficial thrombophlebitis in pregnancy, first trimester**
● ♀ CC **O22.22 Superficial thrombophlebitis in pregnancy, second trimester**
● ♀ CC **O22.23 Superficial thrombophlebitis in pregnancy, third trimester**

\+ **O22.3 Deep phlebothrombosis in pregnancy**
Deep vein thrombosis, antepartum
Use additional code to identify the deep vein thrombosis (I82.4-, I82.5-, I82.62-, I82.72-)

Use additional code, if applicable, for associated long-term (current) use of anticoagulants (Z79.01)
● ♀ CC **O22.30 Deep phlebothrombosis in pregnancy, unspecified trimester**
● ♀ MCC **O22.31 Deep phlebothrombosis in pregnancy, first trimester**
● ♀ MCC **O22.32 Deep phlebothrombosis in pregnancy, second trimester**
● ♀ MCC **O22.33 Deep phlebothrombosis in pregnancy, third trimester**

\+ **O22.4 Hemorrhoids in pregnancy**
● ♀ CC **O22.40 Hemorrhoids in pregnancy, unspecified trimester**
● ♀ CC **O22.41 Hemorrhoids in pregnancy, first trimester**
● ♀ CC **O22.42 Hemorrhoids in pregnancy, second trimester**
● ♀ CC **O22.43 Hemorrhoids in pregnancy, third trimester**

\+ **O22.5 Cerebral venous thrombosis in pregnancy**
Cerebrovenous sinus thrombosis in pregnancy
● ♀ CC **O22.50 Cerebral venous thrombosis in pregnancy, unspecified trimester**
● ♀ CC **O22.51 Cerebral venous thrombosis in pregnancy, first trimester**
● ♀ CC **O22.52 Cerebral venous thrombosis in pregnancy, second trimester**
● ♀ CC **O22.53 Cerebral venous thrombosis in pregnancy, third trimester**

\+ **O22.8 Other venous complications in pregnancy**
\+ **O22.8X Other venous complications in pregnancy**
● ♀ CC **O22.8X1 Other venous complications in pregnancy, first trimester**
● ♀ CC **O22.8X2 Other venous complications in pregnancy, second trimester**
● ♀ CC **O22.8X3 Other venous complications in pregnancy, third trimester**
● ♀ CC **O22.8X9 Other venous complications in pregnancy, unspecified trimester**

\+ **O22.9 Venous complication in pregnancy, unspecified**
Gestational phlebitis NOS
Gestational phlebopathy NOS
Gestational thrombosis NOS
● ♀ CC **O22.90 Venous complication in pregnancy, unspecified, unspecified trimester**
● ♀ **O22.91 Venous complication in pregnancy, unspecified, first trimester**
● ♀ **O22.92 Venous complication in pregnancy, unspecified, second trimester**
● ♀ **O22.93 Venous complication in pregnancy, unspecified, third trimester**

O23 Infections of genitourinary tract in pregnancy

Use additional code to identify organism (B95.-, B96.-)

Excludes2: *gonococcal infections complicating pregnancy, childbirth and the puerperium (O98.2)*
infections with a predominantly sexual mode of transmission NOS complicating pregnancy, childbirth and the puerperium (O98.3)
syphilis complicating pregnancy, childbirth and the puerperium (O98.1)
tuberculosis of genitourinary system complicating pregnancy, childbirth and the puerperium (O98.0)
venereal disease NOS complicating pregnancy, childbirth and the puerperium (O98.3)

\+ **O23.0 Infections of kidney in pregnancy**
Pyelonephritis in pregnancy
● ♀ **O23.00 Infections of kidney in pregnancy, unspecified trimester**
● ♀ CC **O23.01 Infections of kidney in pregnancy, first trimester**
● ♀ CC **O23.02 Infections of kidney in pregnancy, second trimester**
● ♀ CC **O23.03 Infections of kidney in pregnancy, third trimester**

\+ **O23.1 Infections of bladder in pregnancy**
● ♀ **O23.10 Infections of bladder in pregnancy, unspecified trimester**
● ♀ CC **O23.11 Infections of bladder in pregnancy, first trimester**
● ♀ CC **O23.12 Infections of bladder in pregnancy, second trimester**
● ♀ CC **O23.13 Infections of bladder in pregnancy, third trimester**

\+ **O23.2 Infections of urethra in pregnancy**
● ♀ **O23.20 Infections of urethra in pregnancy, unspecified trimester**
● ♀ CC **O23.21 Infections of urethra in pregnancy, first trimester**
● ♀ CC **O23.22 Infections of urethra in pregnancy, second trimester**
● ♀ CC **O23.23 Infections of urethra in pregnancy, third trimester**

\+ **O23.3 Infections of other parts of urinary tract in pregnancy**
● ♀ **O23.30 Infections of other parts of urinary tract in pregnancy, unspecified trimester**
● ♀ CC **O23.31 Infections of other parts of urinary tract in pregnancy, first trimester**
● ♀ CC **O23.32 Infections of other parts of urinary tract in pregnancy, second trimester**
● ♀ CC **O23.33 Infections of other parts of urinary tract in pregnancy, third trimester**

\+ **O23.4 Unspecified infection of urinary tract in pregnancy**
● ♀ **O23.40 Unspecified infection of urinary tract in pregnancy, unspecified trimester**
● ♀ CC **O23.41 Unspecified infection of urinary tract in pregnancy, first trimester**
● ♀ CC **O23.42 Unspecified infection of urinary tract in pregnancy, second trimester**
● ♀ CC **O23.43 Unspecified infection of urinary tract in pregnancy, third trimester**
AHA CC: 2Q, 2018, 20

+ **O23.5 Infections of the genital tract in pregnancy**
  + **O23.51 Infection of cervix in pregnancy**
    - • ♀ CC **O23.511 Infections of cervix in pregnancy, first trimester**
    - • ♀ CC **O23.512 Infections of cervix in pregnancy, second trimester**
    - • ♀ CC **O23.513 Infections of cervix in pregnancy, third trimester**
    - • ♀ **O23.519 Infections of cervix in pregnancy, unspecified trimester**
  + **O23.52 Salpingo-oophoritis in pregnancy**
    Oophoritis in pregnancy
    Salpingitis in pregnancy
    - • ♀ CC **O23.521 Salpingo-oophoritis in pregnancy, first trimester**
    - • ♀ CC **O23.522 Salpingo-oophoritis in pregnancy, second trimester**
    - • ♀ CC **O23.523 Salpingo-oophoritis in pregnancy, third trimester**
    - • ♀ **O23.529 Salpingo-oophoritis in pregnancy, unspecified trimester**
  + **O23.59 Infection of other part of genital tract in pregnancy**
    - • ♀ CC **O23.591 Infection of other part of genital tract in pregnancy, first trimester**
    - • ♀ CC **O23.592 Infection of other part of genital tract in pregnancy, second trimester**
    - • ♀ CC **O23.593 Infection of other part of genital tract in pregnancy, third trimester**
    - • ♀ **O23.599 Infection of other part of genital tract in pregnancy, unspecified trimester**
+ **O23.9 Unspecified genitourinary tract infection in pregnancy**
  Genitourinary tract infection in pregnancy NOS
  - • ♀ **O23.90 Unspecified genitourinary tract infection in pregnancy, unspecified trimester**
  - • ♀ CC **O23.91 Unspecified genitourinary tract infection in pregnancy, first trimester**
  - • ♀ CC **O23.92 Unspecified genitourinary tract infection in pregnancy, second trimester**
  - • ♀ CC **O23.93 Unspecified genitourinary tract infection in pregnancy, third trimester**

O24 Diabetes mellitus in pregnancy, childbirth, and the puerperium
Review coding guideline C.15.g

+ **O24.0 Pre-existing type 1 diabetes mellitus, in pregnancy, childbirth and the puerperium**
  Juvenile onset diabetes mellitus, in pregnancy, childbirth and the puerperium
  Ketosis-prone diabetes mellitus in pregnancy, childbirth and the puerperium
  Use additional code from category E10 to further identify any manifestations
  + **O24.01 Pre-existing type 1 diabetes mellitus, in pregnancy**
    - • ♀ CC **O24.011 Pre-existing type 1 diabetes mellitus, in pregnancy, first trimester**
    - • ♀ CC **O24.012 Pre-existing type 1 diabetes mellitus, in pregnancy, second trimester**
    - • ♀ CC **O24.013 Pre-existing type 1 diabetes mellitus, in pregnancy, third trimester**
    - • ♀ CC **O24.019 Pre-existing type 1 diabetes mellitus, in pregnancy, unspecified trimester**
  - • ♀ MCC **O24.02 Pre-existing type 1 diabetes mellitus, in childbirth**
  - • ♀ CC **O24.03 Pre-existing type 1 diabetes mellitus, in the puerperium**
+ **O24.1 Pre-existing type 2 diabetes mellitus, in pregnancy, childbirth and the puerperium**
  Insulin-resistant diabetes mellitus in pregnancy, childbirth and the puerperium
  Use additional code (for):
  from category E11 to further identify any manifestations
  long-term (current) use of insulin (Z79.4)
  + **O24.11 Pre-existing type 2 diabetes mellitus, in pregnancy**
    - • ♀ CC **O24.111 Pre-existing type 2 diabetes mellitus, in pregnancy, first trimester**
    - • ♀ CC **O24.112 Pre-existing type 2 diabetes mellitus, in pregnancy, second trimester**
    - • ♀ CC **O24.113 Pre-existing type 2 diabetes mellitus, in pregnancy, third trimester**
    - • ♀ CC **O24.119 Pre-existing type 2 diabetes mellitus, in pregnancy, unspecified trimester**
  - • ♀ MCC **O24.12 Pre-existing type 2 diabetes mellitus, in childbirth**
  - • ♀ CC **O24.13 Pre-existing type 2 diabetes mellitus, in the puerperium**
+ **O24.3 Unspecified pre-existing diabetes mellitus in pregnancy, childbirth and the puerperium**
  Use additional code (for):
  from category E11 to further identify any manifestation
  long-term (current) use of insulin (Z79.4)
  + **O24.31 Unspecified pre-existing diabetes mellitus in pregnancy**
    - • ♀ CC **O24.311 Unspecified pre-existing diabetes mellitus in pregnancy, first trimester**
    - • ♀ CC **O24.312 Unspecified pre-existing diabetes mellitus in pregnancy, second trimester**
    - • ♀ CC **O24.313 Unspecified pre-existing diabetes mellitus in pregnancy, third trimester**
    - • ♀ CC **O24.319 Unspecified pre-existing diabetes mellitus in pregnancy, unspecified trimester**
  - • ♀ MCC **O24.32 Unspecified pre-existing diabetes mellitus in childbirth**
  - • ♀ CC **O24.33 Unspecified pre-existing diabetes mellitus in the puerperium**
+ **O24.4 Gestational diabetes mellitus**
  Diabetes mellitus arising in pregnancy
  Gestational diabetes mellitus NOS
  Review coding guideline C.15.i
  AHA CC: 4Q, 2016, 50
  + **O24.41 Gestational diabetes mellitus in pregnancy**
    - • ♀ **O24.410 Gestational diabetes mellitus in pregnancy, diet controlled**
    - • ♀ **O24.414 Gestational diabetes mellitus in pregnancy, insulin controlled**
    - • ♀ **O24.415 Gestational diabetes mellitus in pregnancy, controlled by oral hypoglycemic drugs**
      Gestational diabetes mellitus in pregnancy, controlled by oral antidiabetic drugs
    - • ♀ **O24.419 Gestational diabetes mellitus in pregnancy, unspecified control**
      AHA CC: 4Q, 2015, 34; 3Q, 2020, 30-31
  + **O24.42 Gestational diabetes mellitus in childbirth**
    - • ♀ **O24.420 Gestational diabetes mellitus in childbirth, diet controlled**
    - • ♀ **O24.424 Gestational diabetes mellitus in childbirth, insulin controlled**
    - • ♀ **O24.425 Gestational diabetes mellitus in childbirth, controlled by oral hypoglycemic drugs**
      Gestational diabetes mellitus in childbirth, controlled by oral antidiabetic drugs
    - • ♀ **O24.429 Gestational diabetes mellitus in childbirth, unspecified control**
  + **O24.43 Gestational diabetes mellitus in the puerperium**
    - • ♀ **O24.430 Gestational diabetes mellitus in the puerperium, diet controlled**
    - • ♀ **O24.434 Gestational diabetes mellitus in the puerperium, insulin controlled**
    - • ♀ **O24.435 Gestational diabetes mellitus in puerperium, controlled by oral hypoglycemic drugs**
      Gestational diabetes mellitus in puerperium, controlled by oral antidiabetic drugs
    - • ♀ **O24.439 Gestational diabetes mellitus in the puerperium, unspecified control**
+ **O24.8 Other pre-existing diabetes mellitus in pregnancy, childbirth, and the puerperium**
  Use additional code (for):
  from categories E08, E09 and E13 to further identify any manifestation
  long-term (current) use of insulin (Z79.4)
  + **O24.81 Other pre-existing diabetes mellitus in pregnancy**
    - • ♀ CC **O24.811 Other pre-existing diabetes mellitus in pregnancy, first trimester**
    - • ♀ CC **O24.812 Other pre-existing diabetes mellitus in pregnancy, second trimester**
    - • ♀ CC **O24.813 Other pre-existing diabetes mellitus in pregnancy, third trimester**
    - • ♀ CC **O24.819 Other pre-existing diabetes mellitus in pregnancy, unspecified trimester**
  - • ♀ MCC **O24.82 Other pre-existing diabetes mellitus in childbirth**
  - • ♀ CC **O24.83 Other pre-existing diabetes mellitus in the puerperium**

+ O24.9 Unspecified diabetes mellitus in pregnancy, childbirth and the puerperium
Use additional code for long-term (current) use of insulin (Z79.4)
+ O24.91 Unspecified diabetes mellitus in pregnancy
• ♀ CC O24.911 Unspecified diabetes mellitus in pregnancy, first trimester
• ♀ CC O24.912 Unspecified diabetes mellitus in pregnancy, second trimester
• ♀ CC O24.913 Unspecified diabetes mellitus in pregnancy, third trimester
• ♀ CC O24.919 Unspecified diabetes mellitus in pregnancy, unspecified trimester
• ♀ O24.92 Unspecified diabetes mellitus in childbirth
• ♀ CC O24.93 Unspecified diabetes mellitus in the puerperium

O25 Malnutrition in pregnancy, childbirth and the puerperium
+ O25.1 Malnutrition in pregnancy
• ♀ O25.10 Malnutrition in pregnancy, unspecified trimester
• ♀ O25.11 Malnutrition in pregnancy, first trimester
• ♀ O25.12 Malnutrition in pregnancy, second trimester
• ♀ O25.13 Malnutrition in pregnancy, third trimester
• ♀ O25.2 Malnutrition in childbirth
• ♀ O25.3 Malnutrition in the puerperium

O26 Maternal care for other conditions predominantly related to pregnancy
+ O26.0 Excessive weight gain in pregnancy
Excludes2: *gestational edema (O12.0, O12.2)*
• ♀ O26.00 Excessive weight gain in pregnancy, unspecified trimester
• ♀ O26.01 Excessive weight gain in pregnancy, first trimester
• ♀ O26.02 Excessive weight gain in pregnancy, second trimester
• ♀ O26.03 Excessive weight gain in pregnancy, third trimester
+ O26.1 Low weight gain in pregnancy
• ♀ O26.10 Low weight gain in pregnancy, unspecified trimester
• ♀ O26.11 Low weight gain in pregnancy, first trimester
• ♀ O26.12 Low weight gain in pregnancy, second trimester
• ♀ O26.13 Low weight gain in pregnancy, third trimester
+ O26.2 Pregnancy care for patient with recurrent pregnancy loss
• ♀ O26.20 Pregnancy care for patient with recurrent pregnancy loss, unspecified trimester
• ♀ O26.21 Pregnancy care for patient with recurrent pregnancy loss, first trimester
• ♀ O26.22 Pregnancy care for patient with recurrent pregnancy loss, second trimester
• ♀ O26.23 Pregnancy care for patient with recurrent pregnancy loss, third trimester
+ O26.3 Retained intrauterine contraceptive device in pregnancy
• ♀ O26.30 Retained intrauterine contraceptive device in pregnancy, unspecified trimester
• ♀ O26.31 Retained intrauterine contraceptive device in pregnancy, first trimester
• ♀ O26.32 Retained intrauterine contraceptive device in pregnancy, second trimester
• ♀ O26.33 Retained intrauterine contraceptive device in pregnancy, third trimester
+ O26.4 Herpes gestationis
• ♀ O26.40 Herpes gestationis, unspecified trimester
• ♀ O26.41 Herpes gestationis, first trimester
• ♀ O26.42 Herpes gestationis, second trimester
• ♀ O26.43 Herpes gestationis, third trimester
+ O26.5 Maternal hypotension syndrome
Supine hypotensive syndrome
• ♀ O26.50 Maternal hypotension syndrome, unspecified trimester
• ♀ O26.51 Maternal hypotension syndrome, first trimester
• ♀ O26.52 Maternal hypotension syndrome, second trimester
• ♀ O26.53 Maternal hypotension syndrome, third trimester
+ O26.6 Liver and biliary tract disorders in pregnancy, childbirth and the puerperium
Use additional code to identify the specific disorder
Excludes2: *hepatorenal syndrome following labor and delivery (O90.4)*
+ O26.61 Liver and biliary tract disorders in pregnancy
• ♀ CC O26.611 Liver and biliary tract disorders in pregnancy, first trimester
• ♀ CC O26.612 Liver and biliary tract disorders in pregnancy, second trimester
• ♀ CC O26.613 Liver and biliary tract disorders in pregnancy, third trimester
• ♀ O26.619 Liver and biliary tract disorders in pregnancy, unspecified trimester
• ♀ CC O26.62 Liver and biliary tract disorders in childbirth
• ♀ O26.63 Liver and biliary tract disorders in the puerperium
+ O26.7 Subluxation of symphysis (pubis) in pregnancy, childbirth and the puerperium
Excludes1: *traumatic separation of symphysis (pubis) during childbirth (O71.6)*
+ O26.71 Subluxation of symphysis (pubis) in pregnancy
• ♀ O26.711 Subluxation of symphysis (pubis) in pregnancy, first trimester
• ♀ O26.712 Subluxation of symphysis (pubis) in pregnancy, second trimester
• ♀ O26.713 Subluxation of symphysis (pubis) in pregnancy, third trimester
• ♀ O26.719 Subluxation of symphysis (pubis) in pregnancy, unspecified trimester
• ♀ O26.72 Subluxation of symphysis (pubis) in childbirth
• ♀ O26.73 Subluxation of symphysis (pubis) in the puerperium
+ O26.8 Other specified pregnancy related conditions
+ O26.81 Pregnancy related exhaustion and fatigue
• ♀ O26.811 Pregnancy related exhaustion and fatigue, first trimester
• ♀ O26.812 Pregnancy related exhaustion and fatigue, second trimester
• ♀ O26.813 Pregnancy related exhaustion and fatigue, third trimester
• ♀ O26.819 Pregnancy related exhaustion and fatigue, unspecified trimester
+ O26.82 Pregnancy related peripheral neuritis
• ♀ O26.821 Pregnancy related peripheral neuritis, first trimester
• ♀ O26.822 Pregnancy related peripheral neuritis, second trimester
• ♀ O26.823 Pregnancy related peripheral neuritis, third trimester
• ♀ O26.829 Pregnancy related peripheral neuritis, unspecified trimester
+ O26.83 Pregnancy related renal disease
Use additional code to identify the specific disorder
• ♀ CC O26.831 Pregnancy related renal disease, first trimester
• ♀ CC O26.832 Pregnancy related renal disease, second trimester
• ♀ CC O26.833 Pregnancy related renal disease, third trimester
• ♀ O26.839 Pregnancy related renal disease, unspecified trimester
+ O26.84 Uterine size-date discrepancy complicating pregnancy
Excludes1: *encounter for suspected problem with fetal growth ruled out (Z03.74)*
• ♀ O26.841 Uterine size-date discrepancy, first trimester
• ♀ O26.842 Uterine size-date discrepancy, second trimester
• ♀ O26.843 Uterine size-date discrepancy, third trimester
• ♀ O26.849 Uterine size-date discrepancy, unspecified trimester
+ O26.85 Spotting complicating pregnancy
• ♀ O26.851 Spotting complicating pregnancy, first trimester
• ♀ O26.852 Spotting complicating pregnancy, second trimester
• ♀ O26.853 Spotting complicating pregnancy, third trimester
• ♀ O26.859 Spotting complicating pregnancy, unspecified trimester

• ♀ **O26.86 Pruritic urticarial papules and plaques of pregnancy (PUPPP)**
Polymorphic eruption of pregnancy

\+ **O26.87 Cervical shortening**
Excludes1: *encounter for suspected cervical shortening ruled out (Z03.75)*

• ♀ CC **O26.872 Cervical shortening, second trimester**
• ♀ CC **O26.873 Cervical shortening, third trimester**
• ♀ CC **O26.879 Cervical shortening, unspecified trimester**

\+ **O26.89 Other specified pregnancy related conditions**
• ♀ **O26.891 Other specified pregnancy related conditions, first trimester**
• ♀ **O26.892 Other specified pregnancy related conditions, second trimester**
• ♀ **O26.893 Other specified pregnancy related conditions, third trimester**
AHA CC: 3Q, 2015, 40
• ♀ **O26.899 Other specified pregnancy related conditions, unspecified trimester**

\+ **O26.9 Pregnancy related conditions, unspecified**
• ♀ **O26.90 Pregnancy related conditions, unspecified, unspecified trimester**
• ♀ **O26.91 Pregnancy related conditions, unspecified, first trimester**
• ♀ **O26.92 Pregnancy related conditions, unspecified, second trimester**
• ♀ **O26.93 Pregnancy related conditions, unspecified, third trimester**

O28 Abnormal findings on antenatal screening of mother
Excludes1: *diagnostic findings classified elsewhere - see Alphabetical Index*

• ♀ **O28.0 Abnormal hematological finding on antenatal screening of mother**
• ♀ **O28.1 Abnormal biochemical finding on antenatal screening of mother**
• ♀ **O28.2 Abnormal cytological finding on antenatal screening of mother**
• ♀ **O28.3 Abnormal ultrasonic finding on antenatal screening of mother**
AHA CC: 4Q, 2016, 4-7
• ♀ **O28.4 Abnormal radiological finding on antenatal screening of mother**
• ♀ **O28.5 Abnormal chromosomal and genetic finding on antenatal screening of mother**
• ♀ **O28.8 Other abnormal findings on antenatal screening of mother**
• ♀ **O28.9 Unspecified abnormal findings on antenatal screening of mother**

O29 Complications of anesthesia during pregnancy
Includes: maternal complications arising from the administration of a general, regional or local anesthetic, analgesic or other sedation during pregnancy
Use additional code, if necessary, to identify the complication
Excludes2: *complications of anesthesia during labor and delivery (O74.-)*
complications of anesthesia during the puerperium (O89.-)

\+ **O29.0 Pulmonary complications of anesthesia during pregnancy**
\+ **O29.01 Aspiration pneumonitis due to anesthesia during pregnancy**
Inhalation of stomach contents or secretions NOS due to anesthesia during pregnancy
Mendelson's syndrome due to anesthesia during pregnancy
• ♀ **O29.011 Aspiration pneumonitis due to anesthesia during pregnancy, first trimester**
• ♀ **O29.012 Aspiration pneumonitis due to anesthesia during pregnancy, second trimester**
• ♀ **O29.013 Aspiration pneumonitis due to anesthesia during pregnancy, third trimester**
• ♀ **O29.019 Aspiration pneumonitis due to anesthesia during pregnancy, unspecified trimester**

\+ **O29.02 Pressure collapse of lung due to anesthesia during pregnancy**
• ♀ **O29.021 Pressure collapse of lung due to anesthesia during pregnancy, first trimester**
• ♀ **O29.022 Pressure collapse of lung due to anesthesia during pregnancy, second trimester**
• ♀ **O29.023 Pressure collapse of lung due to anesthesia during pregnancy, third trimester**
• ♀ **O29.029 Pressure collapse of lung due to anesthesia during pregnancy, unspecified trimester**

\+ **O29.09 Other pulmonary complications of anesthesia during pregnancy**
• ♀ **O29.091 Other pulmonary complications of anesthesia during pregnancy, first trimester**
• ♀ **O29.092 Other pulmonary complications of anesthesia during pregnancy, second trimester**
• ♀ **O29.093 Other pulmonary complications of anesthesia during pregnancy, third trimester**
• ♀ **O29.099 Other pulmonary complications of anesthesia during pregnancy, unspecified trimester**

\+ **O29.1 Cardiac complications of anesthesia during pregnancy**
\+ **O29.11 Cardiac arrest due to anesthesia during pregnancy**
• ♀ **O29.111 Cardiac arrest due to anesthesia during pregnancy, first trimester**
• ♀ **O29.112 Cardiac arrest due to anesthesia during pregnancy, second trimester**
• ♀ **O29.113 Cardiac arrest due to anesthesia during pregnancy, third trimester**
• ♀ **O29.119 Cardiac arrest due to anesthesia during pregnancy, unspecified trimester**

\+ **O29.12 Cardiac failure due to anesthesia during pregnancy**
• ♀ **O29.121 Cardiac failure due to anesthesia during pregnancy, first trimester**
• ♀ **O29.122 Cardiac failure due to anesthesia during pregnancy, second trimester**
• ♀ **O29.123 Cardiac failure due to anesthesia during pregnancy, third trimester**
• ♀ **O29.129 Cardiac failure due to anesthesia during pregnancy, unspecified trimester**

\+ **O29.19 Other cardiac complications of anesthesia during pregnancy**
• ♀ **O29.191 Other cardiac complications of anesthesia during pregnancy, first trimester**
• ♀ **O29.192 Other cardiac complications of anesthesia during pregnancy, second trimester**
• ♀ **O29.193 Other cardiac complications of anesthesia during pregnancy, third trimester**
• ♀ **O29.199 Other cardiac complications of anesthesia during pregnancy, unspecified trimester**

\+ **O29.2 Central nervous system complications of anesthesia during pregnancy**
\+ **O29.21 Cerebral anoxia due to anesthesia during pregnancy**
• ♀ **O29.211 Cerebral anoxia due to anesthesia during pregnancy, first trimester**
• ♀ **O29.212 Cerebral anoxia due to anesthesia during pregnancy, second trimester**
• ♀ **O29.213 Cerebral anoxia due to anesthesia during pregnancy, third trimester**
• ♀ **O29.219 Cerebral anoxia due to anesthesia during pregnancy, unspecified trimester**

+ O29.29 **Other central nervous system complications of anesthesia during pregnancy**

• ♀ O29.291 **Other central nervous system complications of anesthesia during pregnancy, first trimester**

• ♀ O29.292 **Other central nervous system complications of anesthesia during pregnancy, second trimester**

• ♀ O29.293 **Other central nervous system complications of anesthesia during pregnancy, third trimester**

• ♀ O29.299 **Other central nervous system complications of anesthesia during pregnancy, unspecified trimester**

+ O29.3 **Toxic reaction to local anesthesia during pregnancy**

+ O29.3X **Toxic reaction to local anesthesia during pregnancy**

• ♀ O29.3X1 **Toxic reaction to local anesthesia during pregnancy, first trimester**

• ♀ O29.3X2 **Toxic reaction to local anesthesia during pregnancy, second trimester**

• ♀ O29.3X3 **Toxic reaction to local anesthesia during pregnancy, third trimester**

• ♀ O29.3X9 **Toxic reaction to local anesthesia during pregnancy, unspecified trimester**

+ O29.4 **Spinal and epidural anesthesia induced headache during pregnancy**

• ♀ O29.40 **Spinal and epidural anesthesia induced headache during pregnancy, unspecified trimester**

• ♀ O29.41 **Spinal and epidural anesthesia induced headache during pregnancy, first trimester**

• ♀ O29.42 **Spinal and epidural anesthesia induced headache during pregnancy, second trimester**

• ♀ O29.43 **Spinal and epidural anesthesia induced headache during pregnancy, third trimester**

+ O29.5 **Other complications of spinal and epidural anesthesia during pregnancy**

+ O29.5X **Other complications of spinal and epidural anesthesia during pregnancy**

• ♀ O29.5X1 **Other complications of spinal and epidural anesthesia during pregnancy, first trimester**

• ♀ O29.5X2 **Other complications of spinal and epidural anesthesia during pregnancy, second trimester**

• ♀ O29.5X3 **Other complications of spinal and epidural anesthesia during pregnancy, third trimester**

• ♀ O29.5X9 **Other complications of spinal and epidural anesthesia during pregnancy, unspecified trimester**

+ O29.6 **Failed or difficult intubation for anesthesia during pregnancy**

• ♀ O29.60 **Failed or difficult intubation for anesthesia during pregnancy, unspecified trimester**

• ♀ O29.61 **Failed or difficult intubation for anesthesia during pregnancy, first trimester**

• ♀ O29.62 **Failed or difficult intubation for anesthesia during pregnancy, second trimester**

• ♀ O29.63 **Failed or difficult intubation for anesthesia during pregnancy, third trimester**

+ O29.8 **Other complications of anesthesia during pregnancy**

+ O29.8X **Other complications of anesthesia during pregnancy**

• ♀ O29.8X1 **Other complications of anesthesia during pregnancy, first trimester**

• ♀ O29.8X2 **Other complications of anesthesia during pregnancy, second trimester**

• ♀ O29.8X3 **Other complications of anesthesia during pregnancy, third trimester**

• ♀ O29.8X9 **Other complications of anesthesia during pregnancy, unspecified trimester**

+ O29.9 **Unspecified complication of anesthesia during pregnancy**

• ♀ O29.90 **Unspecified complication of anesthesia during pregnancy, unspecified trimester**

• ♀ O29.91 **Unspecified complication of anesthesia during pregnancy, first trimester**

• ♀ O29.92 **Unspecified complication of anesthesia during pregnancy, second trimester**

• ♀ O29.93 **Unspecified complication of anesthesia during pregnancy, third trimester**

Maternal care related to the fetus and amniotic cavity and possible delivery problems (O30-O48)

O30 **Multiple gestation**

Code also any complications specific to multiple gestation

+ O30.0 **Twin pregnancy**

+ O30.00 **Twin pregnancy, unspecified number of placenta and unspecified number of amniotic sacs**

• ♀ O30.001 **Twin pregnancy, unspecified number of placenta and unspecified number of amniotic sacs, first trimester**

• ♀ O30.002 **Twin pregnancy, unspecified number of placenta and unspecified number of amniotic sacs, second trimester**

• ♀ O30.003 **Twin pregnancy, unspecified number of placenta and unspecified number of amniotic sacs, third trimester**

• ♀ O30.009 **Twin pregnancy, unspecified number of placenta and unspecified number of amniotic sacs, unspecified trimester**

+ O30.01 **Twin pregnancy, monochorionic/monoamniotic**

Twin pregnancy, one placenta, one amniotic sac

Excludes1: *conjoined twins (O30.02-)*

• ♀ O30.011 **Twin pregnancy, monochorionic/monoamniotic, first trimester**

• ♀ O30.012 **Twin pregnancy, monochorionic/monoamniotic, second trimester**

• ♀ O30.013 **Twin pregnancy, monochorionic/monoamniotic, third trimester**

• ♀ O30.019 **Twin pregnancy, monochorionic/monoamniotic, unspecified trimester**

+ O30.02 **Conjoined twin pregnancy**

• ♀ O30.021 **Conjoined twin pregnancy, first trimester**

• ♀ O30.022 **Conjoined twin pregnancy, second trimester**

• ♀ O30.023 **Conjoined twin pregnancy, third trimester**

• ♀ O30.029 **Conjoined twin pregnancy, unspecified trimester**

+ O30.03 **Twin pregnancy, monochorionic/diamniotic**

Twin pregnancy, one placenta, two amniotic sacs

• ♀ O30.031 **Twin pregnancy, monochorionic/diamniotic, first trimester**

• ♀ O30.032 **Twin pregnancy, monochorionic/diamniotic, second trimester**

• ♀ O30.033 **Twin pregnancy, monochorionic/diamniotic, third trimester**

• ♀ O30.039 **Twin pregnancy, monochorionic/diamniotic, unspecified trimester**

+ O30.04 **Twin pregnancy, dichorionic/diamniotic**

Twin pregnancy, two placentae, two amniotic sacs

• ♀ O30.041 **Twin pregnancy, dichorionic/diamniotic, first trimester**

• ♀ O30.042 **Twin pregnancy, dichorionic/diamniotic, second trimester**

• ♀ O30.043 **Twin pregnancy, dichorionic/diamniotic, third trimester**

• ♀ O30.049 **Twin pregnancy, dichorionic/diamniotic, unspecified trimester**

+ O30.09 **Twin pregnancy, unable to determine number of placenta and number of amniotic sacs**

• ♀ O30.091 **Twin pregnancy, unable to determine number of placenta and number of amniotic sacs, first trimester**

• ♀ O30.092 **Twin pregnancy, unable to determine number of placenta and number of amniotic sacs, second trimester**

• ♀ O30.093 **Twin pregnancy, unable to determine number of placenta and number of amniotic sacs, third trimester**

• ♀ O30.099 **Twin pregnancy, unable to determine number of placenta and number of amniotic sacs, unspecified trimester**

+ **O30.1 Triplet pregnancy**
  + **O30.10 Triplet pregnancy, unspecified number of placenta and unspecified number of amniotic sacs**
    - ● ♀ CC **O30.101 Triplet pregnancy, unspecified number of placenta and unspecified number of amniotic sacs, first trimester**
    - ● ♀ CC **O30.102 Triplet pregnancy, unspecified number of placenta and unspecified number of amniotic sacs, second trimester**
    - ● ♀ CC **O30.103 Triplet pregnancy, unspecified number of placenta and unspecified number of amniotic sacs, third trimester**
      AHA CC: 2Q, 2016, 8
    - ● ♀ **O30.109 Triplet pregnancy, unspecified number of placenta and unspecified number of amniotic sacs, unspecified trimester**
  + **O30.11 Triplet pregnancy with two or more monochorionic fetuses**
    - ● ♀ CC **O30.111 Triplet pregnancy with two or more monochorionic fetuses, first trimester**
    - ● ♀ CC **O30.112 Triplet pregnancy with two or more monochorionic fetuses, second trimester**
    - ● ♀ CC **O30.113 Triplet pregnancy with two or more monochorionic fetuses, third trimester**
    - ● ♀ **O30.119 Triplet pregnancy with two or more monochorionic fetuses, unspecified trimester**
  + **O30.12 Triplet pregnancy with two or more monoamniotic fetuses**
    - ● ♀ CC **O30.121 Triplet pregnancy with two or more monoamniotic fetuses, first trimester**
    - ● ♀ CC **O30.122 Triplet pregnancy with two or more monoamniotic fetuses, second trimester**
    - ● ♀ CC **O30.123 Triplet pregnancy with two or more monoamniotic fetuses, third trimester**
    - ● ♀ **O30.129 Triplet pregnancy with two or more monoamniotic fetuses, unspecified trimester**
  + **O30.13 Triplet pregnancy, trichorionic/trimniotic**
    AHA CC: 4Q, 2018, 22
    - ● ♀ CC **O30.131 Triplet pregnancy, trichorionic/triamniotic, first trimester**
    - ● ♀ CC **O30.132 Triplet pregnancy, trichorionic/triamniotic, second trimester**
    - ● ♀ CC **O30.133 Triplet pregnancy, trichorionic/triamniotic, third trimester**
    - ● ♀ **O30.139 Triplet pregnancy, trichorionic/triamniotic, unspecified trimester**
  + **O30.19 Triplet pregnancy, unable to determine number of placenta and number of amniotic sacs**
    - ● ♀ CC **O30.191 Triplet pregnancy, unable to determine number of placenta and number of amniotic sacs, first trimester**
    - ● ♀ CC **O30.192 Triplet pregnancy, unable to determine number of placenta and number of amniotic sacs, second trimester**
    - ● ♀ CC **O30.193 Triplet pregnancy, unable to determine number of placenta and number of amniotic sacs, third trimester**
    - ● ♀ **O30.199 Triplet pregnancy, unable to determine number of placenta and number of amniotic sacs, unspecified trimester**

+ **O30.2 Quadruplet pregnancy**
  + **O30.20 Quadruplet pregnancy, unspecified number of placenta and unspecified number of amniotic sacs**
    - ● ♀ CC **O30.201 Quadruplet pregnancy, unspecified number of placenta and unspecified number of amniotic sacs, first trimester**
    - ● ♀ CC **O30.202 Quadruplet pregnancy, unspecified number of placenta and unspecified number of amniotic sacs, second trimester**
    - ● ♀ CC **O30.203 Quadruplet pregnancy, unspecified number of placenta and unspecified number of amniotic sacs, third trimester**
    - ● ♀ **O30.209 Quadruplet pregnancy, unspecified number of placenta and unspecified number of amniotic sacs, unspecified trimester**
  + **O30.21 Quadruplet pregnancy with two or more monochorionic fetuses**
    - ● ♀ CC **O30.211 Quadruplet pregnancy with two or more monochorionic fetuses, first trimester**
    - ● ♀ CC **O30.212 Quadruplet pregnancy with two or more monochorionic fetuses, second trimester**
    - ● ♀ CC **O30.213 Quadruplet pregnancy with two or more monochorionic fetuses, third trimester**
    - ● ♀ **O30.219 Quadruplet pregnancy with two or more monochorionic fetuses, unspecified trimester**
  + **O30.22 Quadruplet pregnancy with two or more monoamniotic fetuses**
    - ● ♀ CC **O30.221 Quadruplet pregnancy with two or more monoamniotic fetuses, first trimester**
    - ● ♀ CC **O30.222 Quadruplet pregnancy with two or more monoamniotic fetuses, second trimester**
    - ● ♀ CC **O30.223 Quadruplet pregnancy with two or more monoamniotic fetuses, third trimester**
    - ● ♀ **O30.229 Quadruplet pregnancy with two or more monoamniotic fetuses, unspecified trimester**
  + **O30.23 Quadruplet pregnancy, quadrachorionic/quadra-amniotic**
    AHA CC: 4Q, 2018, 22
    - ● ♀ CC **O30.231 Quadruplet pregnancy, quadrachorionic/quadra-amniotic, first trimester**
    - ● ♀ CC **O30.232 Quadruplet pregnancy, quadrachorionic/quadra-amniotic, second trimester**
    - ● ♀ CC **O30.233 Quadruplet pregnancy, quadrachorionic/quadra-amniotic, third trimester**
    - ● ♀ **O30.239 Quadruplet pregnancy, quadrachorionic/quadra-amniotic, unspecified trimester**
  + **O30.29 Quadruplet pregnancy, unable to determine number of placenta and number of amniotic sacs**
    - ● ♀ CC **O30.291 Quadruplet pregnancy, unable to determine number of placenta and number of amniotic sacs, first trimester**
    - ● ♀ CC **O30.292 Quadruplet pregnancy, unable to determine number of placenta and number of amniotic sacs, second trimester**
    - ● ♀ CC **O30.293 Quadruplet pregnancy, unable to determine number of placenta and number of amniotic sacs, third trimester**
    - ● ♀ **O30.299 Quadruplet pregnancy, unable to determine number of placenta and number of amniotic sacs, unspecified trimester**

+ **O30.8 Other specified multiple gestation**
  Multiple gestation pregnancy greater then quadruplets
  + **O30.80 Other specified multiple gestation, unspecified number of placenta and unspecified number of amniotic sacs**
    - ● ♀ CC **O30.801 Other specified multiple gestation, unspecified number of placenta and unspecified number of amniotic sacs, first trimester**
    - ● ♀ CC **O30.802 Other specified multiple gestation, unspecified number of placenta and unspecified number of amniotic sacs, second trimester**
    - ● ♀ CC **O30.803 Other specified multiple gestation, unspecified number of placenta and unspecified number of amniotic sacs, third trimester**
    - ● ♀ **O30.809 Other specified multiple gestation, unspecified number of placenta and unspecified number of amniotic sacs, unspecified trimester**

+ O30.81 **Other specified multiple gestation with two or more monochorionic fetuses**

● ♀ CC **O30.811 Other specified multiple gestation with two or more monochorionic fetuses, first trimester**

● ♀ CC **O30.812 Other specified multiple gestation with two or more monochorionic fetuses, second trimester**

● ♀ CC **O30.813 Other specified multiple gestation with two or more monochorionic fetuses, third trimester**

● ♀ **O30.819 Other specified multiple gestation with two or more monochorionic fetuses, unspecified trimester**

+ **O30.82 Other specified multiple gestation with two or more monoamniotic fetuses**

● ♀ CC **O30.821 Other specified multiple gestation with two or more monoamniotic fetuses, first trimester**

● ♀ CC **O30.822 Other specified multiple gestation with two or more monoamniotic fetuses, second trimester**

● ♀ CC **O30.823 Other specified multiple gestation with two or more monoamniotic fetuses, third trimester**

● ♀ **O30.829 Other specified multiple gestation with two or more monoamniotic fetuses, unspecified trimester**

+ **O30.83 Other specified multiple gestation, number of chorions and amnions are both equal to the number of fetuses**

Pentachorionic, penta-amniotic pregnancy (quintuplets)

Hexachorionic, hexa-amniotic pregnancy (sextuplets)

Heptachorionic, hepta-amniotic pregnancy (septuplets)

AHA CC: 4Q, 2018, 22

● ♀ CC **O30.831 Other specified multiple gestation, number of chorions and amnions are both equal to the number of fetuses, first trimester**

● ♀ CC **O30.832 Other specified multiple gestation, number of chorions and amnions are both equal to the number of fetuses, second trimester**

● ♀ CC **O30.833 Other specified multiple gestation, number of chorions and amnions are both equal to the number of fetuses, third trimester**

● ♀ **O30.839 Other specified multiple gestation, number of chorions and amnions are both equal to the number of fetuses, unspecified trimester**

+ **O30.89 Other specified multiple gestation, unable to determine number of placenta and number of amniotic sacs**

● ♀ CC **O30.891 Other specified multiple gestation, unable to determine number of placenta and number of amniotic sacs, first trimester**

● ♀ CC **O30.892 Other specified multiple gestation, unable to determine number of placenta and number of amniotic sacs, second trimester**

● ♀ CC **O30.893 Other specified multiple gestation, unable to determine number of placenta and number of amniotic sacs, third trimester**

● ♀ **O30.899 Other specified multiple gestation, unable to determine number of placenta and number of amniotic sacs, unspecified trimester**

+ **O30.9 Multiple gestation, unspecified**

Multiple pregnancy NOS

● ♀ **O30.90 Multiple gestation, unspecified, unspecified trimester**

● ♀ **O30.91 Multiple gestation, unspecified, first trimester**

● ♀ **O30.92 Multiple gestation, unspecified, second trimester**

● ♀ **O30.93 Multiple gestation, unspecified, third trimester**

O31 Complications specific to multiple gestation

Excludes2: *delayed delivery of second twin, triplet, etc. (O63.2)*
malpresentation of one fetus or more (O32.9)
placental transfusion syndromes (O43.0-)

One of the following 7th characters is to be assigned to each code under category O31. 7th character 0 is for single gestations and multiple gestations where the fetus is unspecified. 7th characters 1 through 9 are for cases of multiple gestations to identify the fetus for which the code applies. The appropriate code from category O30, Multiple gestation, must also be assigned when assigning a code from category O31 that has a 7th character of 1 through 9.

0 - not applicable or unspecified
1 - fetus 1
2 - fetus 2
3 - fetus 3
4 - fetus 4
5 - fetus 5
9 - other fetus

+ **O31.0 Papyraceous fetus**

Fetus compressus

● ♀ X+7th **O31.00 Papyraceous fetus, unspecified trimester**

● ♀ X+7th **O31.01 Papyraceous fetus, first trimester**

● ♀ X+7th **O31.02 Papyraceous fetus, second trimester**

● ♀ X+7th **O31.03 Papyraceous fetus, third trimester**

+ **O31.1 Continuing pregnancy after spontaneous abortion of one fetus or more**

● ♀ X+7th **O31.10 Continuing pregnancy after spontaneous abortion of one fetus or more, unspecified trimester**

● ♀ X+7th **O31.11 Continuing pregnancy after spontaneous abortion of one fetus or more, first trimester**

● ♀ X+7th **O31.12 Continuing pregnancy after spontaneous abortion of one fetus or more, second trimester**

● ♀ X+7th **O31.13 Continuing pregnancy after spontaneous abortion of one fetus or more, third trimester**

+ **O31.2 Continuing pregnancy after intrauterine death of one fetus or more**

● ♀ X+7th **O31.20 Continuing pregnancy after intrauterine death of one fetus or more, unspecified trimester**

● ♀ X+7th **O31.21 Continuing pregnancy after intrauterine death of one fetus or more, first trimester**

● ♀ X+7th **O31.22 Continuing pregnancy after intrauterine death of one fetus or more, second trimester**

● ♀ X+7th **O31.23 Continuing pregnancy after intrauterine death of one fetus or more, third trimester**

+ **O31.3 Continuing pregnancy after elective fetal reduction of one fetus or more**

Continuing pregnancy after selective termination of one fetus or more

● ♀ X+7th **O31.30 Continuing pregnancy after elective fetal reduction of one fetus or more, unspecified trimester**

● ♀ X+7th **O31.31 Continuing pregnancy after elective fetal reduction of one fetus or more, first trimester**

● ♀ X+7th **O31.32 Continuing pregnancy after elective fetal reduction of one fetus or more, second trimester**

● ♀ X+7th **O31.33 Continuing pregnancy after elective fetal reduction of one fetus or more, third trimester**

+ **O31.8 Other complications specific to multiple gestation**

+ **O31.8X Other complications specific to multiple gestation**

● ♀ CC +7th **O31.8X1 Other complications specific to multiple gestation, first trimester**

● ♀ +7th **O31.8X2 Other complications specific to multiple gestation, second trimester**

● ♀ +7th **O31.8X3 Other complications specific to multiple gestation, third trimester**

● ♀ +7th **O31.8X9 Other complications specific to multiple gestation, unspecified trimester**

O32 Maternal care for malpresentation of fetus

Includes: the listed conditions as a reason for observation, hospitalization or other obstetric care of the mother, or for cesarean delivery before onset of labor

Excludes1: *malpresentation of fetus with obstructed labor (O64.-)*

One of the following 7th characters is to be assigned to each code under category O32. 7th character 0 is for single gestations and multiple gestations where the fetus is unspecified. 7th characters 1 through 9 are for cases of multiple gestations to identify the fetus for which the code applies. The appropriate code from category O30, Multiple gestation, must also be assigned when assigning a code from category O32 that has a 7th character of 1 through 9.
0 - not applicable or unspecified
1 - fetus 1
2 - fetus 2
3 - fetus 3
4 - fetus 4
5 - fetus 5
9 - other fetus

● ♀ X+7th **O32.0 Maternal care for unstable lie**

● ♀ X+7th **O32.1 Maternal care for breech presentation**
Maternal care for buttocks presentation
Maternal care for complete breech
Maternal care for frank breech
Excludes1: *footling presentation (O32.8)*
incomplete breech (O32.8)

● ♀ X+7th **O32.2 Maternal care for transverse and oblique lie**
Maternal care for oblique presentation
Maternal care for transverse presentation

● ♀ X+7th **O32.3 Maternal care for face, brow and chin presentation**

● ♀ X+7th **O32.4 Maternal care for high head at term**
Maternal care for failure of head to enter pelvic brim

● ♀ X+7th **O32.6 Maternal care for compound presentation**

● ♀ X+7th **O32.8 Maternal care for other malpresentation of fetus**
Maternal care for footling presentation
Maternal care for incomplete breech

● ♀ X+7th **O32.9 Maternal care for malpresentation of fetus, unspecified**

O33 Maternal care for disproportion

Includes: the listed conditions as a reason for observation, hospitalization or other obstetric care of the mother, or for cesarean delivery before onset of labor

Excludes1: *disproportion with obstructed labor (O65-O66)*

● ♀ CC **O33.0 Maternal care for disproportion due to deformity of maternal pelvic bones**
Maternal care for disproportion due to pelvic deformity causing disproportion NOS

● ♀ **O33.1 Maternal care for disproportion due to generally contracted pelvis**
Maternal care for disproportion due to contracted pelvis NOS causing disproportion

● ♀ **O33.2 Maternal care for disproportion due to inlet contraction of pelvis**
Maternal care for disproportion due to inlet contraction (pelvis) causing disproportion

● ♀ +7th **O33.3 Maternal care for disproportion due to outlet contraction of pelvis**
Maternal care for disproportion due to mid-cavity contraction (pelvis)
Maternal care for disproportion due to outlet contraction (pelvis)

One of the following 7th characters is to be assigned to code **O33.3.** 7th character 0 is for single gestations and multiple gestations where the fetus is unspecified. 7th characters 1 through 9 are for cases of multiple gestations to identify the fetus for which the code applies. The appropriate code from category O30, Multiple gestation, must also be assigned when assigning code O33.3 with a 7th character of 1 through 9.
0 - not applicable or unspecified
1 - fetus 1
2 - fetus 2
3 - fetus 3
4 - fetus 4
5 - fetus 5
9 - other fetus

● ♀ X+7th **O33.4 Maternal care for disproportion of mixed maternal and fetal origin**

One of the following 7th characters is to be assigned to code **O33.4.** 7th character 0 is for single gestations and multiple gestations where the fetus is unspecified. 7th characters 1 through 9 are for cases of multiple gestations to identify the fetus for which the code applies. The appropriate code from category O30, Multiple gestation, must also be assigned when assigning code O33.4 with a 7th character of 1 through 9.
0 - not applicable or unspecified
1 - fetus 1
2 - fetus 2
3 - fetus 3
4 - fetus 4
5 - fetus 5
9 - other fetus

● ♀ X+7th **O33.5 Maternal care for disproportion due to unusually large fetus**
Maternal care for disproportion due to disproportion of fetal origin with normally formed fetus
Maternal care for disproportion due to fetal disproportion NOS

One of the following 7th characters is to be assigned to code **O33.5.** 7th character 0 is for single gestations and multiple gestations where the fetus is unspecified. 7th characters 1 through 9 are for cases of multiple gestations to identify the fetus for which the code applies. The appropriate code from category O30, Multiple gestation, must also be assigned when assigning code O33.5 with a 7th character of 1 through 9.
0 - not applicable or unspecified
1 - fetus 1
2 - fetus 2
3 - fetus 3
4 - fetus 4
5 - fetus 5
9 - other fetus

● ♀ X+7th **O33.6 Maternal care for disproportion due to hydrocephalic fetus**

One of the following 7th characters is to be assigned to code **O33.6.** 7th character 0 is for single gestations and multiple gestations where the fetus is unspecified. 7th characters 1 through 9 are for cases of multiple gestations to identify the fetus for which the code applies. The appropriate code from category O30, Multiple gestation, must also be assigned when assigning code O33.6 with a 7th character of 1 through 9.
0 - not applicable or unspecified
1 - fetus 1
2 - fetus 2
3 - fetus 3
4 - fetus 4
5 - fetus 5
9 - other fetus

● ♀ X+7th **O33.7 Maternal care for disproportion due to other fetal deformities**
Maternal care for disproportion due to fetal ascites
Maternal care for disproportion due to fetal hydrops
Maternal care for disproportion due to fetal meningomyelocele
Maternal care for disproportion due to fetal sacral teratoma
Maternal care for disproportion due to fetal tumor
Excludes1: *obstructed labor due to other fetal deformities (O66.3)*
AHA CC: 4Q, 2016, 51

One of the following 7th characters is to be assigned to code **O33.7.** 7th character 0 is for single gestations and multiple gestations where the fetus is unspecified. 7th characters 1 through 9 are for cases of multiple gestations to identify the fetus for which the code applies. The appropriate code from category O30, Multiple gestation, must also be assigned when assigning code O33.7 with a 7th character of 1 through 9.
0 - not applicable or unspecified
1 - fetus 1
2 - fetus 2
3 - fetus 3
4 - fetus 4
5 - fetus 5
9 - other fetus

● ♀ **O33.8 Maternal care for disproportion of other origin**

● ♀ **O33.9 Maternal care for disproportion, unspecified**
Maternal care for disproportion due to cephalopelvic disproportion NOS
Maternal care for disproportion due to fetopelvic disproportion NOS

O34 Maternal care for abnormality of pelvic organs

Includes: the listed conditions as a reason for hospitalization or other obstetric care of the mother, or for cesarean delivery before onset of labor

Code first any associated obstructed labor (O65.5)

Use additional code for specific condition

+ **O34.0 Maternal care for congenital malformation of uterus**
  Maternal care for double uterus
  Maternal care for uterus bicornis
  - • ♀ **O34.00 Maternal care for unspecified congenital malformation of uterus, unspecified trimester**
  - • ♀ **O34.01 Maternal care for unspecified congenital malformation of uterus, first trimester**
  - • ♀ **O34.02 Maternal care for unspecified congenital malformation of uterus, second trimester**
  - • ♀ **O34.03 Maternal care for unspecified congenital malformation of uterus, third trimester**

+ **O34.1 Maternal care for benign tumor of corpus uteri**
  Excludes2: *maternal care for benign tumor of cervix (O34.4-)*
  maternal care for malignant neoplasm of uterus (O9A.1-)
  - • ♀ **O34.10 Maternal care for benign tumor of corpus uteri, unspecified trimester**
  - • ♀ **O34.11 Maternal care for benign tumor of corpus uteri, first trimester**
  - • ♀ **O34.12 Maternal care for benign tumor of corpus uteri, second trimester**
  - • ♀ **O34.13 Maternal care for benign tumor of corpus uteri, third trimester**

+ **O34.2 Maternal care due to uterine scar from previous surgery**
  - + **O34.21 Maternal care for scar from previous cesarean delivery**
    AHA CC: 4Q, 2016, 51-52
    - • ♀ **O34.211 Maternal care for low transverse scar from previous cesarean delivery**
      AHA CC: 3Q, 2018, 23-24
    - • ♀ **O34.212 Maternal care for vertical scar from previous cesarean delivery**
      Maternal care for classical scar from previous cesarean delivery
    - • ♀ **O34.218 Maternal care for other type scar from previous cesarean delivery**
      Mid-transverse T incision
      AHA CC: 4Q, 2020, 36
    - • ♀ **O34.219 Maternal care for unspecified type scar from previous cesarean delivery**
      AHA CC: 3Q, 2018, 23
  - • ♀ **O34.22 Maternal care for cesarean scar defect (isthmocele)**
    AHA CC: 4Q, 2020, 36
  - • ♀ **O34.29 Maternal care due to uterine scar from other previous surgery**
    Maternal care due to uterine scar from other transmural uterine

+ **O34.3 Maternal care for cervical incompetence**
  Maternal care for cerclage with or without cervical incompetence
  Maternal care for Shirodkar suture with or without cervical incompetence
  - • ♀ **O34.30 Maternal care for cervical incompetence, unspecified trimester**
  - • ♀ MCC **O34.31 Maternal care for cervical incompetence, first trimester**
  - • ♀ MCC **O34.32 Maternal care for cervical incompetence, second trimester**
  - • ♀ MCC **O34.33 Maternal care for cervical incompetence, third trimester**

+ **O34.4 Maternal care for other abnormalities of cervix**
  - • ♀ **O34.40 Maternal care for other abnormalities of cervix, unspecified trimester**
  - • ♀ **O34.41 Maternal care for other abnormalities of cervix, first trimester**
  - • ♀ **O34.42 Maternal care for other abnormalities of cervix, second trimester**
  - • ♀ **O34.43 Maternal care for other abnormalities of cervix, third trimester**

+ **O34.5 Maternal care for other abnormalities of gravid uterus**
  - + **O34.51 Maternal care for incarceration of gravid uterus**
    - • ♀ **O34.511 Maternal care for incarceration of gravid uterus, first trimester**
    - • ♀ **O34.512 Maternal care for incarceration of gravid uterus, second trimester**
    - • ♀ **O34.513 Maternal care for incarceration of gravid uterus, third trimester**
    - • ♀ **O34.519 Maternal care for incarceration of gravid uterus, unspecified trimester**
  - + **O34.52 Maternal care for prolapse of gravid uterus**
    - • ♀ **O34.521 Maternal care for prolapse of gravid uterus, first trimester**
    - • ♀ **O34.522 Maternal care for prolapse of gravid uterus, second trimester**
    - • ♀ **O34.523 Maternal care for prolapse of gravid uterus, third trimester**
    - • ♀ **O34.529 Maternal care for prolapse of gravid uterus, unspecified trimester**
  - + **O34.53 Maternal care for retroversion of gravid uterus**
    - • ♀ **O34.531 Maternal care for retroversion of gravid uterus, first trimester**
    - • ♀ **O34.532 Maternal care for retroversion of gravid uterus, second trimester**
    - • ♀ **O34.533 Maternal care for retroversion of gravid uterus, third trimester**
    - • ♀ **O34.539 Maternal care for retroversion of gravid uterus, unspecified trimester**
  - + **O34.59 Maternal care for other abnormalities of gravid uterus**
    - • ♀ **O34.591 Maternal care for other abnormalities of gravid uterus, first trimester**
    - • ♀ **O34.592 Maternal care for other abnormalities of gravid uterus, second trimester**
    - • ♀ **O34.593 Maternal care for other abnormalities of gravid uterus, third trimester**
    - • ♀ **O34.599 Maternal care for other abnormalities of gravid uterus, unspecified trimester**

O34.6 Maternal care for abnormality of vagina
  Excludes2: *maternal care for vaginal varices in pregnancy (O22.1-)*
  - • ♀ **O34.60 Maternal care for abnormality of vagina, unspecified trimester**
  - • ♀ **O34.61 Maternal care for abnormality of vagina, first trimester**
  - • ♀ **O34.62 Maternal care for abnormality of vagina, second trimester**
  - • ♀ **O34.63 Maternal care for abnormality of vagina, third trimester**

+ **O34.7 Maternal care for abnormality of vulva and perineum**
  Excludes2: *maternal care for perineal and vulval varices in pregnancy (O22.1-)*
  - • ♀ **O34.70 Maternal care for abnormality of vulva and perineum, unspecified trimester**
  - • ♀ **O34.71 Maternal care for abnormality of vulva and perineum, first trimester**
  - • ♀ **O34.72 Maternal care for abnormality of vulva and perineum, second trimester**
  - • ♀ **O34.73 Maternal care for abnormality of vulva and perineum, third trimester**

+ **O34.8 Maternal care for other abnormalities of pelvic organs**
  - • ♀ **O34.80 Maternal care for other abnormalities of pelvic organs, unspecified trimester**
  - • ♀ **O34.81 Maternal care for other abnormalities of pelvic organs, first trimester**
  - • ♀ **O34.82 Maternal care for other abnormalities of pelvic organs, second trimester**
  - • ♀ **O34.83 Maternal care for other abnormalities of pelvic organs, third trimester**

+ **O34.9 Maternal care for abnormality of pelvic organ, unspecified**
  - • ♀ **O34.90 Maternal care for abnormality of pelvic organ, unspecified, unspecified trimester**
  - • ♀ **O34.91 Maternal care for abnormality of pelvic organ, unspecified, first trimester**
  - • ♀ **O34.92 Maternal care for abnormality of pelvic organ, unspecified, second trimester**
  - • ♀ **O34.93 Maternal care for abnormality of pelvic organ, unspecified, third trimester**

O35 Maternal care for known or suspected fetal abnormality and damage

Includes: the listed conditions in the fetus as a reason for hospitalization or other obstetric care to the mother, or for termination of pregnancy

Code also any associated maternal condition

Excludes1: *encounter for suspected maternal and fetal conditions ruled out (Z03.7-)*

One of the following 7th characters is to be assigned to each code under category O35. 7th character 0 is for single gestations and multiple gestations where the fetus is unspecified. 7th characters 1 through 9 are for cases of multiple gestations to identify the fetus for which the code applies. The appropriate code from category O30, Multiple gestation, must also be assigned when assigning a code from category O35 that has a 7th character of 1 through 9.
0 - not applicable or unspecified
1 - fetus 1
2 - fetus 2
3 - fetus 3
4 - fetus 4
5 - fetus 5
9 - other fetus

Review coding guideline C.15.e

- • ♀ X+7th **O35.0 Maternal care for (suspected) central nervous system malformation in fetus**
  Maternal care for fetal anencephaly
  Maternal care for fetal hydrocephalus
  Maternal care for fetal spina bifida
  Excludes2: *chromosomal abnormality in fetus (O35.1)*
- • ♀ X+7th **O35.1 Maternal care for (suspected) chromosomal abnormality in fetus**
- • ♀ X+7th **O35.2 Maternal care for (suspected) hereditary disease in fetus**
  Excludes2: *chromosomal abnormality in fetus (O35.1)*
- • ♀ X+7th **O35.3 Maternal care for (suspected) damage to fetus from viral disease in mother**
  Maternal care for damage to fetus from maternal cytomegalovirus infection
  Maternal care for damage to fetus from maternal rubella
  AHA CC: 4Q, 2016, 4-7
- • ♀ X+7th **O35.4 Maternal care for (suspected) damage to fetus from alcohol**
- • ♀ X+7th **O35.5 Maternal care for (suspected) damage to fetus by drugs**
  Maternal care for damage to fetus from drug addiction
- • ♀ X+7th **O35.6 Maternal care for (suspected) damage to fetus by radiation**
- • ♀ X+7th **O35.7 Maternal care for (suspected) damage to fetus by other medical procedures**
  Maternal care for damage to fetus by amniocentesis
  Maternal care for damage to fetus by biopsy procedures
  Maternal care for damage to fetus by hematological investigation
  Maternal care for damage to fetus by intrauterine contraceptive device
  Maternal care for damage to fetus by intrauterine surgery
- • ♀ X+7th **O35.8 Maternal care for other (suspected) fetal abnormality and damage**
  Maternal care for damage to fetus from maternal listeriosis
  Maternal care for damage to fetus from maternal toxoplasmosis
- • ♀ X+7th **O35.9 Maternal care for (suspected) fetal abnormality and damage, unspecified**

O36 Maternal care for other fetal problems

Includes: the listed conditions in the fetus as a reason for hospitalization or other obstetric care of the mother, or for termination of pregnancy

Excludes1: *encounter for suspected maternal and fetal conditions ruled out (Z03.7-)*
placental transfusion syndromes (O43.0-)

Excludes2: *labor and delivery complicated by fetal stress (O77.-)*

One of the following 7th characters is to be assigned to each code under category O36. 7th character 0 is for single gestations and multiple gestations where the fetus is unspecified. 7th characters 1 through 9 are for cases of multiple gestations to identify the fetus for which the code applies. The appropriate code from category O30, Multiple gestation, must also be assigned when assigning a code from category O36 that has a 7th character of 1 through 9.
0 - not applicable or unspecified
1 - fetus 1
2 - fetus 2
3 - fetus 3
4 - fetus 4
5 - fetus 5
9 - other fetus

Review coding guideline C.15.e

+ **O36.0 Maternal care for rhesus isoimmunization**
  Maternal care for Rh incompatibility (with hydrops fetalis)
  + **O36.01 Maternal care for anti-D [Rh] antibodies**
    - • ♀ CC +7th **O36.011 Maternal care for anti-D [Rh] antibodies, first trimester**
    - • ♀ CC +7th **O36.012 Maternal care for anti-D [Rh] antibodies, second trimester**
    - • ♀ CC +7th **O36.013 Maternal care for anti-D [Rh] antibodies, third trimester**
      AHA CC: 4Q, 2014, 17-18
    - • ♀ +7th **O36.019 Maternal care for anti-D [Rh] antibodies, unspecified trimester**
  + **O36.09 Maternal care for other rhesus isoimmunization**
    - • ♀ CC +7th **O36.091 Maternal care for other rhesus isoimmunization, first trimester**
    - • ♀ CC +7th **O36.092 Maternal care for other rhesus isoimmunization, second trimester**
    - • ♀ CC +7th **O36.093 Maternal care for other rhesus isoimmunization, third trimester**
    - • ♀ +7th **O36.099 Maternal care for other rhesus isoimmunization, unspecified trimester**
+ **O36.1 Maternal care for other isoimmunization**
  Maternal care for ABO isoimmunization
  + **O36.11 Maternal care for Anti-A sensitization**
    Maternal care for isoimmunization NOS (with hydrops fetalis)
    - • ♀ +7th **O36.111 Maternal care for Anti-A sensitization, first trimester**
    - • ♀ +7th **O36.112 Maternal care for Anti-A sensitization, second trimester**
    - • ♀ +7th **O36.113 Maternal care for Anti-A sensitization, third trimester**
    - • ♀ +7th **O36.119 Maternal care for Anti-A sensitization, unspecified trimester**
  + **O36.19 Maternal care for other isoimmunization**
    Maternal care for Anti-B sensitization
    - • ♀ +7th **O36.191 Maternal care for other isoimmunization, first trimester**
    - • ♀ +7th **O36.192 Maternal care for other isoimmunization, second trimester**
    - • ♀ +7th **O36.193 Maternal care for other isoimmunization, third trimester**
    - • ♀ +7th **O36.199 Maternal care for other isoimmunization, unspecified trimester**

+ **O36.2 Maternal care for hydrops fetalis**
Maternal care for hydrops fetalis NOS
Maternal care for hydrops fetalis not associated with isoimmunization
Excludes1: *hydrops fetalis associated with ABO isoimmunization (O36.1-)*
hydrops fetalis associated with rhesus isoimmunization (O36.0-)

• ♀ X+7th **O36.20 Maternal care for hydrops fetalis, unspecified trimester**
• ♀ X+7th **O36.21 Maternal care for hydrops fetalis, first trimester**
• ♀ X+7th **O36.22 Maternal care for hydrops fetalis, second trimester**
• ♀ X+7th **O36.23 Maternal care for hydrops fetalis, third trimester**

• ♀ CC X+7th **O36.4 Maternal care for intrauterine death**
Maternal care for intrauterine fetal death NOS
Maternal care for intrauterine fetal death after completion of 20 weeks of gestation
Maternal care for late fetal death
Maternal care for missed delivery
Excludes1: *missed abortion (O02.1)stillbirth (P95)*

+ **O36.5 Maternal care for known or suspected poor fetal growth**
+ **O36.51 Maternal care for known or suspected placental insufficiency**
• ♀ +7th **O36.511 Maternal care for known or suspected placental insufficiency, first trimester**
• ♀ +7th **O36.512 Maternal care for known or suspected placental insufficiency, second trimester**
• ♀ +7th **O36.513 Maternal care for known or suspected placental insufficiency, third trimester**
• ♀ +7th **O36.519 Maternal care for known or suspected placental insufficiency, unspecified trimester**

+ **O36.59 Maternal care for other known or suspected poor fetal growth**
Maternal care for known or suspected light-for-dates NOS
Maternal care for known or suspected small-for-dates NOS
• ♀ +7th **O36.591 Maternal care for other known or suspected poor fetal growth, first trimester**
• ♀ +7th **O36.592 Maternal care for other known or suspected poor fetal growth, second trimester**
• ♀ +7th **O36.593 Maternal care for other known or suspected poor fetal growth, third trimester**
• ♀ +7th **O36.599 Maternal care for other known or suspected poor fetal growth, unspecified trimester**

+ **O36.6 Maternal care for excessive fetal growth**
Maternal care for known or suspected large-for-dates
• ♀ X+7th **O36.60 Maternal care for excessive fetal growth, unspecified trimester**
• ♀ X+7th **O36.61 Maternal care for excessive fetal growth, first trimester**
• ♀ X+7th **O36.62 Maternal care for excessive fetal growth, second trimester**
• ♀ X+7th **O36.63 Maternal care for excessive fetal growth, third trimester**

+ **O36.7 Maternal care for viable fetus in abdominal pregnancy**
• ♀ X+7th **O36.70 Maternal care for viable fetus in abdominal pregnancy, unspecified trimester**
• ♀ X+7th **O36.71 Maternal care for viable fetus in abdominal pregnancy, first trimester**
• ♀ X+7th **O36.72 Maternal care for viable fetus in abdominal pregnancy, second trimester**
• ♀ X+7th **O36.73 Maternal care for viable fetus in abdominal pregnancy, third trimester**

+ **O36.8 Maternal care for other specified fetal problems**
• ♀ X+7th **O36.80 Pregnancy with inconclusive fetal viability**
Encounter to determine fetal viability of pregnancy
AHA CC: 2Q, 2019, 29

+ **O36.81 Decreased fetal movements**
• ♀ +7th **O36.812 Decreased fetal movements, second trimester**
• ♀ +7th **O36.813 Decreased fetal movements, third trimester**
• ♀ +7th **O36.819 Decreased fetal movements, unspecified trimester**

+ **O36.82 Fetal anemia and thrombocytopenia**
• ♀ +7th **O36.821 Fetal anemia and thrombocytopenia, first trimester**
• ♀ +7th **O36.822 Fetal anemia and thrombocytopenia, second trimester**
• ♀ +7th **O36.823 Fetal anemia and thrombocytopenia, third trimester**
• ♀ +7th **O36.829 Fetal anemia and thrombocytopenia, unspecified trimester**

+ **O36.83 Maternal care for abnormalities of the fetal heart rate or rhythm**
Maternal care for depressed fetal heart rate tones
Maternal care for fetal bradycardia
Maternal care for fetal heart rate abnormal variability
Maternal care for fetal heart rate decelerations
Maternal care for fetal heart rate irregularity
Maternal care for fetal tachycardia
Maternal care for non-reassuring fetal heart rate or rhythm
AHA CC: 4Q, 2017, 20
• ♀ +7th **O36.831 Maternal care for abnormalities of the fetal heart rate or rhythm, first trimester**
• ♀ +7th **O36.832 Maternal care for abnormalities of the fetal heart rate or rhythm, second trimester**
• ♀ +7th **O36.833 Maternal care for abnormalities of the fetal heart rate or rhythm, third trimester**
• ♀ +7th **O36.839 Maternal care for abnormalities of the fetal heart rate or rhythm, unspecified trimester**

+ **O36.89 Maternal care for other specified fetal problems**
• ♀ +7th **O36.891 Maternal care for other specified fetal problems, first trimester**
• ♀ +7th **O36.892 Maternal care for other specified fetal problems, second trimester**
• ♀ +7th **O36.893 Maternal care for other specified fetal problems, third trimester**
• ♀ +7th **O36.899 Maternal care for other specified fetal problems, unspecified trimester**

+ **O36.9 Maternal care for fetal problem, unspecified**
• ♀ X+7th **O36.90 Maternal care for fetal problem, unspecified, unspecified trimester**
• ♀ X+7th **O36.91 Maternal care for fetal problem, unspecified, first trimester**
• ♀ X+7th **O36.92 Maternal care for fetal problem, unspecified, second trimester**
• ♀ X+7th **O36.93 Maternal care for fetal problem, unspecified, third trimester**

O40 Polyhydramnios

Includes: hydramnios
Excludes1: *encounter for suspected maternal and fetal conditions ruled out (Z03.7-)*

One of the following 7th characters is to be assigned to each code under category O40. 7th character 0 is for single gestations and multiple gestations where the fetus is unspecified. 7th characters 1 through 9 are for cases of multiple gestations to identify the fetus for which the code applies. The appropriate code from category O30, Multiple gestation, must also be assigned when assigning a code from category O40 that has a 7th character of 1 through 9.
0 - not applicable or unspecified
1 - fetus 1
2 - fetus 2
3 - fetus 3
4 - fetus 4
5 - fetus 5
9 - other fetus

• ♀ X+7th **O40.1 Polyhydramnios, first trimester**
• ♀ X+7th **O40.2 Polyhydramnios, second trimester**
• ♀ X+7th **O40.3 Polyhydramnios, third trimester**
• ♀ X+7th **O40.9 Polyhydramnios, unspecified trimester**

O41 Other disorders of amniotic fluid and membranes

Excludes1: *encounter for suspected maternal and fetal conditions ruled out (Z03.7-)*

One of the following 7th characters is to be assigned to each code under category O41. 7th character 0 is for single gestations and multiple gestations where the fetus is unspecified. 7th characters 1 through 9 are for cases of multiple gestations to identify the fetus for which the code applies. The appropriate code from category O30, Multiple gestation, must also be assigned when assigning a code from category O41 that has a 7th character of 1 through 9.

0 - not applicable or unspecified
1 - fetus 1
2 - fetus 2
3 - fetus 3
4 - fetus 4
5 - fetus 5
9 - other fetus

+ **O41.0 Oligohydramnios**
  Oligohydramnios without rupture of membranes
  - • ♀ X+7th **O41.00 Oligohydramnios, unspecified trimester**
  - • ♀ CC X+7th **O41.01 Oligohydramnios, first trimester**
  - • ♀ CC X+7th **O41.02 Oligohydramnios, second trimester**
  - • ♀ CC X+7th **O41.03 Oligohydramnios, third trimester**
+ **O41.1 Infection of amniotic sac and membranes**
  - + **O41.10 Infection of amniotic sac and membranes, unspecified**
    - • ♀ MCC +7th **O41.101 Infection of amniotic sac and membranes, unspecified, first trimester**
    - • ♀ MCC +7th **O41.102 Infection of amniotic sac and membranes, unspecified, second trimester**
    - • ♀ MCC +7th **O41.103 Infection of amniotic sac and membranes, unspecified, third trimester**
    - • ♀ +7th **O41.109 Infection of amniotic sac and membranes, unspecified, unspecified trimester**
  - + **O41.12 Chorioamnionitis**
    AHA CC: 2Q, 2019, 34-35
    - • ♀ MCC +7th **O41.121 Chorioamnionitis, first trimester**
    - • ♀ MCC +7th **O41.122 Chorioamnionitis, second trimester**
    - • ♀ MCC +7th **O41.123 Chorioamnionitis, third trimester**
    - • ♀ +7th **O41.129 Chorioamnionitis, unspecified trimester**
  - + **O41.14 Placentitis**
    - • ♀ MCC +7th **O41.141 Placentitis, first trimester**
    - • ♀ MCC +7th **O41.142 Placentitis, second trimester**
    - • ♀ MCC +7th **O41.143 Placentitis, third trimester**
    - • ♀ +7th **O41.149 Placentitis, unspecified trimester**
+ **O41.8 Other specified disorders of amniotic fluid and membranes**
  - + **O41.8X Other specified disorders of amniotic fluid and membranes**
    - • ♀ +7th **O41.8X1 Other specified disorders of amniotic fluid and membranes, first trimester**
    - • ♀ +7th **O41.8X2 Other specified disorders of amniotic fluid and membranes, second trimester**
    - • ♀ +7th **O41.8X3 Other specified disorders of amniotic fluid and membranes, third trimester**
    - • ♀ +7th **O41.8X9 Other specified disorders of amniotic fluid and membranes, unspecified trimester**
+ **O41.9 Disorder of amniotic fluid and membranes, unspecified**
  - • ♀ X+7th **O41.90 Disorder of amniotic fluid and membranes, unspecified, unspecified trimester**
  - • ♀ X+7th **O41.91 Disorder of amniotic fluid and membranes, unspecified, first trimester**
  - • ♀ X+7th **O41.92 Disorder of amniotic fluid and membranes, unspecified, second trimester**
  - • ♀ X+7th **O41.93 Disorder of amniotic fluid and membranes, unspecified, third trimester**

O42 Premature rupture of membranes

+ **O42.0 Premature rupture of membranes, onset of labor within 24 hours of rupture**
  - • ♀ **O42.00 Premature rupture of membranes, onset of labor within 24 hours of rupture, unspecified weeks of gestation**
  - + **O42.01 Preterm premature rupture of membranes, onset of labor within 24 hours of rupture**
    Premature rupture of membranes before 37 completed weeks of gestation, onset of labor within 24 hours of rupture
    - • ♀ **O42.011 Preterm premature rupture of membranes, onset of labor within 24 hours of rupture, first trimester**
    - • ♀ **O42.012 Preterm premature rupture of membranes, onset of labor within 24 hours of rupture, second trimester**
    - • ♀ **O42.013 Preterm premature rupture of membranes, onset of labor within 24 hours of rupture, third trimester**
    - • ♀ **O42.019 Preterm premature rupture of membranes, onset of labor within 24 hours of rupture, unspecified trimester**
  - • ♀ **O42.02 Full-term premature rupture of membranes, onset of labor within 24 hours of rupture**
    Premature rupture of membranes at or after 37 completed weeks of gestation, onset of labor within 24 hours of rupture
+ **O42.1 Premature rupture of membranes, onset of labor more than 24 hours following rupture**
  - • ♀ **O42.10 Premature rupture of membranes, onset of labor more than 24 hours following rupture, unspecified weeks of gestation**
  - + **O42.11 Preterm premature rupture of membranes, onset of labor more than 24 hours following rupture**
    Premature rupture of membranes before 37 completed weeks of gestation
    - • ♀ **O42.111 Preterm premature rupture of membranes, onset of labor more than 24 hours following rupture, first trimester**
    - • ♀ **O42.112 Preterm premature rupture of membranes, onset of labor more than 24 hours following rupture, second trimester**
    - • ♀ **O42.113 Preterm premature rupture of membranes, onset of labor more than 24 hours following rupture, third trimester**
    - • ♀ **O42.119 Preterm premature rupture of membranes, onset of labor more than 24 hours following rupture, unspecified trimester**
  - • ♀ **O42.12 Full-term premature rupture of membranes, onset of labor more than 24 hours following rupture**
    Premature rupture of membranes at or after 37 completed weeks of gestation, onset of labor more than 24 hours following rupture
+ **O42.9 Premature rupture of membranes, unspecified as to length of time between rupture and onset of labor**
  - • ♀ **O42.90 Premature rupture of membranes, unspecified as to length of time between rupture and onset of labor, unspecified weeks of gestation**
  - + **O42.91 Preterm premature rupture of membranes, unspecified as to length of time between rupture and onset of labor**
    Premature rupture of membranes before 37 completed weeks of gestation
    - • ♀ **O42.911 Preterm premature rupture of membranes, unspecified as to length of time between rupture and onset of labor, first trimester**
    - • ♀ **O42.912 Preterm premature rupture of membranes, unspecified as to length of time between rupture and onset of labor, second trimester**
    - • ♀ **O42.913 Preterm premature rupture of membranes, unspecified as to length of time between rupture and onset of labor, third trimester**
    - • ♀ **O42.919 Preterm premature rupture of membranes, unspecified as to length of time between rupture and onset of labor, unspecified trimester**

- • ♀ **O42.92 Full-term premature rupture of membranes, unspecified as to length of time between rupture and onset of labor**
  Premature rupture of membranes at or after 37 completed weeks of gestation, unspecified as to length of time between rupture and onset of labor

O43 Placental disorders

Excludes2: *maternal care for poor fetal growth due to placental insufficiency (O36.5-)*
placenta previa (O44.-)
placental polyp (O90.89)
placentitis (O41.14-)
premature separation of placenta [abruptio placentae] (O45.-)

- \+ **O43.0 Placental transfusion syndromes**
  - \+ **O43.01 Fetomaternal placental transfusion syndrome**
    Maternofetal placental transfusion syndrome
    - • ♀ **O43.011 Fetomaternal placental transfusion syndrome, first trimester**
    - • ♀ **O43.012 Fetomaternal placental transfusion syndrome, second trimester**
    - • ♀ **O43.013 Fetomaternal placental transfusion syndrome, third trimester**
    - • ♀ **O43.019 Fetomaternal placental transfusion syndrome, unspecified trimester**
  - \+ **O43.02 Fetus-to-fetus placental transfusion syndrome**
    - • ♀ **O43.021 Fetus-to-fetus placental transfusion syndrome, first trimester**
    - • ♀ **O43.022 Fetus-to-fetus placental transfusion syndrome, second trimester**
    - • ♀ **O43.023 Fetus-to-fetus placental transfusion syndrome, third trimester**
    - • ♀ **O43.029 Fetus-to-fetus placental transfusion syndrome, unspecified trimester**
- \+ **O43.1 Malformation of placenta**
  - \+ **O43.10 Malformation of placenta, unspecified**
    Abnormal placenta NOS
    - • ♀ **O43.101 Malformation of placenta, unspecified, first trimester**
    - • ♀ **O43.102 Malformation of placenta, unspecified, second trimester**
    - • ♀ **O43.103 Malformation of placenta, unspecified, third trimester**
    - • ♀ **O43.109 Malformation of placenta, unspecified, unspecified trimester**
  - \+ **O43.11 Circumvallate placenta**
    - • ♀ **O43.111 Circumvallate placenta, first trimester**
    - • ♀ **O43.112 Circumvallate placenta, second trimester**
    - • ♀ **O43.113 Circumvallate placenta, third trimester**
    - • ♀ **O43.119 Circumvallate placenta, unspecified trimester**
  - \+ **O43.12 Velamentous insertion of umbilical cord**
    - • ♀ **O43.121 Velamentous insertion of umbilical cord, first trimester**
    - • ♀ **O43.122 Velamentous insertion of umbilical cord, second trimester**
    - • ♀ **O43.123 Velamentous insertion of umbilical cord, third trimester**
    - • ♀ **O43.129 Velamentous insertion of umbilical cord, unspecified trimester**
  - \+ **O43.19 Other malformation of placenta**
    - • ♀ **O43.191 Other malformation of placenta, first trimester**
    - • ♀ **O43.192 Other malformation of placenta, second trimester**
    - • ♀ **O43.193 Other malformation of placenta, third trimester**
    - • ♀ **O43.199 Other malformation of placenta, unspecified trimester**
- \+ **O43.2 Morbidly adherent placenta**
  Code also associated third stage postpartum hemorrhage, if applicable (O72.0)
  Excludes1: *retained placenta (O73.-)*
  - MCC + **O43.21 Placenta accreta**
    - • ♀ **O43.211 Placenta accreta, first trimester**
    - • ♀ **O43.212 Placenta accreta, second trimester**
    - • ♀ **O43.213 Placenta accreta, third trimester**
    - • ♀ **O43.219 accreta, unspecified trimester**
  - \+ **O43.22 Placenta increta**
    - • ♀ **O43.221 Placenta increta, first trimester**
    - • ♀ **O43.222 Placenta increta, second trimester**
    - • ♀ **O43.223 Placenta increta, third trimester**
    - • ♀ **O43.229 Placenta increta, unspecified trimester**
  - \+ **O43.23 Placenta percreta**
    - • ♀ **O43.231 Placenta percreta, first trimester**
    - • ♀ **O43.232 Placenta percreta, second trimester**
    - • ♀ **O43.233 Placenta percreta, third trimester**
    - • ♀ **O43.239 Placenta percreta, unspecified trimester**
- \+ **O43.8 Other placental disorders**
  - \+ **O43.81 Placental infarction**
    - • ♀ **O43.811 Placental infarction, first trimester**
    - • ♀ **O43.812 Placental infarction, second trimester**
    - • ♀ **O43.813 Placental infarction, third trimester**
    - • ♀ **O43.819 Placental infarction, unspecified trimester**
  - \+ **O43.89 Other placental disorders**
    Placental dysfunction
    - • ♀ **O43.891 Other placental disorders, first trimester**
    - • ♀ **O43.892 Other placental disorders, second trimester**
    - • ♀ **O43.893 Other placental disorders, third trimester**
    - • ♀ **O43.899 Other placental disorders, unspecified trimester**
- \+ **O43.9 Unspecified placental disorder**
  - • ♀ **O43.90 Unspecified placental disorder, unspecified trimester**
  - • ♀ **O43.91 Unspecified placental disorder, first trimester**
  - • ♀ **O43.92 Unspecified placental disorder, second trimester**
  - • ♀ **O43.93 Unspecified placental disorder, third trimester**

O44 Placenta previa

AHA CC: 4Q, 2016, 52-53

- \+ **O44.0 Complete placenta previa NOS or without hemorrhage**
  Placenta previa NOS
  - • ♀ **O44.00 Complete placenta previa NOS or without hemorrhage, unspecified trimester**
  - • ♀ CC **O44.01 Complete placenta previa NOS or without hemorrhage, first trimester**
  - • ♀ CC **O44.02 Complete placenta previa NOS or without hemorrhage, second trimester**
  - • ♀ CC **O44.03 Complete placenta previa NOS or without hemorrhage, third trimester**
- \+ **O44.1 Complete placenta previa with hemorrhage**
  Excludes1: *labor and delivery complicated by hemorrhage from vasa previa (O69.4)*
  - • ♀ **O44.10 Complete placenta previa with hemorrhage, unspecified trimester**
  - • ♀ MCC **O44.11 Complete placenta previa with hemorrhage, first trimester**
  - • ♀ MCC **O44.12 Complete placenta previa with hemorrhage, second trimester**
  - • ♀ MCC **O44.13 Complete placenta previa with hemorrhage, third trimester**
- \+ **O44.2 Partial placenta previa without hemorrhage**
  Marginal placenta previa, NOS or without hemorrhage
  - • ♀ **O44.20 Partial placenta previa NOS or without hemorrhage, unspecified trimester**
  - • ♀ CC **O44.21 Partial placenta previa NOS or without hemorrhage, first trimester**
  - • ♀ CC **O44.22 Partial placenta previa NOS or without hemorrhage, second trimester**
  - • ♀ CC **O44.23 Partial placenta previa NOS or without hemorrhage, third trimester**
- \+ **O44.3 Partial placenta previa with hemorrhage**
  Marginal placenta previa with hemorrhage
  - • ♀ **O44.30 Partial placenta previa with hemorrhage, unspecified trimester**
  - • ♀ MCC **O44.31 Partial placenta previa with hemorrhage, first trimester**
  - • ♀ MCC **O44.32 Partial placenta previa with hemorrhage, second trimester**
  - • ♀ MCC **O44.33 Partial placenta previa with hemorrhage, third trimester**
- \+ **O44.4 Low lying placenta NOS or without hemorrhage**
  MCCLow implantation of placenta NOS or without hemorrhage
  - • ♀ **O44.40 Low lying placenta NOS or without hemorrhage, unspecified trimester**

- • ♀ CC **O44.41 Low lying placenta NOS or without hemorrhage, first trimester**
- • ♀ CC **O44.42 Low lying placenta NOS or without hemorrhage, second trimester**
- • ♀ CC **O44.43 Low lying placenta NOS or without hemorrhage, third trimester**

\+ **O44.5 Low lying placenta with hemorrhage**

Low implantation of placenta with hemorrhage

- • ♀ **O44.50 Low lying placenta with hemorrhage, unspecified trimester**
- • ♀ MCC **O44.51 Low lying placenta with hemorrhage, first trimester**
- • ♀ MCC **O44.52 Low lying placenta with hemorrhage, second trimester**
- • ♀ MCC **O44.53 Low lying placenta with hemorrhage, third trimester**

O45 Premature separation of placenta [abruptio placentae]

\+ **O45.0 Premature separation of placenta with coagulation defect**

\+ **O45.00 Premature separation of placenta with coagulation defect, unspecified**

- • ♀ MCC **O45.001 Premature separation of placenta with coagulation defect, unspecified, first trimester**
- • ♀ MCC **O45.002 Premature separation of placenta with coagulation defect, unspecified, second trimester**
- • ♀ MCC **O45.003 Premature separation of placenta with coagulation defect, unspecified, third trimester**
- • ♀ **O45.009 Premature separation of placenta with coagulation defect, unspecified, unspecified trimester**

\+ **O45.01 Premature separation of placenta with afibrinogenemia**

Premature separation of placenta with hypofibrinogenemia

- • ♀ MCC **O45.011 Premature separation of placenta with afibrinogenemia, first trimester**
- • ♀ MCC **O45.012 Premature separation of placenta with afibrinogenemia, second trimester**
- • ♀ MCC **O45.013 Premature separation of placenta with afibrinogenemia, third trimester**
- • ♀ **O45.019 Premature separation of placenta with afibrinogenemia, unspecified trimester**

\+ **O45.02 Premature separation of placenta with disseminated intravascular coagulation**

- • ♀ MCC **O45.021 Premature separation of placenta with disseminated intravascular coagulation, first trimester**
- • ♀ MCC **O45.022 Premature separation of placenta with disseminated intravascular coagulation, second trimester**
- • ♀ MCC **O45.023 Premature separation of placenta with disseminated intravascular coagulation, third trimester**
- • ♀ **O45.029 Premature separation of placenta with disseminated intravascular coagulation, unspecified trimester**

O45.09 Premature separation of placenta with other coagulation defect

- • ♀ MCC **O45.091 Premature separation of placenta with other coagulation defect, first trimester**
- • ♀ MCC **O45.092 Premature separation of placenta with other coagulation defect, second trimester**
- • ♀ MCC **O45.093 Premature separation of placenta with other coagulation defect, third trimester**
- • ♀ **O45.099 Premature separation of placenta with other coagulation defect, unspecified trimester**

\+ **O45.8 Other premature separation of placenta**

\+ **O45.8X Other premature separation of placenta**

- • ♀ MCC **O45.8X1 Other premature separation of placenta, first trimester**
- • ♀ MCC **O45.8X2 Other premature separation of placenta, second trimester**
- • ♀ MCC **O45.8X3 Other premature separation of placenta, third trimester**
- • ♀ **O45.8X9 Other premature separation of placenta, unspecified trimester**

\+ **O45.9 Premature separation of placenta, unspecified**

Abruptio placentae NOS

- • ♀ **O45.90 Premature separation of placenta, unspecified, unspecified trimester**
- • ♀ MCC **O45.91 Premature separation of placenta, unspecified, first trimester**
- • ♀ MCC **O45.92 Premature separation of placenta, unspecified, second trimester**
- • ♀ MCC **O45.93 Premature separation of placenta, unspecified, third trimester**

O46 Antepartum hemorrhage, not elsewhere classified

Excludes1: *hemorrhage in early pregnancy (O20.-)*
intrapartum hemorrhage NEC (O67.-)
placenta previa (O44.-)
premature separation of placenta [abruptio placentae] (O45.-)

\+ **O46.0 Antepartum hemorrhage with coagulation defect**

\+ **O46.00 Antepartum hemorrhage with coagulation defect, unspecified**

- • ♀ MCC **O46.001 Antepartum hemorrhage with coagulation defect, unspecified, first trimester**
- • ♀ MCC **O46.002 Antepartum hemorrhage with coagulation defect, unspecified, second trimester**
- • ♀ MCC **O46.003 Antepartum hemorrhage with coagulation defect, unspecified, third trimester**
- • ♀ **O46.009 Antepartum hemorrhage with coagulation defect, unspecified, unspecified trimester**

\+ **O46.01 Antepartum hemorrhage with afibrinogenemia**

Antepartum hemorrhage with hypofibrinogenemia

- • ♀ MCC **O46.011 Antepartum hemorrhage with afibrinogenemia, first trimester**
- • ♀ MCC **O46.012 Antepartum hemorrhage with afibrinogenemia, second trimester**
- • ♀ MCC **O46.013 Antepartum hemorrhage with afibrinogenemia, third trimester**
- • ♀ **O46.019 Antepartum hemorrhage with afibrinogenemia, unspecified trimester**

\+ **O46.02 Antepartum hemorrhage with disseminated intravascular coagulation**

- • ♀ MCC **O46.021 Antepartum hemorrhage with disseminated intravascular coagulation, first trimester**
- • ♀ MCC **O46.022 Antepartum hemorrhage with disseminated intravascular coagulation, second trimester**
- • ♀ MCC **O46.023 Antepartum hemorrhage with disseminated intravascular coagulation, third trimester**
- • ♀ **O46.029 Antepartum hemorrhage with disseminated intravascular coagulation, unspecified trimester**

\+ **O46.09 Antepartum hemorrhage with other coagulation defect**

- • ♀ MCC **O46.091 Antepartum hemorrhage with other coagulation defect, first trimester**
- • ♀ MCC **O46.092 Antepartum hemorrhage with other coagulation defect, second trimester**
- • ♀ MCC **O46.093 Antepartum hemorrhage with other coagulation defect, third trimester**
- • ♀ **O46.099 Antepartum hemorrhage with other coagulation defect, unspecified trimester**

+ O46.8 **Other antepartum hemorrhage**
  + O46.8X **Other antepartum hemorrhage**
    - ● ♀ **O46.8X1 Other antepartum hemorrhage, first trimester**
    - ● ♀ **O46.8X2 Other antepartum hemorrhage, second trimester**
    - ● ♀ **O46.8X3 Other antepartum hemorrhage, third trimester**
    - ● ♀ **O46.8X9 Other antepartum hemorrhage, unspecified trimester**

+ O46.9 **Antepartum hemorrhage, unspecified**
  - ● ♀ **O46.90 Antepartum hemorrhage, unspecified, unspecified trimester**
  - ● ♀ **O46.91 Antepartum hemorrhage, unspecified, first trimester**
  - ● ♀ **O46.92 Antepartum hemorrhage, unspecified, second trimester**
  - ● ♀ **O46.93 Antepartum hemorrhage, unspecified, third trimester**

O47 False labor

Includes: Braxton Hicks contractions
threatened labor

Excludes1: *preterm labor (O60.-)*

+ O47.0 **False labor before 37 completed weeks of gestation**
  - ● ♀ **O47.00 False labor before 37 completed weeks of gestation, unspecified trimester**
  - ● ♀ CC **O47.02 False labor before 37 completed weeks of gestation, second trimester**
  - ● ♀ CC **O47.03 False labor before 37 completed weeks of gestation, third trimester**

● ♀ CC **O47.1 False labor at or after 37 completed weeks of gestation**
AHA CC: 1Q, 2021, 10

● ♀ **O47.9 False labor, unspecified**

O48 Late pregnancy

● ♀ **O48.0 Post-term pregnancy**
Pregnancy over 40 completed weeks to 42 completed weeks gestation

● ♀ **O48.1 Prolonged pregnancy**
Pregnancy which has advanced beyond 42 completed weeks gestation

Complications of labor and delivery (O60-O77)

O60 Preterm labor

Includes: onset (spontaneous) of labor before 37 completed weeks of gestation

Excludes1: *false labor (O47.0-)*
threatened labor NOS (O47.0-)

+ O60.0 **Preterm labor without delivery**
  - ● ♀ **O60.00 Preterm labor without delivery, unspecified trimester**
  - ● ♀ MCC **O60.02 Preterm labor without delivery, second trimester**
  - ● ♀ MCC **O60.03 Preterm labor without delivery, third trimester**

+ O60.1 **Preterm labor with preterm delivery**

One of the following 7th characters is to be assigned to each code under subcategory **O60.1.** 7th character 0 is for single gestations and multiple gestations where the fetus is unspecified. 7th characters 1 through 9 are for cases of multiple gestations to identify the fetus for which the code applies. The appropriate code from category O30, Multiple gestation, must also be assigned when assigning a code from subcategory O60.1 that has a 7th character of 1 through 9.
0 - not applicable or unspecified
1 - fetus 1
2 - fetus 2
3 - fetus 3
4 - fetus 4
5 - fetus 5
9 - other fetus

● ♀ CC X+7th **O60.10 Preterm labor with preterm delivery, unspecified trimester**
Preterm labor with delivery NOS

● ♀ MCC X+7th **O60.12 Preterm labor second trimester with preterm delivery second trimester**

● ♀ MCC X+7th **O60.13 Preterm labor second trimester with preterm delivery third trimester**

● ♀ MCC X+7th **O60.14 Preterm labor third trimester with preterm delivery third trimester**
AHA CC: 2Q, 2016, 10-11

+ O60.2 **Term delivery with preterm labor**

One of the following 7th characters is to be assigned to each code under subcategory **O60.2.** 7th character 0 is for single gestations and multiple gestations where the fetus is unspecified. 7th characters 1 through 9 are for cases of multiple gestations to identify the fetus for which the code applies. The appropriate code from category O30, Multiple gestation, must also be assigned when assigning a code from subcategory O60.2 that has a 7th character of 1 through 9.
0 - not applicable or unspecified
1 - fetus 1
2 - fetus 2
3 - fetus 3
4 - fetus 4
5 - fetus 5
9 - other fetus

● ♀ CC X+7th **O60.20 Term delivery with preterm labor, unspecified trimester**

● ♀ MCC X+7th **O60.22 Term delivery with preterm labor, second trimester**

● ♀ MCC X+7th **O60.23 Term delivery with preterm labor, third trimester**

O61 Failed induction of labor

● ♀ **O61.0 Failed medical induction of labor**
Failed induction (of labor) by oxytocin
Failed induction (of labor) by prostaglandins

● ♀ **O61.1 Failed instrumental induction of labor**
Failed mechanical induction (of labor)
Failed surgical induction (of labor)

● ♀ **O61.8 Other failed induction of labor**

● ♀ **O61.9 Failed induction of labor, unspecified**

O62 Abnormalities of forces of labor

● ♀ **O62.0 Primary inadequate contractions**
Failure of cervical dilatation
Primary hypotonic uterine dysfunction
Uterine inertia during latent phase of labor

● ♀ **O62.1 Secondary uterine inertia**
Arrested active phase of labor
Secondary hypotonic uterine dysfunction

● ♀ **O62.2 Other uterine inertia**
Atony of uterus without hemorrhage
Atony of uterus NOS
Desultory labor
Hypotonic uterine dysfunction NOS
Irregular labor
Poor contractions
Slow slope active phase of labor
Uterine inertia NOS

Excludes1: *atony of uterus with hemorrhage (postpartum) (O72.1)*
postpartum atony of uterus without hemorrhage (O75.89)

● ♀ **O62.3 Precipitate labor**

● ♀ **O62.4 Hypertonic, incoordinate, and prolonged uterine contractions**
Cervical spasm
Contraction ring dystocia
Dyscoordinate labor
Hour-glass contraction of uterus
Hypertonic uterine dysfunction
Incoordinate uterine action
Tetanic contractions
Uterine dystocia NOS
Uterine spasm

Excludes1: *dystocia (fetal) (maternal) NOS (O66.9)*

● ♀ **O62.8 Other abnormalities of forces of labor**

● ♀ **O62.9 Abnormality of forces of labor, unspecified**

O63 Long labor

● ♀ **O63.0 Prolonged first stage (of labor)**

● ♀ **O63.1 Prolonged second stage (of labor)**

● ♀ **O63.2 Delayed delivery of second twin, triplet, etc.**

● ♀ CC **O63.9 Long labor, unspecified**
Prolonged labor NOS

O64 Obstructed labor due to malposition and malpresentation of fetus

One of the following 7th characters is to be assigned to each code under category O64. 7th character 0 is for single gestations and multiple gestations where the fetus is unspecified. 7th characters 1 through 9 are for cases of multiple gestations to identify the fetus for which the code applies. The appropriate code from category O30, Multiple gestation, must also be assigned when assigning a code from category O64 that has a 7th character of 1 through 9.
0 - not applicable or unspecified
1 - fetus 1
2 - fetus 2
3 - fetus 3
4 - fetus 4
5 - fetus 5
9 - other fetus

• ♀ X+7th **O64.0 Obstructed labor due to incomplete rotation of fetal head**
Deep transverse arrest
Obstructed labor due to persistent occipitoiliac (position)
Obstructed labor due to persistent occipitoposterior (position)
Obstructed labor due to persistent occipitosacral (position)
Obstructed labor due to persistent occipitotransverse (position)

• ♀ X+7th **O64.1 Obstructed labor due to breech presentation**
Obstructed labor due to buttocks presentation
Obstructed labor due to complete breech presentation
Obstructed labor due to frank breech presentation

• ♀ X+7th **O64.2 Obstructed labor due to face presentation**
Obstructed labor due to chin presentation

• ♀ X+7th **O64.3 Obstructed labor due to brow presentation**

• ♀ X+7th **O64.4 Obstructed labor due to shoulder presentation**
Prolapsed arm
Excludes1: *impacted shoulders (O66.0)*
shoulder dystocia (O66.0)

• ♀ X+7th **O64.5 Obstructed labor due to compound presentation**

• ♀ X+7th **O64.8 Obstructed labor due to other malposition and malpresentation**
Obstructed labor due to footling presentation
Obstructed labor due to incomplete breech presentation

• ♀ X+7th **O64.9 Obstructed labor due to malposition and malpresentation, unspecified**

O65 Obstructed labor due to maternal pelvic abnormality

• ♀ **O65.0 Obstructed labor due to deformed pelvis**
• ♀ **O65.1 Obstructed labor due to generally contracted pelvis**
• ♀ **O65.2 Obstructed labor due to pelvic inlet contraction**
• ♀ **O65.3 Obstructed labor due to pelvic outlet and mid-cavity contraction**
• ♀ **O65.4 Obstructed labor due to fetopelvic disproportion, unspecified**
Excludes1: *dystocia due to abnormality of fetus (O66.2-O66.3)*

• ♀ **O65.5 Obstructed labor due to abnormality of maternal pelvic organs**
Obstructed labor due to conditions listed in O34.-
Use additional code to identify abnormality of pelvic organs O34.-

• ♀ **O65.8 Obstructed labor due to other maternal pelvic abnormalities**
• ♀ **O65.9 Obstructed labor due to maternal pelvic abnormality, unspecified**

O66 Other obstructed labor

• ♀ **O66.0 Obstructed labor due to shoulder dystocia**
Impacted shoulders
• ♀ **O66.1 Obstructed labor due to locked twins**
• ♀ **O66.2 Obstructed labor due to unusually large fetus**
• ♀ **O66.3 Obstructed labor due to other abnormalities of fetus**
Dystocia due to fetal ascites
Dystocia due to fetal hydrops
Dystocia due to fetal meningomyelocele
Dystocia due to fetal sacral teratoma
Dystocia due to fetal tumor
Dystocia due to hydrocephalic fetus
Use additional code to identify cause of obstruction

\+ **O66.4 Failed trial of labor**
• ♀ **O66.40 Failed trial of labor, unspecified**
• ♀ **O66.41 Failed attempted vaginal birth after previous cesarean delivery**
Code first rupture of uterus, if applicable (O71.0-, O71.1)

• ♀ **O66.5 Attempted application of vacuum extractor and forceps**
Attempted application of vacuum or forceps, with subsequent delivery by forceps or cesarean delivery
• ♀ **O66.6 Obstructed labor due to other multiple fetuses**
• ♀ **O66.8 Other specified obstructed labor**
Use additional code to identify cause of obstruction
• ♀ **O66.9 Obstructed labor, unspecified**
Dystocia NOS
Fetal dystocia NOS
Maternal dystocia NOS

O67 Labor and delivery complicated by intrapartum hemorrhage, not elsewhere classified
Excludes1: *antepartum hemorrhage NEC (O46.-)*
placenta previa (O44.-)
premature separation of placenta [abruptio placentae] (O45.-)
Excludes2: *postpartum hemorrhage (O72.-)*

• ♀ MCC **O67.0 Intrapartum hemorrhage with coagulation defect**
Intrapartum hemorrhage (excessive) associated with afibrinogenemia
Intrapartum hemorrhage (excessive) associated with disseminated intravascular coagulation
Intrapartum hemorrhage (excessive) associated with hyperfibrinolysis
Intrapartum hemorrhage (excessive) associated with hypofibrinogenemia
• ♀ **O67.8 Other intrapartum hemorrhage**
Excessive intrapartum hemorrhage
• ♀ **O67.9 Intrapartum hemorrhage, unspecified**

• ♀ CC **O68 Labor and delivery complicated by abnormality of fetal acid-base balance**
Fetal acidemia complicating labor and delivery
Fetal acidosis complicating labor and delivery
Fetal alkalosis complicating labor and delivery
Fetal metabolic acidemia complicating labor and delivery
Excludes1: *fetal stress NOS (O77.9)*
labor and delivery complicated by electrocardiographic evidence of fetal stress (O77.8)
labor and delivery complicated by ultrasonic evidence of fetal stress (O77.8)
Excludes2: *abnormality in fetal heart rate or rhythm (O76)*
labor and delivery complicated by meconium in amniotic fluid (O77.0)
Valid 3-character code, no further characters required

O69 Labor and delivery complicated by umbilical cord complications

One of the following 7th characters is to be assigned to each code under category O69. 7th character 0 is for single gestations and multiple gestations where the fetus is unspecified. 7th characters 1 through 9 are for cases of multiple gestations to identify the fetus for which the code applies. The appropriate code from category O30, Multiple gestation, must also be assigned when assigning a code from category O69 that has a 7th character of 1 through 9.
0 - not applicable or unspecified
1 - fetus 1
2 - fetus 2
3 - fetus 3
4 - fetus 4
5 - fetus 5
9 - other fetus

• ♀ X+7th **O69.0 Labor and delivery complicated by prolapse of cord**
• ♀ X+7th **O69.1 Labor and delivery complicated by cord around neck, with compression**
Excludes1: *labor and delivery complicated by cord around neck, without compression (O69.81)*
• ♀ X+7th **O69.2 Labor and delivery complicated by other cord entanglement, with compression**
Labor and delivery complicated by compression of cord NOS
Labor and delivery complicated by entanglement of cords of twins in monoamniotic sac
Labor and delivery complicated by knot in cord
Excludes1: *labor and delivery complicated by other cord entanglement, without compression (O69.82)*

• ♀ X+7th **O69.3 Labor and delivery complicated by short cord**
• ♀ X+7th **O69.4 Labor and delivery complicated by vasa previa**
Labor and delivery complicated by hemorrhage from vasa previa
• ♀ X+7th **O69.5 Labor and delivery complicated by vascular lesion of cord**
Labor and delivery complicated by cord bruising
Labor and delivery complicated by cord hematoma
Labor and delivery complicated by thrombosis of umbilical vessels
X+7th **O69.8 Labor and delivery complicated by other cord complications**
• ♀ X+7th **O69.81 Labor and delivery complicated by cord around neck, without compression**
• ♀ X+7th **O69.82 Labor and delivery complicated by other cord entanglement, without compression**
• ♀ X+7th **O69.89 Labor and delivery complicated by other cord complications**
• ♀ X+7th **O69.9 Labor and delivery complicated by cord complication, unspecified**

O70 Perineal laceration during delivery

Includes: episiotomy extended by laceration
Excludes1: *obstetric high vaginal laceration alone (O71.4)*
• ♀ **O70.0 First degree perineal laceration during delivery**
Perineal laceration, rupture or tear involving fourchette during delivery
Perineal laceration, rupture or tear involving labia during delivery
Perineal laceration, rupture or tear involving skin during delivery
Perineal laceration, rupture or tear involving vagina during delivery
Perineal laceration, rupture or tear involving vulva during delivery
Slight perineal laceration, rupture or tear during delivery
• ♀ **O70.1 Second degree perineal laceration during delivery**
Perineal laceration, rupture or tear during delivery as in O70.0, also involving pelvic floor
Perineal laceration, rupture or tear during delivery as in O70.0, also involving perineal muscles
Perineal laceration, rupture or tear during delivery as in O70.0, also involving vaginal muscles
Excludes1: *perineal laceration involving anal sphincter (O70.2)*
AHA CC: 2Q, 2016, 34
\+ **O70.2 Third degree perineal laceration during delivery**
Perineal laceration, rupture or tear during delivery as in O70.1, also involving anal sphincter
Perineal laceration, rupture or tear during delivery as in O70.1, also involving rectovaginal septum
Perineal laceration, rupture or tear during delivery as in O70.1, also involving sphincter NOS
Excludes1: *anal sphincter tear during delivery without third degree perineal laceration (O70.4)*
perineal laceration involving anal or rectal mucosa (O70.3)
AHA CC: 4Q, 2016, 53-54
• ♀ CC **O70.20 Third degree perineal laceration during delivery, unspecified**
• ♀ CC **O70.21 Third degree perineal laceration during delivery, IIIa**
Third degree perineal laceration during delivery with less than 50% of external anal sphincter (EAS) thickness torn
• ♀ CC **O70.22 Third degree perineal laceration during delivery, IIIb**
Third degree perineal laceration during delivery with more than 50% of external anal sphincter (EAS) thickness torn
• ♀ CC **O70.23 Third degree perineal laceration during delivery, IIIc**
Third degree perineal laceration during delivery with both external anal sphincter (EAS) and internal anal sphincter (IAS) torn
• ♀ CC **O70.3 Fourth degree perineal laceration during delivery**
Perineal laceration, rupture or tear during delivery as in O70.2, also involving anal mucosa
Perineal laceration, rupture or tear during delivery as in O70.2, also involving rectal mucosa
• ♀ CC **O70.4 Anal sphincter tear complicating delivery, not associated with third degree laceration**
Excludes1: *anal sphincter tear with third degree perineal laceration (O70.2)*
• ♀ **O70.9 Perineal laceration during delivery, unspecified**

O71 Other obstetric trauma

Includes: obstetric damage from instruments
\+ **O71.0 Rupture of uterus (spontaneous) before onset of labor**
Excludes1: *disruption of (current) cesarean delivery wound (O90.0)*
laceration of uterus, NEC (O71.81)
• ♀ **O71.00 Rupture of uterus before onset of labor, unspecified trimester**
• ♀ MCC **O71.02 Rupture of uterus before onset of labor, second trimester**
• ♀ MCC **O71.03 Rupture of uterus before onset of labor, third trimester**
• ♀ MCC **O71.1 Rupture of uterus during labor**
Rupture of uterus not stated as occurring before onset of labor
Excludes1: *disruption of cesarean delivery wound (O90.0)*
laceration of uterus, NEC (O71.81)
• ♀ CC **O71.2 Postpartum inversion of uterus**
• ♀ CC **O71.3 Obstetric laceration of cervix**
Annular detachment of cervix
• ♀ CC **O71.4 Obstetric high vaginal laceration alone**
Laceration of vaginal wall without perineal laceration
Excludes1: *obstetric high vaginal laceration with perineal laceration (O70.-)*
• ♀ CC **O71.5 Other obstetric injury to pelvic organs**
Obstetric injury to bladder
Obstetric injury to urethra
Excludes2: *obstetric periurethral trauma (O71.82)*
• ♀ CC **O71.6 Obstetric damage to pelvic joints and ligaments**
Obstetric avulsion of inner symphyseal cartilage
Obstetric damage to coccyx
Obstetric traumatic separation of symphysis (pubis)
• ♀ CC **O71.7 Obstetric hematoma of pelvis**
Obstetric hematoma of perineum
Obstetric hematoma of vagina
Obstetric hematoma of vulva
\+ **O71.8 Other specified obstetric trauma**
• ♀ **O71.81 Laceration of uterus, not elsewhere classified**
• ♀ **O71.82 Other specified trauma to perineum and vulva**
Obstetric periurethral trauma
AHA CC: 4Q, 2014, 18-19
• ♀ **O71.89 Other specified obstetric trauma**
• ♀ **O71.9 Obstetric trauma, unspecified**

O72 Postpartum hemorrhage

Includes: hemorrhage after delivery of fetus or infant
• ♀ CC **O72.0 Third-stage hemorrhage**
Hemorrhage associated with retained, trapped or adherent placenta
Retained placenta NOS
Code also type of adherent placenta (O43.2-)
• ♀ CC **O72.1 Other immediate postpartum hemorrhage**
Hemorrhage following delivery of placenta
Postpartum hemorrhage (atonic) NOS
Uterine atony with hemorrhage
Excludes1: *uterine atony NOS (O62.2)*
uterine atony without hemorrhage (O62.2)
postpartum atony of uterus without hemorrhage (O75.89)
• ♀ CC **O72.2 Delayed and secondary postpartum hemorrhage**
Hemorrhage associated with retained portions of placenta or membranes after the first 24 hours following delivery of placenta
Retained products of conception NOS, following delivery
• ♀ **O72.3 Postpartum coagulation defects**
Postpartum afibrinogenemia
Postpartum fibrinolysis

O73 Retained placenta and membranes, without hemorrhage

Excludes1: *placenta accreta (O43.21-)*
placenta increta (O43.22-)
placenta percreta (O43.23-)
• ♀ **O73.0 Retained placenta without hemorrhage**
Adherent placenta, without hemorrhage
Trapped placenta without hemorrhage

• ♀ **O73.1 Retained portions of placenta and membranes, without hemorrhage**

Retained products of conception following delivery, without hemorrhage

O74 Complications of anesthesia during labor and delivery

Includes: maternal complications arising from the administration of a general, regional or local anesthetic, analgesic or other sedation during labor and delivery

Use additional code, if applicable, to identify specific complication

• ♀ **O74.0 Aspiration pneumonitis due to anesthesia during labor and delivery**

Inhalation of stomach contents or secretions NOS due to anesthesia during labor and delivery

Mendelson's syndrome due to anesthesia during labor and delivery

• ♀ **O74.1 Other pulmonary complications of anesthesia during labor and delivery**

• ♀ **O74.2 Cardiac complications of anesthesia during labor and delivery**

• ♀ **O74.3 Central nervous system complications of anesthesia during labor and delivery**

• ♀ **O74.4 Toxic reaction to local anesthesia during labor and delivery**

• ♀ **O74.5 Spinal and epidural anesthesia-induced headache during labor and delivery**

• ♀ **O74.6 Other complications of spinal and epidural anesthesia during labor and delivery**

• ♀ **O74.7 Failed or difficult intubation for anesthesia during labor and delivery**

• ♀ **O74.8 Other complications of anesthesia during labor and delivery**

• ♀ **O74.9 Complication of anesthesia during labor and delivery, unspecified**

O75 Other complications of labor and delivery, not elsewhere classified

Excludes2: *puerperal (postpartum) infection (O86.-)*
puerperal (postpartum) sepsis (O85)

• ♀ **O75.0 Maternal distress during labor and delivery**

• ♀ MCC **O75.1 Shock during or following labor and delivery**

Obstetric shock following labor and delivery

• ♀ CC **O75.2 Pyrexia during labor, not elsewhere classified**

• ♀ MCC **O75.3 Other infection during labor**

Sepsis during labor

Use additional code (B95-B97), to identify infectious agent

Review coding guideline C.15.j

• ♀ **O75.4 Other complications of obstetric surgery and procedures**

Cardiac arrest following obstetric surgery or procedures
Cardiac failure following obstetric surgery or procedures
Cerebral anoxia following obstetric surgery or procedures
Pulmonary edema following obstetric surgery or procedures

Use additional code to identify specific complication

Excludes2: *complications of anesthesia during labor and delivery (O74.-)*
disruption of obstetrical (surgical) wound (O90.0-O90.1)
hematoma of obstetrical (surgical) wound (O90.2)
infection of obstetrical (surgical) wound (O86.0-)

• ♀ **O75.5 Delayed delivery after artificial rupture of membranes**

+ **O75.8 Other specified complications of labor and delivery**

• ♀ **O75.81 Maternal exhaustion complicating labor and delivery**

• ♀ **O75.82 Onset (spontaneous) of labor after 37 completed weeks of gestation but before 39 completed weeks gestation, with delivery by (planned) cesarean section**

Delivery by (planned) cesarean section occurring after 37 completed weeks of gestation but before 39 completed weeks gestation due to (spontaneous) onset of labor

Code first to specify reason for planned cesarean section such as:
cephalopelvic disproportion (normally formed fetus) (O33.9)
previous cesarean delivery (O34.21)

• ♀ **O75.89 Other specified complications of labor and delivery**

• ♀ **O75.9 Complication of labor and delivery, unspecified**

• ♀ **O76 Abnormality in fetal heart rate and rhythm complicating labor and delivery**

Depressed fetal heart rate tones complicating labor and delivery
Fetal bradycardia complicating labor and delivery
Fetal heart rate decelerations complicating labor and delivery
Fetal heart rate irregularity complicating labor and delivery
Fetal heart rate abnormal variability complicating labor and delivery
Fetal tachycardia complicating labor and delivery
Non-reassuring fetal heart rate or rhythm complicating labor and delivery

Excludes1: *fetal stress NOS (O77.9)*
labor and delivery complicated by electrocardiographic evidence of fetal stress (O77.8)
labor and delivery complicated by ultrasonic evidence of fetal stress (O77.8)

Excludes2: *fetal metabolic acidemia (O68)*
other fetal stress (O77.0-O77.1)

AHA CC: 4Q, 2013, 118

Valid 3-character code, no further characters required

O77 Other fetal stress complicating labor and delivery

• ♀ **O77.0 Labor and delivery complicated by meconium in amniotic fluid**

AHA CC: 4Q, 2013, 118

• ♀ **O77.1 Fetal stress in labor or delivery due to drug administration**

• ♀ **O77.8 Labor and delivery complicated by other evidence of fetal stress**

Labor and delivery complicated by electrocardiographic evidence of fetal stress

Labor and delivery complicated by ultrasonic evidence of fetal stress

Excludes1: *abnormality of fetal acid-base balance (O68)*
abnormality in fetal heart rate or rhythm (O76)
fetal metabolic acidemia (O68)

• ♀ **O77.9 Labor and delivery complicated by fetal stress, unspecified**

Excludes1: *abnormality of fetal acid-base balance (O68)*
abnormality in fetal heart rate or rhythm (O76)
fetal metabolic acidemia (O68)

Encounter for delivery (O80-O82)

• ♀ **O80 Encounter for full-term uncomplicated delivery**

Delivery requiring minimal or no assistance, with or without episiotomy, without fetal manipulation [e.g., rotation version] or instrumentation [forceps] of a spontaneous, cephalic, vaginal, full-term, single, live-born infant. This code is for use as a single diagnosis code and is not to be used with any other code from chapter 15.

Use additional code to indicate outcome of delivery (Z37.0)

AHA CC: 2Q, 2014, 9; 4Q, 2016, 150

Review coding guideline C.15.n

Valid 3-character code, no further characters required

• ♀ **O82 Encounter for cesarean delivery without indication**

Use additional code to indicate outcome of delivery (Z37.0)

Valid 3-character code, no further characters required

Complications predominantly related to the puerperium (O85-O92)

Excludes2: *mental and behavioral disorders associated with the puerperium (F53.-)*
obstetrical tetanus (A34)
puerperal osteomalacia (M83.0)

MCC • ♀ **O85 Puerperal sepsis**

Postpartum sepsis
Puerperal peritonitis
Puerperal pyemia

Use additional code (B95-B97), to identify infectious agent

Use additional code (R65.2-) to identify severe sepsis, if applicable

Excludes1: *fever of unknown origin following delivery (O86.4)*
genital tract infection following delivery (O86.1-)
obstetric pyemic and septic embolism (O88.3-)
puerperal septic thrombophlebitis (O86.81)
urinary tract infection following delivery (O86.2-)

Excludes2: *sepsis during labor (O75.3)*

Review coding guideline C.15.k

Valid 3-character code, no further characters required

O86 Other puerperal infections

Use additional code (B95-B97), to identify infectious agent

Excludes2: *infection during labor (O75.3)*
obstetrical tetanus (A34)

\+ **O86.0 Infection of obstetric surgical wound**
Infected cesarean delivery wound following delivery
Infected perineal repair following delivery
Excludes1: *complications of procedures, not elsewhere classified (T81.4-)*
postprocedural fever NOS (R50.82)
postprocedural retroperitoneal abscess (K68.11)
AHA CC: 4Q, 2018, 22-23
Review coding guideline C.1.d.5

• ♀ **O86.00 Infection of obstetric surgical wound, unspecified**

• ♀ **O86.01 Infection of obstetric surgical wound, superficial incisional site**
Subcutaneous abscess following an obstetrical procedure
Stitch abscess following an obstetrical procedure

• ♀ **O86.02 Infection of obstetric surgical wound, deep incisional site**
Intramuscular abscess following an obstetrical procedure
Sub-fascial abscess following an obstetrical procedure
AHA CC: 4Q, 2018, 23; 2Q, 2020, 32-33

• ♀ **O86.03 Infection of obstetric surgical wound, organ and space site**
Intraabdominal abscess following an obstetrical procedure
Subphrenic abscess following an obstetrical procedure

• ♀ MCC **O86.04 Sepsis following an obstetrical procedure**
Use additional code to identify the sepsis
AHA CC: 4Q, 2018, 23; 2Q, 2019, 39; 2Q, 2020, 32-33

• ♀ **O86.09 Infection of obstetric surgical wound, other surgical site**

\+ **O86.1 Other infection of genital tract following delivery**

• ♀ CC **O86.11 Cervicitis following delivery**

• ♀ CC **O86.12 Endometritis following delivery**

• ♀ CC **O86.13 Vaginitis following delivery**

• ♀ CC **O86.19 Other infection of genital tract following delivery**

\+ **O86.2 Urinary tract infection following delivery**

• ♀ CC **O86.20 Urinary tract infection following delivery, unspecified**
Puerperal urinary tract infection NOS

• ♀ CC **O86.21 Infection of kidney following delivery**

• ♀ CC **O86.22 Infection of bladder following delivery**
Infection of urethra following delivery

• ♀ CC **O86.29 Other urinary tract infection following delivery**

• ♀ CC **O86.4 Pyrexia of unknown origin following delivery**
Puerperal infection NOS following delivery
Puerperal pyrexia NOS following delivery
Excludes2: *pyrexia during labor (O75.2)*

\+ **O86.8 Other specified puerperal infections**

• ♀ MCC **O86.81 Puerperal septic thrombophlebitis**

• ♀ MCC **O86.89 Other specified puerperal infections**

O87 Venous complications and hemorrhoids in the puerperium

Includes: venous complications in labor, delivery and the puerperium

Excludes2: *obstetric embolism (O88.-)*
puerperal septic thrombophlebitis (O86.81)
venous complications in pregnancy (O22.-)

• ♀ CC **O87.0 Superficial thrombophlebitis in the puerperium**
Puerperal phlebitis NOS
Puerperal thrombosis NOS

• ♀ MCC **O87.1 Deep phlebothrombosis in the puerperium**
Deep vein thrombosis, postpartum
Pelvic thrombophlebitis, postpartum
Use additional code to identify the deep vein thrombosis (I82.4-, I82.5-, I82.62-, I82.72-)
Use additional code, if applicable, for associated long-term (current) use of anticoagulants (Z79.01)

• ♀ CC **O87.2 Hemorrhoids in the puerperium**

• ♀ CC **O87.3 Cerebral venous thrombosis in the puerperium**
Cerebrovenous sinus thrombosis in the puerperium

• ♀ **O87.4 Varicose veins of lower extremity in the puerperium**

• ♀ CC **O87.8 Other venous complications in the puerperium**
Genital varices in the puerperium

• ♀ **O87.9 Venous complication in the puerperium, unspecified**
Puerperal phlebopathy NOS

O88 Obstetric embolism

Excludes1: *embolism complicating abortion NOS (O03.2)*
embolism complicating ectopic or molar pregnancy (O08.2)
embolism complicating failed attempted abortion (O07.2)
embolism complicating induced abortion (O04.7)
embolism complicating spontaneous abortion (O03.2, O03.7)

\+ **O88.0 Obstetric air embolism**

\+ **O88.01 Obstetric air embolism in pregnancy**

• ♀ MCC **O88.011 Air embolism in pregnancy, first trimester**

• ♀ MCC **O88.012 Air embolism in pregnancy, second trimester**

• ♀ MCC **O88.013 Air embolism in pregnancy, third trimester**

• ♀ **O88.019 Air embolism in pregnancy, unspecified trimester**

• ♀ MCC **O88.02 Air embolism in childbirth**

• ♀ MCC **O88.03 Air embolism in the puerperium**

\+ **O88.1 Amniotic fluid embolism**
Anaphylactoid syndrome in pregnancy

\+ **O88.11 Amniotic fluid embolism in pregnancy**

• ♀ MCC **O88.111 Amniotic fluid embolism in pregnancy, first trimester**

• ♀ MCC **O88.112 Amniotic fluid embolism in pregnancy, second trimester**

• ♀ MCC **O88.113 Amniotic fluid embolism in pregnancy, third trimester**

• ♀ **O88.119 Amniotic fluid embolism in pregnancy, unspecified trimester**

• ♀ MCC **O88.12 Amniotic fluid embolism in childbirth**

• ♀ MCC **O88.13 Amniotic fluid embolism in the puerperium**

\+ **O88.2 Obstetric thromboembolism**

\+ **O88.21 Thromboembolism in pregnancy**
Obstetric (pulmonary) embolism NOS

• ♀ MCC **O88.211 Thromboembolism in pregnancy, first trimester**

• ♀ MCC **O88.212 Thromboembolism in pregnancy, second trimester**

• ♀ MCC **O88.213 Thromboembolism in pregnancy, third trimester**

• ♀ **O88.219 Thromboembolism in pregnancy, unspecified trimester**

• ♀ MCC **O88.22 Thromboembolism in childbirth**

• ♀ MCC **O88.23 Thromboembolism in the puerperium**
Puerperal (pulmonary) embolism NOS

\+ **O88.3 Obstetric pyemic and septic embolism**

\+ **O88.31 Pyemic and septic embolism in pregnancy**

• ♀ MCC **O88.311 Pyemic and septic embolism in pregnancy, first trimester**

• ♀ MCC **O88.312 Pyemic and septic embolism in pregnancy, second trimester**

• ♀ MCC **O88.313 Pyemic and septic embolism in pregnancy, third trimester**

• ♀ **O88.319 Pyemic and septic embolism in pregnancy, unspecified trimester**

• ♀ MCC **O88.32 Pyemic and septic embolism in childbirth**

• ♀ MCC **O88.33 Pyemic and septic embolism in the puerperium**

\+ **O88.8 Other obstetric embolism**
Obstetric fat embolism

\+ **O88.81 Other embolism in pregnancy**

• ♀ MCC **O88.811 Other embolism in pregnancy, first trimester**

• ♀ MCC **O88.812 Other embolism in pregnancy, second trimester**

• ♀ MCC **O88.813 Other embolism in pregnancy, third trimester**

• ♀ CC **O88.819 Other embolism in pregnancy, unspecified trimester**

• ♀ MCC **O88.82 Other embolism in childbirth**

• ♀ MCC **O88.83 Other embolism in the puerperium**

O89 Complications of anesthesia during the puerperium

Includes: maternal complications arising from the administration of a general, regional or local anesthetic, analgesic or other sedation during the puerperium

Use additional code, if applicable, to identify specific complication

+ **O89.0 Pulmonary complications of anesthesia during the puerperium**
  - • ♀ **O89.01 Aspiration pneumonitis due to anesthesia during the puerperium**
    Inhalation of stomach contents or secretions NOS due to anesthesia during the puerperium
    Mendelson's syndrome due to anesthesia during the puerperium
  - • ♀ **O89.09 Other pulmonary complications of anesthesia during the puerperium**
- • ♀ **O89.1 Cardiac complications of anesthesia during the puerperium**
- • ♀ **O89.2 Central nervous system complications of anesthesia during the puerperium**
- • ♀ **O89.3 Toxic reaction to local anesthesia during the puerperium**
- • ♀ **O89.4 Spinal and epidural anesthesia-induced headache during the puerperium**
- • ♀ **O89.5 Other complications of spinal and epidural anesthesia during the puerperium**
- • ♀ **O89.6 Failed or difficult intubation for anesthesia during the puerperium**
- • ♀ **O89.8 Other complications of anesthesia during the puerperium**
- • ♀ **O89.9 Complication of anesthesia during the puerperium, unspecified**

O90 Complications of the puerperium, not elsewhere classified

- • ♀ **O90.0 Disruption of cesarean delivery wound**
  Dehiscence of cesarean delivery wound
  Excludes1: *rupture of uterus (spontaneous) before onset of labor (O71.0-)*
  rupture of uterus during labor (O71.1)
- • ♀ **O90.1 Disruption of perineal obstetric wound**
  Disruption of wound of episiotomy
  Disruption of wound of perineal laceration
  Secondary perineal tear
- • ♀ **O90.2 Hematoma of obstetric wound**
- • ♀ MCC **O90.3 Peripartum cardiomyopathy**
  Conditions in I42.- arising during pregnancy and the puerperium
  Excludes1: *pre-existing heart disease complicating pregnancy and the puerperium (O99.4-)*
  Review coding guideline C.15.o.5
- • ♀ MCC **O90.4 Postpartum acute kidney failure**
  Hepatorenal syndrome following labor and delivery
- • ♀ **O90.5 Postpartum thyroiditis**
- • ♀ **O90.6 Postpartum mood disturbance**
  Postpartum blues
  Postpartum dysphoria
  Postpartum sadness
  Excludes1: *postpartum depression (F53.0)*
  puerperal psychosis (F53.1)
+ **O90.8 Other complications of the puerperium, not elsewhere classified**
  - • ♀ **O90.81 Anemia of the puerperium**
    Postpartum anemia NOS
    Excludes1: *pre-existing anemia complicating the puerperium (O99.03)*
  - • ♀ **O90.89 Other complications of the puerperium, not elsewhere classified**
    Placental polyp
- • ♀ **O90.9 Complication of the puerperium, unspecified**

O91 Infections of breast associated with pregnancy, the puerperium and lactation

Use additional code to identify infection

+ **O91.0 Infection of nipple associated with pregnancy, the puerperium and lactation**
  + **O91.01 Infection of nipple associated with pregnancy**
    Gestational abscess of nipple
    - • ♀ **O91.011 Infection of nipple associated with pregnancy, first trimester**
    - • ♀ **O91.012 Infection of nipple associated with pregnancy, second trimester**
    - • ♀ **O91.013 Infection of nipple associated with pregnancy, third trimester**
    - • ♀ **O91.019 Infection of nipple associated with pregnancy, unspecified trimester**
  - • ♀ **O91.02 Infection of nipple associated with the puerperium**
    Puerperal abscess of nipple
  - • ♀ **O91.03 Infection of nipple associated with lactation**
    Abscess of nipple associated with lactation
+ **O91.1 Abscess of breast associated with pregnancy, the puerperium and lactation**
  + **O91.11 Abscess of breast associated with pregnancy**
    Gestational mammary abscess
    Gestational purulent mastitis
    Gestational subareolar abscess
    - • ♀ **O91.111 Abscess of breast associated with pregnancy, first trimester**
    - • ♀ **O91.112 Abscess of breast associated with pregnancy, second trimester**
    - • ♀ **O91.113 Abscess of breast associated with pregnancy, third trimester**
    - • ♀ **O91.119 Abscess of breast associated with pregnancy, unspecified trimester**
  - • ♀ **O91.12 Abscess of breast associated with the puerperium**
    Puerperal mammary abscess
    Puerperal purulent mastitis
    Puerperal subareolar abscess
  - • ♀ **O91.13 Abscess of breast associated with lactation**
    Mammary abscess associated with lactation
    Purulent mastitis associated with lactation
    Subareolar abscess associated with lactation
+ **O91.2 Nonpurulent mastitis associated with pregnancy, the puerperium and lactation**
  + **O91.21 Nonpurulent mastitis associated with pregnancy**
    Gestational interstitial mastitis
    Gestational lymphangitis of breast
    Gestational mastitis NOS
    Gestational parenchymatous mastitis
    - • ♀ **O91.211 Nonpurulent mastitis associated with pregnancy, first trimester**
    - • ♀ **O91.212 Nonpurulent mastitis associated with pregnancy, second trimester**
    - • ♀ **O91.213 Nonpurulent mastitis associated with pregnancy, third trimester**
    - • ♀ **O91.219 Nonpurulent mastitis associated with pregnancy, unspecified trimester**
  - • ♀ **O91.22 Nonpurulent mastitis associated with the puerperium**
    Puerperal interstitial mastitis
    Puerperal lymphangitis of breast
    Puerperal mastitis NOS
    Puerperal parenchymatous mastitis
  - • ♀ **O91.23 Nonpurulent mastitis associated with lactation**
    Interstitial mastitis associated with lactation
    Lymphangitis of breast associated with lactation
    Mastitis NOS associated with lactation
    Parenchymatous mastitis associated with lactation

O92 Other disorders of breast and disorders of lactation associated with pregnancy and the puerperium

+ **O92.0 Retracted nipple associated with pregnancy, the puerperium, and lactation**
  + **O92.01 Retracted nipple associated with pregnancy**
    - • ♀ **O92.011 Retracted nipple associated with pregnancy, first trimester**
    - • ♀ **O92.012 Retracted nipple associated with pregnancy, second trimester**
    - • ♀ **O92.013 Retracted nipple associated with pregnancy, third trimester**
    - • ♀ **O92.019 Retracted nipple associated with pregnancy, unspecified trimester**
  - • ♀ **O92.02 Retracted nipple associated with the puerperium**
  - • ♀ **O92.03 Retracted nipple associated with lactation**
+ **O92.1 Cracked nipple associated with pregnancy, the puerperium, and lactation**
  Fissure of nipple, gestational or puerperal
  + **O92.11 Cracked nipple associated with pregnancy**
    - • ♀ **O92.111 Cracked nipple associated with pregnancy, first trimester**
    - • ♀ **O92.112 Cracked nipple associated with pregnancy, second trimester**
    - • ♀ **O92.113 Cracked nipple associated with pregnancy, third trimester**
    - • ♀ **O92.119 Cracked nipple associated with pregnancy, unspecified trimester**
  - • ♀ **O92.12 Cracked nipple associated with the puerperium**
  - • ♀ **O92.13 Cracked nipple associated with lactation**

+ **O92.2 Other and unspecified disorders of breast associated with pregnancy and the puerperium**
  - • ♀ **O92.20 Unspecified disorder of breast associated with pregnancy and the puerperium**
  - • ♀ **O92.29 Other disorders of breast associated with pregnancy and the puerperium**

• ♀ **O92.3 Agalactia**
Primary agalactia
Excludes1: *Elective agalactia (O92.5)*
Secondary agalactia (O92.5)
Therapeutic agalactia (O92.5)

• ♀ **O92.4 Hypogalactia**

• ♀ **O92.5 Suppressed lactation**
Elective agalactia
Secondary agalactia
Therapeutic agalactia
Excludes1: *primary agalactia (O92.3)*

• ♀ **O92.6 Galactorrhea**

+ **O92.7 Other and unspecified disorders of lactation**
  - • ♀ **O92.70 Unspecified disorders of lactation**
  - • ♀ **O92.79 Other disorders of lactation**
    Puerperal galactocele

Other obstetric conditions, not elsewhere classified (O94-O9A)

• ♀ **O94 Sequelae of complication of pregnancy, childbirth, and the puerperium**

NOTE This category is to be used to indicate conditions in O00-O77.-, O85-O94 and O98-O9A.- as the cause of late effects. The sequelae include conditions specified as such, or as late effects, which may occur at any time after the puerperium

Code first condition resulting from (sequela) of complication of pregnancy, childbirth, and the puerperium
Review coding guideline C.15.p
Valid 3-character code, no further characters required

O98 Maternal infectious and parasitic diseases classifiable elsewhere but complicating pregnancy, childbirth and the puerperium

Includes: the listed conditions when complicating the pregnant state, when aggravated by the pregnancy, or as a reason for obstetric care

Use additional code (Chapter 1), to identify specific infectious or parasitic disease

Excludes2: *herpes gestationis (O26.4-)*
infectious carrier state (O99.82-, O99.83-)
obstetrical tetanus (A34)
puerperal infection (O86.-)
puerperal sepsis (O85)
when the reason for maternal care is that the disease is known or suspected to have affected the fetus (O35-O36)

+ **O98.0 Tuberculosis complicating pregnancy, childbirth and the puerperium**
  Conditions in A15-A19
  + **O98.01 Tuberculosis complicating pregnancy**
    - • ♀ CC **O98.011 Tuberculosis complicating pregnancy, first trimester**
    - • ♀ CC **O98.012 Tuberculosis complicating pregnancy, second trimester**
    - • ♀ CC **O98.013 Tuberculosis complicating pregnancy, third trimester**
    - • ♀ **O98.019 Tuberculosis complicating pregnancy, unspecified trimester**
  - • ♀ CC **O98.02 Tuberculosis complicating childbirth**
  - • ♀ CC **O98.03 Tuberculosis complicating the puerperium**

+ **O98.1 Syphilis complicating pregnancy, childbirth and the puerperium**
  Conditions in A50-A53
  + **O98.11 Syphilis complicating pregnancy**
    - • ♀ CC **O98.111 Syphilis complicating pregnancy, first trimester**
    - • ♀ CC **O98.112 Syphilis complicating pregnancy, second trimester**
    - • ♀ CC **O98.113 Syphilis complicating pregnancy, third trimester**
    - • ♀ **O98.119 Syphilis complicating pregnancy, unspecified trimester**
  - • ♀ CC **O98.12 Syphilis complicating childbirth**
  - • ♀ CC **O98.13 Syphilis complicating the puerperium**

+ **O98.2 Gonorrhea complicating pregnancy, childbirth and the puerperium**
  Conditions in A54.-
  + **O98.21 Gonorrhea complicating pregnancy**
    - • ♀ CC **O98.211 Gonorrhea complicating pregnancy, first trimester**
    - • ♀ CC **O98.212 Gonorrhea complicating pregnancy, second trimester**
    - • ♀ CC **O98.213 Gonorrhea complicating pregnancy, third trimester**
    - • ♀ **O98.219 Gonorrhea complicating pregnancy, unspecified trimester**
  - • ♀ CC **O98.22 Gonorrhea complicating childbirth**
  - • ♀ CC **O98.23 Gonorrhea complicating the puerperium**

+ **O98.3 Other infections with a predominantly sexual mode of transmission complicating pregnancy, childbirth and the puerperium**
  Conditions in A55-A64
  + **O98.31 Other infections with a predominantly sexual mode of transmission complicating pregnancy**
    - • ♀ CC **O98.311 Other infections with a predominantly sexual mode of transmission complicating pregnancy, first trimester**
    - • ♀ CC **O98.312 Other infections with a predominantly sexual mode of transmission complicating pregnancy, second trimester**
    - • ♀ CC **O98.313 Other infections with a predominantly sexual mode of transmission complicating pregnancy, third trimester**
    - • ♀ **O98.319 Other infections with a predominantly sexual mode of transmission complicating pregnancy, unspecified trimester**
  - • ♀ CC **O98.32 Other infections with a predominantly sexual mode of transmission complicating childbirth**
    AHA CC: 1Q, 2020, 20
  - • ♀ CC **O98.33 Other infections with a predominantly sexual mode of transmission complicating the puerperium**

+ **O98.4 Viral hepatitis complicating pregnancy, childbirth and the puerperium**
  Conditions in B15-B19
  + **O98.41 Viral hepatitis complicating pregnancy**
    - • ♀ CC **O98.411 Viral hepatitis complicating pregnancy, first trimester**
    - • ♀ CC **O98.412 Viral hepatitis complicating pregnancy, second trimester**
    - • ♀ CC **O98.413 Viral hepatitis complicating pregnancy, third trimester**
    - • ♀ **O98.419 Viral hepatitis complicating pregnancy, unspecified trimester**
  - • ♀ CC **O98.42 Viral hepatitis complicating childbirth**
  - • ♀ CC **O98.43 Viral hepatitis complicating the puerperium**

+ **O98.5 Other viral diseases complicating pregnancy, childbirth and the puerperium**
  Conditions in A80-B09, B25-B34, R87.81-, R87.82-
  Excludes1: *human immunodeficiency virus [HIV] disease complicating pregnancy, childbirth and the puerperium (O98.7-)*
  Review coding guideline C.15.s
  + **O98.51 Other viral diseases complicating pregnancy**
    - • ♀ CC **O98.511 Other viral diseases complicating pregnancy, first trimester**
    - • ♀ CC **O98.512 Other viral diseases complicating pregnancy, second trimester**
      AHA CC: 4Q, 2016, 4-7
    - • ♀ CC **O98.513 Other viral diseases complicating pregnancy, third trimester**
      AHA CC: 4Q, 2016, 4-7
    - • ♀ **O98.519 Other viral diseases complicating pregnancy, unspecified trimester**
  - • ♀ CC **O98.52 Other viral diseases complicating childbirth**
  - • ♀ CC **O98.53 Other viral diseases complicating the puerperium**

+ **O98.6 Protozoal diseases complicating pregnancy, childbirth and the puerperium**
  Conditions in B50-B64
  + **O98.61 Protozoal diseases complicating pregnancy**
    - • ♀ CC **O98.611 Protozoal diseases complicating pregnancy, first trimester**
    - • ♀ CC **O98.612 Protozoal diseases complicating pregnancy, second trimester**
    - • ♀ CC **O98.613 Protozoal diseases complicating pregnancy, third trimester**

• ♀ **O98.619 Protozoal diseases complicating pregnancy, unspecified trimester**

• ♀ CC **O98.62 Protozoal diseases complicating childbirth**

• ♀ CC **O98.63 Protozoal diseases complicating the puerperium**

\+ **O98.7 Human immunodeficiency virus [HIV] disease complicating pregnancy, childbirth and the puerperium**

Use additional code to identify the type of HIV disease:
Acquired immune deficiency syndrome (AIDS) (B20)
Asymptomatic HIV status (Z21)
HIV positive NOS (Z21)
Symptomatic HIV disease (B20)

Review coding guideline C.1.a.2.g
Review coding guideline C.15.f

\+ **O98.71 Human immunodeficiency virus [HIV] disease complicating pregnancy**

• ♀ CC **O98.711 Human immunodeficiency virus [HIV] disease complicating pregnancy, first trimester**

• ♀ CC **O98.712 Human immunodeficiency virus [HIV] disease complicating pregnancy, second trimester**

• ♀ CC **O98.713 Human immunodeficiency virus [HIV] disease complicating pregnancy, third trimester**

• ♀ **O98.719 Human immunodeficiency virus [HIV] disease complicating pregnancy, unspecified trimester**

• ♀ CC **O98.72 Human immunodeficiency virus [HIV] disease complicating childbirth**

• ♀ CC **O98.73 Human immunodeficiency virus [HIV] disease complicating the puerperium**

\+ **O98.8 Other maternal infectious and parasitic diseases complicating pregnancy, childbirth and the puerperium**

\+ **O98.81 Other maternal infectious and parasitic diseases complicating pregnancy**

• ♀ CC **O98.811 Other maternal infectious and parasitic diseases complicating pregnancy, first trimester**

• ♀ CC **O98.812 Other maternal infectious and parasitic diseases complicating pregnancy, second trimester**

• ♀ CC **O98.813 Other maternal infectious and parasitic diseases complicating pregnancy, third trimester**

• ♀ **O98.819 Other maternal infectious and parasitic diseases complicating pregnancy, unspecified trimester**

• ♀ CC **O98.82 Other maternal infectious and parasitic diseases complicating childbirth**

AHA CC: 1Q, 2020, 10

• ♀ CC **O98.83 Other maternal infectious and parasitic diseases complicating the puerperium**

\+ **O98.9 Unspecified maternal infectious and parasitic disease complicating pregnancy, childbirth and the puerperium**

\+ **O98.91 Unspecified maternal infectious and parasitic disease complicating pregnancy**

• ♀ CC **O98.911 Unspecified maternal infectious and parasitic disease complicating pregnancy, first trimester**

• ♀ CC **O98.912 Unspecified maternal infectious and parasitic disease complicating pregnancy, second trimester**

• ♀ CC **O98.913 Unspecified maternal infectious and parasitic disease complicating pregnancy, third trimester**

• ♀ **O98.919 Unspecified maternal infectious and parasitic disease complicating pregnancy, unspecified trimester**

• ♀ CC **O98.92 Unspecified maternal infectious and parasitic disease complicating childbirth**

• ♀ CC **O98.93 Unspecified maternal infectious and parasitic disease complicating the puerperium**

O99 Other maternal diseases classifiable elsewhere but complicating pregnancy, childbirth and the puerperium

Includes: conditions which complicate the pregnant state, are aggravated by the pregnancy or are a main reason for obstetric care

Use additional code to identify specific condition

Excludes2: *when the reason for maternal care is that the condition is known or suspected to have affected the fetus (O35-O36)*

\+ **O99.0 Anemia complicating pregnancy, childbirth and the puerperium**

Conditions in D50-D64

Excludes1: *anemia arising in the puerperium (O90.81)*
postpartum anemia NOS (O90.81)

\+ **O99.01 Anemia complicating pregnancy**

• ♀ **O99.011 Anemia complicating pregnancy, first trimester**

• ♀ **O99.012 Anemia complicating pregnancy, second trimester**

• ♀ **O99.013 Anemia complicating pregnancy, third trimester**

• ♀ **O99.019 Anemia complicating pregnancy, unspecified trimester**

• ♀ **O99.02 Anemia complicating childbirth**

• ♀ **O99.03 Anemia complicating the puerperium**

Excludes1: *postpartum anemia not pre-existing prior to delivery (O90.81)*

\+ **O99.1 Other diseases of the blood and blood-forming organs and certain disorders involving the immune mechanism complicating pregnancy, childbirth and the puerperium**

Conditions in D65-D89

Excludes1: *hemorrhage with coagulation defects (O45.-, O46.0-, O67.0, O72.3)*

\+ **O99.11 Other diseases of the blood and blood-forming organs and certain disorders involving the immune mechanism complicating pregnancy**

• ♀ CC **O99.111 Other diseases of the blood and blood-forming organs and certain disorders involving the immune mechanism complicating pregnancy, first trimester**

• ♀ CC **O99.112 Other diseases of the blood and blood-forming organs and certain disorders involving the immune mechanism complicating pregnancy, second trimester**

• ♀ CC **O99.113 Other diseases of the blood and blood-forming organs and certain disorders involving the immune mechanism complicating pregnancy, third trimester**

• ♀ CC **O99.119 Other diseases of the blood and blood-forming organs and certain disorders involving the immune mechanism complicating pregnancy, unspecified trimester**

• ♀ CC **O99.12 Other diseases of the blood and blood-forming organs and certain disorders involving the immune mechanism complicating childbirth**

• ♀ CC **O99.13 Other diseases of the blood and blood-forming organs and certain disorders involving the immune mechanism complicating the puerperium**

\+ **O99.2 Endocrine, nutritional and metabolic diseases complicating pregnancy, childbirth and the puerperium**

Conditions in E00-E89

Excludes2: *diabetes mellitus (O24.-)*
malnutrition (O25.-)
postpartum thyroiditis (O90.5)

\+ **O99.21 Obesity complicating pregnancy, childbirth, and the puerperium**

Use additional code to identify the type of obesity (E66.-)

• ♀ **O99.210 Obesity complicating pregnancy, unspecified trimester**

• ♀ **O99.211 Obesity complicating pregnancy, first trimester**

• ♀ **O99.212 Obesity complicating pregnancy, second trimester**

• ♀ **O99.213 Obesity complicating pregnancy, third trimester**

• ♀ **O99.214 Obesity complicating childbirth**

AHA CC: 4Q, 2018, 80; 2Q, 2021, 10-11

• ♀ **O99.215 Obesity complicating the puerperium**

+ **O99.28 Other endocrine, nutritional and metabolic diseases complicating pregnancy, childbirth and the puerperium**
  - • ♀ **O99.280 Endocrine, nutritional and metabolic diseases complicating pregnancy, unspecified trimester**
  - • ♀ **O99.281 Endocrine, nutritional and metabolic diseases complicating pregnancy, first trimester**
  - • ♀ **O99.282 Endocrine, nutritional and metabolic diseases complicating pregnancy, second trimester**
  - • ♀ **O99.283 Endocrine, nutritional and metabolic diseases complicating pregnancy, third trimester**
  - • ♀ **O99.284 Endocrine, nutritional and metabolic diseases complicating childbirth**
    AHA CC: 1Q, 2021, 8-9
  - • ♀ **O99.285 Endocrine, nutritional and metabolic diseases complicating the puerperium**

+ **O99.3 Mental disorders and diseases of the nervous system complicating pregnancy, childbirth and the puerperium**

+ **O99.31 Alcohol use complicating pregnancy, childbirth, and the puerperium**
  Use additional code(s) from F10 to identify manifestations of the alcohol use
  Review coding guideline C.15.l.1
  - • ♀ **O99.310 Alcohol use complicating pregnancy, unspecified trimester**
  - • ♀ **O99.311 Alcohol use complicating pregnancy, first trimester**
  - • ♀ **O99.312 Alcohol use complicating pregnancy, second trimester**
  - • ♀ **O99.313 Alcohol use complicating pregnancy, third trimester**
  - • ♀ **O99.314 Alcohol use complicating childbirth**
  - • ♀ **O99.315 Alcohol use complicating the puerperium**

+ **O99.32 Drug use complicating pregnancy, childbirth, and the puerperium**
  Use additional code(s) from F11-F16 and F18-F19 to identify manifestations of the drug use
  AHA CC: 2Q, 2018, 10-11
  Review coding guideline C.15.l.3
  - • ♀ **O99.320 Drug use complicating pregnancy, unspecified trimester**
  - • ♀ CC **O99.321 Drug use complicating pregnancy, first trimester**
  - • ♀ CC **O99.322 Drug use complicating pregnancy, second trimester**
  - • ♀ CC **O99.323 Drug use complicating pregnancy, third trimester**
  - • ♀ CC **O99.324 Drug use complicating childbirth**
  - • ♀ CC **O99.325 Drug use complicating the puerperium**

+ **O99.33 Tobacco use disorder complicating pregnancy, childbirth, and the puerperium**
  Smoking complicating pregnancy, childbirth, and the puerperium
  Use additional code from category F17 to identify type of tobacco nicotine dependence
  Review coding guideline C.15.l.2
  - • ♀ **O99.330 Smoking (tobacco) complicating pregnancy, unspecified trimester**
  - • ♀ **O99.331 Smoking (tobacco) complicating pregnancy, first trimester**
  - • ♀ **O99.332 Smoking (tobacco) complicating pregnancy, second trimester**
  - • ♀ **O99.333 Smoking (tobacco) complicating pregnancy, third trimester**
  - • ♀ **O99.334 Smoking (tobacco) complicating childbirth**
  - • ♀ **O99.335 Smoking (tobacco) complicating the puerperium**

+ **O99.34 Other mental disorders complicating pregnancy, childbirth, and the puerperium**
  Conditions in F01-F09, F20-F52 and F54-F99
  Excludes2: *postpartum mood disturbance (O90.6)*
  postnatal psychosis (F53.1)
  puerperal psychosis (F53.1)
  - • ♀ **O99.340 Other mental disorders complicating pregnancy, unspecified trimester**
  - • ♀ **O99.341 Other mental disorders complicating pregnancy, first trimester**
  - • ♀ **O99.342 Other mental disorders complicating pregnancy, second trimester**
  - • ♀ **O99.343 Other mental disorders complicating pregnancy, third trimester**
  - • ♀ **O99.344 Other mental disorders complicating childbirth**
  - • ♀ **O99.345 Other mental disorders complicating the puerperium**
    AHA CC: 4Q, 2018, 8-9

+ **O99.35 Diseases of the nervous system complicating pregnancy, childbirth, and the puerperium**
  Conditions in G00-G99
  Excludes2: *pregnancy related peripheral neuritis (O26.8-)*
  - • ♀ **O99.350 Diseases of the nervous system complicating pregnancy, unspecified trimester**
  - • ♀ **O99.351 Diseases of the nervous system complicating pregnancy, first trimester**
  - • ♀ **O99.352 Diseases of the nervous system complicating pregnancy, second trimester**
  - • ♀ **O99.353 Diseases of the nervous system complicating pregnancy, third trimester**
  - • ♀ CC **O99.354 Diseases of the nervous system complicating childbirth**
  - • ♀ CC **O99.355 Diseases of the nervous system complicating the puerperium**

+ **O99.4 Diseases of the circulatory system complicating pregnancy, childbirth and the puerperium**
  Conditions in I00-I99
  Excludes1: *peripartum cardiomyopathy (O90.3)*
  Excludes2: *hypertensive disorders (O10-O16)*
  obstetric embolism (O88.-)
  venous complications and cerebrovenous sinus thrombosis in labor, childbirth and the puerperium (O87.-)
  venous complications and cerebrovenous sinus thrombosis in pregnancy (O22.-)

+ **O99.41 Diseases of the circulatory system complicating pregnancy**
  AHA CC: 2Q, 2016, 8
  - • ♀ CC **O99.411 Diseases of the circulatory system complicating pregnancy, first trimester**
  - • ♀ CC **O99.412 Diseases of the circulatory system complicating pregnancy, second trimester**
  - • ♀ CC **O99.413 Diseases of the circulatory system complicating pregnancy, third trimester**
  - • ♀ **O99.419 Diseases of the circulatory system complicating pregnancy, unspecified trimester**

• ♀ MCC **O99.42 Diseases of the circulatory system complicating childbirth**

• ♀ CC **O99.43 Diseases of the circulatory system complicating the puerperium**

+ **O99.5 Diseases of the respiratory system complicating pregnancy, childbirth and the puerperium**
  Conditions in J00-J99

+ **O99.51 Diseases of the respiratory system complicating pregnancy**
  - • ♀ **O99.511 Diseases of the respiratory system complicating pregnancy, first trimester**
  - • ♀ **O99.512 Diseases of the respiratory system complicating pregnancy, second trimester**
  - • ♀ **O99.513 Diseases of the respiratory system complicating pregnancy, third trimester**
  - • ♀ **O99.519 Diseases of the respiratory system complicating pregnancy, unspecified trimester**

● ♀ **O99.52 Diseases of the respiratory system complicating childbirth**

● ♀ **O99.53 Diseases of the respiratory system complicating the puerperium**

\+ **O99.6 Diseases of the digestive system complicating pregnancy, childbirth and the puerperium**

Conditions in K00-K93

Excludes2: *liver and biliary tract disorders in pregnancy, childbirth and the puerperium (O26.6-)*
hemorrhoids in pregnancy (O22.4-)

\+ **O99.61 Diseases of the digestive system complicating pregnancy**

● ♀ **O99.611 Diseases of the digestive system complicating pregnancy, first trimester**

● ♀ **O99.612 Diseases of the digestive system complicating pregnancy, second trimester**

● ♀ **O99.613 Diseases of the digestive system complicating pregnancy, third trimester**

● ♀ **O99.619 Diseases of the digestive system complicating pregnancy, unspecified trimester**

● ♀ **O99.62 Diseases of the digestive system complicating childbirth**

● ♀ **O99.63 Diseases of the digestive system complicating the puerperium**

\+ **O99.7 Diseases of the skin and subcutaneous tissue complicating pregnancy, childbirth and the puerperium**

Conditions in L00-L99

Excludes2: *herpes gestationis (O26.4)*
pruritic urticarial papules and plaques of pregnancy (PUPPP) (O26.86)

\+ **O99.71 Diseases of the skin and subcutaneous tissue complicating pregnancy**

● ♀ **O99.711 Diseases of the skin and subcutaneous tissue complicating pregnancy, first trimester**

● ♀ **O99.712 Diseases of the skin and subcutaneous tissue complicating pregnancy, second trimester**

● ♀ **O99.713 Diseases of the skin and subcutaneous tissue complicating pregnancy, third trimester**

● ♀ **O99.719 Diseases of the skin and subcutaneous tissue complicating pregnancy, unspecified trimester**

● ♀ **O99.72 Diseases of the skin and subcutaneous tissue complicating childbirth**

● ♀ **O99.73 Diseases of the skin and subcutaneous tissue complicating the puerperium**

\+ **O99.8 Other specified diseases and conditions complicating pregnancy, childbirth and the puerperium**

Conditions in D00-D48, H00-H95, M00-N99, and Q00-Q99

Use additional code to identify condition

Excludes2: *genitourinary infections in pregnancy (O23.-)*
infection of genitourinary tract following delivery (O86.1-O86.4)
malignant neoplasm complicating pregnancy, childbirth and the puerperium (O9A.1-)
maternal care for known or suspected abnormality of maternal pelvic organs (O34.-)
postpartum acute kidney failure (O90.4)
traumatic injuries in pregnancy (O9A.2-)

\+ **O99.81 Abnormal glucose complicating pregnancy, childbirth and the puerperium**

Excludes1: *gestational diabetes (O24.4-)*

Review coding guideline C.15.i

● ♀ **O99.810 Abnormal glucose complicating pregnancy**

● ♀ **O99.814 Abnormal glucose complicating childbirth**

● ♀ **O99.815 Abnormal glucose complicating the puerperium**

\+ **O99.82 Streptococcus B carrier state complicating pregnancy, childbirth and the puerperium**

Excludes1: *Carrier of streptococcus group B (GBS) in a nonpregnant woman (Z22.330)*

● ♀ **O99.820 Streptococcus B carrier state complicating pregnancy**

● ♀ **O99.824 Streptococcus B carrier state complicating childbirth**

AHA CC: 2Q, 2019, 9

● ♀ **O99.825 Streptococcus B carrier state complicating the puerperium**

\+ **O99.83 Other infection carrier state complicating pregnancy, childbirth and the puerperium**

Use additional code to identify the carrier state (Z22.-)

● ♀ CC **O99.830 Other infection carrier state complicating pregnancy**

● ♀ CC **O99.834 Other infection carrier state complicating childbirth**

● ♀ CC **O99.835 Other infection carrier state complicating the puerperium**

\+ **O99.84 Bariatric surgery status complicating pregnancy, childbirth and the puerperium**

Gastric banding status complicating pregnancy, childbirth and the puerperium
Gastric bypass status for obesity complicating pregnancy, childbirth and the puerperium
Obesity surgery status complicating pregnancy, childbirth and the puerperium

● ♀ **O99.840 Bariatric surgery status complicating pregnancy, unspecified trimester**

● ♀ **O99.841 Bariatric surgery status complicating pregnancy, first trimester**

● ♀ **O99.842 Bariatric surgery status complicating pregnancy, second trimester**

● ♀ **O99.843 Bariatric surgery status complicating pregnancy, third trimester**

● ♀ **O99.844 Bariatric surgery status complicating childbirth**

● ♀ **O99.845 Bariatric surgery status complicating the puerperium**

\+ **O99.89 Other specified diseases and conditions complicating pregnancy, childbirth and the puerperium**

AHA CC: 4Q, 2020, 36-37

● ♀ **O99.891 Other specified diseases and conditions complicating pregnancy**

● ♀ **O99.892 Other specified diseases and conditions complicating childbirth**

● ♀ **O99.893 Other specified diseases and conditions complicating puerperium**

O9A Maternal malignant neoplasms, traumatic injuries and abuse classifiable elsewhere but complicating pregnancy, childbirth and the puerperium

\+ **O9A.1 Malignant neoplasm complicating pregnancy, childbirth and the puerperium**

Conditions in C00-C96

Use additional code to identify neoplasm

Excludes2: *maternal care for benign tumor of corpus uteri (O34.1-)*
maternal care for benign tumor of cervix (O34.4-)

Review coding guideline C.2.l.3

\+ **O9A.11 Malignant neoplasm complicating pregnancy**

● ♀ **O9A.111 Malignant neoplasm complicating pregnancy, first trimester**

● ♀ **O9A.112 Malignant neoplasm complicating pregnancy, second trimester**

● ♀ **O9A.113 Malignant neoplasm complicating pregnancy, third trimester**

● ♀ **O9A.119 Malignant neoplasm complicating pregnancy, unspecified trimester**

● ♀ **O9A.12 Malignant neoplasm complicating childbirth**

● ♀ **O9A.13 Malignant neoplasm complicating the puerperium**

AHA CC: 3Q, 2015, 19-20

+ **O9A.2 Injury, poisoning and certain other consequences of external causes complicating pregnancy, childbirth and the puerperium**
Conditions in S00-T88, except T74 and T76
Use additional code(s) to identify the injury or poisoning
Excludes2: *physical, sexual and psychological abuse complicating pregnancy, childbirth and the puerperium (O9A.3-, O9A.4-, O9A.5-)*
Review coding guideline C.15.m
+ **O9A.21 Injury, poisoning and certain other consequences of external causes complicating pregnancy**
• ♀ **O9A.211 Injury, poisoning and certain other consequences of external causes complicating pregnancy, first trimester**
• ♀ **O9A.212 Injury, poisoning and certain other consequences of external causes complicating pregnancy, second trimester**
• ♀ **O9A.213 Injury, poisoning and certain other consequences of external causes complicating pregnancy, third trimester**
• ♀ **O9A.219 Injury, poisoning and certain other consequences of external causes complicating pregnancy, unspecified trimester**
• ♀ **O9A.22 Injury, poisoning and certain other consequences of external causes complicating childbirth**
• ♀ **O9A.23 Injury, poisoning and certain other consequences of external causes complicating the puerperium**

+ **O9A.3 Physical abuse complicating pregnancy, childbirth and the puerperium**
Conditions in T74.11 or T76.11
Use additional code (if applicable):
to identify any associated current injury due to physical abuse
to identify the perpetrator of abuse (Y07.-)
Excludes2: *sexual abuse complicating pregnancy, childbirth and the puerperium (O9A.4)*
Review coding guideline C.15.r
+ **O9A.31 Physical abuse complicating pregnancy**
• ♀ **O9A.311 Physical abuse complicating pregnancy, first trimester**
• ♀ **O9A.312 Physical abuse complicating pregnancy, second trimester**
• ♀ **O9A.313 Physical abuse complicating pregnancy, third trimester**
• ♀ **O9A.319 Physical abuse complicating pregnancy, unspecified trimester**
• ♀ **O9A.32 Physical abuse complicating childbirth**
• ♀ **O9A.33 Physical abuse complicating the puerperium**

+ **O9A.4 Sexual abuse complicating pregnancy, childbirth and the puerperium**
Conditions in T74.21 or T76.21
Use additional code (if applicable):
to identify any associated current injury due to sexual abuse
to identify the perpetrator of abuse (Y07.-)
Review coding guideline C.15.r
+ **O9A.41 Sexual abuse complicating pregnancy**
• ♀ **O9A.411 Sexual abuse complicating pregnancy, first trimester**
• ♀ **O9A.412 Sexual abuse complicating pregnancy, second trimester**
• ♀ **O9A.413 Sexual abuse complicating pregnancy, third trimester**
• ♀ **O9A.419 Sexual abuse complicating pregnancy, unspecified trimester**
• ♀ **O9A.42 Sexual abuse complicating childbirth**
• ♀ **O9A.43 Sexual abuse complicating the puerperium**

+ **O9A.5 Psychological abuse complicating pregnancy, childbirth and the puerperium**
Conditions in T74.31 or T76.31
Use additional code to identify the perpetrator of abuse (Y07.-)
Review coding guideline C.15.r
+ **O9A.51 Psychological abuse complicating pregnancy**
• ♀ **O9A.511 Psychological abuse complicating pregnancy, first trimester**
• ♀ **O9A.512 Psychological abuse complicating pregnancy, second trimester**
• ♀ **O9A.513 Psychological abuse complicating pregnancy, third trimester**
• ♀ **O9A.519 Psychological abuse complicating pregnancy, unspecified trimester**
• ♀ **O9A.52 Psychological abuse complicating childbirth**
• ♀ **O9A.53 Psychological abuse complicating the puerperium**

Chapter 16: Certain Conditions Originating in the Perinatal Period (P00-P96)

NOTE Codes from this chapter are for use on newborn records only, never on maternal records

Includes: conditions that have their origin in the fetal or perinatal period (before birth through the first 28 days after birth) even if morbidity occurs later

Excludes2: *congenital malformations, deformations and chromosomal abnormalities (Q00-Q99)*
endocrine, nutritional and metabolic diseases (E00-E88)
injury, poisoning and certain other consequences of external causes (S00-T88)
neoplasms (C00-D49)
tetanus neonatorum (A33)

This chapter contains the following category blocks:

P00-P04 Newborn affected by maternal factors and by complications of pregnancy, labor, and delivery
P05-P08 Disorders of newborn related to length of gestation and fetal growth
P09 Abnormal findings on neonatal screening
P10-P15 Birth trauma
P19-P29 Respiratory and cardiovascular disorders specific to the perinatal period
P35-P39 Infections specific to the perinatal period
P50-P61 Hemorrhagic and hematological disorders of newborn
P70-P74 Transitory endocrine and metabolic disorders specific to newborn
P76-P78 Digestive system disorders of newborn
P80-P83 Conditions involving the integument and temperature regulation of newborn
P84 Other problems with newborn
P90-P96 Other disorders originating in the perinatal period

C. Chapter-Specific Coding Guidelines

In addition to general coding guidelines, there are guidelines for specific diagnoses and/or conditions in the classification. Unless otherwise indicated, these guidelines apply to all health care settings. Please refer to Section II for guidelines on the selection of principal diagnosis.

16. Chapter 16: Certain Conditions Originating in the Perinatal Period (P00-P96)

For coding and reporting purposes the perinatal period is defined as before birth through the 28th day following birth. The following guidelines are provided for reporting purposes

a. General Perinatal Rules

1) Use of Chapter 16 Codes

Codes in this chapter are <u>never</u> for use on the maternal record. Codes from Chapter 15, the obstetric chapter, are never permitted on the newborn record. Chapter 16 codes may be used throughout the life of the patient if the condition is still present.

2) Principal Diagnosis for Birth Record

When coding the birth episode in a newborn record, assign a code from category Z38, Liveborn infants according to place of birth and type of delivery, as the principal diagnosis. A code from category Z38 is assigned only once, to a newborn at the time of birth. If a newborn is transferred to another institution, a code from category Z38 should not be used at the receiving hospital.

A code from category Z38 is used only on the newborn record, not on the mother's record.

3) Use of Codes from other Chapters with Codes from Chapter 16

Codes from other chapters may be used with codes from chapter 16 if the codes from the other chapters provide more specific detail. Codes for signs and symptoms may be assigned when a definitive diagnosis has not been established. If the reason for the encounter is a perinatal condition, the code from chapter 16 should be sequenced first.

4) Use of Chapter 16 Codes after the Perinatal Period

Should a condition originate in the perinatal period, and continue throughout the life of the patient, the perinatal code should continue to be used regardless of the patient's age.

5) Birth process or community acquired conditions

If a newborn has a condition that may be either due to the birth process or community acquired and the documentation does not indicate which it is, the default is due to the birth process and the code from Chapter 16 should be used. If the condition is community-acquired, a code from Chapter 16 should not be assigned.

For COVID-19 infection in a newborn, see guideline I.C.16.h

6) Code all clinically significant conditions

All clinically significant conditions noted on routine newborn examination should be coded. A condition is clinically significant if it requires:

- clinical evaluation; or
- therapeutic treatment; or
- diagnostic procedures; or
- extended length of hospital stay; or
- increased nursing care and/or monitoring; or
- has implications for future health care needs

Note: The perinatal guidelines listed above are the same as the general coding guidelines for "additional diagnoses", except for the final point regarding implications for future health care needs. Codes should be assigned for conditions that have been specified by the provider as having implications for future health care needs.

b. Observation and Evaluation of Newborns for Suspected Conditions not Found

1) Use of Z05 codes

Assign a code from category Z05, Observation and evaluation of newborns and infants for suspected conditions ruled out, to identify those instances when a healthy newborn is evaluated for a suspected condition that is determined after study not to be present. Do not use a code from category Z05 when the patient has identified signs or symptoms of a suspected problem; in such cases code the sign or symptom.

2) Z05 on Other than the Birth Record

A code from category Z05 may also be assigned as a principal or first-listed code for readmissions or encounters when the code from category Z38 code no longer applies. Codes from category Z05 are fur use only for healthy newborns and infants for which no condition after study is found to be present.

3) Z05 on a birth record

A code from category Z05 is to be used as a secondary code after the code from category Z38, Liveborn infants according to place of birth and type of delivery.

c. Coding Additional Perinatal Diagnoses

1) Assigning codes for conditions that require treatment

Assign codes for conditions that require treatment or further investigation, prolong the length of stay, or require resource utilization.

2) Codes for conditions specified as having implications for future health care needs

Assign codes for conditions that have been specified by the provider as having implications for future health care needs.

Note: This guideline should not be used for adult patients.

d. Prematurity and Fetal Growth Retardation

Providers utilize different criteria in determining prematurity. A code for prematurity should not be assigned unless it is documented. Assignment of codes in categories P05, Disorders of newborn related to slow fetal growth and fetal malnutrition, and P07, Disorders of newborn related to short gestation and low birth weight, not elsewhere classified, should be based on the recorded birth weight and estimated gestational age.

When both birth weight and gestational age are available, two codes from category P07 should be assigned, with the code for birth weight sequenced before the code for gestational age.

e. Low birth weight and immaturity status

Codes from category P07, Disorders of newborn related to short gestation and low birth weight, not elsewhere classified, are for use for a child or adult who was premature or had a low birth weight as a newborn and this is affecting the patient's current health status.

See Section I.C.21. Factors influencing health status and contact with health services, Status.

f. Bacterial Sepsis of Newborn

Category P36, Bacterial sepsis of newborn, includes congenital sepsis. If a perinate is documented as having sepsis without documentation of congenital or community acquired, the default is congenital and a code from category P36 should be assigned. If the P36 code includes the causal organism, an additional code from category B95, Streptococcus, Staphylococcus, and Enterococcus as the cause of diseases classified elsewhere, or B96, Other bacterial agents as the cause of diseases classified elsewhere, should not be assigned. If the P36 code does not include the causal organism, assign an additional code from category B96. If applicable, use additional codes to identify severe sepsis (R65.2-) and any associated acute organ dysfunction.

g. Stillbirth

Code P95, Stillbirth, is only for use in institutions that maintain separate records for stillbirths. No other code should be used with P95. Code P95 should not be used on the mother's record.

h. COVID-19 Infection in Newborn

For a newborn that tests positive for COVID-19, assign code U07.1, COVID-19, and the appropriate codes for associated manifestation(s) in neonates/newborns in the absence of documentation indicating a specific type of transmission. For a newborn that tests positive for COVID-19 and the provider documents the condition was contracted in utero or during the birth process, assign codes P35.8, Other congenital viral diseases, and U07.1, COVID-19. When coding the birth episode in a newborn record, the appropriate code from category Z38, Liveborn infants according to place of birth and type of delivery, should be assigned as the principal diagnosis.

Newborn affected by maternal factors and by complications of pregnancy, labor, and delivery (P00-P04)

NOTE These codes are for use when the listed maternal conditions are specified as the cause of confirmed morbidity or potential morbidity which have their origin in the perinatal period (before birth through the first 28 days after birth).

AHA CC: 4Q, 2016, 54-55

P00 Newborn affected by maternal conditions that may be unrelated to present pregnancy

Code first any current condition in newborn

Excludes2: *encounter for observation for newborn for suspected diseases and conditions ruled out (Z05.-)*
newborn affected by maternal complications of pregnancy (P01.-)
newborn affected by maternal endocrine and metabolic disorders (P70-P74)
newborn affected by noxious substances transmitted via placenta or breast milk (P04.-)

P00.0 Newborn affected by maternal hypertensive disorders
Newborn affected by maternal conditions classifiable to O10-O11, O13-O16

P00.1 Newborn affected by maternal renal and urinary tract diseases
Newborn affected by maternal conditions classifiable to N00-N39

P00.2 Newborn affected by maternal infectious and parasitic diseases
Newborn affected by maternal infectious disease classifiable to A00-B99, J09 and J10
Excludes1: *maternal genital tract or other localized infections (P00.8)*
Excludes2: *infections specific to the perinatal period (P35-P39)*
newborn affected by (positive) maternal group B streptococcus (GBS) colonization (P00.82)
AHA CC: 3Q, 2015, 20; 2Q, 2019, 10

P00.3 Newborn affected by other maternal circulatory and respiratory diseases
Newborn affected by maternal conditions classifiable to I00-I99, J00-J99, Q20-Q34 and not included in P00.0, P00.2

P00.4 Newborn affected by maternal nutritional disorders
Newborn affected by maternal disorders classifiable to E40-E64
Maternal malnutrition NOS

P00.5 Newborn affected by maternal injury
Newborn affected by maternal conditions classifiable to O9A.2-

P00.6 Newborn affected by surgical procedure on mother
Newborn affected by amniocentesis
Excludes1: *Cesarean delivery for present delivery (P03.4)*
damage to placenta from amniocentesis, Cesarean delivery or surgical induction (P02.1)
previous surgery to uterus or pelvic organs (P03.89)
Excludes2: *newborn affected by complication of (fetal) intrauterine procedure (P96.5)*

P00.7 Newborn affected by other medical procedures on mother, not elsewhere classified
Newborn affected by radiation to mother
Excludes1: *damage to placenta from amniocentesis, cesareandeliveryorsurgicalinduction(P02.1)*
newborn affected by other complications of labor and delivery (P03.-)

\+ **P00.8 Newborn affected by other maternal conditions**

P00.81 Newborn affected by periodontal disease in mother

P00.82 Newborn affected by (positive) maternal group B streptococcus (GBS) colonization
Contact with positive maternal group B streptococcus

P00.89 Newborn affected by other maternal conditions
Newborn affected by conditions classifiable to T80-T88
Newborn affected by maternal genital tract or other localized infections
Newborn affected by maternal systemic lupus erythematosus
Use additional code to identify infectious agent, if known
Excludes2: *newborn affected by positive maternal group B streptococcus (GBS) colonization (P00.82)*
AHA CC: 2Q, 2019, 9

P00.9 Newborn affected by unspecified maternal condition

P01 Newborn affected by maternal complications of pregnancy

Code first any current condition in newborn

Excludes2: *encounter for observation of newborn for suspected diseases and conditions ruled out (Z05.-)*

P01.0 Newborn affected by incompetent cervix

P01.1 Newborn affected by premature rupture of membranes

P01.2 Newborn affected by oligohydramnios
Excludes1: *oligohydramnios due to premature rupture of membranes (P01.1)*

P01.3 Newborn affected by polyhydramnios
Newborn affected by hydramnios

P01.4 Newborn affected by ectopic pregnancy
Newborn affected by abdominal pregnancy

P01.5 Newborn affected by multiple pregnancy
Newborn affected by triplet (pregnancy)
Newborn affected by twin (pregnancy)

P01.6 Newborn affected by maternal death

P01.7 Newborn affected by malpresentation before labor
Newborn affected by breech presentation before labor
Newborn affected by external version before labor
Newborn affected by face presentation before labor
Newborn affected by transverse lie before labor
Newborn affected by unstable lie before labor

P01.8 Newborn affected by other maternal complications of pregnancy

P01.9 Newborn affected by maternal complication of pregnancy, unspecified

P02 Newborn affected by complications of placenta, cord and membranes

Code first any current condition in newborn

Excludes2: *encounter for observation of newborn for suspected diseases and conditions ruled out (Z05.-)*

P02.0 Newborn affected by placenta previa

P02.1 Newborn affected by other forms of placental separation and hemorrhage
Newborn affected by abruptio placenta
Newborn affected by accidental hemorrhage
Newborn affected by antepartum hemorrhage
Newborn affected by damage to placenta from amniocentesis, cesarean delivery or surgical induction
Newborn affected by maternal blood loss
Newborn affected by premature separation of placenta

\+ **P02.2 Newborn affected by other and unspecified morphological and functional abnormalities of placenta**

P02.20 Newborn affected by unspecified morphological and functional abnormalities of placenta

P02.29 Newborn affected by other morphological and functional abnormalities of placenta
Newborn affected by placental dysfunction
Newborn affected by placental infarction
Newborn affected by placental insufficiency

P02.3 Newborn affected by placental transfusion syndromes
Newborn affected by placental and cord abnormalities resulting in twin-to-twin or other transplacental transfusion

P02.4 Newborn affected by prolapsed cord

P02.5 Newborn affected by other compression of umbilical cord
Newborn affected by umbilical cord (tightly) around neck
Newborn affected by entanglement of umbilical cord
Newborn affected by knot in umbilical cord

\+ **P02.6 Newborn affected by other and unspecified conditions of umbilical cord**

P02.60 Newborn affected by unspecified conditions of umbilical cord

P02.69 Newborn affected by other conditions of umbilical cord
Newborn affected by short umbilical cord
Newborn affected by vasa previa
Excludes1: *newborn affected by single umbilical artery (Q27.0)*

+ **P02.7 Newborn affected by chorioamnionitis**
AHA CC: 4Q, 2018, 23-24

P02.70 Newborn affected by fetal inflammatory response syndrome
Newborn affected by FIRS

P02.78 Newborn affected by other conditions from chorioamnionitis
Newborn affected by amnionitis
Newborn affected by membranitis
Newborn affected by placentitis

P02.8 Newborn affected by other abnormalities of membranes

P02.9 Newborn affected by abnormality of membranes, unspecified

P03 Newborn affected by other complications of labor and delivery
Code first any current condition in newborn
Excludes2: *encounter for observation of newborn for suspected diseases and conditions ruled out (Z05.-)*

P03.0 Newborn affected by breech delivery and extraction

P03.1 Newborn affected by other malpresentation, malposition and disproportion during labor and delivery
Newborn affected by contracted pelvis
Newborn affected by conditions classifiable to O64-O66
Newborn affected by persistent occipitoposterior
Newborn affected by transverse lie

P03.2 Newborn affected by forceps delivery

P03.3 Newborn affected by delivery by vacuum extractor [ventouse]

P03.4 Newborn affected by Cesarean delivery

P03.5 Newborn affected by precipitate delivery
Newborn affected by rapid second stage

P03.6 Newborn affected by abnormal uterine contractions
Newborn affected by conditions classifiable to O62.-, except O62.3
Newborn affected by hypertonic labor
Newborn affected by uterine inertia

+ **P03.8 Newborn affected by other specified complications of labor and delivery**

+ **P03.81 Newborn affected by abnormality in fetal (intrauterine) heart rate or rhythm**
Excludes1: *neonatal cardiac dysrhythmia (P29.1-)*

P03.810 Newborn affected by abnormality in fetal (intrauterine) heart rate or rhythm before the onset of labor

P03.811 Newborn affected by abnormality in fetal (intrauterine) heart rate or rhythm during labor

P03.819 Newborn affected by abnormality in fetal (intrauterine) heart rate or rhythm, unspecified as to time of onset

P03.82 Meconium passage during delivery
Excludes1: *meconium aspiration (P24.00, P24.01)*
meconium staining (P96.83)

P03.89 Newborn affected by other specified complications of labor and delivery
Newborn affected by abnormality of maternal soft tissues
Newborn affected by conditions classifiable to O60-O75 and by procedures used in labor and delivery not included in P02.- and P03.0-P03.6
Newborn affected by induction of labor

P03.9 Newborn affected by complication of labor and delivery, unspecified

P04 Newborn affected by noxious substances transmitted via placenta or breast milk
Includes: nonteratogenic effects of substances transmitted via placenta
Code first any current condition in newborn, if applicable
Excludes2: *congenital malformations (Q00-Q99)*
encounter for observation of newborn for suspected diseases and conditions ruled out (Z05.-)
neonatal jaundice from excessive hemolysis due to drugs or toxins transmitted from mother (P58.4)
newborn in contact with and (suspected) exposures hazardous to health not transmitted via placenta or breast milk (Z77.-)
AHA CC: 4Q, 2018, 24-25

P04.0 Newborn affected by maternal anesthesia and analgesia in pregnancy, labor and delivery
Newborn affected by reactions and intoxications from maternal opiates and tranquilizers administered for procedures during pregnancy or labor and delivery
Excludes2: *newborn affected by other maternal medication (P04.1-)*

+ **P04.1 Newborn affected by other maternal medication**
Code first withdrawal symptoms from maternal use of drugs of addiction, if applicable (P96.1)
Excludes1: *dysmorphism due to warfarin (Q86.2)*
fetal hydantoin syndrome (Q86.1)
Excludes2: *maternal anesthesia and analgesia in pregnancy, labor and delivery (P04.0)*
maternal use of drugs of addition (P04.4-)
AHA CC: 4Q, 2016, 54-55; 4Q, 2018, 24-25

P04.11 Newborn affected by maternal antineoplastic chemotherapy

P04.12 Newborn affected by maternal cytotoxic drugs

P04.13 Newborn affected by maternal use of anticonvulsants

P04.14 Newborn affected by maternal use of opiates

P04.15 Newborn affected by maternal use of antidepressants

P04.16 Newborn affected by maternal use of amphetamines

P04.17 Newborn affected by maternal use of sedative-hypnotics

P04.1A Newborn affected by maternal use of anxiolytics

P04.18 Newborn affected by other maternal medication

P04.19 Newborn affected by maternal use of unspecified medication

P04.2 Newborn affected by maternal use of tobacco
Newborn affected by exposure in utero to tobacco smoke
Excludes2: *newborn exposure to environmental tobacco smoke (P96.81)*

P04.3 Newborn affected by maternal use of alcohol
Excludes1: *fetal alcohol syndrome (Q86.0)*

+ **P04.4 Newborn affected by maternal use of drugs of addiction**
AHA CC: 4Q, 2018, 25

P04.40 Newborn affected by maternal use of unspecified drugs of addiction

P04.41 Newborn affected by maternal use of cocaine

P04.42 Newborn affected by maternal use of hallucinogens
Excludes2: *newborn affected by other maternal medication (P04.1-)*

P04.49 Newborn affected by maternal use of other drugs of addiction
Excludes2: *newborn affected by maternal anesthesia and analgesia (P04.0)*
withdrawal symptoms from maternal use
of drugs of addiction (P96.1)

P04.5 Newborn affected by maternal use of nutritional chemical substances

P04.6 Newborn affected by maternal exposure to environmental chemical substances

+ **P04.8 Newborn affected by other maternal noxious substances**
AHA CC: 4Q, 2018, 25

P04.81 Newborn affected by maternal use of cannabis

P04.89 Newborn affected by other maternal noxious substances

P04.9 Newborn affected by maternal noxious substance, unspecified

Disorders of newborn related to length of gestation and fetal growth (P05-P08)

P05 Disorders of newborn related to slow fetal growth and fetal malnutrition

Review coding guideline C.16.d

+ **P05.0 Newborn light for gestational age**
  Newborn light-for-dates
  Weight below but length above 10th percentile for gestational age
  P05.00 Newborn light for gestational age, unspecified weight
  P05.01 Newborn light for gestational age, less than 500 grams
  P05.02 Newborn light for gestational age, 500-749 grams
  P05.03 Newborn light for gestational age, 750-999 grams
  P05.04 Newborn light for gestational age, 1000-1249 grams
  P05.05 Newborn light for gestational age, 1250-1499 grams
  P05.06 Newborn light for gestational age, 1500-1749 grams
  P05.07 Newborn light for gestational age, 1750-1999 grams
  P05.08 Newborn light for gestational age, 2000-2499 grams
  P05.09 Newborn light for gestational age, 2500 grams and over
  Newborn light for gestational age, other
  AHA CC: 4Q, 2016, 55-56

+ **P05.1 Newborn small for gestational age**
  Newborn small-and-light-for-dates
  Newborn small-for-dates
  Weight and length below 10th percentile for gestational age
  P05.10 Newborn small for gestational age, unspecified weight
  P05.11 Newborn small for gestational age, less than 500 grams
  P05.12 Newborn small for gestational age, 500-749 grams
  P05.13 Newborn small for gestational age, 750-999 grams
  P05.14 Newborn small for gestational age, 1000-1249 grams
  P05.15 Newborn small for gestational age, 1250-1499 grams
  P05.16 Newborn small for gestational age, 1500-1749 grams
  P05.17 Newborn small for gestational age, 1750-1999 grams
  P05.18 Newborn small for gestational age, 2000-2499 grams
  P05.19 Newborn small for gestational age, other
  Newborn small for gestational age, 2500 grams and over
  AHA CC: 4Q, 2016, 55-56

P05.2 Newborn affected by fetal (intrauterine) malnutrition not light or small for gestational age
Infant, not light or small for gestational age, showing signs of fetal malnutrition, such as dry, peeling skin and loss of subcutaneous tissue
Excludes1: *newborn affected by fetal malnutrition with light for gestational age (P05.0-)*
newborn affected by fetal malnutrition with small for gestational age (P05.1-)

P05.9 Newborn affected by slow intrauterine growth, unspecified
Newborn affected by fetal growth retardation NOS

P07 Disorders of newborn related to short gestation and low birth weight, not elsewhere classified

NOTE When both birth weight and gestational age of the newborn are available, both should be coded with birth weight sequenced before gestational age

Includes: the listed conditions, without further specification, as the cause of morbidity or additional care, in newborn

Review coding guidelines C.16.d and C.16.e

+ **P07.0 Extremely low birth weight newborn**
  Newborn birth weight 999 g. or less
  Excludes1: low birth weight due to slow fetal growth and fetal malnutrition (P05.-)
  P07.00 Extremely low birth weight newborn, unspecified weight
  P07.01 Extremely low birth weight newborn, less than 500 grams
  P07.02 Extremely low birth weight newborn, 500-749 grams
  P07.03 Extremely low birth weight newborn, 750-999 grams

+ **P07.1 Other low birth weight newborn**
  Newborn birth weight 1000-2499 g.
  Excludes1: low birth weight due to slow fetal growth and fetal malnutrition (P05.-)
  P07.10 Other low birth weight newborn, unspecified weight
  P07.14 Other low birth weight newborn, 1000-1249 grams
  P07.15 Other low birth weight newborn, 1250-1499 grams
  P07.16 Other low birth weight newborn, 1500-1749 grams
  P07.17 Other low birth weight newborn, 1750-1999 grams
  P07.18 Other low birth weight newborn, 2000-2499 grams

+ **P07.2 Extreme immaturity of newborn**
  Less than 28 completed weeks (less than 196 completed days) of gestation.
  P07.20 Extreme immaturity of newborn, unspecified weeks of gestation
  Gestational age less than 28 completed weeks NOS
  P07.21 Extreme immaturity of newborn, gestational age less than 23 completed weeks
  Extreme immaturity of newborn, gestational age less than 23 weeks, 0 days
  P07.22 Extreme immaturity of newborn, gestational age 23 completed weeks
  Extreme immaturity of newborn, gestational age 23 weeks, 0 days through 23 weeks, 6 days
  P07.23 Extreme immaturity of newborn, gestational age 24 completed weeks
  Extreme immaturity of newborn, gestational age 24 weeks, 0 days through 24 weeks, 6 days
  P07.24 Extreme immaturity of newborn, gestational age 25 completed weeks
  Extreme immaturity of newborn, gestational age 25 weeks, 0 days through 25 weeks, 6 days
  P07.25 Extreme immaturity of newborn, gestational age 26 completed weeks
  Extreme immaturity of newborn, gestational age 26 weeks, 0 days through 26 weeks, 6 days
  P07.26 Extreme immaturity of newborn, gestational age 27 completed weeks
  Extreme immaturity of newborn, gestational age 27 weeks, 0 days through 27 weeks, 6 days

+ **P07.3 Preterm [premature] newborn [other]**
  28 completed weeks or more but less than 37 completed weeks (196 completed days but less than 259 completed days) of gestation.
  Prematurity NOS
  P07.30 Preterm newborn, unspecified weeks of gestation
  P07.31 Preterm newborn, gestational age 28 completed weeks
  Preterm newborn, gestational age 28 weeks, 0 days through 28 weeks, 6 days
  P07.32 Preterm newborn, gestational age 29 completed weeks
  Preterm newborn, gestational age 29 weeks, 0 days through 29 weeks, 6 days
  P07.33 Preterm newborn, gestational age 30 completed weeks
  Preterm newborn, gestational age 30 weeks, 0 days through 30 weeks, 6 days
  P07.34 Preterm newborn, gestational age 31 completed weeks
  Preterm newborn, gestational age 31 weeks, 0 days through 31 weeks, 6 days
  P07.35 Preterm newborn, gestational age 32 completed weeks
  Preterm newborn, gestational age 32 weeks, 0 days through 32 weeks, 6 days
  P07.36 Preterm newborn, gestational age 33 completed weeks
  Preterm newborn, gestational age 33 weeks, 0 days through 33 weeks, 6 days
  P07.37 Preterm newborn, gestational age 34 completed weeks
  Preterm newborn, gestational age 34 weeks, 0 days through 34 weeks, 6 days
  AHA CC: 2Q, 2017, 7

P07.38 Preterm newborn, gestational age 35 completed weeks
Preterm newborn, gestational age 35 weeks, 0 days through 35 weeks, 6 days

P07.39 Preterm newborn, gestational age 36 completed weeks
Preterm newborn, gestational age 36 weeks, 0 days through 36 weeks, 6 days
AHA CC: 3Q, 2017, 26

P08 Disorders of newborn related to long gestation and high birth weight

NOTE When both birth weight and gestational age of the newborn are available, priority of assignment should be given to birth weight

Includes: the listed conditions, without further specification, as causes of morbidity or additional care, in newborn

P08.0 Exceptionally large newborn baby
Usually implies a birth weight of 4500 g. or more
Excludes1: *syndrome of infant of diabetic mother (P70.1)*
syndrome of infant of mother with gestational diabetes (P70.0)

P08.1 Other heavy for gestational age newborn
Other newborn heavy- or large-for-dates regardless of period of gestation
Usually implies a birth weight of 4000 g. to 4499 g.
Excludes1: *newborn with a birth weight of 4500 or more (P08.0)*
syndrome of infant of diabetic mother (P70.1)
syndrome of infant of mother with gestational diabetes (P70.0)

+ P08.2 Late newborn, not heavy for gestational age

P08.21 Post-term newborn
Newborn with gestation period over 40 completed weeks to 42 completed weeks
AHA CC: 1Q, 2014, 14

P08.22 Prolonged gestation of newborn
Newborn with gestation period over 42 completed weeks (294 days or more), not heavy- or large-for-dates.
Postmaturity NOS
AHA CC: 1Q, 2014, 14

Abnormal findings on neonatal screening (P09)

P09 Abnormal findings on neonatal screening

Includes: Abnormal findings on state mandated newborn screens
Failed newborn screening
Excludes2: *nonspecific serologic evidence of human immunodeficiency virus [HIV] (R75)*

P09.1 Abnormal findings on neonatal screening for inborn errors of metabolism

P09.2 Abnormal findings on neonatal screening for congenital endocrine disease
Abnormal findings on neonatal screening for congenital adrenal hyperplasia
Abnormal findings on neonatal screening for hypothyroidism screen

P09.3 Abnormal findings on neonatal screening for congenital hematologic disorders
Abnormal findings for hemoglobinothies screen
Abnormal findings on red cell membrane defects screen
Abnormal findings on sickle cell screen

P09.4 Abnormal findings on neonatal screening for cystic fibrosis

P09.5 Abnormal findings on neonatal screening for critical congenital heart disease
Neonatal congenital heart disease screening failure

P09.6 Abnormal findings on neonatal screening for neonatal hearing loss
Excludes2: encounter for hearing examination following failed hearing screening (Z01.110)

P09.8 Other abnormal findings on neonatal screening

P09.9 Abnormal findings on neonatal screening, unspecified

Birth trauma (P10-P15)

P10 Intracranial laceration and hemorrhage due to birth injury

Excludes1: *intracranial hemorrhage of newborn NOS (P52.9)*
intracranial hemorrhage of newborn due to anoxia or hypoxia (P52.-)
nontraumatic intracranial hemorrhage of newborn (P52.-)

MCC **P10.0 Subdural hemorrhage due to birth injury**
Subdural hematoma (localized) due to birth injury
Excludes1: *subdural hemorrhage accompanying tentorial tear (P10.4)*

MCC **P10.1 Cerebral hemorrhage due to birth injury**
CC **P10.2 Intraventricular hemorrhage due to birth injury**
MCC **P10.3 Subarachnoid hemorrhage due to birth injury**
MCC **P10.4 Tentorial tear due to birth injury**
MCC **P10.8 Other intracranial lacerations and hemorrhages due to birth injury**
MCC **P10.9 Unspecified intracranial laceration and hemorrhage due to birth injury**

P11 Other birth injuries to central nervous system

MCC **P11.0 Cerebral edema due to birth injury**
P11.1 Other specified brain damage due to birth injury
MCC **P11.2 Unspecified brain damage due to birth injury**
P11.3 Birth injury to facial nerve
Facial palsy due to birth injury
P11.4 Birth injury to other cranial nerves
P11.5 Birth injury to spine and spinal cord
Fracture of spine due to birth injury
MCC **P11.9 Birth injury to central nervous system, unspecified**

P12 Birth injury to scalp

P12.0 Cephalhematoma due to birth injury
P12.1 Chignon (from vacuum extraction) due to birth injury
CC **P12.2 Epicranial subaponeurotic hemorrhage due to birth injury**
Subgaleal hemorrhage
P12.3 Bruising of scalp due to birth injury
P12.4 Injury of scalp of newborn due to monitoring equipment
Sampling incision of scalp of newborn
Scalp clip (electrode) injury of newborn
+ P12.8 Other birth injuries to scalp
P12.81 Caput succedaneum
P12.89 Other birth injuries to scalp
P12.9 Birth injury to scalp, unspecified

P13 Birth injury to skeleton

Excludes2: *birth injury to spine (P11.5)*
P13.0 Fracture of skull due to birth injury
P13.1 Other birth injuries to skull
Excludes1: *cephalhematoma (P12.0)*
P13.2 Birth injury to femur
P13.3 Birth injury to other long bones
P13.4 Fracture of clavicle due to birth injury
P13.8 Birth injuries to other parts of skeleton
P13.9 Birth injury to skeleton, unspecified

P14 Birth injury to peripheral nervous system

P14.0 Erb's paralysis due to birth injury
P14.1 Klumpke's paralysis due to birth injury
P14.2 Phrenic nerve paralysis due to birth injury
P14.3 Other brachial plexus birth injuries
P14.8 Birth injuries to other parts of peripheral nervous system
P14.9 Birth injury to peripheral nervous system, unspecified

P15 Other birth injuries

P15.0 Birth injury to liver
Rupture of liver due to birth injury
P15.1 Birth injury to spleen
Rupture of spleen due to birth injury
P15.2 Sternomastoid injury due to birth injury
P15.3 Birth injury to eye
Subconjunctival hemorrhage due to birth injury
Traumatic glaucoma due to birth injury
P15.4 Birth injury to face
Facial congestion due to birth injury
P15.5 Birth injury to external genitalia
P15.6 Subcutaneous fat necrosis due to birth injury
P15.8 Other specified birth injuries
P15.9 Birth injury, unspecified

Respiratory and cardiovascular disorders specific to the perinatal period (P19-P29)

P19 Metabolic acidemia in newborn

Includes: metabolic acidemia in newborn

P19.0 Metabolic acidemia in newborn first noted before onset of labor

P19.1 Metabolic acidemia in newborn first noted during labor

P19.2 Metabolic acidemia noted at birth

P19.9 Metabolic acidemia, unspecified

P22 Respiratory distress of newborn

MCC **P22.0 Respiratory distress syndrome of newborn**

Cardiorespiratory distress syndrome of newborn
Hyaline membrane disease
Idiopathic respiratory distress syndrome [IRDS or RDS] of newborn
Pulmonary hypoperfusion syndrome
Respiratory distress syndrome, type I

Excludes2: respiratory arrest of newborn (P28.81)
respiratory failure of newborn NOS (P28.5)

AHA CC: 2Q, 2019, 29

P22.1 Transient tachypnea of newborn

Idiopathic tachypnea of newborn
Respiratory distress syndrome, type II
Wet lung syndrome

P22.8 Other respiratory distress of newborn

Excludes1: respiratory arrest of newborn (P28.81)
respiratory failure of newborn NOS (P28.5)

P22.9 Respiratory distress of newborn, unspecified

Excludes1: respiratory arrest of newborn (P28.81)
respiratory failure of newborn NOS (P28.5)

P23 Congenital pneumonia

Includes: infective pneumonia acquired in utero or during birth

Excludes1: *neonatal pneumonia resulting from aspiration (P24.-)*

MCC **P23.0 Congenital pneumonia due to viral agent**

Use additional code (B97) to identify organism

Excludes1: *congenital rubella pneumonitis (P35.0)*

MCC **P23.1 Congenital pneumonia due to Chlamydia**

MCC **P23.2 Congenital pneumonia due to staphylococcus**

MCC **P23.3 Congenital pneumonia due to streptococcus, group B**

MCC **P23.4 Congenital pneumonia due to Escherichia coli**

P23.5 Congenital pneumonia due to Pseudomonas

MCC **P23.6 Congenital pneumonia due to other bacterial agents**

Congenital pneumonia due to Hemophilus influenzae
Congenital pneumonia due to Klebsiella pneumoniae
Congenital pneumonia due to Mycoplasma
Congenital pneumonia due to Streptococcus, except group B
Use additional code (B95-B96) to identify organism

MCC **P23.8 Congenital pneumonia due to other organisms**

MCC **P23.9 Congenital pneumonia, unspecified**

P24 Neonatal aspiration

Includes: aspiration in utero and during delivery

\+ **P24.0 Meconium aspiration**

Excludes1: *meconium passage (without aspiration) during delivery (P03.82)*
meconium staining (P96.83)

P24.00 Meconium aspiration without respiratory symptoms

Meconium aspiration NOS

MCC **P24.01 Meconium aspiration with respiratory symptoms**

Meconium aspiration pneumonia
Meconium aspiration pneumonitis
Meconium aspiration syndrome NOS
Use additional code to identify any secondary pulmonary hypertension, if applicable (I27.2-)

\+ **P24.1 Neonatal aspiration of (clear) amniotic fluid and mucus**

Neonatal aspiration of liquor (amnii)

P24.10 Neonatal aspiration of (clear) amniotic fluid and mucus without respiratory symptoms

Neonatal aspiration of amniotic fluid and mucus NOS

MCC **P24.11 Neonatal aspiration of (clear) amniotic fluid and mucus with respiratory symptoms**

Neonatal aspiration of amniotic fluid and mucus with pneumonia
Neonatal aspiration of amniotic fluid and mucus with pneumonitis
Use additional code to identify any secondary pulmonary hypertension, if applicable (I27.2-)

\+ **P24.2 Neonatal aspiration of blood**

P24.20 Neonatal aspiration of blood without respiratory symptoms

Neonatal aspiration of blood NOS

MCC **P24.21 Neonatal aspiration of blood with respiratory symptoms**

Neonatal aspiration of blood with pneumonia
Neonatal aspiration of blood with pneumonitis
Use additional code to identify any secondary pulmonary hypertension, if applicable (I27.2-)

\+ **P24.3 Neonatal aspiration of milk and regurgitated food**

Neonatal aspiration of stomach contents

P24.30 Neonatal aspiration of milk and regurgitated food without respiratory symptoms

Neonatal aspiration of milk and regurgitated food NOS

MCC **P24.31 Neonatal aspiration of milk and regurgitated food with respiratory symptoms**

Neonatal aspiration of milk and regurgitated food with pneumonia
Neonatal aspiration of milk and regurgitated food with pneumonitis
Use additional code to identify any secondary pulmonary hypertension, if applicable (I27.2-)

\+ **P24.8 Other neonatal aspiration**

P24.80 Other neonatal aspiration without respiratory symptoms

Neonatal aspiration NEC

MCC **P24.81 Other neonatal aspiration with respiratory symptoms**

Neonatal aspiration pneumonia NEC
Neonatal aspiration with pneumonitis NEC
Neonatal aspiration with pneumonia NOS
Neonatal aspiration with pneumonitis NOS
Use additional code to identify any secondary pulmonary hypertension, if applicable (I27.2-)

P24.9 Neonatal aspiration, unspecified

P25 Interstitial emphysema and related conditions originating in the perinatal period

MCC **P25.0 Interstitial emphysema originating in the perinatal period**

MCC **P25.1 Pneumothorax originating in the perinatal period**

MCC **P25.2 Pneumomediastinum originating in the perinatal period**

MCC **P25.3 Pneumopericardium originating in the perinatal period**

MCC **P25.8 Other conditions related to interstitial emphysema originating in the perinatal period**

P26 Pulmonary hemorrhage originating in the perinatal period

Excludes1: *acute idiopathic hemorrhage in infants over 28 days old (R04.81)*

MCC **P26.0 Tracheobronchial hemorrhage originating in the perinatal period**

MCC **P26.1 Massive pulmonary hemorrhage originating in the perinatal period**

MCC **P26.8 Other pulmonary hemorrhages originating in the perinatal period**

MCC **P26.9 Unspecified pulmonary hemorrhage originating in the perinatal period**

P27 Chronic respiratory disease originating in the perinatal period

Excludes2: *respiratory distress of newborn (P22.0-P22.9)*

MCC **P27.0 Wilson-Mikity syndrome**

Pulmonary dysmaturity

MCC **P27.1 Bronchopulmonary dysplasia originating in the perinatal period**

MCC **P27.8 Other chronic respiratory diseases originating in the perinatal period**

Congenital pulmonary fibrosis
Ventilator lung in newborn

MCC **P27.9 Unspecified chronic respiratory disease originating in the perinatal period**

P28 Other respiratory conditions originating in the perinatal period

Excludes1: *congenital malformations of the respiratory system (Q30-Q34)*

CC **P28.0 Primary atelectasis of newborn**

Primary failure to expand terminal respiratory units
Pulmonary hypoplasia associated with short gestation
Pulmonary immaturity NOS

\+ **P28.1 Other and unspecified atelectasis of newborn**

CC **P28.10 Unspecified atelectasis of newborn**

Atelectasis of newborn NOS

CC **P28.11 Resorption atelectasis without respiratory distress syndrome**
Excludes1: *resorption atelectasis with respiratory distress syndrome (P22.0)*

CC **P28.19 Other atelectasis of newborn**
Partial atelectasis of newborn
Secondary atelectasis of newborn

CC **P28.2 Cyanotic attacks of newborn**
Excludes1: *apnea of newborn (P28.3-P28.4)*

CC **P28.3 Primary sleep apnea of newborn**
Central sleep apnea of newborn
Obstructive sleep apnea of newborn
Sleep apnea of newborn NOS

CC **P28.4 Other apnea of newborn**
Apnea of prematurity
Obstructive apnea of newborn
Excludes1: *obstructive sleep apnea of newborn (P28.3)*

MCC **P28.5 Respiratory failure of newborn**
Excludes1: *respiratory arrest of newborn (P28.81)*
respiratory distress of newborn (P22.0-)
AHA CC: 2Q, 2019, 29

\+ **P28.8 Other specified respiratory conditions of newborn**

MCC **P28.81 Respiratory arrest of newborn**
AHA CC: 2Q, 2017, 6-7

P28.89 Other specified respiratory conditions of newborn
Congenital laryngeal stridor
Sniffles in newborn
Snuffles in newborn
Excludes1: *early congenital syphilitic rhinitis (A50.05)*

P28.9 Respiratory condition of newborn, unspecified
Respiratory depression in newborn

P29 Cardiovascular disorders originating in the perinatal period

Excludes2: *congenital malformations of the circulatory system (Q20-Q28)*

P29.0 Neonatal cardiac failure

\+ **P29.1 Neonatal cardiac dysrhythmia**

P29.11 Neonatal tachycardia

P29.12 Neonatal bradycardia

P29.2 Neonatal hypertension

\+ **P29.3 Persistent fetal circulation**
AHA CC: 4Q, 2017, 20-21

MCC **P29.30 Pulmonary hypertension of newborn**
Persistent pulmonary hypertension of newborn

MCC **P29.38 Other persistent fetal circulation**
Delayed closure of ductus arteriosus

P29.4 Transient myocardial ischemia in newborn

\+ **P29.8 Other cardiovascular disorders originating in the perinatal period**

MCC **P29.81 Cardiac arrest of newborn**

P29.89 Other cardiovascular disorders originating in the perinatal period
AHA CC: 4Q, 2014, 23

P29.9 Cardiovascular disorder originating in the perinatal period, unspecified

Infections specific to the perinatal period (P35-P39)

Infections acquired in utero, during birth via the umbilicus, or during the first 28 days after birth

Excludes2: *asymptomatic human immunodeficiency virus [HIV] infection status (Z21)*
congenital gonococcal infection (A54.-)
congenital pneumonia (P23.-)
congenital syphilis (A50.-)
human immunodeficiency virus [HIV] disease (B20)
infant botulism (A48.51)
infectious diseases not specific to the perinatal period (A00-B99, J09, J10.-)
intestinal infectious disease (A00-A09)
laboratory evidence of human immunodeficiency virus [HIV] (R75)
tetanus neonatorum (A33)

P35 Congenital viral diseases

Includes: infections acquired in utero or during birth

CC **P35.0 Congenital rubella syndrome**
Congenital rubella pneumonitis

MCC **P35.1 Congenital cytomegalovirus infection**

MCC **P35.2 Congenital herpesviral [herpes simplex] infection**

MCC **P35.3 Congenital viral hepatitis**

MCC **P35.4 Congenital Zika virus disease**
Use additional code to identify manifestations of congenital Zika virus disease
AHA CC: 4Q, 2018, 25-26

MCC **P35.8 Other congenital viral diseases**
Congenital varicella [chickenpox]
AHA CC: 4Q, 2016, 4-7; 2Q, 2020, 13
Review coding guideline C.16.h

MCC **P35.9 Congenital viral disease, unspecified**

P36 Bacterial sepsis of newborn

Includes: congenital sepsis
Use additional code(s), if applicable, to identify severe sepsis (R65.2-) and associated acute organ dysfunction(s)
Review coding guideline C.1.d and C.16.f

MCC **P36.0 Sepsis of newborn due to streptococcus, group B**

\+ **P36.1 Sepsis of newborn due to other and unspecified streptococci**

MCC **P36.10 Sepsis of newborn due to unspecified streptococci**

MCC **P36.19 Sepsis of newborn due to other streptococci**

MCC **P36.2 Sepsis of newborn due to Staphylococcus aureus**

\+ **P36.3 Sepsis of newborn due to other and unspecified staphylococci**

MCC **P36.30 Sepsis of newborn due to unspecified staphylococci**

MCC **P36.39 Sepsis of newborn due to other staphylococci**

MCC **P36.4 Sepsis of newborn due to Escherichia coli**

MCC **P36.5 Sepsis of newborn due to anaerobes**

MCC **P36.8 Other bacterial sepsis of newborn**
Use additional code from category B96 to identify organism

MCC **P36.9 Bacterial sepsis of newborn, unspecified**

P37 Other congenital infectious and parasitic diseases

Excludes2: *congenital syphilis (A50.-)*
infectious neonatal diarrhea (A00-A09)
necrotizing enterocolitis in newborn (P77.-)
noninfectious neonatal diarrhea (P78.3)
ophthalmia neonatorum due to gonococcus (A54.31)
tetanus neonatorum (A33)

MCC **P37.0 Congenital tuberculosis**

MCC **P37.1 Congenital toxoplasmosis**
Hydrocephalus due to congenital toxoplasmosis

MCC **P37.2 Neonatal (disseminated) listeriosis**

MCC **P37.3 Congenital falciparum malaria**

MCC **P37.4 Other congenital malaria**

P37.5 Neonatal candidiasis

MCC **P37.8 Other specified congenital infectious and parasitic diseases**

MCC **P37.9 Congenital infectious or parasitic disease, unspecified**

P38 Omphalitis of newborn

Excludes1: *omphalitis not of newborn (L08.82)*
tetanus omphalitis (A33)
umbilical hemorrhage of newborn (P51.-)

CC **P38.1 Omphalitis with mild hemorrhage**

CC **P38.9 Omphalitis without hemorrhage**
Omphalitis of newborn NOS

P39 Other infections specific to the perinatal period

Use additional code to identify organism or specific infection

CC **P39.0 Neonatal infective mastitis**
Excludes1: *breast engorgement of newborn (P83.4)*
noninfective mastitis of newborn (P83.4)

P39.1 Neonatal conjunctivitis and dacryocystitis
Neonatal chlamydial conjunctivitis
Ophthalmia neonatorum NOS
Excludes1: *gonococcal conjunctivitis (A54.31)*

CC **P39.2 Intra-amniotic infection affecting newborn, not elsewhere classified**

CC **P39.3 Neonatal urinary tract infection**

CC **P39.4 Neonatal skin infection**
Neonatal pyoderma
Excludes1: *pemphigus neonatorum (L00)*
staphylococcal scalded skin syndrome (L00)

CC **P39.8 Other specified infections specific to the perinatal period**

CC **P39.9 Infection specific to the perinatal period, unspecified**

Hemorrhagic and hematological disorders of newborn (P50-P61)

Excludes1: *congenital stenosis and stricture of bile ducts (Q44.3)*
Crigler-Najjar syndrome (E80.5)
Dubin-Johnson syndrome (E80.6)
Gilbert syndrome (E80.4)
hereditary hemolytic anemias (D55-D58)

P50 Newborn affected by intrauterine (fetal) blood loss

Excludes1: *congenital anemia from intrauterine (fetal) blood loss (P61.3)*

P50.0 Newborn affected by intrauterine (fetal) blood loss from vasa previa
P50.1 Newborn affected by intrauterine (fetal) blood loss from ruptured cord
P50.2 Newborn affected by intrauterine (fetal) blood loss from placenta
P50.3 Newborn affected by hemorrhage into co-twin
P50.4 Newborn affected by hemorrhage into maternal circulation
P50.5 Newborn affected by intrauterine (fetal) blood loss from cut end of co-twin's cord
P50.8 Newborn affected by other intrauterine (fetal) blood loss
P50.9 Newborn affected by intrauterine (fetal) blood loss, unspecified
Newborn affected by fetal hemorrhage NOS

P51 Umbilical hemorrhage of newborn

Excludes1: *omphalitis with mild hemorrhage (P38.1)*
umbilical hemorrhage from cut end of co-twins cord (P50.5)

P51.0 Massive umbilical hemorrhage of newborn
P51.8 Other umbilical hemorrhages of newborn
Slipped umbilical ligature NOS
P51.9 Umbilical hemorrhage of newborn, unspecified

P52 Intracranial nontraumatic hemorrhage of newborn

Includes: intracranial hemorrhage due to anoxia or hypoxia
Excludes1: *intracranial hemorrhage due to birth injury (P10.-)*
intracranial hemorrhage due to other injury (S06.-)

CC **P52.0 Intraventricular (nontraumatic) hemorrhage, grade 1, of newborn**
Subependymal hemorrhage (without intraventricular extension)
Bleeding into germinal matrix
CC **P52.1 Intraventricular (nontraumatic) hemorrhage, grade 2, of newborn**
Subependymal hemorrhage with intraventricular extension
Bleeding into ventricle
\+ **P52.2 Intraventricular (nontraumatic) hemorrhage, grade 3 and grade 4, of newborn**
MCC **P52.21 Intraventricular (nontraumatic) hemorrhage, grade 3, of newborn**
Subependymal hemorrhage with intraventricular extension with enlargement of ventricle
MCC **P52.22 Intraventricular (nontraumatic) hemorrhage, grade 4, of newborn**
Bleeding into cerebral cortex
Subependymal hemorrhage with intracerebral extension
CC **P52.3 Unspecified intraventricular (nontraumatic) hemorrhage of newborn**
MCC **P52.4 Intracerebral (nontraumatic) hemorrhage of newborn**
MCC **P52.5 Subarachnoid (nontraumatic) hemorrhage of newborn**
MCC **P52.6 Cerebellar (nontraumatic) and posterior fossa hemorrhage of newborn**
MCC **P52.8 Other intracranial (nontraumatic) hemorrhages of newborn**
MCC **P52.9 Intracranial (nontraumatic) hemorrhage of newborn, unspecified**

CC **P53 Hemorrhagic disease of newborn**

Vitamin K deficiency of newborn
Valid 3-character code, no further characters required

P54 Other neonatal hemorrhages

Excludes1: *newborn affected by (intrauterine) blood loss (P50.-)*
pulmonary hemorrhage originating in the perinatal period (P26.-)

P54.0 Neonatal hematemesis
Excludes1: *neonatal hematemesis due to swallowed maternal blood (P78.2)*
MCC **P54.1 Neonatal melena**
Excludes1: *neonatal melena due to swallowed maternal blood (P78.2)*
MCC **P54.2 Neonatal rectal hemorrhage**
MCC **P54.3 Other neonatal gastrointestinal hemorrhage**
CC **P54.4 Neonatal adrenal hemorrhage**
P54.5 Neonatal cutaneous hemorrhage
Neonatal bruising
Neonatal ecchymoses
Neonatal petechiae
Neonatal superficial hematomata
Excludes2: *bruising of scalp due to birth injury (P12.3)*
cephalhematoma due to birth injury (P12.0)
♀ **P54.6 Neonatal vaginal hemorrhage**
Neonatal pseudomenses
P54.8 Other specified neonatal hemorrhages
P54.9 Neonatal hemorrhage, unspecified

P55 Hemolytic disease of newborn

P55.0 Rh isoimmunization of newborn
P55.1 ABO isoimmunization of newborn
AHA CC: 3Q, 2015, 20
P55.8 Other hemolytic diseases of newborn
AHA CC: 3Q, 2018, 24
P55.9 Hemolytic disease of newborn, unspecified

P56 Hydrops fetalis due to hemolytic disease

Excludes1: *hydrops fetalis NOS (P83.2)*

MCC **P56.0 Hydrops fetalis due to isoimmunization**
\+ **P56.9 Hydrops fetalis due to other and unspecified hemolytic disease**
MCC **P56.90 Hydrops fetalis due to unspecified hemolytic disease**
MCC **P56.99 Hydrops fetalis due to other hemolytic disease**

P57 Kernicterus

MCC **P57.0 Kernicterus due to isoimmunization**
MCC **P57.8 Other specified kernicterus**
Excludes1: *Crigler-Najjar syndrome (E80.5)*
MCC **P57.9 Kernicterus, unspecified**

P58 Neonatal jaundice due to other excessive hemolysis

Excludes1: *jaundice due to isoimmunization (P55-P57)*

P58.0 Neonatal jaundice due to bruising
P58.1 Neonatal jaundice due to bleeding
P58.2 Neonatal jaundice due to infection
P58.3 Neonatal jaundice due to polycythemia
\+ **P58.4 Neonatal jaundice due to drugs or toxins transmitted from mother or given to newborn**
Code first poisoning due to drug or toxin, if applicable (T36-T65 with fifth or sixth character 1-4 or 6)
Use additional code for adverse effect, if applicable, to identify drug (T36-T50 with fifth or sixth character 5)
P58.41 Neonatal jaundice due to drugs or toxins transmitted from mother
P58.42 Neonatal jaundice due to drugs or toxins given to newborn
P58.5 Neonatal jaundice due to swallowed maternal blood
P58.8 Neonatal jaundice due to other specified excessive hemolysis
P58.9 Neonatal jaundice due to excessive hemolysis, unspecified

P59 Neonatal jaundice from other and unspecified causes

Excludes1: *jaundice due to inborn errors of metabolism (E70-E88)*
kernicterus (P57.-)

P59.0 Neonatal jaundice associated with preterm delivery
Hyperbilirubinemia of prematurity
Jaundice due to delayed conjugation associated with preterm delivery
MCC **P59.1 Inspissated bile syndrome**
\+ **P59.2 Neonatal jaundice from other and unspecified hepatocellular damage**
Excludes1: *congenital viral hepatitis (P35.3)*
MCC **P59.20 Neonatal jaundice from unspecified hepatocellular damage**
MCC **P59.29 Neonatal jaundice from other hepatocellular damage**
Neonatal giant cell hepatitis
Neonatal (idiopathic) hepatitis
P59.3 Neonatal jaundice from breast milk inhibitor
P59.8 Neonatal jaundice from other specified causes
P59.9 Neonatal jaundice, unspecified
Neonatal physiological jaundice (intense)(prolonged) NOS
AHA CC: 3Q, 2015, 20

P60 Disseminated intravascular coagulation of newborn
MCC
Defibrination syndrome of newborn
Valid 3-character code, no further characters required

P61 Other perinatal hematological disorders
Excludes1: *transient hypogammaglobulinemia of infancy (D80.7)*

MCC **P61.0 Transient neonatal thrombocytopenia**
Neonatal thrombocytopenia due to exchange transfusion
Neonatal thrombocytopenia due to idiopathic maternal thrombocytopenia
Neonatal thrombocytopenia due to isoimmunization

P61.1 Polycythemia neonatorum
CC **P61.2 Anemia of prematurity**
CC **P61.3 Congenital anemia from fetal blood loss**
CC **P61.4 Other congenital anemias, not elsewhere classified**
Congenital anemia NOS
MCC **P61.5 Transient neonatal neutropenia**
Excludes1: *congenital neutropenia (nontransient) (D70.0)*
CC **P61.6 Other transient neonatal disorders of coagulation**
P61.8 Other specified perinatal hematological disorders
P61.9 Perinatal hematological disorder, unspecified

Transitory endocrine and metabolic disorders specific to newborn (P70-P74)

Includes: transitory endocrine and metabolic disturbances caused by the infant's response to maternal endocrine and metabolic factors, or its adjustment to extrauterine environment

P70 Transitory disorders of carbohydrate metabolism specific to newborn

P70.0 Syndrome of infant of mother with gestational diabetes
Newborn (with hypoglycemia) affected by maternal gestational diabetes
Excludes1: *newborn (with hypoglycemia) affected by maternal (pre-existing) diabetes mellitus (P70.1)*
syndrome of infant of a diabetic mother (P70.1)

P70.1 Syndrome of infant of a diabetic mother
Newborn (with hypoglycemia) affected by maternal (pre-existing) diabetes mellitus
Excludes1: *newborn (with hypoglycemia) affected by maternal gestational diabetes (P70.0)*
syndrome of infant of mother with gestational diabetes (P70.0)

CC **P70.2 Neonatal diabetes mellitus**
P70.3 Iatrogenic neonatal hypoglycemia
P70.4 Other neonatal hypoglycemia
Transitory neonatal hypoglycemia
CC **P70.8 Other transitory disorders of carbohydrate metabolism of newborn**
P70.9 Transitory disorder of carbohydrate metabolism of newborn, unspecified

P71 Transitory neonatal disorders of calcium and magnesium metabolism

CC **P71.0 Cow's milk hypocalcemia in newborn**
CC **P71.1 Other neonatal hypocalcemia**
Excludes1: *neonatal hypoparathyroidism (P71.4)*
CC **P71.2 Neonatal hypomagnesemia**
CC **P71.3 Neonatal tetany without calcium or magnesium deficiency**
Neonatal tetany NOS
CC **P71.4 Transitory neonatal hypoparathyroidism**
CC **P71.8 Other transitory neonatal disorders of calcium and magnesium metabolism**
AHA CC: 4Q, 2016, 54-55
CC **P71.9 Transitory neonatal disorder of calcium and magnesium metabolism, unspecified**

P72 Other transitory neonatal endocrine disorders
Excludes1: *congenital hypothyroidism with or without goiter (E03.0-E03.1)*
dyshormogenetic goiter (E07.1)
Pendred's syndrome (E07.1)

CC **P72.0 Neonatal goiter, not elsewhere classified**
Transitory congenital goiter with normal functioning
CC **P72.1 Transitory neonatal hyperthyroidism**
Neonatal thyrotoxicosis
CC **P72.2 Other transitory neonatal disorders of thyroid function, not elsewhere classified**
Transitory neonatal hypothyroidism
CC **P72.8 Other specified transitory neonatal endocrine disorders**
P72.9 Transitory neonatal endocrine disorder, unspecified

P74 Other transitory neonatal electrolyte and metabolic disturbances

MCC **P74.0 Late metabolic acidosis of newborn**
Excludes1: *(fetal) metabolic acidosis of newborn (P19)*
P74.1 Dehydration of newborn
\+ **P74.2 Disturbances of sodium balance of newborn**
AHA CC: 2Q, 2018, 6; 4Q, 2018, 27
P74.21 Hypernatremia of newborn
P74.22 Hyponatremia of newborn
\+ **P74.3 Disturbances of potassium balance of newborn**
AHA CC: 4Q, 2018, 27
P74.31 Hyperkalemia of newborn
P74.32 Hypokalemia of newborn
\+ **P74.4 Other transitory electrolyte disturbances of newborn**
AHA CC: 4Q, 2018, 27
CC **P74.41 Alkalosis of newborn**
Hyperbicarbonatemia
\+ **P74.42 Disturbances of chlorine balance of newborn**
P74.421 Hyperchloremia of newborn
Hyperchloremic metabolic acidosis
Excludes2: *late metatbolic acidosis of the newborn (P74.0)*
P74.422 Hypochloremia of newborn
P74.49 Other transitory electrolyte disturbance of newborn
CC **P74.5 Transitory tyrosinemia of newborn**
CC **P74.6 Transitory hyperammonemia of newborn**
CC **P74.8 Other transitory metabolic disturbances of newborn**
Amino-acid metabolic disorders described as transitory
P74.9 Transitory metabolic disturbance of newborn, unspecified

Digestive system disorders of newborn (P76-P78)

P76 Other intestinal obstruction of newborn

P76.0 Meconium plug syndrome
Meconium ileus NOS
Excludes1: *meconium ileus in cystic fibrosis (E84.11)*
CC **P76.1 Transitory ileus of newborn**
Excludes1: *Hirschsprung's disease (Q43.1)*
P76.2 Intestinal obstruction due to inspissated milk
P76.8 Other specified intestinal obstruction of newborn
Excludes1: *intestinal obstruction classifiable to K56.-*
P76.9 Intestinal obstruction of newborn, unspecified

P77 Necrotizing enterocolitis of newborn

MCC **P77.1 Stage 1 necrotizing enterocolitis in newborn**
Necrotizing enterocolitis without pneumatosis, without perforation
MCC **P77.2 Stage 2 necrotizing enterocolitis in newborn**
Necrotizing enterocolitis with pneumatosis, without perforation
MCC **P77.3 Stage 3 necrotizing enterocolitis in newborn**
Necrotizing enterocolitis with perforation
Necrotizing enterocolitis with pneumatosis and perforation
MCC **P77.9 Necrotizing enterocolitis in newborn, unspecified**
Necrotizing enterocolitis in newborn, NOS

P78 Other perinatal digestive system disorders
Excludes1: *cystic fibrosis (E84.0-E84.9)*
neonatal gastrointestinal hemorrhages (P54.0-P54.3)

MCC **P78.0 Perinatal intestinal perforation**
Meconium peritonitis
P78.1 Other neonatal peritonitis
Neonatal peritonitis NOS
P78.2 Neonatal hematemesis and melena due to swallowed maternal blood
P78.3 Noninfective neonatal diarrhea
Neonatal diarrhea NOS
\+ **P78.8 Other specified perinatal digestive system disorders**
P78.81 Congenital cirrhosis (of liver)
P78.82 Peptic ulcer of newborn
P78.83 Newborn esophageal reflux
Neonatal esophageal reflux

P78.84 **Gestational alloimmune liver disease**
GALD
Neonatal hemochromatosis
Excludes1: *hemochromatosis (E83.11-)*
AHA CC: 4Q, 2017, 21

P78.89 **Other specified perinatal digestive system disorders**

P78.9 **Perinatal digestive system disorder, unspecified**

Conditions involving the integument and temperature regulation of newborn (P80-P83)

P80 Hypothermia of newborn

P80.0 Cold injury syndrome
Severe and usually chronic hypothermia associated with a pink flushed appearance, edema and neurological and biochemical abnormalities.
Excludes1: *mild hypothermia of newborn (P80.8)*

P80.8 Other hypothermia of newborn
Mild hypothermia of newborn

P80.9 Hypothermia of newborn, unspecified

P81 Other disturbances of temperature regulation of newborn

P81.0 Environmental hyperthermia of newborn

P81.8 Other specified disturbances of temperature regulation of newborn

P81.9 Disturbance of temperature regulation of newborn, unspecified
Fever of newborn NOS

P83 Other conditions of integument specific to newborn

Excludes1: *congenital malformations of skin and integument (Q80-Q84)*
hydrops fetalis due to hemolytic disease (P56.-)
neonatal skin infection (P39.4)
staphylococcal scalded skin syndrome (L00)
Excludes2: *cradle cap (L21.0)*
diaper [napkin] dermatitis (L22)

CC **P83.0 Sclerema neonatorum**

P83.1 Neonatal erythema toxicum

MCC **P83.2 Hydrops fetalis not due to hemolytic disease**
Hydrops fetalis NOS

\+ **P83.3 Other and unspecified edema specific to newborn**

CC **P83.30 Unspecified edema specific to newborn**

CC **P83.39 Other edema specific to newborn**

P83.4 Breast engorgement of newborn
Noninfective mastitis of newborn

♂ **P83.5 Congenital hydrocele**

P83.6 Umbilical polyp of newborn

\+ **P83.8 Other specified conditions of integument specific to newborn**
AHA CC: 4Q, 2017, 21-22

P83.81 Umbilical granuloma
Excludes2: *granulomatous disorder of the skin and subcutaneous tissue, unspecified (L92.9)*

P83.88 Other specified conditions of integument specific to newborn
Bronze baby syndrome
Neonatal scleroderma
Urticaria neonatorum

P83.9 Condition of the integument specific to newborn, unspecified

Other problems with newborn (P84)

P84 Other problems with newborn

Acidemia of newborn
Acidosis of newborn
Anoxia of newborn NOS
Asphyxia of newborn NOS
Hypercapnia of newborn
Hypoxemia of newborn
Hypoxia of newborn NOS
Mixed metabolic and respiratory acidosis of newborn
Excludes1: *intracranial hemorrhage due to anoxia or hypoxia (P52.-)*
hypoxic ischemic encephalopathy [HIE] (P91.6-)
late metabolic acidosis of newborn (P74.0)
Valid 3-character code, no further characters required

Other disorders originating in the perinatal period (P90-P96)

MCC **P90 Convulsions of newborn**

Excludes1: *benign myoclonic epilepsy in infancy (G40.3-)*
benign neonatal convulsions (familial) (G40.3-)
Valid 3-character code, no further characters required

P91 Other disturbances of cerebral status of newborn

MCC **P91.0 Neonatal cerebral ischemia**
Excludes1: *Neonatal cerebral infarction (P91.82-)*

MCC **P91.1 Acquired periventricular cysts of newborn**

MCC **P91.2 Neonatal cerebral leukomalacia**
Periventricular leukomalacia

MCC **P91.3 Neonatal cerebral irritability**

MCC **P91.4 Neonatal cerebral depression**

MCC **P91.5 Neonatal coma**

\+ **P91.6 Hypoxic ischemic encephalopathy [HIE]**
Excludes1: *neonatal cerebral depression (P91.4)*
neonatal cerebral irritability (P91.3)
neonatal coma (P91.5)
AHA CC: 4Q, 2017, 22

CC **P91.60 Hypoxic ischemic encephalopathy [HIE], unspecified**

CC **P91.61 Mild hypoxic ischemic encephalopathy [HIE]**

P91.62 Moderate hypoxic ischemic encephalopathy [HIE]

MCC **P91.63 Severe hypoxic ischemic encephalopathy [HIE]**

\+ **P91.8 Other specified disturbances of cerebral status of newborn**

\+ **P91.81 Neonatal encephalopathy**
AHA CC: 4Q, 2017, 22

P91.811 Neonatal encephalopathy in diseases classified elsewhere
Code first underlying condition, if known, such as:
congenital cirrhosis (of liver) (P78.81)
intracranial nontraumatic hemorrhage of newborn (P52.-)
kernicterus (P57.-)

P91.819 Neonatal encephalopathy, unspecified

\+ **P91.82 Neonatal cerebral infarction**
Neonatal stroke
Perinatal arterial ischemic stroke
Perinatal cerebral infarction
Excludes1: *cerebral infarction (I63.-)*
Excludes2: *intracranial hemorrhage of newborn (P52.-)*
AHA CC: 4Q, 2020, 37-38

MCC **P91.821 Neonatal cerebral infarction, right side of brain**

MCC **P91.822 Neonatal cerebral infarction, left side of brain**
AHA CC: 4Q, 2020, 38

MCC **P91.823 Neonatal cerebral infarction, bilateral**

MCC **P91.829 Neonatal cerebral infarction, unspecified side**

P91.88 Other specified disturbances of cerebral status of newborn

P91.9 Disturbance of cerebral status of newborn, unspecified

P92 Feeding problems of newborn

Excludes1: *eating disorders (F50.-)*
Excludes2: *feeding problems in child over 28 days old (R63.3)*

\+ **P92.0 Vomiting of newborn**
Excludes1: *vomiting of child over 28 days old (R11.-)*

MCC **P92.01 Bilious vomiting of newborn**
Excludes1: *bilious vomiting in child over 28 days old (R11.14)*

P92.09 Other vomiting of newborn
Excludes1: *regurgitation of food in newborn (P92.1)*

P92.1 Regurgitation and rumination of newborn

P92.2 Slow feeding of newborn

P92.3 Underfeeding of newborn

P92.4 Overfeeding of newborn

P92.5 Neonatal difficulty in feeding at breast
AHA CC: 3Q, 2016, 19; 1Q, 2017, 28-29

P92.6 Failure to thrive in newborn
Excludes1: *failure to thrive in child over 28 days old (R62.51)*

P92.8 Other feeding problems of newborn

P92.9 Feeding problem of newborn, unspecified

P93 Reactions and intoxications due to drugs administered to newborn

Includes: reactions and intoxications due to drugs administered to fetus affecting newborn

Excludes1: *jaundice due to drugs or toxins transmitted from mother or given to newborn (P58.4-)*
reactions and intoxications from maternal opiates, tranquilizers and other medication (P04.0-P04.1, P04.4-)
withdrawal symptoms from maternal use of drugs of addiction (P96.1)
withdrawal symptoms from therapeutic use of drugs in newborn (P96.2)

CC **P93.0 Grey baby syndrome**
Grey syndrome from chloramphenicol administration in newborn

CC **P93.8 Other reactions and intoxications due to drugs administered to newborn**
Use additional code for adverse effect, if applicable, to identify drug (T36-T50 with fifth or sixth character 5)

P94 Disorders of muscle tone of newborn

CC **P94.0 Transient neonatal myasthenia gravis**
Excludes1: *myasthenia gravis (G70.0)*

P94.1 Congenital hypertonia

P94.2 Congenital hypotonia
Floppy baby syndrome, unspecified

P94.8 Other disorders of muscle tone of newborn

P94.9 Disorder of muscle tone of newborn,unspecified

P95 Stillbirth

Deadborn fetus NOS
Fetal death of unspecified cause
Stillbirth NOS

Excludes1: *maternal care for intrauterine death (O36.4)*
missed abortion (O02.1)
outcome of delivery, stillbirth (Z37.1, Z37.3, Z37.4, Z37.7)

Review coding guideline C.16.g
Valid 3-character code, no further characters required

P96 Other conditions originating in the perinatal period

P96.0 Congenital renal failure
Uremia of newborn

CC **P96.1 Neonatal withdrawal symptoms from maternal use of drugs of addiction**
Drug withdrawal syndrome in infant of dependent mother
Neonatal abstinence syndrome
Excludes1: *reactions and intoxications from maternal opiatesandtranquilizersadministeredduring labor and delivery (P04.0)*
AHA CC: 4Q, 2018, 24-25

CC **P96.2 Withdrawal symptoms from therapeutic use of drugs in newborn**

P96.3 Wide cranial sutures of newborn
Neonatal craniotabes

P96.5 Complication to newborn due to (fetal) intrauterine procedure
Excludes2: *newborn affected by amniocentesis (P00.6)*

\+ **P96.8 Other specified conditions originating in the perinatal period**

P96.81 Exposure to (parental) (environmental) tobacco smoke in the perinatal period
Excludes2: *newborn affected by in utero exposure to tobacco (P04.2)*
exposure to environmental tobacco smoke after the perinatal period (Z77.22)

P96.82 Delayed separation of umbilical cord

P96.83 Meconium staining
Excludes1: *meconium aspiration (P24.00, P24.01)*
meconium passage during delivery (P03.82)

P96.89 Other specified conditions originating in the perinatal period
Use additional code to specify condition

P96.9 Condition originating in the perinatal period, unspecified
Congenital debility NOS

Chapter 17: Congenital Malformations, Deformations and Chromosomal Abnormalities (Q00-Q99)

NOTE Codes from this chapter are not for use on maternal records

Excludes2: *inborn errors of metabolism (E70-E88)*

This chapter contains the following category blocks:

Q00-Q07 Congenital malformations of the nervous system
Q10-Q18 Congenital malformations of eye, ear, face and neck
Q20-Q28 Congenital malformations of the circulatory system
Q30-Q34 Congenital malformations of the respiratory system
Q35-Q37 Cleft lip and cleft palate
Q38-Q45 Other congenital malformations of the digestive system
Q50-Q56 Congenital malformations of genital organs
Q60-Q64 Congenital malformations of the urinary system
Q65-Q79 Congenital malformations and deformations of the musculoskeletal system
Q80-Q89 Other congenital malformations
Q90-Q99 Chromosomal abnormalities, not elsewhere classified

C. Chapter-Specific Coding Guidelines

In addition to general coding guidelines, there are guidelines for specific diagnoses and/or conditions in the classification. Unless otherwise indicated, these guidelines apply to all health care settings. Please refer to Section II for guidelines on the selection of principal diagnosis.

17. Chapter 17: Congenital Malformations, Deformations and Chromosomal Abnormalities (Q00-Q99)

Assign an appropriate code(s) from categories Q00-Q99, Congenital malformations, deformations, and chromosomal abnormalities when a malformation/deformation or chromosomal abnormality is documented. A malformation/deformation or chromosomal abnormality may be the principal/first-listed diagnosis on a record or a secondary diagnosis.

When a malformation/deformation or chromosomal abnormality does not have a unique code assignment, assign additional code(s) for any manifestations that may be present.

When the code assignment specifically identifies the malformation/deformation/or chromosomal abnormality, manifestations that are an inherent component of the anomaly should not be coded separately. Additional codes should be assigned for manifestations that are not an inherent component.

Codes from Chapter 17 may be used throughout the life of the patient. If a congenital malformation or deformity has been corrected, a personal history code should be used to identify the history of the malformation or deformity. Although present at birth, a malformation/deformation or chromosomal abnormality may not be identified until later in life. Whenever the condition is diagnosed by the provider, it is appropriate to assign a code from codes Q00-Q99. For the birth admission, the appropriate code from category Z38, Liveborn infants, according to place of birth and type of delivery, should be sequenced as the principal diagnosis, followed by any congenital anomaly codes, Q00-Q99.

Congenital malformations of the nervous system (Q00-Q07)

Q00 Anencephaly and similar malformations

MCC **Q00.0 Anencephaly**
Acephaly
Acrania
Amyelencephaly
Hemianencephaly
Hemicephaly

MCC **Q00.1 Craniorachischisis**

MCC **Q00.2 Iniencephaly**

Q01 Encephalocele

Includes: Arnold-Chiari syndrome, type III
encephalocystocele
encephalomyelocele
hydroencephalocele
hydromeningocele, cranial
meningocele, cerebral
meningoencephalocele

Excludes1: *Meckel-Gruber syndrome (Q61.9)*

CC **Q01.0 Frontal encephalocele**

CC **Q01.1 Nasofrontal encephalocele**

CC **Q01.2 Occipital encephalocele**

CC **Q01.8 Encephalocele of other sites**

CC **Q01.9 Encephalocele, unspecified**

Q02 Microcephaly

Includes: hydromicrocephaly
micrencephalon

Excludes1: *Meckel-Gruber syndrome (Q61.9)*

Code first, if applicable, congenital Zika virus disease

AHA CC: 4Q, 2016, 4-7; 4Q, 2018, 26

Valid 3-character code, no further characters required

Q03 Congenital hydrocephalus

Includes: hydrocephalus in newborn

Excludes1: *Arnold-Chiari syndrome, type II (Q07.0-)*
acquired hydrocephalus (G91.-)
hydrocephalus due to congenital toxoplasmosis (P37.1)
hydrocephalus with spina bifida (Q05.0-Q05.4)

Q03.0 Malformations of aqueduct of Sylvius
Anomaly of aqueduct of Sylvius
Obstruction of aqueduct of Sylvius, congenital
Stenosis of aqueduct of Sylvius

Q03.1 Atresia of foramina of Magendie and Luschka
Dandy-Walker syndrome

Q03.8 Other congenital hydrocephalus

Q03.9 Congenital hydrocephalus, unspecified

Q04 Other congenital malformations of brain

Excludes1: *cyclopia (Q87.0)*
macrocephaly (Q75.3)

MCC **Q04.0 Congenital malformations of corpus callosum**
Agenesis of corpus callosum

MCC **Q04.1 Arhinencephaly**

MCC **Q04.2 Holoprosencephaly**

MCC **Q04.3 Other reduction deformities of brain**
Absence of part of brain
Agenesis of part of brain
Agyria
Aplasia of part of brain
Hydranencephaly
Hypoplasia of part of brain
Lissencephaly
Microgyria
Pachygyria
Excludes1: *congenital malformations of corpus callosum (Q04.0)*

CC **Q04.4 Septo-optic dysplasia of brain**

CC **Q04.5 Megalencephaly**

CC **Q04.6 Congenital cerebral cysts**
Porencephaly
Schizencephaly
Excludes1: *acquired porencephalic cyst (G93.0)*

CC **Q04.8 Other specified congenital malformations of brain**
Arnold-Chiari syndrome, type IV
Macrogyria

Q04.9 Congenital malformation of brain, unspecified
Congenital anomaly NOS of brain
Congenital deformity NOS of brain
Congenital disease or lesion NOS of brain
Multiple anomalies NOS of brain, congenital

Q05 Spina bifida

Includes: hydromeningocele (spinal)
meningocele (spinal)
meningomyelocele
myelocele
myelomeningocele
rachischisis
spina bifida (aperta)(cystica)
syringomyelocele

Use additional code for any associated paraplegia (paraparesis) (G82.2-)

Excludes1: *Arnold-Chiari syndrome, type II (Q07.0-)*
spina bifida occulta (Q76.0)

CC **Q05.0 Cervical spina bifida with hydrocephalus**

CC **Q05.1 Thoracic spina bifida with hydrocephalus**
Dorsal spina bifida with hydrocephalus
Thoracolumbar spina bifida with hydrocephalus

CC **Q05.2 Lumbar spina bifida with hydrocephalus**
Lumbosacral spina bifida with hydrocephalus

CC **Q05.3 Sacral spina bifida with hydrocephalus**

CC **Q05.4 Unspecified spina bifida with hydrocephalus**

Q05.5 Cervical spina bifida without hydrocephalus

Q05.6 Thoracic spina bifida without hydrocephalus
Dorsal spina bifida NOS
Thoracolumbar spina bifida NOS
Q05.7 Lumbar spina bifida without hydrocephalus
Lumbosacral spina bifida NOS
Q05.8 Sacral spina bifida without hydrocephalus
Q05.9 Spina bifida, unspecified

Q06 Other congenital malformations of spinal cord

Q06.0 Amyelia
Q06.1 Hypoplasia and dysplasia of spinal cord
Atelomyelia
Myelatelia
Myelodysplasia of spinal cord
Q06.2 Diastematomyelia
Q06.3 Other congenital cauda equina malformations
Q06.4 Hydromyelia
Hydrorachis
Q06.8 Other specified congenital malformations of spinal cord
Q06.9 Congenital malformation of spinal cord, unspecified
Congenital anomaly NOS of spinal cord
Congenital deformity NOS of spinal cord
Congenital disease or lesion NOS of spinal cord

Q07 Other congenital malformations of nervous system

Excludes2: *congenital central alveolar hypoventilation syndrome (G47.35)*
familial dysautonomia [Riley-Day] (G90.1)
neurofibromatosis (nonmalignant) (Q85.0-)

\+ **Q07.0 Arnold-Chiari syndrome**
Arnold-Chiari syndrome, type II
Excludes1: *Arnold-Chiari syndrome, type III (Q01.-)*
Arnold-Chiari syndrome, type IV (Q04.8)
Q07.00 Arnold-Chiari syndrome without spina bifida or hydrocephalus
Q07.01 Arnold-Chiari syndrome with spina bifida
CC **Q07.02 Arnold-Chiari syndrome with hydrocephalus**
CC **Q07.03 Arnold-Chiari syndrome with spina bifida and hydrocephalus**
Q07.8 Other specified congenital malformations of nervous system
Agenesis of nerve
Displacement of brachial plexus
Jaw-winking syndrome
Marcus Gunn's syndrome
Q07.9 Congenital malformation of nervous system, unspecified
Congenital anomaly NOS of nervous system
Congenital deformity NOS of nervous system
Congenital disease or lesion NOS of nervous system

Congenital malformations of eye, ear, face and neck (Q10-Q18)

Excludes2: *cleft lip and cleft palate (Q35-Q37)*
congenital malformation of cervical spine (Q05.0, Q05.5, Q67.5, Q76.0-Q76.4)
congenital malformation of larynx (Q31.-)
congenital malformation of lip NEC (Q38.0)
congenital malformation of nose (Q30.-)
congenital malformation of parathyroid gland (Q89.2)
congenital malformation of thyroid gland (Q89.2)

Q10 Congenital malformations of eyelid, lacrimal apparatus and orbit

Excludes1: *cryptophthalmos NOS (Q11.2)*
cryptophthalmos syndrome (Q87.0)

Q10.0 Congenital ptosis
Q10.1 Congenital ectropion
Q10.2 Congenital entropion
Q10.3 Other congenital malformations of eyelid
Ablepharon
Blepharophimosis, congenital
Coloboma of eyelid
Congenital absence or agenesis of cilia
Congenital absence or agenesis of eyelid
Congenital accessory eyelid
Congenital accessory eye muscle
Congenital malformation of eyelid NOS
Q10.4 Absence and agenesis of lacrimal apparatus
Congenital absence of punctum lacrimale
Q10.5 Congenital stenosis and stricture of lacrimal duct
Q10.6 Other congenital malformations of lacrimal apparatus
Congenital malformation of lacrimal apparatus NOS
Q10.7 Congenital malformation of orbit

Q11 Anophthalmos, microphthalmos and macrophthalmos

Q11.0 Cystic eyeball
Q11.1 Other anophthalmos
Anophthalmos NOS
Agenesis of eye
Aplasia of eye
Q11.2 Microphthalmos
Cryptophthalmos NOS
Dysplasia of eye
Hypoplasia of eye
Rudimentary eye
Excludes1: *cryptophthalmos syndrome (Q87.0)*
Q11.3 Macrophthalmos
Excludes1: *macrophthalmos in congenital glaucoma (Q15.0)*

Q12 Congenital lens malformations

CC **Q12.0 Congenital cataract**
CC **Q12.1 Congenital displaced lens**
CC **Q12.2 Coloboma of lens**
Q12.3 Congenital aphakia
Q12.4 Spherophakia
Q12.8 Other congenital lens malformations
Microphakia
Q12.9 Congenital lens malformation, unspecified

Q13 Congenital malformations of anterior segment of eye

Q13.0 Coloboma of iris
Coloboma NOS
Q13.1 Absence of iris
Aniridia
Use additional code for associated glaucoma (H42)
Q13.2 Other congenital malformations of iris
Anisocoria, congenital
Atresia of pupil
Congenital malformation of iris NOS
Corectopia
Q13.3 Congenital corneal opacity
Q13.4 Other congenital corneal malformations
Congenital malformation of cornea NOS
Microcornea
Peter's anomaly
Q13.5 Blue sclera
Q13.8 Other congenital malformations of anterior segment of eye
Q13.81 Rieger's anomaly
Use additional code for associated glaucoma (H42)
Q13.89 Other congenital malformations of anterior segment of eye
Q13.9 Congenital malformation of anterior segment of eye, unspecified

Q14 Congenital malformations of posterior segment of eye

Excludes2: *optic nerve hypoplasia (H47.03-)*
Q14.0 Congenital malformation of vitreous humor
Congenital vitreous opacity
Q14.1 Congenital malformation of retina
Congenital retinal aneurysm
Q14.2 Congenital malformation of optic disc
Coloboma of optic disc
Q14.3 Congenital malformation of choroid
Q14.8 Other congenital malformations of posterior segment of eye
Coloboma of the fundus
Q14.9 Congenital malformation of posterior segment of eye, unspecified

Q15 Other congenital malformations of eye

Excludes1: *congenital nystagmus (H55.01)*
ocular albinism (E70.31-)
optic nerve hypoplasia (H47.03-)
retinitis pigmentosa (H35.52)
Q15.0 Congenital glaucoma
Axenfeld's anomaly
Buphthalmos
Glaucoma of childhood
Glaucoma of newborn
Hydrophthalmos
Keratoglobus, congenital, with glaucoma
Macrocornea with glaucoma
Macrophthalmos in congenital glaucoma
Megalocornea with glaucoma

Q15.8 Other specified congenital malformations of eye
Q15.9 Congenital malformation of eye, unspecified
Congenital anomaly of eye
Congenital deformity of eye

Q16 Congenital malformations of ear causing impairment of hearing
Excludes1: *congenital deafness (H90.-)*
Q16.0 Congenital absence of (ear) auricle
Q16.1 Congenital absence, atresia and stricture of auditory canal (external)
Congenital atresia or stricture of osseous meatus
Q16.2 Absence of eustachian tube
Q16.3 Congenital malformation of ear ossicles
Congenital fusion of ear ossicles
Q16.4 Other congenital malformations of middle ear
Congenital malformation of middle ear NOS
Q16.5 Congenital malformation of inner ear
Congenital anomaly of membranous labyrinth
Congenital anomaly of organ of Corti
Q16.9 Congenital malformation of ear causing impairment of hearing, unspecified
Congenital absence of ear NOS

Q17 Other congenital malformations of ear
Excludes1: *congenital malformations of ear with impairment of hearing (Q16.0-Q16.9)*
preauricular sinus (Q18.1)
Q17.0 Accessory auricle
Accessory tragus
Polyotia
Preauricular appendage or tag
Supernumerary ear
Supernumerary lobule
Q17.1 Macrotia
Q17.2 Microtia
Q17.3 Other misshapen ear
Pointed ear
Q17.4 Misplaced ear
Low-set ears
Excludes1: *cervical auricle (Q18.2)*
Q17.5 Prominent ear
Bat ear
Q17.8 Other specified congenital malformations of ear
Congenital absence of lobe of ear
Q17.9 Congenital malformation of ear, unspecified
Congenital anomaly of ear NOS

Q18 Other congenital malformations of face and neck
Excludes1: *cleft lip and cleft palate (Q35-Q37)*
conditions classified to (Q67.0-Q67.4)
congenital malformations of skull and face bones (Q75.-)
cyclopia (Q87.0)
dentofacial anomalies [including malocclusion] (M26.-)
malformation syndromes affecting facial appearance (Q87.0)
persistent thyroglossal duct (Q89.2)
Q18.0 Sinus, fistula and cyst of branchial cleft
Branchial vestige
Q18.1 Preauricular sinus and cyst
Fistula of auricle, congenital
Cervicoaural fistula
Q18.2 Other branchial cleft malformations
Branchial cleft malformation NOS
Cervical auricle
Otocephaly
Q18.3 Webbing of neck
Pterygium colli
Q18.4 Macrostomia
Q18.5 Microstomia
Q18.6 Macrocheilia
Hypertrophy of lip, congenital
Q18.7 Microcheilia
Q18.8 Other specified congenital malformations of face and neck
Medial cyst of face and neck
Medial fistula of face and neck
Medial sinus of face and neck
Q18.9 Congenital malformation of face and neck, unspecified
Congenital anomaly NOS of face and neck

Congenital malformations of the circulatory system (Q20-Q28)

Q20 Congenital malformations of cardiac chambers and connections
Excludes1: *dextrocardia with situs inversus (Q89.3)*
mirror-image atrial arrangement with situs inversus (Q89.3)
MCC **Q20.0 Common arterial trunk**
Persistent truncus arteriosus
Excludes1: *aortic septal defect (Q21.4)*
MCC **Q20.1 Double outlet right ventricle**
Taussig-Bing syndrome
MCC **Q20.2 Double outlet left ventricle**
MCC **Q20.3 Discordant ventriculoarterial connection**
Dextrotransposition of aorta
Transposition of great vessels (complete)
MCC **Q20.4 Double inlet ventricle**
Common ventricle
Cor triloculare biatriatum
Single ventricle
CC **Q20.5 Discordant atrioventricular connection**
Corrected transposition
Levotransposition
Ventricular inversion
Q20.6 Isomerism of atrial appendages
Isomerism of atrial appendages with asplenia or polysplenia
Q20.8 Other congenital malformations of cardiac chambers and connections
Cor binoculare
Q20.9 Congenital malformation of cardiac chambers and connections, unspecified

Q21 Congenital malformations of cardiac septa
Excludes1: *acquired cardiac septal defect (I51.0)*
CC **Q21.0 Ventricular septal defect**
Roger's disease
CC **Q21.1 Atrial septal defect**
Coronary sinus defect
Patent or persistent foramen ovale
Patent or persistent ostium secundum defect (type II)
Patent or persistent sinus venosus defect
CC **Q21.2 Atrioventricular septal defect**
Common atrioventricular canal
Endocardial cushion defect
Ostium primum atrial septal defect (type I)
MCC **Q21.3 Tetralogy of Fallot**
Ventricular septal defect with pulmonary stenosis or atresia, dextroposition of aorta and hypertrophy of right ventricle.
AHA CC: 3Q, 2014, 16-17
Q21.4 Aortopulmonary septal defect
Aortic septal defect
Aortopulmonary window
Q21.8 Other congenital malformations of cardiac septa
Eisenmenger's defect
Pentalogy of Fallot
Code also, if applicable:
Eisenmenger's complex (I27.83)
Eisenmenger's syndrome (I27.83)
Q21.9 Congenital malformation of cardiac septum, unspecified
Septal (heart) defect NOS

Q22 Congenital malformations of pulmonary and tricuspid valves
MCC **Q22.0 Pulmonary valve atresia**
CC **Q22.1 Congenital pulmonary valve stenosis**
CC **Q22.2 Congenital pulmonary valve insufficiency**
Congenital pulmonary valve regurgitation
CC **Q22.3 Other congenital malformations of pulmonary valve**
Congenital malformation of pulmonary valve NOS
Supernumerary cusps of pulmonary valve
MCC **Q22.4 Congenital tricuspid stenosis**
Congenital tricuspid atresia
MCC **Q22.5 Ebstein's anomaly**
MCC **Q22.6 Hypoplastic right heart syndrome**
MCC **Q22.8 Other congenital malformations of tricuspid valve**
MCC **Q22.9 Congenital malformation of tricuspid valve, unspecified**

Q23 Congenital malformations of aortic and mitral valves

Q23.0 Congenital stenosis of aortic valve
Congenital aortic atresia
Congenital aortic stenosis NOS
Excludes1: *congenital stenosis of aortic valve in hypoplastic left heart syndrome (Q23.4)*
congenital subaortic stenosis (Q24.4)
supravalvular aortic stenosis (congenital) (Q25.3)

Q23.1 Congenital insufficiency of aortic valve
Bicuspid aortic valve
Congenital aortic insufficiency

Q23.2 Congenital mitral stenosis
Congenital mitral atresia

CC **Q23.3 Congenital mitral insufficiency**
MCC **Q23.4 Hypoplastic left heart syndrome**
CC **Q23.8 Other congenital malformations of aortic and mitral valves**
CC **Q23.9 Congenital malformation of aortic and mitral valves, unspecified**

Q24 Other congenital malformations of heart

Excludes1: *endocardial fibroelastosis (I42.4)*

CC **Q24.0 Dextrocardia**
Excludes1: *dextrocardia with situs inversus (Q89.3)*
isomerism of atrial appendages (with asplenia or polysplenia) (Q20.6)
mirror-image atrial arrangement with situs inversus (Q89.3)

CC **Q24.1 Levocardia**
MCC **Q24.2 Cor triatriatum**
CC **Q24.3 Pulmonary infundibular stenosis**
Subvalvular pulmonic stenosis

MCC **Q24.4 Congenital subaortic stenosis**
CC **Q24.5 Malformation of coronary vessels**
Congenital coronary (artery) aneurysm

MCC **Q24.6 Congenital heart block**

Q24.8 Other specified congenital malformations of heart
Congenital diverticulum of left ventricle
Congenital malformation of myocardium
Congenital malformation of pericardium
Malposition of heart
Uhl's disease

Q24.9 Congenital malformation of heart, unspecified
Congenital anomaly of heart
Congenital disease of heart

Q25 Congenital malformations of great arteries

CC **Q25.0 Patent ductus arteriosus**
Patent ductus Botallo
Persistent ductus arteriosus

CC **Q25.1 Coarctation of aorta**
Coarctation of aorta (preductal) (postductal)
Stenosis of aorta
AHA CC: 4Q, 2016, 56-57

\+ **Q25.2 Atresia of aorta**
AHA CC: 4Q, 2016, 56-57

CC **Q25.21 Interruption of aortic arch**
Atresia of aortic arch

CC **Q25.29 Other atresia of aorta**
Atresia of aorta

CC **Q25.3 Supravalvular aortic stenosis**
Excludes1: *congenital aortic stenosis NOS (Q23.0)*
congenital stenosis of aortic valve (Q23.0)

\+ **Q25.4 Other congenital malformations of aorta**
Excludes1: *hypoplasia of aorta in hypoplastic left heart syndrome (Q23.4)*
AHA CC: 4Q, 2016, 57

CC **Q25.40 Congenital malformation of aorta unspecified**
CC **Q25.41 Absence and aplasia of aorta**
CC **Q25.42 Hypoplasia of aorta**
CC **Q25.43 Congenital aneurysm of aorta**
Congenital aneurysm of aortic root
Congenital aneurysm of aortic sinus

CC **Q25.44 Congenital dilation of aorta**
CC **Q25.45 Double aortic arch**
Vascular ring of aorta

CC **Q25.46 Tortuous aortic arch**
Persistent convolutions of aortic arch

CC **Q25.47 Right aortic arch**
Persistent right aortic arch

CC **Q25.48 Anomalous origin of subclavian artery**
CC **Q25.49 Other congenital malformations of aorta**
Aortic arch
Bovine arch

MCC **Q25.5 Atresia of pulmonary artery**
MCC **Q25.6 Stenosis of pulmonary artery**
Supravalvular pulmonary stenosis

\+ **Q25.7 Other congenital malformations of pulmonary artery**
MCC **Q25.71 Coarctation of pulmonary artery**
MCC **Q25.72 Congenital pulmonary arteriovenous malformation**
Congenital pulmonary arteriovenous aneurysm

MCC **Q25.79 Other congenital malformations of pulmonary artery**
Aberrant pulmonary artery
Agenesis of pulmonary artery
Congenital aneurysm of pulmonary artery
Congenital anomaly of pulmonary artery
Hypoplasia of pulmonary artery

Q25.8 Other congenital malformations of other great arteries
CC **Q25.9 Congenital malformation of great arteries, unspecified**

Q26 Congenital malformations of great veins

CC **Q26.0 Congenital stenosis of vena cava**
Congenital stenosis of vena cava (inferior)(superior)

CC **Q26.1 Persistent left superior vena cava**
CC **Q26.2 Total anomalous pulmonary venous connection**
Total anomalous pulmonary venous return [TAPVR], subdiaphragmatic
Total anomalous pulmonary venous return [TAPVR], supradiaphragmatic

CC **Q26.3 Partial anomalous pulmonary venous connection**
Partial anomalous pulmonary venous return

CC **Q26.4 Anomalous pulmonary venous connection, unspecified**
Q26.5 Anomalous portal venous connection
Q26.6 Portal vein-hepatic artery fistula
CC **Q26.8 Other congenital malformations of great veins**
Absence of vena cava (inferior) (superior)
Azygos continuation of inferior vena cava
Persistent left posterior cardinal vein
Scimitar syndrome

CC **Q26.9 Congenital malformation of great vein, unspecified**
Congenital anomaly of vena cava (inferior) (superior) NOS

Q27 Other congenital malformations of peripheral vascular system

Excludes2: *anomalies of cerebral and precerebral vessels (Q28.0-Q28.3)*
anomalies of coronary vessels (Q24.5)
anomalies of pulmonary artery (Q25.5-Q25.7)
congenital retinal aneurysm (Q14.1)
hemangioma and lymphangioma (D18.-)

Q27.0 Congenital absence and hypoplasia of umbilical artery
Single umbilical artery

Q27.1 Congenital renal artery stenosis
Q27.2 Other congenital malformations of renal artery
Congenital malformation of renal artery NOS
Multiple renal arteries

\+ **Q27.3 Arteriovenous malformation (peripheral)**
Arteriovenous aneurysm
Excludes1: *acquired arteriovenous aneurysm (I77.0)*
Excludes2: *arteriovenous malformation of cerebral vessels (Q28.2)*
arteriovenous malformation of precerebral vessels (Q28.0)

CC **Q27.30 Arteriovenous malformation, site unspecified**
Q27.31 Arteriovenous malformation of vessel of upper limb
Q27.32 Arteriovenous malformation of vessel of lower limb
Q27.33 Arteriovenous malformation of digestive system vessel
Q27.34 Arteriovenous malformation of renal vessel
Q27.39 Arteriovenous malformation, other site

CC **Q27.4 Congenital phlebectasia**

Q27.8 Other specified congenital malformations of peripheral vascular system

Absence of peripheral vascular system
Atresia of peripheral vascular system
Congenital aneurysm (peripheral)
Congenital stricture, artery
Congenital varix
Excludes1: *arteriovenous malformation (Q27.3-)*

Q27.9 Congenital malformation of peripheral vascular system, unspecified

Anomaly of artery or vein NOS

Q28 Other congenital malformations of circulatory system

Excludes1: *congenital aneurysm NOS (Q27.8)*
congenital coronary aneurysm (Q24.5)
ruptured cerebral arteriovenous malformation (I60.8)
ruptured malformation of precerebral vessels (I72.0)
Excludes2: *congenital peripheral aneurysm (Q27.8)*
congenital pulmonary aneurysm (Q25.79)
congenital retinal aneurysm (Q14.1)

CC **Q28.0 Arteriovenous malformation of precerebral vessels**

Congenital arteriovenous precerebral aneurysm (nonruptured)

CC **Q28.1 Other malformations of precerebral vessels**

Congenital malformation of precerebral vessels NOS
Congenital precerebral aneurysm (nonruptured)

MCC **Q28.2 Arteriovenous malformation of cerebral vessels**

Arteriovenous malformation of brain NOS
Congenital arteriovenous cerebral aneurysm (nonruptured)

MCC **Q28.3 Other malformations of cerebral vessels**

Congenital cerebral aneurysm (nonruptured)
Congenital malformation of cerebral vessels NOS
Developmental venous anomaly

CC **Q28.8 Other specified congenital malformations of circulatory system**

Congenital aneurysm, specified site NEC
Spinal vessel anomaly

CC **Q28.9 Congenital malformation of circulatory system, unspecified**

Congenital malformations of the respiratory system (Q30-Q34)

Q30 Congenital malformations of nose

Excludes1: *congenital deviation of nasal septum (Q67.4)*

Q30.0 Choanal atresia

Atresia of nares (anterior) (posterior)
Congenital stenosis of nares (anterior) (posterior)

Q30.1 Agenesis and underdevelopment of nose

Congenital absent of nose

Q30.2 Fissured, notched and cleft nose

Q30.3 Congenital perforated nasal septum

Q30.8 Other congenital malformations of nose

Accessory nose
Congenital anomaly of nasal sinus wall

Q30.9 Congenital malformation of nose, unspecified

Q31 Congenital malformations of larynx

Excludes1: *congenital laryngeal stridor NOS (P28.89)*

Q31.0 Web of larynx

Glottic web of larynx
Subglottic web of larynx
Web of larynx NOS

CC **Q31.1 Congenital subglottic stenosis**

CC **Q31.2 Laryngeal hypoplasia**

CC **Q31.3 Laryngocele**

CC **Q31.5 Congenital laryngomalacia**

CC **Q31.8 Other congenital malformations of larynx**

Absence of larynx
Agenesis of larynx
Atresia of larynx
Congenital cleft thyroid cartilage
Congenital fissure of epiglottis
Congenital stenosis of larynx NEC
Posterior cleft of cricoid cartilage

CC **Q31.9 Congenital malformation of larynx, unspecified**

Q32 Congenital malformations of trachea and bronchus

Excludes1: *congenital bronchiectasis (Q33.4)*

CC **Q32.0 Congenital tracheomalacia**

CC **Q32.1 Other congenital malformations of trachea**

Atresia of trachea
Congenital anomaly of tracheal cartilage
Congenital dilatation of trachea
Congenital malformation of trachea
Congenital stenosis of trachea
Congenital tracheocele

CC **Q32.2 Congenital bronchomalacia**

CC **Q32.3 Congenital stenosis of bronchus**

CC **Q32.4 Other congenital malformations of bronchus**

Absence of bronchus
Agenesis of bronchus
Atresia of bronchus
Congenital diverticulum of bronchus
Congenital malformation of bronchus NOS

Q33 Congenital malformations of lung

CC **Q33.0 Congenital cystic lung**

Congenital cystic lung disease
Congenital honeycomb lung
Congenital polycystic lung disease
Excludes1: *cystic fibrosis (E84.0)*
cystic lung disease, acquired or unspecified (J98.4)

Q33.1 Accessory lobe of lung

Azygos lobe (fissured), lung

MCC **Q33.2 Sequestration of lung**

MCC **Q33.3 Agenesis of lung**

Congenital absence of lung (lobe)

CC **Q33.4 Congenital bronchiectasis**

Q33.5 Ectopic tissue in lung

MCC **Q33.6 Congenital hypoplasia and dysplasia of lung**

Excludes1: *pulmonary hypoplasia associated with short gestation (P28.0)*

Q33.8 Other congenital malformations of lung

Q33.9 Congenital malformation of lung, unspecified

Q34 Other congenital malformations of respiratory system

Excludes2: *congenital central alveolar hypoventilation syndrome (G47.35)*

Q34.0 Anomaly of pleura

Q34.1 Congenital cyst of mediastinum

Q34.8 Other specified congenital malformations of respiratory system

Atresia of nasopharynx

Q34.9 Congenital malformation of respiratory system, unspecified

Congenital absence of respiratory system
Congenital anomaly of respiratory system NOS

Cleft lip and cleft palate (Q35-Q37)

Use additional code to identify associated malformation of the nose (Q30.2)

Excludes2: *Robin's syndrome (Q87.0)*

Q35 Cleft palate

Includes: fissure of palate
palatoschisis
Excludes1: *cleft palate with cleft lip (Q37.-)*

Q35.1 Cleft hard palate

Q35.3 Cleft soft palate

Q35.5 Cleft hard palate with cleft soft palate

Q35.7 Cleft uvula

Q35.9 Cleft palate, unspecified

Cleft palate NOS

Q36 Cleft lip

Includes: cheiloschisis
congenital fissure of lip
harelip
labium leporinum
Excludes1: *cleft lip with cleft palate (Q37.-)*

Q36.0 Cleft lip, bilateral

Q36.1 Cleft lip, median

Q36.9 Cleft lip, unilateral

Cleft lip NOS

Q37 Cleft palate with cleft lip

Includes: cheilopalatoschisis

Q37.0 Cleft hard palate with bilateral cleft lip

Q37.1 Cleft hard palate with unilateral cleft lip
Cleft hard palate with cleft lip NOS

Q37.2 Cleft soft palate with bilateral cleft lip

Q37.3 Cleft soft palate with unilateral cleft lip
Cleft soft palate with cleft lip NOS

Q37.4 Cleft hard and soft palate with bilateral cleft lip

Q37.5 Cleft hard and soft palate with unilateral cleft lip
Cleft hard and soft palate with cleft lip NOS

Q37.8 Unspecified cleft palate with bilateral cleft lip

Q37.9 Unspecified cleft palate with unilateral cleft lip
Cleft palate with cleft lip NOS

Other congenital malformations of the digestive system (Q38-Q45)

Q38 Other congenital malformations of tongue, mouth and pharynx

Excludes1: *dentofacial anomalies (M26.-)*
macrostomia (Q18.4)
microstomia (Q18.5)

Q38.0 Congenital malformations of lips, not elsewhere classified
Congenital fistula of lip
Congenital malformation of lip NOS
Van der Woude's syndrome
Excludes1: *cleft lip (Q36.-)*
cleft lip with cleft palate (Q37.-)
macrocheilia (Q18.6)
microcheilia (Q18.7)

Q38.1 Ankyloglossia
Tongue tie

Q38.2 Macroglossia
Congenital hypertrophy of tongue

Q38.3 Other congenital malformations of tongue
Aglossia
Bifid tongue
Congenital adhesion of tongue
Congenital fissure of tongue
Congenital malformation of tongue NOS
Double tongue
Hypoglossia
Hypoplasia of tongue
Microglossia

Q38.4 Congenital malformations of salivary glands and ducts
Atresia of salivary glands and ducts
Congenital absence of salivary glands and ducts
Congenital accessory salivary glands and ducts
Congenital fistula of salivary gland

Q38.5 Congenital malformations of palate, not elsewhere classified
Congenital absence of uvula
Congenital malformation of palate NOS
Congenital high arched palate
Excludes1: *cleft palate (Q35.-)*
cleft palate with cleft lip (Q37.-)

Q38.6 Other congenital malformations of mouth
Congenital malformation of mouth NOS

Q38.7 Congenital pharyngeal pouch
Congenital diverticulum of pharynx
Excludes1: *pharyngeal pouch syndrome (D82.1)*

Q38.8 Other congenital malformations of pharynx
Congenital malformation of pharynx NOS
Imperforate pharynx

Q39 Congenital malformations of esophagus

MCC **Q39.0 Atresia of esophagus without fistula**
Atresia of esophagus NOS

MCC **Q39.1 Atresia of esophagus with tracheo-esophageal fistula**
Atresia of esophagus with broncho-esophageal fistula

MCC **Q39.2 Congenital tracheo-esophageal fistula without atresia**
Congenital tracheo-esophageal fistula NOS

MCC **Q39.3 Congenital stenosis and stricture of esophagus**

MCC **Q39.4 Esophageal web**

CC **Q39.5 Congenital dilatation of esophagus**
Congenital cardiospasm

CC **Q39.6 Congenital diverticulum of esophagus**
Congenital esophageal pouch

CC **Q39.8 Other congenital malformations of esophagus**
Congenital absence of esophagus
Congenital displacement of esophagus
Congenital duplication of esophagus

CC **Q39.9 Congenital malformation of esophagus, unspecified**

Q40 Other congenital malformations of upper alimentary tract

Q40.0 Congenital hypertrophic pyloric stenosis
Congenital or infantile constriction
Congenital or infantile hypertrophy
Congenital or infantile spasm
Congenital or infantile stenosis
Congenital or infantile stricture

Q40.1 Congenital hiatus hernia
Congenital displacement of cardia through esophageal hiatus
Excludes1: *congenital diaphragmatic hernia (Q79.0)*

Q40.2 Other specified congenital malformations of stomach
Congenital displacement of stomach
Congenital diverticulum of stomach
Congenital hourglass stomach
Congenital duplication of stomach
Megalogastria
Microgastria

Q40.3 Congenital malformation of stomach, unspecified

Q40.8 Other specified congenital malformations of upper alimentary tract

Q40.9 Congenital malformation of upper alimentary tract, unspecified
Congenital anomaly of upper alimentary tract
Congenital deformity of upper alimentary tract

Q41 Congenital absence, atresia and stenosis of small intestine

Includes: congenital obstruction, occlusion or stricture of small intestine or intestine NOS

Excludes1: *cystic fibrosis with intestinal manifestation (E84.11)*
meconium ileus NOS (without cystic fibrosis) (P76.0)

CC **Q41.0 Congenital absence, atresia and stenosis of duodenum**

CC **Q41.1 Congenital absence, atresia and stenosis of jejunum**
Apple peel syndrome
Imperforate jejunum

CC **Q41.2 Congenital absence, atresia and stenosis of ileum**

CC **Q41.8 Congenital absence, atresia and stenosis of other specified parts of small intestine**

CC **Q41.9 Congenital absence, atresia and stenosis of small intestine, part unspecified**
Congenital absence, atresia and stenosis of intestine NOS

Q42 Congenital absence, atresia and stenosis of large intestine

Includes: congenital obstruction, occlusion and stricture of large intestine

CC **Q42.0 Congenital absence, atresia and stenosis of rectum with fistula**

CC **Q42.1 Congenital absence, atresia and stenosis of rectum without fistula**
Imperforate rectum

CC **Q42.2 Congenital absence, atresia and stenosis of anus with fistula**

CC **Q42.3 Congenital absence, atresia and stenosis of anus without fistula**
Imperforate anus

CC **Q42.8 Congenital absence, atresia and stenosis of other parts of large intestine**

CC **Q42.9 Congenital absence, atresia and stenosis of large intestine, part unspecified**

Q43 Other congenital malformations of intestine

Q43.0 Meckel's diverticulum (displaced) (hypertrophic)
Persistent omphalomesenteric duct
Persistent vitelline duct

CC **Q43.1 Hirschsprung's disease**
Aganglionosis
Congenital (aganglionic) megacolon

CC **Q43.2 Other congenital functional disorders of colon**
Congenital dilatation of colon

CC **Q43.3 Congenital malformations of intestinal fixation**
Congenital omental, anomalous adhesions [bands]
Congenital peritoneal adhesions [bands]
Incomplete rotation of cecum and colon
Insufficient rotation of cecum and colon
Jackson's membrane
Malrotation of colon
Rotation failure of cecum and colon
Universal mesentery

CC **Q43.4 Duplication of intestine**
CC **Q43.5 Ectopic anus**
CC **Q43.6 Congenital fistula of rectum and anus**
Excludes1: *congenital fistula of anus with absence, atresia and stenosis (Q42.2)*
congenital fistula of rectum with absence, atresia and stenosis (Q42.0)
congenital rectovaginal fistula (Q52.2)
congenital urethrorectal fistula (Q64.73)
pilonidal fistula or sinus (L05.-)
CC **Q43.7 Persistent cloaca**
Cloaca NOS
CC **Q43.8 Other specified congenital malformations of intestine**
Congenital blind loop syndrome
Congenital diverticulitis, colon
Congenital diverticulum, intestine
Dolichocolon
Megaloappendix
Megaloduodenum
Microcolon
Transposition of appendix
Transposition of colon
Transposition of intestine
AHA CC: 2Q, 2013, 31
CC **Q43.9 Congenital malformation of intestine, unspecified**

Q44 Congenital malformations of gallbladder, bile ducts and liver
CC **Q44.0 Agenesis, aplasia and hypoplasia of gallbladder**
Congenital absence of gallbladder
CC **Q44.1 Other congenital malformations of gallbladder**
Congenital malformation of gallbladder NOS
Intrahepatic gallbladder
MCC **Q44.2 Atresia of bile ducts**
MCC **Q44.3 Congenital stenosis and stricture of bile ducts**
CC **Q44.4 Choledochal cyst**
CC **Q44.5 Other congenital malformations of bile ducts**
Accessory hepatic duct
Biliary duct duplication
Congenital malformation of bile duct NOS
Cystic duct duplication
CC **Q44.6 Cystic disease of liver**
Fibrocystic disease of liver
CC **Q44.7 Other congenital malformations of liver**
Accessory liver
Alagille's syndrome
Congenital absence of liver
Congenital hepatomegaly
Congenital malformation of liver NOS

Q45 Other congenital malformations of digestive system
Excludes2: *congenital diaphragmatic hernia (Q79.0)*
congenital hiatus hernia (Q40.1)
CC **Q45.0 Agenesis, aplasia and hypoplasia of pancreas**
Congenital absence of pancreas
CC **Q45.1 Annular pancreas**
CC **Q45.2 Congenital pancreatic cyst**
Q45.3 Other congenital malformations of pancreas and pancreatic duct
Accessory pancreas
Congenital malformation of pancreas or pancreatic duct NOS
Excludes1: *congenital diabetes mellitus (E10.-)*
cystic fibrosis (E84.0-E84.9)
fibrocystic disease of pancreas (E84.-)
neonatal diabetes mellitus (P70.2)
Q45.8 Other specified congenital malformations of digestive system
Absence (complete) (partial) of alimentary tract NOS
Duplication of digestive system
Malposition, congenital of digestive system
Q45.9 Congenital malformation of digestive system, unspecified
Congenital anomaly of digestive system
Congenital deformity of digestive system

Congenital malformations of genital organs (Q50-Q56)

Excludes1: *androgen insensitivity syndrome (E34.5-)*
syndromes associated with anomalies in the number and form of chromosomes (Q90-Q99)

Q50 Congenital malformations of ovaries, fallopian tubes and broad ligaments
+ **Q50.0 Congenital absence of ovary**
Excludes1: *Turner's syndrome (Q96.-)*
♀ **Q50.01 Congenital absence of ovary, unilateral**
♀ **Q50.02 Congenital absence of ovary, bilateral**
♀ **Q50.1 Developmental ovarian cyst**
♀ **Q50.2 Congenital torsion of ovary**
+ **Q50.3 Other congenital malformations of ovary**
♀ **Q50.31 Accessory ovary**
♀ **Q50.32 Ovarian streak**
46, XX with streak gonads
♀ **Q50.39 Other congenital malformation of ovary**
Congenital malformation of ovary NOS
♀ **Q50.4 Embryonic cyst of fallopian tube**
Fimbrial cyst
♀ **Q50.5 Embryonic cyst of broad ligament**
Epoophoron cyst
Parovarian cyst
♀ **Q50.6 Other congenital malformations of fallopian tube and broad ligament**
Absence of fallopian tube and broad ligament
Accessory fallopian tube and broad ligament
Atresia of fallopian tube and broad ligament
Congenital malformation of fallopian tube or broad ligament NOS

Q51 Congenital malformations of uterus and cervix
♀ **Q51.0 Agenesis and aplasia of uterus**
Congenital absence of uterus
+ **Q51.1 Doubling of uterus with doubling of cervix and vagina**
♀ **Q51.10 Doubling of uterus with doubling of cervix and vagina without obstruction**
Doubling of uterus with doubling of cervix and vagina NOS
♀ **Q51.11 Doubling of uterus with doubling of cervix and vagina with obstruction**
+ **Q51.2 Other doubling of uterus**
Doubling of uterus NOS
Septate uterus
AHA CC: 4Q, 2018, 27
♀ **Q51.21 Complete doubling of uterus**
Complete septate uterus
♀ **Q51.22 Partial doubling of uterus**
Partial septate uterus
♀ **Q51.28 Other and unspecified doubling of uterus**
Septate uterus NOS
♀ **Q51.3 Bicornate uterus**
Bicornate uterus, complete or partial
♀ **Q51.4 Unicornate uterus**
Unicornate uterus with or without a separate uterine horn
Uterus with only one functioning horn
♀ **Q51.5 Agenesis and aplasia of cervix**
Congenital absence of cervix
♀ **Q51.6 Embryonic cyst of cervix**
♀ **Q51.7 Congenital fistulae between uterus and digestive and urinary tracts**
+ **Q51.8 Other congenital malformations of uterus and cervix**
+ **Q51.81 Other congenital malformations of uterus**
♀ **Q51.810 Arcuate uterus**
Arcuatus uterus
♀ **Q51.811 Hypoplasia of uterus**
♀ **Q51.818 Other congenital malformations of uterus**
Müllerian anomaly of uterus NEC
+ **Q51.82 Other congenital malformations of cervix**
♀ **Q51.820 Cervical duplication**
♀ **Q51.821 Hypoplasia of cervix**
♀ **Q51.828 Other congenital malformations of cervix**
♀ **Q51.9 Congenital malformation of uterus and cervix, unspecified**

Q52 Other congenital malformations of female genitalia

♀ **Q52.0 Congenital absence of vagina**
Vaginal agenesis, total or partial

+ **Q52.1 Doubling of vagina**
Excludes1: *doubling of vagina with doubling of uterus and cervix (Q51.1-)*

♀ **Q52.10 Doubling of vagina, unspecified**
Septate vagina NOS

♀ **Q52.11 Transverse vaginal septum**

+ **Q52.12 Longitudinal vaginal septum**
AHA CC: 4Q, 2016, 58-59

♀ **Q52.120 Longitudinal vaginal septum, nonobstructing**

♀ **Q52.121 Longitudinal vaginal septum, obstructing, right side**

♀ **Q52.122 Longitudinal vaginal septum, obstructing, left side**

♀ **Q52.123 Longitudinal vaginal septum, microperforate, right side**

♀ **Q52.124 Longitudinal vaginal septum, microperforate, left side**
AHA CC: 4Q, 2016, 58-59

♀ **Q52.129 Other and unspecified longitudinal vaginal septum**

♀ **Q52.2 Congenital rectovaginal fistula**
Excludes1: *cloaca (Q43.7)*

♀ **Q52.3 Imperforate hymen**

♀ **Q52.4 Other congenital malformations of vagina**
Canal of Nuck cyst, congenital
Congenital malformation of vagina NOS
Embryonic vaginal cyst
Gartner's duct cyst

♀ **Q52.5 Fusion of labia**

♀ **Q52.6 Congenital malformation of clitoris**

+ **Q52.7 Other and unspecified congenital malformations of vulva**

♀ **Q52.70 Unspecified congenital malformations of vulva**
Congenital malformation of vulva NOS

♀ **Q52.71 Congenital absence of vulva**

♀ **Q52.79 Other congenital malformations of vulva**
Congenital cyst of vulva

♀ **Q52.8 Other specified congenital malformations of female genitalia**

♀ **Q52.9 Congenital malformation of female genitalia, unspecified**

Q53 Undescended and ectopic testicle

AHA CC: 4Q, 2017, 22-23

+ **Q53.0 Ectopic testis**

♂ **Q53.00 Ectopic testis, unspecified**

♂ **Q53.01 Ectopic testis, unilateral**

♂ **Q53.02 Ectopic testes, bilateral**

+ **Q53.1 Undescended testicle, unilateral**

♂ **Q53.10 Unspecified undescended testicle, unilateral**

+ **Q53.11 Abdominal testis, unilateral**

♂ **Q53.111 Unilateral intraabdominal testis**

♂ **Q53.112 Unilateral inguinal testis**

♂ **Q53.12 Ectopic perineal testis, unilateral**

♂ **Q53.13 Unilateral high scrotal testis**

+ **Q53.2 Undescended testicle, bilateral**

♂ **Q53.20 Undescended testicle, unspecified, bilateral**

+ **Q53.21 Abdominal testis, bilateral**

♂ **Q53.211 Bilateral intraabdominal testes**

♂ **Q53.212 Bilateral inguinal testes**

♂ **Q53.22 Ectopic perineal testis, bilateral**

♂ **Q53.23 Bilateral high scrotal testes**

♂ **Q53.9 Undescended testicle, unspecified**
Cryptorchism NOS

Q54 Hypospadias

Excludes1: *epispadias (Q64.0)*

♂ **Q54.0 Hypospadias, balanic**
Hypospadias, coronal
Hypospadias, glandular

♂ **Q54.1 Hypospadias, penile**

♂ **Q54.2 Hypospadias, penoscrotal**

♂ **Q54.3 Hypospadias, perineal**

♂ **Q54.4 Congenital chordee**
Chordee without hypospadias

♂ **Q54.8 Other hypospadias**
Hypospadias with intersex state

♂ **Q54.9 Hypospadias, unspecified**

Q55 Other congenital malformations of male genital organs

Excludes1: *congenital hydrocele (P83.5)*
hypospadias (Q54.-)

♂ **Q55.0 Absence and aplasia of testis**
Monorchism

♂ **Q55.1 Hypoplasia of testis and scrotum**
Fusion of testes

+ **Q55.2 Other and unspecified congenital malformations of testis and scrotum**

♂ **Q55.20 Unspecified congenital malformations of testis and scrotum**
Congenital malformation of testis or scrotum NOS

♂ **Q55.21 Polyorchism**

♂ **Q55.22 Retractile testis**

♂ **Q55.23 Scrotal transposition**

♂ **Q55.29 Other congenital malformations of testis and scrotum**

♂ **Q55.3 Atresia of vas deferens**
Code first any associated cystic fibrosis (E84.-)

♂ **Q55.4 Other congenital malformations of vas deferens, epididymis, seminal vesicles and prostate**
Absence or aplasia of prostate
Absence or aplasia of spermatic cord
Congenital malformation of vas deferens, epididymis, seminal vesicles or prostate NOS

♂ **Q55.5 Congenital absence and aplasia of penis**

+ **Q55.6 Other congenital malformations of penis**

♂ **Q55.61 Curvature of penis (lateral)**

♂ **Q55.62 Hypoplasia of penis**
Micropenis

♂ **Q55.63 Congenital torsion of penis**
Excludes1: *acquired torsion of penis (N48.82)*

♂ **Q55.64 Hidden penis**
Buried penis
Concealed penis
Excludes1: *acquired buried penis (N48.83)*

♂ **Q55.69 Other congenital malformation of penis**
Congenital malformation of penis NOS

♂ **Q55.7 Congenital vasocutaneous fistula**

♂ **Q55.8 Other specified congenital malformations of male genital organs**

♂ **Q55.9 Congenital malformation of male genital organ, unspecified**
Congenital anomaly of male genital organ
Congenital deformity of male genital organ

Q56 Indeterminate sex and pseudohermaphroditism

Excludes1: *46,XX true hermaphrodite (Q99.1)*
androgen insensitivity syndrome (E34.5-)
chimera 46,XX/46,XY true hermaphrodite (Q99.0)
female pseudohermaphroditism with adrenocortical disorder (E25.-)
pseudohermaphroditism with specified chromosomal anomaly (Q96-Q99)
pure gonadal dysgenesis (Q99.1)

Q56.0 Hermaphroditism, not elsewhere classified
Ovotestis

♂ **Q56.1 Male pseudohermaphroditism, not elsewhere classified**
46, XY with streak gonads
Male pseudohermaphroditism NOS

♀ **Q56.2 Female pseudohermaphroditism, not elsewhere classified**
Female pseudohermaphroditism NOS

Q56.3 Pseudohermaphroditism, unspecified

Q56.4 Indeterminate sex, unspecified
Ambiguous genitalia

Congenital malformations of the urinary system (Q60-Q64)

Q60 Renal agenesis and other reduction defects of kidney

Includes: congenital absence of kidney
congenital atrophy of kidney
infantile atrophy of kidney

CC **Q60.0 Renal agenesis, unilateral**
CC **Q60.1 Renal agenesis, bilateral**
CC **Q60.2 Renal agenesis, unspecified**
CC **Q60.3 Renal hypoplasia, unilateral**
CC **Q60.4 Renal hypoplasia, bilateral**
CC **Q60.5 Renal hypoplasia, unspecified**
CC **Q60.6 Potter's syndrome**

Q61 Cystic kidney disease

Excludes1: *acquired cyst of kidney (N28.1)*
Potter's syndrome (Q60.6)

+ **Q61.0 Congenital renal cyst**
  - CC **Q61.00 Congenital renal cyst, unspecified**
    Cyst of kidney NOS (congenital)
  - CC **Q61.01 Congenital single renal cyst**
  - CC **Q61.02 Congenital multiple renal cysts**

+ **Q61.1 Polycystic kidney, infantile type**
  Polycystic kidney, autosomal recessive
  - CC **Q61.11 Cystic dilatation of collecting ducts**
  - CC **Q61.19 Other polycystic kidney, infantile type**

CC **Q61.2 Polycystic kidney, adult type**
Polycystic kidney, autosomal dominant

CC **Q61.3 Polycystic kidney, unspecified**
AHA CC: 3Q, 2016, 22-23

CC **Q61.4 Renal dysplasia**
Multicystic dysplastic kidney
Multicystic kidney (development)
Multicystic kidney disease
Multicystic renal dysplasia
Excludes1: *polycystic kidney disease (Q61.11-Q61.3)*

CC **Q61.5 Medullary cystic kidney**
Nephronophthisis
Sponge kidney NOS

CC **Q61.8 Other cystic kidney diseases**
Fibrocystic kidney
Fibrocystic renal degeneration or disease

CC **Q61.9 Cystic kidney disease, unspecified**
Meckel-Gruber syndrome

Q62 Congenital obstructive defects of renal pelvis and congenital malformations of ureter

CC **Q62.0 Congenital hydronephrosis**

+ **Q62.1 Congenital occlusion of ureter**
  Atresia and stenosis of ureter
  - CC **Q62.10 Congenital occlusion of ureter, unspecified**
  - CC **Q62.11 Congenital occlusion of ureteropelvic junction**
  - CC **Q62.12 Congenital occlusion of ureterovesical orifice**

Q62.2 Congenital megaureter
Congenital dilatation of ureter

+ **Q62.3 Other obstructive defects of renal pelvis and ureter**
  - CC **Q62.31 Congenital ureterocele, orthotopic**
  - CC **Q62.32 Cecoureterocele**
    Ectopic ureterocele
  - CC **Q62.39 Other obstructive defects of renal pelvis and ureter**
    Ureteropelvic junction obstruction NOS

Q62.4 Agenesis of ureter
Congenital absence ureter

Q62.5 Duplication of ureter
Accessory ureter
Double ureter

+ **Q62.6 Malposition of ureter**
  - **Q62.60 Malposition of ureter, unspecified**
  - **Q62.61 Deviation of ureter**
  - **Q62.62 Displacement of ureter**
  - **Q62.63 Anomalous implantation of ureter**
    Ectopia of ureter
    Ectopic ureter
  - **Q62.69 Other malposition of ureter**

Q62.7 Congenital vesico-uretero-renal reflux

Q62.8 Other congenital malformations of ureter
Anomaly of ureter NOS

Q63 Other congenital malformations of kidney

Excludes1: *congenital nephrotic syndrome (N04.-)*

Q63.0 Accessory kidney

Q63.1 Lobulated, fused and horseshoe kidney

Q63.2 Ectopic kidney
Congenital displaced kidney
Malrotation of kidney

Q63.3 Hyperplastic and giant kidney
Compensatory hypertrophy of kidney

Q63.8 Other specified congenital malformations of kidney
Congenital renal calculi

Q63.9 Congenital malformation of kidney, unspecified

Q64 Other congenital malformations of urinary system

Q64.0 Epispadias
Excludes1: *hypospadias (Q54.-)*

+ **Q64.1 Exstrophy of urinary bladder**
  - CC **Q64.10 Exstrophy of urinary bladder, unspecified**
    Ectopia vesicae
  - CC **Q64.11 Supravesical fissure of urinary bladder**
  - CC **Q64.12 Cloacal exstrophy of urinary bladder**
  - CC **Q64.19 Other exstrophy of urinary bladder**
    Extroversion of bladder

CC **Q64.2 Congenital posterior urethral valves**

+ **Q64.3 Other atresia and stenosis of urethra and bladder neck**
  - CC **Q64.31 Congenital bladder neck obstruction**
    Congenital obstruction of vesicourethral orifice
  - CC **Q64.32 Congenital stricture of urethra**
  - CC **Q64.33 Congenital stricture of urinary meatus**
  - CC **Q64.39 Other atresia and stenosis of urethra and bladder neck**
    Atresia and stenosis of urethra and bladder neck NOS

Q64.4 Malformation of urachus
Cyst of urachus
Patent urachus
Prolapse of urachus

Q64.5 Congenital absence of bladder and urethra

Q64.6 Congenital diverticulum of bladder

+ **Q64.7 Other and unspecified congenital malformations of bladder and urethra**
  Excludes1: *congenital prolapse of bladder (mucosa) (Q79.4)*
  - **Q64.70 Unspecified congenital malformation of bladder and urethra**
    Malformation of bladder or urethra NOS
  - **Q64.71 Congenital prolapse of urethra**
  - **Q64.72 Congenital prolapse of urinary meatus**
  - **Q64.73 Congenital urethrorectal fistula**
  - **Q64.74 Double urethra**
  - **Q64.75 Double urinary meatus**
  - **Q64.79 Other congenital malformations of bladder and urethra**

Q64.8 Other specified congenital malformations of urinary system

Q64.9 Congenital malformation of urinary system, unspecified
Congenital anomaly NOS of urinary system
Congenital deformity NOS of urinary system

Congenital malformations and deformations of the musculoskeletal system (Q65-Q79)

Q65 Congenital deformities of hip

Excludes1: *clicking hip (R29.4)*

+ **Q65.0 Congenital dislocation of hip, unilateral**
  - **Q65.00 Congenital dislocation of unspecified hip, unilateral**
  - **Q65.01 Congenital dislocation of right hip, unilateral**
  - **Q65.02 Congenital dislocation of left hip, unilateral**

Q65.1 Congenital dislocation of hip, bilateral

Q65.2 Congenital dislocation of hip, unspecified

+ **Q65.3 Congenital partial dislocation of hip, unilateral**
  - **Q65.30 Congenital partial dislocation of unspecified hip, unilateral**
  - **Q65.31 Congenital partial dislocation of right hip, unilateral**
  - **Q65.32 Congenital partial dislocation of left hip, unilateral**

Q65.4 Congenital partial dislocation of hip, bilateral

Q65.5 Congenital partial dislocation of hip, unspecified

Q65.6 Congenital unstable hip
Congenital dislocatable hip

+ **Q65.8 Other congenital deformities of hip**
  - **Q65.81 Congenital coxa valga**
  - **Q65.82 Congenital coxa vara**
  - **Q65.89 Other specified congenital deformities of hip**
    Anteversion of femoral neck
    Congenital acetabular dysplasia

Q65.9 Congenital deformity of hip, unspecified

Q66 Congenital deformities of feet

Excludes1: *reduction defects of feet (Q72.-)*
valgus deformities (acquired) (M21.0-)
varus deformities (acquired) (M21.1-)

AHA CC: 4Q, 2019, 13

+ **Q66.0 Congenital talipes equinovarus**
  - **Q66.00 Congenital talipes equinovarus, unspecified foot**
  - **Q66.01 Congenital talipes equinovarus, right foot**
  - **Q66.02 Congenital talipes equinovarus, left foot**

+ **Q66.1 Congenital talipes calcaneovarus**
  - **Q66.10 Congenital talipes calcaneovarus, unspecified foot**
  - **Q66.11 Congenital talipes calcaneovarus, right foot**
  - **Q66.12 Congenital talipes calcaneovarus, left foot**

+ **Q66.2 Congenital metatarsus (primus) varus**

AHA CC: 4Q, 2016, 59

+ **Q66.21 Congenital metatarsus primus varus**
  - **Q66.211 Congenital metatarsus primus varus, right foot**
  - **Q66.212 Congenital metatarsus primus varus, left foot**
  - **Q66.219 Congenital metatarsus primus varus, unspecified foot**

+ **Q66.22 Congenital metatarsus adductus**
  Congenital metatarsus varus
  - **Q66.221 Congenital metatarsus adductus, right foot**
  - **Q66.222 Congenital metatarsus adductus, left foot**
  - **Q66.229 Congenital metatarsus adductus, unspecified foot**

+ **Q66.3 Other congenital varus deformities of feet**
  Hallux varus, congenital
  - **Q66.30 Other congenital varus deformities of feet, unspecified foot**
  - **Q66.31 Other congenital varus deformities of feet, right foot**
  - **Q66.32 Other congenital varus deformities of feet, left foot**

+ **Q66.4 Congenital talipes calcaneovalgus**
  - **Q66.40 Congenital talipes calcaneovalgus, unspecified foot**
  - **Q66.41 Congenital talipes calcaneovalgus, right foot**
  - **Q66.42 Congenital talipes calcaneovalgus, left foot**

+ **Q66.5 Congenital pes planus**
  Congenital flat foot
  Congenital rigid flat foot
  Congenital spastic (everted) flat foot
  Excludes1: *pes planus, acquired (M21.4)*
  - **Q66.50 Congenital pes planus, unspecified foot**
  - **Q66.51 Congenital pes planus, right foot**
  - **Q66.52 Congenital pes planus, left foot**

Q66.6 Other congenital valgus deformities of feet
Congenital metatarsus valgus

+ **Q66.7 Congenital pes cavus**
  - **Q66.70 Congenital pes cavus, unspecified foot**
  - **Q66.71 Congenital pes cavus, right foot**
  - **Q66.72 Congenital pes cavus, left foot**

+ **Q66.8 Other congenital deformities of feet**
  - **Q66.80 Congenital vertical talus deformity, unspecified foot**
  - **Q66.81 Congenital vertical talus deformity, right foot**
  - **Q66.82 Congenital vertical talus deformity, left foot**
  - **Q66.89 Other specified congenital deformities of feet**
    Congenital asymmetric talipes
    Congenital clubfoot NOS
    Congenital talipes NOS
    Congenital tarsal coalition
    Hammer toe, congenital

+ **Q66.9 Congenital deformity of feet, unspecified**
  - **Q66.90 Congenital deformity of feet, unspecified, unspecified foot**
  - **Q66.91 Congenital deformity of feet, unspecified, right foot**
  - **Q66.92 Congenital deformity of feet, unspecified, left foot**

Q67 Congenital musculoskeletal deformities of head, face, spine and chest

Excludes1: *congenital malformation syndromes classified to Q87.-*
Potter's syndrome (Q60.6)

Q67.0 Congenital facial asymmetry
Q67.1 Congenital compression facies
Q67.2 Dolichocephaly
Q67.3 Plagiocephaly
Q67.4 Other congenital deformities of skull, face and jaw
Congenital depressions in skull
Congenital hemifacial atrophy or hypertrophy
Deviation of nasal septum, congenital
Squashed or bent nose, congenital
Excludes1: *dentofacial anomalies [including malocclusion] (M26.-)*
syphilitic saddle nose (A50.5)

CC **Q67.5 Congenital deformity of spine**
Congenital postural scoliosis
Congenital scoliosis NOS
Excludes1: *infantile idiopathic scoliosis (M41.0)*
scoliosis due to congenital bony malformation (Q76.3)

AHA CC: 4Q, 2014, 26

Q67.6 Pectus excavatum
Congenital funnel chest
Q67.7 Pectus carinatum
Congenital pigeon chest
CC **Q67.8 Other congenital deformities of chest**
Congenital deformity of chest wall NOS

Q68 Other congenital musculoskeletal deformities

Excludes1: *reduction defects of limb(s) (Q71-Q73)*
Excludes2: *congenital myotonic chondrodystrophy (G71.13)*

Q68.0 Congenital deformity of sternocleidomastoid muscle
Congenital contracture of sternocleidomastoid (muscle)
Congenital (sternomastoid) torticollis
Sternomastoid tumor (congenital)
CC **Q68.1 Congenital deformity of finger(s) and hand**
Congenital clubfinger
Spade-like hand (congenital)
Q68.2 Congenital deformity of knee
Congenital dislocation of knee
Congenital genu recurvatum
Q68.3 Congenital bowing of femur
Excludes1: *anteversion of femur (neck) (Q65.89)*
Q68.4 Congenital bowing of tibia and fibula
Q68.5 Congenital bowing of long bones of leg, unspecified
Q68.6 Discoid meniscus
Q68.8 Other specified congenital musculoskeletal deformities
Congenital deformity of clavicle
Congenital deformity of elbow
Congenital deformity of forearm
Congenital deformity of scapula
Congenital deformity of wrist
Congenital dislocation of elbow
Congenital dislocation of shoulder
Congenital dislocation of wrist

Q69 Polydactyly

Q69.0 Accessory finger(s)
Q69.1 Accessory thumb(s)
Q69.2 Accessory toe(s)
Accessory hallux
Q69.9 Polydactyly, unspecified
Supernumerary digit(s) NOS

Q70 Syndactyly

+ **Q70.0 Fused fingers**
  Complex syndactyly of fingers with synostosis
  - **Q70.00 Fused fingers, unspecified hand**
  - **Q70.01 Fused fingers, right hand**
  - **Q70.02 Fused fingers, left hand**
  - **Q70.03 Fused fingers, bilateral**

+ **Q70.1 Webbed fingers**
  Simple syndactyly of fingers without synostosis
  - **Q70.10 Webbed fingers, unspecified hand**
  - **Q70.11 Webbed fingers, right hand**
  - **Q70.12 Webbed fingers, left hand**
  - **Q70.13 Webbed fingers, bilateral**

+ **Q70.2 Fused toes**
  Complex syndactyly of toes with synostosis
  - **Q70.20 Fused toes, unspecified foot**
  - **Q70.21 Fused toes, right foot**
  - **Q70.22 Fused toes, left foot**
  - **Q70.23 Fused toes, bilateral**

+ **Q70.3 Webbed toes**
Simple syndactyly of toes without synostosis
Q70.30 Webbed toes, unspecified foot
Q70.31 Webbed toes, right foot
Q70.32 Webbed toes, left foot
Q70.33 Webbed toes, bilateral
Q70.4 Polysyndactyly, unspecified
Excludes1: *specified syndactyly of hand and feet - code to specified conditions (Q70.0-Q70.3-)*
Q70.9 Syndactyly, unspecified
Symphalangy NOS

Q71 Reduction defects of upper limb

+ **Q71.0 Congenital complete absence of upper limb**
Q71.00 Congenital complete absence of unspecified upper limb
Q71.01 Congenital complete absence of right upper limb
Q71.02 Congenital complete absence of left upper limb
Q71.03 Congenital complete absence of upper limb, bilateral
+ **Q71.1 Congenital absence of upper arm and forearm with hand present**
Q71.10 Congenital absence of unspecified upper arm and forearm with hand present
Q71.11 Congenital absence of right upper arm and forearm with hand present
Q71.12 Congenital absence of left upper arm and forearm with hand present
Q71.13 Congenital absence of upper arm and forearm with hand present, bilateral
+ **Q71.2 Congenital absence of both forearm and hand**
Q71.20 Congenital absence of both forearm and hand, unspecified upper limb
Q71.21 Congenital absence of both forearm and hand, right upper limb
Q71.22 Congenital absence of both forearm and hand, left upper limb
Q71.23 Congenital absence of both forearm and hand, bilateral
+ **Q71.3 Congenital absence of hand and finger**
Q71.30 Congenital absence of unspecified hand and finger
Q71.31 Congenital absence of right hand and finger
Q71.32 Congenital absence of left hand and finger
Q71.33 Congenital absence of hand and finger, bilateral
+ **Q71.4 Longitudinal reduction defect of radius**
Clubhand (congenital)
Radial clubhand
Q71.40 Longitudinal reduction defect of unspecified radius
Q71.41 Longitudinal reduction defect of right radius
Q71.42 Longitudinal reduction defect of left radius
Q71.43 Longitudinal reduction defect of radius, bilateral
+ **Q71.5 Longitudinal reduction defect of ulna**
Q71.50 Longitudinal reduction defect of unspecified ulna
Q71.51 Longitudinal reduction defect of right ulna
Q71.52 Longitudinal reduction defect of left ulna
Q71.53 Longitudinal reduction defect of ulna, bilateral
+ **Q71.6 Lobster-claw hand**
Q71.60 Lobster-claw hand, unspecified hand
Q71.61 Lobster-claw right hand
Q71.62 Lobster-claw left hand
Q71.63 Lobster-claw hand, bilateral
+ **Q71.8 Other reduction defects of upper limb**
+ **Q71.81 Congenital shortening of upper limb**
Q71.811 Congenital shortening of right upper limb
Q71.812 Congenital shortening of left upper limb
Q71.813 Congenital shortening of upper limb, bilateral
Q71.819 Congenital shortening of unspecified upper limb
+ **Q71.89 Other reduction defects of upper limb**
Q71.891 Other reduction defects of right upper limb
Q71.892 Other reduction defects of left upper limb
Q71.893 Other reduction defects of upper limb, bilateral
Q71.899 Other reduction defects of unspecified upper limb
+ **Q71.9 Unspecified reduction defect of upper limb**
Q71.90 Unspecified reduction defect of unspecified upper limb
Q71.91 Unspecified reduction defect of right upper limb
Q71.92 Unspecified reduction defect of left upper limb
Q71.93 Unspecified reduction defect of upper limb, bilateral

Q72 Reduction defects of lower limb

+ **Q72.0 Congenital complete absence of lower limb**
Q72.00 Congenital complete absence of unspecified lower limb
Q72.01 Congenital complete absence of right lower limb
Q72.02 Congenital complete absence of left lower limb
Q72.03 Congenital complete absence of lower limb, bilateral
+ **Q72.1 Congenital absence of thigh and lower leg with foot present**
Q72.10 Congenital absence of unspecified thigh and lower leg with foot present
Q72.11 Congenital absence of right thigh and lower leg with foot present
Q72.12 Congenital absence of left thigh and lower leg with foot present
Q72.13 Congenital absence of thigh and lower leg with foot present, bilateral
+ **Q72.2 Congenital absence of both lower leg and foot**
Q72.20 Congenital absence of both lower leg and foot, unspecified lower limb
Q72.21 Congenital absence of both lower leg and foot, right lower limb
Q72.22 Congenital absence of both lower leg and foot, left lower limb
Q72.23 Congenital absence of both lower leg and foot, bilateral
+ **Q72.3 Congenital absence of foot and toe(s)**
Q72.30 Congenital absence of unspecified foot and toe(s)
Q72.31 Congenital absence of right foot and toe(s)
Q72.32 Congenital absence of left foot and toe(s)
Q72.33 Congenital absence of foot and toe(s), bilateral
+ **Q72.4 Longitudinal reduction defect of femur**
Proximal femoral focal deficiency
Q72.40 Longitudinal reduction defect of unspecified femur
Q72.41 Longitudinal reduction defect of right femur
Q72.42 Longitudinal reduction defect of left femur
Q72.43 Longitudinal reduction defect of femur, bilateral
+ **Q72.5 Longitudinal reduction defect of tibia**
Q72.50 Longitudinal reduction defect of unspecified tibia
Q72.51 Longitudinal reduction defect of right tibia
Q72.52 Longitudinal reduction defect of left tibia
Q72.53 Longitudinal reduction defect of tibia, bilateral
+ **Q72.6 Longitudinal reduction defect of fibula**
Q72.60 Longitudinal reduction defect of unspecified fibula
Q72.61 Longitudinal reduction defect of right fibula
Q72.62 Longitudinal reduction defect of left fibula
Q72.63 Longitudinal reduction defect of fibula, bilateral
+ **Q72.7 Split foot**
Q72.70 Split foot, unspecified lower limb
Q72.71 Split foot, right lower limb
Q72.72 Split foot, left lower limb
Q72.73 Split foot, bilateral
+ **Q72.8 Other reduction defects of lower limb**
+ **Q72.81 Congenital shortening of lower limb**
Q72.811 Congenital shortening of right lower limb
Q72.812 Congenital shortening of left lower limb
Q72.813 Congenital shortening of lower limb, bilateral
Q72.819 Congenital shortening of unspecified lower limb
+ **Q72.89 Other reduction defects of lower limb**
Q72.891 Other reduction defects of right lower limb
Q72.892 Other reduction defects of left lower limb
Q72.893 Other reduction defects of lower limb, bilateral
Q72.899 Other reduction defects of unspecified lower limb

\+ **Q72.9 Unspecified reduction defect of lower limb**
Q72.90 Unspecified reduction defect of unspecified lower limb
Q72.91 Unspecified reduction defect of right lower limb
Q72.92 Unspecified reduction defect of left lower limb
Q72.93 Unspecified reduction defect of lower limb, bilateral

Q73 Reduction defects of unspecified limb

Q73.0 Congenital absence of unspecified limb(s)
Amelia NOS
Q73.1 Phocomelia, unspecified limb(s)
Phocomelia NOS
Q73.8 Other reduction defects of unspecified limb(s)
Longitudinal reduction deformity of unspecified limb(s)
Ectromelia of limb NOS
Hemimelia of limb NOS
Reduction defect of limb NOS

Q74 Other congenital malformations of limb(s)

Excludes1: *polydactyly (Q69.-)*
reduction defect of limb (Q71-Q73)
syndactyly (Q70.-)

Q74.0 Other congenital malformations of upper limb(s), including shoulder girdle
Accessory carpal bones
Cleidocranial dysostosis
Congenital pseudarthrosis of clavicle
Macrodactylia (fingers)
Madelung's deformity
Radioulnar synostosis
Sprengel's deformity
Triphalangeal thumb
Q74.1 Congenital malformation of knee
Congenital absence of patella
Congenital dislocation of patella
Congenital genu valgum
Congenital genu varum
Rudimentary patella
Excludes1: *congenital dislocation of knee (Q68.2)*
congenital genu recurvatum (Q68.2)
nail patella syndrome (Q87.2)
Q74.2 Other congenital malformations of lower limb(s), including pelvic girdle
Congenital fusion of sacroiliac joint
Congenital malformation of ankle joint
Congenital malformation of sacroiliac joint
Excludes1: *anteversion of femur (neck) (Q65.89)*
CC **Q74.3 Arthrogryposis multiplex congenita**
Q74.8 Other specified congenital malformations of limb(s)
Q74.9 Unspecified congenital malformation of limb(s)
Congenital anomaly of limb(s) NOS

Q75 Other congenital malformations of skull and face bones

Excludes1: *congenital malformation of face NOS (Q18.-)*
congenital malformation syndromes classified to (Q87.-)
dentofacial anomalies [including malocclusion] (M26.-)
musculoskeletal deformities of head and face (Q67.0-Q67.4)
skull defects associated with congenital anomalies of brain such as:
anencephaly (Q00.0)
encephalocele (Q01.-)
hydrocephalus (Q03.-)
microcephaly (Q02)

Q75.0 Craniosynostosis
Acrocephaly
Imperfect fusion of skull
Oxycephaly
Trigonocephaly
Q75.1 Craniofacial dysostosis
Crouzon's disease
Q75.2 Hypertelorism
Q75.3 Macrocephaly
Q75.4 Mandibulofacial dysostosis
Franceschetti syndrome
Treacher Collins syndrome
Q75.5 Oculomandibular dysostosis
Q75.8 Other specified congenital malformations of skull and face bones
Absence of skull bone, congenital
Congenital deformity of forehead
Platybasia
Q75.9 Congenital malformation of skull and face bones, unspecified
Congenital anomaly of face bones NOS
Congenital anomaly of skull NOS

Q76 Congenital malformations of spine and bony thorax

Excludes1: *congenital musculoskeletal deformities of spine and chest (Q67.5-Q67.8)*

Q76.0 Spina bifida occulta
Excludes1: *meningocele (spinal) (Q05.-)*
spina bifida (aperta) (cystica) (Q05.-)
Q76.1 Klippel-Feil syndrome
Cervical fusion syndrome
Q76.2 Congenital spondylolisthesis
Congenital spondylolysis
Excludes1: *spondylolisthesis (acquired) (M43.1-)*
spondylolysis (acquired) (M43.0-)
CC **Q76.3 Congenital scoliosis due to congenital bony malformation**
Hemivertebra fusion or failure of segmentation with scoliosis
\+ **Q76.4 Other congenital malformations of spine, not associated with scoliosis**
\+ **Q76.41 Congenital kyphosis**
Q76.411 Congenital kyphosis, occipito-atlanto-axial region
Q76.412 Congenital kyphosis, cervical region
Q76.413 Congenital kyphosis, cervicothoracic region
Q76.414 Congenital kyphosis, thoracic region
Q76.415 Congenital kyphosis, thoracolumbar region
Q76.419 Congenital kyphosis, unspecified region
\+ **Q76.42 Congenital lordosis**
CC **Q76.425 Congenital lordosis, thoracolumbar region**
CC **Q76.426 Congenital lordosis, lumbar region**
CC **Q76.427 Congenital lordosis, lumbosacral region**
CC **Q76.428 Congenital lordosis, sacral and sacrococcygeal region**
CC **Q76.429 Congenital lordosis, unspecified region**
Q76.49 Other congenital malformations of spine, not associated with scoliosis
Congenital absence of vertebra NOS
Congenital fusion of spine NOS
Congenital malformation of lumbosacral (joint) (region) NOS
Congenital malformation of spine NOS
Hemivertebra NOS
Malformation of spine NOS
Platyspondylisis NOS
Supernumerary vertebra NOS
Q76.5 Cervical rib
Supernumerary rib in cervical region
CC **Q76.6 Other congenital malformations of ribs**
Accessory rib
Congenital absence of rib
Congenital fusion of ribs
Congenital malformation of ribs NOS
Excludes1: *short rib syndrome (Q77.2)*
CC **Q76.7 Congenital malformation of sternum**
Congenital absence of sternum
Sternum bifidum
CC **Q76.8 Other congenital malformations of bony thorax**
CC **Q76.9 Congenital malformation of bony thorax, unspecified**

Q77 Osteochondrodysplasia with defects of growth of tubular bones and spine

Excludes1: *mucopolysaccharidosis (E76.0-E76.3)*
Excludes2: *congenital myotonic chondrodystrophy (G71.13)*

Q77.0 Achondrogenesis
Hypochondrogenesis
Q77.1 Thanatophoric short stature
CC **Q77.2 Short rib syndrome**
Asphyxiating thoracic dysplasia [Jeune]
Q77.3 Chondrodysplasia punctata
Excludes1: *Rhizomelic chondrodysplasia punctata (E71.43)*
Q77.4 Achondroplasia
Hypochondroplasia
Osteosclerosis congenita
Q77.5 Diastrophic dysplasia
Q77.6 Chondroectodermal dysplasia
Ellis-van Creveld syndrome
Q77.7 Spondyloepiphyseal dysplasia
Q77.8 Other osteochondrodysplasia with defects of growth of tubular bones and spine
Q77.9 Osteochondrodysplasia with defects of growth of tubular bones and spine, unspecified

Q78 Other osteochondrodysplasias

Excludes2: *congenital myotonic chondrodystrophy (G71.13)*

CC **Q78.0 Osteogenesis imperfecta**
Fragilitas ossium
Osteopsathyrosis
Q78.1 Polyostotic fibrous dysplasia
Albright(-McCune)(-Sternberg) syndrome
CC **Q78.2 Osteopetrosis**
Albers-Schönberg syndrome
Osteosclerosis NOS
Q78.3 Progressive diaphyseal dysplasia
Camurati-Engelmann syndrome
Q78.4 Enchondromatosis
Maffucci's syndrome
Ollier's disease
Q78.5 Metaphyseal dysplasia
Pyle's syndrome
Q78.6 Multiple congenital exostoses
Diaphyseal aclasis
Q78.8 Other specified osteochondrodysplasias
Osteopoikilosis
Q78.9 Osteochondrodysplasia, unspecified
Chondrodystrophy NOS
Osteodystrophy NOS

Q79 Congenital malformations of musculoskeletal system, not elsewhere classified

Excludes2: *congenital (sternomastoid) torticollis (Q68.0)*

MCC **Q79.0 Congenital diaphragmatic hernia**
Excludes1: *congenital hiatus hernia (Q40.1)*
MCC **Q79.1 Other congenital malformations of diaphragm**
Absence of diaphragm
Congenital malformation of diaphragm NOS
Eventration of diaphragm
MCC **Q79.2 Exomphalos**
Omphalocele
Excludes1: *umbilical hernia (K42.-)*
MCC **Q79.3 Gastroschisis**
MCC **Q79.4 Prune belly syndrome**
Congenital prolapse of bladder mucosa
Eagle-Barrett syndrome
\+ **Q79.5 Other congenital malformations of abdominal wall**
Excludes1: *umbilical hernia (K42.-)*
MCC **Q79.51 Congenital hernia of bladder**
MCC **Q79.59 Other congenital malformations of abdominal wall**
\+ **Q79.6 Ehlers-Danlos syndromes**
AHA CC: 4Q, 2019, 13-14
CC **Q79.60 Ehlers-Danlos Syndrome, unspecified**
CC **Q79.61 Classical Ehlers-Danlos syndrome**
Classical EDS (cEDS)
CC **Q79.62 Hypermobile Ehlers-Danlos syndrome**
Hypermobile EDS (hEDS)
CC **Q79.63 Vascular Ehlers-Danlas syndrome**
Vascular EDS (vEDS)
CC **Q79.69 Other Ehlers-Danlos syndromes**
Q79.8 Other congenital malformations of musculoskeletal system
Absence of muscle
Absence of tendon
Accessory muscle
Amyotrophia congenita
Congenital constricting bands
Congenital shortening of tendon
Poland syndrome
Q79.9 Congenital malformation of musculoskeletal system, unspecified
Congenital anomaly of musculoskeletal system NOS
Congenital deformity of musculoskeletal system NOS

Other congenital malformations (Q80-Q89)

Q80 Congenital ichthyosis

Excludes1: *Refsum's disease (G60.1)*

Q80.0 Ichthyosis vulgaris
Q80.1 X-linked ichthyosis
Q80.2 Lamellar ichthyosis
Collodion baby
Q80.3 Congenital bullous ichthyosiform erythroderma
Q80.4 Harlequin fetus
Q80.8 Other congenital ichthyosis
Q80.9 Congenital ichthyosis, unspecified

Q81 Epidermolysis bullosa

Q81.0 Epidermolysis bullosa simplex
Excludes1: *Cockayne's syndrome (Q87.19)*
Q81.1 Epidermolysis bullosa letalis
Herlitz' syndrome
Q81.2 Epidermolysis bullosa dystrophica
Q81.8 Other epidermolysis bullosa
Q81.9 Epidermolysis bullosa, unspecified

Q82 Other congenital malformations of skin

Excludes1: *acrodermatitis enteropathica (E83.2)*
congenital erythropoietic porphyria (E80.0)
pilonidal cyst or sinus (L05.-)
Sturge-Weber (-Dimitri) syndrome (Q85.8)

Q82.0 Hereditary lymphedema
Q82.1 Xeroderma pigmentosum
Q82.2 Congenital cutaneous mastocytosis
Congenital diffuse cutaneous mastocytosis
Congenital maculopapular cutaneous mastocytosis
Congenital urticaria pigmentosa
Excludes1: *cutaneous mastocytosis NOS (D47.01)*
diffuse cutaneous mastocytosis (with onset after newborn period) (D47.01)
malignant mastocytosis (C96.2-)
systemic mastocytosis (D47.02)
urticaria pigmentosa (non-congenital) (with onset after newborn period) (D47.01)
AHA CC: 4Q, 2017, 5
Q82.3 Incontinentia pigmenti
Q82.4 Ectodermal dysplasia (anhidrotic)
Excludes1: *Ellis-van Creveld syndrome (Q77.6)*
Q82.5 Congenital non-neoplastic nevus
Birthmark NOS
Flammeus Nevus
Portwine Nevus
Sanguineous Nevus
Strawberry Nevus
Vascular Nevus NOS
Verrucous Nevus
Excludes2: *Café au lait spots (L81.3)*
lentigo (L81.4)
nevus NOS (D22.-)
araneus nevus (I78.1)
melanocytic nevus (D22.-)
pigmented nevus (D22.-)
spider nevus (I78.1)
stellar nevus (I78.1)
Q82.6 Congenital sacral dimple
Parasacral dimple
Excludes2: *pilonidal cyst with abscess (L05.01)*
pilonidal cyst without abscess (L05.91)
AHA CC: 4Q, 2016, 60

Q82.8 Other specified congenital malformations of skin
Abnormal palmar creases
Accessory skin tags
Benign familial pemphigus [Hailey-Hailey]
Congenital poikiloderma
Cutis laxa (hyperelastica)
Dermatoglyphic anomalies
Inherited keratosis palmaris et plantaris
Keratosis follicularis [Darier-White]
Excludes1: *Ehlers-Danlos syndromes (Q79.6-)*
AHA CC: 1Q, 2016, 17

Q82.9 Congenital malformation of skin, unspecified

Q83 Congenital malformations of breast
Excludes2: *absence of pectoral muscle (Q79.8)*
hypoplasia of breast (N64.82)
micromastia (N64.82)

Q83.0 Congenital absence of breast with absent nipple
Q83.1 Accessory breast
Supernumerary breast
Q83.2 Absent nipple
Q83.3 Accessory nipple
Supernumerary nipple
Q83.8 Other congenital malformations of breast
Q83.9 Congenital malformation of breast, unspecified

Q84 Other congenital malformations of integument
Q84.0 Congenital alopecia
Congenital atrichosis
Q84.1 Congenital morphological disturbances of hair, not elsewhere classified
Beaded hair
Monilethrix
Pili annulati
Excludes1: *Menkes' kinky hair syndrome (E83.0)*
Q84.2 Other congenital malformations of hair
Congenital hypertrichosis
Congenital malformation of hair NOS
Persistent lanugo
Q84.3 Anonychia
Excludes1: *nail patella syndrome (Q87.2)*
Q84.4 Congenital leukonychia
Q84.5 Enlarged and hypertrophic nails
Congenital onychauxis
Pachyonychia
Q84.6 Other congenital malformations of nails
Congenital clubnail
Congenital koilonychia
Congenital malformation of nail NOS
Q84.8 Other specified congenital malformations of integument
Aplasia cutis congenita
Q84.9 Congenital malformation of integument, unspecified
Congenital anomaly of integument NOS
Congenital deformity of integument NOS

Q85 Phakomatoses, not elsewhere classified
Excludes1: *ataxia telangiectasia [Louis-Bar] (G11.3)*
familial dysautonomia [Riley-Day] (G90.1)

\+ **Q85.0 Neurofibromatosis (nonmalignant)**
Q85.00 Neurofibromatosis, unspecified
Q85.01 Neurofibromatosis, type 1
Von Recklinghausen disease
Q85.02 Neurofibromatosis, type 2
Acoustic neurofibromatosis
Q85.03 Schwannomatosis
Q85.09 Other neurofibromatosis
CC **Q85.1 Tuberous sclerosis**
Bourneville's disease
Epiloia
CC **Q85.8 Other phakomatoses, not elsewhere classified**
Peutz-Jeghers Syndrome
Sturge-Weber(-Dimitri) syndrome
von Hippel-Lindau syndrome
Excludes1: *Meckel-Gruber syndrome (Q61.9)*
CC **Q85.9 Phakomatosis, unspecified**
Hamartosis NOS

Q86 Congenital malformation syndromes due to known exogenous causes, not elsewhere classified
Excludes2: *iodine-deficiency-related hypothyroidism (E00-E02)*
nonteratogenic effects of substances transmitted via placenta or breast milk (P04.-)

Q86.0 Fetal alcohol syndrome (dysmorphic)
Q86.1 Fetal hydantoin syndrome
Meadow's syndrome
Q86.2 Dysmorphism due to warfarin
Q86.8 Other congenital malformation syndromes due to known exogenous causes

Q87 Other specified congenital malformation syndromes affecting multiple systems
Use additional code(s) to identify all associated manifestations

Q87.0 Congenital malformation syndromes predominantly affecting facial appearance
Acrocephalopolysyndactyly
Acrocephalosyndactyly [Apert]
Cryptophthalmos syndrome
Cyclopia
Goldenhar syndrome
Moebius syndrome
Oro-facial-digital syndrome
Robin syndrome
Whistling face
\+ **Q87.1 Congenital malformation syndromes predominantly associated with short stature**
Excludes1: *Ellis-van Creveld syndrome (Q77.6)*
Smith-Lemli-Opitz syndrome (E78.72)
AHA CC: 4Q, 2019, 14-15
CC **Q87.11 Prader-Willi syndrome**
CC **Q87.19 Other congenital malformation syndromes predominantly associated with short stature**
Aarskog syndrome
Cockayne syndrome
De Lange syndrome
Dubowitz syndrome
Noonan syndrome
Robinow-Silverman-Smith syndrome
Russell-Silver syndrome
Seckel syndrome
CC **Q87.2 Congenital malformation syndromes predominantly involving limbs**
Holt-Oram syndrome
Klippel-Trenaunay-Weber syndrome
Nail patella syndrome
Rubinstein-Taybi syndrome
Sirenomelia syndrome
Thrombocytopenia with absent radius [TAR] syndrome
VATER syndrome
CC **Q87.3 Congenital malformation syndromes involving early overgrowth**
Beckwith-Wiedemann syndrome
Sotos syndrome
Weaver syndrome
\+ **Q87.4 Marfan's syndrome**
CC **Q87.40 Marfan's syndrome, unspecified**
\+ **Q87.41 Marfan's syndrome with cardiovascular manifestations**
CC **Q87.410 Marfan's syndrome with aortic dilation**
CC **Q87.418 Marfan's syndrome with other cardiovascular manifestations**
CC **Q87.42 Marfan's syndrome with ocular manifestations**
CC **Q87.43 Marfan's syndrome with skeletal manifestation**
CC **Q87.5 Other congenital malformation syndromes with other skeletal changes**
\+ **Q87.8 Other specified congenital malformation syndromes, not elsewhere classified**
Excludes1: *Zellweger syndrome (E71.510)*
CC **Q87.81 Alport syndrome**
Use additional code to identify stage of chronic kidney disease (N18.1-N18.6)
CC **Q87.82 Arterial tortuosity syndrome**
AHA CC: 4Q, 2016, 60-61
CC **Q87.89 Other specified congenital malformation syndromes, not elsewhere classified**
Laurence-Moon (-Bardet)-Biedl syndrome

Q89 Other congenital malformations, not elsewhere classified

+ **Q89.0 Congenital absence and malformations of spleen**
  Excludes1: isomerism of atrial appendages (with asplenia or polysplenia) (Q20.6)

CC **Q89.01 Asplenia (congenital)**

CC **Q89.09 Congenital malformations of spleen**
Congenital splenomegaly

Q89.1 Congenital malformations of adrenal gland
Excludes1: adrenogenital disorders (E25.-)
congenital adrenal hyperplasia (E25.0)

Q89.2 Congenital malformations of other endocrine glands
Congenital malformation of parathyroid or thyroid gland
Persistent thyroglossal duct
Thyroglossal cyst
Excludes1: congenital goiter (E03.0)
congenital hypothyroidism (E03.1)

CC **Q89.3 Situs inversus**
Dextrocardia with situs inversus
Mirror-image atrial arrangement with situs inversus
Situs inversus or transversus abdominalis
Situs inversus or transversus thoracis
Transposition of abdominal viscera
Transposition of thoracic viscera
Excludes1: dextrocardia NOS (Q24.0)

MCC **Q89.4 Conjoined twins**
Craniopagus
Dicephaly
Pygopagus
Thoracopagus

CC **Q89.7 Multiple congenital malformations, not elsewhere classified**
Multiple congenital anomalies NOS
Multiple congenital deformities NOS
Excludes1: congenital malformation syndromes affecting multiple systems (Q87.-)

CC **Q89.8 Other specified congenital malformations**
Use additional code(s) to identify all associated manifestations

Q89.9 Congenital malformation, unspecified
Congenital anomaly NOS
Congenital deformity NOS

Chromosomal abnormalities, not elsewhere classified (Q90-Q99)

Excludes2: mitochondrial metabolic disorders (E88.4-)

Q90 Down syndrome

Use additional code(s) to identify any associated physical conditions and degree of intellectual disabilities (F70-F79)

Q90.0 Trisomy 21, nonmosaicism (meiotic nondisjunction)
Q90.1 Trisomy 21, mosaicism (mitotic nondisjunction)
Q90.2 Trisomy 21, translocation
Q90.9 Down syndrome, unspecified
Trisomy 21 NOS

Q91 Trisomy 18 and Trisomy 13

CC **Q91.0 Trisomy 18, nonmosaicism (meiotic nondisjunction)**
CC **Q91.1 Trisomy 18, mosaicism (mitotic nondisjunction)**
CC **Q91.2 Trisomy 18, translocation**
CC **Q91.3 Trisomy 18, unspecified**
CC **Q91.4 Trisomy 13, nonmosaicism (meiotic nondisjunction)**
CC **Q91.5 Trisomy 13, mosaicism (mitotic nondisjunction)**
CC **Q91.6 Trisomy 13, translocation**
CC **Q91.7 Trisomy 13, unspecified**

Q92 Other trisomies and partial trisomies of the autosomes, not elsewhere classified

Includes: unbalanced translocations and insertions
Excludes1: trisomies of chromosomes 13, 18, 21 (Q90-Q91)

Q92.0 Whole chromosome trisomy, nonmosaicism (meiotic nondisjunction)
Q92.1 Whole chromosome trisomy, mosaicism (mitotic nondisjunction)
Q92.2 Partial trisomy
Less than whole arm duplicated
Whole arm or more duplicated
Excludes1: partial trisomy due to unbalanced translocation (Q92.5)

Q92.5 Duplications with other complex rearrangements
Partial trisomy due to unbalanced translocations
Code also any associated deletions due to unbalanced translocations, inversions and insertions (Q93.7)

+ **Q92.6 Marker chromosomes**
Trisomies due to dicentrics
Trisomies due to extra rings
Trisomies due to isochromosomes
Individual with marker heterochromatin

Q92.61 Marker chromosomes in normal individual
Q92.62 Marker chromosomes in abnormal individual

Q92.7 Triploidy and polyploidy
Q92.8 Other specified trisomies and partial trisomies of autosomes
Duplications identified by fluorescence in situ hybridization (FISH)
Duplications identified by in situ hybridization (ISH)
Duplications seen only at prometaphase
Q92.9 Trisomy and partial trisomy of autosomes, unspecified

Q93 Monosomies and deletions from the autosomes, not elsewhere classified

Q93.0 Whole chromosome monosomy, nonmosaicism (meiotic nondisjunction)
Q93.1 Whole chromosome monosomy, mosaicism (mitotic nondisjunction)
Q93.2 Chromosome replaced with ring, dicentric or isochromosome

CC **Q93.3 Deletion of short arm of chromosome 4**
Wolff-Hirschorn syndrome

CC **Q93.4 Deletion of short arm of chromosome 5**
Cri-du-chat syndrome

+ **Q93.5 Other deletions of part of a chromosome**
AHA CC: 4Q, 2018, 28

CC **Q93.51 Angelman syndrome**
CC **Q93.59 Other deletions of part of a chromosome**

CC **Q93.7 Deletions with other complex rearrangements**
Deletions due to unbalanced translocations, inversions and insertions
Code also any associated duplications due to unbalanced translocations, inversions and insertions (Q92.5)

+ **Q93.8 Other deletions from the autosomes**

MCC **Q93.81 Velo-cardio-facial syndrome**
Deletion 22q11.2
AHA CC: 3Q, 2019, 14-15

CC **Q93.82 Williams syndrome**
AHA CC: 4Q, 2018, 28-29

CC **Q93.88 Other microdeletions**
Miller-Dieker syndrome
Smith-Magenis syndrome

CC **Q93.89 Other deletions from the autosomes**
Deletions identified by fluorescence in situ hybridization (FISH)
Deletions identified by in situ hybridization (ISH)
Deletions seen only at prometaphase

CC **Q93.9 Deletion from autosomes, unspecified**

Q95 Balanced rearrangements and structural markers, not elsewhere classified

Includes: Robertsonian and balanced reciprocal translocations and insertions

Q95.0 Balanced translocation and insertion in normal individual
Q95.1 Chromosome inversion in normal individual
Q95.2 Balanced autosomal rearrangement in abnormal individual
Q95.3 Balanced sex/autosomal rearrangement in abnormal individual
Q95.5 Individual with autosomal fragile site
Q95.8 Other balanced rearrangements and structural markers
Q95.9 Balanced rearrangement and structural marker, unspecified

Q96 Turner's syndrome

Excludes1: Noonan syndrome (Q87.19)

♀ **Q96.0 Karyotype 45, X**
♀ **Q96.1 Karyotype 46, X iso (Xq)**
Karyotype 46, isochromosome Xq
♀ **Q96.2 Karyotype 46, X with abnormal sex chromosome, except iso (Xq)**
Karyotype 46, X with abnormal sex chromosome, except isochromosome Xq
♀ **Q96.3 Mosaicism, 45, X/46, XX or XY**
♀ **Q96.4 Mosaicism, 45, X/other cell line(s) with abnormal sex chromosome**
♀ **Q96.8 Other variants of Turner's syndrome**
♀ **Q96.9 Turner's syndrome, unspecified**

Q97 Other sex chromosome abnormalities, female phenotype, not elsewhere classified

Excludes1: *Turner's syndrome (Q96.-)*

- ♀ **Q97.0 Karyotype 47, XXX**
- ♀ **Q97.1 Female with more than three X chromosomes**
- ♀ **Q97.2 Mosaicism, lines with various numbers of X chromosomes**
- ♀ **Q97.3 Female with 46, XY karyotype**
- ♀ **Q97.8 Other specified sex chromosome abnormalities, female phenotype**
- ♀ **Q97.9 Sex chromosome abnormality, female phenotype, unspecified**

Q98 Other sex chromosome abnormalities, male phenotype, not elsewhere classified

- ♂ **Q98.0 Klinefelter syndrome karyotype 47, XXY**
- ♂ **Q98.1 Klinefelter syndrome, male with more than two X chromosomes**
- ♂ **Q98.3 Other male with 46, XX karyotype**
- ♂ **Q98.4 Klinefelter syndrome, unspecified**
- ♂ **Q98.5 Karyotype 47, XYY**
- ♂ **Q98.6 Male with structurally abnormal sex chromosome**
- ♂ **Q98.7 Male with sex chromosome mosaicism**
- ♂ **Q98.8 Other specified sex chromosome abnormalities, male phenotype**
- ♂ **Q98.9 Sex chromosome abnormality, male phenotype, unspecified**

Q99 Other chromosome abnormalities, not elsewhere classified

Q99.0 Chimera 46, XX/46, XY

Chimera 46, XX/46, XY true hermaphrodite

Q99.1 46, XX true hermaphrodite

46, XX with streak gonads
46, XY with streak gonads
Pure gonadal dysgenesis

Q99.2 Fragile X chromosome

Fragile X syndrome

Q99.8 Other specified chromosome abnormalities

Q99.9 Chromosomal abnormality, unspecified

Chapter 18: Symptoms, Signs and Abnormal Clinical and Laboratory Findings, Not Elsewhere Classified (R00-R99)

NOTE This chapter includes symptoms, signs, abnormal results of clinical or other investigative procedures, and ill-defined conditions regarding which no diagnosis classifiable elsewhere is recorded.

Signs and symptoms that point rather definitely to a given diagnosis have been assigned to a category in other chapters of the classification. In general, categories in this chapter include the less well-defined conditions and symptoms that, without the necessary study of the case to establish a final diagnosis, point perhaps equally to two or more diseases or to two or more systems of the body. Practically all categories in the chapter could be designated 'not otherwise specified', 'unknown etiology' or 'transient'. The Alphabetical Index should be consulted to determine which symptoms and signs are to be allocated here and which to other chapters. The residual subcategories, numbered .8, are generally provided for other relevant symptoms that cannot be allocated elsewhere in the classification.

The conditions and signs or symptoms included in categories R00-R94 consist of:
(a) cases for which no more specific diagnosis can be made even after all the facts bearing on the case have been investigated;
(b) signs or symptoms existing at the time of initial encounter that proved to be transient and whose causes could not be determined;
(c) provisional diagnosis in a patient who failed to return for further investigation or care;
(d) cases referred elsewhere for investigation or treatment before the diagnosis was made;
(e) cases in which a more precise diagnosis was not available for any other reason;
(f) certain symptoms, for which supplementary information is provided, that represent important problems in medical care in their own right.

Excludes2: *abnormal findings on antenatal screening of mother (O28.-)*
certain conditions originating in the perinatal period (P04-P96)
signs and symptoms classified in the body system chapters
signs and symptoms of breast (N63, N64.5)

This chapter contains the following category blocks:

R00-R09	Symptoms and signs involving the circulatory and respiratory systems
R10-R19	Symptoms and signs involving the digestive system and abdomen
R20-R23	Symptoms and signs involving the skin and subcutaneous tissue
R25-R29	Symptoms and signs involving the nervous and musculoskeletal systems
R30-R39	Symptoms and signs involving the genitourinary system
R40-R46	Symptoms and signs involving cognition, perception, emotional state and behavior
R47-R49	Symptoms and signs involving speech and voice
R50-R69	General symptoms and signs
R70-R79	Abnormal findings on examination of blood, without diagnosis
R80-R82	Abnormal findings on examination of urine, without diagnosis
R83-R89	Abnormal findings on examination of other body fluids, substances and tissues, without diagnosis
R90-R94	Abnormal findings on diagnostic imaging and in function studies, without diagnosis
R97	Abnormal tumor markers
R99	Ill-defined and unknown cause of mortality

C. Chapter-Specific Coding Guidelines

In addition to general coding guidelines, there are guidelines for specific diagnoses and/or conditions in the classification. Unless otherwise indicated, these guidelines apply to all health care settings. Please refer to Section II for guidelines on the selection of principal diagnosis.

18. Chapter 18: Symptoms, Signs, and Abnormal Clinical and Laboratory Findings, Not Elsewhere Classified (R00-R99)

Chapter 18 includes symptoms, signs, abnormal results of clinical or other investigative procedures, and ill-defined conditions regarding which no diagnosis classifiable elsewhere is recorded. Signs and symptoms that point to a specific diagnosis have been assigned to a category in other chapters of the classification.

a. Use of symptom codes

Codes that describe symptoms and signs are acceptable for reporting purposes when a related definitive diagnosis has not been established (confirmed) by the provider.

b. Use of a symptom code with a definitive diagnosis code

Codes for signs and symptoms may be reported in addition to a related definitive diagnosis when the sign or symptom is not routinely associated with that diagnosis, such as the various signs and symptoms associated with complex syndromes. The definitive diagnosis code should be sequenced before the symptom code.

Signs or symptoms that are associated routinely with a disease process should not be assigned as additional codes, unless otherwise instructed by the classification.

c. Combination codes that include symptoms

ICD-10-CM contains a number of combination codes that identify both the definitive diagnosis and common symptoms of that diagnosis. When using one of these combination codes, an additional code should not be assigned for the symptom.

d. Repeated falls

Code R29.6, Repeated falls, is for use for encounters when a patient has recently fallen and the reason for the fall is being investigated.

Code Z91.81, History of falling, is for use when a patient has fallen in the past and is at risk for future falls. When appropriate, both codes R29.6 and Z91.81 may be assigned together.

e. Coma

Code R40.20, Unspecified coma, may be assigned in conjunction with codes for any medical condition.

Do not report codes for unspecified coma, individual or total Glasgow coma scale scores for a patient with a medically induced coma or a sedated patient.

1) Coma Scale

The coma scale codes (R40.2**1-to R40.24-**) can be used in conjunction with traumatic brain injury codes, acute cerebrovascular disease or sequelae of cerebrovascular disease codes. These codes are primarily for use by trauma registries, but they may be used in any setting where this information is collected. The coma scale codes should be sequenced after the diagnosis code(s).

These codes, one from each subcategory, are needed to complete the scale. The 7th character indicates when the scale was recorded. The 7th character should match for all three codes.

At a minimum, report the initial score documented on presentation at your facility. This may be a score from the emergency medicine technician (EMT) or in the emergency department. If desired, a facility may choose to capture multiple coma scale scores.

Assign code R40.24, Glasgow coma scale, total score, when only the total score is documented in the medical record and not the individual score(s).

If multiple coma scores are captured within the first 24 hours after hospital admission, assign only the code for the score at the time of admission. ICD-10-CM does not classify coma scores that are reported after admission but less than 24 hours later. *See Section I.B.14 for coma scale documentation by clinicians other than the patient's provider.*

f. Functional quadriplegia

GUIDELINE HAS BEEN DELETED EFFECTIVE OCTOBER 1, 2017

g. SIRS due to Non-Infectious Process

The systemic inflammatory response syndrome (SIRS) can develop as a result of certain non-infectious disease processes, such as trauma, malignant neoplasm, or pancreatitis. When SIRS is documented with a noninfectious condition, and no subsequent infection is documented, the code for the underlying condition, such as an injury, should be assigned, followed by code R65.10, Systemic inflammatory response syndrome (SIRS) of non-infectious origin without acute organ dysfunction, or code R65.11, Systemic inflammatory response syndrome (SIRS) of non-infectious origin with acute organ dysfunction. If an associated acute organ dysfunction is documented, the appropriate code(s) for the specific type of organ dysfunction(s) should be assigned in addition to code R65.11. If acute organ dysfunction is documented, but it cannot be determined if the acute organ dysfunction is associated with SIRS or due to another condition (e.g., directly due to the trauma), the provider should be queried.

h. Death NOS

Code R99, Ill-defined and unknown cause of mortality, is only for use in the very limited circumstance when a patient who has already died is brought into an emergency department or other healthcare facility and is pronounced dead upon arrival. It does not represent the discharge disposition of death.

i. NIHSS Stroke Scale

The NIH stroke scale (NIHSS) codes (R29.7--) can be used in conjunction with acute stroke codes (I63) to identify the patient's neurological status and the severity of the stroke. The stroke scale codes should be sequenced after the acute stroke diagnosis code(s).

At a minimum, report the initial score documented. If desired, a facility may choose to capture multiple stroke scale scores.

See Section I.B.14 for NIHSS stroke scale documentation by clinicians other than patient's provider.

Symptoms and signs involving the circulatory and respiratory systems (R00-R09)

R00 Abnormalities of heart beat

Excludes1: *abnormalities originating in the perinatal period (P29.1-)*

Excludes2: *specified arrhythmias (I47-I49)*

R00.0 Tachycardia, unspecified

Rapid heart beat
Sinoauricular tachycardia NOS
Sinus [sinusal] tachycardia NOS

Excludes1: *neonatal tachycardia (P29.11)*
paroxysmal tachycardia (I47.-)

R00.1 Bradycardia, unspecified

Sinoatrial bradycardia
Sinus bradycardia
Slow heart beat
Systolic murmur NOS
Vagal bradycardia
Use additional code for adverse effect, if applicable, to identify drug (T36-T50 with fifth or sixth character 5)

Excludes1: *neonatal bradycardia (P29.12)*

AHA CC: 2Q, 2020, 23-24

R00.2 Palpitations

Awareness of heart beat

R00.8 Other abnormalities of heart beat

R00.9 Unspecified abnormalities of heart beat

R01 Cardiac murmurs and other cardiac sounds

Excludes1: *cardiac murmurs and sounds originating in the perinatal period (P29.8)*

R01.0 Benign and innocent cardiac murmurs

Functional cardiac murmur

R01.1 Cardiac murmur, unspecified

Cardiac bruit NOS
Heart murmur NOS
Systolic murmur NOS

R01.2 Other cardiac sounds

Cardiac dullness, increased or decreased
Precordial friction

R03 Abnormal blood-pressure reading, without diagnosis

R03.0 Elevated blood-pressure reading, without diagnosis of hypertension

NOTE This category is to be used to record an episode of elevated blood pressure in a patient in whom no formal diagnosis of hypertension has been made, or as an isolated incidental finding.

Review coding guideline C.9.a.7

R03.1 Nonspecific low blood-pressure reading

Excludes1: *hypotension (I95.-)*
maternal hypotension syndrome (O26.5-)
neurogenic orthostatic hypotension (G90.3)

R04 Hemorrhage from respiratory passages

R04.0 Epistaxis

Hemorrhage from nose
Nosebleed

AHA CC: 4Q, 2018, 38

R04.1 Hemorrhage from throat

Excludes2: *hemoptysis (R04.2)*

CC **R04.2 Hemoptysis**

Blood-stained sputum
Cough with hemorrhage

AHA CC: 4Q, 2013, 118

\+ **R04.8 Hemorrhage from other sites in respiratory passages**

• CC **R04.81 Acute idiopathic pulmonary hemorrhage in infants**

AIPHI
Acute idiopathic hemorrhage in infants over 28 days old

Excludes1: *perinatal pulmonary hemorrhage (P26.-)*
von Willebrand's disease (D68.0)

CC **R04.89 Hemorrhage from other sites in respiratory passages**

Pulmonary hemorrhage NOS

CC **R04.9 Hemorrhage from respiratory passages, unspecified**

R05 Cough

Excludes1: *paroxysmal cough due to Bordetella pertussis (A37.0-)*
smoker's cough (J41.0)

Excludes2: *cough with hemorrhage (R04.2)*

AHA CC: 2Q, 2016, 34; 1Q, 2020, 34-36

R05.1 Acute cough

R05.2 Subacute cough

R05.3 Chronic cough

Persistent cough
Refractory cough
Unexplained cough

R05.4 Cough syncope

Code first syncope and collapse (R55)

R05.8 Other specified cough

R05.9 Cough, unspecified

R06 Abnormalities of breathing

Excludes1: *acute respiratory distress syndrome (J80)*
respiratory arrest (R09.2)
respiratory arrest of newborn (P28.81)
respiratory distress syndrome of newborn (P22.-)
respiratory failure (J96.-)
respiratory failure of newborn (P28.5)

\+ **R06.0 Dyspnea**

Excludes1: *tachypnea NOS (R06.82)*
transient tachypnea of newborn (P22.1)

R06.00 Dyspnea, unspecified

AHA CC: 1Q, 2017, 26-27

R06.01 Orthopnea

R06.02 Shortness of breath

AHA CC: 1Q, 2020, 34-36

R06.03 Acute respiratory distress

AHA CC: 4Q, 2017, 23

R06.09 Other forms of dyspnea

R06.1 Stridor

Excludes1: *congenital laryngeal stridor (P28.89)*
laryngismus (stridulus) (J38.5)

R06.2 Wheezing

Excludes1: *Asthma (J45.-)*

AHA CC: 2Q, 2016, 34

CC **R06.3 Periodic breathing**

Cheyne-Stokes breathing

R06.4 Hyperventilation

Excludes1: *psychogenic hyperventilation (F45.8)*

R06.5 Mouth breathing

Excludes2: *dry mouth NOS (R68.2)*

R06.6 Hiccough

Excludes1: *psychogenic hiccough (F45.8)*

R06.7 Sneezing

\+ **R06.8 Other abnormalities of breathing**

R06.81 Apnea, not elsewhere classified

Apnea NOS

Excludes1: *apnea (of) newborn (P28.4)*
sleep apnea (G47.3-)
sleep apnea of newborn (primary) (P28.3)

R06.82 Tachypnea, not elsewhere classified

Tachypnea NOS

Excludes1: *transitory tachypnea of newborn (P22.1)*

R06.83 Snoring

R06.89 Other abnormalities of breathing

Breath-holding (spells)
Sighing

R06.9 Unspecified abnormalities of breathing

R07 Pain in throat and chest

Excludes1: *epidemic myalgia (B33.0)*
Excludes2: *jaw pain (R68.84)*
pain in breast (N64.4)

R07.0 Pain in throat
Excludes1: *chronic sore throat (J31.2)*
sore throat (acute) NOS (J02.9)
Excludes2: *dysphagia (R13.1-)*
pain in neck (M54.2)

R07.1 Chest pain on breathing
Painful respiration

R07.2 Precordial pain

+ **R07.8 Other chest pain**

R07.81 Pleurodynia
Pleurodynia NOS
Excludes1: *epidemic pleurodynia (B33.0)*

R07.82 Intercostal pain

R07.89 Other chest pain
Anterior chest-wall pain NOS
AHA CC: 1Q, 2021, 42

R07.9 Chest pain, unspecified

R09 Other symptoms and signs involving the circulatory and respiratory system

Excludes1: *acute respiratory distress syndrome (J80)*
respiratory arrest of newborn (P28.81)
respiratory distress syndrome of newborn (P22.0)
respiratory failure (J96.-)
respiratory failure of newborn (P28.5)

+ **R09.0 Asphyxia and hypoxemia**
Excludes1: *asphyxia due to carbon monoxide (T58.-)*
asphyxia due to foreign body in respiratory tract (T17.-)
birth (intrauterine) asphyxia (P84)
hyperventilation (R06.4)
traumatic asphyxia (T71-)
Excludes2: *hypercapnia (R06.89)*

CC **R09.01 Asphyxia**

R09.02 Hypoxemia
AHA CC: 3Q, 2019, 15

R09.1 Pleurisy
Excludes1: *pleurisy with effusion (J90)*

MCC **R09.2 Respiratory arrest**
Cardiorespiratory failure
Excludes1: *cardiac arrest (I46.-)*
respiratory arrest of newborn (P28.81)
respiratory distress of newborn (P22.0)
respiratory failure (J96.-)
respiratory failure of newborn (P28.5)
respiratory insufficiency (R06.89)
respiratory insufficiency of newborn (P28.5)

R09.3 Abnormal sputum
Abnormal amount of sputum
Abnormal color of sputum
Abnormal odor of sputum
Excessive sputum
Excludes1: *blood-stained sputum (R04.2)*

+ **R09.8 Other specified symptoms and signs involving the circulatory and respiratory systems**

R09.81 Nasal congestion

R09.82 Postnasal drip

R09.89 Other specified symptoms and signs involving the circulatory and respiratory systems
Bruit (arterial)
Abnormal chest percussion
Feeling of foreign body in throat
Friction sounds in chest
Chest tympany
Choking sensation
Rales
Weak pulse
Excludes2: *foreign body in throat (T17.2-)*
wheezing (R06.2)
AHA CC: 1Q, 2021, 42

Symptoms and signs involving the digestive system and abdomen (R10-R19)

Excludes2: *congenital or infantile pylorospasm (Q40.0)*
gastrointestinal hemorrhage (K92.0-K92.2)
intestinal obstruction (K56.-)
newborn gastrointestinal hemorrhage (P54.0-P54.3)
newborn intestinal obstruction (P76.-)
pylorospasm (K31.3)
signs and symptoms involving the urinary system (R30-R39)
symptoms referable to female genital organs (N94.-)
symptoms referable to male genital organs male (N48-N50)

R10 Abdominal and pelvic pain

Excludes1: *renal colic (N23)*
Excludes2: *dorsalgia (M54.-)*
flatulence and related conditions (R14.-)

R10.0 Acute abdomen
Severe abdominal pain (generalized) (with abdominal rigidity)
Excludes1: *abdominal rigidity NOS (R19.3)*
generalized abdominal pain NOS (R10.84)
localized abdominal pain (R10.1-R10.3-)

+ **R10.1 Pain localized to upper abdomen**

R10.10 Upper abdominal pain, unspecified

R10.11 Right upper quadrant pain

R10.12 Left upper quadrant pain

R10.13 Epigastric pain
Dyspepsia
Excludes1: *functional dyspepsia (K30)*

R10.2 Pelvic and perineal pain
Excludes1: *vulvodynia (N94.81)*

+ **R10.3 Pain localized to other parts of lower abdomen**

R10.30 Lower abdominal pain, unspecified

R10.31 Right lower quadrant pain

R10.32 Left lower quadrant pain

R10.33 Periumbilical pain

+ **R10.8 Other abdominal pain**

+ **R10.81 Abdominal tenderness**
Abdominal tenderness NOS

R10.811 Right upper quadrant abdominal tenderness

R10.812 Left upper quadrant abdominal tenderness

R10.813 Right lower quadrant abdominal tenderness

R10.814 Left lower quadrant abdominal tenderness

R10.815 Periumbilic abdominal tenderness

R10.816 Epigastric abdominal tenderness

R10.817 Generalized abdominal tenderness

R10.819 Abdominal tenderness, unspecified site

+ **R10.82 Rebound abdominal tenderness**

R10.821 Right upper quadrant rebound abdominal tenderness

R10.822 Left upper quadrant rebound abdominal tenderness

R10.823 Right lower quadrant rebound abdominal tenderness

R10.824 Left lower quadrant rebound abdominal tenderness

R10.825 Periumbilic rebound abdominal tenderness

R10.826 Epigastric rebound abdominal tenderness

R10.827 Generalized rebound abdominal tenderness

R10.829 Rebound abdominal tenderness, unspecified site

• **R10.83 Colic**
Colic NOS
Infantile colic
Excludes1: *colic in adult and child over 12 months old (R10.84)*

R10.84 Generalized abdominal pain
Excludes1: *generalized abdominal pain associated with acute abdomen (R10.0)*

R10.9 Unspecified abdominal pain

R11 Nausea and vomiting

Excludes1: *cyclical vomiting associated with migraine (G43.A-)*
excessive vomiting in pregnancy (O21.-)
hematemesis (K92.0)
neonatal hematemesis (P54.0)
newborn vomiting (P92.0-)
psychogenic vomiting (F50.89)
vomiting associated with bulimia nervosa (F50.2)
vomiting following gastrointestinal surgery (K91.0)
AHA CC: 1Q, 2017, 28

R11.0 Nausea
Nausea NOS
Nausea without vomiting

+ **R11.1 Vomiting**
R11.10 Vomiting, unspecified
Vomiting NOS
R11.11 Vomiting without nausea
R11.12 Projectile vomiting
R11.13 Vomiting of fecal matter
R11.14 Bilious vomiting
Bilious emesis
R11.15 Cyclical vomiting syndrome unrelated to migraine
Cyclic vomiting syndrome NOS
Persistent vomiting
Excludes1: *cyclical vomiting in migraine (G43.A-)*
Excludes2: *bulimia nervosa (F50.2)*
diabetes mellitus due to underlying condition (E08.-)
AHA CC: 4Q, 2019, 15

R11.2 Nausea with vomiting, unspecified
Persistent nausea with vomiting NOS
AHA CC: 1Q, 2020, 8

R12 Heartburn

Excludes1: *dyspepsia NOS (R10.13)*
functional dyspepsia (K30)
Valid 3-character code, no further characters required

R13 Aphagia and dysphagia

R13.0 Aphagia
Inability to swallow
Excludes1: *psychogenic aphagia (F50.9)*

+ **R13.1 Dysphagia**
Code first if applicable, dysphagia following cerebrovascular disease (I69. with final characters -91)
Excludes1: *psychogenic dysphagia (F45.8)*
R13.10 Dysphagia, unspecified
Difficulty in swallowing NOS
R13.11 Dysphagia, oral phase
R13.12 Dysphagia, oropharyngeal phase
R13.13 Dysphagia, pharyngeal phase
R13.14 Dysphagia, pharyngoesophageal phase
R13.19 Other dysphagia
Cervical dysphagia
Neurogenic dysphagia

R14 Flatulence and related conditions

Excludes1: *psychogenic aerophagy (F45.8)*

R14.0 Abdominal distension (gaseous)
Bloating
Tympanites (abdominal) (intestinal)
R14.1 Gas pain
R14.2 Eructation
R14.3 Flatulence

R15 Fecal incontinence

Includes: encopresis NOS
Excludes1: *fecal incontinence of nonorganic origin (F98.1)*

R15.0 Incomplete defecation
Excludes1: *constipation (K59.0-)*
fecal impaction (K56.41)
R15.1 Fecal smearing
Fecal soiling
R15.2 Fecal urgency
R15.9 Full incontinence of feces
Fecal incontinence NOS

R16 Hepatomegaly and splenomegaly, not elsewhere classified

R16.0 Hepatomegaly, not elsewhere classified
Hepatomegaly NOS
R16.1 Splenomegaly, not elsewhere classified
Splenomegaly NOS
R16.2 Hepatomegaly with splenomegaly, not elsewhere classified
Hepatosplenomegaly NOS

R17 Unspecified jaundice

Excludes1: *neonatal jaundice (P55, P57-P59)*
Valid 3-character code, no further characters required

CC **R18 Ascites**

Includes: fluid in peritoneal cavity
Excludes1: *ascites in alcoholic cirrhosis (K70.31)*
ascites in alcoholic hepatitis (K70.11)
ascites in toxic liver disease with chronic active hepatitis (K71.51)

CC **R18.0 Malignant ascites**
Code first malignancy, such as:
malignant neoplasm of ovary (C56.-)
secondary malignant neoplasm of retroperitoneum and peritoneum (C78.6)

CC **R18.8 Other ascites**
Ascites NOS
Peritoneal effusion (chronic)
AHA CC: 1Q, 2018, 4-5

R19 Other symptoms and signs involving the digestive system and abdomen

Excludes1: *acute abdomen (R10.0)*

+ **R19.0 Intra-abdominal and pelvic swelling, mass and lump**
Excludes1: *abdominal distension (gaseous) (R14.-)*
ascites (R18.-)
R19.00 Intra-abdominal and pelvic swelling, mass and lump, unspecified site
R19.01 Right upper quadrant abdominal swelling, mass and lump
R19.02 Left upper quadrant abdominal swelling, mass and lump
R19.03 Right lower quadrant abdominal swelling, mass and lump
R19.04 Left lower quadrant abdominal swelling, mass and lump
R19.05 Periumbilic swelling, mass or lump
Diffuse or generalized umbilical swelling or mass
R19.06 Epigastric swelling, mass or lump
R19.07 Generalized intra-abdominal and pelvic swelling, mass and lump
Diffuse or generalized intra-abdominal swelling or mass NOS
Diffuse or generalized pelvic swelling or mass NOS
R19.09 Other intra-abdominal and pelvic swelling, mass and lump

+ **R19.1 Abnormal bowel sounds**
R19.11 Absent bowel sounds
R19.12 Hyperactive bowel sounds
R19.15 Other abnormal bowel sounds
Abnormal bowel sounds NOS

R19.2 Visible peristalsis
Hyperperistalsis

+ **R19.3 Abdominal rigidity**
Excludes1: *abdominal rigidity with severe abdominal pain (R10.0)*
R19.30 Abdominal rigidity, unspecified site
R19.31 Right upper quadrant abdominal rigidity
R19.32 Left upper quadrant abdominal rigidity
R19.33 Right lower quadrant abdominal rigidity
R19.34 Left lower quadrant abdominal rigidity
R19.35 Periumbilic abdominal rigidity
R19.36 Epigastric abdominal rigidity
R19.37 Generalized abdominal rigidity

R19.4 Change in bowel habit
Excludes1: *constipation (K59.0-)*
functional diarrhea (K59.1)

R19.5 Other fecal abnormalities
Abnormal stool color
Bulky stools
Mucus in stools
Occult blood in feces
Occult blood in stools
Excludes1: *melena (K92.1)*
neonatal melena (P54.1)
AHA CC: 1Q, 2019, 32; 1Q, 2021, 9-10

R19.6 Halitosis

R19.7 Diarrhea, unspecified
Diarrhea NOS
Excludes1: *functional diarrhea (K59.1)*
neonatal diarrhea (P78.3)
psychogenic diarrhea (F45.8)
R19.8 Other specified symptoms and signs involving the digestive system and abdomen

Symptoms and signs involving the skin and subcutaneous tissue (R20-R23)

Excludes2: *symptoms relating to breast (N64.4-N64.5)*

R20 Disturbances of skin sensation

Excludes1: *dissociative anesthesia and sensory loss (F44.6)*
psychogenic disturbances (F45.8)

R20.0 Anesthesia of skin
R20.1 Hypoesthesia of skin
R20.2 Paresthesia of skin
Formication
Pins and needles
Tingling skin
Excludes1: *acroparesthesia (I73.8)*
R20.3 Hyperesthesia
R20.8 Other disturbances of skin sensation
R20.9 Unspecified disturbances of skin sensation

R21 Rash and other nonspecific skin eruption

Includes: rash NOS
Excludes1: *specified type of rash- code to condition vesicular eruption (R23.8)*
Valid 3-character code, no further characters required

R22 Localized swelling, mass and lump of skin and subcutaneous tissue

Includes: subcutaneous nodules (localized)(superficial)
Excludes1: *abnormal findings on diagnostic imaging (R90-R93)*
edema (R60.-)
enlarged lymph nodes (R59.-)
localized adiposity (E65)
swelling of joint (M25.4-)

R22.0 Localized swelling, mass and lump, head
R22.1 Localized swelling, mass and lump, neck
R22.2 Localized swelling, mass and lump, trunk
Excludes1: *intra-abdominal or pelvic mass and lump (R19.0-)*
intra-abdominal or pelvic swelling (R19.0-)
Excludes2: *breast mass and lump (N63)*
\+ **R22.3 Localized swelling, mass and lump, upper limb**
R22.30 Localized swelling, mass and lump, unspecified upper limb
R22.31 Localized swelling, mass and lump, right upper limb
R22.32 Localized swelling, mass and lump, left upper limb
R22.33 Localized swelling, mass and lump, upper limb, bilateral
\+ **R22.4 Localized swelling, mass and lump, lower limb**
R22.40 Localized swelling, mass and lump, unspecified lower limb
R22.41 Localized swelling, mass and lump, right lower limb
R22.42 Localized swelling, mass and lump, left lower limb
R22.43 Localized swelling, mass and lump, lower limb, bilateral
R22.9 Localized swelling, mass and lump, unspecified

R23 Other skin changes

R23.0 Cyanosis
Excludes1: *acrocyanosis (I73.8)*
cyanotic attacks of newborn (P28.2)
R23.1 Pallor
Clammy skin
R23.2 Flushing
Excessive blushing
Code first, if applicable, menopausal and female climacteric states (N95.1)
R23.3 Spontaneous ecchymoses
Petechiae
Excludes1: *ecchymoses of newborn (P54.5)*
purpura (D69.-)
R23.4 Changes in skin texture
Desquamation of skin
Induration of skin
Scaling of skin
Excludes1: *epidermal thickening NOS (L85.9)*
R23.8 Other skin changes
R23.9 Unspecified skin changes

Symptoms and signs involving the nervous and musculoskeletal systems (R25-R29)

R25 Abnormal involuntary movements

Excludes1: *specific movement disorders (G20-G26)*
stereotyped movement disorders (F98.4)
tic disorders (F95.-)

R25.0 Abnormal head movements
R25.1 Tremor, unspecified
Excludes1: *chorea NOS (G25.5)*
essential tremor (G25.0)
hysterical tremor (F44.4)
intention tremor (G25.2)
R25.2 Cramp and spasm
Excludes2: *carpopedal spasm (R29.0)*
charley-horse (M62.831)
infantile spasms (G40.4-)
muscle spasm of back (M62.830)
muscle spasm of calf (M62.831)
R25.3 Fasciculation
Twitching NOS
R25.8 Other abnormal involuntary movements
R25.9 Unspecified abnormal involuntary movements

R26 Abnormalities of gait and mobility

Excludes1: *ataxia NOS (R27.0)*
hereditary ataxia (G11.-)
locomotor (syphilitic) ataxia (A52.11)
immobility syndrome (paraplegic) (M62.3)

R26.0 Ataxic gait
Staggering gait
R26.1 Paralytic gait
Spastic gait
R26.2 Difficulty in walking, not elsewhere classified
Excludes1: *falling (R29.6)*
unsteadiness on feet (R26.81)
AHA CC: 2Q, 2016, 7
R26.8 Other abnormalities of gait and mobility
R26.81 Unsteadiness on feet
R26.89 Other abnormalities of gait and mobility
AHA CC: 2Q, 2020, 29
R26.9 Unspecified abnormalities of gait and mobility

R27 Other lack of coordination

Excludes1: *ataxic gait (R26.0)*
hereditary ataxia (G11.-)
vertigo NOS (R42)

R27.0 Ataxia, unspecified
Excludes1: *ataxia following cerebrovascular disease (I69. with final characters -93)*
R27.8 Other lack of coordination
R27.9 Unspecified lack of coordination

R29 Other symptoms and signs involving the nervous and musculoskeletal systems

CC **R29.0 Tetany**
Carpopedal spasm
Excludes1: *hysterical tetany (F44.5)*
neonatal tetany (P71.3)
parathyroid tetany (E20.9)
post-thyroidectomy tetany (E89.2)
CC **R29.1 Meningismus**
R29.2 Abnormal reflex
Excludes2: *abnormal pupillary reflex (H57.0)*
hyperactive gag reflex (J39.2)
vasovagal reaction or syncope (R55)
R29.3 Abnormal posture
R29.4 Clicking hip
Excludes1: *congenital deformities of hip (Q65.-)*

CC **R29.5 Transient paralysis**
Code first any associated spinal cord injury (S14.0, S14.1-, S24.0, S24.1-, S34.0-, S34.1-)
Excludes1: *transient ischemic attack (G45.9)*

R29.6 Repeated falls
Falling
Tendency to fall
Excludes2: *at risk for falling (Z91.81)*
history of falling (Z91.81)
Review coding guideline C.18.d
AHA CC: 2Q, 2016, 6-7

\+ **R29.7 National Institutes of Health Stroke Scale (NIHSS) score**
Code first the type of cerebral infarction (I63.-)
Review coding guidelines B.14 and C.18.i
AHA CC: 4Q, 2016, 61-62

\+ **R29.70 NIHSS score 0-9**
R29.700 NIHSS score 0
R29.701 NIHSS score 1
R29.702 NIHSS score 2
R29.703 NIHSS score 3
R29.704 NIHSS score 4
R29.705 NIHSS score 5
R29.706 NIHSS score 6
R29.707 NIHSS score 7
R29.708 NIHSS score 8
R29.709 NIHSS score 9

\+ **R29.71 NIHSS score 10-19**
R29.710 NIHSS score 10
R29.711 NIHSS score 11
R29.712 NIHSS score 12
R29.713 NIHSS score 13
R29.714 NIHSS score 14
R29.715 NIHSS score 15
R29.716 NIHSS score 16
R29.717 NIHSS score 17
R29.718 NIHSS score 18
R29.719 NIHSS score 19

\+ **R29.72 NIHSS score 20-29**
R29.720 NIHSS score 20
R29.721 NIHSS score 21
R29.722 NIHSS score 22
R29.723 NIHSS score 23
R29.724 NIHSS score 24
R29.725 NIHSS score 25
R29.726 NIHSS score 26
R29.727 NIHSS score 27
R29.728 NIHSS score 28
R29.729 NIHSS score 29

\+ **R29.73 NIHSS score 30-39**
R29.730 NIHSS score 30
AHA CC: 4Q, 2016, 61-62
R29.731 NIHSS score 31
R29.732 NIHSS score 32
R29.733 NIHSS score 33
R29.734 NIHSS score 34
R29.735 NIHSS score 35
R29.736 NIHSS score 36
R29.737 NIHSS score 37
R29.738 NIHSS score 38
R29.739 NIHSS score 39

\+ **R29.74 NIHSS score 40-42**
R29.740 NIHSS score 40
R29.741 NIHSS score 41
R29.742 NIHSS score 42

\+ **R29.8 Other symptoms and signs involving the nervous and musculoskeletal systems**

\+ **R29.81 Other symptoms and signs involving the nervous system**
R29.810 Facial weakness
Facial droop
Excludes1: *Bell's palsy (G51.0)*
facial weakness following cerebrovascular disease (I69. with final characters -92)
R29.818 Other symptoms and signs involving the nervous system

\+ **R29.89 Other symptoms and signs involving the musculoskeletal system**
Excludes2: *pain in limb (M79.6-)*
R29.890 Loss of height
Excludes1: *osteoporosis (M80-M81)*
R29.891 Ocular torticollis
Excludes1: *congenital (sternomastoid) torticollis (Q68.0)*
psychogenic torticollis (F45.8)
spasmodic torticollis (G24.3)
torticollis due to birth injury (P15.8)
torticollis NOS (M43.6)
R29.898 Other symptoms and signs involving the musculoskeletal system

\+ **R29.9 Unspecified symptoms and signs involving the nervous and musculoskeletal systems**
R29.90 Unspecified symptoms and signs involving the nervous system
R29.91 Unspecified symptoms and signs involving the musculoskeletal system

Symptoms and signs involving the genitourinary system (R30-R39)

R30 Pain associated with micturition
Excludes1: *psychogenic pain associated with micturition (F45.8)*
R30.0 Dysuria
Strangury
R30.1 Vesical tenesmus
R30.9 Painful micturition, unspecified
Painful urination NOS

R31 Hematuria
Excludes1: *hematuria included with underlying conditions, such as:*
acute cystitis with hematuria (N30.01)
recurrent and persistent hematuria in glomerular diseases (N02.-)
R31.0 Gross hematuria
AHA CC: 1Q, 2017, 17-18
R31.1 Benign essential microscopic hematuria
\+ **R31.2 Other microscopic hematuria**
AHA CC: 4Q, 2016, 62
R31.21 Asymptomatic microscopic hematuria
AMH
AHA CC: 4Q, 2016, 62
R31.29 Other microscopic hematuria
R31.9 Hematuria, unspecified
AHA CC: 1Q, 2017, 6

R32 Unspecified urinary incontinence
Enuresis NOS
Excludes1: *functional urinary incontinence (R39.81)*
nonorganic enuresis (F98.0)
stress incontinence and other specified urinary incontinence (N39.3-N39.4-)
urinary incontinence associated with cognitive impairment (R39.81)
Valid 3-character code, no further characters required

R33 Retention of urine
Excludes1: *psychogenic retention of urine (F45.8)*
R33.0 Drug induced retention of urine
Use additional code for adverse effect, if applicable, to identify drug (T36-T50 with fifth or sixth character 5)
R33.8 Other retention of urine
Code first if applicable, any causal condition, such as: enlarged prostate (N40.1)
R33.9 Retention of urine, unspecified

R34 Anuria and oliguria
Excludes1: *anuria and oliguria complicating abortion or ectopic or molar pregnancy (O00-O07, O08.4)*
anuria and oliguria complicating pregnancy (O26.83-)
anuria and oliguria complicating the puerperium (O90.4)
Valid 3-character code, no further characters required

R35 Polyuria

Code first if applicable, any causal condition, such as:
enlarged prostate (N40.1)

Excludes1: *psychogenic polyuria (F45.8)*

R35.0 Frequency of micturition

R35.1 Nocturia

\+ **R35.8 Other polyuria**

R35.81 Nocturnal polyuria

Excludes2: *nocturnal enuresis (N39.44)*

R35.89 Other polyuria

Polyuria NOS

R36 Urethral discharge

R36.0 Urethral discharge without blood

♂ **R36.1 Hematospermia**

R36.9 Urethral discharge, unspecified

Penile discharge NOS
Urethrorrhea

R37 Sexual dysfunction, unspecified

Valid 3-character code, no further characters required

R39 Other and unspecified symptoms and signs involving the genitourinary system

CC **R39.0 Extravasation of urine**

\+ **R39.1 Other difficulties with micturition**

Code first if applicable, any causal condition, such as:
enlarged prostate (N40.1)

R39.11 Hesitancy of micturition

R39.12 Poor urinary stream

Weak urinary steam

R39.13 Splitting of urinary stream

R39.14 Feeling of incomplete bladder emptying

R39.15 Urgency of urination

Excludes1: *urge incontinence (N39.41, N39.46)*

R39.16 Straining to void

\+ **R39.19 Other difficulties with micturition**

AHA CC: 4Q, 2016, 63

R39.191 Need to immediately re-void

R39.192 Position dependent micturition

R39.198 Other difficulties with micturition

R39.2 Extrarenal uremia

Prerenal uremia

Excludes1: *uremia NOS (N19)*

\+ **R39.8 Other symptoms and signs involving the genitourinary system**

AHA CC: 4Q, 2016, 64

R39.81 Functional urinary incontinence

Urinary incontinence due to cognitive impairment, or severe physical disability or immobility

Excludes1: *stress incontinence and other specified urinary incontinence (N39.3-N39.4-)*
urinary incontinence NOS (R32)

R39.82 Chronic bladder pain

AHA CC: 4Q, 2016, 64

♂ **R39.83 Unilateral non-palpable testicle**

AHA CC: 4Q, 2017, 22-23

♂ **R39.84 Bilateral non-palpable testicles**

AHA CC: 4Q, 2017, 22-23

R39.89 Other symptoms and signs involving the genitourinary system

R39.9 Unspecified symptoms and signs involving the genitourinary system

Symptoms and signs involving cognition, perception, emotional state and behavior (R40-R46)

Excludes2: *symptoms and signs constituting part of a pattern of mental disorder (F01-F99)*

R40 Somnolence, stupor and coma

Excludes1: *neonatal coma (P91.5)*
somnolence, stupor and coma in diabetes (E08-E13)
somnolence, stupor and coma in hepatic failure (K72.-)
somnolence, stupor and coma in hypoglycemia (nondiabetic) (E15)

R40.0 Somnolence

Drowsiness

Excludes1: *coma (R40.2-)*

R40.1 Stupor

Catatonic stupor
Semicoma

Excludes1: *catatonic schizophrenia (F20.2)*
coma (R40.2-)
depressive stupor (F31-F33)
dissociative stupor (F44.2)
manic stupor (F30.2)

\+ **R40.2 Coma**

Code first any associated:
fracture of skull (S02.-)
intracranial injury (S06.-)

NOTE One code from each subcategory, R40.21-R40.23, is required to complete the coma scale

Review coding guidelines B.14 and C.18.e

AHA CC: 1Q, 2014, 19-20; 2Q, 2015, 17-18

MCC X+7th **R40.20 Unspecified coma**

Coma NOS
Unconsciousness NOS

AHA CC: 2Q, 2021, 5

\+ **R40.21 Coma scale, eyes open**

AHA CC: 4Q, 2017, 25

The appropriate 7th character is to be added to each code from subcategory **R40.21-**:
0 unspecified time
1 in the field [EMT or ambulance]
2 at arrival to emergency department
3 at hospital admission
4 24 hours or more after hospital admission

MCC +7th **R40.211 Coma scale, eyes open, never**

Coma scale eye opening score of 1

MCC +7th **R40.212 Coma scale, eyes open, to pain**

Coma scale eye opening score of 2

+7th **R40.213 Coma scale, eyes open, to sound**

Coma scale eye opening score of 3

+7th **R40.214 Coma scale, eyes open, spontaneous**

Coma scale eye opening score of 4

\+ **R40.22 Coma scale, best verbal response**

AHA CC: 4Q, 2017, 23-25

The appropriate 7th character is to be added to each code from subcategory **R40.22-**:
0 unspecified time
1 in the field [EMT or ambulance]
2 at arrival to emergency department
3 at hospital admission
4 24 hours or more after hospital admission

MCC +7th **R40.221 Coma scale, best verbal response, none**

Coma scale verbal score of 1

MCC +7th **R40.222 Coma scale, best verbal response, incomprehensible words**

Coma scale verbal score of 2
Incomprehensible sounds (2-5 years of age)
Moans/grunts to pain (<2 years of age)

+7th **R40.223 Coma scale, best verbal response, inappropriate words**

Coma scale verbal score of 3
Inappropriate crying or screaming (<2 years of age)
Screaming (2-5 years of age)

+7th **R40.224 Coma scale, best verbal response, confused conversation**

Coma scale verbal score of 4
Inappropriate words (2-5 years of age)
Irritable cries (<2 years of age)

+7th **R40.225 Coma scale, best verbal response, oriented**

Coma scale verbal score of 5
Cooing or babbling or crying appropriately (<2 years of age)
Uses appropriate words (2-5 years of age)

+ **R40.23 Coma scale, best motor response**
AHA CC: 4Q, 2017, 23-25

The appropriate 7th character is to be added to each code from subcategory **R40.23-**:
0 unspecified time
1 in the field [EMT or ambulance]
2 at arrival to emergency department
3 at hospital admission
4 24 hours or more after hospital admission

MCC +7th **R40.231 Coma scale, best motor response, none**
Coma scale motor score of 1

MCC +7th **R40.232 Coma scale, best motor response, extension**
Abnormal extensor posturing to pain or noxious stimuli (<2 years of age)
Coma scale motor score of 2
Extensor posturing to pain or noxious stimuli (2-5 years of age)

+7th **R40.233 Coma scale, best motor response, abnormal flexion**
Abnormal flexure posturing to pain or noxious stimuli (2-5 years of age)
Coma scale motor score of 3
Flexion/decorticate posturing (<2 years of age)

MCC +7th **R40.234 Coma scale, best motor response, flexion withdrawal**
Coma scale motor score of 4
Withdraws from pain or noxious stimuli (2-5 years of age)

+7th **R40.235 Coma scale, best motor response, localizes pain**
Coma scale motor score of 5
Localizes pain (2-5 years of age)
Withdraws to touch (<2 years of age)

+7th **R40.236 Coma scale, best motor response, obeys commands**
Coma scale motor score of 6
Normal or spontaneous movement (<2 years of age)
Obeys commands (2-5 years of age)

+ **R40.24 Glasgow coma scale, total score**
NOTE Assign a code from subcategory R40.24, when only the total coma score is documented.
AHA CC: 4Q, 2016, 64-65

The appropriate 7th character is to be added to each code from subcategory **R40.24-**:
0 unspecified time
1 in the field [EMT or ambulance]
2 at arrival to emergency department
3 at hospital admission
4 24 hours or more after hospital admission

+7th **R40.241 Glasgow coma scale score 13-15**
+7th **R40.242 Glasgow coma scale score 9-12**
+7th **R40.243 Glasgow coma scale score 3-8**
+7th **R40.244 Other coma, without documented Glasgow coma scale score, or with partial score reported**
AHA CC: 3Q, 2020, 46

CC **R40.3 Persistent vegetative state**
R40.4 Transient alteration of awareness
AHA CC: 2Q, 2020, 24

R41 Other symptoms and signs involving cognitive functions and awareness
Excludes1: *dissociative [conversion] disorders (F44.-)*
mild cognitive impairment, so stated (G31.84)

R41.0 Disorientation, unspecified
Confusion NOS
Delirium NOS
AHA CC: 4Q, 2016, 74-76; 2Q, 2019, 34

R41.1 Anterograde amnesia
R41.2 Retrograde amnesia
R41.3 Other amnesia
Amnesia NOS
Memory loss NOS
Excludes1: *amnestic disorder due to known physiologic condition (F04)*
amnestic syndrome due to psychoactive substance use (F10-F19 with 5th character .6)
mild memory disturbance due to known physiological condition (F06.8)
transient global amnesia (G45.4)

CC **R41.4 Neurologic neglect syndrome**
Asomatognosia
Hemi-akinesia
Hemi-inattention
Hemispatial neglect
Left-sided neglect
Sensory neglect
Visuospatial neglect
Excludes1: *visuospatial deficit (R41.842)*

+ **R41.8 Other symptoms and signs involving cognitive functions and awareness**

● **R41.81 Age-related cognitive decline**
Senility NOS

R41.82 Altered mental status, unspecified
Change in mental status NOS
Excludes1: *altered level of consciousness (R40.-)*
altered mental status due to known condition - code to condition
delirium NOS (R41.0)
AHA CC: 4Q, 2012, 98

R41.83 Borderline intellectual functioning
IQ level 71 to 84
Excludes1: *intellectual disabilities (F70-F79)*

+ **R41.84 Other specified cognitive deficit**
Excludes1: *cognitive deficits as sequelae of cerebrovascular disease (I69.01-, I69.11-, I19.21-, I69.31-, I59.81-, I69.91-)*

R41.840 Attention and concentration deficit
Excludes1: *attention-deficit hyperactivity disorders (F90.-)*

R41.841 Cognitive communication deficit
R41.842 Visuospatial deficit
R41.843 Psychomotor deficit
R41.844 Frontal lobe and executive function deficit

R41.89 Other symptoms and signs involving cognitive functions and awareness
Anosognosia

R41.9 Unspecified symptoms and signs involving cognitive functions and awareness
Unspecified neurocognitive disorder

R42 Dizziness and giddiness
Light-headedness
Vertigo NOS
Excludes1: *vertiginous syndromes (H81.-)*
vertigo from infrasound (T75.23)
Valid 3-character code, no further characters required

R43 Disturbances of smell and taste
R43.0 Anosmia
R43.1 Parosmia
R43.2 Parageusia
R43.8 Other disturbances of smell and taste
Mixed disturbance of smell and taste
R43.9 Unspecified disturbances of smell and taste

R44 Other symptoms and signs involving general sensations and perceptions

Excludes1: *alcoholic hallucinations (F10.151, F10.251, F10.951)*
hallucinations in drug psychosis (F11-F19 with fifth to sixth characters 51)
hallucinations in mood disorders with psychotic symptoms (F30.2, F31.5, F32.3, F33.3)
hallucinations in schizophrenia, schizotypal and delusional disorders (F20-F29)

Excludes2: *disturbances of skin sensation (R20.-)*

CC **R44.0 Auditory hallucinations**
R44.1 Visual hallucinations
CC **R44.2 Other hallucinations**
CC **R44.3 Hallucinations, unspecified**
R44.8 Other symptoms and signs involving general sensations and perceptions
R44.9 Unspecified symptoms and signs involving general sensations and perceptions

R45 Symptoms and signs involving emotional state

R45.0 Nervousness
Nervous tension
R45.1 Restlessness and agitation
R45.2 Unhappiness
R45.3 Demoralization and apathy
Excludes1: *anhedonia (R45.84)*
R45.4 Irritability and anger
R45.5 Hostility
R45.6 Violent behavior
R45.7 State of emotional shock and stress, unspecified
\+ **R45.8 Other symptoms and signs involving emotional state**
R45.81 Low self-esteem
R45.82 Worries
R45.83 Excessive crying of child, adolescent or adult
Excludes1: *excessive crying of infant (baby) (R68.11)*
R45.84 Anhedonia
\+ **R45.85 Homicidal and suicidal ideations**
Excludes1: *suicide attempt (T14.91)*
R45.850 Homicidal ideations
CC **R45.851 Suicidal ideations**
R45.86 Emotional lability
R45.87 Impulsiveness
R45.88 Nonsuicidal self-harm
Nonsuicidal self-injury
Nonsuicidal self-mutilation
Self-inflicted injury without suicidal intent
Code also injury, if known
R45.89 Other symptoms and signs involving emotional state

R46 Symptoms and signs involving appearance and behavior

Excludes1: *appearance and behavior in schizophrenia, schizotypal and delusional disorders (F20-F29)*
mental and behavioral disorders (F01-F99)

R46.0 Very low level of personal hygiene
R46.1 Bizarre personal appearance
R46.2 Strange and inexplicable behavior
R46.3 Overactivity
R46.4 Slowness and poor responsiveness
Excludes1: *stupor (R40.1)*
R46.5 Suspiciousness and marked evasiveness
R46.6 Undue concern and preoccupation with stressful events
R46.7 Verbosity and circumstantial detail obscuring reason for contact
\+ **R46.8 Other symptoms and signs involving appearance and behavior**
R46.81 Obsessive-compulsive behavior
Excludes1: *obsessive-compulsive disorder (F42.-)*
R46.89 Other symptoms and signs involving appearance and behavior

Symptoms and signs involving speech and voice (R47-R49)

R47 Speech disturbances, not elsewhere classified

Excludes1: *autism (F84.0)*
cluttering (F80.81)
specific developmental disorders of speech and language (F80.-)
stuttering (F80.81)

\+ **R47.0 Dysphasia and aphasia**
CC **R47.01 Aphasia**
Excludes1: *aphasia following cerebrovascular disease (I69. with final characters -20)*
progressive isolated aphasia (G31.01)
R47.02 Dysphasia
Excludes1: *dysphasia following cerebrovascular disease (I69. with final characters -21)*
R47.1 Dysarthria and anarthria
Excludes1: *dysarthria following cerebrovascular disease (I69. with final characters -22)*
\+ **R47.8 Other speech disturbances**
Excludes1: *dysarthria following cerebrovascular disease (I69. with final characters -28)*
R47.81 Slurred speech
R47.82 Fluency disorder in conditions classified elsewhere
Stuttering in conditions classified elsewhere
Code first underlying disease or condition, such as:
Parkinson's disease (G20)
Excludes1: *adult onset fluency disorder (F98.5)*
childhood onset fluency disorder (F80.81)
fluency disorder (stuttering) following cerebrovascular disease (I69. with final characters -23)
R47.89 Other speech disturbances
R47.9 Unspecified speech disturbances

R48 Dyslexia and other symbolic dysfunctions, not elsewhere classified

Excludes1: *specific developmental disorders of scholastic skills (F81.-)*

R48.0 Dyslexia and alexia
R48.1 Agnosia
Astereognosia (astereognosis)
Autotopagnosia
Excludes1: *visual object agnosia (R48.3)*
R48.2 Apraxia
Excludes1: *apraxia following cerebrovascular disease (I69. with final characters -90)*
R48.3 Visual agnosia
Prosopagnosia
Simultanagnosia (asimultagnosia)
R48.8 Other symbolic dysfunctions
Acalculia
Agraphia
AHA CC: 1Q, 2017, 27-28
R48.9 Unspecified symbolic dysfunctions

R49 Voice and resonance disorders

Excludes1: *psychogenic voice and resonance disorders (F44.4)*

R49.0 Dysphonia
Hoarseness
R49.1 Aphonia
Loss of voice
\+ **R49.2 Hypernasality and hyponasality**
R49.21 Hypernasality
R49.22 Hyponasality
R49.8 Other voice and resonance disorders
R49.9 Unspecified voice and resonance disorder
Change in voice NOS
Resonance disorder NOS

General symptoms and signs (R50-R69)

R50 Fever of other and unknown origin

Excludes1: *chills without fever (R68.83)*
febrile convulsions (R56.0-)
fever of unknown origin during labor (O75.2)
fever of unknown origin in newborn (P81.9)
hypothermia due to illness (R68.0)
malignant hyperthermia due to anesthesia (T88.3)
puerperal pyrexia NOS (O86.4)

R50.2 Drug induced fever

Use additional code for adverse effect, if applicable, to identify drug (T36-T50 with fifth or sixth character 5)

Excludes1: *postvaccination (postimmunization) fever (R50.83)*

+ **R50.8 Other specified fever**

R50.81 Fever presenting with conditions classified elsewhere

Code first underlying condition when associated fever is present, such as with:
leukemia (C91-C95)
neutropenia (D70.-)
sickle-cell disease (D57.-)

AHA CC: 4Q, 2014, 22-23; 2Q, 2019, 24-25; 3Q, 2020, 22-23

R50.82 Postprocedural fever

Excludes1: *postprocedural infection (T81.4-)*
posttransfusion fever (R50.84)
postvaccination (postimmunization) fever (R50.83)

R50.83 Postvaccination fever

Postimmunization fever

R50.84 Febrile nonhemolytic transfusion reaction

FNHTR
Posttransfusion fever

R50.9 Fever, unspecified

Fever NOS
Fever of unknown origin [FUO]
Fever with chills
Fever with rigors
Hyperpyrexia NOS
Persistent fever
Pyrexia NOS

AHA CC: 1Q, 2020, 34-36

R51 Headache

Excludes2: *atypical face pain (G50.1)*
migraine and other headache syndromes (G43-G44)
trigeminal neuralgia (G50.0)

AHA CC: 4Q, 2020, 38-39

R51.0 Headache with orthostatic component, not elsewhere classified

Headache with positional component, not elsewhere classified

R51.9 Headache, unspecified

Facial pain NOS

R52 Pain, unspecified

Acute pain NOS
Generalized pain NOS
Pain NOS

Excludes1: *acute and chronic pain, not elsewhere classified (G89.-)*
localized pain, unspecified type - code to pain by site, such as:
abdomen pain (R10.-)
back pain (M54.9)
breast pain (N64.4)
chest pain (R07.1-R07.9)
ear pain (H92.0-)
eye pain (H57.1)
headache (R51.9)
joint pain (M25.5-)
limb pain (M79.6-)
lumbar region pain (M54.5-)
pelvic and perineal pain (R10.2)
shoulder pain (M25.51-)
spine pain (M54.-)
throat pain (R07.0)
tongue pain (K14.6)
tooth pain (K08.8)
renal colic (N23)
pain disorders exclusively related to psychological factors (F45.41)

Valid 3-character code, no further characters required

R53 Malaise and fatigue

R53.0 Neoplastic (malignant) related fatigue

Code first associated neoplasm

R53.1 Weakness

Asthenia NOS

Excludes1: *age-related weakness (R54)*
muscle weakness (generalized) (M62.81)
sarcopenia (M62.84)
senile asthenia (R54)

AHA CC: 1Q, 2017, 7

MCC **R53.2 Functional quadriplegia**

Complete immobility due to severe physical disability or frailty

Excludes1: *frailty NOS (R54)*
hysterical paralysis (F44.4)
immobility syndrome (M62.3)
neurologic quadriplegia (G82.5-)
quadriplegia (G82.50)

Review coding guideline C.18.f

AHA CC: 2Q, 2016, 6

+ **R53.8 Other malaise and fatigue**

Excludes1: *combat exhaustion and fatigue (F43.0)*
congenital debility (P96.9)
exhaustion and fatigue due to excessive exertion (T73.3)
exhaustion and fatigue due to exposure (T73.2)
exhaustion and fatigue due to heat (T67.-)
exhaustion and fatigue due to pregnancy (O26.8-)
exhaustion and fatigue due to recurrent depressive episode (F33)
exhaustion and fatigue due to senile debility (R54)

R53.81 Other malaise

Chronic debility
Debility NOS
General physical deterioration
Malaise NOS
Nervous debility

Excludes1: *age-related physical debility (R54)*

AHA CC: 1Q, 2021, 43

R53.82 Chronic fatigue, unspecified

Chronic fatigue syndrome NOS

Excludes1: *postviral fatigue syndrome (G93.3)*

R53.83 Other fatigue

Fatigue NOS
Lack of energy
Lethargy
Tiredness

Excludes2: *exhaustion and fatigue due to depressive episode (F32.-)*

AHA CC: 1Q, 2017, 7

• **R54 Age-related physical debility**

Frailty
Old age
Senescence
Senile asthenia
Senile debility
Excludes1: *age-related cognitive decline (R41.81)*
sarcopenia (M62.84)
senile psychosis (F03)
senility NOS (R41.81)
Valid 3-character code, no further characters required

R55 Syncope and collapse

Blackout
Fainting
Vasovagal attack
Excludes1: *cardiogenic shock (R57.0)*
carotid sinus syncope (G90.01)
heat syncope (T67.1)
neurocirculatory asthenia (F45.8)
neurogenic orthostatic hypotension (G90.3)
orthostatic hypotension (I95.1)
postprocedural shock (T81.1-)
psychogenic syncope (F48.8)
shock NOS (R57.9)
shock complicating or following abortion or ectopic or molar pregnancy (O00-O07, O08.3)
shock complicating or following labor and delivery (O75.1)
Stokes-Adams attack (I45.9)
unconsciousness NOS (R40.2-)
Valid 3-character code, no further characters required

R56 Convulsions, not elsewhere classified

Excludes1: *dissociative convulsions and seizures (F44.5)*
epileptic convulsions and seizures (G40.-)
newborn convulsions and seizures (P90)

\+ **R56.0 Febrile convulsions**

CC **R56.00 Simple febrile convulsions**
Febrile convulsion NOS
Febrile seizure NOS

CC **R56.01 Complex febrile convulsions**
Atypical febrile seizure
Complex febrile seizure
Complicated febrile seizure
Excludes1: *status epilepticus (G40.901)*

CC **R56.1 Post traumatic seizures**
Excludes1: *post traumatic epilepsy (G40.-)*

R56.9 Unspecified convulsions
Convulsion disorder
Fit NOS
Recurrent convulsions
Seizure(s) (convulsive) NOS
AHA CC: 4Q, 2019, 17-18; 1Q, 2021, 3

R57 Shock, not elsewhere classified

Excludes1: *anaphylactic shock NOS (T78.2)*
anaphylactic reaction or shock due to adverse food reaction (T78.0-)
anaphylactic shock due to adverse effect of correct drug or medicament properly administered (T88.6)
anaphylactic shock due to serum (T80.5-)
electric shock (T75.4)
obstetric shock (O75.1)
postprocedural shock (T81.1-)
psychic shock (F43.0)
shock complicating or following ectopic or molar pregnancy (O00-O07, O08.3)
shock due to anesthesia (T88.2)
shock due to lightning (T75.01)
traumatic shock (T79.4)
toxic shock syndrome (A48.3)

MCC **R57.0 Cardiogenic shock**
Excludes2: *septic shock (R65.21)*
AHA CC: 3Q, 2020, 26

MCC **R57.1 Hypovolemic shock**
AHA CC: 2Q, 2019, 7-8

MCC **R57.8 Other shock**

CC **R57.9 Shock, unspecified**
Failure of peripheral circulation NOS

R58 Hemorrhage, not elsewhere classified

Hemorrhage NOS
Excludes1: *hemorrhage included with underlying conditions, such as:*
acute duodenal ulcer with hemorrhage (K26.0)
acute gastritis with bleeding (K29.01)
ulcerative enterocolitis with rectal bleeding (K51.01)
Valid 3-character code, no further characters required

R59 Enlarged lymph nodes

Includes: swollen glands
Excludes1: *lymphadenitis NOS (I88.9)*
acute lymphadenitis (L04.-)
chronic lymphadenitis (I88.1)
mesenteric (acute) (chronic) lymphadenitis (I88.0)

R59.0 Localized enlarged lymph nodes
R59.1 Generalized enlarged lymph nodes
Lymphadenopathy NOS
R59.9 Enlarged lymph nodes, unspecified

R60 Edema, not elsewhere classified

Excludes1: *angioneurotic edema (T78.3)*
ascites (R18.-)
cerebral edema (G93.6)
cerebral edema due to birth injury (P11.0)
edema of larynx (J38.4)
edema of nasopharynx (J39.2)
edema of pharynx (J39.2)
gestational edema (O12.0-)
hereditary edema (Q82.0)
hydrops fetalis NOS (P83.2)
hydrothorax (J94.8)
hydrops fetalis NOS (P83.2)
newborn edema (P83.3)
pulmonary edema (J81.-)

R60.0 Localized edema
R60.1 Generalized edema
Excludes2: *nutritional edema (E40-E46)*
R60.9 Edema, unspecified
Fluid retention NOS

R61 Generalized hyperhidrosis

Excessive sweating
Night sweats
Secondary hyperhidrosis
Code first if applicable, menopausal and female climacteric states (N95.1)
Excludes1: *focal (primary) (secondary) hyperhidrosis (L74.5-)*
Frey's syndrome (L74.52)
localized (primary) (secondary) hyperhidrosis (L74.5-)
Valid 3-character code, no further characters required

R62 Lack of expected normal physiological development in childhood and adults

Excludes1: *delayed puberty (E30.0)*
gonadal dysgenesis (Q99.1)
hypopituitarism (E23.0)

• **R62.0 Delayed milestone in childhood**
Delayed attainment of expected physiological developmental stage
Late talker
Late walker

\+ **R62.5 Other and unspecified lack of expected normal physiological development in childhood**
Excludes1: *HIV disease resulting in failure to thrive (B20)*
physical retardation due to malnutrition (E45)

R62.50 Unspecified lack of expected normal physiological development in childhood
Infantilism NOS

• **R62.51 Failure to thrive (child)**
Failure to gain weight
Excludes1: *failure to thrive in child under 28 days old (P92.6)*
AHA CC: 4Q, 2018, 82

R62.52 Short stature (child)
Lack of growth
Physical retardation
Short stature NOS
Excludes1: *short stature due to endocrine disorder (E34.3)*

R62.59 Other lack of expected normal physiological development in childhood

• **R62.7 Adult failure to thrive**

Sepsis

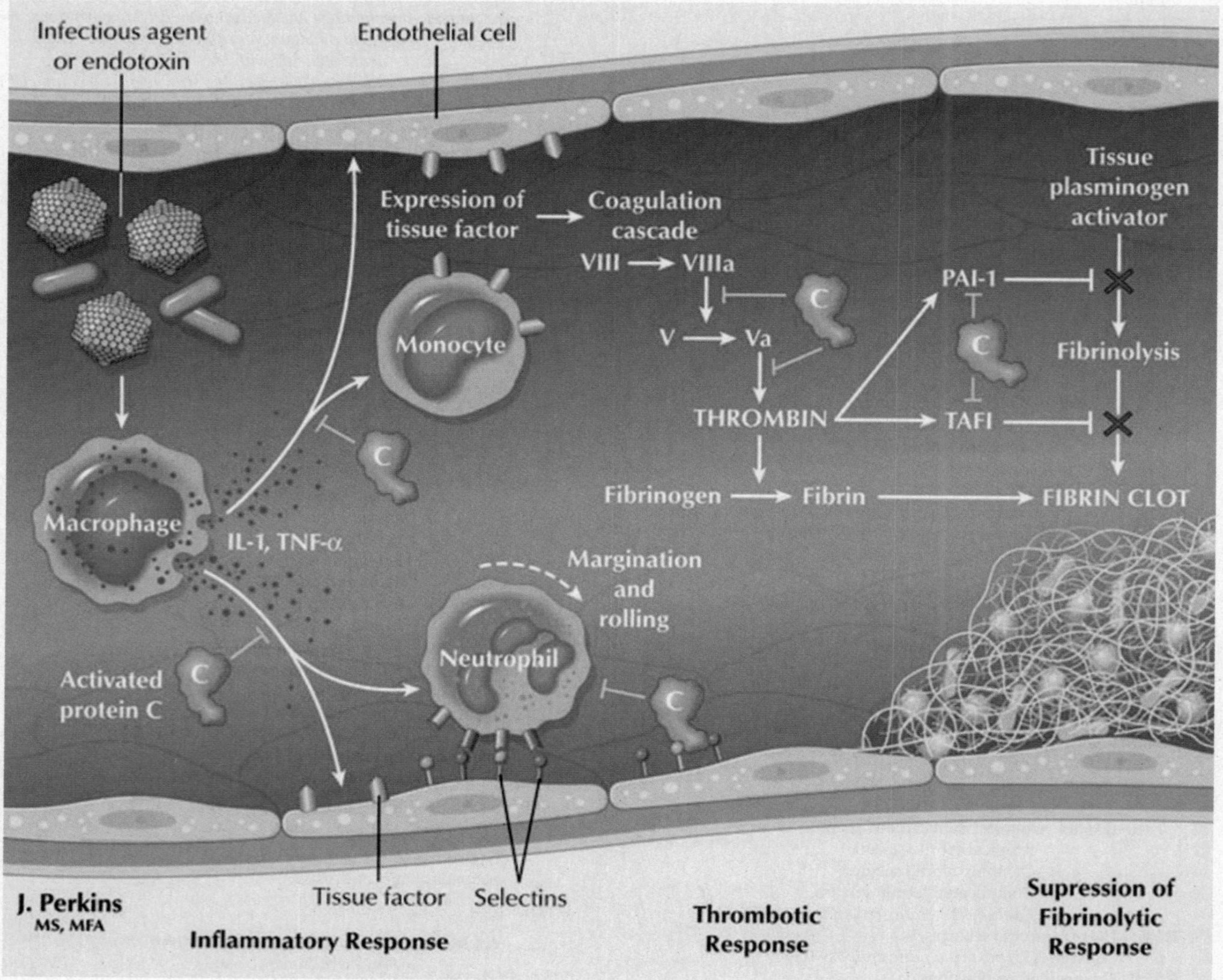

R63 Symptoms and signs concerning food and fluid intake

Excludes1: *bulimia NOS (F50.2)*

R63.0 Anorexia

Loss of appetite

Excludes1: *anorexia nervosa (F50.0-)*
loss of appetite of nonorganic origin (F50.89)

R63.1 Polydipsia

Excessive thirst

R63.2 Polyphagia

Excessive eating
Hyperalimentation NOS

\+ **R63.3 Feeding difficulties**

Excludes2: *eating disorders (F50.-)*
feeding problems of newborn (P92.-)
infant feeding disorder of nonorganic origin (F98.2-)

R63.30 Feeding difficulties, unspecified

● **R63.31 Pediatric feeding disorder, acute**

Pediatric feeding dysfunction, acute
Code also, if applicable, associated conditions such as:
aspiration pneumonia (J69.0)
dysphagia (R13.1-)
gastro-esophageal reflux disease (K21.-)
malnutrition (E40-E46)

● **R63.32 Pediatric feeding disorder, chronic**

Pediatric feeding dysfunction, chronic
Code also, if applicable, associated conditions such as:
aspiration pneumonia (J69.0)
dysphagia (R13.1-)
gastro-esophageal reflux disease (K21.-)
malnutrition (E40-E46)

R63.39 Other feeding difficulties

Feeding problem (elderly) (infant) NOS
Picky eater

R63.4 Abnormal weight loss

R63.5 Abnormal weight gain

Excludes1: *excessive weight gain in pregnancy (O26.0-)*
obesity (E66.-)

R63.6 Underweight

Use additional code to identify body mass index (BMI), if known (Z68.-)

Excludes1: *abnormal weight loss (R63.4)*
anorexia nervosa (F50.0-)
malnutrition (E40-E46)

R63.8 Other symptoms and signs concerning food and fluid intake

CC **R64 Cachexia**

Wasting syndrome
Code first underlying condition, if known

Excludes1: *abnormal weight loss (R63.4)*
nutritional marasmus (E41)

AHA CC: 3Q, 2017, 24-25

Valid 3-character code, no further characters required

R65 Symptoms and signs specifically associated with systemic inflammation and infection
See page 966 for Sepsis illustration.

+ **R65.1 Systemic inflammatory response syndrome (SIRS) of non-infectious origin**
  Code first underlying condition, such as:
  heatstroke (T67.0-)
  injury and trauma (S00-T88)
  Excludes1: *sepsis- code to infection*
  severe sepsis (R65.2)

CC **R65.10 Systemic inflammatory response syndrome (SIRS) of non-infectious origin without acute organ dysfunction**
  Systemic inflammatory response syndrome (SIRS) NOS
  AHA CC: 2Q, 2019, 24-26, 38
  Review coding guideline C.18.g

MCC **R65.11 Systemic inflammatory response syndrome (SIRS) of non-infectious origin with acute organ dysfunction**
  Use additional code to identify specific acute organ dysfunction, such as:
  acute kidney failure (N17.-)
  acute respiratory failure (J96.0-)
  critical illness myopathy (G72.81)
  critical illness polyneuropathy (G62.81)
  disseminated intravascular coagulopathy [DIC] (D65)
  encephalopathy (metabolic) (septic) (G93.41)
  hepatic failure (K72.0-)
  Review coding guideline C.18.g

+ **R65.2 Severe sepsis**
  Infection with associated acute organ dysfunction
  Sepsis with acute organ dysfunction
  Sepsis with multiple organ dysfunction
  Systemic inflammatory response syndrome due to infectious process with acute organ dysfunction
  Code first underlying infection, such as:
  infection following a procedure (T81.4-)
  infections following infusion, transfusion and therapeutic injection (T80.2-)
  puerperal sepsis (O85)
  sepsis following complete or unspecified spontaneous abortion (O03.87)
  sepsis following ectopic and molar pregnancy (O08.82)
  sepsis following incomplete spontaneous abortion (O03.37)
  sepsis following (induced) termination of pregnancy (O04.87)
  sepsis NOS (A41.9)

  Use additional code to identify specific acute organ dysfunction, such as:
  acute kidney failure (N17.-)
  acute respiratory failure (J96.0-)
  critical illness myopathy (G72.81)
  critical illness polyneuropathy (G62.81)
  disseminated intravascular coagulopathy [DIC] (D65)
  encephalopathy (metabolic) (septic) (G93.41)
  hepatic failure (K72.0-)
  AHA CC: 4Q, 2017, 98-99
  Review coding guideline C.1.d

MCC **R65.20 Severe sepsis without septic shock**
  Severe sepsis NOS
  AHA CC: 3Q, 2016, 14; 2Q, 2020, 17-18

MCC **R65.21 Severe sepsis with septic shock**
  Review coding guideline C.1.d.2 and C.1.d.5.c

R68 Other general symptoms and signs

R68.0 Hypothermia, not associated with low environmental temperature
  Excludes1: *hypothermia NOS (accidental) (T68)*
  hypothermia due to anesthesia (T88.51)
  hypothermia due to low environmental temperature (T68)
  newborn hypothermia (P80.-)

+ **R68.1 Nonspecific symptoms peculiar to infancy**
  Excludes1: *colic, infantile (R10.83)*
  neonatal cerebral irritability (P91.3)
  teething syndrome (K00.7)

• **R68.11 Excessive crying of infant (baby)**
  Excludes1: *excessive crying of child, adolescent, or adult (R45.83)*

• **R68.12 Fussy infant (baby)**
  Irritable infant

• **R68.13 Apparent life threatening event in infant (ALTE)**
  Apparent life threatening event in newborn
  Brief resolved unexplained event (BRUE)
  Code first confirmed diagnosis, if known

  Use additional code(s) for associated signs and symptoms if no confirmed diagnosis established, or if signs and symptoms are not associated routinely with confirmed diagnosis, or provide additional information for cause of ALTE

• **R68.19 Other nonspecific symptoms peculiar to infancy**

R68.2 Dry mouth, unspecified
  Excludes1: *dry mouth due to dehydration (E86.0)*
  dry mouth due to Sjögren syndrome (M35.0-)
  salivary gland hyposecretion (K11.7)

R68.3 Clubbing of fingers
  Clubbing of nails
  Excludes1: *congenital clubfinger (Q68.1)*

+ **R68.8 Other general symptoms and signs**

R68.81 Early satiety

• **R68.82 Decreased libido**
  Decreased sexual desire

R68.83 Chills (without fever)
  Chills NOS
  Excludes1: *chills with fever (R50.9)*

R68.84 Jaw pain
  Mandibular pain
  Maxilla pain
  Excludes1: *temporomandibular joint arthralgia (M26.62-)*

R68.89 Other general symptoms and signs

R69 Illness, unspecified
  Unknown and unspecified cases of morbidity
  Valid 3-character code, no further characters required

Abnormal findings on examination of blood, without diagnosis (R70-R79)

Excludes2: *abnormal findings on antenatal screening of mother (O28.-)*
abnormalities of lipids (E78.-)
abnormalities of platelets and thrombocytes (D69.-)
abnormalities of white blood cells classified elsewhere (D70-D72)
coagulation hemorrhagic disorders (D65-D68)
diagnostic abnormal findings classified elsewhere - see Alphabetic Index
hemorrhagic and hematological disorders of newborn (P50-P61)

R70 Elevated erythrocyte sedimentation rate and abnormality of plasma viscosity

R70.0 Elevated erythrocyte sedimentation rate

R70.1 Abnormal plasma viscosity

R71 Abnormality of red blood cells
  Excludes1: *anemias (D50-D64)*
  anemia of premature infant (P61.2)
  benign (familial) polycythemia (D75.0)
  congenital anemias (P61.2-P61.4)
  newborn anemia due to isoimmunization (P55.-)
  polycythemia neonatorum (P61.1)
  polycythemia NOS (D75.1)
  polycythemia vera (D45)
  secondary polycythemia (D75.1)

CC **R71.0 Precipitous drop in hematocrit**
  Drop (precipitous) in hemoglobin
  Drop in hematocrit

R71.8 Other abnormality of red blood cells
  Abnormal red-cell morphology NOS
  Abnormal red-cell volume NOS
  Anisocytosis
  Poikilocytosis

R73 Elevated blood glucose level

Excludes1: *diabetes mellitus (E08-E13)*
diabetes mellitus in pregnancy, childbirth and the puerperium (O24.-)
neonatal disorders (P70.0-P70.2)
postsurgical hypoinsulinemia (E89.1)

+ **R73.0 Abnormal glucose**

Excludes1: *abnormal glucose in pregnancy (O99.81-)*
diabetes mellitus (E08-E13)
dysmetabolic syndrome X (E88.81)
gestational diabetes (O24.4-)
glycosuria (R81)
hypoglycemia (E16.2)

R73.01 Impaired fasting glucose
Elevated fasting glucose

R73.02 Impaired glucose tolerance (oral)
Elevated glucose tolerance

R73.03 Prediabetes
Latent diabetes
AHA CC: 4Q, 2016, 65

R73.09 Other abnormal glucose
Abnormal glucose NOS
Abnormal non-fasting glucose tolerance

R73.9 Hyperglycemia, unspecified

R74 Abnormal serum enzyme levels

+ **R74.0 Nonspecific elevation of levels of transaminase and lactic acid dehydrogenase [LDH]**
AHA CC: 4Q, 2020, 39

R74.01 Elevation of levels of liver transaminase levels
Elevation of levels of alanine transaminase (ALT)
Elevation of levels of aspartate transaminase (AST)

R74.02 Elevation of levels of lactic acid dehydrogenase [LDH]

R74.8 Abnormal levels of other serum enzymes
Abnormal level of acid phosphatase
Abnormal level of alkaline phosphatase
Abnormal level of amylase
Abnormal level of lipase [triacylglycerol lipase]
AHA CC: 2Q, 2019, 6

R74.9 Abnormal serum enzyme level, unspecified

R75 Inconclusive laboratory evidence of human immunodeficiency virus [HIV]

Nonconclusive HIV-test finding in infants
Excludes1: *asymptomatic human immunodeficiency virus [HIV] infection status (Z21)*
human immunodeficiency virus [HIV] disease (B20)
Review coding guidelines C.1.a.2.e and C.1.a.2.f
Valid 3-character code, no further characters required

R76 Other abnormal immunological findings in serum

R76.0 Raised antibody titer
Excludes1: *isoimmunization in pregnancy (O36.0-O36.1)*
isoimmunization affecting newborn (P55.-)
AHA CC: 1Q, 2021, 6-7

+ **R76.1 Nonspecific reaction to test for tuberculosis**

R76.11 Nonspecific reaction to tuberculin skin test without active tuberculosis
Abnormal result of Mantoux test
PPD positive
Tuberculin (skin test) positive
Tuberculin (skin test) reactor
Excludes1: *nonspecific reaction to cell mediated immunity measurement of gamma interferon antigen response without active tuberculosis (R76.12)*

R76.12 Nonspecific reaction to cell mediated immunity measurement of gamma interferon antigen response without active tuberculosis
Nonspecific reaction to QuantiFERON-TB test (QFT) without active tuberculosis
Excludes1: *nonspecific reaction to tuberculin skin test without active tuberculosis (R76.11)*
positive tuberculin skin test (R76.11)

R76.8 Other specified abnormal immunological findings in serum
Raised level of immunoglobulins NOS
AHA CC: 1Q, 2021, 6-7

R76.9 Abnormal immunological finding in serum, unspecified

R77 Other abnormalities of plasma proteins

Excludes1: *disorders of plasma-protein metabolism (E88.0-)*

R77.0 Abnormality of albumin

R77.1 Abnormality of globulin
Hyperglobulinemia NOS

R77.2 Abnormality of alphafetoprotein

R77.8 Other specified abnormalities of plasma proteins

R77.9 Abnormality of plasma protein, unspecified
AHA CC: 2Q, 2019, 6

R78 Findings of drugs and other substances, not normally found in blood

Use additional code to identify the any retained foreign body, if applicable (Z18.-)
Excludes1: *mental or behavioral disorders due to psychoactive substance use (F10-F19)*

R78.0 Finding of alcohol in blood
external cause code (Y90.-), for detail regarding alcohol level.

R78.1 Finding of opiate drug in blood

R78.2 Finding of cocaine in blood

R78.3 Finding of hallucinogen in blood

R78.4 Finding of other drugs of addictive potential in blood

R78.5 Finding of other psychotropic drug in blood

R78.6 Finding of steroid agent in blood

+ **R78.7 Finding of abnormal level of heavy metals in blood**

R78.71 Abnormal lead level in blood
Excludes1: *lead poisoning (T56.0-)*

R78.79 Finding of abnormal level of heavy metals in blood

+ **R78.8 Finding of other specified substances, not normally found in blood**

CC **R78.81 Bacteremia**
Excludes1: *sepsis-code to specified infection*

R78.89 Finding of other specified substances, not normally found in blood
Finding of abnormal level of lithium in blood

R78.9 Finding of unspecified substance, not normally found in blood

R79 Other abnormal findings of blood chemistry

Use additional code to identify any retained foreign body, if applicable (Z18.-)
Excludes1: *asymptomatic hyperuricemia (E79.0)*
hyperglycemia NOS (R73.9)
hypoglycemia NOS (E16.2)
neonatal hypoglycemia (P70.3-P70.4)
specific findings indicating disorder of amino-acid metabolism (E70-E72)
specific findings indicating disorder of carbohydrate metabolism (E73-E74)
specific findings indicating disorder of lipid metabolism (E75.-)

R79.0 Abnormal level of blood mineral
Abnormal blood level of cobalt
Abnormal blood level of copper
Abnormal blood level of iron
Abnormal blood level of magnesium
Abnormal blood level of mineral NEC
Abnormal blood level of zinc
Excludes1: *abnormal level of lithium (R78.89)*
disorders of mineral metabolism (E83.-)
neonatal hypomagnesemia (P71.2)
nutritional mineral deficiency (E58-E61)

R79.1 Abnormal coagulation profile
Abnormal or prolonged bleeding time
Abnormal or prolonged coagulation time
Abnormal or prolonged partial thromboplastin time [PTT]
Abnormal or prolonged prothrombin time [PT]
Excludes2: *abnormality of fluid, electrolyte or acid-base balance (E86-E87)*
coagulation defects (D68.-)

+ **R79.8 Other specified abnormal findings of blood chemistry**
R79.81 Abnormal blood-gas level
R79.82 Elevated C-reactive protein (CRP)
R79.83 Abnormal findings of blood amino-acid level
Homocysteinemia
Excludes1: *disorders of amino-acid metabolism (E70-E72)*
R79.89 Other specified abnormal findings of blood chemistry
AHA CC: 2Q, 2019, 6
R79.9 Abnormal finding of blood chemistry, unspecified

Abnormal findings on examination of urine, without diagnosis (R80-R82)

Excludes1: *abnormal findings on antenatal screening of mother (O28.-)*
diagnostic abnormal findings classified elsewhere - see Alphabetical Index
specific findings indicating disorder of amino-acid metabolism (E70-E72)
specific findings indicating disorder of carbohydrate metabolism (E73-E74)

R80 Proteinuria
Excludes1: *gestational proteinuria (O12.1-)*
R80.0 Isolated proteinuria
Idiopathic proteinuria
Excludes1: *isolated proteinuria with specific morphological lesion (N06.-)*
R80.1 Persistent proteinuria, unspecified
R80.2 Orthostatic proteinuria, unspecified
Postural proteinuria
R80.3 Bence Jones proteinuria
R80.8 Other proteinuria
R80.9 Proteinuria, unspecified
Albuminuria NOS

R81 Glycosuria
Excludes1: *renal glycosuria (E74.818)*
Valid 3-character code, no further characters required

R82 Other and unspecified abnormal findings in urine
Includes: chromoabnormalities in urine
Use additional code to identify any retained foreign body, if applicable (Z18.-)
Excludes2: *hematuria (R31.-)*
CC **R82.0 Chyluria**
Excludes1: *filarial chyluria (B74.-)*
CC **R82.1 Myoglobinuria**
R82.2 Biliuria
R82.3 Hemoglobinuria
Excludes1: *hemoglobinuria due to hemolysis from external causes NEC (D59.6)*
hemoglobinuria due to paroxysmal nocturnal [Marchiafava-Micheli] (D59.5)
R82.4 Acetonuria
Ketonuria
R82.5 Elevated urine levels of drugs, medicaments and biological substances
Elevated urine levels of catecholamines
Elevated urine levels of indoleacetic acid
Elevated urine levels of 17-ketosteroids
Elevated urine levels of steroids
R82.6 Abnormal urine levels of substances chiefly nonmedicinal as to source
Abnormal urine level of heavy metals
+ **R82.7 Abnormal findings on microbiological examination of urine**
Excludes1: *colonization status (Z22.-)*
AHA CC: 4Q, 2016, 65
R82.71 Bacteriuria
R82.79 Other abnormal findings on microbiological examination of urine
Positive culture findings of urine
+ **R82.8 Abnormal findings on cytological and histological examination of urine**
AHA CC: 4Q, 2019, 16
R82.81 Pyuria
Sterile pyuria
AHA CC: 4Q, 2019, 16
R82.89 Other abnormal findings on cytological and histological examination of urine
+ **R82.9 Other and unspecified abnormal findings in urine**
R82.90 Unspecified abnormal findings in urine
R82.91 Other chromoabnormalities of urine
Chromoconversion (dipstick)
Idiopathic dipstick converts positive for blood with no cellular forms in sediment
Excludes1: *hemoglobinuria (R82.3)*
myoglobinuria (R82.1)
+ **R82.99 Other abnormal findings in urine**
AHA CC: 4Q, 2018, 29-30
R82.991 Hypocitraturia
R82.992 Hyperoxaluria
Excludes1: *Primary hyperoxaluria (E72.53)*
R82.993 Hyperuricosuria
R82.994 Hypercalciuria
Idiopathic hypercalciuria
R82.998 Other abnormal findings in urine
Cells and casts in urine
Crystalluria
Melanuria

Abnormal findings on examination of other body fluids, substances and tissues, without diagnosis (R83-R89)

Excludes1: *abnormal findings on antenatal screening of mother (O28.-)*
diagnostic abnormal findings classified elsewhere - see Alphabetical Index

Excludes2: *abnormal findings on examination of blood, without diagnosis (R70-R79)*
abnormal findings on examination of urine, without diagnosis (R80-R82)
abnormal tumor markers (R97.-)

R83 Abnormal findings in cerebrospinal fluid
R83.0 Abnormal level of enzymes in cerebrospinal fluid
R83.1 Abnormal level of hormones in cerebrospinal fluid
R83.2 Abnormal level of other drugs, medicaments and biological substances in cerebrospinal fluid
R83.3 Abnormal level of substances chiefly nonmedicinal as to source in cerebrospinal fluid
R83.4 Abnormal immunological findings in cerebrospinal fluid
R83.5 Abnormal microbiological findings in cerebrospinal fluid
Positive culture findings in cerebrospinal fluid
Excludes1: *colonization status (Z22.-)*
R83.6 Abnormal cytological findings in cerebrospinal fluid
R83.8 Other abnormal findings in cerebrospinal fluid
Abnormal chromosomal findings in cerebrospinal fluid
R83.9 Unspecified abnormal finding in cerebrospinal fluid

R84 Abnormal findings in specimens from respiratory organs and thorax
Includes: abnormal findings in bronchial washings
abnormal findings in nasal secretions
abnormal findings in pleural fluid
abnormal findings in sputum
abnormal findings in throat scrapings
Excludes1: *blood-stained sputum (R04.2)*
R84.0 Abnormal level of enzymes in specimens from respiratory organs and thorax
R84.1 Abnormal level of hormones in specimens from respiratory organs and thorax
R84.2 Abnormal level of other drugs, medicaments and biological substances in specimens from respiratory organs and thorax
R84.3 Abnormal level of substances chiefly nonmedicinal as to source in specimens from respiratory organs and thorax
R84.4 Abnormal immunological findings in specimens from respiratory organs and thorax
R84.5 Abnormal microbiological findings in specimens from respiratory organs and thorax
Positive culture findings in specimens from respiratory organs and thorax
Excludes1: *colonization status (Z22.-)*
R84.6 Abnormal cytological findings in specimens from respiratory organs and thorax
R84.7 Abnormal histological findings in specimens from respiratory organs and thorax

R84.8 Other abnormal findings in specimens from respiratory organs and thorax
Abnormal chromosomal findings in specimens from respiratory organs and thorax
R84.9 Unspecified abnormal finding in specimens from respiratory organs and thorax

R85 Abnormal findings in specimens from digestive organs and abdominal cavity
Includes: abnormal findings in peritoneal fluid
abnormal findings in saliva
Excludes1: *cloudy peritoneal dialysis effluent (R88.0)*
fecal abnormalities (R19.5)
R85.0 Abnormal level of enzymes in specimens from digestive organs and abdominal cavity
R85.1 Abnormal level of hormones in specimens from digestive organs and abdominal cavity
R85.2 Abnormal level of other drugs, medicaments and biological substances in specimens from digestive organs and abdominal cavity
R85.3 Abnormal level of substances chiefly nonmedicinal as to source in specimens from digestive organs and abdominal cavity
R85.4 Abnormal immunological findings in specimens from digestive organs and abdominal cavity
R85.5 Abnormal microbiological findings in specimens from digestive organs and abdominal cavity
Positive culture findings in specimens from digestive organs and abdominal cavity
Excludes1: *colonization status (Z22.-)*
+ **R85.6 Abnormal cytological findings in specimens from digestive organs and abdominal cavity**
+ **R85.61 Abnormal cytologic smear of anus**
Excludes1: *abnormal cytological findings in specimens from other digestive organs and abdominal cavity (R85.69)*
carcinoma in situ of anus (histologically confirmed) (D01.3)
anal intraepithelial neoplasia I [AIN I] (K62.82)
anal intraepithelial neoplasia II [AIN II] (K62.82)
anal intraepithelial neoplasia III [AIN III] (D01.3)
dysplasia (mild) (moderate) of anus (histologically confirmed) (K62.82)
severe dysplasia of anus (histologically confirmed) (D01.3)
Excludes2: *anal high risk human papillomavirus (HPV) DNA test positive (R85.81)*
anal low risk human papillomavirus (HPV) DNA test positive (R85.82)
R85.610 Atypical squamous cells of undetermined significance on cytologic smear of anus (ASC-US)
R85.611 Atypical squamous cells cannot exclude high grade squamous intraepithelial lesion on cytologic smear of anus (ASC-H)
R85.612 Low grade squamous intraepithelial lesion on cytologic smear of anus (LGSIL)
R85.613 High grade squamous intraepithelial lesion on cytologic smear of anus (HGSIL)
R85.614 Cytologic evidence of malignancy on smear of anus
R85.615 Unsatisfactory cytologic smear of anus
Inadequate sample of cytologic smear of anus
R85.616 Satisfactory anal smear but lacking transformation zone
R85.618 Other abnormal cytological findings on specimens from anus
R85.619 Unspecified abnormal cytological findings in specimens from anus
Abnormal anal cytology NOS
Atypical glandular cells of anus NOS
R85.69 Abnormal cytological findings in specimens from other digestive organs and abdominal cavity
R85.7 Abnormal histological findings in specimens from digestive organs and abdominal cavity
+ **R85.8 Other abnormal findings in specimens from digestive organs and abdominal cavity**
R85.81 Anal high risk human papillomavirus (HPV) DNA test positive
Excludes1: *anogenital warts due to human papillomavirus (HPV) (A63.0)*
condyloma acuminatum (A63.0)
R85.82 Anal low risk human papillomavirus (HPV) DNA test positive
Use additional code for associated human papillomavirus (B97.7)
R85.89 Other abnormal findings in specimens from digestive organs and abdominal cavity
Abnormal chromosomal findings in specimens from digestive organs and abdominal cavity
R85.9 Unspecified abnormal finding in specimens from digestive organs and abdominal cavity

R86 Abnormal findings in specimens from male genital organs
Includes: abnormal findings in prostatic secretions
abnormal findings in semen, seminal fluid
abnormal spermatozoa
Excludes1: *azoospermia (N46.0-)*
oligospermia (N46.1-)
♂ **R86.0 Abnormal level of enzymes in specimens from male genital organs**
♂ **R86.1 Abnormal level of hormones in specimens from male genital organs**
♂ **R86.2 Abnormal level of other drugs, medicaments and biological substances in specimens from male genital organs**
♂ **R86.3 Abnormal level of substances chiefly nonmedicinal as to source in specimens from male genital organs**
♂ **R86.4 Abnormal immunological findings in specimens from male genital organs**
♂ **R86.5 Abnormal microbiological findings in specimens from male genital organs**
Positive culture findings in specimens from male genital organs
Excludes1: *colonization status (Z22.-)*
♂ **R86.6 Abnormal cytological findings in specimens from male genital organs**
♂ **R86.7 Abnormal histological findings in specimens from male genital organs**
♂ **R86.8 Other abnormal findings in specimens from male genital organs**
Abnormal chromosomal findings in specimens from male genital organs
♂ **R86.9 Unspecified abnormal finding in specimens from male genital organs**

R87 Abnormal findings in specimens from female genital organs
Includes: abnormal findings in secretion and smears from cervix uteri
abnormal findings in secretion and smears from vagina
abnormal findings in secretion and smears from vulva
♀ **R87.0 Abnormal level of enzymes in specimens from female genital organs**
♀ **R87.1 Abnormal level of hormones in specimens from female genital organs**
♀ **R87.2 Abnormal level of other drugs, medicaments and biological substances in specimens from female genital organs**
♀ **R87.3 Abnormal level of substances chiefly nonmedicinal as to source in specimens from female genital organs**
♀ **R87.4 Abnormal immunological findings in specimens from female genital organs**
♀ **R87.5 Abnormal microbiological findings in specimens from female genital organs**
Positive culture findings in specimens from female genital organs
Excludes1: *colonization status (Z22.-)*

+ **R87.6 Abnormal cytological findings in specimens from female genital organs**

+ **R87.61 Abnormal cytological findings in specimens from cervix uteri**

Excludes1: *abnormal cytological findings in specimens from other female genital organs (R87.69)*
abnormal cytological findings in specimens from vagina (R87.62-)
carcinoma in situ of cervix uteri (histologically confirmed) (D06.-)
cervical intraepithelial neoplasia I [CIN I] (N87.0)
cervical intraepithelial neoplasia II [CIN II] (N87.1)
cervical intraepithelial neoplasia III [CIN III] (D06.-)
dysplasia (mild) (moderate) of cervix uteri (histologically confirmed) (N87.-)
severe dysplasia of cervix uteri (histologically confirmed) (D06.-)

Excludes2: *cervical high risk human papillomavirus (HPV) DNA test positive (R87.810)*
cervical low risk human papillomavirus (HPV) DNA test positive (R87.820)

♀ **R87.610 Atypical squamous cells of undetermined significance on cytologic smear of cervix (ASC-US)**

♀ **R87.611 Atypical squamous cells cannot exclude high grade squamous intraepithelial lesion on cytologic smear of cervix (ASC-H)**

♀ **R87.612 Low grade squamous intraepithelial lesion on cytologic smear of cervix (LGSIL)**

♀ **R87.613 High grade squamous intraepithelial lesion on cytologic smear of cervix (HGSIL)**

♀ **R87.614 Cytologic evidence of malignancy on smear of cervix**

♀ **R87.615 Unsatisfactory cytologic smear of cervix**
Inadequate sample of cytologic smear of cervix

♀ **R87.616 Satisfactory cervical smear but lacking transformation zone**

♀ **R87.618 Other abnormal cytological findings on specimens from cervix uteri**

♀ **R87.619 Unspecified abnormal cytological findings in specimens from cervix uteri**
Abnormal cervical cytology NOS
Abnormal Papanicolaou smear of cervix NOS
Abnormal thin preparation smear of cervix NOS
Atypical endocervial cells of cervix NOS
Atypical endometrial cells of cervix NOS
Atypical glandular cells of cervix NOS

+ **R87.62 Abnormal cytological findings in specimens from vagina**
Use additional code to identify acquired absence of uterus and cervix, if applicable (Z90.71-)

Excludes1: *abnormal cytological findings in specimens from cervix uteri (R87.61-)*
abnormal cytological findings in specimens from other female genital organs (R87.69)
carcinoma in situ of vagina (histologically confirmed) (D07.2)
vaginal intraepithelial neoplasia I [VAIN I] (N89.0)
vaginal intraepithelial neoplasia II [VAIN II] (N89.1)
vaginal intraepithelial neoplasia III [VAIN III] (D07.2)
dysplasia (mild) (moderate) of vagina (histologically confirmed) (N89.-)
severe dysplasia of vagina (histologically confirmed) (D07.2)

Excludes2: *vaginal high risk human papillomavirus (HPV) DNA test positive (R87.811)*
vaginal low risk human papillomavirus (HPV) DNA test positive (R87.821)

♀ **R87.620 Atypical squamous cells of undetermined significance on cytologic smear of vagina (ASC-US)**

♀ **R87.621 Atypical squamous cells cannot exclude high grade squamous intraepithelial lesion on cytologic smear of vagina (ASC-H)**

♀ **R87.622 Low grade squamous intraepithelial lesion on cytologic smear of vagina (LGSIL)**

♀ **R87.623 High grade squamous intraepithelial lesion on cytologic smear of vagina (HGSIL)**

♀ **R87.624 Cytologic evidence of malignancy on smear of vagina**

♀ **R87.625 Unsatisfactory cytologic smear of vagina**
Inadequate sample of cytologic smear of vagina

♀ **R87.628 Other abnormal cytological findings on specimens from vagina**

♀ **R87.629 Unspecified abnormal cytological findings in specimens from vagina**
Abnormal Papanicolaou smear of vagina NOS
Abnormal thin preparation smear of vagina NOS
Abnormal vaginal cytology NOS
Atypical endocervical cells of vagina NOS
Atypical endometrial cells of vagina NOS
Atypical glandular cells of vagina NOS

♀ **R87.69 Abnormal cytological findings in specimens from other female genital organs**
Abnormal cytological findings in specimens from female genital organs NOS

Excludes1: *dysplasia of vulva (histologically confirmed) (N90.0-N90.3)*

♀ **R87.7 Abnormal histological findings in specimens from female genital organs**

Excludes1: *carcinoma in situ (histologically confirmed) of female genital organs (D06-D07.3)*
cervical intraepithelial neoplasia I [CIN I] (N87.0)
cervical intraepithelial neoplasia II [CIN II] (N87.1)
cervical intraepithelial neoplasia III [CIN III] (D06.-)
dysplasia (mild) (moderate) of cervix uteri (histologically confirmed) (N87.-)
dysplasia (mild) (moderate) of vagina (histologically confirmed) (N89.-)
vaginal intraepithelial neoplasia I [VAIN I] (N89.0)
vaginal intraepithelial neoplasia II [VAIN II] (N89.1)
vaginal intraepithelial neoplasia III [VAIN III] (D07.2)
severe dysplasia of cervix uteri (histologically confirmed) (D06.-)
severe dysplasia of vagina (histologically confirmed) (D07.2)

+ **R87.8 Other abnormal findings in specimens from female genital organs**

+ **R87.81 High risk human papillomavirus (HPV) DNA test positive from female genital organs**

Excludes1: *anogenital warts due to human papillomavirus (HPV) (A63.0)*
condyloma acuminatum (A63.0)

♀ **R87.810 Cervical high risk human papillomavirus (HPV) DNA test positive**

♀ **R87.811 Vaginal high risk human papillomavirus (HPV) DNA test positive**

+ **R87.82 Low risk human papillomavirus (HPV) DNA test positive from female genital organs**

Use additional code for associated human papillomavirus (B97.7)

♀ **R87.820 Cervical low risk human papillomavirus (HPV) DNA test positive**

♀ **R87.821 Vaginal low risk human papillomavirus (HPV) DNA test positive**

♀ **R87.89 Other abnormal findings in specimens from female genital organs**

Abnormal chromosomal findings in specimens from female genital organs

♀ **R87.9 Unspecified abnormal finding in specimens from female genital organs**

R88 Abnormal findings in other body fluids and substances

R88.0 Cloudy (hemodialysis) (peritoneal) dialysis effluent

R88.8 Abnormal findings in other body fluids and substances

R89 Abnormal findings in specimens from other organs, systems and tissues

Includes: abnormal findings in nipple discharge
abnormal findings in synovial fluid
abnormal findings in wound secretions

R89.0 Abnormal level of enzymes in specimens from other organs, systems and tissues

R89.1 Abnormal level of hormones in specimens from other organs, systems and tissues

R89.2 Abnormal level of other drugs, medicaments and biological substances in specimens from other organs, systems and tissues

R89.3 Abnormal level of substances chiefly nonmedicinal as to source in specimens from other organs, systems and tissues

R89.4 Abnormal immunological findings in specimens from other organs, systems and tissues

R89.5 Abnormal microbiological findings in specimens from other organs, systems and tissues

Positive culture findings in specimens from other organs, systems and tissues

Excludes1: *colonization status (Z22.-)*

R89.6 Abnormal cytological findings in specimens from other organs, systems and tissues

R89.7 Abnormal histological findings in specimens from other organs, systems and tissues

R89.8 Other abnormal findings in specimens from other organs, systems and tissues

Abnormal chromosomal findings in specimens from other organs, systems and tissues

R89.9 Unspecified abnormal finding in specimens from other organs, systems and tissues

Abnormal findings on diagnostic imaging and in function studies, without diagnosis (R90-R94)

Includes: nonspecific abnormal findings on diagnostic imaging by computerized axial tomography [CAT scan]
nonspecific abnormal findings on diagnostic imaging by magnetic resonance imaging [MRI][NMR]
nonspecific abnormal findings on diagnostic imaging by positron emission tomography [PET scan]
nonspecific abnormal findings on diagnostic imaging by thermography
nonspecific abnormal findings on diagnostic imaging by ultrasound [echogram]
nonspecific abnormal findings on diagnostic imaging by X-ray examination

Excludes1: *abnormal findings on antenatal screening of mother (O28.-)*
diagnostic abnormal findings classified elsewhere - see Alphabetical Index

R90 Abnormal findings on diagnostic imaging of central nervous system

R90.0 Intracranial space-occupying lesion found on diagnostic imaging of central nervous system

+ **R90.8 Other abnormal findings on diagnostic imaging of central nervous system**

R90.81 Abnormal echoencephalogram

R90.82 White matter disease, unspecified

R90.89 Other abnormal findings on diagnostic imaging of central nervous system

Other cerebrovascular abnormality found on diagnostic imaging of central nervous system

R91 Abnormal findings on diagnostic imaging of lung

R91.1 Solitary pulmonary nodule

Coin lesion lung
Solitary pulmonary nodule, subsegmental branch of the bronchial tree

R91.8 Other nonspecific abnormal finding of lung field

Lung mass NOS found on diagnostic imaging of lung
Pulmonary infiltrate NOS
Shadow, lung

R92 Abnormal and inconclusive findings on diagnostic imaging of breast

R92.0 Mammographic microcalcification found on diagnostic imaging of breast

Excludes2: *mammographic calcification (calculus) found on diagnostic imaging of breast (R92.1)*

R92.1 Mammographic calcification found on diagnostic imaging of breast

Mammographic calculus found on diagnostic imaging of breast

R92.2 Inconclusive mammogram

Dense breasts NOS
Inconclusive mammogram NEC
Inconclusive mammography due to dense breasts
Inconclusive mammography NEC
AHA CC: 1Q, 2015, 24

R92.8 Other abnormal and inconclusive findings on diagnostic imaging of breast

R93 Abnormal findings on diagnostic imaging of other body structures

R93.0 Abnormal findings on diagnostic imaging of skull and head, not elsewhere classified

Excludes1: *intracranial space-occupying lesion found on diagnostic imaging (R90.0)*

R93.1 Abnormal findings on diagnostic imaging of heart and coronary circulation

Abnormal echocardiogram NOS
Abnormal heart shadow

R93.2 Abnormal findings on diagnostic imaging of liver and biliary tract

Nonvisualization of gallbladder

R93.3 **Abnormal findings on diagnostic imaging of other parts of digestive tract**

+ R93.4 **Abnormal findings on diagnostic imaging of urinary organs**

Excludes2: *hypertrophy of kidney (N28.81)*

AHA CC: 4Q, 2016, 66

R93.41 **Abnormal radiologic findings on diagnostic imaging of of renal pelvis, ureter, or bladder**

Filling defect of bladder found on diagnostic imaging

Filling defect of renal pelvis found on diagnostic imaging

Filling defect of ureter found on diagnostic imaging

+ R93.42 **Abnormal radiologic findings on diagnostic imaging of kidney**

R93.421 **Abnormal radiologic findings on diagnostic imaging of right kidney**

R93.422 **Abnormal radiologic findings on diagnostic imaging of left kidney**

R93.429 **Abnormal radiologic findings on diagnostic imaging of unspecified kidney**

R93.49 **Abnormal radiologic findings on diagnostic imaging of other urinary organs**

R93.5 **Abnormal findings on diagnostic imaging of other abdominal regions, including retroperitoneum**

R93.6 **Abnormal findings on diagnostic imaging of limbs**

Excludes2: *abnormal finding in skin and subcutaneous tissue (R93.8-)*

AHA CC: 1Q, 2020, 14-15

R93.7 **Abnormal findings on diagnostic imaging of other parts of musculoskeletal system**

Excludes2: *abnormal findings on diagnostic imaging of skull (R93.0)*

+ R93.8 **Abnormal findings on diagnostic imaging of other specified body structures**

AHA CC: 4Q, 2018, 30

+ R93.81 **Abnormal radiologic findings on diagnostic imaging of testis**

♂ R93.811 **Abnormal radiologic findings on diagnostic imaging of right testicle**

♂ R93.812 **Abnormal radiologic findings on diagnostic imaging of left testicle**

♂ R93.813 **Abnormal radiologic findings on diagnostic imaging of testicles, bilateral**

♂ R93.819 **Abnormal radiologic findings on diagnostic imaging of unspecified testicle**

R93.89 **Abnormal findings on diagnostic imaging of other specified body structures**

Abnormal findings by radioisotope localization of placenta

Abnormal radiological finding in skin and subcutaneous tissue

Mediastinal shift

R93.9 **Diagnostic imaging inconclusive due to excess body fat of patient**

R94 **Abnormal results of function studies**

Includes: abnormal results of radionuclide [radioisotope] uptake studies

abnormal results of scintigraphy

+ R94.0 **Abnormal results of function studies of central nervous system**

R94.01 **Abnormal electroencephalogram [EEG]**

R94.02 **Abnormal brain scan**

R94.09 **Abnormal results of other function studies of central nervous system**

+ R94.1 **Abnormal results of function studies of peripheral nervous system and special senses**

+ R94.11 **Abnormal results of function studies of eye**

R94.110 **Abnormal electro-oculogram [EOG]**

R94.111 **Abnormal electroretinogram [ERG]**

Abnormal retinal function study

R94.112 **Abnormal visually evoked potential [VEP]**

R94.113 **Abnormal oculomotor study**

R94.118 **Abnormal results of other function studies of eye**

+ R94.12 **Abnormal results of function studies of ear and other special senses**

R94.120 **Abnormal auditory function study**

AHA CC: 3Q, 2016, 17

R94.121 **Abnormal vestibular function study**

R94.128 **Abnormal results of other function studies of ear and other special senses**

+ R94.13 **Abnormal results of function studies of peripheral nervous system**

R94.130 **Abnormal response to nerve stimulation, unspecified**

R94.131 **Abnormal electromyogram [EMG]**

Excludes1: *electromyogram of eye (R94.113)*

R94.138 **Abnormal results of other function studies of peripheral nervous system**

R94.2 **Abnormal results of pulmonary function studies**

Reduced ventilatory capacity

Reduced vital capacity

+ R94.3 **Abnormal results of cardiovascular function studies**

R94.30 **Abnormal result of cardiovascular function study, unspecified**

R94.31 **Abnormal electrocardiogram [ECG] [EKG]**

Excludes1: *long QT syndrome (I45.81)*

R94.39 **Abnormal result of other cardiovascular function study**

Abnormal electrophysiological intracardiac studies

Abnormal phonocardiogram

Abnormal vectorcardiogram

R94.4 **Abnormal results of kidney function studies**

Abnormal renal function test

R94.5 **Abnormal results of liver function studies**

R94.6 **Abnormal results of thyroid function studies**

R94.7 **Abnormal results of other endocrine function studies**

Excludes2: *abnormal glucose (R73.0-)*

R94.8 **Abnormal results of function studies of other organs and systems**

Abnormal basal metabolic rate [BMR]

Abnormal bladder function test

Abnormal splenic function test

Abnormal tumor markers (R97)

R97 **Abnormal tumor markers**

Elevated tumor associated antigens [TAA]

Elevated tumor specific antigens [TSA]

R97.0 **Elevated carcinoembryonic antigen [CEA]**

R97.1 **Elevated cancer antigen 125 [CA 125]**

+ R97.2 **Elevated prostate specific antigen [PSA]**

AHA CC: 4Q, 2016, 66

• ♂ R97.20 **Elevated prostate specific antigen [PSA]**

• ♂ R97.21 **Rising PSA following treatment for malignant neoplasm of prostate**

R97.8 **Other abnormal tumor markers**

Ill-defined and unknown cause of mortality (R99)

R99 **Ill-defined and unknown cause of mortality**

Death (unexplained) NOS

Unspecified cause of mortality

Review coding guideline C.18.h

Valid 3-character code, no further characters required

Muscles

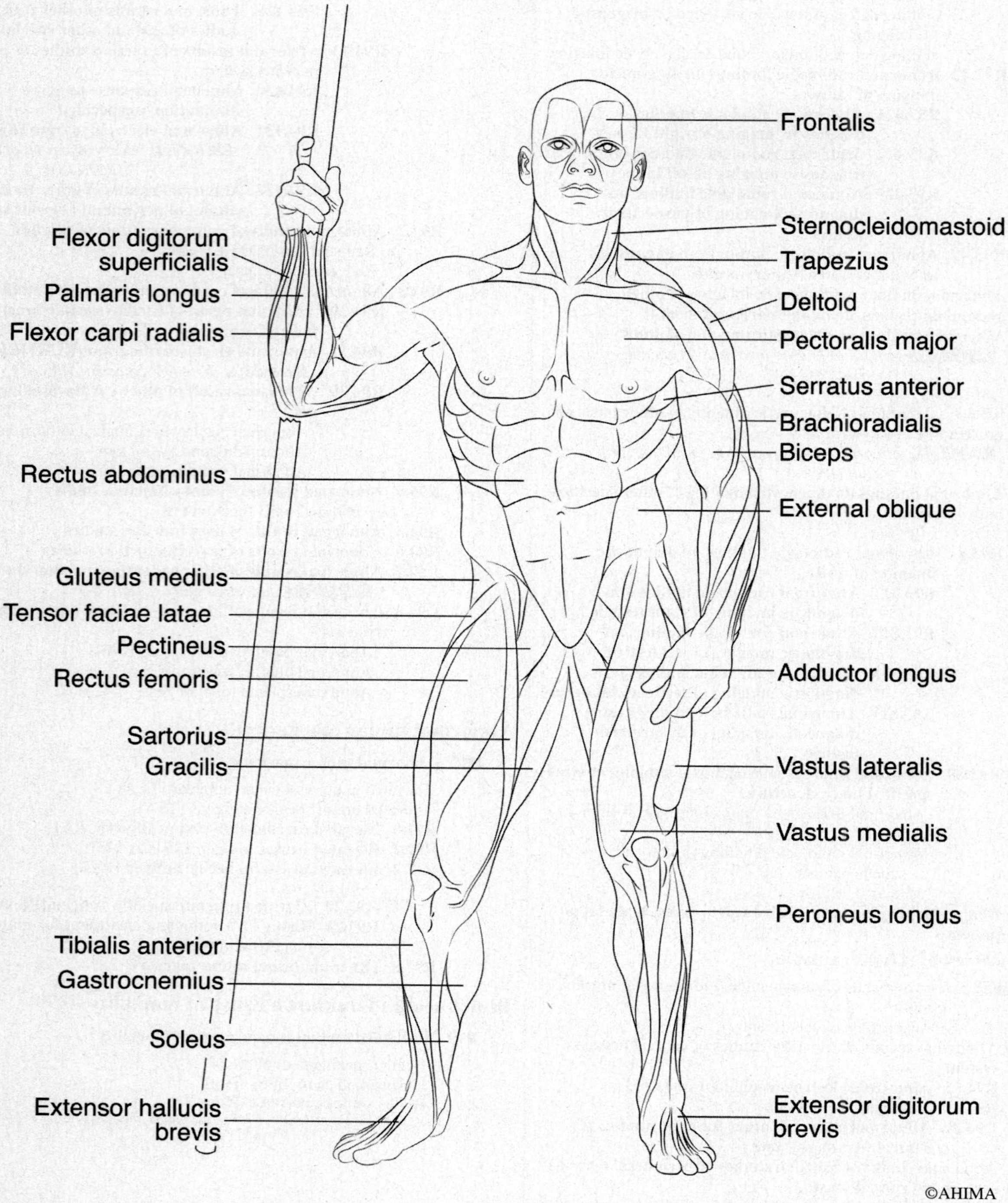
Frontalis
Flexor digitorum superficialis
Sternocleidomastoid
Trapezius
Palmaris longus
Deltoid
Flexor carpi radialis
Pectoralis major
Serratus anterior
Brachioradialis
Biceps
Rectus abdominus
External oblique
Gluteus medius
Tensor faciae latae
Pectineus
Adductor longus
Rectus femoris
Sartorius
Gracilis
Vastus lateralis
Vastus medialis
Peroneus longus
Tibialis anterior
Gastrocnemius
Soleus
Extensor hallucis brevis
Extensor digitorum brevis

Skeleton - Front and Side Views

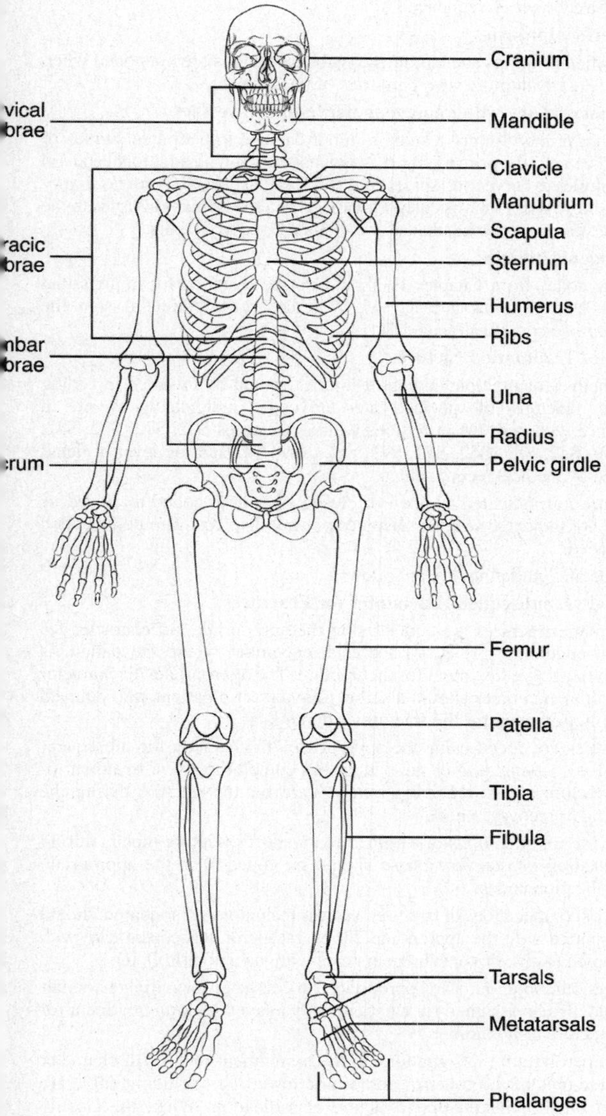

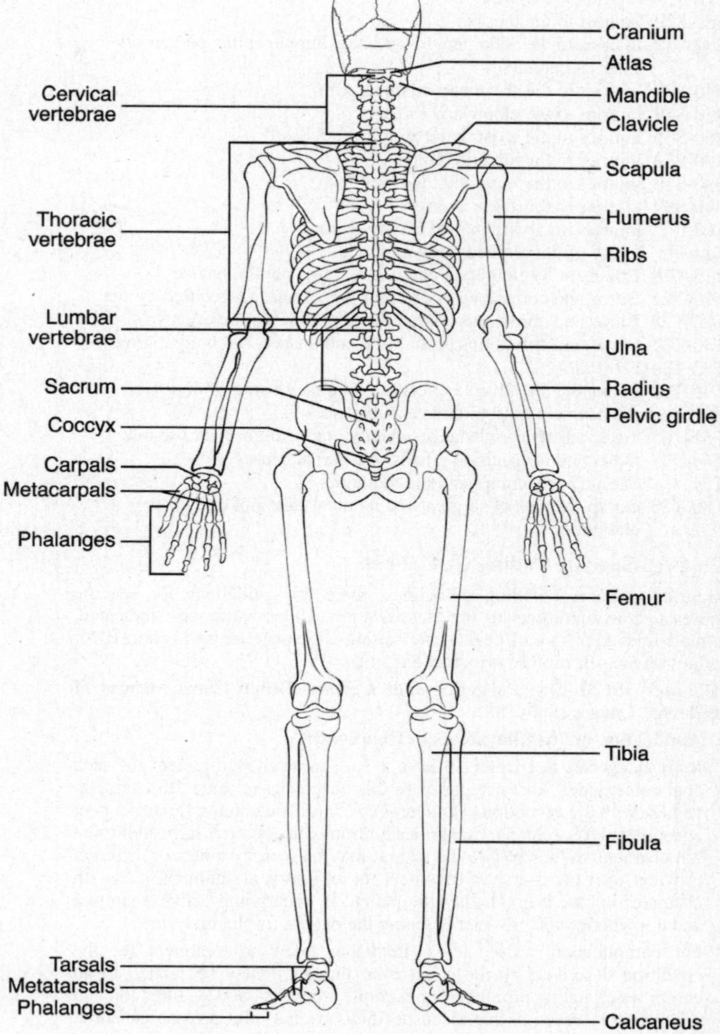

Chapter 19: Injury, Poisoning and Certain Other Consequences of External Causes (S00-T88)

NOTE Use secondary code(s) from Chapter 20, External causes of morbidity, to indicate cause of injury. Codes within the T-section that include the external cause do not require an additional external cause code

Use additional code to identify any retained foreign body, if applicable (Z18.-)

Excludes1: *birth trauma (P10-P15)*
obstetric trauma (O70-O71)

NOTE The chapter uses the S-section for coding different types of injuries related to single body regions and the T-section to cover injuries to unspecified body regions as well as poisoning and certain other consequences of external causes.
AHA CC: 1Q, 2015, 3-21

This chapter contains the following category blocks:

S00-S09	Injuries to the head
S10-S19	Injuries to the neck
S20-S29	Injuries to the thorax
S30-S39	Injuries to the abdomen, lower back, lumbar spine, pelvis and external genitals
S40-S49	Injuries to the shoulder and upper arm
S50-S59	Injuries to the elbow and forearm
S60-S69	Injuries to the wrist, hand and fingers
S70-S79	Injuries to the hip and thigh
S80-S89	Injuries to the knee and lower leg
S90-S99	Injuries to the ankle and foot
T07	Injuries involving multiple body regions
T14	Injury of unspecified body region
T15-T19	Effects of foreign body entering through natural orifice
T20-T25	Burns and corrosions of external body surface, specified by site
T26-T28	Burns and corrosions confined to eye and internal organs
T30-T32	Burns and corrosions of multiple and unspecified body regions
T33-T34	Frostbite
T36-T50	Poisoning by, adverse effect of and underdosing of drugs, medicaments and biological substances
T51-T65	Toxic effects of substances chiefly nonmedicinal as to source
T66-T78	Other and unspecified effects of external causes
T79	Certain early complications of trauma
T80-T88	Complications of surgical and medical care, not elsewhere classified

C. Chapter-Specific Coding Guidelines

In addition to general coding guidelines, there are guidelines for specific diagnoses and/or conditions in the classification. Unless otherwise indicated, these guidelines apply to all health care settings. Please refer to Section II for guidelines on the selection of principal diagnosis.

19. Chapter 19: Injury, Poisoning and Certain Other Consequences of External Causes (S00-T88)

a. Application of 7th Characters in Chapter 19

Most categories in chapter 19 have a 7th character requirement for each applicable code. Most categories in this chapter have three 7th character values (with the exception of fractures): A, initial encounter, D, subsequent encounter and S, sequela. Categories for traumatic fractures have additional 7th character values. While the patient may be seen by a new or different provider over the course of treatment for an injury, assignment of the 7th character is based on whether the patient is undergoing active treatment and not whether the provider is seeing the patient for the first time.

For complication codes, active treatment refers to treatment for the condition described by the code, even though it may be related to an earlier precipitating problem. For example, code T84.50XA, Infection and inflammatory reaction due to unspecified internal joint prosthesis, initial encounter, is used when active treatment is provided for the infection, even though the condition relates to the prosthetic device, implant or graft that was placed at a previous encounter.

7th character "A", initial encounter is used for each encounter where the patient is receiving active treatment for the condition.

7th character "D" subsequent encounter is used for encounters after the patient has completed active treatment of the condition and is receiving routine care for the condition during the healing or recovery phase.

The aftercare Z codes should not be used for aftercare for conditions such as injuries or poisonings, where 7th characters are provided to identify subsequent care. For example, for aftercare of an injury, assign the acute injury code with the 7th character "D" (subsequent encounter).

7th character "S", sequela, is for use for complications or conditions that arise as a direct result of a condition, such as scar formation after a burn. The scars are sequelae of the burn. When using 7th character "S", it is necessary to use both the injury code that precipitated the sequela and the code for the sequela itself. The "S" is added only to the injury code, not the sequela code. The 7th character "S" identifies the injury responsible for the sequela. The specific type of sequela (e.g. scar) is sequenced first, followed by the injury code.

See Section I.B.10 Sequela (Late Effects)

b. Coding of Injuries

When coding injuries, assign separate codes for each injury unless a combination code is provided, in which case the combination code is assigned. Codes from category T07, Unspecified multiple injuries should not be assigned in the inpatient setting unless information for a more specific code is not available. Traumatic injury codes (S00-T14.9) are not to be used for normal, healing surgical wounds or to identify complications of surgical wounds.

The code for the most serious injury, as determined by the provider and the focus of treatment, is sequenced first.

1) Superficial injuries

Superficial injuries such as abrasions or contusions are not coded when associated with more severe injuries of the same site.

2) Primary injury with damage to nerves/blood vessels

When a primary injury results in minor damage to peripheral nerves or blood vessels, the primary injury is sequenced first with additional code(s) for injuries to nerves and spinal cord (such as category S04), and/or injury to blood vessels (such as category S15). When the primary injury is to the blood vessels or nerves, that injury should be sequenced first.

3) Iatrogenic injuries

Injury codes from Chapter 19 should not be assigned for injuries that occur during, or as a result of, a medical intervention. Assign the appropriate complication code(s).

c. Coding of Traumatic Fractures

The principles of multiple coding of injuries should be followed in coding fractures. Fractures of specified sites are coded individually by site in accordance with both the provisions within categories S02, S12, S22, S32, S42, S49, S52, S59, S62, S72, S79, S82, S89, S92 and the level of detail furnished by medical record content.

A fracture not indicated as open or closed should be coded to closed. A fracture not indicated whether displaced or not displaced should be coded to displaced.

More specific guidelines are as follows:

1) Initial vs. Subsequent Encounter for Fractures

Traumatic fractures are coded using the appropriate 7th character for initial encounter (A, B, C) for each encounter where the patient is receiving active treatment for the fracture. The appropriate 7th character for initial encounter should also be assigned for a patient who delayed seeking treatment for the fracture or nonunion.

Fractures are coded using the appropriate 7th character for subsequent care for encounters after the patient has completed active treatment of the fracture and is receiving routine care for the fracture during the healing or recovery phase.

Care for complications of surgical treatment for fracture repairs during the healing or recovery phase should be coded with the appropriate complication codes.

Care of complications of fractures, such as malunion and nonunion, should be reported with the appropriate 7th character for subsequent care with nonunion (K, M, N,) or subsequent care with malunion (P, Q, R).

Malunion/nonunion: The appropriate 7th character for initial encounter should also be assigned for a patient who delayed seeking treatment for the fracture or nonunion.

The open fracture designations in the assignment of the 7th character for fractures of the forearm, femur and lower leg, including ankle are based on the Gustilo open fracture classification. When the Gustilo classification type is not specified for an open fracture, the 7th character for open fracture type I or II should be assigned (B, E, H, M, Q).

A code from category M80, not a traumatic fracture code, should be used for any patient with known osteoporosis who suffers a fracture, even if the patient had a minor fall or trauma, if that fall or trauma would not usually break a normal, healthy bone.

See Section I.C.13. Osteoporosis.

The aftercare Z codes should not be used for aftercare for traumatic fractures. For aftercare of a traumatic fracture, assign the acute fracture code with the appropriate 7th character.

2) Multiple fractures sequencing

Multiple fractures are sequenced in accordance with the severity of the fracture.

3) Physeal fractures

For physeal fractures, assign only the code identifying the type of physeal fracture. Do not assign a separate code to identify the specific bone that is fractured.

d. Coding of Burns and Corrosions

The ICD-10-CM makes a distinction between burns and corrosions. The burn codes are for thermal burns, except sunburns, that come from a heat source, such as a fire or hot appliance. The burn codes are also for burns resulting from electricity and radiation. Corrosions are burns due to chemicals. The guidelines are the same for burns and corrosions.

Current burns (T20-T25) are classified by depth, extent and by agent (X code). Burns are classified by depth as first degree (erythema), second degree (blistering), and third degree (full-thickness involvement). Burns of the eye and internal organs (T26-T28) are classified by site, but not by degree.

1) Sequencing of burn and related condition codes

Sequence first the code that reflects the highest degree of burn when more than one burn is present.

a. When the reason for the admission or encounter is for treatment of external multiple burns, sequence first the code that reflects the burn of the highest degree.

b. When a patient has both internal and external burns, the circumstances of admission govern the selection of the principal diagnosis or first-listed diagnosis.

c. When a patient is admitted for burn injuries and other related conditions such as smoke inhalation and/or respiratory failure, the circumstances of admission govern the selection of the principal or first-listed diagnosis.

2) Burns of the same anatomical site

Classify burns of the same anatomical site and on the same site but of different degrees to the subcategory identifying the highest degree recorded in the diagnosis (e.g., for second and third degree burns of right thigh, assign only code T24.311-).

3) Non-healing burns

Non-healing burns are coded as acute burns.

Necrosis of burned skin should be coded as a non-healed burn.

4) Infected Burn

For any documented infected burn site, use an additional code for the infection.

5) Assign separate codes for each burn site

When coding burns, assign separate codes for each burn site. Category T30, Burn and corrosion, body region unspecified is extremely vague and should rarely be used.

Codes for burns of "multiple sites" should only be assigned when the medical record documentation does not specify the individual sites.

6) Burns and Corrosions Classified According to Extent of Body Surface Involved

Assign codes from category T31, Burns classified according to extent of body surface involved, or T32, Corrosions classified according to extent of body surface involved, **for acute burns or corrosions** when the site of the burn **or corrosion** is not specified or when there is a need for additional data. It is advisable to use category T31 as additional coding when needed to provide data for evaluating burn mortality, such as that needed by burn units. It is also advisable to use category T31 as an additional code for reporting purposes when there is mention of a third-degree burn involving 20 percent or more of the body surface. **Codes from categories T31 and T32 should not be used for sequelae of burns or corrosions.**

Categories T31 and T32 are based on the classic "rule of nines" in estimating body surface involved: head and neck are assigned nine percent, each arm nine percent, each leg 18 percent, the anterior trunk 18 percent, posterior trunk 18 percent, and genitalia one percent. Providers may change these percentage assignments where necessary to accommodate infants and children who have proportionately larger heads than adults, and patients who have large buttocks, thighs, or abdomen that involve burns.

7) Encounters for treatment of sequela of burns

Encounters for the treatment of the late effects of burns or corrosions (i.e., scars or joint contractures) should be coded with a burn or corrosion code with the 7th character "S" for sequela.

8) Sequelae with a late effect code and current burn

When appropriate, both a code for a current burn or corrosion with 7th character "A" or "D" and a burn or corrosion code with 7th character "S" may be assigned on the same record (when both a current burn and sequelae of an old burn exist). Burns and corrosions do not heal at the same rate and a current healing wound may still exist with sequela of a healed burn or corrosion. *See Section I.B.10 Sequela (Late Effects)*

9) Use of an external cause code with burns and corrosions

An external cause code should be used with burns and corrosions to identify the source and intent of the burn, as well as the place where it occurred.

e. Adverse Effects, Poisoning, Underdosing and Toxic Effects

Codes in categories T36-T65 are combination codes that include the substance that was taken as well as the intent. No additional external cause code is required for poisonings, toxic effects, adverse effects and underdosing codes.

1) Do not code directly from the Table of Drugs

Do not code directly from the Table of Drugs and Chemicals. Always refer back to the Tabular List.

2) Use as many codes as necessary to describe

Use as many codes as necessary to describe completely all drugs, medicinal or biological substances.

3) If the same code would describe the causative agent

If the same code would describe the causative agent for more than one adverse reaction, poisoning, toxic effect or underdosing, assign the code only once.

4) If two or more drugs, medicinal or biological substances

If two or more drugs, medicinal or biological substances are taken, code each individually unless a combination code is listed in the Table of Drugs and Chemicals.

If multiple unspecified drugs, medicinal or biological substances were taken, assign the appropriate code from subcategory T50.91, Poisoning by, adverse effect of and underdosing of multiple unspecified drugs, medicaments and biological substances.

5) The occurrence of drug toxicity is classified in ICD-10-CM as follows:

(a) Adverse Effect

When coding an adverse effect of a drug that has been correctly prescribed and properly administered, assign the appropriate code for the nature of the adverse effect followed by the appropriate code for the adverse effect of the drug (T36-T50). The code for the drug should have a 5th or 6th character "5" (for example T36.0X5-) Examples of the nature of an adverse effect are tachycardia, delirium, gastrointestinal hemorrhaging, vomiting, hypokalemia, hepatitis, renal failure, or respiratory failure.

(b) Poisoning

When coding a poisoning or reaction to the improper use of a medication (e.g., overdose, wrong substance given or taken in error, wrong route of administration), first assign the appropriate code from categories T36-T50. The poisoning codes have an associated intent as their 5th or 6th character (accidental, intentional self-harm, assault and undetermined.) If the intent of the poisoning is unknown or unspecified, code the intent as accidental intent. The undetermined intent is only for use if the documentation in the record specifies that the intent cannot be determined. Use additional code(s) for all manifestations of poisonings.

If there is also a diagnosis of abuse or dependence of the substance, the abuse or dependence is assigned as an additional code.

Examples of poisoning include:

(i) Error was made in drug prescription

Errors made in drug prescription or in the administration of the drug by provider, nurse, patient, or other person.

(ii) Overdose of a drug intentionally taken

If an overdose of a drug was intentionally taken or administered and resulted in drug toxicity, it would be coded as a poisoning.

(iii) Nonprescribed drug taken with correctly prescribed and properly administered drug

If a nonprescribed drug or medicinal agent was taken in combination with a correctly prescribed and properly administered drug, any drug toxicity or other reaction resulting from the interaction of the two drugs would be classified as a poisoning.

(iv) Interaction of drug(s) and alcohol

When a reaction results from the interaction of a drug(s) and alcohol, this would be classified as poisoning.

See Section I.C.4. if poisoning is the result of insulin pump malfunctions.

(c) Underdosing

Underdosing refers to taking less of a medication than is prescribed by a provider or a manufacturer's instruction. Discontinuing the use of a prescribed medication on the patient's own initiative (not directed by the patient's provider) is also classified as an underdosing. For underdosing, assign the code from categories T36-T50 (fifth or sixth character "6").

Codes for underdosing should never be assigned as principal or first-listed codes. If a patient has a relapse or exacerbation of the medical condition for which the drug is prescribed because of the reduction in dose, then the medical condition itself should be coded.

Noncompliance (Z91.12-, Z91.13- and Z91.14-) or complication of care (Y63.6-Y63.9) codes are to be used with an underdosing code to indicate intent, if known.

(d) Toxic Effects

When a harmful substance is ingested or comes in contact with a person, this is classified as a toxic effect. The toxic effect codes are in categories T51-T65.

Toxic effect codes have an associated intent: accidental, intentional self-harm, assault and undetermined.

f. Adult and child abuse, neglect and other maltreatment

Sequence first the appropriate code from categories T74.- (Adult and child abuse, neglect and other maltreatment, confirmed) or T76.- (Adult and child abuse, neglect and other maltreatment, suspected) for abuse, neglect and other maltreatment, followed by any accompanying mental health or injury code(s).

If the documentation in the medical record states abuse or neglect it is coded as confirmed (T74.-). It is coded as suspected if it is documented as suspected (T76.-).

For cases of confirmed abuse or neglect an external cause code from the assault section (X92-Y09) should be added to identify the cause of any physical injuries. A perpetrator code (Y07) should be added when the perpetrator of the abuse is known. For suspected cases of abuse or neglect, do not report external cause or perpetrator code.

If a suspected case of abuse, neglect or mistreatment is ruled out during an encounter code Z04.71, Encounter for examination and observation following alleged physical adult abuse, ruled out, or code Z04.72, Encounter for examination and observation following alleged child physical abuse, ruled out, should be used, not a code from T76.

If a suspected case of alleged rape or sexual abuse is ruled out during an encounter code Z04.41, Encounter for examination and observation following alleged adult rape or code Z04.42, Encounter for examination and observation following alleged child rape, should be used, not a code from T76.

If a suspected case of forced sexual exploitation or forced labor exploitation is ruled out during an encounter, code Z04.81, Encounter for examination and observation of victim following forced sexual exploitation, or code Z04.82, Encounter for examination and observation of victim following forced labor exploitation, should be used, not a code from T76.

See Section I.C.15. Abuse in a pregnant patient.

g. Complications of care

1) General guidelines for complications of care

(a) Documentation of complications of care

See Section I.B.16. for information on documentation of complications of care.

2) Pain due to medical devices

Pain associated with devices, implants or grafts left in a surgical site (for example painful hip prosthesis) is assigned to the appropriate code(s) found in Chapter 19, Injury, poisoning, and certain other consequences of external causes. Specific codes for pain due to medical devices are found in the T code section of the ICD-10-CM. Use additional code(s) from category G89 to identify acute or chronic pain due to presence of the device, implant or graft (G89.18 or G89.28).

3) Transplant complications

(a) Transplant complications other than kidney

Codes under category T86, Complications of transplanted organs and tissues, are for use for both complications and rejection of transplanted organs. A transplant complication code is only assigned if the complication affects the function of the transplanted organ. Two codes are required to fully describe a transplant complication: the appropriate code from category T86 and a secondary code that identifies the complication.

Pre-existing conditions or conditions that develop after the transplant are not coded as complications unless they affect the function of the transplanted organs.

See I.C.21. for transplant organ removal status.

See I.C.2. for malignant neoplasm associated with transplanted organ.

(b) Kidney transplant complications

Patients who have undergone kidney transplant may still have some form of chronic kidney disease (CKD) because the kidney transplant may not fully restore kidney function. Code T86.1- should be assigned for documented complications of a kidney transplant, such as transplant failure or rejection or other transplant complication. Code T86.1- should not be assigned for post kidney transplant patients who have chronic kidney (CKD) unless a transplant complication such as transplant failure or rejection is documented. If the documentation is unclear as to whether the patient has a complication of the transplant, query the provider.

Conditions that affect the function of the transplanted kidney, other than CKD, should be assigned a code from subcategory T86.1, Complications of transplanted organ, Kidney, and a secondary code that identifies the complication.

For patients with CKD following a kidney transplant, but who do not have a complication such as failure or rejection, *see section I.C.14. Chronic kidney disease and kidney transplant status.*

4) Complication codes that include the external cause

As with certain other T codes, some of the complications of care codes have the external cause included in the code. The code includes the nature of the complication as well as the type of procedure that caused the complication. No external cause code indicating the type of procedure is necessary for these codes.

5) Complications of care codes within the body system chapters

Intraoperative and postprocedural complication codes are found within the body system chapters with codes specific to the organs and structures of that body system. These codes should be sequenced first, followed by a code(s) for the specific complication, if applicable.

Complication codes from the body system chapters should be assigned for intraoperative and postprocedural complications (e.g., the appropriate complication code from chapter 9 would be assigned for a vascular intraoperative or postprocedural complication) unless the complication is specifically indexed to a T code in chapter 19.

Injuries to the head (S00-S09)

Includes: *injuries of ear*
injuries of eye
injuries of face [any part]
injuries of gum
injuries of jaw
injuries of oral cavity
injuries of palate
injuries of periocular area
injuries of scalp
injuries of temporomandibular joint area
injuries of tongue
injuries of tooth

Code also for any associated infection

Excludes2: *burns and corrosions (T20-T32)*
effects of foreign body in ear (T16)
effects of foreign body in larynx (T17.3)
effects of foreign body in mouth NOS (T18.0)
effects of foreign body in nose (T17.0-T17.1)
effects of foreign body in pharynx (T17.2)
effects of foreign body on external eye (T15.-)
frostbite (T33-T34)
insect bite or sting, venomous (T63.4)

S00 Superficial injury of head

Excludes1: *diffuse cerebral contusion (S06.2-)*
focal cerebral contusion (S06.3-)
injury of eye and orbit (S05.-)
open wound of head (S01.-)

The appropriate 7th character is to be added to each code from category S00
A initial encounter
D subsequent encounter
S sequela

+ **S00.0 Superficial injury of scalp**
X+7th **S00.00 Unspecified superficial injury of scalp**
X+7th **S00.01 Abrasion of scalp**
X+7th **S00.02 Blister (nonthermal) of scalp**
X+7th **S00.03 Contusion of scalp**
Bruise of scalp
Hematoma of scalp
X+7th **S00.04 External constriction of part of scalp**
X+7th **S00.05 Superficial foreign body of scalp**
Splinter in the scalp
X+7th **S00.06 Insect bite (nonvenomous) of scalp**
X+7th **S00.07 Other superficial bite of scalp**
Excludes1: *open bite of scalp (S01.05)*
+ **S00.1 Contusion of eyelid and periocular area**
Black eye
Excludes2: *contusion of eyeball and orbital tissues (S05.1-)*
X+7th **S00.10 Contusion of unspecified eyelid and periocular area**
X+7th **S00.11 Contusion of right eyelid and periocular area**
X+7th **S00.12 Contusion of left eyelid and periocular area**
+ **S00.2 Other and unspecified superficial injuries of eyelid and periocular area**
Excludes2: *superficial injury of conjunctiva and cornea (S05.0-)*
+ **S00.20 Unspecified superficial injury of eyelid and periocular area**
+7th **S00.201 Unspecified superficial injury of right eyelid and periocular area**
+7th **S00.202 Unspecified superficial injury of left eyelid and periocular area**
+7th **S00.209 Unspecified superficial injury of unspecified eyelid and periocular area**
+ **S00.21 Abrasion of eyelid and periocular area**
+7th **S00.211 Abrasion of right eyelid and periocular area**
+7th **S00.212 Abrasion of left eyelid and periocular area**
+7th **S00.219 Abrasion of unspecified eyelid and periocular area**
+ **S00.22 Blister (nonthermal) of eyelid and periocular area**
+7th **S00.221 Blister (nonthermal) of right eyelid and periocular area**
+7th **S00.222 Blister (nonthermal) of left eyelid and periocular area**
+7th **S00.229 Blister (nonthermal) of unspecified eyelid and periocular area**
+ **S00.24 External constriction of eyelid and periocular area**
+7th **S00.241 External constriction of right eyelid and periocular area**
+7th **S00.242 External constriction of left eyelid and periocular area**
+7th **S00.249 External constriction of unspecified eyelid and periocular area**
+ **S00.25 Superficial foreign body of eyelid and periocular area**
Splinter of eyelid and periocular area
Excludes2: *retained foreign body in eyelid (H02.81-)*
+7th **S00.251 Superficial foreign body of right eyelid and periocular area**
+7th **S00.252 Superficial foreign body of left eyelid and periocular area**
+7th **S00.259 Superficial foreign body of unspecified eyelid and periocular area**
+ **S00.26 Insect bite (nonvenomous) of eyelid and periocular area**
+7th **S00.261 Insect bite (nonvenomous) of right eyelid and periocular area**
+7th **S00.262 Insect bite (nonvenomous) of left eyelid and periocular area**
+7th **S00.269 Insect bite (nonvenomous) of unspecified eyelid and periocular area**
+ **S00.27 Other superficial bite of eyelid and periocular area**
Excludes1: *open bite of eyelid and periocular area (S01.15)*
+7th **S00.271 Other superficial bite of right eyelid and periocular area**
+7th **S00.272 Other superficial bite of left eyelid and periocular area**
+7th **S00.279 Other superficial bite of unspecified eyelid and periocular area**
+ **S00.3 Superficial injury of nose**
X+7th **S00.30 Unspecified superficial injury of nose**
X+7th **S00.31 Abrasion of nose**
X+7th **S00.32 Blister (nonthermal) of nose**
X+7th **S00.33 Contusion of nose**
Bruise of nose
Hematoma of nose
X+7th **S00.34 External constriction of nose**
X+7th **S00.35 Superficial foreign body of nose**
Splinter in the nose
X+7th **S00.36 Insect bite (nonvenomous) of nose**
X+7th **S00.37 Other superficial bite of nose**
Excludes1: *open bite of nose (S01.25)*
+ **S00.4 Superficial injury of ear**
+ **S00.40 Unspecified superficial injury of ear**
+7th **S00.401 Unspecified superficial injury of right ear**
+7th **S00.402 Unspecified superficial injury of left ear**
+7th **S00.409 Unspecified superficial injury of unspecified ear**
+ **S00.41 Abrasion of ear**
+7th **S00.411 Abrasion of right ear**
+7th **S00.412 Abrasion of left ear**
+7th **S00.419 Abrasion of unspecified ear**
+ **S00.42 Blister (nonthermal) of ear**
+7th **S00.421 Blister (nonthermal) of right ear**
+7th **S00.422 Blister (nonthermal) of left ear**
+7th **S00.429 Blister (nonthermal) of unspecified ear**
+ **S00.43 Contusion of ear**
Bruise of ear
Hematoma of ear
+7th **S00.431 Contusion of right ear**
+7th **S00.432 Contusion of left ear**
+7th **S00.439 Contusion of unspecified ear**
+ **S00.44 External constriction of ear**
+7th **S00.441 External constriction of right ear**
+7th **S00.442 External constriction of left ear**
+7th **S00.449 External constriction of unspecified ear**
+ **S00.45 Superficial foreign body of ear**
Splinter in the ear
+7th **S00.451 Superficial foreign body of right ear**
+7th **S00.452 Superficial foreign body of left ear**
+7th **S00.459 Superficial foreign body of unspecified ear**
+ **S00.46 Insect bite (nonvenomous) of ear**
+7th **S00.461 Insect bite (nonvenomous) of right ear**
+7th **S00.462 Insect bite (nonvenomous) of left ear**
+7th **S00.469 Insect bite (nonvenomous) of unspecified ear**
+ **S00.47 Other superficial bite of ear**
Excludes1: *open bite of ear (S01.35)*
+7th **S00.471 Other superficial bite of right ear**
+7th **S00.472 Other superficial bite of left ear**
+7th **S00.479 Other superficial bite of unspecified ear**
+ **S00.5 Superficial injury of lip and oral cavity**
+ **S00.50 Unspecified superficial injury of lip and oral cavity**
+7th **S00.501 Unspecified superficial injury of lip**
+7th **S00.502 Unspecified superficial injury of oral cavity**
+ **S00.51 Abrasion of lip and oral cavity**
+7th **S00.511 Abrasion of lip**
+7th **S00.512 Abrasion of oral cavity**
+ **S00.52 Blister (nonthermal) of lip and oral cavity**
+7th **S00.521 Blister (nonthermal) of lip**
+7th **S00.522 Blister (nonthermal) of oral cavity**
+ **S00.53 Contusion of lip and oral cavity**
+7th **S00.531 Contusion of lip**
Bruise of lip
Hematoma of lip
+7th **S00.532 Contusion of oral cavity**
Bruise of oral cavity
Hematoma of oral cavity
+ **S00.54 External constriction of lip and oral cavity**
+7th **S00.541 External constriction of lip**
+7th **S00.542 External constriction of oral cavity**
+ **S00.55 Superficial foreign body of lip and oral cavity**
+7th **S00.551 Superficial foreign body of lip**
Splinter of lip and oral cavity
+7th **S00.552 Superficial foreign body of oral cavity**
Splinter of lip and oral cavity

+ **S00.56 Insect bite (nonvenomous) of lip and oral cavity**
  - +7th **S00.561 Insect bite (nonvenomous) of lip**
  - +7th **S00.562 Insect bite (nonvenomous) of oral cavity**
+ **S00.57 Other superficial bite of lip and oral cavity**
  - +7th **S00.571 Other superficial bite of lip**
    - ***Excludes1:*** *open bite of lip (S01.551)*
  - +7th **S00.572 Other superficial bite of oral cavity**
    - ***Excludes1:*** *open bite of oral cavity (S01.552)*

+ **S00.8 Superficial injury of other parts of head**
  - Superficial injuries of face [any part]
  - X+7th **S00.80 Unspecified superficial injury of other part of head**
  - X+7th **S00.81 Abrasion of other part of head**
  - X+7th **S00.82 Blister (nonthermal) of other part of head**
  - X+7th **S00.83 Contusion of other part of head**
    - Bruise of other part of head
    - Hematoma of other part of head
  - X+7th **S00.84 External constriction of other part of head**
  - X+7th **S00.85 Superficial foreign body of other part of head**
    - Splinter in other part of head
  - X+7th **S00.86 Insect bite (nonvenomous) of other part of head**
  - X+7th **S00.87 Other superficial bite of other part of head**
    - ***Excludes1:*** *open bite of other part of head (S01.85)*

+ **S00.9 Superficial injury of unspecified part of head**
  - X+7th **S00.90 Unspecified superficial injury of unspecified part of head**
  - X+7th **S00.91 Abrasion of unspecified part of head**
  - X+7th **S00.92 Blister (nonthermal) of unspecified part of head**
  - X+7th **S00.93 Contusion of unspecified part of head**
    - Bruise of head
    - Hematoma of head
  - X+7th **S00.94 External constriction of unspecified part of head**
  - X+7th **S00.95 Superficial foreign body of unspecified part of head**
    - Splinter of head
  - X+7th **S00.96 Insect bite (nonvenomous) of unspecified part of head**
  - X+7th **S00.97 Other superficial bite of unspecified part of head**
    - ***Excludes1:*** *open bite of head (S01.95)*

S01 Open wound of head

Code also any associated:
injury of cranial nerve (S04.-)
injury of muscle and tendon of head (S09.1-)
intracranial injury (S06.-)
wound infection

Excludes1: *open skull fracture (S02.- with 7th character B)*
Excludes2: *injury of eye and orbit (S05.-)*
traumatic amputation of part of head (S08.-)

The appropriate 7th character is to be added to each code from category S01
A initial encounter
D subsequent encounter
S sequela

+ **S01.0 Open wound of scalp**
  - ***Excludes1:*** *avulsion of scalp (S08.0-)*
  - X+7th **S01.00 Unspecified open wound of scalp**
  - X+7th **S01.01 Laceration without foreign body of scalp**
  - X+7th **S01.02 Laceration with foreign body of scalp**
    - *AHA CC: 1Q, 2015, 3-21*
  - X+7th **S01.03 Puncture wound without foreign body of scalp**
  - X+7th **S01.04 Puncture wound with foreign body of scalp**
  - X+7th **S01.05 Open bite of scalp**
    - Bite of scalp NOS
    - ***Excludes1:*** *superficial bite of scalp (S00.06, S00.07-)*

+ **S01.1 Open wound of eyelid and periocular area**
  - Open wound of eyelid and periocular area with or without involvement of lacrimal passages
  + **S01.10 Unspecified open wound of eyelid and periocular area**
    - CC +7th **S01.101 Unspecified open wound of right eyelid and periocular area**
    - CC +7th **S01.102 Unspecified open wound of left eyelid and periocular area**
    - CC +7th **S01.109 Unspecified open wound of unspecified eyelid and periocular area**
  + **S01.11 Laceration without foreign body of eyelid and periocular area**
    - +7th **S01.111 Laceration without foreign body of right eyelid and periocular area**
    - +7th **S01.112 Laceration without foreign body of left eyelid and periocular area**
    - +7th **S01.119 Laceration without foreign body of unspecified eyelid and periocular area**
  + **S01.12 Laceration with foreign body of eyelid and periocular area**
    - +7th **S01.121 Laceration with foreign body of right eyelid and periocular area**
    - +7th **S01.122 Laceration with foreign body of left eyelid and periocular area**
    - +7th **S01.129 Laceration with foreign body of unspecified eyelid and periocular area**
  + **S01.13 Puncture wound without foreign body of eyelid and periocular area**
    - +7th **S01.131 Puncture wound without foreign body of right eyelid and periocular area**
    - +7th **S01.132 Puncture wound without foreign body of left eyelid and periocular area**
    - +7th **S01.139 Puncture wound without foreign body of unspecified eyelid and periocular area**
  + **S01.14 Puncture wound with foreign body of eyelid and periocular area**
    - +7th **S01.141 Puncture wound with foreign body of right eyelid and periocular area**
    - +7th **S01.142 Puncture wound with foreign body of left eyelid and periocular area**
    - +7th **S01.149 Puncture wound with foreign body of unspecified eyelid and periocular area**
  + **S01.15 Open bite of eyelid and periocular area**
    - Bite of eyelid and periocular area NOS
    - ***Excludes1:*** *superficial bite of eyelid and periocular area (S00.26, S00.27)*
    - +7th **S01.151 Open bite of right eyelid and periocular area**
    - +7th **S01.152 Open bite of left eyelid and periocular area**
    - +7th **S01.159 Open bite of unspecified eyelid and periocular area**

+ **S01.2 Open wound of nose**
  - X+7th **S01.20 Unspecified open wound of nose**
  - X+7th **S01.21 Laceration without foreign body of nose**
    - *AHA CC: 1Q, 2015, 3-21*
  - X+7th **S01.22 Laceration with foreign body of nose**
  - X+7th **S01.23 Puncture wound without foreign body of nose**
  - X+7th **S01.24 Puncture wound with foreign body of nose**
  - X+7th **S01.25 Open bite of nose**
    - Bite of nose NOS
    - ***Excludes1:*** *superficial bite of nose (S00.36, S00.37)*

+ **S01.3 Open wound of ear**
  + **S01.30 Unspecified open wound of ear**
    - +7th **S01.301 Unspecified open wound of right ear**
    - +7th **S01.302 Unspecified open wound of left ear**
    - +7th **S01.309 Unspecified open wound of unspecified ear**
  + **S01.31 Laceration without foreign body of ear**
    - +7th **S01.311 Laceration without foreign body of right ear**
    - +7th **S01.312 Laceration without foreign body of left ear**
    - +7th **S01.319 Laceration without foreign body of unspecified ear**
  + **S01.32 Laceration with foreign body of ear**
    - +7th **S01.321 Laceration with foreign body of right ear**
    - +7th **S01.322 Laceration with foreign body of left ear**
    - +7th **S01.329 Laceration with foreign body of unspecified ear**
  + **S01.33 Puncture wound without foreign body of ear**
    - +7th **S01.331 Puncture wound without foreign body of right ear**
    - +7th **S01.332 Puncture wound without foreign body of left ear**
    - +7th **S01.339 Puncture wound without foreign body of unspecified ear**

+ **S01.34 Puncture wound with foreign body of ear**
  - +7th **S01.341 Puncture wound with foreign body of right ear**
  - +7th **S01.342 Puncture wound with foreign body of left ear**
  - +7th **S01.349 Puncture wound with foreign body of unspecified ear**

+ **S01.35 Open bite of ear**
  Bite of ear NOS
  Excludes1: *superficial bite of ear (S00.46, S00.47)*
  - +7th **S01.351 Open bite of right ear**
  - +7th **S01.352 Open bite of left ear**
  - +7th **S01.359 Open bite of unspecified ear**

+ **S01.4 Open wound of cheek and temporomandibular area**

+ **S01.40 Unspecified open wound of cheek and temporomandibular area**
  - +7th **S01.401 Unspecified open wound of right cheek and temporomandibular area**
  - +7th **S01.402 Unspecified open wound of left cheek and temporomandibular area**
  - +7th **S01.409 Unspecified open wound of unspecified cheek and temporomandibular area**

+ **S01.41 Laceration without foreign body of cheek and temporomandibular area**
  - +7th **S01.411 Laceration without foreign body of right cheek and temporomandibular area**
    AHA CC: 1Q, 2015, 3-21
  - +7th **S01.412 Laceration without foreign body of left cheek and temporomandibular area**
  - +7th **S01.419 Laceration without foreign body of unspecified cheek and temporomandibular area**

+ **S01.42 Laceration with foreign body of cheek and temporomandibular area**
  - +7th **S01.421 Laceration with foreign body of right cheek and temporomandibular area**
  - +7th **S01.422 Laceration with foreign body of left cheek and temporomandibular area**
  - +7th **S01.429 Laceration with foreign body of unspecified cheek and temporomandibular area**

+ **S01.43 Puncture wound without foreign body of cheek and temporomandibular area**
  - +7th **S01.431 Puncture wound without foreign body of right cheek and temporomandibular area**
  - +7th **S01.432 Puncture wound without foreign body of left cheek and temporomandibular area**
  - +7th **S01.439 Puncture wound without foreign body of unspecified cheek and temporomandibular area**

+ **S01.44 Puncture wound with foreign body of cheek and temporomandibular area**
  - +7th **S01.441 Puncture wound with foreign body of right cheek and temporomandibular area**
  - +7th **S01.442 Puncture wound with foreign body of left cheek and temporomandibular area**
  - +7th **S01.449 Puncture wound with foreign body of unspecified cheek and temporomandibular area**

+ **S01.45 Open bite of cheek and temporomandibular area**
  Bite of cheek and temporomandibular area NOS
  Excludes2: *superficial bite of cheek and temporomandibular area (S00.86, S00.87)*
  - +7th **S01.451 Open bite of right cheek and temporomandibular area**
  - +7th **S01.452 Open bite of left cheek and temporomandibular area**
  - +7th **S01.459 Open bite of unspecified cheek and temporomandibular area**

+ **S01.5 Open wound of lip and oral cavity**
  Excludes2: *tooth dislocation (S03.2)*
  tooth fracture (S02.5)

+ **S01.50 Unspecified open wound of lip and oral cavity**
  - +7th **S01.501 Unspecified open wound of lip**
  - +7th **S01.502 Unspecified open wound of oral cavity**

+ **S01.51 Laceration of lip and oral cavity without foreign body**
  - +7th **S01.511 Laceration without foreign body of lip**
  - +7th **S01.512 Laceration without foreign body of oral cavity**

+ **S01.52 Laceration of lip and oral cavity with foreign body**
  - +7th **S01.521 Laceration with foreign body of lip**
  - +7th **S01.522 Laceration with foreign body of oral cavity**

+ **S01.53 Puncture wound of lip and oral cavity without foreign body**
  - +7th **S01.531 Puncture wound without foreign body of lip**
  - +7th **S01.532 Puncture wound without foreign body of oral cavity**

+ **S01.54 Puncture wound of lip and oral cavity with foreign body**
  - +7th **S01.541 Puncture wound with foreign body of lip**
  - +7th **S01.542 Puncture wound with foreign body of oral cavity**

+ **S01.55 Open bite of lip and oral cavity**
  - +7th **S01.551 Open bite of lip**
    Bite of lip NOS
    Excludes1: *superficial bite of lip (S00.571)*
  - +7th **S01.552 Open bite of oral cavity**
    Bite of oral cavity NOS
    Excludes1: *superficial bite of oral cavity (S00.572)*

+ **S01.8 Open wound of other parts of head**
  - X+7th **S01.80 Unspecified open wound of other part of head**
  - X+7th **S01.81 Laceration without foreign body of other part of head**
  - X+7th **S01.82 Laceration with foreign body of other part of head**
  - X+7th **S01.83 Puncture wound without foreign body of other part of head**
  - X+7th **S01.84 Puncture wound with foreign body of other part of head**
  - X+7th **S01.85 Open bite of other part of head**
    Bite of other part of head NOS
    Excludes1: *superficial bite of other part of head (S00.87)*

+ **S01.9 Open wound of unspecified part of head**
  - X+7th **S01.90 Unspecified open wound of unspecified part of head**
  - X+7th **S01.91 Laceration without foreign body of unspecified part of head**
  - X+7th **S01.92 Laceration with foreign body of unspecified part of head**
  - X+7th **S01.93 Puncture wound without foreign body of unspecified part of head**
  - X+7th **S01.94 Puncture wound with foreign body of unspecified part of head**
  - X+7th **S01.95 Open bite of unspecified part of head**
    Bite of head NOS
    Excludes1: *superficial bite of head NOS (S00.97)*

Head and Facial Bones - Side View

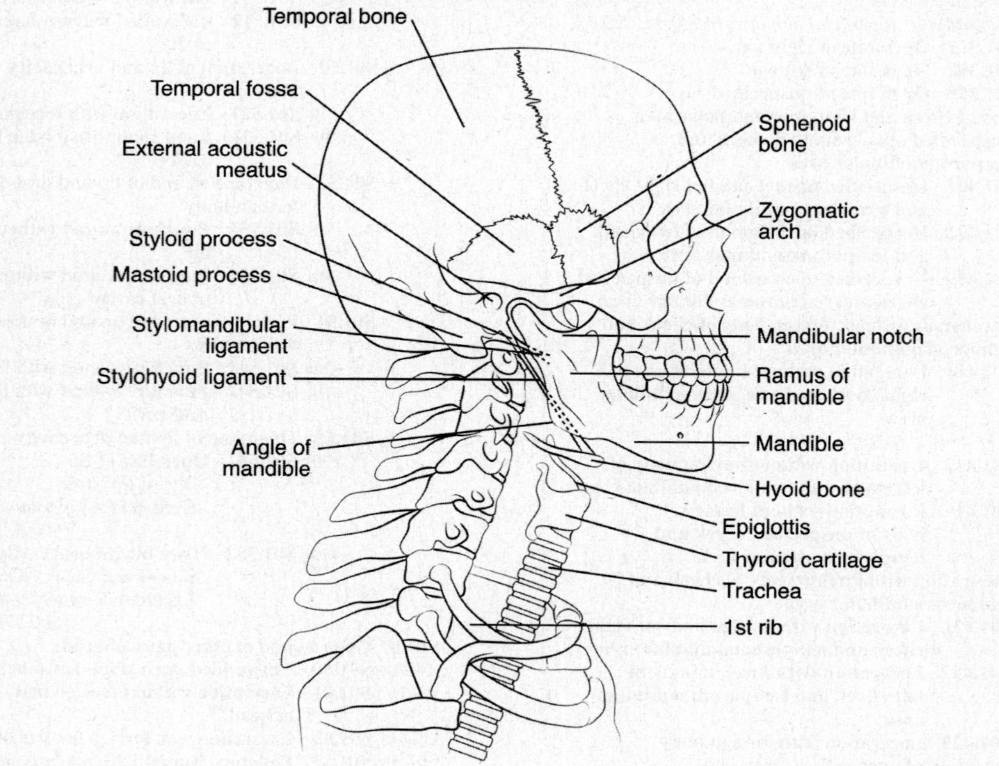

Head and Facial Bones - Side View

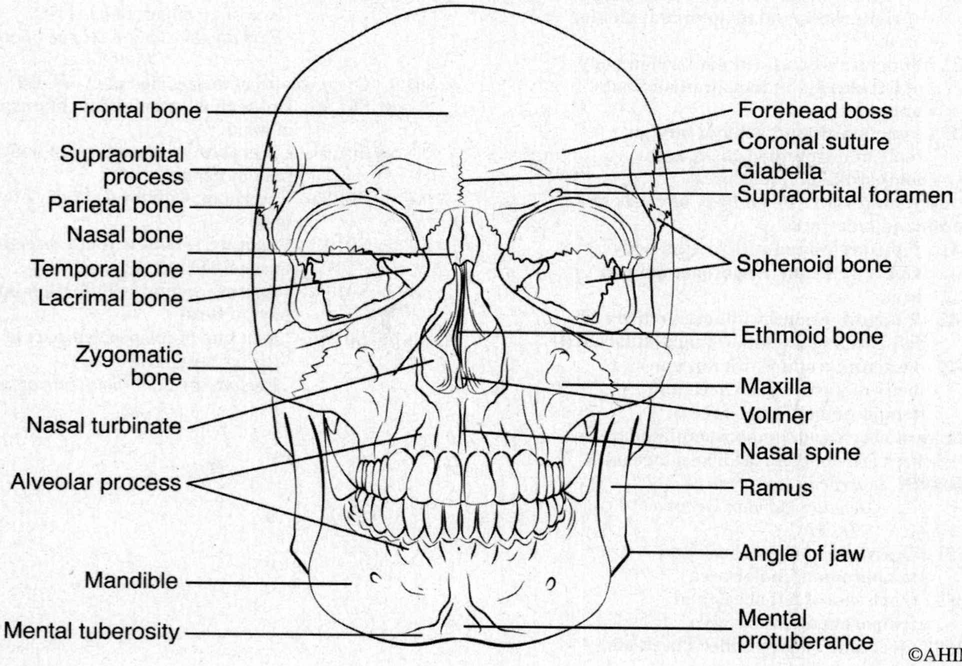

S02 Fracture of skull and facial bones

NOTE A fracture not indicated as open or closed should be coded to closed

Code also any associated intracranial injury (S06.-)

Review coding guideline C.19.c

AHA CC: 4Q, 2016, 66-67

The appropriate 7th character is to be added to each code from category S02
- A initial encounter for closed fracture
- B initial encounter for open fracture
- D subsequent encounter for fracture with routine healing
- G subsequent encounter for fracture with delayed healing
- K subsequent encounter for fracture with nonunion
- S sequela

X+7th CC MCC **S02.0 Fracture of vault of skull**
Fracture of frontal bone
Fracture of parietal bone
HAC 7th characters A & B see Appendix B for HAC conditional logic

\+ **S02.1 Fracture of base of skull**
Excludes2: *lateral orbital wall (S02.84-)*
medial orbital wall (S02.83-)
orbital floor (S02.3-)
AHA CC: 4Q, 2019, 16

\+ **S02.10 Unspecified fracture of base of skull**

CC MCC +7th **S02.101 Fracture of base of skull, right side**
HAC 7th characters A & B see Appendix B for HAC conditional logic

CC MCC +7th **S02.102 Fracture of base of skull, left side**
HAC 7th characters A & B see Appendix B for HAC conditional logic

CC MCC +7th **S02.109 Fracture of base of skull, unspecified side**
HAC 7th characters A & B see Appendix B for HAC conditional logic

\+ **S02.11 Fracture of occiput**

CC MCC +7th **S02.110 Type I occipital condyle fracture, unspecified side**
HAC 7th characters A & B see Appendix B for HAC conditional logic

CC MCC +7th **S02.111 Type II occipital condyle fracture, unspecified side**
HAC 7th characters A & B see Appendix B for HAC conditional logic

CC MCC +7th **S02.112 Type III occipital condyle fracture, unspecified side**
HAC 7th characters A & B see Appendix B for HAC conditional logic

CC MCC +7th **S02.113 Unspecified occipital condyle fracture**
HAC 7th characters A & B see Appendix B for HAC conditional logic

CC MCC +7th **S02.118 Other fracture of occiput, unspecified side**
HAC 7th characters A & B see Appendix B for HAC conditional logic

CC MCC +7th **S02.119 Unspecified fracture of occiput**
HAC 7th characters A & B see Appendix B for HAC conditional logic

CC MCC +7th **S02.11A Type I occipital condyle fracture, right side**
HAC 7th characters A & B see Appendix B for HAC conditional logic

CC MCC +7th **S02.11B Type I occipital condyle fracture, left side**
HAC 7th characters A & B see Appendix B for HAC conditional logic

CC MCC +7th **S02.11C Type II occipital condyle fracture, right side**
HAC 7th characters A & B see Appendix B for HAC conditional logic

CC MCC +7th **S02.11D Type II occipital condyle fracture, left side**
HAC 7th characters A & B see Appendix B for HAC conditional logic

CC MCC +7th **S02.11E Type III occipital condyle fracture, right side**
HAC 7th characters A & B see Appendix B for HAC conditional logic

CC MCC +7th **S02.11F Type III occipital condyle fracture, left side**
HAC 7th characters A & B see Appendix B for HAC conditional logic

CC MCC +7th **S02.11G Other fracture or occiput, right side**
HAC 7th characters A & B see Appendix B for HAC conditional logic

CC MCC +7th **S02.11H Other fracture or occiput, left side**
HAC 7th characters A & B see Appendix B for HAC conditional logic

\+ **S02.12 Fracture of orbital roof**

CC MCC **S02.121 Fracture of orbital roof, right side**
HAC 7th characters A & B see Appendix B for HAC conditional logic

CC MCC **S02.122 Fracture of orbital roof, left side**
HAC 7th characters A & B see Appendix B for HAC conditional logic

CC MCC **S02.129 Fracture of orbital roof, unspecified side**
HAC 7th characters A & B see Appendix B for HAC conditional logic

CC MCC X+7th **S02.19 Other fracture of base of skull**
Fracture of anterior fossa of base of skull
Fracture of ethmoid sinus
Fracture of frontal sinus
Fracture of middle fossa of base of skull
Fracture of posterior fossa of base of skull
Fracture of sphenoid
Fracture of temporal bone
HAC 7th characters A & B see Appendix B for HAC conditional logic

CC X+7th **S02.2 Fracture of nasal bones**
HAC 7th character B see Appendix B for HAC conditional logic

\+ **S02.3 Fracture of orbital floor**
Excludes1: *orbit NOS (S02.85)*
Excludes2: *lateral orbital wall (S02.84-)*
medial orbital wall (S02.83-)
orbital roof (S02.1-)

CC X+7th **S02.30 Fracture of orbital floor, unspecified side**
HAC 7th characters A & B see Appendix B for HAC conditional logic

CC X+7th **S02.31 Fracture of orbital floor, right side**
HAC 7th characters A & B see Appendix B for HAC conditional logic

CC X+7th **S02.32 Fracture of orbital floor, left side**
HAC 7th characters A & B see Appendix B for HAC conditional logic

\+ **S02.4 Fracture of malar, maxillary and zygoma bones**
Fracture of superior maxilla
Fracture of upper jaw (bone)
Fracture of zygomatic process of temporal bone

\+ **S02.40 Fracture of malar, maxillary and zygoma bones, unspecified**

CC +7th **S02.400 Malar fracture, unspecified side**
HAC 7th characters A & B see Appendix B for HAC conditional logic

CC +7th **S02.401 Maxillary fracture, unspecified side**
HAC 7th characters A & B see Appendix B for HAC conditional logic

CC +7th **S02.402 Zygomatic fracture, unspecified side**
HAC 7th characters A & B see Appendix B for HAC conditional logic

CC +7th **S02.40A Malar fracture, right side**
HAC 7th characters A & B see Appendix B for HAC conditional logic

CC +7th **S02.40B Malar fracture, left side**
HAC 7th characters A & B see Appendix B for HAC conditional logic

CC +7th **S02.40C Maxillary fracture, right side**
HAC 7th characters A & B see Appendix B for HAC conditional logic

CC +7th **S02.40D Maxillary fracture, left side**
HAC 7th characters A & B see Appendix B for HAC conditional logic

CC +7th **S02.40E Zygomatic fracture, right side**
HAC 7th characters A & B see Appendix B for HAC conditional logic

CC +7th **S02.40F Zygomatic fracture, left side**
HAC 7th characters A & B see Appendix B for HAC conditional logic

\+ **S02.41 LeFort fracture**

CC +7th **S02.411 LeFort I fracture**
HAC 7th characters A & B see Appendix B for HAC conditional logic

CC +7th **S02.412 LeFort II fracture**
HAC 7th characters A & B see Appendix B for HAC conditional logic

CC +7th **S02.413 LeFort III fracture**
HAC 7th characters A & B see Appendix B for HAC conditional logic

CC X+7th **S02.42 Fracture of alveolus of maxilla**
HAC 7th characters A & B see Appendix B for HAC conditional logic

CC X+7th **S02.5 Fracture of tooth (traumatic)**
Broken tooth
Excludes1: *cracked tooth (nontraumatic) (K03.81)*

\+ **S02.6 Fracture of mandible**
Fracture of lower jaw (bone)

\+ **S02.60 Fracture of mandible, unspecified**

CC+7th **S02.600 Fracture of unspecified part of body of mandible, unspecified side**
HAC 7th characters A & B see Appendix B for HAC conditional logic

CC +7th **S02.601 Fracture of unspecified part of body of right mandible**
HAC 7th characters A & B see Appendix B for HAC conditional logic

CC +7th **S02.602 Fracture of unspecified part of body of left mandible**
HAC 7th characters A & B see Appendix B for HAC conditional logic

CC X+7th **S02.609 Fracture of mandible, unspecified**
HAC 7th characters A & B see Appendix B for HAC conditional logic

\+ **S02.61 Fracture of condylar process of mandible**

CC +7th **S02.610 Fracture of condylar process of mandible, unspecified side**
HAC 7th characters A & B see Appendix B for HAC conditional logic

CC +7th **S02.611 Fracture of condylar process of right mandible**
AHA CC: 1Q, 2021, 6
HAC 7th characters A & B see Appendix B for HAC conditional logic

CC +7th **S02.612 Fracture of condylar process of left mandible**
HAC 7th characters A & B see Appendix B for HAC conditional logic

\+ **S02.62 Fracture of subcondylar process of mandible**

CC +7th **S02.620 Fracture of subcondylar process of mandible, unspecified side**
HAC 7th characters A & B see Appendix B for HAC conditional logic

CC +7th **S02.621 Fracture of subcondylar process of right mandible**
HAC 7th characters A & B see Appendix B for HAC conditional logic

CC +7th **S02.622 Fracture of subcondylar process of left mandible**
HAC 7th characters A & B see Appendix B for HAC conditional logic

\+ **S02.63 Fracture of coronoid process of mandible**

CC +7th **S02.630 Fracture of coronoid process of mandible, unspecified side**
HAC 7th characters A & B see Appendix B for HAC conditional logic

CC +7th **S02.631 Fracture of coronoid process of right mandible**
HAC 7th characters A & B see Appendix B for HAC conditional logic

CC +7th **S02.632 Fracture of coronoid process of left mandible**
HAC 7th characters A & B see Appendix B for HAC conditional logic

\+ **S02.64 Fracture of ramus of mandible**

CC +7th **S02.640 Fracture of ramus of mandible, unspecified side**
HAC 7th characters A & B see Appendix B for HAC conditional logic

CC +7th **S02.641 Fracture of ramus of right mandible**
HAC 7th characters A & B see Appendix B for HAC conditional logic

CC +7th **S02.642 Fracture of ramus of left mandible**
HAC 7th characters A & B see Appendix B for HAC conditional logic

\+ **S02.65 Fracture of angle of mandible**

CC +7th **S02.650 Fracture of angle of mandible, unspecified side**
HAC 7th characters A & B see Appendix B for HAC conditional logic

CC +7th **S02.651 Fracture of angle of right mandible**
HAC 7th characters A & B see Appendix B for HAC conditional logic

CC +7th **S02.652 Fracture of angle of left mandible**
HAC 7th characters A & B see Appendix B for HAC conditional logic

CC X+7th **S02.66 Fracture of symphysis of mandible**
AHA CC: 1Q, 2021, 6
HAC 7th characters A & B see Appendix B for HAC conditional logic

\+ **S02.67 Fracture of alveolus of mandible**

CC +7th **S02.670 Fracture of alveolus of mandible, unspecified side**
HAC 7th characters A & B see Appendix B for HAC conditional logic

CC +7th **S02.671 Fracture of alveolus of right mandible**
HAC 7th characters A & B see Appendix B for HAC conditional logic

CC +7th **S02.672 Fracture of alveolus of left mandible**
HAC 7th characters A & B see Appendix B for HAC conditional logic

CC X+7th **S02.69 Fracture of mandible of other specified site**
HAC 7th characters A & B see Appendix B for HAC conditional logic

\+ **S02.8 Fractures of other specified skull and facial bones**
Fracture of palate
Excludes2: *fracture of orbital floor (S02.3-)*
fracture of orbital roof (S02.12-)
AHA CC: 4Q, 2019, 16-17

CC X+7th **S02.80 Fracture of other specified skull and facial bones, unspecified side**
HAC 7th characters A & B see Appendix B for HAC conditional logic

CC X+7th **S02.81 Fracture of other specified skull and facial bones, right side**
HAC 7th characters A & B see Appendix B for HAC conditional logic

CC X+7th **S02.82 Fracture of other specified skull and facial bones, left side**
HAC 7th characters A & B see Appendix B for HAC conditional logic

\+ **S02.83 Fracture of medial orbital wall**
Excludes2: *orbital floor (S02.3-)*
orbital roof (S02.12-)

CC **S02.831 Fracture of medial orbital wall, right side**
HAC 7th characters A & B see Appendix B for HAC conditional logic

CC **S02.832 Fracture of medical orbital wall, left side**
HAC 7th characters A & B see Appendix B for HAC conditional logic

CC **S03.839 Fracture of medical orbital wall, unspecified side**
HAC 7th characters A & B see Appendix B for HAC conditional logic

\+ **S02.84 Fracture of lateral orbital wall**
Excludes2: *orbital floor (S02.3-)*
orbital roof (S02.12-)

CC **S02.841 Fracture of lateral orbital wall, right side**
HAC 7th characters A & B see Appendix B for HAC conditional logic

CC **S02.842 Fracture of lateral orbital wall, left side**
HAC 7th characters A & B see Appendix B for HAC conditional logic

CC **S02.849 Fracture of lateral orbital wall, unspecified side**
HAC 7th characters A & B see Appendix B for HAC conditional logic

CC **S02.85 Fracture of orbit, unspecified**
Fracture of orbit NOS
Fracture of orbit wall NOS
Excludes1: *lateral orbital wall (S02.84-)*
medial orbital wall (S02.83-)
orbital floor (S02.3-)
orbital roof (S02.12-)
HAC 7th characters A & B see Appendix B for HAC conditional logic

\+ **S02.9 Fracture of unspecified skull and facial bones**

CC MCC X+7th **S02.91 Unspecified fracture of skull**
AHA CC: 2Q, 2020, 24
HAC 7th characters A & B see Appendix B for HAC conditional logic

CC X+7th **S02.92 Unspecified fracture of facial bones**
HAC 7th characters A & B see Appendix B for HAC conditional logic

S03 Dislocation and sprain of joints and ligaments of head

Includes: avulsion of joint (capsule) or ligament of head
laceration of cartilage, joint (capsule) or ligament of head
sprain of cartilage, joint (capsule) or ligament of head
traumatic hemarthrosis of joint or ligament of head
traumatic rupture of joint or ligament of head
traumatic subluxation of joint or ligament of head
traumatic tear of joint or ligament of head

Code also any associated open wound

Excludes2: *Strain of muscle or tendon of head (S09.1)*

The appropriate 7th character is to be added to each code from category S03
A initial encounter
D subsequent encounter
S sequela

\+ **S03.0 Dislocation of jaw**
Dislocation of jaw (cartilage) (meniscus)
Dislocation of mandible
Dislocation of temporomandibular (joint)
AHA CC: 4Q, 2016, 67

X+7th **S03.00 Dislocation of jaw, unspecified side**
X+7th **S03.01 Dislocation of jaw, right side**
X+7th **S03.02 Dislocation of jaw, left side**
X+7th **S03.03 Dislocation of jaw, bilateral**

X+7th **S03.1 Dislocation of septal cartilage of nose**
X+7th **S03.2 Dislocation of tooth**

\+ **S03.4 Sprain of jaw**
Sprain of temporomandibular (joint) (ligament)
AHA CC: 4Q, 2016, 67

X+7th **S03.40 Sprain of jaw, unspecified side**
X+7th **S03.41 Sprain of jaw, right side**
X+7th **S03.42 Sprain of jaw, left side**
X+7th **S03.43 Sprain of jaw, bilateral**

X+7th **S03.8 Sprain of joints and ligaments of other parts of head**
X+7th **S03.9 Sprain of joints and ligaments of unspecified parts of head**

S04 Injury of cranial nerve

The selection of side should be based on the side of the body being affected

Code first any associated intracranial injury (S06.-)

Code also any associated:
open wound of head (S01.-)
skull fracture (S02.-)

The appropriate 7th character is to be added to each code from category S04
A initial encounter
D subsequent encounter
S sequela

\+ **S04.0 Injury of optic nerve and pathways**
Use additional code to identify any visual field defect or blindness (H53.4-, H54.-)

\+ **S04.01 Injury of optic nerve**
Injury of 2nd cranial nerve

CC +7th **S04.011 Injury of optic nerve, right eye**
CC +7th **S04.012 Injury of optic nerve, left eye**
CC +7th **S04.019 Injury of optic nerve, unspecified eye**
Injury of optic nerve NOS

CC X+7th **S04.02 Injury of optic chiasm**

\+ **S04.03 Injury of optic tract and pathways**
Injury of optic radiation

CC +7th **S04.031 Injury of optic tract and pathways, right side**
CC +7th **S04.032 Injury of optic tract and pathways, left side**
CC +7th **S04.039 Injury of optic tract and pathways, unspecified side**
Injury of optic tract and pathways NOS

\+ **S04.04 Injury of visual cortex**

CC +7th **S04.041 Injury of visual cortex, right side**
CC +7th **S04.042 Injury of visual cortex, left side**
CC +7th **S04.049 Injury of visual cortex, unspecified side**
Injury of visual cortex NOS

\+ **S04.1 Injury of oculomotor nerve**
Injury of 3rd cranial nerve

CC X+7th **S04.10 Injury of oculomotor nerve, unspecified side**
CC X+7th **S04.11 Injury of oculomotor nerve, right side**
CC X+7th **S04.12 Injury of oculomotor nerve, left side**

\+ **S04.2 Injury of trochlear nerve**
Injury of 4th cranial nerve

CC X+7th **S04.20 Injury of trochlear nerve, unspecified side**
CC X+7th **S04.21 Injury of trochlear nerve, right side**
CC X+7th **S04.22 Injury of trochlear nerve, left side**

\+ **S04.3 Injury of trigeminal nerve**
Injury of 5th cranial nerve

CC X+7th **S04.30 Injury of trigeminal nerve, unspecified side**
CC X+7th **S04.31 Injury of trigeminal nerve, right side**
CC X+7th **S04.32 Injury of trigeminal nerve, left side**

\+ **S04.4 Injury of abducent nerve**
Injury of 6th cranial nerve

CC X+7th **S04.40 Injury of abducent nerve, unspecified side**
CC X+7th **S04.41 Injury of abducent nerve, right side**
CC X+7th **S04.42 Injury of abducent nerve, left side**

\+ **S04.5 Injury of facial nerve**
Injury of 7th cranial nerve

CC X+7th **S04.50 Injury of facial nerve, unspecified side**
CC X+7th **S04.51 Injury of facial nerve, right side**
CC X+7th **S04.52 Injury of facial nerve, left side**

\+ **S04.6 Injury of acoustic nerve**
Injury of auditory nerve
Injury of 8th cranial nerve

CC X+7th **S04.60 Injury of acoustic nerve, unspecified side**
CC X+7th **S04.61 Injury of acoustic nerve, right side**
CC X+7th **S04.62 Injury of acoustic nerve, left side**

\+ **S04.7 Injury of accessory nerve**
Injury of 11th cranial nerve

CC X+7th **S04.70 Injury of accessory nerve, unspecified side**
CC X+7th **S04.71 Injury of accessory nerve, right side**
CC X+7th **S04.72 Injury of accessory nerve, left side**

\+ **S04.8 Injury of other cranial nerves**

\+ **S04.81 Injury of olfactory [1st] nerve**

CC +7th **S04.811 Injury of olfactory [1st] nerve, right side**
CC +7th **S04.812 Injury of olfactory [1st] nerve, left side**
CC +7th **S04.819 Injury of olfactory [1st] nerve, unspecified side**

\+ **S04.89 Injury of other cranial nerves**
Injury of vagus [10th] nerve

CC +7th **S04.891 Injury of other cranial nerves, right side**
CC +7th **S04.892 Injury of other cranial nerves, left side**
CC +7th **S04.899 Injury of other cranial nerves, unspecified side**

CC X+7th **S04.9 Injury of unspecified cranial nerve**

S05 Injury of eye and orbit

Includes: open wound of eye and orbit

Excludes2: *2nd cranial [optic] nerve injury (S04.0-)*
3rd cranial [oculomotor] nerve injury (S04.1-)
open wound of eyelid and periocular area (S01.1-)
orbital bone fracture (S02.1-, S02.3-, S02.8-)
superficial injury of eyelid (S00.1-S00.2)

The appropriate 7th character is to be added to each code from category S05
A initial encounter
D subsequent encounter
S sequela

\+ **S05.0 Injury of conjunctiva and corneal abrasion without foreign body**

Excludes1: *foreign body in conjunctival sac (T15.1)*
foreign body in cornea (T15.0)

X+7th **S05.00 Injury of conjunctiva and corneal abrasion without foreign body, unspecified eye**
X+7th **S05.01 Injury of conjunctiva and corneal abrasion without foreign body, right eye**
X+7th **S05.02 Injury of conjunctiva and corneal abrasion without foreign body, left eye**

\+ **S05.1 Contusion of eyeball and orbital tissues**
Traumatic hyphema

Excludes2: *black eye NOS (S00.1)*
contusion of eyelid and periocular area (S00.1)

X+7th **S05.10 Contusion of eyeball and orbital tissues, unspecified eye**
X+7th **S05.11 Contusion of eyeball and orbital tissues, right eye**
X+7th **S05.12 Contusion of eyeball and orbital tissues, left eye**

\+ **S05.2 Ocular laceration and rupture with prolapse or loss of intraocular tissue**

CC X+7th **S05.20 Ocular laceration and rupture with prolapse or loss of intraocular tissue, unspecified eye**

CC X+7th **S05.21 Ocular laceration and rupture with prolapse or loss of intraocular tissue, right eye**

CC X+7th **S05.22 Ocular laceration and rupture with prolapse or loss of intraocular tissue, left eye**

\+ **S05.3 Ocular laceration without prolapse or loss of intraocular tissue**

Laceration of eye NOS

CC X+7th **S05.30 Ocular laceration without prolapse or loss of intraocular tissue, unspecified eye**

CC X+7th **S05.31 Ocular laceration without prolapse or loss of intraocular tissue, right eye**

CC X+7th **S05.32 Ocular laceration without prolapse or loss of intraocular tissue, left eye**

\+ **S05.4 Penetrating wound of orbit with or without foreign body**

Excludes2: *retained (old) foreign body following penetrating wound in orbit (H05.5-)*

CC X+7th **S05.40 Penetrating wound of orbit with or without foreign body, unspecified eye**

CC X+7th **S05.41 Penetrating wound of orbit with or without foreign body, right eye**

CC X+7th **S05.42 Penetrating wound of orbit with or without foreign body, left eye**

\+ **S05.5 Penetrating wound with foreign body of eyeball**

Excludes2: *retained (old) intraocular foreign body (H44.6-, H44.7)*

CC X+7th **S05.50 Penetrating wound with foreign body of unspecified eyeball**

CC X+7th **S05.51 Penetrating wound with foreign body of right eyeball**

CC X+7th **S05.52 Penetrating wound with foreign body of left eyeball**

\+ **S05.6 Penetrating wound without foreign body of eyeball**

Ocular penetration NOS

X+7th **S05.60 Penetrating wound without foreign body of unspecified eyeball**

X+7th **S05.61 Penetrating wound without foreign body of right eyeball**

X+7th **S05.62 Penetrating wound without foreign body of left eyeball**

\+ **S05.7 Avulsion of eye**

Traumatic enucleation

CC X+7th **S05.70 Avulsion of unspecified eye**

CC X+7th **S05.71 Avulsion of right eye**

CC X+7th **S05.72 Avulsion of left eye**

CC + **S05.8 Other injuries of eye and orbit**

Lacrimal duct injury

\+ **S05.8X Other injuries of eye and orbit**

+7th **S05.8X1 Other injuries of right eye and orbit**

+7th **S05.8X2 Other injuries of left eye and orbit**

+7th **S05.8X9 Other injuries of unspecified eye and orbit**

\+ **S05.9 Unspecified injury of eye and orbit**

Injury of eye NOS

X+7th **S05.90 Unspecified injury of unspecified eye and orbit**

CC X+7th **S05.91 Unspecified injury of right eye and orbit**

CC X+7th **S05.92 Unspecified injury of left eye and orbit**

S06 Intracranial injury

Includes: traumatic brain injury

Code also any associated:

open wound of head (S01.-)

skull fracture (S02.-)

Excludes1: *head injury NOS (S09.90)*

AHA CC: 4Q, 2017, 25

The appropriate 7th character is to be added to each code from category S06
- A initial encounter
- D subsequent encounter
- S sequela

NOTE 7th characters D and S do not apply to codes in category S06 with 6th character 7 - death due to brain injury prior to regaining consciousness, or 8 - death due to other cause prior to regaining consciousness.

\+ **S06.0 Concussion**

Commotio cerebri

Excludes1: *concussion with other intracranial injuries classified in category S06.1- to S06.6-, S06.81- and S06.82- code to specified intracranial injury*

AHA CC: 4Q, 2016, 67-68

\+ **S06.0X Concussion**

+7th **S06.0X0 Concussion without loss of consciousness**

HAC 7th character A see Appendix B for HAC conditional logic

CC +7th **S06.0X1 Concussion with loss of consciousness of 30 minutes or less**

HAC 7th character A see Appendix B for HAC conditional logic

CC +7th **S06.0X9 Concussion with loss of consciousness of unspecified duration**

Concussion NOS

HAC 7th character A see Appendix B for HAC conditional logic

\+ **S06.1 Traumatic cerebral edema**

Diffuse traumatic cerebral edema

Focal traumatic cerebral edema

\+ **S06.1X Traumatic cerebral edema**

MCC +7th **S06.1X0 Traumatic cerebral edema without loss of consciousness**

HAC 7th character A see Appendix B for HAC conditional logic

AHA CC: 1Q, 2015, 3-21

MCC +7th **S06.1X1 Traumatic cerebral edema with loss of consciousness of 30 minutes or less**

HAC 7th character A see Appendix B for HAC conditional logic

MCC +7th **S06.1X2 Traumatic cerebral edema with loss of consciousness of 31 minutes to 59 minutes**

HAC 7th character A see Appendix B for HAC conditional logic

MCC +7th **S06.1X3 Traumatic cerebral edema with loss of consciousness of 1 hour to 5 hours 59 minutes**

HAC 7th character A see Appendix B for HAC conditional logic

MCC +7th **S06.1X4 Traumatic cerebral edema with loss of consciousness of 6 hours to 24 hours**

HAC 7th character A see Appendix B for HAC conditional logic

MCC +7th **S06.1X5 Traumatic cerebral edema with loss of consciousness greater than 24 hours with return to pre-existing conscious level**

HAC 7th character A see Appendix B for HAC conditional logic

MCC +7th **S06.1X6 Traumatic cerebral edema with loss of consciousness greater than 24 hours without return to pre-existing conscious level with patient surviving**

HAC 7th character A see Appendix B for HAC conditional logic

MCC +7th **S06.1X7 Traumatic cerebral edema with loss of consciousness of any duration with death due to brain injury prior to regaining consciousness**

HAC 7th character A see Appendix B for HAC conditional logic

MCC +7th **S06.1X8 Traumatic cerebral edema with loss of consciousness of any duration with death due to other cause prior to regaining consciousness**

HAC 7th character A see Appendix B for HAC conditional logic

MCC +7th **S06.1X9 Traumatic cerebral edema with loss of consciousness of unspecified duration**

Traumatic cerebral edema NOS

HAC 7th character A see Appendix B for HAC conditional logic

CC + **S06.2 Diffuse traumatic brain injury**
Diffuse axonal brain injury
Use additional code, if applicable, for traumatic brain compression or herniation (S06.A-)
Excludes1: *traumatic diffuse cerebral edema (S06.1X-)*

+ **S06.2X Diffuse traumatic brain injury**

+7th **S06.2X0 Diffuse traumatic brain injury without loss of consciousness**
HAC 7th character A see Appendix B for HAC conditional logic

+7th **S06.2X1 Diffuse traumatic brain injury with loss of consciousness of 30 minutes or less**
HAC 7th character A see Appendix B for HAC conditional logic

+7th **S06.2X2 Diffuse traumatic brain injury with loss of consciousness of 31 minutes to 59 minutes**
HAC 7th character A see Appendix B for HAC conditional logic

+7th **S06.2X3 Diffuse traumatic brain injury with loss of consciousness of 1 hour to 5 hours 59 minutes**
HAC 7th character A see Appendix B for HAC conditional logic

+7th **S06.2X4 Diffuse traumatic brain injury with loss of consciousness of 6 hours to 24 hours**
HAC 7th character A see Appendix B for HAC conditional logic

+7th **S06.2X5 Diffuse traumatic brain injury with loss of consciousness greater than 24 hours with return to pre-existing conscious levels**
HAC 7th character A see Appendix B for HAC conditional logic

MCC +7th **S06.2X6 Diffuse traumatic brain injury with loss of consciousness greater than 24 hours without return to pre-existing conscious level with patient surviving**
HAC 7th character A see Appendix B for HAC conditional logic

MCC +7th **S06.2X7 Diffuse traumatic brain injury with loss of consciousness of any duration with death due to brain injury prior to regaining consciousness**
HAC 7th character A see Appendix B for HAC conditional logic

MCC +7th **S06.2X8 Diffuse traumatic brain injury with loss of consciousness of any duration with death due to other cause prior to regaining consciousness**
HAC 7th character A see Appendix B for HAC conditional logic

+7th **S06.2X9 Diffuse traumatic brain injury with loss of consciousness of unspecified duration**
Diffuse traumatic brain injury NOS
HAC 7th character A see Appendix B for HAC conditional logic

+ **S06.3 Focal traumatic brain injury**
Use additional code, if applicable, for traumatic brain compression or herniation (S06.A-)
Excludes1: *any condition classifiable to S06.4-S06.6*
Excludes2: *focal cerebral edema (S06.1)*

+ **S06.30 Unspecified focal traumatic brain injury**

+7th **S06.300 Unspecified focal traumatic brain injury without loss of consciousness**

CC +7th **S06.301 Unspecified focal traumatic brain injury with loss of consciousness of 30 minutes or less**
HAC 7th character A see Appendix B for HAC conditional logic

CC +7th **S06.302 Unspecified focal traumatic brain injury with loss of consciousness of 31 minutes to 59 minutes**
HAC 7th character A see Appendix B for HAC conditional logic

CC +7th **S06.303 Unspecified focal traumatic brain injury with loss of consciousness of 1 hour to 5 hours 59 minutes**
HAC 7th character A see Appendix B for HAC conditional logic

CC +7th **S06.304 Unspecified focal traumatic brain injury with loss of consciousness of 6 hours to 24 hours**
HAC 7th character A see Appendix B for HAC conditional logic

CC +7th **S06.305 Unspecified focal traumatic brain injury with loss of consciousness greater than 24 hours with return to pre-existing conscious level**
HAC 7th character A see Appendix B for HAC conditional logic

MCC +7th **S06.306 Unspecified focal traumatic brain injury with loss of consciousness greater than 24 hours without return to pre-existing conscious level with patient surviving**
HAC 7th character A see Appendix B for HAC conditional logic

MCC +7th **S06.307 Unspecified focal traumatic brain injury with loss of consciousness of any duration with death due to brain injury prior to regaining consciousness**
HAC 7th character A see Appendix B for HAC conditional logic

MCC +7th **S06.308 Unspecified focal traumatic brain injury with loss of consciousness of any duration with death due to other cause prior to regaining consciousness**
HAC 7th character A see Appendix B for HAC conditional logic

CC +7th **S06.309 Unspecified focal traumatic brain injury with loss of consciousness of unspecified duration**
Unspecified focal traumatic brain injury NOS
HAC 7th character A see Appendix B for HAC conditional logic

+ **S06.31 Contusion and laceration of right cerebrum**

MCC +7th **S06.310 Contusion and laceration of right cerebrum without loss of consciousness**
HAC 7th character A see Appendix B for HAC conditional logic

MCC +7th **S06.311 Contusion and laceration of right cerebrum with loss of consciousness of 30 minutes or less**
HAC 7th character A see Appendix B for HAC conditional logic

MCC +7th **S06.312 Contusion and laceration of right cerebrum with loss of consciousness of 31 minutes to 59 minutes**
HAC 7th character A see Appendix B for HAC conditional logic

MCC +7th **S06.313 Contusion and laceration of right cerebrum with loss of consciousness of 1 hour to 5 hours 59 minutes**
HAC 7th character A see Appendix B for HAC conditional logic

MCC +7th **S06.314 Contusion and laceration of right cerebrum with loss of consciousness of 6 hours to 24 hours**
HAC 7th character A see Appendix B for HAC conditional logic

MCC +7th **S06.315 Contusion and laceration of right cerebrum with loss of consciousness greater than 24 hours with return to pre-existing conscious level**
HAC 7th character A see Appendix B for HAC conditional logic

MCC +7th **S06.316 Contusion and laceration of right cerebrum with loss of consciousness greater than 24 hours without return to pre-existing conscious level with patient surviving**
HAC 7th character A see Appendix B for HAC conditional logic

MCC +7th **S06.317 Contusion and laceration of right cerebrum with loss of consciousness of any duration with death due to brain injury prior to regaining consciousness**
HAC 7th character A see Appendix B for HAC conditional logic

MCC +7th **S06.318 Contusion and laceration of right cerebrum with loss of consciousness of any duration with death due to other cause prior to regaining consciousness**
HAC 7th character A see Appendix B for HAC conditional logic

MCC +7th **S06.319 Contusion and laceration of right cerebrum with loss of consciousness of unspecified duration**
Contusion and laceration of right cerebrum NOS
HAC 7th character A see Appendix B for HAC conditional logic

\+ **S06.32 Contusion and laceration of left cerebrum**

MCC +7th **S06.320 Contusion and laceration of left cerebrum without loss of consciousness**
HAC 7th character A see Appendix B for HAC conditional logic

MCC +7th **S06.321 Contusion and laceration of left cerebrum with loss of consciousness of 30 minutes or less**
HAC 7th character A see Appendix B for HAC conditional logic

MCC +7th **S06.322 Contusion and laceration of left cerebrum with loss of consciousness of 31 minutes to 59 minutes**
HAC 7th character A see Appendix B for HAC conditional logic

MCC +7th **S06.323 Contusion and laceration of left cerebrum with loss of consciousness of 1 hour to 5 hours 59 minutes**
HAC 7th character A see Appendix B for HAC conditional logic

MCC +7th **S06.324 Contusion and laceration of left cerebrum with loss of consciousness of 6 hours to 24 hours**
HAC 7th character A see Appendix B for HAC conditional logic

MCC +7th **S06.325 Contusion and laceration of left cerebrum with loss of consciousness greater than 24 hours with return to pre-existing conscious level**
HAC 7th character A see Appendix B for HAC conditional logic

MCC +7th **S06.326 Contusion and laceration of left cerebrum with loss of consciousness greater than 24 hours without return to pre-existing conscious level with patient surviving**
HAC 7th character A see Appendix B for HAC conditional logic

MCC +7th **S06.327 Contusion and laceration of left cerebrum with loss of consciousness of any duration with death due to brain injury prior to regaining consciousness**
HAC 7th character A see Appendix B for HAC conditional logic

MCC +7th **S06.328 Contusion and laceration of left cerebrum with loss of consciousness of any duration with death due to other cause prior to regaining consciousness**
HAC 7th character A see Appendix B for HAC conditional logic

MCC +7th **S06.329 Contusion and laceration of left cerebrum with loss of consciousness of unspecified duration**
Contusion and laceration of left cerebrum NOS
HAC 7th character A see Appendix B for HAC conditional logic

\+ **S06.33 Contusion and laceration of cerebrum, unspecified**

MCC +7th **S06.330 Contusion and laceration of cerebrum, unspecified, without loss of consciousness**
HAC 7th character A see Appendix B for HAC conditional logic

MCC +7th **S06.331 Contusion and laceration of cerebrum, unspecified, with loss of consciousness of 30 minutes or less**
HAC 7th character A see Appendix B for HAC conditional logic

MCC +7th **S06.332 Contusion and laceration of cerebrum, unspecified, with loss of consciousness of 31 minutes to 59 minutes**
HAC 7th character A see Appendix B for HAC conditional logic

MCC +7th **S06.333 Contusion and laceration of cerebrum, unspecified, with loss of consciousness of 1 hour to 5 hours 59 minutes**
HAC 7th character A see Appendix B for HAC conditional logic

MCC +7th **S06.334 Contusion and laceration of cerebrum, unspecified, with loss of consciousness of 6 hours to 24 hours**
HAC 7th character A see Appendix B for HAC conditional logic

MCC +7th **S06.335 Contusion and laceration of cerebrum, unspecified, with loss of consciousness greater than 24 hours with return to pre-existing conscious level**
HAC 7th character A see Appendix B for HAC conditional logic

MCC +7th **S06.336 Contusion and laceration of cerebrum, unspecified, with loss of consciousness greater than 24 hours without return to pre-existing conscious level with patient surviving**
HAC 7th character A see Appendix B for HAC conditional logic

MCC +7th **S06.337 Contusion and laceration of cerebrum, unspecified, with loss of consciousness of any duration with death due to brain injury prior to regaining consciousness**
HAC 7th character A see Appendix B for HAC conditional logic

MCC +7th **S06.338 Contusion and laceration of cerebrum, unspecified, with loss of consciousness of any duration with death due to other cause prior to regaining consciousness**
HAC 7th character A see Appendix B for HAC conditional logic

MCC +7th **S06.339 Contusion and laceration of cerebrum, unspecified, with loss of consciousness of unspecified duration**
Contusion and laceration of cerebrum NOS
HAC 7th character A see Appendix B for HAC conditional logic

\+ **S06.34 Traumatic hemorrhage of right cerebrum**
Traumatic intracerebral hemorrhage and hematoma of right cerebrum

MCC +7th **S06.340 Traumatic hemorrhage of right cerebrum without loss of consciousness**
HAC 7th character A see Appendix B for HAC conditional logic
AHA CC: 1Q, 2015, 3-21

MCC +7th **S06.341 Traumatic hemorrhage of right cerebrum with loss of consciousness of 30 minutes or less**
HAC 7th character A see Appendix B for HAC conditional logic

MCC +7th **S06.342 Traumatic hemorrhage of right cerebrum with loss of consciousness of 31 minutes to 59 minutes**
HAC 7th character A see Appendix B for HAC conditional logic

MCC +7th **S06.343 Traumatic hemorrhage of right cerebrum with loss of consciousness of 1 hours to 5 hours 59 minutes**
HAC 7th character A see Appendix B for HAC conditional logic

MCC +7th **S06.344 Traumatic hemorrhage of right cerebrum with loss of consciousness of 6 hours to 24 hours**
HAC 7th character A see Appendix B for HAC conditional logic

MCC +7th **S06.345 Traumatic hemorrhage of right cerebrum with loss of consciousness greater than 24 hours with return to pre-existing conscious level**
HAC 7th character A see Appendix B for HAC conditional logic

MCC +7th **S06.346 Traumatic hemorrhage of right cerebrum with loss of consciousness greater than 24 hours without return to pre-existing conscious level with patient surviving**
HAC 7th character A see Appendix B for HAC conditional logic

MCC +7th **S06.347** **Traumatic hemorrhage of right cerebrum with loss of consciousness of any duration with death due to brain injury prior to regaining consciousness**
HAC 7th character A see Appendix B for HAC conditional logic

MCC +7th **S06.348** **Traumatic hemorrhage of right cerebrum with loss of consciousness of any duration with death due to other cause prior to regaining consciousness**
HAC 7th character A see Appendix B for HAC conditional logic

MCC +7th **S06.349** **Traumatic hemorrhage of right cerebrum with loss of consciousness of unspecified duration**
Traumatic hemorrhage of right cerebrum NOS
HAC 7th character A see Appendix B for HAC conditional logic

+ **S06.35** **Traumatic hemorrhage of left cerebrum**
Traumatic intracerebral hemorrhage and hematoma of left cerebrum

MCC +7th **S06.350** **Traumatic hemorrhage of left cerebrum without loss of consciousness**
HAC 7th character A see Appendix B for HAC conditional logic

MCC +7th **S06.351** **Traumatic hemorrhage of left cerebrum with loss of consciousness of 30 minutes or less**
HAC 7th character A see Appendix B for HAC conditional logic

MCC +7th **S06.352** **Traumatic hemorrhage of left cerebrum with loss of consciousness of 31 minutes to 59 minutes**
HAC 7th character A see Appendix B for HAC conditional logic

MCC +7th **S06.353** **Traumatic hemorrhage of left cerebrum with loss of consciousness of 1 hours to 5 hours 59 minutes**
HAC 7th character A see Appendix B for HAC conditional logic

MCC +7th **S06.354** **Traumatic hemorrhage of left cerebrum with loss of consciousness of 6 hours to 24 hours**
HAC 7th character A see Appendix B for HAC conditional logic

MCC +7th **S06.355** **Traumatic hemorrhage of left cerebrum with loss of consciousness greater than 24 hours with return to pre-existing conscious level**
HAC 7th character A see Appendix B for HAC conditional logic

MCC +7th **S06.356** **Traumatic hemorrhage of left cerebrum with loss of consciousness greater than 24 hours without return to pre-existing conscious level with patient surviving**
HAC 7th character A see Appendix B for HAC conditional logic

MCC +7th **S06.357** **Traumatic hemorrhage of left cerebrum with loss of consciousness of≈any duration with death due to brain injury prior to regaining consciousness**
HAC 7th character A see Appendix B for HAC conditional logic

MCC +7th **S06.358** **Traumatic hemorrhage of left cerebrum with loss of consciousness of any duration with death due to other cause prior to regaining consciousness**
HAC 7th character A see Appendix B for HAC conditional logic

MCC +7th **S06.359** **Traumatic hemorrhage of left cerebrum with loss of consciousness of unspecified duration**
Traumatic hemorrhage of left cerebrum NOS
HAC 7th character A see Appendix B for HAC conditional logic

+ **S06.36** **Traumatic hemorrhage of cerebrum, unspecified**
Traumatic intracerebral hemorrhage and hematoma, unspecified

MCC +7th **S06.360** **Traumatic hemorrhage of cerebrum, unspecified, without loss of consciousness**
HAC 7th character A see Appendix B for HAC conditional logic

MCC +7th **S06.361** **Traumatic hemorrhage of cerebrum, unspecified, with loss of consciousness of 30 minutes or less**
HAC 7th character A see Appendix B for HAC conditional logic

MCC +7th **S06.362** **Traumatic hemorrhage of cerebrum, unspecified, with loss of consciousness of 31 minutes to 59 minutes**
HAC 7th character A see Appendix B for HAC conditional logic

MCC +7th **S06.363** **Traumatic hemorrhage of cerebrum, unspecified, with loss of consciousness of 1 hours to 5 hours 59 minutes**
HAC 7th character A see Appendix B for HAC conditional logic

MCC +7th **S06.364** **Traumatic hemorrhage of cerebrum, unspecified, with loss of consciousness of 6 hours to 24 hours**
HAC 7th character A see Appendix B for HAC conditional logic

MCC +7th **S06.365** **Traumatic hemorrhage of cerebrum, unspecified, with loss of consciousness greater than 24 hours with return to pre-existing conscious level**
HAC 7th character A see Appendix B for HAC conditional logic

MCC +7th **S06.366** **Traumatic hemorrhage of cerebrum, unspecified, with loss of consciousness greater than 24 hours without return to pre-existing conscious level with patient surviving**
HAC 7th character A see Appendix B for HAC conditional logic

MCC +7th **S06.367** **Traumatic hemorrhage of cerebrum, unspecified, with loss of consciousness of any duration with death due to brain injury prior to regaining consciousness**
HAC 7th character A see Appendix B for HAC conditional logic

MCC +7th **S06.368** **Traumatic hemorrhage of cerebrum, unspecified, with loss of consciousness of any duration with death due to other cause prior to regaining consciousness**
HAC 7th character A see Appendix B for HAC conditional logic

MCC +7th **S06.369** **Traumatic hemorrhage of cerebrum, unspecified, with loss of consciousness of unspecified duration**
Traumatic hemorrhage of cerebrum NOS
HAC 7th character A see Appendix B for HAC conditional logic

+ **S06.37** **Contusion, laceration, and hemorrhage of cerebellum**

MCC +7th **S06.370** **Contusion, laceration, and hemorrhage of cerebellum without loss of consciousness**
HAC 7th character A see Appendix B for HAC conditional logic

CC +7th **S06.371** **Contusion, laceration, and hemorrhage of cerebellum with loss of consciousness of 30 minutes or less**
HAC 7th character A see Appendix B for HAC conditional logic

CC +7th **S06.372** **Contusion, laceration, and hemorrhage of cerebellum with loss of consciousness of 31 minutes to 59 minutes**
HAC 7th character A see Appendix B for HAC conditional logic

CC +7th **S06.373** **Contusion, laceration, and hemorrhage of cerebellum with loss of consciousness of 1 hour to 5 hours 59 minutes**
HAC 7th character A see Appendix B for HAC conditional logic

CC +7th **S06.374** **Contusion, laceration, and hemorrhage of cerebellum with loss of consciousness of 6 hours to 24 hours**
HAC 7th character A see Appendix B for HAC conditional logic

CC +7th **S06.375** **Contusion, laceration, and hemorrhage of cerebellum with loss of consciousness greater than 24 hours with return to pre-existing conscious level**
HAC 7th character A see Appendix B for HAC conditional logic

MCC +7th **S06.376** **Contusion, laceration, and hemorrhage of cerebellum with loss of consciousness greater than 24 hours without return to pre-existing conscious level with patient surviving**
HAC 7th character A see Appendix B for HAC conditional logic

MCC +7th **S06.377** **Contusion, laceration, and hemorrhage of cerebellum with loss of consciousness of any duration with death due to brain injury prior to regaining consciousness**
HAC 7th character A see Appendix B for HAC conditional logic

MCC +7th **S06.378** **Contusion, laceration, and hemorrhage of cerebellum with loss of consciousness of any duration with death due to other cause prior to regaining consciousness**
HAC 7th character A see Appendix B for HAC conditional logic

CC +7th **S06.379** **Contusion, laceration, and hemorrhage of cerebellum with loss of consciousness of unspecified duration**
Contusion, laceration, and hemorrhage of cerebellum NOS
HAC 7th character A see Appendix B for HAC conditional logic

+ **S06.38** **Contusion, laceration, and hemorrhage of brainstem**

MCC +7th **S06.380** **Contusion, laceration, and hemorrhage of brainstem without loss of consciousness**
HAC 7th character A see Appendix B for HAC conditional logic

CC +7th **S06.381** **Contusion, laceration, and hemorrhage of brainstem with loss of consciousness of 30 minutes or less**
HAC 7th character A see Appendix B for HAC conditional logic

CC +7th **S06.382** **Contusion, laceration, and hemorrhage of brainstem with loss of consciousness of 31 minutes to 59 minutes**
HAC 7th character A see Appendix B for HAC conditional logic

CC +7th **S06.383** **Contusion, laceration, and hemorrhage of brainstem with loss of consciousness of 1 hour to 5 hours 59 minutes**
HAC 7th character A see Appendix B for HAC conditional logic

CC +7th **S06.384** **Contusion, laceration, and hemorrhage of brainstem with loss of consciousness of 6 hours to 24 hours**
HAC 7th character A see Appendix B for HAC conditional logic

CC +7th **S06.385** **Contusion, laceration, and hemorrhage of brainstem with loss of consciousness greater than 24 hours with return to pre-existing conscious level**
HAC 7th character A see Appendix B for HAC conditional logic

MCC +7th **S06.386** **Contusion, laceration, and hemorrhage of brainstem with loss of consciousness greater than 24 hours without return to pre-existing conscious level with patient surviving**
HAC 7th character A see Appendix B for HAC conditional logic

MCC +7th **S06.387** **Contusion, laceration, and hemorrhage of brainstem with loss of consciousness of any duration with death due to brain injury prior to regaining consciousness**
HAC 7th character A see Appendix B for HAC conditional logic

MCC +7th **S06.388** **Contusion, laceration, and hemorrhage of brainstem with loss of consciousness of any duration with death due to other cause prior to regaining consciousness**
HAC 7th character A see Appendix B for HAC conditional logic

CC +7th **S06.389** **Contusion, laceration, and hemorrhage of brainstem with loss of consciousness of unspecified duration**
Contusion, laceration, and hemorrhage of brainstem NOS
HAC 7th character A see Appendix B for HAC conditional logic

+ **S06.4** **Epidural hemorrhage**
Extradural hemorrhage NOS
Extradural hemorrhage (traumatic)

+ **S06.4X** **Epidural hemorrhage**

MCC +7th **S06.4X0** **Epidural hemorrhage without loss of consciousness**
HAC 7th character A see Appendix B for HAC conditional logic

MCC +7th **S06.4X1** **Epidural hemorrhage with loss of consciousness of 30 minutes or less**
HAC 7th character A see Appendix B for HAC conditional logic

MCC +7th **S06.4X2** **Epidural hemorrhage with loss of consciousness of 31 minutes to 59 minutes**
HAC 7th character A see Appendix B for HAC conditional logic

MCC +7th **S06.4X3** **Epidural hemorrhage with loss of consciousness of 1 hour to 5 hours 59 minutes**
HAC 7th character A see Appendix B for HAC conditional logic

MCC +7th **S06.4X4** **Epidural hemorrhage with loss of consciousness of 6 hours to 24 hours**
HAC 7th character A see Appendix B for HAC conditional logic

MCC +7th **S06.4X5** **Epidural hemorrhage with loss of consciousness greater than 24 hours with return to pre-existing conscious level**
HAC 7th character A see Appendix B for HAC conditional logic

MCC +7th **S06.4X6** **Epidural hemorrhage with loss of consciousness greater than 24 hours without return to pre-existing conscious level with patient surviving**
HAC 7th character A see Appendix B for HAC conditional logic

MCC +7th **S06.4X7** **Epidural hemorrhage with loss of consciousness of any duration with death due to brain injury prior to regaining consciousness**
HAC 7th character A see Appendix B for HAC conditional logic

MCC +7th **S06.4X8** **Epidural hemorrhage with loss of consciousness of any duration with death due to other causes prior to regaining consciousness**
HAC 7th character A see Appendix B for HAC conditional logic

MCC +7th **S06.4X9** **Epidural hemorrhage with loss of consciousness of unspecified duration**
Epidural hemorrhage NOS
HAC 7th character A see Appendix B for HAC conditional logic

+ **S06.5** **Traumatic subdural hemorrhage**
Use additional code, if applicable, for traumatic brain compression or herniation (S06.A-)

+ **S06.5X** **Traumatic subdural hemorrhage**

MCC +7th **S06.5X0** **Traumatic subdural hemorrhage without loss of consciousness**
HAC 7th character A see Appendix B for HAC conditional logic
AHA CC: 3Q, 2015, 37; 2Q, 2018, 13; 1Q, 2021, 4-5

MCC +7th **S06.5X1** **Traumatic subdural hemorrhage with loss of consciousness of 30 minutes or less**
HAC 7th character A see Appendix B for HAC conditional logic

MCC +7th **S06.5X2** **Traumatic subdural hemorrhage with loss of consciousness of 31 minutes to 59 minutes**
HAC 7th character A see Appendix B for HAC conditional logic

MCC +7th **S06.5X3** **Traumatic subdural hemorrhage with loss of consciousness of 1 hour to 5 hours 59 minutes**
HAC 7th character A see Appendix B for HAC conditional logic

MCC +7th **S06.5X4** **Traumatic subdural hemorrhage with loss of consciousness of 6 hours to 24 hours**
HAC 7th character A see Appendix B for HAC conditional logic

MCC +7th **S06.5X5** **Traumatic subdural hemorrhage with loss of consciousness greater than 24 hours with return to pre-existing conscious level**
HAC 7th character A see Appendix B for HAC conditional logic

MCC +7th **S06.5X6** **Traumatic subdural hemorrhage with loss of consciousness greater than 24 hours without return to pre-existing conscious level with patient surviving**
AHA CC: 2Q, 2021, 5
HAC 7th character A see Appendix B for HAC conditional logic

MCC +7th **S06.5X7** **Traumatic subdural hemorrhage with loss of consciousness of any duration with death due to brain injury before regaining consciousness**
HAC 7th character A see Appendix B for HAC conditional logic

MCC +7th **S06.5X8** **Traumatic subdural hemorrhage with loss of consciousness of any duration with death due to other cause before regaining consciousness**
HAC 7th character A see Appendix B for HAC conditional logic

MCC +7th **S06.5X9** **Traumatic subdural hemorrhage with loss of consciousness of unspecified duration**
Traumatic subdural hemorrhage NOS
HAC 7th character A see Appendix B for HAC conditional logic

\+ **S06.6** **Traumatic subarachnoid hemorrhage**
Use additional code, if applicable, for traumatic brain compression or herniation (S06.A-)

\+ **S06.6X** **Traumatic subarachnoid hemorrhage**

MCC +7th **S06.6X0** **Traumatic subarachnoid hemorrhage without loss of consciousness**
HAC 7th character A see Appendix B for HAC conditional logic
AHA CC: 3Q, 2015, 37

MCC +7th **S06.6X1** **Traumatic subarachnoid hemorrhage with loss of consciousness of 30 minutes or less**
HAC 7th character A see Appendix B for HAC conditional logic

MCC +7th **S06.6X2** **Traumatic subarachnoid hemorrhage with loss of consciousness of 31 minutes to 59 minutes**
HAC 7th character A see Appendix B for HAC conditional logic

MCC +7th **S06.6X3** **Traumatic subarachnoid hemorrhage with loss of consciousness of 1 hour to 5 hours 59 minutes**
HAC 7th character A see Appendix B for HAC conditional logic

MCC +7th **S06.6X4** **Traumatic subarachnoid hemorrhage with loss of consciousness of 6 hours to 24 hours**
HAC 7th character A see Appendix B for HAC conditional logic

MCC +7th **S06.6X5** **Traumatic subarachnoid hemorrhage with loss of consciousness greater than 24 hours with return to pre-existing conscious level**
HAC 7th character A see Appendix B for HAC conditional logic

MCC +7th **S06.6X6** **Traumatic subarachnoid hemorrhage with loss of consciousness greater than 24 hours without return to pre-existing conscious level with patient surviving**
AHA CC: 2Q, 2021, 5
HAC 7th character A see Appendix B for HAC conditional logic

MCC +7th **S06.6X7** **Traumatic subarachnoid hemorrhage with loss of consciousness of any duration with death due to brain injury prior to regaining consciousness**
HAC 7th character A see Appendix B for HAC conditional logic

MCC +7th **S06.6X8** **Traumatic subarachnoid hemorrhage with loss of consciousness of any duration with death due to other cause prior to regaining consciousness**
HAC 7th character A see Appendix B for HAC conditional logic

MCC +7th **S06.6X9** **Traumatic subarachnoid hemorrhage with loss of consciousness of unspecified duration**
Traumatic subarachnoid hemorrhage NOS
HAC 7th character A see Appendix B for HAC conditional logic

\+ **S06.8** **Other specified intracranial injuries**

\+ **S06.81** **Injury of right internal carotid artery, intracranial portion, not elsewhere classified**

+7th **S06.810** **Injury of right internal carotid artery, intracranial portion, not elsewhere classified without loss of consciousness**

CC +7th **S06.811** **Injury of right internal carotid artery, intracranial portion, not elsewhere classified with loss of consciousness of 30 minutes or less**
HAC 7th character A see Appendix B for HAC conditional logic

CC +7th **S06.812** **Injury of right internal carotid artery, intracranial portion, not elsewhere classified with loss of consciousness of 31 minutes to 59 minutes**
HAC 7th character A see Appendix B for HAC conditional logic

CC +7th **S06.813** **Injury of right internal carotid artery, intracranial portion, not elsewhere classified with loss of consciousness of 1 hour to 5 hours 59 minutes**
HAC 7th character A see Appendix B for HAC conditional logic

CC +7th **S06.814** **Injury of right internal carotid artery, intracranial portion, not elsewhere classified with loss of consciousness of 6 hours to 24 hours**
HAC 7th character A see Appendix B for HAC conditional logic

CC +7th **S06.815** **Injury of right internal carotid artery, intracranial portion, not elsewhere classified with loss of consciousness greater than 24 hours with return to pre-existing conscious level**
HAC 7th character A see Appendix B for HAC conditional logic

MCC +7th **S06.816** **Injury of right internal carotid artery, intracranial portion, not elsewhere classified with loss of consciousness greater than 24 hours without return to pre-existing conscious level with patient surviving**
HAC 7th character A see Appendix B for HAC conditional logic

MCC +7th **S06.817** **Injury of right internal carotid artery, intracranial portion, not elsewhere classified with loss of consciousness of any duration with death due to brain injury prior to regaining consciousness**
HAC 7th character A see Appendix B for HAC conditional logic

MCC +7th **S06.818** **Injury of right internal carotid artery, intracranial portion, not elsewhere classified with loss of consciousness of any duration with death due to other cause prior to regaining consciousness**
HAC 7th character A see Appendix B for HAC conditional logic

CC +7th **S06.819** **Injury of right internal carotid artery, intracranial portion, not elsewhere classified with loss of consciousness of unspecified duration**
Injury of right internal carotid artery, intracranial portion, not elsewhere classified NOS
HAC 7th character A see Appendix B for HAC conditional logic

\+ **S06.82** **Injury of left internal carotid artery, intracranial portion, not elsewhere classified**

+7th **S06.820** **Injury of left internal carotid artery, intracranial portion, not elsewhere classified without loss of consciousness**

CC +7th **S06.821** **Injury of left internal carotid artery, intracranial portion, not elsewhere classified with loss of consciousness of 30 minutes or less**
HAC 7th character A see Appendix B for HAC conditional logic

CC +7th **S06.822** **Injury of left internal carotid artery, intracranial portion, not elsewhere classified with loss of consciousness of 31 minutes to 59 minutes**
HAC 7th character A see Appendix B for HAC conditional logic

CC +7th **S06.823** **Injury of left internal carotid artery, intracranial portion, not elsewhere classified with loss of consciousness of 1 hour to 5 hours 59 minutes**
HAC 7th character A see Appendix B for HAC conditional logic

CC +7th **S06.824** **Injury of left internal carotid artery, intracranial portion, not elsewhere classified with loss of consciousness of 6 hours to 24 hours**
HAC 7th character A see Appendix B for HAC conditional logic

CC +7th **S06.825** **Injury of left internal carotid artery, intracranial portion, not elsewhere classified with loss of consciousness greater than 24 hours with return to pre-existing conscious level**
HAC 7th character A see Appendix B for HAC conditional logic

MCC +7th **S06.826** **Injury of left internal carotid artery, intracranial portion, not elsewhere classified with loss of consciousness greater than 24 hours without return to pre-existing conscious level with patient surviving**
HAC 7th character A see Appendix B for HAC conditional logic

MCC +7th **S06.827** **Injury of left internal carotid artery, intracranial portion, not elsewhere classified with loss of consciousness of any duration with death due to brain injury prior to regaining consciousness**
HAC 7th character A see Appendix B for HAC conditional logic

MCC +7th **S06.828** **Injury of left internal carotid artery, intracranial portion, not elsewhere classified with loss of consciousness of any duration with death due to other cause prior to regaining consciousness**
HAC 7th character A see Appendix B for HAC conditional logic

CC +7th **S06.829** **Injury of left internal carotid artery, intracranial portion, not elsewhere classified with loss of consciousness of unspecified duration**
Injury of left internal carotid artery, intracranial portion, not elsewhere classified NOS
HAC 7th character A see Appendix B for HAC conditional logic

\+ **S06.89** **Other specified intracranial injury**
Excludes1: *concussion (S06.0X-)*

+7th **S06.890** **Other specified intracranial injury without loss of consciousness**

CC +7th **S06.891** **Other specified intracranial injury with loss of consciousness of 30 minutes or less**
HAC 7th character A see Appendix B for HAC conditional logic

CC +7th **S06.892** **Other specified intracranial injury with loss of consciousness of 31 minutes to 59 minutes**
HAC 7th character A see Appendix B for HAC conditional logic

CC +7th **S06.893** **Other specified intracranial injury with loss of consciousness of 1 hour to 5 hours 59 minutes**
HAC 7th character A see Appendix B for HAC conditional logic

CC +7th **S06.894** **Other specified intracranial injury with loss of consciousness of 6 hours to 24 hours**
HAC 7th character A see Appendix B for HAC conditional logic

CC +7th **S06.895** **Other specified intracranial injury with loss of consciousness greater than 24 hours with return to pre-existing conscious level**
HAC 7th character A see Appendix B for HAC conditional logic

MCC +7th **S06.896** **Other specified intracranial injury with loss of consciousness greater than 24 hours without return to pre-existing conscious level with patient surviving**
HAC 7th character A see Appendix B for HAC conditional logic

MCC +7th **S06.897** **Other specified intracranial injury with loss of consciousness of any duration with death due to brain injury prior to regaining consciousness**
HAC 7th character A see Appendix B for HAC conditional logic

MCC +7th **S06.898** **Other specified intracranial injury with loss of consciousness of any duration with death due to other cause prior to regaining consciousness**
HAC 7th character A see Appendix B for HAC conditional logic

CC +7th **S06.899** **Other specified intracranial injury with loss of consciousness of unspecified duration**
HAC 7th character A see Appendix B for HAC conditional logic

CC + **S06.9** **Unspecified intracranial injury**
Brain injury NOS
Head injury NOS with loss of consciousness
Traumatic brain injury NOS
Excludes1: *conditions classifiable to S06.0- to S06.8- code to specified intracranial injury*
head injury NOS (S09.90)

\+ **S06.9X** **Unspecified intracranial injury**

+7th **S06.9X0** **Unspecified intracranial injury without loss of consciousness**
AHA CC: 2Q, 2020, 31
HAC 7th character A see Appendix B for HAC conditional logic

+7th **S06.9X1** **Unspecified intracranial injury with loss of consciousness of 30 minutes or less**
HAC 7th character A see Appendix B for HAC conditional logic

+7th **S06.9X2** **Unspecified intracranial injury with loss of consciousness of 31 minutes to 59 minutes**
HAC 7th character A see Appendix B for HAC conditional logic

+7th **S06.9X3 Unspecified intracranial injury with loss of consciousness of 1 hour to 5 hours 59 minutes**
HAC 7th character A see Appendix B for HAC conditional logic

+7th **S06.9X4 Unspecified intracranial injury with loss of consciousness of 6 hours to 24 hours**
HAC 7th character A see Appendix B for HAC conditional logic

+7th **S06.9X5 Unspecified intracranial injury with loss of consciousness greater than 24 hours with return to pre-existing conscious level**
HAC 7th character A see Appendix B for HAC conditional logic

MCC +7th **S06.9X6 Unspecified intracranial injury with loss of consciousness greater than 24 hours without return to pre-existing conscious level with patient surviving**
HAC 7th character A see Appendix B for HAC conditional logic

MCC +7th **S06.9X7 Unspecified intracranial injury with loss of consciousness of any duration with death due to brain injury prior to regaining consciousness**
HAC 7th character A see Appendix B for HAC conditional logic

MCC +7th **S06.9X8 Unspecified intracranial injury with loss of consciousness of any duration with death due to other cause prior to regaining consciousness**
HAC 7th character A see Appendix B for HAC conditional logic

+7th **S06.9X9 Unspecified intracranial injury with loss of consciousness of unspecified duration**
HAC 7th character A see Appendix B for HAC conditional logic

+ **S06.A Traumatic brain compression and herniation**
Traumatic cerebral compression
Code first the underlying traumatic brain injury, such as:
diffuse traumatic brain injury (S06.2-)
focal traumatic brain injury (S06.3-)
traumatic subdural hemorrhage (S06.5-)
traumatic subarachnoid hemorrhage (S06.6-)

MCC **S06.A0 Traumatic brain compression without herniation**
Traumatic brain compression NOS
Traumatic cerebral compression NOS

MCC **S06.A1 Traumatic brain compression with herniation**
Traumatic brain herniation
Traumatic brainstem compression with herniation
Traumatic cerebellar compression with herniation
Traumatic cerebral compression with herniation

S07 Crushing injury of head

Use additional code for all associated injuries, such as:
intracranial injuries (S06.-)
skull fractures (S02.-)

The appropriate 7th character is to be added to each code from category S07
A initial encounter
D subsequent encounter
S sequela

CC X+7th **S07.0 Crushing injury of face**
HAC 7th character A see Appendix B for HAC conditional logic

CC X+7th **S07.1 Crushing injury of skull**
HAC 7th character A see Appendix B for HAC conditional logic

CC X+7th **S07.8 Crushing injury of other parts of head**
HAC 7th character A see Appendix B for HAC conditional logic

CC X+7th **S07.9 Crushing injury of head, part unspecified**
HAC 7th character A see Appendix B for HAC conditional logic

S08 Avulsion and traumatic amputation of part of head

An amputation not identified as partial or complete should be coded to complete

The appropriate 7th character is to be added to each code from category S08
A initial encounter
D subsequent encounter
S sequela

X+7th **S08.0 Avulsion of scalp**
+ **S08.1 Traumatic amputation of ear**
+ **S08.11 Complete traumatic amputation of ear**
+7th **S08.111 Complete traumatic amputation of right ear**
+7th **S08.112 Complete traumatic amputation of left ear**
+7th **S08.119 Complete traumatic amputation of unspecified ear**
+ **S08.12 Partial traumatic amputation of ear**
+7th **S08.121 Partial traumatic amputation of right ear**
+7th **S08.122 Partial traumatic amputation of left ear**
+7th **S08.129 Partial traumatic amputation of unspecified ear**
+ **S08.8 Traumatic amputation of other parts of head**
+ **S08.81 Traumatic amputation of nose**
+7th **S08.811 Complete traumatic amputation of nose**
+7th **S08.812 Partial traumatic amputation of nose**
X+7th **S08.89 Traumatic amputation of other parts of head**

S09 Other and unspecified injuries of head

The appropriate 7th character is to be added to each code from category S09
A initial encounter
D subsequent encounter
S sequela

CC X+7th **S09.0 Injury of blood vessels of head, not elsewhere classified**
Excludes1: *injury of cerebral blood vessels (S06.-)*
injury of precerebral blood vessels (S15.-)

+ **S09.1 Injury of muscle and tendon of head**
Code also any associated open wound (S01.-)
Excludes2: *sprain to joints and ligament of head (S03.9)*

X+7th **S09.10 Unspecified injury of muscle and tendon of head**
Injury of muscle and tendon of head NOS
X+7th **S09.11 Strain of muscle and tendon of head**
X+7th **S09.12 Laceration of muscle and tendon of head**
X+7th **S09.19 Other specified injury of muscle and tendon of head**

+ **S09.2 Traumatic rupture of ear drum**
Excludes1: *traumatic rupture of ear drum due to blast injury (S09.31-)*

CC X+7th **S09.20 Traumatic rupture of unspecified ear drum**
CC X+7th **S09.21 Traumatic rupture of right ear drum**
CC X+7th **S09.22 Traumatic rupture of left ear drum**

+ **S09.3 Other specified and unspecified injury of middle and inner ear**
Excludes1: *injury to ear NOS (S09.91-)*
Excludes2: *injury to external ear (S00.4-, S01.3-, S08.1-)*

+ **S09.30 Unspecified injury of middle and inner ear**
CC +7th **S09.301 Unspecified injury of right middle and inner ear**
CC +7th **S09.302 Unspecified injury of left middle and inner ear**
CC +7th **S09.309 Unspecified injury of unspecified middle and inner ear**
+ **S09.31 Primary blast injury of ear**
Blast injury of ear NOS
CC +7th **S09.311 Primary blast injury of right ear**
CC +7th **S09.312 Primary blast injury of left ear**
CC +7th **S09.313 Primary blast injury of ear, bilateral**
CC +7th **S09.319 Primary blast injury of unspecified ear**
+ **S09.39 Other specified injury of middle and inner ear**
Secondary blast injury to ear
CC +7th **S09.391 Other specified injury of right middle and inner ear**
CC +7th **S09.392 Other specified injury of left middle and inner ear**
CC +7th **S09.399 Other specified injury of unspecified middle and inner ear**

Vertebrae

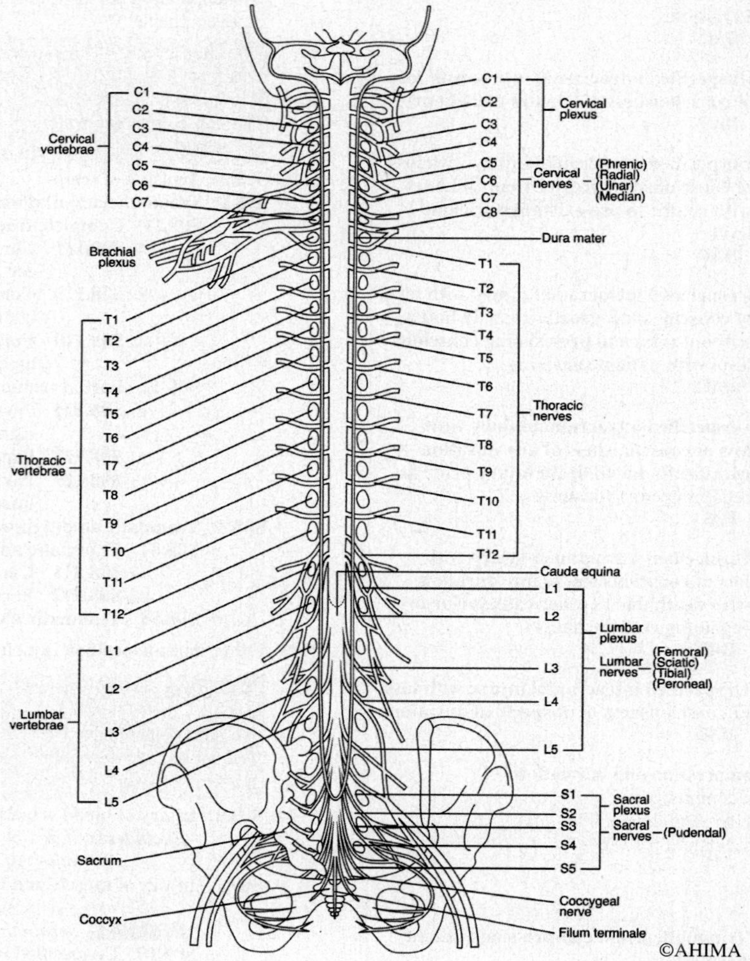

©AHIMA

X+7th **S09.8 Other specified injuries of head**

\+ **S09.9 Unspecified injury of face and head**

X+7th **S09.90 Unspecified injury of head**

Head injury NOS

Excludes1: *brain injury NOS (S06.9-)*
head injury NOS with loss of consciousness (S06.9-)
intracranial injury NOS (S06.9-)

X+7th **S09.91 Unspecified injury of ear**

Injury of ear NOS

X+7th **S09.92 Unspecified injury of nose**

Injury of nose NOS

X+7th **S09.93 Unspecified injury of face**

Injury of face NOS

Injuries to the neck (S10-S19)

Includes: injuries of nape
injuries of supraclavicular region
injuries of throat

Excludes2: *burns and corrosions (T20-T32)*
effects of foreign body in esophagus (T18.1)
effects of foreign body in larynx (T17.3)
effects of foreign body in pharynx (T17.2)
effects of foreign body in trachea (T17.4)
frostbite (T33-T34)
insect bite or sting, venomous (T63.4)

S10 Superficial injury of neck

The appropriate 7th character is to be added to each code from category S10
A initial encounter
D subsequent encounter
S sequela

X+7th **S10.0 Contusion of throat**

Contusion of cervical esophagus
Contusion of larynx
Contusion of pharynx
Contusion of trachea

\+ **S10.1 Other and unspecified superficial injuries of throat**

X+7th **S10.10 Unspecified superficial injuries of throat**

X+7th **S10.11 Abrasion of throat**

X+7th **S10.12 Blister (nonthermal) of throat**

X+7th **S10.14 External constriction of part of throat**

X+7th **S10.15 Superficial foreign body of throat**

Splinter in the throat

X+7th **S10.16 Insect bite (nonvenomous) of throat**

X+7th **S10.17 Other superficial bite of throat**

Excludes1: *open bite of throat (S11.85)*

\+ **S10.8 Superficial injury of other specified parts of neck**

X+7th **S10.80 Unspecified superficial injury of other specified part of neck**

X+7th **S10.81 Abrasion of other specified part of neck**

X+7th **S10.82 Blister (nonthermal) of other specified part of neck**

X+7th **S10.83 Contusion of other specified part of neck**

X+7th **S10.84 External constriction of other specified part of neck**

X+7th **S10.85 Superficial foreign body of other specified part of neck**

Splinter in other specified part of neck

X+7th **S10.86 Insect bite of other specified part of neck**
X+7th **S10.87 Other superficial bite of other specified part of neck**
Excludes1: *open bite of other specified parts of neck (S11.85)*

\+ **S10.9 Superficial injury of unspecified part of neck**
X+7th **S10.90 Unspecified superficial injury of unspecified part of neck**
X+7th **S10.91 Abrasion of unspecified part of neck**
X+7th **S10.92 Blister (nonthermal) of unspecified part of neck**
X+7th **S10.93 Contusion of unspecified part of neck**
X+7th **S10.94 External constriction of unspecified part of neck**
X+7th **S10.95 Superficial foreign body of unspecified part of neck**
X+7th **S10.96 Insect bite of unspecified part of neck**
X+7th **S10.97 Other superficial bite of unspecified part of neck**

S11 Open wound of neck

Code also any associated:
spinal cord injury (S14.0, S14.1-)
wound infection

Excludes2: *open fracture of vertebra (S12.- with 7th character B)*

The appropriate 7th character is to be added to each code from category S11
A initial encounter
D subsequent encounter
S sequela

\+ **S11.0 Open wound of larynx and trachea**
\+ **S11.01 Open wound of larynx**
Excludes2: *open wound of vocal cord (S11.03)*
MCC +7th **S11.011 Laceration without foreign body of larynx**
MCC +7th **S11.012 Laceration with foreign body of larynx**
MCC +7th **S11.013 Puncture wound without foreign body of larynx**
MCC +7th **S11.014 Puncture wound with foreign body of larynx**
MCC +7th **S11.015 Open bite of larynx**
Bite of larynx NOS
MCC +7th **S11.019 Unspecified open wound of larynx**
\+ **S11.02 Open wound of trachea**
Open wound of cervical trachea
Open wound of trachea NOS
Excludes2: *open wound of thoracic trachea (S27.5-)*
MCC +7th **S11.021 Laceration without foreign body of trachea**
MCC +7th **S11.022 Laceration with foreign body of trachea**
MCC +7th **S11.023 Puncture wound without foreign body of trachea**
MCC +7th **S11.024 Puncture wound with foreign body of trachea**
MCC +7th **S11.025 Open bite of trachea**
Bite of trachea NOS
MCC +7th **S11.029 Unspecified open wound of trachea**
\+ **S11.03 Open wound of vocal cord**
MCC +7th **S11.031 Laceration without foreign body of vocal cord**
MCC +7th **S11.032 Laceration with foreign body of vocal cord**
MCC +7th **S11.033 Puncture wound without foreign body of vocal cord**
MCC +7th **S11.034 Puncture wound with foreign body of vocal cord**
MCC +7th **S11.035 Open bite of vocal cord**
Bite of vocal cord NOS
MCC +7th **S11.039 Unspecified open wound of vocal cord**

\+ **S11.1 Open wound of thyroid gland**
CC X+7th **S11.10 Unspecified open wound of thyroid gland**
CC X+7th **S11.11 Laceration without foreign body of thyroid gland**
CC X+7th **S11.12 Laceration with foreign body of thyroid gland**
CC X+7th **S11.13 Puncture wound without foreign body of thyroid gland**
CC X+7th **S11.14 Puncture wound with foreign body of thyroid gland**
CC X+7th **S11.15 Open bite of thyroid gland**
Bite of thyroid gland NOS

\+ **S11.2 Open wound of pharynx and cervical esophagus**
Excludes1: *open wound of esophagus NOS (S27.8-)*
CC X+7th **S11.20 Unspecified open wound of pharynx and cervical esophagus**
CC X+7th **S11.21 Laceration without foreign body of pharynx and cervical esophagus**
CC X+7th **S11.22 Laceration with foreign body of pharynx and cervical esophagus**
CC X+7th **S11.23 Puncture wound without foreign body of pharynx and cervical esophagus**
CC X+7th **S11.24 Puncture wound with foreign body of pharynx and cervical esophagus**
CC X+7th **S11.25 Open bite of pharynx and cervical esophagus**
Bite of pharynx and cervical esophagus NOS

\+ **S11.8 Open wound of other specified parts of neck**
X+7th **S11.80 Unspecified open wound of other specified part of neck**
X+7th **S11.81 Laceration without foreign body of other specified part of neck**
X+7th **S11.82 Laceration with foreign body of other specified part of neck**
X+7th **S11.83 Puncture wound without foreign body of other specified part of neck**
X+7th **S11.84 Puncture wound with foreign body of other specified part of neck**
X+7th **S11.85 Open bite of other specified part of neck**
Bite of other specified part of neck NOS
Excludes1: *superficial bite of other specified part of neck (S10.87)*
X+7th **S11.89 Other open wound of other specified part of neck**

\+ **S11.9 Open wound of unspecified part of neck**
X+7th **S11.90 Unspecified open wound of unspecified part of neck**
X+7th **S11.91 Laceration without foreign body of unspecified part of neck**
X+7th **S11.92 Laceration with foreign body of unspecified part of neck**
X+7th **S11.93 Puncture wound without foreign body of unspecified part of neck**
X+7th **S11.94 Puncture wound with foreign body of unspecified part of neck**
X+7th **S11.95 Open bite of unspecified part of neck**
Bite of neck NOS
Excludes1: *superficial bite of neck (S10.97)*

S12 Fracture of cervical vertebra and other parts of neck

NOTE A fracture not indicated as displaced or nondisplaced should be coded to displaced
A fracture not indicated as open or closed should be coded to closed

Includes: fracture of cervical neural arch
fracture of cervical spine
fracture of cervical spinous process
fracture of cervical transverse process
fracture of cervical vertebral arch
fracture of neck

Code first any associated cervical spinal cord injury (S14.0, S14.1-)

The appropriate 7th character is to be added to all codes from subcategories **S12.0-S12.6**
A initial encounter for closed fracture
B initial encounter for open fracture
D subsequent encounter for fracture with routine healing
G subsequent encounter for fracture with delayed healing
K subsequent encounter for fracture with nonunion
S sequela

Review coding guideline C.19.c

\+ **S12.0 Fracture of first cervical vertebra**
Atlas
\+ **S12.00 Unspecified fracture of first cervical vertebra**
CC MCC +7th **S12.000 Unspecified displaced fracture of first cervical vertebra**
HAC 7th characters A & B see Appendix B for HAC conditional logic
CC MCC +7th **S12.001 Unspecified nondisplaced fracture of first cervical vertebra**
HAC 7th characters A & B see Appendix B for HAC conditional logic
CC MCC X+7th **S12.01 Stable burst fracture of first cervical vertebra**
HAC 7th characters A & B see Appendix B for HAC conditional logic
CC MCC X+7th **S12.02 Unstable burst fracture of first cervical vertebra**
HAC 7th characters A & B see Appendix B for HAC conditional logic

+ S12.03 **Posterior arch fracture of first cervical vertebra**

CC MCC +7th **S12.030** **Displaced posterior arch fracture of first cervical vertebra**
HAC 7th characters A & B see Appendix B for HAC conditional logic

CC MCC +7th **S12.031** **Nondisplaced posterior arch fracture of first cervical vertebra**
HAC 7th characters A & B see Appendix B for HAC conditional logic

+ S12.04 **Lateral mass fracture of first cervical vertebra**

CC MCC +7th **S12.040** **Displaced lateral mass fracture of first cervical vertebra**
HAC 7th characters A & B see Appendix B for HAC conditional logic

CC MCC +7th **S12.041** **Nondisplaced lateral mass fracture of first cervical vertebra**
HAC 7th characters A & B see Appendix B for HAC conditional logic

+ S12.09 **Other fracture of first cervical vertebra**

CC MCC +7th **S12.090** **Other displaced fracture of first cervical vertebra**
HAC 7th characters A & B see Appendix B for HAC conditional logic

CC MCC +7th **S12.091** **Other nondisplaced fracture of first cervical vertebra**
HAC 7th characters A & B see Appendix B for HAC conditional logic

+ S12.1 **Fracture of second cervical vertebra**
Axis

+ S12.10 **Unspecified fracture of second cervical vertebra**

CC MCC +7th **S12.100** **Unspecified displaced fracture of second cervical vertebra**
HAC 7th characters A & B see Appendix B for HAC conditional logic

CC MCC +7th **S12.101** **Unspecified nondisplaced fracture of second cervical vertebra**
HAC 7th characters A & B see Appendix B for HAC conditional logic

+ S12.11 **Type II dens fracture**

CC MCC +7th **S12.110** **Anterior displaced Type II dens fracture**
HAC 7th characters A & B see Appendix B for HAC conditional logic

CC MCC +7th **S12.111** **Posterior displaced Type II dens fracture**
HAC 7th characters A & B see Appendix B for HAC conditional logic

CC MCC +7th **S12.112** **Nondisplaced Type II dens fracture**
HAC 7th characters A & B see Appendix B for HAC conditional logic

+ S12.12 **Other dens fracture**

CC MCC +7th **S12.120** **Other displaced dens fracture**
HAC 7th characters A & B see Appendix B for HAC conditional logic

CC MCC +7th **S12.121** **Other nondisplaced dens fracture**
HAC 7th characters A & B see Appendix B for HAC conditional logic

+ S12.13 **Unspecified traumatic spondylolisthesis of second cervical vertebra**

CC MCC +7th **S12.130** **Unspecified traumatic displaced spondylolisthesis of second cervical vertebra**
HAC 7th characters A & B see Appendix B for HAC conditional logic

CC MCC +7th **S12.131** **Unspecified traumatic nondisplaced spondylolisthesis of second cervical vertebra**
HAC 7th characters A & B see Appendix B for HAC conditional logic

CC MCC X+7th **S12.14** **Type III traumatic spondylolisthesis of second cervical vertebra**
HAC 7th characters A & B see Appendix B for HAC conditional logic

+ S12.15 **Other traumatic spondylolisthesis of second cervical vertebra**

CC MCC +7th **S12.150** **Other traumatic displaced spondylolisthesis of second cervical vertebra**
HAC 7th characters A & B see Appendix B for HAC conditional logic

CC MCC +7th **S12.151** **Other traumatic nondisplaced spondylolisthesis of second cervical vertebra**
HAC 7th characters A & B see Appendix B for HAC conditional logic

+ S12.19 **Other fracture of second cervical vertebra**

CC MCC +7th **S12.190** **Other displaced fracture of second cervical vertebra**
HAC 7th characters A & B see Appendix B for HAC conditional logic

CC MCC +7th **S12.191** **Other nondisplaced fracture of second cervical vertebra**
HAC 7th characters A & B see Appendix B for HAC conditional logic

+ S12.2 **Fracture of third cervical vertebra**

+ S12.20 **Unspecified fracture of third cervical vertebra**

CC MCC +7th **S12.200** **Unspecified displaced fracture of third cervical vertebra**
HAC 7th characters A & B see Appendix B for HAC conditional logic

CC MCC +7th **S12.201** **Unspecified nondisplaced fracture of third cervical vertebra**
HAC 7th characters A & B see Appendix B for HAC conditional logic

+ S12.23 **Unspecified traumatic spondylolisthesis of third cervical vertebra**

CC MCC +7th **S12.230** **Unspecified traumatic displaced spondylolisthesis of third cervical vertebra**
HAC 7th characters A & B see Appendix B for HAC conditional logic

CC MCC +7th **S12.231** **Unspecified traumatic nondisplaced spondylolisthesis of third cervical vertebra**
HAC 7th characters A & B see Appendix B for HAC conditional logic

CC MCC X+7th **S12.24** **Type III traumatic spondylolisthesis of third cervical vertebra**
HAC 7th characters A & B see Appendix B for HAC conditional logic

+ S12.25 **Other traumatic spondylolisthesis of third cervical vertebra**

CC MCC +7th **S12.250** **Other traumatic displaced spondylolisthesis of third cervical vertebra**
HAC 7th characters A & B see Appendix B for HAC conditional logic

CC MCC +7th **S12.251** **Other traumatic nondisplaced spondylolisthesis of third cervical vertebra**
HAC 7th characters A & B see Appendix B for HAC conditional logic

+ S12.29 **Other fracture of third cervical vertebra**

CC MCC +7th **S12.290** **Other displaced fracture of third cervical vertebra**
HAC 7th characters A & B see Appendix B for HAC conditional logic

CC MCC +7th **S12.291** **Other nondisplaced fracture of third cervical vertebra**
HAC 7th characters A & B see Appendix B for HAC conditional logic

+ S12.3 **Fracture of fourth cervical vertebra**

+ S12.30 **Unspecified fracture of fourth cervical vertebra**

CC MCC +7th **S12.300** **Unspecified displaced fracture of fourth cervical vertebra**
HAC 7th characters A & B see Appendix B for HAC conditional logic

CC MCC +7th **S12.301** **Unspecified nondisplaced fracture of fourth cervical vertebra**
HAC 7th characters A & B see Appendix B for HAC conditional logic

+ S12.33 **Unspecified traumatic spondylolisthesis of fourth cervical vertebra**

CC MCC +7th **S12.330** **Unspecified traumatic displaced spondylolisthesis of fourth cervical vertebra**
HAC 7th characters A & B see Appendix B for HAC conditional logic

CC MCC +7th **S12.331** **Unspecified traumatic nondisplaced spondylolisthesis of fourth cervical vertebra**
HAC 7th characters A & B see Appendix B for HAC conditional logic

CC MCC X+7th **S12.34** **Type III traumatic spondylolisthesis of fourth cervical vertebra**
HAC 7th characters A & B see Appendix B for HAC conditional logic

+ **S12.35 Other traumatic spondylolisthesis of fourth cervical vertebra**

CC MCC +7th **S12.350 Other traumatic displaced spondylolisthesis of fourth cervical vertebra**
HAC 7th characters A & B see Appendix B for HAC conditional logic

CC MCC +7th **S12.351 Other traumatic nondisplaced spondylolisthesis of fourth cervical vertebra**
HAC 7th characters A & B see Appendix B for HAC conditional logic

+ **S12.39 Other fracture of fourth cervical vertebra**

CC MCC +7th **S12.390 Other displaced fracture of fourth cervical vertebra**
HAC 7th characters A & B see Appendix B for HAC conditional logic

CC MCC +7th **S12.391 Other nondisplaced fracture of fourth cervical vertebra**
HAC 7th characters A & B see Appendix B for HAC conditional logic

+ **S12.4 Fracture of fifth cervical vertebra**

+ **S12.40 Unspecified fracture of fifth cervical vertebra**

CC MCC +7th **S12.400 Unspecified displaced fracture of fifth cervical vertebra**
HAC 7th characters A & B see Appendix B for HAC conditional logic

CC MCC +7th **S12.401 Unspecified nondisplaced fracture of fifth cervical vertebra**
HAC 7th characters A & B see Appendix B for HAC conditional logic

+ **S12.43 Unspecified traumatic spondylolisthesis of fifth cervical vertebra**

CC MCC +7th **S12.430 Unspecified traumatic displaced spondylolisthesis of fifth cervical vertebra**
HAC 7th characters A & B see Appendix B for HAC conditional logic

CC MCC +7th **S12.431 Unspecified traumatic nondisplaced spondylolisthesis of fifth cervical vertebra**
HAC 7th characters A & B see Appendix B for HAC conditional logic

CC MCC X+7th **S12.44 Type III traumatic spondylolisthesis of fifth cervical vertebra**
HAC 7th characters A & B see Appendix B for HAC conditional logic

+ **S12.45 Other traumatic spondylolisthesis of fifth cervical vertebra**

CC MCC +7th **S12.450 Other traumatic displaced spondylolisthesis of fifth cervical vertebra**
HAC 7th characters A & B see Appendix B for HAC conditional logic

CC MCC +7th **S12.451 Other traumatic nondisplaced spondylolisthesis of fifth cervical vertebra**
HAC 7th characters A & B see Appendix B for HAC conditional logic

+ **S12.49 Other fracture of fifth cervical vertebra**

CC MCC +7th **S12.490 Other displaced fracture of fifth cervical vertebra**
HAC 7th characters A & B see Appendix B for HAC conditional logic

CC MCC +7th **S12.491 Other nondisplaced fracture of fifth cervical vertebra**
HAC 7th characters A & B see Appendix B for HAC conditional logic

+ **S12.5 Fracture of sixth cervical vertebra**

+ **S12.50 Unspecified fracture of sixth cervical vertebra**

CC MCC +7th **S12.500 Unspecified displaced fracture of sixth cervical vertebra**
HAC 7th characters A & B see Appendix B for HAC conditional logic

CC MCC +7th **S12.501 Unspecified nondisplaced fracture of sixth cervical vertebra**
HAC 7th characters A & B see Appendix B for HAC conditional logic

+ **S12.53 Unspecified traumatic spondylolisthesis of sixth cervical vertebra**

CC MCC +7th **S12.530 Unspecified traumatic displaced spondylolisthesis of sixth cervical vertebra**
HAC 7th characters A & B see Appendix B for HAC conditional logic

CC MCC +7th **S12.531 Unspecified traumatic nondisplaced spondylolisthesis of sixth cervical vertebra**
HAC 7th characters A & B see Appendix B for HAC conditional logic

CC MCC X+7th **S12.54 Type III traumatic spondylolisthesis of sixth cervical vertebra**
HAC 7th characters A & B see Appendix B for HAC conditional logic

+ **S12.55 Other traumatic spondylolisthesis of sixth cervical vertebra**

CC MCC +7th **S12.550 Other traumatic displaced spondylolisthesis of sixth cervical vertebra**
HAC 7th characters A & B see Appendix B for HAC conditional logic

CC MCC +7th **S12.551 Other traumatic nondisplaced spondylolisthesis of sixth cervical vertebra**
HAC 7th characters A & B see Appendix B for HAC conditional logic

+ **S12.59 Other fracture of sixth cervical vertebra**

CC MCC +7th **S12.590 Other displaced fracture of sixth cervical vertebra**
HAC 7th characters A & B see Appendix B for HAC conditional logic

CC MCC +7th **S12.591 Other nondisplaced fracture of sixth cervical vertebra**
HAC 7th characters A & B see Appendix B for HAC conditional logic

+ **S12.6 Fracture of seventh cervical vertebra**

+ **S12.60 Unspecified fracture of seventh cervical vertebra**

CC MCC +7th **S12.600 Unspecified displaced fracture of seventh cervical vertebra**
HAC 7th characters A & B see Appendix B for HAC conditional logic

CC MCC +7th **S12.601 Unspecified nondisplaced fracture of seventh cervical vertebra**
HAC 7th characters A & B see Appendix B for HAC conditional logic

+ **S12.63 Unspecified traumatic spondylolisthesis of seventh cervical vertebra**

CC MCC +7th **S12.630 Unspecified traumatic displaced spondylolisthesis of seventh cervical vertebra**
HAC 7th characters A & B see Appendix B for HAC conditional logic

CC MCC +7th **S12.631 Unspecified traumatic nondisplaced spondylolisthesis of seventh cervical vertebra**
HAC 7th characters A & B see Appendix B for HAC conditional logic

CC MCC X+7th **S12.64 Type III traumatic spondylolisthesis of seventh cervical vertebra**
HAC 7th characters A & B see Appendix B for HAC conditional logic

+ **S12.65 Other traumatic spondylolisthesis of seventh cervical vertebra**

CC MCC +7th **S12.650 Other traumatic displaced spondylolisthesis of seventh cervical vertebra**
HAC 7th characters A & B see Appendix B for HAC conditional logic

CC MCC +7th **S12.651 Other traumatic nondisplaced spondylolisthesis of seventh cervical vertebra**
HAC 7th characters A & B see Appendix B for HAC conditional logic

+ **S12.69 Other fracture of seventh cervical vertebra**

CC MCC +7th **S12.690 Other displaced fracture of seventh cervical vertebra**
HAC 7th characters A & B see Appendix B for HAC conditional logic

CC MCC +7th **S12.691 Other nondisplaced fracture of seventh cervical vertebra**
HAC 7th characters A & B see Appendix B for HAC conditional logic

X+7th MCC **S12.8 Fracture of other parts of neck**

The appropriate 7th character is to be added to code **S12.8**
A initial encounter
D subsequent encounter
S sequela

Hyoid bone
Larynx
Thyroid cartilage
Trachea
HAC 7th character A see Appendix B for HAC conditional logic

CC X+7th **S12.9 Fracture of neck, unspecified**

The appropriate 7th character is to be added to code **S12.9**
A initial encounter
D subsequent encounter
S sequela

Fracture of neck NOS
Fracture of cervical spine NOS
Fracture of cervical vertebra NOS
HAC 7th character A see Appendix B for HAC conditional logic

S13 Dislocation and sprain of joints and ligaments at neck level

Includes: avulsion of joint or ligament at neck level
laceration of cartilage, joint or ligament at neck level
sprain of cartilage, joint or ligament at neck level
traumatic hemarthrosis of joint or ligament at neck level
traumatic rupture of joint or ligament at neck level
traumatic subluxation of joint or ligament at neck level
traumatic tear of joint or ligament at neck level

Code also any associated open wound

Excludes2: *strain of muscle or tendon at neck level (S16.1)*

The appropriate 7th character is to be added to each code from category S13
A initial encounter
D subsequent encounter
S sequela

CC X+7th **S13.0 Traumatic rupture of cervical intervertebral disc**
Excludes1: *rupture or displacement (nontraumatic) of cervical intervertebral disc NOS (M50.-)*
HAC 7th character A see Appendix B for HAC conditional logic

\+ **S13.1 Subluxation and dislocation of cervical vertebrae**
Code also any associated:
open wound of neck (S11.-)
spinal cord injury (S14.1-)
Excludes2: *fracture of cervical vertebrae (S12.0-S12.3-)*

\+ **S13.10 Subluxation and dislocation of unspecified cervical vertebrae**

CC +7th **S13.100 Subluxation of unspecified cervical vertebrae**
HAC 7th character A see Appendix B for HAC conditional logic

CC +7th **S13.101 Dislocation of unspecified cervical vertebrae**
HAC 7th character A see Appendix B for HAC conditional logic

\+ **S13.11 Subluxation and dislocation of C0/C1 cervical vertebrae**
Subluxation and dislocation of atlantooccipital joint
Subluxation and dislocation of atloidooccipital joint
Subluxation and dislocation of occipitoatloid joint

CC +7th **S13.110 Subluxation of C0/C1 cervical vertebrae**
HAC 7th character A see Appendix B for HAC conditional logic

CC +7th **S13.111 Dislocation of C0/C1 cervical vertebrae**
HAC 7th character A see Appendix B for HAC conditional logic

\+ **S13.12 Subluxation and dislocation of C1/C2 cervical vertebrae**
Subluxation and dislocation of atlantoaxial joint

CC +7th **S13.120 Subluxation of C1/C2 cervical vertebrae**
HAC 7th character A see Appendix B for HAC conditional logic

CC +7th **S13.121 Dislocation of C1/C2 cervical vertebrae**
HAC 7th character A see Appendix B for HAC conditional logic

\+ **S13.13 Subluxation and dislocation of C2/C3 cervical vertebrae**

CC +7th **S13.130 Subluxation of C2/C3 cervical vertebrae**
HAC 7th character A see Appendix B for HAC conditional logic

CC +7th **S13.131 Dislocation of C2/C3 cervical vertebrae**
HAC 7th character A see Appendix B for HAC conditional logic

\+ **S13.14 Subluxation and dislocation of C3/C4 cervical vertebrae**

CC +7th **S13.140 Subluxation of C3/C4 cervical vertebrae**
HAC 7th character A see Appendix B for HAC conditional logic

CC +7th **S13.141 Dislocation of C3/C4 cervical vertebrae**
HAC 7th character A see Appendix B for HAC conditional logic

\+ **S13.15 Subluxation and dislocation of C4/C5 cervical vertebrae**

CC +7th **S13.150 Subluxation of C4/C5 cervical vertebrae**
HAC 7th character A see Appendix B for HAC conditional logic

CC +7th **S13.151 Dislocation of C4/C5 cervical vertebrae**
HAC 7th character A see Appendix B for HAC conditional logic

\+ **S13.16 Subluxation and dislocation of C5/C6 cervical vertebrae**

CC +7th **S13.160 Subluxation of C5/C6 cervical vertebrae**
HAC 7th character A see Appendix B for HAC conditional logic

CC +7th **S13.161 Dislocation of C5/C6 cervical vertebrae**
HAC 7th character A see Appendix B for HAC conditional logic

\+ **S13.17 Subluxation and dislocation of C6/C7 cervical vertebrae**

CC +7th **S13.170 Subluxation of C6/C7 cervical vertebrae**
HAC 7th character A see Appendix B for HAC conditional logic

CC +7th **S13.171 Dislocation of C6/C7 cervical vertebrae**
HAC 7th character A see Appendix B for HAC conditional logic

\+ **S13.18 Subluxation and dislocation of C7/T1 cervical vertebrae**

CC +7th **S13.180 Subluxation of C7/T1 cervical vertebrae**
HAC 7th character A see Appendix B for HAC conditional logic

CC +7th **S13.181 Dislocation of C7/T1 cervical vertebrae**
HAC 7th character A see Appendix B for HAC conditional logic

\+ **S13.2 Dislocation of other and unspecified parts of neck**

CC X+7th **S13.20 Dislocation of unspecified parts of neck**
HAC 7th character A see Appendix B for HAC conditional logic

CC X+7th **S13.29 Dislocation of other parts of neck**
HAC 7th character A see Appendix B for HAC conditional logic

X+7th **S13.4 Sprain of ligaments of cervical spine**
Sprain of anterior longitudinal (ligament), cervical
Sprain of atlanto-axial (joints)
Sprain of atlanto-occipital (joints)
Whiplash injury of cervical spine

X+7th **S13.5 Sprain of thyroid region**
Sprain of cricoarytenoid (joint) (ligament)
Sprain of cricothyroid (joint) (ligament)
Sprain of thyroid cartilage

X+7th **S13.8 Sprain of joints and ligaments of other parts of neck**

X+7th **S13.9 Sprain of joints and ligaments of unspecified parts of neck**

S14 Injury of nerves and spinal cord at neck level

NOTE Code to highest level of cervical cord injury

Code also any associated:
fracture of cervical vertebra (S12.0--S12.6.-)
open wound of neck (S11.-)
transient paralysis (R29.5)

The appropriate 7th character is to be added to each code from category S14
A initial encounter
D subsequent encounter
S sequela

MCC X+7th **S14.0 Concussion and edema of cervical spinal cord**

\+ **S14.1 Other and unspecified injuries of cervical spinal cord**

\+ **S14.10 Unspecified injury of cervical spinal cord**

MCC +7th **S14.101 Unspecified injury at C1 level of cervical spinal cord**
HAC 7th character A see Appendix B for HAC conditional logic

MCC +7th **S14.102 Unspecified injury at C2 level of cervical spinal cord**
HAC 7th character A see Appendix B for HAC conditional logic

MCC +7th **S14.103 Unspecified injury at C3 level of cervical spinal cord**
HAC 7th character A see Appendix B for HAC conditional logic

MCC +7th **S14.104** **Unspecified injury at C4 level of cervical spinal cord**
HAC 7th character A see Appendix B for HAC conditional logic

MCC +7th **S14.105** **Unspecified injury at C5 level of cervical spinal cord**
HAC 7th character A see Appendix B for HAC conditional logic

MCC +7th **S14.106** **Unspecified injury at C6 level of cervical spinal cord**
HAC 7th character A see Appendix B for HAC conditional logic

MCC +7th **S14.107** **Unspecified injury at C7 level of cervical spinal cord**
HAC 7th character A see Appendix B for HAC conditional logic

MCC +7th **S14.108** **Unspecified injury at C8 level of cervical spinal cord**

+7th **S14.109** **Unspecified injury at unspecified level of cervical spinal cord**
Injury of cervical spinal cord NOS
HAC 7th character A see Appendix B for HAC conditional logic

+ S14.11 Complete lesion of cervical spinal cord

MCC +7th **S14.111** **Complete lesion at C1 level of cervical spinal cord**
HAC 7th character A see Appendix B for HAC conditional logic

MCC +7th **S14.112** **Complete lesion at C2 level of cervical spinal cord**
HAC 7th character A see Appendix B for HAC conditional logic

MCC +7th **S14.113** **Complete lesion at C3 level of cervical spinal cord**
HAC 7th character A see Appendix B for HAC conditional logic

MCC +7th **S14.114** **Complete lesion at C4 level of cervical spinal cord**
HAC 7th character A see Appendix B for HAC conditional logic

MCC +7th **S14.115** **Complete lesion at C5 level of cervical spinal cord**
HAC 7th character A see Appendix B for HAC conditional logic

MCC +7th **S14.116** **Complete lesion at C6 level of cervical spinal cord**
HAC 7th character A see Appendix B for HAC conditional logic

MCC +7th **S14.117** **Complete lesion at C7 level of cervical spinal cord**
HAC 7th character A see Appendix B for HAC conditional logic

MCC +7th **S14.118** **Complete lesion at C8 level of cervical spinal cord**

+7th **S14.119** **Complete lesion at unspecified level of cervical spinal cord**

+ S14.12 Central cord syndrome of cervical spinal cord

MCC +7th **S14.121** **Central cord syndrome at C1 level of cervical spinal cord**
HAC 7th character A see Appendix B for HAC conditional logic

MCC +7th **S14.122** **Central cord syndrome at C2 level of cervical spinal cord**
HAC 7th character A see Appendix B for HAC conditional logic

MCC +7th **S14.123** **Central cord syndrome at C3 level of cervical spinal cord**
HAC 7th character A see Appendix B for HAC conditional logic

MCC +7th **S14.124** **Central cord syndrome at C4 level of cervical spinal cord**
HAC 7th character A see Appendix B for HAC conditional logic

MCC +7th **S14.125** **Central cord syndrome at C5 level of cervical spinal cord**
HAC 7th character A see Appendix B for HAC conditional logic

MCC +7th **S14.126** **Central cord syndrome at C6 level of cervical spinal cord**
HAC 7th character A see Appendix B for HAC conditional logic

MCC +7th **S14.127** **Central cord syndrome at C7 level of cervical spinal cord**
HAC 7th character A see Appendix B for HAC conditional logic

MCC +7th **S14.128** **Central cord syndrome at C8 level of cervical spinal cord**

+7th **S14.129** **Central cord syndrome at unspecified level of cervical spinal cord**

+ S14.13 Anterior cord syndrome of cervical spinal cord

MCC +7th **S14.131** **Anterior cord syndrome at C1 level of cervical spinal cord**
HAC 7th character A see Appendix B for HAC conditional logic

MCC +7th **S14.132** **Anterior cord syndrome at C2 level of cervical spinal cord**
HAC 7th character A see Appendix B for HAC conditional logic

MCC +7th **S14.133** **Anterior cord syndrome at C3 level of cervical spinal cord**
HAC 7th character A see Appendix B for HAC conditional logic

MCC +7th **S14.134** **Anterior cord syndrome at C4 level of cervical spinal cord**
HAC 7th character A see Appendix B for HAC conditional logic

MCC +7th **S14.135** **Anterior cord syndrome at C5 level of cervical spinal cord**
HAC 7th character A see Appendix B for HAC conditional logic

MCC +7th **S14.136** **Anterior cord syndrome at C6 level of cervical spinal cord**
HAC 7th character A see Appendix B for HAC conditional logic

MCC +7th **S14.137** **Anterior cord syndrome at C7 level of cervical spinal cord**
HAC 7th character A see Appendix B for HAC conditional logic

MCC +7th **S14.138** **Anterior cord syndrome at C8 level of cervical spinal cord**

+7th **S14.139** **Anterior cord syndrome at unspecified level of cervical spinal cord**

+ S14.14 Brown-Séquard syndrome of cervical spinal cord

MCC +7th **S14.141** **Brown-Séquard syndrome at C1 level of cervical spinal cord**

MCC +7th **S14.142** **Brown-Séquard syndrome at C2 level of cervical spinal cord**

MCC +7th **S14.143** **Brown-Séquard syndrome at C3 level of cervical spinal cord**

MCC +7th **S14.144** **Brown-Séquard syndrome at C4 level of cervical spinal cord**

MCC +7th **S14.145** **Brown-Séquard syndrome at C5 level of cervical spinal cord**

MCC +7th **S14.146** **Brown-Séquard syndrome at C6 level of cervical spinal cord**

MCC +7th **S14.147** **Brown-Séquard syndrome at C7 level of cervical spinal cord**

MCC +7th **S14.148** **Brown-Séquard syndrome at C8 level of cervical spinal cord**

+7th **S14.149** **Brown-Séquard syndrome at unspecified level of cervical spinal cord**

+ S14.15 Other incomplete lesions of cervical spinal cord
Incomplete lesion of cervical spinal cord NOS
Posterior cord syndrome of cervical spinal cord

MCC +7th **S14.151** **Other incomplete lesion at C1 level of cervical spinal cord**
HAC 7th character A see Appendix B for HAC conditional logic

MCC +7th **S14.152** **Other incomplete lesion at C2 level of cervical spinal cord**
HAC 7th character A see Appendix B for HAC conditional logic

MCC +7th **S14.153** **Other incomplete lesion at C3 level of cervical spinal cord**
HAC 7th character A see Appendix B for HAC conditional logic

MCC +7th **S14.154** **Other incomplete lesion at C4 level of cervical spinal cord**
HAC 7th character A see Appendix B for HAC conditional logic

MCC +7th **S14.155** **Other incomplete lesion at C5 level of cervical spinal cord**
HAC 7th character A see Appendix B for HAC conditional logic

MCC +7th **S14.156** **Other incomplete lesion at C6 level of cervical spinal cord**
HAC 7th character A see Appendix B for HAC conditional logic

MCC +7th **S14.157** **Other incomplete lesion at C7 level of cervical spinal cord**
HAC 7th character A see Appendix B for HAC conditional logic

MCC +7th **S14.158** **Other incomplete lesion at C8 level of cervical spinal cord**

+7th **S14.159** **Other incomplete lesion at unspecified level of cervical spinal cord**

X+7th **S14.2** **Injury of nerve root of cervical spine**
X+7th **S14.3** **Injury of brachial plexus**
X+7th **S14.4** **Injury of peripheral nerves of neck**
X+7th **S14.5** **Injury of cervical sympathetic nerves**
X+7th **S14.8** **Injury of other specified nerves of neck**
X+7th **S14.9** **Injury of unspecified nerves of neck**

S15 **Injury of blood vessels at neck level**
Code also any associated open wound (S11.-)

The appropriate 7th character is to be added to each code from category S15
A initial encounter
D subsequent encounter
S sequela

\+ **S15.0** **Injury of carotid artery of neck**
Injury of carotid artery (common) (external) (internal, extracranial portion)
Injury of carotid artery NOS
Excludes1: *injury of internal carotid artery, intracranial portion (S06.8)*

\+ **S15.00** **Unspecified injury of carotid artery**
CC +7th **S15.001** **Unspecified injury of right carotid artery**
CC +7th **S15.002** **Unspecified injury of left carotid artery**
CC +7th **S15.009** **Unspecified injury of unspecified carotid artery**

\+ **S15.01** **Minor laceration of carotid artery**
Incomplete transection of carotid artery
Laceration of carotid artery NOS
Superficial laceration of carotid artery
CC +7th **S15.011** **Minor laceration of right carotid artery**
CC +7th **S15.012** **Minor laceration of left carotid artery**
CC +7th **S15.019** **Minor laceration of unspecified carotid artery**

\+ **S15.02** **Major laceration of carotid artery**
Complete transection of carotid artery
Traumatic rupture of carotid artery
CC +7th **S15.021** **Major laceration of right carotid artery**
CC +7th **S15.022** **Major laceration of left carotid artery**
CC +7th **S15.029** **Major laceration of unspecified carotid artery**

\+ **S15.09** **Other specified injury of carotid artery**
CC +7th **S15.091** **Other specified injury of right carotid artery**
CC +7th **S15.092** **Other specified injury of left carotid artery**
CC +7th **S15.099** **Other specified injury of unspecified carotid artery**

\+ **S15.1** **Injury of vertebral artery**

\+ **S15.10** **Unspecified injury of vertebral artery**
CC +7th **S15.101** **Unspecified injury of right vertebral artery**
CC +7th **S15.102** **Unspecified injury of left vertebral artery**
CC +7th **S15.109** **Unspecified injury of unspecified vertebral artery**

\+ **S15.11** **Minor laceration of vertebral artery**
Incomplete transection of vertebral artery
Laceration of vertebral artery NOS
Superficial laceration of vertebral artery
CC +7th **S15.111** **Minor laceration of right vertebral artery**
CC +7th **S15.112** **Minor laceration of left vertebral artery**
CC +7th **S15.119** **Minor laceration of unspecified vertebral artery**

\+ **S15.12** **Major laceration of vertebral artery**
Complete transection of vertebral artery
Traumatic rupture of vertebral artery
CC +7th **S15.121** **Major laceration of right vertebral artery**
CC +7th **S15.122** **Major laceration of left vertebral artery**
CC +7th **S15.129** **Major laceration of unspecified vertebral artery**

\+ **S15.19** **Other specified injury of vertebral artery**
CC +7th **S15.191** **Other specified injury of right vertebral artery**
CC +7th **S15.192** **Other specified injury of left vertebral artery**
CC +7th **S15.199** **Other specified injury of unspecified vertebral artery**

\+ **S15.2** **Injury of external jugular vein**

\+ **S15.20** **Unspecified injury of external jugular vein**
CC +7th **S15.201** **Unspecified injury of right external jugular vein**
CC +7th **S15.202** **Unspecified injury of left external jugular vein**
CC +7th **S15.209** **Unspecified injury of unspecified external jugular vein**

\+ **S15.21** **Minor laceration of external jugular vein**
Incomplete transection of external jugular vein
Laceration of external jugular vein NOS
Superficial laceration of external jugular vein
CC +7th **S15.211** **Minor laceration of right external jugular vein**
CC +7th **S15.212** **Minor laceration of left external jugular vein**
CC +7th **S15.219** **Minor laceration of unspecified external jugular vein**

\+ **S15.22** **Major laceration of external jugular vein**
Complete transection of external jugular vein
Traumatic rupture of external jugular vein
CC +7th **S15.221** **Major laceration of right external jugular vein**
CC +7th **S15.222** **Major laceration of left external jugular vein**
CC +7th **S15.229** **Major laceration of unspecified external jugular vein**

\+ **S15.29** **Other specified injury of external jugular vein**
CC +7th **S15.291** **Other specified injury of right external jugular vein**
CC +7th **S15.292** **Other specified injury of left external jugular vein**
CC +7th **S15.299** **Other specified injury of unspecified external jugular vein**

\+ **S15.3** **Injury of internal jugular vein**

\+ **S15.30** **Unspecified injury of internal jugular vein**
CC +7th **S15.301** **Unspecified injury of right internal jugular vein**
CC +7th **S15.302** **Unspecified injury of left internal jugular vein**
CC +7th **S15.309** **Unspecified injury of unspecified internal jugular vein**

\+ **S15.31** **Minor laceration of internal jugular vein**
Incomplete transection of internal jugular vein
Laceration of internal jugular vein NOS
Superficial laceration of internal jugular vein
CC +7th **S15.311** **Minor laceration of right internal jugular vein**
CC +7th **S15.312** **Minor laceration of left internal jugular vein**
CC +7th **S15.319** **Minor laceration of unspecified internal jugular vein**

\+ **S15.32** **Major laceration of internal jugular vein**
Complete transection of internal jugular vein
Traumatic rupture of internal jugular vein
CC +7th **S15.321** **Major laceration of right internal jugular vein**
CC +7th **S15.322** **Major laceration of left internal jugular vein**
CC +7th **S15.329** **Major laceration of unspecified internal jugular vein**

+ **S15.39 Other specified injury of internal jugular vein**
  - CC +7th **S15.391 Other specified injury of right internal jugular vein**
  - CC +7th **S15.392 Other specified injury of left internal jugular vein**
  - CC +7th **S15.399 Other specified injury of unspecified internal jugular vein**

CC **S15.8 Injury of other specified blood vessels at neck level**
CC **S15.9 Injury of unspecified blood vessel at neck level**

S16 Injury of muscle, fascia and tendon at neck level

Code also any associated open wound (S11.-)

Excludes2: *sprain of joint or ligament at neck level (S13.9)*

The appropriate 7th character is to be added to each code from category S16
A initial encounter
D subsequent encounter
S sequela

X+7th **S16.1 Strain of muscle, fascia and tendon at neck level**
X+7th **S16.2 Laceration of muscle, fascia and tendon at neck level**
X+7th **S16.8 Other specified injury of muscle, fascia and tendon at neck level**
X+7th **S16.9 Unspecified injury of muscle, fascia and tendon at neck level**

S17 Crushing injury of neck

Use additional code for all associated injuries, such as:
injury of blood vessels (S15.-)
open wound of neck (S11.-)
spinal cord injury (S14.0, S14.1-)
vertebral fracture (S12.0--S12.3-)

The appropriate 7th character is to be added to each code from category S17
A initial encounter
D subsequent encounter
S sequela

CC X+7th **S17.0 Crushing injury of larynx and trachea**
HAC 7th character A see Appendix B for HAC conditional logic
CC X+7th **S17.8 Crushing injury of other specified parts of neck**
HAC 7th character A see Appendix B for HAC conditional logic
CC X+7th **S17.9 Crushing injury of neck, part unspecified**
HAC 7th character A see Appendix B for HAC conditional logic

S19 Other specified and unspecified injuries of neck

The appropriate 7th character is to be added to each code from category S19
A initial encounter
D subsequent encounter
S sequela

+ **S19.8 Other specified injuries of neck**
  - X+7th **S19.80 Other specified injuries of unspecified part of neck**
  - X+7th **S19.81 Other specified injuries of larynx**
  - X+7th **S19.82 Other specified injuries of cervical trachea**
    Excludes2: *other specified injury of thoracic trachea (S27.5-)*
  - X+7th **S19.83 Other specified injuries of vocal cord**
  - X+7th **S19.84 Other specified injuries of thyroid gland**
  - X+7th **S19.85 Other specified injuries of pharynx and cervical esophagus**
  - X+7th **S19.89 Other specified injuries of other specified part of neck**

X+7th **S19.9 Unspecified injury of neck**

Injuries to the thorax (S20-S29)

Includes: injuries of breast
injuries of chest (wall)
injuries of interscapular area

Excludes2: *burns and corrosions (T20-T32)*
effects of foreign body in bronchus (T17.5)
effects of foreign body in esophagus (T18.1)
effects of foreign body in lung (T17.8)
effects of foreign body in trachea (T17.4)
frostbite (T33-T34)
injuries of axilla
injuries of clavicle
injuries of scapular region
injuries of shoulder
insect bite or sting, venomous (T63.4)

S20 Superficial injury of thorax

The appropriate 7th character is to be added to each code from category S20
A initial encounter
D subsequent encounter
S sequela

AHA CC: 4Q, 2020, 39

+ **S20.0 Contusion of breast**
  - X+7th **S20.00 Contusion of breast, unspecified breast**
  - X+7th **S20.01 Contusion of right breast**
  - X+7th **S20.02 Contusion of left breast**
+ **S20.1 Other and unspecified superficial injuries of breast**
  + **S20.10 Unspecified superficial injuries of breast**
    - +7th **S20.101 Unspecified superficial injuries of breast, right breast**
    - +7th **S20.102 Unspecified superficial injuries of breast, left breast**
    - +7th **S20.109 Unspecified superficial injuries of breast, unspecified breast**
  + **S20.11 Abrasion of breast**
    - +7th **S20.111 Abrasion of breast, right breast**
    - +7th **S20.112 Abrasion of breast, left breast**
    - +7th **S20.119 Abrasion of breast, unspecified breast**
  + **S20.12 Blister (nonthermal) of breast**
    - +7th **S20.121 Blister (nonthermal) of breast, right breast**
    - +7th **S20.122 Blister (nonthermal) of breast, left breast**
    - +7th **S20.129 Blister (nonthermal) of breast, unspecified breast**
  + **S20.14 External constriction of part of breast**
    - +7th **S20.141 External constriction of part of breast, right breast**
    - +7th **S20.142 External constriction of part of breast, left breast**
    - +7th **S20.149 External constriction of part of breast, unspecified breast**
  + **S20.15 Superficial foreign body of breast**
    Splinter in the breast
    - +7th **S20.151 Superficial foreign body of breast, right breast**
    - +7th **S20.152 Superficial foreign body of breast, left breast**
    - +7th **S20.159 Superficial foreign body of breast, unspecified breast**
  + **S20.16 Insect bite (nonvenomous) of breast**
    - +7th **S20.161 Insect bite (nonvenomous) of breast, right breast**
    - +7th **S20.162 Insect bite (nonvenomous) of breast, left breast**
    - +7th **S20.169 Insect bite (nonvenomous) of breast, unspecified breast**
  + **S20.17 Other superficial bite of breast**
    Excludes1: *open bite of breast (S21.05-)*
    - +7th **S20.171 Other superficial bite of breast, right breast**
    - +7th **S20.172 Other superficial bite of breast, left breast**
    - +7th **S20.179 Other superficial bite of breast, unspecified breast**

+ **S20.2 Contusion of thorax**
  X+7th **S20.20 Contusion of thorax, unspecified**
  + **S20.21 Contusion of front wall of thorax**
    +7th **S20.211 Contusion of right front wall of thorax**
    +7th **S20.212 Contusion of left front wall of thorax**
    +7th **S20.213 Contusion of bilateral front wall of thorax**
    +7th **S20.214 Contusion of middle front wall of thorax**
    +7th **S20.219 Contusion of unspecified front wall of thorax**
  + **S20.22 Contusion of back wall of thorax**
    +7th **S20.221 Contusion of right back wall of thorax**
    +7th **S20.222 Contusion of left back wall of thorax**
    +7th **S20.223 Contusion of bilateral back wall of thorax**
    +7th **S20.224 Contusion of middle back wall of thorax**
    +7th **S20.229 Contusion of unspecified back wall of thorax**

+ **S20.3 Other and unspecified superficial injuries of front wall of thorax**
  + **S20.30 Unspecified superficial injuries of front wall of thorax**
    +7th **S20.301 Unspecified superficial injuries of right front wall of thorax**
    +7th **S20.302 Unspecified superficial injuries of left front wall of thorax**
    +7th **S20.303 Unspecified superficial injuries of bilateral front wall of thorax**
    +7th **S20.304 Unspecified superficial injuries of middle front wall of thorax**
    +7th **S20.309 Unspecified superficial injuries of unspecified front wall of thorax**
  + **S20.31 Abrasion of front wall of thorax**
    +7th **S20.311 Abrasion of right front wall of thorax**
    +7th **S20.312 Abrasion of left front wall of thorax**
    +7th **S20.313 Abrasion of bilateral front wall of thorax**
    +7th **S20.314 Abrasion of middle front wall of thorax**
    +7th **S20.319 Abrasion of unspecified front wall of thorax**
  + **S20.32 Blister (nonthermal) of front wall of thorax**
    +7th **S20.321 Blister (nonthermal) of right front wall of thorax**
    +7th **S20.322 Blister (nonthermal) of left front wall of thorax**
    +7th **S20.323 Blister (nonthermal) of bilateral front wall of thorax**
    +7th **S20.324 Blister (nonthermal) of middle front wall of thorax**
    +7th **S20.329 Blister (nonthermal) of unspecified front wall of thorax**
  + **S20.34 External constriction of front wall of thorax**
    +7th **S20.341 External constriction of right front wall of thorax**
    +7th **S20.342 External constriction of left front wall of thorax**
    +7th **S20.343 External constriction of bilateral front wall of thorax**
    +7th **S20.344 External constriction of middle front wall of thorax**
    +7th **S20.349 External constriction of unspecified front wall of thorax**
  + **S20.35 Superficial foreign body of front wall of thorax**
    Splinter in front wall of thorax
    +7th **S20.351 Superficial foreign body of right front wall of thorax**
    +7th **S20.352 Superficial foreign body of left front wall of thorax**
    +7th **S20.353 Superficial foreign body of bilateral front wall of thorax**
    +7th **S20.354 Superficial foreign body of middle front wall of thorax**
    +7th **S20.359 Superficial foreign body of unspecified front wall of thorax**
  + **S20.36 Insect bite (nonvenomous) of front wall of thorax**
    +7th **S20.361 Insect bite (nonvenomous) of right front wall of thorax**
    +7th **S20.362 Insect bite (nonvenomous) of left front wall of thorax**
    +7th **S20.363 Insect bite (nonvenomous) of bilateral front wall of thorax**
    +7th **S20.364 Insect bite (nonvenomous) of middle front wall of thorax**
    +7th **S20.369 Insect bite (nonvenomous) of unspecified front wall of thorax**
  + **S20.37 Other superficial bite of front wall of thorax**
    Excludes1: *open bite of front wall of thorax (S21.14)*
    +7th **S20.371 Other superficial bite of right front wall of thorax**
    +7th **S20.372 Other superficial bite of left front wall of thorax**
    +7th **S20.373 Other superficial bite of bilateral front wall of thorax**
    +7th **S20.374 Other superficial bite of middle front wall of thorax**
    +7th **S20.379 Other superficial bite of unspecified front wall of thorax**

+ **S20.4 Other and unspecified superficial injuries of back wall of thorax**
  + **S20.40 Unspecified superficial injuries of back wall of thorax**
    +7th **S20.401 Unspecified superficial injuries of right back wall of thorax**
    +7th **S20.402 Unspecified superficial injuries of left back wall of thorax**
    +7th **S20.409 Unspecified superficial injuries of unspecified back wall of thorax**
  + **S20.41 Abrasion of back wall of thorax**
    +7th **S20.411 Abrasion of right back wall of thorax**
    +7th **S20.412 Abrasion of left back wall of thorax**
    +7th **S20.419 Abrasion of unspecified back wall of thorax**
  + **S20.42 Blister (nonthermal) of back wall of thorax**
    +7th **S20.421 Blister (nonthermal) of right back wall of thorax**
    +7th **S20.422 Blister (nonthermal) of left back wall of thorax**
    +7th **S20.429 Blister (nonthermal) of unspecified back wall of thorax**
  + **S20.44 External constriction of back wall of thorax**
    +7th **S20.441 External constriction of right back wall of thorax**
    +7th **S20.442 External constriction of left back wall of thorax**
    +7th **S20.449 External constriction of unspecified back wall of thorax**
  + **S20.45 Superficial foreign body of back wall of thorax**
    Splinter of back wall of thorax
    +7th **S20.451 Superficial foreign body of right back wall of thorax**
    +7th **S20.452 Superficial foreign body of left back wall of thorax**
    +7th **S20.459 Superficial foreign body of unspecified back wall of thorax**
  + **S20.46 Insect bite (nonvenomous) of back wall of thorax**
    +7th **S20.461 Insect bite (nonvenomous) of right back wall of thorax**
    +7th **S20.462 Insect bite (nonvenomous) of left back wall of thorax**
    +7th **S20.469 Insect bite (nonvenomous) of unspecified back wall of thorax**
  + **S20.47 Other superficial bite of back wall of thorax**
    Excludes1: *open bite of back wall of thorax (S21.24)*
    +7th **S20.471 Other superficial bite of right back wall of thorax**
    +7th **S20.472 Other superficial bite of left back wall of thorax**
    +7th **S20.479 Other superficial bite of unspecified back wall of thorax**

+ **S20.9 Superficial injury of unspecified parts of thorax**
  Excludes1: *contusion of thorax NOS (S20.20)*
  X+7th **S20.90 Unspecified superficial injury of unspecified parts of thorax**
    Superficial injury of thoracic wall NOS
  X+7th **S20.91 Abrasion of unspecified parts of thorax**
  X+7th **S20.92 Blister (nonthermal) of unspecified parts of thorax**

X+7th **S20.94 External constriction of unspecified parts of thorax**

X+7th **S20.95 Superficial foreign body of unspecified parts of thorax**

Splinter in thorax NOS

X+7th **S20.96 Insect bite (nonvenomous) of unspecified parts of thorax**

X+7th **S20.97 Other superficial bite of unspecified parts of thorax**

Excludes1: *open bite of thorax NOS (S21.95)*

S21 Open wound of thorax

Code also any associated injury, such as:
injury of heart (S26.-)
injury of intrathoracic organs (S27.-)
rib fracture (S22.3-, S22.4-)
spinal cord injury (S24.0-, S24.1-)
traumatic hemothorax (S27.1)
traumatic hemopneumothorax (S27.3)
traumatic pneumothorax (S27.0)
wound infection

Excludes1: *traumatic amputation (partial) of thorax (S28.1)*

The appropriate 7th character is to be added to each code from category S21
A initial encounter
D subsequent encounter
S sequela

\+ **S21.0 Open wound of breast**

\+ **S21.00 Unspecified open wound of breast**

+7th **S21.001 Unspecified open wound of right breast**

+7th **S21.002 Unspecified open wound of left breast**

+7th **S21.009 Unspecified open wound of unspecified breast**

\+ **S21.01 Laceration without foreign body of breast**

+7th **S21.011 Laceration without foreign body of right breast**

+7th **S21.012 Laceration without foreign body of left breast**

+7th **S21.019 Laceration without foreign body of unspecified breast**

\+ **S21.02 Laceration with foreign body of breast**

+7th **S21.021 Laceration with foreign body of right breast**

+7th **S21.022 Laceration with foreign body of left breast**

+7th **S21.029 Laceration with foreign body of unspecified breast**

\+ **S21.03 Puncture wound without foreign body of breast**

+7th **S21.031 Puncture wound without foreign body of right breast**

+7th **S21.032 Puncture wound without foreign body of left breast**

+7th **S21.039 Puncture wound without foreign body of unspecified breast**

\+ **S21.04 Puncture wound with foreign body of breast**

+7th **S21.041 Puncture wound with foreign body of right breast**

+7th **S21.042 Puncture wound with foreign body of left breast**

+7th **S21.049 Puncture wound with foreign body of unspecified breast**

\+ **S21.05 Open bite of breast**

Bite of breast NOS

Excludes1: *superficial bite of breast (S20.17)*

S21.051 Open bite of right breast

S21.052 Open bite of left breast

S21.059 Open bite of unspecified breast

\+ **S21.1 Open wound of front wall of thorax without penetration into thoracic cavity**

Open wound of chest without penetration into thoracic cavity

\+ **S21.10 Unspecified open wound of front wall of thorax without penetration into thoracic cavity**

CC +7th **S21.101 Unspecified open wound of right front wall of thorax without penetration into thoracic cavity**

CC +7th **S21.102 Unspecified open wound of left front wall of thorax without penetration into thoracic cavity**

CC +7th **S21.109 Unspecified open wound of unspecified front wall of thorax without penetration into thoracic cavity**

\+ **S21.11 Laceration without foreign body of front wall of thorax without penetration into thoracic cavity**

CC +7th **S21.111 Laceration without foreign body of right front wall of thorax without penetration into thoracic cavity**

CC +7th **S21.112 Laceration without foreign body of left front wall of thorax without penetration into thoracic cavity**

CC +7th **S21.119 Laceration without foreign body of unspecified front wall of thorax without penetration into thoracic cavity**

\+ **S21.12 Laceration with foreign body of front wall of thorax without penetration into thoracic cavity**

CC +7th **S21.121 Laceration with foreign body of right front wall of thorax without penetration into thoracic cavity**

CC +7th **S21.122 Laceration with foreign body of left front wall of thorax without penetration into thoracic cavity**

CC +7th **S21.129 Laceration with foreign body of unspecified front wall of thorax without penetration into thoracic cavity**

\+ **S21.13 Puncture wound without foreign body of front wall of thorax without penetration into thoracic cavity**

CC +7th **S21.131 Puncture wound without foreign body of right front wall of thorax without penetration into thoracic cavity**

CC +7th **S21.132 Puncture wound without foreign body of left front wall of thorax without penetration into thoracic cavity**

CC +7th **S21.139 Puncture wound without foreign body of unspecified front wall of thorax without penetration into thoracic cavity**

\+ **S21.14 Puncture wound with foreign body of front wall of thorax without penetration into thoracic cavity**

CC +7th **S21.141 Puncture wound with foreign body of right front wall of thorax without penetration into thoracic cavity**

CC +7th **S21.142 Puncture wound with foreign body of left front wall of thorax without penetration into thoracic cavity**

CC +7th **S21.149 Puncture wound with foreign body of unspecified front wall of thorax without penetration into thoracic cavity**

\+ **S21.15 Open bite of front wall of thorax without penetration into thoracic cavity**

Bite of front wall of thorax NOS

Excludes1: *superficial bite of front wall of thorax (S20.37)*

CC +7th **S21.151 Open bite of right front wall of thorax without penetration into thoracic cavity**

CC +7th **S21.152 Open bite of left front wall of thorax without penetration into thoracic cavity**

CC +7th **S21.159 Open bite of unspecified front wall of thorax without penetration into thoracic cavity**

\+ **S21.2 Open wound of back wall of thorax without penetration into thoracic cavity**

\+ **S21.20 Unspecified open wound of back wall of thorax without penetration into thoracic cavity**

+7th **S21.201 Unspecified open wound of right back wall of thorax without penetration into thoracic cavity**

+7th **S21.202 Unspecified open wound of left back wall of thorax without penetration into thoracic cavity**

+7th **S21.209 Unspecified open wound of unspecified back wall of thorax without penetration into thoracic cavity**

\+ **S21.21 Laceration without foreign body of back wall of thorax without penetration into thoracic cavity**

+7th **S21.211 Laceration without foreign body of right back wall of thorax without penetration into thoracic cavity**

+7th **S21.212 Laceration without foreign body of left back wall of thorax without penetration into thoracic cavity**

+7th **S21.219 Laceration without foreign body of unspecified back wall of thorax without penetration into thoracic cavity**

+ **S21.22 Laceration with foreign body of back wall of thorax without penetration into thoracic cavity**

+7th **S21.221 Laceration with foreign body of right back wall of thorax without penetration into thoracic cavity**

+7th **S21.222 Laceration with foreign body of left back wall of thorax without penetration into thoracic cavity**

+7th **S21.229 Laceration with foreign body of unspecified back wall of thorax without penetration into thoracic cavity**

+ **S21.23 Puncture wound without foreign body of back wall of thorax without penetration into thoracic cavity**

+7th **S21.231 Puncture wound without foreign body of right back wall of thorax without penetration into thoracic cavity**

+7th **S21.232 Puncture wound without foreign body of left back wall of thorax without penetration into thoracic cavity**

+7th **S21.239 Puncture wound without foreign body of unspecified back wall of thorax without penetration into thoracic cavity**

+ **S21.24 Puncture wound with foreign body of back wall of thorax without penetration into thoracic cavity**

+7th **S21.241 Puncture wound with foreign body of right back wall of thorax without penetration into thoracic cavity**

+7th **S21.242 Puncture wound with foreign body of left back wall of thorax without penetration into thoracic cavity**

+7th **S21.249 Puncture wound with foreign body of unspecified back wall of thorax without penetration into thoracic cavity**

+ **S21.25 Open bite of back wall of thorax without penetration into thoracic cavity**

Bite of back wall of thorax NOS

Excludes1: *superficial bite of back wall of thorax (S20.47)*

+7th **S21.251 Open bite of right back wall of thorax without penetration into thoracic cavity**

+7th **S21.252 Open bite of left back wall of thorax without penetration into thoracic cavity**

+7th **S21.259 Open bite of unspecified back wall of thorax without penetration into thoracic cavity**

+ **S21.3 Open wound of front wall of thorax with penetration into thoracic cavity**

Open wound of chest with penetration into thoracic cavity

+ **S21.30 Unspecified open wound of front wall of thorax with penetration into thoracic cavity**

MCC +7th **S21.301 Unspecified open wound of right front wall of thorax with penetration into thoracic cavity**

MCC +7th **S21.302 Unspecified open wound of left front wall of thorax with penetration into thoracic cavity**

MCC +7th **S21.309 Unspecified open wound of unspecified front wall of thorax with penetration into thoracic cavity**

+ **S21.31 Laceration without foreign body of front wall of thorax with penetration into thoracic cavity**

MCC +7th **S21.311 Laceration without foreign body of right front wall of thorax with penetration into thoracic cavity**

MCC +7th **S21.312 Laceration without foreign body of left front wall of thorax with penetration into thoracic cavity**

MCC +7th **S21.319 Laceration without foreign body of unspecified front wall of thorax with penetration into thoracic cavity**

+ **S21.32 Laceration with foreign body of front wall of thorax with penetration into thoracic cavity**

MCC +7th **S21.321 Laceration with foreign body of right front wall of thorax with penetration into thoracic cavity**

MCC +7th **S21.322 Laceration with foreign body of left front wall of thorax with penetration into thoracic cavity**

MCC +7th **S21.329 Laceration with foreign body of unspecified front wall of thorax with penetration into thoracic cavity**

+ **S21.33 Puncture wound without foreign body of front wall of thorax with penetration into thoracic cavity**

MCC +7th **S21.331 Puncture wound without foreign body of right front wall of thorax with penetration into thoracic cavity**

MCC +7th **S21.332 Puncture wound without foreign body of left front wall of thorax with penetration into thoracic cavity**

MCC +7th **S21.339 Puncture wound without foreign body of unspecified front wall of thorax with penetration into thoracic cavity**

+ **S21.34 Puncture wound with foreign body of front wall of thorax with penetration into thoracic cavity**

MCC +7th **S21.341 Puncture wound with foreign body of right front wall of thorax with penetration into thoracic cavity**

MCC +7th **S21.342 Puncture wound with foreign body of left front wall of thorax with penetration into thoracic cavity**

MCC +7th **S21.349 Puncture wound with foreign body of unspecified front wall of thorax with penetration into thoracic cavity**

+ **S21.35 Open bite of front wall of thorax with penetration into thoracic cavity**

Excludes1: *superficial bite of front wall of thorax (S20.37)*

MCC +7th **S21.351 Open bite of right front wall of thorax with penetration into thoracic cavity**

MCC +7th **S21.352 Open bite of left front wall of thorax with penetration into thoracic cavity**

MCC +7th **S21.359 Open bite of unspecified front wall of thorax with penetration into thoracic cavity**

+ **S21.4 Open wound of back wall of thorax with penetration into thoracic cavity**

+ **S21.40 Unspecified open wound of back wall of thorax with penetration into thoracic cavity**

MCC +7th **S21.401 Unspecified open wound of right back wall of thorax with penetration into thoracic cavity**

MCC +7th **S21.402 Unspecified open wound of left back wall of thorax with penetration into thoracic cavity**

MCC +7th **S21.409 Unspecified open wound of unspecified back wall of thorax with penetration into thoracic cavity**

+ **S21.41 Laceration without foreign body of back wall of thorax with penetration into thoracic cavity**

MCC +7th **S21.411 Laceration without foreign body of right back wall of thorax with penetration into thoracic cavity**

MCC +7th **S21.412 Laceration without foreign body of left back wall of thorax with penetration into thoracic cavity**

MCC +7th **S21.419 Laceration without foreign body of unspecified back wall of thorax with penetration into thoracic cavity**

+ **S21.42 Laceration with foreign body of back wall of thorax with penetration into thoracic cavity**

MCC +7th **S21.421 Laceration with foreign body of right back wall of thorax with penetration into thoracic cavity**

MCC +7th **S21.422 Laceration with foreign body of left back wall of thorax with penetration into thoracic cavity**

MCC +7th S21.429 **Laceration with foreign body of unspecified back wall of thorax with penetration into thoracic cavity**

+ S21.43 **Puncture wound without foreign body of back wall of thorax with penetration into thoracic cavity**

MCC +7th S21.431 **Puncture wound without foreign body of right back wall of thorax with penetration into thoracic cavity**

MCC +7th S21.432 **Puncture wound without foreign body of left back wall of thorax with penetration into thoracic cavity**

MCC +7th S21.439 **Puncture wound without foreign body of unspecified back wall of thorax with penetration into thoracic cavity**

+ S21.44 **Puncture wound with foreign body of back wall of thorax with penetration into thoracic cavity**

MCC +7th S21.441 **Puncture wound with foreign body of right back wall of thorax with penetration into thoracic cavity**

MCC +7th S21.442 **Puncture wound with foreign body of left back wall of thorax with penetration into thoracic cavity**

MCC +7th S21.449 **Puncture wound with foreign body of unspecified back wall of thorax with penetration into thoracic cavity**

+ S21.45 **Open bite of back wall of thorax with penetration into thoracic cavity**

Bite of back wall of thorax NOS

Excludes1: *superficial bite of back wall of thorax (S20.47)*

MCC +7th S21.451 **Open bite of right back wall of thorax with penetration into thoracic cavity**

MCC +7th S21.452 **Open bite of left back wall of thorax with penetration into thoracic cavity**

MCC +7th S21.459 **Open bite of unspecified back wall of thorax with penetration into thoracic cavity**

+ S21.9 **Open wound of unspecified part of thorax**

Open wound of thoracic wall NOS

CC X+7th S21.90 **Unspecified open wound of unspecified part of thorax**

CC X+7th S21.91 **Laceration without foreign body of unspecified part of thorax**

CC X+7th S21.92 **Laceration with foreign body of unspecified part of thorax**

CC X+7th S21.93 **Puncture wound without foreign body of unspecified part of thorax**

CC X+7th S21.94 **Puncture wound with foreign body of unspecified part of thorax**

CC X+7th S21.95 **Open bite of unspecified part of thorax**

Excludes1: *superficial bite of thorax (S20.97)*

See page 994 for Vertebrae Illustration.

S22 Fracture of rib(s), sternum and thoracic spine

NOTE A fracture not indicated as displaced or nondisplaced should be coded to displaced

A fracture not indicated as open or closed should be coded to closed

Includes: fracture of thoracic neural arch
fracture of thoracic spinous process
fracture of thoracic transverse process
fracture of thoracic vertebra
fracture of thoracic vertebral arch

Code first any associated:
injury of intrathoracic organ (S27.-)
spinal cord injury (S24.0-, S24.1-)

Excludes1: *transection of thorax (S28.1)*

Excludes2: *fracture of clavicle (S42.0-)*
fracture of scapula (S42.1-)

The appropriate 7th character is to be added to each code from category S22

- A initial encounter for closed fracture
- B initial encounter for open fracture
- D subsequent encounter for fracture with routine healing
- G subsequent encounter for fracture with delayed healing
- K subsequent encounter for fracture with nonunion
- S sequela

Review coding guideline C.19.c

+ S22.0 **Fracture of thoracic vertebra**

+ S22.00 **Fracture of unspecified thoracic vertebra**

CC MCC +7th **S22.000** **Wedge compression fracture of unspecified thoracic vertebra**

HAC 7th characters A & B see Appendix B for HAC conditional logic

CC MCC +7th **S22.001** **Stable burst fracture of unspecified thoracic vertebra**

HAC 7th characters A & B see Appendix B for HAC conditional logic

CC MCC +7th **S22.002** **Unstable burst fracture of unspecified thoracic vertebra**

HAC 7th characters A & B see Appendix B for HAC conditional logic

CC MCC +7th **S22.008** **Other fracture of unspecified thoracic vertebra**

HAC 7th characters A & B see Appendix B for HAC conditional logic

CC MCC +7th **S22.009** **Unspecified fracture of unspecified thoracic vertebra**

HAC 7th characters A & B see Appendix B for HAC conditional logic

+ S22.01 **Fracture of first thoracic vertebra**

CC MCC +7th **S22.010** **Wedge compression fracture of first thoracic vertebra**

HAC 7th characters A & B see Appendix B for HAC conditional logic

CC MCC +7th **S22.011** **Stable burst fracture of first thoracic vertebra**

HAC 7th characters A & B see Appendix B for HAC conditional logic

CC MCC +7th **S22.012** **Unstable burst fracture of first thoracic vertebra**

HAC 7th characters A & B see Appendix B for HAC conditional logic

CC MCC +7th **S22.018** **Other fracture of first thoracic vertebra**

HAC 7th characters A & B see Appendix B for HAC conditional logic

CC MCC +7th **S22.019** **Unspecified fracture of first thoracic vertebra**

HAC 7th characters A & B see Appendix B for HAC conditional logic

+ S22.02 **Fracture of second thoracic vertebra**

CC MCC +7th **S22.020** **Wedge compression fracture of second thoracic vertebra**

HAC 7th characters A & B see Appendix B for HAC conditional logic

CC MCC +7th **S22.021** **Stable burst fracture of second thoracic vertebra**

HAC 7th characters A & B see Appendix B for HAC conditional logic

CC MCC +7th **S22.022** **Unstable burst fracture of second thoracic vertebra**

HAC 7th characters A & B see Appendix B for HAC conditional logic

CC MCC +7th **S22.028** **Other fracture of second thoracic vertebra**

HAC 7th characters A & B see Appendix B for HAC conditional logic

CC MCC +7th **S22.029** **Unspecified fracture of second thoracic vertebra**

HAC 7th characters A & B see Appendix B for HAC conditional logic

+ S22.03 **Fracture of third thoracic vertebra**

CC MCC +7th **S22.030** **Wedge compression fracture of third thoracic vertebra**

HAC 7th characters A & B see Appendix B for HAC conditional logic

CC MCC +7th **S22.031** **Stable burst fracture of third thoracic vertebra**

HAC 7th characters A & B see Appendix B for HAC conditional logic

CC MCC +7th **S22.032** **Unstable burst fracture of third thoracic vertebra**

HAC 7th characters A & B see Appendix B for HAC conditional logic

CC MCC +7th **S22.038** **Other fracture of third thoracic vertebra**

HAC 7th characters A & B see Appendix B for HAC conditional logic

CC MCC +7th **S22.039** **Unspecified fracture of third thoracic vertebra**

HAC 7th characters A & B see Appendix B for HAC conditional logic

+ **S22.04 Fracture of fourth thoracic vertebra**

CC MCC +7th **S22.040 Wedge compression fracture of fourth thoracic vertebra**
HAC 7th characters A & B see Appendix B for HAC conditional logic

CC MCC +7th **S22.041 Stable burst fracture of fourth thoracic vertebra**
HAC 7th characters A & B see Appendix B for HAC conditional logic

CC MCC +7th **S22.042 Unstable burst fracture of fourth thoracic vertebra**
HAC 7th characters A & B see Appendix B for HAC conditional logic

CC MCC +7th **S22.048 Other fracture of fourth thoracic vertebra**
HAC 7th characters A & B see Appendix B for HAC conditional logic

CC MCC +7th **S22.049 Unspecified fracture of fourth thoracic vertebra**
HAC 7th characters A & B see Appendix B for HAC conditional logic

+ **S22.05 Fracture of T5-T6 vertebra**

CC MCC +7th **S22.050 Wedge compression fracture of T5-T6 vertebra**
HAC 7th characters A & B see Appendix B for HAC conditional logic

CC MCC +7th **S22.051 Stable burst fracture of T5-T6 vertebra**
HAC 7th characters A & B see Appendix B for HAC conditional logic

CC MCC +7th **S22.052 Unstable burst fracture of T5-T6 vertebra**
HAC 7th characters A & B see Appendix B for HAC conditional logic

CC MCC +7th **S22.058 Other fracture of T5-T6 vertebra**
HAC 7th characters A & B see Appendix B for HAC conditional logic

CC MCC +7th **S22.059 Unspecified fracture of T5-T6 vertebra**
HAC 7th characters A & B see Appendix B for HAC conditional logic

+ **S22.06 Fracture of T7-T8 vertebra**

CC MCC +7th **S22.060 Wedge compression fracture of T7-T8 vertebra**
HAC 7th characters A & B see Appendix B for HAC conditional logic

CC MCC +7th **S22.061 Stable burst fracture of T7-T8 vertebra**
HAC 7th characters A & B see Appendix B for HAC conditional logic

CC MCC +7th **S22.062 Unstable burst fracture of T7-T8 vertebra**
HAC 7th characters A & B see Appendix B for HAC conditional logic

CC MCC +7th **S22.068 Other fracture of T7-T8 thoracic vertebra**
HAC 7th characters A & B see Appendix B for HAC conditional logic

CC MCC +7th **S22.069 Unspecified fracture of T7-T8 vertebra**
HAC 7th characters A & B see Appendix B for HAC conditional logic

+ **S22.07 Fracture of T9-T10 vertebra**

CC MCC +7th **S22.070 Wedge compression fracture of T9-T10 vertebra**
HAC 7th characters A & B see Appendix B for HAC conditional logic

CC MCC +7th **S22.071 Stable burst fracture of T9-T10 vertebra**
HAC 7th characters A & B see Appendix B for HAC conditional logic

CC MCC +7th **S22.072 Unstable burst fracture of T9-T10 vertebra**
HAC 7th characters A & B see Appendix B for HAC conditional logic

CC MCC +7th **S22.078 Other fracture of T9-T10 vertebra**
HAC 7th characters A & B see Appendix B for HAC conditional logic

CC MCC +7th **S22.079 Unspecified fracture of T9-T10 vertebra**
HAC 7th characters A & B see Appendix B for HAC conditional logic

+ **S22.08 Fracture of T11-T12 vertebra**

CC MCC +7th **S22.080 Wedge compression fracture of T11-T12 vertebra**
HAC 7th characters A & B see Appendix B for HAC conditional logic

CC MCC +7th **S22.081 Stable burst fracture of T11-T12 vertebra**
HAC 7th characters A & B see Appendix B for HAC conditional logic

CC MCC +7th **S22.082 Unstable burst fracture of T11-T12 vertebra**
HAC 7th characters A & B see Appendix B for HAC conditional logic

CC MCC +7th **S22.088 Other fracture of T11-T12 vertebra**
HAC 7th characters A & B see Appendix B for HAC conditional logic

CC MCC +7th **S22.089 Unspecified fracture of T11-T12 vertebra**
HAC 7th characters A & B see Appendix B for HAC conditional logic

+ **S22.2 Fracture of sternum**

MCC X+7th **S22.20 Unspecified fracture of sternum**
HAC 7th characters A & B see Appendix B for HAC conditional logic

CC MCC X+7th **S22.21 Fracture of manubrium**
HAC 7th characters A & B see Appendix B for HAC conditional logic

CC MCC X+7th **S22.22 Fracture of body of sternum**
HAC 7th characters A & B see Appendix B for HAC conditional logic

CC MCC X+7th **S22.23 Sternal manubrial dissociation**
HAC 7th characters A & B see Appendix B for HAC conditional logic

CC MCC X+7th **S22.24 Fracture of xiphoid process**
HAC 7th characters A & B see Appendix B for HAC conditional logic

+ **S22.3 Fracture of one rib**

CC MCC X+7th **S22.31 Fracture of one rib, right side**
HAC 7th characters A & B see Appendix B for HAC conditional logic

CC MCC X+7th **S22.32 Fracture of one rib, left side**
HAC 7th characters A & B see Appendix B for HAC conditional logic

CC MCC X+7th **S22.39 Fracture of one rib, unspecified side**
HAC 7th characters A & B see Appendix B for HAC conditional logic

+ **S22.4 Multiple fractures of ribs**
Fractures of two or more ribs
Excludes1: *flail chest (S22.5-)*

CC MCC X+7th **S22.41 Multiple fractures of ribs, right side**
HAC 7th characters A & B see Appendix B for HAC conditional logic

CC MCC X+7th **S22.42 Multiple fractures of ribs, left side**
HAC 7th characters A & B see Appendix B for HAC conditional logic

CC MCC X+7th **S22.43 Multiple fractures of ribs, bilateral**
HAC 7th characters A & B see Appendix B for HAC conditional logic

CC MCC X+7th **S22.49 Multiple fractures of ribs, unspecified side**
HAC 7th characters A & B see Appendix B for HAC conditional logic

X+7th **S22.5 Flail chest**
HAC 7th characters A & B see Appendix B for HAC conditional logic

X+7th **S22.9 Fracture of bony thorax, part unspecified**
HAC 7th characters A & B see Appendix B for HAC conditional logic

S23 Dislocation and sprain of joints and ligaments of thorax

Includes: avulsion of joint or ligament of thorax
laceration of cartilage, joint or ligament of thorax
sprain of cartilage, joint or ligament of thorax
traumatic hemarthrosis of joint or ligament of thorax
traumatic rupture of joint or ligament of thorax
traumatic subluxation of joint or ligament of thorax
traumatic tear of joint or ligament of thorax

Code also any associated open wound

Excludes2: *dislocation, sprain of sternoclavicular joint (S43.2, S43.6)*
strain of muscle or tendon of thorax (S29.01-)

The appropriate 7th character is to be added to each code from category S23
A initial encounter
D subsequent encounter
S sequela

X+7th **S23.0 Traumatic rupture of thoracic intervertebral disc**
Excludes1: *rupture or displacement (nontraumatic) of thoracic intervertebral disc NOS (M51.- with fifth character 4)*

+ **S23.1 Subluxation and dislocation of thoracic vertebra**
Code also any associated:
open wound of thorax (S21.-)
spinal cord injury (S24.0-, S24.1-)
Excludes2: *fracture of thoracic vertebrae (S22.0-)*
+ **S23.10 Subluxation and dislocation of unspecified thoracic vertebra**
+7th **S23.100 Subluxation of unspecified thoracic vertebra**
+7th **S23.101 Dislocation of unspecified thoracic vertebra**
+ **S23.11 Subluxation and dislocation of T1/T2 thoracic vertebra**
+7th **S23.110 Subluxation of T1/T2 thoracic vertebra**
+7th **S23.111 Dislocation of T1/T2 thoracic vertebra**
+ **S23.12 Subluxation and dislocation of T2/T3-T3/T4 thoracic vertebra**
+7th **S23.120 Subluxation of T2/T3 thoracic vertebra**
+7th **S23.121 Dislocation of T2/T3 thoracic vertebra**
+7th **S23.122 Subluxation of T3/T4 thoracic vertebra**
+7th **S23.123 Dislocation of T3/T4 thoracic vertebra**
+ **S23.13 Subluxation and dislocation of T4/T5-T5/T6 thoracic vertebra**
+7th **S23.130 Subluxation of T4/T5 thoracic vertebra**
+7th **S23.131 Dislocation of T4/T5 thoracic vertebra**
+7th **S23.132 Subluxation of T5/T6 thoracic vertebra**
+7th **S23.133 Dislocation of T5/T6 thoracic vertebra**
+ **S23.14 Subluxation and dislocation of T6/T7-T7/T8 thoracic vertebra**
+7th **S23.140 Subluxation of T6/T7 thoracic vertebra**
+7th **S23.141 Dislocation of T6/T7 thoracic vertebra**
+7th **S23.142 Subluxation of T7/T8 thoracic vertebra**
+7th **S23.143 Dislocation of T7/T8 thoracic vertebra**
+ **S23.15 Subluxation and dislocation of T8/T9-T9/T10 thoracic vertebra**
+7th **S23.150 Subluxation of T8/T9 thoracic vertebra**
+7th **S23.151 Dislocation of T8/T9 thoracic vertebra**
+7th **S23.152 Subluxation of T9/T10 thoracic vertebra**
+7th **S23.153 Dislocation of T9/T10 thoracic vertebra**
+ **S23.16 Subluxation and dislocation of T10/T11-T11/T12 thoracic vertebra**
+7th **S23.160 Subluxation of T10/T11 thoracic vertebra**
+7th **S23.161 Dislocation of T10/T11 thoracic vertebra**
+7th **S23.162 Subluxation of T11/T12 thoracic vertebra**
+7th **S23.163 Dislocation of T11/T12 thoracic vertebra**
+ **S23.17 Subluxation and dislocation of T12/L1 thoracic vertebra**
+7th **S23.170 Subluxation of T12/L1 thoracic vertebra**
+7th **S23.171 Dislocation of T12/L1 thoracic vertebra**
+ **S23.2 Dislocation of other and unspecified parts of thorax**
X+7th **S23.20 Dislocation of unspecified part of thorax**
X+7th **S23.29 Dislocation of other parts of thorax**
X+7th **S23.3 Sprain of ligaments of thoracic spine**
+ **S23.4 Sprain of ribs and sternum**
X+7th **S23.41 Sprain of ribs**
+ **S23.42 Sprain of sternum**
+7th **S23.420 Sprain of sternoclavicular (joint) (ligament)**
+7th **S23.421 Sprain of chondrosternal joint**
+7th **S23.428 Other sprain of sternum**
+7th **S23.429 Unspecified sprain of sternum**
X+7th **S23.8 Sprain of other specified parts of thorax**
X+7th **S23.9 Sprain of unspecified parts of thorax**

S24 Injury of nerves and spinal cord at thorax level
NOTE Code to highest level of thoracic spinal cord injury
Injuries to the spinal cord (S24.0 and S24.1) refer to the cord level and not bone level injury, and can affect nerve roots at and below the level given.
Code also any associated:
fracture of thoracic vertebra (S22.0-)
open wound of thorax (S21.-)
transient paralysis (R29.5)
Excludes2: *injury of brachial plexus (S14.3)*

The appropriate 7th character is to be added to each code from category S24
A initial encounter
D subsequent encounter
S sequela

MCC X+7th **S24.0 Concussion and edema of thoracic spinal cord**
+ **S24.1 Other and unspecified injuries of thoracic spinal cord**
+ **S24.10 Unspecified injury of thoracic spinal cord**
MCC +7th **S24.101 Unspecified injury at T1 level of thoracic spinal cord**
HAC 7th character A see Appendix B for HAC conditional logic
MCC +7th **S24.102 Unspecified injury at T2-T6 level of thoracic spinal cord**
HAC 7th character A see Appendix B for HAC conditional logic
MCC +7th **S24.103 Unspecified injury at T7-T10 level of thoracic spinal cord**
HAC 7th character A see Appendix B for HAC conditional logic
MCC +7th **S24.104 Unspecified injury at T11-T12 level of thoracic spinal cord**
HAC 7th character A see Appendix B for HAC conditional logic
+7th **S24.109 Unspecified injury at unspecified level of thoracic spinal cord**
Injury of thoracic spinal cord NOS
HAC 7th character A see Appendix B for HAC conditional logic
+ **S24.11 Complete lesion of thoracic spinal cord**
MCC +7th **S24.111 Complete lesion at T1 level of thoracic spinal cord**
HAC 7th character A see Appendix B for HAC conditional logic
MCC +7th **S24.112 Complete lesion at T2-T6 level of thoracic spinal cord**
HAC 7th character A see Appendix B for HAC conditional logic
MCC +7th **S24.113 Complete lesion at T7-T10 level of thoracic spinal cord**
HAC 7th character A see Appendix B for HAC conditional logic
MCC +7th **S24.114 Complete lesion at T11-T12 level of thoracic spinal cord**
HAC 7th character A see Appendix B for HAC conditional logic
+7th **S24.119 Complete lesion at unspecified level of thoracic spinal cord**
+ **S24.13 Anterior cord syndrome of thoracic spinal cord**
MCC +7th **S24.131 Anterior cord syndrome at T1 level of thoracic spinal cord**
HAC 7th character A see Appendix B for HAC conditional logic
MCC +7th **S24.132 Anterior cord syndrome at T2-T6 level of thoracic spinal cord**
HAC 7th character A see Appendix B for HAC conditional logic
MCC +7th **S24.133 Anterior cord syndrome at T7-T10 level of thoracic spinal cord**
HAC 7th character A see Appendix B for HAC conditional logic
MCC +7th **S24.134 Anterior cord syndrome at T11-T12 level of thoracic spinal cord**
HAC 7th character A see Appendix B for HAC conditional logic
+7th **S24.139 Anterior cord syndrome at unspecified level of thoracic spinal cord**

+ **S24.14 Brown-Séquard syndrome of thoracic spinal cord**
MCC +7th **S24.141 Brown-Séquard syndrome at T1 level of thoracic spinal cord**
MCC +7th **S24.142 Brown-Séquard syndrome at T2-T6 level of thoracic spinal cord**
MCC +7th **S24.143 Brown-Séquard syndrome at T7-T10 level of thoracic spinal cord**
MCC +7th **S24.144 Brown-Séquard syndrome at T11-T12 level of thoracic spinal cord**
+7th **S24.149 Brown-Séquard syndrome at unspecified level of thoracic spinal cord**
+ **S24.15 Other incomplete lesions of thoracic spinal cord**
Incomplete lesion of thoracic spinal cord NOS
Posterior cord syndrome of thoracic spinal cord
MCC +7th **S24.151 Other incomplete lesion at T1 level of thoracic spinal cord**
HAC 7th character A see Appendix B for HAC conditional logic
MCC +7th **S24.152 Other incomplete lesion at T2-T6 level of thoracic spinal cord**
HAC 7th character A see Appendix B for HAC conditional logic
MCC +7th **S24.153 Other incomplete lesion at T7-T10 level of thoracic spinal cord**
HAC 7th character A see Appendix B for HAC conditional logic
MCC +7th **S24.154 Other incomplete lesion at T11-T12 level of thoracic spinal cord**
HAC 7th character A see Appendix B for HAC conditional logic
+7th **S24.159 Other incomplete lesion at unspecified level of thoracic spinal cord**
X+7th **S24.2 Injury of nerve root of thoracic spine**
X+7th **S24.3 Injury of peripheral nerves of thorax**
X+7th **S24.4 Injury of thoracic sympathetic nervous system**
Injury of cardiac plexus
Injury of esophageal plexus
Injury of pulmonary plexus
Injury of stellate ganglion
Injury of thoracic sympathetic ganglion
X+7th **S24.8 Injury of other specified nerves of thorax**
X+7th **S24.9 Injury of unspecified nerve of thorax**

S25 Injury of blood vessels of thorax
Code also any associated open wound (S21.-)

The appropriate 7th character is to be added to each code from category S25
A initial encounter
D subsequent encounter
S sequela

+ **S25.0 Injury of thoracic aorta**
Injury of aorta NOS
MCC X+7th **S25.00 Unspecified injury of thoracic aorta**
MCC X+7th **S25.01 Minor laceration of thoracic aorta**
Incomplete transection of thoracic aorta
Laceration of thoracic aorta NOS
Superficial laceration of thoracic aorta
MCC X+7th **S25.02 Major laceration of thoracic aorta**
Complete transection of thoracic aorta
Traumatic rupture of thoracic aorta
MCC X+7th **S25.09 Other specified injury of thoracic aorta**
+ **S25.1 Injury of innominate or subclavian artery**
+ **S25.10 Unspecified injury of innominate or subclavian artery**
MCC +7th **S25.101 Unspecified injury of right innominate or subclavian artery**
MCC +7th **S25.102 Unspecified injury of left innominate or subclavian artery**
MCC +7th **S25.109 Unspecified injury of unspecified innominate or subclavian artery**
+ **S25.11 Minor laceration of innominate or subclavian artery**
Incomplete transection of innominate or subclavian artery
Laceration of innominate or subclavian artery NOS
Superficial laceration of innominate or subclavian artery
MCC +7th **S25.111 Minor laceration of right innominate or subclavian artery**
MCC +7th **S25.112 Minor laceration of left innominate or subclavian artery**
MCC +7th **S25.119 Minor laceration of unspecified innominate or subclavian artery**
+ **S25.12 Major laceration of innominate or subclavian artery**
Complete transection of innominate or subclavian artery
Traumatic rupture of innominate or subclavian artery
MCC +7th **S25.121 Major laceration of right innominate or subclavian artery**
MCC +7th **S25.122 Major laceration of left innominate or subclavian artery**
MCC +7th **S25.129 Major laceration of unspecified innominate or subclavian artery**
+ **S25.19 Other specified injury of innominate or subclavian artery**
MCC +7th **S25.191 Other specified injury of right innominate or subclavian artery**
MCC +7th **S25.192 Other specified injury of left innominate or subclavian artery**
MCC +7th **S25.199 Other specified injury of unspecified innominate or subclavian artery**
+ **S25.2 Injury of superior vena cava**
Injury of vena cava NOS
MCC X+7th **S25.20 Unspecified injury of superior vena cava**
MCC X+7th **S25.21 Minor laceration of superior vena cava**
Incomplete transection of superior vena cava
Laceration of superior vena cava NOS
Superficial laceration of superior vena cava
MCC X+7th **S25.22 Major laceration of superior vena cava**
Complete transection of superior vena cava
Traumatic rupture of superior vena cava
MCC X+7th **S25.29 Other specified injury of superior vena cava**
+ **S25.3 Injury of innominate or subclavian vein**
+ **S25.30 Unspecified injury of innominate or subclavian vein**
MCC +7th **S25.301 Unspecified injury of right innominate or subclavian vein**
MCC +7th **S25.302 Unspecified injury of left innominate or subclavian vein**
MCC +7th **S25.309 Unspecified injury of unspecified innominate or subclavian vein**
+ **S25.31 Minor laceration of innominate or subclavian vein**
Incomplete transection of innominate or subclavian vein
Laceration of innominate or subclavian vein NOS
Superficial laceration of innominate or subclavian vein
MCC +7th **S25.311 Minor laceration of right innominate or subclavian vein**
MCC +7th **S25.312 Minor laceration of left innominate or subclavian vein**
MCC +7th **S25.319 Minor laceration of unspecified innominate or subclavian vein**
+ **S25.32 Major laceration of innominate or subclavian vein**
Complete transection of innominate or subclavian vein
Traumatic rupture of innominate or subclavian vein
MCC +7th **S25.321 Major laceration of right innominate or subclavian vein**
MCC +7th **S25.322 Major laceration of left innominate or subclavian vein**
MCC +7th **S25.329 Major laceration of unspecified innominate or subclavian vein**
+ **S25.39 Other specified injury of innominate or subclavian vein**
MCC +7th **S25.391 Other specified injury of right innominate or subclavian vein**
MCC +7th **S25.392 Other specified injury of left innominate or subclavian vein**
MCC +7th **S25.399 Other specified injury of unspecified innominate or subclavian vein**

+ **S25.4 Injury of pulmonary blood vessels**

+ **S25.40 Unspecified injury of pulmonary blood vessels**

MCC +7th **S25.401 Unspecified injury of right pulmonary blood vessels**

MCC +7th **S25.402 Unspecified injury of left pulmonary blood vessels**

MCC +7th **S25.409 Unspecified injury of unspecified pulmonary blood vessels**

+ **S25.41 Minor laceration of pulmonary blood vessels**

Incomplete transection of pulmonary blood vessels
Laceration of pulmonary blood vessels NOS
Superficial laceration of pulmonary blood vessels

MCC +7th **S25.411 Minor laceration of right pulmonary blood vessels**

MCC +7th **S25.412 Minor laceration of left pulmonary blood vessels**

MCC +7th **S25.419 Minor laceration of unspecified pulmonary blood vessels**

+ **S25.42 Major laceration of pulmonary blood vessels**

Complete transection of pulmonary blood vessels
Traumatic rupture of pulmonary blood vessels

MCC +7th **S25.421 Major laceration of right pulmonary blood vessels**

MCC +7th **S25.422 Major laceration of left pulmonary blood vessels**

MCC +7th **S25.429 Major laceration of unspecified pulmonary blood vessels**

+ **S25.49 Other specified injury of pulmonary blood vessels**

MCC +7th **S25.491 Other specified injury of right pulmonary blood vessels**

MCC +7th **S25.492 Other specified injury of left pulmonary blood vessels**

MCC +7th **S25.499 Other specified injury of unspecified pulmonary blood vessels**

+ **S25.5 Injury of intercostal blood vessels**

+ **S25.50 Unspecified injury of intercostal blood vessels**

CC +7th **S25.501 Unspecified injury of intercostal blood vessels, right side**

CC +7th **S25.502 Unspecified injury of intercostal blood vessels, left side**

CC +7th **S25.509 Unspecified injury of intercostal blood vessels, unspecified side**

+ **S25.51 Laceration of intercostal blood vessels**

CC +7th **S25.511 Laceration of intercostal blood vessels, right side**

CC +7th **S25.512 Laceration of intercostal blood vessels, left side**

CC +7th **S25.519 Laceration of intercostal blood vessels, unspecified side**

+ **S25.59 Other specified injury of intercostal blood vessels**

CC +7th **S25.591 Other specified injury of intercostal blood vessels, right side**

CC +7th **S25.592 Other specified injury of intercostal blood vessels, left side**

CC +7th **S25.599 Other specified injury of intercostal blood vessels, unspecified side**

+ **S25.8 Injury of other blood vessels of thorax**

Injury of azygos vein
Injury of mammary artery or vein

+ **S25.80 Unspecified injury of other blood vessels of thorax**

CC +7th **S25.801 Unspecified injury of other blood vessels of thorax, right side**

CC +7th **S25.802 Unspecified injury of other blood vessels of thorax, left side**

CC +7th **S25.809 Unspecified injury of other blood vessels of thorax, unspecified side**

+ **S25.81 Laceration of other blood vessels of thorax**

CC +7th **S25.811 Laceration of other blood vessels of thorax, right side**

CC +7th **S25.812 Laceration of other blood vessels of thorax, left side**

CC +7th **S25.819 Laceration of other blood vessels of thorax, unspecified side**

+ **S25.89 Other specified injury of other blood vessels of thorax**

CC +7th **S25.891 Other specified injury of other blood vessels of thorax, right side**

CC +7th **S25.892 Other specified injury of other blood vessels of thorax, left side**

CC +7th **S25.899 Other specified injury of other blood vessels of thorax, unspecified side**

+ **S25.9 Injury of unspecified blood vessel of thorax**

CC X+7th **S25.90 Unspecified injury of unspecified blood vessel of thorax**

CC X+7th **S25.91 Laceration of unspecified blood vessel of thorax**

CC X+7th **S25.99 Other specified injury of unspecified blood vessel of thorax**

S26 Injury of heart

Code also any associated:
open wound of thorax (S21.-)
traumatic hemopneumothorax (S27.2)
traumatic hemothorax (S27.1)
traumatic pneumothorax (S27.0)

The appropriate 7th character is to be added to each code from category S26
A initial encounter
D subsequent encounter
S sequela

+ **S26.0 Injury of heart with hemopericardium**

CC X+7th **S26.00 Unspecified injury of heart with hemopericardium**

CC X+7th **S26.01 Contusion of heart with hemopericardium**

+ **S26.02 Laceration of heart with hemopericardium**

MCC +7th **S26.020 Mild laceration of heart with hemopericardium**

Laceration of heart without penetration of heart chamber

MCC +7th **S26.021 Moderate laceration of heart with hemopericardium**

Laceration of heart with penetration of heart chamber

MCC +7th **S26.022 Major laceration of heart with hemopericardium**

Laceration of heart with penetration of multiple heart chambers

CC X+7th **S26.09 Other injury of heart with hemopericardium**

+ **S26.1 Injury of heart without hemopericardium**

CC X+7th **S26.10 Unspecified injury of heart without hemopericardium**

CC X+7th **S26.11 Contusion of heart without hemopericardium**

MCC X+7th **S26.12 Laceration of heart without hemopericardium**

CC X+7th **S26.19 Other injury of heart without hemopericardium**

+ **S26.9 Injury of heart, unspecified with or without hemopericardium**

CC X+7th **S26.90 Unspecified injury of heart, unspecified with or without hemopericardium**

CC X+7th **S26.91 Contusion of heart, unspecified with or without hemopericardium**

MCC X+7th **S26.92 Laceration of heart, unspecified with or without hemopericardium**

Laceration of heart NOS

CC X+7th **S26.99 Other injury of heart, unspecified with or without hemopericardium**

S27 Injury of other and unspecified intrathoracic organs

Code also associated open wound of thorax (S21.-)

Excludes2: *injury of cervical esophagus (S10-S19)*
injury of trachea (cervical) (S10-S19)

The appropriate 7th character is to be added to each code from category S27
A initial encounter
D subsequent encounter
S sequela

CC X+7th **S27.0 Traumatic pneumothorax**

Excludes1: *spontaneous pneumothorax (J93.-)*

MCC **S27.1 Traumatic hemothorax**

MCC **S27.2 Traumatic hemopneumothorax**

S27.3 Other and unspecified injuries of lung
+ S27.30 Unspecified injury of lung
CC +7th S27.301 Unspecified injury of lung, unilateral
CC +7th S27.302 Unspecified injury of lung, bilateral
CC +7th S27.309 Unspecified injury of lung, unspecified
+ S27.31 Primary blast injury of lung
Blast injury of lung NOS
CC +7th S27.311 Primary blast injury of lung, unilateral
CC +7th S27.312 Primary blast injury of lung, bilateral
CC +7th S27.319 Primary blast injury of lung, unspecified
+ S27.32 Contusion of lung
CC +7th S27.321 Contusion of lung, unilateral
CC +7th S27.322 Contusion of lung, bilateral
CC +7th S27.329 Contusion of lung, unspecified
+ S27.33 Laceration of lung
MCC +7th S27.331 Laceration of lung, unilateral
MCC +7th S27.332 Laceration of lung, bilateral
MCC +7th S27.339 Laceration of lung, unspecified
+ S27.39 Other injuries of lung
Secondary blast injury of lung
CC +7th S27.391 Other injuries of lung, unilateral
CC +7th S27.392 Other injuries of lung, bilateral
CC +7th S27.399 Other injuries of lung, unspecified

S27.4 Injury of bronchus
+ S27.40 Unspecified injury of bronchus
MCC +7th S27.401 Unspecified injury of bronchus, unilateral
MCC +7th S27.402 Unspecified injury of bronchus, bilateral
MCC +7th S27.409 Unspecified injury of bronchus, unspecified
+ S27.41 Primary blast injury of bronchus
Blast injury of bronchus NOS
MCC +7th S27.411 Primary blast injury of bronchus, unilateral
MCC +7th S27.412 Primary blast injury of bronchus, bilateral
MCC +7th S27.419 Primary blast injury of bronchus, unspecified
+ S27.42 Contusion of bronchus
MCC +7th S27.421 Contusion of bronchus, unilateral
MCC +7th S27.422 Contusion of bronchus, bilateral
MCC +7th S27.429 Contusion of bronchus, unspecified
+ S27.43 Laceration of bronchus
MCC +7th S27.431 Laceration of bronchus, unilateral
MCC +7th S27.432 Laceration of bronchus, bilateral
MCC +7th S27.439 Laceration of bronchus, unspecified
+ S27.49 Other injury of bronchus
Secondary blast injury of bronchus
MCC +7th S27.491 Other injury of bronchus, unilateral
MCC +7th S27.492 Other injury of bronchus, bilateral
MCC +7th S27.499 Other injury of bronchus, unspecified

+ S27.5 Injury of thoracic trachea
CC X+7th S27.50 Unspecified injury of thoracic trachea
CC X+7th S27.51 Primary blast injury of thoracic trachea
Blast injury of thoracic trachea NOS
CC X+7th S27.52 Contusion of thoracic trachea
CC X+7th S27.53 Laceration of thoracic trachea
CC X+7th S27.59 Other injury of thoracic trachea
Secondary blast injury of thoracic trachea

+ S27.6 Injury of pleura
CC X+7th S27.60 Unspecified injury of pleura
CC X+7th S27.63 Laceration of pleura
CC X+7th S27.69 Other injury of pleura

+ S27.8 Injury of other specified intrathoracic organs
+ S27.80 Injury of diaphragm
CC +7th S27.802 Contusion of diaphragm
CC +7th S27.803 Laceration of diaphragm
CC +7th S27.808 Other injury of diaphragm
CC +7th S27.809 Unspecified injury of diaphragm
+ S27.81 Injury of esophagus (thoracic part)
MCC +7th S27.812 Contusion of esophagus (thoracic part)
MCC +7th S27.813 Laceration of esophagus (thoracic part)
MCC +7th S27.818 Other injury of esophagus (thoracic part)
MCC +7th S27.819 Unspecified injury of esophagus (thoracic part)
+ S27.89 Injury of other specified intrathoracic organs
Injury of lymphatic thoracic duct
Injury of thymus gland
CC +7th S27.892 Contusion of other specified intrathoracic organs
CC +7th S27.893 Laceration of other specified intrathoracic organs
CC +7th S27.898 Other injury of other specified intrathoracic organs
CC +7th S27.899 Unspecified injury of other specified intrathoracic organs

CC X+7th S27.9 Injury of unspecified intrathoracic organ

S28 Crushing injury of thorax, and traumatic amputation of part of thorax

The appropriate 7th character is to be added to each code from category S28
A initial encounter
D subsequent encounter
S sequela

X+7th S28.0 Crushed chest
Use additional code for all associated injuries
Excludes1: *flail chest (S22.5)*

CC X+7th S28.1 Traumatic amputation (partial) of part of thorax, except breast
+ S28.2 Traumatic amputation of breast
+ S28.21 Complete traumatic amputation of breast
Traumatic amputation of breast NOS
+7th S28.211 Complete traumatic amputation of right breast
+7th S28.212 Complete traumatic amputation of left breast
+7th S28.219 Complete traumatic amputation of unspecified breast
+ S28.22 Partial traumatic amputation of breast
+7th S28.221 Partial traumatic amputation of right breast
+7th S28.222 Partial traumatic amputation of left breast
+7th S28.229 Partial traumatic amputation of unspecified breast

S29 Other and unspecified injuries of thorax

Code also any associated open wound (S21.-)

The appropriate 7th character is to be added to each code from category S29
A initial encounter
D subsequent encounter
S sequela

+ S29.0 Injury of muscle and tendon at thorax level
+ S29.00 Unspecified injury of muscle and tendon of thorax
+7th S29.001 Unspecified injury of muscle and tendon of front wall of thorax
+7th S29.002 Unspecified injury of muscle and tendon of back wall of thorax
+7th S29.009 Unspecified injury of muscle and tendon of unspecified wall of thorax
+ S29.01 Strain of muscle and tendon of thorax
+7th S29.011 Strain of muscle and tendon of front wall of thorax
+7th S29.012 Strain of muscle and tendon of back wall of thorax
+7th S29.019 Strain of muscle and tendon of unspecified wall of thorax
+ S29.02 Laceration of muscle and tendon of thorax
CC +7th S29.021 Laceration of muscle and tendon of front wall of thorax
+7th S29.022 Laceration of muscle and tendon of back wall of thorax
CC +7th S29.029 Laceration of muscle and tendon of unspecified wall of thorax
+ S29.09 Other injury of muscle and tendon of thorax
+7th S29.091 Other injury of muscle and tendon of front wall of thorax
+7th S29.092 Other injury of muscle and tendon of back wall of thorax
+7th S29.099 Other injury of muscle and tendon of unspecified wall of thorax

X+7th S29.8 Other specified injuries of thorax
X+7th S29.9 Unspecified injury of thorax

Injuries to the abdomen, lower back, lumbar spine, pelvis and external genitals (S30-S39)

Includes: injuries to the abdominal wall
injuries to the anus
injuries to the buttock
injuries to the external genitalia
injuries to the flank
injuries to the groin

Excludes2: *burns and corrosions (T20-T32)*
effects of foreign body in anus and rectum (T18.5)
effects of foreign body in genitourinary tract (T19.-)
effects of foreign body in stomach, small intestine and colon (T18.2-T18.4)
frostbite (T33-T34)
insect bite or sting, venomous (T63.4)

S30 Superficial injury of abdomen, lower back, pelvis and external genitals
Excludes2: *superficial injury of hip (S70.-)*

The appropriate 7th character is to be added to each code from category S30
A initial encounter
D subsequent encounter
S sequela

X+7th **S30.0 Contusion of lower back and pelvis**
Contusion of buttock
X+7th **S30.1 Contusion of abdominal wall**
Contusion of flank
Contusion of groin
\+ **S30.2 Contusion of external genital organs**
\+ **S30.20 Contusion of unspecified external genital organ**
♂ +7th **S30.201 Contusion of unspecified external genital organ, male**
♀ +7th **S30.202 Contusion of unspecified external genital organ, female**
♂ X+7th **S30.21 Contusion of penis**
♂ X+7th **S30.22 Contusion of scrotum and testes**
♀ X+7th **S30.23 Contusion of vagina and vulva**
X+7th **S30.3 Contusion of anus**
\+ **S30.8 Other superficial injuries of abdomen, lower back, pelvis and external genitals**
\+ **S30.81 Abrasion of abdomen, lower back, pelvis and external genitals**
+7th **S30.810 Abrasion of lower back and pelvis**
+7th **S30.811 Abrasion of abdominal wall**
♂ +7th **S30.812 Abrasion of penis**
♂ +7th **S30.813 Abrasion of scrotum and testes**
♀ +7th **S30.814 Abrasion of vagina and vulva**
♂ +7th **S30.815 Abrasion of unspecified external genital organs, male**
♀ +7th **S30.816 Abrasion of unspecified external genital organs, female**
+7th **S30.817 Abrasion of anus**
\+ **S30.82 Blister (nonthermal) of abdomen, lower back, pelvis and external genitals**
+7th **S30.820 Blister (nonthermal) of lower back and pelvis**
+7th **S30.821 Blister (nonthermal) of abdominal wall**
♂ +7th **S30.822 Blister (nonthermal) of penis**
♂ +7th **S30.823 Blister (nonthermal) of scrotum and testes**
♀ +7th **S30.824 Blister (nonthermal) of vagina and vulva**
♂ +7th **S30.825 Blister (nonthermal) of unspecified external genital organs, male**
♀ +7th **S30.826 Blister (nonthermal) of unspecified external genital organs, female**
+7th **S30.827 Blister (nonthermal) of anus**
\+ **S30.84 External constriction of abdomen, lower back, pelvis and external genitals**
+7th **S30.840 External constriction of lower back and pelvis**
+7th **S30.841 External constriction of abdominal wall**
♂ +7th **S30.842 External constriction of penis**
Hair tourniquet syndrome of penis
Use additional cause code to identify the constricting item (W49.0-)
♂ +7th **S30.843 External constriction of scrotum and testes**
♀ +7th **S30.844 External constriction of vagina and vulva**
♂ +7th **S30.845 External constriction of unspecified external genital organs, male**
♀ +7th **S30.846 External constriction of unspecified external genital organs, female**
\+ **S30.85 Superficial foreign body of abdomen, lower back, pelvis and external genitals**
Splinter in the abdomen, lower back, pelvis and external genitals
+7th **S30.850 Superficial foreign body of lower back and pelvis**
+7th **S30.851 Superficial foreign body of abdominal wall**
♂ +7th **S30.852 Superficial foreign body of penis**
♂ +7th **S30.853 Superficial foreign body of scrotum and testes**
♀ +7th **S30.854 Superficial foreign body of vagina and vulva**
♂ +7th **S30.855 Superficial foreign body of unspecified external genital organs, male**
♀ +7th **S30.856 Superficial foreign body of unspecified external genital organs, female**
+7th **S30.857 Superficial foreign body of anus**
\+ **S30.86 Insect bite (nonvenomous) of abdomen, lower back, pelvis and external genitals**
+7th **S30.860 Insect bite (nonvenomous) of lower back and pelvis**
+7th **S30.861 Insect bite (nonvenomous) of abdominal wall**
♂ +7th **S30.862 Insect bite (nonvenomous) of penis**
♂ +7th **S30.863 Insect bite (nonvenomous) of scrotum and testes**
♀ +7th **S30.864 Insect bite (nonvenomous) of vagina and vulva**
♂ +7th **S30.865 Insect bite (nonvenomous) of unspecified external genital organs, male**
♀ +7th **S30.866 Insect bite (nonvenomous) of unspecified external genital organs, female**
+7th **S30.867 Insect bite (nonvenomous) of anus**
\+ **S30.87 Other superficial bite of abdomen, lower back, pelvis and external genitals**
Excludes1: *open bite of abdomen, lower back, pelvis and external genitals (S31.05, S31.15, S31.25, S31.35, S31.45, S31.55)*
+7th **S30.870 Other superficial bite of lower back and pelvis**
+7th **S30.871 Other superficial bite of abdominal wall**
♂ +7th **S30.872 Other superficial bite of penis**
♂ +7th **S30.873 Other superficial bite of scrotum and testes**
♀ +7th **S30.874 Other superficial bite of vagina and vulva**
♂ +7th **S30.875 Other superficial bite of unspecified external genital organs, male**
♀ +7th **S30.876 Other superficial bite of unspecified external genital organs, female**
+7th **S30.877 Other superficial bite of anus**
\+ **S30.9 Unspecified superficial injury of abdomen, lower back, pelvis and external genitals**
X+7th **S30.91 Unspecified superficial injury of lower back and pelvis**
X+7th **S30.92 Unspecified superficial injury of abdominal wall**
♂ X+7th **S30.93 Unspecified superficial injury of penis**
♂ X+7th **S30.94 Unspecified superficial injury of scrotum and testes**
♀ X+7th **S30.95 Unspecified superficial injury of vagina and vulva**
♂ X+7th **S30.96 Unspecified superficial injury of unspecified external genital organs, male**
♀ X+7th **S30.97 Unspecified superficial injury of unspecified external genital organs, female**
X+7th **S30.98 Unspecified superficial injury of anus**

S31 Open wound of abdomen, lower back, pelvis and external genitals

Code also any associated:
spinal cord injury (S24.0, S24.1-, S34.0-, S34.1-)
wound infection

Excludes1: *traumatic amputation of part of abdomen, lower back and pelvis (S38.2-, S38.3)*

Excludes2: *open wound of hip (S71.00-S71.02)*
open fracture of pelvis (S32.1--S32.9 with 7th character B)

The appropriate 7th character is to be added to each code from category S31
A initial encounter
D subsequent encounter
S sequela

+ **S31.0 Open wound of lower back and pelvis**
+ **S31.00 Unspecified open wound of lower back and pelvis**
+7th **S31.000 Unspecified open wound of lower back and pelvis without penetration into retroperitoneum**
Unspecified open wound of lower back and pelvis NOS
MCC +7th **S31.001 Unspecified open wound of lower back and pelvis with penetration into retroperitoneum**
+ **S31.01 Laceration without foreign body of lower back and pelvis**
+7th **S31.010 Laceration without foreign body of lower back and pelvis without penetration into retroperitoneum**
Laceration without foreign body of lower back and pelvis NOS
MCC +7th **S31.011 Laceration without foreign body of lower back and pelvis with penetration into retroperitoneum**
+ **S31.02 Laceration with foreign body of lower back and pelvis**
+7th **S31.020 Laceration with foreign body of lower back and pelvis without penetration into retroperitoneum**
Laceration with foreign body of lower back and pelvis NOS
MCC +7th **S31.021 Laceration with foreign body of lower back and pelvis with penetration into retroperitoneum**
+ **S31.03 Puncture wound without foreign body of lower back and pelvis**
+7th **S31.030 Puncture wound without foreign body of lower back and pelvis without penetration into retroperitoneum**
Puncture wound without foreign body of lower back and pelvis NOS
MCC +7th **S31.031 Puncture wound without foreign body of lower back and pelvis with penetration into retroperitoneum**
+ **S31.04 Puncture wound with foreign body of lower back and pelvis**
+7th **S31.040 Puncture wound with foreign body of lower back and pelvis without penetration into retroperitoneum**
Puncture wound with foreign body of lower back and pelvis NOS
MCC +7th **S31.041 Puncture wound with foreign body of lower back and pelvis with penetration into retroperitoneum**
+ **S31.05 Open bite of lower back and pelvis**
Bite of lower back and pelvis NOS
Excludes1: *superficial bite of lower back and pelvis (S30.860, S30.870)*
+7th **S31.050 Open bite of lower back and pelvis without penetration into retroperitoneum**
Open bite of lower back and pelvis NOS
MCC +7th **S31.051 Open bite of lower back and pelvis with penetration into retroperitoneum**

+ **S31.1 Open wound of abdominal wall without penetration into peritoneal cavity**
Open wound of abdominal wall NOS
Excludes2: *open wound of abdominal wall with penetration into peritoneal cavity (S31.6-)*
+ **S31.10 Unspecified open wound of abdominal wall without penetration into peritoneal cavity**
+7th **S31.100 Unspecified open wound of abdominal wall, right upper quadrant without penetration into peritoneal cavity**
+7th **S31.101 Unspecified open wound of abdominal wall, left upper quadrant without penetration into peritoneal cavity**
+7th **S31.102 Unspecified open wound of abdominal wall, epigastric region without penetration into peritoneal cavity**
+7th **S31.103 Unspecified open wound of abdominal wall, right lower quadrant without penetration into peritoneal cavity**
+7th **S31.104 Unspecified open wound of abdominal wall, left lower quadrant without penetration into peritoneal cavity**
+7th **S31.105 Unspecified open wound of abdominal wall, periumbilic region without penetration into peritoneal cavity**
+7th **S31.109 Unspecified open wound of abdominal wall, unspecified quadrant without penetration into peritoneal cavity**
Unspecified open wound of abdominal wall NOS
+ **S31.11 Laceration without foreign body of abdominal wall without penetration into peritoneal cavity**
+7th **S31.110 Laceration without foreign body of abdominal wall, right upper quadrant without penetration into peritoneal cavity**
+7th **S31.111 Laceration without foreign body of abdominal wall, left upper quadrant without penetration into peritoneal cavity**
+7th **S31.112 Laceration without foreign body of abdominal wall, epigastric region without penetration into peritoneal cavity**
+7th **S31.113 Laceration without foreign body of abdominal wall, right lower quadrant without penetration into peritoneal cavity**
+7th **S31.114 Laceration without foreign body of abdominal wall, left lower quadrant without penetration into peritoneal cavity**
+7th **S31.115 Laceration without foreign body of abdominal wall, periumbilic region without penetration into peritoneal cavity**
+7th **S31.119 Laceration without foreign body of abdominal wall, unspecified quadrant without penetration into peritoneal cavity**
+ **S31.12 Laceration with foreign body of abdominal wall without penetration into peritoneal cavity**
+7th **S31.120 Laceration of abdominal wall with foreign body, right upper quadrant without penetration into peritoneal cavity**
+7th **S31.121 Laceration of abdominal wall with foreign body, left upper quadrant without penetration into peritoneal cavity**
+7th **S31.122 Laceration of abdominal wall with foreign body, epigastric region without penetration into peritoneal cavity**
+7th **S31.123 Laceration of abdominal wall with foreign body, right lower quadrant without penetration into peritoneal cavity**
+7th **S31.124 Laceration of abdominal wall with foreign body, left lower quadrant without penetration into peritoneal cavity**

+7th **S31.125** **Laceration of abdominal wall with foreign body, periumbilic region without penetration into peritoneal cavity**

+7th **S31.129** **Laceration of abdominal wall with foreign body, unspecified quadrant without penetration into peritoneal cavity**

+ **S31.13** **Puncture wound of abdominal wall without foreign body without penetration into peritoneal cavity**

+7th **S31.130** **Puncture wound of abdominal wall without foreign body, right upper quadrant without penetration into peritoneal cavity**

+7th **S31.131** **Puncture wound of abdominal wall without foreign body, left upper quadrant without penetration into peritoneal cavity**

+7th **S31.132** **Puncture wound of abdominal wall without foreign body, epigastric region without penetration into peritoneal cavity**

+7th **S31.133** **Puncture wound of abdominal wall without foreign body, right lower quadrant without penetration into peritoneal cavity**

+7th **S31.134** **Puncture wound of abdominal wall without foreign body, left lower quadrant without penetration into peritoneal cavity**

+7th **S31.135** **Puncture wound of abdominal wall without foreign body, periumbilic region without penetration into peritoneal cavity**

+7th **S31.139** **Puncture wound of abdominal wall without foreign body, unspecified quadrant without penetration into peritoneal cavity**

+ **S31.14** **Puncture wound of abdominal wall with foreign body without penetration into peritoneal cavity**

+7th **S31.140** **Puncture wound of abdominal wall with foreign body, right upper quadrant without penetration into peritoneal cavity**

+7th **S31.141** **Puncture wound of abdominal wall with foreign body, left upper quadrant without penetration into peritoneal cavity**

+7th **S31.142** **Puncture wound of abdominal wall with foreign body, epigastric region without penetration into peritoneal cavity**

+7th **S31.143** **Puncture wound of abdominal wall with foreign body, right lower quadrant without penetration into peritoneal cavity**

+7th **S31.144** **Puncture wound of abdominal wall with foreign body, left lower quadrant without penetration into peritoneal cavity**

+7th **S31.145** **Puncture wound of abdominal wall with foreign body, periumbilic region without penetration into peritoneal cavity**

+7th **S31.149** **Puncture wound of abdominal wall with foreign body, unspecified quadrant without penetration into peritoneal cavity**

+ **S31.15** **Open bite of abdominal wall without penetration into peritoneal cavity**

Bite of abdominal wall NOS

Excludes1: *superficial bite of abdominal wall (S30.871)*

+7th **S31.150** **Open bite of abdominal wall, right upper quadrant without penetration into peritoneal cavity**

+7th **S31.151** **Open bite of abdominal wall, left upper quadrant without penetration into peritoneal cavity**

+7th **S31.152** **Open bite of abdominal wall, epigastric region without penetration into peritoneal cavity**

+7th **S31.153** **Open bite of abdominal wall, right lower quadrant without penetration into peritoneal cavity**

+7th **S31.154** **Open bite of abdominal wall, left lower quadrant without penetration into peritoneal cavity**

+7th **S31.155** **Open bite of abdominal wall, periumbilic region without penetration into peritoneal cavity**

+7th **S31.159** **Open bite of abdominal wall, unspecified quadrant without penetration into peritoneal cavity**

+ **S31.2** **Open wound of penis**

♂ X+7th **S31.20** **Unspecified open wound of penis**

♂ X+7th **S31.21** **Laceration without foreign body of penis**

♂ X+7th **S31.22** **Laceration with foreign body of penis**

♂ X+7th **S31.23** **Puncture wound without foreign body of penis**

♂ X+7th **S31.24** **Puncture wound with foreign body of penis**

♂ X+7th **S31.25** **Open bite of penis**

Bite of penis NOS

Excludes1: *superficial bite of penis (S30.862, S30.872)*

+ **S31.3** **Open wound of scrotum and testes**

♂ X+7th **S31.30** **Unspecified open wound of scrotum and testes**

♂ X+7th **S31.31** **Laceration without foreign body of scrotum and testes**

♂ X+7th **S31.32** **Laceration with foreign body of scrotum and testes**

♂ X+7th **S31.33** **Puncture wound without foreign body of scrotum and testes**

♂ X+7th **S31.34** **Puncture wound with foreign body of scrotum and testes**

♂ X+7th **S31.35** **Open bite of scrotum and testes**

Bite of scrotum and testes NOS

Excludes1: *superficial bite of scrotum and testes (S30.863, S30.873)*

+ **S31.4** **Open wound of vagina and vulva**

Excludes1: *injury to vagina and vulva during delivery (O70.-, O71.4)*

♀ X+7th **S31.40** **Unspecified open wound of vagina and vulva**

♀ X+7th **S31.41** **Laceration without foreign body of vagina and vulva**

♀ X+7th **S31.42** **Laceration with foreign body of vagina and vulva**

♀ X+7th **S31.43** **Puncture wound without foreign body of vagina and vulva**

♀ X+7th **S31.44** **Puncture wound with foreign body of vagina and vulva**

♀ X+7th **S31.45** **Open bite of vagina and vulva**

Bite of vagina and vulva NOS

Excludes1: *superficial bite of vagina and vulva (S30.864, S30.874)*

+ **S31.5** **Open wound of unspecified external genital organs**

Excludes1: *traumatic amputation of external genital organs (S38.21, S38.22)*

+ **S31.50** **Unspecified open wound of unspecified external genital organs**

♂ +7th **S31.501** **Unspecified open wound of unspecified external genital organs, male**

♀ +7th **S31.502** **Unspecified open wound of unspecified external genital organs, female**

+ **S31.51** **Laceration without foreign body of unspecified external genital organs**

♂ +7th **S31.511** **Laceration without foreign body of unspecified external genital organs, male**

♀ +7th **S31.512** **Laceration without foreign body of unspecified external genital organs, female**

+ **S31.52** **Laceration with foreign body of unspecified external genital organs**

♂ +7th **S31.521** **Laceration with foreign body of unspecified external genital organs, male**

♀ +7th **S31.522** **Laceration with foreign body of unspecified external genital organs, female**

+ **S31.53 Puncture wound without foreign body of unspecified external genital organs**
  - ♂ +7th **S31.531 Puncture wound without foreign body of unspecified external genital organs, male**
  - ♀ +7th **S31.532 Puncture wound without foreign body of unspecified external genital organs, female**

+ **S31.54 Puncture wound with foreign body of unspecified external genital organs**
  - ♂ +7th **S31.541 Puncture wound with foreign body of unspecified external genital organs, male**
  - ♀ +7th **S31.542 Puncture wound with foreign body of unspecified external genital organs, female**

+ **S31.55 Open bite of unspecified external genital organs**
  Bite of unspecified external genital organs NOS
  Excludes1: *superficial bite of unspecified external genital organs (S30.865, S30.866, S30.875, S30.876)*
  - ♂ +7th **S31.551 Open bite of unspecified external genital organs, male**
  - ♀ +7th **S31.552 Open bite of unspecified external genital organs, female**

+ **S31.6 Open wound of abdominal wall with penetration into peritoneal cavity**

+ **S31.60 Unspecified open wound of abdominal wall with penetration into peritoneal cavity**
  - MCC +7th **S31.600 Unspecified open wound of abdominal wall, right upper quadrant with penetration into peritoneal cavity**
  - MCC +7th **S31.601 Unspecified open wound of abdominal wall, left upper quadrant with penetration into peritoneal cavity**
  - MCC +7th **S31.602 Unspecified open wound of abdominal wall, epigastric region with penetration into peritoneal cavity**
  - MCC +7th **S31.603 Unspecified open wound of abdominal wall, right lower quadrant with penetration into peritoneal cavity**
  - MCC +7th **S31.604 Unspecified open wound of abdominal wall, left lower quadrant with penetration into peritoneal cavity**
  - MCC +7th **S31.605 Unspecified open wound of abdominal wall, periumbilic region with penetration into peritoneal cavity**
  - MCC +7th **S31.609 Unspecified open wound of abdominal wall, unspecified quadrant with penetration into peritoneal cavity**

+ **S31.61 Laceration without foreign body of abdominal wall with penetration into peritoneal cavity**
  - MCC +7th **S31.610 Laceration without foreign body of abdominal wall, right upper quadrant with penetration into peritoneal cavity**
  - MCC +7th **S31.611 Laceration without foreign body of abdominal wall, left upper quadrant with penetration into peritoneal cavity**
  - MCC +7th **S31.612 Laceration without foreign body of abdominal wall, epigastric region with penetration into peritoneal cavity**
  - MCC +7th **S31.613 Laceration without foreign body of abdominal wall, right lower quadrant with penetration into peritoneal cavity**
    AHA CC: 4Q, 2015, 37-38
  - MCC +7th **S31.614 Laceration without foreign body of abdominal wall, left lower quadrant with penetration into peritoneal cavity**
  - MCC +7th **S31.615 Laceration without foreign body of abdominal wall, periumbilic region with penetration into peritoneal cavity**
  - MCC +7th **S31.619 Laceration without foreign body of abdominal wall, unspecified quadrant with penetration into peritoneal cavity**

+ **S31.62 Laceration with foreign body of abdominal wall with penetration into peritoneal cavity**
  - MCC +7th **S31.620 Laceration with foreign body of abdominal wall, right upper quadrant with penetration into peritoneal cavity**
  - MCC +7th **S31.621 Laceration with foreign body of abdominal wall, left upper quadrant with penetration into peritoneal cavity**
  - MCC +7th **S31.622 Laceration with foreign body of abdominal wall, epigastric region with penetration into peritoneal cavity**
  - MCC +7th **S31.623 Laceration with foreign body of abdominal wall, right lower quadrant with penetration into peritoneal cavity**
  - MCC +7th **S31.624 Laceration with foreign body of abdominal wall, left lower quadrant with penetration into peritoneal cavity**
  - MCC +7th **S31.625 Laceration with foreign body of abdominal wall, periumbilic region with penetration into peritoneal cavity**
  - MCC +7th **S31.629 Laceration with foreign body of abdominal wall, unspecified quadrant with penetration into peritoneal cavity**

+ **S31.63 Puncture wound without foreign body of abdominal wall with penetration into peritoneal cavity**
  - MCC +7th **S31.630 Puncture wound without foreign body of abdominal wall, right upper quadrant with penetration into peritoneal cavity**
  - MCC +7th **S31.631 Puncture wound without foreign body of abdominal wall, left upper quadrant with penetration into peritoneal cavity**
  - MCC +7th **S31.632 Puncture wound without foreign body of abdominal wall, epigastric region with penetration into peritoneal cavity**
  - MCC +7th **S31.633 Puncture wound without foreign body of abdominal wall, right lower quadrant with penetration into peritoneal cavity**
  - MCC +7th **S31.634 Puncture wound without foreign body of abdominal wall, left lower quadrant with penetration into peritoneal cavity**
  - MCC +7th **S31.635 Puncture wound without foreign body of abdominal wall, periumbilic region with penetration into peritoneal cavity**
  - MCC +7th **S31.639 Puncture wound without foreign body of abdominal wall, unspecified quadrant with penetration into peritoneal cavity**

+ **S31.64 Puncture wound with foreign body of abdominal wall with penetration into peritoneal cavity**
  - MCC +7th **S31.640 Puncture wound with foreign body of abdominal wall, right upper quadrant with penetration into peritoneal cavity**
  - MCC +7th **S31.641 Puncture wound with foreign body of abdominal wall, left upper quadrant with penetration into peritoneal cavity**
  - MCC +7th **S31.642 Puncture wound with foreign body of abdominal wall, epigastric region with penetration into peritoneal cavity**
  - MCC +7th **S31.643 Puncture wound with foreign body of abdominal wall, right lower quadrant with penetration into peritoneal cavity**
  - MCC +7th **S31.644 Puncture wound with foreign body of abdominal wall, left lower quadrant with penetration into peritoneal cavity**
  - MCC +7th **S31.645 Puncture wound with foreign body of abdominal wall, periumbilic region with penetration into peritoneal cavity**

MCC +7th **S31.649 Puncture wound with foreign body of abdominal wall, unspecified quadrant with penetration into peritoneal cavity**

+ **S31.65 Open bite of abdominal wall with penetration into peritoneal cavity**

Excludes1: *superficial bite of abdominal wall (S30.861, S30.871)*

MCC +7th **S31.650 Open bite of abdominal wall, right upper quadrant with penetration into peritoneal cavity**

MCC +7th **S31.651 Open bite of abdominal wall, left upper quadrant with penetration into peritoneal cavity**

MCC +7th **S31.652 Open bite of abdominal wall, epigastric region with penetration into peritoneal cavity**

MCC +7th **S31.653 Open bite of abdominal wall, right lower quadrant with penetration into peritoneal cavity**

MCC +7th **S31.654 Open bite of abdominal wall, left lower quadrant with penetration into peritoneal cavity**

MCC +7th **S31.655 Open bite of abdominal wall, periumbilic region with penetration into peritoneal cavity**

MCC +7th **S31.659 Open bite of abdominal wall, unspecified quadrant with penetration into peritoneal cavity**

+ **S31.8 Open wound of other parts of abdomen, lower back and pelvis**

+ **S31.80 Open wound of unspecified buttock**

+7th **S31.801 Laceration without foreign body of unspecified buttock**

+7th **S31.802 Laceration with foreign body of unspecified buttock**

+7th **S31.803 Puncture wound without foreign body of unspecified buttock**

+7th **S31.804 Puncture wound with foreign body of unspecified buttock**

+7th **S31.805 Open bite of unspecified buttock**

Bite of buttock NOS

Excludes1: *superficial bite of buttock (S30.870)*

+7th **S31.809 Unspecified open wound of unspecified buttock**

+ **S31.81 Open wound of right buttock**

+7th **S31.811 Laceration without foreign body of right buttock**

+7th **S31.812 Laceration with foreign body of right buttock**

+7th **S31.813 Puncture wound without foreign body of right buttock**

+7th **S31.814 Puncture wound with foreign body of right buttock**

+7th **S31.815 Open bite of right buttock**

Bite of right buttock NOS

Excludes1: *superficial bite of buttock (S30.870)*

+7th **S31.819 Unspecified open wound of right buttock**

+ **S31.82 Open wound of left buttock**

+7th **S31.821 Laceration without foreign body of left buttock**

+7th **S31.822 Laceration with foreign body of left buttock**

+7th **S31.823 Puncture wound without foreign body of left buttock**

+7th **S31.824 Puncture wound with foreign body of left buttock**

+7th **S31.825 Open bite of left buttock**

Bite of left buttock NOS

Excludes1: *superficial bite of buttock (S30.870)*

+7th **S31.829 Unspecified open wound of left buttock**

+ **S31.83 Open wound of anus**

+7th **S31.831 Laceration without foreign body of anus**

+7th **S31.832 Laceration with foreign body of anus**

+7th **S31.833 Puncture wound without foreign body of anus**

+7th **S31.834 Puncture wound with foreign body of anus**

+7th **S31.835 Open bite of anus**

Bite of anus NOS

Excludes1: *superficial bite of anus (S30.877)*

+7th **S31.839 Unspecified open wound of anus**

See page 994 for Vertebrae Illustration.

S32 Fracture of lumbar spine and pelvis

NOTE A fracture not indicated as displaced or nondisplaced should be coded to displaced

A fracture not indicated as opened or closed should be coded to closed

Includes: fracture of lumbosacral neural arch
fracture of lumbosacral spinous process
fracture of lumbosacral transverse process
fracture of lumbosacral vertebra
fracture of lumbosacral vertebral arch

Code first any associated spinal cord and spinal nerve injury (S34.-)

Excludes1: *transection of abdomen (S38.3)*

Excludes2: *fracture of hip NOS (S72.0-)*

The appropriate 7th character is to be added to each code from category S32
- A initial encounter for closed fracture
- B initial encounter for open fracture
- D subsequent encounter for fracture with routine healing
- G subsequent encounter for fracture with delayed healing
- K subsequent encounter for fracture with nonunion
- S sequela

Review coding guideline C.19.c

+ **S32.0 Fracture of lumbar vertebra**

Fracture of lumbar spine NOS

+ **S32.00 Fracture of unspecified lumbar vertebra**

CC MCC +7th **S32.000 Wedge compression fracture of unspecified lumbar vertebra**

HAC 7th characters A & B see Appendix B for HAC conditional logic

CC MCC +7th **S32.001 Stable burst fracture of unspecified lumbar vertebra**

HAC 7th characters A & B see Appendix B for HAC conditional logic

CC MCC +7th **S32.002 Unstable burst fracture of unspecified lumbar vertebra**

HAC 7th characters A & B see Appendix B for HAC conditional logic

CC MCC +7th **S32.008 Other fracture of unspecified lumbar vertebra**

HAC 7th characters A & B see Appendix B for HAC conditional logic

CC MCC +7th **S32.009 Unspecified fracture of unspecified lumbar vertebra**

HAC 7th characters A & B see Appendix B for HAC conditional logic

+ **S32.01 Fracture of first lumbar vertebra**

CC MCC +7th **S32.010 Wedge compression fracture of first lumbar vertebra**

HAC 7th characters A & B see Appendix B for HAC conditional logic

CC MCC +7th **S32.011 Stable burst fracture of first lumbar vertebra**

HAC 7th characters A & B see Appendix B for HAC conditional logic

CC MCC +7th **S32.012 Unstable burst fracture of first lumbar vertebra**

HAC 7th characters A & B see Appendix B for HAC conditional logic

CC MCC +7th **S32.018 Other fracture of first lumbar vertebra**

HAC 7th characters A & B see Appendix B for HAC conditional logic

CC MCC +7th **S32.019 Unspecified fracture of first lumbar vertebra**

HAC 7th characters A & B see Appendix B for HAC conditional logic

+ **S32.02 Fracture of second lumbar vertebra**

CC MCC +7th **S32.020 Wedge compression fracture of second lumbar vertebra**

HAC 7th characters A & B see Appendix B for HAC conditional logic

CC MCC +7th **S32.021** **Stable burst fracture of second lumbar vertebra**
HAC 7th characters A & B see Appendix B for HAC conditional logic

CC MCC +7th **S32.022** **Unstable burst fracture of second lumbar vertebra**
HAC 7th characters A & B see Appendix B for HAC conditional logic

CC MCC +7th **S32.028** **Other fracture of second lumbar vertebra**
HAC 7th characters A & B see Appendix B for HAC conditional logic

CC MCC +7th **S32.029** **Unspecified fracture of second lumbar vertebra**
HAC 7th characters A & B see Appendix B for HAC conditional logic

+ **S32.03** **Fracture of third lumbar vertebra**

CC MCC +7th **S32.030** **Wedge compression fracture of third lumbar vertebra**
HAC 7th characters A & B see Appendix B for HAC conditional logic

CC MCC +7th **S32.031** **Stable burst fracture of third lumbar vertebra**
HAC 7th characters A & B see Appendix B for HAC conditional logic

CC MCC +7th **S32.032** **Unstable burst fracture of third lumbar vertebra**
HAC 7th characters A & B see Appendix B for HAC conditional logic

CC MCC +7th **S32.038** **Other fracture of third lumbar vertebra**
HAC 7th characters A & B see Appendix B for HAC conditional logic

CC MCC +7th **S32.039** **Unspecified fracture of third lumbar vertebra**
HAC 7th characters A & B see Appendix B for HAC conditional logic

+ **S32.04** **Fracture of fourth lumbar vertebra**

CC MCC +7th **S32.040** **Wedge compression fracture of fourth lumbar vertebra**
HAC 7th characters A & B see Appendix B for HAC conditional logic

CC MCC +7th **S32.041** **Stable burst fracture of fourth lumbar vertebra**
HAC 7th characters A & B see Appendix B for HAC conditional logic

CC MCC +7th **S32.042** **Unstable burst fracture of fourth lumbar vertebra**
HAC 7th characters A & B see Appendix B for HAC conditional logic

CC MCC +7th **S32.048** **Other fracture of fourth lumbar vertebra**
HAC 7th characters A & B see Appendix B for HAC conditional logic

CC MCC +7th **S32.049** **Unspecified fracture of fourth lumbar vertebra**
HAC 7th characters A & B see Appendix B for HAC conditional logic

+ **S32.05** **Fracture of fifth lumbar vertebra**

CC MCC +7th **S32.050** **Wedge compression fracture of fifth lumbar vertebra**
HAC 7th characters A & B see Appendix B for HAC conditional logic

CC MCC +7th **S32.051** **Stable burst fracture of fifth lumbar vertebra**
HAC 7th characters A & B see Appendix B for HAC conditional logic

CC MCC +7th **S32.052** **Unstable burst fracture of fifth lumbar vertebra**
HAC 7th characters A & B see Appendix B for HAC conditional logic

CC MCC +7th **S32.058** **Other fracture of fifth lumbar vertebra**
HAC 7th characters A & B see Appendix B for HAC conditional logic

CC MCC +7th **S32.059** **Unspecified fracture of fifth lumbar vertebra**
HAC 7th characters A & B see Appendix B for HAC conditional logic

+ **S32.1** **Fracture of sacrum**
NOTE For vertical fractures, code to most medial fracture extension
Use two codes if both a vertical and transverse fracture are present

Code also any associated fracture of pelvic ring (S32.8-)

CC MCC X+7th **S32.10** **Unspecified fracture of sacrum**
HAC 7th characters A & B see Appendix B for HAC conditional logic

+ **S32.11** **Zone I fracture of sacrum**
Vertical sacral ala fracture of sacrum

CC MCC +7th **S32.110** **Nondisplaced Zone I fracture of sacrum**
HAC 7th characters A & B see Appendix B for HAC conditional logic

CC MCC +7th **S32.111** **Minimally displaced Zone I fracture of sacrum**
HAC 7th characters A & B see Appendix B for HAC conditional logic

CC MCC +7th **S32.112** **Severely displaced Zone I fracture of sacrum**
HAC 7th characters A & B see Appendix B for HAC conditional logic

CC MCC +7th **S32.119** **Unspecified Zone I fracture of sacrum**
HAC 7th characters A & B see Appendix B for HAC conditional logic

+ **S32.12** **Zone II fracture of sacrum**
Vertical foraminal region fracture of sacrum

CC MCC +7th **S32.120** **Nondisplaced Zone II fracture of sacrum**
HAC 7th characters A & B see Appendix B for HAC conditional logic

CC MCC +7th **S32.121** **Minimally displaced Zone II fracture of sacrum**
HAC 7th characters A & B see Appendix B for HAC conditional logic

CC MCC +7th **S32.122** **Severely displaced Zone II fracture of sacrum**
HAC 7th characters A & B see Appendix B for HAC conditional logic

CC MCC +7th **S32.129** **Unspecified Zone II fracture of sacrum**
HAC 7th characters A & B see Appendix B for HAC conditional logic

+ **S32.13** **Zone III fracture of sacrum**
Vertical fracture into spinal canal region of sacrum

CC MCC +7th **S32.130** **Nondisplaced Zone III fracture of sacrum**
HAC 7th characters A & B see Appendix B for HAC conditional logic

CC MCC +7th **S32.131** **Minimally displaced Zone III fracture of sacrum**
HAC 7th characters A & B see Appendix B for HAC conditional logic

CC MCC +7th **S32.132** **Severely displaced Zone III fracture of sacrum**
HAC 7th characters A & B see Appendix B for HAC conditional logic

CC MCC +7th **S32.139** **Unspecified Zone III fracture of sacrum**
HAC 7th characters A & B see Appendix B for HAC conditional logic

CC MCC X+7th **S32.14** **Type 1 fracture of sacrum**
Transverse flexion fracture of sacrum without displacement
HAC 7th characters A & B see Appendix B for HAC conditional logic

CC MCC X+7th **S32.15** **Type 2 fracture of sacrum**
Transverse flexion fracture of sacrum with posterior displacement
HAC 7th characters A & B see Appendix B for HAC conditional logic

CC MCC X+7th **S32.16** **Type 3 fracture of sacrum**
Transverse extension fracture of sacrum with anterior displacement
HAC 7th characters A & B see Appendix B for HAC conditional logic

CC MCC X+7th **S32.17** **Type 4 fracture of sacrum**
Transverse segmental comminution of upper sacrum
HAC 7th characters A & B see Appendix B for HAC conditional logic

CC MCC X+7th **S32.19** **Other fracture of sacrum**
HAC 7th characters A & B see Appendix B for HAC conditional logic

X+7th **S32.2 Fracture of coccyx**
HAC 7th characters A & B see Appendix B for HAC conditional logic

+ **S32.3 Fracture of ilium**
Excludes1: fracture of ilium with associated disruption of pelvic ring (S32.8-)

+ **S32.30 Unspecified fracture of ilium**

CC MCC +7th **S32.301 Unspecified fracture of right ilium**
HAC 7th characters A & B see Appendix B for HAC conditional logic

CC MCC +7th **S32.302 Unspecified fracture of left ilium**
HAC 7th characters A & B see Appendix B for HAC conditional logic

CC MCC +7th **S32.309 Unspecified fracture of unspecified ilium**
HAC 7th characters A & B see Appendix B for HAC conditional logic

+ **S32.31 Avulsion fracture of ilium**

CC MCC +7th **S32.311 Displaced avulsion fracture of right ilium**
HAC 7th characters A & B see Appendix B for HAC conditional logic

CC MCC +7th **S32.312 Displaced avulsion fracture of left ilium**
HAC 7th characters A & B see Appendix B for HAC conditional logic

CC MCC +7th **S32.313 Displaced avulsion fracture of unspecified ilium**
HAC 7th characters A & B see Appendix B for HAC conditional logic

CC MCC +7th **S32.314 Nondisplaced avulsion fracture of right ilium**
HAC 7th characters A & B see Appendix B for HAC conditional logic

CC MCC +7th **S32.315 Nondisplaced avulsion fracture of left ilium**
HAC 7th characters A & B see Appendix B for HAC conditional logic

CC MCC +7th **S32.316 Nondisplaced avulsion fracture of unspecified ilium**
HAC 7th characters A & B see Appendix B for HAC conditional logic

+ **S32.39 Other fracture of ilium**

CC MCC +7th **S32.391 Other fracture of right ilium**
HAC 7th characters A & B see Appendix B for HAC conditional logic

CC MCC +7th **S32.392 Other fracture of left ilium**
HAC 7th characters A & B see Appendix B for HAC conditional logic

CC MCC +7th **S32.399 Other fracture of unspecified ilium**
HAC 7th characters A & B see Appendix B for HAC conditional logic

+ **S32.4 Fracture of acetabulum**
Code also any associated fracture of pelvic ring (S32.8-)

+ **S32.40 Unspecified fracture of acetabulum**

CC +7th **S32.401 Unspecified fracture of right acetabulum**
HAC 7th characters A & B see Appendix B for HAC conditional logic

CC +7th **S32.402 Unspecified fracture of left acetabulum**
HAC 7th characters A & B see Appendix B for HAC conditional logic

CC +7th **S32.409 Unspecified fracture of unspecified acetabulum**
HAC 7th characters A & B see Appendix B for HAC conditional logic

S32.41 Fracture of anterior wall of acetabulum

CC MCC +7th **S32.411 Displaced fracture of anterior wall of right acetabulum**
HAC 7th characters A & B see Appendix B for HAC conditional logic

CC MCC +7th **S32.412 Displaced fracture of anterior wall of left acetabulum**
HAC 7th characters A & B see Appendix B for HAC conditional logic

CC MCC +7th **S32.413 Displaced fracture of anterior wall of unspecified acetabulum**
HAC 7th characters A & B see Appendix B for HAC conditional logic

CC MCC +7th **S32.414 Nondisplaced fracture of anterior wall of right acetabulum**
HAC 7th characters A & B see Appendix B for HAC conditional logic

CC MCC +7th **S32.415 Nondisplaced fracture of anterior wall of left acetabulum**
HAC 7th characters A & B see Appendix B for HAC conditional logic

CC MCC +7th **S32.416 Nondisplaced fracture of anterior wall of unspecified acetabulum**
HAC 7th characters A & B see Appendix B for HAC conditional logic

+ **S32.42 Fracture of posterior wall of acetabulum**

CC MCC +7th **S32.421 Displaced fracture of posterior wall of right acetabulum**
HAC 7th characters A & B see Appendix B for HAC conditional logic

CC MCC +7th **S32.422 Displaced fracture of posterior wall of left acetabulum**
HAC 7th characters A & B see Appendix B for HAC conditional logic

CC MCC +7th **S32.423 Displaced fracture of posterior wall of unspecified acetabulum**
HAC 7th characters A & B see Appendix B for HAC conditional logic

CC MCC +7th **S32.424 Nondisplaced fracture of posterior wall of right acetabulum**
HAC 7th characters A & B see Appendix B for HAC conditional logic

CC MCC +7th **S32.425 Nondisplaced fracture of posterior wall of left acetabulum**
HAC 7th characters A & B see Appendix B for HAC conditional logic

CC MCC +7th **S32.426 Nondisplaced fracture of posterior wall of unspecified acetabulum**
HAC 7th characters A & B see Appendix B for HAC conditional logic

+ **S32.43 Fracture of anterior column [iliopubic] of acetabulum**

CC MCC +7th **S32.431 Displaced fracture of anterior column [iliopubic] of right acetabulum**
HAC 7th characters A & B see Appendix B for HAC conditional logic

CC MCC +7th **S32.432 Displaced fracture of anterior column [iliopubic] of left acetabulum**
HAC 7th characters A & B see Appendix B for HAC conditional logic

CC MCC +7th **S32.433 Displaced fracture of anterior column [iliopubic] of unspecified acetabulum**
HAC 7th characters A & B see Appendix B for HAC conditional logic

CC MCC +7th **S32.434 Nondisplaced fracture of anterior column [iliopubic] of right acetabulum**
HAC 7th characters A & B see Appendix B for HAC conditional logic

CC MCC +7th **S32.435 Nondisplaced fracture of anterior column [iliopubic] of left acetabulum**
HAC 7th characters A & B see Appendix B for HAC conditional logic

CC MCC +7th **S32.436 Nondisplaced fracture of anterior column [iliopubic] of unspecified acetabulum**
HAC 7th characters A & B see Appendix B for HAC conditional logic

+ **S32.44 Fracture of posterior column [ilioischial] of acetabulum**

CC MCC +7th **S32.441 Displaced fracture of posterior column [ilioischial] of right acetabulum**
HAC 7th characters A & B see Appendix B for HAC conditional logic

CC MCC +7th **S32.442 Displaced fracture of posterior column [ilioischial] of left acetabulum**
HAC 7th characters A & B see Appendix B for HAC conditional logic

CC MCC +7th **S32.443 Displaced fracture of posterior column [ilioischial] of unspecified acetabulum**
HAC 7th characters A & B see Appendix B for HAC conditional logic

CC MCC +7th **S32.444 Nondisplaced fracture of posterior column [ilioischial] of right acetabulum**
HAC 7th characters A & B see Appendix B for HAC conditional logic

CC MCC +7th **S32.445 Nondisplaced fracture of posterior column [ilioischial] of left acetabulum**
HAC 7th characters A & B see Appendix B for HAC conditional logic

CC MCC +7th **S32.446 Nondisplaced fracture of posterior column [ilioischial] of unspecified acetabulum**
HAC 7th characters A & B see Appendix B for HAC conditional logic

+ **S32.45 Transverse fracture of acetabulum**

CC MCC +7th **S32.451 Displaced transverse fracture of right acetabulum**
HAC 7th characters A & B see Appendix B for HAC conditional logic

CC MCC +7th **S32.452 Displaced transverse fracture of left acetabulum**
HAC 7th characters A & B see Appendix B for HAC conditional logic

CC MCC +7th **S32.453 Displaced transverse fracture of unspecified acetabulum**
HAC 7th characters A & B see Appendix B for HAC conditional logic

CC MCC +7th **S32.454 Nondisplaced transverse fracture of right acetabulum**
HAC 7th characters A & B see Appendix B for HAC conditional logic

CC MCC +7th **S32.455 Nondisplaced transverse fracture of left acetabulum**
HAC 7th characters A & B see Appendix B for HAC conditional logic

CC MCC +7th **S32.456 Nondisplaced transverse fracture of unspecified acetabulum**
HAC 7th characters A & B see Appendix B for HAC conditional logic

+ **S32.46 Associated transverse-posterior fracture of acetabulum**

CC MCC +7th **S32.461 Displaced associated transverse-posterior fracture of right acetabulum**
HAC 7th characters A & B see Appendix B for HAC conditional logic

CC MCC +7th **S32.462 Displaced associated transverse-posterior fracture of left acetabulum**
HAC 7th characters A & B see Appendix B for HAC conditional logic

CC MCC +7th **S32.463 Displaced associated transverse-posterior fracture of unspecified acetabulum**
HAC 7th characters A & B see Appendix B for HAC conditional logic

CC MCC +7th **S32.464 Nondisplaced associated transverse-posterior fracture of right acetabulum**
HAC 7th characters A & B see Appendix B for HAC conditional logic

CC MCC +7th **S32.465 Nondisplaced associated transverse-posterior fracture of left acetabulum**
HAC 7th characters A & B see Appendix B for HAC conditional logic

CC MCC +7th **S32.466 Nondisplaced associated transverse-posterior fracture of unspecified acetabulum**
HAC 7th characters A & B see Appendix B for HAC conditional logic

+ **S32.47 Fracture of medial wall of acetabulum**

CC MCC +7th **S32.471 Displaced fracture of medial wall of right acetabulum**
HAC 7th characters A & B see Appendix B for HAC conditional logic

CC MCC +7th **S32.472 Displaced fracture of medial wall of left acetabulum**
HAC 7th characters A & B see Appendix B for HAC conditional logic

CC MCC +7th **S32.473 Displaced fracture of medial wall of unspecified acetabulum**
HAC 7th characters A & B see Appendix B for HAC conditional logic

CC MCC +7th **S32.474 Nondisplaced fracture of medial wall of right acetabulum**
HAC 7th characters A & B see Appendix B for HAC conditional logic

CC MCC +7th **S32.475 Nondisplaced fracture of medial wall of left acetabulum**
HAC 7th characters A & B see Appendix B for HAC conditional logic

CC MCC +7th **S32.476 Nondisplaced fracture of medial wall of unspecified acetabulum**
HAC 7th characters A & B see Appendix B for HAC conditional logic

+ **S32.48 Dome fracture of acetabulum**

CC MCC +7th **S32.481 Displaced dome fracture of right acetabulum**
HAC 7th characters A & B see Appendix B for HAC conditional logic

CC MCC +7th **S32.482 Displaced dome fracture of left acetabulum**
HAC 7th characters A & B see Appendix B for HAC conditional logic

CC MCC +7th **S32.483 Displaced dome fracture of unspecified acetabulum**
HAC 7th characters A & B see Appendix B for HAC conditional logic

CC MCC +7th **S32.484 Nondisplaced dome fracture of right acetabulum**
HAC 7th characters A & B see Appendix B for HAC conditional logic

CC MCC +7th **S32.485 Nondisplaced dome fracture of left acetabulum**
HAC 7th characters A & B see Appendix B for HAC conditional logic

CC MCC +7th **S32.486 Nondisplaced dome fracture of unspecified acetabulum**
HAC 7th characters A & B see Appendix B for HAC conditional logic

+ **S32.49 Other specified fracture of acetabulum**

CC MCC +7th **S32.491 Other specified fracture of right acetabulum**
HAC 7th characters A & B see Appendix B for HAC conditional logic

CC MCC +7th **S32.492 Other specified fracture of left acetabulum**
HAC 7th characters A & B see Appendix B for HAC conditional logic

CC MCC +7th **S32.499 Other specified fracture of unspecified acetabulum**
HAC 7th characters A & B see Appendix B for HAC conditional logic

+ **S32.5 Fracture of pubis**
Excludes1: *fracture of pubis with associated disruption of pelvic ring (S32.8-)*

+ **S32.50 Unspecified fracture of pubis**

CC MCC +7th **S32.501 Unspecified fracture of right pubis**
HAC 7th characters A & B see Appendix B for HAC conditional logic

CC MCC +7th **S32.502 Unspecified fracture of left pubis**
HAC 7th characters A & B see Appendix B for HAC conditional logic

CC MCC +7th **S32.509 Unspecified fracture of unspecified pubis**
HAC 7th characters A & B see Appendix B for HAC conditional logic

+ **S32.51 Fracture of superior rim of pubis**

CC MCC +7th **S32.511 Fracture of superior rim of right pubis**
HAC 7th characters A & B see Appendix B for HAC conditional logic

CC MCC +7th **S32.512 Fracture of superior rim of left pubis**
HAC 7th characters A & B see Appendix B for HAC conditional logic

CC MCC +7th **S32.519 Fracture of superior rim of unspecified pubis**
HAC 7th characters A & B see Appendix B for HAC conditional logic

+ **S32.59 Other specified fracture of pubis**

CC MCC +7th **S32.591 Other specified fracture of right pubis**
HAC 7th characters A & B see Appendix B for HAC conditional logic

CC MCC +7th **S32.592 Other specified fracture of left pubis**
HAC 7th characters A & B see Appendix B for HAC conditional logic

CC MCC +7th **S32.599 Other specified fracture of unspecified pubis**
HAC 7th characters A & B see Appendix B for HAC conditional logic

+ **S32.6 Fracture of ischium**
Excludes1: *fracture of ischium with associated disruption of pelvic ring (S32.8-)*

+ **S32.60 Unspecified fracture of ischium**

CC MCC +7th **S32.601 Unspecified fracture of right ischium**
HAC 7th characters A & B see Appendix B for HAC conditional logic

CC MCC +7th **S32.602 Unspecified fracture of left ischium**
HAC 7th characters A & B see Appendix B for HAC conditional logic

CC MCC +7th **S32.609 Unspecified fracture of unspecified ischium**
HAC 7th characters A & B see Appendix B for HAC conditional logic

+ **S32.61 Avulsion fracture of ischium**

CC MCC +7th **S32.611 Displaced avulsion fracture of right ischium**
HAC 7th characters A & B see Appendix B for HAC conditional logic

CC MCC +7th **S32.612 Displaced avulsion fracture of left ischium**
HAC 7th characters A & B see Appendix B for HAC conditional logic

CC MCC +7th **S32.613 Displaced avulsion fracture of unspecified ischium**
HAC 7th characters A & B see Appendix B for HAC conditional logic

CC MCC +7th **S32.614 Nondisplaced avulsion fracture of right ischium**
HAC 7th characters A & B see Appendix B for HAC conditional logic

CC MCC +7th **S32.615 Nondisplaced avulsion fracture of left ischium**
HAC 7th characters A & B see Appendix B for HAC conditional logic

CC MCC +7th **S32.616 Nondisplaced avulsion fracture of unspecified ischium**
HAC 7th characters A & B see Appendix B for HAC conditional logic

+ **S32.69 Other specified fracture of ischium**

CC MCC +7th **S32.691 Other specified fracture of right ischium**
HAC 7th characters A & B see Appendix B for HAC conditional logic

CC MCC +7th **S32.692 Other specified fracture of left ischium**
HAC 7th characters A & B see Appendix B for HAC conditional logic

+ **S32.8 Fracture of other parts of pelvis**
Code also any associated:
fracture of acetabulum (S32.4-)
sacral fracture (S32.1-)

+ **S32.81 Multiple fractures of pelvis with disruption of pelvic ring**
Multiple pelvic fractures with disruption of pelvic circle

CC MCC +7th **S32.810 Multiple fractures of pelvis with stable disruption of pelvic ring**
HAC 7th characters A & B see Appendix B for HAC conditional logic

CC MCC +7th **S32.811 Multiple fractures of pelvis with unstable disruption of pelvic ring**
HAC 7th characters A & B see Appendix B for HAC conditional logic

CC MCC X+7th **S32.82 Multiple fractures of pelvis without disruption of pelvic ring**
Multiple pelvic fractures without disruption of pelvic circle
HAC 7th characters A & B see Appendix B for HAC conditional logic

CC MCC X+7th **S32.89 Fracture of other parts of pelvis**
HAC 7th characters A & B see Appendix B for HAC conditional logic

X+7th MCC CC **S32.9 Fracture of unspecified parts of lumbosacral spine and pelvis**
Fracture of lumbosacral spine NOS
Fracture of pelvis NOS
HAC 7th characters A & B see Appendix B for HAC conditional logic

S33 Dislocation and sprain of joints and ligaments of lumbar spine and pelvis

Includes: avulsion of joint or ligament of lumbar spine and pelvis
laceration of cartilage, joint or ligament of lumbar spine and pelvis
sprain of cartilage, joint or ligament of lumbar spine and pelvis
traumatic hemarthrosis of joint or ligament of lumbar spine and pelvis
traumatic rupture of joint or ligament of lumbar spine and pelvis
traumatic subluxation of joint or ligament of lumbar spine and pelvis
traumatic tear of joint or ligament of lumbar spine and pelvis

Code also any associated open wound

Excludes1: *nontraumatic rupture or displacement of lumbar intervertebral disc NOS (M51.-)*
obstetric damage to pelvic joints and ligaments (O71.6)

Excludes2: *dislocation and sprain of joints and ligaments of hip (S73.-)*
strain of muscle of lower back and pelvis (S39.01-)

The appropriate 7th character is to be added to each code from category S33
A initial encounter
D subsequent encounter
S sequela

X+7th **S33.0 Traumatic rupture of lumbar intervertebral disc**
Excludes1: *rupture or displacement (nontraumatic) of lumbar intervertebral disc NOS (M51.- with fifth character 6)*

+ **S33.1 Subluxation and dislocation of lumbar vertebra**
Code also any associated:
open wound of abdomen, lower back and pelvis (S31)
spinal cord injury (S24.0, S24.1-, S34.0-, S34.1-)
Excludes2: *fracture of lumbar vertebrae (S32.0-)*

+ **S33.10 Subluxation and dislocation of unspecified lumbar vertebra**
+7th **S33.100 Subluxation of unspecified lumbar vertebra**
+7th **S33.101 Dislocation of unspecified lumbar vertebra**

+ **S33.11 Subluxation and dislocation of L1/L2 lumbar vertebra**
+7th **S33.110 Subluxation of L1/L2 lumbar vertebra**
+7th **S33.111 Dislocation of L1/L2 lumbar vertebra**

+ **S33.12 Subluxation and dislocation of L2/L3 lumbar vertebra**
+7th **S33.120 Subluxation of L2/L3 lumbar vertebra**
+7th **S33.121 Dislocation of L2/L3 lumbar vertebra**

+ **S33.13 Subluxation and dislocation of L3/L4 lumbar vertebra**
+7th **S33.130 Subluxation of L3/L4 lumbar vertebra**
+7th **S33.131 Dislocation of L3/L4 lumbar vertebra**

+ **S33.14 Subluxation and dislocation of L4/L5 lumbar vertebra**
+7th **S33.140 Subluxation of L4/L5 lumbar vertebra**
+7th **S33.141 Dislocation of L4/L5 lumbar vertebra**

X+7th **S33.2 Dislocation of sacroiliac and sacrococcygeal joint**

+ **S33.3 Dislocation of other and unspecified parts of lumbar spine and pelvis**
X+7th **S33.30 Dislocation of unspecified parts of lumbar spine and pelvis**
X+7th **S33.39 Dislocation of other parts of lumbar spine and pelvis**

X+7th **S33.4 Traumatic rupture of symphysis pubis**
X+7th **S33.5 Sprain of ligaments of lumbar spine**
X+7th **S33.6 Sprain of sacroiliac joint**
X+7th **S33.8 Sprain of other parts of lumbar spine and pelvis**
X+7th **S33.9 Sprain of unspecified parts of lumbar spine and pelvis**

S34 Injury of lumbar and sacral spinal cord and nerves at abdomen, lower back and pelvis level

NOTE Code to highest level of lumbar cord injury
Injuries to the spinal cord (S34.0 and S34.1) refer to the cord level and not bone level injury, and can affect nerve roots at and below the level given.

Code also any associated:
fracture of vertebra (S22.0-, S32.0-)
open wound of abdomen, lower back and pelvis (S31.-)
transient paralysis (R29.5)

The appropriate 7th character is to be added to each code from category S34
A initial encounter
D subsequent encounter
S sequela

+ **S34.0 Concussion and edema of lumbar and sacral spinal cord**
MCC X+7th **S34.01 Concussion and edema of lumbar spinal cord**
MCC X+7th **S34.02 Concussion and edema of sacral spinal cord**
Concussion and edema of conus medullaris

+ **S34.1 Other and unspecified injury of lumbar and sacral spinal cord**

+ **S34.10 Unspecified injury to lumbar spinal cord**

MCC +7th **S34.101 Unspecified injury to L1 level of lumbar spinal cord**
Unspecified injury to lumbar spinal cord level 1
HAC 7th character A see Appendix B for HAC conditional logic

MCC +7th **S34.102 Unspecified injury to L2 level of lumbar spinal cord**
Unspecified injury to lumbar spinal cord level 2
HAC 7th character A see Appendix B for HAC conditional logic

MCC +7th **S34.103 Unspecified injury to L3 level of lumbar spinal cord**
Unspecified injury to lumbar spinal cord level 3
HAC 7th character A see Appendix B for HAC conditional logic

MCC +7th **S34.104 Unspecified injury to L4 level of lumbar spinal cord**
Unspecified injury to lumbar spinal cord level 4
HAC 7th character A see Appendix B for HAC conditional logic

MCC +7th **S34.105 Unspecified injury to L5 level of lumbar spinal cord**
Unspecified injury to lumbar spinal cord level 5
HAC 7th character A see Appendix B for HAC conditional logic

MCC +7th **S34.109 Unspecified injury to unspecified level of lumbar spinal cord**
HAC 7th character A see Appendix B for HAC conditional logic

+ **S34.11 Complete lesion of lumbar spinal cord**

MCC +7th **S34.111 Complete lesion of L1 level of lumbar spinal cord**
Complete lesion of lumbar spinal cord level 1
HAC 7th character A see Appendix B for HAC conditional logic

MCC +7th **S34.112 Complete lesion of L2 level of lumbar spinal cord**
Complete lesion of lumbar spinal cord level 2
HAC 7th character A see Appendix B for HAC conditional logic

MCC +7th **S34.113 Complete lesion of L3 level of lumbar spinal cord**
Complete lesion of lumbar spinal cord level 3
HAC 7th character A see Appendix B for HAC conditional logic

MCC +7th **S34.114 Complete lesion of L4 level of lumbar spinal cord**
Complete lesion of lumbar spinal cord level 4
HAC 7th character A see Appendix B for HAC conditional logic

MCC +7th **S34.115 Complete lesion of L5 level of lumbar spinal cord**
Complete lesion of lumbar spinal cord level 5
HAC 7th character A see Appendix B for HAC conditional logic

MCC +7th **S34.119 Complete lesion of unspecified level of lumbar spinal cord**
HAC 7th character A see Appendix B for HAC conditional logic

+ **S34.12 Incomplete lesion of lumbar spinal cord**

MCC +7th **S34.121 Incomplete lesion of L1 level of lumbar spinal cord**
Incomplete lesion of lumbar spinal cord level 1
HAC 7th character A see Appendix B for HAC conditional logic

MCC +7th **S34.122 Incomplete lesion of L2 level of lumbar spinal cord**
Incomplete lesion of lumbar spinal cord level 2
HAC 7th character A see Appendix B for HAC conditional logic

MCC +7th **S34.123 Incomplete lesion of L3 level of lumbar spinal cord**
Incomplete lesion of lumbar spinal cord level 3
HAC 7th character A see Appendix B for HAC conditional logic

MCC +7th **S34.124 Incomplete lesion of L4 level of lumbar spinal cord**
Incomplete lesion of lumbar spinal cord level 4
HAC 7th character A see Appendix B for HAC conditional logic

MCC +7th **S34.125 Incomplete lesion of L5 level of lumbar spinal cord**
Incomplete lesion of lumbar spinal cord level 5
HAC 7th character A see Appendix B for HAC conditional logic

MCC +7th **S34.129 Incomplete lesion of unspecified level of lumbar spinal cord**
HAC 7th character A see Appendix B for HAC conditional logic

+ **S34.13 Other and unspecified injury to sacral spinal cord**
Other injury to conus medullaris

MCC +7th **S34.131 Complete lesion of sacral spinal cord**
Complete lesion of conus medullaris
HAC 7th character A see Appendix B for HAC conditional logic

MCC +7th **S34.132 Incomplete lesion of sacral spinal cord**
Incomplete lesion of conus medullaris
HAC 7th character A see Appendix B for HAC conditional logic

MCC +7th **S34.139 Unspecified injury to sacral spinal cord**
Unspecified injury of conus medullaris
HAC 7th character A see Appendix B for HAC conditional logic

+ **S34.2 Injury of nerve root of lumbar and sacral spine**

X+7th **S34.21 Injury of nerve root of lumbar spine**

X+7th **S34.22 Injury of nerve root of sacral spine**

MCC X+7th **S34.3 Injury of cauda equina**
HAC 7th character A see Appendix B for HAC conditional logic

X+7th **S34.4 Injury of lumbosacral plexus**

X+7th **S34.5 Injury of lumbar, sacral and pelvic sympathetic nerves**
Injury of celiac ganglion or plexus
Injury of hypogastric plexus
Injury of mesenteric plexus (inferior) (superior)
Injury of splanchnic nerve

X+7th **S34.6 Injury of peripheral nerve(s) at abdomen, lower back and pelvis level**

X+7th **S34.8 Injury of other nerves at abdomen, lower back and pelvis level**

X+7th **S34.9 Injury of unspecified nerves at abdomen, lower back and pelvis level**

S35 Injury of blood vessels at abdomen, lower back and pelvis level

Code also any associated open wound (S31.-)

The appropriate 7th character is to be added to each code from category S35
A initial encounter
D subsequent encounter
S sequela

+ **S35.0 Injury of abdominal aorta**
Excludes1: *injury of aorta NOS (S25.0)*

MCC X+7th **S35.00 Unspecified injury of abdominal aorta**

MCC X+7th **S35.01 Minor laceration of abdominal aorta**
Incomplete transection of abdominal aorta
Laceration of abdominal aorta NOS
Superficial laceration of abdominal aorta

MCC X+7th **S35.02 Major laceration of abdominal aorta**
Complete transection of abdominal aorta
Traumatic rupture of abdominal aorta

MCC X+7th **S35.09 Other injury of abdominal aorta**

+ **S35.1 Injury of inferior vena cava**
Injury of hepatic vein
Excludes1: *injury of vena cava NOS (S25.2)*

MCC X+7th **S35.10 Unspecified injury of inferior vena cava**

MCC X+7th **S35.11 Minor laceration of inferior vena cava**
Incomplete transection of inferior vena cava
Laceration of inferior vena cava NOS
Superficial laceration of inferior vena cava

MCC X+7th **S35.12 Major laceration of inferior vena cava**
Complete transection of inferior vena cava
Traumatic rupture of inferior vena cava
MCC X+7th **S35.19 Other injury of inferior vena cava**
+ **S35.2 Injury of celiac or mesenteric artery and branches**
+ **S35.21 Injury of celiac artery**
MCC +7th **S35.211 Minor laceration of celiac artery**
Incomplete transection of celiac artery
Laceration of celiac artery NOS
Superficial laceration of celiac artery
MCC +7th **S35.212 Major laceration of celiac artery**
Complete transection of celiac artery
Traumatic rupture of celiac artery
MCC +7th **S35.218 Other injury of celiac artery**
MCC +7th **S35.219 Unspecified injury of celiac artery**
+ **S35.22 Injury of superior mesenteric artery**
MCC +7th **S35.221 Minor laceration of superior mesenteric artery**
Incomplete transection of superior mesenteric artery
Laceration of superior mesenteric artery NOS
Superficial laceration of superior mesenteric artery
MCC +7th **S35.222 Major laceration of superior mesenteric artery**
Complete transection of superior mesenteric artery
Traumatic rupture of superior mesenteric artery
MCC +7th **S35.228 Other injury of superior mesenteric artery**
MCC +7th **S35.229 Unspecified injury of superior mesenteric artery**
+ **S35.23 Injury of inferior mesenteric artery**
MCC +7th **S35.231 Minor laceration of inferior mesenteric artery**
Incomplete transection of inferior mesenteric artery
Laceration of inferior mesenteric artery NOS
Superficial laceration of inferior mesenteric artery
MCC +7th **S35.232 Major laceration of inferior mesenteric artery**
Complete transection of inferior mesenteric artery
Traumatic rupture of inferior mesenteric artery
MCC +7th **S35.238 Other injury of inferior mesenteric artery**
MCC +7th **S35.239 Unspecified injury of inferior mesenteric artery**
+ **S35.29 Injury of branches of celiac and mesenteric artery**
Injury of gastric artery
Injury of gastroduodenal artery
Injury of hepatic artery
Injury of splenic artery
MCC +7th **S35.291 Minor laceration of branches of celiac and mesenteric artery**
Incomplete transection of branches of celiac and mesenteric artery
Laceration of branches of celiac and mesenteric artery NOS
Superficial laceration of branches of celiac and mesenteric artery
MCC +7th **S35.292 Major laceration of branches of celiac and mesenteric artery**
Complete transection of branches of celiac and mesenteric artery
Traumatic rupture of branches of celiac and mesenteric artery
MCC +7th **S35.298 Other injury of branches of celiac and mesenteric artery**
MCC +7th **S35.299 Unspecified injury of branches of celiac and mesenteric artery**
+ **S35.3 Injury of portal or splenic vein and branches**
+ **S35.31 Injury of portal vein**
MCC +7th **S35.311 Laceration of portal vein**
MCC +7th **S35.318 Other specified injury of portal vein**
MCC +7th **S35.319 Unspecified injury of portal vein**
+ **S35.32 Injury of splenic vein**
MCC +7th **S35.321 Laceration of splenic vein**
MCC +7th **S35.328 Other specified injury of splenic vein**
MCC +7th **S35.329 Unspecified injury of splenic vein**
+ **S35.33 Injury of superior mesenteric vein**
MCC +7th **S35.331 Laceration of superior mesenteric vein**
MCC +7th **S35.338 Other specified injury of superior mesenteric vein**
MCC +7th **S35.339 Unspecified injury of superior mesenteric vein**
+ **S35.34 Injury of inferior mesenteric vein**
MCC +7th **S35.341 Laceration of inferior mesenteric vein**
MCC +7th **S35.348 Other specified injury of inferior mesenteric vein**
MCC +7th **S35.349 Unspecified injury of inferior mesenteric vein**
+ **S35.4 Injury of renal blood vessels**
+ **S35.40 Unspecified injury of renal blood vessel**
MCC +7th **S35.401 Unspecified injury of right renal artery**
MCC +7th **S35.402 Unspecified injury of left renal artery**
MCC +7th **S35.403 Unspecified injury of unspecified renal artery**
MCC +7th **S35.404 Unspecified injury of right renal vein**
MCC +7th **S35.405 Unspecified injury of left renal vein**
MCC +7th **S35.406 Unspecified injury of unspecified renal vein**
+ **S35.41 Laceration of renal blood vessel**
MCC +7th **S35.411 Laceration of right renal artery**
MCC +7th **S35.412 Laceration of left renal artery**
MCC +7th **S35.413 Laceration of unspecified renal artery**
MCC +7th **S35.414 Laceration of right renal vein**
MCC +7th **S35.415 Laceration of left renal vein**
MCC +7th **S35.416 Laceration of unspecified renal vein**
+ **S35.49 Other specified injury of renal blood vessel**
MCC +7th **S35.491 Other specified injury of right renal artery**
MCC +7th **S35.492 Other specified injury of left renal artery**
MCC +7th **S35.493 Other specified injury of unspecified renal artery**
MCC +7th **S35.494 Other specified injury of right renal vein**
MCC +7th **S35.495 Other specified injury of left renal vein**
MCC +7th **S35.496 Other specified injury of unspecified renal vein**
+ **S35.5 Injury of iliac blood vessels**
MCC X+7th **S35.50 Injury of unspecified iliac blood vessel(s)**
+ **S35.51 Injury of iliac artery or vein**
Injury of hypogastric artery or vein
MCC +7th **S35.511 Injury of right iliac artery**
MCC +7th **S35.512 Injury of left iliac artery**
MCC +7th **S35.513 Injury of unspecified iliac artery**
MCC +7th **S35.514 Injury of right iliac vein**
MCC +7th **S35.515 Injury of left iliac vein**
MCC +7th **S35.516 Injury of unspecified iliac vein**
+ **S35.53 Injury of uterine artery or vein**
♀ CC +7th **S35.531 Injury of right uterine artery**
♀ CC +7th **S35.532 Injury of left uterine artery**
♀ CC +7th **S35.533 Injury of unspecified uterine artery**
♀ CC +7th **S35.534 Injury of right uterine vein**
♀ CC +7th **S35.535 Injury of left uterine vein**
♀ CC +7th **S35.536 Injury of unspecified uterine vein**
MCC X+7th **S35.59 Injury of other iliac blood vessels**
CC + **S35.8 Injury of other blood vessels at abdomen, lower back and pelvis level**
Injury of ovarian artery or vein
+ **S35.8X Injury of other blood vessels at abdomen, lower back and pelvis level**
+7th **S35.8X1 Laceration of other blood vessels at abdomen, lower back and pelvis level**
+7th **S35.8X8 Other specified injury of other blood vessels at abdomen, lower back and pelvis level**
+7th **S35.8X9 Unspecified injury of other blood vessels at abdomen, lower back and pelvis level**
+ **S35.9 Injury of unspecified blood vessel at abdomen, lower back and pelvis level**
CC X+7th **S35.90 Unspecified injury of unspecified blood vessel at abdomen, lower back and pelvis level**

CC X+7th **S35.91 Laceration of unspecified blood vessel at abdomen, lower back and pelvis level**

CC X+7th **S35.99 Other specified injury of unspecified blood vessel at abdomen, lower back and pelvis level**

S36 Injury of intra-abdominal organs

Code also any associated open wound (S31.-)

The appropriate 7th character is to be added to each code from category S36
A initial encounter
D subsequent encounter
S sequela

\+ **S36.0 Injury of spleen**
CC X+7th **S36.00 Unspecified injury of spleen**
\+ **S36.02 Contusion of spleen**
CC +7th **S36.020 Minor contusion of spleen**
Contusion of spleen less than 2 cm
CC +7th **S36.021 Major contusion of spleen**
Contusion of spleen greater than 2 cm
CC +7th **S36.029 Unspecified contusion of spleen**
\+ **S36.03 Laceration of spleen**
CC +7th **S36.030 Superficial (capsular) laceration of spleen**
Laceration of spleen less than 1 cm
Minor laceration of spleen
AHA CC: 1Q, 2015, 3-21
MCC +7th **S36.031 Moderate laceration of spleen**
Laceration of spleen 1 to 3 cm
AHA CC: 1Q, 2015, 3-21
MCC +7th **S36.032 Major laceration of spleen**
Avulsion of spleen
Laceration of spleen greater than 3 cm
Massive laceration of spleen
Multiple moderate lacerations of spleen
Stellate laceration of spleen
CC +7th **S36.039 Unspecified laceration of spleen**
CC X+7th **S36.09 Other injury of spleen**
\+ **S36.1 Injury of liver and gallbladder and bile duct**
\+ **S36.11 Injury of liver**
CC +7th **S36.112 Contusion of liver**
CC +7th **S36.113 Laceration of liver, unspecified degree**
CC +7th **S36.114 Minor laceration of liver**
Laceration involving capsule only, or, without significant involvement of hepatic parenchyma [i.e., less than 1 cmdeep]
MCC +7th **S36.115 Moderate laceration of liver**
Laceration involving parenchyma but without major disruption of parenchyma [i.e., less than 10 cm long and less than 3 cm deep]
MCC +7th **S36.116 Major laceration of liver**
Laceration with significant disruption of hepatic parenchyma [i.e., greater than 10 cm long and 3 cm deep]
Multiple moderate lacerations, with or without hematoma
Stellate laceration of liver
CC +7th **S36.118 Other injury of liver**
CC +7th **S36.119 Unspecified injury of liver**
\+ **S36.12 Injury of gallbladder**
CC +7th **S36.122 Contusion of gallbladder**
CC +7th **S36.123 Laceration of gallbladder**
CC +7th **S36.128 Other injury of gallbladder**
CC +7th **S36.129 Unspecified injury of gallbladder**
CC X+7th **S36.13 Injury of bile duct**
\+ **S36.2 Injury of pancreas**
\+ **S36.20 Unspecified injury of pancreas**
CC +7th **S36.200 Unspecified injury of head of pancreas**
CC +7th **S36.201 Unspecified injury of body of pancreas**
CC +7th **S36.202Unspecified injury of tail of pancreas**
CC +7th **S36.209 Unspecified injury of unspecified part of pancreas**
\+ **S36.22 Contusion of pancreas**
CC **S36.220 Contusion of head of pancreas**
CC **S36.221 Contusion of body of pancreas**
CC **S36.222 Contusion of tail of pancreas**
CC **S36.229 Contusion of unspecified part of pancreas**
\+ **S36.23 Laceration of pancreas, unspecified degree**
CC +7th **S36.230 Laceration of head of pancreas, unspecified degree**
CC +7th **S36.231 Laceration of body of pancreas, unspecified degree**
CC +7th **S36.232 Laceration of tail of pancreas, unspecified degree**
CC +7th **S36.239 Laceration of unspecified part of pancreas, unspecified degree**
\+ **S36.24 Minor laceration of pancreas**
CC +7th **S36.240 Minor laceration of head of pancreas**
CC +7th **S36.241 Minor laceration of body of pancreas**
CC +7th **S36.242 Minor laceration of tail of pancreas**
CC +7th **S36.249 Minor laceration of unspecified part of pancreas**
\+ **S36.25 Moderate laceration of pancreas**
CC +7th **S36.250 Moderate laceration of head of pancreas**
CC +7th **S36.251 Moderate laceration of body of pancreas**
CC +7th **S36.252 Moderate laceration of tail of pancreas**
CC +7th **S36.259 Moderate laceration of unspecified part of pancreas**
\+ **S36.26 Major laceration of pancreas**
CC +7th **S36.260 Major laceration of head of pancreas**
CC +7th **S36.261 Major laceration of body of pancreas**
CC +7th **S36.262 Major laceration of tail of pancreas**
CC +7th **S36.269 Major laceration of unspecified part of pancreas**
\+ **S36.29 Other injury of pancreas**
CC +7th **S36.290 Other injury of head of pancreas**
CC +7th **S36.291 Other injury of body of pancreas**
CC +7th **S36.292 Other injury of tail of pancreas**
CC +7th **S36.299 Other injury of unspecified part of pancreas**
\+ **S36.3 Injury of stomach**
CC X+7th **S36.30 Unspecified injury of stomach**
CC X+7th **S36.32 Contusion of stomach**
CC X+7th **S36.33 Laceration of stomach**
CC X+7th **S36.39 Other injury of stomach**
\+ **S36.4 Injury of small intestine**
\+ **S36.40 Unspecified injury of small intestine**
CC +7th **S36.400 Unspecified injury of duodenum**
CC +7th **S36.408 Unspecified injury of other part of small intestine**
CC +7th **S36.409 Unspecified injury of unspecified part of small intestine**
\+ **S36.41 Primary blast injury of small intestine**
Blast injury of small intestine NOS
CC +7th **S36.410 Primary blast injury of duodenum**
CC +7th **S36.418 Primary blast injury of other part of small intestine**
CC +7th **S36.419 Primary blast injury of unspecified part of small intestine**
\+ **S36.42 Contusion of small intestine**
CC +7th **S36.420 Contusion of duodenum**
CC +7th **S36.428 Contusion of other part of small intestine**
CC +7th **S36.429 Contusion of unspecified part of small intestine**
\+ **S36.43 Laceration of small intestine**
CC +7th **S36.430 Laceration of duodenum**
CC +7th **S36.438 Laceration of other part of small intestine**
CC +7th **S36.439 Laceration of unspecified part of small intestine**
\+ **S36.49 Other injury of small intestine**
CC +7th **S36.490 Other injury of duodenum**
CC +7th **S36.498 Other injury of other part of small intestine**
CC +7th **S36.499 Other injury of unspecified part of small intestine**
S36.5 Injury of colon
Excludes2: *injury of rectum (S36.6-)*
\+ **S36.50 Unspecified injury of colon**
CC +7th **S36.500 Unspecified injury of ascending [right] colon**
CC +7th **S36.501 Unspecified injury of transverse colon**
CC +7th **S36.502 Unspecified injury of descending [left] colon**
CC +7th **S36.503 Unspecified injury of sigmoid colon**
CC +7th **S36.508 Unspecified injury of other part of colon**
CC +7th **S36.509 Unspecified injury of unspecified part of colon**

Shoulder

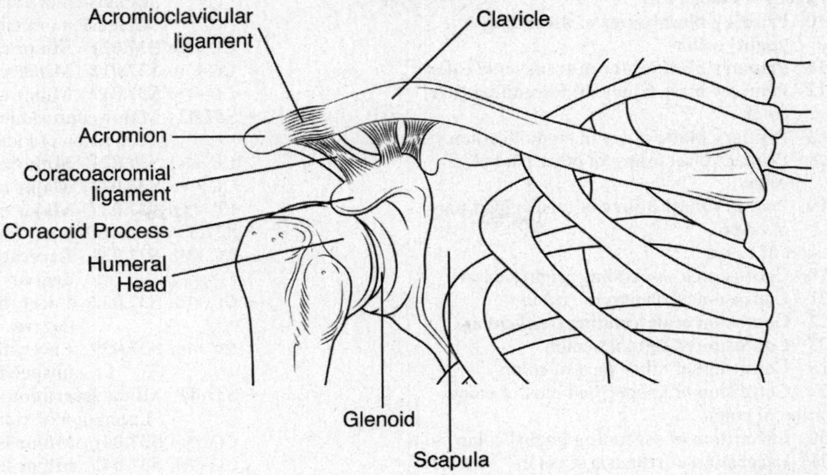

Shoulder Tendons

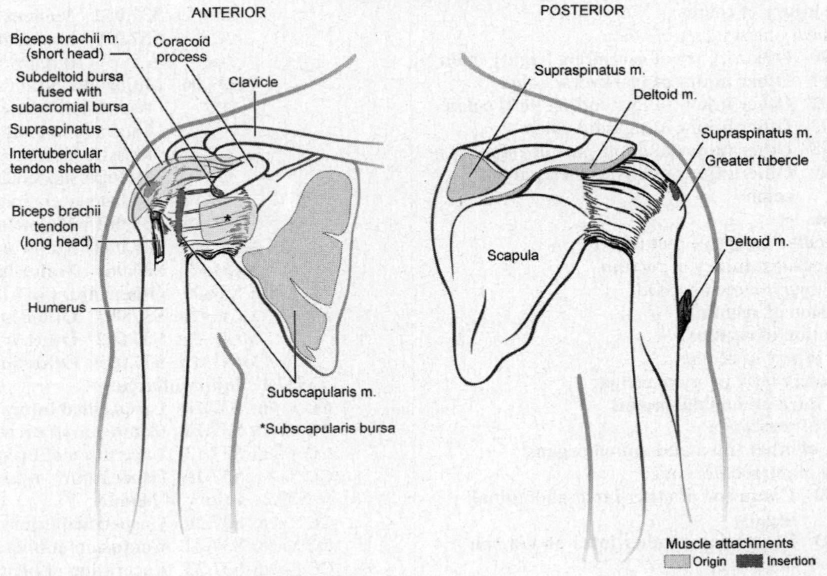

Shoulder Ligaments

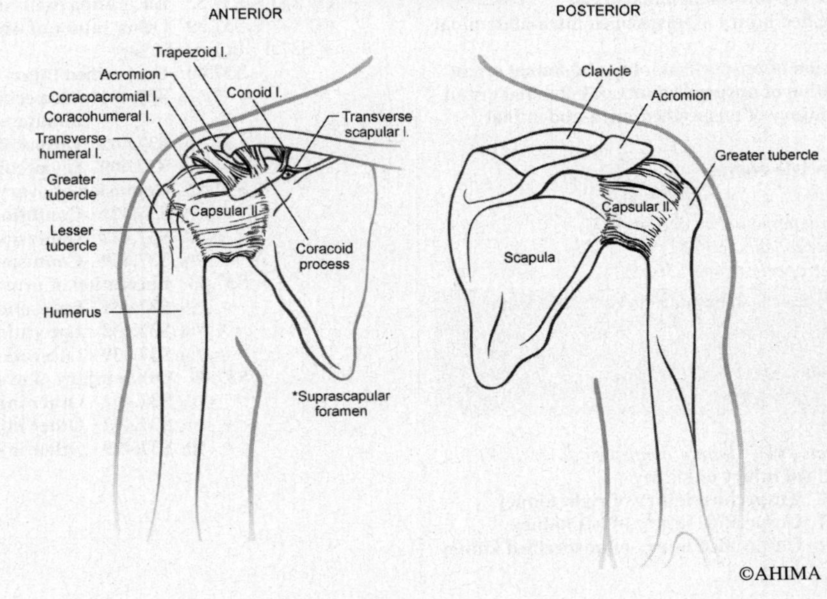

+ **S36.51 Primary blast injury of colon**
Blast injury of colon NOS
CC +7th **S36.510 Primary blast injury of ascending [right] colon**
CC +7th **S36.511 Primary blast injury of transverse colon**
CC +7th **S36.512 Primary blast injury of descending [left] colon**
CC +7th **S36.513 Primary blast injury of sigmoid colon**
CC +7th **S36.518 Primary blast injury of other part of colon**
CC +7th **S36.519 Primary blast injury of unspecified part of colon**
+ **S36.52 Contusion of colon**
CC +7th **S36.520 Contusion of ascending [right] colon**
CC +7th **S36.521 Contusion of transverse colon**
CC +7th **S36.522 Contusion of descending [left] colon**
CC +7th **S36.523 Contusion of sigmoid colon**
CC +7th **S36.528 Contusion of other part of colon**
CC +7th **S36.529 Contusion of unspecified part of colon**
+ **S36.53 Laceration of colon**
CC +7th **S36.530 Laceration of ascending [right] colon**
CC +7th **S36.531 Laceration of transverse colon**
CC +7th **S36.532 Laceration of descending [left] colon**
CC +7th **S36.533 Laceration of sigmoid colon**
CC +7th **S36.538 Laceration of other part of colon**
CC +7th **S36.539 Laceration of unspecified part of colon**
+ **S36.59 Other injury of colon**
Secondary blast injury of colon
CC +7th **S36.590 Other injury of ascending [right] colon**
CC +7th **S36.591 Other injury of transverse colon**
CC +7th **S36.592 Other injury of descending [left] colon**
CC +7th **S36.593 Other injury of sigmoid colon**
CC +7th **S36.598 Other injury of other part of colon**
CC +7th **S36.599 Other injury of unspecified part of colon**
+ **S36.6 Injury of rectum**
CC X+7th **S36.60 Unspecified injury of rectum**
CC X+7th **S36.61 Primary blast injury of rectum**
Blast injury of rectum NOS
CC X+7th **S36.62 Contusion of rectum**
CC X+7th **S36.63 Laceration of rectum**
CC X+7th **S36.69 Other injury of rectum**
Secondary blast injury of rectum
+ **S36.8 Injury of other intra-abdominal organs**
CC X+7th **S36.81 Injury of peritoneum**
+ **S36.89 Injury of other intra-abdominal organs**
Injury of retroperitoneum
CC +7th **S36.892 Contusion of other intra-abdominal organs**
CC +7th **S36.893 Laceration of other intra-abdominal organs**
CC +7th **S36.898 Other injury of other intra-abdominal organs**
CC +7th **S36.899 Unspecified injury of other intra-abdominal organs**
+ **S36.9 Injury of unspecified intra-abdominal organ**
CC X+7th **S36.90 Unspecified injury of unspecified intra-abdominal organ**
CC X+7th **S36.92 Contusion of unspecified intra-abdominal organ**
CC X+7th **S36.93 Laceration of unspecified intra-abdominal organ**
CC X+7th **S36.99 Other injury of unspecified intra-abdominal organ**

S37 Injury of urinary and pelvic organs

Code also any associated open wound (S31.-)
Excludes1: *obstetric trauma to pelvic organs (O71.-)*
Excludes2: *injury of peritoneum (S36.81)*
injury of retroperitoneum (S36.89-)

The appropriate 7th character is to be added to each code from category S37
A initial encounter
D subsequent encounter
S sequela

+ **S37.0 Injury of kidney**
Excludes2: *acute kidney injury (nontraumatic) (N17.9)*
+ **S37.00 Unspecified injury of kidney**
CC +7th **S37.001 Unspecified injury of right kidney**
CC +7th **S37.002 Unspecified injury of left kidney**
CC +7th **S37.009 Unspecified injury of unspecified kidney**
+ **S37.01 Minor contusion of kidney**
Contusion of kidney less than 2 cm
Contusion of kidney NOS
CC +7th **S37.011 Minor contusion of right kidney**
CC +7th **S37.012 Minor contusion of left kidney**
CC +7th **S37.019 Minor contusion of unspecified kidney**
+ **S37.02 Major contusion of kidney**
Contusion of kidney greater than 2 cm
CC +7th **S37.021 Major contusion of right kidney**
CC +7th **S37.022 Major contusion of left kidney**
CC +7th **S37.029 Major contusion of unspecified kidney**
+ **S37.03 Laceration of kidney, unspecified degree**
CC +7th **S37.031 Laceration of right kidney, unspecified degree**
CC +7th **S37.032 Laceration of left kidney, unspecified degree**
CC +7th **S37.039 Laceration of unspecified kidney, unspecified degree**
+ **S37.04 Minor laceration of kidney**
Laceration of kidney less than 1 cm
CC +7th **S37.041 Minor laceration of right kidney**
CC +7th **S37.042 Minor laceration of left kidney**
CC +7th **S37.049 Minor laceration of unspecified kidney**
+ **S37.05 Moderate laceration of kidney**
Laceration of kidney 1 to 3 cm
CC +7th **S37.051 Moderate laceration of right kidney**
CC +7th **S37.052 Moderate laceration of left kidney**
CC +7th **S37.059 Moderate laceration of unspecified kidney**
+ **S37.06 Major laceration of kidney**
Avulsion of kidney
Laceration of kidney greater than 3 cm
Massive laceration of kidney
Multiple moderate lacerations of kidney
Stellate laceration of kidney
MCC +7th **S37.061 Major laceration of right kidney**
MCC +7th **S37.062 Major laceration of left kidney**
MCC +7th **S37.069 Major laceration of unspecified kidney**
+ **S37.09 Other injury of kidney**
MCC +7th **S37.091 Other injury of right kidney**
MCC +7th **S37.092 Other injury of left kidney**
MCC +7th **S37.099 Other injury of unspecified kidney**
+ **S37.1 Injury of ureter**
CC X+7th **S37.10 Unspecified injury of ureter**
CC X+7th **S37.12 Contusion of ureter**
CC X+7th **S37.13 Laceration of ureter**
CC X+7th **S37.19 Other injury of ureter**
+ **S37.2 Injury of bladder**
CC X+7th **S37.20 Unspecified injury of bladder**
CC X+7th **S37.22 Contusion of bladder**
CC X+7th **S37.23 Laceration of bladder**
CC X+7th **S37.29 Other injury of bladder**
+ **S37.3 Injury of urethra**
CC X+7th **S37.30 Unspecified injury of urethra**
CC X+7th **S37.32 Contusion of urethra**
CC X+7th **S37.33 Laceration of urethra**
CC X+7th **S37.39 Other injury of urethra**
+ **S37.4 Injury of ovary**
+ **S37.40 Unspecified injury of ovary**
♀ +7th **S37.401 Unspecified injury of ovary, unilateral**
♀ +7th **S37.402 Unspecified injury of ovary, bilateral**
♀ +7th **S37.409 Unspecified injury of ovary, unspecified**
+ **S37.42 Contusion of ovary**
♀ +7th **S37.421 Contusion of ovary, unilateral**
♀ +7th **S37.422 Contusion of ovary, bilateral**
♀ +7th **S37.429 Contusion of ovary, unspecified**
+ **S37.43 Laceration of ovary**
♀ +7th **S37.431 Laceration of ovary, unilateral**
♀ +7th **S37.432 Laceration of ovary, bilateral**
♀ +7th **S37.439 Laceration of ovary, unspecified**
+ **S37.49 Other injury of ovary**
♀ +7th **S37.491 Other injury of ovary, unilateral**
♀ +7th **S37.492 Other injury of ovary, bilateral**
♀ +7th **S37.499 Other injury of ovary, unspecified**

+ S37.5 **Injury of fallopian tube**
+ S37.50 **Unspecified injury of fallopian tube**
♀ +7th S37.501 **Unspecified injury of fallopian tube, unilateral**
♀ +7th S37.502 **Unspecified injury of fallopian tube, bilateral**
♀ +7th S37.509 **Unspecified injury of fallopian tube, unspecified**
+ S37.51 **Primary blast injury of fallopian tube**
Blast injury of fallopian tube NOS
♀ +7th S37.511 **Primary blast injury of fallopian tube, unilateral**
♀ +7th S37.512 **Primary blast injury of fallopian tube, bilateral**
♀ +7th S37.519 **Primary blast injury of fallopian tube, unspecified**
+ S37.52 **Contusion of fallopian tube**
♀ +7th S37.521 **Contusion of fallopian tube, unilateral**
♀ +7th S37.522 **Contusion of fallopian tube, bilateral**
♀ +7th S37.529 **Contusion of fallopian tube, unspecified**
+ S37.53 **Laceration of fallopian tube**
♀ +7th S37.531 **Laceration of fallopian tube, unilateral**
♀ +7th S37.532 **Laceration of fallopian tube, bilateral**
♀ +7th S37.539 **Laceration of fallopian tube, unspecified**
+ S37.59 **Other injury of fallopian tube**
Secondary blast injury of fallopian tube
♀ +7th S37.591 **Other injury of fallopian tube, unilateral**
♀ +7th S37.592 **Other injury of fallopian tube, bilateral**
♀ +7th S37.599 **Other injury of fallopian tube, unspecified**
+ S37.6 **Injury of uterus**
Excludes1: *injury to gravid uterus (O9A.2-)*
injury to uterus during delivery (O71.-)
♀ CC X+7th S37.60 **Unspecified injury of uterus**
♀ CC X+7th S37.62 **Contusion of uterus**
♀ CC X+7th S37.63 **Laceration of uterus**
♀ CC X+7th S37.69 **Other injury of uterus**
+ S37.8 **Injury of other urinary and pelvic organs**
+ S37.81 **Injury of adrenal gland**
CC +7th S37.812 **Contusion of adrenal gland**
CC +7th S37.813 **Laceration of adrenal gland**
CC +7th S37.818 **Other injury of adrenal gland**
CC +7th S37.819 **Unspecified injury of adrenal gland**
+ S37.82 **Injury of prostate**
♂ +7th S37.822 **Contusion of prostate**
♂ +7th S37.823 **Laceration of prostate**
♂ +7th S37.828 **Other injury of prostate**
♂ +7th S37.829 **Unspecified injury of prostate**
+ S37.89 **Injury of other urinary and pelvic organ**
CC +7th S37.892 **Contusion of other urinary and pelvic organ**
CC +7th S37.893 **Laceration of other urinary and pelvic organ**
CC +7th S37.898 **Other injury of other urinary and pelvic organ**
CC +7th S37.899 **Unspecified injury of other urinary and pelvic organ**
+ S37.9 **Injury of unspecified urinary and pelvic organ**
CC X+7th S37.90 **Unspecified injury of unspecified urinary and pelvic organ**
CC X+7th S37.92 **Contusion of unspecified urinary and pelvic organ**
CC X+7th S37.93 **Laceration of unspecified urinary and pelvic organ**
CC X+7th S37.99 **Other injury of unspecified urinary and pelvic organ**

S38 **Crushing injury and traumatic amputation of abdomen, lower back, pelvis and external genitals**

An amputation not identified as partial or complete should be coded to complete

The appropriate 7th character is to be added to each code from category S38
A initial encounter
D subsequent encounter
S sequela

+ S38.0 **Crushing injury of external genital organs**
Use additional code for any associated injuries
+ S38.00 **Crushing injury of unspecified external genital organs**
♂ +7th S38.001 **Crushing injury of unspecified external genital organs, male**
♀ +7th S38.002 **Crushing injury of unspecified external genital organs, female**
♂ X+7th S38.01 **Crushing injury of penis**
♂ X+7th S38.02 **Crushing injury of scrotum and testis**
♀ X+7th S38.03 **Crushing injury of vulva**
X+7th S38.1 **Crushing injury of abdomen, lower back, and pelvis**
Use additional code for all associated injuries, such as:
fracture of thoracic or lumbar spine and pelvis (S22.0-, S32.-)
injury to intra-abdominal organs (S36.-)
injury to urinary and pelvic organs (S37.-)
open wound of abdominal wall (S31.-)
spinal cord injury (S34.0, S34.1-)
Excludes2: *crushing injury of external genital organs (S38.0-)*
+ S38.2 **Traumatic amputation of external genital organs**
+ S38.21 **Traumatic amputation of female external genital organs**
Traumatic amputation of clitoris
Traumatic amputation of labium (majus) (minus)
Traumatic amputation of vulva
♀ +7th S38.211 **Complete traumatic amputation of female external genital organs**
♀ +7th S38.212 **Partial traumatic amputation of female external genital organs**
+ S38.22 **Traumatic amputation of penis**
♂ +7th S38.221 **Complete traumatic amputation of penis**
♂ +7th S38.222 **Partial traumatic amputation of penis**
+ S38.23 **Traumatic amputation of scrotum and testis**
♂ +7th S38.231 **Complete traumatic amputation of scrotum and testis**
♂ +7th S38.232 **Partial traumatic amputation of scrotum and testis**
X+7th S38.3 **Transection (partial) of abdomen**

S39 **Other and unspecified injuries of abdomen, lower back, pelvis and external genitals**

Code also any associated open wound (S31.-)
Excludes2: *sprain of joints and ligaments of lumbar spine and pelvis (S33.-)*

The appropriate 7th character is to be added to each code from category S39
A initial encounter
D subsequent encounter
S sequela

+ S39.0 **Injury of muscle, fascia and tendon of abdomen, lower back and pelvis**
+ S39.00 **Unspecified injury of muscle, fascia and tendon of abdomen, lower back and pelvis**
+7th S39.001 **Unspecified injury of muscle, fascia and tendon of abdomen**
+7th S39.002 **Unspecified injury of muscle, fascia and tendon of lower back**
+7th S39.003 **Unspecified injury of muscle, fascia and tendon of pelvis**

+ **S39.01 Strain of muscle, fascia and tendon of abdomen, lower back and pelvis**
  - +7th **S39.011 Strain of muscle, fascia and tendon of abdomen**
  - +7th **S39.012 Strain of muscle, fascia and tendon of lower back**
    AHA CC: 4Q, 2016, 73-74
  - +7th **S39.013 Strain of muscle, fascia and tendon of pelvis**
+ **S39.02 Laceration of muscle, fascia and tendon of abdomen, lower back and pelvis**
  - +7th **S39.021 Laceration of muscle, fascia and tendon of abdomen**
  - +7th **S39.022 Laceration of muscle, fascia and tendon of lower back**
  - +7th **S39.023 Laceration of muscle, fascia and tendon of pelvis**
+ **S39.09 Other injury of muscle, fascia and tendon of abdomen, lower back and pelvis**
  - +7th **S39.091 Other injury of muscle, fascia and tendon of abdomen**
  - +7th **S39.092 Other injury of muscle, fascia and tendon of lower back**
  - +7th **S39.093 Other injury of muscle, fascia and tendon of pelvis**

+ **S39.8 Other specified injuries of abdomen, lower back, pelvis and external genitals**
  - X+7th **S39.81 Other specified injuries of abdomen**
  - X+7th **S39.82 Other specified injuries of lower back**
  - X+7th **S39.83 Other specified injuries of pelvis**
  - + **S39.84 Other specified injuries of external genitals**
    - ♂ X+7th **S39.840 Fracture of corpus cavernosum penis**
    - X+7th **S39.848 Other specified injuries of external genitals**
+ **S39.9 Unspecified injury of abdomen, lower back, pelvis and external genitals**
  - X+7th **S39.91 Unspecified injury of abdomen**
  - X+7th **S39.92 Unspecified injury of lower back**
  - X+7th **S39.93 Unspecified injury of pelvis**
  - X+7th **S39.94 Unspecified injury of external genitals**

Injuries to the shoulder and upper arm (S40-S49)

Includes: injuries of axilla
injuries of scapular region

Excludes2: *and corrosions (T20-T32)*
frostbite (T33-T34)
injuries of elbow (S50-S59)
insect bite or sting, venomous (T63.4)

S40 Superficial injury of shoulder and upper arm

> The appropriate 7th character is to be added to each code from category S40
> A initial encounter
> D subsequent encounter
> S sequela

+ **S40.0 Contusion of shoulder and upper arm**
  - + **S40.01 Contusion of shoulder**
    - +7th **S40.011 Contusion of right shoulder**
    - +7th **S40.012 Contusion of left shoulder**
    - +7th **S40.019 Contusion of unspecified shoulder**
  - + **S40.02 Contusion of upper arm**
    - +7th **S40.021 Contusion of right upper arm**
    - +7th **S40.022 Contusion of left upper arm**
    - +7th **S40.029 Contusion of unspecified upper arm**
+ **S40.2 Other superficial injuries of shoulder**
  - + **S40.21 Abrasion of shoulder**
    - +7th **S40.211 Abrasion of right shoulder**
    - +7th **S40.212 Abrasion of left shoulder**
    - +7th **S40.219 Abrasion of unspecified shoulder**
  - + **S40.22 Blister (nonthermal) of shoulder**
    - +7th **S40.221 Blister (nonthermal) of right shoulder**
    - +7th **S40.222 Blister (nonthermal) of left shoulder**
    - +7th **S40.229 Blister (nonthermal) of unspecified shoulder**
  - + **S40.24 External constriction of shoulder**
    - +7th **S40.241 External constriction of right shoulder**
    - +7th **S40.242 External constriction of left shoulder**
    - +7th **S40.249 External constriction of unspecified shoulder**
  - + **S40.25 Superficial foreign body of shoulder**
    Splinter in the shoulder
    - +7th **S40.251 Superficial foreign body of right shoulder**
    - +7th **S40.252 Superficial foreign body of left shoulder**
    - +7th **S40.259 Superficial foreign body of unspecified shoulder**
  - + **S40.26 Insect bite (nonvenomous) of shoulder**
    - +7th **S40.261 Insect bite (nonvenomous) of right shoulder**
    - +7th **S40.262 Insect bite (nonvenomous) of left shoulder**
    - +7th **S40.269 Insect bite (nonvenomous) of unspecified shoulder**
  - + **S40.27 Other superficial bite of shoulder**
    Excludes1: *open bite of shoulder (S41.05)*
    - +7th **S40.271 Other superficial bite of right shoulder**
    - +7th **S40.272 Other superficial bite of left shoulder**
    - +7th **S40.279 Other superficial bite of unspecified shoulder**
+ **S40.8 Other superficial injuries of upper arm**
  - + **S40.81 Abrasion of upper arm**
    - +7th **S40.811 Abrasion of right upper arm**
    - +7th **S40.812 Abrasion of left upper arm**
    - +7th **S40.819 Abrasion of unspecified upper arm**
  - + **S40.82 Blister (nonthermal) of upper arm**
    - +7th **S40.821 Blister (nonthermal) of right upper arm**
    - +7th **S40.822 Blister (nonthermal) of left upper arm**
    - +7th **S40.829 Blister (nonthermal) of unspecified upper arm**
  - + **S40.84 External constriction of upper arm**
    - +7th **S40.841 External constriction of right upper arm**
    - +7th **S40.842 External constriction of left upper arm**
    - +7th **S40.849 External constriction of unspecified upper arm**
  - + **S40.85 Superficial foreign body of upper arm**
    Splinter in the upper arm
    - +7th **S40.851 Superficial foreign body of right upper arm**
    - +7th **S40.852 Superficial foreign body of left upper arm**
    - +7th **S40.859 Superficial foreign body of unspecified upper arm**
  - + **S40.86 Insect bite (nonvenomous) of upper arm**
    - +7th **S40.861 Insect bite (nonvenomous) of right upper arm**
    - +7th **S40.862 Insect bite (nonvenomous) of left upper arm**
    - +7th **S40.869 Insect bite (nonvenomous) of unspecified upper arm**
  - + **S40.87 Other superficial bite of upper arm**
    Excludes1: *open bite of upper arm (S41.14)*
    Excludes2: *other superficial bite of shoulder (S40.27-)*
    - +7th **S40.871 Other superficial bite of right upper arm**
    - +7th **S40.872 Other superficial bite of left upper arm**
    - +7th **S40.879 Other superficial bite of unspecified upper arm**
+ **S40.9 Unspecified superficial injury of shoulder and upper arm**
  - + **S40.91 Unspecified superficial injury of shoulder**
    - +7th **S40.911 Unspecified superficial injury of right shoulder**
    - +7th **S40.912 Unspecified superficial injury of left shoulder**
    - +7th **S40.919 Unspecified superficial injury of unspecified shoulder**
  - + **S40.92 Unspecified superficial injury of upper arm**
    - +7th **S40.921 Unspecified superficial injury of right upper arm**
    - +7th **S40.922 Unspecified superficial injury of left upper arm**
    - +7th **S40.929 Unspecified superficial injury of unspecified upper arm**

S41 Open wound of shoulder and upper arm

Code also any associated wound infection

Excludes1: *traumatic amputation of shoulder and upper arm (S48.-)*

Excludes2: *open fracture of shoulder and upper arm (S42.- with 7th character B or C)*

The appropriate 7th character is to be added to each code from category S41
A initial encounter
D subsequent encounter
S sequela

+ **S41.0 Open wound of shoulder**
  + **S41.00 Unspecified open wound of shoulder**
    - +7th **S41.001 Unspecified open wound of right shoulder**
    - +7th **S41.002 Unspecified open wound of left shoulder**
    - +7th **S41.009 Unspecified open wound of unspecified shoulder**
  + **S41.01 Laceration without foreign body of shoulder**
    - +7th **S41.011 Laceration without foreign body of right shoulder**
    - +7th **S41.012 Laceration without foreign body of left shoulder**
    - +7th **S41.019 Laceration without foreign body of unspecified shoulder**
  + **S41.02 Laceration with foreign body of shoulder**
    - +7th **S41.021 Laceration with foreign body of right shoulder**
    - +7th **S41.022 Laceration with foreign body of left shoulder**
    - +7th **S41.029 Laceration with foreign body of unspecified shoulder**
  + **S41.03 Puncture wound without foreign body of shoulder**
    - +7th **S41.031 Puncture wound without foreign body of right shoulder**
    - +7th **S41.032 Puncture wound without foreign body of left shoulder**
    - +7th **S41.039 Puncture wound without foreign body of unspecified shoulder**
  + **S41.04 Puncture wound with foreign body of shoulder**
    - +7th **S41.041 Puncture wound with foreign body of right shoulder**
    - +7th **S41.042 Puncture wound with foreign body of left shoulder**
    - +7th **S41.049 Puncture wound with foreign body of unspecified shoulder**
  + **S41.05 Open bite of shoulder**
    Bite of shoulder NOS
    Excludes1: *superficial bite of shoulder (S40.27)*
    - +7th **S41.051 Open bite of right shoulder**
    - +7th **S41.052 Open bite of left shoulder**
    - +7th **S41.059 Open bite of unspecified shoulder**
+ **S41.1 Open wound of upper arm**
  + **S41.10 Unspecified open wound of upper arm**
    - +7th **S41.101 Unspecified open wound of right upper arm**
    - +7th **S41.102 Unspecified open wound of left upper arm**
    - +7th **S41.109 Unspecified open wound of unspecified upper arm**
  + **S41.11 Laceration without foreign body of upper arm**
    - **S41.111 Laceration without foreign body of right upper arm**
    - **S41.112 Laceration without foreign body of left upper arm**
    - **S41.119 Laceration without foreign body of unspecified upper arm**
  + **S41.12 Laceration with foreign body of upper arm**
    - +7th **S41.121 Laceration with foreign body of right upper arm**
    - +7th **S41.122 Laceration with foreign body of left upper arm**
    - +7th **S41.129 Laceration with foreign body of unspecified upper arm**
  + **S41.13 Puncture wound without foreign body of upper arm**
    - +7th **S41.131 Puncture wound without foreign body of right upper arm**
    - +7th **S41.132 Puncture wound without foreign body of left upper arm**
    - +7th **S41.139 Puncture wound without foreign body of unspecified upper arm**
  + **S41.14 Puncture wound with foreign body of upper arm**
    - +7th **S41.141 Puncture wound with foreign body of right upper arm**
    - +7th **S41.142 Puncture wound with foreign body of left upper arm**
    - +7th **S41.149 Puncture wound with foreign body of unspecified upper arm**
  + **S41.15 Open bite of upper arm**
    Bite of upper arm NOS
    Excludes1: *superficial bite of upper arm (S40.87)*
    - +7th **S41.151 Open bite of right upper arm**
    - +7th **S41.152 Open bite of left upper arm**
    - +7th **S41.159 Open bite of unspecified upper arm**

S42 Fracture of shoulder and upper arm

NOTE A fracture not indicated as displaced or nondisplaced should be coded to displaced
A fracture not indicated as open or closed should be coded to closed unless otherwise indicated.

Excludes1: *traumatic amputation of shoulder and upper arm (S48.-)*

The appropriate 7th character is to be added to all codes from category S42
A initial encounter for closed fracture
B initial encounter for open fracture
D subsequent encounter for fracture with routine healing
G subsequent encounter for fracture with delayed healing
K subsequent encounter for fracture with nonunion
P subsequent encounter for fracture with malunion
S sequela

Review coding guideline C.19.c

+ **S42.0 Fracture of clavicle**
  + **S42.00 Fracture of unspecified part of clavicle**
    - CC +7th **S42.001 Fracture of unspecified part of right clavicle**
      HAC 7th character B see Appendix B for HAC conditional logic
    - CC +7th **S42.002 Fracture of unspecified part of left clavicle**
      HAC 7th character B see Appendix B for HAC conditional logic
    - CC +7th **S42.009 Fracture of unspecified part of unspecified clavicle**
      HAC 7th character B see Appendix B for HAC conditional logic
  + **S42.01 Fracture of sternal end of clavicle**
    - CC +7th **S42.011 Anterior displaced fracture of sternal end of right clavicle**
      HAC 7th character B see Appendix B for HAC conditional logic
    - CC +7th **S42.012 Anterior displaced fracture of sternal end of left clavicle**
      HAC 7th character B see Appendix B for HAC conditional logic
    - CC +7th **S42.013 Anterior displaced fracture of sternal end of unspecified clavicle**
      Displaced fracture of sternal end of clavicle NOS
      HAC 7th character B see Appendix B for HAC conditional logic
    - CC +7th **S42.014 Posterior displaced fracture of sternal end of right clavicle**
      HAC 7th character B see Appendix B for HAC conditional logic
    - CC +7th **S42.015 Posterior displaced fracture of sternal end of left clavicle**
      HAC 7th character B see Appendix B for HAC conditional logic
    - CC +7th **S42.016 Posterior displaced fracture of sternal end of unspecified clavicle**
      HAC 7th character B see Appendix B for HAC conditional logic

CC +7th **S42.017** **Nondisplaced fracture of sternal end of right clavicle**
HAC 7th character B see Appendix B for HAC conditional logic

CC +7th **S42.018** **Nondisplaced fracture of sternal end of left clavicle**
HAC 7th character B see Appendix B for HAC conditional logic

CC +7th **S42.019** **Nondisplaced fracture of sternal end of unspecified clavicle**
HAC 7th character B see Appendix B for HAC conditional logic

\+ **S42.02** **Fracture of shaft of clavicle**

CC +7th **S42.021** **Displaced fracture of shaft of right clavicle**
HAC 7th character B see Appendix B for HAC conditional logic

CC +7th **S42.022** **Displaced fracture of shaft of left clavicle**
HAC 7th character B see Appendix B for HAC conditional logic

CC +7th **S42.023** **Displaced fracture of shaft of unspecified clavicle**
HAC 7th character B see Appendix B for HAC conditional logic

CC +7th **S42.024** **Nondisplaced fracture of shaft of right clavicle**
HAC 7th character B see Appendix B for HAC conditional logic

CC +7th **S42.025** **Nondisplaced fracture of shaft of left clavicle**
HAC 7th character B see Appendix B for HAC conditional logic

CC +7th **S42.026** **Nondisplaced fracture of shaft of unspecified clavicle**
HAC 7th character B see Appendix B for HAC conditional logic

\+ **S42.03** **Fracture of lateral end of clavicle**
Fracture of acromial end of clavicle

CC +7th **S42.031** **Displaced fracture of lateral end of right clavicle**
HAC 7th character B see Appendix B for HAC conditional logic

CC +7th **S42.032** **Displaced fracture of lateral end of left clavicle**
HAC 7th character B see Appendix B for HAC conditional logic

CC +7th **S42.033** **Displaced fracture of lateral end of unspecified clavicle**
HAC 7th character B see Appendix B for HAC conditional logic

CC +7th **S42.034** **Nondisplaced fracture of lateral end of right clavicle**
HAC 7th character B see Appendix B for HAC conditional logic

CC +7th **S42.035** **Nondisplaced fracture of lateral end of left clavicle**
HAC 7th character B see Appendix B for HAC conditional logic

CC +7th **S42.036** **Nondisplaced fracture of lateral end of unspecified clavicle**
HAC 7th character B see Appendix B for HAC conditional logic

\+ **S42.1** **Fracture of scapula**

\+ **S42.10** **Fracture of unspecified part of scapula**

CC +7th **S42.101** **Fracture of unspecified part of scapula, right shoulder**
HAC 7th character B see Appendix B for HAC conditional logic

CC +7th **S42.102** **Fracture of unspecified part of scapula, left shoulder**
HAC 7th character B see Appendix B for HAC conditional logic

CC +7th **S42.109** **Fracture of unspecified part of scapula, unspecified shoulder**
HAC 7th character B see Appendix B for HAC conditional logic

\+ **S42.11** **Fracture of body of scapula**

CC +7th **S42.111** **Displaced fracture of body of scapula, right shoulder**
HAC 7th character B see Appendix B for HAC conditional logic

CC +7th **S42.112** **Displaced fracture of body of scapula, left shoulder**
HAC 7th character B see Appendix B for HAC conditional logic

CC +7th **S42.113** **Displaced fracture of body of scapula, unspecified shoulder**
HAC 7th character B see Appendix B for HAC conditional logic

CC +7th **S42.114** **Nondisplaced fracture of body of scapula, right shoulder**
HAC 7th character B see Appendix B for HAC conditional logic

CC +7th **S42.115** **Nondisplaced fracture of body of scapula, left shoulder**
HAC 7th character B see Appendix B for HAC conditional logic

CC +7th **S42.116** **Nondisplaced fracture of body of scapula, unspecified shoulder**
HAC 7th character B see Appendix B for HAC conditional logic

\+ **S42.12** **Fracture of acromial process**

CC +7th **S42.121** **Displaced fracture of acromial process, right shoulder**
HAC 7th character B see Appendix B for HAC conditional logic

CC +7th **S42.122** **Displaced fracture of acromial process, left shoulder**
HAC 7th character B see Appendix B for HAC conditional logic

CC +7th **S42.123** **Displaced fracture of acromial process, unspecified shoulder**
HAC 7th character B see Appendix B for HAC conditional logic

CC +7th **S42.124** **Nondisplaced fracture of acromial process, right shoulder**
HAC 7th character B see Appendix B for HAC conditional logic

CC +7th **S42.125** **Nondisplaced fracture of acromial process, left shoulder**
HAC 7th character B see Appendix B for HAC conditional logic

CC +7th **S42.126** **Nondisplaced fracture of acromial process, unspecified shoulder**
HAC 7th character B see Appendix B for HAC conditional logic

\+ **S42.13** **Fracture of coracoid process**

CC +7th **S42.131** **Displaced fracture of coracoid process, right shoulder**
HAC 7th character B see Appendix B for HAC conditional logic

CC +7th **S42.132** **Displaced fracture of coracoid process, left shoulder**
HAC 7th character B see Appendix B for HAC conditional logic

CC +7th **S42.133** **Displaced fracture of coracoid process, unspecified shoulder**
HAC 7th character B see Appendix B for HAC conditional logic

CC +7th **S42.134** **Nondisplaced fracture of coracoid process, right shoulder**
HAC 7th character B see Appendix B for HAC conditional logic

CC +7th **S42.135** **Nondisplaced fracture of coracoid process, left shoulder**
HAC 7th character B see Appendix B for HAC conditional logic

CC +7th **S42.136** **Nondisplaced fracture of coracoid process, unspecified shoulder**
HAC 7th character B see Appendix B for HAC conditional logic

\+ **S42.14** **Fracture of glenoid cavity of scapula**

CC +7th **S42.141** **Displaced fracture of glenoid cavity of scapula, right shoulder**
HAC 7th character B see Appendix B for HAC conditional logic

CC +7th **S42.142** **Displaced fracture of glenoid cavity of scapula, left shoulder**
HAC 7th character B see Appendix B for HAC conditional logic

CC +7th **S42.143** **Displaced fracture of glenoid cavity of scapula, unspecified shoulder**
HAC 7th character B see Appendix B for HAC conditional logic

CC +7th **S42.144** **Nondisplaced fracture of glenoid cavity of scapula, right shoulder**
HAC 7th character B see Appendix B for HAC conditional logic

CC +7th **S42.145 Nondisplaced fracture of glenoid cavity of scapula, left shoulder**
HAC 7th character B see Appendix B for HAC conditional logic

CC +7th **S42.146 Nondisplaced fracture of glenoid cavity of scapula, unspecified shoulder**
HAC 7th character B see Appendix B for HAC conditional logic

+ **S42.15 Fracture of neck of scapula**

CC +7th **S42.151 Displaced fracture of neck of scapula, right shoulder**
HAC 7th character B see Appendix B for HAC conditional logic

CC +7th **S42.152 Displaced fracture of neck of scapula, left shoulder**
HAC 7th character B see Appendix B for HAC conditional logic

CC +7th **S42.153 Displaced fracture of neck of scapula, unspecified shoulder**
HAC 7th character B see Appendix B for HAC conditional logic

CC +7th **S42.154 Nondisplaced fracture of neck of scapula, right shoulder**
HAC 7th character B see Appendix B for HAC conditional logic

CC +7th **S42.155 Nondisplaced fracture of neck of scapula, left shoulder**
HAC 7th character B see Appendix B for HAC conditional logic

CC +7th **S42.156 Nondisplaced fracture of neck of scapula, unspecified shoulder**
HAC 7th character B see Appendix B for HAC conditional logic

+ **S42.19 Fracture of other part of scapula**

CC +7th **S42.191 Fracture of other part of scapula, right shoulder**
HAC 7th character B see Appendix B for HAC conditional logic

CC +7th **S42.192 Fracture of other part of scapula, left shoulder**
HAC 7th character B see Appendix B for HAC conditional logic

CC +7th **S42.199 Fracture of other part of scapula, unspecified shoulder**
HAC 7th character B see Appendix B for HAC conditional logic

+ **S42.2 Fracture of upper end of humerus**
Fracture of proximal end of humerus
Excludes2: *fracture of shaft of humerus (S42.3-)*
physeal fracture of upper end of humerus (S49.0-)

+ **S42.20 Unspecified fracture of upper end of humerus**

CC MCC +7th **S42.201 Unspecified fracture of upper end of right humerus**
HAC 7th characters A & B see Appendix B for HAC conditional logic

CC MCC +7th **S42.202 Unspecified fracture of upper end of left humerus**
HAC 7th characters A & B see Appendix B for HAC conditional logic

CC MCC +7th **S42.209 Unspecified fracture of upper end of unspecified humerus**
HAC 7th characters A & B see Appendix B for HAC conditional logic

+ **S42.21 Unspecified fracture of surgical neck of humerus**
Fracture of neck of humerus NOS

CC MCC +7th **S42.211 Unspecified displaced fracture of surgical neck of right humerus**
HAC 7th characters A & B see Appendix B for HAC conditional logic

CC MCC +7th **S42.212 Unspecified displaced fracture of surgical neck of left humerus**

CC MCC +7th **S42.213 Unspecified displaced fracture of surgical neck of unspecified humerus**
HAC 7th characters A & B see Appendix B for HAC conditional logic

CC MCC +7th **S42.214 Unspecified nondisplaced fracture of surgical neck of right humerus**
HAC 7th characters A & B see Appendix B for HAC conditional logic

CC MCC +7th **S42.215 Unspecified nondisplaced fracture of surgical neck of left humerus**
HAC 7th characters A & B see Appendix B for HAC conditional logic

CC MCC +7th **S42.216 Unspecified nondisplaced fracture of surgical neck of unspecified humerus**
HAC 7th characters A & B see Appendix B for HAC conditional logic

+ **S42.22 2-part fracture of surgical neck of humerus**

CC MCC +7th **S42.221 2-part displaced fracture of surgical neck of right humerus**
HAC 7th characters A & B see Appendix B for HAC conditional logic

CC MCC +7th **S42.222 2-part displaced fracture of surgical neck of left humerus**
HAC 7th characters A & B see Appendix B for HAC conditional logic

CC MCC +7th **S42.223 2-part displaced fracture of surgical neck of unspecified humerus**
HAC 7th characters A & B see Appendix B for HAC conditional logic

CC MCC +7th **S42.224 2-part nondisplaced fracture of surgical neck of right humerus**
HAC 7th characters A & B see Appendix B for HAC conditional logic

CC MCC +7th **S42.225 2-part nondisplaced fracture of surgical neck of left humerus**
HAC 7th characters A & B see Appendix B for HAC conditional logic

CC MCC +7th **S42.226 2-part nondisplaced fracture of surgical neck of unspecified humerus**
HAC 7th characters A & B see Appendix B for HAC conditional logic

+ **S42.23 3-part fracture of surgical neck of humerus**

CC MCC +7th **S42.231 3-part fracture of surgical neck of right humerus**
HAC 7th characters A & B see Appendix B for HAC conditional logic

CC MCC +7th **S42.232 3-part fracture of surgical neck of left humerus**
HAC 7th characters A & B see Appendix B for HAC conditional logic

CC MCC +7th **S42.239 3-part fracture of surgical neck of unspecified humerus**
HAC 7th characters A & B see Appendix B for HAC conditional logic

+ **S42.24 4-part fracture of surgical neck of humerus**

CC MCC +7th **S42.241 4-part fracture of surgical neck of right humerus**
HAC 7th characters A & B see Appendix B for HAC conditional logic

CC MCC +7th **S42.242 4-part fracture of surgical neck of left humerus**
HAC 7th characters A & B see Appendix B for HAC conditional logic

CC MCC +7th **S42.249 4-part fracture of surgical neck of unspecified humerus**
HAC 7th characters A & B see Appendix B for HAC conditional logic

+ **S42.25 Fracture of greater tuberosity of humerus**

CC MCC +7th **S42.251 Displaced fracture of greater tuberosity of right humerus**
HAC 7th characters A & B see Appendix B for HAC conditional logic

CC MCC +7th **S42.252 Displaced fracture of greater tuberosity of left humerus**
HAC 7th characters A & B see Appendix B for HAC conditional logic

CC MCC +7th **S42.253 Displaced fracture of greater tuberosity of unspecified humerus**
HAC 7th characters A & B see Appendix B for HAC conditional logic

CC MCC +7th **S42.254 Nondisplaced fracture of greater tuberosity of right humerus**
HAC 7th characters A & B see Appendix B for HAC conditional logic

CC MCC +7th **S42.255 Nondisplaced fracture of greater tuberosity of left humerus**
HAC 7th characters A & B see Appendix B for HAC conditional logic

CC MCC +7th **S42.256 Nondisplaced fracture of greater tuberosity of unspecified humerus**
HAC 7th characters A & B see Appendix B for HAC conditional logic

+ **S42.26 Fracture of lesser tuberosity of humerus**

CC MCC +7th **S42.261 Displaced fracture of lesser tuberosity of right humerus**
HAC 7th characters A & B see Appendix B for HAC conditional logic

CC MCC +7th **S42.262 Displaced fracture of lesser tuberosity of left humerus**
HAC 7th characters A & B see Appendix B for HAC conditional logic

CC MCC +7th **S42.263 Displaced fracture of lesser tuberosity of unspecified humerus**
HAC 7th characters A & B see Appendix B for HAC conditional logic

CC MCC +7th **S42.264 Nondisplaced fracture of lesser tuberosity of right humerus**
HAC 7th characters A & B see Appendix B for HAC conditional logic

CC MCC +7th **S42.265 Nondisplaced fracture of lesser tuberosity of left humerus**
HAC 7th characters A & B see Appendix B for HAC conditional logic

CC MCC +7th **S42.266 Nondisplaced fracture of lesser tuberosity of unspecified humerus**
HAC 7th characters A & B see Appendix B for HAC conditional logic

+ **S42.27 Torus fracture of upper end of humerus**

The appropriate 7th character is to be added to all codes in subcategory **S42.27**
A initial encounter for closed fracture
D subsequent encounter for fracture with routine healing
G subsequent encounter for fracture with delayed healing
K subsequent encounter for fracture with nonunion
P subsequent encounter for fracture with malunion
S sequela

CC +7th **S42.271 Torus fracture of upper end of right humerus**
HAC 7th character A see Appendix B for HAC conditional logic

CC +7th **S42.272 Torus fracture of upper end of left humerus**
HAC 7th character A see Appendix B for HAC conditional logic

CC +7th **S42.279 Torus fracture of upper end of unspecified humerus**
HAC 7th character A see Appendix B for HAC conditional logic

+ **S42.29 Other fracture of upper end of humerus**
Fracture of anatomical neck of humerus
Fracture of articular head of humerus

CC MCC +7th **S42.291 Other displaced fracture of upper end of right humerus**
HAC 7th characters A & B see Appendix B for HAC conditional logic

CC MCC +7th **S42.292 Other displaced fracture of upper end of left humerus**
HAC 7th characters A & B see Appendix B for HAC conditional logic

CC MCC +7th **S42.293 Other displaced fracture of upper end of unspecified humerus**
HAC 7th characters A & B see Appendix B for HAC conditional logic

CC MCC +7th **S42.294 Other nondisplaced fracture of upper end of right humerus**
HAC 7th characters A & B see Appendix B for HAC conditional logic

CC MCC +7th **S42.295 Other nondisplaced fracture of upper end of left humerus**
AHA CC: 1Q, 2019, 18-19
HAC 7th characters A & B see Appendix B for HAC conditional logic

CC MCC +7th **S42.296 Other nondisplaced fracture of upper end of unspecified humerus**
HAC 7th characters A & B see Appendix B for HAC conditional logic

+ **S42.3 Fracture of shaft of humerus**
Fracture of humerus NOS
Fracture of upper arm NOS
Excludes2: *physeal fractures of upper end of humerus (S49.0-)*
physeal fractures of lower end of humerus (S49.1-)

+ **S42.30 Unspecified fracture of shaft of humerus**

CC MCC +7th **S42.301 Unspecified fracture of shaft of humerus, right arm**
HAC 7th characters A & B see Appendix B for HAC conditional logic

CC MCC +7th **S42.302 Unspecified fracture of shaft of humerus, left arm**
HAC 7th characters A & B see Appendix B for HAC conditional logic

CC MCC +7th **S42.309 Unspecified fracture of shaft of humerus, unspecified arm**
HAC 7th characters A & B see Appendix B for HAC conditional logic

+ **S42.31 Greenstick fracture of shaft of humerus**

The appropriate 7th character is to be added to all codes in subcategory **S42.31**
A initial encounter for closed fracture
D subsequent encounter for fracture with routine healing
G subsequent encounter for fracture with delayed healing
K subsequent encounter for fracture with nonunion
P subsequent encounter for fracture with malunion
S sequela

CC +7th **S42.311 Greenstick fracture of shaft of humerus, right arm**
HAC 7th character A see Appendix B for HAC conditional logic

CC +7th **S42.312 Greenstick fracture of shaft of humerus, left arm**
HAC 7th character A see Appendix B for HAC conditional logic

CC +7th **S42.319 Greenstick fracture of shaft of humerus, unspecified arm**
HAC 7th character A see Appendix B for HAC conditional logic

+ **S42.32 Transverse fracture of shaft of humerus**

CC MCC +7th **S42.321 Displaced transverse fracture of shaft of humerus, right arm**
HAC 7th characters A & B see Appendix B for HAC conditional logic

CC MCC +7th **S42.322 Displaced transverse fracture of shaft of humerus, left arm**
HAC 7th characters A & B see Appendix B for HAC conditional logic

CC MCC +7th **S42.323 Displaced transverse fracture of shaft of humerus, unspecified arm**
HAC 7th characters A & B see Appendix B for HAC conditional logic

CC MCC +7th **S42.324 Nondisplaced transverse fracture of shaft of humerus, right arm**
HAC 7th characters A & B see Appendix B for HAC conditional logic

CC MCC +7th **S42.325 Nondisplaced transverse fracture of shaft of humerus, left arm**
HAC 7th characters A & B see Appendix B for HAC conditional logic

CC MCC +7th **S42.326 Nondisplaced transverse fracture of shaft of humerus, unspecified arm**
HAC 7th characters A & B see Appendix B for HAC conditional logic

+ **S42.33 Oblique fracture of shaft of humerus**

CC MCC +7th **S42.331 Displaced oblique fracture of shaft of humerus, right arm**
HAC 7th characters A & B see Appendix B for HAC conditional logic

CC MCC +7th **S42.332 Displaced oblique fracture of shaft of humerus, left arm**
HAC 7th characters A & B see Appendix B for HAC conditional logic

CC MCC +7th **S42.333 Displaced oblique fracture of shaft of humerus, unspecified arm**
HAC 7th characters A & B see Appendix B for HAC conditional logic

CC MCC +7th **S42.334 Nondisplaced oblique fracture of shaft of humerus, right arm**
HAC 7th characters A & B see Appendix B for HAC conditional logic

CC MCC +7th **S42.335 Nondisplaced oblique fracture of shaft of humerus, left arm**
HAC 7th characters A & B see Appendix B for HAC conditional logic

CC MCC +7th **S42.336 Nondisplaced oblique fracture of shaft of humerus, unspecified arm**
HAC 7th characters A & B see Appendix B for HAC conditional logic

+ **S42.34 Spiral fracture of shaft of humerus**

CC MCC +7th **S42.341 Displaced spiral fracture of shaft of humerus, right arm**
HAC 7th characters A & B see Appendix B for HAC conditional logic

CC MCC +7th **S42.342 Displaced spiral fracture of shaft of humerus, left arm**
HAC 7th characters A & B see Appendix B for HAC conditional logic

CC MCC +7th **S42.343 Displaced spiral fracture of shaft of humerus, unspecified arm**
HAC 7th characters A & B see Appendix B for HAC conditional logic

CC MCC +7th **S42.344 Nondisplaced spiral fracture of shaft of humerus, right arm**
HAC 7th characters A & B see Appendix B for HAC conditional logic

CC MCC +7th **S42.345 Nondisplaced spiral fracture of shaft of humerus, left arm**
HAC 7th characters A & B see Appendix B for HAC conditional logic

CC MCC +7th **S42.346 Nondisplaced spiral fracture of shaft of humerus, unspecified arm**
HAC 7th characters A & B see Appendix B for HAC conditional logic

+ **S42.35 Comminuted fracture of shaft of humerus**

CC MCC +7th **S42.351 Displaced comminuted fracture of shaft of humerus, right arm**
HAC 7th characters A & B see Appendix B for HAC conditional logic

CC MCC +7th **S42.352 Displaced comminuted fracture of shaft of humerus, left arm**
HAC 7th characters A & B see Appendix B for HAC conditional logic

CC MCC +7th **S42.353 Displaced comminuted fracture of shaft of humerus, unspecified arm**
HAC 7th characters A & B see Appendix B for HAC conditional logic

CC MCC +7th **S42.354 Nondisplaced comminuted fracture of shaft of humerus, right arm**
HAC 7th characters A & B see Appendix B for HAC conditional logic

CC MCC +7th **S42.355 Nondisplaced comminuted fracture of shaft of humerus, left arm**
HAC 7th characters A & B see Appendix B for HAC conditional logic

CC MCC +7th **S42.356 Nondisplaced comminuted fracture of shaft of humerus, unspecified arm**
HAC 7th characters A & B see Appendix B for HAC conditional logic

+ **S42.36 Segmental fracture of shaft of humerus**

CC MCC +7th **S42.361 Displaced segmental fracture of shaft of humerus, right arm**
HAC 7th characters A & B see Appendix B for HAC conditional logic

CC MCC +7th **S42.362 Displaced segmental fracture of shaft of humerus, left arm**
HAC 7th characters A & B see Appendix B for HAC conditional logic

CC MCC +7th **S42.363 Displaced segmental fracture of shaft of humerus, unspecified arm**
HAC 7th characters A & B see Appendix B for HAC conditional logic

CC MCC +7th **S42.364 Nondisplaced segmental fracture of shaft of humerus, right arm**
HAC 7th characters A & B see Appendix B for HAC conditional logic

CC MCC +7th **S42.365 Nondisplaced segmental fracture of shaft of humerus, left arm**
HAC 7th characters A & B see Appendix B for HAC conditional logic

CC MCC +7th **S42.366 Nondisplaced segmental fracture of shaft of humerus, unspecified arm**
HAC 7th characters A & B see Appendix B for HAC conditional logic

+ **S42.39 Other fracture of shaft of humerus**

CC MCC +7th **S42.391 Other fracture of shaft of right humerus**
HAC 7th characters A & B see Appendix B for HAC conditional logic

CC MCC +7th **S42.392 Other fracture of shaft of left humerus**
HAC 7th characters A & B see Appendix B for HAC conditional logic

CC MCC +7th **S42.399 Other fracture of shaft of unspecified humerus**
HAC 7th characters A & B see Appendix B for HAC conditional logic

+ **S42.4 Fracture of lower end of humerus**
Fracture of distal end of humerus
Excludes2: *fracture of shaft of humerus (S42.3-)*
physeal fracture of lower end of humerus (S49.1-)

+ **S42.40 Unspecified fracture of lower end of humerus**
Fracture of elbow NOS

CC MCC +7th **S42.401 Unspecified fracture of lower end of right humerus**
HAC 7th characters A & B see Appendix B for HAC conditional logic

CC MCC +7th **S42.402 Unspecified fracture of lower end of left humerus**
HAC 7th characters A & B see Appendix B for HAC conditional logic

CC MCC +7th **S42.409 Unspecified fracture of lower end of unspecified humerus**
HAC 7th characters A & B see Appendix B for HAC conditional logic

+ **S42.41 Simple supracondylar fracture without intercondylar fracture of humerus**

CC MCC +7th **S42.411 Displaced simple supracondylar fracture without intercondylar fracture of right humerus**
HAC 7th characters A & B see Appendix B for HAC conditional logic

CC MCC +7th **S42.412 Displaced simple supracondylar fracture without intercondylar fracture of left humerus**
HAC 7th characters A & B see Appendix B for HAC conditional logic

CC MCC +7th **S42.413 Displaced simple supracondylar fracture without intercondylar fracture of unspecified humerus**
HAC 7th characters A & B see Appendix B for HAC conditional logic

CC MCC +7th **S42.414 Nondisplaced simple supracondylar fracture without intercondylar fracture of right humerus**
HAC 7th characters A & B see Appendix B for HAC conditional logic

CC MCC +7th **S42.415 Nondisplaced simple supracondylar fracture without intercondylar fracture of left humerus**
HAC 7th characters A & B see Appendix B for HAC conditional logic

CC MCC +7th **S42.416 Nondisplaced simple supracondylar fracture without intercondylar fracture of unspecified humerus**
HAC 7th characters A & B see Appendix B for HAC conditional logic

+ **S42.42 Comminuted supracondylar fracture without intercondylar fracture of humerus**

CC MCC +7th **S42.421 Displaced comminuted supracondylar fracture without intercondylar fracture of right humerus**
HAC 7th characters A & B see Appendix B for HAC conditional logic

CC MCC +7th **S42.422 Displaced comminuted supracondylar fracture without intercondylar fracture of left humerus**
HAC 7th characters A & B see Appendix B for HAC conditional logic

CC MCC +7th **S42.423 Displaced comminuted supracondylar fracture without intercondylar fracture of unspecified humerus**
HAC 7th characters A & B see Appendix B for HAC conditional logic

CC MCC +7th **S42.424 Nondisplaced comminuted supracondylar fracture without intercondylar fracture of right humerus**
HAC 7th characters A & B see Appendix B for HAC conditional logic

CC MCC +7th **S42.425 Nondisplaced comminuted supracondylar fracture without intercondylar fracture of left humerus**
HAC 7th characters A & B see Appendix B for HAC conditional logic

CC MCC +7th **S42.426** **Nondisplaced comminuted supracondylar fracture without intercondylar fracture of unspecified humerus**
HAC 7th characters A & B see Appendix B for HAC conditional logic

+ **S42.43** **Fracture (avulsion) of lateral epicondyle of humerus**

CC MCC +7th **S42.431** **Displaced fracture (avulsion) of lateral epicondyle of right humerus**
HAC 7th characters A & B see Appendix B for HAC conditional logic

CC MCC +7th **S42.432** **Displaced fracture (avulsion) of lateral epicondyle of left humerus**
HAC 7th characters A & B see Appendix B for HAC conditional logic

CC MCC +7th **S42.433** **Displaced fracture (avulsion) of lateral epicondyle of unspecified humerus**
HAC 7th characters A & B see Appendix B for HAC conditional logic

CC MCC +7th **S42.434** **Nondisplaced fracture (avulsion) of lateral epicondyle of right humerus**
HAC 7th characters A & B see Appendix B for HAC conditional logic

CC MCC +7th **S42.435** **Nondisplaced fracture (avulsion) of lateral epicondyle of left humerus**
HAC 7th characters A & B see Appendix B for HAC conditional logic

CC MCC +7th **S42.436** **Nondisplaced fracture (avulsion) of lateral epicondyle of unspecified humerus**
HAC 7th characters A & B see Appendix B for HAC conditional logic

+ **S42.44** **Fracture (avulsion) of medial epicondyle of humerus**

CC MCC +7th **S42.441** **Displaced fracture (avulsion) of medial epicondyle of right humerus**
HAC 7th characters A & B see Appendix B for HAC conditional logic

CC MCC +7th **S42.442** **Displaced fracture (avulsion) of medial epicondyle of left humerus**
HAC 7th characters A & B see Appendix B for HAC conditional logic

CC MCC +7th **S42.443** **Displaced fracture (avulsion) of medial epicondyle of unspecified humerus**
HAC 7th characters A & B see Appendix B for HAC conditional logic

CC MCC +7th **S42.444** **Nondisplaced fracture (avulsion) of medial epicondyle of right humerus**
HAC 7th characters A & B see Appendix B for HAC conditional logic

CC MCC +7th **S42.445** **Nondisplaced fracture (avulsion) of medial epicondyle of left humerus**
HAC 7th characters A & B see Appendix B for HAC conditional logic

CC MCC +7th **S42.446** **Nondisplaced fracture (avulsion) of medial epicondyle of unspecified humerus**
HAC 7th characters A & B see Appendix B for HAC conditional logic

CC MCC +7th **S42.447** **Incarcerated fracture (avulsion) of medial epicondyle of right humerus**
HAC 7th characters A & B see Appendix B for HAC conditional logic

CC MCC +7th **S42.448** **Incarcerated fracture (avulsion) of medial epicondyle of left humerus**
HAC 7th characters A & B see Appendix B for HAC conditional logic

CC MCC +7th **S42.449** **Incarcerated fracture (avulsion) of medial epicondyle of unspecified humerus**
HAC 7th characters A & B see Appendix B for HAC conditional logic

+ **S42.45** **Fracture of lateral condyle of humerus**
Fracture of capitellum of humerus

CC MCC +7th **S42.451** **Displaced fracture of lateral condyle of right humerus**
HAC 7th characters A & B see Appendix B for HAC conditional logic

CC MCC +7th **S42.452** **Displaced fracture of lateral condyle of left humerus**
HAC 7th characters A & B see Appendix B for HAC conditional logic

CC MCC +7th **S42.453** **Displaced fracture of lateral condyle of unspecified humerus**
HAC 7th characters A & B see Appendix B for HAC conditional logic

CC MCC +7th **S42.454** **Nondisplaced fracture of lateral condyle of right humerus**
HAC 7th characters A & B see Appendix B for HAC conditional logic

CC MCC +7th **S42.455** **Nondisplaced fracture of lateral condyle of left humerus**
HAC 7th characters A & B see Appendix B for HAC conditional logic

CC MCC +7th **S42.456** **Nondisplaced fracture of lateral condyle of unspecified humerus**
HAC 7th characters A & B see Appendix B for HAC conditional logic

+ **S42.46** **Fracture of medial condyle of humerus**
Trochlea fracture of humerus

CC MCC +7th **S42.461** **Displaced fracture of medial condyle of right humerus**
HAC 7th characters A & B see Appendix B for HAC conditional logic

CC MCC +7th **S42.462** **Displaced fracture of medial condyle of left humerus**
HAC 7th characters A & B see Appendix B for HAC conditional logic

CC MCC +7th **S42.463** **Displaced fracture of medial condyle of unspecified humerus**
HAC 7th characters A & B see Appendix B for HAC conditional logic

CC MCC +7th **S42.464** **Nondisplaced fracture of medial condyle of right humerus**
HAC 7th characters A & B see Appendix B for HAC conditional logic

CC MCC +7th **S42.465** **Nondisplaced fracture of medial condyle of left humerus**
HAC 7th characters A & B see Appendix B for HAC conditional logic

CC MCC +7th **S42.466** **Nondisplaced fracture of medial condyle of unspecified humerus**
HAC 7th characters A & B see Appendix B for HAC conditional logic

+ **S42.47** **Transcondylar fracture of humerus**

CC MCC +7th **S42.471** **Displaced transcondylar fracture of right humerus**
HAC 7th characters A & B see Appendix B for HAC conditional logic

CC MCC +7th **S42.472** **Displaced transcondylar fracture of left humerus**
HAC 7th characters A & B see Appendix B for HAC conditional logic

CC MCC +7th **S42.473** **Displaced transcondylar fracture of unspecified humerus**
HAC 7th characters A & B see Appendix B for HAC conditional logic

CC MCC +7th **S42.474** **Nondisplaced transcondylar fracture of right humerus**
HAC 7th characters A & B see Appendix B for HAC conditional logic

CC MCC +7th **S42.475** **Nondisplaced transcondylar fracture of left humerus**
HAC 7th characters A & B see Appendix B for HAC conditional logic

CC MCC +7th **S42.476** **Nondisplaced transcondylar fracture of unspecified humerus**
HAC 7th characters A & B see Appendix B for HAC conditional logic

+ **S42.48** **Torus fracture of lower end of humerus**

The appropriate 7th character is to be added to all codes in subcategory **S42.48**
A initial encounter for closed fracture
D subsequent encounter for fracture with routine healing
G subsequent encounter for fracture with delayed healing
K subsequent encounter for fracture with nonunion
P subsequent encounter for fracture with malunion
S sequela

CC +7th **S42.481** **Torus fracture of lower end of right humerus**
HAC 7th character A see Appendix B for HAC conditional logic

CC +7th **S42.482 Torus fracture of lower end of left humerus**
HAC 7th character A see Appendix B for HAC conditional logic

CC +7th **S42.489 Torus fracture of lower end of unspecified humerus**
HAC 7th character A see Appendix B for HAC conditional logic

+ **S42.49 Other fracture of lower end of humerus**

CC MCC +7th **S42.491 Other displaced fracture of lower end of right humerus**
HAC 7th characters A & B see Appendix B for HAC conditional logic

CC MCC +7th **S42.492 Other displaced fracture of lower end of left humerus**
HAC 7th characters A & B see Appendix B for HAC conditional logic

CC MCC +7th **S42.493 Other displaced fracture of lower end of unspecified humerus**
HAC 7th characters A & B see Appendix B for HAC conditional logic

CC MCC +7th **S42.494 Other nondisplaced fracture of lower end of right humerus**
HAC 7th characters A & B see Appendix B for HAC conditional logic

CC MCC +7th **S42.495 Other nondisplaced fracture of lower end of left humerus**
HAC 7th characters A & B see Appendix B for HAC conditional logic

CC MCC +7th **S42.496 Other nondisplaced fracture of lower end of unspecified humerus**
HAC 7th characters A & B see Appendix B for HAC conditional logic

+ **S42.9 Fracture of shoulder girdle, part unspecified**
Fracture of shoulder NOS

CC MCC X+7th **S42.90 Fracture of unspecified shoulder girdle, part unspecified**
HAC 7th characters A & B see Appendix B for HAC conditional logic

CC MCC X+7th **S42.91 Fracture of right shoulder girdle, part unspecified**
HAC 7th characters A & B see Appendix B for HAC conditional logic

CC MCC X+7th **S42.92 Fracture of left shoulder girdle, part unspecified**
HAC 7th characters A & B see Appendix B for HAC conditional logic

S43 Dislocation and sprain of joints and ligaments of shoulder girdle

Includes: avulsion of joint or ligament of shoulder girdle
laceration of cartilage, joint or ligament of shoulder girdle
sprain of cartilage, joint or ligament of shoulder girdle
traumatic hemarthrosis of joint or ligament of shoulder girdle
traumatic rupture of joint or ligament of shoulder girdle
traumatic subluxation of joint or ligament of shoulder girdle
traumatic tear of joint or ligament of shoulder girdle

Code also any associated open wound

Excludes2: *strain of muscle, fascia and tendon of shoulder and upper arm (S46.-)*

The appropriate 7th character is to be added to each code from category S43
A initial encounter
D subsequent encounter
S sequela

+ **S43.0 Subluxation and dislocation of shoulder joint**
Dislocation of glenohumeral joint
Subluxation of glenohumeral joint

+ **S43.00 Unspecified subluxation and dislocation of shoulder joint**
Dislocation of humerus NOS
Subluxation of humerus NOS

+7th **S43.001 Unspecified subluxation of right shoulder joint**
+7th **S43.002 Unspecified subluxation of left shoulder joint**
+7th **S43.003 Unspecified subluxation of unspecified shoulder joint**
+7th **S43.004 Unspecified dislocation of right shoulder joint**
+7th **S43.005 Unspecified dislocation of left shoulder joint**
+7th **S43.006 Unspecified dislocation of unspecified shoulder joint**

+ **S43.01 Anterior subluxation and dislocation of humerus**
+7th **S43.011 Anterior subluxation of right humerus**
+7th **S43.012 Anterior subluxation of left humerus**
+7th **S43.013 Anterior subluxation of unspecified humerus**
+7th **S43.014 Anterior dislocation of right humerus**
+7th **S43.015 Anterior dislocation of left humerus**
+7th **S43.016 Anterior dislocation of unspecified humerus**

+ **S43.02 Posterior subluxation and dislocation of humerus**
+7th **S43.021 Posterior subluxation of right humerus**
+7th **S43.022 Posterior subluxation of left humerus**
+7th **S43.023 Posterior subluxation of unspecified humerus**
+7th **S43.024 Posterior dislocation of right humerus**
+7th **S43.025 Posterior dislocation of left humerus**
+7th **S43.026 Posterior dislocation of unspecified humerus**

+ **S43.03 Inferior subluxation and dislocation of humerus**
+7th **S43.031 Inferior subluxation of right humerus**
+7th **S43.032 Inferior subluxation of left humerus**
+7th **S43.033 Inferior subluxation of unspecified humerus**
+7th **S43.034 Inferior dislocation of right humerus**
+7th **S43.035 Inferior dislocation of left humerus**
+7th **S43.036 Inferior dislocation of unspecified humerus**

+ **S43.08 Other subluxation and dislocation of shoulder joint**
+7th **S43.081 Other subluxation of right shoulder joint**
+7th **S43.082 Other subluxation of left shoulder joint**
+7th **S43.083 Other subluxation of unspecified shoulder joint**
+7th **S43.084 Other dislocation of right shoulder joint**
+7th **S43.085 Other dislocation of left shoulder joint**
+7th **S43.086 Other dislocation of unspecified shoulder joint**

+ **S43.1 Subluxation and dislocation of acromioclavicular joint**

+ **S43.10 Unspecified dislocation of acromioclavicular joint**
+7th **S43.101 Unspecified dislocation of right acromioclavicular joint**
+7th **S43.102 Unspecified dislocation of left acromioclavicular joint**
+7th **S43.109 Unspecified dislocation of unspecified acromioclavicular joint**

+ **S43.11 Subluxation of acromioclavicular joint**
+7th **S43.111 Subluxation of right acromioclavicular joint**
+7th **S43.112 Subluxation of left acromioclavicular joint**
+7th **S43.119 Subluxation of unspecified acromioclavicular joint**

+ **S43.12 Dislocation of acromioclavicular joint, 100%-200% displacement**
+7th **S43.121 Dislocation of right acromioclavicular joint, 100%-200% displacement**
+7th **S43.122 Dislocation of left acromioclavicular joint, 100%-200% displacement**
+7th **S43.129 Dislocation of unspecified acromioclavicular joint, 100%-200% displacement**

+ **S43.13 Dislocation of acromioclavicular joint, greater than 200% displacement**
+7th **S43.131 Dislocation of right acromioclavicular joint, greater than 200% displacement**
+7th **S43.132 Dislocation of left acromioclavicular joint, greater than 200% displacement**
+7th **S43.139 Dislocation of unspecified acromioclavicular joint, greater than 200% displacement**

+ **S43.14 Inferior dislocation of acromioclavicular joint**
+7th **S43.141 Inferior dislocation of right acromioclavicular joint**
+7th **S43.142 Inferior dislocation of left acromioclavicular joint**
+7th **S43.149 Inferior dislocation of unspecified acromioclavicular joint**

\+ **S43.15 Posterior dislocation of acromioclavicular joint**
+7th **S43.151 Posterior dislocation of right acromioclavicular joint**
+7th **S43.152 Posterior dislocation of left acromioclavicular joint**
+7th **S43.159 Posterior dislocation of unspecified acromioclavicular joint**

\+ **S43.2 Subluxation and dislocation of sternoclavicular joint**

\+ **S43.20 Unspecified subluxation and dislocation of sternoclavicular joint**
CC +7th **S43.201 Unspecified subluxation of right sternoclavicular joint**
HAC 7th character A see Appendix B for HAC conditional logic
CC +7th **S43.202 Unspecified subluxation of left sternoclavicular joint**
HAC 7th character A see Appendix B for HAC conditional logic
CC +7th **S43.203 Unspecified subluxation of unspecified sternoclavicular joint**
HAC 7th character A see Appendix B for HAC conditional logic
CC +7th **S43.204 Unspecified dislocation of right sternoclavicular joint**
HAC 7th character A see Appendix B for HAC conditional logic
CC +7th **S43.205 Unspecified dislocation of left sternoclavicular joint**
HAC 7th character A see Appendix B for HAC conditional logic
CC +7th **S43.206 Unspecified dislocation of unspecified sternoclavicular joint**
HAC 7th character A see Appendix B for HAC conditional logic

\+ **S43.21 Anterior subluxation and dislocation of sternoclavicular joint**
CC +7th **S43.211 Anterior subluxation of right sternoclavicular joint**
HAC 7th character A see Appendix B for HAC conditional logic
CC +7th **S43.212 Anterior subluxation of left sternoclavicular joint**
HAC 7th character A see Appendix B for HAC conditional logic
CC +7th **S43.213 Anterior subluxation of unspecified sternoclavicular joint**
HAC 7th character A see Appendix B for HAC conditional logic
CC +7th **S43.214 Anterior dislocation of right sternoclavicular joint**
HAC 7th character A see Appendix B for HAC conditional logic
CC +7th **S43.215 Anterior dislocation of left sternoclavicular joint**
HAC 7th character A see Appendix B for HAC conditional logic
CC +7th **S43.216 Anterior dislocation of unspecified sternoclavicular joint**
HAC 7th character A see Appendix B for HAC conditional logic

\+ **S43.22 Posterior subluxation and dislocation of sternoclavicular joint**
CC +7th **S43.221 Posterior subluxation of right sternoclavicular joint**
HAC 7th character A see Appendix B for HAC conditional logic
CC +7th **S43.222 Posterior subluxation of left sternoclavicular joint**
HAC 7th character A see Appendix B for HAC conditional logic
CC +7th **S43.223 Posterior subluxation of unspecified sternoclavicular joint**
HAC 7th character A see Appendix B for HAC conditional logic
CC +7th **S43.224 Posterior dislocation of right sternoclavicular joint**
HAC 7th character A see Appendix B for HAC conditional logic
CC +7th **S43.225 Posterior dislocation of left sternoclavicular joint**
HAC 7th character A see Appendix B for HAC conditional logic
CC +7th **S43.226 Posterior dislocation of unspecified sternoclavicular joint**

\+ **S43.3 Subluxation and dislocation of other and unspecified parts of shoulder girdle**

\+ **S43.30 Subluxation and dislocation of unspecified parts of shoulder girdle**
Dislocation of shoulder girdle NOS
Subluxation of shoulder girdle NOS
+7th **S43.301 Subluxation of unspecified parts of right shoulder girdle**
+7th **S43.302 Subluxation of unspecified parts of left shoulder girdle**
+7th **S43.303 Subluxation of unspecified parts of unspecified shoulder girdle**
+7th **S43.304 Dislocation of unspecified parts of right shoulder girdle**
+7th **S43.305 Dislocation of unspecified parts of left shoulder girdle**
+7th **S43.306 Dislocation of unspecified parts of unspecified shoulder girdle**

\+ **S43.31 Subluxation and dislocation of scapula**
+7th **S43.311 Subluxation of right scapula**
+7th **S43.312 Subluxation of left scapula**
+7th **S43.313 Subluxation of unspecified scapula**
+7th **S43.314 Dislocation of right scapula**
+7th **S43.315 Dislocation of left scapula**
+7th **S43.316 Dislocation of unspecified scapula**

\+ **S43.39 Subluxation and dislocation of other parts of shoulder girdle**
+7th **S43.391 Subluxation of other parts of right shoulder girdle**
+7th **S43.392 Subluxation of other parts of left shoulder girdle**
+7th **S43.393 Subluxation of other parts of unspecified shoulder girdle**
+7th **S43.394 Dislocation of other parts of right shoulder girdle**
+7th **S43.395 Dislocation of other parts of left shoulder girdle**
+7th **S43.396 Dislocation of other parts of unspecified shoulder girdle**

\+ **S43.4 Sprain of shoulder joint**

\+ **S43.40 Unspecified sprain of shoulder joint**
+7th **S43.401 Unspecified sprain of right shoulder joint**
+7th **S43.402 Unspecified sprain of left shoulder joint**
+7th **S43.409 Unspecified sprain of unspecified shoulder joint**

\+ **S43.41 Sprain of coracohumeral (ligament)**
+7th **S43.411 Sprain of right coracohumeral (ligament)**
+7th **S43.412 Sprain of left coracohumeral (ligament)**
+7th **S43.419 Sprain of unspecified coracohumeral (ligament)**

\+ **S43.42 Sprain of rotator cuff capsule**
Excludes1: *rotator cuff syndrome (complete) (incomplete), not specified as traumatic (M75.1-)*
Excludes2: *injury of tendon of rotator cuff (S46.0-)*
+7th **S43.421 Sprain of right rotator cuff capsule**
+7th **S43.422 Sprain of left rotator cuff capsule**
+7th **S43.429 Sprain of unspecified rotator cuff capsule**

\+ **S43.43 Superior glenoid labrum lesion**
SLAP lesion
AHA CC: 2Q, 2019, 26-27
+7th **S43.431 Superior glenoid labrum lesion of right shoulder**
+7th **S43.432 Superior glenoid labrum lesion of left shoulder**
+7th **S43.439 Superior glenoid labrum lesion of unspecified shoulder**

\+ **S43.49 Other sprain of shoulder joint**
S43.491 Other sprain of right shoulder joint
S43.492 Other sprain of left shoulder joint
S43.499 Other sprain of unspecified shoulder joint

\+ **S43.5 Sprain of acromioclavicular joint**
Sprain of acromioclavicular ligament
X+7th **S43.50 Sprain of unspecified acromioclavicular joint**
X+7th **S43.51 Sprain of right acromioclavicular joint**
X+7th **S43.52 Sprain of left acromioclavicular joint**

+ **S43.6 Sprain of sternoclavicular joint**
 X+7th **S43.60 Sprain of unspecified sternoclavicular joint**
 X+7th **S43.61 Sprain of right sternoclavicular joint**
 X+7th **S43.62 Sprain of left sternoclavicular joint**
+ **S43.8 Sprain of other specified parts of shoulder girdle**
 X+7th **S43.80 Sprain of other specified parts of unspecified shoulder girdle**
 X+7th **S43.81 Sprain of other specified parts of right shoulder girdle**
 X+7th **S43.82 Sprain of other specified parts of left shoulder girdle**
+ **S43.9 Sprain of unspecified parts of shoulder girdle**
 X+7th **S43.90 Sprain of unspecified parts of unspecified shoulder girdle**
 Sprain of shoulder girdle NOS
 X+7th **S43.91 Sprain of unspecified parts of right shoulder girdle**
 X+7th **S43.92 Sprain of unspecified parts of left shoulder girdle**

S44 Injury of nerves at shoulder and upper arm level

Code also any associated open wound (S41.-)

Excludes2: *injury of brachial plexus (S14.3-)*

The appropriate 7th character is to be added to each code from category S44
A initial encounter
D subsequent encounter
S sequela

+ **S44.0 Injury of ulnar nerve at upper arm level**
 Excludes1: *ulnar nerve NOS (S54.0)*
 X+7th **S44.00 Injury of ulnar nerve at upper arm level, unspecified arm**
 X+7th **S44.01 Injury of ulnar nerve at upper arm level, right arm**
 X+7th **S44.02 Injury of ulnar nerve at upper arm level, left arm**
+ **S44.1 Injury of median nerve at upper arm level**
 Excludes1: *median nerve NOS (S54.1)*
 X+7th **S44.10 Injury of median nerve at upper arm level, unspecified arm**
 X+7th **S44.11 Injury of median nerve at upper arm level, right arm**
 X+7th **S44.12 Injury of median nerve at upper arm level, left arm**
+ **S44.2 Injury of radial nerve at upper arm level**
 Excludes1: *radial nerve NOS (S54.2)*
 X+7th **S44.20 Injury of radial nerve at upper arm level, unspecified arm**
 X+7th **S44.21 Injury of radial nerve at upper arm level, right arm**
 X+7th **S44.22 Injury of radial nerve at upper arm level, left arm**
+ **S44.3 Injury of axillary nerve**
 X+7th **S44.30 Injury of axillary nerve, unspecified arm**
 X+7th **S44.31 Injury of axillary nerve, right arm**
 X+7th **S44.32 Injury of axillary nerve, left arm**
+ **S44.4 Injury of musculocutaneous nerve**
 X+7th **S44.40 Injury of musculocutaneous nerve, unspecified arm**
 X+7th **S44.41 Injury of musculocutaneous nerve, right arm**
 X+7th **S44.42 Injury of musculocutaneous nerve, left arm**
+ **S44.5 Injury of cutaneous sensory nerve at shoulder and upper arm level**
 X+7th **S44.50 Injury of cutaneous sensory nerve at shoulder and upper arm level, unspecified arm**
 X+7th **S44.51 Injury of cutaneous sensory nerve at shoulder and upper arm level, right arm**
 X+7th **S44.52 Injury of cutaneous sensory nerve at shoulder and upper arm level, left arm**
+ **S44.8 Injury of other nerves at shoulder and upper arm level**
 + **S44.8X Injury of other nerves at shoulder and upper arm level**
 +7th **S44.8X1 Injury of other nerves at shoulder and upper arm level, right arm**
 +7th **S44.8X2 Injury of other nerves at shoulder and upper arm level, left arm**
 +7th **S44.8X9 Injury of other nerves at shoulder and upper arm level, unspecified arm**
+ **S44.9 Injury of unspecified nerve at shoulder and upper arm level**
 X+7th **S44.90 Injury of unspecified nerve at shoulder and upper arm level, unspecified arm**
 X+7th **S44.91 Injury of unspecified nerve at shoulder and upper arm level, right arm**
 X+7th **S44.92 Injury of unspecified nerve at shoulder and upper arm level, left arm**

S45 Injury of blood vessels at shoulder and upper arm level

Code also any associated open wound (S41.-)

Excludes2: *injury of subclavian artery (S25.1)*
injury of subclavian vein (S25.3)

The appropriate 7th character is to be added to each code from category S45
A initial encounter
D subsequent encounter
S sequela

+ **S45.0 Injury of axillary artery**
 + **S45.00 Unspecified injury of axillary artery**
 MCC +7th **S45.001 Unspecified injury of axillary artery, right side**
 MCC +7th **S45.002 Unspecified injury of axillary artery, left side**
 MCC +7th **S45.009 Unspecified injury of axillary artery, unspecified side**
 + **S45.01 Laceration of axillary artery**
 MCC +7th **S45.011 Laceration of axillary artery, right side**
 MCC +7th **S45.012 Laceration of axillary artery, left side**
 MCC +7th **S45.019 Laceration of axillary artery, unspecified side**
 + **S45.09 Other specified injury of axillary artery**
 MCC +7th **S45.091 Other specified injury of axillary artery, right side**
 MCC +7th **S45.092 Other specified injury of axillary artery, left side**
 MCC +7th **S45.099 Other specified injury of axillary artery, unspecified side**
+ **S45.1 Injury of brachial artery**
 + **S45.10 Unspecified injury of brachial artery**
 CC +7th **S45.101 Unspecified injury of brachial artery, right side**
 CC +7th **S45.102 Unspecified injury of brachial artery, left side**
 CC +7th **S45.109 Unspecified injury of brachial artery, unspecified side**
 + **S45.11 Laceration of brachial artery**
 CC +7th **S45.111 Laceration of brachial artery, right side**
 CC +7th **S45.112 Laceration of brachial artery, left side**
 CC +7th **S45.119 Laceration of brachial artery, unspecified side**
 + **S45.19 Other specified injury of brachial artery**
 CC +7th **S45.191 Other specified injury of brachial artery, right side**
 CC +7th **S45.192 Other specified injury of brachial artery, left side**
 CC +7th **S45.199 Other specified injury of brachial artery, unspecified side**
+ **S45.2 Injury of axillary or brachial vein**
 + **S45.20 Unspecified injury of axillary or brachial vein**
 CC +7th **S45.201 Unspecified injury of axillary or brachial vein, right side**
 CC +7th **S45.202 Unspecified injury of axillary or brachial vein, left side**
 CC +7th **S45.209 Unspecified injury of axillary or brachial vein, unspecified side**
 + **S45.21 Laceration of axillary or brachial vein**
 CC +7th **S45.211 Laceration of axillary or brachial vein, right side**
 CC +7th **S45.212 Laceration of axillary or brachial vein, left side**
 CC +7th **S45.219 Laceration of axillary or brachial vein, unspecified side**
 + **S45.29 Other specified injury of axillary or brachial vein**
 CC +7th **S45.291 Other specified injury of axillary or brachial vein, right side**
 CC +7th **S45.292 Other specified injury of axillary or brachial vein, left side**
 CC +7th **S45.299 Other specified injury of axillary or brachial vein, unspecified side**

+ S45.3 Injury of superficial vein at shoulder and upper arm level

+ S45.30 Unspecified injury of superficial vein at shoulder and upper arm level

CC +7th **S45.301 Unspecified injury of superficial vein at shoulder and upper arm level, right arm**

CC +7th **S45.302 Unspecified injury of superficial vein at shoulder and upper arm level, left arm**

CC +7th **S45.309 Unspecified injury of superficial vein at shoulder and upper arm level, unspecified arm**

+ S45.31 Laceration of superficial vein at shoulder and upper arm level

CC +7th **S45.311 Laceration of superficial vein at shoulder and upper arm level, right arm**

CC +7th **S45.312 Laceration of superficial vein at shoulder and upper arm level, left arm**

CC +7th **S45.319 Laceration of superficial vein at shoulder and upper arm level, unspecified arm**

+ S45.39 Other specified injury of superficial vein at shoulder and upper arm level

CC +7th **S45.391 Other specified injury of superficial vein at shoulder and upper arm level, right arm**

CC +7th **S45.392 Other specified injury of superficial vein at shoulder and upper arm level, left arm**

CC +7th **S45.399 Other specified injury of superficial vein at shoulder and upper arm level, unspecified arm**

+ S45.8 Injury of other specified blood vessels at shoulder and upper arm level

+ S45.80 Unspecified injury of other specified blood vessels at shoulder and upper arm level

CC +7th **S45.801 Unspecified injury of other specified blood vessels at shoulder and upper arm level, right arm**

CC +7th **S45.802 Unspecified injury of other specified blood vessels at shoulder and upper arm level, left arm**

CC +7th **S45.809 Unspecified injury of other specified blood vessels at shoulder and upper arm level, unspecified arm**

+ S45.81 Laceration of other specified blood vessels at shoulder and upper arm level

CC +7th **S45.811 Laceration of other specified blood vessels at shoulder and upper arm level, right arm**

CC +7th **S45.812 Laceration of other specified blood vessels at shoulder and upper arm level, left arm**

CC +7th **S45.819 Laceration of other specified blood vessels at shoulder and upper arm level, unspecified arm**

+ S45.89 Other specified injury of other specified blood vessels at shoulder and upper arm level

CC +7th **S45.891 Other specified injury of other specified blood vessels at shoulder and upper arm level, right arm**

CC +7th **S45.892 Other specified injury of other specified blood vessels at shoulder and upper arm level, left arm**

CC +7th **S45.899 Other specified injury of other specified blood vessels at shoulder and upper arm level, unspecified arm**

+ S45.9 Injury of unspecified blood vessel at shoulder and upper arm level

+ S45.90 Unspecified injury of unspecified blood vessel at shoulder and upper arm level

CC +7th **S45.901 Unspecified injury of unspecified blood vessel at shoulder and upper arm level, right arm**

CC +7th **S45.902 Unspecified injury of unspecified blood vessel at shoulder and upper arm level, left arm**

CC +7th **S45.909 Unspecified injury of unspecified blood vessel at shoulder and upper arm level, unspecified arm**

+ S45.91 Laceration of unspecified blood vessel at shoulder and upper arm level

CC +7th **S45.911 Laceration of unspecified blood vessel at shoulder and upper arm level, right arm**

CC +7th **S45.912 Laceration of unspecified blood vessel at shoulder and upper arm level, left arm**

CC +7th **S45.919 Laceration of unspecified blood vessel at shoulder and upper arm level, unspecified arm**

+ S45.99 Other specified injury of unspecified blood vessel at shoulder and upper arm level

CC +7th **S45.991 Other specified injury of unspecified blood vessel at shoulder and upper arm level, right arm**

CC +7th **S45.992 Other specified injury of unspecified blood vessel at shoulder and upper arm level, left arm**

CC +7th **S45.999 Other specified injury of unspecified blood vessel at shoulder and upper arm level, unspecified arm**

S46 Injury of muscle, fascia and tendon at shoulder and upper arm level

Code also any associated open wound (S41.-)

Excludes2: *injury of muscle, fascia and tendon at elbow (S56.-)*
sprain of joints and ligaments of shoulder girdle (S43.9)

The appropriate 7th character is to be added to each code from category S46
A initial encounter
D subsequent encounter
S sequela

+ S46.0 Injury of muscle(s) and tendon(s) of the rotator cuff of shoulder

+ S46.00 Unspecified injury of muscle(s) and tendon(s) of the rotator cuff of shoulder

+7th **S46.001 Unspecified injury of muscle(s) and tendon(s) of the rotator cuff of right shoulder**

+7th **S46.002 Unspecified injury of muscle(s) and tendon(s) of the rotator cuff of left shoulder**

+7th **S46.009 Unspecified injury of muscle(s) and tendon(s) of the rotator cuff of unspecified shoulder**

+ S46.01 Strain of muscle(s) and tendon(s) of the rotator cuff of shoulder

+7th **S46.011 Strain of muscle(s) and tendon(s) of the rotator cuff of right shoulder**

+7th **S46.012 Strain of muscle(s) and tendon(s) of the rotator cuff of left shoulder**

+7th **S46.019 Strain of muscle(s) and tendon(s) of the rotator cuff of unspecified shoulder**

+ S46.02 Laceration of muscle(s) and tendon(s) of the rotator cuff of shoulder

CC +7th **S46.021 Laceration of muscle(s) and tendon(s) of the rotator cuff of right shoulder**

CC +7th **S46.022 Laceration of muscle(s) and tendon(s) of the rotator cuff of left shoulder**

CC +7th **S46.029 Laceration of muscle(s) and tendon(s) of the rotator cuff of unspecified shoulder**

+ S46.09 Other injury of muscle(s) and tendon(s) of the rotator cuff of shoulder

+7th **S46.091 Other injury of muscle(s) and tendon(s) of the rotator cuff of right shoulder**

+7th **S46.092 Other injury of muscle(s) and tendon(s) of the rotator cuff of left shoulder**

+7th **S46.099 Other injury of muscle(s) and tendon(s) of the rotator cuff of unspecified shoulder**

+ S46.1 Injury of muscle, fascia and tendon of long head of biceps

+ S46.10 Unspecified injury of muscle, fascia and tendon of long head of biceps

+7th **S46.101 Unspecified injury of muscle, fascia and tendon of long head of biceps, right arm**

+7th **S46.102 Unspecified injury of muscle, fascia and tendon of long head of biceps, left arm**

+7th **S46.109 Unspecified injury of muscle, fascia and tendon of long head of biceps, unspecified arm**

+ **S46.11** **Strain of muscle, fascia and tendon of long head of biceps**

AHA CC: 2Q, 2019, 27

+7th **S46.111** **Strain of muscle, fascia and tendon of long head of biceps, right arm**

+7th **S46.112** **Strain of muscle, fascia and tendon of long head of biceps, left arm**

+7th **S46.119** **Strain of muscle, fascia and tendon of long head of biceps, unspecified arm**

+ **S46.12** **Laceration of muscle, fascia and tendon of long head of biceps**

CC +7th **S46.121** **Laceration of muscle, fascia and tendon of long head of biceps, right arm**

CC +7th **S46.122** **Laceration of muscle, fascia and tendon of long head of biceps, left arm**

CC +7th **S46.129** **Laceration of muscle, fascia and tendon of long head of biceps, unspecified arm**

+ **S46.19** **Other injury of muscle, fascia and tendon of long head of biceps**

+7th **S46.191** **Other injury of muscle, fascia and tendon of long head of biceps, right arm**

+7th **S46.192** **Other injury of muscle, fascia and tendon of long head of biceps, left arm**

+7th **S46.199** **Other injury of muscle, fascia and tendon of long head of biceps, unspecified arm**

+ **S46.2** **Injury of muscle, fascia and tendon of other parts of biceps**

+ **S46.20** **Unspecified injury of muscle, fascia and tendon of other parts of biceps**

+7th **S46.201** **Unspecified injury of muscle, fascia and tendon of other parts of biceps, right arm**

+7th **S46.202** **Unspecified injury of muscle, fascia and tendon of other parts of biceps, left arm**

+7th **S46.209** **Unspecified injury of muscle, fascia and tendon of other parts of biceps, unspecified arm**

+ **S46.21** **Strain of muscle, fascia and tendon of other parts of biceps**

+7th **S46.211** **Strain of muscle, fascia and tendon of other parts of biceps, right arm**

+7th **S46.212** **Strain of muscle, fascia and tendon of other parts of biceps, left arm**

+7th **S46.219** **Strain of muscle, fascia and tendon of other parts of biceps, unspecified arm**

+ **S46.22** **Laceration of muscle, fascia and tendon of other parts of biceps**

CC +7th **S46.221** **Laceration of muscle, fascia and tendon of other parts of biceps, right arm**

CC +7th **S46.222** **Laceration of muscle, fascia and tendon of other parts of biceps, left arm**

CC +7th **S46.229** **Laceration of muscle, fascia and tendon of other parts of biceps, unspecified arm**

+ **S46.29** **Other injury of muscle, fascia and tendon of other parts of biceps**

+7th **S46.291** **Other injury of muscle, fascia and tendon of other parts of biceps, right arm**

+7th **S46.292** **Other injury of muscle, fascia and tendon of other parts of biceps, left arm**

+7th **S46.299** **Other injury of muscle, fascia and tendon of other parts of biceps, unspecified arm**

+ **S46.3** **Injury of muscle, fascia and tendon of triceps**

+ **S46.30** **Unspecified injury of muscle, fascia and tendon of triceps**

+7th **S46.301** **Unspecified injury of muscle, fascia and tendon of triceps, right arm**

+7th **S46.302** **Unspecified injury of muscle, fascia and tendon of triceps, left arm**

+7th **S46.309** **Unspecified injury of muscle, fascia and tendon of triceps, unspecified arm**

+ **S46.31** **Strain of muscle, fascia and tendon of triceps**

+7th **S46.311** **Strain of muscle, fascia and tendon of triceps, right arm**

+7th **S46.312** **Strain of muscle, fascia and tendon of triceps, left arm**

+7th **S46.319** **Strain of muscle, fascia and tendon of triceps, unspecified arm**

+ **S46.32** **Laceration of muscle, fascia and tendon of triceps**

CC +7th **S46.321** **Laceration of muscle, fascia and tendon of triceps, right arm**

CC +7th **S46.322** **Laceration of muscle, fascia and tendon of triceps, left arm**

CC +7th **S46.329** **Laceration of muscle, fascia and tendon of triceps, unspecified arm**

+ **S46.39** **Other injury of muscle, fascia and tendon of triceps**

+7th **S46.391** **Other injury of muscle, fascia and tendon of triceps, right arm**

+7th **S46.392** **Other injury of muscle, fascia and tendon of triceps, left arm**

+7th **S46.399** **Other injury of muscle, fascia and tendon of triceps, unspecified arm**

+ **S46.8** **Injury of other muscles, fascia and tendons at shoulder and upper arm level**

+ **S46.80** **Unspecified injury of other muscles, fascia and tendons at shoulder and upper arm level**

+7th **S46.801** **Unspecified injury of other muscles, fascia and tendons at shoulder and upper arm level, right arm**

+7th **S46.802** **Unspecified injury of other muscles, fascia and tendons at shoulder and upper arm level, left arm**

+7th **S46.809** **Unspecified injury of other muscles, fascia and tendons at shoulder and upper arm level, unspecified arm**

+ **S46.81** **Strain of other muscles, fascia and tendons at shoulder and upper arm level**

+7th **S46.811** **Strain of other muscles, fascia and tendons at shoulder and upper arm level, right arm**

+7th **S46.812** **Strain of other muscles, fascia and tendons at shoulder and upper arm level, left arm**

+7th **S46.819** **Strain of other muscles, fascia and tendons at shoulder and upper arm level, unspecified arm**

+ **S46.82** **Laceration of other muscles, fascia and tendons at shoulder and upper arm level**

CC +7th **S46.821** **Laceration of other muscles, fascia and tendons at shoulder and upper arm level, right arm**

CC +7th **S46.822** **Laceration of other muscles, fascia and tendons at shoulder and upper arm level, left arm**

CC +7th **S46.829** **Laceration of other muscles, fascia and tendons at shoulder and upper arm level, unspecified arm**

+ **S46.89** **Other injury of other muscles, fascia and tendons at shoulder and upper arm level**

+7th **S46.891** **Other injury of other muscles, fascia and tendons at shoulder and upper arm level, right arm**

+7th **S46.892** **Other injury of other muscles, fascia and tendons at shoulder and upper arm level, left arm**

+7th **S46.899** **Other injury of other muscles, fascia and tendons at shoulder and upper arm level, unspecified arm**

+ **S46.9** **Injury of unspecified muscle, fascia and tendon at shoulder and upper arm level**

+ **S46.90** **Unspecified injury of unspecified muscle, fascia and tendon at shoulder and upper arm level**

+7th **S46.901** **Unspecified injury of unspecified muscle, fascia and tendon at shoulder and upper arm level, right arm**

+7th **S46.902** **Unspecified injury of unspecified muscle, fascia and tendon at shoulder and upper arm level, left arm**

+7th **S46.909** **Unspecified injury of unspecified muscle, fascia and tendon at shoulder and upper arm level, unspecified arm**

Injury to Growth Plate (Salter-Harris Classification, Rang Modification)

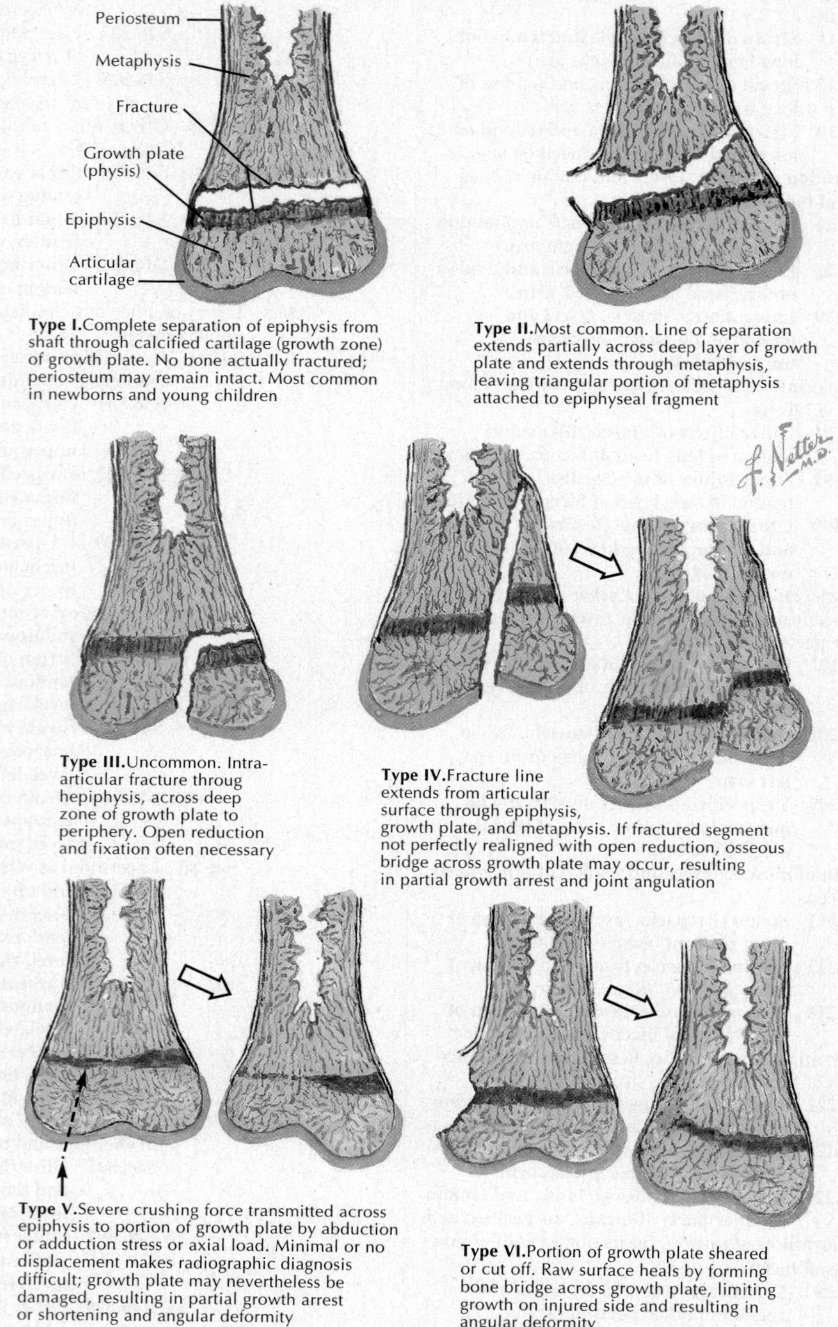

Type I. Complete separation of epiphysis from shaft through calcified cartilage (growth zone) of growth plate. No bone actually fractured; periosteum may remain intact. Most common in newborns and young children

Type II. Most common. Line of separation extends partially across deep layer of growth plate and extends through metaphysis, leaving triangular portion of metaphysis attached to epiphyseal fragment

Type III. Uncommon. Intra-articular fracture throug hepiphysis, across deep zone of growth plate to periphery. Open reduction and fixation often necessary

Type IV. Fracture line extends from articular surface through epiphysis, growth plate, and metaphysis. If fractured segment not perfectly realigned with open reduction, osseous bridge across growth plate may occur, resulting in partial growth arrest and joint angulation

Type V. Severe crushing force transmitted across epiphysis to portion of growth plate by abduction or adduction stress or axial load. Minimal or no displacement makes radiographic diagnosis difficult; growth plate may nevertheless be damaged, resulting in partial growth arrest or shortening and angular deformity

Type VI. Portion of growth plate sheared or cut off. Raw surface heals by forming bone bridge across growth plate, limiting growth on injured side and resulting in angular deformity

+ **S46.91 Strain of unspecified muscle, fascia and tendon at shoulder and upper arm level**
  - +7th **S46.911 Strain of unspecified muscle, fascia and tendon at shoulder and upper arm level, right arm**
  - +7th **S46.912 Strain of unspecified muscle, fascia and tendon at shoulder and upper arm level, left arm**
  - +7th **S46.919 Strain of unspecified muscle, fascia and tendon at shoulder and upper arm level, unspecified arm**

+ **S46.92 Laceration of unspecified muscle, fascia and tendon at shoulder and upper arm level**
  - CC +7th **S46.921 Laceration of unspecified muscle, fascia and tendon at shoulder and upper arm level, right arm**
  - CC +7th **S46.922 Laceration of unspecified muscle, fascia and tendon at shoulder and upper arm level, left arm**
  - CC +7th **S46.929 Laceration of unspecified muscle, fascia and tendon at shoulder and upper arm level, unspecified arm**

+ **S46.99 Other injury of unspecified muscle, fascia and tendon at shoulder and upper arm level**
  - +7th **S46.991 Other injury of unspecified muscle, fascia and tendon at shoulder and upper arm level, right arm**
  - +7th **S46.992 Other injury of unspecified muscle, fascia and tendon at shoulder and upper arm level, left arm**
  - +7th **S46.999 Other injury of unspecified muscle, fascia and tendon at shoulder and upper arm level, unspecified arm**

Elbow

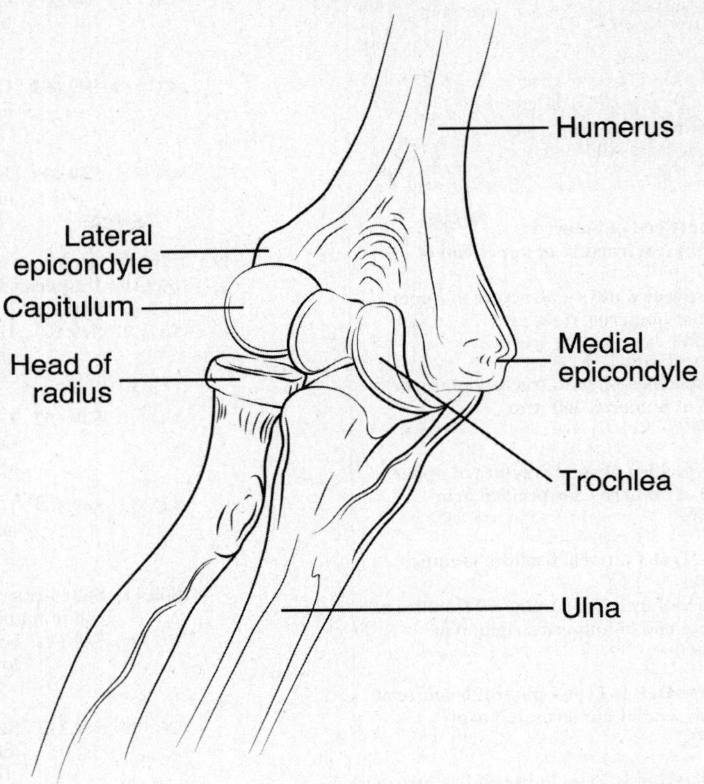

S47 Crushing injury of shoulder and upper arm

Use additional code for all associated injuries

Excludes2: *crushing injury of elbow (S57.0-)*

The appropriate 7th character is to be added to each code from category S47
A initial encounter
D subsequent encounter
S sequela

X+7th **S47.1 Crushing injury of right shoulder and upper arm**
X+7th **S47.2 Crushing injury of left shoulder and upper arm**
X+7th **S47.9 Crushing injury of shoulder and upper arm, unspecified arm**

S48 Traumatic amputation of shoulder and upper arm

An amputation not identified as partial or complete should be coded to complete

Excludes1: *traumatic amputation at elbow level (S58.0)*

The appropriate 7th character is to be added to each code from category S48
A initial encounter
D subsequent encounter
S sequela

\+ **S48.0 Traumatic amputation at shoulder joint**
\+ **S48.01 Complete traumatic amputation at shoulder joint**
CC +7th **S48.011 Complete traumatic amputation at right shoulder joint**
CC +7th **S48.012 Complete traumatic amputation at left shoulder joint**
CC +7th **S48.019 Complete traumatic amputation at unspecified shoulder joint**
\+ **S48.02 Partial traumatic amputation at shoulder joint**
CC +7th **S48.021 Partial traumatic amputation at right shoulder joint**
CC +7th **S48.022 Partial traumatic amputation at left shoulder joint**
CC +7th **S48.029 Partial traumatic amputation at unspecified shoulder joint**

\+ **S48.1 Traumatic amputation at level between shoulder and elbow**
\+ **S48.11 Complete traumatic amputation at level between shoulder and elbow**
CC +7th **S48.111 Complete traumatic amputation at level between right shoulder and elbow**
CC +7th **S48.112 Complete traumatic amputation at level between left shoulder and elbow**
CC +7th **S48.119 Complete traumatic amputation at level between unspecified shoulder and elbow**
\+ **S48.12 Partial traumatic amputation at level between shoulder and elbow**
CC +7th **S48.121 Partial traumatic amputation at level between right shoulder and elbow**
CC +7th **S48.122 Partial traumatic amputation at level between left shoulder and elbow**
CC +7th **S48.129 Partial traumatic amputation at level between unspecified shoulder and elbow**
\+ **S48.9 Traumatic amputation of shoulder and upper arm, level unspecified**
\+ **S48.91 Complete traumatic amputation of shoulder and upper arm, level unspecified**
CC +7th **S48.911 Complete traumatic amputation of right shoulder and upper arm, level unspecified**
CC +7th **S48.912 Complete traumatic amputation of left shoulder and upper arm, level unspecified**
CC +7th **S48.919 Complete traumatic amputation of unspecified shoulder and upper arm, level unspecified**
\+ **S48.92 Partial traumatic amputation of shoulder and upper arm, level unspecified**
CC +7th **S48.921 Partial traumatic amputation of right shoulder and upper arm, level unspecified**
CC +7th **S48.922 Partial traumatic amputation of left shoulder and upper arm, level unspecified**
CC +7th **S48.929 Partial traumatic amputation of unspecified shoulder and upper arm, level unspecified**

S49 Other and unspecified injuries of shoulder and upper arm

The appropriate 7th character is to be added to each code from subcategories **S49.0** and **S49.1**
A initial encounter for closed fracture
D subsequent encounter for fracture with routine healing
G subsequent encounter for fracture with delayed healing
K subsequent encounter for fracture with nonunion
P subsequent encounter for fracture with malunion
S sequela

Review coding guideline C.19.c

+ S49.0 Physeal fracture of upper end of humerus

+ S49.00 Unspecified physeal fracture of upper end of humerus

CC +7th **S49.001 Unspecified physeal fracture of upper end of humerus, right arm**
HAC 7th character A see Appendix B for HAC conditional logic

CC +7th **S49.002 Unspecified physeal fracture of upper end of humerus, left arm**
HAC 7th character A see Appendix B for HAC conditional logic

CC +7th **S49.009 Unspecified physeal fracture of upper end of humerus, unspecified arm**
HAC 7th character A see Appendix B for HAC conditional logic

+ S49.01 Salter-Harris Type I physeal fracture of upper end of humerus

CC +7th **S49.011 Salter-Harris Type I physeal fracture of upper end of humerus, right arm**
HAC 7th character A see Appendix B for HAC conditional logic

CC +7th **S49.012 Salter-Harris Type I physeal fracture of upper end of humerus, left arm**
HAC 7th character A see Appendix B for HAC conditional logic

CC +7th **S49.019 Salter-Harris Type I physeal fracture of upper end of humerus, unspecified arm**
HAC 7th character A see Appendix B for HAC conditional logic

+ S49.02 Salter-Harris Type II physeal fracture of upper end of humerus

CC +7th **S49.021 Salter-Harris Type II physeal fracture of upper end of humerus, right arm**
HAC 7th character A see Appendix B for HAC conditional logic

CC +7th **S49.022 Salter-Harris Type II physeal fracture of upper end of humerus, left arm**
HAC 7th character A see Appendix B for HAC conditional logic

CC +7th **S49.029 Salter-Harris Type II physeal fracture of upper end of humerus, unspecified arm**
HAC 7th character A see Appendix B for HAC conditional logic

+ S49.03 Salter-Harris Type III physeal fracture of upper end of humerus

CC +7th **S49.031 Salter-Harris Type III physeal fracture of upper end of humerus, right arm**
HAC 7th character A see Appendix B for HAC conditional logic

CC +7th **S49.032 Salter-Harris Type III physeal fracture of upper end of humerus, left arm**
HAC 7th character A see Appendix B for HAC conditional logic

CC +7th **S49.039 Salter-Harris Type III physeal fracture of upper end of humerus, unspecified arm**
HAC 7th character A see Appendix B for HAC conditional logic

+ S49.04 Salter-Harris Type IV physeal fracture of upper end of humerus

CC +7th **S49.041 Salter-Harris Type IV physeal fracture of upper end of humerus, right arm**
HAC 7th character A see Appendix B for HAC conditional logic

CC +7th **S49.042 Salter-Harris Type IV physeal fracture of upper end of humerus, left arm**
HAC 7th character A see Appendix B for HAC conditional logic

CC +7th **S49.049 Salter-Harris Type IV physeal fracture of upper end of humerus, unspecified arm**
HAC 7th character A see Appendix B for HAC conditional logic

+ S49.09 Other physeal fracture of upper end of humerus

CC +7th **S49.091 Other physeal fracture of upper end of humerus, right arm**
HAC 7th character A see Appendix B for HAC conditional logic

CC +7th **S49.092 Other physeal fracture of upper end of humerus, left arm**
HAC 7th character A see Appendix B for HAC conditional logic

CC +7th **S49.099 Other physeal fracture of upper end of humerus, unspecified arm**
HAC 7th character A see Appendix B for HAC conditional logic

+ S49.1 Physeal fracture of lower end of humerus

+ S49.10 Unspecified physeal fracture of lower end of humerus

CC +7th **S49.101 Unspecified physeal fracture of lower end of humerus, right arm**
HAC 7th character A see Appendix B for HAC conditional logic

CC +7th **S49.102 Unspecified physeal fracture of lower end of humerus, left arm**
HAC 7th character A see Appendix B for HAC conditional logic

CC +7th **S49.109 Unspecified physeal fracture of lower end of humerus, unspecified arm**
HAC 7th character A see Appendix B for HAC conditional logic

+ S49.11 Salter-Harris Type I physeal fracture of lower end of humerus

CC +7th **S49.111 Salter-Harris Type I physeal fracture of lower end of humerus, right arm**
HAC 7th character A see Appendix B for HAC conditional logic

CC +7th **S49.112 Salter-Harris Type I physeal fracture of lower end of humerus, left arm**
HAC 7th character A see Appendix B for HAC conditional logic

CC +7th **S49.119 Salter-Harris Type I physeal fracture of lower end of humerus, unspecified arm**
HAC 7th character A see Appendix B for HAC conditional logic

+ S49.12 Salter-Harris Type II physeal fracture of lower end of humerus

CC +7th **S49.121 Salter-Harris Type II physeal fracture of lower end of humerus, right arm**
HAC 7th character A see Appendix B for HAC conditional logic

CC +7th **S49.122 Salter-Harris Type II physeal fracture of lower end of humerus, left arm**
HAC 7th character A see Appendix B for HAC conditional logic

CC +7th **S49.129 Salter-Harris Type II physeal fracture of lower end of humerus, unspecified arm**
HAC 7th character A see Appendix B for HAC conditional logic

+ S49.13 Salter-Harris Type III physeal fracture of lower end of humerus

CC +7th **S49.131 Salter-Harris Type III physeal fracture of lower end of humerus, right arm**
HAC 7th character A see Appendix B for HAC conditional logic

CC +7th **S49.132 Salter-Harris Type III physeal fracture of lower end of humerus, left arm**
HAC 7th character A see Appendix B for HAC conditional logic

CC +7th **S49.139 Salter-Harris Type III physeal fracture of lower end of humerus, unspecified arm**
HAC 7th character A see Appendix B for HAC conditional logic

+ S49.14 Salter-Harris Type IV physeal fracture of lower end of humerus

CC +7th **S49.141 Salter-Harris Type IV physeal fracture of lower end of humerus, right arm**
HAC 7th character A see Appendix B for HAC conditional logic

CC +7th **S49.142 Salter-Harris Type IV physeal fracture of lower end of humerus, left arm**
HAC 7th character A see Appendix B for HAC conditional logic

CC +7th **S49.149 Salter-Harris Type IV physeal fracture of lower end of humerus, unspecified arm**
HAC 7th character A see Appendix B for HAC conditional logic

\+ **S49.19 Other physeal fracture of lower end of humerus**

CC +7th **S49.191 Other physeal fracture of lower end of humerus, right arm**
HAC 7th character A see Appendix B for HAC conditional logic

CC +7th **S49.192 Other physeal fracture of lower end of humerus, left arm**
HAC 7th character A see Appendix B for HAC conditional logic

CC +7th **S49.199 Other physeal fracture of lower end of humerus, unspecified arm**
HAC 7th character A see Appendix B for HAC conditional logic

\+ **S49.8 Other specified injuries of shoulder and upper arm**

The appropriate 7th character is to be added to each code in subcategory **S49.8**
A initial encounter
D subsequent encounter
S sequela

X+7th **S49.80 Other specified injuries of shoulder and upper arm, unspecified arm**
X+7th **S49.81 Other specified injuries of right shoulder and upper arm**
X+7th **S49.82 Other specified injuries of left shoulder and upper arm**

\+ **S49.9 Unspecified injury of shoulder and upper arm**

The appropriate 7th character is to be added to each code in subcategory **S49.9**
A initial encounter
D subsequent encounter
S sequela

X+7th **S49.90 Unspecified injury of shoulder and upper arm, unspecified arm**
X+7th **S49.91 Unspecified injury of right shoulder and upper arm**
X+7th **S49.92 Unspecified injury of left shoulder and upper arm**

Injuries to the elbow and forearm (S50-S59)

Excludes2: *burns and corrosions (T20-T32)*
frostbite (T33-T34)
injuries of wrist and hand (S60-S69)
insect bite or sting, venomous (T63.4)

S50 Superficial injury of elbow and forearm

Excludes2: *superficial injury of wrist and hand (S60.-)*

The appropriate 7th character is to be added to each code from category S50
A initial encounter
D subsequent encounter
S sequela

\+ **S50.0 Contusion of elbow**
X+7th **S50.00 Contusion of unspecified elbow**
X+7th **S50.01 Contusion of right elbow**
X+7th **S50.02 Contusion of left elbow**

\+ **S50.1 Contusion of forearm**
X+7th **S50.10 Contusion of unspecified forearm**
X+7th **S50.11 Contusion of right forearm**
X+7th **S50.12 Contusion of left forearm**

\+ **S50.3 Other superficial injuries of elbow**

\+ **S50.31 Abrasion of elbow**
+7th **S50.311 Abrasion of right elbow**
+7th **S50.312 Abrasion of left elbow**
+7th **S50.319 Abrasion of unspecified elbow**

\+ **S50.32 Blister (nonthermal) of elbow**
+7th **S50.321 Blister (nonthermal) of right elbow**
+7th **S50.322 Blister (nonthermal) of left elbow**
+7th **S50.329 Blister (nonthermal) of unspecified elbow**

\+ **S50.34 External constriction of elbow**
+7th **S50.341 External constriction of right elbow**
+7th **S50.342 External constriction of left elbow**
+7th **S50.349 External constriction of unspecified elbow**

\+ **S50.35 Superficial foreign body of elbow**
Splinter in the elbow
+7th **S50.351 Superficial foreign body of right elbow**
+7th **S50.352 Superficial foreign body of left elbow**
+7th **S50.359 Superficial foreign body of unspecified elbow**

\+ **S50.36 Insect bite (nonvenomous) of elbow**
+7th **S50.361 Insect bite (nonvenomous) of right elbow**
+7th **S50.362 Insect bite (nonvenomous) of left elbow**
+7th **S50.369 Insect bite (nonvenomous) of unspecified elbow**

\+ **S50.37 Other superficial bite of elbow**
Excludes1: *open bite of elbow (S51.04)*
+7th **S50.371 Other superficial bite of right elbow**
+7th **S50.372 Other superficial bite of left elbow**
+7th **S50.379 Other superficial bite of unspecified elbow**

\+ **S50.8 Other superficial injuries of forearm**

\+ **S50.81 Abrasion of forearm**
+7th **S50.811 Abrasion of right forearm**
+7th **S50.812 Abrasion of left forearm**
+7th **S50.819 Abrasion of unspecified forearm**

\+ **S50.82 Blister (nonthermal) of forearm**
+7th **S50.821 Blister (nonthermal) of right forearm**
+7th **S50.822 Blister (nonthermal) of left forearm**
+7th **S50.829 Blister (nonthermal) of unspecified forearm**

\+ **S50.84 External constriction of forearm**
+7th **S50.841 External constriction of right forearm**
+7th **S50.842 External constriction of left forearm**
+7th **S50.849 External constriction of unspecified forearm**

\+ **S50.85 Superficial foreign body of forearm**
Splinter in the forearm
+7th **S50.851 Superficial foreign body of right forearm**
+7th **S50.852 Superficial foreign body of left forearm**
+7th **S50.859 Superficial foreign body of unspecified forearm**

\+ **S50.86 Insect bite (nonvenomous) of forearm**
+7th **S50.861 Insect bite (nonvenomous) of right forearm**
+7th **S50.862 Insect bite (nonvenomous) of left forearm**
+7th **S50.869 Insect bite (nonvenomous) of unspecified forearm**

\+ **S50.87 Other superficial bite of forearm**
Excludes1: *open bite of forearm (S51.84)*
+7th **S50.871 Other superficial bite of right forearm**
+7th **S50.872 Other superficial bite of left forearm**
+7th **S50.879 Other superficial bite of unspecified forearm**

\+ **S50.9 Unspecified superficial injury of elbow and forearm**

\+ **S50.90 Unspecified superficial injury of elbow**
+7th **S50.901 Unspecified superficial injury of right elbow**
+7th **S50.902 Unspecified superficial injury of left elbow**
+7th **S50.909 Unspecified superficial injury of unspecified elbow**

\+ **S50.91 Unspecified superficial injury of forearm**
S50.911 Unspecified superficial injury of right forearm
S50.912 Unspecified superficial injury of left forearm
S50.919 Unspecified superficial injury of unspecified forearm

S51 Open wound of elbow and forearm

Code also any associated wound infection

Excludes1: *open fracture of elbow and forearm (S52.- with open fracture 7th character)*
traumatic amputation of elbow and forearm (S58.-)

Excludes2: *open wound of wrist and hand (S61.-)*

The appropriate 7th character is to be added to each code from category S51
A initial encounter
D subsequent encounter
S sequela

+ **S51.0 Open wound of elbow**
  + **S51.00 Unspecified open wound of elbow**
    +7th **S51.001 Unspecified open wound of right elbow**
    AHA CC: 4Q, 2012, 108
    +7th **S51.002 Unspecified open wound of left elbow**
    +7th **S51.009 Unspecified open wound of unspecified elbow**
    Open wound of elbow NOS
  + **S51.01 Laceration without foreign body of elbow**
    +7th **S51.011 Laceration without foreign body of right elbow**
    +7th **S51.012 Laceration without foreign body of left elbow**
    +7th **S51.019 Laceration without foreign body of unspecified elbow**
  + **S51.02 Laceration with foreign body of elbow**
    +7th **S51.021 Laceration with foreign body of right elbow**
    +7th **S51.022 Laceration with foreign body of left elbow**
    +7th **S51.029 Laceration with foreign body of unspecified elbow**
  + **S51.03 Puncture wound without foreign body of elbow**
    +7th **S51.031 Puncture wound without foreign body of right elbow**
    +7th **S51.032 Puncture wound without foreign body of left elbow**
    +7th **S51.039 Puncture wound without foreign body of unspecified elbow**
  + **S51.04 Puncture wound with foreign body of elbow**
    +7th **S51.041 Puncture wound with foreign body of right elbow**
    +7th **S51.042 Puncture wound with foreign body of left elbow**
    +7th **S51.049 Puncture wound with foreign body of unspecified elbow**
  + **S51.05 Open bite of elbow**
    Bite of elbow NOS
    Excludes1: *superficial bite of elbow (S50.36, S50.37)*
    +7th **S51.051 Open bite, right elbow**
    +7th **S51.052 Open bite, left elbow**
    +7th **S51.059 Open bite, unspecified elbow**
+ **S51.8 Open wound of forearm**
  Excludes2: *open wound of elbow (S51.0-)*
  + **S51.80 Unspecified open wound of forearm**
    +7th **S51.801 Unspecified open wound of right forearm**
    +7th **S51.802 Unspecified open wound of left forearm**
    +7th **S51.809 Unspecified open wound of unspecified forearm**
    Open wound of forearm NOS
  + **S51.81 Laceration without foreign body of forearm**
    +7th **S51.811 Laceration without foreign body of right forearm**
    +7th **S51.812 Laceration without foreign body of left forearm**
    +7th **S51.819 Laceration without foreign body of unspecified forearm**
  + **S51.82 Laceration with foreign body of forearm**
    +7th **S51.821 Laceration with foreign body of right forearm**
    +7th **S51.822 Laceration with foreign body of left forearm**
    +7th **S51.829 Laceration with foreign body of unspecified forearm**
  + **S51.83 Puncture wound without foreign body of forearm**
    +7th **S51.831 Puncture wound without foreign body of right forearm**
    +7th **S51.832 Puncture wound without foreign body of left forearm**
    +7th **S51.839 Puncture wound without foreign body of unspecified forearm**
  + **S51.84 Puncture wound with foreign body of forearm**
    +7th **S51.841 Puncture wound with foreign body of right forearm**
    +7th **S51.842 Puncture wound with foreign body of left forearm**
    +7th **S51.849 Puncture wound with foreign body of unspecified forearm**
  + **S51.85 Open bite of forearm**
    Bite of forearm NOS
    Excludes1: *superficial bite of forearm (S50.86, S50.87)*
    +7th **S51.851 Open bite of right forearm**
    +7th **S51.852 Open bite of left forearm**
    +7th **S51.859 Open bite of unspecified forearm**

S52 Fracture of forearm

NOTE A fracture not indicated as displaced or nondisplaced should be coded to displaced
A fracture not indicated as open or closed should be coded to closed
The open fracture designations are based on the Gustilo open fracture classification

Excludes1: *traumatic amputation of forearm (S58.-)*

Excludes2: *fracture at wrist and hand level (S62.-)*

The appropriate 7th character is to be added to all codes from category S52
A initial encounter for closed fracture
B initial encounter for open fracture type I or II initial encounter for open fracture NOS
C initial encounter for open fracture type IIIA, IIIB, or IIIC
D subsequent encounter for closed fracture with routine healing
E subsequent encounter for open fracture type I or II with routine healing
F subsequent encounter for open fracture type IIIA, IIIB, or IIIC with routine healing
G subsequent encounter for closed fracture with delayed healing
H subsequent encounter for open fracture type I or II with delayed healing
J subsequent encounter for open fracture type IIIA, IIIB, or IIIC with delayed healing
K subsequent encounter for closed fracture with nonunion
M subsequent encounter for open fracture type I or II with nonunion
N subsequent encounter for open fracture type IIIA, IIIB, or IIIC with nonunion
P subsequent encounter for closed fracture with malunion
Q subsequent encounter for open fracture type I or II with malunion
R subsequent encounter for open fracture type IIIA, IIIB, or IIIC with malunion
S sequela

Review coding guideline C.19.c

+ **S52.0 Fracture of upper end of ulna**
  Fracture of proximal end of ulna
  Excludes2: *fracture of elbow NOS (S42.40-)*
  fractures of shaft of ulna (S52.2-)
  + **S52.00 Unspecified fracture of upper end of ulna**
    CC MCC +7th **S52.001 Unspecified fracture of upper end of right ulna**
    HAC 7th characters B & C see Appendix B for HAC conditional logic
    CC MCC +7th **S52.002 Unspecified fracture of upper end of left ulna**
    HAC 7th characters B & C see Appendix B for HAC conditional logic
    CC MCC +7th **S52.009 Unspecified fracture of upper end of unspecified ulna**
    HAC 7th characters B & C see Appendix B for HAC conditional logic

+ S52.01 Torus fracture of upper end of ulna

The appropriate 7th character is to be added to all codes in subcategory **S52.01**
A initial encounter for closed fracture
D subsequent encounter for fracture with routine healing
G subsequent encounter for fracture with delayed healing
K subsequent encounter for fracture with nonunion
P - subsequent encounter for fracture with malunion
S - sequela

CC +7th **S52.011 Torus fracture of upper end of right ulna**
HAC 7th character A see Appendix B for HAC conditional logic

CC +7th **S52.012 Torus fracture of upper end of left ulna**
HAC 7th character A see Appendix B for HAC conditional logic

CC +7th **S52.019 Torus fracture of upper end of unspecified ulna**
HAC 7th character A see Appendix B for HAC conditional logic

+ S52.02 Fracture of olecranon process without intraarticular extension of ulna

CC MCC +7th **S52.021 Displaced fracture of olecranon process without intraarticular extension of right ulna**
HAC 7th characters B & C see Appendix B for HAC conditional logic

CC MCC +7th **S52.022 Displaced fracture of olecranon process without intraarticular extension of left ulna**
HAC 7th characters B & C see Appendix B for HAC conditional logic

CC MCC +7th **S52.023 Displaced fracture of olecranon process without intraarticular extension of unspecified ulna**
HAC 7th characters B & C see Appendix B for HAC conditional logic

CC MCC +7th **S52.024 Nondisplaced fracture of olecranon process without intraarticular extension of right ulna**
HAC 7th characters B & C see Appendix B for HAC conditional logic

CC MCC +7th **S52.025 Nondisplaced fracture of olecranon process without intraarticular extension of left ulna**
HAC 7th characters B & C see Appendix B for HAC conditional logic

CC MCC +7th **S52.026 Nondisplaced fracture of olecranon process without intraarticular extension of unspecified ulna**
HAC 7th characters B & C see Appendix B for HAC conditional logic

+ S52.03 Fracture of olecranon process with intraarticular extension of ulna

CC MCC +7th **S52.031 Displaced fracture of olecranon process with intraarticular extension of right ulna**
HAC 7th characters B & C see Appendix B for HAC conditional logic

CC MCC +7th **S52.032 Displaced fracture of olecranon process with intraarticular extension of left ulna**
HAC 7th characters B & C see Appendix B for HAC conditional logic

CC MCC +7th **S52.033 Displaced fracture of olecranon process with intraarticular extension of unspecified ulna**
HAC 7th characters B & C see Appendix B for HAC conditional logic

CC MCC +7th **S52.034 Nondisplaced fracture of olecranon process with intraarticular extension of right ulna**
HAC 7th characters B & C see Appendix B for HAC conditional logic

CC MCC +7th **S52.035 Nondisplaced fracture of olecranon process with intraarticular extension of left ulna**
HAC 7th characters B & C see Appendix B for HAC conditional logic

CC MCC +7th **S52.036 Nondisplaced fracture of olecranon process with intraarticular extension of unspecified ulna**
HAC 7th characters B & C see Appendix B for HAC conditional logic

+ S52.04 Fracture of coronoid process of ulna

CC MCC +7th **S52.041 Displaced fracture of coronoid process of right ulna**
HAC 7th characters B & C see Appendix B for HAC conditional logic

CC MCC +7th **S52.042 Displaced fracture of coronoid process of left ulna**
HAC 7th characters B & C see Appendix B for HAC conditional logic

CC MCC +7th **S52.043 Displaced fracture of coronoid process of unspecified ulna**
HAC 7th characters B & C see Appendix B for HAC conditional logic

CC MCC +7th **S52.044 Nondisplaced fracture of coronoid process of right ulna**
HAC 7th characters B & C see Appendix B for HAC conditional logic

CC MCC +7th **S52.045 Nondisplaced fracture of coronoid process of left ulna**
HAC 7th characters B & C see Appendix B for HAC conditional logic

CC MCC +7th **S52.046 Nondisplaced fracture of coronoid process of unspecified ulna**
HAC 7th characters B & C see Appendix B for HAC conditional logic

+ S52.09 Other fracture of upper end of ulna

CC MCC +7th **S52.091 Other fracture of upper end of right ulna**
HAC 7th characters B & C see Appendix B for HAC conditional logic

CC MCC +7th **S52.092 Other fracture of upper end of left ulna**
HAC 7th characters B & C see Appendix B for HAC conditional logic

CC MCC +7th **S52.099 Other fracture of upper end of unspecified ulna**
HAC 7th characters B & C see Appendix B for HAC conditional logic

+ S52.1 Fracture of upper end of radius

Fracture of proximal end of radius

Excludes2: *physeal fractures of upper end of radius (S59.2-)*
fracture of shaft of radius (S52.3-)

+ S52.10 Unspecified fracture of upper end of radius

CC MCC +7th **S52.101 Unspecified fracture of upper end of right radius**
HAC 7th characters B & C see Appendix B for HAC conditional logic

CC MCC +7th **S52.102 Unspecified fracture of upper end of left radius**
HAC 7th characters B & C see Appendix B for HAC conditional logic

CC MCC +7th **S52.109 Unspecified fracture of upper end of unspecified radius**
HAC 7th characters B & C see Appendix B for HAC conditional logic

+ S52.11 Torus fracture of upper end of radius

The appropriate 7th character is to be added to all codes in subcategory **S52.11**
A initial encounter for closed fracture
D subsequent encounter for fracture with routine healing
G subsequent encounter for fracture with delayed healing
K subsequent encounter for fracture with nonunion
P subsequent encounter for fracture with malunion
S sequela

CC +7th **S52.111 Torus fracture of upper end of right radius**
HAC 7th character A see Appendix B for HAC conditional logic

CC +7th **S52.112 Torus fracture of upper end of left radius**
HAC 7th character A see Appendix B for HAC conditional logic

CC +7th **S52.119 Torus fracture of upper end of unspecified radius**
HAC 7th character A see Appendix B for HAC conditional logic

+ S52.12 Fracture of head of radius

CC MCC +7th **S52.121 Displaced fracture of head of right radius**
HAC 7th characters B & C see Appendix B for HAC conditional logic

CC MCC +7th **S52.122 Displaced fracture of head of left radius**
HAC 7th characters B & C see Appendix B for HAC conditional logic

CC MCC +7th **S52.123 Displaced fracture of head of unspecified radius**
HAC 7th characters B & C see Appendix B for HAC conditional logic

CC MCC +7th **S52.124 Nondisplaced fracture of head of right radius**
HAC 7th characters B & C see Appendix B for HAC conditional logic

CC MCC +7th **S52.125 Nondisplaced fracture of head of left radius**
HAC 7th characters B & C see Appendix B for HAC conditional logic

CC MCC +7th **S52.126 Nondisplaced fracture of head of unspecified radius**
HAC 7th characters B & C see Appendix B for HAC conditional logic

\+ **S52.13 Fracture of neck of radius**

CC MCC +7th **S52.131 Displaced fracture of neck of right radius**
HAC 7th characters B & C see Appendix B for HAC conditional logic

CC MCC +7th **S52.132 Displaced fracture of neck of left radius**
HAC 7th characters B & C see Appendix B for HAC conditional logic

CC MCC +7th **S52.133 Displaced fracture of neck of unspecified radius**
HAC 7th characters B & C see Appendix B for HAC conditional logic

CC MCC +7th **S52.134 Nondisplaced fracture of neck of right radius**
HAC 7th characters B & C see Appendix B for HAC conditional logic

CC MCC +7th **S52.135 Nondisplaced fracture of neck of left radius**
HAC 7th characters B & C see Appendix B for HAC conditional logic

CC MCC +7th **S52.136 Nondisplaced fracture of neck of unspecified radius**
HAC 7th characters B & C see Appendix B for HAC conditional logic

\+ **S52.18 Other fracture of upper end of radius**

CC MCC +7th **S52.181 Other fracture of upper end of right radius**
HAC 7th characters B & C see Appendix B for HAC conditional logic

CC MCC +7th **S52.182 Other fracture of upper end of left radius**
HAC 7th characters B & C see Appendix B for HAC conditional logic

CC MCC +7th **S52.189 Other fracture of upper end of unspecified radius**
HAC 7th characters B & C see Appendix B for HAC conditional logic

\+ **S52.2 Fracture of shaft of ulna**

\+ **S52.20 Unspecified fracture of shaft of ulna**
Fracture of ulna NOS

CC MCC +7th **S52.201 Unspecified fracture of shaft of right ulna**
HAC 7th characters A - C see Appendix B for HAC conditional logic

CC MCC +7th **S52.202 Unspecified fracture of shaft of left ulna**
HAC 7th characters A - C see Appendix B for HAC conditional logic

CC MCC +7th **S52.209 Unspecified fracture of shaft of unspecified ulna**
HAC 7th characters A - C see Appendix B for HAC conditional logic

\+ **S52.21 Greenstick fracture of shaft of ulna**

The appropriate 7th character is to be added to all codes in subcategory **S52.21**
A initial encounter for closed fracture
D subsequent encounter for fracture with routine healing
G subsequent encounter for fracture with delayed healing
K subsequent encounter for fracture with nonunion
P subsequent encounter for fracture with malunion
S sequela

CC +7th **S52.211 Greenstick fracture of shaft of right ulna**
HAC 7th character A see Appendix B for HAC conditional logic

CC +7th **S52.212 Greenstick fracture of shaft of left ulna**
HAC 7th character A see Appendix B for HAC conditional logic

CC +7th **S52.219 Greenstick fracture of shaft of unspecified ulna**
HAC 7th character A see Appendix B for HAC conditional logic

\+ **S52.22 Transverse fracture of shaft of ulna**

CC MCC +7th **S52.221 Displaced transverse fracture of shaft of right ulna**
HAC 7th characters A - C see Appendix B for HAC conditional logic

CC MCC +7th **S52.222 Displaced transverse fracture of shaft of left ulna**
HAC 7th characters A - C see Appendix B for HAC conditional logic

CC MCC +7th **S52.223 Displaced transverse fracture of shaft of unspecified ulna**
HAC 7th characters A - C see Appendix B for HAC conditional logic

CC MCC +7th **S52.224 Nondisplaced transverse fracture of shaft of right ulna**
HAC 7th characters A - C see Appendix B for HAC conditional logic

CC MCC +7th **S52.225 Nondisplaced transverse fracture of shaft of left ulna**
HAC 7th characters A - C see Appendix B for HAC conditional logic

CC MCC +7th **S52.226 Nondisplaced transverse fracture of shaft of unspecified ulna**
HAC 7th characters A - C see Appendix B for HAC conditional logic

\+ **S52.23 Oblique fracture of shaft of ulna**

CC MCC +7th **S52.231 Displaced oblique fracture of shaft of right ulna**
HAC 7th characters A - C see Appendix B for HAC conditional logic

CC MCC +7th **S52.232 Displaced oblique fracture of shaft of left ulna**
HAC 7th characters A - C see Appendix B for HAC conditional logic

CC MCC +7th **S52.233 Displaced oblique fracture of shaft of unspecified ulna**
HAC 7th characters A - C see Appendix B for HAC conditional logic

CC MCC +7th **S52.234 Nondisplaced oblique fracture of shaft of right ulna**
HAC 7th characters A - C see Appendix B for HAC conditional logic

CC MCC +7th **S52.235 Nondisplaced oblique fracture of shaft of left ulna**
HAC 7th characters A - C see Appendix B for HAC conditional logic

CC MCC +7th **S52.236 Nondisplaced oblique fracture of shaft of unspecified ulna**
HAC 7th characters A - C see Appendix B for HAC conditional logic

\+ **S52.24 Spiral fracture of shaft of ulna**

CC MCC +7th **S52.241 Displaced spiral fracture of shaft of ulna, right arm**
HAC 7th characters A - C see Appendix B for HAC conditional logic

CC MCC +7th **S52.242 Displaced spiral fracture of shaft of ulna, left arm**
HAC 7th characters A - C see Appendix B for HAC conditional logic

CC MCC +7th **S52.243 Displaced spiral fracture of shaft of ulna, unspecified arm**
HAC 7th characters A - C see Appendix B for HAC conditional logic

CC MCC +7th **S52.244 Nondisplaced spiral fracture of shaft of ulna, right arm**
HAC 7th characters A - C see Appendix B for HAC conditional logic

CC MCC +7th **S52.245 Nondisplaced spiral fracture of shaft of ulna, left arm**
HAC 7th characters A - C see Appendix B for HAC conditional logic

CC MCC +7th **S52.246 Nondisplaced spiral fracture of shaft of ulna, unspecified arm**
HAC 7th characters A - C see Appendix B for HAC conditional logic

+ S52.25 Comminuted fracture of shaft of ulna

CC MCC +7th **S52.251 Displaced comminuted fracture of shaft of ulna, right arm**
HAC 7th characters A - C see Appendix B for HAC conditional logic

CC MCC +7th **S52.252 Displaced comminuted fracture of shaft of ulna, left arm**
HAC 7th characters A - C see Appendix B for HAC conditional logic

CC MCC +7th **S52.253 Displaced comminuted fracture of shaft of ulna, unspecified arm**
HAC 7th characters A - C see Appendix B for HAC conditional logic

CC MCC +7th **S52.254 Nondisplaced comminuted fracture of shaft of ulna, right arm**
HAC 7th characters A - C see Appendix B for HAC conditional logic

CC MCC +7th **S52.255 Nondisplaced comminuted fracture of shaft of ulna, left arm**
HAC 7th characters A - C see Appendix B for HAC conditional logic

CC MCC +7th **S52.256 Nondisplaced comminuted fracture of shaft of ulna, unspecified arm**
HAC 7th characters A - C see Appendix B for HAC conditional logic

+ S52.26 Segmental fracture of shaft of ulna

CC MCC +7th **S52.261 Displaced segmental fracture of shaft of ulna, right arm**
HAC 7th characters A - C see Appendix B for HAC conditional logic

CC MCC +7th **S52.262 Displaced segmental fracture of shaft of ulna, left arm**
HAC 7th characters A - C see Appendix B for HAC conditional logic

CC MCC +7th **S52.263 Displaced segmental fracture of shaft of ulna, unspecified arm**
HAC 7th characters A - C see Appendix B for HAC conditional logic

CC MCC +7th **S52.264 Nondisplaced segmental fracture of shaft of ulna, right arm**
HAC 7th characters A - C see Appendix B for HAC conditional logic

CC MCC +7th **S52.265 Nondisplaced segmental fracture of shaft of ulna, left arm**
HAC 7th characters A - C see Appendix B for HAC conditional logic

CC MCC +7th **S52.266 Nondisplaced segmental fracture of shaft of ulna, unspecified arm**
HAC 7th characters A - C see Appendix B for HAC conditional logic

+ S52.27 Monteggia's fracture of ulna
Fracture of upper shaft of ulna with dislocation of radial head

CC MCC +7th **S52.271 Monteggia's fracture of right ulna**
HAC 7th characters B & C see Appendix B for HAC conditional logic

CC MCC +7th **S52.272 Monteggia's fracture of left ulna**
HAC 7th characters B & C see Appendix B for HAC conditional logic

CC MCC +7th **S52.279 Monteggia's fracture of unspecified ulna**
HAC 7th characters B & C see Appendix B for HAC conditional logic

+ S52.28 Bent bone of ulna

CC MCC +7th **S52.281 Bent bone of right ulna**
HAC 7th characters A - C see Appendix B for HAC conditional logic

CC MCC +7th **S52.282 Bent bone of left ulna**
HAC 7th characters A - C see Appendix B for HAC conditional logic

CC MCC +7th **S52.283 Bent bone of unspecified ulna**
HAC 7th characters A - C see Appendix B for HAC conditional logic

+ S52.29 Other fracture of shaft of ulna

CC MCC +7th **S52.291 Other fracture of shaft of right ulna**
HAC 7th characters A - C see Appendix B for HAC conditional logic

CC MCC +7th **S52.292 Other fracture of shaft of left ulna**
HAC 7th characters A - C see Appendix B for HAC conditional logic

CC MCC +7th **S52.299 Other fracture of shaft of unspecified ulna**
HAC 7th characters A - C see Appendix B for HAC conditional logic

+ S52.3 Fracture of shaft of radius

+ S52.30 Unspecified fracture of shaft of radius

CC MCC +7th **S52.301 Unspecified fracture of shaft of right radius**
HAC 7th characters A - C see Appendix B for HAC conditional logic

CC MCC +7th **S52.302 Unspecified fracture of shaft of left radius**
HAC 7th characters A - C see Appendix B for HAC conditional logic

CC MCC +7th **S52.309 Unspecified fracture of shaft of unspecified radius**
HAC 7th characters A - C see Appendix B for HAC conditional logic

+ S52.31 Greenstick fracture of shaft of radius

The appropriate 7th character is to be added to all codes in subcategory **S52.31**
A initial encounter for closed fracture
D subsequent encounter for fracture with routine healing
G subsequent encounter for fracture with delayed healing
K subsequent encounter for fracture with nonunion
P subsequent encounter for fracture with malunion
S sequela

CC +7th **S52.311 Greenstick fracture of shaft of radius, right arm**
HAC 7th character A see Appendix B for HAC conditional logic

CC +7th **S52.312 Greenstick fracture of shaft of radius, left arm**
HAC 7th character A see Appendix B for HAC conditional logic

CC +7th **S52.319 Greenstick fracture of shaft of radius, unspecified arm**
HAC 7th character A see Appendix B for HAC conditional logic

+ S52.32 Transverse fracture of shaft of radius

CC MCC +7th **S52.321 Displaced transverse fracture of shaft of right radius**
HAC 7th characters A - C see Appendix B for HAC conditional logic

CC MCC +7th **S52.322 Displaced transverse fracture of shaft of left radius**
HAC 7th characters A - C see Appendix B for HAC conditional logic

CC MCC +7th **S52.323 Displaced transverse fracture of shaft of unspecified radius**
HAC 7th characters A - C see Appendix B for HAC conditional logic

CC MCC +7th **S52.324 Nondisplaced transverse fracture of shaft of right radius**
HAC 7th characters A - C see Appendix B for HAC conditional logic

CC MCC +7th **S52.325 Nondisplaced transverse fracture of shaft of left radius**
HAC 7th characters A - C see Appendix B for HAC conditional logic

CC MCC +7th **S52.326 Nondisplaced transverse fracture of shaft of unspecified radius**
HAC 7th characters A - C see Appendix B for HAC conditional logic

+ **S52.33 Oblique fracture of shaft of radius**

CC MCC +7th **S52.331 Displaced oblique fracture of shaft of right radius**
HAC 7th characters A - C see Appendix B for HAC conditional logic

CC MCC +7th **S52.332 Displaced oblique fracture of shaft of left radius**
HAC 7th characters A - C see Appendix B for HAC conditional logic

CC MCC +7th **S52.333 Displaced oblique fracture of shaft of unspecified radius**
HAC 7th characters A - C see Appendix B for HAC conditional logic

CC MCC +7th **S52.334 Nondisplaced oblique fracture of shaft of right radius**
HAC 7th characters A - C see Appendix B for HAC conditional logic

CC MCC +7th **S52.335 Nondisplaced oblique fracture of shaft of left radius**
HAC 7th characters A - C see Appendix B for HAC conditional logic

CC MCC +7th **S52.336 Nondisplaced oblique fracture of shaft of unspecified radius**
HAC 7th characters A - C see Appendix B for HAC conditional logic

+ **S52.34 Spiral fracture of shaft of radius**

CC MCC +7th **S52.341 Displaced spiral fracture of shaft of radius, right arm**
HAC 7th characters A - C see Appendix B for HAC conditional logic

CC MCC +7th **S52.342 Displaced spiral fracture of shaft of radius, left arm**
HAC 7th characters A - C see Appendix B for HAC conditional logic

CC MCC +7th **S52.343 Displaced spiral fracture of shaft of radius, unspecified arm**
HAC 7th characters A - C see Appendix B for HAC conditional logic

CC MCC +7th **S52.344 Nondisplaced spiral fracture of shaft of radius, right arm**
HAC 7th characters A - C see Appendix B for HAC conditional logic

CC MCC +7th **S52.345 Nondisplaced spiral fracture of shaft of radius, left arm**
HAC 7th characters A - C see Appendix B for HAC conditional logic

CC MCC +7th **S52.346 Nondisplaced spiral fracture of shaft of radius, unspecified arm**
HAC 7th characters A - C see Appendix B for HAC conditional logic

+ **S52.35 Comminuted fracture of shaft of radius**

CC MCC +7th **S52.351 Displaced comminuted fracture of shaft of radius, right arm**
HAC 7th characters A - C see Appendix B for HAC conditional logic

CC MCC +7th **S52.352 Displaced comminuted fracture of shaft of radius, left arm**
HAC 7th characters A - C see Appendix B for HAC conditional logic

CC MCC +7th **S52.353 Displaced comminuted fracture of shaft of radius, unspecified arm**
HAC 7th characters A - C see Appendix B for HAC conditional logic

CC MCC +7th **S52.354 Nondisplaced comminuted fracture of shaft of radius, right arm**
HAC 7th characters A - C see Appendix B for HAC conditional logic

CC MCC +7th **S52.355 Nondisplaced comminuted fracture of shaft of radius, left arm**
HAC 7th characters A - C see Appendix B for HAC conditional logic

CC MCC +7th **S52.356 Nondisplaced comminuted fracture of shaft of radius, unspecified arm**
HAC 7th characters A - C see Appendix B for HAC conditional logic

+ **S52.36 Segmental fracture of shaft of radius**

CC MCC +7th **S52.361 Displaced segmental fracture of shaft of radius, right arm**
HAC 7th characters A - C see Appendix B for HAC conditional logic

CC MCC +7th **S52.362 Displaced segmental fracture of shaft of radius, left arm**
HAC 7th characters A - C see Appendix B for HAC conditional logic

CC MCC +7th **S52.363 Displaced segmental fracture of shaft of radius, unspecified arm**
HAC 7th characters A - C see Appendix B for HAC conditional logic

CC MCC +7th **S52.364 Nondisplaced segmental fracture of shaft of radius, right arm**
HAC 7th characters A - C see Appendix B for HAC conditional logic

CC MCC +7th **S52.365 Nondisplaced segmental fracture of shaft of radius, left arm**
HAC 7th characters A - C see Appendix B for HAC conditional logic

CC MCC +7th **S52.366 Nondisplaced segmental fracture of shaft of radius, unspecified arm**
HAC 7th characters A - C see Appendix B for HAC conditional logic

+ **S52.37 Galeazzi's fracture**
Fracture of lower shaft of radius with radioulnar joint dislocation

CC MCC +7th **S52.371 Galeazzi's fracture of right radius**
HAC 7th characters A - C see Appendix B for HAC conditional logic

CC MCC +7th **S52.372 Galeazzi's fracture of left radius**
HAC 7th characters A - C see Appendix B for HAC conditional logic

CC MCC +7th **S52.379 Galeazzi's fracture of unspecified radius**
HAC 7th characters A - C see Appendix B for HAC conditional logic

+ **S52.38 Bent bone of radius**

CC MCC +7th **S52.381 Bent bone of right radius**
HAC 7th characters A - C see Appendix B for HAC conditional logic

CC MCC +7th **S52.382 Bent bone of left radius**
HAC 7th characters A - C see Appendix B for HAC conditional logic

CC MCC +7th **S52.389 Bent bone of unspecified radius**
HAC 7th characters A - C see Appendix B for HAC conditional logic

+ **S52.39 Other fracture of shaft of radius**

CC MCC +7th **S52.391 Other fracture of shaft of radius, right arm**
HAC 7th characters A - C see Appendix B for HAC conditional logic

CC MCC +7th **S52.392 Other fracture of shaft of radius, left arm**
HAC 7th characters A - C see Appendix B for HAC conditional logic

CC MCC +7th **S52.399 Other fracture of shaft of radius, unspecified arm**
HAC 7th characters A - C see Appendix B for HAC conditional logic

+ **S52.5 Fracture of lower end of radius**
Fracture of distal end of radius
Excludes2: *physeal fractures of lower end of radius (S59.2-)*

+ **S52.50 Unspecified fracture of the lower end of radius**

CC MCC +7th **S52.501 Unspecified fracture of the lower end of right radius**
HAC 7th characters A - C see Appendix B for HAC conditional logic

CC MCC +7th **S52.502 Unspecified fracture of the lower end of left radius**
HAC 7th characters A - C see Appendix B for HAC conditional logic

CC MCC +7th **S52.509 Unspecified fracture of the lower end of unspecified radius**
HAC 7th characters A - C see Appendix B for HAC conditional logic

+ **S52.51 Fracture of radial styloid process**

CC MCC +7th **S52.511 Displaced fracture of right radial styloid process**
HAC 7th characters A - C see Appendix B for HAC conditional logic

CC MCC +7th **S52.512 Displaced fracture of left radial styloid process**
HAC 7th characters A - C see Appendix B for HAC conditional logic

CC MCC +7th **S52.513 Displaced fracture of unspecified radial styloid process**
HAC 7th characters A - C see Appendix B for HAC conditional logic

CC MCC +7th **S52.514 Nondisplaced fracture of right radial styloid process**
HAC 7th characters A - C see Appendix B for HAC conditional logic

CC MCC +7th **S52.515 Nondisplaced fracture of left radial styloid process**
HAC 7th characters A - C see Appendix B for HAC conditional logic

CC MCC +7th **S52.516 Nondisplaced fracture of unspecified radial styloid process**
HAC 7th characters A - C see Appendix B for HAC conditional logic

+ S52.52 Torus fracture of lower end of radius

The appropriate 7th character is to be added to all codes in subcategory **S52.52**
- A initial encounter for closed fracture
- D subsequent encounter for fracture with routine healing
- G subsequent encounter for fracture with delayed healing
- K subsequent encounter for fracture with nonunion
- P subsequent encounter for fracture with malunion
- S sequela

CC +7th **S52.521 Torus fracture of lower end of right radius**
HAC 7th character A see Appendix B for HAC conditional logic

CC +7th **S52.522 Torus fracture of lower end of left radius**
HAC 7th character A see Appendix B for HAC conditional logic

CC +7th **S52.529 Torus fracture of lower end of unspecified radius**
HAC 7th character A see Appendix B for HAC conditional logic

+ S52.53 Colles' fracture

CC MCC +7th **S52.531 Colles' fracture of right radius**
HAC 7th characters A - C see Appendix B for HAC conditional logic

CC MCC +7th **S52.532 Colles' fracture of left radius**
AHA CC: 2Q, 2016, 4-5
HAC 7th characters A - C see Appendix B for HAC conditional logic

CC MCC +7th **S52.539 Colles' fracture of unspecified radius**
HAC 7th characters A - C see Appendix B for HAC conditional logic

+ S52.54 Smith's fracture

CC MCC +7th **S52.541 Smith's fracture of right radius**
HAC 7th characters A - C see Appendix B for HAC conditional logic

CC MCC +7th **S52.542 Smith's fracture of left radius**
HAC 7th characters A - C see Appendix B for HAC conditional logic

CC MCC +7th **S52.549 Smith's fracture of unspecified radius**
HAC 7th characters A - C see Appendix B for HAC conditional logic

+ S52.55 Other extraarticular fracture of lower end of radius

CC MCC +7th **S52.551 Other extraarticular fracture of lower end of right radius**
HAC 7th characters A - C see Appendix B for HAC conditional logic

CC MCC +7th **S52.552 Other extraarticular fracture of lower end of left radius**
HAC 7th characters A - C see Appendix B for HAC conditional logic

CC MCC +7th **S52.559 Other extraarticular fracture of lower end of unspecified radius**
HAC 7th characters A - C see Appendix B for HAC conditional logic

+ S52.56 Barton's fracture

CC MCC +7th **S52.561 Barton's fracture of right radius**
HAC 7th characters A - C see Appendix B for HAC conditional logic

CC MCC +7th **S52.562 Barton's fracture of left radius**
HAC 7th characters A - C see Appendix B for HAC conditional logic

CC MCC +7th **S52.569 Barton's fracture of unspecified radius**
HAC 7th characters A - C see Appendix B for HAC conditional logic

+ S52.57 Other intraarticular fracture of lower end of radius

CC MCC +7th **S52.571 Other intraarticular fracture of lower end of right radius**
HAC 7th characters A - C see Appendix B for HAC conditional logic

CC MCC +7th **S52.572 Other intraarticular fracture of lower end of left radius**
HAC 7th characters A - C see Appendix B for HAC conditional logic

CC MCC +7th **S52.579 Other intraarticular fracture of lower end of unspecified radius**
HAC 7th characters A - C see Appendix B for HAC conditional logic

+ S52.59 Other fractures of lower end of radius

CC MCC +7th **S52.591 Other fractures of lower end of right radius**
AHA CC: 3Q, 2019, 9-10
HAC 7th characters A - C see Appendix B for HAC conditional logic

CC MCC +7th **S52.592 Other fractures of lower end of left radius**
HAC 7th characters A - C see Appendix B for HAC conditional logic

CC MCC +7th **S52.599 Other fractures of lower end of unspecified radius**
HAC 7th characters A - C see Appendix B for HAC conditional logic

+ S52.6 Fracture of lower end of ulna

+ S52.60 Unspecified fracture of lower end of ulna

CC MCC +7th **S52.601 Unspecified fracture of lower end of right ulna**
HAC 7th characters A - C see Appendix B for HAC conditional logic

CC MCC +7th **S52.602 Unspecified fracture of lower end of left ulna**
HAC 7th characters A - C see Appendix B for HAC conditional logic

CC MCC +7th **S52.609 Unspecified fracture of lower end of unspecified ulna**
HAC 7th characters A - C see Appendix B for HAC conditional logic

+ S52.61 Fracture of ulna styloid process

CC MCC +7th **S52.611 Displaced fracture of right ulna styloid process**
HAC 7th characters A - C see Appendix B for HAC conditional logic

CC MCC +7th **S52.612 Displaced fracture of left ulna styloid process**
HAC 7th characters A - C see Appendix B for HAC conditional logic

CC MCC +7th **S52.613 Displaced fracture of unspecified ulna styloid process**
HAC 7th characters A - C see Appendix B for HAC conditional logic

CC MCC +7th **S52.614 Nondisplaced fracture of right ulna styloid process**
HAC 7th characters A - C see Appendix B for HAC conditional logic

CC MCC +7th **S52.615 Nondisplaced fracture of left ulna styloid process**
HAC 7th characters A - C see Appendix B for HAC conditional logic

CC MCC +7th **S52.616 Nondisplaced fracture of unspecified ulna styloid process**
HAC 7th characters A - C see Appendix B for HAC conditional logic

+ S52.62 Torus fracture of lower end of ulna

The appropriate 7th character is to be added to all codes in subcategory **S52.62**
- A initial encounter for closed fracture
- D subsequent encounter for fracture with routine healing
- G subsequent encounter for fracture with delayed healing
- K subsequent encounter for fracture with nonunion
- P subsequent encounter for fracture with malunion
- S sequela

CC +7th **S52.621 Torus fracture of lower end of right ulna**
HAC 7th character A see Appendix B for HAC conditional logic

CC +7th **S52.622 Torus fracture of lower end of left ulna**
HAC 7th character A see Appendix B for HAC conditional logic

CC +7th **S52.629 Torus fracture of lower end of unspecified ulna**
HAC 7th character A see Appendix B for HAC conditional logic

\+ **S52.69 Other fracture of lower end of ulna**

CC MCC +7th **S52.691 Other fracture of lower end of right ulna**
AHA CC: 3Q, 2019, 9-10
HAC 7th characters A - C see Appendix B for HAC conditional logic

CC MCC +7th **S52.692 Other fracture of lower end of left ulna**
HAC 7th characters A - C see Appendix B for HAC conditional logic

CC MCC +7th **S52.699 Other fracture of lower end of unspecified ulna**
HAC 7th characters A - C see Appendix B for HAC conditional logic

\+ **S52.9 Unspecified fracture of forearm**

CC MCC X+7th **S52.90 Unspecified fracture of unspecified forearm**
HAC 7th characters A - C see Appendix B for HAC conditional logic

CC MCC X+7th **S52.91 Unspecified fracture of right forearm**
HAC 7th characters A - C see Appendix B for HAC conditional logic

CC MCC X+7th **S52.92 Unspecified fracture of left forearm**
HAC 7th characters A - C see Appendix B for HAC conditional logic

S53 Dislocation and sprain of joints and ligaments of elbow

Includes: avulsion of joint or ligament of elbow
laceration of cartilage, joint or ligament of elbow
sprain of cartilage, joint or ligament of elbow
traumatic hemarthrosis of joint or ligament of elbow
traumatic rupture of joint or ligament of elbow
traumatic subluxation of joint or ligament of elbow
traumatic tear of joint or ligament of elbow

Code also any associated open wound

Excludes2: *strain of muscle, fascia and tendon at forearm level (S56.-)*

The appropriate 7th character is to be added to each code from category S53
A initial encounter
D subsequent encounter
S sequela

\+ **S53.0 Subluxation and dislocation of radial head**
Dislocation of radiohumeral joint
Subluxation of radiohumeral joint
Excludes1: *Monteggia's fracture-dislocation (S52.27-)*

\+ **S53.00 Unspecified subluxation and dislocation of radial head**

+7th **S53.001 Unspecified subluxation of right radial head**

+7th **S53.002 Unspecified subluxation of left radial head**

+7th **S53.003 Unspecified subluxation of unspecified radial head**

+7th **S53.004 Unspecified dislocation of right radial head**

+7th **S53.005 Unspecified dislocation of left radial head**

+7th **S53.006 Unspecified dislocation of unspecified radial head**

\+ **S53.01 Anterior subluxation and dislocation of radial head**
Anteriomedial subluxation and dislocation of radial head

+7th **S53.011 Anterior subluxation of right radial head**

+7th **S53.012 Anterior subluxation of left radial head**

+7th **S53.013 Anterior subluxation of unspecified radial head**

+7th **S53.014 Anterior dislocation of right radial head**

+7th **S53.015 Anterior dislocation of left radial head**

+7th **S53.016 Anterior dislocation of unspecified radial head**

\+ **S53.02 Posterior subluxation and dislocation of radial head**
Posteriolateral subluxation and dislocation of radial head

+7th **S53.021 Posterior subluxation of right radial head**

+7th **S53.022 Posterior subluxation of left radial head**

+7th **S53.023 Posterior subluxation of unspecified radial head**

+7th **S53.024 Posterior dislocation of right radial head**

+7th **S53.025 Posterior dislocation of left radial head**

+7th **S53.026 Posterior dislocation of unspecified radial head**

\+ **S53.03 Nursemaid's elbow**

+7th **S53.031 Nursemaid's elbow, right elbow**
AHA CC: 1Q, 2015, 3-21

+7th **S53.032 Nursemaid's elbow, left elbow**

+7th **S53.033 Nursemaid's elbow, unspecified elbow**

\+ **S53.09 Other subluxation and dislocation of radial head**

+7th **S53.091 Other subluxation of right radial head**

+7th **S53.092 Other subluxation of left radial head**

+7th **S53.093 Other subluxation of unspecified radial head**

+7th **S53.094 Other dislocation of right radial head**

+7th **S53.095 Other dislocation of left radial head**

+7th **S53.096 Other dislocation of unspecified radial head**

\+ **S53.1 Subluxation and dislocation of ulnohumeral joint**
Subluxation and dislocation of elbow NOS
Excludes1: *dislocation of radial head alone (S53.0-)*

\+ **S53.10 Unspecified subluxation and dislocation of ulnohumeral joint**

+7th **S53.101 Unspecified subluxation of right ulnohumeral joint**

+7th **S53.102 Unspecified subluxation of left ulnohumeral joint**

+7th **S53.103 Unspecified subluxation of unspecified ulnohumeral joint**

+7th **S53.104 Unspecified dislocation of right ulnohumeral joint**

+7th **S53.105 Unspecified dislocation of left ulnohumeral joint**

+7th **S53.106 Unspecified dislocation of unspecified ulnohumeral joint**

\+ **S53.11 Anterior subluxation and dislocation of ulnohumeral joint**

+7th **S53.111 Anterior subluxation of right ulnohumeral joint**

+7th **S53.112 Anterior subluxation of left ulnohumeral joint**

+7th **S53.113 Anterior subluxation of unspecified ulnohumeral joint**

+7th **S53.114 Anterior dislocation of right ulnohumeral joint**
AHA CC: 4Q, 2012, 108

+7th **S53.115 Anterior dislocation of left ulnohumeral joint**

+7th **S53.116 Anterior dislocation of unspecified ulnohumeral joint**

\+ **S53.12 Posterior subluxation and dislocation of ulnohumeral joint**

+7th **S53.121 Posterior subluxation of right ulnohumeral joint**

+7th **S53.122 Posterior subluxation of left ulnohumeral joint**

+7th **S53.123 Posterior subluxation of unspecified ulnohumeral joint**

+7th **S53.124 Posterior dislocation of right ulnohumeral joint**

+7th **S53.125 Posterior dislocation of left ulnohumeral joint**

+7th **S53.126 Posterior dislocation of unspecified ulnohumeral joint**

\+ **S53.13 Medial subluxation and dislocation of ulnohumeral joint**

+7th **S53.131 Medial subluxation of right ulnohumeral joint**

+7th **S53.132 Medial subluxation of left ulnohumeral joint**

+7th **S53.133 Medial subluxation of unspecified ulnohumeral joint**
+7th **S53.134 Medial dislocation of right ulnohumeral joint**
+7th **S53.135 Medial dislocation of left ulnohumeral joint**
+7th **S53.136 Medial dislocation of unspecified ulnohumeral joint**
+ **S53.14 Lateral subluxation and dislocation of ulnohumeral joint**
+7th **S53.141 Lateral subluxation of right ulnohumeral joint**
+7th **S53.142 Lateral subluxation of left ulnohumeral joint**
+7th **S53.143 Lateral subluxation of unspecified ulnohumeral joint**
+7th **S53.144 Lateral dislocation of right ulnohumeral joint**
+7th **S53.145 Lateral dislocation of left ulnohumeral joint**
+7th **S53.146 Lateral dislocation of unspecified ulnohumeral joint**
+ **S53.19 Other subluxation and dislocation of ulnohumeral joint**
+7th **S53.191 Other subluxation of right ulnohumeral joint**
+7th **S53.192 Other subluxation of left ulnohumeral joint**
+7th **S53.193 Other subluxation of unspecified ulnohumeral joint**
+7th **S53.194 Other dislocation of right ulnohumeral joint**
+7th **S53.195 Other dislocation of left ulnohumeral joint**
+7th **S53.196 Other dislocation of unspecified ulnohumeral joint**
+ **S53.2 Traumatic rupture of radial collateral ligament**
Excludes1: *sprain of radial collateral ligament NOS (S53.43-)*
X+7th **S53.20 Traumatic rupture of unspecified radial collateral ligament**
X+7th **S53.21 Traumatic rupture of right radial collateral ligament**
X+7th **S53.22 Traumatic rupture of left radial collateral ligament**
+ **S53.3 Traumatic rupture of ulnar collateral ligament**
Excludes1: *sprain of ulnar collateral ligament (S53.44-)*
X+7th **S53.30 Traumatic rupture of unspecified ulnar collateral ligament**
X+7th **S53.31 Traumatic rupture of right ulnar collateral ligament**
X+7th **S53.32 Traumatic rupture of left ulnar collateral ligament**
+ **S53.4 Sprain of elbow**
Excludes2: *traumatic rupture of radial collateral ligament (S53.2-)*
traumatic rupture of ulnar collateral ligament (S53.3-)
+ **S53.40 Unspecified sprain of elbow**
+7th **S53.401 Unspecified sprain of right elbow**
+7th **S53.402 Unspecified sprain of left elbow**
+7th **S53.409 Unspecified sprain of unspecified elbow**
Sprain of elbow NOS
+ **S53.41 Radiohumeral (joint) sprain**
+7th **S53.411 Radiohumeral (joint) sprain of right elbow**
+7th **S53.412 Radiohumeral (joint) sprain of left elbow**
+7th **S53.419 Radiohumeral (joint) sprain of unspecified elbow**
+ **S53.42 Ulnohumeral (joint) sprain**
+7th **S53.421 Ulnohumeral (joint) sprain of right elbow**
+7th **S53.422 Ulnohumeral (joint) sprain of left elbow**
+7th **S53.429 Ulnohumeral (joint) sprain of unspecified elbow**
+ **S53.43 Radial collateral ligament sprain**
+7th **S53.431 Radial collateral ligament sprain of right elbow**
+7th **S53.432 Radial collateral ligament sprain of left elbow**
+7th **S53.439 Radial collateral ligament sprain of unspecified elbow**
+ **S53.44 Ulnar collateral ligament sprain**
+7th **S53.441 Ulnar collateral ligament sprain of right elbow**
+7th **S53.442 Ulnar collateral ligament sprain of left elbow**
+7th **S53.449 Ulnar collateral ligament sprain of unspecified elbow**
+ **S53.49 Other sprain of elbow**
+7th **S53.491 Other sprain of right elbow**
+7th **S53.492 Other sprain of left elbow**
+7th **S53.499 Other sprain of unspecified elbow**

S54 Injury of nerves at forearm level
Code also any associated open wound (S51.-)
Excludes2: *injury of nerves at wrist and hand level (S64.-)*

The appropriate 7th character is to be added to each code from category S54
A initial encounter
D subsequent encounter
S sequela

+ **S54.0 Injury of ulnar nerve at forearm level**
Injury of ulnar nerve NOS
X+7th **S54.00 Injury of ulnar nerve at forearm level, unspecified arm**
X+7th **S54.01 Injury of ulnar nerve at forearm level, right arm**
X+7th **S54.02 Injury of ulnar nerve at forearm level, left arm**
+ **S54.1 Injury of median nerve at forearm level**
Injury of median nerve NOS
X+7th **S54.10 Injury of median nerve at forearm level, unspecified arm**
X+7th **S54.11 Injury of median nerve at forearm level, right arm**
X+7th **S54.12 Injury of median nerve at forearm level, left arm**
+ **S54.2 Injury of radial nerve at forearm level**
Injury of radial nerve NOS
X+7th **S54.20 Injury of radial nerve at forearm level, unspecified arm**
X+7th **S54.21 Injury of radial nerve at forearm level, right arm**
X+7th **S54.22 Injury of radial nerve at forearm level, left arm**
+ **S54.3 Injury of cutaneous sensory nerve at forearm level**
X+7th **S54.30 Injury of cutaneous sensory nerve at forearm level, unspecified arm**
X+7th **S54.31 Injury of cutaneous sensory nerve at forearm level, right arm**
X+7th **S54.32 Injury of cutaneous sensory nerve at forearm level, left arm**
+ **S54.8 Injury of other nerves at forearm level**
+ **S54.8X Injury of other nerves at forearm level**
+7th **S54.8X1 Injury of other nerves at forearm level, right arm**
+7th **S54.8X2 Injury of other nerves at forearm level, left arm**
+7th **S54.8X9 Injury of other nerves at forearm level, unspecified arm**
+ **S54.9 Injury of unspecified nerve at forearm level**
X+7th **S54.90 Injury of unspecified nerve at forearm level, unspecified arm**
X+7th **S54.91 Injury of unspecified nerve at forearm level, right arm**
X+7th **S54.92 Injury of unspecified nerve at forearm level, left arm**

S55 Injury of blood vessels at forearm level

Code also any associated open wound (S51.-)

Excludes2: *injury of blood vessels at wrist and hand level (S65.-)*
injury of brachial vessels (S45.1-S45.2)

The appropriate 7th character is to be added to each code from category S55
A initial encounter
D subsequent encounter
S sequela

+ S55.0 Injury of ulnar artery at forearm level
+ S55.00 Unspecified injury of ulnar artery at forearm level
CC +7th **S55.001 Unspecified injury of ulnar artery at forearm level, right arm**
CC +7th **S55.002 Unspecified injury of ulnar artery at forearm level, left arm**
CC +7th **S55.009 Unspecified injury of ulnar artery at forearm level, unspecified arm**
+ S55.01 Laceration of ulnar artery at forearm level
CC +7th **S55.011 Laceration of ulnar artery at forearm level, right arm**
CC +7th **S55.012 Laceration of ulnar artery at forearm level, left arm**
CC +7th **S55.019 Laceration of ulnar artery at forearm level, unspecified arm**
+ S55.09 Other specified injury of ulnar artery at forearm level
CC +7th **S55.091 Other specified injury of ulnar artery at forearm level, right arm**
CC +7th **S55.092 Other specified injury of ulnar artery at forearm level, left arm**
CC +7th **S55.099 Other specified injury of ulnar artery at forearm level, unspecified arm**

+ S55.1 Injury of radial artery at forearm level
+ S55.10 Unspecified injury of radial artery at forearm level
CC +7th **S55.101 Unspecified injury of radial artery at forearm level, right arm**
CC +7th **S55.102 Unspecified injury of radial artery at forearm level, left arm**
CC +7th **S55.109 Unspecified injury of radial artery at forearm level, unspecified arm**
+ S55.11 Laceration of radial artery at forearm level
CC +7th **S55.111 Laceration of radial artery at forearm level, right arm**
CC +7th **S55.112 Laceration of radial artery at forearm level, left arm**
CC +7th **S55.119 Laceration of radial artery at forearm level, unspecified arm**
+ S55.19 Other specified injury of radial artery at forearm level
CC +7th **S55.191 Other specified injury of radial artery at forearm level, right arm**
CC +7th **S55.192 Other specified injury of radial artery at forearm level, left arm**
CC +7th **S55.199 Other specified injury of radial artery at forearm level, unspecified arm**

+ S55.2 Injury of vein at forearm level
+ S55.20 Unspecified injury of vein at forearm level
CC +7th **S55.201 Unspecified injury of vein at forearm level, right arm**
CC +7th **S55.202 Unspecified injury of vein at forearm level, left arm**
CC +7th **S55.209 Unspecified injury of vein at forearm level, unspecified arm**
+ S55.21 Laceration of vein at forearm level
CC +7th **S55.211 Laceration of vein at forearm level, right arm**
CC +7th **S55.212 Laceration of vein at forearm level, left arm**
CC +7th **S55.219 Laceration of vein at forearm level, unspecified arm**
+ S55.29 Other specified injury of vein at forearm level
CC +7th **S55.291 Other specified injury of vein at forearm level, right arm**
CC +7th **S55.292 Other specified injury of vein at forearm level, left arm**
CC +7th **S55.299 Other specified injury of vein at forearm level, unspecified arm**

+ S55.8 Injury of other blood vessels at forearm level
+ S55.80 Unspecified injury of other blood vessels at forearm level
CC +7th **S55.801 Unspecified injury of other blood vessels at forearm level, right arm**
CC +7th **S55.802 Unspecified injury of other blood vessels at forearm level, left arm**
CC +7th **S55.809 Unspecified injury of other blood vessels at forearm level, unspecified arm**
+ S55.81 Laceration of other blood vessels at forearm level
CC +7th **S55.811 Laceration of other blood vessels at forearm level, right arm**
CC +7th **S55.812 Laceration of other blood vessels at forearm level, left arm**
CC +7th **S55.819 Laceration of other blood vessels at forearm level, unspecified arm**
+ S55.89 Other specified injury of other blood vessels at forearm level
CC +7th **S55.891 Other specified injury of other blood vessels at forearm level, right arm**
CC +7th **S55.892 Other specified injury of other blood vessels at forearm level, left arm**
CC +7th **S55.899 Other specified injury of other blood vessels at forearm level, unspecified arm**

+ S55.9 Injury of unspecified blood vessel at forearm level
+ S55.90 Unspecified injury of unspecified blood vessel at forearm level
CC +7th **S55.901 Unspecified injury of unspecified blood vessel at forearm level, right arm**
CC +7th **S55.902 Unspecified injury of unspecified blood vessel at forearm level, left arm**
CC +7th **S55.909 Unspecified injury of unspecified blood vessel at forearm level, unspecified arm**
+ S55.91 Laceration of unspecified blood vessel at forearm level
CC +7th **S55.911 Laceration of unspecified blood vessel at forearm level, right arm**
CC +7th **S55.912 Laceration of unspecified blood vessel at forearm level, left arm**
CC +7th **S55.919 Laceration of unspecified blood vessel at forearm level, unspecified arm**
+ S55.99 Other specified injury of unspecified blood vessel at forearm level
CC +7th **S55.991 Other specified injury of unspecified blood vessel at forearm level, right arm**
CC +7th **S55.992 Other specified injury of unspecified blood vessel at forearm level, left arm**
CC +7th **S55.999 Other specified injury of unspecified blood vessel at forearm level, unspecified arm**

S56 Injury of muscle, fascia and tendon at forearm level

Code also any associated open wound (S51.-)

Excludes2: *injury of muscle, fascia and tendon at or below wrist (S66.-)*
sprain of joints and ligaments of elbow (S53.4-)

The appropriate 7th character is to be added to each code from category S56
A initial encounter
D subsequent encounter
S sequela

+ S56.0 Injury of flexor muscle, fascia and tendon of thumb at forearm level
+ S56.00 Unspecified injury of flexor muscle, fascia and tendon of thumb at forearm level
+7th **S56.001 Unspecified injury of flexor muscle, fascia and tendon of right thumb at forearm level**
+7th **S56.002 Unspecified injury of flexor muscle, fascia and tendon of left thumb at forearm level**
+7th **S56.009 Unspecified injury of flexor muscle, fascia and tendon of unspecified thumb at forearm level**

+ **S56.01** Strain of flexor muscle, fascia and tendon of thumb at forearm level
+7th **S56.011** Strain of flexor muscle, fascia and tendon of right thumb at forearm level
+7th **S56.012** Strain of flexor muscle, fascia and tendon of left thumb at forearm level
+7th **S56.019** Strain of flexor muscle, fascia and tendon of unspecified thumb at forearm level

+ **S56.02** Laceration of flexor muscle, fascia and tendon of thumb at forearm level
CC +7th **S56.021** Laceration of flexor muscle, fascia and tendon of right thumb at forearm level
CC +7th **S56.022** Laceration of flexor muscle, fascia and tendon of left thumb at forearm level
CC +7th **S56.029** Laceration of flexor muscle, fascia and tendon of unspecified thumb at forearm level

+ **S56.09** Other injury of flexor muscle, fascia and tendon of thumb at forearm level
+7th **S56.091** Other injury of flexor muscle, fascia and tendon of right thumb at forearm level
+7th **S56.092** Other injury of flexor muscle, fascia and tendon of left thumb at forearm level
+7th **S56.099** Other injury of flexor muscle, fascia and tendon of unspecified thumb at forearm level

+ **S56.1** Injury of flexor muscle, fascia and tendon of other and unspecified finger at forearm level

+ **S56.10** Unspecified injury of flexor muscle, fascia and tendon of other and unspecified finger at forearm level
+7th **S56.101** Unspecified injury of flexor muscle, fascia and tendon of right index finger at forearm level
+7th **S56.102** Unspecified injury of flexor muscle, fascia and tendon of left index finger at forearm level
+7th **S56.103** Unspecified injury of flexor muscle, fascia and tendon of right middle finger at forearm level
+7th **S56.104** Unspecified injury of flexor muscle, fascia and tendon of left middle finger at forearm level
+7th **S56.105** Unspecified injury of flexor muscle, fascia and tendon of right ring finger at forearm level
+7th **S56.106** Unspecified injury of flexor muscle, fascia and tendon of left ring finger at forearm level
+7th **S56.107** Unspecified injury of flexor muscle, fascia and tendon of right little finger at forearm level
+7th **S56.108** Unspecified injury of flexor muscle, fascia and tendon of left little finger at forearm level
+7th **S56.109** Unspecified injury of flexor muscle, fascia and tendon of unspecified finger at forearm level

+ **S56.11** Strain of flexor muscle, fascia and tendon of other and unspecified finger at forearm level
+7th **S56.111** Strain of flexor muscle, fascia and tendon of right index finger at forearm level
+7th **S56.112** Strain of flexor muscle, fascia and tendon of left index finger at forearm level
+7th **S56.113** Strain of flexor muscle, fascia and tendon of right middle finger at forearm level
+7th **S56.114** Strain of flexor muscle, fascia and tendon of left middle finger at forearm level
+7th **S56.115** Strain of flexor muscle, fascia and tendon of right ring finger at forearm level
+7th **S56.116** Strain of flexor muscle, fascia and tendon of left ring finger at forearm level
+7th **S56.117** Strain of flexor muscle, fascia and tendon of right little finger at forearm level
+7th **S56.118** Strain of flexor muscle, fascia and tendon of left little finger at forearm level
+7th **S56.119** Strain of flexor muscle, fascia and tendon of finger of unspecified finger at forearm level

+ **S56.12** Laceration of flexor muscle, fascia and tendon of other and unspecified finger at forearm level
CC +7th **S56.121** Laceration of flexor muscle, fascia and tendon of right index finger at forearm level
CC +7th **S56.122** Laceration of flexor muscle, fascia and tendon of left index finger at forearm level
CC +7th **S56.123** Laceration of flexor muscle, fascia and tendon of right middle finger at forearm level
CC +7th **S56.124** Laceration of flexor muscle, fascia and tendon of left middle finger at forearm level
CC +7th **S56.125** Laceration of flexor muscle, fascia and tendon of right ring finger at forearm level
CC +7th **S56.126** Laceration of flexor muscle, fascia and tendon of left ring finger at forearm level
CC +7th **S56.127** Laceration of flexor muscle, fascia and tendon of right little finger at forearm level
CC +7th **S56.128** Laceration of flexor muscle, fascia and tendon of left little finger at forearm level
CC +7th **S56.129** Laceration of flexor muscle, fascia and tendon of unspecified finger at forearm level

+ **S56.19** Other injury of flexor muscle, fascia and tendon of other and unspecified finger at forearm level
+7th **S56.191** Other injury of flexor muscle, fascia and tendon of right index finger at forearm level
+7th **S56.192** Other injury of flexor muscle, fascia and tendon of left index finger at forearm level
+7th **S56.193** Other injury of flexor muscle, fascia and tendon of right middle finger at forearm level
+7th **S56.194** Other injury of flexor muscle, fascia and tendon of left middle finger at forearm level
+7th **S56.195** Other injury of flexor muscle, fascia and tendon of right ring finger at forearm level
+7th **S56.196** Other injury of flexor muscle, fascia and tendon of left ring finger at forearm level
+7th **S56.197** Other injury of flexor muscle, fascia and tendon of right little finger at forearm level
+7th **S56.198** Other injury of flexor muscle, fascia and tendon of left little finger at forearm level
+7th **S56.199** Other injury of flexor muscle, fascia and tendon of unspecified finger at forearm level

+ **S56.2** Injury of other flexor muscle, fascia and tendon at forearm level

+ **S56.20** Unspecified injury of other flexor muscle, fascia and tendon at forearm level
+7th **S56.201** Unspecified injury of other flexor muscle, fascia and tendon at forearm level, right arm
+7th **S56.202** Unspecified injury of other flexor muscle, fascia and tendon at forearm level, left arm
+7th **S56.209** Unspecified injury of other flexor muscle, fascia and tendon at forearm level, unspecified arm

+ **S56.21 Strain of other flexor muscle, fascia and tendon at forearm level**
  - +7th **S56.211 Strain of other flexor muscle, fascia and tendon at forearm level, right arm**
  - +7th **S56.212 Strain of other flexor muscle, fascia and tendon at forearm level, left arm**
  - +7th **S56.219 Strain of other flexor muscle, fascia and tendon at forearm level, unspecified arm**
+ **S56.22 Laceration of other flexor muscle, fascia and tendon at forearm level**
  - CC +7th **S56.221 Laceration of other flexor muscle, fascia and tendon at forearm level, right arm**
  - CC +7th **S56.222 Laceration of other flexor muscle, fascia and tendon at forearm level, left arm**
  - CC +7th **S56.229 Laceration of other flexor muscle, fascia and tendon at forearm level, unspecified arm**
+ **S56.29 Other injury of other flexor muscle, fascia and tendon at forearm level**
  - +7th **S56.291 Other injury of other flexor muscle, fascia and tendon at forearm level, right arm**
  - +7th **S56.292 Other injury of other flexor muscle, fascia and tendon at forearm level, left arm**
  - +7th **S56.299 Other injury of other flexor muscle, fascia and tendon at forearm level, unspecified arm**

+ **S56.3 Injury of extensor or abductor muscles, fascia and tendons of thumb at forearm level**
  + **S56.30 Unspecified injury of extensor or abductor muscles, fascia and tendons of thumb at forearm level**
    - +7th **S56.301 Unspecified injury of extensor or abductor muscles, fascia and tendons of right thumb at forearm level**
    - +7th **S56.302 Unspecified injury of extensor or abductor muscles, fascia and tendons of left thumb at forearm level**
    - +7th **S56.309 Unspecified injury of extensor or abductor muscles, fascia and tendons of unspecified thumb at forearm level**
  + **S56.31 Strain of extensor or abductor muscles, fascia and tendons of thumb at forearm level**
    - +7th **S56.311 Strain of extensor or abductor muscles, fascia and tendons of right thumb at forearm level**
    - +7th **S56.312 Strain of extensor or abductor muscles, fascia and tendons of left thumb at forearm level**
    - +7th **S56.319 Strain of extensor or abductor muscles, fascia and tendons of unspecified thumb at forearm level**
  + **S56.32 Laceration of extensor or abductor muscles, fascia and tendons of thumb at forearm level**
    - CC +7th **S56.321 Laceration of extensor or abductor muscles, fascia and tendons of right thumb at forearm level**
    - CC +7th **S56.322 Laceration of extensor or abductor muscles, fascia and tendons of left thumb at forearm level**
    - CC +7th **S56.329 Laceration of extensor or abductor muscles, fascia and tendons of unspecified thumb at forearm level**
  + **S56.39 Other injury of extensor or abductor muscles, fascia and tendons of thumb at forearm level**
    - +7th **S56.391 Other injury of extensor or abductor muscles, fascia and tendons of right thumb at forearm level**
    - +7th **S56.392 Other injury of extensor or abductor muscles, fascia and tendons of left thumb at forearm level**
    - +7th **S56.399 Other injury of extensor or abductor muscles, fascia and tendons of unspecified thumb at forearm level**

+ **S56.4 Injury of extensor muscle, fascia and tendon of other and unspecified finger at forearm level**
  + **S56.40 Unspecified injury of extensor muscle, fascia and tendon of other and unspecified finger at forearm level**
    - +7th **S56.401 Unspecified injury of extensor muscle, fascia and tendon of right index finger at forearm level**
    - +7th **S56.402 Unspecified injury of extensor muscle, fascia and tendon of left index finger at forearm level**
    - +7th **S56.403 Unspecified injury of extensor muscle, fascia and tendon of right middle finger at forearm level**
    - +7th **S56.404 Unspecified injury of extensor muscle, fascia and tendon of left middle finger at forearm level**
    - +7th **S56.405 Unspecified injury of extensor muscle, fascia and tendon of right ring finger at forearm level**
    - +7th **S56.406 Unspecified injury of extensor muscle, fascia and tendon of left ring finger at forearm level**
    - +7th **S56.407 Unspecified injury of extensor muscle, fascia and tendon of right little finger at forearm level**
    - +7th **S56.408 Unspecified injury of extensor muscle, fascia and tendon of left little finger at forearm level**
    - +7th **S56.409 Unspecified injury of extensor muscle, fascia and tendon of unspecified finger at forearm level**
  + **S56.41 Strain of extensor muscle, fascia and tendon of other and unspecified finger at forearm level**
    - +7th **S56.411 Strain of extensor muscle, fascia and tendon of right index finger at forearm level**
    - +7th **S56.412 Strain of extensor muscle, fascia and tendon of left index finger at forearm level**
    - +7th **S56.413 Strain of extensor muscle, fascia and tendon of right middle finger at forearm level**
    - +7th **S56.414 Strain of extensor muscle, fascia and tendon of left middle finger at forearm level**
    - +7th **S56.415 Strain of extensor muscle, fascia and tendon of right ring finger at forearm level**
    - +7th **S56.416 Strain of extensor muscle, fascia and tendon of left ring finger at forearm level**
    - +7th **S56.417 Strain of extensor muscle, fascia and tendon of right little finger at forearm level**
    - +7th **S56.418 Strain of extensor muscle, fascia and tendon of left little finger at forearm level**
    - +7th **S56.419 Strain of extensor muscle, fascia and tendon of finger, unspecified finger at forearm level**
  + **S56.42 Laceration of extensor muscle, fascia and tendon of other and unspecified finger at forearm level**
    - CC +7th **S56.421 Laceration of extensor muscle, fascia and tendon of right index finger at forearm level**
    - CC +7th **S56.422 Laceration of extensor muscle, fascia and tendon of left index finger at forearm level**
    - CC +7th **S56.423 Laceration of extensor muscle, fascia and tendon of right middle finger at forearm level**
    - CC +7th **S56.424 Laceration of extensor muscle, fascia and tendon of left middle finger at forearm level**
    - CC +7th **S56.425 Laceration of extensor muscle, fascia and tendon of right ring finger at forearm level**
    - CC +7th **S56.426 Laceration of extensor muscle, fascia and tendon of left ring finger at forearm level**

CC +7th **S56.427** Laceration of extensor muscle, fascia and tendon of right little finger at forearm level

CC +7th **S56.428** Laceration of extensor muscle, fascia and tendon of left little finger at forearm level

CC +7th **S56.429** Laceration of extensor muscle, fascia and tendon of unspecified finger at forearm level

\+ **S56.49** Other injury of extensor muscle, fascia and tendon of other and unspecified finger at forearm level

+7th **S56.491** Other injury of extensor muscle, fascia and tendon of right index finger at forearm level

+7th **S56.492** Other injury of extensor muscle, fascia and tendon of left index finger at forearm level

+7th **S56.493** Other injury of extensor muscle, fascia and tendon of right middle finger at forearm level

+7th **S56.494** Other injury of extensor muscle, fascia and tendon of left middle finger at forearm level

+7th **S56.495** Other injury of extensor muscle, fascia and tendon of right ring finger at forearm level

+7th **S56.496** Other injury of extensor muscle, fascia and tendon of left ring finger at forearm level

+7th **S56.497** Other injury of extensor muscle, fascia and tendon of right little finger at forearm level

+7th **S56.498** Other injury of extensor muscle, fascia and tendon of left little finger at forearm level

+7th **S56.499** Other injury of extensor muscle, fascia and tendon of unspecified finger at forearm level

\+ **S56.5** Injury of other extensor muscle, fascia and tendon at forearm level

\+ **S56.50** Unspecified injury of other extensor muscle, fascia and tendon at forearm level

+7th **S56.501** Unspecified injury of other extensor muscle, fascia and tendon at forearm level, right arm

+7th **S56.502** Unspecified injury of other extensor muscle, fascia and tendon at forearm level, left arm

+7th **S56.509** Unspecified injury of other extensor muscle, fascia and tendon at forearm level, unspecified arm

\+ **S56.51** Strain of other extensor muscle, fascia and tendon at forearm level

+7th **S56.511** Strain of other extensor muscle, fascia and tendon at forearm level, right arm

+7th **S56.512** Strain of other extensor muscle, fascia≈and tendon at forearm level, left arm

+7th **S56.519** Strain of other extensor muscle, fascia and tendon at forearm level, unspecified arm

\+ **S56.52** Laceration of other extensor muscle, fascia and tendon at forearm level

CC +7th **S56.521** Laceration of other extensor muscle, fascia and tendon at forearm level, right arm

CC +7th **S56.522** Laceration of other extensor muscle, fascia and tendon at forearm level, left arm

CC +7th **S56.529** Laceration of other extensor muscle, fascia and tendon at forearm level, unspecified arm

\+ **S56.59** Other injury of other extensor muscle, fascia and tendon at forearm level

+7th **S56.591** Other injury of other extensor muscle, fascia and tendon at forearm level, right arm

+7th **S56.592** Other injury of other extensor muscle, fascia and tendon at forearm level, left arm

+7th **S56.599** Other injury of other extensor muscle, fascia and tendon at forearm level, unspecified arm

\+ **S56.8** Injury of other muscles, fascia and tendons at forearm level

\+ **S56.80** Unspecified injury of other muscles, fascia and tendons at forearm level

+7th **S56.801** Unspecified injury of other muscles, fascia and tendons at forearm level, right arm

+7th **S56.802** Unspecified injury of other muscles, fascia and tendons at forearm level, left arm

+7th **S56.809** Unspecified injury of other muscles, fascia and tendons at forearm level, unspecified arm

\+ **S56.81** Strain of other muscles, fascia and tendons at forearm level

+7th **S56.811** Strain of other muscles, fascia and tendons at forearm level, right arm

+7th **S56.812** Strain of other muscles, fascia and tendons at forearm level, left arm

+7th **S56.819** Strain of other muscles, fascia and tendons at forearm level, unspecified arm

\+ **S56.82** Laceration of other muscles, fascia and tendons at forearm level

CC +7th **S56.821** Laceration of other muscles, fascia and tendons at forearm level, right arm

CC +7th **S56.822** Laceration of other muscles, fascia and tendons at forearm level, left arm

CC +7th **S56.829** Laceration of other muscles, fascia and tendons at forearm level, unspecified arm

\+ **S56.89** Other injury of other muscles, fascia and tendons at forearm level

+7th **S56.891** Other injury of other muscles, fascia and tendons at forearm level, right arm

+7th **S56.892** Other injury of other muscles, fascia and tendons at forearm level, left arm

+7th **S56.899** Other injury of other muscles, fascia and tendons at forearm level, unspecified arm

\+ **S56.9** Injury of unspecified muscles, fascia and tendons at forearm level

\+ **S56.90** Unspecified injury of unspecified muscles, fascia and tendons at forearm level

+7th **S56.901** Unspecified injury of unspecified muscles, fascia and tendons at forearm level, right arm

+7th **S56.902** Unspecified injury of unspecified muscles, fascia and tendons at forearm level, left arm

+7th **S56.909** Unspecified injury of unspecified muscles, fascia and tendons at forearm level, unspecified arm

\+ **S56.91** Strain of unspecified muscles, fascia and tendons at forearm level

+7th **S56.911** Strain of unspecified muscles, fascia and tendons at forearm level, right arm

+7th **S56.912** Strain of unspecified muscles, fascia and tendons at forearm level, left arm

+7th **S56.919** Strain of unspecified muscles, fascia and tendons at forearm level, unspecified arm

\+ **S56.92** Laceration of unspecified muscles, fascia and tendons at forearm level

CC +7th **S56.921** Laceration of unspecified muscles, fascia and tendons at forearm level, right arm

CC +7th **S56.922** Laceration of unspecified muscles, fascia and tendons at forearm level, left arm

CC +7th **S56.929** Laceration of unspecified muscles, fascia and tendons at forearm level, unspecified arm

+ **S56.99 Other injury of unspecified muscles, fascia and tendons at forearm level**
  - +7th **S56.991 Other injury of unspecified muscles, fascia and tendons at forearm level, right arm**
  - +7th **S56.992 Other injury of unspecified muscles, fascia and tendons at forearm level, left arm**
  - +7th **S56.999 Other injury of unspecified muscles, fascia and tendons at forearm level, unspecified arm**

S57 Crushing injury of elbow and forearm

Use additional code(s) for all associated injuries

Excludes2: *crushing injury of wrist and hand (S67.-)*

The appropriate 7th character is to be added to each code from category S57
A initial encounter
D subsequent encounter
S sequela

+ **S57.0 Crushing injury of elbow**
  - X+7th **S57.00 Crushing injury of unspecified elbow**
  - X+7th **S57.01 Crushing injury of right elbow**
  - X+7th **S57.02 Crushing injury of left elbow**
+ **S57.8 Crushing injury of forearm**
  - X+7th **S57.80 Crushing injury of unspecified forearm**
  - X+7th **S57.81 Crushing injury of right forearm**
  - X+7th **S57.82 Crushing injury of left forearm**

S58 Traumatic amputation of elbow and forearm

An amputation not identified as partial or complete should be coded to complete

Excludes1: *traumatic amputation of wrist and hand (S68.-)*

The appropriate 7th character is to be added to each code from category S58
A initial encounter
D subsequent encounter
S sequela

+ **S58.0 Traumatic amputation at elbow level**
  + **S58.01 Complete traumatic amputation at elbow level**
    - CC +7th **S58.011 Complete traumatic amputation at elbow level, right arm**
    - CC +7th **S58.012 Complete traumatic amputation at elbow level, left arm**
    - CC +7th **S58.019 Complete traumatic amputation at elbow level, unspecified arm**
  + **S58.02 Partial traumatic amputation at elbow level**
    - CC +7th **S58.021 Partial traumatic amputation at elbow level, right arm**
    - CC +7th **S58.022 Partial traumatic amputation at elbow level, left arm**
    - CC +7th **S58.029 Partial traumatic amputation at elbow level, unspecified arm**
+ **S58.1 Traumatic amputation at level between elbow and wrist**
  + **S58.11 Complete traumatic amputation at level between elbow and wrist**
    - CC +7th **S58.111 Complete traumatic amputation at level between elbow and wrist, right arm**
    - CC +7th **S58.112 Complete traumatic amputation at level between elbow and wrist, left arm**
    - CC +7th **S58.119 Complete traumatic amputation at level between elbow and wrist, unspecified arm**
  + **S58.12 Partial traumatic amputation at level between elbow and wrist**
    - CC +7th **S58.121 Partial traumatic amputation at level between elbow and wrist, right arm**
    - CC +7th **S58.122 Partial traumatic amputation at level between elbow and wrist, left arm**
    - CC +7th **S58.129 Partial traumatic amputation at level between elbow and wrist, unspecified arm**
+ **S58.9 Traumatic amputation of forearm, level unspecified**

  Excludes1: *traumatic amputation of wrist (S68.-)*
  + **S58.91 Complete traumatic amputation of forearm, level unspecified**
    - CC +7th **S58.911 Complete traumatic amputation of right forearm, level unspecified**
    - CC +7th **S58.912 Complete traumatic amputation of left forearm, level unspecified**
    - CC +7th **S58.919 Complete traumatic amputation of unspecified forearm, level unspecified**
  + **S58.92 Partial traumatic amputation of forearm, level unspecified**
    - CC +7th **S58.921 Partial traumatic amputation of right forearm, level unspecified**
    - CC +7th **S58.922 Partial traumatic amputation of left forearm, level unspecified**
    - CC +7th **S58.929 Partial traumatic amputation of unspecified forearm, level unspecified**

S59 Other and unspecified injuries of elbow and forearm

Excludes2: *other and unspecified injuries of wrist and hand (S69.-)*

The appropriate 7th character is to be added to each code from subcategories **S59.0, S59.1, and S59.2**
A initial encounter for closed fracture
D subsequent encounter for fracture with routine healing
G subsequent encounter for fracture with delayed healing
K subsequent encounter for fracture with nonunion
P subsequent encounter for fracture with malunion
S sequela

Review coding guideline C.19.c

+ **S59.0 Physeal fracture of lower end of ulna**
  + **S59.00 Unspecified physeal fracture of lower end of ulna**
    - CC +7th **S59.001 Unspecified physeal fracture of lower end of ulna, right arm**
      HAC 7th character A see Appendix B for HAC conditional logic
    - CC +7th **S59.002 Unspecified physeal fracture of lower end of ulna, left arm**
      HAC 7th character A see Appendix B for HAC conditional logic
    - CC +7th **S59.009 Unspecified physeal fracture of lower end of ulna, unspecified arm**
      HAC 7th character A see Appendix B for HAC conditional logic
  + **S59.01 Salter-Harris Type I physeal fracture of lower end of ulna**
    - CC +7th **S59.011 Salter-Harris Type I physeal fracture of lower end of ulna, right arm**
      HAC 7th character A see Appendix B for HAC conditional logic
    - CC +7th **S59.012 Salter-Harris Type I physeal fracture of lower end of ulna, left arm**
      HAC 7th character A see Appendix B for HAC conditional logic
    - CC +7th **S59.019 Salter-Harris Type I physeal fracture of lower end of ulna, unspecified arm**
      HAC 7th character A see Appendix B for HAC conditional logic
  + **S59.02 Salter-Harris Type II physeal fracture of lower end of ulna**
    - CC +7th **S59.021 Salter-Harris Type II physeal fracture of lower end of ulna, right arm**
      HAC 7th character A see Appendix B for HAC conditional logic
    - CC +7th **S59.022 Salter-Harris Type II physeal fracture of lower end of ulna, left arm**
      HAC 7th character A see Appendix B for HAC conditional logic
    - CC +7th **S59.029 Salter-Harris Type II physeal fracture of lower end of ulna, unspecified arm**
      HAC 7th character A see Appendix B for HAC conditional logic
  + **S59.03 Salter-Harris Type III physeal fracture of lower end of ulna**
    - CC +7th **S59.031 Salter-Harris Type III physeal fracture of lower end of ulna, right arm**
      HAC 7th character A see Appendix B for HAC conditional logic
    - CC +7th **S59.032 Salter-Harris Type III physeal fracture of lower end of ulna, left arm**
      HAC 7th character A see Appendix B for HAC conditional logic
    - CC +7th **S59.039 Salter-Harris Type III physeal fracture of lower end of ulna, unspecified arm**
      HAC 7th character A see Appendix B for HAC conditional logic

+ **S59.04 Salter-Harris Type IV physeal fracture of lower end of ulna**
  - CC +7th **S59.041 Salter-Harris Type IV physeal fracture of lower end of ulna, right arm**
    HAC 7th character A see Appendix B for HAC conditional logic
  - CC +7th **S59.042 Salter-Harris Type IV physeal fracture of lower end of ulna, left arm**
    HAC 7th character A see Appendix B for HAC conditional logic
  - CC +7th **S59.049 Salter-Harris Type IV physeal fracture of lower end of ulna, unspecified arm**
    HAC 7th character A see Appendix B for HAC conditional logic

+ **S59.09 Other physeal fracture of lower end of ulna**
  - CC +7th **S59.091 Other physeal fracture of lower end of ulna, right arm**
    HAC 7th character A see Appendix B for HAC conditional logic
  - CC +7th **S59.092 Other physeal fracture of lower end of ulna, left arm**
    HAC 7th character A see Appendix B for HAC conditional logic
  - CC +7th **S59.099 Other physeal fracture of lower end of ulna, unspecified arm**
    HAC 7th character A see Appendix B for HAC conditional logic

+ **S59.1 Physeal fracture of upper end of radius**

+ **S59.10 Unspecified physeal fracture of upper end of radius**
  - CC +7th **S59.101 Unspecified physeal fracture of upper end of radius, right arm**
  - CC +7th **S59.102 Unspecified physeal fracture of upper end of radius, left arm**
  - CC +7th **S59.109 Unspecified physeal fracture of upper end of radius, unspecified arm**

+ **S59.11 Salter-Harris Type I physeal fracture of upper end of radius**
  - CC +7th **S59.111 Salter-Harris Type I physeal fracture of upper end of radius, right arm**
  - CC +7th **S59.112 Salter-Harris Type I physeal fracture of upper end of radius, left arm**
  - CC +7th **S59.119 Salter-Harris Type I physeal fracture of upper end of radius, unspecified arm**

+ **S59.12 Salter-Harris Type II physeal fracture of upper end of radius**
  - CC +7th **S59.121 Salter-Harris Type II physeal fracture of upper end of radius, right arm**
  - CC +7th **S59.122 Salter-Harris Type II physeal fracture of upper end of radius, left arm**
  - CC +7th **S59.129 Salter-Harris Type II physeal fracture of upper end of radius, unspecified arm**

+ **S59.13 Salter-Harris Type III physeal fracture of upper end of radius**
  - CC +7th **S59.131 Salter-Harris Type III physeal fracture of upper end of radius, right arm**
  - CC +7th **S59.132 Salter-Harris Type III physeal fracture of upper end of radius, left arm**
  - CC +7th **S59.139 Salter-Harris Type III physeal fracture of upper end of radius, unspecified arm**

+ **S59.14 Salter-Harris Type IV physeal fracture of upper end of radius**
  - CC +7th **S59.141 Salter-Harris Type IV physeal fracture of upper end of radius, right arm**
  - CC +7th **S59.142 Salter-Harris Type IV physeal fracture of upper end of radius, left arm**
  - CC +7th **S59.149 Salter-Harris Type IV physeal fracture of upper end of radius, unspecified arm**

+ **S59.19 Other physeal fracture of upper end of radius**
  - CC +7th **S59.191 Other physeal fracture of upper end of radius, right arm**
  - CC +7th **S59.192 Other physeal fracture of upper end of radius, left arm**
  - CC +7th **S59.199 Other physeal fracture of upper end of radius, unspecified arm**

+ **S59.2 Physeal fracture of lower end of radius**

+ **S59.20 Unspecified physeal fracture of lower end of radius**
  - CC +7th **S59.201 Unspecified physeal fracture of lower end of radius, right arm**
    HAC 7th character A see Appendix B for HAC conditional logic
  - CC +7th **S59.202 Unspecified physeal fracture of lower end of radius, left arm**
    HAC 7th character A see Appendix B for HAC conditional logic
  - CC +7th **S59.209 Unspecified physeal fracture of lower end of radius, unspecified arm**
    HAC 7th character A see Appendix B for HAC conditional logic

+ **S59.21 Salter-Harris Type I physeal fracture of lower end of radius**
  - CC +7th **S59.211 Salter-Harris Type I physeal fracture of lower end of radius, right arm**
    HAC 7th character A see Appendix B for HAC conditional logic
  - CC +7th **S59.212 Salter-Harris Type I physeal fracture of lower end of radius, left arm**
    HAC 7th character A see Appendix B for HAC conditional logic
  - CC +7th **S59.219 Salter-Harris Type I physeal fracture of lower end of radius, unspecified arm**
    HAC 7th character A see Appendix B for HAC conditional logic

+ **S59.22 Salter-Harris Type II physeal fracture of lower end of radius**
  - CC +7th **S59.221 Salter-Harris Type II physeal fracture of lower end of radius, right arm**
    HAC 7th character A see Appendix B for HAC conditional logic
  - CC +7th **S59.222 Salter-Harris Type II physeal fracture of lower end of radius, left arm**
    HAC 7th character A see Appendix B for HAC conditional logic
  - CC +7th **S59.229 Salter-Harris Type II physeal fracture of lower end of radius, unspecified arm**
    HAC 7th character A see Appendix B for HAC conditional logic

+ **S59.23 Salter-Harris Type III physeal fracture of lower end of radius**
  - CC +7th **S59.231 Salter-Harris Type III physeal fracture of lower end of radius, right arm**
    HAC 7th character A see Appendix B for HAC conditional logic
  - CC +7th **S59.232 Salter-Harris Type III physeal fracture of lower end of radius, left arm**
    HAC 7th character A see Appendix B for HAC conditional logic
  - CC +7th **S59.239 Salter-Harris Type III physeal fracture of lower end of radius, unspecified arm**
    HAC 7th character A see Appendix B for HAC conditional logic

+ **S59.24 Salter-Harris Type IV physeal fracture of lower end of radius**
  - CC +7th **S59.241 Salter-Harris Type IV physeal fracture of lower end of radius, right arm**
    HAC 7th character A see Appendix B for HAC conditional logic
  - CC +7th **S59.242 Salter-Harris Type IV physeal fracture of lower end of radius, left arm**
    HAC 7th character A see Appendix B for HAC conditional logic
  - CC +7th **S59.249 Salter-Harris Type IV physeal fracture of lower end of radius, unspecified arm**
    HAC 7th character A see Appendix B for HAC conditional logic

Wrist

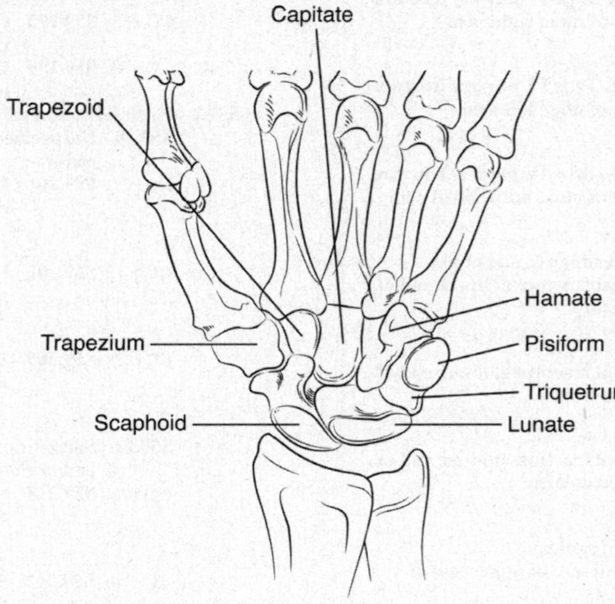

©AHIMA

Bones of the Hand

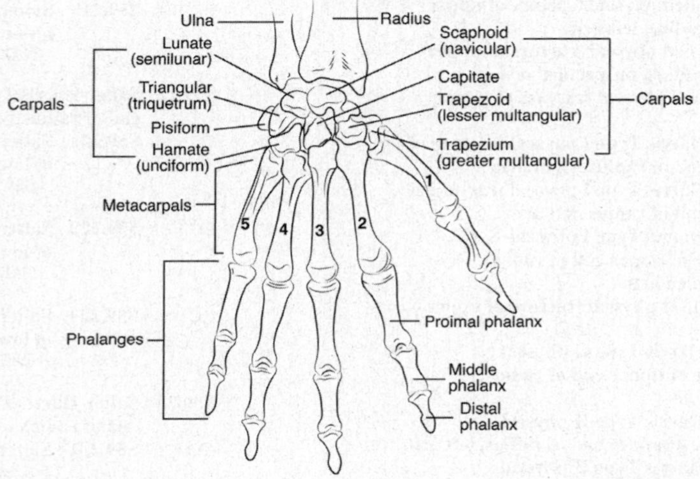

©AHIMA

Muscles of the Hand

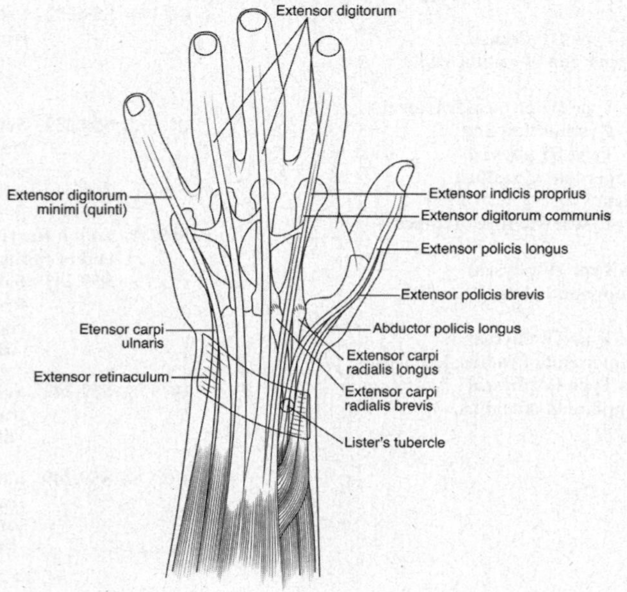

©AHIMA

+ **S59.29** **Other physeal fracture of lower end of radius**
  - CC +7th **S59.291** **Other physeal fracture of lower end of radius, right arm**
    HAC 7th character A see Appendix B for HAC conditional logic
  - CC +7th **S59.292** **Other physeal fracture of lower end of radius, left arm**
    HAC 7th character A see Appendix B for HAC conditional logic
  - CC +7th **S59.299** **Other physeal fracture of lower end of radius, unspecified arm**
    HAC 7th character A see Appendix B for HAC conditional logic

+ **S59.8** **Other specified injuries of elbow and forearm**

> The appropriate 7th character is to be added to each code in subcategory **S59.8**
> A initial encounter
> D subsequent encounter
> S sequela

+ **S59.80** **Other specified injuries of elbow**
  - +7th **S59.801** **Other specified injuries of right elbow**
  - +7th **S59.802** **Other specified injuries of left elbow**
  - +7th **S59.809** **Other specified injuries of unspecified elbow**
+ **S59.81** **Other specified injuries of forearm**
  - +7th **S59.811** **Other specified injuries right forearm**
  - +7th **S59.812** **Other specified injuries left forearm**
  - +7th **S59.819** **Other specified injuries unspecified forearm**

+ **S59.9** **Unspecified injury of elbow and forearm**

> The appropriate 7th character is to be added to each code in subcategory **S59.9**
> A initial encounter
> D subsequent encounter
> S sequela

+ **S59.90** **Unspecified injury of elbow**
  - +7th **S59.901** **Unspecified injury of right elbow**
  - +7th **S59.902** **Unspecified injury of left elbow**
  - +7th **S59.909** **Unspecified injury of unspecified elbow**
+ **S59.91** **Unspecified injury of forearm**
  - +7th **S59.911** **Unspecified injury of right forearm**
  - +7th **S59.912** **Unspecified injury of left forearm**
  - +7th **S59.919** **Unspecified injury of unspecified forearm**

Injuries to the wrist, hand and fingers (S60-S69)

Excludes2: *burns and corrosions (T20-T32)*
frostbite (T33-T34)
insect bite or sting, venomous (T63.4)

S60 Superficial injury of wrist, hand and fingers

> The appropriate 7th character is to be added to each code from category S60
> A initial encounter
> D subsequent encounter
> S sequela

+ **S60.0** **Contusion of finger without damage to nail**
  Excludes1: *contusion involving nail (matrix) (S60.1)*
  - X+7th **S60.00** **Contusion of unspecified finger without damage to nail**
    Contusion of finger(s) NOS
  + **S60.01** **Contusion of thumb without damage to nail**
    - +7th **S60.011** **Contusion of right thumb without damage to nail**
    - +7th **S60.012** **Contusion of left thumb without damage to nail**
    - +7th **S60.019** **Contusion of unspecified thumb without damage to nail**
  + **S60.02** **Contusion of index finger without damage to nail**
    - +7th **S60.021** **Contusion of right index finger without damage to nail**
    - +7th **S60.022** **Contusion of left index finger without damage to nail**
    - +7th **S60.029** **Contusion of unspecified index finger without damage to nail**
  + **S60.03** **Contusion of middle finger without damage to nail**
    - +7th **S60.031** **Contusion of right middle finger without damage to nail**
    - +7th **S60.032** **Contusion of left middle finger without damage to nail**
    - +7th **S60.039** **Contusion of unspecified middle finger without damage to nail**
  + **S60.04** **Contusion of ring finger without damage to nail**
    - +7th **S60.041** **Contusion of right ring finger without damage to nail**
    - +7th **S60.042** **Contusion of left ring finger without damage to nail**
    - +7th **S60.049** **Contusion of unspecified ring finger without damage to nail**
  + **S60.05** **Contusion of little finger without damage to nail**
    - +7th **S60.051** **Contusion of right little finger without damage to nail**
    - +7th **S60.052** **Contusion of left little finger without damage to nail**
    - +7th **S60.059** **Contusion of unspecified little finger without damage to nail**

+ **S60.1** **Contusion of finger with damage to nail**
  - X+7th **S60.10** **Contusion of unspecified finger with damage to nail**
  + **S60.11** **Contusion of thumb with damage to nail**
    - +7th **S60.111** **Contusion of right thumb with damage to nail**
    - +7th **S60.112** **Contusion of left thumb with damage to nail**
    - +7th **S60.119** **Contusion of unspecified thumb with damage to nail**
  + **S60.12** **Contusion of index finger with damage to nail**
    - +7th **S60.121** **Contusion of right index finger with damage to nail**
    - +7th **S60.122** **Contusion of left index finger with damage to nail**
    - +7th **S60.129** **Contusion of unspecified index finger with damage to nail**
  + **S60.13** **Contusion of middle finger with damage to nail**
    - +7th **S60.131** **Contusion of right middle finger with damage to nail**
    - +7th **S60.132** **Contusion of left middle finger with damage to nail**
    - +7th **S60.139** **Contusion of unspecified middle finger with damage to nail**
  + **S60.14** **Contusion of ring finger with damage to nail**
    - +7th **S60.141** **Contusion of right ring finger with damage to nail**
    - +7th **S60.142** **Contusion of left ring finger with damage to nail**
    - +7th **S60.149** **Contusion of unspecified ring finger with damage to nail**
  + **S60.15** **Contusion of little finger with damage to nail**
    - +7th **S60.151** **Contusion of right little finger with damage to nail**
    - +7th **S60.152** **Contusion of left little finger with damage to nail**
    - +7th **S60.159** **Contusion of unspecified little finger with damage to nail**

+ **S60.2** **Contusion of wrist and hand**
  Excludes2: *contusion of fingers (S60.0-, S60.1-)*
  + **S60.21** **Contusion of wrist**
    - +7th **S60.211** **Contusion of right wrist**
    - +7th **S60.212** **Contusion of left wrist**
    - +7th **S60.219** **Contusion of unspecified wrist**
  + **S60.22** **Contusion of hand**
    - +7th **S60.221** **Contusion of right hand**
    - +7th **S60.222** **Contusion of left hand**
    - +7th **S60.229** **Contusion of unspecified hand**

+ **S60.3** **Other superficial injuries of thumb**
  + **S60.31** **Abrasion of thumb**
    - +7th **S60.311** **Abrasion of right thumb**
    - +7th **S60.312** **Abrasion of left thumb**
    - +7th **S60.319** **Abrasion of unspecified thumb**
  + **S60.32** **Blister (nonthermal) of thumb**
    - +7th **S60.321** **Blister (nonthermal) of right thumb**
    - +7th **S60.322** **Blister (nonthermal) of left thumb**
    - +7th **S60.329** **Blister (nonthermal) of unspecified thumb**

+ **S60.34 External constriction of thumb**
  Hair tourniquet syndrome of thumb
  Use additional cause code to identify the constricting item (W49.0-)
  - +7th **S60.341 External constriction of right thumb**
  - +7th **S60.342 External constriction of left thumb**
  - +7th **S60.349 External constriction of unspecified thumb**
+ **S60.35 Superficial foreign body of thumb**
  Splinter in the thumb
  - +7th **S60.351 Superficial foreign body of right thumb**
  - +7th **S60.352 Superficial foreign body of left thumb**
  - +7th **S60.359 Superficial foreign body of unspecified thumb**
+ **S60.36 Insect bite (nonvenomous) of thumb**
  - +7th **S60.361 Insect bite (nonvenomous) of right thumb**
  - +7th **S60.362 Insect bite (nonvenomous) of left thumb**
  - +7th **S60.369 Insect bite (nonvenomous) of unspecified thumb**
+ **S60.37 Other superficial bite of thumb**
  Excludes1: *open bite of thumb (S61.05-, S61.15-)*
  - +7th **S60.371 Other superficial bite of right thumb**
  - +7th **S60.372 Other superficial bite of left thumb**
  - +7th **S60.379 Other superficial bite of unspecified thumb**
+ **S60.39 Other superficial injuries of thumb**
  - +7th **S60.391 Other superficial injuries of right thumb**
  - +7th **S60.392 Other superficial injuries of left thumb**
  - +7th **S60.399 Other superficial injuries of unspecified thumb**

+ **S60.4 Other superficial injuries of other fingers**
+ **S60.41 Abrasion of fingers**
  - +7th **S60.410 Abrasion of right index finger**
  - +7th **S60.411 Abrasion of left index finger**
  - +7th **S60.412 Abrasion of right middle finger**
  - +7th **S60.413 Abrasion of left middle finger**
  - +7th **S60.414 Abrasion of right ring finger**
  - +7th **S60.415 Abrasion of left ring finger**
  - +7th **S60.416 Abrasion of right little finger**
  - +7th **S60.417 Abrasion of left little finger**
  - +7th **S60.418 Abrasion of other finger**
    Abrasion of specified finger with unspecified laterality
  - +7th **S60.419 Abrasion of unspecified finger**
+ **S60.42 Blister (nonthermal) of fingers**
  - +7th **S60.420 Blister (nonthermal) of right index finger**
  - +7th **S60.421 Blister (nonthermal) of left index finger**
  - +7th **S60.422 Blister (nonthermal) of right middle finger**
  - +7th **S60.423 Blister (nonthermal) of left middle finger**
  - +7th **S60.424 Blister (nonthermal) of right ring finger**
  - +7th **S60.425 Blister (nonthermal) of left ring finger**
  - +7th **S60.426 Blister (nonthermal) of right little finger**
  - +7th **S60.427 Blister (nonthermal) of left little finger**
  - +7th **S60.428 Blister (nonthermal) of other finger**
    Blister (nonthermal) of specified finger with unspecified laterality
  - +7th **S60.429 Blister (nonthermal) of unspecified finger**
+ **S60.44 External constriction of fingers**
  Hair tourniquet syndrome of finger
  Use additional cause code to identify the constricting item (W49.0-)
  - +7th **S60.440 External constriction of right index finger**
  - +7th **S60.441 External constriction of left index finger**
  - +7th **S60.442 External constriction of right middle finger**
  - +7th **S60.443 External constriction of left middle finger**
  - +7th **S60.444 External constriction of right ring finger**
  - +7th **S60.445 External constriction of left ring finger**
  - +7th **S60.446 External constriction of right little finger**
  - +7th **S60.447 External constriction of left little finger**
  - +7th **S60.448 External constriction of other finger**
    External constriction of specified finger with unspecified laterality
  - +7th **S60.449 External constriction of unspecified finger**
+ **S60.45 Superficial foreign body of fingers**
  Splinter in the finger(s)
  - +7th **S60.450 Superficial foreign body of right index finger**
  - +7th **S60.451 Superficial foreign body of left index finger**
  - +7th **S60.452 Superficial foreign body of right middle finger**
  - +7th **S60.453 Superficial foreign body of left middle finger**
  - +7th **S60.454 Superficial foreign body of right ring finger**
  - +7th **S60.455 Superficial foreign body of left ring finger**
  - +7th **S60.456 Superficial foreign body of right little finger**
  - +7th **S60.457 Superficial foreign body of left little finger**
  - +7th **S60.458 Superficial foreign body of other finger**
    Superficial foreign body of specified finger with unspecified laterality
  - +7th **S60.459 Superficial foreign body of unspecified finger**
+ **S60.46 Insect bite (nonvenomous) of fingers**
  - +7th **S60.460 Insect bite (nonvenomous) of right index finger**
  - +7th **S60.461 Insect bite (nonvenomous) of left index finger**
  - +7th **S60.462 Insect bite (nonvenomous) of right middle finger**
  - +7th **S60.463 Insect bite (nonvenomous) of left middle finger**
  - +7th **S60.464 Insect bite (nonvenomous) of right ring finger**
  - +7th **S60.465 Insect bite (nonvenomous) of left ring finger**
  - +7th **S60.466 Insect bite (nonvenomous) of right little finger**
  - +7th **S60.467 Insect bite (nonvenomous) of left little finger**
  - +7th **S60.468 Insect bite (nonvenomous) of other finger**
    Insect bite (nonvenomous) of specified finger with unspecified laterality
  - +7th **S60.469 Insect bite (nonvenomous) of unspecified finger**
+ **S60.47 Other superficial bite of fingers**
  Excludes1: *open bite of fingers (S61.25-, S61.35-)*
  - +7th **S60.470 Other superficial bite of right index finger**
  - +7th **S60.471 Other superficial bite of left index finger**
  - +7th **S60.472 Other superficial bite of right middle finger**
  - +7th **S60.473 Other superficial bite of left middle finger**
  - +7th **S60.474 Other superficial bite of right ring finger**
  - +7th **S60.475 Other superficial bite of left ring finger**
  - +7th **S60.476 Other superficial bite of right little finger**
  - +7th **S60.477 Other superficial bite of left little finger**
  - +7th **S60.478 Other superficial bite of other finger**
    Other superficial bite of specified finger with unspecified laterality
  - +7th **S60.479 Other superficial bite of unspecified finger**

+ **S60.5 Other superficial injuries of hand**
  Excludes2: *superficial injuries of fingers (S60.3-, S60.4-)*
+ **S60.51 Abrasion of hand**
  - +7th **S60.511 Abrasion of right hand**
  - +7th **S60.512 Abrasion of left hand**
  - +7th **S60.519 Abrasion of unspecified hand**
+ **S60.52 Blister (nonthermal) of hand**
  - +7th **S60.521 Blister (nonthermal) of right hand**

+7th **S60.522** **Blister (nonthermal) of left hand**
+7th **S60.529** **Blister (nonthermal) of unspecified hand**
+ **S60.54** **External constriction of hand**
+7th **S60.541** **External constriction of right hand**
+7th **S60.542** **External constriction of left hand**
+7th **S60.549** **External constriction of unspecified hand**
+ **S60.55** **Superficial foreign body of hand**
Splinter in the hand
+7th **S60.551** **Superficial foreign body of right hand**
+7th **S60.552** **Superficial foreign body of left hand**
+7th **S60.559** **Superficial foreign body of unspecified hand**
+ **S60.56** **Insect bite (nonvenomous) of hand**
+7th **S60.561** **Insect bite (nonvenomous) of right hand**
+7th **S60.562** **Insect bite (nonvenomous) of left hand**
+7th **S60.569** **Insect bite (nonvenomous) of unspecified hand**
+ **S60.57** **Other superficial bite of hand**
Excludes1: *open bite of hand (S61.45-)*
+7th **S60.571** **Other superficial bite of hand of right hand**
+7th **S60.572** **Other superficial bite of hand of left hand**
+7th **S60.579** **Other superficial bite of hand of unspecified hand**
+ **S60.8** **Other superficial injuries of wrist**
+ **S60.81** **Abrasion of wrist**
+7th **S60.811** **Abrasion of right wrist**
+7th **S60.812** **Abrasion of left wrist**
+7th **S60.819** **Abrasion of unspecified wrist**
+ **S60.82** **Blister (nonthermal) of wrist**
+7th **S60.821** **Blister (nonthermal) of right wrist**
+7th **S60.822** **Blister (nonthermal) of left wrist**
+7th **S60.829** **Blister (nonthermal) of unspecified wrist**
+ **S60.84** **External constriction of wrist**
+7th **S60.841** **External constriction of right wrist**
+7th **S60.842** **External constriction of left wrist**
+7th **S60.849** **External constriction of unspecified wrist**
+ **S60.85** **Superficial foreign body of wrist**
Splinter in the wrist
+7th **S60.851** **Superficial foreign body of right wrist**
+7th **S60.852** **Superficial foreign body of left wrist**
+7th **S60.859** **Superficial foreign body of unspecified wrist**
+ **S60.86** **Insect bite (nonvenomous) of wrist**
+7th **S60.861** **Insect bite (nonvenomous) of right wrist**
+7th **S60.862** **Insect bite (nonvenomous) of left wrist**
+7th **S60.869** **Insect bite (nonvenomous) of unspecified wrist**
+ **S60.87** **Other superficial bite of wrist**
Excludes1: *open bite of wrist (S61.55)*
+7th **S60.871** **Other superficial bite of right wrist**
+7th **S60.872** **Other superficial bite of left wrist**
+7th **S60.879** **Other superficial bite of unspecified wrist**
+ **S60.9** **Unspecified superficial injury of wrist, hand and fingers**
+ **S60.91** **Unspecified superficial injury of wrist**
+7th **S60.911** **Unspecified superficial injury of right wrist**
+7th **S60.912** **Unspecified superficial injury of left wrist**
+7th **S60.919** **Unspecified superficial injury of unspecified wrist**
+ **S60.92** **Unspecified superficial injury of hand**
+7th **S60.921** **Unspecified superficial injury of right hand**
+7th **S60.922** **Unspecified superficial injury of left hand**
+7th **S60.929** **Unspecified superficial injury of unspecified hand**
+ **S60.93** **Unspecified superficial injury of thumb**
+7th **S60.931** **Unspecified superficial injury of right thumb**
+7th **S60.932** **Unspecified superficial injury of left thumb**
+7th **S60.939** **Unspecified superficial injury of unspecified thumb**
+ **S60.94** **Unspecified superficial injury of other fingers**
+7th **S60.940** **Unspecified superficial injury of right index finger**
+7th **S60.941** **Unspecified superficial injury of left index finger**
+7th **S60.942** **Unspecified superficial injury of right middle finger**
+7th **S60.943** **Unspecified superficial injury of left middle finger**
+7th **S60.944** **Unspecified superficial injury of right ring finger**
+7th **S60.945** **Unspecified superficial injury of left ring finger**
+7th **S60.946** **Unspecified superficial injury of right little finger**
+7th **S60.947** **Unspecified superficial injury of left little finger**
+7th **S60.948** **Unspecified superficial injury of other finger**
Unspecified superficial injury of specified finger with unspecified laterality
+7th **S60.949** **Unspecified superficial injury of unspecified finger**

S61 **Open wound of wrist, hand and fingers**
Code also any associated wound infection
Excludes1: *open fracture of wrist, hand and finger (S62.- with 7th character B)*
traumatic amputation of wrist and hand (S68.-)

The appropriate 7th character is to be added to each code from category S61 A initial encounter D subsequent encounter S sequela

+ **S61.0** **Open wound of thumb without damage to nail**
Excludes1: *open wound of thumb with damage to nail (S61.1-)*
+ **S61.00** **Unspecified open wound of thumb without damage to nail**
+7th **S61.001** **Unspecified open wound of right thumb without damage to nail**
+7th **S61.002** **Unspecified open wound of left thumb without damage to nail**
+7th **S61.009** **Unspecified open wound of unspecified thumb without damage to nail**
+ **S61.01** **Laceration without foreign body of thumb without damage to nail**
+7th **S61.011** **Laceration without foreign body of right thumb without damage to nail**
+7th **S61.012** **Laceration without foreign body of left thumb without damage to nail**
+7th **S61.019** **Laceration without foreign body of unspecified thumb without damage to nail**
+ **S61.02** **Laceration with foreign body of thumb without damage to nail**
+7th **S61.021** **Laceration with foreign body of right thumb without damage to nail**
+7th **S61.022** **Laceration with foreign body of left thumb without damage to nail**
+7th **S61.029** **Laceration with foreign body of unspecified thumb without damage to nail**
+ **S61.03** **Puncture wound without foreign body of thumb without damage to nail**
+7th **S61.031** **Puncture wound without foreign body of right thumb without damage to nail**
+7th **S61.032** **Puncture wound without foreign body of left thumb without damage to nail**
+7th **S61.039** **Puncture wound without foreign body of unspecified thumb without damage to nail**
+ **S61.04** **Puncture wound with foreign body of thumb without damage to nail**
+7th **S61.041** **Puncture wound with foreign body of right thumb without damage to nail**
+7th **S61.042** **Puncture wound with foreign body of left thumb without damage to nail**
+7th **S61.049** **Puncture wound with foreign body of unspecified thumb without damage to nail**

+ **S61.05** **Open bite of thumb without damage to nail**
  Bite of thumb NOS
  Excludes1: *superficial bite of thumb (S60.36-, S60.37-)*
  - +7th **S61.051** **Open bite of right thumb without damage to nail**
  - +7th **S61.052** **Open bite of left thumb without damage to nail**
  - +7th **S61.059** **Open bite of unspecified thumb without damage to nail**

+ **S61.1** **Open wound of thumb with damage to nail**
+ **S61.10** **Unspecified open wound of thumb with damage to nail**
  - +7th **S61.101** **Unspecified open wound of right thumb with damage to nail**
  - +7th **S61.102** **Unspecified open wound of left thumb with damage to nail**
  - +7th **S61.109** **Unspecified open wound of unspecified thumb with damage to nail**
+ **S61.11** **Laceration without foreign body of thumb with damage to nail**
  - +7th **S61.111** **Laceration without foreign body of right thumb with damage to nail**
  - +7th **S61.112** **Laceration without foreign body of left thumb with damage to nail**
  - +7th **S61.119** **Laceration without foreign body of unspecified thumb with damage to nail**
+ **S61.12** **Laceration with foreign body of thumb with damage to nail**
  - +7th **S61.121** **Laceration with foreign body of right thumb with damage to nail**
  - +7th **S61.122** **Laceration with foreign body of left thumb with damage to nail**
  - +7th **S61.129** **Laceration with foreign body of unspecified thumb with damage to nail**
+ **S61.13** **Puncture wound without foreign body of thumb with damage to nail**
  - +7th **S61.131** **Puncture wound without foreign body of right thumb with damage to nail**
  - +7th **S61.132** **Puncture wound without foreign body of left thumb with damage to nail**
  - +7th **S61.139** **Puncture wound without foreign body of unspecified thumb with damage to nail**
+ **S61.14** **Puncture wound with foreign body of thumb with damage to nail**
  - +7th **S61.141** **Puncture wound with foreign body of right thumb with damage to nail**
  - +7th **S61.142** **Puncture wound with foreign body of left thumb with damage to nail**
  - +7th **S61.149** **Puncture wound with foreign body of unspecified thumb with damage to nail**
+ **S61.15** **Open bite of thumb with damage to nail**
  Bite of thumb with damage to nail NOS
  Excludes1: *superficial bite of thumb (S60.36-, S60.37-)*
  - +7th **S61.151** **Open bite of right thumb with damage to nail**
  - +7th **S61.152** **Open bite of left thumb with damage to nail**
  - +7th **S61.159** **Open bite of unspecified thumb with damage to nail**

+ **S61.2** **Open wound of other finger without damage to nail**
  Excludes1: *open wound of finger involving nail (matrix) (S61.3-)*
  Excludes2: *open wound of thumb without damage to nail (S61.0-)*
+ **S61.20** **Unspecified open wound of other finger without damage to nail**
  - +7th **S61.200** **Unspecified open wound of right index finger without damage to nail**
  - +7th **S61.201** **Unspecified open wound of left index finger without damage to nail**
  - +7th **S61.202** **Unspecified open wound of right middle finger without damage to nail**
  - +7th **S61.203** **Unspecified open wound of left middle finger without damage to nail**
  - +7th **S61.204** **Unspecified open wound of right ring finger without damage to nail**
  - +7th **S61.205** **Unspecified open wound of left ring finger without damage to nail**
  - +7th **S61.206** **Unspecified open wound of right little finger without damage to nail**
  - +7th **S61.207** **Unspecified open wound of left little finger without damage to nail**
  - +7th **S61.208** **Unspecified open wound of other finger without damage to nail**
    Unspecified open wound of specified finger with unspecified laterality without damage to nail
  - +7th **S61.209** **Unspecified open wound of unspecified finger without damage to nail**
+ **S61.21** **Laceration without foreign body of finger without damage to nail**
  - +7th **S61.210** **Laceration without foreign body of right index finger without damage to nail**
  - +7th **S61.211** **Laceration without foreign body of left index finger without damage to nail**
  - +7th **S61.212** **Laceration without foreign body of right middle finger without damage to nail**
  - +7th **S61.213** **Laceration without foreign body of left middle finger without damage to nail**
  - +7th **S61.214** **Laceration without foreign body of right ring finger without damage to nail**
  - +7th **S61.215** **Laceration without foreign body of left ring finger without damage to nail**
  - +7th **S61.216** **Laceration without foreign body of right little finger without damage to nail**
  - +7th **S61.217** **Laceration without foreign body of left little finger without damage to nail**
  - +7th **S61.218** **Laceration without foreign body of other finger without damage to nail**
    Laceration without foreign body of specified finger with unspecified laterality without damage to nail
  - +7th **S61.219** **Laceration without foreign body of unspecified finger without damage to nail**
+ **S61.22** **Laceration with foreign body of finger without damage to nail**
  - +7th **S61.220** **Laceration with foreign body of right index finger without damage to nail**
  - +7th **S61.221** **Laceration with foreign body of left index finger without damage to nail**
  - +7th **S61.222** **Laceration with foreign body of right middle finger without damage to nail**
  - +7th **S61.223** **Laceration with foreign body of left middle finger without damage to nail**
  - +7th **S61.224** **Laceration with foreign body of right ring finger without damage to nail**
  - +7th **S61.225** **Laceration with foreign body of left ring finger without damage to nail**
  - +7th **S61.226** **Laceration with foreign body of right little finger without damage to nail**
  - +7th **S61.227** **Laceration with foreign body of left little finger without damage to nail**
  - +7th **S61.228** **Laceration with foreign body of other finger without damage to nail**
    Laceration with foreign body of specified finger with unspecified laterality without damage to nail
  - +7th **S61.229** **Laceration with foreign body of unspecified finger without damage to nail**
+ **S61.23** **Puncture wound without foreign body of finger without damage to nail**
  - +7th **S61.230** **Puncture wound without foreign body of right index finger without damage to nail**
  - +7th **S61.231** **Puncture wound without foreign body of left index finger without damage to nail**

+7th **S61.232 Puncture wound without foreign body of right middle finger without damage to nail**

+7th **S61.233 Puncture wound without foreign body of left middle finger without damage to nail**

+7th **S61.234 Puncture wound without foreign body of right ring finger without damage to nail**

+7th **S61.235 Puncture wound without foreign body of left ring finger without damage to nail**

+7th **S61.236 Puncture wound without foreign body of right little finger without damage to nail**

+7th **S61.237 Puncture wound without foreign body of left little finger without damage to nail**

+7th **S61.238 Puncture wound without foreign body of other finger without damage to nail**
Puncture wound without foreign body of specified finger with unspecified laterality without damage to nail

+7th **S61.239 Puncture wound without foreign body of unspecified finger without damage to nail**

\+ **S61.24 Puncture wound with foreign body of finger without damage to nail**

+7th **S61.240 Puncture wound with foreign body of right index finger without damage to nail**

+7th **S61.241 Puncture wound with foreign body of left index finger without damage to nail**

+7th **S61.242 Puncture wound with foreign body of right middle finger without damage to nail**

+7th **S61.243 Puncture wound with foreign body of left middle finger without damage to nail**

+7th **S61.244 Puncture wound with foreign body of right ring finger without damage to nail**

+7th **S61.245 Puncture wound with foreign body of left ring finger without damage to nail**

+7th **S61.246 Puncture wound with foreign body of right little finger without damage to nail**

+7th **S61.247 Puncture wound with foreign body of left little finger without damage to nail**

+7th **S61.248 Puncture wound with foreign body of other finger without damage to nail**
Puncture wound with foreign body of specified finger with unspecified laterality without damage to nail

+7th **S61.249 Puncture wound with foreign body of unspecified finger without damage to nail**

\+ **S61.25 Open bite of finger without damage to nail**
Bite of finger without damage to nail NOS
Excludes1: *superficial bite of finger (S60.46-, S60.47-)*

+7th **S61.250 Open bite of right index finger without damage to nail**

+7th **S61.251 Open bite of left index finger without damage to nail**

+7th **S61.252 Open bite of right middle finger without damage to nail**

+7th **S61.253 Open bite of left middle finger without damage to nail**

+7th **S61.254 Open bite of right ring finger without damage to nail**

+7th **S61.255 Open bite of left ring finger without damage to nail**

+7th **S61.256 Open bite of right little finger without damage to nail**

+7th **S61.257 Open bite of left little finger without damage to nail**

+7th **S61.258 Open bite of other finger without damage to nail**
Open bite of specified finger with unspecified laterality without damage to nail

+7th **S61.259 Open bite of unspecified finger without damage to nail**

\+ **S61.3 Open wound of other finger with damage to nail**

\+ **S61.30 Unspecified open wound of finger with damage to nail**

+7th **S61.300 Unspecified open wound of right index finger with damage to nail**

+7th **S61.301 Unspecified open wound of left index finger with damage to nail**

+7th **S61.302 Unspecified open wound of right middle finger with damage to nail**

+7th **S61.303 Unspecified open wound of left middle finger with damage to nail**

+7th **S61.304 Unspecified open wound of right ring finger with damage to nail**

+7th **S61.305 Unspecified open wound of left ring finger with damage to nail**

+7th **S61.306 Unspecified open wound of right little finger with damage to nail**

+7th **S61.307 Unspecified open wound of left little finger with damage to nail**

+7th **S61.308 Unspecified open wound of other finger with damage to nail**
Unspecified open wound of specified finger with unspecified laterality with damage to nail

+7th **S61.309 Unspecified open wound of unspecified finger with damage to nail**

\+ **S61.31 Laceration without foreign body of finger with damage to nail**

+7th **S61.310 Laceration without foreign body of right index finger with damage to nail**

+7th **S61.311 Laceration without foreign body of left index finger with damage to nail**

+7th **S61.312 Laceration without foreign body of right middle finger with damage to nail**

+7th **S61.313 Laceration without foreign body of left middle finger with damage to nail**

+7th **S61.314 Laceration without foreign body of right ring finger with damage to nail**

+7th **S61.315 Laceration without foreign body of left ring finger with damage to nail**

+7th **S61.316 Laceration without foreign body of right little finger with damage to nail**

+7th **S61.317 Laceration without foreign body of left little finger with damage to nail**

+7th **S61.318 Laceration without foreign body of other finger with damage to nail**
Laceration without foreign body of specified finger with unspecified laterality with damage to nail

+7th **S61.319 Laceration without foreign body of unspecified finger with damage to nail**

\+ **S61.32 Laceration with foreign body of finger with damage to nail**

+7th **S61.320 Laceration with foreign body of right index finger with damage to nail**

+7th **S61.321 Laceration with foreign body of left index finger with damage to nail**

+7th **S61.322 Laceration with foreign body of right middle finger with damage to nail**

+7th **S61.323 Laceration with foreign body of left middle finger with damage to nail**

+7th **S61.324 Laceration with foreign body of right ring finger with damage to nail**

+7th **S61.325 Laceration with foreign body of left ring finger with damage to nail**

+7th **S61.326 Laceration with foreign body of right little finger with damage to nail**

+7th **S61.327 Laceration with foreign body of left little finger with damage to nail**

+7th **S61.328 Laceration with foreign body of other finger with damage to nail**
Laceration with foreign body of specified finger with unspecified laterality with damage to nail

+7th **S61.329 Laceration with foreign body of unspecified finger with damage to nail**

\+ **S61.33 Puncture wound without foreign body of finger with damage to nail**

+7th **S61.330 Puncture wound without foreign body of right index finger with damage to nail**

+7th **S61.331 Puncture wound without foreign body of left index finger with damage to nail**
+7th **S61.332 Puncture wound without foreign body of right middle finger with damage to nail**
+7th **S61.333 Puncture wound without foreign body of left middle finger with damage to nail**
+7th **S61.334 Puncture wound without foreign body of right ring finger with damage to nail**
+7th **S61.335 Puncture wound without foreign body of left ring finger with damage to nail**
+7th **S61.336 Puncture wound without foreign body of right little finger with damage to nail**
+7th **S61.337 Puncture wound without foreign body of left little finger with damage to nail**
+7th **S61.338 Puncture wound without foreign body of other finger with damage to nail**
Puncture wound without foreign body of specified finger with unspecified laterality with damage to nail
+7th **S61.339 Puncture wound without foreign body of unspecified finger with damage to nail**

\+ **S61.34 Puncture wound with foreign body of finger with damage to nail**
+7th **S61.340 Puncture wound with foreign body of right index finger with damage to nail**
+7th **S61.341 Puncture wound with foreign body of left index finger with damage to nail**
+7th **S61.342 Puncture wound with foreign body of right middle finger with damage to nail**
+7th **S61.343 Puncture wound with foreign body of left middle finger with damage to nail**
+7th **S61.344 Puncture wound with foreign body of right ring finger with damage to nail**
+7th **S61.345 Puncture wound with foreign body of left ring finger with damage to nail**
+7th **S61.346 Puncture wound with foreign body of right little finger with damage to nail**
+7th **S61.347 Puncture wound with foreign body of left little finger with damage to nail**
+7th **S61.348 Puncture wound with foreign body of other finger with damage to nail**
Puncture wound with foreign body of specified finger with unspecified laterality with damage to nail
+7th **S61.349 Puncture wound with foreign body of unspecified finger with damage to nail**

\+ **S61.35 Open bite of finger with damage to nail**
Bite of finger with damage to nail NOS
Excludes1: *superficial bite of finger (S60.46-, S60.47-)*
+7th **S61.350 Open bite of right index finger with damage to nail**
+7th **S61.351 Open bite of left index finger with damage to nail**
+7th **S61.352 Open bite of right middle finger with damage to nail**
+7th **S61.353 Open bite of left middle finger with damage to nail**
+7th **S61.354 Open bite of right ring finger with damage to nail**
+7th **S61.355 Open bite of left ring finger with damage to nail**
+7th **S61.356 Open bite of right little finger with damage to nail**
+7th **S61.357 Open bite of left little finger with damage to nail**
+7th **S61.358 Open bite of other finger with damage to nail**
Open bite of specified finger with unspecified laterality with damage to nail
+7th **S61.359 Open bite of unspecified finger with damage to nail**

\+ **S61.4 Open wound of hand**
\+ **S61.40 Unspecified open wound of hand**
+7th **S61.401 Unspecified open wound of right hand**
+7th **S61.402 Unspecified open wound of left hand**
+7th **S61.409 Unspecified open wound of unspecified hand**

\+ **S61.41 Laceration without foreign body of hand**
+7th **S61.411 Laceration without foreign body of right hand**
+7th **S61.412 Laceration without foreign body of left hand**
+7th **S61.419 Laceration without foreign body of unspecified hand**
\+ **S61.42 Laceration with foreign body of hand**
+7th **S61.421 Laceration with foreign body of right hand**
+7th **S61.422 Laceration with foreign body of left hand**
+7th **S61.429 Laceration with foreign body of unspecified hand**
\+ **S61.43 Puncture wound without foreign body of hand**
+7th **S61.431 Puncture wound without foreign body of right hand**
+7th **S61.432 Puncture wound without foreign body of left hand**
+7th **S61.439 Puncture wound without foreign body of unspecified hand**
\+ **S61.44 Puncture wound with foreign body of hand**
+7th **S61.441 Puncture wound with foreign body of right hand**
+7th **S61.442 Puncture wound with foreign body of left hand**
+7th **S61.449 Puncture wound with foreign body of unspecified hand**
\+ **S61.45 Open bite of hand**
Bite of hand NOS
Excludes1: *superficial bite of hand (S60.56-, S60.57-)*
+7th **S61.451 Open bite of right hand**
+7th **S61.452 Open bite of left hand**
+7th **S61.459 Open bite of unspecified hand**

\+ **S61.5 Open wound of wrist**
\+ **S61.50 Unspecified open wound of wrist**
+7th **S61.501 Unspecified open wound of right wrist**
+7th **S61.502 Unspecified open wound of left wrist**
+7th **S61.509 Unspecified open wound of unspecified wrist**
\+ **S61.51 Laceration without foreign body of wrist**
+7th **S61.511 Laceration without foreign body of right wrist**
+7th **S61.512 Laceration without foreign body of left wrist**
+7th **S61.519 Laceration without foreign body of unspecified wrist**
\+ **S61.52 Laceration with foreign body of wrist**
+7th **S61.521 Laceration with foreign body of right wrist**
+7th **S61.522 Laceration with foreign body of left wrist**
+7th **S61.529 Laceration with foreign body of unspecified wrist**
\+ **S61.53 Puncture wound without foreign body of wrist**
+7th **S61.531 Puncture wound without foreign body of right wrist**
+7th **S61.532 Puncture wound without foreign body of left wrist**
+7th **S61.539 Puncture wound without foreign body of unspecified wrist**
\+ **S61.54 Puncture wound with foreign body of wrist**
+7th **S61.541 Puncture wound with foreign body of right wrist**
+7th **S61.542 Puncture wound with foreign body of left wrist**
+7th **S61.549 Puncture wound with foreign body of unspecified wrist**
\+ **S61.55 Open bite of wrist**
Bite of wrist NOS
Excludes1: *superficial bite of wrist (S60.86-, S60.87-)*
+7th **S61.551 Open bite of right wrist**
+7th **S61.552 Open bite of left wrist**
+7th **S61.559 Open bite of unspecified wrist**

S62 Fracture at wrist and hand level

NOTE A fracture not indicated as displaced or nondisplaced should be coded to displaced
A fracture not indicated as open or closed should be coded to closed

Excludes1: *traumatic amputation of wrist and hand (S68.-)*
Excludes2: *fracture of distal parts of ulna and radius (S52.-)*

The appropriate 7th character is to be added to each code from category S62
A initial encounter for closed fracture
B initial encounter for open fracture
D subsequent encounter for fracture with routine healing
G subsequent encounter for fracture with delayed healing
K subsequent encounter for fracture with nonunion
P subsequent encounter for fracture with malunion
S sequela

Review coding guideline C.19.c

\+ **S62.0 Fracture of navicular [scaphoid] bone of wrist**

\+ **S62.00 Unspecified fracture of navicular [scaphoid] bone of wrist**

CC +7th **S62.001 Unspecified fracture of navicular [scaphoid] bone of right wrist**
HAC 7th character B see Appendix B for HAC conditional logic

CC +7th **S62.002 Unspecified fracture of navicular [scaphoid] bone of left wrist**
AHA CC: 4Q, 2012, 106
HAC 7th character B see Appendix B for HAC conditional logic

CC +7th **S62.009 Unspecified fracture of navicular [scaphoid] bone of unspecified wrist**
HAC 7th character B see Appendix B for HAC conditional logic

\+ **S62.01 Fracture of distal pole of navicular [scaphoid] bone of wrist**
Fracture of volar tuberosity of navicular [scaphoid] bone of wrist

CC +7th **S62.011 Displaced fracture of distal pole of navicular [scaphoid] bone of right wrist**
HAC 7th character B see Appendix B for HAC conditional logic

CC +7th **S62.012 Displaced fracture of distal pole of navicular [scaphoid] bone of left wrist**
HAC 7th character B see Appendix B for HAC conditional logic

CC +7th **S62.013 Displaced fracture of distal pole of navicular [scaphoid] bone of unspecified wrist**
HAC 7th character B see Appendix B for HAC conditional logic

CC +7th **S62.014 Nondisplaced fracture of distal pole of navicular [scaphoid] bone of right wrist**
HAC 7th character B see Appendix B for HAC conditional logic

CC +7th **S62.015 Nondisplaced fracture of distal pole of navicular [scaphoid] bone of left wrist**
HAC 7th character B see Appendix B for HAC conditional logic

CC +7th **S62.016 Nondisplaced fracture of distal pole of navicular [scaphoid] bone of unspecified wrist**
HAC 7th character B see Appendix B for HAC conditional logic

\+ **S62.02 Fracture of middle third of navicular [scaphoid] bone of wrist**

CC +7th **S62.021 Displaced fracture of middle third of navicular [scaphoid] bone of right wrist**
HAC 7th character B see Appendix B for HAC conditional logic

CC +7th **S62.022 Displaced fracture of middle third of navicular [scaphoid] bone of left wrist**
HAC 7th character B see Appendix B for HAC conditional logic

CC +7th **S62.023 Displaced fracture of middle third of navicular [scaphoid] bone of unspecified wrist**
HAC 7th character B see Appendix B for HAC conditional logic

CC +7th **S62.024 Nondisplaced fracture of middle third of navicular [scaphoid] bone of right wrist**
HAC 7th character B see Appendix B for HAC conditional logic

CC +7th **S62.025 Nondisplaced fracture of middle third of navicular [scaphoid] bone of left wrist**
HAC 7th character B see Appendix B for HAC conditional logic

CC +7th **S62.026 Nondisplaced fracture of middle third of navicular [scaphoid] bone of unspecified wrist**
HAC 7th character B see Appendix B for HAC conditional logic

\+ **S62.03 Fracture of proximal third of navicular [scaphoid] bone of wrist**

CC +7th **S62.031 Displaced fracture of proximal third of navicular [scaphoid] bone of right wrist**
HAC 7th character B see Appendix B for HAC conditional logic

CC +7th **S62.032 Displaced fracture of proximal third of navicular [scaphoid] bone of left wrist**
HAC 7th character B see Appendix B for HAC conditional logic

CC +7th **S62.033 Displaced fracture of proximal third of navicular [scaphoid] bone of unspecified wrist**
HAC 7th character B see Appendix B for HAC conditional logic

CC +7th **S62.034 Nondisplaced fracture of proximal third of navicular [scaphoid] bone of right wrist**
HAC 7th character B see Appendix B for HAC conditional logic

CC +7th **S62.035 Nondisplaced fracture of proximal third of navicular [scaphoid] bone of left wrist**
HAC 7th character B see Appendix B for HAC conditional logic

CC +7th **S62.036 Nondisplaced fracture of proximal third of navicular [scaphoid] bone of unspecified wrist**
HAC 7th character B see Appendix B for HAC conditional logic

\+ **S62.1 Fracture of other and unspecified carpal bone(s)**
Excludes2: *fracture of scaphoid of wrist (S62.0-)*

\+ **S62.10 Fracture of unspecified carpal bone**
Fracture of wrist NOS

CC +7th **S62.101 Fracture of unspecified carpal bone, right wrist**
HAC 7th character B see Appendix B for HAC conditional logic

CC +7th **S62.102 Fracture of unspecified carpal bone, left wrist**
AHA CC: 4Q, 2012, 95-96
HAC 7th character B see Appendix B for HAC conditional logic

CC +7th **S62.109 Fracture of unspecified carpal bone, unspecified wrist**
HAC 7th character B see Appendix B for HAC conditional logic

\+ **S62.11 Fracture of triquetrum [cuneiform] bone of wrist**

CC +7th **S62.111 Displaced fracture of triquetrum [cuneiform] bone, right wrist**
HAC 7th character B see Appendix B for HAC conditional logic

CC +7th **S62.112 Displaced fracture of triquetrum [cuneiform] bone, left wrist**
HAC 7th character B see Appendix B for HAC conditional logic

CC +7th **S62.113 Displaced fracture of triquetrum [cuneiform] bone, unspecified wrist**
HAC 7th character B see Appendix B for HAC conditional logic

CC +7th **S62.114 Nondisplaced fracture of triquetrum [cuneiform] bone, right wrist**
HAC 7th character B see Appendix B for HAC conditional logic

CC +7th **S62.115 Nondisplaced fracture of triquetrum [cuneiform] bone, left wrist**
HAC 7th character B see Appendix B for HAC conditional logic

CC +7th **S62.116 Nondisplaced fracture of triquetrum [cuneiform] bone, unspecified wrist**
HAC 7th character B see Appendix B for HAC conditional logic

+ **S62.12 Fracture of lunate [semilunar]**

CC +7th **S62.121 Displaced fracture of lunate [semilunar], right wrist**
HAC 7th character B see Appendix B for HAC conditional logic

CC +7th **S62.122 Displaced fracture of lunate [semilunar], left wrist**
HAC 7th character B see Appendix B for HAC conditional logic

CC +7th **S62.123 Displaced fracture of lunate [semilunar], unspecified wrist**
HAC 7th character B see Appendix B for HAC conditional logic

CC +7th **S62.124 Nondisplaced fracture of lunate [semilunar], right wrist**
HAC 7th character B see Appendix B for HAC conditional logic

CC +7th **S62.125 Nondisplaced fracture of lunate [semilunar], left wrist**
HAC 7th character B see Appendix B for HAC conditional logic

CC +7th **S62.126 Nondisplaced fracture of lunate [semilunar], unspecified wrist**
HAC 7th character B see Appendix B for HAC conditional logic

+ **S62.13 Fracture of capitate [os magnum] bone**

CC +7th **S62.131 Displaced fracture of capitate [os magnum] bone, right wrist**
HAC 7th character B see Appendix B for HAC conditional logic

CC +7th **S62.132 Displaced fracture of capitate [os magnum] bone, left wrist**
HAC 7th character B see Appendix B for HAC conditional logic

CC +7th **S62.133 Displaced fracture of capitate [os magnum] bone, unspecified wrist**
HAC 7th character B see Appendix B for HAC conditional logic

CC +7th **S62.134 Nondisplaced fracture of capitate [os magnum] bone, right wrist**
HAC 7th character B see Appendix B for HAC conditional logic

CC +7th **S62.135 Nondisplaced fracture of capitate [os magnum] bone, left wrist**
HAC 7th character B see Appendix B for HAC conditional logic

CC +7th **S62.136 Nondisplaced fracture of capitate [os magnum] bone, unspecified wrist**
HAC 7th character B see Appendix B for HAC conditional logic

+ **S62.14 Fracture of body of hamate [unciform] bone**
Fracture of hamate [unciform] bone NOS

CC +7th **S62.141 Displaced fracture of body of hamate [unciform] bone, right wrist**
HAC 7th character B see Appendix B for HAC conditional logic

CC +7th **S62.142 Displaced fracture of body of hamate [unciform] bone, left wrist**
HAC 7th character B see Appendix B for HAC conditional logic

CC +7th **S62.143 Displaced fracture of body of hamate [unciform] bone, unspecified wrist**
HAC 7th character B see Appendix B for HAC conditional logic

CC +7th **S62.144 Nondisplaced fracture of body of hamate [unciform] bone, right wrist**
HAC 7th character B see Appendix B for HAC conditional logic

CC +7th **S62.145 Nondisplaced fracture of body of hamate [unciform] bone, left wrist**
HAC 7th character B see Appendix B for HAC conditional logic

CC +7th **S62.146 Nondisplaced fracture of body of hamate [unciform] bone, unspecified wrist**
HAC 7th character B see Appendix B for HAC conditional logic

+ **S62.15 Fracture of hook process of hamate [unciform] bone**
Fracture of unciform process of hamate [unciform] bone

CC +7th **S62.151 Displaced fracture of hook process of hamate [unciform] bone, right wrist**
HAC 7th character B see Appendix B for HAC conditional logic

CC +7th **S62.152 Displaced fracture of hook process of hamate [unciform] bone, left wrist**
HAC 7th character B see Appendix B for HAC conditional logic

CC +7th **S62.153 Displaced fracture of hook process of hamate [unciform] bone, unspecified wrist**
HAC 7th character B see Appendix B for HAC conditional logic

CC +7th **S62.154 Nondisplaced fracture of hook process of hamate [unciform] bone, right wrist**
HAC 7th character B see Appendix B for HAC conditional logic

CC +7th **S62.155 Nondisplaced fracture of hook process of hamate [unciform] bone, left wrist**
HAC 7th character B see Appendix B for HAC conditional logic

CC +7th **S62.156 Nondisplaced fracture of hook process of hamate [unciform] bone, unspecified wrist**
HAC 7th character B see Appendix B for HAC conditional logic

+ **S62.16 Fracture of pisiform**

CC +7th **S62.161 Displaced fracture of pisiform, right wrist**
HAC 7th character B see Appendix B for HAC conditional logic

CC +7th **S62.162 Displaced fracture of pisiform, left wrist**
HAC 7th character B see Appendix B for HAC conditional logic

CC +7th **S62.163 Displaced fracture of pisiform, unspecified wrist**
HAC 7th character B see Appendix B for HAC conditional logic

CC +7th **S62.164 Nondisplaced fracture of pisiform, right wrist**
HAC 7th character B see Appendix B for HAC conditional logic

CC +7th **S62.165 Nondisplaced fracture of pisiform, left wrist**
HAC 7th character B see Appendix B for HAC conditional logic

CC +7th **S62.166 Nondisplaced fracture of pisiform, unspecified wrist**
HAC 7th character B see Appendix B for HAC conditional logic

+ **S62.17 Fracture of trapezium [larger multangular]**

CC +7th **S62.171 Displaced fracture of trapezium [larger multangular], right wrist**
HAC 7th character B see Appendix B for HAC conditional logic

CC +7th **S62.172 Displaced fracture of trapezium [larger multangular], left wrist**
HAC 7th character B see Appendix B for HAC conditional logic

CC +7th **S62.173 Displaced fracture of trapezium [larger multangular], unspecified wrist**
HAC 7th character B see Appendix B for HAC conditional logic

CC +7th **S62.174 Nondisplaced fracture of trapezium [larger multangular], right wrist**
HAC 7th character B see Appendix B for HAC conditional logic

CC +7th **S62.175 Nondisplaced fracture of trapezium [larger multangular], left wrist**
HAC 7th character B see Appendix B for HAC conditional logic

CC +7th **S62.176 Nondisplaced fracture of trapezium [larger multangular], unspecified wrist**
HAC 7th character B see Appendix B for HAC conditional logic

+ **S62.18 Fracture of trapezoid [smaller multangular]**

CC +7th **S62.181 Displaced fracture of trapezoid [smaller multangular], right wrist**
HAC 7th character B see Appendix B for HAC conditional logic

CC +7th **S62.182 Displaced fracture of trapezoid [smaller multangular], left wrist**
HAC 7th character B see Appendix B for HAC conditional logic

CC +7th **S62.183 Displaced fracture of trapezoid [smaller multangular], unspecified wrist**
HAC 7th character B see Appendix B for HAC conditional logic

CC +7th **S62.184 Nondisplaced fracture of trapezoid [smaller multangular], right wrist**
HAC 7th character B see Appendix B for HAC conditional logic

CC +7th **S62.185 Nondisplaced fracture of trapezoid [smaller multangular], left wrist**
HAC 7th character B see Appendix B for HAC conditional logic

CC +7th **S62.186 Nondisplaced fracture of trapezoid [smaller multangular], unspecified wrist**
HAC 7th character B see Appendix B for HAC conditional logic

\+ **S62.2 Fracture of first metacarpal bone**

\+ **S62.20 Unspecified fracture of first metacarpal bone**

CC +7th **S62.201 Unspecified fracture of first metacarpal bone, right hand**
HAC 7th character B see Appendix B for HAC conditional logic

CC +7th **S62.202 Unspecified fracture of first metacarpal bone, left hand**
HAC 7th character B see Appendix B for HAC conditional logic

CC +7th **S62.209 Unspecified fracture of first metacarpal bone, unspecified hand**
HAC 7th character B see Appendix B for HAC conditional logic

\+ **S62.21 Bennett's fracture**

CC +7th **S62.211 Bennett's fracture, right hand**
HAC 7th character B see Appendix B for HAC conditional logic

CC +7th **S62.212 Bennett's fracture, left hand**
HAC 7th character B see Appendix B for HAC conditional logic

CC +7th **S62.213 Bennett's fracture, unspecified hand**
HAC 7th character B see Appendix B for HAC conditional logic

\+ **S62.22 Rolando's fracture**

CC +7th **S62.221 Displaced Rolando's fracture, right hand**
HAC 7th character B see Appendix B for HAC conditional logic

CC +7th **S62.222 Displaced Rolando's fracture, left hand**
HAC 7th character B see Appendix B for HAC conditional logic

CC +7th **S62.223 Displaced Rolando's fracture, unspecified hand**
HAC 7th character B see Appendix B for HAC conditional logic

CC +7th **S62.224 Nondisplaced Rolando's fracture, right hand**
HAC 7th character B see Appendix B for HAC conditional logic

CC +7th **S62.225 Nondisplaced Rolando's fracture, left hand**
HAC 7th character B see Appendix B for HAC conditional logic

CC +7th **S62.226 Nondisplaced Rolando's fracture, unspecified hand**
HAC 7th character B see Appendix B for HAC conditional logic

\+ **S62.23 Other fracture of base of first metacarpal bone**

CC +7th **S62.231 Other displaced fracture of base of first metacarpal bone, right hand**
HAC 7th character B see Appendix B for HAC conditional logic

CC +7th **S62.232 Other displaced fracture of base of first metacarpal bone, left hand**
HAC 7th character B see Appendix B for HAC conditional logic

CC +7th **S62.233 Other displaced fracture of base of first metacarpal bone, unspecified hand**
HAC 7th character B see Appendix B for HAC conditional logic

CC +7th **S62.234 Other nondisplaced fracture of base of first metacarpal bone, right hand**
HAC 7th character B see Appendix B for HAC conditional logic

CC +7th **S62.235 Other nondisplaced fracture of base of first metacarpal bone, left hand**
HAC 7th character B see Appendix B for HAC conditional logic

CC +7th **S62.236 Other nondisplaced fracture of base of first metacarpal bone, unspecified hand**
HAC 7th character B see Appendix B for HAC conditional logic

\+ **S62.24 Fracture of shaft of first metacarpal bone**

CC +7th **S62.241 Displaced fracture of shaft of first metacarpal bone, right hand**
HAC 7th character B see Appendix B for HAC conditional logic

CC +7th **S62.242 Displaced fracture of shaft of first metacarpal bone, left hand**
HAC 7th character B see Appendix B for HAC conditional logic

CC +7th **S62.243 Displaced fracture of shaft of first metacarpal bone, unspecified hand**
HAC 7th character B see Appendix B for HAC conditional logic

CC +7th **S62.244 Nondisplaced fracture of shaft of first metacarpal bone, right hand**
HAC 7th character B see Appendix B for HAC conditional logic

CC +7th **S62.245 Nondisplaced fracture of shaft of first metacarpal bone, left hand**
HAC 7th character B see Appendix B for HAC conditional logic

CC +7th **S62.246 Nondisplaced fracture of shaft of first metacarpal bone, unspecified hand**
HAC 7th character B see Appendix B for HAC conditional logic

\+ **S62.25 Fracture of neck of first metacarpal bone**

CC +7th **S62.251 Displaced fracture of neck of first metacarpal bone, right hand**
HAC 7th character B see Appendix B for HAC conditional logic

CC +7th **S62.252 Displaced fracture of neck of first metacarpal bone, left hand**
HAC 7th character B see Appendix B for HAC conditional logic

CC +7th **S62.253 Displaced fracture of neck of first metacarpal bone, unspecified hand**
HAC 7th character B see Appendix B for HAC conditional logic

CC +7th **S62.254 Nondisplaced fracture of neck of first metacarpal bone, right hand**
HAC 7th character B see Appendix B for HAC conditional logic

CC +7th **S62.255 Nondisplaced fracture of neck of first metacarpal bone, left hand**
HAC 7th character B see Appendix B for HAC conditional logic

CC +7th **S62.256 Nondisplaced fracture of neck of first metacarpal bone, unspecified hand**
HAC 7th character B see Appendix B for HAC conditional logic

\+ **S62.29 Other fracture of first metacarpal bone**

CC +7th **S62.291 Other fracture of first metacarpal bone, right hand**
HAC 7th character B see Appendix B for HAC conditional logic

CC +7th **S62.292 Other fracture of first metacarpal bone, left hand**
HAC 7th character B see Appendix B for HAC conditional logic

CC +7th **S62.299 Other fracture of first metacarpal bone, unspecified hand**
HAC 7th character B see Appendix B for HAC conditional logic

\+ **S62.3 Fracture of other and unspecified metacarpal bone**
Excludes2: *fracture of first metacarpal bone (S62.2-)*

\+ **S62.30 Unspecified fracture of other metacarpal bone**

CC +7th **S62.300 Unspecified fracture of second metacarpal bone, right hand**
HAC 7th character B see Appendix B for HAC conditional logic

CC +7th **S62.301 Unspecified fracture of second metacarpal bone, left hand**
HAC 7th character B see Appendix B for HAC conditional logic

CC +7th **S62.302 Unspecified fracture of third metacarpal bone, right hand**
HAC 7th character B see Appendix B for HAC conditional logic

CC +7th **S62.303 Unspecified fracture of third metacarpal bone, left hand**
HAC 7th character B see Appendix B for HAC conditional logic

CC +7th **S62.304 Unspecified fracture of fourth metacarpal bone, right hand**
HAC 7th character B see Appendix B for HAC conditional logic

CC +7th **S62.305 Unspecified fracture of fourth metacarpal bone, left hand**
HAC 7th character B see Appendix B for HAC conditional logic

CC +7th **S62.306 Unspecified fracture of fifth metacarpal bone, right hand**
HAC 7th character B see Appendix B for HAC conditional logic

CC +7th **S62.307 Unspecified fracture of fifth metacarpal bone, left hand**
HAC 7th character B see Appendix B for HAC conditional logic

CC +7th **S62.308 Unspecified fracture of other metacarpal bone**
Unspecified fracture of specified metacarpal bone with unspecified laterality
HAC 7th character B see Appendix B for HAC conditional logic

CC +7th **S62.309 Unspecified fracture of unspecified metacarpal bone**
HAC 7th character B see Appendix B for HAC conditional logic

\+ **S62.31 Displaced fracture of base of other metacarpal bone**

CC +7th **S62.310 Displaced fracture of base of second metacarpal bone, right hand**
HAC 7th character B see Appendix B for HAC conditional logic

CC +7th **S62.311 Displaced fracture of base of second metacarpal bone, left hand**
HAC 7th character B see Appendix B for HAC conditional logic

CC +7th **S62.312 Displaced fracture of base of third metacarpal bone, right hand**
HAC 7th character B see Appendix B for HAC conditional logic

CC +7th **S62.313 Displaced fracture of base of third metacarpal bone, left hand**
HAC 7th character B see Appendix B for HAC conditional logic

CC +7th **S62.314 Displaced fracture of base of fourth metacarpal bone, right hand**
HAC 7th character B see Appendix B for HAC conditional logic

CC +7th **S62.315 Displaced fracture of base of fourth metacarpal bone, left hand**
HAC 7th character B see Appendix B for HAC conditional logic

CC +7th **S62.316 Displaced fracture of base of fifth metacarpal bone, right hand**
HAC 7th character B see Appendix B for HAC conditional logic

CC +7th **S62.317 Displaced fracture of base of fifth metacarpal bone, left hand**
HAC 7th character B see Appendix B for HAC conditional logic

CC +7th **S62.318 Displaced fracture of base of other metacarpal bone**
Displaced fracture of base of specified metacarpal bone with unspecified laterality
HAC 7th character B see Appendix B for HAC conditional logic

CC +7th **S62.319 Displaced fracture of base of unspecified metacarpal bone**
HAC 7th character B see Appendix B for HAC conditional logic

\+ **S62.32 Displaced fracture of shaft of other metacarpal bone**

CC +7th **S62.320 Displaced fracture of shaft of second metacarpal bone, right hand**
HAC 7th character B see Appendix B for HAC conditional logic

CC +7th **S62.321 Displaced fracture of shaft of second metacarpal bone, left hand**
HAC 7th character B see Appendix B for HAC conditional logic

CC +7th **S62.322 Displaced fracture of shaft of third metacarpal bone, right hand**
HAC 7th character B see Appendix B for HAC conditional logic

CC +7th **S62.323 Displaced fracture of shaft of third metacarpal bone, left hand**
HAC 7th character B see Appendix B for HAC conditional logic

CC +7th **S62.324 Displaced fracture of shaft of fourth metacarpal bone, right hand**
HAC 7th character B see Appendix B for HAC conditional logic

CC +7th **S62.325 Displaced fracture of shaft of fourth metacarpal bone, left hand**
HAC 7th character B see Appendix B for HAC conditional logic

CC +7th **S62.326 Displaced fracture of shaft of fifth metacarpal bone, right hand**
HAC 7th character B see Appendix B for HAC conditional logic

CC +7th **S62.327 Displaced fracture of shaft of fifth metacarpal bone, left hand**
HAC 7th character B see Appendix B for HAC conditional logic

CC +7th **S62.328 Displaced fracture of shaft of other metacarpal bone**
Displaced fracture of shaft of specified metacarpal bone with unspecified laterality
HAC 7th character B see Appendix B for HAC conditional logic

CC +7th **S62.329 Displaced fracture of shaft of unspecified metacarpal bone**
HAC 7th character B see Appendix B for HAC conditional logic

\+ **S62.33 Displaced fracture of neck of other metacarpal bone**

CC +7th **S62.330 Displaced fracture of neck of second metacarpal bone, right hand**
HAC 7th character B see Appendix B for HAC conditional logic

CC +7th **S62.331 Displaced fracture of neck of second metacarpal bone, left hand**
HAC 7th character B see Appendix B for HAC conditional logic

CC +7th **S62.332 Displaced fracture of neck of third metacarpal bone, right hand**
HAC 7th character B see Appendix B for HAC conditional logic

CC +7th **S62.333 Displaced fracture of neck of third metacarpal bone, left hand**
HAC 7th character B see Appendix B for HAC conditional logic

CC +7th **S62.334 Displaced fracture of neck of fourth metacarpal bone, right hand**
HAC 7th character B see Appendix B for HAC conditional logic

CC +7th **S62.335 Displaced fracture of neck of fourth metacarpal bone, left hand**
HAC 7th character B see Appendix B for HAC conditional logic

CC +7th **S62.336 Displaced fracture of neck of fifth metacarpal bone, right hand**
HAC 7th character B see Appendix B for HAC conditional logic

CC +7th **S62.337 Displaced fracture of neck of fifth metacarpal bone, left hand**
HAC 7th character B see Appendix B for HAC conditional logic

CC +7th **S62.338 Displaced fracture of neck of other metacarpal bone**
Displaced fracture of neck of specified metacarpal bone with unspecified laterality
HAC 7th character B see Appendix B for HAC conditional logic

CC +7th **S62.339 Displaced fracture of neck of unspecified metacarpal bone**
HAC 7th character B see Appendix B for HAC conditional logic

+ **S62.34 Nondisplaced fracture of base of other metacarpal bone**

CC +7th **S62.340 Nondisplaced fracture of base of second metacarpal bone, right hand**
HAC 7th character B see Appendix B for HAC conditional logic

CC +7th **S62.341 Nondisplaced fracture of base of second metacarpal bone, left hand**
HAC 7th character B see Appendix B for HAC conditional logic

CC +7th **S62.342 Nondisplaced fracture of base of third metacarpal bone, right hand**
HAC 7th character B see Appendix B for HAC conditional logic

CC +7th **S62.343 Nondisplaced fracture of base of third metacarpal bone, left hand**
HAC 7th character B see Appendix B for HAC conditional logic

CC +7th **S62.344 Nondisplaced fracture of base of fourth metacarpal bone, right hand**
HAC 7th character B see Appendix B for HAC conditional logic

CC +7th **S62.345 Nondisplaced fracture of base of fourth metacarpal bone, left hand**
HAC 7th character B see Appendix B for HAC conditional logic

CC +7th **S62.346 Nondisplaced fracture of base of fifth metacarpal bone, right hand**
HAC 7th character B see Appendix B for HAC conditional logic

CC +7th **S62.347 Nondisplaced fracture of base of fifth metacarpal bone, left hand**
HAC 7th character B see Appendix B for HAC conditional logic

CC +7th **S62.348 Nondisplaced fracture of base of other metacarpal bone**
Nondisplaced fracture of base of specified metacarpal bone with unspecified laterality
HAC 7th character B see Appendix B for HAC conditional logic

CC +7th **S62.349 Nondisplaced fracture of base of unspecified metacarpal bone**
HAC 7th character B see Appendix B for HAC conditional logic

+ **S62.35 Nondisplaced fracture of shaft of other metacarpal bone**

CC +7th **S62.350 Nondisplaced fracture of shaft of second metacarpal bone, right hand**
HAC 7th character B see Appendix B for HAC conditional logic

CC +7th **S62.351 Nondisplaced fracture of shaft of second metacarpal bone, left hand**
HAC 7th character B see Appendix B for HAC conditional logic

CC +7th **S62.352 Nondisplaced fracture of shaft of third metacarpal bone, right hand**
HAC 7th character B see Appendix B for HAC conditional logic

CC +7th **S62.353 Nondisplaced fracture of shaft of third metacarpal bone, left hand**
HAC 7th character B see Appendix B for HAC conditional logic

CC +7th **S62.354 Nondisplaced fracture of shaft of fourth metacarpal bone, right hand**
HAC 7th character B see Appendix B for HAC conditional logic

CC +7th **S62.355 Nondisplaced fracture of shaft of fourth metacarpal bone, left hand**
HAC 7th character B see Appendix B for HAC conditional logic

CC +7th **S62.356 Nondisplaced fracture of shaft of fifth metacarpal bone, right hand**
HAC 7th character B see Appendix B for HAC conditional logic

CC +7th **S62.357 Nondisplaced fracture of shaft of fifth metacarpal bone, left hand**
HAC 7th character B see Appendix B for HAC conditional logic

CC +7th **S62.358 Nondisplaced fracture of shaft of other metacarpal bone**
Nondisplaced fracture of shaft of specified metacarpal bone with unspecified laterality
HAC 7th character B see Appendix B for HAC conditional logic

CC +7th **S62.359 Nondisplaced fracture of shaft of unspecified metacarpal bone**
HAC 7th character B see Appendix B for HAC conditional logic

+ **S62.36 Nondisplaced fracture of neck of other metacarpal bone**

CC +7th **S62.360 Nondisplaced fracture of neck of second metacarpal bone, right hand**
HAC 7th character B see Appendix B for HAC conditional logic

CC +7th **S62.361 Nondisplaced fracture of neck of second metacarpal bone, left hand**
HAC 7th character B see Appendix B for HAC conditional logic

CC +7th **S62.362 Nondisplaced fracture of neck of third metacarpal bone, right hand**
HAC 7th character B see Appendix B for HAC conditional logic

CC +7th **S62.363 Nondisplaced fracture of neck of third metacarpal bone, left hand**
HAC 7th character B see Appendix B for HAC conditional logic

CC +7th **S62.364 Nondisplaced fracture of neck of fourth metacarpal bone, right hand**
HAC 7th character B see Appendix B for HAC conditional logic

CC +7th **S62.365 Nondisplaced fracture of neck of fourth metacarpal bone, left hand**
HAC 7th character B see Appendix B for HAC conditional logic

CC +7th **S62.366 Nondisplaced fracture of neck of fifth metacarpal bone, right hand**
HAC 7th character B see Appendix B for HAC conditional logic

CC +7th **S62.367 Nondisplaced fracture of neck of fifth metacarpal bone, left hand**
HAC 7th character B see Appendix B for HAC conditional logic

CC +7th **S62.368 Nondisplaced fracture of neck of other metacarpal bone**
Nondisplaced fracture of neck of specified metacarpal bone with unspecified laterality
HAC 7th character B see Appendix B for HAC conditional logic

CC +7th **S62.369 Nondisplaced fracture of neck of unspecified metacarpal bone**
HAC 7th character B see Appendix B for HAC conditional logic

+ **S62.39 Other fracture of other metacarpal bone**

CC +7th **S62.390 Other fracture of second metacarpal bone, right hand**
HAC 7th character B see Appendix B for HAC conditional logic

CC +7th **S62.391 Other fracture of second metacarpal bone, left hand**
HAC 7th character B see Appendix B for HAC conditional logic

CC +7th **S62.392 Other fracture of third metacarpal bone, right hand**
HAC 7th character B see Appendix B for HAC conditional logic

CC +7th **S62.393 Other fracture of third metacarpal bone, left hand**
HAC 7th character B see Appendix B for HAC conditional logic

CC +7th **S62.394 Other fracture of fourth metacarpal bone, right hand**
HAC 7th character B see Appendix B for HAC conditional logic

CC +7th **S62.395 Other fracture of fourth metacarpal bone, left hand**
HAC 7th character B see Appendix B for HAC conditional logic

CC +7th **S62.396 Other fracture of fifth metacarpal bone, right hand**
HAC 7th character B see Appendix B for HAC conditional logic

CC +7th **S62.397 Other fracture of fifth metacarpal bone, left hand**
HAC 7th character B see Appendix B for HAC conditional logic

CC +7th **S62.398 Other fracture of other metacarpal bone**
Other fracture of specified metacarpal bone with unspecified laterality
HAC 7th character B see Appendix B for HAC conditional logic

CC +7th **S62.399 Other fracture of unspecified metacarpal bone**
HAC 7th character B see Appendix B for HAC conditional logic

+ S62.5 Fracture of thumb

+ S62.50 Fracture of unspecified phalanx of thumb

CC +7th **S62.501 Fracture of unspecified phalanx of right thumb**
HAC 7th character B see Appendix B for HAC conditional logic

CC +7th **S62.502 Fracture of unspecified phalanx of left thumb**
HAC 7th character B see Appendix B for HAC conditional logic

CC +7th **S62.509 Fracture of unspecified phalanx of unspecified thumb**
HAC 7th character B see Appendix B for HAC conditional logic

+ S62.51 Fracture of proximal phalanx of thumb

CC +7th **S62.511 Displaced fracture of proximal phalanx of right thumb**
HAC 7th character B see Appendix B for HAC conditional logic

CC +7th **S62.512 Displaced fracture of proximal phalanx of left thumb**
HAC 7th character B see Appendix B for HAC conditional logic

CC +7th **S62.513 Displaced fracture of proximal phalanx of unspecified thumb**
HAC 7th character B see Appendix B for HAC conditional logic

CC +7th **S62.514 Nondisplaced fracture of proximal phalanx of right thumb**
HAC 7th character B see Appendix B for HAC conditional logic

CC +7th **S62.515 Nondisplaced fracture of proximal phalanx of left thumb**
HAC 7th character B see Appendix B for HAC conditional logic

CC +7th **S62.516 Nondisplaced fracture of proximal phalanx of unspecified thumb**
HAC 7th character B see Appendix B for HAC conditional logic

+ S62.52 Fracture of distal phalanx of thumb

CC +7th **S62.521 Displaced fracture of distal phalanx of right thumb**
HAC 7th character B see Appendix B for HAC conditional logic

CC +7th **S62.522 Displaced fracture of distal phalanx of left thumb**
HAC 7th character B see Appendix B for HAC conditional logic

CC +7th **S62.523 Displaced fracture of distal phalanx of unspecified thumb**
HAC 7th character B see Appendix B for HAC conditional logic

CC +7th **S62.524 Nondisplaced fracture of distal phalanx of right thumb**
HAC 7th character B see Appendix B for HAC conditional logic

CC +7th **S62.525 Nondisplaced fracture of distal phalanx of left thumb**
HAC 7th character B see Appendix B for HAC conditional logic

CC +7th **S62.526 Nondisplaced fracture of distal phalanx of unspecified thumb**
HAC 7th character B see Appendix B for HAC conditional logic

+ S62.6 Fracture of other and unspecified finger(s)
Excludes2: *fracture of thumb (S62.5-)*

+ S62.60 Fracture of unspecified phalanx of finger

CC +7th **S62.600 Fracture of unspecified phalanx of right index finger**
HAC 7th character B see Appendix B for HAC conditional logic

CC +7th **S62.601 Fracture of unspecified phalanx of left index finger**
HAC 7th character B see Appendix B for HAC conditional logic

CC +7th **S62.602 Fracture of unspecified phalanx of right middle finger**
HAC 7th character B see Appendix B for HAC conditional logic

CC +7th **S62.603 Fracture of unspecified phalanx of left middle finger**
HAC 7th character B see Appendix B for HAC conditional logic

CC +7th **S62.604 Fracture of unspecified phalanx of right ring finger**
HAC 7th character B see Appendix B for HAC conditional logic

CC +7th **S62.605 Fracture of unspecified phalanx of left ring finger**
HAC 7th character B see Appendix B for HAC conditional logic

CC +7th **S62.606 Fracture of unspecified phalanx of right little finger**
HAC 7th character B see Appendix B for HAC conditional logic

CC +7th **S62.607 Fracture of unspecified phalanx of left little finger**
HAC 7th character B see Appendix B for HAC conditional logic

CC +7th **S62.608 Fracture of unspecified phalanx of other finger**
Fracture of unspecified phalanx of specified finger with unspecified laterality
HAC 7th character B see Appendix B for HAC conditional logic

CC +7th **S62.609 Fracture of unspecified phalanx of unspecified finger**
HAC 7th character B see Appendix B for HAC conditional logic

+ S62.61 Displaced fracture of proximal phalanx of finger

CC +7th **S62.610 Displaced fracture of proximal phalanx of right index finger**
HAC 7th character B see Appendix B for HAC conditional logic

CC +7th **S62.611 Displaced fracture of proximal phalanx of left index finger**
HAC 7th character B see Appendix B for HAC conditional logic

CC +7th **S62.612 Displaced fracture of proximal phalanx of right middle finger**
HAC 7th character B see Appendix B for HAC conditional logic

CC +7th **S62.613 Displaced fracture of proximal phalanx of left middle finger**
HAC 7th character B see Appendix B for HAC conditional logic

CC +7th **S62.614 Displaced fracture of proximal phalanx of right ring finger**
HAC 7th character B see Appendix B for HAC conditional logic

CC +7th **S62.615 Displaced fracture of proximal phalanx of left ring finger**
HAC 7th character B see Appendix B for HAC conditional logic

CC +7th **S62.616 Displaced fracture of proximal phalanx of right little finger**
HAC 7th character B see Appendix B for HAC conditional logic

CC +7th **S62.617 Displaced fracture of proximal phalanx of left little finger**
HAC 7th character B see Appendix B for HAC conditional logic

CC +7th **S62.618 Displaced fracture of proximal phalanx of other finger**
Displaced fracture of proximal phalanx of specified finger with unspecified laterality
HAC 7th character B see Appendix B for HAC conditional logic

CC +7th **S62.619 Displaced fracture of proximal phalanx of unspecified finger**
HAC 7th character B see Appendix B for HAC conditional logic

+ S62.62 Displaced fracture of middle phalanx of finger

CC +7th **S62.620 Displaced fracture of middle phalanx of right index finger**
HAC 7th character B see Appendix B for HAC conditional logic

CC +7th **S62.621** **Displaced fracture of middle phalanx of left index finger**
HAC 7th character B see Appendix B for HAC conditional logic

CC +7th **S62.622** **Displaced fracture of middle phalanx of right middle finger**
HAC 7th character B see Appendix B for HAC conditional logic

CC +7th **S62.623** **Displaced fracture of middle phalanx of left middle finger**
HAC 7th character B see Appendix B for HAC conditional logic

CC +7th **S62.624** **Displaced fracture of middle phalanx of right ring finger**
HAC 7th character B see Appendix B for HAC conditional logic

CC +7th **S62.625** **Displaced fracture of middle phalanx of left ring finger**
HAC 7th character B see Appendix B for HAC conditional logic

CC +7th **S62.626** **Displaced fracture of middle phalanx of right little finger**
HAC 7th character B see Appendix B for HAC conditional logic

CC +7th **S62.627** **Displaced fracture of middle phalanx of left little finger**
HAC 7th character B see Appendix B for HAC conditional logic

CC +7th **S62.628** **Displaced fracture of middle phalanx of other finger**
Displaced fracture of middle phalanx of specified finger with unspecified laterality
HAC 7th character B see Appendix B for HAC conditional logic

CC +7th **S62.629** **Displaced fracture of middle phalanx of unspecified finger**
HAC 7th character B see Appendix B for HAC conditional logic

\+ **S62.63** **Displaced fracture of distal phalanx of finger**

CC +7th **S62.630** **Displaced fracture of distal phalanx of right index finger**
HAC 7th character B see Appendix B for HAC conditional logic

CC +7th **S62.631** **Displaced fracture of distal phalanx of left index finger**
HAC 7th character B see Appendix B for HAC conditional logic

CC +7th **S62.632** **Displaced fracture of distal phalanx of right middle finger**
HAC 7th character B see Appendix B for HAC conditional logic

CC +7th **S62.633** **Displaced fracture of distal phalanx of left middle finger**
HAC 7th character B see Appendix B for HAC conditional logic

CC +7th **S62.634** **Displaced fracture of distal phalanx of right ring finger**
HAC 7th character B see Appendix B for HAC conditional logic

CC +7th **S62.635** **Displaced fracture of distal phalanx of left ring finger**
HAC 7th character B see Appendix B for HAC conditional logic

CC +7th **S62.636** **Displaced fracture of distal phalanx of right little finger**
HAC 7th character B see Appendix B for HAC conditional logic

CC +7th **S62.637** **Displaced fracture of distal phalanx of left little finger**
HAC 7th character B see Appendix B for HAC conditional logic

CC +7th **S62.638** **Displaced fracture of distal phalanx of other finger**
Displaced fracture of distal phalanx of specified finger with unspecified laterality
HAC 7th character B see Appendix B for HAC conditional logic

CC +7th **S62.639** **Displaced fracture of distal phalanx of unspecified finger**
HAC 7th character B see Appendix B for HAC conditional logic

\+ **S62.64** **Nondisplaced fracture of proximal phalanx of finger**

CC +7th **S62.640** **Nondisplaced fracture of proximal phalanx of right index finger**
HAC 7th character B see Appendix B for HAC conditional logic

CC +7th **S62.641** **Nondisplaced fracture of proximal phalanx of left index finger**
HAC 7th character B see Appendix B for HAC conditional logic

CC +7th **S62.642** **Nondisplaced fracture of proximal phalanx of right middle finger**
HAC 7th character B see Appendix B for HAC conditional logic

CC +7th **S62.643** **Nondisplaced fracture of proximal phalanx of left middle finger**
HAC 7th character B see Appendix B for HAC conditional logic

CC +7th **S62.644** **Nondisplaced fracture of proximal phalanx of right ring finger**
HAC 7th character B see Appendix B for HAC conditional logic

CC +7th **S62.645** **Nondisplaced fracture of proximal phalanx of left ring finger**
HAC 7th character B see Appendix B for HAC conditional logic

CC +7th **S62.646** **Nondisplaced fracture of proximal phalanx of right little finger**
HAC 7th character B see Appendix B for HAC conditional logic

CC +7th **S62.647** **Nondisplaced fracture of proximal phalanx of left little finger**
HAC 7th character B see Appendix B for HAC conditional logic

CC +7th **S62.648** **Nondisplaced fracture of proximal phalanx of other finger**
Nondisplaced fracture of proximal phalanx of specified finger with unspecified laterality
HAC 7th character B see Appendix B for HAC conditional logic

CC +7th **S62.649** **Nondisplaced fracture of proximal phalanx of unspecified finger**
HAC 7th character B see Appendix B for HAC conditional logic

\+ **S62.65** **Nondisplaced fracture of middle phalanx of finger**

CC +7th **S62.650** **Nondisplaced fracture of middle phalanx of right index finger**
HAC 7th character B see Appendix B for HAC conditional logic

CC +7th **S62.651** **Nondisplaced fracture of middle phalanx of left index finger**
HAC 7th character B see Appendix B for HAC conditional logic

CC +7th **S62.652** **Nondisplaced fracture of middle phalanx of right middle finger**
HAC 7th character B see Appendix B for HAC conditional logic

CC +7th **S62.653** **Nondisplaced fracture of middle phalanx of left middle finger**
HAC 7th character B see Appendix B for HAC conditional logic

CC +7th **S62.654** **Nondisplaced fracture of middle phalanx of right ring finger**
HAC 7th character B see Appendix B for HAC conditional logic

CC +7th **S62.655** **Nondisplaced fracture of middle phalanx of left ring finger**
HAC 7th character B see Appendix B for HAC conditional logic

CC +7th **S62.656** **Nondisplaced fracture of middle phalanx of right little finger**
HAC 7th character B see Appendix B for HAC conditional logic

CC +7th **S62.657** **Nondisplaced fracture of middle phalanx of left little finger**
HAC 7th character B see Appendix B for HAC conditional logic

CC +7th **S62.658 Nondisplaced fracture of middle phalanx of other finger**
Nondisplaced fracture of middle phalanx of specified finger with unspecified laterality
HAC 7th character B see Appendix B for HAC conditional logic

CC +7th **S62.659 Nondisplaced fracture of middle phalanx of unspecified finger**
HAC 7th character B see Appendix B for HAC conditional logic

+ **S62.66 Nondisplaced fracture of distal phalanx of finger**

CC +7th **S62.660 Nondisplaced fracture of distal phalanx of right index finger**
HAC 7th character B see Appendix B for HAC conditional logic

CC +7th **S62.661 Nondisplaced fracture of distal phalanx of left index finger**
HAC 7th character B see Appendix B for HAC conditional logic

CC +7th **S62.662 Nondisplaced fracture of distal phalanx of right middle finger**
HAC 7th character B see Appendix B for HAC conditional logic

CC +7th **S62.663 Nondisplaced fracture of distal phalanx of left middle finger**
HAC 7th character B see Appendix B for HAC conditional logic

CC +7th **S62.664 Nondisplaced fracture of distal phalanx of right ring finger**
HAC 7th character B see Appendix B for HAC conditional logic

CC +7th **S62.665 Nondisplaced fracture of distal phalanx of left ring finger**
HAC 7th character B see Appendix B for HAC conditional logic

CC +7th **S62.666 Nondisplaced fracture of distal phalanx of right little finger**
HAC 7th character B see Appendix B for HAC conditional logic

CC +7th **S62.667 Nondisplaced fracture of distal phalanx of left little finger**
HAC 7th character B see Appendix B for HAC conditional logic

CC +7th **S62.668 Nondisplaced fracture of distal phalanx of other finger**
Nondisplaced fracture of distal phalanx of specified finger with unspecified laterality
HAC 7th character B see Appendix B for HAC conditional logic

CC +7th **S62.669 Nondisplaced fracture of distal phalanx of unspecified finger**
HAC 7th character B see Appendix B for HAC conditional logic

+ **S62.9 Unspecified fracture of wrist and hand**

CC X+7th **S62.90 Unspecified fracture of unspecified wrist and hand**
HAC 7th character B see Appendix B for HAC conditional logic

CC X+7th **S62.91 Unspecified fracture of right wrist and hand**
HAC 7th character B see Appendix B for HAC conditional logic

CC X+7th **S62.92 Unspecified fracture of left wrist and hand**
HAC 7th character B see Appendix B for HAC conditional logic

S63 Dislocation and sprain of joints and ligaments at wrist and hand level

Includes: avulsion of joint or ligament at wrist and hand level
laceration of cartilage, joint or ligament at wrist and hand level
sprain of cartilage, joint or ligament at wrist and hand level
traumatic hemarthrosis of joint or ligament at wrist and hand level
traumatic rupture of joint or ligament at wrist and hand level
traumatic subluxation of joint or ligament at wrist and hand level
traumatic tear of joint or ligament at wrist and hand level

Code also any associated open wound

Excludes2: *strain of muscle, fascia and tendon of wrist and hand (S66.-)*

The appropriate 7th character is to be added to each code from category S63
A initial encounter
D subsequent encounter
S sequela

+ **S63.0 Subluxation and dislocation of wrist and hand joints**

+ **S63.00 Unspecified subluxation and dislocation of wrist and hand**
Dislocation of carpal bone NOS
Dislocation of distal end of radius NOS
Subluxation of carpal bone NOS
Subluxation of distal end of radius NOS

+7th **S63.001 Unspecified subluxation of right wrist and hand**

+7th **S63.002 Unspecified subluxation of left wrist and hand**

+7th **S63.003 Unspecified subluxation of unspecified wrist and hand**

+7th **S63.004 Unspecified dislocation of right wrist and hand**

+7th **S63.005 Unspecified dislocation of left wrist and hand**

+7th **S63.006 Unspecified dislocation of unspecified wrist and hand**

+ **S63.01 Subluxation and dislocation of distal radioulnar joint**

+7th **S63.011 Subluxation of distal radioulnar joint of right wrist**

+7th **S63.012 Subluxation of distal radioulnar joint of left wrist**

+7th **S63.013 Subluxation of distal radioulnar joint of unspecified wrist**

+7th **S63.014 Dislocation of distal radioulnar joint of right wrist**

+7th **S63.015 Dislocation of distal radioulnar joint of left wrist**

+7th **S63.016 Dislocation of distal radioulnar joint of unspecified wrist**

+ **S63.02 Subluxation and dislocation of radiocarpal joint**

+7th **S63.021 Subluxation of radiocarpal joint of right wrist**

+7th **S63.022 Subluxation of radiocarpal joint of left wrist**

+7th **S63.023 Subluxation of radiocarpal joint of unspecified wrist**

+7th **S63.024 Dislocation of radiocarpal joint of right wrist**

+7th **S63.025 Dislocation of radiocarpal joint of left wrist**

+7th **S63.026 Dislocation of radiocarpal joint of unspecified wrist**

+ **S63.03 Subluxation and dislocation of midcarpal joint**

+7th **S63.031 Subluxation of midcarpal joint of right wrist**

+7th **S63.032 Subluxation of midcarpal joint of left wrist**

+7th **S63.033 Subluxation of midcarpal joint of unspecified wrist**

+7th **S63.034 Dislocation of midcarpal joint of right wrist**

+7th **S63.035 Dislocation of midcarpal joint of left wrist**

+7th **S63.036 Dislocation of midcarpal joint of unspecified wrist**

+ **S63.04 Subluxation and dislocation of carpometacarpal joint of thumb**

Excludes2: *interphalangeal subluxation and dislocation of thumb (S63.1-)*

+7th **S63.041 Subluxation of carpometacarpal joint of right thumb**

+7th **S63.042 Subluxation of carpometacarpal joint of left thumb**

+7th **S63.043 Subluxation of carpometacarpal joint of unspecified thumb**

+7th **S63.044 Dislocation of carpometacarpal joint of right thumb**

+7th **S63.045 Dislocation of carpometacarpal joint of left thumb**

+7th **S63.046 Dislocation of carpometacarpal joint of unspecified thumb**

+ **S63.05 Subluxation and dislocation of other carpometacarpal joint**

Excludes2: *subluxation and dislocation of carpometacarpal joint of thumb (S63.04-)*

+7th **S63.051 Subluxation of other carpometacarpal joint of right hand**

+7th **S63.052** **Subluxation of other carpometacarpal joint of left hand**
+7th **S63.053** **Subluxation of other carpometacarpal joint of unspecified hand**
+7th **S63.054** **Dislocation of other carpometacarpal joint of right hand**
+7th **S63.055** **Dislocation of other carpometacarpal joint of left hand**
+7th **S63.056** **Dislocation of other carpometacarpal joint of unspecified hand**

\+ **S63.06** **Subluxation and dislocation of metacarpal (bone), proximal end**
+7th **S63.061** **Subluxation of metacarpal (bone), proximal end of right hand**
+7th **S63.062** **Subluxation of metacarpal (bone), proximal end of left hand**
+7th **S63.063** **Subluxation of metacarpal (bone), proximal end of unspecified hand**
+7th **S63.064** **Dislocation of metacarpal (bone), proximal end of right hand**
+7th **S63.065** **Dislocation of metacarpal (bone), proximal end of left hand**
+7th **S63.066** **Dislocation of metacarpal (bone), proximal end of unspecified hand**

\+ **S63.07** **Subluxation and dislocation of distal end of ulna**
+7th **S63.071** **Subluxation of distal end of right ulna**
+7th **S63.072** **Subluxation of distal end of left ulna**
+7th **S63.073** **Subluxation of distal end of unspecified ulna**
+7th **S63.074** **Dislocation of distal end of right ulna**
+7th **S63.075** **Dislocation of distal end of left ulna**
+7th **S63.076** **Dislocation of distal end of unspecified ulna**

\+ **S63.09** **Other subluxation and dislocation of wrist and hand**
+7th **S63.091** **Other subluxation of right wrist and hand**
+7th **S63.092** **Other subluxation of left wrist and hand**
+7th **S63.093** **Other subluxation of unspecified wrist and hand**
+7th **S63.094** **Other dislocation of right wrist and hand**
+7th **S63.095** **Other dislocation of left wrist and hand**
+7th **S63.096** **Other dislocation of unspecified wrist and hand**

\+ **S63.1** **Subluxation and dislocation of thumb**

\+ **S63.10** **Unspecified subluxation and dislocation of thumb**
+7th **S63.101** **Unspecified subluxation of right thumb**
+7th **S63.102** **Unspecified subluxation of left thumb**
+7th **S63.103** **Unspecified subluxation of unspecified thumb**
+7th **S63.104** **Unspecified dislocation of right thumb**
+7th **S63.105** **Unspecified dislocation of left thumb**
+7th **S63.106** **Unspecified dislocation of unspecified thumb**

\+ **S63.11** **Subluxation and dislocation of metacarpophalangeal joint of thumb**
+7th **S63.111** **Subluxation of metacarpophalangeal joint of right thumb**
+7th **S63.112** **Subluxation of metacarpophalangeal joint of left thumb**
+7th **S63.113** **Subluxation of metacarpophalangeal joint of unspecified thumb**
+7th **S63.114** **Dislocation of metacarpophalangeal joint of right thumb**
+7th **S63.115** **Dislocation of metacarpophalangeal joint of left thumb**
+7th **S63.116** **Dislocation of metacarpophalangeal joint of unspecified thumb**

\+ **S63.12** **Subluxation and dislocation of interphalangeal joint of thumb**
+7th **S63.121** **Subluxation of interphalangeal joint of right thumb**
+7th **S63.122** **Subluxation of interphalangeal joint of left thumb**
+7th **S63.123** **Subluxation of interphalangeal joint of unspecified thumb**
+7th **S63.124** **Dislocation of interphalangeal joint of right thumb**
+7th **S63.125** **Dislocation of interphalangeal joint of left thumb**
+7th **S63.126** **Dislocation of interphalangeal joint of unspecified thumb**

\+ **S63.2** **Subluxation and dislocation of other finger(s)**
Excludes2: *subluxation and dislocation of thumb (S63.1-)*

\+ **S63.20** **Unspecified subluxation of other finger**
+7th **S63.200** **Unspecified subluxation of right index finger**
+7th **S63.201** **Unspecified subluxation of left index finger**
+7th **S63.202** **Unspecified subluxation of right middle finger**
+7th **S63.203** **Unspecified subluxation of left middle finger**
+7th **S63.204** **Unspecified subluxation of right ring finger**
+7th **S63.205** **Unspecified subluxation of left ring finger**
+7th **S63.206** **Unspecified subluxation of right little finger**
+7th **S63.207** **Unspecified subluxation of left little finger**
+7th **S63.208** **Unspecified subluxation of other finger**
Unspecified subluxation of specified finger with unspecified laterality
+7th **S63.209** **Unspecified subluxation of unspecified finger**

\+ **S63.21** **Subluxation of metacarpophalangeal joint of finger**
+7th **S63.210** **Subluxation of metacarpophalangeal joint of right index finger**
+7th **S63.211** **Subluxation of metacarpophalangeal joint of left index finger**
+7th **S63.212** **Subluxation of metacarpophalangeal joint of right middle finger**
+7th **S63.213** **Subluxation of metacarpophalangeal joint of left middle finger**
+7th **S63.214** **Subluxation of metacarpophalangeal joint of right ring finger**
+7th **S63.215** **Subluxation of metacarpophalangeal joint of left ring finger**
+7th **S63.216** **Subluxation of metacarpophalangeal joint of right little finger**
+7th **S63.217** **Subluxation of metacarpophalangeal joint of left little finger**
+7th **S63.218** **Subluxation of metacarpophalangeal joint of other finger**
Subluxation of metacarpophalangeal joint of specified finger with unspecified laterality
+7th **S63.219** **Subluxation of metacarpophalangeal joint of unspecified finger**

\+ **S63.22** **Subluxation of unspecified interphalangeal joint of finger**
+7th **S63.220** **Subluxation of unspecified interphalangeal joint of right index finger**
+7th **S63.221** **Subluxation of unspecified interphalangeal joint of left index finger**
+7th **S63.222** **Subluxation of unspecified interphalangeal joint of right middle finger**
+7th **S63.223** **Subluxation of unspecified interphalangeal joint of left middle finger**
+7th **S63.224** **Subluxation of unspecified interphalangeal joint of right ring finger**
+7th **S63.225** **Subluxation of unspecified interphalangeal joint of left ring finger**
+7th **S63.226** **Subluxation of unspecified interphalangeal joint of right little finger**
+7th **S63.227** **Subluxation of unspecified interphalangeal joint of left little finger**
+7th **S63.228** **Subluxation of unspecified interphalangeal joint of other finger**
Subluxation of unspecified interphalangeal joint of specified finger with unspecified laterality
+7th **S63.229** **Subluxation of unspecified interphalangeal joint of unspecified finger**

+ S63.23 Subluxation of proximal interphalangeal joint of finger

+7th S63.230 Subluxation of proximal interphalangeal joint of right index finger

+7th S63.231 Subluxation of proximal interphalangeal joint of left index finger

+7th S63.232 Subluxation of proximal interphalangeal joint of right middle finger

+7th S63.233 Subluxation of proximal interphalangeal joint of left middle finger

+7th S63.234 Subluxation of proximal interphalangeal joint of right ring finger

+7th S63.235 Subluxation of proximal interphalangeal joint of left ring finger

+7th S63.236 Subluxation of proximal interphalangeal joint of right little finger

+7th S63.237 Subluxation of proximal interphalangeal joint of left little finger

+7th S63.238 Subluxation of proximal interphalangeal joint of other finger

Subluxation of proximal interphalangeal joint of specified finger with unspecified laterality

+7th S63.239 Subluxation of proximal interphalangeal joint of unspecified finger

+ S63.24 Subluxation of distal interphalangeal joint of finger

+7th S63.240 Subluxation of distal interphalangeal joint of right index finger

+7th S63.241 Subluxation of distal interphalangeal joint of left index finger

+7th S63.242 Subluxation of distal interphalangeal joint of right middle finger

+7th S63.243 Subluxation of distal interphalangeal joint of left middle finger

+7th S63.244 Subluxation of distal interphalangeal joint of right ring finger

+7th S63.245 Subluxation of distal interphalangeal joint of left ring finger

+7th S63.246 Subluxation of distal interphalangeal joint of right little finger

+7th S63.247 Subluxation of distal interphalangeal joint of left little finger

+7th S63.248 Subluxation of distal interphalangeal joint of other finger

Subluxation of distal interphalangeal joint of specified finger with unspecified laterality

+7th S63.249 Subluxation of distal interphalangeal joint of unspecified finger

+ S63.25 Unspecified dislocation of other finger

+7th S63.250 Unspecified dislocation of right index finger

+7th S63.251 Unspecified dislocation of left index finger

+7th S63.252 Unspecified dislocation of right middle finger

+7th S63.253 Unspecified dislocation of left middle finger

+7th S63.254 Unspecified dislocation of right ring finger

+7th S63.255 Unspecified dislocation of left ring finger

+7th S63.256 Unspecified dislocation of right little finger

+7th S63.257 Unspecified dislocation of left little finger

+7th S63.258 Unspecified dislocation of other finger

Unspecified dislocation of specified finger with unspecified laterality

+7th S63.259 Unspecified dislocation of unspecified finger

Unspecified dislocation of unspecified finger with unspecified laterality

+ S63.26 Dislocation of metacarpophalangeal joint of finger

+7th S63.260 Dislocation of metacarpophalangeal joint of right index finger

+7th S63.261 Dislocation of metacarpophalangeal joint of left index finger

+7th S63.262 Dislocation of metacarpophalangeal joint of right middle finger

+7th S63.263 Dislocation of metacarpophalangeal joint of left middle finger

+7th S63.264 Dislocation of metacarpophalangeal joint of right ring finger

+7th S63.265 Dislocation of metacarpophalangeal joint of left ring finger

+7th S63.266 Dislocation of metacarpophalangeal joint of right little finger

+7th S63.267 Dislocation of metacarpophalangeal joint of left little finger

+7th S63.268 Dislocation of metacarpophalangeal joint of other finger

Dislocation of metacarpophalangeal joint of specified finger with unspecified laterality

+7th S63.269 Dislocation of metacarpophalangeal joint of unspecified finger

+ S63.27 Dislocation of unspecified interphalangeal joint of finger

+7th S63.270 Dislocation of unspecified interphalangeal joint of right index finger

+7th S63.271 Dislocation of unspecified interphalangeal joint of left index finger

+7th S63.272 Dislocation of unspecified interphalangeal joint of right middle finger

+7th S63.273 Dislocation of unspecified interphalangeal joint of left middle finger

+7th S63.274 Dislocation of unspecified interphalangeal joint of right ring finger

+7th S63.275 Dislocation of unspecified interphalangeal joint of left ring finger

+7th S63.276 Dislocation of unspecified interphalangeal joint of right little finger

+7th S63.277 Dislocation of unspecified interphalangeal joint of left little finger

+7th S63.278 Dislocation of unspecified interphalangeal joint of other finger

Dislocation of unspecified interphalangeal joint of specified finger with unspecified laterality

+7th S63.279 Dislocation of unspecified interphalangeal joint of unspecified finger

Dislocation of unspecified interphalangeal joint of unspecified finger without specified laterality

+ S63.28 Dislocation of proximal interphalangeal joint of finger

+7th S63.280 Dislocation of proximal interphalangeal joint of right index finger

+7th S63.281 Dislocation of proximal interphalangeal joint of left index finger

+7th S63.282 Dislocation of proximal interphalangeal joint of right middle finger

+7th S63.283 Dislocation of proximal interphalangeal joint of left middle finger

+7th S63.284 Dislocation of proximal interphalangeal joint of right ring finger

+7th S63.285 Dislocation of proximal interphalangeal joint of left ring finger

+7th S63.286 Dislocation of proximal interphalangeal joint of right little finger

+7th S63.287 Dislocation of proximal interphalangeal joint of left little finger

+7th S63.288 Dislocation of proximal interphalangeal joint of other finger

Dislocation of proximal interphalangeal joint of specified finger with unspecified laterality

+7th S63.289 Dislocation of proximal interphalangeal joint of unspecified finger

+ S63.29 Dislocation of distal interphalangeal joint of finger
- **+7th S63.290 Dislocation of distal interphalangeal joint of right index finger**
- **+7th S63.291 Dislocation of distal interphalangeal joint of left index finger**
- **+7th S63.292 Dislocation of distal interphalangeal joint of right middle finger**
- **+7th S63.293 Dislocation of distal interphalangeal joint of left middle finger**
- **+7th S63.294 Dislocation of distal interphalangeal joint of right ring finger**
- **+7th S63.295 Dislocation of distal interphalangeal joint of left ring finger**
- **+7th S63.296 Dislocation of distal interphalangeal joint of right little finger**
- **+7th S63.297 Dislocation of distal interphalangeal joint of left little finger**
- **+7th S63.298 Dislocation of distal interphalangeal joint of other finger**
  Dislocation of distal interphalangeal joint of specified finger with unspecified laterality
- **+7th S63.299 Dislocation of distal interphalangeal joint of unspecified finger**

+ S63.3 Traumatic rupture of ligament of wrist

+ S63.30 Traumatic rupture of unspecified ligament of wrist
- **+7th S63.301 Traumatic rupture of unspecified ligament of right wrist**
- **+7th S63.302 Traumatic rupture of unspecified ligament of left wrist**
- **+7th S63.309 Traumatic rupture of unspecified ligament of unspecified wrist**

+ S63.31 Traumatic rupture of collateral ligament of wrist
- **+7th S63.311 Traumatic rupture of collateral ligament of right wrist**
- **+7th S63.312 Traumatic rupture of collateral ligament of left wrist**
- **+7th S63.319 Traumatic rupture of collateral ligament of unspecified wrist**

+ S63.32 Traumatic rupture of radiocarpal ligament
- **+7th S63.321 Traumatic rupture of right radiocarpal ligament**
- **+7th S63.322 Traumatic rupture of left radiocarpal ligament**
- **+7th S63.329 Traumatic rupture of unspecified radiocarpal ligament**

+ S63.33 Traumatic rupture of ulnocarpal (palmar) ligament
- **+7th S63.331 Traumatic rupture of right ulnocarpal (palmar) ligament**
- **+7th S63.332 Traumatic rupture of left ulnocarpal (palmar) ligament**
- **+7th S63.339 Traumatic rupture of unspecified ulnocarpal (palmar) ligament**

+ S63.39 Traumatic rupture of other ligament of wrist
- **+7th S63.391 Traumatic rupture of other ligament of right wrist**
- **+7th S63.392 Traumatic rupture of other ligament of left wrist**
- **+7th S63.399 Traumatic rupture of other ligament of unspecified wrist**

+ S63.4 Traumatic rupture of ligament of finger at metacarpophalangeal and interphalangeal joint(s)

+ S63.40 Traumatic rupture of unspecified ligament of finger at metacarpophalangeal and interphalangeal joint
- **+7th S63.400 Traumatic rupture of unspecified ligament of right index finger at metacarpophalangeal and interphalangeal joint**
- **+7th S63.401 Traumatic rupture of unspecified ligament of left index finger at metacarpophalangeal and interphalangeal joint**
- **+7th S63.402 Traumatic rupture of unspecified ligament of right middle finger at metacarpophalangeal and interphalangeal joint**
- **+7th S63.403 Traumatic rupture of unspecified ligament of left middle finger at metacarpophalangeal and interphalangeal joint**
- **+7th S63.404 Traumatic rupture of unspecified ligament of right ring finger at metacarpophalangeal and interphalangeal joint**
- **+7th S63.405 Traumatic rupture of unspecified ligament of left ring finger at metacarpophalangeal and interphalangeal joint**
- **+7th S63.406 Traumatic rupture of unspecified ligament of right little finger at metacarpophalangeal and interphalangeal joint**
- **+7th S63.407 Traumatic rupture of unspecified ligament of left little finger at metacarpophalangeal and interphalangeal joint**
- **+7th S63.408 Traumatic rupture of unspecified ligament of other finger at metacarpophalangeal and interphalangeal joint**
  Traumatic rupture of unspecified ligament of specified finger with unspecified laterality at metacarpophalangeal and interphalangeal joint
- **+7th S63.409 Traumatic rupture of unspecified ligament of unspecified finger at metacarpophalangeal and interphalangeal joint**

+ S63.41 Traumatic rupture of collateral ligament of finger at metacarpophalangeal and interphalangeal joint
- **+7th S63.410 Traumatic rupture of collateral ligament of right index finger at metacarpophalangeal and interphalangeal joint**
- **+7th S63.411 Traumatic rupture of collateral ligament of left index finger at metacarpophalangeal and interphalangeal joint**
- **+7th S63.412 Traumatic rupture of collateral ligament of right middle finger at metacarpophalangeal and interphalangeal joint**
- **+7th S63.413 Traumatic rupture of collateral ligament of left middle finger at metacarpophalangeal and interphalangeal joint**
- **+7th S63.414 Traumatic rupture of collateral ligament of right ring finger at metacarpophalangeal and interphalangeal joint**
- **+7th S63.415 Traumatic rupture of collateral ligament of left ring finger at metacarpophalangeal and interphalangeal joint**
- **+7th S63.416 Traumatic rupture of collateral ligament of right little finger at metacarpophalangeal and interphalangeal joint**
- **+7th S63.417 Traumatic rupture of collateral ligament of left little finger at metacarpophalangeal and interphalangeal joint**
- **+7th S63.418 Traumatic rupture of collateral ligament of other finger at metacarpophalangeal and interphalangeal joint**
  Traumatic rupture of collateral ligament of specified finger with unspecified laterality at metacarpophalangeal and interphalangeal joint
- **+7th S63.419 Traumatic rupture of collateral ligament of unspecified finger at metacarpophalangeal and interphalangeal joint**

+ **S63.42 Traumatic rupture of palmar ligament of finger at metacarpophalangeal and interphalangeal joint**
  - +7th **S63.420 Traumatic rupture of palmarligament of right index finger at metacarpophalangeal and interphalangeal joint**
  - +7th **S63.421 Traumatic rupture of palmar ligament of left index finger at metacarpophalangeal and interphalangeal joint**
  - +7th **S63.422 Traumatic rupture of palmar ligament of right middle finger at metacarpophalangeal and interphalangeal joint**
  - +7th **S63.423 Traumatic rupture of palmar ligament of left middle finger at metacarpophalangeal and interphalangeal joint**
  - +7th **S63.424 Traumatic rupture of palmar ligament of right ring finger at metacarpophalangeal and interphalangeal joint**
  - +7th **S63.425 Traumatic rupture of palmar ligament of left ring finger at metacarpophalangeal and interphalangeal joint**
  - +7th **S63.426 Traumatic rupture of palmar ligament of right little finger at metacarpophalangeal and interphalangeal joint**
  - +7th **S63.427 Traumatic rupture of palmar ligament of left little finger at metacarpophalangeal and interphalangeal joint**
  - +7th **S63.428 Traumatic rupture of palmar ligament of other finger at metacarpophalangeal and interphalangeal joint**
    Traumatic rupture of palmar ligament of specified finger with unspecified laterality at metacarpophalangeal and interphalangeal joint
  - +7th **S63.429 Traumatic rupture of palmar ligament of unspecified finger at metacarpophalangeal and interphalangeal joint**

+ **S63.43 Traumatic rupture of volar plate of finger at metacarpophalangeal and interphalangeal joint**
  - +7th **S63.430 Traumatic rupture of volar plate of right index finger at metacarpophalangeal and interphalangeal joint**
  - +7th **S63.431 Traumatic rupture of volar plate of left index finger at metacarpophalangeal and interphalangeal joint**
  - +7th **S63.432 Traumatic rupture of volar plate of right middle finger at metacarpophalangeal and interphalangeal joint**
  - +7th **S63.433 Traumatic rupture of volar plate of left middle finger at metacarpophalangeal and interphalangeal joint**
  - +7th **S63.434 Traumatic rupture of volar plate of right ring finger at metacarpophalangeal and interphalangeal joint**
  - +7th **S63.435 Traumatic rupture of volar plate of left ring finger at metacarpophalangeal and interphalangeal joint**
  - +7th **S63.436 Traumatic rupture of volar plate of right little finger at metacarpophalangeal and interphalangeal joint**
  - +7th **S63.437 Traumatic rupture of volar plate of left little finger at metacarpophalangeal and interphalangeal joint**
  - +7th **S63.438 Traumatic rupture of volar plate of other finger at metacarpophalangeal and interphalangeal joint**
    Traumatic rupture of volar plate of specified finger with unspecified laterality at metacarpophalangeal and interphalangeal joint
  - +7th **S63.439 Traumatic rupture of volar plate of unspecified finger at metacarpophalangeal and interphalangeal joint**

+ **S63.49 Traumatic rupture of other ligament of finger at metacarpophalangeal and interphalangeal joint**
  - +7th **S63.490 Traumatic rupture of other ligament of right index finger at metacarpophalangeal and interphalangeal joint**
  - +7th **S63.491 Traumatic rupture of other ligament of left index finger at metacarpophalangeal and interphalangeal joint**
  - +7th **S63.492 Traumatic rupture of other ligament of right middle finger at metacarpophalangeal and interphalangeal joint**
  - +7th **S63.493 Traumatic rupture of other ligament of left middle finger at metacarpophalangeal and interphalangeal joint**
  - +7th **S63.494 Traumatic rupture of other ligament of right ring finger at metacarpophalangeal and interphalangeal joint**
  - +7th **S63.495 Traumatic rupture of other ligament of left ring finger at metacarpophalangeal and interphalangeal joint**
  - +7th **S63.496 Traumatic rupture of other ligament of right little finger at metacarpophalangeal and interphalangeal joint**
  - +7th **S63.497 Traumatic rupture of other ligament of left little finger at metacarpophalangeal and interphalangeal joint**
  - +7th **S63.498 Traumatic rupture of other ligament of other finger at metacarpophalangeal and interphalangeal joint**
    Traumatic rupture of ligament of specified finger with unspecified laterality at metacarpophalangeal and interphalangeal joint
  - +7th **S63.499 Traumatic rupture of other ligament of unspecified finger at metacarpophalangeal and interphalangeal joint**

+ **S63.5 Other and unspecified sprain of wrist**
  + **S63.50 Unspecified sprain of wrist**
    - +7th **S63.501 Unspecified sprain of right wrist**
    - +7th **S63.502 Unspecified sprain of left wrist**
    - +7th **S63.509 Unspecified sprain of unspecified wrist**
  + **S63.51 Sprain of carpal (joint)**
    - +7th **S63.511 Sprain of carpal joint of right wrist**
    - +7th **S63.512 Sprain of carpal joint of left wrist**
    - +7th **S63.519 Sprain of carpal joint of unspecified wrist**
  + **S63.52 Sprain of radiocarpal joint**
    Excludes1: *traumatic rupture of radiocarpal ligament (S63.32-)*
    - +7th **S63.521 Sprain of radiocarpal joint of right wrist**
    - +7th **S63.522 Sprain of radiocarpal joint of left wrist**
    - +7th **S63.529 Sprain of radiocarpal joint of unspecified wrist**
  + **S63.59 Other specified sprain of wrist**
    - +7th **S63.591 Other specified sprain of right wrist**
    - +7th **S63.592 Other specified sprain of left wrist**
    - +7th **S63.599 Other specified sprain of unspecified wrist**

+ **S63.6 Other and unspecified sprain of finger(s)**

Excludes1: *traumatic rupture of ligament of finger at metacarpophalangeal and interphalangeal joint(s) (S63.4-)*

+ **S63.60 Unspecified sprain of thumb**
  - +7th **S63.601 Unspecified sprain of right thumb**
  - +7th **S63.602 Unspecified sprain of left thumb**
  - +7th **S63.609 Unspecified sprain of unspecified thumb**
+ **S63.61 Unspecified sprain of other and unspecified finger(s)**
  - +7th **S63.610 Unspecified sprain of right index finger**
  - +7th **S63.611 Unspecified sprain of left index finger**
  - +7th **S63.612 Unspecified sprain of right middle finger**
  - +7th **S63.613 Unspecified sprain of left middle finger**
  - +7th **S63.614 Unspecified sprain of right ring finger**
  - +7th **S63.615 Unspecified sprain of left ring finger**
  - +7th **S63.616 Unspecified sprain of right little finger**
  - +7th **S63.617 Unspecified sprain of left little finger**
  - +7th **S63.618 Unspecified sprain of other finger**
    Unspecified sprain of specified finger with unspecified laterality
  - +7th **S63.619 Unspecified sprain of unspecified finger**
+ **S63.62 Sprain of interphalangeal joint of thumb**
  - +7th **S63.621 Sprain of interphalangeal joint of right thumb**
  - +7th **S63.622 Sprain of interphalangeal joint of left thumb**
  - +7th **S63.629 Sprain of interphalangeal joint of unspecified thumb**
+ **S63.63 Sprain of interphalangeal joint of other and unspecified finger(s)**
  - +7th **S63.630 Sprain of interphalangeal joint of right index finger**
  - +7th **S63.631 Sprain of interphalangeal joint of left index finger**
  - +7th **S63.632 Sprain of interphalangeal joint of right middle finger**
  - +7th **S63.633 Sprain of interphalangeal joint of left middle finger**
  - +7th **S63.634 Sprain of interphalangeal joint of right ring finger**
  - +7th **S63.635 Sprain of interphalangeal joint of left ring finger**
  - +7th **S63.636 Sprain of interphalangeal joint of right little finger**
  - +7th **S63.637 Sprain of interphalangeal joint of left little finger**
  - +7th **S63.638 Sprain of interphalangeal joint of other finger**
  - +7th **S63.639 Sprain of interphalangeal joint of unspecified finger**
+ **S63.64 Sprain of metacarpophalangeal joint of thumb**
  - +7th **S63.641 Sprain of metacarpophalangeal joint of right thumb**
  - +7th **S63.642 Sprain of metacarpophalangeal joint of left thumb**
  - +7th **S63.649 Sprain of metacarpophalangeal joint of unspecified thumb**
+ **S63.65 Sprain of metacarpophalangeal joint of other and unspecified finger(s)**
  - +7th **S63.650 Sprain of metacarpophalangeal joint of right index finger**
  - +7th **S63.651 Sprain of metacarpophalangeal joint of left index finger**
  - +7th **S63.652 Sprain of metacarpophalangeal joint of right middle finger**
  - +7th **S63.653 Sprain of metacarpophalangeal joint of left middle finger**
  - +7th **S63.654 Sprain of metacarpophalangeal joint of right ring finger**
  - +7th **S63.655 Sprain of metacarpophalangeal joint of left ring finger**
  - +7th **S63.656 Sprain of metacarpophalangeal joint of right little finger**
  - +7th **S63.657 Sprain of metacarpophalangeal joint of left little finger**
  - +7th **S63.658 Sprain of metacarpophalangeal joint of other finger**
    Sprain of metacarpophalangeal joint of specified finger with unspecified laterality
  - +7th **S63.659 Sprain of metacarpophalangeal joint of unspecified finger**
+ **S63.68 Other sprain of thumb**
  - +7th **S63.681 Other sprain of right thumb**
  - +7th **S63.682 Other sprain of left thumb**
  - +7th **S63.689 Other sprain of unspecified thumb**
+ **S63.69 Other sprain of other and unspecified finger(s)**
  - +7th **S63.690 Other sprain of right index finger**
  - +7th **S63.691 Other sprain of left index finger**
  - +7th **S63.692 Other sprain of right middle finger**
  - +7th **S63.693 Other sprain of left middle finger**
  - +7th **S63.694 Other sprain of right ring finger**
  - +7th **S63.695 Other sprain of left ring finger**
  - +7th **S63.696 Other sprain of right little finger**
  - +7th **S63.697 Other sprain of left little finger**
  - +7th **S63.698 Other sprain of other finger**
    Other sprain of specified finger with unspecified laterality
  - +7th **S63.699 Other sprain of unspecified finger**

+ **S63.8 Sprain of other part of wrist and hand**
  + **S63.8X Sprain of other part of wrist and hand**
    - +7th **S63.8X1 Sprain of other part of right wrist and hand**
    - +7th **S63.8X2 Sprain of other part of left wrist and hand**
    - +7th **S63.8X9 Sprain of other part of unspecified wrist and hand**
+ **S63.9 Sprain of unspecified part of wrist and hand**
  - X+7th **S63.90 Sprain of unspecified part of unspecified wrist and hand**
  - X+7th **S63.91 Sprain of unspecified part of right wrist and hand**
  - X+7th **S63.92 Sprain of unspecified part of left wrist and hand**

S64 Injury of nerves at wrist and hand level

Code also any associated open wound (S61.-)

The appropriate 7th character is to be added to each code from category S64
A initial encounter
D subsequent encounter
S sequela

+ **S64.0 Injury of ulnar nerve at wrist and hand level**
  - X+7th **S64.00 Injury of ulnar nerve at wrist and hand level of unspecified arm**
  - X+7th **S64.01 Injury of ulnar nerve at wrist and hand level of right arm**
  - X+7th **S64.02 Injury of ulnar nerve at wrist and hand level of left arm**
+ **S64.1 Injury of median nerve at wrist and hand level**
  - X+7th **S64.10 Injury of median nerve at wrist and hand level of unspecified arm**
  - X+7th **S64.11 Injury of median nerve at wrist and hand level of right arm**
  - X+7th **S64.12 Injury of median nerve at wrist and hand level of left arm**
+ **S64.2 Injury of radial nerve at wrist and hand level**
  - X+7th **S64.20 Injury of radial nerve at wrist and hand level of unspecified arm**
  - X+7th **S64.21 Injury of radial nerve at wrist and hand level of right arm**
  - X+7th **S64.22 Injury of radial nerve at wrist and hand level of left arm**
+ **S64.3 Injury of digital nerve of thumb**
  - X+7th **S64.30 Injury of digital nerve of unspecified thumb**
  - X+7th **S64.31 Injury of digital nerve of right thumb**
  - X+7th **S64.32 Injury of digital nerve of left thumb**
+ **S64.4 Injury of digital nerve of other and unspecified finger**
  - X+7th **S64.40 Injury of digital nerve of unspecified finger**
  + **S64.49 Injury of digital nerve of other finger**
    - +7th **S64.490 Injury of digital nerve of right index finger**
    - +7th **S64.491 Injury of digital nerve of left index finger**
    - +7th **S64.492 Injury of digital nerve of right middle finger**

+7th **S64.493** **Injury of digital nerve of left middle finger**
+7th **S64.494** **Injury of digital nerve of right ring finger**
+7th **S64.495** **Injury of digital nerve of left ring finger**
+7th **S64.496** **Injury of digital nerve of right little finger**
+7th **S64.497** **Injury of digital nerve of left little finger**
+7th **S64.498** **Injury of digital nerve of other finger**
Injury of digital nerve of specified finger with unspecified laterality

\+ **S64.8** **Injury of other nerves at wrist and hand level**
\+ **S64.8X** **Injury of other nerves at wrist and hand level**
+7th **S64.8X1** **Injury of other nerves at wrist and hand level of right arm**
+7th **S64.8X2** **Injury of other nerves at wrist and hand level of left arm**
+7th **S64.8X9** **Injury of other nerves at wrist and hand level of unspecified arm**

\+ **S64.9** **Injury of unspecified nerve at wrist and hand level**
X+7th **S64.90** **Injury of unspecified nerve at wrist and hand level of unspecified arm**
X+7th **S64.91** **Injury of unspecified nerve at wrist and hand level of right arm**
X+7th **S64.92** **Injury of unspecified nerve at wrist and hand level of left arm**

S65 **Injury of blood vessels at wrist and hand level**
Code also any associated open wound (S61.-)

The appropriate 7th character is to be added to each code from category S65
A initial encounter
D subsequent encounter
S sequela

\+ **S65.0** **Injury of ulnar artery at wrist and hand level**
\+ **S65.00** **Unspecified injury of ulnar artery at wrist and hand level**
CC +7th **S65.001** **Unspecified injury of ulnar artery at wrist and hand level of right arm**
CC +7th **S65.002** **Unspecified injury of ulnar artery at wrist and hand level of left arm**
CC +7th **S65.009** **Unspecified injury of ulnar artery at wrist and hand level of unspecified arm**
\+ **S65.01** **Laceration of ulnar artery at wrist and hand level**
CC +7th **S65.011** **Laceration of ulnar artery at wrist and hand level of right arm**
CC +7th **S65.012** **Laceration of ulnar artery at wrist and hand level of left arm**
CC +7th **S65.019** **Laceration of ulnar artery at wrist and hand level of unspecified arm**
\+ **S65.09** **Other specified injury of ulnar artery at wrist and hand level**
CC +7th **S65.091** **Other specified injury of ulnar artery at wrist and hand level of right arm**
CC +7th **S65.092** **Other specified injury of ulnar artery at wrist and hand level of left arm**
CC +7th **S65.099** **Other specified injury of ulnar artery at wrist and hand level of unspecified arm**

\+ **S65.1** **Injury of radial artery at wrist and hand level**
\+ **S65.10** **Unspecified injury of radial artery at wrist and hand level**
CC +7th **S65.101** **Unspecified injury of radial artery at wrist and hand level of right arm**
CC +7th **S65.102** **Unspecified injury of radial artery at wrist and hand level of left arm**
CC +7th **S65.109** **Unspecified injury of radial artery at wrist and hand level of unspecified arm**
\+ **S65.11** **Laceration of radial artery at wrist and hand level**
CC +7th **S65.111** **Laceration of radial artery at wrist and hand level of right arm**
CC +7th **S65.112** **Laceration of radial artery at wrist and hand level of left arm**
CC +7th **S65.119** **Laceration of radial artery at wrist and hand level of unspecified arm**
\+ **S65.19** **Other specified injury of radial artery at wrist and hand level**
CC +7th **S65.191** **Other specified injury of radial artery at wrist and hand level of right arm**
CC +7th **S65.192** **Other specified injury of radial artery at wrist and hand level of left arm**
CC +7th **S65.199** **Other specified injury of radial artery at wrist and hand level of unspecified arm**

\+ **S65.2** **Injury of superficial palmar arch**
\+ **S65.20** **Unspecified injury of superficial palmar arch**
CC +7th **S65.201** **Unspecified injury of superficial palmar arch of right hand**
CC +7th **S65.202** **Unspecified injury of superficial palmar arch of left hand**
CC +7th **S65.209** **Unspecified injury of superficial palmar arch of unspecified hand**
\+ **S65.21** **Laceration of superficial palmar arch**
CC +7th **S65.211** **Laceration of superficial palmar arch of right hand**
CC +7th **S65.212** **Laceration of superficial palmar arch of left hand**
CC +7th **S65.219** **Laceration of superficial palmar arch of unspecified hand**
\+ **S65.29** **Other specified injury of superficial palmar arch**
CC +7th **S65.291** **Other specified injury of superficial palmar arch of right hand**
CC +7th **S65.292** **Other specified injury of superficial palmar arch of left hand**
CC +7th **S65.299** **Other specified injury of superficial palmar arch of unspecified hand**

\+ **S65.3** **Injury of deep palmar arch**
\+ **S65.30** **Unspecified injury of deep palmar arch**
CC +7th **S65.301** **Unspecified injury of deep palmar arch of right hand**
CC +7th **S65.302** **Unspecified injury of deep palmar arch of left hand**
CC +7th **S65.309** **Unspecified injury of deep palmar arch of unspecified hand**
\+ **S65.31** **Laceration of deep palmar arch**
CC +7th **S65.311** **Laceration of deep palmar arch of right hand**
CC +7th **S65.312** **Laceration of deep palmar arch of left hand**
CC +7th **S65.319** **Laceration of deep palmar arch of unspecified hand**
\+ **S65.39** **Other specified injury of deep palmar arch**
CC +7th **S65.391** **Other specified injury of deep palmar arch of right hand**
CC +7th **S65.392** **Other specified injury of deep palmar arch of left hand**
CC +7th **S65.399** **Other specified injury of deep palmar arch of unspecified hand**

\+ **S65.4** **Injury of blood vessel of thumb**
\+ **S65.40** **Unspecified injury of blood vessel of thumb**
CC +7th **S65.401** **Unspecified injury of blood vessel of right thumb**
CC +7th **S65.402** **Unspecified injury of blood vessel of left thumb**
CC +7th **S65.409** **Unspecified injury of blood vessel of unspecified thumb**
\+ **S65.41** **Laceration of blood vessel of thumb**
CC +7th **S65.411** **Laceration of blood vessel of right thumb**
CC +7th **S65.412** **Laceration of blood vessel of left thumb**
CC +7th **S65.419** **Laceration of blood vessel of unspecified thumb**
\+ **S65.49** **Other specified injury of blood vessel of thumb**
CC +7th **S65.491** **Other specified injury of blood vessel of right thumb**
CC +7th **S65.492** **Other specified injury of blood vessel of left thumb**
CC +7th **S65.499** **Other specified injury of blood vessel of unspecified thumb**

\+ **S65.5** **Injury of blood vessel of other and unspecified finger**
\+ **S65.50** **Unspecified injury of blood vessel of other and unspecified finger**
CC +7th **S65.500** **Unspecified injury of blood vessel of right index finger**
CC +7th **S65.501** **Unspecified injury of blood vessel of left index finger**
CC +7th **S65.502** **Unspecified injury of blood vessel of right middle finger**
CC +7th **S65.503** **Unspecified injury of blood vessel of left middle finger**

CC +7th **S65.504** **Unspecified injury of blood vessel of right ring finger**

CC +7th **S65.505** **Unspecified injury of blood vessel of left ring finger**

CC +7th **S65.506** **Unspecified injury of blood vessel of right little finger**

CC +7th **S65.507** **Unspecified injury of blood vessel of left little finger**

CC +7th **S65.508** **Unspecified injury of blood vessel of other finger**

Unspecified injury of blood vessel of specified finger with unspecified laterality

CC +7th **S65.509** **Unspecified injury of blood vessel of unspecified finger**

+ **S65.51** **Laceration of blood vessel of other and unspecified finger**

CC +7th **S65.510** **Laceration of blood vessel of right index finger**

CC +7th **S65.511** **Laceration of blood vessel of left index finger**

CC +7th **S65.512** **Laceration of blood vessel of right middle finger**

CC +7th **S65.513** **Laceration of blood vessel of left middle finger**

CC +7th **S65.514** **Laceration of blood vessel of right ring finger**

CC +7th **S65.515** **Laceration of blood vessel of left ring finger**

CC +7th **S65.516** **Laceration of blood vessel of right little finger**

CC +7th **S65.517** **Laceration of blood vessel of left little finger**

CC +7th **S65.518** **Laceration of blood vessel of other finger**

Laceration of blood vessel of specified finger with unspecified laterality

CC +7th **S65.519** **Laceration of blood vessel of unspecified finger**

+ **S65.59** **Other specified injury of blood vessel of other and unspecified finger**

CC +7th **S65.590** **Other specified injury of blood vessel of right index finger**

CC +7th **S65.591** **Other specified injury of blood vessel of left index finger**

CC +7th **S65.592** **Other specified injury of blood vessel of right middle finger**

CC +7th **S65.593** **Other specified injury of blood vessel of left middle finger**

CC +7th **S65.594** **Other specified injury of blood vessel of right ring finger**

CC +7th **S65.595** **Other specified injury of blood vessel of left ring finger**

CC +7th **S65.596** **Other specified injury of blood vessel of right little finger**

CC +7th **S65.597** **Other specified injury of blood vessel of left little finger**

CC +7th **S65.598** **Other specified injury of blood vessel of other finger**

Other specified injury of blood vessel of specified finger with unspecified laterality

CC +7th **S65.599** **Other specified injury of blood vessel of unspecified finger**

+ **S65.8** **Injury of other blood vessels at wrist and hand level**

+ **S65.80** **Unspecified injury of other blood vessels at wrist and hand level**

CC +7th **S65.801** **Unspecified injury of other blood vessels at wrist and hand level of right arm**

CC +7th **S65.802** **Unspecified injury of other blood vessels at wrist and hand level of left arm**

CC +7th **S65.809** **Unspecified injury of other blood vessels at wrist and hand level of unspecified arm**

+ **S65.81** **Laceration of other blood vessels at wrist and hand level**

CC +7th **S65.811** **Laceration of other blood vessels at wrist and hand level of right arm**

CC +7th **S65.812** **Laceration of other blood vessels at wrist and hand level of left arm**

CC +7th **S65.819** **Laceration of other blood vessels at wrist and hand level of unspecified arm**

+ **S65.89** **Other specified injury of other blood vessels at wrist and hand level**

CC +7th **S65.891** **Other specified injury of other blood vessels at wrist and hand level of right arm**

CC +7th **S65.892** **Other specified injury of other blood vessels at wrist and hand level of left arm**

CC +7th **S65.899** **Other specified injury of other blood vessels at wrist and hand level of unspecified arm**

+ **S65.9** **Injury of unspecified blood vessel at wrist and hand level**

+ **S65.90** **Unspecified injury of unspecified blood vessel at wrist and hand level**

CC +7th **S65.901** **Unspecified injury of unspecified blood vessel at wrist and hand level of right arm**

CC +7th **S65.902** **Unspecified injury of unspecified blood vessel at wrist and hand level of left arm**

CC +7th **S65.909** **Unspecified injury of unspecified blood vessel at wrist and hand level of unspecified arm**

+ **S65.91** **Laceration of unspecified blood vessel at wrist and hand level**

CC +7th **S65.911** **Laceration of unspecified blood vessel at wrist and hand level of right arm**

CC +7th **S65.912** **Laceration of unspecified blood vessel at wrist and hand level of left arm**

CC +7th **S65.919** **Laceration of unspecified blood vessel at wrist and hand level of unspecified arm**

+ **S65.99** **Other specified injury of unspecified blood vessel at wrist and hand level**

CC +7th **S65.991** **Other specified injury of unspecified blood vessel at wrist and hand of right arm**

CC +7th **S65.992** **Other specified injury of unspecified blood vessel at wrist and hand of left arm**

CC +7th **S65.999** **Other specified injury of unspecified blood vessel at wrist and hand of unspecified arm**

S66 **Injury of muscle, fascia and tendon at wrist and hand level**

Code also any associated open wound (S61.-)

Excludes2: *sprain of joints and ligaments of wrist and hand (S63.-)*

The appropriate 7th character is to be added to each code from category S66
A initial encounter
D subsequent encounter
S sequela

+ **S66.0** **Injury of long flexor muscle, fascia and tendon of thumb at wrist and hand level**

+ **S66.00** **Unspecified injury of long flexor muscle, fascia and tendon of thumb at wrist and hand level**

+7th **S66.001** **Unspecified injury of long flexor muscle, fascia and tendon of right thumb at wrist and hand level**

+7th **S66.002** **Unspecified injury of long flexor muscle, fascia and tendon of left thumb at wrist and hand level**

+7th **S66.009** **Unspecified injury of long flexor muscle, fascia and tendon of unspecified thumb at wrist and hand level**

+ **S66.01** **Strain of long flexor muscle, fascia and tendon of thumb at wrist and hand level**

+7th **S66.011** **Strain of long flexor muscle, fascia and tendon of right thumb at wrist and hand level**

+7th **S66.012** **Strain of long flexor muscle, fascia and tendon of left thumb at wrist and hand level**

+7th **S66.019** **Strain of long flexor muscle, fascia and tendon of unspecified thumb at wrist and hand level**

+ **S66.02 Laceration of long flexor muscle, fascia and tendon of thumb at wrist and hand level**

CC +7th **S66.021 Laceration of long flexor muscle, fascia and tendon of right thumb at wrist and hand level**

CC +7th **S66.022 Laceration of long flexor muscle, fascia and tendon of left thumb at wrist and hand level**

CC +7th **S66.029 Laceration of long flexor muscle, fascia and tendon of unspecified thumb at wrist and hand level**

+ **S66.09 Other specified injury of long flexor muscle, fascia and tendon of thumb at wrist and hand level**

+7th **S66.091 Other specified injury of long flexor muscle, fascia and tendon of right thumb at wrist and hand level**

+7th **S66.092 Other specified injury of long flexor muscle, fascia and tendon of left thumb at wrist and hand level**

+7th **S66.099 Other specified injury of long flexor muscle, fascia and tendon of unspecified thumb at wrist and hand level**

+ **S66.1 Injury of flexor muscle, fascia and tendon of other and unspecified finger at wrist and hand level**

Excludes2: *Injury of long flexor muscle, fascia and tendon of thumb at wrist and hand level (S66.0-)*

+ **S66.10 Unspecified injury of flexor muscle, fascia and tendon of other and unspecified finger at wrist and hand level**

+7th **S66.100 Unspecified injury of flexor muscle, fascia and tendon of right index finger at wrist and hand level**

+7th **S66.101 Unspecified injury of flexor muscle, fascia and tendon of left index finger at wrist and hand level**

+7th **S66.102 Unspecified injury of flexor muscle, fascia and tendon of right middle finger at wrist and hand level**

+7th **S66.103 Unspecified injury of flexor muscle, fascia and tendon of left middle finger at wrist and hand level**

+7th **S66.104 Unspecified injury of flexor muscle, fascia and tendon of right ring finger at wrist and hand level**

+7th **S66.105 Unspecified injury of flexor muscle, fascia and tendon of left ring finger at wrist and hand level**

+7th **S66.106 Unspecified injury of flexor muscle, fascia and tendon of right little finger at wrist and hand level**

+7th **S66.107 Unspecified injury of flexor muscle, fascia and tendon of left little finger at wrist and hand level**

+7th **S66.108 Unspecified injury of flexor muscle, fascia and tendon of other finger at wrist and hand level**

Unspecified injury of flexor muscle, fascia and tendon of specified finger with unspecified laterality at wrist and hand level

+7th **S66.109 Unspecified injury of flexor muscle, fascia and tendon of unspecified finger at wrist and hand level**

+ **S66.11 Strain of flexor muscle, fascia and tendon of other and unspecified finger at wrist and hand level**

+7th **S66.110 Strain of flexor muscle, fascia and tendon of right index finger at wrist and hand level**

+7th **S66.111 Strain of flexor muscle, fascia and tendon of left index finger at wrist and hand level**

+7th **S66.112 Strain of flexor muscle, fascia and tendon of right middle finger at wrist and hand level**

+7th **S66.113 Strain of flexor muscle, fascia and tendon of left middle finger at wrist and hand level**

+7th **S66.114 Strain of flexor muscle, fascia and tendon of right ring finger at wrist and hand level**

+7th **S66.115 Strain of flexor muscle, fascia and tendon of left ring finger at wrist and hand level**

+7th **S66.116 Strain of flexor muscle, fascia and tendon of right little finger at wrist and hand level**

+7th **S66.117 Strain of flexor muscle, fascia and tendon of left little finger at wrist and hand level**

+7th **S66.118 Strain of flexor muscle, fascia and tendon of other finger at wrist and hand level**

Strain of flexor muscle, fascia and tendon of specified finger with unspecified laterality at wrist and hand level

+7th **S66.119 Strain of flexor muscle, fascia and tendon of unspecified finger at wrist and hand level**

+ **S66.12 Laceration of flexor muscle, fascia and tendon of other and unspecified finger at wrist and hand level**

CC +7th **S66.120 Laceration of flexor muscle, fascia and tendon of right index finger at wrist and hand level**

CC +7th **S66.121 Laceration of flexor muscle, fascia and tendon of left index finger at wrist and hand level**

CC +7th **S66.122 Laceration of flexor muscle, fascia and tendon of right middle finger at wrist and hand level**

CC +7th **S66.123 Laceration of flexor muscle, fascia and tendon of left middle finger at wrist and hand level**

CC +7th **S66.124 Laceration of flexor muscle, fascia and tendon of right ring finger at wrist and hand level**

CC +7th **S66.125 Laceration of flexor muscle, fascia and tendon of left ring finger at wrist and hand level**

CC +7th **S66.126 Laceration of flexor muscle, fascia and tendon of right little finger at wrist and hand level**

CC +7th **S66.127 Laceration of flexor muscle, fascia and tendon of left little finger at wrist and hand level**

CC +7th **S66.128 Laceration of flexor muscle, fascia and tendon of other finger at wrist and hand level**

Laceration of flexor muscle, fascia and tendon of specified finger with unspecified laterality at wrist and hand level

CC +7th **S66.129 Laceration of flexor muscle, fascia and tendon of unspecified finger at wrist and hand level**

+ **S66.19 Other injury of flexor muscle, fascia and tendon of other and unspecified finger at wrist and hand level**

+7th **S66.190 Other injury of flexor muscle, fascia and tendon of right index finger at wrist and hand level**

+7th **S66.191 Other injury of flexor muscle, fascia and tendon of left index finger at wrist and hand level**

+7th **S66.192 Other injury of flexor muscle, fascia and tendon of right middle finger at wrist and hand level**

+7th **S66.193 Other injury of flexor muscle, fascia and tendon of left middle finger at wrist and hand level**

+7th **S66.194 Other injury of flexor muscle, fascia and tendon of right ring finger at wrist and hand level**

+7th **S66.195 Other injury of flexor muscle, fascia and tendon of left ring finger at wrist and hand level**

+7th **S66.196 Other injury of flexor muscle, fascia and tendon of right little finger at wrist and hand level**

+7th **S66.197 Other injury of flexor muscle, fascia and tendon of left little finger at wrist and hand level**

+7th **S66.198** **Other injury of flexor muscle, fascia and tendon of other finger at wrist and hand level**
Other injury of flexor muscle, fascia and tendon of specified finger with unspecified laterality at wrist and hand level

+7th **S66.199** **Other injury of flexor muscle, fascia and tendon of unspecified finger at wrist and hand level**

\+ **S66.2** **Injury of extensor muscle, fascia and tendon of thumb at wrist and hand level**

\+ **S66.20** **Unspecified injury of extensor muscle, fascia and tendon of thumb at wrist and hand level**

+7th **S66.201** **Unspecified injury of extensor muscle, fascia and tendon of right thumb at wrist and hand level**

+7th **S66.202** **Unspecified injury of extensor muscle, fascia and tendon of left thumb at wrist and hand level**

+7th **S66.209** **Unspecified injury of extensor muscle, fascia and tendon of unspecified thumb at wrist and hand level**

\+ **S66.21** **Strain of extensor muscle, fascia and tendon of thumb at wrist and hand level**

+7th **S66.211** **Strain of extensor muscle, fascia and tendon of right thumb at wrist and hand level**

+7th **S66.212** **Strain of extensor muscle, fascia and tendon of left thumb at wrist and hand level**

+7th **S66.219** **Strain of extensor muscle, fascia and tendon of unspecified thumb at wrist and hand level**

\+ **S66.22** **Laceration of extensor muscle, fascia and tendon of thumb at wrist and hand level**

CC +7th **S66.221** **Laceration of extensor muscle, fascia and tendon of right thumb at wrist and hand level**

CC +7th **S66.222** **Laceration of extensor muscle, fascia and tendon of left thumb at wrist and hand level**

CC +7th **S66.229** **Laceration of extensor muscle, fascia and tendon of unspecified thumb at wrist and hand level**

\+ **S66.29** **Other specified injury of extensor muscle, fascia and tendon of thumb at wrist and hand level**

+7th **S66.291** **Other specified injury of extensor muscle, fascia and tendon of right thumb at wrist and hand level**

+7th **S66.292** **Other specified injury of extensor muscle, fascia and tendon of left thumb at wrist and hand level**

+7th **S66.299** **Other specified injury of extensor muscle, fascia and tendon of unspecified thumb at wrist and hand level**

\+ **S66.3** **Injury of extensor muscle, fascia and tendon of other and unspecified finger at wrist and hand level**

Excludes2: *Injury of extensor muscle, fascia and tendon of thumb at wrist and hand level (S66.2-)*

\+ **S66.30** **Unspecified injury of extensor muscle, fascia and tendon of other and unspecified finger at wrist and hand level**

+7th **S66.300** **Unspecified injury of extensor muscle, fascia and tendon of right index finger at wrist and hand level**

+7th **S66.301** **Unspecified injury of extensor muscle, fascia and tendon of left index finger at wrist and hand level**

+7th **S66.302** **Unspecified injury of extensor muscle, fascia and tendon of right middle finger at wrist and hand level**

+7th **S66.303** **Unspecified injury of extensor muscle, fascia and tendon of left middle finger at wrist and hand level**

+7th **S66.304** **Unspecified injury of extensor muscle, fascia and tendon of right ring finger at wrist and hand level**

+7th **S66.305** **Unspecified injury of extensor muscle, fascia and tendon of left ring finger at wrist and hand level**

+7th **S66.306** **Unspecified injury of extensor muscle, fascia and tendon of right little finger at wrist and hand level**

+7th **S66.307** **Unspecified injury of extensor muscle, fascia and tendon of left little finger at wrist and hand level**

+7th **S66.308** **Unspecified injury of extensor muscle, fascia and tendon of other finger at wrist and hand level**
Unspecified injury of extensor muscle, fascia and tendon of specified finger with unspecified laterality at wrist and hand level

+7th **S66.309** **Unspecified injury of extensor muscle, fascia and tendon of unspecified finger at wrist and hand level**

\+ **S66.31** **Strain of extensor muscle, fascia and tendon of other and unspecified finger at wrist and hand level**

+7th **S66.310** **Strain of extensor muscle, fascia and tendon of right index finger at wrist and hand level**

+7th **S66.311** **Strain of extensor muscle, fascia and tendon of left index finger at wrist and hand level**

+7th **S66.312** **Strain of extensor muscle, fascia and tendon of right middle finger at wrist and hand level**

+7th **S66.313** **Strain of extensor muscle, fascia and tendon of left middle finger at wrist and hand level**

+7th **S66.314** **Strain of extensor muscle, fascia and tendon of right ring finger at wrist and hand level**

+7th **S66.315** **Strain of extensor muscle, fascia and tendon of left ring finger at wrist and hand level**

+7th **S66.316** **Strain of extensor muscle, fascia and tendon of right little finger at wrist and hand level**

+7th **S66.317** **Strain of extensor muscle, fascia and tendon of left little finger at wrist and hand level**

+7th **S66.318** **Strain of extensor muscle, fascia and tendon of other finger at wrist and hand level**
Strain of extensor muscle, fascia and tendon of specified finger with unspecified laterality at wrist and hand level

+7th **S66.319** **Strain of extensor muscle, fascia and tendon of unspecified finger at wrist and hand level**

\+ **S66.32** **Laceration of extensor muscle, fascia and tendon of other and unspecified finger at wrist and hand level**

CC +7th **S66.320** **Laceration of extensor muscle, fascia and tendon of right index finger at wrist and hand level**

CC +7th **S66.321** **Laceration of extensor muscle, fascia and tendon of left index finger at wrist and hand level**

CC +7th **S66.322** **Laceration of extensor muscle, fascia and tendon of right middle finger at wrist and hand level**

CC +7th **S66.323** **Laceration of extensor muscle, fascia and tendon of left middle finger at wrist and hand level**

CC +7th **S66.324** **Laceration of extensor muscle, fascia and tendon of right ring finger at wrist and hand level**

CC +7th **S66.325** **Laceration of extensor muscle, fascia and tendon of left ring finger at wrist and hand level**

CC +7th **S66.326** **Laceration of extensor muscle, fascia and tendon of right little finger at wrist and hand level**

CC +7th **S66.327** **Laceration of extensor muscle, fascia and tendon of left little finger at wrist and hand level**

CC +7th **S66.328 Laceration of extensor muscle, fascia and tendon of other finger at wrist and hand level**
Laceration of extensor muscle, fascia and tendon of specified finger with unspecified laterality at wrist and hand level

CC +7th **S66.329 Laceration of extensor muscle, fascia and tendon of unspecified finger at wrist and hand level**

\+ **S66.39 Other injury of extensor muscle, fascia and tendon of other and unspecified finger at wrist and hand level**

+7th **S66.390 Other injury of extensor muscle, fascia and tendon of right index finger at wrist and hand level**

+7th **S66.391 Other injury of extensor muscle, fascia and tendon of left index finger at wrist and hand level**

+7th **S66.392 Other injury of extensor muscle, fascia and tendon of right middle finger at wrist and hand level**

+7th **S66.393 Other injury of extensor muscle, fascia and tendon of left middle finger at wrist and hand level**

+7th **S66.394 Other injury of extensor muscle, fascia and tendon of right ring finger at wrist and hand level**

+7th **S66.395 Other injury of extensor muscle, fascia and tendon of left ring finger at wrist and hand level**

+7th **S66.396 Other injury of extensor muscle, fascia and tendon of right little finger at wrist and hand level**

+7th **S66.397 Other injury of extensor muscle, fascia and tendon of left little finger at wrist and hand level**

+7th **S66.398 Other injury of extensor muscle, fascia and tendon of other finger at wrist and hand level**
Other injury of extensor muscle, fascia and tendon of specified finger with unspecified laterality at wrist and hand level

+7th **S66.399 Other injury of extensor muscle, fascia and tendon of unspecified finger at wrist and hand level**

\+ **S66.4 Injury of intrinsic muscle, fascia and tendon of thumb at wrist and hand level**

\+ **S66.40 Unspecified injury of intrinsic muscle, fascia and tendon of thumb at wrist and hand level**

+7th **S66.401 Unspecified injury of intrinsic muscle, fascia and tendon of right thumb at wrist and hand level**

+7th **S66.402 Unspecified injury of intrinsic muscle, fascia and tendon of left thumb at wrist and hand level**

+7th **S66.409 Unspecified injury of intrinsic muscle, fascia and tendon of unspecified thumb at wrist and hand level**

\+ **S66.41 Strain of intrinsic muscle, fascia and tendon of thumb at wrist and hand level**

+7th **S66.411 Strain of intrinsic muscle, fascia and tendon of right thumb at wrist and hand level**

+7th **S66.412 Strain of intrinsic muscle, fascia and tendon of left thumb at wrist and hand level**

+7th **S66.419 Strain of intrinsic muscle, fascia and tendon of unspecified thumb at wrist and hand level**

\+ **S66.42 Laceration of intrinsic muscle, fascia and tendon of thumb at wrist and hand level**

CC +7th **S66.421 Laceration of intrinsic muscle, fascia and tendon of right thumb at wrist and hand level**

CC +7th **S66.422 Laceration of intrinsic muscle, fascia and tendon of left thumb at wrist and hand level**

CC +7th **S66.429 Laceration of intrinsic muscle, fascia and tendon of unspecified thumb at wrist and hand level**

\+ **S66.49 Other specified injury of intrinsic muscle, fascia and tendon of thumb at wrist and hand level**

+7th **S66.491 Other specified injury of intrinsic muscle, fascia and tendon of right thumb at wrist and hand level**

+7th **S66.492 Other specified injury of intrinsic muscle, fascia and tendon of left thumb at wrist and hand level**

+7th **S66.499 Other specified injury of intrinsic muscle, fascia and tendon of unspecified thumb at wrist and hand level**

\+ **S66.5 Injury of intrinsic muscle, fascia and tendon of other and unspecified finger at wrist and hand level**
Excludes2: *injury of intrinsic muscle, fascia and tendon of thumb at wrist and hand level (S66.4-)*

\+ **S66.50 Unspecified injury of intrinsic muscle, fascia and tendon of other and unspecified finger at wrist and hand level**

+7th **S66.500 Unspecified injury of intrinsic muscle, fascia and tendon of right index finger at wrist and hand level**

+7th **S66.501 Unspecified injury of intrinsic muscle, fascia and tendon of left index finger at wrist and hand level**

+7th **S66.502 Unspecified injury of intrinsic muscle, fascia and tendon of right middle finger at wrist and hand level**

+7th **S66.503 Unspecified injury of intrinsic muscle, fascia and tendon of left middle finger at wrist and hand level**

+7th **S66.504 Unspecified injury of intrinsic muscle, fascia and tendon of right ring finger at wrist and hand level**

+7th **S66.505 Unspecified injury of intrinsic muscle, fascia and tendon of left ring finger at wrist and hand level**

+7th **S66.506 Unspecified injury of intrinsic muscle, fascia and tendon of right little finger at wrist and hand level**

+7th **S66.507 Unspecified injury of intrinsic muscle, fascia and tendon of left little finger at wrist and hand level**

+7th **S66.508 Unspecified injury of intrinsic muscle, fascia and tendon of other finger at wrist and hand level**
Unspecified injury of intrinsic muscle, fascia and tendon of specified finger with unspecified laterality at wrist and hand level

+7th **S66.509 Unspecified injury of intrinsic muscle, fascia and tendon of unspecified finger at wrist and hand level**

\+ **S66.51 Strain of intrinsic muscle, fascia and tendon of other and unspecified finger at wrist and hand level**

+7th **S66.510 Strain of intrinsic muscle, fascia and tendon of right index finger at wrist and hand level**

+7th **S66.511 Strain of intrinsic muscle, fascia and tendon of left index finger at wrist and hand level**

+7th **S66.512 Strain of intrinsic muscle, fascia and tendon of right middle finger at wrist and hand level**

+7th **S66.513 Strain of intrinsic muscle, fascia and tendon of left middle finger at wrist and hand level**

+7th **S66.514 Strain of intrinsic muscle, fascia and tendon of right ring finger at wrist and hand level**

+7th **S66.515 Strain of intrinsic muscle, fascia and tendon of left ring finger at wrist and hand level**

+7th **S66.516 Strain of intrinsic muscle, fascia and tendon of right little finger at wrist and hand level**

+7th **S66.517 Strain of intrinsic muscle, fascia and tendon of left little finger at wrist and hand level**

+7th **S66.518** **Strain of intrinsic muscle, fascia and tendon of other finger at wrist and hand level**
Strain of intrinsic muscle, fascia and tendon of specified finger with unspecified laterality at wrist and hand level

+7th **S66.519** **Strain of intrinsic muscle, fascia and tendon of unspecified finger at wrist and hand level**

\+ **S66.52** **Laceration of intrinsic muscle, fascia and tendon of other and unspecified finger at wrist and hand level**

CC +7th **S66.520** **Laceration of intrinsic muscle, fascia and tendon of right index finger at wrist and hand level**

CC +7th **S66.521** **Laceration of intrinsic muscle, fascia and tendon of left index finger at wrist and hand level**

CC +7th **S66.522** **Laceration of intrinsic muscle, fascia and tendon of right middle finger at wrist and hand level**

CC +7th **S66.523** **Laceration of intrinsic muscle, fascia and tendon of left middle finger at wrist and hand level**

CC +7th **S66.524** **Laceration of intrinsic muscle, fascia and tendon of right ring finger at wrist and hand level**

CC +7th **S66.525** **Laceration of intrinsic muscle, fascia and tendon of left ring finger at wrist and hand level**

CC +7th **S66.526** **Laceration of intrinsic muscle, fascia and tendon of right little finger at wrist and hand level**

CC +7th **S66.527** **Laceration of intrinsic muscle, fascia and tendon of left little finger at wrist and hand level**

CC +7th **S66.528** **Laceration of intrinsic muscle, fascia and tendon of other finger at wrist and hand level**
Laceration of intrinsic muscle, fascia and tendon of specified finger with unspecified laterality at wrist and hand level

CC +7th **S66.529** **Laceration of intrinsic muscle, fascia and tendon of unspecified finger at wrist and hand level**

\+ **S66.59** **Other injury of intrinsic muscle, fascia and tendon of other and unspecified finger at wrist and hand level**

+7th **S66.590** **Other injury of intrinsic muscle, fascia and tendon of right index finger at wrist and hand level**

+7th **S66.591** **Other injury of intrinsic muscle, fascia and tendon of left index finger at wrist and hand level**

+7th **S66.592** **Other injury of intrinsic muscle, fascia and tendon of right middle finger at wrist and hand level**

+7th **S66.593** **Other injury of intrinsic muscle, fascia and tendon of left middle finger at wrist and hand level**

+7th **S66.594** **Other injury of intrinsic muscle, fascia and tendon of right ring finger at wrist and hand level**

+7th **S66.595** **Other injury of intrinsic muscle, fascia and tendon of left ring finger at wrist and hand level**

+7th **S66.596** **Other injury of intrinsic muscle, fascia and tendon of right little finger at wrist and hand level**

+7th **S66.597** **Other injury of intrinsic muscle, fascia and tendon of left little finger at wrist and hand level**

+7th **S66.598** **Other injury of intrinsic muscle, fascia and tendon of other finger at wrist and hand level**
Other injury of intrinsic muscle, fascia and tendon of specified finger with unspecified laterality at wrist and hand level

+7th **S66.599** **Other injury of intrinsic muscle, fascia and tendon of unspecified finger at wrist and hand level**

\+ **S66.8** **Injury of other specified muscles, fascia and tendons at wrist and hand level**

\+ **S66.80** **Unspecified injury of other specified muscles, fascia and tendons at wrist and hand level**

+7th **S66.801** **Unspecified injury of other specified muscles, fascia and tendons at wrist and hand level, right hand**

+7th **S66.802** **Unspecified injury of other specified muscles, fascia and tendons at wrist and hand level, left hand**

+7th **S66.809** **Unspecified injury of other specified muscles, fascia and tendons at wrist and hand level, unspecified hand**

\+ **S66.81** **Strain of other specified muscles, fascia and tendons at wrist and hand level**

+7th **S66.811** **Strain of other specified muscles, fascia and tendons at wrist and hand level, right hand**

+7th **S66.812** **Strain of other specified muscles, fascia and tendons at wrist and hand level, left hand**

+7th **S66.819** **Strain of other specified muscles, fascia and tendons at wrist and hand level, unspecified hand**

\+ **S66.82** **Laceration of other specified muscles, fascia and tendons at wrist and hand level**

CC +7th **S66.821** **Laceration of other specified muscles, fascia and tendons at wrist and hand level, right hand**

CC +7th **S66.822** **Laceration of other specified muscles, fascia and tendons at wrist and hand level, left hand**

CC +7th **S66.829** **Laceration of other specified muscles, fascia and tendons at wrist and hand level, unspecified hand**

\+ **S66.89** **Other injury of other specified muscles, fascia and tendons at wrist and hand level**

+7th **S66.891** **Other injury of other specified muscles, fascia and tendons at wrist and hand level, right hand**

+7th **S66.892** **Other injury of other specified muscles, fascia and tendons at wrist and hand level, left hand**

+7th **S66.899** **Other injury of other specified muscles, fascia and tendons at wrist and hand level, unspecified hand**

\+ **S66.9** **Injury of unspecified muscle, fascia and tendon at wrist and hand level**

\+ **S66.90** **Unspecified injury of unspecified muscle, fascia and tendon at wrist and hand level**

+7th **S66.901** **Unspecified injury of unspecified muscle, fascia and tendon at wrist and hand level, right hand**

+7th **S66.902** **Unspecified injury of unspecified muscle, fascia and tendon at wrist and hand level, left hand**

+7th **S66.909** **Unspecified injury of unspecified muscle, fascia and tendon at wrist and hand level, unspecified hand**

\+ **S66.91** **Strain of unspecified muscle, fascia and tendon at wrist and hand level**

+7th **S66.911** **Strain of unspecified muscle, fascia and tendon at wrist and hand level, right hand**

+7th **S66.912** **Strain of unspecified muscle, fascia and tendon at wrist and hand level, left hand**

+7th **S66.919** **Strain of unspecified muscle, fascia and tendon at wrist and hand level, unspecified hand**

\+ **S66.92** **Laceration of unspecified muscle, fascia and tendon at wrist and hand level**

CC +7th **S66.921** **Laceration of unspecified muscle, fascia and tendon at wrist and hand level, right hand**

CC +7th **S66.922** **Laceration of unspecified muscle, fascia and tendon at wrist and hand level, left hand**

CC +7th **S66.929** **Laceration of unspecified muscle, fascia and tendon at wrist and hand level, unspecified hand**

\+ **S66.99 Other injury of unspecified muscle, fascia and tendon at wrist and hand level**

+7th **S66.991 Other injury of unspecified muscle, fascia and tendon at wrist and hand level, right hand**

+7th **S66.992 Other injury of unspecified muscle, fascia and tendon at wrist and hand level, left hand**

+7th **S66.999 Other injury of unspecified muscle, fascia and tendon at wrist and hand level, unspecified hand**

S67 Crushing injury of wrist, hand and fingers

Use additional code for all associated injuries, such as:
fracture of wrist and hand (S62.-)
open wound of wrist and hand (S61.-)

The appropriate 7th character is to be added to each code from category S67
A initial encounter
D subsequent encounter
S sequela

\+ **S67.0 Crushing injury of thumb**

X+7th **S67.00 Crushing injury of unspecified thumb**

X+7th **S67.01 Crushing injury of right thumb**

X+7th **S67.02 Crushing injury of left thumb**

\+ **S67.1 Crushing injury of other and unspecified finger(s)**

Excludes2: *crushing injury of thumb (S67.0-)*

X+7th **S67.10 Crushing injury of unspecified finger(s)**

\+ **S67.19 Crushing injury of other finger(s)**

+7th **S67.190 Crushing injury of right index finger**

+7th **S67.191 Crushing injury of left index finger**

+7th **S67.192 Crushing injury of right middle finger**

+7th **S67.193 Crushing injury of left middle finger**

+7th **S67.194 Crushing injury of right ring finger**

+7th **S67.195 Crushing injury of left ring finger**

+7th **S67.196 Crushing injury of right little finger**

+7th **S67.197 Crushing injury of left little finger**

+7th **S67.198 Crushing injury of other finger**

Crushing injury of specified finger with unspecified laterality

\+ **S67.2 Crushing injury of hand**

Excludes2: *crushing injury of fingers (S67.1-)*
crushing injury of thumb (S67.0-)

X+7th **S67.20 Crushing injury of unspecified hand**

X+7th **S67.21 Crushing injury of right hand**

X+7th **S67.22 Crushing injury of left hand**

\+ **S67.3 Crushing injury of wrist**

X+7th **S67.30 Crushing injury of unspecified wrist**

X+7th **S67.31 Crushing injury of right wrist**

X+7th **S67.32 Crushing injury of left wrist**

\+ **S67.4 Crushing injury of wrist and hand**

Excludes1: *crushing injury of hand alone (S67.2-)*
crushing injury of wrist alone (S67.3-)

Excludes2: *crushing injury of fingers (S67.1-)*
crushing injury of thumb (S67.0-)

X+7th **S67.40 Crushing injury of unspecified wrist and hand**

X+7th **S67.41 Crushing injury of right wrist and hand**

X+7th **S67.42 Crushing injury of left wrist and hand**

\+ **S67.9 Crushing injury of unspecified part(s) of wrist, hand and fingers**

X+7th **S67.90 Crushing injury of unspecified part(s) of unspecified wrist, hand and fingers**

X+7th **S67.91 Crushing injury of unspecified part(s) of right wrist, hand and fingers**

X+7th **S67.92 Crushing injury of unspecified part(s) of left wrist, hand and fingers**

S68 Traumatic amputation of wrist, hand and fingers

An amputation not identified as partial or complete should be coded to complete

The appropriate 7th character is to be added to each code from category S68
A initial encounter
D subsequent encounter
S sequela

\+ **S68.0 Traumatic metacarpophalangeal amputation of thumb**

Traumatic amputation of thumb NOS

\+ **S68.01 Complete traumatic metacarpophalangeal amputation of thumb**

+7th **S68.011 Complete traumatic metacarpophalangeal amputation of right thumb**

+7th **S68.012 Complete traumatic metacarpophalangeal amputation of left thumb**

+7th **S68.019 Complete traumatic metacarpophalangeal amputation of unspecified thumb**

\+ **S68.02 Partial traumatic metacarpophalangeal amputation of thumb**

+7th **S68.021 Partial traumatic metacarpophalangeal amputation of right thumb**

+7th **S68.022 Partial traumatic metacarpophalangeal amputation of left thumb**

+7th **S68.029 Partial traumatic metacarpophalangeal amputation of unspecified thumb**

\+ **S68.1 Traumatic metacarpophalangeal amputation of other and unspecified finger**

Traumatic amputation of finger NOS

Excludes2: *traumatic metacarpophalangeal amputation of thumb (S68.0-)*

\+ **S68.11 Complete traumatic metacarpophalangeal amputation of other and unspecified finger**

+7th **S68.110 Complete traumatic metacarpophalangeal amputation of right index finger**

+7th **S68.111 Complete traumatic metacarpophalangeal amputation of left index finger**

+7th **S68.112 Complete traumatic metacarpophalangeal amputation of right middle finger**

+7th **S68.113 Complete traumatic metacarpophalangeal amputation of left middle finger**

+7th **S68.114 Complete traumatic metacarpophalangeal amputation of right ring finger**

+7th **S68.115 Complete traumatic metacarpophalangeal amputation of left ring finger**

+7th **S68.116 Complete traumatic metacarpophalangeal amputation of right little finger**

+7th **S68.117 Complete traumatic metacarpophalangeal amputation of left little finger**

+7th **S68.118 Complete traumatic metacarpophalangeal amputation of other finger**

Complete traumatic metacarpophalangeal amputation of specified finger with unspecified laterality

+7th **S68.119 Complete traumatic metacarpophalangeal amputation of unspecified finger**

\+ **S68.12 Partial traumatic metacarpophalangeal amputation of other and unspecified finger**

+7th **S68.120 Partial traumatic metacarpophalangeal amputation of right index finger**

+7th **S68.121 Partial traumatic metacarpophalangeal amputation of left index finger**

+7th **S68.122 Partial traumatic metacarpophalangeal amputation of right middle finger**

+7th **S68.123 Partial traumatic metacarpophalangeal amputation of left middle finger**

+7th **S68.124 Partial traumatic metacarpophalangeal amputation of right ring finger**
+7th **S68.125 Partial traumatic metacarpophalangeal amputation of left ring finger**
+7th **S68.126 Partial traumatic metacarpophalangeal amputation of right little finger**
+7th **S68.127 Partial traumatic metacarpophalangeal amputation of left little finger**
+7th **S68.128 Partial traumatic metacarpophalangeal amputation of other finger**
Partial traumatic metacarpophalangeal amputation of specified finger with unspecified laterality
+7th **S68.129 Partial traumatic metacarpophalangeal amputation of unspecified finger**

+ **S68.4 Traumatic amputation of hand at wrist level**
Traumatic amputation of hand NOS
Traumatic amputation of wrist
+ **S68.41 Complete traumatic amputation of hand at wrist level**
CC +7th **S68.411 Complete traumatic amputation of right hand at wrist level**
CC +7th **S68.412 Complete traumatic amputation of left hand at wrist level**
CC +7th **S68.419 Complete traumatic amputation of unspecified hand at wrist level**
+ **S68.42 Partial traumatic amputation of hand at wrist level**
CC +7th **S68.421 Partial traumatic amputation of right hand at wrist level**
CC +7th **S68.422 Partial traumatic amputation of left hand at wrist level**
CC +7th **S68.429 Partial traumatic amputation of unspecified hand at wrist level**

+ **S68.5 Traumatic transphalangeal amputation of thumb**
Traumatic interphalangeal joint amputation of thumb
+ **S68.51 Complete traumatic transphalangeal amputation of thumb**
+7th **S68.511 Complete traumatic transphalangeal amputation of right thumb**
+7th **S68.512 Complete traumatic transphalangeal amputation of left thumb**
+7th **S68.519 Complete traumatic transphalangeal amputation of unspecified thumb**
+ **S68.52 Partial traumatic transphalangeal amputation of thumb**
+7th **S68.521 Partial traumatic transphalangeal amputation of right thumb**
+7th **S68.522 Partial traumatic transphalangeal amputation of left thumb**
+7th **S68.529 Partial traumatic transphalangeal amputation of unspecified thumb**

+ **S68.6 Traumatic transphalangeal amputation of other and unspecified finger**
+ **S68.61 Complete traumatic transphalangeal amputation of other and unspecified finger(s)**
+7th **S68.610 Complete traumatic transphalangeal amputation of right index finger**
+7th **S68.611 Complete traumatic transphalangeal amputation of left index finger**
+7th **S68.612 Complete traumatic transphalangeal amputation of right middle finger**
+7th **S68.613 Complete traumatic transphalangeal amputation of left middle finger**
+7th **S68.614 Complete traumatic transphalangeal amputation of right ring finger**
+7th **S68.615 Complete traumatic transphalangeal amputation of left ring finger**
+7th **S68.616 Complete traumatic transphalangeal amputation of right little finger**
+7th **S68.617 Complete traumatic transphalangeal amputation of left little finger**
+7th **S68.618 Complete traumatic transphalangeal amputation of other finger**
Complete traumatic transphalangeal amputation of specified finger with unspecified laterality
+7th **S68.619 Complete traumatic transphalangeal amputation of unspecified finger**
+ **S68.62 Partial traumatic transphalangeal amputation of other and unspecified finger**
+7th **S68.620 Partial traumatic transphalangeal amputation of right index finger**
+7th **S68.621 Partial traumatic transphalangeal amputation of left index finger**
+7th **S68.622 Partial traumatic transphalangeal amputation of right middle finger**
+7th **S68.623 Partial traumatic transphalangeal amputation of left middle finger**
+7th **S68.624 Partial traumatic transphalangeal amputation of right ring finger**
+7th **S68.625 Partial traumatic transphalangeal amputation of left ring finger**
+7th **S68.626 Partial traumatic transphalangeal amputation of right little finger**
+7th **S68.627 Partial traumatic transphalangeal amputation of left little finger**
+7th **S68.628 Partial traumatic transphalangeal amputation of other finger**
Partial traumatic transphalangeal amputation of specified finger with unspecified laterality
+7th **S68.629 Partial traumatic transphalangeal amputation of unspecified finger**

+ **S68.7 Traumatic transmetacarpal amputation of hand**
+ **S68.71 Complete traumatic transmetacarpal amputation of hand**
CC +7th **S68.711 Complete traumatic transmetacarpal amputation of right hand**
CC +7th **S68.712 Complete traumatic transmetacarpal amputation of left hand**
CC +7th **S68.719 Complete traumatic transmetacarpal amputation of unspecified hand**
+ **S68.72 Partial traumatic transmetacarpal amputation of hand**
CC +7th **S68.721 Partial traumatic transmetacarpal amputation of right hand**
CC +7th **S68.722 Partial traumatic transmetacarpal amputation of left hand**
CC +7th **S68.729 Partial traumatic transmetacarpal amputation of unspecified hand**

S69 Other and unspecified injuries of wrist, hand and finger(s)

The appropriate 7th character is to be added to each code from category S69
A initial encounter
D subsequent encounter
S sequela

+ **S69.8 Other specified injuries of wrist, hand and finger(s)**
X+7th **S69.80 Other specified injuries of unspecified wrist, hand and finger(s)**
X+7th **S69.81 Other specified injuries of right wrist, hand and finger(s)**
X+7th **S69.82 Other specified injuries of left wrist, hand and finger(s)**
+ **S69.9 Unspecified injury of wrist, hand and finger(s)**
X+7th **S69.90 Unspecified injury of unspecified wrist, hand and finger(s)**
X+7th **S69.91 Unspecified injury of right wrist, hand and finger(s)**
X+7th **S69.92 Unspecified injury of left wrist, hand and finger(s)**

Injuries to the hip and thigh (S70-S79)

Excludes2: *burns and corrosions (T20-T32)*
frostbite (T33-T34)
snake bite (T63.0-)
venomous insect bite or sting (T63.4-)

S70 Superficial injury of hip and thigh

The appropriate 7th character is to be added to each code from category S70
A initial encounter
D subsequent encounter
S sequela

+ **S70.0 Contusion of hip**
X+7th **S70.00 Contusion of unspecified hip**
X+7th **S70.01 Contusion of right hip**
X+7th **S70.02 Contusion of left hip**

+ **S70.1 Contusion of thigh**
  - X+7th **S70.10 Contusion of unspecified thigh**
  - X+7th **S70.11 Contusion of right thigh**
  - X+7th **S70.12 Contusion of left thigh**

+ **S70.2 Other superficial injuries of hip**
  - + **S70.21 Abrasion of hip**
    - +7th **S70.211 Abrasion, right hip**
    - +7th **S70.212 Abrasion, left hip**
    - +7th **S70.219 Abrasion, unspecified hip**
  - + **S70.22 Blister (nonthermal) of hip**
    - +7th **S70.221 Blister (nonthermal), right hip**
    - +7th **S70.222 Blister (nonthermal), left hip**
    - +7th **S70.229 Blister (nonthermal), unspecified hip**
  - + **S70.24 External constriction of hip**
    - +7th **S70.241 External constriction, right hip**
    - +7th **S70.242 External constriction, left hip**
    - +7th **S70.249 External constriction, unspecified hip**
  - + **S70.25 Superficial foreign body of hip**
    Splinter in the hip
    - +7th **S70.251 Superficial foreign body, right hip**
    - +7th **S70.252 Superficial foreign body, left hip**
    - +7th **S70.259 Superficial foreign body, unspecified hip**
  - + **S70.26 Insect bite (nonvenomous) of hip**
    - +7th **S70.261 Insect bite (nonvenomous), right hip**
    - +7th **S70.262 Insect bite (nonvenomous), left hip**
    - +7th **S70.269 Insect bite (nonvenomous), unspecified hip**
  - + **S70.27 Other superficial bite of hip**
    Excludes1: *open bite of hip (S71.05-)*
    - +7th **S70.271 Other superficial bite of hip, right hip**
    - +7th **S70.272 Other superficial bite of hip, left hip**
    - +7th **S70.279 Other superficial bite of hip, unspecified hip**

+ **S70.3 Other superficial injuries of thigh**
  - + **S70.31 Abrasion of thigh**
    - +7th **S70.311 Abrasion, right thigh**
    - +7th **S70.312 Abrasion, left thigh**
    - +7th **S70.319 Abrasion, unspecified thigh**
  - + **S70.32 Blister (nonthermal) of thigh**
    - +7th **S70.321 Blister (nonthermal), right thigh**
    - +7th **S70.322 Blister (nonthermal), left thigh**
    - +7th **S70.329 Blister (nonthermal), unspecified thigh**
  - + **S70.34 External constriction of thigh**
    - +7th **S70.341 External constriction, right thigh**
    - +7th **S70.342 External constriction, left thigh**
    - +7th **S70.349 External constriction, unspecified thigh**
  - + **S70.35 Superficial foreign body of thigh**
    Splinter in the thigh
    - +7th **S70.351 Superficial foreign body, right thigh**
    - +7th **S70.352 Superficial foreign body, left thigh**
    - +7th **S70.359 Superficial foreign body, unspecified thigh**
  - + **S70.36 Insect bite (nonvenomous) of thigh**
    - +7th **S70.361 Insect bite (nonvenomous), right thigh**
    - +7th **S70.362 Insect bite (nonvenomous), left thigh**
    - +7th **S70.369 Insect bite (nonvenomous), unspecified thigh**
  - + **S70.37 Other superficial bite of thigh**
    Excludes1: *open bite of thigh (S71.15)*
    - +7th **S70.371 Other superficial bite of right thigh**
    - +7th **S70.372 Other superficial bite of left thigh**
    - +7th **S70.379 Other superficial bite of unspecified thigh**

+ **S70.9 Unspecified superficial injury of hip and thigh**
  - + **S70.91 Unspecified superficial injury of hip**
    - +7th **S70.911 Unspecified superficial injury of right hip**
    - +7th **S70.912 Unspecified superficial injury of left hip**
    - +7th **S70.919 Unspecified superficial injury of unspecified hip**
  - + **S70.92 Unspecified superficial injury of thigh**
    - +7th **S70.921 Unspecified superficial injury of right thigh**
    - +7th **S70.922 Unspecified superficial injury of left thigh**
    - +7th **S70.929 Unspecified superficial injury of unspecified thigh**

S71 Open wound of hip and thigh

Code also any associated wound infection

Excludes1: *open fracture of hip and thigh (S72.-)*
traumatic amputation of hip and thigh (S78.-)

Excludes2: *bite of venomous animal (T63.-)*
open wound of ankle, foot and toes (S91.-)
open wound of knee and lower leg (S81.-)

> The appropriate 7th character is to be added to each code from category S71
> A initial encounter
> D subsequent encounter
> S sequela

+ **S71.0 Open wound of hip**
  - + **S71.00 Unspecified open wound of hip**
    - +7th **S71.001 Unspecified open wound, right hip**
    - +7th **S71.002 Unspecified open wound, left hip**
    - +7th **S71.009 Unspecified open wound, unspecified hip**
  - + **S71.01 Laceration without foreign body of hip**
    - +7th **S71.011 Laceration without foreign body, right hip**
    - +7th **S71.012 Laceration without foreign body, left hip**
    - +7th **S71.019 Laceration without foreign body, unspecified hip**
  - + **S71.02 Laceration with foreign body of hip**
    - +7th **S71.021 Laceration with foreign body, right hip**
    - +7th **S71.022 Laceration with foreign body, left hip**
    - +7th **S71.029 Laceration with foreign body, unspecified hip**
  - + **S71.03 Puncture wound without foreign body of hip**
    - +7th **S71.031 Puncture wound without foreign body, right hip**
    - +7th **S71.032 Puncture wound without foreign body, left hip**
    - +7th **S71.039 Puncture wound without foreign body, unspecified hip**
  - + **S71.04 Puncture wound with foreign body of hip**
    - +7th **S71.041 Puncture wound with foreign body, right hip**
    - +7th **S71.042 Puncture wound with foreign body, left hip**
    - +7th **S71.049 Puncture wound with foreign body, unspecified hip**
  - + **S71.05 Open bite of hip**
    Bite of hip NOS
    Excludes1: *superficial bite of hip (S70.26, S70.27)*
    - +7th **S71.051 Open bite, right hip**
    - +7th **S71.052 Open bite, left hip**
    - +7th **S71.059 Open bite, unspecified hip**

+ **S71.1 Open wound of thigh**
  - + **S71.10 Unspecified open wound of thigh**
    - +7th **S71.101 Unspecified open wound, right thigh**
    - +7th **S71.102 Unspecified open wound, left thigh**
    - +7th **S71.109 Unspecified open wound, unspecified thigh**
  - + **S71.11 Laceration without foreign body of thigh**
    - +7th **S71.111 Laceration without foreign body, right thigh**
    - +7th **S71.112 Laceration without foreign body, left thigh**
    - +7th **S71.119 Laceration without foreign body, unspecified thigh**
  - + **S71.12 Laceration with foreign body of thigh**
    - +7th **S71.121 Laceration with foreign body, right thigh**
    - +7th **S71.122 Laceration with foreign body, left thigh**
    - +7th **S71.129 Laceration with foreign body, unspecified thigh**
  - + **S71.13 Puncture wound without foreign body of thigh**
    - +7th **S71.131 Puncture wound without foreign body, right thigh**
    - +7th **S71.132 Puncture wound without foreign body, left thigh**
    - +7th **S71.139 Puncture wound without foreign body, unspecified thigh**

+ S71.14 **Puncture wound with foreign body of thigh**
  - +7th S71.141 **Puncture wound with foreign body, right thigh**
  - +7th S71.142 **Puncture wound with foreign body, left thigh**
  - +7th S71.149 **Puncture wound with foreign body, unspecified thigh**

+ S71.15 **Open bite of thigh**
  Bite of thigh NOS
  Excludes1: *superficial bite of thigh (S70.37-)*
  - +7th S71.151 **Open bite, right thigh**
  - +7th S71.152 **Open bite, left thigh**
  - +7th S71.159 **Open bite, unspecified thigh**

S72 Fracture of femur

NOTE A fracture not indicated as displaced or nondisplaced should be coded to displaced
A fracture not indicated as open or closed should be coded to closed
The open fracture designations are based on the Gustilo open fracture classification

Excludes1: *traumatic amputation of hip and thigh (S78.-)*
Excludes2: *fracture of lower leg and ankle (S82.-)*
fracture of foot (S92.-)
periprosthetic fracture of prosthetic implant of hip (M97.0-)

The appropriate 7th character is to be added to all codes from category S72
- A initial encounter for closed fracture
- B initial encounter for open fracture type I or II
  initial encounter for open fracture NOS
- C initial encounter for open fracture type IIIA, IIIB, or IIIC
- D subsequent encounter for closed fracture with routine healing
- E subsequent encounter for open fracture type I or II with routine healing
- F subsequent encounter for open fracture type IIIA, IIIB, or IIIC with routine healing
- G subsequent encounter for closed fracture with delayed healing
- H subsequent encounter for open fracture type I or II with delayed healing
- J subsequent encounter for open fracture type IIIA, IIIB, or IIIC with delayed healing
- K subsequent encounter for closed fracture with nonunion
- M subsequent encounter for open fracture type I or II with nonunion
- N subsequent encounter for open fracture type IIIA, IIIB, or IIIC with nonunion
- P subsequent encounter for closed fracture with malunion
- Q subsequent encounter for open fracture type I or II with malunion
- R subsequent encounter for open fracture type IIIA, IIIB, or IIIC with malunion
- S sequela

Review coding guideline C.19.c

+ S72.0 **Fracture of head and neck of femur**
  Excludes2: *physeal fracture of upper end of femur (S79.0-)*

+ S72.00 **Fracture of unspecified part of neck of femur**
  Fracture of hip NOS
  Fracture of neck of femur NOS
  - CC MCC +7th S72.001 **Fracture of unspecified part of neck of right femur**
    HAC 7th characters A - C see Appendix B for HAC conditional logic
  - CC MCC +7th S72.002 **Fracture of unspecified part of neck of left femur**
    HAC 7th characters A - C see Appendix B for HAC conditional logic
    AHA CC: 1Q, 2015, 3-21; 4Q, 2015, 36-37
  - CC MCC +7th S72.009 **Fracture of unspecified part of neck of unspecified femur**
    HAC 7th characters A - C see Appendix B for HAC conditional logic

+ S72.01 **Unspecified intracapsular fracture of femur**
  Subcapital fracture of femur
  - CC +7th S72.011 **Unspecified intracapsular fracture of right femur**
    HAC 7th characters A - C see Appendix B for HAC conditional logic
  - CC +7th S72.012 **Unspecified intracapsular fracture of left femur**
    HAC 7th characters A - C see Appendix B for HAC conditional logic
  - CC +7th S72.019 **Unspecified intracapsular fracture of unspecified femur**
    HAC 7th characters A - C see Appendix B for HAC conditional logic

+ S72.02 **Fracture of epiphysis (separation) (upper) of femur**
  Transepiphyseal fracture of femur
  Excludes1: *capital femoral epiphyseal fracture (pediatric) of femur (S79.01-)*
  Salter-Harris Type I physeal fracture of upper end of femur (S79.01-)
  - CC MCC +7th S72.021 **Displaced fracture of epiphysis (separation) (upper) of right femur**
    HAC 7th characters A - C see Appendix B for HAC conditional logic
  - CC MCC +7th S72.022 **Displaced fracture of epiphysis (separation) (upper) of left femur**
    HAC 7th characters A - C see Appendix B for HAC conditional logic
  - CC MCC +7th S72.023 **Displaced fracture of epiphysis (separation) (upper) of unspecified femur**
    HAC 7th characters A - C see Appendix B for HAC conditional logic
  - CC MCC +7th S72.024 **Nondisplaced fracture of epiphysis (separation) (upper) of right femur**
    HAC 7th characters A - C see Appendix B for HAC conditional logic
  - CC MCC +7th S72.025 **Nondisplaced fracture of epiphysis (separation) (upper) of left femur**
    HAC 7th characters A - C see Appendix B for HAC conditional logic
  - CC MCC +7th S72.026 **Nondisplaced fracture of epiphysis (separation) (upper) of unspecified femur**
    HAC 7th characters A - C see Appendix B for HAC conditional logic

+ S72.03 **Midcervical fracture of femur**
  Transcervical fracture of femur NOS
  - CC MCC +7th S72.031 **Displaced midcervical fracture of right femur**
    HAC 7th characters A - C see Appendix B for HAC conditional logic
  - CC MCC +7th S72.032 **Displaced midcervical fracture of left femur**
    HAC 7th characters A - C see Appendix B for HAC conditional logic
  - CC MCC +7th S72.033 **Displaced midcervical fracture of unspecified femur**
    HAC 7th characters A - C see Appendix B for HAC conditional logic
  - CC MCC +7th S72.034 **Nondisplaced midcervical fracture of right femur**
    HAC 7th characters A - C see Appendix B for HAC conditional logic
  - CC MCC +7th S72.035 **Nondisplaced midcervical fracture of left femur**
    HAC 7th characters A - C see Appendix B for HAC conditional logic
  - CC MCC +7th S72.036 **Nondisplaced midcervical fracture of unspecified femur**
    HAC 7th characters A - C see Appendix B for HAC conditional logic

+ S72.04 **Fracture of base of neck of femur**
  Cervicotrochanteric fracture of femur
  - CC MCC +7th S72.041 **Displaced fracture of base of neck of right femur**
    HAC 7th characters A - C see Appendix B for HAC conditional logic
  - CC MCC +7th S72.042 **Displaced fracture of base of neck of left femur**
    HAC 7th characters A - C see Appendix B for HAC conditional logic
  - CC MCC +7th S72.043 **Displaced fracture of base of neck of unspecified femur**
    HAC 7th characters A - C see Appendix B for HAC conditional logic
  - CC MCC +7th S72.044 **Nondisplaced fracture of base of neck of right femur**
    HAC 7th characters A - C see Appendix B for HAC conditional logic

CC MCC +7th **S72.045** **Nondisplaced fracture of base of neck of left femur**
HAC 7th characters A - C see Appendix B for HAC conditional logic

CC MCC +7th **S72.046** **Nondisplaced fracture of base of neck of unspecified femur**
HAC 7th characters A - C see Appendix B for HAC conditional logic

+ **S72.05** **Unspecified fracture of head of femur**
Fracture of head of femur NOS

CC MCC +7th **S72.051** **Unspecified fracture of head of right femur**
HAC 7th characters A - C see Appendix B for HAC conditional logic

CC MCC +7th **S72.052** **Unspecified fracture of head of left femur**
HAC 7th characters A - C see Appendix B for HAC conditional logic

CC MCC +7th **S72.059** **Unspecified fracture of head of unspecified femur**
HAC 7th characters A - C see Appendix B for HAC conditional logic

+ **S72.06** **Articular fracture of head of femur**

CC MCC +7th **S72.061** **Displaced articular fracture of head of right femur**
HAC 7th characters A - C see Appendix B for HAC conditional logic

CC MCC +7th **S72.062** **Displaced articular fracture of head of left femur**
HAC 7th characters A - C see Appendix B for HAC conditional logic

CC MCC +7th **S72.063** **Displaced articular fracture of head of unspecified femur**
HAC 7th characters A - C see Appendix B for HAC conditional logic

CC MCC +7th **S72.064** **Nondisplaced articular fracture of head of right femur**
HAC 7th characters A - C see Appendix B for HAC conditional logic

CC MCC +7th **S72.065** **Nondisplaced articular fracture of head of left femur**
HAC 7th characters A - C see Appendix B for HAC conditional logic

CC MCC +7th **S72.066** **Nondisplaced articular fracture of head of unspecified femur**
HAC 7th characters A - C see Appendix B for HAC conditional logic

+ **S72.09** **Other fracture of head and neck of femur**

CC MCC +7th **S72.091** **Other fracture of head and neck of right femur**
HAC 7th characters A - C see Appendix B for HAC conditional logic

CC MCC +7th **S72.092** **Other fracture of head and neck of left femur**
HAC 7th characters A - C see Appendix B for HAC conditional logic

CC MCC +7th **S72.099** **Other fracture of head and neck of unspecified femur**
HAC 7th characters A - C see Appendix B for HAC conditional logic

+ **S72.1** **Pertrochanteric fracture**

+ **S72.10** **Unspecified trochanteric fracture of femur**
Fracture of trochanter NOS

CC MCC **S72.101** **Unspecified trochanteric fracture of right femur**
HAC 7th characters A - C see Appendix B for HAC conditional logic

CC MCC **S72.102** **Unspecified trochanteric fracture of left femur**
HAC 7th characters A - C see Appendix B for HAC conditional logic

CC MCC **S72.109** **Unspecified trochanteric fracture of unspecified femur**
HAC 7th characters A - C see Appendix B for HAC conditional logic

+ **S72.11** **Fracture of greater trochanter of femur**

CC +7th **S72.111** **Displaced fracture of greater trochanter of right femur**
HAC 7th characters A - C see Appendix B for HAC conditional logic

CC +7th **S72.112** **Displaced fracture of greater trochanter of left femur**
HAC 7th characters A - C see Appendix B for HAC conditional logic

CC +7th **S72.113** **Displaced fracture of greater trochanter of unspecified femur**
HAC 7th characters A - C see Appendix B for HAC conditional logic

CC +7th **S72.114** **Nondisplaced fracture of greater trochanter of right femur**
HAC 7th characters A - C see Appendix B for HAC conditional logic

CC +7th **S72.115** **Nondisplaced fracture of greater trochanter of left femur**
HAC 7th characters A - C see Appendix B for HAC conditional logic

CC +7th **S72.116** **Nondisplaced fracture of greater trochanter of unspecified femur**
HAC 7th characters A - C see Appendix B for HAC conditional logic

+ **S72.12** **Fracture of lesser trochanter of femur**

CC +7th **S72.121** **Displaced fracture of lesser trochanter of right femur**
HAC 7th characters A - C see Appendix B for HAC conditional logic

CC +7th **S72.122** **Displaced fracture of lesser trochanter of left femur**
HAC 7th characters A - C see Appendix B for HAC conditional logic

CC +7th **S72.123** **Displaced fracture of lesser trochanter of unspecified femur**
HAC 7th characters A - C see Appendix B for HAC conditional logic

CC +7th **S72.124** **Nondisplaced fracture of lesser trochanter of right femur**
HAC 7th characters A - C see Appendix B for HAC conditional logic

CC +7th **S72.125** **Nondisplaced fracture of lesser trochanter of left femur**
HAC 7th characters A - C see Appendix B for HAC conditional logic

CC +7th **S72.126** **Nondisplaced fracture of lesser trochanter of unspecified femur**
HAC 7th characters A - C see Appendix B for HAC conditional logic

+ **S72.13** **Apophyseal fracture of femur**
Excludes1: *chronic (nontraumatic) slipped upper femoral epiphysis (M93.0-)*

CC +7th **S72.131** **Displaced apophyseal fracture of right femur**
HAC 7th characters A - C see Appendix B for HAC conditional logic

CC +7th **S72.132** **Displaced apophyseal fracture of left femur**
HAC 7th characters A - C see Appendix B for HAC conditional logic

CC +7th **S72.133** **Displaced apophyseal fracture of unspecified femur**
HAC 7th characters A - C see Appendix B for HAC conditional logic

CC +7th **S72.134** **Nondisplaced apophyseal fracture of right femur**
HAC 7th characters A - C see Appendix B for HAC conditional logic

CC +7th **S72.135** **Nondisplaced apophyseal fracture of left femur**
HAC 7th characters A - C see Appendix B for HAC conditional logic

CC +7th **S72.136** **Nondisplaced apophyseal fracture of unspecified femur**
HAC 7th characters A - C see Appendix B for HAC conditional logic

+ **S72.14** **Intertrochanteric fracture of femur**

CC +7th **S72.141** **Displaced intertrochanteric fracture of right femur**
AHA CC: 4Q, 2013, 128-129; 3Q, 2016, 16-17
HAC 7th characters A - C see Appendix B for HAC conditional logic

CC +7th **S72.142** **Displaced intertrochanteric fracture of left femur**
HAC 7th characters A - C see Appendix B for HAC conditional logic

CC +7th **S72.143** **Displaced intertrochanteric fracture of unspecified femur**
HAC 7th characters A - C see Appendix B for HAC conditional logic

CC +7th **S72.144** **Nondisplaced intertrochanteric fracture of right femur**
HAC 7th characters A - C see Appendix B for HAC conditional logic

CC +7th **S72.145 Nondisplaced intertrochanteric fracture of left femur**
HAC 7th characters A - C see Appendix B for HAC conditional logic

CC +7th **S72.146 Nondisplaced intertrochanteric fracture of unspecified femur**
HAC 7th characters A - C see Appendix B for HAC conditional logic

\+ **S72.2 Subtrochanteric fracture of femur**

CC X+7th **S72.21 Displaced subtrochanteric fracture of right femur**
HAC 7th characters A - C see Appendix B for HAC conditional logic

CC X+7th **S72.22 Displaced subtrochanteric fracture of left femur**
HAC 7th characters A - C see Appendix B for HAC conditional logic

CC X+7th **S72.23 Displaced subtrochanteric fracture of unspecified femur**
HAC 7th characters A - C see Appendix B for HAC conditional logic

CC X+7th **S72.24 Nondisplaced subtrochanteric fracture of right femur**
HAC 7th characters A - C see Appendix B for HAC conditional logic

CC X+7th **S72.25 Nondisplaced subtrochanteric fracture of left femur**
HAC 7th characters A - C see Appendix B for HAC conditional logic

CC X+7th **S72.26 Nondisplaced subtrochanteric fracture of unspecified femur**
HAC 7th characters A - C see Appendix B for HAC conditional logic

\+ **S72.3 Fracture of shaft of femur**

\+ **S72.30 Unspecified fracture of shaft of femur**

CC +7th **S72.301 Unspecified fracture of shaft of right femur**
AHA CC: 2Q, 2018, 12
HAC 7th characters A - C see Appendix B for HAC conditional logic

CC +7th **S72.302 Unspecified fracture of shaft of left femur**
HAC 7th characters A - C see Appendix B for HAC conditional logic

CC +7th **S72.309 Unspecified fracture of shaft of unspecified femur**
HAC 7th characters A - C see Appendix B for HAC conditional logic

\+ **S72.32 Transverse fracture of shaft of femur**

CC MCC +7th **S72.321 Displaced transverse fracture of shaft of right femur**
HAC 7th characters A - C see Appendix B for HAC conditional logic

CC MCC +7th **S72.322 Displaced transverse fracture of shaft of left femur**
HAC 7th characters A - C see Appendix B for HAC conditional logic

CC MCC +7th **S72.323 Displaced transverse fracture of shaft of unspecified femur**
HAC 7th characters A - C see Appendix B for HAC conditional logic

CC MCC +7th **S72.324 Nondisplaced transverse fracture of shaft of right femur**
HAC 7th characters A - C see Appendix B for HAC conditional logic

CC MCC +7th **S72.325 Nondisplaced transverse fracture of shaft of left femur**
HAC 7th characters A - C see Appendix B for HAC conditional logic

CC MCC +7th **S72.326 Nondisplaced transverse fracture of shaft of unspecified femur**
HAC 7th characters A - C see Appendix B for HAC conditional logic

\+ **S72.33 Oblique fracture of shaft of femur**

CC MCC +7th **S72.331 Displaced oblique fracture of shaft of right femur**
HAC 7th characters A - C see Appendix B for HAC conditional logic

CC MCC +7th **S72.332 Displaced oblique fracture of shaft of left femur**
HAC 7th characters A - C see Appendix B for HAC conditional logic

CC MCC +7th **S72.333 Displaced oblique fracture of shaft of unspecified femur**
HAC 7th characters A - C see Appendix B for HAC conditional logic

CC MCC +7th **S72.334 Nondisplaced oblique fracture of shaft of right femur**
HAC 7th characters A - C see Appendix B for HAC conditional logic

CC MCC +7th **S72.335 Nondisplaced oblique fracture of shaft of left femur**
HAC 7th characters A - C see Appendix B for HAC conditional logic

CC MCC +7th **S72.336 Nondisplaced oblique fracture of shaft of unspecified femur**
HAC 7th characters A - C see Appendix B for HAC conditional logic

\+ **S72.34 Spiral fracture of shaft of femur**

CC MCC +7th **S72.341 Displaced spiral fracture of shaft of right femur**
HAC 7th characters A - C see Appendix B for HAC conditional logic

CC MCC +7th **S72.342 Displaced spiral fracture of shaft of left femur**
HAC 7th characters A - C see Appendix B for HAC conditional logic

CC MCC +7th **S72.343 Displaced spiral fracture of shaft of unspecified femur**
HAC 7th characters A - C see Appendix B for HAC conditional logic

CC MCC +7th **S72.344 Nondisplaced spiral fracture of shaft of right femur**
HAC 7th characters A - C see Appendix B for HAC conditional logic

CC MCC +7th **S72.345 Nondisplaced spiral fracture of shaft of left femur**
HAC 7th characters A - C see Appendix B for HAC conditional logic

CC MCC +7th **S72.346 Nondisplaced spiral fracture of shaft of unspecified femur**
HAC 7th characters A - C see Appendix B for HAC conditional logic

\+ **S72.35 Comminuted fracture of shaft of femur**

CC MCC +7th **S72.351 Displaced comminuted fracture of shaft of right femur**
HAC 7th characters A - C see Appendix B for HAC conditional logic

CC MCC +7th **S72.352 Displaced comminuted fracture of shaft of left femur**
HAC 7th characters A - C see Appendix B for HAC conditional logic

CC MCC +7th **S72.353 Displaced comminuted fracture of shaft of unspecified femur**
HAC 7th characters A - C see Appendix B for HAC conditional logic

CC MCC +7th **S72.354 Nondisplaced comminuted fracture of shaft of right femur**
HAC 7th characters A - C see Appendix B for HAC conditional logic

CC MCC +7th **S72.355 Nondisplaced comminuted fracture of shaft of left femur**
HAC 7th characters A - C see Appendix B for HAC conditional logic

CC MCC +7th **S72.356 Nondisplaced comminuted fracture of shaft of unspecified femur**
HAC 7th characters A - C see Appendix B for HAC conditional logic

\+ **S72.36 Segmental fracture of shaft of femur**

CC MCC +7th **S72.361 Displaced segmental fracture of shaft of right femur**
HAC 7th characters A - C see Appendix B for HAC conditional logic

CC MCC +7th **S72.362 Displaced segmental fracture of shaft of left femur**
HAC 7th characters A - C see Appendix B for HAC conditional logic

CC MCC +7th **S72.363 Displaced segmental fracture of shaft of unspecified femur**
HAC 7th characters A - C see Appendix B for HAC conditional logic

CC MCC +7th **S72.364 Nondisplaced segmental fracture of shaft of right femur**
HAC 7th characters A - C see Appendix B for HAC conditional logic

CC MCC +7th **S72.365 Nondisplaced segmental fracture of shaft of left femur**
HAC 7th characters A - C see Appendix B for HAC conditional logic

CC MCC +7th **S72.366 Nondisplaced segmental fracture of shaft of unspecified femur**
HAC 7th characters A - C see Appendix B for HAC conditional logic

\+ **S72.39 Other fracture of shaft of femur**

CC MCC +7th **S72.391 Other fracture of shaft of right femur**
HAC 7th characters A - C see Appendix B for HAC conditional logic

CC MCC +7th **S72.392 Other fracture of shaft of left femur**
HAC 7th characters A - C see Appendix B for HAC conditional logic

CC MCC +7th **S72.399 Other fracture of shaft of unspecified femur**
HAC 7th characters A - C see Appendix B for HAC conditional logic

\+ **S72.4 Fracture of lower end of femur**
Fracture of distal end of femur
Excludes2: *fracture of shaft of femur (S72.3-)*
physeal fracture of lower end of femur (S79.1-)

\+ **S72.40 Unspecified fracture of lower end of femur**

CC MCC +7th **S72.401 Unspecified fracture of lower end of right femur**
AHA CC: 4Q, 2016, 42-43
HAC 7th characters A - C see Appendix B for HAC conditional logic

CC MCC +7th **S72.402 Unspecified fracture of lower end of left femur**
HAC 7th characters A - C see Appendix B for HAC conditional logic

CC MCC +7th **S72.409 Unspecified fracture of lower end of unspecified femur**
HAC 7th characters A - C see Appendix B for HAC conditional logic

\+ **S72.41 Unspecified condyle fracture of lower end of femur**
Condyle fracture of femur NOS

CC MCC +7th **S72.411 Displaced unspecified condyle fracture of lower end of right femur**
HAC 7th characters A - C see Appendix B for HAC conditional logic

CC MCC +7th **S72.412 Displaced unspecified condyle fracture of lower end of left femur**
HAC 7th characters A - C see Appendix B for HAC conditional logic

CC MCC +7th **S72.413 Displaced unspecified condyle fracture of lower end of unspecified femur**
HAC 7th characters A - C see Appendix B for HAC conditional logic

CC MCC +7th **S72.414 Nondisplaced unspecified condyle fracture of lower end of right femur**
HAC 7th characters A - C see Appendix B for HAC conditional logic

CC MCC +7th **S72.415 Nondisplaced unspecified condyle fracture of lower end of left femur**
HAC 7th characters A - C see Appendix B for HAC conditional logic

CC MCC +7th **S72.416 Nondisplaced unspecified condyle fracture of lower end of unspecified femur**
HAC 7th characters A - C see Appendix B for HAC conditional logic

\+ **S72.42 Fracture of lateral condyle of femur**

CC MCC +7th **S72.421 Displaced fracture of lateral condyle of right femur**
HAC 7th characters A - C see Appendix B for HAC conditional logic

CC MCC +7th **S72.422 Displaced fracture of lateral condyle of left femur**
HAC 7th characters A - C see Appendix B for HAC conditional logic

CC MCC +7th **S72.423 Displaced fracture of lateral condyle of unspecified femur**
HAC 7th characters A - C see Appendix B for HAC conditional logic

CC MCC +7th **S72.424 Nondisplaced fracture of lateral condyle of right femur**
HAC 7th characters A - C see Appendix B for HAC conditional logic

CC MCC +7th **S72.425 Nondisplaced fracture of lateral condyle of left femur**
HAC 7th characters A - C see Appendix B for HAC conditional logic

CC MCC +7th **S72.426 Nondisplaced fracture of lateral condyle of unspecified femur**
HAC 7th characters A - C see Appendix B for HAC conditional logic

\+ **S72.43 Fracture of medial condyle of femur**

CC MCC +7th **S72.431 Displaced fracture of medial condyle of right femur**
HAC 7th characters A - C see Appendix B for HAC conditional logic

CC MCC +7th **S72.432 Displaced fracture of medial condyle of left femur**
HAC 7th characters A - C see Appendix B for HAC conditional logic

CC MCC +7th **S72.433 Displaced fracture of medial condyle of unspecified femur**
HAC 7th characters A - C see Appendix B for HAC conditional logic

CC MCC +7th **S72.434 Nondisplaced fracture of medial condyle of right femur**
HAC 7th characters A - C see Appendix B for HAC conditional logic

CC MCC +7th **S72.435 Nondisplaced fracture of medial condyle of left femur**
HAC 7th characters A - C see Appendix B for HAC conditional logic

CC MCC +7th **S72.436 Nondisplaced fracture of medial condyle of unspecified femur**
HAC 7th characters A - C see Appendix B for HAC conditional logic

\+ **S72.44 Fracture of lower epiphysis (separation) of femur**
Excludes1: *Salter-Harris Type I physeal fracture of lower end of femur (S79.11-)*

CC MCC +7th **S72.441 Displaced fracture of lower epiphysis (separation) of right femur**
HAC 7th characters A - C see Appendix B for HAC conditional logic

CC MCC +7th **S72.442 Displaced fracture of lower epiphysis (separation) of left femur**
HAC 7th characters A - C see Appendix B for HAC conditional logic

CC MCC +7th **S72.443 Displaced fracture of lower epiphysis (separation) of unspecified femur**
HAC 7th characters A - C see Appendix B for HAC conditional logic

CC MCC +7th **S72.444 Nondisplaced fracture of lower epiphysis (separation) of right femur**
HAC 7th characters A - C see Appendix B for HAC conditional logic

CC MCC +7th **S72.445 Nondisplaced fracture of lower epiphysis (separation) of left femur**
HAC 7th characters A - C see Appendix B for HAC conditional logic

CC MCC +7th **S72.446 Nondisplaced fracture of lower epiphysis (separation) of unspecified femur**
HAC 7th characters A - C see Appendix B for HAC conditional logic

\+ **S72.45 Supracondylar fracture without intracondylar extension of lower end of femur**
Supracondylar fracture of lower end of femur NOS
Excludes1: *supracondylar fracture with intracondylar extension of lower end of femur (S72.46-)*

CC MCC +7th **S72.451 Displaced supracondylar fracture without intracondylar extension of lower end of right femur**
HAC 7th characters A - C see Appendix B for HAC conditional logic

CC MCC +7th **S72.452 Displaced supracondylar fracture without intracondylar extension of lower end of left femur**
HAC 7th characters A - C see Appendix B for HAC conditional logic

CC MCC +7th **S72.453 Displaced supracondylar fracture without intracondylar extension of lower end of unspecified femur**
HAC 7th characters A - C see Appendix B for HAC conditional logic

CC MCC +7th **S72.454** **Nondisplaced supracondylar fracture without intracondylar extension of lower end of right femur**
HAC 7th characters A - C see Appendix B for HAC conditional logic

CC MCC +7th **S72.455** **Nondisplaced supracondylar fracture without intracondylar extension of lower end of left femur**
HAC 7th characters A - C see Appendix B for HAC conditional logic

CC MCC +7th **S72.456** **Nondisplaced supracondylar fracture without intracondylar extension of lower end of unspecified femur**
HAC 7th characters A - C see Appendix B for HAC conditional logic

+ **S72.46** **Supracondylar fracture with intracondylar extension of lower end of femur**
Excludes1: *supracondylar fracture without intracondylarextensionoflowerend of femur (S72.45-)*

CC MCC +7th **S72.461** **Displaced supracondylar fracture with intracondylar extension of lower end of right femur**
HAC 7th characters A - C see Appendix B for HAC conditional logic

CC MCC +7th **S72.462** **Displaced supracondylar fracture with intracondylar extension of lower end of left femur**
HAC 7th characters A - C see Appendix B for HAC conditional logic

CC MCC +7th **S72.463** **Displaced supracondylar fracture with intracondylar extension of lower end of unspecified femur**
HAC 7th characters A - C see Appendix B for HAC conditional logic

CC MCC +7th **S72.464** **Nondisplaced supracondylar fracture with intracondylar extension of lower end of right femur**
HAC 7th characters A - C see Appendix B for HAC conditional logic

CC MCC +7th **S72.465** **Nondisplaced supracondylar fracture with intracondylar extension of lower end of left femur**
HAC 7th characters A - C see Appendix B for HAC conditional logic

CC MCC +7th **S72.466** **Nondisplaced supracondylar fracture with intracondylar extension of lower end of unspecified femur**
HAC 7th characters A - C see Appendix B for HAC conditional logic

+ **S72.47** **Torus fracture of lower end of femur**

The appropriate 7th character is to be added to all codes in subcategory **S72.47**
A initial encounter for closed fracture
D subsequent encounter for fracture with routine healing
G subsequent encounter for fracture with delayed healing
K subsequent encounter for fracture with nonunion
P subsequent encounter for fracture with malunion
S sequela

CC +7th **S72.471** **Torus fracture of lower end of right femur**
HAC 7th character A see Appendix B for HAC conditional logic

CC +7th **S72.472** **Torus fracture of lower end of left femur**
HAC 7th character A see Appendix B for HAC conditional logic

CC +7th **S72.479** **Torus fracture of lower end of unspecified femur**
HAC 7th character A see Appendix B for HAC conditional logic

+ **S72.49** **Other fracture of lower end of femur**

CC MCC +7th **S72.491** **Other fracture of lower end of right femur**
HAC 7th characters A - C see Appendix B for HAC conditional logic

CC MCC +7th **S72.492** **Other fracture of lower end of left femur**
HAC 7th characters A - C see Appendix B for HAC conditional logic

CC MCC +7th **S72.499** **Other fracture of lower end of unspecified femur**
HAC 7th characters A - C see Appendix B for HAC conditional logic

MCC + **S72.8** **Other fracture of femur**
HAC 7th characters A - C see Appendix B for HAC conditional logic

+ **S72.8X** **Other fracture of femur**
+7th **S72.8X1** **Other fracture of right femur**
+7th **S72.8X2** **Other fracture of left femur**
+7th **S72.8X9** **Other fracture of unspecified femur**

+ **S72.9** **Unspecified fracture of femur**
Fracture of thigh NOS
Fracture of upper leg NOS
Excludes1: *fracture of hip NOS (S72.00-, S72.01-)*

CC MCC X+7th **S72.90** **Unspecified fracture of unspecified femur**
AHA CC: 4Q, 2012, 93-94
HAC 7th characters A - C see Appendix B for HAC conditional logic

CC MCC X+7th **S72.91** **Unspecified fracture of right femur**
HAC 7th characters A - C see Appendix B for HAC conditional logic

CC MCC X+7th **S72.92** **Unspecified fracture of left femur**
HAC 7th characters A - C see Appendix B for HAC conditional logic

S73 Dislocation and sprain of joint and ligaments of hip

Includes: avulsion of joint or ligament of hip
lacervw ation of cartilage, joint or ligament of hip
sprain of cartilage, joint or ligament of hip
traumatic hemarthrosis of joint or ligament of hip
traumatic rupture of joint or ligament of hip
traumatic subluxation of joint or ligament of hip
traumatic tear of joint or ligament of hip

Code also any associated open wound
Excludes2: *strain of muscle, fascia and tendon of hip and thigh (S76.-)*

The appropriate 7th character is to be added to each code from category S73
A initial encounter
D subsequent encounter
S sequela

+ **S73.0** **Subluxation and dislocation of hip**
Excludes2: *dislocation and subluxation of hip prosthesis (T84.020, T84.021)*

+ **S73.00** **Unspecified subluxation and dislocation of hip**
Dislocation of hip NOS
Subluxation of hip NOS

CC +7th **S73.001** **Unspecified subluxation of right hip**
HAC 7th character A see Appendix B for HAC conditional logic

CC +7th **S73.002** **Unspecified subluxation of left hip**
HAC 7th character A see Appendix B for HAC conditional logic

CC +7th **S73.003** **Unspecified subluxation of unspecified hip**
HAC 7th character A see Appendix B for HAC conditional logic

CC +7th **S73.004** **Unspecified dislocation of right hip**
HAC 7th character A see Appendix B for HAC conditional logic

CC +7th **S73.005** **Unspecified dislocation of left hip**
HAC 7th character A see Appendix B for HAC conditional logic

CC +7th **S73.006** **Unspecified dislocation of unspecified hip**
HAC 7th character A see Appendix B for HAC conditional logic

+ **S73.01** **Posterior subluxation and dislocation of hip**

CC +7th **S73.011** **Posterior subluxation of right hip**
HAC 7th character A see Appendix B for HAC conditional logic

CC +7th **S73.012** **Posterior subluxation of left hip**
HAC 7th character A see Appendix B for HAC conditional logic

CC +7th **S73.013** **Posterior subluxation of unspecified hip**
HAC 7th character A see Appendix B for HAC conditional logic

CC +7th **S73.014** **Posterior dislocation of right hip**
HAC 7th character A see Appendix B for HAC conditional logic

CC +7th **S73.015** **Posterior dislocation of left hip**
HAC 7th character A see Appendix B for HAC conditional logic

CC +7th **S73.016 Posterior dislocation of unspecified hip**
HAC 7th character A see Appendix B for HAC conditional logic

+ **S73.02 Obturator subluxation and dislocation of hip**

CC +7th **S73.021 Obturator subluxation of right hip**
HAC 7th character A see Appendix B for HAC conditional logic

CC +7th **S73.022 Obturator subluxation of left hip**
HAC 7th character A see Appendix B for HAC conditional logic

CC +7th **S73.023 Obturator subluxation of unspecified hip**
HAC 7th character A see Appendix B for HAC conditional logic

CC +7th **S73.024 Obturator dislocation of right hip**
HAC 7th character A see Appendix B for HAC conditional logic

CC +7th **S73.025 Obturator dislocation of left hip**
HAC 7th character A see Appendix B for HAC conditional logic

CC +7th **S73.026 Obturator dislocation of unspecified hip**
HAC 7th character A see Appendix B for HAC conditional logic

+ **S73.03 Other anterior subluxation and dislocation of hip**

CC +7th **S73.031 Other anterior subluxation of right hip**
HAC 7th character A see Appendix B for HAC conditional logic

CC +7th **S73.032 Other anterior subluxation of left hip**
HAC 7th character A see Appendix B for HAC conditional logic

CC +7th **S73.033 Other anterior subluxation of unspecified hip**
HAC 7th character A see Appendix B for HAC conditional logic

CC +7th **S73.034 Other anterior dislocation of right hip**
HAC 7th character A see Appendix B for HAC conditional logic

CC +7th **S73.035 Other anterior dislocation of left hip**
HAC 7th character A see Appendix B for HAC conditional logic

CC +7th **S73.036 Other anterior dislocation of unspecified hip**
HAC 7th character A see Appendix B for HAC conditional logic

+ **S73.04 Central subluxation and dislocation of hip**

CC +7th **S73.041 Central subluxation of right hip**
HAC 7th character A see Appendix B for HAC conditional logic

CC +7th **S73.042 Central subluxation of left hip**
HAC 7th character A see Appendix B for HAC conditional logic

CC +7th **S73.043 Central subluxation of unspecified hip**
HAC 7th character A see Appendix B for HAC conditional logic

CC +7th **S73.044 Central dislocation of right hip**
HAC 7th character A see Appendix B for HAC conditional logic

CC +7th **S73.045 Central dislocation of left hip**
HAC 7th character A see Appendix B for HAC conditional logic

CC +7th **S73.046 Central dislocation of unspecified hip**
HAC 7th character A see Appendix B for HAC conditional logic

+ **S73.1 Sprain of hip**

+ **S73.10 Unspecified sprain of hip**

+7th **S73.101 Unspecified sprain of right hip**

+7th **S73.102 Unspecified sprain of left hip**

+7th **S73.109 Unspecified sprain of unspecified hip**

+ **S73.11 Iliofemoral ligament sprain of hip**

+7th **S73.111 Iliofemoral ligament sprain of right hip**

+7th **S73.112 Iliofemoral ligament sprain of left hip**

+7th **S73.119 Iliofemoral ligament sprain of unspecified hip**

+ **S73.12 Ischiocapsular (ligament) sprain of hip**

+7th **S73.121 Ischiocapsular ligament sprain of right hip**

+7th **S73.122 Ischiocapsular ligament sprain of left hip**

+7th **S73.129 Ischiocapsular ligament sprain of unspecified hip**

+ **S73.19 Other sprain of hip**

+7th **S73.191 Other sprain of right hip**

+7th **S73.192 Other sprain of left hip**
AHA CC: 4Q, 2014, 25

+7th **S73.199 Other sprain of unspecified hip**

S74 Injury of nerves at hip and thigh level

Code also any associated open wound (S71.-)

Excludes2: *injury of nerves at ankle and foot level (S94.-)*
injury of nerves at lower leg level (S84.-)

The appropriate 7th character is to be added to each code from category S74
A initial encounter
D subsequent encounter
S sequela

+ **S74.0 Injury of sciatic nerve at hip and thigh level**

X+7th **S74.00 Injury of sciatic nerve at hip and thigh level, unspecified leg**

X+7th **S74.01 Injury of sciatic nerve at hip and thigh level, right leg**

X+7th **S74.02 Injury of sciatic nerve at hip and thigh level, left leg**

+ **S74.1 Injury of femoral nerve at hip and thigh level**

X+7th **S74.10 Injury of femoral nerve at hip and thigh level, unspecified leg**

X+7th **S74.11 Injury of femoral nerve at hip and thigh level, right leg**

X+7th **S74.12 Injury of femoral nerve at hip and thigh level, left leg**

+ **S74.2 Injury of cutaneous sensory nerve at hip and thigh level**

X+7th **S74.20 Injury of cutaneous sensory nerve at hip and thigh level, unspecified leg**

X+7th **S74.21 Injury of cutaneous sensory nerve at hip and high level, right leg**

X+7th **S74.22 Injury of cutaneous sensory nerve at hip and thigh level, left leg**

+ **S74.8 Injury of other nerves at hip and thigh level**

+ **S74.8X Injury of other nerves at hip and thigh level**

+7th **S74.8X1 Injury of other nerves at hip and thigh level, right leg**

+7th **S74.8X2 Injury of other nerves at hip and thigh level, left leg**

+7th **S74.8X9 Injury of other nerves at hip and thigh level, unspecified leg**

+ **S74.9 Injury of unspecified nerve at hip and thigh level**

X+7th **S74.90 Injury of unspecified nerve at hip and thigh level, unspecified leg**

X+7th **S74.91 Injury of unspecified nerve at hip and thigh level, right leg**

X+7th **S74.92 Injury of unspecified nerve at hip and thigh level, left leg**

S75 Injury of blood vessels at hip and thigh level

Code also any associated open wound (S71.-)

Excludes2: *injury of blood vessels at lower leg level (S85.-)*
injury of popliteal artery (S85.0)

The appropriate 7th character is to be added to each code from category S75
A initial encounter
D subsequent encounter
S sequela

+ **S75.0 Injury of femoral artery**

+ **S75.00 Unspecified injury of femoral artery**

MCC +7th **S75.001 Unspecified injury of femoral artery, right leg**

MCC +7th **S75.002 Unspecified injury of femoral artery, left leg**

MCC +7th **S75.009 Unspecified injury of femoral artery, unspecified leg**

+ **S75.01 Minor laceration of femoral artery**
Incomplete transection of femoral artery
Laceration of femoral artery NOS
Superficial laceration of femoral artery

MCC +7th **S75.011 Minor laceration of femoral artery, right leg**

MCC +7th **S75.012 Minor laceration of femoral artery, left leg**

MCC +7th **S75.019 Minor laceration of femoral artery, unspecified leg**

+ **S75.02 Major laceration of femoral artery**
Complete transection of femoral artery
Traumatic rupture of femoral artery

MCC +7th **S75.021 Major laceration of femoral artery, right leg**

MCC +7th **S75.022 Major laceration of femoral artery, left leg**
MCC +7th **S75.029 Major laceration of femoral artery, unspecified leg**
+ **S75.09 Other specified injury of femoral artery**
MCC +7th **S75.091 Other specified injury of femoral artery, right leg**
MCC +7th **S75.092 Other specified injury of femoral artery, left leg**
MCC +7th **S75.099 Other specified injury of femoral artery, unspecified leg**

+ **S75.1 Injury of femoral vein at hip and thigh level**
+ **S75.10 Unspecified injury of femoral vein at hip and thigh level**
MCC +7th **S75.101 Unspecified injury of femoral vein at hip and thigh level, right leg**
MCC +7th **S75.102 Unspecified injury of femoral vein at hip and thigh level, left leg**
MCC +7th **S75.109 Unspecified injury of femoral vein at hip and thigh level, unspecified leg**
+ **S75.11 Minor laceration of femoral vein at hip and thigh level**
Incomplete transection of femoral vein at hip and thigh level
Laceration of femoral vein at hip and thigh level NOS
Superficial laceration of femoral vein at hip and thigh level
MCC +7th **S75.111 Minor laceration of femoral vein at hip and thigh level, right leg**
MCC +7th **S75.112 Minor laceration of femoral vein at hip and thigh level, left leg**
MCC +7th **S75.119 Minor laceration of femoral vein at hip and thigh level, unspecified leg**
+ **S75.12 Major laceration of femoral vein at hip and thigh level**
Complete transection of femoral vein at hip and thigh level
Traumatic rupture of femoral vein at hip and thigh level
MCC +7th **S75.121 Major laceration of femoral vein at hip and thigh level, right leg**
MCC +7th **S75.122 Major laceration of femoral vein at hip and thigh level, left leg**
MCC +7th **S75.129 Major laceration of femoral vein at hip and thigh level, unspecified leg**
+ **S75.19 Other specified injury of femoral vein at hip and thigh level**
MCC +7th **S75.191 Other specified injury of femoral vein at hip and thigh level, right leg**
MCC +7th **S75.192 Other specified injury of femoral vein at hip and thigh level, left leg**
MCC +7th **S75.199 Other specified injury of femoral vein at hip and thigh level, unspecified leg**

+ **S75.2 Injury of greater saphenous vein at hip and thigh level**
Excludes1: *greater saphenous vein NOS (S85.3)*
+ **S75.20 Unspecified injury of greater saphenous vein at hip and thigh level**
CC +7th **S75.201 Unspecified injury of greater saphenous vein at hip and thigh level, right leg**
CC +7th **S75.202 Unspecified injury of greater saphenous vein at hip and thigh level, left leg**
CC +7th **S75.209 Unspecified injury of greater saphenous vein at hip and thigh level, unspecified leg**
+ **S75.21 Minor laceration of greater saphenous vein at hip and thigh level**
Incomplete transection of greater saphenous vein at hip and thigh level
Laceration of greater saphenous vein at hip and thigh level NOS
Superficial laceration of greater saphenous vein at hip and thigh level
CC +7th **S75.211 Minor laceration of greater saphenous vein at hip and thigh level, right leg**
CC +7th **S75.212 Minor laceration of greater saphenous vein at hip and thigh level, left leg**
CC +7th **S75.219 Minor laceration of greater saphenous vein at hip and thigh level, unspecified leg**
+ **S75.22 Major laceration of greater saphenous vein at hip and thigh level**
Complete transection of greater saphenous vein at hip and thigh level
Traumatic rupture of greater saphenous vein at hip and thigh level
CC +7th **S75.221 Major laceration of greater saphenous vein at hip and thigh level, right leg**
CC +7th **S75.222 Major laceration of greater saphenous vein at hip and thigh level, left leg**
CC +7th **S75.229 Major laceration of greater saphenous vein at hip and thigh level, unspecified leg**
+ **S75.29 Other specified injury of greater saphenous vein at hip and thigh level**
CC +7th **S75.291 Other specified injury of greater saphenous vein at hip and thigh level, right leg**
CC +7th **S75.292 Other specified injury of greater saphenous vein at hip and thigh level, left leg**
CC +7th **S75.299 Other specified injury of greater saphenous vein at hip and thigh level, unspecified leg**

+ **S75.8 Injury of other blood vessels at hip and thigh level**
+ **S75.80 Unspecified injury of other blood vessels at hip and thigh level**
CC +7th **S75.801 Unspecified injury of other blood vessels at hip and thigh level, right leg**
CC +7th **S75.802 Unspecified injury of other blood vessels at hip and thigh level, left leg**
CC +7th **S75.809 Unspecified injury of other blood vessels at hip and thigh level, unspecified leg**
+ **S75.81 Laceration of other blood vessels at hip and thigh level**
CC +7th **S75.811 Laceration of other blood vessels at hip and thigh level, right leg**
CC +7th **S75.812 Laceration of other blood vessels at hip and thigh level, left leg**
CC +7th **S75.819 Laceration of other blood vessels at hip and thigh level, unspecified leg**
+ **S75.89 Other specified injury of other blood vessels at hip and thigh level**
CC +7th **S75.891 Other specified injury of other blood vessels at hip and thigh level, right leg**
CC +7th **S75.892 Other specified injury of other blood vessels at hip and thigh level, left leg**
CC +7th **S75.899 Other specified injury of other blood vessels at hip and thigh level, unspecified leg**

+ **S75.9 Injury of unspecified blood vessel at hip and thigh level**
+ **S75.90 Unspecified injury of unspecified blood vessel at hip and thigh level**
CC +7th **S75.901 Unspecified injury of unspecified blood vessel at hip and thigh level, right leg**
CC +7th **S75.902 Unspecified injury of unspecified blood vessel at hip and thigh level, left leg**
CC +7th **S75.909 Unspecified injury of unspecified blood vessel at hip and thigh level, unspecified leg**
+ **S75.91 Laceration of unspecified blood vessel at hip and thigh level**
CC +7th **S75.911 Laceration of unspecified blood vessel at hip and thigh level, right leg**
CC +7th **S75.912 Laceration of unspecified blood vessel at hip and thigh level, left leg**
CC +7th **S75.919 Laceration of unspecified blood vessel at hip and thigh level, unspecified leg**
+ **S75.99 Other specified injury of unspecified blood vessel at hip and thigh level**
CC +7th **S75.991 Other specified injury of unspecified blood vessel at hip and thigh level, right leg**
CC +7th **S75.992 Other specified injury of unspecified blood vessel at hip and thigh level, left leg**
CC +7th **S75.999 Other specified injury of unspecified blood vessel at hip and thigh level, unspecified leg**

S76 Injury of muscle, fascia and tendon at hip and thigh level

Code also any associated open wound (S71.-)

Excludes2: *injury of muscle, fascia and tendon at lower leg level (S86)*
sprain of joint and ligament of hip (S73.1)

The appropriate 7th character is to be added to each code from category S76
A initial encounter
D subsequent encounter
S sequela

+ **S76.0 Injury of muscle, fascia and tendon of hip**
+ **S76.00 Unspecified injury of muscle, fascia and tendon of hip**
+7th **S76.001 Unspecified injury of muscle, fascia and tendon of right hip**
+7th **S76.002 Unspecified injury of muscle, fascia and tendon of left hip**
+7th **S76.009 Unspecified injury of muscle, fascia and tendon of unspecified hip**
+ **S76.01 Strain of muscle, fascia and tendon of hip**
+7th **S76.011 Strain of muscle, fascia and tendon of right hip**
+7th **S76.012 Strain of muscle, fascia and tendon of left hip**
+7th **S76.019 Strain of muscle, fascia and tendon of unspecified hip**
+ **S76.02 Laceration of muscle, fascia and tendon of hip**
CC +7th **S76.021 Laceration of muscle, fascia and tendon of right hip**
CC +7th **S76.022 Laceration of muscle, fascia and tendon of left hip**
CC +7th **S76.029 Laceration of muscle, fascia and tendon of unspecified hip**
+ **S76.09 Other specified injury of muscle, fascia and tendon of hip**
+7th **S76.091 Other specified injury of muscle, fascia and tendon of right hip**
+7th **S76.092 Other specified injury of muscle, fascia and tendon of left hip**
+7th **S76.099 Other specified injury of muscle, fascia and tendon of unspecified hip**
+ **S76.1 Injury of quadriceps muscle, fascia and tendon**
Injury of patellar ligament (tendon)
+ **S76.10 Unspecified injury of quadriceps muscle, fascia and tendon**
+7th **S76.101 Unspecified injury of right quadriceps muscle, fascia and tendon**
+7th **S76.102 Unspecified injury of left quadriceps muscle, fascia and tendon**
+7th **S76.109 Unspecified injury of unspecified quadriceps muscle, fascia and tendon**
+ **S76.11 Strain of quadriceps muscle, fascia and tendon**
+7th **S76.111 Strain of right quadriceps muscle, fascia and tendon**
+7th **S76.112 Strain of left quadriceps muscle, fascia and tendon**
+7th **S76.119 Strain of unspecified quadriceps muscle, fascia and tendon**
+ **S76.12 Laceration of quadriceps muscle, fascia and tendon**
CC +7th **S76.121 Laceration of right quadriceps muscle, fascia and tendon**
CC +7th **S76.122 Laceration of left quadriceps muscle, fascia and tendon**
CC +7th **S76.129 Laceration of unspecified quadriceps muscle, fascia and tendon**
+ **S76.19 Other specified injury of quadriceps muscle, fascia and tendon**
+7th **S76.191 Other specified injury of right quadriceps muscle, fascia and tendon**
+7th **S76.192 Other specified injury of left quadriceps muscle, fascia and tendon**
+7th **S76.199 Other specified injury of unspecified quadriceps muscle, fascia and tendon**
+ **S76.2 Injury of adductor muscle, fascia and tendon of thigh**
+ **S76.20 Unspecified injury of adductor muscle, fascia and tendon of thigh**
+7th **S76.201 Unspecified injury of adductor muscle, fascia and tendon of right thigh**
+7th **S76.202 Unspecified injury of adductor muscle, fascia and tendon of left thigh**
+7th **S76.209 Unspecified injury of adductor muscle, fascia and tendon of unspecified thigh**
+ **S76.21 Strain of adductor muscle, fascia and tendon of thigh**
+7th **S76.211 Strain of adductor muscle, fascia and tendon of right thigh**
+7th **S76.212 Strain of adductor muscle, fascia and tendon of left thigh**
+7th **S76.219 Strain of adductor muscle, fascia and tendon of unspecified thigh**
+ **S76.22 Laceration of adductor muscle, fascia and tendon of thigh**
CC +7th **S76.221 Laceration of adductor muscle, fascia and tendon of right thigh**
CC +7th **S76.222 Laceration of adductor muscle, fascia and tendon of left thigh**
CC +7th **S76.229 Laceration of adductor muscle, fascia and tendon of unspecified thigh**
+ **S76.29 Other injury of adductor muscle, fascia and tendon of thigh**
+7th **S76.291 Other injury of adductor muscle, fascia and tendon of right thigh**
+7th **S76.292 Other injury of adductor muscle, fascia and tendon of left thigh**
+7th **S76.299 Other injury of adductor muscle, fascia and tendon of unspecified thigh**
+ **S76.3 Injury of muscle, fascia and tendon of the posterior muscle group at thigh level**
+ **S76.30 Unspecified injury of muscle, fascia and tendon of the posterior muscle group at thigh level**
+7th **S76.301 Unspecified injury of muscle, fascia and tendon of the posterior muscle group at thigh level, right thigh**
+7th **S76.302 Unspecified injury of muscle, fascia and tendon of the posterior muscle group at thigh level, left thigh**
+7th **S76.309 Unspecified injury of muscle, fascia and tendon of the posterior muscle group at thigh level, unspecified thigh**
+ **S76.31 Strain of muscle, fascia and tendon of the posterior muscle group at thigh level**
+7th **S76.311 Strain of muscle, fascia and tendon of the posterior muscle group at thigh level, right thigh**
+7th **S76.312 Strain of muscle, fascia and tendon of the posterior muscle group at thigh level, left thigh**
+7th **S76.319 Strain of muscle, fascia and tendon of the posterior muscle group at thigh level, unspecified thigh**
+ **S76.32 Laceration of muscle, fascia and tendon of the posterior muscle group at thigh level**
CC +7th **S76.321 Laceration of muscle, fascia and tendon of the posterior muscle group at thigh level, right thigh**
CC +7th **S76.322 Laceration of muscle, fascia and tendon of the posterior muscle group at thigh level, left thigh**
CC +7th **S76.329 Laceration of muscle, fascia and tendon of the posterior muscle group at thigh level, unspecified thigh**
+ **S76.39 Other specified injury of muscle, fascia and tendon of the posterior muscle group at thigh level**
+7th **S76.391 Other specified injury of muscle, fascia and tendon of the posterior muscle group at thigh level, right thigh**
+7th **S76.392 Other specified injury of muscle, fascia and tendon of the posterior muscle group at thigh level, left thigh**
+7th **S76.399 Other specified injury of muscle, fascia and tendon of the posterior muscle group at thigh level, unspecified thigh**
+ **S76.8 Injury of other specified muscles, fascia and tendons at thigh level**
+ **S76.80 Unspecified injury of other specified muscles, fascia and tendons at thigh level**
+7th **S76.801 Unspecified injury of other specified muscles, fascia and tendons at thigh level, right thigh**

+7th **S76.802** **Unspecified injury of other specified muscles, fascia and tendons at thigh level, left thigh**
+7th **S76.809** **Unspecified injury of other specified muscles, fascia and tendons at thigh level, unspecified thigh**
+ **S76.81** **Strain of other specified muscles, fascia and tendons at thigh level**
+7th **S76.811** **Strain of other specified muscles, fascia and tendons at thigh level, right thigh**
+7th **S76.812** **Strain of other specified muscles, fascia and tendons at thigh level, left thigh**
+7th **S76.819** **Strain of other specified muscles, fascia and tendons at thigh level, unspecified thigh**
+ **S76.82** **Laceration of other specified muscles, fascia and tendons at thigh level**
CC +7th **S76.821** **Laceration of other specified muscles, fascia and tendons at thigh level, right thigh**
CC +7th **S76.822** **Laceration of other specified muscles, fascia and tendons at thigh level, left thigh**
CC +7th **S76.829** **Laceration of other specified muscles, fascia and tendons at thigh level, unspecified thigh**
+ **S76.89** **Other injury of other specified muscles, fascia and tendons at thigh level**
+7th **S76.891** **Other injury of other specified muscles, fascia and tendons at thigh level, right thigh**
+7th **S76.892** **Other injury of other specified muscles, fascia and tendons at thigh level, left thigh**
+7th **S76.899** **Other injury of other specified muscles, fascia and tendons at thigh level, unspecified thigh**
+ **S76.9** **Injury of unspecified muscles, fascia and tendons at thigh level**
+ **S76.90** **Unspecified injury of unspecified muscles, fascia and tendons at thigh level**
+7th **S76.901** **Unspecified injury of unspecified muscles, fascia and tendons at thigh level, right thigh**
+7th **S76.902** **Unspecified injury of unspecified muscles, fascia and tendons at thigh level, left thigh**
+7th **S76.909** **Unspecified injury of unspecified muscles, fascia and tendons at thigh level, unspecified thigh**
+ **S76.91** **Strain of unspecified muscles, fascia and tendons at thigh level**
+7th **S76.911** **Strain of unspecified muscles, fascia and tendons at thigh level, right thigh**
+7th **S76.912** **Strain of unspecified muscles, fascia and tendons at thigh level, left thigh**
+7th **S76.919** **Strain of unspecified muscles, fascia and tendons at thigh level, unspecified thigh**
+ **S76.92** **Laceration of unspecified muscles, fascia and tendons at thigh level**
CC +7th **S76.921** **Laceration of unspecified muscles, fascia and tendons at thigh level, right thigh**
CC +7th **S76.922** **Laceration of unspecified muscles, fascia and tendons at thigh level, left thigh**
CC +7th **S76.929** **Laceration of unspecified muscles, fascia and tendons at thigh level, unspecified thigh**
+ **S76.99** **Other specified injury of unspecified muscles, fascia and tendons at thigh level**
+7th **S76.991** **Other specified injury of unspecified muscles, fascia and tendons at thigh level, right thigh**
+7th **S76.992** **Other specified injury of unspecified muscles, fascia and tendons at thigh level, left thigh**
+7th **S76.999** **Other specified injury of unspecified muscles, fascia and tendons at thigh level, unspecified thigh**

S77 Crushing injury of hip and thigh

Use additional code(s) for all associated injuries

Excludes2: *crushing injury of ankle and foot (S97.-)*
crushing injury of lower leg (S87.-)

The appropriate 7th character is to be added to each code from category S77
A initial encounter
D subsequent encounter
S sequela

+ **S77.0** **Crushing injury of hip**
CC X+7th **S77.00** **Crushing injury of unspecified hip**
HAC 7th character A see Appendix B for HAC conditional logic
CC X+7th **S77.01** **Crushing injury of right hip**
HAC 7th character A see Appendix B for HAC conditional logic
CC X+7th **S77.02** **Crushing injury of left hip**
HAC 7th character A see Appendix B for HAC conditional logic
+ **S77.1** **Crushing injury of thigh**
CC X+7th **S77.10** **Crushing injury of unspecified thigh**
HAC 7th character A see Appendix B for HAC conditional logic
CC X+7th **S77.11** **Crushing injury of right thigh**
HAC 7th character A see Appendix B for HAC conditional logic
CC X+7th **S77.12** **Crushing injury of left thigh**
HAC 7th character A see Appendix B for HAC conditional logic
+ **S77.2** **Crushing injury of hip with thigh**
X+7th **S77.20** **Crushing injury of unspecified hip with thigh**
X+7th **S77.21** **Crushing injury of right hip with thigh**
X+7th **S77.22** **Crushing injury of left hip with thigh**

S78 Traumatic amputation of hip and thigh

An amputation not identified as partial or complete should be coded to complete

Excludes1: *traumatic amputation of knee (S88.0-)*

The appropriate 7th character is to be added to each code from category S78
A initial encounter
D subsequent encounter
S sequela

+ **S78.0** **Traumatic amputation at hip joint**
+ **S78.01** **Complete traumatic amputation at hip joint**
CC +7th **S78.011** **Complete traumatic amputation at right hip joint**
CC +7th **S78.012** **Complete traumatic amputation at left hip joint**
CC +7th **S78.019** **Complete traumatic amputation at unspecified hip joint**
+ **S78.02** **Partial traumatic amputation at hip joint**
CC +7th **S78.021** **Partial traumatic amputation at right hip joint**
CC +7th **S78.022** **Partial traumatic amputation at left hip joint**
CC +7th **S78.029** **Partial traumatic amputation at unspecified hip joint**
+ **S78.1** **Traumatic amputation at level between hip and knee**
Excludes1: *traumatic amputation of knee (S88.0-)*
+ **S78.11** **Complete traumatic amputation at level between hip and knee**
CC +7th **S78.111** **Complete traumatic amputation at level between right hip and knee**
CC +7th **S78.112** **Complete traumatic amputation at level between left hip and knee**
CC +7th **S78.119** **Complete traumatic amputation at level between unspecified hip and knee**
+ **S78.12** **Partial traumatic amputation at level between hip and knee**
CC +7th **S78.121** **Partial traumatic amputation at level between right hip and knee**
CC +7th **S78.122** **Partial traumatic amputation at level between left hip and knee**
CC +7th **S78.129** **Partial traumatic amputation at level between unspecified hip and knee**

+ S78.9 **Traumatic amputation of hip and thigh, level unspecified**
  + S78.91 **Complete traumatic amputation of hip and thigh, level unspecified**
    - CC +7th **S78.911** **Complete traumatic amputation of right hip and thigh, level unspecified**
    - CC +7th **S78.912** **Complete traumatic amputation of left hip and thigh, level unspecified**
    - CC +7th **S78.919** **Complete traumatic amputation of unspecified hip and thigh, level unspecified**
  + S78.92 **Partial traumatic amputation of hip and thigh, level unspecified**
    - CC +7th **S78.921** **Partial traumatic amputation of right hip and thigh, level unspecified**
    - CC +7th **S78.922** **Partial traumatic amputation of left hip and thigh, level unspecified**
    - CC +7th **S78.929** **Partial traumatic amputation of unspecified hip and thigh, level unspecified**

S79 Other and unspecified injuries of hip and thigh

NOTE A fracture not indicated as open or closed should be coded to closed

The appropriate 7th character is to be added to each code from subcategories **S79.0** and **S79.1**
A initial encounter for closed fracture
D subsequent encounter for fracture with routine healing
G subsequent encounter for fracture with delayed healing
K subsequent encounter for fracture with nonunion
P subsequent encounter for fracture with malunion
S sequela

Review coding guideline C.19.c

+ S79.0 **Physeal fracture of upper end of femur**
  Excludes1: *apophyseal fracture of upper end of femur (S72.13-)*
  nontraumatic slipped upper femoral epiphysis (M93.0-)
  + S79.00 **Unspecified physeal fracture of upper end of femur**
    - CC MCC +7th **S79.001** **Unspecified physeal fracture of upper end of right femur**
      HAC 7th character A see Appendix B for HAC conditional logic
    - CC MCC +7th **S79.002** **Unspecified physeal fracture of upper end of left femur**
      HAC 7th character A see Appendix B for HAC conditional logic
    - CC MCC +7th **S79.009** **Unspecified physeal fracture of upper end of unspecified femur**
      HAC 7th character A see Appendix B for HAC conditional logic
  + S79.01 **Salter-Harris Type I physeal fracture of upper end of femur**
    Acute on chronic slipped capital femoral epiphysis (traumatic)
    Acute slipped capital femoral epiphysis (traumatic)
    Capital femoral epiphyseal fracture
    Excludes1: *chronic slipped upper femoral epiphysis(nontraumatic)(M93.02-)*
    - CC MCC +7th **S79.011** **Salter-Harris Type I physeal fracture of upper end of right femur**
      HAC 7th character A see Appendix B for HAC conditional logic
    - CC MCC +7th **S79.012** **Salter-Harris Type I physeal fracture of upper end of left femur**
      HAC 7th character A see Appendix B for HAC conditional logic
    - CC MCC +7th **S79.019** **Salter-Harris Type I physeal fracture of upper end of unspecified femur**
      HAC 7th character A see Appendix B for HAC conditional logic
  + S79.09 **Other physeal fracture of upper end of femur**
    - CC MCC +7th **S79.091** **Other physeal fracture of upper end of right femur**
      HAC 7th character A see Appendix B for HAC conditional logic
    - CC MCC +7th **S79.092** **Other physeal fracture of upper end of left femur**
      HAC 7th character A see Appendix B for HAC conditional logic
    - CC MCC +7th **S79.099** **Other physeal fracture of upper end of unspecified femur**
      HAC 7th character A see Appendix B for HAC conditional logic

+ S79.1 **Physeal fracture of lower end of femur**
  + S79.10 **Unspecified physeal fracture of lower end of femur**
    - CC +7th **S79.101** **Unspecified physeal fracture of lower end of right femur**
      HAC 7th character A see Appendix B for HAC conditional logic
    - CC +7th **S79.102** **Unspecified physeal fracture of lower end of left femur**
      HAC 7th character A see Appendix B for HAC conditional logic
    - CC +7th **S79.109** **Unspecified physeal fracture of lower end of unspecified femur**
      HAC 7th character A see Appendix B for HAC conditional logic
  + S79.11 **Salter-Harris Type I physeal fracture of lower end of femur**
    - CC +7th **S79.111** **Salter-Harris Type I physeal fracture of lower end of right femur**
      HAC 7th character A see Appendix B for HAC conditional logic
    - CC +7th **S79.112** **Salter-Harris Type I physeal fracture of lower end of left femur**
      HAC 7th character A see Appendix B for HAC conditional logic
    - CC +7th **S79.119** **Salter-Harris Type I physeal fracture of lower end of unspecified femur**
      HAC 7th character A see Appendix B for HAC conditional logic
  + S79.12 **Salter-Harris Type II physeal fracture of lower end of femur**
    - CC +7th **S79.121** **Salter-Harris Type II physeal fracture of lower end of right femur**
      HAC 7th character A see Appendix B for HAC conditional logic
    - CC +7th **S79.122** **Salter-Harris Type II physeal fracture of lower end of left femur**
      HAC 7th character A see Appendix B for HAC conditional logic
    - CC +7th **S79.129** **Salter-Harris Type II physeal fracture of lower end of unspecified femur**
      HAC 7th character A see Appendix B for HAC conditional logic
  + S79.13 **Salter-Harris Type III physeal fracture of lower end of femur**
    - CC +7th **S79.131** **Salter-Harris Type III physeal fracture of lower end of right femur**
      HAC 7th character A see Appendix B for HAC conditional logic
    - CC +7th **S79.132** **Salter-Harris Type III physeal fracture of lower end of left femur**
      HAC 7th character A see Appendix B for HAC conditional logic
    - CC +7th **S79.139** **Salter-Harris Type III physeal fracture of lower end of unspecified femur**
      HAC 7th character A see Appendix B for HAC conditional logic
  + S79.14 **Salter-Harris Type IV physeal fracture of lower end of femur**
    - CC +7th **S79.141** **Salter-Harris Type IV physeal fracture of lower end of right femur**
      HAC 7th character A see Appendix B for HAC conditional logic
    - CC +7th **S79.142** **Salter-Harris Type IV physeal fracture of lower end of left femur**
      HAC 7th character A see Appendix B for HAC conditional logic
    - CC +7th **S79.149** **Salter-Harris Type IV physeal fracture of lower end of unspecified femur**
      HAC 7th character A see Appendix B for HAC conditional logic
  + S79.19 **Other physeal fracture of lower end of femur**
    - CC +7th **S79.191** **Other physeal fracture of lower end of right femur**
      HAC 7th character A see Appendix B for HAC conditional logic

CC +7th **S79.192 Other physeal fracture of lower end of left femur**
HAC 7th character A see Appendix B for HAC conditional logic

CC +7th **S79.199 Other physeal fracture of lower end of unspecified femur**
HAC 7th character A see Appendix B for HAC conditional logic

\+ **S79.8 Other specified injuries of hip and thigh**

The appropriate 7th character is to be added to each code in subcategory **S79.8**
A initial encounter
D subsequent encounter
S sequela

\+ **S79.81 Other specified injuries of hip**
+7th **S79.811 Other specified injuries of right hip**
+7th **S79.812 Other specified injuries of left hip**
+7th **S79.819 Other specified injuries of unspecified hip**

\+ **S79.82 Other specified injuries of thigh**
+7th **S79.821 Other specified injuries of right thigh**
+7th **S79.822 Other specified injuries of left thigh**
+7th **S79.829 Other specified injuries of unspecified thigh**

\+ **S79.9 Unspecified injury of hip and thigh**

The appropriate 7th character is to be added to each code in subcategory **S79.9**
A - initial encounter
D - subsequent encounter
S - sequela

\+ **S79.91 Unspecified injury of hip**
+7th **S79.911 Unspecified injury of right hip**
+7th **S79.912 Unspecified injury of left hip**
+7th **S79.919 Unspecified injury of unspecified hip**

\+ **S79.92 Unspecified injury of thigh**
+7th **S79.921 Unspecified injury of right thigh**
+7th **S79.922 Unspecified injury of left thigh**
+7th **S79.929 Unspecified injury of unspecified thigh**

Injuries to the knee and lower leg (S80-S89)

Excludes2: *burns and corrosions (T20-T32)*
frostbite (T33-T34)
injuries of ankle and foot, except fracture of ankle and malleolus (S90-S99)
insect bite or sting, venomous (T63.4)

S80 Superficial injury of knee and lower leg

Excludes2: *superficial injury of ankle and foot (S90.-)*

The appropriate 7th character is to be added to each code from category S80
A initial encounter
D subsequent encounter
S sequela

\+ **S80.0 Contusion of knee**
X+7th **S80.00 Contusion of unspecified knee**
X+7th **S80.01 Contusion of right knee**
X+7th **S80.02 Contusion of left knee**

\+ **S80.1 Contusion of lower leg**
X+7th **S80.10 Contusion of unspecified lower leg**
X+7th **S80.11 Contusion of right lower leg**
X+7th **S80.12 Contusion of left lower leg**

\+ **S80.2 Other superficial injuries of knee**

\+ **S80.21 Abrasion of knee**
+7th **S80.211 Abrasion, right knee**
+7th **S80.212 Abrasion, left knee**
+7th **S80.219 Abrasion, unspecified knee**

\+ **S80.22 Blister (nonthermal) of knee**
+7th **S80.221 Blister (nonthermal), right knee**
+7th **S80.222 Blister (nonthermal), left knee**
+7th **S80.229 Blister (nonthermal), unspecified knee**

\+ **S80.24 External constriction of knee**
+7th **S80.241 External constriction, right knee**
+7th **S80.242 External constriction, left knee**
+7th **S80.249 External constriction, unspecified knee**

\+ **S80.25 Superficial foreign body of knee**
Splinter in the knee
+7th **S80.251 Superficial foreign body, right knee**
+7th **S80.252 Superficial foreign body, left knee**
+7th **S80.259 Superficial foreign body, unspecified knee**

\+ **S80.26 Insect bite (nonvenomous) of knee**
+7th **S80.261 Insect bite (nonvenomous), right knee**
+7th **S80.262 Insect bite (nonvenomous), left knee**
+7th **S80.269 Insect bite (nonvenomous), unspecified knee**

\+ **S80.27 Other superficial bite of knee**
Excludes1: *open bite of knee (S81.05-)*
+7th **S80.271 Other superficial bite of right knee**
+7th **S80.272 Other superficial bite of left knee**
+7th **S80.279 Other superficial bite of unspecified knee**

\+ **S80.8 Other superficial injuries of lower leg**

\+ **S80.81 Abrasion of lower leg**
+7th **S80.811 Abrasion, right lower leg**
+7th **S80.812 Abrasion, left lower leg**
+7th **S80.819 Abrasion, unspecified lower leg**

\+ **S80.82 Blister (nonthermal) of lower leg**
+7th **S80.821 Blister (nonthermal), right lower leg**
+7th **S80.822 Blister (nonthermal), left lower leg**
+7th **S80.829 Blister (nonthermal), unspecified lower leg**

\+ **S80.84 External constriction of lower leg**
+7th **S80.841 External constriction, right lower leg**
+7th **S80.842 External constriction, left lower leg**
+7th **S80.849 External constriction, unspecified lower leg**

\+ **S80.85 Superficial foreign body of lower leg**
Splinter in the lower leg
+7th **S80.851 Superficial foreign body, right lower leg**
+7th **S80.852 Superficial foreign body, left lower leg**
+7th **S80.859 Superficial foreign body, unspecified lower leg**

\+ **S80.86 Insect bite (nonvenomous) of lower leg**
+7th **S80.861 Insect bite (nonvenomous), right lower leg**
+7th **S80.862 Insect bite (nonvenomous), left lower leg**
+7th **S80.869 Insect bite (nonvenomous), unspecified lower leg**

\+ **S80.87 Other superficial bite of lower leg**
Excludes1: *open bite of lower leg (S81.85-)*
+7th **S80.871 Other superficial bite, right lower leg**
+7th **S80.872 Other superficial bite, left lower leg**
+7th **S80.879 Other superficial bite, unspecified lower leg**

\+ **S80.9 Unspecified superficial injury of knee and lower leg**

\+ **S80.91 Unspecified superficial injury of knee**
+7th **S80.911 Unspecified superficial injury of right knee**
+7th **S80.912 Unspecified superficial injury of left knee**
+7th **S80.919 Unspecified superficial injury of unspecified knee**

\+ **S80.92 Unspecified superficial injury of lower leg**
+7th **S80.921 Unspecified superficial injury of right lower leg**
+7th **S80.922 Unspecified superficial injury of left lower leg**
+7th **S80.929 Unspecified superficial injury of unspecified lower leg**

S81 Open wound of knee and lower leg

Code also any associated wound infection

Excludes1: *open fracture of knee and lower leg (S82.-)*
traumatic amputation of lower leg (S88.-)

Excludes2: *open wound of ankle and foot (S91.-)*

The appropriate 7th character is to be added to each code from category S81
A initial encounter
D subsequent encounter
S sequela

+ **S81.0 Open wound of knee**
  + **S81.00 Unspecified open wound of knee**
    - +7th **S81.001 Unspecified open wound, right knee**
    - +7th **S81.002 Unspecified open wound, left knee**
    - +7th **S81.009 Unspecified open wound, unspecified knee**
  + **S81.01 Laceration without foreign body of knee**
    - +7th **S81.011 Laceration without foreign body, right knee**
    - +7th **S81.012 Laceration without foreign body, left knee**
    - +7th **S81.019 Laceration without foreign body, unspecified knee**
  + **S81.02 Laceration with foreign body of knee**
    - +7th **S81.021 Laceration with foreign body, right knee**
    - +7th **S81.022 Laceration with foreign body, left knee**
    - +7th **S81.029 Laceration with foreign body, unspecified knee**
  + **S81.03 Puncture wound without foreign body of knee**
    - +7th **S81.031 Puncture wound without foreign body, right knee**
    - +7th **S81.032 Puncture wound without foreign body, left knee**
    - +7th **S81.039 Puncture wound without foreign body, unspecified knee**
  + **S81.04 Puncture wound with foreign body of knee**
    - +7th **S81.041 Puncture wound with foreign body, right knee**
    - +7th **S81.042 Puncture wound with foreign body, left knee**
    - +7th **S81.049 Puncture wound with foreign body, unspecified knee**
  + **S81.05 Open bite of knee**
    Bite of knee NOS
    Excludes1: *superficial bite of knee (S80.27-)*
    - +7th **S81.051 Open bite, right knee**
    - +7th **S81.052 Open bite, left knee**
    - +7th **S81.059 Open bite, unspecified knee**
+ **S81.8 Open wound of lower leg**
  + **S81.80 Unspecified open wound of lower leg**
    - +7th **S81.801 Unspecified open wound, right lower leg**
    - +7th **S81.802 Unspecified open wound, left lower leg**
    - +7th **S81.809 Unspecified open wound, unspecified lower leg**
  + **S81.81 Laceration without foreign body of lower leg**
    - +7th **S81.811 Laceration without foreign body, right lower leg**
    - +7th **S81.812 Laceration without foreign body, left lower leg**
    - +7th **S81.819 Laceration without foreign body, unspecified lower leg**
  + **S81.82 Laceration with foreign body of lower leg**
    - +7th **S81.821 Laceration with foreign body, right lower leg**
    - +7th **S81.822 Laceration with foreign body, left lower leg**
    - +7th **S81.829 Laceration with foreign body, unspecified lower leg**
  + **S81.83 Puncture wound without foreign body of lower leg**
    - +7th **S81.831 Puncture wound without foreign body, right lower leg**
    - +7th **S81.832 Puncture wound without foreign body, left lower leg**
    - +7th **S81.839 Puncture wound without foreign body, unspecified lower leg**
  + **S81.84 Puncture wound with foreign body of lower leg**
    - +7th **S81.841 Puncture wound with foreign body, right lower leg**
      AHA CC: 3Q, 2016, 24
    - +7th **S81.842 Puncture wound with foreign body, left lower leg**
    - +7th **S81.849 Puncture wound with foreign body, unspecified lower leg**
  + **S81.85 Open bite of lower leg**
    Bite of lower leg NOS
    Excludes1: *superficial bite of lower leg (S80.86-, S80.87-)*
    - +7th **S81.851 Open bite, right lower leg**
    - +7th **S81.852 Open bite, left lower leg**
    - +7th **S81.859 Open bite, unspecified lower leg**

S82 Fracture of lower leg, including ankle

NOTE A fracture not indicated as displaced or nondisplaced should be coded to displaced
A fracture not indicated as open or closed should be coded to closed
The open fracture designations are based on the Gustilo open fracture classification

Includes: fracture of malleolus

Excludes1: *traumatic amputation of lower leg (S88.-)*

Excludes2: *fracture of foot, except ankle (S92.-)*
periprosthetic fracture around internal prosthetic implant of knee joint (M97.1-)

The appropriate 7th character is to be added to all codes from category S82
A initial encounter for closed fracture
B initial encounter for open fracture type I or II
initial encounter for open fracture NOS
C initial encounter for open fracture type IIIA, IIIB, or IIIC
D subsequent encounter for closed fracture with routine healing
E subsequent encounter for open fracture type I or II with routine healing
F subsequent encounter for open fracture type IIIA, IIIB, or IIIC with routine healing
G subsequent encounter for closed fracture with delayed healing
H subsequent encounter for open fracture type I or II with delayed healing
J subsequent encounter for open fracture type IIIA, IIIB, or IIIC with delayed healing
K subsequent encounter for closed fracture with nonunion
M subsequent encounter for open fracture type I or II with nonunion
N subsequent encounter for open fracture type IIIA, IIIB, or IIIC with nonunion
P subsequent encounter for closed fracture with malunion
Q subsequent encounter for open fracture type I or II with malunion
R subsequent encounter for open fracture type IIIA, IIIB, or IIIC with malunion
S sequela

Review coding guideline C.19.c

+ **S82.0 Fracture of patella**
  Knee cap
  + **S82.00 Unspecified fracture of patella**
    - CC +7th **S82.001 Unspecified fracture of right patella**
      HAC 7th characters A - C see Appendix B for HAC conditional logic
    - CC +7th **S82.002 Unspecified fracture of left patella**
      HAC 7th characters A - C see Appendix B for HAC conditional logic
    - CC +7th **S82.009 Unspecified fracture of unspecified patella**
      HAC 7th characters A - C see Appendix B for HAC conditional logic

+ **S82.01 Osteochondral fracture of patella**

CC +7th **S82.011 Displaced osteochondral fracture of right patella**
HAC 7th characters A - C see Appendix B for HAC conditional logic

CC +7th **S82.012 Displaced osteochondral fracture of left patella**
HAC 7th characters A - C see Appendix B for HAC conditional logic

CC +7th **S82.013 Displaced osteochondral fracture of unspecified patella**
HAC 7th characters A - C see Appendix B for HAC conditional logic

CC +7th **S82.014 Nondisplaced osteochondral fracture of right patella**
HAC 7th characters A - C see Appendix B for HAC conditional logic

CC +7th **S82.015 Nondisplaced osteochondral fracture of left patella**
HAC 7th characters A - C see Appendix B for HAC conditional logic

CC +7th **S82.016 Nondisplaced osteochondral fracture of unspecified patella**
HAC 7th characters A - C see Appendix B for HAC conditional logic

+ **S82.02 Longitudinal fracture of patella**

CC +7th **S82.021 Displaced longitudinal fracture of right patella**
HAC 7th characters A - C see Appendix B for HAC conditional logic

CC +7th **S82.022 Displaced longitudinal fracture of left patella**
HAC 7th characters A - C see Appendix B for HAC conditional logic

CC +7th **S82.023 Displaced longitudinal fracture of unspecified patella**
HAC 7th characters A - C see Appendix B for HAC conditional logic

CC +7th **S82.024 Nondisplaced longitudinal fracture of right patella**
HAC 7th characters A - C see Appendix B for HAC conditional logic

CC +7th **S82.025 Nondisplaced longitudinal fracture of left patella**
HAC 7th characters A - C see Appendix B for HAC conditional logic

CC +7th **S82.026 Nondisplaced longitudinal fracture of unspecified patella**
HAC 7th characters A - C see Appendix B for HAC conditional logic

+ **S82.03 Transverse fracture of patella**

CC +7th **S82.031 Displaced transverse fracture of right patella**
HAC 7th characters A - C see Appendix B for HAC conditional logic

CC +7th **S82.032 Displaced transverse fracture of left patella**
HAC 7th characters A - C see Appendix B for HAC conditional logic

CC +7th **S82.033 Displaced transverse fracture of unspecified patella**
HAC 7th characters A - C see Appendix B for HAC conditional logic

CC +7th **S82.034 Nondisplaced transverse fracture of right patella**
HAC 7th characters A - C see Appendix B for HAC conditional logic

CC +7th **S82.035 Nondisplaced transverse fracture of left patella**
HAC 7th characters A - C see Appendix B for HAC conditional logic

CC +7th **S82.036 Nondisplaced transverse fracture of unspecified patella**
HAC 7th characters A - C see Appendix B for HAC conditional logic

+ **S82.04 Comminuted fracture of patella**

CC +7th **S82.041 Displaced comminuted fracture of right patella**
HAC 7th characters A - C see Appendix B for HAC conditional logic

CC +7th **S82.042 Displaced comminuted fracture of left patella**
HAC 7th characters A - C see Appendix B for HAC conditional logic

CC +7th **S82.043 Displaced comminuted fracture of unspecified patella**
HAC 7th characters A - C see Appendix B for HAC conditional logic

CC +7th **S82.044 Nondisplaced comminuted fracture of right patella**
HAC 7th characters A - C see Appendix B for HAC conditional logic

CC +7th **S82.045 Nondisplaced comminuted fracture of left patella**
HAC 7th characters A - C see Appendix B for HAC conditional logic

CC +7th **S82.046 Nondisplaced comminuted fracture of unspecified patella**
HAC 7th characters A - C see Appendix B for HAC conditional logic

+ **S82.09 Other fracture of patella**

CC +7th **S82.091 Other fracture of right patella**
HAC 7th characters A - C see Appendix B for HAC conditional logic

CC +7th **S82.092 Other fracture of left patella**
HAC 7th characters A - C see Appendix B for HAC conditional logic

CC +7th **S82.099 Other fracture of unspecified patella**
HAC 7th characters A - C see Appendix B for HAC conditional logic

+ **S82.1 Fracture of upper end of tibia**
Fracture of proximal end of tibia
Excludes2: *fracture of shaft of tibia (S82.2-)*
physeal fracture of upper end of tibia (S89.0-)

+ **S82.10 Unspecified fracture of upper end of tibia**

CC MCC +7th **S82.101 Unspecified fracture of upper end of right tibia**
HAC 7th characters A - C see Appendix B for HAC conditional logic

CC MCC +7th **S82.102 Unspecified fracture of upper end of left tibia**
HAC 7th characters A - C see Appendix B for HAC conditional logic

CC MCC +7th **S82.109 Unspecified fracture of upper end of unspecified tibia**
HAC 7th characters A - C see Appendix B for HAC conditional logic

+ **S82.11 Fracture of tibial spine**

CC MCC +7th **S82.111 Displaced fracture of right tibial spine**
HAC 7th characters A - C see Appendix B for HAC conditional logic

CC MCC +7th **S82.112 Displaced fracture of left tibial spine**
HAC 7th characters A - C see Appendix B for HAC conditional logic

CC MCC +7th **S82.113 Displaced fracture of unspecified tibial spine**
HAC 7th characters A - C see Appendix B for HAC conditional logic

CC MCC +7th **S82.114 Nondisplaced fracture of right tibial spine**
HAC 7th characters A - C see Appendix B for HAC conditional logic

CC MCC +7th **S82.115 Nondisplaced fracture of left tibial spine**
HAC 7th characters A - C see Appendix B for HAC conditional logic

CC MCC +7th **S82.116 Nondisplaced fracture of unspecified tibial spine**
HAC 7th characters A - C see Appendix B for HAC conditional logic

+ **S82.12 Fracture of lateral condyle of tibia**

CC MCC +7th **S82.121 Displaced fracture of lateral condyle of right tibia**
HAC 7th characters A - C see Appendix B for HAC conditional logic

CC MCC +7th **S82.122 Displaced fracture of lateral condyle of left tibia**
HAC 7th characters A - C see Appendix B for HAC conditional logic

CC MCC +7th **S82.123 Displaced fracture of lateral condyle of unspecified tibia**
HAC 7th characters A - C see Appendix B for HAC conditional logic

CC MCC +7th **S82.124 Nondisplaced fracture of lateral condyle of right tibia**
HAC 7th characters A - C see Appendix B for HAC conditional logic

CC MCC +7th **S82.125 Nondisplaced fracture of lateral condyle of left tibia**
HAC 7th characters A - C see Appendix B for HAC conditional logic

CC MCC +7th **S82.126 Nondisplaced fracture of lateral condyle of unspecified tibia**
HAC 7th characters A - C see Appendix B for HAC conditional logic

+ **S82.13 Fracture of medial condyle of tibia**

CC MCC +7th **S82.131 Displaced fracture of medial condyle of right tibia**
HAC 7th characters A - C see Appendix B for HAC conditional logic

CC MCC +7th **S82.132 Displaced fracture of medial condyle of left tibia**
HAC 7th characters A - C see Appendix B for HAC conditional logic

CC MCC +7th **S82.133 Displaced fracture of medial condyle of unspecified tibia**
HAC 7th characters A - C see Appendix B for HAC conditional logic

CC MCC +7th **S82.134 Nondisplaced fracture of medial condyle of right tibia**
HAC 7th characters A - C see Appendix B for HAC conditional logic

CC MCC +7th **S82.135 Nondisplaced fracture of medial condyle of left tibia**
HAC 7th characters A - C see Appendix B for HAC conditional logic

CC MCC +7th **S82.136 Nondisplaced fracture of medial condyle of unspecified tibia**
HAC 7th characters A - C see Appendix B for HAC conditional logic

+ **S82.14 Bicondylar fracture of tibia**
Fracture of tibial plateau NOS

CC MCC +7th **S82.141 Displaced bicondylar fracture of right tibia**
HAC 7th characters A - C see Appendix B for HAC conditional logic

CC MCC +7th **S82.142 Displaced bicondylar fracture of left tibia**
HAC 7th characters A - C see Appendix B for HAC conditional logic

CC MCC +7th **S82.143 Displaced bicondylar fracture of unspecified tibia**
HAC 7th characters A - C see Appendix B for HAC conditional logic

CC MCC +7th **S82.144 Nondisplaced bicondylar fracture of right tibia**
HAC 7th characters A - C see Appendix B for HAC conditional logic

CC MCC +7th **S82.145 Nondisplaced bicondylar fracture of left tibia**
HAC 7th characters A - C see Appendix B for HAC conditional logic

CC MCC +7th **S82.146 Nondisplaced bicondylar fracture of unspecified tibia**
HAC 7th characters A - C see Appendix B for HAC conditional logic

+ **S82.15 Fracture of tibial tuberosity**

CC MCC +7th **S82.151 Displaced fracture of right tibial tuberosity**
HAC 7th characters A - C see Appendix B for HAC conditional logic

CC MCC +7th **S82.152 Displaced fracture of left tibial tuberosity**
HAC 7th characters A - C see Appendix B for HAC conditional logic

CC MCC +7th **S82.153 Displaced fracture of unspecified tibial tuberosity**
HAC 7th characters A - C see Appendix B for HAC conditional logic

CC MCC +7th **S82.154 Nondisplaced fracture of right tibial tuberosity**
HAC 7th characters A - C see Appendix B for HAC conditional logic

CC MCC +7th **S82.155 Nondisplaced fracture of left tibial tuberosity**
HAC 7th characters A - C see Appendix B for HAC conditional logic

CC MCC +7th **S82.156 Nondisplaced fracture of unspecified tibial tuberosity**
HAC 7th characters A - C see Appendix B for HAC conditional logic

+ **S82.16 Torus fracture of upper end of tibia**

The appropriate 7th character is to be added to all codes in subcategory **S82.16**
A initial encounter for closed fracture
D subsequent encounter for fracture with routine healing
G subsequent encounter for fracture with delayed healing
K subsequent encounter for fracture with nonunion
P subsequent encounter for fracture with malunion
S sequela

CC +7th **S82.161 Torus fracture of upper end of right tibia**
HAC 7th character A see Appendix B for HAC conditional logic

CC +7th **S82.162 Torus fracture of upper end of left tibia**
HAC 7th character A see Appendix B for HAC conditional logic

CC +7th **S82.169 Torus fracture of upper end of unspecified tibia**
HAC 7th character A see Appendix B for HAC conditional logic

+ **S82.19 Other fracture of upper end of tibia**

CC MCC +7th **S82.191 Other fracture of upper end of right tibia**
HAC 7th characters A - C see Appendix B for HAC conditional logic

CC MCC +7th **S82.192 Other fracture of upper end of left tibia**
HAC 7th characters A - C see Appendix B for HAC conditional logic

CC MCC +7th **S82.199 Other fracture of upper end of unspecified tibia**
HAC 7th characters A - C see Appendix B for HAC conditional logic

+ **S82.2 Fracture of shaft of tibia**

+ **S82.20 Unspecified fracture of shaft of tibia**
Fracture of tibia NOS

CC MCC +7th **S82.201 Unspecified fracture of shaft of right tibia**
HAC 7th characters A - C see Appendix B for HAC conditional logic

CC MCC +7th **S82.202 Unspecified fracture of shaft of left tibia**
HAC 7th characters A - C see Appendix B for HAC conditional logic

CC MCC +7th **S82.209 Unspecified fracture of shaft of unspecified tibia**
HAC 7th characters A - C see Appendix B for HAC conditional logic

+ **S82.22 Transverse fracture of shaft of tibia**

CC MCC +7th **S82.221 Displaced transverse fracture of shaft of right tibia**
HAC 7th characters A - C see Appendix B for HAC conditional logic

CC MCC +7th **S82.222 Displaced transverse fracture of shaft of left tibia**
HAC 7th characters A - C see Appendix B for HAC conditional logic

CC MCC +7th **S82.223 Displaced transverse fracture of shaft of unspecified tibia**
HAC 7th characters A - C see Appendix B for HAC conditional logic

CC MCC +7th **S82.224 Nondisplaced transverse fracture of shaft of right tibia**
HAC 7th characters A - C see Appendix B for HAC conditional logic

CC MCC +7th **S82.225 Nondisplaced transverse fracture of shaft of left tibia**
HAC 7th characters A - C see Appendix B for HAC conditional logic

CC MCC +7th **S82.226 Nondisplaced transverse fracture of shaft of unspecified tibia**
HAC 7th characters A - C see Appendix B for HAC conditional logic

\+ **S82.23 Oblique fracture of shaft of tibia**

CC MCC +7th **S82.231 Displaced oblique fracture of shaft of right tibia**
HAC 7th characters A - C see Appendix B for HAC conditional logic

CC MCC +7th **S82.232 Displaced oblique fracture of shaft of left tibia**
HAC 7th characters A - C see Appendix B for HAC conditional logic

CC MCC +7th **S82.233 Displaced oblique fracture of shaft of unspecified tibia**
HAC 7th characters A - C see Appendix B for HAC conditional logic

CC MCC +7th **S82.234 Nondisplaced oblique fracture of shaft of right tibia**
HAC 7th characters A - C see Appendix B for HAC conditional logic
AHA CC: 1Q, 2015, 3-21

CC MCC +7th **S82.235 Nondisplaced oblique fracture of shaft of left tibia**
HAC 7th characters A - C see Appendix B for HAC conditional logic

CC MCC +7th **S82.236 Nondisplaced oblique fracture of shaft of unspecified tibia**
HAC 7th characters A - C see Appendix B for HAC conditional logic

\+ **S82.24 Spiral fracture of shaft of tibia**
Toddler fracture

CC MCC +7th **S82.241 Displaced spiral fracture of shaft of right tibia**
HAC 7th characters A - C see Appendix B for HAC conditional logic

CC MCC +7th **S82.242 Displaced spiral fracture of shaft of left tibia**
HAC 7th characters A - C see Appendix B for HAC conditional logic

CC MCC +7th **S82.243 Displaced spiral fracture of shaft of unspecified tibia**
HAC 7th characters A - C see Appendix B for HAC conditional logic

CC MCC +7th **S82.244 Nondisplaced spiral fracture of shaft of right tibia**
HAC 7th characters A - C see Appendix B for HAC conditional logic

CC MCC +7th **S82.245 Nondisplaced spiral fracture of shaft of left tibia**
HAC 7th characters A - C see Appendix B for HAC conditional logic

CC MCC +7th **S82.246 Nondisplaced spiral fracture of shaft of unspecified tibia**
HAC 7th characters A - C see Appendix B for HAC conditional logic

\+ **S82.25 Comminuted fracture of shaft of tibia**

CC MCC +7th **S82.251 Displaced comminuted fracture of shaft of right tibia**
HAC 7th characters A - C see Appendix B for HAC conditional logic
AHA CC: 2Q, 2015, 6-7

CC MCC +7th **S82.252 Displaced comminuted fracture of shaft of left tibia**
HAC 7th characters A - C see Appendix B for HAC conditional logic

CC MCC +7th **S82.253 Displaced comminuted fracture of shaft of unspecified tibia**
HAC 7th characters A - C see Appendix B for HAC conditional logic

CC MCC +7th **S82.254 Nondisplaced comminuted fracture of shaft of right tibia**
HAC 7th characters A - C see Appendix B for HAC conditional logic

CC MCC +7th **S82.255 Nondisplaced comminuted fracture of shaft of left tibia**
HAC 7th characters A - C see Appendix B for HAC conditional logic

CC MCC +7th **S82.256 Nondisplaced comminuted fracture of shaft of unspecified tibia**
HAC 7th characters A - C see Appendix B for HAC conditional logic

\+ **S82.26 Segmental fracture of shaft of tibia**

CC MCC +7th **S82.261 Displaced segmental fracture of shaft of right tibia**
HAC 7th characters A - C see Appendix B for HAC conditional logic

CC MCC +7th **S82.262 Displaced segmental fracture of shaft of left tibia**
HAC 7th characters A - C see Appendix B for HAC conditional logic

CC MCC +7th **S82.263 Displaced segmental fracture of shaft of unspecified tibia**
HAC 7th characters A - C see Appendix B for HAC conditional logic

CC MCC +7th **S82.264 Nondisplaced segmental fracture of shaft of right tibia**
HAC 7th characters A - C see Appendix B for HAC conditional logic

CC MCC +7th **S82.265 Nondisplaced segmental fracture of shaft of left tibia**
HAC 7th characters A - C see Appendix B for HAC conditional logic

CC MCC +7th **S82.266 Nondisplaced segmental fracture of shaft of unspecified tibia**
HAC 7th characters A - C see Appendix B for HAC conditional logic

\+ **S82.29 Other fracture of shaft of tibia**

CC MCC +7th **S82.291 Other fracture of shaft of right tibia**
HAC 7th characters A - C see Appendix B for HAC conditional logic

CC MCC +7th **S82.292 Other fracture of shaft of left tibia**
HAC 7th characters A - C see Appendix B for HAC conditional logic

CC MCC +7th **S82.299 Other fracture of shaft of unspecified tibia**
HAC 7th characters A - C see Appendix B for HAC conditional logic

+ **S82.3 Fracture of lower end of tibia**
Excludes1: *bimalleolar fracture of lower leg (S82.84-)*
fracture of medial malleolus alone (S82.5-)
Maisonneuve's fracture (S82.86-)
pilon fracture of distal tibia (S82.87-)
trimalleolar fractures of lower leg (S82.85-)

+ **S82.30 Unspecified fracture of lower end of tibia**

CC +7th **S82.301 Unspecified fracture of lower end of right tibia**
HAC 7th characters B & C see Appendix B for HAC conditional logic

CC +7th **S82.302 Unspecified fracture of lower end of left tibia**
HAC 7th characters B & C see Appendix B for HAC conditional logic

CC +7th **S82.309 Unspecified fracture of lower end of unspecified tibia**
HAC 7th characters B & C see Appendix B for HAC conditional logic

+ **S82.31 Torus fracture of lower end of tibia**

The appropriate 7th character is to be added to all codes in subcategory **S82.31**
A initial encounter for closed fracture
D subsequent encounter for fracture with routine healing
G subsequent encounter for fracture with delayed healing
K subsequent encounter for fracture with nonunion
P subsequent encounter for fracture with malunion
S sequela

CC +7th **S82.311 Torus fracture of lower end of right tibia**
HAC 7th character A see Appendix B for HAC conditional logic

CC +7th **S82.312 Torus fracture of lower end of left tibia**
HAC 7th character A see Appendix B for HAC conditional logic

CC +7th **S82.319 Torus fracture of lower end of unspecified tibia**
HAC 7th character A see Appendix B for HAC conditional logic

+ **S82.39 Other fracture of lower end of tibia**

CC +7th **S82.391 Other fracture of lower end of right tibia**
HAC 7th characters B & C see Appendix B for HAC conditional logic

CC +7th **S82.392 Other fracture of lower end of left tibia**
HAC 7th characters B & C see Appendix B for HAC conditional logic
AHA CC: 1Q, 2015, 25

CC +7th **S82.399 Other fracture of lower end of unspecified tibia**
HAC 7th characters B & C see Appendix B for HAC conditional logic

+ **S82.4 Fracture of shaft of fibula**
Excludes2: *fracture of lateral malleolus alone (S82.6-)*

+ **S82.40 Unspecified fracture of shaft of fibula**

CC MCC +7th **S82.401 Unspecified fracture of shaft of right fibula**
HAC 7th characters B & C see Appendix B for HAC conditional logic

CC MCC +7th **S82.402 Unspecified fracture of shaft of left fibula**
HAC 7th characters B & C see Appendix B for HAC conditional logic

CC MCC +7th **S82.409 Unspecified fracture of shaft of unspecified fibula**
HAC 7th characters B & C see Appendix B for HAC conditional logic

+ **S82.42 Transverse fracture of shaft of fibula**

CC MCC +7th **S82.421 Displaced transverse fracture of shaft of right fibula**
HAC 7th characters B & C see Appendix B for HAC conditional logic

CC MCC +7th **S82.422 Displaced transverse fracture of shaft of left fibula**
HAC 7th characters B & C see Appendix B for HAC conditional logic

CC MCC +7th **S82.423 Displaced transverse fracture of shaft of unspecified fibula**
HAC 7th characters B & C see Appendix B for HAC conditional logic

CC MCC +7th **S82.424 Nondisplaced transverse fracture of shaft of right fibula**
HAC 7th characters B & C see Appendix B for HAC conditional logic

CC MCC +7th **S82.425 Nondisplaced transverse fracture of shaft of left fibula**
HAC 7th characters B & C see Appendix B for HAC conditional logic

CC MCC +7th **S82.426 Nondisplaced transverse fracture of shaft of unspecified fibula**
HAC 7th characters B & C see Appendix B for HAC conditional logic

+ **S82.43 Oblique fracture of shaft of fibula**

CC MCC +7th **S82.431 Displaced oblique fracture of shaft of right fibula**
HAC 7th characters B & C see Appendix B for HAC conditional logic

CC MCC +7th **S82.432 Displaced oblique fracture of shaft of left fibula**
HAC 7th characters B & C see Appendix B for HAC conditional logic

CC MCC +7th **S82.433 Displaced oblique fracture of shaft of unspecified fibula**
HAC 7th characters B & C see Appendix B for HAC conditional logic

CC MCC +7th **S82.434 Nondisplaced oblique fracture of shaft of right fibula**
HAC 7th characters B & C see Appendix B for HAC conditional logic

CC MCC +7th **S82.435 Nondisplaced oblique fracture of shaft of left fibula**
HAC 7th characters B & C see Appendix B for HAC conditional logic

CC MCC +7th **S82.436 Nondisplaced oblique fracture of shaft of unspecified fibula**
HAC 7th characters B & C see Appendix B for HAC conditional logic

+ **S82.44 Spiral fracture of shaft of fibula**

CC MCC +7th **S82.441 Displaced spiral fracture of shaft of right fibula**
HAC 7th characters B & C see Appendix B for HAC conditional logic

CC MCC +7th **S82.442 Displaced spiral fracture of shaft of left fibula**
HAC 7th characters B & C see Appendix B for HAC conditional logic

CC MCC +7th **S82.443 Displaced spiral fracture of shaft of unspecified fibula**
HAC 7th characters B & C see Appendix B for HAC conditional logic

CC MCC +7th **S82.444 Nondisplaced spiral fracture of shaft of right fibula**
HAC 7th characters B & C see Appendix B for HAC conditional logic

CC MCC +7th **S82.445 Nondisplaced spiral fracture of shaft of left fibula**
HAC 7th characters B & C see Appendix B for HAC conditional logic

CC MCC +7th **S82.446 Nondisplaced spiral fracture of shaft of unspecified fibula**
HAC 7th characters B & C see Appendix B for HAC conditional logic

+ **S82.45 Comminuted fracture of shaft of fibula**

CC MCC +7th **S82.451 Displaced comminuted fracture of shaft of right fibula**
HAC 7th characters B & C see Appendix B for HAC conditional logic

CC MCC +7th **S82.452 Displaced comminuted fracture of shaft of left fibula**
HAC 7th characters B & C see Appendix B for HAC conditional logic

CC MCC +7th **S82.453 Displaced comminuted fracture of shaft of unspecified fibula**
HAC 7th characters B & C see Appendix B for HAC conditional logic

CC MCC +7th **S82.454 Nondisplaced comminuted fracture of shaft of right fibula**
HAC 7th characters B & C see Appendix B for HAC conditional logic

CC MCC +7th **S82.455 Nondisplaced comminuted fracture of shaft of left fibula**
HAC 7th characters B & C see Appendix B for HAC conditional logic

CC MCC +7th **S82.456 Nondisplaced comminuted fracture of shaft of unspecified fibula**
HAC 7th characters B & C see Appendix B for HAC conditional logic

\+ **S82.46 Segmental fracture of shaft of fibula**

CC MCC +7th **S82.461 Displaced segmental fracture of shaft of right fibula**
HAC 7th characters B & C see Appendix B for HAC conditional logic

CC MCC +7th **S82.462 Displaced segmental fracture of shaft of left fibula**
HAC 7th characters B & C see Appendix B for HAC conditional logic

CC MCC +7th **S82.463 Displaced segmental fracture of shaft of unspecified fibula**
HAC 7th characters B & C see Appendix B for HAC conditional logic

CC MCC +7th **S82.464 Nondisplaced segmental fracture of shaft of right fibula**
HAC 7th characters B & C see Appendix B for HAC conditional logic

CC MCC +7th **S82.465 Nondisplaced segmental fracture of shaft of left fibula**
HAC 7th characters B & C see Appendix B for HAC conditional logic

CC MCC +7th **S82.466 Nondisplaced segmental fracture of shaft of unspecified fibula**
HAC 7th characters B & C see Appendix B for HAC conditional logic

\+ **S82.49 Other fracture of shaft of fibula**

CC MCC +7th **S82.491 Other fracture of shaft of right fibula**
HAC 7th characters B & C see Appendix B for HAC conditional logic

CC MCC +7th **S82.492 Other fracture of shaft of left fibula**
HAC 7th characters B & C see Appendix B for HAC conditional logic

CC MCC +7th **S82.499 Other fracture of shaft of unspecified fibula**
HAC 7th characters B & C see Appendix B for HAC conditional logic

\+ **S82.5 Fracture of medial malleolus**
Excludes1: *pilon fracture of distal tibia (S82.87-)*
Salter-Harris type III of lower end of tibia (S89.13-)
Salter-Harris type IV of lower end of tibia (S89.14-)

CC X+7th **S82.51 Displaced fracture of medial malleolus of right tibia**
HAC 7th characters B & C see Appendix B for HAC conditional logic

CC X+7th **S82.52 Displaced fracture of medial malleolus of left tibia**
HAC 7th characters B & C see Appendix B for HAC conditional logic

CC X+7th **S82.53 Displaced fracture of medial malleolus of unspecified tibia**
HAC 7th characters B & C see Appendix B for HAC conditional logic

CC X+7th **S82.54 Nondisplaced fracture of medial malleolus of right tibia**
HAC 7th characters B & C see Appendix B for HAC conditional logic

CC X+7th **S82.55 Nondisplaced fracture of medial malleolus of left tibia**
HAC 7th characters B & C see Appendix B for HAC conditional logic

CC X+7th **S82.56 Nondisplaced fracture of medial malleolus of unspecified tibia**
HAC 7th characters B & C see Appendix B for HAC conditional logic

\+ **S82.6 Fracture of lateral malleolus**
Excludes1: *pilon fracture of distal tibia (S82.87-)*

CC X+7th **S82.61 Displaced fracture of lateral malleolus of right fibula**
HAC 7th characters B & C see Appendix B for HAC conditional logic

CC X+7th **S82.62 Displaced fracture of lateral malleolus of left fibula**
HAC 7th characters B & C see Appendix B for HAC conditional logic

CC X+7th **S82.63 Displaced fracture of lateral malleolus of unspecified fibula**
HAC 7th characters B & C see Appendix B for HAC conditional logic

CC X+7th **S82.64 Nondisplaced fracture of lateral malleolus of right fibula**
HAC 7th characters B & C see Appendix B for HAC conditional logic

CC X+7th **S82.65 Nondisplaced fracture of lateral malleolus of left fibula**
HAC 7th characters B & C see Appendix B for HAC conditional logic

CC X+7th **S82.66 Nondisplaced fracture of lateral malleolus of unspecified fibula**
HAC 7th characters B & C see Appendix B for HAC conditional logic

\+ **S82.8 Other fractures of lower leg**

\+ **S82.81 Torus fracture of upper end of fibula**

The appropriate 7th character is to be added to all codes in subcategory **S82.81**
A initial encounter for closed fracture
D subsequent encounter for fracture with routine healing
G subsequent encounter for fracture with delayed healing
K subsequent encounter for fracture with nonunion
P subsequent encounter for fracture with malunion
S sequela

CC +7th **S82.811 Torus fracture of upper end of right fibula**

CC +7th **S82.812 Torus fracture of upper end of left fibula**

CC +7th **S82.819 Torus fracture of upper end of unspecified fibula**

\+ **S82.82 Torus fracture of lower end of fibula**

The appropriate 7th character is to be added to all codes in subcategory **S82.82**
A initial encounter for closed fracture
D subsequent encounter for fracture with routine healing
G subsequent encounter for fracture with delayed healing
K subsequent encounter for fracture with nonunion
P subsequent encounter for fracture with malunion
S sequela

CC +7th **S82.821 Torus fracture of lower end of right fibula**

CC +7th **S82.822 Torus fracture of lower end of left fibula**

CC +7th **S82.829 Torus fracture of lower end of unspecified fibula**

\+ **S82.83 Other fracture of upper and lower end of fibula**

CC MCC +7th **S82.831 Other fracture of upper and lower end of right fibula**
HAC 7th characters B & C see Appendix B for HAC conditional logic

CC MCC +7th **S82.832 Other fracture of upper and lower end of left fibula**
HAC 7th characters B & C see Appendix B for HAC conditional logic
AHA CC: 1Q, 2015, 25

CC MCC +7th **S82.839 Other fracture of upper and lower end of unspecified fibula**
HAC 7th characters B & C see Appendix B for HAC conditional logic

Tears of Meniscus

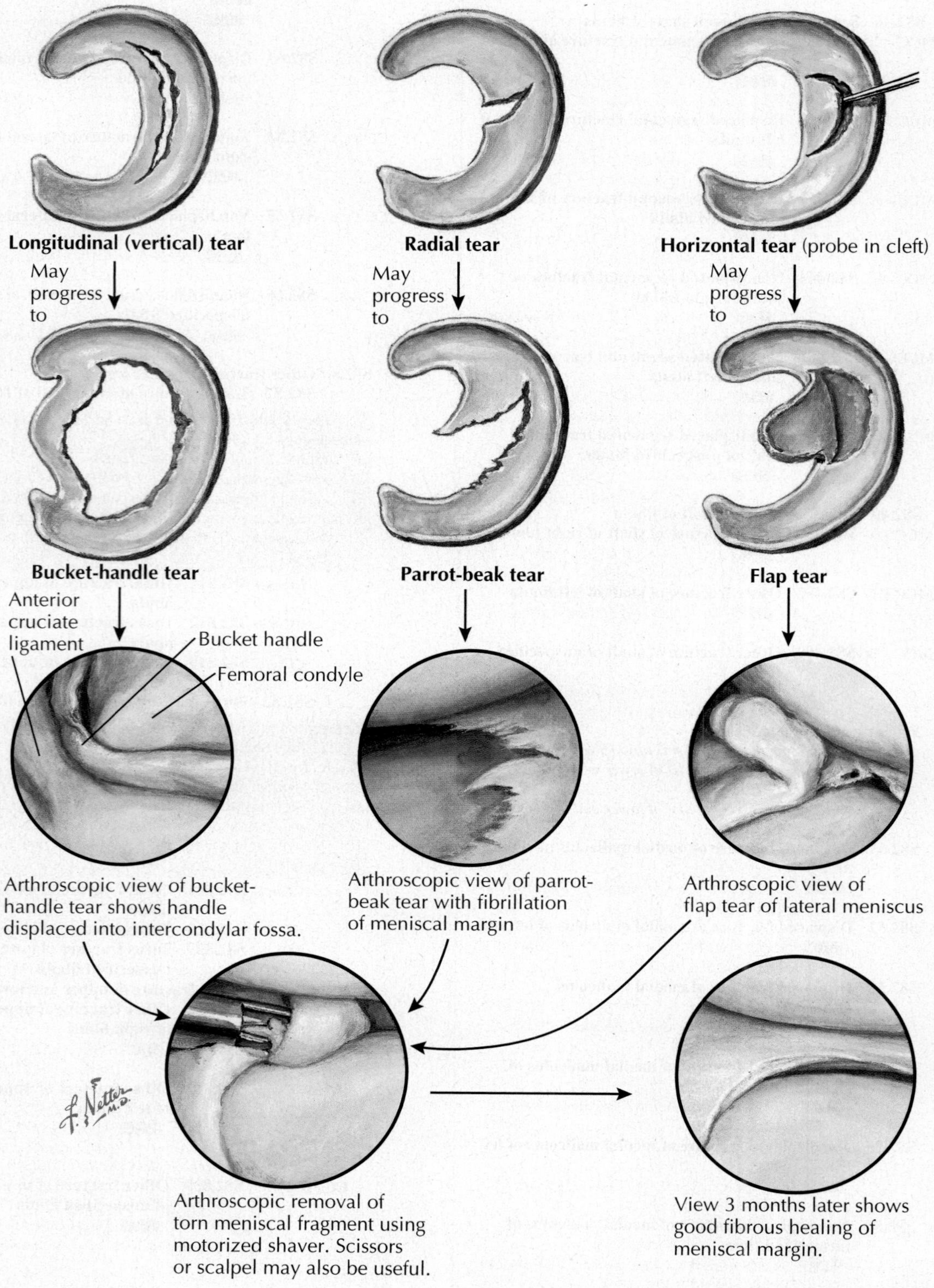

+ **S82.84 Bimalleolar fracture of lower leg**

CC +7th **S82.841 Displaced bimalleolar fracture of right lower leg**
HAC 7th characters B & C see Appendix B for HAC conditional logic

CC +7th **S82.842 Displaced bimalleolar fracture of left lower leg**
HAC 7th characters B & C see Appendix B for HAC conditional logic

CC +7th **S82.843 Displaced bimalleolar fracture of unspecified lower leg**
HAC 7th characters B & C see Appendix B for HAC conditional logic

CC +7th **S82.844 Nondisplaced bimalleolar fracture of right lower leg**
HAC 7th characters B & C see Appendix B for HAC conditional logic

CC +7th **S82.845 Nondisplaced bimalleolar fracture of left lower leg**
HAC 7th characters B & C see Appendix B for HAC conditional logic

CC +7th **S82.846 Nondisplaced bimalleolar fracture of unspecified lower leg**
HAC 7th characters B & C see Appendix B for HAC conditional logic

+ **S82.85 Trimalleolar fracture of lower leg**

CC +7th **S82.851 Displaced trimalleolar fracture of right lower leg**
HAC 7th characters B & C see Appendix B for HAC conditional logic

CC +7th **S82.852 Displaced trimalleolar fracture of left lower leg**
HAC 7th characters B & C see Appendix B for HAC conditional logic

CC +7th **S82.853 Displaced trimalleolar fracture of unspecified lower leg**
HAC 7th characters B & C see Appendix B for HAC conditional logic

CC +7th **S82.854 Nondisplaced trimalleolar fracture of right lower leg**
HAC 7th characters B & C see Appendix B for HAC conditional logic

CC +7th **S82.855 Nondisplaced trimalleolar fracture of left lower leg**
HAC 7th characters B & C see Appendix B for HAC conditional logic

CC +7th **S82.856 Nondisplaced trimalleolar fracture of unspecified lower leg**
HAC 7th characters B & C see Appendix B for HAC conditional logic

+ **S82.86 Maisonneuve's fracture**

CC MCC +7th **S82.861 Displaced Maisonneuve's fracture of right leg**
HAC 7th characters B & C see Appendix B for HAC conditional logic

CC MCC +7th **S82.862 Displaced Maisonneuve's fracture of left leg**
HAC 7th characters B & C see Appendix B for HAC conditional logic

CC MCC +7th **S82.863 Displaced Maisonneuve's fracture of unspecified leg**
HAC 7th characters B & C see Appendix B for HAC conditional logic

CC MCC +7th **S82.864 Nondisplaced Maisonneuve's fracture of right leg**
HAC 7th characters B & C see Appendix B for HAC conditional logic

CC MCC +7th **S82.865 Nondisplaced Maisonneuve's fracture of left leg**
HAC 7th characters B & C see Appendix B for HAC conditional logic

CC MCC +7th **S82.866 Nondisplaced Maisonneuve's fracture of unspecified leg**
HAC 7th characters B & C see Appendix B for HAC conditional logic

+ **S82.87 Pilon fracture of tibia**

CC +7th **S82.871 Displaced pilon fracture of right tibia**
HAC 7th characters B & C see Appendix B for HAC conditional logic

CC +7th **S82.872 Displaced pilon fracture of left tibia**
HAC 7th characters B & C see Appendix B for HAC conditional logic

CC +7th **S82.873 Displaced pilon fracture of unspecified tibia**
HAC 7th characters B & C see Appendix B for HAC conditional logic

CC +7th **S82.874 Nondisplaced pilon fracture of right tibia**
HAC 7th characters B & C see Appendix B for HAC conditional logic

CC +7th **S82.875 Nondisplaced pilon fracture of left tibia**
HAC 7th characters B & C see Appendix B for HAC conditional logic

CC +7th **S82.876 Nondisplaced pilon fracture of unspecified tibia**
HAC 7th characters B & C see Appendix B for HAC conditional logic

+ **S82.89 Other fractures of lower leg**
Fracture of ankle NOS

CC +7th **S82.891 Other fracture of right lower leg**
HAC 7th characters B & C see Appendix B for HAC conditional logic

CC +7th **S82.892 Other fracture of left lower leg**
HAC 7th characters B & C see Appendix B for HAC conditional logic

CC +7th **S82.899 Other fracture of unspecified lower leg**
HAC 7th characters B & C see Appendix B for HAC conditional logic

+ **S82.9 Unspecified fracture of lower leg**

CC X+7th **S82.90 Unspecified fracture of unspecified lower leg**
HAC 7th characters B & C see Appendix B for HAC conditional logic

CC X+7th **S82.91 Unspecified fracture of right lower leg**
HAC 7th characters B & C see Appendix B for HAC conditional logic

CC X+7th **S82.92 Unspecified fracture of left lower leg**
HAC 7th characters B & C see Appendix B for HAC conditional logic

S83 Dislocation and sprain of joints and ligaments of knee

Includes: avulsion of joint or ligament of knee
laceration of cartilage, joint or ligament of knee
sprain of cartilage, joint or ligament of knee
traumatic hemarthrosis of joint or ligament of knee
traumatic rupture of joint or ligament of knee
traumatic subluxation of joint or ligament of knee
traumatic tear of joint or ligament of knee

Code also any associated open wound

Excludes2: *derangement of patella (M22.0-M22.3)*
injury of patellar ligament (tendon) (S76.1-)
internal derangement of knee (M23.-)
old dislocation of knee (M24.36)
pathological dislocation of knee (M24.36)
recurrent dislocation of knee (M22.0)
strain of muscle, fascia and tendon of lower leg (S86.-)

The appropriate 7th character is to be added to each code from category S83
A initial encounter
D subsequent encounter
S sequela

+ **S83.0 Subluxation and dislocation of patella**

+ **S83.00 Unspecified subluxation and dislocation of patella**

+7th **S83.001 Unspecified subluxation of right patella**
+7th **S83.002 Unspecified subluxation of left patella**
+7th **S83.003 Unspecified subluxation of unspecified patella**
+7th **S83.004 Unspecified dislocation of right patella**
+7th **S83.005 Unspecified dislocation of left patella**
+7th **S83.006 Unspecified dislocation of unspecified patella**

+ **S83.01 Lateral subluxation and dislocation of patella**
  - +7th **S83.011 Lateral subluxation of right patella**
  - +7th **S83.012 Lateral subluxation of left patella**
  - +7th **S83.013 Lateral subluxation of unspecified patella**
  - +7th **S83.014 Lateral dislocation of right patella**
  - +7th **S83.015 Lateral dislocation of left patella**
  - +7th **S83.016 Lateral dislocation of unspecified patella**

+ **S83.09 Other subluxation and dislocation of patella**
  - +7th **S83.091 Other subluxation of right patella**
  - +7th **S83.092 Other subluxation of left patella**
  - +7th **S83.093 Other subluxation of unspecified patella**
  - +7th **S83.094 Other dislocation of right patella**
  - +7th **S83.095 Other dislocation of left patella**
  - +7th **S83.096 Other dislocation of unspecified patella**

+ **S83.1 Subluxation and dislocation of knee**
  Excludes2: *instability of knee prosthesis (T84.022, T84.023)*

+ **S83.10 Unspecified subluxation and dislocation of knee**
  - +7th **S83.101 Unspecified subluxation of right knee**
  - +7th **S83.102 Unspecified subluxation of left knee**
  - +7th **S83.103 Unspecified subluxation of unspecified knee**
  - +7th **S83.104 Unspecified dislocation of right knee**
  - +7th **S83.105 Unspecified dislocation of left knee**
  - +7th **S83.106 Unspecified dislocation of unspecified knee**

+ **S83.11 Anterior subluxation and dislocation of proximal end of tibia**
  Posterior subluxation and dislocation of distal end of femur
  - +7th **S83.111 Anterior subluxation of proximal end of tibia, right knee**
  - +7th **S83.112 Anterior subluxation of proximal end of tibia, left knee**
  - +7th **S83.113 Anterior subluxation of proximal end of tibia, unspecified knee**
  - +7th **S83.114 Anterior dislocation of proximal end of tibia, right knee**
  - +7th **S83.115 Anterior dislocation of proximal end of tibia, left knee**
  - +7th **S83.116 Anterior dislocation of proximal end of tibia, unspecified knee**

+ **S83.12 Posterior subluxation and dislocation of proximal end of tibia**
  Anterior dislocation of distal end of femur
  - +7th **S83.121 Posterior subluxation of proximal end of tibia, right knee**
  - +7th **S83.122 Posterior subluxation of proximal end of tibia, left knee**
  - +7th **S83.123 Posterior subluxation of proximal end of tibia, unspecified knee**
  - +7th **S83.124 Posterior dislocation of proximal end of tibia, right knee**
  - +7th **S83.125 Posterior dislocation of proximal end of tibia, left knee**
  - +7th **S83.126 Posterior dislocation of proximal end of tibia, unspecified knee**

+ **S83.13 Medial subluxation and dislocation of proximal end of tibia**
  - +7th **S83.131 Medial subluxation of proximal end of tibia, right knee**
  - +7th **S83.132 Medial subluxation of proximal end of tibia, left knee**
  - +7th **S83.133 Medial subluxation of proximal end of tibia, unspecified knee**
  - +7th **S83.134 Medial dislocation of proximal end of tibia, right knee**
  - +7th **S83.135 Medial dislocation of proximal end of tibia, left knee**
  - +7th **S83.136 Medial dislocation of proximal end of tibia, unspecified knee**

+ **S83.14 Lateral subluxation and dislocation of proximal end of tibia**
  - +7th **S83.141 Lateral subluxation of proximal end of tibia, right knee**
  - +7th **S83.142 Lateral subluxation of proximal end of tibia, left knee**
  - +7th **S83.143 Lateral subluxation of proximal end of tibia, unspecified knee**
  - +7th **S83.144 Lateral dislocation of proximal end of tibia, right knee**
  - +7th **S83.145 Lateral dislocation of proximal end of tibia, left knee**
  - +7th **S83.146 Lateral dislocation of proximal end of tibia, unspecified knee**

+ **S83.19 Other subluxation and dislocation of knee**
  - +7th **S83.191 Other subluxation of right knee**
  - +7th **S83.192 Other subluxation of left knee**
  - +7th **S83.193 Other subluxation of unspecified knee**
  - +7th **S83.194 Other dislocation of right knee**
  - +7th **S83.195 Other dislocation of left knee**
  - +7th **S83.196 Other dislocation of unspecified knee**

+ **S83.2 Tear of meniscus, current injury**
  Excludes1: *old bucket-handle tear (M23.2)*

+ **S83.20 Tear of unspecified meniscus, current injury**
  Tear of meniscus of knee NOS
  - +7th **S83.200 Bucket-handle tear of unspecified meniscus, current injury, right knee**
  - +7th **S83.201 Bucket-handle tear of unspecified meniscus, current injury, left knee**
  - +7th **S83.202 Bucket-handle tear of unspecified meniscus, current injury, unspecified knee**
  - +7th **S83.203 Other tear of unspecified meniscus, current injury, right knee**
  - +7th **S83.204 Other tear of unspecified meniscus, current injury, left knee**
  - +7th **S83.205 Other tear of unspecified meniscus, current injury, unspecified knee**
  - +7th **S83.206 Unspecified tear of unspecified meniscus, current injury, right knee**
  - +7th **S83.207 Unspecified tear of unspecified meniscus, current injury, left knee**
  - +7th **S83.209 Unspecified tear of unspecified meniscus, current injury, unspecified knee**

+ **S83.21 Bucket-handle tear of medial meniscus, current injury**
  - +7th **S83.211 Bucket-handle tear of medial meniscus, current injury, right knee**
  - +7th **S83.212 Bucket-handle tear of medial meniscus, current injury, left knee**
  - +7th **S83.219 Bucket-handle tear of medial meniscus, current injury, unspecified knee**

+ **S83.22 Peripheral tear of medial meniscus, current injury**
  - +7th **S83.221 Peripheral tear of medial meniscus, current injury, right knee**
  - +7th **S83.222 Peripheral tear of medial meniscus, current injury, left knee**
  - +7th **S83.229 Peripheral tear of medial meniscus, current injury, unspecified knee**

+ **S83.23 Complex tear of medial meniscus, current injury**
  - +7th **S83.231 Complex tear of medial meniscus, current injury, right knee**
  - +7th **S83.232 Complex tear of medial meniscus, current injury, left knee**
    AHA CC: 2Q, 2019, 26
  - +7th **S83.239 Complex tear of medial meniscus, current injury, unspecified knee**

+ **S83.24 Other tear of medial meniscus, current injury**
  - +7th **S83.241 Other tear of medial meniscus, current injury, right knee**
  - +7th **S83.242 Other tear of medial meniscus, current injury, left knee**
  - +7th **S83.249 Other tear of medial meniscus, current injury, unspecified knee**

+ **S83.25 Bucket-handle tear of lateral meniscus, current injury**
+7th **S83.251 Bucket-handle tear of lateral meniscus, current injury, right knee**
+7th **S83.252 Bucket-handle tear of lateral meniscus, current injury, left knee**
+7th **S83.259 Bucket-handle tear of lateral meniscus, current injury, unspecified knee**
+ **S83.26 Peripheral tear of lateral meniscus, current injury**
+7th **S83.261 Peripheral tear of lateral meniscus, current injury, right knee**
+7th **S83.262 Peripheral tear of lateral meniscus, current injury, left knee**
+7th **S83.269 Peripheral tear of lateral meniscus, current injury, unspecified knee**
+ **S83.27 Complex tear of lateral meniscus, current injury**
+7th **S83.271 Complex tear of lateral meniscus, current injury, right knee**
+7th **S83.272 Complex tear of lateral meniscus, current injury, left knee**
+7th **S83.279 Complex tear of lateral meniscus, current injury, unspecified knee**
+ **S83.28 Other tear of lateral meniscus, current injury**
+7th **S83.281 Other tear of lateral meniscus, current injury, right knee**
+7th **S83.282 Other tear of lateral meniscus, current injury, left knee**
+7th **S83.289 Other tear of lateral meniscus, current injury, unspecified knee**
+ **S83.3 Tear of articular cartilage of knee, current**
X+7th **S83.30 Tear of articular cartilage of unspecified knee, current**
X+7th **S83.31 Tear of articular cartilage of right knee, current**
X+7th **S83.32 Tear of articular cartilage of left knee, current**
+ **S83.4 Sprain of collateral ligament of knee**
+ **S83.40 Sprain of unspecified collateral ligament of knee**
+7th **S83.401 Sprain of unspecified collateral ligament of right knee**
+7th **S83.402 Sprain of unspecified collateral ligament of left knee**
+7th **S83.409 Sprain of unspecified collateral ligament of unspecified knee**
+ **S83.41 Sprain of medial collateral ligament of knee**
Sprain of tibial collateral ligament
+7th **S83.411 Sprain of medial collateral ligament of right knee**
+7th **S83.412 Sprain of medial collateral ligament of left knee**
+7th **S83.419 Sprain of medial collateral ligament of unspecified knee**
+ **S83.42 Sprain of lateral collateral ligament of knee**
Sprain of fibular collateral ligament
+7th **S83.421 Sprain of lateral collateral ligament of right knee**
+7th **S83.422 Sprain of lateral collateral ligament of left knee**
+7th **S83.429 Sprain of lateral collateral ligament of unspecified knee**
+ **S83.5 Sprain of cruciate ligament of knee**
+ **S83.50 Sprain of unspecified cruciate ligament of knee**
+7th **S83.501 Sprain of unspecified cruciate ligament of right knee**
+7th **S83.502 Sprain of unspecified cruciate ligament of left knee**
+7th **S83.509 Sprain of unspecified cruciate ligament of unspecified knee**
+ **S83.51 Sprain of anterior cruciate ligament of knee**
+7th **S83.511 Sprain of anterior cruciate ligament of right knee**
AHA CC: 2Q, 2016, 3–4
+7th **S83.512 Sprain of anterior cruciate ligament of left knee**
+7th **S83.519 Sprain of anterior cruciate ligament of unspecified knee**
+ **S83.52 Sprain of posterior cruciate ligament of knee**
+7th **S83.521 Sprain of posterior cruciate ligament of right knee**
+7th **S83.522 Sprain of posterior cruciate ligament of left knee**
+7th **S83.529 Sprain of posterior cruciate ligament of unspecified knee**
+ **S83.6 Sprain of the superior tibiofibular joint and ligament**
X+7th **S83.60 Sprain of the superior tibiofibular joint and ligament, unspecified knee**
X+7th **S83.61 Sprain of the superior tibiofibular joint and ligament, right knee**
X+7th **S83.62 Sprain of the superior tibiofibular joint and ligament, left knee**
+ **S83.8 Sprain of other specified parts of knee**
+ **S83.8X Sprain of other specified parts of knee**
+7th **S83.8X1 Sprain of other specified parts of right knee**
+7th **S83.8X2 Sprain of other specified parts of left knee**
+7th **S83.8X9 Sprain of other specified parts of unspecified knee**
+ **S83.9 Sprain of unspecified site of knee**
X+7th **S83.90 Sprain of unspecified site of unspecified knee**
X+7th **S83.91 Sprain of unspecified site of right knee**
X+7th **S83.92 Sprain of unspecified site of left knee**

S84 Injury of nerves at lower leg level
Code also any associated open wound (S81.-)
Excludes2: *injury of nerves at ankle and foot level (S94.-)*

The appropriate 7th character is to be added to each code from category S84
A initial encounter
D subsequent encounter
S sequela

+ **S84.0 Injury of tibial nerve at lower leg level**
X+7th **S84.00 Injury of tibial nerve at lower leg level, unspecified leg**
X+7th **S84.01 Injury of tibial nerve at lower leg level, right leg**
X+7th **S84.02 Injury of tibial nerve at lower leg level, left leg**
+ **S84.1 Injury of peroneal nerve at lower leg level**
X+7th **S84.10 Injury of peroneal nerve at lower leg level, unspecified leg**
X+7th **S84.11 Injury of peroneal nerve at lower leg level, right leg**
X+7th **S84.12 Injury of peroneal nerve at lower leg level, left leg**
+ **S84.2 Injury of cutaneous sensory nerve at lower leg level**
X+7th **S84.20 Injury of cutaneous sensory nerve at lower leg level, unspecified leg**
X+7th **S84.21 Injury of cutaneous sensory nerve at lower leg level, right leg**
X+7th **S84.22 Injury of cutaneous sensory nerve at lower leg level, left leg**
+ **S84.8 Injury of other nerves at lower leg level**
+ **S84.80 Injury of other nerves at lower leg level**
+7th **S84.801 Injury of other nerves at lower leg level, right leg**
+7th **S84.802 Injury of other nerves at lower leg level, left leg**
+7th **S84.809 Injury of other nerves at lower leg level, unspecified leg**
+ **S84.9 Injury of unspecified nerve at lower leg level**
X+7th **S84.90 Injury of unspecified nerve at lower leg level, unspecified leg**
X+7th **S84.91 Injury of unspecified nerve at lower leg level, right leg**
X+7th **S84.92 Injury of unspecified nerve at lower leg level, left leg**

S85 Injury of blood vessels at lower leg level

Code also any associated open wound (S81.-)

Excludes2: *injury of blood vessels at ankle and foot level (S95.-)*

The appropriate 7th character is to be added to each code from category S85
A initial encounter
D subsequent encounter
S sequela

\+ **S85.0 Injury of popliteal artery**
\+ **S85.00 Unspecified injury of popliteal artery**
MCC +7th **S85.001 Unspecified injury of popliteal artery, right leg**
MCC +7th **S85.002 Unspecified injury of popliteal artery, left leg**
MCC +7th **S85.009 Unspecified injury of popliteal artery, unspecified leg**
\+ **S85.01 Laceration of popliteal artery**
MCC +7th **S85.011 Laceration of popliteal artery, right leg**
MCC +7th **S85.012 Laceration of popliteal artery, left leg**
MCC +7th **S85.019 Laceration of popliteal artery, unspecified leg**
\+ **S85.09 Other specified injury of popliteal artery**
MCC +7th **S85.091 Other specified injury of popliteal artery, right leg**
MCC +7th **S85.092 Other specified injury of popliteal artery, left leg**
MCC +7th **S85.099 Other specified injury of popliteal artery, unspecified leg**
\+ **S85.1 Injury of tibial artery**
\+ **S85.10 Unspecified injury of unspecified tibial artery**
Injury of tibial artery NOS
CC +7th **S85.101 Unspecified injury of unspecified tibial artery, right leg**
CC +7th **S85.102 Unspecified injury of unspecified tibial artery, left leg**
CC +7th **S85.109 Unspecified injury of unspecified tibial artery, unspecified leg**
\+ **S85.11 Laceration of unspecified tibial artery**
CC +7th **S85.111 Laceration of unspecified tibial artery, right leg**
CC +7th **S85.112 Laceration of unspecified tibial artery, left leg**
CC +7th **S85.119 Laceration of unspecified tibial artery, unspecified leg**
\+ **S85.12 Other specified injury of unspecified tibial artery**
CC +7th **S85.121 Other specified injury of unspecified tibial artery, right leg**
CC +7th **S85.122 Other specified injury of unspecified tibial artery, left leg**
CC +7th **S85.129 Other specified injury of unspecified tibial artery, unspecified leg**
\+ **S85.13 Unspecified injury of anterior tibial artery**
CC +7th **S85.131 Unspecified injury of anterior tibial artery, right leg**
CC +7th **S85.132 Unspecified injury of anterior tibial artery, left leg**
CC +7th **S85.139 Unspecified injury of anterior tibial artery, unspecified leg**
\+ **S85.14 Laceration of anterior tibial artery**
CC +7th **S85.141 Laceration of anterior tibial artery, right leg**
CC +7th **S85.142 Laceration of anterior tibial artery, left leg**
CC +7th **S85.149 Laceration of anterior tibial artery, unspecified leg**
\+ **S85.15 Other specified injury of anterior tibial artery**
CC +7th **S85.151 Other specified injury of anterior tibial artery, right leg**
CC +7th **S85.152 Other specified injury of anterior tibial artery, left leg**
CC +7th **S85.159 Other specified injury of anterior tibial artery, unspecified leg**
\+ **S85.16 Unspecified injury of posterior tibial artery**
CC +7th **S85.161 Unspecified injury of posterior tibial artery, right leg**
CC +7th **S85.162 Unspecified injury of posterior tibial artery, left leg**
CC +7th **S85.169 Unspecified injury of posterior tibial artery, unspecified leg**
\+ **S85.17 Laceration of posterior tibial artery**
CC +7th **S85.171 Laceration of posterior tibial artery, right leg**
CC +7th **S85.172 Laceration of posterior tibial artery, left leg**
CC +7th **S85.179 Laceration of posterior tibial artery, unspecified leg**
\+ **S85.18 Other specified injury of posterior tibial artery**
CC +7th **S85.181 Other specified injury of posterior tibial artery, right leg**
CC +7th **S85.182 Other specified injury of posterior tibial artery, left leg**
CC +7th **S85.189 Other specified injury of posterior tibial artery, unspecified leg**
\+ **S85.2 Injury of peroneal artery**
\+ **S85.20 Unspecified injury of peroneal artery**
CC +7th **S85.201 Unspecified injury of peroneal artery, right leg**
CC +7th **S85.202 Unspecified injury of peroneal artery, left leg**
CC +7th **S85.209 Unspecified injury of peroneal artery, unspecified leg**
\+ **S85.21 Laceration of peroneal artery**
CC +7th **S85.211 Laceration of peroneal artery, right leg**
CC +7th **S85.212 Laceration of peroneal artery, left leg**
CC +7th **S85.219 Laceration of peroneal artery, unspecified leg**
\+ **S85.29 Other specified injury of peroneal artery**
CC +7th **S85.291 Other specified injury of peroneal artery, right leg**
CC +7th **S85.292 Other specified injury of peroneal artery, left leg**
CC +7th **S85.299 Other specified injury of peroneal artery, unspecified leg**
\+ **S85.3 Injury of greater saphenous vein at lower leg level**
Injury of greater saphenous vein NOS
Injury of saphenous vein NOS
\+ **S85.30 Unspecified injury of greater saphenous vein at lower leg level**
CC +7th **S85.301 Unspecified injury of greater saphenous vein at lower leg level, right leg**
CC +7th **S85.302 Unspecified injury of greater saphenous vein at lower leg level, left leg**
CC +7th **S85.309 Unspecified injury of greater saphenous vein at lower leg level, unspecified leg**
\+ **S85.31 Laceration of greater saphenous vein at lower leg level**
CC +7th **S85.311 Laceration of greater saphenous vein at lower leg level, right leg**
CC +7th **S85.312 Laceration of greater saphenous vein at lower leg level, left leg**
CC +7th **S85.319 Laceration of greater saphenous vein at lower leg level, unspecified leg**
\+ **S85.39 Other specified injury of greater saphenous vein at lower leg level**
CC +7th **S85.391 Other specified injury of greater saphenous vein at lower leg level, right leg**
CC +7th **S85.392 Other specified injury of greater saphenous vein at lower leg level, left leg**
CC +7th **S85.399 Other specified injury of greater saphenous vein at lower leg level, unspecified leg**
\+ **S85.4 Injury of lesser saphenous vein at lower leg level**
\+ **S85.40 Unspecified injury of lesser saphenous vein at lower leg level**
CC +7th **S85.401 Unspecified injury of lesser saphenous vein at lower leg level, right leg**
CC +7th **S85.402 Unspecified injury of lesser saphenous vein at lower leg level, left leg**
CC +7th **S85.409 Unspecified injury of lesser saphenous vein at lower leg level, unspecified leg**
\+ **S85.41 Laceration of lesser saphenous vein at lower leg level**
CC +7th **S85.411 Laceration of lesser saphenous vein at lower leg level, right leg**
CC +7th **S85.412 Laceration of lesser saphenous vein at lower leg level, left leg**
CC +7th **S85.419 Laceration of lesser saphenous vein at lower leg level, unspecified leg**

+ **S85.49 Other specified injury of lesser saphenous vein at lower leg level**
  - CC +7th **S85.491 Other specified injury of lesser saphenous vein at lower leg level, right leg**
  - CC +7th **S85.492 Other specified injury of lesser saphenous vein at lower leg level, left leg**
  - CC +7th **S85.499 Other specified injury of lesser saphenous vein at lower leg level, unspecified leg**

+ **S85.5 Injury of popliteal vein**
  + **S85.50 Unspecified injury of popliteal vein**
    - MCC +7th **S85.501 Unspecified injury of popliteal vein, right leg**
    - MCC +7th **S85.502 Unspecified injury of popliteal vein, left leg**
    - MCC +7th **S85.509 Unspecified injury of popliteal vein, unspecified leg**
  + **S85.51 Laceration of popliteal vein**
    - MCC +7th **S85.511 Laceration of popliteal vein, right leg**
    - MCC +7th **S85.512 Laceration of popliteal vein, left leg**
    - MCC +7th **S85.519 Laceration of popliteal vein, unspecified leg**
  + **S85.59 Other specified injury of popliteal vein**
    - MCC +7th **S85.591 Other specified injury of popliteal vein, right leg**
    - MCC +7th **S85.592 Other specified injury of popliteal vein, left leg**
    - MCC +7th **S85.599 Other specified injury of popliteal vein, unspecified leg**

+ **S85.8 Injury of other blood vessels at lower leg level**
  + **S85.80 Unspecified injury of other blood vessels at lower leg level**
    - CC +7th **S85.801 Unspecified injury of other blood vessels at lower leg level, right leg**
    - CC +7th **S85.802 Unspecified injury of other blood vessels at lower leg level, left leg**
    - CC +7th **S85.809 Unspecified injury of other blood vessels at lower leg level, unspecified leg**
  + **S85.81 Laceration of other blood vessels at lower leg level**
    - CC +7th **S85.811 Laceration of other blood vessels at lower leg level, right leg**
    - CC +7th **S85.812 Laceration of other blood vessels at lower leg level, left leg**
    - CC +7th **S85.819 Laceration of other blood vessels at lower leg level, unspecified leg**
  + **S85.89 Other specified injury of other blood vessels at lower leg level**
    - CC +7th **S85.891 Other specified injury of other blood vessels at lower leg level, right leg**
    - CC +7th **S85.892 Other specified injury of other blood vessels at lower leg level, left leg**
    - CC +7th **S85.899 Other specified injury of other blood vessels at lower leg level, unspecified leg**

+ **S85.9 Injury of unspecified blood vessel at lower leg level**
  + **S85.90 Unspecified injury of unspecified blood vessel at lower leg level**
    - CC +7th **S85.901 Unspecified injury of unspecified blood vessel at lower leg level, right leg**
    - CC +7th **S85.902 Unspecified injury of unspecified blood vessel at lower leg level, left leg**
    - CC +7th **S85.909 Unspecified injury of unspecified blood vessel at lower leg level, unspecified leg**
  + **S85.91 Laceration of unspecified blood vessel at lower leg level**
    - CC +7th **S85.911 Laceration of unspecified blood vessel at lower leg level, right leg**
    - CC +7th **S85.912 Laceration of unspecified blood vessel at lower leg level, left leg**
    - CC +7th **S85.919 Laceration of unspecified blood vessel at lower leg level, unspecified leg**
  + **S85.99 Other specified injury of unspecified blood vessel at lower leg level**
    - CC +7th **S85.991 Other specified injury of unspecified blood vessel at lower leg level, right leg**
    - CC +7th **S85.992 Other specified injury of unspecified blood vessel at lower leg level, left leg**
    - CC +7th **S85.999 Other specified injury of unspecified blood vessel at lower leg level, unspecified leg**

S86 Injury of muscle, fascia and tendon at lower leg level

Code also any associated open wound (S81.-)

Excludes2: *injury of muscle, fascia and tendon at ankle (S96.-)*
injury of patellar ligament (tendon) (S76.1-)
sprain of joints and ligaments of knee (S83.-)

The appropriate 7th character is to be added to each code from category S86
- A initial encounter
- D subsequent encounter
- S sequela

+ **S86.0 Injury of Achilles tendon**
  + **S86.00 Unspecified injury of Achilles tendon**
    - +7th **S86.001 Unspecified injury of right Achilles tendon**
    - +7th **S86.002 Unspecified injury of left Achilles tendon**
    - +7th **S86.009 Unspecified injury of unspecified Achilles tendon**
  + **S86.01 Strain of Achilles tendon**
    - +7th **S86.011 Strain of right Achilles tendon**
    - +7th **S86.012 Strain of left Achilles tendon**
    - +7th **S86.019 Strain of unspecified Achilles tendon**
  + **S86.02 Laceration of Achilles tendon**
    - CC +7th **S86.021 Laceration of right Achilles tendon**
    - CC +7th **S86.022 Laceration of left Achilles tendon**
    - CC +7th **S86.029 Laceration of unspecified Achilles tendon**
  + **S86.09 Other specified injury of Achilles tendon**
    - +7th **S86.091 Other specified injury of right Achilles tendon**
    - +7th **S86.092 Other specified injury of left Achilles tendon**
    - +7th **S86.099 Other specified injury of unspecified Achilles tendon**

+ **S86.1 Injury of other muscle(s) and tendon(s) of posterior muscle group at lower leg level**
  + **S86.10 Unspecified injury of other muscle(s) and tendon(s) of posterior muscle group at lower leg level**
    - +7th **S86.101 Unspecified injury of other muscle(s) and tendon(s) of posterior muscle group at lower leg level, right leg**
    - +7th **S86.102 Unspecified injury of other muscle(s) and tendon(s) of posterior muscle group at lower leg level, left leg**
    - +7th **S86.109 Unspecified injury of other muscle(s) and tendon(s) of posterior muscle group at lower leg level, unspecified leg**
  + **S86.11 Strain of other muscle(s) and tendon(s) of posterior muscle group at lower leg level**
    - +7th **S86.111 Strain of other muscle(s) and tendon(s) of posterior muscle group at lower leg level, right leg**
    - +7th **S86.112 Strain of other muscle(s) and tendon(s) of posterior muscle group at lower leg level, left leg**
    - +7th **S86.119 Strain of other muscle(s) and tendon(s) of posterior muscle group at lower leg level, unspecified leg**
  + **S86.12 Laceration of other muscle(s) and tendon(s) of posterior muscle group at lower leg level**
    - CC +7th **S86.121 Laceration of other muscle(s) and tendon(s) of posterior muscle group at lower leg level, right leg**
    - CC +7th **S86.122 Laceration of other muscle(s) and tendon(s) of posterior muscle group at lower leg level, left leg**
    - CC +7th **S86.129 Laceration of other muscle(s) and tendon(s) of posterior muscle group at lower leg level, unspecified leg**
  + **S86.19 Other injury of other muscle(s) and tendon(s) of posterior muscle group at lower leg level**
    - +7th **S86.191 Other injury of other muscle(s) and tendon(s) of posterior muscle group at lower leg level, right leg**
    - +7th **S86.192 Other injury of other muscle(s) and tendon(s) of posterior muscle group at lower leg level, left leg**
    - +7th **S86.199 Other injury of other muscle(s) and tendon(s) of posterior muscle group at lower leg level, unspecified leg**

+ **S86.2** Injury of muscle(s) and tendon(s) of anterior muscle group at lower leg level
  + **S86.20** Unspecified injury of muscle(s) and tendon(s) of anterior muscle group at lower leg level
    - +7th **S86.201** Unspecified injury of muscle(s) and tendon(s) of anterior muscle group at lower leg level, right leg
    - +7th **S86.202** Unspecified injury of muscle(s) and tendon(s) of anterior muscle group at lower leg level, left leg
    - +7th **S86.209** Unspecified injury of muscle(s) and tendon(s) of anterior muscle group at lower leg level, unspecified leg
  + **S86.21** Strain of muscle(s) and tendon(s) of anterior muscle group at lower leg level
    - +7th **S86.211** Strain of muscle(s) and tendon(s) of anterior muscle group at lower leg level, right leg
    - +7th **S86.212** Strain of muscle(s) and tendon(s) of anterior muscle group at lower leg level, left leg
    - +7th **S86.219** Strain of muscle(s) and tendon(s) of anterior muscle group at lower leg level, unspecified leg
  + **S86.22** Laceration of muscle(s) and tendon(s) of anterior muscle group at lower leg level
    - CC +7th **S86.221** Laceration of muscle(s) and tendon(s) of anterior muscle group at lower leg level, right leg
    - CC +7th **S86.222** Laceration of muscle(s) and tendon(s) of anterior muscle group at lower leg level, left leg
    - CC +7th **S86.229** Laceration of muscle(s) and tendon(s) of anterior muscle group at lower leg level, unspecified leg
  + **S86.29** Other injury of muscle(s) and tendon(s) of anterior muscle group at lower leg level
    - +7th **S86.291** Other injury of muscle(s) and tendon(s) of anterior muscle group at lower leg level, right leg
    - +7th **S86.292** Other injury of muscle(s) and tendon(s) of anterior muscle group at lower leg level, left leg
    - +7th **S86.299** Other injury of muscle(s) and tendon(s) of anterior muscle group at lower leg level, unspecified leg

+ **S86.3** Injury of muscle(s) and tendon(s) of peroneal muscle group at lower leg level
  + **S86.30** Unspecified injury of muscle(s) and tendon(s) of peroneal muscle group at lower leg level
    - +7th **S86.301** Unspecified injury of muscle(s) and tendon(s) of peroneal muscle group at lower leg level, right leg
    - +7th **S86.302** Unspecified injury of muscle(s) and tendon(s) of peroneal muscle group at lower leg level, left leg
    - +7th **S86.309** Unspecified injury of muscle(s) and tendon(s) of peroneal muscle group at lower leg level, unspecified leg
  + **S86.31** Strain of muscle(s) and tendon(s) of peroneal muscle group at lower leg level
    - +7th **S86.311** Strain of muscle(s) and tendon(s) of peroneal muscle group at lower leg level, right leg
    - +7th **S86.312** Strain of muscle(s) and tendon(s) of peroneal muscle group at lower leg level, left leg
    - +7th **S86.319** Strain of muscle(s) and tendon(s) of peroneal muscle group at lower leg level, unspecified leg
  + **S86.32** Laceration of muscle(s) and tendon(s) of peroneal muscle group at lower leg level
    - CC +7th **S86.321** Laceration of muscle(s) and tendon(s) of peroneal muscle group at lower leg level, right leg
    - CC +7th **S86.322** Laceration of muscle(s) and tendon(s) of peroneal muscle group at lower leg level, left leg
    - CC +7th **S86.329** Laceration of muscle(s) and tendon(s) of peroneal muscle group at lower leg level, unspecified leg
  + **S86.39** Other injury of muscle(s) and tendon(s) of peroneal muscle group at lower leg level
    - +7th **S86.391** Other injury of muscle(s) and tendon(s) of peroneal muscle group at lower leg level, right leg
    - +7th **S86.392** Other injury of muscle(s) and tendon(s) of peroneal muscle group at lower leg level, left leg
    - +7th **S86.399** Other injury of muscle(s) and tendon(s) of peroneal muscle group at lower leg level, unspecified leg

+ **S86.8** Injury of other muscles and tendons at lower leg level
  + **S86.80** Unspecified injury of other muscles and tendons at lower leg level
    - + **S86.801** Unspecified injury of other muscle(s) and tendon(s) at lower leg level, right leg
    - + **S86.802** Unspecified injury of other muscle(s) and tendon(s) at lower leg level, left leg
    - + **S86.809** Unspecified injury of other muscle(s) and tendon(s) at lower leg level, unspecified leg
  + **S86.81** Strain of other muscles and tendons at lower leg level
    - +7th **S86.811** Strain of other muscle(s) and tendon(s) at lower leg level, right leg
    - +7th **S86.812** Strain of other muscle(s) and tendon(s) at lower leg level, left leg
    - +7th **S86.819** Strain of other muscle(s) and tendon(s) at lower leg level, unspecified leg
  + **S86.82** Laceration of other muscles and tendons at lower leg level
    - CC +7th **S86.821** Laceration of other muscle(s) and tendon(s) at lower leg level, right leg
    - CC +7th **S86.822** Laceration of other muscle(s) and tendon(s) at lower leg level, left leg
    - CC +7th **S86.829** Laceration of other muscle(s) and tendon(s) at lower leg level, unspecified leg
  + **S86.89** Other injury of other muscles and tendons at lower leg level
    - +7th **S86.891** Other injury of other muscle(s) and tendon(s) at lower leg level, right leg
    - +7th **S86.892** Other injury of other muscle(s) and tendon(s) at lower leg level, left leg
    - +7th **S86.899** Other injury of other muscle(s) and tendon(s) at lower leg level, unspecified leg

+ **S86.9** Injury of unspecified muscle and tendon at lower leg level
  + **S86.90** Unspecified injury of unspecified muscle and tendon at lower leg level
    - +7th **S86.901** Unspecified injury of unspecified muscle(s) and tendon(s) at lower leg level, right leg
    - +7th **S86.902** Unspecified injury of unspecified muscle(s) and tendon(s) at lower leg level, left leg
    - +7th **S86.909** Unspecified injury of unspecified muscle(s) and tendon(s) at lower leg level, unspecified leg
  + **S86.91** Strain of unspecified muscle and tendon at lower leg level
    - +7th **S86.911** Strain of unspecified muscle(s) and tendon(s) at lower leg level, right leg
    - +7th **S86.912** Strain of unspecified muscle(s) and tendon(s) at lower leg level, left leg
    - +7th **S86.919** Strain of unspecified muscle(s) and tendon(s) at lower leg level, unspecified leg
  + **S86.92** Laceration of unspecified muscle and tendon at lower leg level
    - CC +7th **S86.921** Laceration of unspecified muscle(s) and tendon(s) at lower leg level, right leg
    - CC +7th **S86.922** Laceration of unspecified muscle(s) and tendon(s) at lower leg level, left leg
    - CC +7th **S86.929** Laceration of unspecified muscle(s) and tendon(s) at lower leg level, unspecified leg

\+ **S86.99 Other injury of unspecified muscle and tendon at lower leg level**

+7th **S86.991 Other injury of unspecified muscle(s) and tendon(s) at lower leg level, right leg**

+7th **S86.992 Other injury of unspecified muscle(s) and tendon(s) at lower leg level, left leg**

+7th **S86.999 Other injury of unspecified muscle(s) and tendon(s) at lower leg level, unspecified leg**

S87 Crushing injury of lower leg

Use additional code(s) for all associated injuries

Excludes2: *crushing injury of ankle and foot (S97.-)*

The appropriate 7th character is to be added to each code from category S87
A initial encounter
D subsequent encounter
S sequela

\+ **S87.0 Crushing injury of knee**

X+7th **S87.00 Crushing injury of unspecified knee**

X+7th **S87.01 Crushing injury of right knee**

X+7th **S87.02 Crushing injury of left knee**

\+ **S87.8 Crushing injury of lower leg**

X+7th **S87.80 Crushing injury of unspecified lower leg**

X+7th **S87.81 Crushing injury of right lower leg**

X+7th **S87.82 Crushing injury of left lower leg**

S88 Traumatic amputation of lower leg

NOTE An amputation not identified as partial or complete should be coded to complete

Excludes1: *traumatic amputation of ankle and foot (S98.-)*

The appropriate 7th character is to be added to each code from category S88
A initial encounter
D subsequent encounter
S sequela

\+ **S88.0 Traumatic amputation at knee level**

\+ **S88.01 Complete traumatic amputation at knee level**

CC +7th **S88.011 Complete traumatic amputation at knee level, right lower leg**

CC +7th **S88.012 Complete traumatic amputation at knee level, left lower leg**

CC +7th **S88.019 Complete traumatic amputation at knee level, unspecified lower leg**

\+ **S88.02 Partial traumatic amputation at knee level**

CC +7th **S88.021 Partial traumatic amputation at knee level, right lower leg**

CC +7th **S88.022 Partial traumatic amputation at knee level, left lower leg**

CC +7th **S88.029 Partial traumatic amputation at knee level, unspecified lower leg**

\+ **S88.1 Traumatic amputation at level between knee and ankle**

\+ **S88.11 Complete traumatic amputation at level between knee and ankle**

CC +7th **S88.111 Complete traumatic amputation at level between knee and ankle, right lower leg**

CC +7th **S88.112 Complete traumatic amputation at level between knee and ankle, left lower leg**

CC +7th **S88.119 Complete traumatic amputation at level between knee and ankle, unspecified lower leg**

\+ **S88.12 Partial traumatic amputation at level between knee and ankle**

CC +7th **S88.121 Partial traumatic amputation at level between knee and ankle, right lower leg**

CC +7th **S88.122 Partial traumatic amputation at level between knee and ankle, left lower leg**

CC +7th **S88.129 Partial traumatic amputation at level between knee and ankle, unspecified lower leg**

\+ **S88.9 Traumatic amputation of lower leg, level unspecified**

\+ **S88.91 Complete traumatic amputation of lower leg, level unspecified**

CC +7th **S88.911 Complete traumatic amputation of right lower leg, level unspecified**

CC +7th **S88.912 Complete traumatic amputation of left lower leg, level unspecified**

CC +7th **S88.919 Complete traumatic amputation of unspecified lower leg, level unspecified**

\+ **S88.92 Partial traumatic amputation of lower leg, level unspecified**

CC +7th **S88.921 Partial traumatic amputation of right lower leg, level unspecified**

CC +7th **S88.922 Partial traumatic amputation of left lower leg, level unspecified**

CC +7th **S88.929 Partial traumatic amputation of unspecified lower leg, level unspecified**

S89 Other and unspecified injuries of lower leg

NOTE A fracture not indicated as open or closed should be coded to closed

Excludes2: *other and unspecified injuries of ankle and foot (S99.-)*

The appropriate 7th character is to be added to each code from subcategories **S89.0, S89.1, S89.2,** and **S89.3**
A initial encounter for closed fracture
D subsequent encounter for fracture with routine healing
G subsequent encounter for fracture with delayed healing
K subsequent encounter for fracture with nonunion
P subsequent encounter for fracture with malunion
S sequela

Review coding guideline C.19.c

\+ **S89.0 Physeal fracture of upper end of tibia**

\+ **S89.00 Unspecified physeal fracture of upper end of tibia**

CC +7th **S89.001 Unspecified physeal fracture of upper end of right tibia**
HAC 7th character A see Appendix B for HAC conditional logic

CC +7th **S89.002 Unspecified physeal fracture of upper end of left tibia**
HAC 7th character A see Appendix B for HAC conditional logic

CC +7th **S89.009 Unspecified physeal fracture of upper end of unspecified tibia**
HAC 7th character A see Appendix B for HAC conditional logic

\+ **S89.01 Salter-Harris Type I physeal fracture of upper end of tibia**

CC +7th **S89.011 Salter-Harris Type I physeal fracture of upper end of right tibia**
HAC 7th character A see Appendix B for HAC conditional logic

CC +7th **S89.012 Salter-Harris Type I physeal fracture of upper end of left tibia**
HAC 7th character A see Appendix B for HAC conditional logic

CC +7th **S89.019 Salter-Harris Type I physeal fracture of upper end of unspecified tibia**
HAC 7th character A see Appendix B for HAC conditional logic

\+ **S89.02 Salter-Harris Type II physeal fracture of upper end of tibia**

CC +7th **S89.021 Salter-Harris Type II physeal fracture of upper end of right tibia**
HAC 7th character A see Appendix B for HAC conditional logic

CC +7th **S89.022 Salter-Harris Type II physeal fracture of upper end of left tibia**
HAC 7th character A see Appendix B for HAC conditional logic

CC +7th **S89.029 Salter-Harris Type II physeal fracture of upper end of unspecified tibia**
HAC 7th character A see Appendix B for HAC conditional logic

\+ **S89.03 Salter-Harris Type III physeal fracture of upper end of tibia**

CC +7th **S89.031 Salter-Harris Type III physeal fracture of upper end of right tibia**
HAC 7th character A see Appendix B for HAC conditional logic

CC +7th **S89.032 Salter-Harris Type III physeal fracture of upper end of left tibia**
HAC 7th character A see Appendix B for HAC conditional logic

CC +7th **S89.039 Salter-Harris Type III physeal fracture of upper end of unspecified tibia**
HAC 7th character A see Appendix B for HAC conditional logic

+ **S89.04 Salter-Harris Type IV physeal fracture of upper end of tibia**
  - CC +7th **S89.041 Salter-Harris Type IV physeal fracture of upper end of right tibia**
    - HAC 7th character A see Appendix B for HAC conditional logic
  - CC +7th **S89.042 Salter-Harris Type IV physeal fracture of upper end of left tibia**
    - HAC 7th character A see Appendix B for HAC conditional logic
  - CC +7th **S89.049 Salter-Harris Type IV physeal fracture of upper end of unspecified tibia**
    - HAC 7th character A see Appendix B for HAC conditional logic
+ **S89.09 Other physeal fracture of upper end of tibia**
  - CC +7th **S89.091 Other physeal fracture of upper end of right tibia**
    - HAC 7th character A see Appendix B for HAC conditional logic
  - CC +7th **S89.092 Other physeal fracture of upper end of left tibia**
    - HAC 7th character A see Appendix B for HAC conditional logic
  - CC +7th **S89.099 Other physeal fracture of upper end of unspecified tibia**
    - HAC 7th character A see Appendix B for HAC conditional logic

+ **S89.1 Physeal fracture of lower end of tibia**
  + **S89.10 Unspecified physeal fracture of lower end of tibia**
    - CC +7th **S89.101 Unspecified physeal fracture of lower end of right tibia**
    - CC +7th **S89.102 Unspecified physeal fracture of lower end of left tibia**
    - CC +7th **S89.109 Unspecified physeal fracture of lower end of unspecified tibia**
  + **S89.11 Salter-Harris Type I physeal fracture of lower end of tibia**
    - CC +7th **S89.111 Salter-Harris Type I physeal fracture of lower end of right tibia**
    - CC +7th **S89.112 Salter-Harris Type I physeal fracture of lower end of left tibia**
    - CC +7th **S89.119 Salter-Harris Type I physeal fracture of lower end of unspecified tibia**
  + **S89.12 Salter-Harris Type II physeal fracture of lower end of tibia**
    - CC +7th **S89.121 Salter-Harris Type II physeal fracture of lower end of right tibia**
    - CC +7th **S89.122 Salter-Harris Type II physeal fracture of lower end of left tibia**
    - CC +7th **S89.129 Salter-Harris Type II physeal fracture of lower end of unspecified tibia**
  + **S89.13 Salter-Harris Type III physeal fracture of lower end of tibia**
    - ***Excludes1:*** *fracture of medial malleolus (adult) (S82.5-)*
    - CC +7th **S89.131 Salter-Harris Type III physeal fracture of lower end of right tibia**
    - CC +7th **S89.132 Salter-Harris Type III physeal fracture of lower end of left tibia**
    - CC +7th **S89.139 Salter-Harris Type III physeal fracture of lower end of unspecified tibia**
  + **S89.14 Salter-Harris Type IV physeal fracture of lower end of tibia**
    - ***Excludes1:*** *fracture of medial malleolus (adult) (S82.5-)*
    - CC +7th **S89.141 Salter-Harris Type IV physeal fracture of lower end of right tibia**
    - CC +7th **S89.142 Salter-Harris Type IV physeal fracture of lower end of left tibia**
    - CC +7th **S89.149 Salter-Harris Type IV physeal fracture of lower end of unspecified tibia**
  + **S89.19 Other physeal fracture of lower end of tibia**
    - CC +7th **S89.191 Other physeal fracture of lower end of right tibia**
    - CC +7th **S89.192 Other physeal fracture of lower end of left tibia**
    - CC +7th **S89.199 Other physeal fracture of lower end of unspecified tibia**

+ **S89.2 Physeal fracture of upper end of fibula**
  + **S89.20 Unspecified physeal fracture of upper end of fibula**
    - CC +7th **S89.201 Unspecified physeal fracture of upper end of right fibula**
    - CC +7th **S89.202 Unspecified physeal fracture of upper end of left fibula**
    - CC +7th **S89.209 Unspecified physeal fracture of upper end of unspecified fibula**
  + **S89.21 Salter-Harris Type I physeal fracture of upper end of fibula**
    - CC +7th **S89.211 Salter-Harris Type I physeal fracture of upper end of right fibula**
    - CC +7th **S89.212 Salter-Harris Type I physeal fracture of upper end of left fibula**
    - CC +7th **S89.219 Salter-Harris Type I physeal fracture of upper end of unspecified fibula**
  + **S89.22 Salter-Harris Type II physeal fracture of upper end of fibula**
    - CC +7th **S89.221 Salter-Harris Type II physeal fracture of upper end of right fibula**
    - CC +7th **S89.222 Salter-Harris Type II physeal fracture of upper end of left fibula**
    - CC +7th **S89.229 Salter-Harris Type II physeal fracture of upper end of unspecified fibula**
  + **S89.29 Other physeal fracture of upper end of fibula**
    - CC +7th **S89.291 Other physeal fracture of upper end of right fibula**
    - CC +7th **S89.292 Other physeal fracture of upper end of left fibula**
    - CC +7th **S89.299 Other physeal fracture of upper end of unspecified fibula**

+ **S89.3 Physeal fracture of lower end of fibula**
  + **S89.30 Unspecified physeal fracture of lower end of fibula**
    - CC +7th **S89.301 Unspecified physeal fracture of lower end of right fibula**
    - CC +7th **S89.302 Unspecified physeal fracture of lower end of left fibula**
    - CC +7th **S89.309 Unspecified physeal fracture of lower end of unspecified fibula**
  + **S89.31 Salter-Harris Type I physeal fracture of lower end of fibula**
    - CC +7th **S89.311 Salter-Harris Type I physeal fracture of lower end of right fibula**
    - CC +7th **S89.312 Salter-Harris Type I physeal fracture of lower end of left fibula**
    - CC +7th **S89.319 Salter-Harris Type I physeal fracture of lower end of unspecified fibula**
  + **S89.32 Salter-Harris Type II physeal fracture of lower end of fibula**
    - CC +7th **S89.321 Salter-Harris Type II physeal fracture of lower end of right fibula**
    - CC +7th **S89.322 Salter-Harris Type II physeal fracture of lower end of left fibula**
    - CC +7th **S89.329 Salter-Harris Type II physeal fracture of lower end of unspecified fibula**
  + **S89.39 Other physeal fracture of lower end of fibula**
    - CC +7th **S89.391 Other physeal fracture of lower end of right fibula**
    - CC +7th **S89.392 Other physeal fracture of lower end of left fibula**
    - CC +7th **S89.399 Other physeal fracture of lower end of unspecified fibula**

+ **S89.8 Other specified injuries of lower leg**

> The appropriate 7th character is to be added to each code in subcategory **S89.8**
> A initial encounter
> D subsequent encounter
> S sequela

  - X+7th **S89.80 Other specified injuries of unspecified lower leg**
  - X+7th **S89.81 Other specified injuries of right lower leg**
  - X+7th **S89.82 Other specified injuries of left lower leg**

+ **S89.9 Unspecified injury of lower leg**

> The appropriate 7th character is to be added to each code in subcategory **S89.9**
> A initial encounter
> D subsequent encounter
> S sequela

  - X+7th **S89.90 Unspecified injury of unspecified lower leg**
  - X+7th **S89.91 Unspecified injury of right lower leg**
  - X+7th **S89.92 Unspecified injury of left lower leg**

Injuries to the ankle and foot (S90-S99)

Excludes2: *burns and corrosions (T20-T32)*
fracture of ankle and malleolus (S82.-)
frostbite (T33-T34)
insect bite or sting, venomous (T63.4)

S90 Superficial injury of ankle, foot and toes

The appropriate 7th character is to be added to each code from category S90
A initial encounter
D subsequent encounter
S sequela

+ **S90.0 Contusion of ankle**
  - X+7th **S90.00 Contusion of unspecified ankle**
  - X+7th **S90.01 Contusion of right ankle**
  - X+7th **S90.02 Contusion of left ankle**

+ **S90.1 Contusion of toe without damage to nail**
  + **S90.11 Contusion of great toe without damage to nail**
    - +7th **S90.111 Contusion of right great toe without damage to nail**
    - +7th **S90.112 Contusion of left great toe without damage to nail**
    - +7th **S90.119 Contusion of unspecified great toe without damage to nail**
  + **S90.12 Contusion of lesser toe without damage to nail**
    - +7th **S90.121 Contusion of right lesser toe(s) without damage to nail**
    - +7th **S90.122 Contusion of left lesser toe(s) without damage to nail**
    - +7th **S90.129 Contusion of unspecified lesser toe(s) without damage to nail**
      Contusion of toe NOS

+ **S90.2 Contusion of toe with damage to nail**
  + **S90.21 Contusion of great toe with damage to nail**
    - +7th **S90.211 Contusion of right great toe with damage to nail**
    - +7th **S90.212 Contusion of left great toe with damage to nail**
    - +7th **S90.219 Contusion of unspecified great toe with damage to nail**
  + **S90.22 Contusion of lesser toe with damage to nail**
    - +7th **S90.221 Contusion of right lesser toe(s) with damage to nail**
    - +7th **S90.222 Contusion of left lesser toe(s) with damage to nail**
    - +7th **S90.229 Contusion of unspecified lesser toe(s) with damage to nail**

+ **S90.3 Contusion of foot**
  Excludes2: *contusion of toes (S90.1-, S90.2-)*
  - X+7th **S90.30 Contusion of unspecified foot**
    Contusion of foot NOS
  - X+7th **S90.31 Contusion of right foot**
  - X+7th **S90.32 Contusion of left foot**

+ **S90.4 Other superficial injuries of toe**
  + **S90.41 Abrasion of toe**
    - +7th **S90.411 Abrasion, right great toe**
    - +7th **S90.412 Abrasion, left great toe**
    - +7th **S90.413 Abrasion, unspecified great toe**
    - +7th **S90.414 Abrasion, right lesser toe(s)**
    - +7th **S90.415 Abrasion, left lesser toe(s)**
    - +7th **S90.416 Abrasion, unspecified lesser toe(s)**
  + **S90.42 Blister (nonthermal) of toe**
    - +7th **S90.421 Blister (nonthermal), right great toe**
    - +7th **S90.422 Blister (nonthermal), left great toe**
    - +7th **S90.423 Blister (nonthermal), unspecified great toe**
    - +7th **S90.424 Blister (nonthermal), right lesser toe(s)**
    - +7th **S90.425 Blister (nonthermal), left lesser toe(s)**
    - +7th **S90.426 Blister (nonthermal), unspecified lesser toe(s)**
  + **S90.44 External constriction of toe**
    Hair tourniquet syndrome of toe
    - +7th **S90.441 External constriction, right great toe**
    - +7th **S90.442 External constriction, left great toe**
    - +7th **S90.443 External constriction, unspecified great toe**
    - +7th **S90.444 External constriction, right lesser toe(s)**
    - +7th **S90.445 External constriction, left lesser toe(s)**
    - +7th **S90.446 External constriction, unspecified lesser toe(s)**
  + **S90.45 Superficial foreign body of toe**
    Splinter in the toe
    - +7th **S90.451 Superficial foreign body, right great toe**
    - +7th **S90.452 Superficial foreign body, left great toe**
    - +7th **S90.453 Superficial foreign body, unspecified great toe**
    - +7th **S90.454 Superficial foreign body, right lesser toe(s)**
    - +7th **S90.455 Superficial foreign body, left lesser toe(s)**
    - +7th **S90.456 Superficial foreign body, unspecified lesser toe(s)**
  + **S90.46 Insect bite (nonvenomous) of toe**
    - +7th **S90.461 Insect bite (nonvenomous), right great toe**
    - +7th **S90.462 Insect bite (nonvenomous), left great toe**
    - +7th **S90.463 Insect bite (nonvenomous), unspecified great toe**
    - +7th **S90.464 Insect bite (nonvenomous), right lesser toe(s)**
    - +7th **S90.465 Insect bite (nonvenomous), left lesser toe(s)**
    - +7th **S90.466 Insect bite (nonvenomous), unspecified lesser toe(s)**
  + **S90.47 Other superficial bite of toe**
    Excludes1: *open bite of toe (S91.15-, S91.25-)*
    - +7th **S90.471 Other superficial bite of right great toe**
    - +7th **S90.472 Other superficial bite of left great toe**
    - +7th **S90.473 Other superficial bite of unspecified great toe**
    - +7th **S90.474 Other superficial bite of right lesser toe(s)**
    - +7th **S90.475 Other superficial bite of left lesser toe(s)**
    - +7th **S90.476 Other superficial bite of unspecified lesser toe(s)**

+ **S90.5 Other superficial injuries of ankle**
  + **S90.51 Abrasion of ankle**
    - +7th **S90.511 Abrasion, right ankle**
    - +7th **S90.512 Abrasion, left ankle**
    - +7th **S90.519 Abrasion, unspecified ankle**
  + **S90.52 Blister (nonthermal) of ankle**
    - +7th **S90.521 Blister (nonthermal), right ankle**
    - +7th **S90.522 Blister (nonthermal), left ankle**
    - +7th **S90.529 Blister (nonthermal), unspecified ankle**
  + **S90.54 External constriction of ankle**
    - +7th **S90.541 External constriction, right ankle**
    - +7th **S90.542 External constriction, left ankle**
    - +7th **S90.549 External constriction, unspecified ankle**
  + **S90.55 Superficial foreign body of ankle**
    Splinter in the ankle
    - +7th **S90.551 Superficial foreign body, right ankle**
    - +7th **S90.552 Superficial foreign body, left ankle**
    - +7th **S90.559 Superficial foreign body, unspecified ankle**
  + **S90.56 Insect bite (nonvenomous) of ankle**
    - +7th **S90.561 Insect bite (nonvenomous), right ankle**
    - +7th **S90.562 Insect bite (nonvenomous), left ankle**
    - +7th **S90.569 Insect bite (nonvenomous), unspecified ankle**
  + **S90.57 Other superficial bite of ankle**
    Excludes1: *open bite of ankle (S91.05-)*
    - +7th **S90.571 Other superficial bite of ankle, right ankle**
    - +7th **S90.572 Other superficial bite of ankle, left ankle**
    - +7th **S90.579 Other superficial bite of ankle, unspecified ankle**

+ **S90.8 Other superficial injuries of foot**
  + **S90.81 Abrasion of foot**
    - +7th **S90.811 Abrasion, right foot**
    - +7th **S90.812 Abrasion, left foot**
    - +7th **S90.819 Abrasion, unspecified foot**
  + **S90.82 Blister (nonthermal) of foot**
    - +7th **S90.821 Blister (nonthermal), right foot**
    - +7th **S90.822 Blister (nonthermal), left foot**
    - +7th **S90.829 Blister (nonthermal), unspecified foot**
  + **S90.84 External constriction of foot**
    - +7th **S90.841 External constriction, right foot**
    - +7th **S90.842 External constriction, left foot**
    - +7th **S90.849 External constriction, unspecified foot**

Ankle

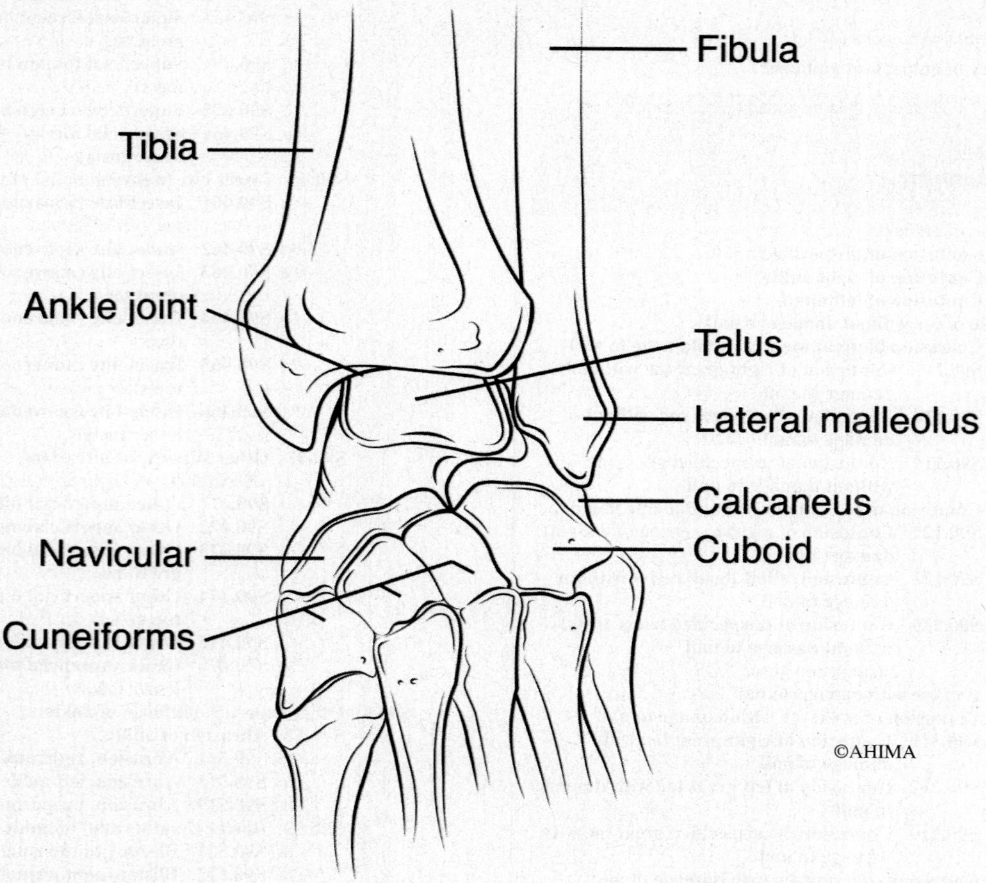

Muscles of the Foot

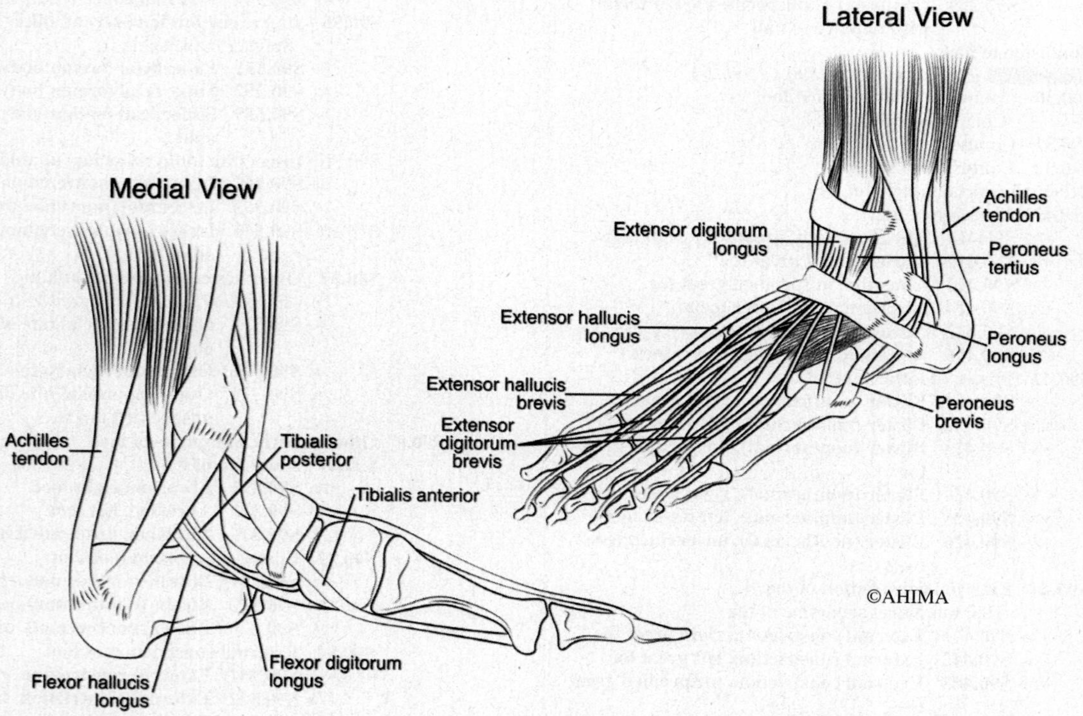

+ **S90.85 Superficial foreign body of foot**
  Splinter in the foot
  - +7th **S90.851 Superficial foreign body, right foot**
  - +7th **S90.852 Superficial foreign body, left foot**
  - +7th **S90.859 Superficial foreign body, unspecified foot**
+ **S90.86 Insect bite (nonvenomous) of foot**
  - +7th **S90.861 Insect bite (nonvenomous), right foot**
  - +7th **S90.862 Insect bite (nonvenomous), left foot**
  - +7th **S90.869 Insect bite (nonvenomous), unspecified foot**
+ **S90.87 Other superficial bite of foot**
  Excludes1: *open bite of foot (S91.35-)*
  - +7th **S90.871 Other superficial bite of right foot**
  - +7th **S90.872 Other superficial bite of left foot**
  - +7th **S90.879 Other superficial bite of unspecified foot**

+ **S90.9 Unspecified superficial injury of ankle, foot and toe**
+ **S90.91 Unspecified superficial injury of ankle**
  - +7th **S90.911 Unspecified superficial injury of right ankle**
  - +7th **S90.912 Unspecified superficial injury of left ankle**
  - +7th **S90.919 Unspecified superficial injury of unspecified ankle**
+ **S90.92 Unspecified superficial injury of foot**
  - +7th **S90.921 Unspecified superficial injury of right foot**
  - +7th **S90.922 Unspecified superficial injury of left foot**
  - +7th **S90.929 Unspecified superficial injury of unspecified foot**
+ **S90.93 Unspecified superficial injury of toes**
  - +7th **S90.931 Unspecified superficial injury of right great toe**
  - +7th **S90.932 Unspecified superficial injury of left great toe**
  - +7th **S90.933 Unspecified superficial injury of unspecified great toe**
  - +7th **S90.934 Unspecified superficial injury of right lesser toe(s)**
  - +7th **S90.935 Unspecified superficial injury of left lesser toe(s)**
  - +7th **S90.936 Unspecified superficial injury of unspecified lesser toe(s)**

S91 Open wound of ankle, foot and toes

Code also any associated wound infection

Excludes1: *open fracture of ankle, foot and toes (S92.-with 7th character B)*
traumatic amputation of ankle and foot (S98.-)

The appropriate 7th character is to be added to each code from category S91
A initial encounter
D subsequent encounter
S sequela

+ **S91.0 Open wound of ankle**
+ **S91.00 Unspecified open wound of ankle**
  - +7th **S91.001 Unspecified open wound, right ankle**
  - +7th **S91.002 Unspecified open wound, left ankle**
  - +7th **S91.009 Unspecified open wound, unspecified ankle**
+ **S91.01 Laceration without foreign body of ankle**
  - +7th **S91.011 Laceration without foreign body, right ankle**
  - +7th **S91.012 Laceration without foreign body, left ankle**
    AHA CC: 1Q, 2021, 7-8
  - +7th **S91.019 Laceration without foreign body, unspecified ankle**
+ **S91.02 Laceration with foreign body of ankle**
  - +7th **S91.021 Laceration with foreign body, right ankle**
  - +7th **S91.022 Laceration with foreign body, left ankle**
  - +7th **S91.029 Laceration with foreign body, unspecified ankle**
+ **S91.03 Puncture wound without foreign body of ankle**
  - +7th **S91.031 Puncture wound without foreign body, right ankle**
  - +7th **S91.032 Puncture wound without foreign body, left ankle**
  - +7th **S91.039 Puncture wound without foreign body, unspecified ankle**
+ **S91.04 Puncture wound with foreign body of ankle**
  - +7th **S91.041 Puncture wound with foreign body, right ankle**
  - +7th **S91.042 Puncture wound with foreign body, left ankle**
  - +7th **S91.049 Puncture wound with foreign body, unspecified ankle**
+ **S91.05 Open bite of ankle**
  Excludes1: *superficial bite of ankle (S90.56-, S90.57-)*
  - +7th **S91.051 Open bite, right ankle**
  - +7th **S91.052 Open bite, left ankle**
  - +7th **S91.059 Open bite, unspecified ankle**

+ **S91.1 Open wound of toe without damage to nail**
+ **S91.10 Unspecified open wound of toe without damage to nail**
  - +7th **S91.101 Unspecified open wound of right great toe without damage to nail**
  - +7th **S91.102 Unspecified open wound of left great toe without damage to nail**
  - +7th **S91.103 Unspecified open wound of unspecified great toe without damage to nail**
  - +7th **S91.104 Unspecified open wound of right lesser toe(s) without damage to nail**
  - +7th **S91.105 Unspecified open wound of left lesser toe(s) without damage to nail**
  - +7th **S91.106 Unspecified open wound of unspecified lesser toe(s) without damage to nail**
  - +7th **S91.109 Unspecified open wound of unspecified toe(s) without damage to nail**
+ **S91.11 Laceration without foreign body of toe without damage to nail**
  - +7th **S91.111 Laceration without foreign body of right great toe without damage to nail**
  - +7th **S91.112 Laceration without foreign body of left great toe without damage to nail**
  - +7th **S91.113 Laceration without foreign body of unspecified great toe without damage to nail**
  - +7th **S91.114 Laceration without foreign body of right lesser toe(s) without damage to nail**
  - +7th **S91.115 Laceration without foreign body of left lesser toe(s) without damage to nail**
  - +7th **S91.116 Laceration without foreign body of unspecified lesser toe(s) without damage to nail**
  - +7th **S91.119 Laceration without foreign body of unspecified toe without damage to nail**
+ **S91.12 Laceration with foreign body of toe without damage to nail**
  - +7th **S91.121 Laceration with foreign body of right great toe without damage to nail**
  - +7th **S91.122 Laceration with foreign body of left great toe without damage to nail**
  - +7th **S91.123 Laceration with foreign body of unspecified great toe without damage to nail**
  - +7th **S91.124 Laceration with foreign body of right lesser toe(s) without damage to nail**
  - +7th **S91.125 Laceration with foreign body of left lesser toe(s) without damage to nail**
  - +7th **S91.126 Laceration with foreign body of unspecified lesser toe(s) without damage to nail**
  - +7th **S91.129 Laceration with foreign body of unspecified toe(s) without damage to nail**

\+ **S91.13 Puncture wound without foreign body of toe without damage to nail**

+7th **S91.131 Puncture wound without foreign body of right great toe without damage to nail**

+7th **S91.132 Puncture wound without foreign body of left great toe without damage to nail**

+7th **S91.133 Puncture wound without foreign body of unspecified great toe without damage to nail**

+7th **S91.134 Puncture wound without foreign body of right lesser toe(s) without damage to nail**

+7th **S91.135 Puncture wound without foreign body of left lesser toe(s) without damage to nail**

+7th **S91.136 Puncture wound without foreign body of unspecified lesser toe(s) without damage to nail**

+7th **S91.139 Puncture wound without foreign body of unspecified toe(s) without damage to nail**

\+ **S91.14 Puncture wound with foreign body of toe without damage to nail**

+7th **S91.141 Puncture wound with foreign body of right great toe without damage to nail**

+7th **S91.142 Puncture wound with foreign body of left great toe without damage to nail**

+7th **S91.143 Puncture wound with foreign body of unspecified great toe without damage to nail**

+7th **S91.144 Puncture wound with foreign body of right lesser toe(s) without damage to nail**

+7th **S91.145 Puncture wound with foreign body of left lesser toe(s) without damage to nail**

+7th **S91.146 Puncture wound with foreign body of unspecified lesser toe(s) without damage to nail**

+7th **S91.149 Puncture wound with foreign body of unspecified toe(s) without damage to nail**

\+ **S91.15 Open bite of toe without damage to nail**

Bite of toe NOS

Excludes1: *superficial bite of toe (S90.46-,S90.47-)*

+7th **S91.151 Open bite of right great toe without damage to nail**

+7th **S91.152 Open bite of left great toe without damage to nail**

+7th **S91.153 Open bite of unspecified great toe without damage to nail**

+7th **S91.154 Open bite of right lesser toe(s) without damage to nail**

+7th **S91.155 Open bite of left lesser toe(s) without damage to nail**

+7th **S91.156 Open bite of unspecified lesser toe(s) without damage to nail**

+7th **S91.159 Open bite of unspecified toe(s) without damage to nail**

\+ **S91.2 Open wound of toe with damage to nail**

\+ **S91.20 Unspecified open wound of toe with damage to nail**

+7th **S91.201 Unspecified open wound of right great toe with damage to nail**

+7th **S91.202 Unspecified open wound of left great toe with damage to nail**

+7th **S91.203 Unspecified open wound of unspecified great toe with damage to nail**

+7th **S91.204 Unspecified open wound of right lesser toe(s) with damage to nail**

+7th **S91.205 Unspecified open wound of left lesser toe(s) with damage to nail**

+7th **S91.206 Unspecified open wound of unspecified lesser toe(s) with damage to nail**

+7th **S91.209 Unspecified open wound of unspecified toe(s) with damage to nail**

\+ **S91.21 Laceration without foreign body of toe with damage to nail**

+7th **S91.211 Laceration without foreign body of right great toe with damage to nail**

+7th **S91.212 Laceration without foreign body of left great toe with damage to nail**

+7th **S91.213 Laceration without foreign body of unspecified great toe with damage to nail**

+7th **S91.214 Laceration without foreign body of right lesser toe(s) with damage to nail**

+7th **S91.215 Laceration without foreign body of left lesser toe(s) with damage to nail**

+7th **S91.216 Laceration without foreign body of unspecified lesser toe(s) with damage to nail**

+7th **S91.219 Laceration without foreign body of unspecified toe(s) with damage to nail**

\+ **S91.22 Laceration with foreign body of toe with damage to nail**

+7th **S91.221 Laceration with foreign body of right great toe with damage to nail**

+7th **S91.222 Laceration with foreign body of left great toe with damage to nail**

+7th **S91.223 Laceration with foreign body of unspecified great toe with damage to nail**

+7th **S91.224 Laceration with foreign body of right lesser toe(s) with damage to nail**

+7th **S91.225 Laceration with foreign body of left lesser toe(s) with damage to nail**

+7th **S91.226 Laceration with foreign body of unspecified lesser toe(s) with damage to nail**

+7th **S91.229 Laceration with foreign body of unspecified toe(s) with damage to nail**

\+ **S91.23 Puncture wound without foreign body of toe with damage to nail**

+7th **S91.231 Puncture wound without foreign body of right great toe with damage to nail**

+7th **S91.232 Puncture wound without foreign body of left great toe with damage to nail**

+7th **S91.233 Puncture wound without foreign body of unspecified great toe with damage to nail**

+7th **S91.234 Puncture wound without foreign body of right lesser toe(s) with damage to nail**

+7th **S91.235 Puncture wound without foreign body of left lesser toe(s) with damage to nail**

+7th **S91.236 Puncture wound without foreign body of unspecified lesser toe(s) with damage to nail**

+7th **S91.239 Puncture wound without foreign body of unspecified toe(s) with damage to nail**

\+ **S91.24 Puncture wound with foreign body of toe with damage to nail**

+7th **S91.241 Puncture wound with foreign body of right great toe with damage to nail**

+7th **S91.242 Puncture wound with foreign body of left great toe with damage to nail**

+7th **S91.243 Puncture wound with foreign body of unspecified great toe with damage to nail**

+7th **S91.244 Puncture wound with foreign body of right lesser toe(s) with damage to nail**

+7th **S91.245 Puncture wound with foreign body of left lesser toe(s) with damage to nail**

+7th **S91.246 Puncture wound with foreign body of unspecified lesser toe(s) with damage to nail**

+7th **S91.249 Puncture wound with foreign body of unspecified toe(s) with damage to nail**

+ **S91.25 Open bite of toe with damage to nail**
Bite of toe with damage to nail NOS
Excludes1: *superficial bite of toe (S90.46-, S90.47-)*
+7th **S91.251 Open bite of right great toe with damage to nail**
+7th **S91.252 Open bite of left great toe with damage to nail**
+7th **S91.253 Open bite of unspecified great toe with damage to nail**
+7th **S91.254 Open bite of right lesser toe(s) with damage to nail**
+7th **S91.255 Open bite of left lesser toe(s) with damage to nail**
+7th **S91.256 Open bite of unspecified lesser toe(s) with damage to nail**
+7th **S91.259 Open bite of unspecified toe(s) with damage to nail**

+ **S91.3 Open wound of foot**
+ **S91.30 Unspecified open wound of foot**
+7th **S91.301 Unspecified open wound, right foot**
+7th **S91.302 Unspecified open wound, left foot**
+7th **S91.309 Unspecified open wound, unspecified foot**
+ **S91.31 Laceration without foreign body of foot**
+7th **S91.311 Laceration without foreign body, right foot**
+7th **S91.312 Laceration without foreign body, left foot**
+7th **S91.319 Laceration without foreign body, unspecified foot**
+ **S91.32 Laceration with foreign body of foot**
+7th **S91.321 Laceration with foreign body, right foot**
+7th **S91.322 Laceration with foreign body, left foot**
+7th **S91.329 Laceration with foreign body, unspecified foot**
+ **S91.33 Puncture wound without foreign body of foot**
+7th **S91.331 Puncture wound without foreign body, right foot**
+7th **S91.332 Puncture wound without foreign body, left foot**
+7th **S91.339 Puncture wound without foreign body, unspecified foot**
+ **S91.34 Puncture wound with foreign body of foot**
+7th **S91.341 Puncture wound with foreign body, right foot**
+7th **S91.342 Puncture wound with foreign body, left foot**
+7th **S91.349 Puncture wound with foreign body, unspecified foot**
+ **S91.35 Open bite of foot**
Excludes1: *superficial bite of foot (S90.86-, S90.87-)*
+7th **S91.351 Open bite, right foot**
+7th **S91.352 Open bite, left foot**
+7th **S91.359 Open bite, unspecified foot**

S92 Fracture of foot and toe, except ankle

NOTE A fracture not indicated as displaced or nondisplaced should be coded to displaced
A fracture not indicated as open or closed should be coded to closed

Excludes2: *fracture of ankle (S82.-)*
fracture of malleolus (S82.-)
traumatic amputation of ankle and foot (S98.-)

The appropriate 7th character is to be added to each code from category S92
A initial encounter for closed fracture
B initial encounter for open fracture
D subsequent encounter for fracture with routine healing
G subsequent encounter for fracture with delayed healing
K subsequent encounter for fracture with nonunion
P subsequent encounter for fracture with malunion
S sequela

Review coding guideline C.19.c

+ **S92.0 Fracture of calcaneus**
Heel bone
Os calcis
Excludes2: *Physeal fracture of calcaneus (S99.0-)*
+ **S92.00 Unspecified fracture of calcaneus**
CC +7th **S92.001 Unspecified fracture of right calcaneus**
HAC 7th character B see Appendix B for HAC conditional logic
CC +7th **S92.002 Unspecified fracture of left calcaneus**
HAC 7th character B see Appendix B for HAC conditional logic
CC +7th **S92.009 Unspecified fracture of unspecified calcaneus**
HAC 7th character B see Appendix B for HAC conditional logic
+ **S92.01 Fracture of body of calcaneus**
CC +7th **S92.011 Displaced fracture of body of right calcaneus**
HAC 7th character B see Appendix B for HAC conditional logic
CC +7th **S92.012 Displaced fracture of body of left calcaneus**
HAC 7th character B see Appendix B for HAC conditional logic
CC +7th **S92.013 Displaced fracture of body of unspecified calcaneus**
HAC 7th character B see Appendix B for HAC conditional logic
CC +7th **S92.014 Nondisplaced fracture of body of right calcaneus**
HAC 7th character B see Appendix B for HAC conditional logic
CC +7th **S92.015 Nondisplaced fracture of body of left calcaneus**
HAC 7th character B see Appendix B for HAC conditional logic
CC +7th **S92.016 Nondisplaced fracture of body of unspecified calcaneus**
HAC 7th character B see Appendix B for HAC conditional logic
+ **S92.02 Fracture of anterior process of calcaneus**
CC +7th **S92.021 Displaced fracture of anterior process of right calcaneus**
HAC 7th character B see Appendix B for HAC conditional logic
CC +7th **S92.022 Displaced fracture of anterior process of left calcaneus**
HAC 7th character B see Appendix B for HAC conditional logic
CC +7th **S92.023 Displaced fracture of anterior process of unspecified calcaneus**
HAC 7th character B see Appendix B for HAC conditional logic
CC +7th **S92.024 Nondisplaced fracture of anterior process of right calcaneus**
HAC 7th character B see Appendix B for HAC conditional logic
CC +7th **S92.025 Nondisplaced fracture of anterior process of left calcaneus**
HAC 7th character B see Appendix B for HAC conditional logic
CC +7th **S92.026 Nondisplaced fracture of anterior process of unspecified calcaneus**
HAC 7th character B see Appendix B for HAC conditional logic

+ **S92.03 Avulsion fracture of tuberosity of calcaneus**

CC +7th **S92.031 Displaced avulsion fracture of tuberosity of right calcaneus**
HAC 7th character B see Appendix B for HAC conditional logic

CC +7th **S92.032 Displaced avulsion fracture of tuberosity of left calcaneus**
HAC 7th character B see Appendix B for HAC conditional logic

CC +7th **S92.033 Displaced avulsion fracture of tuberosity of unspecified calcaneus**
HAC 7th character B see Appendix B for HAC conditional logic

CC +7th **S92.034 Nondisplaced avulsion fracture of tuberosity of right calcaneus**
HAC 7th character B see Appendix B for HAC conditional logic

CC +7th **S92.035 Nondisplaced avulsion fracture of tuberosity of left calcaneus**
HAC 7th character B see Appendix B for HAC conditional logic

CC +7th **S92.036 Nondisplaced avulsion fracture of tuberosity of unspecified calcaneus**
HAC 7th character B see Appendix B for HAC conditional logic

+ **S92.04 Other fracture of tuberosity of calcaneus**

CC +7th **S92.041 Displaced other fracture of tuberosity of right calcaneus**
HAC 7th character B see Appendix B for HAC conditional logic

CC +7th **S92.042 Displaced other fracture of tuberosity of left calcaneus**
HAC 7th character B see Appendix B for HAC conditional logic

CC +7th **S92.043 Displaced other fracture of tuberosity of unspecified calcaneus**
HAC 7th character B see Appendix B for HAC conditional logic

CC +7th **S92.044 Nondisplaced other fracture of tuberosity of right calcaneus**
HAC 7th character B see Appendix B for HAC conditional logic

CC +7th **S92.045 Nondisplaced other fracture of tuberosity of left calcaneus**
HAC 7th character B see Appendix B for HAC conditional logic

CC +7th **S92.046 Nondisplaced other fracture of tuberosity of unspecified calcaneus**
HAC 7th character B see Appendix B for HAC conditional logic

+ **S92.05 Other extraarticular fracture of calcaneus**

CC +7th **S92.051 Displaced other extraarticular fracture of right calcaneus**
HAC 7th character B see Appendix B for HAC conditional logic

CC +7th **S92.052 Displaced other extraarticular fracture of left calcaneus**
HAC 7th character B see Appendix B for HAC conditional logic

CC +7th **S92.053 Displaced other extraarticular fracture of unspecified calcaneus**
HAC 7th character B see Appendix B for HAC conditional logic

CC +7th **S92.054 Nondisplaced other extraarticular fracture of right calcaneus**
HAC 7th character B see Appendix B for HAC conditional logic

CC +7th **S92.055 Nondisplaced other extraarticular fracture of left calcaneus**
HAC 7th character B see Appendix B for HAC conditional logic

CC +7th **S92.056 Nondisplaced other extraarticular fracture of unspecified calcaneus**
HAC 7th character B see Appendix B for HAC conditional logic

+ **S92.06 Intraarticular fracture of calcaneus**

CC +7th **S92.061 Displaced intraarticular fracture of right calcaneus**
HAC 7th character B see Appendix B for HAC conditional logic

CC +7th **S92.062 Displaced intraarticular fracture of left calcaneus**
HAC 7th character B see Appendix B for HAC conditional logic

CC +7th **S92.063 Displaced intraarticular fracture of unspecified calcaneus**
HAC 7th character B see Appendix B for HAC conditional logic

CC +7th **S92.064 Nondisplaced intraarticular fracture of right calcaneus**
HAC 7th character B see Appendix B for HAC conditional logic

CC +7th **S92.065 Nondisplaced intraarticular fracture of left calcaneus**
HAC 7th character B see Appendix B for HAC conditional logic

CC +7th **S92.066 Nondisplaced intraarticular fracture of unspecified calcaneus**
HAC 7th character B see Appendix B for HAC conditional logic

+ **S92.1 Fracture of talus**
Astragalus

+ **S92.10 Unspecified fracture of talus**

CC +7th **S92.101 Unspecified fracture of right talus**
HAC 7th character B see Appendix B for HAC conditional logic

CC +7th **S92.102 Unspecified fracture of left talus**
HAC 7th character B see Appendix B for HAC conditional logic

CC +7th **S92.109 Unspecified fracture of unspecified talus**
HAC 7th character B see Appendix B for HAC conditional logic

+ **S92.11 Fracture of neck of talus**

CC +7th **S92.111 Displaced fracture of neck of right talus**
HAC 7th character B see Appendix B for HAC conditional logic

CC +7th **S92.112 Displaced fracture of neck of left talus**

CC +7th **S92.113 Displaced fracture of neck of unspecified talus**
HAC 7th character B see Appendix B for HAC conditional logic

CC +7th **S92.114 Nondisplaced fracture of neck of right talus**
HAC 7th character B see Appendix B for HAC conditional logic

CC +7th **S92.115 Nondisplaced fracture of neck of left talus**
HAC 7th character B see Appendix B for HAC conditional logic

CC +7th **S92.116 Nondisplaced fracture of neck of unspecified talus**
HAC 7th character B see Appendix B for HAC conditional logic

+ **S92.12 Fracture of body of talus**

CC +7th **S92.121 Displaced fracture of body of right talus**
HAC 7th character B see Appendix B for HAC conditional logic

CC +7th **S92.122 Displaced fracture of body of left talus**
HAC 7th character B see Appendix B for HAC conditional logic

CC +7th **S92.123 Displaced fracture of body of unspecified talus**
HAC 7th character B see Appendix B for HAC conditional logic

CC +7th **S92.124 Nondisplaced fracture of body of right talus**
HAC 7th character B see Appendix B for HAC conditional logic

CC +7th **S92.125 Nondisplaced fracture of body of left talus**
HAC 7th character B see Appendix B for HAC conditional logic

CC +7th **S92.126 Nondisplaced fracture of body of unspecified talus**
HAC 7th character B see Appendix B for HAC conditional logic

+ **S92.13 Fracture of posterior process of talus**

CC +7th **S92.131 Displaced fracture of posterior process of right talus**
HAC 7th character B see Appendix B for HAC conditional logic

CC +7th **S92.132 Displaced fracture of posterior process of left talus**
HAC 7th character B see Appendix B for HAC conditional logic

CC +7th **S92.133 Displaced fracture of posterior process of unspecified talus**
HAC 7th character B see Appendix B for HAC conditional logic

CC +7th **S92.134 Nondisplaced fracture of posterior process of right talus**
HAC 7th character B see Appendix B for HAC conditional logic

CC +7th **S92.135 Nondisplaced fracture of posterior process of left talus**
HAC 7th character B see Appendix B for HAC conditional logic

CC +7th **S92.136 Nondisplaced fracture of posterior process of unspecified talus**
HAC 7th character B see Appendix B for HAC conditional logic

+ **S92.14 Dome fracture of talus**
Excludes1: *osteochondritis dissecans (M93.2)*

CC +7th **S92.141 Displaced dome fracture of right talus**
HAC 7th character B see Appendix B for HAC conditional logic

CC +7th **S92.142 Displaced dome fracture of left talus**
HAC 7th character B see Appendix B for HAC conditional logic

CC +7th **S92.143 Displaced dome fracture of unspecified talus**
HAC 7th character B see Appendix B for HAC conditional logic

CC +7th **S92.144 Nondisplaced dome fracture of right talus**
HAC 7th character B see Appendix B for HAC conditional logic

CC +7th **S92.145 Nondisplaced dome fracture of left talus**
HAC 7th character B see Appendix B for HAC conditional logic

CC +7th **S92.146 Nondisplaced dome fracture of unspecified talus**
HAC 7th character B see Appendix B for HAC conditional logic

+ **S92.15 Avulsion fracture (chip fracture) of talus**

CC +7th **S92.151 Displaced avulsion fracture (chip fracture) of right talus**
HAC 7th character B see Appendix B for HAC conditional logic

CC +7th **S92.152 Displaced avulsion fracture (chip fracture) of left talus**
HAC 7th character B see Appendix B for HAC conditional logic

CC +7th **S92.153 Displaced avulsion fracture (chip fracture) of unspecified talus**
HAC 7th character B see Appendix B for HAC conditional logic

CC +7th **S92.154 Nondisplaced avulsion fracture (chip fracture) of right talus**
HAC 7th character B see Appendix B for HAC conditional logic

CC +7th **S92.155 Nondisplaced avulsion fracture (chip fracture) of left talus**
HAC 7th character B see Appendix B for HAC conditional logic

CC +7th **S92.156 Nondisplaced avulsion fracture (chip fracture) of unspecified talus**
HAC 7th character B see Appendix B for HAC conditional logic

+ **S92.19 Other fracture of talus**

CC +7th **S92.191 Other fracture of right talus**
HAC 7th character B see Appendix B for HAC conditional logic

CC +7th **S92.192 Other fracture of left talus**
HAC 7th character B see Appendix B for HAC conditional logic

CC +7th **S92.199 Other fracture of unspecified talus**
HAC 7th character B see Appendix B for HAC conditional logic

+ **S92.2 Fracture of other and unspecified tarsal bone(s)**

+ **S92.20 Fracture of unspecified tarsal bone(s)**

CC +7th **S92.201 Fracture of unspecified tarsal bone(s) of right foot**
HAC 7th character B see Appendix B for HAC conditional logic

CC +7th **S92.202 Fracture of unspecified tarsal bone(s) of left foot**
HAC 7th character B see Appendix B for HAC conditional logic

CC +7th **S92.209 Fracture of unspecified tarsal bone(s) of unspecified foot**
HAC 7th character B see Appendix B for HAC conditional logic

+ **S92.21 Fracture of cuboid bone**

CC +7th **S92.211 Displaced fracture of cuboid bone of right foot**
HAC 7th character B see Appendix B for HAC conditional logic

CC +7th **S92.212 Displaced fracture of cuboid bone of left foot**
HAC 7th character B see Appendix B for HAC conditional logic

CC +7th **S92.213 Displaced fracture of cuboid bone of unspecified foot**
HAC 7th character B see Appendix B for HAC conditional logic

CC +7th **S92.214 Nondisplaced fracture of cuboid bone of right foot**
HAC 7th character B see Appendix B for HAC conditional logic

CC +7th **S92.215 Nondisplaced fracture of cuboid bone of left foot**
HAC 7th character B see Appendix B for HAC conditional logic

CC +7th **S92.216 Nondisplaced fracture of cuboid bone of unspecified foot**
HAC 7th character B see Appendix B for HAC conditional logic

+ **S92.22 Fracture of lateral cuneiform**

CC +7th **S92.221 Displaced fracture of lateral cuneiform of right foot**
HAC 7th character B see Appendix B for HAC conditional logic

CC +7th **S92.222 Displaced fracture of lateral cuneiform of left foot**
HAC 7th character B see Appendix B for HAC conditional logic

CC +7th **S92.223 Displaced fracture of lateral cuneiform of unspecified foot**
HAC 7th character B see Appendix B for HAC conditional logic

CC +7th **S92.224 Nondisplaced fracture of lateral cuneiform of right foot**
HAC 7th character B see Appendix B for HAC conditional logic

CC +7th **S92.225 Nondisplaced fracture of lateral cuneiform of left foot**
HAC 7th character B see Appendix B for HAC conditional logic

CC +7th **S92.226 Nondisplaced fracture of lateral cuneiform of unspecified foot**
HAC 7th character B see Appendix B for HAC conditional logic

+ **S92.23 Fracture of intermediate cuneiform**
  - CC +7th **S92.231 Displaced fracture of intermediate cuneiform of right foot**
    HAC 7th character B see Appendix B for HAC conditional logic
  - CC +7th **S92.232 Displaced fracture of intermediate cuneiform of left foot**
    HAC 7th character B see Appendix B for HAC conditional logic
  - CC +7th **S92.233 Displaced fracture of intermediate cuneiform of unspecified foot**
    HAC 7th character B see Appendix B for HAC conditional logic
  - CC +7th **S92.234 Nondisplaced fracture of intermediate cuneiform of right foot**
    HAC 7th character B see Appendix B for HAC conditional logic
  - CC +7th **S92.235 Nondisplaced fracture of intermediate cuneiform of left foot**
    HAC 7th character B see Appendix B for HAC conditional logic
  - CC +7th **S92.236 Nondisplaced fracture of intermediate cuneiform of unspecified foot**
    HAC 7th character B see Appendix B for HAC conditional logic

+ **S92.24 Fracture of medial cuneiform**
  - CC +7th **S92.241 Displaced fracture of medial cuneiform of right foot**
    HAC 7th character B see Appendix B for HAC conditional logic
  - CC +7th **S92.242 Displaced fracture of medial cuneiform of left foot**
    HAC 7th character B see Appendix B for HAC conditional logic
  - CC +7th **S92.243 Displaced fracture of medial cuneiform of unspecified foot**
    HAC 7th character B see Appendix B for HAC conditional logic
  - CC +7th **S92.244 Nondisplaced fracture of medial cuneiform of right foot**
    HAC 7th character B see Appendix B for HAC conditional logic
  - CC +7th **S92.245 Nondisplaced fracture of medial cuneiform of left foot**
    HAC 7th character B see Appendix B for HAC conditional logic
  - CC +7th **S92.246 Nondisplaced fracture of medial cuneiform of unspecified foot**
    HAC 7th character B see Appendix B for HAC conditional logic

+ **S92.25 Fracture of navicular [scaphoid] of foot**
  - CC +7th **S92.251 Displaced fracture of navicular [scaphoid] of right foot**
    HAC 7th character B see Appendix B for HAC conditional logic
  - CC +7th **S92.252 Displaced fracture of navicular [scaphoid] of left foot**
    HAC 7th character B see Appendix B for HAC conditional logic
  - CC +7th **S92.253 Displaced fracture of navicular [scaphoid] of unspecified foot**
    HAC 7th character B see Appendix B for HAC conditional logic
  - CC +7th **S92.254 Nondisplaced fracture of navicular [scaphoid] of right foot**
    HAC 7th character B see Appendix B for HAC conditional logic
  - CC +7th **S92.255 Nondisplaced fracture of navicular [scaphoid] of left foot**
    HAC 7th character B see Appendix B for HAC conditional logic
  - CC +7th **S92.256 Nondisplaced fracture of navicular [scaphoid] of unspecified foot**
    HAC 7th character B see Appendix B for HAC conditional logic

+ **S92.3 Fracture of metatarsal bone(s)**
  Excludes2: *Physeal fracture of metatarsal (S99.1-)*

+ **S92.30 Fracture of unspecified metatarsal bone(s)**
  - CC +7th **S92.301 Fracture of unspecified metatarsal bone(s), right foot**
    HAC 7th character B see Appendix B for HAC conditional logic
  - CC +7th **S92.302 Fracture of unspecified metatarsal bone(s), left foot**
    HAC 7th character B see Appendix B for HAC conditional logic
  - CC +7th **S92.309 Fracture of unspecified metatarsal bone(s), unspecified foot**

+ **S92.31 Fracture of first metatarsal bone**
  - CC +7th **S92.311 Displaced fracture of first metatarsal bone, right foot**
    HAC 7th character B see Appendix B for HAC conditional logic
  - CC +7th **S92.312 Displaced fracture of first metatarsal bone, left foot**
    HAC 7th character B see Appendix B for HAC conditional logic
  - CC +7th **S92.313 Displaced fracture of first metatarsal bone, unspecified foot**
    HAC 7th character B see Appendix B for HAC conditional logic
  - CC +7th **S92.314 Nondisplaced fracture of first metatarsal bone, right foot**
    HAC 7th character B see Appendix B for HAC conditional logic
  - CC +7th **S92.315 Nondisplaced fracture of first metatarsal bone, left foot**
    HAC 7th character B see Appendix B for HAC conditional logic
  - CC +7th **S92.316 Nondisplaced fracture of first metatarsal bone, unspecified foot**
    HAC 7th character B see Appendix B for HAC conditional logic

+ **S92.32 Fracture of second metatarsal bone**
  - CC +7th **S92.321 Displaced fracture of second metatarsal bone, right foot**
    HAC 7th character B see Appendix B for HAC conditional logic
  - CC +7th **S92.322 Displaced fracture of second metatarsal bone, left foot**
    HAC 7th character B see Appendix B for HAC conditional logic
  - CC +7th **S92.323 Displaced fracture of second metatarsal bone, unspecified foot**
    HAC 7th character B see Appendix B for HAC conditional logic
  - CC +7th **S92.324 Nondisplaced fracture of second metatarsal bone, right foot**
    HAC 7th character B see Appendix B for HAC conditional logic
  - CC +7th **S92.325 Nondisplaced fracture of second metatarsal bone, left foot**
    HAC 7th character B see Appendix B for HAC conditional logic
  - CC +7th **S92.326 Nondisplaced fracture of second metatarsal bone, unspecified foot**
    HAC 7th character B see Appendix B for HAC conditional logic

+ **S92.33 Fracture of third metatarsal bone**
  AHA CC: 1Q, 2018, 3
  - CC +7th **S92.331 Displaced fracture of third metatarsal bone, right foot**
    HAC 7th character B see Appendix B for HAC conditional logic
  - CC +7th **S92.332 Displaced fracture of third metatarsal bone, left foot**
    HAC 7th character B see Appendix B for HAC conditional logic
  - CC +7th **S92.333 Displaced fracture of third metatarsal bone, unspecified foot**
    HAC 7th character B see Appendix B for HAC conditional logic

CC +7th **S92.334** **Nondisplaced fracture of third metatarsal bone, right foot**
HAC 7th character B see Appendix B for HAC conditional logic

CC +7th **S92.335** **Nondisplaced fracture of third metatarsal bone, left foot**
HAC 7th character B see Appendix B for HAC conditional logic

CC +7th **S92.336** **Nondisplaced fracture of third metatarsal bone, unspecified foot**
HAC 7th character B see Appendix B for HAC conditional logic

\+ **S92.34** **Fracture of fourth metatarsal bone**

CC +7th **S92.341** **Displaced fracture of fourth metatarsal bone, right foot**
HAC 7th character B see Appendix B for HAC conditional logic

CC +7th **S92.342** **Displaced fracture of fourth metatarsal bone, left foot**
HAC 7th character B see Appendix B for HAC conditional logic

CC +7th **S92.343** **Displaced fracture of fourth metatarsal bone, unspecified foot**
HAC 7th character B see Appendix B for HAC conditional logic

CC +7th **S92.344** **Nondisplaced fracture of fourth metatarsal bone, right foot**
HAC 7th character B see Appendix B for HAC conditional logic

CC +7th **S92.345** **Nondisplaced fracture of fourth metatarsal bone, left foot**
HAC 7th character B see Appendix B for HAC conditional logic

CC +7th **S92.346** **Nondisplaced fracture of fourth metatarsal bone, unspecified foot**
HAC 7th character B see Appendix B for HAC conditional logic

\+ **S92.35** **Fracture of fifth metatarsal bone**

CC +7th **S92.351** **Displaced fracture of fifth metatarsal bone, right foot**
HAC 7th character B see Appendix B for HAC conditional logic

CC +7th **S92.352** **Displaced fracture of fifth metatarsal bone, left foot**
HAC 7th character B see Appendix B for HAC conditional logic

CC +7th **S92.353** **Displaced fracture of fifth metatarsal bone, unspecified foot**
HAC 7th character B see Appendix B for HAC conditional logic

CC +7th **S92.354** **Nondisplaced fracture of fifth metatarsal bone, right foot**
HAC 7th character B see Appendix B for HAC conditional logic

CC +7th **S92.355** **Nondisplaced fracture of fifth metatarsal bone, left foot**
HAC 7th character B see Appendix B for HAC conditional logic

CC +7th **S92.356** **Nondisplaced fracture of fifth metatarsal bone, unspecified foot**
HAC 7th character B see Appendix B for HAC conditional logic

\+ **S92.4** **Fracture of great toe**

Excludes2: *Physeal fracture of phalanx of toe (S99.2-)*

\+ **S92.40** **Unspecified fracture of great toe**

CC +7th **S92.401** **Displaced unspecified fracture of right great toe**

CC +7th **S92.402** **Displaced unspecified fracture of left great toe**

CC +7th **S92.403** **Displaced unspecified fracture of unspecified great toe**

CC +7th **S92.404** **Nondisplaced unspecified fracture of right great toe**

CC +7th **S92.405** **Nondisplaced unspecified fracture of left great toe**

CC +7th **S92.406** **Nondisplaced unspecified fracture of unspecified great toe**

\+ **S92.41** **Fracture of proximal phalanx of great toe**

CC +7th **S92.411** **Displaced fracture of proximal phalanx of right great toe**

CC +7th **S92.412** **Displaced fracture of proximal phalanx of left great toe**

CC +7th **S92.413** **Displaced fracture of proximal phalanx of unspecified great toe**

CC +7th **S92.414** **Nondisplaced fracture of proximal phalanx of right great toe**

CC +7th **S92.415** **Nondisplaced fracture of proximal phalanx of left great toe**

CC +7th **S92.416** **Nondisplaced fracture of proximal phalanx of unspecified great toe**

\+ **S92.42** **Fracture of distal phalanx of great toe**

CC +7th **S92.421** **Displaced fracture of distal phalanx of right great toe**

CC +7th **S92.422** **Displaced fracture of distal phalanx of left great toe**

CC +7th **S92.423** **Displaced fracture of distal phalanx of unspecified great toe**

CC +7th **S92.424** **Nondisplaced fracture of distal phalanx of right great toe**

CC +7th **S92.425** **Nondisplaced fracture of distal phalanx of left great toe**

CC +7th **S92.426** **Nondisplaced fracture of distal phalanx of unspecified great toe**

\+ **S92.49** **Other fracture of great toe**

CC +7th **S92.491** **Other fracture of right great toe**

CC +7th **S92.492** **Other fracture of left great toe**

CC +7th **S92.499** **Other fracture of unspecified great toe**

\+ **S92.5** **Fracture of lesser toe(s)**

Excludes2: *Physeal fracture of phalanx of toe (S99.2-)*

\+ **S92.50** **Unspecified fracture of lesser toe(s)**

CC +7th **S92.501** **Displaced unspecified fracture of right lesser toe(s)**

CC +7th **S92.502** **Displaced unspecified fracture of left lesser toe(s)**

CC +7th **S92.503** **Displaced unspecified fracture of unspecified lesser toe(s)**

CC +7th **S92.504** **Nondisplaced unspecified fracture of right lesser toe(s)**

CC +7th **S92.505** **Nondisplaced unspecified fracture of left lesser toe(s)**

CC +7th **S92.506** **Nondisplaced unspecified fracture of unspecified lesser toe(s)**

\+ **S92.51** **Fracture of proximal phalanx of lesser toe(s)**

CC +7th **S92.511** **Displaced fracture of proximal phalanx of right lesser toe(s)**

CC +7th **S92.512** **Displaced fracture of proximal phalanx of left lesser toe(s)**

CC +7th **S92.513** **Displaced fracture of proximal phalanx of unspecified lesser toe(s)**

CC +7th **S92.514** **Nondisplaced fracture of proximal phalanx of right lesser toe(s)**

CC +7th **S92.515** **Nondisplaced fracture of proximal phalanx of left lesser toe(s)**

CC +7th **S92.516** **Nondisplaced fracture of proximal phalanx of unspecified lesser toe(s)**

\+ **S92.52** **Fracture of middle phalanx of lesser toe(s)**

CC +7th **S92.521** **Displaced fracture of middle phalanx of right lesser toe(s)**

CC +7th **S92.522** **Displaced fracture of middle phalanx of left lesser toe(s)**

CC +7th **S92.523** **Displaced fracture of middle phalanx of unspecified lesser toe(s)**

CC +7th **S92.524** **Nondisplaced fracture of middle phalanx of right lesser toe(s)**

CC +7th **S92.525** **Nondisplaced fracture of middle phalanx of left lesser toe(s)**

CC +7th **S92.526** **Nondisplaced fracture of middle phalanx of unspecified lesser toe(s)**

+ **S92.53 Fracture of distal phalanx of lesser toe(s)**
  - CC +7th **S92.531 Displaced fracture of distal phalanx of right lesser toe(s)**
  - CC +7th **S92.532 Displaced fracture of distal phalanx of left lesser toe(s)**
  - CC +7th **S92.533 Displaced fracture of distal phalanx of unspecified lesser toe(s)**
  - CC +7th **S92.534 Nondisplaced fracture of distal phalanx of right lesser toe(s)**
  - CC +7th **S92.535 Nondisplaced fracture of distal phalanx of left lesser toe(s)**
  - CC +7th **S92.536 Nondisplaced fracture of distal phalanx of unspecified lesser toe(s)**

+ **S92.59 Other fracture of lesser toe(s)**
  - CC +7th **S92.591 Other fracture of right lesser toe(s)**
  - CC +7th **S92.592 Other fracture of left lesser toe(s)**
  - CC +7th **S92.599 Other fracture of unspecified lesser toe(s)**

+ **S92.8 Other fracture of foot, except ankle**

+ **S92.81 Other fracture of foot**

  Sesamoid fracture of foot

  AHA CC: 4Q, 2016, 68

  - CC +7th **S92.811 Other fracture of right foot**

    HAC 7th character B see Appendix B for HAC conditional logic
  - CC +7th **S92.812 Other fracture of left foot**

    HAC 7th character B see Appendix B for HAC conditional logic
  - CC +7th **S92.819 Other fracture of unspecified foot**

    HAC 7th character B see Appendix B for HAC conditional logic

+ **S92.9 Unspecified fracture of foot and toe**

+ **S92.90 Unspecified fracture of foot**
  - CC +7th **S92.901 Unspecified fracture of right foot**

    HAC 7th character B see Appendix B for HAC conditional logic
  - CC +7th **S92.902 Unspecified fracture of left foot**

    HAC 7th character B see Appendix B for HAC conditional logic
  - CC +7th **S92.909 Unspecified fracture of unspecified foot**

    HAC 7th character B see Appendix B for HAC conditional logic

+ **S92.91 Unspecified fracture of toe**
  - CC +7th **S92.911 Unspecified fracture of right toe(s)**
  - CC +7th **S92.912 Unspecified fracture of left toe(s)**
  - CC +7th **S92.919 Unspecified fracture of unspecified toe(s)**

S93 Dislocation and sprain of joints and ligaments at ankle, foot and toe level

Includes: avulsion of joint or ligament of ankle, foot and toe
laceration of cartilage, joint or ligament of ankle, foot and toe
sprain of cartilage, joint or ligament of ankle, foot and toe
traumatic hemarthrosis of joint or ligament of ankle, foot and toe
traumatic rupture of joint or ligament of ankle, foot and toe
traumatic subluxation of joint or ligament of ankle, foot and toe
traumatic tear of joint or ligament of ankle, foot and toe

Code also any associated open wound

Excludes2: *strain of muscle and tendon of ankle and foot (S96.-)*

The appropriate 7th character is to be added to each code from category S93
- A initial encounter
- D subsequent encounter
- S sequela

+ **S93.0 Subluxation and dislocation of ankle joint**

  Subluxation and dislocation of astragalus

  Subluxation and dislocation of fibula, lower end

  Subluxation and dislocation of talus

  Subluxation and dislocation of tibia, lower end
  - X+7th **S93.01 Subluxation of right ankle joint**
  - X+7th **S93.02 Subluxation of left ankle joint**
  - X+7th **S93.03 Subluxation of unspecified ankle joint**
  - X+7th **S93.04 Dislocation of right ankle joint**
  - X+7th **S93.05 Dislocation of left ankle joint**
  - X+7th **S93.06 Dislocation of unspecified ankle joint**

+ **S93.1 Subluxation and dislocation of toe**

+ **S93.10 Unspecified subluxation and dislocation of toe**

  Dislocation of toe NOS

  Subluxation of toe NOS
  - +7th **S93.101 Unspecified subluxation of right toe(s)**
  - +7th **S93.102 Unspecified subluxation of left toe(s)**
  - +7th **S93.103 Unspecified subluxation of unspecified toe(s)**
  - +7th **S93.104 Unspecified dislocation of right toe(s)**
  - +7th **S93.105 Unspecified dislocation of left toe(s)**
  - +7th **S93.106 Unspecified dislocation of unspecified toe(s)**

+ **S93.11 Dislocation of interphalangeal joint**
  - +7th **S93.111 Dislocation of interphalangeal joint of right great toe**
  - +7th **S93.112 Dislocation of interphalangeal joint of left great toe**
  - +7th **S93.113 Dislocation of interphalangeal joint of unspecified great toe**
  - +7th **S93.114 Dislocation of interphalangeal joint of right lesser toe(s)**
  - +7th **S93.115 Dislocation of interphalangeal joint of left lesser toe(s)**
  - +7th **S93.116 Dislocation of interphalangeal joint of unspecified lesser toe(s)**
  - +7th **S93.119 Dislocation of interphalangeal joint of unspecified toe(s)**

+ **S93.12 Dislocation of metatarsophalangeal joint**
  - +7th **S93.121 Dislocation of metatarsophalangeal joint of right great toe**
  - +7th **S93.122 Dislocation of metatarsophalangeal joint of left great toe**
  - +7th **S93.123 Dislocation of metatarsophalangeal joint of unspecified great toe**
  - +7th **S93.124 Dislocation of metatarsophalangeal joint of right lesser toe(s)**
  - +7th **S93.125 Dislocation of metatarsophalangeal joint of left lesser toe(s)**
  - +7th **S93.126 Dislocation of metatarsophalangeal joint of unspecified lesser toe(s)**
  - +7th **S93.129 Dislocation of metatarsophalangeal joint of unspecified toe(s)**

+ **S93.13 Subluxation of interphalangeal joint**
  - +7th **S93.131 Subluxation of interphalangeal joint of right great toe**
  - +7th **S93.132 Subluxation of interphalangeal joint of left great toe**
  - +7th **S93.133 Subluxation of interphalangeal joint of unspecified great toe**
  - +7th **S93.134 Subluxation of interphalangeal joint of right lesser toe(s)**
  - +7th **S93.135 Subluxation of interphalangeal joint of left lesser toe(s)**
  - +7th **S93.136 Subluxation of interphalangeal joint of unspecified lesser toe(s)**
  - +7th **S93.139 Subluxation of interphalangeal joint of unspecified toe(s)**

+ **S93.14 Subluxation of metatarsophalangeal joint**
  - +7th **S93.141 Subluxation of metatarsophalangeal joint of right great toe**
  - +7th **S93.142 Subluxation of metatarsophalangeal joint of left great toe**
  - +7th **S93.143 Subluxation of metatarsophalangeal joint of unspecified great toe**
  - +7th **S93.144 Subluxation of metatarsophalangeal joint of right lesser toe(s)**
  - +7th **S93.145 Subluxation of metatarsophalangeal joint of left lesser toe(s)**
  - +7th **S93.146 Subluxation of metatarsophalangeal joint of unspecified lesser toe(s)**
  - +7th **S93.149 Subluxation of metatarsophalangeal joint of unspecified toe(s)**

+ **S93.3 Subluxation and dislocation of foot**
Excludes2: *dislocation of toe (S93.1-)*
+ **S93.30 Unspecified subluxation and dislocation of foot**
Dislocation of foot NOS
Subluxation of foot NOS
+7th **S93.301 Unspecified subluxation of right foot**
+7th **S93.302 Unspecified subluxation of left foot**
+7th **S93.303 Unspecified subluxation of unspecified foot**
+7th **S93.304 Unspecified dislocation of right foot**
+7th **S93.305 Unspecified dislocation of left foot**
+7th **S93.306 Unspecified dislocation of unspecified foot**
+ **S93.31 Subluxation and dislocation of tarsal joint**
+7th **S93.311 Subluxation of tarsal joint of right foot**
+7th **S93.312 Subluxation of tarsal joint of left foot**
+7th **S93.313 Subluxation of tarsal joint of unspecified foot**
+7th **S93.314 Dislocation of tarsal joint of right foot**
+7th **S93.315 Dislocation of tarsal joint of left foot**
+7th **S93.316 Dislocation of tarsal joint of unspecified foot**
+ **S93.32 Subluxation and dislocation of tarsometatarsal joint**
+7th **S93.321 Subluxation of tarsometatarsal joint of right foot**
+7th **S93.322 Subluxation of tarsometatarsal joint of left foot**
+7th **S93.323 Subluxation of tarsometatarsal joint of unspecified foot**
+7th **S93.324 Dislocation of tarsometatarsal joint of right foot**
+7th **S93.325 Dislocation of tarsometatarsal joint of left foot**
+7th **S93.326 Dislocation of tarsometatarsal joint of unspecified foot**
+ **S93.33 Other subluxation and dislocation of foot**
+7th **S93.331 Other subluxation of right foot**
+7th **S93.332 Other subluxation of left foot**
+7th **S93.333 Other subluxation of unspecified foot**
+7th **S93.334 Other dislocation of right foot**
+7th **S93.335 Other dislocation of left foot**
+7th **S93.336 Other dislocation of unspecified foot**
+ **S93.4 Sprain of ankle**
Excludes2: *injury of Achilles tendon (S86.0-)*
+ **S93.40 Sprain of unspecified ligament of ankle**
Sprain of ankle NOS
Sprained ankle NOS
+7th **S93.401 Sprain of unspecified ligament of right ankle**
+7th **S93.402 Sprain of unspecified ligament of left ankle**
+7th **S93.409 Sprain of unspecified ligament of unspecified ankle**
+ **S93.41 Sprain of calcaneofibular ligament**
+7th **S93.411 Sprain of calcaneofibular ligament of right ankle**
+7th **S93.412 Sprain of calcaneofibular ligament of left ankle**
+7th **S93.419 Sprain of calcaneofibular ligament of unspecified ankle**
+ **S93.42 Sprain of deltoid ligament**
+7th **S93.421 Sprain of deltoid ligament of right ankle**
+7th **S93.422 Sprain of deltoid ligament of left ankle**
+7th **S93.429 Sprain of deltoid ligament of unspecified ankle**
+ **S93.43 Sprain of tibiofibular ligament**
+7th **S93.431 Sprain of tibiofibular ligament of right ankle**
+7th **S93.432 Sprain of tibiofibular ligament of left ankle**
+7th **S93.439 Sprain of tibiofibular ligament of unspecified ankle**
+ **S93.49 Sprain of other ligament of ankle**
Sprain of internal collateral ligament
Sprain of talofibular ligament
+7th **S93.491 Sprain of other ligament of right ankle**
+7th **S93.492 Sprain of other ligament of left ankle**
+7th **S93.499 Sprain of other ligament of unspecified ankle**
+ **S93.5 Sprain of toe**
+ **S93.50 Unspecified sprain of toe**
+7th **S93.501 Unspecified sprain of right great toe**
+7th **S93.502 Unspecified sprain of left great toe**
+7th **S93.503 Unspecified sprain of unspecified great toe**
+7th **S93.504 Unspecified sprain of right lesser toe(s)**
+7th **S93.505 Unspecified sprain of left lesser toe(s)**
+7th **S93.506 Unspecified sprain of unspecified lesser toe(s)**
+7th **S93.509 Unspecified sprain of unspecified toe(s)**
+ **S93.51 Sprain of interphalangeal joint of toe**
+7th **S93.511 Sprain of interphalangeal joint of right great toe**
+7th **S93.512 Sprain of interphalangeal joint of left great toe**
+7th **S93.513 Sprain of interphalangeal joint of unspecified great toe**
+7th **S93.514 Sprain of interphalangeal joint of right lesser toe(s)**
+7th **S93.515 Sprain of interphalangeal joint of left lesser toe(s)**
+7th **S93.516 Sprain of interphalangeal joint of unspecified lesser toe(s)**
+7th **S93.519 Sprain of interphalangeal joint of unspecified toe(s)**
+ **S93.52 Sprain of metatarsophalangeal joint of toe**
+7th **S93.521 Sprain of metatarsophalangeal joint of right great toe**
+7th **S93.522 Sprain of metatarsophalangeal joint of left great toe**
+7th **S93.523 Sprain of metatarsophalangeal joint of unspecified great toe**
+7th **S93.524 Sprain of metatarsophalangeal joint of right lesser toe(s)**
+7th **S93.525 Sprain of metatarsophalangeal joint of left lesser toe(s)**
+7th **S93.526 Sprain of metatarsophalangeal joint of unspecified lesser toe(s)**
+7th **S93.529 Sprain of metatarsophalangeal joint of unspecified toe(s)**
+ **S93.6 Sprain of foot**
Excludes2: *sprain of metatarsophalangeal joint of toe (S93.52-) sprain of toe (S93.5-)*
+ **S93.60 Unspecified sprain of foot**
+7th **S93.601 Unspecified sprain of right foot**
+7th **S93.602 Unspecified sprain of left foot**
+7th **S93.609 Unspecified sprain of unspecified foot**
+ **S93.61 Sprain of tarsal ligament of foot**
+7th **S93.611 Sprain of tarsal ligament of right foot**
+7th **S93.612 Sprain of tarsal ligament of left foot**
+7th **S93.619 Sprain of tarsal ligament of unspecified foot**
+ **S93.62 Sprain of tarsometatarsal ligament of foot**
+7th **S93.621 Sprain of tarsometatarsal ligament of right foot**
+7th **S93.622 Sprain of tarsometatarsal ligament of left foot**
+7th **S93.629 Sprain of tarsometatarsal ligament of unspecified foot**
+ **S93.69 Other sprain of foot**
+7th **S93.691 Other sprain of right foot**
+7th **S93.692 Other sprain of left foot**
+7th **S93.699 Other sprain of unspecified foot**

S94 Injury of nerves at ankle and foot level
Code also any associated open wound (S91.-)

The appropriate 7th character is to be added to each code from category S94
A initial encounter
D subsequent encounter
S sequela

+ **S94.0 Injury of lateral plantar nerve**
X+7th **S94.00 Injury of lateral plantar nerve, unspecified leg**
X+7th **S94.01 Injury of lateral plantar nerve, right leg**
X+7th **S94.02 Injury of lateral plantar nerve, left leg**
+ **S94.1 Injury of medial plantar nerve**
X+7th **S94.10 Injury of medial plantar nerve, unspecified leg**
X+7th **S94.11 Injury of medial plantar nerve, right leg**
X+7th **S94.12 Injury of medial plantar nerve, left leg**

+ **S94.2 Injury of deep peroneal nerve at ankle and foot level**
  Injury of terminal, lateral branch of deep peroneal nerve
  - X+7th **S94.20 Injury of deep peroneal nerve at ankle and foot level, unspecified leg**
  - X+7th **S94.21 Injury of deep peroneal nerve at ankle and foot level, right leg**
  - X+7th **S94.22 Injury of deep peroneal nerve at ankle and foot level, left leg**

+ **S94.3 Injury of cutaneous sensory nerve at ankle and foot level**
  - X+7th **S94.30 Injury of cutaneous sensory nerve at ankle and foot level, unspecified leg**
  - X+7th **S94.31 Injury of cutaneous sensory nerve at ankle and foot level, right leg**
  - X+7th **S94.32 Injury of cutaneous sensory nerve at ankle and foot level, left leg**

+ **S94.8 Injury of other nerves at ankle and foot level**
  - + **S94.8X Injury of other nerves at ankle and foot level**
    - +7th **S94.8X1 Injury of other nerves at ankle and foot level, right leg**
    - +7th **S94.8X2 Injury of other nerves at ankle and foot level, left leg**
    - +7th **S94.8X9 Injury of other nerves at ankle and foot level, unspecified leg**

+ **S94.9 Injury of unspecified nerve at ankle and foot level**
  - X+7th **S94.90 Injury of unspecified nerve at ankle and foot level, unspecified leg**
  - X+7th **S94.91 Injury of unspecified nerve at ankle and foot level, right leg**
  - X+7th **S94.92 Injury of unspecified nerve at ankle and foot level, left leg**

S95 Injury of blood vessels at ankle and foot level

Code also any associated open wound (S91.-)

Excludes2: *injury of posterior tibial artery and vein (S85.1-, S85.8-)*

The appropriate 7th character is to be added to each code from category S95
A initial encounter
D subsequent encounter
S sequela

+ **S95.0 Injury of dorsal artery of foot**
  - + **S95.00 Unspecified injury of dorsal artery of foot**
    - CC +7th **S95.001 Unspecified injury of dorsal artery of right foot**
    - CC +7th **S95.002 Unspecified injury of dorsal artery of left foot**
    - CC +7th **S95.009 Unspecified injury of dorsal artery of unspecified foot**
  - + **S95.01 Laceration of dorsal artery of foot**
    - CC +7th **S95.011 Laceration of dorsal artery of right foot**
    - CC +7th **S95.012 Laceration of dorsal artery of left foot**
    - CC +7th **S95.019 Laceration of dorsal artery of unspecified foot**
  - + **S95.09 Other specified injury of dorsal artery of foot**
    - CC +7th **S95.091 Other specified injury of dorsal artery of right foot**
    - CC +7th **S95.092 Other specified injury of dorsal artery of left foot**
    - CC +7th **S95.099 Other specified injury of dorsal artery of unspecified foot**

+ **S95.1 Injury of plantar artery of foot**
  - + **S95.10 Unspecified injury of plantar artery of foot**
    - CC +7th **S95.101 Unspecified injury of plantar artery of right foot**
    - CC +7th **S95.102 Unspecified injury of plantar artery of left foot**
    - CC +7th **S95.109 Unspecified injury of plantar artery of unspecified foot**
  - + **S95.11 Laceration of plantar artery of foot**
    - CC +7th **S95.111 Laceration of plantar artery of right foot**
    - CC +7th **S95.112 Laceration of plantar artery of left foot**
    - CC +7th **S95.119 Laceration of plantar artery of unspecified foot**
  - + **S95.19 Other specified injury of plantar artery of foot**
    - CC +7th **S95.191 Other specified injury of plantar artery of right foot**
    - CC +7th **S95.192 Other specified injury of plantar artery of left foot**
    - CC +7th **S95.199 Other specified injury of plantar artery of unspecified foot**

+ **S95.2 Injury of dorsal vein of foot**
  - + **S95.20 Unspecified injury of dorsal vein of foot**
    - CC +7th **S95.201 Unspecified injury of dorsal vein of right foot**
    - CC +7th **S95.202 Unspecified injury of dorsal vein of left foot**
    - CC +7th **S95.209 Unspecified injury of dorsal vein of unspecified foot**
  - + **S95.21 Laceration of dorsal vein of foot**
    - CC +7th **S95.211 Laceration of dorsal vein of right foot**
    - CC +7th **S95.212 Laceration of dorsal vein of left foot**
    - CC +7th **S95.219 Laceration of dorsal vein of unspecified foot**
  - + **S95.29 Other specified injury of dorsal vein of foot**
    - CC +7th **S95.291 Other specified injury of dorsal vein of right foot**
    - CC +7th **S95.292 Other specified injury of dorsal vein of left foot**
    - CC +7th **S95.299 Other specified injury of dorsal vein of unspecified foot**

S95.8 Injury of other blood vessels at ankle and foot level
  - + **S95.80 Unspecified injury of other blood vessels at ankle and foot level**
    - CC +7th **S95.801 Unspecified injury of other blood vessels at ankle and foot level, right leg**
    - CC +7th **S95.802 Unspecified injury of other blood vessels at ankle and foot level, left leg**
    - CC +7th **S95.809 Unspecified injury of other blood vessels at ankle and foot level, unspecified leg**
  - + **S95.81 Laceration of other blood vessels at ankle and foot level**
    - CC +7th **S95.811 Laceration of other blood vessels at ankle and foot level, right leg**
    - CC +7th **S95.812 Laceration of other blood vessels at ankle and foot level, left leg**
    - CC +7th **S95.819 Laceration of other blood vessels at ankle and foot level, unspecified leg**
  - + **S95.89 Other specified injury of other blood vessels at ankle and foot level**
    - CC +7th **S95.891 Other specified injury of other blood vessels at ankle and foot level, right leg**
    - CC +7th **S95.892 Other specified injury of other blood vessels at ankle and foot level, left leg**
    - CC +7th **S95.899 Other specified injury of other blood vessels at ankle and foot level, unspecified leg**

+ **S95.9 Injury of unspecified blood vessel at ankle and foot level**
  - + **S95.90 Unspecified injury of unspecified blood vessel at ankle and foot level**
    - CC +7th **S95.901 Unspecified injury of unspecified blood vessel at ankle and foot level, right leg**
    - CC +7th **S95.902 Unspecified injury of unspecified blood vessel at ankle and foot level, left leg**
    - CC +7th **S95.909 Unspecified injury of unspecified blood vessel at ankle and foot level, unspecified leg**
  - + **S95.91 Laceration of unspecified blood vessel at ankle and foot level**
    - CC +7th **S95.911 Laceration of unspecified blood vessel at ankle and foot level, right leg**
    - CC +7th **S95.912 Laceration of unspecified blood vessel at ankle and foot level, left leg**
    - CC +7th **S95.919 Laceration of unspecified blood vessel at ankle and foot level, unspecified leg**
  - + **S95.99 Other specified injury of unspecified blood vessel at ankle and foot level**
    - CC +7th **S95.991 Other specified injury of unspecified blood vessel at ankle and foot level, right leg**
    - CC +7th **S95.992 Other specified injury of unspecified blood vessel at ankle and foot level, left leg**
    - CC +7th **S95.999 Other specified injury of unspecified blood vessel at ankle and foot level, unspecified leg**

S96 Injury of muscle and tendon at ankle and foot level

Code also any associated open wound (S91.-)

Excludes2: *injury of Achilles tendon (S86.0-)*
sprain of joints and ligaments of ankle and foot (S93.-)

The appropriate 7th character is to be added to each code from category S96
A initial encounter
D subsequent encounter
S sequela

\+ **S96.0 Injury of muscle and tendon of long flexor muscle of toe at ankle and foot level**

\+ **S96.00 Unspecified injury of muscle and tendon of long flexor muscle of toe at ankle and foot level**

+7th **S96.001 Unspecified injury of muscle and tendon of long flexor muscle of toe at ankle and foot level, right foot**

+7th **S96.002 Unspecified injury of muscle and tendon of long flexor muscle of toe at ankle and foot level, left foot**

+7th **S96.009 Unspecified injury of muscle and tendon of long flexor muscle of toe at ankle and foot level, unspecified foot**

\+ **S96.01 Strain of muscle and tendon of long flexor muscle of toe at ankle and foot level**

+7th **S96.011 Strain of muscle and tendon of long flexor muscle of toe at ankle and foot level, right foot**

+7th **S96.012 Strain of muscle and tendon of long flexor muscle of toe at ankle and foot level, left foot**

+7th **S96.019 Strain of muscle and tendon of long flexor muscle of toe at ankle and foot level, unspecified foot**

\+ **S96.02 Laceration of muscle and tendon of long flexor muscle of toe at ankle and foot level**

CC +7th **S96.021 Laceration of muscle and tendon of long flexor muscle of toe at ankle and foot level, right foot**

CC +7th **S96.022 Laceration of muscle and tendon of long flexor muscle of toe at ankle and foot level, left foot**

CC +7th **S96.029 Laceration of muscle and tendon of long flexor muscle of toe at ankle and foot level, unspecified foot**

\+ **S96.09 Other injury of muscle and tendon of long flexor muscle of toe at ankle and foot level**

+7th **S96.091 Other injury of muscle and tendon of long flexor muscle of toe at ankle and foot level, right foot**

+7th **S96.092 Other injury of muscle and tendon of long flexor muscle of toe at ankle and foot level, left foot**

+7th **S96.099 Other injury of muscle and tendon of long flexor muscle of toe at ankle and foot level, unspecified foot**

\+ **S96.1 Injury of muscle and tendon of long extensor muscle of toe at ankle and foot level**

\+ **S96.10 Unspecified injury of muscle and tendon of long extensor muscle of toe at ankle and foot level**

+7th **S96.101 Unspecified injury of muscle and tendon of long extensor muscle of toe at ankle and foot level, right foot**

+7th **S96.102 Unspecified injury of muscle and tendon of long extensor muscle of toe at ankle and foot level, left foot**

+7th **S96.109 Unspecified injury of muscle and tendon of long extensor muscle of toe at ankle and foot level, unspecified foot**

\+ **S96.11 Strain of muscle and tendon of long extensor muscle of toe at ankle and foot level**

+7th **S96.111 Strain of muscle and tendon of long extensor muscle of toe at ankle and foot level, right foot**

+7th **S96.112 Strain of muscle and tendon of long extensor muscle of toe at ankle and foot level, left foot**

+7th **S96.119 Strain of muscle and tendon of long extensor muscle of toe at ankle and foot level, unspecified foot**

\+ **S96.12 Laceration of muscle and tendon of long extensor muscle of toe at ankle and foot level**

CC +7th **S96.121 Laceration of muscle and tendon of long extensor muscle of toe at ankle and foot level, right foot**

CC +7th **S96.122 Laceration of muscle and tendon of long extensor muscle of toe at ankle and foot level, left foot**

CC +7th **S96.129 Laceration of muscle and tendon of long extensor muscle of toe at ankle and foot level, unspecified foot**

\+ **S96.19 Other specified injury of muscle and tendon of long extensor muscle of toe at ankle and foot level**

+7th **S96.191 Other specified injury of muscle and tendon of long extensor muscle of toe at ankle and foot level, right foot**

+7th **S96.192 Other specified injury of muscle and tendon of long extensor muscle of toe at ankle and foot level, left foot**

+7th **S96.199 Other specified injury of muscle and tendon of long extensor muscle of toe at ankle and foot level, unspecified foot**

\+ **S96.2 Injury of intrinsic muscle and tendon at ankle and foot level**

\+ **S96.20 Unspecified injury of intrinsic muscle and tendon at ankle and foot level**

+7th **S96.201 Unspecified injury of intrinsic muscle and tendon at ankle and foot level, right foot**

+7th **S96.202 Unspecified injury of intrinsic muscle and tendon at ankle and foot level, left foot**

+7th **S96.209 Unspecified injury of intrinsic muscle and tendon at ankle and foot level, unspecified foot**

\+ **S96.21 Strain of intrinsic muscle and tendon at ankle and foot level**

+7th **S96.211 Strain of intrinsic muscle and tendon at ankle and foot level, right foot**

+7th **S96.212 Strain of intrinsic muscle and tendon at ankle and foot level, left foot**

+7th **S96.219 Strain of intrinsic muscle and tendon at ankle and foot level, unspecified foot**

\+ **S96.22 Laceration of intrinsic muscle and tendon at ankle and foot level**

CC +7th **S96.221 Laceration of intrinsic muscle and tendon at ankle and foot level, right foot**

CC +7th **S96.222 Laceration of intrinsic muscle and tendon at ankle and foot level, left foot**

CC +7th **S96.229 Laceration of intrinsic muscle and tendon at ankle and foot level, unspecified foot**

\+ **S96.29 Other specified injury of intrinsic muscle and tendon at ankle and foot level**

+7th **S96.291 Other specified injury of intrinsic muscle and tendon at ankle and foot level, right foot**

+7th **S96.292 Other specified injury of intrinsic muscle and tendon at ankle and foot level, left foot**

+7th **S96.299 Other specified injury of intrinsic muscle and tendon at ankle and foot level, unspecified foot**

\+ **S96.8 Injury of other specified muscles and tendons at ankle and foot level**

\+ **S96.80 Unspecified injury of other specified muscles and tendons at ankle and foot level**

+7th **S96.801 Unspecified injury of other specified muscles and tendons at ankle and foot level, right foot**

+7th **S96.802 Unspecified injury of other specified muscles and tendons at ankle and foot level, left foot**

+7th **S96.809 Unspecified injury of other specified muscles and tendons at ankle and foot level, unspecified foot**

\+ **S96.81 Strain of other specified muscles and tendons at ankle and foot level**

+7th **S96.811 Strain of other specified muscles and tendons at ankle and foot level, right foot**

+7th **S96.812 Strain of other specified muscles and tendons at ankle and foot level, left foot**

+7th **S96.819 Strain of other specified muscles and tendons at ankle and foot level, unspecified foot**

+ **S96.82 Laceration of other specified muscles and tendons at ankle and foot level**
  - CC +7th **S96.821 Laceration of other specified muscles and tendons at ankle and foot level, right foot**
  - CC +7th **S96.822 Laceration of other specified muscles and tendons at ankle and foot level, left foot**
  - CC +7th **S96.829 Laceration of other specified muscles and tendons at ankle and foot level, unspecified foot**

+ **S96.89 Other specified injury of other specified muscles and tendons at ankle and foot level**
  - +7th **S96.891 Other specified injury of other specified muscles and tendons at ankle and foot level, right foot**
  - +7th **S96.892 Other specified injury of other specified muscles and tendons at ankle and foot level, left foot**
  - +7th **S96.899 Other specified injury of other specified muscles and tendons at ankle and foot level, unspecified foot**

+ **S96.9 Injury of unspecified muscle and tendon at ankle and foot level**
  + **S96.90 Unspecified injury of unspecified muscle and tendon at ankle and foot level**
    - +7th **S96.901 Unspecified injury of unspecified muscle and tendon at ankle and foot level, right foot**
    - +7th **S96.902 Unspecified injury of unspecified muscle and tendon at ankle and foot level, left foot**
    - +7th **S96.909 Unspecified injury of unspecified muscle and tendon at ankle and foot level, unspecified foot**
  + **S96.91 Strain of unspecified muscle and tendon at ankle and foot level**
    - +7th **S96.911 Strain of unspecified muscle and tendon at ankle and foot level, right foot**
    - +7th **S96.912 Strain of unspecified muscle and tendon at ankle and foot level, left foot**
    - +7th **S96.919 Strain of unspecified muscle and tendon at ankle and foot level, unspecified foot**
  + **S96.92 Laceration of unspecified muscle and tendon at ankle and foot level**
    - CC +7th **S96.921 Laceration of unspecified muscle and tendon at ankle and foot level, right foot**
    - CC +7th **S96.922 Laceration of unspecified muscle and tendon at ankle and foot level, left foot**
    - CC +7th **S96.929 Laceration of unspecified muscle and tendon at ankle and foot level, unspecified foot**
  + **S96.99 Other specified injury of unspecified muscle and tendon at ankle and foot level**
    - +7th **S96.991 Other specified injury of unspecified muscle and tendon at ankle and foot level, right foot**
    - +7th **S96.992 Other specified injury of unspecified muscle and tendon at ankle and foot level, left foot**
    - +7th **S96.999 Other specified injury of unspecified muscle and tendon at ankle and foot level, unspecified foot**

S97 Crushing injury of ankle and foot

Use additional code(s) for all associated injuries

The appropriate 7th character is to be added to each code from category S97
- A initial encounter
- D subsequent encounter
- S sequela

+ **S97.0 Crushing injury of ankle**
  - X+7th **S97.00 Crushing injury of unspecified ankle**
  - X+7th **S97.01 Crushing injury of right ankle**
  - X+7th **S97.02 Crushing injury of left ankle**

+ **S97.1 Crushing injury of toe**
  + **S97.10 Crushing injury of unspecified toe(s)**
    - +7th **S97.101 Crushing injury of unspecified right toe(s)**
    - +7th **S97.102 Crushing injury of unspecified left toe(s)**
    - +7th **S97.109 Crushing injury of unspecified toe(s)**
      Crushing injury of toe NOS
  + **S97.11 Crushing injury of great toe**
    - +7th **S97.111 Crushing injury of right great toe**
    - +7th **S97.112 Crushing injury of left great toe**
    - +7th **S97.119 Crushing injury of unspecified great toe**
  + **S97.12 Crushing injury of lesser toe(s)**
    - +7th **S97.121 Crushing injury of right lesser toe(s)**
    - +7th **S97.122 Crushing injury of left lesser toe(s)**
    - +7th **S97.129 Crushing injury of unspecified lesser toe(s)**

+ **S97.8 Crushing injury of foot**
  - X+7th **S97.80 Crushing injury of unspecified foot**
    Crushing injury of foot NOS
  - X+7th **S97.81 Crushing injury of right foot**
  - X+7th **S97.82 Crushing injury of left foot**

S98 Traumatic amputation of ankle and foot

NOTE An amputation not identified as partial or complete should be coded to complete

The appropriate 7th character is to be added to each code from category S98
- A initial encounter
- D subsequent encounter
- S sequela

+ **S98.0 Traumatic amputation of foot at ankle level**
  + **S98.01 Complete traumatic amputation of foot at ankle level**
    - CC +7th **S98.011 Complete traumatic amputation of right foot at ankle level**
    - CC +7th **S98.012 Complete traumatic amputation of left foot at ankle level**
    - CC +7th **S98.019 Complete traumatic amputation of unspecified foot at ankle level**
  + **S98.02 Partial traumatic amputation of foot at ankle level**
    - CC +7th **S98.021 Partial traumatic amputation of right foot at ankle level**
    - CC +7th **S98.022 Partial traumatic amputation of left foot at ankle level**
    - CC +7th **S98.029 Partial traumatic amputation of unspecified foot at ankle level**

+ **S98.1 Traumatic amputation of one toe**
  + **S98.11 Complete traumatic amputation of great toe**
    - +7th **S98.111 Complete traumatic amputation of right great toe**
    - +7th **S98.112 Complete traumatic amputation of left great toe**
    - +7th **S98.119 Complete traumatic amputation of unspecified great toe**
  + **S98.12 Partial traumatic amputation of great toe**
    - +7th **S98.121 Partial traumatic amputation of right great toe**
    - +7th **S98.122 Partial traumatic amputation of left great toe**
    - +7th **S98.129 Partial traumatic amputation of unspecified great toe**
  + **S98.13 Complete traumatic amputation of one lesser toe**
    Traumatic amputation of toe NOS
    - +7th **S98.131 Complete traumatic amputation of one right lesser toe**
    - +7th **S98.132 Complete traumatic amputation of one left lesser toe**
    - +7th **S98.139 Complete traumatic amputation of one unspecified lesser toe**
  + **S98.14 Partial traumatic amputation of one lesser toe**
    - +7th **S98.141 Partial traumatic amputation of one right lesser toe**
    - +7th **S98.142 Partial traumatic amputation of one left lesser toe**
    - +7th **S98.149 Partial traumatic amputation of one unspecified lesser toe**

+ S98.2 Traumatic amputation of two or more lesser toes
  + S98.21 Complete traumatic amputation of two or more lesser toes
    +7th S98.211 Complete traumatic amputation of two or more right lesser toes
    +7th S98.212 Complete traumatic amputation of two or more left lesser toes
    +7th S98.219 Complete traumatic amputation of two or more unspecified lesser toes
  + S98.22 Partial traumatic amputation of two or more lesser toes
    +7th S98.221 Partial traumatic amputation of two or more right lesser toes
    +7th S98.222 Partial traumatic amputation of two or more left lesser toes
    +7th S98.229 Partial traumatic amputation of two or more unspecified lesser toes
+ S98.3 Traumatic amputation of midfoot
  + S98.31 Complete traumatic amputation of midfoot
    CC +7th S98.311 Complete traumatic amputation of right midfoot
    CC +7th S98.312 Complete traumatic amputation of left midfoot
    CC +7th S98.319 Complete traumatic amputation of unspecified midfoot
  + S98.32 Partial traumatic amputation of midfoot
    CC +7th S98.321 Partial traumatic amputation of right midfoot
    CC +7th S98.322 Partial traumatic amputation of left midfoot
    CC +7th S98.329 Partial traumatic amputation of unspecified midfoot
+ S98.9 Traumatic amputation of foot, level unspecified
  + S98.91 Complete traumatic amputation of foot, level unspecified
    CC +7th S98.911 Complete traumatic amputation of right foot, level unspecified
    CC +7th S98.912 Complete traumatic amputation of left foot, level unspecified
    CC +7th S98.919 Complete traumatic amputation of unspecified foot, level unspecified
  + S98.92 Partial traumatic amputation of foot, level unspecified
    CC +7th S98.921 Partial traumatic amputation of right foot, level unspecified
    CC +7th S98.922 Partial traumatic amputation of left foot, level unspecified
    CC +7th S98.929 Partial traumatic amputation of unspecified foot, level unspecified

S99 Other and unspecified injuries of ankle and foot

+ S99.0 Physeal fracture of calcaneus
  AHA CC: 4Q, 2016, 68-69

The appropriate 7th character is to be added to each code in subcategory **S99.0**

A initial encounter for closed fracture
B initial encounter for open fracture
D subsequent encounter for fracture with routine healing
G subsequent encounter for fracture with delayed healing
K subsequent encounter for fracture with nonunion
P subsequent encounter for fracture with malunion
S sequela

  + S99.00 Unspecified physeal fracture of calcaneus
    Unspecified physeal fracture of calcaneus
    +7th S99.001 Unspecified physeal fracture of right calcaneus
    +7th S99.002 Unspecified physeal fracture of left calcaneus
    +7th S99.009 Unspecified physeal fracture of unspecified calcaneus
  + S99.01 Salter-Harris Type I physeal fracture of calcaneus
    +7th S99.011 Salter-Harris Type I physeal fracture of right calcaneus
    +7th S99.012 Salter-Harris Type I physeal fracture of left calcaneus
    +7th S99.019 Salter-Harris Type I physeal fracture of unspecified calcaneus
  + S99.02 Salter-Harris Type II physeal fracture of calcaneus
    +7th S99.021 Salter-Harris Type II physeal fracture of right calcaneus
    +7th S99.022 Salter-Harris Type II physeal fracture of left calcaneus
    +7th S99.029 Salter-Harris Type II physeal fracture of unspecified calcaneus
  + S99.03 Salter-Harris Type III physeal fracture of calcaneus
    +7th S99.031 Salter-Harris Type III physeal fracture of right calcaneus
    +7th S99.032 Salter-Harris Type III physeal fracture of left calcaneus
    +7th S99.039 Salter-Harris Type III physeal fracture of unspecified calcaneus
  + S99.04 Salter-Harris Type IV physeal fracture of calcaneus
    +7th S99.041 Salter-Harris Type IV physeal fracture of right calcaneus
    +7th S99.042 Salter-Harris Type IV physeal fracture of left calcaneus
    +7th S99.049 Salter-Harris Type IV physeal fracture of unspecified calcaneus
  + S99.09 Other physeal fracture of calcaneus
    +7th S99.091 Other physeal fracture of right calcaneus
    +7th S99.092 Other physeal fracture of left calcaneus
    +7th S99.099 Other physeal fracture of unspecified calcaneus

+ S99.1 Physeal fracture of metatarsal

The appropriate 7th character is to be added to each code in subcategory **S99.1**

A initial encounter for closed fracture
B initial encounter for open fracture
D subsequent encounter for fracture with routine healing
G subsequent encounter for fracture with delayed healing
K subsequent encounter for fracture with nonunion
P subsequent encounter for fracture with malunion
S sequela

  + S99.10 Unspecified physeal fracture of metatarsal
    +7th S99.101 Unspecified physeal fracture of right metatarsal
    +7th S99.102 Unspecified physeal fracture of left metatarsal
    +7th S99.109 Unspecified physeal fracture of unspecified metatarsal
  + S99.11 Salter-Harris Type I physeal fracture of metatarsal
    +7th S99.111 Salter-Harris Type I physeal fracture of right metatarsal
    +7th S99.112 Salter-Harris Type I physeal fracture of left metatarsal
      AHA CC: 1Q, 2018, 3
    +7th S99.119 Salter-Harris Type I physeal fracture of unspecified metatarsal
  + S99.12 Salter-Harris Type II physeal fracture of metatarsal
    +7th S99.121 Salter-Harris Type II physeal fracture of right metatarsal
    +7th S99.122 Salter-Harris Type II physeal fracture of left metatarsal
    +7th S99.129 Salter-Harris Type II physeal fracture of unspecified metatarsal
  + S99.13 Salter-Harris Type III physeal fracture of metatarsal
    +7th S99.131 Salter-Harris Type III physeal fracture of right metatarsal
    +7th S99.132 Salter-Harris Type III physeal fracture of left metatarsal
    +7th S99.139 Salter-Harris Type III physeal fracture of unspecified metatarsal
  + S99.14 Salter-Harris Type IV physeal fracture of metatarsal
    +7th S99.141 Salter-Harris Type IV physeal fracture of right metatarsal
    +7th S99.142 Salter-Harris Type IV physeal fracture of left metatarsal
    +7th S99.149 Salter-Harris Type IV physeal fracture of unspecified metatarsal

\+ **S99.19 Other physeal fracture of metatarsal**
+7th **S99.191 Other physeal fracture of right metatarsal**
+7th **S99.192 Other physeal fracture of left metatarsal**
+7th **S99.199 Other physeal fracture of unspecified metatarsal**

\+ **S99.2 Phseal fracture of phalanx of toe**

The appropriate 7th character is to be added to each code in subcategory **S99.2**
A initial encounter for closed fracture
B initial encounter for open fracture
D subsequent encounter for fracture with routine healing
G subsequent encounter for fracture with delayed healing
K subsequent encounter for fracture with nonunion
P subsequent encounter for fracture with malunion
S sequela

\+ **S99.20 Unspecified physeal fracture of phalanx of toe**
+7th **S99.201 Unspecified physeal fracture of phalanx of right toe**
+7th **S99.202 Unspecified physeal fracture of phalanx of left toe**
+7th **S99.209 Unspecified physeal fracture of phalanx of unspecified toe**
\+ **S99.21 Salter-Harris Type I physeal fracture of phalanx of toe**
+7th **S99.211 Salter-Harris Type I physeal fracture of phalanx of right toe**
+7th **S99.212 Salter-Harris Type I physeal fracture of phalanx of left toe**
+7th **S99.219 Salter-Harris Type I physeal fracture of phalanx of unspecified toe**
\+ **S99.22 Salter-Harris Type II physeal fracture of phalanx of toe**
+7th **S99.221 Salter-Harris Type II physeal fracture of phalanx of right toe**
+7th **S99.222 Salter-Harris Type II physeal fracture of phalanx of left toe**
+7th **S99.229 Salter-Harris Type II physeal fracture of phalanx of unspecified toe**
\+ **S99.23 Salter-Harris Type III physeal fracture of phalanx of toe**
+7th **S99.231 Salter-Harris Type III physeal fracture of phalanx of right toe**
+7th **S99.232 Salter-Harris Type III physeal fracture of phalanx of left toe**
+7th **S99.239 Salter-Harris Type III physeal fracture of phalanx of unspecified toe**
\+ **S99.24 Salter-Harris Type IV physeal fracture of phalanx of toe**
+7th **S99.241 Salter-Harris Type IV physeal fracture of phalanx of right toe**
+7th **S99.242 Salter-Harris Type IV physeal fracture of phalanx of left toe**
+7th **S99.249 Salter-Harris Type IV physeal fracture of phalanx of unspecified toe**
\+ **S99.29 Other physeal fracture of phalanx of toe**
+7th **S99.291 Other physeal fracture of phalanx of right toe**
+7th **S99.292 Other physeal fracture of phalanx of left toe**
+7th **S99.299 Other physeal fracture of phalanx of unspecified toe**

\+ **S99.8 Other specified injuries of ankle and foot**

The appropriate 7th character is to be added to each code from category **S99.8**
A initial encounter
D subsequent encounter
S sequela

\+ **S99.81 Other specified injuries of ankle**
+7th **S99.811 Other specified injuries of right ankle**
+7th **S99.812 Other specified injuries of left ankle**
+7th **S99.819 Other specified injuries of unspecified ankle**
\+ **S99.82 Other specified injuries of foot**
+7th **S99.821 Other specified injuries of right foot**
+7th **S99.822 Other specified injuries of left foot**
+7th **S99.829 Other specified injuries of unspecified foot**

\+ **S99.9 Unspecified injury of ankle and foot**

The appropriate 7th character is to be added to each code from category **S99.9**
A initial encounter
D subsequent encounter
S sequela

\+ **S99.91 Unspecified injury of ankle**
+7th **S99.911 Unspecified injury of right ankle**
+7th **S99.912 Unspecified injury of left ankle**
+7th **S99.919 Unspecified injury of unspecified ankle**
\+ **S99.92 Unspecified injury of foot**
+7th **S99.921 Unspecified injury of right foot**
+7th **S99.922 Unspecified injury of left foot**
+7th **S99.929 Unspecified injury of unspecified foot**

INJURY, POISONING AND CERTAIN OTHER CONSEQUENCES OF EXTERNAL CAUSES (T07-T88)

Injuries involving multiple body regions (T07)

Excludes1: *burns and corrosions (T20-T32)*
frostbite (T33-T34)
insect bite or sting, venomous (T63.4)
sunburn (L55.-)

T07 Unspecified multiple injuries

The appropriate 7th character is to be added to each code from category T07
A initial encounter
D subsequent encounter
S sequela

Excludes1: *injury NOS (T14.90)*
AHA CC: 4Q, 2017, 26
Review coding guideline C.19.b

Injury of unspecified body region (T14)

T14 Injury of unspecified body region

The appropriate 7th character is to be added to each code from category T14
A initial encounter
D subsequent encounter
S sequela

Excludes1: *multiple unspecified injuries (T07)*
AHA CC: 4Q, 2017, 26

T14.8 Other injury of unspecified body region
Abrasion NOS
Contusion NOS
Crush injury NOS
Fracture NOS
Skin injury NOS
Vascular injury NOS
Wound NOS
\+ **T14.9 Unspecified injury**
T14.90 Injury, unspecified
Injury NOS
T14.91 Suicide attempt
Attempted suicide NOS

Effects of foreign body entering through natural orifice (T15-T19)

Excludes2: *foreign body accidentally left in operation wound (T81.5-)*
foreign body in penetrating wound - See open wound by body region
residual foreign body in soft tissue (M79.5)
splinter, without open wound - See superficial injury by body region

T15 Foreign body on external eye

Excludes2: *foreign body in penetrating wound of orbit and eye ball (S05.4-, S05.5-)*
open wound of eyelid and periocular area (S01.1-)
retained foreign body in eyelid (H02.8-)
retained (old) foreign body in penetrating wound of orbit and eye ball (H05.5-, H44.6-, H44.7-)
superficial foreign body of eyelid and periocular area (S00.25-)

The appropriate 7th character is to be added to each code from category T15
A initial encounter
D subsequent encounter
S sequela

+ **T15.0 Foreign body in cornea**
  - X+7th **T15.00 Foreign body in cornea, unspecified eye**
  - X+7th **T15.01 Foreign body in cornea, right eye**
  - X+7th **T15.02 Foreign body in cornea, left eye**
+ **T15.1 Foreign body in conjunctival sac**
  - X+7th **T15.10 Foreign body in conjunctival sac, unspecified eye**
  - X+7th **T15.11 Foreign body in conjunctival sac, right eye**
  - X+7th **T15.12 Foreign body in conjunctival sac, left eye**
+ **T15.8 Foreign body in other and multiple parts of external eye**
  Foreign body in lacrimal punctum
  - X+7th **T15.80 Foreign body in other and multiple parts of external eye, unspecified eye**
  - X+7th **T15.81 Foreign body in other and multiple parts of external eye, right eye**
  - X+7th **T15.82 Foreign body in other and multiple parts of external eye, left eye**
+ **T15.9 Foreign body on external eye, part unspecified**
  - X+7th **T15.90 Foreign body on external eye, part unspecified, unspecified eye**
  - X+7th **T15.91 Foreign body on external eye, part unspecified, right eye**
  - X+7th **T15.92 Foreign body on external eye, part unspecified, left eye**

T16 Foreign body in ear

Includes: foreign body in auditory canal

The appropriate 7th character is to be added to each code from category T16
A initial encounter
D subsequent encounter
S sequela

X+7th **T16.1 Foreign body in right ear**
X+7th **T16.2 Foreign body in left ear**
X+7th **T16.9 Foreign body in ear, unspecified ear**

T17 Foreign body in respiratory tract

The appropriate 7th character is to be added to each code from category T17
A initial encounter
D subsequent encounter
S sequela

X+7th **T17.0 Foreign body in nasal sinus**
X+7th **T17.1 Foreign body in nostril**
  Foreign body in nose NOS
+ **T17.2 Foreign body in pharynx**
  Foreign body in nasopharynx
  Foreign body in throat NOS
  + **T17.20 Unspecified foreign body in pharynx**
    - +7th **T17.200 Unspecified foreign body in pharynx causing asphyxiation**
    - +7th **T17.208 Unspecified foreign body in pharynx causing other injury**
  + **T17.21 Gastric contents in pharynx**
    Aspiration of gastric contents into pharynx
    Vomitus in pharynx
    - +7th **T17.210 Gastric contents in pharynx causing asphyxiation**
    - +7th **T17.218 Gastric contents in pharynx causing other injury**
  + **T17.22 Food in pharynx**
    Bones in pharynx
    Seeds in pharynx
    - +7th **T17.220 Food in pharynx causing asphyxiation**
    - +7th **T17.228 Food in pharynx causing other injury**
  + **T17.29 Other foreign object in pharynx**
    - +7th **T17.290 Other foreign object in pharynx causing asphyxiation**
    - +7th **T17.298 Other foreign object in pharynx causing other injury**
+ **T17.3 Foreign body in larynx**
  + **T17.30 Unspecified foreign body in larynx**
    - +7th **T17.300 Unspecified foreign body in larynx causing asphyxiation**
    - +7th **T17.308 Unspecified foreign body in larynx causing other injury**
  + **T17.31 Gastric contents in larynx**
    Aspiration of gastric contents into larynx
    Vomitus in larynx
    - +7th **T17.310 Gastric contents in larynx causing asphyxiation**
    - +7th **T17.318 Gastric contents in larynx causing other injury**
  + **T17.32 Food in larynx**
    Bones in larynx
    Seeds in larynx
    - +7th **T17.320 Food in larynx causing asphyxiation**
    - +7th **T17.328 Food in larynx causing other injury**
  + **T17.39 Other foreign object in larynx**
    - +7th **T17.390 Other foreign object in larynx causing asphyxiation**
    - +7th **T17.398 Other foreign object in larynx causing other injury**
+ **T17.4 Foreign body in trachea**
  + **T17.40 Unspecified foreign body in trachea**
    - CC +7th **T17.400 Unspecified foreign body in trachea causing asphyxiation**
    - CC +7th **T17.408 Unspecified foreign body in trachea causing other injury**
  + **T17.41 Gastric contents in trachea**
    Aspiration of gastric contents into trachea
    Vomitus in trachea
    - CC +7th **T17.410 Gastric contents in trachea causing asphyxiation**
    - CC +7th **T17.418 Gastric contents in trachea causing other injury**
  + **T17.42 Food in trachea**
    Bones in trachea
    Seeds in trachea
    - CC +7th **T17.420 Food in trachea causing asphyxiation**
    - CC +7th **T17.428 Food in trachea causing other injury**
  + **T17.49 Other foreign object in trachea**
    - CC +7th **T17.490 Other foreign object in trachea causing asphyxiation**
    - CC +7th **T17.498 Other foreign object in trachea causing other injury**
+ **T17.5 Foreign body in bronchus**
  + **T17.50 Unspecified foreign body in bronchus**
    - CC +7th **T17.500 Unspecified foreign body in bronchus causing asphyxiation**
    - CC +7th **T17.508 Unspecified foreign body in bronchus causing other injury**
  + **T17.51 Gastric contents in bronchus**
    Aspiration of gastric contents into bronchus
    Vomitus in bronchus
    - CC +7th **T17.510 Gastric contents in bronchus causing asphyxiation**
    - CC +7th **T17.518 Gastric contents in bronchus causing other injury**
  + **T17.52 Food in bronchus**
    Bones in bronchus
    Seeds in bronchus
    - CC +7th **T17.520 Food in bronchus causing asphyxiation**
    - CC +7th **T17.528 Food in bronchus causing other injury**
  + **T17.59 Other foreign object in bronchus**
    - CC +7th **T17.590 Other foreign object in bronchus causing asphyxiation**
    - CC +7th **T17.598 Other foreign object in bronchus causing other injury**
+ **T17.8 Foreign body in other parts of respiratory tract**
  Foreign body in bronchioles
  Foreign body in lung
  + **T17.80 Unspecified foreign body in other parts of respiratory tract**
    - CC +7th **T17.800 Unspecified foreign body in other parts of respiratory tract causing asphyxiation**
    - CC +7th **T17.808 Unspecified foreign body in other parts of respiratory tract causing other injury**

+ **T17.81 Gastric contents in other parts of respiratory tract**
Aspiration of gastric contents into other parts of respiratory tract
Vomitus in other parts of respiratory tract
CC +7th **T17.810 Gastric contents in other parts of respiratory tract causing asphyxiation**
CC +7th **T17.818 Gastric contents in other parts of respiratory tract causing other injury**
+ **T17.82 Food in other parts of respiratory tract**
Bones in other parts of respiratory tract
Seeds in other parts of respiratory tract
CC +7th **T17.820 Food in other parts of respiratory tract causing asphyxiation**
CC +7th **T17.828 Food in other parts of respiratory tract causing other injury**
+ **T17.89 Other foreign object in other parts of respiratory tract**
CC +7th **T17.890 Other foreign object in other parts of respiratory tract causing asphyxiation**
CC +7th **T17.898 Other foreign object in other parts of respiratory tract causing other injury**

T17.9 Foreign body in respiratory tract, part unspecified
+ **T17.90 Unspecified foreign body in respiratory tract, part unspecified**
+7th **T17.900 Unspecified foreign body in respiratory tract, part unspecified causing asphyxiation**
+7th **T17.908 Unspecified foreign body in respiratory tract, part unspecified causing other injury**
+ **T17.91 Gastric contents in respiratory tract, part unspecified**
Aspiration of gastric contents into respiratory tract, part unspecified
Vomitus in trachea respiratory tract, part unspecified
+7th **T17.910 Gastric contents in respiratory tract, part unspecified causing asphyxiation**
+7th **T17.918 Gastric contents in respiratory tract, part unspecified causing other injury**
+ **T17.92 Food in respiratory tract, part unspecified**
Bones in respiratory tract, part unspecified
Seeds in respiratory tract, part unspecified
+7th **T17.920 Food in respiratory tract, part unspecified causing asphyxiation**
+7th **T17.928 Food in respiratory tract, part unspecified causing other injury**
+ **T17.99 Other foreign object in respiratory tract, part unspecified**
+7th **T17.990 Other foreign object in respiratory tract, part unspecified in causing asphyxiation**
+7th **T17.998 Other foreign object in respiratory tract, part unspecified causing other injury**

T18 Foreign body in alimentary tract
Excludes2: *foreign body in pharynx (T17.2-)*

The appropriate 7th character is to be added to each code from category T18
A initial encounter
D subsequent encounter
S sequela

X+7th **T18.0 Foreign body in mouth**
+ **T18.1 Foreign body in esophagus**
Excludes2: *foreign body in respiratory tract (T17.-)*
+ **T18.10 Unspecified foreign body in esophagus**
+7th **T18.100 Unspecified foreign body in esophagus causing compression of trachea**
Unspecified foreign body in esophagus causing obstruction of respiration
+7th **T18.108 Unspecified foreign body in esophagus causing other injury**
+ **T18.11 Gastric contents in esophagus**
Vomitus in esophagus
+7th **T18.110 Gastric contents in esophagus causing compression of trachea**
Gastric contents in esophagus causing obstruction of respiration
+7th **T18.118 Gastric contents in esophagus causing other injury**
+ **T18.12 Food in esophagus**
Bones in esophagus
Seeds in esophagus
+7th **T18.120 Food in esophagus causing compression of trachea**
Food in esophagus causing obstruction of respiration
+7th **T18.128 Food in esophagus causing other injury**
+ **T18.19 Other foreign object in esophagus**
+7th **T18.190 Other foreign object in esophagus causing compression of trachea**
Other foreign body in esophagus causing obstruction of respiration
AHA CC: 1Q, 2015, 23-24
+7th **T18.198 Other foreign object in esophagus causing other injury**
AHA CC: 1Q, 2015, 23-24

X+7th **T18.2 Foreign body in stomach**
X+7th **T18.3 Foreign body in small intestine**
X+7th **T18.4 Foreign body in colon**
X+7th **T18.5 Foreign body in anus and rectum**
Foreign body in rectosigmoid (junction)
X+7th **T18.8 Foreign body in other parts of alimentary tract**
X+7th **T18.9 Foreign body of alimentary tract, part unspecified**
Foreign body in digestive system NOS
Swallowed foreign body NOS

T19 Foreign body in genitourinary tract
Excludes2: *complications due to implanted mesh (T83.7-)*
mechanical complications of contraceptive device (intrauterine) (vaginal) (T83.3-)
presence of contraceptive device (intrauterine) (vaginal) (Z97.5)

The appropriate 7th character is to be added to each code from category T19
A initial encounter
D subsequent encounter
S sequela

X+7th **T19.0 Foreign body in urethra**
X+7th **T19.1 Foreign body in bladder**
♀ X+7th **T19.2 Foreign body in vulva and vagina**
♀ X+7th **T19.3 Foreign body in uterus**
♂ X+7th **T19.4 Foreign body in penis**
X+7th **T19.8 Foreign body in other parts of genitourinary tract**
X+7th **T19.9 Foreign body in genitourinary tract, part unspecified**

BURNS AND CORROSIONS (T20-T32)

Includes: burns (thermal) from electrical heating appliances
burns (thermal) from electricity
burns (thermal) from flame
burns (thermal) from friction
burns (thermal) from hot air and hot gases
burns (thermal) from hot objects
burns (thermal) from lightning
burns (thermal) from radiation
chemical burn [corrosion] (external) (internal)
scalds

Excludes2: *erythema [dermatitis] ab igne (L59.0)*
radiation-related disorders of the skin and subcutaneous tissue (L55-L59)
sunburn (L55.-)

Burns and corrosions of external body surface, specified by site (T20-T25)

Includes: burns and corrosions of first degree [erythema]
burns and corrosions of second degree [blisters][epidermal loss]
burns and corrosions of third degree [deep necrosis of underlying tissue] [full- thickness skin loss]

Use additional code from category T31 or T32 to identify extent of body surface involved

Review coding guideline C.19.d

T20 Burn and corrosion of head, face, and neck

Excludes2: *burn and corrosion of ear drum (T28.41, T28.91)*
burn and corrosion of eye and adnexa (T26.-)
burn and corrosion of mouth and pharynx (T28.0)

The appropriate 7th character is to be added to each code from category T20
A initial encounter
D subsequent encounter
S sequela

\+ **T20.0 Burn of unspecified degree of head, face, and neck**
Use additional external cause code to identify the source, place and intent of the burn (X00-X19, X75-X77, X96-X98, Y92)

X+7th **T20.00 Burn of unspecified degree of head, face, and neck, unspecified site**

\+ **T20.01 Burn of unspecified degree of ear [any part, except ear drum]**
Excludes2: *burn of ear drum (T28.41-)*

+7th **T20.011 Burn of unspecified degree of right ear [any part, except ear drum]**

+7th **T20.012 Burn of unspecified degree of left ear [any part, except ear drum]**

+7th **T20.019 Burn of unspecified degree of unspecified ear [any part, except ear drum]**

X+7th **T20.02 Burn of unspecified degree of lip(s)**

X+7th **T20.03 Burn of unspecified degree of chin**

X+7th **T20.04 Burn of unspecified degree of nose (septum)**

X+7th **T20.05 Burn of unspecified degree of scalp [any part]**

X+7th **T20.06 Burn of unspecified degree of forehead and cheek**

X+7th **T20.07 Burn of unspecified degree of neck**

X+7th **T20.09 Burn of unspecified degree of multiple sites of head, face, and neck**

\+ **T20.1 Burn of first degree of head, face, and neck**
Use additional external cause code to identify the source, place and intent of the burn (X00-X19, X75-X77, X96-X98, Y92)

X+7th **T20.10 Burn of first degree of head, face, and neck, unspecified site**

\+ **T20.11 Burn of first degree of ear [any part, except ear drum]**
Excludes2: *burn of ear drum (T28.41-)*

+7th **T20.111 Burn of first degree of right ear [any part, except ear drum]**

+7th **T20.112 Burn of first degree of left ear [any part, except ear drum]**

+7th **T20.119 Burn of first degree of unspecified ear [any part, except ear drum]**

X+7th **T20.12 Burn of first degree of lip(s)**

X+7th **T20.13 Burn of first degree of chin**

X+7th **T20.14 Burn of first degree of nose (septum)**

X+7th **T20.15 Burn of first degree of scalp [any part]**

X+7th **T20.16 Burn of first degree of forehead and cheek**

X+7th **T20.17 Burn of first degree of neck**

X+7th **T20.19 Burn of first degree of multiple sites of head, face, and neck**

\+ **T20.2 Burn of second degree of head, face, and neck**
Use additional external cause code to identify the source, place and intent of the burn (X00-X19, X75-X77, X96-X98, Y92)

X+7th **T20.20 Burn of second degree of head, face, and neck, unspecified site**

\+ **T20.21 Burn of second degree of ear [any part, except ear drum]**
Excludes2: *burn of ear drum (T28.41-)*

+7th **T20.211 Burn of second degree of right ear [any part, except ear drum]**

+7th **T20.212 Burn of second degree of left ear [any part, except ear drum]**

+7th **T20.219 Burn of second degree of unspecified ear [any part, except ear drum]**

X+7th **T20.22 Burn of second degree of lip(s)**

X+7th **T20.23 Burn of second degree of chin**

X+7th **T20.24 Burn of second degree of nose (septum)**

X+7th **T20.25 Burn of second degree of scalp [any part]**
AHA CC: 1Q, 2015, 3-21

X+7th **T20.26 Burn of second degree of forehead and cheek**

X+7th **T20.27 Burn of second degree of neck**

X+7th **T20.29 Burn of second degree of multiple sites of head, face, and neck**

\+ **T20.3 Burn of third degree of head, face, and neck**
Use additional external cause code to identify the source, place and intent of the burn (X00-X19, X75-X77, X96-X98, Y92)

CC X+7th **T20.30 Burn of third degree of head, face, and neck, unspecified site**
HAC 7th character A see Appendix B for HAC conditional logic

\+ **T20.31 Burn of third degree of ear [any part, except ear drum]**
Excludes2: *burn of ear drum (T28.41-)*

CC +7th **T20.311 Burn of third degree of right ear [any part, except ear drum]**
HAC 7th character A see Appendix B for HAC conditional logic

CC +7th **T20.312 Burn of third degree of left ear [any part, except ear drum]**
HAC 7th character A see Appendix B for HAC conditional logic
AHA CC: 1Q, 2015, 3-21

CC +7th **T20.319 Burn of third degree of unspecified ear [any part, except ear drum]**
HAC 7th character A see Appendix B for HAC conditional logic

CC X+7th **T20.32 Burn of third degree of lip(s)**
HAC 7th character A see Appendix B for HAC conditional logic

CC X+7th **T20.33 Burn of third degree of chin**
HAC 7th character A see Appendix B for HAC conditional logic

CC X+7th **T20.34 Burn of third degree of nose (septum)**
HAC 7th character A see Appendix B for HAC conditional logic

CC X+7th **T20.35 Burn of third degree of scalp [any part]**
HAC 7th character A see Appendix B for HAC conditional logic

CC X+7th **T20.36 Burn of third degree of forehead and cheek**
HAC 7th character A see Appendix B for HAC conditional logic

CC X+7th **T20.37 Burn of third degree of neck**
HAC 7th character A see Appendix B for HAC conditional logic

CC X+7th **T20.39 Burn of third degree of multiple sites of head, face, and neck**
HAC 7th character A see Appendix B for HAC conditional logic

\+ **T20.4 Corrosion of unspecified degree of head, face, and neck**
Code first (T51-T65) to identify chemical and intent external cause code to identify place (Y92)

X+7th **T20.40 Corrosion of unspecified degree of head, face, and neck, unspecified site**

+ **T20.41 Corrosion of unspecified degree of ear [any part, except ear drum]**
  Excludes2: *corrosion of ear drum (T28.91-)*
  +7th **T20.411 Corrosion of unspecified degree of right ear [any part, except ear drum]**
  +7th **T20.412 Corrosion of unspecified degree of left ear [any part, except ear drum]**
  +7th **T20.419 Corrosion of unspecified degree of unspecified ear [any part, except ear drum]**
X+7th **T20.42 Corrosion of unspecified degree of lip(s)**
X+7th **T20.43 Corrosion of unspecified degree of chin**
X+7th **T20.44 Corrosion of unspecified degree of nose (septum)**
X+7th **T20.45 Corrosion of unspecified degree of scalp [any part]**
X+7th **T20.46 Corrosion of unspecified degree of forehead and cheek**
X+7th **T20.47 Corrosion of unspecified degree of neck**
X+7th **T20.49 Corrosion of unspecified degree of multiple sites of head, face, and neck**

+ **T20.5 Corrosion of first degree of head, face, and neck**
  Code first (T51-T65) to identify chemical and intent

  Use additional external cause code to identify place (Y92)
X+7th **T20.50 Corrosion of first degree of head, face, and neck, unspecified site**
+ **T20.51 Corrosion of first degree of ear [any part, except ear drum]**
  Excludes2: *corrosion of ear drum (T28.91-)*
  +7th **T20.511 Corrosion of first degree of right ear [any part, except ear drum]**
  +7th **T20.512 Corrosion of first degree of left ear [any part, except ear drum]**
  +7th **T20.519 Corrosion of first degree of unspecified ear [any part, except ear drum]**
X+7th **T20.52 Corrosion of first degree of lip(s)**
X+7th **T20.53 Corrosion of first degree of chin**
X+7th **T20.54 Corrosion of first degree of nose (septum)**
X+7th **T20.55 Corrosion of first degree of scalp [any part]**
X+7th **T20.56 Corrosion of first degree of forehead and cheek**
X+7th **T20.57 Corrosion of first degree of neck**
X+7th **T20.59 Corrosion of first degree of multiple sites of head, face, and neck**

+ **T20.6 Corrosion of second degree of head, face, and neck**
  Code first (T51-T65) to identify chemical and intent

  Use additional external cause code to identify place (Y92)
X+7th **T20.60 Corrosion of second degree of head, face, and neck, unspecified site**
+ **T20.61 Corrosion of second degree of ear [any part, except ear drum]**
  Excludes2: *corrosion of ear drum (T28.91-)*
  +7th **T20.611 Corrosion of second degree of right ear [any part, except ear drum]**
  +7th **T20.612 Corrosion of second degree of left ear [any part, except ear drum]**
  +7th **T20.619 Corrosion of second degree of unspecified ear [any part, except ear drum]**
X+7th **T20.62 Corrosion of second degree of lip(s)**
X+7th **T20.63 Corrosion of second degree of chin**
X+7th **T20.64 Corrosion of second degree of nose (septum)**
X+7th **T20.65 Corrosion of second degree of scalp [any part]**
X+7th **T20.66 Corrosion of second degree of forehead and cheek**
X+7th **T20.67 Corrosion of second degree of neck**
X+7th **T20.69 Corrosion of second degree of multiple sites of head, face, and neck**

+ **T20.7 Corrosion of third degree of head, face, and neck**
  Code first (T51-T65) to identify chemical and intent

  Use additional external cause code to identify place (Y92)
CC X+7th **T20.70 Corrosion of third degree of head, face, and neck, unspecified site**
  HAC 7th character A see Appendix B for HAC conditional logic
+ **T20.71 Corrosion of third degree of ear [any part, except ear drum]**
  Excludes2: *corrosion of ear drum (T28.91-)*
  CC +7th **T20.711 Corrosion of third degree of right ear [any part, except ear drum]**
    HAC 7th character A see Appendix B for HAC conditional logic
  CC +7th **T20.712 Corrosion of third degree of left ear [any part, except ear drum]**
    HAC 7th character A see Appendix B for HAC conditional logic
  CC +7th **T20.719 Corrosion of third degree of unspecified ear [any part, except ear drum]**
    HAC 7th character A see Appendix B for HAC conditional logic
CC X+7th **T20.72 Corrosion of third degree of lip(s)**
  HAC 7th character A see Appendix B for HAC conditional logic
CC X+7th **T20.73 Corrosion of third degree of chin**
  HAC 7th character A see Appendix B for HAC conditional logic
CC X+7th **T20.74 Corrosion of third degree of nose (septum)**
  HAC 7th character A see Appendix B for HAC conditional logic
CC X+7th **T20.75 Corrosion of third degree of scalp [any part]**
  HAC 7th character A see Appendix B for HAC conditional logic
CC X+7th **T20.76 Corrosion of third degree of forehead and cheek**
  HAC 7th character A see Appendix B for HAC conditional logic
CC X+7th **T20.77 Corrosion of third degree of neck**
  HAC 7th character A see Appendix B for HAC conditional logic
CC X+7th **T20.79 Corrosion of third degree of multiple sites of head, face, and neck**
  HAC 7th character A see Appendix B for HAC conditional logic

T21 Burn and corrosion of trunk

Includes: burns and corrosion of hip region
Excludes2: *burns and corrosion of axilla (T22.- with fifth character 4)*
burns and corrosion of scapular region (T22.- with fifth character 6)
burns and corrosion of shoulder (T22.- with fifth character 5)

The appropriate 7th character is to be added to each code from category T21
A initial encounter
D subsequent encounter
S sequela

+ **T21.0 Burn of unspecified degree of trunk**
  Use external cause code to identify the source, place and intent of the burn (X00-X19, X75-X77, X96-X98, Y92)
X+7th **T21.00 Burn of unspecified degree of trunk, unspecified site**
X+7th **T21.01 Burn of unspecified degree of chest wall**
  Burn of unspecified degree of breast
X+7th **T21.02 Burn of unspecified degree of abdominal wall**
  Burn of unspecified degree of flank
  Burn of unspecified degree of groin
X+7th **T21.03 Burn of unspecified degree of upper back**
  Burn of unspecified degree of interscapular region
X+7th **T21.04 Burn of unspecified degree of lower back**
X+7th **T21.05 Burn of unspecified degree of buttock**
  Burn of unspecified degree of anus
♂ X+7th **T21.06 Burn of unspecified degree of male genital region**
  Burn of unspecified degree of penis
  Burn of unspecified degree of scrotum
  Burn of unspecified degree of testis
♀ X+7th **T21.07 Burn of unspecified degree of female genital region**
  Burn of unspecified degree of labium (majus) (minus)
  Burn of unspecified degree of perineum
  Burn of unspecified degree of vulva
  Excludes2: *burn of vagina (T28.3)*
X+7th **T21.09 Burn of unspecified degree of other site of trunk**

+ **T21.1 Burn of first degree of trunk**
Use external cause code to identify the source, place and intent of the burn (X00-X19, X75-X77, X96-X98, Y92)
X+7th **T21.10 Burn of first degree of trunk, unspecified site**
X+7th **T21.11 Burn of first degree of chest wall**
Burn of first degree of breast
X+7th **T21.12 Burn of first degree of abdominal wall**
Burn of first degree of flank
Burn of first degree of groin
X+7th **T21.13 Burn of first degree of upper back**
Burn of first degree of interscapular region
X+7th **T21.14 Burn of first degree of lower back**
X+7th **T21.15 Burn of first degree of buttock**
Burn of first degree of anus
♂ X+7th **T21.16 Burn of first degree of male genital region**
Burn of first degree of penis
Burn of first degree of scrotum
Burn of first degree of testis
♀ X+7th **T21.17 Burn of first degree of female genital region**
Burn of first degree of labium (majus) (minus)
Burn of first degree of perineum
Burn of first degree of vulva
Excludes2: *burn of vagina (T28.3)*
X+7th **T21.19 Burn of first degree of other site of trunk**
+ **T21.2 Burn of second degree of trunk**
Use external cause code to identify the source, place and intent of the burn (X00-X19, X75-X77, X96-X98, Y92)
X+7th **T21.20 Burn of second degree of trunk, unspecified site**
X+7th **T21.21 Burn of second degree of chest wall**
Burn of second degree of breast
X+7th **T21.22 Burn of second degree of abdominal wall**
Burn of second degree of flank
Burn of second degree of groin
X+7th **T21.23 Burn of second degree of upper back**
Burn of second degree of interscapular region
X+7th **T21.24 Burn of second degree of lower back**
X+7th **T21.25 Burn of second degree of buttock**
Burn of second degree of anus
♂ X+7th **T21.26 Burn of second degree of male genital region**
Burn of second degree of penis
Burn of second degree of scrotum
Burn of second degree of testis
♀ X+7th **T21.27 Burn of second degree of female genital region**
Burn of second degree of labium (majus) (minus)
Burn of second degree of perineum
Burn of second degree of vulva
Excludes2: *burn of vagina (T28.3)*
X+7th **T21.29 Burn of second degree of other site of trunk**
+ **T21.3 Burn of third degree of trunk**
Use additional external cause code to identify the source, place and intent of the burn (X00-X19, X75-X77, X96-X98, Y92)
CC X+7th **T21.30 Burn of third degree of trunk, unspecified site**
HAC 7th character A see Appendix B for HAC conditional logic
CC X+7th **T21.31 Burn of third degree of chest wall**
Burn of third degree of breast
AHA CC: 2Q, 2016, 5-6
HAC 7th character A see Appendix B for HAC conditional logic
CC X+7th **T21.32 Burn of third degree of abdominal wall**
Burn of third degree of flank
Burn of third degree of groin
HAC 7th character A see Appendix B for HAC conditional logic
CC X+7th **T21.33 Burn of third degree of upper back**
Burn of third degree of interscapular region
HAC 7th character A see Appendix B for HAC conditional logic
CC X+7th **T21.34 Burn of third degree of lower back**
HAC 7th character A see Appendix B for HAC conditional logic
CC X+7th **T21.35 Burn of third degree of buttock**
Burn of third degree of anus
HAC 7th character A see Appendix B for HAC conditional logic
CC X+7th **T21.36 Burn of third degree of male genital region**
Burn of third degree of penis
Burn of third degree of scrotum
Burn of third degree of testis
HAC 7th character A see Appendix B for HAC conditional logic
CC X+7th **T21.37 Burn of third degree of female genital region**
Burn of third degree of labium (majus) (minus)
Burn of third degree of perineum
Burn of third degree of vulva
Excludes2: *burn of vagina (T28.3)*
HAC 7th character A see Appendix B for HAC conditional logic
CC X+7th **T21.39 Burn of third degree of other site of trunk**
HAC 7th character A see Appendix B for HAC conditional logic
+ **T21.4 Corrosion of unspecified degree of trunk**
Code first (T51-T65) to identify chemical and intent
Use additional external cause code to identify place (Y92)
X+7th **T21.40 Corrosion of unspecified degree of trunk, unspecified site**
X+7th **T21.41 Corrosion of unspecified degree of chest wall**
Corrosion of unspecified degree of breast
X+7th **T21.42 Corrosion of unspecified degree of abdominal wall**
Corrosion of unspecified degree of flank
Corrosion of unspecified degree of groin
X+7th **T21.43 Corrosion of unspecified degree of upper back**
Corrosion of unspecified degree of interscapular region
X+7th **T21.44 Corrosion of unspecified degree of lower back**
X+7th **T21.45 Corrosion of unspecified degree of buttock**
Corrosion of unspecified degree of anus
♂ X+7th **T21.46 Corrosion of unspecified degree of male genital region**
Corrosion of unspecified degree of penis
Corrosion of unspecified degree of scrotum
Corrosion of unspecified degree of testis
♀ X+7th **T21.47 Corrosion of unspecified degree of female genital region**
Corrosion of unspecified degree of labium (majus) (minus)
Corrosion of unspecified degree of perineum
Corrosion of unspecified degree of vulva
Excludes2: *corrosion of vagina (T28.8)*
X+7th **T21.49 Corrosion of unspecified degree of other site of trunk**
+ **T21.5 Corrosion of first degree of trunk**
Code first (T51-T65) to identify chemical and intent
Use additional external cause code to identify place (Y92)
X+7th **T21.50 Corrosion of first degree of trunk, unspecified site**
X+7th **T21.51 Corrosion of first degree of chest wall**
Corrosion of first degree of breast
X+7th **T21.52 Corrosion of first degree of abdominal wall**
Corrosion of first degree of flank
Corrosion of first degree of groin
X+7th **T21.53 Corrosion of first degree of upper back**
Corrosion of first degree of interscapular region
X+7th **T21.54 Corrosion of first degree of lower back**
X+7th **T21.55 Corrosion of first degree of buttock**
Corrosion of first degree of anus
♂ X+7th **T21.56 Corrosion of first degree of male genital region**
Corrosion of first degree of penis
Corrosion of first degree of scrotum
Corrosion of first degree of testis
♀ X+7th **T21.57 Corrosion of first degree of female genital region**
Corrosion of first degree of labium (majus) (minus)
Corrosion of first degree of perineum
Corrosion of first degree of vulva
Excludes2: *corrosion of vagina (T28.8)*
X+7th **T21.59 Corrosion of first degree of other site of trunk**

\+ **T21.6 Corrosion of second degree of trunk**
Code first (T51-T65) to identify chemical and intent
Use additional external cause code to identify place (Y92)

X+7th **T21.60 Corrosion of second degree of trunk, unspecified site**

X+7th **T21.61 Corrosion of second degree of chest wall**
Corrosion of second degree of breast

X+7th **T21.62 Corrosion of second degree of abdominal wall**
Corrosion of second degree of flank
Corrosion of second degree of groin

X+7th **T21.63 Corrosion of second degree of upper back**
Corrosion of second degree of interscapular region

X+7th **T21.64 Corrosion of second degree of lower back**

X+7th **T21.65 Corrosion of second degree of buttock**
Corrosion of second degree of anus

♂ X+7th **T21.66 Corrosion of second degree of male genital region**
Corrosion of second degree of penis
Corrosion of second degree of scrotum
Corrosion of second degree of testis

♀ X+7th **T21.67 Corrosion of second degree of female genital region**
Corrosion of second degree of labium (majus) (minus)
Corrosion of second degree of perineum
Corrosion of second degree of vulva
Excludes2: *corrosion of vagina (T28.8)*

X+7th **T21.69 Corrosion of second degree of other site of trunk**

\+ **T21.7 Corrosion of third degree of trunk**
Code first (T51-T65) to identify chemical and intent
Use additional external cause code to identify place (Y92)

CC X+7th **T21.70 Corrosion of third degree of trunk, unspecified site**
HAC 7th character A see Appendix B for HAC conditional logic

CC X+7th **T21.71 Corrosion of third degree of chest wall**
Corrosion of third degree of breast
HAC 7th character A see Appendix B for HAC conditional logic

CC X+7th **T21.72 Corrosion of third degree of abdominal wall**
Corrosion of third degree of flank
Corrosion of third degree of groin
HAC 7th character A see Appendix B for HAC conditional logic

CC X+7th **T21.73 Corrosion of third degree of upper back**
Corrosion of third degree of interscapular region
HAC 7th character A see Appendix B for HAC conditional logic

CC X+7th **T21.74 Corrosion of third degree of lower back**
HAC 7th character A see Appendix B for HAC conditional logic

CC X+7th **T21.75 Corrosion of third degree of buttock**
Corrosion of third degree of anus
HAC 7th character A see Appendix B for HAC conditional logic

CC X+7th **T21.76 Corrosion of third degree of male genital region**
Corrosion of third degree of penis
Corrosion of third degree of scrotum
Corrosion of third degree of testis
HAC 7th character A see Appendix B for HAC conditional logic

CC X+7th **T21.77 Corrosion of third degree of female genital region**
Corrosion of third degree of labium (majus) (minus)
Corrosion of third degree of perineum
Corrosion of third degree of vulva
Excludes2: *corrosion of vagina (T28.8)*
HAC 7th character A see Appendix B for HAC conditional logic

CC X+7th **T21.79 Corrosion of third degree of other site of trunk**
HAC 7th character A see Appendix B for HAC conditional logic

T22 Burn and corrosion of shoulder and upper limb, except wrist and hand

Excludes2: *burn and corrosion of interscapular region (T21.-)*
burn and corrosion of wrist and hand (T23.-)

The appropriate 7th character is to be added to each code from category T22
- A initial encounter
- D subsequent encounter
- S sequela

\+ **T22.0 Burn of unspecified degree of shoulder and upper limb, except wrist and hand**
Use additional external cause code to identify the source, place and intent of the burn (X00-X19, X75-X77, X96-X98, Y92)

X+7th **T22.00 Burn of unspecified degree of shoulder and upper limb, except wrist and hand, unspecified site**

\+ **T22.01 Burn of unspecified degree of forearm**
- +7th **T22.011 Burn of unspecified degree of right forearm**
- +7th **T22.012 Burn of unspecified degree of left forearm**
- +7th **T22.019 Burn of unspecified degree of unspecified forearm**

\+ **T22.02 Burn of unspecified degree of elbow**
- +7th **T22.021 Burn of unspecified degree of right elbow**
- +7th **T22.022 Burn of unspecified degree of left elbow**
- +7th **T22.029 Burn of unspecified degree of unspecified elbow**

\+ **T22.03 Burn of unspecified degree of upper arm**
- +7th **T22.031 Burn of unspecified degree of right upper arm**
- +7th **T22.032 Burn of unspecified degree of left upper arm**
- +7th **T22.039 Burn of unspecified degree of unspecified upper arm**

\+ **T22.04 Burn of unspecified degree of axilla**
- +7th **T22.041 Burn of unspecified degree of right axilla**
- +7th **T22.042 Burn of unspecified degree of left axilla**
- +7th **T22.049 Burn of unspecified degree of unspecified axilla**

\+ **T22.05 Burn of unspecified degree of shoulder**
- +7th **T22.051 Burn of unspecified degree of right shoulder**
- +7th **T22.052 Burn of unspecified degree of left shoulder**
- +7th **T22.059 Burn of unspecified degree of unspecified shoulder**

\+ **T22.06 Burn of unspecified degree of scapular region**
- +7th **T22.061 Burn of unspecified degree of right scapular region**
- +7th **T22.062 Burn of unspecified degree of left scapular region**
- +7th **T22.069 Burn of unspecified degree of unspecified scapular region**

\+ **T22.09 Burn of unspecified degree of multiple sites of shoulder and upper limb, except wrist and hand**
- +7th **T22.091 Burn of unspecified degree of multiple sites of right shoulder and upper limb, except wrist and hand**
- +7th **T22.092 Burn of unspecified degree of multiple sites of left shoulder and upper limb, except wrist and hand**
- +7th **T22.099 Burn of unspecified degree of multiple sites of unspecified shoulder and upper limb, except wrist and hand**

\+ **T22.1 Burn of first degree of shoulder and upper limb, except wrist and hand**
Use additional external cause code to identify the source, place and intent of the burn (X00-X19, X75-X77, X96-X98, Y92)

X+7th **T22.10 Burn of first degree of shoulder and upper limb, except wrist and hand, unspecified site**

\+ **T22.11 Burn of first degree of forearm**
- +7th **T22.111 Burn of first degree of right forearm**
- +7th **T22.112 Burn of first degree of left forearm**
- +7th **T22.119 Burn of first degree of unspecified forearm**

\+ **T22.12 Burn of first degree of elbow**
- +7th **T22.121 Burn of first degree of right elbow**
- +7th **T22.122 Burn of first degree of left elbow**
- +7th **T22.129 Burn of first degree of unspecified elbow**

\+ **T22.13 Burn of first degree of upper arm**
- +7th **T22.131 Burn of first degree of right upper arm**
- +7th **T22.132 Burn of first degree of left upper arm**
- +7th **T22.139 Burn of first degree of unspecified upper arm**

+ **T22.14 Burn of first degree of axilla**
  - +7th **T22.141 Burn of first degree of right axilla**
  - +7th **T22.142 Burn of first degree of left axilla**
  - +7th **T22.149 Burn of first degree of unspecified axilla**

+ **T22.15 Burn of first degree of shoulder**
  - +7th **T22.151 Burn of first degree of right shoulder**
  - +7th **T22.152 Burn of first degree of left shoulder**
  - +7th **T22.159 Burn of first degree of unspecified shoulder**

+ **T22.16 Burn of first degree of scapular region**
  - +7th **T22.161 Burn of first degree of right scapular region**
  - +7th **T22.162 Burn of first degree of left scapular region**
  - +7th **T22.169 Burn of first degree of unspecified scapular region**

+ **T22.19 Burn of first degree of multiple sites of shoulder and upper limb, except wrist and hand**
  - +7th **T22.191 Burn of first degree of multiple sites of right shoulder and upper limb, except wrist and hand**
  - +7th **T22.192 Burn of first degree of multiple sites of left shoulder and upper limb, except wrist and hand**
  - +7th **T22.199 Burn of first degree of multiple sites of unspecified shoulder and upper limb, except wrist and hand**

+ **T22.2 Burn of second degree of shoulder and upper limb, except wrist and hand**

  Use additional external cause code to identify the source, place and intent of the burn (X00-X19, X75-X77, X96-X98, Y92)

  - X+7th **T22.20 Burn of second degree of shoulder and upper limb, except wrist and hand, unspecified site**

+ **T22.21 Burn of second degree of forearm**
  - +7th **T22.211 Burn of second degree of right forearm**
  - +7th **T22.212 Burn of second degree of left forearm**
  - +7th **T22.219 Burn of second degree of unspecified forearm**

+ **T22.22 Burn of second degree of elbow**
  - +7th **T22.221 Burn of second degree of right elbow**
  - +7th **T22.222 Burn of second degree of left elbow**
  - +7th **T22.229 Burn of second degree of unspecified elbow**

+ **T22.23 Burn of second degree of upper arm**
  - +7th **T22.231 Burn of second degree of right upper arm**
  - +7th **T22.232 Burn of second degree of left upper arm**
  - +7th **T22.239 Burn of second degree of unspecified upper arm**

+ **T22.24 Burn of second degree of axilla**
  - +7th **T22.241 Burn of second degree of right axilla**
  - +7th **T22.242 Burn of second degree of left axilla**
  - +7th **T22.249 Burn of second degree of unspecified axilla**

+ **T22.25 Burn of second degree of shoulder**
  - +7th **T22.251 Burn of second degree of right shoulder**
  - +7th **T22.252 Burn of second degree of left shoulder**
  - +7th **T22.259 Burn of second degree of unspecified shoulder**

+ **T22.26 Burn of second degree of scapular region**
  - +7th **T22.261 Burn of second degree of right scapular region**
  - +7th **T22.262 Burn of second degree of left scapular region**
  - +7th **T22.269 Burn of second degree of unspecified scapular region**

+ **T22.29 Burn of second degree of multiple sites of shoulder and upper limb, except wrist and hand**
  - +7th **T22.291 Burn of second degree of multiple sites of right shoulder and upper limb, except wrist and hand**
  - +7th **T22.292 Burn of second degree of multiple sites of left shoulder and upper limb, except wrist and hand**
  - +7th **T22.299 Burn of second degree of multiple sites of unspecified shoulder and upper limb, except wrist and hand**

+ **T22.3 Burn of third degree of shoulder and upper limb, except wrist and hand**

  Use additional external cause code to identify the source, place and intent of the burn (X00-X19, X75-X77, X96-X98, Y92)

  - CC X+7th **T22.30 Burn of third degree of shoulder and upper limb, except wrist and hand, unspecified site**
    HAC 7th character A see Appendix B for HAC conditional logic

+ **T22.31 Burn of third degree of forearm**
  - CC +7th **T22.311 Burn of third degree of right forearm**
    HAC 7th character A see Appendix B for HAC conditional logic
  - CC +7th **T22.312 Burn of third degree of left forearm**
    HAC 7th character A see Appendix B for HAC conditional logic
  - CC +7th **T22.319 Burn of third degree of unspecified forearm**
    HAC 7th character A see Appendix B for HAC conditional logic

+ **T22.32 Burn of third degree of elbow**
  - CC +7th **T22.321 Burn of third degree of right elbow**
    HAC 7th character A see Appendix B for HAC conditional logic
  - CC +7th **T22.322 Burn of third degree of left elbow**
    HAC 7th character A see Appendix B for HAC conditional logic
  - CC +7th **T22.329 Burn of third degree of unspecified elbow**
    HAC 7th character A see Appendix B for HAC conditional logic

+ **T22.33 Burn of third degree of upper arm**
  - CC +7th **T22.331 Burn of third degree of right upper arm**
    HAC 7th character A see Appendix B for HAC conditional logic
  - CC +7th **T22.332 Burn of third degree of left upper arm**
    HAC 7th character A see Appendix B for HAC conditional logic
  - CC +7th **T22.339 Burn of third degree of unspecified upper arm**
    HAC 7th character A see Appendix B for HAC conditional logic

+ **T22.34 Burn of third degree of axilla**
  - CC +7th **T22.341 Burn of third degree of right axilla**
    HAC 7th character A see Appendix B for HAC conditional logic
  - CC +7th **T22.342 Burn of third degree of left axilla**
    HAC 7th character A see Appendix B for HAC conditional logic
  - CC +7th **T22.349 Burn of third degree of unspecified axilla**
    HAC 7th character A see Appendix B for HAC conditional logic

+ **T22.35 Burn of third degree of shoulder**
  - CC +7th **T22.351 Burn of third degree of right shoulder**
    HAC 7th character A see Appendix B for HAC conditional logic
  - CC +7th **T22.352 Burn of third degree of left shoulder**
    HAC 7th character A see Appendix B for HAC conditional logic
  - CC +7th **T22.359 Burn of third degree of unspecified shoulder**
    HAC 7th character A see Appendix B for HAC conditional logic

+ **T22.36 Burn of third degree of scapular region**
  - CC +7th **T22.361 Burn of third degree of right scapular region**
    HAC 7th character A see Appendix B for HAC conditional logic
  - CC +7th **T22.362 Burn of third degree of left scapular region**
    HAC 7th character A see Appendix B for HAC conditional logic
  - CC +7th **T22.369 Burn of third degree of unspecified scapular region**
    HAC 7th character A see Appendix B for HAC conditional logic

+ **T22.39 Burn of third degree of multiple sites of shoulder and upper limb, except wrist and hand**
  - CC +7th **T22.391 Burn of third degree of multiple sites of right shoulder and upper limb, except wrist and hand**
    HAC 7th character A see Appendix B for HAC conditional logic
  - CC +7th **T22.392 Burn of third degree of multiple sites of left shoulder and upper limb, except wrist and hand**
    HAC 7th character A see Appendix B for HAC conditional logic
  - CC +7th **T22.399 Burn of third degree of multiple sites of unspecified shoulder and upper limb, except wrist and hand**
    HAC 7th character A see Appendix B for HAC conditional logic

+ **T22.4 Corrosion of unspecified degree of shoulder and upper limb, except wrist and hand**
  Code first (T51-T65) to identify chemical and intent
  Use additional external cause code to identify place (Y92)
  - X+7th **T22.40 Corrosion of unspecified degree of shoulder and upper limb, except wrist and hand, unspecified site**
  - + **T22.41 Corrosion of unspecified degree of forearm**
    - +7th **T22.411 Corrosion of unspecified degree of right forearm**
    - +7th **T22.412 Corrosion of unspecified degree of left forearm**
    - +7th **T22.419 Corrosion of unspecified degree of unspecified forearm**
  - + **T22.42 Corrosion of unspecified degree of elbow**
    - +7th **T22.421 Corrosion of unspecified degree of right elbow**
    - +7th **T22.422 Corrosion of unspecified degree of left elbow**
    - +7th **T22.429 Corrosion of unspecified degree of unspecified elbow**
  - + **T22.43 Corrosion of unspecified degree of upper arm**
    - +7th **T22.431 Corrosion of unspecified degree of right upper arm**
    - +7th **T22.432 Corrosion of unspecified degree of left upper arm**
    - +7th **T22.439 Corrosion of unspecified degree of unspecified upper arm**
  - + **T22.44 Corrosion of unspecified degree of axilla**
    - +7th **T22.441 Corrosion of unspecified degree of right axilla**
    - +7th **T22.442 Corrosion of unspecified degree of left axilla**
    - +7th **T22.449 Corrosion of unspecified degree of unspecified axilla**
  - + **T22.45 Corrosion of unspecified degree of shoulder**
    - +7th **T22.451 Corrosion of unspecified degree of right shoulder**
    - +7th **T22.452 Corrosion of unspecified degree of left shoulder**
    - +7th **T22.459 Corrosion of unspecified degree of unspecified shoulder**
  - + **T22.46 Corrosion of unspecified degree of scapular region**
    - +7th **T22.461 Corrosion of unspecified degree of right scapular region**
    - +7th **T22.462 Corrosion of unspecified degree of left scapular region**
    - +7th **T22.469 Corrosion of unspecified degree of unspecified scapular region**
  - + **T22.49 Corrosion of unspecified degree of multiple sites of shoulder and upper limb, except wrist and hand**
    - +7th **T22.491 Corrosion of unspecified degree of multiple sites of right shoulder and upper limb, except wrist and hand**
    - +7th **T22.492 Corrosion of unspecified degree of multiple sites of left shoulder and upper limb, except wrist and hand**
    - +7th **T22.499 Corrosion of unspecified degree of multiple sites of unspecified shoulder and upper limb, except wrist and hand**

+ **T22.5 Corrosion of first degree of shoulder and upper limb, except wrist and hand**
  Code first (T51-T65) to identify chemical and intent
  Use additional external cause code to identify place (Y92)
  - X+7th **T22.50 Corrosion of first degree of shoulder and upper limb, except wrist and hand unspecified site**
  - + **T22.51 Corrosion of first degree of forearm**
    - +7th **T22.511 Corrosion of first degree of right forearm**
    - +7th **T22.512 Corrosion of first degree of left forearm**
    - +7th **T22.519 Corrosion of first degree of unspecified forearm**
  - + **T22.52 Corrosion of first degree of elbow**
    - +7th **T22.521 Corrosion of first degree of right elbow**
    - +7th **T22.522 Corrosion of first degree of left elbow**
    - +7th **T22.529 Corrosion of first degree of unspecified elbow**
  - + **T22.53 Corrosion of first degree of upper arm**
    - +7th **T22.531 Corrosion of first degree of right upper arm**
    - +7th **T22.532 Corrosion of first degree of left upper arm**
    - +7th **T22.539 Corrosion of first degree of unspecified upper arm**
  - + **T22.54 Corrosion of first degree of axilla**
    - +7th **T22.541 Corrosion of first degree of right axilla**
    - +7th **T22.542 Corrosion of first degree of left axilla**
    - +7th **T22.549 Corrosion of first degree of unspecified axilla**
  - + **T22.55 Corrosion of first degree of shoulder**
    - +7th **T22.551 Corrosion of first degree of right shoulder**
    - +7th **T22.552 Corrosion of first degree of left shoulder**
    - +7th **T22.559 Corrosion of first degree of unspecified shoulder**
  - + **T22.56 Corrosion of first degree of scapular region**
    - +7th **T22.561 Corrosion of first degree of right scapular region**
    - +7th **T22.562 Corrosion of first degree of left scapular region**
    - +7th **T22.569 Corrosion of first degree of unspecified scapular region**
  - + **T22.59 Corrosion of first degree of multiple sites of shoulder and upper limb, except wrist and hand**
    - +7th **T22.591 Corrosion of first degree of multiple sites of right shoulder and upper limb, except wrist and hand**
    - +7th **T22.592 Corrosion of first degree of multiple sites of left shoulder and upper limb, except wrist and hand**
    - +7th **T22.599 Corrosion of first degree of multiple sites of unspecified shoulder and upper limb, except wrist and hand**

+ **T22.6 Corrosion of second degree of shoulder and upper limb, except wrist and hand**
  Code first (T51-T65) to identify chemical and intent
  Use additional external cause code to identify place (Y92)
  - X+7th **T22.60 Corrosion of second degree of shoulder and upper limb, except wrist and hand, unspecified site**
  - + **T22.61 Corrosion of second degree of forearm**
    - +7th **T22.611 Corrosion of second degree of right forearm**
    - +7th **T22.612 Corrosion of second degree of left forearm**
    - +7th **T22.619 Corrosion of second degree of unspecified forearm**
  - + **T22.62 Corrosion of second degree of elbow**
    - +7th **T22.621 Corrosion of second degree of right elbow**
    - +7th **T22.622 Corrosion of second degree of left elbow**
    - +7th **T22.629 Corrosion of second degree of unspecified elbow**
  - + **T22.63 Corrosion of second degree of upper arm**
    - +7th **T22.631 Corrosion of second degree of right upper arm**
    - +7th **T22.632 Corrosion of second degree of left upper arm**
    - +7th **T22.639 Corrosion of second degree of unspecified upper arm**

+ **T22.64 Corrosion of second degree of axilla**
  - +7th **T22.641 Corrosion of second degree of right axilla**
  - +7th **T22.642 Corrosion of second degree of left axilla**
  - +7th **T22.649 Corrosion of second degree of unspecified axilla**

+ **T22.65 Corrosion of second degree of shoulder**
  - +7th **T22.651 Corrosion of second degree of right shoulder**
  - +7th **T22.652 Corrosion of second degree of left shoulder**
  - +7th **T22.659 Corrosion of second degree of unspecified shoulder**

+ **T22.66 Corrosion of second degree of scapular region**
  - +7th **T22.661 Corrosion of second degree of right scapular region**
  - +7th **T22.662 Corrosion of second degree of left scapular region**
  - +7th **T22.669 Corrosion of second degree of unspecified scapular region**

+ **T22.69 Corrosion of second degree of multiple sites of shoulder and upper limb, except wrist and hand**
  - +7th **T22.691 Corrosion of second degree of multiple sites of right shoulder and upper limb, except wrist and hand**
  - +7th **T22.692 Corrosion of second degree of multiple sites of left shoulder and upper limb, except wrist and hand**
  - +7th **T22.699 Corrosion of second degree of multiple sites of unspecified shoulder and upper limb, except wrist and hand**

+ **T22.7 Corrosion of third degree of shoulder and upper limb, except wrist and hand**

  Code first (T51-T65) to identify chemical and intent external cause code to identify place (Y92)

  - CC X+7th **T22.70 Corrosion of third degree of shoulder and upper limb, except wrist and hand, unspecified site**
    HAC 7th character A see Appendix B for HAC conditional logic

+ **T22.71 Corrosion of third degree of forearm**
  - CC +7th **T22.711 Corrosion of third degree of right forearm**
    HAC 7th character A see Appendix B for HAC conditional logic
  - CC +7th **T22.712 Corrosion of third degree of left forearm**
    HAC 7th character A see Appendix B for HAC conditional logic
  - CC +7th **T22.719 Corrosion of third degree of unspecified forearm**
    HAC 7th character A see Appendix B for HAC conditional logic

+ **T22.72 Corrosion of third degree of elbow**
  - CC +7th **T22.721 Corrosion of third degree of right elbow**
    HAC 7th character A see Appendix B for HAC conditional logic
  - CC +7th **T22.722 Corrosion of third degree of left elbow**
    HAC 7th character A see Appendix B for HAC conditional logic
  - CC +7th **T22.729 Corrosion of third degree of unspecified elbow**
    HAC 7th character A see Appendix B for HAC conditional logic

+ **T22.73 Corrosion of third degree of upper arm**
  - CC +7th **T22.731 Corrosion of third degree of right upper arm**
    HAC 7th character A see Appendix B for HAC conditional logic
  - CC +7th **T22.732 Corrosion of third degree of left upper arm**
    HAC 7th character A see Appendix B for HAC conditional logic
  - CC +7th **T22.739 Corrosion of third degree of unspecified upper arm**
    HAC 7th character A see Appendix B for HAC conditional logic

+ **T22.74 Corrosion of third degree of axilla**
  - CC +7th **T22.741 Corrosion of third degree of right axilla**
    HAC 7th character A see Appendix B for HAC conditional logic
  - CC +7th **T22.742 Corrosion of third degree of left axilla**
    HAC 7th character A see Appendix B for HAC conditional logic
  - CC +7th **T22.749 Corrosion of third degree of unspecified axilla**
    HAC 7th character A see Appendix B for HAC conditional logic

+ **T22.75 Corrosion of third degree of shoulder**
  - CC +7th **T22.751 Corrosion of third degree of right shoulder**
    HAC 7th character A see Appendix B for HAC conditional logic
  - CC +7th **T22.752 Corrosion of third degree of left shoulder**
    HAC 7th character A see Appendix B for HAC conditional logic
  - CC +7th **T22.759 Corrosion of third degree of unspecified shoulder**
    HAC 7th character A see Appendix B for HAC conditional logic

+ **T22.76 Corrosion of third degree of scapular region**
  - CC +7th **T22.761 Corrosion of third degree of right scapular region**
    HAC 7th character A see Appendix B for HAC conditional logic
  - CC +7th **T22.762 Corrosion of third degree of left scapular region**
    HAC 7th character A see Appendix B for HAC conditional logic
  - CC +7th **T22.769 Corrosion of third degree of unspecified scapular region**
    HAC 7th character A see Appendix B for HAC conditional logic

+ **T22.79 Corrosion of third degree of multiple sites of shoulder and upper limb, except wrist and hand**
  - CC +7th **T22.791 Corrosion of third degree of multiple sites of right shoulder and upper limb, except wrist and hand**
    HAC 7th character A see Appendix B for HAC conditional logic
  - CC +7th **T22.792 Corrosion of third degree of multiple sites of left shoulder and upper limb, except wrist and hand**
    HAC 7th character A see Appendix B for HAC conditional logic
  - CC +7th **T22.799 Corrosion of third degree of multiple sites of unspecified shoulder and upper limb, except wrist and hand**
    HAC 7th character A see Appendix B for HAC conditional logic

T23 Burn and corrosion of wrist and hand

The appropriate 7th character is to be added to each code from category T23
A initial encounter
D subsequent encounter
S sequela

+ **T23.0 Burn of unspecified degree of wrist and hand**

  Use additional external cause code to identify the source, place and intent of the burn (X00-X19, X75-X77, X96-X98, Y92)

  + **T23.00 Burn of unspecified degree of hand, unspecified site**
    - +7th **T23.001 Burn of unspecified degree of right hand, unspecified site**
    - +7th **T23.002 Burn of unspecified degree of left hand, unspecified site**
    - +7th **T23.009 Burn of unspecified degree of unspecified hand, unspecified site**

+ **T23.01 Burn of unspecified degree of thumb (nail)**
  - +7th **T23.011 Burn of unspecified degree of right thumb (nail)**
  - +7th **T23.012 Burn of unspecified degree of left thumb (nail)**
  - +7th **T23.019 Burn of unspecified degree of unspecified thumb (nail)**
+ **T23.02 Burn of unspecified degree of single finger (nail) except thumb**
  - +7th **T23.021 Burn of unspecified degree of single right finger (nail) except thumb**
  - +7th **T23.022 Burn of unspecified degree of single left finger (nail) except thumb**
  - +7th **T23.029 Burn of unspecified degree of unspecified single finger (nail) except thumb**
+ **T23.03 Burn of unspecified degree of multiple fingers (nail), not including thumb**
  - +7th **T23.031 Burn of unspecified degree of multiple right fingers (nail), not including thumb**
  - +7th **T23.032 Burn of unspecified degree of multiple left fingers (nail), not including thumb**
  - +7th **T23.039 Burn of unspecified degree of unspecified multiple fingers (nail), not including thumb**
+ **T23.04 Burn of unspecified degree of multiple fingers (nail), including thumb**
  - +7th **T23.041 Burn of unspecified degree of multiple right fingers (nail), including thumb**
  - +7th **T23.042 Burn of unspecified degree of multiple left fingers (nail), including thumb**
  - +7th **T23.049 Burn of unspecified degree of unspecified multiple fingers (nail), including thumb**
+ **T23.05 Burn of unspecified degree of palm**
  - +7th **T23.051 Burn of unspecified degree of right palm**
  - +7th **T23.052 Burn of unspecified degree of left palm**
  - +7th **T23.059 Burn of unspecified degree of unspecified palm**
+ **T23.06 Burn of unspecified degree of back of hand**
  - +7th **T23.061 Burn of unspecified degree of back of right hand**
  - +7th **T23.062 Burn of unspecified degree of back of left hand**
  - +7th **T23.069 Burn of unspecified degree of back of unspecified hand**
+ **T23.07 Burn of unspecified degree of wrist**
  - +7th **T23.071 Burn of unspecified degree of right wrist**
  - +7th **T23.072 Burn of unspecified degree of left wrist**
  - +7th **T23.079 Burn of unspecified degree of unspecified wrist**
+ **T23.09 Burn of unspecified degree of multiple sites of wrist and hand**
  - +7th **T23.091 Burn of unspecified degree of multiple sites of right wrist and hand**
  - +7th **T23.092 Burn of unspecified degree of multiple sites of left wrist and hand**
  - +7th **T23.099 Burn of unspecified degree of multiple sites of unspecified wrist and hand**

+ **T23.1 Burn of first degree of wrist and hand**

  Use additional external cause code to identify the source, place and intent of the burn (X00-X19, X75-X77, X96-X98, Y92)

+ **T23.10 Burn of first degree of hand, unspecified site**
  - +7th **T23.101 Burn of first degree of right hand, unspecified site**
  - +7th **T23.102 Burn of first degree of left hand, unspecified site**
  - +7th **T23.109 Burn of first degree of unspecified hand, unspecified site**
+ **T23.11 Burn of first degree of thumb (nail)**
  - +7th **T23.111 Burn of first degree of right thumb (nail)**
  - +7th **T23.112 Burn of first degree of left thumb (nail)**
  - +7th **T23.119 Burn of first degree of unspecified thumb (nail)**
+ **T23.12 Burn of first degree of single finger (nail) except thumb**
  - +7th **T23.121 Burn of first degree of single right finger (nail) except thumb**
  - +7th **T23.122 Burn of first degree of single left finger (nail) except thumb**
  - +7th **T23.129 Burn of first degree of unspecified single finger (nail) except thumb**
+ **T23.13 Burn of first degree of multiple fingers (nail), not including thumb**
  - +7th **T23.131 Burn of first degree of multiple right fingers (nail), not including thumb**
  - +7th **T23.132 Burn of first degree of multiple left fingers (nail), not including thumb**
  - +7th **T23.139 Burn of first degree of unspecified multiple fingers (nail), not including thumb**
+ **T23.14 Burn of first degree of multiple fingers (nail), including thumb**
  - +7th **T23.141 Burn of first degree of multiple right fingers (nail), including thumb**
  - +7th **T23.142 Burn of first degree of multiple left fingers (nail), including thumb**
  - +7th **T23.149 Burn of first degree of unspecified multiple fingers (nail), including thumb**
+ **T23.15 Burn of first degree of palm**
  - +7th **T23.151 Burn of first degree of right palm**
  - +7th **T23.152 Burn of first degree of left palm**
  - +7th **T23.159 Burn of first degree of unspecified palm**
+ **T23.16 Burn of first degree of back of hand**
  - +7th **T23.161 Burn of first degree of back of right hand**
  - +7th **T23.162 Burn of first degree of back of left hand**
  - +7th **T23.169 Burn of first degree of back of unspecified hand**
+ **T23.17 Burn of first degree of wrist**
  - +7th **T23.171 Burn of first degree of right wrist**
  - +7th **T23.172 Burn of first degree of left wrist**
  - +7th **T23.179 Burn of first degree of unspecified wrist**
+ **T23.19 Burn of first degree of multiple sites of wrist and hand**
  - +7th **T23.191 Burn of first degree of multiple sites of right wrist and hand**
  - +7th **T23.192 Burn of first degree of multiple sites of left wrist and hand**
  - +7th **T23.199 Burn of first degree of multiple sites of unspecified wrist and hand**

+ **T23.2 Burn of second degree of wrist and hand**

  Use additional external cause code to identify the source, place and intent of the burn (X00-X19, X75-X77, X96-X98, Y92)

+ **T23.20 Burn of second degree of hand, unspecified site**
  - +7th **T23.201 Burn of second degree of right hand, unspecified site**
  - +7th **T23.202 Burn of second degree of left hand, unspecified site**
  - +7th **T23.209 Burn of second degree of unspecified hand, unspecified site**
+ **T23.21 Burn of second degree of thumb (nail)**
  - +7th **T23.211 Burn of second degree of right thumb (nail)**
  - +7th **T23.212 Burn of second degree of left thumb (nail)**
  - +7th **T23.219 Burn of second degree of unspecified thumb (nail)**
+ **T23.22 Burn of second degree of single finger (nail) except thumb**
  - +7th **T23.221 Burn of second degree of single right finger (nail) except thumb**
  - +7th **T23.222 Burn of second degree of single left finger (nail) except thumb**
  - +7th **T23.229 Burn of second degree of unspecified single finger (nail) except thumb**
+ **T23.23 Burn of second degree of multiple fingers (nail), not including thumb**
  - +7th **T23.231 Burn of second degree of multiple right fingers (nail), not including thumb**
  - +7th **T23.232 Burn of second degree of multiple left fingers (nail), not including thumb**
  - +7th **T23.239 Burn of second degree of unspecified multiple fingers (nail), not including thumb**

+ **T23.24 Burn of second degree of multiple fingers (nail), including thumb**
  - +7th **T23.241 Burn of second degree of multiple right fingers (nail), including thumb**
  - +7th **T23.242 Burn of second degree of multiple left fingers (nail), including thumb**
  - +7th **T23.249 Burn of second degree of unspecified multiple fingers (nail), including thumb**

+ **T23.25 Burn of second degree of palm**
  - +7th **T23.251 Burn of second degree of right palm**
  - +7th **T23.252 Burn of second degree of left palm**
  - +7th **T23.259 Burn of second degree of unspecified palm**

+ **T23.26 Burn of second degree of back of hand**
  - +7th **T23.261 Burn of second degree of back of right hand**
  - +7th **T23.262 Burn of second degree of back of left hand**
  - +7th **T23.269 Burn of second degree of back of unspecified hand**

+ **T23.27 Burn of second degree of wrist**
  - +7th **T23.271 Burn of second degree of right wrist**
  - +7th **T23.272 Burn of second degree of left wrist**
  - +7th **T23.279 Burn of second degree of unspecified wrist**

+ **T23.29 Burn of second degree of multiple sites of wrist and hand**
  - +7th **T23.291 Burn of second degree of multiple sites of right wrist and hand**
  - +7th **T23.292 Burn of second degree of multiple sites of left wrist and hand**
  - +7th **T23.299 Burn of second degree of multiple sites of unspecified wrist and hand**

+ **T23.3 Burn of third degree of wrist and hand**

  Use additional external cause code to identify the source, place and intent of the burn (X00-X19, X75-X77, X96-X98, Y92)

+ **T23.30 Burn of third degree of hand, unspecified site**
  - CC +7th **T23.301 Burn of third degree of right hand, unspecified site**
    AHA CC: 1Q, 2015, 3-21
    HAC 7th character A see Appendix B for HAC conditional logic
  - CC +7th **T23.302 Burn of third degree of left hand, unspecified site**
    AHA CC: 2Q, 2016, 5
    HAC 7th character A see Appendix B for HAC conditional logic
  - CC +7th **T23.309 Burn of third degree of unspecified hand, unspecified site**
    HAC 7th character A see Appendix B for HAC conditional logic

+ **T23.31 Burn of third degree of thumb (nail)**
  - CC +7th **T23.311 Burn of third degree of right thumb (nail)**
    HAC 7th character A see Appendix B for HAC conditional logic
  - CC +7th **T23.312 Burn of third degree of left thumb (nail)**
    HAC 7th character A see Appendix B for HAC conditional logic
  - CC +7th **T23.319 Burn of third degree of unspecified thumb (nail)**
    HAC 7th character A see Appendix B for HAC conditional logic

+ **T23.32 Burn of third degree of single finger (nail) except thumb**
  - CC +7th **T23.321 Burn of third degree of single right finger (nail) except thumb**
    HAC 7th character A see Appendix B for HAC conditional logic
  - CC +7th **T23.322 Burn of third degree of single left finger (nail) except thumb**
    HAC 7th character A see Appendix B for HAC conditional logic
  - CC +7th **T23.329 Burn of third degree of unspecified single finger (nail) except thumb**
    HAC 7th character A see Appendix B for HAC conditional logic

+ **T23.33 Burn of third degree of multiple fingers (nail), not including thumb**
  - CC +7th **T23.331 Burn of third degree of multiple right fingers (nail), not including thumb**
    HAC 7th character A see Appendix B for HAC conditional logic
  - CC +7th **T23.332 Burn of third degree of multiple left fingers (nail), not including thumb**
    HAC 7th character A see Appendix B for HAC conditional logic
  - CC +7th **T23.339 Burn of third degree of unspecified multiple fingers (nail), not including thumb**

+ **T23.34 Burn of third degree of multiple fingers (nail), including thumb**
  - CC +7th **T23.341 Burn of third degree of multiple right fingers (nail), including thumb**
    HAC 7th character A see Appendix B for HAC conditional logic
  - CC +7th **T23.342 Burn of third degree of multiple left fingers (nail), including thumb**
    HAC 7th character A see Appendix B for HAC conditional logic
  - CC +7th **T23.349 Burn of third degree of unspecified multiple fingers (nail), including thumb**
    HAC 7th character A see Appendix B for HAC conditional logic

+ **T23.35 Burn of third degree of palm**
  - CC +7th **T23.351 Burn of third degree of right palm**
    HAC 7th character A see Appendix B for HAC conditional logic
  - CC +7th **T23.352 Burn of third degree of left palm**
    HAC 7th character A see Appendix B for HAC conditional logic
  - CC +7th **T23.359 Burn of third degree of unspecified palm**
    HAC 7th character A see Appendix B for HAC conditional logic

+ **T23.36 Burn of third degree of back of hand**
  - CC +7th **T23.361 Burn of third degree of back of right hand**
    HAC 7th character A see Appendix B for HAC conditional logic
  - CC +7th **T23.362 Burn of third degree of back of left hand**
    HAC 7th character A see Appendix B for HAC conditional logic
  - CC +7th **T23.369 Burn of third degree of back of unspecified hand**
    HAC 7th character A see Appendix B for HAC conditional logic

+ **T23.37 Burn of third degree of wrist**
  - CC +7th **T23.371 Burn of third degree of right wrist**
    HAC 7th character A see Appendix B for HAC conditional logic
  - CC +7th **T23.372 Burn of third degree of left wrist**
    HAC 7th character A see Appendix B for HAC conditional logic
  - CC +7th **T23.379 Burn of third degree of unspecified wrist**
    HAC 7th character A see Appendix B for HAC conditional logic

+ **T23.39 Burn of third degree of multiple sites of wrist and hand**
  - CC +7th **T23.391 Burn of third degree of multiple sites of right wrist and hand**
    HAC 7th character A see Appendix B for HAC conditional logic
  - CC +7th **T23.392 Burn of third degree of multiple sites of left wrist and hand**
    HAC 7th character A see Appendix B for HAC conditional logic
  - CC +7th **T23.399 Burn of third degree of multiple sites of unspecified wrist and hand**
    HAC 7th character A see Appendix B for HAC conditional logic

+ **T23.4 Corrosion of unspecified degree of wrist and hand**
  Code first (T51-T65) to identify chemical and intent
  Use additional external cause code to identify place (Y92)
  + **T23.40 Corrosion of unspecified degree of hand, unspecified site**
    - +7th **T23.401 Corrosion of unspecified degree of right hand, unspecified site**
    - +7th **T23.402 Corrosion of unspecified degree of left hand, unspecified site**
    - +7th **T23.409 Corrosion of unspecified degree of unspecified hand, unspecified site**
  + **T23.41 Corrosion of unspecified degree of thumb (nail)**
    - +7th **T23.411 Corrosion of unspecified degree of right thumb (nail)**
    - +7th **T23.412 Corrosion of unspecified degree of left thumb (nail)**
    - +7th **T23.419 Corrosion of unspecified degree of unspecified thumb (nail)**
  + **T23.42 Corrosion of unspecified degree of single finger (nail) except thumb**
    - +7th **T23.421 Corrosion of unspecified degree of single right finger (nail) except thumb**
    - +7th **T23.422 Corrosion of unspecified degree of single left finger (nail) except thumb**
    - +7th **T23.429 Corrosion of unspecified degree of unspecified single finger (nail) except thumb**
  + **T23.43 Corrosion of unspecified degree of multiple fingers (nail), not including thumb**
    - +7th **T23.431 Corrosion of unspecified degree of multiple right fingers (nail), not including thumb**
    - +7th **T23.432 Corrosion of unspecified degree of multiple left fingers (nail), not including thumb**
    - +7th **T23.439 Corrosion of unspecified degree of unspecified multiple fingers (nail), not including thumb**
  + **T23.44 Corrosion of unspecified degree of multiple fingers (nail), including thumb**
    - +7th **T23.441 Corrosion of unspecified degree of multiple right fingers (nail), including thumb**
    - +7th **T23.442 Corrosion of unspecified degree of multiple left fingers (nail), including thumb**
    - +7th **T23.449 Corrosion of unspecified degree of unspecified multiple fingers (nail), including thumb**
  + **T23.45 Corrosion of unspecified degree of palm**
    - +7th **T23.451 Corrosion of unspecified degree of right palm**
    - +7th **T23.452 Corrosion of unspecified degree of left palm**
    - +7th **T23.459 Corrosion of unspecified degree of unspecified palm**
  + **T23.46 Corrosion of unspecified degree of back of hand**
    - +7th **T23.461 Corrosion of unspecified degree of back of right hand**
    - +7th **T23.462 Corrosion of unspecified degree of back of left hand**
    - +7th **T23.469 Corrosion of unspecified degree of back of unspecified hand**
  + **T23.47 Corrosion of unspecified degree of wrist**
    - +7th **T23.471 Corrosion of unspecified degree of right wrist**
    - +7th **T23.472 Corrosion of unspecified degree of left wrist**
    - +7th **T23.479 Corrosion of unspecified degree of unspecified wrist**
  + **T23.49 Corrosion of unspecified degree of multiple sites of wrist and hand**
    - +7th **T23.491 Corrosion of unspecified degree of multiple sites of right wrist and hand**
    - +7th **T23.492 Corrosion of unspecified degree of multiple sites of left wrist and hand**
    - +7th **T23.499 Corrosion of unspecified degree of multiple sites of unspecified wrist and hand**

+ **T23.5 Corrosion of first degree of wrist and hand**
  Code first (T51-T65) to identify chemical and intent
  Use additional external cause code to identify place (Y92)
  + **T23.50 Corrosion of first degree of hand, unspecified site**
    - +7th **T23.501 Corrosion of first degree of right hand, unspecified site**
    - +7th **T23.502 Corrosion of first degree of left hand, unspecified site**
    - +7th **T23.509 Corrosion of first degree of unspecified hand, unspecified site**
  + **T23.51 Corrosion of first degree of thumb (nail)**
    - +7th **T23.511 Corrosion of first degree of right thumb (nail)**
    - +7th **T23.512 Corrosion of first degree of left thumb (nail)**
    - +7th **T23.519 Corrosion of first degree of unspecified thumb (nail)**
  + **T23.52 Corrosion of first degree of single finger (nail) except thumb**
    - +7th **T23.521 Corrosion of first degree of single right finger (nail) except thumb**
    - +7th **T23.522 Corrosion of first degree of single left finger (nail) except thumb**
    - +7th **T23.529 Corrosion of first degree of unspecified single finger (nail) except thumb**
  + **T23.53 Corrosion of first degree of multiple fingers (nail), not including thumb**
    - +7th **T23.531 Corrosion of first degree of multiple right fingers (nail), not including thumb**
    - +7th **T23.532 Corrosion of first degree of multiple left fingers (nail), not including thumb**
    - +7th **T23.539 Corrosion of first degree of unspecified multiple fingers (nail), not including thumb**
  + **T23.54 Corrosion of first degree of multiple fingers (nail), including thumb**
    - +7th **T23.541 Corrosion of first degree of multiple right fingers (nail), including thumb**
    - +7th **T23.542 Corrosion of first degree of multiple left fingers (nail), including thumb**
    - +7th **T23.549 Corrosion of first degree of unspecified multiple fingers (nail), including thumb**
  + **T23.55 Corrosion of first degree of palm**
    - +7th **T23.551 Corrosion of first degree of right palm**
    - +7th **T23.552 Corrosion of first degree of left palm**
    - +7th **T23.559 Corrosion of first degree of unspecified palm**
  + **T23.56 Corrosion of first degree of back of hand**
    - +7th **T23.561 Corrosion of first degree of back of right hand**
    - +7th **T23.562 Corrosion of first degree of back of left hand**
    - +7th **T23.569 Corrosion of first degree of back of unspecified hand**
  + **T23.57 Corrosion of first degree of wrist**
    - +7th **T23.571 Corrosion of first degree of right wrist**
    - +7th **T23.572 Corrosion of first degree of left wrist**
    - +7th **T23.579 Corrosion of first degree of unspecified wrist**
  + **T23.59 Corrosion of first degree of multiple sites of wrist and hand**
    - +7th **T23.591 Corrosion of first degree of multiple sites of right wrist and hand**
    - +7th **T23.592 Corrosion of first degree of multiple sites of left wrist and hand**
    - +7th **T23.599 Corrosion of first degree of multiple sites of unspecified wrist and hand**

+ **T23.6 Corrosion of second degree of wrist and hand**
Code first (T51-T65) to identify chemical and intent
Use additionalexternal cause code to identify place (Y92)

+ **T23.60 Corrosion of second degree of hand, unspecified site**
+7th **T23.601 Corrosion of second degree of right hand, unspecified site**
+7th **T23.602 Corrosion of second degree of left hand, unspecified site**
+7th **T23.609 Corrosion of second degree of unspecified hand, unspecified site**

+ **T23.61 Corrosion of second degree of thumb (nail)**
+7th **T23.611 Corrosion of second degree of right thumb (nail)**
+7th **T23.612 Corrosion of second degree of left thumb (nail)**
+7th **T23.619 Corrosion of second degree of unspecified thumb (nail)**

+ **T23.62 Corrosion of second degree of single finger (nail) except thumb**
+7th **T23.621 Corrosion of second degree of single right finger (nail) except thumb**
+7th **T23.622 Corrosion of second degree of single left finger (nail) except thumb**
+7th **T23.629 Corrosion of second degree of unspecified single finger (nail) except thumb**

+ **T23.63 Corrosion of second degree of multiple fingers (nail), not including thumb**
+7th **T23.631 Corrosion of second degree of multiple right fingers (nail), not including thumb**
+7th **T23.632 Corrosion of second degree of multiple left fingers (nail), not including thumb**
+7th **T23.639 Corrosion of second degree of unspecified multiple fingers (nail), not including thumb**

+ **T23.64 Corrosion of second degree of multiple fingers (nail), including thumb**
+7th **T23.641 Corrosion of second degree of multiple right fingers (nail), including thumb**
+7th **T23.642 Corrosion of second degree of multiple left fingers (nail), including thumb**
+7th **T23.649 Corrosion of second degree of unspecified multiple fingers (nail), including thumb**

+ **T23.65 Corrosion of second degree of palm**
+7th **T23.651 Corrosion of second degree of right palm**
+7th **T23.652 Corrosion of second degree of left palm**
+7th **T23.659 Corrosion of second degree of unspecified palm**

+ **T23.66 Corrosion of second degree of back of hand**
+7th **T23.661 Corrosion of second degree back of right hand**
+7th **T23.662 Corrosion of second degree back of left hand**
+7th **T23.669 Corrosion of second degree back of unspecified hand**

+ **T23.67 Corrosion of second degree of wrist**
+7th **T23.671 Corrosion of second degree of right wrist**
+7th **T23.672 Corrosion of second degree of left wrist**
+7th **T23.679 Corrosion of second degree of unspecified wrist**

+ **T23.69 Corrosion of second degree of multiple sites of wrist and hand**
+7th **T23.691 Corrosion of second degree of multiple sites of right wrist and hand**
+7th **T23.692 Corrosion of second degree of multiple sites of left wrist and hand**
+7th **T23.699 Corrosion of second degree of multiple sites of unspecified wrist and hand**

+ **T23.7 Corrosion of third degree of wrist and hand**
Code first (T51-T65) to identify chemical and intent
Use additional external cause code to identify place (Y92)

+ **T23.70 Corrosion of third degree of hand, unspecified site**
CC +7th **T23.701 Corrosion of third degree of right hand, unspecified site**
HAC 7th character A see Appendix B for HAC conditional logic
CC +7th **T23.702 Corrosion of third degree of left hand, unspecified site**
HAC 7th character A see Appendix B for HAC conditional logic
CC +7th **T23.709 Corrosion of third degree of unspecified hand, unspecified site**
HAC 7th character A see Appendix B for HAC conditional logic

+ **T23.71 Corrosion of third degree of thumb (nail)**
CC +7th **T23.711 Corrosion of third degree of right thumb (nail)**
HAC 7th character A see Appendix B for HAC conditional logic
CC +7th **T23.712 Corrosion of third degree of left thumb (nail)**
HAC 7th character A see Appendix B for HAC conditional logic
CC +7th **T23.719 Corrosion of third degree of unspecified thumb (nail)**
HAC 7th character A see Appendix B for HAC conditional logic

+ **T23.72 Corrosion of third degree of single finger (nail) except thumb**
CC +7th **T23.721 Corrosion of third degree of single right finger (nail) except thumb**
HAC 7th character A see Appendix B for HAC conditional logic
CC +7th **T23.722 Corrosion of third degree of single left finger (nail) except thumb**
HAC 7th character A see Appendix B for HAC conditional logic
CC +7th **T23.729 Corrosion of third degree of unspecified single finger (nail) except thumb**
HAC 7th character A see Appendix B for HAC conditional logic

+ **T23.73 Corrosion of third degree of multiple fingers (nail), not including thumb**
CC +7th **T23.731 Corrosion of third degree of multiple right fingers (nail), not including thumb**
HAC 7th character A see Appendix B for HAC conditional logic
CC +7th **T23.732 Corrosion of third degree of multiple left fingers (nail), not including thumb**
HAC 7th character A see Appendix B for HAC conditional logic
CC +7th **T23.739 Corrosion of third degree of unspecified multiple fingers (nail), not including thumb**
HAC 7th character A see Appendix B for HAC conditional logic

+ **T23.74 Corrosion of third degree of multiple fingers (nail), including thumb**
CC +7th **T23.741 Corrosion of third degree of multiple right fingers (nail), including thumb**
HAC 7th character A see Appendix B for HAC conditional logic
CC +7th **T23.742 Corrosion of third degree of multiple left fingers (nail), including thumb**
HAC 7th character A see Appendix B for HAC conditional logic
CC +7th **T23.749 Corrosion of third degree of unspecified multiple fingers (nail), including thumb**
HAC 7th character A see Appendix B for HAC conditional logic

+ **T23.75 Corrosion of third degree of palm**
  - CC +7th **T23.751 Corrosion of third degree of right palm**
    HAC 7th character A see Appendix B for HAC conditional logic
  - CC +7th **T23.752 Corrosion of third degree of left palm**
    HAC 7th character A see Appendix B for HAC conditional logic
  - CC +7th **T23.759 Corrosion of third degree of unspecified palm**
    HAC 7th character A see Appendix B for HAC conditional logic

+ **T23.76 Corrosion of third degree of back of hand**
  - CC +7th **T23.761 Corrosion of third degree of back of right hand**
    HAC 7th character A see Appendix B for HAC conditional logic
  - CC +7th **T23.762 Corrosion of third degree of back of left hand**
    HAC 7th character A see Appendix B for HAC conditional logic
  - CC +7th **T23.769 Corrosion of third degree back of unspecified hand**
    HAC 7th character A see Appendix B for HAC conditional logic

+ **T23.77 Corrosion of third degree of wrist**
  - CC +7th **T23.771 Corrosion of third degree of right wrist**
    HAC 7th character A see Appendix B for HAC conditional logic
  - CC +7th **T23.772 Corrosion of third degree of left wrist**
    HAC 7th character A see Appendix B for HAC conditional logic
  - CC +7th **T23.779 Corrosion of third degree of unspecified wrist**
    HAC 7th character A see Appendix B for HAC conditional logic

+ **T23.79 Corrosion of third degree of multiple sites of wrist and hand**
  - CC +7th **T23.791 Corrosion of third degree of multiple sites of right wrist and hand**
    HAC 7th character A see Appendix B for HAC conditional logic
  - CC +7th **T23.792 Corrosion of third degree of multiple sites of left wrist and hand**
    HAC 7th character A see Appendix B for HAC conditional logic
  - CC +7th **T23.799 Corrosion of third degree of multiple sites of unspecified wrist and hand**
    HAC 7th character A see Appendix B for HAC conditional logic

T24 Burn and corrosion of lower limb, except ankle and foot

Excludes2: *burn and corrosion of ankle and foot (T25.-)*
burn and corrosion of hip region (T21.-)

The appropriate 7th character is to be added to each code from category T24
A initial encounter
D subsequent encounter
S sequela

+ **T24.0 Burn of unspecified degree of lower limb, except ankle and foot**
  Use additional external cause code to identify the source, place and intent of the burn (X00-X19, X75-X77, X96-X98, Y92)

+ **T24.00 Burn of unspecified degree of unspecified site of lower limb, except ankle and foot**
  - +7th **T24.001 Burn of unspecified degree of unspecified site of right lower limb, except ankle and foot**
  - +7th **T24.002 Burn of unspecified degree of unspecified site of left lower limb, except ankle and foot**
  - +7th **T24.009 Burn of unspecified degree of unspecified site of unspecified lower limb, except ankle and foot**

+ **T24.01 Burn of unspecified degree of thigh**
  - +7th **T24.011 Burn of unspecified degree of right thigh**
  - +7th **T24.012 Burn of unspecified degree of left thigh**
  - +7th **T24.019 Burn of unspecified degree of unspecified thigh**

+ **T24.02 Burn of unspecified degree of knee**
  - +7th **T24.021 Burn of unspecified degree of right knee**
  - +7th **T24.022 Burn of unspecified degree of left knee**
  - +7th **T24.029 Burn of unspecified degree of unspecified knee**

+ **T24.03 Burn of unspecified degree of lower leg**
  - +7th **T24.031 Burn of unspecified degree of right lower leg**
  - +7th **T24.032 Burn of unspecified degree of left lower leg**
  - +7th **T24.039 Burn of unspecified degree of unspecified lower leg**

+ **T24.09 Burn of unspecified degree of multiple sites of lower limb, except ankle and foot**
  - +7th **T24.091 Burn of unspecified degree of multiple sites of right lower limb, except ankle and foot**
  - +7th **T24.092 Burn of unspecified degree of multiple sites of left lower limb, except ankle and foot**
  - +7th **T24.099 Burn of unspecified degree of multiple sites of unspecified lower limb, except ankle and foot**

+ **T24.1 Burn of first degree of lower limb, except ankle and foot**
  Use additional external cause code to identify the source, place and intent of the burn (X00-X19, X75-X77, X96-X98, Y92)

+ **T24.10 Burn of first degree of unspecified site of lower limb, except ankle and foot**
  - +7th **T24.101 Burn of first degree of unspecified site of right lower limb, except ankle and foot**
  - +7th **T24.102 Burn of first degree of unspecified site of left lower limb, except ankle and foot**
  - +7th **T24.109 Burn of first degree of unspecified site of unspecified lower limb, except ankle and foot**

+ **T24.11 Burn of first degree of thigh**
  - +7th **T24.111 Burn of first degree of right thigh**
  - +7th **T24.112 Burn of first degree of left thigh**
  - +7th **T24.119 Burn of first degree of unspecified thigh**

+ **T24.12 Burn of first degree of knee**
  - +7th **T24.121 Burn of first degree of right knee**
  - +7th **T24.122 Burn of first degree of left knee**
  - +7th **T24.129 Burn of first degree of unspecified knee**

+ **T24.13 Burn of first degree of lower leg**
  - +7th **T24.131 Burn of first degree of right lower leg**
  - +7th **T24.132 Burn of first degree of left lower leg**
  - +7th **T24.139 Burn of first degree of unspecified lower leg**

+ **T24.19 Burn of first degree of multiple sites of lower limb, except ankle and foot**
  - +7th **T24.191 Burn of first degree of multiple sites of right lower limb, except ankle and foot**
  - +7th **T24.192 Burn of first degree of multiple sites of left lower limb, except ankle and foot**
  - +7th **T24.199 Burn of first degree of multiple sites of unspecified lower limb, except ankle and foot**

+ **T24.2 Burn of second degree of lower limb, except ankle and foot**
  Use additional external cause code to identify the source, place and intent of the burn (X00-X19, X75-X77, X96-X98, Y92)
  + **T24.20 Burn of second degree of unspecified site of lower limb, except ankle and foot**
    - +7th **T24.201 Burn of second degree of unspecified site of right lower limb, except ankle and foot**
    - +7th **T24.202 Burn of second degree of unspecified site of left lower limb, except ankle and foot**
    - +7th **T24.209 Burn of second degree of unspecified site of unspecified lower limb, except ankle and foot**
  + **T24.21 Burn of second degree of thigh**
    - +7th **T24.211 Burn of second degree of right thigh**
    - +7th **T24.212 Burn of second degree of left thigh**
    - +7th **T24.219 Burn of second degree of unspecified thigh**
  + **T24.22 Burn of second degree of knee**
    - +7th **T24.221 Burn of second degree of right knee**
    - +7th **T24.222 Burn of second degree of left knee**
    - +7th **T24.229 Burn of second degree of unspecified knee**
  + **T24.23 Burn of second degree of lower leg**
    - +7th **T24.231 Burn of second degree of right lower leg**
    - +7th **T24.232 Burn of second degree of left lower leg**
    - +7th **T24.239 Burn of second degree of unspecified lower leg**
  + **T24.29 Burn of second degree of multiple sites of lower limb, except ankle and foot**
    - +7th **T24.291 Burn of second degree of multiple sites of right lower limb, except ankle and foot**
    - +7th **T24.292 Burn of second degree of multiple sites of left lower limb, except ankle and foot**
    - +7th **T24.299 Burn of second degree of multiple sites of unspecified lower limb, except ankle and foot**

+ **T24.3 Burn of third degree of lower limb, except ankle and foot**
  Use additional external cause code to identify the source, place and intent of the burn (X00-X19, X75-X77, X96-X98, Y92)
  + **T24.30 Burn of third degree of unspecified site of lower limb, except ankle and foot**
    - CC +7th **T24.301 Burn of third degree of unspecified site of right lower limb, except ankle and foot**
      HAC 7th character A see Appendix B for HAC conditional logic
    - CC +7th **T24.302 Burn of third degree of unspecified site of left lower limb, except ankle and foot**
      HAC 7th character A see Appendix B for HAC conditional logic
    - CC +7th **T24.309 Burn of third degree of unspecified site of unspecified lower limb, except ankle and foot**
      HAC 7th character A see Appendix B for HAC conditional logic
  + **T24.31 Burn of third degree of thigh**
    - CC +7th **T24.311 Burn of third degree of right thigh**
      HAC 7th character A see Appendix B for HAC conditional logic
    - CC +7th **T24.312 Burn of third degree of left thigh**
      HAC 7th character A see Appendix B for HAC conditional logic
    - CC +7th **T24.319 Burn of third degree of unspecified thigh**
      HAC 7th character A see Appendix B for HAC conditional logic
  + **T24.32 Burn of third degree of knee**
    - CC +7th **T24.321 Burn of third degree of right knee**
      HAC 7th character A see Appendix B for HAC conditional logic
    - CC +7th **T24.322 Burn of third degree of left knee**
      HAC 7th character A see Appendix B for HAC conditional logic
    - CC +7th **T24.329 Burn of third degree of unspecified knee**
      HAC 7th character A see Appendix B for HAC conditional logic
  + **T24.33 Burn of third degree of lower leg**
    - CC +7th **T24.331 Burn of third degree of right lower leg**
      HAC 7th character A see Appendix B for HAC conditional logic
    - CC +7th **T24.332 Burn of third degree of left lower leg**
      HAC 7th character A see Appendix B for HAC conditional logic
    - CC +7th **T24.339 Burn of third degree of unspecified lower leg**
      HAC 7th character A see Appendix B for HAC conditional logic
  + **T24.39 Burn of third degree of multiple sites of lower limb, except ankle and foot**
    - CC +7th **T24.391 Burn of third degree of multiple sites of right lower limb, except ankle and foot**
      AHA CC: 2Q, 2016, 4
      HAC 7th character A see Appendix B for HAC conditional logic
    - CC +7th **T24.392 Burn of third degree of multiple sites of left lower limb, except ankle and foot**
      AHA CC: 2Q, 2016, 4
      HAC 7th character A see Appendix B for HAC conditional logic
    - CC +7th **T24.399 Burn of third degree of multiple sites of unspecified lower limb, except ankle and foot**
      HAC 7th character A see Appendix B for HAC conditional logic

+ **T24.4 Corrosion of unspecified degree of lower limb, except ankle and foot**
  Code first (T51-T65) to identify chemical and intent
  Use additional external cause code to identify place (Y92)
  + **T24.40 Corrosion of unspecified degree of unspecified site of lower limb, except ankle and foot**
    - +7th **T24.401 Corrosion of unspecified degree of unspecified site of right lower limb, except ankle and foot**
    - +7th **T24.402 Corrosion of unspecified degree of unspecified site of left lower limb, except ankle and foot**
    - +7th **T24.409 Corrosion of unspecified degree of unspecified site of unspecified lower limb, except ankle and foot**
  + **T24.41 Corrosion of unspecified degree of thigh**
    - +7th **T24.411 Corrosion of unspecified degree of right thigh**
    - +7th **T24.412 Corrosion of unspecified degree of left thigh**
    - +7th **T24.419 Corrosion of unspecified degree of unspecified thigh**
  + **T24.42 Corrosion of unspecified degree of knee**
    - +7th **T24.421 Corrosion of unspecified degree of right knee**
    - +7th **T24.422 Corrosion of unspecified degree of left knee**
    - +7th **T24.429 Corrosion of unspecified degree of unspecified knee**
  + **T24.43 Corrosion of unspecified degree of lower leg**
    - +7th **T24.431 Corrosion of unspecified degree of right lower leg**
    - +7th **T24.432 Corrosion of unspecified degree of left lower leg**
    - +7th **T24.439 Corrosion of unspecified degree of unspecified lower leg**
  + **T24.49 Corrosion of unspecified degree of multiple sites of lower limb, except ankle and foot**
    - +7th **T24.491 Corrosion of unspecified degree of multiple sites of right lower limb, except ankle and foot**
    - +7th **T24.492 Corrosion of unspecified degree of multiple sites of left lower limb, except ankle and foot**
    - +7th **T24.499 Corrosion of unspecified degree of multiple sites of unspecified lower limb, except ankle and foot**

+ **T24.5 Corrosion of first degree of lower limb, except ankle and foot**
  Code first (T51-T65) to identify chemical and intent
  Use additional external cause code to identify place (Y92)
+ **T24.50 Corrosion of first degree of unspecified site of lower limb, except ankle and foot**
  - +7th **T24.501 Corrosion of first degree of unspecified site of right lower limb, except ankle and foot**
  - +7th **T24.502 Corrosion of first degree of unspecified site of left lower limb, except ankle and foot**
  - +7th **T24.509 Corrosion of first degree of unspecified site of unspecified lower limb, except ankle and foot**
+ **T24.51 Corrosion of first degree of thigh**
  - +7th **T24.511 Corrosion of first degree of right thigh**
  - +7th **T24.512 Corrosion of first degree of left thigh**
  - +7th **T24.519 Corrosion of first degree of unspecified thigh**
+ **T24.52 Corrosion of first degree of knee**
  - +7th **T24.521 Corrosion of first degree of right knee**
  - +7th **T24.522 Corrosion of first degree of left knee**
  - +7th **T24.529 Corrosion of first degree of unspecified knee**
+ **T24.53 Corrosion of first degree of lower leg**
  - +7th **T24.531 Corrosion of first degree of right lower leg**
  - +7th **T24.532 Corrosion of first degree of left lower leg**
  - +7th **T24.539 Corrosion of first degree of unspecified lower leg**
+ **T24.59 Corrosion of first degree of multiple sites of lower limb, except ankle and foot**
  - +7th **T24.591 Corrosion of first degree of multiple sites of right lower limb, except ankle and foot**
  - +7th **T24.592 Corrosion of first degree of multiple sites of left lower limb, except ankle and foot**
  - +7th **T24.599 Corrosion of first degree of multiple sites of unspecified lower limb, except ankle and foot**
+ **T24.6 Corrosion of second degree of lower limb, except ankle and foot**
  Code first (T51-T65) to identify chemical and intent
  Use additional external cause code to identify place (Y92)
+ **T24.60 Corrosion of second degree of unspecified site of lower limb, except ankle and foot**
  - +7th **T24.601 Corrosion of second degree of unspecified site of right lower limb, except ankle and foot**
  - +7th **T24.602 Corrosion of second degree of unspecified site of left lower limb, except ankle and foot**
  - +7th **T24.609 Corrosion of second degree of unspecified site of unspecified lower limb, except ankle and foot**
+ **T24.61 Corrosion of second degree of thigh**
  - +7th **T24.611 Corrosion of second degree of right thigh**
  - +7th **T24.612 Corrosion of second degree of left thigh**
  - +7th **T24.619 Corrosion of second degree of unspecified thigh**
+ **T24.62 Corrosion of second degree of knee**
  - +7th **T24.621 Corrosion of second degree of right knee**
  - +7th **T24.622 Corrosion of second degree of left knee**
  - +7th **T24.629 Corrosion of second degree of unspecified knee**
+ **T24.63 Corrosion of second degree of lower leg**
  - +7th **T24.631 Corrosion of second degree of right lower leg**
  - +7th **T24.632 Corrosion of second degree of left lower leg**
  - +7th **T24.639 Corrosion of second degree of unspecified lower leg**
+ **T24.69 Corrosion of second degree of multiple sites of lower limb, except ankle and foot**
  - +7th **T24.691 Corrosion of second degree of multiple sites of right lower limb, except ankle and foot**
  - +7th **T24.692 Corrosion of second degree of multiple sites of left lower limb, except ankle and foot**
  - +7th **T24.699 Corrosion of second degree of multiple sites of unspecified lower limb, except ankle and foot**
+ **T24.7 Corrosion of third degree of lower limb, except ankle and foot**
  Code first (T51-T65) to identify chemical and intent
  Use additional external cause code to identify place (Y92)
+ **T24.70 Corrosion of third degree of unspecified site of lower limb, except ankle and foot**
  - CC +7th **T24.701 Corrosion of third degree of unspecified site of right lower limb, except ankle and foot**
    HAC 7th character A see Appendix B for HAC conditional logic
  - CC +7th **T24.702 Corrosion of third degree of unspecified site of left lower limb, except ankle and foot**
    HAC 7th character A see Appendix B for HAC conditional logic
  - CC +7th **T24.709 Corrosion of third degree of unspecified site of unspecified lower limb, except ankle and foot**
    HAC 7th character A see Appendix B for HAC conditional logic
+ **T24.71 Corrosion of third degree of thigh**
  - CC +7th **T24.711 Corrosion of third degree of right thigh**
    HAC 7th character A see Appendix B for HAC conditional logic
  - CC +7th **T24.712 Corrosion of third degree of left thigh**
    HAC 7th character A see Appendix B for HAC conditional logic
  - CC +7th **T24.719 Corrosion of third degree of unspecified thigh**
    HAC 7th character A see Appendix B for HAC conditional logic
+ **T24.72 Corrosion of third degree of knee**
  - CC +7th **T24.721 Corrosion of third degree of right knee**
    HAC 7th character A see Appendix B for HAC conditional logic
  - CC +7th **T24.722 Corrosion of third degree of left knee**
    HAC 7th character A see Appendix B for HAC conditional logic
  - CC +7th **T24.729 Corrosion of third degree of unspecified knee**
    HAC 7th character A see Appendix B for HAC conditional logic
+ **T24.73 Corrosion of third degree of lower leg**
  - CC +7th **T24.731 Corrosion of third degree of right lower leg**
    HAC 7th character A see Appendix B for HAC conditional logic
  - CC +7th **T24.732 Corrosion of third degree of left lower leg**
    HAC 7th character A see Appendix B for HAC conditional logic
  - CC +7th **T24.739 Corrosion of third degree of unspecified lower leg**
    HAC 7th character A see Appendix B for HAC conditional logic
+ **T24.79 Corrosion of third degree of multiple sites of lower limb, except ankle and foot**
  - CC +7th **T24.791 Corrosion of third degree of multiple sites of right lower limb, except ankle and foot**
    HAC 7th character A see Appendix B for HAC conditional logic

CC +7th **T24.792 Corrosion of third degree of multiple sites of left lower limb, except ankle and foot**
HAC 7th character A see Appendix B for HAC conditional logic

CC +7th **T24.799 Corrosion of third degree of multiple sites of unspecified lower limb, except ankle and foot**
HAC 7th character A see Appendix B for HAC conditional logic

T25 Burn and corrosion of ankle and foot

The appropriate 7th character is to be added to each code from category T25
A initial encounter
D subsequent encounter
S sequela

\+ **T25.0 Burn of unspecified degree of ankle and foot**
Use additional external cause code to identify the source, place and intent of the burn (X00-X19, X75-X77, X96-X98, Y92)

\+ **T25.01 Burn of unspecified degree of ankle**
+7th **T25.011 Burn of unspecified degree of right ankle**
+7th **T25.012 Burn of unspecified degree of left ankle**
+7th **T25.019 Burn of unspecified degree of unspecified ankle**

\+ **T25.02 Burn of unspecified degree of foot**
Excludes2: *burn of unspecified degree of toe(s) (nail) (T25.03-)*
+7th **T25.021 Burn of unspecified degree of right foot**
+7th **T25.022 Burn of unspecified degree of left foot**
+7th **T25.029 Burn of unspecified degree of unspecified foot**

\+ **T25.03 Burn of unspecified degree of toe(s) (nail)**
+7th **T25.031 Burn of unspecified degree of right toe(s) (nail)**
+7th **T25.032 Burn of unspecified degree of left toe(s) (nail)**
+7th **T25.039 Burn of unspecified degree of unspecified toe(s) (nail)**

\+ **T25.09 Burn of unspecified degree of multiple sites of ankle and foot**
+7th **T25.091 Burn of unspecified degree of multiple sites of right ankle and foot**
+7th **T25.092 Burn of unspecified degree of multiple sites of left ankle and foot**
+7th **T25.099 Burn of unspecified degree of multiple sites of unspecified ankle and foot**

\+ **T25.1 Burn of first degree of ankle and foot**
Use additional external cause code to identify the source, place and intent of the burn (X00-X19, X75-X77, X96-X98, Y92)

\+ **T25.11 Burn of first degree of ankle**
+7th **T25.111 Burn of first degree of right ankle**
+7th **T25.112 Burn of first degree of left ankle**
+7th **T25.119 Burn of first degree of unspecified ankle**

\+ **T25.12 Burn of first degree of foot**
Excludes2: *burn of first degree of toe(s) (nail) (T25.13-)*
+7th **T25.121 Burn of first degree of right foot**
+7th **T25.122 Burn of first degree of left foot**
+7th **T25.129 Burn of first degree of unspecified foot**

\+ **T25.13 Burn of first degree of toe(s) (nail)**
+7th **T25.131 Burn of first degree of right toe(s) (nail)**
+7th **T25.132 Burn of first degree of left toe(s) (nail)**
+7th **T25.139 Burn of first degree of unspecified toe(s) (nail)**

\+ **T25.19 Burn of first degree of multiple sites of ankle and foot**
+7th **T25.191 Burn of first degree of multiple sites of right ankle and foot**
+7th **T25.192 Burn of first degree of multiple sites of left ankle and foot**
+7th **T25.199 Burn of first degree of multiple sites of unspecified ankle and foot**

\+ **T25.2 Burn of second degree of ankle and foot**
Use additional external cause code to identify the source, place and intent of the burn (X00-X19, X75-X77, X96-X98, Y92)

\+ **T25.21 Burn of second degree of ankle**
+7th **T25.211 Burn of second degree of right ankle**
+7th **T25.212 Burn of second degree of left ankle**
+7th **T25.219 Burn of second degree of unspecified ankle**

\+ **T25.22 Burn of second degree of foot**
Excludes2: *burn of second degree of toe(s) (nail) (T25.23-)*
+7th **T25.221 Burn of second degree of right foot**
+7th **T25.222 Burn of second degree of left foot**
+7th **T25.229 Burn of second degree of unspecified foot**

\+ **T25.23 Burn of second degree of toe(s) (nail)**
+7th **T25.231 Burn of second degree of right toe(s) (nail)**
+7th **T25.232 Burn of second degree of left toe(s) (nail)**
+7th **T25.239 Burn of second degree of unspecified toe(s) (nail)**

\+ **T25.29 Burn of second degree of multiple sites of ankle and foot**
+7th **T25.291 Burn of second degree of multiple sites of right ankle and foot**
+7th **T25.292 Burn of second degree of multiple sites of left ankle and foot**
+7th **T25.299 Burn of second degree of multiple sites of unspecified ankle and foot**

\+ **T25.3 Burn of third degree of ankle and foot**
Use external cause code to identify the source, place and intent of the burn (X00-X19, X75-X77, X96-X98, Y92)

\+ **T25.31 Burn of third degree of ankle**
CC +7th **T25.311 Burn of third degree of right ankle**
HAC 7th character A see Appendix B for HAC conditional logic
CC +7th **T25.312 Burn of third degree of left ankle**
HAC 7th character A see Appendix B for HAC conditional logic
CC +7th **T25.319 Burn of third degree of unspecified ankle**
HAC 7th character A see Appendix B for HAC conditional logic

\+ **T25.32 Burn of third degree of foot**
Excludes2: *burn of third degree of toe(s) (nail) (T25.33-)*
CC +7th **T25.321 Burn of third degree of right foot**
HAC 7th character A see Appendix B for HAC conditional logic
CC +7th **T25.322 Burn of third degree of left foot**
HAC 7th character A see Appendix B for HAC conditional logic
CC +7th **T25.329 Burn of third degree of unspecified foot**
HAC 7th character A see Appendix B for HAC conditional logic

\+ **T25.33 Burn of third degree of toe(s) (nail)**
CC +7th **T25.331 Burn of third degree of right toe(s) (nail)**
HAC 7th character A see Appendix B for HAC conditional logic
CC +7th **T25.332 Burn of third degree of left toe(s) (nail)**
HAC 7th character A see Appendix B for HAC conditional logic
CC +7th **T25.339 Burn of third degree of unspecified toe(s) (nail)**
HAC 7th character A see Appendix B for HAC conditional logic

\+ **T25.39 Burn of third degree of multiple sites of ankle and foot**
CC +7th **T25.391 Burn of third degree of multiple sites of right ankle and foot**
HAC 7th character A see Appendix B for HAC conditional logic
CC +7th **T25.392 Burn of third degree of multiple sites of left ankle and foot**
HAC 7th character A see Appendix B for HAC conditional logic

CC +7th **T25.399 Burn of third degree of multiple sites of unspecified ankle and foot**
HAC 7th character A see Appendix B for HAC conditional logic

\+ **T25.4 Corrosion of unspecified degree of ankle and foot**
Code first (T51-T65) to identify chemical and intent
Use additional external cause code to identify place (Y92)

\+ **T25.41 Corrosion of unspecified degree of ankle**
+7th **T25.411 Corrosion of unspecified degree of right ankle**
+7th **T25.412 Corrosion of unspecified degree of left ankle**
+7th **T25.419 Corrosion of unspecified degree of unspecified ankle**

\+ **T25.42 Corrosion of unspecified degree of foot**
Excludes2: *corrosion of unspecified degree of toe(s) (nail) (T25.43-)*
+7th **T25.421 Corrosion of unspecified degree of right foot**
+7th **T25.422 Corrosion of unspecified degree of left foot**
+7th **T25.429 Corrosion of unspecified degree of unspecified foot**

\+ **T25.43 Corrosion of unspecified degree of toe(s) (nail)**
+7th **T25.431 Corrosion of unspecified degree of right toe(s) (nail)**
+7th **T25.432 Corrosion of unspecified degree of left toe(s) (nail)**
+7th **T25.439 Corrosion of unspecified degree of unspecified toe(s) (nail)**

\+ **T25.49 Corrosion of unspecified degree of multiple sites of ankle and foot**
+7th **T25.491 Corrosion of unspecified degree of multiple sites of right ankle and foot**
+7th **T25.492 Corrosion of unspecified degree of multiple sites of left ankle and foot**
+7th **T25.499 Corrosion of unspecified degree of multiple sites of unspecified ankle and foot**

\+ **T25.5 Corrosion of first degree of ankle and foot**
Code first (T51-T65) to identify chemical and intent
Use additional external cause code to identify place (Y92)

\+ **T25.51 Corrosion of first degree of ankle**
+7th **T25.511 Corrosion of first degree of right ankle**
+7th **T25.512 Corrosion of first degree of left ankle**
+7th **T25.519 Corrosion of first degree of unspecified ankle**

\+ **T25.52 Corrosion of first degree of foot**
Excludes2: *corrosion of first degree of toe(s) (nail) (T25.53-)*
+7th **T25.521 Corrosion of first degree of right foot**
+7th **T25.522 Corrosion of first degree of left foot**
+7th **T25.529 Corrosion of first degree of unspecified foot**

\+ **T25.53 Corrosion of first degree of toe(s) (nail)**
+7th **T25.531 Corrosion of first degree of right toe(s) (nail)**
+7th **T25.532 Corrosion of first degree of left toe(s) (nail)**
+7th **T25.539 Corrosion of first degree of unspecified toe(s) (nail)**

\+ **T25.59 Corrosion of first degree of multiple sites of ankle and foot**
+7th **T25.591 Corrosion of first degree of multiple sites of right ankle and foot**
+7th **T25.592 Corrosion of first degree of multiple sites of left ankle and foot**
+7th **T25.599 Corrosion of first degree of multiple sites of unspecified ankle and foot**

\+ **T25.6 Corrosion of second degree of ankle and foot**
Code first (T51-T65) to identify chemical and intent
Use additional external cause code to identify place (Y92)

\+ **T25.61 Corrosion of second degree of ankle**
+7th **T25.611 Corrosion of second degree of right ankle**
+7th **T25.612 Corrosion of second degree of left ankle**
+7th **T25.619 Corrosion of second degree of unspecified ankle**

\+ **T25.62 Corrosion of second degree of foot**
Excludes2: *corrosion of second degree of toe(s) (nail) (T25.63-)*
+7th **T25.621 Corrosion of second degree of right foot**
+7th **T25.622 Corrosion of second degree of left foot**
+7th **T25.629 Corrosion of second degree of unspecified foot**

\+ **T25.63 Corrosion of second degree of toe(s) (nail)**
+7th **T25.631 Corrosion of second degree of right toe(s) (nail)**
+7th **T25.632 Corrosion of second degree of left toe(s) (nail)**
+7th **T25.639 Corrosion of second degree of unspecified toe(s) (nail)**

\+ **T25.69 Corrosion of second degree of multiple sites of ankle and foot**
+7th **T25.691 Corrosion of second degree of right ankle and foot**
+7th **T25.692 Corrosion of second degree of left ankle and foot**
+7th **T25.699 Corrosion of second degree of unspecified ankle and foot**

\+ **T25.7 Corrosion of third degree of ankle and foot**
Code first (T51-T65) to identify chemical and intent
Use additional external cause code to identify place (Y92)

\+ **T25.71 Corrosion of third degree of ankle**
CC +7th **T25.711 Corrosion of third degree of right ankle**
HAC 7th character A see Appendix B for HAC conditional logic
CC +7th **T25.712 Corrosion of third degree of left ankle**
HAC 7th character A see Appendix B for HAC conditional logic
CC +7th **T25.719 Corrosion of third degree of unspecified ankle**
HAC 7th character A see Appendix B for HAC conditional logic

\+ **T25.72 Corrosion of third degree of foot**
Excludes2: *corrosion of third degree of toe(s) (nail) (T25.73-)*
CC +7th **T25.721 Corrosion of third degree of right foot**
HAC 7th character A see Appendix B for HAC conditional logic
CC +7th **T25.722 Corrosion of third degree of left foot**
HAC 7th character A see Appendix B for HAC conditional logic
CC +7th **T25.729 Corrosion of third degree of unspecified foot**
HAC 7th character A see Appendix B for HAC conditional logic

\+ **T25.73 Corrosion of third degree of toe(s) (nail)**
CC +7th **T25.731 Corrosion of third degree of right toe(s) (nail)**
HAC 7th character A see Appendix B for HAC conditional logic
CC +7th **T25.732 Corrosion of third degree of left toe(s) (nail)**
HAC 7th character A see Appendix B for HAC conditional logic
CC +7th **T25.739 Corrosion of third degree of unspecified toe(s) (nail)**
HAC 7th character A see Appendix B for HAC conditional logic

\+ **T25.79 Corrosion of third degree of multiple sites of ankle and foot**
CC +7th **T25.791 Corrosion of third degree of multiple sites of right ankle and foot**
HAC 7th character A see Appendix B for HAC conditional logic
CC +7th **T25.792 Corrosion of third degree of multiple sites of left ankle and foot**
HAC 7th character A see Appendix B for HAC conditional logic
CC +7th **T25.799 Corrosion of third degree of multiple sites of unspecified ankle and foot**
HAC 7th character A see Appendix B for HAC conditional logic

Burns and corrosions confined to eye and internal organs (T26-T28)

Review coding guideline C.19.d

T26 Burn and corrosion confined to eye and adnexa

The appropriate 7th character is to be added to each code from category T26
A initial encounter
D subsequent encounter
S sequela

\+ **T26.0 Burn of eyelid and periocular area**
Use additional external cause code to identify the source, place and intent of the burn (X00-X19, X75-X77, X96-X98, Y92)
X+7th **T26.00 Burn of unspecified eyelid and periocular area**
X+7th **T26.01 Burn of right eyelid and periocular area**
X+7th **T26.02 Burn of left eyelid and periocular area**

\+ **T26.1 Burn of cornea and conjunctival sac**
Use additional external cause code to identify the source, place and intent of the burn (X00-X19, X75-X77, X96-X98, Y92)
X+7th **T26.10 Burn of cornea and conjunctival sac, unspecified eye**
X+7th **T26.11 Burn of cornea and conjunctival sac, right eye**
X+7th **T26.12 Burn of cornea and conjunctival sac, left eye**

\+ **T26.2 Burn with resulting rupture and destruction of eyeball**
Use additional external cause code to identify the source, place and intent of the burn (X00-X19, X75-X77, X96-X98, Y92)
CC X+7th **T26.20 Burn with resulting rupture and destruction of unspecified eyeball**
HAC 7th character A see Appendix B for HAC conditional logic
CC X+7th **T26.21 Burn with resulting rupture and destruction of right eyeball**
HAC 7th character A see Appendix B for HAC conditional logic
CC X+7th **T26.22 Burn with resulting rupture and destruction of left eyeball**
HAC 7th character A see Appendix B for HAC conditional logic

\+ **T26.3 Burns of other specified parts of eye and adnexa**
Use additional external cause code to identify the source, place and intent of the burn (X00-X19, X75-X77, X96-X98, Y92)
X+7th **T26.30 Burns of other specified parts of unspecified eye and adnexa**
X+7th **T26.31 Burns of other specified parts of right eye and adnexa**
X+7th **T26.32 Burns of other specified parts of left eye and adnexa**

\+ **T26.4 Burn of eye and adnexa, part unspecified**
Use additional external cause code to identify the source, place and intent of the burn (X00-X19, X75-X77, X96-X98, Y92)
X+7th **T26.40 Burn of unspecified eye and adnexa, part unspecified**
X+7th **T26.41 Burn of right eye and adnexa, part unspecified**
X+7th **T26.42 Burn of left eye and adnexa, part unspecified**

\+ **T26.5 Corrosion of eyelid and periocular area**
Code first (T51-T65) to identify chemical and intent

Use additional external cause code to identify place (Y92)
X+7th **T26.50 Corrosion of unspecified eyelid and periocular area**
X+7th **T26.51 Corrosion of right eyelid and periocular area**
X+7th **T26.52 Corrosion of left eyelid and periocular area**

\+ **T26.6 Corrosion of cornea and conjunctival sac**
Code first (T51-T65) to identify chemical and intent

Use additional external cause code to identify place (Y92)
X+7th **T26.60 Corrosion of cornea and conjunctival sac, unspecified eye**
X+7th **T26.61 Corrosion of cornea and conjunctival sac, right eye**
X+7th **T26.62 Corrosion of cornea and conjunctival sac, left eye**

\+ **T26.7 Corrosion with resulting rupture and destruction of eyeball**
Code first (T51-T65) to identify chemical and intent

Use additional external cause code to identify place (Y92)
CC X+7th **T26.70 Corrosion with resulting rupture and destruction of unspecified eyeball**
HAC 7th character A see Appendix B for HAC conditional logic
CC X+7th **T26.71 Corrosion with resulting rupture and destruction of right eyeball**
HAC 7th character A see Appendix B for HAC conditional logic
CC X+7th **T26.72 Corrosion with resulting rupture and destruction of left eyeball**
HAC 7th character A see Appendix B for HAC conditional logic

\+ **T26.8 Corrosions of other specified parts of eye and adnexa**
Code first (T51-T65) to identify chemical and intent

Use add itional external cause code to identify place (Y92)
X+7th **T26.80 Corrosions of other specified parts of unspecified eye and adnexa**
X+7th **T26.81 Corrosions of other specified parts of right eye and adnexa**
X+7th **T26.82 Corrosions of other specified parts of left eye and adnexa**

\+ **T26.9 Corrosion of eye and adnexa, part unspecified**
Code first (T51-T65) to identify chemical and intent

Use additional external cause code to identify place (Y92)
X+7th **T26.90 Corrosion of unspecified eye and adnexa, part unspecified**
X+7th **T26.91 Corrosion of right eye and adnexa, part unspecified**
X+7th **T26.92 Corrosion of left eye and adnexa, part unspecified**

T27 Burn and corrosion of respiratory tract
Use additional external cause code to identify the source and intent of the burn (X00-X19, X75-X77, X96-X98)

Use external cause code to identify place (Y92)

The appropriate 7th character is to be added to each code from category T27
A initial encounter
D subsequent encounter
S sequela

CC X+7th **T27.0 Burn of larynx and trachea**
HAC 7th character A see Appendix B for HAC conditional logic
CC X+7th **T27.1 Burn involving larynx and trachea with lung**
HAC 7th character A see Appendix B for HAC conditional logic
CC X+7th **T27.2 Burn of other parts of respiratory tract**
Burn of thoracic cavity
HAC 7th character A see Appendix B for HAC conditional logic
CC X+7th **T27.3 Burn of respiratory tract, part unspecified**
HAC 7th character A see Appendix B for HAC conditional logic
CC X+7th **T27.4 Corrosion of larynx and trachea**
Code first (T51-T65) to identify chemical and intent
HAC 7th character A see Appendix B for HAC conditional logic
CC X+7th **T27.5 Corrosion involving larynx and trachea with lung**
Code first (T51-T65) to identify chemical and intent
HAC 7th character A see Appendix B for HAC conditional logic
CC X+7th **T27.6 Corrosion of other parts of respiratory tract**
Code first (T51-T65) to identify chemical and intent
HAC 7th character A see Appendix B for HAC conditional logic
CC X+7th **T27.7 Corrosion of respiratory tract, part unspecified**
Code first (T51-T65) to identify chemical and intent
HAC 7th character A see Appendix B for HAC conditional logic

T28 Burn and corrosion of other internal organs
Use additional external cause code to identify the source and intent of the burn (X00-X19, X75-X77, X96-X98)

Use external cause code to identify place (Y92)

The appropriate 7th character is to be added to each code from category T28
A initial encounter
D subsequent encounter
S sequela

X+7th **T28.0 Burn of mouth and pharynx**
CC X+7th **T28.1 Burn of esophagus**
HAC 7th character A see Appendix B for HAC conditional logic
CC X+7th **T28.2 Burn of other parts of alimentary tract**
HAC 7th character A see Appendix B for HAC conditional logic

X+7th **T28.3 Burn of internal genitourinary organs**

\+ **T28.4 Burns of other and unspecified internal organs**

X+7th **T28.40 Burn of unspecified internal organ**

\+ **T28.41 Burn of ear drum**

+7th **T28.411 Burn of right ear drum**

+7th **T28.412 Burn of left ear drum**

+7th **T28.419 Burn of unspecified ear drum**

X+7th **T28.49 Burn of other internal organ**

X+7th **T28.5 Corrosion of mouth and pharynx**

Code first (T51-T65) to identify chemical and intent

CC X+7th **T28.6 Corrosion of esophagus**

Code first (T51-T65) to identify chemical and intent

HAC 7th character A see Appendix B for HAC conditional logic

CC X+7th **T28.7 Corrosion of other parts of alimentary tract**

Code first (T51-T65) to identify chemical and intent

HAC 7th character A see Appendix B for HAC conditional logic

X+7th **T28.8 Corrosion of internal genitourinary organs**

Code first (T51-T65) to identify chemical and intent

\+ **T28.9 Corrosions of other and unspecified internal organs**

Code first (T51-T65) to identify chemical and intent

X+7th **T28.90 Corrosions of unspecified internal organs**

\+ **T28.91 Corrosions of ear drum**

+7th **T28.911 Corrosions of right ear drum**

+7th **T28.912 Corrosions of left ear drum**

+7th **T28.919 Corrosions of unspecified ear drum**

X+7th **T28.99 Corrosions of other internal organs**

Burns and corrosions of multiple and unspecified body regions (T30-T32)

T30 Burn and corrosion, body region unspecified

Review coding guideline C.19.d.5

T30.0 Burn of unspecified body region, unspecified degree

This code is not for inpatient use. Code to specified site and degree of burns

Burn NOS

Multiple burns NOS

T30.4 Corrosion of unspecified body region, unspecified degree

This code is not for inpatient use. Code to specified site and degree of corrosion

Corrosion NOS

Multiple corrosion NOS

T31 Burns classified according to extent of body surface involved

NOTE This category is to be used as the primary code only when the site of the burn is unspecified. It should be used as a supplementary code with categories T20-T25 when the site is specified.

Review coding guideline C.19.d.6

T31.0 Burns involving less than 10% of body surface

\+ **T31.1 Burns involving 10-19% of body surface**

CC **T31.10 Burns involving 10-19% of body surface with 0% to 9% third degree burns**

Burns involving 10-19% of body surface NOS

HAC see Appendix B for HAC conditional logic

CC **T31.11 Burns involving 10-19% of body surface with 10-19% third degree burns**

HAC see Appendix B for HAC conditional logic

\+ **T31.2 Burns involving 20-29% of body surface**

CC **T31.20 Burns involving 20-29% of body surface with 0% to 9% third degree burns**

Burns involving 20-29% of body surface NOS

HAC see Appendix B for HAC conditional logic

MCC **T31.21 Burns involving 20-29% of body surface with 10-19% third degree burns**

HAC see Appendix B for HAC conditional logic

MCC **T31.22 Burns involving 20-29% of body surface with 20-29% third degree burns**

HAC see Appendix B for HAC conditional logic

\+ **T31.3 Burns involving 30-39% of body surface**

CC **T31.30 Burns involving 30-39% of body surface with 0% to 9% third degree burns**

Burns involving 30-39% of body surface NOS

HAC see Appendix B for HAC conditional logic

MCC **T31.31 Burns involving 30-39% of body surface with 10-19% third degree burns**

HAC see Appendix B for HAC conditional logic

MCC **T31.32 Burns involving 30-39% of body surface with 20-29% third degree burns**

HAC see Appendix B for HAC conditional logic

MCC **T31.33 Burns involving 30-39% of body surface with 30-39% third degree burns**

HAC see Appendix B for HAC conditional logic

\+ **T31.4 Burns involving 40-49% of body surface**

CC **T31.40 Burns involving 40-49% of body surface with 0% to 9% third degree burns**

Burns involving 40-49% of body surface NOS

HAC see Appendix B for HAC conditional logic

MCC **T31.41 Burns involving 40-49% of body surface with 10-19% third degree burns**

HAC see Appendix B for HAC conditional logic

MCC **T31.42 Burns involving 40-49% of body surface with 20-29% third degree burns**

HAC see Appendix B for HAC conditional logic

MCC **T31.43 Burns involving 40-49% of body surface with 30-39% third degree burns**

HAC see Appendix B for HAC conditional logic

MCC **T31.44 Burns involving 40-49% of body surface with 40-49% third degree burns**

HAC see Appendix B for HAC conditional logic

\+ **T31.5 Burns involving 50-59% of body surface**

CC **T31.50 Burns involving 50-59% of body surface with 0% to 9% third degree burns**

Burns involving 50-59% of body surface NOS

HAC see Appendix B for HAC conditional logic

MCC **T31.51 Burns involving 50-59% of body surface with 10-19% third degree burns**

HAC see Appendix B for HAC conditional logic

MCC **T31.52 Burns involving 50-59% of body surface with 20-29% third degree burns**

HAC see Appendix B for HAC conditional logic

MCC **T31.53 Burns involving 50-59% of body surface with 30-39% third degree burns**

HAC see Appendix B for HAC conditional logic

MCC **T31.54 Burns involving 50-59% of body surface with 40-49% third degree burns**

HAC see Appendix B for HAC conditional logic

MCC **T31.55 Burns involving 50-59% of body surface with 50-59% third degree burns**

HAC see Appendix B for HAC conditional logic

\+ **T31.6 Burns involving 60-69% of body surface**

CC **T31.60 Burns involving 60-69% of body surface with 0% to 9% third degree burns**

Burns involving 60-69% of body surface NOS

HAC see Appendix B for HAC conditional logic

MCC **T31.61 Burns involving 60-69% of body surface with 10-19% third degree burns**

HAC see Appendix B for HAC conditional logic

MCC **T31.62 Burns involving 60-69% of body surface with 20-29% third degree burns**

HAC see Appendix B for HAC conditional logic

MCC **T31.63 Burns involving 60-69% of body surface with 30-39% third degree burns**

HAC see Appendix B for HAC conditional logic

MCC **T31.64 Burns involving 60-69% of body surface with 40-49% third degree burns**

HAC see Appendix B for HAC conditional logic

MCC **T31.65 Burns involving 60-69% of body surface with 50-59% third degree burns**

HAC see Appendix B for HAC conditional logic

MCC **T31.66 Burns involving 60-69% of body surface with 60-69% third degree burns**

HAC see Appendix B for HAC conditional logic

\+ **T31.7 Burns involving 70-79% of body surface**

CC **T31.70 Burns involving 70-79% of body surface with 0% to 9% third degree burns**

Burns involving 70-79% of body surface NOS

HAC see Appendix B for HAC conditional logic

MCC **T31.71 Burns involving 70-79% of body surface with 10-19% third degree burns**

HAC see Appendix B for HAC conditional logic

MCC **T31.72 Burns involving 70-79% of body surface with 20-29% third degree burns**

HAC see Appendix B for HAC conditional logic

MCC T31.73 **Burns involving 70-79% of body surface with 30-39% third degree burns**
HAC see Appendix B for HAC conditional logic

MCC T31.74 **Burns involving 70-79% of body surface with 40-49% third degree burns**
HAC see Appendix B for HAC conditional logic

MCC T31.75 **Burns involving 70-79% of body surface with 50-59% third degree burns**
HAC see Appendix B for HAC conditional logic

MCC T31.76 **Burns involving 70-79% of body surface with 60-69% third degree burns**
HAC see Appendix B for HAC conditional logic

MCC T31.77 **Burns involving 70-79% of body surface with 70-79% third degree burns**
HAC see Appendix B for HAC conditional logic

+ T31.8 **Burns involving 80-89% of body surface**

CC T31.80 **Burns involving 80-89% of body surface with 0% to 9% third degree burns**
Burns involving 80-89% of body surface NOS
HAC see Appendix B for HAC conditional logic

MCC T31.81 **Burns involving 80-89% of body surface with 10-19% third degree burns**
HAC see Appendix B for HAC conditional logic

MCC T31.82 **Burns involving 80-89% of body surface with 20-29% third degree burns**
HAC see Appendix B for HAC conditional logic

MCC T31.83 **Burns involving 80-89% of body surface with 30-39% third degree burns**
HAC see Appendix B for HAC conditional logic

MCC T31.84 **Burns involving 80-89% of body surface with 40-49% third degree burns**
HAC see Appendix B for HAC conditional logic

MCC T31.85 **Burns involving 80-89% of body surface with 50-59% third degree burns**
HAC see Appendix B for HAC conditional logic

MCC T31.86 **Burns involving 80-89% of body surface with 60-69% third degree burns**
HAC see Appendix B for HAC conditional logic

MCC T31.87 **Burns involving 80-89% of body surface with 70-79% third degree burns**
HAC see Appendix B for HAC conditional logic

MCC T31.88 **Burns involving 80-89% of body surface with 80-89% third degree burns**
HAC see Appendix B for HAC conditional logic

+ T31.9 **Burns involving 90% or more of body surface**

CC T31.90 **Burns involving 90% or more of body surface with 0% to 9% third degree burns**
Burns involving 90% or more of body surface NOS
HAC see Appendix B for HAC conditional logic

MCC T31.91 **Burns involving 90% or more of body surface with 10-19% third degree burns**
HAC see Appendix B for HAC conditional logic

MCC T31.92 **Burns involving 90% or more of body surface with 20-29% third degree burns**
HAC see Appendix B for HAC conditional logic

MCC T31.93 **Burns involving 90% or more of body surface with 30-39% third degree burns**
HAC see Appendix B for HAC conditional logic

MCC T31.94 **Burns involving 90% or more of body surface with 40-49% third degree burns**
HAC see Appendix B for HAC conditional logic

MCC T31.95 **Burns involving 90% or more of body surface with 50-59% third degree burns**
HAC see Appendix B for HAC conditional logic

MCC T31.96 **Burns involving 90% or more of body surface with 60-69% third degree burns**
HAC see Appendix B for HAC conditional logic

MCC T31.97 **Burns involving 90% or more of body surface with 70-79% third degree burns**
HAC see Appendix B for HAC conditional logic

MCC T31.98 **Burns involving 90% or more of body surface with 80-89% third degree burns**
HAC see Appendix B for HAC conditional logic

MCC T31.99 **Burns involving 90% or more of body surface with 90% or more third degree burns**
HAC see Appendix B for HAC conditional logic

T32 Corrosions classified according to extent of body surface involved

NOTE This category is to be used as the primary code only when the site of the corrosion is unspecified. It may be used as a supplementary code with categories T20-T25 when the site is specified.

Review coding guideline C.19.d.6

T32.0 **Corrosions involving less than 10% of body surface**

+ T32.1 **Corrosions involving 10-19% of body surface**

CC T32.10 **Corrosions involving 10-19% of body surface with 0% to 9% third degree corrosion**
Corrosions involving 10-19% of body surface NOS
HAC see Appendix B for HAC conditional logic

CC T32.11 **Corrosions involving 10-19% of body surface with 10-19% third degree corrosion**
HAC see Appendix B for HAC conditional logic

+ T32.2 **Corrosions involving 20-29% of body surface**

CC T32.20 **Corrosions involving 20-29% of body surface with 0% to 9% third degree corrosion**
HAC see Appendix B for HAC conditional logic

MCC T32.21 **Corrosions involving 20-29% of body surface with 10-19% third degree corrosion**
HAC see Appendix B for HAC conditional logic

MCC T32.22 **Corrosions involving 20-29% of body surface with 20-29% third degree corrosion**
HAC see Appendix B for HAC conditional logic

+ T32.3 **Corrosions involving 30-39% of body surface**

CC T32.30 **Corrosions involving 30-39% of body surface with 0% to 9% third degree corrosion**
HAC see Appendix B for HAC conditional logic

MCC T32.31 **Corrosions involving 30-39% of body surface with 10-19% third degree corrosion**
HAC see Appendix B for HAC conditional logic

MCC T32.32 **Corrosions involving 30-39% of body surface with 20-29% third degree corrosion**
HAC see Appendix B for HAC conditional logic

MCC T32.33 **Corrosions involving 30-39% of body surface with 30-39% third degree corrosion**
HAC see Appendix B for HAC conditional logic

+ T32.4 **Corrosions involving 40-49% of body surface**

CC T32.40 **Corrosions involving 40-49% of body surface with 0% to 9% third degree corrosion**
HAC see Appendix B for HAC conditional logic

MCC T32.41 **Corrosions involving 40-49% of body surface with 10-19% third degree corrosion**
HAC see Appendix B for HAC conditional logic

MCC T32.42 **Corrosions involving 40-49% of body surface with 20-29% third degree corrosion**
HAC see Appendix B for HAC conditional logic

MCC T32.43 **Corrosions involving 40-49% of body surface with 30-39% third degree corrosion**
HAC see Appendix B for HAC conditional logic

MCC T32.44 **Corrosions involving 40-49% of body surface with 40-49% third degree corrosion**
HAC see Appendix B for HAC conditional logic

+ T32.5 **Corrosions involving 50-59% of body surface**

CC T32.50 **Corrosions involving 50-59% of body surface with 0% to 9% third degree corrosion**
HAC see Appendix B for HAC conditional logic

MCC T32.51 **Corrosions involving 50-59% of body surface with 10-19% third degree corrosion**
HAC see Appendix B for HAC conditional logic

MCC T32.52 **Corrosions involving 50-59% of body surface with 20-29% third degree corrosion**
HAC see Appendix B for HAC conditional logic

MCC T32.53 **Corrosions involving 50-59% of body surface with 30-39% third degree corrosion**
HAC see Appendix B for HAC conditional logic

MCC T32.54 **Corrosions involving 50-59% of body surface with 40-49% third degree corrosion**
HAC see Appendix B for HAC conditional logic

MCC T32.55 **Corrosions involving 50-59% of body surface with 50-59% third degree corrosion**
HAC see Appendix B for HAC conditional logic

+ **T32.6 Corrosions involving 60-69% of body surface**
  - CC **T32.60 Corrosions involving 60-69% of body surface with 0% to 9% third degree corrosion**
    HAC see Appendix B for HAC conditional logic
  - MCC **T32.61 Corrosions involving 60-69% of body surface with 10-19% third degree corrosion**
    HAC see Appendix B for HAC conditional logic
  - MCC **T32.62 Corrosions involving 60-69% of body surface with 20-29% third degree corrosion**
    HAC see Appendix B for HAC conditional logic
  - MCC **T32.63 Corrosions involving 60-69% of body surface with 30-39% third degree corrosion**
    HAC see Appendix B for HAC conditional logic
  - MCC **T32.64 Corrosions involving 60-69% of body surface with 40-49% third degree corrosion**
    HAC see Appendix B for HAC conditional logic
  - MCC **T32.65 Corrosions involving 60-69% of body surface with 50-59% third degree corrosion**
    HAC see Appendix B for HAC conditional logic
  - MCC **T32.66 Corrosions involving 60-69% of body surface with 60-69% third degree corrosion**
    HAC see Appendix B for HAC conditional logic

+ **T32.7 Corrosions involving 70-79% of body surface**
  - CC **T32.70 Corrosions involving 70-79% of body surface with 0% to 9% third degree corrosion**
    HAC see Appendix B for HAC conditional logic
  - MCC **T32.71 Corrosions involving 70-79% of body surface with 10-19% third degree corrosion**
    HAC see Appendix B for HAC conditional logic
  - MCC **T32.72 Corrosions involving 70-79% of body surface with 20-29% third degree corrosion**
    HAC see Appendix B for HAC conditional logic
  - MCC **T32.73 Corrosions involving 70-79% of body surface with 30-39% third degree corrosion**
    HAC see Appendix B for HAC conditional logic
  - MCC **T32.74 Corrosions involving 70-79% of body surface with 40-49% third degree corrosion**
    HAC see Appendix B for HAC conditional logic
  - MCC **T32.75 Corrosions involving 70-79% of body surface with 50-59% third degree corrosion**
    HAC see Appendix B for HAC conditional logic
  - MCC **T32.76 Corrosions involving 70-79% of body surface with 60-69% third degree corrosion**
    HAC see Appendix B for HAC conditional logic
  - MCC **T32.77 Corrosions involving 70-79% of body surface with 70-79% third degree corrosion**
    HAC see Appendix B for HAC conditional logic

+ **T32.8 Corrosions involving 80-89% of body surface**
  - CC **T32.80 Corrosions involving 80-89% of body surface with 0% to 9% third degree corrosion**
    HAC see Appendix B for HAC conditional logic
  - MCC **T32.81 Corrosions involving 80-89% of body surface with 10-19% third degree corrosion**
    HAC see Appendix B for HAC conditional logic
  - MCC **T32.82 Corrosions involving 80-89% of body surface with 20-29% third degree corrosion**
    HAC see Appendix B for HAC conditional logic
  - MCC **T32.83 Corrosions involving 80-89% of body surface with 30-39% third degree corrosion**
    HAC see Appendix B for HAC conditional logic
  - MCC **T32.84 Corrosions involving 80-89% of body surface with 40-49% third degree corrosion**
    HAC see Appendix B for HAC conditional logic
  - MCC **T32.85 Corrosions involving 80-89% of body surface with 50-59% third degree corrosion**
    HAC see Appendix B for HAC conditional logic
  - MCC **T32.86 Corrosions involving 80-89% of body surface with 60-69% third degree corrosion**
    HAC see Appendix B for HAC conditional logic
  - MCC **T32.87 Corrosions involving 80-89% of body surface with 70-79% third degree corrosion**
    HAC see Appendix B for HAC conditional logic
  - MCC **T32.88 Corrosions involving 80-89% of body surface with 80-89% third degree corrosion**
    HAC see Appendix B for HAC conditional logic

+ **T32.9 Corrosions involving 90% or more of body surface**
  - CC **T32.90 Corrosions involving 90% or more of body surface with 0% to 9% third degree corrosion**
    HAC see Appendix B for HAC conditional logic
  - MCC **T32.91 Corrosions involving 90% or more of body surface with 10-19% third degree corrosion**
    HAC see Appendix B for HAC conditional logic
  - MCC **T32.92 Corrosions involving 90% or more of body surface with 20-29% third degree corrosion**
    HAC see Appendix B for HAC conditional logic
  - MCC **T32.93 Corrosions involving 90% or more of body surface with 30-39% third degree corrosion**
    HAC see Appendix B for HAC conditional logic
  - MCC **T32.94 Corrosions involving 90% or more of body surface with 40-49% third degree corrosion**
    HAC see Appendix B for HAC conditional logic
  - MCC **T32.95 Corrosions involving 90% or more of body surface with 50-59% third degree corrosion**
    HAC see Appendix B for HAC conditional logic
  - MCC **T32.96 Corrosions involving 90% or more of body surface with 60-69% third degree corrosion**
    HAC see Appendix B for HAC conditional logic
  - MCC **T32.97 Corrosions involving 90% or more of body surface with 70-79% third degree corrosion**
    HAC see Appendix B for HAC conditional logic
  - MCC **T32.98 Corrosions involving 90% or more of body surface with 80-89% third degree corrosion**
    HAC see Appendix B for HAC conditional logic
  - MCC **T32.99 Corrosions involving 90% or more of body surface with 90% or more third degree corrosion**
    HAC see Appendix B for HAC conditional logic

Frostbite (T33-T34)

Excludes2: *hypothermia and other effects of reduced temperature (T68, T69.-)*

T33 Superficial frostbite

Includes: frostbite with partial thickness skin loss

> The appropriate 7th character is to be added to each code from category T33
> A initial encounter
> D subsequent encounter
> S sequela

+ **T33.0 Superficial frostbite of head**
  + **T33.01 Superficial frostbite of ear**
    - CC +7th **T33.011 Superficial frostbite of right ear**
      HAC 7th character A see Appendix B for HAC conditional logic
    - CC +7th **T33.012 Superficial frostbite of left ear**
      HAC 7th character A see Appendix B for HAC conditional logic
    - CC +7th **T33.019 Superficial frostbite of unspecified ear**
      HAC 7th character A see Appendix B for HAC conditional logic
  - CC X+7th **T33.02 Superficial frostbite of nose**
    HAC 7th character A see Appendix B for HAC conditional logic
  - CC X+7th **T33.09 Superficial frostbite of other part of head**
    HAC 7th character A see Appendix B for HAC conditional logic
- CC X+7th **T33.1 Superficial frostbite of neck**
  HAC 7th character A see Appendix B for HAC conditional logic
- CC X+7th **T33.2 Superficial frostbite of thorax**
  HAC 7th character A see Appendix B for HAC conditional logic
- CC X+7th **T33.3 Superficial frostbite of abdominal wall, lower back and pelvis**
  HAC 7th character A see Appendix B for HAC conditional logic
+ **T33.4 Superficial frostbite of arm**
  Excludes2: *superficial frostbite of wrist and hand (T33.5-)*
  - CC X+7th **T33.40 Superficial frostbite of unspecified arm**
    HAC 7th character A see Appendix B for HAC conditional logic
  - CC X+7th **T33.41 Superficial frostbite of right arm**
    HAC 7th character A see Appendix B for HAC conditional logic
  - CC X+7th **T33.42 Superficial frostbite of left arm**
    HAC 7th character A see Appendix B for HAC conditional logic

+ T33.5 **Superficial frostbite of wrist, hand, and fingers**

+ T33.51 **Superficial frostbite of wrist**

CC +7th T33.511 **Superficial frostbite of right wrist**
HAC 7th character A see Appendix B for HAC conditional logic

CC +7th T33.512 **Superficial frostbite of left wrist**
HAC 7th character A see Appendix B for HAC conditional logic

CC +7th T33.519 **Superficial frostbite of unspecified wrist**
HAC 7th character A see Appendix B for HAC conditional logic

+ T33.52 **Superficial frostbite of hand**
Excludes2: *superficial frostbite of fingers (T33.53-)*

CC +7th T33.521 **Superficial frostbite of right hand**
HAC 7th character A see Appendix B for HAC conditional logic

CC +7th T33.522 **Superficial frostbite of left hand**
HAC 7th character A see Appendix B for HAC conditional logic

CC +7th T33.529 **Superficial frostbite of unspecified hand**
HAC 7th character A see Appendix B for HAC conditional logic

+ T33.53 **Superficial frostbite of finger(s)**

CC +7th T33.531 **Superficial frostbite of right finger(s)**
HAC 7th character A see Appendix B for HAC conditional logic

CC +7th T33.532 **Superficial frostbite of left finger(s)**
HAC 7th character A see Appendix B for HAC conditional logic

CC +7th T33.539 **Superficial frostbite of unspecified finger(s)**
HAC 7th character A see Appendix B for HAC conditional logic

+ T33.6 **Superficial frostbite of hip and thigh**

CC X+7th T33.60 **Superficial frostbite of unspecified hip and thigh**
HAC 7th character A see Appendix B for HAC conditional logic

CC X+7th T33.61 **Superficial frostbite of right hip and thigh**
HAC 7th character A see Appendix B for HAC conditional logic

CC X+7th T33.62 **Superficial frostbite of left hip and thigh**
HAC 7th character A see Appendix B for HAC conditional logic

+ T33.7 **Superficial frostbite of knee and lower leg**
Excludes2: *superficial frostbite of ankle and foot (T33.8-)*

CC X+7th T33.70 **Superficial frostbite of unspecified knee and lower leg**
HAC 7th character A see Appendix B for HAC conditional logic

CC X+7th T33.71 **Superficial frostbite of right knee and lower leg**
HAC 7th character A see Appendix B for HAC conditional logic

CC X+7th T33.72 **Superficial frostbite of left knee and lower leg**
HAC 7th character A see Appendix B for HAC conditional logic

+ T33.8 **Superficial frostbite of ankle, foot, and toe(s)**

+ T33.81 **Superficial frostbite of ankle**

CC +7th T33.811 **Superficial frostbite of right ankle**
HAC 7th character A see Appendix B for HAC conditional logic

CC +7th T33.812 **Superficial frostbite of left ankle**
HAC 7th character A see Appendix B for HAC conditional logic

CC +7th T33.819 **Superficial frostbite of unspecified ankle**
HAC 7th character A see Appendix B for HAC conditional logic

+ T33.82 **Superficial frostbite of foot**

CC +7th T33.821 **Superficial frostbite of right foot**
HAC 7th character A see Appendix B for HAC conditional logic

CC +7th T33.822 **Superficial frostbite of left foot**
HAC 7th character A see Appendix B for HAC conditional logic

CC +7th T33.829 **Superficial frostbite of unspecified foot**
HAC 7th character A see Appendix B for HAC conditional logic

+ T33.83 **Superficial frostbite of toe(s)**

CC +7th T33.831 **Superficial frostbite of right toe(s)**
HAC 7th character A see Appendix B for HAC conditional logic

CC +7th T33.832 **Superficial frostbite of left toe(s)**
HAC 7th character A see Appendix B for HAC conditional logic

CC +7th T33.839 **Superficial frostbite of unspecified toe(s)**
HAC 7th character A see Appendix B for HAC conditional logic

+ T33.9 **Superficial frostbite of other and unspecified sites**

CC X+7th T33.90 **Superficial frostbite of unspecified sites**
Superficial frostbite NOS
HAC 7th character A see Appendix B for HAC conditional logic

CC X+7th T33.99 **Superficial frostbite of other sites**
Superficial frostbite of leg NOS
Superficial frostbite of trunk NOS
HAC 7th character A see Appendix B for HAC conditional logic

T34 Frostbite with tissue necrosis

The appropriate 7th character is to be added to each code from category T34
A initial encounter
D subsequent encounter
S sequela

+ T34.0 **Frostbite with tissue necrosis of head**

+ T34.01 **Frostbite with tissue necrosis of ear**

CC +7th T34.011 **Frostbite with tissue necrosis of right ear**
HAC 7th character A see Appendix B for HAC conditional logic

CC +7th T34.012 **Frostbite with tissue necrosis of left ear**
HAC 7th character A see Appendix B for HAC conditional logic

CC +7th T34.019 **Frostbite with tissue necrosis of unspecified ear**
HAC 7th character A see Appendix B for HAC conditional logic

CC X+7th T34.02 **Frostbite with tissue necrosis of nose**
HAC 7th character A see Appendix B for HAC conditional logic

CC X+7th T34.09 **Frostbite with tissue necrosis of other part of head**
HAC 7th character A see Appendix B for HAC conditional logic

CC X+7th T34.1 **Frostbite with tissue necrosis of neck**
HAC 7th character A see Appendix B for HAC conditional logic

CC X+7th T34.2 **Frostbite with tissue necrosis of thorax**
HAC 7th character A see Appendix B for HAC conditional logic

CC X+7th T34.3 **Frostbite with tissue necrosis of abdominal wall, lower back and pelvis**
HAC 7th character A see Appendix B for HAC conditional logic

+ T34.4 **Frostbite with tissue necrosis of arm**
Excludes2: *frostbite with tissue necrosis of wrist and hand (T34.5-)*

CC X+7th T34.40 **Frostbite with tissue necrosis of unspecified arm**
HAC 7th character A see Appendix B for HAC conditional logic

CC X+7th T34.41 **Frostbite with tissue necrosis of right arm**
HAC 7th character A see Appendix B for HAC conditional logic

CC X+7th T34.42 **Frostbite with tissue necrosis of left arm**
HAC 7th character A see Appendix B for HAC conditional logic

+ T34.5 **Frostbite with tissue necrosis of wrist, hand, and finger(s)**

+ T34.51 **Frostbite with tissue necrosis of wrist**

CC +7th T34.511 **Frostbite with tissue necrosis of right wrist**
HAC 7th character A see Appendix B for HAC conditional logic

CC +7th T34.512 **Frostbite with tissue necrosis of left wrist**
HAC 7th character A see Appendix B for HAC conditional logic

CC +7th T34.519 **Frostbite with tissue necrosis of unspecified wrist**
HAC 7th character A see Appendix B for HAC conditional logic

+ **T34.52 Frostbite with tissue necrosis of hand**
Excludes2: *frostbite with tissue necrosis of finger(s) (T34.53-)*
CC +7th **T34.521 Frostbite with tissue necrosis of right hand**
HAC 7th character A see Appendix B for HAC conditional logic
CC +7th **T34.522 Frostbite with tissue necrosis of left hand**
HAC 7th character A see Appendix B for HAC conditional logic
CC +7th **T34.529 Frostbite with tissue necrosis of unspecified hand**
HAC 7th character A see Appendix B for HAC conditional logic
+ **T34.53 Frostbite with tissue necrosis of finger(s)**
CC +7th **T34.531 Frostbite with tissue necrosis of right finger(s)**
HAC 7th character A see Appendix B for HAC conditional logic
CC +7th **T34.532 Frostbite with tissue necrosis of left finger(s)**
HAC 7th character A see Appendix B for HAC conditional logic
CC +7th **T34.539 Frostbite with tissue necrosis of unspecified finger(s)**
HAC 7th character A see Appendix B for HAC conditional logic
+ **T34.6 Frostbite with tissue necrosis of hip and thigh**
CC X+7th **T34.60 Frostbite with tissue necrosis of unspecified hip and thigh**
HAC 7th character A see Appendix B for HAC conditional logic
CC X+7th **T34.61 Frostbite with tissue necrosis of right hip and thigh**
HAC 7th character A see Appendix B for HAC conditional logic
CC X+7th **T34.62 Frostbite with tissue necrosis of left hip and thigh**
HAC 7th character A see Appendix B for HAC conditional logic
+ **T34.7 Frostbite with tissue necrosis of knee and lower leg**
Excludes2: *frostbite with tissue necrosis of ankle and foot (T34.8-)*
CC X+7th **T34.70 Frostbite with tissue necrosis of unspecified knee and lower leg**
HAC 7th character A see Appendix B for HAC conditional logic
CC X+7th **T34.71 Frostbite with tissue necrosis of right knee and lower leg**
HAC 7th character A see Appendix B for HAC conditional logic
CC X+7th **T34.72 Frostbite with tissue necrosis of left knee and lower leg**
HAC 7th character A see Appendix B for HAC conditional logic
+ **T34.8 Frostbite with tissue necrosis of ankle, foot, and toe(s)**
+ **T34.81 Frostbite with tissue necrosis of ankle**
CC +7th **T34.811 Frostbite with tissue necrosis of right ankle**
HAC 7th character A see Appendix B for HAC conditional logic
CC +7th **T34.812 Frostbite with tissue necrosis of left ankle**
HAC 7th character A see Appendix B for HAC conditional logic
CC +7th **T34.819 Frostbite with tissue necrosis of unspecified ankle**
HAC 7th character A see Appendix B for HAC conditional logic
+ **T34.82 Frostbite with tissue necrosis of foot**
CC +7th **T34.821 Frostbite with tissue necrosis of right foot**
HAC 7th character A see Appendix B for HAC conditional logic
CC +7th **T34.822 Frostbite with tissue necrosis of left foot**
HAC 7th character A see Appendix B for HAC conditional logic
CC +7th **T34.829 Frostbite with tissue necrosis of unspecified foot**
HAC 7th character A see Appendix B for HAC conditional logic
+ **T34.83 Frostbite with tissue necrosis of toe(s)**
CC +7th **T34.831 Frostbite with tissue necrosis of right toe(s)**
HAC 7th character A see Appendix B for HAC conditional logic
CC +7th **T34.832 Frostbite with tissue necrosis of left toe(s)**
HAC 7th character A see Appendix B for HAC conditional logic
CC +7th **T34.839 Frostbite with tissue necrosis of unspecified toe(s)**
HAC 7th character A see Appendix B for HAC conditional logic
+ **T34.9 Frostbite with tissue necrosis of other and unspecified sites**
CC X+7th **T34.90 Frostbite with tissue necrosis of unspecified sites**
Frostbite with tissue necrosis NOS
HAC 7th character A see Appendix B for HAC conditional logic
CC X+7th **T34.99 Frostbite with tissue necrosis of other sites**
Frostbite with tissue necrosis of leg NOS
Frostbite with tissue necrosis of trunk NOS
HAC 7th character A see Appendix B for HAC conditional logic

Poisoning by, adverse effects of and underdosing of drugs, medicaments and biological substances (T36-T50)

Includes: adverse effect of correct substance properly administered
poisoning by overdose of substance
poisoning by wrong substance given or taken in error
underdosing by (inadvertently) (deliberately) taking less substance than prescribed or instructed

Code first: for adverse effects, the nature of the adverse effect, such as:
adverse effect NOS (T88.7)
aspirin gastritis (K29.-)
blood disorders (D56-D76)
contact dermatitis (L23-L25)
dermatitis due to substances taken internally (L27.-)
nephropathy (N14.0-N14.2)

NOTE The drug giving rise to the adverse effect should be identified by use of codes from categories T36-T50 with fifth or sixth character 5.

Use additional: code(s) to specify:
manifestations of poisoning
underdosing or failure in dosage during medical and surgical care (Y63.6, Y63.8-Y63.9)
underdosing of medication regimen (Z91.12-, Z91.13-)

Excludes1: *toxic reaction to local anesthesia in pregnancy (O29.3-)*

Excludes2: *abuse and dependence of psychoactive substances (F10-F19)*
abuse of non-dependence-producing substances (F55.-)
drug reaction and poisoning affecting newborn (P00-P96)
immunodeficiency due to drugs (D84.821)
pathological drug intoxication (inebriation) (F10-F19)

Review coding guideline C.19.e

T36 Poisoning by, adverse effect of and underdosing of systemic antibiotics

Excludes1: *antineoplastic antibiotics (T45.1-)*
locally applied antibiotic NEC (T49.0)
topically used antibiotic for ear, nose and throat (T49.6)
topically used antibiotic for eye (T49.5)

The appropriate 7th character is to be added to each code from category T36
A initial encounter
D subsequent encounter
S sequela

+ **T36.0 Poisoning by, adverse effect of and underdosing of penicillins**
+ **T36.0X Poisoning by, adverse effect of and underdosing of penicillins**
+7th **T36.0X1 Poisoning by penicillins, accidental (unintentional)**
Poisoning by penicillins NOS
+7th **T36.0X2 Poisoning by penicillins, intentional self-harm**
+7th **T36.0X3 Poisoning by penicillins, assault**
+7th **T36.0X4 Poisoning by penicillins, undetermined**
+7th **T36.0X5 Adverse effect of penicillins**
+7th **T36.0X6 Underdosing of penicillins**

+ T36.1 Poisoning by, adverse effect of and underdosing of cephalosporins and other beta-lactam antibiotics

+ T36.1X Poisoning by, adverse effect of and underdosing of cephalosporins and other beta-lactam antibiotics

+7th **T36.1X1 Poisoning by cephalosporins and other beta-lactam antibiotics, accidental (unintentional)**
Poisoning by cephalosporins and other beta-lactam antibiotics NOS

+7th **T36.1X2 Poisoning by cephalosporins and other beta-lactam antibiotics, intentional self-harm**

+7th **T36.1X3 Poisoning by cephalosporins and other beta-lactam antibiotics, assault**

+7th **T36.1X4 Poisoning by cephalosporins and other beta-lactam antibiotics, undetermined**

+7th **T36.1X5 Adverse effect of cephalosporins and other beta-lactam antibiotics**

+7th **T36.1X6 Underdosing of cephalosporins and other beta-lactam antibiotics**

+ T36.2 Poisoning by, adverse effect of and underdosing of chloramphenicol group

+ T36.2X Poisoning by, adverse effect of and underdosing of chloramphenicol group

+7th **T36.2X1 Poisoning by chloramphenicol group, accidental (unintentional)**
Poisoning by chloramphenicol group NOS

+7th **T36.2X2 Poisoning by chloramphenicol group, intentional self-harm**

+7th **T36.2X3 Poisoning by chloramphenicol group, assault**

+7th **T36.2X4 Poisoning by chloramphenicol group, undetermined**

+7th **T36.2X5 Adverse effect of chloramphenicol group**

+7th **T36.2X6 Underdosing of chloramphenicol group**

+ T36.3 Poisoning by, adverse effect of and underdosing of macrolides

+ T36.3X Poisoning by, adverse effect of and underdosing of macrolides

+7th **T36.3X1 Poisoning by macrolides, accidental (unintentional)**
Poisoning by macrolides NOS

+7th **T36.3X2 Poisoning by macrolides, intentional self-harm**

+7th **T36.3X3 Poisoning by macrolides, assault**

+7th **T36.3X4 Poisoning by macrolides, undetermined**

+7th **T36.3X5 Adverse effect of macrolides**

+7th **T36.3X6 Underdosing of macrolides**

+ T36.4 Poisoning by, adverse effect of and underdosing of tetracyclines

+ T36.4X Poisoning by, adverse effect of and underdosing of tetracyclines

+7th **T36.4X1 Poisoning by tetracyclines, accidental (unintentional)**
Poisoning by tetracyclines NOS

+7th **T36.4X2 Poisoning by tetracyclines, intentional self-harm**

+7th **T36.4X3 Poisoning by tetracyclines, assault**

+7th **T36.4X4 Poisoning by tetracyclines, undetermined**

+7th **T36.4X5 Adverse effect of tetracyclines**

+7th **T36.4X6 Underdosing of tetracyclines**

+ T36.5 Poisoning by, adverse effect of and underdosing of aminoglycosides
Poisoning by, adverse effect of and underdosing of streptomycin

+ T36.5X Poisoning by, adverse effect of and underdosing of aminoglycosides

+7th **T36.5X1 Poisoning by aminoglycosides, accidental (unintentional)**
Poisoning by aminoglycosides NOS

+7th **T36.5X2 Poisoning by aminoglycosides, intentional self-harm**

+7th **T36.5X3 Poisoning by aminoglycosides, assault**

+7th **T36.5X4 Poisoning by aminoglycosides, undetermined**

+7th **T36.5X5 Adverse effect of aminoglycosides**

+7th **T36.5X6 Underdosing of aminoglycosides**

+ T36.6 Poisoning by, adverse effect of and underdosing of rifampicins

+ T36.6X Poisoning by, adverse effect of and underdosing of rifampicins

+7th **T36.6X1 Poisoning by rifampicins, accidental (unintentional)**
Poisoning by rifampicins NOS

+7th **T36.6X2 Poisoning by rifampicins, intentional self-harm**

+7th **T36.6X3 Poisoning by rifampicins, assault**

+7th **T36.6X4 Poisoning by rifampicins, undetermined**

+7th **T36.6X5 Adverse effect of rifampicins**

+7th **T36.6X6 Underdosing of rifampicins**

+ T36.7 Poisoning by, adverse effect of and underdosing of antifungal antibiotics, systemically used

+ T36.7X Poisoning by, adverse effect of and underdosing of antifungal antibiotics, systemically used

+7th **T36.7X1 Poisoning by antifungal antibiotics, systemically used, accidental (unintentional)**
Poisoning by antifungal antibiotics, systemically used NOS

+7th **T36.7X2 Poisoning by antifungal antibiotics, systemically used, intentional self-harm**

+7th **T36.7X3 Poisoning by antifungal antibiotics, systemically used, assault**

+7th **T36.7X4 Poisoning by antifungal antibiotics, systemically used, undetermined**

+7th **T36.7X5 Adverse effect of antifungal antibiotics, systemically used**

+7th **T36.7X6 Underdosing of antifungal antibiotics, systemically used**

+ T36.8 Poisoning by, adverse effect of and underdosing of other systemic antibiotics

+ T36.8X Poisoning by, adverse effect of and underdosing of other systemic antibiotics

+7th **T36.8X1 Poisoning by other systemic antibiotics, accidental (unintentional)**
Poisoning by other systemic antibiotics NOS

+7th **T36.8X2 Poisoning by other systemic antibiotics, intentional self-harm**

+7th **T36.8X3 Poisoning by other systemic antibiotics, assault**

+7th **T36.8X4 Poisoning by other systemic antibiotics, undetermined**

+7th **T36.8X5 Adverse effect of other systemic antibiotics**
AHA CC: 1Q, 2017, 39

+7th **T36.8X6 Underdosing of other systemic antibiotics**

+ T36.9 Poisoning by, adverse effect of and underdosing of unspecified systemic antibiotic

X+7th **T36.91 Poisoning by unspecified systemic antibiotic, accidental (unintentional)**
Poisoning by systemic antibiotic NOS

X+7th **T36.92 Poisoning by unspecified systemic antibiotic, intentional self-harm**

X+7th **T36.93 Poisoning by unspecified systemic antibiotic, assault**

X+7th **T36.94 Poisoning by unspecified systemic antibiotic, undetermined**

X+7th **T36.95 Adverse effect of unspecified systemic antibiotic**

X+7th **T36.96 Underdosing of unspecified systemic antibiotic**

T37 Poisoning by, adverse effect of and underdosing of other systemic anti-infectives and antiparasitics

Excludes1: *anti-infectives topically used for ear, nose and throat (T49.6-)*
anti-infectives topically used for eye (T49.5-)
locally applied anti-infectives NEC (T49.0-)

The appropriate 7th character is to be added to each code from category T37
A initial encounter
D subsequent encounter
S sequela

+ **T37.0 Poisoning by, adverse effect of and underdosing of sulfonamides**
  + **T37.0X Poisoning by, adverse effect of and underdosing of sulfonamides**
    - +7th **T37.0X1 Poisoning by sulfonamides, accidental (unintentional)**
      Poisoning by sulfonamides NOS
    - +7th **T37.0X2 Poisoning by sulfonamides, intentional self-harm**
    - +7th **T37.0X3 Poisoning by sulfonamides, assault**
    - +7th **T37.0X4 Poisoning by sulfonamides, undetermined**
    - +7th **T37.0X5 Adverse effect of sulfonamides**
    - +7th **T37.0X6 Underdosing of sulfonamides**

+ **T37.1 Poisoning by, adverse effect of and underdosing of antimycobacterial drugs**
  Excludes1: *rifampicins (T36.6-)*
  streptomycin (T36.5-)
  + **T37.1X Poisoning by, adverse effect of and underdosing of antimycobacterial drugs**
    - +7th **T37.1X1 Poisoning by antimycobacterial drugs, accidental (unintentional)**
      Poisoning by antimycobacterial drugs NOS
    - +7th **T37.1X2 Poisoning by antimycobacterial drugs, intentional self-harm**
    - +7th **T37.1X3 Poisoning by antimycobacterial drugs, assault**
    - +7th **T37.1X4 Poisoning by antimycobacterial drugs, undetermined**
    - +7th **T37.1X5 Adverse effect of antimycobacterial drugs**
    - +7th **T37.1X6 Underdosing of antimycobacterial drugs**

+ **T37.2 Poisoning by, adverse effect of and underdosing of antimalarials and drugs acting on other blood protozoa**
  Excludes1: *hydroxyquinoline derivatives (T37.8-)*
  + **T37.2X Poisoning by, adverse effect of and underdosing of antimalarials and drugs acting on other blood protozoa**
    - +7th **T37.2X1 Poisoning by antimalarials and drugs acting on other blood protozoa, accidental (unintentional)**
      Poisoning by antimalarials and drugs acting on other blood protozoa NOS
    - +7th **T37.2X2 Poisoning by antimalarials and drugs acting on other blood protozoa, intentional self-harm**
    - +7th **T37.2X3 Poisoning by antimalarials and drugs acting on other blood protozoa, assault**
    - +7th **T37.2X4 Poisoning by antimalarials and drugs acting on other blood protozoa, undetermined**
    - +7th **T37.2X5 Adverse effect of antimalarials and drugs acting on other blood protozoa**
    - +7th **T37.2X6 Underdosing of antimalarials and drugs acting on other blood protozoa**

+ **T37.3 Poisoning by, adverse effect of and underdosing of other antiprotozoal drugs**
  + **T37.3X Poisoning by, adverse effect of and underdosing of other antiprotozoal drugs**
    - +7th **T37.3X1 Poisoning by other antiprotozoal drugs, accidental (unintentional)**
      Poisoning by other antiprotozoal drugs NOS
    - +7th **T37.3X2 Poisoning by other antiprotozoal drugs, intentional self-harm**
    - +7th **T37.3X3 Poisoning by other antiprotozoal drugs, assault**
    - +7th **T37.3X4 Poisoning by other antiprotozoal drugs, undetermined**
    - +7th **T37.3X5 Adverse effect of other antiprotozoal drugs**
    - +7th **T37.3X6 Underdosing of other antiprotozoal drugs**

+ **T37.4 Poisoning by, adverse effect of and underdosing of anthelminthics**
  + **T37.4X Poisoning by, adverse effect of and underdosing of anthelminthics**
    - +7th **T37.4X1 Poisoning by anthelminthics, accidental (unintentional)**
      Poisoning by anthelminthics NOS
    - +7th **T37.4X2 Poisoning by anthelminthics, intentional self-harm**
    - +7th **T37.4X3 Poisoning by anthelminthics, assault**
    - +7th **T37.4X4 Poisoning by anthelminthics, undetermined**
    - +7th **T37.4X5 Adverse effect of anthelminthics**
    - +7th **T37.4X6 Underdosing of anthelminthics**

+ **T37.5 Poisoning by, adverse effect of and underdosing of antiviral drugs**
  Excludes1: *amantadine (T42.8-)*
  cytarabine (T45.1-)
  + **T37.5X Poisoning by, adverse effect of and underdosing of antiviral drugs**
    - +7th **T37.5X1 Poisoning by antiviral drugs, accidental (unintentional)**
      Poisoning by antiviral drugs NOS
    - +7th **T37.5X2 Poisoning by antiviral drugs, intentional self-harm**
    - +7th **T37.5X3 Poisoning by antiviral drugs, assault**
    - +7th **T37.5X4 Poisoning by antiviral drugs, undetermined**
    - +7th **T37.5X5 Adverse effect of antiviral drugs**
    - +7th **T37.5X6 Underdosing of antiviral drugs**

+ **T37.8 Poisoning by, adverse effect of and underdosing of other specified systemic anti-infectives and antiparasitics**
  Poisoning by, adverse effect of and underdosing of hydroxyquinoline derivatives
  Excludes1: *antimalarial drugs (T37.2-)*
  + **T37.8X Poisoning by, adverse effect of and underdosing of other specified systemic anti-infectives and antiparasitics**
    - +7th **T37.8X1 Poisoning by other specified systemic anti-infectives and antiparasitics, accidental (unintentional)**
      Poisoning by other specified systemic anti-infectives and antiparasitics NOS
    - +7th **T37.8X2 Poisoning by other specified systemic anti-infectives and antiparasitics, intentional self-harm**
    - +7th **T37.8X3 Poisoning by other specified systemic anti-infectives and antiparasitics, assault**
    - +7th **T37.8X4 Poisoning by other specified systemic anti-infectives and antiparasitics, undetermined**
    - +7th **T37.8X5 Adverse effect of other specified systemic anti-infectives and antiparasitics**
    - +7th **T37.8X6 Underdosing of other specified systemic anti-infectives and antiparasitics**

+ **T37.9 Poisoning by, adverse effect of and underdosing of unspecified systemic anti-infective and antiparasitics**
  - X+7th **T37.91 Poisoning by unspecified systemic anti-infective and antiparasitics, accidental (unintentional)**
    Poisoning by, adverse effect of and underdosing of systemic anti-infective and antiparasitics NOS
  - X+7th **T37.92 Poisoning by unspecified systemic anti-infective and antiparasitics, intentional self-harm**
  - X+7th **T37.93 Poisoning by unspecified systemic anti-infective and antiparasitics, assault**
  - X+7th **T37.94 Poisoning by unspecified systemic anti-infective and antiparasitics, undetermined**
  - X+7th **T37.95 Adverse effect of unspecified systemic anti-infective and antiparasitic**
  - X+7th **T37.96 Underdosing of unspecified systemic anti-infectives and antiparasitics**

T38 Poisoning by, adverse effect of and underdosing of hormones and their synthetic substitutes and antagonists, not elsewhere classified

Excludes1: *mineralocorticoids and their antagonists (T50.0-)*
oxytocic hormones (T48.0-)
parathyroid hormones and derivatives (T50.9-)

The appropriate 7th character is to be added to each code from category T38
A initial encounter
D subsequent encounter
S sequela

\+ **T38.0 Poisoning by, adverse effect of and underdosing of glucocorticoids and synthetic analogues**
Excludes1: *glucocorticoids, topically used (T49.-)*
\+ **T38.0X Poisoning by, adverse effect of and underdosing of glucocorticoids and synthetic analogues**
+7th **T38.0X1 Poisoning by glucocorticoids and synthetic analogues, accidental (unintentional)**
Poisoning by glucocorticoids and synthetic analogues NOS
+7th **T38.0X2 Poisoning by glucocorticoids and synthetic analogues, intentional self-harm**
+7th **T38.0X3 Poisoning by glucocorticoids and synthetic analogues, assault**
+7th **T38.0X4 Poisoning by glucocorticoids and synthetic analogues, undetermined**
+7th **T38.0X5 Adverse effect of glucocorticoids and synthetic analogues**
+7th **T38.0X6 Underdosing of glucocorticoids and synthetic analogues**

\+ **T38.1 Poisoning by, adverse effect of and underdosing of thyroid hormones and substitutes**
\+ **T38.1X Poisoning by, adverse effect of and underdosing of thyroid hormones and substitutes**
+7th **T38.1X1 Poisoning by thyroid hormones and substitutes, accidental (unintentional)**
Poisoning by thyroid hormones and substitutes NOS
+7th **T38.1X2 Poisoning by thyroid hormones and substitutes, intentional self-harm**
+7th **T38.1X3 Poisoning by thyroid hormones and substitutes, assault**
+7th **T38.1X4 Poisoning by thyroid hormones and substitutes, undetermined**
+7th **T38.1X5 Adverse effect of thyroid hormones and substitutes**
+7th **T38.1X6 Underdosing of thyroid hormones and substitutes**

\+ **T38.2 Poisoning by, adverse effect of and underdosing of antithyroid drugs**
\+ **T38.2X Poisoning by, adverse effect of and underdosing of antithyroid drugs**
+7th **T38.2X1 Poisoning by antithyroid drugs, accidental (unintentional)**
Poisoning by antithyroid drugs NOS
+7th **T38.2X2 Poisoning by antithyroid drugs, intentional self-harm**
+7th **T38.2X3 Poisoning by antithyroid drugs, assault**
+7th **T38.2X4 Poisoning by antithyroid drugs, undetermined**
+7th **T38.2X5 Adverse effect of antithyroid drugs**
+7th **T38.2X6 Underdosing of antithyroid drugs**

\+ **T38.3 Poisoning by, adverse effect of and underdosing of insulin and oral hypoglycemic [antidiabetic] drugs**
\+ **T38.3X Poisoning by, adverse effect of and underdosing of insulin and oral hypoglycemic [antidiabetic] drugs**
+7th **T38.3X1 Poisoning by insulin and oral hypoglycemic [antidiabetic] drugs, accidental (unintentional)**
Poisoning by insulin and oral hypoglycemic [antidiabetic] drugs NOS
Review coding guideline C.4.a.5.b
+7th **T38.3X2 Poisoning by insulin and oral hypoglycemic [antidiabetic] drugs, intentional self-harm**
+7th **T38.3X3 Poisoning by insulin and oral hypoglycemic [antidiabetic] drugs, assault**
+7th **T38.3X4 Poisoning by insulin and oral hypoglycemic [antidiabetic] drugs, undetermined**
+7th **T38.3X5 Adverse effect of insulin and oral hypoglycemic [antidiabetic] drugs**
+7th **T38.3X6 Underdosing of insulin and oral hypoglycemic [antidiabetic] drugs**
Review coding guideline C.4.a.5.a

\+ **T38.4 Poisoning by, adverse effect of and underdosing of oral contraceptives**
Poisoning by, adverse effect of and underdosing of multiple- and single-ingredient oral contraceptive preparations
\+ **T38.4X Poisoning by, adverse effect of and underdosing of oral contraceptives**
+7th **T38.4X1 Poisoning by oral contraceptives, accidental (unintentional)**
Poisoning by oral contraceptives NOS
+7th **T38.4X2 Poisoning by oral contraceptives, intentional self-harm**
+7th **T38.4X3 Poisoning by oral contraceptives, assault**
+7th **T38.4X4 Poisoning by oral contraceptives, undetermined**
+7th **T38.4X5 Adverse effect of oral contraceptives**
+7th **T38.4X6 Underdosing of oral contraceptives**

\+ **T38.5 Poisoning by, adverse effect of and underdosing of other estrogens and progestogens**
Poisoning by, adverse effect of and underdosing of estrogens and progestogens mixtures and substitutes
\+ **T38.5X Poisoning by, adverse effect of and underdosing of other estrogens and progestogens**
+7th **T38.5X1 Poisoning by other estrogens and progestogens, accidental (unintentional)**
Poisoning by other estrogens and progestogens NOS
+7th **T38.5X2 Poisoning by other estrogens and progestogens, intentional self-harm**
+7th **T38.5X3 Poisoning by other estrogens and progestogens, assault**
+7th **T38.5X4 Poisoning by other estrogens and progestogens, undetermined**
+7th **T38.5X5 Adverse effect of other estrogens and progestogens**
+7th **T38.5X6 Underdosing of other estrogens and progestogens**

\+ **T38.6 Poisoning by, adverse effect of and underdosing of antigonadotrophins, antiestrogens, antiandrogens, not elsewhere classified**
Poisoning by, adverse effect of and underdosing of tamoxifen
\+ **T38.6X Poisoning by, adverse effect of and underdosing of antigonadotrophins, antiestrogens, antiandrogens, not elsewhere classified**
+7th **T38.6X1 Poisoning by antigonadotrophins, antiestrogens, antiandrogens, not elsewhere classified, accidental (unintentional)**
Poisoning by antigonadotrophins, antiestrogens, antiandrogens, not elsewhere classified NOS
+7th **T38.6X2 Poisoning by antigonadotrophins, antiestrogens, antiandrogens, not elsewhere classified, intentional self-harm**
+7th **T38.6X3 Poisoning by antigonadotrophins, antiestrogens, antiandrogens, not elsewhere classified, assault**
+7th **T38.6X4 Poisoning by antigonadotrophins, antiestrogens, antiandrogens, not elsewhere classified, undetermined**
+7th **T38.6X5 Adverse effect of antigonadotrophins, antiestrogens, antiandrogens, not elsewhere classified**
+7th **T38.6X6 Underdosing of antigonadotrophins, antiestrogens, antiandrogens, not elsewhere classified**

+ T38.7 Poisoning by, adverse effect of and underdosing of androgens and anabolic congeners

+ T38.7X Poisoning by, adverse effect of and underdosing of androgens and anabolic congeners

+7th **T38.7X1 Poisoning by androgens and anabolic congeners, accidental (unintentional)**
Poisoning by androgens and anabolic congeners NOS

+7th **T38.7X2 Poisoning by androgens and anabolic congeners, intentional self-harm**

+7th **T38.7X3 Poisoning by androgens and anabolic congeners, assault**

+7th **T38.7X4 Poisoning by androgens and anabolic congeners, undetermined**

+7th **T38.7X5 Adverse effect of androgens and anabolic congeners**

+7th **T38.7X6 Underdosing of androgens and anabolic congeners**

+ T38.8 Poisoning by, adverse effect of and underdosing of other and unspecified hormones and synthetic substitutes

+ T38.80 Poisoning by, adverse effect of and underdosing of unspecified hormones and synthetic substitutes

+7th **T38.801 Poisoning by unspecified hormones and synthetic substitutes, accidental (unintentional)**
Poisoning by unspecified hormones and synthetic substitutes NOS

+7th **T38.802 Poisoning by unspecified hormones and synthetic substitutes, intentional self-harm**

+7th **T38.803 Poisoning by unspecified hormones and synthetic substitutes, assault**

+7th **T38.804 Poisoning by unspecified hormones and synthetic substitutes, undetermined**

+7th **T38.805 Adverse effect of unspecified hormones and synthetic substitutes**

+7th **T38.806 Underdosing of unspecified hormones and synthetic substitutes**

+ T38.81 Poisoning by, adverse effect of and underdosing of anterior pituitary [adenohypophyseal] hormones

+7th **T38.811 Poisoning by anterior pituitary [adenohypophyseal] hormones, accidental (unintentional)**
Poisoning by anterior pituitary [adenohypophyseal] hormones NOS

+7th **T38.812 Poisoning by anterior pituitary [adenohypophyseal] hormones, intentional self-harm**

+7th **T38.813 Poisoning by anterior pituitary [adenohypophyseal] hormones, assault**

+7th **T38.814 Poisoning by anterior pituitary [adenohypophyseal] hormones, undetermined**

+7th **T38.815 Adverse effect of anterior pituitary [adenohypophyseal] hormones**

+7th **T38.816 Underdosing of anterior pituitary [adenohypophyseal] hormones**

+ T38.89 Poisoning by, adverse effect of and underdosing of other hormones and synthetic substitutes

+7th **T38.891 Poisoning by other hormones and synthetic substitutes, accidental (unintentional)**
Poisoning by other hormones and synthetic substitutes NOS

+7th **T38.892 Poisoning by other hormones and synthetic substitutes, intentional self-harm**

+7th **T38.893 Poisoning by other hormones and synthetic substitutes, assault**

+7th **T38.894 Poisoning by other hormones and synthetic substitutes, undetermined**

+7th **T38.895 Adverse effect of other hormones and synthetic substitutes**

+7th **T38.896 Underdosing of other hormones and synthetic substitutes**

+ T38.9 Poisoning by, adverse effect of and underdosing of other and unspecified hormone antagonists

+ T38.90 Poisoning by, adverse effect of and underdosing of unspecified hormone antagonists

+7th **T38.901 Poisoning by unspecified hormone antagonists, accidental (unintentional)**
Poisoning by unspecified hormone antagonists NOS

+7th **T38.902 Poisoning by unspecified hormone antagonists, intentional self-harm**

+7th **T38.903 Poisoning by unspecified hormone antagonists, assault**

+7th **T38.904 Poisoning by unspecified hormone antagonists, undetermined**

+7th **T38.905 Adverse effect of unspecified hormone antagonists**

+7th **T38.906 Underdosing of unspecified hormone antagonists**

+ T38.99 Poisoning by, adverse effect of and underdosing of other hormone antagonists

+7th **T38.991 Poisoning by other hormone antagonists, accidental (unintentional)**
Poisoning by other hormone antagonists NOS

+7th **T38.992 Poisoning by other hormone antagonists, intentional self-harm**

+7th **T38.993 Poisoning by other hormone antagonists, assault**

+7th **T38.994 Poisoning by other hormone antagonists, undetermined**

+7th **T38.995 Adverse effect of other hormone antagonists**

+7th **T38.996 Underdosing of other hormone antagonists**

T39 Poisoning by, adverse effect of and underdosing of nonopioid analgesics, antipyretics and antirheumatics

The appropriate 7th character is to be added to each code from category T39
A initial encounter
D subsequent encounter
S sequela

+ T39.0 Poisoning by, adverse effect of and underdosing of salicylates

+ T39.01 Poisoning by, adverse effect of and underdosing of aspirin
Poisoning by, adverse effect of and underdosing of acetylsalicylic acid

+7th **T39.011 Poisoning by aspirin, accidental (unintentional)**

+7th **T39.012 Poisoning by aspirin, intentional self-harm**

+7th **T39.013 Poisoning by aspirin, assault**

+7th **T39.014 Poisoning by aspirin, undetermined**

+7th **T39.015 Adverse effect of aspirin**
AHA CC: 1Q, 2016, 15

+7th **T39.016 Underdosing of aspirin**

+ T39.09 Poisoning by, adverse effect of and underdosing of other salicylates

+7th **T39.091 Poisoning by salicylates, accidental (unintentional)**
Poisoning by salicylates NOS

+7th **T39.092 Poisoning by salicylates, intentional self-harm**

+7th **T39.093 Poisoning by salicylates, assault**

+7th **T39.094 Poisoning by salicylates, undetermined**

+7th **T39.095 Adverse effect of salicylates**

+7th **T39.096 Underdosing of salicylates**

+ T39.1 Poisoning by, adverse effect of and underdosing of 4-Aminophenol derivatives

+ T39.1X Poisoning by, adverse effect of and underdosing of 4-Aminophenol derivatives

+7th **T39.1X1 Poisoning by 4-Aminophenol derivatives, accidental (unintentional)**
Poisoning by 4-Aminophenol derivatives NOS

+7th **T39.1X2 Poisoning by 4-Aminophenol derivatives, intentional self-harm**

+7th **T39.1X3 Poisoning by 4-Aminophenol derivatives, assault**

+7th **T39.1X4 Poisoning by 4-Aminophenol derivatives, undetermined**

+7th **T39.1X5 Adverse effect of 4-Aminophenol derivatives**

+7th **T39.1X6 Underdosing of 4-Aminophenol derivatives**

+ **T39.2 Poisoning by, adverse effect of and underdosing of pyrazolone derivatives**

+ **T39.2X Poisoning by, adverse effect of and underdosing of pyrazolone derivatives**

+7th **T39.2X1 Poisoning by pyrazolone derivatives, accidental (unintentional)**

Poisoning by pyrazolone derivatives NOS

+7th **T39.2X2 Poisoning by pyrazolone derivatives, intentional self-harm**

+7th **T39.2X3 Poisoning by pyrazolone derivatives, assault**

+7th **T39.2X4 Poisoning by pyrazolone derivatives, undetermined**

+7th **T39.2X5 Adverse effect of pyrazolone derivatives**

+7th **T39.2X6 Underdosing of pyrazolone derivatives**

+ **T39.3 Poisoning by, adverse effect of and underdosing of other nonsteroidal anti-inflammatory drugs [NSAID]**

+ **T39.31 Poisoning by, adverse effect of and underdosing of propionic acid derivatives**

Poisoning by, adverse effect of and underdosing of fenoprofen

Poisoning by, adverse effect of and underdosing of flurbiprofen

Poisoning by, adverse effect of and underdosing of ibuprofen

Poisoning by, adverse effect of and underdosing of ketoprofen

Poisoning by, adverse effect of and underdosing of naproxen

Poisoning by, adverse effect of and underdosing of oxaprozin

+7th **T39.311 Poisoning by propionic acid derivatives, accidental (unintentional)**

+7th **T39.312 Poisoning by propionic acid derivatives, intentional self-harm**

+7th **T39.313 Poisoning by propionic acid derivatives, assault**

+7th **T39.314 Poisoning by propionic acid derivatives, undetermined**

+7th **T39.315 Adverse effect of propionic acid derivatives**

+7th **T39.316 Underdosing of propionic acid derivatives**

+ **T39.39 Poisoning by, adverse effect of and underdosing of other nonsteroidal anti-inflammatory drugs [NSAID]**

+7th **T39.391 Poisoning by other nonsteroidal anti-inflammatory drugs [NSAID], accidental (unintentional)**

Poisoning by other nonsteroidal anti-inflammatory drugs NOS

+7th **T39.392 Poisoning by other nonsteroidal anti-inflammatory drugs [NSAID], intentional self-harm**

+7th **T39.393 Poisoning by other nonsteroidal anti-inflammatory drugs [NSAID], assault**

+7th **T39.394 Poisoning by other nonsteroidal anti-inflammatory drugs [NSAID], undetermined**

+7th **T39.395 Adverse effect of other nonsteroidal anti-inflammatory drugs [NSAID]**

+7th **T39.396 Underdosing of other nonsteroidal anti-inflammatory drugs [NSAID]**

+ **T39.4 Poisoning by, adverse effect of and underdosing of antirheumatics, not elsewhere classified**

Excludes1: *poisoning by, adverse effect of and underdosing of glucocorticoids (T38.0-)*
poisoning by, adverse effect of and underdosing of salicylates (T39.0-)

+ **T39.4X Poisoning by, adverse effect of and underdosing of antirheumatics, not elsewhere classified**

+7th **T39.4X1 Poisoning by antirheumatics, not elsewhere classified, accidental (unintentional)**

Poisoning by antirheumatics, not elsewhere classified NOS

+7th **T39.4X2 Poisoning by antirheumatics, not elsewhere classified, intentional self-harm**

+7th **T39.4X3 Poisoning by antirheumatics, not elsewhere classified, assault**

+7th **T39.4X4 Poisoning by antirheumatics, not elsewhere classified, undetermined**

+7th **T39.4X5 Adverse effect of antirheumatics, not elsewhere classified**

+7th **T39.4X6 Underdosing of antirheumatics, not elsewhere classified**

+ **T39.8 Poisoning by, adverse effect of and underdosing of other nonopioid analgesics and antipyretics, not elsewhere classified**

+ **T39.8X Poisoning by, adverse effect of and underdosing of other nonopioid analgesics and antipyretics, not elsewhere classified**

+7th **T39.8X1 Poisoning by other nonopioid analgesics and antipyretics, not elsewhere classified, accidental (unintentional)**

Poisoning by other nonopioid analgesics and antipyretics, not elsewhere classified NOS

+7th **T39.8X2 Poisoning by other nonopioid analgesics and antipyretics, not elsewhere classified, intentional self-harm**

+7th **T39.8X3 Poisoning by other nonopioid analgesics and antipyretics, not elsewhere classified, assault**

+7th **T39.8X4 Poisoning by other nonopioid analgesics and antipyretics, not elsewhere classified, undetermined**

+7th **T39.8X5 Adverse effect of other nonopioid analgesics and antipyretics, not elsewhere classified**

+7th **T39.8X6 Underdosing of other nonopioid analgesics and antipyretics, not elsewhere classified**

+ **T39.9 Poisoning by, adverse effect of and underdosing of unspecified nonopioid analgesic, antipyretic and antirheumatic**

x+7th **T39.91 Poisoning by unspecified nonopioid analgesic, antipyretic and antirheumatic, accidental (unintentional)**

Poisoning by nonopioid analgesic, antipyretic and antirheumatic NOS

x+7th **T39.92 Poisoning by unspecified nonopioid analgesic, antipyretic and antirheumatic, intentional self-harm**

x+7th **T39.93 Poisoning by unspecified nonopioid analgesic, antipyretic and antirheumatic, assault**

x+7th **T39.94 Poisoning by unspecified nonopioid analgesic, antipyretic and antirheumatic, undetermined**

x+7th **T39.95 Adverse effect of unspecified nonopioid analgesic, antipyretic and antirheumatic**

x+7th **T39.96 Underdosing of unspecified nonopioid analgesic, antipyretic and antirheumatic**

T40 Poisoning by, adverse effect of and underdosing of narcotics and psychodysleptics [hallucinogens]

Excludes2: *drug dependence and related mental and behavioral disorders due to psychoactive substance use (F10.-F19.-)*

The appropriate 7th character is to be added to each code from category T40
A initial encounter
D subsequent encounter
S sequela

+ **T40.0 Poisoning by, adverse effect of and underdosing of opium**

+ **T40.0X Poisoning by, adverse effect of and underdosing of opium**

+7th **T40.0X1 Poisoning by opium, accidental (unintentional)**

Poisoning by opium NOS

+7th **T40.0X2 Poisoning by opium, intentional self-harm**
+7th **T40.0X3 Poisoning by opium, assault**
+7th **T40.0X4 Poisoning by opium, undetermined**
+7th **T40.0X5 Adverse effect of opium**
+7th **T40.0X6 Underdosing of opium**

+ **T40.1 Poisoning by and adverse effect of heroin**
+ **T40.1X Poisoning by and adverse effect of heroin**
+7th **T40.1X1 Poisoning by heroin, accidental (unintentional)**
Poisoning by heroin NOS
+7th **T40.1X2 Poisoning by heroin, intentional self-harm**
+7th **T40.1X3 Poisoning by heroin, assault**
+7th **T40.1X4 Poisoning by heroin, undetermined**

+ **T40.2 Poisoning by, adverse effect of and underdosing of other opioids**
+ **T40.2X Poisoning by, adverse effect of and underdosing of other opioids**
+7th **T40.2X1 Poisoning by other opioids, accidental (unintentional)**
Poisoning by other opioids NOS
+7th **T40.2X2 Poisoning by other opioids, intentional self-harm**
+7th **T40.2X3 Poisoning by other opioids, assault**
+7th **T40.2X4 Poisoning by other opioids, undetermined**
+7th **T40.2X5 Adverse effect of other opioids**
AHA CC: 2Q, 2020, 24
+7th **T40.2X6 Underdosing of other opioids**

+ **T40.3 Poisoning by, adverse effect of and underdosing of methadone**
+ **T40.3X Poisoning by, adverse effect of and underdosing of methadone**
+7th **T40.3X1 Poisoning by methadone, accidental (unintentional)**
Poisoning by methadone NOS
+7th **T40.3X2 Poisoning by methadone, intentional self-harm**
+7th **T40.3X3 Poisoning by methadone, assault**
+7th **T40.3X4 Poisoning by methadone, undetermined**
+7th **T40.3X5 Adverse effect of methadone**
+7th **T40.3X6 Underdosing of methadone**

+ **T40.4 Poisoning by, adverse effect of and underdosing of other synthetic narcotics**
AHA CC: 4Q, 2020, 40
+ **T40.41 Poisoning by, adverse effect of and underdosing of fentanyl or fentanyl analogs**
+7th **T40.411 Poisoning by fentanyl or fentanyl analogs, accidental (unintentional)**
+7th **T40.412 Poisoning by fentanyl or fentanyl analogs, intentional self-harm**
+7th **T40.413 Poisoning by fentanyl or fentanyl analogs, assault**
+7th **T40.414 Poisoning by fentanyl or fentanyl analogs, undetermined**
+7th **T40.415 Adverse effect of fentanyl or fentanyl analogs**
+7th **T40.416 Underdosing of fentanyl or fentanyl analogs**
+ **T40.42 Poisoning by, adverse effect of and underdosing of tramadol**
+7th **T40.421 Poisoning by tramadol, accidental (unintentional)**
+7th **T40.422 Poisoning by tramadol, intentional self-harm**
+7th **T40.423 Poisoning by tramadol, assault**
+7th **T40.424 Poisoning by tramadol, undetermined**
+7th **T40.425 Adverse effect of tramadol**
+7th **T40.426 Underdosing of tramadol**
+ **T40.49 Poisoning by, adverse effect of and underdosing of other synthetic narcotics**
+7th **T40.491 Poisoning by other synthetic narcotics, accidental (unintentional)**
+7th **T40.492 Poisoning by other synthetic narcotics, intentional self-harm**
+7th **T40.493 Poisoning by other synthetic narcotics, assault**
+7th **T40.494 Poisoning by other synthetic narcotics, undetermined**
+7th **T40.495 Adverse effect of other synthetic narcotics**
+7th **T40.496 Underdosing of other synthetic narcotics**

+ **T40.5 Poisoning by, adverse effect of and underdosing of cocaine**
+ **T40.5X Poisoning by, adverse effect of and underdosing of cocaine**
+7th **T40.5X1 Poisoning by cocaine, accidental (unintentional)**
Poisoning by cocaine NOS
AHA CC: 2Q, 2016, 8-9
+7th **T40.5X2 Poisoning by cocaine, intentional self-harm**
+7th **T40.5X3 Poisoning by cocaine, assault**
+7th **T40.5X4 Poisoning by cocaine, undetermined**
+7th **T40.5X5 Adverse effect of cocaine**
+7th **T40.5X6 Underdosing of cocaine**

+ **T40.6 Poisoning by, adverse effect of and underdosing of other and unspecified narcotics**
+ **T40.60 Poisoning by, adverse effect of and underdosing of unspecified narcotics**
+7th **T40.601 Poisoning by unspecified narcotics, accidental (unintentional)**
Poisoning by narcotics NOS
+7th **T40.602 Poisoning by unspecified narcotics, intentional self-harm**
+7th **T40.603 Poisoning by unspecified narcotics, assault**
+7th **T40.604 Poisoning by unspecified narcotics, undetermined**
+7th **T40.605 Adverse effect of unspecified narcotics**
+7th **T40.606 Underdosing of unspecified narcotics**
+ **T40.69 Poisoning by, adverse effect of and underdosing of other narcotics**
+7th **T40.691 Poisoning by other narcotics, accidental (unintentional)**
Poisoning by other narcotics NOS
+7th **T40.692 Poisoning by other narcotics, intentional self-harm**
+7th **T40.693 Poisoning by other narcotics, assault**
+7th **T40.694 Poisoning by other narcotics, undetermined**
+7th **T40.695 Adverse effect of other narcotics**
+7th **T40.696 Underdosing of other narcotics**

+ **T40.7 Poisoning by, adverse effect of and underdosing of cannabis (derivatives)**
AHA CC: 1Q, 2020, 8
+ **T40.71 Poisoning by, adverse effect of and underdosing of cannabis (derivatives)**
+7th **T40.711 Poisoning by cannabis, accidental (unintentional)**
+7th **T40.712 Poisoning by cannabis, intentional self-harm**
+7th **T40.713 Poisoning by cannabis, assault**
+7th **T40.714 Poisoning by cannabis, undetermined**
+7th **T40.715 Adverse effect of cannabis**
+7th **T40.716 Underdosing of cannabis**
+ **T40.72 Poisoning by, adverse effect of and underdosing of synthetic cannabinoids**
+7th **T40.721 Poisoning by synthetic cannabinoids, accidental (unintentional)**
+7th **T40.722 Poisoning by synthetic cannabinoids, intentional self-harm**
+7th **T40.723 Poisoning by synthetic cannabinoids, assault**
+7th **T40.724 Poisoning by synthetic cannabinoids, undetermined**
+7th **T40.725 Adverse effect of synthetic cannabinoids**
+7th **T40.726 Underdosing of synthetic cannabinoids**

+ **T40.8 Poisoning by and adverse effect of lysergide [LSD]**
+ **T40.8X Poisoning by and adverse effect of lysergide [LSD]**
+7th **T40.8X1 Poisoning by lysergide [LSD], accidental (unintentional)**
Poisoning by lysergide [LSD] NOS
+7th **T40.8X2 Poisoning by lysergide [LSD], intentional self-harm**
+7th **T40.8X3 Poisoning by lysergide [LSD], assault**
+7th **T40.8X4 Poisoning by lysergide [LSD], undetermined**

+ **T40.9 Poisoning by, adverse effect of and underdosing of other and unspecified psychodysleptics [hallucinogens]**
+ **T40.90 Poisoning by, adverse effect of and underdosing of unspecified psychodysleptics [hallucinogens]**
+7th **T40.901 Poisoning by unspecified psychodysleptics [hallucinogens], accidental (unintentional)**
+7th **T40.902 Poisoning by unspecified psychodysleptics [hallucinogens], intentional self-harm**
+7th **T40.903 Poisoning by unspecified psychodysleptics [hallucinogens], assault**
+7th **T40.904 Poisoning by unspecified psychodysleptics [hallucinogens], undetermined**
+7th **T40.905 Adverse effect of unspecified psychodysleptics [hallucinogens]**
+7th **T40.906 Underdosing of unspecified psychodysleptics [hallucinogens]**
+ **T40.99 Poisoning by, adverse effect of and underdosing of other psychodysleptics [hallucinogens]**
+7th **T40.991 Poisoning by other psychodysleptics [hallucinogens], accidental (unintentional)**
Poisoning by other psychodysleptics [hallucinogens] NOS
+7th **T40.992 Poisoning by other psychodysleptics [hallucinogens], intentional self-harm**
+7th **T40.993 Poisoning by other psychodysleptics [hallucinogens], assault**
+7th **T40.994 Poisoning by other psychodysleptics [hallucinogens], undetermined**
+7th **T40.995 Adverse effect of other psychodysleptics [hallucinogens]**
+7th **T40.996 Underdosing of other psychodysleptics [hallucinogens]**

T41 Poisoning by, adverse effect of and underdosing of anesthetics and therapeutic gases

Excludes1: *benzodiazepines (T42.4-)*
cocaine (T40.5-)
complications of anesthesia during pregnancy (O29.-)
complications of anesthesia during labor and delivery (O74.-)
complications of anesthesia during the puerperium (O89.-)
opioids (T40.0-T40.2-)

The appropriate 7th character is to be added to each code from category T41
A initial encounter
D subsequent encounter
S sequela

+ **T41.0 Poisoning by, adverse effect of and underdosing of inhaled anesthetics**
Excludes1: *oxygen (T41.5-)*
+ **T41.0X Poisoning by, adverse effect of and underdosing of inhaled anesthetics**
+7th **T41.0X1 Poisoning by inhaled anesthetics, accidental (unintentional)**
Poisoning by inhaled anesthetics NOS
+7th **T41.0X2 Poisoning by inhaled anesthetics, intentional self-harm**
+7th **T41.0X3 Poisoning by inhaled anesthetics, assault**
+7th **T41.0X4 Poisoning by inhaled anesthetics, undetermined**
+7th **T41.0X5 Adverse effect of inhaled anesthetics**
+7th **T41.0X6 Underdosing of inhaled anesthetics**
+ **T41.1 Poisoning by, adverse effect of and underdosing of intravenous anesthetics**
Poisoning by, adverse effect of and underdosing of thiobarbiturates
+ **T41.1X Poisoning by, adverse effect of and underdosing of intravenous anesthetics**
+7th **T41.1X1 Poisoning by intravenous anesthetics, accidental (unintentional)**
Poisoning by intravenous anesthetics NOS
+7th **T41.1X2 Poisoning by intravenous anesthetics, intentional self-harm**
+7th **T41.1X3 Poisoning by intravenous anesthetics, assault**
+7th **T41.1X4 Poisoning by intravenous anesthetics, undetermined**
+7th **T41.1X5 Adverse effect of intravenous anesthetics**
+7th **T41.1X6 Underdosing of intravenous anesthetics**
+ **T41.2 Poisoning by, adverse effect of and underdosing of other and unspecified general anesthetics**
+ **T41.20 Poisoning by, adverse effect of and underdosing of unspecified general anesthetics**
+7th **T41.201 Poisoning by unspecified general anesthetics, accidental (unintentional)**
Poisoning by general anesthetics NOS
+7th **T41.202 Poisoning by unspecified general anesthetics, intentional self-harm**
+7th **T41.203 Poisoning by unspecified general anesthetics, assault**
+7th **T41.204 Poisoning by unspecified general anesthetics, undetermined**
+7th **T41.205 Adverse effect of unspecified general anesthetics**
AHA CC: 4Q, 2016, 72-73
+7th **T41.206 Underdosing of unspecified general anesthetics**
+ **T41.29 Poisoning by, adverse effect of and underdosing of other general anesthetics**
+7th **T41.291 Poisoning by other general anesthetics, accidental (unintentional)**
Poisoning by other general anesthetics NOS
+7th **T41.292 Poisoning by other general anesthetics, intentional self-harm**
+7th **T41.293 Poisoning by other general anesthetics, assault**
+7th **T41.294 Poisoning by other general anesthetics, undetermined**
+7th **T41.295 Adverse effect of other general anesthetics**
+7th **T41.296 Underdosing of other general anesthetics**
+ **T41.3 Poisoning by, adverse effect of and underdosing of local anesthetics**
Cocaine (topical)
Excludes2: *poisoning by cocaine used as a central nervous system stimulant (T40.5X1-T40.5X4)*
+ **T41.3X Poisoning by, adverse effect of and underdosing of local anesthetics**
+7th **T41.3X1 Poisoning by local anesthetics, accidental (unintentional)**
Poisoning by local anesthetics NOS
+7th **T41.3X2 Poisoning by local anesthetics, intentional self-harm**
+7th **T41.3X3 Poisoning by local anesthetics, assault**
+7th **T41.3X4 Poisoning by local anesthetics, undetermined**
+7th **T41.3X5 Adverse effect of local anesthetics**
+7th **T41.3X6 Underdosing of local anesthetics**
+ **T41.4 Poisoning by, adverse effect of and underdosing of unspecified anesthetic**
X+7th **T41.41 Poisoning by unspecified anesthetic, accidental (unintentional)**
Poisoning by anesthetic NOS
X+7th **T41.42 Poisoning by unspecified anesthetic, intentional self-harm**
X+7th **T41.43 Poisoning by unspecified anesthetic, assault**
X+7th **T41.44 Poisoning by unspecified anesthetic, undetermined**
X+7th **T41.45 Adverse effect of unspecified anesthetic**
X+7th **T41.46 Underdosing of unspecified anesthetics**
+ **T41.5 Poisoning by, adverse effect of and underdosing of therapeutic gases**
+ **T41.5X Poisoning by, adverse effect of and underdosing of therapeutic gases**
+7th **T41.5X1 Poisoning by therapeutic gases, accidental (unintentional)**
Poisoning by therapeutic gases NOS
+7th **T41.5X2 Poisoning by therapeutic gases, intentional self-harm**
+7th **T41.5X3 Poisoning by therapeutic gases, assault**
+7th **T41.5X4 Poisoning by therapeutic gases, undetermined**
+7th **T41.5X5 Adverse effect of therapeutic gases**
+7th **T41.5X6 Underdosing of therapeutic gases**

T42 Poisoning by, adverse effect of and underdosing of antiepileptic, sedative- hypnotic and antiparkinsonism drugs

Excludes2: *drug dependence and related mental and behavioral disorders due to psychoactive substance use (F10.--F19.-)*

The appropriate 7th character is to be added to each code from category T42
A initial encounter
D subsequent encounter
S sequela

\+ **T42.0 Poisoning by, adverse effect of and underdosing of hydantoin derivatives**

\+ **T42.0X Poisoning by, adverse effect of and underdosing of hydantoin derivatives**

+7th **T42.0X1 Poisoning by hydantoin derivatives, accidental (unintentional)**
Poisoning by hydantoin derivatives NOS

+7th **T42.0X2 Poisoning by hydantoin derivatives, intentional self-harm**

+7th **T42.0X3 Poisoning by hydantoin derivatives, assault**

+7th **T42.0X4 Poisoning by hydantoin derivatives, undetermined**

+7th **T42.0X5 Adverse effect of hydantoin derivatives**

+7th **T42.0X6 Underdosing of hydantoin derivatives**

\+ **T42.1 Poisoning by, adverse effect of and underdosing of iminostilbenes**
Poisoning by, adverse effect of and underdosing of carbamazepine

\+ **T42.1X Poisoning by, adverse effect of and underdosing of iminostilbenes**

+7th **T42.1X1 Poisoning by iminostilbenes, accidental (unintentional)**
Poisoning by iminostilbenes NOS

+7th **T42.1X2 Poisoning by iminostilbenes, intentional self-harm**

+7th **T42.1X3 Poisoning by iminostilbenes, assault**

+7th **T42.1X4 Poisoning by iminostilbenes, undetermined**

+7th **T42.1X5 Adverse effect of iminostilbenes**

+7th **T42.1X6 Underdosing of iminostilbenes**

\+ **T42.2 Poisoning by, adverse effect of and underdosing of succinimides and oxazolidinediones**

\+ **T42.2X Poisoning by, adverse effect of and underdosing of succinimides and oxazolidinediones**

+7th **T42.2X1 Poisoning by succinimides and oxazolidinediones, accidental (unintentional)**
Poisoning by succinimides and oxazolidinediones NOS

+7th **T42.2X2 Poisoning by succinimides and oxazolidinediones, intentional self-harm**

+7th **T42.2X3 Poisoning by succinimides and oxazolidinediones, assault**

+7th **T42.2X4 Poisoning by succinimides and oxazolidinediones, undetermined**

+7th **T42.2X5 Adverse effect of succinimides and oxazolidinediones**

+7th **T42.2X6 Underdosing of succinimides and oxazolidinediones**

\+ **T42.3 Poisoning by, adverse effect of and underdosing of barbiturates**

Excludes1: *poisoning by, adverse effect of and underdosing of thiobarbiturates (T41.1-)*

\+ **T42.3X Poisoning by, adverse effect of and underdosing of barbiturates**

+7th **T42.3X1 Poisoning by barbiturates, accidental (unintentional)**
Poisoning by barbiturates NOS

+7th **T42.3X2 Poisoning by barbiturates, intentional self-harm**

+7th **T42.3X3 Poisoning by barbiturates, assault**

+7th **T42.3X4 Poisoning by barbiturates, undetermined**

+7th **T42.3X5 Adverse effect of barbiturates**

+7th **T42.3X6 Underdosing of barbiturates**

\+ **T42.4 Poisoning by, adverse effect of and underdosing of benzodiazepines**

\+ **T42.4X Poisoning by, adverse effect of and underdosing of benzodiazepines**

+7th **T42.4X1 Poisoning by benzodiazepines, accidental (unintentional)**
Poisoning by benzodiazepines NOS

+7th **T42.4X2 Poisoning by benzodiazepines, intentional self-harm**

+7th **T42.4X3 Poisoning by benzodiazepines, assault**

+7th **T42.4X4 Poisoning by benzodiazepines, undetermined**

+7th **T42.4X5 Adverse effect of benzodiazepines**

+7th **T42.4X6 Underdosing of benzodiazepines**

\+ **T42.5 Poisoning by, adverse effect of and underdosing of mixed antiepileptics**

\+ **T42.5X Poisoning by, adverse effect of and underdosing of antiepileptics**

+7th **T42.5X1 Poisoning by mixed antiepileptics, accidental (unintentional)**
Poisoning by mixed antiepileptics NOS

+7th **T42.5X2 Poisoning by mixed antiepileptics, intentional self-harm**

+7th **T42.5X3 Poisoning by mixed antiepileptics, assault**

+7th **T42.5X4 Poisoning by mixed antiepileptics, undetermined**

+7th **T42.5X5 Adverse effect of mixed antiepileptics**

+7th **T42.5X6 Underdosing of mixed antiepileptics**

\+ **T42.6 Poisoning by, adverse effect of and underdosing of other antiepileptic and sedative-hypnotic drugs**
Poisoning by, adverse effect of and underdosing of methaqualone
Poisoning by, adverse effect of and underdosing of valproic acid

Excludes1: *poisoning by, adverse effect of and underdosing of carbamazepine (T42.1-)*

\+ **T42.6X Poisoning by, adverse effect of and underdosing of other antiepileptic and sedative-hypnotic drugs**

+7th **T42.6X1 Poisoning by other antiepileptic and sedative-hypnotic drugs, accidental (unintentional)**
Poisoning by other antiepileptic and sedative-hypnotic drugs NOS

+7th **T42.6X2 Poisoning by other antiepileptic and sedative-hypnotic drugs, intentional self-harm**

+7th **T42.6X3 Poisoning by other antiepileptic and sedative-hypnotic drugs, assault**

+7th **T42.6X4 Poisoning by other antiepileptic and sedative-hypnotic drugs, undetermined**

+7th **T42.6X5 Adverse effect of other antiepileptic and sedative-hypnotic drugs**

+7th **T42.6X6 Underdosing of other antiepileptic and sedative-hypnotic drugs**

\+ **T42.7 Poisoning by, adverse effect of and underdosing of unspecified antiepileptic and sedative-hypnotic drugs**

X+7th **T42.71 Poisoning by unspecified antiepileptic and sedative-hypnotic drugs, accidental (unintentional)**
Poisoning by antiepileptic and sedative-hypnotic drugs NOS

X+7th **T42.72 Poisoning by unspecified antiepileptic and sedative-hypnotic drugs, intentional self-harm**

X+7th **T42.73 Poisoning by unspecified antiepileptic and sedative-hypnotic drugs, assault**

X+7th **T42.74 Poisoning by unspecified antiepileptic and sedative-hypnotic drugs, undetermined**

X+7th **T42.75 Adverse effect of unspecified antiepileptic and sedative-hypnotic drugs**

X+7th **T42.76 Underdosing of unspecified antiepileptic and sedative-hypnotic drugs**

+ **T42.8 Poisoning by, adverse effect of and underdosing of antiparkinsonism drugs and other central muscle-tone depressants**
  Poisoning by, adverse effect of and underdosing of amantadine
  + **T42.8X Poisoning by, adverse effect of and underdosing of antiparkinsonism drugs and other central muscle-tone depressants**
    +7th **T42.8X1 Poisoning by antiparkinsonism drugs and other central muscle-tone depressants, accidental (unintentional)**
      Poisoning by antiparkinsonism drugs and other central muscle-tone depressants NOS
    +7th **T42.8X2 Poisoning by antiparkinsonism drugs and other central muscle-tone depressants, intentional self-harm**
    +7th **T42.8X3 Poisoning by antiparkinsonism drugs and other central muscle-tone depressants, assault**
    +7th **T42.8X4 Poisoning by antiparkinsonism drugs and other central muscle-tone depressants, undetermined**
    +7th **T42.8X5 Adverse effect of antiparkinsonism drugs and other central muscle-tone depressants**
    +7th **T42.8X6 Underdosing of antiparkinsonism drugs and other central muscle-tone depressants**

T43 Poisoning by, adverse effect of and underdosing of psychotropic drugs, not elsewhere classified

Excludes1: *appetite depressants (T50.5-)*
barbiturates (T42.3-)
benzodiazepines (T42.4-)
methaqualone (T42.6-)
psychodysleptics [hallucinogens] (T40.7-T40.9-)

Excludes2: *drug dependence and related mental and behavioral disorders due to psychoactive substance use (F10.- -F19.-)*

The appropriate 7th character is to be added to each code from category T43
A initial encounter
D subsequent encounter
S sequela

+ **T43.0 Poisoning by, adverse effect of and underdosing of tricyclic and tetracyclic antidepressants**
  + **T43.01 Poisoning by, adverse effect of and underdosing of tricyclic antidepressants**
    +7th **T43.011 Poisoning by tricyclic antidepressants, accidental (unintentional)**
      Poisoning by tricyclic antidepressants NOS
    +7th **T43.012 Poisoning by tricyclic antidepressants, intentional self-harm**
    +7th **T43.013 Poisoning by tricyclic antidepressants, assault**
    +7th **T43.014 Poisoning by tricyclic antidepressants, undetermined**
    +7th **T43.015 Adverse effect of tricyclic antidepressants**
    +7th **T43.016 Underdosing of tricyclic antidepressants**
  + **T43.02 Poisoning by, adverse effect of and underdosing of tetracyclic antidepressants**
    +7th **T43.021 Poisoning by tetracyclic antidepressants, accidental (unintentional)**
      Poisoning by tetracyclic antidepressants NOS
    +7th **T43.022 Poisoning by tetracyclic antidepressants, intentional self-harm**
    +7th **T43.023 Poisoning by tetracyclic antidepressants, assault**
    +7th **T43.024 Poisoning by tetracyclic antidepressants, undetermined**
    +7th **T43.025 Adverse effect of tetracyclic antidepressants**
    +7th **T43.026 Underdosing of tetracyclic antidepressants**

+ **T43.1 Poisoning by, adverse effect of and underdosing of monoamine-oxidase-inhibitor antidepressants**
  + **T43.1X Poisoning by, adverse effect of and underdosing of monoamine-oxidase-inhibitor antidepressants**
    +7th **T43.1X1 Poisoning by monoamine-oxidase-inhibitor antidepressants, accidental (unintentional)**
      Poisoning by monoamine-oxidase-inhibitor antidepressants NOS
    +7th **T43.1X2 Poisoning by monoamine-oxidase-inhibitor antidepressants, intentional self-harm**
    +7th **T43.1X3 Poisoning by monoamine-oxidase-inhibitor antidepressants, assault**
    +7th **T43.1X4 Poisoning by monoamine-oxidase-inhibitor antidepressants, undetermined**
    +7th **T43.1X5 Adverse effect of monoamine-oxidase-inhibitor antidepressants**
    +7th **T43.1X6 Underdosing of monoamine-oxidase-inhibitor antidepressants**
+ **T43.2 Poisoning by, adverse effect of and underdosing of other and unspecified antidepressants**
  + **T43.20 Poisoning by, adverse effect of and underdosing of unspecified antidepressants**
    +7th **T43.201 Poisoning by unspecified antidepressants, accidental (unintentional)**
      Poisoning by antidepressants NOS
    +7th **T43.202 Poisoning by unspecified antidepressants, intentional self-harm**
    +7th **T43.203 Poisoning by unspecified antidepressants, assault**
    +7th **T43.204 Poisoning by unspecified antidepressants, undetermined**
    +7th **T43.205 Adverse effect of unspecified antidepressants**
      Antidepressant discontinuation syndrome
    +7th **T43.206 Underdosing of unspecified antidepressants**
  + **T43.21 Poisoning by, adverse effect of and underdosing of selective serotonin and norepinephrine reuptake inhibitors**
    Poisoning by, adverse effect of and underdosing of SSNRI antidepressants
    +7th **T43.211 Poisoning by selective serotonin and norepinephrine reuptake inhibitors, accidental (unintentional)**
    +7th **T43.212 Poisoning by selective serotonin and norepinephrine reuptake inhibitors, intentional self-harm**
    +7th **T43.213 Poisoning by selective serotonin and norepinephrine reuptake inhibitors, assault**
    +7th **T43.214 Poisoning by selective serotonin and norepinephrine reuptake inhibitors, undetermined**
    +7th **T43.215 Adverse effect of selective serotonin and norepinephrine reuptake inhibitors**
    +7th **T43.216 Underdosing of selective serotonin and norepinephrine reuptake inhibitors**
  + **T43.22 Poisoning by, adverse effect of and underdosing of selective serotonin reuptake inhibitors**
    Poisoning by, adverse effect of and underdosing of SSRI antidepressants
    +7th **T43.221 Poisoning by selective serotonin reuptake inhibitors, accidental (unintentional)**
    +7th **T43.222 Poisoning by selective serotonin reuptake inhibitors, intentional self-harm**
    +7th **T43.223 Poisoning by selective serotonin reuptake inhibitors, assault**
    +7th **T43.224 Poisoning by selective serotonin reuptake inhibitors, undetermined**
    +7th **T43.225 Adverse effect of selective serotonin reuptake inhibitors**
    +7th **T43.226 Underdosing of selective serotonin reuptake inhibitors**

+ **T43.29 Poisoning by, adverse effect of and underdosing of other antidepressants**
  - +7th **T43.291 Poisoning by other antidepressants, accidental (unintentional)**
    Poisoning by other antidepressants NOS
  - +7th **T43.292 Poisoning by other antidepressants, intentional self-harm**
  - +7th **T43.293 Poisoning by other antidepressants, assault**
  - +7th **T43.294 Poisoning by other antidepressants, undetermined**
  - +7th **T43.295 Adverse effect of other antidepressants**
  - +7th **T43.296 Underdosing of other antidepressants**

+ **T43.3 Poisoning by, adverse effect of and underdosing of phenothiazine antipsychotics and neuroleptics**

+ **T43.3X Poisoning by, adverse effect of and underdosing of phenothiazine antipsychotics and neuroleptics**
  - +7th **T43.3X1 Poisoning by phenothiazine antipsychotics and neuroleptics, accidental (unintentional)**
    Poisoning by phenothiazine antipsychotics and neuroleptics NOS
  - +7th **T43.3X2 Poisoning by phenothiazine antipsychotics and neuroleptics, intentional self-harm**
  - +7th **T43.3X3 Poisoning by phenothiazine antipsychotics and neuroleptics, assault**
  - +7th **T43.3X4 Poisoning by phenothiazine antipsychotics and neuroleptics, undetermined**
  - +7th **T43.3X5 Adverse effect of phenothiazine antipsychotics and neuroleptics**
  - +7th **T43.3X6 Underdosing of phenothiazine antipsychotics and neuroleptics**

+ **T43.4 Poisoning by, adverse effect of and underdosing of butyrophenone and thiothixene neuroleptics**

+ **T43.4X Poisoning by, adverse effect of and underdosing of butyrophenone and thiothixene neuroleptics**
  - +7th **T43.4X1 Poisoning by butyrophenone and thiothixene neuroleptics, accidental (unintentional)**
    Poisoning by butyrophenone and thiothixene neuroleptics NOS
  - +7th **T43.4X2 Poisoning by butyrophenone and thiothixene neuroleptics, intentional self-harm**
  - +7th **T43.4X3 Poisoning by butyrophenone and thiothixene neuroleptics, assault**
  - +7th **T43.4X4 Poisoning by butyrophenone and thiothixene neuroleptics, undetermined**
  - +7th **T43.4X5 Adverse effect of butyrophenone and thiothixene neuroleptics**
  - +7th **T43.4X6 Underdosing of butyrophenone and thiothixene neuroleptics**

+ **T43.5 Poisoning by, adverse effect of and underdosing of other and unspecified antipsychotics and neuroleptics**
  Excludes1: *poisoning by, adverse effect of and underdosing of rauwolfia (T46.5-)*

+ **T43.50 Poisoning by, adverse effect of and underdosing of unspecified antipsychotics and neuroleptics**
  - +7th **T43.501 Poisoning by unspecified antipsychotics and neuroleptics, accidental (unintentional)**
    Poisoning by antipsychotics and neuroleptics NOS
  - +7th **T43.502 Poisoning by unspecified antipsychotics and neuroleptics, intentional self-harm**
  - +7th **T43.503 Poisoning by unspecified antipsychotics and neuroleptics, assault**
  - +7th **T43.504 Poisoning by unspecified antipsychotics and neuroleptics, undetermined**
  - +7th **T43.505 Adverse effect of unspecified antipsychotics and neuroleptics**
  - +7th **T43.506 Underdosing of unspecified antipsychotics and neuroleptics**

+ **T43.59 Poisoning by, adverse effect of and underdosing of other antipsychotics and neuroleptics**
  - +7th **T43.591 Poisoning by other antipsychotics and neuroleptics, accidental (unintentional)**
    Poisoning by other antipsychotics and neuroleptics NOS
  - +7th **T43.592 Poisoning by other antipsychotics and neuroleptics, intentional self-harm**
    AHA CC: 1Q, 2017, 40
  - +7th **T43.593 Poisoning by other antipsychotics and neuroleptics, assault**
  - +7th **T43.594 Poisoning by other antipsychotics and neuroleptics, undetermined**
  - +7th **T43.595 Adverse effect of other antipsychotics and neuroleptics**
  - +7th **T43.596 Underdosing of other antipsychotics and neuroleptics**

+ **T43.6 Poisoning by, adverse effect of and underdosing of psychostimulants**
  Excludes1: *poisoning by, adverse effect of and underdosing of cocaine (T40.5-)*

+ **T43.60 Poisoning by, adverse effect of and underdosing of unspecified psychostimulant**
  - +7th **T43.601 Poisoning by unspecified psychostimulants, accidental (unintentional)**
    Poisoning by psychostimulants NOS
  - +7th **T43.602 Poisoning by unspecified psychostimulants, intentional self-harm**
  - +7th **T43.603 Poisoning by unspecified psychostimulants, assault**
  - +7th **T43.604 Poisoning by unspecified psychostimulants, undetermined**
  - +7th **T43.605 Adverse effect of unspecified psychostimulants**
  - +7th **T43.606 Underdosing of unspecified psychostimulants**

+ **T43.61 Poisoning by, adverse effect of and underdosing of caffeine**
  - +7th **T43.611 Poisoning by caffeine, accidental (unintentional)**
    Poisoning by caffeine NOS
  - +7th **T43.612 Poisoning by caffeine, intentional self-harm**
  - +7th **T43.613 Poisoning by caffeine, assault**
  - +7th **T43.614 Poisoning by caffeine, undetermined**
  - +7th **T43.615 Adverse effect of caffeine**
  - +7th **T43.616 Underdosing of caffeine**

+ **T43.62 Poisoning by, adverse effect of and underdosing of amphetamines**
  Poisoning by, adverse effect of and underdosing of methamphetamines
  - +7th **T43.621 Poisoning by amphetamines, accidental (unintentional)**
    Poisoning by amphetamines NOS
  - +7th **T43.622 Poisoning by amphetamines, intentional self-harm**
  - +7th **T43.623 Poisoning by amphetamines, assault**
  - +7th **T43.624 Poisoning by amphetamines, undetermined**
  - +7th **T43.625 Adverse effect of amphetamines**
  - +7th **T43.626 Underdosing of amphetamines**

+ **T43.63 Poisoning by, adverse effect of and underdosing of methylphenidate**
  - +7th **T43.631 Poisoning by methylphenidate, accidental (unintentional)**
    Poisoning by methylphenidate NOS
  - +7th **T43.632 Poisoning by methylphenidate, intentional self-harm**
  - +7th **T43.633 Poisoning by methylphenidate, assault**
  - +7th **T43.634 Poisoning by methylphenidate, undetermined**
  - +7th **T43.635 Adverse effect of methylphenidate**
  - +7th **T43.636 Underdosing of methylphenidate**

+ T43.64 **Poisoning by ecstasy**
Poisoning by MDMA
Poisoning by 3,4-methylenedioxymethamphetamine
AHA CC: 4Q, 2018, 30-31

+7th **T43.641 Poisoning by ecstasy, accidental (unintentional)**
Poisoning by ecstasy NOS
AHA CC: 4Q, 2018, 31

+7th **T43.642 Poisoning by ecstasy, intentional self-harm**

+7th **T43.643 Poisoning by ecstasy, assault**

+7th **T43.644 Poisoning by ecstasy, undetermined**

+ **T43.69 Poisoning by, adverse effect of and underdosing of other psychostimulants**

+7th **T43.691 Poisoning by other psychostimulants, accidental (unintentional)**
Poisoning by other psychostimulants NOS

+7th **T43.692 Poisoning by other psychostimulants, intentional self-harm**

+7th **T43.693 Poisoning by other psychostimulants, assault**

+7th **T43.694 Poisoning by other psychostimulants, undetermined**

+7th **T43.695 Adverse effect of other psychostimulants**

+7th **T43.696 Underdosing of other psychostimulants**

+ **T43.8 Poisoning by, adverse effect of and underdosing of other psychotropic drugs**

+ **T43.8X Poisoning by, adverse effect of and underdosing of other psychotropic drugs**

+7th **T43.8X1 Poisoning by other psychotropic drugs, accidental (unintentional)**
Poisoning by other psychotropic drugs NOS

+7th **T43.8X2 Poisoning by other psychotropic drugs, intentional self-harm**

+7th **T43.8X3 Poisoning by other psychotropic drugs, assault**

+7th **T43.8X4 Poisoning by other psychotropic drugs, undetermined**

+7th **T43.8X5 Adverse effect of other psychotropic drugs**

+7th **T43.8X6 Underdosing of other psychotropic drugs**

+ **T43.9 Poisoning by, adverse effect of and underdosing of unspecified psychotropic drug**

X+7th **T43.91 Poisoning by unspecified psychotropic drug, accidental (unintentional)**
Poisoning by psychotropic drug NOS

X+7th **T43.92 Poisoning by unspecified psychotropic drug, intentional self-harm**

X+7th **T43.93 Poisoning by unspecified psychotropic drug, assault**

X+7th **T43.94 Poisoning by unspecified psychotropic drug, undetermined**

X+7th **T43.95 Adverse effect of unspecified psychotropic drug**

X+7th **T43.96 Underdosing of unspecified psychotropic drug**

T44 Poisoning by, adverse effect of and underdosing of drugs primarily affecting the autonomic nervous system

The appropriate 7th character is to be added to each code from category T44
A initial encounter
D subsequent encounter
S sequela

+ **T44.0 Poisoning by, adverse effect of and underdosing of anticholinesterase agents**

+ **T44.0X Poisoning by, adverse effect of and underdosing of anticholinesterase agents**

+7th **T44.0X1 Poisoning by anticholinesterase agents, accidental (unintentional)**
Poisoning by anticholinesterase agents NOS

+7th **T44.0X2 Poisoning by anticholinesterase agents, intentional self-harm**

+7th **T44.0X3 Poisoning by anticholinesterase agents, assault**

+7th **T44.0X4 Poisoning by anticholinesterase agents, undetermined**

+7th **T44.0X5 Adverse effect of anticholinesterase agents**

+7th **T44.0X6 Underdosing of anticholinesterase agents**

+ **T44.1 Poisoning by, adverse effect of and underdosing of other parasympathomimetics [cholinergics]**

+ **T44.1X Poisoning by, adverse effect of and underdosing of other parasympathomimetics [cholinergics]**

+7th **T44.1X1 Poisoning by other parasympathomimetics [cholinergics], accidental (unintentional)**
Poisoning by other parasympathomimetics [cholinergics] NOS

+7th **T44.1X2 Poisoning by other parasympathomimetics [cholinergics], intentional self-harm**

+7th **T44.1X3 Poisoning by other parasympathomimetics [cholinergics], assault**

+7th **T44.1X4 Poisoning by other parasympathomimetics [cholinergics], undetermined**

+7th **T44.1X5 Adverse effect of other parasympathomimetics [cholinergics]**

+7th **T44.1X6 Underdosing of other parasympathomimetics [cholinergics]**

+ **T44.2 Poisoning by, adverse effect of and underdosing of ganglionic blocking drugs**

+ **T44.2X Poisoning by, adverse effect of and underdosing of ganglionic blocking drugs**

+7th **T44.2X1 Poisoning by ganglionic blocking drugs, accidental (unintentional)**
Poisoning by ganglionic blocking drugs NOS

+7th **T44.2X2 Poisoning by ganglionic blocking drugs, intentional self-harm**

+7th **T44.2X3 Poisoning by ganglionic blocking drugs, assault**

+7th **T44.2X4 Poisoning by ganglionic blocking drugs, undetermined**

+7th **T44.2X5 Adverse effect of ganglionic blocking drugs**

+7th **T44.2X6 Underdosing of ganglionic blocking drugs**

+ **T44.3 Poisoning by, adverse effect of and underdosing of other parasympatholytics [anticholinergics and antimuscarinics] and spasmolytics**
Poisoning by, adverse effect of and underdosing of papaverine

+ **T44.3X Poisoning by, adverse effect of and underdosing of other parasympatholytics [anticholinergics and antimuscarinics] and spasmolytics**

+7th **T44.3X1 Poisoning by other parasympatholytics [anticholinergics and antimuscarinics] and spasmolytics, accidental (unintentional)**
Poisoning by other parasympatholytics [anticholinergics and antimuscarinics] and spasmolytics NOS

+7th **T44.3X2 Poisoning by other parasympatholytics [anticholinergics and antimuscarinics] and spasmolytics, intentional self-harm**

+7th **T44.3X3 Poisoning by other parasympatholytics [anticholinergics and antimuscarinics] and spasmolytics, assault**

+7th **T44.3X4 Poisoning by other parasympatholytics [anticholinergics and antimuscarinics] and spasmolytics, undetermined**

+7th **T44.3X5 Adverse effect of other parasympatholytics [anticholinergics and antimuscarinics] and spasmolytics**

+7th **T44.3X6 Underdosing of other parasympatholytics [anticholinergics and antimuscarinics] and spasmolytics**

+ **T44.4 Poisoning by, adverse effect of and underdosing of predominantly alpha-adrenoreceptor agonists**
Poisoning by, adverse effect of and underdosing of metaraminol
+ **T44.4X Poisoning by, adverse effect of and underdosing of predominantly alpha-adrenoreceptor agonists**
+7th **T44.4X1 Poisoning by predominantly alpha-adrenoreceptor agonists, accidental (unintentional)**
Poisoning by predominantly alpha-adrenoreceptor agonists NOS
+7th **T44.4X2 Poisoning by predominantly alpha-adrenoreceptor agonists, intentional self-harm**
+7th **T44.4X3 Poisoning by predominantly alpha-adrenoreceptor agonists, assault**
+7th **T44.4X4 Poisoning by predominantly alpha-adrenoreceptor agonists, undetermined**
+7th **T44.4X5 Adverse effect of predominantly alpha-adrenoreceptor agonists**
+7th **T44.4X6 Underdosing of predominantly alpha-adrenoreceptor agonists**
+ **T44.5 Poisoning by, adverse effect of and underdosing of predominantly beta-adrenoreceptor agonists**
Excludes1: *poisoning by, adverse effect of and underdosing of beta-adrenoreceptor agonists used in asthma therapy (T48.6-)*
+ **T44.5X Poisoning by, adverse effect of and underdosing of predominantly beta-adrenoreceptor agonists**
+7th **T44.5X1 Poisoning by predominantly beta-adrenoreceptor agonists, accidental (unintentional)**
Poisoning by predominantly beta-adrenoreceptor agonists NOS
+7th **T44.5X2 Poisoning by predominantly beta-adrenoreceptor agonists, intentional self-harm**
+7th **T44.5X3 Poisoning by predominantly beta-adrenoreceptor agonists, assault**
+7th **T44.5X4 Poisoning by predominantly beta-adrenoreceptor agonists, undetermined**
+7th **T44.5X5 Adverse effect of predominantly beta-adrenoreceptor agonists**
+7th **T44.5X6 Underdosing of predominantly beta-adrenoreceptor agonists**
+ **T44.6 Poisoning by, adverse effect of and underdosing of alpha-adrenoreceptor antagonists**
Excludes1: *poisoning by, adverse effect of and underdosing of ergot alkaloids (T48.0)*
+ **T44.6X Poisoning by, adverse effect of and underdosing of alpha-adrenoreceptor antagonists**
+7th **T44.6X1 Poisoning by alpha-adrenoreceptor antagonists, accidental (unintentional)**
Poisoning by alpha-adrenoreceptor antagonists NOS
+7th **T44.6X2 Poisoning by alpha-adrenoreceptor antagonists, intentional self-harm**
+7th **T44.6X3 Poisoning by alpha-adrenoreceptor antagonists, assault**
+7th **T44.6X4 Poisoning by alpha-adrenoreceptor antagonists, undetermined**
+7th **T44.6X5 Adverse effect of alpha-adrenoreceptor antagonists**
+7th **T44.6X6 Underdosing of alpha-adrenoreceptor antagonists**
+ **T44.7 Poisoning by, adverse effect of and underdosing of beta-adrenoreceptor antagonists**
+ **T44.7X Poisoning by, adverse effect of and underdosing of beta-adrenoreceptor antagonists**
+7th **T44.7X1 Poisoning by beta-adrenoreceptor antagonists, accidental (unintentional)**
Poisoning by beta-adrenoreceptor antagonists NOS
+7th **T44.7X2 Poisoning by beta-adrenoreceptor antagonists, intentional self-harm**
+7th **T44.7X3 Poisoning by beta-adrenoreceptor antagonists, assault**
+7th **T44.7X4 Poisoning by beta-adrenoreceptor antagonists, undetermined**
+7th **T44.7X5 Adverse effect of beta-adrenoreceptor antagonists**
+7th **T44.7X6 Underdosing of beta-adrenoreceptor antagonists**
+ **T44.8 Poisoning by, adverse effect of and underdosing of centrally-acting and adrenergic-neuron- blocking agents**
Excludes2: *poisoning by, adverse effect of and underdosing of clonidine (T46.5)*
poisoning by, adverse effect of and underdosing of guanethidine (T46.5)
+ **T44.8X Poisoning by, adverse effect of and underdosing of centrally-acting and adrenergic- neuron-blocking agents**
+7th **T44.8X1 Poisoning by centrally-acting and adrenergic-neuron-blocking agents, accidental (unintentional)**
Poisoning by centrally-acting and adrenergic-neuron-blocking agents NOS
+7th **T44.8X2 Poisoning by centrally-acting and adrenergic-neuron-blocking agents, intentional self-harm**
+7th **T44.8X3 Poisoning by centrally-acting and adrenergic-neuron-blocking agents, assault**
+7th **T44.8X4 Poisoning by centrally-acting and adrenergic-neuron-blocking agents, undetermined**
+7th **T44.8X5 Adverse effect of centrally-acting and adrenergic-neuron-blocking agents**
+7th **T44.8X6 Underdosing of centrally-acting and adrenergic-neuron-blocking agents**
+ **T44.9 Poisoning by, adverse effect of and underdosing of other and unspecified drugs primarily affecting the autonomic nervous system**
Poisoning by, adverse effect of and underdosing of drug stimulating both alpha and beta-adrenoreceptors
+ **T44.90 Poisoning by, adverse effect of and underdosing of unspecified drugs primarily affecting the autonomic nervous system**
+7th **T44.901 Poisoning by unspecified drugs primarily affecting the autonomic nervous system, accidental (unintentional)**
Poisoning by unspecified drugs primarily affecting the autonomic nervous system NOS
+7th **T44.902 Poisoning by unspecified drugs primarily affecting the autonomic nervous system, intentional self-harm**
+7th **T44.903 Poisoning by unspecified drugs primarily affecting the autonomic nervous system, assault**
+7th **T44.904 Poisoning by unspecified drugs primarily affecting the autonomic nervous system, undetermined**
+7th **T44.905 Adverse effect of unspecified drugs primarily affecting the autonomic nervous system**
+7th **T44.906 Underdosing of unspecified drugs primarily affecting the autonomic nervous system**
+ **T44.99 Poisoning by, adverse effect of and underdosing of other drugs primarily affecting the autonomic nervous system**
+7th **T44.991 Poisoning by other drug primarily affecting the autonomic nervous system, accidental (unintentional)**
Poisoning by other drugs primarily affecting the autonomic nervous system NOS
+7th **T44.992 Poisoning by other drug primarily affecting the autonomic nervous system, intentional self-harm**
+7th **T44.993 Poisoning by other drug primarily affecting the autonomic nervous system, assault**
+7th **T44.994 Poisoning by other drug primarily affecting the autonomic nervous system, undetermined**
+7th **T44.995 Adverse effect of other drug primarily affecting the autonomic nervous system**
+7th **T44.996 Underdosing of other drug primarily affecting the autonomic nervous system**

T45 Poisoning by, adverse effect of and underdosing of primarily systemic and hematological agents, not elsewhere classified

The appropriate 7th character is to be added to each code from category T45
A initial encounter
D subsequent encounter
S sequela

\+ **T45.0 Poisoning by, adverse effect of and underdosing of antiallergic and antiemetic drugs**
Excludes1: *poisoning by, adverse effect of and underdosing of phenothiazine-based neuroleptics (T43.3)*

\+ **T45.0X Poisoning by, adverse effect of and underdosing of antiallergic and antiemetic drugs**

+7th **T45.0X1 Poisoning by antiallergic and antiemetic drugs, accidental (unintentional)**
Poisoning by antiallergic and antiemetic drugs NOS

+7th **T45.0X2 Poisoning by antiallergic and antiemetic drugs, intentional self-harm**

+7th **T45.0X3 Poisoning by antiallergic and antiemetic drugs, assault**

+7th **T45.0X4 Poisoning by antiallergic and antiemetic drugs, undetermined**

+7th **T45.0X5 Adverse effect of antiallergic and antiemetic drugs**

+7th **T45.0X6 Underdosing of antiallergic and antiemetic drugs**

\+ **T45.1 Poisoning by, adverse effect of and underdosing of antineoplastic and immunosuppressive drugs**
Excludes1: *poisoning by, adverse effect of and underdosing of tamoxifen (T38.6)*

\+ **T45.1X Poisoning by, adverse effect of and underdosing of antineoplastic and immunosuppressive drugs**

+7th **T45.1X1 Poisoning by antineoplastic and immunosuppressive drugs, accidental (unintentional)**
Poisoning by antineoplastic and immunosuppressive drugs NOS

+7th **T45.1X2 Poisoning by antineoplastic and immunosuppressive drugs, intentional self-harm**

+7th **T45.1X3 Poisoning by antineoplastic and immunosuppressive drugs, assault**

+7th **T45.1X4 Poisoning by antineoplastic and immunosuppressive drugs, undetermined**

+7th **T45.1X5 Adverse effect of antineoplastic and immunosuppressive drugs**
Review coding guideline C.2.c.2
AHA CC: 4Q, 2014, 22-23; 1Q, 2019, 17, 20-21; 2Q, 2019, 24-26, 28; 3Q, 2020, 22-23; 4Q, 2020, 11-12

+7th **T45.1X6 Underdosing of antineoplastic and immunosuppressive drugs**

\+ **T45.2 Poisoning by, adverse effect of and underdosing of vitamins**
Excludes2: *poisoning by, adverse effect of and underdosing of nicotinic acid (derivatives) (T46.7)*
poisoning by, adverse effect of and underdosing of iron (T45.4)
poisoning by, adverse effect of and underdosing of vitamin K (T45.7)

\+ **T45.2X Poisoning by, adverse effect of and underdosing of vitamins**

+7th **T45.2X1 Poisoning by vitamins, accidental (unintentional)**
Poisoning by vitamins NOS

+7th **T45.2X2 Poisoning by vitamins, intentional self-harm**

+7th **T45.2X3 Poisoning by vitamins, assault**

+7th **T45.2X4 Poisoning by vitamins, undetermined**

+7th **T45.2X5 Adverse effect of vitamins**

+7th **T45.2X6 Underdosing of vitamins**
Excludes1: *vitamin deficiencies (E50-E56)*

\+ **T45.3 Poisoning by, adverse effect of and underdosing of enzymes**

\+ **T45.3X Poisoning by, adverse effect of and underdosing of enzymes**

+7th **T45.3X1 Poisoning by enzymes, accidental (unintentional)**
Poisoning by enzymes NOS

+7th **T45.3X2 Poisoning by enzymes, intentional self-harm**

+7th **T45.3X3 Poisoning by enzymes, assault**

+7th **T45.3X4 Poisoning by enzymes, undetermined**

+7th **T45.3X5 Adverse effect of enzymes**

+7th **T45.3X6 Underdosing of enzymes**

\+ **T45.4 Poisoning by, adverse effect of and underdosing of iron and its compounds**

\+ **T45.4X Poisoning by, adverse effect of and underdosing of iron and its compounds**

+7th **T45.4X1 Poisoning by iron and its compounds, accidental (unintentional)**
Poisoning by iron and its compounds NOS

+7th **T45.4X2 Poisoning by iron and its compounds, intentional self-harm**

+7th **T45.4X3 Poisoning by iron and its compounds, assault**

+7th **T45.4X4 Poisoning by iron and its compounds, undetermined**

+7th **T45.4X5 Adverse effect of iron and its compounds**

+7th **T45.4X6 Underdosing of iron and its compounds**
Excludes1: *iron deficiency (E61.1)*

\+ **T45.5 Poisoning by, adverse effect of and underdosing of anticoagulants and antithrombotic drugs**

\+ **T45.51 Poisoning by, adverse effect of and underdosing of anticoagulants**

+7th **T45.511 Poisoning by anticoagulants, accidental (unintentional)**
Poisoning by anticoagulants NOS

+7th **T45.512 Poisoning by anticoagulants, intentional self-harm**

+7th **T45.513 Poisoning by anticoagulants, assault**

+7th **T45.514 Poisoning by anticoagulants, undetermined**

+7th **T45.515 Adverse effect of anticoagulants**
AHA CC: 2Q, 2013, 34-35; 1Q, 2016, 14-15; 1Q, 2021, 4-5

+7th **T45.516 Underdosing of anticoagulants**

\+ **T45.52 Poisoning by, adverse effect of and underdosing of antithrombotic drugs**
Poisoning by, adverse effect of and underdosing of antiplatelet drugs
Excludes2: *poisoning by, adverse effect of and underdosing of aspirin (T39.01-)*
poisoning by, adverse effect of and underdosing of acetylsalicylic acid (T39.01-)

+7th **T45.521 Poisoning by antithrombotic drugs, accidental (unintentional)**
Poisoning by antithrombotic drug NOS

+7th **T45.522 Poisoning by antithrombotic drugs, intentional self-harm**

+7th **T45.523 Poisoning by antithrombotic drugs, assault**

+7th **T45.524 Poisoning by antithrombotic drugs, undetermined**

+7th **T45.525 Adverse effect of antithrombotic drugs**
AHA CC: 1Q, 2016, 15

+7th **T45.526 Underdosing of antithrombotic drugs**

\+ **T45.6 Poisoning by, adverse effect of and underdosing of fibrinolysis-affecting drugs**

\+ **T45.60 Poisoning by, adverse effect of and underdosing of unspecified fibrinolysis-affecting drugs**

+7th **T45.601 Poisoning by unspecified fibrinolysis-affecting drugs, accidental (unintentional)**
Poisoning by fibrinolysis-affecting drug NOS

+7th **T45.602 Poisoning by unspecified fibrinolysis-affecting drugs, intentional self-harm**

+7th **T45.603 Poisoning by unspecified fibrinolysis-affecting drugs, assault**

+7th **T45.604 Poisoning by unspecified fibrinolysis-affecting drugs, undetermined**

+7th **T45.605 Adverse effect of unspecified fibrinolysis-affecting drugs**

+7th **T45.606 Underdosing of unspecified fibrinolysis-affecting drugs**

+ **T45.61 Poisoning by, adverse effect of and underdosing of thrombolytic drugs**

+7th **T45.611 Poisoning by thrombolytic drug, accidental (unintentional)**

Poisoning by thrombolytic drug NOS

+7th **T45.612 Poisoning by thrombolytic drug, intentional self-harm**

+7th **T45.613 Poisoning by thrombolytic drug, assault**

+7th **T45.614 Poisoning by thrombolytic drug, undetermined**

+7th **T45.615 Adverse effect of thrombolytic drugs**

AHA CC: 2Q, 2017, 9-10

+7th **T45.616 Underdosing of thrombolytic drugs**

+ **T45.62 Poisoning by, adverse effect of and underdosing of hemostatic drugs**

+7th **T45.621 Poisoning by hemostatic drug, accidental (unintentional)**

Poisoning by hemostatic drug NOS

+7th **T45.622 Poisoning by hemostatic drug, intentional self-harm**

+7th **T45.623 Poisoning by hemostatic drug, assault**

+7th **T45.624 Poisoning by hemostatic drug, undetermined**

+7th **T45.625 Adverse effect of hemostatic drug**

+7th **T45.626 Underdosing of hemostatic drugs**

+ **T45.69 Poisoning by, adverse effect of and underdosing of other fibrinolysis-affecting drugs**

+7th **T45.691 Poisoning by other fibrinolysis-affecting drugs, accidental (unintentional)**

Poisoning by other fibrinolysis-affecting drug NOS

+7th **T45.692 Poisoning by other fibrinolysis-affecting drugs, intentional self-harm**

+7th **T45.693 Poisoning by other fibrinolysis-affecting drugs, assault**

+7th **T45.694 Poisoning by other fibrinolysis-affecting drugs, undetermined**

+7th **T45.695 Adverse effect of other fibrinolysis-affecting drugs**

+7th **T45.696 Underdosing of other fibrinolysis-affecting drugs**

+ **T45.7 Poisoning by, adverse effect of and underdosing of anticoagulant antagonists, vitamin K and other coagulants**

+ **T45.7X Poisoning by, adverse effect of and underdosing of anticoagulant antagonists, vitamin K and other coagulants**

+7th **T45.7X1 Poisoning by anticoagulant antagonists, vitamin K and other coagulants, accidental (unintentional)**

Poisoning by anticoagulant antagonists, vitamin K and other coagulants NOS

+7th **T45.7X2 Poisoning by anticoagulant antagonists, vitamin K and other coagulants, intentional self-harm**

+7th **T45.7X3 Poisoning by anticoagulant antagonists, vitamin K and other coagulants, assault**

+7th **T45.7X4 Poisoning by anticoagulant antagonists, vitamin K and other coagulants, undetermined**

+7th **T45.7X5 Adverse effect of anticoagulant antagonists, vitamin K and other coagulants**

+7th **T45.7X6 Underdosing of anticoagulant antagonist, vitamin K and other coagulants**

Excludes1: *vitamin K deficiency (E56.1)*

+ **T45.8 Poisoning by, adverse effect of and underdosing of other primarily systemic and hematological agents**

Poisoning by, adverse effect of and underdosing of liver preparations and other antianemic agents

Poisoning by, adverse effect of and underdosing of natural blood and blood products

Poisoning by, adverse effect of and underdosing of plasma substitute

Excludes2: *poisoning by, adverse effect of and underdosing of immunoglobulin (T50.Z1)*
poisoning by, adverse effect of and underdosing of iron (T45.4)
transfusion reactions (T80.-)

+ **T45.8X Poisoning by, adverse effect of and underdosing of other primarily systemic and hematological agents**

+7th **T45.8X1 Poisoning by other primarily systemic and hematological agents, accidental (unintentional)**

Poisoning by other primarily systemic and hematological agents NOS

+7th **T45.8X2 Poisoning by other primarily systemic and hematological agents, intentional self-harm**

+7th **T45.8X3 Poisoning by other primarily systemic and hematological agents, assault**

+7th **T45.8X4 Poisoning by other primarily systemic and hematological agents, undetermined**

+7th **T45.8X5 Adverse effect of other primarily systemic and hematological agents**

AHA CC: 4Q, 2016, 41-42

+7th **T45.8X6 Underdosing of other primarily systemic and hematological agents**

+ **T45.9 Poisoning by, adverse effect of and underdosing of unspecified primarily systemic and hematological agent**

X+7th **T45.91 Poisoning by unspecified primarily systemic and hematological agent, accidental (unintentional)**

Poisoning by primarily systemic and hematological agent NOS

X+7th **T45.92 Poisoning by unspecified primarily systemic and hematological agent, intentional self-harm**

X+7th **T45.93 Poisoning by unspecified primarily systemic and hematological agent, assault**

X+7th **T45.94 Poisoning by unspecified primarily systemic and hematological agent, undetermined**

X+7th **T45.95 Adverse effect of unspecified primarily systemic and hematological agent**

X+7th **T45.96 Underdosing of unspecified primarily systemic and hematological agent**

T46 Poisoning by, adverse effect of and underdosing of agents primarily affecting the cardiovascular system

Excludes1: *poisoning by, adverse effect of and underdosing of metaraminol (T44.4)*

The appropriate 7th character is to be added to each code from category T46
A initial encounter
D subsequent encounter
S sequela

+ **T46.0 Poisoning by, adverse effect of and underdosing of cardiac-stimulant glycosides and drugs of similar action**

+ **T46.0X Poisoning by, adverse effect of and underdosing of cardiac-stimulant glycosides and drugs of similar action**

+7th **T46.0X1 Poisoning by cardiac-stimulant glycosides and drugs of similar action, accidental (unintentional)**

Poisoning by cardiac-stimulant glycosides and drugs of similar action NOS

+7th **T46.0X2 Poisoning by cardiac-stimulant glycosides and drugs of similar action, intentional self-harm**

+7th **T46.0X3 Poisoning by cardiac-stimulant glycosides and drugs of similar action, assault**

+7th **T46.0X4** **Poisoning by cardiac-stimulant glycosides and drugs of similar action, undetermined**

+7th **T46.0X5** **Adverse effect of cardiac-stimulant glycosides and drugs of similar action**

+7th **T46.0X6** **Underdosing of cardiac-stimulant glycosides and drugs of similar action**

\+ **T46.1** **Poisoning by, adverse effect of and underdosing of calcium-channel blockers**

\+ **T46.1X** **Poisoning by, adverse effect of and underdosing of calcium-channel blockers**

+7th **T46.1X1** **Poisoning by calcium-channel blockers, accidental (unintentional)**

Poisoning by calcium-channel blockers NOS

+7th **T46.1X2** **Poisoning by calcium-channel blockers, intentional self-harm**

+7th **T46.1X3** **Poisoning by calcium-channel blockers, assault**

+7th **T46.1X4** **Poisoning by calcium-channel blockers, undetermined**

+7th **T46.1X5** **Adverse effect of calcium-channel blockers**

+7th **T46.1X6** **Underdosing of calcium-channel blockers**

\+ **T46.2** **Poisoning by, adverse effect of and underdosing of other antidysrhythmic drugs, not elsewhere classified**

Excludes1: *poisoning by, adverse effect of and underdosing of beta-adrenoreceptor antagonists (T44.7-)*

\+ **T46.2X** **Poisoning by, adverse effect of and underdosing of other antidysrhythmic drugs**

+7th **T46.2X1** **Poisoning by other antidysrhythmic drugs, accidental (unintentional)**

Poisoning by other antidysrhythmic drugs NOS

+7th **T46.2X2** **Poisoning by other antidysrhythmic drugs, intentional self-harm**

+7th **T46.2X3** **Poisoning by other antidysrhythmic drugs, assault**

+7th **T46.2X4** **Poisoning by other antidysrhythmic drugs, undetermined**

+7th **T46.2X5** **Adverse effect of other antidysrhythmic drugs**

+7th **T46.2X6** **Underdosing of other antidysrhythmic drugs**

\+ **T46.3** **Poisoning by, adverse effect of and underdosing of coronary vasodilators**

Poisoning by, adverse effect of and underdosing of dipyridamole

Excludes1: *poisoning by, adverse effect of and underdosing of calcium-channel blockers (T46.1)*

\+ **T46.3X** **Poisoning by, adverse effect of and underdosing of coronary vasodilators**

+7th **T46.3X1** **Poisoning by coronary vasodilators, accidental (unintentional)**

Poisoning by coronary vasodilators NOS

+7th **T46.3X2** **Poisoning by coronary vasodilators, intentional self-harm**

+7th **T46.3X3** **Poisoning by coronary vasodilators, assault**

+7th **T46.3X4** **Poisoning by coronary vasodilators, undetermined**

+7th **T46.3X5** **Adverse effect of coronary vasodilators**

+7th **T46.3X6** **Underdosing of coronary vasodilators**

\+ **T46.4** **Poisoning by, adverse effect of and underdosing of angiotensin-converting-enzyme inhibitors**

\+ **T46.4X** **Poisoning by, adverse effect of and underdosing of angiotensin-converting-enzyme inhibitors**

+7th **T46.4X1** **Poisoning by angiotensin-converting-enzyme inhibitors, accidental (unintentional)**

Poisoning by angiotensin-converting-enzyme inhibitors NOS

+7th **T46.4X2** **Poisoning by angiotensin-converting-enzyme inhibitors, intentional self-harm**

+7th **T46.4X3** **Poisoning by angiotensin-converting-enzyme inhibitors, assault**

+7th **T46.4X4** **Poisoning by angiotensin-converting-enzyme inhibitors, undetermined**

+7th **T46.4X5** **Adverse effect of angiotensin-converting-enzyme inhibitors**

+7th **T46.4X6** **Underdosing of angiotensin-converting-enzyme inhibitors**

\+ **T46.5** **Poisoning by, adverse effect of and underdosing of other antihypertensive drugs**

Excludes2: *poisoning by, adverse effect of and underdosing of beta-adrenoreceptor antagonists (T44.7)*
poisoning by, adverse effect of and underdosing of calcium-channel blockers (T46.1)
poisoning by, adverse effect of and underdosing of diuretics (T50.0-T50.2)

\+ **T46.5X** **Poisoning by, adverse effect of and underdosing of other antihypertensive drugs**

+7th **T46.5X1** **Poisoning by other antihypertensive drugs, accidental (unintentional)**

Poisoning by other antihypertensive drugs NOS

+7th **T46.5X2** **Poisoning by other antihypertensive drugs, intentional self-harm**

+7th **T46.5X3** **Poisoning by other antihypertensive drugs, assault**

+7th **T46.5X4** **Poisoning by other antihypertensive drugs, undetermined**

+7th **T46.5X5** **Adverse effect of other antihypertensive drugs**

+7th **T46.5X6** **Underdosing of other antihypertensive drugs**

\+ **T46.6** **Poisoning by, adverse effect of and underdosing of antihyperlipidemic and antiarteriosclerotic drugs**

\+ **T46.6X** **Poisoning by, adverse effect of and underdosing of antihyperlipidemic and antiarteriosclerotic drugs**

+7th **T46.6X1** **Poisoning by antihyperlipidemic and antiarteriosclerotic drugs, accidental (unintentional)**

Poisoning by antihyperlipidemic and antiarteriosclerotic drugs NOS

+7th **T46.6X2** **Poisoning by antihyperlipidemic and antiarteriosclerotic drugs, intentional self-harm**

+7th **T46.6X3** **Poisoning by antihyperlipidemic and antiarteriosclerotic drugs, assault**

+7th **T46.6X4** **Poisoning by antihyperlipidemic and antiarteriosclerotic drugs, undetermined**

+7th **T46.6X5** **Adverse effect of antihyperlipidemic and antiarteriosclerotic drugs**

+7th **T46.6X6** **Underdosing of antihyperlipidemic and antiarteriosclerotic drugs**

\+ **T46.7** **Poisoning by, adverse effect of and underdosing of peripheral vasodilators**

Poisoning by, adverse effect of and underdosing of nicotinic acid (derivatives)

Excludes1: *poisoning by, adverse effect of and underdosing of papaverine (T44.3)*

\+ **T46.7X** **Poisoning by, adverse effect of and underdosing of peripheral vasodilators**

+7th **T46.7X1** **Poisoning by peripheral vasodilators, accidental (unintentional)**

Poisoning by peripheral vasodilators NOS

+7th **T46.7X2** **Poisoning by peripheral vasodilators, intentional self-harm**

+7th **T46.7X3** **Poisoning by peripheral vasodilators, assault**

+7th **T46.7X4** **Poisoning by peripheral vasodilators, undetermined**

+7th **T46.7X5** **Adverse effect of peripheral vasodilators**

+7th **T46.7X6** **Underdosing of peripheral vasodilators**

+ T46.8 Poisoning by, adverse effect of and underdosing of antivaricose drugs, including sclerosing agents

+ T46.8X Poisoning by, adverse effect of and underdosing of antivaricose drugs, including sclerosing agents

+7th **T46.8X1 Poisoning by antivaricose drugs, including sclerosing agents, accidental (unintentional)**

Poisoning by antivaricose drugs, including sclerosing agents NOS

+7th **T46.8X2 Poisoning by antivaricose drugs, including sclerosing agents, intentional self-harm**

+7th **T46.8X3 Poisoning by antivaricose drugs, including sclerosing agents, assault**

+7th **T46.8X4 Poisoning by antivaricose drugs, including sclerosing agents, undetermined**

+7th **T46.8X5 Adverse effect of antivaricose drugs, including sclerosing agents**

+7th **T46.8X6 Underdosing of antivaricose drugs, including sclerosing agents**

+ T46.9 Poisoning by, adverse effect of and underdosing of other and unspecified agents primarily affecting the cardiovascular system

+ T46.90 Poisoning by, adverse effect of and underdosing of unspecified agents primarily affecting the cardiovascular system

+7th **T46.901 Poisoning by unspecified agents primarily affecting the cardiovascular system, accidental (unintentional)**

+7th **T46.902 Poisoning by unspecified agents primarily affecting the cardiovascular system, intentional self-harm**

+7th **T46.903 Poisoning by unspecified agents primarily affecting the cardiovascular system, assault**

+7th **T46.904 Poisoning by unspecified agents primarily affecting the cardiovascular system, undetermined**

+7th **T46.905 Adverse effect of unspecified agents primarily affecting the cardiovascular system**

+7th **T46.906 Underdosing of unspecified agents primarily affecting the cardiovascular system**

+ T46.99 Poisoning by, adverse effect of and underdosing of other agents primarily affecting the cardiovascular system

+7th **T46.991 Poisoning by other agents primarily affecting the cardiovascular system, accidental (unintentional)**

+7th **T46.992 Poisoning by other agents primarily affecting the cardiovascular system, intentional self-harm**

+7th **T46.993 Poisoning by other agents primarily affecting the cardiovascular system, assault**

+7th **T46.994 Poisoning by other agents primarily affecting the cardiovascular system, undetermined**

+7th **T46.995 Adverse effect of other agents primarily affecting the cardiovascular system**

+7th **T46.996 Underdosing of other agents primarily affecting the cardiovascular system**

T47 Poisoning by, adverse effect of and underdosing of agents primarily affecting the gastrointestinal system

The appropriate 7th character is to be added to each code from category T47
A initial encounter
D subsequent encounter
S sequela

+ T47.0 Poisoning by, adverse effect of and underdosing of histamine H2-receptor blockers

+ T47.0X Poisoning by, adverse effect of and underdosing of histamine H2-receptor blockers

+7th **T47.0X1 Poisoning by histamine H2-receptor blockers, accidental (unintentional)**

Poisoning by histamine H2-receptor blockers NOS

+7th **T47.0X2 Poisoning by histamine H2-receptor blockers, intentional self-harm**

+7th **T47.0X3 Poisoning by histamine H2-receptor blockers, assault**

+7th **T47.0X4 Poisoning by histamine H2-receptor blockers, undetermined**

+7th **T47.0X5 Adverse effect of histamine H2-receptor blockers**

+7th **T47.0X6 Underdosing of histamine H2-receptor blockers**

+ T47.1 Poisoning by, adverse effect of and underdosing of other antacids and anti-gastric-secretion drugs

+ T47.1X Poisoning by, adverse effect of and underdosing of other antacids and anti-gastric-secretion drugs

+7th **T47.1X1 Poisoning by other antacids and anti-gastric-secretion drugs, accidental (unintentional)**

Poisoning by other antacids and anti-gastric-secretion drugs NOS

+7th **T47.1X2 Poisoning by other antacids and anti-gastric-secretion drugs, intentional self-harm**

+7th **T47.1X3 Poisoning by other antacids and anti-gastric-secretion drugs, assault**

+7th **T47.1X4 Poisoning by other antacids and anti-gastric-secretion drugs, undetermined**

+7th **T47.1X5 Adverse effect of other antacids and anti-gastric-secretion drugs**

+7th **T47.1X6 Underdosing of other antacids and anti-gastric-secretion drugs**

+ T47.2 Poisoning by, adverse effect of and underdosing of stimulant laxatives

+ T47.2X Poisoning by, adverse effect of and underdosing of stimulant laxatives

+7th **T47.2X1 Poisoning by stimulant laxatives, accidental (unintentional)**

Poisoning by stimulant laxatives NOS

+7th **T47.2X2 Poisoning by stimulant laxatives, intentional self-harm**

+7th **T47.2X3 Poisoning by stimulant laxatives, assault**

+7th **T47.2X4 Poisoning by stimulant laxatives, undetermined**

+7th **T47.2X5 Adverse effect of stimulant laxatives**

+7th **T47.2X6 Underdosing of stimulant laxatives**

+ T47.3 Poisoning by, adverse effect of and underdosing of saline and osmotic laxatives

+ T47.3X Poisoning by and adverse effect of saline and osmotic laxatives

+7th **T47.3X1 Poisoning by saline and osmotic laxatives, accidental (unintentional)**

Poisoning by saline and osmotic laxatives NOS

+7th **T47.3X2 Poisoning by saline and osmotic laxatives, intentional self-harm**

+7th **T47.3X3 Poisoning by saline and osmotic laxatives, assault**

+7th **T47.3X4 Poisoning by saline and osmotic laxatives, undetermined**

+7th **T47.3X5 Adverse effect of saline and osmotic laxatives**

+7th **T47.3X6 Underdosing of saline and osmotic laxatives**

+ T47.4 **Poisoning by, adverse effect of and underdosing of other laxatives**

+ T47.4X **Poisoning by, adverse effect of and underdosing of other laxatives**

+7th T47.4X1 **Poisoning by other laxatives, accidental (unintentional)**

Poisoning by other laxatives NOS

+7th T47.4X2 **Poisoning by other laxatives, intentional self-harm**

+7th T47.4X3 **Poisoning by other laxatives, assault**

+7th T47.4X4 **Poisoning by other laxatives, undetermined**

+7th T47.4X5 **Adverse effect of other l axatives**

+7th T47.4X6 **Underdosing of other laxatives**

+ T47.5 **Poisoning by, adverse effect of and underdosing of digestants**

+ T47.5X **Poisoning by, adverse effect of and underdosing of digestants**

+7th T47.5X1 **Poisoning by digestants, accidental (unintentional)**

Poisoning by digestants NOS

+7th T47.5X2 **Poisoning by digestants, intentional self-harm**

+7th T47.5X3 **Poisoning by digestants, assault**

+7th T47.5X4 **Poisoning by digestants, undetermined**

+7th T47.5X5 **Adverse effect of digestants**

+7th T47.5X6 **Underdosing of digestants**

+ T47.6 **Poisoning by, adverse effect of and underdosing of antidiarrheal drugs**

Excludes2: *poisoning by, adverse effect of and underdosing of systemic antibiotics and other anti-infectives (T36-T37)*

+ T47.6X **Poisoning by, adverse effect of and underdosing of antidiarrheal drugs**

+7th T47.6X1 **Poisoning by antidiarrheal drugs, accidental (unintentional)**

Poisoning by antidiarrheal drugs NOS

+7th T47.6X2 **Poisoning by antidiarrheal drugs, intentional self-harm**

+7th T47.6X3 **Poisoning by antidiarrheal drugs, assault**

+7th T47.6X4 **Poisoning by antidiarrheal drugs, undetermined**

+7th T47.6X5 **Adverse effect of antidiarrheal drugs**

+7th T47.6X6 **Underdosing of antidiarrheal drugs**

+ T47.7 **Poisoning by, adverse effect of and underdosing of emetics**

+ T47.7X **Poisoning by, adverse effect of and underdosing of emetics**

+7th T47.7X1 **Poisoning by emetics, accidental (unintentional)**

Poisoning by emetics NOS

+7th T47.7X2 **Poisoning by emetics, intentional self-harm**

+7th T47.7X3 **Poisoning by emetics, assault**

+7th T47.7X4 **Poisoning by emetics, undetermined**

+7th T47.7X5 **Adverse effect of emetics**

+7th T47.7X6 **Underdosing of emetics**

+ T47.8 **Poisoning by, adverse effect of and underdosing of other agents primarily affecting gastrointestinal system**

+ T47.8X **Poisoning by, adverse effect of and underdosing of other agents primarily affecting gastrointestinal system**

+7th T47.8X1 **Poisoning by other agents primarily affecting gastrointestinal system, accidental (unintentional)**

Poisoning by other agents primarily affecting gastrointestinal system NOS

+7th T47.8X2 **Poisoning by other agents primarily affecting gastrointestinal system, intentional self-harm**

+7th T47.8X3 **Poisoning by other agents primarily affecting gastrointestinal system, assault**

+7th T47.8X4 **Poisoning by other agents primarily affecting gastrointestinal system, undetermined**

+7th T47.8X5 **Adverse effect of other agents primarily affecting gastrointestinal system**

+7th T47.8X6 **Underdosing of other agents primarily affecting gastrointestinal system**

+ T47.9 **Poisoning by, adverse effect of and underdosing of unspecified agents primarily affecting the gastrointestinal system**

X+7th T47.91 **Poisoning by unspecified agents primarily affecting the gastrointestinal system, accidental (unintentional)**

Poisoning by agents primarily affecting the gastrointestinal system NOS

X+7th T47.92 **Poisoning by unspecified agents primarily affecting the gastrointestinal system, intentional self-harm**

X+7th T47.93 **Poisoning by unspecified agents primarily affecting the gastrointestinal system, assault**

X+7th T47.94 **Poisoning by unspecified agents primarily affecting the gastrointestinal system, undetermined**

X+7th T47.95 **Adverse effect of unspecified agents primarily affecting the gastrointestinal system**

X+7th T47.96 **Underdosing of unspecified agents primarily affecting the gastrointestinal system**

T48 Poisoning by, adverse effect of and underdosing of agents primarily acting on smooth and skeletal muscles and the respiratory system

The appropriate 7th character is to be added to each code from category T48
A initial encounter
D subsequent encounter
S sequela

+ T48.0 **Poisoning by, adverse effect of and underdosing of oxytocic drugs**

Excludes1: *poisoning by, adverse effect of and underdosing of estrogens, progestogens and antagonists (T38.4-T38.6)*

+ T48.0X **Poisoning by, adverse effect of and underdosing of oxytocic drugs**

+7th T48.0X1 **Poisoning by oxytocic drugs, accidental (unintentional)**

Poisoning by oxytocic drugs NOS

+7th T48.0X2 **Poisoning by oxytocic drugs, intentional self-harm**

+7th T48.0X3 **Poisoning by oxytocic drugs, assault**

+7th T48.0X4 **Poisoning by oxytocic drugs, undetermined**

+7th T48.0X5 **Adverse effect of oxytocic drugs**

+7th T48.0X6 **Underdosing of oxytocic drugs**

+ T48.1 **Poisoning by, adverse effect of and underdosing of skeletal muscle relaxants [neuromuscular blocking agents]**

+ T48.1X **Poisoning by, adverse effect of and underdosing of skeletal muscle relaxants [neuromuscular blocking agents]**

+7th T48.1X1 **Poisoning by skeletal muscle relaxants [neuromuscular blocking agents], accidental (unintentional)**

Poisoning by skeletal muscle relaxants [neuromuscular blocking agents] NOS

+7th T48.1X2 **Poisoning by skeletal muscle relaxants [neuromuscular blocking agents], intentional self-harm**

+7th T48.1X3 **Poisoning by skeletal muscle relaxants [neuromuscular blocking agents], assault**

+7th T48.1X4 **Poisoning by skeletal muscle relaxants [neuromuscular blocking agents], undetermined**

+7th T48.1X5 **Adverse effect of skeletal muscle relaxants [neuromuscular blocking agents]**

+7th T48.1X6 **Underdosing of skeletal muscle relaxants [neuromuscular blocking agents]**

+ T48.2 **Poisoning by, adverse effect of and underdosing of other and unspecified drugs acting on muscles**

+ T48.20 **Poisoning by, adverse effect of and underdosing of unspecified drugs acting on muscles**

+7th T48.201 **Poisoning by unspecified drugs acting on muscles, accidental (unintentional)**

Poisoning by unspecified drugs acting on muscles NOS

+7th T48.202 **Poisoning by unspecified drugs acting on muscles, intentional self-harm**

+7th **T48.203 Poisoning by unspecified drugs acting on muscles, assault**

+7th **T48.204 Poisoning by unspecified drugs acting on muscles, undetermined**

+7th **T48.205 Adverse effect of unspecified drugs acting on muscles**

+7th **T48.206 Underdosing of unspecified drugs acting on muscles**

\+ **T48.29 Poisoning by, adverse effect of and underdosing of other drugs acting on muscles**

+7th **T48.291 Poisoning by other drugs acting on muscles, accidental (unintentional)**

Poisoning by other drugs acting on muscles NOS

+7th **T48.292 Poisoning by other drugs acting on muscles, intentional self-harm**

+7th **T48.293 Poisoning by other drugs acting on muscles, assault**

+7th **T48.294 Poisoning by other drugs acting on muscles, undetermined**

+7th **T48.295 Adverse effect of other drugs acting on muscles**

+7th **T48.296 Underdosing of other drugs acting on muscles**

\+ **T48.3 Poisoning by, adverse effect of and underdosing of antitussives**

\+ **T48.3X Poisoning by, adverse effect of and underdosing of antitussives**

+7th **T48.3X1 Poisoning by antitussives, accidental (unintentional)**

Poisoning by antitussives NOS

+7th **T48.3X2 Poisoning by antitussives, intentional self-harm**

+7th **T48.3X3 Poisoning by antitussives, assault**

+7th **T48.3X4 Poisoning by antitussives, undetermined**

+7th **T48.3X5 Adverse effect of antitussives**

+7th **T48.3X6 Underdosing of antitussives**

\+ **T48.4 Poisoning by, adverse effect of and underdosing of expectorants**

\+ **T48.4X Poisoning by, adverse effect of and underdosing of expectorants**

+7th **T48.4X1 Poisoning by expectorants, accidental (unintentional)**

Poisoning by expectorants NOS

+7th **T48.4X2 Poisoning by expectorants, intentional self-harm**

+7th **T48.4X3 Poisoning by expectorants, assault**

+7th **T48.4X4 Poisoning by expectorants, undetermined**

+7th **T48.4X5 Adverse effect of expectorants**

+7th **T48.4X6 Underdosing of expectorants**

\+ **T48.5 Poisoning by, adverse effect of and underdosing of other anti-common-cold drugs**

Poisoning by, adverse effect of and underdosing of decongestants

Excludes2: *poisoning by, adverse effect of and underdosing of antipyretics, NEC (T39.9-)*
poisoning by, adverse effect of and underdosing of non-steroidal antiinflammatory drugs (T39.3-)
poisoning by, adverse effect of and underdosing of salicylates (T39.0-)

\+ **T48.5X Poisoning by, adverse effect of and underdosing of other anti-common-cold drugs**

+7th **T48.5X1 Poisoning by other anti-common-cold drugs, accidental (unintentional)**

Poisoning by other anti-common-cold drugs NOS

+7th **T48.5X2 Poisoning by other anti-common-cold drugs, intentional self-harm**

+7th **T48.5X3 Poisoning by other anti-common-cold drugs, assault**

+7th **T48.5X4 Poisoning by other anti-common-cold drugs, undetermined**

+7th **T48.5X5 Adverse effect of other anti-common-cold drugs**

+7th **T48.5X6 Underdosing of other anti-common-cold drugs**

\+ **T48.6 Poisoning by, adverse effect of and underdosing of antiasthmatics, not elsewhere classified**

Poisoning by, adverse effect of and underdosing of beta-adrenoreceptor agonists used in asthma therapy

Excludes1: *poisoning by, adverse effect of and underdosing of beta-adrenoreceptor agonists not used in asthma therapy (T44.5)*
poisoning by, adverse effect of and underdosing of anterior pituitary [adenohypophyseal] hormones (T38.8)

\+ **T48.6X Poisoning by, adverse effect of and underdosing of antiasthmatics**

+7th **T48.6X1 Poisoning by antiasthmatics, accidental (unintentional)**

Poisoning by antiasthmatics NOS

+7th **T48.6X2 Poisoning by antiasthmatics, intentional self-harm**

+7th **T48.6X3 Poisoning by antiasthmatics, assault**

+7th **T48.6X4 Poisoning by antiasthmatics, undetermined**

+7th **T48.6X5 Adverse effect of antiasthmatics**

+7th **T48.6X6 Underdosing of antiasthmatics**

\+ **T48.9 Poisoning by, adverse effect of and underdosing of other and unspecified agents primarily acting on the respiratory system**

\+ **T48.90 Poisoning by, adverse effect of and underdosing of unspecified agents primarily acting on the respiratory system**

+7th **T48.901 Poisoning by unspecified agents primarily acting on the respiratory system, accidental (unintentional)**

+7th **T48.902 Poisoning by unspecified agents primarily acting on the respiratory system, intentional self-harm**

+7th **T48.903 Poisoning by unspecified agents primarily acting on the respiratory system, assault**

+7th **T48.904 Poisoning by unspecified agents primarily acting on the respiratory system, undetermined**

+7th **T48.905 Adverse effect of unspecified agents primarily acting on the respiratory system**

+7th **T48.906 Underdosing of unspecified agents primarily acting on the respiratory system**

\+ **T48.99 Poisoning by, adverse effect of and underdosing of other agents primarily acting on the respiratory system**

+7th **T48.991 Poisoning by other agents primarily acting on the respiratory system, accidental (unintentional)**

+7th **T48.992 Poisoning by other agents primarily acting on the respiratory system, intentional self-harm**

+7th **T48.993 Poisoning by other agents primarily acting on the respiratory system, assault**

+7th **T48.994 Poisoning by other agents primarily acting on the respiratory system, undetermined**

+7th **T48.995 Adverse effect of other agents primarily acting on the respiratory system**

+7th **T48.996 Underdosing of other agents primarily acting on the respiratory system**

T49 Poisoning by, adverse effect of and underdosing of topical agents primarily affecting skin and mucous membrane and by ophthalmological, otorhinolaryngological and dental drugs

Includes: poisoning by, adverse effect of and underdosing of glucocorticoids, topically used

The appropriate 7th character is to be added to each code from category T49
A initial encounter
D subsequent encounter
S sequela

+ **T49.0 Poisoning by, adverse effect of and underdosing of local antifungal, anti-infective and anti-inflammatory drugs**

+ **T49.0X Poisoning by, adverse effect of and underdosing of local antifungal, anti-infective and anti-inflammatory drugs**

+7th **T49.0X1 Poisoning by local antifungal, anti-infective and anti-inflammatory drugs, accidental (unintentional)**

Poisoning by local antifungal, anti-infective and anti-inflammatory drugs NOS

+7th **T49.0X2 Poisoning by local antifungal, anti-infective and anti-inflammatory drugs, intentional self-harm**

+7th **T49.0X3 Poisoning by local antifungal, anti-infective and anti-inflammatory drugs, assault**

+7th **T49.0X4 Poisoning by local antifungal, anti-infective and anti-inflammatory drugs, undetermined**

+7th **T49.0X5 Adverse effect of local antifungal, anti-infective and anti-inflammatory drugs**

+7th **T49.0X6 Underdosing of local antifungal, anti-infective and anti-inflammatory drugs**

+ **T49.1 Poisoning by, adverse effect of and underdosing of antipruritics**

+ **T49.1X Poisoning by, adverse effect of and underdosing of antipruritics**

+7th **T49.1X1 Poisoning by antipruritics, accidental (unintentional)**

Poisoning by antipruritics NOS

+7th **T49.1X2 Poisoning by antipruritics, intentional self-harm**

+7th **T49.1X3 Poisoning by antipruritics, assault**

+7th **T49.1X4 Poisoning by antipruritics, undetermined**

+7th **T49.1X5 Adverse effect of antipruritics**

+7th **T49.1X6 Underdosing of antipruritics**

+ **T49.2 Poisoning by, adverse effect of and underdosing of local astringents and local detergents**

+ **T49.2X Poisoning by, adverse effect of and underdosing of local astringents and local detergents**

+7th **T49.2X1 Poisoning by local astringents and local detergents, accidental (unintentional)**

Poisoning by local astringents and local detergents NOS

+7th **T49.2X2 Poisoning by local astringents and local detergents, intentional self-harm**

+7th **T49.2X3 Poisoning by local astringents and local detergents, assault**

+7th **T49.2X4 Poisoning by local astringents and local detergents, undetermined**

+7th **T49.2X5 Adverse effect of local astringents and local detergents**

+7th **T49.2X6 Underdosing of local astringents and local detergents**

+ **T49.3 Poisoning by, adverse effect of and underdosing of emollients, demulcents and protectants**

+ **T49.3X Poisoning by, adverse effect of and underdosing of emollients, demulcents and protectants**

+7th **T49.3X1 Poisoning by emollients, demulcents and protectants, accidental (unintentional)**

Poisoning by emollients, demulcents and protectants NOS

+7th **T49.3X2 Poisoning by emollients, demulcents and protectants, intentional self-harm**

+7th **T49.3X3 Poisoning by emollients, demulcents and protectants, assault**

+7th **T49.3X4 Poisoning by emollients, demulcents and protectants, undetermined**

+7th **T49.3X5 Adverse effect of emollients, demulcents and protectants**

+7th **T49.3X6 Underdosing of emollients, demulcents and protectants**

+ **T49.4 Poisoning by, adverse effect of and underdosing of keratolytics, keratoplastics, and other hair treatment drugs and preparations**

+ **T49.4X Poisoning by, adverse effect of and underdosing of keratolytics, keratoplastics, and other hair treatment drugs and preparations**

+7th **T49.4X1 Poisoning by keratolytics, keratoplastics, and other hair treatment drugs and preparations, accidental (unintentional)**

Poisoning by keratolytics, keratoplastics, and other hair treatment drugs and preparations NOS

+7th **T49.4X2 Poisoning by keratolytics, keratoplastics, and other hair treatment drugs and preparations, intentional self-harm**

+7th **T49.4X3 Poisoning by keratolytics, keratoplastics, and other hair treatment drugs and preparations, assault**

+7th **T49.4X4 Poisoning by keratolytics, keratoplastics, and other hair treatment drugs and preparations, undetermined**

+7th **T49.4X5 Adverse effect of keratolytics, keratoplastics, and other hair treatment drugs and preparations**

+7th **T49.4X6 Underdosing of keratolytics, keratoplastics, and other hair treatment drugs and preparations**

+ **T49.5 Poisoning by, adverse effect of and underdosing of ophthalmological drugs and preparations**

+ **T49.5X Poisoning by, adverse effect of and underdosing of ophthalmological drugs and preparations**

+7th **T49.5X1 Poisoning by ophthalmological drugs and preparations, accidental (unintentional)**

Poisoning by ophthalmological drugs and preparations NOS

+7th **T49.5X2 Poisoning by ophthalmological drugs and preparations, intentional self-harm**

+7th **T49.5X3 Poisoning by ophthalmological drugs and preparations, assault**

+7th **T49.5X4 Poisoning by ophthalmological drugs and preparations, undetermined**

+7th **T49.5X5 Adverse effect of ophthalmological drugs and preparations**

+7th **T49.5X6 Underdosing of ophthalmological drugs and preparations**

+ **T49.6 Poisoning by, adverse effect of and underdosing of otorhinolaryngological drugs and preparations**

+ **T49.6X Poisoning by, adverse effect of and underdosing of otorhinolaryngological drugs and preparations**

+7th **T49.6X1 Poisoning by otorhinolaryngological drugs and preparations, accidental (unintentional)**

Poisoning by otorhinolaryngological drugs and preparations NOS

+7th **T49.6X2 Poisoning by otorhinolaryngological drugs and preparations, intentional self-harm**

+7th **T49.6X3 Poisoning by otorhinolaryngological drugs and preparations, assault**

+7th **T49.6X4 Poisoning by otorhinolaryngological drugs and preparations, undetermined**

+7th **T49.6X5 Adverse effect of otorhinolaryngological drugs and preparations**

+7th **T49.6X6 Underdosing of otorhinolaryngological drugs and preparations**

+ **T49.7 Poisoning by, adverse effect of and underdosing of dental drugs, topically applied**

+ **T49.7X Poisoning by, adverse effect of and underdosing of dental drugs, topically applied**

+7th **T49.7X1 Poisoning by dental drugs, topically applied, accidental (unintentional)**

Poisoning by dental drugs, topically applied NOS

+7th **T49.7X2 Poisoning by dental drugs, topically applied, intentional self-harm**

+7th **T49.7X3 Poisoning by dental drugs, topically applied, assault**

+7th **T49.7X4 Poisoning by dental drugs, topically applied, undetermined**

+7th **T49.7X5 Adverse effect of dental drugs, topically applied**

+7th **T49.7X6 Underdosing of dental drugs, topically applied**

\+ **T49.8 Poisoning by, adverse effect of and underdosing of other topical agents**

Poisoning by, adverse effect of and underdosing of spermicides

\+ **T49.8X Poisoning by, adverse effect of and underdosing of other topical agents**

+7th **T49.8X1 Poisoning by other topical agents, accidental (unintentional)**

Poisoning by other topical agents NOS

+7th **T49.8X2 Poisoning by other topical agents, intentional self-harm**

+7th **T49.8X3 Poisoning by other topical agents, assault**

+7th **T49.8X4 Poisoning by other topical agents, undetermined**

+7th **T49.8X5 Adverse effect of other topical agents**

+7th **T49.8X6 Underdosing of other topical agents**

\+ **T49.9 Poisoning by, adverse effect of and underdosing of unspecified topical agent**

X+7th **T49.91 Poisoning by unspecified topical agent, accidental (unintentional)**

X+7th **T49.92 Poisoning by unspecified topical agent, intentional self-harm**

X+7th **T49.93 Poisoning by unspecified topical agent, assault**

X+7th **T49.94 Poisoning by unspecified topical agent, undetermined**

X+7th **T49.95 Adverse effect of unspecified topical agent**

X+7th **T49.96 Underdosing of unspecified topical agent**

T50 Poisoning by, adverse effect of and underdosing of diuretics and other and unspecified drugs, medicaments and biological substances

The appropriate 7th character is to be added to each code from category T50
A initial encounter
D subsequent encounter
S sequela

\+ **T50.0 Poisoning by, adverse effect of and underdosing of mineralocorticoids and their antagonists**

\+ **T50.0X Poisoning by, adverse effect of and underdosing of mineralocorticoids and their antagonists**

+7th **T50.0X1 Poisoning by mineralocorticoids and their antagonists, accidental (unintentional)**

Poisoning by mineralocorticoids and their antagonists NOS

+7th **T50.0X2 Poisoning by mineralocorticoids and their antagonists, intentional self-harm**

+7th **T50.0X3 Poisoning by mineralocorticoids and their antagonists, assault**

+7th **T50.0X4 Poisoning by mineralocorticoids and their antagonists, undetermined**

+7th **T50.0X5 Adverse effect of mineralocorticoids and their antagonists**

+7th **T50.0X6 Underdosing of mineralocorticoids and their antagonists**

\+ **T50.1 Poisoning by, adverse effect of and underdosing of loop [high-ceiling] diuretics**

\+ **T50.1X Poisoning by, adverse effect of and underdosing of loop [high-ceiling] diuretics**

+7th **T50.1X1 Poisoning by loop [high-ceiling] diuretics, accidental (unintentional)**

Poisoning by loop [high-ceiling] diuretics NOS

+7th **T50.1X2 Poisoning by loop [high-ceiling] diuretics, intentional self-harm**

+7th **T50.1X3 Poisoning by loop [high-ceiling] diuretics, assault**

+7th **T50.1X4 Poisoning by loop [high-ceiling] diuretics, undetermined**

+7th **T50.1X5 Adverse effect of loop [high-ceiling] diuretics**

+7th **T50.1X6 Underdosing of loop [high-ceiling] diuretics**

\+ **T50.2 Poisoning by, adverse effect of and underdosing of carbonic-anhydrase inhibitors, benzothiadiazides and other diuretics**

Poisoning by, adverse effect of and underdosing of acetazolamide

\+ **T50.2X Poisoning by, adverse effect of and underdosing of carbonic-anhydrase inhibitors, benzothiadiazides and other diuretics**

+7th **T50.2X1 Poisoning by carbonic-anhydrase inhibitors, benzothiadiazides and other diuretics, accidental (unintentional)**

Poisoning by carbonic-anhydrase inhibitors, benzothiadiazides and other diuretics NOS

+7th **T50.2X2 Poisoning by carbonic-anhydrase inhibitors, benzothiadiazides and other diuretics, intentional self-harm**

+7th **T50.2X3 Poisoning by carbonic-anhydrase inhibitors, benzothiadiazides and other diuretics, assault**

+7th **T50.2X4 Poisoning by carbonic-anhydrase inhibitors, benzothiadiazides and other diuretics, undetermined**

+7th **T50.2X5 Adverse effect of carbonic-anhydrase inhibitors, benzothiadiazides and other diuretics**

+7th **T50.2X6 Underdosing of carbonic-anhydrase inhibitors, benzothiadiazides and other diuretics**

\+ **T50.3 Poisoning by, adverse effect of and underdosing of electrolytic, caloric and water-balance agents**

Poisoning by, adverse effect of and underdosing of oral rehydration salts

\+ **T50.3X Poisoning by, adverse effect of and underdosing of electrolytic, caloric and water-balance agents**

+7th **T50.3X1 Poisoning by electrolytic, caloric and water-balance agents, accidental (unintentional)**

Poisoning by electrolytic, caloric and water-balance agents NOS

+7th **T50.3X2 Poisoning by electrolytic, caloric and water-balance agents, intentional self-harm**

+7th **T50.3X3 Poisoning by electrolytic, caloric and water-balance agents, assault**

+7th **T50.3X4 Poisoning by electrolytic, caloric and water-balance agents, undetermined**

+7th **T50.3X5 Adverse effect of electrolytic, caloric and water-balance agents**

+7th **T50.3X6 Underdosing of electrolytic, caloric and water-balance agents**

\+ **T50.4 Poisoning by, adverse effect of and underdosing of drugs affecting uric acid metabolism**

\+ **T50.4X Poisoning by, adverse effect of and underdosing of drugs affecting uric acid metabolism**

+7th **T50.4X1 Poisoning by drugs affecting uric acid metabolism, accidental (unintentional)**

Poisoning by drugs affecting uric acid metabolism NOS

+7th **T50.4X2 Poisoning by drugs affecting uric acid metabolism, intentional self-harm**

+7th **T50.4X3 Poisoning by drugs affecting uric acid metabolism, assault**

+7th **T50.4X4 Poisoning by drugs affecting uric acid metabolism, undetermined**

+7th **T50.4X5 Adverse effect of drugs affecting uric acid metabolism**

+7th **T50.4X6 Underdosing of drugs affecting uric acid metabolism**

\+ **T50.5 Poisoning by, adverse effect of and underdosing of appetite depressants**

\+ **T50.5X Poisoning by, adverse effect of and underdosing of appetite depressants**

+7th **T50.5X1 Poisoning by appetite depressants, accidental (unintentional)**

Poisoning by appetite depressants NOS

+7th **T50.5X2 Poisoning by appetite depressants, intentional self-harm**

+7th **T50.5X3 Poisoning by appetite depressants, assault**

+7th **T50.5X4 Poisoning by appetite depressants, undetermined**

+7th **T50.5X5 Adverse effect of appetite depressants**

+7th **T50.5X6 Underdosing of appetite depressants**

+ **T50.6 Poisoning by, adverse effect of and underdosing of antidotes and chelating agents**
Poisoning by, adverse effect of and underdosing of alcohol deterrents
+ **T50.6X Poisoning by, adverse effect of and underdosing of antidotes and chelating agents**
+7th **T50.6X1 Poisoning by antidotes and chelatingagents, accidental (unintentional)**
Poisoning by antidotes and chelating agents NOS
+7th **T50.6X2 Poisoning by antidotes and chelating agents, intentional self-harm**
+7th **T50.6X3 Poisoning by antidotes and chelating agents, assault**
+7th **T50.6X4 Poisoning by antidotes and chelating agents, undetermined**
+7th **T50.6X5 Adverse effect of antidotes and chelating agents**
+7th **T50.6X6 Underdosing of antidotes and chelating agents**
+ **T50.7 Poisoning by, adverse effect of and underdosing of analeptics and opioid receptor antagonists**
+ **T50.7X Poisoning by, adverse effect of and underdosing of analeptics and opioid receptor antagonists**
+7th **T50.7X1 Poisoning by analeptics and opioid receptor antagonists, accidental (unintentional)**
Poisoning by analeptics and opioid receptor antagonists NOS
+7th **T50.7X2 Poisoning by analeptics and opioid receptor antagonists, intentional self-harm**
+7th **T50.7X3 Poisoning by analeptics and opioid receptor antagonists, assault**
+7th **T50.7X4 Poisoning by analeptics and opioid receptor antagonists, undetermined**
+7th **T50.7X5 Adverse effect of analeptics and opioid receptor antagonists**
+7th **T50.7X6 Underdosing of analeptics and opioid receptor antagonists**
+ **T50.8 Poisoning by, adverse effect of and underdosing of diagnostic agents**
+ **T50.8X Poisoning by, adverse effect of and underdosing of diagnostic agents**
+7th **T50.8X1 Poisoning by diagnostic agents, accidental (unintentional)**
Poisoning by diagnostic agents NOS
+7th **T50.8X2 Poisoning by diagnostic agents, intentional self-harm**
+7th **T50.8X3 Poisoning by diagnostic agents, assault**
+7th **T50.8X4 Poisoning by diagnostic agents, undetermined**
+7th **T50.8X5 Adverse effect of diagnostic agents**
+7th **T50.8X6 Underdosing of diagnostic agents**
+ **T50.A Poisoning by, adverse effect of and underdosing of bacterial vaccines**
+ **T50.A1 Poisoning by, adverse effect of and underdosing of pertussis vaccine, including combinations with a pertussis component**
+7th **T50.A11 Poisoning by pertussis vaccine, including combinations with a pertussis component, accidental (unintentional)**
+7th **T50.A12 Poisoning by pertussis vaccine, including combinations with a pertussis component, intentional self-harm**
+7th **T50.A13 Poisoning by pertussis vaccine, including combinations with a pertussis component, assault**
+7th **T50.A14 Poisoning by pertussis vaccine, including combinations with a pertussis component, undetermined**
+7th **T50.A15 Adverse effect of pertussis vaccine, including combinations with a pertussis component**
+7th **T50.A16 Underdosing of pertussis vaccine, including combinations with a pertussis component**
+ **T50.A2 Poisoning by, adverse effect of and underdosing of mixed bacterial vaccines without a pertussis component**
+7th **T50.A21 Poisoning by mixed bacterial vaccines without a pertussis component, accidental (unintentional)**
+7th **T50.A22 Poisoning by mixed bacterial vaccines without a pertussis component, intentional self-harm**
+7th **T50.A23 Poisoning by mixed bacterial vaccines without a pertussis component, assault**
+7th **T50.A24 Poisoning by mixed bacterial vaccines without a pertussis component, undetermined**
+7th **T50.A25 Adverse effect of mixed bacterial vaccines without a pertussis component**
+7th **T50.A26 Underdosing of mixed bacterial vaccines without a pertussis component**
+ **T50.A9 Poisoning by, adverse effect of and underdosing of other bacterial vaccines**
+7th **T50.A91 Poisoning by other bacterial vaccines, accidental (unintentional)**
+7th **T50.A92 Poisoning by other bacterial vaccines, intentional self-harm**
+7th **T50.A93 Poisoning by other bacterial vaccines, assault**
+7th **T50.A94 Poisoning by other bacterial vaccines, undetermined**
+7th **T50.A95 Adverse effect of other bacterial vaccines**
+7th **T50.A96 Underdosing of other bacterial vaccines**
+ **T50.B Poisoning by, adverse effect of and underdosing of viral vaccines**
+ **T50.B1 Poisoning by, adverse effect of and underdosing of smallpox vaccines**
+7th **T50.B11 Poisoning by smallpox vaccines, accidental (unintentional)**
+7th **T50.B12 Poisoning by smallpox vaccines, intentional self-harm**
+7th **T50.B13 Poisoning by smallpox vaccines, assault**
+7th **T50.B14 Poisoning by smallpox vaccines, undetermined**
+7th **T50.B15 Adverse effect of smallpox vaccines**
+7th **T50.B16 Underdosing of smallpox vaccines**
+ **T50.B9 Poisoning by, adverse effect of and underdosing of other viral vaccines**
+7th **T50.B91 Poisoning by other viral vaccines, accidental (unintentional)**
+7th **T50.B92 Poisoning by other viral vaccines, intentional self-harm**
+7th **T50.B93 Poisoning by other viral vaccines, assault**
+7th **T50.B94 Poisoning by other viral vaccines, undetermined**
+7th **T50.B95 Adverse effect of other viral vaccines**
AHA CC: 1Q, 2021, 43-44
+7th **T50.B96 Underdosing of other viral vaccines**
+ **T50.Z Poisoning by, adverse effect of and underdosing of other vaccines and biological substances**
+ **T50.Z1 Poisoning by, adverse effect of and underdosing of immunoglobulin**
+7th **T50.Z11 Poisoning by immunoglobulin, accidental (unintentional)**
+7th **T50.Z12 Poisoning by immunoglobulin, intentional self-harm**
+7th **T50.Z13 Poisoning by immunoglobulin, assault**
+7th **T50.Z14 Poisoning by immunoglobulin, undetermined**
+7th **T50.Z15 Adverse effect of immunoglobulin**
+7th **T50.Z16 Underdosing of immunoglobulin**
+ **T50.Z9 Poisoning by, adverse effect of and underdosing of other vaccines and biological substances**
+7th **T50.Z91 Poisoning by other vaccines and biological substances, accidental (unintentional)**
+7th **T50.Z92 Poisoning by other vaccines and biological substances, intentional self-harm**
+7th **T50.Z93 Poisoning by other vaccines and biological substances, assault**
+7th **T50.Z94 Poisoning by other vaccines and biological substances, undetermined**
+7th **T50.Z95 Adverse effect of other vaccines and biological substances**
AHA CC: 1Q, 2020, 18-19
+7th **T50.Z96 Underdosing of other vaccines and biological substances**

+ T50.9 Poisoning by, adverse effect of and underdosing of other and unspecified drugs, medicaments and biological substances

+ T50.90 Poisoning by, adverse effect of and underdosing of unspecified drugs, medicaments and biological substances

+7th **T50.901 Poisoning by unspecified drugs, medicaments and biological substances, accidental (unintentional)**

AHA CC: 1Q, 2015, 3-21

+7th **T50.902 Poisoning by unspecified drugs, medicaments and biological substances, intentional self-harm**

+7th **T50.903 Poisoning by unspecified drugs, medicaments and biological substances, assault**

+7th **T50.904 Poisoning by unspecified drugs, medicaments and biological substances, undetermined**

+7th **T50.905 Adverse effect of unspecified drugs, medicaments and biological substances**

+7th **T50.906 Underdosing of unspecified drugs, medicaments and biological substances**

+ T50.91 Poisoning by, adverse effect of and underdosing of multiple unspecified drugs, medicaments and biological substances

Multiple drug ingestion NOS

Code also any specific drugs, medicaments and biological substances

AHA CC: 4Q, 2019, 17

T50.911 Poisoning by multiple unspecified drugs, medicaments and biological substances, accidental (unintentional)

T50.912 Poisoning by multiple unspecified drugs, medicaments and biological substances, intentional self-harm

T50.913 Poisoning by multiple unspecified drugs, medicaments and biological substances, assault

T50.914 Poisoning by multiple unspecified drugs, medicaments and biological substances, undetermined

T50.915 Adverse effect of multiple unspecified drugs, medicaments and biological substances

T50.916 Underdosing of multiple unspecified drugs, medicaments and biological substance

+ T50.99 Poisoning by, adverse effect of and underdosing of other drugs, medicaments and biological substances

+7th **T50.991 Poisoning by other drugs, medicaments and biological substances, accidental (unintentional)**

+7th **T50.992 Poisoning by other drugs, medicaments and biological substances, intentional self-harm**

+7th **T50.993 Poisoning by other drugs, medicaments and biological substances, assault**

+7th **T50.994 Poisoning by other drugs, medicaments and biological substances, undetermined**

+7th **T50.995 Adverse effect of other drugs, medicaments and biological substances**

+7th **T50.996 Underdosing of other drugs, medicaments and biological substances**

Toxic effects of substances chiefly nonmedicinal as to source (T51-T65)

NOTE When no intent is indicated code to accidental. Undetermined intent is only for use when there is specific documentation in the record that the intent of the toxic effect cannot be determined.

Use additional code(s):
- for all associated manifestations of toxic effect, such as: respiratory conditions due to external agents (J60-J70)
- personal history of foreign body fully removed (Z87.821)
- to identify any retained foreign body, if applicable (Z18.-)

Excludes1: *contact with and (suspected) exposure to toxic substances (Z77.-)*

Review coding guideline C.19.e

T51 Toxic effect of alcohol

The appropriate 7th character is to be added to each code from category T51
A initial encounter
D subsequent encounter
S sequela

+ T51.0 Toxic effect of ethanol

Toxic effect of ethyl alcohol

Excludes2: acute alcohol intoxication or 'hangover' effects
drunkenness (F10.129, F10.229, F10.929)
pathological (F10.129, F10.229, F10.929)
alcohol intoxication (F10.129, F10.229, F10.929)

+ T51.0X Toxic effect of ethanol

+7th **T51.0X1 Toxic effect of ethanol, accidental (unintentional)**

Toxic effect of ethanol NOS

+7th **T51.0X2 Toxic effect of ethanol, intentional self-harm**

+7th **T51.0X3 Toxic effect of ethanol, assault**

+7th **T51.0X4 Toxic effect of ethanol, undetermined**

+ T51.1 Toxic effect of methanol

Toxic effect of methyl alcohol

+ T51.1X Toxic effect of methanol

+7th **T51.1X1 Toxic effect of methanol, accidental (unintentional)**

Toxic effect of methanol NOS

+7th **T51.1X2 Toxic effect of methanol, intentional self-harm**

+7th **T51.1X3 Toxic effect of methanol, assault**

+7th **T51.1X4 Toxic effect of methanol, undetermined**

+ T51.2 Toxic effect of 2-Propanol

Toxic effect of isopropyl alcohol

+ T51.2X Toxic effect of 2-Propanol

+7th **T51.2X1 Toxic effect of 2-Propanol, accidental (unintentional)**

Toxic effect of 2-Propanol NOS

+7th **T51.2X2 Toxic effect of 2-Propanol, intentional self-harm**

+7th **T51.2X3 Toxic effect of 2-Propanol, assault**

+7th **T51.2X4 Toxic effect of 2-Propanol, undetermined**

+ T51.3 Toxic effect of fusel oil

Toxic effect of amyl alcohol
Toxic effect of butyl [1-butanol] alcohol
Toxic effect of propyl [1-propanol] alcohol

+ T51.3X Toxic effect of fusel oil

+7th **T51.3X1 Toxic effect of fusel oil, accidental (unintentional)**

Toxic effect of fusel oil NOS

+7th **T51.3X2 Toxic effect of fusel oil, intentional self-harm**

+7th **T51.3X3 Toxic effect of fusel oil, assault**

+7th **T51.3X4 Toxic effect of fusel oil, undetermined**

+ T51.8 Toxic effect of other alcohols

+ T51.8X Toxic effect of other alcohols

+7th **T51.8X1 Toxic effect of other alcohols, accidental (unintentional)**

Toxic effect of other alcohols NOS

+7th **T51.8X2 Toxic effect of other alcohols, intentional self-harm**

+7th **T51.8X3 Toxic effect of other alcohols, assault**

+7th **T51.8X4 Toxic effect of other alcohols, undetermined**

+ T51.9 Toxic effect of unspecified alcohol

X+7th **T51.91 Toxic effect of unspecified alcohol, accidental (unintentional)**

X+7th **T51.92 Toxic effect of unspecified alcohol, intentional self-harm**

X+7th **T51.93 Toxic effect of unspecified alcohol, assault**

X+7th **T51.94 Toxic effect of unspecified alcohol, undetermined**

T52 Toxic effect of organic solvents

Excludes1: *halogen derivatives of aliphatic and aromatic hydrocarbons (T53.-)*

The appropriate 7th character is to be added to each code from category T52
A initial encounter
D subsequent encounter
S sequela

+ T52.0 Toxic effects of petroleum products
Toxic effects of gasoline [petrol]
Toxic effects of kerosene [paraffin oil]
Toxic effects of paraffin wax
Toxic effects of ether petroleum
Toxic effects of naphtha petroleum
Toxic effects of spirit petroleum

+ T52.0X Toxic effects of petroleum products
+7th **T52.0X1 Toxic effect of petroleum products, accidental (unintentional)**
Toxic effects of petroleum products NOS
+7th **T52.0X2 Toxic effect of petroleum products, intentional self-harm**
+7th **T52.0X3 Toxic effect of petroleum products, assault**
+7th **T52.0X4 Toxic effect of petroleum products, undetermined**

+ T52.1 Toxic effects of benzene
Excludes1: homologues of benzene (T52.2)
nitroderivatives and aminoderivatives of benzene and its homologues (T65.3)

+ T52.1X Toxic effects of benzene
+7th **T52.1X1 Toxic effect of benzene, accidental (unintentional)**
Toxic effects of benzene NOS
+7th **T52.1X2 Toxic effect of benzene, intentional self-harm**
+7th **T52.1X3 Toxic effect of benzene, assault**
+7th **T52.1X4 Toxic effect of benzene, undetermined**

+ T52.2 Toxic effects of homologues of benzene
Toxic effects of toluene [methylbenzene]
Toxic effects of xylene [dimethylbenzene]

+ T52.2X Toxic effects of homologues of benzene
+7th **T52.2X1 Toxic effect of homologues of benzene, accidental (unintentional)**
Toxic effects of homologues of benzene NOS
+7th **T52.2X2 Toxic effect of homologues of benzene, intentional self-harm**
+7th **T52.2X3 Toxic effect of homologues of benzene, assault**
+7th **T52.2X4 Toxic effect of homologues of benzene, undetermined**

+ T52.3 Toxic effects of glycols

+ T52.3X Toxic effects of glycols
+7th **T52.3X1 Toxic effect of glycols, accidental (unintentional)**
Toxic effects of glycols NOS
+7th **T52.3X2 Toxic effect of glycols, intentional self-harm**
+7th **T52.3X3 Toxic effect of glycols, assault**
+7th **T52.3X4 Toxic effect of glycols, undetermined**

+ T52.4 Toxic effects of ketones

+ T52.4X Toxic effects of ketones
+7th **T52.4X1 Toxic effect of ketones, accidental (unintentional)**
Toxic effects of ketones NOS
+7th **T52.4X2 Toxic effect of ketones, intentional self-harm**
+7th **T52.4X3 Toxic effect of ketones, assault**
+7th **T52.4X4 Toxic effect of ketones, undetermined**

+ T52.8 Toxic effects of other organic solvents

+ T52.8X Toxic effects of other organic solvents
+7th **T52.8X1 Toxic effect of other organic solvents, accidental (unintentional)**
Toxic effects of other organic solvents NOS
+7th **T52.8X2 Toxic effect of other organic solvents, intentional self-harm**
+7th **T52.8X3 Toxic effect of other organic solvents, assault**
+7th **T52.8X4 Toxic effect of other organic solvents, undetermined**

+ T52.9 Toxic effects of unspecified organic solvent
X+7th **T52.91 Toxic effect of unspecified organic solvent, accidental (unintentional)**
X+7th **T52.92 Toxic effect of unspecified organic solvent, intentional self-harm**
X+7th **T52.93 Toxic effect of unspecified organic solvent, assault**
X+7th **T52.94 Toxic effect of unspecified organic solvent, undetermined**

T53 Toxic effect of halogen derivatives of aliphatic and aromatic hydrocarbons

The appropriate 7th character is to be added to each code from category T53
A initial encounter
D subsequent encounter
S sequela

+ T53.0 Toxic effects of carbon tetrachloride
Toxic effects of tetrachloromethane

+ T53.0X Toxic effects of carbon tetrachloride
+7th **T53.0X1 Toxic effect of carbon tetrachloride, accidental (unintentional)**
Toxic effects of carbon tetrachloride NOS
+7th **T53.0X2 Toxic effect of carbon tetrachloride, intentional self-harm**
+7th **T53.0X3 Toxic effect of carbon tetrachloride, assault**
+7th **T53.0X4 Toxic effect of carbon tetrachloride, undetermined**

+ T53.1 Toxic effects of chloroform
Toxic effects of trichloromethane

+ T53.1X Toxic effects of chloroform
+7th **T53.1X1 Toxic effect of chloroform, accidental (unintentional)**
Toxic effects of chloroform NOS
+7th **T53.1X2 Toxic effect of chloroform, intentional self-harm**
+7th **T53.1X3 Toxic effect of chloroform, assault**
+7th **T53.1X4 Toxic effect of chloroform, undetermined**

+ T53.2 Toxic effects of trichloroethylene
Toxic effects of trichloroethene

+ T53.2X Toxic effects of trichloroethylene
+7th **T53.2X1 Toxic effect of trichloroethylene, accidental (unintentional)**
Toxic effects of trichloroethylene NOS
+7th **T53.2X2 Toxic effect of trichloroethylene, intentional self-harm**
+7th **T53.2X3 Toxic effect of trichloroethylene, assault**
+7th **T53.2X4 Toxic effect of trichloroethylene, undetermined**

+ **T53.3 Toxic effects of tetrachloroethylene**
  Toxic effects of perchloroethylene
  Toxic effect of tetrachloroethene
  + **T53.3X Toxic effects of tetrachloroethylene**
    +7th **T53.3X1 Toxic effect of tetrachloroethylene, accidental (unintentional)**
      Toxic effects of tetrachloroethylene NOS
    +7th **T53.3X2 Toxic effect of tetrachloroethylene, intentional self-harm**
    +7th **T53.3X3 Toxic effect of tetrachloroethylene, assault**
    +7th **T53.3X4 Toxic effect of tetrachloroethylene, undetermined**
+ **T53.4 Toxic effects of dichloromethane**
  Toxic effects of methylene chloride
  + **T53.4X Toxic effects of dichloromethane**
    +7th **T53.4X1 Toxic effect of dichloromethane, accidental (unintentional)**
      Toxic effects of dichloromethane NOS
    +7th **T53.4X2 Toxic effect of dichloromethane, intentional self-harm**
    +7th **T53.4X3 Toxic effect of dichloromethane, assault**
    +7th **T53.4X4 Toxic effect of dichloromethane, undetermined**
+ **T53.5 Toxic effects of chlorofluorocarbons**
  + **T53.5X Toxic effects of chlorofluorocarbons**
    +7th **T53.5X1 Toxic effect of chlorofluorocarbons, accidental (unintentional)**
      Toxic effects of chlorofluorocarbons NOS
    +7th **T53.5X2 Toxic effect of chlorofluorocarbons, intentional self-harm**
    +7th **T53.5X3 Toxic effect of chlorofluorocarbons, assault**
    +7th **T53.5X4 Toxic effect of chlorofluorocarbons, undetermined**
+ **T53.6 Toxic effects of other halogen derivatives of aliphatic hydrocarbons**
  + **T53.6X Toxic effects of other halogen derivatives of aliphatic hydrocarbons**
    +7th **T53.6X1 Toxic effect of other halogen derivatives of aliphatic hydrocarbons, accidental (unintentional)**
      Toxic effects of other halogen derivatives of aliphatic hydrocarbons NOS
    +7th **T53.6X2 Toxic effect of other halogen derivatives of aliphatic hydrocarbons, intentional self-harm**
    +7th **T53.6X3 Toxic effect of other halogen derivatives of aliphatic hydrocarbons, assault**
    +7th **T53.6X4 Toxic effect of other halogen derivatives of aliphatic hydrocarbons, undetermined**
+ **T53.7 Toxic effects of other halogen derivatives of aromatic hydrocarbons**
  + **T53.7X Toxic effects of other halogen derivatives of aromatic hydrocarbons**
    +7th **T53.7X1 Toxic effect of other halogen derivatives of aromatic hydrocarbons, accidental (unintentional)**
      Toxic effects of other halogen derivatives of aromatic hydrocarbons NOS
    +7th **T53.7X2 Toxic effect of other halogen derivatives of aromatic hydrocarbons, intentional self-harm**
    +7th **T53.7X3 Toxic effect of other halogen derivatives of aromatic hydrocarbons, assault**
    +7th **T53.7X4 Toxic effect of other halogen derivatives of aromatic hydrocarbons, undetermined**
+ **T53.9 Toxic effects of unspecified halogen derivatives of aliphatic and aromatic hydrocarbons**
  X+7th **T53.91 Toxic effect of unspecified halogen derivatives of aliphatic and aromatic hydrocarbons, accidental (unintentional)**
  X+7th **T53.92 Toxic effect of unspecified halogen derivatives of aliphatic and aromatic hydrocarbons, intentional self-harm**
  X+7th **T53.93 Toxic effect of unspecified halogen derivatives of aliphatic and aromatic hydrocarbons, assault**
  X+7th **T53.94 Toxic effect of unspecified halogen derivatives of aliphatic and aromatic hydrocarbons, undetermined**

T54 Toxic effect of corrosive substances

The appropriate 7th character is to be added to each code from category T54
A initial encounter
D subsequent encounter
S sequela

+ **T54.0 Toxic effects of phenol and phenol homologues**
  + **T54.0X Toxic effects of phenol and phenol homologues**
    +7th **T54.0X1 Toxic effect of phenol and phenol homologues, accidental (unintentional)**
      Toxic effects of phenol and phenol homologues NOS
    +7th **T54.0X2 Toxic effect of phenol and phenol homologues, intentional self-harm**
    +7th **T54.0X3 Toxic effect of phenol and phenol homologues, assault**
    +7th **T54.0X4 Toxic effect of phenol and phenol homologues, undetermined**
+ **T54.1 Toxic effects of other corrosive organic compounds**
  + **T54.1X Toxic effects of other corrosive organic compounds**
    +7th **T54.1X1 Toxic effect of other corrosive organic compounds, accidental (unintentional)**
      Toxic effects of other corrosive organic compounds NOS
    +7th **T54.1X2 Toxic effect of other corrosive organic compounds, intentional self-harm**
    +7th **T54.1X3 Toxic effect of other corrosive organic compounds, assault**
    +7th **T54.1X4 Toxic effect of other corrosive organic compounds, undetermined**
+ **T54.2 Toxic effects of corrosive acids and acid-like substances**
  Toxic effects of hydrochloric acid
  Toxic effects of sulfuric acid
  + **T54.2X Toxic effects of corrosive acids and acid-like substances**
    +7th **T54.2X1 Toxic effect of corrosive acids and acid-like substances, accidental (unintentional)**
      Toxic effects of corrosive acids and acid-like substances NOS
    +7th **T54.2X2 Toxic effect of corrosive acids and acid-like substances, intentional self-harm**
    +7th **T54.2X3 Toxic effect of corrosive acids and acid-like substances, assault**
    +7th **T54.2X4 Toxic effect of corrosive acids and acid-like substances, undetermined**
+ **T54.3 Toxic effects of corrosive alkalis and alkali-like substances**
  Toxic effects of potassium hydroxide
  Toxic effects of sodium hydroxide
  + **T54.3X Toxic effects of corrosive alkalis and alkali-like substances**
    +7th **T54.3X1 Toxic effect of corrosive alkalis and alkali-like substances, accidental (unintentional)**
      Toxic effects of corrosive alkalis and alkali-like substances NOS
    +7th **T54.3X2 Toxic effect of corrosive alkalis and alkali-like substances, intentional self-harm**
    +7th **T54.3X3 Toxic effect of corrosive alkalis and alkali-like substances, assault**
    +7th **T54.3X4 Toxic effect of corrosive alkalis and alkali-like substances, undetermined**
+ **T54.9 Toxic effects of unspecified corrosive substance**
  X+7th **T54.91 Toxic effect of unspecified corrosive substance, accidental (unintentional)**
  X+7th **T54.92 Toxic effect of unspecified corrosive substance, intentional self-harm**
  X+7th **T54.93 Toxic effect of unspecified corrosive substance, assault**
  X+7th **T54.94 Toxic effect of unspecified corrosive substance, undetermined**

T55 Toxic effect of soaps and detergents

The appropriate 7th character is to be added to each code from category T55
A initial encounter
D subsequent encounter
S sequela

+ T55.0 Toxic effect of soaps
+ T55.0X Toxic effect of soaps
+7th T55.0X1 Toxic effect of soaps, accidental (unintentional)
Toxic effect of soaps NOS
+7th T55.0X2 Toxic effect of soaps, intentional self-harm
+7th T55.0X3 Toxic effect of soaps, assault
+7th T55.0X4 Toxic effect of soaps, undetermined
+ T55.1 Toxic effect of detergents
+ T55.1X Toxic effect of detergents
+7th T55.1X1 Toxic effect of detergents, accidental (unintentional)
Toxic effect of detergents NOS
+7th T55.1X2 Toxic effect of detergents, intentional self-harm
+7th T55.1X3 Toxic effect of detergents, assault
+7th T55.1X4 Toxic effect of detergents, undetermined

T56 Toxic effect of metals

Includes: toxic effects of fumes and vapors of metals
toxic effects of metals from all sources, except medicinal substances

Use additional code to identify any retained metal foreign body, if applicable (Z18.0-, T18.1-)

Excludes1: *arsenic and its compounds (T57.0)*
manganese and its compounds (T57.2)

The appropriate 7th character is to be added to each code from category T56
A initial encounter
D subsequent encounter
S sequela

+ T56.0 Toxic effects of lead and its compounds
+ T56.0X Toxic effects of lead and its compounds
+7th T56.0X1 Toxic effect of lead and its compounds, accidental (unintentional)
Toxic effects of lead and its compounds NOS
+7th T56.0X2 Toxic effect of lead and its compounds, intentional self-harm
+7th T56.0X3 Toxic effect of lead and its compounds, assault
+7th T56.0X4 Toxic effect of lead and its compounds, undetermined
+ T56.1 Toxic effects of mercury and its compounds
+ T56.1X Toxic effects of mercury and its compounds
+7th T56.1X1 Toxic effect of mercury and its compounds, accidental (unintentional)
Toxic effects of mercury and its compounds NOS
+7th T56.1X2 Toxic effect of mercury and its compounds, intentional self-harm
+7th T56.1X3 Toxic effect of mercury and its compounds, assault
+7th T56.1X4 Toxic effect of mercury and its compounds, undetermined
+ T56.2 Toxic effects of chromium and its compounds
+ T56.2X Toxic effects of chromium and its compounds
+7th T56.2X1 Toxic effect of chromium and its compounds, accidental (unintentional)
Toxic effects of chromium and its compounds NOS
+7th T56.2X2 Toxic effect of chromium and its compounds, intentional self-harm
+7th T56.2X3 Toxic effect of chromium and its compounds, assault
+7th T56.2X4 Toxic effect of chromium and its compounds, undetermined
+ T56.3 Toxic effects of cadmium and its compounds
+ T56.3X Toxic effects of cadmium and its compounds
+7th T56.3X1 Toxic effect of cadmium and its compounds, accidental (unintentional)
Toxic effects of cadmium and its compounds NOS
+7th T56.3X2 Toxic effect of cadmium and its compounds, intentional self-harm
+7th T56.3X3 Toxic effect of cadmium and its compounds, assault
+7th T56.3X4 Toxic effect of cadmium and its compounds, undetermined
+ T56.4 Toxic effects of copper and its compounds
+ T56.4X Toxic effects of copper and its compounds
+7th T56.4X1 Toxic effect of copper and its compounds, accidental (unintentional)
Toxic effects of copper and its compounds NOS
+7th T56.4X2 Toxic effect of copper and its compounds, intentional self-harm
+7th T56.4X3 Toxic effect of copper and its compounds, assault
+7th T56.4X4 Toxic effect of copper and its compounds, undetermined
+ T56.5 Toxic effects of zinc and its compounds
+ T56.5X Toxic effects of zinc and its compounds
+7th T56.5X1 Toxic effect of zinc and its compounds, accidental (unintentional)
Toxic effects of zinc and its compounds NOS
+7th T56.5X2 Toxic effect of zinc and its compounds, intentional self-harm
+7th T56.5X3 Toxic effect of zinc and its compounds, assault
+7th T56.5X4 Toxic effect of zinc and its compounds, undetermined
+ T56.6 Toxic effects of tin and its compounds
+ T56.6X Toxic effects of tin and its compounds
+7th T56.6X1 Toxic effect of tin and its compounds, accidental (unintentional)
Toxic effects of tin and its compounds NOS
+7th T56.6X2 Toxic effect of tin and its compounds, intentional self-harm
+7th T56.6X3 Toxic effect of tin and its compounds, assault
+7th T56.6X4 Toxic effect of tin and its compounds, undetermined
+ T56.7 Toxic effects of beryllium and its compounds
+ T56.7X Toxic effects of beryllium and its compounds
+7th T56.7X1 Toxic effect of beryllium and its compounds, accidental (unintentional)
Toxic effects of beryllium and its compounds NOS
+7th T56.7X2 Toxic effect of beryllium and its compounds, intentional self-harm
+7th T56.7X3 Toxic effect of beryllium and its compounds, assault
+7th T56.7X4 Toxic effect of beryllium and its compounds, undetermined
+ T56.8 Toxic effects of other metals
+ T56.81 Toxic effect of thallium
+7th T56.811 Toxic effect of thallium, accidental (unintentional)
Toxic effect of thallium NOS
+7th T56.812 Toxic effect of thallium, intentional self-harm
+7th T56.813 Toxic effect of thallium, assault
+7th T56.814 Toxic effect of thallium, undetermined
+ T56.89 Toxic effects of other metals
+7th T56.891 Toxic effect of other metals, accidental (unintentional)
Toxic effects of other metals NOS
+7th T56.892 Toxic effect of other metals, intentional self-harm
+7th T56.893 Toxic effect of other metals, assault
+7th T56.894 Toxic effect of other metals, undetermined
+ T56.9 Toxic effects of unspecified metal
X+7th T56.91 Toxic effect of unspecified metal, accidental (unintentional)
X+7th T56.92 Toxic effect of unspecified metal, intentional self-harm
X+7th T56.93 Toxic effect of unspecified metal, assault
X+7th T56.94 Toxic effect of unspecified metal, undetermined

T57 Toxic effect of other inorganic substances

The appropriate 7th character is to be added to each code from category T57
A initial encounter
D subsequent encounter
S sequela

+ T57.0 **Toxic effect of arsenic and its compounds**
  + T57.0X **Toxic effect of arsenic and its compounds**
    +7th T57.0X1 **Toxic effect of arsenic and its compounds, accidental (unintentional)**
    Toxic effect of arsenic and its compounds NOS
    +7th T57.0X2 **Toxic effect of arsenic and its compounds, intentional self-harm**
    +7th T57.0X3 **Toxic effect of arsenic and its compounds, assault**
    +7th T57.0X4 **Toxic effect of arsenic and its compounds, undetermined**

+ T57.1 **Toxic effect of phosphorus and its compounds**
  Excludes1: *organophosphate insecticides (T60.0)*
  + T57.1X **Toxic effect of phosphorus and its compounds**
    +7th T57.1X1 **Toxic effect of phosphorus and its compounds, accidental (unintentional)**
    Toxic effect of phosphorus and its compounds NOS
    +7th T57.1X2 **Toxic effect of phosphorus and its compounds, intentional self-harm**
    +7th T57.1X3 **Toxic effect of phosphorus and its compounds, assault**
    +7th T57.1X4 **Toxic effect of phosphorus and its compounds, undetermined**

+ T57.2 **Toxic effect of manganese and its compounds**
  + T57.2X **Toxic effect of manganese and its compounds**
    +7th T57.2X1 **Toxic effect of manganese and its compounds, accidental (unintentional)**
    Toxic effect of manganese and its compounds NOS
    +7th T57.2X2 **Toxic effect of manganese and its compounds, intentional self-harm**
    +7th T57.2X3 **Toxic effect of manganese and its compounds, assault**
    +7th T57.2X4 **Toxic effect of manganese and its compounds, undetermined**

+ T57.3 **Toxic effect of hydrogen cyanide**
  + T57.3X **Toxic effect of hydrogen cyanide**
    +7th T57.3X1 **Toxic effect of hydrogen cyanide, accidental (unintentional)**
    Toxic effect of hydrogen cyanide NOS
    +7th T57.3X2 **Toxic effect of hydrogen cyanide, intentional self-harm**
    +7th T57.3X3 **Toxic effect of hydrogen cyanide, assault**
    +7th T57.3X4 **Toxic effect of hydrogen cyanide, undetermined**

+ T57.8 **Toxic effect of other specified inorganic substances**
  + T57.8X **Toxic effect of other specified inorganic substances**
    +7th T57.8X1 **Toxic effect of other specified inorganic substances, accidental (unintentional)**
    Toxic effect of other specified inorganic substances NOS
    +7th T57.8X2 **Toxic effect of other specified inorganic substances, intentional self-harm**
    +7th T57.8X3 **Toxic effect of other specified inorganic substances, assault**
    +7th T57.8X4 **Toxic effect of other specified inorganic substances, undetermined**

+ T57.9 **Toxic effect of unspecified inorganic substance**
  X+7th T57.91 **Toxic effect of unspecified inorganic substance, accidental (unintentional)**
  X+7th T57.92 **Toxic effect of unspecified inorganic substance, intentional self-harm**
  X+7th T57.93 **Toxic effect of unspecified inorganic substance, assault**
  X+7th T57.94 **Toxic effect of unspecified inorganic substance, undetermined**

T58 Toxic effect of carbon monoxide

Includes: asphyxiation from carbon monoxide
toxic effect of carbon monoxide from all sources

The appropriate 7th character is to be added to each code from category T58
A initial encounter
D subsequent encounter
S sequela

+ T58.0 **Toxic effect of carbon monoxide from motor vehicle exhaust**
  Toxic effect of exhaust gas from gas engine
  Toxic effect of exhaust gas from motor pump
  X+7th T58.01 **Toxic effect of carbon monoxide from motor vehicle exhaust, accidental (unintentional)**
  X+7th T58.02 **Toxic effect of carbon monoxide from motor vehicle exhaust, intentional self-harm**
  X+7th T58.03 **Toxic effect of carbon monoxide from motor vehicle exhaust, assault**
  X+7th T58.04 **Toxic effect of carbon monoxide from motor vehicle exhaust, undetermined**

+ T58.1 **Toxic effect of carbon monoxide from utility gas**
  Toxic effect of acetylene
  Toxic effect of gas NOS used for lighting, heating, cooking
  Toxic effect of water gas
  X+7th T58.11 **Toxic effect of carbon monoxide from utility gas, accidental (unintentional)**
  X+7th T58.12 **Toxic effect of carbon monoxide from utility gas, intentional self-harm**
  X+7th T58.13 **Toxic effect of carbon monoxide from utility gas, assault**
  X+7th T58.14 **Toxic effect of carbon monoxide from utility gas, undetermined**

+ T58.2 **Toxic effect of carbon monoxide from incomplete combustion of other domestic fuels**
  Toxic effect of carbon monoxide from incomplete combustion of coal, coke, kerosene, wood
  + T58.2X **Toxic effect of carbon monoxide from incomplete combustion of other domestic fuels**
    +7th T58.2X1 **Toxic effect of carbon monoxide from incomplete combustion of other domestic fuels, accidental (unintentional)**
    +7th T58.2X2 **Toxic effect of carbon monoxide from incomplete combustion of other domestic fuels, intentional self-harm**
    +7th T58.2X3 **Toxic effect of carbon monoxide from incomplete combustion of other domestic fuels, assault**
    +7th T58.2X4 **Toxic effect of carbon monoxide from incomplete combustion of other domestic fuels, undetermined**

+ T58.8 **Toxic effect of carbon monoxide from other source**
  Toxic effect of carbon monoxide from blast furnace gas
  Toxic effect of carbon monoxide from fuels in industrial use
  Toxic effect of carbon monoxide from kiln vapor
  + T58.8X **Toxic effect of carbon monoxide from other source**
    +7th T58.8X1 **Toxic effect of carbon monoxide from other source, accidental (unintentional)**
    +7th T58.8X2 **Toxic effect of carbon monoxide from other source, intentional self-harm**
    +7th T58.8X3 **Toxic effect of carbon monoxide from other source, assault**
    +7th T58.8X4 **Toxic effect of carbon monoxide from other source, undetermined**

+ T58.9 **Toxic effect of carbon monoxide from unspecified source**
  X+7th T58.91 **Toxic effect of carbon monoxide from unspecified source, accidental (unintentional)**
  X+7th T58.92 **Toxic effect of carbon monoxide from unspecified source, intentional self-harm**
  X+7th T58.93 **Toxic effect of carbon monoxide from unspecified source, assault**
  X+7th T58.94 **Toxic effect of carbon monoxide from unspecified source, undetermined**

T59 Toxic effect of other gases, fumes and vapors

Includes: aerosol propellants
Excludes1: *chlorofluorocarbons (T53.5)*

The appropriate 7th character is to be added to each code from category T59
A initial encounter
D subsequent encounter
S sequela

+ T59.0 Toxic effect of nitrogen oxides
+ T59.0X Toxic effect of nitrogen oxides
+7th T59.0X1 Toxic effect of nitrogen oxides, accidental (unintentional)
Toxic effect of nitrogen oxides NOS
+7th T59.0X2 Toxic effect of nitrogen oxides, intentional self-harm
+7th T59.0X3 Toxic effect of nitrogen oxides, assault
+7th T59.0X4 Toxic effect of nitrogen oxides, undetermined
+ T59.1 Toxic effect of sulfur dioxide
+ T59.1X Toxic effect of sulfur dioxide
+7th T59.1X1 Toxic effect of sulfur dioxide, accidental (unintentional)
Toxic effect of sulfur dioxide NOS
+7th T59.1X2 Toxic effect of sulfur dioxide, intentional self-harm
+7th T59.1X3 Toxic effect of sulfur dioxide, assault
+7th T59.1X4 Toxic effect of sulfur dioxide, undetermined
+ T59.2 Toxic effect of formaldehyde
+ T59.2X Toxic effect of formaldehyde
+7th T59.2X1 Toxic effect of formaldehyde, accidental (unintentional)
Toxic effect of formaldehyde NOS
+7th T59.2X2 Toxic effect of formaldehyde, intentional self-harm
+7th T59.2X3 Toxic effect of formaldehyde, assault
+7th T59.2X4 Toxic effect of formaldehyde, undetermined
+ T59.3 Toxic effect of lacrimogenic gas
Toxic effect of tear gas
+ T59.3X Toxic effect of lacrimogenic gas
+7th T59.3X1 Toxic effect of lacrimogenic gas, accidental (unintentional)
Toxic effect of lacrimogenic gas NOS
+7th T59.3X2 Toxic effect of lacrimogenic gas, intentional self-harm
+7th T59.3X3 Toxic effect of lacrimogenic gas, assault
+7th T59.3X4 Toxic effect of lacrimogenic gas, undetermined
+ T59.4 Toxic effect of chlorine gas
+ T59.4X Toxic effect of chlorine gas
+7th T59.4X1 Toxic effect of chlorine gas, accidental (unintentional)
Toxic effect of chlorine gas NOS
+7th T59.4X2 Toxic effect of chlorine gas, intentional self-harm
+7th T59.4X3 Toxic effect of chlorine gas, assault
+7th T59.4X4 Toxic effect of chlorine gas, undetermined
+ T59.5 Toxic effect of fluorine gas and hydrogen fluoride
+ T59.5X Toxic effect of fluorine gas and hydrogen fluoride
+7th T59.5X1 Toxic effect of fluorine gas and hydrogen fluoride, accidental (unintentional)
Toxic effect of fluorine gas and hydrogen fluoride NOS
+7th T59.5X2 Toxic effect of fluorine gas and hydrogen fluoride, intentional self-harm
+7th T59.5X3 Toxic effect of fluorine gas and hydrogen fluoride, assault
+7th T59.5X4 Toxic effect of fluorine gas and hydrogen fluoride, undetermined
+ T59.6 Toxic effect of hydrogen sulfide
+ T59.6X Toxic effect of hydrogen sulfide
+7th T59.6X1 Toxic effect of hydrogen sulfide, accidental (unintentional)
Toxic effect of hydrogen sulfide NOS
+7th T59.6X2 Toxic effect of hydrogen sulfide, intentional self-harm
+7th T59.6X3 Toxic effect of hydrogen sulfide, assault
+7th T59.6X4 Toxic effect of hydrogen sulfide, undetermined
+ T59.7 Toxic effect of carbon dioxide
+ T59.7X Toxic effect of carbon dioxide
+7th T59.7X1 Toxic effect of carbon dioxide, accidental (unintentional)
Toxic effect of carbon dioxide NOS
+7th T59.7X2 Toxic effect of carbon dioxide, intentional self-harm
+7th T59.7X3 Toxic effect of carbon dioxide, assault
+7th T59.7X4 Toxic effect of carbon dioxide, undetermined
+ T59.8 Toxic effect of other specified gases, fumes and vapors
+ T59.81 Toxic effect of smoke
Smoke inhalation
Excludes2: *toxic effect of cigarette (tobacco) smoke (T65.22-)*
+7th T59.811 Toxic effect of smoke, accidental (unintentional)
Toxic effect of smoke NOS
+7th T59.812 Toxic effect of smoke, intentional self-harm
+7th T59.813 Toxic effect of smoke, assault
+7th T59.814 Toxic effect of smoke, undetermined
+ T59.89 Toxic effect of other specified gases, fumes and vapors
+7th T59.891 Toxic effect of other specified gases, fumes and vapors, accidental (unintentional)
+7th T59.892 Toxic effect of other specified gases, fumes and vapors, intentional self-harm
+7th T59.893 Toxic effect of other specified gases, fumes and vapors, assault
+7th T59.894 Toxic effect of other specified gases, fumes and vapors, undetermined
+ T59.9 Toxic effect of unspecified gases, fumes and vapors
X+7th T59.91 Toxic effect of unspecified gases, fumes and vapors, accidental (unintentional)
X+7th T59.92 Toxic effect of unspecified gases, fumes and vapors, intentional self-harm
X+7th T59.93 Toxic effect of unspecified gases, fumes and vapors, assault
X+7th T59.94 Toxic effect of unspecified gases, fumes and vapors, undetermined

T60 Toxic effect of pesticides
Includes: toxic effect of wood preservatives

The appropriate 7th character is to be added to each code from category T60
A initial encounter
D subsequent encounter
S sequela

+ T60.0 Toxic effect of organophosphate and carbamate insecticides
+ T60.0X Toxic effect of organophosphate and carbamate insecticides
+7th T60.0X1 Toxic effect of organophosphate and carbamate insecticides, accidental (unintentional)
Toxic effect of organophosphate and carbamate insecticides NOS
+7th T60.0X2 Toxic effect of organophosphate and carbamate insecticides, intentional self-harm
+7th T60.0X3 Toxic effect of organophosphate and carbamate insecticides, assault
+7th T60.0X4 Toxic effect of organophosphate and carbamate insecticides, undetermined
+ T60.1 Toxic effect of halogenated insecticides
Excludes1: *chlorinated hydrocarbon (T53.-)*
+ T60.1X Toxic effect of halogenated insecticides
+7th T60.1X1 Toxic effect of halogenated insecticides, accidental (unintentional)
Toxic effect of halogenated insecticides NOS
+7th T60.1X2 Toxic effect of halogenated insecticides, intentional self-harm
+7th T60.1X3 Toxic effect of halogenated insecticides, assault
+7th T60.1X4 Toxic effect of halogenated insecticides, undetermined
+ T60.2 Toxic effect of other insecticides
+ T60.2X Toxic effect of other insecticides
+7th T60.2X1 Toxic effect of other insecticides, accidental (unintentional)
Toxic effect of other insecticides NOS
+7th T60.2X2 Toxic effect of other insecticides, intentional self-harm
+7th T60.2X3 Toxic effect of other insecticides, assault
+7th T60.2X4 Toxic effect of other insecticides, undetermined

+ **T60.3 Toxic effect of herbicides and fungicides**
  + **T60.3X Toxic effect of herbicides and fungicides**
    - +7th **T60.3X1 Toxic effect of herbicides and fungicides, accidental (unintentional)**
      Toxic effect of herbicides and fungicides NOS
    - +7th **T60.3X2 Toxic effect of herbicides and fungicides, intentional self-harm**
    - +7th **T60.3X3 Toxic effect of herbicides and fungicides, assault**
    - +7th **T60.3X4 Toxic effect of herbicides and fungicides, undetermined**

+ **T60.4 Toxic effect of rodenticides**
  Excludes1: *strychnine and its salts (T65.1)*
  thallium (T56.81-)
  + **T60.4X Toxic effect of rodenticides**
    - +7th **T60.4X1 Toxic effect of rodenticides, accidental (unintentional)**
      Toxic effect of rodenticides NOS
    - +7th **T60.4X2 Toxic effect of rodenticides, intentional self-harm**
    - +7th **T60.4X3 Toxic effect of rodenticides, assault**
    - +7th **T60.4X4 Toxic effect of rodenticides, undetermined**

+ **T60.8 Toxic effect of other pesticides**
  + **T60.8X Toxic effect of other pesticides**
    - +7th **T60.8X1 Toxic effect of other pesticides, accidental (unintentional)**
      Toxic effect of other pesticides NOS
    - +7th **T60.8X2 Toxic effect of other pesticides, intentional self-harm**
    - +7th **T60.8X3 Toxic effect of other pesticides, assault**
    - +7th **T60.8X4 Toxic effect of other pesticides, undetermined**

+ **T60.9 Toxic effect of unspecified pesticide**
  - X+7th **T60.91 Toxic effect of unspecified pesticide, accidental (unintentional)**
  - X+7th **T60.92 Toxic effect of unspecified pesticide, intentional self-harm**
  - X+7th **T60.93 Toxic effect of unspecified pesticide, assault**
  - X+7th **T60.94 Toxic effect of unspecified pesticide, undetermined**

T61 Toxic effect of noxious substances eaten as seafood

Excludes1: *allergic reaction to food, such as:*
anaphylactic reaction or shock due to adverse food reaction (T78.0-)
bacterial foodborne intoxications (A05.-)
dermatitis (L23.6, L25.4, L27.2)
food protein-induced enterocolitis syndrome (K52.21)
food protein-induced enteropathy (K52.22)
gastroenteritis (noninfective) (K52.29)
toxic effect of aflatoxin and other mycotoxins (T64)
toxic effect of cyanides (T65.0-)
toxic effect of harmful algae bloom (T65.82-)
toxic effect of hydrogen cyanide (T57.3-)
toxic effect of mercury (T56.1-)
toxic effect of red tide (T65.82-)

The appropriate 7th character is to be added to each code from category T61
A initial encounter
D subsequent encounter
S sequela

+ **T61.0 Ciguatera fish poisoning**
  - X+7th **T61.01 Ciguatera fish poisoning, accidental (unintentional)**
  - X+7th **T61.02 Ciguatera fish poisoning, intentional self-harm**
  - X+7th **T61.03 Ciguatera fish poisoning, assault**
  - X+7th **T61.04 Ciguatera fish poisoning, undetermined**

+ **T61.1 Scombroid fish poisoning**
  Histamine-like syndrome
  - X+7th **T61.11 Scombroid fish poisoning, accidental (unintentional)**
  - X+7th **T61.12 Scombroid fish poisoning, intentional self-harm**
  - X+7th **T61.13 Scombroid fish poisoning, assault**
  - X+7th **T61.14 Scombroid fish poisoning, undetermined**

+ **T61.7 Other fish and shellfish poisoning**
  + **T61.77 Other fish poisoning**
    - +7th **T61.771 Other fish poisoning, accidental (unintentional)**
    - +7th **T61.772 Other fish poisoning, intentional self-harm**
    - +7th **T61.773 Other fish poisoning, assault**
    - +7th **T61.774 Other fish poisoning, undetermined**
  + **T61.78 Other shellfish poisoning**
    - +7th **T61.781 Other shellfish poisoning, accidental (unintentional)**
    - +7th **T61.782 Other shellfish poisoning, intentional self-harm**
    - +7th **T61.783 Other shellfish poisoning, assault**
    - +7th **T61.784 Other shellfish poisoning, undetermined**

+ **T61.8 Toxic effect of other seafood**
  + **T61.8X Toxic effect of other seafood**
    - +7th **T61.8X1 Toxic effect of other seafood, accidental (unintentional)**
    - +7th **T61.8X2 Toxic effect of other seafood, intentional self-harm**
    - +7th **T61.8X3 Toxic effect of other seafood, assault**
    - +7th **T61.8X4 Toxic effect of other seafood, undetermined**

+ **T61.9 Toxic effect of unspecified seafood**
  - X+7th **T61.91 Toxic effect of unspecified seafood, accidental (unintentional)**
  - X+7th **T61.92 Toxic effect of unspecified seafood, intentional self-harm**
  - X+7th **T61.93 Toxic effect of unspecified seafood, assault**
  - X+7th **T61.94 Toxic effect of unspecified seafood, undetermined**

T62 Toxic effect of other noxious substances eaten as food

Excludes1: *allergic reaction to food, such as:*
anaphylactic shock (reaction) due to adverse food reaction (T78.0-)
bacterial food borne intoxications (A05.-)
dermatitis (L23.6, L25.4, L27.2)
food protein-induced enterocolitis syndrome (K52.21)
food protein-induced enteropathy (K52.22)
gastroenteritis (noninfective) (K52.29)
toxic effect of aflatoxin and other mycotoxins (T64)
toxic effect of cyanides (T65.0-)
toxic effect of hydrogen cyanide (T57.3-)
toxic effect of mercury (T56.1-)

The appropriate 7th character is to be added to each code from category T62
A initial encounter
D subsequent encounter
S sequela

+ **T62.0 Toxic effect of ingested mushrooms**
  + **T62.0X Toxic effect of ingested mushrooms**
    - +7th **T62.0X1 Toxic effect of ingested mushrooms, accidental (unintentional)**
      Toxic effect of ingested mushrooms NOS
    - +7th **T62.0X2 Toxic effect of ingested mushrooms, intentional self-harm**
    - +7th **T62.0X3 Toxic effect of ingested mushrooms, assault**
    - +7th **T62.0X4 Toxic effect of ingested mushrooms, undetermined**

+ **T62.1 Toxic effect of ingested berries**
  + **T62.1X Toxic effect of ingested berries**
    - +7th **T62.1X1 Toxic effect of ingested berries, accidental (unintentional)**
      Toxic effect of ingested berries NOS
    - +7th **T62.1X2 Toxic effect of ingested berries, intentional self-harm**
    - +7th **T62.1X3 Toxic effect of ingested berries, assault**
    - +7th **T62.1X4 Toxic effect of ingested berries, undetermined**

+ **T62.2 Toxic effect of other ingested (parts of) plant(s)**
+ **T62.2X Toxic effect of other ingested (parts of) plant(s)**
+7th **T62.2X1 Toxic effect of other ingested (parts of) plant(s), accidental (unintentional)**
Toxic effect of other ingested (parts of) plant(s) NOS
+7th **T62.2X2 Toxic effect of other ingested (parts of) plant(s), intentional self-harm**
+7th **T62.2X3 Toxic effect of other ingested (parts of) plant(s), assault**
+7th **T62.2X4 Toxic effect of other ingested (parts of) plant(s), undetermined**
+ **T62.8 Toxic effect of other specified noxious substances eaten as food**
+ **T62.8X Toxic effect of other specified noxious substances eaten as food**
+7th **T62.8X1 Toxic effect of other specified noxious substances eaten as food, accidental (unintentional)**
Toxic effect of other specified noxious substances eaten as food NOS
+7th **T62.8X2 Toxic effect of other specified noxious substances eaten as food, intentional self-harm**
+7th **T62.8X3 Toxic effect of other specified noxious substances eaten as food, assault**
+7th **T62.8X4 Toxic effect of other specified noxious substances eaten as food, undetermined**
+ **T62.9 Toxic effect of unspecified noxious substance eaten as food**
X+7th **T62.91 Toxic effect of unspecified noxious substance eaten as food, accidental (unintentional)**
Toxic effect of unspecified noxious substance eaten as food NOS
X+7th **T62.92 Toxic effect of unspecified noxious substance eaten as food, intentional self-harm**
X+7th **T62.93 Toxic effect of unspecified noxious substance eaten as food, assault**
X+7th **T62.94 Toxic effect of unspecified noxious substance eaten as food, undetermined**

T63 Toxic effect of contact with venomous animals and plants

Includes: bite or touch of venomous animal
pricked or stuck by thorn or leaf

Excludes2: *ingestion of toxic animal or plant (T61.-, T62.-)*

The appropriate 7th character is to be added to each code from category T63
A initial encounter
D subsequent encounter
S sequela

+ **T63.0 Toxic effect of snake venom**
+ **T63.00 Toxic effect of unspecified snake venom**
+7th **T63.001 Toxic effect of unspecified snake venom, accidental (unintentional)**
Toxic effect of unspecified snake venom NOS
+7th **T63.002 Toxic effect of unspecified snake venom, intentional self-harm**
+7th **T63.003 Toxic effect of unspecified snake venom, assault**
+7th **T63.004 Toxic effect of unspecified snake venom, undetermined**
+ **T63.01 Toxic effect of rattlesnake venom**
+7th **T63.011 Toxic effect of rattlesnake venom, accidental (unintentional)**
Toxic effect of rattlesnake venom NOS
+7th **T63.012 Toxic effect of rattlesnake venom, intentional self-harm**
+7th **T63.013 Toxic effect of rattlesnake venom, assault**
+7th **T63.014 Toxic effect of rattlesnake venom, undetermined**
+ **T63.02 Toxic effect of coral snake venom**
+7th **T63.021 Toxic effect of coral snake venom, accidental (unintentional)**
Toxic effect of coral snake venom NOS
+7th **T63.022 Toxic effect of coral snake venom, intentional self-harm**
+7th **T63.023 Toxic effect of coral snake venom, assault**
+7th **T63.024 Toxic effect of coral snake venom, undetermined**
+ **T63.03 Toxic effect of taipan venom**
+7th **T63.031 Toxic effect of taipan venom, accidental (unintentional)**
Toxic effect of taipan venom NOS
+7th **T63.032 Toxic effect of taipan venom, intentional self-harm**
+7th **T63.033 Toxic effect of taipan venom, assault**
+7th **T63.034 Toxic effect of taipan venom, undetermined**
+ **T63.04 Toxic effect of cobra venom**
+7th **T63.041 Toxic effect of cobra venom, accidental (unintentional)**
Toxic effect of cobra venom NOS
+7th **T63.042 Toxic effect of cobra venom, intentional self-harm**
+7th **T63.043 Toxic effect of cobra venom, assault**
+7th **T63.044 Toxic effect of cobra venom, undetermined**
+ **T63.06 Toxic effect of venom of other North and South American snake**
+7th **T63.061 Toxic effect of venom of other North and South American snake, accidental (unintentional)**
Toxic effect of venom of other North and South American snake NOS
+7th **T63.062 Toxic effect of venom of other North and South American snake, intentional self-harm**
+7th **T63.063 Toxic effect of venom of other North and South American snake, assault**
+7th **T63.064 Toxic effect of venom of other North and South American snake, undetermined**
+ **T63.07 Toxic effect of venom of other Australian snake**
+7th **T63.071 Toxic effect of venom of other Australian snake, accidental (unintentional)**
Toxic effect of venom of other Australian snake NOS
+7th **T63.072 Toxic effect of venom of other Australian snake, intentional self-harm**
+7th **T63.073 Toxic effect of venom of other Australian snake, assault**
+7th **T63.074 Toxic effect of venom of other Australian snake, undetermined**
+ **T63.08 Toxic effect of venom of other African and Asian snake**
+7th **T63.081 Toxic effect of venom of other African and Asian snake, accidental (unintentional)**
Toxic effect of venom of other African and Asian snake NOS
+7th **T63.082 Toxic effect of venom of other African and Asian snake, intentional self-harm**
+7th **T63.083 Toxic effect of venom of other African and Asian snake, assault**
+7th **T63.084 Toxic effect of venom of other African and Asian snake, undetermined**
+ **T63.09 Toxic effect of venom of other snake**
+7th **T63.091 Toxic effect of venom of other snake, accidental (unintentional)**
Toxic effect of venom of other snake NOS
+7th **T63.092 Toxic effect of venom of other snake, intentional self-harm**
+7th **T63.093 Toxic effect of venom of other snake, assault**
+7th **T63.094 Toxic effect of venom of other snake, undetermined**
+ **T63.1 Toxic effect of venom of other reptiles**
+ **T63.11 Toxic effect of venom of gila monster**
+7th **T63.111 Toxic effect of venom of gila monster, accidental (unintentional)**
Toxic effect of venom of gila monster NOS
+7th **T63.112 Toxic effect of venom of gila monster, intentional self-harm**
+7th **T63.113 Toxic effect of venom of gila monster, assault**
+7th **T63.114 Toxic effect of venom of gila monster, undetermined**

+ **T63.12 Toxic effect of venom of other venomous lizard**
  - +7th **T63.121 Toxic effect of venom of other venomous lizard, accidental (unintentional)**
    - Toxic effect of venom of other venomous lizard NOS
  - +7th **T63.122 Toxic effect of venom of other venomous lizard, intentional self-harm**
  - +7th **T63.123 Toxic effect of venom of other venomous lizard, assault**
  - +7th **T63.124 Toxic effect of venom of other venomous lizard, undetermined**

+ **T63.19 Toxic effect of venom of other reptiles**
  - +7th **T63.191 Toxic effect of venom of other reptiles, accidental (unintentional)**
    - Toxic effect of venom of other reptiles NOS
  - +7th **T63.192 Toxic effect of venom of other reptiles, intentional self-harm**
  - +7th **T63.193 Toxic effect of venom of other reptiles, assault**
  - +7th **T63.194 Toxic effect of venom of other reptiles, undetermined**

+ **T63.2 Toxic effect of venom of scorpion**

+ **T63.2X Toxic effect of venom of scorpion**
  - +7th **T63.2X1 Toxic effect of venom of scorpion, accidental (unintentional)**
    - Toxic effect of venom of scorpion NOS
  - +7th **T63.2X2 Toxic effect of venom of scorpion, intentional self-harm**
  - +7th **T63.2X3 Toxic effect of venom of scorpion, assault**
  - +7th **T63.2X4 Toxic effect of venom of scorpion, undetermined**

+ **T63.3 Toxic effect of venom of spider**

+ **T63.30 Toxic effect of unspecified spider venom**
  - +7th **T63.301 Toxic effect of unspecified spider venom, accidental (unintentional)**
  - +7th **T63.302 Toxic effect of unspecified spider venom, intentional self-harm**
  - +7th **T63.303 Toxic effect of unspecified spider venom, assault**
  - +7th **T63.304 Toxic effect of unspecified spider venom, undetermined**

+ **T63.31 Toxic effect of venom of black widow spider**
  - +7th **T63.311 Toxic effect of venom of black widow spider, accidental (unintentional)**
  - +7th **T63.312 Toxic effect of venom of black widow spider, intentional self-harm**
  - +7th **T63.313 Toxic effect of venom of black widow spider, assault**
  - +7th **T63.314 Toxic effect of venom of black widow spider, undetermined**

+ **T63.32 Toxic effect of venom of tarantula**
  - +7th **T63.321 Toxic effect of venom of tarantula, accidental (unintentional)**
  - +7th **T63.322 Toxic effect of venom of tarantula, intentional self-harm**
  - +7th **T63.323 Toxic effect of venom of tarantula, assault**
  - +7th **T63.324 Toxic effect of venom of tarantula, undetermined**

+ **T63.33 Toxic effect of venom of brown recluse spider**
  - +7th **T63.331 Toxic effect of venom of brown recluse spider, accidental (unintentional)**
  - +7th **T63.332 Toxic effect of venom of brown recluse spider, intentional self-harm**
  - +7th **T63.333 Toxic effect of venom of brown recluse spider, assault**
  - +7th **T63.334 Toxic effect of venom of brown recluse spider, undetermined**

+ **T63.39 Toxic effect of venom of other spider**
  - +7th **T63.391 Toxic effect of venom of other spider, accidental (unintentional)**
  - +7th **T63.392 Toxic effect of venom of other spider, intentional self-harm**
  - +7th **T63.393 Toxic effect of venom of other spider, assault**
  - +7th **T63.394 Toxic effect of venom of other spider, undetermined**

+ **T63.4 Toxic effect of venom of other arthropods**

+ **T63.41 Toxic effect of venom of centipedes and venomous millipedes**
  - +7th **T63.411 Toxic effect of venom of centipedes and venomous millipedes, accidental (unintentional)**
  - +7th **T63.412 Toxic effect of venom of centipedes and venomous millipedes, intentional self-harm**
  - +7th **T63.413 Toxic effect of venom of centipedes and venomous millipedes, assault**
  - +7th **T63.414 Toxic effect of venom of centipedes and venomous millipedes, undetermined**

+ **T63.42 Toxic effect of venom of ants**
  - +7th **T63.421 Toxic effect of venom of ants, accidental (unintentional)**
  - +7th **T63.422 Toxic effect of venom of ants, intentional self-harm**
  - +7th **T63.423 Toxic effect of venom of ants, assault**
  - +7th **T63.424 Toxic effect of venom of ants, undetermined**

+ **T63.43 Toxic effect of venom of caterpillars**
  - +7th **T63.431 Toxic effect of venom of caterpillars, accidental (unintentional)**
  - +7th **T63.432 Toxic effect of venom of caterpillars, intentional self-harm**
  - +7th **T63.433 Toxic effect of venom of caterpillars, assault**
  - +7th **T63.434 Toxic effect of venom of caterpillars, undetermined**

+ **T63.44 Toxic effect of venom of bees**
  - +7th **T63.441 Toxic effect of venom of bees, accidental (unintentional)**
  - +7th **T63.442 Toxic effect of venom of bees, intentional self-harm**
  - +7th **T63.443 Toxic effect of venom of bees, assault**
  - +7th **T63.444 Toxic effect of venom of bees, undetermined**

+ **T63.45 Toxic effect of venom of hornets**
  - +7th **T63.451 Toxic effect of venom of hornets, accidental (unintentional)**
  - +7th **T63.452 Toxic effect of venom of hornets, intentional self-harm**
  - +7th **T63.453 Toxic effect of venom of hornets, assault**
  - +7th **T63.454 Toxic effect of venom of hornets, undetermined**

+ **T63.46 Toxic effect of venom of wasps**
  - Toxic effect of yellow jacket
  - +7th **T63.461 Toxic effect of venom of wasps, accidental (unintentional)**
  - +7th **T63.462 Toxic effect of venom of wasps, intentional self-harm**
  - +7th **T63.463 Toxic effect of venom of wasps, assault**
  - +7th **T63.464 Toxic effect of venom of wasps, undetermined**

+ **T63.48 Toxic effect of venom of other arthropod**
  - +7th **T63.481 Toxic effect of venom of other arthropod, accidental (unintentional)**
  - +7th **T63.482 Toxic effect of venom of other arthropod, intentional self-harm**
  - +7th **T63.483 Toxic effect of venom of other arthropod, assault**
  - +7th **T63.484 Toxic effect of venom of other arthropod, undetermined**

+ **T63.5 Toxic effect of contact with venomous fish**
  - ***Excludes2:*** *poisoning by ingestion of fish (T61.-)*

+ **T63.51 Toxic effect of contact with stingray**
  - +7th **T63.511 Toxic effect of contact with stingray, accidental (unintentional)**
  - +7th **T63.512 Toxic effect of contact with stingray, intentional self-harm**
  - +7th **T63.513 Toxic effect of contact with stingray, assault**
  - +7th **T63.514 Toxic effect of contact with stingray, undetermined**

+ **T63.59 Toxic effect of contact with other venomous fish**
  - +7th **T63.591 Toxic effect of contact with other venomous fish, accidental (unintentional)**
  - +7th **T63.592 Toxic effect of contact with other venomous fish, intentional self-harm**
  - +7th **T63.593 Toxic effect of contact with other venomous fish, assault**
  - +7th **T63.594 Toxic effect of contact with other venomous fish, undetermined**

+ **T63.6 Toxic effect of contact with other venomous marine animals**
  Excludes1: *sea-snake venom (T63.09)*
  Excludes2: *poisoning by ingestion of shellfish (T61.78-)*

+ **T63.61 Toxic effect of contact with Portuguese Man-o-war**
  Toxic effect of contact with bluebottle
  - +7th **T63.611 Toxic effect of contact with Portuguese Man-o-war, accidental (unintentional)**
  - +7th **T63.612 Toxic effect of contact with Portuguese Man-o-war, intentional self-harm**
  - +7th **T63.613 Toxic effect of contact with Portuguese Man-o-war, assault**
  - +7th **T63.614 Toxic effect of contact with Portuguese Man-o-war, undetermined**

+ **T63.62 Toxic effect of contact with other jellyfish**
  - +7th **T63.621 Toxic effect of contact with other jellyfish, accidental (unintentional)**
  - +7th **T63.622 Toxic effect of contact with other jellyfish, intentional self-harm**
  - +7th **T63.623 Toxic effect of contact with other jellyfish, assault**
  - +7th **T63.624 Toxic effect of contact with other jellyfish, undetermined**

+ **T63.63 Toxic effect of contact with sea anemone**
  - +7th **T63.631 Toxic effect of contact with sea anemone, accidental (unintentional)**
  - +7th **T63.632 Toxic effect of contact with sea anemone, intentional self-harm**
  - +7th **T63.633 Toxic effect of contact with sea anemone, assault**
  - +7th **T63.634 Toxic effect of contact with sea anemone, undetermined**

+ **T63.69 Toxic effect of contact with other venomous marine animals**
  - +7th **T63.691 Toxic effect of contact with other venomous marine animals, accidental (unintentional)**
  - +7th **T63.692 Toxic effect of contact with other venomous marine animals, intentional self-harm**
  - +7th **T63.693 Toxic effect of contact with other venomous marine animals, assault**
  - +7th **T63.694 Toxic effect of contact with other venomous marine animals, undetermined**

+ **T63.7 Toxic effect of contact with venomous plant**

+ **T63.71 Toxic effect of contact with venomous marine plant**
  - +7th **T63.711 Toxic effect of contact with venomous marine plant, accidental (unintentional)**
  - +7th **T63.712 Toxic effect of contact with venomous marine plant, intentional self-harm**
  - +7th **T63.713 Toxic effect of contact with venomous marine plant, assault**
  - +7th **T63.714 Toxic effect of contact with venomous marine plant, undetermined**

+ **T63.79 Toxic effect of contact with other venomous plant**
  - +7th **T63.791 Toxic effect of contact with other venomous plant, accidental (unintentional)**
  - +7th **T63.792 Toxic effect of contact with other venomous plant, intentional self-harm**
  - +7th **T63.793 Toxic effect of contact with other venomous plant, assault**
  - +7th **T63.794 Toxic effect of contact with other venomous plant, undetermined**

+ **T63.8 Toxic effect of contact with other venomous animals**

+ **T63.81 Toxic effect of contact with venomous frog**
  Excludes1: *contact with nonvenomous frog (W62.0)*
  - +7th **T63.811 Toxic effect of contact with venomous frog, accidental (unintentional)**
  - +7th **T63.812 Toxic effect of contact with venomous frog, intentional self-harm**
  - +7th **T63.813 Toxic effect of contact with venomous frog, assault**
  - +7th **T63.814 Toxic effect of contact with venomous frog, undetermined**

+ **T63.82 Toxic effect of contact with venomous toad**
  Excludes1: *contact with nonvenomous toad (W62.1)*
  - +7th **T63.821 Toxic effect of contact with venomous toad, accidental (unintentional)**
  - +7th **T63.822 Toxic effect of contact with venomous toad, intentional self-harm**
  - +7th **T63.823 Toxic effect of contact with venomous toad, assault**
  - +7th **T63.824 Toxic effect of contact with venomous toad, undetermined**

+ **T63.83 Toxic effect of contact with other venomous amphibian**
  Excludes1: *contact with nonvenomous amphibian (W62.9)*
  - +7th **T63.831 Toxic effect of contact with other venomous amphibian, accidental (unintentional)**
  - +7th **T63.832 Toxic effect of contact with other venomous amphibian, intentional self-harm**
  - +7th **T63.833 Toxic effect of contact with other venomous amphibian, assault**
  - +7th **T63.834 Toxic effect of contact with other venomous amphibian, undetermined**

+ **T63.89 Toxic effect of contact with other venomous animals**
  - +7th **T63.891 Toxic effect of contact with other venomous animals, accidental (unintentional)**
  - +7th **T63.892 Toxic effect of contact with other venomous animals, intentional self-harm**
  - +7th **T63.893 Toxic effect of contact with other venomous animals, assault**
  - +7th **T63.894 Toxic effect of contact with other venomous animals, undetermined**

+ **T63.9 Toxic effect of contact with unspecified venomous animal**
  - X+7th **T63.91 Toxic effect of contact with unspecified venomous animal, accidental (unintentional)**
  - X+7th **T63.92 Toxic effect of contact with unspecified venomous animal, intentional self-harm**
  - X+7th **T63.93 Toxic effect of contact with unspecified venomous animal, assault**
  - X+7th **T63.94 Toxic effect of contact with unspecified venomous animal, undetermined**

T64 Toxic effect of aflatoxin and other mycotoxin food contaminants

> The appropriate 7th character is to be added to each code from category T64
> A initial encounter
> D subsequent encounter
> S sequela

+ **T64.0 Toxic effect of aflatoxin**
  - X+7th **T64.01 Toxic effect of aflatoxin, accidental (unintentional)**
  - X+7th **T64.02 Toxic effect of aflatoxin, intentional self-harm**
  - X+7th **T64.03 Toxic effect of aflatoxin, assault**
  - X+7th **T64.04 Toxic effect of aflatoxin, undetermined**

+ **T64.8 Toxic effect of other mycotoxin food contaminants**
  - X+7th **T64.81 Toxic effect of other mycotoxin food contaminants, accidental (unintentional)**
  - X+7th **T64.82 Toxic effect of other mycotoxin food contaminants, intentional self-harm**
  - X+7th **T64.83 Toxic effect of other mycotoxin food contaminants, assault**
  - X+7th **T64.84 Toxic effect of other mycotoxin food contaminants, undetermined**

T65 Toxic effect of other and unspecified substances

The appropriate 7th character is to be added to each code from category T65
A initial encounter
D subsequent encounter
S sequela

+ **T65.0 Toxic effect of cyanides**
Excludes1: *hydrogen cyanide (T57.3-)*
+ **T65.0X Toxic effect of cyanides**
+7th **T65.0X1 Toxic effect of cyanides, accidental (unintentional)**
Toxic effect of cyanides NOS
+7th **T65.0X2 Toxic effect of cyanides, intentional self-harm**
+7th **T65.0X3 Toxic effect of cyanides, assault**
+7th **T65.0X4 Toxic effect of cyanides, undetermined**
+ **T65.1 Toxic effect of strychnine and its salts**
+ **T65.1X Toxic effect of strychnine and its salts**
+7th **T65.1X1 Toxic effect of strychnine and its salts, accidental (unintentional)**
Toxic effect of strychnine and its salts NOS
+7th **T65.1X2 Toxic effect of strychnine and its salts, intentional self-harm**
+7th **T65.1X3 Toxic effect of strychnine and its salts, assault**
+7th **T65.1X4 Toxic effect of strychnine and its salts, undetermined**
+ **T65.2 Toxic effect of tobacco and nicotine**
Excludes2: *nicotine dependence (F17.-)*
+ **T65.21 Toxic effect of chewing tobacco**
+7th **T65.211 Toxic effect of chewing tobacco, accidental (unintentional)**
Toxic effect of chewing tobacco NOS
+7th **T65.212 Toxic effect of chewing tobacco, intentional self-harm**
+7th **T65.213 Toxic effect of chewing tobacco, assault**
+7th **T65.214 Toxic effect of chewing tobacco, undetermined**
+ **T65.22 Toxic effect of tobacco cigarettes**
Toxic effect of tobacco smoke
Use additional code for exposure to second hand tobacco smoke (Z57.31, Z77.22)
+7th **T65.221 Toxic effect of tobacco cigarettes, accidental (unintentional)**
Toxic effect of tobacco cigarettes NOS
+7th **T65.222 Toxic effect of tobacco cigarettes, intentional self-harm**
+7th **T65.223 Toxic effect of tobacco cigarettes, assault**
+7th **T65.224 Toxic effect of tobacco cigarettes, undetermined**
+ **T65.29 Toxic effect of other tobacco and nicotine**
+7th **T65.291 Toxic effect of other tobacco and nicotine, accidental (unintentional)**
Toxic effect of other tobacco and nicotine NOS
+7th **T65.292 Toxic effect of other tobacco and nicotine, intentional self-harm**
+7th **T65.293 Toxic effect of other tobacco and nicotine, assault**
+7th **T65.294 Toxic effect of other tobacco and nicotine, undetermined**
+ **T65.3 Toxic effect of nitroderivatives and aminoderivatives of benzene and its homologues**
Toxic effect of anilin [benzenamine]
Toxic effect of nitrobenzene
Toxic effect of trinitrotoluene
+ **T65.3X Toxic effect of nitroderivatives and aminoderivatives of benzene and its homologues**
+7th **T65.3X1 Toxic effect of nitroderivatives and aminoderivatives of benzene and its homologues, accidental (unintentional)**
Toxic effect of nitroderivatives and aminoderivatives of benzene and its homologues NOS
+7th **T65.3X2 Toxic effect of nitroderivatives and aminoderivatives of benzene and its homologues, intentional self-harm**
+7th **T65.3X3 Toxic effect of nitroderivatives and aminoderivatives of benzene and its homologues, assault**
+7th **T65.3X4 Toxic effect of nitroderivatives and aminoderivatives of benzene and its homologues, undetermined**
+ **T65.4 Toxic effect of carbon disulfide**
+ **T65.4X Toxic effect of carbon disulfide**
+7th **T65.4X1 Toxic effect of carbon disulfide, accidental (unintentional)**
Toxic effect of carbon disulfide NOS
+7th **T65.4X2 Toxic effect of carbon disulfide, intentional self-harm**
+7th **T65.4X3 Toxic effect of carbon disulfide, assault**
+7th **T65.4X4 Toxic effect of carbon disulfide, undetermined**
+ **T65.5 Toxic effect of nitroglycerin and other nitric acids and esters**
Toxic effect of 1,2,3-Propanetriol trinitrate
+ **T65.5X Toxic effect of nitroglycerin and other nitric acids and esters**
+7th **T65.5X1 Toxic effect of nitroglycerin and other nitric acids and esters, accidental (unintentional)**
Toxic effect of nitroglycerin and other nitric acids and esters NOS
+7th **T65.5X2 Toxic effect of nitroglycerin and other nitric acids and esters, intentional self-harm**
+7th **T65.5X3 Toxic effect of nitroglycerin and other nitric acids and esters, assault**
+7th **T65.5X4 Toxic effect of nitroglycerin and other nitric acids and esters, undetermined**
+ **T65.6 Toxic effect of paints and dyes, not elsewhere classified**
+ **T65.6X Toxic effect of paints and dyes, not elsewhere classified**
+7th **T65.6X1 Toxic effect of paints and dyes, not elsewhere classified, accidental (unintentional)**
Toxic effect of paints and dyes NOS
+7th **T65.6X2 Toxic effect of paints and dyes, not elsewhere classified, intentional self-harm**
+7th **T65.6X3 Toxic effect of paints and dyes, not elsewhere classified, assault**
+7th **T65.6X4 Toxic effect of paints and dyes, not elsewhere classified, undetermined**
+ **T65.8 Toxic effect of other specified substances**
+ **T65.81 Toxic effect of latex**
+7th **T65.811 Toxic effect of latex, accidental (unintentional)**
Toxic effect of latex NOS
+7th **T65.812 Toxic effect of latex, intentional self-harm**
+7th **T65.813 Toxic effect of latex, assault**
+7th **T65.814 Toxic effect of latex, undetermined**
+ **T65.82 Toxic effect of harmful algae and algae toxins**
Toxic effect of (harmful) algae bloom NOS
Toxic effect of blue-green algae bloom
Toxic effect of brown tide
Toxic effect of cyanobacteria bloom
Toxic effect of Florida red tide
Toxic effect of pfiesteria piscicida
Toxic effect of red tide
+7th **T65.821 Toxic effect of harmful algae and algae toxins, accidental (unintentional)**
Toxic effect of harmful algae and algae toxins NOS
+7th **T65.822 Toxic effect of harmful algae and algae toxins, intentional self-harm**
+7th **T65.823 Toxic effect of harmful algae and algae toxins, assault**
+7th **T65.824 Toxic effect of harmful algae and algae toxins, undetermined**

+ **T65.83 Toxic effect of fiberglass**
  - +7th **T65.831 Toxic effect of fiberglass, accidental (unintentional)**
    Toxic effect of fiberglass NOS
  - +7th **T65.832 Toxic effect of fiberglass, intentional self-harm**
  - +7th **T65.833 Toxic effect of fiberglass, assault**
  - +7th **T65.834 Toxic effect of fiberglass, undetermined**

+ **T65.89 Toxic effect of other specified substances**
  - +7th **T65.891 Toxic effect of other specified substances, accidental (unintentional)**
    Toxic effect of other specified substances NOS
    AHA CC: 1Q, 2018, 5
  - +7th **T65.892 Toxic effect of other specified substances, intentional self-harm**
  - +7th **T65.893 Toxic effect of other specified substances, assault**
  - +7th **T65.894 Toxic effect of other specified substances, undetermined**

+ **T65.9 Toxic effect of unspecified substance**
  - X+7th **T65.91 Toxic effect of unspecified substance, accidental (unintentional)**
    Poisoning NOS
  - X+7th **T65.92 Toxic effect of unspecified substance, intentional self-harm**
  - X+7th **T65.93 Toxic effect of unspecified substance, assault**
  - X+7th **T65.94 Toxic effect of unspecified substance, undetermined**

Other and unspecified effects of external causes (T66-T78)

T66 Radiation sickness, unspecified
X+7th

Excludes1: *specified adverse effects of radiation, such as:*
burns (T20-T31)
leukemia (C91-C95)
radiation gastroenteritis and colitis (K52.0)
radiation pneumonitis (J70.0)
radiation related disorders of the skin and subcutaneous tissue (L55-L59)
sunburn (L55.-)

The appropriate 7th character is to be added to code T66
A initial encounter
D subsequent encounter
S sequela

T67 Effects of heat and light

Excludes1: *erythema [dermatitis] ab igne (L59.0)*
malignant hyperpyrexia due to anesthesia (T88.3)
radiation-related disorders of the skin and subcutaneous tissue (L55-L59)

Excludes2: *burns (T20-T31)*
sunburn (L55.-)
sweat disorder due to heat (L74-L75)

The appropriate 7th character is to be added to each code from category T67
A initial encounter
D subsequent encounter
S sequela

+ **T67.0 Heatstroke and sunstroke**
  Use additional code(s) to identify any associated complications of heatstroke, such as:
  coma and stupor (R40.-)
  rhabdomyolysis (M62.82)
  systemic inflammatory response syndrome (R65.1-)
  AHA CC: 4Q, 2019, 17-18
  HAC 7th character A see Appendix B for HAC conditional logic
  - CC X+7th **T67.01 Heatstroke and sunstroke**
    Heat apoplexy
    Heat pyrexia
    Siriasis
    Thermoplegia
    HAC 7th character A see Appendix B for HAC conditional logic
  - CC X+7th **T67.02 Exertional heatstroke**
    AHA CC: 4Q, 2019, 17-18
    HAC 7th character A see Appendix B for HAC conditional logic
  - CC X+7th **T67.09 Other heatstroke and sunstroke**
    HAC 7th character A see Appendix B for HAC conditional logic

X+7th **T67.1 Heat syncope**
Heat collapse

X+7th **T67.2 Heat cramp**

X+7th **T67.3 Heat exhaustion, anhydrotic**
Heat prostration due to water depletion
Excludes1: *heat exhaustion due to salt depletion (T67.4)*

X+7th **T67.4 Heat exhaustion due to salt depletion**
Heat prostration due to salt (and water) depletion

X+7th **T67.5 Heat exhaustion, unspecified**
Heat prostration NOS

X+7th **T67.6 Heat fatigue, transient**

X+7th **T67.7 Heat edema**

X+7th **T67.8 Other effects of heat and light**

X+7th **T67.9 Effect of heat and light, unspecified**

T68 Hypothermia
X+7th

Accidental hypothermia
Hypothermia NOS
Use additional code to identify source of exposure:
Exposure to excessive cold of man-made origin (W93)
Exposure to excessive cold of natural origin (X31)

Excludes1: *hypothermia following anesthesia (T88.51)*
hypothermia not associated with low environmental temperature (R68.0)
hypothermia of newborn (P80.-)

Excludes2: *frostbite (T33-T34)*

The appropriate 7th character is to be added to code T68
A initial encounter
D subsequent encounter
S sequela

T69 Other effects of reduced temperature

Use additional code to identify source of exposure:
Exposure to excessive cold of man-made origin (W93)
Exposure to excessive cold of natural origin (X31)

Excludes2: *frostbite (T33-T34)*

The appropriate 7th character is to be added to each code from category T69
A initial encounter
D subsequent encounter
S sequela

+ **T69.0 Immersion hand and foot**
  + **T69.01 Immersion hand**
    - +7th **T69.011 Immersion hand, right hand**
    - +7th **T69.012 Immersion hand, left hand**
    - +7th **T69.019 Immersion hand, unspecified hand**
  + **T69.02 Immersion foot**
    Trench foot
    - CC +7th **T69.021 Immersion foot, right foot**
      HAC 7th character A see Appendix B for HAC conditional logic
    - CC +7th **T69.022 Immersion foot, left foot**
      HAC 7th character A see Appendix B for HAC conditional logic
    - CC +7th **T69.029 Immersion foot, unspecified foot**
      HAC 7th character A see Appendix B for HAC conditional logic

X+7th **T69.1 Chilblains**

X+7th **T69.8 Other specified effects of reduced temperature**

X+7th **T69.9 Effect of reduced temperature, unspecified**

T70 Effects of air pressure and water pressure

The appropriate 7th character is to be added to each code from category T70
A initial encounter
D subsequent encounter
S sequela

X+7th **T70.0 Otitic barotrauma**
Aero-otitis media
Effects of change in ambient atmospheric pressure or water pressure on ears

X+7th **T70.1 Sinus barotrauma**
Aerosinusitis
Effects of change in ambient atmospheric pressure on sinuses

+ **T70.2 Other and unspecified effects of high altitude**
Excludes2: polycythemia due to high altitude (D75.1)
X+7th **T70.20 Unspecified effects of high altitude**
X+7th **T70.29 Other effects of high altitude**
Alpine sickness
Anoxia due to high altitude
Barotrauma NOS
Hypobaropathy
Mountain sickness
CC X+7th **T70.3 Caisson disease [decompression sickness]**
Compressed-air disease
Diver's palsy or paralysis
HAC 7th character A see Appendix B for HAC conditional logic
X+7th **T70.4 Effects of high-pressure fluids**
Hydraulic jet injection (industrial)
Pneumatic jet injection (industrial)
Traumatic jet injection (industrial)
X+7th **T70.8 Other effects of air pressure and water pressure**
X+7th **T70.9 Effect of air pressure and water pressure, unspecified**

T71 Asphyxiation
Mechanical suffocation
Traumatic suffocation
Excludes1: acute respiratory distress (syndrome) (J80)
anoxia due to high altitude (T70.2)
asphyxia NOS (R09.01)
asphyxia from carbon monoxide (T58.-)
asphyxia from inhalation of food or foreign body (T17.-)
asphyxia from other gases, fumes and vapors (T59.-)
respiratory distress (syndrome) in newborn (P22.-)

The appropriate 7th character is to be added to each code from category T71
A initial encounter
D subsequent encounter
S sequela

+ **T71.1 Asphyxiation due to mechanical threat to breathing**
Suffocation due to mechanical threat to breathing
+ **T71.11 Asphyxiation due to smothering under pillow**
CC +7th **T71.111 Asphyxiation due to smothering under pillow, accidental**
Asphyxiation due to smothering under pillow NOS
HAC 7th character A see Appendix B for HAC conditional logic
CC +7th **T71.112 Asphyxiation due to smothering under pillow, intentional self-harm**
HAC 7th character A see Appendix B for HAC conditional logic
CC +7th **T71.113 Asphyxiation due to smothering under pillow, assault**
HAC 7th character A see Appendix B for HAC conditional logic
CC +7th **T71.114 Asphyxiation due to smothering under pillow, undetermined**
HAC 7th character A see Appendix B for HAC conditional logic
+ **T71.12 Asphyxiation due to plastic bag**
CC +7th **T71.121 Asphyxiation due to plastic bag, accidental**
Asphyxiation due to plastic bag NOS
HAC 7th character A see Appendix B for HAC conditional logic
CC +7th **T71.122 Asphyxiation due to plastic bag, intentional self-harm**
HAC 7th character A see Appendix B for HAC conditional logic
CC +7th **T71.123 Asphyxiation due to plastic bag, assault**
HAC 7th character A see Appendix B for HAC conditional logic
CC +7th **T71.124 Asphyxiation due to plastic bag, undetermined**
HAC 7th character A see Appendix B for HAC conditional logic
+ **T71.13 Asphyxiation due to being trapped in bed linens**
CC +7th **T71.131 Asphyxiation due to being trapped in bed linens, accidental**
Asphyxiation due to being trapped in bed linens NOS
HAC 7th character A see Appendix B for HAC conditional logic
CC +7th **T71.132 Asphyxiation due to being trapped in bed linens, intentional self-harm**
HAC 7th character A see Appendix B for HAC conditional logic
CC +7th **T71.133 Asphyxiation due to being trapped in bed linens, assault**
HAC 7th character A see Appendix B for HAC conditional logic
CC +7th **T71.134 Asphyxiation due to being trapped in bed linens, undetermined**
HAC 7th character A see Appendix B for HAC conditional logic
+ **T71.14 Asphyxiation due to smothering under another person's body (in bed)**
CC +7th **T71.141 Asphyxiation due to smothering under another person's body (in bed), accidental**
Asphyxiation due to smothering under another person's body (in bed) NOS
HAC 7th character A see Appendix B for HAC conditional logic
CC +7th **T71.143 Asphyxiation due to smothering under another person's body (in bed), assault**
HAC 7th character A see Appendix B for HAC conditional logic
CC +7th **T71.144 Asphyxiation due to smothering under another person's body (in bed), undetermined**
HAC 7th character A see Appendix B for HAC conditional logic
+ **T71.15 Asphyxiation due to smothering in furniture**
CC +7th **T71.151 Asphyxiation due to smothering in furniture, accidental**
Asphyxiation due to smothering in furniture NOS
HAC 7th character A see Appendix B for HAC conditional logic
CC +7th **T71.152 Asphyxiation due to smothering in furniture, intentional self-harm**
HAC 7th character A see Appendix B for HAC conditional logic
CC +7th **T71.153 Asphyxiation due to smothering in furniture, assault**
HAC 7th character A see Appendix B for HAC conditional logic
CC +7th **T71.154 Asphyxiation due to smothering in furniture, undetermined**
HAC 7th character A see Appendix B for HAC conditional logic
+ **T71.16 Asphyxiation due to hanging**
Hanging by window shade cord
Use additional code for any associated injuries, such as:
crushing injury of neck (S17.-)
fracture of cervical vertebrae (S12.0-S12.2-)
open wound of neck (S11.-)
CC +7th **T71.161 Asphyxiation due to hanging, accidental**
Asphyxiation due to hanging NOS
Hanging NOS
HAC 7th character A see Appendix B for HAC conditional logic
CC +7th **T71.162 Asphyxiation due to hanging, intentional self-harm**
HAC 7th character A see Appendix B for HAC conditional logic
CC +7th **T71.163 Asphyxiation due to hanging, assault**
HAC 7th character A see Appendix B for HAC conditional logic
CC +7th **T71.164 Asphyxiation due to hanging, undetermined**
HAC 7th character A see Appendix B for HAC conditional logic

+ **T71.19 Asphyxiation due to mechanical threat to breathing due to other causes**

CC +7th **T71.191 Asphyxiation due to mechanical threat to breathing due to other causes, accidental**

Asphyxiation due to other causes NOS

AHA CC: 4Q, 2016, 74-76

HAC 7th character A see Appendix B for HAC conditional logic

CC +7th **T71.192 Asphyxiation due to mechanical threat to breathing due to other causes, intentional self-harm**

HAC 7th character A see Appendix B for HAC conditional logic

CC +7th **T71.193 Asphyxiation due to mechanical threat to breathing due to other causes, assault**

HAC 7th character A see Appendix B for HAC conditional logic

CC +7th **T71.194 Asphyxiation due to mechanical threat to breathing due to other causes, undetermined**

HAC 7th character A see Appendix B for HAC conditional logic

+ **T71.2 Asphyxiation due to systemic oxygen deficiency due to low oxygen content in ambient air**

Suffocation due to systemic oxygen deficiency due to low oxygen content in ambient air

CC X+7th **T71.20 Asphyxiation due to systemic oxygen deficiency due to low oxygen content in ambient air due to unspecified cause**

HAC 7th character A see Appendix B for HAC conditional logic

CC X+7th **T71.21 Asphyxiation due to cave-in or falling earth**

Use additional code for any associated cataclysm (X34-X38)

HAC 7th character A see Appendix B for HAC conditional logic

+ **T71.22 Asphyxiation due to being trapped in a car trunk**

CC +7th **T71.221 Asphyxiation due to being trapped in a car trunk, accidental**

CC +7th **T71.222 Asphyxiation due to being trapped in a car trunk, intentional self-harm**

CC +7th **T71.223 Asphyxiation due to being trapped in a car trunk, assault**

CC +7th **T71.224 Asphyxiation due to being trapped in a car trunk, undetermined**

+ **T71.23 Asphyxiation due to being trapped in a (discarded) refrigerator**

CC +7th **T71.231 Asphyxiation due to being trapped in a (discarded) refrigerator, accidental**

CC +7th **T71.232 Asphyxiation due to being trapped in a (discarded) refrigerator, intentional self-harm**

CC +7th **T71.233 Asphyxiation due to being trapped in a (discarded) refrigerator, assault**

CC +7th **T71.234 Asphyxiation due to being trapped in a (discarded) refrigerator, undetermined**

CC X+7th **T71.29 Asphyxiation due to being trapped in other low oxygen environment**

HAC 7th character A see Appendix B for HAC conditional logic

CC X+7th **T71.9 Asphyxiation due to unspecified cause**

Suffocation (by strangulation) due to unspecified cause

Suffocation NOS

Systemic oxygen deficiency due to low oxygen content in ambient air due to unspecified cause

Systemic oxygen deficiency due to mechanical threat to breathing due to unspecified cause

Traumatic asphyxia NOS

HAC 7th character A see Appendix B for HAC conditional logic

T73 Effects of other deprivation

The appropriate 7th character is to be added to each code from category T73
- A initial encounter
- D subsequent encounter
- S sequela

X+7th **T73.0 Starvation**

Deprivation of food

X+7th **T73.1 Deprivation of water**

X+7th **T73.2 Exhaustion due to exposure**

X+7th **T73.3 Exhaustion due to excessive exertion**

Exhaustion due to overexertion

X+7th **T73.8 Other effects of deprivation**

X+7th **T73.9 Effect of deprivation, unspecified**

T74 Adult and child abuse, neglect and other maltreatment, confirmed

Use additional code, if applicable, to identify any associated current injury.

Use additional external cause code to identify perpetrator, if known (Y07.-)

Excludes1: *abuse and maltreatment in pregnancy (O9A.3-, O9A.4-, O9A.5-)*
adult and child maltreatment, suspected (T76.-)

AHA CC: 4Q, 2018, 9

The appropriate 7th character is to be added to each code from category T74
- A initial encounter
- D subsequent encounter
- S sequela

Review coding guidelines C.5.c and C.19.f

+ **T74.0 Neglect or abandonment, confirmed**

• CC X+7th **T74.01 Adult neglect or abandonment, confirmed**

• CC X+7th **T74.02 Child neglect or abandonment, confirmed**

+ **T74.1 Physical abuse, confirmed**

Excludes2: *sexual abuse (T74.2-)*

• CC X+7th **T74.11 Adult physical abuse, confirmed**

• CC X+7th **T74.12 Child physical abuse, confirmed**

Excludes2: *shaken infant syndrome (T74.4)*

+ **T74.2 Sexual abuse, confirmed**

Rape, confirmed

Sexual assault, confirmed

• CC X+7th **T74.21 Adult sexual abuse, confirmed**

• CC X+7th **T74.22 Child sexual abuse, confirmed**

+ **T74.3 Psychological abuse, confirmed**

Bullying and intimidation, confirmed

Intimidation through social media, confirmed

• X+7th **T74.31 Adult psychological abuse, confirmed**

• CC X+7th **T74.32 Child psychological abuse, confirmed**

• CC X+7th **T74.4 Shaken infant syndrome**

+ **T74.5 Forced sexual exploitation, confirmed**

AHA CC: 4Q, 2018, 32-33

• CC X+7th **T74.51 Adult forced sexual exploitation, confirmed**

• CC X+7th **T74.52 Child sexual exploitation, confirmed**

+ **T74.6 Forced labor exploitation, confirmed**

AHA CC: 4Q, 2018, 32-33

• CC X+7th **T74.61 Adult forced labor exploitation, confirmed**

• CC X+7th **T74.62 Child forced labor exploitation, confirmed**

+ **T74.9 Unspecified maltreatment, confirmed**

• CC X+7th **T74.91 Unspecified adult maltreatment, confirmed**

• CC X+7th **T74.92 Unspecified child maltreatment, confirmed**

T75 Other and unspecified effects of other external causes

Excludes1: *adverse effects NEC (T78.-)*

Excludes2: *burns (electric) (T20-T31)*

The appropriate 7th character is to be added to each code from category T75
- A initial encounter
- D subsequent encounter
- S sequela

+ **T75.0 Effects of lightning**

Struck by lightning

X+7th **T75.00 Unspecified effects of lightning**

Struck by lightning NOS

X+7th **T75.01 Shock due to being struck by lightning**

X+7th **T75.09 Other effects of lightning**

Use additional code for other effects of lightning

CC X+7th **T75.1 Unspecified effects of drowning and nonfatal submersion**
Immersion
Excludes1: *specified effects of drowning- code to effects*
HAC 7th character A see Appendix B for HAC conditional logic

\+ **T75.2 Effects of vibration**
X+7th **T75.20 Unspecified effects of vibration**
X+7th **T75.21 Pneumatic hammer syndrome**
X+7th **T75.22 Traumatic vasospastic syndrome**
X+7th **T75.23 Vertigo from infrasound**
Excludes1: *vertigo NOS (R42)*
X+7th **T75.29 Other effects of vibration**

X+7th **T75.3 Motion sickness**
Airsickness
Seasickness
Travel sickness
Use additional external cause code to identify vehicle or type of motion (Y92.81-, Y93.5-)

X+7th **T75.4 Electrocution**
Shock from electric current
Shock from electroshock gun (taser)

\+ **T75.8 Other specified effects of external causes**
X+7th **T75.81 Effects of abnormal gravitation [G] forces**
X+7th **T75.82 Effects of weightlessness**
X+7th **T75.89 Other specified effects of external causes**

T76 Adult and child abuse, neglect and other maltreatment, suspected
Use additional code, if applicable, to identify any associated current injury
Excludes1: adult and child maltreatment, confirmed (T74.-)
suspected abuse and maltreatment in pregnancy (O9A.3-, O9A.4-, O9A.5-)
suspected adult physical abuse, ruled out (Z04.71)
suspected adult sexual abuse, ruled out (Z04.41)
suspected child physical abuse, ruled out (Z04.72)
suspected child sexual abuse, ruled out (Z04.42)
AHA CC: 4Q, 2018, 9

The appropriate 7th character is to be added to each code from category T76
A initial encounter
D subsequent encounter
S sequela

Review coding guidelines C.5.c and C.19.f

\+ **T76.0 Neglect or abandonment, suspected**
● CC X+7th **T76.01 Adult neglect or abandonment, suspected**
● CC X+7th **T76.02 Child neglect or abandonment, suspected**

\+ **T76.1 Physical abuse, suspected**
● CC X+7th **T76.11 Adult physical abuse, suspected**
● CC X+7th **T76.12 Child physical abuse, suspected**
AHA CC: 2Q, 2019, 12

\+ **T76.2 Sexual abuse, suspected**
Rape, suspected
Excludes1: *alleged abuse, ruled out (Z04.7)*
● CC X+7th **T76.21 Adult sexual abuse, suspected**
● CC X+7th **T76.22 Child sexual abuse, suspected**

\+ **T76.3 Psychological abuse, suspected**
Bullying and intimidation, suspected
Intimidation through social medial, suspected
● X+7th **T76.31 Adult psychological abuse, suspected**
● CC X+7th **T76.32 Child psychological abuse, suspected**

\+ **T76.5 Forced sexual exploitation, suspected**
AHA CC: 4Q, 2018, 32-33
● CC X+7th **T76.51 Adult forced sexual exploitation, suspected**
● CC X+7th **T76.52 Child sexual exploitation, suspected**

\+ **T76.6 Forced labor exploitation, suspected**
AHA CC: 4Q, 2018, 32-33
● CC X+7th **T76.61 Adult forced labor exploitation, suspected**
● CC X+7th **T76.62 Child forced labor exploitation, suspected**

\+ **T76.9 Unspecified maltreatment, suspected**
● CC X+7th **T76.91 Unspecified adult maltreatment, suspected**
● CC X+7th **T76.92 Unspecified child maltreatment, suspected**

T78 Adverse effects, not elsewhere classified
Excludes2: *complications of surgical and medical care NEC (T80-T88)*

The appropriate 7th character is to be added to each code from category T78
A initial encounter
D subsequent encounter
S sequela

\+ **T78.0 Anaphylactic reaction due to food**
Anaphylactic reaction due to adverse food reaction
Anaphylactic shock or reaction due to nonpoisonous foods
Anaphylactoid reaction due to food
CC X+7th **T78.00 Anaphylactic reaction due to unspecified food**
CC X+7th **T78.01 Anaphylactic reaction due to peanuts**
CC X+7th **T78.02 Anaphylactic reaction due to shellfish (crustaceans)**
CC X+7th **T78.03 Anaphylactic reaction due to other fish**
CC X+7th **T78.04 Anaphylactic reaction due to fruits and vegetables**
CC X+7th **T78.05 Anaphylactic reaction due to tree nuts and seeds**
Excludes2: *anaphylactic reaction due to peanuts (T78.01)*
CC X+7th **T78.06 Anaphylactic reaction due to food additives**
CC X+7th **T78.07 Anaphylactic reaction due to milk and dairy products**
CC X+7th **T78.08 Anaphylactic reaction due to eggs**
CC X+7th **T78.09 Anaphylactic reaction due to other food products**

X+7th **T78.1 Other adverse food reactions, not elsewhere classified**
Use additional code to identify the type of reaction, if applicable
Excludes1: *anaphylactic reaction or shock due to adverse food reaction (T78.0-)*
anaphylactic reaction due to food (T78.0-)
bacterial food borne intoxications (A05.-)
Excludes2: *allergic and dietetic gastroenteritis and colitis (K52.29)*
allergic rhinitis due to food (J30.5)
dermatitis due to food in contact with skin (L23.6, L24.6, L25.4)
dermatitis due to ingested food (L27.2)
food protein-induced entercolitis syndrome (K52.21)
food protein-induced enteropathy (K52.22)

CC X+7th **T78.2 Anaphylactic shock, unspecified**
Allergic shock
Anaphylactic reaction
Anaphylaxis
Excludes1: *anaphylactic reaction or shock due to adverse effectofcorrectmedicinalsubstanceproperly administered (T88.6)*
anaphylactic reaction or shock due to adverse food reaction (T78.0-)
anaphylactic reaction or shock due to serum (T80.5-)

X+7th **T78.3 Angioneurotic edema**
Allergic angioedema
Giant urticaria
Quincke's edema
Excludes1: *serum urticaria (T80.6-)*
urticaria (L50.-)

\+ **T78.4 Other and unspecified allergy**
Excludes1: *specified types of allergic reaction such as:*
allergic diarrhea (K52.29)
allergic gastroenteritis and colitis (K52.29)
dermatitis (L23-L25, L27.-)
food protein-induced entercolitis syndrome (K52.21)
food protein-induced enteropathy (K52.22)
hay fever (J30.1)
X+7th **T78.40 Allergy, unspecified**
Allergic reaction NOS
Hypersensitivity NOS
X+7th **T78.41 Arthus phenomenon**
Arthus reaction
X+7th **T78.49 Other allergy**
AHA CC: 1Q, 2021, 42

X+7th **T78.8 Other adverse effects, not elsewhere classified**

Certain early complications of trauma (T79)

T79 Certain early complications of trauma, not elsewhere classified

Excludes2: *acute respiratory distress syndrome (J80)*
complications occurring during or following medical procedures (T80-T88)
complications of surgical and medical care NEC (T80-T88)
newborn respiratory distress syndrome (P22.0)

The appropriate 7th character is to be added to each code from category T79
A initial encounter
D subsequent encounter
S sequela

MCC X+7th **T79.0 Air embolism (traumatic)**
Excludes1: *air embolism complicating abortion or ectopic or molar pregnancy (O00-O07, O08.2)*
air embolism complicating pregnancy, childbirth and the puerperium (O88.0)
air embolism following infusion, transfusion, and therapeutic injection (T80.0)
air embolism following procedure NEC (T81.7-)

MCC X+7th **T79.1 Fat embolism (traumatic)**
Excludes1: *fat embolism complicating:*
abortion or ectopic or molar pregnancy (O00-O07, O08.2)
pregnancy, childbirth and the puerperium (O88.8)

CC X+7th **T79.2 Traumatic secondary and recurrent hemorrhage and seroma**

MCC X+7th **T79.4 Traumatic shock**
Shock (immediate) (delayed) following injury
Excludes1: *anaphylactic shock due to adverse food reaction (T78.0-)*
anaphylactic shock due to correct medicinal substance properly administered (T88.6)
anaphylactic shock due to serum (T80.5-)
anaphylactic shock NOS (T78.2)
electric shock (T75.4)
nontraumatic shock NEC (R57.-)
obstetric shock (O75.1)
postprocedural shock (T81.1-)
septic shock (R65.21)
shock complicating abortion or ectopic or molar pregnancy (O00-O07, O08.3)
shock due to anesthesia (T88.2)
shock due to lightning (T75.01)
shock NOS (R57.9)

MCC X+7th **T79.5 Traumatic anuria**
Crush syndrome
Renal failure following crushing

X+7th **T79.6 Traumatic ischemia of muscle**
Traumatic rhabdomyolysis
Volkmann's ischemic contracture
Excludes2: *anterior tibial syndrome (M76.8)*
compartment syndrome (traumatic) (T79.A-)
nontraumatic ischemia of muscle (M62.2-)

CC X+7th **T79.7 Traumatic subcutaneous emphysema**
Excludes2: *emphysema NOS (J43)*
emphysema (subcutaneous) resulting from a procedure (T81.82)

\+ **T79.A Traumatic compartment syndrome**
Excludes1: *fibromyalgia (M79.7)*
nontraumatic compartment syndrome (M79.A-)
Excludes2: *traumatic ischemic infarction of muscle (T79.6)*

CC X+7th **T79.A0 Compartment syndrome, unspecified**
Compartment syndrome NOS

\+ **T79.A1 Traumatic compartment syndrome of upper extremity**
Traumatic compartment syndrome of shoulder, arm, forearm, wrist, hand, and fingers

CC +7th **T79.A11 Traumatic compartment syndrome of right upper extremity**

CC +7th **T79.A12 Traumatic compartment syndrome of left upper extremity**

CC +7th **T79.A19 Traumatic compartment syndrome of unspecified upper extremity**

\+ **T79.A2 Traumatic compartment syndrome of lower extremity**
Traumatic compartment syndrome of hip, buttock, thigh, leg, foot, and toes

CC +7th **T79.A21 Traumatic compartment syndrome of right lower extremity**

CC +7th **T79.A22 Traumatic compartment syndrome of left lower extremity**

CC +7th **T79.A29 Traumatic compartment syndrome of unspecified lower extremity**

CC X+7th **T79.A3 Traumatic compartment syndrome of abdomen**

CC X+7th **T79.A9 Traumatic compartment syndrome of other sites**

X+7th **T79.8 Other early complications of trauma**

X+7th **T79.9 Unspecified early complication of trauma**

Complications of surgical and medical care, not elsewhere classified (T80-T88)

Use additional code for adverse effect, if applicable, to identify drug (T36-T50 with fifth or sixth character 5)

Use additional code(s) to identify the specified condition resulting from the complication

Use additional code to identify devices involved and details of circumstances (Y62-Y82)

Excludes2: *any encounters with medical care for postprocedural conditions in which no complications are present, such as:*
artificial opening status (Z93.-)
closure of external stoma (Z43.-)
fitting and adjustment of external prosthetic device (Z44.-)
burns and corrosions from local applications and irradiation (T20-T32)
complications of surgical procedures during pregnancy, childbirth and the puerperium (O00-O9A)
mechanical complication of respirator [ventilator] (J95.850)
poisoning and toxic effects of drugs and chemicals (T36-T65 with fifth or sixth character 1-4 or 6)
postprocedural fever (R50.82)
specified complications classified elsewhere, such as:
cerebrospinal fluid leak from spinal puncture (G97.0)
colostomy malfunction (K94.0-)
disorders of fluid and electrolyte imbalance (E86-E87)
functional disturbances following cardiac surgery (I97.0-I97.1)
intraoperative and postprocedural complications of specified body systems (D78.-, E36.-, E89.-, G97.3-, G97.4, H59.3-, H59.-, H95.2-, H95.3, I97.4-, I97.5, J95.6-, J95.7, K91.6-, L76.-, M96.-, N99.-)
ostomy complications (J95.0-, K94.-, N99.5-)
postgastric surgery syndromes (K91.1)
postlaminectomy syndrome NEC (M96.1)
postmastectomy lymphedema syndrome (I97.2)
postsurgical blind-loop syndrome (K91.2)
ventilator associated pneumonia (J95.851)

T80 Complications following infusion, transfusion and therapeutic injection

Includes: complications following perfusion
Excludes2: *bone marrow transplant rejection (T86.01)*
febrile nonhemolytic transfusion reaction (R50.84)
fluid overload due to transfusion (E87.71)
posttransfusion purpura (D69.51)
transfusion associated circulatory overload (TACO) (E87.71)
transfusion (red blood cell) associated hemochromatosis (E83.111)
transfusion related acute lung injury (TRALI) (J95.84)

The appropriate 7th character is to be added to each code from category T80
A initial encounter
D subsequent encounter
S sequela

MCC X+7th **T80.0 Air embolism following infusion, transfusion and therapeutic injection**
HAC 7th character A see Appendix B for HAC conditional logic

CC X+7th **T80.1 Vascular complications following infusion, transfusion and therapeutic injection**
Use additional code to identify the vascular complication
Excludes2: *extravasation of vesicant agent (T80.81-)*
infiltration of vesicant agent (T80.81-)
vascular complications specified as due to prosthetic devices, implants and grafts (T82.8-, T83.8-, T84.8-, T85.8-)
postprocedural vascular complications (T81.7-)

\+ **T80.2 Infections following infusion, transfusion and therapeutic injection**
Use additional code to identify the specific infection, such as: sepsis (A41.9)
Use additional code (R65.2-) to identify severe sepsis, if applicable
Excludes2: *infections specified as due to prosthetic devices, implants and grafts (T82.6-T82.7, T83.5-T83.6, T84.5-T84.7, T85.7)*
postprocedural infections (T81.4-)
Review coding guideline C.1.d.5

\+ **T80.21 Infection due to central venous catheter**
Infection due to pulmonary artery catheter (Swan-Ganz catheter)

CC +7th **T80.211 Bloodstream infection due to central venous catheter**
Catheter-related bloodstream infection (CRBSI) NOS
Central line-associated bloodstream infection (CLABSI)
Bloodstream infection due to Hickman catheter
Bloodstream infection due to peripherally inserted central catheter (PICC)
Bloodstream infection due to portacath (port-a-cath)
Bloodstream infection due to pulmonary artery catheter
Bloodstream infection due to triple lumen catheter
Bloodstream infection due to umbilical venous catheter
AHA CC: 4Q, 2018, 89; 1Q, 2019, 14
HAC 7th character A see Appendix B for HAC conditional logic

CC +7th **T80.212 Local infection due to central venous catheter**
Exit or insertion site infection
Local infection due to Hickman catheter
Local infection due to peripherally inserted central catheter (PICC)
Local infection due to portacath (port-a-cath)
Local infection due to pulmonary artery catheter
Local infection due to triple lumen catheter
Local infection due to umbilical venous catheter
Port or reservoir infection
Tunnel infection
HAC 7th character A see Appendix B for HAC conditional logic

CC +7th **T80.218 Other infection due to central venous catheter**
Other central line-associated infection
Other infection due to Hickman catheter
Other infection due to peripherally inserted central catheter (PICC)
Other infection due to portacath (port-a-cath)
Other infection due to pulmonary artery catheter
Other infection due to triple lumen catheter
Other infection due to umbilical venous catheter
HAC 7th character A see Appendix B for HAC conditional logic

CC +7th **T80.219 Unspecified infection due to central venous catheter**
Central line-associated infection NOS
Unspecified infection due to Hickman catheter
Unspecified infection due to peripherally inserted central catheter (PICC)
Unspecified infection due to portacath (port-a-cath)
Unspecified infection due to pulmonary artery catheter
Unspecified infection due to triple lumen catheter
Unspecified infection due to umbilical venous catheter
HAC 7th character A see Appendix B for HAC conditional logic

CC X+7th **T80.22 Acute infection following transfusion, infusion, or injection of blood and blood products**

CC X+7th **T80.29 Infection following other infusion, transfusion and therapeutic injection**

\+ **T80.3 ABO incompatibility reaction due to transfusion of blood or blood products**
Excludes1: *minor blood group antigens reactions (Duffy) (E) (K) (Kell) (Kidd) (Lewis) (M) (N) (P) (S) (T80.A-)*

CC X+7th **T80.30 ABO incompatibility reaction due to transfusion of blood or blood products, unspecified**
ABO incompatibility blood transfusion NOS
Reaction to ABO incompatibility from transfusion NOS
HAC 7th character A see Appendix B for HAC conditional logic

\+ **T80.31 ABO incompatibility with hemolytic transfusion reaction**

CC +7th **T80.310 ABO incompatibility with acute hemolytic transfusion reaction**
ABO incompatibility with hemolytic transfusion reaction less than 24 hours after transfusion
Acute hemolytic transfusion reaction (AHTR) due to ABO incompatibility
HAC 7th character A see Appendix B for HAC conditional logic

CC +7th **T80.311 ABO incompatibility with delayed hemolytic transfusion reaction**
ABO incompatibility with hemolytic transfusion reaction 24 hours or more after transfusion
Delayed hemolytic transfusion reaction (DHTR) due to ABO incompatibility
HAC 7th character A see Appendix B for HAC conditional logic

CC +7th **T80.319 ABO incompatibility with hemolytic transfusion reaction, unspecified**
ABO incompatibility with hemolytic transfusion reaction at unspecified time after transfusion
Hemolytic transfusion reaction (HTR) due to ABO incompatibility NOS
HAC 7th character A see Appendix B for HAC conditional logic

CC X+7th **T80.39 Other ABO incompatibility reaction due to transfusion of blood or blood products**
Delayed serologic transfusion reaction (DSTR) from ABO incompatibility
Other ABO incompatible blood transfusion
Other reaction to ABO incompatible blood transfusion
HAC 7th character A see Appendix B for HAC conditional logic

\+ **T80.4 Rh incompatibility reaction due to transfusion of blood or blood products**
Reaction due to incompatibility of Rh antigens (C) (c) (D) (E) (e)

CC X+7th **T80.40 Rh incompatibility reaction due to transfusion of blood or blood products, unspecified**
Reaction due to Rh factor in transfusion NOS
Rh incompatible blood transfusion NOS

\+ **T80.41 Rh incompatibility with hemolytic transfusion reaction**

CC +7th **T80.410 Rh incompatibility with acute hemolytic transfusion reaction**
Acute hemolytic transfusion reaction (AHTR) due to Rh incompatibility
Rh incompatibility with hemolytic transfusion reaction less than 24 hours after transfusion

CC +7th **T80.411 Rh incompatibility with delayed hemolytic transfusion reaction**
Delayed hemolytic transfusion reaction (DHTR) due to Rh incompatibility
Rh incompatibility with hemolytic transfusion reaction 24 hours or more after transfusion

CC +7th **T80.419 Rh incompatibility with hemolytic transfusion reaction, unspecified**
Rh incompatibility with hemolytic transfusion reaction at unspecified time after transfusion
Hemolytic transfusion reaction (HTR) due to Rh incompatibility NOS

CC X+7th **T80.49 Other Rh incompatibility reaction due to transfusion of blood or blood products**
Delayed serologic transfusion reaction (DSTR) from Rh incompatibility
Other reaction to Rh incompatible blood transfusion

\+ **T80.A Non-ABO incompatibility reaction due to transfusion of blood or blood products**
Reaction due to incompatibility of minor antigens (Duffy) (Kell) (Kidd) (Lewis) (M) (N) (P) (S)

CC X+7th **T80.A0 Non-ABO incompatibility reaction due to transfusion of blood or blood products, unspecified**
Non-ABO antigen incompatibility reaction from transfusion NOS

\+ **T80.A1 Non-ABO incompatibility with hemolytic transfusion reaction**

CC +7th **T80.A10 Non-ABO incompatibility with acute hemolytic transfusion reaction**
Acute hemolytic transfusion reaction (AHTR) due to non-ABO incompatibility
Non-ABO incompatibility with hemolytic transfusion reaction less than 24 hours after transfusion

CC +7th **T80.A11 Non-ABO incompatibility with delayed hemolytic transfusion reaction**
Delayed hemolytic transfusion reaction (DHTR) due to non-ABO incompatibility
Non-ABO incompatibility with hemolytic transfusion reaction 24 or more hours after transfusion

CC +7th **T80.A19 Non-ABO incompatibility with hemolytic transfusion reaction, unspecified**
Hemolytic transfusion reaction (HTR) due to non-ABO incompatibility NOS
Non-ABO incompatibility with hemolytic transfusion reaction at unspecified time after transfusion

CC X+7th **T80.A9 Other non-ABO incompatibility reaction due to transfusion of blood or blood products**
Delayed serologic transfusion reaction (DSTR) from non-ABO incompatibility
Other reaction to non-ABO incompatible blood transfusion

\+ **T80.5 Anaphylactic reaction due to serum**
Allergic shock due to serum
Anaphylactic shock due to serum
Anaphylactoid reaction due to serum
Anaphylaxis due to serum
Excludes1: *ABO incompatibility reaction due to transfusion of blood or blood products (T80.3-)*
allergic reaction or shock NOS (T78.2)
anaphylactic reaction or shock NOS (T78.2)
anaphylactic reaction or shock due to adverse effect of correct medicinal substance properly administered (T88.6)
other serum reaction (T80.6-)

CC X+7th **T80.51 Anaphylactic reaction due to administration of blood and blood products**

CC X+7th **T80.52 Anaphylactic reaction due to vaccination**
AHA CC: 1Q, 2021, 43

CC X+7th **T80.59 Anaphylactic reaction due to other serum**

\+ **T80.6 Other serum reactions**
Intoxication by serum
Protein sickness
Serum rash
Serum sickness
Serum urticaria
Excludes2: *serum hepatitis (B16-B19)*

CC X+7th **T80.61 Other serum reaction due to administration of blood and blood products**

CC X+7th **T80.62 Other serum reaction due to vaccination**
AHA CC: 1Q, 2021, 42

CC X+7th **T80.69 Other serum reaction due to other serum**
Code also, if applicable, arthropathy in hypersensitivity reactions classified elsewhere (M36.4)

\+ **T80.8 Other complications following infusion, transfusion and therapeutic injection**

\+ **T80.81 Extravasation of vesicant agent**
Infiltration of vesicant agent

CC +7th **T80.810 Extravasation of vesicant antineoplastic chemotherapy**
Infiltration of vesicant antineoplastic chemotherapy

CC +7th **T80.818 Extravasation of other vesicant agent**
Infiltration of other vesicant agent

T80.82 Complication of immune effector cellular therapy
Complication of chimeric antigen receptor (CAR-T) cell therapy
Complication of IEC therapy
Excludes2: *complication of bone marrow transplant (T86.0)*
complication of stem cell transplant (T86.5)
Use additional code to identify the specific complication, such as:
cytokine release syndrome (D89.83-)
immune effector cell-associated neurotoxicity syndrome (G92.0-)

X+7th **T80.89 Other complications following infusion, transfusion and therapeutic injection**
Delayed serologic transfusion reaction (DSTR), unspecified incompatibility
Use additional code to identify graft-versus-host reaction, if applicable, (D89.81-)
AHA CC: 4Q, 2020, 14-15

\+ **T80.9 Unspecified complication following infusion, transfusion and therapeutic injection**

X+7th **T80.90 Unspecified complication following infusion and therapeutic injection**

\+ **T80.91 Hemolytic transfusion reaction, unspecified incompatibility**
Excludes1: *ABO incompatibility with hemolytic transfusion reaction (T80.31-)*
Non-ABO incompatibility with hemolytic transfusion reaction (T80.A1-)
Rh incompatibility with hemolytic transfusion reaction (T80.41-)

CC +7th **T80.910 Acute hemolytic transfusion reaction, unspecified incompatibility**

CC +7th **T80.911 Delayed hemolytic transfusion reaction, unspecified incompatibility**

CC +7th **T80.919 Hemolytic transfusion reaction, unspecified incompatibility, unspecified as acute or delayed**
Hemolytic transfusion reaction NOS

X+7th **T80.92 Unspecified transfusion reaction**
Transfusion reaction NOS

T81 Complications of procedures, not elsewhere classified
Use additional code for adverse effect, if applicable, to identify drug (T36-T50 with fifth or sixth character 5)
Excludes2: *complications following immunization (T88.0-T88.1)*
complications following infusion, transfusion and therapeutic injection (T80.-)
complications of transplanted organs and tissue (T86.-)
specified complications classified elsewhere, such as:
complication of prosthetic devices, implants and grafts (T82-T85)
dermatitis due to drugs and medicaments (L23.3, L24.4, L25.1, L27.0-L27.1)
endosseous dental implant failure (M27.6-)
floppy iris syndrome (IFIS) (intraoperative) H21.81
intraoperative and postprocedural complications of specific body system (D78.-, E36.-, E89.-, G97.3-, G97.4, H59.3-, H59.-, H95.2-, H95.3, I97.4-, I97.5, J95, K91.-, L76.-, M96.-, N99.-)
ostomy complications (J95.0-, K94.-, N99.5-)
plateau iris syndrome (post-iridectomy) (postprocedural) (H21.82)
poisoning and toxic effects of drugs and chemicals (T36-T65 with fifth or sixth character 1-4 or 6)

The appropriate 7th character is to be added to each code from category T81
A initial encounter
D subsequent encounter
S sequela

\+ **T81.1 Postprocedural shock**
Shock during or resulting from a procedure, not elsewhere classified
Excludes1: *anaphylactic shock NOS (T78.2)*
anaphylactic shock due to correct substance properly administered (T88.6)
anaphylactic shock due to serum (T80.5-)
electric shock (T75.4)
obstetric shock (O75.1)
septic shock (R65.21)
shock due to anesthesia (T88.2)
shock following abortion or ectopic or molar pregnancy (O00-O07, O08.3)
traumatic shock (T79.4)

CC X+7th **T81.10 Postprocedural shock unspecified**
Collapse NOS during or resulting from a procedure, not elsewhere classified
Postprocedural failure of peripheral circulation
Postprocedural shock NOS

MCC X+7th **T81.11 Postprocedural cardiogenic shock**

MCC X+7th **T81.12 Postprocedural septic shock**
Postprocedural endotoxic shock resulting from a procedure, not elsewhere classified
Postprocedural gram-negative shock resulting from a procedure, not elsewhere classified
Code first underlying infection
Use additional code, to identify any associated acute organ dysfunction, if applicable
Review coding guideline C.1.d.2 and C.1.d.5.c

MCC X+7th **T81.19 Other postprocedural shock**
Postprocedural hypovolemic shock
AHA CC: 1Q, 2021, 13-14

\+ **T81.3 Disruption of wound, not elsewhere classified**
Disruption of any suture materials or other closure methods
Excludes1: *breakdown (mechanical) of permanent sutures (T85.612)*
displacement of permanent sutures (T85.622)
disruption of cesarean delivery wound (O90.0)
disruption of perineal obstetric wound (O90.1)
mechanical complication of permanent sutures NEC (T85.692)
AHA.CC: 1Q, 2014, 23

CC X+7th **T81.30 Disruption of wound, unspecified**
Disruption of wound NOS

CC X+7th **T81.31 Disruption of external operation (surgical) wound, not elsewhere classified**
Dehiscence of operation wound NOS
Disruption of operation wound NOS
Disruption or dehiscence of closure of cornea
Disruption or dehiscence of closure of mucosa
Disruption or dehiscence of closure of skin and subcutaneous tissue
Full-thickness skin disruption or dehiscence
Superficial disruption or dehiscence of operation wound
Excludes1: *dehiscence of amputation stump (T87.81)*
AHA CC: 1Q, 2015, 3-21

CC X+7th **T81.32 Disruption of internal operation (surgical) wound, not elsewhere classified**
Deep disruption or dehiscence of operation wound NOS
Disruption or dehiscence of closure of internal organ or other internal tissue
Disruption or dehiscence of closure of muscle or muscle flap
Disruption or dehiscence of closure of ribs or rib cage
Disruption or dehiscence of closure of skull or craniotomy
Disruption or dehiscence of closure of sternum or sternotomy
Disruption or dehiscence of closure of tendon or ligament
Disruption or dehiscence of closure of superficial or muscular fascia
AHA CC: 3Q, 2017, 4; 2Q, 2020, 22-23

CC X+7th **T81.33 Disruption of traumatic injury wound repair**
Disruption or dehiscence of closure of traumatic laceration (external) (internal)

\+ **T81.4 Infection following a procedure**
Wound abscess following a procedure
Use additional code to identify infection
Use additional code (R65.2-) to identify severe sepsis, if applicable
Excludes2: *bleb associated endophthalmitis (H59.4-)*
infection due to infusion, transfusion and therapeutic injection (T80.2-)
infection due to prosthetic devices, implants and grafts (T82.6-T82.7, T83.5-T83.6, T84.5-T84.7, T85.7)
obstetric surgical wound infection (O86.0-)
postprocedural fever NOS (R50.82)
postprocedural retroperitoneal abscess (K68.11)
AHA CC: 1Q, 2014, 23; 4Q, 2015, 37; 4Q, 2018, 33-34
Review coding guidelines C.1.d.5.b and C.1.d.5

CC X+7th **T81.40 Infection following a procedure, unspecified**
HAC 7th character A see Appendix B for HAC conditional logic

CC X+7th **T81.41 Infection following a procedure, superficial incisional surgical site**
Subcutaneous abscess following a procedure
Stitch abscess following a procedure
HAC 7th character A see Appendix B for HAC conditional logic
AHA CC: 4Q, 2018, 34

CC X+7th **T81.42 Infection following a procedure, deep incisional surgical site**
Intra-muscular abscess following a procedure
HAC 7th character A see Appendix B for HAC conditional logic

CC X+7th **T81.43 Infection following a procedure, organ and space surgical site**
Intra-abdominal abscess following a procedure
Subphrenic abscess following a procedure
HAC 7th character A see Appendix B for HAC conditional logic

CC X+7th **T81.44 Sepsis following a procedure**
Use additional code to identify the sepsis
HAC 7th character A see Appendix B for HAC conditional logic

CC X+7th **T81.49 Infection following a procedure, other surgical site**
HAC 7th character A see Appendix B for HAC conditional logic

+ T81.5 Complications of foreign body accidentally left in body following procedure

+ T81.50 Unspecified complication of foreign body accidentally left in body following procedure

CC +7th **T81.500 Unspecified complication of foreign body accidentally left in body following surgical operation**
HAC 7th character A see Appendix B for HAC conditional logic

CC +7th **T81.501 Unspecified complication of foreign body accidentally left in body following infusion or transfusion**
HAC 7th character A see Appendix B for HAC conditional logic

CC +7th **T81.502 Unspecified complication of foreign body accidentally left in body following kidney dialysis**
HAC 7th character A see Appendix B for HAC conditional logic

CC +7th **T81.503 Unspecified complication of foreign body accidentally left in body following injection or immunization**
HAC 7th character A see Appendix B for HAC conditional logic

CC +7th **T81.504 Unspecified complication of foreign body accidentally left in body following endoscopic examination**
HAC 7th character A see Appendix B for HAC conditional logic

CC +7th **T81.505 Unspecified complication of foreign body accidentally left in body following heart catheterization**
HAC 7th character A see Appendix B for HAC conditional logic

CC +7th **T81.506 Unspecified complication of foreign body accidentally left in body following aspiration, puncture or other catheterization**
HAC 7th character A see Appendix B for HAC conditional logic

CC +7th **T81.507 Unspecified complication of foreign body accidentally left in body following removal of catheter or packing**
HAC 7th character A see Appendix B for HAC conditional logic

CC +7th **T81.508 Unspecified complication of foreign body accidentally left in body following other procedure**
HAC 7th character A see Appendix B for HAC conditional logic

CC +7th **T81.509 Unspecified complication of foreign body accidentally left in body following unspecified procedure**
HAC 7th character A see Appendix B for HAC conditional logic

+ T81.51 Adhesions due to foreign body accidentally left in body following procedure

CC +7th **T81.510 Adhesions due to foreign body accidentally left in body following surgical operation**
HAC 7th character A see Appendix B for HAC conditional logic

CC +7th **T81.511 Adhesions due to foreign body accidentally left in body following infusion or transfusion**
HAC 7th character A see Appendix B for HAC conditional logic

CC +7th **T81.512 Adhesions due to foreign body accidentally left in body following kidney dialysis**
HAC 7th character A see Appendix B for HAC conditional logic

CC +7th **T81.513 Adhesions due to foreign body accidentally left in body following injection or immunization**
HAC 7th character A see Appendix B for HAC conditional logic

CC +7th **T81.514 Adhesions due to foreign body accidentally left in body following endoscopic examination**
HAC 7th character A see Appendix B for HAC conditional logic

CC +7th **T81.515 Adhesions due to foreign body accidentally left in body following heart catheterization**
HAC 7th character A see Appendix B for HAC conditional logic

CC +7th **T81.516 Adhesions due to foreign body accidentally left in body following aspiration, puncture or other catheterization**
HAC 7th character A see Appendix B for HAC conditional logic

CC +7th **T81.517 Adhesions due to foreign body accidentally left in body following removal of catheter or packing**
HAC 7th character A see Appendix B for HAC conditional logic

CC +7th **T81.518 Adhesions due to foreign body accidentally left in body following other procedure**
HAC 7th character A see Appendix B for HAC conditional logic

CC +7th **T81.519 Adhesions due to foreign body accidentally left in body following unspecified procedure**
HAC 7th character A see Appendix B for HAC conditional logic

+ T81.52 Obstruction due to foreign body accidentally left in body following procedure

CC +7th **T81.520 Obstruction due to foreign body accidentally left in body following surgical operation**
HAC 7th character A see Appendix B for HAC conditional logic

CC +7th **T81.521 Obstruction due to foreign body accidentally left in body following infusion or transfusion**
HAC 7th character A see Appendix B for HAC conditional logic

CC +7th **T81.522 Obstruction due to foreign body accidentally left in body following kidney dialysis**
HAC 7th character A see Appendix B for HAC conditional logic

CC +7th **T81.523 Obstruction due to foreign body accidentally left in body following injection or immunization**
HAC 7th character A see Appendix B for HAC conditional logic

CC +7th **T81.524 Obstruction due to foreign body accidentally left in body following endoscopic examination**
HAC 7th character A see Appendix B for HAC conditional logic

CC +7th **T81.525 Obstruction due to foreign body accidentally left in body following heart catheterization**
HAC 7th character A see Appendix B for HAC conditional logic

CC +7th **T81.526 Obstruction due to foreign body accidentally left in body following aspiration, puncture or other catheterization**
HAC 7th character A see Appendix B for HAC conditional logic

CC +7th **T81.527 Obstruction due to foreign body accidentally left in body following removal of catheter or packing**
HAC 7th character A see Appendix B for HAC conditional logic

CC +7th **T81.528 Obstruction due to foreign body accidentally left in body following other procedure**
HAC 7th character A see Appendix B for HAC conditional logic

CC +7th **T81.529 Obstruction due to foreign body accidentally left in body following unspecified procedure**
HAC 7th character A see Appendix B for HAC conditional logic

+ **T81.53 Perforation due to foreign body accidentally left in body following procedure**

CC +7th **T81.530 Perforation due to foreign body accidentally left in body following surgical operation**
HAC 7th character A see Appendix B for HAC conditional logic

CC +7th **T81.531 Perforation due to foreign body accidentally left in body following infusion or transfusion**
HAC 7th character A see Appendix B for HAC conditional logic

+7th **T81.532 Perforation due to foreign body accidentally left in body following kidney dialysis**
HAC 7th character A see Appendix B for HAC conditional logic

CC +7th **T81.533 Perforation due to foreign body accidentally left in body following injection or immunization**
HAC 7th character A see Appendix B for HAC conditional logic

CC +7th **T81.534 Perforation due to foreign body accidentally left in body following endoscopic examination**
HAC 7th character A see Appendix B for HAC conditional logic

CC +7th **T81.535 Perforation due to foreign body accidentally left in body following heart catheterization**
HAC 7th character A see Appendix B for HAC conditional logic

CC +7th **T81.536 Perforation due to foreign body accidentally left in body following aspiration, puncture or other catheterization**
HAC 7th character A see Appendix B for HAC conditional logic

CC +7th **T81.537 Perforation due to foreign body accidentally left in body following removal of catheter or packing**
HAC 7th character A see Appendix B for HAC conditional logic

CC +7th **T81.538 Perforation due to foreign body accidentally left in body following other procedure**
HAC 7th character A see Appendix B for HAC conditional logic

CC +7th **T81.539 Perforation due to foreign body accidentally left in body following unspecified procedure**
HAC 7th character A see Appendix B for HAC conditional logic

+ **T81.59 Other complications of foreign body accidentally left in body following procedure**
Excludes2: *obstruction or perforation due to prosthetic devices and implants intentionally left in body (T82.0-T82.5, T83.0-T83.4, T83.7, T84.0-T84.4, T85.0-T85.6)*

CC +7th **T81.590 Other complications of foreign body accidentally left in body following surgical operation**
HAC 7th character A see Appendix B for HAC conditional logic
AHA CC: 4Q, 2014, 24

CC +7th **T81.591 Other complications of foreign body accidentally left in body following infusion or transfusion**
HAC 7th character A see Appendix B for HAC conditional logic

CC +7th **T81.592 Other complications of foreign body accidentally left in body following kidney dialysis**
HAC 7th character A see Appendix B for HAC conditional logic

CC +7th **T81.593 Other complications of foreign body accidentally left in body following injection or immunization**
HAC 7th character A see Appendix B for HAC conditional logic

CC +7th **T81.594 Other complications of foreign body accidentally left in body following endoscopic examination**
HAC 7th character A see Appendix B for HAC conditional logic

CC +7th **T81.595 Other complications of foreign body accidentally left in body following heart catheterization**
HAC 7th character A see Appendix B for HAC conditional logic

CC +7th **T81.596 Other complications of foreign body accidentally left in body following aspiration, puncture or other catheterization**
HAC 7th character A see Appendix B for HAC conditional logic

CC +7th **T81.597 Other complications of foreign body accidentally left in body following removal of catheter or packing**
HAC 7th character A see Appendix B for HAC conditional logic

CC +7th **T81.598 Other complications of foreign body accidentally left in body following other procedure**
HAC 7th character A see Appendix B for HAC conditional logic

CC +7th **T81.599 Other complications of foreign body accidentally left in body following unspecified procedure**
HAC 7th character A see Appendix B for HAC conditional logic

+ **T81.6 Acute reaction to foreign substance accidentally left during a procedure**
Excludes2: *complications of foreign body accidentally left in body cavity or operation wound following procedure (T81.5-)*

CC X+7th **T81.60 Unspecified acute reaction to foreign substance accidentally left during a procedure**
HAC 7th character A see Appendix B for HAC conditional logic

CC X+7th **T81.61 Aseptic peritonitis due to foreign substance accidentally left during a procedure**
Chemical peritonitis
HAC 7th character A see Appendix B for HAC conditional logic

CC X+7th **T81.69 Other acute reaction to foreign substance accidentally left during a procedure**
HAC 7th character A see Appendix B for HAC conditional logic

+ **T81.7 Vascular complications following a procedure, not elsewhere classified**
Air embolism following procedure NEC
Phlebitis or thrombophlebitis resulting from a procedure
Excludes1: *embolism complicating abortion or ectopic or molar pregnancy (O00-O07, O08.2)*
embolism complicating pregnancy, childbirth and the puerperium (O88.-)
traumatic embolism (T79.0)
Excludes2: *embolism due to prosthetic devices, implants and grafts (T82.8-, T83.81, T84.8-, T85.81-)*
embolism following infusion, transfusion and therapeutic injection (T80.0)

+ **T81.71 Complication of artery following a procedure, not elsewhere classified**

CC +7th **T81.710 Complication of mesenteric artery following a procedure, not elsewhere classified**

CC +7th **T81.711 Complication of renal artery following a procedure, not elsewhere classified**

CC +7th **T81.718 Complication of other artery following a procedure, not elsewhere classified**
AHA CC: 2Q, 2019, 21-23

CC +7th **T81.719 Complication of unspecified artery following a procedure, not elsewhere classified**

CC X+7th **T81.72 Complication of vein following a procedure, not elsewhere classified**

+ T81.8 **Other complications of procedures, not elsewhere classified**
Excludes2: hypothermia following anesthesia (T88.51)
malignant hyperpyrexia due to anesthesia (T88.3)

X+7th T81.81 **Complication of inhalation therapy**

X+7th T81.82 **Emphysema (subcutaneous) resulting from a procedure**

CC X+7th T81.83 **Persistent postprocedural fistula**
AHA CC: 3Q, 2017, 3-5

X+7th T81.89 **Other complications of procedures, not elsewhere classified**
Use additional code to specify complication, such as:
postprocedural delirium (F05)
AHA CC: 1Q, 2014, 23

X+7th T81.9 **Unspecified complication of procedure**

T82 **Complications of cardiac and vascular prosthetic devices, implants and grafts**
Excludes2: failure and rejection of transplanted organs and tissue (T86.-)
AHA CC: 3Q, 2020, 36

The appropriate 7th character is to be added to each code from category T82
A initial encounter
D subsequent encounter
S sequela

+ T82.0 **Mechanical complication of heart valve prosthesis**
Mechanical complication of artificial heart valve
Excludes1: mechanical complication of biological heart valve graft (T82.22-)

CC X+7th T82.01 **Breakdown (mechanical) of heart valve prosthesis**

CC X+7th T82.02 **Displacement of heart valve prosthesis**
Malposition of heart valve prosthesis

CC X+7th T82.03 **Leakage of heart valve prosthesis**

CC X+7th T82.09 **Other mechanical complication of heart valve prosthesis**
Obstruction (mechanical) of heart valve prosthesis
Perforation of heart valve prosthesis
Protrusion of heart valve prosthesis

+ T82.1 **Mechanical complication of cardiac electronic device**

+ T82.11 **Breakdown (mechanical) of cardiac electronic device**

CC +7th T82.110 **Breakdown (mechanical) of cardiac electrode**

CC +7th T82.111 **Breakdown (mechanical) of cardiac pulse generator (battery)**

CC +7th T82.118 **Breakdown (mechanical) of other cardiac electronic device**

CC +7th T82.119 **Breakdown (mechanical) of unspecified cardiac electronic device**

+ T82.12 **Displacement of cardiac electronic device**
Malposition of cardiac electronic device

CC +7th T82.120 **Displacement of cardiac electrode**

CC +7th T82.121 **Displacement of cardiac pulse generator (battery)**

CC +7th T82.128 **Displacement of other cardiac electronic device**

CC +7th T82.129 **Displacement of unspecified cardiac electronic device**

+ T82.19 **Other mechanical complication of cardiac electronic device**
Leakage of cardiac electronic device
Obstruction of cardiac electronic device
Perforation of cardiac electronic device
Protrusion of cardiac electronic device

CC +7th T82.190 **Other mechanical complication of cardiac electrode**

CC +7th T82.191 **Other mechanical complication of cardiac pulse generator (battery)**

CC +7th T82.198 **Other mechanical complication of other cardiac electronic device**

CC +7th T82.199 **Other mechanical complication of unspecified cardiac device**

+ T82.2 **Mechanical complication of coronary artery bypass graft and biological heart valve graft**
Excludes1: mechanical complication of artificial heart valve prosthesis (T82.0-)

+ T82.21 **Mechanical complication of coronary artery bypass graft**

CC +7th T82.211 **Breakdown (mechanical) of coronary artery bypass graft**

CC +7th T82.212 **Displacement of coronary artery bypass graft**
Malposition of coronary artery bypass graft

CC +7th T82.213 **Leakage of coronary artery bypass graft**

CC +7th T82.218 **Other mechanical complication of coronary artery bypass graft**
Obstruction, mechanical of coronary artery bypass graft
Perforation of coronary artery bypass graft
Protrusion of coronary artery bypass graft

+ T82.22 **Mechanical complication of biological heart valve graft**

CC +7th T82.221 **Breakdown (mechanical) of biological heart valve graft**

CC +7th T82.222 **Displacement of biological heart valve graft**
Malposition of biological heart valve graft

CC +7th T82.223 **Leakage of biological heart valve graft**

CC +7th T82.228 **Other mechanical complication of biological heart valve graft**
Obstruction of biological heart valve graft
Perforation of biological heart valve graft
Protrusion of biological heart valve graft

+ T82.3 **Mechanical complication of other vascular grafts**

+ T82.31 **Breakdown (mechanical) of other vascular grafts**

CC +7th T82.310 **Breakdown (mechanical) of aortic (bifurcation) graft (replacement)**
AHA CC: 3Q, 2020, 3-7

CC +7th T82.311 **Breakdown (mechanical) of carotid arterial graft (bypass)**

CC +7th T82.312 **Breakdown (mechanical) of femoral arterial graft (bypass)**

CC +7th T82.318 **Breakdown (mechanical) of other vascular grafts**

CC +7th T82.319 **Breakdown (mechanical) of unspecified vascular grafts**

+ T82.32 **Displacement of other vascular grafts**
Malposition of other vascular grafts

CC +7th T82.320 **Displacement of aortic (bifurcation) graft (replacement)**

CC +7th T82.321 **Displacement of carotid arterial graft (bypass)**

CC +7th T82.322 **Displacement of femoral arterial graft (bypass)**

CC +7th T82.328 **Displacement of other vascular grafts**

CC +7th T82.329 **Displacement of unspecified vascular grafts**

+ T82.33 **Leakage of other vascular grafts**

CC +7th T82.330 **Leakage of aortic (bifurcation) graft (replacement)**
AHA CC: 3Q, 2020, 4-7

CC +7th T82.331 **Leakage of carotid arterial graft (bypass)**

CC +7th T82.332 **Leakage of femoral arterial graft (bypass)**

CC +7th T82.338 **Leakage of other vascular grafts**

CC +7th T82.339 **Leakage of unspecified vascular graft**

+ T82.39 **Other mechanical complication of other vascular grafts**
Obstruction (mechanical) of other vascular grafts
Perforation of other vascular grafts
Protrusion of other vascular grafts

CC +7th T82.390 **Other mechanical complication of aortic (bifurcation) graft (replacement)**
AHA CC: 3Q, 2020, 5

CC +7th T82.391 **Other mechanical complication of carotid arterial graft (bypass)**

CC +7th T82.392 **Other mechanical complication of femoral arterial graft (bypass)**

CC +7th T82.398 **Other mechanical complication of other vascular grafts**

CC +7th T82.399 **Other mechanical complication of unspecified vascular grafts**

+ **T82.4 Mechanical complication of vascular dialysis catheter**
Mechanical complication of hemodialysis catheter
Excludes1: *mechanical complication of intraperitoneal dialysis catheter (T85.62)*

CC X+7th **T82.41 Breakdown (mechanical) of vascular dialysis catheter**

CC X+7th **T82.42 Displacement of vascular dialysis catheter**
Malposition of vascular dialysis catheter

CC X+7th **T82.43 Leakage of vascular dialysis catheter**

CC X+7th **T82.49 Other complication of vascular dialysis catheter**
Obstruction (mechanical) of vascular dialysis catheter
Perforation of vascular dialysis catheter
Protrusion of vascular dialysis catheter

+ **T82.5 Mechanical complication of other cardiac and vascular devices and implants**
Excludes2: *mechanical complication of epidural and subdural infusion catheter (T85.61)*

+ **T82.51 Breakdown (mechanical) of other cardiac and vascular devices and implants**

CC +7th **T82.510 Breakdown (mechanical) of surgically created arteriovenous fistula**
AHA CC: 3Q, 2020, 36

CC +7th **T82.511 Breakdown (mechanical) of surgically created arteriovenous shunt**
AHA CC: 3Q, 2020, 37

CC +7th **T82.512 Breakdown (mechanical) of artificial heart**

CC +7th **T82.513 Breakdown (mechanical) of balloon (counterpulsation) device**

CC +7th **T82.514 Breakdown (mechanical) of infusion catheter**

CC +7th **T82.515 Breakdown (mechanical) of umbrella device**

CC +7th **T82.518 Breakdown (mechanical) of other cardiac and vascular devices and implants**

CC +7th **T82.519 Breakdown (mechanical) of unspecified cardiac and vascular devices and implants**

+ **T82.52 Displacement of other cardiac and vascular devices and implants**
Malposition of other cardiac and vascular devices and implants

CC +7th **T82.520 Displacement of surgically created arteriovenous fistula**

CC +7th **T82.521 Displacement of surgically created arteriovenous shunt**

CC +7th **T82.522 Displacement of artificial heart**

CC +7th **T82.523 Displacement of balloon (counterpulsation) device**

CC +7th **T82.524 Displacement of infusion catheter**
AHA CC: 3Q, 2019, 15-16; 2Q, 2020, 21-22

CC +7th **T82.525 Displacement of umbrella device**

CC +7th **T82.528 Displacement of other cardiac and vascular devices and implants**

CC +7th **T82.529 Displacement of unspecified cardiac and vascular devices and implants**

+ **T82.53 Leakage of other cardiac and vascular devices and implants**

CC +7th **T82.530 Leakage of surgically created arteriovenous fistula**

CC +7th **T82.531 Leakage of surgically created arteriovenous shunt**

CC +7th **T82.532 Leakage of artificial heart**

CC +7th **T82.533 Leakage of balloon (counterpulsation) device**

CC +7th **T82.534 Leakage of infusion catheter**

CC +7th **T82.535 Leakage of umbrella device**

CC +7th **T82.538 Leakage of other cardiac and vascular devices and implants**

CC +7th **T82.539 Leakage of unspecified cardiac and vascular devices and implants**

+ **T82.59 Other mechanical complication of other cardiac and vascular devices and implants**
Obstruction (mechanical) of other cardiac and vascular devices and implants
Perforation of other cardiac and vascular devices and implants
Protrusion of other cardiac and vascular devices and implants

CC +7th **T82.590 Other mechanical complication of surgically created arteriovenous fistula**

CC +7th **T82.591 Other mechanical complication of surgically created arteriovenous shunt**

CC +7th **T82.592 Other mechanical complication of artificial heart**

CC +7th **T82.593 Other mechanical complication of balloon (counterpulsation) device**

CC +7th **T82.594 Other mechanical complication of infusion catheter**

CC +7th **T82.595 Other mechanical complication of umbrella device**

CC +7th **T82.598 Other mechanical complication of other cardiac and vascular devices and implants**

CC +7th **T82.599 Other mechanical complication of unspecified cardiac and vascular devices and implants**

CC X+7th **T82.6 Infection and inflammatory reaction due to cardiac valve prosthesis**
Use additional code to identify infection
HAC 7th character A see Appendix B for HAC conditional logic

CC X+7th **T82.7 Infection and inflammatory reaction due to other cardiac and vascular devices, implants and grafts**
Use additional code to identify infection
HAC 7th character A see Appendix B for HAC conditional logic
AHA CC: 1Q, 2015, 3-21; 4Q, 2018, 89; 1Q, 2019, 13-14

+ **T82.8 Other specified complications due to cardiac and vascular prosthetic devices, implants and grafts**

+ **T82.81 Embolism due to cardiac and vascular prosthetic devices, implants and grafts**

CC +7th **T82.817 Embolism due to cardiac prosthetic devices, implants and grafts**

CC +7th **T82.818 Embolism due to vascular prosthetic devices, implants and grafts**

+ **T82.82 Fibrosis due to cardiac and vascular prosthetic devices, implants and grafts**

CC +7th **T82.827 Fibrosis due to cardiac prosthetic devices, implants and grafts**

CC +7th **T82.828 Fibrosis due to vascular prosthetic devices, implants and grafts**

+ **T82.83 Hemorrhage due to cardiac and vascular prosthetic devices, implants and grafts**

CC +7th **T82.837 Hemorrhage due to cardiac prosthetic devices, implants and grafts**

CC +7th **T82.838 Hemorrhage due to vascular prosthetic devices, implants and grafts**
AHA CC: 3Q, 2020, 36-37

+ **T82.84 Pain due to cardiac and vascular prosthetic devices, implants and grafts**

CC +7th **T82.847 Pain due to cardiac prosthetic devices, implants and grafts**

CC +7th **T82.848 Pain due to vascular prosthetic devices, implants and grafts**

+ **T82.85 Stenosis due to cardiac and vascular prosthetic devices, implants and grafts**

CC +7th **T82.855 Stenosis of coronary artery stent**
In-stent stenosis (restenosis) of coronary artery stent
Restenosis of coronary artery stent
AHA CC: 4Q, 2016, 69

CC +7th **T82.856 Stenosis of peripheral vascular stent**
In-stent stenosis (restenosis) of peripheral vascular stent
Restenosis of peripheral vascular stent
AHA CC: 4Q, 2016, 69

CC +7th **T82.857 Stenosis of other cardiac prosthetic devices, implants and grafts**

CC +7th **T82.858 Stenosis of other vascular prosthetic devices, implants and grafts**

+ **T82.86 Thrombosis due to cardiac and vascular prosthetic devices, implants and grafts**

CC +7th **T82.867 Thrombosis due to cardiac prosthetic devices, implants and grafts**

AHA CC: 2Q, 2019, 32-33

CC +7th **T82.868 Thrombosis due to vascular prosthetic devices, implants and grafts**

+ **T82.89 Other specified complication of cardiac and vascular prosthetic devices, implants and grafts**

CC +7th **T82.897 Other specified complication of cardiac prosthetic devices, implants and grafts**

CC +7th **T82.898 Other specified complication of vascular prosthetic devices, implants and grafts**

AHA CC: 3Q, 2020, 3

CC X+7th **T82.9 Unspecified complication of cardiac and vascular prosthetic device, implant and graft**

T83 Complications of genitourinary prosthetic devices, implants and grafts

Excludes2: *failure and rejection of transplanted organs and tissue (T86.-)*

AHA CC: 4Q, 2016, 70-71

The appropriate 7th character is to be added to each code from category T83
A initial encounter
D subsequent encounter
S sequela

+ **T83.0 Mechanical complication of urinary catheter**

Excludes2: *complications of stoma of urinary tract (N99.5-)*

+ **T83.01 Breakdown (mechanical) of urinary catheter**

CC +7th **T83.010 Breakdown (mechanical) of cystostomy catheter**

+7th **T83.011 Breakdown (mechanical) of indwelling urethral catheter**

+7th **T83.012 Breakdown (mechanical) of nephrostomy catheter**

+7th **T83.018 Breakdown (mechanical) of other urinary catheter**

Breakdown (mechanical) of Hopkins catheter

Breakdown (mechanical) of ileostomy catheter

Breakdown (mechanical) of urostomy catheter

+ **T83.02 Displacement of urinary catheter**

Malposition of urinary catheter

CC +7th **T83.020 Displacement of cystostomy catheter**

+7th **T83.021 Displacement of indwelling urethral catheter**

+7th **T83.022 Displacement of nephrostomy catheter**

+7th **T83.028 Displacement of other urinary catheter**

Displacement of Hopkins catheter

Displacement of ileostomy catheter

Displacement of urostomy catheter

+ **T83.03 Leakage of urinary catheter**

CC +7th **T83.030 Leakage of cystostomy catheter**

+7th **T83.031 Leakage of indwelling urethral catheter**

+7th **T83.032 Leakage of nephrostomy catheter**

+7th **T83.038 Leakage of other urinary catheter**

Leakage of Hopkins catheter

Leakage of ileostomy catheter

Leakage of urostomy catheter

+ **T83.09 Other mechanical complication of urinary catheter**

Obstruction (mechanical) of urinary catheter

Perforation of urinary catheter

Protrusion of urinary catheter

CC +7th **T83.090 Other mechanical complication of cystostomy catheter**

+7th **T83.091 Other mechanical complication of indwelling urethral catheter**

+7th **T83.092 Other mechanical complication of nephrostomy catheter**

+7th **T83.098 Other mechanical complication of other urinary catheter**

Other mechanical complication of Hopkins catheter

Other mechanical complication of ileostomy catheter

Other mechanical complication of urostomy catheter

+ **T83.1 Mechanical complication of other urinary devices and implants**

+ **T83.11 Breakdown (mechanical) of other urinary devices and implants**

CC +7th **T83.110 Breakdown (mechanical) of urinary electronic stimulator device**

Excludes2: *breakdown (mechanical) of electrode(lead)forsacral nerve neurostimulator (T85.111)*

breakdown (mechanical) of implanted electronic sacral neurostimulator, pulse generator or receiver (T85.113)

CC +7th **T83.111 Breakdown (mechanical) of implanted urinary sphincter**

CC +7th **T83.112 Breakdown (mechanical) of indwelling ureteral stent**

CC +7th **T83.113 Breakdown (mechanical) of other urinary stents**

Breakdown (mechanical) of ileal conduit stent

Breakdown (mechanical) of nephroureteral stent

CC +7th **T83.118 Breakdown (mechanical) of other urinary devices and implants**

+ **T83.12 Displacement of other urinary devices and implants**

Malposition of other urinary devices and implants

CC +7th **T83.120 Displacement of urinary electronic stimulator device**

Excludes2: *displacement of electrode (lead) for sacral nerve neurostimulator(T85.121)*

displacement of implanted electronic sacral neurostimulator, pulse generator or receiver (T85.123)

CC +7th **T83.121 Displacement of implanted urinary sphincter**

CC +7th **T83.122 Displacement of indwelling ureteral stent**

CC +7th **T83.123 Displacement of other urinary stents**

Displacement of ileal conduit stent

Displacement of nephroureteral stent

CC +7th **T83.128 Displacement of other urinary devices and implants**

+ **T83.19 Other mechanical complication of other urinary devices and implants**

Leakage of other urinary devices and implants

Obstruction (mechanical) of other urinary devices and implants

Perforation of other urinary devices and implants

Protrusion of other urinary devices and implants

CC +7th **T83.190 Other mechanical complication of urinary electronic stimulator device**

Excludes2: *other mechanical complicationofelectrode (lead) for sacral nerve neurostimulator(T85.191)*

other mechanical complication of implanted electronic sacral neurostimulator, pulse generator or receiver (T85.193)

CC +7th **T83.191 Other mechanical complication of implanted urinary sphincter**

CC +7th **T83.192 Other mechanical complication of indwelling ureteral stent**

CC +7th **T83.193 Other mechanical complication of other urinary stent**

Other mechanical complication of ileal conduit stent

Other mechanical complication of nephroureteral stent

CC +7th **T83.198 Other mechanical complication of other urinary devices and implants**

+ **T83.2 Mechanical complication of graft of urinary organ**

CC X+7th **T83.21 Breakdown (mechanical) of graft of urinary organ**

CC X+7th **T83.22 Displacement of graft of urinary organ**
Malposition of graft of urinary organ

CC X+7th **T83.23 Leakage of graft of urinary organ**

CC X+7th **T83.24 Erosion of graft of urinary organ**

CC X+7th **T83.25 Exposure of graft of urinary organ**

CC X+7th **T83.29 Other mechanical complication of graft of urinary organ**
Obstruction (mechanical) of graft of urinary organ
Perforation of graft of urinary organ
Protrusion of graft of urinary organ

+ **T83.3 Mechanical complication of intrauterine contraceptive device**

♀ X+7th **T83.31 Breakdown (mechanical) of intrauterine contraceptive device**

♀ X+7th **T83.32 Displacement of intrauterine contraceptive device**
Malposition of intrauterine contraceptive device
Missing string of intrauterine contraceptive device

♀ X+7th **T83.39 Other mechanical complication of intrauterine contraceptive device**
Leakage of intrauterine contraceptive device
Obstruction (mechanical) of intrauterine contraceptive device
Perforation of intrauterine contraceptive device
Protrusion of intrauterine contraceptive device

+ **T83.4 Mechanical complication of other prosthetic devices, implants and grafts of genital tract**

+ **T83.41 Breakdown (mechanical) of other prosthetic devices, implants and grafts of genital tract**

♂ CC +7th **T83.410 Breakdown (mechanical) of implanted penile prosthesis**
Breakdown (mechanical) of penile prosthesis cylinder
Breakdown (mechanical) of penile prosthesis pump
Breakdown (mechanical) of penile prosthesis reservoir

CC +7th **T83.411 Breakdown (mechanical) of implanted testicular prosthesis**

CC +7th **T83.418 Breakdown (mechanical) of other prosthetic devices, implants and grafts of genital tract**

+ **T83.42 Displacement of other prosthetic devices, implants and grafts of genital tract**
Malposition of other prosthetic devices, implants and grafts of genital tract

♂ CC +7th **T83.420 Displacement of implanted penile prosthesis**
Displacement of penile prosthesis cylinder
Displacement of penile prosthesis pump
Displacement of penile prosthesis reservoir

CC +7th **T83.421 Displacement of implanted testicular prosthesis**

CC +7th **T83.428 Displacement of other prosthetic devices, implants and grafts of genital tract**
AHA CC: 1Q, 2018, 5-6

+ **T83.49 Other mechanical complication of other prosthetic devices, implants and grafts of genital tract**
Leakage of other prosthetic devices, implants and grafts of genital tract
Obstruction, mechanical of other prosthetic devices, implants and grafts of genital tract
Perforation of other prosthetic devices, implants and grafts of genital tract
Protrusion of other prosthetic devices, implants and grafts of genital tract

♂ CC +7th **T83.490 Other mechanical complication of implanted penile prosthesis**
Other mechanical complication of penile prosthesis cylinder
Other mechanical complication of penile prosthesis pump
Other mechanical complication of penile prosthesis reservoir

CC +7th **T83.491 Other mechanical complication of implanted testicular prosthesis**

CC +7th **T83.498 Other mechanical complication of other prosthetic devices, implants and grafts of genital tract**

+ **T83.5 Infection and inflammatory reaction due to prosthetic device, implant and graft in urinary system**
Use additional code to identify infection

+ **T83.51 Infection and inflammatory reaction due to urinary catheter**
Excludes2: *complications of stoma of urinary tract (N99.5-)*

CC +7th **T83.510 Infection and inflammatory reaction due to cystostomy catheter**

CC +7th **T83.511 Infection and inflammatory reaction due to indwelling urethral catheter**
HAC 7th character A see Appendix B for HAC conditional logic

CC +7th **T83.512 Infection and inflammatory reaction due to nephrostomy catheter**

CC +7th **T83.518 Infection and inflammatory reaction due to other urinary catheter**
Infection and inflammatory reaction due to Hopkins catheter
Infection and inflammatory reaction due to ileostomy catheter
Infection and inflammatory reaction due to urostomy catheter
HAC 7th character A see Appendix B for HAC conditional logic

+ **T83.59 Infection and inflammatory reaction due to prosthetic device, implant and graft in urinary system**

CC +7th **T83.590 Infection and inflammatory reaction due to implanted urinary neurostimulation device**
Excludes2: *infection and inflammatory reaction due to electrode lead of sacral nerve neurostimulator (T85.732)*
infection and inflammatory reaction due to pulse generator or receiver of sacralnerveneurostimulator (T85.734)

CC +7th **T83.591 Infection and inflammatory reaction due to implanted urinary sphincter**

CC +7th **T83.592 Infection and inflammatory reaction due to indwelling ureteral stent**

CC +7th **T83.593 Infection and inflammatory reaction due to other urinary stents**
Infection and inflammatory reaction due to ileal conduit stents
Infection and inflammatory reaction due to nephroureteral stent

CC +7th **T83.598 Infection and inflammatory reaction due to other prosthetic device, implant and graft in urinary system**
AHA CC: 3Q, 2020, 25-26

+ **T83.6 Infection and inflammatory reaction due to prosthetic device, implant and graft in genital tract**
Use additional code to identify infection

CC X+7th **T83.61 Infection and inflammatory reaction due to implanted penile prosthesis**
Infection and inflammatory reaction due to penile prosthesis cylinder
Infection and inflammatory reaction due to penile prosthesis pump
Infection and inflammatory reaction due to penile prosthesis reservoir

CC X+7th **T83.62 Infection and inflammatory reaction due to implanted testicular prosthesis**

CC X+7th **T83.69 Infection and inflammatory reaction due to other prosthetic device, implant and graft in genital tract**

+ T83.7 **Complications due to implanted mesh and other prosthetic materials**

+ T83.71 **Erosion of implanted mesh and other prosthetic materials to surrounding organ or tissue**

♀ +7th **T83.711** **Erosion of implanted vaginal mesh to surrounding organ or tissue**

Erosion of implanted vaginal mesh into pelvic floor muscles

CC +7th **T83.712** **Erosion of implanted urethral mesh to surrounding organ or tissue**

Erosion of implanted female urethral sling

Erosion of implanted male urethral sling

Erosion of implanted urethral mesh into pelvic floor muscles

CC +7th **T83.713** **Erosion of implanted urethral bulking agent to surrounding organ or tissue**

CC +7th **T83.714** **Erosion of implanted ureteral bulking agent to surrounding organ or tissue**

CC +7th **T83.718** **Erosion of other implanted mesh to organ or tissue**

CC +7th **T83.719** **Erosion of other prosthetic materials to surrounding organ or tissue**

+ T83.72 **Exposure of implanted mesh and other prosthetic materials into surrounding organ or tissue**

Extrusion of implanted mesh

♀ +7th **T83.721** **Exposure of implanted vaginal mesh into vagina**

Exposure of implanted vaginal mesh through vaginal wall

CC +7th **T83.722** **Exposure of implanted urethral mesh into urethra**

Exposure of implanted female urethral sling

Exposure of implanted male urethral sling

Exposure of implanted urethral mesh through urethral wall

CC +7th **T83.723** **Exposure of implanted urethral bulking agent into urethra**

CC +7th **T83.724** **Exposure of implanted ureteral bulking agent into ureter**

CC +7th **T83.728** **Exposure of other implanted mesh into organ or tissue**

CC +7th **T83.729** **Exposure of other prosthetic materials into organ or tissue**

CC X+7th **T83.79** **Other specified complications due to other genitourinary prosthetic materials**

+ T83.8 **Other specified complications of genitourinary prosthetic devices, implants and grafts**

CC X+7th **T83.81** **Embolism due to genitourinary prosthetic devices, implants and grafts**

CC X+7th **T83.82** **Fibrosis due to genitourinary prosthetic devices, implants and grafts**

CC X+7th **T83.83** **Hemorrhage due to genitourinary prosthetic devices, implants and grafts**

CC X+7th **T83.84** **Pain due to genitourinary prosthetic devices, implants and grafts**

CC X+7th **T83.85** **Stenosis due to genitourinary prosthetic devices, implants and grafts**

CC X+7th **T83.86** **Thrombosis due to genitourinary prosthetic devices, implants and grafts**

CC X+7th **T83.89** **Other specified complication of genitourinary prosthetic devices, implants and grafts**

CC X+7th **T83.9** **Unspecified complication of genitourinary prosthetic device, implant and graft**

T84 **Complications of internal orthopedic prosthetic devices, implants and grafts**

Excludes2: *failure and rejection of transplanted organs and tissues (T86.-)*

fracture of bone following insertion of orthopedic implant, joint prosthesis or bone plate (M96.6)

The appropriate 7th character is to be added to each code from category T84

A initial encounter

D subsequent encounter

S sequela

+ T84.0 **Mechanical complication of internal joint prosthesis**

+ T84.01 **Broken internal joint prosthesis**

Breakage (fracture) of prosthetic joint

Broken prosthetic joint implant

Excludes1: *periprosthetic joint implant fracture (M97.-)*

CC +7th **T84.010** **Broken internal right hip prosthesis**

CC +7th **T84.011** **Broken internal left hip prosthesis**

CC +7th **T84.012** **Broken internal right knee prosthesis**

AHA CC: 2Q, 2019, 27-28

CC +7th **T84.013** **Broken internal left knee prosthesis**

CC +7th **T84.018** **Broken internal joint prosthesis, other site**

Use additional code to identify the joint (Z96.6-)

CC +7th **T84.019** **Broken internal joint prosthesis, unspecified site**

+ T84.02 **Dislocation of internal joint prosthesis**

Instability of internal joint prosthesis

Subluxation of internal joint prosthesis

CC +7th **T84.020** **Dislocation of internal right hip prosthesis**

CC +7th **T84.021** **Dislocation of internal left hip prosthesis**

CC +7th **T84.022** **Instability of internal right knee prosthesis**

CC +7th **T84.023** **Instability of internal left knee prosthesis**

CC +7th **T84.028** **Dislocation of other internal joint prosthesis**

Use additional code to identify the joint (Z96.6-)

CC +7th **T84.029** **Dislocation of unspecified internal joint prosthesis**

+ T84.03 **Mechanical loosening of internal prosthetic joint**

Aseptic loosening of prosthetic joint

CC +7th **T84.030** **Mechanical loosening of internal right hip prosthetic joint**

CC +7th **T84.031** **Mechanical loosening of internal left hip prosthetic joint**

CC +7th **T84.032** **Mechanical loosening of internal right knee prosthetic joint**

CC +7th **T84.033** **Mechanical loosening of internal left knee prosthetic joint**

CC +7th **T84.038** **Mechanical loosening of other internal prosthetic joint**

Use additional code to identify the joint (Z96.6-)

CC +7th **T84.039** **Mechanical loosening of unspecified internal prosthetic joint**

+ T84.05 **Periprosthetic osteolysis of internal prosthetic joint**

Use additional code to identify major osseous defect, if applicable (M89.7-)

CC +7th **T84.050** **Periprosthetic osteolysis of internal prosthetic right hip joint**

CC +7th **T84.051** **Periprosthetic osteolysis of internal prosthetic left hip joint**

CC +7th **T84.052** **Periprosthetic osteolysis of internal prosthetic right knee joint**

CC +7th **T84.053** **Periprosthetic osteolysis of internal prosthetic left knee joint**

CC +7th **T84.058** **Periprosthetic osteolysis of other internal prosthetic joint**

Use additional code to identify the joint (Z96.6-)

CC +7th **T84.059** **Periprosthetic osteolysis of unspecified internal prosthetic joint**

+ **T84.06 Wear of articular bearing surface of internal prosthetic joint**
- CC +7th **T84.060 Wear of articular bearing surface of internal prosthetic right hip joint**
- CC +7th **T84.061 Wear of articular bearing surface of internal prosthetic left hip joint**
- CC +7th **T84.062 Wear of articular bearing surface of internal prosthetic right knee joint**
- CC +7th **T84.063 Wear of articular bearing surface of internal prosthetic left knee joint**
- CC +7th **T84.068 Wear of articular bearing surface of other internal prosthetic joint**
  Use additional code to identify the joint (Z96.6-)
- CC +7th **T84.069 Wear of articular bearing surface of unspecified internal prosthetic joint**

+ **T84.09 Other mechanical complication of internal joint prosthesis**
  Prosthetic joint implant failure NOS
- CC +7th **T84.090 Other mechanical complication of internal right hip prosthesis**
  AHA CC: 1Q, 2019, 20
- CC +7th **T84.091 Other mechanical complication of internal left hip prosthesis**
- CC +7th **T84.092 Other mechanical complication of internal right knee prosthesis**
- CC +7th **T84.093 Other mechanical complication of internal left knee prosthesis**
- CC +7th **T84.098 Other mechanical complication of other internal joint prosthesis**
  Use additional code to identify the joint (Z96.6-)
- CC +7th **T84.099 Other mechanical complication of unspecified internal joint prosthesis**

+ **T84.1 Mechanical complication of internal fixation device of bones of limb**
  Excludes2: *mechanical complication of internal fixation device of bones of feet (T84.2-)*
  mechanical complication of internal fixation device of bones of fingers (T84.2-)
  mechanical complication of internal fixation device of bones of hands (T84.2-)
  mechanical complication of internal fixation device of bones of toes (T84.2-)

+ **T84.11 Breakdown (mechanical) of internal fixation device of bones of limb**
- CC +7th **T84.110 Breakdown (mechanical) of internal fixation device of right humerus**
- CC +7th **T84.111 Breakdown (mechanical) of internal fixation device of left humerus**
- CC +7th **T84.112 Breakdown (mechanical) of internal fixation device of bone of right forearm**
- CC +7th **T84.113 Breakdown (mechanical) of internal fixation device of bone of left forearm**
- CC +7th **T84.114 Breakdown (mechanical) of internal fixation device of right femur**
- CC +7th **T84.115 Breakdown (mechanical) of internal fixation device of left femur**
- CC +7th **T84.116 Breakdown (mechanical) of internal fixation device of bone of right lower leg**
- CC +7th **T84.117 Breakdown (mechanical) of internal fixation device of bone of left lower leg**
- CC +7th **T84.119 Breakdown (mechanical) of internal fixation device of unspecified bone of limb**

+ **T84.12 Displacement of internal fixation device of bones of limb**
  Malposition of internal fixation device of bones of limb
- CC +7th **T84.120 Displacement of internal fixation device of right humerus**
- CC +7th **T84.121 Displacement of internal fixation device of left humerus**
- CC +7th **T84.122 Displacement of internal fixation device of bone of right forearm**
- CC +7th **T84.123 Displacement of internal fixation device of bone of left forearm**
- CC +7th **T84.124 Displacement of internal fixation device of right femur**
- CC +7th **T84.125 Displacement of internal fixation device of left femur**
- CC +7th **T84.126 Displacement of internal fixation device of bone of right lower leg**
- CC +7th **T84.127 Displacement of internal fixation device of bone of left lower leg**
- CC +7th **T84.129 Displacement of internal fixation device of unspecified bone of limb**

+ **T84.19 Other mechanical complication of internal fixation device of bones of limb**
  Obstruction (mechanical) of internal fixation device of bones of limb
  Perforation of internal fixation device of bones of limb
  Protrusion of internal fixation device of bones of limb
- CC +7th **T84.190 Other mechanical complication of internal fixation device of right humerus**
- CC +7th **T84.191 Other mechanical complication of internal fixation device of left humerus**
- CC +7th **T84.192 Other mechanical complication of internal fixation device of bone of right forearm**
- CC +7th **T84.193 Other mechanical complication of internal fixation device of bone of left forearm**
- CC +7th **T84.194 Other mechanical complication of internal fixation device of right femur**
- CC +7th **T84.195 Other mechanical complication of internal fixation device of left femur**
- CC +7th **T84.196 Other mechanical complication of internal fixation device of bone of right lower leg**
- CC +7th **T84.197 Other mechanical complication of internal fixation device of bone of left lower leg**
- CC +7th **T84.199 Other mechanical complication of internal fixation device of unspecified bone of limb**

+ **T84.2 Mechanical complication of internal fixation device of other bones**

+ **T84.21 Breakdown (mechanical) of internal fixation device of other bones**
- CC +7th **T84.210 Breakdown (mechanical) of internal fixation device of bones of hand and fingers**
- CC +7th **T84.213 Breakdown (mechanical) of internal fixation device of bones of foot and toes**
- CC +7th **T84.216 Breakdown (mechanical) of internal fixation device of vertebrae**
- CC +7th **T84.218 Breakdown (mechanical) of internal fixation device of other bones**

+ **T84.22 Displacement of internal fixation device of other bones**
  Malposition of internal fixation device of other bones
- CC +7th **T84.220 Displacement of internal fixation device of bones of hand and fingers**
- CC +7th **T84.223 Displacement of internal fixation device of bones of foot and toes**
- CC +7th **T84.226 Displacement of internal fixation device of vertebrae**
- CC +7th **T84.228 Displacement of internal fixation device of other bones**

+ **T84.29 Other mechanical complication of internal fixation device of other bones**
Obstruction (mechanical) of internal fixation device of other bones
Perforation of internal fixation device of other bones
Protrusion of internal fixation device of other bones

CC +7th **T84.290 Other mechanical complication of internal fixation device of bones of hand and fingers**

CC +7th **T84.293 Other mechanical complication of internal fixation device of bones of foot and toes**

CC +7th **T84.296 Other mechanical complication of internal fixation device of vertebrae**

CC +7th **T84.298 Other mechanical complication of internal fixation device of other bones**

+ **T84.3 Mechanical complication of other bone devices, implants and grafts**
Excludes2: *other complications of bone graft (T86.83-)*

+ **T84.31 Breakdown (mechanical) of other bone devices, implants and grafts**

CC +7th **T84.310 Breakdown (mechanical) of electronic bone stimulator**

CC +7th **T84.318 Breakdown (mechanical) of other bone devices, implants and grafts**

+ **T84.32 Displacement of other bone devices, implants and grafts**
Malposition of other bone devices, implants and grafts

CC +7th **T84.320 Displacement of electronic bone stimulator**

CC +7th **T84.328 Displacement of other bone devices, implants and grafts**
AHA CC: 4Q, 2014, 28-29

+ **T84.39 Other mechanical complication of other bone devices, implants and grafts**
Obstruction (mechanical) of other bone devices, implants and grafts
Perforation of other bone devices, implants and grafts
Protrusion of other bone devices, implants and grafts

CC +7th **T84.390 Other mechanical complication of electronic bone stimulator**

CC +7th **T84.398 Other mechanical complication of other bone devices, implants and grafts**

+ **T84.4 Mechanical complication of other internal orthopedic devices, implants and grafts**

+ **T84.41 Breakdown (mechanical) of other internal orthopedic devices, implants and grafts**

CC +7th **T84.410 Breakdown (mechanical) of muscle and tendon graft**

CC +7th **T84.418 Breakdown (mechanical) of other internal orthopedic devices, implants and grafts**

+ **T84.42 Displacement of other internal orthopedic devices, implants and grafts**
Malposition of other internal orthopedic devices, implants and grafts

CC +7th **T84.420 Displacement of muscle and tendon graft**

CC +7th **T84.428 Displacement of other internal orthopedic devices, implants and grafts**

+ **T84.49 Other mechanical complication of other internal orthopedic devices, implants and grafts**
Mechanical complication of other internal orthopedic devices, implants and grafts NOS
Obstruction (mechanical) of other internal orthopedic devices, implants and grafts
Perforation of other internal orthopedic devices, implants and grafts
Protrusion of other internal orthopedic devices, implants and grafts

CC +7th **T84.490 Other mechanical complication of muscle and tendon graft**

CC +7th **T84.498 Other mechanical complication of other internal orthopedic devices, implants and grafts**

+ **T84.5 Infection and inflammatory reaction due to internal joint prosthesis**
Use additional code to identify infection

CC X+7th **T84.50 Infection and inflammatory reaction due to unspecified internal joint prosthesis**

CC X+7th **T84.51 Infection and inflammatory reaction due to internal right hip prosthesis**
AHA CC: 4Q, 2015, 36

CC X+7th **T84.52 Infection and inflammatory reaction due to internal left hip prosthesis**
AHA CC: 1Q, 2015, 3-21

CC X+7th **T84.53 Infection and inflammatory reaction due to internal right knee prosthesis**

CC X+7th **T84.54 Infection and inflammatory reaction due to internal left knee prosthesis**

CC X+7th **T84.59 Infection and inflammatory reaction due to other internal joint prosthesis**

+ **T84.6 Infection and inflammatory reaction due to internal fixation device**
Use additional code to identify infection

CC X+7th **T84.60 Infection and inflammatory reaction due to internal fixation device of unspecified site**
HAC 7th character A see Appendix B for HAC conditional logic

+ **T84.61 Infection and inflammatory reaction due to internal fixation device of arm**

CC +7th **T84.610 Infection and inflammatory reaction due to internal fixation device of right humerus**
HAC 7th character A see Appendix B for HAC conditional logic

CC +7th **T84.611 Infection and inflammatory reaction due to internal fixation device of left humerus**
HAC 7th character A see Appendix B for HAC conditional logic

CC +7th **T84.612 Infection and inflammatory reaction due to internal fixation device of right radius**
HAC 7th character A see Appendix B for HAC conditional logic

CC +7th **T84.613 Infection and inflammatory reaction due to internal fixation device of left radius**
HAC 7th character A see Appendix B for HAC conditional logic

CC +7th **T84.614 Infection and inflammatory reaction due to internal fixation device of right ulna**
HAC 7th character A see Appendix B for HAC conditional logic

CC +7th **T84.615 Infection and inflammatory reaction due to internal fixation device of left ulna**
HAC 7th character A see Appendix B for HAC conditional logic

CC +7th **T84.619 Infection and inflammatory reaction due to internal fixation device of unspecified bone of arm**
HAC 7th character A see Appendix B for HAC conditional logic

+ **T84.62 Infection and inflammatory reaction due to internal fixation device of leg**

CC +7th **T84.620 Infection and inflammatory reaction due to internal fixation device of right femur**

CC +7th **T84.621 Infection and inflammatory reaction due to internal fixation device of left femur**

CC +7th **T84.622 Infection and inflammatory reaction due to internal fixation device of right tibia**

CC +7th **T84.623 Infection and inflammatory reaction due to internal fixation device of left tibia**

CC +7th **T84.624 Infection and inflammatory reaction due to internal fixation device of right fibula**

CC +7th **T84.625 Infection and inflammatory reaction due to internal fixation device of left fibula**

CC +7th **T84.629 Infection and inflammatory reaction due to internal fixation device of unspecified bone of leg**

CC X+7th **T84.63 Infection and inflammatory reaction due to internal fixation device of spine**
HAC 7th character A see Appendix B for HAC conditional logic

CC X+7th **T84.69 Infection and inflammatory reaction due to internal fixation device of other site**
HAC 7th character A see Appendix B for HAC conditional logic

CC X+7th **T84.7 Infection and inflammatory reaction due to other internal orthopedic prosthetic devices, implants and grafts**
Use additional code to identify infection
HAC 7th character A see Appendix B for HAC conditional logic

+ **T84.8 Other specified complications of internal orthopedic prosthetic devices, implants and grafts**

CC X+7th **T84.81 Embolism due to internal orthopedic prosthetic devices, implants and grafts**

CC X+7th **T84.82 Fibrosis due to internal orthopedic prosthetic devices, implants and grafts**

CC X+7th **T84.83 Hemorrhage due to internal orthopedic prosthetic devices, implants and grafts**

CC X+7th **T84.84 Pain due to internal orthopedic prosthetic devices, implants and grafts**

CC X+7th **T84.85 Stenosis due to internal orthopedic prosthetic devices, implants and grafts**

CC X+7th **T84.86 Thrombosis due to internal orthopedic prosthetic devices, implants and grafts**

CC X+7th **T84.89 Other specified complication of internal orthopedic prosthetic devices, implants and grafts**

CC X+7th **T84.9 Unspecified complication of internal orthopedic prosthetic device, implant and graft**

T85 Complications of other internal prosthetic devices, implants and grafts

Excludes2: *failure and rejection of transplanted organs and tissue (T86.-)*

AHA CC: 4Q, 2016, 71-72

The appropriate 7th character is to be added to each code from category T85
A initial encounter
D subsequent encounter
S sequela

+ **T85.0 Mechanical complication of ventricular intracranial (communicating) shunt**

CC X+7th **T85.01 Breakdown (mechanical) of ventricular intracranial (communicating) shunt**

CC X+7th **T85.02 Displacement of ventricular intracranial (communicating) shunt**
Malposition of ventricular intracranial (communicating) shunt

CC X+7th **T85.03 Leakage of ventricular intracranial (communicating) shunt**

CC X+7th **T85.09 Other mechanical complication of ventricular intracranial (communicating) shunt**
Obstruction (mechanical) of ventricular intracranial (communicating) shunt
Perforation of ventricular intracranial (communicating) shunt
Protrusion of ventricular intracranial (communicating) shunt

+ **T85.1 Mechanical complication of implanted electronic stimulator of nervous system**

+ **T85.11 Breakdown (mechanical) of implanted electronic stimulator of nervous system**

CC +7th **T85.110 Breakdown (mechanical) of implanted electronic neurostimulator of brain electrode (lead)**

CC +7th **T85.111 Breakdown (mechanical) of implanted electronic neurostimulator of peripheral nerve electrode (lead)**
Breakdown of electrode (lead) for cranial nerve neurostimulators
Breakdown of electrode (lead) for gastric neurostimulators
Breakdown of electrode (lead) for sacral nerve neurostimulators
Breakdown of electrode (lead) for vagal nerve neurostimulators

CC +7th **T85.112 Breakdown (mechanical) of implanted electronic neurostimulator of spinal cord electrode (lead)**

CC +7th **T85.113 Breakdown (mechanical) of implanted electronic neurostimulator, generator**
Breakdown (mechanical) of implanted electronic neurostimulator generator, brain, peripheral, gastric, spinal
Breakdown (mechanical) of implanted electronic sacral neurostimulator, pulse generator receiver

CC +7th **T85.118 Breakdown (mechanical) of other implanted electronic stimulator of nervous system**

+ **T85.12 Displacement of implanted electronic stimulator of nervous system**
Malposition of implanted electronic stimulator of nervous system

CC +7th **T85.120 Displacement of implanted electronic neurostimulator of brain electrode (lead)**

CC +7th **T85.121 Displacement of implanted electronic neurostimulator of peripheral nerve electrode (lead)**
Displacement of electrode (lead) for cranial nerve neurostimulators
Displacement of electrode (lead) for gastric neurostimulators
Displacement of electrode (lead) for sacral nerve neurostimulators
Displacement of electrode (lead) for vagal nerve neurostimulators

CC +7th **T85.122 Displacement of implanted electronic neurostimulator of spinal cord electrode (lead)**

CC +7th **T85.123 Displacement of implanted electronic neurostimulator, generator**
Displacement of implanted electronic neurostimulator generator, brain, peripheral, gastric, spinal
Displacement of implanted electronic sacral neurostimulator, pulse generator receiver

CC +7th **T85.128 Displacement of other implanted electronic stimulator of nervous system**

+ **T85.19 Other mechanical complication of implanted electronic stimulator of nervous system**
Leakage of implanted electronic stimulator of nervous system
Obstruction (mechanical) of implanted electronic stimulator of nervous system
Perforation of implanted electronic stimulator of nervous system
Protrusion of implanted electronic stimulator of nervous system

CC +7th **T85.190 Other mechanical complication of implanted electronic neurostimulator of brain electrode (lead)**

CC +7th **T85.191 Other mechanical complication of implanted electronic neurostimulator of peripheral nerve electrode (lead)**
Other mechanical complication of electrode (lead) for cranial nerve neurostimulators
Other mechanical complication of electrode (lead) for gastric neurostimulators
Other mechanical complication of electrode (lead) for sacral nerve neurostimulators
Other mechanical complication of electrode (lead) for vagal nerve neurostimulators

CC +7th **T85.192 Other mechanical complication of implanted electronic neurostimulator of spinal cord electrode (lead)**

CC +7th **T85.193 Other mechanical complication of implanted electronic neurostimulator, generator**
Other mechanical complication of implanted electronic neurostimulator generator, brain, peripheral, gastric, spinal
Other mechanical complication of implanted electronic sacral neurostimulator, pulse generator receiver

CC +7th **T85.199 Other mechanical complication of other implanted electronic stimulator of nervous system**

\+ **T85.2 Mechanical complication of intraocular lens**

CC X+7th **T85.21 Breakdown (mechanical) of intraocular lens**

CC X+7th **T85.22 Displacement of intraocular lens**
Malposition of intraocular lens

CC X+7th **T85.29 Other mechanical complication of intraocular lens**
Obstruction (mechanical) of intraocular lens
Perforation of intraocular lens
Protrusion of intraocular lens

\+ **T85.3 Mechanical complication of other ocular prosthetic devices, implants and grafts**
Excludes2: *other complications of corneal graft (T86.84-)*

\+ **T85.31 Breakdown (mechanical) of other ocular prosthetic devices, implants and grafts**

CC +7th **T85.310 Breakdown (mechanical) of prosthetic orbit of right eye**

CC +7th **T85.311 Breakdown (mechanical) of prosthetic orbit of left eye**

CC +7th **T85.318 Breakdown (mechanical) of other ocular prosthetic devices, implants and grafts**

\+ **T85.32 Displacement of other ocular prosthetic devices, implants and grafts**
Malposition of other ocular prosthetic devices, implants and grafts

CC +7th **T85.320 Displacement of prosthetic orbit of right eye**

CC +7th **T85.321 Displacement of prosthetic orbit of left eye**

+7th **T85.328 Displacement of other ocular prosthetic devices, implants and grafts**

\+ **T85.39 Other mechanical complication of other ocular prosthetic devices, implants and grafts**
Obstruction (mechanical) of other ocular prosthetic devices, implants and grafts
Perforation of other ocular prosthetic devices, implants and grafts
Protrusion of other ocular prosthetic devices, implants and grafts

CC +7th **T85.390 Other mechanical complication of prosthetic orbit of right eye**

CC +7th **T85.391 Other mechanical complication of prosthetic orbit of left eye**

+7th **T85.398 Other mechanical complication of other ocular prosthetic devices, implants and grafts**

\+ **T85.4 Mechanical complication of breast prosthesis and implant**

CC X+7th **T85.41 Breakdown (mechanical) of breast prosthesis and implant**

CC X+7th **T85.42 Displacement of breast prosthesis and implant**
Malposition of breast prosthesis and implant

CC X+7th **T85.43 Leakage of breast prosthesis and implant**

CC X+7th **T85.44 Capsular contracture of breast implant**

CC X+7th **T85.49 Other mechanical complication of breast prosthesis and implant**
Obstruction (mechanical) of breast prosthesis and implant
Perforation of breast prosthesis and implant
Protrusion of breast prosthesis and implant

\+ **T85.5 Mechanical complication of gastrointestinal prosthetic devices, implants and grafts**

\+ **T85.51 Breakdown (mechanical) of gastrointestinal prosthetic devices, implants and grafts**

CC +7th **T85.510 Breakdown (mechanical) of bile duct prosthesis**

CC +7th **T85.511 Breakdown (mechanical) of esophageal anti-reflux device**

CC +7th **T85.518 Breakdown (mechanical) of other gastrointestinal prosthetic devices, implants and grafts**

\+ **T85.52 Displacement of gastrointestinal prosthetic devices, implants and grafts**
Malposition of gastrointestinal prosthetic devices, implants and grafts

CC +7th **T85.520 Displacement of bile duct prosthesis**

CC +7th **T85.521 Displacement of esophageal anti-reflux device**

CC +7th **T85.528 Displacement of other gastrointestinal prosthetic devices, implants and grafts**

\+ **T85.59 Other mechanical complication of gastrointestinal prosthetic devices, implants and**
Obstruction, mechanical of gastrointestinal prosthetic devices, implants and grafts
Perforation of gastrointestinal prosthetic devices, implants and grafts
Protrusion of gastrointestinal prosthetic devices, implants and grafts

CC +7th **T85.590 Other mechanical complication of bile duct prosthesis**

CC +7th **T85.591 Other mechanical complication of esophageal anti-reflux device**

CC +7th **T85.598 Other mechanical complication of other gastrointestinal prosthetic devices, implants and grafts**

\+ **T85.6 Mechanical complication of other specified internal and external prosthetic devices, implants and grafts**
Review coding guidelines C.4.a.5.a and C.4.a.5.b

\+ **T85.61 Breakdown (mechanical) of other specified internal prosthetic devices, implants and grafts**

CC +7th **T85.610 Breakdown (mechanical) of cranial or spinal infusion catheter**
Breakdown (mechanical) of epidural infusion catheter
Breakdown (mechanical) of intrathecal infusion catheter
Breakdown (mechanical) of subarachnoid infusion catheter
Breakdown (mechanical) of subdural infusion catheter

CC +7th **T85.611 Breakdown (mechanical) of intraperitoneal dialysis catheter**
Excludes1: *mechanical complication of vascular dialysis catheter (T82.4-)*

CC +7th **T85.612 Breakdown (mechanical) of permanent sutures**
Excludes1: *mechanical complication of permanent (wire) suture used in bone repair (T84.1-T84.2)*

CC +7th **T85.613 Breakdown (mechanical) of artificial skin graft and decellularized allodermis**
Failure of artificial skin graft and decellularized allodermis
Non-adherence of artificial skin graft and decellularized allodermis
Poor incorporation of artificial skin graft and decellularized allodermis
Shearing of artificial skin graft and decellularized allodermis

CC +7th **T85.614 Breakdown (mechanical) of insulin pump**

CC +7th **T85.615 Breakdown (mechanical) of other nervous system device, implant or graft**
Breakdown (mechanical) of intrathecal infusion pump

CC +7th **T85.618 Breakdown (mechanical) of other specified internal prosthetic devices, implants and grafts**

+ **T85.62 Displacement of other specified internal prosthetic devices, implants and grafts**
Malposition of other specified internal prosthetic devices, implants and grafts

CC +7th **T85.620 Displacement of cranial or spinal infusion catheter**
Displacement of epidural infusion catheter
Displacement of intrathecal infusion catheter
Displacement of subarachnoid infusion catheter
Displacement of subdural infusion catheter

CC +7th **T85.621 Displacement of intraperitoneal dialysis catheter**
Excludes1: *mechanical complication of vasculardialysiscatheter (T82.4-)*

CC +7th **T85.622 Displacement of permanent sutures**
Excludes1: *mechanical complication of permanent (wire) sutureusedinbonerepair (T84.1-T84.2)*

CC +7th **T85.623 Displacement of artificial skin graft and decellularized allodermis**
Dislodgement of artificial skin graft and decellularized allodermis

CC +7th **T85.624 Displacement of insulin pump**

CC +7th **T85.625 Displacement of other nervous system device, implant or graft**
Displacement of intrathecal infusion pump

CC +7th **T85.628 Displacement of other specified internal prosthetic devices, implants and grafts**
AHA CC: 1Q, 2015, 3-21

+ **T85.63 Leakage of other specified internal prosthetic devices, implants and grafts**

CC +7th **T85.630 Leakage of cranial or spinal infusion catheter**
Leakage of epidural infusion catheter
Leakage of intrathecal infusion catheter
Leakage of subarachnoid infusion catheter
Leakage of subdural infusion catheter

CC +7th **T85.631 Leakage of intraperitoneal dialysis catheter**
Excludes1: *mechanical complication of vasculardialysiscatheter (T82.4)*

CC +7th **T85.633 Leakage of insulin pump**

CC +7th **T85.635 Leakage of other nervous system device, implant or graft**
Leakage of intrathecal infusion pump

CC +7th **T85.638 Leakage of other specified internal prosthetic devices, implants and grafts**

+ **T85.69 Other mechanical complication of other specified internal prosthetic devices, implants and grafts**
Obstruction, mechanical of other specified internal prosthetic devices, implants and grafts
Perforation of other specified internal prosthetic devices, implants and grafts
Protrusion of other specified internal prosthetic devices, implants and grafts

CC +7th **T85.690 Other mechanical complication of cranial or spinal infusion catheter**
Other mechanical complication of epidural infusion catheter
Other mechanical complication of intrathecal infusion catheter
Other mechanical complication of subarachnoid infusion catheter
Other mechanical complication of subdural infusion catheter

CC +7th **T85.691 Other mechanical complication of intraperitoneal dialysis catheter**
Excludes1: *mechanical complication of vasculardialysiscatheter (T82.4)*

CC +7th **T85.692 Other mechanical complication of permanent sutures**
Excludes1: *mechanical complication of permanent (wire) sutureusedinbonerepair (T84.1-T84.2)*

CC +7th **T85.693 Other mechanical complication of artificial skin graft and decellularized allodermis**

CC +7th **T85.694 Other mechanical complication of insulin pump**

CC +7th **T85.695 Other mechanical complication of other nervous system device, implant or graft**
Other mechanical complication of intrathecal infusion pump

CC +7th **T85.698 Other mechanical complication of other specified internal prosthetic devices, implants and grafts**
Mechanical complication of nonabsorbable surgical material NOS

+ **T85.7 Infection and inflammatory reaction due to other internal prosthetic devices, implants and grafts**
Use additional code to identify infection

CC X+7th **T85.71 Infection and inflammatory reaction due to peritoneal dialysis catheter**

CC X+7th **T85.72 Infection and inflammatory reaction due to insulin pump**

+ **T85.73 Infection and inflammatory reaction due to nervous system devices, implants and graft**

CC +7th **T85.730 Infection and inflammatory reaction due to ventricular intracranial (communicating) shunt**

CC +7th **T85.731 Infection and inflammatory reaction due to implanted electronic neurostimulator of brain, electrode (lead)**

CC +7th **T85.732 Infection and inflammatory reaction due to implanted electronic neurostimulator of peripheral nerve, electrode (lead)**
Infection and inflammatory reaction due to electrode (lead) for cranial nerve neurostimulators
Infection and inflammatory reaction due to electrode (lead) for gastric neurostimulators
Infection and inflammatory reaction due to electrode (lead) for sacral nerve neurostimulators
Infection and inflammatory reaction due to electrode (lead) for vagal nerve neurostimulators

CC +7th **T85.733 Infection and inflammatory reaction due to implanted electronic neurostimulator of spinal cord, electrode (lead)**

CC +7th **T85.734 Infection and inflammatory reaction due to implanted electronic neurostimulator, generator**
Generator pocket infection

CC +7th **T85.735 Infection and inflammatory reaction due to cranial or spinal infusion catheter**
Infection and inflammatory reaction due to epidural catheter
Infection and inflammatory reaction due to intrathecal infsuion catheter
Infection and inflammatory reaction due to subarachnoid catheter
Infection and inflammatory reaction due to subdural catheter

CC +7th **T85.738 Infection and inflammatory reaction due to other nervous system device, implant or graft**
Infection and inflammatory reaction due to intrathecal infusion pump

CC X+7th **T85.79 Infection and inflammatory reaction due to other internal prosthetic devices, implants and grafts**

+ **T85.8 Other specified complications of internal prosthetic devices, implants and grafts, not elsewhere classified**

+ **T85.81 Embolism due to internal prosthetic devices, implants and grafts, not elsewhere classified**

CC +7th **T85.810 Embolism due to nervous system prosthetic devices, implants and grafts**

+7th **T85.818 Embolism due to other internal prosthetic devices, implants and grafts**

+ **T85.82 Fibrosis due to internal prosthetic devices, implants and grafts, not elsewhere classified**

CC +7th **T85.820 Fibrosis due to nervous system prosthetic devices, implants and grafts**

+7th **T85.828 Fibrosis due to other internal prosthetic devices, implants and grafts**

+ **T85.83 Hemorrhage due to internal prosthetic devices, implants and grafts, not elsewhere classified**

CC +7th **T85.830 Hemorrhage due to nervous system prosthetic devices, implants and grafts**

+7th **T85.838 Hemorrhage due to other internal prosthetic devices, implants and grafts**

+ **T85.84 Pain due to internal prosthetic devices, implants and grafts, not elsewhere classified**

CC +7th **T85.840 Pain due to nervous system prosthetic devices, implants and grafts**

+7th **T85.848 Pain due to other internal prosthetic devices, implants and grafts**

+ **T85.85 Stenosis due to internal prosthetic devices, implants and grafts, not elsewhere classified**

CC +7th **T85.850 Stenosis due to nervous system prosthetic devices, implants and grafts**

+7th **T85.858 Stenosis due to other internal prosthetic devices, implants and grafts**

+ **T85.86 Thrombosis due to internal prosthetic devices, implants and grafts, not elsewhere classified**

CC +7th **T85.860 Thrombosis due to nervous system prosthetic devices, implants and grafts**

+7th **T85.868 Thrombosis due to other internal prosthetic devices, implants and grafts**

+ **T85.89 Other specified complication of internal prosthetic devices, implants and grafts, not elsewhere classified**

Erosion or breakdown of subcutaneous device pocket

CC +7th **T85.890 Other specified complication of nervous system prosthetic devices, implants and grafts**

+7th **T85.898 Other specified complication of other internal prosthetic devices, implants and grafts**

X+7th **T85.9 Unspecified complication of internal prosthetic device, implant and graft**

Complication of internal prosthetic device, implant and graft NOS

T86 Complications of transplanted organs and tissue

Use additional code to identify other transplant complications, such as:
graft-versus-host disease (D89.81-)
malignancy associated with organ transplant (C80.2)
post-transplant lymphoproliferative disorders (PTLD) (D47.Z1)

Review coding guideline C.2.r
Review coding guideline C.19.g.3

+ **T86.0 Complications of bone marrow transplant**

CC **T86.00 Unspecified complication of bone marrow transplant**
CC **T86.01 Bone marrow transplant rejection**
CC **T86.02 Bone marrow transplant failure**
CC **T86.03 Bone marrow transplant infection**
CC **T86.09 Other complications of bone marrow transplant**

+ **T86.1 Complications of kidney transplant**

Review coding guideline C.19.g.3.b

CC **T86.10 Unspecified complication of kidney transplant**
CC **T86.11 Kidney transplant rejection**
CC **T86.12 Kidney transplant failure**
AHA CC: 1Q, 2014, 24
CC **T86.13 Kidney transplant infection**
Use additional code to specify infection
CC **T86.19 Other complication of kidney transplant**
AHA CC: 2Q, 2019, 7

+ **T86.2 Complications of heart transplant**

Excludes1: *complication of:*
artificial heart device (T82.5-)
heart-lung transplant (T86.3-)

CC **T86.20 Unspecified complication of heart transplant**
CC **T86.21 Heart transplant rejection**
CC **T86.22 Heart transplant failure**
CC **T86.23 Heart transplant infection**
Use additional code to specify infection

+ **T86.29 Other complications of heart transplant**

CC **T86.290 Cardiac allograft vasculopathy**
Excludes1: *atherosclerosis of coronary arteries(I25.75-, I25.76-, I25.81-)*
CC **T86.298 Other complications of heart transplant**

+ **T86.3 Complications of heart-lung transplant**

CC **T86.30 Unspecified complication of heart-lung transplant**
CC **T86.31 Heart-lung transplant rejection**
CC **T86.32 Heart-lung transplant failure**
CC **T86.33 Heart-lung transplant infection**
Use additional code to specify infection
CC **T86.39 Other complications of heart-lung transplant**

+ **T86.4 Complications of liver transplant**

CC **T86.40 Unspecified complication of liver transplant**
CC **T86.41 Liver transplant rejection**
CC **T86.42 Liver transplant failure**
CC **T86.43 Liver transplant infection**
Use additional code to identify infection, such as:
Cytomegalovirus (CMV) infection (B25.-)
CC **T86.49 Other complications of liver transplant**

CC **T86.5 Complications of stem cell transplant**

Complications from stem cells from peripheral blood
Complications from stem cells from umbilical cord
AHA CC: 4Q, 2020, 14

+ **T86.8 Complications of other transplanted organs and tissues**

+ **T86.81 Complications of lung transplant**

Excludes1: *complication of heart-lung transplant (T86.3-)*

CC **T86.810 Lung transplant rejection**
CC **T86.811 Lung transplant failure**
CC **T86.812 Lung transplant infection**
Use additional code to specify infection
CC **T86.818 Other complications of lung transplant**
AHA CC: 2Q, 2019, 6-7
CC **T86.819 Unspecified complication of lung transplant**

+ **T86.82 Complications of skin graft (allograft) (autograft)**

Excludes2: *complication of artificial skin graft (T85.693)*

CC **T86.820 Skin graft (allograft) rejection**
CC **T86.821 Skin graft (allograft) (autograft) failure**
CC **T86.822 Skin graft (allograft) (autograft) infection**
Use additional code to specify infection
CC **T86.828 Other complications of skin graft (allograft) (autograft)**
CC **T86.829 Unspecified complication of skin graft (allograft) (autograft)**

+ **T86.83 Complications of bone graft**

Excludes2: *mechanical complications of bone graft (T84.3-)*

CC **T86.830 Bone graft rejection**
CC **T86.831 Bone graft failure**
CC **T86.832 Bone graft infection**
Use additional code to specify infection
CC **T86.838 Other complications of bone graft**
CC **T86.839 Unspecified complication of bone graft**

+ **T86.84 Complications of corneal transplant**

Excludes2: *mechanical complications of corneal graft (T85.3-)*
AHA CC: 4Q, 2020, 40

+ **T86.840 Corneal transplant rejection**

CC **T86.8401 Corneal transplant rejection, right eye**
CC **T86.8402 Corneal transplant rejection, left eye**
CC **T86.8403 Corneal transplant rejection, bilateral**
CC **T86.8409 Corneal transplant rejection, unspecified eye**

+ T86.841 Corneal transplant failure
  - CC T86.8411 Corneal transplant failure, right eye
  - CC T86.8412 Corneal transplant failure, left eye
  - CC T86.8413 Corneal transplant failure, bilateral
  - CC T86.8419 Corneal transplant failure, unspecified eye

+ T86.842 Corneal transplant infection
  - CC T86.8421 Corneal transplant infection, right eye
  - CC T86.8422 Corneal transplant infection, left eye
  - CC T86.8423 Corneal transplant infection, bilateral
  - CC T86.8429 Corneal transplant infection, unspecified eye

  Use additional code to specify infection

+ T86.848 Other complications of corneal transplant
  - CC T86.8481 Other complications of corneal transplant, right eye
  - CC T86.8482 Other complications of corneal transplant, left eye
  - CC T86.8483 Other complications of corneal transplant, bilateral
  - CC T86.8489 Other complications of corneal transplant, unspecified eye

+ T86.849 Unspecified complication of corneal transplant
  - CC T86.8491 Unspecified complication of corneal transplant, right eye
  - CC T86.8492 Unspecified complication of corneal transplant, left eye
  - CC T86.8493 Unspecified complication of corneal transplant, bilateral
  - CC T86.8499 Unspecified complication of corneal transplant, unspecified eye

+ T86.85 Complication of intestine transplant
  - CC T86.850 Intestine transplant rejection
  - CC T86.851 Intestine transplant failure
  - CC T86.852 Intestine transplant infection

    Use additional code to specify infection
  - CC T86.858 Other complications of intestine transplant
  - CC T86.859 Unspecified complication of intestine transplant

+ T86.89 Complications of other transplanted tissue

  Transplant failure or rejection of pancreas
  - CC T86.890 Other transplanted tissue rejection
  - CC T86.891 Other transplanted tissue failure
  - CC T86.892 Other transplanted tissue infection

    Use additional code to specify infection
  - CC T86.898 Other complications of other transplanted tissue
  - CC T86.899 Unspecified complication of other transplanted tissue

+ T86.9 Complication of unspecified transplanted organ and tissue
  - CC T86.90 Unspecified complication of unspecified transplanted organ and tissue
  - CC T86.91 Unspecified transplanted organ and tissue rejection
  - CC T86.92 Unspecified transplanted organ and tissue failure
  - CC T86.93 Unspecified transplanted organ and tissue infection

    Use additional code to specify infection
  - CC T86.99 Other complications of unspecified transplanted organ and tissue

T87 Complications peculiar to reattachment and amputation

+ T87.0 Complications of reattached (part of) upper extremity
  + T87.0X Complications of reattached (part of) upper extremity
    - CC T87.0X1 Complications of reattached (part of) right upper extremity
    - CC T87.0X2 Complications of reattached (part of) left upper extremity
    - CC T87.0X9 Complications of reattached (part of) unspecified upper extremity

+ T87.1 Complications of reattached (part of) lower extremity
  + T87.1X Complications of reattached (part of) lower extremity
    - CC T87.1X1 Complications of reattached (part of) right lower extremity
    - CC T87.1X2 Complications of reattached (part of) left lower extremity
    - CC T87.1X9 Complications of reattached (part of) unspecified lower extremity

CC T87.2 Complications of other reattached body part

+ T87.3 Neuroma of amputation stump
  - T87.30 Neuroma of amputation stump, unspecified extremity
  - T87.31 Neuroma of amputation stump, right upper extremity
  - T87.32 Neuroma of amputation stump, left upper extremity
  - T87.33 Neuroma of amputation stump, right lower extremity
  - T87.34 Neuroma of amputation stump, left lower extremity

+ T87.4 Infection of amputation stump
  - CC T87.40 Infection of amputation stump, unspecified extremity
  - CC T87.41 Infection of amputation stump, right upper extremity
  - CC T87.42 Infection of amputation stump, left upper extremity
  - CC T87.43 Infection of amputation stump, right lower extremity
  - CC T87.44 Infection of amputation stump, left lower extremity

+ T87.5 Necrosis of amputation stump
  - T87.50 Necrosis of amputation stump, unspecified extremity
  - T87.51 Necrosis of amputation stump, right upper extremity
  - T87.52 Necrosis of amputation stump, left upper extremity
  - T87.53 Necrosis of amputation stump, right lower extremity
  - T87.54 Necrosis of amputation stump, left lower extremity

+ T87.8 Other complications of amputation stump
  - T87.81 Dehiscence of amputation stump
  - T87.89 Other complications of amputation stump

    Amputation stump contracture

    Amputation stump contracture of next proximal joint

    Amputation stump flexion

    Amputation stump edema

    Amputation stump hematoma

    Excludes2: *phantom limb syndrome (G54.6-G54.7)*

T87.9 Unspecified complications of amputation stump

T88 Other complications of surgical and medical care, not elsewhere classified

Excludes2: *complication following infusion, transfusion and therapeutic injection (T80.-)*
complication following procedure NEC (T81.-)
complications of anesthesia in labor and delivery (O74.-)
complications of anesthesia in pregnancy (O29.-)
complications of anesthesia in puerperium (O89.-)
complications of devices, implants and grafts (T82-T85)
complications of obstetric surgery and procedure (O75.4)
dermatitis due to drugs and medicaments (L23.3, L24.4, L25.1, L27.0-L27.1)
poisoning and toxic effects of drugs and chemicals (T36-T65 with fifth or sixth character 1-4 or 6)
specified complications classified elsewhere

AHA CC: 4Q, 2018, 89-90

The appropriate 7th character is to be added to each code from category T88
A initial encounter
D subsequent encounter
S sequela

CC X+7th **T88.0 Infection following immunization**
Sepsis following immunization
Review coding guideline C.1.d.5

CC X+7th **T88.1 Other complications following immunization, not elsewhere classified**
Generalized vaccinia
Rash following immunization
Excludes1: *vaccinia not from vaccine (B08.011)*
Excludes2: *anaphylactic shock due to serum (T80.5-)*
other serum reactions (T80.6-)
postimmunization arthropathy (M02.2)
postimmunization encephalitis (G04.02)
postimmunization fever (R50.83)

CC X+7th **T88.2 Shock due to anesthesia**
Use additional code for adverse effect, if applicable, to identify drug (T41.- with fifth or sixth character 5)
Excludes1: *complications of anesthesia (in):*
labor and delivery (O74.-)
pregnancy (O29.-)
puerperium (O89.-)
postprocedural shock NOS (T81.1-)

CC X+7th **T88.3 Malignant hyperthermia due to anesthesia**
Use additional code for adverse effect, if applicable, to identify drug (T41.- with fifth or sixth character 5)

X+7th **T88.4 Failed or difficult intubation**

\+ **T88.5 Other complications of anesthesia**
Use additional code for adverse effect, if applicable, to identify drug (T41.- with fifth or sixth character 5)
AHA CC: 4Q, 2016, 72-73

X+7th **T88.51 Hypothermia following anesthesia**

X+7th **T88.52 Failed moderate sedation during procedure**
Failed conscious sedation during procedure
Excludes2: *personal history of failed moderate sedation (Z92.83)*

X+7th **T88.53 Unintended awareness under general anesthesia during procedure**
Excludes2: *personal history of unintended awareness under general anesthesia (Z92.84)*
AHA CC: 4Q, 2016, 72-73

X+7th **T88.59 Other complications of anesthesia**

CC X+7th **T88.6 Anaphylactic reaction due to adverse effect of correct drug or medicament properly administered**
Anaphylactic shock due to adverse effect of correct drug or medicament properly administered
Anaphylactoid reaction NOS
Use additional code for adverse effect, if applicable, to identify drug (T36-T50 with fifth or sixth character 5)
Excludes1: *anaphylactic reaction due to serum (T80.5-)*
anaphylactic shock or reaction due to adverse food reaction (T78.0-)
AHA CC: 1Q, 2020, 18-19

X+7th **T88.7 Unspecified adverse effect of drug or medicament**
Drug hypersensitivity NOS
Drug reaction NOS
Use additional code for adverse effect, if applicable, to identify drug (T36-T50 with fifth or sixth character 5)
Excludes1: *specified adverse effects of drugs and medicaments (A00-R94 and T80-T88.6, T88.8)*

X+7th **T88.8 Other specified complications of surgical and medical care, not elsewhere classified**
Use additional code to identify the complication

X+7th **T88.9 Complication of surgical and medical care, unspecified**

Chapter 20: External Causes of Morbidity (V00-Y99)

NOTE This chapter permits the classification of environmental events and circumstances as the cause of injury, and other adverse effects. Where a code from this section is applicable, it is intended that it shall be used secondary to a code from another chapter of the Classification indicating the nature of the condition. Most often, the condition will be classifiable to Chapter 19, Injury, poisoning and certain other consequences of external causes (S00-T88). Other conditions that may be stated to be due to external causes are classified in Chapters 1 to 18. For these conditions, codes from Chapter 20 should be used to provide additional information as to the cause of the condition.

AHA CC: 1Q, 2015, 3-21

This chapter contains the following category blocks:

V00-X58	Accidents
V00-V99	Transport accidents
V00-V09	Pedestrian injured in transport accident
V10-V19	Pedal cycle rider injured in transport accident
V20-V29	Motorcycle rider injured in transport accident
V30-V39	Occupant of three-wheeled motor vehicle injured in transport accident
V40-V49	Car occupant injured in transport accident
V50-V59	Occupant of pick-up truck or van injured in transport accident
V60-V69	Occupant of heavy transport vehicle injured in transport accident
V70-V79	Bus occupant injured in transport accident
V80-V89	Other land transport accidents
V90-V94	Water transport accidents
V95-V97	Air and space transport accidents
V98-V99	Other and unspecified transport accidents
W00-X58	Other external causes of accidental injury
W00-W19	Slipping, tripping, stumbling and falls
W20-W49	Exposure to inanimate mechanical forces
W50-W64	Exposure to animate mechanical forces
W65-W74	Accidental non-transport drowning and submersion
W85-W99	Exposure to electric current, radiation and extreme ambient air temperature and pressure
X00-X08	Exposure to smoke, fire and flames
X10-X19	Contact with heat and hot substances
X30-X39	Exposure to forces of nature
X50	Overexertion and strenuous or repetitive movements
X52-X58	Accidental exposure to other specified factors
X71-X83	Intentional self-harm
X92-Y09	Assault
Y21-Y33	Event of undetermined intent
Y35-Y38	Legal intervention, operations of war, military operations, and terrorism
Y62-Y84	Complications of medical and surgical care
Y62-Y69	Misadventures to patients during surgical and medical care
Y70-Y82	Medical devices associated with adverse incidents in diagnostic and therapeutic use
Y83-Y84	Surgical and other medical procedures as the cause of abnormal reaction of the patient, or of later complication, without mention of misadventure at the time of the procedure
Y90-Y99	Supplementary factors related to causes of morbidity classified elsewhere

C. Chapter-Specific Coding Guidelines

In addition to general coding guidelines, there are guidelines for specific diagnoses and/or conditions in the classification. Unless otherwise indicated, these guidelines apply to all health care settings. Please refer to Section II for guidelines on the selection of principal diagnosis.

20. Chapter 20: External Causes of Morbidity (V00-Y99)

The external causes of morbidity codes should never be sequenced as the first-listed or principal diagnosis.

External cause codes are intended to provide data for injury research and evaluation of injury prevention strategies. These codes capture how the injury or health condition happened (cause), the intent (unintentional or accidental; or intentional, such as suicide or assault), the place where the event occurred the activity of the patient at the time of the event, and the person's status (e.g., civilian, military).

There is no national requirement for mandatory ICD-10-CM external cause code reporting. Unless a provider is subject to a state-based external cause code reporting mandate or these codes are required by a particular payer, reporting of ICD-10-CM codes in Chapter 20, External Causes of Morbidity, is not required. In the absence of a mandatory reporting requirement, providers are encouraged to voluntarily report external cause codes, as they provide valuable data for injury research and evaluation of injury prevention strategies.

a. General External Cause Coding Guidelines

1) Used with any code in the range of A00.0-T88.9, Z00-Z99

An external cause code may be used with any code in the range of A00.0-T88.9, Z00-Z99, classification that represents a health condition due to an external cause. Though they are most applicable to injuries, they are also valid for use with such things as infections or diseases due to an external source, and other health conditions, such as a heart attack that occurs during strenuous physical activity.

2) External cause code used for length of treatment

Assign the external cause code, with the appropriate 7th character (initial encounter, subsequent encounter or sequela) for each encounter for which the injury or condition is being treated.

Most categories in chapter 20 have a 7th character requirement for each applicable code. Most categories in this chapter have three 7th character values: A, initial encounter, D, subsequent encounter and S, sequela. While the patient may be seen by a new or different provider over the course of treatment for an injury or condition, assignment of the 7th character for external cause should match the 7th character of the code assigned for the associated injury or condition for the encounter.

3) Use the full range of external cause codes

Use the full range of external cause codes to completely describe the cause, the intent, the place of occurrence, and if applicable, the activity of the patient at the time of the event, and the patient's status, for all injuries, and other health conditions due to an external cause.

4) Assign as many external cause codes as necessary

Assign as many external cause codes as necessary to fully explain each cause. If only one external code can be recorded, assign the code most related to the principal diagnosis.

5) The selection of the appropriate external cause code

The selection of the appropriate external cause code is guided by the Alphabetic Index of External Causes and by Inclusion and Exclusion notes in the Tabular List.

6) External cause code can never be a principal diagnosis

An external cause code can never be a principal (first-listed) diagnosis.

7) Combination external cause codes

Certain of the external cause codes are combination codes that identify sequential events that result in an injury, such as a fall which results in striking against an object. The injury may be due to either event or both. The combination external cause code used should correspond to the sequence of events regardless of which caused the most serious injury.

8) No external cause code needed in certain circumstances

No external cause code from Chapter 20 is needed if the external cause and intent are included in a code from another chapter (e.g. T36.0X1- Poisoning by penicillins, accidental (unintentional)).

b. Place of Occurrence Guideline

Codes from category Y92, Place of occurrence of the external cause, are secondary codes for use after other external cause codes to identify the location of the patient at the time of injury or other condition.

Generally, a place of occurrent code is assigned only once, at the initial encounter for treatment. However, in the rare instance that a new injury occurs during hospitalization, an additional place of occurrence code may be assigned. No 7th characters are used for Y92.

Do not use place of occurrence code Y92.9 if the place is not stated or is not applicable.

c. Activity Code

Assign a code from category Y93, Activity code, to describe the activity of the patient at the time the injury or other health condition occurred.

An activity code is used only once, at the initial encounter for treatment. Only one code from Y93 should be recorded on a medical record.

The activity codes are not applicable to poisonings, adverse effects, misadventures or sequela.

Do not assign Y93.9, Unspecified activity, if the activity is not stated.

A code from category Y93 is appropriate for use with external cause and intent codes if identifying the activity provides additional information about the event.

d. Place of Occurrence, Activity, and Status Codes Used with other External Cause Code

When applicable, place of occurrence, activity, and external cause status codes are sequenced after the main external cause code(s). Regardless of the number of external cause codes assigned, generally there should be only one place of occurrence code, one activity code, and one external cause status code assigned to an encounter. However, in the rare instance that a new injury occurs during hospitalization, an additional place of occurrence code may be assigned.

e. If the Reporting Format Limits the Number of External Cause Codes

If the reporting format limits the number of external cause codes that can be used in reporting clinical data, report the code for the cause/intent most related to the principal diagnosis. If the format permits capture of additional external cause codes, the cause/intent, including medical misadventures, of the additional events should be reported rather than the codes for place, activity, or external status.

f. Multiple External Cause Coding Guidelines

More than one external cause code is required to fully describe the external cause of an illness or injury. The assignment of external cause codes should be sequenced in the following priority:

If two or more events cause separate injuries, an external cause code should be assigned for each cause. The first-listed external cause code will be selected in the following order:

External codes for child and adult abuse take priority over all other external cause codes.

See Section I.C.19., Child and Adult abuse guidelines.

External cause codes for terrorism events take priority over all other external cause codes except child and adult abuse.

External cause codes for cataclysmic events take priority over all other external cause codes except child and adult abuse and terrorism.

External cause codes for transport accidents take priority over all other external cause codes except cataclysmic events, child and adult abuse and terrorism.

Activity and external cause status codes are assigned following all causal (intent) external cause codes.

The first-listed external cause code should correspond to the cause of the most serious diagnosis due to an assault, accident, or self-harm, following the order of hierarchy listed above.

g. Child and Adult Abuse Guideline

Adult and child abuse, neglect and maltreatment are classified as assault. Any of the assault codes may be used to indicate the external cause of any injury resulting from the confirmed abuse.

For confirmed cases of abuse, neglect and maltreatment, when the perpetrator is known, a code from Y07, Perpetrator of maltreatment and neglect, should accompany any other assault codes.

See Section I.C.19. Adult and child abuse, neglect and other maltreatment

h. Unknown or Undetermined Intent Guideline

If the intent (accident, self-harm, assault) of the cause of an injury or other condition is unknown or unspecified, code the intent as accidental intent. All transport accident categories assume accidental intent.

1) Use of undetermined intent

External cause codes for events of undetermined intent are only for use if the documentation in the record specifies that the intent cannot be determined.

i. Sequelae (Late Effects) of External Cause Guidelines

1) Sequelae external cause codes

Sequela are reported using the external cause code with the 7th character "S" for sequela. These codes should be used with any report of a late effect or sequela resulting from a previous injury.

See Section I.B.10 Sequela (Late Effects)

2) Sequela external cause code with a related current injury

A sequela external cause code should never be used with a related current nature of injury code.

3) Use of sequela external cause codes for subsequent visits

Use a late effect external cause code for subsequent visits when a late effect of the initial injury is being treated. Do not use a late effect external cause code for subsequent visits for follow- up care (e.g., to assess healing, to receive rehabilitative therapy) of the injury when no late effect of the injury has been documented.

j. Terrorism Guidelines

1) Cause of injury identified by the Federal Government (FBI) as terrorism

When the cause of an injury is identified by the Federal Government (FBI) as terrorism, the first-listed external cause code should be a code from category Y38, Terrorism. The definition of terrorism employed by the FBI is found at the inclusion note at the beginning of category Y38. Use additional code for place of occurrence (Y92.-). More than one Y38 code may be assigned if the injury is the result of more than one mechanism of terrorism.

2) Cause of an injury is suspected to be the result of terrorism

When the cause of an injury is suspected to be the result of terrorism a code from category Y38 should not be assigned. Suspected cases should be classified as assault.

3) Code Y38.9, Terrorism, secondary effects

Assign code Y38.9, Terrorism, secondary effects, for conditions occurring subsequent to the terrorist event. This code should not be assigned for conditions that are due to the initial terrorist act.

It is acceptable to assign code Y38.9 with another code from Y38 if there is an injury due to the initial terrorist event and an injury that is a subsequent result of the terrorist event.

k. External cause status

A code from category Y99, External cause status, should be assigned whenever any other external cause code is assigned for an encounter, including an Activity code, except for the events noted below. Assign a code from category Y99, External cause status, to indicate the work status of the person at the time the event occurred. The status code indicates whether the event occurred during military activity, whether a non-military person was at work, whether an individual including a student or volunteer was involved in a non-work activity at the time of the causal event.

A code from Y99, External cause status, should be assigned, when applicable, with other external cause codes, such as transport accidents and falls. The external cause status codes are not applicable to poisonings, adverse effects, misadventures or late effects. Do not assign a code from category Y99 if no other external cause codes (cause, activity) are applicable for the encounter.

An external cause status code is used only once, at the initial encounter for treatment. Only one code from Y99 should be recorded on a medical record.

Do not assign code Y99.9, Unspecified external cause status, if the status is not stated.

Accidents (V00-X58)

Transport accidents (V00-V99)

NOTE This section is structured in 12 groups. Those relating to land transport accidents (V00-V89) reflect the victim's mode of transport and are subdivided to identify the victim's 'counterpart' or the type of event. The vehicle of which the injured person is an occupant is identified in the first two characters since it is seen as the most important factor to identify for prevention purposes. A transport accident is one in which the vehicle involved must be moving or running or in use for transport purposes at the time of the accident.

Use additional code to identify:
Airbag injury (W22.1)
Type of street or road (Y92.4-)
Use of cellular telephone and other electronic equipment at the time of the transport accident (Y93.C-)

Excludes1: *agricultural vehicles in stationary use or maintenance (W31.-)*
assault by crashing of motor vehicle (Y03.-)
automobile or motor cycle in stationary use or maintenance- code to type of accident
crashing of motor vehicle, undetermined intent (Y32)
intentional self-harm by crashing of motor vehicle (X82)

Excludes2: *transport accidents due to cataclysm (X34-X38)*

NOTE Definitions related to transport accidents:

(a) A transport accident (V00-V99) is any accident involving a device designed primarily for, or used at the time primarily for, conveying persons or goods from one place to another.

(b) A public highway [trafficway] or street is the entire width between property lines (or other boundary lines) of land open to the public as a matter of right or custom for purposes of moving persons or property from one place to another. A roadway is that part of the public highway designed, improved and customarily used for vehicular traffic.

(c) A traffic accident is any vehicle accident occurring on the public highway [i.e. originating on, terminating on, or involving a vehicle partially on the highway]. A vehicle accident is assumed to have occurred on the public highway unless another place is specified, except i the case of accidents involving only off-road motor vehicles, which are classified as nontraffic accidents unless the contrary is stated.

(d) A nontraffic accident is any vehicle accident that occurs entirely in any place other than a public highway.

(e) A pedestrian is any person involved in an accident who was not at the time of the accident riding in or on a motor vehicle, railway train, streetcar or animal-drawn or other vehicle, or on a pedal cycle or animal. This includes, a person changing a tire, working on a parked care, or a person on foot. It also includes the user of a pedestrian conveyance such as a baby stroller, ice-skates, skis, sled, roller skates, a skateboard, nonmotorized or motorized wheelchair, motorized mobility scooter, or nonmotorized scooter.
(f) A driver is an occupant of a transport vehicle who is operating or intending to operate it.
(g) A passenger is any occupant of a transport vehicle other than the driver, except a person traveling on the outside of the vehicle.
(h) A person on the outside of a vehicle is any person being transported by a vehicle but not occupying the space normally reserved for the driver or passengers, or the space intended for the transport of property. This includes a person travailing on the bodywork, bumper, fender, roof, running board or step of a vehicle, as well as, hanging on the outside of the vehicle.
(i) A pedal cycle is any land transport vehicle operated solely by nonmotorized pedals including a bicycle or tricycle.
(j) A pedal cyclist is any person riding a pedal cycle or in a sidecar or trailer attached to a pedal cycle.
(k) A motorcycle is a two-wheeled motor vehicle with one or two riding saddles and sometimes with a third wheel for the support of a sidecar. The sidecar is considered part of the motorcycle. This includes a moped, motor scooter, or motorized bicycle.
(l) A motorcycle rider is any person riding a motorcycle or in a sidecar or trailer attached to the motorcycle.
(m) A three-wheeled motor vehicle is a motorized tricycle designed primarily for on-road use. This includes a motor-driven tricycle, a motorized rickshaw, or a three-wheeled motor car.
(n) A car [automobile] is a four-wheeled motor vehicle designed primarily for carrying up to 7 persons. A trailer being towed by the car is considered par of the car. It does not include a van or minivan - see definition (o)
(o) A pick-up truck or van is a four or six-wheeled motor vehicle designed for carrying passengers as well as property or cargo weighing less than the local limit for classification as a heavy goods vehicle, and not requiring a special driver's license. this includes a minivan and a sport-utility vehicle (SUV)
(p) A heavy transport vehicle is a motor vehicle designed primarily for carrying property, meeting local criteria for classification as a heavy goods vehicle in terms of weight and requiring a special driver's license.
(q) A bus (coach) is a motor vehicle designed or adapted primarily for carrying more than 10 passengers, and requiring a special driver's license.
(r) A railway train or railway vehicle is any device, with or without freight or passenger cars couple to it, designed for traffic on a railway track. This includes subterranean (subways) or elevated trains.
(s) A streetcar, is a device designed and used primarily for transporting passengers within a municipality, running on rails, usually subject to normal traffic control signals, and operated principally on a right-of-way that forms part of the roadway. This includes a tram or trolley that runs on rails. A trailer being towed by a streetcar is considered part of the streetcar.
(t) A special vehicle mainly used on industrial premises is a motor vehicle designed primarily for use within the building and premises of industrial or commercial establishments. This includes battery-powered airport passenger vehicles or baggage/mail trucks, forklifts, coal-cars in a coal min, logging cars and trucks used in mines or quarries.
(u) A special vehicle mainly used in agriculture is a motor vehicle designed specifically for use in farming and agriculture (horticulture), to work the land, tend and harvest crops and transport materials on the farm. This includes harvesters, farm machinery and tractor and trailers.
(v) A special construction vehicle is a motor vehicle designed specifically for use on construction and demolition sites. This includes bulldozers, diggers, earth levellers, dump trucks, backhoes, front-end loaders, pavers, and mechanical shovels.
(w) A special all-terrain vehicle is a motor vehicle of special design to enable it to negotiate over rough or soft terrain, snow or sand. Examples of special design are high construction, special wheels and tires, tracks, and support on a cushion of air. This includes snow mobiles, All terrain vehicles (ATV), and dune buggies. It does not include passenger vehicle designated as Sport Utility Vehicles (SUV).
(x) A water craft is any device designed for transporting passengers or goods on water. This includes motor or sail boats, ships, and hovercraft.
(y) An aircraft is any device for transporting passengers or goods in the air. This includes hot-air balloons, gliders, helicopters and airplanes.
(z) A military vehicle is any motorized vehicle operating on a public roadway owned by the military and being operated by a member of the military.

Pedestrian injured in transport accident (V00-V09)

Includes: person changing tire on transport vehicle
person examining engine of vehicle broken down in (on side of) road

Excludes1: *fall due to non-transport collision with other person (W03)*
pedestrian on foot falling (slipping) on ice and snow (W00.-)
struck or bumped by another person (W51)

AHA CC: 4Q, 2020, 41

V00 Pedestrian conveyance accident

Use additional place of occurrence and activity external cause codes, if known (Y92.-, Y93.-)

Excludes1: *collision with another person without fall (W51)*
fall due to person on foot colliding with another person on foot (W03)
fall from non-moving wheelchair, nonmotorized scooter and motorized mobility scooter without collision (W05.-)
pedestrian (conveyance) collision with other land transport vehicle (V01-V09)
pedestrian on foot falling (slipping) on ice and snow (W00.-)

The appropriate 7th character is to be added to each code from category V00
A initial encounter
D subsequent encounter
S sequela

+ **V00.0 Pedestrian on foot injured in collision with pedestrian conveyance**
  - X+7th **V00.01 Pedestrian on foot injured in collision with roller-skater**
  - X+7th **V00.02 Pedestrian on foot injured in collision with skateboarder**
  - + **V00.03 Pedestrian on foot injured in collision with pedestrian conveyance**
    - +7th **V00.031 Pedestrian on foot injured in collision with rider of standing electric scooter**
    - +7th **V00.038 Pedestrian on foot injured in collision with rider of other standing micro-mobility pedestrian conveyance**
      Pedestrian on foot injured in collision with rider of hoverboard
      Pedestrian on foot injured in collision with rider of segway
  - X+7th **V00.09 Pedestrian on foot injured in collision with other pedestrian conveyance**

+ **V00.1 Rolling-type pedestrian conveyance accident**

  Excludes1: *accident with baby stroller (V00.82-)*
  accident with wheelchair (powered) (V00.81-)
  accident with motorized mobility scooter (V00.83-)

  - + **V00.11 In-line roller-skate accident**
    - +7th **V00.111 Fall from in-line roller-skates**
    - +7th **V00.112 In-line roller-skater colliding with stationary object**
    - +7th **V00.118 Other in-line roller-skate accident**
      Excludes1: *roller-skater collision with other land transport vehicle(V01-V09with5th character 1)*
  - + **V00.12 Non-in- line roller-skate accident**
    - +7th **V00.121 Fall from non-in-line roller-skates**
    - +7th **V00.122 Non-in-line roller-skater colliding with stationary object**
    - +7th **V00.128 Other non-in-line roller-skating accident**
      Excludes1: *roller-skater collision with other land transport vehicle(V01-V09with5th character 1)*

+ **V00.13 Skateboard accident**
  - +7th **V00.131 Fall from skateboard**
  - +7th **V00.132 Skateboarder colliding with stationary object**
  - +7th **V00.138 Other skateboard accident**
    Excludes1: *skateboarder collision with other land transport vehicle(V01-V09with5th character 2)*
+ **V00.14 Scooter (nonmotorized) accident**
  Excludes1: *motor scooter accident (V20-V29)*
  - +7th **V00.141 Fall from scooter (nonmotorized)**
  - +7th **V00.142 Scooter (nonmotorized) colliding with stationary object**
  - +7th **V00.148 Other scooter (nonmotorized) accident**
    Excludes1: *scooter (nonmotorized) collision with other land transport vehicle (V01-V09 with fifth character 9)*
+ **V00.15 Heelies accident**
  Rolling shoe
  Wheeled shoe
  Wheelies accident
  - +7th **V00.151 Fall from heelies**
  - +7th **V00.152 Heelies colliding with stationary object**
  - +7th **V00.158 Other heelies accident**
+ **V00.18 Accident on other rolling-type pedestrian conveyance**
  - +7th **V00.181 Fall from other rolling-type pedestrian conveyance**
  - +7th **V00.182 Pedestrian on other rolling-type pedestrian conveyance colliding with stationary object**
  - +7th **V00.188 Other accident on other rolling-type pedestrian conveyance**

+ **V00.2 Gliding-type pedestrian conveyance accident**
+ **V00.21 Ice-skates accident**
  - +7th **V00.211 Fall from ice-skates**
  - +7th **V00.212 Ice-skater colliding with stationary object**
  - +7th **V00.218 Other ice-skates accident**
    Excludes1: *ice-skater collision with other land transport vehicle(V01-V09with5th character 9)*
+ **V00.22 Sled accident**
  - +7th **V00.221 Fall from sled**
  - +7th **V00.222 Sledder colliding with stationary object**
  - +7th **V00.228 Other sled accident**
    Excludes1: *sled collision with other land transport vehicle (V01-V09 with 5th character 9)*
+ **V00.28 Other gliding-type pedestrian conveyance accident**
  - +7th **V00.281 Fall from other gliding-type pedestrian conveyance**
  - +7th **V00.282 Pedestrian on other gliding-type pedestrian conveyance colliding with stationary object**
  - +7th **V00.288 Other accident on other gliding-type pedestrian conveyance**
    Excludes1: *gliding-type pedestrian conveyance collision with other land transport vehicle(V01-V09with5th character 9)*

+ **V00.3 Flat-bottomed pedestrian conveyance accident**
+ **V00.31 Snowboard accident**
  - +7th **V00.311 Fall from snowboard**
  - +7th **V00.312 Snowboarder colliding with stationary object**
  - +7th **V00.318 Other snowboard accident**
    Excludes1: *snowboarder collision with other land transport vehicle(V01-V09with5th character 9)*
+ **V00.32 Snow-ski accident**
  - +7th **V00.321 Fall from snow-skis**
    AHA CC: 1Q, 2015, 3-21
  - +7th **V00.322 Snow-skier colliding with stationary object**
  - +7th **V00.328 Other snow-ski accident**
    Excludes1: *snow-skier collision with other land transport vehicle(V01-V09with5th character 9)*
+ **V00.38 Other flat-bottomed pedestrian conveyance accident**
  - +7th **V00.381 Fall from other flat-bottomed pedestrian conveyance**
  - +7th **V00.382 Pedestrian on other flat-bottomed pedestrian conveyance colliding with stationary object**
  - +7th **V00.388 Other accident on other flat-bottomed pedestrian conveyance**

+ **V00.8 Accident on other pedestrian conveyance**
+ **V00.81 Accident with wheelchair (powered)**
  - +7th **V00.811 Fall from moving wheelchair (powered)**
    Excludes1: *fall from non-moving wheelchair (W05.0)*
  - +7th **V00.812 Wheelchair (powered) colliding with stationary object**
  - +7th **V00.818 Other accident with wheelchair (powered)**
+ **V00.82 Accident with baby stroller**
  - +7th **V00.821 Fall from baby stroller**
  - +7th **V00.822 Baby stroller colliding with stationary object**
  - +7th **V00.828 Other accident with baby stroller**
+ **V00.83 Accident with motorized mobility scooter**
  - +7th **V00.831 Fall from motorized mobility scooter**
    Excludes1: *fall from non-moving motorized mobility scooter (W05.2)*
  - +7th **V00.832 Motorized mobility scooter colliding with stationary object**
  - +7th **V00.838 Other accident with motorized mobility scooter**
+ **V00.84 Accident with standing micro-mobility pedestrian conveyance**
  - +7th **V00.841 Fall from standing electric scooter**
  - +7th **V00.842 Pedestrian on standing electric scooter colliding with stationary object**
  - +7th **V00.848 Other accident with standing micro-mobility pedestrian conveyance**
    Accident with hoverboard
    Accident with segway
+ **V00.89 Accident on other pedestrian conveyance**
  - +7th **V00.891 Fall from other pedestrian conveyance**
  - +7th **V00.892 Pedestrian on other pedestrian conveyance colliding with stationary object**
  - +7th **V00.898 Other accident on other pedestrian conveyance**
    Excludes1: *other pedestrian (conveyance) collision with other land transport vehicle(V01-V09with5th character 9)*

V01 Pedestrian injured in collision with pedal cycle

> The appropriate 7th character is to be added to each code from category V01
> A initial encounter
> D subsequent encounter
> S sequela

+ **V01.0 Pedestrian injured in collision with pedal cycle in nontraffic accident**
  - X+7th **V01.00 Pedestrian on foot injured in collision with pedal cycle in nontraffic accident**
    Pedestrian NOS injured in collision with pedal cycle in nontraffic accident
  - X+7th **V01.01 Pedestrian on roller-skates injured in collision with pedal cycle in nontraffic accident**
  - X+7th **V01.02 Pedestrian on skateboard injured in collision with pedal cycle in nontraffic accident**
  - + **V01.03 Pedestrian on standing micro-mobility pedestrian conveyance injured in collision with pedal cycle in nontraffic accident**
    - +7th **V01.031 Pedestrian on standing electric scooter injured in collision with pedal cycle in nontraffic accident**

+7th **V01.038 Pedestrian on other standing micro-mobility pedestrian conveyance injured in collision with pedal cycle in nontraffic accident**
Pedestrian on hoverboard injured in collision with pedal cycle in nontraffic accident
Pedestrian on segway injured in collision with pedal cycle in nontraffic accident

X+7th **V01.09 Pedestrian with other conveyance injured in collision with pedal cycle in nontraffic accident**
Pedestrian with baby stroller injured in collision with pedal cycle in nontraffic accident
Pedestrian on ice-skates injured in collision with pedal cycle in nontraffic accident
Pedestrian on nonmotorized scooter injured in collision with pedal cycle in nontraffic accident
Pedestrian on sled injured in collision with pedal cycle in nontraffic accident
Pedestrian on snowboard injured in collision with pedal cycle in nontraffic accident
Pedestrian on snow-skis injured in collision with pedal cycle in nontraffic accident
Pedestrian in wheelchair (powered) injured in collision with pedal cycle in nontraffic accident
Pedestrian in motorized mobility scooter injured in collision with pedal cycle in nontraffic accident

+ **V01.1 Pedestrian injured in collision with pedal cycle in traffic accident**

X+7th **V01.10 Pedestrian on foot injured in collision with pedal cycle in traffic accident**
Pedestrian NOS injured in collision with pedal cycle in traffic accident

X+7th **V01.11 Pedestrian on roller-skates injured in collision with pedal cycle in traffic accident**

X+7th **V01.12 Pedestrian on skateboard injured in collision with pedal cycle in traffic accident**

+ **V01.13 Pedestrian on standing micro-mobility pedestrian conveyance injured in collision with pedal cycle in traffic accident**

+7th **V01.131 Pedestrian on standing electric scooter injured in collision with pedal cycle in traffic accident**

+7th **V01.138 Pedestrian on other standing micro-mobility pedestrian conveyance injured in collision with pedal cycle in traffic accident**
Pedestrian on hoverboard injured in collision with pedal cycle in traffic accident
Pedestrian on segway injured in collisiion with pedal cycle in traffic accident

X+7th **V01.19 Pedestrian with other conveyance injured in collision with pedal cycle in traffic accident**
Pedestrian with baby stroller injured in collision with pedal cycle in traffic accident
Pedestrian on ice-skates injured in collision with pedal cycle in traffic accident
Pedestrian on nonmotorized scooter injured in collision with pedal cycle in traffic accident
Pedestrian on sled injured in collision with pedal cycle in traffic accident
Pedestrian on snowboard injured in collision with pedal cycle in traffic accident
Pedestrian on snow-skis injured in collision with pedal cycle in traffic accident
Pedestrian in wheelchair (powered) injured in collision with pedal cycle in traffic accident
Pedestrian in motorized mobility scooter injured in collision with pedal cycle in traffic accident

+ **V01.9 Pedestrian injured in collision with pedal cycle, unspecified whether traffic or nontraffic accident**

X+7th **V01.90 Pedestrian on foot injured in collision with pedal cycle, unspecified whether traffic or nontraffic accident**
Pedestrian NOS injured in collision with pedal cycle, unspecified whether traffic or nontraffic accident

X+7th **V01.91 Pedestrian on roller-skates injured in collision with pedal cycle, unspecified whether traffic or nontraffic accident**

X+7th **V01.92 Pedestrian on skateboard injured in collision with pedal cycle, unspecified whether traffic or nontraffic accident**

+ **V01.93 Pedestrian on standing micro-mobility pedestrian conveyance injured in collision with pedal cycle, unspecified whether traffic or nontraffic accident**

+7th **V01.931 Pedestrian on standing electric scooter injured in collision with pedal cycle, unspecified whether traffic or nontraffic accident**

+7th **V01.938 Pedestrian on other standing micro-mobility pedestrian conveyance injured in collision with pedal cycle, unspecified whether traffic or nontraffic accident**
Pedestrian on hoverboard injured in collision with pedal cycle, unspecified whether traffic or nontraffic accident
Pedestrian on segway injured in collision with pedal cycle, unspecified whether traffic or nontraffic accident

X+7th **V01.99 Pedestrian with other conveyance injured in collision with pedal cycle, unspecified whether traffic or nontraffic accident**
Pedestrian with baby stroller injured in collision with pedal cycle, unspecified whether traffic or nontraffic accident
Pedestrian on ice-skates injured in collision with pedal cycle unspecified, whether traffic or nontraffic accident
Pedestrian on nonmotorized scooter injured in collision with pedal cycle, unspecified whether traffic or nontraffic accident
Pedestrian on sled injured in collision with pedal cycle unspecified, whether traffic or nontraffic accident
Pedestrian on snowboard injured in collision with pedal cycle, unspecified whether traffic or nontraffic accident
Pedestrian on snow-skis injured in collision with pedal cycle, unspecified whether traffic or nontraffic accident
Pedestrian in wheelchair (powered) injured in collision with pedal cycle, unspecified whether traffic or nontraffic accident
Pedestrian in motorized mobility scooter injured in collision with pedal cycle, unspecified whether traffic or nontraffic accident

V02 Pedestrian injured in collision with two- or three-wheeled motor vehicle

The appropriate 7th character is to be added to each code from category V02
A initial encounter
D subsequent encounter
S sequela

+ **V02.0 Pedestrian injured in collision with two- or three-wheeled motor vehicle in nontraffic accident**

X+7th **V02.00 Pedestrian on foot injured in collision with two- or three-wheeled motor vehicle in nontraffic accident**
Pedestrian NOS injured in collision with two- or three-wheeled motor vehicle in nontraffic accident

X+7th **V02.01 Pedestrian on roller-skates injured in collision with two- or three-wheeled motor vehicle in nontraffic accident**

X+7th **V02.02 Pedestrian on skateboard injured in collision with two- or three-wheeled motor vehicle in nontraffic accident**

+ **V02.03 Pedestrian on standing micro-mobility pedestrian conveyance injured in collision with two- or three-wheeled motor vehicle in nontraffic accident**

+7th **V02.031 Pedestrian on standing electric scooter injured in collision with two- or three-wheeled motor vehicle in nontraffic accident**

+7th **V02.038 Pedestrian on other standing micro-mobility pedestrian conveyance injured in collision with two- or three-wheeled motor vehicle in nontraffic accident**
Pedestrian on hoverboard injured in collision with two- or three-wheeled motor vehicle in nontraffic accident
Pedestrian on segway injured in collision with two- or three-wheeled motor vehicle in nontraffic accident

X+7th **V02.09 Pedestrian with other conveyance injured in collision with two- or three-wheeled motor vehicle in nontraffic accident**
Pedestrian with baby stroller injured in collision with two- or three-wheeled motor vehicle in nontraffic accident
Pedestrian on ice-skates injured in collision with two- or three-wheeled motor vehicle in nontraffic accident
Pedestrian on nonmotorized scooter injured in collision with two- or three-wheeled motor vehicle in nontraffic accident
Pedestrian on sled injured in collision with two- or three-wheeled motor vehicle in nontraffic accident
Pedestrian on snowboard injured in collision with two- or three-wheeled motor vehicle in nontraffic accident
Pedestrian on snow-skis injured in collision with two- or three-wheeled motor vehicle in nontraffic accident
Pedestrian in wheelchair (powered) injured in collision with two- or three-wheeled motor vehicle in nontraffic accident
Pedestrian in motorized mobility scooter injured in collision with two- or three-wheeled motor vehicle in nontraffic accident

\+ **V02.1 Pedestrian injured in collision with two- or three-wheeled motor vehicle in traffic accident**

X+7th **V02.10 Pedestrian on foot injured in collision with two- or three-wheeled motor vehicle in traffic accident**
Pedestrian NOS injured in collision with two- or three-wheeled motor vehicle in traffic accident

X+7th **V02.11 Pedestrian on roller-skates injured in collision with two- or three-wheeled motor vehicle in traffic accident**

X+7th **V02.12 Pedestrian on skateboard injured in collision with two- or three-wheeled motor vehicle in traffic accident**

\+ **V02.13 Pedestrian on standing micro-mobility pedestrian conveyance injured in collision with two- or three-wheeled motor vehicle in traffic accident**

X+7th **V02.131 Pedestrian on standing electric scooter injured in collision with two- or three-wheeled motor vehicle in traffic accident**

X+7th **V02.138 Pedestrian on other standing micro-mobility pedestrian conveyance injured in collision with two- or three-wheeled motor vehicle in traffic accident**
Pedestrian on hoverboard injured in collision with two- or three-wheeled motor vehicle in traffic accident
Pedestrian on segway injured in collision with two- or three-wheeled motor vehicle in traffic accident

X+7th **V02.19 Pedestrian with other conveyance injured in collision with two- or three-wheeled motor vehicle in traffic accident**
Pedestrian with baby stroller injured in collision with two- or three-wheeled motor vehicle in traffic accident
Pedestrian on ice-skates injured in collision with two- or three-wheeled motor vehicle in traffic accident
Pedestrian on nonmotorized scooter injured in collision with two- or three-wheeled motor vehicle in traffic accident
Pedestrian on sled injured in collision with two- or three-wheeled motor vehicle in traffic accident
Pedestrian on snowboard injured in collision with two- or three-wheeled motor vehicle in traffic accident
Pedestrian on snow-skis injured in collision with two- or three-wheeled motor vehicle in traffic accident
Pedestrian in wheelchair (powered) injured in collision with two- or three-wheeled motor vehicle in traffic accident
Pedestrian in motorized mobility scooter injured in collision with two- or three-wheeled motor vehicle in traffic accident

\+ **V02.9 Pedestrian injured in collision with two- or three-wheeled motor vehicle, unspecified whether traffic or nontraffic accident**

X+7th **V02.90 Pedestrian on foot injured in collision with two- or three-wheeled motor vehicle, unspecified whether traffic or nontraffic accident**
Pedestrian NOS injured in collision with two- or three-wheeled motor vehicle, unspecified whether traffic or nontraffic accident

X+7th **V02.91 Pedestrian on roller-skates injured in collision with two- or three-wheeled motor vehicle, unspecified whether traffic or nontraffic accident**

X+7th **V02.92 Pedestrian on skateboard injured in collision with two- or three-wheeled motor vehicle, unspecified whether traffic or nontraffic accident**

\+ **V02.93 Pedestrian on standing micro-mobility pedestrian conveyance injured in collision with two- or three wheeled motor vehicle, unspecified whether traffic or nontraffic accident**

+7th **V02.931 Pedestrian on standing electric scooter injured in collision with two- or three wheeled motor vehicle, unspecified whether traffic or nontraffic accident**

+7th **V02.938 Pedestrian on other standing micro-mobility pedestrian conveyance injured in collision with two- or three wheeled motor vehicle, unspecified whether traffic or nontraffic accident**
Pedestrian on hoverbaord injured in collision with two- or three wheeled motor vehicle, unspecified whether traffic or nontraffic accident
Pedestrian on segway injured in collision with two- or three wheeled motor vehicle, unspecified whether traffic or nontraffic accident

X+7th **V02.99 Pedestrian with other conveyance injured in collision with two- or three-wheeled motor vehicle, unspecified whether traffic or nontraffic accident**
Pedestrian with baby stroller injured in collision with two- or three-wheeled motor vehicle, unspecified whether traffic or nontraffic accident
Pedestrian on ice-skates injured in collision with two- or three-wheeled motor vehicle, unspecified whether traffic or nontraffic accident
Pedestrian on nonmotorized scooter injured in collision with two- or three-wheeled motor vehicle, unspecified whether traffic or nontraffic accident
Pedestrian on sled injured in collision with two- or three-wheeled motor vehicle, unspecified whether traffic or nontraffic accident
Pedestrian on snowboard injured in collision with two- or three-wheeled motor vehicle, unspecified whether traffic or nontraffic accident
Pedestrian on snow-skis injured in collision with two- or three-wheeled motor vehicle, unspecified whether traffic or nontraffic accident
Pedestrian in wheelchair (powered) injured in collision with two- or three-wheeled motor vehicle, unspecified whether traffic or nontraffic accident
Pedestrian in motorized mobility scooter injured in collision with two- or three-wheeled motor vehicle, unspecified whether traffic or nontraffic accident

V03 Pedestrian injured in collision with car, pick-up truck or van

The appropriate 7th character is to be added to each code from category V03
A initial encounter
D subsequent encounter
S sequela

+ V03.0 Pedestrian injured in collision with car, pick-up truck or van in nontraffic accident

X+7th V03.00 Pedestrian on foot injured in collision with car, pick-up truck or van in nontraffic accident
Pedestrian NOS injured in collision with car, pick-up truck or van in nontraffic accident

X+7th V03.01 Pedestrian on roller-skates injured in collision with car, pick-up truck or van in nontraffic accident

X+7th V03.02 Pedestrian on skateboard injured in collision with car, pick-up truck or van in nontraffic accident

+ V03.03 Pedestrian on standing micro-mobility pedestrian conveyance injured in collision with car, pick-up or van in nontraffic accident

+7th V03.031 Pedestrian on standing electric scooter injured in collision with car, pick-up or van in nontraffic accident

+7th V03.038 Pedestrian on other standing micro-mobility pedestrian conveyance injured in collision with car, pick-up or van in nontraffic accident
Pedestrian on hoverboard injured in collision with car, pick-up or van in nontraffic accident
Pedestrian on segway injured in collision with car, pick-up or van in nontraffic accident

X+7th V03.09 Pedestrian with other conveyance injured in collision with car, pick-up truck or van in nontraffic accident
Pedestrian with baby stroller injured in collision with car, pick-up truck or van in nontraffic accident
Pedestrian on ice-skates injured in collision with car, pick-up truck or van in nontraffic accident
Pedestrian on nonmotorized scooter injured in collision with car, pick-up truck or van in nontraffic accident
Pedestrian on sled injured in collision with car, pick-up truck or van in nontraffic accident
Pedestrian on snowboard injured in collision with car, pick-up truck or van in nontraffic accident
Pedestrian on snow-skis injured in collision with car, pick-up truck or van in nontraffic accident
Pedestrian in wheelchair (powered) injured in collision with car, pick-up truck or van in nontraffic accident
Pedestrian in motorized mobility scooter injured in collision with car, pick-up truck or van in nontraffic accident

+ V03.1 Pedestrian injured in collision with car, pick-up truck or van in traffic accident

X+7th V03.10 Pedestrian on foot injured in collision with car, pick-up truck or van in traffic accident
Pedestrian NOS injured in collision with car, pick-up truck or van in traffic accident

X+7th V03.11 Pedestrian on roller-skates injured in collision with car, pick-up truck or van in traffic accident

X+7th V03.12 Pedestrian on skateboard injured in collision with car, pick-up truck or van in traffic accident

+ V03.13 Pedestrian on standing micro-mobility pedestrian conveyance injured in collision with car, pick-up or van in traffic accident

+7th V03.131 Pedestrian on standing electric scooter injured in collision with car, pick-up or van in traffic accident

+7th V03.138 Pedestrian on other standing micro-mobility pedestrian conveyance injured in collision with car, pick-up or van in traffic accident
Pedestrian on hoverboard injured in collision with car, pick-up or van in traffic accident
Pedestrian on segway injured in collision with car, pick-up or van in traffic accident

X+7th V03.19 Pedestrian with other conveyance injured in collision with car, pick-up truck or van in traffic accident
Pedestrian with baby stroller injured in collision with car, pick-up truck or van in traffic accident
Pedestrian on ice-skates injured in collision with car, pick-up truck or van in traffic accident
Pedestrian on nonmotorized scooter injured in collision with car, pick-up truck or van in traffic accident
Pedestrian on sled injured in collision with car, pick-up truck or van in traffic accident
Pedestrian on snowboard injured in collision with car, pick-up truck or van in traffic accident
Pedestrian on snow-skis injured in collision with car, pick-up truck or van in traffic accident
Pedestrian in wheelchair (powered) injured in collision with car, pick-up truck or van in traffic accident
Pedestrian in motorized mobility scooter injured in collision with car, pick-up truck or van in traffic accident

+ V03.9 Pedestrian injured in collision with car, pick-up truck or van, unspecified whether traffic or nontraffic accident

X+7th V03.90 Pedestrian on foot injured in collision with car, pick-up truck or van, unspecified whether traffic or nontraffic accident
Pedestrian NOS injured in collision with car, pick-up truck or van, unspecified whether traffic or nontraffic accident

X+7th V03.91 Pedestrian on roller-skates injured in collision with car, pick-up truck or van, unspecified whether traffic or nontraffic accident

X+7th V03.92 Pedestrian on skateboard injured in collision with car, pick-up truck or van, unspecified whether traffic or nontraffic accident

+ V03.93 Pedestrian on standing micro-mobility pedestrian conveyance injured in collision with car, pick-up or van, unspecified whether traffic or nontraffic accident

+7th V03.931 Pedestrian on standing electric scooter injured in collision with car, pick-up or van, unspecified whether traffic or nontraffic accident

+7th V03.938 Pedestrian on other standing micro-mobility pedestrian conveyance injured in collision with car, pick-up or van, unspecified whether traffic or nontraffic accident
Pedestrian on hoverboard injured in collision with car, pick-up or van, unspecified whether traffic or nontraffic accident
Pedestrian on segway injured in collision with car, pick-up or van, unspecified whether traffic or nontraffic accident

X+7th V03.99 Pedestrian with other conveyance injured in collision with car, pick-up truck or van, unspecified whether traffic or nontraffic accident
Pedestrian with baby stroller injured in collision with car, pick-up truck or van, unspecified whether traffic or nontraffic accident
Pedestrian on ice-skates injured in collision with car, pick-up truck or van, unspecified whether traffic or nontraffic accident
Pedestrian on nonmotorized scooter injured in collision with car, pick-up truck or van, unspecified whether traffic or nontraffic accident
Pedestrian on sled injured in collision with car, pick-up truck or van in nontraffic accident
Pedestrian on snowboard injured in collision with car, pick-up truck or van, unspecified whether traffic or nontraffic accident

Pedestrian on snow-skis injured in collision with car, pick-up truck or van, unspecified whether traffic or nontraffic accident
Pedestrian in wheelchair (powered) injured in collision with car, pick-up truck or van, unspecified whether traffic or nontraffic accident
Pedestrian in motorized mobility scooter injured in collision with car, pick-up truck or van, unspecified whether traffic or nontraffic accident

V04 Pedestrian injured in collision with heavy transport vehicle or bus

Excludes1: *pedestrian injured in collision with military vehicle (V09.01, V09.21)*

The appropriate 7th character is to be added to each code from category V04
A initial encounter
D subsequent encounter
S sequela

\+ **V04.0 Pedestrian injured in collision with heavy transport vehicle or bus in nontraffic accident**

X+7th **V04.00 Pedestrian on foot injured in collision with heavy transport vehicle or bus in nontraffic accident**
Pedestrian NOS injured in collision with heavy transport vehicle or bus in nontraffic accident

X+7th **V04.01 Pedestrian on roller-skates injured in collision with heavy transport vehicle or bus in nontraffic accident**

X+7th **V04.02 Pedestrian on skateboard injured in collision with heavy transport vehicle or bus in nontraffic accident**

\+ **V04.03 Pedestrian on standing micro-mobility pedestrian conveyance injured in collision with heavy transport vehicle or bus in nontraffic accident**

+7th **V04.031 Pedestrian on standing electric scooter injured in collision with heavy transport vehicle or bus in nontraffic accident**

+7th **V04.038 Pedestrian on other standing micro-mobility pedestrian conveyance injured in collision with heavy transport vehicle or bus in nontraffic accident**
Pedestrian on hoverboard injured in collision with heavy transport vehicle or bus in nontraffic accident
Pedestrian on segway injured in collision with heavy transport vehicle or bus in nontraffic accident

X+7th **V04.09 Pedestrian with other conveyance injured in collision with heavy transport vehicle or bus in nontraffic accident**
Pedestrian with baby stroller injured in collision with heavy transport vehicle or bus in nontraffic accident
Pedestrian on ice-skates injured in collision with heavy transport vehicle or bus in nontraffic accident
Pedestrian on nonmotorized scooter injured in collision with heavy transport vehicle or bus in nontraffic accident
Pedestrian on sled injured in collision with heavy transport vehicle or bus in nontraffic accident
Pedestrian on snowboard injured in collision with heavy transport vehicle or bus in nontraffic accident
Pedestrian on snow-skis injured in collision with heavy transport vehicle or bus in nontraffic accident
Pedestrian in wheelchair (powered) injured in collision with heavy transport vehicle or bus in nontraffic accident
Pedestrian in motorized mobility scooter injured in collision with heavy transport vehicle or bus in nontraffic accident

\+ **V04.1 Pedestrian injured in collision with heavy transport vehicle or bus in traffic accident**

X+7th **V04.10 Pedestrian on foot injured in collision with heavy transport vehicle or bus in traffic accident**
Pedestrian NOS injured in collision with heavy transport vehicle or bus in traffic accident

X+7th **V04.11 Pedestrian on roller-skates injured in collision with heavy transport vehicle or bus in traffic accident**

X+7th **V04.12 Pedestrian on skateboard injured in collision with heavy transport vehicle or bus in traffic accident**

\+ **V04.13 Pedestrian on standing micro-mobility pedestrian conveyance injured in collision with heavy transport vehicle or bus in traffic accident**

+7th **V04.131 Pedestrian on standing electric scooter injured in collision with heavy transport vehicle or bus in traffic accident**

+7th **V04.138 Pedestrian on other standing micro-mobility pedestrian conveyance injured in collision with heavy transport vehicle or bus in traffic accident**
Pedestrian on hoverboard injured in collision with heavy transport vehicle or bus in traffic accident
Pedestrian on segway injured in collision with heavy transport vehicle or bus in traffic accident

X+7th **V04.19 Pedestrian with other conveyance injured in collision with heavy transport vehicle or bus in traffic accident**
Pedestrian with baby stroller injured in collision with heavy transport vehicle or bus in traffic accident
Pedestrian on ice-skates injured in collision with heavy transport vehicle or bus in traffic accident
Pedestrian on nonmotorized scooter injured in collision with heavy transport vehicle or bus in traffic accident
Pedestrian on sled injured in collision with heavy transport vehicle or bus in traffic accident
Pedestrian on snowboard injured in collision with heavy transport vehicle or bus in traffic accident
Pedestrian on snow-skis injured in collision with heavy transport vehicle or bus in traffic accident
Pedestrian in wheelchair (powered) injured in collision with heavy transport vehicle or bus in traffic accident
Pedestrian in motorized mobility scooter injured in collision with heavy transport vehicle or bus in traffic accident

\+ **V04.9 Pedestrian injured in collision with heavy transport vehicle or bus, unspecified whether traffic or nontraffic accident**

X+7th **V04.90 Pedestrian on foot injured in collision with heavy transport vehicle or bus, unspecified whether traffic or nontraffic accident**
Pedestrian NOS injured in collision with heavy transport vehicle or bus, unspecified whether traffic or nontraffic accident

X+7th **V04.91 Pedestrian on roller-skates injured in collision with heavy transport vehicle or bus, unspecified whether traffic or nontraffic accident**

X+7th **V04.92 Pedestrian on skateboard injured in collision with heavy transport vehicle or bus, unspecified whether traffic or nontraffic accident**

\+ **V04.93 Pedestrian on standing micro-mobility pedestrian conveyance injured in collision with heavy transport vehicle or bus, unspecified whether traffic or nontraffic accident**

+7th **V04.931 Pedestrian on standing electric scooter injured in collision with heavy transport vehicle or bus, unspecified whether traffic or nontraffic accident**

+7th **V04.938 Pedestrian on other standing micro-mobility pedestrian conveyance injured in collision with heavy transport vehicle or bus, unspecified whether traffic or nontraffic accident**
Pedestrian on hoverboard injured in collision with heavy transport vehicle or bus, unspecified whether traffic or nontraffic accident
Pedestrian on segway injured in collision with heavy transport vehicle or bus, unspecified whether traffic or nontraffic accident

X+7th V04.99 Pedestrian with other conveyance injured in collision with heavy transport vehicle or bus, unspecified whether traffic or nontraffic accident

Pedestrian with baby stroller injured in collision with heavy transport vehicle or bus, unspecified whether traffic or nontraffic accident

Pedestrian on ice-skates injured in collision with heavy transport vehicle or bus, unspecified whether traffic or nontraffic accident

Pedestrian on nonmotorized scooter injured in collision with heavy transport vehicle or bus, unspecified whether traffic or nontraffic accident

Pedestrian on sled injured in collision with heavy transport vehicle or bus, unspecified whether traffic or nontraffic accident

Pedestrian on snowboard injured in collision with heavy transport vehicle or bus, unspecified whether traffic or nontraffic accident

Pedestrian on snow-skis injured in collision with heavy transport vehicle or bus, unspecified whether traffic or nontraffic accident

Pedestrian in wheelchair (powered) injured in collision with heavy transport vehicle or bus, unspecified whether traffic or nontraffic accident

Pedestrian in motorized mobility scooter injured in collision with heavy transport vehicle or bus, unspecified whether traffic or nontraffic accident

V05 Pedestrian injured in collision with railway train or railway vehicle

The appropriate 7th character is to be added to each code from category V05
A initial encounter
D subsequent encounter
S sequela

+ V05.0 Pedestrian injured in collision with railway train or railway vehicle in nontraffic accident

X+7th V05.00 Pedestrian on foot injured in collision with railway train or railway vehicle in nontraffic accident

Pedestrian NOS injured in collision with railway train or railway vehicle in nontraffic accident

X+7th V05.01 Pedestrian on roller-skates injured in collision with railway train or railway vehicle in nontraffic accident

X+7th V05.02 Pedestrian on skateboard injured in collision with railway train or railway vehicle in nontraffic accident

+ V05.03 Pedestrian on standing micro-mobility pedestrian conveyance injured in collision with railway train or railway vehicle in nontraffic accident

+7th V05.031 Pedestrian on standing electric scooter injured in collision with railway train or railway vehicle in nontraffic accident

+7th V05.038 Pedestrian on other standing micro-mobility pedestrian conveyance injured in collision with railway train or railway vehicle in nontraffic accident

Pedestrian on hoverboard injured in collision with railway train or railway vehicle in nontraffic accident

Pedestrian on segway injured in collision with railway train or railway vehicle in nontraffic accident

X+7th V05.09 Pedestrian with other conveyance injured in collision with railway train or railway vehicle in nontraffic accident

Pedestrian with baby stroller injured in collision with railway train or railway vehicle in nontraffic accident

Pedestrian on ice-skates injured in collision with railway train or railway vehicle in nontraffic accident

Pedestrian on nonmotorized scooter injured in collision with railway train or railway vehicle in nontraffic accident

Pedestrian on sled injured in collision with railway train or railway vehicle in nontraffic accident

Pedestrian on snowboard injured in collision with railway train or railway vehicle in nontraffic accident

Pedestrian on snow-skis injured in collision with railway train or railway vehicle in nontraffic accident

Pedestrian in wheelchair (powered) injured in collision with railway train or railway vehicle in nontraffic accident

Pedestrian in motorized mobility scooter injured in collision with railway train or railway vehicle in nontraffic accident

+ V05.1 Pedestrian injured in collision with railway train or railway vehicle in traffic accident

X+7th V05.10 Pedestrian on foot injured in collision with railway train or railway vehicle in traffic accident

Pedestrian NOS injured in collision with railway train or railway vehicle in traffic accident

X+7th V05.11 Pedestrian on roller-skates injured in collision with railway train or railway vehicle in traffic accident

X+7th V05.12 Pedestrian on skateboard injured in collision with railway train or railway vehicle in traffic accident

+ V05.13 Pedestrian on standing micro-mobility pedestrian conveyance injured in collision with railway train or railway vehicle in traffic accident

+7th V05.131 Pedestrian on standing electric scooter injured in collision with railway train or railway vehicle in traffic accident

+7th V05.138 Pedestrian on other standing micro-mobility pedestrian conveyance injured in collision with railway train or railway vehicle in traffic accident

Pedestrian on hoverboard injured in collision with railway train or railway vehicle in traffic accident

Pedestrian on segway injured in collision with railway train or railway vehicle in traffic accident

X+7th V05.19 Pedestrian with other conveyance injured in collision with railway train or railway vehicle in traffic accident

Pedestrian with baby stroller injured in collision with railway train or railway vehicle in traffic accident

Pedestrian on ice-skates injured in collision with railway train or railway vehicle in traffic accident

Pedestrian on nonmotorized scooter injured in collision with railway train or railway vehicle in traffic accident

Pedestrian on sled injured in collision with railway train or railway vehicle in traffic accident

Pedestrian on snowboard injured in collision with railway train or railway vehicle in traffic accident

Pedestrian on snow-skis injured in collision with railway train or railway vehicle in traffic accident

Pedestrian in wheelchair (powered) injured in collision with railway train or railway vehicle in traffic accident

Pedestrian in motorized mobility scooter injured in collision with railway train or railway vehicle in traffic accident

+ V05.9 Pedestrian injured in collision with railway train or railway vehicle, unspecified whether traffic or nontraffic accident

X+7th V05.90 Pedestrian on foot injured in collision with railway train or railway vehicle, unspecified whether traffic or nontraffic accident

Pedestrian NOS injured in collision with railway train or railway vehicle, unspecified whether traffic or nontraffic accident

X+7th V05.91 Pedestrian on roller-skates injured in collision with railway train or railway vehicle, unspecified whether traffic or nontraffic accident

X+7th V05.92 Pedestrian on skateboard injured in collision with railway train or railway vehicle, unspecified whether traffic or nontraffic accident

+ V05.93 Pedestrian on standing micro-mobility pedestrian conveyance injured in collision with railway train or railway vehicle, unspecified whether traffic or nontraffic accident

+7th V05.931 Pedestrian on standing electric scooter injured in collision with railway train or railway vehicle, unspecified whether traffic or nontraffic accident

+7th **V05.938 Pedestrian on other standing micro-mobility pedestrian conveyance injured in collision with railway train or railway vehicle, unspecified whether traffic or nontraffic accident**

Pedestrian on hoverboard injured in collision with railway train or railway vehicle, unspecified whether traffic or nontraffic accident

Pedestrian on segway injured in collision with railway train or railway vehicle, unspecified whether traffic or nontraffic accident

X+7th **V05.99 Pedestrian with other conveyance injured in collision with railway train or railway vehicle, unspecified whether traffic or nontraffic accident**

Pedestrian with baby stroller injured in collision with railway train or railway vehicle, unspecified whether traffic or nontraffic

Pedestrian on ice-skates injured in collision with railway train or railway vehicle, unspecified whether traffic or nontraffic

Pedestrian on nonmotorized scooter injured in collision with railway train or railway vehicle, unspecified whether traffic or nontraffic

Pedestrian on sled injured in collision with railway train or railway vehicle, unspecified whether traffic or nontraffic

Pedestrian on snowboard injured in collision with railway train or railway vehicle, unspecified whether traffic or nontraffic

Pedestrian on snow-skis injured in collision with railway train or railway vehicle, unspecified whether traffic or nontraffic

Pedestrian in wheelchair (powered) injured in collision with railway train or railway vehicle, unspecified whether traffic or nontraffic

Pedestrian in motorized mobility scooter injured in collision with railway train or railway vehicle, unspecified whether traffic or nontraffic

V06 Pedestrian injured in collision with other nonmotor vehicle

Includes: collision with animal-drawn vehicle, animal being ridden, nonpowered streetcar

Excludes1: *pedestrian injured in collision with pedestrian conveyance (V00.0-)*

The appropriate 7th character is to be added to each code from category V06
A initial encounter
D subsequent encounter
S sequela

\+ **V06.0 Pedestrian injured in collision with other nonmotor vehicle in nontraffic accident**

X+7th **V06.00 Pedestrian on foot injured in collision with other nonmotor vehicle in nontraffic accident**

Pedestrian NOS injured in collision with other nonmotor vehicle in nontraffic accident

X+7th **V06.01 Pedestrian on roller-skates injured in collision with other nonmotor vehicle in nontraffic accident**

X+7th **V06.02 Pedestrian on skateboard injured in collision with other nonmotor vehicle in nontraffic accident**

\+ **V06.03 Pedestrian on standing micro-mobility pedestrian conveyance injured in collision with other nonmotor vehicle in nontraffic accident**

+7th **V06.031 Pedestrian on standing electric scooter injured in collision with other nonmotor vehicle in nontraffic accident**

+7th **V06.038 Pedestrian on other standing micro-mobility pedestrian conveyance injured in collision with other nonmotor vehicle in nontraffic accident**

Pedestrian on hoverboard injured in collision with other nonmotor vehicle in nontraffic accident

Pedestrian on segway injured in collision with other nonmotor vehicle in nontraffic accident

X+7th **V06.09 Pedestrian with other conveyance injured in collision with other nonmotor vehicle in nontraffic accident**

Pedestrian with baby stroller injured in collision with other nonmotor vehicle in nontraffic accident

Pedestrian on ice-skates injured in collision with other nonmotor vehicle in nontraffic accident

Pedestrian on nonmotorized scooter injured in collision with other nonmotor vehicle in nontraffic accident

Pedestrian on sled injured in collision with other nonmotor vehicle in nontraffic accident

Pedestrian on snowboard injured in collision with other nonmotor vehicle in nontraffic accident

Pedestrian on snow-skis injured in collision with other nonmotor vehicle in nontraffic accident

Pedestrian in wheelchair (powered) injured in collision with other nonmotor vehicle in nontraffic accident

Pedestrian in motorized mobility scooter injured in collision with other nonmotor vehicle in nontraffic accident

\+ **V06.1 Pedestrian injured in collision with other nonmotor vehicle in traffic accident**

X+7th **V06.10 Pedestrian on foot injured in collision with other nonmotor vehicle in traffic accident**

Pedestrian NOS injured in collision with other nonmotor vehicle in traffic accident

X+7th **V06.11 Pedestrian on roller-skates injured in collision with other nonmotor vehicle in traffic accident**

X+7th **V06.12 Pedestrian on skateboard injured in collision with other nonmotor vehicle in traffic accident**

\+ **V06.13 Pedestrian on standing micro-mobility pedestrian conveyance injured in collision with other nonmotor vehicle in traffic accident**

+7th **V06.131 Pedestrian on standing electric scooter injured in collision with other nonmotor vehicle in traffic accident**

+7th **V06.138 Pedestrian on other standing micro-mobility pedestrian conveyance injured in collision with other nonmotor vehicle in traffic accident**

Pedestrian on hoverboard injured in collision with other nonmotor vehicle in traffic accident

Pedestrian on segway injured in collision with other nonmotor vehicle in traffic accident

X+7th **V06.19 Pedestrian with other conveyance injured in collision with other nonmotor vehicle in traffic accident**

Pedestrian with baby stroller injured in collision with other nonmotor vehicle in nontraffic accident

Pedestrian on ice-skates injured in collision with other nonmotor vehicle in traffic accident

Pedestrian on nonmotorized scooter injured in collision with other nonmotor vehicle in traffic accident

Pedestrian on sled injured in collision with other nonmotor vehicle in traffic accident

Pedestrian on snowboard injured in collision with other nonmotor vehicle in traffic accident

Pedestrian on snow-skis injured in collision with other nonmotor vehicle in traffic accident

Pedestrian in wheelchair (powered) injured in collision with other nonmotor vehicle in traffic accident

Pedestrian in motorized mobility scooter injured in collision with other nonmotor vehicle in traffic accident

\+ **V06.9 Pedestrian injured in collision with other nonmotor vehicle, unspecified whether traffic or nontraffic accident**

X+7th **V06.90 Pedestrian on foot injured in collision with other nonmotor vehicle, unspecified whether traffic or nontraffic accident**

Pedestrian NOS injured in collision with other nonmotor vehicle, unspecified whether traffic or nontraffic accident

X+7th **V06.91 Pedestrian on roller-skates injured in collision with other nonmotor vehicle, unspecified whether traffic or nontraffic accident**

X+7th **V06.92 Pedestrian on skateboard injured in collision with other nonmotor vehicle, unspecified whether traffic or nontraffic accident**

+ **V06.93 Pedestrian on standing micro-mobility pedestrian conveyance injured in collision with other nonmotor vehicle, unspecified whether traffic or nontraffic accident**

+7th **V06.931 Pedestrian on standing electric scooter injured in collision with other nonmotor vehicle, unspecified whether traffic or nontraffic accident**

+7th **V06.938 Pedestrian on other standing micro-mobility pedestrian conveyance injured in collision with other nonmotor vehicle, unspecified whether traffic or nontraffic accident**

Pedestrian on hoverboard injured in collision with other nonmotor vehicle, unspecified whether traffic or nontraffic accident

Pedestrian on other segway injured in collision with other nonmotor vehicle, unspecified whether traffic or nontraffic accident

X+7th **V06.99 Pedestrian with other conveyance injured in collision with other nonmotor vehicle, unspecified whether traffic or nontraffic accident**

Pedestrian with baby stroller injured in collision with other nonmotor vehicle, unspecified whether traffic or nontraffic accident

Pedestrian on ice-skates injured in collision with other nonmotor vehicle, unspecified whether traffic or nontraffic accident

Pedestrian on nonmotorized scooter injured in collision with other nonmotor vehicle, unspecified whether traffic or nontraffic accident

Pedestrian on sled injured in collision with other nonmotor vehicle, unspecified whether traffic or nontraffic accident

Pedestrian on snowboard injured in collision with other nonmotor vehicle, unspecified whether traffic or nontraffic accident

Pedestrian on snow-skis injured in collision with other nonmotor vehicle, unspecified whether traffic or nontraffic accident

Pedestrian in wheelchair (powered) injured in collision with other nonmotor vehicle, unspecified whether traffic or nontraffic accident

Pedestrian in motorized mobility scooter injured in collision with other nonmotor vehicle, unspecified whether traffic or nontraffic accident

V09 Pedestrian injured in other and unspecified transport accidents

The appropriate 7th character is to be added to each code from category V09
A initial encounter
D subsequent encounter
S sequela

+ **V09.0 Pedestrian injured in nontraffic accident involving other and unspecified motor vehicles**

X+7th **V09.00 Pedestrian injured in nontraffic accident involving unspecified motor vehicles**

X+7th **V09.01 Pedestrian injured in nontraffic accident involving military vehicle**

X+7th **V09.09 Pedestrian injured in nontraffic accident involving other motor vehicles**

Pedestrian injured in nontraffic accident by special vehicle

X+7th **V09.1 Pedestrian injured in unspecified nontraffic accident**

+ **V09.2 Pedestrian injured in traffic accident involving other and unspecified motor vehicles**

X+7th **V09.20 Pedestrian injured in traffic accident involving unspecified motor vehicles**

X+7th **V09.21 Pedestrian injured in traffic accident involving military vehicle**

X+7th **V09.29 Pedestrian injured in traffic accident involving other motor vehicles**

X+7th **V09.3 Pedestrian injured in unspecified traffic accident**

X+7th **V09.9 Pedestrian injured in unspecified transport accident**

Pedal cycle rider injured in transport accident (V10-V19)

Includes: any non-motorized vehicle, excluding an animal-drawn vehicle, or a sidecar or trailer attached to the pedal cycle

Excludes2: *rupture of pedal cycle tire (W37.0)*

V10 Pedal cycle rider injured in collision with pedestrian or animal

Excludes1: *pedal cycle rider collision with animal-drawn vehicle or animal being ridden (V16.-)*

The appropriate 7th character is to be added to each code from category V10
A initial encounter
D subsequent encounter
S sequela

X+7th **V10.0 Pedal cycle driver injured in collision with pedestrian or animal in nontraffic accident**

X+7th **V10.1 Pedal cycle passenger injured in collision with pedestrian or animal in nontraffic accident**

X+7th **V10.2 Unspecified pedal cyclist injured in collision with pedestrian or animal in nontraffic accident**

X+7th **V10.3 Person boarding or alighting a pedal cycle injured in collision with pedestrian or animal**

X+7th **V10.4 Pedal cycle driver injured in collision with pedestrian or animal in traffic accident**

X+7th **V10.5 Pedal cycle passenger injured in collision with pedestrian or animal in traffic accident**

X+7th **V10.9 Unspecified pedal cyclist injured in collision with pedestrian or animal in traffic accident**

V11 Pedal cycle rider injured in collision with other pedal cycle

The appropriate 7th character is to be added to each code from category V11
A initial encounter
D subsequent encounter
S sequela

X+7th **V11.0 Pedal cycle driver injured in collision with other pedal cycle in nontraffic accident**

X+7th **V11.1 Pedal cycle passenger injured in collision with other pedal cycle in nontraffic accident**

X+7th **V11.2 Unspecified pedal cyclist injured in collision with other pedal cycle in nontraffic accident**

X+7th **V11.3 Person boarding or alighting a pedal cycle injured in collision with other pedal cycle**

X+7th **V11.4 Pedal cycle driver injured in collision with other pedal cycle in traffic accident**

X+7th **V11.5 Pedal cycle passenger injured in collision with other pedal cycle in traffic accident**

X+7th **V11.9 Unspecified pedal cyclist injured in collision with other pedal cycle in traffic accident**

V12 Pedal cycle rider injured in collision with two- or three-wheeled motor vehicle

The appropriate 7th character is to be added to each code from category V12
A initial encounter
D subsequent encounter
S sequela

X+7th **V12.0 Pedal cycle driver injured in collision with two- or three-wheeled motor vehicle in nontraffic accident**

X+7th **V12.1 Pedal cycle passenger injured in collision with two- or three-wheeled motor vehicle in nontraffic accident**

X+7th **V12.2 Unspecified pedal cyclist injured in collision with two- or three-wheeled motor vehicle in nontraffic accident**

X+7th **V12.3 Person boarding or alighting a pedal cycle injured in collision with two- or three-wheeled motor vehicle**

X+7th **V12.4 Pedal cycle driver injured in collision with two- or three-wheeled motor vehicle in traffic accident**

X+7th **V12.5 Pedal cycle passenger injured in collision with two- or three-wheeled motor vehicle in traffic accident**

X+7th **V12.9 Unspecified pedal cyclist injured in collision with two- or three-wheeled motor vehicle in traffic accident**

V13 Pedal cycle rider injured in collision with car, pick-up truck or van

The appropriate 7th character is to be added to each code from category V13
A initial encounter
D subsequent encounter
S sequela

X+7th **V13.0 Pedal cycle driver injured in collision with car, pick-up truck or van in nontraffic accident**
X+7th **V13.1 Pedal cycle passenger injured in collision with car, pick-up truck or van in nontraffic accident**
X+7th **V13.2 Unspecified pedal cyclist injured in collision with car, pick-up truck or van in nontraffic accident**
X+7th **V13.3 Person boarding or alighting a pedal cycle injured in collision with car, pick-up truck or van**
X+7th **V13.4 Pedal cycle driver injured in collision with car, pick-up truck or van in traffic accident**
X+7th **V13.5 Pedal cycle passenger injured in collision with car, pick-up truck or van in traffic accident**
X+7th **V13.9 Unspecified pedal cyclist injured in collision with car, pick-up truck or van in traffic accident**

V14 Pedal cycle rider injured in collision with heavy transport vehicle or bus

Excludes1: *pedal cycle rider injured in collision with military vehicle (V19.81)*

The appropriate 7th character is to be added to each code from category V14
A initial encounter
D subsequent encounter
S sequela

X+7th **V14.0 Pedal cycle driver injured in collision with heavy transport vehicle or bus in nontraffic accident**
X+7th **V14.1 Pedal cycle passenger injured in collision with heavy transport vehicle or bus in nontraffic accident**
X+7th **V14.2 Unspecified pedal cyclist injured in collision with heavy transport vehicle or bus in nontraffic accident**
X+7th **V14.3 Person boarding or alighting a pedal cycle injured in collision with heavy transport vehicle or bus**
X+7th **V14.4 Pedal cycle driver injured in collision with heavy transport vehicle or bus in traffic accident**
X+7th **V14.5 Pedal cycle passenger injured in collision with heavy transport vehicle or bus in traffic accident**
X+7th **V14.9 Unspecified pedal cyclist injured in collision with heavy transport vehicle or bus in traffic accident**

V15 Pedal cycle rider injured in collision with railway train or railway vehicle

The appropriate 7th character is to be added to each code from category V15
A initial encounter
D subsequent encounter
S sequela

X+7th **V15.0 Pedal cycle driver injured in collision with railway train or railway vehicle in nontraffic accident**
X+7th **V15.1 Pedal cycle passenger injured in collision with railway train or railway vehicle in nontraffic accident**
X+7th **V15.2 Unspecified pedal cyclist injured in collision with railway train or railway vehicle in nontraffic accident**
X+7th **V15.3 Person boarding or alighting a pedal cycle injured in collision with railway train or railway vehicle**
X+7th **V15.4 Pedal cycle driver injured in collision with railway train or railway vehicle in traffic accident**
X+7th **V15.5 Pedal cycle passenger injured in collision with railway train or railway vehicle in traffic accident**
X+7th **V15.9 Unspecified pedal cyclist injured in collision with railway train or railway vehicle in traffic accident**

V16 Pedal cycle rider injured in collision with other nonmotor vehicle

Includes: collision with animal-drawn vehicle, animal being ridden, streetcar

The appropriate 7th character is to be added to each code from category V16
A initial encounter
D subsequent encounter
S sequela

X+7th **V16.0 Pedal cycle driver injured in collision with other nonmotor vehicle in nontraffic accident**
X+7th **V16.1 Pedal cycle passenger injured in collision with other nonmotor vehicle in nontraffic accident**
X+7th **V16.2 Unspecified pedal cyclist injured in collision with other nonmotor vehicle in nontraffic accident**
X+7th **V16.3 Person boarding or alighting a pedal cycle injured in collision with other nonmotor vehicle in nontraffic accident**
X+7th **V16.4 Pedal cycle driver injured in collision with other nonmotor vehicle in traffic accident**
X+7th **V16.5 Pedal cycle passenger injured in collision with other nonmotor vehicle in traffic accident**
X+7th **V16.9 Unspecified pedal cyclist injured in collision with other nonmotor vehicle in traffic accident**

V17 Pedal cycle rider injured in collision with fixed or stationary object

The appropriate 7th character is to be added to each code from category V17
A initial encounter
D subsequent encounter
S sequela

X+7th **V17.0 Pedal cycle driver injured in collision with fixed or stationary object in nontraffic accident**
X+7th **V17.1 Pedal cycle passenger injured in collision with fixed or stationary object in nontraffic accident**
X+7th **V17.2 Unspecified pedal cyclist injured in collision with fixed or stationary object in nontraffic accident**
X+7th **V17.3 Person boarding or alighting a pedal cycle injured in collision with fixed or stationary object**
X+7th **V17.4 Pedal cycle driver injured in collision with fixed or stationary object in traffic accident**
X+7th **V17.5 Pedal cycle passenger injured in collision with fixed or stationary object in traffic accident**
X+7th **V17.9 Unspecified pedal cyclist injured in collision with fixed or stationary object in traffic accident**

V18 Pedal cycle rider injured in noncollision transport accident

Includes: fall or thrown from pedal cycle (without antecedent collision)
overturning pedal cycle NOS
overturning pedal cycle without collision

The appropriate 7th character is to be added to each code from category V18
A initial encounter
D subsequent encounter
S sequela

X+7th **V18.0 Pedal cycle driver injured in noncollision transport accident in nontraffic accident**
X+7th **V18.1 Pedal cycle passenger injured in noncollision transport accident in nontraffic accident**
X+7th **V18.2 Unspecified pedal cyclist injured in noncollision transport accident in nontraffic accident**
X+7th **V18.3 Person boarding or alighting a pedal cycle injured in noncollision transport accident**
X+7th **V18.4 Pedal cycle driver injured in noncollision transport accident in traffic accident**
X+7th **V18.5 Pedal cycle passenger injured in noncollision transport accident in traffic accident**
X+7th **V18.9 Unspecified pedal cyclist injured in noncollision transport accident in traffic accident**

V19 Pedal cycle rider injured in other and unspecified transport accidents

The appropriate 7th character is to be added to each code from category V19
A initial encounter
D subsequent encounter
S sequela

\+ **V19.0 Pedal cycle driver injured in collision with other and unspecified motor vehicles in nontraffic accident**
X+7th **V19.00 Pedal cycle driver injured in collision with unspecified motor vehicles in nontraffic accident**
X+7th **V19.09 Pedal cycle driver injured in collision with other motor vehicles in nontraffic accident**
\+ **V19.1 Pedal cycle passenger injured in collision with other and unspecified motor vehicles in nontraffic accident**
X+7th **V19.10 Pedal cycle passenger injured in collision with unspecified motor vehicles in nontraffic accident**
X+7th **V19.19 Pedal cycle passenger injured in collision with other motor vehicles in nontraffic accident**

+ **V19.2 Unspecified pedal cyclist injured in collision with other and unspecified motor vehicles in nontraffic accident**
  - X+7th **V19.20 Unspecified pedal cyclist injured in collision with unspecified motor vehicles in nontraffic accident**
    Pedal cycle collision NOS, nontraffic
  - X+7th **V19.29 Unspecified pedal cyclist injured in collision with other motor vehicles in nontraffic accident**

X+7th **V19.3 Pedal cyclist (driver) (passenger) injured in unspecified nontraffic accident**
  Pedal cycle accident NOS, nontraffic
  Pedal cyclist injured in nontraffic accident NOS

+ **V19.4 Pedal cycle driver injured in collision with other and unspecified motor vehicles in traffic accident**
  - X+7th **V19.40 Pedal cycle driver injured in collision with unspecified motor vehicles in traffic accident**
  - X+7th **V19.49 Pedal cycle driver injured in collision with other motor vehicles in traffic accident**

+ **V19.5 Pedal cycle passenger injured in collision with other and unspecified motor vehicles in traffic accident**
  - X+7th **V19.50 Pedal cycle passenger injured in collision with unspecified motor vehicles in traffic accident**
  - X+7th **V19.59 Pedal cycle passenger injured in collision with other motor vehicles in traffic accident**

+ **V19.6 Unspecified pedal cyclist injured in collision with other and unspecified motor vehicles in traffic accident**
  - X+7th **V19.60 Unspecified pedal cyclist injured in collision with unspecified motor vehicles in traffic accident**
    Pedal cycle collision NOS (traffic)
  - X+7th **V19.69 Unspecified pedal cyclist injured in collision with other motor vehicles in traffic accident**

+ **V19.8 Pedal cyclist (driver) (passenger) injured in other specified transport accidents**
  - X+7th **V19.81 Pedal cyclist (driver) (passenger) injured in transport accident with military vehicle**
  - X+7th **V19.88 Pedal cyclist (driver) (passenger) injured in other specified transport accidents**

X+7th **V19.9 Pedal cyclist (driver) (passenger) injured in unspecified traffic accident**
  Pedal cycle accident NOS

Motorcycle rider injured in transport accident (V20-V29)

Includes: moped
motorcycle with sidecar
motorized bicycle
motor scooter

Excludes1: *three-wheeled motor vehicle (V30-V39)*

V20 Motorcycle rider injured in collision with pedestrian or animal

Excludes1: *motorcycle rider collision with animal-drawn vehicle or animal being ridden (V26.-)*

The appropriate 7th character is to be added to each code from category V20
A initial encounter
D subsequent encounter
S sequela

- X+7th **V20.0 Motorcycle driver injured in collision with pedestrian or animal in nontraffic accident**
- X+7th **V20.1 Motorcycle passenger injured in collision with pedestrian or animal in nontraffic accident**
- X+7th **V20.2 Unspecified motorcycle rider injured in collision with pedestrian or animal in nontraffic accident**
- X+7th **V20.3 Person boarding or alighting a motorcycle injured in collision with pedestrian or animal**
- X+7th **V20.4 Motorcycle driver injured in collision with pedestrian or animal in traffic accident**
- X+7th **V20.5 Motorcycle passenger injured in collision with pedestrian or animal in traffic accident**
- X+7th **V20.9 Unspecified motorcycle rider injured in collision with pedestrian or animal in traffic accident**

V21 Motorcycle rider injured in collision with pedal cycle

The appropriate 7th character is to be added to each code from category V21
A initial encounter
D subsequent encounter
S sequela

- X+7th **V21.0 Motorcycle driver injured in collision with pedal cycle in nontraffic accident**
- X+7th **V21.1 Motorcycle passenger injured in collision with pedal cycle in nontraffic accident**
- X+7th **V21.2 Unspecified motorcycle rider injured in collision with pedal cycle in nontraffic accident**
- X+7th **V21.3 Person boarding or alighting a motorcycle injured in collision with pedal cycle**
- X+7th **V21.4 Motorcycle driver injured in collision with pedal cycle in traffic accident**
- X+7th **V21.5 Motorcycle passenger injured in collision with pedal cycle in traffic accident**
- X+7th **V21.9 Unspecified motorcycle rider injured in collision with pedal cycle in traffic accident**

V22 Motorcycle rider injured in collision with two- or three-wheeled motor vehicle

The appropriate 7th character is to be added to each code from category V22
A initial encounter
D subsequent encounter
S sequela

- X+7th **V22.0 Motorcycle driver injured in collision with two- or three-wheeled motor vehicle in nontraffic accident**
- X+7th **V22.1 Motorcycle passenger injured in collision with two- or three-wheeled motor vehicle in nontraffic accident**
- X+7th **V22.2 Unspecified motorcycle rider injured in collision with two- or three-wheeled motor vehicle in nontraffic accident**
- X+7th **V22.3 Person boarding or alighting a motorcycle injured in collision with two- or three-wheeled motor vehicle**
- X+7th **V22.4 Motorcycle driver injured in collision with two- or three-wheeled motor vehicle in traffic accident**
- X+7th **V22.5 Motorcycle passenger injured in collision with two- or three-wheeled motor vehicle in traffic accident**
- X+7th **V22.9 Unspecified motorcycle rider injured in collision with two- or three-wheeled motor vehicle in traffic accident**

V23 Motorcycle rider injured in collision with car, pick-up truck or van

The appropriate 7th character is to be added to each code from category V23
A initial encounter
D subsequent encounter
S sequela

- X+7th **V23.0 Motorcycle driver injured in collision with car, pick-up truck or van in nontraffic accident**
- X+7th **V23.1 Motorcycle passenger injured in collision with car, pick-up truck or van in nontraffic accident**
- X+7th **V23.2 Unspecified motorcycle rider injured in collision with car, pick-up truck or van in nontraffic accident**
- X+7th **V23.3 Person boarding or alighting a motorcycle injured in collision with car, pick-up truck or van**
- X+7th **V23.4 Motorcycle driver injured in collision with car, pick-up truck or van in traffic accident**
- X+7th **V23.5 Motorcycle passenger injured in collision with car, pick-up truck or van in traffic accident**
- X+7th **V23.9 Unspecified motorcycle rider injured in collision with car, pick-up truck or van in traffic accident**

V24 Motorcycle rider injured in collision with heavy transport vehicle or bus

Excludes1: *motorcycle rider injured in collision with military vehicle (V29.81)*

The appropriate 7th character is to be added to each code from category V24
A initial encounter
D subsequent encounter
S sequela

- X+7th **V24.0 Motorcycle driver injured in collision with heavy transport vehicle or bus in nontraffic accident**
- X+7th **V24.1 Motorcycle passenger injured in collision with heavy transport vehicle or bus in nontraffic accident**
- X+7th **V24.2 Unspecified motorcycle rider injured in collision with heavy transport vehicle or bus in nontraffic accident**
- X+7th **V24.3 Person boarding or alighting a motorcycle injured in collision with heavy transport vehicle or bus**
- X+7th **V24.4 Motorcycle driver injured in collision with heavy transport vehicle or bus in traffic accident**
- X+7th **V24.5 Motorcycle passenger injured in collision with heavy transport vehicle or bus in traffic accident**
- X+7th **V24.9 Unspecified motorcycle rider injured in collision with heavy transport vehicle or bus in traffic accident**

V25 Motorcycle rider injured in collision with railway train or railway vehicle

The appropriate 7th character is to be added to each code from category V25
A initial encounter
D subsequent encounter
S sequela

X+7th **V25.0 Motorcycle driver injured in collision with railway train or railway vehicle in nontraffic accident**
X+7th **V25.1 Motorcycle passenger injured in collision with railway train or railway vehicle in nontraffic accident**
X+7th **V25.2 Unspecified motorcycle rider injured in collision with railway train or railway vehicle in nontraffic accident**
X+7th **V25.3 Person boarding or alighting a motorcycle injured in collision with railway train or railway vehicle**
X+7th **V25.4 Motorcycle driver injured in collision with railway train or railway vehicle in traffic accident**
X+7th **V25.5 Motorcycle passenger injured in collision with railway train or railway vehicle in traffic accident**
X+7th **V25.9 Unspecified motorcycle rider injured in collision with railway train or railway vehicle in traffic accident**

V26 Motorcycle rider injured in collision with other nonmotor vehicle

Includes: collision with animal-drawn vehicle, animal being ridden, streetcar

The appropriate 7th character is to be added to each code from category V26
A initial encounter
D subsequent encounter
S sequela

X+7th **V26.0 Motorcycle driver injured in collision with other nonmotor vehicle in nontraffic accident**
X+7th **V26.1 Motorcycle passenger injured in collision with other nonmotor vehicle in nontraffic accident**
X+7th **V26.2 Unspecified motorcycle rider injured in collision with other nonmotor vehicle in nontraffic accident**
X+7th **V26.3 Person boarding or alighting a motorcycle injured in collision with other nonmotor vehicle**
X+7th **V26.4 Motorcycle driver injured in collision with other nonmotor vehicle in traffic accident**
X+7th **V26.5 Motorcycle passenger injured in collision with other nonmotor vehicle in traffic accident**
X+7th **V26.9 Unspecified motorcycle rider injured in collision with other nonmotor vehicle in traffic accident**

V27 Motorcycle rider injured in collision with fixed or stationary object

The appropriate 7th character is to be added to each code from category V27
A initial encounter
D subsequent encounter
S sequela

X+7th **V27.0 Motorcycle driver injured in collision with fixed or stationary object in nontraffic accident**
X+7th **V27.1 Motorcycle passenger injured in collision with fixed or stationary object in nontraffic accident**
X+7th **V27.2 Unspecified motorcycle rider injured in collision with fixed or stationary object in nontraffic accident**
X+7th **V27.3 Person boarding or alighting a motorcycle injured in collision with fixed or stationary object**
X+7th **V27.4 Motorcycle driver injured in collision with fixed or stationary object in traffic accident**
X+7th **V27.5 Motorcycle passenger injured in collision with fixed or stationary object in traffic accident**
X+7th **V27.9 Unspecified motorcycle rider injured in collision with fixed or stationary object in traffic accident**

V28 Motorcycle rider injured in noncollision transport accident

Includes: fall or thrown from motorcycle (without antecedent collision)
overturning motorcycle NOS
overturning motorcycle without collision

The appropriate 7th character is to be added to each code from category V28
A initial encounter
D subsequent encounter
S sequela

X+7th **V28.0 Motorcycle driver injured in noncollision transport accident in nontraffic accident**
X+7th **V28.1 Motorcycle passenger injured in noncollision transport accident in nontraffic accident**
X+7th **V28.2 Unspecified motorcycle rider injured in noncollision transport accident in nontraffic accident**
X+7th **V28.3 Person boarding or alighting a motorcycle injured in noncollision transport accident**
X+7th **V28.4 Motorcycle driver injured in noncollision transport accident in traffic accident**
X+7th **V28.5 Motorcycle passenger injured in noncollision transport accident in traffic accident**
X+7th **V28.9 Unspecified motorcycle rider injured in noncollision transport accident in traffic accident**

V29 Motorcycle rider injured in other and unspecified transport accidents

The appropriate 7th character is to be added to each code from category V29
A initial encounter
D subsequent encounter
S sequela

\+ **V29.0 Motorcycle driver injured in collision with other and unspecified motor vehicles in nontraffic accident**
X+7th **V29.00 Motorcycle driver injured in collision with unspecified motor vehicles in nontraffic accident**
X+7th **V29.09 Motorcycle driver injured in collision with other motor vehicles in nontraffic accident**
\+ **V29.1 Motorcycle passenger injured in collision with other and unspecified motor vehicles in nontraffic accident**
X+7th **V29.10 Motorcycle passenger injured in collision with unspecified motor vehicles in nontraffic accident**
X+7th **V29.19 Motorcycle passenger injured in collision with other motor vehicles in nontraffic accident**
\+ **V29.2 Unspecified motorcycle rider injured in collision with other and unspecified motor vehicles in nontraffic accident**
X+7th **V29.20 Unspecified motorcycle rider injured in collision with unspecified motor vehicles in nontraffic accident**
Motorcycle collision NOS, nontraffic
X+7th **V29.29 Unspecified motorcycle rider injured in collision with other motor vehicles in nontraffic accident**
X+7th **V29.3 Motorcycle rider (driver) (passenger) injured in unspecified nontraffic accident**
Motorcycle accident NOS, nontraffic
Motorcycle rider injured in nontraffic accident NOS
\+ **V29.4 Motorcycle driver injured in collision with other and unspecified motor vehicles in traffic accident**
X+7th **V29.40 Motorcycle driver injured in collision with unspecified motor vehicles in traffic accident**
X+7th **V29.49 Motorcycle driver injured in collision with other motor vehicles in traffic accident**
\+ **V29.5 Motorcycle passenger injured in collision with other and unspecified motor vehicles in traffic accident**
X+7th **V29.50 Motorcycle passenger injured in collision with unspecified motor vehicles in traffic accident**
X+7th **V29.59 Motorcycle passenger injured in collision with other motor vehicles in traffic accident**
\+ **V29.6 Unspecified motorcycle rider injured in collision with other and unspecified motor vehicles in traffic accident**
X+7th **V29.60 Unspecified motorcycle rider injured in collision with unspecified motor vehicles in traffic accident**
Motorcycle collision NOS (traffic)
X+7th **V29.69 Unspecified motorcycle rider injured in collision with other motor vehicles in traffic accident**
\+ **V29.8 Motorcycle rider (driver) (passenger) injured in other specified transport accidents**
X+7th **V29.81 Motorcycle rider (driver) (passenger) injured in transport accident with military vehicle**
X+7th **V29.88 Motorcycle rider (driver) (passenger) injured in other specified transport accidents**
X+7th **V29.9 Motorcycle rider (driver) (passenger) injured in unspecified traffic accident**
Motorcycle accident NOS

Occupant of three-wheeled motor vehicle injured in transport accident (V30-V39)

Includes: motorized tricycle
motorized rickshaw
three-wheeled motor car

Excludes1: *all-terrain vehicles (V86.-)*
motorcycle with sidecar (V20-V29)
vehicle designed primarily for off-road use (V86.-)

V30 Occupant of three-wheeled motor vehicle injured in collision with pedestrian or animal

Excludes1: *three-wheeled motor vehicle collision with animal-drawn vehicle or animal being ridden (V36.-)*

The appropriate 7th character is to be added to each code from category V30
A initial encounter
D subsequent encounter
S sequela

X+7th **V30.0 Driver of three-wheeled motor vehicle injured in collision with pedestrian or animal in nontraffic accident**
X+7th **V30.1 Passenger in three-wheeled motor vehicle injured in collision with pedestrian or animal in nontraffic accident**
X+7th **V30.2 Person on outside of three-wheeled motor vehicle injured in collision with pedestrian or animal in nontraffic accident**
X+7th **V30.3 Unspecified occupant of three-wheeled motor vehicle injured in collision with pedestrian or animal in nontraffic accident**
X+7th **V30.4 Person boarding or alighting a three-wheeled motor vehicle injured in collision with pedestrian or animal**
X+7th **V30.5 Driver of three-wheeled motor vehicle injured in collision with pedestrian or animal in traffic accident**
X+7th **V30.6 Passenger in three-wheeled motor vehicle injured in collision with pedestrian or animal in traffic accident**
X+7th **V30.7 Person on outside of three-wheeled motor vehicle injured in collision with pedestrian or animal in traffic accident**
X+7th **V30.9 Unspecified occupant of three-wheeled motor vehicle injured in collision with pedestrian or animal in traffic accident**

V31 Occupant of three-wheeled motor vehicle injured in collision with pedal cycle

The appropriate 7th character is to be added to each code from category V31
A initial encounter
D subsequent encounter
S sequela

X+7th **V31.0 Driver of three-wheeled motor vehicle injured in collision with pedal cycle in nontraffic accident**
X+7th **V31.1 Passenger in three-wheeled motor vehicle injured in collision with pedal cycle in nontraffic accident**
X+7th **V31.2 Person on outside of three-wheeled motor vehicle injured in collision with pedal cycle in nontraffic accident**
X+7th **V31.3 Unspecified occupant of three-wheeled motor vehicle injured in collision with pedal cycle in nontraffic accident**
X+7th **V31.4 Person boarding or alighting a three-wheeled motor vehicle injured in collision with pedal cycle**
X+7th **V31.5 Driver of three-wheeled motor vehicle injured in collision with pedal cycle in traffic accident**
X+7th **V31.6 Passenger in three-wheeled motor vehicle injured in collision with pedal cycle in traffic accident**
X+7th **V31.7 Person on outside of three-wheeled motor vehicle injured in collision with pedal cycle in traffic accident**
X+7th **V31.9 Unspecified occupant of three-wheeled motor vehicle injured in collision with pedal cycle in traffic accident**

V32 Occupant of three-wheeled motor vehicle injured in collision with two- or three-wheeled motor vehicle

The appropriate 7th character is to be added to each code from category V32
A initial encounter
D subsequent encounter
S sequela

X+7th **V32.0 Driver of three-wheeled motor vehicle injured in collision with two- or three-wheeled motor vehicle in nontraffic accident**
X+7th **V32.1 Passenger in three-wheeled motor vehicle injured in collision with two- or three-wheeled motor vehicle in nontraffic accident**
X+7th **V32.2 Person on outside of three-wheeled motor vehicle injured in collision with two- or three-wheeled motor vehicle in nontraffic accident**
X+7th **V32.3 Unspecified occupant of three-wheeled motor vehicle injured in collision with two- or three-wheeled motor vehicle in nontraffic accident**
X+7th **V32.4 Person boarding or alighting a three-wheeled motor vehicle injured in collision with two- or three-wheeled motor vehicle**
X+7th **V32.5 Driver of three-wheeled motor vehicle injured in collision with two- or three-wheeled motor vehicle in traffic accident**
X+7th **V32.6 Passenger in three-wheeled motor vehicle injured in collision with two- or three-wheeled motor vehicle in traffic accident**
X+7th **V32.7 Person on outside of three-wheeled motor vehicle injured in collision with two- or three-wheeled motor vehicle in traffic accident**
X+7th **V32.9 Unspecified occupant of three-wheeled motor vehicle injured in collision with two- or three-wheeled motor vehicle in traffic accident**

V33 Occupant of three-wheeled motor vehicle injured in collision with car, pick-up truck or van

The appropriate 7th character is to be added to each code from category V33
A initial encounter
D subsequent encounter
S sequela

X+7th **V33.0 Driver of three-wheeled motor vehicle injured in collision with car, pick-up truck or van in nontraffic accident**
X+7th **V33.1 Passenger in three-wheeled motor vehicle injured in collision with car, pick-up truck or van in nontraffic accident**
X+7th **V33.2 Person on outside of three-wheeled motor vehicle injured in collision with car, pick-up truck or van in nontraffic accident**
X+7th **V33.3 Unspecified occupant of three-wheeled motor vehicle injured in collision with car, pick-up truck or van in nontraffic accident**
X+7th **V33.4 Person boarding or alighting a three-wheeled motor vehicle injured in collision with car, pick-up truck or van**
X+7th **V33.5 Driver of three-wheeled motor vehicle injured in collision with car, pick-up truck or van in traffic accident**
X+7th **V33.6 Passenger in three-wheeled motor vehicle injured in collision with car, pick-up truck or van in traffic accident**
X+7th **V33.7 Person on outside of three-wheeled motor vehicle injured in collision with car, pick-up truck or van in traffic accident**
X+7th **V33.9 Unspecified occupant of three-wheeled motor vehicle injured in collision with car, pick-up truck or van in traffic accident**

V34 Occupant of three-wheeled motor vehicle injured in collision with heavy transport vehicle or bus

Excludes1: *occupant of three-wheeled motor vehicle injured in collision with military vehicle (V39.81)*

The appropriate 7th character is to be added to each code from category V34
A initial encounter
D subsequent encounter
S sequela

X+7th **V34.0 Driver of three-wheeled motor vehicle injured in collision with heavy transport vehicle or bus in nontraffic accident**
X+7th **V34.1 Passenger in three-wheeled motor vehicle injured in collision with heavy transport vehicle or bus in nontraffic accident**
X+7th **V34.2 Person on outside of three-wheeled motor vehicle injured in collision with heavy transport vehicle or bus in nontraffic accident**
X+7th **V34.3 Unspecified occupant of three-wheeled motor vehicle injured in collision with heavy transport vehicle or bus in nontraffic accident**
X+7th **V34.4 Person boarding or alighting a three-wheeled motor vehicle injured in collision with heavy transport vehicle or bus**
X+7th **V34.5 Driver of three-wheeled motor vehicle injured in collision with heavy transport vehicle or bus in traffic accident**
X+7th **V34.6 Passenger in three-wheeled motor vehicle injured in collision with heavy transport vehicle or bus in traffic accident**
X+7th **V34.7 Person on outside of three-wheeled motor vehicle injured in collision with heavy transport vehicle or bus in traffic accident**
X+7th **V34.9 Unspecified occupant of three-wheeled motor vehicle injured in collision with heavy transport vehicle or bus in traffic accident**

V35 Occupant of three-wheeled motor vehicle injured in collision with railway train or railway vehicle

The appropriate 7th character is to be added to each code from category V35
A initial encounter
D subsequent encounter
S sequela

X+7th **V35.0 Driver of three-wheeled motor vehicle injured in collision with railway train or railway vehicle in nontraffic accident**
X+7th **V35.1 Passenger in three-wheeled motor vehicle injured in collision with railway train or railway vehicle in nontraffic accident**
X+7th **V35.2 Person on outside of three-wheeled motor vehicle injured in collision with railway train or railway vehicle in nontraffic accident**
X+7th **V35.3 Unspecified occupant of three-wheeled motor vehicle injured in collision with railway train or railway vehicle in nontraffic accident**
X+7th **V35.4 Person boarding or alighting a three-wheeled motor vehicle injured in collision with railway train or railway vehicle**
X+7th **V35.5 Driver of three-wheeled motor vehicle injured in collision with railway train or railway vehicle in traffic accident**
X+7th **V35.6 Passenger in three-wheeled motor vehicle injured in collision with railway train or railway vehicle in traffic accident**
X+7th **V35.7 Person on outside of three-wheeled motor vehicle injured in collision with railway train or railway vehicle in traffic accident**
X+7th **V35.9 Unspecified occupant of three-wheeled motor vehicle injured in collision with railway train or railway vehicle in traffic accident**

V36 Occupant of three-wheeled motor vehicle injured in collision with other nonmotor vehicle

Includes: collision with animal-drawn vehicle, animal being ridden, streetcar

The appropriate 7th character is to be added to each code from category V36
A initial encounter
D subsequent encounter
S sequela

X+7th **V36.0 Driver of three-wheeled motor vehicle injured in collision with other nonmotor vehicle in nontraffic accident**
X+7th **V36.1 Passenger in three-wheeled motor vehicle injured in collision with other nonmotor vehicle in nontraffic accident**
X+7th **V36.2 Person on outside of three-wheeled motor vehicle injured in collision with other nonmotor vehicle in nontraffic accident**
X+7th **V36.3 Unspecified occupant of three-wheeled motor vehicle injured in collision with other nonmotor vehicle in nontraffic accident**
X+7th **V36.4 Person boarding or alighting a three-wheeled motor vehicle injured in collision with other nonmotor vehicle**
X+7th **V36.5 Driver of three-wheeled motor vehicle injured in collision with other nonmotor vehicle in traffic accident**
X+7th **V36.6 Passenger in three-wheeled motor vehicle injured in collision with other nonmotor vehicle in traffic accident**
X+7th **V36.7 Person on outside of three-wheeled motor vehicle injured in collision with other nonmotor vehicle in traffic accident**
X+7th **V36.9 Unspecified occupant of three-wheeled motor vehicle injured in collision with other nonmotor vehicle in traffic accident**

V37 Occupant of three-wheeled motor vehicle injured in collision with fixed or stationary object

The appropriate 7th character is to be added to each code from category V37
A initial encounter
D subsequent encounter
S sequela

X+7th **V37.0 Driver of three-wheeled motor vehicle injured in collision with fixed or stationary object in nontraffic accident**
X+7th **V37.1 Passenger in three-wheeled motor vehicle injured in collision with fixed or stationary object in nontraffic accident**
X+7th **V37.2 Person on outside of three-wheeled motor vehicle injured in collision with fixed or stationary object in nontraffic accident**
X+7th **V37.3 Unspecified occupant of three-wheeled motor vehicle injured in collision with fixed or stationary object in nontraffic accident**
X+7th **V37.4 Person boarding or alighting a three-wheeled motor vehicle injured in collision with fixed or stationary object**
X+7th **V37.5 Driver of three-wheeled motor vehicle injured in collision with fixed or stationary object in traffic accident**
X+7th **V37.6 Passenger in three-wheeled motor vehicle injured in collision with fixed or stationary object in traffic accident**
X+7th **V37.7 Person on outside of three-wheeled motor vehicle injured in collision with fixed or stationary object in traffic accident**
X+7th **V37.9 Unspecified occupant of three-wheeled motor vehicle injured in collision with fixed or stationary object in traffic accident**

V38 Occupant of three-wheeled motor vehicle injured in noncollision transport accident

Includes: fall or thrown from three-wheeled motor vehicle
overturning of three-wheeled motor vehicle NOS
overturning of three-wheeled motor vehicle without collision

The appropriate 7th character is to be added to each code from category V38
A initial encounter
D subsequent encounter
S sequela

X+7th **V38.0 Driver of three-wheeled motor vehicle injured in noncollision transport accident in nontraffic accident**
X+7th **V38.1 Passenger in three-wheeled motor vehicle injured in noncollision transport accident in nontraffic accident**
X+7th **V38.2 Person on outside of three-wheeled motor vehicle injured in noncollision transport accident in nontraffic accident**
X+7th **V38.3 Unspecified occupant of three-wheeled motor vehicle injured in noncollision transport accident in nontraffic accident**
X+7th **V38.4 Person boarding or alighting a three-wheeled motor vehicle injured in noncollision transport accident**
X+7th **V38.5 Driver of three-wheeled motor vehicle injured in noncollision transport accident in traffic accident**
X+7th **V38.6 Passenger in three-wheeled motor vehicle injured in noncollision transport accident in traffic accident**
X+7th **V38.7 Person on outside of three-wheeled motor vehicle injured in noncollision transport accident in traffic accident**
X+7th **V38.9 Unspecified occupant of three-wheeled motor vehicle injured in noncollision transport accident in traffic accident**

V39 Occupant of three-wheeled motor vehicle injured in other and unspecified transport accidents

The appropriate 7th character is to be added to each code from category V39
A initial encounter
D subsequent encounter
S sequela

+ **V39.0 Driver of three-wheeled motor vehicle injured in collision with other and unspecified motor vehicles in nontraffic accident**
  - X+7th **V39.00 Driver of three-wheeled motor vehicle injured in collision with unspecified motor vehicles in nontraffic accident**
  - X+7th **V39.09 Driver of three-wheeled motor vehicle injured in collision with other motor vehicles in nontraffic accident**
+ **V39.1 Passenger in three-wheeled motor vehicle injured in collision with other and unspecified motor vehicles in nontraffic accident**
  - X+7th **V39.10 Passenger in three-wheeled motor vehicle injured in collision with unspecified motor vehicles in nontraffic accident**
  - X+7th **V39.19 Passenger in three-wheeled motor vehicle injured in collision with other motor vehicles in nontraffic accident**
+ **V39.2 Unspecified occupant of three-wheeled motor vehicle injured in collision with other and unspecified motor vehicles in nontraffic accident**
  - X+7th **V39.20 Unspecified occupant of three-wheeled motor vehicle injured in collision with unspecified motor vehicles in nontraffic accident**
    Collision NOS involving three-wheeled motor vehicle, nontraffic
  - X+7th **V39.29 Unspecified occupant of three-wheeled motor vehicle injured in collision with other motor vehicles in nontraffic accident**

X+7th **V39.3 Occupant (driver) (passenger) of three-wheeled motor vehicle injured in unspecified nontraffic accident**
Accident NOS involving three-wheeled motor vehicle, nontraffic
Occupant of three-wheeled motor vehicle injured in nontraffic accident NOS

\+ **V39.4 Driver of three-wheeled motor vehicle injured in collision with other and unspecified motor vehicles in traffic accident**

X+7th **V39.40 Driver of three-wheeled motor vehicle injured in collision with unspecified motor vehicles in traffic accident**

X+7th **V39.49 Driver of three-wheeled motor vehicle injured in collision with other motor vehicles in traffic accident**

\+ **V39.5 Passenger in three-wheeled motor vehicle injured in collision with other and unspecified motor vehicles in traffic accident**

X+7th **V39.50 Passenger in three-wheeled motor vehicle injured in collision with unspecified motor vehicles in traffic accident**

X+7th **V39.59 Passenger in three-wheeled motor vehicle injured in collision with other motor vehicles in traffic accident**

\+ **V39.6 Unspecified occupant of three-wheeled motor vehicle injured in collision with other and unspecified motor vehicles in traffic accident**

X+7th **V39.60 Unspecified occupant of three-wheeled motor vehicle injured in collision with unspecified motor vehicles in traffic accident**
Collision NOS involving three-wheeled motor vehicle (traffic)

X+7th **V39.69 Unspecified occupant of three-wheeled motor vehicle injured in collision with other motor vehicles in traffic accident**

\+ **V39.8 Occupant (driver) (passenger) of three-wheeled motor vehicle injured in other specified transport accidents**

X+7th **V39.81 Occupant (driver) (passenger) of three-wheeled motor vehicle injured in transport accident with military vehicle**

X+7th **V39.89 Occupant (driver) (passenger) of three-wheeled motor vehicle injured in other specified transport accidents**

X+7th **V39.9 Occupant (driver) (passenger) of three-wheeled motor vehicle injured in unspecified traffic accident**
Accident NOS involving three-wheeled motor vehicle

Car occupant injured in transport accident (V40-V49)

Includes: a four-wheeled motor vehicle designed primarily for carrying passengers
automobile (pulling a trailer or camper)

Excludes1: *bus (V50-V59)*
minibus (V50-V59)
minivan (V50-V59)
motorcoach (V70-V79)
pick-up truck (V50-V59)
sport utility vehicle (SUV) (V50-V59)

V40 Car occupant injured in collision with pedestrian or animal

Excludes1: *car collision with animal-drawn vehicle or animal being ridden (V46.-)*

The appropriate 7th character is to be added to each code from category V40
A initial encounter
D subsequent encounter
S sequela

X+7th **V40.0 Car driver injured in collision with pedestrian or animal in nontraffic accident**

X+7th **V40.1 Car passenger injured in collision with pedestrian or animal in nontraffic accident**

X+7th **V40.2 Person on outside of car injured in collision with pedestrian or animal in nontraffic accident**

X+7th **V40.3 Unspecified car occupant injured in collision with pedestrian or animal in nontraffic accident**

X+7th **V40.4 Person boarding or alighting a car injured in collision with pedestrian or animal**

X+7th **V40.5 Car driver injured in collision with pedestrian or animal in traffic accident**

X+7th **V40.6 Car passenger injured in collision with pedestrian or animal in traffic accident**

X+7th **V40.7 Person on outside of car injured in collision with pedestrian or animal in traffic accident**

X+7th **V40.9 Unspecified car occupant injured in collision with pedestrian or animal in traffic accident**

V41 Car occupant injured in collision with pedal cycle

The appropriate 7th character is to be added to each code from category V41
A initial encounter
D subsequent encounter
S sequela

X+7th **V41.0 Car driver injured in collision with pedal cycle in nontraffic accident**

X+7th **V41.1 Car passenger injured in collision with pedal cycle in nontraffic accident**

X+7th **V41.2 Person on outside of car injured in collision with pedal cycle in nontraffic accident**

X+7th **V41.3 Unspecified car occupant injured in collision with pedal cycle in nontraffic accident**

X+7th **V41.4 Person boarding or alighting a car injured in collision with pedal cycle**

X+7th **V41.5 Car driver injured in collision with pedal cycle in traffic accident**

X+7th **V41.6 Car passenger injured in collision with pedal cycle in traffic accident**

X+7th **V41.7 Person on outside of car injured in collision with pedal cycle in traffic accident**

X+7th **V41.9 Unspecified car occupant injured in collision with pedal cycle in traffic accident**

V42 Car occupant injured in collision with two- or three-wheeled motor vehicle

The appropriate 7th character is to be added to each code from category V42
A initial encounter
D subsequent encounter
S sequela

X+7th **V42.0 Car driver injured in collision with two- or three-wheeled motor vehicle in nontraffic accident**

X+7th **V42.1 Car passenger injured in collision with two- or three-wheeled motor vehicle in nontraffic accident**

X+7th **V42.2 Person on outside of car injured in collision with two- or three-wheeled motor vehicle in nontraffic accident**

X+7th **V42.3 Unspecified car occupant injured in collision with two- or three-wheeled motor vehicle in nontraffic accident**

X+7th **V42.4 Person boarding or alighting a car injured in collision with two- or three-wheeled motor vehicle**

X+7th **V42.5 Car driver injured in collision with two- or three-wheeled motor vehicle in traffic accident**

X+7th **V42.6 Car passenger injured in collision with two- or three-wheeled motor vehicle in traffic accident**

X+7th **V42.7 Person on outside of car injured in collision with two- or three-wheeled motor vehicle in traffic accident**

X+7th **V42.9 Unspecified car occupant injured in collision with two- or three-wheeled motor vehicle in traffic accident**

V43 Car occupant injured in collision with car, pick-up truck or van

The appropriate 7th character is to be added to each code from category V43
A initial encounter
D subsequent encounter
S sequela

\+ **V43.0 Car driver injured in collision with car, pick-up truck or van in nontraffic accident**

X+7th **V43.01 Car driver injured in collision with sport utility vehicle in nontraffic accident**

X+7th **V43.02 Car driver injured in collision with other type car in nontraffic accident**

X+7th **V43.03 Car driver injured in collision with pick-up truck in nontraffic accident**

X+7th **V43.04 Car driver injured in collision with van in nontraffic accident**

+ **V43.1 Car passenger injured in collision with car, pick-up truck or van in nontraffic accident**

X+7th **V43.11 Car passenger injured in collision with sport utility vehicle in nontraffic accident**

X+7th **V43.12 Car passenger injured in collision with other type car in nontraffic accident**

X+7th **V43.13 Car passenger injured in collision with pick-up truck in nontraffic accident**

X+7th **V43.14 Car passenger injured in collision with van in nontraffic accident**

+ **V43.2 Person on outside of car injured in collision with car, pick-up truck or van in nontraffic accident**

X+7th **V43.21 Person on outside of car injured in collision with sport utility vehicle in nontraffic accident**

X+7th **V43.22 Person on outside of car injured in collision with other type car in nontraffic accident**

X+7th **V43.23 Person on outside of car injured in collision with pick-up truck in nontraffic accident**

X+7th **V43.24 Person on outside of car injured in collision with van in nontraffic accident**

+ **V43.3 Unspecified car occupant injured in collision with car, pick-up truck or van in nontraffic accident**

X+7th **V43.31 Unspecified car occupant injured in collision with sport utility vehicle in nontraffic accident**

X+7th **V43.32 Unspecified car occupant injured in collision with other type car in nontraffic accident**

X+7th **V43.33 Unspecified car occupant injured in collision with pick-up truck in nontraffic accident**

X+7th **V43.34 Unspecified car occupant injured in collision with van in nontraffic accident**

+ **V43.4 Person boarding or alighting a car injured in collision with car, pick-up truck or van**

X+7th **V43.41 Person boarding or alighting a car injured in collision with sport utility vehicle**

X+7th **V43.42 Person boarding or alighting a car injured in collision with other type car**

X+7th **V43.43 Person boarding or alighting a car injured in collision with pick-up truck**

X+7th **V43.44 Person boarding or alighting a car injured in collision with van**

+ **V43.5 Car driver injured in collision with car, pick-up truck or van in traffic accident**

X+7th **V43.51 Car driver injured in collision with sport utility vehicle in traffic accident**

X+7th **V43.52 Car driver injured in collision with other type car in traffic accident**

X+7th **V43.53 Car driver injured in collision with pick-up truck in traffic accident**

X+7th **V43.54 Car driver injured in collision with van in traffic accident**

+ **V43.6 Car passenger injured in collision with car, pick-up truck or van in traffic accident**

X+7th **V43.61 Car passenger injured in collision with sport utility vehicle in traffic accident**

AHA CC: 1Q, 2015, 3-21

X+7th **V43.62 Car passenger injured in collision with other type car in traffic accident**

X+7th **V43.63 Car passenger injured in collision with pick-up truck in traffic accident**

X+7th **V43.64 Car passenger injured in collision with van in traffic accident**

+ **V43.7 Person on outside of car injured in collision with car, pick-up truck or van in traffic accident**

X+7th **V43.71 Person on outside of car injured in collision with sport utility vehicle in traffic accident**

X+7th **V43.72 Person on outside of car injured in collision with other type car in traffic accident**

X+7th **V43.73 Person on outside of car injured in collision with pick-up truck in traffic accident**

X+7th **V43.74 Person on outside of car injured in collision with van in traffic accident**

+ **V43.9 Unspecified car occupant injured in collision with car, pick-up truck or van in traffic accident**

X+7th **V43.91 Unspecified car occupant injured in collision with sport utility vehicle in traffic accident**

X+7th **V43.92 Unspecified car occupant injured in collision with other type car in traffic accident**

X+7th **V43.93 Unspecified car occupant injured in collision with pick-up truck in traffic accident**

X+7th **V43.94 Unspecified car occupant injured in collision with van in traffic accident**

V44 Car occupant injured in collision with heavy transport vehicle or bus

Excludes1: *car occupant injured in collision with military vehicle (V49.81)*

The appropriate 7th character is to be added to each code from category V44
A initial encounter
D subsequent encounter
S sequela

X+7th **V44.0 Car driver injured in collision with heavy transport vehicle or bus in nontraffic accident**

X+7th **V44.1 Car passenger injured in collision with heavy transport vehicle or bus in nontraffic accident**

X+7th **V44.2 Person on outside of car injured in collision with heavy transport vehicle or bus in nontraffic accident**

X+7th **V44.3 Unspecified car occupant injured in collision with heavy transport vehicle or bus in nontraffic accident**

X+7th **V44.4 Person boarding or alighting a car injured in collision with heavy transport vehicle or bus**

X+7th **V44.5 Car driver injured in collision with heavy transport vehicle or bus in traffic accident**

X+7th **V44.6 Car passenger injured in collision with heavy transport vehicle or bus in traffic accident**

X+7th **V44.7 Person on outside of car injured in collision with heavy transport vehicle or bus in traffic accident**

X+7th **V44.9 Unspecified car occupant injured in collision with heavy transport vehicle or bus in traffic accident**

V45 Car occupant injured in collision with railway train or railway vehicle

The appropriate 7th character is to be added to each code from category V45
A initial encounter
D subsequent encounter
S sequela

X+7th **V45.0 Car driver injured in collision with railway train or railway vehicle in nontraffic accident**

X+7th **V45.1 Car passenger injured in collision with railway train or railway vehicle in nontraffic accident**

X+7th **V45.2 Person on outside of car injured in collision with railway train or railway vehicle in nontraffic accident**

X+7th **V45.3 Unspecified car occupant injured in collision with railway train or railway vehicle in nontraffic accident**

X+7th **V45.4 Person boarding or alighting a car injured in collision with railway train or railway vehicle**

X+7th **V45.5 Car driver injured in collision with railway train or railway vehicle in traffic accident**

X+7th **V45.6 Car passenger injured in collision with railway train or railway vehicle in traffic accident**

X+7th **V45.7 Person on outside of car injured in collision with railway train or railway vehicle in traffic accident**

X+7th **V45.9 Unspecified car occupant injured in collision with railway train or railway vehicle in traffic accident**

V46 Car occupant injured in collision with other nonmotor vehicle

Includes: collision with animal-drawn vehicle, animal being ridden, streetcar

The appropriate 7th character is to be added to each code from category V46
A initial encounter
D subsequent encounter
S sequela

X+7th **V46.0 Car driver injured in collision with other nonmotor vehicle in nontraffic accident**

X+7th **V46.1 Car passenger injured in collision with other nonmotor vehicle in nontraffic accident**

X+7th **V46.2 Person on outside of car injured in collision with other nonmotor vehicle in nontraffic accident**

X+7th **V46.3 Unspecified car occupant injured in collision with other nonmotor vehicle in nontraffic accident**

X+7th **V46.4 Person boarding or alighting a car injured in collision with other nonmotor vehicle**

X+7th **V46.5 Car driver injured in collision with other nonmotor vehicle in traffic accident**

X+7th **V46.6 Car passenger injured in collision with other nonmotor vehicle in traffic accident**

X+7th **V46.7 Person on outside of car injured in collision with other nonmotor vehicle in traffic accident**

X+7th **V46.9 Unspecified car occupant injured in collision with other nonmotor vehicle in traffic accident**

V47 Car occupant injured in collision with fixed or stationary object

AHA CC: 4Q, 2016, 73

The appropriate 7th character is to be added to each code from category V47
A initial encounter
D subsequent encounter
S sequela

X+7th **V47.0 Car driver injured in collision with fixed or stationary object in nontraffic accident**

X+7th **V47.1 Car passenger injured in collision with fixed or stationary object in nontraffic accident**

X+7th **V47.2 Person on outside of car injured in collision with fixed or stationary object in nontraffic accident**

X+7th **V47.3 Unspecified car occupant injured in collision with fixed or stationary object in nontraffic accident**

X+7th **V47.4 Person boarding or alighting a car injured in collision with fixed or stationary object**

X+7th **V47.5 Car driver injured in collision with fixed or stationary object in traffic accident**

X+7th **V47.6 Car passenger injured in collision with fixed or stationary object in traffic accident**

X+7th **V47.7 Person on outside of car injured in collision with fixed or stationary object in traffic accident**

X+7th **V47.9 Unspecified car occupant injured in collision with fixed or stationary object in traffic accident**

V48 Car occupant injured in noncollision transport accident

Includes: overturning car NOS
overturning car without collision

The appropriate 7th character is to be added to each code from category V48
A initial encounter
D subsequent encounter
S sequela

X+7th **V48.0 Car driver injured in noncollision transport accident in nontraffic accident**

X+7th **V48.1 Car passenger injured in noncollision transport accident in nontraffic accident**

X+7th **V48.2 Person on outside of car injured in noncollision transport accident in nontraffic accident**

X+7th **V48.3 Unspecified car occupant injured in noncollision transport accident in nontraffic accident**

X+7th **V48.4 Person boarding or alighting a car injured in noncollision transport accident**

X+7th **V48.5 Car driver injured in noncollision transport accident in traffic accident**

X+7th **V48.6 Car passenger injured in noncollision transport accident in traffic accident**

X+7th **V48.7 Person on outside of car injured in noncollision transport accident in traffic accident**

X+7th **V48.9 Unspecified car occupant injured in noncollision transport accident in traffic accident**

V49 Car occupant injured in other and unspecified transport accidents

The appropriate 7th character is to be added to each code from category V49
A initial encounter
D subsequent encounter
S sequela

\+ **V49.0 Driver injured in collision with other and unspecified motor vehicles in nontraffic accident**

X+7th **V49.00 Driver injured in collision with unspecified motor vehicles in nontraffic accident**

X+7th **V49.09 Driver injured in collision with other motor vehicles in nontraffic accident**

\+ **V49.1 Passenger injured in collision with other and unspecified motor vehicles in nontraffic accident**

X+7th **V49.10 Passenger injured in collision with unspecified motor vehicles in nontraffic accident**

X+7th **V49.19 Passenger injured in collision with other motor vehicles in nontraffic accident**

\+ **V49.2 Unspecified car occupant injured in collision with other and unspecified motor vehicles in nontraffic accident**

X+7th **V49.20 Unspecified car occupant injured in collision with unspecified motor vehicles in nontraffic accident**
Car collision NOS, nontraffic

X+7th **V49.29 Unspecified car occupant injured in collision with other motor vehicles in nontraffic accident**

X+7th **V49.3 Car occupant (driver) (passenger) injured in unspecified nontraffic accident**
Car accident NOS, nontraffic
Car occupant injured in nontraffic accident NOS

\+ **V49.4 Driver injured in collision with other and unspecified motor vehicles in traffic accident**

X+7th **V49.40 Driver injured in collision with unspecified motor vehicles in traffic accident**

X+7th **V49.49 Driver injured in collision with other motor vehicles in traffic accident**

\+ **V49.5 Passenger injured in collision with other and unspecified motor vehicles in traffic accident**

X+7th **V49.50 Passenger injured in collision with unspecified motor vehicles in traffic accident**

X+7th **V49.59 Passenger injured in collision with other motor vehicles in traffic accident**

\+ **V49.6 Unspecified car occupant injured in collision with other and unspecified motor vehicles in traffic accident**

X+7th **V49.60 Unspecified car occupant injured in collision with unspecified motor vehicles in traffic accident**
Car collision NOS (traffic)

X+7th **V49.69 Unspecified car occupant injured in collision with other motor vehicles in traffic accident**

\+ **V49.8 Car occupant (driver) (passenger) injured in other specified transport accidents**

X+7th **V49.81 Car occupant (driver) (passenger) injured in transport accident with military vehicle**

X+7th **V49.88 Car occupant (driver) (passenger) injured in other specified transport accidents**

X+7th **V49.9 Car occupant (driver) (passenger) injured in unspecified traffic accident**
Car accident NOS
AHA CC: 1Q, 2015, 3-21

Occupant of pick-up truck or van injured in transport accident (V50-V59)

Includes: a four or six wheel motor vehicle designed primarily for carrying passengers and property but weighing less than the local limit for classification as a heavy goods vehicle
minibus
minivan
sport utility vehicle (SUV)
truck
van

Excludes1: *heavy transport vehicle (V60-V69)*

V50 Occupant of pick-up truck or van injured in collision with pedestrian or animal

Excludes1: *pick-up truck or van collision with animal-drawn vehicle or animal being ridden (V56.-)*

The appropriate 7th character is to be added to each code from category V50
A initial encounter
D subsequent encounter
S sequela

X+7th **V50.0 Driver of pick-up truck or van injured in collision with pedestrian or animal in nontraffic accident**

X+7th **V50.1 Passenger in pick-up truck or van injured in collision with pedestrian or animal in nontraffic accident**

X+7th **V50.2 Person on outside of pick-up truck or van injured in collision with pedestrian or animal in nontraffic accident**

X+7th **V50.3 Unspecified occupant of pick-up truck or van injured in collision with pedestrian or animal in nontraffic accident**

X+7th **V50.4 Person boarding or alighting a pick-up truck or van injured in collision with pedestrian or animal**

X+7th **V50.5 Driver of pick-up truck or van injured in collision with pedestrian or animal in traffic accident**

X+7th **V50.6 Passenger in pick-up truck or van injured in collision with pedestrian or animal in traffic accident**

X+7th **V50.7 Person on outside of pick-up truck or van injured in collision with pedestrian or animal in traffic accident**

X+7th **V50.9 Unspecified occupant of pick-up truck or van injured in collision with pedestrian or animal in traffic accident**

V51 Occupant of pick-up truck or van injured in collision with pedal cycle

The appropriate 7th character is to be added to each code from category V51
A initial encounter
D subsequent encounter
S sequela

X+7th **V51.0** **Driver of pick-up truck or van injured in collision with pedal cycle in nontraffic accident**

X+7th **V51.1** **Passenger in pick-up truck or van injured in collision with pedal cycle in nontraffic accident**

X+7th **V51.2** **Person on outside of pick-up truck or van injured in collision with pedal cycle in nontraffic accident**

X+7th **V51.3** **Unspecified occupant of pick-up truck or van injured in collision with pedal cycle in nontraffic accident**

X+7th **V51.4** **Person boarding or alighting a pick-up truck or van injured in collision with pedal cycle**

X+7th **V51.5** **Driver of pick-up truck or van injured in collision with pedal cycle in traffic accident**

X+7th **V51.6** **Passenger in pick-up truck or van injured in collision with pedal cycle in traffic accident**

X+7th **V51.7** **Person on outside of pick-up truck or van injured in collision with pedal cycle in traffic accident**

X+7th **V51.9** **Unspecified occupant of pick-up truck or van injured in collision with pedal cycle in traffic accident**

V52 **Occupant of pick-up truck or van injured in collision with two- or three-wheeled motor vehicle**

The appropriate 7th character is to be added to each code from category V52
A initial encounter
D subsequent encounter
S sequela

X+7th **V52.0** **Driver of pick-up truck or van injured in collision with two- or three-wheeled motor vehicle in nontraffic accident**

X+7th **V52.1** **Passenger in pick-up truck or van injured in collision with two- or three-wheeled motor vehicle in nontraffic accident**

X+7th **V52.2** **Person on outside of pick-up truck or van injured in collision with two- or three-wheeled motor vehicle in nontraffic accident**

X+7th **V52.3** **Unspecified occupant of pick-up truck or van injured in collision with two- or three-wheeled motor vehicle in nontraffic accident**

X+7th **V52.4** **Person boarding or alighting a pick-up truck or van injured in collision with two- or three-wheeled motor vehicle**

X+7th **V52.5** **Driver of pick-up truck or van injured in collision with two- or three-wheeled motor vehicle in traffic accident**

X+7th **V52.6** **Passenger in pick-up truck or van injured in collision with two- or three-wheeled motor vehicle in traffic accident**

X+7th **V52.7** **Person on outside of pick-up truck or van injured in collision with two- or three-wheeled motor vehicle in traffic accident**

X+7th **V52.9** **Unspecified occupant of pick-up truck or van injured in collision with two- or three-wheeled motor vehicle in traffic accident**

V53 **Occupant of pick-up truck or van injured in collision with car, pick-up truck or van**

The appropriate 7th character is to be added to each code from category V53
A initial encounter
D subsequent encounter
S sequela

X+7th **V53.0** **Driver of pick-up truck or van injured in collision with car, pick-up truck or van in nontraffic accident**

X+7th **V53.1** **Passenger in pick-up truck or van injured in collision with car, pick-up truck or van in nontraffic accident**

X+7th **V53.2** **Person on outside of pick-up truck or van injured in collision with car, pick-up truck or van in nontraffic accident**

X+7th **V53.3** **Unspecified occupant of pick-up truck or van injured in collision with car, pick-up truck or van in nontraffic accident**

X+7th **V53.4** **Person boarding or alighting a pick-up truck or van injured in collision with car, pick-up truck or van**

X+7th **V53.5** **Driver of pick-up truck or van injured in collision with car, pick-up truck or van in traffic accident**

X+7th **V53.6** **Passenger in pick-up truck or van injured in collision with car, pick-up truck or van in traffic accident**

X+7th **V53.7** **Person on outside of pick-up truck or van injured in collision with car, pick-up truck or van in traffic accident**

X+7th **V53.9** **Unspecified occupant of pick-up truck or van injured in collision with car, pick-up truck or van in traffic accident**

V54 **Occupant of pick-up truck or van injured in collision with heavy transport vehicle or bus**

Excludes1: *occupant of pick-up truck or van injured in collision with military vehicle (V59.81)*

The appropriate 7th character is to be added to each code from category V54
A initial encounter
D subsequent encounter
S sequela

X+7th **V54.0** **Driver of pick-up truck or van injured in collision with heavy transport vehicle or bus in nontraffic accident**

X+7th **V54.1** **Passenger in pick-up truck or van injured in collision with heavy transport vehicle or bus in nontraffic accident**

X+7th **V54.2** **Person on outside of pick-up truck or van injured in collision with heavy transport vehicle or bus in nontraffic accident**

X+7th **V54.3** **Unspecified occupant of pick-up truck or van injured in collision with heavy transport vehicle or bus in nontraffic accident**

X+7th **V54.4** **Person boarding or alighting a pick-up truck or van injured in collision with heavy transport vehicle or bus**

X+7th **V54.5** **Driver of pick-up truck or van injured in collision with heavy transport vehicle or bus in traffic accident**

X+7th **V54.6** **Passenger in pick-up truck or van injured in collision with heavy transport vehicle or bus in traffic accident**

X+7th **V54.7** **Person on outside of pick-up truck or van injured in collision with heavy transport vehicle or bus in traffic accident**

X+7th **V54.9** **Unspecified occupant of pick-up truck or van injured in collision with heavy transport vehicle or bus in traffic accident**

V55 **Occupant of pick-up truck or van injured in collision with railway train or railway vehicle**

The appropriate 7th character is to be added to each code from category V55
A initial encounter
D subsequent encounter
S sequela

X+7th **V55.0** **Driver of pick-up truck or van injured in collision with railway train or railway vehicle in nontraffic accident**

X+7th **V55.1** **Passenger in pick-up truck or van injured in collision with railway train or railway vehicle in nontraffic accident**

X+7th **V55.2** **Person on outside of pick-up truck or van injured in collision with railway train or railway vehicle in nontraffic accident**

X+7th **V55.3** **Unspecified occupant of pick-up truck or van injured in collision with railway train or railway vehicle in nontraffic accident**

X+7th **V55.4** **Person boarding or alighting a pick-up truck or van injured in collision with railway train or railway vehicle**

X+7th **V55.5** **Driver of pick-up truck or van injured in collision with railway train or railway vehicle in traffic accident**

X+7th **V55.6** **Passenger in pick-up truck or van injured in collision with railway train or railway vehicle in traffic accident**

X+7th **V55.7** **Person on outside of pick-up truck or van injured in collision with railway train or railway vehicle in traffic accident**

X+7th **V55.9** **Unspecified occupant of pick-up truck or van injured in collision with railway train or railway vehicle in traffic accident**

V56 **Occupant of pick-up truck or van injured in collision with other nonmotor vehicle**

Includes: collision with animal-drawn vehicle, animal being ridden, streetcar

The appropriate 7th character is to be added to each code from category V56
A initial encounter
D subsequent encounter
S sequela

X+7th **V56.0** **Driver of pick-up truck or van injured in collision with other nonmotor vehicle in nontraffic accident**

X+7th **V56.1** **Passenger in pick-up truck or van injured in collision with other nonmotor vehicle in nontraffic accident**

X+7th **V56.2** **Person on outside of pick-up truck or van injured in collision with other nonmotor vehicle in nontraffic accident**

X+7th **V56.3** **Unspecified occupant of pick-up truck or van injured in collision with other nonmotor vehicle in nontraffic accident**

X+7th **V56.4** **Person boarding or alighting a pick-up truck or van injured in collision with other nonmotor vehicle**

X+7th **V56.5** **Driver of pick-up truck or van injured in collision with other nonmotor vehicle in traffic accident**

X+7th **V56.6** **Passenger in pick-up truck or van injured in collision with other nonmotor vehicle in traffic accident**

X+7th **V56.7** **Person on outside of pick-up truck or van injured in collision with other nonmotor vehicle in traffic accident**

X+7th **V56.9** **Unspecified occupant of pick-up truck or van injured in collision with other nonmotor vehicle in traffic accident**

V57 **Occupant of pick-up truck or van injured in collision with fixed or stationary object**

The appropriate 7th character is to be added to each code from category V57
A initial encounter
D subsequent encounter
S sequela

X+7th **V57.0** **Driver of pick-up truck or van injured in collision with fixed or stationary object in nontraffic accident**

X+7th **V57.1** **Passenger in pick-up truck or van injured in collision with fixed or stationary object in nontraffic accident**

X+7th **V57.2** **Person on outside of pick-up truck or van injured in collision with fixed or stationary object in nontraffic accident**

X+7th **V57.3** **Unspecified occupant of pick-up truck or van injured in collision with fixed or stationary object in nontraffic accident**

X+7th **V57.4** **Person boarding or alighting a pick-up truck or van injured in collision with fixed or stationary object**

X+7th **V57.5** **Driver of pick-up truck or van injured in collision with fixed or stationary object in traffic accident**

X+7th **V57.6** **Passenger in pick-up truck or van injured in collision with fixed or stationary object in traffic accident**

X+7th **V57.7** **Person on outside of pick-up truck or van injured in collision with fixed or stationary object in traffic accident**

X+7th **V57.9** **Unspecified occupant of pick-up truck or van injured in collision with fixed or stationary object in traffic accident**

V58 **Occupant of pick-up truck or van injured in noncollision transport accident**

Includes: overturning pick-up truck or van NOS
overturning pick-up truck or van without collision

The appropriate 7th character is to be added to each code from category V58
A initial encounter
D subsequent encounter
S sequela

X+7th **V58.0** **Driver of pick-up truck or van injured in noncollision transport accident in nontraffic accident**

X+7th **V58.1** **Passenger in pick-up truck or van injured in noncollision transport accident in nontraffic accident**

X+7th **V58.2** **Person on outside of pick-up truck or van injured in noncollision transport accident in nontraffic accident**

X+7th **V58.3** **Unspecified occupant of pick-up truck or van injured in noncollision transport accident in nontraffic accident**

X+7th **V58.4** **Person boarding or alighting a pick-up truck or van injured in noncollision transport accident**

X+7th **V58.5** **Driver of pick-up truck or van injured in noncollision transport accident in traffic accident**

X+7th **V58.6** **Passenger in pick-up truck or van injured in noncollision transport accident in traffic accident**

X+7th **V58.7** **Person on outside of pick-up truck or van injured in noncollision transport accident in traffic accident**

X+7th **V58.9** **Unspecified occupant of pick-up truck or van injured in noncollision transport accident in traffic accident**

V59 **Occupant of pick-up truck or van injured in other and unspecified transport accidents**

The appropriate 7th character is to be added to each code from category V59
A initial encounter
D subsequent encounter
S sequela

+ **V59.0** **Driver of pick-up truck or van injured in collision with other and unspecified motor vehicles in nontraffic accident**

X+7th **V59.00** **Driver of pick-up truck or van injured in collision with unspecified motor vehicles in nontraffic accident**

X+7th **V59.09** **Driver of pick-up truck or van injured in collision with other motor vehicles in nontraffic accident**

+ **V59.1** **Passenger in pick-up truck or van injured in collision with other and unspecified motor vehicles in nontraffic accident**

X+7th **V59.10** **Passenger in pick-up truck or van injured in collision with unspecified motor vehicles in nontraffic accident**

X+7th **V59.19** **Passenger in pick-up truck or van injured in collision with other motor vehicles in nontraffic accident**

+ **V59.2** **Unspecified occupant of pick-up truck or van injured in collision with other and unspecified motor vehicles in nontraffic accident**

X+7th **V59.20** **Unspecified occupant of pick-up truck or van injured in collision with unspecified motor vehicles in nontraffic accident**
Collision NOS involving pick-up truck or van, nontraffic

X+7th **V59.29** **Unspecified occupant of pick-up truck or van injured in collision with other motor vehicles in nontraffic accident**

X+7th **V59.3** **Occupant (driver) (passenger) of pick-up truck or van injured in unspecified nontraffic accident**
Accident NOS involving pick-up truck or van, nontraffic
Occupant of pick-up truck or van injured in nontraffic accident NOS

+ **V59.4** **Driver of pick-up truck or van injured in collision with other and unspecified motor vehicles in traffic accident**

X+7th **V59.40** **Driver of pick-up truck or van injured in collision with unspecified motor vehicles in traffic accident**

X+7th **V59.49** **Driver of pick-up truck or van injured in collision with other motor vehicles in traffic accident**

+ **V59.5** **Passenger in pick-up truck or van injured in collision with other and unspecified motor vehicles in traffic accident**

X+7th **V59.50** **Passenger in pick-up truck or van injured in collision with unspecified motor vehicles in traffic accident**

X+7th **V59.59** **Passenger in pick-up truck or van injured in collision with other motor vehicles in traffic accident**

+ **V59.6** **Unspecified occupant of pick-up truck or van injured in collision with other and unspecified motor vehicles in traffic accident**

X+7th **V59.60** **Unspecified occupant of pick-up truck or van injured in collision with unspecified motor vehicles in traffic accident**
Collision NOS involving pick-up truck or van (traffic)

X+7th **V59.69** **Unspecified occupant of pick-up truck or van injured in collision with other motor vehicles in traffic accident**

+ **V59.8** **Occupant (driver) (passenger) of pick-up truck or van injured in other specified transport accidents**

X+7th **V59.81** **Occupant (driver) (passenger) of pick-up truck or van injured in transport accident with military vehicle**

X+7th **V59.88** **Occupant (driver) (passenger) of pick-up truck or van injured in other specified transport accidents**

X+7th **V59.9** **Occupant (driver) (passenger) of pick-up truck or van injured in unspecified traffic accident**
Accident NOS involving pick-up truck or van

Occupant of heavy transport vehicle injured in transport accident (V60-V69)

Includes: 18 wheeler
armored car
panel truck

Excludes1: *bus*
motorcoach

V60 **Occupant of heavy transport vehicle injured in collision with pedestrian or animal**

Excludes1: *heavy transport vehicle collision with animal-drawn vehicle or animal being ridden (V66.-)*

The appropriate 7th character is to be added to each code from category V60
A initial encounter
D subsequent encounter
S sequela

X+7th **V60.0** **Driver of heavy transport vehicle injured in collision with pedestrian or animal in nontraffic accident**

X+7th **V60.1** **Passenger in heavy transport vehicle injured in collision with pedestrian or animal in nontraffic accident**

X+7th **V60.2** **Person on outside of heavy transport vehicle injured in collision with pedestrian or animal in nontraffic accident**

X+7th **V60.3** **Unspecified occupant of heavy transport vehicle injured in collision with pedestrian or animal in nontraffic accident**

X+7th V60.4 **Person boarding or alighting a heavy transport vehicle injured in collision with pedestrian or animal**

X+7th V60.5 **Driver of heavy transport vehicle injured in collision with pedestrian or animal in traffic accident**

X+7th V60.6 **Passenger in heavy transport vehicle injured in collision with pedestrian or animal in traffic accident**

X+7th V60.7 **Person on outside of heavy transport vehicle injured in collision with pedestrian or animal in traffic accident**

X+7th V60.9 **Unspecified occupant of heavy transport vehicle injured in collision with pedestrian or animal in traffic accident**

V61 Occupant of heavy transport vehicle injured in collision with pedal cycle

The appropriate 7th character is to be added to each code from category V61
A initial encounter
D subsequent encounter
S sequela

X+7th V61.0 **Driver of heavy transport vehicle injured in collision with pedal cycle in nontraffic accident**

X+7th V61.1 **Passenger in heavy transport vehicle injured in collision with pedal cycle in nontraffic accident**

X+7th V61.2 **Person on outside of heavy transport vehicle injured in collision with pedal cycle in nontraffic accident**

X+7th V61.3 **Unspecified occupant of heavy transport vehicle injured in collision with pedal cycle in nontraffic accident**

X+7th V61.4 **Person boarding or alighting a heavy transport vehicle injured in collision with pedal cycle while boarding or alighting**

X+7th V61.5 **Driver of heavy transport vehicle injured in collision with pedal cycle in traffic accident**

X+7th V61.6 **Passenger in heavy transport vehicle injured in collision with pedal cycle in traffic accident**

X+7th V61.7 **Person on outside of heavy transport vehicle injured in collision with pedal cycle in traffic accident**

X+7th V61.9 **Unspecified occupant of heavy transport vehicle injured in collision with pedal cycle in traffic accident**

V62 Occupant of heavy transport vehicle injured in collision with two- or three-wheeled motor vehicle

The appropriate 7th character is to be added to each code from category V62
A initial encounter
D subsequent encounter
S sequela

X+7th V62.0 **Driver of heavy transport vehicle injured in collision with two- or three-wheeled motor vehicle in nontraffic accident**

X+7th V62.1 **Passenger in heavy transport vehicle injured in collision with two- or three-wheeled motor vehicle in nontraffic accident**

X+7th V62.2 **Person on outside of heavy transport vehicle injured in collision with two- or three-wheeled motor vehicle in nontraffic accident**

X+7th V62.3 **Unspecified occupant of heavy transport vehicle injured in collision with two- or three-wheeled motor vehicle in nontraffic accident**

X+7th V62.4 **Person boarding or alighting a heavy transport vehicle injured in collision with two- or three-wheeled motor vehicle**

X+7th V62.5 **Driver of heavy transport vehicle injured in collision with two- or three-wheeled motor vehicle in traffic accident**

X+7th V62.6 **Passenger in heavy transport vehicle injured in collision with two- or three-wheeled motor vehicle in traffic accident**

X+7th V62.7 **Person on outside of heavy transport vehicle injured in collision with two- or three-wheeled motor vehicle in traffic accident**

X+7th V62.9 **Unspecified occupant of heavy transport vehicle injured in collision with two- or three-wheeled motor vehicle in traffic accident**

V63 Occupant of heavy transport vehicle injured in collision with car, pick-up truck or van

The appropriate 7th character is to be added to each code from category V63
A initial encounter
D subsequent encounter
S sequela

X+7th V63.0 **Driver of heavy transport vehicle injured in collision with car, pick-up truck or van in nontraffic accident**

X+7th V63.1 **Passenger in heavy transport vehicle injured in collision with car, pick-up truck or van in nontraffic accident**

X+7th V63.2 **Person on outside of heavy transport vehicle injured in collision with car, pick-up truck or van in nontraffic accident**

X+7th V63.3 **Unspecified occupant of heavy transport vehicle injured in collision with car, pick-up truck or van in nontraffic accident**

X+7th V63.4 **Person boarding or alighting a heavy transport vehicle injured in collision with car, pick-up truck or van**

X+7th V63.5 **Driver of heavy transport vehicle injured in collision with car, pick-up truck or van in traffic accident**

X+7th V63.6 **Passenger in heavy transport vehicle injured in collision with car, pick-up truck or van in traffic accident**

X+7th V63.7 **Person on outside of heavy transport vehicle injured in collision with car, pick-up truck or van in traffic accident**

X+7th V63.9 **Unspecified occupant of heavy transport vehicle injured in collision with car, pick-up truck or van in traffic accident**

V64 Occupant of heavy transport vehicle injured in collision with heavy transport vehicle or bus

Excludes1: *occupant of heavy transport vehicle injured in collision with military vehicle (V69.81)*

The appropriate 7th character is to be added to each code from category V64
A initial encounter
D subsequent encounter
S sequela

X+7th V64.0 **Driver of heavy transport vehicle injured in collision with heavy transport vehicle or bus in nontraffic accident**

X+7th V64.1 **Passenger in heavy transport vehicle injured in collision with heavy transport vehicle or bus in nontraffic accident**

X+7th V64.2 **Person on outside of heavy transport vehicle injured in collision with heavy transport vehicle or bus in nontraffic accident**

X+7th V64.3 **Unspecified occupant of heavy transport vehicle injured in collision with heavy transport vehicle or bus in nontraffic accident**

X+7th V64.4 **Person boarding or alighting a heavy transport vehicle injured in collision with heavy transport vehicle or bus while boarding or alighting**

X+7th V64.5 **Driver of heavy transport vehicle injured in collision with heavy transport vehicle or bus in traffic accident**

X+7th V64.6 **Passenger in heavy transport vehicle injured in collision with heavy transport vehicle or bus in traffic accident**

X+7th V64.7 **Person on outside of heavy transport vehicle injured in collision with heavy transport vehicle or bus in traffic accident**

X+7th V64.9 **Unspecified occupant of heavy transport vehicle injured in collision with heavy transport vehicle or bus in traffic accident**

V65 Occupant of heavy transport vehicle injured in collision with railway train or railway vehicle

The appropriate 7th character is to be added to each code from category V65
A initial encounter
D subsequent encounter
S sequela

X+7th V65.0 **Driver of heavy transport vehicle injured in collision with railway train or railway vehicle in nontraffic accident**

X+7th V65.1 **Passenger in heavy transport vehicle injured in collision with railway train or railway vehicle in nontraffic accident**

X+7th V65.2 **Person on outside of heavy transport vehicle injured in collision with railway train or railway vehicle in nontraffic accident**

X+7th V65.3 **Unspecified occupant of heavy transport vehicle injured in collision with railway train or railway vehicle in nontraffic accident**

X+7th V65.4 **Person boarding or alighting a heavy transport vehicle injured in collision with railway train or railway vehicle**

X+7th V65.5 **Driver of heavy transport vehicle injured in collision with railway train or railway vehicle in traffic accident**

X+7th V65.6 **Passenger in heavy transport vehicle injured in collision with railway train or railway vehicle in traffic accident**

X+7th V65.7 **Person on outside of heavy transport vehicle injured in collision with railway train or railway vehicle in traffic accident**

X+7th V65.9 **Unspecified occupant of heavy transport vehicle injured in collision with railway train or railway vehicle in traffic accident**

V66 Occupant of heavy transport vehicle injured in collision with other nonmotor vehicle

Includes: collision with animal-drawn vehicle, animal being ridden, streetcar

The appropriate 7th character is to be added to each code from category V66
A initial encounter
D subsequent encounter
S sequela

X+7th **V66.0 Driver of heavy transport vehicle injured in collision with other nonmotor vehicle in nontraffic accident**
X+7th **V66.1 Passenger in heavy transport vehicle injured in collision with other nonmotor vehicle in nontraffic accident**
X+7th **V66.2 Person on outside of heavy transport vehicle injured in collision with other nonmotor vehicle in nontraffic accident**
X+7th **V66.3 Unspecified occupant of heavy transport vehicle injured in collision with other nonmotor vehicle in nontraffic accident**
X+7th **V66.4 Person boarding or alighting a heavy transport vehicle injured in collision with other nonmotor vehicle**
X+7th **V66.5 Driver of heavy transport vehicle injured in collision with other nonmotor vehicle in traffic accident**
X+7th **V66.6 Passenger in heavy transport vehicle injured in collision with other nonmotor vehicle in traffic accident**
X+7th **V66.7 Person on outside of heavy transport vehicle injured in collision with other nonmotor vehicle in traffic accident**
X+7th **V66.9 Unspecified occupant of heavy transport vehicle injured in collision with other nonmotor vehicle in traffic accident**

V67 Occupant of heavy transport vehicle injured in collision with fixed or stationary object

The appropriate 7th character is to be added to each code from category V67
A initial encounter
D subsequent encounter
S sequela

X+7th **V67.0 Driver of heavy transport vehicle injured in collision with fixed or stationary object in nontraffic accident**
X+7th **V67.1 Passenger in heavy transport vehicle injured in collision with fixed or stationary object in nontraffic accident**
X+7th **V67.2 Person on outside of heavy transport vehicle injured in collision with fixed or stationary object in nontraffic accident**
X+7th **V67.3 Unspecified occupant of heavy transport vehicle injured in collision with fixed or stationary object in nontraffic accident**
X+7th **V67.4 Person boarding or alighting a heavy transport vehicle injured in collision with fixed or stationary object**
X+7th **V67.5 Driver of heavy transport vehicle injured in collision with fixed or stationary object in traffic accident**
X+7th **V67.6 Passenger in heavy transport vehicle injured in collision with fixed or stationary object in traffic accident**
X+7th **V67.7 Person on outside of heavy transport vehicle injured in collision with fixed or stationary object in traffic accident**
X+7th **V67.9 Unspecified occupant of heavy transport vehicle injured in collision with fixed or stationary object in traffic accident**

V68 Occupant of heavy transport vehicle injured in noncollision transport accident

Includes: overturning heavy transport vehicle NOS
overturning heavy transport vehicle without collision

The appropriate 7th character is to be added to each code from category V68
A initial encounter
D subsequent encounter
S sequela

X+7th **V68.0 Driver of heavy transport vehicle injured in noncollision transport accident in nontraffic accident**
X+7th **V68.1 Passenger in heavy transport vehicle injured in noncollision transport accident in nontraffic accident**
X+7th **V68.2 Person on outside of heavy transport vehicle injured in noncollision transport accident in nontraffic accident**
X+7th **V68.3 Unspecified occupant of heavy transport vehicle injured in noncollision transport accident in nontraffic accident**
X+7th **V68.4 Person boarding or alighting a heavy transport vehicle injured in noncollision transport accident**
X+7th **V68.5 Driver of heavy transport vehicle injured in noncollision transport accident in traffic accident**
X+7th **V68.6 Passenger in heavy transport vehicle injured in noncollision transport accident in traffic accident**
X+7th **V68.7 Person on outside of heavy transport vehicle injured in noncollision transport accident in traffic accident**
X+7th **V68.9 Unspecified occupant of heavy transport vehicle injured in noncollision transport accident in traffic accident**

V69 Occupant of heavy transport vehicle injured in other and unspecified transport accidents

The appropriate 7th character is to be added to each code from category V69
A initial encounter
D subsequent encounter
S sequela

\+ **V69.0 Driver of heavy transport vehicle injured in collision with other and unspecified motor vehicles in nontraffic accident**
X+7th **V69.00 Driver of heavy transport vehicle injured in collision with unspecified motor vehicles in nontraffic accident**
X+7th **V69.09 Driver of heavy transport vehicle injured in collision with other motor vehicles in nontraffic accident**
\+ **V69.1 Passenger in heavy transport vehicle injured in collision with other and unspecified motor vehicles in nontraffic accident**
X+7th **V69.10 Passenger in heavy transport vehicle injured in collision with unspecified motor vehicles in nontraffic accident**
X+7th **V69.19 Passenger in heavy transport vehicle injured in collision with other motor vehicles in nontraffic accident**
\+ **V69.2 Unspecified occupant of heavy transport vehicle injured in collision with other and unspecified motor vehicles in nontraffic accident**
X+7th **V69.20 Unspecified occupant of heavy transport vehicle injured in collision with unspecified motor vehicles in nontraffic accident**
Collision NOS involving heavy transport vehicle, nontraffic
X+7th **V69.29 Unspecified occupant of heavy transport vehicle injured in collision with other motor vehicles in nontraffic accident**
X+7th **V69.3 Occupant (driver) (passenger) of heavy transport vehicle injured in unspecified nontraffic accident**
Accident NOS involving heavy transport vehicle, nontraffic
Occupant of heavy transport vehicle injured in nontraffic accident NOS
\+ **V69.4 Driver of heavy transport vehicle injured in collision with other and unspecified motor vehicles in traffic accident**
X+7th **V69.40 Driver of heavy transport vehicle injured in collision with unspecified motor vehicles in traffic accident**
X+7th **V69.49 Driver of heavy transport vehicle injured in collision with other motor vehicles in traffic accident**
\+ **V69.5 Passenger in heavy transport vehicle injured in collision with other and unspecified motor vehicles in traffic accident**
X+7th **V69.50 Passenger in heavy transport vehicle injured in collision with unspecified motor vehicles in traffic accident**
X+7th **V69.59 Passenger in heavy transport vehicle injured in collision with other motor vehicles in traffic accident**
\+ **V69.6 Unspecified occupant of heavy transport vehicle injured in collision with other and unspecified motor vehicles in traffic accident**
X+7th **V69.60 Unspecified occupant of heavy transport vehicle injured in collision with unspecified motor vehicles in traffic accident**
Collision NOS involving heavy transport vehicle (traffic)
X+7th **V69.69 Unspecified occupant of heavy transport vehicle injured in collision with other motor vehicles in traffic accident**
\+ **V69.8 Occupant (driver) (passenger) of heavy transport vehicle injured in other specified transport accidents**
X+7th **V69.81 Occupant (driver) (passenger) of heavy transport vehicle injured in transport accidents with military vehicle**
X+7th **V69.88 Occupant (driver) (passenger) of heavy transport vehicle injured in other specified transport accidents**
X+7th **V69.9 Occupant (driver) (passenger) of heavy transport vehicle injured in unspecified traffic accident**
Accident NOS involving heavy transport vehicle

Bus occupant injured in transport accident (V70-V79)

Includes: motorcoach

Excludes1: *minibus (V50-V59)*

V70 Bus occupant injured in collision with pedestrian or animal

The appropriate 7th character is to be added to each code from category V70
A initial encounter
D subsequent encounter
S sequela

Excludes1: *bus collision with animal-drawn vehicle or animal being ridden (V76.-)*

X+7th **V70.0 Driver of bus injured in collision with pedestrian or animal in nontraffic accident**
X+7th **V70.1 Passenger on bus injured in collision with pedestrian or animal in nontraffic accident**
X+7th **V70.2 Person on outside of bus injured in collision with pedestrian or animal in nontraffic accident**
X+7th **V70.3 Unspecified occupant of bus injured in collision with pedestrian or animal in nontraffic accident**
X+7th **V70.4 Person boarding or alighting from bus injured in collision with pedestrian or animal**
X+7th **V70.5 Driver of bus injured in collision with pedestrian or animal in traffic accident**
X+7th **V70.6 Passenger on bus injured in collision with pedestrian or animal in traffic accident**
X+7th **V70.7 Person on outside of bus injured in collision with pedestrian or animal in traffic accident**
X+7th **V70.9 Unspecified occupant of bus injured in collision with pedestrian or animal in traffic accident**

V71 Bus occupant injured in collision with pedal cycle

The appropriate 7th character is to be added to each code from category V71
A initial encounter
D subsequent encounter
S sequela

X+7th **V71.0 Driver of bus injured in collision with pedal cycle in nontraffic accident**
X+7th **V71.1 Passenger on bus injured in collision with pedal cycle in nontraffic accident**
X+7th **V71.2 Person on outside of bus injured in collision with pedal cycle in nontraffic accident**
X+7th **V71.3 Unspecified occupant of bus injured in collision with pedal cycle in nontraffic accident**
X+7th **V71.4 Person boarding or alighting from bus injured in collision with pedal cycle**
X+7th **V71.5 Driver of bus injured in collision with pedal cycle in traffic accident**
X+7th **V71.6 Passenger on bus injured in collision with pedal cycle in traffic accident**
X+7th **V71.7 Person on outside of bus injured in collision with pedal cycle in traffic accident**
X+7th **V71.9 Unspecified occupant of bus injured in collision with pedal cycle in traffic accident**

V72 Bus occupant injured in collision with two- or three-wheeled motor vehicle

The appropriate 7th character is to be added to each code from category V72
A initial encounter
D subsequent encounter
S sequela

X+7th **V72.0 Driver of bus injured in collision with two- or three-wheeled motor vehicle in nontraffic accident**
X+7th **V72.1 Passenger on bus injured in collision with two- or three-wheeled motor vehicle in nontraffic accident**
X+7th **V72.2 Person on outside of bus injured in collision with two- or three-wheeled motor vehicle in nontraffic accident**
X+7th **V72.3 Unspecified occupant of bus injured in collision with two- or three-wheeled motor vehicle in nontraffic accident**
X+7th **V72.4 Person boarding or alighting from bus injured in collision with two- or three-wheeled motor vehicle**
X+7th **V72.5 Driver of bus injured in collision with two- or three-wheeled motor vehicle in traffic accident**
X+7th **V72.6 Passenger on bus injured in collision with two- or three-wheeled motor vehicle in traffic accident**
X+7th **V72.7 Person on outside of bus injured in collision with two- or three-wheeled motor vehicle in traffic accident**
X+7th **V72.9 Unspecified occupant of bus injured in collision with two- or three-wheeled motor vehicle in traffic accident**

V73 Bus occupant injured in collision with car, pick-up truck or van

The appropriate 7th character is to be added to each code from category V73
A initial encounter
D subsequent encounter
S sequela

X+7th **V73.0 Driver of bus injured in collision with car, pick-up truck or van in nontraffic accident**
X+7th **V73.1 Passenger on bus injured in collision with car, pick-up truck or van in nontraffic accident**
X+7th **V73.2 Person on outside of bus injured in collision with car, pick-up truck or van in nontraffic accident**
X+7th **V73.3 Unspecified occupant of bus injured in collision with car, pick-up truck or van in nontraffic accident**
X+7th **V73.4 Person boarding or alighting from bus injured in collision with car, pick-up truck or van**
X+7th **V73.5 Driver of bus injured in collision with car, pick-up truck or van in traffic accident**
X+7th **V73.6 Passenger on bus injured in collision with car, pick-up truck or van in traffic accident**
X+7th **V73.7 Person on outside of bus injured in collision with car, pick-up truck or van in traffic accident**
X+7th **V73.9 Unspecified occupant of bus injured in collision with car, pick-up truck or van in traffic accident**

V74 Bus occupant injured in collision with heavy transport vehicle or bus

Excludes1: *bus occupant injured in collision with military vehicle (V79.81)*

The appropriate 7th character is to be added to each code from category V74
A initial encounter
D subsequent encounter
S sequela

X+7th **V74.0 Driver of bus injured in collision with heavy transport vehicle or bus in nontraffic accident**
X+7th **V74.1 Passenger on bus injured in collision with heavy transport vehicle or bus in nontraffic accident**
X+7th **V74.2 Person on outside of bus injured in collision with heavy transport vehicle or bus in nontraffic accident**
X+7th **V74.3 Unspecified occupant of bus injured in collision with heavy transport vehicle or bus in nontraffic accident**
X+7th **V74.4 Person boarding or alighting from bus injured in collision with heavy transport vehicle or bus**
X+7th **V74.5 Driver of bus injured in collision with heavy transport vehicle or bus in traffic accident**
X+7th **V74.6 Passenger on bus injured in collision with heavy transport vehicle or bus in traffic accident**
X+7th **V74.7 Person on outside of bus injured in collision with heavy transport vehicle or bus in traffic accident**
X+7th **V74.9 Unspecified occupant of bus injured in collision with heavy transport vehicle or bus in traffic accident**

V75 Bus occupant injured in collision with railway train or railway vehicle

The appropriate 7th character is to be added to each code from category V75
A initial encounter
D subsequent encounter
S sequela

X+7th **V75.0 Driver of bus injured in collision with railway train or railway vehicle in nontraffic accident**
X+7th **V75.1 Passenger on bus injured in collision with railway train or railway vehicle in nontraffic accident**
X+7th **V75.2 Person on outside of bus injured in collision with railway train or railway vehicle in nontraffic accident**
X+7th **V75.3 Unspecified occupant of bus injured in collision with railway train or railway vehicle in nontraffic accident**
X+7th **V75.4 Person boarding or alighting from bus injured in collision with railway train or railway vehicle**
X+7th **V75.5 Driver of bus injured in collision with railway train or railway vehicle in traffic accident**
X+7th **V75.6 Passenger on bus injured in collision with railway train or railway vehicle in traffic accident**
X+7th **V75.7 Person on outside of bus injured in collision with railway train or railway vehicle in traffic accident**
X+7th **V75.9 Unspecified occupant of bus injured in collision with railway train or railway vehicle in traffic accident**

V76 Bus occupant injured in collision with other nonmotor vehicle

Includes: collision with animal-drawn vehicle, animal being ridden, streetcar

The appropriate 7th character is to be added to each code from category V76
A initial encounter
D subsequent encounter
S sequela

X+7th **V76.0 Driver of bus injured in collision with other nonmotor vehicle in nontraffic accident**
X+7th **V76.1 Passenger on bus injured in collision with other nonmotor vehicle in nontraffic accident**
X+7th **V76.2 Person on outside of bus injured in collision with other nonmotor vehicle in nontraffic accident**
X+7th **V76.3 Unspecified occupant of bus injured in collision with other nonmotor vehicle in nontraffic accident**
X+7th **V76.4 Person boarding or alighting from bus injured in collision with other nonmotor vehicle**
X+7th **V76.5 Driver of bus injured in collision with other nonmotor vehicle in traffic accident**
X+7th **V76.6 Passenger on bus injured in collision with other nonmotor vehicle in traffic accident**
X+7th **V76.7 Person on outside of bus injured in collision with other nonmotor vehicle in traffic accident**
X+7th **V76.9 Unspecified occupant of bus injured in collision with other nonmotor vehicle in traffic accident**

V77 Bus occupant injured in collision with fixed or stationary object

The appropriate 7th character is to be added to each code from category V77
A initial encounter
D subsequent encounter
S sequela

X+7th **V77.0 Driver of bus injured in collision with fixed or stationary object in nontraffic accident**
X+7th **V77.1 Passenger on bus injured in collision with fixed or stationary object in nontraffic accident**
X+7th **V77.2 Person on outside of bus injured in collision with fixed or stationary object in nontraffic accident**
X+7th **V77.3 Unspecified occupant of bus injured in collision with fixed or stationary object in nontraffic accident**
X+7th **V77.4 Person boarding or alighting from bus injured in collision with fixed or stationary object**
X+7th **V77.5 Driver of bus injured in collision with fixed or stationary object in traffic accident**
X+7th **V77.6 Passenger on bus injured in collision with fixed or stationary object in traffic accident**
X+7th **V77.7 Person on outside of bus injured in collision with fixed or stationary object in traffic accident**
X+7th **V77.9 Unspecified occupant of bus injured in collision with fixed or stationary object in traffic accident**

V78 Bus occupant injured in noncollision transport accident

Includes: overturning bus NOS
overturning bus without collision

The appropriate 7th character is to be added to each code from category V78
A initial encounter
D subsequent encounter
S sequela

X+7th **V78.0 Driver of bus injured in noncollision transport accident in nontraffic accident**
X+7th **V78.1 Passenger on bus injured in noncollision transport accident in nontraffic accident**
X+7th **V78.2 Person on outside of bus injured in noncollision transport accident in nontraffic accident**
X+7th **V78.3 Unspecified occupant of bus injured in noncollision transport accident in nontraffic accident**
X+7th **V78.4 Person boarding or alighting from bus injured in noncollision transport accident**
X+7th **V78.5 Driver of bus injured in noncollision transport accident in traffic accident**
X+7th **V78.6 Passenger on bus injured in noncollision transport accident in traffic accident**
X+7th **V78.7 Person on outside of bus injured in noncollision transport accident in traffic accident**
X+7th **V78.9 Unspecified occupant of bus injured in noncollision transport accident in traffic accident**

V79 Bus occupant injured in other and unspecified transport accidents

The appropriate 7th character is to be added to each code from category V79
A initial encounter
D subsequent encounter
S sequela

\+ **V79.0 Driver of bus injured in collision with other and unspecified motor vehicles in nontraffic accident**
X+7th **V79.00 Driver of bus injured in collision with unspecified motor vehicles in nontraffic accident**
X+7th **V79.09 Driver of bus injured in collision with other motor vehicles in nontraffic accident**
\+ **V79.1 Passenger on bus injured in collision with other and unspecified motor vehicles in nontraffic accident**
X+7th **V79.10 Passenger on bus injured in collision with unspecified motor vehicles in nontraffic accident**
X+7th **V79.19 Passenger on bus injured in collision with other motor vehicles in nontraffic accident**
\+ **V79.2 Unspecified bus occupant injured in collision with other and unspecified motor vehicles in nontraffic accident**
X+7th **V79.20 Unspecified bus occupant injured in collision with unspecified motor vehicles in nontraffic accident**
Bus collision NOS, nontraffic
X+7th **V79.29 Unspecified bus occupant injured in collision with other motor vehicles in nontraffic accident**
X+7th **V79.3 Bus occupant (driver) (passenger) injured in unspecified nontraffic accident**
Bus accident NOS, nontraffic
Bus occupant injured in nontraffic accident NOS
\+ **V79.4 Driver of bus injured in collision with other and unspecified motor vehicles in traffic accident**
X+7th **V79.40 Driver of bus injured in collision with unspecified motor vehicles in traffic accident**
X+7th **V79.49 Driver of bus injured in collision with other motor vehicles in traffic accident**
\+ **V79.5 Passenger on bus injured in collision with other and unspecified motor vehicles in traffic accident**
X+7th **V79.50 Passenger on bus injured in collision with unspecified motor vehicles in traffic accident**
X+7th **V79.59 Passenger on bus injured in collision with other motor vehicles in traffic accident**
\+ **V79.6 Unspecified bus occupant injured in collision with other and unspecified motor vehicles in traffic accident**
X+7th **V79.60 Unspecified bus occupant injured in collision with unspecified motor vehicles in traffic accident**
Bus collision NOS (traffic)
X+7th **V79.69 Unspecified bus occupant injured in collision with other motor vehicles in traffic accident**
\+ **V79.8 Bus occupant (driver) (passenger) injured in other specified transport accidents**
X+7th **V79.81 Bus occupant (driver) (passenger) injured in transport accidents with military vehicle**
X+7th **V79.88 Bus occupant (driver) (passenger) injured in other specified transport accidents**
X+7th **V79.9 Bus occupant (driver) (passenger) injured in unspecified traffic accident**
Bus accident NOS

Other land transport accidents (V80-V89)

V80 Animal-rider or occupant of animal-drawn vehicle injured in transport accident

The appropriate 7th character is to be added to each code from category V80
A initial encounter
D subsequent encounter
S sequela

\+ **V80.0 Animal-rider or occupant of animal drawn vehicle injured by fall from or being thrown from animal or animal-drawn vehicle in noncollision accident**
\+ **V80.01 Animal-rider injured by fall from or being thrown from animal in noncollision accident**
+7th **V80.010 Animal-rider injured by fall from or being thrown from horse in noncollision accident**
+7th **V80.018 Animal-rider injured by fall from or being thrown from other animal in noncollision accident**

X+7th **V80.02 Occupant of animal-drawn vehicle injured by fall from or being thrown from animal-drawn vehicle in noncollision accident**
Overturning animal-drawn vehicle NOS
Overturning animal-drawn vehicle without collision

\+ **V80.1 Animal-rider or occupant of animal-drawn vehicle injured in collision with pedestrian or animal**
Excludes1: *animal-rider or animal-drawn vehicle collision with animal-drawn vehicle or animal being ridden (V80.7)*

X+7th **V80.11 Animal-rider injured in collision with pedestrian or animal**

X+7th **V80.12 Occupant of animal-drawn vehicle injured in collision with pedestrian or animal**

\+ **V80.2 Animal-rider or occupant of animal-drawn vehicle injured in collision with pedal cycle**

X+7th **V80.21 Animal-rider injured in collision with pedal cycle**

X+7th **V80.22 Occupant of animal-drawn vehicle injured in collision with pedal cycle**

\+ **V80.3 Animal-rider or occupant of animal-drawn vehicle injured in collision with two- or three-wheeled motor vehicle**

X+7th **V80.31 Animal-rider injured in collision with two- or three-wheeled motor vehicle**

X+7th **V80.32 Occupant of animal-drawn vehicle injured in collision with two- or three-wheeled motor vehicle**

\+ **V80.4 Animal-rider or occupant of animal-drawn vehicle injured in collision with car, pick-up truck, van, heavy transport vehicle or bus**
Excludes1: *animal-rider injured in collision with military vehicle (V80.910)*
occupant of animal-drawn vehicle injured in collision with military vehicle (V80.920)

X+7th **V80.41 Animal-rider injured in collision with car, pick-up truck, van, heavy transport vehicle or bus**

X+7th **V80.42 Occupant of animal-drawn vehicle injured in collision with car, pick-up truck, van, heavy transport vehicle or bus**

\+ **V80.5 Animal-rider or occupant of animal-drawn vehicle injured in collision with other specified motor vehicle**

X+7th **V80.51 Animal-rider injured in collision with other specified motor vehicle**

X+7th **V80.52 Occupant of animal-drawn vehicle injured in collision with other specified motor vehicle**

\+ **V80.6 Animal-rider or occupant of animal-drawn vehicle injured in collision with railway train or railway vehicle**

X+7th **V80.61 Animal-rider injured in collision with railway train or railway vehicle**

X+7th **V80.62 Occupant of animal-drawn vehicle injured in collision with railway train or railway vehicle**

\+ **V80.7 Animal-rider or occupant of animal-drawn vehicle injured in collision with other nonmotor vehicles**

X+7th **V80.71 Animal-rider or occupant of animal-drawn vehicle injured in collision with animal being ridden**

X+7th **V80.710 Animal-rider injured in collision with other animal being ridden**

X+7th **V80.711 Occupant of animal-drawn vehicle injured in collision with animal being ridden**

X+7th **V80.72 Animal-rider or occupant of animal-drawn vehicle injured in collision with other animal-drawn vehicle**

X+7th **V80.720 Animal-rider injured in collision with animal-drawn vehicle**

X+7th **V80.721 Occupant of animal-drawn vehicle injured in collision with other animal-drawn vehicle**

\+ **V80.73 Animal-rider or occupant of animal-drawn vehicle injured in collision with streetcar**

X+7th **V80.730 Animal-rider injured in collision with streetcar**

X+7th **V80.731 Occupant of animal-drawn vehicle injured in collision with streetcar**

X+7th **V80.79 Animal-rider or occupant of animal-drawn vehicle injured in collision with other nonmotor vehicles**

X+7th **V80.790 Animal-rider injured in collision with other nonmotor vehicles**

X+7th **V80.791 Occupant of animal-drawn vehicle injured in collision with other nonmotor vehicles**

\+ **V80.8 Animal-rider or occupant of animal-drawn vehicle injured in collision with fixed or stationary object**

X+7th **V80.81 Animal-rider injured in collision with fixed or stationary object**

X+7th **V80.82 Occupant of animal-drawn vehicle injured in collision with fixed or stationary object**

\+ **V80.9 Animal-rider or occupant of animal-drawn vehicle injured in other and unspecified transport accidents**

\+ **V80.91 Animal-rider injured in other and unspecified transport accidents**

+7th **V80.910 Animal-rider injured in transport accident with military vehicle**

+7th **V80.918 Animal-rider injured in other transport accident**

+7th **V80.919 Animal-rider injured in unspecified transport accident**
Animal rider accident NOS

\+ **V80.92 Occupant of animal-drawn vehicle injured in other and unspecified transport accidents**

+7th **V80.920 Occupant of animal-drawn vehicle injured in transport accident with military vehicle**

+7th **V80.928 Occupant of animal-drawn vehicle injured in other transport accident**

+7th **V80.929 Occupant of animal-drawn vehicle injured in unspecified transport accident**
Animal-drawn vehicle accident NOS

V81 Occupant of railway train or railway vehicle injured in transport accident

Includes: derailment of railway train or railway vehicle
person on outside of train
Excludes1: *streetcar (V82.-)*

The appropriate 7th character is to be added to each code from category V81
A initial encounter
D subsequent encounter
S sequela

X+7th **V81.0 Occupant of railway train or railway vehicle injured in collision with motor vehicle in nontraffic accident**
Excludes1: *Occupant of railway train or railway vehicle injured due to collision with military vehicle (V81.83)*

X+7th **V81.1 Occupant of railway train or railway vehicle injured in collision with motor vehicle in traffic accident**
Excludes1: *Occupant of railway train or railway vehicle injured due to collision with military vehicle (V81.83)*

X+7th **V81.2 Occupant of railway train or railway vehicle injured in collision with or hit by rolling stock**

X+7th **V81.3 Occupant of railway train or railway vehicle injured in collision with other object**
Railway collision NOS

X+7th **V81.4 Person injured while boarding or alighting from railway train or railway vehicle**

X+7th **V81.5 Occupant of railway train or railway vehicle injured by fall in railway train or railway vehicle**

X+7th **V81.6 Occupant of railway train or railway vehicle injured by fall from railway train or railway vehicle**

X+7th **V81.7 Occupant of railway train or railway vehicle injured in derailment without antecedent collision**

\+ **V81.8 Occupant of railway train or railway vehicle injured in other specified railway accidents**

X+7th **V81.81 Occupant of railway train or railway vehicle injured due to explosion or fire on train**

X+7th **V81.82 Occupant of railway train or railway vehicle injured due to object falling onto train**
Occupant of railway train or railway vehicle injured due to falling earth onto train
Occupant of railway train or railway vehicle injured due to falling rocks onto train
Occupant of railway train or railway vehicle injured due to falling snow onto train
Occupant of railway train or railway vehicle injured due to falling trees onto train

X+7th **V81.83 Occupant of railway train or railway vehicle injured due to collision with military vehicle**

X+7th **V81.89 Occupant of railway train or railway vehicle injured due to other specified railway accident**

X+7th **V81.9 Occupant of railway train or railway vehicle injured in unspecified railway accident**
Railway accident NOS

V82 Occupant of powered streetcar injured in transport accident

Includes: interurban electric car
person on outside of streetcar
tram (car)
trolley (car)

Excludes1: *bus (V70-V79)*
motorcoach (V70-V79)
nonpowered streetcar (V76.-)
train (V81.-)

The appropriate 7th character is to be added to each code from category V82
A initial encounter
D subsequent encounter
S sequela

X+7th **V82.0 Occupant of streetcar injured in collision with motor vehicle in nontraffic accident**

X+7th **V82.1 Occupant of streetcar injured in collision with motor vehicle in traffic accident**

X+7th **V82.2 Occupant of streetcar injured in collision with or hit by rolling stock**

X+7th **V82.3 Occupant of streetcar injured in collision with other object**
Excludes1: *collision with animal-drawn vehicle or animal being ridden (V82.8)*

X+7th **V82.4 Person injured while boarding or alighting from streetcar**

X+7th **V82.5 Occupant of streetcar injured by fall in streetcar**
Excludes1: *fall in streetcar:*
while boarding or alighting (V82.4)
with antecedent collision (V82.0-V82.3)

X+7th **V82.6 Occupant of streetcar injured by fall from streetcar**
Excludes1: *fall from streetcar:*
while boarding or alighting (V82.4)
with antecedent collision (V82.0-V82.3)

X+7th **V82.7 Occupant of streetcar injured in derailment without antecedent collision**
Excludes1: *occupant of streetcar injured in derailment with antecedent collision (V82.0-V82.3)*

X+7th **V82.8 Occupant of streetcar injured in other specified transport accidents**
Streetcar collision with military vehicle
Streetcar collision with train or nonmotor vehicles

X+7th **V82.9 Occupant of streetcar injured in unspecified traffic accident**
Streetcar accident NOS

V83 Occupant of special vehicle mainly used on industrial premises injured in transport accident

Includes: battery-powered airport passenger vehicle
battery-powered truck (baggage) (mail)
coal-car in mine
forklift (truck)
logging car
self-propelled industrial truck
station baggage truck (powered)
tram, truck, or tub (powered) in mine or quarry

Excludes1: *special construction vehicles (V85.-)*
special industrial vehicle in stationary use or maintenance (W31.-)

The appropriate 7th character is to be added to each code from category V83
A initial encounter
D subsequent encounter
S sequela

X+7th **V83.0 Driver of special industrial vehicle injured in traffic accident**

X+7th **V83.1 Passenger of special industrial vehicle injured in traffic accident**

X+7th **V83.2 Person on outside of special industrial vehicle injured in traffic accident**

X+7th **V83.3 Unspecified occupant of special industrial vehicle injured in traffic accident**

X+7th **V83.4 Person injured while boarding or alighting from special industrial vehicle**

X+7th **V83.5 Driver of special industrial vehicle injured in nontraffic accident**

X+7th **V83.6 Passenger of special industrial vehicle injured in nontraffic accident**

X+7th **V83.7 Person on outside of special industrial vehicle injured in nontraffic accident**

X+7th **V83.9 Unspecified occupant of special industrial vehicle injured in nontraffic accident**
Special-industrial-vehicle accident NOS

V84 Occupant of special vehicle mainly used in agriculture injured in transport accident

Includes: self-propelled farm machinery
tractor (and trailer)

Excludes1: *animal-powered farm machinery accident (W30.8-)*
contact with combine harvester (W30.0)
special agricultural vehicle in stationary use or maintenance (W30.-)

The appropriate 7th character is to be added to each code from category V84
A initial encounter
D subsequent encounter
S sequela

X+7th **V84.0 Driver of special agricultural vehicle injured in traffic accident**

X+7th **V84.1 Passenger of special agricultural vehicle injured in traffic accident**

X+7th **V84.2 Person on outside of special agricultural vehicle injured in traffic accident**

X+7th **V84.3 Unspecified occupant of special agricultural vehicle injured in traffic accident**

X+7th **V84.4 Person injured while boarding or alighting from special agricultural vehicle**

X+7th **V84.5 Driver of special agricultural vehicle injured in nontraffic accident**

X+7th **V84.6 Passenger of special agricultural vehicle injured in nontraffic accident**

X+7th **V84.7 Person on outside of special agricultural vehicle injured in nontraffic accident**

X+7th **V84.9 Unspecified occupant of special agricultural vehicle injured in nontraffic accident**
Special-agricultural vehicle accident NOS

V85 Occupant of special construction vehicle injured in transport accident

Includes: bulldozer
digger
dump truck
earth-leveller
mechanical shovel
road-roller

Excludes1: *special industrial vehicle (V83.-)*
special construction vehicle in stationary use or maintenance (W31.-)

The appropriate 7th character is to be added to each code from category V85
A initial encounter
D subsequent encounter
S sequela

X+7th **V85.0 Driver of special construction vehicle injured in traffic accident**

X+7th **V85.1 Passenger of special construction vehicle injured in traffic accident**

X+7th **V85.2 Person on outside of special construction vehicle injured in traffic accident**

X+7th **V85.3 Unspecified occupant of special construction vehicle injured in traffic accident**

X+7th **V85.4 Person injured while boarding or alighting from special construction vehicle**

X+7th **V85.5 Driver of special construction vehicle injured in nontraffic accident**

X+7th **V85.6 Passenger of special construction vehicle injured in nontraffic accident**

X+7th **V85.7 Person on outside of special construction vehicle injured in nontraffic accident**

X+7th **V85.9 Unspecified occupant of special construction vehicle injured in nontraffic accident**
Special-construction-vehicle accident NOS

V86 Occupant of special all-terrain or other off-road motor vehicle, injured in transport accident

Excludes1: *special all-terrain vehicle in stationary use or maintenance (W31.-)*
sport-utility vehicle (V50-V59)
three-wheeled motor vehicle designed for on-road use (V30-V39)

AHA CC: 4Q, 2017, 26

The appropriate 7th character is to be added to each code from category V86
A initial encounter
D subsequent encounter
S sequela

+ **V86.0 Driver of special all-terrain or other off-road motor vehicle injured in traffic accident**
- +7th **V86.01 Driver of ambulance or fire engine injured in traffic accident**
- +7th **V86.02 Driver of snowmobile injured in traffic accident**
- +7th **V86.03 Driver of dune buggy injured in traffic accident**
- +7th **V86.04 Driver of military vehicle injured in traffic accident**
- +7th **V86.05 Driver of 3- or 4- wheeled all-terrain vehicle (ATV) injured in traffic accident**
- +7th **V86.06 Driver of dirt bike or motor/cross bike injured in traffic accident**
- +7th **V86.09 Driver of other special all-terrain or other off-road motor vehicle injured in traffic accident**
  Driver of go cart injured in traffic accident
  Driver of golf cart injured in traffic accident

+ **V86.1 Passenger of special all-terrain or other off-road motor vehicle injured in traffic accident**
- +7th **V86.11 Passenger of ambulance or fire engine injured in traffic accident**
- +7th **V86.12 Passenger of snowmobile injured in traffic accident**
- +7th **V86.13 Passenger of dune buggy injured in traffic accident**
- +7th **V86.14 Passenger of military vehicle injured in traffic accident**
- +7th **V86.15 Passenger of 3- or 4- wheeled all-terrain vehicle (ATV) injured in traffic accident**
- +7th **V86.16 Passenger of dirt bike or motor/cross bike injured in traffic accident**
- +7th **V86.19 Passenger of other special all-terrain or other off-road motor vehicle injured in traffic accident**
  Passenger of go cart injured in traffic accident
  Passenger of golf cart injured in traffic accident

+ **V86.2 Person on outside of special all-terrain or other off-road motor vehicle injured in traffic accident**
- +7th **V86.21 Person on outside of ambulance or fire engine injured in traffic accident**
- +7th **V86.22 Person on outside of snowmobile injured in traffic accident**
- +7th **V86.23 Person on outside of dune buggy injured in traffic accident**
- +7th **V86.24 Person on outside of military vehicle injured in traffic accident**
- +7th **V86.25 Person on outside of 3- or 4- wheeled all-terrain vehicle (ATV) injured in traffic accident**
- +7th **V86.26 Person on outside of dirt bike or motor/cross bike injured in traffic accident**
- +7th **V86.29 Person on outside of other special all-terrain or other off-road motor vehicle injured in traffic accident**
  Person on outside of go cart in traffic accident
  Person on outside of golf cart injured in traffic accident

+ **V86.3 Unspecified occupant of special all-terrain or other off-road motor vehicle injured in traffic accident**
- +7th **V86.31 Unspecified occupant of ambulance or fire engine injured in traffic accident**
- +7th **V86.32 Unspecified occupant of snowmobile injured in traffic accident**
- +7th **V86.33 Unspecified occupant of dune buggy injured in traffic accident**
- +7th **V86.34 Unspecified occupant of military vehicle injured in traffic accident**
- +7th **V86.35 Unspecified occupant of 3- or 4- wheeled all-terrain vehicle (ATV) injured in traffic accident**
- +7th **V86.36 Unspecified occupant of dirt bike or motor/cross bike injured in traffic accident**
- +7th **V86.39 Unspecified occupant of other special all-terrain or other off-road motor vehicle injured in traffic accident**
  Unspecified occupant of go cart injured in traffic accident
  Unspecified occupant of golf cart injured in traffic accident

+ **V86.4 Person injured while boarding or alighting from special all-terrain or other off-road motor vehicle**
- +7th **V86.41 Person injured while boarding or alighting from ambulance or fire engine**
- +7th **V86.42 Person injured while boarding or alighting from snowmobile**
- +7th **V86.43 Person injured while boarding or alighting from dune buggy**
- +7th **V86.44 Person injured while boarding or alighting from military vehicle**
- +7th **V86.45 Person injured while boarding or alighting from a 3- or 4- wheeled all-terrain vehicle (ATV)**
- +7th **V86.46 Person injured while boarding or alighting from a dirt bike or motor/cross bike**
- +7th **V86.49 Person injured while boarding or alighting from other special all-terrain or other off-road motor vehicle**
  Person injured while boarding or alighting from go cart
  Person injured while boarding or alighting from golf cart

+ **V86.5 Driver of special all-terrain or other off-road motor vehicle injured in nontraffic accident**
- +7th **V86.51 Driver of ambulance or fire engine injured in nontraffic accident**
- +7th **V86.52 Driver of snowmobile injured in nontraffic accident**
- +7th **V86.53 Driver of dune buggy injured in nontraffic accident**
- +7th **V86.54 Driver of military vehicle injured in nontraffic accident**
- +7th **V86.55 Driver of 3- or 4- wheeled all-terrain vehicle (ATV) injured in nontraffic accident**
- +7th **V86.56 Driver of dirt bike or motor/cross bike injured in nontraffic accident, initial encounter**
- +7th **V86.59 Driver of other special all-terrain or other off-road motor vehicle injured in nontraffic accident**
  Driver of go cart injured in nontraffic accident
  Driver of golf cart injured in nontraffic accident

+ **V86.6 Passenger of special all-terrain or other off-road motor vehicle injured in nontraffic accident**
- +7th **V86.61 Passenger of ambulance or fire engine injured in nontraffic accident**
- +7th **V86.62 Passenger of snowmobile injured in nontraffic accident**
- +7th **V86.63 Passenger of dune buggy injured in nontraffic accident**
- +7th **V86.64 Passenger of military vehicle injured in nontraffic accident**
- +7th **V86.65 Passenger of 3- or 4- wheeled all-terrain vehicle (ATV) injured in nontraffic accident**
- +7th **V86.66 Passenger of dirt bike or motor/cross bike injured in nontraffic accident**
- +7th **V86.69 Passenger of other special all-terrain or other off-road motor vehicle injured in nontraffic accident**
  Passenger of go cart injured in nontraffic accident
  Passenger of golf cart injured in nontraffic accident

+ **V86.7 Person on outside of special all-terrain or other off-road motor vehicle injured in nontraffic accident**
- +7th **V86.71 Person on outside of ambulance or fire engine injured in nontraffic accident**
- +7th **V86.72 Person on outside of snowmobile injured in nontraffic accident**
- +7th **V86.73 Person on outside of dune buggy injured in nontraffic accident**
- +7th **V86.74 Person on outside of military vehicle injured in nontraffic accident**
- +7th **V86.75 Person on outside of 3- or 4- wheeled all-terrain vehicle (ATV) injured in nontraffic accident**
- +7th **V86.76 Person on outside of dirt bike or motor/cross bike injured in nontraffic accident**

+7th **V86.79 Person on outside of other special all-terrain or other off-road motor vehicles injured in nontraffic accident**
Person on outside of go cart injured in nontraffic accident
Person on outside of golf cart injured in nontraffic accident

\+ **V86.9 Unspecified occupant of special all-terrain or other off-road motor vehicle injured in nontraffic accident**

+7th **V86.91 Unspecified occupant of ambulance or fire engine injured in nontraffic accident**

+7th **V86.92 Unspecified occupant of snowmobile injured in nontraffic accident**

+7th **V86.93 Unspecified occupant of dune buggy injured in nontraffic accident**

+7th **V86.94 Unspecified occupant of military vehicle injured in nontraffic accident**

+7th **V86.95 Unspecified occupant of 3- or 4- wheeled all-terrain vehicle (ATV) injured in nontraffic accident**

+7th **V86.96 Unspecified occupant of dirt bike or motor/cross bike injured in nontraffic accident**

+7th **V86.99 Unspecified occupant of other special all-terrain or other off-road motor vehicle injured in nontraffic accident**
Off-road motor-vehicle accident NOS
Other motor-vehicle accident NOS
Unspecified occupant of go cart injured in nontraffic accident
Unspecified occupant of golf cart injured in nontraffic accident

V87 Traffic accident of specified type but victim's mode of transport unknown

Excludes1: *collision involving:*
pedal cycle (V10-V19)
pedestrian (V01-V09)

The appropriate 7th character is to be added to each code from category V87
A initial encounter
D subsequent encounter
S sequela

X+7th **V87.0 Person injured in collision between car and two- or three-wheeled powered vehicle (traffic)**

X+7th **V87.1 Person injured in collision between other motor vehicle and two- or three-wheeled motor vehicle (traffic)**

X+7th **V87.2 Person injured in collision between car and pick-up truck or van (traffic)**

X+7th **V87.3 Person injured in collision between car and bus (traffic)**

X+7th **V87.4 Person injured in collision between car and heavy transport vehicle (traffic)**

X+7th **V87.5 Person injured in collision between heavy transport vehicle and bus (traffic)**

X+7th **V87.6 Person injured in collision between railway train or railway vehicle and car (traffic)**

X+7th **V87.7 Person injured in collision between other specified motor vehicles (traffic)**

X+7th **V87.8 Person injured in other specified noncollision transport accidents involving motor vehicle (traffic)**

X+7th **V87.9 Person injured in other specified (collision) (noncollision) transport accidents involving nonmotor vehicle (traffic)**

V88 Nontraffic accident of specified type but victim's mode of transport unknown

Excludes1: *collision involving:*
pedal cycle (V10-V19)
pedestrian (V01-V09)

The appropriate 7th character is to be added to each code from category V88
A initial encounter
D subsequent encounter
S sequela

X+7th **V88.0 Person injured in collision between car and two- or three-wheeled motor vehicle, nontraffic**

X+7th **V88.1 Person injured in collision between other motor vehicle and two- or three-wheeled motor vehicle, nontraffic**

X+7th **V88.2 Person injured in collision between car and pick-up truck or van, nontraffic**

X+7th **V88.3 Person injured in collision between car and bus, nontraffic**

X+7th **V88.4 Person injured in collision between car and heavy transport vehicle, nontraffic**

X+7th **V88.5 Person injured in collision between heavy transport vehicle and bus, nontraffic**

X+7th **V88.6 Person injured in collision between railway train or railway vehicle and car, nontraffic**

X+7th **V88.7 Person injured in collision between other specified motor vehicle, nontraffic**

X+7th **V88.8 Person injured in other specified noncollision transport accidents involving motor vehicle, nontraffic**

X+7th **V88.9 Person injured in other specified (collision)(noncollision) transport accidents involving nonmotor vehicle, nontraffic**

V89 Motor- or nonmotor-vehicle accident, type of vehicle unspecified

The appropriate 7th character is to be added to each code from category V89
A initial encounter
D subsequent encounter
S sequela

X+7th **V89.0 Person injured in unspecified motor-vehicle accident, nontraffic**
Motor-vehicle accident NOS, nontraffic

X+7th **V89.1 Person injured in unspecified nonmotor-vehicle accident, nontraffic**
Nonmotor-vehicle accident NOS (nontraffic)

X+7th **V89.2 Person injured in unspecified motor-vehicle accident, traffic**
Motor-vehicle accident [MVA] NOS
Road (traffic) accident [RTA] NOS

X+7th **V89.3 Person injured in unspecified nonmotor-vehicle accident, traffic**
Nonmotor-vehicle traffic accident NOS

X+7th **V89.9 Person injured in unspecified vehicle accident**
Collision NOS

Water transport accidents (V90-V94)

V90 Drowning and submersion due to accident to watercraft

Excludes1: *civilian water transport accident involving military watercraft (V94.81-)*
fall into water not from watercraft (W16.-)
military watercraft accident in military or war operations (Y36.0-, Y37.0-)
water-transport-related drowning or submersion without accident to watercraft (V92.-)

The appropriate 7th character is to be added to each code from category V90
A initial encounter
D subsequent encounter
S sequela

\+ **V90.0 Drowning and submersion due to watercraft overturning**

X+7th **V90.00 Drowning and submersion due to merchant ship overturning**

X+7th **V90.01 Drowning and submersion due to passenger ship overturning**
Drowning and submersion due to Ferry-boat overturning
Drowning and submersion due to Liner overturning

X+7th **V90.02 Drowning and submersion due to fishing boat overturning**

X+7th **V90.03 Drowning and submersion due to other powered watercraft overturning**
Drowning and submersion due to Hovercraft (on open water) overturning
Drowning and submersion due to Jet ski overturning

X+7th **V90.04 Drowning and submersion due to sailboat overturning**

X+7th **V90.05 Drowning and submersion due to canoe or kayak overturning**

X+7th **V90.06 Drowning and submersion due to (nonpowered) inflatable craft overturning**

X+7th **V90.08 Drowning and submersion due to other unpowered watercraft overturning**
Drowning and submersion due to windsurfer overturning

X+7th **V90.09 Drowning and submersion due to unspecified watercraft overturning**
Drowning and submersion due to boat NOS overturning
Drowning and submersion due to ship NOS overturning
Drowning and submersion due to watercraft NOS overturning

\+ **V90.1 Drowning and submersion due to watercraft sinking**

X+7th **V90.10 Drowning and submersion due to merchant ship sinking**

X+7th **V90.11 Drowning and submersion due to passenger ship sinking**
Drowning and submersion due to Ferry-boat sinking
Drowning and submersion due to Liner sinking

X+7th **V90.12 Drowning and submersion due to fishing boat sinking**

X+7th **V90.13 Drowning and submersion due to other powered watercraft sinking**
Drowning and submersion due to Hovercraft (on open water) sinking
Drowning and submersion due to Jet ski sinking

X+7th **V90.14 Drowning and submersion due to sailboat sinking**

X+7th **V90.15 Drowning and submersion due to canoe or kayak sinking**

X+7th **V90.16 Drowning and submersion due to (nonpowered) inflatable craft sinking**

X+7th **V90.18 Drowning and submersion due to other unpowered watercraft sinking**

X+7th **V90.19 Drowning and submersion due to unspecified watercraft sinking**
Drowning and submersion due to boat NOS sinking
Drowning and submersion due to ship NOS sinking
Drowning and submersion due to watercraft NOS sinking

\+ **V90.2 Drowning and submersion due to falling or jumping from burning watercraft**

X+7th **V90.20 Drowning and submersion due to falling or jumping from burning merchant ship**

X+7th **V90.21 Drowning and submersion due to falling or jumping from burning passenger ship**
Drowning and submersion due to falling or jumping from burning Ferry-boat
Drowning and submersion due to falling or jumping from burning Liner

X+7th **V90.22 Drowning and submersion due to falling or jumping from burning fishing boat**

X+7th **V90.23 Drowning and submersion due to falling or jumping from other burning powered watercraft**
Drowning and submersion due to falling and jumping from burning Hovercraft (on open water)
Drowning and submersion due to falling and jumping from burning Jet ski

X+7th **V90.24 Drowning and submersion due to falling or jumping from burning sailboat**

X+7th **V90.25 Drowning and submersion due to falling or jumping from burning canoe or kayak**

X+7th **V90.26 Drowning and submersion due to falling or jumping from burning (nonpowered) inflatable craft**

X+7th **V90.27 Drowning and submersion due to falling or jumping from burning water-skis**

X+7th **V90.28 Drowning and submersion due to falling or jumping from other burning unpowered watercraft**
Drowning and submersion due to falling and jumping from burning surf-board
Drowning and submersion due to falling and jumping from burning windsurfer

X+7th **V90.29 Drowning and submersion due to falling or jumping from unspecified burning watercraft**
Drowning and submersion due to falling or jumping from burning boat NOS
Drowning and submersion due to falling or jumping from burning ship NOS
Drowning and submersion due to falling or jumping from burning watercraft NOS

\+ **V90.3 Drowning and submersion due to falling or jumping from crushed watercraft**

X+7th **V90.30 Drowning and submersion due to falling or jumping from crushed merchant ship**

X+7th **V90.31 Drowning and submersion due to falling or jumping from crushed passenger ship**
Drowning and submersion due to falling and jumping from crushed Ferry boat
Drowning and submersion due to falling and jumping from crushed Liner

X+7th **V90.32 Drowning and submersion due to falling or jumping from crushed fishing boat**

X+7th **V90.33 Drowning and submersion due to falling or jumping from other crushed powered watercraft**
Drowning and submersion due to falling and jumping from crushed Hovercraft
Drowning and submersion due to falling and jumping from crushed Jet ski

X+7th **V90.34 Drowning and submersion due to falling or jumping from crushed sailboat**

X+7th **V90.35 Drowning and submersion due to falling or jumping from crushed canoe or kayak**

X+7th **V90.36 Drowning and submersion due to falling or jumping from crushed (nonpowered) inflatable craft**

X+7th **V90.37 Drowning and submersion due to falling or jumping from crushed water-skis**

X+7th **V90.38 Drowning and submersion due to falling or jumping from other crushed unpowered watercraft**
Drowning and submersion due to falling and jumping from crushed surf-board
Drowning and submersion due to falling and jumping from crushed windsurfer

X+7th **V90.39 Drowning and submersion due to falling or jumping from crushed unspecified watercraft**
Drowning and submersion due to falling and jumping from crushed boat NOS
Drowning and submersion due to falling and jumping from crushed ship NOS
Drowning and submersion due to falling and jumping from crushed watercraft NOS

\+ **V90.8 Drowning and submersion due to other accident to watercraft**

X+7th **V90.80 Drowning and submersion due to other accident to merchant ship**

X+7th **V90.81 Drowning and submersion due to other accident to passenger ship**
Drowning and submersion due to other accident to Ferry-boat
Drowning and submersion due to other accident to Liner

X+7th **V90.82 Drowning and submersion due to other accident to fishing boat**

X+7th **V90.83 Drowning and submersion due to other accident to other powered watercraft**
Drowning and submersion due to other accident to Hovercraft (on open water)
Drowning and submersion due to other accident to Jet ski

X+7th **V90.84 Drowning and submersion due to other accident to sailboat**

X+7th **V90.85 Drowning and submersion due to other accident to canoe or kayak**

X+7th **V90.86 Drowning and submersion due to other accident to (nonpowered) inflatable craft**

X+7th **V90.87 Drowning and submersion due to other accident to water-skis**

X+7th **V90.88 Drowning and submersion due to other accident to other unpowered watercraft**

Drowning and submersion due to other accident to surf-board

Drowning and submersion due to other accident to windsurfer

X+7th **V90.89 Drowning and submersion due to other accident to unspecified watercraft**

Drowning and submersion due to other accident to boat NOS

Drowning and submersion due to other accident to ship NOS

Drowning and submersion due to other accident to watercraft NOS

V91 Other injury due to accident to watercraft

Includes: any injury except drowning and submersion as a result of an accident to watercraft

Excludes1: *civilian water transport accident involving military watercraft (V94.81-)*

military watercraft accident in military or war operations (Y36, Y37.-)

Excludes2: *drowning and submersion due to accident to watercraft (V90.-)*

The appropriate 7th character is to be added to each code from category V91
A initial encounter
D subsequent encounter
S sequela

\+ **V91.0 Burn due to watercraft on fire**

Excludes1: *burn from localized fire or explosion on board ship without accident to watercraft (V93.-)*

X+7th **V91.00 Burn due to merchant ship on fire**

X+7th **V91.01 Burn due to passenger ship on fire**

Burn due to Ferry-boat on fire

Burn due to Liner on fire

X+7th **V91.02 Burn due to fishing boat on fire**

X+7th **V91.03 Burn due to other powered watercraft on fire**

Burn due to Hovercraft (on open water) on fire

Burn due to Jet ski on fire

X+7th **V91.04 Burn due to sailboat on fire**

X+7th **V91.05 Burn due to canoe or kayak on fire**

X+7th **V91.06 Burn due to (nonpowered) inflatable craft on fire**

X+7th **V91.07 Burn due to water-skis on fire**

X+7th **V91.08 Burn due to other unpowered watercraft on fire**

X+7th **V91.09 Burn due to unspecified watercraft on fire**

Burn due to boat NOS on fire

Burn due to ship NOS on fire

Burn due to watercraft NOS on fire

\+ **V91.1 Crushed between watercraft and other watercraft or other object due to collision**

Crushed by lifeboat after abandoning ship in a collision

NOTE Select the specified type of watercraft that the victim was on at the time of the collision

X+7th **V91.10 Crushed between merchant ship and other watercraft or other object due to collision**

X+7th **V91.11 Crushed between passenger ship and other watercraft or other object due to collision**

Crushed between Ferry-boat and other watercraft or other object due to collision

Crushed between Liner and other watercraft or other object due to collision

X+7th **V91.12 Crushed between fishing boat and other watercraft or other object due to collision**

X+7th **V91.13 Crushed between other powered watercraft and other watercraft or other object due to collision**

Crushed between Hovercraft (on open water) and other watercraft or other object due to collision

Crushed between Jet ski and other watercraft or other object due to collision

X+7th **V91.14 Crushed between sailboat and other watercraft or other object due to collision**

X+7th **V91.15 Crushed between canoe or kayak and other watercraft or other object due to collision**

X+7th **V91.16 Crushed between (nonpowered) inflatable craft and other watercraft or other object due to collision**

X+7th **V91.18 Crushed between other unpowered watercraft and other watercraft or other object due to collision**

Crushed between surfboard and other watercraft or other object due to collision

Crushed between windsurfer and other watercraft or other object due to collision

X+7th **V91.19 Crushed between unspecified watercraft and other watercraft or other object due to collision**

Crushed between boat NOS and other watercraft or other object due to collision

Crushed between ship NOS and other watercraft or other object due to collision

Crushed between watercraft NOS and other watercraft or other object due to collision

\+ **V91.2 Fall due to collision between watercraft and other watercraft or other object**

Fall while remaining on watercraft after collision

NOTE Select the specified type of watercraft that the victim was on at the time of the collision

Excludes1: *crushed between watercraft and other watercraft and other object due to collision (V91.1-)*

drowning and submersion due to falling from crushed watercraft (V90.3-)

X+7th **V91.20 Fall due to collision between merchant ship and other watercraft or other object**

X+7th **V91.21 Fall due to collision between passenger ship and other watercraft or other object**

Fall due to collision between Ferry-boat and other watercraft or other object

Fall due to collision between Liner and other watercraft or other object

X+7th **V91.22 Fall due to collision between fishing boat and other watercraft or other object**

X+7th **V91.23 Fall due to collision between other powered watercraft and other watercraft or other object**

Fall due to collision between Hovercraft (on open water) and other watercraft or other object

Fall due to collision between Jet ski and other watercraft or other object

X+7th **V91.24 Fall due to collision between sailboat and other watercraft or other object**

X+7th **V91.25 Fall due to collision between canoe or kayak and other watercraft or other object**

X+7th **V91.26 Fall due to collision between (nonpowered) inflatable craft and other watercraft or other object**

X+7th **V91.29 Fall due to collision between unspecified watercraft and other watercraft or other object**

Fall due to collision between boat NOS and other watercraft or other object

Fall due to collision between ship NOS and other watercraft or other object

Fall due to collision between watercraft NOS and other watercraft or other object

\+ **V91.3 Hit or struck by falling object due to accident to watercraft**

Hit or struck by falling object (part of damaged watercraft or other object) after falling or jumping from damaged watercraft

Excludes2: *drowning or submersion due to fall or jumping from damaged watercraft (V90.2-, V90.3-)*

X+7th **V91.30 Hit or struck by falling object due to accident to merchant ship**

X+7th **V91.31 Hit or struck by falling object due to accident to passenger ship**

Hit or struck by falling object due to accident to Ferry-boat

Hit or struck by falling object due to accident to Liner

X+7th **V91.32 Hit or struck by falling object due to accident to fishing boat**

X+7th **V91.33 Hit or struck by falling object due to accident to other powered watercraft**

Hit or struck by falling object due to accident to Hovercraft (on open water)

Hit or struck by falling object due to accident to Jet ski

X+7th **V91.34 Hit or struck by falling object due to accident to sailboat**

X+7th **V91.35 Hit or struck by falling object due to accident to canoe or kayak**

X+7th **V91.36 Hit or struck by falling object due to accident to (nonpowered) inflatable craft**

X+7th **V91.37 Hit or struck by falling object due to accident to water-skis**
Hit by water-skis after jumping off of waterskis

X+7th **V91.38 Hit or struck by falling object due to accident to other unpowered watercraft**
Hit or struck by surf-board after falling off damaged surf-board
Hit or struck by object after falling off damaged windsurfer

X+7th **V91.39 Hit or struck by falling object due to accident to unspecified watercraft**
Hit or struck by falling object due to accident to boat NOS
Hit or struck by falling object due to accident to ship NOS
Hit or struck by falling object due to accident to watercraft NOS

\+ **V91.8 Other injury due to other accident to watercraft**

X+7th **V91.80 Other injury due to other accident to merchant ship**

X+7th **V91.81 Other injury due to other accident to passenger ship**
Other injury due to other accident to Ferry-boat
Other injury due to other accident to Liner

X+7th **V91.82 Other injury due to other accident to fishing boat**

X+7th **V91.83 Other injury due to other accident to other powered watercraft**
Other injury due to other accident to Hovercraft (on open water)
Other injury due to other accident to Jet ski

X+7th **V91.84 Other injury due to other accident to sailboat**

X+7th **V91.85 Other injury due to other accident to canoe or kayak**

X+7th **V91.86 Other injury due to other accident to (nonpowered) inflatable craft**

X+7th **V91.87 Other injury due to other accident to water-skis**

X+7th **V91.88 Other injury due to other accident to other unpowered watercraft**
Other injury due to other accident to surf-board
Other injury due to other accident to windsurfer

X+7th **V91.89 Other injury due to other accident to unspecified watercraft**
Other injury due to other accident to boat NOS
Other injury due to other accident to ship NOS
Other injury due to other accident to watercraft NOS

V92 Drowning and submersion due to accident on board watercraft, without accident to watercraft

Excludes1: *civilian water transport accident involving military watercraft (V94.81-)*
drowning or submersion due to accident to watercraft (V90-V91)
drowning or submersion of diver who voluntarily jumps from boat not involved in an accident (W16.711, W16.721)
fall into water without watercraft (W16.-)
military watercraft accident in military or war operations (Y36, Y37)

The appropriate 7th character is to be added to each code from category V92
A initial encounter
D subsequent encounter
S sequela

\+ **V92.0 Drowning and submersion due to fall off watercraft**
Drowning and submersion due to fall from gangplank of watercraft
Drowning and submersion due to fall overboard watercraft
Excludes2: *hitting head on object or bottom of body of water due to fall from watercraft (V94.0-)*

X+7th **V92.00 Drowning and submersion due to fall off merchant ship**

X+7th **V92.01 Drowning and submersion due to fall off passenger ship**
Drowning and submersion due to fall off Ferry-boat
Drowning and submersion due to fall off Liner

X+7th **V92.02 Drowning and submersion due to fall off fishing boat**

X+7th **V92.03 Drowning and submersion due to fall off other powered watercraft**
Drowning and submersion due to fall off Hovercraft (on open water)
Drowning and submersion due to fall off Jet ski

X+7th **V92.04 Drowning and submersion due to fall off sailboat**

X+7th **V92.05 Drowning and submersion due to fall off canoe or kayak**

X+7th **V92.06 Drowning and submersion due to fall off (nonpowered) inflatable craft**

X+7th **V92.07 Drowning and submersion due to fall off water-skis**
Excludes1: *drowning and submersion due to falling off burning water-skis (V90.27)*
drowning and submersion due to falling off crushed water-skis (V90.37)
hit by boat while water-skiing NOS (V94.X)

X+7th **V92.08 Drowning and submersion due to fall off other unpowered watercraft**
Drowning and submersion due to fall off surf-board
Drowning and submersion due to fall off windsurfer
Excludes1: *drowning and submersion due to fall off burning unpowered watercraft (V90.28)*
drowning and submersion due to fall off crushed unpowered watercraft (V90.38)
drowning and submersion due to fall off damaged unpowered watercraft (V90.88)
drowning and submersion due to rider of nonpowered watercraft being hit by other watercraft (V94.-)
other injury due to rider of nonpowered watercraft being hit by other watercraft (V94.-)

X+7th **V92.09 Drowning and submersion due to fall off unspecified watercraft**
Drowning and submersion due to fall off boat NOS
Drowning and submersion due to fall off ship
Drowning and submersion due to fall off watercraft NOS

\+ **V92.1 Drowning and submersion due to being thrown overboard by motion of watercraft**
Excludes1: *drowning and submersion due to fall off surf-board (V92.08)*
drowning and submersion due to fall off water-skis (V92.07)
drowning and submersion due to fall off windsurfer (V92.08)

X+7th **V92.10 Drowning and submersion due to being thrown overboard by motion of merchant ship**

X+7th **V92.11 Drowning and submersion due to being thrown overboard by motion of passenger ship**
Drowning and submersion due to being thrown overboard by motion of Ferry-boat
Drowning and submersion due to being thrown overboard by motion of Liner

X+7th **V92.12 Drowning and submersion due to being thrown overboard by motion of fishing boat**

X+7th **V92.13 Drowning and submersion due to being thrown overboard by motion of other powered watercraft**
Drowning and submersion due to being thrown overboard by motion of Hovercraft

X+7th **V92.14 Drowning and submersion due to being thrown overboard by motion of sailboat**

X+7th **V92.15 Drowning and submersion due to being thrown overboard by motion of canoe or kayak**

X+7th **V92.16 Drowning and submersion due to being thrown overboard by motion of (nonpowered) inflatable craft**

X+7th **V92.19 Drowning and submersion due to being thrown overboard by motion of unspecified watercraft**
Drowning and submersion due to being thrown overboard by motion of boat NOS
Drowning and submersion due to being thrown overboard by motion of ship NOS
Drowning and submersion due to being thrown overboard by motion of watercraft NOS

\+ **V92.2 Drowning and submersion due to being washed overboard from watercraft**
Code first any associated cataclysm (X37.0-)

X+7th **V92.20 Drowning and submersion due to being washed overboard from merchant ship**

X+7th **V92.21 Drowning and submersion due to being washed overboard from passenger ship**
Drowning and submersion due to being washed overboard from Ferry-boat
Drowning and submersion due to being washed overboard from Liner

X+7th **V92.22 Drowning and submersion due to being washed overboard from fishing boat**

X+7th **V92.23 Drowning and submersion due to being washed overboard from other powered watercraft**
Drowning and submersion due to being washed overboard from Hovercraft (on open water)
Drowning and submersion due to being washed overboard from Jet ski

X+7th **V92.24 Drowning and submersion due to being washed overboard from sailboat**

X+7th **V92.25 Drowning and submersion due to being washed overboard from canoe or kayak**

X+7th **V92.26 Drowning and submersion due to being washed overboard from (nonpowered) inflatable craft**

X+7th **V92.27 Drowning and submersion due to being washed overboard from water-skis**
Excludes1: *drowning and submersion due to fall off water-skis (V92.07)*

X+7th **V92.28 Drowning and submersion due to being washed overboard from other unpowered watercraft**
Drowning and submersion due to being washed overboard from surf-board
Drowning and submersion due to being washed overboard from windsurfer

X+7th **V92.29 Drowning and submersion due to being washed overboard from unspecified watercraft**
Drowning and submersion due to being washed overboard from boat NOS
Drowning and submersion due to being washed overboard from ship NOS
Drowning and submersion due to being washed overboard from watercraft NOS

V93 Other injury due to accident on board watercraft, without accident to watercraft
Excludes1: *civilian water transport accident involving military watercraft (V94.81-)*
other injury due to accident to watercraft (V91.-)
military watercraft accident in military or war operations (Y36, Y37.-)
Excludes2: *drowning and submersion due to accident on board watercraft, without accident to watercraft (V92.-)*

The appropriate 7th character is to be added to each code from category V93
A initial encounter
D subsequent encounter
S sequela

\+ **V93.0 Burn due to localized fire on board watercraft**
Excludes1: *burn due to watercraft on fire (V91.0-)*

X+7th **V93.00 Burn due to localized fire on board merchant vessel**

X+7th **V93.01 Burn due to localized fire on board passenger vessel**
Burn due to localized fire on board Ferry-boat
Burn due to localized fire on board Liner

X+7th **V93.02 Burn due to localized fire on board fishing boat**

X+7th **V93.03 Burn due to localized fire on board other powered watercraft**
Burn due to localized fire on board Hovercraft
Burn due to localized fire on board Jet ski

X+7th **V93.04 Burn due to localized fire on board sailboat**

X+7th **V93.09 Burn due to localized fire on board unspecified watercraft**
Burn due to localized fire on board boat NOS
Burn due to localized fire on board ship NOS
Burn due to localized fire on board watercraft NOS

\+ **V93.1 Other burn on board watercraft**
Burn due to source other than fire on board watercraft
Excludes1: *burn due to watercraft on fire (V91.0-)*

X+7th **V93.10 Other burn on board merchant vessel**

X+7th **V93.11 Other burn on board passenger vessel**
Other burn on board Ferry-boat
Other burn on board Liner

X+7th **V93.12 Other burn on board fishing boat**

X+7th **V93.13 Other burn on board other powered watercraft**
Other burn on board Hovercraft
Other burn on board Jet ski

X+7th **V93.14 Other burn on board sailboat**

X+7th **V93.19 Other burn on board unspecified watercraft**
Other burn on board boat NOS
Other burn on board ship NOS
Other burn on board watercraft NOS

\+ **V93.2 Heat exposure on board watercraft**
Excludes1: *exposure to man-made heat not aboard watercraft (W92)*
exposure to natural heat while on board watercraft (X30)
exposure to sunlight while on board watercraft (X32)
Excludes2: *burn due to fire on board watercraft (V93.0-)*

X+7th **V93.20 Heat exposure on board merchant ship**

X+7th **V93.21 Heat exposure on board passenger ship**
Heat exposure on board Ferry-boat
Heat exposure on board Liner

X+7th **V93.22 Heat exposure on board fishing boat**

X+7th **V93.23 Heat exposure on board other powered watercraft**
Heat exposure on board hovercraft

X+7th **V93.24 Heat exposure on board sailboat**

X+7th **V93.29 Heat exposure on board unspecified watercraft**
Heat exposure on board boat NOS
Heat exposure on board ship NOS
Heat exposure on board watercraft NOS

\+ **V93.3 Fall on board watercraft**
Excludes1: *fall due to collision of watercraft (V91.2-)*

X+7th **V93.30 Fall on board merchant ship**

X+7th **V93.31 Fall on board passenger ship**
Fall on board Ferry-boat
Fall on board Liner

X+7th **V93.32 Fall on board fishing boat**

X+7th **V93.33 Fall on board other powered watercraft**
Fall on board Hovercraft (on open water)
Fall on board Jet ski

X+7th **V93.34 Fall on board sailboat**

X+7th **V93.35 Fall on board canoe or kayak**

X+7th **V93.36 Fall on board (nonpowered) inflatable craft**

X+7th **V93.38 Fall on board other unpowered watercraft**

X+7th **V93.39 Fall on board unspecified watercraft**
Fall on board boat NOS
Fall on board ship NOS
Fall on board watercraft NOS

\+ **V93.4 Struck by falling object on board watercraft**
Hit by falling object on board watercraft
Excludes1: *struck by falling object due to accident to watercraft (V91.3)*

X+7th **V93.40 Struck by falling object on merchant ship**

X+7th **V93.41 Struck by falling object on passenger ship**
Struck by falling object on Ferry-boat
Struck by falling object on Liner

X+7th **V93.42 Struck by falling object on fishing boat**

X+7th **V93.43 Struck by falling object on other powered watercraft**
Struck by falling object on Hovercraft

X+7th **V93.44 Struck by falling object on sailboat**

X+7th **V93.48 Struck by falling object on other unpowered watercraft**

X+7th **V93.49 Struck by falling object on unspecified watercraft**

\+ **V93.5 Explosion on board watercraft**
Boiler explosion on steamship
Excludes2: *fire on board watercraft (V93.0-)*

X+7th **V93.50 Explosion on board merchant ship**
X+7th **V93.51 Explosion on board passenger ship**
Explosion on board Ferry-boat
Explosion on board Liner
X+7th **V93.52 Explosion on board fishing boat**
X+7th **V93.53 Explosion on board other powered watercraft**
Explosion on board Hovercraft
Explosion on board Jet ski
X+7th **V93.54 Explosion on board sailboat**
X+7th **V93.59 Explosion on board unspecified watercraft**
Explosion on board boat NOS
Explosion on board ship NOS
Explosion on board watercraft NOS
\+ **V93.6 Machinery accident on board watercraft**
Excludes1: *machinery explosion on board watercraft (V93.4-)*
machinery fire on board watercraft (V93.0-)
X+7th **V93.60 Machinery accident on board merchant ship**
X+7th **V93.61 Machinery accident on board passenger ship**
Machinery accident on board Ferry-boat
Machinery accident on board Liner
X+7th **V93.62 Machinery accident on board fishing boat**
X+7th **V93.63 Machinery accident on board other powered watercraft**
Machinery accident on board Hovercraft
X+7th **V93.64 Machinery accident on board sailboat**
X+7th **V93.69 Machinery accident on board unspecified watercraft**
Machinery accident on board boat NOS
Machinery accident on board ship NOS
Machinery accident on board watercraft NOS
\+ **V93.8 Other injury due to other accident on board watercraft**
Accidental poisoning by gases or fumes on watercraft
X+7th **V93.80 Other injury due to other accident on board merchant ship**
X+7th **V93.81 Other injury due to other accident on board passenger ship**
Other injury due to other accident on board Ferry-boat
Other injury due to other accident on board Liner
X+7th **V93.82 Other injury due to other accident on board fishing boat**
X+7th **V93.83 Other injury due to other accident on board other powered watercraft**
Other injury due to other accident on board Hovercraft
Other injury due to other accident on board Jet ski
X+7th **V93.84 Other injury due to other accident on board sailboat**
X+7th **V93.85 Other injury due to other accident on board canoe or kayak**
X+7th **V93.86 Other injury due to other accident on board (nonpowered) inflatable craft**
X+7th **V93.87 Other injury due to other accident on board water-skis**
Hit or struck by object while waterskiing
X+7th **V93.88 Other injury due to other accident on board other unpowered watercraft**
Hit or struck by object while surfing
Hit or struck by object while on board windsurfer
X+7th **V93.89 Other injury due to other accident on board unspecified watercraft**
Other injury due to other accident on board boat NOS
Other injury due to other accident on board ship NOS
Other injury due to other accident on board watercraft NOS

V94 Other and unspecified water transport accidents
Excludes1: *military watercraft accidents in military or war operations (Y36, Y37)*

The appropriate 7th character is to be added to each code from category V94
A initial encounter
D subsequent encounter
S sequela

X+7th **V94.0 Hitting object or bottom of body of water due to fall from watercraft**
Excludes2: *drowning and submersion due to fall from watercraft (V92.0-)*
\+ **V94.1 Bather struck by watercraft**
Swimmer hit by watercraft
X+7th **V94.11 Bather struck by powered watercraft**
X+7th **V94.12 Bather struck by nonpowered watercraft**
\+ **V94.2 Rider of nonpowered watercraft struck by other watercraft**
X+7th **V94.21 Rider of nonpowered watercraft struck by other nonpowered watercraft**
Canoer hit by other nonpowered watercraft
Surfer hit by other nonpowered watercraft
Windsurfer hit by other nonpowered watercraft
X+7th **V94.22 Rider of nonpowered watercraft struck by powered watercraft**
Canoer hit by motorboat
Surfer hit by motorboat
Windsurfer hit by motorboat
\+ **V94.3 Injury to rider of (inflatable) watercraft being pulled behind other watercraft**
X+7th **V94.31 Injury to rider of (inflatable) recreational watercraft being pulled behind other watercraft**
Injury to rider of inner-tube pulled behind motor boat
X+7th **V94.32 Injury to rider of non-recreational watercraft being pulled behind other watercraft**
Injury to occupant of dingy being pulled behind boat or ship
Injury to occupant of life-raft being pulled behind boat or ship
X+7th **V94.4 Injury to barefoot water-skier**
Injury to person being pulled behind boat or ship
\+ **V94.8 Other water transport accident**
\+ **V94.81 Water transport accident involving military watercraft**
+7th **V94.810 Civilian watercraft involved in water transport accident with military watercraft**
Passenger on civilian watercraft injured due to accident with military watercraft
+7th **V94.811 Civilian in water injured by military watercraft**
+7th **V94.818 Other water transport accident involving military watercraft**
X+7th **V94.89 Other water transport accident**
X+7th **V94.9 Unspecified water transport accident**
Water transport accident NOS

Air and space transport accidents (V95-V97)

Excludes1: *military aircraft accidents in military or war operations (Y36, Y37.-)*

V95 Accident to powered aircraft causing injury to occupant

The appropriate 7th character is to be added to each code from category V95
A initial encounter
D subsequent encounter
S sequela

\+ **V95.0 Helicopter accident injuring occupant**
X+7th **V95.00 Unspecified helicopter accident injuring occupant**
X+7th **V95.01 Helicopter crash injuring occupant**
X+7th **V95.02 Forced landing of helicopter injuring occupant**
X+7th **V95.03 Helicopter collision injuring occupant**
Helicopter collision with any object, fixed, movable or moving
X+7th **V95.04 Helicopter fire injuring occupant**
X+7th **V95.05 Helicopter explosion injuring occupant**
X+7th **V95.09 Other helicopter accident injuring occupant**
\+ **V95.1 Ultralight, microlight or powered-glider accident injuring occupant**
X+7th **V95.10 Unspecified ultralight, microlight or powered-glider accident injuring occupant**
X+7th **V95.11 Ultralight, microlight or powered-glider crash injuring occupant**
X+7th **V95.12 Forced landing of ultralight, microlight or powered-glider injuring occupant**
X+7th **V95.13 Ultralight, microlight or powered-glider collision injuring occupant**
Ultralight, microlight or powered-glider collision with any object, fixed, movable or moving
X+7th **V95.14 Ultralight, microlight or powered-glider fire injuring occupant**

X+7th **V95.15 Ultralight, microlight or powered-glider explosion injuring occupant**

X+7th **V95.19 Other ultralight, microlight or powered-glider accident injuring occupant**

\+ **V95.2 Other private fixed-wing aircraft accident injuring occupant**

X+7th **V95.20 Unspecified accident to other private fixed-wing aircraft, injuring occupant**

X+7th **V95.21 Other private fixed-wing aircraft crash injuring occupant**

X+7th **V95.22 Forced landing of other private fixed-wing aircraft injuring occupant**

X+7th **V95.23 Other private fixed-wing aircraft collision injuring occupant**

Other private fixed-wing aircraft collision with any object, fixed, movable or moving

X+7th **V95.24 Other private fixed-wing aircraft fire injuring occupant**

X+7th **V95.25 Other private fixed-wing aircraft explosion injuring occupant**

X+7th **V95.29 Other accident to other private fixed-wing aircraft injuring occupant**

\+ **V95.3 Commercial fixed-wing aircraft accident injuring occupant**

X+7th **V95.30 Unspecified accident to commercial fixed-wing aircraft injuring occupant**

X+7th **V95.31 Commercial fixed-wing aircraft crash injuring occupant**

X+7th **V95.32 Forced landing of commercial fixed-wing aircraft injuring occupant**

X+7th **V95.33 Commercial fixed-wing aircraft collision injuring occupant**

Commercial fixed-wing aircraft collision with any object, fixed, movable or moving

X+7th **V95.34 Commercial fixed-wing aircraft fire injuring occupant**

X+7th **V95.35 Commercial fixed-wing aircraft explosion injuring occupant**

X+7th **V95.39 Other accident to commercial fixed-wing aircraft injuring occupant**

\+ **V95.4 Spacecraft accident injuring occupant**

X+7th **V95.40 Unspecified spacecraft accident injuring occupant**

X+7th **V95.41 Spacecraft crash injuring occupant**

X+7th **V95.42 Forced landing of spacecraft injuring occupant**

X+7th **V95.43 Spacecraft collision injuring occupant**

Spacecraft collision with any object, fixed, moveable or moving

X+7th **V95.44 Spacecraft fire injuring occupant**

X+7th **V95.45 Spacecraft explosion injuring occupant**

X+7th **V95.49 Other spacecraft accident injuring occupant**

X+7th **V95.8 Other powered aircraft accidents injuring occupant**

X+7th **V95.9 Unspecified aircraft accident injuring occupant**

Aircraft accident NOS

Air transport accident NOS

V96 Accident to nonpowered aircraft causing injury to occupant

The appropriate 7th character is to be added to each code from category V96
- A initial encounter
- D subsequent encounter
- S sequela

\+ **V96.0 Balloon accident injuring occupant**

X+7th **V96.00 Unspecified balloon accident injuring occupant**

X+7th **V96.01 Balloon crash injuring occupant**

X+7th **V96.02 Forced landing of balloon injuring occupant**

X+7th **V96.03 Balloon collision injuring occupant**

Balloon collision with any object, fixed, moveable or moving

X+7th **V96.04 Balloon fire injuring occupant**

X+7th **V96.05 Balloon explosion injuring occupant**

X+7th **V96.09 Other balloon accident injuring occupant**

\+ **V96.1 Hang-glider accident injuring occupant**

X+7th **V96.10 Unspecified hang-glider accident injuring occupant**

X+7th **V96.11 Hang-glider crash injuring occupant**

X+7th **V96.12 Forced landing of hang-glider injuring occupant**

X+7th **V96.13 Hang-glider collision injuring occupant**

Hang-glider collision with any object, fixed, moveable or moving

X+7th **V96.14 Hang-glider fire injuring occupant**

X+7th **V96.15 Hang-glider explosion injuring occupant**

X+7th **V96.19 Other hang-glider accident injuring occupant**

\+ **V96.2 Glider (nonpowered) accident injuring occupant**

X+7th **V96.20 Unspecified glider (nonpowered) accident injuring occupant**

X+7th **V96.21 Glider (nonpowered) crash injuring occupant**

X+7th **V96.22 Forced landing of glider (nonpowered) injuring occupant**

X+7th **V96.23 Glider (nonpowered) collision injuring occupant**

Glider (nonpowered) collision with any object, fixed, moveable or moving

X+7th **V96.24 Glider (nonpowered) fire injuring occupant**

V96.25 Glider (nonpowered) explosion injuring occupant

X+7th **V96.29 Other glider (nonpowered) accident injuring occupant**

X+7th **V96.8 Other nonpowered-aircraft accidents injuring occupant**

Kite carrying a person accident injuring occupant

X+7th **V96.9 Unspecified nonpowered-aircraft accident injuring occupant**

Nonpowered-aircraft accident NOS

V97 Other specified air transport accidents

The appropriate 7th character is to be added to each code from category V97
- A initial encounter
- D subsequent encounter
- S sequela

X+7th **V97.0 Occupant of aircraft injured in other specified air transport accidents**

Fall in, on or from aircraft in air transport accident

Excludes1: *accident while boarding or alighting aircraft (V97.1)*

X+7th **V97.1 Person injured while boarding or alighting from aircraft**

\+ **V97.2 Parachutist accident**

X+7th **V97.21 Parachutist entangled in object**

Parachutist landing in tree

X+7th **V97.22 Parachutist injured on landing**

X+7th **V97.29 Other parachutist accident**

\+ **V97.3 Person on ground injured in air transport accident**

X+7th **V97.31 Hit by object falling from aircraft**

Hit by crashing aircraft

Injured by aircraft hitting house

Injured by aircraft hitting car

X+7th **V97.32 Injured by rotating propeller**

X+7th **V97.33 Sucked into jet engine**

X+7th **V97.39 Other injury to person on ground due to air transport accident**

\+ **V97.8 Other air transport accidents, not elsewhere classified**

Excludes1: *aircraft accident NOS (V95.9)*

exposure to changes in air pressure during ascent or descent (W94.-)

\+ **V97.81 Air transport accident involving military aircraft**

+7th **V97.810 Civilian aircraft involved in air transport accident with military aircraft**

Passenger in civilian aircraft injured due to accident with military aircraft

+7th **V97.811 Civilian injured by military aircraft**

+7th **V97.818 Other air transport accident involving military aircraft**

X+7th **V97.89 Other air transport accidents, not elsewhere classified**

Injury from machinery on aircraft

Other and unspecified transport accidents (V98-V99)

Excludes1: *vehicle accident, type of vehicle unspecified (V89.-)*

V98 Other specified transport accidents

The appropriate 7th character is to be added to each code from category V98
- A initial encounter
- D subsequent encounter
- S sequela

X+7th **V98.0 Accident to, on or involving cable-car, not on rails**

Caught or dragged by cable-car, not on rails

Fall or jump from cable-car, not on rails

Object thrown from or in cable-car, not on rails

X+7th **V98.1 Accident to, on or involving land-yacht**

X+7th **V98.2 Accident to, on or involving ice yacht**

X+7th **V98.3 Accident to, on or involving ski lift**
Accident to, on or involving ski chair-lift
Accident to, on or involving ski-lift with gondola

X+7th **V98.8 Other specified transport accidents**

V99 Unspecified transport accident
X+7th
The appropriate 7th character is to be added to code V99
A initial encounter
D subsequent encounter
S sequela

Other external causes of accidental injury (W00-X58)

Slipping, tripping, stumbling and falls (W00-W19)

Excludes1: *assault involving a fall (Y01-Y02)*
fall from animal (V80.-)
fall (in) (from) machinery (in operation) (W28-W31)
fall (in) (from) transport vehicle (V01-V99)
intentional self-harm involving a fall (X80-X81)

Excludes2: *at risk for fall (history of fall) (Z91.81)*
fall (in) (from) burning building (X00.-)
fall into fire (X00-X04, X08)

W00 Fall due to ice and snow

Includes: pedestrian on foot falling (slipping) on ice and snow
Excludes1: *fall on (from) ice and snow involving pedestrian conveyance (V00.-)*
fall from stairs and steps not due to ice and snow (W10.-)

The appropriate 7th character is to be added to each code from category W00
A initial encounter
D subsequent encounter
S sequela

X+7th **W00.0 Fall on same level due to ice and snow**
AHA CC: 2Q, 2016, 4-5

X+7th **W00.1 Fall from stairs and steps due to ice and snow**
X+7th **W00.2 Other fall from one level to another due to ice and snow**
X+7th **W00.9 Unspecified fall due to ice and snow**

W01 Fall on same level from slipping, tripping and stumbling

Includes: fall on moving sidewalk
Excludes1: *fall due to bumping (striking) against object (W18.0-)*
fall in shower or bathtub (W18.2-)
fall on same level NOS (W18.30)
fall on same level from slipping, tripping and stumbling due to ice or snow (W00.0)
fall off or from toilet (W18.1-)
slipping, tripping and stumbling NOS (W18.40)
slipping, tripping and stumbling without falling (W18.4-)

The appropriate 7th character is to be added to each code from category W01
A initial encounter
D subsequent encounter
S sequela

X+7th **W01.0 Fall on same level from slipping, tripping and stumbling without subsequent striking against object**
Falling over animal

\+ **W01.1 Fall on same level from slipping, tripping and stumbling with subsequent striking against object**

X+7th **W01.10 Fall on same level from slipping, tripping and stumbling with subsequent striking against unspecified object**

\+ **W01.11 Fall on same level from slipping, tripping and stumbling with subsequent striking against sharp object**

+7th **W01.110 Fall on same level from slipping, tripping and stumbling with subsequent striking against sharp glass**

+7th **W01.111 Fall on same level from slipping, tripping and stumbling with subsequent striking against power tool or machine**

+7th **W01.118 Fall on same level from slipping, tripping and stumbling with subsequent striking against other sharp object**

+7th **W01.119 Fall on same level from slipping, tripping and stumbling with subsequent striking against unspecified sharp object**

\+ **W01.19 Fall on same level from slipping, tripping and stumbling with subsequent striking against other object**

+7th **W01.190 Fall on same level from slipping, tripping and stumbling with subsequent striking against furniture**
AHA CC: 1Q, 2021, 4-5

+7th **W01.198 Fall on same level from slipping, tripping and stumbling with subsequent striking against other object**

W03 Other fall on same level due to collision with another person
X+7th
Fall due to non-transport collision with other person
Excludes1: *collision with another person without fall (W51)*
crushed or pushed by a crowd or human stampede (W52)
fall involving pedestrian conveyance (V00-V09)
fall due to ice or snow (W00)
fall on same level NOS (W18.30)
AHA CC: 4Q, 2012, 108; 1Q, 2015, 3-21

The appropriate 7th character is to be added to code W03
A initial encounter
D subsequent encounter
S sequela

W04 Fall while being carried or supported by other persons
X+7th
Accidentally dropped while being carried

The appropriate 7th character is to be added to code W04
A initial encounter
D subsequent encounter
S sequela

W05 Fall from non-movitng wheelchair, nonmotorized scooter and motorized mobility scooter

Excludes1: *fall from moving wheelchair (powered) (V00.811)*
fall from moving motorized mobility scooter (V00.831)
fall from nonmotorized scooter (V00.141)
AHA CC: 2Q, 2019, 27-28

The appropriate 7th character is to be added to each code from category W05
A initial encounter
D subsequent encounter
S sequela

X+7th **W05.0 Fall from non-moving wheelchair**
X+7th **W05.1 Fall from non-moving nonmotorized scooter**
X+7th **W05.2 Fall from non-moving motorized mobility scooter**

W06 Fall from bed
X+7th
The appropriate 7th character is to be added to code W06
A initial encounter
D subsequent encounter
S sequela
AHA CC: 4Q, 2020, 33

W07 Fall from chair
X+7th
The appropriate 7th character is to be added to code W07
A initial encounter
D subsequent encounter
S sequela

W08 Fall from other furniture
X+7th
The appropriate 7th character is to be added to code W08
A initial encounter
D subsequent encounter
S sequela

W09 Fall on and from playground equipment

Excludes1: *fall involving recreational machinery (W31)*

The appropriate 7th character is to be added to each code from category W09
A initial encounter
D subsequent encounter
S sequela

X+7th **W09.0 Fall on or from playground slide**
X+7th **W09.1 Fall from playground swing**
X+7th **W09.2 Fall on or from jungle gym**
X+7th **W09.8 Fall on or from other playground equipment**

W10 Fall on and from stairs and steps

Excludes1: *Fall from stairs and steps due to ice and snow (W00.1)*

The appropriate 7th character is to be added to each code from category W10
A initial encounter
D subsequent encounter
S sequela

X+7th **W10.0 Fall (on)(from) escalator**
X+7th **W10.1 Fall (on)(from) sidewalk curb**
X+7th **W10.2 Fall (on)(from) incline**
Fall (on) (from) ramp
X+7th **W10.8 Fall (on) (from) other stairs and steps**
X+7th **W10.9 Fall (on) (from) unspecified stairs and steps**

W11 Fall on and from ladder
X+7th
The appropriate 7th character is to be added to code W11
A initial encounter
D subsequent encounter
S sequela

W12 Fall on and from scaffolding
X+7th
The appropriate 7th character is to be added to code W12
A initial encounter
D subsequent encounter
S sequela

W13 Fall from, out of or through building or structure

The appropriate 7th character is to be added to each code from category W13
A initial encounter
D subsequent encounter
S sequela

X+7th **W13.0 Fall from, out of or through balcony**
Fall from, out of or through railing
X+7th **W13.1 Fall from, out of or through bridge**
X+7th **W13.2 Fall from, out of or through roof**
X+7th **W13.3 Fall through floor**
X+7th **W13.4 Fall from, out of or through window**
Excludes2: *fall with subsequent striking against sharp glass (W01.110-)*
X+7th **W13.8 Fall from, out of or through other building or structure**
Fall from, out of or through viaduct
Fall from, out of or through wall
Fall from, out of or through flag-pole
X+7th **W13.9 Fall from, out of or through building, not otherwise specified**
Excludes1: *collapse of a building or structure (W20.-)*
fall or jump from burning building or structure (X00.-)

W14 Fall from tree
X+7th
The appropriate 7th character is to be added to code W14
A initial encounter
D subsequent encounter
S sequela

W15 Fall from cliff
X+7th
The appropriate 7th character is to be added to code W15
A initial encounter
D subsequent encounter
S sequela

W16 Fall, jump or diving into water

Excludes1: *accidental non-watercraft drowning and submersion not involving fall (W65-W74)*
effects of air pressure from diving (W94.-)
fall into water from watercraft (V90-V94)
hitting an object or against bottom when falling from watercraft (V94.0)
Excludes2: *striking or hitting diving board (W21.4)*

The appropriate 7th character is to be added to each code from category W16
A initial encounter
D subsequent encounter
S sequela

\+ **W16.0 Fall into swimming pool**
Fall into swimming pool NOS
Excludes1: *fall into empty swimming pool (W17.3)*
\+ **W16.01 Fall into swimming pool striking water surface**
+7th **W16.011 Fall into swimming pool striking water surface causing drowning and submersion**
Excludes1: *drowning and submersion while in swimming pool without fall (W67)*
+7th **W16.012 Fall into swimming pool striking water surface causing other injury**
\+ **W16.02 Fall into swimming pool striking bottom**
+7th **W16.021 Fall into swimming pool striking bottom causing drowning and submersion**
Excludes1: *drowning and submersion while in swimming pool without fall (W67)*
+7th **W16.022 Fall into swimming pool striking bottom causing other injury**
\+ **W16.03 Fall into swimming pool striking wall**
+7th **W16.031 Fall into swimming pool striking wall causing drowning and submersion**
Excludes1: *drowning and submersion while in swimming pool without fall (W67)*
+7th **W16.032 Fall into swimming pool striking wall causing other injury**
\+ **W16.1 Fall into natural body of water**
Fall into lake
Fall into open sea
Fall into river
Fall into stream
\+ **W16.11 Fall into natural body of water striking water surface**
+7th **W16.111 Fall into natural body of water striking water surface causing drowning and submersion**
Excludes1: *drowning and submersion while in natural body of water without fall (W69)*
+7th **W16.112 Fall into natural body of water striking water surface causing other injury**
\+ **W16.12 Fall into natural body of water striking bottom**
+7th **W16.121 Fall into natural body of water striking bottom causing drowning and submersion**
Excludes1: *drowning and submersion while in natural body of water without fall (W69)*
+7th **W16.122 Fall into natural body of water striking bottom causing other injury**
\+ **W16.13 Fall into natural body of water striking side**
+7th **W16.131 Fall into natural body of water striking side causing drowning and submersion**
Excludes1: *drowning and submersion while in natural body of water without fall (W69)*
+7th **W16.132 Fall into natural body of water striking side causing other injury**
\+ **W16.2 Fall in (into) filled bathtub or bucket of water**
\+ **W16.21 Fall in (into) filled bathtub**
Excludes1: *fall into empty bathtub (W18.2)*
+7th **W16.211 Fall in (into) filled bathtub causing drowning and submersion**
Excludes1: *drowning and submersion while in filled bathtub without fall (W65)*
+7th **W16.212 Fall in (into) filled bathtub causing other injury**
\+ **W16.22 Fall in (into) bucket of water**
+7th **W16.221 Fall in (into) bucket of water causing drowning and submersion**
+7th **W16.222 Fall in (into) bucket of water causing other injury**
\+ **W16.3 Fall into other water**
Fall into fountain
Fall into reservoir
\+ **W16.31 Fall into other water striking water surface**
+7th **W16.311 Fall into other water striking water surface causing drowning and submersion**
Excludes1: *drowning and submersion while in other water without fall (W73)*
+7th **W16.312 Fall into other water striking water surface causing other injury**

+ **W16.32 Fall into other water striking bottom**
  +7th **W16.321 Fall into other water striking bottom causing drowning and submersion**
  Excludes1: *drowning and submersion while in other water without fall (W73)*
  +7th **W16.322 Fall into other water striking bottom causing other injury**
+ **W16.33 Fall into other water striking wall**
  +7th **W16.331 Fall into other water striking wall causing drowning and submersion**
  Excludes1: *drowning and submersion while in other water without fall (W73)*
  +7th **W16.332 Fall into other water striking wall causing other injury**

+ **W16.4 Fall into unspecified water**
  X+7th **W16.41 Fall into unspecified water causing drowning and submersion**
  X+7th **W16.42 Fall into unspecified water causing other injury**

+ **W16.5 Jumping or diving into swimming pool**
+ **W16.51 Jumping or diving into swimming pool striking water surface**
  +7th **W16.511 Jumping or diving into swimming pool striking water surface causing drowning and submersion**
  Excludes1: *drowning and submersion while in swimming pool withoutjumpingordiving (W67)*
  +7th **W16.512 Jumping or diving into swimming pool striking water surface causing other injury**
+ **W16.52 Jumping or diving into swimming pool striking bottom**
  +7th **W16.521 Jumping or diving into swimming pool striking bottom causing drowning and submersion**
  Excludes1: *drowning and submersion while in swimming pool withoutjumpingordiving (W67)*
  +7th **W16.522 Jumping or diving into swimming pool striking bottom causing other injury**
+ **W16.53 Jumping or diving into swimming pool striking wall**
  +7th **W16.531 Jumping or diving into swimming pool striking wall causing drowning and submersion**
  Excludes1: *drowning and submersion while in swimming pool withoutjumpingordiving (W67)*
  +7th **W16.532 Jumping or diving into swimming pool striking wall causing other injury**

+ **W16.6 Jumping or diving into natural body of water**
  Jumping or diving into lake
  Jumping or diving into open sea
  Jumping or diving into river
  Jumping or diving into stream
+ **W16.61 Jumping or diving into natural body of water striking water surface**
  +7th **W16.611 Jumping or diving into natural body of water striking water surface causing drowning and submersion**
  Excludes1: *drowning and submersion while in natural body of water without jumping or diving (W69)*
  +7th **W16.612 Jumping or diving into natural body of water striking water surface causing other injury**
+ **W16.62 Jumping or diving into natural body of water striking bottom**
  +7th **W16.621 Jumping or diving into natural body of water striking bottom causing drowning and submersion**
  Excludes1: *drowning and submersion while in natural body of water without jumping or diving (W69)*
  +7th **W16.622 Jumping or diving into natural body of water striking bottom causing other injury**

+ **W16.7 Jumping or diving from boat**
  Excludes1: *Fall from boat into water -see watercraft accident (V90-V94)*
+ **W16.71 Jumping or diving from boat striking water surface**
  +7th **W16.711 Jumping or diving from boat striking water surface causing drowning and submersion**
  +7th **W16.712 Jumping or diving from boat striking water surface causing other injury**
+ **W16.72 Jumping or diving from boat striking bottom**
  +7th **W16.721 Jumping or diving from boat striking bottom causing drowning and submersion**
  +7th **W16.722 Jumping or diving from boat striking bottom causing other injury**

+ **W16.8 Jumping or diving into other water**
  Jumping or diving into fountain
  Jumping or diving into reservoir
+ **W16.81 Jumping or diving into other water striking water surface**
  +7th **W16.811 Jumping or diving into other water striking water surface causing drowning and submersion**
  Excludes1: *drowning and submersion while in other water withoutjumpingordiving (W73)*
  +7th **W16.812 Jumping or diving into other water striking water surface causing other injury**
+ **W16.82 Jumping or diving into other water striking bottom**
  +7th **W16.821 Jumping or diving into other water striking bottom causing drowning and submersion**
  Excludes1: *drowning and submersion while in other water withoutjumpingordiving (W73)*
  +7th **W16.822 Jumping or diving into other water striking bottom causing other injury**
+ **W16.83 Jumping or diving into other water striking wall**
  +7th **W16.831 Jumping or diving into other water striking wall causing drowning and submersion**
  Excludes1: *drowning and submersion while in other water withoutjumpingordiving (W73)*
  +7th **W16.832 Jumping or diving into other water striking wall causing other injury**

+ **W16.9 Jumping or diving into unspecified water**
  X+7th **W16.91 Jumping or diving into unspecified water causing drowning and submersion**
  X+7th **W16.92 Jumping or diving into unspecified water causing other injury**

W17 Other fall from one level to another

The appropriate 7th character is to be added to each code from category W17
A initial encounter
D subsequent encounter
S sequela

X+7th **W17.0 Fall into well**
X+7th **W17.1 Fall into storm drain or manhole**
X+7th **W17.2 Fall into hole**
Fall into pit
X+7th **W17.3 Fall into empty swimming pool**
Excludes1: *fall into filled swimming pool (W16.0-)*
X+7th **W17.4 Fall from dock**
+ **W17.8 Other fall from one level to another**
X+7th **W17.81 Fall down embankment (hill)**
X+7th **W17.82 Fall from (out of) grocery cart**
Fall due to grocery cart tipping over
X+7th **W17.89 Other fall from one level to another**
Fall from cherry picker
Fall from lifting device
Fall from mobile elevated work platform [MEWP]
Fall from sky lift
AHA CC: 2Q, 2015, 6-7

W18 Other slipping, tripping and stumbling and falls

The appropriate 7th character is to be added to each code from category W18
A initial encounter
D subsequent encounter
S sequela

+ **W18.0 Fall due to bumping against object**
Striking against object with subsequent fall
Excludes1: *fall on same level due to slipping, tripping, or stumbling with subsequent striking against object (W01.1-)*
X+7th **W18.00 Striking against unspecified object with subsequent fall**
X+7th **W18.01 Striking against sports equipment with subsequent fall**
X+7th **W18.02 Striking against glass with subsequent fall**
X+7th **W18.09 Striking against other object with subsequent fall**
+ **W18.1 Fall from or off toilet**
X+7th **W18.11 Fall from or off toilet without subsequent striking against object**
Fall from (off) toilet NOS
X+7th **W18.12 Fall from or off toilet with subsequent striking against object**
X+7th **W18.2 Fall in (into) shower or empty bathtub**
Excludes1: *fall in full bathtub causing drowning or submersion (W16.21-)*
+ **W18.3 Other and unspecified fall on same level**
X+7th **W18.30 Fall on same level, unspecified**
X+7th **W18.31 Fall on same level due to stepping on an object**
Fall on same level due to stepping on an animal
Excludes1: *slipping, tripping and stumbling without fall due to stepping on animal (W18.41)*
X+7th **W18.39 Other fall on same level**
+ **W18.4 Slipping, tripping and stumbling without falling**
Excludes1: *collision with another person without fall (W51)*
X+7th **W18.40 Slipping, tripping and stumbling without falling, unspecified**
X+7th **W18.41 Slipping, tripping and stumbling without falling due to stepping on object**
Slipping, tripping and stumbling without falling due to stepping on animal
Excludes1: *slipping, tripping and stumbling with fall due to stepping on animal (W18.31)*
X+7th **W18.42 Slipping, tripping and stumbling without falling due to stepping into hole or opening**
X+7th **W18.43 Slipping, tripping and stumbling without falling due to stepping from one level to another**
X+7th **W18.49 Other slipping, tripping and stumbling without falling**

W19 Unspecified fall
X+7th
Accidental fall NOS
AHA CC: 4Q, 2012, 95-96; 2Q, 2021, 5

The appropriate 7th character is to be added to code W19
A initial encounter
D subsequent encounter
S sequela

Exposure to inanimate mechanical forces (W20-W49)

Excludes1: *assault (X92-Y09)*
contact or collision with animals or persons (W50-W64)
exposure to inanimate mechanical forces involving military or war operations (Y36.-, Y37.-)
intentional self-harm (X71-X83)

W20 Struck by thrown, projected or falling object

Code first any associated:
cataclysm (X34-X39)
lightning strike (T75.00)
Excludes1: *falling object in machinery accident (W24, W28-W31)*
falling object in transport accident (V01-V99)
object set in motion by explosion (W35-W40)
object set in motion by firearm (W32-W34)
struck by thrown sports equipment (W21.-)

The appropriate 7th character is to be added to each code from category W20
A initial encounter
D subsequent encounter
S sequela

X+7th **W20.0 Struck by falling object in cave-in**
Excludes2: *asphyxiation due to cave-in (T71.21)*
X+7th **W20.1 Struck by object due to collapse of building**
Excludes1: *struck by object due to collapse of burning building (X00.2, X02.2)*
X+7th **W20.8 Other cause of strike by thrown, projected or falling object**
Excludes1: *struck by thrown sports equipment (W21.-)*

W21 Striking against or struck by sports equipment

Excludes1: *assault with sports equipment (Y08.0-)*
striking against or struck by sports equipment with subsequent fall (W18.01)

The appropriate 7th character is to be added to each code from category W21
A initial encounter
D subsequent encounter
S sequela

+ **W21.0 Struck by hit or thrown ball**
X+7th **W21.00 Struck by hit or thrown ball, unspecified type**
X+7th **W21.01 Struck by football**
X+7th **W21.02 Struck by soccer ball**
X+7th **W21.03 Struck by baseball**
X+7th **W21.04 Struck by golf ball**
X+7th **W21.05 Struck by basketball**
X+7th **W21.06 Struck by volleyball**
X+7th **W21.07 Struck by softball**
X+7th **W21.09 Struck by other hit or thrown ball**
+ **W21.1 Struck by bat, racquet or club**
X+7th **W21.11 Struck by baseball bat**
X+7th **W21.12 Struck by tennis racquet**
X+7th **W21.13 Struck by golf club**
X+7th **W21.19 Struck by other bat, racquet or club**
+ **W21.2 Struck by hockey stick or puck**
+ **W21.21 Struck by hockey stick**
+7th **W21.210 Struck by ice hockey stick**
+7th **W21.211 Struck by field hockey stick**
+ **W21.22 Struck by hockey puck**
X+7th **W21.220 Struck by ice hockey puck**
X+7th **W21.221 Struck by field hockey puck**
+ **W21.3 Struck by sports foot wear**
X+7th **W21.31 Struck by shoe cleats**
Stepped on by shoe cleats
X+7th **W21.32 Struck by skate blades**
Skated over by skate blades
X+7th **W21.39 Struck by other sports foot wear**

X+7th **W21.4 Striking against diving board**
Use additional code for subsequent falling into water, if applicable (W16.-)

\+ **W21.8 Striking against or struck by other sports equipment**
X+7th **W21.81 Striking against or struck by football helmet**
X+7th **W21.89 Striking against or struck by other sports equipment**

X+7th **W21.9 Striking against or struck by unspecified sports equipment**

W22 Striking against or struck by other objects

Excludes1: *striking against or struck by object with subsequent fall (W18.09)*

The appropriate 7th character is to be added to each code from category W22
A initial encounter
D subsequent encounter
S sequela

\+ **W22.0 Striking against stationary object**
Excludes1: *striking against stationary sports equipment (W21.8)*
X+7th **W22.01 Walked into wall**
X+7th **W22.02 Walked into lamppost**
X+7th **W22.03 Walked into furniture**
\+ **W22.04 Striking against wall of swimming pool**
+7th **W22.041 Striking against wall of swimming pool causing drowning and submersion**
Excludes1: *drowning and submersion while swimming without striking against wall (W67)*
+7th **W22.042 Striking against wall of swimming pool causing other injury**
X+7th **W22.09 Striking against other stationary object**

\+ **W22.1 Striking against or struck by automobile airbag**
X+7th **W22.10 Striking against or struck by unspecified automobile airbag**
X+7th **W22.11 Striking against or struck by driver side automobile airbag**
X+7th **W22.12 Striking against or struck by front passenger side automobile airbag**
X+7th **W22.19 Striking against or struck by other automobile airbag**

X+7th **W22.8 Striking against or struck by other objects**
Striking against or struck by object NOS
Excludes1: *struck by thrown, projected or falling object (W20.-)*

W23 Caught, crushed, jammed or pinched in or between objects

Excludes1: *injury caused by cutting or piercing instruments (W25-W27)*
injury caused by firearms malfunction (W32.1, W33.1-, W34.1-)
injury caused by lifting and transmission devices (W24.-)
injury caused by machinery (W28-W31)
injury caused by nonpowered hand tools (W27.-)
injury caused by transport vehicle being used as a means of transportation (V01-V99)
injury caused by struck by thrown, projected or falling object (W20.-)

The appropriate 7th character is to be added to each code from category W23
A initial encounter
D subsequent encounter
S sequela

X+7th **W23.0 Caught, crushed, jammed, or pinched between moving objects**
X+7th **W23.1 Caught, crushed, jammed, or pinched between stationary objects**

W24 Contact with lifting and transmission devices, not elsewhere classified

Excludes1: *transport accidents (V01-V99)*

The appropriate 7th character is to be added to each code from category W24
A initial encounter
D subsequent encounter
S sequela

X+7th **W24.0 Contact with lifting devices, not elsewhere classified**
Contact with chain hoist
Contact with drive belt
Contact with pulley (block)
X+7th **W24.1 Contact with transmission devices, not elsewhere classified**
Contact with transmission belt or cable

W25 Contact with sharp glass
X+7th
Code first any associated:
injury due to flying glass from explosion or firearm discharge (W32-W40)
transport accident (V00-V99)
Excludes1: *fall on same level due to slipping, tripping and stumbling with subsequent striking against sharp glass (W01.110-)*
striking against sharp glass with subsequent fall (W18.02-)
Excludes2: *glass embedded in skin (W45.-)*

The appropriate 7th character is to be added to code W25
A initial encounter
D subsequent encounter
S sequela

W26 Contact with other sharp objects

Excludes2: *sharp object(s) embedded in skin (W45.-)*
AHA CC: 4Q, 2016, 73

The appropriate 7th character is to be added to each code from category W26
A initial encounter
D subsequent encounter
S sequela

X+7th **W26.0 Contact with knife**
Excludes1: *contact with electric knife (W29.1)*
X+7th **W26.1 Contact with sword or dagger**
X+7th **W26.2 Contact with edge of stiff paper**
Paper cut
X+7th **W26.8 Contact with other sharp object(s), not elsewhere classified**
Contact with tin can lid
X+7th **W26.9 Contact with unspecified sharp object(s)**

W27 Contact with nonpowered hand tool

The appropriate 7th character is to be added to each code from category W27
A initial encounter
D subsequent encounter
S sequela

X+7th **W27.0 Contact with workbench tool**
Contact with auger
Contact with axe
Contact with chisel
Contact with handsaw
Contact with screwdriver
X+7th **W27.1 Contact with garden tool**
Contact with hoe
Contact with nonpowered lawn mower
Contact with pitchfork
Contact with rake
X+7th **W27.2 Contact with scissors**
X+7th **W27.3 Contact with needle (sewing)**
Excludes1: *contact with hypodermic needle (W46.-)*
X+7th **W27.4 Contact with kitchen utensil**
Contact with fork
Contact with ice-pick
Contact with can-opener NOS

X+7th **W27.5 Contact with paper-cutter**
X+7th **W27.8 Contact with other nonpowered hand tool**
Contact with nonpowered sewing machine
Contact with shovel

W28 Contact with powered lawn mower
X+7th
Powered lawn mower (commercial) (residential)
Excludes1: *contact with nonpowered lawn mower (W27.1)*
Excludes2: *exposure to electric current (W86.-)*

The appropriate 7th character is to be added to code W28
A initial encounter
D subsequent encounter
S sequela

W29 Contact with other powered hand tools and household machinery

Excludes1: *contact with commercial machinery (W31.82)*
contact with hot household appliance (X15)
contact with nonpowered hand tool (W27.-)
exposure to electric current (W86)

The appropriate 7th character is to be added to each code from category W29
A initial encounter
D subsequent encounter
S sequela

X+7th **W29.0 Contact with powered kitchen appliance**
Contact with blender
Contact with can-opener
Contact with garbage disposal
Contact with mixer
X+7th **W29.1 Contact with electric knife**
X+7th **W29.2 Contact with other powered household machinery**
Contact with electric fan
Contact with powered dryer (clothes) (powered) (spin)
Contact with washing-machine
Contact with sewing machine
X+7th **W29.3 Contact with powered garden and outdoor hand tools and machinery**
Contact with chainsaw
Contact with edger
Contact with garden cultivator (tiller)
Contact with hedge trimmer
Contact with other powered garden tool
Excludes1: *contact with powered lawn mower (W28)*
X+7th **W29.4 Contact with nail gun**
X+7th **W29.8 Contact with other powered hand tools and household machinery**
Contact with do-it-yourself tool NOS

W30 Contact with agricultural machinery

Includes: animal-powered farm machine
Excludes1: *agricultural transport vehicle accident (V01-V99)*
explosion of grain store (W40.8)
exposure to electric current (W86.-)

The appropriate 7th character is to be added to each code from category W30
A initial encounter
D subsequent encounter
S sequela

X+7th **W30.0 Contact with combine harvester**
Contact with reaper
Contact with thresher
X+7th **W30.1 Contact with power take-off devices (PTO)**
X+7th **W30.2 Contact with hay derrick**
X+7th **W30.3 Contact with grain storage elevator**
Excludes1: *explosion of grain store (W40.8)*
\+ **W30.8 Contact with other specified agricultural machinery**
X+7th **W30.81 Contact with agricultural transport vehicle in stationary use**
Contact with agricultural transport vehicle under repair, not on public roadway
Excludes1: *agricultural transport vehicle accident (V01-V99)*
X+7th **W30.89 Contact with other specified agricultural machinery**
X+7th **W30.9 Contact with unspecified agricultural machinery**
Contact with farm machinery NOS

W31 Contact with other and unspecified machinery

Excludes1: *contact with agricultural machinery (W30.-)*
contact with machinery in transport under own power or being towed by a vehicle (V01-V99)
exposure to electric current (W86)

The appropriate 7th character is to be added to each code from category W31
A initial encounter
D subsequent encounter
S sequela

X+7th **W31.0 Contact with mining and earth-drilling machinery**
Contact with bore or drill (land) (seabed)
Contact with shaft hoist
Contact with shaft lift
Contact with undercutter
X+7th **W31.1 Contact with metalworking machines**
Contact with abrasive wheel
Contact with forging machine
Contact with lathe
Contact with mechanical shears
Contact with metal drilling machine
Contact with milling machine
Contact with power press
Contact with rolling-mill
Contact with metal sawing machine
X+7th **W31.2 Contact with powered woodworking and forming machines**
Contact with band saw
Contact with bench saw
Contact with circular saw
Contact with molding machine
Contact with overhead plane
Contact with powered saw
Contact with radial saw
Contact with sander
Excludes1: *nonpowered woodworking tools (W27.0)*
X+7th **W31.3 Contact with prime movers**
Contact with gas turbine
Contact with internal combustion engine
Contact with steam engine
Contact with water driven turbine
\+ **W31.8 Contact with other specified machinery**
X+7th **W31.81 Contact with recreational machinery**
Contact with roller coaster
X+7th **W31.82 Contact with other commercial machinery**
Contact with commercial electric fan
Contact with commercial kitchen appliances
Contact with commercial powered dryer (clothes) (powered) (spin)
Contact with commercial washing-machine
Contact with commercial sewing machine
Excludes1: *contact with household machinery (W29.-)*
contact with powered lawn mower (W28)
X+7th **W31.83 Contact with special construction vehicle in stationary use**
Contact with special construction vehicle under repair, not on public roadway
Excludes1: *special construction vehicle accident (V01-V99)*
X+7th **W31.89 Contact with other specified machinery**
X+7th **W31.9 Contact with unspecified machinery**
Contact with machinery NOS

W32 Accidental handgun discharge and malfunction

Includes: accidental discharge and malfunction of gun for single hand use
accidental discharge and malfunction of pistol
accidental discharge and malfunction of revolver
Handgun discharge and malfunction NOS
Excludes1: *accidental airgun discharge and malfunction (W34.010, W34.110)*
accidental BB gun discharge and malfunction (W34.010, W34.110)
accidental pellet gun discharge and malfunction (W34.010, W34.110)
accidental shotgun discharge and malfunction (W33.01, W33.11)

assault by handgun discharge (X93)
handgun discharge involving legal intervention (Y35.0-)
handgun discharge involving military or war operations (Y36.4-)
intentional self-harm by handgun discharge (X72)
Very pistol discharge and malfunction (W34.09, W34.19)

The appropriate 7th character is to be added to each code from category W32
A initial encounter
D subsequent encounter
S sequela

X+7th **W32.0 Accidental handgun discharge**
X+7th **W32.1 Accidental handgun malfunction**
Injury due to explosion of handgun (parts)
Injury due to malfunction of mechanism or component of handgun
Injury due to recoil of handgun
Powder burn from handgun

W33 Accidental rifle, shotgun and larger firearm discharge and malfunction

Includes: rifle, shotgun and larger firearm discharge and malfunction NOS

Excludes1: *accidental airgun discharge and malfunction (W34.010, W34.110)*
accidental BB gun discharge and malfunction (W34.010, W34.110)
accidental handgun discharge and malfunction (W32.-)
accidental pellet gun discharge and malfunction (W34.010, W34.110)
assault by rifle, shotgun and larger firearm discharge (X94)
firearm discharge involving legal intervention (Y35.0-)
firearm discharge involving military or war operations (Y36.4-)
intentional self-harm by rifle, shotgun and larger firearm discharge (X73)

The appropriate 7th character is to be added to each code from category W33
A initial encounter
D subsequent encounter
S sequela

\+ **W33.0 Accidental rifle, shotgun and larger firearm discharge**
X+7th **W33.00 Accidental discharge of unspecified larger firearm**
Discharge of unspecified larger firearm NOS
X+7th **W33.01 Accidental discharge of shotgun**
Discharge of shotgun NOS
X+7th **W33.02 Accidental discharge of hunting rifle**
Discharge of hunting rifle NOS
X+7th **W33.03 Accidental discharge of machine gun**
Discharge of machine gun NOS
X+7th **W33.09 Accidental discharge of other larger firearm**
Discharge of other larger firearm NOS
\+ **W33.1 Accidental rifle, shotgun and larger firearm malfunction**
Injury due to explosion of rifle, shotgun and larger firearm (parts)
Injury due to malfunction of mechanism or component of rifle, shotgun and larger firearm
Injury due to piercing, cutting, crushing or pinching due to (by) slide trigger mechanism, scope or other gun part
Injury due to recoil of rifle, shotgun and larger firearm
Powder burn from rifle, shotgun and larger firearm
X+7th **W33.10 Accidental malfunction of unspecified larger firearm**
Malfunction of unspecified larger firearm NOS
X+7th **W33.11 Accidental malfunction of shotgun**
Malfunction of shotgun NOS
X+7th **W33.12 Accidental malfunction of hunting rifle**
Malfunction of hunting rifle NOS
X+7th **W33.13 Accidental malfunction of machine gun**
Malfunction of machine gun NOS
X+7th **W33.19 Accidental malfunction of other larger firearm**
Malfunction of other larger firearm NOS

W34 Accidental discharge and malfunction from other and unspecified firearms and guns

The appropriate 7th character is to be added to each code from category W34
A initial encounter
D subsequent encounter
S sequela

\+ **W34.0 Accidental discharge from other and unspecified firearms and guns**
X+7th **W34.00 Accidental discharge from unspecified firearms or gun**
Discharge from firearm NOS
Gunshot wound NOS
Shot NOS
AHA CC: 1Q, 2015, 3-21
\+ **W34.01 Accidental discharge of gas, air or spring-operated guns**
+7th **W34.010 Accidental discharge of airgun**
Accidental discharge of BB gun
Accidental discharge of pellet gun
+7th **W34.011 Accidental discharge of paintball gun**
Accidental injury due to paintball discharge
+7th **W34.018 Accidental discharge of other gas, air or spring-operated gun**
X+7th **W34.09 Accidental discharge from other specified firearms**
Accidental discharge from Very pistol [flare]
\+ **W34.1 Accidental malfunction from other and unspecified firearms and guns**
X+7th **W34.10 Accidental malfunction from unspecified firearms or gun**
Firearm malfunction NOS
\+ **W34.11 Accidental malfunction of gas, air or spring-operated guns**
+7th **W34.110 Accidental malfunction of airgun**
Accidental malfunction of BB gun
Accidental malfunction of pellet gun
+7th **W34.111 Accidental malfunction of paintball gun**
Accidental injury due to paintball gun malfunction
+7th **W34.118 Accidental malfunction of other gas, air or spring-operated gun**
X+7th **W34.19 Accidental malfunction from other specified firearms**
Accidental malfunction from Very pistol [flare]

W35 Explosion and rupture of boiler
X+7th

Excludes1: *explosion and rupture of boiler on watercraft (V93.4)*

The appropriate 7th character is to be added to code W35
A initial encounter
D subsequent encounter
S sequela

W36 Explosion and rupture of gas cylinder

The appropriate 7th character is to be added to each code from category W36
A initial encounter
D subsequent encounter
S sequela

X+7th **W36.1 Explosion and rupture of aerosol can**
X+7th **W36.2 Explosion and rupture of air tank**
X+7th **W36.3 Explosion and rupture of pressurized-gas tank**
X+7th **W36.8 Explosion and rupture of other gas cylinder**
X+7th **W36.9 Explosion and rupture of unspecified gas cylinder**

W37 Explosion and rupture of pressurized tire, pipe or hose

The appropriate 7th character is to be added to each code from category W37
A initial encounter
D subsequent encounter
S sequela

X+7th **W37.0 Explosion of bicycle tire**
X+7th **W37.8 Explosion and rupture of other pressurized tire, pipe or hose**

W38 Explosion and rupture of other specified pressurized devices
X+7th

The appropriate 7th character is to be added to code W38
A initial encounter
D subsequent encounter
S sequela

W39 Discharge of firework
X+7th

The appropriate 7th character is to be added to code W39
A initial encounter
D subsequent encounter
S sequela

W40 Explosion of other materials

Excludes1: *assault by explosive material (X96)*
explosion involving legal intervention (Y35.1-)
explosion involving military or war operations (Y36.0-, Y36.2-)
intentional self-harm by explosive material (X75)

The appropriate 7th character is to be added to each code from category W40
A initial encounter
D subsequent encounter
S sequela

X+7th **W40.0 Explosion of blasting material**
Explosion of blasting cap
Explosion of detonator
Explosion of dynamite
Explosion of explosive (any) used in blasting operations

X+7th **W40.1 Explosion of explosive gases**
Explosion of acetylene
Explosion of butane
Explosion of coal gas
Explosion in mine NOS
Explosion of explosive gas
Explosion of fire damp
Explosion of gasoline fumes
Explosion of methane
Explosion of propane

X+7th **W40.8 Explosion of other specified explosive materials**
Explosion in dump NOS
Explosion in factory NOS
Explosion in grain store
Explosion in munitions
Excludes1: *explosion involving legal intervention (Y35.1-)*
explosion involving military or war operations (Y36.0-, Y36.2-)

X+7th **W40.9 Explosion of unspecified explosive materials**
Explosion NOS

W42 Exposure to noise

The appropriate 7th character is to be added to each code from category W42
A initial encounter
D subsequent encounter
S sequela

X+7th **W42.0 Exposure to supersonic waves**
X+7th **W42.9 Exposure to other noise**
Exposure to sound waves NOS

W45 Foreign body or object entering through skin

Includes: foreign body or object embedded in skin
nail embedded in skin
Excludes2: *contact with hand tools (nonpowered) (powered) (W27-W29)*
contact with other sharp object(s) (W26.-)
contact with sharp glass (W25.-)
struck by objects (W20-W22)

The appropriate 7th character is to be added to each code from category W45
A initial encounter
D subsequent encounter
S sequela

X+7th **W45.0 Nail entering through skin**
X+7th **W45.8 Other foreign body or object entering through skin**
Splinter in skin NOS

W46 Contact with hypodermic needle

The appropriate 7th character is to be added to each code from category W46
A initial encounter
D subsequent encounter
S sequela

X+7th **W46.0 Contact with hypodermic needle**
Hypodermic needle stick NOS
X+7th **W46.1 Contact with contaminated hypodermic needle**

W49 Exposure to other inanimate mechanical forces

Includes: exposure to abnormal gravitational [G] forces
exposure to inanimate mechanical forces NEC
Excludes1: *exposure to inanimate mechanical forces involving military or war operations (Y36.-, Y37.-)*

The appropriate 7th character is to be added to each code from category W49
A initial encounter
D subsequent encounter
S sequela

+ **W49.0 Item causing external constriction**
X+7th **W49.01 Hair causing external constriction**
X+7th **W49.02 String or thread causing external constriction**
X+7th **W49.03 Rubber band causing external constriction**
X+7th **W49.04 Ring or other jewelry causing external constriction**
X+7th **W49.09 Other specified item causing external constriction**
X+7th **W49.9 Exposure to other inanimate mechanical forces**

Exposure to animate mechanical forces (W50-W64)

Excludes1: *Toxic effect of contact with venomous animals and plants (T63.-)*

W50 Accidental hit, strike, kick, twist, bite or scratch by another person

Includes: hit, strike, kick, twist, bite, or scratch by another person NOS
Excludes1: *assault by bodily force (Y04)*
struck by objects (W20-W22)

The appropriate 7th character is to be added to each code from category W50
A initial encounter
D subsequent encounter
S sequela

X+7th **W50.0 Accidental hit or strike by another person**
Hit or strike by another person NOS
X+7th **W50.1 Accidental kick by another person**
Kick by another person NOS
X+7th **W50.2 Accidental twist by another person**
Twist by another person NOS
AHA CC: 1Q, 2015, 3-21
X+7th **W50.3 Accidental bite by another person**
Human bite
Bite by another person NOS
X+7th **W50.4 Accidental scratch by another person**
Scratch by another person NOS

W51 Accidental striking against or bumped into by another person
X+7th
Excludes1: *assault by striking against or bumping into by another person (Y04.2)*
fall due to collision with another person (W03)

The appropriate 7th character is to be added to code W51
A initial encounter
D subsequent encounter
S sequela

W52 Crushed, pushed or stepped on by crowd or human stampede
X+7th
Crushed, pushed or stepped on by crowd or human stampede with or without fall

The appropriate 7th character is to be added to code W52
A initial encounter
D subsequent encounter
S sequela

+ **W53 Contact with rodent**

Includes: contact with saliva, feces or urine of rodent

The appropriate 7th character is to be added to each code from category W53
A initial encounter
D subsequent encounter
S sequela

+ **W53.0 Contact with mouse**
  - X+7th **W53.01 Bitten by mouse**
  - X+7th **W53.09 Other contact with mouse**
+ **W53.1 Contact with rat**
  - X+7th **W53.11 Bitten by rat**
  - X+7th **W53.19 Other contact with rat**
+ **W53.2 Contact with squirrel**
  - X+7th **W53.21 Bitten by squirrel**
  - X+7th **W53.29 Other contact with squirrel**
+ **W53.8 Contact with other rodent**
  - X+7th **W53.81 Bitten by other rodent**
  - X+7th **W53.89 Other contact with other rodent**

W54 Contact with dog

Includes: contact with saliva, feces or urine of dog

The appropriate 7th character is to be added to each code from category W54
A initial encounter
D subsequent encounter
S sequela

X+7th **W54.0 Bitten by dog**
AHA CC: 4Q, 2017, 112-114
Review coding guideline B.19.c

X+7th **W54.1 Struck by dog**
Knocked over by dog

X+7th **W54.8 Other contact with dog**

W55 Contact with other mammals

Includes: contact with saliva, feces or urine of mammal
Excludes1: *animal being ridden- see transport accidents*
bitten or struck by dog (W54)
bitten or struck by rodent (W53.-)
contact with marine mammals (W56.-)

The appropriate 7th character is to be added to each code from category W55
A initial encounter
D subsequent encounter
S sequela

+ **W55.0 Contact with cat**
  - X+7th **W55.01 Bitten by cat**
  - X+7th **W55.03 Scratched by cat**
  - X+7th **W55.09 Other contact with cat**
+ **W55.1 Contact with horse**
  - X+7th **W55.11 Bitten by horse**
  - X+7th **W55.12 Struck by horse**
  - X+7th **W55.19 Other contact with horse**
+ **W55.2 Contact with cow**
  Contact with bull
  - X+7th **W55.21 Bitten by cow**
  - X+7th **W55.22 Struck by cow**
    Gored by bull
  - X+7th **W55.29 Other contact with cow**
+ **W55.3 Contact with other hoof stock**
  Contact with goats
  Contact with sheep
  - X+7th **W55.31 Bitten by other hoof stock**
  - X+7th **W55.32 Struck by other hoof stock**
    Gored by goat
    Gored by ram
  - X+7th **W55.39 Other contact with other hoof stock**
+ **W55.4 Contact with pig**
  - X+7th **W55.41 Bitten by pig**
  - X+7th **W55.42 Struck by pig**
  - X+7th **W55.49 Other contact with pig**
+ **W55.5 Contact with raccoon**
  - X+7th **W55.51 Bitten by raccoon**
  - X+7th **W55.52 Struck by raccoon**
  - X+7th **W55.59 Other contact with raccoon**
+ **W55.8 Contact with other mammals**
  - X+7th **W55.81 Bitten by other mammals**
  - X+7th **W55.82 Struck by other mammals**
  - X+7th **W55.89 Other contact with other mammals**

W56 Contact with nonvenomous marine animal

Excludes1: *contact with venomous marine animal (T63.-)*

The appropriate 7th character is to be added to each code from category W56
A initial encounter
D subsequent encounter
S sequela

+ **W56.0 Contact with dolphin**
  - X+7th **W56.01 Bitten by dolphin**
  - X+7th **W56.02 Struck by dolphin**
  - X+7th **W56.09 Other contact with dolphin**
+ **W56.1 Contact with sea lion**
  - X+7th **W56.11 Bitten by sea lion**
  - X+7th **W56.12 Struck by sea lion**
  - X+7th **W56.19 Other contact with sea lion**
+ **W56.2 Contact with orca**
  Contact with killer whale
  - X+7th **W56.21 Bitten by orca**
  - X+7th **W56.22 Struck by orca**
  - X+7th **W56.29 Other contact with orca**
+ **W56.3 Contact with other marine mammals**
  - X+7th **W56.31 Bitten by other marine mammals**
  - X+7th **W56.32 Struck by other marine mammals**
  - X+7th **W56.39 Other contact with other marine mammals**
+ **W56.4 Contact with shark**
  - X+7th **W56.41 Bitten by shark**
  - X+7th **W56.42 Struck by shark**
  - X+7th **W56.49 Other contact with shark**
+ **W56.5 Contact with other fish**
  - X+7th **W56.51 Bitten by other fish**
  - X+7th **W56.52 Struck by other fish**
  - X+7th **W56.59 Other contact with other fish**
+ **W56.8 Contact with other nonvenomous marine animals**
  - X+7th **W56.81 Bitten by other nonvenomous marine animals**
  - X+7th **W56.82 Struck by other nonvenomous marine animals**
  - X+7th **W56.89 Other contact with other nonvenomous marine animals**

W57 X+7th **Bitten or stung by nonvenomous insect and other nonvenomous arthropods**

Excludes1: *contact with venomous insects and arthropods (T63.2-, T63.3-, T63.4-)*

The appropriate 7th character is to be added to code W57
A initial encounter
D subsequent encounter
S sequela

W58 Contact with crocodile or alligator

The appropriate 7th character is to be added to each code from category W58
A initial encounter
D subsequent encounter
S sequela

+ **W58.0 Contact with alligator**
  - X+7th **W58.01 Bitten by alligator**
  - X+7th **W58.02 Struck by alligator**
  - X+7th **W58.03 Crushed by alligator**
  - X+7th **W58.09 Other contact with alligator**
+ **W58.1 Contact with crocodile**
  - X+7th **W58.11 Bitten by crocodile**
  - X+7th **W58.12 Struck by crocodile**
  - X+7th **W58.13 Crushed by crocodile**
  - X+7th **W58.19 Other contact with crocodile**

W59 Contact with other nonvenomous reptiles

Excludes1: *contact with venomous reptile (T63.0-, T63.1-)*

The appropriate 7th character is to be added to each code from category W59
A initial encounter
D subsequent encounter
S sequela

+ **W59.0 Contact with nonvenomous lizards**
  - X+7th **W59.01 Bitten by nonvenomous lizards**
  - X+7th **W59.02 Struck by nonvenomous lizards**
  - X+7th **W59.09 Other contact with nonvenomous lizards**
    Exposure to nonvenomous lizards
+ **W59.1 Contact with nonvenomous snakes**
  - X+7th **W59.11 Bitten by nonvenomous snake**
  - X+7th **W59.12 Struck by nonvenomous snake**

X+7th **W59.13 Crushed by nonvenomous snake**
X+7th **W59.19 Other contact with nonvenomous snake**
+ **W59.2 Contact with turtles**

Excludes1: *contact with tortoises (W59.8-)*

X+7th **W59.21 Bitten by turtle**
X+7th **W59.22 Struck by turtle**
X+7th **W59.29 Other contact with turtle**
Exposure to turtles
+ **W59.8 Contact with other nonvenomous reptiles**
X+7th **W59.81 Bitten by other nonvenomous reptiles**
X+7th **W59.82 Struck by other nonvenomous reptiles**
X+7th **W59.83 Crushed by other nonvenomous reptiles**
X+7th **W59.89 Other contact with other nonvenomous reptiles**

W60 Contact with nonvenomous plant thorns and spines and sharp leaves X+7th

Excludes1: *Contact with venomous plants (T63.7-)*

The appropriate 7th character is to be added to code W60
A initial encounter
D subsequent encounter
S sequela

W61 Contact with birds (domestic) (wild)

Includes: contact with excreta of birds

The appropriate 7th character is to be added to each code from category W61
A initial encounter
D subsequent encounter
S sequela

+ **W61.0 Contact with parrot**
X+7th **W61.01 Bitten by parrot**
X+7th **W61.02 Struck by parrot**
X+7th **W61.09 Other contact with parrot**
Exposure to parrots
+ **W61.1 Contact with macaw**
X+7th **W61.11 Bitten by macaw**
X+7th **W61.12 Struck by macaw**
X+7th **W61.19 Other contact with macaw**
Exposure to macaws
+ **W61.2 Contact with other psittacines**
X+7th **W61.21 Bitten by other psittacines**
X+7th **W61.22 Struck by other psittacines**
X+7th **W61.29 Other contact with other psittacines**
Exposure to other psittacines
+ **W61.3 Contact with chicken**
X+7th **W61.32 Struck by chicken**
X+7th **W61.33 Pecked by chicken**
X+7th **W61.39 Other contact with chicken**
Exposure to chickens
+ **W61.4 Contact with turkey**
X+7th **W61.42 Struck by turkey**
X+7th **W61.43 Pecked by turkey**
X+7th **W61.49 Other contact with turkey**
+ **W61.5 Contact with goose**
X+7th **W61.51 Bitten by goose**
X+7th **W61.52 Struck by goose**
X+7th **W61.59 Other contact with goose**
+ **W61.6 Contact with duck**
X+7th **W61.61 Bitten by duck**
X+7th **W61.62 Struck by duck**
X+7th **W61.69 Other contact with duck**
+ **W61.9 Contact with other birds**
X+7th **W61.91 Bitten by other birds**
X+7th **W61.92 Struck by other birds**
X+7th **W61.99 Other contact with other birds**
Contact with bird NOS

W62 Contact with nonvenomous amphibians

Excludes1: *contact with venomous amphibians (T63.81-R63.83)*

The appropriate 7th character is to be added to each code from category W62
A initial encounter
D subsequent encounter
S sequela

X+7th **W62.0 Contact with nonvenomous frogs**
X+7th **W62.1 Contact with nonvenomous toads**
X+7th **W62.9 Contact with other nonvenomous amphibians**

W64 Exposure to other animate mechanical forces X+7th

Includes: exposure to nonvenomous animal NOS
Excludes1: *contact with venomous animal (T63.-)*

The appropriate 7th character is to be added to code W64
A initial encounter
D subsequent encounter
S sequela

Accidental non-transport drowning and submersion (W65-W74)

Excludes1: *accidental drowning and submersion due to fall into water (W16.-)*
accidental drowning and submersion due to water transport accident (V90.-, V92.-)

Excludes2: *accidental drowning and submersion due to cataclysm (X34-X39)*

W65 Accidental drowning and submersion while in bath-tub X+7th

Excludes1: *accidental drowning and submersion due to fall in (into) bathtub (W16.211)*

The appropriate 7th character is to be added to code W65
A initial encounter
D subsequent encounter
S sequela

W67 Accidental drowning and submersion while in swimming-pool X+7th

Excludes1: *accidental drowning and submersion due to fall into swimming pool (W16.011, W16.021, W16.031)*
accidental drowning and submersion due to striking into wall of swimming pool (W22.041)

The appropriate 7th character is to be added to code W67
A initial encounter
D subsequent encounter
S sequela

W69 Accidental drowning and submersion while in natural water X+7th

Accidental drowning and submersion while in lake
Accidental drowning and submersion while in open sea
Accidental drowning and submersion while in river
Accidental drowning and submersion while in stream

Excludes1: *accidental drowning and submersion due to fall into natural body of water (W16.111, W16.121, W16.131)*

The appropriate 7th character is to be added to code W69
A initial encounter
D subsequent encounter
S sequela

W73 Other specified cause of accidental non-transport drowning and submersion X+7th

Accidental drowning and submersion while in quenching tank
Accidental drowning and submersion while in reservoir

Excludes1: *accidental drowning and submersion due to fall into other water (W16.311, W16.321, W16.331)*

The appropriate 7th character is to be added to code W73
A initial encounter
D subsequent encounter
S sequela

W74 Unspecified cause of accidental drowning and submersion X+7th

Drowning NOS

The appropriate 7th character is to be added to code W74
A initial encounter
D subsequent encounter
S sequela

Exposure to electric current, radiation and extreme ambient air temperature and pressure (W85-W99)

Excludes1: *exposure to:*
failure in dosage of radiation or temperature during surgical and medical care (Y63.2-Y63.5)
lightning (T75.0-)
natural cold (X31)
natural heat (X30)
natural radiation NOS (X39)
radiological procedure and radiotherapy (Y84.2)
sunlight (X32)

W85 Exposure to electric transmission lines
X+7th
Broken power line

The appropriate 7th character is to be added to code W85
A initial encounter
D subsequent encounter
S sequela

W86 Exposure to other specified electric current

The appropriate 7th character is to be added to each code from category W86
A initial encounter
D subsequent encounter
S sequela

X+7th **W86.0 Exposure to domestic wiring and appliances**
X+7th **W86.1 Exposure to industrial wiring, appliances and electrical machinery**
Exposure to conductors
Exposure to control apparatus
Exposure to electrical equipment and machinery
Exposure to transformers
X+7th **W86.8 Exposure to other electric current**
Exposure to wiring and appliances in or on farm (not farmhouse)
Exposure to wiring and appliances outdoors
Exposure to wiring and appliances in or on public building
Exposure to wiring and appliances in or on residential institutions
Exposure to wiring and appliances in or on schools

W88 Exposure to ionizing radiation

Excludes1: *exposure to sunlight (X32)*

The appropriate 7th character is to be added to each code from category W88
A initial encounter
D subsequent encounter
S sequela

X+7th **W88.0 Exposure to X-rays**
X+7th **W88.1 Exposure to radioactive isotopes**
X+7th **W88.8 Exposure to other ionizing radiation**

W89 Exposure to man-made visible and ultraviolet light

Includes: exposure to welding light (arc)
Excludes2: *exposure to sunlight (X32)*

The appropriate 7th character is to be added to each code from category W89
A initial encounter
D subsequent encounter
S sequela

X+7th **W89.0 Exposure to welding light (arc)**
X+7th **W89.1 Exposure to tanning bed**
X+7th **W89.8 Exposure to other man-made visible and ultraviolet light**
X+7th **W89.9 Exposure to unspecified man-made visible and ultraviolet light**

W90 Exposure to other nonionizing radiation

Excludes2: *exposure to sunlight (X32)*

The appropriate 7th character is to be added to each code from category W90
A initial encounter
D subsequent encounter
S sequela

X+7th **W90.0 Exposure to radiofrequency**
X+7th **W90.1 Exposure to infrared radiation**
X+7th **W90.2 Exposure to laser radiation**
X+7th **W90.8 Exposure to other nonionizing radiation**

W92 Exposure to excessive heat of man-made origin
X+7th

The appropriate 7th character is to be added to code W92
A initial encounter
D subsequent encounter
S sequela

W93 Exposure to excessive cold of man-made origin

The appropriate 7th character is to be added to each code from category W93
A initial encounter
D subsequent encounter
S sequela

\+ **W93.0 Contact with or inhalation of dry ice**
X+7th **W93.01 Contact with dry ice**
X+7th **W93.02 Inhalation of dry ice**
\+ **W93.1 Contact with or inhalation of liquid air**
X+7th **W93.11 Contact with liquid air**
Contact with liquid hydrogen
Contact with liquid nitrogen
X+7th **W93.12 Inhalation of liquid air**
Inhalation of liquid hydrogen
Inhalation of liquid nitrogen
X+7th **W93.2 Prolonged exposure in deep freeze unit or refrigerator**
X+7th **W93.8 Exposure to other excessive cold of man-made origin**

W94 Exposure to high and low air pressure and changes in air pressure

The appropriate 7th character is to be added to each code from category W94
A initial encounter
D subsequent encounter
S sequela

X+7th **W94.0 Exposure to prolonged high air pressure**
\+ **W94.1 Exposure to prolonged low air pressure**
X+7th **W94.11 Exposure to residence or prolonged visit at high altitude**
X+7th **W94.12 Exposure to other prolonged low air pressure**
\+ **W94.2 Exposure to rapid changes in air pressure during ascent**
X+7th **W94.21 Exposure to reduction in atmospheric pressure while surfacing from deep-water diving**
X+7th **W94.22 Exposure to reduction in atmospheric pressure while surfacing from underground**
X+7th **W94.23 Exposure to sudden change in air pressure in aircraft during ascent**
X+7th **W94.29 Exposure to other rapid changes in air pressure during ascent**
\+ **W94.3 Exposure to rapid changes in air pressure during descent**
X+7th **W94.31 Exposure to sudden change in air pressure in aircraft during descent**
X+7th **W94.32 Exposure to high air pressure from rapid descent in water**
X+7th **W94.39 Exposure to other rapid changes in air pressure during descent**

W99 Exposure to other man-made environmental factors
X+7th

The appropriate 7th character is to be added to code W99
A initial encounter
D subsequent encounter
S sequela

Exposure to smoke, fire and flames (X00-X08)

Excludes1: *arson (X97)*

Excludes2: *explosions (W35-W40)*
lightning (T75.0-)
transport accident (V01-V99)

X00 Exposure to uncontrolled fire in building or structure

Includes: conflagration in building or structure
Code first any associated cataclysm
Excludes2: *Exposure to ignition or melting of nightwear (X05)*
Exposure to ignition or melting of other clothing and apparel (X06.-)
Exposure to other specified smoke, fire and flames (X08.-)

The appropriate 7th character is to be added to each code from category X00
A initial encounter
D subsequent encounter
S sequela

X+7th **X00.0 Exposure to flames in uncontrolled fire in building or structure**
AHA CC: 1Q, 2015, 3-21; 2Q, 2016, 5-6
X+7th **X00.1 Exposure to smoke in uncontrolled fire in building or structure**
X+7th **X00.2 Injury due to collapse of burning building or structure in uncontrolled fire**
Excludes1: *injury due to collapse of building not on fire (W20.1)*
X+7th **X00.3 Fall from burning building or structure in uncontrolled fire**

X+7th **X00.4 Hit by object from burning building or structure in uncontrolled fire**
X+7th **X00.5 Jump from burning building or structure in uncontrolled fire**
X+7th **X00.8 Other exposure to uncontrolled fire in building or structure**

X01 Exposure to uncontrolled fire, not in building or structure

Includes: exposure to forest fire

The appropriate 7th character is to be added to each code from category X01
A initial encounter
D subsequent encounter
S sequela

X+7th **X01.0 Exposure to flames in uncontrolled fire, not in building or structure**
X+7th **X01.1 Exposure to smoke in uncontrolled fire, not in building or structure**
X+7th **X01.3 Fall due to uncontrolled fire, not in building or structure**
X+7th **X01.4 Hit by object due to uncontrolled fire, not in building or structure**
X+7th **X01.8 Other exposure to uncontrolled fire, not in building or structure**

X02 Exposure to controlled fire in building or structure

Includes: exposure to fire in fireplace
exposure to fire in stove

The appropriate 7th character is to be added to each code from category X02
A initial encounter
D subsequent encounter
S sequela

X+7th **X02.0 Exposure to flames in controlled fire in building or structure**
X+7th **X02.1 Exposure to smoke in controlled fire in building or structure**
X+7th **X02.2 Injury due to collapse of burning building or structure in controlled fire**
Excludes1: *injury due to collapse of building not on fire (W20.1)*
X+7th **X02.3 Fall from burning building or structure in controlled fire**
X+7th **X02.4 Hit by object from burning building or structure in controlled fire**
X+7th **X02.5 Jump from burning building or structure in controlled fire**
X+7th **X02.8 Other exposure to controlled fire in building or structure**

X03 Exposure to controlled fire, not in building or structure

Includes: exposure to bon fire
exposure to camp-fire
exposure to trash fire

The appropriate 7th character is to be added to each code from category X03
A initial encounter
D subsequent encounter
S sequela

X+7th **X03.0 Exposure to flames in controlled fire, not in building or structure**
AHA CC: 1Q, 2015, 3-21
X+7th **X03.1 Exposure to smoke in controlled fire, not in building or structure**
X+7th **X03.3 Fall due to controlled fire, not in building or structure**
X+7th **X03.4 Hit by object due to controlled fire, not in building or structure**
X+7th **X03.8 Other exposure to controlled fire, not in building or structure**

X04 Exposure to ignition of highly flammable material
X+7th
Exposure to ignition of gasoline
Exposure to ignition of kerosene
Exposure to ignition of petrol
Excludes2: *exposure to ignition or melting of nightwear (X05)*
exposure to ignition or melting of other clothing and apparel (X06)
AHA CC: 2Q, 2016, 4

The appropriate 7th character is to be added to code X04
A initial encounter
D subsequent encounter
S sequela

X05 Exposure to ignition or melting of nightwear
X+7th
Excludes2: *exposure to uncontrolled fire in building or structure (X00.-)*
exposure to uncontrolled fire, not in building or structure (X01.-)
exposure to controlled fire in building or structure (X02.-)
exposure to controlled fire, not in building or structure (X03.-)
exposure to ignition of highly flammable materials (X04.-)

The appropriate 7th character is to be added to code X05
A initial encounter
D subsequent encounter
S sequela

X06 Exposure to ignition or melting of other clothing and apparel

Excludes2: *exposure to uncontrolled fire in building or structure (X00.-)*
exposure to uncontrolled fire, not in building or structure (X01.-)
exposure to controlled fire in building or structure (X02.-)
exposure to controlled fire, not in building or structure (X03.-)
exposure to ignition of highly flammable materials (X04.-)

The appropriate 7th character is to be added to each code from category X06
A initial encounter
D subsequent encounter
S sequela

X+7th **X06.0 Exposure to ignition of plastic jewelry**
X+7th **X06.1 Exposure to melting of plastic jewelry**
X+7th **X06.2 Exposure to ignition of other clothing and apparel**
X+7th **X06.3 Exposure to melting of other clothing and apparel**

X08 Exposure to other specified smoke, fire and flames

The appropriate 7th character is to be added to each code from category X08
A initial encounter
D subsequent encounter
S sequela

\+ **X08.0 Exposure to bed fire**
Exposure to mattress fire
X+7th **X08.00 Exposure to bed fire due to unspecified burning material**
X+7th **X08.01 Exposure to bed fire due to burning cigarette**
AHA CC: 1Q, 2015, 3-21
X+7th **X08.09 Exposure to bed fire due to other burning material**
\+ **X08.1 Exposure to sofa fire**
X+7th **X08.10 Exposure to sofa fire due to unspecified burning material**
X+7th **X08.11 Exposure to sofa fire due to burning cigarette**
X+7th **X08.19 Exposure to sofa fire due to other burning material**
\+ **X08.2 Exposure to other furniture fire**
X+7th **X08.20 Exposure to other furniture fire due to unspecified burning material**
X+7th **X08.21 Exposure to other furniture fire due to burning cigarette**
X+7th **X08.29 Exposure to other furniture fire due to other burning material**
X+7th **X08.8 Exposure to other specified smoke, fire and flames**

Contact with heat and hot substances (X10-X19)

Excludes1: *exposure to excessive natural heat (X30)*
exposure to fire and flames (X00-X08)

X10 Contact with hot drinks, food, fats and cooking oils

The appropriate 7th character is to be added to each code from category X10
A initial encounter
D subsequent encounter
S sequela

X+7th **X10.0 Contact with hot drinks**
X+7th **X10.1 Contact with hot food**
X+7th **X10.2 Contact with fats and cooking oils**

X11 Contact with hot tap-water

Includes: contact with boiling tap-water
contact with boiling water NOS

Excludes1: *contact with water heated on stove (X12)*

The appropriate 7th character is to be added to each code from category X11
A initial encounter
D subsequent encounter
S sequela

X+7th **X11.0 Contact with hot water in bath or tub**

Excludes1: *contact with running hot water in bath or tub (X11.1)*

X+7th **X11.1 Contact with running hot water**

Contact with hot water running out of hose
Contact with hot water running out of tap

X+7th **X11.8 Contact with other hot tap-water**

Contact with hot water in bucket
Contact with hot tap-water NOS

X12 Contact with other hot fluids
X+7th

Contact with water heated on stove

Excludes1: *hot (liquid) metals (X18)*

The appropriate 7th character is to be added to code X12
A initial encounter
D subsequent encounter
S sequela

X13 Contact with steam and other hot vapors

The appropriate 7th character is to be added to each code from category X13
A initial encounter
D subsequent encounter
S sequela

X+7th **X13.0 Inhalation of steam and other hot vapors**
X+7th **X13.1 Other contact with steam and other hot vapors**

X14 Contact with hot air and other hot gases

The appropriate 7th character is to be added to each code from category X14
A initial encounter
D subsequent encounter
S sequela

X+7th **X14.0 Inhalation of hot air and gases**
X+7th **X14.1 Other contact with hot air and other hot gases**

X15 Contact with hot household appliances

Excludes1: *contact with heating appliances (X16)*
contact with powered household appliances (W29.-)
exposure to controlled fire in building or structure due to household appliance (X02.8)
exposure to household appliances electrical current (W86.0)

The appropriate 7th character is to be added to each code from category X15
A initial encounter
D subsequent encounter
S sequela

X+7th **X15.0 Contact with hot stove (kitchen)**
X+7th **X15.1 Contact with hot toaster**
X+7th **X15.2 Contact with hotplate**
X+7th **X15.3 Contact with hot saucepan or skillet**
X+7th **X15.8 Contact with other hot household appliances**

Contact with cooker
Contact with kettle
Contact with light bulbs

X16 Contact with hot heating appliances, radiators and pipes
X+7th

Excludes1: *contact with powered appliances (W29.-)*
exposure to controlled fire in building or structure due to appliance (X02.8)
exposure to industrial appliances electrical current (W86.1)

The appropriate 7th character is to be added to code X16
A initial encounter
D subsequent encounter
S sequela

X17 Contact with hot engines, machinery and tools
X+7th

Excludes1: *contact with hot heating appliances, radiators and pipes (X16)*
contact with hot household appliances (X15)

The appropriate 7th character is to be added to code X17
A initial encounter
D subsequent encounter
S sequela

X18 Contact with other hot metals
X+7th

Contact with liquid metal

The appropriate 7th character is to be added to code X18
A initial encounter
D subsequent encounter
S sequela

X19 Contact with other heat and hot substances
X+7th

Excludes1: *objects that are not normally hot, e.g., an object made hot by a house fire (X00-X08)*

The appropriate 7th character is to be added to code X19
A initial encounter
D subsequent encounter
S sequela

Exposure to forces of nature (X30-X39)

X30 Exposure to excessive natural heat
X+7th

Exposure to excessive heat as the cause of sunstroke
Exposure to heat NOS

Excludes1: *excessive heat of man-made origin (W92)*
exposure to man-made radiation (W89)
exposure to sunlight (X32)
exposure to tanning bed (W89)

AHA CC: 4Q, 2017, 112-114
Review coding guideline B.19.c

The appropriate 7th character is to be added to code X30
A initial encounter
D subsequent encounter
S sequela

X31 Exposure to excessive natural cold
X+7th

Excessive cold as the cause of chilblains NOS
Excessive cold as the cause of immersion foot or hand
Exposure to cold NOS
Exposure to weather conditions

Excludes1: *cold of man-made origin (W93.-)*
contact with or inhalation of dry ice (W93.-)
contact with or inhalation of liquefied gas (W93.-)

AHA CC: 4Q, 2017, 112-114
Review coding guideline B.19.c

The appropriate 7th character is to be added to code X31
A initial encounter
D subsequent encounter
S sequela

X32 Exposure to sunlight
X+7th

Excludes1: *man-made radiation (tanning bed) (W89)*
Excludes2: *radiation-related disorders of the skin and subcutaneous tissue (L55-L59)*

The appropriate 7th character is to be added to code X32
A initial encounter
D subsequent encounter
S sequela

X34 Earthquake
X+7th

Excludes2: *tidal wave (tsunami) due to earthquake (X37.41)*

The appropriate 7th character is to be added to code X34
A initial encounter
D subsequent encounter
S sequela

X35 Volcanic eruption
X+7th

Excludes2: *tidal wave (tsunami) due to volcanic eruption (X37.41)*

The appropriate 7th character is to be added to code X35
A initial encounter
D subsequent encounter
S sequela

X36 Avalanche, landslide and other earth movements
X+7th
Includes: victim of mudslide of cataclysmic nature
Excludes1: *earthquake (X34)*
Excludes2: *transport accident involving collision with avalanche or landslide not in motion (V01-V99)*

The appropriate 7th character is to be added to each code from category X36
A initial encounter
D subsequent encounter
S sequela

X36.0 Collapse of dam or man-made structure causing earth movement
AHA CC: 4Q, 2017, 112-114
Review coding guideline B.19.b
X36.1 Avalanche, landslide, or mudslide

X37 Cataclysmic storm

The appropriate 7th character is to be added to each code from category X37
A initial encounter
D subsequent encounter
S sequela

X+7th **X37.0 Hurricane**
Storm surge
Typhoon
AHA CC: 4Q, 2017, 112-114
Review coding guideline B.19
X+7th **X37.1 Tornado**
Cyclone
Twister
X+7th **X37.2 Blizzard (snow)(ice)**
X+7th **X37.3 Dust storm**
\+ **X37.4 Tidalwave**
X+7th **X37.41 Tidal wave due to earthquake or volcanic eruption**
Tidal wave NOS
Tsunami
X+7th **X37.42 Tidal wave due to storm**
X+7th **X37.43 Tidal wave due to landslide**
X+7th **X37.8 Other cataclysmic storms**
Cloudburst
Torrential rain
Excludes2: *flood (X38)*
X+7th **X37.9 Unspecified cataclysmic storm**
Storm NOS
Excludes1: *collapse of dam or man-made structure causing earth movement (X36.0)*

X38 Flood
X+7th
Flood arising from remote storm
Flood of cataclysmic nature arising from melting snow
Flood resulting directly from storm
Excludes1: *collapse of dam or man-made structure causing earth movement (X36.0)*
tidal wave NOS (X37.41)
tidal wave caused by storm (X37.42)
AHA CC: 4Q, 2017, 112-114
Review coding guideline B.19

The appropriate 7th character is to be added to code X38
A initial encounter
D subsequent encounter
S sequela

X39 Exposure to other forces of nature

The appropriate 7th character is to be added to each code from category X39
A initial encounter
D subsequent encounter
S sequela

\+ **X39.0 Exposure to natural radiation**
Excludes1: *contact with and (suspected) exposure to radon and other naturally occurring radiation (Z77.123)*
exposure to man-made radiation (W88-W90)
exposure to sunlight (X32)
X+7th **X39.01 Exposure to radon**
X+7th **X39.08 Exposure to other natural radiation**
X+7th **X39.8 Other exposure to forces of nature**

Overexertion and strenuous or repetitive movements (X50)

X50 Overexertion and strenuous or repetitive movements
AHA CC: 4Q, 2016, 73-74

The appropriate 7th character is to be added to each code from category X50
A initial encounter
D subsequent encounter
S sequela

X+7th **X50.0 Overexertion from strenuous movement or load**
Lifting heavy objects
Lifting weights
X+7th **X50.1 Overexertion from prolonged static or awkward postures**
Prolonged bending
Prolonged kneeling
Prolonged reaching
Prolonged sitting
Prolonged standing
Prolonged twisting
Static bending
Static kneeling
Static reaching
Static sitting
Static standing
Static twisting
X+7th **X50.3 Overexertion from repetitive movements**
Use of hand as hammer.
Excludes2: Overuse from prolonged static or awkward postures (X50.1)
X+7th **X50.9 Other and unspecified overexertion or strenuous movements or postures**
Contact pressure
Contact stress

Accidental exposure to other specified factors (X52-X58)

X52 Prolonged stay in weightless environment
X+7th
Weightlessness in spacecraft (simulator)

The appropriate 7th character is to be added to code X52
A initial encounter
D subsequent encounter
S sequela

X58 Exposure to other specified factors
X+7th
Accident NOS
Exposure NOS

The appropriate 7th character is to be added to code X58
A initial encounter
D subsequent encounter
S sequela

Intentional self-harm (X71-X83)

Purposely self-inflicted injury
Suicide (attempted)

X71 Intentional self-harm by drowning and submersion

The appropriate 7th character is to be added to each code from category X71
A initial encounter
D subsequent encounter
S sequela

X+7th **X71.0 Intentional self-harm by drowning and submersion while in bathtub**
X+7th **X71.1 Intentional self-harm by drowning and submersion while in swimming pool**
X+7th **X71.2 Intentional self-harm by drowning and submersion after jump into swimming pool**
X+7th **X71.3 Intentional self-harm by drowning and submersion in natural water**
X+7th **X71.8 Other intentional self-harm by drowning and submersion**
X+7th **X71.9 Intentional self-harm by drowning and submersion, unspecified**

X72 Intentional self-harm by handgun discharge
X+7th
Intentional self-harm by gun for single hand use
Intentional self-harm by pistol
Intentional self-harm by revolver
Excludes1: *Very pistol (X74.8)*

The appropriate 7th character is to be added to code X72
A initial encounter
D subsequent encounter
S sequela

X73 Intentional self-harm by rifle, shotgun and larger firearm discharge
X+7th

Excludes1: *airgun (X74.01)*

The appropriate 7th character is to be added to each code from category X73
A initial encounter
D subsequent encounter
S sequela

X+7th **X73.0 Intentional self-harm by shotgun discharge**
X+7th **X73.1 Intentional self-harm by hunting rifle discharge**
X+7th **X73.2 Intentional self-harm by machine gun discharge**
X+7th **X73.8 Intentional self-harm by other larger firearm discharge**
X+7th **X73.9 Intentional self-harm by unspecified larger firearm discharge**

X74 Intentional self-harm by other and unspecified firearm and gun discharge

The appropriate 7th character is to be added to each code from category X74
A initial encounter
D subsequent encounter
S sequela

+ **X74.0 Intentional self-harm by gas, air or spring-operated guns**
X+7th **X74.01 Intentional self-harm by airgun**
Intentional self-harm by BB gun discharge
Intentional self-harm by pellet gun discharge
X+7th **X74.02 Intentional self-harm by paintball gun**
X+7th **X74.09 Intentional self-harm by other gas, air or spring-operated gun**
X+7th **X74.8 Intentional self-harm by other firearm discharge**
Intentional self-harm by Very pistol [flare] discharge
X+7th **X74.9 Intentional self-harm by unspecified firearm discharge**

X75 Intentional self-harm by explosive material
X+7th

The appropriate 7th character is to be added to code X75
A initial encounter
D subsequent encounter
S sequela

X76 Intentional self-harm by smoke, fire and flames
X+7th

The appropriate 7th character is to be added to code X76
A initial encounter
D subsequent encounter
S sequela

X77 Intentional self-harm by steam, hot vapors and hot objects

The appropriate 7th character is to be added to each code from category X77
A initial encounter
D subsequent encounter
S sequela

X+7th **X77.0 Intentional self-harm by steam or hot vapors**
X+7th **X77.1 Intentional self-harm by hot tap water**
X+7th **X77.2 Intentional self-harm by other hot fluids**
X+7th **X77.3 Intentional self-harm by hot household appliances**
X+7th **X77.8 Intentional self-harm by other hot objects**
X+7th **X77.9 Intentional self-harm by unspecified hot objects**

X78 Intentional self-harm by sharp object

The appropriate 7th character is to be added to each code from category X78
A initial encounter
D subsequent encounter
S sequela

X+7th **X78.0 Intentional self-harm by sharp glass**
X+7th **X78.1 Intentional self-harm by knife**
X+7th **X78.2 Intentional self-harm by sword or dagger**
X+7th **X78.8 Intentional self-harm by other sharp object**
X+7th **X78.9 Intentional self-harm by unspecified sharp object**

X79 Intentional self-harm by blunt object
X+7th

The appropriate 7th character is to be added to code X79
A initial encounter
D subsequent encounter
S sequela

X80 Intentional self-harm by jumping from a high place
X+7th
Intentional fall from one level to another

The appropriate 7th character is to be added to code X80
A initial encounter
D subsequent encounter
S sequela

X81 Intentional self-harm by jumping or lying in front of moving object

The appropriate 7th character is to be added to each code from category X81
A initial encounter
D subsequent encounter
S sequela

X+7th **X81.0 Intentional self-harm by jumping or lying in front of motor vehicle**
X+7th **X81.1 Intentional self-harm by jumping or lying in front of (subway) train**
X+7th **X81.8 Intentional self-harm by jumping or lying in front of other moving object**

X82 Intentional self-harm by crashing of motor vehicle

The appropriate 7th character is to be added to each code from category X82
A initial encounter
D subsequent encounter
S sequela

X+7th **X82.0 Intentional collision of motor vehicle with other motor vehicle**
X+7th **X82.1 Intentional collision of motor vehicle with train**
X+7th **X82.2 Intentional collision of motor vehicle with tree**
X+7th **X82.8 Other intentional self-harm by crashing of motor vehicle**

X83 Intentional self-harm by other specified means

Excludes1: *intentional self-harm by poisoning or contact with toxic substance- See Table of Drugs and Chemicals*

The appropriate 7th character is to be added to each code from category X83
A initial encounter
D subsequent encounter
S sequela

X+7th **X83.0 Intentional self-harm by crashing of aircraft**
X+7th **X83.1 Intentional self-harm by electrocution**
X+7th **X83.2 Intentional self-harm by exposure to extremes of cold**
X+7th **X83.8 Intentional self-harm by other specified means**

Assault (X92-Y09)

Includes: homicide
injuries inflicted by another person with intent to injure or kill, by any means

Excludes1: *injuries due to legal intervention (Y35.-)*
injuries due to operations of war (Y36.-)
injuries due to terrorism (Y38.-)

Review coding guideline C.19.f

X92 Assault by drowning and submersion

The appropriate 7th character is to be added to each code from category X92
A initial encounter
D subsequent encounter
S sequela

X+7th **X92.0 Assault by drowning and submersion while in bathtub**
X+7th **X92.1 Assault by drowning and submersion while in swimming pool**
X+7th **X92.2 Assault by drowning and submersion after push into swimming pool**
X+7th **X92.3 Assault by drowning and submersion in natural water**
X+7th **X92.8 Other assault by drowning and submersion**
X+7th **X92.9 Assault by drowning and submersion, unspecified**

X93 Assault by handgun discharge
X+7th
Assault by discharge of gun for single hand use
Assault by discharge of pistol
Assault by discharge of revolver
Excludes1: *Very pistol (X95.8)*

The appropriate 7th character is to be added to code X93
A initial encounter
D subsequent encounter
S sequela

X94 Assault by rifle, shotgun and larger firearm discharge

Excludes1: *airgun (X95.01)*

The appropriate 7th character is to be added to each code from category X94
A initial encounter
D subsequent encounter
S sequela

X+7th **X94.0 Assault by shotgun**
X+7th **X94.1 Assault by hunting rifle**
X+7th **X94.2 Assault by machine gun**
X+7th **X94.8 Assault by other larger firearm discharge**
X+7th **X94.9 Assault by unspecified larger firearm discharge**

X95 Assault by other and unspecified firearm and gun discharge

The appropriate 7th character is to be added to each code from category X95
A initial encounter
D subsequent encounter
S sequela

\+ **X95.0 Assault by gas, air or spring-operated guns**
X+7th **X95.01 Assault by airgun discharge**
Assault by BB gun discharge
Assault by pellet gun discharge
X+7th **X95.02 Assault by paintball gun discharge**
X+7th **X95.09 Assault by other gas, air or spring-operated gun**
X+7th **X95.8 Assault by other firearm discharge**
Assault by very pistol [flare] discharge
X+7th **X95.9 Assault by unspecified firearm discharge**
AHA CC: 3Q, 2016, 24

X96 Assault by explosive material

Excludes1: *incendiary device (X97)*
terrorism involving explosive material (Y38.2-)

The appropriate 7th character is to be added to each code from category X96
A initial encounter
D subsequent encounter
S sequela

X+7th **X96.0 Assault by antipersonnel bomb**
Excludes1: *antipersonnel bomb use in military or war (Y36.2-)*
X+7th **X96.1 Assault by gasoline bomb**
X+7th **X96.2 Assault by letter bomb**
X+7th **X96.3 Assault by fertilizer bomb**
X+7th **X96.4 Assault by pipe bomb**
X+7th **X96.8 Assault by other specified explosive**
X+7th **X96.9 Assault by unspecified explosive**

X97 Assault by smoke, fire and flames X+7th

Assault by arson
Assault by cigarettes
Assault by incendiary device

The appropriate 7th character is to be added to code X97
A initial encounter
D subsequent encounter
S sequela

X98 Assault by steam, hot vapors and hot objects

The appropriate 7th character is to be added to each code from category X98
A initial encounter
D subsequent encounter
S sequela

X+7th **X98.0 Assault by steam or hot vapors**
X+7th **X98.1 Assault by hot tap water**
X+7th **X98.2 Assault by hot fluids**
X+7th **X98.3 Assault by hot household appliances**
X+7th **X98.8 Assault by other hot objects**
X+7th **X98.9 Assault by unspecified hot objects**

X99 Assault by sharp object

Excludes1: *assault by strike by sports equipment (Y08.0-)*

The appropriate 7th character is to be added to each code from category X99
A initial encounter
D subsequent encounter
S sequela

X+7th **X99.0 Assault by sharp glass**
X+7th **X99.1 Assault by knife**
X+7th **X99.2 Assault by sword or dagger**
X+7th **X99.8 Assault by other sharp object**
X+7th **X99.9 Assault by unspecified sharp object**
Assault by stabbing NOS

Y00 Assault by blunt object X+7th

Excludes1: *assault by strike by sports equipment (Y08.0-)*

The appropriate 7th character is to be added to code Y00
A initial encounter
D subsequent encounter
S sequela

Y01 Assault by pushing from high place X+7th

The appropriate 7th character is to be added to code Y01
A initial encounter
D subsequent encounter
S sequela

Y02 Assault by pushing or placing victim in front of moving object

The appropriate 7th character is to be added to each code from category Y02
A initial encounter
D subsequent encounter
S sequela

X+7th **Y02.0 Assault by pushing or placing victim in front of motor vehicle**
X+7th **Y02.1 Assault by pushing or placing victim in front of (subway) train**
X+7th **Y02.8 Assault by pushing or placing victim in front of other moving object**

Y03 Assault by crashing of motor vehicle

The appropriate 7th character is to be added to each code from category Y03
A initial encounter
D subsequent encounter
S sequela

X+7th **Y03.0 Assault by being hit or run over by motor vehicle**
X+7th **Y03.8 Other assault by crashing of motor vehicle**

Y04 Assault by bodily force

Excludes1: *assault by:*
submersion (X92.-)
use of weapon (X93-X95, X99, Y00)

The appropriate 7th character is to be added to each code from category Y04
A initial encounter
D subsequent encounter
S sequela

X+7th **Y04.0 Assault by unarmed brawl or fight**
X+7th **Y04.1 Assault by human bite**
X+7th **Y04.2 Assault by strike against or bumped into by another person**
X+7th **Y04.8 Assault by other bodily force**
Assault by bodily force NOS

Y07 Perpetrator of assault, maltreatment and neglect

NOTE Codes from this category are for use only in cases of confirmed abuse (T74.-)
Selection of the correct perpetrator code is based on the relationship between the perpetrator and the victim

Includes: perpetrator of abandonment
perpetrator of emotional neglect
perpetrator of mental cruelty
perpetrator of physical abuse
perpetrator of physical neglect
perpetrator of sexual abuse
perpetrator of torture

Review coding guideline C.20.g
AHA CC: 4Q, 2018, 32-33

\+ **Y07.0 Spouse or partner, perpetrator of maltreatment and neglect**
Spouse or partner, perpetrator of maltreatment and neglect against spouse or partner
Y07.01 Husband, perpetrator of maltreatment and neglect
Y07.02 Wife, perpetrator of maltreatment and neglect

Y07.03 **Male partner, perpetrator of maltreatment and neglect**

Y07.04 **Female partner, perpetrator of maltreatment and neglect**

\+ **Y07.1 Parent (adoptive) (biological), perpetrator of maltreatment and neglect**

Y07.11 Biological father, perpetrator of maltreatment and neglect

Y07.12 Biological mother, perpetrator of maltreatment and neglect

Y07.13 Adoptive father, perpetrator of maltreatment and neglect

Y07.14 Adoptive mother, perpetrator of maltreatment and neglect

\+ **Y07.4 Other family member, perpetrator of maltreatment and neglect**

\+ **Y07.41 Sibling, perpetrator of maltreatment and neglect**

Excludes1: *stepsibling, perpetrator of maltreatmentandneglect(Y07.435, Y07.436)*

Y07.410 Brother, perpetrator of maltreatment and neglect

Y07.411 Sister, perpetrator of maltreatment and neglect

\+ **Y07.42 Foster parent, perpetrator of maltreatment and neglect**

Y07.420 Foster father, perpetrator of maltreatment and neglect

Y07.421 Foster mother, perpetrator of maltreatment and neglect

\+ **Y07.43 Stepparent or stepsibling, perpetrator of maltreatment and neglect**

Y07.430 Stepfather, perpetrator of maltreatment and neglect

Y07.432 Male friend of parent (co-residing in household), perpetrator of maltreatment and neglect

Y07.433 Stepmother, perpetrator of maltreatment and neglect

Y07.434 Female friend of parent (co-residing in household), perpetrator of maltreatment and neglect

Y07.435 Stepbrother, perpetrator or maltreatment and neglect

Y07.436 Stepsister, perpetrator of maltreatment and neglect

\+ **Y07.49 Other family member, perpetrator of maltreatment and neglect**

Y07.490 Male cousin, perpetrator of maltreatment and neglect

Y07.491 Female cousin, perpetrator of maltreatment and neglect

Y07.499 Other family member, perpetrator of maltreatment and neglect

\+ **Y07.5 Non-family member, perpetrator of maltreatment and neglect**

Y07.50 Unspecified non-family member, perpetrator of maltreatment and neglect

\+ **Y07.51 Daycare provider, perpetrator of maltreatment and neglect**

Y07.510 At-home childcare provider, perpetrator of maltreatment and neglect

Y07.511 Daycare center childcare provider, perpetrator of maltreatment and neglect

Y07.512 At-home adultcare provider, perpetrator of maltreatment and neglect

Y07.513 Adultcare center provider, perpetrator of maltreatment and neglect

Y07.519 Unspecified daycare provider, perpetrator of maltreatment and neglect

\+ **Y07.52 Healthcare provider, perpetrator of maltreatment and neglect**

Y07.521 Mental health provider, perpetrator of maltreatment and neglect

Y07.528 Other therapist or healthcare provider, perpetrator of maltreatment and neglect

Nurse perpetrator of maltreatment and neglect

Occupational therapist perpetrator of maltreatment and neglect

Physical therapist perpetrator of maltreatment and neglect

Speech therapist perpetrator of maltreatment and neglect

Y07.529 Unspecified healthcare provider, perpetrator of maltreatment and neglect

Y07.53 Teacher or instructor, perpetrator of maltreatment and neglect

Coach, perpetrator of maltreatment and neglect

Y07.59 Other non-family member, perpetrator of maltreatment and neglect

Y07.6 Multiple perpetrators of maltreatment and neglect

AHA CC: 4Q, 2018, 32-33

Y07.9 Unspecified perpetrator of maltreatment and neglect

Y08 Assault by other specified means

The appropriate 7th character is to be added to each code from category Y08
A initial encounter
D subsequent encounter
S sequela

\+ **Y08.0 Assault by strike by sport equipment**

X+7th **Y08.01 Assault by strike by hockey stick**

X+7th **Y08.02 Assault by strike by baseball bat**

X+7th **Y08.09 Assault by strike by other specified type of sport equipment**

\+ **Y08.8 Assault by other specified means**

X+7th **Y08.81 Assault by crashing of aircraft**

X+7th **Y08.89 Assault by other specified means**

Y09 Assault by unspecified means

Assassination (attempted) NOS
Homicide (attempted) NOS
Manslaughter (attempted) NOS
Murder (attempted) NOS

Valid 3-character code, no further characters required

Event of undetermined intent (Y21-Y33)

Undetermined intent is only for use when there is specific documentation in the record that the intent of the injury cannot be determined. If no such documentation is present, code to accidental (unintentional)

Y21 Drowning and submersion, undetermined intent

The appropriate 7th character is to be added to each code from category Y21
A initial encounter
D subsequent encounter
S sequela

X+7th **Y21.0 Drowning and submersion while in bathtub, undetermined intent**

X+7th **Y21.1 Drowning and submersion after fall into bathtub, undetermined intent**

X+7th **Y21.2 Drowning and submersion while in swimming pool, undetermined intent**

X+7th **Y21.3 Drowning and submersion after fall into swimming pool, undetermined intent**

X+7th **Y21.4 Drowning and submersion in natural water, undetermined intent**

X+7th **Y21.8 Other drowning and submersion, undetermined intent**

X+7th **Y21.9 Unspecified drowning and submersion, undetermined intent**

X+7th **Y22 Handgun discharge, undetermined intent**

Discharge of gun for single hand use, undetermined intent
Discharge of pistol, undetermined intent
Discharge of revolver, undetermined intent

Excludes2: *very pistol (Y24.8)*

The appropriate 7th character is to be added to code Y22
A initial encounter
D subsequent encounter
S sequela

Y23 Rifle, shotgun and larger firearm discharge, undetermined intent

Excludes2: *airgun (Y24.0)*

The appropriate 7th character is to be added to each code from category Y23
A initial encounter
D subsequent encounter
S sequela

X+7th **Y23.0 Shotgun discharge, undetermined intent**
X+7th **Y23.1 Hunting rifle discharge, undetermined intent**
X+7th **Y23.2 Military firearm discharge, undetermined intent**
X+7th **Y23.3 Machine gun discharge, undetermined intent**
X+7th **Y23.8 Other larger firearm discharge, undetermined intent**
X+7th **Y23.9 Unspecified larger firearm discharge, undetermined intent**

Y24 Other and unspecified firearm discharge, undetermined intent

The appropriate 7th character is to be added to each code from category Y24
A initial encounter
D subsequent encounter
S sequela

X+7th **Y24.0 Airgun discharge, undetermined intent**
BB gun discharge, undetermined intent
Pellet gun discharge, undetermined intent
X+7th **Y24.8 Other firearm discharge, undetermined intent**
Paintball gun discharge, undetermined intent
Very pistol [flare] discharge, undetermined intent
X+7th **Y24.9 Unspecified firearm discharge, undetermined intent**

Y25 Contact with explosive material, undetermined intent
X+7th

The appropriate 7th character is to be added to code Y25
A initial encounter
D subsequent encounter
S sequela

Y26 Exposure to smoke, fire and flames, undetermined intent
X+7th

The appropriate 7th character is to be added to code Y26
A initial encounter
D subsequent encounter
S sequela

Y27 Contact with steam, hot vapors and hot objects, undetermined intent

The appropriate 7th character is to be added to each code from category Y27
A initial encounter
D subsequent encounter
S sequela

X+7th **Y27.0 Contact with steam and hot vapors, undetermined intent**
X+7th **Y27.1 Contact with hot tap water, undetermined intent**
X+7th **Y27.2 Contact with hot fluids, undetermined intent**
X+7th **Y27.3 Contact with hot household appliance, undetermined intent**
X+7th **Y27.8 Contact with other hot objects, undetermined intent**
X+7th **Y27.9 Contact with unspecified hot objects, undetermined intent**

Y28 Contact with sharp object, undetermined intent

The appropriate 7th character is to be added to each code from category Y28
A initial encounter
D subsequent encounter
S sequela

X+7th **Y28.0 Contact with sharp glass, undetermined intent**
X+7th **Y28.1 Contact with knife, undetermined intent**
X+7th **Y28.2 Contact with sword or dagger, undetermined intent**
X+7th **Y28.8 Contact with other sharp object, undetermined intent**
X+7th **Y28.9 Contact with unspecified sharp object, undetermined intent**

Y29 Contact with blunt object, undetermined intent
X+7th

The appropriate 7th character is to be added to code Y29
A initial encounter
D subsequent encounter
S sequela

Y30 Falling, jumping or pushed from a high place, undetermined intent
X+7th

Victim falling from one level to another, undetermined intent

The appropriate 7th character is to be added to code Y30
A initial encounter
D subsequent encounter
S sequela

Y31 Falling, lying or running before or into moving object, undetermined intent
X+7th

The appropriate 7th character is to be added to code Y31
A initial encounter
D subsequent encounter
S sequela

Y32 Crashing of motor vehicle, undetermined intent
X+7th

The appropriate 7th character is to be added to code Y32
A initial encounter
D subsequent encounter
S sequela

Y33 Other specified events, undetermined intent
X+7th

The appropriate 7th character is to be added to code Y33
A initial encounter
D subsequent encounter
S sequela

Legal intervention, operations of war, military operations, and terrorism (Y35-Y38)

Y35 Legal intervention

Includes: any injury sustained as a result of an encounter with any law enforcement official, serving in any capacity at the time of the encounter, whether on-duty or off-duty. Includes: a injury to law enforcement official, suspect and bystander

The appropriate 7th character is to be added to each code from category Y35
A initial encounter
D subsequent encounter
S sequela

AHA CC: 4Q, 2019, 18-19

\+ **Y35.0 Legal intervention involving firearm discharge**
\+ **Y35.00 Legal intervention involving unspecified firearm discharge**
Legal intervention involving gunshot wound
Legal intervention involving shot NOS
+7th **Y35.001 Legal intervention involving unspecified firearm discharge, law enforcement official injured**
+7th **Y35.002 Legal intervention involving unspecified firearm discharge, bystander injured**
+7th **Y35.003 Legal intervention involving unspecified firearm discharge, suspect injured**
+7th **Y35.009 Legal intervention involving unspecified firearm discharge, unspecified person injured**
\+ **Y35.01 Legal intervention involving injury by machine gun**
+7th **Y35.011 Legal intervention involving injury by machine gun, law enforcement official injured**
+7th **Y35.012 Legal intervention involving injury by machine gun, bystander injured**
+7th **Y35.013 Legal intervention involving injury by machine gun, suspect injured**
+7th **Y35.019 Legal intervention involving injury by machine gun, unspecified person injured**
\+ **Y35.02 Legal intervention involving injury by handgun**
+7th **Y35.021 Legal intervention involving injury by handgun, law enforcement official injured**
+7th **Y35.022 Legal intervention involving injury by handgun, bystander injured**
+7th **Y35.023 Legal intervention involving injury by handgun, suspect injured**
+7th **Y35.029 Legal intervention involving injury by handgun, unspecified person injured**
\+ **Y35.03 Legal intervention involving injury by rifle pellet**
+7th **Y35.031 Legal intervention involving injury by rifle pellet, law enforcement official injured**
+7th **Y35.032 Legal intervention involving injury by rifle pellet, bystander injured**
+7th **Y35.033 Legal intervention involving injury by rifle pellet, suspect injured**
+7th **Y35.039 Legal intervention involving injury by rifle pellet, unspecified person injured**
\+ **Y35.04 Legal intervention involving injury by rubber bullet**
+7th **Y35.041 Legal intervention involving injury by rubber bullet, law enforcement official injured**

+7th **Y35.042** **Legal intervention involving injury by rubber bullet, bystander injured**
+7th **Y35.043** **Legal intervention involving injury by rubber bullet, suspect injured**
+7th **Y35.049** **Legal intervention involving injury by rubber bullet, unspecified person injured**
+ **Y35.09** **Legal intervention involving other firearm discharge**
+7th **Y35.091** **Legal intervention involving other firearm discharge, law enforcement official injured**
+7th **Y35.092** **Legal intervention involving other firearm discharge, bystander injured**
+7th **Y35.093** **Legal intervention involving other firearm discharge, suspect injured**
+7th **Y35.099** **Legal intervention involving injury other firearm discharge, unspecified person injured**
+ **Y35.1** **Legal intervention involving explosives**
+ **Y35.10** **Legal intervention involving unspecified explosives**
+7th **Y35.101** **Legal intervention involving unspecified explosives, law enforcement official injured**
+7th **Y35.102** **Legal intervention involving unspecified explosives, bystander injured**
+7th **Y35.103** **Legal intervention involving unspecified explosives, suspect injured**
+7th **Y35.109** **Legal intervention involving unspecified explosives, unspecified person injured**
+ **Y35.11** **Legal intervention involving injury by dynamite**
+7th **Y35.111** **Legal intervention involving injury by dynamite, law enforcement official injured**
+7th **Y35.112** **Legal intervention involving injury by dynamite, bystander injured**
+7th **Y35.113** **Legal intervention involving injury by dynamite, suspect injured**
+7th **Y35.119** **Legal intervention involving injury by dynamite, unspecified person injured**
+ **Y35.12** **Legal intervention involving injury by explosive shell**
+7th **Y35.121** **Legal intervention involving injury by explosive shell, law enforcement official injured**
+7th **Y35.122** **Legal intervention involving injury by explosive shell, bystander injured**
+7th **Y35.123** **Legal intervention involving injury by explosive shell, suspect injured**
+7th **Y35.129** **Legal intervention involving injury by explosive shell, unspecified person injured**
+ **Y35.19** **Legal intervention involving other explosives**
Legal intervention involving injury by grenade
Legal intervention involving injury by mortar bomb
+7th **Y35.191** **Legal intervention involving other explosives, law enforcement official injured**
+7th **Y35.192** **Legal intervention involving other explosives, bystander injured**
+7th **Y35.193** **Legal intervention involving other explosives, suspect injured**
+7th **Y35.199** **Legal intervention involving other explosives, unspecified person injured**
+ **Y35.2** **Legal intervention involving gas**
Legal intervention involving asphyxiation by gas
Legal intervention involving poisoning by gas
+ **Y35.20** **Legal intervention involving unspecified gas**
+7th **Y35.201** **Legal intervention involving unspecified gas, law enforcement official injured**
+7th **Y35.202** **Legal intervention involving unspecified gas, bystander injured**
+7th **Y35.203** **Legal intervention involving unspecified gas, suspect injured**
+7th **Y35.209** **Legal intervention involving unspecified gas, unspecified person injured**
+ **Y35.21** **Legal intervention involving injury by tear gas**
+7th **Y35.211** **Legal intervention involving injury by tear gas, law enforcement official injured**
+7th **Y35.212** **Legal intervention involving injury by tear gas, bystander injured**
+7th **Y35.213** **Legal intervention involving injury by tear gas, suspect injured**
+7th **Y35.219** **Legal intervention involving injury by tear gas, unspecified person injured**
+ **Y35.29** **Legal intervention involving other gas**
+7th **Y35.291** **Legal intervention involving other gas, law enforcement official injured**
+7th **Y35.292** **Legal intervention involving other gas, bystander injured**
+7th **Y35.293** **Legal intervention involving other gas, suspect injured**
+7th **Y35.299** **Legal intervention involving other gas, unspecified person injured**
+ **Y35.3** **Legal intervention involving blunt objects**
Legal intervention involving being hit or struck by blunt object
+ **Y35.30** **Legal intervention involving unspecified blunt objects**
+7th **Y35.301** **Legal intervention involving unspecified blunt objects, law enforcement official injured**
+7th **Y35.302** **Legal intervention involving unspecified blunt objects, bystander injured**
+7th **Y35.303** **Legal intervention involving unspecified blunt objects, suspect injured**
+7th **Y35.309** **Legal intervention involving unspecified blunt objects, unspecified person injured**
+ **Y35.31** **Legal intervention involving baton**
+7th **Y35.311** **Legal intervention involving baton, law enforcement official injured**
+7th **Y35.312** **Legal intervention involving baton, bystander injured**
+7th **Y35.313** **Legal intervention involving baton, suspect injured**
+7th **Y35.319** **Legal intervention involving baton, unspecified person injured**
+ **Y35.39** **Legal intervention involving other blunt objects**
+7th **Y35.391** **Legal intervention involving other blunt objects, law enforcement official injured**
+7th **Y35.392** **Legal intervention involving other blunt objects, bystander injured**
+7th **Y35.393** **Legal intervention involving other blunt objects, suspect injured**
+7th **Y35.399** **Legal intervention involving other blunt objects, unspecified person injured**
+ **Y35.4** **Legal intervention involving sharp objects**
Legal intervention involving being cut by sharp objects
Legal intervention involving being stabbed by sharp objects
+ **Y35.40** **Legal intervention involving unspecified sharp objects**
+7th **Y35.401** **Legal intervention involving unspecified sharp objects, law enforcement official injured**
+7th **Y35.402** **Legal intervention involving unspecified sharp objects, bystander injured**
+7th **Y35.403** **Legal intervention involving unspecified sharp objects, suspect injured**
+7th **Y35.409** **Legal intervention involving unspecified sharp objects, unspecified person injured**
+ **Y35.41** **Legal intervention involving bayonet**
+7th **Y35.411** **Legal intervention involving bayonet, law enforcement official injured**
+7th **Y35.412** **Legal intervention involving bayonet, bystander injured**
+7th **Y35.413** **Legal intervention involving bayonet, suspect injured**
+7th **Y35.419** **Legal intervention involving bayonet, unspecified person injured**

+ Y35.49 Legal intervention involving other sharp objects
+7th Y35.491 Legal intervention involving other sharp objects, law enforcement official injured
+7th Y35.492 Legal intervention involving other sharp objects, bystander injured
+7th Y35.493 Legal intervention involving other sharp objects, suspect injured
+7th Y35.499 Legal intervention involving other sharp objects, unspecified person injured
+ Y35.8 Legal intervention involving other specified means
+ Y35.81 Legal intervention involving manhandling
+7th Y35.811 Legal intervention involving manhandling, law enforcement official injured
+7th Y35.812 Legal intervention involving manhandling, bystander injured
+7th Y35.813 Legal intervention involving manhandling, suspect injured
+7th Y35.819 Legal intervention involving manhandling, unspecified person injured
+ Y35.83 Legal intervention involving a conducted energy device
Electroshock device (taser)
Stun gun
+7th Y35.831 Legal intervention involving a conducted energy device, law enforcement official injured
+7th Y35.832 Legal intervention involving a conducted energy device, bystander injured
+7th Y35.833 Legal intervention involving a conducted energy device, suspect injured
+7th Y35.839 Legal intervention involving a conducted energy device, unspecified person injured
+ Y35.89 Legal intervention involving other specified means
+7th Y35.891 Legal intervention involving other specified means, law enforcement official injured
+7th Y35.892 Legal intervention involving other specified means, bystanderinjured
+7th Y35.893 Legal intervention involving other specified means, suspect injured
AHA CC: 1Q, 2018, 5
+7th Y35.899 Legal intervention involving other specified means, unspecified person
+ Y35.9 Legal intervention, means unspecified
X+7th Y35.91 Legal intervention, means unspecified, law enforcement official injured
X+7th Y35.92 Legal intervention, means unspecified, bystander injured
X+7th Y35.93 Legal intervention, means unspecified, suspect injured
X+7th Y35.99 Legal intervention, means unspecified, unspecified person injured

Y36 Operations of war

Includes: injuries to military personnel and civilians caused by war, civil insurrection, and peacekeeping missions

Excludes1: *injury to military personnel occurring during peacetime military operations (Y37.-)*
military vehicles involved in transport accidents with non-military vehicle during peacetime (V09.01, V09.21, V19.81, V29.81, V39.81, V49.81, V59.81, V69.81, V79.81)

AHA CC: 3Q, 2014, 4-5

The appropriate 7th character is to be added to each code from category Y36
A initial encounter
D subsequent encounter
S sequela

+ Y36.0 War operations involving explosion of marine weapons
+ Y36.00 War operations involving explosion of unspecified marine weapon
War operations involving underwater blast NOS
+7th Y36.000 War operations involving explosion of unspecified marine weapon, military personnel
+7th Y36.001 War operations involving explosion of unspecified marine weapon, civilian
+ Y36.01 War operations involving explosion of depth-charge
+7th Y36.010 War operations involving explosion of depth-charge, military personnel
+7th Y36.011 War operations involving explosion of depth-charge, civilian
+ Y36.02 War operations involving explosion of marine mine
War operations involving explosion of marine mine, at sea or in harbor
+7th Y36.020 War operations involving explosion of marine mine, military personnel
+7th Y36.021 War operations involving explosion of marine mine, civilian
+ Y36.03 War operations involving explosion of sea-based artillery shell
+7th Y36.030 War operations involving explosion of sea-based artillery shell, military personnel
+7th Y36.031 War operations involving explosion of sea-based artillery shell, civilian
+ Y36.04 War operations involving explosion of torpedo
+7th Y36.040 War operations involving explosion of torpedo, military personnel
+7th Y36.041 War operations involving explosion of torpedo, civilian
+ Y36.05 War operations involving accidental detonation of onboard marine weapons
+7th Y36.050 War operations involving accidental detonation of onboard marine weapons, military personnel
+7th Y36.051 War operations involving accidental detonation of onboard marine weapons, civilian
+ Y36.09 War operations involving explosion of other marine weapons
+7th Y36.090 War operations involving explosion of other marine weapons, military personnel
+7th Y36.091 War operations involving explosion of other marine weapons, civilian
+ Y36.1 War operations involving destruction of aircraft
+ Y36.10 War operations involving unspecified destruction of aircraft
+7th Y36.100 War operations involving unspecified destruction of aircraft, military personnel
+7th Y36.101 War operations involving unspecified destruction of aircraft, civilian
+ Y36.11 War operations involving destruction of aircraft due to enemy fire or explosives
War operations involving destruction of aircraft due to air to air missile
War operations involving destruction of aircraft due to explosive placed on aircraft
War operations involving destruction of aircraft due to rocket propelled grenade [RPG]
War operations involving destruction of aircraft due to small arms fire
War operations involving destruction of aircraft due to surface to air missile
+7th Y36.110 War operations involving destruction of aircraft due to enemy fire or explosives, military personnel
+7th Y36.111 War operations involving destruction of aircraft due to enemy fire or explosives, civilian
+ Y36.12 War operations involving destruction of aircraft due to collision with other aircraft
+7th Y36.120 War operations involving destruction of aircraft due to collision with other aircraft, military personnel
+7th Y36.121 War operations involving destruction of aircraft due to collision with other aircraft, civilian
+ Y36.13 War operations involving destruction of aircraft due to onboard fire
+7th Y36.130 War operations involving destruction of aircraft due to onboard fire, military personnel
+7th Y36.131 War operations involving destruction of aircraft due to onboard fire, civilian

+ **Y36.14 War operations involving destruction of aircraft due to accidental detonation of onboard munitions and explosives**

+7th **Y36.140 War operations involving destruction of aircraft due to accidental detonation of onboard munitions and explosives, military personnel**

+7th **Y36.141 War operations involving destruction of aircraft due to accidental detonation of onboard munitions and explosives, civilian**

+ **Y36.19 War operations involving other destruction of aircraft**

+7th **Y36.190 War operations involving other destruction of aircraft, military personnel**

+7th **Y36.191 War operations involving other destruction of aircraft, civilian**

+ **Y36.2 War operations involving other explosions and fragments**

Excludes1: *war operations involving explosion of aircraft (Y36.1-)*
war operations involving explosion of marine weapons (Y36.0-)
war operations involving explosion of nuclear weapons (Y36.5-)
war operations involving explosion occurring after cessation of hostilities (Y36.8-)

+ **Y36.20 War operations involving unspecified explosion and fragments**

War operations involving air blast NOS
War operations involving blast NOS
War operations involving blast fragments NOS
War operations involving blast wave NOS
War operations involving blast wind NOS
War operations involving explosion NOS
War operations involving explosion of bomb NOS

+7th **Y36.200 War operations involving unspecified explosion and fragments, military personnel**

+7th **Y36.201 War operations involving unspecified explosion and fragments, civilian**

+ **Y36.21 War operations involving explosion of aerial bomb**

+7th **Y36.210 War operations involving explosion of aerial bomb, military personnel**

+7th **Y36.211 War operations involving explosion of aerial bomb, civilian**

+ **Y36.22 War operations involving explosion of guided missile**

+7th **Y36.220 War operations involving explosion of guided missile, military personnel**

+7th **Y36.221 War operations involving explosion of guided missile, civilian**

+ **Y36.23 War operations involving explosion of improvised explosive device [IED]**

War operations involving explosion of person-borne improvised explosive device [IED]
War operations involving explosion of vehicle-borne improvised explosive device [IED]
War operations involving explosion of roadside improvised explosive device [IED]

+7th **Y36.230 War operations involving explosion of improvised explosive device [IED], military personnel**

+7th **Y36.231 War operations involving explosion of improvised explosive device [IED], civilian**

+ **Y36.24 War operations involving explosion due to accidental detonation and discharge of own munitions or munitions launch device**

+7th **Y36.240 War operations involving explosion due to accidental detonation and discharge of own munitions or munitions launch device, military personnel**

+7th **Y36.241 War operations involving explosion due to accidental detonation and discharge of own munitions or munitions launch device, civilian**

+ **Y36.25 War operations involving fragments from munitions**

+7th **Y36.250 War operations involving fragments from munitions, military personnel**

+7th **Y36.251 War operations involving fragments from munitions, civilian**

+ **Y36.26 War operations involving fragments of improvised explosive device [IED]**

War operations involving fragments of person-borne improvised explosive device [IED]
War operations involving fragments of vehicle-borne improvised explosive device [IED]
War operations involving fragments of roadside improvised explosive device [IED]

+7th **Y36.260 War operations involving fragments of improvised explosive device [IED], military personnel**

+7th **Y36.261 War operations involving fragments of improvised explosive device [IED], civilian**

+ **Y36.27 War operations involving fragments from weapons**

+7th **Y36.270 War operations involving fragments from weapons, military personnel**

+7th **Y36.271 War operations involving fragments from weapons, civilian**

+ **Y36.29 War operations involving other explosions and fragments**

War operations involving explosion of grenade
War operations involving explosions of land mine
War operations involving shrapnel NOS

+7th **Y36.290 War operations involving other explosions and fragments, military personnel**

+7th **Y36.291 War operations involving other explosions and fragments, civilian**

+ **Y36.3 War operations involving fires, conflagrations and hot substances**

War operations involving smoke, fumes, and heat from fires, conflagrations and hot substances

Excludes1: *war operations involving fires and conflagrations aboard military aircraft (Y36.1-)*
war operations involving fires and conflagrations aboard military watercraft (Y36.0-)
war operations involving fires and conflagrations caused indirectly by conventional weapons (Y36.2-)
war operations involving fires and thermal effects of nuclear weapons (Y36.53-)

+ **Y36.30 War operations involving unspecified fire, conflagration and hot substance**

+7th **Y36.300 War operations involving unspecified fire, conflagration and hot substance, military personnel**

+7th **Y36.301 War operations involving unspecified fire, conflagration and hot substance, civilian**

+ **Y36.31 War operations involving gasoline bomb**

War operations involving incendiary bomb
War operations involving petrol bomb

+7th **Y36.310 War operations involving gasoline bomb, military personnel**

+7th **Y36.311 War operations involving gasoline bomb, civilian**

+ **Y36.32 War operations involving incendiary bullet**

+7th **Y36.320 War operations involving incendiary bullet, military personnel**

+7th **Y36.321 War operations involving incendiary bullet, civilian**

+ **Y36.33 War operations involving flamethrower**

+7th **Y36.330 War operations involving flamethrower, military personnel**

+7th **Y36.331 War operations involving flamethrower, civilian**

+ **Y36.39 War operations involving other fires, conflagrations and hot substances**
  - +7th **Y36.390 War operations involving other fires, conflagrations and hot substances, military personnel**
  - +7th **Y36.391 War operations involving other fires, conflagrations and hot substances, civilian**

+ **Y36.4 War operations involving firearm discharge and other forms of conventional warfare**

+ **Y36.41 War operations involving rubber bullets**
  - +7th **Y36.410 War operations involving rubber bullets, military personnel**
  - +7th **Y36.411 War operations involving rubber bullets, civilian**

+ **Y36.42 War operations involving firearms pellets**
  - +7th **Y36.420 War operations involving firearms pellets, military personnel**
  - +7th **Y36.421 War operations involving firearms pellets, civilian**

+ **Y36.43 War operations involving other firearms discharge**

  War operations involving bullets NOS

  Excludes1: *war operations involving munitions fragments (Y36.25-)*
  war operations involving incendiary bullets (Y36.32-)
  - +7th **Y36.430 War operations involving other firearms discharge, military personnel**
  - +7th **Y36.431 War operations involving other firearms discharge, civilian**

+ **Y36.44 War operations involving unarmed hand to hand combat**

  Excludes1: *war operations involving combat using blunt or piercing object (Y36.45-)*
  war operations involving intentional restriction of air and airway (Y36.46-)
  war operations involving unintentional restriction of air and airway (Y36.47-)
  - +7th **Y36.440 War operations involving unarmed hand to hand combat, military personnel**
  - +7th **Y36.441 War operations involving unarmed hand to hand combat, civilian**

+ **Y36.45 War operations involving combat using blunt or piercing object**
  - +7th **Y36.450 War operations involving combat using blunt or piercing object, military personnel**
  - +7th **Y36.451 War operations involving combat using blunt or piercing object, civilian**

+ **Y36.46 War operations involving intentional restriction of air and airway**
  - +7th **Y36.460 War operations involving intentional restriction of air and airway, military personnel**
  - +7th **Y36.461 War operations involving intentional restriction of air and airway, civilian**

+ **Y36.47 War operations involving unintentional restriction of air and airway**
  - +7th **Y36.470 War operations involving unintentional restriction of air and airway, military personnel**
  - +7th **Y36.471 War operations involving unintentional restriction of air and airway, civilian**

+ **Y36.49 War operations involving other forms of conventional warfare**
  - +7th **Y36.490 War operations involving other forms of conventional warfare, military personnel**
  - +7th **Y36.491 War operations involving other forms of conventional warfare, civilian**

+ **Y36.5 War operations involving nuclear weapons**

  War operations involving dirty bomb NOS

+ **Y36.50 War operations involving unspecified effect of nuclear weapon**
  - +7th **Y36.500 War operations involving unspecified effect of nuclear weapon, military personnel**
  - +7th **Y36.501 War operations involving unspecified effect of nuclear weapon, civilian**

+ **Y36.51 War operations involving direct blast effect of nuclear weapon**

  War operations involving blast pressure of nuclear weapon
  - +7th **Y36.510 War operations involving direct blast effect of nuclear weapon, military personnel**
  - +7th **Y36.511 War operations involving direct blast effect of nuclear weapon, civilian**

+ **Y36.52 War operations involving indirect blast effect of nuclear weapon**

  War operations involving being thrown by blast of nuclear weapon

  War operations involving being struck or crushed by blast debris of nuclear weapon
  - +7th **Y36.520 War operations involving indirect blast effect of nuclear weapon, military personnel**
  - +7th **Y36.521 War operations involving indirect blast effect of nuclear weapon, civilian**

+ **Y36.53 War operations involving thermal radiation effect of nuclear weapon**

  War operations involving direct heat from nuclear weapon

  War operation involving fireball effects from nuclear weapon
  - +7th **Y36.530 War operations involving thermal radiation effect of nuclear weapon, military personnel**
  - +7th **Y36.531 War operations involving thermal radiation effect of nuclear weapon, civilian**

+ **Y36.54 War operation involving nuclear radiation effects of nuclear weapon**

  War operation involving acute radiation exposure from nuclear weapon

  War operation involving exposure to immediate ionizing radiation from nuclear weapon

  War operation involving fallout exposure from nuclear weapon

  War operation involving secondary effects of nuclear weapons
  - +7th **Y36.540 War operation involving nuclear radiation effects of nuclear weapon, military personnel**
  - +7th **Y36.541 War operation involving nuclear radiation effects of nuclear weapon, civilian**

+ **Y36.59 War operation involving other effects of nuclear weapons**
  - +7th **Y36.590 War operation involving other effects of nuclear weapons, military personnel**
  - +7th **Y36.591 War operation involving other effects of nuclear weapons, civilian**

+ **Y36.6 War operations involving biological weapons**

+ **Y36.6X War operations involving biological weapons**
  - +7th **Y36.6X0 War operations involving biological weapons, military personnel**
  - +7th **Y36.6X1 War operations involving biological weapons, civilian**

+ **Y36.7 War operations involving chemical weapons and other forms of unconventional warfare**

  Excludes1: *war operations involving incendiary devices (Y36.3-, Y36.5-)*

+ Y36.7X War operations involving chemical weapons and other forms of unconventional warfare
  - +7th Y36.7X0 War operations involving chemical weapons and other forms of unconventional warfare, military personnel
  - +7th Y36.7X1 War operations involving chemical weapons and other forms of unconventional warfare, civilian

+ Y36.8 War operations occurring after cessation of hostilities
  War operations classifiable to categories Y36.0-Y36.8 but occurring after cessation of hostilities
  + Y36.81 Explosion of mine placed during war operations but exploding after cessation of hostilities
    - +7th Y36.810 Explosion of mine placed during war operations but exploding after cessation of hostilities, military personnel
    - +7th Y36.811 Explosion of mine placed during war operations but exploding after cessation of hostilities, civilian
  + Y36.82 Explosion of bomb placed during war operations but exploding after cessation of hostilities
    - +7th Y36.820 Explosion of bomb placed during war operations but exploding after cessation of hostilities, military personnel
    - +7th Y36.821 Explosion of bomb placed during war operations but exploding after cessation of hostilities, civilian
  + Y36.88 Other war operations occurring after cessation of hostilities
    - +7th Y36.880 Other war operations occurring after cessation of hostilities, military personnel
    - +7th Y36.881 Other war operations occurring after cessation of hostilities, civilian
  + Y36.89 Unspecified war operations occurring after cessation of hostilities
    - +7th Y36.890 Unspecified war operations occurring after cessation of hostilities, military personnel
    - +7th Y36.891 Unspecified war operations occurring after cessation of hostilities, civilian

+ Y36.9 Other and unspecified war operations
  - X+7th Y36.90 War operations, unspecified
  - X+7th Y36.91 War operations involving unspecified weapon of mass destruction [WMD]
  - X+7th Y36.92 War operations involving friendly fire

Y37 Military operations

Includes: injuries to military personnel and civilians occurring during peacetime on military property and during routine military exercises and operations

Excludes1: *military aircraft involved in aircraft accident with civilian aircraft (V97.81-)*
military vehicles involved in transport accident with civilian vehicle (V09.01, V09.21, V19.81, V29.81, V39.81, V49.81, V59.81, V69.81, V79.81)
military watercraft involved in water transport accident with civilian watercraft (V94.81-)
war operations (Y36.-)

The appropriate 7th character is to be added to each code from category Y37
A initial encounter
D subsequent encounter
S sequela

+ Y37.0 Military operations involving explosion of marine weapons
  + Y37.00 Military operations involving explosion of unspecified marine weapon
    Military operations involving underwater blast NOS
    - +7th Y37.000 Military operations involving explosion of unspecified marine weapon, military personnel
    - +7th Y37.001 Military operations involving explosion of unspecified marine weapon, civilian
  + Y37.01 Military operations involving explosion of depth-charge
    - +7th Y37.010 Military operations involving explosion of depth-charge, military personnel
    - +7th Y37.011 Military operations involving explosion of depth-charge, civilian
  + Y37.02 Military operations involving explosion of marine mine
    Military operations involving explosion of marine mine, at sea or in harbor
    - +7th Y37.020 Military operations involving explosion of marine mine, military personnel
    - +7th Y37.021 Military operations involving explosion of marine mine, civilian
  + Y37.03 Military operations involving explosion of sea-based artillery shell
    - +7th Y37.030 Military operations involving explosion of sea-based artillery shell, military personnel
    - +7th Y37.031 Military operations involving explosion of sea-based artillery shell, civilian
  + Y37.04 Military operations involving explosion of torpedo
    - +7th Y37.040 Military operations involving explosion of torpedo, military personnel
    - +7th Y37.041 Military operations involving explosion of torpedo, civilian
  + Y37.05 Military operations involving accidental detonation of onboard marine weapons
    - +7th Y37.050 Military operations involving accidental detonation of onboard marine weapons, military personnel
    - +7th Y37.051 Military operations involving accidental detonation of onboard marine weapons, civilian
  + Y37.09 Military operations involving explosion of other marine weapons
    - +7th Y37.090 Military operations involving explosion of other marine weapons, military personnel
    - +7th Y37.091 Military operations involving explosion of other marine weapons, civilian

+ Y37.1 Military operations involving destruction of aircraft
  + Y37.10 Military operations involving unspecified destruction of aircraft
    - +7th Y37.100 Military operations involving unspecified destruction of aircraft, military personnel
    - +7th Y37.101 Military operations involving unspecified destruction of aircraft, civilian
  + Y37.11 Military operations involving destruction of aircraft due to enemy fire or explosives
    Military operations involving destruction of aircraft due to air to air missile
    Military operations involving destruction of aircraft due to explosive placed on aircraft
    Military operations involving destruction of aircraft due to rocket propelled grenade [RPG]
    Military operations involving destruction of aircraft due to small arms fire
    Military operations involving destruction of aircraft due to surface to air missile
    - +7th Y37.110 Military operations involving destruction of aircraft due to enemy fire or explosives, military personnel
    - +7th Y37.111 Military operations involving destruction of aircraft due to enemy fire or explosives, civilian
  + Y37.12 Military operations involving destruction of aircraft due to collision with other aircraft
    - +7th Y37.120 Military operations involving destruction of aircraft due to collision with other aircraft, military personnel
    - +7th Y37.121 Military operations involving destruction of aircraft due to collision with other aircraft, civilian
  + Y37.13 Military operations involving destruction of aircraft due to onboard fire
    - +7th Y37.130 Military operations involving destruction of aircraft due to onboard fire, military personnel
    - +7th Y37.131 Military operations involving destruction of aircraft due to onboard fire, civilian

+ **Y37.14 Military operations involving destruction of aircraft due to accidental detonation of onboard munitions and explosives**
  - +7th **Y37.140 Military operations involving destruction of aircraft due to accidental detonation of onboard munitions and explosives, military personnel**
  - +7th **Y37.141 Military operations involving destruction of aircraft due to accidental detonation of onboard munitions and explosives, civilian**
+ **Y37.19 Military operations involving other destruction of aircraft**
  - +7th **Y37.190 Military operations involving other destruction of aircraft, military personnel**
  - +7th **Y37.191 Military operations involving other destruction of aircraft, civilian**

+ **Y37.2 Military operations involving other explosions and fragments**

Excludes1: *military operations involving explosion of aircraft (Y37.1-)*
military operations involving explosion of marine weapons (Y37.0-)
military operations involving explosion of nuclear weapons (Y37.5-)

+ **Y37.20 Military operations involving unspecified explosion and fragments**
  Military operations involving air blast NOS
  Military operations involving blast NOS
  Military operations involving blast fragments NOS
  Military operations involving blast wave NOS
  Military operations involving blast wind NOS
  Military operations involving explosion NOS
  Military operations involving explosion of bomb NOS
  - +7th **Y37.200 Military operations involving unspecified explosion and fragments, military personnel**
  - +7th **Y37.201 Military operations involving unspecified explosion and fragments, civilian**
+ **Y37.21 Military operations involving explosion of aerial bomb**
  - +7th **Y37.210 Military operations involving explosion of aerial bomb, military personnel**
  - +7th **Y37.211 Military operations involving explosion of aerial bomb, civilian**
+ **Y37.22 Military operations involving explosion of guided missile**
  - +7th **Y37.220 Military operations involving explosion of guided missile, military personnel**
  - +7th **Y37.221 Military operations involving explosion of guided missile, civilian**
+ **Y37.23 Military operations involving explosion of improvised explosive device [IED]**
  Military operations involving explosion of person-borne improvised explosive device [IED]
  Military operations involving explosion of vehicle-borne improvised explosive device [IED]
  Military operations involving explosion of roadside improvised explosive device [IED]
  - +7th **Y37.230 Military operations involving explosion of improvised explosive device [IED], military personnel**
  - +7th **Y37.231 Military operations involving explosion of improvised explosive device [IED], civilian**
+ **Y37.24 Military operations involving explosion due to accidental detonation and discharge of own munitions or munitions launch device**
  - +7th **Y37.240 Military operations involving explosion due to accidental detonation and discharge of own munitions or munitions launch device, military personnel**
  - +7th **Y37.241 Military operations involving explosion due to accidental detonation and discharge of own munitions or munitions launch device, civilian**
+ **Y37.25 Military operations involving fragments from munitions**
  - +7th **Y37.250 Military operations involving fragments from munitions, military personnel**
  - +7th **Y37.251 Military operations involving fragments from munitions, civilian**
+ **Y37.26 Military operations involving fragments of improvised explosive device [IED]**
  Military operations involving fragments of person-borne improvised explosive device [IED]
  Military operations involving fragments of vehicle-borne improvised explosive device [IED]
  Military operations involving fragments of roadside improvised explosive device [IED]
  - +7th **Y37.260 Military operations involving fragments of improvised explosive device [IED], military personnel**
  - +7th **Y37.261 Military operations involving fragments of improvised explosive device [IED], civilian**
+ **Y37.27 Military operations involving fragments from weapons**
  - +7th **Y37.270 Military operations involving fragments from weapons, military personnel**
  - +7th **Y37.271 Military operations involving fragments from weapons, civilian**
+ **Y37.29 Military operations involving other explosions and fragments**
  Military operations involving explosion of grenade
  Military operations involving explosions of land mine
  Military operations involving shrapnel NOS
  - +7th **Y37.290 Military operations involving other explosions and fragments, military personnel**
  - +7th **Y37.291 Military operations involving other explosions and fragments,civilian**

+ **Y37.3 Military operations involving fires, conflagrations and hot substances**

Military operations involving smoke, fumes, and heat from fires, conflagrations and hot substances

Excludes1: *military operations involving fires and conflagrations aboard military aircraft (Y37.1-)*
military operations involving fires and conflagrations aboard military watercraft (Y37.0-)
military operations involving fires and conflagrations caused indirectly by conventional weapons (Y37.2-)
military operations involving fires and thermal effects of nuclear weapons (Y36.53-)

+ **Y37.30 Military operations involving unspecified fire, conflagration and hot substance**
  - +7th **Y37.300 Military operations involving unspecified fire, conflagration and hot substance, military personnel**
  - +7th **Y37.301 Military operations involving unspecified fire, conflagration and hot substance, civilian**
+ **Y37.31 Military operations involving gasoline bomb**
  Military operations involving incendiary bomb
  Military operations involving petrol bomb
  - +7th **Y37.310 Military operations involving gasoline bomb, military personnel**
  - +7th **Y37.311 Military operations involving gasoline bomb, civilian**
+ **Y37.32 Military operations involving incendiary bullet**
  - +7th **Y37.320 Military operations involving incendiary bullet, military personnel**
  - +7th **Y37.321 Military operations involving incendiary bullet, civilian**
+ **Y37.33 Military operations involving flamethrower**
  - +7th **Y37.330 Military operations involving flamethrower, military personnel**
  - +7th **Y37.331 Military operations involving flamethrower, civilian**

+ **Y37.39 Military operations involving other fires, conflagrations and hot substances**

+7th **Y37.390 Military operations involving other fires, conflagrations and hot substances, military personnel**

+7th **Y37.391 Military operations involving other fires, conflagrations and hot substances, civilian**

+ **Y37.4 Military operations involving firearm discharge and other forms of conventional warfare**

+ **Y37.41 Military operations involving rubber bullets**

+7th **Y37.410 Military operations involving rubber bullets, military personnel**

+7th **Y37.411 Military operations involving rubber bullets, civilian**

+ **Y37.42 Military operations involving firearms pellets**

+7th **Y37.420 Military operations involving firearms pellets, military personnel**

+7th **Y37.421 Military operations involving firearms pellets, civilian**

+ **Y37.43 Military operations involving other firearms discharge**

Military operations involving bullets NOS

Excludes1: *military operations involving munitions fragments (Y37.25-)*
military operations involving incendiary bullets (Y37.32-)

+7th **Y37.430 Military operations involving other firearms discharge, military personnel**

+7th **Y37.431 Military operations involving other firearms discharge, civilian**

+ **Y37.44 Military operations involving unarmed hand to hand combat**

Excludes1: *military operations involving combat using blunt or piercing object (Y37.45-)*
military operations involving intentional restriction of air and airway (Y37.46-)
military operations involving unintentional restriction of air and airway (Y37.47-)

+7th **Y37.440 Military operations involving unarmed hand to hand combat, military personnel**

+7th **Y37.441 Military operations involving unarmed hand to hand combat, civilian**

+ **Y37.45 Military operations involving combat using blunt or piercing object**

+7th **Y37.450 Military operations involving combat using blunt or piercing object, military personnel**

+7th **Y37.451 Military operations involving combat using blunt or piercing object, civilian**

+ **Y37.46 Military operations involving intentional restriction of air and airway**

+7th **Y37.460 Military operations involving intentional restriction of air and airway, military personnel**

+7th **Y37.461 Military operations involving intentional restriction of air and airway, civilian**

+ **Y37.47 Military operations involving unintentional restriction of air and airway**

+7th **Y37.470 Military operations involving unintentional restriction of air and airway, military personnel**

+7th **Y37.471 Military operations involving unintentional restriction of air and airway, civilian**

+ **Y37.49 Military operations involving other forms of conventional warfare**

+7th **Y37.490 Military operations involving other forms of conventional warfare, military personnel**

+7th **Y37.491 Military operations involving other forms of conventional warfare, civilian**

+ **Y37.5 Military operations involving nuclear weapons**

Military operation involving dirty bomb NOS

+ **Y37.50 Military operations involving unspecified effect of nuclear weapon**

+7th **Y37.500 Military operations involving unspecified effect of nuclear weapon, military personnel**

+7th **Y37.501 Military operations involving unspecified effect of nuclear weapon, civilian**

+ **Y37.51 Military operations involving direct blast effect of nuclear weapon**

Military operations involving blast pressure of nuclear weapon

+7th **Y37.510 Military operations involving direct blast effect of nuclear weapon, military personnel**

+7th **Y37.511 Military operations involving direct blast effect of nuclear weapon, civilian**

+ **Y37.52 Military operations involving indirect blast effect of nuclear weapon**

Military operations involving being thrown by blast of nuclear weapon

Military operations involving being struck or crushed by blast debris of nuclear weapon

+7th **Y37.520 Military operations involving indirect blast effect of nuclear weapon, military personnel**

+7th **Y37.521 Military operations involving indirect blast effect of nuclear weapon, civilian**

+ **Y37.53 Military operations involving thermal radiation effect of nuclear weapon**

Military operations involving direct heat from nuclear weapon

Military operation involving fireball effects from nuclear weapon

+7th **Y37.530 Military operations involving thermal radiation effect of nuclear weapon, military personnel**

+7th **Y37.531 Military operations involving thermal radiation effect of nuclear weapon, civilian**

+ **Y37.54 Military operation involving nuclear radiation effects of nuclear weapon**

Military operation involving acute radiation exposure from nuclear weapon

Military operation involving exposure to immediate ionizing radiation from nuclear weapon

Military operation involving fallout exposure from nuclear weapon

Military operation involving secondary effects of nuclear weapons

+7th **Y37.540 Military operation involving nuclear radiation effects of nuclear weapon, military personnel**

+7th **Y37.541 Military operation involving nuclear radiation effects of nuclear weapon, civilian**

+ **Y37.59 Military operation involving other effects of nuclear weapons**

+7th **Y37.590 Military operation involving other effects of nuclear weapons, military personnel**

+7th **Y37.591 Military operation involving other effects of nuclear weapons, civilian**

+ **Y37.6 Military operations involving biological weapons**

+ **Y37.6X Military operations involving biological weapons**

+7th **Y37.6X0 Military operations involving biological weapons, military personnel**

+7th **Y37.6X1 Military operations involving biological weapons, civilian**

+ **Y37.7 Military operations involving chemical weapons and other forms of unconventional warfare**

Excludes1: *military operations involving incendiary devices (Y36.3-, Y36.5-)*

+ **Y37.7X Military operations involving chemical weapons and other forms of unconventional warfare**
  - +7th **Y37.7X0 Military operations involving chemical weapons and other forms of unconventional warfare, military personnel**
  - +7th **Y37.7X1 Military operations involving chemical weapons and other forms of unconventional warfare, civilian**

+ **Y37.9 Other and unspecified military operations**
  - X+7th **Y37.90 Military operations, unspecified**
  - X+7th **Y37.91 Military operations involving unspecified weapon of mass destruction [WMD]**
  - X+7th **Y37.92 Military operations involving friendly fire**

Y38 Terrorism

These codes are for use to identify injuries resulting from the unlawful use of force or violence against persons or property to intimidate or coerce a Government, the civilian population, or any segment thereof, in furtherance of political or social objective

Use additional code for place of occurrence (Y92.-)

The appropriate 7th character is to be added to each code from category Y38
- A initial encounter
- D subsequent encounter
- S sequela

Review coding guideline C.20.j

+ **Y38.0 Terrorism involving explosion of marine weapons**
  Terrorism involving depth-charge
  Terrorism involving marine mine
  Terrorism involving mine NOS, at sea or in harbor
  Terrorism involving sea-based artillery shell
  Terrorism involving torpedo
  Terrorism involving underwater blast
  + **Y38.0X Terrorism involving explosion of marine weapons**
    - +7th **Y38.0X1 Terrorism involving explosion of marine weapons, public safety official injured**
    - +7th **Y38.0X2 Terrorism involving explosion of marine weapons, civilian injured**
    - +7th **Y38.0X3 Terrorism involving explosion of marine weapons, terrorist injured**

+ **Y38.1 Terrorism involving destruction of aircraft**
  Terrorism involving aircraft burned
  Terrorism involving aircraft exploded
  Terrorism involving aircraft being shot down
  Terrorism involving aircraft used as a weapon
  + **Y38.1X Terrorism involving destruction of aircraft**
    - +7th **Y38.1X1 Terrorism involving destruction of aircraft, public safety official injured**
    - +7th **Y38.1X2 Terrorism involving destruction of aircraft, civilian injured**
    - +7th **Y38.1X3 Terrorism involving destruction of aircraft, terrorist injured**

+ **Y38.2 Terrorism involving other explosions and fragments**
  Terrorism involving antipersonnel (fragments) bomb
  Terrorism involving blast NOS
  Terrorism involving explosion NOS
  Terrorism involving explosion of breech block
  Terrorism involving explosion of cannon block
  Terrorism involving explosion (fragments) of artillery shell
  Terrorism involving explosion (fragments) of bomb
  Terrorism involving explosion (fragments) of grenade
  Terrorism involving explosion (fragments) of guided missile
  Terrorism involving explosion (fragments) of land mine
  Terrorism involving explosion of mortar bomb
  Terrorism involving explosion of munitions
  Terrorism involving explosion (fragments) of rocket
  Terrorism involving explosion (fragments) of shell
  Terrorism involving shrapnel
  Terrorism involving mine NOS, on land
  Excludes1: *terrorism involving explosion of nuclear weapon (Y38.5)*
  terrorism involving suicide bomber (Y38.81)
  + **Y38.2X Terrorism involving other explosions and fragments**
    - +7th **Y38.2X1 Terrorism involving other explosions and fragments, public safety official injured**
    - +7th **Y38.2X2 Terrorism involving other explosions and fragments, civilian injured**
    - +7th **Y38.2X3 Terrorism involving other explosions and fragments, terrorist injured**

+ **Y38.3 Terrorism involving fires, conflagration and hot substances**
  Terrorism involving conflagration NOS
  Terrorism involving fire NOS
  Terrorism involving petrol bomb
  Excludes1: *terrorism involving fire or heat of nuclear weapon (Y38.5)*
  + **Y38.3X Terrorism involving fires, conflagration and hot substances**
    - +7th **Y38.3X1 Terrorism involving fires, conflagration and hot substances, public safety official injured**
    - +7th **Y38.3X2 Terrorism involving fires, conflagration and hot substances, civilian injured**
    - +7th **Y38.3X3 Terrorism involving fires, conflagration and hot substances, terrorist injured**

+ **Y38.4 Terrorism involving firearms**
  Terrorism involving carbine bullet
  Terrorism involving machine gun bullet
  Terrorism involving pellets (shotgun)
  Terrorism involving pistol bullet
  Terrorism involving rifle bullet
  Terrorism involving rubber (rifle) bullet
  + **Y38.4X Terrorism involving firearms**
    - +7th **Y38.4X1 Terrorism involving firearms, public safety official injured**
    - +7th **Y38.4X2 Terrorism involving firearms, civilian injured**
    - +7th **Y38.4X3 Terrorism involving firearms, terrorist injured**

+ **Y38.5 Terrorism involving nuclear weapons**
  Terrorism involving blast effects of nuclear weapon
  Terrorism involving exposure to ionizing radiation from nuclear weapon
  Terrorism involving fireball effect of nuclear weapon
  Terrorism involving heat from nuclear weapon
  + **Y38.5X Terrorism involving nuclear weapons**
    - +7th **Y38.5X1 Terrorism involving nuclear weapons, public safety official injured**
    - +7th **Y38.5X2 Terrorism involving nuclear weapons, civilian injured**
    - +7th **Y38.5X3 Terrorism involving nuclear weapons, terrorist injured**

+ **Y38.6 Terrorism involving biological weapons**
  Terrorism involving anthrax
  Terrorism involving cholera
  Terrorism involving smallpox
  + **Y38.6X Terrorism involving biological weapons**
    - +7th **Y38.6X1 Terrorism involving biological weapons, public safety official injured**
    - +7th **Y38.6X2 Terrorism involving biological weapons, civilian injured**
    - +7th **Y38.6X3 Terrorism involving biological weapons, terrorist injured**

+ **Y38.7 Terrorism involving chemical weapons**
  Terrorism involving gases, fumes, chemicals
  Terrorism involving hydrogen cyanide
  Terrorism involving phosgene
  Terrorism involving sarin
  + **Y38.7X Terrorism involving chemical weapons**
    - +7th **Y38.7X1 Terrorism involving chemical weapons, public safety official injured**
    - +7th **Y38.7X2 Terrorism involving chemical weapons, civilian injured**
    - +7th **Y38.7X3 Terrorism involving chemical weapons, terrorist injured**

+ **Y38.8 Terrorism involving other and unspecified means**
  - X+7th **Y38.80 Terrorism involving unspecified means**
    Terrorism NOS
  + **Y38.81 Terrorism involving suicide bomber**
    - +7th **Y38.811 Terrorism involving suicide bomber, public safety official injured**
    - +7th **Y38.812 Terrorism involving suicide bomber, civilian injured**
  + **Y38.89 Terrorism involving other means**
    Terrorism involving drowning and submersion
    Terrorism involving lasers
    Terrorism involving piercing or stabbing instruments
    - +7th **Y38.891 Terrorism involving other means, public safety official injured**

+7th Y38.892 **Terrorism involving other means, civilian injured**

+7th Y38.893 **Terrorism involving other means, terrorist injured**

+ Y38.9 **Terrorism, secondary effects**

NOTE This code is for use to identify conditions occurring subsequent to a terrorist attack not those that are due to the initial terrorist attack

+ Y38.9X **Terrorism, secondary effects**

+7th Y38.9X1 **Terrorism, secondary effects, public safety official injured**

+7th Y38.9X2 **Terrorism, secondary effects, civilian injured**

Complications of medical and surgical care (Y62-Y84)

Includes: complications of medical devices surgical and medical procedures as the cause of abnormal reaction of the patient, or of later complication, without mention of misadventure at the time of the procedure

Misadventures to patients during surgical and medical care (Y62-Y69)

Excludes1: *surgical and medical procedures as the cause of abnormal reaction of the patient, without mention of misadventure at the time of the procedure (Y83-Y84)*

Excludes2: *breakdown or malfunctioning of medical device (during procedure) (after implantation) (ongoing use) (Y70-Y82)*

Y62 Failure of sterile precautions during surgical and medical care

- **Y62.0 Failure of sterile precautions during surgical operation**
- **Y62.1 Failure of sterile precautions during infusion or transfusion**
- **Y62.2 Failure of sterile precautions during kidney dialysis and other perfusion**
- **Y62.3 Failure of sterile precautions during injection or immunization**
- **Y62.4 Failure of sterile precautions during endoscopic examination**
- **Y62.5 Failure of sterile precautions during heart catheterization**
- **Y62.6 Failure of sterile precautions during aspiration, puncture and other catheterization**
- **Y62.8 Failure of sterile precautions during other surgical and medical care**
- **Y62.9 Failure of sterile precautions during unspecified surgical and medical care**

Y63 Failure in dosage during surgical and medical care

Excludes2: *accidental overdose of drug or wrong drug given in error (T36-T50)*

- **Y63.0 Excessive amount of blood or other fluid given during transfusion or infusion**
- **Y63.1 Incorrect dilution of fluid used during infusion**
- **Y63.2 Overdose of radiation given during therapy**
- **Y63.3 Inadvertent exposure of patient to radiation during medical care**
- **Y63.4 Failure in dosage in electroshock or insulin-shock therapy**
- **Y63.5 Inappropriate temperature in local application and packing**
- **Y63.6 Underdosing and nonadministration of necessary drug, medicament or biological substance**
  Review coding guideline C.19.e.5.c
- **Y63.8 Failure in dosage during other surgical and medical care**
  Review coding guideline C.19.e.5.c
- **Y63.9 Failure in dosage during unspecified surgical and medical care**
  Review coding guideline C.19.e.5.c

Y64 Contaminated medical or biological substances

- **Y64.0 Contaminated medical or biological substance, transfused or infused**
- **Y64.1 Contaminated medical or biological substance, injected or used for immunization**
- **Y64.8 Contaminated medical or biological substance administered by other means**
- **Y64.9 Contaminated medical or biological substance administered by unspecified means**
  Administered contaminated medical or biological substance NOS

Y65 Other misadventures during surgical and medical care

- **Y65.0 Mismatched blood in transfusion**
- **Y65.1 Wrong fluid used in infusion**
- **Y65.2 Failure in suture or ligature during surgical operation**
- **Y65.3 Endotracheal tube wrongly placed during anesthetic procedure**
- **Y65.4 Failure to introduce or to remove other tube or instrument**
- + **Y65.5 Performance of wrong procedure (operation)**
  - **Y65.51 Performance of wrong procedure (operation) on correct patient**
    Wrong device implanted into correct surgical site
    Excludes1: *performance of correct procedure (operation) on wrong side or body part (Y65.53)*
  - **Y65.52 Performance of procedure (operation) on patient not scheduled for surgery**
    Performance of procedure (operation) intended for another patient
    Performance of procedure (operation) on wrong patient
  - **Y65.53 Performance of correct procedure (operation) on wrong side or body part**
    Performance of correct procedure (operation) on wrong side
    Performance of correct procedure (operation) on wrong site
- **Y65.8 Other specified misadventures during surgical and medical care**
  AHA CC: 2Q, 2019, 24

Y66 Nonadministration of surgical and medical care

Premature cessation of surgical and medical care

Excludes1: *DNR status (Z66)*
palliative care (Z51.5)

Valid 3-character code, no further characters required

Y69 Unspecified misadventure during surgical and medical care

Valid 3-character code, no further characters required

Medical devices associated with adverse incidents in diagnostic and therapeutic use (Y70-Y82)

Includes: breakdown or malfunction of medical devices (during use) (after implantation) (ongoing use)

Excludes2: *later complications following use of medical devices without breakdown or malfunctioning of device (Y83-Y84)*
misadventure to patients during surgical and medical care, classifiable to (Y62-Y69)
surgical and other medical procedures as the cause of abnormal reaction of the patient, or of later complication, without mention of misadventure at the time of the procedure (Y83-Y84)

Y70 Anesthesiology devices associated with adverse incidents

- **Y70.0 Diagnostic and monitoring anesthesiology devices associated with adverse incidents**
- **Y70.1 Therapeutic (nonsurgical) and rehabilitative anesthesiology devices associated with adverse incidents**
- **Y70.2 Prosthetic and other implants, materials and accessory anesthesiology devices associated with adverse incidents**
- **Y70.3 Surgical instruments, materials and anesthesiology devices (including sutures) associated with adverse incidents**
- **Y70.8 Miscellaneous anesthesiology devices associated with adverse incidents, not elsewhere classified**

Y71 Cardiovascular devices associated with adverse incidents

- **Y71.0 Diagnostic and monitoring cardiovascular devices associated with adverse incidents**
- **Y71.1 Therapeutic (nonsurgical) and rehabilitative cardiovascular devices associated with adverse incidents**
- **Y71.2 Prosthetic and other implants, materials and accessory cardiovascular devices associated with adverse incidents**
- **Y71.3 Surgical instruments, materials and cardiovascular devices (including sutures) associated with adverse incidents**
- **Y71.8 Miscellaneous cardiovascular devices associated with adverse incidents, not elsewhere classified**

Y72 Otorhinolaryngological devices associated with adverse incidents

- **Y72.0 Diagnostic and monitoring otorhinolaryngological devices associated with adverse incidents**
- **Y72.1 Therapeutic (nonsurgical) and rehabilitative otorhinolaryngological devices associated with adverse incidents**
- **Y72.2 Prosthetic and other implants, materials and accessory otorhinolaryngological devices associated with adverse incidents**

Y72.3 **Surgical instruments, materials and otorhinolaryngological devices (including sutures) associated with adverse incidents**

Y72.8 **Miscellaneous otorhinolaryngological devices associated with adverse incidents, not elsewhere classified**

Y73 Gastroenterology and urology devices associated with adverse incidents

Y73.0 **Diagnostic and monitoring gastroenterology and urology devices associated with adverse incidents**

Y73.1 **Therapeutic (nonsurgical) and rehabilitative gastroenterology and urology devices associated with adverse incidents**

Y73.2 **Prosthetic and other implants, materials and accessory gastroenterology and urology devices associated with adverse incidents**

Y73.3 **Surgical instruments, materials and gastroenterology and urology devices (including sutures) associated with adverse incidents**

Y73.8 **Miscellaneous gastroenterology and urology devices associated with adverse incidents, not elsewhere classified**

Y74 General hospital and personal-use devices associated with adverse incidents

Y74.0 **Diagnostic and monitoring general hospital and personal-use devices associated with adverse incidents**

Y74.1 **Therapeutic (nonsurgical) and rehabilitative general hospital and personal-use devices associated with adverse incidents**

Y74.2 **Prosthetic and other implants, materials and accessory general hospital and personal-use devices associated with adverse incidents**

Y74.3 **Surgical instruments, materials and general hospital and personal-use devices (including sutures) associated with adverse incidents**

Y74.8 **Miscellaneous general hospital and personal-use devices associated with adverse incidents, not elsewhere classified**

Y75 Neurological devices associated with adverse incidents

Y75.0 **Diagnostic and monitoring neurological devices associated with adverse incidents**

Y75.1 **Therapeutic (nonsurgical) and rehabilitative neurological devices associated with adverse incidents**

Y75.2 **Prosthetic and other implants, materials and neurological devices associated with adverse incidents**

Y75.3 **Surgical instruments, materials and neurological devices (including sutures) associated with adverse incidents**

Y75.8 **Miscellaneous neurological devices associated with adverse incidents, not elsewhere classified**

Y76 Obstetric and gynecological devices associated with adverse incidents

♀ Y76.0 **Diagnostic and monitoring obstetric and gynecological devices associated with adverse incidents**

♀ Y76.1 **Therapeutic (nonsurgical) and rehabilitative obstetric and gynecological devices associated with adverse incidents**

♀ Y76.2 **Prosthetic and other implants, materials and accessory obstetric and gynecological devices associated with adverse incidents**

♀ Y76.3 **Surgical instruments, materials and obstetric and gynecological devices (including sutures) associated with adverse incidents**

♀ Y76.8 **Miscellaneous obstetric and gynecological devices associated with adverse incidents, not elsewhere classified**

Y77 Ophthalmic devices associated with adverse incidents

Y77.0 **Diagnostic and monitoring ophthalmic devices associated with adverse incidents**

\+ Y77.1 **Therapeutic (nonsurgical) and rehabilitative ophthalmic devices associated with adverse incidents**

AHA CC: 4Q, 2020, 41

Y77.11 **Contact lens associated with adverse incidents**

Rigid gas permeable contact lens associated with adverse incidents

Soft (hydrophilic) contact lens associated with adverse incidents

Y77.19 **Other therapeutic (nonsurgical) and rehabilitative ophthalmic devices associated with adverse incidents**

Y77.2 **Prosthetic and other implants, materials and accessory ophthalmic devices associated with adverse incidents**

Y77.3 **Surgical instruments, materials and ophthalmic devices (including sutures) associated with adverse incidents**

Y77.8 **Miscellaneous ophthalmic devices associated with adverse incidents, not elsewhere classified**

Y78 Radiological devices associated with adverse incidents

Y78.0 **Diagnostic and monitoring radiological devices associated with adverse incidents**

Y78.1 **Therapeutic (nonsurgical) and rehabilitative radiological devices associated with adverse incidents**

Y78.2 **Prosthetic and other implants, materials and accessory radiological devices associated with adverse incidents**

Y78.3 **Surgical instruments, materials and radiological devices (including sutures) associated with adverse incidents**

Y78.8 **Miscellaneous radiological devices associated with adverse incidents, not elsewhere classified**

Y79 Orthopedic devices associated with adverse incidents

Y79.0 **Diagnostic and monitoring orthopedic devices associated with adverse incidents**

Y79.1 **Therapeutic (nonsurgical) and rehabilitative orthopedic devices associated with adverse incidents**

Y79.2 **Prosthetic and other implants, materials and accessory orthopedic devices associated with adverse incidents**

Y79.3 **Surgical instruments, materials and orthopedic devices (including sutures) associated with adverse incidents**

Y79.8 **Miscellaneous orthopedic devices associated with adverse incidents, not elsewhere classified**

Y80 Physical medicine devices associated with adverse incidents

Y80.0 **Diagnostic and monitoring physical medicine devices associated with adverse incidents**

Y80.1 **Therapeutic (nonsurgical) and rehabilitative physical medicine devices associated with adverse incidents**

Y80.2 **Prosthetic and other implants, materials and accessory physical medicine devices associated with adverse incidents**

Y80.3 **Surgical instruments, materials and physical medicine devices (including sutures) associated with adverse incidents**

Y80.8 **Miscellaneous physical medicine devices associated with adverse incidents, not elsewhere classified**

Y81 General- and plastic-surgery devices associated with adverse incidents

Y81.0 **Diagnostic and monitoring general- and plastic-surgery devices associated with adverse incidents**

Y81.1 **Therapeutic (nonsurgical) and rehabilitative general- and plastic-surgery devices associated with adverse incidents**

Y81.2 **Prosthetic and other implants, materials and accessory general- and plastic-surgery devices associated with adverse incidents**

Y81.3 **Surgical instruments, materials and general- and plastic-surgery devices (including sutures) associated with adverse incidents**

Y81.8 **Miscellaneous general- and plastic-surgery devices associated with adverse incidents, not elsewhere classified**

Y82 Other and unspecified medical devices associated with adverse incidents

Y82.8 **Other medical devices associated with adverse incidents**

Y82.9 **Unspecified medical devices associated with adverse incidents**

Surgical and other medical procedures as the cause of abnormal reaction of the patient, or of later complication, without mention of misadventure at the time of the procedure (Y83-Y84)

Excludes1: *misadventures to patients during surgical and medical care, classifiable to (Y62-Y69)*

Excludes2: *breakdown or malfunctioning of medical device (after implantation) (during procedure) (ongoing use) (Y70-Y82)*

Y83 Surgical operation and other surgical procedures as the cause of abnormal reaction of the patient, or of later complication, without mention of misadventure at the time of the procedure

Y83.0 Surgical operation with transplant of whole organ as the cause of abnormal reaction of the patient, or of later complication, without mention of misadventure at the time of the procedure

Y83.1 Surgical operation with implant of artificial internal device as the cause of abnormal reaction of the patient, or of later complication, without mention of misadventure at the time of the procedure

Y83.2 Surgical operation with anastomosis, bypass or graft as the cause of abnormal reaction of the patient, or of later complication, without mention of misadventure at the time of the procedure

Y83.3 Surgical operation with formation of external stoma as the cause of abnormal reaction of the patient, or of later complication, without mention of misadventure at the time of the procedure

Y83.4 Other reconstructive surgery as the cause of abnormal reaction of the patient, or of later complication, without mention of misadventure at the time of the procedure

Y83.5 Amputation of limb(s) as the cause of abnormal reaction of the patient, or of later complication, without mention of misadventure at the time of the procedure

Y83.6 Removal of other organ (partial) (total) as the cause of abnormal reaction of the patient, or of later complication, without mention of misadventure at the time of the procedure

Y83.8 Other surgical procedures as the cause of abnormal reaction of the patient, or of later complication, without mention of misadventure at the time of the procedure

Y83.9 Surgical procedure, unspecified as the cause of abnormal reaction of the patient, or of later complication, without mention of misadventure at the time of the procedure

Y84 Other medical procedures as the cause of abnormal reaction of the patient, or of later complication, without mention of misadventure at the time of the procedure

Y84.0 Cardiac catheterization as the cause of abnormal reaction of the patient, or of later complication, without mention of misadventure at the time of the procedure

Y84.1 Kidney dialysis as the cause of abnormal reaction of the patient, or of later complication, without mention of misadventure at the time of the procedure

Y84.2 Radiological procedure and radiotherapy as the cause of abnormal reaction of the patient, or of later complication, without mention of misadventure at the time of the procedure

AHA CC: 1Q, 2019, 21

Review coding guideline C.2.c.2

Y84.3 Shock therapy as the cause of abnormal reaction of the patient, or of later complication, without mention of misadventure at the time of the procedure

Y84.4 Aspiration of fluid as the cause of abnormal reaction of the patient, or of later complication, without mention of misadventure at the time of the procedure

Y84.5 Insertion of gastric or duodenal sound as the cause of abnormal reaction of the patient, or of later complication, without mention of misadventure at the time of the procedure

Y84.6 Urinary catheterization as the cause of abnormal reaction of the patient, or of later complication, without mention of misadventure at the time of the procedure

Y84.7 Blood-sampling as the cause of abnormal reaction of the patient, or of later complication, without mention of misadventure at the time of the procedure

Y84.8 Other medical procedures as the cause of abnormal reaction of the patient, or of later complication, without mention of misadventure at the time of the procedure

AHA CC: 4Q, 2014, 24; 1Q, 2021, 5-6

Y84.9 Medical procedure, unspecified as the cause of abnormal reaction of the patient, or of later complication, without mention of misadventure at the time of the procedure

Supplementary factors related to causes of morbidity classified elsewhere (Y90-Y99)

NOTE These categories may be used to provide supplementary information concerning causes of morbidity. They are not to be used for single-condition coding.

Y90 Evidence of alcohol involvement determined by blood alcohol level

Code first any associated alcohol related disorders (F10)

Y90.0 Blood alcohol level of less than 20 mg/100 ml
Y90.1 Blood alcohol level of 20-39 mg/100 ml
Y90.2 Blood alcohol level of 40-59 mg/100 ml
Y90.3 Blood alcohol level of 60-79 mg/100 ml
Y90.4 Blood alcohol level of 80-99 mg/100 ml
Y90.5 Blood alcohol level of 100-119 mg/100 ml
Y90.6 Blood alcohol level of 120-199 mg/100 ml
Y90.7 Blood alcohol level of 200-239 mg/100 ml
Y90.8 Blood alcohol level of 240 mg/100 ml or more
Y90.9 Presence of alcohol in blood, level not specified

Y92 Place of occurrence of the external cause

The following category is for use, when relevant, to identify the place of occurrence of the external cause. Use in conjunction with an activity code.

Place of occurrence should be recorded only at the initial encounter for treatment

Review coding guideline C.20.b

+ **Y92.0 Non-institutional (private) residence as the place of occurrence of the external cause**

Excludes1: *abandoned or derelict house (Y92.89)*
home under construction but not yet occupied (Y92.6-)
institutional place of residence (Y92.1-)

+ **Y92.00 Unspecified non-institutional (private) residence as the place of occurrence of the external cause**

Y92.000 Kitchen of unspecified non-institutional (private) residence as the place of occurrence of the external cause

Y92.001 Dining room of unspecified non-institutional (private) residence as the place of occurrence of the external cause

Y92.002 Bathroom of unspecified non-institutional (private) residence as the place of occurrence of the external cause

Y92.003 Bedroom of unspecified non-institutional (private) residence as the place of occurrence of the external cause

Y92.007 Garden or yard of unspecified non-institutional (private) residence as the place of occurrence of the external cause

Y92.008 Other place in unspecified non-institutional (private) residence as the place of occurrence of the external cause

Y92.009 Unspecified place in unspecified non-institutional (private) residence as the place of occurrence of the external cause

Home (NOS) as the place of occurrence of the external cause

AHA CC: 2Q, 2021, 5

+ **Y92.01 Single-family non-institutional (private) house as the place of occurrence of the external cause**

Farmhouse as the place of occurrence of the external cause

Excludes1: *barn (Y92.71)*
chicken coop or hen house (Y92.72)
farm field (Y92.73)
orchard (Y92.74)
single family mobile home or trailer (Y92.02-)
slaughter house (Y92.86)

Y92.010 Kitchen of single-family (private) house as the place of occurrence of the external cause

Y92.011 Dining room of single-family (private) house as the place of occurrence of the external cause

Y92.012 Bathroom of single-family (private) house as the place of occurrence of the external cause

Y92.013 Bedroom of single-family (private) house as the place of occurrence of the external cause

Y92.014 Private driveway to single-family (private) house as the place of occurrence of the external cause

Y92.015 Private garage of single-family (private) house as the place of occurrence of the external cause

Y92.016 **Swimming-pool in single-family (private) house or garden as the place of occurrence of the external cause**

Y92.017 **Garden or yard in single-family (private) house as the place of occurrence of the external cause**

Y92.018 **Other place in single-family (private) house as the place of occurrence of the external cause**

Y92.019 **Unspecified place in single-family (private) house as the place of occurrence of the external cause**

+ Y92.02 **Mobile home as the place of occurrence of the external cause**

Y92.020 **Kitchen in mobile home as the place of occurrence of the external cause**

Y92.021 **Dining room in mobile home as the place of occurrence of the external cause**

Y92.022 **Bathroom in mobile home as the place of occurrence of the external cause**

Y92.023 **Bedroom in mobile home as the place of occurrence of the external cause**

Y92.024 **Driveway of mobile home as the place of occurrence of the external cause**

Y92.025 **Garage of mobile home as the place of occurrence of the external cause**

Y92.026 **Swimming-pool of mobile home as the place of occurrence of the external cause**

Y92.027 **Garden or yard of mobile home as the place of occurrence of the external cause**

Y92.028 **Other place in mobile home as the place of occurrence of the external cause**

Y92.029 **Unspecified place in mobile home as the place of occurrence of the external cause**

+ Y92.03 **Apartment as the place of occurrence of the external cause**

Condominium as the place of occurrence of the external cause

Co-op apartment as the place of occurrence of the external cause

Y92.030 **Kitchen in apartment as the place of occurrence of the external cause**

Y92.031 **Bathroom in apartment as the place of occurrence of the external cause**

Y92.032 **Bedroom in apartment as the place of occurrence of the external cause**

Y92.038 **Other place in apartment as the place of occurrence of the external cause**

Y92.039 **Unspecified place in apartment as the place of occurrence of the external cause**

+ Y92.04 **Boarding-house as the place of occurrence of the external cause**

Y92.040 **Kitchen in boarding-house as the place of occurrence of the external cause**

Y92.041 **Bathroom in boarding-house as the place of occurrence of the external cause**

Y92.042 **Bedroom in boarding-house as the place of occurrence of the external cause**

Y92.043 **Driveway of boarding-house as the place of occurrence of the external cause**

Y92.044 **Garage of boarding-house as the place of occurrence of the external cause**

Y92.045 **Swimming-pool of boarding-house as the place of occurrence of the external cause**

Y92.046 **Garden or yard of boarding-house as the place of occurrence of the external cause**

Y92.048 **Other place in boarding-house as the place of occurrence of the external cause**

Y92.049 **Unspecified place in boarding-house as the place of occurrence of the external cause**

+ Y92.09 **Other non-institutional residence as the place of occurrence of the external cause**

Y92.090 **Kitchen in other non-institutional residence as the place of occurrence of the external cause**

Y92.091 **Bathroom in other non-institutional residence as the place of occurrence of the external cause**

Y92.092 **Bedroom in other non-institutional residence as the place of occurrence of the external cause**

Y92.093 **Driveway of other non-institutional residence as the place of occurrence of the external cause**

Y92.094 **Garage of other non-institutional residence as the place of occurrence of the external cause**

Y92.095 **Swimming-pool of other non-institutional residence as the place of occurrence of the external cause**

Y92.096 **Garden or yard of other non-institutional residence as the place of occurrence of the external cause**

Y92.098 **Other place in other non-institutional residence as the place of occurrence of the external cause**

AHA CC: 2Q, 2017, 10-11

Y92.099 **Unspecified place in other non-institutional residence as the place of occurrence of the external cause**

+ Y92.1 **Institutional (nonprivate) residence as the place of occurrence of the external cause**

Y92.10 **Unspecified residential institution as the place of occurrence of the external cause**

+ Y92.11 **Children's home and orphanage as the place of occurrence of the external cause**

Y92.110 **Kitchen in children's home and orphanage as the place of occurrence of the external cause**

Y92.111 **Bathroom in children's home and orphanage as the place of occurrence of the external cause**

Y92.112 **Bedroom in children's home and orphanage as the place of occurrence of the external cause**

Y92.113 **Driveway of children's home and orphanage as the place of occurrence of the external cause**

Y92.114 **Garage of children's home and orphanage as the place of occurrence of the external cause**

Y92.115 **Swimming-pool of children's home and orphanage as the place of occurrence of the external cause**

Y92.116 **Garden or yard of children's home and orphanage as the place of occurrence of the external cause**

Y92.118 **Other place in children's home and orphanage as the place of occurrence of the external cause**

Y92.119 **Unspecified place in children's home and orphanage as the place of occurrence of the external cause**

+ Y92.12 **Nursing home as the place of occurrence of the external cause**

Home for the sick as the place of occurrence of the external cause

Hospice as the place of occurrence of the external cause

Y92.120 **Kitchen in nursing home as the place of occurrence of the external cause**

Y92.121 **Bathroom in nursing home as the place of occurrence of the external cause**

Y92.122 **Bedroom in nursing home as the place of occurrence of the external cause**

AHA CC: 4Q, 2020, 33

Y92.123 **Driveway of nursing home as the place of occurrence of the external cause**

Y92.124 **Garage of nursing home as the place of occurrence of the external cause**

Y92.125 **Swimming-pool of nursing home as the place of occurrence of the external cause**

Y92.126 **Garden or yard of nursing home as the place of occurrence of the external cause**

Y92.128 **Other place in nursing home as the place of occurrence of the external cause**

Y92.129 **Unspecified place in nursing home as the place of occurrence of the external cause**

+ **Y92.13 Military base as the place of occurrence of the external cause**

Excludes1: military training grounds (Y92.83)

Y92.130 Kitchen on military base as the place of occurrence of the external cause

Y92.131 Mess hall on military base as the place of occurrence of the external cause

Y92.133 Barracks on military base as the place of occurrence of the external cause

Y92.135 Garage on military base as the place of occurrence of the external cause

Y92.136 Swimming-pool on military base as the place of occurrence of the external cause

Y92.137 Garden or yard on military base as the place of occurrence of the external cause

Y92.138 Other place on military base as the place of occurrence of the external cause

Y92.139 Unspecified place military base as the place of occurrence of the external cause

+ **Y92.14 Prison as the place of occurrence of the external cause**

Y92.140 Kitchen in prison as the place of occurrence of the external cause

Y92.141 Dining room in prison as the place of occurrence of the external cause

Y92.142 Bathroom in prison as the place of occurrence of the external cause

Y92.143 Cell of prison as the place of occurrence of the external cause

Y92.146 Swimming-pool of prison as the place of occurrence of the external cause

Y92.147 Courtyard of prison as the place of occurrence of the external cause

Y92.148 Other place in prison as the place of occurrence of the external cause

Y92.149 Unspecified place in prison as the place of occurrence of the external cause

+ **Y92.15 Reform school as the place of occurrence of the external cause**

Y92.150 Kitchen in reform school as the place of occurrence of the external cause

Y92.151 Dining room in reform school as the place of occurrence of the external cause

Y92.152 Bathroom in reform school as the place of occurrence of the external cause

Y92.153 Bedroom in reform school as the place of occurrence of the external cause

Y92.154 Driveway of reform school as the place of occurrence of the external cause

Y92.155 Garage of reform school as the place of occurrence of the external cause

Y92.156 Swimming-pool of reform school as the place of occurrence of the external cause

Y92.157 Garden or yard of reform school as the place of occurrence of the external cause

Y92.158 Other place in reform school as the place of occurrence of the external cause

Y92.159 Unspecified place in reform school as the place of occurrence of the external cause

+ **Y92.16 School dormitory as the place of occurrence of the external cause**

Excludes1: reform school as the place of occurrence of the external cause (Y92.15-)
school buildings and grounds as the place of occurrence of the external cause (Y92.2-)
school sports and athletic areas as the place of occurrence of the external cause (Y92.3-)

Y92.160 Kitchen in school dormitory as the place of occurrence of the external cause

Y92.161 Dining room in school dormitory as the place of occurrence of the external cause

Y92.162 Bathroom in school dormitory as the place of occurrence of the external cause

Y92.163 Bedroom in school dormitory as the place of occurrence of the external cause

Y92.168 Other place in school dormitory as the place of occurrence of the external cause

Y92.169 Unspecified place in school dormitory as the place of occurrence of the external cause

+ **Y92.19 Other specified residential institution as the place of occurrence of the external cause**

Y92.190 Kitchen in other specified residential institution as the place of occurrence of the external cause

Y92.191 Dining room in other specified residential institution as the place of occurrence of the external cause

Y92.192 Bathroom in other specified residential institution as the place of occurrence of the external cause

Y92.193 Bedroom in other specified residential institution as the place of occurrence of the external cause

Y92.194 Driveway of other specified residential institution as the place of occurrence of the external cause

Y92.195 Garage of other specified residential institution as the place of occurrence of the external cause

Y92.196 Pool of other specified residential institution as the place of occurrence of the external cause

Y92.197 Garden or yard of other specified residential institution as the place of occurrence of the external cause

Y92.198 Other place in other specified residential institution as the place of occurrence of the external cause

Y92.199 Unspecified place in other specified residential institution as the place of occurrence of the external cause

+ **Y92.2 School, other institution and public administrative area as the place of occurrence of the external cause**

Building and adjacent grounds used by the general public or by a particular group of the public

Excludes1: building under construction as the place of occurrence of the external cause (Y92.6)
residential institution as the place of occurrence of the external cause (Y92.1)
school dormitory as the place of occurrence of the external cause (Y92.16-)
sports and athletics area of schools as the place of occurrence of the external cause (Y92.3-)

+ **Y92.21 School (private) (public) (state) as the place of occurrence of the external cause**

Y92.210 Daycare center as the place of occurrence of the external cause

Y92.211 Elementary school as the place of occurrence of the external cause

Kindergarten as the place of occurrence of the external cause

Y92.212 Middle school as the place of occurrence of the external cause

Y92.213 High school as the place of occurrence of the external cause

AHA CC: 4Q, 2012, 108

Y92.214 College as the place of occurrence of the external cause

University as the place of occurrence of the external cause

Y92.215 Trade school as the place of occurrence of the external cause

Y92.218 Other school as the place of occurrence of the external cause

Y92.219 Unspecified school as the place of occurrence of the external cause

Y92.22 Religious institution as the place of occurrence of the external cause

Church as the place of occurrence of the external cause

Mosque as the place of occurrence of the external cause

Synagogue as the place of occurrence of the external cause

+ Y92.23 Hospital as the place of occurrence of the external cause

Excludes1: *ambulatory (outpatient) health services establishments (Y92.53-)*
home for the sick as the place of occurrence of the external cause (Y92.12-)
hospice as the place of occurrence of the external cause (Y92.12-)
nursing home as the place of occurrence of the external cause (Y92.12-)

Y92.230 Patient room in hospital as the place of occurrence of the external cause

Y92.231 Patient bathroom in hospital as the place of occurrence of the external cause

Y92.232 Corridor of hospital as the place of occurrence of the external cause

Y92.233 Cafeteria of hospital as the place of occurrence of the external cause

Y92.234 Operating room of hospital as the place of occurrence of the external cause

Y92.238 Other place in hospital as the place of occurrence of the external cause

Y92.239 Unspecified place in hospital as the place of occurrence of the external cause

+ Y92.24 Public administrative building as the place of occurrence of the external cause

Y92.240 Courthouse as the place of occurrence of the external cause

Y92.241 Library as the place of occurrence of the external cause

Y92.242 Post office as the place of occurrence of the external cause

Y92.243 City hall as the place of occurrence of the external cause

Y92.248 Other public administrative building as the place of occurrence of the external cause

+ Y92.25 Cultural building as the place of occurrence of the external cause

Y92.250 Art Gallery as the place of occurrence of the external cause

Y92.251 Museum as the place of occurrence of the external cause

Y92.252 Music hall as the place of occurrence of the external cause

Y92.253 Opera house as the place of occurrence of the external cause

Y92.254 Theater (live) as the place of occurrence of the external cause

Y92.258 Other cultural public building as the place of occurrence of the external cause

Y92.26 Movie house or cinema as the place of occurrence of the external cause

Y92.29 Other specified public building as the place of occurrence of the external cause

Assembly hall as the place of occurrence of the external cause
Clubhouse as the place of occurrence of the external cause

+ Y92.3 Sports and athletics area as the place of occurrence of the external cause

+ Y92.31 Athletic court as the place of occurrence of the external cause

Excludes1: *tennis court in private home or garden (Y92.09)*

Y92.310 Basketball court as the place of occurrence of the external cause

Y92.311 Squash court as the place of occurrence of the external cause

Y92.312 Tennis court as the place of occurrence of the external cause

Y92.318 Other athletic court as the place of occurrence of the external cause

+ Y92.32 Athletic field as the place of occurrence of the external cause

Y92.320 Baseball field as the place of occurrence of the external cause

Y92.321 Football field as the place of occurrence of the external cause

Y92.322 Soccer field as the place of occurrence of the external cause

Y92.328 Other athletic field as the place of occurrence of the external cause

Cricket field as the place of occurrence of the external cause
Hockey field as the place of occurrence of the external cause

+ Y92.33 Skating rink as the place of occurrence of the external cause

Y92.330 Ice skating rink (indoor) (outdoor) as the place of occurrence of the external cause

Y92.331 Roller skating rink as the place of occurrence of the external cause

Y92.34 Swimming pool (public) as the place of occurrence of the external cause

Excludes1: *swimming pool in private home or garden (Y92.016)*

Y92.39 Other specified sports and athletic area as the place of occurrence of the external cause

Golf-course as the place of occurrence of the external cause
Gymnasium as the place of occurrence of the external cause
Riding-school as the place of occurrence of the external cause
Stadium as the place of occurrence of the external cause

+ Y92.4 Street, highway and other paved roadways as the place of occurrence of the external cause

Excludes1: *private driveway of residence (Y92.014, Y92.024, Y92.043, Y92.093, Y92.113, Y92.123, Y92.154, Y92.194)*

+ Y92.41 Street and highway as the place of occurrence of the external cause

Y92.410 Unspecified street and highway as the place of occurrence of the external cause

Road NOS as the place of occurrence of the external cause

Y92.411 Interstate highway as the place of occurrence of the external cause

Freeway as the place of occurrence of the external cause
Motorway as the place of occurrence of the external cause

Y92.412 Parkway as the place of occurrence of the external cause

Y92.413 State road as the place of occurrence of the external cause

Y92.414 Local residential or business street as the place of occurrence of the external cause

Y92.415 Exit ramp or entrance ramp of street or highway as the place of occurrence of the external cause

+ Y92.48 Other paved roadways as the place of occurrence of the external cause

Y92.480 Sidewalk as the place of occurrence of the external cause

Y92.481 Parking lot as the place of occurrence of the external cause

Y92.482 Bike path as the place of occurrence of the external cause

Y92.488 Other paved roadways as the place of occurrence of the external cause

+ Y92.5 Trade and service area as the place of occurrence of the external cause

Excludes1: *garage in private home (Y92.015)*
schools and other public administration buildings (Y92.2-)

+ Y92.51 Private commercial establishments as the place of occurrence of the external cause

Y92.510 Bank as the place of occurrence of the external cause

Y92.511 Restaurant or café as the place of occurrence of the external cause

Y92.512 Supermarket, store or market as the place of occurrence of the external cause

Y92.513 Shop (commercial) as the place of occurrence of the external cause

+ **Y92.52 Service areas as the place of occurrence of the external cause**
  - **Y92.520 Airport as the place of occurrence of the external cause**
  - **Y92.521 Bus station as the place of occurrence of the external cause**
  - **Y92.522 Railway station as the place of occurrence of the external cause**
  - **Y92.523 Highway rest stop as the place of occurrence of the external cause**
  - **Y92.524 Gas station as the place of occurrence of the external cause**
    - Petroleum station as the place of occurrence of the external cause
    - Service station as the place of occurrence of the external cause

+ **Y92.53 Ambulatory health services establishments as the place of occurrence of the external cause**
  - **Y92.530 Ambulatory surgery center as the place of occurrence of the external cause**
    - Outpatient surgery center, including that connected with a hospital as the place of occurrence of the external cause
    - Same day surgery center, including that connected with a hospital as the place of occurrence of the external cause
  - **Y92.531 Health care provider office as the place of occurrence of the external cause**
    - Physician office as the place of occurrence of the external cause
  - **Y92.532 Urgent care center as the place of occurrence of the external cause**
  - **Y92.538 Other ambulatory health services establishments as the place of occurrence of the external cause**
    - *AHA CC: 1Q, 2019, 21*

Y92.59 Other trade areas as the place of occurrence of the external cause
- Office building as the place of occurrence of the external cause
- Casino as the place of occurrence of the external cause
- Garage (commercial) as the place of occurrence of the external cause
- Hotel as the place of occurrence of the external cause
- Radio or television station as the place of occurrence of the external cause
- Shopping mall as the place of occurrence of the external cause
- Warehouse as the place of occurrence of the external cause

+ **Y92.6 Industrial and construction area as the place of occurrence of the external cause**
  - **Y92.61 Building [any] under construction as the place of occurrence of the external cause**
  - **Y92.62 Dock or shipyard as the place of occurrence of the external cause**
    - Dockyard as the place of occurrence of the external cause
    - Dry dock as the place of occurrence of the external cause
    - Shipyard as the place of occurrence of the external cause
  - **Y92.63 Factory as the place of occurrence of the external cause**
    - Factory building as the place of occurrence of the external cause
    - Factory premises as the place of occurrence of the external cause
    - Industrial yard as the place of occurrence of the external cause
  - **Y92.64 Mine or pit as the place of occurrence of the external cause**
    - Mine as the place of occurrence of the external cause
  - **Y92.65 Oil rig as the place of occurrence of the external cause**
    - Pit (coal) (gravel) (sand) as the place of occurrence of the external cause
  - **Y92.69 Other specified industrial and construction area as the place of occurrence of the external cause**
    - Gasworks as the place of occurrence of the external cause
    - Power-station (coal) (nuclear) (oil) as the place of occurrence of the external cause
    - Tunnel under construction as the place of occurrence of the external cause
    - Workshop as the place of occurrence of the external cause

+ **Y92.7 Farm as the place of occurrence of the external cause**
  - Ranch as the place of occurrence of the external cause
  - ***Excludes1:*** *farmhouse and home premises of farm (Y92.01-)*
  - **Y92.71 Barn as the place of occurrence of the external cause**
  - **Y92.72 Chicken coop as the place of occurrence of the external cause**
    - Hen house as the place of occurrence of the external cause
  - **Y92.73 Farm field as the place of occurrence of the external cause**
  - **Y92.74 Orchard as the place of occurrence of the external cause**
  - **Y92.79 Other farm location as the place of occurrence of the external cause**

+ **Y92.8 Other places as the place of occurrence of the external cause**
  + **Y92.81 Transport vehicle as the place of occurrence of the external cause**
    - ***Excludes1:*** *transport accidents (V00-V99)*
    - **Y92.810 Car as the place of occurrence of the external cause**
    - **Y92.811 Bus as the place of occurrence of the external cause**
    - **Y92.812 Truck as the place of occurrence of the external cause**
    - **Y92.813 Airplane as the place of occurrence of the external cause**
    - **Y92.814 Boat as the place of occurrence of the external cause**
    - **Y92.815 Train as the place of occurrence of the external cause**
    - **Y92.816 Subway car as the place of occurrence of the external cause**
    - **Y92.818 Other transport vehicle as the place of occurrence of the external cause**
  + **Y92.82 Wilderness area**
    - **Y92.820 Desert as the place of occurrence of the external cause**
    - **Y92.821 Forest as the place of occurrence of the external cause**
    - **Y92.828 Other wilderness area as the place of occurrence of the external cause**
      - Swamp as the place of occurrence of the external cause
      - Mountain as the place of occurrence of the external cause
      - Marsh as the place of occurrence of the external cause
      - Prairie as the place of occurrence of the external cause
  + **Y92.83 Recreation area as the place of occurrence of the external cause**
    - **Y92.830 Public park as the place of occurrence of the external cause**
    - **Y92.831 Amusement park as the place of occurrence of the external cause**

Y92.832 Beach as the place of occurrence of the external cause
Seashore as the place of occurrence of the external cause
Y92.833 Campsite as the place of occurrence of the external cause
Y92.834 Zoological garden (Zoo) as the place of occurrence of the external cause
Y92.838 Other recreation area as the place of occurrence of the external cause
Y92.84 Military training ground as the place of occurrence of the external cause
Y92.85 Railroad track as the place of occurrence of the external cause
Y92.86 Slaughter house as the place of occurrence of the external cause
Y92.89 Other specified places as the place of occurrence of the external cause
Derelict house as the place of occurrence of the external cause
Y92.9 Unspecified place or not applicable

Y93 Activity codes

NOTE Category Y93 is provided for use to indicate the activity of the person seeking healthcare for an injury or health condition, such as a heart attack while shoveling snow, which resulted from, or was contributed to, by the activity. These codes are appropriate for use for both acute injuries, such as those from chapter 19, and conditions that are due to the long-term, cumulative effects of an activity, such as those from chapter 13. They are also appropriate for use with external cause codes for cause and intent if identifying the activity provides additional information on the event. These codes should be used in conjunction with codes for external cause status (Y99) and place of occurrence (Y92).

This section contains the following broad activity categories:
Y93.0 Activities involving walking and running
Y93.1 Activities involving water and water craft
Y93.2 Activities involving ice and snow
Y93.3 Activities involving climbing, rappelling, and jumping off
Y93.4 Activities involving dancing and other rhythmic movement
Y93.5 Activities involving other sports and athletics played individually
Y93.6 Activities involving other sports and athletics played as a team or group
Y93.7 Activities involving other specified sports and athletics
Y93.A Activities involving other cardiorespiratory exercise
Y93.B Activities involving other muscle strengthening exercises
Y93.C Activities involving computer technology and electronic devices
Y93.D Activities involving arts and handcrafts
Y93.E Activities involving personal hygiene and interior property and clothing maintenance
Y93.F Activities involving caregiving
Y93.G Activities involving food preparation, cooking and grilling
Y93.H Activities involving exterior property and land maintenance, building and construction
Y93.I Activities involving roller coasters and other types of external motion
Y93.J Activities involving playing musical instrument
Y93.K Activities involving animal care
Y93.8 Activities, other specified
Y93.9 Activity, unspecified

Review coding guideline C.20.c

+ Y93.0 Activities involving walking and running
Excludes1: *activity, walking an animal (Y93.K1)*
activity, walking or running on a treadmill (Y93.A1)
Y93.01 Activity, walking, marching and hiking
Activity, walking, marching and hiking on level or elevated terrain
Excludes1: *activity, mountain climbing (Y93.31)*
Y93.02 Activity, running

+ Y93.1 Activities involving water and water craft
Excludes1: *activities involving ice (Y93.2-)*
Y93.11 Activity, swimming
Y93.12 Activity, springboard and platform diving
Y93.13 Activity, water polo
Y93.14 Activity, water aerobics and water exercise
Y93.15 Activity, underwater diving and snorkeling
Activity, SCUBA diving
Y93.16 Activity, rowing, canoeing, kayaking, rafting and tubing
Activity, canoeing, kayaking, rafting and tubing in calm and turbulent water
Y93.17 Activity, water skiing and wake boarding
Y93.18 Activity, surfing, windsurfing and boogie boarding
Activity, water sliding
Y93.19 Activity, other involving water and watercraft
Activity involving water NOS
Activity, parasailing
Activity, water survival training and testing

+ Y93.2 Activities involving ice and snow
Excludes1: *activity, shoveling ice and snow (Y93.H1)*
Y93.21 Activity, ice skating
Activity, figure skating (singles) (pairs)
Activity, ice dancing
Excludes1: *activity, ice hockey (Y93.22)*
Y93.22 Activity, ice hockey
Y93.23 Activity, snow (alpine) (downhill) skiing, snowboarding, sledding, tobogganing and snow tubing
Excludes1: *activity, cross country skiing (Y93.24)*
Y93.24 Activity, cross country skiing
Activity, nordic skiing
Y93.29 Activity, other involving ice and snow
Activity involving ice and snow NOS

+ Y93.3 Activities involving climbing, rappelling and jumping off
Excludes1: *activity, hiking on level or elevated terrain (Y93.01)*
activity, jumping rope (Y93.56)
activity, trampoline jumping (Y93.44)
Y93.31 Activity, mountain climbing, rock climbing and wall climbing
Y93.32 Activity, rappelling
Y93.33 Activity, BASE jumping
Activity, Building, Antenna, Span, Earth jumping
Y93.34 Activity, bungee jumping
Y93.35 Activity, hang gliding
Y93.39 Activity, other involving climbing, rappelling and jumping off

+ Y93.4 Activities involving dancing and other rhythmic movement
Excludes1: *activity, martial arts (Y93.75)*
Y93.41 Activity, dancing
AHA CC: 4Q, 2012, 108
Y93.42 Activity, yoga
Y93.43 Activity, gymnastics
Activity, rhythmic gymnastics
Excludes1: *activity, trampolining (Y93.44)*
Y93.44 Activity, trampolining
Y93.45 Activity, cheerleading
Y93.49 Activity, other involving dancing and other rhythmic movements

+ Y93.5 Activities involving other sports and athletics played individually
Excludes1: *activity, dancing (Y93.41)*
activity, gymnastic (Y93.43)
activity, trampolining (Y93.44)
activity, yoga (Y93.42)
Y93.51 Activity, roller skating (inline) and skateboarding
Y93.52 Activity, horseback riding
Y93.53 Activity, golf
Y93.54 Activity, bowling
Y93.55 Activity, bike riding
Y93.56 Activity, jumping rope
Y93.57 Activity, non-running track and field events
Excludes1: *activity, running (any form) (Y93.02)*

Y93.59 Activity, other involving other sports and athletics played individually
Excludes1: *activities involving climbing, rappelling, and jumping (Y93.3-)*
activities involving ice and snow (Y93.2-)
activities involving walking and running (Y93.0-)
activities involving water and watercraft (Y93.1-)

+ Y93.6 Activities involving other sports and athletics played as a team or group
Excludes1: *activity, ice hockey (Y93.22)*
activity, water polo (Y93.13)

Y93.61 Activity, american tackle football
Activity, football NOS
Y93.62 Activity, american flag or touch football
Y93.63 Activity, rugby
Y93.64 Activity, baseball
Activity, softball
Y93.65 Activity, lacrosse and field hockey
AHA CC: 1Q, 2015, 3-21
Y93.66 Activity, soccer
Y93.67 Activity, basketball
AHA CC: 4Q, 2019, 17-18
Y93.68 Activity, volleyball (beach) (court)
Y93.6A Activity, physical games generally associated with school recess, summer camp and children
Activity, capture the flag
Activity, dodge ball
Activity, four square
Activity, kickball
Y93.69 Activity, other involving other sports and athletics played as a team or group
Activity, cricket

+ Y93.7 Activities involving other specified sports and athletics
Y93.71 Activity, boxing
Y93.72 Activity, wrestling
Y93.73 Activity, racquet and hand sports
Activity, handball
Activity, racquetball
Activity, squash
Activity, tennis
Y93.74 Activity, frisbee
Activity, ultimate frisbee
Y93.75 Activity, martial arts
Activity, combatives
Y93.79 Activity, other specified sports and athletics
Excludes1: *sports and athletics activities specified in categories Y93.0-Y93.6*

+ Y93.A Activities involving other cardiorespiratory exercise
Activities involving physical training
Y93.A1 Activity, exercise machines primarily for cardiorespiratory conditioning
Activity, elliptical and stepper machines
Activity, stationary bike
Activity, treadmill
Y93.A2 Activity, calisthenics
Activity, jumping jacks
Activity, warm up and cool down
Y93.A3 Activity, aerobic and step exercise
Y93.A4 Activity, circuit training
Y93.A5 Activity, obstacle course
Activity, challenge course
Activity, confidence course
Y93.A6 Activity, grass drills
Activity, guerilla drills
Y93.A9 Activity, other involving cardiorespiratory exercise
Excludes1: *activities involving cardiorespiratory exercise specified in categories Y93.0-Y93.7*

+ Y93.B Activities involving other muscle strengthening exercises
Y93.B1 Activity, exercise machines primarily for muscle strengthening
Y93.B2 Activity, push-ups, pull-ups, sit-ups
Y93.B3 Activity, free weights
Activity, barbells
Activity, dumbbells
Y93.B4 Activity, pilates
Y93.B9 Activity, other involving muscle strengthening exercises
Excludes1: *activities involving muscle strengthening specified in categories Y93.0-Y93.A*

+ Y93.C Activities involving computer technology and electronic devices
Excludes1: *activity, electronic musical keyboard or instruments (Y93.J-)*
Y93.C1 Activity, computer keyboarding
Activity, electronic game playing using keyboard or other stationary device
Y93.C2 Activity, hand held interactive electronic device
Activity, cellular telephone and communication device
Activity, electronic game playing using interactive device
Excludes1: *activity, electronic game playing using keyboard or other stationary device (Y93.C1)*
Y93.C9 Activity, other involving computer technology and electronic devices

+ Y93.D Activities involving arts and handcrafts
Excludes1: *activities involving playing musical instrument (Y93.J-)*
Y93.D1 Activity, knitting and crocheting
Y93.D2 Activity, sewing
Y93.D3 Activity, furniture building and finishing
Activity, furniture repair
Y93.D9 Activity, other involving arts and handcrafts

+ Y93.E Activities involving personal hygiene and interior property and clothing maintenance
Excludes1: *activities involving cooking and grilling (Y93.G-)*
activities involving exterior property and land maintenance, building and construction (Y93.H-)
activities involving caregiving (Y93.F-)
activity, dishwashing (Y93.G1)
activity, food preparation (Y93.G1)
activity, gardening (Y93.H2)
Y93.E1 Activity, personal bathing and showering
Y93.E2 Activity, laundry
Y93.E3 Activity, vacuuming
Y93.E4 Activity, ironing
Y93.E5 Activity, floor mopping and cleaning
Y93.E6 Activity, residential relocation
Activity, packing up and unpacking involved in moving to a new residence
Y93.E8 Activity, other personal hygiene
Y93.E9 Activity, other interior property and clothing maintenance

+ Y93.F Activities involving caregiving
Activity involving the provider of caregiving
Y93.F1 Activity, caregiving, bathing
Y93.F2 Activity, caregiving, lifting
AHA CC: 4Q, 2016, 73-74
Y93.F9 Activity, other caregiving

+ Y93.G Activities involving food preparation, cooking and grilling
Y93.G1 Activity, food preparation and clean up
Activity, dishwashing
Y93.G2 Activity, grilling and smoking food
Y93.G3 Activity, cooking and baking
Activity, use of stove, oven and microwave oven
Y93.G9 Activity, other involving cooking and grilling

+ Y93.H Activities involving exterior property and land maintenance, building and construction
Y93.H1 Activity, digging, shoveling and raking
Activity, dirt digging
Activity, raking leaves
Activity, snow shoveling
Y93.H2 Activity, gardening and landscaping
Activity, pruning, trimming shrubs, weeding
Y93.H3 Activity, building and construction
Y93.H9 Activity, other involving exterior property and land maintenance, building and construction

+ **Y93.I Activities involving roller coasters and other types of external motion**
  - **Y93.I1 Activity, roller coaster riding**
  - **Y93.I9 Activity, other involving external motion**

+ **Y93.J Activities involving playing musical instrument**
  Activity involving playing electric musical instrument
  - **Y93.J1 Activity, piano playing**
    Activity, musical keyboard (electronic) playing
  - **Y93.J2 Activity, drum and other percussion instrument playing**
  - **Y93.J3 Activity, string instrument playing**
  - **Y93.J4 Activity, winds and brass instrument playing**

+ **Y93.K Activities involving animal care**
  Excludes1: *activity, horseback riding (Y93.52)*
  - **Y93.K1 Activity, walking an animal**
  - **Y93.K2 Activity, milking an animal**
  - **Y93.K3 Activity, grooming and shearing an animal**
  - **Y93.K9 Activity, other involving animal care**

+ **Y93.8 Activities, other specified**
  - **Y93.81 Activity, refereeing a sports activity**
  - **Y93.82 Activity, spectator at an event**
  - **Y93.83 Activity, rough housing and horseplay**
    AHA CC: 1Q, 2015, 3-21
  - **Y93.84 Activity, sleeping**
  - **Y93.85 Activity, choking game**
    Activity, blackout game
    Activity, fainting game
    Activity, pass out game
    AHA CC: 4Q, 2016, 74-76
  - **Y93.89 Activity, other specified**

Y93.9 Activity, unspecified

Y95 Nosocomial condition
Valid 3-character code, no further characters required
AHA CC: 4Q, 2013, 119

Y99 External cause status

NOTE A single code from category Y99 should be used in conjunction with the external cause code(s) assigned to a record to indicate the status of the person at the time the event occurred.

Review coding guideline C.20.k

Y99.0 Civilian activity done for income or pay
Civilian activity done for financial or other compensation
Excludes1: *military activity (Y99.1)*
volunteer activity (Y99.2)
AHA CC: 4Q, 2016, 73-74

Y99.1 Military activity
Excludes1: *activity of off duty military personnel (Y99.8)*

Y99.2 Volunteer activity
Excludes1: *activity of child or other family member assisting in compensated work of other family member (Y99.8)*

Y99.8 Other external cause status
Activity NEC
Activity of child or other family member assisting in compensated work of other family member
Hobby not done for income
Leisure activity
Off-duty activity of military personnel
Recreation or sport not for income or while a student
Student activity
Excludes1: *civilian activity done for income or compensation (Y99.0)*
military activity (Y99.1)
AHA CC: 4Q, 2012, 108

Y99.9 Unspecified external cause status

Chapter 21: Factors Influencing Health Status and Contact with Health Services (Z00-Z99)

NOTE Z codes represent reasons for encounters. A corresponding procedure code must accompany a Z code if a procedure is performed.
Categories Z00-Z99 are provided for occasions when circumstances other than a disease, injury or external cause classifiable to categories A00-Y89 are recorded as 'diagnoses' or 'problems'. This can arise in two main ways:
(a) When a person who may or may not be sick encounters the health services for some specific purpose, such as to receive limited care or service for a current condition, to donate an organ or tissue, to receive prophylactic vaccination (immunization), or to discuss a problem which is in itself not a disease or injury.
(b) When some circumstance or problem is present which influences the person's health status but is not in itself a current illness or injury.

This chapter contains the following category blocks:

Z00-Z13	Persons encountering health services for examinations
Z14-Z15	Genetic carrier and genetic susceptibility to disease
Z16	Resistance to antimicrobial drugs
Z17	Estrogen receptor status
Z18	Retained foreign body fragments
Z19	Hormone sensitivity malignancy status
Z20-Z29	Persons with potential health hazards related to communicable diseases
Z30-Z39	Persons encountering health services in circumstances related to reproduction
Z40-Z53	Encounters for other specific health care
Z55-Z65	Persons with potential health hazards related to socioeconomic and psychosocial circumstances
Z66	Do not resuscitate status
Z67	Blood type
Z68	Body mass index (BMI)
Z69-Z76	Persons encountering health services in other circumstances
Z77-Z99	Persons with potential health hazards related to family and personal history and certain conditions influencing health status

C. Chapter-Specific Coding Guidelines

In addition to general coding guidelines, there are guidelines for specific diagnoses and/or conditions in the classification. Unless otherwise indicated, these guidelines apply to all health care settings. Please refer to Section II for guidelines on the selection of principal diagnosis.

21. Chapter 21: Factors Influencing Health Status and Contact with Health Services (Z00-Z99)

NOTE The chapter specific guidelines provide additional information about the use of Z codes for specified encounters.

a. Use of Z codes in any healthcare setting

Z codes are for use in any healthcare setting. Z codes may be used as either a first-listed (principal diagnosis code in the inpatient setting) or secondary code, depending on the circumstances of the encounter. Certain Z codes may only be used as first-listed or principal diagnosis.

b. Z Codes indicate a reason for an encounter *or Provide Additional Information about a Patient Encounter*

Z codes are not procedure codes. A corresponding procedure code must accompany a Z code to describe any procedure performed.

c. Categories of Z Codes

1) Contact/Exposure

Category Z20 indicates contact with, and suspected exposure to, communicable diseases. These codes are for patients who do not show any sign or symptom of a disease but are suspected to have been exposed to it by close personal contact with an infected individual or are in an area where a disease is epidemic.

Category Z77, Other contact with and (suspected) exposures hazardous to health, indicates contact with and suspected exposures hazardous to health.

Contact/exposure codes may be used as a first-listed code to explain an encounter for testing, or, more commonly, as a secondary code to identify a potential risk.

2) Inoculations and vaccinations

Code Z23 is for encounters for inoculations and vaccinations. It indicates that a patient is being seen to receive a prophylactic inoculation against a disease. Procedure codes are required to identify the actual administration of the injection and the type(s) of immunizations given. Code Z23 may be used as a secondary code if the inoculation is given as a routine part of preventive health care, such as a well-baby visit.

3) Status

Status codes indicate that a patient is either a carrier of a disease or has the sequelae or residual of a past disease or condition. This includes such things as the presence of prosthetic or mechanical devices resulting from past treatment. A status code is informative, because the status may affect the course of treatment and its outcome. A status code is distinct from a history code. The history code indicates that the patient no longer has the condition.

A status code should not be used with a diagnosis code from one of the body system chapters, if the diagnosis code includes the information provided by the status code. For example, code Z94.1, Heart transplant status, should not be used with a code from subcategory T86.2, Complications of heart transplant. The status code does not provide additional information. The complication code indicates that the patient is a heart transplant patient.

For encounters for weaning from a mechanical ventilator, assign a code from subcategory J96.1, Chronic respiratory failure, followed by code Z99.11, Dependence on respirator [ventilator] status.

The status Z codes/categories are:

Z14 Genetic carrier
Genetic carrier status indicates that a person carries a gene, associated with a particular disease, which may be passed to offspring who may develop that disease. The person does not have the disease and is not at risk of developing the disease.

Z15 Genetic susceptibility to disease
Genetic susceptibility indicates that a person has a gene that increases the risk of that person developing the disease.

Codes from category Z15 should not be used as principal or first-listed codes. If the patient has the condition to which he/she is susceptible, and that condition is the reason for the encounter, the code for the current condition should be sequenced first. If the patient is being seen for follow-up after completed treatment for this condition, and the condition no longer exists, a follow-up code should be sequenced first, followed by the appropriate personal history and genetic susceptibility codes. If the purpose of the encounter is genetic counseling associated with procreative management, code Z31.5, Encounter for genetic counseling, should be assigned as the first-listed code, followed by a code from category Z15. Additional codes should be assigned for any applicable family or personal history.

Z16 Resistance to antimicrobial drugs
This code indicates that a patient has a condition that is resistant to antimicrobial drug treatment. Sequence the infection code first.

Z17 Estrogen receptor status

Z18 Retained foreign body fragments

Z19 Hormone sensitivity malignancy status

Z21 Asymptomatic HIV infection status
This code indicates that a patient has tested positive for HIV but has manifested no signs or symptoms of the disease.

Z22 Carrier of infectious disease
Carrier status indicates that a person harbors the specific organisms of a disease without manifest symptoms and is capable of transmitting the infection.

Z28.3 Underimmunization status

Z33.1 Pregnant state, incidental
This code is a secondary code only for use when the pregnancy is in no way complicating the reason for visit. Otherwise, a code from the obstetric chapter is required.

Z66 Do not resuscitate
This code may be used when it is documented by the provider that a patient is on do not resuscitate status at any time during the stay.

Z67 Blood type

Z68 Body mass index (BMI)
BMI codes should only be assigned when there is an associated, reportable diagnosis (such as obesity). Do not assign BMI codes during pregnancy.
See Section I.B.14 for BMI documentation by clinicians other than the patient's provider.

Z74.01 Bed confinement status

Z76.82 Awaiting organ transplant status

Z78 Other specified health status
Code Z78.1, Physical restraint status, may be used when it is documented by the provider that a patient has been put in restraints during the current encounter. Please note that this code should not be reported when it is documented by the provider that a patient is temporarily restrained during a procedure.

Z79 Long-term (current) drug therapy

Codes from this category indicate a patient's continuous use of a prescribed drug (including such things as aspirin therapy) for the long-term treatment of a condition or for prophylactic use. It is not for use for patients who have addictions to drugs. This subcategory is not for use of medications for detoxification or maintenance programs to prevent withdrawal symptoms in patients with drug dependence (e.g., methadone maintenance for opiate dependence). Assign the appropriate code for the drug dependence instead.

Assign a code from Z79 if the patient is receiving a medication for an extended period as a prophylactic measure (such as for the prevention of deep vein thrombosis) or as treatment of a chronic condition (such as arthritis) or a disease requiring a lengthy course of treatment (such as cancer). Do not assign a code from category Z79 for medication being administered for a brief period of time to treat an acute illness or injury (such as a course of antibiotics to treat acute bronchitis).

Z88 Allergy status to drugs, medicaments and biological substances
Except: Z88.9, Allergy status to unspecified drugs, medicaments and biological substances status

Z89 Acquired absence of limb

Z90 Acquired absence of organs, not elsewhere classified

Z91.0- Allergy status, other than to drugs and biological substances

Z92.82 Status post administration of tPA (rtPA) in a different facility within the last 24 hours prior to admission to a current facility

Assign code Z92.82, Status post administration of tPA (rtPA) in a different facility within the last 24 hours prior to admission to current facility, as a secondary diagnosis when a patient is received by transfer into a facility and documentation indicates they were administered tissue plasminogen activator (tPA) within the last 24 hours prior to admission to the current facility.

This guideline applies even if the patient is still receiving the tPA at the time they are received into the current facility.

The appropriate code for the condition for which the tPA was administered (such as cerebrovascular disease or myocardial infarction) should be assigned first.

Code Z92.82 is only applicable to the receiving facility record and not to the transferring facility record.

Z93 Artificial opening status

Z94 Transplanted organ and tissue status

Z95 Presence of cardiac and vascular implants and grafts

Z96 Presence of other functional implants

Z97 Presence of other devices

Z98 Other postprocedural states

Assign code Z98.85, Transplanted organ removal status, to indicate that a transplanted organ has been previously removed. This code should not be assigned for the encounter in which the transplanted organ is removed. The complication necessitating removal of the transplant organ should be assigned for that encounter.

See section I.C19. for information on the coding of organ transplant complications.

Z99 Dependence on enabling machines and devices, not elsewhere classified

NOTE Categories Z89-Z90 and Z93-Z99 are for use only if there are no complications or malfunctions of the organ or tissue replaced, the amputation site or the equipment on which the patient is dependent.

4) History (of)

There are two types of history Z codes, personal and family. Personal history codes explain a patient's past medical condition that no longer exists and is not receiving any treatment, but that has the potential for recurrence, and therefore may require continued monitoring.

Family history codes are for use when a patient has a family member(s) who has had a particular disease that causes the patient to be at higher risk of also contracting the disease.

Personal history codes may be used in conjunction with follow-up codes and family history codes may be used in conjunction with screening codes to explain the need for a test or procedure. History codes are also acceptable on any medical record regardless of the reason for visit. A history of an illness, even if no longer present, is important information that may alter the type of treatment ordered. **The reason for the encounter (for example, screening or counseling) should be sequenced first and the appropriate personal and/or family history code(s) should be assigned as additional diagnos(es).**

The history Z code categories are:

Z80 Family history of primary malignant neoplasm

Z81 Family history of mental and behavioral disorders

Z82 Family history of certain disabilities and chronic diseases (leading to disablement)

Z83 Family history of other specific disorders

Z84 Family history of other conditions

Z85 Personal history of malignant neoplasm

Z86 Personal history of certain other diseases

Z87 Personal history of other diseases and conditions

Z91.4- Personal history of psychological trauma, not elsewhere classified

Z91.5 Personal history of self-harm

Z91.81 History of falling

Z91.82 Personal history of military deployment

Z92 Personal history of medical treatment
Except: Z92.0, Personal history of contraception Except: Z92.82, Status post administration of tPA (rtPA) in a different facility within the last 24 hours prior to admission to a current facility

5) Screening

Screening is the testing for disease or disease precursors in seemingly well individuals so that early detection and treatment can be provided for those who test positive for the disease (e.g., screening mammogram).

The testing of a person to rule out or confirm a suspected diagnosis because the patient has some sign or symptom is a diagnostic examination, not a screening. In these cases, the sign or symptom is used to explain the reason for the test.

A screening code may be a first-listed code if the reason for the visit is specifically the screening exam. It may also be used as an additional code if the screening is done during an office visit for other health problems. A screening code is not necessary if the screening is inherent to a routine examination, such as a pap smear done during a routine pelvic examination.

Should a condition be discovered during the screening then the code for the condition may be assigned as an additional diagnosis.

The Z code indicates that a screening exam is planned. A procedure code is required to confirm that the screening was performed.

The screening Z codes/categories:

Z11 Encounter for screening for infectious and parasitic diseases

Z12 Encounter for screening for malignant neoplasms

Z13 Encounter for screening for other diseases and disorders
Except: Z13.9, Encounter for screening, unspecified

Z36 Encounter for antenatal screening for mother

6) Observation

There are three observation Z code categories. They are for use in very limited circumstances when a person is being observed for a suspected condition that is ruled out. The observation codes are not for use if an injury or illness or any signs or symptoms related to the suspected condition are present. In such cases the diagnosis/symptom code is used with the corresponding external cause code.

The observation codes are primarily to be used as principal/first-listed diagnosis. An observation code may be assigned as a secondary diagnosis code when the patient is being observed for a condition that is ruled out and is unrelated to the principal/first-listed diagnosis (e.g., patient presents for treatment following injuries sustained in a motor vehicle accident and is also observed for suspected COVID-19 infection that is subsequently ruled out). Also, when the principal diagnosis is required to be a code from category Z38, Liveborn infants according to place of birth and type of delivery, then a code form category Z05, Encounter for observation and evaluation of newborn for suspected diseases and conditions ruled out, is sequenced after the Z38 code. Additional codes may be used in addition to the observation code but only if they are unrelated to the suspected condition being observed.

Codes from subcategory Z03.7, Encounter for suspected maternal and fetal conditions ruled out, may either be used as a first-listed or as an additional code assignment depending on the case. They are for use in very limited circumstances on a maternal record when an encounter is for a suspected maternal or fetal condition that is ruled out during that encounter (for example, a maternal or fetal condition may be suspected due to an abnormal test result). These codes should not be used when the condition is confirmed. In those cases, the confirmed condition should be coded. In addition, these codes are not for use if an illness or any signs or symptoms related to the suspected condition or problem are present. In such cases the diagnosis/symptom code is used.

Additional codes may be used in addition to the code from subcategory Z03.7, but only if they are unrelated to the suspected condition being evaluated.

Codes from subcategory Z03.7 may not be used for encounters for antenatal screening of mother. *See Section I.C.21. Screening.*

For encounters for suspected fetal condition that are inconclusive following testing and evaluation, assign the appropriate code from category O35, O36, O40 or O41.

The observation Z code categories:

Z03	Encounter for medical observation for suspected diseases and conditions ruled out
Z04	Encounter for examination and observation for other reasons Except: Z04.9, Encounter for examination and observation for unspecified reason
Z05	Encounter for observation and evaluation of newborn for suspected diseases and conditions ruled out

7) Aftercare

Aftercare visit codes cover situations when the initial treatment of a disease has been performed and the patient requires continued care during the healing or recovery phase, or for the long-term consequences of the disease. The aftercare Z code should not be used if treatment is directed at a current, acute disease. The diagnosis code is to be used in these cases. Exceptions to this rule are codes Z51.0, Encounter for antineoplastic radiation therapy, and codes from subcategory Z51.1, Encounter for antineoplastic chemotherapy and immunotherapy. These codes are to be first-listed, followed by the diagnosis code when a patient's encounter is solely to receive radiation therapy, chemotherapy, or immunotherapy for the treatment of a neoplasm. If the reason for the encounter is more than one type of antineoplastic therapy, code Z51.0 and a code from subcategory Z51.1 may be assigned together, in which case one of these codes would be reported as a secondary diagnosis.

The aftercare Z codes should also not be used for aftercare for injuries. For aftercare of an injury, assign the acute injury code with the appropriate 7th character (for subsequent encounter).

The aftercare codes are generally first-listed to explain the specific reason for the encounter. An aftercare code may be used as an additional code when some type of aftercare is provided in addition to the reason for admission and no diagnosis code is applicable. An example of this would be the closure of a colostomy during an encounter for treatment of another condition.

Aftercare codes should be used in conjunction with other aftercare codes or diagnosis codes to provide better detail on the specifics of an aftercare encounter visit, unless otherwise directed by the classification. Should a patient receive multiple types of antineoplastic therapy during the same encounter, code Z51.0, Encounter for antineoplastic radiation therapy, and codes from subcategory Z51.1, Encounter for antineoplastic chemotherapy and immunotherapy, may be used together on a record. The sequencing of multiple aftercare codes depends on the circumstances of the encounter.

Certain aftercare Z code categories need a secondary diagnosis code to describe the resolving condition or sequelae. For others, the condition is included in the code title.

Additional Z code aftercare category terms include fitting and adjustment, and attention to artificial openings.

Status Z codes may be used with aftercare Z codes to indicate the nature of the aftercare. For example code Z95.1, Presence of aortocoronary bypass graft, may be used with code Z48.812, Encounter for surgical aftercare following surgery on the circulatory system, to indicate the surgery for which the aftercare is being performed. A status code should not be used when the aftercare code indicates the type of status, such as using Z43.0, Encounter for attention to tracheostomy, with Z93.0, Tracheostomy status.

The aftercare Z category/codes:

Z42	Encounter for plastic and reconstructive surgery following medical procedure or healed injury
Z43	Encounter for attention to artificial openings
Z44	Encounter for fitting and adjustment of external prosthetic device
Z45	Encounter for adjustment and management of implanted device
Z46	Encounter for fitting and adjustment of other devices
Z47	Orthopedic aftercare
Z48	Encounter for other postprocedural aftercare
Z49	Encounter for care involving renal dialysis
Z51	Encounter for other aftercare and medical care

8) Follow-up

The follow-up codes are used to explain continuing surveillance following completed treatment of a disease, condition, or injury. They imply that the condition has been fully treated and no longer exists. They should not be confused with aftercare codes, or injury codes with a 7th character for subsequent encounter, that explain ongoing care of a healing condition or its sequelae. Follow-up codes may be used in conjunction with history codes to provide the full picture of the healed condition and its treatment. The follow-up code is sequenced first, followed by the history code.

A follow-up code may be used to explain multiple visits. Should a condition be found to have recurred on the follow-up visit, then the diagnosis code for the condition should be assigned in place of the follow-up code.

The follow-up Z code categories:

Z08	Encounter for follow-up examination after completed treatment for malignant neoplasm
Z09	Encounter for follow-up examination after completed treatment for conditions other than malignant neoplasm
Z39	Encounter for maternal postpartum care and examination

9) Donor

Codes in category Z52, Donors of organs and tissues, are used for living individuals who are donating blood or other body tissue. These codes are only for individuals donating for others, not for self-donations. They are not used to identify cadaveric donations.

10) Counseling

Counseling Z codes are used when a patient or family member receives assistance in the aftermath of an illness or injury, or when support is required in coping with family or social problems.

The counseling Z codes/categories:

Z30.0-	Encounter for general counseling and advice on contraception
Z31.5	Encounter for procreative genetic counseling
Z31.6-	Encounter for general counseling and advice on procreation
Z32.2	Encounter for childbirth instruction
Z32.3	Encounter for childcare instruction
Z69	Encounter for mental health services for victim and perpetrator of abuse
Z70	Counseling related to sexual attitude, behavior and orientation
Z71	Persons encountering health services for other counseling and medical advice, not elsewhere classified

NOTE Code Z71.84, Encounter for health counseling related to travel, is to be used for health risk and safety counseling for future travel purposes.

Code Z71.85, Encounter for immunization safety counseling, is to be used for counseling of the patient or caregiver regarding the safety of a vaccine. This code should not be used for the provision of general information regarding risks and potential side effects during routine encounters for the administration of vaccines.

Z76.81	Expectant mother prebirth pediatrician visit

11) Encounters for Obstetrical and Reproductive Services

See Section I.C.15. Pregnancy, Childbirth, and the Puerperium, for further instruction on the use of these codes.

Z codes for pregnancy are for use in those circumstances when none of the problems or complications included in the codes from the Obstetrics chapter exist (a routine prenatal visit or postpartum care). Codes in category Z34, Encounter for supervision of normal pregnancy, are always first-listed and are not to be used with any other code from the OB chapter.

Codes in category Z3A, Weeks of gestation, may be assigned to provide additional information about the pregnancy. Category Z3A codes should not be assigned for pregnancies with abortive outcomes (categories O00-O08), elective termination of pregnancy (code Z33.2), nor for postpartum conditions, as category Z3A is not applicable to these conditions. The date of the admission should be used to determine weeks of gestation for inpatient admissions that encompass more than one gestational week.

The outcome of delivery, category Z37, should be included on all maternal delivery records. It is always a secondary code. Codes in category Z37 should not be used on the newborn record.

Z codes for family planning (contraceptive) or procreative management and counseling should be included on an obstetric record either during the pregnancy or the postpartum stage, if applicable.

Z codes/categories for obstetrical and reproductive services:

Z30	Encounter for contraceptive management
Z31	Encounter for procreative management
Z32.2	Encounter for childbirth instruction
Z32.3	Encounter for childcare instruction
Z33	Pregnant state
Z34	Encounter for supervision of normal pregnancy
Z36	Encounter for antenatal screening of mother
Z3A	Weeks of gestation
Z37	Outcome of delivery

Z39	Encounter for maternal postpartum care and examination
Z76.81	Expectant mother prebirth pediatrician visit

12) Newborns and Infants

See Section I.C.16. Newborn (Perinatal) Guidelines, for further instruction on the use of these codes.

Newborn Z codes/categories:

Z76.1	Encounter for health supervision and care of foundling
Z00.1-	Encounter for routine child health examination
Z38	Liveborn infants according to place of birth and type of delivery

13) Routine and administrative examinations

The Z codes allow for the description of encounters for routine examinations, such as, a general check-up, or, examinations for administrative purposes, such as, a pre-employment physical. The codes are not to be used if the examination is for diagnosis of a suspected condition or for treatment purposes. In such cases the diagnosis code is used. During a routine exam, should a diagnosis or condition be discovered, it should be coded as an additional code. Pre-existing and chronic conditions and history codes may also be included as additional codes as long as the examination is for administrative purposes and not focused on any particular condition.

Some of the codes for routine health examinations distinguish between "with" and "without" abnormal findings. Code assignment depends on the information that is known at the time the encounter is being coded. For example, if no abnormal findings were found during the examination, but the encounter is being coded before test results are back, it is acceptable to assign the code for "without abnormal findings." When assigning a code for "with abnormal findings," additional code(s) should be assigned to identify the specific abnormal finding(s).

Pre-operative examination and pre-procedural laboratory examination Z codes are for use only in those situations when a patient is being cleared for a procedure or surgery and no treatment is given.

The Z codes/categories for routine and administrative examinations:

Z00	Encounter for general examination without complaint, suspected or reported diagnosis
Z01	Encounter for other special examination without complaint, suspected or reported diagnosis
Z02	Encounter for administrative examination Except: Z02.9, Encounter for administrative examinations, unspecified
Z32.0-	Encounter for pregnancy test

14) Miscellaneous Z codes

The miscellaneous Z codes capture a number of other health care encounters that do not fall into one of the other categories. Certain of these codes identify the reason for the encounter; others are for use as additional codes that provide useful information on circumstances that may affect a patient's care and treatment.

Prophylactic Organ Removal

For encounters specifically for prophylactic removal of an organ (such as prophylactic removal of breasts due to a genetic susceptibility to cancer or a family history of cancer), the principal or first-listed code should be a code from category Z40, Encounter for prophylactic surgery, followed by the appropriate codes to identify the associated risk factor (such as genetic susceptibility or family history).

If the patient has a malignancy of one site and is having prophylactic removal at another site to prevent either a new primary malignancy or metastatic disease, a code for the malignancy should also be assigned in addition to a code from subcategory Z40.0, Encounter for prophylactic surgery for risk factors related to malignant neoplasms. A Z40.0 code should not be assigned if the patient is having organ removal for treatment of a malignancy, such as the removal of the testes for the treatment of prostate cancer.

Miscellaneous Z codes/categories:

Z28	Immunization not carried out Except: Z28.3, Underimmunization status
Z29	Encounter for other prophylactic measures
Z40	Encounter for prophylactic surgery
Z41	Encounter for procedures for purposes other than remedying health state Except: Z41.9, Encounter for procedure for purposes other than remedying health state, unspecified
Z53	Persons encountering health services for specific procedures and treatment, not carried out
Z55	Problems related to education and literacy
Z56	Problems related to employment and unemployment
Z57	Occupational exposure to risk factors
Z58	Problems related to physical environment
Z59	Problems related to housing and economic circumstances
Z60	Problems related to social environment
Z62	Problems related to upbringing
Z63	Other problems related to primary support group, including family circumstances
Z64	Problems related to certain psychosocial circumstances
Z65	Problems related to other psychosocial circumstances
Z72	Problems related to lifestyle Note: These codes should be assigned only when the documentation specifies that the patient has an associated problem.
Z73	Problems related to life management difficulty
Z74	Problems related to care provider dependency Except: Z74.01, Bed confinement status
Z75	Problems related to medical facilities and other health care
Z76.0	Encounter for issue of repeat prescription
Z76.3	Healthy person accompanying sick person
Z76.4	Other boarder to healthcare facility
Z76.5	Malingerer [conscious simulation]
Z91.1-	Patient's noncompliance with medical treatment and regimen
Z91.83	Wandering in diseases classified elsewhere
Z91.84-	Oral health risk factors
Z91.89	Other specified personal risk factors, not elsewhere classified

See Section I.B.14 for Z55-Z65 Persons with potential health hazards related to socioeconomic and psychosocial circumstances, documentation by clinicians other than the patient's provider.

15) Nonspecific Z codes

Certain Z codes are so non-specific, or potentially redundant with other codes in the classification, that there can be little justification for their use in the inpatient setting. Their use in the outpatient setting should be limited to those instances when there is no further documentation to permit more precise coding. Otherwise, any sign or symptom or any other reason for visit that is captured in another code should be used.

Nonspecific Z codes/categories:

Z02.9	Encounter for administrative examinations, unspecified
Z04.9	Encounter for examination and observation for unspecified reason
Z13.9	Encounter for screening, unspecified
Z41.9	Encounter for procedure for purposes other than remedying health state, unspecified
Z52.9	Donor of unspecified organ or tissue
Z86.59	Personal history of other mental and behavioral disorders
Z88.9	Allergy status to unspecified drugs, medicaments and biological substances status
Z92.0	Personal history of contraception

16) Z Codes That May Only be Principal/First-Listed Diagnosis

The following Z codes/categories may only be reported as the principal/first-listed diagnosis, except when there are multiple encounters on the same day and the medical records for the encounters are combined:

Z00	Encounter for general examination without complaint, suspected or reported diagnosis Except: Z00.6
Z01	Encounter for other special examination without complaint, suspected or reported diagnosis
Z02	Encounter for administrative examination
Z03	Encounter for medical observation for suspected diseases and conditions ruled out
Z04	Encounter for examination and observation for other reasons
Z33.2	Encounter for elective termination of pregnancy
Z31.81	Encounter for male factor infertility in female patient
Z31.83	Encounter for assisted reproductive fertility procedure cycle
Z31.84	Encounter for fertility preservation procedure
Z34	Encounter for supervision of normal pregnancy
Z39	Encounter for maternal postpartum care and examination
Z38	Liveborn infants according to place of birth and type of delivery
Z40	Encounter for prophylactic surgery
Z42	Encounter for plastic and reconstructive surgery following medical procedure or healed injury
Z51.0	Encounter for antineoplastic radiation therapy
Z51.1-	Encounter for antineoplastic chemotherapy and immunotherapy
Z52	Donors of organs and tissues Except: Z52.9, Donor of unspecified organ or tissue
Z76.1	Encounter for health supervision and care of foundling
Z76.2	Encounter for health supervision and care of other healthy infant and child
Z99.12	Encounter for respirator [ventilator] dependence during power failure

17) **Social Determinants of Health**

Codes describing social determinants of health (SDOH) should be assigned when this information is documented.

For social determinants of health, such as information found in categories Z55-Z65, Persons with potential health hazards related to socioeconomic and psychosocial circumstances, code assignment may be based on medical record documentation from clinicians involved in the care of the patient who are not the patient's provider since this information represents social information, rather than medical diagnoses. **For example, coding professionals may utilize documentation of social information from social workers, community health workers, case managers, or nurses, if their documentation is included in the official medical record.**

Patient self-reported documentation may be used to assign codes for social determinants of health, as long as the patient self-reported information is signed-off by and incorporated into the medical record by either a clinician or provider.

Social determinants of health codes are located primarily in these Z code categories:

Z55 Problems related to education and literacy
Z56 Problems related to employment and unemployment
Z57 Occupational exposure to risk factors
Z58 Problems related to physical environment
Z59 Problems related to housing and economic circumstances
Z60 Problems related to social environment
Z62 Problems related to upbringing
Z63 Other problems related to primary support group, including family circumstances
Z64 Problems related to certain psychosocial circumstances
Z65 Problems related to other psychosocial circumstances

See Section I.B.14. Documentation by Clinicians Other than the Patient's Provider.

Persons encountering health services for examinations (Z00-Z13)

NOTE Nonspecific abnormal findings disclosed at the time of these examinations are classified to categories R70-R94.

Excludes1: *examinations related to pregnancy and reproduction (Z30-Z36, Z39.-)*

Z00 Encounter for general examination without complaint, suspected or reported diagnosis

Excludes1: *encounter for examination for administrative purposes (Z02.-)*
Excludes2: *encounter for pre-procedural examinations (Z01.81-)*
special screening examinations (Z11-Z13)
Review coding guidelines C.21.c.13 and C.21.c.16

+ **Z00.0 Encounter for general adult medical examination**
Encounter for adult periodic examination (annual) (physical) and any associated laboratory and radiologic examinations
Excludes1: *encounter for examination of sign or symptom- code to sign or symptom*
general health check-up of infant orchild (Z00.12.-)

• **Z00.00 Encounter for general adult medical examination without abnormal findings**
Encounter for adult health check-up NOS
AHA CC: 1Q, 2016, 36-37; 4Q, 2017, 95-96

• **Z00.01 Encounter for general adult medical examination with abnormal findings**
Use additional code to identify abnormal findings
AHA CC: 1Q, 2016, 35-36

+ **Z00.1 Encounter for newborn, infant and child health examinations**
Review coding guideline C.21.c.12

+ **Z00.11 Newborn health examination**
Health check for child under 29 days old
Use additional code to identify any abnormal findings
Excludes1: *health check for child over 28 days old (Z00.12-)*

• **Z00.110 Health examination for newborn under 8 days old**
Health check for newborn under 8 days old

• **Z00.111 Health examination for newborn 8 to 28 days old**
Health check for newborn 8 to 28 days old
Newborn weight check

+ **Z00.12 Encounter for routine child health examination**
Health check (routine) for child over 28 days old
Immunizations appropriate for age
Routine developmental screening of infant or child
Routine vision and hearing testing
Excludes1: *health check for child under 29 days old (Z00.11-)*
health supervision of foundling or other healthy infant or child (Z76.1-Z76.2)
newborn health examination (Z00.11-)

• **Z00.121 Encounter for routine child health examination with abnormal findings**
Use additional code to identify abnormal findings
AHA CC: 1Q, 2016, 34-35; 4Q, 2017, 95-96

• **Z00.129 Encounter for routine child health examination without abnormal findings**
Encounter for routine child health examination NOS
AHA CC: 1Q, 2016, 34-35

• **Z00.2 Encounter for examination for period of rapid growth in childhood**

• **Z00.3 Encounter for examination for adolescent development state**
Encounter for puberty development state

Z00.5 Encounter for examination of potential donor of organ and tissue

Z00.6 Encounter for examination for normal comparison and control in clinical research program
Examination of participant or control in clinical research program

+ **Z00.7 Encounter for examination for period of delayed growth in childhood**

• **Z00.70 Encounter for examination for period of delayed growth in childhood without abnormal findings**

• **Z00.71 Encounter for examination for period of delayed growth in childhood with abnormal findings**
Use additional code to identify abnormal findings

Z00.8 Encounter for other general examination
Encounter for health examination in population surveys

Z01 Encounter for other special examination without complaint, suspected or reported diagnosis

Includes: routine examination of specific system
NOTE Codes from category Z01 represent the reason for the encounter. A separate procedure code is required to identify any examinations or procedures performed
Excludes1: *encounter for examination for administrative purposes (Z02.-)*
encounter for examination for suspected conditions, proven not to exist (Z03.-)
encounter for laboratory and radiologic examinations as a component of general medical examinations (Z00.0-)
encounter for laboratory, radiologic and imaging examinations for sign(s) and symptom(s) - code to the sign(s) or symptom(s)
Excludes2: *screening examinations (Z11-Z13)*
Review coding guidelines C.21.c.13 and C.21.c.16

+ **Z01.0 Encounter for examination of eyes and vision**
Excludes1: *examination for driving license (Z02.4)*

Z01.00 Encounter for examination of eyes and vision without abnormal findings
Encounter for examination of eyes and vision NOS

Z01.01 Encounter for examination of eyes and vision with abnormal findings
Use additional code to identify abnormal findings
AHA CC: 4Q, 2016, 21

+ **Z01.02 Encounter for examination of eyes and vision following failed vision screening**
Excludes1: *encounter for examination of eyes and vision with abnormal findings (Z01.01)*
encounter for examination of eyes and vision without abnormal findings (Z01.00)
AHA CC: 4Q, 2019, 20

Z01.020 Examination for examination of eyes and vision following failed vision screening without abnormal findings

Z01.021 Examination for examination of eyes and vision following failed vision screening with abnormal findings
Use additional code to identify abnormal findings

+ Z01.1 **Encounter for examination of ears and hearing**

Z01.10 **Encounter for examination of ears and hearing without abnormal findings**

Encounter for examination of ears and hearing NOS

AHA CC: 4Q, 2016, 21

+ Z01.11 **Encounter for examination of ears and hearing with abnormal findings**

Z01.110 **Encounter for hearing examination following failed hearing screening**

AHA CC: 3Q, 2016, 18-19

Z01.118 **Encounter for examination of ears and hearing with other abnormal findings**

Use additional code to identify abnormal findings

AHA CC: 3Q, 2016, 17

Z01.12 **Encounter for hearing conservation and treatment**

+ Z01.2 **Encounter for dental examination and cleaning**

Z01.20 **Encounter for dental examination and cleaning without abnormal findings**

Encounter for dental examination and cleaning NOS

Z01.21 **Encounter for dental examination and cleaning with abnormal findings**

Use additional code to identify abnormal findings

+ Z01.3 **Encounter for examination of blood pressure**

Z01.30 **Encounter for examination of blood pressure without abnormal findings**

Encounter for examination of blood pressure NOS

Z01.31 **Encounter for examination of blood pressure with abnormal findings**

Use additional code to identify abnormal findings

+ Z01.4 **Encounter for gynecological examination**

Excludes2: *pregnancy examination or test (Z32.0-)*
routine examination for contraceptive maintenance (Z30.4-)

+ Z01.41 **Encounter for routine gynecological examination**

Encounter for general gynecological examination with or without cervical smear

Encounter for gynecological examination (general) (routine) NOS

Encounter for pelvic examination (annual) (periodic)

Use additional code:
for screening for human papillomavirus, if applicable, (Z11.51)
for screening vaginal pap smear, if applicable (Z12.72)
to identify acquired absence of uterus, if applicable (Z90.71-)

Excludes1: *gynecologic examination status-post hysterectomy for malignant condition (Z08)*
screening cervical pap smear not a part of a routine gynecological examination (Z12.4)

♀ Z01.411 **Encounter for gynecological examination (general) (routine) with abnormal findings**

Use additional code to identify abnormal findings.

♀ Z01.419 **Encounter for gynecological examination (general) (routine) without abnormal findings**

♀ Z01.42 **Encounter for cervical smear to confirm findings of recent normal smear following initial abnormal smear**

+ Z01.8 **Encounter for other specified special examinations**

+ Z01.81 **Encounter for preprocedural examinations**

Encounter for preoperative examinations

Encounter for radiological and imaging examinations as part of preprocedural examination

Z01.810 **Encounter for preprocedural cardiovascular examination**

Z01.811 **Encounter for preprocedural respiratory examination**

Z01.812 **Encounter for preprocedural laboratory examination**

Blood and urine tests prior to treatment or procedure

AHA CC: 3Q, 2020, 14-15; 1Q, 2021, 37-38

Z01.818 **Encounter for other preprocedural examination**

Encounter for preprocedural examination NOS

Encounter for examinations prior to antineoplastic chemotherapy

Z01.82 **Encounter for allergy testing**

Excludes1: *encounter for antibody response examination (Z01.84)*

Z01.83 **Encounter for blood typing**

Encounter for Rh typing

Z01.84 **Encounter for antibody response examination**

Encounter for immunity status testing

Excludes1: *encounter for allergy testing (Z01.82)*

AHA CC: 2Q, 2020, 11

Review coding guideline C.1.g.1.k

Z01.89 **Encounter for other specified special examinations**

Z02 **Encounter for administrative examination**

Review coding guidelines C.21.c.13 and C.21.c.16

Z02.0 **Encounter for examination for admission to educational institution**

Encounter for examination for admission to preschool (education)

Encounter for examination for re-admission to school following illness or medical treatment

Z02.1 **Encounter for pre-employment examination**

Z02.2 **Encounter for examination for admission to residential institution**

Excludes1: *examination for admission to prison (Z02.89)*

Z02.3 **Encounter for examination for recruitment to armed forces**

Z02.4 **Encounter for examination for driving license**

Z02.5 **Encounter for examination for participation in sport**

Excludes1: *blood-alcohol and blood-drug test (Z02.83)*

Z02.6 **Encounter for examination for insurance purposes**

+ Z02.7 **Encounter for issue of medical certificate**

Excludes1: *encounter for general medical examination (Z00-Z01, Z02.0-Z02.6, Z02.8-Z02.9)*

Z02.71 **Encounter for disability determination**

Encounter for issue of medical certificate of incapacity

Encounter for issue of medical certificate of invalidity

Z02.79 **Encounter for issue of other medical certificate**

+ Z02.8 **Encounter for other administrative examinations**

Z02.81 **Encounter for paternity testing**

Z02.82 **Encounter for adoption services**

Z02.83 **Encounter for blood-alcohol and blood-drug test**

Use additional code for findings of alcohol or drugs in blood (R78.-)

Z02.89 **Encounter for other administrative examinations**

Encounter for examination for admission to prison

Encounter for examination for admission to summer camp

Encounter for immigration examination

Encounter for naturalization examination

Encounter for premarital examination

Excludes1: *health supervision of foundling or other healthy infant or child (Z76.1-Z76.2)*

Z02.9 **Encounter for administrative examinations, unspecified**

Z03 Encounter for medical observation for suspected diseases and conditions ruled out

This category is to be used when a person without a diagnosis is suspected of having an abnormal condition, without signs or symptoms, which requires study, but after examination and observation, is ruled out. This category is also for use for administrative and legal observation status.

Excludes1: *contact with and (suspected) exposures hazardous to health (Z77.-)*
encounter for observation and evaluation of newborn for suspected diseases and conditions, ruled out (Z05.-)
person with feared complaint in whom no diagnosis is made (Z71.1)
signs or symptoms under study- code to signs or symptoms

AHA CC: 4Q, 2017, 27
Review coding guidelines C.21.c.6 and C.21.c.16

Z03.6 Encounter for observation for suspected toxic effect from ingested substance ruled out
Encounter for observation for suspected adverse effect from drug
Encounter for observation for suspected poisoning

\+ **Z03.7 Encounter for suspected maternal and fetal conditions ruled out**
Encounter for suspected maternal and fetal conditions not found
Excludes1: *known or suspected fetal anomalies affecting management of mother, not ruled out (O26.-, O35.-, O36.-, O40.-, O41.-)*

● ♀ **Z03.71 Encounter for suspected problem with amniotic cavity and membrane ruled out**
Encounter for suspected oligohydramnios ruled out
Encounter for suspected polyhydramnios ruled out

● ♀ **Z03.72 Encounter for suspected placental problem ruled out**

● ♀ **Z03.73 Encounter for suspected fetal anomaly ruled out**
AHA CC: 4Q, 2016, 4-7

● ♀ **Z03.74 Encounter for suspected problem with fetal growth ruled out**

● ♀ **Z03.75 Encounter for suspected cervical shortening ruled out**

● ♀ **Z03.79 Encounter for other suspected maternal and fetal conditions ruled out**
AHA CC: 4Q, 2016, 4-7

\+ **Z03.8 Encounter for observation for other suspected diseases and conditions ruled out**

Z03.81 Encounter for observation for suspected exposure to biological agents ruled out

Z03.810 Encounter for observation for suspected exposure to anthrax ruled out

Z03.818 Encounter for observation for suspected exposure to other biological agents ruled out
AHA CC: 1Q, 2020, 34-36; 2Q, 2020, 8-9

\+ **Z03.82 Encounter for observation for suspected foreign body ruled out**
Excludes1: *retained foreign body (Z18.-)*
retained foreign body in eyelid (H02.81)
residual foreign body in soft tissue (M79.5)
Excludes2: *confirmed foreign body ingestion or aspiration including*
foreign body in alimentary tract (T18)
foreign body in ear (T16)
foreign body on external eye (T15)
foreign body in respiratory tract (T17)
AHA CC: 4Q, 2020, 42

Z03.821 Encounter for observation for suspected ingested foreign body ruled out

Z03.822 Encounter for observation for suspected aspirated (inhaled) foreign body ruled out

Z03.823 Encounter for observation for suspected inserted (injected) foreign body ruled out
Encounter for observation for suspected inserted (injected) foreign body in eye ruled out
Encounter for observation for suspected inserted (injected) foreign body in orifice ruled out
Encounter for observation for suspected inserted (injected) foreign body in skin ruled out

Z03.89 Encounter for observation for other suspected diseases and conditions ruled out

Z04 Encounter for examination and observation for other reasons

Includes: encounter for examination for medicolegal reasons
This category is to be used when a person without a diagnosis is suspected of having an abnormal condition, without signs or symptoms, which requires study, but after examination and observation, is ruled-out. This category is also for use for administrative and legal observation status.

Review coding guidelines C.21.c.6 and C.21.c.16

Z04.1 Encounter for examination and observation following transport accident
Excludes1: *encounter for examination and observation following work accident (Z04.2)*
AHA CC: 2Q, 2018, 8; 2Q, 2019, 11

Z04.2 Encounter for examination and observation following work accident

Z04.3 Encounter for examination and observation following other accident
AHA CC: 2Q, 2018, 7-8

\+ **Z04.4 Encounter for examination and observation following alleged rape**
Encounter for examination and observation of victim following alleged rape
Encounter for examination and observation of victim following alleged sexual abuse

● **Z04.41 Encounter for examination and observation following alleged adult rape**
Suspected adult rape, ruled out
Suspected adult sexual abuse, ruled out
Review coding guideline C.19.f

● **Z04.42 Encounter for examination and observation following alleged child rape**
Suspected child rape, ruled out
Suspected child sexual abuse, ruled out
Review coding guideline C.19.f

Z04.6 Encounter for general psychiatric examination, requested by authority

\+ **Z04.7 Encounter for examination and observation following alleged physical abuse**

● **Z04.71 Encounter for examination and observation following alleged adult physical abuse**
Suspected adult physical abuse, ruled out
Excludes1: *confirmed case of adult physical abuse (T74.-)*
encounter for examination and observation following alleged adult sexual abuse (Z04.41)
suspected case of adult physical abuse, not ruled out (T76.-)
Review coding guideline C.19.f

● **Z04.72 Encounter for examination and observation following alleged child physical abuse**
Suspected child physical abuse, ruled out
Excludes1: *confirmed case of child physical abuse (T74.-)*
encounter for examination and observation following alleged child sexual abuse (Z04.42)
suspected case of child physical abuse, not ruled out (T76.-)
Review coding guideline C.19.f

+ **Z04.8 Encounter for examination and observation for other specified reasons**
  Encounter for examination and observation for request for expert evidence
  Review coding guideline C.19.f
  Z04.81 Encounter for examination and observation of victim following forced sexual exploitation
  AHA CC: 4Q, 2018, 32-33, 35
  Z04.82 Encounter for examination and observation of victim following forced labor exploitation
  AHA CC: 4Q, 2018, 32-33, 35
  Z04.89 Encounter for examination and observation for other specified reasons
  AHA CC: 4Q, 2018, 35

Z04.9 Encounter for examination and observation for unspecified reason
  Encounter for observation NOS

Z05 Encounter for observation and evaluation of newborn for suspected diseases and conditions ruled out

NOTE This category is to be used for newborns, within the neonatal period (the first 28 days of life), who are suspected of having an abnormal condition, but without signs or symptoms, and which, after examination and observation, is ruled out.
Review coding guideline C.16.b
Review coding guideline C.21.c.6
AHA CC: 4Q, 2016, 77; 4Q, 2017, 27

• **Z05.0 Observation and evaluation of newborn for suspected cardiac condition ruled out**
• **Z05.1 Observation and evaluation of newborn for suspected infectious condition ruled out**
  AHA CC: 2Q, 2019, 10-11
• **Z05.2 Observation and evaluation of newborn for suspected neurological condition ruled out**
• **Z05.3 Observation and evaluation of newborn for suspected respiratory condition ruled out**
+ **Z05.4 Observation and evaluation of newborn for suspected genetic, metabolic or immunologic condition ruled out**
  • **Z05.41 Observation and evaluation of newborn for suspected genetic condition ruled out**
    AHA CC: 4Q, 2016, 54-55
  • **Z05.42 Observation and evaluation of newborn for suspected metabolic condition ruled out**
  • **Z05.43 Observation and evaluation of newborn for suspected immunologic condition ruled out**
• **Z05.5 Observation and evaluation of newborn for suspected gastrointestinal condition ruled out**
• **Z05.6 Observation and evaluation of newborn for suspected genitourinary condition ruled out**
+ **Z05.7 Observation and evaluation of newborn for suspected skin, subcutaneous, musculoskeletal and connective tissue condition ruled out**
  • **Z05.71 Observation and evaluation of newborn for suspected skin and subcutaneous tissue condition ruled out**
  • **Z05.72 Observation and evaluation of newborn for suspected musculoskeletal condition ruled out**
  • **Z05.73 Observation and evaluation of newborn for suspected connective tissue condition ruled out**
• **Z05.8 Observation and evaluation of newborn for other specified suspected condition ruled out**
• **Z05.9 Observation and evaluation of newborn for unspecified suspected condition ruled out**

Z08 Encounter for follow-up examination after completed treatment for malignant neoplasm
  Medical surveillance following completed treatment
  Use additional code to identify any acquired absence of organs (Z90.-)
  Use additional code to identify the personal history of malignant neoplasm (Z85.-)
  Excludes1: *aftercare following medical care (Z43-Z49, Z51)*
  AHA CC: 3Q, 2020, 30
  Review coding guideline C.21.c.8
  Valid 3-character code, no further characters required

Z09 Encounter for follow-up examination after completed treatment for conditions other than malignant neoplasm
  Medical surveillance following completed treatment
  Use additional code to identify any applicable history of disease code (Z86.-, Z87.-)
  Excludes1: *aftercare following medical care (Z43-Z49, Z51)*
  surveillance of contraception (Z30.4-)
  surveillance of prosthetic and other medical devices (Z44-Z46)
  Review coding guideline C.1.g.1.j
  Review coding guideline C.21.c.8
  AHA CC: 1Q, 2017, 9; 2Q, 2020, 10-11; 1Q, 2021, 33-34
  Valid 3-character code, no further characters required

Z11 Encounter for screening for infectious and parasitic diseases
  Screening is the testing for disease or disease precursors in asymptomatic individuals so that early detection and treatment can be provided for those who test positive for the disease.
  Excludes1: *encounter for diagnostic examination-code to sign or symptom*
  Review coding guideline C.21.c.5
  Z11.0 Encounter for screening for intestinal infectious diseases
  Z11.1 Encounter for screening for respiratory tuberculosis
    Encounter for screening for active tuberculosis disease
  Z11.2 Encounter for screening for other bacterial diseases
  Z11.3 Encounter for screening for infections with a predominantly sexual mode of transmission
    Excludes2: *encounter for screening for human immunodeficiency virus [HIV] (Z11.4)*
    encounter for screening for human papillomavirus (Z11.51)
  Z11.4 Encounter for screening for human immunodeficiency virus [HIV]
    Review coding guideline C.1.a.2.h
+ **Z11.5 Encounter for screening for other viral diseases**
    Excludes2: *encounter for screening for viral intestinal disease (Z11.0)*
    Z11.51 Encounter for screening for human papillomavirus (HPV)
    Z11.52 Encounter for screening for COVID-19
    AHA CC: 1Q, 2021, 41-42
    Z11.59 Encounter for screening for other viral diseases
  Z11.6 Encounter for screening for other protozoal diseases and helminthiases
    Excludes2: *encounter for screening for protozoal intestinal disease (Z11.0)*
  Z11.7 Encounter for testing for latent tuberculosis infection
    AHA CC: 4Q, 2019, 20
  Z11.8 Encounter for screening for other infectious and parasitic diseases
    Encounter for screening for chlamydia
    Encounter for screening for rickettsial
    Encounter for screening for spirochetal
    Encounter for screening for mycoses
  Z11.9 Encounter for screening for infectious and parasitic diseases, unspecified

Z12 Encounter for screening for malignant neoplasms
  Screening is the testing for disease or disease precursors in asymptomatic individuals so that early detection and treatment can be provided for those who test positive for the disease.
  Use additional code to identify any family history of malignant neoplasm (Z80.-)
  Excludes1: *encounter for diagnostic examination-code to sign or symptom*
  Review coding guideline C.21.c.5
  Z12.0 Encounter for screening for malignant neoplasm of stomach
+ **Z12.1 Encounter for screening for malignant neoplasm of intestinal tract**
    Z12.10 Encounter for screening for malignant neoplasm of intestinal tract, unspecified
    Z12.11 Encounter for screening for malignant neoplasm of colon
      Encounter for screening colonoscopy NOS
      AHA CC: 1Q, 2017, 8-9; 1Q, 2018, 6-7
    Z12.12 Encounter for screening for malignant neoplasm of rectum
    Z12.13 Encounter for screening for malignant neoplasm of small intestine

Z12.2 Encounter for screening for malignant neoplasm of respiratory organs

+ **Z12.3 Encounter for screening for malignant neoplasm of breast**

Z12.31 Encounter for screening mammogram for malignant neoplasm of breast

Excludes1: *inconclusive mammogram (R92.2)*

AHA CC: 1Q, 2015, 24

Z12.39 Encounter for other screening for malignant neoplasm of breast

♀ **Z12.4 Encounter for screening for malignant neoplasm of cervix**

Encounter for screening pap smear for malignant neoplasm of cervix

Excludes1: *when screening is part of general gynecological examination (Z01.4-)*

Excludes2: *encounter for screening for human papillomavirus (Z11.51)*

♂ **Z12.5 Encounter for screening for malignant neoplasm of prostate**

Z12.6 Encounter for screening for malignant neoplasm of bladder

+ **Z12.7 Encounter for screening for malignant neoplasm of other genitourinary organs**

♂ **Z12.71 Encounter for screening for malignant neoplasm of testis**

♀ **Z12.72 Encounter for screening for malignant neoplasm of vagina**

Vaginal pap smear status-post hysterectomy for non-malignant condition

Use additional code to identify acquired absence of uterus (Z90.71-)

Excludes1: *vaginal pap smear status-post hysterectomy for malignant conditions (Z08)*

♀ **Z12.73 Encounter for screening for malignant neoplasm of ovary**

Z12.79 Encounter for screening for malignant neoplasm of other genitourinary organs

+ **Z12.8 Encounter for screening for malignant neoplasm of other sites**

Z12.81 Encounter for screening for malignant neoplasm of oral cavity

Z12.82 Encounter for screening for malignant neoplasm of nervous system

Z12.83 Encounter for screening for malignant neoplasm of skin

Z12.89 Encounter for screening for malignant neoplasm of other sites

AHA CC: 1Q, 2021, 14-15

Z12.9 Encounter for screening for malignant neoplasm, site unspecified

Z13 Encounter for screening for other diseases and disorders

Screening is the testing for disease or disease precursors in asymptomatic individuals so that early detection and treatment can be provided for those who test positive for the disease.

Excludes1: *encounter for diagnostic examination-code to sign or symptom*

Review coding guideline C.21.c.5

Z13.0 Encounter for screening for diseases of the blood and blood-forming organs and certain disorders involving the immune mechanism

Z13.1 Encounter for screening for diabetes mellitus

+ **Z13.2 Encounter for screening for nutritional, metabolic and other endocrine disorders**

Z13.21 Encounter for screening for nutritional disorder

+ **Z13.22 Encounter for screening for metabolic disorder**

Z13.220 Encounter for screening for lipoid disorders

Encounter for screening for cholesterol level

Encounter for screening for hypercholesterolemia

Encounter for screening for hyperlipidemia

Z13.228 Encounter for screening for other metabolic disorders

Z13.29 Encounter for screening for other suspected endocrine disorder

Excludes2: *encounter for screening for diabetes mellitus (Z13.1)*

+ **Z13.3 Encounter for screening examination for mental health and behavioral disorders**

AHA CC: 4Q, 2018, 35-36

Z13.30 Encounter for screening examination for mental health and behavioral disorders, unspecified

Z13.31 Encounter for screening for depression

Encounter for screening for depression, adult

Encounter for screening for depression for child or adolescent

♀ **Z13.32 Encounter for screening for maternal depression**

Encounter for screening for perinatal depression

Z13.39 Encounter for screening examination for other mental health and behavioral disorders

Encounter for screening for alcoholism

Encounter for screening for intellectual disabilities

+ **Z13.4 Encounter for screening for certain developmental disorders in childhood**

Encounter for development testing of infant or child

Encounter for screening for developmental handicaps in early childhood

Excludes2: encounter for routine child health examination (Z00.12-)

AHA CC: 4Q, 2018, 36

Z13.40 Encounter for screening for unspecified developmental delays

Z13.41 Encounter for autism screening

Z13.42 Encounter for screening for global developmental delays (milestones)

Encounter for screening for developmental handicaps in early childhood

Z13.49 Encounter for screening for other developmental delays

Z13.5 Encounter for screening for eye and ear disorders

Excludes2: *encounter for general hearing examination (Z01.1-)*

encounter for general vision examination (Z01.0-)

AHA CC: 3Q, 2016, 17

Z13.6 Encounter for screening for cardiovascular disorders

+ **Z13.7 Encounter for screening for genetic and chromosomal anomalies**

Excludes1: *genetic testing for procreative management (Z31.4-)*

Z13.71 Encounter for nonprocreative screening for genetic disease carrier status

Z13.79 Encounter for other screening for genetic and chromosomal anomalies

+ **Z13.8 Encounter for screening for other specified diseases and disorders**

Excludes2: *screening for malignant neoplasms (Z12.-)*

+ **Z13.81 Encounter for screening for digestive system disorders**

Z13.810 Encounter for screening for upper gastrointestinal disorder

Z13.811 Encounter for screening for lower gastrointestinal disorder

Excludes1: *encounter for screening for intestinal infectious disease (Z11.0)*

Z13.818 Encounter for screening for other digestive system disorders

+ **Z13.82 Encounter for screening for musculoskeletal disorder**

Z13.820 Encounter for screening for osteoporosis

Z13.828 Encounter for screening for other musculoskeletal disorder

Z13.83 Encounter for screening for respiratory disorder NEC

Excludes1: *encounter for screening for respiratory tuberculosis (Z11.1)*

Z13.84 Encounter for screening for dental disorders

+ **Z13.85 Encounter for screening for nervous system disorders**

Z13.850 Encounter for screening for traumatic brain injury

Z13.858 Encounter for screening for other nervous system disorders

Z13.88 **Encounter for screening for disorder due to exposure to contaminants**
Excludes1: *those exposed to contaminants without suspected disorders (Z57.-, Z77.-)*
Z13.89 **Encounter for screening for other disorder**
Encounter for screening for genitourinary disorders
Z13.9 **Encounter for screening, unspecified**

Genetic carrier and genetic susceptibility to disease (Z14-Z15)

Z14 Genetic carrier
Review coding guideline C.21.c.3
\+ **Z14.0** **Hemophilia A carrier**
Z14.01 **Asymptomatic hemophilia A carrier**
Z14.02 **Symptomatic hemophilia A carrier**
Z14.1 **Cystic fibrosis carrier**
Z14.8 **Genetic carrier of other disease**

Z15 Genetic susceptibility to disease
Includes: confirmed abnormal gene
Use additional code, if applicable, for any associated family history of the disease (Z80-Z84)
Excludes1: *chromosomal anomalies (Q90-Q99)*
Review coding guideline C.21.c.3
\+ **Z15.0** **Genetic susceptibility to malignant neoplasm**
Code first , if applicable, any current malignant neoplasm (C00-C75, C81-C96)
Use additional code, if applicable, for any personal history of malignant neoplasm (Z85.-)
Z15.01 **Genetic susceptibility to malignant neoplasm of breast**
♀ **Z15.02** **Genetic susceptibility to malignant neoplasm of ovary**
♂ **Z15.03** **Genetic susceptibility to malignant neoplasm of prostate**
♀ **Z15.04** **Genetic susceptibility to malignant neoplasm of endometrium**
Z15.09 **Genetic susceptibility to other malignant neoplasm**
AHA CC: 1Q, 2021, 14-15
\+ **Z15.8** **Genetic susceptibility to other disease**
Z15.81 **Genetic susceptibility to multiple endocrine neoplasia [MEN]**
Excludes1: *multiple endocrine neoplasia [MEN] syndromes (E31.2-)*
Z15.89 **Genetic susceptibility to other disease**

Resistance to antimicrobial drugs (Z16)

Z16 Resistance to antimicrobial drugs
NOTE The codes in this category are provided for use as additional codes to identify the resistance and non-responsiveness of a condition to antimicrobial drugs.
Code first the infection
Excludes1: *Methicillin resistant Staphylococcus aureus infection (A49.02)*
Methicillin resistant Staphylococcus aureus pneumonia (J15.212)
Sepsis due to Methicillin resistant Staphylococcus aureus (A41.02)
Review coding guideline C.1.c
Review coding guideline C.21.c.3
\+ **Z16.1** **Resistance to beta lactam antibiotics**
CC **Z16.10** **Resistance to unspecified beta lactam antibiotics**
CC **Z16.11** **Resistance to penicillins**
Resistance to amoxicillin
Resistance to ampicillin
Review coding guidelines C.1.e.1.a and C.1.e.1.b
CC **Z16.12** **Extended spectrum beta lactamase (ESBL) resistance**
Excludes2: *Methicillin resistant Staphylococcus aureus infection in diseases classified elsewhere (B95.62)*
CC **Z16.19** **Resistance to other specified beta lactam antibiotics**
Resistance to cephalosporins

\+ **Z16.2** **Resistance to other antibiotics**
CC **Z16.20** **Resistance to unspecified antibiotic**
Resistance to antibiotics NOS
CC **Z16.21** **Resistance to vancomycin**
CC **Z16.22** **Resistance to vancomycin related antibiotics**
CC **Z16.23** **Resistance to quinolones and fluoroquinolones**
CC **Z16.24** **Resistance to multiple antibiotics**
CC **Z16.29** **Resistance to other single specified antibiotic**
Resistance to aminoglycosides
Resistance to macrolides
Resistance to sulfonamides
Resistance to tetracyclines
\+ **Z16.3** **Resistance to other antimicrobial drugs**
Excludes1: *resistance to antibiotics (Z16.1-, Z16.2-)*
CC **Z16.30** **Resistance to unspecified antimicrobial drugs**
Drug resistance NOS
CC **Z16.31** **Resistance to antiparasitic drug(s)**
Resistance to quinine and related compounds
CC **Z16.32** **Resistance to antifungal drug(s)**
CC **Z16.33** **Resistance to antiviral drug(s)**
\+ **Z16.34** **Resistance to antimycobacterial drug(s)**
Resistance to tuberculostatics
CC **Z16.341** **Resistance to single antimycobacterial drug**
Resistance to antimycobacterial drug NOS
CC **Z16.342** **Resistance to multiple antimycobacterial drugs**
CC **Z16.35** **Resistance to multiple antimicrobial drugs**
Excludes1: *Resistance to multiple antibiotics only (Z16.24)*
CC **Z16.39** **Resistance to other specified antimicrobial drug**

Estrogen receptor status (Z17)

Z17 Estrogen receptor status
Code first malignant neoplasm of breast (C50.-)
Review coding guideline C.21.c.3
Z17.0 **Estrogen receptor positive status [ER+]**
Z17.1 **Estrogen receptor negative status [ER-]**

Retained foreign body fragments (Z18)

Z18 Retained foreign body fragments
Includes: embedded fragment (status)
embedded splinter (status)
retained foreign body status
Excludes1: *artificial joint prosthesis status (Z96.6-)*
foreign body accidentally left during a procedure (T81.5-)
foreign body entering through orifice (T15-T19)
in situ cardiac device (Z95.-)
organ or tissue replaced by means other than transplant (Z96.-, Z97.-)
organ or tissue replaced by transplant (Z94.-)
personal history of retained foreign body fully removed (Z87.821)
superficial foreign body (non-embedded splinter) - code to superficial foreign body, by site
Review coding guideline C.21.c.3
\+ **Z18.0** **Retained radioactive fragments**
Z18.01 **Retained depleted uranium fragments**
Z18.09 **Other retained radioactive fragments**
Other retained depleted isotope fragments
Retained nontherapeutic radioactive fragments
\+ **Z18.1** **Retained metal fragments**
Excludes1: *retained radioactive metal fragments (Z18.01-Z18.09)*
Z18.10 **Retained metal fragments, unspecified**
Retained metal fragment NOS
Z18.11 **Retained magnetic metal fragments**
Z18.12 **Retained nonmagnetic metal fragments**
Z18.2 **Retained plastic fragments**
Acrylics fragments
Diethylhexyl phthalates fragments
Isocyanate fragments
\+ **Z18.3** **Retained organic fragments**
Z18.31 **Retained animal quills or spines**
Z18.32 **Retained tooth**
Z18.33 **Retained wood fragments**
Z18.39 **Other retained organic fragments**

+ Z18.8 **Other specified retained foreign body**

Z18.81 Retained glass fragments

Z18.83 Retained stone or crystalline fragments

Retained concrete or cement fragments

Z18.89 Other specified retained foreign body fragments

AHA CC: 3Q, 2016, 24

Z18.9 Retained foreign body fragments, unspecified material

Hormone sensitivity malignancy status (Z19)

Z19 **Hormone sensitivity malignancy status**

Code first malignant neoplasm - see Table of Neoplasms, by site, malignant

Review coding guideline C.21.c.3

AHA CC: 4Q, 2016, 76

Z19.1 Hormone sensitive malignancy status

Z19.2 Hormone resistant malignancy status

Castrate resistant prostate malignancy status

Persons with potential health hazards related to communicable diseases (Z20-Z29)

Z20 **Contact with and (suspected) exposure to communicable diseases**

Excludes1: *carrier of infectious disease (Z22.-)*
diagnosed current infectious or parasitic disease -see Alphabetic Index

Excludes2: *personal history of infectious and parasitic diseases (Z86.1-)*

Review coding guideline C.21.c.1

+ Z20.0 **Contact with and (suspected) exposure to intestinal infectious diseases**

Z20.01 Contact with and (suspected) exposure to intestinal infectious diseases due to Escherichia coli (E. coli)

Z20.09 Contact with and (suspected) exposure to other intestinal infectious diseases

Z20.1 Contact with and (suspected) exposure to tuberculosis

Z20.2 Contact with and (suspected) exposure to infections with a predominantly sexual mode of transmission

Z20.3 Contact with and (suspected) exposure to rabies

Z20.4 Contact with and (suspected) exposure to rubella

Z20.5 Contact with and (suspected) exposure to viral hepatitis

Z20.6 Contact with and (suspected) exposure to human immunodeficiency virus [HIV]

Excludes1: *asymptomatic human immunodeficiency virus [HIV]*
HIV infection status (Z21)

Z20.7 Contact with and (suspected) exposure to pediculosis, acariasis and other infestations

+ Z20.8 **Contact with and (suspected) exposure to other communicable diseases**

+ Z20.81 **Contact with and (suspected) exposure to other bacterial communicable diseases**

Z20.810 Contact with and (suspected) exposure to anthrax

Z20.811 Contact with and (suspected) exposure to meningococcus

Z20.818 Contact with and (suspected) exposure to other bacterial communicable diseases

AHA CC: 2Q, 2019, 10-11

+ Z20.82 **Contact with and (suspected) exposure to other viral communicable diseases**

AHA CC: 4Q, 2018, 35

Z20.820 Contact with and (suspected) exposure to varicella

Z20.821 Contact with and (suspected) exposure to Zika virus

Review coding guideline C.1.f

Z20.822 Contact with and (suspected) exposure to COVID-19

Contact with and (suspected) exposure to SARS-CoV-2

AHA CC: 1Q, 2021, 37-39, 41-42

Z20.828 Contact with and (suspected) exposure to other viral communicable diseases

AHA CC: 4Q, 2016, 4-7; 1Q, 2020, 34-36; 2Q, 2020, 4-5, 8-9; 3Q, 2020, 14-16; 1Q, 2021, 37-39

Review coding guidelines C.1.g.1.e and C.1.g.1.g

Z20.89 Contact with and (suspected) exposure to other communicable diseases

Z20.9 Contact with and (suspected) exposure to unspecified communicable disease

Z21 Asymptomatic human immunodeficiency virus [HIV] infection status

HIV positive NOS

Code first Human immunodeficiency virus [HIV] disease complicating pregnancy, childbirth and the puerperium, if applicable (O98.7-)

Excludes1: *acquired immunodeficiency syndrome (B20)*
contact with human immunodeficiency virus [HIV] (Z20.6)
exposure to human immunodeficiency virus [HIV] (Z20.6)
human immunodeficiency virus [HIV] disease (B20)
inconclusive laboratory evidence of human immunodeficiency virus [HIV] (R75)

Review coding guidelines C.1.a.2.d, C.1.a.2.f and C.1.a.2.g

Review coding guideline C.15.f

Review coding guideline C.21.c.3

AHA CC: 1Q, 2019, 10-11

Valid 3-character code, no further characters required

Z22 **Carrier of infectious disease**

Includes: colonization status
suspected carrier

Excludes2: *carrier of viral hepatitis (B18.-)*

Review coding guideline C.21.c.3

Z22.0 Carrier of typhoid

Z22.1 Carrier of other intestinal infectious diseases

Z22.2 Carrier of diphtheria

+ Z22.3 **Carrier of other specified bacterial diseases**

Z22.31 Carrier of bacterial disease due to meningococci

+ Z22.32 **Carrier of bacterial disease due to staphylococci**

Z22.321 Carrier or suspected carrier of Methicillin susceptible Staphylococcus aureus

MSSA colonization

Review coding guidelines C.1.e.1.c and C.1.e.1.d

Z22.322 Carrier or suspected carrier of Methicillin resistant Staphylococcus aureus

MRSA colonization

Review coding guidelines C.1.e.1.c and C.1.e.1.d

+ Z22.33 **Carrier of bacterial disease due to streptococci**

Z22.330 Carrier of Group B streptococcus

Excludes1: *carrier of streptococcus group B (GBS) complicating pregnancy, childbirth and the puerperium (O99.82-)*

Z22.338 Carrier of other streptococcus

Z22.39 Carrier of other specified bacterial diseases

Z22.4 Carrier of infections with a predominantly sexual mode of transmission

Z22.6 Carrier of human T-lymphotropic virus type-1 [HTLV-1] infection

Z22.7 Latent tuberculosis

Latent tuberculosis infection (LTBI)

Excludes1: *nonspecific reaction to cell mediated immunity measurement of gamma interferon antigen response without active tuberculosis (R76.12)*
nonspecific reaction to tuberculin skin test without active tuberculosis (R76.11)

AHA CC: 4Q, 2019, 19

Z22.8 Carrier of other infectious diseases

Z22.9 Carrier of infectious disease, unspecified

Z23 Encounter for immunization

Code also, if applicable, encounter for immunization safety counseling (Z71.85)

Code first any routine childhood examination

NOTE Procedure codes are required to identify the types of immunizations given

Review coding guideline C.21.c.2

Valid 3-character code, no further characters required

Z28 Immunization not carried out and underimmunization status

Includes: vaccination not carried out

Code also, if applicable, encounter for immunization safety counseling (Z71.85)

+ **Z28.0 Immunization not carried out because of contraindication**
  - **Z28.01 Immunization not carried out because of acute illness of patient**
  - **Z28.02 Immunization not carried out because of chronic illness or condition of patient**
  - **Z28.03 Immunization not carried out because of immune compromised state of patient**
  - **Z28.04 Immunization not carried out because of patient allergy to vaccine or component**
  - **Z28.09 Immunization not carried out because of other contraindication**

Z28.1 Immunization not carried out because of patient decision for reasons of belief or group pressure

Immunization not carried out because of religious belief

+ **Z28.2 Immunization not carried out because of patient decision for other and unspecified reason**
  - **Z28.20 Immunization not carried out because of patient decision for unspecified reason**
  - **Z28.21 Immunization not carried out because of patient refusal**
  - **Z28.29 Immunization not carried out because of patient decision for other reason**

Z28.3 Underimmunization status

Delinquent immunization status

Lapsed immunization schedule status

Review coding guideline C.21.c.3

+ **Z28.8 Immunization not carried out for other reason**
  - **Z28.81 Immunization not carried out due to patient having had the disease**
  - **Z28.82 Immunization not carried out because of caregiver refusal**

    Immunization not carried out because of guardian refusal

    Immunization not carried out because of parent refusal

    Excludes1: *immunization not carried out because of caregiver refusal because of religious belief (Z28.1)*
  - **Z28.83 Immunization not carried out due to unavailability of vaccine**

    Delay in delivery of vaccine

    Lack of availability of vaccine

    Manufacturer delay of vaccine

    AHA CC: 4Q, 2018, 36
  - **Z28.89 Immunization not carried out for other reason**

Z28.9 Immunization not carried out for unspecified reason

Z29 Encounter for other prophylactic measures

Excludes1: *desensitization to allergens (Z51.6)*
prophylactic surgery (Z40.-)

Review coding guideline C.21.c.14

AHA CC: 4Q, 2016, 78-79

+ **Z29.1 Encounter for prophylactic immunotherapy**

  Encounter for administration of immunoglobulin
  - **Z29.11 Encounter for prophylactic immunotherapy for respiratory syncytial virus (RSV)**
  - **Z29.12 Encounter for prophylactic antivenin**
  - **Z29.13 Encounter for prophylactic Rho(D) immune globulin**

    AHA CC: 3Q, 2019, 5
  - **Z29.14 Encounter for prophylactic rabies immune globin**

Z29.3 Encounter for prophylactic fluoride administration

Z29.8 Encounter for other specified prophylactic measures

Z29.9 Encounter for prophylactic measures, unspecified

Persons encountering health services in circumstances related to reproduction (Z30-Z39)

Z30 Encounter for contraceptive management

Review coding guideline C.21.c.11

AHA CC: 4Q, 2016, 78

+ **Z30.0 Encounter for general counseling and advice on contraception**

  Review coding guideline C.21.c.10

  + **Z30.01 Encounter for initial prescription of contraceptives**

    Excludes1: *encounter for surveillance of contraceptives (Z30.4-)*
    - ♀ **Z30.011 Encounter for initial prescription of contraceptive pills**
    - ♀ **Z30.012 Encounter for prescription of emergency contraception**

      Encounter for postcoital contraception
    - ♀ **Z30.013 Encounter for initial prescription of injectable contraceptive**
    - ♀ **Z30.014 Encounter for initial prescription of intrauterine contraceptive device**

      Excludes1: *encounter for insertion of intrauterinecontraceptive device (Z30.430, Z30.432)*
    - ♀ **Z30.015 Encounter for initial prescription of vaginal ring hormonal contraceptive**
    - **Z30.016 Encounter for initial prescription of transdermal patch hormonal contraceptive device**
    - **Z30.017 Encounter for initial prescription of implantable subdermal contraceptive**
    - ♀ **Z30.018 Encounter for initial prescription of other contraceptives**

      Encounter for initial prescription of barrier contraception

      Encounter for initial prescription of diaphragm
    - ♀ **Z30.019 Encounter for initial prescription of contraceptives, unspecified**

  Z30.02 Counseling and instruction in natural family planning to avoid pregnancy

  Z30.09 Encounter for other general counseling and advice on contraception

  Encounter for family planning advice NOS

Z30.2 Encounter for sterilization

+ **Z30.4 Encounter for surveillance of contraceptives**
  - **Z30.40 Encounter for surveillance of contraceptives, unspecified**
  - ♀ **Z30.41 Encounter for surveillance of contraceptive pills**

    Encounter for repeat prescription for contraceptive pill
  - ♀ **Z30.42 Encounter for surveillance of injectable contraceptive**
  - + **Z30.43 Encounter for surveillance of intrauterine contraceptive device**
    - ♀ **Z30.430 Encounter for insertion of intrauterine contraceptive device**
    - ♀ **Z30.431 Encounter for routine checking of intrauterine contraceptive device**
    - ♀ **Z30.432 Encounter for removal of intrauterine contraceptive device**
    - ♀ **Z30.433 Encounter for removal and reinsertion of intrauterine contraceptive device**

      Encounter for replacement of intrauterine contraceptive device
  - ♀ **Z30.44 Encounter for surveillance of vaginal ring hormonal contraceptive device**
  - ♀ **Z30.45 Encounter for surveillance of transdermal patch hormonal contraceptive device**
  - ♀ **Z30.46 Encounter for surveillance of implantable subdermal contraceptive**

    Encounter for checking, reinsertion or removal of implantable subdermal contraceptive
  - ♀ **Z30.49 Encounter for surveillance of other contraceptives**

    Encounter for surveillance of barrier contraception

    Encounter for surveillance of diaphragm

Z30.8 Encounter for other contraceptive management
Encounter for postvasectomy sperm count
Encounter for routine examination for contraceptive maintenance
Excludes1: *sperm count following sterilization reversal (Z31.42)*
sperm count for fertility testing (Z31.41)

Z30.9 Encounter for contraceptive management, unspecified

Z31 Encounter for procreative management
Excludes2: *complications associated with artificial fertilization (N98.-)*
female infertility (N97.-)
male infertility (N46.-)
Review coding guideline C.21.c.11

Z31.0 Encounter for reversal of previous sterilization

+ **Z31.4 Encounter for procreative investigation and testing**
Excludes1: *postvasectomy sperm count (Z30.8)*

Z31.41 Encounter for fertility testing
Encounter for fallopian tube patency testing
Encounter for sperm count for fertility testing

Z31.42 Aftercare following sterilization reversal
Sperm count following sterilization reversal

+ **Z31.43 Encounter for genetic testing of female for procreative management**
Use additional code for recurrent pregnancy loss, if applicable (N96, O26.2-)
Excludes1: *nonprocreative genetic testing (Z13.7-)*

♀ **Z31.430 Encounter of female for testing for genetic disease carrier status for procreative management**

♀ **Z31.438 Encounter for other genetic testing of female for procreative management**

+ **Z31.44 Encounter for genetic testing of male for procreative management**
Excludes1: *nonprocreative genetic testing (Z13.7-)*

♂ **Z31.440 Encounter of male for testing for genetic disease carrier status for procreative management**

● ♂ **Z31.441 Encounter for testing of male partner of patient with recurrent pregnancy loss**

● ♂ **Z31.448 Encounter for other genetic testing of male for procreative management**

Z31.49 Encounter for other procreative investigation and testing

Z31.5 Encounter for procreative genetic counseling
AHA CC: 4Q, 2017, 27
Review coding guideline C.21.c.10

+ **Z31.6 Encounter for general counseling and advice on procreation**
Review coding guideline C.21.c.10

Z31.61 Procreative counseling and advice using natural family planning

Z31.62 Encounter for fertility preservation counseling
Encounter for fertility preservation counseling prior to cancer therapy
Encounter for fertility preservation counseling prior to surgical removal of gonads

Z31.69 Encounter for other general counseling and advice on procreation

♀ **Z31.7 Encounter for procreative management and counseling for gestational carrier**
Excludes1: *pregnant state, gestational carrier (Z33.3)*
AHA CC: 4Q, 2016, 78

+ **Z31.8 Encounter for other procreative management**

♀ **Z31.81 Encounter for male factor infertility in female patient**
Review coding guideline C.21.c.16

♀ **Z31.82 Encounter for Rh incompatibility status**
Review coding guideline C.21.c.16
AHA CC: 4Q, 2014, 17

♀ **Z31.83 Encounter for assisted reproductive fertility procedure cycle**
Patient undergoing in vitro fertilization cycle
Use additional code to identify the type of infertility
Excludes1: *pre-cycle diagnosis and testing - code to reason for encounter*
Review coding guideline C.21.c.16

Z31.84 Encounter for fertility preservation procedure
Encounter for fertility preservation procedure prior to cancer therapy
Encounter for fertility preservation procedure prior to surgical removal of gonads
Review coding guideline C.21.c.16

Z31.89 Encounter for other procreative management

Z31.9 Encounter for procreative management, unspecified

Z32 Encounter for pregnancy test and childbirth and childcare instruction

+ **Z32.0 Encounter for pregnancy test**
Review coding guideline C.21.c.13

♀ **Z32.00 Encounter for pregnancy test, result unknown**
Encounter for pregnancy test NOS

● ♀ **Z32.01 Encounter for pregnancy test, result positive**

♀ **Z32.02 Encounter for pregnancy test, result negative**

Z32.2 Encounter for childbirth instruction
Review coding guidelines C.21.c.10 and C.21.c.11

Z32.3 Encounter for childcare instruction
Encounter for prenatal or postpartum childcare instruction
Review coding guidelines C.21.c.10 and C.21.c.11

Z33 Pregnant state
Review coding guideline C.21.c.11
AHA CC: 4Q, 2016, 78

● ♀ **Z33.1 Pregnant state, incidental**
Pregnancy NOS
Pregnant state NOS
Excludes1: *complications of pregnancy (O00-O9A)*
pregnant state, gestational carrier (Z33.3)
Review coding guideline C.15.a.1
Review coding guidelines C.21.c.3

● ♀ **Z33.2 Encounter for elective termination of pregnancy**
Excludes1: *early fetal death with retention of dead fetus (O02.1)*
late fetal death (O36.4)
spontaneous abortion (O03)
Review coding guidelines C.15.q.1 and C.15.q.2
Review coding guidelines C.21.c.16

● ♀ **Z33.3 Pregnant state, gestational carrier**
Excludes1: *encounter for procreative management and counseling for gestational carrier (Z31.7)*

Z34 Encounter for supervision of normal pregnancy
Excludes1: *any complication of pregnancy (O00-O9A)*
encounter for pregnancy test (Z32.0-)
encounter for supervision of high risk pregnancy (O09.-)
Review coding guideline C.15.b.1
Review coding guidelines C.21.c.11 and C.21.c.16
AHA CC: 4Q, 2016, 4-7

+ **Z34.0 Encounter for supervision of normal first pregnancy**

● ♀ **Z34.00 Encounter for supervision of normal first pregnancy, unspecified trimester**

● ♀ **Z34.01 Encounter for supervision of normal first pregnancy, first trimester**

● ♀ **Z34.02 Encounter for supervision of normal first pregnancy, second trimester**

● ♀ **Z34.03 Encounter for supervision of normal first pregnancy, third trimester**

+ **Z34.8 Encounter for supervision of other normal pregnancy**

● ♀ **Z34.80 Encounter for supervision of other normal pregnancy, unspecified trimester**

● ♀ **Z34.81 Encounter for supervision of other normal pregnancy, first trimester**

● ♀ **Z34.82 Encounter for supervision of other normal pregnancy, second trimester**

● ♀ **Z34.83 Encounter for supervision of other normal pregnancy, third trimester**
AHA CC: 4Q, 2014, 17

+ **Z34.9 Encounter for supervision of normal pregnancy, unspecified**

● ♀ **Z34.90 Encounter for supervision of normal pregnancy, unspecified, unspecified trimester**

● ♀ **Z34.91 Encounter for supervision of normal pregnancy, unspecified, first trimester**

● ♀ **Z34.92 Encounter for supervision of normal pregnancy, unspecified, second trimester**

● ♀ **Z34.93 Encounter for supervision of normal pregnancy, unspecified, third trimester**

Z36 Encounter for antenatal screening of mother

Includes: Encounter for placental sample (taken vaginally)
Screening is the testing for disease or disease precursors in asymptomatic individuals so that early detection and treatment can be provided for those who test positive for the disease.

Excludes1: *diagnostic examination- code to sign or symptom*
encounter for suspected maternal and fetal conditions ruled out (Z03.7-)
suspected fetal condition affecting management of pregnancy - code to condition in Chapter 15

Excludes2: *abnormal findings on antenatal screening of mother (O28.-)*
genetic counseling and testing (Z31.43-, Z31.5)
routine prenatal care (Z34)

AHA CC: 4Q, 2017, 28

Review coding guidelines C.21.c.5 and C.21.c.11

- ● ♀ **Z36.0 Encounter for antenatal screening for chromosomal anomalies**
- ● ♀ **Z36.1 Encounter for antenatal screening for raised alphafetoprotein level**
  Encounter for antenatal screening for elevated maternal serum alphafetoprotein level
- ● ♀ **Z36.2 Encounter for other antenatal screening follow-up**
  Non-visualized anatomy on a previous scan
- ● ♀ **Z36.3 Encounter for antenatal screening for malformations**
  Screening for suspected anomaly
- ● ♀ **Z36.4 Encounter for antenatal screening for fetal growth retardation**
  Intrauterine growth restriction (IUGR)/small-for-dates
- ● ♀ **Z36.5 Encounter for antenatal screening for isoimmunization**
- \+ **Z36.8 Encounter for other antenatal screening**
  - ● ♀ **Z36.81 Encounter for antenatal screening for hydrops fetalis**
  - ● ♀ **Z36.82 Encounter for antenatal screening fornuchal translucency**
  - ● ♀ **Z36.83 Encounter for antenatal screening for congenital cardiac abnormalities**
  - ● ♀ **Z36.84 Encounter for antenatal screening for fetal lung maturity**
  - ● ♀ **Z36.85 Encounter for antenatal screening for Streptococcus B**
  - ● ♀ **Z36.86 Encounter for antenatal screening for for cervical length**
    Screening for risk of pre-term labor
  - ● ♀ **Z36.87 Encounter for antenatal screening for uncertain dates**
  - ● ♀ **Z36.88 Encounter for antenatal screening for fetal macrosomia**
    Screening for large-for-dates
  - ● ♀ **Z36.89 Encounter for other specified antenatal screening**
  - ● ♀ **Z36.8A Encounter for antenatal screening for other genetic defects**
- ● ♀ **Z36.9 Encounter for antenatal screening, unspecified**

Z3A Weeks of gestation

NOTE Codes from category Z3A are for use, only on the maternal record, to indicate the weeks of gestation of the pregnancy, if known.

Code first obstetric condition or encounter for delivery (O09-O60, O80-O82)

Review coding guideline C.21.c.11

- \+ **Z3A.0 Weeks of gestation of pregnancy, unspecified or less than 10 weeks**
  - ● ♀ **Z3A.00 Weeks of gestation of pregnancy not specified**
  - ● ♀ **Z3A.01 Less than 8 weeks gestation of pregnancy**
  - ● ♀ **Z3A.08 8 weeks gestation of pregnancy**
  - ● ♀ **Z3A.09 9 weeks gestation of pregnancy**
- \+ **Z3A.1 Weeks of gestation of pregnancy, weeks 10-19**
  - ● ♀ **Z3A.10 10 weeks gestation of pregnancy**
  - ● ♀ **Z3A.11 11 weeks gestation of pregnancy**
  - ● ♀ **Z3A.12 12 weeks gestation of pregnancy**
  - ● ♀ **Z3A.13 13 weeks gestation of pregnancy**
  - ● ♀ **Z3A.14 14 weeks gestation of pregnancy**
  - ● ♀ **Z3A.15 15 weeks gestation of pregnancy**
  - ● ♀ **Z3A.16 16 weeks gestation of pregnancy**
    AHA CC: 4Q, 2016, 4-7
  - ● ♀ **Z3A.17 17 weeks gestation of pregnancy**
  - ● ♀ **Z3A.18 18 weeks gestation of pregnancy**
    AHA CC: 2Q, 2019, 11
  - ● ♀ **Z3A.19 19 weeks gestation of pregnancy**
- \+ **Z3A.2 Weeks of gestation of pregnancy, weeks 20-29**
  - ● ♀ **Z3A.20 20 weeks gestation of pregnancy**
    AHA CC: 4Q, 2016, 4-7
  - ● ♀ **Z3A.21 21 weeks gestation of pregnancy**
  - ● ♀ **Z3A.22 22 weeks gestation of pregnancy**
    AHA CC: 4Q, 2016, 4-7
  - ● ♀ **Z3A.23 23 weeks gestation of pregnancy**
  - ● ♀ **Z3A.24 24 weeks gestation of pregnancy**
  - ● ♀ **Z3A.25 25 weeks gestation of pregnancy**
  - ● ♀ **Z3A.26 26 weeks gestation of pregnancy**
  - ● ♀ **Z3A.27 27 weeks gestation of pregnancy**
  - ● ♀ **Z3A.28 28 weeks gestation of pregnancy**
  - ● ♀ **Z3A.29 29 weeks gestation of pregnancy**
- \+ **Z3A.3 Weeks of gestation of pregnancy, weeks 30-39**
  - ● ♀ **Z3A.30 30 weeks gestation of pregnancy**
  - ● ♀ **Z3A.31 31 weeks gestation of pregnancy**
  - ● ♀ **Z3A.32 32 weeks gestation of pregnancy**
    AHA CC: 4Q, 2016, 4-7
  - ● ♀ **Z3A.33 33 weeks gestation of pregnancy**
  - ● ♀ **Z3A.34 34 weeks gestation of pregnancy**
  - ● ♀ **Z3A.35 35 weeks gestation of pregnancy**
  - ● ♀ **Z3A.36 36 weeks gestation of pregnancy**
  - ● ♀ **Z3A.37 37 weeks gestation of pregnancy**
  - ● ♀ **Z3A.38 38 weeks gestation of pregnancy**
    AHA CC: 2Q, 2016, 34
  - ● ♀ **Z3A.39 39 weeks gestation of pregnancy**
- \+ **Z3A.4 Weeks of gestation of pregnancy, weeks 40 or greater**
  - ● ♀ **Z3A.40 40 weeks gestation of pregnancy**
    AHA CC: 2Q, 2014, 9
  - ● ♀ **Z3A.41 41 weeks gestation of pregnancy**
  - ● ♀ **Z3A.42 42 weeks gestation of pregnancy**
    AHA CC: 4Q, 2014, 23
  - ● ♀ **Z3A.49 Greater than 42 weeks gestation of pregnancy**

Z37 Outcome of delivery

This category is intended for use as an additional code to identify the outcome of delivery on the mother's record. It is not for use on the newborn record.

Excludes1: *stillbirth (P95)*

Review coding guidelines C.15.b.5
Review coding guidelines C.15.n.3 and C.15.q.1
Review coding guidelines C.21.c.11

- ● ♀ **Z37.0 Single live birth**
  AHA CC: 2Q, 2014, 9; 4Q, 2014, 17-18; 2Q, 2016, 34
- ● ♀ **Z37.1 Single stillbirth**
- ● ♀ **Z37.2 Twins, both liveborn**
- ● ♀ **Z37.3 Twins, one liveborn and one stillborn**
- ● ♀ **Z37.4 Twins, both stillborn**
- \+ **Z37.5 Other multiple births, all liveborn**
  - ● ♀ **Z37.50 Multiple births, unspecified, all liveborn**
  - ● ♀ **Z37.51 Triplets, all liveborn**
  - ● ♀ **Z37.52 Quadruplets, all liveborn**
  - ● ♀ **Z37.53 Quintuplets, all liveborn**
  - ● ♀ **Z37.54 Sextuplets, all liveborn**
  - ● ♀ **Z37.59 Other multiple births, all liveborn**
- \+ **Z37.6 Other multiple births, some liveborn**
  - ● ♀ **Z37.60 Multiple births, unspecified, some liveborn**
  - ● ♀ **Z37.61 Triplets, some liveborn**
  - ● ♀ **Z37.62 Quadruplets, some liveborn**
  - ● ♀ **Z37.63 Quintuplets, some liveborn**
  - ● ♀ **Z37.64 Sextuplets, some liveborn**
  - ● ♀ **Z37.69 Other multiple births, some liveborn**
- ● ♀ **Z37.7 Other multiple births, all stillborn**
- ● ♀ **Z37.9 Outcome of delivery, unspecified**
  Multiple birth NOS
  Single birth NOS

Z38 Liveborn infants according to place of birth and type of delivery

This category is for use as the principal code on the initial record of a newborn baby. It is to be used for the initial birth record only. It is not to be used on the mother's record.

Review coding guideline C.16.a.2 and C.16.h
Review coding guideline C.17
Review coding guidelines C.21.c.6, C.21.c.12 and C.21.c.16
AHA CC: 2Q, 2015, 15; 4Q, 2016, 4-7, 54-55; 2Q, 2020, 13

\+ **Z38.0 Single liveborn infant, born in hospital**
Single liveborn infant, born in birthing center or other health care facility
AHA CC: 2Q, 2017, 5-7
- • **Z38.00 Single liveborn infant, delivered vaginally**
AHA CC: 4Q, 2018, 26; 4Q, 2020, 38
- • **Z38.01 Single liveborn infant, delivered by cesarean**
AHA CC: 3Q, 2016, 18

• **Z38.1 Single liveborn infant, born outside hospital**
• **Z38.2 Single liveborn infant, unspecified as to place of birth**
Single liveborn infant NOS
\+ **Z38.3 Twin liveborn infant, born in hospital**
- • **Z38.30 Twin liveborn infant, delivered vaginally**
- • **Z38.31 Twin liveborn infant, delivered by cesarean**

• **Z38.4 Twin liveborn infant, born outside hospital**
• **Z38.5 Twin liveborn infant, unspecified as to place of birth**
\+ **Z38.6 Other multiple liveborn infant, born in hospital**
- • **Z38.61 Triplet liveborn infant, delivered vaginally**
- • **Z38.62 Triplet liveborn infant, delivered by cesarean**
- • **Z38.63 Quadruplet liveborn infant, delivered vaginally**
- • **Z38.64 Quadruplet liveborn infant, delivered by cesarean**
- • **Z38.65 Quintuplet liveborn infant, delivered vaginally**
- • **Z38.66 Quintuplet liveborn infant, delivered by cesarean**
- • **Z38.68 Other multiple liveborn infant, delivered vaginally**
- • **Z38.69 Other multiple liveborn infant, delivered by cesarean**

• **Z38.7 Other multiple liveborn infant, born outside hospital**
• **Z38.8 Other multiple liveborn infant, unspecified as to place of birth**

Z39 Encounter for maternal postpartum care and examination

Review coding guidelines C.21.c.8, C.21.c.11 and C.21.c.16

• ♀ **Z39.0 Encounter for care and examination of mother immediately after delivery**
Care and observation in uncomplicated cases when the delivery occurs outside a healthcare facility
Excludes1: *care for postpartum complication- see Alphabetic index*
Review coding guideline C.15.o.4

• ♀ **Z39.1 Encounter for care and examination of lactating mother**
Encounter for supervision of lactation
Excludes1: *disorders of lactation (O92.-)*

• ♀ **Z39.2 Encounter for routine postpartum follow-up**

Encounters for other specific health care (Z40-Z53)

Categories Z40-Z53 are intended for use to indicate a reason for care. They may be used for patients who have already been treated for a disease or injury, but who are receiving aftercare or prophylactic care, or care to consolidate the treatment, or to deal with a residual state

Excludes2: *follow-up examination for medical surveillance after treatment (Z08-Z09)*

Z40 Encounter for prophylactic surgery

Excludes1: *organ donations (Z52.-)*
therapeutic organ removal-code to condition
Review coding guideline C.21.c.14 and C21.c.16

\+ **Z40.0 Encounter for prophylactic surgery for risk factors related to malignant neoplasms**
Admission for prophylactic organ removal
Use additional code to identify risk factor
- **Z40.00 Encounter for prophylactic removal of unspecified organ**
- **Z40.01 Encounter for prophylactic removal of breast**
- ♀ **Z40.02 Encounter for prophylactic removal of ovary(s)**
Encounter for prophylactic removal of ovary(s) and fallopian tube(s)
- ♀ **Z40.03 Encounter for prophylactic removal of fallopian tube(s)**
AHA CC: 4Q, 2017, 28
- **Z40.09 Encounter for prophylactic removal of other organ**

Z40.8 Encounter for other prophylactic surgery
Z40.9 Encounter for prophylactic surgery, unspecified

Z41 Encounter for procedures for purposes other than remedying health state

Z41.1 Encounter for cosmetic surgery
Encounter for cosmetic breast implant
Encounter for cosmetic procedure
Excludes1: *encounter for plastic and reconstructive surgery following medical procedure or healed injury (Z42.-)*
encounter for post-mastectomy breast implantation (Z42.1)

♂ **Z41.2 Encounter for routine and ritual male circumcision**
AHA CC: 3Q, 2018, 15

Z41.3 Encounter for ear piercing
Z41.8 Encounter for other procedures for purposes other than remedying health state
Z41.9 Encounter for procedure for purposes other than remedying health state, unspecified

Z42 Encounter for plastic and reconstructive surgery following medical procedure or healed injury

Excludes1: *encounter for cosmetic plastic surgery (Z41.1)*
encounter for plastic surgery for treatment of current injury - code to relevent injury
Review coding guidelines C.21.c.7 and C.21.c.16

• **Z42.1 Encounter for breast reconstruction following mastectomy**
Excludes1: *deformity and disproportion of reconstructed breast (N65.1-)*

Z42.8 Encounter for other plastic and reconstructive surgery following medical procedure or healed injury
AHA CC: 1Q, 2017, 42-43

Z43 Encounter for attention to artificial openings

Includes: closure of artificial openings
passage of sounds or bougies through artificial openings
reforming artificial openings
removal of catheter from artificial openings
toilet or cleansing of artificial openings
Excludes1: *complications of external stoma (J95.0-, K94.-, N99.5-)*
Excludes2: *fitting and adjustment of prosthetic and other devices (Z44-Z46)*
Review coding guideline C.21.c.7

Z43.0 Encounter for attention to tracheostomy
CC **Z43.1 Encounter for attention to gastrostomy**
Excludes2: *artificial opening status only, without need for care (Z93.-)*
Z43.2 Encounter for attention to ileostomy
AHA CC: 3Q, 2016, 5
Z43.3 Encounter for attention to colostomy
Z43.4 Encounter for attention to other artificial openings of digestive tract
Z43.5 Encounter for attention to cystostomy
Z43.6 Encounter for attention to other artificial openings of urinary tract
Encounter for attention to nephrostomy
Encounter for attention to ureterostomy
Encounter for attention to urethrostomy
Z43.7 Encounter for attention to artificial vagina
Z43.8 Encounter for attention to other artificial openings
Z43.9 Encounter for attention to unspecified artificial opening

Z44 Encounter for fitting and adjustment of external prosthetic device

Includes: removal or replacement of external prosthetic device

Excludes1: *malfunction or other complications of device - see Alphabetical Index*

presence of prosthetic device (Z97.-)

Review coding guideline C.21.c.7

\+ **Z44.0 Encounter for fitting and adjustment of artificial arm**

\+ **Z44.00 Encounter for fitting and adjustment of unspecified artificial arm**

Z44.001 Encounter for fitting and adjustment of unspecified right artificial arm

Z44.002 Encounter for fitting and adjustment of unspecified left artificial arm

Z44.009 Encounter for fitting and adjustment of unspecified artificial arm, unspecified arm

\+ **Z44.01 Encounter for fitting and adjustment of complete artificial arm**

Z44.011 Encounter for fitting and adjustment of complete right artificial arm

Z44.012 Encounter for fitting and adjustment of complete left artificial arm

Z44.019 Encounter for fitting and adjustment of complete artificial arm, unspecified arm

\+ **Z44.02 Encounter for fitting and adjustment of partial artificial arm**

Z44.021 Encounter for fitting and adjustment of partial artificial right arm

Z44.022 Encounter for fitting and adjustment of partial artificial left arm

Z44.029 Encounter for fitting and adjustment of partial artificial arm, unspecified arm

\+ **Z44.1 Encounter for fitting and adjustment of artificial leg**

\+ **Z44.10 Encounter for fitting and adjustment of unspecified artificial leg**

Z44.101 Encounter for fitting and adjustment of unspecified right artificial leg

Z44.102 Encounter for fitting and adjustment of unspecified left artificial leg

Z44.109 Encounter for fitting and adjustment of unspecified artificial leg, unspecified leg

\+ **Z44.11 Encounter for fitting and adjustment of complete artificial leg**

Z44.111 Encounter for fitting and adjustment of complete right artificial leg

Z44.112 Encounter for fitting and adjustment of complete left artificial leg

Z44.119 Encounter for fitting and adjustment of complete artificial leg, unspecified leg

\+ **Z44.12 Encounter for fitting and adjustment of partial artificial leg**

Z44.121 Encounter for fitting and adjustment of partial artificial right leg

Z44.122 Encounter for fitting and adjustment of partial artificial left leg

Z44.129 Encounter for fitting and adjustment of partial artificial leg, unspecified leg

\+ **Z44.2 Encounter for fitting and adjustment of artificial eye**

Excludes1: *mechanical complication of ocular prosthesis (T85.3)*

Z44.20 Encounter for fitting and adjustment of artificial eye, unspecified

Z44.21 Encounter for fitting and adjustment of artificial right eye

Z44.22 Encounter for fitting and adjustment of artificial left eye

\+ **Z44.3 Encounter for fitting and adjustment of external breast prosthesis**

Excludes1: *complications of breast implant (T85.4-)*

encounter for adjustment or removal of breast implant (Z45.81-)

encounter for initial breast implant insertion for cosmetic breast augmentation (Z41.1)

encounter for breast reconstruction following mastectomy (Z42.1)

Z44.30 Encounter for fitting and adjustment of external breast prosthesis, unspecified breast

Z44.31 Encounter for fitting and adjustment of external right breast prosthesis

Z44.32 Encounter for fitting and adjustment of external left breast prosthesis

Z44.8 Encounter for fitting and adjustment of other external prosthetic devices

Z44.9 Encounter for fitting and adjustment of unspecified external prosthetic device

Z45 Encounter for adjustment and management of implanted device

Includes: removal or replacement of implanted device

Excludes1: *malfunction or other complications of device - see Alphabetical Index*

Excludes2: *encounter for fitting and adjustment of non-implanted device (Z46.-)*

Review coding guideline C.21.c.7

\+ **Z45.0 Encounter for adjustment and management of cardiac device**

\+ **Z45.01 Encounter for adjustment and management of cardiac pacemaker**

Encounter for adjustment and management of cardiac resynchronization therapy pacemaker (CRT-P)

Excludes1: *encounter for adjustment and management of automatic implantable cardiac defibrillator with synchronous cardiac pacemaker (Z45.02)*

Z45.010 Encounter for checking and testing of cardiac pacemaker pulse generator [battery]

Encounter for replacing cardiac pacemaker pulse generator [battery]

Z45.018 Encounter for adjustment and management of other part of cardiac pacemaker

Excludes1: *presence of other part of cardiac pacemaker (Z95.0)*

Excludes2: *presence of prosthetic and other devices (Z95.1-Z95.5, Z95.811-Z97)*

Z45.02 Encounter for adjustment and management of automatic implantable cardiac defibrillator

Encounter for adjustment and management of automatic implantable cardiac defibrillator with synchronous cardiac pacemaker

Encounter for adjustment and management of cardiac resynchronization therapy defibrillator (CRT-D)

Z45.09 Encounter for adjustment and management of other cardiac device

Z45.1 Encounter for adjustment and management of infusion pump

Z45.2 Encounter for adjustment and management of vascular access device

Encounter for adjustment and management of vascular catheters

Excludes1: *encounter for adjustment and management of renal dialysis catheter (Z49.01)*

AHA CC: 3Q, 2018, 20-21; 2Q, 2020, 21-22

+ **Z45.3 Encounter for adjustment and management of implanted devices of the special senses**
  - **Z45.31 Encounter for adjustment and management of implanted visual substitution device**
  - + **Z45.32 Encounter for adjustment and management of implanted hearing device**
    - **Excludes1:** *Encounter for fitting and adjustment of hearing aide (Z46.1)*
    - **Z45.320 Encounter for adjustment and management of bone conduction device**
    - **Z45.321 Encounter for adjustment and management of cochlear device**
    - **Z45.328 Encounter for adjustment and management of other implanted hearing device**

+ **Z45.4 Encounter for adjustment and management of implanted nervous system device**
  - **Z45.41 Encounter for adjustment and management of cerebrospinal fluid drainage device**
    - Encounter for adjustment and management of cerebral ventricular (communicating) shunt
  - **Z45.42 Encounter for adjustment and management of neurostimulator**
    - Encounter for adjustment and management of brain neurostimulator
    - Encounter for adjustment and management of gastric neurostimulator
    - Encounter for adjustment and management of peripheral nerve neurostimulator
    - Encounter for adjustment and management of sacral nerve neurostimulator
    - Encounter for adjustment and management of spinal cord neurostimulator
    - Encounter for adjustment and management of vagus nerve neurostimulator
  - **Z45.49 Encounter for adjustment and management of other implanted nervous system device**
    - *AHA CC: 3Q, 2014, 19-20*

+ **Z45.8 Encounter for adjustment and management of other implanted devices**
  - + **Z45.81 Encounter for adjustment or removal of breast implant**
    - Encounter for elective implant exchange (different material) (different size)
    - Encounter for removal of tissue expander with or without synchronous insertion of permanent implant
    - **Excludes1:** *complications of breast implant (T85.4-)*
      encounter for initial breast implant insertion for cosmetic breast augmentation (Z41.1)
      encounter for breast reconstruction following mastectomy (Z42.1)
    - **Z45.811 Encounter for adjustment or removal of right breast implant**
    - **Z45.812 Encounter for adjustment or removal of left breast implant**
    - **Z45.819 Encounter for adjustment or removal of unspecified breast implant**
  - **Z45.82 Encounter for adjustment or removal of myringotomy device (stent) (tube)**
  - **Z45.89 Encounter for adjustment and management of other implanted devices**
    - *AHA CC: 4Q, 2014, 26-28*

Z45.9 Encounter for adjustment and management of unspecified implanted device

Z46 Encounter for fitting and adjustment of other devices

Includes: removal or replacement of other device
Excludes1: *malfunction or other complications of device - see Alphabetical Index*
Excludes2: *encounter for fitting and management of implanted devices (Z45.-)*
issue of repeat prescription only (Z76.0)
presence of prosthetic and other devices (Z95-Z97)
Review coding guideline C.21.c.7

- **Z46.0 Encounter for fitting and adjustment of spectacles and contact lenses**
- **Z46.1 Encounter for fitting and adjustment of hearing aid**
  - **Excludes1:** *encounter for adjustment and management of implanted hearing device (Z45.32-)*
- **Z46.2 Encounter for fitting and adjustment of other devices related to nervous system and special senses**
  - **Excludes2:** *encounter for adjustment and management of implanted nervous system device (Z45.4-)*
    encounter for adjustment and management of implanted visual substitution device (Z45.31)
- **Z46.3 Encounter for fitting and adjustment of dental prosthetic device**
  - Encounter for fitting and adjustment of dentures
- **Z46.4 Encounter for fitting and adjustment of orthodontic device**
- + **Z46.5 Encounter for fitting and adjustment of other gastrointestinal appliance and device**
  - **Excludes1:** *encounter for attention to artificial openings of digestive tract (Z43.1-Z43.4)*
  - **Z46.51 Encounter for fitting and adjustment of gastric lap band**
  - **Z46.59 Encounter for fitting and adjustment of other gastrointestinal appliance and device**
- **Z46.6 Encounter for fitting and adjustment of urinary device**
  - **Excludes2:** *attention to artificial openings of urinary tract (Z43.5, Z43.6)*
- + **Z46.8 Encounter for fitting and adjustment of other specified devices**
  - **Z46.81 Encounter for fitting and adjustment of insulin pump**
    - Encounter for insulin pump titration
    - Encounter for insulin pump instruction and training
  - **Z46.82 Encounter for fitting and adjustment of non-vascular catheter**
  - **Z46.89 Encounter for fitting and adjustment of other specified devices**
    - Encounter for fitting and adjustment of wheelchair
- **Z46.9 Encounter for fitting and adjustment of unspecified device**

Z47 Orthopedic aftercare

Excludes1: *aftercare for healing fracture-code to fracture with 7th character D*
Review coding guideline C.21.c.7

- **Z47.1 Aftercare following joint replacement surgery**
  - Use additional code to identify the joint (Z96.6-)
  - *AHA CC: 1Q, 2020, 23-24*
- **Z47.2 Encounter for removal of internal fixation device**
  - **Excludes1:** *encounter for adjustment of internal fixation device for fracture treatment- code to fracture with appropriate 7th character*
    encounter for removal of external fixation device- code to fracture with 7th character D
    infection or inflammatory reaction to internal fixation device (T84.6-)
    mechanical complication of internal fixation device (T84.1-)
- + **Z47.3 Aftercare following explantation of joint prosthesis**
  - Aftercare following explantation of joint prosthesis, staged procedure
  - Encounter for joint prosthesis insertion following prior explantation of joint prosthesis
  - *AHA CC: 1Q, 2020, 23-24*
  - **Z47.31 Aftercare following explantation of shoulder joint prosthesis**
    - **Excludes1:** *acquired absence of shoulder joint following prior explantation of shoulder joint prosthesis (Z89.23-)*
      shoulder joint prosthesis explantation status (Z89.23-)
  - **Z47.32 Aftercare following explantation of hip joint prosthesis**
    - **Excludes1:** *acquired absence of hip joint following prior explantation of hip joint prosthesis (Z89.62-)*
      hip joint prosthesis explantation status (Z89.62-)
    - *AHA CC: 1Q, 2015, 16-17*

Z47.33 Aftercare following explantation of knee joint prosthesis

Excludes1: *acquired absence of knee joint following prior explantation of knee prosthesis (Z89.52-*
knee joint prosthesis explantation status (Z89.52-)

+ Z47.8 Encounter for other orthopedic aftercare

Z47.81 Encounter for orthopedic aftercare following surgical amputation

Use additional code to identify the limb amputated (Z89.-)

Z47.82 Encounter for orthopedic aftercare following scoliosis surgery

Z47.89 Encounter for other orthopedic aftercare

Z48 Encounter for other postprocedural aftercare

Excludes1: *encounter for aftercare following injury - code to Injury, by site, with appropriate 7th character for subsequent encounter*
encounter for follow-up examination after completed treatment (Z08-Z09)

Excludes2: *encounter for attention to artificial openings (Z43.-)*
encounter for fitting and adjustment of prosthetic and other devices (Z44-Z46)

Review coding guideline C.21.c.7

+ Z48.0 Encounter for attention to dressings, sutures and drains

Excludes1: *encounter for planned postprocedural wound closure (Z48.1)*

Z48.00 Encounter for change or removal of nonsurgical wound dressing

Encounter for change or removal of wound dressing NOS

Z48.01 Encounter for change or removal of surgical wound dressing

AHA CC: 4Q, 2015, 38; 2Q, 2019, 33

Z48.02 Encounter for removal of sutures

Encounter for removal of staples

Z48.03 Encounter for change or removal of drains

Z48.1 Encounter for planned postprocedural wound closure

Excludes1: *encounter for attention to dressings and sutures (Z48.0-)*

+ Z48.2 Encounter for aftercare following organ transplant

CC **Z48.21 Encounter for aftercare following heart transplant**

CC **Z48.22 Encounter for aftercare following kidney transplant**

CC **Z48.23 Encounter for aftercare following liver transplant**

CC **Z48.24 Encounter for aftercare following lung transplant**

+ Z48.28 Encounter for aftercare following multiple organ transplant

CC **Z48.280 Encounter for aftercare following heart-lung transplant**

Z48.288 Encounter for aftercare following multiple organ transplant

+ Z48.29 Encounter for aftercare following other organ transplant

CC **Z48.290 Encounter for aftercare following bone marrow transplant**

Z48.298 Encounter for aftercare following other organ transplant

Z48.3 Aftercare following surgery for neoplasm

Use additional code to identify the neoplasm

+ Z48.8 Encounter for other specified postprocedural aftercare

+ Z48.81 Encounter for surgical aftercare following surgery on specified body systems

These codes identify the body system requiring aftercare. They are for use in conjunction with other aftercare codes to fully explain the aftercare encounter. The condition treated should also be coded if still present.

Excludes1: *aftercare for injury- code the injury with 7th character D*
aftercare following surgery for neoplasm (Z48.3)

Excludes2: *aftercare following organ transplant (Z48.2-)*
orthopedic aftercare (Z47.-)

Z48.810 Encounter for surgical aftercare following surgery on the sense organs

Z48.811 Encounter for surgical aftercare following surgery on the nervous system

Excludes2: *encounter for surgical aftercare following surgery on the sense organs (Z48.810)*

Z48.812 Encounter for surgical aftercare following surgery on the circulatory system

AHA CC: 4Q, 2012, 96-97

Z48.813 Encounter for surgical aftercare following surgery on the respiratory system

AHA CC: 2Q, 2019, 33

Z48.814 Encounter for surgical aftercare following surgery on the teeth or oral cavity

Z48.815 Encounter for surgical aftercare following surgery on the digestive system

AHA CC: 4Q, 2015, 38

Z48.816 Encounter for surgical aftercare following surgery on the genitourinary system

Excludes1: *encounter for aftercare following sterilization reversal (Z31.42)*

Z48.817 Encounter for surgical aftercare following surgery on the skin and subcutaneous tissue

Z48.89 Encounter for other specified surgical aftercare

Z49 Encounter for5 care involving renal dialysis

Code also associated end stage renal disease (N18.6)

Review coding guideline C.21.c.7

+ Z49.0 Preparatory care for renal dialysis

Encounter for dialysis instruction and training

Z49.01 Encounter for fitting and adjustment of extracorporeal dialysis catheter

Removal or replacement of renal dialysis catheter

Toilet or cleansing of renal dialysis catheter

Z49.02 Encounter for fitting and adjustment of peritoneal dialysis catheter

+ Z49.3 Encounter for adequacy testing for dialysis

Z49.31 Encounter for adequacy testing for hemodialysis

Z49.32 Encounter for adequacy testing for peritoneal dialysis

Encounter for peritoneal equilibration test

Z51 Encounter for other aftercare and medical care

Code also condition requiring care

Excludes1: *follow-up examination after treatment (Z08-Z09)*

Review coding guidelines C.2.a, C.2.e.2 and C.2.e.3

Review coding guideline C.21.c.7

Z51.0 Encounter for antineoplastic radiation therapy

Review coding guidelines C.21.c.7 and C.21.c.16

+ Z51.1 Encounter for antineoplastic chemotherapy and immunotherapy

Excludes2: *encounter for chemotherapy and immunotherapy for nonneoplastic condition- code to condition*

Review coding guidelines C.21.c.7 and C21.c.16

Z51.11 Encounter for antineoplastic chemotherapy

AHA CC: 3Q, 2015, 19-20

Z51.12 Encounter for antineoplastic immunotherapy

Z51.5 Encounter for palliative care

AHA CC: 1Q, 2017, 48-49; 4Q, 2020, 98

Z51.6 Encounter for desensitization to allergens

AHA CC: 4Q, 2016, 77

+ Z51.8 Encounter for other specified aftercare

Excludes1: *holiday relief care (Z75.5)*

Z51.81 Encounter for therapeutic drug level monitoring

Code also any long-term (current) drug therapy (Z79.-)

Excludes1: *encounter for blood-drug test for administrative or medicolegal reasons (Z02.83)*

Z51.89 Encounter for other specified aftercare
AHA CC: 4Q, 2012, 96-97
NOTE Z51.89 is an acceptable PDX when reported with a secondary diagnosis.

Z52 Donors of organs and tissues
Includes: autologous and other living donors
Excludes1: *cadaveric donor - omit code*
examination of potential donor (Z00.5)
Review coding guidelines C.21.c.9 and C.21.c.16
+ **Z52.0 Blood donor**
+ **Z52.00 Unspecified blood donor**
Z52.000 Unspecified donor, whole blood
Z52.001 Unspecified donor, stem cells
Z52.008 Unspecified donor, other blood
+ **Z52.01 Autologous blood donor**
Z52.010 Autologous donor, whole blood
Z52.011 Autologous donor, stem cells
Z52.018 Autologous donor, other blood
+ **Z52.09 Other blood donor**
Volunteer donor
Z52.090 Other blood donor, whole blood
Z52.091 Other blood donor, stem cells
Z52.098 Other blood donor, other blood
+ **Z52.1 Skin donor**
Z52.10 Skin donor, unspecified
Z52.11 Skin donor, autologous
Z52.19 Skin donor, other
+ **Z52.2 Bone donor**
Z52.20 Bone donor, unspecified
Z52.21 Bone donor, autologous
Z52.29 Bone donor, other
Z52.3 Bone marrow donor
Z52.4 Kidney donor
Z52.5 Cornea donor
Z52.6 Liver donor
+ **Z52.8 Donor of other specified organs or tissues**
+ **Z52.81 Egg (Oocyte) donor**
♀ **Z52.810 Egg (Oocyte) donor under age 35, anonymous recipient**
Egg donor under age 35 NOS
♀ **Z52.811 Egg (Oocyte) donor under age 35, designated recipient**
♀ **Z52.812 Egg (Oocyte) donor age 35 and over, anonymous recipient**
Egg donor age 35 and over NOS
♀ **Z52.813 Egg (Oocyte) donor age 35 and over, designated recipient**
♀ **Z52.819 Egg (Oocyte) donor, unspecified**
Z52.89 Donor of other specified organs or tissues
Z52.9 Donor of unspecified organ or tissue
Donor NOS

Z53 Persons encountering health services for specific procedures and treatment, not carried out
+ **Z53.0 Procedure and treatment not carried out because of contraindication**
Z53.01 Procedure and treatment not carried out due to patient smoking
Z53.09 Procedure and treatment not carried out because of other contraindication
Z53.1 Procedure and treatment not carried out because of patient's decision for reasons of belief and group pressure
+ **Z53.2 Procedure and treatment not carried out because of patient's decision for other and unspecified reasons**
Z53.20 Procedure and treatment not carried out because of patient's decision for unspecified reasons
Z53.21 Procedure and treatment not carried out due to patient leaving prior to being seen by health care provider
Z53.29 Procedure and treatment not carried out because of patient's decision for other reasons
+ **Z53.3 Procedure converted to open procedure**
AHA CC: 4Q, 2016, 79
Z53.31 Laparoscopic surgical procedure converted to open procedure
AHA CC: 4Q, 2016, 100-101
Z53.32 Thoracoscopic surgical procedure converted to open procedure
Z53.33 Arthroscopic surgical procedure converted to open procedure
Z53.39 Other specified procedure converted to open procedure
Z53.8 Procedure and treatment not carried out for other reasons
Z53.9 Procedure and treatment not carried out, unspecified reason

Persons with potential health hazards related to socioeconomic and psychosocial circumstances (Z55-Z65)

AHA CC: 1Q, 2018, 18
Review coding guideline B.14

Z55 Problems related to education and literacy
Excludes1: *disorders of psychological development (F80-F89)*
Z55.0 Illiteracy and low-level literacy
Z55.1 Schooling unavailable and unattainable
Z55.2 Failed school examinations
Z55.3 Underachievement in school
Z55.4 Educational maladjustment and discord with teachers and classmates
Z55.5 Less than a high school diploma
No general equivalence degree (GED)
Z55.8 Other problems related to education and literacy
Problems related to inadequate teaching
Z55.9 Problems related to education and literacy, unspecified
Academic problems NOS

Z56 Problems related to employment and unemployment
Excludes2: *occupational exposure to risk factors (Z57.-)*
problems related to housing and economic circumstances (Z59.-)
Z56.0 Unemployment, unspecified
● **Z56.1 Change of job**
Z56.2 Threat of job loss
Z56.3 Stressful work schedule
Z56.4 Discord with boss and workmates
Z56.5 Uncongenial work environment
Difficult conditions at work
Z56.6 Other physical and mental strain related to work
+ **Z56.8 Other problems related to employment**
Z56.81 Sexual harassment on the job
Z56.82 Military deployment status
Individual (civilian or military) currently deployed in theater or in support of military war, peacekeeping and humanitarian operations
Z56.89 Other problems related to employment
Z56.9 Unspecified problems related to employment
Occupational problems NOS

Z57 Occupational exposure to risk factors
Z57.0 Occupational exposure to noise
Z57.1 Occupational exposure to radiation
Z57.2 Occupational exposure to dust
+ **Z57.3 Occupational exposure to other air contaminants**
Z57.31 Occupational exposure to environmental tobacco smoke
Excludes2: *exposure to environmental tobacco smoke (Z77.22)*
Z57.39 Occupational exposure to other air contaminants
Z57.4 Occupational exposure to toxic agents in agriculture
Occupational exposure to solids, liquids, gases or vapors in agriculture
Z57.5 Occupational exposure to toxic agents in other industries
Occupational exposure to solids, liquids, gases or vapors in other industries
Z57.6 Occupational exposure to extreme temperature
Z57.7 Occupational exposure to vibration
Z57.8 Occupational exposure to other risk factors
Z57.9 Occupational exposure to unspecified risk factor

Z58 Problems related to physical environment
Excludes2: *occupational exposure (Z57.-)*
Z58.6 Inadequate drinking-water supply
Lack of safe drinking water
Excludes2: deprivation of water (T73.1)

Z59 Problems related to housing and economic circumstances

Excludes2: *problems related to upbringing (Z62.-)*

+ **Z59.0 Homelessness**
  AHA CC: 4Q, 2017, 112-114
  Review coding guideline B.19.d
  - **Z59.00 Homelessness unspecified**
  - **Z59.01 Sheltered homelessness**
    Doubled up
    Living in a shelter such as: motel, scattered site housing, temporary or transitional living situation
  - **Z59.02 Unsheltered homelessness**
    Residing in place not meant for human inhabitation such as: abandoned buildings, cars, parks, sidewalk
    Residing on the street
- **Z59.1 Inadequate housing**
  Lack of heating
  Restriction of space
  Technical defects in home preventing adequate care
  Unsatisfactory surroundings
  Excludes1: *problems related to the natural and physical environment (Z77.1-)*
  AHA CC: 4Q, 2017, 112-114
  Review coding guideline B.19.d
- **Z59.2 Discord with neighbors, lodgers and landlord**
- **Z59.3 Problems related to living in residential institution**
  Boarding-school resident
  Excludes1: *institutional upbringing (Z62.2)*

+ **Z59.4 Lack of adequate food**
  Excludes2: *deprivation of food (T73.0)*
  effects of hunger (T73.0)
  inappropriate diet or eating habits (Z72.4)
  malnutrition (E40-E46)
  - **Z59.41 Food insecurity**
  - **Z59.48 Other specified lack of adequate food**
    Inadequate food
    Lack of food
- **Z59.5 Extreme poverty**
  AHA CC: 4Q, 2017, 112-114
  Review coding guideline B.19.d
- **Z59.6 Low income**
- **Z59.7 Insufficient social insurance and welfare support**

+ **Z59.8 Other problems related to housing and economic circumstances**
  + **Z59.81 Housing instability, housed**
    Foreclosure on home loan
    Past due on rent or mortgage
    Unwanted multiple moves in the last 12 months
    - **Z59.811 Housing instability, housed, with risk of homelessness**
      Imminent risk of homelessness
    - **Z59.812 Housing instability, housed, homelessness in past 12 months**
    - **Z59.819 Housing instability, housed unspecified**
  - **Z59.89 Other problems related to housing and economic circumstances**
    Foreclosure on loan
    Isolated dwelling
    Problems with creditors
- **Z59.9 Problem related to housing and economic circumstances, unspecified**

Z60 Problems related to social environment

- **Z60.0 Problems of adjustment to life-cycle transitions**
  Empty nest syndrome
  Phase of life problem
  Problem with adjustment to retirement [pension]
- **Z60.2 Problems related to living alone**
- **Z60.3 Acculturation difficulty**
  Problem with migration
  Problem with social transplantation
- **Z60.4 Social exclusion and rejection**
  Exclusion and rejection on the basis of personal characteristics, such as unusual physical appearance, illness or behavior.
  Excludes1: *target of adverse discrimination such as for racial or religious reasons (Z60.5)*
- **Z60.5 Target of (perceived) adverse discrimination and persecution**
  Excludes1: *social exclusion and rejection (Z60.4)*
- **Z60.8 Other problems related to social environment**
- **Z60.9 Problem related to social environment, unspecified**

Z62 Problems related to upbringing

Includes: current and past negative life events in childhood
current and past problems of a child related to upbringing

Excludes2: *maltreatment syndrome (T74.-)*
problems related to housing and economic circumstances (Z59.-)

- **Z62.0 Inadequate parental supervision and control**
- **Z62.1 Parental overprotection**

+ **Z62.2 Upbringing away from parents**
  Excludes1: *problems with boarding school (Z59.3)*
  - ● **Z62.21 Child in welfare custody**
    Child in care of non-parental family member
    Child in foster care
    Excludes2: *problem for parent due to child in welfare custody (Z63.5)*
  - **Z62.22 Institutional upbringing**
    Child living in orphanage or group home
  - **Z62.29 Other upbringing away from parents**
- ● **Z62.3 Hostility towards and scapegoating of child**
- **Z62.6 Inappropriate (excessive) parental pressure**

+ **Z62.8 Other specified problems related to upbringing**
  + **Z62.81 Personal history of abuse in childhood**
    - **Z62.810 Personal history of physical and sexual abuse in childhood**
      Excludes1: *current child physical abuse (T74.12, T76.12)*
      current child sexual abuse (T74.22, T76.22)
    - **Z62.811 Personal history of psychological abuse in childhood**
      Excludes1: *current child psychological abuse (T74.32, T76.32)*
    - **Z62.812 Personal history of neglect in childhood**
      Excludes1: *current child neglect (T74.02, T76.02)*
    - **Z62.813 Personal history of forced labor or sexual exploitation in childhood**
      AHA CC: 4Q, 2018, 32-33, 35
    - **Z62.819 Personal history of unspecified abuse in childhood**
      Excludes1: *current child abuse NOS (T74.92, T76.92)*
  + **Z62.82 Parent-child conflict**
    - **Z62.820 Parent-biological child conflict**
      Parent-child problem NOS
    - **Z62.821 Parent-adopted child conflict**
    - **Z62.822 Parent-foster child conflict**
  + **Z62.89 Other specified problems related to upbringing**
    - **Z62.890 Parent-child estrangement NEC**
    - **Z62.891 Sibling rivalry**
    - **Z62.898 Other specified problems related to upbringing**
- **Z62.9 Problem related to upbringing, unspecified**

Z63 Other problems related to primary support group, including family circumstances

Excludes2: *maltreatment syndrome (T74.-, T76)*
parent-child problems (Z62.-)
problems related to negative life events in childhood (Z62.-)
problems related to upbringing (Z62.-)

- **Z63.0 Problems in relationship with spouse or partner**
  Relationship distress with spouse or intimate partner
  Excludes1: *counseling for spousal or partner abuse problems (Z69.1)*
  counseling related to sexual attitude, behavior, and orientation (Z70.-)
- **Z63.1 Problems in relationship with in-laws**

+ **Z63.3 Absence of family member**
  Excludes1: *absence of family member due to disappearance and death (Z63.4)*
  absence of family member due to separation and divorce (Z63.5)
  - **Z63.31 Absence of family member due to military deployment**
    Individual or family affected by other family member being on military deployment
    Excludes1: *family disruption due to return of family member from military deployment (Z63.71)*
  - **Z63.32 Other absence of family member**

Z63.4 Disappearance and death of family member
Assumed death of family member
Bereavement
AHA CC: 1Q, 2014, 25

Z63.5 Disruption of family by separation and divorce
Marital estrangement

Z63.6 Dependent relative needing care at home

+ **Z63.7 Other stressful life events affecting family and household**

Z63.71 Stress on family due to return of family member from military deployment
Individual or family affected by family member having returned from military deployment (current or past conflict)

Z63.72 Alcoholism and drug addiction in family

Z63.79 Other stressful life events affecting family and household
Anxiety (normal) about sick person in family
Health problems within family
Ill or disturbed family member
Isolated family

Z63.8 Other specified problems related to primary support group
Family discord NOS
Family estrangement NOS
High expressed emotional level within family
Inadequate family support NOS
Inadequate or distorted communication within family

Z63.9 Problem related to primary support group, unspecified
Relationship disorder NOS

Z64 Problems related to certain psychosocial circumstances

♀ **Z64.0 Problems related to unwanted pregnancy**

♀ **Z64.1 Problems related to multiparity**

Z64.4 Discord with counselors
Discord with probation officer
Discord with social worker

Z65 Problems related to other psychosocial circumstances

Z65.0 Conviction in civil and criminal proceedings without imprisonment

Z65.1 Imprisonment and other incarceration

Z65.2 Problems related to release from prison

Z65.3 Problems related to other legal circumstances
Arrest
Child custody or support proceedings
Litigation
Prosecution

Z65.4 Victim of crime and terrorism
Victim of torture

• **Z65.5 Exposure to disaster, war and other hostilities**
Excludes1: *target of perceived discrimination or persecution (Z60.5)*

Z65.8 Other specified problems related to psychosocial circumstances
Religious or spiritual problem

Z65.9 Problem related to unspecified psychosocial circumstances

Do not resuscitate status (Z66)

Z66 Do not resuscitate
DNR status
Review coding guideline C.21.c.3
Valid 3-character code, no further characters required

Blood type (Z67)

Z67 Blood type
Review coding guideline C.21.c.3
AHA CC: 3Q, 2015, 40

+ **Z67.1 Type A blood**
Z67.10 Type A blood, Rh positive
Z67.11 Type A blood, Rh negative

+ **Z67.2 Type B blood**
Z67.20 Type B blood, Rh positive
Z67.21 Type B blood, Rh negative

+ **Z67.3 Type AB blood**
Z67.30 Type AB blood, Rh positive
Z67.31 Type AB blood, Rh negative

+ **Z67.4 Type O blood**
Z67.40 Type O blood, Rh positive
Z67.41 Type O blood, Rh negative

+ **Z67.9 Unspecified blood type**
Z67.90 Unspecified blood type, Rh positive
Z67.91 Unspecified blood type, Rh negative

Body mass index [BMI] (Z68)

Z68 Body mass index [BMI]
Kilograms per meters squared
NOTE BMI adult codes are for use for persons 20 years of age or older
BMI pediatric codes are for use for persons 2-19 years of age. These percentiles are based on the growth charts published by the Centers for Disease Control and Prevention (CDC)
Review coding guidelines B.14 and C.21.c.3
AHA CC: 4Q, 2018, 77-83; 4Q, 2019, 19

• CC **Z68.1 Body mass index [BMI] 19.9 or less, adult**
AHA CC: 1Q, 2017, 39

+ **Z68.2 Body mass index [BMI] 20-29, adult**
• **Z68.20 Body mass index [BMI] 20.0-20.9, adult**
• **Z68.21 Body mass index [BMI] 21.0-21.9, adult**
• **Z68.22 Body mass index [BMI] 22.0-22.9, adult**
• **Z68.23 Body mass index [BMI] 23.0-23.9, adult**
• **Z68.24 Body mass index [BMI] 24.0-24.9, adult**
• **Z68.25 Body mass index [BMI] 25.0-25.9, adult**
• **Z68.26 Body mass index [BMI] 26.0-26.9, adult**
• **Z68.27 Body mass index [BMI] 27.0-27.9, adult**
• **Z68.28 Body mass index [BMI] 28.0-28.9, adult**
• **Z68.29 Body mass index [BMI] 29.0-29.9, adult**

+ **Z68.3 Body mass index [BMI] 30-39, adult**
• **Z68.30 Body mass index [BMI] 30.0-30.9, adult**
• **Z68.31 Body mass index [BMI] 31.0-31.9, adult**
• **Z68.32 Body mass index [BMI] 32.0-32.9, adult**
• **Z68.33 Body mass index [BMI] 33.0-33.9, adult**
• **Z68.34 Body mass index [BMI] 34.0-34.9, adult**
• **Z68.35 Body mass index [BMI] 35.0-35.9, adult**
• **Z68.36 Body mass index [BMI] 36.0-36.9, adult**
• **Z68.37 Body mass index [BMI] 37.0-37.9, adult**
• **Z68.38 Body mass index [BMI] 38.0-38.9, adult**
• **Z68.39 Body mass index [BMI] 39.0-39.9, adult**

+ **Z68.4 Body mass index [BMI] 40 or greater, adult**
• CC **Z68.41 Body mass index [BMI] 40.0-44.9, adult**
• CC **Z68.42 Body mass index [BMI] 45.0-49.9, adult**
• CC **Z68.43 Body mass index [BMI] 50.0-59.9, adult**
• CC **Z68.44 Body mass index [BMI] 60.0-69.9, adult**
• CC **Z68.45 Body mass index [BMI] 70 or greater, adult**

+ **Z68.5 Body mass index [BMI] pediatric**
AHA CC: 4Q, 2018, 81
Z68.51 Body mass index [BMI] pediatric, less than 5th percentile for age
AHA CC: 4Q, 2018, 82
Z68.52 Body mass index [BMI] pediatric, 5th percentile to less than 85th percentile for age
Z68.53 Body mass index [BMI] pediatric, 85th percentile to less than 95th percentile for age
Z68.54 Body mass index [BMI] pediatric, greater than or equal to 95th percentile for age

Persons encountering health services in other circumstances (Z69-Z76)

Z69 Encounter for mental health services for victim and perpetrator of abuse
Includes: counseling for victims and perpetrators of abuse
Review coding guideline C.21.c.10

+ **Z69.0 Encounter for mental health services for child abuse problems**

+ **Z69.01 Encounter for mental health services for parental child abuse**

• **Z69.010 Encounter for mental health services for victim of parental child abuse**
Encounter for mental health services for victim of child abuse by parent
Encounter for mental health services for victim of child neglect by parent
Encounter for mental health services for victim of child psychological abuse by parent
Encounter for mental health services for victim of child sexual abuse by parent

Z69.011 Encounter for mental health services for perpetrator of parental child abuse
Encounter for mental health services for perpetrator of parental child neglect
Encounter for mental health services for perpetrator of parental child psychological abuse
Encounter for mental health services for perpetrator of parental child sexual abuse
Excludes1: *encounter for mental health services for non-parental child abuse (Z69.02-)*

\+ **Z69.02 Encounter for mental health services for non-parental child abuse**
● **Z69.020 Encounter for mental health services for victim of non-parental child abuse**
Encounter for mental health services for victim of non-parental child neglect
Encounter for mental health services for victim of non-parental child psychological abuse
Encounter for mental health services for victim of non-parental child sexual abuse
Z69.021 Encounter for mental health services for perpetrator of non-parental child abuse
Encounter for mental health services for perpetrator of non-parental child neglect
Encounter for mental health services for perpetrator of non-parental child psychological abuse
Encounter for mental health services for perpetrator of non-parental child sexual abuse

\+ **Z69.1 Encounter for mental health services for spousal or partner abuse problems**
Z69.11 Encounter for mental health services for victim of spousal or partner abuse
Encounter for mental health services for victim of spouse or partner neglect
Encounter for mental health services for victim of spouse or partner psychological abuse
Encounter for mental health services for victim of spouse or partner violence, physical
Z69.12 Encounter for mental health services for perpetrator of spousal or partner abuse
Encounter for mental health services for perpetrator of spouse or partner neglect
Encounter for mental health services for perpetrator of spouse or partner psychological abuse
Encounter for mental health services for perpetrator of spouse or partner violence, physical

\+ **Z69.8 Encounter for mental health services for victim or perpetrator of other abuse**
Z69.81 Encounter for mental health services for victim of other abuse
Encounter for mental health services for victim of non-spousal adult abuse
Encounter for mental health services for victim of spouse or partner violence, sexual
Encounter for rape victim counseling
Z69.82 Encounter for mental health services for perpetrator of other abuse
Encounter for mental health services for perpetrator of non-spousal adult abuse

Z70 Counseling related to sexual attitude, behavior and orientation
Includes: encounter for mental health services for sexual attitude, behavior and orientation
Excludes2: *contraceptive or procreative counseling (Z30-Z31)*
Review coding guideline C.21.c.10
Z70.0 Counseling related to sexual attitude
Z70.1 Counseling related to patient's sexual behavior and orientation
Patient concerned regarding impotence
Patient concerned regarding non-responsiveness
Patient concerned regarding promiscuity
Patient concerned regarding sexual orientation
Z70.2 Counseling related to sexual behavior and orientation of third party
Advice sought regarding sexual behavior and orientation of child
Advice sought regarding sexual behavior and orientation of partner
Advice sought regarding sexual behavior and orientation of spouse
Z70.3 Counseling related to combined concerns regarding sexual attitude, behavior and orientation
Z70.8 Other sex counseling
Encounter for sex education
Z70.9 Sex counseling, unspecified

Z71 Persons encountering health services for other counseling and medical advice, not elsewhere classified
Excludes2: *contraceptive or procreation counseling (Z30-Z31)*
sex counseling (Z70.-)
Review coding guideline C.21.c.10
Z71.0 Person encountering health services to consult on behalf of another person
Person encountering health services to seek advice or treatment for non-attending third party
Excludes2: *anxiety (normal) about sick person in family (Z63.7)*
expectant (adoptive) parent(s) pre-birth pediatrician visit (Z76.81)
Z71.1 Person with feared health complaint in whom no diagnosis is made
Person encountering health services with feared condition which was not demonstrated
Person encountering health services in which problem was normal state
'Worried well'
Excludes1: *medical observation for suspected diseases and conditions proven not to exist (Z03.-)*
AHA CC: 4Q, 2016, 4-7
Z71.2 Person consulting for explanation of examination or test findings
Z71.3 Dietary counseling and surveillance
Use additional code for any associated underlying medical condition
Use additional code to identify body mass index (BMI), if known (Z68.-)
\+ **Z71.4 Alcohol abuse counseling and surveillance**
Use additional code for alcohol abuse or dependence (F10.-)
Z71.41 Alcohol abuse counseling and surveillance of alcoholic
Z71.42 Counseling for family member of alcoholic
Counseling for significant other, partner, or friend of alcoholic
\+ **Z71.5 Drug abuse counseling and surveillance**
Use additional code for drug abuse or dependence (F11-F16, F18-F19)
Z71.51 Drug abuse counseling and surveillance of drug abuser
Z71.52 Counseling for family member of drug abuser
Counseling for significant other, partner, or friend of drug abuser
Z71.6 Tobacco abuse counseling
Use additional code for nicotine dependence (F17.-)
Z71.7 Human immunodeficiency virus [HIV] counseling
Review coding guideline C.1.a.2.h
\+ **Z71.8 Other specified counseling**
Excludes2: *counseling for contraception (Z30.0-)*
Z71.81 Spiritual or religious counseling
Z71.82 Exercise counseling
AHA CC: 4Q, 2017, 27
Z71.83 Encounter for nonprocreative genetic counseling
Exludes1: *counseling for procreative genetics (Z31.5)*
counseling for procreative management (Z31.6)
AHA CC: 4Q, 2017, 27

Z71.84 Encounter for health counseling related to travel
Encounter for health risk and safety counseling for (international) travel
Code also, if applicable, encounter for immunization (Z23)
Excludes2: *encounter for administrative examination (Z02.-)*
encounter for other special examination without complaint, suspected or reported diagnosis (Z01.-)
AHA CC: 4Q, 2019, 20

Z71.85 Encounter for immunization safety counseling
Encounter for vaccine product safety counseling
Code also, if applicable, encounter for immunization (Z23)
Code also, if applicable, immunization not carried out (Z28.-)
Excludes1: *encounter for health counseling related to travel (Z71.84)*

Z71.89 Other specified counseling

Z71.9 Counseling, unspecified
Encounter for medical advice NOS

Z72 Problems related to lifestyle
Excludes2: *problems related to life-management difficulty (Z73.-)*
problems related to socioeconomic and psychosocial circumstances (Z55-Z65)
Review coding guideline C.21.c.14

Z72.0 Tobacco use
Tobacco use NOS
Excludes1: *history of tobacco dependence (Z87.891)*
nicotine dependence (F17.2-)
tobacco dependence (F17.2-)
tobacco use during pregnancy (O99.33-)
Review coding guideline C.15.l.2

Z72.3 Lack of physical exercise

Z72.4 Inappropriate diet and eating habits
Excludes1: *behavioral eating disorders of infancy or childhood (F98.2-F98.3)*
eating disorders (F50.-)
lack of adequate food (Z59.48)
malnutrition and other nutritional deficiencies (E40-E64)

+ **Z72.5 High risk sexual behavior**
Promiscuity
Excludes1: *paraphilias (F65)*

Z72.51 High risk heterosexual behavior

Z72.52 High risk homosexual behavior

Z72.53 High risk bisexual behavior

Z72.6 Gambling and betting
Excludes1: *compulsive or pathological gambling (F63.0)*

+ **Z72.8 Other problems related to lifestyle**

+ **Z72.81 Antisocial behavior**
Excludes1: *conduct disorders (F91.-)*

• **Z72.810 Child and adolescent antisocial behavior**
Antisocial behavior (child) (adolescent) without manifest psychiatric disorder
Delinquency NOS
Group delinquency
Offenses in the context of gang membership
Stealing in company with others
Truancy from school

• **Z72.811 Adult antisocial behavior**
Adult antisocial behavior without manifest psychiatric disorder

+ **Z72.82 Problems related to sleep**

Z72.820 Sleep deprivation
Lack of adequate sleep
Excludes1: *insomnia (G47.0-)*

Z72.821 Inadequate sleep hygiene
Bad sleep habits
Irregular sleep habits
Unhealthy sleep wake schedule
Excludes1: *insomnia (F51.0-, G47.0-)*

Z72.89 Other problems related to lifestyle
Self-damaging behavior

Z72.9 Problem related to lifestyle, unspecified

Z73 Problems related to life management difficulty
Excludes2: *problems related to socioeconomic and psychosocial circumstances (Z55-Z65)*

Z73.0 Burn-out

Z73.1 Type A behavior pattern

Z73.2 Lack of relaxation and leisure

Z73.3 Stress, not elsewhere classified
Physical and mental strain NOS
Excludes1: *stress related to employment or unemployment (Z56.-)*

Z73.4 Inadequate social skills, not elsewhere classified

Z73.5 Social role conflict, not elsewhere classified

Z73.6 Limitation of activities due to disability
Excludes1: *care-provider dependency (Z74.-)*

+ **Z73.8 Other problems related to life management difficulty**

+ **Z73.81 Behavioral insomnia of childhood**

• **Z73.810 Behavioral insomnia of childhood, sleep-onset association type**

• **Z73.811 Behavioral insomnia of childhood, limit setting type**

• **Z73.812 Behavioral insomnia of childhood, combined type**

• **Z73.819 Behavioral insomnia of childhood, unspecified type**

Z73.82 Dual sensory impairment

Z73.89 Other problems related to life management difficulty

Z73.9 Problem related to life management difficulty, unspecified

Z74 Problems related to care provider dependency
Excludes2: *dependence on enabling machines or devices NEC (Z99.-)*

+ **Z74.0 Reduced mobility**

Z74.01 Bed confinement status
Bedridden
Review coding guideline C.21.c.3

Z74.09 Other reduced mobility
Chairridden
Reduced mobility NOS
Excludes2: *wheelchair dependence (Z99.3)*

Z74.1 Need for assistance with personal care

Z74.2 Need for assistance at home and no other household member able to render care

Z74.3 Need for continuous supervision

Z74.8 Other problems related to care provider dependency

Z74.9 Problem related to care provider dependency, unspecified

Z75 Problems related to medical facilities and other health care

Z75.0 Medical services not available in home
Excludes1: *no other household member able to render care (Z74.2)*

Z75.1 Person awaiting admission to adequate facility elsewhere
AHA CC: 4Q, 2017, 112-114
Review coding guideline B.19.d

Z75.2 Other waiting period for investigation and treatment

Z75.3 Unavailability and inaccessibility of health-care facilities
Excludes1: *bed unavailable (Z75.1)*
AHA CC: 4Q, 2017, 112-114
Review coding guideline B.19.d

Z75.4 Unavailability and inaccessibility of other helping agencies
AHA CC: 4Q, 2017, 112-114
Review coding guideline B.19.d

Z75.5 Holiday relief care

Z75.8 Other problems related to medical facilities and other health care

Z75.9 Unspecified problem related to medical facilities and other health care

Z76 Persons encountering health services in other circumstances

Z76.0 Encounter for issue of repeat prescription
Encounter for issue of repeat prescription for appliance
Encounter for issue of repeat prescription for medicaments
Encounter for issue of repeat prescription for spectacles
Excludes2: *issue of medical certificate (Z02.7)*
repeat prescription for contraceptive (Z30.4-)

Z76.1 Encounter for health supervision and care of foundling
Review coding guidelines C.21.c.12 and C.21.c.16

● **Z76.2 Encounter for health supervision and care of other healthy infant and child**
Encounter for medical or nursing care or supervision of healthy infant under circumstances such as adverse socioeconomic conditions at home
Encounter for medical or nursing care or supervision of healthy infant under circumstances such as awaiting foster or adoptive placement
Encounter for medical or nursing care or supervision of healthy infant under circumstances such as maternal illness
Encounter for medical or nursing care or supervision of healthy infant under circumstances such as number of children at home preventing or interfering with normal care
AHA CC: 4Q, 2017, 112-114
Review coding guidelines B.19.d and C.21.c.16

Z76.3 Healthy person accompanying sick person

Z76.4 Other boarder to healthcare facility
Excludes1: *homelessness (Z59.0-)*

Z76.5 Malingerer [conscious simulation]
Person feigning illness (with obvious motivation)
Excludes1: *factitious disorder (F68.1-, F68.A)*
peregrinating patient (F68.1-)

+ **Z76.8 Persons encountering health services in other specified circumstances**

Z76.81 Expectant parent(s) prebirth pediatrician visit
Pre-adoption pediatrician visit for adoptive parent(s)
Review coding guideline C.21.c.10

Z76.82 Awaiting organ transplant status
Patient waiting for organ availability
Review coding guideline C.21.c.3

Z76.89 Persons encountering health services in other specified circumstances
Persons encountering health services NOS
AHA CC: 2Q, 2014, 10

Persons with potential health hazards related to family and personal history and certain conditions influencing health status (Z77-Z99)

Code also any follow-up examination (Z08-Z09)

Z77 Other contact with and (suspected) exposures hazardous to health

Includes: contact with and (suspected) exposures to potential hazards to health
Excludes2: *contact with and (suspected) exposure to communicable diseases (Z20.-)*
exposure to (parental) (environmental) tobacco smoke in the perinatal period (P96.81)
newborn affected by noxious substances transmitted via placenta or breast milk (P04.-)
occupational exposure to risk factors (Z57.-)
retained foreign body (Z18.-)
retained foreign body fully removed (Z87.821)
toxic effects of substances chiefly nonmedicinal as to source (T51-T65)
Review coding guideline C.21.c.1

+ **Z77.0 Contact with and (suspected) exposure to hazardous, chiefly nonmedicinal, chemicals**

+ **Z77.01 Contact with and (suspected) exposure to hazardous metals**

Z77.010 Contact with and (suspected) exposure to arsenic

Z77.011 Contact with and (suspected) exposure to lead

Z77.012 Contact with and (suspected) exposure to uranium
Excludes1: *retained depleted uranium fragments (Z18.01)*

Z77.018 Contact with and (suspected) exposure to other hazardous metals
Contact with and (suspected) exposure to chromium compounds
Contact with and (suspected) exposure to nickel dust

+ **Z77.02 Contact with and (suspected) exposure to hazardous aromatic compounds**

Z77.020 Contact with and (suspected) exposure to aromatic amines

Z77.021 Contact with and (suspected) exposure to benzene

Z77.028 Contact with and (suspected) exposure to other hazardous aromatic compounds
Aromatic dyes NOS
Polycyclic aromatic hydrocarbons

+ **Z77.09 Contact with and (suspected) exposure to other hazardous, chiefly nonmedicinal, chemicals**

Z77.090 Contact with and (suspected) exposure to asbestos

Z77.098 Contact with and (suspected) exposure to other hazardous, chiefly nonmedicinal, chemicals
Dyes NOS

+ **Z77.1 Contact with and (suspected) exposure to environmental pollution and hazards in the physical environment**

+ **Z77.11 Contact with and (suspected) exposure to environmental pollution**

Z77.110 Contact with and (suspected) exposure to air pollution

Z77.111 Contact with and (suspected) exposure to water pollution

Z77.112 Contact with and (suspected) exposure to soil pollution

Z77.118 Contact with and (suspected) exposure to other environmental pollution

+ **Z77.12 Contact with and (suspected) exposure to hazards in the physical environment**

Z77.120 Contact with and (suspected) exposure to mold (toxic)

Z77.121 Contact with and (suspected) exposure to harmful algae and algae toxins
Contact with and (suspected) exposure to (harmful) algae bloom NOS
Contact with and (suspected) exposure to blue-green algae bloom
Contact with and (suspected) exposure to brown tide
Contact with and (suspected) exposure to cyanobacteria bloom
Contact with and (suspected) exposure to Florida red tide
Contact with and (suspected) exposure to pfiesteria piscicida
Contact with and (suspected) exposure to red tide

Z77.122 Contact with and (suspected) exposure to noise

Z77.123 Contact with and (suspected) exposure to radon and other naturally occurring radiation
Excludes2: *radiation exposure as the cause of a confirmed condition (W88-W90, X39.0-)*
radiation sickness NOS (T66)

Z77.128 Contact with and (suspected) exposure to other hazards in the physical environment

+ **Z77.2 Contact with and (suspected) exposure to other hazardous substances**

Z77.21 Contact with and (suspected) exposure to potentially hazardous body fluids

Z77.22 Contact with and (suspected) exposure to environmental tobacco smoke (acute) (chronic)
Exposure to second hand tobacco smoke (acute) (chronic)
Passive smoking (acute) (chronic)
Excludes1: *nicotine dependence (F17.-)*
tobacco use (Z72.0)
Excludes2: *occupational exposure to environmental tobacco smoke (Z57.31)*

Z77.29 Contact with and (suspected) exposure to other hazardous substances
AHA CC: 2Q, 2016, 34

Z77.9 Other contact with and (suspected) exposures hazardous to health

Z78 Other specified health status

Excludes2: *asymptomatic human immunodeficiency virus [HIV] infection status (Z21)*
postprocedural status (Z93-Z99)
sex reassignment status (Z87.890)

Review coding guideline C.21.c.3

● ♀ **Z78.0 Asymptomatic menopausal state**
Menopausal state NOS
Postmenopausal status NOS
Excludes2: *symptomatic menopausal state (N95.1)*

Z78.1 Physical restraint status
Excludes1: *physical restraint due to a procedure - omit code*

Z78.9 Other specified health status

Z79 Long term (current) drug therapy

Includes: long term (current) drug use for prophylactic purposes
Code also any therapeutic drug level monitoring (Z51.81)
Excludes2: *drug abuse and dependence (F11-F19)*
drug use complicating pregnancy, childbirth, and the puerperium (O99.32-)

AHA CC: 1Q, 2021, 12-13
Review coding guideline C.21.c.3

\+ **Z79.0 Long term (current) use of anticoagulants and antithrombotics/antiplatelets**
Excludes2: *long term (current) use of aspirin (Z79.82)*

Z79.01 Long term (current) use of anticoagulants
AHA CC: 2Q, 2020, 20-21; 1Q, 2021, 4-5

Z79.02 Long term (current) use of antithrombotics/antiplatelets

Z79.1 Long term (current) use of non-steroidal anti-inflammatories (NSAID)
Excludes2: *long term (current) use of aspirin (Z79.82)*

Z79.2 Long term (current) use of antibiotics

Z79.3 Long term (current) use of hormonal contraceptives
Long term (current) use of birth control pill or patch

Z79.4 Long term (current) use of insulin
Excludes2: *long term (current) use of oral antidiabetic drugs (Z79.84)*
long term (current) use of oral hypoglycemic drugs (Z79.84)

AHA CC: 3Q, 2020, 31
Review coding guidelines C.4.a.3 and C.4.a.6
Review coding guidelines C.15.h and C.15.i

\+ **Z79.5 Long term (current) use of steroids**

Z79.51 Long term (current) use of inhaled steroids

Z79.52 Long term (current) use of systemic steroids

\+ **Z79.8 Other long term (current) drug therapy**

\+ **Z79.81 Long term (current) use of agents affecting estrogen receptors and estrogen levels**
Code first if applicable:
malignant neoplasm of breast (C50.-)
malignant neoplasm of prostate (C61)

Use additional code, if applicable, to identify:
estrogen receptor positive status (Z17.0)
family history of breast cancer (Z80.3)
genetic susceptibility to malignant neoplasm (cancer) (Z15.0-)
personal history of breast cancer (Z85.3)
personal history of prostate cancer (Z85.46)
postmenopausal status (Z78.0)
Excludes1: *hormone replacement therapy (Z79.890)*

Z79.810 Long term (current) use of selective estrogen receptor modulators (SERMs)
Long term (current) use of raloxifene (Evista)
Long term (current) use of tamoxifen (Nolvadex)
Long term (current) use of toremifene (Fareston)

Z79.811 Long term (current) use of aromatase inhibitors
Long term (current) use of anastrozole (Arimidex)
Long term (current) use of exemestane (Aromasin)
Long term (current) use of letrozole (Femara)

Z79.818 Long term (current) use of other agents affecting estrogen receptors and estrogen levels
Long term (current) use of estrogen receptor downregulators
Long term (current) use of fulvestrant (Faslodex)
Long term (current) use of gonadotropin-releasing hormone (GnRH) agonist
Long term (current) use of goserelin acetate (Zoladex)
Long term (current) use of leuprolide acetate (leuprorelin) (Lupron)
Long term (current) use of megestrol acetate (Megace)

Z79.82 Long term (current) use of aspirin

Z79.83 Long term (current) use of bisphosphonates
AHA CC: 4Q, 2016, 21

Z79.84 Long term (current) use of oral hypoglycemic drugs
Long term (current) use of oral antidiabetic drugs
Excludes2: *long term (current) use of insulin (Z79.4)*

Review coding guidelines C.4.a.e and C.4.a.6
Review coding guidelines C.15.h and C.15.i
AHA CC: 4Q, 2016, 76; 3Q, 2020, 31

\+ **Z79.89 Other long term (current) drug therapy**

Z79.890 Hormone replacement therapy

Z79.891 Long term (current) use of opiate analgesic
Long term (current) use of methadone for pain management
Excludes1: *methodone use NOS (F11.9-)*
use of methodone for treatment of heroin addiction (F11.2-)

Z79.899 Other long term (current) drug therapy
AHA CC: 3Q, 2015, 21-22; 4Q, 2015, 34; 2Q, 2020, 14-15; 3Q, 2020, 31; 4Q, 2020, 11-12
Review coding guideline C.4.a.3

Z80 Family history of primary malignant neoplasm

Review coding guideline C.21.c.4

Z80.0 Family history of malignant neoplasm of digestive organs
Conditions classifiable to C15-C26
AHA CC: 1Q, 2018, 6-7

Z80.1 Family history of malignant neoplasm of trachea, bronchus and lung
Conditions classifiable to C33-C34

Z80.2 Family history of malignant neoplasm of other respiratory and intrathoracic organs
Conditions classifiable to C30-C32, C37-C39

Z80.3 Family history of malignant neoplasm of breast
Conditions classifiable to C50.-

\+ **Z80.4 Family history of malignant neoplasm of genital organs**
Conditions classifiable to C51-C63

Z80.41 Family history of malignant neoplasm of ovary

Z80.42 Family history of malignant neoplasm of prostate

Z80.43 Family history of malignant neoplasm of testis

Z80.49 Family history of malignant neoplasm of other genital organs

\+ **Z80.5 Family history of malignant neoplasm of urinary tract**
Conditions classifiable to C64-C68

Z80.51 Family history of malignant neoplasm of kidney

Z80.52 Family history of malignant neoplasm of bladder

Z80.59 Family history of malignant neoplasm of other urinary tract organ

Z80.6 Family history of leukemia
Conditions classifiable to C91-C95

Z80.7 Family history of other malignant neoplasms of lymphoid, hematopoietic and related tissues
Conditions classifiable to C81-C90, C96.-

Z80.8 Family history of malignant neoplasm of other organs or systems
Conditions classifiable to C00-C14, C40-C49, C69-C79

Z80.9 Family history of malignant neoplasm, unspecified
Conditions classifiable to C80.1

Z81 Family history of mental and behavioral disorders
Review coding guideline C.21.c.4
Z81.0 Family history of intellectual disabilities
Conditions classifiable to F70-F79
Z81.1 Family history of alcohol abuse and dependence
Conditions classifiable to F10.-
Z81.2 Family history of tobacco abuse and dependence
Conditions classifiable to F17.-
Z81.3 Family history of other psychoactive substance abuse and dependence
Conditions classifiable to F11-F16, F18-F19
Z81.4 Family history of other substance abuse and dependence
Conditions classifiable to F55
Z81.8 Family history of other mental and behavioral disorders
Conditions classifiable elsewhere in F01-F99

Z82 Family history of certain disabilities and chronic diseases (leading to disablement)
Review coding guideline C.21.c.4
Z82.0 Family history of epilepsy and other diseases of the nervous system
Conditions classifiable to G00-G99
Z82.1 Family history of blindness and visual loss
Conditions classifiable to H54.-
Z82.2 Family history of deafness and hearing loss
Conditions classifiable to H90-H91
Z82.3 Family history of stroke
Conditions classifiable to I60-I64
+ **Z82.4 Family history of ischemic heart disease and other diseases of the circulatory system**
Conditions classifiable to I00-I5A, I65-I99
Z82.41 Family history of sudden cardiac death
Z82.49 Family history of ischemic heart disease and other diseases of the circulatory system
Z82.5 Family history of asthma and other chronic lower respiratory diseases
Conditions classifiable to J40-J47
Excludes2: *family history of other diseases of the respiratory system (Z83.6)*
+ **Z82.6 Family history of arthritis and other diseases of the musculoskeletal system and connective tissue**
Conditions classifiable to M00-M99
Z82.61 Family history of arthritis
Z82.62 Family history of osteoporosis
Z82.69 Family history of other diseases of the musculoskeletal system and connective tissue
+ **Z82.7 Family history of congenital malformations, deformations and chromosomal abnormalities**
Conditions classifiable to Q00-Q99
Z82.71 Family history of polycystic kidney
Z82.79 Family history of other congenital malformations, deformations and chromosomal abnormalities
Z82.8 Family history of other disabilities and chronic diseases leading to disablement, not elsewhere classified

Z83 Family history of other specific disorders
Excludes2: *contact with and (suspected) exposure to communicable disease in the family (Z20.-)*
Review coding guideline C.21.c.4
Z83.0 Family history of human immunodeficiency virus [HIV] disease
Conditions classifiable to B20
Z83.1 Family history of other infectious and parasitic diseases
Conditions classifiable to A00-B19, B25-B94, B99
Z83.2 Family history of diseases of the blood and blood-forming organs and certain disorders involving the immune mechanism
Conditions classifiable to D50-D89
Z83.3 Family history of diabetes mellitus
Conditions classifiable to E08-E13
+ **Z83.4 Family history of other endocrine, nutritional and metabolic diseases**
Conditions classifiable to E00-E07, E15-E88
Z83.41 Family history of multiple endocrine neoplasia [MEN] syndrome
Z83.42 Family history of familial hypercholesterolemia
AHA CC: 4Q, 2016, 77
+ **Z83.43 Family history of other disorder of lipoprotein metabolism and other lipidemias**
AHA CC: 4Q, 2018, 6
Z83.430 Family history of elevated lipoprotein(a)
Family history of elevated Lp(a)
Z83.438 Family history of other disorder of lipoprotein metabolism and other lipidemia
Family history of familial combined hyperlipidemia
Z83.49 Family history of other endocrine, nutritional and metabolic diseases
+ **Z83.5 Family history of eye and ear disorders**
+ **Z83.51 Family history of eye disorders**
Conditions classifiable to H00-H53, H55-H59
Excludes2: *family history of blindness and visual loss (Z82.1)*
Z83.511 Family history of glaucoma
Z83.518 Family history of other specified eye disorder
Z83.52 Family history of ear disorders
Conditions classifiable to H60-H83, H92-H95
Excludes2: *family history of deafness and hearing loss (Z82.2)*
Z83.6 Family history of other diseases of the respiratory system
Conditions classifiable to J00-J39, J60-J99
Excludes2: *family history of asthma and other chronic lower respiratory diseases (Z82.5)*
+ **Z83.7 Family history of diseases of the digestive system**
Conditions classifiable to K00-K93
Z83.71 Family history of colonic polyps
Excludes2: *family history of malignant neoplasm of digestive organs (Z80.0)*
AHA CC: 1Q, 2021, 14-15
Z83.79 Family history of other diseases of the digestive system

Z84 Family history of other conditions
Review coding guideline C.21.c.4
Z84.0 Family history of diseases of the skin and subcutaneous tissue
Conditions classifiable to L00-L99
Z84.1 Family history of disorders of kidney and ureter
Conditions classifiable to N00-N29
Z84.2 Family history of other diseases of the genitourinary system
Conditions classifiable to N30-N99
Z84.3 Family history of consanguinity
+ **Z84.8 Family history of other specified conditions**
Z84.81 Family history of carrier of genetic disease
AHA CC: 1Q, 2021, 14-15
Z84.82 Family history of sudden infant death syndrome
Family history of SIDS
AHA CC: 4Q, 2016, 77
Z84.89 Family history of other specified conditions

Z85 Personal history of malignant neoplasm
Code first any follow-up examination after treatment of malignant neoplasm (Z08)
Use additional code to identify:
alcohol use and dependence (F10.-)
exposure to environmental tobacco smoke (Z77.22)
history of tobacco dependence (Z87.891)
occupational exposure to environmental tobacco smoke (Z57.31)
tobacco dependence (F17.-)
tobacco use (Z72.0)
Excludes2: *personal history of benign neoplasm (Z86.01-)*
personal history of carcinoma-in-situ (Z86.00-)
Review coding guidelines C.2.d and C.2.m
Review coding guideline C.21.c.4
+ **Z85.0 Personal history of malignant neoplasm of digestive organs**
Z85.00 Personal history of malignant neoplasm of unspecified digestive organ
Z85.01 Personal history of malignant neoplasm of esophagus
Conditions classifiable to C15

+ Z85.02 **Personal history of malignant neoplasm of stomach**
  - Z85.020 **Personal history of malignant carcinoid tumor of stomach**
    Conditions classifiable to C7A.092
  - Z85.028 **Personal history of other malignant neoplasm of stomach**
    Conditions classifiable to C16

+ Z85.03 **Personal history of malignant neoplasm of large intestine**
  - Z85.030 **Personal history of malignant carcinoid tumor of large intestine**
    Conditions classifiable to C7A.022-C7A.025, C7A.029
  - Z85.038 **Personal history of other malignant neoplasm of large intestine**
    Conditions classifiable to C18

+ Z85.04 **Personal history of malignant neoplasm of rectum, rectosigmoid junction, and anus**
  - Z85.040 **Personal history of malignant carcinoid tumor of rectum**
    Conditions classifiable to C7A.026
  - Z85.048 **Personal history of other malignant neoplasm of rectum, rectosigmoid junction, and anus**
    Conditions classifiable to C19-C21

Z85.05 **Personal history of malignant neoplasm of liver**
Conditions classifiable to C22

+ Z85.06 **Personal history of malignant neoplasm of small intestine**
  - Z85.060 **Personal history of malignant carcinoid tumor of small intestine**
    Conditions classifiable to C7A.01-
  - Z85.068 **Personal history of other malignant neoplasm of small intestine**
    Conditions classifiable to C17

Z85.07 **Personal history of malignant neoplasm of pancreas**
Conditions classifiable to C25

Z85.09 **Personal history of malignant neoplasm of other digestive organs**

+ Z85.1 **Personal history of malignant neoplasm of trachea, bronchus and lung**

+ Z85.11 **Personal history of malignant neoplasm of bronchus and lung**
  - Z85.110 **Personal history of malignant carcinoid tumor of bronchus and lung**
    Conditions classifiable to C7A.090
  - Z85.118 **Personal history of other malignant neoplasm of bronchus and lung**
    Conditions classifiable to C34

Z85.12 **Personal history of malignant neoplasm of trachea**
Conditions classifiable to C33

+ Z85.2 **Personal history of malignant neoplasm of other respiratory and intrathoracic organs**

Z85.20 **Personal history of malignant neoplasm of unspecified respiratory organ**

Z85.21 **Personal history of malignant neoplasm of larynx**
Conditions classifiable to C32

Z85.22 **Personal history of malignant neoplasm of nasal cavities, middle ear, and accessory sinuses**
Conditions classifiable to C30-C31

+ Z85.23 **Personal history of malignant neoplasm of thymus**
  - Z85.230 **Personal history of malignant carcinoid tumor of thymus**
    Conditions classifiable to C7A.091
  - Z85.238 **Personal history of other malignant neoplasm of thymus**
    Conditions classifiable to C37

Z85.29 **Personal history of malignant neoplasm of other respiratory and intrathoracic organs**

Z85.3 **Personal history of malignant neoplasm of breast**
Conditions classifiable to C50.-
AHA CC: 3Q, 2020, 30

+ Z85.4 **Personal history of malignant neoplasm of genital organs**
Conditions classifiable to C51-C63

♀ Z85.40 **Personal history of malignant neoplasm of unspecified female genital organ**

♀ Z85.41 **Personal history of malignant neoplasm of cervix uteri**

♀ Z85.42 **Personal history of malignant neoplasm of other parts of uterus**

♀ Z85.43 **Personal history of malignant neoplasm of ovary**

♀ Z85.44 **Personal history of malignant neoplasm of other female genital organs**

♂ Z85.45 **Personal history of malignant neoplasm of unspecified male genital organ**

♂ Z85.46 **Personal history of malignant neoplasm of prostate**

♂ Z85.47 **Personal history of malignant neoplasm of testis**

♂ Z85.48 **Personal history of malignant neoplasm of epididymis**

♂ Z85.49 **Personal history of malignant neoplasm of other male genital organs**

+ Z85.5 **Personal history of malignant neoplasm of urinary tract**
Conditions classifiable to C64-C68

Z85.50 **Personal history of malignant neoplasm of unspecified urinary tract organ**

Z85.51 **Personal history of malignant neoplasm of bladder**

+ Z85.52 **Personal history of malignant neoplasm of kidney**
Excludes1: *personal history of malignant neoplasm of renal pelvis (Z85.53)*
  - Z85.520 **Personal history of malignant carcinoid tumor of kidney**
    Conditions classifiable to C7A.093
  - Z85.528 **Personal history of other malignant neoplasm of kidney**
    Conditions classifiable to C64

Z85.53 **Personal history of malignant neoplasm of renal pelvis**

Z85.54 **Personal history of malignant neoplasm of ureter**

Z85.59 **Personal history of malignant neoplasm of other urinary tract organ**

Z85.6 **Personal history of leukemia**
Conditions classifiable to C91-C95
Excludes1: *leukemia in remission C91.0-C95.9 with 5th character 1*
Review coding guideline C.2.n

+ Z85.7 **Personal history of other malignant neoplasms of lymphoid, hematopoietic and related tissues**

Z85.71 **Personal history of Hodgkin lymphoma**
Conditions classifiable to C81

Z85.72 **Personal history of non-Hodgkin lymphomas**
Conditions classifiable to C82-C85

Z85.79 **Personal history of other malignant neoplasms of lymphoid, hematopoietic and related tissues**
Conditions classifiable to C88-C90, C96
Excludes1: *multiple myeloma in remission (C90.01)*
plasma cell leukemia in remission (C90.11)
plasmacytoma in remission (C90.21)
Review coding guideline C.2.n

+ Z85.8 **Personal history of malignant neoplasms of other organs and systems**
Conditions classifiable to C00-C14, C40-C49, C69-C75, C7A.098, C76-C79

+ Z85.81 **Personal history of malignant neoplasm of lip, oral cavity, and pharynx**
Conditions classifiable to C00-C14
  - Z85.810 **Personal history of malignant neoplasm of tongue**
  - Z85.818 **Personal history of malignant neoplasm of other sites of lip, oral cavity, and pharynx**
  - Z85.819 **Personal history of malignant neoplasm of unspecified site of lip, oral cavity, and pharynx**

+ Z85.82 **Personal history of malignant neoplasm of skin**
  - Z85.820 **Personal history of malignant melanoma of skin**
    Conditions classifiable to C43
  - Z85.821 **Personal history of Merkel cell carcinoma**
    Conditions classifiable to C4A
  - Z85.828 **Personal history of other malignant neoplasm of skin**
    Conditions classifiable to C44

+ **Z85.83 Personal history of malignant neoplasm of bone and soft tissue**
  Conditions classifiable to C40-C41; C45-C49
  Z85.830 Personal history of malignant neoplasm of bone
  Z85.831 Personal history of malignant neoplasm of soft tissue
  Excludes2: *personal history of malignant neoplasm of skin (Z85.82-)*
+ **Z85.84 Personal history of malignant neoplasm of eye and nervous tissue**
  Conditions classifiable to C69-C72
  Z85.840 Personal history of malignant neoplasm of eye
  Z85.841 Personal history of malignant neoplasm of brain
  Z85.848 Personal history of malignant neoplasm of other parts of nervous tissue
+ **Z85.85 Personal history of malignant neoplasm of endocrine glands**
  Conditions classifiable to C73-C75
  Z85.850 Personal history of malignant neoplasm of thyroid
  Z85.858 Personal history of malignant neoplasm of other endocrine glands
Z85.89 Personal history of malignant neoplasm of other organs and systems
  Conditions classifiable to C7A.098, C76, C77-C79
Z85.9 Personal history of malignant neoplasm, unspecified
  Conditions classifiable to C7A.00, C80.1

Z86 Personal history of certain other diseases
Code first any follow-up examination after treatment (Z09)
AHA CC: 4Q, 2019, 20
Review coding guideline C.21.c.4

+ **Z86.0 Personal history of in-situ and benign neoplasms and neoplasms of uncertain behavior**
  Excludes2: *personal history of malignant neoplasms (Z85.-)*
+ **Z86.00 Personal history of in-situ neoplasm**
  Conditions classifiable to D00-D09
  Z86.000 Personal history of in-situ neoplasm of breast
  Conditions classifiable to D05
  ♀ **Z86.001 Personal history of in-situ neoplasm of cervix uteri**
  Conditions classifiable to D06
  Personal history of cervical intraepithelial neoplasia III [CINIII]
  Z86.002 Personal history of in-situ neoplasm of other and unspecified genital organs
  Conditions classifiable to D07
  Personal history of high-grade prostatic intraepithelial neoplasia III [HGPIN III]
  Personal history of vaginal intraepithelial neoplasia III [VAIN III]
  Personal history of vulvar intraepithelial neoplasia III [VAN III]
  Z86.003 Personal history of in-situ neoplasm of oral cavity, esophagus and stomach
  Conditions classifiable to D00
  Z86.004 Personal history of in-situ neoplasm of other and unspecified digestive organs
  Conditions classifiable to D01
  Personal history of anal intraepithelial neoplasia III [AIN III]
  Z86.005 Personal history of in-situ neoplasm of middle ear and respiratory system
  Conditions classifiable to D02
  Z86.006 Personal history of melanoma in-situ
  Conditions classifiable to D03
  Excludes2: *sites other than skin - code to personal history of in-situ neoplasm of the site*
  Z86.007 Personal history of in-situ neoplasm of skin
  Conditions classifiable to D04
  Personal history of carcinoma in-situ of skin
  Z86.008 Personal history of in-situ neoplasm of other site
  Conditions classifiable to D09
+ **Z86.01 Personal history of benign neoplasm**
  Z86.010 Personal history of colonic polyps
  AHA CC: 1Q, 2017, 9; 1Q, 2021, 14-15
  Z86.011 Personal history of benign neoplasm of the brain
  Z86.012 Personal history of benign carcinoid tumor
  Z86.018 Personal history of other benign neoplasm
Z86.03 Personal history of neoplasm of uncertain behavior
+ **Z86.1 Personal history of infectious and parasitic diseases**
  Conditions classifiable to A00-B89, B99
  Excludes1: *personal history of infectious diseases specific to a body system*
  sequelae of infectious and parasitic diseases (B90-B94)
  AHA CC: 4Q, 2016, 4-7
  Z86.11 Personal history of tuberculosis
  Z86.12 Personal history of poliomyelitis
  Z86.13 Personal history of malaria
  Z86.14 Personal history of Methicillin resistant Staphylococcus aureus infection
  Personal history of MRSA infection
  Z86.15 Personal history of latent tuberculosis infection
  Z86.16 Personal history of COVID-19
  Excludes1: *post COVID-19 condition (U09.9)*
  AHA CC: 1Q, 2021, 33-35, 40-42
  Z86.19 Personal history of other infectious and parasitic diseases
  AHA CC: 2Q, 2020, 10-12; 3Q, 2020, 13; 1Q, 2021, 33-35, 40-41
  Review coding guideline C.1.g.1.i
Z86.2 Personal history of diseases of the blood and blood-forming organs and certain disorders involving the immune mechanism
  Conditions classifiable to D50-D89
+ **Z86.3 Personal history of endocrine, nutritional and metabolic diseases**
  Conditions classifiable to E00-E88
  Z86.31 Personal history of diabetic foot ulcer
  Excludes2: *current diabetic foot ulcer (E08.621, E09.621, E10.621, E11.621, E13.621)*
  ♀ **Z86.32 Personal history of gestational diabetes**
  Personal history of conditions classifiable to O24.4-
  Excludes1: *gestational diabetes mellitus in current pregnancy (O24.4-)*
  Z86.39 Personal history of other endocrine, nutritional and metabolic disease
  AHA CC: 1Q, 2020, 12-13
+ **Z86.5 Personal history of mental and behavioral disorders**
  Conditions classifiable to F40-F59
  • **Z86.51 Personal history of combat and operational stress reaction**
  Z86.59 Personal history of other mental and behavioral disorders
+ **Z86.6 Personal history of diseases of the nervous system and sense organs**
  Conditions classifiable to G00-G99, H00-H95
  Z86.61 Personal history of infections of the central nervous system
  Personal history of encephalitis
  Personal history of meningitis
  Z86.69 Personal history of other diseases of the nervous system and sense organs
  AHA CC: 4Q, 2016, 21
+ **Z86.7 Personal history of diseases of the circulatory system**
  Conditions classifiable to I00-I99
  Excludes2: *old myocardial infarction (I25.2)*
  personal history of anaphylactic shock (Z87.892)
  postmyocardial infarction syndrome (I24.1)
+ **Z86.71 Personal history of venous thrombosis and embolism**
  Z86.711 Personal history of pulmonary embolism
  Z86.718 Personal history of other venous thrombosis and embolism
  AHA CC: 2Q, 2020, 20-21

Z86.72 **Personal history of thrombophlebitis**

Z86.73 **Personal history of transient ischemic attack (TIA), and cerebral infarction without residual deficits**

Personal history of prolonged reversible ischemic neurological deficit (PRIND)

Personal history of stroke NOS without residual deficits

Excludes1: *personal history of traumatic brain injury (Z87.820)*

sequelae of cerebrovascular disease (I69.-)

Review coding guideline C.9.d.3

Z86.74 **Personal history of sudden cardiac arrest**

Personal history of sudden cardiac death successfully resuscitated

Z86.79 **Personal history of other diseases of the circulatory system**

AHA CC: 1Q, 2020, 12-13

Z87 **Personal history of other diseases and conditions**

Code first any follow-up examination after treatment (Z09)

Review coding guideline C.21.c.4

+ **Z87.0** **Personal history of diseases of the respiratory system**

Conditions classifiable to J00-J99

Z87.01 **Personal history of pneumonia (recurrent)**

Z87.09 **Personal history of other diseases of the respiratory system**

+ **Z87.1** **Personal history of diseases of the digestive system**

Conditions classifiable to K00-K93

Z87.11 **Personal history of peptic ulcer disease**

Z87.19 **Personal history of other diseases of the digestive system**

AHA CC: 1Q, 2017, 14-15

Z87.2 **Personal history of diseases of the skin and subcutaneous tissue**

Conditions classifiable to L00-L99

Excludes2: *personal history of diabetic foot ulcer (Z86.31)*

+ **Z87.3** **Personal history of diseases of the musculoskeletal system and connective tissue**

Conditions classifiable to M00-M99

Excludes2: *personal history of (healed) traumatic fracture (Z87.81)*

+ **Z87.31** **Personal history of (healed) nontraumatic fracture**

Z87.310 **Personal history of (healed) osteoporosis fracture**

Personal history of (healed) fragility fracture

Personal history of (healed) collapsed vertebra due to osteoporosis

Review coding guideline C.13.d.1

Z87.311 **Personal history of (healed) other pathological fracture**

Personal history of (healed) collapsed vertebra NOS

Excludes2: *personal history of osteoporosis fracture (Z87.310)*

Z87.312 **Personal history of (healed) stress fracture**

Personal history of (healed) fatigue fracture

Z87.39 **Personal history of other diseases of the musculoskeletal system and connective tissue**

+ **Z87.4** **Personal history of diseases of genitourinary system**

Conditions classifiable to N00-N99

+ **Z87.41** **Personal history of dysplasia of the female genital tract**

Excludes1: *personal history of malignant neoplasm of female genital tract (Z85.40-Z85.44)*

personal history of intraepithelial neoplasia III of female genital tract (Z86.001, Z86.008)

♀ **Z87.410** **Personal history of cervical dysplasia**

♀ **Z87.411** **Personal history of vaginal dysplasia**

♀ **Z87.412** **Personal history of vulvar dysplasia**

♀ **Z87.42** **Personal history of other diseases of the female genital tract**

+ **Z87.43** **Personal history of diseases of male genital organs**

♂ **Z87.430** **Personal history of prostatic dysplasia**

Excludes1: *personal history of malignant neoplasm of prostate (Z85.46)*

♂ **Z87.438** **Personal history of other diseases of male genital organs**

+ **Z87.44** **Personal history of diseases of urinary system**

Excludes1: *personal history of malignant neoplasm of cervix uteri (Z85.41)*

Z87.440 **Personal history of urinary (tract) infections**

Z87.441 **Personal history of nephrotic syndrome**

Z87.442 **Personal history of urinary calculi**

Personal history of kidney stones

Z87.448 **Personal history of other diseases of urinary system**

+ **Z87.5** **Personal history of complications of pregnancy, childbirth and the puerperium**

Conditions classifiable to O00-O9A

Excludes2: *recurrent pregnancy loss (N96)*

♀ **Z87.51** **Personal history of pre-term labor**

Excludes1: *current pregnancy with history of pre-term labor (O09.21-)*

♀ **Z87.59** **Personal history of other complications of pregnancy, childbirth and the puerperium**

Personal history of trophoblastic disease

+ **Z87.7** **Personal history of (corrected) congenital malformations**

Conditions classifiable to Q00-Q89 that have been repaired or corrected

Excludes1: *congenital malformations that have been partially corrected or repair but which still require medical treatment - code to condition*

Excludes2: *other postprocedural states (Z98.-)*

personal history of medical treatment (Z92.-)

presence of cardiac and vascular implants and grafts (Z95.-)

presence of other devices (Z97.-)

presence of other functional implants (Z96.-)

transplanted organ and tissue status (Z94.-)

+ **Z87.71** **Personal history of (corrected) congenital malformations of genitourinary system**

♂ **Z87.710** **Personal history of (corrected) hypospadias**

Z87.718 **Personal history of other specified (corrected) congenital malformations of genitourinary system**

+ **Z87.72** **Personal history of (corrected) congenital malformations of nervous system and sense organs**

Z87.720 **Personal history of (corrected) congenital malformations of eye**

Z87.721 **Personal history of (corrected) congenital malformations of ear**

Z87.728 **Personal history of other specified (corrected) congenital malformations of nervous system and sense organs**

+ **Z87.73** **Personal history of (corrected) congenital malformations of digestive system**

Z87.730 **Personal history of (corrected) cleft lip and palate**

Z87.738 **Personal history of other specified (corrected) congenital malformations of digestive system**

Z87.74 **Personal history of (corrected) congenital malformations of heart and circulatory system**

Z87.75 **Personal history of (corrected) congenital malformations of respiratory system**

Z87.76 **Personal history of (corrected) congenital malformations of integument, limbs and musculoskeletal system**

+ **Z87.79** **Personal history of other (corrected) congenital malformations**

Z87.790 **Personal history of (corrected) congenital malformations of face and neck**

Z87.798 **Personal history of other (corrected) congenital malformations**

+ **Z87.8 Personal history of other specified conditions**
  Excludes2: *personal history of self harm (Z91.5-)*
  - **Z87.81 Personal history of (healed) traumatic fracture**
    Excludes2: *personal history of (healed) nontraumatic fracture (Z87.31-)*
  - + **Z87.82 Personal history of other (healed) physical injury and trauma**
    Conditions classifiable to S00-T88, except traumatic fractures
    - **Z87.820 Personal history of traumatic brain injury**
      Excludes1: *personal history of transient ischemicattack(TIA),and cerebralinfarctionwithout residual deficits (Z86.73)*
    - **Z87.821 Personal history of retained foreign body fully removed**
    - **Z87.828 Personal history of other (healed) physical injury and trauma**
  - + **Z87.89 Personal history of other specified conditions**
    - **Z87.890 Personal history of sex reassignment**
    - **Z87.891 Personal history of nicotine dependence**
      Excludes1: *current nicotine dependence (F17.2-)*
      AHA CC: 2Q, 2017, 26-28
    - **Z87.892 Personal history of anaphylaxis**
      Code also allergy status such as:
      allergy status to drugs, medicaments and biological substances (Z88.-)
      allergy status, other than to drugs and biological substances (Z91.0-)
    - **Z87.898 Personal history of other specified conditions**
      AHA CC: 1Q, 2013, 21

Z88 Allergy status to drugs, medicaments and biological substances
Excludes2: *Allergy status, other than to drugs and biological substances (Z91.0-)*
Review coding guideline C.21.c.3
- **Z88.0 Allergy status to penicillin**
- **Z88.1 Allergy status to other antibiotic agents**
- **Z88.2 Allergy status to sulfonamides**
  AHA CC: 3Q, 2015, 23
- **Z88.3 Allergy status to other anti-infective agents**
- **Z88.4 Allergy status to anesthetic agent**
- **Z88.5 Allergy status to narcotic agent**
- **Z88.6 Allergy status to analgesic agent**
- **Z88.7 Allergy status to serum and vaccine**
- **Z88.8 Allergy status to other drugs, medicaments and biological substances**
- **Z88.9 Allergy status to unspecified drugs, medicaments and biological substances**

Z89 Acquired absence of limb
Includes: amputation status
postprocedural loss of limb
post-traumatic loss of limb
Excludes1: *acquired deformities of limbs (M20-M21)*
congenital absence of limbs (Q71-Q73)
Review coding guideline C.21.c.3
+ **Z89.0 Acquired absence of thumb and other finger(s)**
  - + **Z89.01 Acquired absence of thumb**
    - **Z89.011 Acquired absence of right thumb**
    - **Z89.012 Acquired absence of left thumb**
    - **Z89.019 Acquired absence of unspecified thumb**
  - + **Z89.02 Acquired absence of other finger(s)**
    Excludes2: *acquired absence of thumb (Z89.01-)*
    - **Z89.021 Acquired absence of right finger(s)**
    - **Z89.022 Acquired absence of left finger(s)**
    - **Z89.029 Acquired absence of unspecified finger(s)**
+ **Z89.1 Acquired absence of hand and wrist**
  - + **Z89.11 Acquired absence of hand**
    - **Z89.111 Acquired absence of right hand**
    - **Z89.112 Acquired absence of left hand**
    - **Z89.119 Acquired absence of unspecified hand**
  - + **Z89.12 Acquired absence of wrist**
    Disarticulation at wrist
    - **Z89.121 Acquired absence of right wrist**
    - **Z89.122 Acquired absence of left wrist**
    - **Z89.129 Acquired absence of unspecified wrist**
+ **Z89.2 Acquired absence of upper limb above wrist**
  - + **Z89.20 Acquired absence of upper limb, unspecified level**
    - **Z89.201 Acquired absence of right upper limb, unspecified level**
    - **Z89.202 Acquired absence of left upper limb, unspecified level**
    - **Z89.209 Acquired absence of unspecified upper limb, unspecified level**
      Acquired absence of arm NOS
  - + **Z89.21 Acquired absence of upper limb below elbow**
    - **Z89.211 Acquired absence of right upper limb below elbow**
    - **Z89.212 Acquired absence of left upper limb below elbow**
    - **Z89.219 Acquired absence of unspecified upper limb below elbow**
  - + **Z89.22 Acquired absence of upper limb above elbow**
    Disarticulation at elbow
    - **Z89.221 Acquired absence of right upper limb above elbow**
    - **Z89.222 Acquired absence of left upper limb above elbow**
    - **Z89.229 Acquired absence of unspecified upper limb above elbow**
  - + **Z89.23 Acquired absence of shoulder**
    Acquired absence of shoulder joint following explantation of shoulder joint prosthesis, with or without presence of antibiotic-impregnated cement spacer
    - **Z89.231 Acquired absence of right shoulder**
    - **Z89.232 Acquired absence of left shoulder**
    - **Z89.239 Acquired absence of unspecified shoulder**
+ **Z89.4 Acquired absence of toe(s), foot, and ankle**
  - + **Z89.41 Acquired absence of great toe**
    - **Z89.411 Acquired absence of right great toe**
    - **Z89.412 Acquired absence of left great toe**
    - **Z89.419 Acquired absence of unspecified great toe**
  - + **Z89.42 Acquired absence of other toe(s)**
    Excludes2: *acquired absence of great toe (Z89.41-)*
    - **Z89.421 Acquired absence of other right toe(s)**
    - **Z89.422 Acquired absence of other left toe(s)**
    - **Z89.429 Acquired absence of other toe(s), unspecified side**
  - + **Z89.43 Acquired absence of foot**
    - **Z89.431 Acquired absence of right foot**
    - **Z89.432 Acquired absence of left foot**
    - **Z89.439 Acquired absence of unspecified foot**
  - + **Z89.44 Acquired absence of ankle**
    Disarticulation of ankle
    - **Z89.441 Acquired absence of right ankle**
    - **Z89.442 Acquired absence of left ankle**
    - **Z89.449 Acquired absence of unspecified ankle**
+ **Z89.5 Acquired absence of leg below knee**
  - + **Z89.51 Acquired absence of leg below knee**
    - **Z89.511 Acquired absence of right leg below knee**
    - **Z89.512 Acquired absence of left leg below knee**
    - **Z89.519 Acquired absence of unspecified leg below knee**
  - + **Z89.52 Acquired absence of knee**
    Acquired absence of knee joint following explantation of knee joint prosthesis, with or without presence of antibiotic-impregnated cement spacer
    - **Z89.521 Acquired absence of right knee**
    - **Z89.522 Acquired absence of left knee**
    - **Z89.529 Acquired absence of unspecified knee**
+ **Z89.6 Acquired absence of leg above knee**
  - + **Z89.61 Acquired absence of leg above knee**
    Acquired absence of leg NOS
    Disarticulation at knee
    - **Z89.611 Acquired absence of right leg above knee**
    - **Z89.612 Acquired absence of left leg above knee**
    - **Z89.619 Acquired absence of unspecified leg above knee**

+ **Z89.62 Acquired absence of hip**

Acquired absence of hip joint following explantation of hip joint prosthesis, with or without presence of antibiotic-impregnated cement spacer

Disarticulation at hip

Z89.621 Acquired absence of right hip joint

Z89.622 Acquired absence of left hip joint

Z89.629 Acquired absence of unspecified hip joint

Z89.9 Acquired absence of limb, unspecified

Z90 Acquired absence of organs, not elsewhere classified

Includes: postprocedural or post-traumatic loss of body part NEC

Excludes1: *congenital absence - see Alphabetical Index*

Excludes2: *postprocedural absence of endocrine glands (E89.-)*

Review coding guideline C.21.c.3

+ **Z90.0 Acquired absence of part of head and neck**

Z90.01 Acquired absence of eye

Z90.02 Acquired absence of larynx

Z90.09 Acquired absence of other part of head and neck

Acquired absence of nose

Excludes2: *teeth (K08.1)*

+ **Z90.1 Acquired absence of breast and nipple**

Z90.10 Acquired absence of unspecified breast and nipple

Z90.11 Acquired absence of right breast and nipple

Z90.12 Acquired absence of left breast and nipple

Z90.13 Acquired absence of bilateral breasts and nipples

Z90.2 Acquired absence of lung [part of]

Z90.3 Acquired absence of stomach [part of]

+ **Z90.4 Acquired absence of other specified parts of digestive tract**

+ **Z90.41 Acquired absence of pancreas**

Code also exocrine pancreatic insufficiency (K86.81)

Use additional code to identify any associated: diabetes mellitus, postpancreatectomy (E13.-) insulin use (Z79.4)

Review coding guideline C.4.a.6.b.i

Z90.410 Acquired total absence of pancreas

Acquired absence of pancreas NOS

Z90.411 Acquired partial absence of pancreas

Z90.49 Acquired absence of other specified parts of digestive tract

Z90.5 Acquired absence of kidney

Z90.6 Acquired absence of other parts of urinary tract

Acquired absence of bladder

+ **Z90.7 Acquired absence of genital organ(s)**

Excludes1: *personal history of sex reassignment (Z87.890)*

Excludes2: *female genital mutilation status (N90.81-)*

+ **Z90.71 Acquired absence of cervix and uterus**

♀ **Z90.710 Acquired absence of both cervix and uterus**

Acquired absence of uterus NOS

Status post total hysterectomy

♀ **Z90.711 Acquired absence of uterus with remaining cervical stump**

Status post partial hysterectomy with remaining cervical stump

♀ **Z90.712 Acquired absence of cervix with remaining uterus**

+ **Z90.72 Acquired absence of ovaries**

♀ **Z90.721 Acquired absence of ovaries, unilateral**

♀ **Z90.722 Acquired absence of ovaries, bilateral**

Z90.79 Acquired absence of other genital organ(s)

+ **Z90.8 Acquired absence of other organs**

Z90.81 Acquired absence of spleen

Z90.89 Acquired absence of other organs

Z91 Personal risk factors, not elsewhere classified

Excludes2: *contact with and (suspected) exposures hazardous to health (Z77.-)*

exposure to pollution and other problems related to physical environment (Z77.1-)

female genital mutilation status (N90.81-)

personal history of physical injury and trauma (Z87.81, Z87.82-)

occupational exposure to risk factors (Z57.-)

+ **Z91.0 Allergy status, other than to drugs and biological substances**

Excludes2: *Allergy status to drugs, medicaments, and biological substances (Z88.-)*

Review coding guideline C.21.c.3

+ **Z91.01 Food allergy status**

Excludes2: *food additives allergy status (Z91.02)*

Z91.010 Allergy to peanuts

Z91.011 Allergy to milk products

Excludes1: *lactose intolerance (E73.-)*

Z91.012 Allergy to eggs

Z91.013 Allergy to seafood

Allergy to shellfish

Allergy to octopus or squid ink

Z91.014 Allergy to mammalian meats

Allergy to beef

Allergy to lamb

Allergy to pork

Allergy to red meats

Z91.018 Allergy to other foods

Allergy to nuts other than peanuts

Z91.02 Food additives allergy status

+ **Z91.03 Insect allergy status**

Z91.030 Bee allergy status

Z91.038 Other insect allergy status

+ **Z91.04 Nonmedicinal substance allergy status**

Z91.040 Latex allergy status

Latex sensitivity status

Z91.041 Radiographic dye allergy status

Allergy status to contrast media used for diagnostic X-ray procedure

Z91.048 Other nonmedicinal substance allergy status

Z91.09 Other allergy status, other than to drugs and biological substances

+ **Z91.1 Patient's noncompliance with medical treatment and regimen**

Z91.11 Patient's noncompliance with dietary regimen

+ **Z91.12 Patient's intentional underdosing of medication regimen**

Code first underdosing of medication (T36-T50) with fifth or sixth character 6

Excludes1: *adverse effect of prescribed drug taken as directed- code to adverse effect poisoning (overdose) -code to poisoning*

Review coding guideline C.19.e.5.c

Z91.120 Patient's intentional underdosing of medication regimen due to financial hardship

Z91.128 Patient's intentional underdosing of medication regimen for other reason

+ **Z91.13 Patient's unintentional underdosing of medication regimen**

Code first underdosing of medication (T36-T50) with fifth or sixth character 6

Excludes1: *adverse effect of prescribed drug taken as directed- code to adverse effect poisoning (overdose) -code to poisoning*

Review coding guideline C.19.e.5.c

Z91.130 Patient's unintentional underdosing of medication regimen due to age-related debility

Z91.138 Patient's unintentional underdosing of medication regimen for other reason

Z91.14 Patient's other noncompliance with medication regimen

Patient's underdosing of medication NOS

Review coding guideline C.19.e.5.c

Z91.15 Patient's noncompliance with renal dialysis
Z91.19 Patient's noncompliance with other medical treatment and regimen
Nonadherence to medical treatment

+ **Z91.4 Personal history of psychological trauma, not elsewhere classified**
Review coding guideline C.21.c.4

+ **Z91.41 Personal history of adult abuse**
Excludes2: *personal history of abuse in childhood (Z62.81-)*

• **Z91.410 Personal history of adult physical and sexual abuse**
Excludes1: *current adult physical abuse (T74.11, T76.11)*
current adult sexual abuse (T74.21-T76.11)

• **Z91.411 Personal history of adult psychological abuse**

• **Z91.412 Personal history of adult neglect**
Excludes1: *current adult neglect (T74.01, T76.01)*

• **Z91.419 Personal history of unspecified adult abuse**

Z91.42 Personal history of forced labor or sexual exploitation
AHA CC: 4Q, 2018, 32-33, 35

Z91.49 Other personal history of psychological trauma, not elsewhere classified

+ **Z91.5 Personal history of self-harm**
Code also mental health disorder, if known.
Review coding guideline C.21.c.4

Z91.51 Personal history of suicidal behavior
Personal history of parasuicide
Personal history of self-poisoning
Personal history of suicide attempt

Z91.52 Personal history of nonsuicidal self-harm
Personal history of nonsuicidal self-injury
Personal history of self-inflicted injury without suicidal intent
Personal history of self-mutilation

+ **Z91.8 Other specified personal risk factors, not elsewhere classified**
Review coding guideline C.21.c.4

Z91.81 History of falling
At risk for falling
Review coding guideline C.18.d and C21.c.4

• **Z91.82 Personal history of military deployment**
Individual (civilian or military) with past history of military war, peacekeeping and humanitarian deployment (current or past conflict)
Returned from military deployment
Review coding guideline C.21.c.4

Z91.83 Wandering in diseases classified elsewhere
Code first underlying disorder such as:
Alzheimer's disease (G30.-)
autism or pervasive developmental disorder (F84.-)
intellectual disabilities (F70-F79)
unspecified dementia with behavioral disturbance (F03.9-)

+ **Z91.84 Oral health risk factors**
AHA CC: 4Q, 2017, 29
Review coding guideline C.21.c.14

Z91.841 Risk for dental caries, low
Z91.842 Risk for dental caries, moderate
Z91.843 Risk for dental caries, high
Z91.849 Unspecified risk for dental caries

Z91.89 Other specified personal risk factors, not elsewhere classified
AHA CC: 1Q, 2017, 45-46

Z92 Personal history of medical treatment

Excludes2: *postprocedural states (Z98.-)*
Review coding guideline C.21.c.4

Z92.0 Personal history of contraception
Excludes1: *counseling or management of current contraceptive practices (Z30.-)*
long term (current) use of contraception (Z79.3)
presence of (intrauterine) contraceptive device (Z97.5)

+ **Z92.2 Personal history of drug therapy**
Excludes2: *long term (current) drug therapy (Z79.-)*

Z92.21 Personal history of antineoplastic chemotherapy
Z92.22 Personal history of monoclonal drug therapy
Z92.23 Personal history of estrogen therapy

+ **Z92.24 Personal history of steroid therapy**
Z92.240 Personal history of inhaled steroid therapy
Z92.241 Personal history of systemic steroid therapy
Personal history of steroid therapy NOS

Z92.25 Personal history of immunosuppression therapy
Excludes2: *personal history of steroid therapy (Z92.24)*

Z92.29 Personal history of other drug therapy

Z92.3 Personal history of irradiation
Personal history of exposure to therapeutic radiation
Excludes1: *exposure to radiation in the physical environment (Z77.12)*
occupational exposure to radiation (Z57.1)

+ **Z92.8 Personal history of other medical treatment**

Z92.81 Personal history of extracorporeal membrane oxygenation (ECMO)

Z92.82 Status post administration of tPA (rtPA) in a different facility within the last 24 hours prior to admission to current facility
Code first condition requiring tPA administration, such as:
acute cerebral infarction (I63.-)
acute myocardial infarction (I21.-, I22.-)
AHA CC: 4Q, 2013, 124
Review coding guideline C.21.c.3

Z92.83 Personal history of failed moderate sedation
Personal history of failed conscious sedation
Excludes2: *failed moderate sedation during procedure (T88.52)*

Z92.84 Personal history of unintended awareness under general anesthesia
Excludes2: *unintended awareness under general anesthesia during procedure (T88.53)*
AHA CC: 4Q, 2016, 72-73, 77

+ **Z92.85 Personal history of cellular therapy**
Z92.850 Personal history of Chimeric Antigen Receptor T-cell therapy
Personal history of CAR-T cell therapy
Z92.858 Personal history of other cellular therapy
Z92.859 Personal history of cellular therapy, unspecified

Z92.86 Personal history of gene therapy
Z92.89 Personal history of other medical treatment
AHA CC: 1Q, 2020, 18

Z93 Artificial opening status

Excludes1: *artificial openings requiring attention or management (Z43.-)*
complications of external stoma (J95.0-, K94.-, N99.5-)
Review coding guideline C.21.c.3

Z93.0 Tracheostomy status
AHA CC: 4Q, 2013, 129
Z93.1 Gastrostomy status
Z93.2 Ileostomy status
Z93.3 Colostomy status
Z93.4 Other artificial openings of gastrointestinal tract status

+ **Z93.5 Cystostomy status**
Z93.50 Unspecified cystostomy status
Z93.51 Cutaneous-vesicostomy status
Z93.52 Appendico-vesicostomy status
Z93.59 Other cystostomy status

Z93.6 Other artificial openings of urinary tract status
Nephrostomy status
Ureterostomy status
Urethrostomy status

Z93.8 Other artificial opening status
Z93.9 Artificial opening status, unspecified

Z94 Transplanted organ and tissue status

Includes: organ or tissue replaced by heterogenous or homogenous transplant

Excludes1: *complications of transplanted organ or tissue - see Alphabetical Index*

Excludes2: *presence of vascular grafts (Z95.-)*

Review coding guideline C.21.c.3

CC **Z94.0 Kidney transplant status**

Review coding guideline C.14.a.2

CC **Z94.1 Heart transplant status**

Excludes1: *artificial heart status (Z95.812)*
heart-valve replacement status (Z95.2-Z95.4)

CC **Z94.2 Lung transplant status**

CC **Z94.3 Heart and lungs transplant status**

CC **Z94.4 Liver transplant status**

Z94.5 Skin transplant status

Autogenous skin transplant status

Z94.6 Bone transplant status

Z94.7 Corneal transplant status

\+ **Z94.8 Other transplanted organ and tissue status**

CC **Z94.81 Bone marrow transplant status**

CC **Z94.82 Intestine transplant status**

CC **Z94.83 Pancreas transplant status**

CC **Z94.84 Stem cells transplant status**

Z94.89 Other transplanted organ and tissue status

Z94.9 Transplanted organ and tissue status, unspecified

Z95 Presence of cardiac and vascular implants and grafts

Excludes2: *complications of cardiac and vascular devices, implants and grafts (T82.-)*

Review coding guideline C.21.c.3

Z95.0 Presence of cardiac pacemaker

Presence of cardiac resynchronization therapy (CRT-P) pacemaker

Excludes1: *adjustment or management of cardiac device (Z45.0-)*
adjustment or management of cardiac pacemaker (Z45.0)
presence of automatic (implantable) cardiac defibrillator with synchronous cardiac pacemaker (Z95.810)

AHA CC: 1Q, 2019, 33-34

Z95.1 Presence of aortocoronary bypass graft

Presence of coronary artery bypass graft

Z95.2 Presence of prosthetic heart valve

Presence of heart valve NOS

Z95.3 Presence of xenogenic heart valve

Z95.4 Presence of other heart-valve replacement

Z95.5 Presence of coronary angioplasty implant and graft

Excludes1: *coronary angioplasty status without implant and graft (Z98.61)*

\+ **Z95.8 Presence of other cardiac and vascular implants and grafts**

\+ **Z95.81 Presence of other cardiac implants and grafts**

Z95.810 Presence of automatic (implantable) cardiac defibrillator

Presence of automatic (implantable) cardiac defibillator with synchronous cardiac pacemaker

Presence of cardiac resynchronization therapy defibillator (CRT-D)

Present of cardioverter-defibillator (ICD)

CC **Z95.811 Presence of heart assist device**

CC **Z95.812 Presence of fully implantable artificial heart**

Z95.818 Presence of other cardiac implants and grafts

\+ **Z95.82 Presence of other vascular implants and grafts**

Z95.820 Peripheral vascular angioplasty status with implants and grafts

Excludes1: *peripheral vascular angioplasty without implantandgraft(Z98.62)*

Z95.828 Presence of other vascular implants and grafts

Presence of intravascular prosthesis NEC

Z95.9 Presence of cardiac and vascular implant and graft, unspecified

Z96 Presence of other functional implants

Excludes2: *complications of internal prosthetic devices, implants and grafts (T82-T85)*
fitting and adjustment of prosthetic and other devices (Z44-Z46)

Review coding guideline C.21.c.3

Z96.0 Presence of urogenital implants

Z96.1 Presence of intraocular lens

Presence of pseudophakia

\+ **Z96.2 Presence of otological and audiological implants**

Z96.20 Presence of otological and audiological implant, unspecified

Z96.21 Cochlear implant status

Z96.22 Myringotomy tube(s) status

Z96.29 Presence of other otological and audiological implants

Presence of bone-conduction hearing device

Presence of eustachian tube stent

Stapes replacement

Z96.3 Presence of artificial larynx

\+ **Z96.4 Presence of endocrine implants**

Z96.41 Presence of insulin pump (external) (internal)

Z96.49 Presence of other endocrine implants

Z96.5 Presence of tooth-root and mandibular implants

\+ **Z96.6 Presence of orthopedic joint implants**

Z96.60 Presence of unspecified orthopedic joint implant

\+ **Z96.61 Presence of artificial shoulder joint**

Z96.611 Presence of right artificial shoulder joint

Z96.612 Presence of left artificial shoulder joint

Z96.619 Presence of unspecified artificial shoulder joint

\+ **Z96.62 Presence of artificial elbow joint**

Z96.621 Presence of right artificial elbow joint

Z96.622 Presence of left artificial elbow joint

Z96.629 Presence of unspecified artificial elbow joint

\+ **Z96.63 Presence of artificial wrist joint**

Z96.631 Presence of right artificial wrist joint

Z96.632 Presence of left artificial wrist joint

Z96.639 Presence of unspecified artificial wrist joint

\+ **Z96.64 Presence of artificial hip joint**

Hip-joint replacement (partial) (total)

Z96.641 Presence of right artificial hip joint

AHA CC: 3Q, 2016, 16-17

Z96.642 Presence of left artificial hip joint

AHA CC: 1Q, 2015, 16-17

Z96.643 Presence of artificial hip joint, bilateral

Z96.649 Presence of unspecified artificial hip joint

\+ **Z96.65 Presence of artificial knee joint**

Z96.651 Presence of right artificial knee joint

Z96.652 Presence of left artificial knee joint

AHA CC: 3Q, 2019, 16-17

Z96.653 Presence of artificial knee joint, bilateral

Z96.659 Presence of unspecified artificial knee joint

\+ **Z96.66 Presence of artificial ankle joint**

Z96.661 Presence of right artificial ankle joint

Z96.662 Presence of left artificial ankle joint

Z96.669 Presence of unspecified artificial ankle joint

\+ **Z96.69 Presence of other orthopedic joint implants**

Z96.691 Finger-joint replacement of right hand

Z96.692 Finger-joint replacement of left hand

Z96.693 Finger-joint replacement, bilateral

Z96.698 Presence of other orthopedic joint implants

Z96.7 Presence of other bone and tendon implants

Presence of skull plate

+ **Z96.8 Presence of other specified functional implants**
  - **Z96.81 Presence of artificial skin**
  - **Z96.82 Presence of neurostimulator**
    Presence of brain neurostimulator
    Presence of gastric neurostimulator
    Presence of peripheral nerve neurostimulator
    Presence of sacral nerve neurostimulator
    Presence of spinal cord neurostimulator
    Presence of vagus nerve neurostimulator
    AHA CC: 4Q, 2019, 19
  - **Z96.89 Presence of other specified functional implants**
- **Z96.9 Presence of functional implant, unspecified**

Z97 Presence of other devices

Excludes1: *complications of internal prosthetic devices, implants and grafts (T82-T85)*

Excludes2: *fitting and adjustment of prosthetic and other devices (Z44-Z46)*
presence of cerebrospinal fluid drainage device (Z98.2)

Review coding guideline C.21.c.3

- **Z97.0 Presence of artificial eye**
- + **Z97.1 Presence of artificial limb (complete) (partial)**
  - **Z97.10 Presence of artificial limb (complete) (partial), unspecified**
  - **Z97.11 Presence of artificial right arm (complete) (partial)**
  - **Z97.12 Presence of artificial left arm (complete) (partial)**
  - **Z97.13 Presence of artificial right leg (complete) (partial)**
  - **Z97.14 Presence of artificial left leg (complete) (partial)**
  - **Z97.15 Presence of artificial arms, bilateral (complete) (partial)**
  - **Z97.16 Presence of artificial legs, bilateral (complete) (partial)**
- **Z97.2 Presence of dental prosthetic device (complete) (partial)**
  Presence of dentures (complete) (partial)
- **Z97.3 Presence of spectacles and contact lenses**
- **Z97.4 Presence of external hearing-aid**
- ♀ **Z97.5 Presence of (intrauterine) contraceptive device**
  Excludes1: *checking, reinsertion or removal of implantable subdermal contraceptive (Z30.46)*
  checking, reinsertion or removal of intrauterine contraceptive device (Z30.43-)
- **Z97.8 Presence of other specified devices**

Z98 Other postprocedural states

Excludes2: *aftercare (Z43-Z49, Z51)*
follow-up medical care (Z08-Z09)
postprocedural complication - see Alphabetical Index

Review coding guideline C.21.c.3

- **Z98.0 Intestinal bypass and anastomosis status**
  Excludes2: *bariatric surgery status (Z98.84)*
  gastric bypass status (Z98.84)
  obesity surgery status (Z98.84)
- **Z98.1 Arthrodesis status**
- **Z98.2 Presence of cerebrospinal fluid drainage device**
  Presence of CSF shunt
- **Z98.3 Post therapeutic collapse of lung status**
  Code first underlying disease
- + **Z98.4 Cataract extraction status**
  Use additional code to identify intraocular lens implant status (Z96.1)
  Excludes1: *aphakia (H27.0)*
  - **Z98.41 Cataract extraction status, right eye**
  - **Z98.42 Cataract extraction status, left eye**
  - **Z98.49 Cataract extraction status, unspecified eye**
- + **Z98.5 Sterilization status**
  Excludes1: *female infertility (N97.-)*
  male infertility (N46.-)
  - ♀ **Z98.51 Tubal ligation status**
  - ● ♂ **Z98.52 Vasectomy status**
- + **Z98.6 Angioplasty status**
  - **Z98.61 Coronary angioplasty status**
    Excludes1: *coronary angioplasty status with implant and graft (Z95.5)*
  - **Z98.62 Peripheral vascular angioplasty status**
    Excludes1: *peripheral vascular angioplasty status with implant and graft (Z95.820)*
- + **Z98.8 Other specified postprocedural states**
  AHA CC: 4Q, 2016, 76
  - + **Z98.81 Dental procedure status**
    - **Z98.810 Dental sealant status**
    - **Z98.811 Dental restoration status**
      Dental crown status
      Dental fillings status
    - **Z98.818 Other dental procedure status**
  - **Z98.82 Breast implant status**
    Excludes1: *breast implant removal status (Z98.86)*
  - **Z98.83 Filtering (vitreous) bleb after glaucoma surgery status**
    Excludes1: *Inflammation (infection) of postprocedural bleb (H59.4-)*
    AHA CC: 3Q, 2020, 29
  - **Z98.84 Bariatric surgery status**
    Gastric banding status
    Gastric bypass status for obesity
    Obesity surgery status
    Excludes1: *bariatric surgery status complicating pregnancy, childbirth, or the puerperium (O99.84)*
    Excludes2: *intestinal bypass and anastomosis status (Z98.0)*
    AHA CC: 1Q, 2020, 12
  - **Z98.85 Transplanted organ removal status**
    Transplanted organ previously removed due to complication, failure, rejection or infection
    Excludes1: *encounter for removal of transplanted organ -code to complication of transplanted organ (T86.-)*
  - **Z98.86 Personal history of breast implant removal**
  - + **Z98.87 Personal history of in utero procedure**
    - ♀ **Z98.870 Personal history of in utero procedure during pregnancy**
      Excludes2: *complications from in utero procedure for current pregnancy (O35.7)*
      supervision of current pregnancy with history of in utero procedure during previous pregnancy (O09.82-)
    - **Z98.871 Personal history of in utero procedure while a fetus**
  - + **Z98.89 Other specified postprocedural states**
    - **Z98.890 Other specified postprocedural states**
      Personal history of surgery, note elsewhere classified
    - ♀ **Z98.891 History of uterine scar from previous surgery**
      Excludes1: *Maternal care due to uterine scar from previous surgery (O34.2-)*
      AHA CC: 4Q, 2016, 51-52

Z99 Dependence on enabling machines and devices, not elsewhere classified

AHA CC: 1Q, 2020, 11

Review coding guideline C.21.c.3

- **Z99.0 Dependence on aspirator**
- + **Z99.1 Dependence on respirator**
  Dependence on ventilator
  - CC **Z99.11 Dependence on respirator [ventilator] status**
    AHA CC: 1Q, 2015, 21
  - CC **Z99.12 Encounter for respirator [ventilator] dependence during power failure**
    Excludes1: *mechanical complication of respirator [ventilator] (J95.850)*
    AHA CC: 4Q, 2017, 112-114
    Review coding guidelines B19.d and C.21.c.16

Z99.2 Dependence on renal dialysis
Hemodialysis status
Peritoneal dialysis status
Presence of arteriovenous shunt for dialysis
Renal dialysis status NOS
Excludes1: *encounter for fitting and adjustment of dialysis catheter (Z49.0-)*
Excludes2: *noncompliance with renal dialysis (Z91.15)*

Z99.3 Dependence on wheelchair
Wheelchair confinement status
Code first cause of dependence, such as:
muscular dystrophy (G71.0-)
obesity (E66.-)

+ Z99.8 Dependence on other enabling machines and devices

Z99.81 Dependence on supplemental oxygen
Dependence on long-term oxygen
AHA CC: 4Q, 2013, 129

Z99.89 Dependence on other enabling machines and devices
Dependence on machine or device NOS

Chapter 22: Codes for Special Purposes (U00-U85)

This chapter contains the following blocks:

U00-U49 Provisional assignment of new diseases of uncertain etiology or emergency use

C. Chapter-Specific Coding Guidelines

In addition to general coding guidelines, there are guidelines for specific diagnoses and/or conditions in the classification. Unless otherwise indicated, these guidelines apply to all health care settings. Please refer to Section II for guidelines on the selection of the principal diagnosis.

22. Chapter 22: Codes for Special Purposes (U00-U85)

U07.0 Vaping-related disorder (*see Section I.C.10.e, Vaping-related disorders*)

U07.1 COVID-19 (*see Section I.C.1.g.1., COVID-19 infection*)

U09.9 Post COVID-19 condition, unspecified (see Section I.C.1.g.1.m)

Provisional assignment of new diseases of uncertain etiology or emergency use (U00-U49)

U07 Emergency use of U07

U07.0 Vaping related disorder (*see Section I.C.10.e, Vaping-related disorders*)

Dabbing related lung damage
Dabbing related lung injury
E-cigarette, or vaping, product use associated lung injury [EVALI]
Electronic cigarette related lung damage
Electronic cigarette related lung injury

Use additional code to identify manifestations, such as:
abdominal pain (R10.84)
acute respiratory distress syndrome (J80)
diarrhea (R19.7)
drug-induced interstitial lung disorder (J70.4)
lipoid pneumonia (J69.1)
weight loss (R63.4)

AHA CC: 1Q, 2020, 3-4

Review coding guideline C.11.3

MCC **U07.1 COVID-19 (*see Section I.C.1.g.1., COVID-19 infection*)**

Use additional code to identify pneumonia or other manifestations, such as: pneumonia due to COVID-19 (J12.82)

Excludes2: *coronavirus as the cause of diseases classified elsewhere (B97.2-)*
coronavirus infection, unspecified (B34.2)
pneumonia due to SARS-associated coronavirus (J12.81)

AHA CC: 2Q, 2020, 3-13; 3Q, 2020, 9-16; 4Q, 2020, 14; 1Q, 2021, 31-33, 36-40, 46-49

Review coding guideline C.15.s
Review coding guideline C.16.h

U09 Post COVID-19 condition

U09.9 Post COVID-19 condition, unspecified

NOTE This code enables establishment of a link with COVID-19.
This code is not to be used in cases that are still presenting with active COVID-19.
However, an exception is made in cases of re-infection with COVID-19, occurring with a condition related to prior COVID-19.
Post-acute sequela of COVID-19

Code first the specific condition related to COVID-19 if known, such as:
chronic respiratory failure (J96.1-)
loss of smell (R43.8)
loss of taste (R43.8)
multisystem inflammatory syndrome (M35.81)
pulmonary embolism (I26.-)
pulmonary fibrosis (J84.10)

Appendix A: CC/MCC Principal Diagnosis Collections and Exclusion Lists

Appendix A is provided online in a format suitable for spreadsheet and/or database use. Go to http://ahimapress.org/casto8437, click the "Online Resources" link, and enter case-sensitive password AHIMAQq27sP2022 to download the files.

Appendix B: Hospital-Acquired Conditions (HAC) List

Appendix B is provided online in a format suitable for spreadsheet and/or database use. Go to http://ahimapress.org/casto8437, click the "Online Resources" link, and enter case-sensitive password AHIMAQq27sP2022 to download the files.

Appendix C: New ICD-10-CM Codes FY2022

Appendix C is provided online in a format suitable for spreadsheet and/or database use. Go to http://ahimapress.org/casto8437, click the "Online Resources" link, and enter case sensitive password AHIMAQq27sP2022 to download files.

Appendix D: Deleted ICD-10-CM Codes FY2022

Appendix D is provided online in a format suitable for spreadsheet and/or database use. Go to http://ahimapress.org/casto8437, click the "Online Resources" link, and enter case sensitive password AHIMAQq27sP2022 to download files.